Kathy VandenBerg PhD.

D1505295

Avery's
Neonatology
Pathophysiology & Management of the Newborn

6th Edition

Avery's
Neonatology
Pathophysiology & Management of the Newborn

6th Edition

EDITED BY

■ **Mhairi G. MacDonald, M.B.Ch.B., F.R.C.P.(E.), F.R.C.P.C.H., D.C.H.**
Professor of Pediatrics
George Washington University School of Medicine and Health Sciences
Washington, District of Columbia

■ **Mary M. K. Seshia, M.B.Ch.B., F.R.C.P.(E.), F.R.C.P.C.H., D.C.H.**
Professor of Pediatrics
Head, Section of Neonatology
Health Sciences Centre
University of Manitoba
Winnipeg, Manitoba

■ **Martha D. Mullett, M.D., M.P.H.**
Professor of Pediatrics
Robert C. Byrd Health Sciences Center
West Virginia University
Department of Pediatrics
Morgantown, West Virginia

◆ LIPPINCOTT WILLIAMS & WILKINS
A **Wolters Kluwer** Company
Philadelphia • Baltimore • New York • London
Buenos Aires • Hong Kong • Sydney • Tokyo

Acquisitions Editor: Anne M. Sydor
Developmental Editor: Jenny Kim
Project Manager: Alicia Jackson
Senior Manufacturing Manager: Benjamin Rivera
Marketing Manager: Kathy Neely
Cover Designer: Andrew Gatto
Production Service: TechBooks
Printer: Quebecor World-Taunton

© 2005 by LIPPINCOTT WILLIAMS & WILKINS
530 Walnut Street
Philadelphia, PA 19106 USA
LWW.com

1st Edition, ©1975 J.B. Lippincott
2nd Edition, ©1981 J.B. Lippincott
3rd Edition, ©1987 J.B. Lippincott
4th Edition, ©1994 J.B. Lippincott
5th Edition, ©1999 Lippincott William & Wilkins

All rights reserved. This book is protected by copyright. No part of this book may
be reproduced in any form by any means, including photocopying, or utilized by
any information storage and retrieval system without written permission from the
copyright owner, except for brief quotations embodied in critical articles and
reviews. Materials appearing in this book prepared by individuals as part of their
official duties as U.S. government employees are not covered by the above-
mentioned copyright.

Printed in the USA

Library of Congress Cataloging-in-Publication Data

Avery's neonatology : pathophysiology & management of the newborn/edited
by Mhairi G. MacDonald, Mary M.K. Seshia, Martha D. Mullett.—6th ed.
    p. ; cm.
    Rev. ed. of: Neonatology / edited by Gordon B. Avery, Mary Ann Fletcher,
Mhairi G. MacDonald. c1999.
    Includes bibliographical references and index.
    ISBN 0-7817-4643-4
    1. Infants (Newborn)—Diseases. 2. Neonatology. I. Avery, Gordon B.
II. MacDonald, Mhairi G. III. Seshia, Mary M. K. IV. Mullett, Martha D.
V. Neonatology. VI. Title: Neonatology. [DNLM: 1. Infant, Newborn,
Diseases—physiopathology. 2. Infant, Newborn, Diseases—therapy.
3. Prenatal Diagnosis. WS 421 A9556 2005]
RJ254.N46 2005
618.92'01—dc22

                                        2005004348

Care has been taken to confirm the accuracy of the information presented and to
describe generally accepted practices. However, the authors, editors, and publisher
are not responsible for errors or omissions or for any consequences from application
of the information in this book and make no warranty, expressed or implied, with
respect to the currency, completeness, or accuracy of the contents of the publication.
Application of the information in a particular situation remains the professional
responsibility of the practitioner.

The authors, editors, and publisher have exerted every effort to ensure that drug
selection and dosage set forth in this text are in accordance with current
recommendations and practice at the time of publication. However, in view of
ongoing research, changes in government regulations, and the constant flow of
information relating to drug therapy and drug reactions, the reader is urged to check
the package insert for each drug for any change in indications and dosage and for
added warnings and precautions. This is particularly important when the
recommended agent is a new or infrequently employed drug.

Some drugs and medical devices presented in the publication have Food and
Drug Administration (FDA) clearance for limited use in restricted research settings. It
is the responsibility of the health care provider to ascertain the FDA status of each
drug or device planned for use in their clinical practice.

                                        10 9 8 7 6 5 4 3 2

Contents

Contributors vii
Foreword xiii
Preface xv
Color Insert

PART I: GENERAL CONSIDERATIONS 1

1 Neonatology: Past, Present, and Future 2
Gordon B. Avery

2 Current Moral Priorities and Decision Making in Neonatal-Perinatal Medicine 8
Robert J. Boyle and John C. Fletcher

3 Neonatology in the United States: Scope and Organization 24
Richard L. Bucciarelli

4 Neonatal Transport 40
Karen S. Wood and Carl L. Bose

5 Telehealth in Neonatology 54
Sarah C. Muttitt, Mary M. K. Seshia, and Liz Loewen

6 Newborn Intensive Care Unit Design: Scientific and Practical Considerations 64
Robert D. White, Gilbert I. Martin, Judith Smith, and Stanley N. Graven

7 Organization of Care and Quality in the NICU 76
Richard Powers and Carolyn Houska Lund

8 Law, Quality Assurance and Risk Management in the Practice of Neonatology 89
Harold M. Ginzburg and Mhairi G. MacDonald

9 The Vulnerable Neonate and the Neonatal Intensive Care Environment 111
Penny Glass

PART II: THE FETAL PATIENT 129

10 Prenatal Diagnosis in the Molecular Age— Indications, Procedures, and Laboratory Techniques 130
Arie Drugan, Nelson B. Isada, and Mark I. Evans

11 Feto-Maternal Interactions: Placental Physiology, the In Utero Environment, and Fetal Determinants of Adult Disease 149
Gabriella Pridjian

12 Fetal Imaging: Ultrasound and Magnetic Resonance Imaging 166
Dorothy I. Bulas

13 Fetal Therapy 186
Mark I. Evans, Mark P. Johnson, Alan W. Flake, Yuval Yaron, and Michael R. Harrison

14 The Impact of Maternal Illness on the Neonate 202
Helain J. Landy

15 The Effects of Maternal Drugs on the Developing Fetus 224
David A. Beckman, Lynda B. Fawcett, and Robert L. Brent

16 Obstetric Anesthesia and Analgesia: Effects on the Fetus and Newborn 260
Judith Littleford

PART III: TRANSITION AND STABILIZATION 283

17 Cardiorespiratory Adjustments at Birth 284
Ruben E. Alvaro and Henrique Rigatto

18 Delivery Room Management 304
Virender K. Rehan and Roderic H. Phibbs

19 Physical Assessment and Classification 327
Michael Narvey and Mary Ann Fletcher

20 General Care 351
Ian Laing

21 Fluid and Electrolyte Management 362
Edward F. Bell and William Oh

22 Nutrition 380
Michael K. Georgieff

23 Breastfeeding and the Use of Human Milk in the Neonatal Intensive Care Unit 413
Kathleen A. Marinelli and Kathy Hamelin

24 Thermal Regulation 445
Michael Friedman and Stephen Baumgart

PART IV: THE LOW-BIRTH-WEIGHT INFANT 458

25 The Extremely Low-Birth-Weight Infant 459
Apostolos Papageorgiou, Ermelinda Pelausa, and Lajos Kovacs

26 Intrauterine Growth Restriction and the Small-For-Gestational-Age Infant 490
Marianne S. Anderson and William W. Hay

27   Multiple Gestations 523
     Mary E. Revenis and Lauren A. Johnson-Robbins

PART V: THE NEWBORN INFANT 534

28   Control of Breathing: Development, Apnea of
     Prematurity, Apparent Life-Threatening Events,
     Sudden Infant Death Syndrome 535
     Mark W. Thompson and Carl E. Hunt

29   Acute Respiratory Disorders 553
     *Jeffrey A. Whitsett, Ward R. Rice, Barbara B. Warner,
     Susan E. Wert, and Gloria S. Pryhuber*

30   Bronchopulmonary Dysplasia 578
     Jonathan M. Davis and Warren N. Rosenfeld

31   Principles of Management of Respiratory Problems 600
     William E. Truog and Sergio G. Golombek

32   Extracorporeal Membrane Oxygenation 622
     Billie Lou Short

33   Cardiac Disease 633
     *Michael F. Flanagan, Scott B. Yeager, and
     Steven N. Weindling*

34   Preoperative and Postoperative Care of the Infant
     with Critical Congenital Heart Disease 710
     John M. Costello and Wayne H. Franklin

35   Jaundice 768
     M. Jeffrey Maisels

36   Calcium and Magnesium Homeostasis 847
     Winston W. K. Koo and Reginald C. Tsang

37   Carbohydrate Homeostasis 876
     Edward S. Ogata

38   Congenital Anomalies 892
     Scott Douglas McLean

39   Endocrine Disorders of the Newborn 914
     Mary M. Lee and Thomas Moshang, Jr.

40   Gastrointestinal Disease 940
     Jon A. Vanderhoof, Terence L. Zach, and Thomas E. Adrian

41   Inherited Metabolic Disorders 965
     Barbara K. Burton

42   Renal Disease 981
     *Suhas M. Nafday, Luc P. Brion, Corinne Benchimol, Lisa M.
     Satlin, Joseph T. Flynn, and Chester M. Edelmann, Jr.*

43   Structural Abnormalities of the Genitourinary
     Tract 1066
     George W. Kaplan and Irene M. McAleer

44   Surgical Care of Conditions Presenting in the
     Newborn 1097
     *Gary E. Hartman, Michael J. Boyajian, Sukgi S. Choi,
     Martin R. Eichelberger, Kurt D. Newman, and
     David M. Powell*

45   Immunology of the Fetus and Newborn 1135
     Joseph A. Bellanti, Barbara J. Zeligs, and Yung-Hao Pung

46   Hematology 1169
     Victor Blanchette, Yigal Dror, and Anthony Chan

47   Bacterial and Fungal Infections 1235
     *Robert L. Schelonka, Bishara J. Freij, and George H.
     McCracken, Jr.*

48   Viral and Protozoal Infections 1274
     Bishara J. Freij and John L. Sever

49   Healthcare-Associated Infections 1357
     Jukka K. Korpela, Joyce Campbell, and Nalini Singh

50   Neurological and Neuromuscular Disorders 1384
     Alan Hill

51   Neurosurgery of the Newborn 1410
     Joseph R. Madsen, David M. Frim, and Anne R. Hansen

52   Orthopedics 1428
     William W. Robertson, Jr.

53   Neoplasia 1444
     Robert J. Arceci and Howard J. Weinstein

54   Eye Disorders 1469
     Sherwin J. Isenberg

55   Dermatologic Conditions 1485
     James G. H. Dinulos and Gary L. Darmstadt

PART VI: PHARMACOLOGY 1506

56   Drug Therapy in the Newborn 1507
     Robert M. Ward and Ralph A. Lugo

57   Anesthesia and Analgesia in the Neonate 1557
     Sally H. Vitali, Anthony J. Camerota, and John H. Arnold

58   The Infant of the Drug-Dependent Mother 1572
     *Enrique M. Ostrea, Jr., J. Edgar Winston Cruz Posecion,
     and Maria Esterlita-Uy T. Villanueva*

PART VII: BEYOND THE NURSERY 1617

59   Medical Care After Discharge 1618
     Judy Bernbaum

60   Developmental Outcome 1632
     Forrest C. Bennett

Appendix A   The Healthcare Matrix 1653
Appendix B   Hemoglobin–Oxygen Dissociation Curves
             1655
Appendix C   Breast Milk in the NICU 1656
Appendix D   Growth Parameters 1659
Appendix E   Jaundice 1670
Appendix F   Blood Pressure 1672
Appendix G   Renal and Urinary Tract Anomalies 1676
Appendix H   Drug Formulary 1688
Appendix I   Nutritional Values 1702
Appendix J   Technical Procedures 1704
Index 1707

Contributors

THOMAS E. ADRIAN, Ph.D., F.R.C.Path. Professor, Department of Biomedical Sciences, Creighton University School of Medicine, Omaha, Nebraska.

RUBEN E. ALVARO, M.D., F.A.A.P. Associate Professor, Department of Pediatrics, University of Manitoba, Acting Head of Neonatology, Department of Pediatrics, St. Boniface General Hospital, Winnipeg, Manitoba, Canada.

MARIANNE S. ANDERSON Associate Professor of Pediatrics and Neonatology, Perinatal Research Center, University of Colorado HSC, Denver, Colorado.

ROBERT J. ARCECI, M.D., Ph.D. Director and King Fahd Professor of Pediatric Oncology, Professor of Pediatrics and Oncology, Sidney Kimmel Comprehensive Cancer Center at Johns Hopkins, Baltimore, Maryland.

JOHN H. ARNOLD, M.D. Assistant Professor, Department of Anaesthesia (Pediatrics), Harvard Medical School; and Senior Associate, Anesthesia and Critical Care, Children's Hospital, Boston, Massachusetts.

GORDON B. AVERY, M.D., Ph.D. Emeritus Professor of Pediatrics, Retired Chair, Department of Pediatrics, The George Washington University School of Medicine and Health Sciences; and Chief Academic Officer, Emeritus, Department of Pediatrics and Neonatology, Children's National Medical Center, Washington, D.C.

STEPHEN BAUMGART, M.D. Professor of Pediatrics Elect, George Washington University School of Medicine, Senior Staff Physician, Department of Neonatology, Children's Hospital National Medical Center, Washington, D.C.

DAVID A. BECKMAN, Ph.D. Associate Professor, Department of Pediatrics, Thomas Jefferson University; and Nemours Research Programs, Alfred I. duPont Hospital for Children, Wilmington, Delaware.

EDWARD F. BELL, M.D. Professor, Department of Pediatrics, University of Iowa; and Director, Divison of Neonatology, Children's Hospital of Iowa, Iowa City, Iowa.

JOSEPH A. BELLANTI, M.D. Professor, Department of Pediatrics and Microbiology-Immunology, Georgetown University Medical Center, Washington, D.C.

CORINNE BENCHIMOL, D.O. Clinical Assistant Professor, Department of Pediatrics, Mount Sinai School of Medicine, Clinical Assistant Professor, Department of Pediatrics, Mount Sinai Hospital, New York, New York.

FORREST C. BENNETT, M.D. Professor, Department of Pediatrics, University of Washington School of Medicine, Seattle, Washington.

JUDY BERNBAUM, M.D. Professor, Department of Pediatrics, University of Pennsylvania School of Medicine; and Director, Neonatal Follow-Up Program, The Children's Hospital of Philadelphia, Philadelphia, Pennsylvania.

VICTOR BLANCHETTE, M.D., B.Ch., F.R.C.P. Professor, Department of Pediatrics, University of Toronto; and Chief, Division of Hematology/Oncology, The Hospital for Sick Children, Toronto, Ontario, Canada.

CARL L. BOSE, M.D. Professor, Department of Pediatrics, University of North Carolina at Chapel Hill; and Chief Division of Neonatal-Perinatal Medicine, UNC Hospitals, Chapel Hill, North Carolina.

MICHAEL J. BOYAJIAN Program director—plastic and reconstructive surgery, Director—craniofacial surgery program, Division: plastic and reconstructive surgery, Children's National Medical Center, Washington, D.C.

ROBERT J. BOYLE, M.D. Professor of Pediatrics, University of Virginia Health System, Charlottesville, Virginia.

ROBERT L. BRENT, M.D., Ph.D., D.Sc. Distinguished Professor of Pediatrics, Radiology, and Pathology, Department of Pediatrics, Jefferson Medical College, Philadelphia, Pennsylvania; and Head, Clinical and Environmental Teratology Laboratory, Nemours Research Programs, Alfred I. duPont Hospital for Children, Wilmington, Delaware.

LUC P. BRION, M.D. Professor, Department of Pediatrics, Albert Einstein College of Medicine and Attending Neonatologist, Department of Pediatrics, Children's Hospital at Montefiore, Bronx, New York.

RICHARD L. BUCCIARELLI, M.D. Associate Vice President for Health Affairs and Professor of Pediatrics, Department of Pediatrics, University of Florida, Neonatologist, Department of Pediatrics and Neonatology, Shands at University of Florida, Gainesville, Florida.

DOROTHY I. BULAS, M.D. Professor of Pediatrics and Radiology, Departments of Radiology and Pediatrics, The George Washington University Medical Center; and Director, Program in Diagnostic Imaging, Division of Diagnostic Imaging, Children's National Medical Center, Washington, D.C.

BARBARA K. BURTON, M.D. Professor and Head, Division of Genetics and Metabolism, Department of Pediatrics, University of Illinois College of Medicine; and Director, Center for Medical and Reproductive Genetics, Michael Reese Hospital, Chicago, Illinois.

ANTHONY J. CAMEROTA, M.D.   Department of Critical Care Medicine, Naval Regional Center, Portsmith, Virginia.

JOYCE CAMPBELL, R.N., M.S.   Service Director, Emergency Department, Infection Control Practitioner, Children's National Medical Center, Washington, D.C.

ANTHONY CHAN, M.B.B.S., F.R.C.P.C.   Professor of Pediatrics, McMaster University, Hamilton, Canada; and Consultant, Coagulation Laboratory, Department of Pediatric Laboratory Medicine, The Hospital for Sick Children, Toronto, Canada.

SUKGI S. CHOI, M.D.   Associate Professor, Department of Otolaryngology and Pediatrics, The George Washington University School of Medicine; and Vice Chairman, Department of Otolaryngology, Children's National Medical Center, Washington, D.C.

JOHN M. COSTELLO, M.D.   Instructor, Department of Pediatrics, Harvard Medical School, Division of Cardiac Intensive Care, Department of Cardiology, Children's Hospital Boston, Boston, Massachusetts.

GARY L. DARMSTADT, M.D.   Assistant Director, Department of International Health, Bloomberg School of Public Health, Johns Hopkins University, Baltimore, Maryland; and Senior Research Advisor, Saving Newborn Lives Initiative, Office of Health, Save the Children Federation-USA, Washington, D.C.

JONATHAN M. DAVIS, M.D.   Professor, Department of Pediatrics, State University of New York at Stony Brook School of Medicine, Stony Brook; and Director, Neonatology, Director, Cardiopulmonary Research Institute, Department of Pediatrics, Winthrop-University Hospital, Mineola, New York.

JAMES G.H. DINULOS, M.D.   Assistant Professor of Medicine and Pediatrics (Dermatology), Children's Hospital at Dartmouth, Dartmouth Medical School, Lebanon, New Hampshire.

YIGAL DROR, M.D.   Division of Hematology/Oncology and Bone Marrow Transplantation, Director, Marrow Failure and Myelodysplasia Program, Scientist Track, Research Institute, The Hospital for Sick Children, University of Toronto, Canada.

ARIE DRUGAN, M.D.   Associate Professor, Department of Obstetrics and Gynecology, Wayne State University, Hutzel Hospital, Detroit, Michigan; and Vice-Chairman, Department of Obstetrics and Gynecology, Rambam Medical Center, Haifa, Israel.

CHESTER M. EDELMANN, Jr., M.D.   Professor, Department of Pediatrics, Albert Einstein College of Medicine, Attending Physician, Department of Pediatrics, Montefiore Medical Center, Bronx, New York.

MARTIN R. EICHELBERGER, M.D.   Professor, Department of Surgery and Pediatrics, The George Washington University School of Medicine; and Director, Emergency Trauma Services, Children's National Medical Center, Washington, D.C.

MARK I. EVANS, M.D.   Professor, Department of Obstetrics and Gynecology, Mount Sinai School of Medicine, Director, Institute for Genetics, New York, New York.

LYNDA B. FAWCETT, Ph.D.   Assistant Professor of Pediatrics, Department of Pediatrics, Jefferson Medical College, Philadelphia, Pennsylvania; and Assistant Professor, Nemours Biomedical Research, Alfred I. duPont Hospital for Children, Wilmington, Delaware.

MICHAEL F. FLANAGAN, M.D.   Department of Pediatrics, Section of Pediatrics Cardiology, Dartmouth Medical School; and Dartmouth–Hitchcock Medical Center, Lebanon, New Hampshire.

ALAN W. FLAKE, M.D.   Department of Pediatric Surgery, Children's Hospital of Philadelphia, Philadelphia, Pennsylvania.

JOHN C. FLETCHER, Ph.D.   Deceased, Prior Professor Emeritus of Biomedical Ethics, Department of Internal Medicine, University of Virginia School of Medicine, Charlottesville, Virginia.

MARY ANN FLETCHER, M.D.   Clinical Professor of Pediatrics, The George Washington University School of Medicine and Health Sciences, Washington, D.C.

JOSEPH T. FLYNN, M.D., M.Sc.   Associate Professor of Clinical Pediatrics, Department of Pediatrics, Albert Einstein College of Medicine; and Director, Pediatric Hypertension Program, Department of Pediatric Nephrology, Montefiore Medical Center, New York, New York.

WAYNE H. FRANKLIN, M.D., M.P.H.   Associate Professor, Department of Pediatrics, Feinberg School of Medicine at Northwestern University, Division of Pediatric Cardiology, Children's Memorial Hospital, Chicago, Illinois.

BISHARA J. FREIJ, M.D.   Clinical Professor of Pediatrics, Department of Pediatrics, Wayne State University School of Medicine; and Chief, Division of Infectious Diseases, Department of Pediatrics, William Beaumont Hospital, Royal Oak, Detroit, Michigan.

MICHAEL FRIEDMAN, M.D.   Assistant Professor of Pediatrics, Division of Neonatology, Stoneybrook University; and Senior Staff Physician, Department of Neonatology, Stoneybrook University Hospital, Stoneybrook, New York.

DAVID M. FRIM, M.D., Ph.D.   Assistant Professor, Department of Surgery and Pediatrics, The University of Chicago; and Chief, Section of Pediatric Neurosurgery, The University of Chicago Children's Hospital, Chicago, Illinois.

MICHAEL K. GEORGIEFF, M.D.   Professor, Department of Pediatrics, University of Minnesota; and Staff Neonatologist, Department of Pediatrics, Fairview-University Medical Center, Minneapolis, Minnesota.

HAROLD M. GINZBURG, M.D., J.D., M.P.H.   Clinical Professor, Departments of Psychiatry and Neurology, Tulane Medical Center; and Clinical Professor, Department of Psychiatry, Louisiana State University, New Orleans, Louisiana.

PENNY GLASS, Ph.D. Associate Professor of Pediatrics, Department of Pediatrics, George Washington University School of Medicine and Health Sciences; and Director, Child Development Program, Department of Psychology, Children's National Medical Center, Washington, D.C.

SERGIO G. GOLOMBEK, M.D. Associate Professor of Pediatrics, Department of Pediatrics, Division of Neonatology, Westchester Medical Center, New York Medical College, Valhalla, New York.

STANLEY N. GRAVEN, M.D. Professor, Community and Family Health, Department of Pediatrics, University of South Florida; and Staff Physician, Department of Pediatrics, Tampa General Hospital, Tampa, Florida.

KATHY HAMELIN, R.N. B.A, M.N., I.B.C.L.C. Clinical Nurse Specialist, Lactation Consultant, Women's Health Program, Health Sciences Centre, Adjunct Professor, Faculty of Nursing, University of Manitoba, Winnipeg, Manitoba, Canada.

ANNE R. HANSEN, M.D. Assistant Professor, Department of Pediatrics, Harvard Medical School; and Medical Director Neonatal Intensive Care Unit, Department of Medicine, Children's Hospital Boston, Boston, Massachusetts.

MICHAEL R. HARRISON, M.D. Department of Pediatric Surgery, University of California, San Francisco, San Francisco, California.

GARY E. HARTMAN, M.D. Professor of Surgery and Pediatrics, Department of Surgery, The George Washington University School of Medicine; and Chairman, Department of Pediatric Surgery, Children's National Medical Center, Washington, D.C.

WILLIAM W. HAY, Jr., M.D. Professor, Department of Pediatrics, University of Colorado Health Sciences Center, Aurora, Colorado.

ALAN HILL, M.D., Ph.D. Professor, Department of Pediatrics, University of British Columbia; and Head, Division of Neurology, Department of Pediatrics, British Columbia's Children's Hospital, Vancouver, British Columbia, Canada.

CARL E. HUNT, M.D. Department of Pediatrics, Medical College of Ohio, Toledo, Ohio; and Director, National Center on Sleep Disorders Research, National Heart, Lung, and Blood Institute, Bethesda, Maryland.

NELSON B. ISADA, M.D. Alaska Perinatology Associates, Anchorage, Alaska.

SHERWIN J. ISENBERG, M.D. Lantz Professor of Pediatric Ophthalmology and Vice-Chairman, Department of Ophthalmology, Jules Stein Eye Institute, Harbor–UCLA School of Medicine, Los Angeles, California.

MARK P. JOHNSON, M.D. Associate Professor, Departments of Obstetrics/Gynecology, Pathology, Molecular Medicine, and Genetics, Wayne State University; and Associate Director, Reproductive Genetics, Department of Obstetrics and Gynecology, Hutzel Hospital/The Detroit Medical Center, Detroit, Michigan.

LAUREN A. JOHNSON-ROBBINS, M.D. Assistant Professor, Department of Pediatrics, Albany Medical College; and Attending Neonatologist, Albany Medical Center, Albany, New York.

GEORGE W. KAPLAN, M.D., M.S., F.A.A.P., F.A.C.S. Clinical Professor, Department of Surgery and Pediatrics, School of Medicine, University of California, San Diego; and Chairman, Division of Urology, Children's Hospital, San Diego, California.

WINSTON W. K. KOO, M.B.B.S. Professor, Department of Pediatrics, Wayne State University; and Neonatologist, Department of Pediatrics, Hutzel Hospital, Detroit, Michigan.

LAJOS KOVACS, M.D.C.M., F.R.C.P.C., F.A.A.P. Associate Professor, Department of Pediatrics, Faculty of Medicine, McGill University; and Staff Neonatologist, Department of Neonatology, Sir Mortimer B. Davis Jewish General Hospital, Montreal, Quebec, Canada.

JUKKA K. KORPELA, M.D., Ph.D. Adjunct Professor of Pediatrics, Department of Infectious Diseases, The George Washington University Medical Center; and Faculty, Department of Infectious Diseases, Children's National Medical Center, Washington, D.C.

IAN LAING, M.D., F.R.C.P.C.H., F.R.C.P.E. Clinical Director, Neonatal Unit, Simpson Centre for Reproductive Health, Royal Infirmary, Edinburgh, Great Britain.

HELAIN J. LANDY, M.D. Professor and Chair, Department of Obstetrics and Gynecology, Georgetown University; and Chief, Department of Obstetrics and Gynecology, Georgetown University Hospital, Washington, D.C.

MARY M. LEE, M.D. Associate Professor of Pediatrics, Department of Pediatrics, Duke University Medical Center, Durham, North Carolina.

JUDITH LITTLEFORD, M.D., B.Sc., F.R.C.P.C. Associate Professor, Department of Anesthesia, University of Manitoba; and Section Head, Women's Hospital of Anesthesia, Department of Anesthesia, Winnipeg, Manitoba, Canada.

LIZ LOEWEN, R.N., B.F.A., M.N. Lecturer, Faculty of Nursing, University of Manitoba; and Network Researcher, MB Telehealth, Winnipeg, Regional Health Authority, Winnipeg, Manitoba, Canada.

RALPH A. LUGO, M.D. Associate Professor, Department of Pharmacotherapy, University of Utah College of Pharmacy, Salt Lake City, Utah.

CAROLYN HOUSKA LUND, R.N., M.S.N, F.A.A.N. Intensive Care Nursery, Children's Hospital, Oakland, California.

GEORGE H. McCRACKEN, Jr., M.D. Professor, The Sarah M. and Charles E. Seay Chair in Pediatric Infectious Diseases, Department of Pediatrics, University of Texas, Southwestern Medical Center; and Attending Physician, Children's Medical Center, Dallas, Texas.

MHAIRI G. MacDONALD, M.B.Ch.B., F.R.C.P.(E.), F.R.C.P.C.H., D.C.H. Professor of Pediatrics, The George Washington University School of Medicine and Health Sciences, Washington, D.C.

JOSEPH R. MADSEN, M.D. Assistant Professor, Department of Surgery, Harvard Medical School; and Associate Professor, Department of Neurosurgery, Children's Hospital, Boston, Massachusetts.

M. JEFFREY MAISELS, M.B., B.Ch. Clinical Professor of Pediatrics, Wayne State University School of Medicine, University of Michigan Medical Center; and Chairman, Department of Pediatrics, William Beaumont Hospital, Royal Oak, Michigan.

KATHLEEN A. MARINELLI, M.D., T.R.C.L.C., F.A.B.M. Associate Professor of Pediatrics, Department of Pediatrics, University of Connecticut School of Medicine, Hartford, Connecticut.

GILBERT I. MARTIN, M.D. Clinical Professor, Department of Pediatrics, University of California, Irvine, Irvine; and Director, Neonatal Intensive Care Unit, Citrus Valley Medical Center, West Covina, California.

IRENE M. McALEER, M.D. Department of Surgery, School of Medicine, University of California, San Diego; and Division of Urology, Children's Hospital, San Diego, California.

SCOTT DOUGLAS McLEAN, M.D. Assistant Professor, Department of Pediatrics, Uniformed Services University of the Health Sciences, Bethesda, Maryland; and Chief, Medical Genetics, San Antonio Military Pediatrics Center, Brooke Army Medical Center, Ft. Sam Houston, Texas.

THOMAS MOSHANG, Jr., M.D. Professor, Department of Pediatrics, University of Pennsylvania; and Chief, Department of Pediatrics, Children's Hospital of Philadelphia, Philadelphia, Pennsylvania.

MARTHA D. MULLETT, M.D. Professor of Pediatrics, Robert C. Byrd Health Sciences Center, West Virginia University, Department of Pediatrics, Morgantown, West Virginia.

SARAH C. MUTTITT, M.D., F.R.C.P.C., F.A.A.P., M.B.A. Assistant Professor, Department of Pediatrics and Child Health, University of Manitoba; and Director, MB Telehealth, Winnipeg RHA, Winnipeg, Manitoba, Canada.

SUHAS M. NAFDAY, M.D., M.R.C.P.I., F.A.A.P. Assistant Professor, Department of Pediatrics, Albert Einstein College of Medicine; and Attending Neonatologist, Section of Neonatology, Children's Hospital at Montefiore, Bronx, New York.

MICHAEL NARVEY, M.D., F.R.C.P.C. Neonatal Fellow, Department of Pediatrics, University of Alberta, Edmonton, Alberta, Canada.

KURT D. NEWMAN, M.D. Departments of Surgery and Pediatrics, The George Washington University School of Medicine, Department of Pediatric Surgery, Children's National Medical Center, Washington, D.C.

EDWARD S. OGATA, M.D., M.M. Professor, Department of Pediatrics, Northwestern University Medical School; and Chief Medical Officer, Children's Memorial Hospital, Chicago, Illinois.

WILLIAM OH, M.D. Professor, Department of Pediatrics, Brown Medical School, Attending Neonatologist, Department of Pediatrics, Women and Infants' Hospital, Providence, Rhode Island.

ENRIQUE M. OSTREA, Jr., M.D. Professor, Department of Pediatrics, Wayne State University School of Medicine; and Neonatologist, Department of Neonatology, Hutzel Women's Hospital, Detroit, Michigan.

APOSTOLOS PAPAGEORGIOU, M.D., F.R.C.P.C., F.A.A.P. Professor, Departments of Pediatrics and Obstetrics and Gynecology, McGill University; and Chief, Department of Pediatrics and Neonatology, Sir Mortimer B. Davis Jewish General Hospital, Montreal, Quebec, Canada.

ERMELINDA PELAUSA, M.D., F.R.C.P.C. Assistant Professor of Pediatrics (Neonatology), McGill University Faculty of Medicine; and Staff Neonatologist, Medical Director (Neonatal Follow-up), Department of Neonatology, Sir Mortimer B. Davis Jewish General Hospital, Montreal, Quebec, Canada.

RODERIC H. PHIBBS, M.D. Department of Pediatrics, University of California, San Francisco, San Francisco, California.

J. EDGAR WINSTON CRUZ POSECION, M.D. Division of Neonatal–Perinatal Medicine, Department of Pediatrics, Wayne State University School of Medicine, Hutzel Hospital; and Children's Hospital of Michigan, Detroit, Michigan.

DAVID M. POWELL, M.D. Assistant Professor, Department of Surgery, The George Washington University School of Medicine; and Attending Surgeon, Department of Pediatric Surgery, Children's National Medical Center, Washington, D.C.

RICHARD POWERS, M.D. Associate Neonatologist, Division of Neonatology, Children's Hospital and Research Center at Oakland, Oakland, California.

GABRIELLA PRIDJIAN, M.D. Professor and Chairman, The Ernest A. and Elizabeth Miller-Robin Chair in Obstetrics and Gynecology, Tulane University School of Medicine; and Assistant Dean, Lakeside Hospital and Clinic, Adjunct Professor of Pediatrics, Clinical Geneticist in Human Genetics Program, New Orleans, Louisiana.

GLORIA S. PRYHUBER, M.D. Associate Professor of Pediatrics (Neonatology) and Environmental Medicine Associate; and Director, Neonatal-Perinatal Fellowship Program, Golisano Children's Hospital at Strong, Rochester, New York.

YUNG-HAO PUNG, M.D., M.P.H. Assistant Professor, Department of Pediatrics, Georgetown University School of Medicine, Washington, D.C.

VIRENDER K. REHAN, M.D., M.R.C.P. (UK), M.R.C.P.I. (DUBLIN) Associate Professor, Department of Pediatrics, David Geffen School of Medicine at UCLA; and Director, Neonatal Intensive Care, Department of Pediatrics, Harbor UCLA Medical Center, Torrance, California.

MARY E. REVENIS, M.D. Assistant Professor of Pediatrics, Department of Neonatology, The George Washington University School of Medicine and Health Sciences, and Children's National Medical Center, Washington, D.C.

WARD R. RICE, M.D., Ph.D. Associate Professor of Pediatrics, University of Cincinnati College of Medicine, Children's Hospital Medical Center, Cincinnati, Ohio.

HENRIQUE RIGATTO, M.D. Professor, Department of Pediatrics, Physiology and Reproductive Medicine, University of Manitoba–Winnipeg; and Director of Neonatal Research, Health Sciences Centre, Winnepeg, Manitoba, Canada.

WILLIAM W. ROBERTSON, Jr., M.D. Professor, Departments of Orthopaedic Surgery and Pediatrics, The George Washington University School of Medicine, Washington, D.C.

WARREN N. ROSENFELD, M.D. Professor, Department of Pediatrics, State University of New York at Stony Brook School of Medicine, Stony Brook; and Chairman, Department of Pediatrics, Winthrop-University Hospital, Mineola, New York.

LISA M. SATLIN, M.D. Professor, Department of Pediatrics, Mount Sinai School of Medicine, Chief, Division of Pediatric Nephrology, Department of Pediatrics, Mount Sinai Medical Center, New York, New York.

ROBERT L. SCHELONKA, M.D. Assistant Professor, Department of Pediatrics, University of Alabama at Birmingham; and Associate Medical Director, Regional Newborn Intensive Care Unit, Division of Neonatology, University of Alabama at Birmingham, Birmingham, Alabama.

MARY M. K. SESHIA, M.B.Ch.B., F.R.C.P.(E.), F.R.C.P.C.H., D.C.H. Professor of Pediatrics, Head, Section of Neonatology, University of Manitoba, Winnipeg, Manitoba, Canada.

JOHN L. SEVER, M.D., Ph.D. Professor, Departments of Pediatrics, Obstetrics and Gynecology, The George Washington University School of Medicine; and Professor, Department of Infectious Disease, Children's National Medical Center, Washington, D.C.

BILLIE LOU SHORT, M.D. Chief, Division of Neonatology, Children's National Medical Center, Washington, D.C.

NALINI SINGH, M.D., M.P.H. Professor, George Washington School of Medicine and Health Sciences, and Division Director, Pediatric Infectious Diseases, Children's National Medical Center, Washington, D.C.

JUDITH SMITH, M.H.A. Principal, Smith Hager Bajo, Inc., Ashburn, Virginia.

MARK W. THOMPSON, M.D. Assistant Professor of Pediatrics, Uniformed Services University of the Health Sciences Bethesda, Maryland; and Director, Neonatal Fellowship Program, Tripler Army Medical Center, Kapiólani Medical Center for Women and Children, Honolulu, Hawaii.

WILLIAM E. TRUOG, M.D. Professor, Department of Pediatrics, University of Missouri–Kansas City School of Medicine, Sosland Endorsed Chair in Neonatal Research, Section of Neonatology, Children's Mercy Hospitals and Clinics, Kansas City, Missouri.

REGINALD C. TSANG, M.D., M.B.B.S. Emeritus Professor of Pediatrics, Department of Neonatology, Cincinnati Children's Hospital Medical Center, Cincinnati, Ohio.

JON A. VANDERHOOF, M.D. Professor, Director, Pediatric Gastroenterology and Nutrition, University of Nebraska Medical Center, Omaha, Nebraska.

MARIA ESTERLITA-UY T. VILLANUEVA, M.D. Division of Neonatal–Perinatal Medicine, Department of Pediatrics, Wayne State University School of Medicine, Hutzel Hospital; and Children's Hospital of Michigan, Detroit, Michigan.

SALLY H. VITALI, M.D. Instructor, Department of Anesthesia, Harvard Medical School, Assistant in Critical Care Medicine, Department of Anesthesia, Perioperative and Pain Medicine, Childrens' Hospital Boston, Boston, Massachusetts.

ROBERT M. WARD, M.D. Professor, Director, Pediatric Pharmacology Program, University of Utah, Attending Neonatologist, Department of Neonatology, Primary Children's Medical Center, Salt Lake City, Utah.

BARBARA B. WARNER, M.D. William Cooper Proctor Research Scholar, University of Cincinnati College of Medicine, Children's Hospital Medical Center, Cincinnati, Ohio.

STEVEN N. WEINDLING, M.D. Department of Pediatrics, Section of Pediatric Cardiology, Dartmouth Medical School; and Dartmouth–Hitchcock Medical Center, Lebanon, New Hampshire.

HOWARD J. WEINSTEIN, M.D. Associate Professor, Division of Hematology and Oncology, Children's Hospital Medical Center, Cincinnati, Ohio; and Massachusetts General Hospital, Boston, Massachusetts

SUSAN E. WERT, Ph.D.   Research Associate, Divisions of Neonatology and Pulmonary Biology, Department of Pediatrics; Research Scholar, University of Cincinnati College of Medicine; and Director, Morphology Care, Division of Pulmonary Biology, Children's Hospital Research Foundation, Cincinnati, Ohio.

ROBERT D. WHITE, M.D.   Clinical Assistant Professor, Department of Pediatrics, Indiana University School of Medicine, Notre Dame, Indianapolis, Director, Regional Newborn Program, Memorial Hospital, South Bend, Indiana.

JEFFREY A. WHITSETT, M.D.   Professor, Department of Pediatrics, University of Cincinnati College of Medicine; and Director, Division of Pulmonary Biology, Children's Hospital Medical Center, Cincinnati, Ohio.

KAREN S. WOOD, M.D.   Assistant Professor, Department of Pediatrics, University of North Carolina at Chapel Hill, Medical Director, Pediatric Transport, Carolina Air Care, UNC Hospitals, Chapel Hill, North Carolina.

YUVAL YARON, M.D.   Sourasly Medical Center, Tel Aviv, Israel.

SCOTT B. YEAGER, M.D.   Associate Professor, Department of Pediatrics, University of Vermont; and Chief, Division of Pediatric Cardiology, Medical Center Hospital of Vermont, Burlington, Vermont.

TERENCE L. ZACH, M.D.   Associate Professor, Department of Pediatrics, Creighton University, Omaha, Nebraska.

BARBARA J. ZELIGS   Research Associate, Department of Pediatrics, Georgetown University School of Medicine; and International Center for Interdisciplinary Studies of Immunology, Washington, D.C.

Foreword

It was in 1972 that I began planning the first edition of *Neonatology: Pathophysiology and Management of the Newborn*. In the preface of the first edition, I wrote that "Knowledge in this area has so expanded that it now seems important to collect this material in a multi-author reference work . . . . The newborn is heir to so many problems, and his or her physiology is so unique and rapidly changing, that all conditions in the newborn should come within the concern of the new and expanding discipline of neonatology." This thinking still guides the sixth edition, which you hold in your hands.

In the meantime, science and practice in neonatology have grown so rapidly that it is impossible for anyone to retain all the information that this text contains. It is more an anthology, a collection of major state-of-the-art papers, than a single book. We just do not have enough personal disk space and RAM to encompass it all. Many neonatologists have become sub-sub-specialists, while still retaining a broad view of the field. We also have become adept at using remote information, via electronic searches and consultation. Perhaps one of our all-too-frequent weaknesses rests in failing to fulfill the role of the general practitioner who puts it all together for individual families. In this respect, the chapter on ethical considerations has been an important aspect of each edition. As we go to publication, we mourn the death of John C. Fletcher, a pioneer and leader in medical ethics and co-author of the current Ethical Considerations chapter, who died May 27, 2004, at the age of 72. Dr. Fletcher was an Episcopal priest—a man of deep personal convictions—who was chief ethics officer at the NIH Clinical Center and a member of the faculty of the Virginia Theological Seminary. He served on many NIH committees as an ethicist, and he was a frequent consultant, author, and lecturer on ethics. We have learned much from his wisdom and compassion, and we offer him our admiration and respect.

There are 60 chapters in the current edition. All of those previously published have been extensively rewritten. Eight chapters have new authors, and there are three entirely new chapters regarding breast feeding, infection control in the NICU, and telehealth. "Something old, something new, something borrowed, something blue," as the saying goes. Concerns about thermoregulation, delivery room resuscitation, nutrition, and infection have been there since the beginning. New contributions regarding molecular genetics, imaging and monitoring technology, and respiratory support are now important. Borrowed information comes from experts in perinatal obstetrics, radiology and imaging technology, pharmacology, laboratory medicine, cardiology, surgery, and outcomes research. And something blue is still with us: the critical problems of oxygenation attending delivery, lung immaturity, cardiac malformations, and pulmonary hypertension.

This is my last hurrah with this textbook. I have long been out of the nursery, even longer out of the laboratory, and I find life as an Emeritus Professor pleasant indeed. But I still delight in the wonderful interplay of science and art in the now-robust field of neonatology. Permit me, then, a few predictions. We will devote more energy to understanding and preventing preterm birth. We will find ways to deal with adverse behaviors that result in poor outcomes for the neonate: smoking, alcohol, drugs, poor prenatal care, inadequate nutrition, excess stress, prenatal infections, and others not yet described. We will apply health outcomes research to provide efficient feedback loops so that our best practices will be more quickly adopted, and variation among NICUs will be reduced. We will understand how to use our new molecular biology tools to modify growth and aid healing and repair. We will become more adept at neuroprotection and will intervene in destructive spirals such as reperfusion injury to the brain. And most importantly, we will learn wonderful and unexpected things about the plasticity of the brain and nervous system. Geoffrey Raisman, a founder of the concept of neuroplasticity, has said that current theory is the enemy of new scientific discovery. We need to marvel at the feats of regeneration achieved by salamanders, for one, and not rest until we understand which factors turn on, and which inhibit, regrowth of neural tissue. If newts can do it, we can do it. Enjoy!!

Gordon B. Avery, M.D., Ph.D.

Preface

Early in the 1970s, the major medical postgraduate examining bodies in the United Kingdom, the Royal College of Physicians and the Royal College of Surgeons, recognized two specialties: adult medicine and general surgery. Pediatrics could be practiced only after completion of training and examination in adult medicine. The subspecialty of neonatology did not yet exist, and newborns weighing less than 1500 grams at birth were considered unlikely to survive. In the United States, subspecialty apprenticeships (fellowships) were available in neonatology; however, the treatment provided to sick newborn infants was largely extrapolated by miniaturization of that provided to adults and larger children. Earlier misadventures with "benign" therapeutic agents, such as oxygen, had resulted in calamitous complications, leading to the concept that premature infants stood a greater chance of intact survival if interventions were limited to the minimum.

In 1972, when the founding editor of *Neonatology: Pathophysiology and Management of the Newborn*, Gordon B. Avery, M.D. Ph.D., was planning the first edition, Dr. Mhairi MacDonald was in residency training in Edinburgh, Scotland; Dr. Martha Mullett in Morgantown, West Virginia, USA; Dr. Molly Seshia was practicing pediatrics in India. By the time that Drs. MacDonald and Mary Ann Fletcher joined Dr. Avery as co-editors for the fourth edition in the early 1990s, neonatology was an established pediatric subspecialty in both the United Kingdom and the United States, with a track record at once admirable for the pace of advancement of knowledge and technology and cautionary for the significant incidence of long-term morbidity in NICU survivors.

As the sixth edition goes to press, with two new editors, Drs. Mullett and Seshia, it is clear that the optimal practice of neonatology continues to require a careful balance between the aggressive use of modern therapeutic technology and the prevention of unintended damage to a fragile organism. The prefaces to previous editions reflect an ongoing concern with ethical issues surrounding the increasing ability to treat newborns previously considered nonviable.

The Accreditation Council for Graduate Medicine (ACGME) in the United States has defined 6 general medical competencies that must be achieved by trainees in any branch of clinical medicine and surgery; namely: patient care (appropriate, effective, and compassionate), clinical science (application of evolving biomedical and clinical science to patient care), practice-based learning and improvement (ongoing investigation, evaluation, and improvement of patient care practices), interpersonal skills and communication (with patients, patients' families, and other members of the healthcare team), professionalism (vocation, ethical practice, self-evaluation, demeanor), and systems-based medicine (having the awareness that all healthcare is provided in the context of a larger system and the ability to effectively utilize system resources to support the care of patients). We hope that the sixth edition of this text will substantially assist those in training to acquire all six competencies. ACGME emphasis on communication skills and systems-based medicine, in particular, provides a timely reminder that the NICU team cannot exist in a vacuum; sound decisions must be made with the assistance of consultants in the community, and follow-up care for NICU graduates must be planned and monitored as carefully as acute intensive care.

In this edition of *Neonatology* there are three new chapters and eight new first authors. The addition of the chapter on telemedicine is based on advances in knowledge and technology. The addition of the chapters on breast feeding and infection control in the NICU are long overdue.

Mhairi G. MacDonald,
M.B.Ch.B., F.R.C.P.(E.), F.R.C.P.C.H., F.A.A.P., D.C.H.
Martha D. Mullett,
M.D., M.P.H.
Mary M. K. Seshia,
M.B.Ch.B., F.R.C.P.(E.), F.R.C.P.C.H., D.C.H.

Preface to the First Edition

Neonatology means knowledge of the human newborn. The term was coined by Alexander Schaffer, whose book on the subject, *Diseases of the Newborn,* was first published in 1960. This book, together with Clement Smith's *Physiology of the Newborn Infant,* formed cornerstones of the developing field. In the past fifteen years, neonatology has grown from the preoccupation of a handful of pioneers to a major subspecialty of pediatrics. Knowledge in this area has so expanded that it now seems important to collect this material into a multiauthor reference work.

Although the perinatal mortality rate has declined over the past fifty years, the best presently attainable survival rates have not been achieved throughout the world, and indeed the United States lags behind fifteen other countries, despite its vast resources. New knowledge and improvement in the coordination of services for mother and child are needed to drive down perinatal mortality further. And finally, far greater emphasis must be placed on morbidity, so that surviving infants can lead full and productive lives. One hopes that in the future the yardstick of success will be the quality of life and not the mere fact of life itself.

In this past decade, neonatology, as a recognized subspeciality of pediatrics, has come into being around the intensive care-premature nursery. Needless to say, the problems of prematurity are far from solved. But neonatology is ripe for a broadening-out from its prematurity-hyaline membrane disease beginnings. The newborn is heir to so many problems, and his or her physiology is so unique and rapidly changing that all conditions of the newborn should come within the concern of the new and expanding discipline of neonatology. It has long since become standard practice to admit to premature nurseries other high-risk infants such as those of diabetic or toxemic mothers. Here the criterion is the need for intensive care. However, the neonatologist's specialized knowledge should give him a significant role in the care of other infants in the first two to three months of life, whether they require intensive care and whether they are readmitted for problems unrelated to prematurity and birth itself. Detailed knowledge of newborn physiology can assist in the management of congenital anomalies, surgical conditions of the neonate, failure to thrive, nutritional problems, genetic, neurologic, and biochemical diseases, and a host of conditions involving delayed maturation. Thus one can conceive of a subspecialty sharply limited in age to early infancy but broad in its study of the interaction of normal physiology and disease processes.

Neonatology must also grow in its relationship to obstetrics and fetal biology. In the best centers, an active partnership has developed between obstetrics and pediatrics around the management of high-risk pregnancies and newborns. Sometimes training has been cooperative, but in only a few instances have basic scientists concerned with fetal biology been brought into this effort. Important beginnings have been made in studying the fetomaternal unit, such as the endocrine studies of Egon Diczfalusy, the cardiopulmonary studies of Geoffrey Dawes, and the immunologic studies of Arther Silverstein. But fundamental processes such as the controls of fetal growth and the onset of labor are not understood at this time. Centers or institutes bringing together workers of diverse points of view are needed to wrestle with the profound problems of fetal biology. At the clinical level, the interdependence of obstetrics and neonatology is obvious. As an ultimate development, these two specialties may one day be joined as a new entity-perinatology-at least at the level of training and certification. In the meantime, far greater mutual understanding and daily interaction are needed for the optimal care of mothers and their infants.

This book is organized around problems as they occur, as well as by organ systems. It hopes to achieve a balance between presentation of the basic science on which rational management must rest, and the advice concerning patient care which experts in each subarea are qualified to give. Individual chapter authors have approached their subjects in various ways, and no attempt has been made to achieve a completely uniform format. In some instances, there is overlap of subject material, but the somewhat different viewpoints presented, and the desire to spare the reader from hopscotching through the book after cross references, have persuaded me to leave small overlaps undisturbed.

It is appreciated that no volume such as this can have more than a finite useful lifetime. Yet while its currency lasts, I hope it will serve as a practical guide to therapy and an aid in the understanding of pathophysiology for those active in the care of newborns.

Gordon B. Avery, M.D., Ph.D.

Avery's
Neonatology
Pathophysiology &
Management of
the Newborn

6th Edition

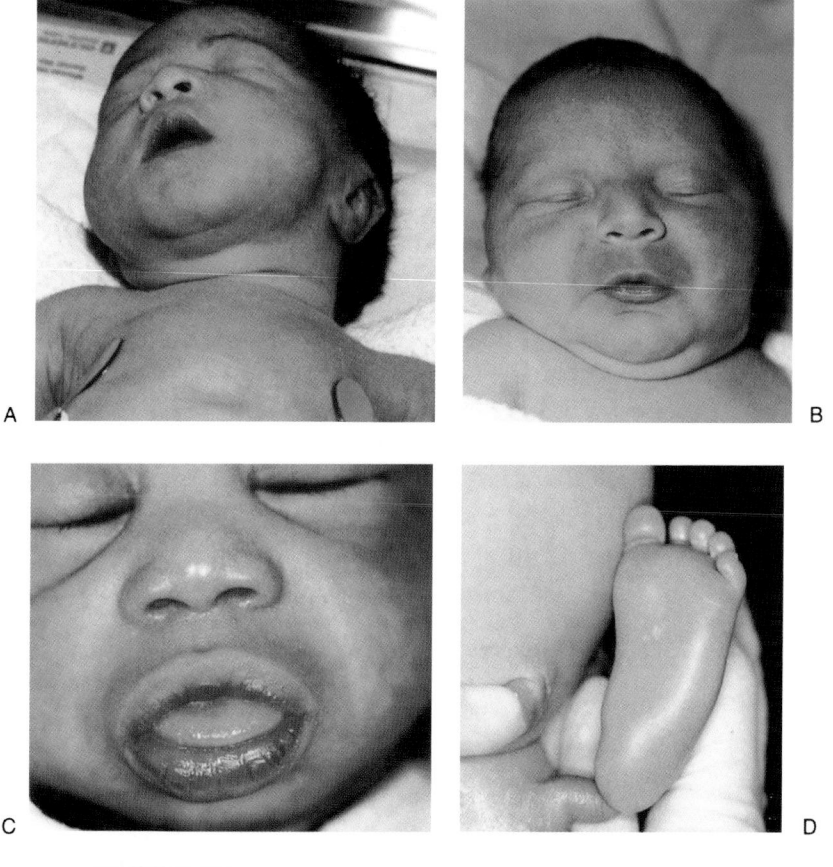

Cyanosis. **A.** Generalized cyanosis due to total anomalous pulmonary venous return with an oxygen saturation level of 80%. **B.** Perioral cyanosis. The mucous membranes and area over the chest remain pink in the presence of mild cyanosis above the lips. Petechiae make the forehead area appear blue. **C.** Lips appear blue from normal pigment deposition in vermilion border but the mucous membranes are pink. **D.** Acrocyanosis in the first half hour of life in a 32-week infant. **E.** Cyanosis localized to the abdominal wall. The blue color is caused by meconium peritonitis after an intrauterine bowel perforation. If peritoneal meconium is of long enough standing, a flat plat of the abdomen would show calcifications.

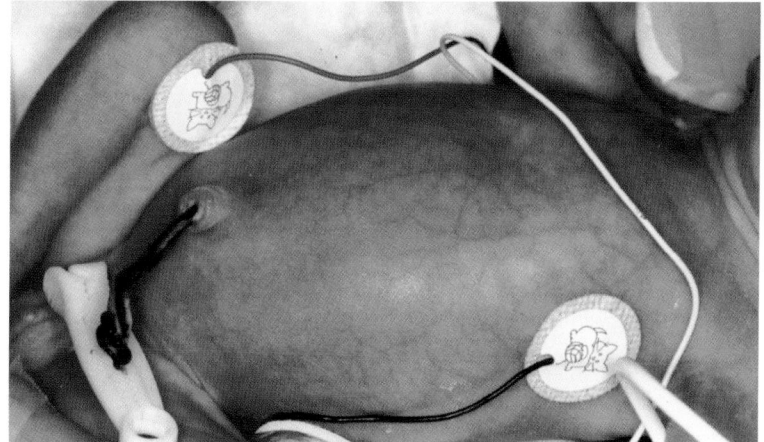

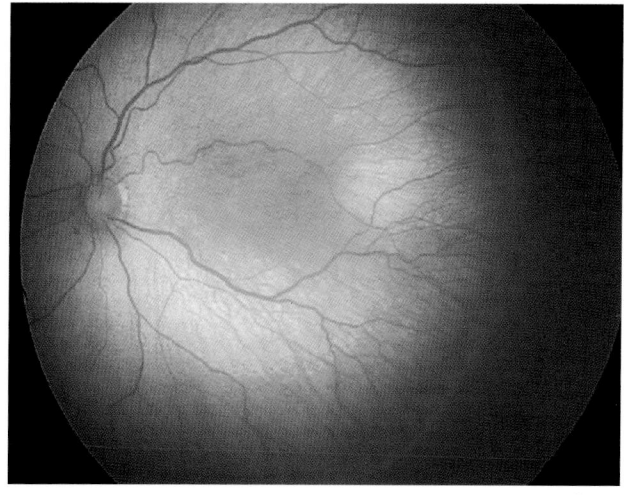

Figure 5-3 This image of an infant with ROP demonstrates the wide-field imaging capability of the RetCamII.

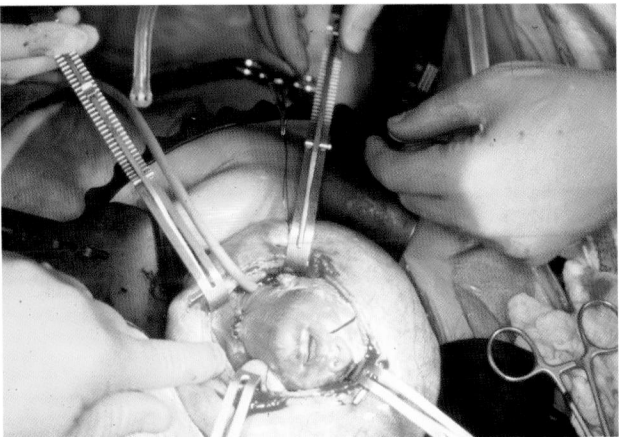

Figure 13-3 Surgical isolation of the fetal trachea prior to placement of hemoclips in a tracheal occlusion procedure for congenital diaphragmatic hernia.

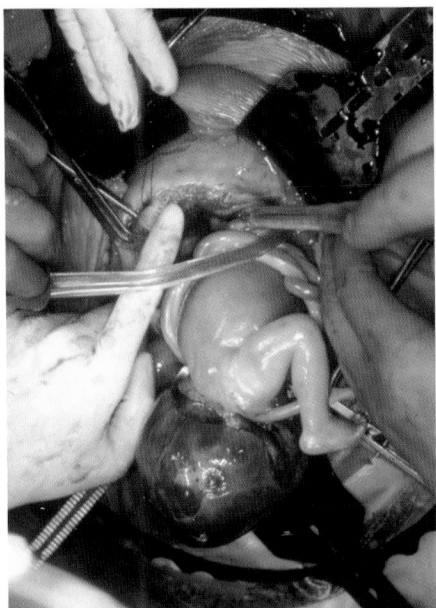

Figure 13-5 Saccrococcygeal teratoma in a fetus.

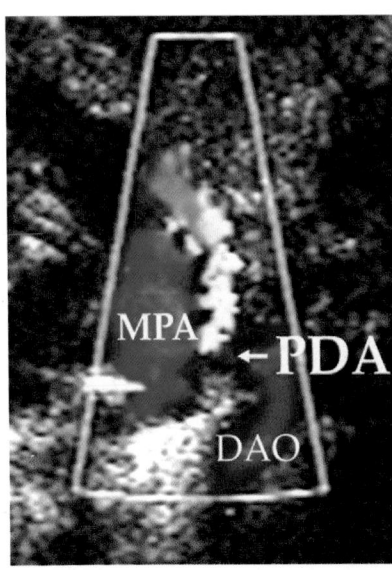

Figure 33-15 **A:** Echocardiographic apical four-chamber view in systole. Color Doppler analysis of the right heart demonstrates a jet of tricuspid regurgitation depicted by the blue flow jet (white arrow).

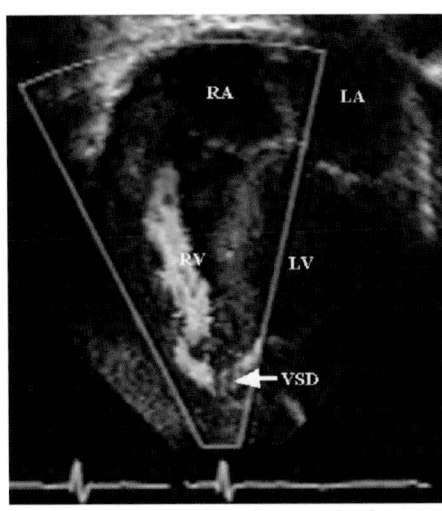

Figure 33-39 Echocardiogram 4 chamber view with color Doppler analysis demonstrates an apical musular ventricular septal defect. (LA, left atrium; LV, left ventricle; RA, right atrium; RV, right ventricle; VSD, ventricular septal defect.)

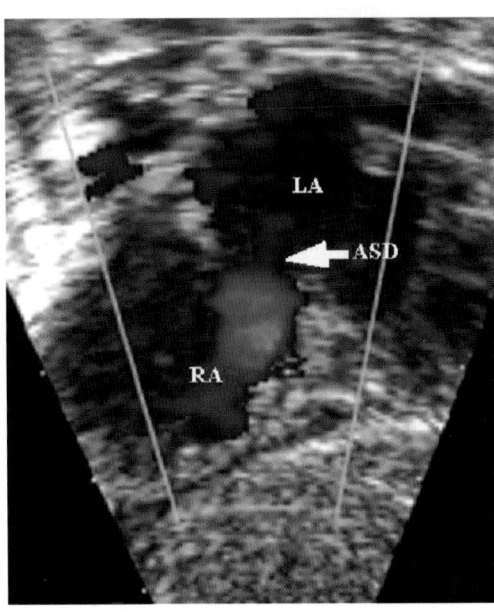

Figure 33-40 Echocardiogram 4 subcostal view with color Doppler analysis demonstrates an secundum atrial septal defect. (ASD, ventricular septal defect; LA, left atrium; RA, right atrium.)

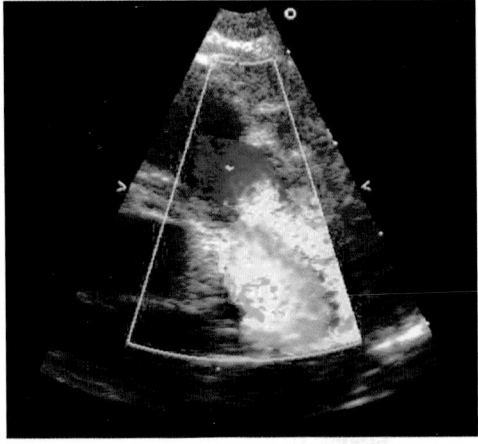

Figure 34-1 Critical pulmonary valve stenosis. **B.** Application of color Doppler during ventricular systole demonstrates a turbulent flow jet originating at the pulmonary valve leaflets and extending into the main pulmonary artery.

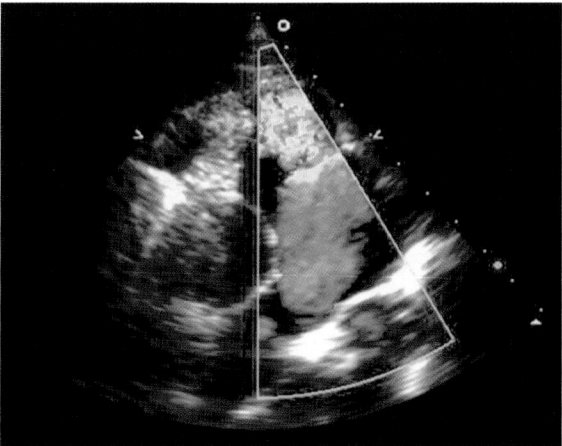

B

Figure 34-2 Tetralogy of Fallot with absent pulmonary valve. **B.** Application of color Doppler during ventricular diastole revealing free regurgitation from the main pulmonary artery into the right ventricular outflow tract. MPA, main pulmonary artery; PV, pulmonary valve; RVOT, right ventricular outflow tract.

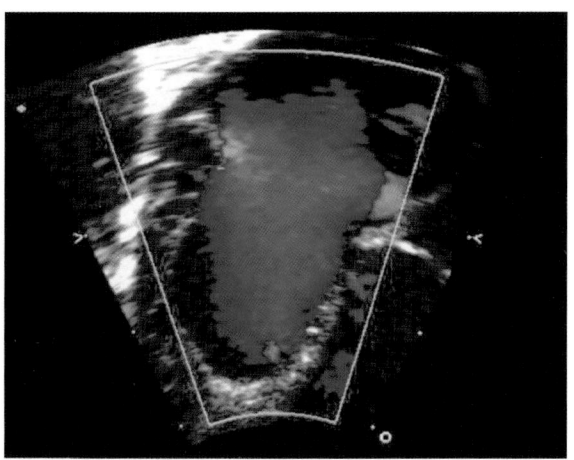

B

Figure 34-3 Ebstein's anomaly of the tricuspid valve. **B.** During ventricular diastole, color Doppler demonstrating free retrograde flow across the tricuspid valve annulus. ARV, atrialized right ventricle; LA, left atrium; LV, left ventricle; RA, right atrium; TV, tricuspid valve.

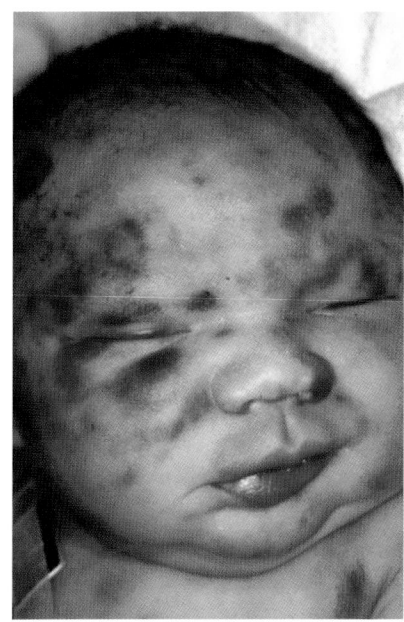

Figure 53-1 Congenital acute monocytic leukemia with skin nodules.

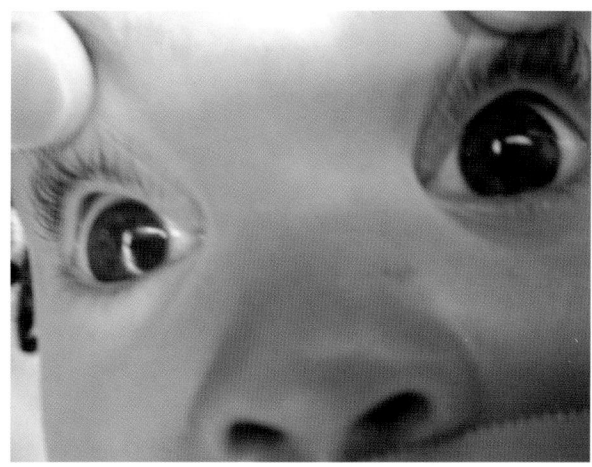

Figure 54-1 When the corneal diameter exceeds 11 mm in a neonate, a differential diagnosis must be considered.

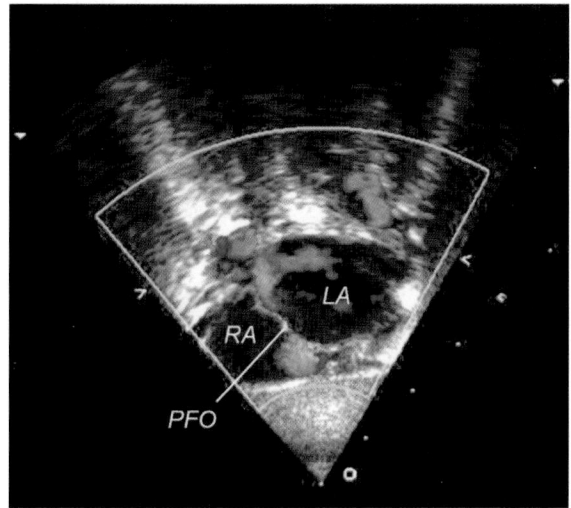

A

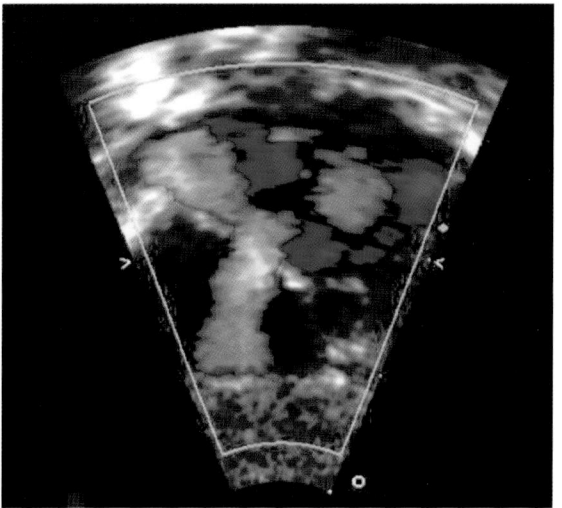

B

Figure 34-12 Restrictive atrial septum in a newborn with transposition of the great arteries. **A.** Two-dimensional echocardiogram with color Doppler from the subcostal window demonstrating a tiny patent foramen ovale with left to right flow across the atrial septum. **B.** Following successful balloon atrial septostomy, a wide communication now exists between the left and right atria. LA, left atrium; PFO, patent foramen ovale; RA, right atrium.

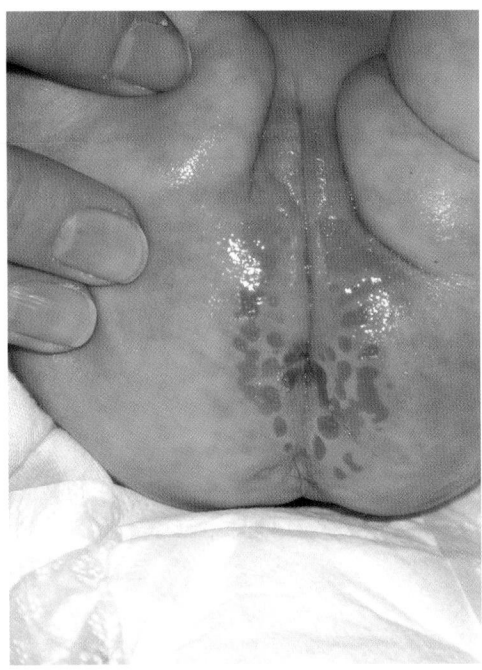

Figure 55-1 Erosive dermatitis.

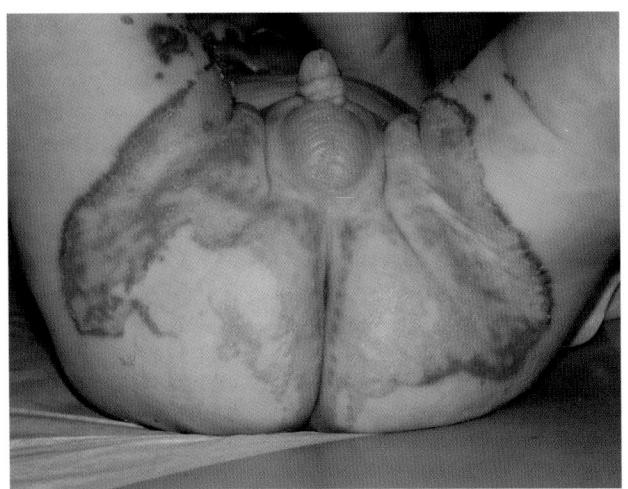

Figure 55-5 Acrodermatitis enteropathica.

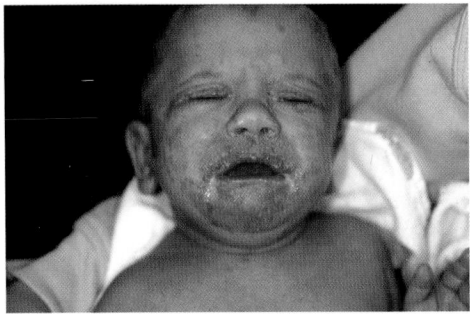

Figure 55-6 Staphylococcal scalded skin syndrome.

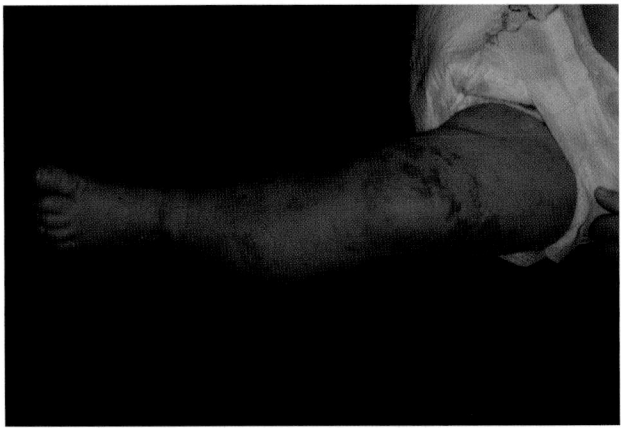

Figure 55-10 Incontinentia pigmenti.

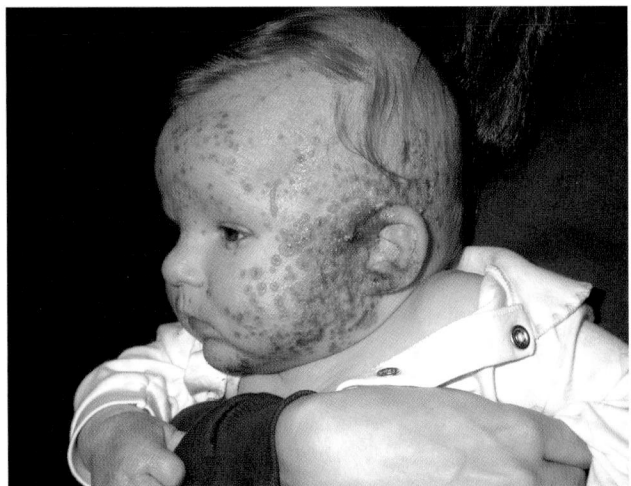

Figure 55-13 Eczema herpeticum.

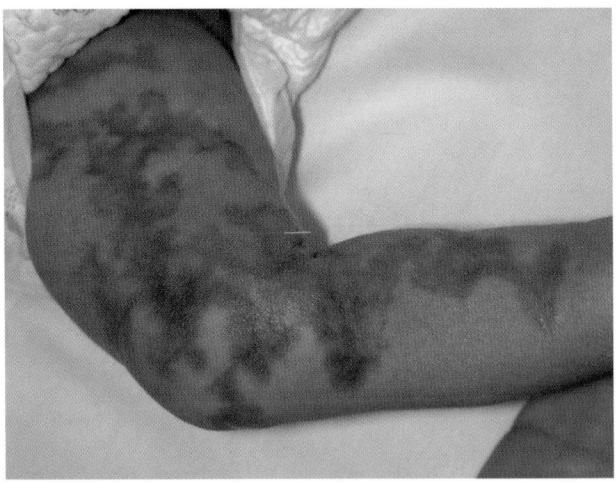

Figure 55-19 Cutis marmorata telangiectatica congenita.

General Considerations

Neonatology: Past, Present and Future

Gordon B. Avery

Rapid change has characterized neonatology since the name was coined in 1960 by Alexander Schaffer. Structurally, it can be compared with a tree (Fig. 1-1). Its *roots*—obstetrics, pediatrics, and physiology—began at the turn of the century. A sturdy *trunk* has developed in the intensive care nurseries (ICNs) scattered across the United States and around the world. The *branches* have spread so widely that it is difficult for a single person to be expert in all the areas of activity required for a tertiary neonatology service. Important interactions have gone beyond allied disciplines such as obstetrics, anesthesiology, cardiology, radiology, and surgery. Neonatologists today struggle with hospital administrators, pediatric training program directors, legislatures, Congress, the courts, the federal government, malpractice lawyers, right-to-life groups, and ethicists in an effort to determine their proper roles and limits. Caught in a cross-fire between strenuous cost-containment measures and regulations mandating the vigorous treatment of all newborns regardless of prognosis, many neonatologists wonder when a stable situation will be reached. Yet stimulating growth has occurred, mainly since 1960.

PAST: THE ROOTS

One of the main roots from which neonatology grew was supplied by obstetricians such as Pierre Budin and Sir Dugald Baird, who were interested in the babies they delivered and not merely in the immediate welfare of the mother. It may be a serious oversimplification to imply that, in former times, obstetricians were content if the baby was born alive. Childbirth, however, was the cause of a significant number of maternal deaths and for many was a fearful experience. Premature infants were expected to die, as were most neonates with malformations. There was a feeling that natural selection should be allowed to discard the "runt of the litter," as suggested by the designation of premature babies as *weaklings*. It was Budin and his pupil

Couney who pioneered incubator care of premature infants and thus helped change some of the early, pessimistic attitudes toward these babies.

Another significant root of neonatology can be found in the "quiet premature nursery," such as that operated by Julius Hess and Evelyn Lundeen in Chicago in the early 1900s (1). Only premature infants were admitted to these nurseries, and gentleness with minimal intervention was the policy. To prevent infection, staff wore gowns, caps, and masks and set up a scrub routine that excluded parents and minimized traffic in the area. Feedings of breast milk by eyedropper were delayed for up to 72 hours, and the infants were handled as little as possible. Yet the supportive conditions needed to allow the body to recover, as described by Florence Nightingale, were present: "warmth, rest, diet, quiet, sanitation, space, and others" (2). Perhaps some of the high-tech nurseries of today could benefit from an infusion of this superb nurturing orientation.

Physiology is a taproot of neonatology. Advances in neonatal care rest directly on descriptions of the changing body processes of the newborn infant. Men such as Barcroft and Dawes began delineation of fetal circulation and placental function. These studies in turn led to the establishment of the fetal lamb model, which subsequently was widely exploited. Neonatal metabolic, gastrointestinal, respiratory, and central nervous system functions were studied by Levine, Smith, Peiper, and others. The 1945 publication of the first edition of Clement Smith's textbook, *The Physiology of the Newborn Infant*, was a signal event in our evolving ability to care for sick newborns in a rational manner (3).

A final anchoring root of neonatology is the therapeutic trial. Innumerable traditional teachings about premature infants eventually have been proved false. Without scientific testing as a guide, neonatologists would constantly be off course. As it is, several dangerous misadventures have been averted by clinical trials. An example is prophylactic sulfonamide treatment of premature infants, which was

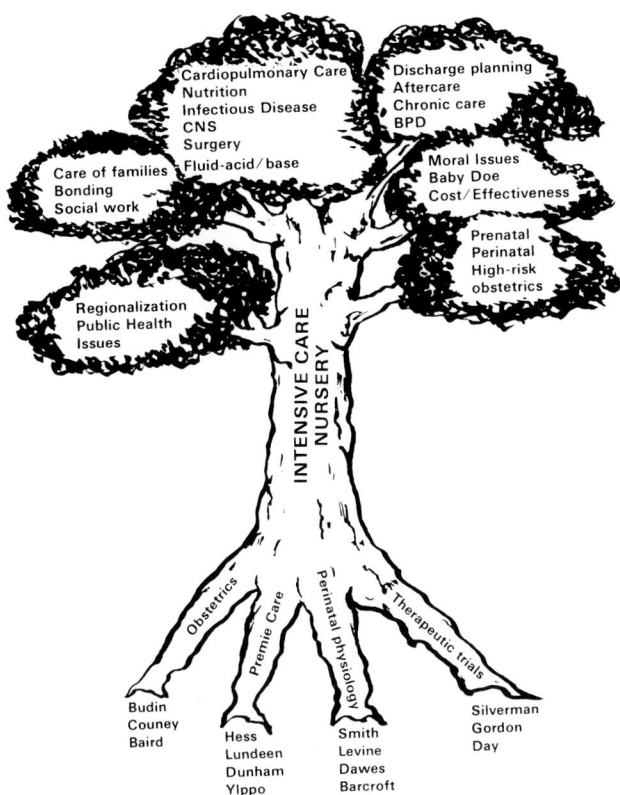

Figure 1-1 The neonatal-perinatal tree shows the roots, trunk, and branches of the specialty.

found to cause increased kernicterus (4). Silverman, Gordon, and Day were pioneers who insisted on rigor in such trials.

PRESENT: THE TRUNK

The ICN is the institution that forms the sturdy trunk of endeavors in neonatology. The ICN is a therapeutic environment, a collection of equipment, and a multidisciplinary team that is guided by dedicated leadership, by a group of specific protocols, and by a body of relevant scientific knowledge. It is the ICN as an integrated organism, rather than any single person or collection of people, that takes care of the sick neonate—in a sense, this is holistic medicine turned inside out. The ICN is very effective in the care of desperately ill babies, but its rationale remains difficult to explain to hospital administrators, insurance companies, and the U.S. Congress.

Over the years, there has been a steady increase in the intensity of illness observed in the ICN. With this rise has come an increase in the number and variety of personnel and the amount of technically sophisticated equipment. In the 1950s, premature care was a major concern. The principal interventions were resuscitation, thermoregulation, careful feeding, simple and exchange transfusion, and supportive care of respiratory distress. By the 1960s, electronic monitors came into use, and blood gases began to be measured. Feedings were aided by nasogastric tubes, and in-

creased laboratory monitoring became possible. Antibiotics became available for treatment of neonatal sepsis.

By the 1970s, the use of umbilical catheters and arterial pressure transducers was routine, and respirator therapy for hyaline membrane disease began to succeed. Nutritional support for sick infants was aided by transpyloric feeding tubes and finally by complete intravenous alimentation. Microchemistry tests for most necessary parameters became widely available. Neonatal surgery was shown to be feasible for many congenital abnormalities, including serious cardiac defects. With the 1980s came the advent of computed tomography and ultrasonography. Significant concern centered around ventricular hemorrhages and consequent posthemorrhagic hydrocephalus in small premature infants. Transcutaneous electrodes became available first for measurement of oxygen and then for carbon dioxide. Pulse oximetry was used increasingly for continuous physiologic monitoring. Nutritional and metabolic supports were significantly refined. Surfactant replacement has reduced the severity of lung disease in premature infants. Extracorporeal membrane oxygenation permitted the survival of some previously unsalvageable infants. In the 1990s, magnetic resonance imaging improved visualization of lesions, and positron emission tomography and magnetic resonance spectroscopy promise to reveal the physiology of the intact brain. As survival has become common for infants who weigh as little as 600 g (1.3 lb) at birth, increased attention has swung to assuring intact survival, and the 1990s have been dubbed the decade of the brain.

THE BRANCHES

Perinatology

A body of specialized knowledge, a group of subspecialized professionals, the advent of technically advanced equipment, and the formation of special care units all contributed to the development of neonatology. In obstetrics, these same elements came together approximately 10 years later and resulted in the specialty of maternofetal medicine. Perinatologists developed high-risk prenatal clinics and special delivery facilities for unstable patients. A steadily growing body of literature from animal and clinical investigations allowed improved management of pregnancy complications and monitoring of fetal status. Ultrasonography detected fetal abnormalities and determined fetal size, anatomy, activity, breathing, and response to stress. For the first time, mothers were given drugs designed to treat fetal conditions, and intrauterine transfusions were performed in cases of threatened hydrops. Fetal surgery has yet to find its proper place, but prenatal shunts have been inserted for hydrocephalus, obstructed urinary tracts have been drained, and diaphragmatic hernia repair has been attempted.

In many major teaching hospitals, perinatal obstetric and neonatal services have joined forces to form perinatal centers. Often with codirectors from the two disciplines, these centers foster cooperation in the best interests of the high-risk patient. Integrated planning and management in optimal cases consist of a high-risk prenatal clinic, timing and management of labor and delivery, resuscitation, and intensive care in the nursery. Statistics on morbidity and mortality, reviewed in periodic joint conferences, permit constant refinement of policy and technique. These centers facilitate training programs in both perinatology and neonatology and are important sources for research. They demonstrate the best survival rates for small premature and other categories of infants at highest risk, and they provide the standard by which perinatal care is judged.

The natural alliance between perinatal obstetrics and neonatology is so great that some have suggested it receive department status within the medical complex. In some ways, the perinatal center accomplishes this on an ad hoc basis. However, perinatologists and neonatologists are parts of traditional departments of obstetrics and pediatrics, with surgical and medical orientations, respectively. Allocation of resources and ranking of faculty occur predominantly through the parent departments, where the priorities of the chairpersons are paramount.

Regional Connections

The medical community found that to optimize function of the perinatal center, it was necessary to form complex relationships among hospitals and community resources (see Chapter 3). First, neonatal and then maternal transport services were developed to move patients safely and efficiently to the center and back. Hot lines were established to provide consultation and bed allocation, which could be coordinated through a single phone number. Affiliations for continuing education were formed, and standard protocols for referral were worked out. In some instances, exchange of personnel and joint review of statistics helped cement the connection.

Government agencies extended a helping hand in this networking. Some state legislatures were convinced early of the public health advantage of regional systems. The government began to award grants to perinatal centers to underwrite some of the cost of outreach and system activities. Training and research grants from the federal government often were given to the same perinatal centers and served to buttress the resources of these centers. With passage of the National Health Planning and Resources Development Act (Public Law 93-641) in 1974, the federal government mandated regional planning of expensive resources in the interest of efficiency and economy. Designation of care levels I, II, and III was adopted, and publication of regional plans for perinatal care became widespread.

Unfortunately, during the 1980s regionalization suffered striking reversals. The mandated state health planning mechanisms were emasculated. Hospitals became increasingly competitive and wished to offer full services to prepaid health plans. Large numbers of neonatologists moved into suburban hospitals and set up level II nurseries.

The result was a decentralization of perinatal high-risk care, with loss of efficiency and economy of scale.

Finally, I wish to call attention to the involvement of neonatologists in a mixture of educational, administrative, and political activities that have been very taxing and time-consuming. Although neonatology training has emphasized bedside care, a business school or public health degree would be directly useful to today's neonatologist. A thorough training in counseling, group dynamics, and law also would be invaluable.

THE PRESENT

Ethics

During the newborn period, babies with congenital malformations, asphyxia, and extreme immaturity are seen. Modern, powerful life-support systems provide the technology for relatively prolonged continuation of futile care. These circumstances have thrust neonatologists into the center of a national debate on medical ethics. In the midst of all this, neonatologists must keep their heads and care for babies and their families as best they can. Chapter 2 deals extensively with the moral issues raised by neonatal intensive care.

Care of the Family

In general, there has been striking improvement in care of the distressed families of critically ill newborn infants. Formerly excluded from the ICN because of fear of infection, parents are brought to the bedside and encouraged to touch their babies. Limited sibling visitation often is permitted. Nurses help parents get used to intrusive medical equipment, and, as soon as possible, parents perform simple caretaking procedures with their child. Social workers, parent support groups, chaplains, and literature for parents have become increasingly available. Starting with the work of Klaus and Kennell, a growing body of publications has appeared that suggests that bonding of parents to the newborn infant is important to later functioning of the family unit. The change of the title of Klaus and Kennell's monograph from *Maternal-Infant Bonding* (5) in 1976 to *Parent-Infant Bonding* (6) in 1982 reflects recognition of the role of fathers in the parenting of neonates.

Home Care

The aftercare of discharged high-risk newborns has become an increasingly important area of concern for neonatologists. Although many problems are resolved quickly and require only routine follow-up, a significant number of babies with chronic problems are taken home from the ICN. As a small premature infant approaches discharge, it becomes clear that parent instruction; sleep apnea testing; cardiopulmonary resuscitation training; concern with feeding and growth; schedules for testing sight, hearing, and speech; physical medicine; and developmental psychology foreshadow a first year of life crowded with clinic visits and special needs. Infants with chronic lung disease often go home on oxygen therapy, multiple medications, and special feeding regimens. During the first year or two of life, intercurrent infections may require several readmissions. The best outcomes have been achieved with early diagnosis of developmental difficulties and the mobilization of community resources. All this necessitates input from a physician with appreciation of the stormy neonatal period and an understanding of the continuing problems of infants born prematurely with other perinatal insults. Often, a multidisciplinary team at the tertiary center collaborates with the family's pediatrician to provide this special care. Although oriented to neonatal intensive care, neonatologists have begun to assume responsibility in this aftercare.

The Intensive Care Nursery as a Space Station

The quiet, simple, gentle premature nursery of 50 years ago has been transformed into a bustling space station. Suspended halfway up a tall building, too often it is drenched in bright light and alive with activity throughout the night. The tiny baby in the incubator is dwarfed by a procedure light, a respirator, a multichannel monitor, four intravenous pumps, and a transcutaneous oxygen module. The baby's chest is covered with electrodes, and tubes lead into and out of his or her body at several points. Eight to 12 electrical cords, 2 oxygen lines, and a suction catheter attach to the bedside console. Medications and flush solutions are drawn up in syringes close at hand. A resuscitation bag is at the head of the baby's bed in case he or she should stop breathing. Alarms sound, knots of people move busily about, and large machines are pushed among the incubators. Ultrasonography elements are touched to the infant's head, chest, and abdomen. Images flash on a screen and are recorded on tape for later analysis. House officers speak rapidly in an acronymic code barely intelligible to residents who graduated 2 years previously. Hess and Lundeen, coming some morning for a visit, might wonder if they had missed the address and arrived on the wrong planet!

At such a bedside, today's neonatologist must cope with a constantly enlarging body of new literature on cardiopulmonary physiology; nutritional and metabolic support; new antibiotics and infectious disease conditions; ventricular hemorrhage and asphyxial syndromes; and surgical, genetic, and cardiac problems. It is no longer possible for a physician to read all the new publications, even when restricted to the area of neonatology. New therapeutic approaches are proposed much faster than they can be tested in an orderly way; many such theories never will be tested.

THE FUTURE

In the future, I believe neonatology will move in two divergent directions. In the realm of neonatal intensive care, the contributions of basic science, and particularly genetics, will produce powerful diagnostic and therapeutic tools, which will significantly improve results. However, the global and public health dimensions of dealing with distressed newborns will require simpler, less expensive interventions that can be applied in developing nations. Clearly, the *bang for the buck* in neonatology is greatest where care is the least developed, and is least where the standard of care is already high. The challenge will be to keep the locomotive moving forward without leaving the caboose too far behind.

Of course, I cannot report to you with any precision what new developments in neonatology will occur in the next 20 years. Nevertheless, Table 1-1 is offered to illustrate, side by side, several areas of practice: past, present, and future. A few themes are highlighted. The past was characterized by minimum intervention and a nurturing sort of care dominated by gentle bedside nursing. The present era seizes on maintenance of normal physiologic and biochemical parameters. The baby—beset with indwelling lines, ventilators, and monitors, who "dies in balance"—is in line with this approach. The future will include accepting or deliberately producing some abnormal values in recognition of the baby's unique disease state. Examples include cooling for neuroprotection, hyperthermia for tumor inhibition, permissive hypercapnia to minimize pulmonary barotrauma, and cardiovascular unloading to treat neonatal lung failure. We will develop gene products and receptor blockers as medications, and use gene promoters and inhibitors to manipulate the cell's own genetic apparatus to treat diseases. Examples are the use of vascular endothelial growth factor (VEGF) and elastase inhibitors for reducing chronic lung disease (7–9).

Worldwide, measures to combat perinatal and neonatal infections, lower the incidence of prematurity, and reduce maternal malnutrition will benefit outcomes without the need for new technology. The impact of basic public health measures is so dramatic that one World Health Organization (WHO) official described infant mortality as "a public health problem with medical aspects, not a medical problem with public health aspects" (10,11).

Finally, the way we learn will evolve in the years ahead. Our scientific method emphasizes comparisons of groups differing by a single variable, ideally in a single disease state. Studies using tissue culture or the laboratory mouse are the models we try to approximate in the intensive care nursery. But our babies typically have many abnormal states simultaneously, and many therapies running at the same time. The staff is caring for many infants at the same time, and sometimes several investigative protocols are running alongside one another. The research study is never the first priority where life-and-death illness is involved. While all this is going on, there are changes in policy and equipment that affect care in the whole neonatal intensive care unit (NICU), across all diseases and birth weights.

We will need new types of statistics to aid in benchmarking interventions and studies of the impact of benchmarking practices. Large, computer-supported databases will help with hypothesis generation. We will become more adept at recognizing secular trends in NICU care

TABLE 1-1

NEONATOLOGY—PAST, PRESENT, AND FUTURE. THE AUTHOR'S THOUGHTS AND REPRESENTATIVE EXAMPLES

	PAST	PRESENT	FUTURE
Temperature	Physical bundling Laissez-Faire	Thermoneutral maintenance Servocontrols	Cooling for brain protection Hyperthermia for tumor inhibition
Nutrition	Small frequent feeds Nasal spoon Human milk	Early tiny feeds: priming I-V alimentatiaon gavage/gastrostomy	Growth factors Gene manipulation anti-stress endocrine adjustment
Infection	Isolation Aseptic technique	Antibiotics Some anitvirals	Immunotherapy Gene manipulation
Brain injury	Resuscitation triage	Trials of phenobarb, Mg, cooling DR resuscitation, support	Anti-oxidants, reduce reperfusion injury Gene manipulation; inhibitors and expression triggers Reduce programmed cell death
Metabolic funct	Minimal lab work Minimal intervention	Microchemistries Adjust towards normal values	patterns of gene activation microarrays, 10,000 genes → RNA inhibitors, releasers, gene products
Gene function	Errors of metabolism described	Enzyme ontogeny Neonatal pharmacology	Selective gene activation Rx with gene products or inhibitors Ontogeny of gene activation
Birth defects	Description and observation Support	Neonatal surgery Fetal ultrasound Dx	Preconception risk identification Intrapartum management of risk Fetal genetic diagnosis and treatment Molecular study of normal/abnormal development
Lung function	oxygen humidity	respirators, HFO inhaled nitrous oxide surfactant replacement ECMO	Vascular endothelial growth factor (VEGF) VEGF activation or instillation elastase inhibitors chronic inhaled NO cardiovascular unloading
Scope of practice	One patient, one doctor One disease, one transaction The controlling unit nurse	NICU: large team of attendings and support Multiple abnormal conditions simultaneously Multiple subspecialities, consultants Support services: lab, imaging, social work Ethics, legal requirements, HMOs Funding, privacy regulations Family rights, autonomy, advocacy	World-wide, public health point of view Cutting edge bio-technical vs simple, practical Prevention vs drastic support (prematurity, infections, malnutrition Low tech, lay trainee interventions Education, change of traditional practices Benchmarking, care systems research Telemedicine, regional centers
How we learn	Laboratory models: animals, tissue culture, reports of institutional results The published series Focus on a single variable Physiologic research	Multi-institutional controlled clinical trials Fundamental basic lab research Molecular mechanisms dominate grants Outcome studies	Dealing with multiple variables and secular change New statistical methodology for benchmarking Large outcome databases The computer in the NICU: care, record keeping, study Multiple levels of phenomenology The single variable in a single disease state The impact of changed practices across diseases The result of societal pressures on practice The impact of pre-hospitalization care The impact of post-hospitalization care Public health and health of the baby It takes a village to raise a child

versus the specific interventions we intend to study. And some of our interventions will be outside the nursery, in programs of education and/or pre- and post-NICU care. The years ahead will be as fast paced and challenging as those that have gone before.

REFERENCES

1. Hess JH, Lundeen EC. *The premature infant: its medical and nursing care.* Philadelphia: JB Lippincott, 1941.
2. Nightingale F. *Notes on nursing: what it is and what it is not.* (A facsimile of the first edition printed in London, 1859, with a foreword by Annie W. Goodrich.) Philadelphia: JB Lippincott, 1969.
3. Smith CA. *The physiology of the newborn infant.* Springfield, IL: Charles C Thomas, 1945.
4. Silverman WA, Anderson DH, et al. A difference in mortality rate and incidence of kernicterus among premature infants allotted to two prophylactic antibiotic regimens. *Pediatrics* 1956;18:614–624.
5. Klaus MH, Kennell JH. *Maternal-infant bonding.* St. Louis: CV Mosby, 1976.
6. Klaus MH, Kennell JH. *Parent-infant bonding.* St. Louis: CV Mosby, 1982.
7. Rabinovitch M, Bland M. Novel notions on newborn lung disease. *Nat Med* 2002;8:664–666.
8. Zaidi SH, You XM, Ciura S Husain M, et al. Overexpression of the serine protease elafin protects transgenic mice from hypoxic pulmonary hypertension. *Circulation* 2002;105:516–521.
9. O'Blenes SB, Fischer S, McIntyre B, et al. Hemodynamic unloading leads to regression of pulmonary vascular disease in rats. *J Thorac Cardiovasc Surg* 2001;121:279–289.
10. Vidyasagar D. A global view of advancing neonatal health and survival. *J Perinatol* 2002;22:513–515.
11. Coco G, Darmstadt GL, Kelley LM, et al. Perinatal and neonatal health interventions research. *J Perinatol* 2002;22:S1–S4.

Current Moral Priorities and Decision Making in Neonatal-Perinatal Medicine

Robert J. Boyle   *John C. Fletcher (deceased)*

GOALS OF NEONATAL-PERINATAL MEDICINE

The first part of this chapter discusses broad goals and moral priorities of neonatal-perinatal medicine (NPM) in relation to patients, American society, and developing nations. The second part reviews some specific ethical issues that frequently arise in clinical decision making in the neonatal period.

Medicine is a goal-oriented profession. One approach might argue that healing is the sole and overriding goal of medicine. This view is unconvincing, because some valid goals of medicine (e.g., prevention) cannot be collapsed into healing. The practice of NPM illustrates that medicine has multiple, complex, and sometimes conflicting goals:

- To save life and cure disease
- To relieve pain, suffering, and disability
- To rehabilitate and restore function
- To prevent disease
- To improve the quality of living and dying
- To seek new knowledge

The highest moral priority of these subspecialties is to implement medicine's goals in the perinatal period. In a recent review, Carter and Stahlman broadly discuss the successes (and limits) of neonatal intensive care in the United States over the past 40 years (1).

SOCIETAL AND PROFESSIONAL ISSUES

Medicine is also accountable to society and to the international community. Critics may validly argue that American medicine and public policy have neglected primary prevention and fostered the technological imperative. To counter these criticisms, the moral priorities of NPM specialists need to include advocacy for comprehensive prenatal care, improved nutrition, prevention of premature delivery and appropriate family support and services for the infant after discharge. NPM in the United States is also part of a global community of science, medicine, and humanitarian outreach. The moral priorities of the field ought to include commitment to global infant health. An editorial by Sidney Brenner, a leading figure in genetics, also applies to neonatal medicine. He wrote: "Somehow, in our abstruse discussions about the high technology of the developed world, we need to balance the equation by thinking about the rest of the world as well" (2). Nations where newborns are in greatest danger of death or lifelong disability could benefit from transferable knowledge and technology, for example, maternal folic acid supplementation, prevention of HIV transmission, vitamin K prophylaxis, eye prophylaxis for gonorrhea, and prevention of neonatal tetanus.

Preterm delivery—live birth prior to 37 completed weeks' gestation—grew in the United States from 8.9% in 1980 to 11.9% in 2001, more than 476,000 annual preterm births (3,4). The increase is caused by an 11% rise in moderately preterm births (32 to 36 weeks' gestation) in the 1990's. In 2001; charges for hospital stays for prematurity-related illness reached $13.6 billion. There are large differences in preterm births by race and ethnicity, although non-Hispanic white women give birth to the majority of the 4 million annual live births.

Paradoxically, both poverty and economic success are harmful to many infants. Poverty, race, class, and substance abuse are linked to a large percentage of prematurity, extremely low-birth-weight, and brain injury. However, multifetal pregnancies after assisted reproductive technologies (ART) and non-ART procedures have reached epidemic proportions (5–8). Epidemiologic studies also suggest an increased risk of major birth defects after assisted reproduction (9). Neonatologists see first hand the human damage and costs of these polar social determinants of gestational harm. Infertile individuals who want their own genetic child suffer psychologically and spiritually. Fertility treatments have allowed literally millions of women to have children who otherwise would not have been able to conceive. The primary responsibility to reduce these harms falls on reproductive medicine and policy makers. NPM specialists can facilitate research and remedies for the problem. To date, reliance on professional self-regulation has not been effective in reducing multifetal pregnancy in the United States. There is currently a debate about whether social controls of infertility treatment and research are fitting for a pluralistic society that highly values reproductive liberty. The President's Council on Bioethics is now considering a set of very strong federal controls to protect human embryos and constrain infertility treatment (8). At this point, all could agree that women undergoing ART should be informed about the risks of multiple gestation and preterm delivery.

What perspective ought to be taken on the social ethics of the medical profession and its mission? Many in the United States believe that the *'answer'* is simply to let markets work in the interests of liberty (10). In this model, health care is a two-tiered marketplace. The costs for those who can pay include a pool of money and charity care for those who cannot pay. When the overriding value is justice, medicine ought to be a largely subsidized service in a society that guarantees security in health care for all to increase solidarity among its people. However, even when health policy guarantees universal access, disparities persist in disease and health care that reflect class, race, and sex.

Following Buchanan, we propose that in a pluralistic democracy, the relation between society and medicine ought to be understood as a self-correcting contract or bargain (11). Instead of resting on one supreme value easily captured by ideology, the contract reflects a commonwealth of values. These values govern the complex goals of medicine and interests of society in health. A commonwealth has a primary locus of loyalty. In this society, the preeminent value is fidelity to patients or loyalty to the patient at hand. Using the right procedural principles, patient-centered medicine is not inconsistent with viewing the patient in a population with needs for a finite supply of expensive community health care resources. (12) Within constraints of fidelity to patients and their rights, physicians ought to promote the welfare of the many, to practice fairness in access and distribution of resources, and to be efficient and effective in their practices. Physicians in this society are also members of a scientific community with a high standard of evidence in practicing medicine. Guided by these values, society grants the profession a privileged place, permits its members to earn high incomes, and subsidizes their training. In return, society expects the net health benefits of pursuit of the goals of medicine to outweigh the net costs.

In the United States, the increasing investment in perinatal-neonatal care has not produced proportional improvements in crude infant survival and low-birth-weight. Thompson and associates (13) compared the neonatal intensive care (NICU) resources of the United States with those of Australia, Canada, and the United Kingdom. Compared to the other three nations, the United States has far greater resources but higher rates of low-birth-weight and death among newborns. The United States has 6.1 neonatologists per 10,000 live births compared with 3.7, 3.3, and 2.7 in the other nations, respectively. NICU beds in the United States are 3.3 per 10,000 live births, compared with 2.6 in the first two nations and 0.67 in the UK. Resources are not linked with low-birth-weight. In the United States, 1.45% of all neonates have a very low-birth-weight (<1500 g) compared with approximately 1% in the other nations. Newborns weighing less than 2500 g are born more frequently in the United States. Low-birth-weight is the single most accurate predictor of neonatal death. The crude neonatal mortality rate is 4.7% deaths per 1000 births in the United States, compared with 3.0% in Australia, 3.7% in Canada, and 3.8% in England and Wales.

Why does success not follow from greater resources? Thompson and associates (13) point to cultural and political differences between the nations. Australia, Canada, and the United Kingdom provide health insurance for all children under 18 years of age and all women ages 18 to 44 years. In the United States only 86% of children and 78% of women had health insurance at the time of the study. These three nations provide free family planning advice and prenatal and perinatal care, and the United States does not. The influence of race, poverty, and poor nutrition must also be factored into the answers. Longstanding recommendations of the Committee on Perinatal Health to address the root problems have not been implemented (14). The current March of Dimes campaign on prematurity is a valuable step but does not replace missing federal support (3).

ETHICS AND MORAL DELIBERATION

Ethics is a body of practical knowledge comprised of principles and values, judgments about cases and policies, and beliefs and theories about the world and persons (15). John Dewey's view of the main purpose of ethics is integration of beliefs about the world with beliefs about the values and purposes that should direct human conduct (16). Decision making for infants and children should follow the same general approaches taken for all patients who are unable to make decisions for themselves.

John Dewey wrote, "life is a moving affair in which old truth ceases to apply" (16). Making judgments in novel situations can lead to change of background beliefs and practices. Since the advent of modern neonatal care in the 1960's, rapid advances in technology and aggressive care of smaller and sicker neonates have focused philosophical, theological, professional, legal, consumer, and media attention (both positive and negative) on the use of technology and the processes for decision making in life or death choices for newborns. One can trace changes in background beliefs and values in the history of ethics in neonatal decision making using the "landmark" cases in which medical decisions for infants have been scrutinized by the United States govern-

ment or the legal system. Table 2-1 gives samples of important cases, events, articles, and studies in that history. In addition, several recent reviews trace this evolution and multinational differences in approach (1,17–19).

Neonatologists, nurses, and parents of newborns today stand on the cumulative moral experience of the past. The

TABLE 2-1

LANDMARK CASES IN NEONATAL ETHICS

Year	Name of Case, Event	Clinical Issues	Outcome
1963	Hopkins Baby[a]	Trisomy 21, duodenal atresia; parental refusal of surgery.	Died after 15 days of no feeding/hydration.
1974	Baby Houle[b,c]	Muliple malformations; parental refusal.	Court orders surgery; infant died.
1973	Duff & Campbell[d]	Selective nontreatment of multiple infants with variety of medical conditions.	Controversial report from a NICU.
1981	The Danville Twins[e]	Siamese twins, joined at the abdomen, with three legs and a common pelvis. The parents and physicians were criminally charged with ordering that the infants not be fed.	The parents and physicians were found not guilty.
1981	Stinson baby[f]	Premature infant; 800 g, 26 wks; parents object to unwanted treatment.	Infant dies at 6 mo.
1982	Bloomington Baby (Baby Doe)[g]	Trisomy 21, tracheal esophageal fistula; parental refusal of surgery.	Indiana Supreme Court rules for parents.
1983	Baby Jane Doe[h]	Spina bifida, hydrocephalus, and *microcephaly*; parental refusal of surgery.	NY Court of Appeals rules for parents.
1983	Baby Doe regulations[i]	U.S. Dept. of HHS issues regulations.	Requires life-sustaining treatment for every infant.
1983	President's Commission[j]	Clarifies decisions to forgo treatment in newborns.	More moderate than U.S. Dept. of HHS regulations.
1984	Child Abuse Protection Act[k]	Federal law.	To receive federal funds for child protection, states must have procedures for such cases.
1990	Baby K[l–n]	Anencephaly.	Mother demands life supports and federal courts rule for her.
1994	Messenger[o–q]	Premature infant; 780 g, 25 wk. Parents request no resuscitation.	Father disconnects respirator and jury finds not guilty of manslaughter.
2000	HCA v. Miller[r,s]	Premature (629 g, 23 wk) infant resuscitated against parents wishes.	Court of Appeals reverses prior judgment awarding parents $60 million.

[a] Gustafson JM. Mongolism, parental desires, and the right to life. *Perspect in Bio Med* 1973;16:524.
[b] Maine Medical Center v Houle, No 74–145, 1974 (Super. Ct. Cumberland Co. Me. Feb. 14, 1974).
[c] McCormick RA. To save or let die: the dilemma of modern medicine. *JAMA* 1974;229:172.
[d] Duff RS, Campbell AGM, Moral and ethical dilemmas in the special care nursery. *N Engl J Med* 1973;289:890.
[e] Stinson R, Stinson P. The long dying of Baby Andrew. Boston, MA: Little Brown, 1983.
[f] Murray TH, Caplan AL. Beyond Babies Doe. In: Murray TH, Caplan AL, eds. *Which babies shall live: humanistic dimensions of the care of imperiled newborns*. Clifton, NJ: Humana Press, 1985:3.
[g] State ex rel. Infant Doe v Baker, No. 482 S 140 (Ind. May 27, 1982).
[h] Weber v Stony Brook Hosp, 476 NY.S. 2d 685, 686 (App. Div.); Bowen v American Hospital Association, 476 US. 610 at 611(1986).
[i] U.S. Department of Health and Human Services. Nondiscrimination on the basis of handicaps: procedures and guidelines relating to health care for handicapped infants. *Federal Register* 1984 Jan 12:49:622–654.
[j] U.S. President's Commission for the Study of Ethical Problems in Medicine and Biomedical and Behavioral Research. Seriously ill newborns, in deciding to forego life-sustaining treatment: a report on the ethical, medical, and legal issues in treatment decisions. Washington: US. Government Printing Office; 1983;197.
[k] Child Abuse Protection Act, 42 U.S.C. § 5103 (1982).
[l] In re Baby K, 832 F. Supp. 1022 (E.D. Va. 1993); In re Baby K, 16 F. 3d 5900 (4th Cir.).
[m] Annas G. Asking the courts to set the standard of emergency care—the case of Baby K. *N Engl J Med* 1994;330:1542.
[n] Paris JJ, Crone RK, Reardon FE. Physician refusal of requested treatment: the case of Baby K. *N Engl J Med* 1990;322:1012.
[o] State v Messenger, file 94–67694-FY, Clerk of the Cir. Ct. County of Ingram, Mich.
[p] Clark FI. Making sense of State v Messenger. *Pediatrics* 1996;97:579.
[q] Paris JJ. Manslaughter or a legitimate parental decision? The Messenger case. *J Perinatol* 1996;16:60.
[r] HCA v Miller, 2000 WL 1867775, Tex. App. Hous. (Dec. 28, 2000).
[s] Paris JJ, Schreiber MD, Reardon F. The "emergent circumstances" exception to the need for consent: the Texas Supreme Court ruling in Miller v HCA. *J Perinatol* 2004;24:337.
Abbreviations: HHS, Health and Human Services; NICU, neonatal intensive care unit.

process for decision making in NPM is more transparent and shared between clinicians and parents than in the past. However, it is never immune from confusion, especially when cultural beliefs about medicine collide. Practitioners are arguably better trained to identify ethical issues, participate in shared decision making, and seek help with ethical problems. For example, most try to be empathetic, non-biased, and honest in disclosing a poor or uncertain prognosis to anxious parents.

Neonatologists, nurses, and their colleagues are fallible. They have made serious mistakes in excluding parents from decisions and imputing guilt to them for wanting to withdraw treatment (20). Some events and cases test the limits of moral concepts, for example, the best interests of the infant, parental autonomy, professional integrity, futility, and fairness in use of resources, or quality of life. These cases brew storms that can throw experienced neonatologists, nurses, other staff, parents, and administrators off balance and into conflict with one another. In these situations, Martin Buber's metaphor of a "narrow rocky ridge between the gulfs" (21) can ring true. Ethics helps human beings to keep enough balance, when taking hazardous, puzzling, or new paths in social and personal life, to maintain moral insight and equilibrium. It is a self-correcting, constantly evolving body of practical knowledge about human problems—conflicts of moral principles, duties, or loyalties in relationships.

CULTURAL AND RELIGIOUS DIVERSITY

Because ethics is a self-correcting body of knowledge, open societies require a public process of debate about continuity and change in the moral aspects of social and professional practices. The United States is now the world's most diverse religious and cultural society. These differences are very difficult to sort out in debate about ethics. To change public policy in this society, faith-based reasons standing alone are insufficient. Secular and presumably rational reasons are required to persuade a court, legislature, or commission. In debatable health care decisions, we see cases involving newborns that break down the limits of rationality. For example, should physicians continue to respect parents' faith-based rejection of futility of treatment when the baby has total intestinal necrosis or renal agenesis and pulmonary hypoplasia? In our view, the case of Baby K (22) shows that the federal courts can approve parental faith-based demands as a legally justified reason to continue futile treatment of an anencephalic newborn, because the society has been unwilling to ration resources for this category of newborns.

Cross-cultural issues deeply complicate debate on ethics. For example, should any moral weight be given to a request to withdraw life support if the parents of a neonate are immigrants from a society with very different moral beliefs about medicine and what constitutes a seriously impaired newborn? What if the parents' culture requires that a traditional healer participate in the care of the infant? Should weight be given to parents' religious views when the infant is in pain and not benefiting from additional procedures and the parents flatly reject the concept of futility? What is best, all things considered, for the infant? Does concern for the infant absolutely override competing concerns?

The authors take a broadly pragmatic approach to ethics and to cross-cultural issues in ethical debates. Moral norms and ways of life are, in fact, relative to culture and personality. However, cultural and psychological relativity does not drain ethics of content or moral force. Although ethics is a phenomenon within and not independent of human experience, it has objectivity in two senses. First, ethics is objective as a growing and evolving body of knowledge about practices in society and the professions. Secondly, the basic imperatives of ethics are "no less objective than law or medicine" (23) when it comes to destructive acts like murder, torture, genocide, rape, cruelty for its own sake, and so forth. Such acts "violate our most basic convictions" about the intrinsic value of human life and community. As Benjamin writes, "If these things aren't wrong, nothing is" (24). Some argue that moral judgments are not binding across cultural boundaries or that ethics is "merely" a matter of personal taste. If ethics is merely subjective or relative, there is no basis for a moral judgment about any horrific act that occurs in subcultures or beyond one's own culture, such as forcing children to wage war against their own people or to suffer loss of limb or life. The case of Baby K ought not be judged as "horrific acts" because the parents' intentions are loving and not destructive. The moral failure in these cases is societal in its failure to assume responsibility for setting democratically debated limits on health care resources. Societal failures can result in horrific consequences, but the parents and staff involved in these cases do not deserve moral blame.

Working Through Ethical Problems

Although important moral values and principles are binding, there is no prefabricated way to work through ethical problems in cases or events when principles collide. Different methods of moral deliberation compete for selection. When compared with highly theoretical or case-by-case approaches, the method of "wide reflective equilibrium" (25) has proven useful in bioethics. In this approach, one weighs ethical problems in cases by creating a dialogue (internally or externally) that moves between three interactive elements: the values and principles at stake, the problem at hand, and relevant background beliefs and theories.

"Principlism" is a dialectical method that analyzes ethical problems in a framework of *prima facie* principles of biomedical ethics (10). This approach is widely used in ethics courses and in the literature of neonatal ethics. In our view, a method that moves only between values or principles and the problem at hand lacks larger constraints and correctives. Cultural influences and personal bias are at work in selecting principles and putting them to work in cases. Judgments made in past cases, such as Baby K (22)

and Baby Doe (26), are fallible and need evaluation. Background beliefs and theories are sources of critical distance and constraint—beliefs and theories about the nature of personhood, community, the world as revealed by science and metaphysics, human psychology, sociology, and political and economic behavior; the nature of nonhuman animals, and so forth. In short, our uses of principles and judgments in cases ought to make sense in terms of intelligible background beliefs and in-depth knowledge of the issues at hand.

When parents and clinicians are unable to reach agreement on an approach to care, additional resources should be available to assist the process. Many "ethical conflicts" are actually problems in communication and misunderstanding. Involvement of social workers, chaplains, parent support groups, or other clinical staff often improves the interaction and leads to a resolution of the conflict. One of the outcomes of the Baby Doe controversy (27) in the early 1980's was the recommendation that infant bioethics review committees be established to prospectively and retrospectively review cases where life-sustaining therapy was withheld or withdrawn. While the function of these committees was short-lived, they were the forerunners of the current ethics committees in most institutions. Ethics committees serve multiple functions including policy development and review, staff education, and review of difficult cases brought to them. In many institutions, both medical staff and families may bring cases to the committee. Committee process varies widely from institution to institution in terms of membership, involvement of family, and decision-making models (28–30). Other institutions use a less intimidating model of an ethics consultation service, where an individual consultant, or, more often, a team of consultants (who usually have multidisciplinary backgrounds), will review the situation with those involved, provide background or policy information, facilitate communication, and, when necessary, bring the parties together to work toward a consensus. In most institutions the committee or consultation service recommendations are advisory rather than binding. Finally, when consensus is cannot be reached and the clinician, family or institution feels the issues are sufficiently serious, the court system can be petitioned to intervene. While the court system is seen as the voice of society weighing in on a difficult issue, this is often a time-consuming, not necessarily objective process that by its nature is adversarial and may negatively impact the relationship between the clinician and parents. A court decision may be appealed and overturned or may result in an outcome that with greater societal scrutiny may be seen as questionable. Most would argue that approaching the court should be a last resort.

Moral Status of the Newborn

Part of the evolution in clinical ethics in neonatal-perinatal medicine has involved ascribing greater moral status and protection at birth to seriously ill newborns. There has been a dramatic transition from frequent nontreatment of

trisomy 21 (31) to the Baby Doe Rules (22) and support for appropriate assessment of extremely low-birth-weight (ELBW) infants.(32) However, there remains a philosophical impression that decisions to withhold or withdraw treatment for newborns, especially the extremely premature newborn, may be less troublesome than decisions for older children and adults, because the newborn does not have the same moral worth or is not fully a person. Tooley (33) argued that because a newborn lacks advanced brain function, has no self-consciousness, ability to suffer, or sense of the future, it should not be considered a person. Engelhardt (34) agrees that neonates are not persons in the strict sense at the time but affirms that they are persons in a social and cultural sense. Others have further defined this view, identifying the bonding, affection, and care given newborns by parents and other adults (35).

While detailed plans for conception, antenatal ultrasound, and fetal movement may support parental attachment early in and progressing through gestation, it cannot be denied these emotions are not as strong in the perinatal period, especially when the infant is extremely preterm, as they are at several months or years of age. In addition, many preterm infants are the result of unplanned, often unwanted, or sometimes unknown pregnancies. Blustein describes the neonate as "not born into the family circle so much as outside it, awaiting inclusion or exclusion. The moral problem the family must confront is whether the child should become part of the family unit" (36). Ross notes that respect for the person is "owed to all individuals on the basis of the individual's personhood (and developing personhood) … proportionate to the actualized capacities of the individual and his or her potential to attain full personhood" (37). It is therefore problematic that the infant's moral worth is variable, dependent on acceptance by its family rather than on any innate socially or even legally accepted character. This worth may change over a short period of time, and this change may then affect differences in or difficulties with decision making prior to birth versus at a week or month of life. Decisions made in the labor room regarding a child who has never been seen by the parent and who may have an increased risk of mental retardation become much more difficult when the 6-month-old child has confirmed severe developmental delay.

Decision Making

Sound clinical decision making should be based on sound data, a careful and thorough diagnostic assessment, and, based on that diagnostic assessment, accurate prognostic estimates. Sometimes this is relatively easily accomplished: chromosomal analysis has documented trisomy 13 and the natural history of this disease is well-known. In other situations the diagnosis may not be well-defined or the prognosis is uncertain. For both the ELBW infant about to be born or the premature infant with grade III intraventricular hemorrhage, there is an increased statistical risk of developmental delay, but it is not certain how this particular infant will progress. Rhoden (38) has defined strategies that have been or might be used when there is uncertainty about prognosis:

- Wait until certain: Continue until the patient is actually dying or will survive but with definite severe disability. There is an underlying discomfort with infants, admittedly few in number, who are dying but who might survive with aggressive care. There is little attention paid to suffering, burden-benefit ratios, or the number of infants needed to be treated for one additional intact survivor.
- Statistical prognosis: Use statistical cutoffs and aggressively treat all those selected. This might be described as the "evidence-based approach." Selection might be by birth weight or gestational age. This approach may be used when resources are limited. Professional, regional, or national guidelines might exist to define these cutoffs. This approach ignores individual variation and may sacrifice some potentially normal infants who may behave outside of the norm. It relies on data that may or may not accurately reflect the clinical situation at hand. Decision making is psychologically *"easier,"* because it is allegedly *"objective."* Most clinicians justifiably use some criteria for limiting treatment for some populations, for example, resuscitation at 21 to 22 weeks gestation.
- Individualized prognosis: Decide for each infant using the available data, the present condition, and a benefit-burden analysis. This approach allows for clinical change, evaluation and reevaluation, and ongoing communication. There is more of a role for the family in decision making. It also can be a source of confusion, uncertainty, error, and agony. However, Rhoden believes that this is justified, given the tragic nature of the situations. Fischer and Stevenson (39), and more recently Kraybill (40), have expanded on this approach beginning with a "nonprobabilistic paradigm" of attempting to save every ELBW infant's life ("provisional intensive care for all") modified by an "individualized prognostic strategy" when prognosis could be better defined. The American Academy of Pediatrics has endorsed this approach (41).

Withholding/Withdrawing

Most agree that it is ethically superior to withdraw a therapy compared to withholding it (42,43). If therapy is begun and is effective, the patient benefits. If the therapy is begun but is not effective, it can be stopped. If the therapy is never initiated, the patient can never benefit. Initiation of therapy also provides the clinician with additional time to collect data, which may lead to a more accurate diagnosis and therefore more reliable prognosis and allows the family more time to understand the situation. While a preference to withdrawing rather than withholding is sound philosophically, in actual clinical settings there are often emotional responses and in some settings religious restrictions to withdrawal of a therapy. It is much easier emotionally to be passive than to make an active decision to withdraw aggressive care. "Pulling the plug" and "killing my baby" are

not infrequently heard. "Letting God decide" and "waiting for a miracle" are examples of the same phenomenon. Doron and associates (44) document the relatively frequent disagreement of parents when clinicians recommend withholding aggressive care. There is a potential for weeks or months of care, and possible pain and suffering, before the infant's death or an eventual decision to withdraw. The clinical situation may reach the point that there is no aggressive care to withdraw, and the outcome is poor. Some clinicians are reluctant, based on this experience, to initiate care as freely. If a clinician is less willing to withdraw care than not to initiate it because of uncertainty or philosophical reasons, this should influence their decision process and be made clear during discussions with parents.

Clinically the withdrawal of life-sustaining therapy does not require that the patient have multiorgan system failure or meet criteria for brain death. If the organ that has failed or been irreversibly injured is a vital one, decision making should be based on the infant's prognosis for recovery, long-term survival, quality of life, and so forth. Technology would be withdrawn, and the infant would be allowed to die. "Brain death" or "death by neurological criteria" is a clinical and legal definition of a type of death. Criteria for brain death in the newborn are somewhat different than for older children and adults (45–47). Some jurisdictions allow for a religious exemption. However, in most circumstances, once the criteria have been met, the patient is pronounced dead. These families need to be compassionately informed about what this means ethically and legally and appropriately prepared for withdrawal of the ventilator. There should be no discussion of removing "life-sustaining treatment" or "keeping the baby alive" because the patient is legally dead.

The term *"euthanasia"* generates a great deal of confusion and debate in legal, legislative, media, and clinical spheres. Active versus passive euthanasia, voluntary versus involuntary euthanasia, physician-assisted suicide, and other descriptors have created unfortunate ambiguity about the actual issue at hand. If one defines euthanasia or active euthanasia as directly and actively causing the death of a patient who may not be imminently dying or is dependent on life-sustaining technology, usually by administering a lethal dose of a drug, most state law and policies of the American Medical Association and the American Academy of Pediatrics would prohibit that action (48,49). How often active euthanasia of neonates actually occurs in the United States is not known. However, there is a significantly different approach in Europe. Recent studies suggest that while active euthanasia is illegal and rarely occurs in most countries, it appears to be acceptable practice in the Netherlands and France. Approximately 70% of neonatal physicians in France and 45% in the Netherlands have been involved in a decision of active euthanasia (50). Confusion arises when the term "passive euthanasia" is used for decisions to withdraw life-sustaining therapy with the expectation that the patient will die (51). The use of medication to treat symptoms of pain or dyspnea or other suffering in the context of comfort or palliative care further compounds the confusion, in spite of an ethical duty to provide this type of care. Some would argue that the overall intention may be the same as or may certainly blur into "active euthanasia." However, others would suggest that intention is an important determinant (52). Describing what actually is being considered as a plan of care and avoiding the terminology may prevent the confusion and the associated emotion.

The Role of Parents

Parents are the decision makers for their children. This role is understood to have social, legal, and ethical facets; some are better defined than others, some are potentially in conflict with others. Parents should be in the best position to judge what is in their child's best interest. They will be the ones who will continue to raise the child after the newborn period. Numerous studies and commentaries have reflected on the difficulties families may have to face following the birth of an infant who will have long-term medical and educational needs and how they perceive their situations (53–56). They will be the ones who will have to deal with the consequences of the decisions. Ethically, this right and responsibility of parents has been the focus of considerable analysis and commentary since the Baby Doe era. The extremes of "no one, including parents, should make these decisions" and "absolute right of parents to make medical decisions" are simplistic and unrealistic (57). Parents should be seen as guardians of their child's welfare, not owners.

Bartholome (58) suggests using the language of "permission," a term somewhat less rigid than "consent." He sees the parents' role as a duty rather than a right, a duty to ensure the provision of necessary medical care. "Parental permission for interventions into children's lives must not be seen as the unconditional right to demand or refuse a particular intervention because it is a proper exercise of parental authority over the lives of children. That children are largely dependent, at least for a time, on their parents is to be affirmed, but that dependency does not warrant the second-class social standing implied by a parental right of *'consent'* in decisions affecting the health care of their children." Child abuse and neglect statutes frequently result in challenges to parental decision and control. Finally, decision making for another individual is not identical to making decisions for oneself. While the legal system and ethical consensus give an adult patient's personal decisions wide leeway, surrogate decision making for the adult patient requires that decisions be solely in the patient's best interests or what the patient would have wanted. Surrogates are often questioned, especially when life-sustaining therapies are at issue. The infant and child should be afforded this same protection.

Weir (59) proposes that the parents as decision makers should:

- Have relevant knowledge and information about medical facts, prognosis, and family setting
- Be impartial
- Be emotionally stable
- Be consistent

This final quality should assure that the process ends with the same result in similar cases. However, what information the parents receive and from whom may clearly impact their decision. The clinician has an obligation to present accurate, up-to-date information. The story of Baby Doe resulted, in part, from outdated impressions about Down syndrome (26). The large number of studies, many now outdated, with small sample sizes or preselected samples, clouds prognostication about extremely premature infants. Several studies document the different prognoses presented by obstetricians versus pediatricians/neonatologists for the extremely premature infant (60). Others reflect major differences in clinical approach and parental counsel between intensivists and rehabilitation physicians for children who are or might become ventilator dependent (61).

Other issues complicate the process relative to the parents' emotional stability and consistency. Especially in the immediate newborn period, the infant and parents—especially the mother—may have been separated, sometimes by hundreds of miles. In some cases the parents may not even have seen the baby before it was transferred to a neonatal unit. The mother may at times be ill herself or recovering from anesthesia. The parents may have varying degrees of support from other family members. The father of the baby may or may not be involved. The birth of a critically ill or severely malformed infant is often seen as a loss (of the normal-term infant they expected); the family may actually be grieving or dealing with anger, depression, denial, or fear. Often the information presented to the family is complex and difficult to understand, especially at first hearing. Time constraints may further complicate the process, for example, in the delivery suite or for surgical emergencies.

Standards for Decision Making

The usual broad standard for decision making for this population is to decide what is "in the child's "best interests."" However, defining *"best interests"* can be difficult and reflects a basic problem with the use of terms that may carry very different meanings for different individuals.

Weir and Bale (62) suggest eight variables for evaluating "best interest":

1. The severity of the patient's medical condition
2. The achievability of curative or corrective treatment
3. The important medical goals in the case (such as prolongation of life, relief of pain, or amelioration of disabling conditions)
4. The presence of serious neurologic impairments
5. The extent of the infant's suffering
6. The multiplicity of other serious medical problems
7. The life expectancy of the infant
8. The proportionality of treatment-related benefits and burdens

Is the "best-interests" standard not, in fact, quite subjective; potentially defined differently by clinicians and family? How do we define how much potential pain and suffering is acceptable for a given outcome, especially when the outcome may not be precisely predicted? How do we define an *"acceptable"* outcome? Is being alive but vegetative "acceptable"? Is a 20% or 40% or 70% risk of death or developmental disability acceptable? Is it in the best interests of a child with trisomy 21 to have surgery for duodenal atresia, or the child with trisomy 18 to have open heart repair for congenital heart disease? How differently should one consider a 25% risk of a poor outcome (e.g., for the very-low-birth-weight [VLBW] infant) versus a known, defined poor prognosis (e.g., for trisomy 13)? Silverman (63,64) has proposed abandoning the term *"best interests"* and adopting the concept of a "standard of reasonableness" proposed by Veatch. Here the issue is how far the technology is pursued to "accomplish reasonable ends defined by those most directly affected by the decisions—the parents." Well-being extends beyond organic and physiologic function into the realms of social, legal, occupational, religious, aesthetic, and other aspects of life.

Are *"best interest"* or *"reasonableness"* standards the same as *"quality of life"* standards? The latter term is often viewed negatively because of the even greater subjective element. How does one define a good or bad quality of life? Does defining a ""quality of life that is "poor" reflect potential for discrimination against individuals with disabilities? In response to the death of an infant with trisomy 21 whose parents refused surgery for tracheoesophageal fistula, the federal government in 1982, under pressure from right-to-life advocates and advocacy groups for the handicapped, proposed regulations to prohibit hospitals from withholding care from newborns. "The Baby Doe" rules stated:

1. All such disabled infants must, under all circumstances, receive appropriate nutrition, hydration, and medication.
2. All such disabled infants must be given medically indicated treatment.
3. There are three exceptions to the requirement that all disabled infants must receive treatment, or, stated in other terms, three circumstances in which treatment is not considered "medically indicated." These circumstances are:
   a. The infant is chronically and irreversibly comatose.
   b. The provision of such treatment would merely prolong dying, not be effective in ameliorating or correcting all of the infant's life-threatening conditions, or otherwise be futile in terms of the survival of the infant.
   c. The provision of such treatment would be virtually futile in terms of the survival of the infant, and the treatment itself under such circumstances would be inhumane.
4. The physician's *"reasonable* medical judgment" concerning the medically indicated treatment must be one that would be made by a reasonably prudent physician who is knowledgeable about the case and the treatment possibilities with respect to the medical conditions involved. It is not to be based on subjective *"quality of life"* or other abstract concepts (27).

In the commentary for the rules, certain conditions were identified as not requiring treatment, including anencephaly, trisomy 13, and extremely low-birth-weight.

"Quality-of-life" terminology carries negative connotations from the Baby Doe era. "Quality of life," just as "best interests," can be very subjective; what one clinician sees as a good quality of life may be unacceptable to another professional or a parent. A family may see the life of a child who is profoundly visually handicapped but with normal intelligence as qualitatively poor. Although many families do not feel burdened with a moderately mentally retarded child, others consider learning disability with normal intelligence unacceptable. Clinicians who work with developmentally impaired children often have a very different appraisal than do laypersons of the quality of life in this patient population.

However, it may be possible to use quality of life as a basis for decision making when considering more fundamental issues. Richard McCormick (65) proposes a minimal condition for defining *"quality"*: the capacity for experience or social interrelating. If the condition is not met, as with anencephaly, treatment is not required. Coulter and associates (66) define interests that would constitute a "minimal quality of life" as:

- Freedom from intractable pain and suffering. Mental retardation, paralysis, cerebral palsy would not be considered physical suffering; dyspnea or intractable physical pain would.
- Capacity to experience and enjoy life—the ability to enjoy food, warmth, or the caring touch of another; the ability to give or receive love.
- Expectation of continued life—heroic treatment, when death will likely occur in a few weeks or months, may be cruel.

There has been considerable debate about how much attention should be paid in the decision-making process to interests other than the child's. Parents may be overwhelmed with the prospects of chronic medical care, financial burdens, difficulty in raising a handicapped child, need for special education, and harm to other children in the family. Some parents may focus on their own psychological and financial interests, protecting their lifestyle and other children at home. Fost (67) suggests, "The history of childhood is one that does not support idyllic notions of parents as decision makers for their children. "It is naïve to posit an identity of interest between infant and parent [in all situations]. Parents guard their own interests, those of the family as a unit, and those of current and future siblings—all of which may be gravely threatened by the newborn" (68). Most would argue that the parents should not refuse treatment that would be in the infant's interests in order to avoid burdens to the family (59,69,70). These considerations are rarely allowed to play a role in surrogate decisions for older children and adults. Others suggest that the impact of a decision on the welfare of the family may be taken into account. Silverman (71) comments, "parents of a badly damaged baby often resent that their family is required to pass a sacrifice test to satisfy the moral expectations of those who do not live, day by day, with the consequences of diffuse idealism. It is easy … to demand prolongation of each … life that requires none of [the clinician's] own resources to maintain that life later." Ross (72), using the concept of the "intimate family," proposes a model of "constrained parental autonomy," where the parent should be guided by the child's well being, but is not obligated to disregard all personal interests of themselves or other children in order to fulfill the child's needs and interests. This is an issue that requires sensitivity to the parents and family situation, but at the same time balancing the short- and long-term needs of the child. A New York Academy of Medicine conference reached the following conclusion:

> Although parents may have legitimate concerns about the effect of treatment decisions on themselves and their other children, the desire to avoid emotional, financial or other hardships cannot justify the denial of clearly beneficial medical care to an ill or injured child.… If parents are unable or unwilling to provide essential medical treatment, healthcare professionals should first assure that social counseling and supports are made available to the family to assist them. If the parents remain unwilling to consent to the needed medical treatment, then we must utilize legal mechanisms to ensure social support or supervision to provide those treatments which are clearly in the best interests of the child." (73)

What is the clinician's role in decision making for the infant? Do pediatric practitioners have a stronger responsibility for the decisions made for the child than the clinician caring for an adult patient? Bartholome (74) defines a role that imposes "legal and ethical duties and obligations which exist independently of any parental wishes, desires or consentings." The New York Academy of Medicine states the clinician "must maintain an independent obligation to protect the child's interest" (73). The Academy of Pediatrics defines providers' responsibilities as follows:

> "Proxy consent poses serious problems for … providers. [They] have legal and ethical duties to their child patients to render competent medical care based on what the patient needs, not what someone else expresses … The pediatrician's responsibilities to his or her patient exist independent of parental desires or proxy consent" (75).

Futility

Conflict also may arise when the parents demand care that the clinician feels is inappropriate, futile, and potentially harmful to the child. The clinician should not be required to provide care that he or she considers harmful or unethical. The problem again is one of definition: What is futile care? Who defines futility? What may be futile in the eyes of the clinician may be beneficial for the child from the parents' point of view (76). Being kept alive on the ventilator with no chance of recovery and minimal or no social interaction may be sufficient for the parents to continue. The case of

Baby K complicated this question even further when the federal court upheld the mother's demand for resuscitation and aggressive treatment of her anencephalic infant (22). While the application of this case to other futility cases may be limited—because the court's decision was based on the Federal Emergency Treatment and Labor Act, which requires emergency care for life-threatening situations—it has clearly raised the level of sensitivity to parental demands. Again, ethics consultation or ethics committee involvement may facilitate resolution. The clinician may transfer the patient to another clinician (or institution) who is willing to provide the care. Some institutions have developed procedures for case review that may conclude that life-sustaining treatments can be withdrawn, even against the objections of the family (77). As noted earlier, the health care system and society have usually been unwilling to consider the important justice issues of the financial costs to society, both immediate and long-term, and of limitation of resources.

The Extremely Low-birth-weight Infant

Infants who are born at gestational ages of less than 27 weeks or who weigh less than 800 g have been the focus of considerable professional, legal, and media debate about withholding resuscitation in the delivery room, parental requests for aggressive care or no resuscitation, mortality rates, and quality of outcome (both short-term into later infancy and long-term to school age). There are hundreds of outcome studies and reviews regarding this population, several of which highlight the critical issues for this population (78–80). The problems of decision making (discussed previously) are painfully apparent. For example, the clinician has an obligation to accurately inform the parents expecting an ELBW infant about the clinical situation, prognosis, anticipated clinical course, and so forth. While there is certainly no lack of outcome data, it is clear that there are wide variations in outcome from one study to another. The studies are also faulted by the sample size of infants at any gestation, by the selection criteria (were all live born infants included or only those admitted to the NICU, inborn or outborn, etc), and by decisions about viability and nonresuscitation that then impact mortality of the sample as a whole. Mortality will, by definition, be higher if most infants were not resuscitated because of clinician or family preference. Drop out and incomplete followup, small numbers, and variation in definitions of morbidity impact the usefulness of long-term outcome studies. With such a wide range of study results, there is a risk or tendency for an individual clinician to choose those that support his or her philosophical approach (conservative or aggressive). Fortunately, there are several large, collaborative studies now available that lessen the impact of uncontrolled variables and provide more reliable outcome data (81–86). El-Metwally and associates (87) report significantly different survival rates when all ELBW infants are aggressively managed. Ideally, clinicians should have mortality and morbidity data for their own institution in addition to national statistics to share with the parents.

Use of gestational criteria for decision making is reasonable because studies show a very dramatic correlation to survival (81,82,88–95). Each additional gestational week adds a significant increase in survival percentage. However, in many cases both obstetrical estimates using ultrasound and neonatal estimates using physical exam scoring are not accurate enough to define 23 versus 24 or 24 versus 25 weeks gestation (96–98). The current practice of quoting gestational age in fractions of a week (e.g., 23 5/7) provides a sense of accuracy that is not justified by the existing data.

Birth weights are accurately measured and have been correlated to outcome (35,88,89,99–103). However, for gestations in the 22- to 25-week range, there is an extremely wide variation in birth weights. Using birth weights also ignores the impact of intrauterine growth restriction. If study populations include growth-restricted infants, outcome data may be overly optimistic. If the decision makers consider only birth weight, the predicted prognosis may be overly pessimistic.

Guidelines for Resuscitation/Care

Several professional groups have developed criteria or guidelines for decision making for this population. In 1994, the Canadian Paediatric Society and the Society of Obstetricians and Gynaecologists of Canada defined relatively specific recommendations:

> At 22 completed weeks of gestation, they suggest "treatment should be started only at the request of fully informed parents or if it appears that the gestational age has been underestimated." At 23 to 24 completed weeks of gestation, they emphasize a significant role for parental wishes, the option of resuscitation, and the importance of discussion with parents about the "need for flexibility in deciding to start or withhold resuscitation, depending on the infant's condition at birth." Finally, at 25 weeks gestation they state "resuscitation should be attempted for all infants ... without fatal anomalies" (104).

Discussions by neonatologists in Colorado, in collaboration with the Colorado Collective for Medical Decisions, developed guidelines that define comfort care as the only appropriate choice for the 22 weeks' gestation infant. At 23 weeks, most would advise comfort care; but, if the parents understood the high risks involved, would be willing to initiate a course of intensive care. At 24 weeks, the neonatologists were able to support either decision, as long as a collaborative process with good information occurred. At 25 weeks, they were uncomfortable with withholding intensive care, and some, but not all, were willing to support a parental request for comfort care, if there had been a good parent education process and an effort to collaborate with the parents (Hulac P. Colorado Collective for Medical Decisions, personal communication, January 2000). Tyson and associates (80) have suggested developing fairly detailed guidelines based on outcome data. Female and/or small-for-gestational-age infants would be resuscitated at lower birth weights than male and/or appropriately grown infants. Antenatal steroids would lower the recommended weight further. They recommend mandatory resuscitation when the data reveal a greater

than 50% chance of survival without severe sequelae and optional resuscitation when the chance is 25% to 49%. Resuscitation for infants with a less than 25% chance of survival without severe sequelae would be seen as investigational. Neonatal Resuscitation Program, which is supported by the American Academy of Pediatrics and the American Heart Association, suggests that noninitiation of resuscitation for newborns of less than 23 weeks' gestational age and/or 400 g in birth weight is appropriate (105). Interestingly, clinicians have overinterpreted these criteria as either demanding resuscitation at 23 weeks or 400 g or as stating it is inappropriate to resuscitate at less than 23 weeks or 400 g (80).

Discussions with the family should include the uncertainty of gestational age if that is at issue, the advantage of assessing and then making decisions, the possibility of withdrawal of support if it is apparent that there will be a bad outcome, and the importance of ongoing assessment and ongoing communication. To avoid confusion and conflict, the obstetrician and the pediatrician/neonatologist should coordinate their approaches. For the extremely immature infant, the parents should be aware that there may be nothing that can be done. There may be physical limitations to the resuscitation. In most circumstances, firm decisions about how to proceed should be avoided. Likewise, vague terms such as "no heroic measures" or "do everything" can cause confusion and conflict. Several recent papers have discussed the importance of antenatal and intrapartum discussions (106,107). When possible, the use of educational materials, tours of the NICU, or videos of NICU experiences may further the parents understanding of the situation. The Colorado Collective for Medical Decisions has developed a video especially for the parents of an ELBW infant (108).

Infants with Severe Encephalopathy/Brain Death

Infants with perinatal hypoxic-ischemic injury may have lethal multisystem failure. However, more often they are able to survive despite severe central nervous system (CNS) injury. Prolonged, difficult-to-control seizures, hypotonia; poor feeding; apnea; and inability to maintain body temperature are poor prognostic signs for developmental outcome. Imaging studies (computed tomography [CT], magnetic resonance imaging [MRI]) as well as an electroencephalogram (EEG) may add additional prognostic data. Some may be ventilator dependent because of poor respiratory drive. Others may require gastrostomy feedings. Prognosticating may be difficult early after the insult, but in some circumstances the clinical data convincingly show that the prognosis is extremely poor. Do not resuscitate orders and/or withdrawal from the ventilator are appropriate decisions at this time.

Infants with Severe Congenital Malformations/Chromosomal Anomalies

In a series of articles and commentaries beginning in 1973, pediatricians Duff and Campbell (20) reported on a practice of selective nontreatment at Yale-New Haven Hospital that resulted in the deaths of 43 infants over a period of 30 months. Physicians and parents decided together, with the physicians sometimes yielding to parental wishes. Surveys at that time confirmed that many pediatricians and pediatric surgeons accepted selective nontreatment of seriously impaired newborns. In a survey of New England pediatricians, 54% did not recommend surgery for an infant with Down syndrome and duodenal atresia, and 66% would not recommend surgery for an infant with a severe case of spina bifida (109). Twenty-two percent of surveyed pediatricians in the San Francisco area favored nontreatment for infants with trisomy 21 who had no complications, and more than 50% recommended nontreatment for Down syndrome with duodenal atresia (110). With the Baby Doe case, advocates for the handicapped, developmental pediatricians, and family support groups promoted a change in approach for infants with trisomy 21 and meningomyelocele. Treatment and approaches to rehabilitation and special education have improved; the current standard of care in the United States is that infants with trisomy 21 receive the same treatment that is indicated for a child with a similar medical or surgical condition who does not have trisomy 21.

There are other conditions associated with extremely poor prognoses for survival or for reasonable "quality of life", including anencephaly and other severe CNS developmental anomalies, trisomy 13, and trisomy 18 (111). Most of these infants will not survive beyond the first few months of life. Those who do survive have severe neurodevelopmental delays. Many have life-threatening conditions in the immediate newborn period and require life-sustaining treatment to prolong survival. Most would agree that a recommendation to withdraw or withhold aggressive therapy and provide comfort care is appropriate. The Neonatal Resuscitation Program guidelines suggest that noninitiation of resuscitation is appropriate for confirmed diagnoses of anencephaly or trisomies 13 or 18 (105). Hopefully, every parent of such an infant would have appropriate counseling about the diagnosis; and in this circumstance, a definite plan for care in the delivery room (including no cesarean section for fetal distress) and during the newborn period can be very helpful and comforting to the parent. Again, the guideline does not state that it is inappropriate to resuscitate. When a condition is not diagnosed until after birth, there is the usual obligation for the clinician to provide the parents with appropriate, accurate information in a timely fashion. Some families wish to pursue aggressive treatment, and their wishes should be considered. Internet sites and parent support groups have expanded the options available to families for treatment (112). While cardiac surgery for infants with trisomy 18 was formerly quite uncommon, there are now increasing requests for such procedures. The parents should be well informed, and a plan should be developed for the care, including how to proceed if the infant does not tolerate the procedure, becomes ventilator dependent, and so forth. If the clinician is not willing to offer this level of care, efforts should be made to transfer care to another physician or facility.

Artificial Nutrition and Hydration

While most agree that withdrawing artificial nutrition and hydration from hopelessly ill, persistently vegetative or dying patients may be appropriate (113,114), this issue becomes less well-defined in the newborn population, who are all dependent on others for feeding and where tube feeding is the standard of care for many until they develop the ability to feed. There are circumstances, however, where discontinuing intravenous nutrition or tube feedings may be appropriate (115–118). If the infant is actively dying, there is no benefit to feeding or hydration, and experience would suggest that there may be less suffering from excess secretions if the patient is somewhat dehydrated (113). Coma and persistent vegetative state are rarely defined in the newborn, but severe neurologic impairment is, unfortunately, not rare. However, exact prognostication about recovery is difficult, and some infants who need feeding support initially may develop the ability to feed normally after a period of recovery. When clinical evaluation strongly suggests an extremely poor neurologic outcome, it may be reasonable to withhold feedings (118). Factors to consider include whether the infant is able to feed at all or whether the infant demonstrates hunger or satiety. Infants may have medical conditions that preclude enteral feeding (e.g., short gut syndrome), and, therefore, they are dependent on total parenteral nutrition (TPN). TPN has many potential complications including loss of venous access, infection, and liver toxicity. If the possibility of slow recovery of absorptive ability or successful bowel transplant is poor, withdrawal of TPN may be an option after consideration of the criteria discussed earlier. Withdrawal of feeding often presents more psychological and emotional angst than withdrawal of other life-sustaining technology because of the cultural connotations of "feeding" and "starving" (119). While the "Baby Doe" regulations specifically list hydration and nutrition as "required," the term "appropriate" is also used and therefore open to interpretation.

Palliative/Comfort Care and Pain Control

When aggressive care or life-sustaining technology is withheld or withdrawn, care does not stop. The clinician has an obligation to the patient and the parents to provide comfort care, warmth, feedings, if desired, and emotional support. The clinical staff must attend to relief of symptoms and pain control (120). Care may in fact become more "intensive" in terms of time spent with the family. Catlin and Carter (121) have developed a protocol for neonatal end-of-life palliative care. Clinicians and, more recently, regulators have highlighted the importance clinically and ethically of identification and treatment of pain in the neonate (122–124).

High-Technology Home Care

With technological advances in the hospital has come the use of this same technology in the home—tube feedings, oxygen, and mechanical ventilators. This development has raised numerous ethical issues both on an individual patient basis and related to the general issues of resource allocation, funding, and health planning (125, 126). How a family and the clinician reach the conclusion to proceed or not proceed with long-term home care, especially mechanical ventilation, requires careful attention to the details of adequate information, parent education and training, planning for professional assistance in the home, adequate support and funding, opportunity for respite care, and so forth. Studies suggest that there is wide variation in physician practice regarding offering home ventilation, with families then receiving unbalanced information (61). With the growing incidence of ventilator use in the home, parent support groups and the Internet offer a very positive bias. Physicians may feel that this is fiscally inappropriate, or that the child's quality of life may be poor, or that the family will be unable to manage at home. Home ventilation for older children and adults with a variety of diseases provides a great deal of satisfaction for many of them (127). Every child and family is unique in their clinical situation, prognosis, family goals and stamina, and resources. On the other hand, just because the technology for home ventilation is now available does not require its use in every circumstance. If the family is unable or unwilling to provide less intensive care in the home (e.g., tube feeding or oxygen), other options must be identified. It is inappropriate to discharge an infant with heavy ongoing health care needs home to a family that is ill prepared and does not have adequate support from outside services.

HIV SCREENING OF PREGNANT WOMEN AND NEWBORN INFANTS

The diagnosis and treatment of HIV infection has changed dramatically in a short time period. A decade ago, diagnosis often involved a screening test with confirmation testing to follow; diagnosis can now be quite accurately made in an hour or less. Antibody testing of the newborn is, in reality, antibody testing of the mother; it is now possible to test the newborn for viral DNA. The critical treatment element relates to the ability to prevent transmission of infection from mother to baby, by treatment of the mother during the pregnancy and labor and of the newborn in the first several weeks after birth. There is also evidence that treatment limited to labor and the postnatal period only, or even to the infant postnatally, may significantly decrease the risk of transmission. It has therefore become significantly more important to know the mother's HIV status early in the gestation and certainly during labor. Public Health recommendations promote universal, voluntary, routine testing of the mother, using an "opt-out" strategy for consent—"we will test you for HIV unless you specifically say you refuse" (128–131). Mandatory testing potentially violates the mother's rights to privacy and self-determination and, even today, may expose her to social consequences and discrimination. Being pregnant should not require an individual to

forgo rights. Once the infant has been born, some would argue that the advantages of early diagnosis and treatment outweigh the risks to the mother. Some jurisdictions have mandated newborn screening if the mother's status is not known. However, most professionals would recommend routine, but voluntary, testing. The mother's status will be defined, but the benefits to the baby would outweigh the risks to the mother (131).

SUBSTANCE ABUSE IN PREGNANCY

Substance abuse during pregnancy has incited a great deal of media and legal attention. Prosecutors and governmental agencies have charged mothers with homicide and child abuse, imprisoned them for the duration of their pregnancies, and removed their children from their custody (132,133,134). Complicating the ethical and legal issues is a wide range of scientific opinion about the short- and long-term effects of drug exposure in utero on the child (135,136). Recent studies suggest that the rearing environment is much more critical for the child's development (135). Routine drug screening of pregnant women without their consent has been ruled unconstitutional (137). Punitive approaches in general are counterproductive, potentially keeping women away from prenatal care (132). Routine screening of newborns should be limited to situations in which there is a clinical history or signs or symptoms compatible with drug exposure or withdrawal. Testing infants solely to identify substance-abusing mothers should be avoided. The approach to mothers and babies should be supportive, voluntary, and nonpunitive (138).

GENETIC TESTING

In the past two decades, there has been a dramatic increase in knowledge about the human genome and the ability to screen for the presence of certain genetic diseases, carrier states, traits, or predispositions to disease. Genetic testing of a newborn raises different issues than routine medical testing performed as part of clinical care. The genetic information relates not only to the individual tested but also to other members of the family. Results of testing may have psychological (guilt, anxiety), social (stigmatization, discrimination), and financial impact (insurability, employment considerations) with long-term consequences. Some genetic information defines risks only and does not predict with any certitude a specific condition or outcome. Finally, many defined conditions do not necessarily have effective therapy. For these reasons, concerned professional organizations have developed policies and guidelines related to these issues. Testing should involve effective counseling, informed consent, and attention to confidentiality. Genetic testing to confirm a medical diagnosis would be an appropriate component of medical care, for example, DNA analysis for cystic fibrosis in an infant with meconium ileus or chromosomal analysis for a newborn with clinical features of Down syndrome. Testing for conditions that may benefit from monitoring, prophylaxis, or treatment in an otherwise healthy individual (e.g., familial hyperlipidemia) may also be in the child's best interest. However, carrier screening for diseases with no risk to the pediatric patient should be avoided. Likewise, screening for adult-onset conditions should be deferred until adulthood or until the mature adolescent is able to consent (139–140).

MAKING DECISIONS REGARDING THE APPROPRIATENESS OF INTER-INSTITUTIONAL TRANSFER

The transfer of neonates from referring to referral hospitals potentially adds an additional layer of ambiguity to the process of ethical decision making, particularly if there is uncertainty on the part of the NPM team at the referral hospital regarding the level of treatment received by the infant since birth. For example, a 25-week gestation premature infant who has been *'set aside'* as nonviable but is found gasping 1 hour later and resuscitated is unlikely to benefit from transfer to another institution for aggressive support.

A regional network of hospitals can reduce this problem by having a common set of criteria for delivery room practices and inter-institutional referral. Fletcher and Paris (141) suggested the following mnemonics to assist in formulating these policies:

1. **ACUTE (Acute, Critical, Unexpected, Treatable, and Easily diagnosed)**. Infants included in this group are those with prematurity and respiratory distress syndrome; ELBW infants of gestational age known to be 25 weeks or greater; term or preterm infants with sepsis, pneumonia, or meningitis; and infants with surgically correctable malformations.

    The authors place these infants in a *'definite'* category for transfer to an NICU capable of providing the level of care required.
2. **UNSURE (UNknown disease, SUspected REsponse)**. This group includes preterms of 23 to 24 weeks gestational age or with very low-birth-weight and uncertain gestational age, infants with severe birth asphyxia, and any infant with an unexplained disease or syndrome that requires further diagnostic efforts. Within this group there will be a significant number of infants for whom the response to treatment will be unpredictable. These infants should be given full medical care until the diagnosis has been made or the response to treatment is clear; decisions to omit care or not to transfer should not be made precipitously.
3. **KNOT (Known, NOt Treatable)**. Although only a small number of infants fit into this category, treatment decisions for this group frequently take a disproportionate amount of time. This group includes neonates with anencephaly and those with lethal genetic disorders such as trisomy 13 and trisomy 18.

Transfer of neonates with anencephaly for aggressive support is not indicated; transfer of those with lethal genetic defects is not indicated if there are facilities for accurate diagnosis 'and appropriate care and counseling at the hospital of birth. When diagnostic facilities are not available at the birth hospital, onsite consultation by a specialist from the referral hospital is an appropriate alternative to transferring the infant.

REFERENCES

1. Carter BS, Stahlman M. Reflections on neonatal intensive care in the US: limited success or success with limits. *J Clin Ethics* 2001;12:215–222.
2. Brenner S. Humanity as the model system. *Science* 2003;302:533.
3. Martin JA, Hamilton BE, Ventura SJ, et al. Births: final data for 2001. National Center for Vital Statistics Reports 2002;51:1.
4. National Foundation March of Dimes. Available online at www.marchofdimes.com
5. Olivennes F, Fanchin R, Ledee N, et al. Perinatal outcome and developmental studies on children born after IVF. *Human Repro Update* 2002;8:117–128.
6. Keith LG, Oleszczuk JJ, Keith DM. Multiple gestation: reflections on epidemiology, causes and consequences. *Int J Fert Womens Med* 2000;45:206–209.
7. Schieve LA, Meikle SF, Ferre C, et al. Low and very low-birth-weight infants conceived with use of assisted reproductive technology. *N Engl J Med* 2002;346:731–737.
8. The President's Council on Bioethics. Reproduction and responsibility: the regulation of new biotechnologies. 2004. Available online at http://bioethics.gov/reports/productionandresponsibility
9. Hansen M, Kurinczuk JJ, Bower C, et al. The risk of major birth defects after intracytoplasmic sperm injection and in vitro fertilization. *N Engl J Med* 2002;346:725–730.
10. Beauchamp TL, Childress JF. *Principles of biomedical ethics.* 5th ed. New York: Oxford University Press, 2001:231.
11. Buchanan AE. Is there a medical profession in the house? In: Spece RG, Shimm DS, Buchanan AE, eds. *Conflict of interest in clinical practice and research.* New York: Oxford University Press, 1996:105.
12. Emanuel EJ. *The ends of human life: medical ethics in a liberal polity.* Cambridge, MA: Harvard University Press, 1991.
13. Thompson LA, Goodman DC, Little GA. Is more neonatal intensive care always better? Insights from a cross-national comparison of reproductive care. *Pediatrics* 2002;109:1036–1043.
14. Committee on Perinatal Health. *Toward improving the outcome of pregnancy: recommendations for the regional development of maternal and perinatal health services.* White Plains, NY: National Foundation March of Dimes, 1976.
15. Benjamin M. *Philosophy and this actual world.* Lanham, MD: Rowman & Littlefield, 2003:112.
16. Dewey J. *Human nature and conduct.* Carbondale, IL: Southern Illinois University Press, 1988:164.
17. Paris JJ, Ferranti J, Reardon F. From the Johns Hopkins Baby to Baby Miller: what have we learned from four decades of reflection on neonatal cases. *J Clin Ethics* 2001;12:207.
18. Howe EG. Helping infants by seeing the invisible. *J Clin Ethics* 2001;12:191–204.
19. Cuttini M and the Euronic Study Group. The European Union collaborative project on ethical decision making in neonatal intensive care (Euronic): findings from 11 countries. *J Clin Ethics* 2001;12:290–296.
20. Stinson R, Stinson P. The long dying of Baby Andrew. Boston, MA: Little Brown, 1983.
21. Buber M. *Between man and man.* New York: Macmillan, 1965:164. Smith RG, translator.
22. In re Baby K, 832 F. Supp. 1022 (E.D. Va. 1993); In re Baby K, 16 F. 3d 5900 (4th Cir.).
23. Benjamin M. *Philosophy and this actual world.* Lanham, MD: Rowman & Littlefield, 2003:119.
24. Benjamin M. *Philosophy and this actual world.* Lanham, MD: Rowman & Littlefield, 2003:115.

25. Brown-Ballard J. Consistency, common morality, and reflective equilibrium. Kennedy Inst Ethics J. 2003;13:231–258.
26. State ex rel. Infant Doe v Baker, No. 482 S 140 (Ind. May 27, 1982).
27. U.S. Department of Health and Human Services. Nondiscrimination on the basis of handicaps: procedures and guidelines relating to health care for handicapped infants. *Federal Register* 1984 Jan 12:49:622–654.
28. Leikin S, Moreno JD. Pediatrics ethics committees. In: Cassidy RC, Fleischman AR, eds. *Pediatric ethics—from principles to practice.* Amsterdam: Harwood Academic Publishers, 1996:51.
29. Lo B. Behind closed doors: promises and pitfalls of ethics committees. *N Engl J Med* 1987;317:46–50.
30. Weir RF. Pediatric ethics committees: ethical advisers or legal watchdogs? Law Med & Hlth Care 1987;15:99–109.
31. Duff RS, Campbell AGM. Moral and ethical dilemmas in the special care nursery. *N Engl J Med* 1973;289:890–894.
32. Paris JJ, Schreiber MD, Reardon F. The "emergent circumstances" exception to the need for consent: the Texas Supreme Court ruling in Miller v HCA. *J Perinatol* 2004;24:337–342.
33. Tooley M: Abortion and infanticide. Philosophy and Public Affairs 1972;2:37–65.
34. Engelhardt HT: *The foundations of bioethics.* New York, Oxford University Press, 1986:116–119.
35. May WF. Parenting, bonding, and valuing the retarded. In: Kopelman LM, Moskop JC, eds. *Ethics and mental retardation.* Dordrecht, The Netherlands: D Reidel, 1984;141–160.
36. Blustein J. The rights approach and the intimacy approach: family suffering and care of defective newborns *Mount Sinai J Med* 1989;56:164–167.
37. Ross LF: *Children, families and health care decision-making.* Oxford, England: Clarendon Press, 1998:47.
38. Rhoden NK. Treating Baby Doe: the ethics of uncertainty. *Hastings Cent Rep* 1986;16:34–42.
39. Fischer AF, Stevenson DK. The consequences of uncertainty: an empirical approach to medical decision making in neonatal intensive care. *JAMA* 1987;258:1929–1931.
40. Kraybill EN. Ethical issues in the care of extremely low-birth-weight infants. *Semin Perinatol* 1998;22:207–215.
41. Committee on Fetus and Newborn, American Academy of Pediatrics."The initiation or withdrawal of treatment for high-risk newborns." *Pediatrics* 1995;96:362–363.
42. Beauchamp TL, Childress JF. *Principles of medical ethics,* 5th ed. New York: Oxford University Press, 2001:120.
43. Fletcher JC: The decision to forgo life-sustaining treatment when the patient is incapacitated. In: Fletcher JC, Lombardo PA, Marshall MF, et al., eds. *Introduction to clinical ethics.* Frederick, MD: University Publishing Group, 1997:158.
44. Doran MW, Vaness-Meehan KA, Margolis LH, et al. Delivery room resuscitation decisions for extremely premature infants. *Pediatrics* 1998;102:574–582.
45. Volpe JJ. Guidelines for the determination of brain death in children. *Pediatrics* 1987;80:293–297.
46. Farrell MM, Levin DL. Brain death in the pediatric patient: historical, medical, religious, cultural, legal and ethical considerations. *Crit Care Med* 1993;21:1951–1965.
47. Ashwal S. Brain death in the newborn. *Clin Perinatol* 1997; 24:859–882.
48. Council on Ethical and Judicial Affairs, America Medical Association. Euthanasia. In: *Code of medical ethics: current opinions with annotations.* Chicago American Medical Association, 2002:83.
49. Committee on Bioethics, Committee on Hospital Care, American Academy of Pediatrics. Palliative care for children. *Pediatrics* 2000;106:351–357.
50. Cuttini M, Casotto V, Kaminski M, et al. Should euthanasia be legal? An international survey of neonatal intensive care units staff. *Arch Dis Child Fetal Neonatal Ed* 2004;89:F19–F24.
51. Sklansky M. Neonatal euthanasia: moral considerations and criminal liability. *J Med Ethics* 2001;27:5–11.
52. Edwards SJ. The distinction between withdrawing life-sustaining treatment under the influence of paralyzing agents and euthanasia. The doctrine of double effect is difficult but not impossible to apply. *BMJ* 2001;323:390–391.
53. Harrison H. Making lemonade: a parent's view of "quality of life" studies. *J Clin Ethics* 2001;12:239–250.
54. Saigal S. Perception of health status and quality of life of extremely low-birth weight survivors. The consumer, the provider, and the child. *Clin Perinatol* 2000;27:403–419.
55. Saigal S, Burrows E, Stoskopf BL, et al. Impact of extreme prematurity on families of adolescent children. *J Pediatr* 2000;137:701–706.
56. Saigal S, Pinelli J, Hoult L, et al. Psychopathology and social competencies of adolescents who were extremely low-birth-weight. *Pediatrics* 2003;111:969–975.
57. Paris JJ, Schreiber MD. Parental discretion in refusal of treatment for newborns: a real but limited right. *Clin Perinatol* 1996;23:573–581.
58. Bartholome WG, The Child-Patient: Do Parents Have the "Right to Decide." In Spicker SF, Healey JM, and Engelhardt HT, eds. The Law-Medicine Relation: A Philosophical Exploration. Boston, MA: Reidel, 1981:271.
59. Weir R: *Selective treatment of handicapped newborns: moral dilemmas in neonatal medicine.* New York: Oxford University Press, 1984.
60. Haywood JL, Goldenberg RL, Bronstein J, et al. Comparison of perceived and actual rates of survival and freedom from handicap in premature infants. *Am J Obstet Gynecol* 1994;171:432–439.
61. Hardart MKM, Truog RD. Spinal muscular atrophy—type 1. Arch Dis Child 2003;88:848–850.
62. Weir RF, Bale JF Jr. Selective nontreatment of neurologically impaired neonates. *Neurol Clin* 1989;7:807–821.
63. Silverman WA, Medical decisions: an appeal for reasonableness. *Pediatrics* 1996;98:1182–1184.
64. Veatch RM. Abandoning informed consent. *Hastings Cent Rep* 1995;25:5–12.
65. McCormick RA. To save or let die: the dilemma of modern medicine. *JAMA* 1974;229:172–176.
66. Coulter DL, Murray TH, Cerreto MC. Practical ethics in pediatrics. *Curr Probl Pediatr* 1988;18:168–169.
67. Fost N. Parents as decision makers for children. *Prim Care* 1986;13:285–293.
68. Dellinger AM, Kuszler PC. Infants: public-policy and legal issues. In: Reich WT, ed. *Encyclopedia of bioethics.* New York: Simon & Schuster and MacMillan, 1995:1214.
69. Beauchamp TL, Childress JF. Principles of biomedical ethics. 5th ed. New York, Oxford University Press, 2001:137.
70. Fleischman AR, Nolan K, Dubler NN, et al. Caring for gravely ill children. *Pediatrics* 1992;94:422–439.
71. Silverman W. Overtreatment of neonates? A personal perspective. *Pediatrics* 1992;90:971–976.
72. Ross LF. Children, families and health care decision-making. Oxford, England: Clarendon Press, 1998:51.
73. Fleischman AR, Nolan K, Dubler NN, et al. Caring for gravely ill children. *Pediatrics* 1992;94:422–439.
74. Bartholome WG. Withholding/withdrawing life-sustaining treatment. In: Burgess MM, Woodrow BE, eds. *Contemporary issues in pediatric ethics.* Lewiston NY: Edwin Mellen Press, 1991:17.
75. Committee on Bioethics, American Academy of Pediatrics. Informed consent, parental permission, and assent in pediatric practice. *Pediatrics* 1995;95:314–317.
76. Carter BS, Sandling J. Decision making in the NICU: the question of medical futility. *J Clin Ethics* 1992;3:142–143.
77. Truog RD. Futility in pediatrics: from case to policy. *J Clin Ethics* 2000;11(2):136–141.
78. Boyle RJ, Kattwinkel J. Ethical issues surrounding resuscitation. *Clin Perinatol* 1999;26:779–792.
79. Meadow W, Lantos JD. Ethics at the limit of viability: a premie's progress. *NeoReviews* 2003;4:e157.
80. Tyson JE, Stoll BJ. Evidence-based ethics and the care and outcome of extremely premature infants. *Clin Perinatol* 2003;30:363–387.
81. Wood NS, Marlow N, Costeloe K, et al. Neurologic and developmental disability after extremely preterm birth. *N Eng J Med* 2000;343:378–384.
82. Costeloe K, Hennessy E, Gibson T, et al. The EPICure study: outcomes to discharge from hospital for infants born at the threshold of viability. *Pediatrics* 2000;106(4):659–671.
83. Lemons JA, Bauer CR, Oh W, et al. Very low-birth-weight outcomes of the National Institute of Child Health and Human Development Neonatal Research Network, January 1995 through December 1996. *Pediatrics* 2001;107(1):e1.
84. Horbar JD, Badger GJ, Carpenter JH, et al. Trends in mortality and morbidity for very low-birth-weight infants, 1991–1999. *Pediatrics* 2002;110(1 pt 1):143–151.
85. Vohr BR, Wright LL, Dusick AM, et al. Neurodevelopmental and functional outcomes of extremely low-birth-weight infants in the

National Institute of Child Health and Human Development Neonatal Research network, 1993–1994. *Pediatrics* 2000;105: 1216–1226.

86. Yu VYH. Developmental outcome of extremely preterm infants. *Amer J Perinatol* 2000;17:57–61.

87. El-Metwally D, Vohr B, Tucker R. Survival and neonatal morbidity at the limits of viability in the mid 1990s: 22 to 25 weeks. *J Pediatr* 2000;137:616–622.

88. Fanaroff AA, Wright LL, Stevenson DK, et al. Very-low-birth-weight outcomes of the National Institutue of Child Health and Human Development Neonatal Research Network, May 1991 through December 1992. *Am J Obstet Gynecol* 1995;173: 1423–1431.

89. Hack M, Friedman H, Fanaroff AA. Outcomes of extremely low-birth-weight infants. *Pediatrics* 1998;98:931–937.

90. Kilpatrick SJ, Schlueter MA, Piecuch R, et al. Outcome of infants born at 24–26 weeks' gestation: I. survival and cost. *Obstet Gynecol* 1997;90:803–808.

91. O'Shea TM, Klinepeter KL, Goldstein DJ, et al. Survival and developmental disability in infants with birth weights of 501 to 800 grams, born between 1979 and 1994. *Pediatrics* 1997;100: 982–986.

92. Emsley HCA, Wardle SP, Sims DG, et al. Increased survival and deteriorating developmental outcome in 23 to 25 week old gestation infants. 1990–4 compared with 1984–9. *Arch Dis Child Fetal Neonatal Ed* 1998;78:F99–F104.

93. Larroque B, Breart G, Kaminski M, et al. On behalf of the EPI-PAGE study group. Survival of very preterm infants: Epipage, a population based cohort study. *Arch Dis Child Fetal Neonatal Ed* 2004;89:F139.

94. Lefebvre F, Glorieux J, St-Laurent-Gagnon T. Neonatal survival and disability rate at 18 months for infants born between 23 and 28 weeks of gestation. *Am J Obstet Gynecol* 1996;174:833.

95. Levene M. Is intensive care for very immature babies justified? *Acta Paediatr* 2004;93:144–149.

96. Haidet KR, Kurtz AB. Routine ultrasound evaluation of the uncomplicated pregnancy. In: Spitzer AR, ed. *Intensive care of the fetus and neonate*. St. Louis, MO: Mosby-Year Book, 1996:45.

97. American Academy of Pediatrics, Committee on Fetus and Newborn, American College of Obstetricians and Gynecologists, Committee on Obstetric Practice. Perinatal care at the threshold of viability. *Pediatrics* 1995;96:974–976.

98. Donovan EF, Tyson JE, Ehrenkranz RA, et al. Inaccuracy of Ballard scores before 28 weeks gestation. *J Pediatr* 1999;135: 147–152.

99. Lucey JF, Rowan CA, Shiono P, et al. Fetal infants: the fate of 4172 infants with birth weights of 401–500 grams—the Vermont Oxford Network experience (1996–2000). *Pediatrics* 2004;113: 1559–1566.

100. Sauve RS, Robertson C, Etches P, et al. Before viability: a geographically based outcome study of infants weighing 500 grams or less at birth. *Pediatrics* 1998;101:438–445.

101. Hack M, Horbar JD, Malloy MH, et al. Very low-birth-weight outcomes of the National Institute of Child Health and Human Development Neonatal Network. *Pediatrics* 1991;87:587–597.

102. Piecuch RE, Leonard CH, Cooper BA, et al. Outcome of extremely low-birth-weight infants (500 to 999 grams) over a 12-year period. *Pediatrics* 1997;100:633–639.

103. Tyson JE, Younes N, Verter J, et al. Viability, morbidity and resource use among newborns of 501–800-g birth weight. *JAMA* 1996;276:1645–1651.

104. Fetus and Newborn Committee, Canadian Paediatric Society; Maternal Fetal Medicine Committee, Society of Obstetricians and Gynaecologists of Canada. Management of the woman with threshold birth of an infant of extremely low gestational age. *CMAJ* 1994;151:547–553.

105. American Academy of Pediatrics. Special considerations. In: Braner D, Kattwinkel J, Denson S, et al., eds. *Textbook of neonatal resuscitation*, 4th ed. Elk Grove Village, IL: 2000:7.

106. Halamek LP. Prenatal consultation at the limits of viability. *NeoReviews* 2003;4:e153.

107. Munro M, Yu VYH, Partridge JC, et al. Antenatal counseling, resuscitation practices and attitudes among Australian neonatologists towards life support in extreme prematurity. *Aust N Z J Obstet Gynaecol* 2001;41:275–280.

108. Hulac P. Creation and use of "You are not alone," a video for parents facing difficult decisions. *J Clin Ethics* 2001;12:251–252.

109. Todres ID, Krane D, Howell MC, et al. "Pediatricians' attitudes affecting decision-making in defective newborns." *Pediatrics* 1977;60:197–201.

110. Treating the defective newborn: a survey of physicians' attitudes. *Hastings Cent Rep* 1976;6:2.

111. Rasmussen SA, Wong LY, Yang Q, et al. Population-based analyses of mortality in trisomy 13 and trisomy 18. *Pediatrics* 2003;111: 777–784.

112. Support Organization for Trisomy 18, 13 and Related Disorders. Available online at www.trisomy.org

113. Lynn J, Childress JF. Must patients always be given food and water? *Hastings Cent Rep* 1983;13:17–21.

114. American Academy of Pediatrics, Committee on Bioethics. Guidelines for forgoing life-sustaining medical treatment. *Pediatrics* 1994;93:532–536.

115. Nelson LJ, Rushton CH, Cranford RE, et al. Forgoing medically provided nutrition and hydration in pediatric patients. *J Law Med Ethics* 1995;23:33–46.

116. Cranford RE. Withdrawing artificial feeding from children with brain damage is not the same as euthanasia or assisted suicide. *BMJ* 1995;311:464–465.

117. Johnson J, Mitchell C. Responding to parental requests to forego pediatric nutrition and hydration. *J Clin Ethics* 2000;11: 128–135.

118. Carter BS, Leuthner SR. The ethics of withholding/withdrawing nutrition in the newborn. *Semin Perinatol* 2003;27:480–487.

119. Miraie ED. Withholding nutrition from seriously ill newborn infants: a parent's perspective. *J Pediatr* 1988;113:262–265.

120. Field MJ, Behrman RE, eds. *When children die: improving palliative and end-of-life care for children and their families*. Washington, DC: The National Academies Press, 2003.

121. Catlin A, Carter B. Creation of a neonatal end-of-life protocol. *J Perinatol* 2002;22:184–195.

122. Franck L, Lefrak L. For crying out loud: the ethical treatment of infants' pain. *J Clin Ethics* 2001;12:275–281.

123. American Academy of Pediatrics and Canadian Pediatric Society. Prevention and management of pain and stress in the newborn. *Pediatrics* 2000;105:454–461.

124. Anand KJ, International Evidence-Based Group for Neonatal Pain. Consensus statement for the prevention and management of pain in the newborn. *Arch Pediatr Adolesc Med* 2001;155: 173–180.

125. Lantos JD, Kohrman AF. Ethical aspects of pediatric home care. *Pediatrics* 1992;89:920–924.

126. Goldberg AI, Faure EAM, O'Callaghan JJ. High-technology home care: critical issues and ethical choices. In: Monagle JF, Thomasma DC, eds. *Health care ethics: critical issues for the 21st century*. Gaithersburg, MD: Aspen Publications, 1998:146.

127. Bach JR, Campagnolo D, Hoeman S. Life satisfaction of individuals with Duchenne muscular dystrophy using long-term mechanical ventilatory support. *Am J Phys Med Rehabil* 1991; 70:129–135.

128. Institute of Medicine, National Research Council. *Reducing the odds: preventing perinatal transmission of HIV in the United States*. Washington, DC: National Academy Press, 1999.

129. American College of Obstetricians and Gynecologists. Human immunodeficiency virus screening. Joint statement of the American Academy of Pediatrics and the American College of Obstetricians and Gynecologists. *Pediatrics* 1999;104:128.

130. Centers for Disease Control and Prevention. Revised recommendations for HIV screening of pregnant women. *MMWR* 2001;50(RR19):59.

131. Mofenson LM, Committee on Pediatric AIDS, AAP. Technical report: perinatal Human Immunodeficiency Virus testing and the prevention of transmission. *Pediatrics* 2000;106:e88.

132. Acuff K. Perinatal drug use: state interventions and the implications for HIV-infected women. In: Faden RR, Kass NE, eds. *HIV, AIDS and childbearing: public policy, private lives*. New York: Oxford University Press, 1996:214.

133. American Academy of Pediatrics, Committee on Substance Abuse. Drug-exposed infants. *Pediatrics* 1995;96:364.

134. DeVille KA, Kopelman LM. Substance abuse in pregnancy: moral and social issues regarding pregnant women who use and abuse drugs. Obstet Gynecol Clin 1998;25:237.

135. Jos PH, Marshall MF, Perlmutter M. The Charleston policy on cocaine use during pregnancy: a cautionary tale. *J Law Med Ethics* 1995;23:120–128.

136. Frank DA, Augustyn M, Knight WG, et al. Growth, development, and behavior in early childhood following cocaine exposure: a systematic review. *JAMA* 2001;285:1613.
137. Chavkin W. Cocaine and pregnancy—time to look at the evidence. *JAMA* 2001;285:1626.
138. Ferguson v Charleston 532 U.S. 67 (2001).
139. The American Society of Human Genetics Board of Directors and The American College of Medical Genetics Board of Directors, "Points to Consider: Ethical, Legal and Psychological Implications of Genetic Testing in Children and Adolescents," *American Journal of Human Genetics* 1995;57:1233–1241.
140. American Academy of Pediatrics, Committee on Bioethics, "Ethical Issues with Genetic Testing in Pediatrics," *Pediatrics* 2001;107:1451–1455.
141. Fletcher AB, Paris JJ. Bioethical issues surrounding transport of neonates. In: Mhairi G. MacDonald, eds., Miller MK, assoc. ed. *Emergency transport of the perinatal patient* Boston: Little Brown & Company, 1989:173.
142. DELGustafson JM. Mongolism, parental desires, and the right to life. Perspect in Bio Med 1973;16:524.
143. DELMaine Medical Center v Houle, No. 74–145, 1974 (Superior Ct, Cumberland Co, Me. Feb 14, 1974).
144. DELWeber v Stony Brook Hosp, 476 NY.S. 2d 685, 686 (App. Div.); Bowen v American Hospital Association, 476 US. 610 at 611 (1986).
145. DELU.S. President's Commission for the Study of Ethical Problems in Medicine and Biomedical and Behavioral Research. Seriously ill newborns, in deciding to forego life-sustaining treatment: a report on the ethical, medical, and legal issues in treatment decisions. Washington: US. Government Printing Office; 1983; 197.
146. Child Abuse Protection Act, 42 U.S.C. § 5103 (1982).
147. Annas G. Asking the courts to set the standard of emergency care—the case of Baby K. *N Engl J Med* 1994;330:1542.
148. Paris JJ, Crone RK, Reardon FE. Physician refusal of requested treatment: the case of Baby K. *N Engl J Med* 1990;322:1012.
149. State v Messenger, file 94–67694-FY, Clerk of the Cir. Ct. County of Ingram, Mich.
150. Clark FI. Making sense of State v Messenger. *Pediatrics* 1996; 97:579.
151. Paris JJ. Manslaughter or a legitimate parental decision? The Messenger case. *J Perinatol* 1996;16:60.
152. HCA v Miller, 2000 WL 1867775, Tex. App. Hous. (Dec. 28, 2000).

Neonatology in the United States: Scope and Organization

Richard L. Bucciarelli

The practice of neonatal and perinatal medicine has changed enormously since its recognition as a distinct subspecialty in 1975. The development of technologies as complex as extracorporeal membrane oxygenation and as simple as the administration of exogenous surfactant, has resulted in the survival of many infants who would have succumbed to their illnesses just a few years ago. In addition, an ever-increasing awareness of the benefits of inter-pregnancy and prenatal care has lead to significant behavior modification among many pregnant women, resulting in a reduction in the occurrences of conditions such as fetal alcohol syndrome and neural tube defects (1). Early diagnosis and peripartum therapy has decreased the risk of the vertical transmission of diseases such as hepatitis B and HIV (2). Despite erosions in health insurance coverage for women and the general population, fewer pregnant women are uninsured than nonpregnant women (13% versus 28%), and recent expansions in eligibility for coverage under Medicaid may reduce this number even further (1). In 2000, 83.2% of women received early prenatal care, up from 75.8% in 1990 (Fig. 3-1) (3). Teen birth rate has reached an all time low at 27 per 1,000 females ages 15 to 17 years, compared to 39 per 1,000 in 1991 (Fig. 3-2) (4).

Notwithstanding these positive trends, the rate of preterm, very preterm, low-birth-weight (LBW), and very-low-birth-weight (VLBW) deliveries in the United States has not changed significantly in more than a decade and remains far below the Healthy People 2010 goals (1). In 1998 the United States reported an infant mortality rate of 7.2 per 1,000 live births, resulting in a ranking of 28th in the world behind Cuba and just ahead of Slovakia (Table 3-1) (5). Even more troubling is the existence of significant racial and ethnic disparities in every indicator of perinatal health outcome, with neonatal and infant mortality for African Americans exceeding twice that of whites and three times the year 2010 goal (1).

This poor performance of the United States is not because of an unwillingness to commit significant resources to the delivery of perinatal care. In 1985, expenditures for obstetric and neonatal care approached $15 billion. Today this figure exceeds $40 billion, with the incremental costs for hospitalization for preterm labor reaching $820 million (6).

The stark contrast between the enormous economic investment in perinatal care and the relatively static outcome statistics suggests that while the United States has concentrated on developing the world's most sophisticated high-tech care, we have done little to understand the biological and societal issues responsible for producing high-risk infants. Perhaps this is a statement of our health care system's superb ability to care for the individual patient, in this case a high-risk infant after delivery, while failing to develop systems that integrate resources to provide efficient, cost-effective preventive care that could reduce human suffering and conserve vast resources.

In this chapter, the current size and scope of the practice of neonatology in the United States is reviewed, emphasizing how resources are currently used to deliver neonatal care. Issues are presented in an attempt to identify potential areas of focus for those involved in developing future perinatal public policy.

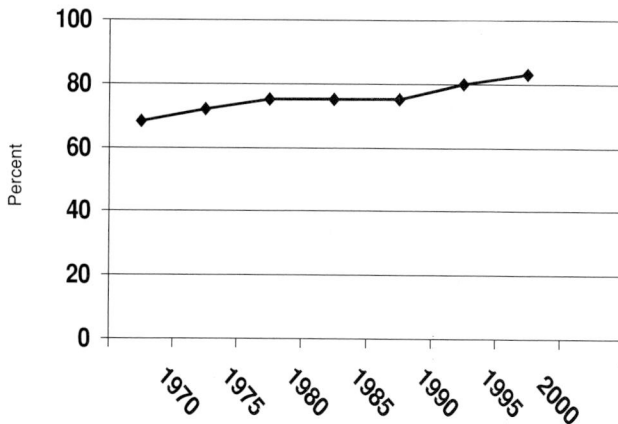

Figure 3-1 Early prenatal care among mothers: United States, 1970–2000. Early prenatal care begins during the first trimester of pregnancy. This figure is related to the *Healthy People 2010* leading health indicators on access to health care. (From *Chartbook on trends in the health of Americans 2002*. Centers for Disease Control and Prevention, National Center for Health Statistics, National Vital Statistics System. Redrawn from table 6, with permission.)

THE CAPACITY TO DELIVER IN-HOSPITAL NEONATAL CARE

Neonatal Hospital Bed Capacity

Because there is no national database defining or inventorying special-care neonatal beds, the exact capacity for providing neonatal intensive care unit (NICU) services in the United States is unknown. The estimates of capacity are further complicated by the fact that the definition for levels of inpatient NICU services varies greatly from state to state. Although clearly outlined by the Committee on Perinatal Health (COPH) of the March of Dimes Birth Defects Foundation in 1970 (revised in 1980 and 1993), financial, marketing, medical–legal, and community demands have

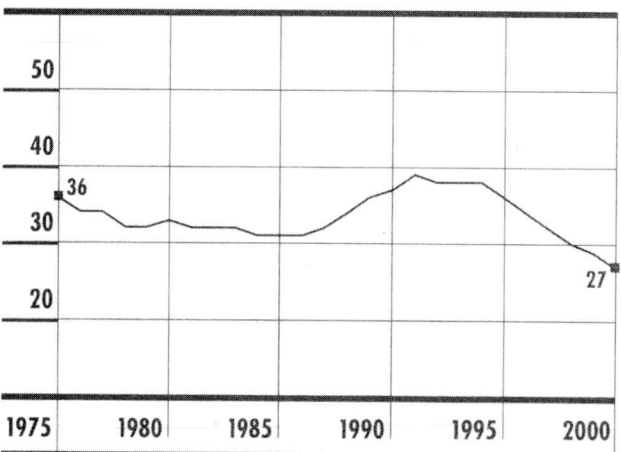

Figure 3-2 Teen birth rate (births per 1,000 females ages 15 to 17 years), 1975–2000. Note: Teenage childbearing has declined steadily since rising to 39 births per 1,000 teen girls in 1991. At 27 births per 1,000 in 2000, the teen birth rate has reached its lowest level ever. (From The Annie E. Casey Foundation, *Kids count data book, 2003 a pocket guide*. Baltimore, MD: The Annie E. Casey Foundation, 2003:7, with permission.)

TABLE 3-1
INFANT MORTALITY RATES, BY COUNTRY, 1998

Rank	Country	Rate
1	Hong Kong	3.2
2	Sweden	3.5
3	Japan	3.6
4	Norway	4.0
5	Finland	4.1
6	Singapore	4.2
7	France	4.6
7	Germany	4.6
9	Denmark	4.7
10	Switzerland	4.8
11	Austria	4.9
12	Australia	5.0
13	Czech Republic	5.2
13	Netherlands	5.2
15	Canada	5.3
15	Italy	5.3
17	New Zealand	5.5
17	Scotland	5.5
19	Belgium	5.6
19	Northern Ireland	5.6
21	England and Wales	5.7
21	Greece	5.7
21	Israel	5.7
21	Spain	5.7
25	Portugal	5.9
26	Ireland	6.2
27	Cuba	7.1
28	**United States**	**7.2**
29	Slovakia	8.8
30	Kuwait	9.4

Note: Differences in data and definitions limit international comparisons. For more information, see National Center for Health Statistics, 2002. Table 26, p. 114.
From Pastor PN, Makuc DM, Reuben C, et al. *Chartbook on trends in the health of Americans 2002*. Hyattsville, MD: National Center for Health Statistics, 2002, with permission.
March of Dimes. *March of Dimes data book for policy makers*, Washington, DC: March of Dimes Office of Government Affairs 2003, with permission.

encouraged many hospitals to elevate the level of select perinatal services, focusing on the provision of services locally with little regard to regional needs (7,8). As a result, there has been a significant increase in the number of hospitals providing NICU care, as well as blending neonatal services available primarily at basic care (level I) and specialty care (level II) centers (8).

In 1996, the National Perinatal Information Center reported an extensive survey of the supply and distribution of obstetric and neonatal services. While the number of hospitals offering obstetric services had declined, the numbers offering NICU services had increased dramatically by 64% such that one third of all hospitals with obstetric services were also operating an NICU. When the investigators adjusted for the number of live births, they discovered that the number of neonatal special care beds had increased significantly from 3.0 per 1,000 live births to 4.3 per 1,000 live births over the 10-year period of the study (9). More recent information suggests that this ratio has climbed

TABLE 3-2
NEONATAL CARE: PHYSICIAN AND HOSPITAL CAPACITY

	United States	Australia	Canada	United Kingdom
Annual deliveries (in thousands)	3942	256	349	636
Physicians* (per 10,000 live births):				
Pediatricians	144.7	34.2	59.7	20.0
Neonatologists	6.1	3.7	3.3	2.7
Neonatologists per 1,000 low-birth-weight infants	8.0	5.7	5.5	3.7
Obstetricians/gynecologists	100.2	42.2	45.3	24.3
Maternal/fetal specialists	3.2	0.4	NA	NA
Family practitioners	169.7	813.9	816.7	597.7
Number level III units* (per 10,000 live births)	1.21	0.90	0.72	2.92
Neonatal hospital beds* (per 1,000 live births) Intensive care beds	3.3	NA	NA	0.67
Intensive beds per 1,000 low birth weight	43.4	NA	NA	9.3
Intensive + intermediate care beds	5.1	2.6	2.6	NA
Intensive + intermediate care beds per 1,000 low-birth-weight infants	67.1	39.4	44.8	NA

From Thompson LA, Goodman DC, Little GA. Is more neonatal intensive care always better? Insights from a cross-national comparison of reproductive care. *Pediatrics* 2002; 109:1036–1043, with permission.

even further to 5.1 per 1,000 live births, exceeding the calculated demand by a factor of between 2 and 3 (10,11). In 2002, Thompson and associates (11) compared the capacity for in-hospital neonatal intensive care in the United States with that of the United Kingdom, Australia, and Canada (countries with similar neonatal practices). It is no surprise that the United States leads the way with an NICU bed capacity equal to five times that of the United Kingdom and twice that of Australia and Canada. Further, this difference remains even if the capacity is adjusted for the incidence of LBW infants (Table 3-2). The authors also point out that despite this huge capital investment, the United States trails all three countries in reported neonatal and infant mortality rates.

Although the United States has an in-hospital neonatal bed capacity that exceeds that of any other nation, its distribution across our nation is not homogenous and does not seem to follow any identifiable pattern, ranging from a low of 14 per 10,000 live births to a high of 59 per 10,000 live births (from 71 to 1,319 total births per NICU bed). Once again there was no correlation between the number of beds in a region with the incidence of LBW or neonatal mortality (12).

Size and Effectiveness of the Neonatologist Workforce

In an attempt to address the capacity issue more accurately, investigation recently has focused on the size and distribution of the neonatal work force as a potentially more accurate proxy for our capacity to deliver in-hospital neonatal care in the United States. Clearly, neonatologists are the catalysts that create a hospital environment, resulting in the creation of NICU beds and ultimately in the desire to provide higher risk obstetrical and neonatal care within that institution. Because a neonatologist can utilize a broad array of neonatal health care specialists to provide

services at several institutions simultaneously, the ratio of neonatologists to both high- and low-risk deliveries and their distribution within the region may more accurately define the capacity for in-hospital neonatal care.

In 1975, the American Board of Pediatrics' sub-Board of Neonatal and Perinatal Medicine certified 355 physicians as the first neonatologists in the United States. Since then, the American Board of Pediatrics has certified an additional 3,531 candidates. Currently there are 3,886 neonatologists certified by the Board, including the results of the latest certifying examination in 2001 (Fig. 3-3) (13). It is of interest to note that between 1987 and 1999, an average of 300 candidates was certified with each examination. In 2001, the number dropped to 182, the lowest number ever certified during a single examination. The average age at certification is 32 years, while the average age of all certified neonatologists is 51 years. During the early years of certification, males dominated by almost 3:1. In more recent years, the gender distribution approached 1:1, with

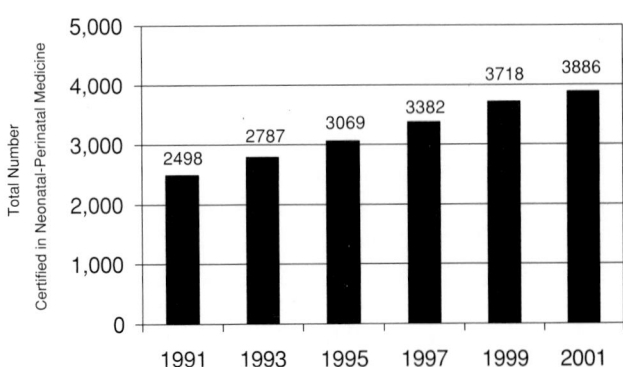

Figure 3-3 Cumulative total of specialists in neonatal and perinatal medicine certified by the American Board of Pediatrics, 1991–2001. (From American Board of Pediatrics. American Board of Pediatrics Neonatal-Perinatal Medicine qualifying examination statistics. Chapel Hill, NC: American Board of Pediatrics. Available online at http://www.abp.org/stats/WRKFRC/neostat.htm.)

TABLE 3-3

BIRTHS PER EACH CLINICALLY ACTIVE NEONATOLOGIST AND PEDIATRICIAN IN UNITED STATES, 1981–1996

	Number of Birth (millions)*	Number of Neonatologists†	Births per Neonatologist			
			All Births	Low-Birth-Weight (<2500 g)	Very-Low-Birth-Weight (<1500 g)	Extremely Low-Birth-Weight (1000 g)
1981	3.63	504	7201	490	83	39
1985	3.76	952	3951	266	48	24
1989	4.04	1507	2681	189	34	17
1992	4.07	1866	2178	154	28	14
1996	3.90	2311	1687	123	23	11

*Birth from U.S. Vital Statistics; 1995 births substituted for 1996.
†Physician numbers used for calculation exclude residents and fellows (N = 304), and those predominantly engaged in teaching (N = 106), administration (N = 97), and research (N = 232). From AMA Physician Masterfile (December 31 of calendar year). For comparison, the *United States Directory of Neonatologists 1996* listed 2,635 board-certified, 652 board admissible, and 230 others practicing in neonatology; the professional activities (clinical care, teaching, etc) of the neonatologists are not available.
From Goodman DC, Little GA. General pediatrics, neonatology and the law of diminishing returns. *Pediatrics* 1998;102:396–399, with permission.

more females certified during the 2001 certification (97 females, 85 males). Although the attrition rate for neonatologists was once believed to be quite high, it has remained low at 1% to 2% over a 10-year period. Additionally, it appears that almost 1,000 physicians actively engaged in the practice of neonatology are physicians who have not completed sub-Board certification or are pediatricians with special training in neonatology who concentrate their efforts on caring for neonates with special needs (14,15). Thus, the total neonatal physician workforce approaches 5,500, having doubled in the last decade and more than tripled since 1985 (13–15).

Concerns about a physician workforce devoted to neonatology, its distribution, its affect on regionalization, and, most importantly, its affect on outcome measures have been raised several times (16). In 1981, there were 83 very-low-birth-weight (less than 1,500 g) and 39 additional extremely low-birth-weight (ELBW [less than 1,000 g]) infants for every neonatologist. By 1996 these numbers dropped to 23 VLBW infants and 11 ELBW infants for every active neonatologist (Table 3-3) (17). In its statement on the neonatal workforce, the American Academy of Pediatrics Committee on the Fetus and Newborn (COFN) recommended that the neonatologist:live birth ratio be 1:2,569 live births—which is 3.9 neonatologists per 10,000 live births (16). In 1996, the ratio was calculated to be 1:1,687 live births—which is 5.9 neonatologists per 10,000 live births, 1.5 times the original target. In addition, 50% of the neonatologists surveyed in this study reported that a very significant portion of their practice was devoted to the care of normal newborn infants (18).

Similar to the in-hospital bed capacity analysis, Goodman and associates (18) report wide variations in the availability of neonatologists, ranging from 1.2 per 10,000 live births to a high of 25.6 per 10,000 live births (a range of 390–8,197 births per neonatologist) (Figs. 3-4a, 3-4b).

Regional variations were unexplained by differences in LBW, number of high-risk pregnancies, or use of mid-level providers. Regions with an average of 2.7 neonatologists per 10,000 live births or less experienced a slight, but significant increase in mortality only for infants with birth weights of 500 to 999 g. Once birth weight exceeds 999 g or the number of neonatologists exceeds 4.3 per 10,000 live births, there are no additional improvements seen in neonatal mortality (19).

Lessons Learned

The attempt to correlate outcome with either NICU in-hospital bed capacity or the number and distribution of neonatologists presents several dilemmas. First, gross outcome of neonatal care, such as the incidence of LBW or neonatal and infant mortality, may be insensitive to regional changes in resource availability. It is entirely possible that there exists a yet-to-be-defined threshold above which the impact of additional available resources is no longer obvious. Alternatively, it is well established that birth weight is a reflection of socioeconomic status and quality of care before delivery and is not directly influenced by postnatal medical interventions (12,20). As the COPH stated in 1993, appropriate preconception and prenatal care may contribute significantly to increasing birth weight and decreasing neonatal mortality (7).

COSTS OF DELIVERING NEONATAL CARE

Acute Care In-Hospital Costs

Estimates suggest that the total expenditures for perinatal care in the United States exceed $6,850 per mother–infant pair (7). This represents 4.5% of personal health care

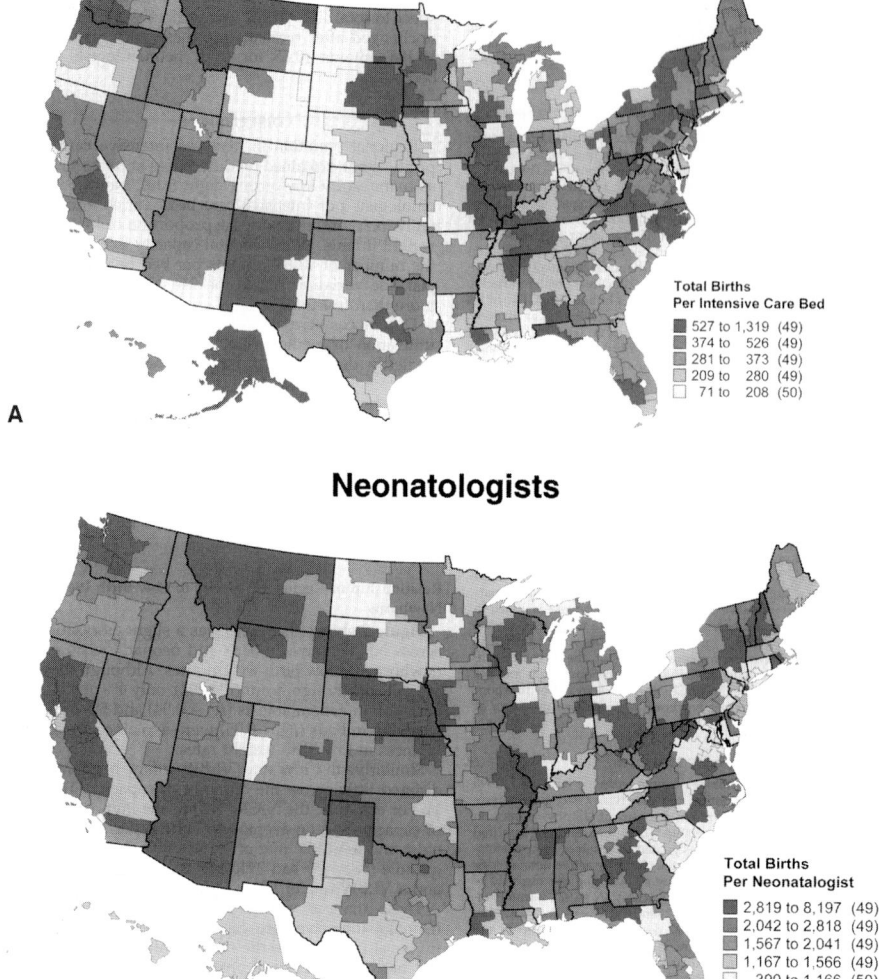

Neonatal Intensive Care Beds

Total Births
Per Intensive Care Bed
■ 527 to 1,319 (49)
■ 374 to   526 (49)
■ 281 to   373 (49)
□ 209 to   280 (49)
□ 71 to   208 (50)

A

Neonatologists

Total Births
Per Neonatalogist
■ 2,819 to 8,197 (49)
■ 2,042 to 2,818 (49)
■ 1,567 to 2,041 (49)
□ 1,167 to 1,566 (49)
□   390 to 1,166 (50)

B

Figure 3-4   Total birth figures. **A:** Total births per intensive care bed. **B:** Total births per neonatologist. (From Goodman DC Fisher ES, Little GA. Are neonatal intensive care resources located according to need? Regional variations in neonatologists, beds, and low birth weight newborns. *Pediatrics*: 2001;108:426, with permission.)

spending by all Americans and 7% of health care spending by the population younger than 65 years of age. Most of these resources are spent on acute, high-tech care of the critically ill neonate, with daily charges easily reaching $1,000 to $2,500 for hospital services and an additional $300 to $450 each day for physician services (21). Of the four million births predicted in 2003, 280,000 will be premature, with an estimated cost of $12 billion for acute in-hospital neonatal care. Approximately one third of these expenditures, $4 billion, would be used to provide care for infants weighing between 500 and 700 g (22). An additional $1 billion would be spent on hospitalizations for preterm labor in an attempt to delay delivery as long as possible. Because the costs for complicated births (ranging from $20,000 to $400,000) are many fold greater than the costs of an uncomplicated delivery (averaging $6,400), the investment in delaying delivery as long as possible is entirely justified (6).

Charges associated with specific perinatal diagnoses rank among the highest of all hospital diagnoses (Table 3-4). A 1999 report by the Health Care Cost and Utilization Project's Nationwide Inpatient Sample listed neonatal respiratory distress syndrome as the most expensive diagnosis, with a mean charge of $82,648 and a mean length of stay of 27.8 days. Other diagnoses included in the top 10 categories were:

- Low-birth-weight (mean charge of $56,942)
- Cardiac anomalies (mean charge of $49,858)
- Intrauterine hypoxia and birth asphyxia (mean charge of $36,954) (23)

In analyzing data from 3,288 VLBW infants from 25 NICUs, Rogowski (24) reported that treatment costs vary inversely with birth weight, with a median treatment cost of $89,546 for infants weighing between 501 g and 750 g and $32,531 for infants weighing between 1,251 g and 1500 g.

TABLE 3-4

MOST COMMON HOSPITAL DISCHARGE DIAGNOSES WITH MEAN CHARGES AND MEAN LENGTH OF STAY

Rank	Principal Diagnosis	Mean Charges*	Mean Length of Stay (days)
1	Respiratory distress syndrome	82,648	27.8
2	Spinal cord injury	58,690	12.4
3	Short gestation, low-birth-weight, and fetal growth retardation	56,942	22.7
4	Leukemias	53,252	13.8
5	Heart valve disorders	51,292	8.8
6	Cardiac and circulatory congenital anomalies	49,858	7.8
7	Other CNS infection and poliomyelitis aneurysms	44,060	12.6
8	Aortic, peripheral, and visceral artery	42,461	8.7
9	Intrauterine hypoxia and birth asphyxia	36,954	12.1
10	Cancer of stomach	35,426	10.8

*Charges are for acute hospital care and do not include physician and other professional fees, rehabilitation expenses, or costs associated with follow-up or home care.
CNS, central nervous system.
From March of Dimes Perinatal Data Centers. *Economic costs of prenatal care—Health Care Utilization Project nationwide inpatient sample.* 1999, White Plains, NY: March of Dimes, 2002, with permission.

In this analysis, she included costs of accommodation (room and personnel costs) and ancillary services (respiratory therapy, laboratory, radiology, pharmacy, and medical supplies). While accommodation costs varied by a factor of two when comparing the largest and smallest VLBW infants, ancillary costs varied by almost five fold, with laboratory and respiratory services showing the widest variation. When costs were corrected for length of stay, the costs per day were surprisingly similar, varying by only $552 per day between infants weighing 1,251 to 1,500 g at birth and those weighing 501 to 750 g at birth (Table 3-5).

Because physician services are billed separately from the hospital, most studies do not include them in the analysis and, as a result, the true picture of the cost of neonatal care is somewhat distorted. This distortion can be significant when one considers that the cost of physician services in the NICU approaches 15% of the total hospital bill (21).

Although these data are valuable and serve as a rough estimate of expenditures, caution must be used when attempting to apply them to actual expenditures for neonatal care at the local or state level. By and large, these data are derived from in-hospital data as reported on state and federal cost reports, which reflect charges and not the true costs of delivering care. Further, many studies report individual hospital, state, or regional experiences that vary greatly based on the accounting principles used by that facility.

In many instances, hospital estimates of disease and patient-specific expenditures are based on small samples, resulting in wide variations within and between studies. Expenditure comparisons are complicated further by regional variations in costs, charges, standards of care, differences in patient population demographics, and intensity of illness. Finally, much of the available information is derived from urban level III NICUs or state-funded perinatal programs, which include a high percentage of publicly funded patients. Because these patients often represent the highest perinatal risks, disease-specific expenditures may be skewed by overrepresentation of the most complex patients in the database, resulting in higher cost estimates when compared to private-sector spending.

In an attempt to control expenditures for neonatal services, both public and private payers have developed

TABLE 3-5a

MEDIAN TREATMENT COSTS AND LENGTH OF STAY FOR VERY-LOW-BIRTH-WEIGHT INFANTS

	N	Total Cost	Accommodation Cost	Ancillary Cost	Length (days) of Stay	Cost per Day
All infants	3288	$49,457	$35,521	$13,872	49	$1115
Birth weight						
501–750 g	601	$89,546	$59,318	$28,094	79	$1483
751–1000 g	811	$78,455	$54,259	$23,288	72	$1200
1001–1250 g	861	$49,097	$35,460	$13,376	49	$1059
1251–1500 g	1015	$31,531	$24,609	$ 6,224	35	$ 932

TABLE 3-5b

MEDIAN ANCILLARY COSTS FOR VERY-LOW-BIRTH-WEIGHT INFANTS

Cost Per Day	N	Total Ancillary Cost	Respiratory Therapy	Laboratory	Radiology	Pharmacy	Other	Ancillary
All infants	3288	$13,872	$3112	$3308	$ 942	$2258	2474	$323
Birth Weight								
501–750 g	601	$28,094	$8678	$6550	$1671	$3717	4054	$546
751–1000 g	811	$23,288	$7421	$5494	$1475	$3668	3726	$382
1001–1250 g	861	$13,376	$2884	$3205	$ 900	$2195	2554	$301
1251–1500 g	1015	$ 6,224	$1044	$1720	$ 473	$1101	1382	$194

From Rogowski J. Measuring the cost of neonatal and perinatal care. *Pediatrics* 1999;103:329–335, with permission.

prospective payment systems, which place providers of neonatal care at risk for managing costs generated by their patients. Payment systems such as the Florida Neonatal Care Groups and the APR-DRGs (all patient refined-diagnostic care groups) have proved to be acceptable ways to provide appropriate reimbursement for services while controlling costs for public and private payers (21,25). With the recent Medicaid expansions and many states enrolling more and more patients in Medicaid managed care plans, fixed rather than cost-based reimbursement is becoming more common, leading many institutions to explore new ways to control NICU costs.

Without a doubt, NICU care is one of the most expensive services available because of the high technology and the prolonged length of stay. If we are going to be able to continue to provide every patient the full range of services, neonatal health care professionals will need to ensure that the available resources are used in the most cost-effective manner to provide the highest quality of care. To achieve this goal, neonatal providers should become aware of the costs and hospital cost structures associated with the care they are providing. Richardson and associates (26) published a detailed analysis of the types of costs generated by an inpatient (Fig. 3-5). Understanding how fixed, variable, direct, and indirect costs are derived will help the neonatal team identify items that can be considered part of cost reduction and those that are unaffected by census or acuity. Although we must strive to be sure that every neonate has access to a full range of therapies, resources used inappropriately on one or a group of patients may deny full access to care to others (27).

Acute Medical Care Post Discharge

Graduation from the NICU does not herald the end of increased capital investment in the surviving infant. In a series from the United Kingdom, Stevenson and associates (28) determined that the mean cost per LBW infant, born at less than 1,500 g and surviving without major disability, was 13 times greater than that of an infant weighing between 1,501 and 2,000 g; and the cost per infant weighing less than 1,000 g at birth was 55 times control. Further, LBW infants continued to utilize hospital and practioner services at a greater rate than control until age 8 to 9. Similarly, Rogowski

(29) reported in 1998 that, on average, the VLBW who is an NICU graduate will require almost $1,400 in outpatient services and be hospitalized twice with an average length of stay of 11 days at a cost of almost $12,000. In many instance these outpatient visits and pharmaceuticals are either not covered by traditional payers or they have significant copayments and deductibles, resulting in significant financial hardships for families. Thus, additional acute medical costs after discharge from the NICU are of major concern to private and public payers as well as parents.

Long-Term Costs

Because LBW infants are at high risk for long-term sequelae, the resources dedicated to providing acute care must be supplemented with the continued investment of resources for long-term followup. With the realization that the long-term outcome of LBW infants is enhanced by developmental followup, including multidisciplinary intervention programs, postdischarge costs per NICU graduate have become substantial (30). In a study reported from Helsinki, Finland, the costs for 71 ELBW infants during

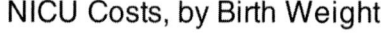

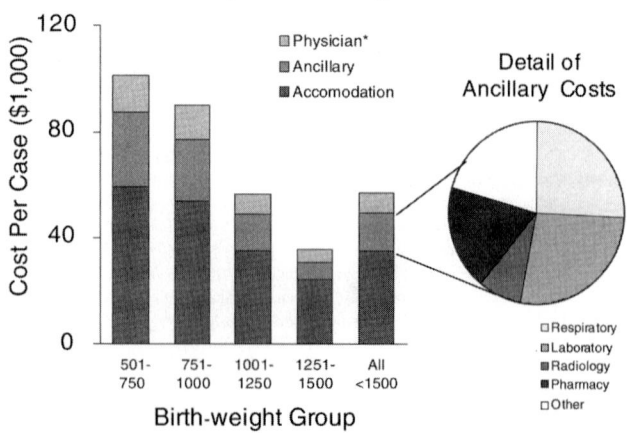

Figure 3-5 Total hospital costs for newborns greater than 1500 g birth weight, by birth-weight group. (From Richardson DK, Zupancic JA, Escobar GJ, et al. A critical review of cost reduction in the neonatal intensive care unit. I. The structure of costs. *J Perinatol* 2001;21:107, with permission.)

the first 2 years after discharge from an NICU averaged $34,529 compared to $1,034 for term, control infants (31). Although this study attempted to identify total post-discharge costs, family out-of-pocket expenses were not estimated. A recent survey indicates that these expenses for children with special health care needs can exceed 15% of annual family income (32).

The increased survival of ELBW infants presents several challenges to our educational system. Stevenson and colleagues (28) report that 52% of the long-term expenditures related to LBW are related to special education needs. Lewit and colleagues (33) report that health care, education, and child care for the more than 4 million children ages 0 to 15 born at LBW and VLBW cost between $5.5 and $6.0 billion more than they would have if these children had been born at a normal birth weight.

Beyond the Costs of Acute Neonatal Care

When long-term cost–benefit ratios were calculated in each of the past 3 decades, the provision of neonatal care appeared extremely cost-effective. This is still true, because high-quality neonatal care decreases the incidence of significant morbidity in almost all weight groups. However, the increased number of surviving ELBW infants with their financial, social, and educational impacts has led several researchers to raise significant ethical and moral questions about future therapeutic directions as we approach the limits of viability for some of our smallest patients. While the cost–benefit ratio for ELBW infants is of obvious concern, the more fundamental ethical and moral issues deal with whether or not high-tech care should be provided to infants whose very survival is extremely unlikely, and the long-term consequences for those who survive are significant. How should we approach these infants? Who should decide what therapies should and should not be given? What is the role of the neonatal team, the family, the payers in the decision-making process? There appear to be few, if any, consensus answers to these critical questions because the ethical, legal, and moral considerations involving the extremely premature infant have not kept pace with the advancement of technology. Our nation has only recently been willing to admit that even the richest country in the world cannot afford to buy all that science has to offer. Prioritizing therapies and making very difficult decisions about the use of resources must be discussed more in years to come (34).

Missed Opportunities

One cannot consider the magnitude of these costs and the amount of human suffering involved in the delivery of a high-risk infant without wondering why the United States continues to expend enormous resources on postnatal care when half of the ELBW deliveries could be avoided with early prenatal care (1). The benefit of $1,000 of prenatal care instead of $150,000 for each surviving LBW infant is obvious. Almost 2 decades ago, the Institute of Medicine

reported that for every $1 spent on prenatal care, $3 were saved in the first year of life, and $10 more were saved over a lifetime (35). This relationship between prenatal care and downstream costs appears to be true today as well. A recent report by Lu and associates (36) shows that for every $1 reduction in prenatal care provided by public programs there was an increase of $3.33 in postnatal care costs and a $4.63 increase in long-term morbidity costs. The average cost of long-term care (medical, child care, and special education) for women without prenatal care is $4,839 compared to $1,592 for women with prenatal care.

Fortunately, today 83% of women receive prenatal care and begin that care within the first trimester (3). Financial access to care combined with comprehensive prepregnancy and prenatal programs, including good nutrition and avoidance of high-risk lifestyles, have been identified as key in reducing LBW with its attendant costs and human loss (7). Of major concern, however, is the remaining economic and noneconomic barriers confronting minority populations, resulting in late or no prenatal care rates, which are three to four times that of whites (1).

Major Payers of Perinatal Care

There are four major payers for perinatal care in the United States:

1. Private health insurance, purchased through employers or directly by individuals
2. Public programs including Medicaid and other federal, state, and local programs
3. Special perinatal demonstration projects, both public and private
4. Self-pay or uninsured

None of the major payers completely cover the costs of high-risk obstetric and neonatal care, especially for the complicated ELBW infant. A significant portion of the uncompensated care created by underpayment by public payers and the uninsured is often shifted to other subscribers in the form of increased charges. One study suggests that as much as 27% of total costs of NICU care were shifted to paying patients who are responsible for generating 60% of total revenues while accounting for only 33% of costs (37). In recent years, payments under fee-for-service plans have been replaced by capitated managed care and discounted plans, reducing the ability of NICUs to shift cost and placing many in financial jeopardy.

Private Health Insurance

Only 72% of women of childbearing age are covered by employer or privately purchased insurance (Fig. 3-6A). Women are less likely than men to have employer-based coverage because they are more likely to be employed less than full time, to work for small employers who do not offer insurance, or have spouses who work for employers who do not offer dependent coverage (1). Even for those with health insurance, 7% of plans offered in 2000 by

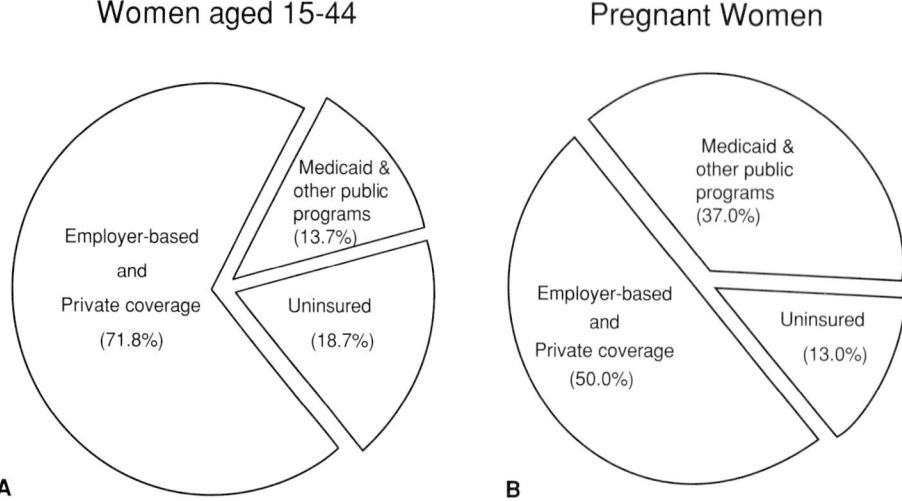

Figure 3-6   Insurance status of **(A)** women ages 15 to 44 years and **(B)** pregnant women in the United States, 2002. (From U.S. Department of Health and Human Services. Retrieved July 1, 2003, from http://www.hhs.gov/budget/docbudget.htm.)

small employers (10 to 24 workers) did not cover prenatal care or delivery expenses. Plans providing maternity benefits often impose substantial cost-sharing arrangements, which can become a significant barrier to care, resulting in limited prenatal care and increasing the chance of a high-risk delivery. Similar limitations are often seen in coverage of high-risk neonates after delivery (38). Cost-sharing arrangements with lifetime caps on policy benefits can be financially devastating to families. For example, a 20% copayment responsibility on a combined hospital and physician bill of $250,000 for an LBW infant results in a family out-of-pocket expense of $50,000, an amount that would be impossible for most families to pay. Many policies carry a $250,000 to $500,000 lifetime cap. In this case the infant would use all or half of the entire lifetime benefit at discharge from the NICU.

Medicaid

Medicaid is the largest public program for the financing of prenatal and neonatal care. Authorized as Title XIX of the Social Security Act in 1965, Medicaid is a federal–state partnership that finances care for 51 million low-income pregnant women, children, the elderly, the blind, and the disabled. In 2002, it surpassed Medicare to become the nation's largest health insurance program in numbers of people served and in expenditures, totaling $259 billion and outspending Medicare by $2 billion (39). During the past several years, the federal–state match has remained relatively constant, with federal funds accounting for an average of 56.9% of total fiscal-year program expenditures. The exact level of federal funding is determined from a formula reflecting the state's per capita income and varies between 50% and 80% of the state's total Medicaid expenditures.

Today, 51% of the targeted population consists of pregnant women and children; however, only 15% of total program expenditures are directed toward them (40). With the

exception of the matching requirements for federal funds and the required compliance with specific federal mandates, each state has the responsibility for developing and administering its own Medicaid program. This includes setting eligibility and coverage standards within broad federal guidelines. As a result, there is considerable variation among states in eligibility, range of services offered, limitations on services, and reimbursement policies.

Over the past several years, Congress has been successful in extending Medicaid eligibility to more pregnant women and children. Beginning in 1989, all states were required to cover pregnant women and children younger than 6 years of age with family incomes below 133% of the federal poverty level (FPL) and had the option of extending benefits to pregnant women and infants younger than 1 year of age with family incomes below 185% of the FPL. The State Children's Health Insurance Program, under Title XXI of the Social Security Act, enacted in 1997, gave states new latitude in identifying eligible patients and allows states to expand coverage for children and pregnant women up to 200% of the FPL, with some states using additional funds to reach 300% of the FPL (37,40).

In 2001, Medicaid was the source of payment for 1.6 million births, 37% of the nation's deliveries, ranging from a low of 9% in Hawaii (the only state with universal health coverage) to a high of 56% of all births in New Mexico (1,40,41). As a result of this expanded eligibility, many women drop more expensive employer-based and private coverage and enroll in Medicaid. Thus, employer-based and private coverage among pregnant women has dropped to 50% with 13.0% remaining uninsured (Fig. 3-6B) (37).

Title V Maternal and Child Health Block Grant Program

Located within the Health Resources and Services Administration (HRSA) of the Department of Health and

Human Services (HHS), the Maternal and Child Health (MCH) Block Grant Program was authorized by Title V of the Social Security Act to provide grants to states for a variety of preventive and primary care services to women and children, including prenatal care, immunizations, and rehabilitative services for children with special needs. Although fiscal year 2002 funding for this program exceeded $930 million, it accounts for less than 1% of the HHS budget (42). Current funding levels allow less than half of eligible women access to prenatal care under the program.

Community Health Centers, Migrant Health Centers, and the National Health Service Corps

As part of HRSA, $1.4 billion for community health centers, migrant health centers, and programs of the National Health Service Corps are directed toward providing primary preventive care, including prenatal and well-child care, for those served in urban community health centers and in rural areas of the United States (42).

Special Demonstration Projects

Because prevention of low-birth-weight infants can positively affect perinatal outcome, many public (e.g., state, county, and municipal governments) and private (e.g., March of Dimes, Robert Wood Johnson, Pew Foundation) organizations have dedicated significant resources to study how to reach high-risk populations more effectively to reduce the mortality and morbidity related to premature deliveries. Although most of these projects are small and contribute little to covering the total costs of perinatal care, many are highly successful, improve outcomes for individual patients, and add significantly to our understanding of the perinatal health care system and the delivery of health care to special populations. A major problem with these projects is that targeted patients are highly selected, making it difficult to apply program results to larger populations. Many programs are funded for a limited time, creating the problem of how to continue to provide services after funding has expired.

Uninsured, Self-Paying Patients

Many of the uninsured are in young families working for small business or are in the service industry and are not provided employer-based health insurance. Sixty percent of young families of childbearing age are two-parent families, and 85% of them have at least one member employed full- or part-time. Most uninsured families have limited resources, with incomes between $30,000 and $32,000 annually. Sixty-one percent of uninsured women have family incomes below 200% of the FPL, making it very difficult to pay out of pocket for medical expenses or even for prenatal care (37).

More than a decade ago, the National Commission on Children found that being uninsured during pregnancy is the greatest barrier to receiving prenatal care, and it results

in the highest risk for delivering an LBW infant, approximately three to five times the rate for women with even minimal prenatal care (43). Fortunately, this barrier to access to prenatal care seems to have been significantly reduced. As a result of enhanced eligibility under Medicaid, only 13% of pregnant women (422,000) are uninsured during pregnancy and up to 1 year following delivery (Fig. 3-6B) (1).

Although enhanced coverage for pregnant women ensures access to prenatal care, the loss of eligibility 1 year after delivery presents major problems for continued care between pregnancies and makes preparation for subsequent healthy pregnancies problematic. As many as 20 million women have their insurance interrupted for at least 2 months over a 24-month period, and data indicate that 26% of women are uninsured when they conceive (44).

MAJOR MEASURES OF OUTCOME

Infant Mortality Rate

The infant mortality rate (IMR) is defined by the National Center for Health Statistics and by the World Health Organization as the number of deaths occurring within the first year of life per 1,000 live births. Infant mortality can be divided further into neonatal mortality (i.e., death before 29 days of age) and postneonatal mortality (i.e., death between 29 days and 1 year of age). Neonatal mortality generally is the result of factors related to pregnancy and birth, while postneonatal mortality generally is the result of environmental factors (e.g., trauma, infection, nutrition, sudden infant death syndrome) (41).

Infant mortality in the United States has declined substantially since 1975. Initially, the largest declines were seen in the neonatal mortality rate (NMR), but more recently these advances have been matched by similar declines in the postneonatal mortality rate (PNMR). Between 1980 and 2001, the IMR dropped from 12.5 deaths per 1,000 live births to 6.9 deaths per 1,000 live births as a result of a 45% decline in the NMR (Fig. 3-7) (41). Despite these achievements the current IMR exceeds the Healthy People 2010 goal of 4.5 by 35% (1,3).

Of major concern is the persistent disparity in the IMR between white and African American infants. Although all race groups have experienced a decrease in IMR, the rate for African American infants fell by only 36.5%, which is 12.1% less than that of whites. Recently published 2000 rates show an IMR for white infants at 5.7 per 1,000 live births, whereas that of African American infants is reported to be 14.1 deaths per 1,000 live births, a ratio of 2.5:1 (Fig. 3-8). The infant mortality rate for Hispanics is slightly better than that for whites at 5.6 per 1,000 live births (41,44).

Neonatal Mortality Rate

Although the IMR reflects the general health of a community, separate examination of early and late infant deaths

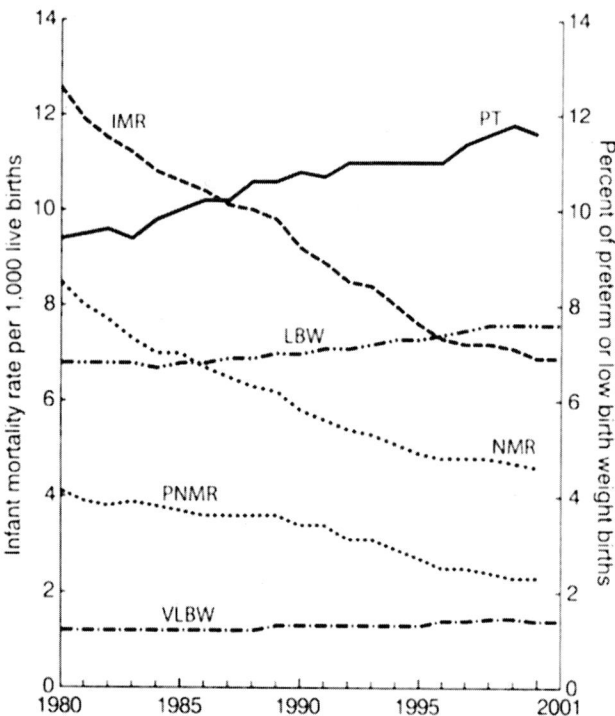

Figure 3-7 Infant, neonatal, and postneonatal mortality for low-birth-weight (LBW), very-low-birth-weight (VLBW), and preterm (PT) delivery in the United States from 1980–2001. Infant mortality rate (IMR) indicates infant deaths per 1,000 live births; neonatal mortality rate (NMR) indicates neonatal deaths per 1,000 live births; postneonatal mortality rate (PNMR) indicates postneonatal deaths per 1,000 live births; LBW indicates percent low-birth-weight (<2500 g); VLBW indicates percent very-low-birth-weight (<1500 g); PT indicates percent preterm (<37 weeks of gestation). (From MacDorman MF, Minino AM, Strobino DM, et al. Annual summary of vital statistics 2001. *Pediatrics* 2002;110:1037, with permission.)

can further pinpoint problems. The NMR equals the number of deaths occurring at less than 29 days after birth per 1,000 live births (39). These account for approximately 67% of all infant deaths. Half of all neonatal deaths can be attributed to four leading causes:

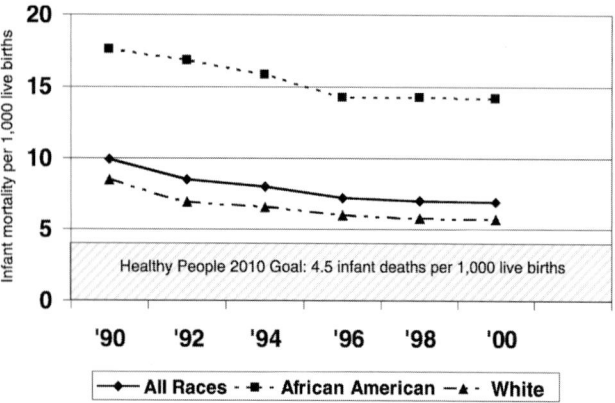

Figure 3-8 Infant mortality in the United States from 1990 to 2000 by race. Infant mortality constitutes deaths that occur before 1 year of age. (From U.S. Department of Health and Human Services. Retrieved July 1, 2003, from http://www.hhs.gov/budget/dccbudget.htm)

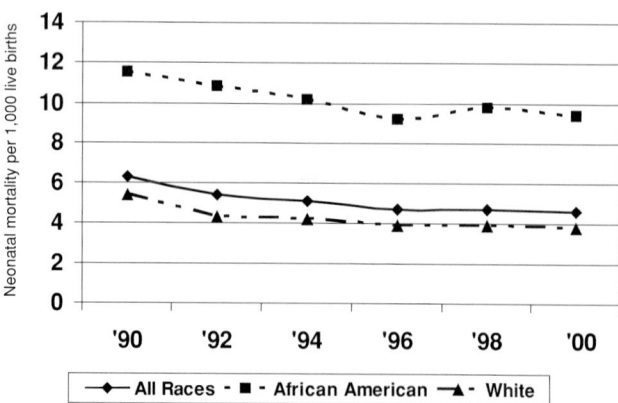

Figure 3-9 Neonatal mortality in the United States from 1990 to 2000 by race. Neonatal mortality constitutes deaths that occur before 28 days of age. (From U.S. Department of Health and Human Services. Retrieved July 1, 2003, from http://www.hhs.gov/budget/dccbudget.htm)

1. LBW
2. Acute perinatal asphyxia
3. Congenital anomalies
4. Perinatal infections

Between 1980 and 2001, the NMR declined by 45%. The 2000 rate of 4.6 deaths per 1,000 live births is thought to be a reflection of the marked improvement in the treatment of respiratory illnesses in term and preterm infants. Once again the rate for African Americans (9.4 deaths per 1,000 live births) parallels the IMR and is considerably higher than the white NMR, with an NMR ratio of African Americans to whites of 2.5:1 (Fig. 3-9). These differences appear to be primarily because of the higher incidence of LBW (less than 2,500 g) and VLBW (less than 1,500 g) infants born to African American women and a higher NMR for African American infants weighing more than 2,500 g (1.2 deaths per 1,000 live births for African Americans compared to 0.9 deaths per 1,000 live births for whites). NMR for Hispanics is slightly better than for whites at 3.7 deaths per 1,000 live births (41).

Perinatal Mortality Rate

The perinatal mortality rate (PMR) is defined by the National Center for Health Statistics as the number of late fetal deaths (i.e., fetal deaths of 28 weeks or more gestation) plus early neonatal deaths (i.e., deaths of infants 0 to 6 days of age) per 1,000 live births (41).

Most fetal deaths are a result of chronic asphyxia (60% to 70%); congenital malformations (20% to 25%); superimposed complications of pregnancy, such as placental abruption, diabetes mellitus, intrauterine infection (5% to 10%); and unexplained deaths (5% to 10%) (43). Although the incidence of congenital malformations has remained relatively constant over the last few years, improvements in the management of pregnancy-related complications, combined with improved early neonatal survival, has resulted in

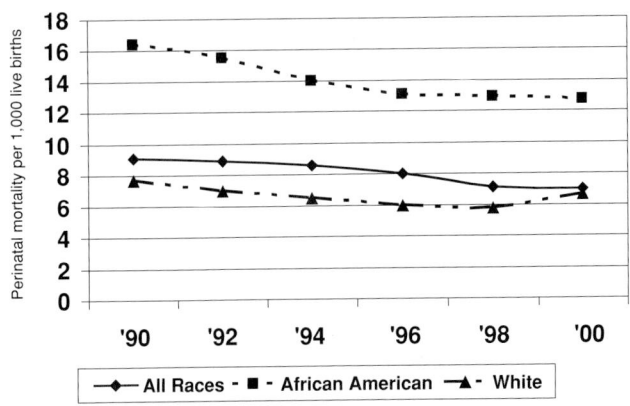

Figure 3-10 Perinatal mortality in the United States from 1990 to 2000 by race. Perinatal mortality constitutes fetal death before 28 weeks of gestation plus infant deaths at 0 to 6 days of age. (From U.S. Department of Health and Human Services. Retrieved July 1, 2003, from http://www.hhs.gov/budget/dccbudget.htm)

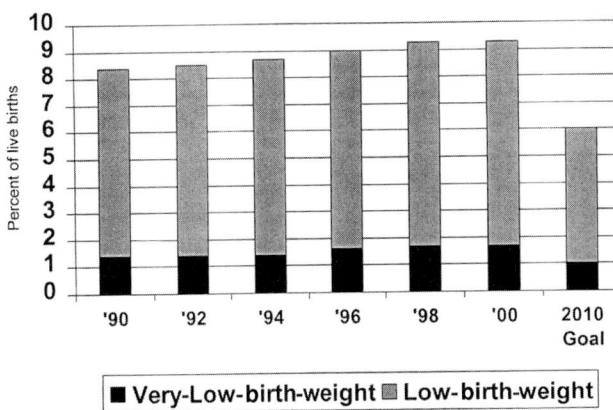

Figure 3-12 Incidence of low-birth-weight and very-low-birth-weight births as a percent of all live births in the United States from 1990 to 2000. (From March of Dimes. *March of Dimes data book for policy makers*, Washington, DC: March of Dimes Office of Government Affairs, 2003, with permission.)

a significant decrease in PMR to 7.0 deaths per 1,000 live births for 2000. Race variations in PMR are slightly better than those seen in IMR and NMR (Fig. 3-10). PMR in African American women is less than twice that of whites (12.7 deaths per 1,000 live births compared to 6.7 deaths per 1,000 live births). The reported PMR for Hispanics for 2000 is 6.0 deaths per 1,000 live births and is considerably less than the 6.7 deaths per 1,000 live births reported for whites (41).

MAJOR MORBIDITIES

Preterm Birth

The preterm birth rate is defined as births from pregnancies that have completed less than 37 weeks of gestation. In 2000 there were 467,201 (11.6% of live births) preterm births recorded, only 40% of which were also low-birth-weight (Fig. 3-11). This is the first time there has been a decline in the rate of preterm births in the United States since 1992, declining from 11.8% of live births in 1999 to 11.6% of live births in 2000 (1). Although recent trends are encouraging, the 2000 preterm rate still exceeds that of the

Healthy People 2010 goal of 7.6% of live births by 50%. The decrease in preterm births form 10.5% to 10.4% of live births among non-Hispanic whites is the first decrease in a decade, during which rates steadily rose from 8.5% of live births. The preterm birth rate in African Americans remains high at 17.3% of live births, but has trended downward since peaking at 18.9% of live births in 1991. The very preterm rate (less than 32 completed weeks of gestation) remains unchanged from the 1981 rate of 1.93% of live births, and is more than twice the Healthy People 2010 goal of 0.9 % of live births (3).

Low-Birth-Weight

LBW is responsible for 66% of the U.S. IMR and carries a six-fold increased risk of death for infants weighing between 1,500 and 2,499 g, a 98-fold increased risk of death for infants weighing less than 1,500 g, and a two- to three-fold increase in the chance of long-term disability (41). Considering these realities, the prevention of LBW has been one of the nation's top priorities in its effort to reduce infant mortality and morbidity. Despite this focus, no progress has been made in reducing the incidence of LBW over the last decade. In 2000, more than 300,000 infants (7.6% of live births) were born at LBW, which is the highest recorded in the previous 20 years and exceeds the Healthy People 2010 goal by 52% (Fig. 3-12) (1). Currently, the LBW rate among African Americans, at 13.0 % of live births, is 1.7 times that of whites. Examination of annual LBW statistics reveals a slow but continued increase in the overall number of infants born at LBW since 1990 (Fig. 3-13) (41,45). However, the greatest rise in LBW occurred between 1990 and 1995, coincident to a dramatic increase in the number of births to teens (Fig. 3-2). This association is not surprising when one realizes that teen pregnancy carries a very significant increase in the risk of having an LBW infant.

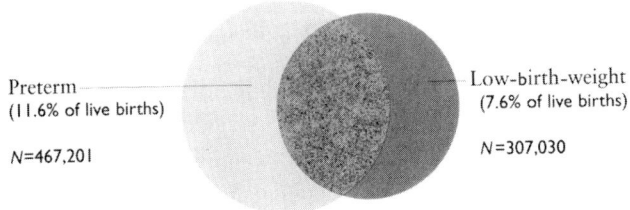

Figure 3-11 Incidence of preterm and low-birth-weight births in 2000. (From March of Dimes. *March of Dimes data book for policy makers*, Washington, DC: March of Dimes Office of Government Affairs, 2003, with permission.)

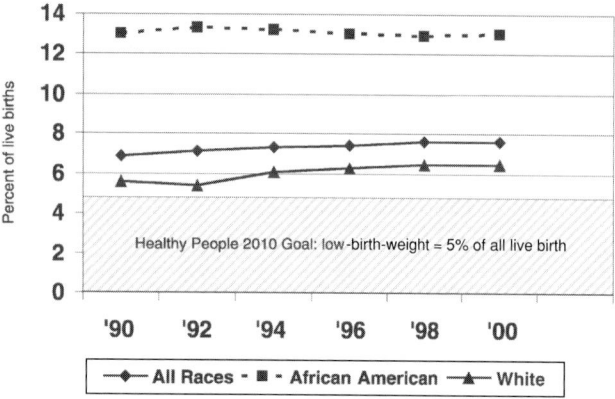

Figure 3-13 Trends in low-birth-weight births (less than 2500 g) by race as a percentage of all births, United States 1990–2000. (From U.S. Department of Health and Human Services. Retrieved July 1, 2003, from http://www.hhs.gov/budget/dccbudget.htm)

Multiple Births

The twin birth rate has risen by 55% since 1980. This is of major health significance because half of all twin gestations and the great majority of triplet births are high risk. In fact, twins are 5 times as likely to be premature and 9.5 times as likely to be of VLBW than singleton deliveries. As such, they are responsible for some of the continued trends in U.S. perinatal statistics and consume significant resources (41). However, this increase in use of perinatal resources is directly related to prematurity and low-birth-weight rather than the twin gestation *per se* (46). It appears that this increase in multiple births is related to two trends in American society. First, more and more women are delivering later in life. In 2000, birth rates for women in their thirties reached their highest levels in 30 years. Birth rates for women 40 to 44 years of age also rose in 2000 and have more than doubled since 1981 (41). These increases are related to the growing tendency for many women to postpone childbearing. Secondly, the use of assisted reproductive technology, ovulation-inducing drugs, and *in vitro* fertilization, have long been associated with a higher risk of multiple births (47,48). The real potential for multiple births and their attendant increased risk for LBW (with its increased mortality and morbidity) should be considered when either delay in childbearing and/or assisted reproduction are being considered.

Lifestyle Choices

Some of the perinatal risk factors associated with LBW and poor perinatal outcome are not within a pregnant woman's immediate control. However, many of the factors associated with lifestyle choices are (49).

Cigarette Smoking

Cigarette smoking during pregnancy is the single largest modifiable risk factor for LBW (up to 20%) and infant mortality. Babies born to mothers who smoke are, on average,

200 g lighter than those born to mothers who do not smoke. In a recent review, Eyler and Behnke (48) reported that infants exposed to tobacco *in utero* demonstrated abnormal behavior up to 14 days after delivery. Abnormalities included poor auditory habituation, and disorders of orientation and autonomic regulation. Although implications of these findings are unclear, they do suggest that smoking during pregnancy carries significant long-term behavioral risks in addition to those associated with a low-birth-weight.

Despite these and other well-publicized risks of smoking during pregnancy, a March of Dimes survey reports that 20% of pregnant women 15 to 44 years of age stated that they had been smoking cigarettes regularly, and smoking during pregnancy was common with women under 20 years of age. Of the 10% to 15% of smoking women who stop smoking during pregnancy, two thirds resume smoking within 1 year of delivery, exposing the infant to secondhand smoke (1). Because most of these infants are term and near-term LBW infants, their prognosis is good and their medical costs are only moderate. Nonetheless, reduction of smoking during pregnancy can decrease the incidence of LBW and reduce the risk of long-term development delays (1,49,50).

Alcohol

The use of alcohol during pregnancy has been associated with both short- and long-term morbidity. Fetal alcohol syndrome is a well-recognized consequence of excessive consumption of alcohol during pregnancy, occurring in 1 per 1,000 live births. However, several studies report an increase in LBW babies born to women who consume between one and three drinks per day, resulting in an average decrease in birth weight of between 28 and 141 g. Almost 5% of pregnant women report "binge" alcohol use (five or more drinks on the same occasion or the same day) (1,49). Recent studies performed in older alcohol-exposed infants show an increase in the number of speech and language delays, which seem to be directly related to the amount of alcohol consumed during pregnancy. In this study, the decreased mental developmental index in these infants also appears to be dose dependent (50). These data and that of others strongly suggest that the avoidance of alcohol during pregnancy can significantly improve perinatal outcome.

Illicit Drug Use

The exact incidence of illicit drug use during pregnancy is unknown, but several researchers report perinatal cocaine exposure rates of between 0.4% and 27%, depending on the region of the country and the population demographics (49–51). A myriad of neonatal complications have been reported as a result of cocaine exposure, ranging from none to antenatal cerebral infarction. The estimated short-term costs of perinatal cocaine exposure are between $33 million and $650 million (51). The long-term neurodevelopmental effects of perinatal illicit drug exposure are just now being studied carefully. Many studies in newborns have shown irritability and lability of state, decreases in alertness and orientation, and abnormal muscle tone and reflexes. However, one third of newborn behavioral studies have found no demonstrable effect of perinatal exposure. Further, studies performed in older infants have failed to show significant effects of perinatal cocaine exposure on either the mental developmental index or the physical developmental index (50).

Although perinatal exposure to any drug cannot accurately predict long-term outcome, such exposure often exposes a child to multiple risks—physical, developmental, and psychosocial. If we can eliminate these risks, we have every reason to believe that perinatal outcome will be enhanced.

Neurodevelopmental Sequelae

With survival rates approaching 95% for premature infants weighing between 1,200 and 2,500 g and 60% for those between 500 and 750 g, the incidence and magnitude of the neurodevelopmental sequelae related to the treatment of premature and critically ill neonates has become increasingly important (52). Long-term outcome of infants treated in the NICU has an enormous impact on many aspects of society. Even though the vast majority of children treated in the NICU survive intact, those who experience significant sequelae will need considerable additional resources from the family, state, and federal government in order for them to achieve their full potential. This impact is felt in the form of financial pressures placed on the family and public programs to provide necessary medical services and on schools as they attempt to provide an appropriate learning environment (53). The greatest risks of sequelae occur in the ELBW infants (less than 1,000 g birth weight) and in large infants experiencing perinatal hypoxic-ischemic encephalopathy. These issues are discussed in detail in other chapters; however, it is important to realize that after discharge from the NICU, infants with significant neurodevelopmental sequelae need a system that not only provides long-term support for specialty medical care, but also provides a lifetime of financial, social, and educational support for such children and their families (54). Clearly, the best way to deal with these problems is to prevent them from occurring in the future.

REGIONALIZATION TODAY

Regionalization of perinatal care has been lauded by many as the single most important factor influencing the birth-weight–specific neonatal mortality. Outlined in 1977 by the Committee on Perinatal Health of the National Foundation of the March of Dimes in its landmark report, *Toward Improving the Outcome of Pregnancy: Recommendations for the Regional Development of Maternal and Perinatal Health Services*, this concept served as the guide for the development of perinatal services for the last 2 decades (7). The

Committee's concept of regionalization was based on the geographic concentration of neonatal intensive care services supported by cooperative arrangements among hospitals within a region to provide, as a network, the necessary levels of care defined in the document as level I, II, and III services. Although quite intuitive and logical, this concept of cooperation is rather foreign to the American health care system, which is built on the philosophy of free market, free enterprise, and competition. The level of planning and cooperation necessary to make regionalization work is often resisted by all levels of health care providers. How then did regionalization take hold? Many observers think that it came at the right time, when knowledge of high-risk mothers and neonates was advancing rapidly. It came when the transfer of technology was confined to larger urban teaching hospitals and academic centers. It came at a time when other hospital services were running at near capacity.

Under the plan, regions were not defined strictly by geography, but by tradition and the organizational skills of a small number of highly respected early leaders in neonatology. This informal approach to the organization of perinatal care worked well as long as cooperation was seen as mutually beneficial to all involved. In the late 1970s and early 1980s, the health care environment began to change significantly. Driven by dramatic changes in the public financing of health care, the fragile alliance built on cooperation was being replaced by a drive for competition (55).

Medicare's replacement of fee-for-service reimbursement with a prospective payment system caused hospital inpatient census to drop as adult care was shifted to the outpatient clinics and ambulatory surgical centers. Declining hospital margins with excess capacity in the form of empty beds began to drive competition. The diffusion of technology into the community in conjunction with increased numbers of available neonatologists made competition for neonatal patients a possibility. Managed care plans captured an increasing share of the traditional indemnity plan markets and required hospitals to be full-service providers, making competition even more of a reality. Obstetric and newborn services, once seen as avoidable losses, became a requirement of participation in health plans. In some parts of the country, other factors hastened the move to competition. The medical liability crisis of the 1980s and 1990s, with the huge legal awards for poor neonatal outcome, particularly in the southern United States, increased the desire to have a neonatologist present at almost every delivery. At the same time, the presence of a hospital-based neonatologist presented the opportunity and the necessity to expand neonatal services beyond the delivery room into newly acquired NICU beds in an attempt to cover the costs of the neonatologist and to present appropriate clinical challenges to him or her and the nursery staff. In other regions, the overcrowding of level III units and the need to back transport convalescing neonates provided additional opportunity for community hospitals to begin neonatal programs. The differences in the levels of care, as defined by the COPH and by the American

Academy of Pediatrics, became blurred. A comprehensive study of regionalization revealed a general weakening of structures and relationships, with many hospitals and physicians working outside the designed networks (55). As a result, the COPH was reconvened in 1990 to respond to the changing health care environment and to make recommendations for the regionalization of perinatal care in the 1990s and beyond. The COPH's report reinforced the concept of regionalization of perinatal services, emphasizing the need for developing systems that integrate all levels of care within the region into a matrix with specific mechanisms for quality review and accountability between and among the various components. To facilitate this integration, the COPH suggested the formation of state and regional perinatal boards, with the authority and responsibility for providing or coordinating regional planning, monitoring access and data collection, and providing education (7). The plan's foundation appeared to be very regulatory in nature at a time when competition and the market were still very strong. As a result, very little progress has been made on the implementation of its recommendations.

So where are we today? It appears that regionalization of perinatal care still exists; however, its focus has evolved from level III units to the level II units, which have expanded their roles. Many neonatologists at level II units are providing labor room resuscitation and stabilization, as well as normal newborn and low-risk neonatal care at level I hospitals in their community. If these infants need more acute care, they are often transported to the local level II facility instead of the regional level III one. The availability of exogenous surfactant therapy, safer mechanical ventilators, and expanded roles for members of the neonatal provider team have allowed more of the LBW and VLBW infants to remain in level II facilities. Although this is troubling to some, the limited outcome information on LBW and VLBW neonates treated at level II rather than level III facilities fail to show any adverse outcomes as a result (56–58). It appears that the level III units have become the regional referral centers for ELBW infants, for larger infants in need of high frequency ventilation—extracorporeal membrane oxygenation (ECMO)—and for those in need of medical and surgical subspecialists. This redefinition of regionalization is not too far from the 1993 recommendations. What's missing is the development of specific relationships outlined in the report and the requirement that the various levels of care enter into formal agreements for referral, data transfer, outcomes review, and followup.

What are the inherent concerns about the evolved system? There is a danger that smaller and smaller infants will receive care at level II units as technology advances further. The guiding principle here should be the need for, and availability of, pediatric specialists as well as the availability of postdischarge specialty care and followup. Few level II units have sufficient numbers of critically ill neonates to justify on-site subspecialty coverage, and very few have enough ELBW or VLBW infants to justify investment in posthospital care; however, both are required to provide quality care for this population. Another concern is the

effect that changes in referral patterns have on level III regional referral centers. LBW and VLBW infants tend to be less expensive to care for than ELBW infants, those with birth defects, and those in need of specialty care. As a result, the level III units are experiencing more and more financial pressures as they receive the smallest, most complex patients with the smallest reimbursement-to-cost ratio. Because public programs, which routinely are among the poorest payers, cover so many premature infants, shifting the intensity of the level III units to even higher levels of acuity could result in more financial stress for many. Although the primary goal of regionalization is to provide the best, most cost effective care to today's neonates, we must remember that neonatology has evolved to where we are today because of the discovery of new therapies and the training of the next generation of neonatologists and neonatal specialists. A rational system of regionalized care must recognize that institutions dedicated to the development of future therapies and the future providers of neonatal care cannot always survive in a competitive environment. Our few truly educational and research institutions must continue to have a sufficient resources and a patient population representative of all levels of care in order to develop the workforce and therapies of tomorrow, today.

REFERENCES

1. March of Dimes. *March of Dimes data book for policy makers*, Washington, DC: March of Dimes Office of Government Affairs, 2003.
2. Pickering LK, ed. *Red book*: 2003 report of the Committee on Infectious Diseases, 26th ed. Elk Grove Village, IL: American Academy of Pediatrics, 2003:320–321.
3. Pastor PN, Makuc DM, Reuben C, et al. *Chartbook on trends in the health of Americans 2002.* Hyattsville, MD: National Center for Health Statistics, 2002.
4. The Annie E. Casey Foundation, *Kids count data book, 2003 a pocket guide.* Baltimore, MD: The Annie E. Casey Foundation, 2003:7.
5. U.S. Department of Health and Human Services, Center for Disease Control and Prevention. *Infant mortality rate by country* Hyattsville, MD: National Center for Health Statistics, 1998:114.
6. Nicholson WK, Frick KD, Powe NR. Economic burden of hospitalization for preterm labor in the United States. *Obstet. Gynecol* 2000;96:95.
7. Committee on Perinatal Health. *Toward improving the outcome of pregnancy: the 90's and beyond*, White Plains, NY: The National Foundation—March of Dimes, 1993.
8. Gilstrap LC, ed. *Guidelines for perinatal care*, 5th ed. Elk Grove, IL and Washington, DC: American Academy of Pediatrics, American College of Obstetrics and Gynecology, March of Dimes, 2003:17.
9. National Perinatal Information Center. American Hospital Association survey data tapes 1985–1988. *National Perinatal Information Center Newsletter* 1990;Fall:1.
10. Schartz RM. Supply and demand for neonatal intensive care beds: trends and implications. *J. Perinatol* 1996;16:483.
11. Thompson LA, Goodman DC, Little GA. Is more neonatal intensive care always better? Insights from a cross-national comparison of reproductive care. *Pediatrics* 2002;109:1036.
12. Goodman DC, Fisher ES, Little GA, et al. The relation between the availability of neonatal intensive care and neonatal mortality. *NEJM* 2002;346:1538.
13. American Board of Pediatrics Neonatal-Perinatal Medicine qualifying examination statistics Chapel Hill, NC: American Board of Pediatrics. Retrieved June 28, 2003, from http://www.abp.org/stats/WRKFRC/neostat.htm

14. Bhatt DR, Escobeda M, Kattwinkel J, et al. *1998 US neonatologist directory, perinatal pediatrics section.* Elk Grove, IL: American Academy of Pediatrics, 1996.
15. Pollak LD, Ratner IM, Lund GC. United States neonatology practice survey: personnel, practice, hospital and neonatal intensive care unit characteristics. *Pediatrics* 1998;101:398.
16. American Academy of Pediatrics Committee on Fetus and Newborns. Manpower needs in neonatal pediatrics. *Pediatrics* 1985;76:312.
17. Goodman DC, Little GA. General pediatrics, neonatology and the law of diminishing returns. *Pediatrics* 1998;102:396.
18. Goodman DC, Fisher ES, Little GA. Are neonatal intensive care resources located according to need? Regional variations in neonatologists, beds, and low birth weight newborns. *Pediatrics*: 2001;108:426.
19. Goodman DC, Fisher ES, Little GA, et al. The uneven landscape of newborn intensive care services: variations in the neonatology workforce. *Eff. Clin. Pract.* 2001;4:143.
20. Shiono PH, Behman RE. Low birth weight: analysis and recommendations. *Future Child.* 1995;5:4.
21. Resnick MB, Eitzman DV, Dickman H, et al. Data base management for Children's Medical Services Regional Perinatal Intensive Care Centers program. *JFMA* 1983;70:718.
22. Sills J. Understanding catastrophic health care exposures. neonatal intensive care—How did we get here and where are we going? Retrieved June 28, 2003, from http://www.amre.com/hc2003/summaries/sills.htm
23. March of Dimes Perinatal Data Centers. *Economic costs of prenatal care—Health Care Utilization Project nationwide inpatient sample, 1999.* White Plains, NY: March of Dimes, 2002.
24. Rogowski J. Measuring the cost of neonatal and perinatal care. *Pediatrics* 1999;103:329.
25. Muldoon J. Florida profiles its hospitals. In: *Today.* National Association of Children's Hospitals and Related Institutions, Alexandria, VA: 1996;Summer:10.
26. Richardson DK, Zupancic JA, Escobar GJ, et al. A critical review of cost reduction in the neonatal intensive care unit. I. The structure of costs. *J. Perinatol* 2001;21:107.
27. Mugford M, Richardson DK, Zupancic, JA, et al. Response to Hugh MacDonald, letter to the editor. *J Perinatol* 2002;22:336.
28. Stevenson RC, Pharoal PO, Stevenson CJ, et al. Cost of care for a geographically determined population of low birth weight infants to age 8–9 years. II: Children with disability. *Arch Dis Child* 1996; 74:F118.
29. Rogowski J. Cost-effectiveness of care for very low birth weight infants. *Pediatrics* 1998;102:35.
30. Resnick MD, Eyler FD, Nelson RM, et al. Developmental intervention for low birth weight infants: Improved early developmental outcomes. *Pediatrics* 1987;80:68.
31. Tommiska V, Trominen R, Fellman V. Economic costs of care in extremely low birth weight infants during the first 2 years of life. *Pediatr Crit Care Med* 2003;4:157.
32. Committee on Children, Health Insurance, and Access to Care. *Health insurance and access to care for children.* Washington, DC: The Institute of Medicine, National Academies Press, 1998.
33. Lewit EM, Baker, LS, Corman H, et al. The direct cost of low birth weight. *Future Child* 1995;5:35.
34. MacDonald H, American Academy of Pediatrics, Committee on Fetus and Newborn. Perinatal care at the threshold of viability. *Pediatrics* 2002;110:1024.
35. Committee to Study the Prevention of Low Birth Weight. *Preventing low birth weight.* Washington, DC: National Academy Press, 1985.
36. Lu MC, Lin YG, Prietto NM, et al. Elimination of public funding of prenatal care for undocumented immigrants in California: a cost/benefit analysis. *Am J. Obstet Gynecol* 2000;181:233.
37. Imershein AW, Turner C, Wells JC, et al. Covering the costs of care in the neonatal intensive care units. *Pediatrics* 1992;89:56.
38. Committee on the Consequences of Uninsurance. *Health insurance is a family matter.* Washington, DC: The Institute of Medicine, National Academies Press, 2002:47.
39. Iglehart JK. The dilemma of Medicaid. *NEJM* 2003:2140.
40. Rosenbaum S. Medicaid. *NEJM* 2002;346:635.
41. MacDorman MF, Minino AM, Strobino DM, et al. Annual summary of vital statistics 2001. *Pediatrics* 2002;110:1037.
42. U.S. Department of Health and Human Services. Retrieved July 1, 2003, from http://www.hhs.gov/budget/dccbudget.htm
43. National Commission on Children. *Beyond rhetoric: a new American agenda for children and families.* Washington, DC: National Commission on Children, 1991:127.
44. U.S. Department of Health and Human Services, Center for Disease Control and Prevention. *National Vital Statistics Reports* 2002;50(12):3.
45. Luke B, Bigger HR, Leugans S, et al. The cost of prematurity: a case-control study of twins vs. singletons. *Am J Public Health* 1996;86:809.
46. Centers for Disease Control and Prevention. Contribution of assisted reproduction technology and ovulation-inducing drugs to triplet and higher-order multiple births—US 1980–1997. *MMRW* 2000;49:535.
47. Chromitz VR, Cherry L, Lieberman E. The roll of lifestyle in preventing low birth weight. *Future Child* 1995;5:121.
48. Eyler FD, Behnke ML. Early development of infants exposed to drugs perinatally. *Clin Perinatol* 1999;26:107.
49. Phibbs C. The economic implications of perinatal substance exposure. *Future Child* 1991;1:113.
50. Sweet MP, Hodgman JE, Pena I, et al. Two-year outcome of infants weighing 600 grams or less at birth and born 1994 through 1998. *Obstet Gynecol* 2003;101:18.
51. Hanke C, Lohaus A, Gawrilow C, et al. Preschool development of very low birth weight children born 1994–1995. *Eur J Pediatr* 2003;162:159.
52. Resnick MB, Gomatam S, Carter RL, et al. Educational disabilities of neonatal intensive care graduates. *Pediatrics* 1998;102:308.
53. Gagnon DE, Allison-Cook S, Schwartz RM. Perinatal care: the threat of de-regionalization. *Pediatr Ann* 1988;17:447.
54. LeFevre M, Sanner L, Anderson MA, et al. The relationship between neonatal mortality and hospital level. *J Fam Pract* 1992;35:259.
55. Phibbs CS, Branstein JM, Buxtan E. The effects of patient volume and level of care that the hospital of birth on neonatal mortality. *JAMA* 1996;276:1054.
56. Yeast JD, Poskin M, Stockbauer JW, et al. Changing patterns in regionalization of perinatal care and the impact on neonatal mortality. *Am J Obstet Gynecol* 1998;178:131.
57. Mathews TJ, Menacher F, MacDorman MF. Infant mortality statistics from the 2000 linked birth/infant death data set. *National Vital Statistics Reports* 2002;50:10.
58. Martin JA, Park NM. Trends in twins and triplet births 1980–1997. *National Vital Statistics Reports* 1999;47:27.

Neonatal Transport

Karen S. Wood   Carl L. Bose

HISTORY

Neonatal transport began in 1900 with the development of the first mobile incubator for premature infants by Dr. Joseph DeLee of the Chicago Lying-In Hospital (1). This "hand ambulance" provided warmth while transporting premature infants to the hospital following home birth. The development acknowledged the need to create a controlled environment for the transport of infants that simulated the inpatient setting. In 1934, the first dedicated neonatal transport vehicle in the United States was donated to the Chicago Department of Health by Dr. Martin Couney (2), following the closure of the Chicago World's Fair where the vehicle was used to transport premature babies to the exhibit. The first organized transport program in the United States began in 1948 with the development of the New York Premature Infant Transport Service by the New York Department of Health in conjunction with area hospitals (3,4). This remarkable system, created more than a decade before the evolution of neonatal intensive care units (NICUs), incorporated many of the features of modern neonatal transport programs, including around-the-clock staffing by specially trained nurses, dedicated vehicles, a clerk to receive referral calls, and equipment designed specifically for neonatal transport. During a two-year period, this program transported 1,209 patients, of whom 194 weighed less than 1,000 g (4).

Neonatal transport took to the air in 1958 with the first fixed-wing transport of a newborn infant by the Colorado Air National Guard (2). The 1967 flight of a premature baby to St. Francis Hospital in Peoria, Illinois using the *Peoria Journal Star* helicopter marked the first rotor-wing neonatal transport (2). Routine use of air transportation for neonatal patients began in 1972 with Flight for Life of Denver's St. Anthony Hospital (5).

Proliferation of organized transport programs occurred in the late 1970s, in conjunction with regionalization of perinatal care. Regionalization initially minimized the number of infants requiring transport by promoting maternal–fetal transport. Regionalization also shifted the responsibility for transporting infants born in outside centers to the tertiary care center. Subsequently, the next decade saw improvements in perinatal mortality (6) and neonatal morbidity (7) as the percentage of very-low-birth-weight (VLBW) infants delivered in level III hospitals increased.

Since the late 1980s patterns of referral dictated by schemes of regionalization deteriorated in many areas (8), coincident with an increase in level II hospitals capable of providing some degree of neonatal intensive care. As a result, increasing numbers of infants deliver at centers without subspecialists or the necessary support services demanded by some VLBW infants. Community-based neonatal intensive care creates a need to transport infants at a critical time in their illness, occasionally while receiving therapies such as high-frequency ventilation or inhaled nitric oxide, which are not easily portable. Even in areas where regionalized perinatal care persists and prenatal risk assessment is routine, unpredictable, emergent events may precipitate the delivery of an infant in an unsuitable hospital. Collectively these situations mandate increasingly sophisticated neonatal transport systems.

ORGANIZATION AND ADMINISTRATION

Neonatal transport can be performed by either the community hospital referring the patient (one-way transport) or by the tertiary center receiving the patient (two-way transport). Two-way transport offers an economic advantage, generally more highly skilled and experienced transport personnel (9), and may result in improved survival (10,11). The American Academy of Pediatrics supports two-way transport (12), and in most perinatal regions tertiary centers have assumed this responsibility. Of note the major disadvantage of two-way transport is the time delay in getting the transport crew to the referring hospital. The remainder of this chapter discusses two-way transport exclusively.

Administrative Personnel

The components of a transport program include those related to medical care and the nonmedical components such as transportation, communications, finances, and

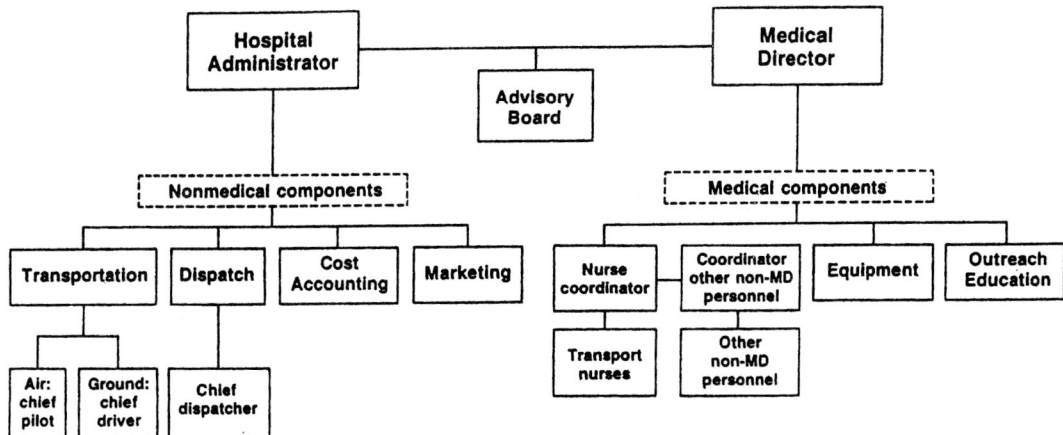

Figure 4-1 The administrative structure of a typical neonatal transport program.

marketing. The medical components must fall under the direction of a physician who is credentialed to supervise the patients served by the program. Direction of the nonmedical components and ultimate responsibility for the program often rests with a hospital administration staff person (Fig. 4-1). The following is a brief discussion of each of the potential contributors to the administration of a transport program (13).

Hospital Administrator

Generally, a hospital administrator manages aspects of the program that are not directly related to patient care. Many decisions regarding program operation require a cost–benefit analysis. While medical personnel are relied on to provide an estimate of benefit, the hospital administrator must assess financial impact. Therefore, the hospital administrator should be prepared to receive advice from medical personnel and develop the nonmedical components of the program in consideration of the financial resources of the institution.

Medical Director

The medical director of a neonatal transport program is usually a neonatologist with expertise or a special interest in transport. The medical director is ultimately responsible for the quality of care provided by the transport team; this is particularly true if physicians do not participate directly in transport. The medical director assumes responsibility for developing and updating training programs, equipment procurement, and treatment protocols. The medical director, in conjunction with the coordinator of nonphysician personnel, must ensure that all personnel have completed training requirements successfully and have satisfied the regulations of the agencies that govern the various professional groups. The director also must develop and maintain a system for reviewing the quality of care provided during transport.

Coordinator of Nonphysician Personnel

Each group of professionals (e.g., nurses, respiratory therapists, paramedics) on the transport team should have a designated coordinator. The coordinator supervises the selection and training of personnel and develops systems of peer review. Additional coordinator responsibilities include scheduling personnel, organizing continuing medical education, ordering supplies and equipment, monitoring documentation standards, promoting effective internal dynamics, and identifying the needs of team members. It is advisable to designate a single person to coordinate team activities who will interface closely with the medical director and, in some programs, the hospital administrator as well.

Consulting Neonatologists and Other Subspecialists

During the transport of a patient, it is important, and often mandated by state law, that a physician provides consultation to the transport team. This physician, known as the medical control officer (MCO), is typically the physician receiving the patient and often has already discussed the patient's care with the referring physician and made recommendations about interim management. Given this broad consultative role to both the referring physician and to the transport team, the MCO should be a person with extensive training, at a level in excess of that available in the community hospital, such as a neonatologist, a trained pediatric subspecialist, or a postdoctoral fellow. In addition, the MCO must be aware of the handicaps and hazards imposed by the transport environment and must be familiar with the operational aspects of the program.

The Advisory Board

A neonatal transport program should be considered an extension of the inpatient unit to which it delivers patients.

Therefore, the operation of the program should be reviewed periodically by representatives of all services interfacing with the inpatient unit. These representatives, comprising the advisory board, might include the following:

- Medical Director of the NICU
- Director of the Neonatal Division
- Respiratory Therapy Administrator
- Nursing Administrator
- Outreach Education Coordinator
- Director of Public Relations
- Representatives of community hospitals involved in transport

Advice should be solicited from the advisory board about all major program changes because of the impact these changes may have on their respective services.

The Transport Team

A variety of personnel participate in the inpatient care of infants, and all should be considered candidates for caretakers during neonatal transport. These personnel include the following:

- Neonatologists
- Neonatal fellows
- Pediatric house staff
- Nurse practitioners
- Transport nurses
- Respiratory therapists
- NICU staff nurses
- Paramedics

The selection of the type of personnel used by each program is based on the unique aspects of that program; however, some general principles apply that determine the relative desirability of various professionals. As the number of transports increases, it becomes less practical to send physicians on transport. Neonatologists rarely have the time to devote to frequent transports, and reimbursement is not sufficient to justify their presence. Although participation in transport can be very educational, in high-volume programs, time spent on transport by house staff and fellows potentially competes with other aspects of training. In addition, the interest in participation and expertise may vary considerably among trainees. This is a particular problem if participation is mandated. Pediatric residents who participate in transport should be senior-level trainees under close supervision.

Most high-volume programs choose to use nonphysician personnel as attendants during transport. The use of neonatal nurse practitioners offers an attractive alternative to physician attendance (14,15). Nurse practitioners are highly skilled in neonatal stabilization and care and provide a consistency of expertise not usually encountered in other professional groups. They are licensed in most states to perform all the diagnostic and therapeutic procedures required during transport. The greatest disadvantages to

the use of neonatal nurse practitioners in some regions are their scarcity and high cost. They are also rarely trained, or willing, to transport patients other than neonates.

As a cost-effective alternative to nurse practitioners, many centers train readily available NICU staff nurses to participate in transport. In addition, most states permit them to perform invasive procedures as an extension of their inpatient nursing role under guidelines and protocols approved by the Boards of Nursing. Therefore, NICU staff nurses can be trained to provide all the care required by a critically ill neonate during transport. This training often is extensive, however, because the cognitive knowledge necessary to diagnose disorders and the experience to perform invasive procedures must be mastered. This extensive training must be considered when estimating the cost of using staff nurses as compared to nurse practitioners. The requirement of training is particularly burdensome when there is a high personnel turnover rate.

Most patients transported to the NICU have either respiratory failure requiring mechanical ventilation or are receiving supplemental oxygen. Respiratory therapists should be considered when selecting transport personnel because of their expertise in the use and maintenance of respiratory care equipment. The therapists' ability to adapt this equipment to the unique environment of transport can be lifesaving, particularly in circumstances when unexpected events occur. The only disadvantage of using therapists is the narrow focus of their usual training. Further education and cross-training allows their scope of practice to be expanded.

Eliminating physicians from attendance during transport can create problems that must be anticipated. For example, leadership of the team is not defined by the usual medical model in which a physician assumes this role. Designating one member of the transport team as the leader—who is accountable for communication, decision making, and documentation—solves this problem.

Advisory personnel at the tertiary center, particularly physicians, often are unwilling to endorse a patient care program that does not mandate initial evaluation by a physician. This resistance usually stems from a concern for the well-being of the patient and can be overcome by the selection and training of competent nonphysician personnel. The support and endorsement of an involved medical director may also be critical. A similar attitude may prevail in community hospitals. Referring physicians may find it unacceptable to relinquish care of a critically ill patient to nonphysician personnel. In an environment in which tertiary centers compete for patients, this may be a motivation for maintaining physician attendance during transport. Most referring physicians, however, are concerned only with transferring their patients in a safe and timely fashion. Anecdotal experience, as well as retrospective and prospective studies, suggests that properly selected and trained nurses provide a level of care during transport that approximates the level provided by physicians (5,16–18). Once a nonphysician team demonstrates competence and efficiency, the concerns of most referring physicians vanish.

Because the use of specially trained nonphysician personnel represents both a safe and economic alternative to physician participation in neonatal transport, most programs now rely on nonphysician personnel for patient care.

Transport personnel must be proficient in cognitive knowledge of neonatal diseases, management principles of acute problems, and technical skills. The method and extent of training necessary to reach proficiency will depend on the type of personnel; however, the pattern of preparation will be similar for all professionals (19). Cognitive knowledge is best provided in didactic sessions in conjunction with self-study exercises. Management principles may also be taught in a didactic setting, but refinement of these skills requires repeated experiences in the inpatient setting. Laboratory simulation of technical skills, such as intubation, umbilical vessel catheterization, and thoracostomy tube placement, provides a good introduction to these procedures. These skills can then be refined in the inpatient setting under supervision. Demonstration of proficiency in these areas should be ensured by examination or observation by a qualified supervisor. After initial preparation, a period of training should be provided, during which the trainee accompanies a more experienced team member on transport. Final certification of competence should be awarded by both the medical director and the coordinator for the trainee's professional group.

Communication

The quality of the communication system that supports a transport program may be the key determinant for its success. The communication system serves two basic functions: to provide a point of access for referring physicians, and to coordinate the activities of the transport team (20). A single call by the referring physician should provide access to all of the neonatal services of the tertiary center. The use of a toll-free hot line, often associated with a memorable acronym, is favored by some centers (21). Alternatively, referring physicians can call the NICU directly. If consultation is requested, the referring physician should be connected in a timely fashion with a consultant of appropriate training. If transfer is requested and deemed appropriate, an available bed in the NICU of the tertiary center, or an alternate center if necessary, should be identified. Bed procurement and all subsequent details of the transport should occur without additional calls by the referring physician.

Locating an available and appropriate site of care may be difficult because of a shortage of NICU beds or the lack of availability of subspecialty support in some areas. These regions often benefit from an organized system of identifying available resources. Several such programs exist and are of two varieties. In some areas, sophisticated computerized communication networks link neighboring centers (22). An alternative is an operator-assisted central referral or bed locator system. These systems speed the referral of patients and relieve both the referring physician and the physician at the tertiary center of the burden of placing numerous calls to locate a bed.

Once the decision is made to transport the patient and an admission bed is located, the role of the communications system shifts to dispatching the team and disseminating information about the transport. In this role, the system is best served by a communication center that is staffed and equipped for emergency medical service functions. The referring hospital should be informed of the estimated time of arrival and of any necessary preparations for the arrival of the vehicle. The receiving unit should be notified and be provided with medical information necessary for admission of the patient.

During the conduct of the transport, periodic communication between the dispatch center and the vehicle operator is advisable. Unexpected delays or mishaps are identified promptly and appropriate action taken. Some high-volume transport programs use satellite-tracking systems to monitor the movement of their transport vehicles, which can be exceedingly useful if diversion is necessary. When the transport team does not include a physician, the team should have the capability of communicating directly with the consulting physician at all times. This level of communication is mandated by some states' nurse practice acts. Communication capabilities are usually a trivial problem while in the referring hospital, however they can present a challenge during transit. The gravity of this problem declines each year with the improvement of telecommunications equipment. Cellular phones are typically used during ground transport because of the broad coverage in most areas and the general familiarity of medical personnel with this type of communication. The use of VHF and UHF radios with patching devices to phone lines is an alternative during flight. Typically, air traffic control, medical control, and general communications have separate frequencies.

Many communication centers are equipped with automated devices that record all communications. Although not essential, the recorded transmissions may be valuable educational tools and aids in identifying system errors; in addition, they are often critical if a medicolegal question arises.

Communication should not end with the conclusion of the transport. The transport team should contact both the patient's family and the referring facility to relate the events of the transport. The receiving physician should update the referring physician following admission and give further followup information at regular intervals, including at the patient's discharge. This update should be expedited if an acute event occurs and should occur immediately in the event of death. Even with the ease of communication systems, failure to effectively communicate followup information remains one of the most common criticisms of tertiary care centers.

Financial Considerations

Subjecting a transport program to periodic cost–benefit analyses is a critical aspect of the program's operation. The following elements should be included in the cost of operation:

1. Medical components
   - Nonphysician personnel salaries/benefits
   - Salary support of the medical director
   - Equipment and supplies
   - Medication
   - Expenses related to education of personnel
2. Nonmedical components
   - Administrative overhead
   - Vehicle operation, maintenance, insurance
   - Communications
   - Educational and marketing material

Identifying the costs associated with the program may be difficult if its operation is financially integrated into the operation of the NICU. For example, personnel costs often are difficult to quantify because, except in very high-volume programs, transport personnel usually contribute to inpatient services during transport duty time. Therefore, the cost allocated to the transport program should be discounted based on this contribution. The proportion of time devoted by the medical director is even more difficult to quantify and often is ignored in the financial analysis. The cost of equipment most easily separates from the cost of inpatient services as transport equipment rarely is used for other purposes. Included in estimates of equipment costs should be allowances for depreciation and maintenance.

The nonmedical components of a program are often more costly than the medical components because of expenses related to transportation. This is particularly true when air transportation is used. Sharing resources with other hospitals or agencies can minimize these expenses. Ground ambulances can be shared with local emergency medical service agencies or be used for convalescent transport. Aircraft can be used by a consortium of hospitals. The major disadvantage of the shared approach is the possibility of a vehicle being unavailable at the time of a request for transport; however, the potential for this occasional conflict may be far outweighed by the cost reductions.

The revenues of a transport program come from three general sources: reimbursement, support from governmental agencies, and support from other extramural organizations (23). Support from government and charitable organizations is unusual in the United States, and hospitals are increasingly dependent on reimbursement to support transport programs. Most third-party payers will reimburse the majority of the initial transport as long as the care rendered at the receiving hospital was unavailable at the referring hospital. Reimbursement for back transports is less consistent. In general, the cost of a transport program exceeds its revenues. Subsistence of the program, therefore, depends on financial assistance from the sponsor hospital.

The decision to fund a transport program usually is based on a favorable cost–benefit analysis. Providing a service that is unavailable at the outside hospital is clearly of benefit to the patient. Benefit can be quantified by reductions in mortality, morbidity, and length of hospital stay. Among low-birth-weight (LBW) infants with respiratory disease, one study has demonstrated that the services of a hospital-based neonatal transport team reduce hypothermia and acidosis, the greatest prognostic indicators of mortality (10). However, beyond this study little evidence exists to support the benefits of neonatal transport teams. In an attempt to quantify the benefits of a neonatal transport program, the most prudent approach may be to scrutinize carefully the type of patients being transported to ensure potential benefit from transport. These benefits should be combined with nonmedical benefits to the institution, such as improved public relations and the recruitment of new patients. Ultimately, many institutions in the United States elect to support a neonatal transport program, despite its financial disincentives, in order to increase occupancy of NICU beds.

A potential economy for transport programs may be to combine services, either within a program or between programs. An example of the former would be to cross-train members of specialty transport teams (e.g., pediatric, neonatal, and adult) such that the total number of personnel can be reduced. This strategy invariably results in some loss of expertise but may be necessary to ensure financial viability. Collaboration between programs may include sharing vehicles or teams. Smaller institutions may benefit from outsourcing entirely by contracting with larger medical centers for the provision of all transport services.

TECHNICAL ASPECTS

The Transport Environment

The principles of care provided during transport resemble the principles of inpatient care. Any differences in practice arise from the unique features of the transport environment (24). Many features—including excessive noise, vibration, improper lighting, variable ambient temperature and humidity, changes in barometric pressure, confined space and limited support services—can create problems during transport. The impact of these environmental factors relative to the mode of transportation is summarized in Fig. 4-2.

	GROUND	ROTOR	FIXED WING
Acceleration	−	−	+
Vibration	+	+	+/−
Noise	+	+	+/−
Heat Loss	+/−	+/−	+/−
Hypoxia	−	+/−	+/−
Gas expansion	−	+/−	+/−
EMI	+/−	+	+

EMI = Electromagnetic interference

Figure 4-2 Environmental factors and their impact relative to different modes of transportation.

Noise

High sound levels, in the range of 60 to 70 decibels, are inherent to the NICU (25–27); but levels recorded on transport are significantly higher, on the order of 90 to 110 decibels (28,29). The effects of exposure to high sound levels on the neonate are not known, but the possibility of physiologic changes is suggested by studies of hospitalized infants (30,31). Brief exposure to high sound levels probably has little long-term effect on transport personnel; however, repeated exposure over time may result in hearing loss. Personnel should protect themselves from exposure by using sound-attenuating devices. Probably the most significant problem resulting from high sound levels is the inability to use auscultation to assess the patient. This handicap must be recognized before transport, and alternative methods for assessing heart rate and respiratory sufficiency must be available during transport.

Vibration

Vibration exposure is a problem unique to the transport environment (29,32,33). The physiologic consequences in patients of this exposure are not known. Animal studies and investigations using healthy adults suggest that negative effects on the autonomic and central nervous system may occur (34–36). The vibrational effects on transport personnel are potentially important. For example, a typical helicopter transport results in vibration exposure associated with reduced personnel efficiency (37). The overt symptoms of motion sickness resulting from low-frequency vibration may be incapacitating. A more subtle manifestation of motion sickness, termed the sopite syndrome, also may affect transport team members (38,39). The symptoms associated with this syndrome include drowsiness, inability to concentrate, and disinclination to communicate with others. The sopite syndrome is common among crew members during transport, regardless of the mode of transportation (40). The impact on patient care is poorly understood but may be significant.

The effect of vibration on equipment also poses a major problem. Monitor artifact is a common phenomenon. Personnel should be familiar with monitor artifact and with the use of alternative monitoring techniques. The selection of equipment should be made in consideration of resistance to the effects of vibration. Premature failure of equipment secondary to vibrational damage should be anticipated, and preventive maintenance should be on an accelerated schedule.

Poor Lighting

Improper lighting in transport vehicles is a common problem. The patient care compartment should have illumination to 400 lux (41). In addition, high-intensity directional lighting (1,000–1,500 lux) should be available for procedures. The eyes of the patient, as well as those of the driver or pilot, should be screened from these light sources.

Heat Loss

The difficulties in maintaining a neutral thermal environment are accentuated during transport because of the increased opportunities for heat loss. Hypothermia can be a significant problem during transport and has been linked to increased mortality (10). Heat loss in the transport environment usually occurs by two mechanisms: convection and radiation. Heat loss can be minimized by use of a double-walled isolette, avoiding opening of the isolette, heating the transport vehicle, creating barriers between the isolette and cold surfaces and limiting time in transit.

Variable Humidity

Transport teams often elect not to humidify respiratory gases both for simplicity and to eliminate the negative effects of water vapor pressure on infants in respiratory failure. This is a reasonable approach assuming short transport times; however, long-term effects of poor humidification include dehydration and increased tenacity of secretions. Therefore, gas humidification and close attention to hydration are desirable for longer transports.

Variable Altitude

Changes in altitude that occur during air transport present a potential hazard to an acutely ill neonate because of the phenomena that occur during ascent. As altitude increases the following occur:

- Air temperature decreases
- Partial pressure of gases decreases
- Total atmospheric pressure decreases

For the change in altitude to be clinically important, ascent must be of significant magnitude (in excess of 5,000 feet). At constant temperature, gas volume expands as atmospheric pressure decreases:

$$P_1 V_1 = P_2 V_2$$

where
P_1 = initial pressure
P_2 = final pressure
V_1 = initial volume
V_2 = final volume

Therefore, gases contained in spaces not in continuity with the atmosphere—such as those in cuffed endotracheal tubes, sinuses, middle ear canals, pneumothoraces, pneumatoses, intrapulmonary cysts, pulmonary interstitial emphysema, intracranial and intraglobal air, and air spaces distal to obstructed bronchi—can all expand as atmospheric pressure declines. Attempts should be made to ventilate closed-space gas to the atmosphere when significant changes in altitude are expected. Also, the impact of gas expansion during ascent can be minimized by the use of pressurized aircraft if a significant change in altitude during the conduct of a transport is anticipated.

Confined Space

Space limitations in transport vehicles may impact care. The recommended floor space for the care of a critically ill neonate in an NICU setting is 150 square feet (42); however, the standard ambulance has approximately 47 square feet and aeromedical helicopters have 22 to 36 square feet of workspace. Personnel must remain seated and restrained while the vehicle is in motion; therefore, typically only one provider has any access to the patient in transit.

An appreciation of the problems created by the transport environment and strategies to minimize their impact are essential for safe transport. Some general principles include the following:

- *Prepare the transport vehicle.* The vehicle should be retrofitted to simulate the inpatient environment as much as is possible and practical. This generally requires the addition of supplemental lighting, sound insulation, and a regulated heating–cooling system.
- *Assess and stabilize the patient extensively before transport.* Other than surgical emergencies, neonates have problems that can be managed adequately by the transport team. There is rarely urgency in returning to the tertiary center, and time spent in the community hospital preparing the patient for transport is not time wasted. Stabilization will prepare the patient for the highest risk period, the time in transit between hospitals.
- *Monitor electronically all possible physiologic parameters.* Because of the dynamic nature of the diseases in most transported patients and the inability to assess patients by physical examination in transit, electronic monitoring is critical to the identification of significant changes in physiology.
- *Anticipate deterioration.* All possible forms of deterioration should be anticipated before transport, and strategies to support the patient in the event of deterioration should be planned. Application of this principle can result in the performance of procedures or therapies that may not be necessary in the inpatient setting.

Equipment

Considerable effort has been devoted to the development of devices specifically for neonatal transport, resulting in greater safety and efficacy. The following is a list of the major pieces of equipment used during transport:

1. **Essential equipment**
   - Portable incubator
   - Mechanical ventilator
   - Cardiorespiratory monitor
   - Blood pressure transducer
   - Transcutaneous O_2 monitor or pulse oximeter
   - Intravascular infusion pumps
   - Air–oxygen blender
   - Suction apparatus
2. **Desirable equipment**
   - Body temperature monitor
   - Transcutaneous CO_2 or end-tidal CO_2 monitor
   - Noninvasive blood pressure monitor
   - Airway humidification system
   - Blood gas/glucose analyzer

Although these devices can be purchased individually and either carried separately or attached to the incubator, it usually is advisable, and often more economical, to purchase a modular incubator that includes many of the devices listed. Modular transport incubators have been designed to minimize space and weight. They also use a common battery power supply for most devices. Several transport incubators are commercially available. The logical choice for each program often depends on the size, weight, and heating capability of the unit.

With the increased use of inhaled nitric oxide, many transport teams have acquired the ability to provide this gas during transport. The inhaled nitric oxide delivery system can be cumbersome. Some transport teams use a small, portable, commercially available device, while other teams have constructed their own system for transport (43).

Small accessory equipment and supplies can be divided into respiratory care supplies and nursing supplies. These supplies can be carried in packs or equipment bags (Tables 4.1 through 4.4). They should be organized in a recognized and reproducible fashion. This technique will aid in rapidly locating an item during transport and assist in restocking after use.

Transport Vehicles

An essential component of neonatal transport is rapid, safe transportation. The types of vehicles in use include standard ambulances, specially prepared ground ambulances, rotor-wing aircraft, and fixed-wing aircraft. The selection of one or more of these vehicles to support a neonatal transport program usually is based on patient population, resources, geography, and practical issues, such as the use of the vehicle by other hospital-based services (44,45).

Ambulances are economical, available, and least affected by weather; however, they generally require retrofitting to make them acceptable for neonatal transport. Extensive retrofitting, including the addition of radiant heat and a blood gas analyzer, improves patient care capabilities but dramatically increases costs and decreases usefulness for other services. The major disadvantage of ground ambulance transport is time consumption, which can be prohibitive if frequent long transports are anticipated.

Rotor-wing aircraft minimize transit time and, within a 150-mile radius, usually provide the fastest service. The major disadvantages of helicopter transportation are the constraints of the patient care environment, the high cost of operation, and the inherent safety risks (46,47) of helicopter flight. The cost of rotor-wing transportation usually cannot be justified unless the vehicle can be shared by other emergency medical services.

Fixed-wing aircraft are more economical, spacious, quiet, and efficient as compared to rotor-wing aircraft; however, they must travel between airports and therefore

TABLE 4-1
NEONATAL NURSING PACK

Equipment	Amount	Equipment	Amount
Chest tube insertion kit	1	Disposable transducer	2
Omphalocele bag, sterile	1	Scissors	1
Sterile lancets	4	Hemostat	1
Blood culture bottle	1	Tape measure	1
Angiocath		Lubricant	2
18 gauge	2	Disposable blood pressure	
22 gauge	2	cuffs sizes 2, 3, 4, and 5	1 each
24 gauge	9	Pacifier	1
Intraosseous needles	2	Bulb syringe	1
IV limb board	2	Sterile gauze	2
Rubber bands	6	Stopcocks	2
Safety pins	6	Extension tubing	1
Tape		Thoracostomy tubes	
Silk	1 roll	10 French	2
Dermaclear	1 roll	12 French	2
Stethoscope	1	Digital thermometer	1
IV fluids		Umbilical catheters	
$D_{10}W$	1 500-mL bag	3.5 French	2
D_5W	1 500-mL bag	5.0 French	2
LR	1 1000-ml bag	Heimlich valves	2
NS	1 100-mL bag	Alcohol and Betadine swabs	10 each
Masks	2	IV extension T-connectors	2
Syringes		Butterfly needles	
20-mL Luer Lok	2	19 gauge	2
60-mL Luer Lok	4	23 gauge	2
Transilluminator	1	25 gauge	3
Gloves, sterile		Syringes	
Size 6½	2 pairs	10 mL	3
Size 7½	2 pairs	3 mL	9
Suction catheters, sterile		1 mL	9
Size 6 French	2	60-cc catheter tip syringe	1
Size 8 French	2	60-cc luer lock syringe	4
Stockinette for caps	2	Needles, 19 gauge	10
Cotton balls	4	Tubing adapters (blunt needles)	2
Feeding tubes		Replogle, 10 French	2
8 French	2	Tubing	
5 French	2	Mini-volume extension	1
Gowns	2	Low-volume extension	4
Blood gas syringe	2	Blood component and filter set	1
Tegaderm	1	IV ext. double "T"-connector	1
Protocol Manual	1		

cc, cubic centimeter; D_5W, 5% dextrose in water; $D_{10}W$, 10% aqueous dextrose solution; IV, intravenous; LR, lactated ringer; NS, normal saline.

additional transfers are required. These shuttles between the hospital and airport often are troublesome and increase the likelihood of mishap. For these reasons, transportation by fixed-wing aircraft usually is advantageous only for distances between hospitals in excess of 150 miles.

DOCUMENTATION

Transport programs typically maintain record-keeping systems that are distinct from the inpatient record. An accurate, thorough record of each transport is essential to provide permanent documentation of the care rendered. The transport record should adhere to the standards of documentation of the sponsor institution. The record also is a valuable tool for quality assurance and education. The critical components of a typical transport record include the following:

- Medical necessity documentation/referral form
- Transport medical record
- Parental consent form
- Billing form

The trend in transport documentation, just as with inpatient charting, has been toward computerized medical records using laptops or personal digital assistants in transport.

TABLE 4-2
NEONATAL RESPIRATORY THERAPY PACK

Equipment	Amount	Equipment	Amount
EXTERIOR POCKETS		Silicone adapter	2
Oxygen tubing	2	O₂ flowmeter nipple	2
Infant nasal cannula	1	One-way valve	1
Complete ventilation setup with exhalation	1 valve (plus one in isolette)	Set of EKG lead wires	2
		23G, 25G, ½-inch butterfly	3 each
Spare exhalation valve	1	Breath Tracker	1
Face tent	1	Albuterol	1
Treatment setup	1	Racemic epinephrine	1
Space blanket	1	Tape measure	1
Thermal hats	2	Infant MVB bag, O₂ tubing, PEEP valve	1 (plus one in isolette)
Pulse oximeter sensors (N-25 and I-20)	2 each	Infant oral airway	2
Suction catheters		Normal saline	4 vials
6 Fr, 8 Fr, 10 Fr	3 each	Silk tape	1 roll
NCPAP prongs (#1,#2)	1 each	Oxygen connectors	2
Luekens trap	1	Hemostat	1
		Briggs T-adapters	2
INTERIOR OF BAG		15-mm adapter	2
Airway supplies		O₂ connectors (NCG, OES, P-B)	1 each
Laerdal masks		Air connectors (NCG, P-B)	1 each
No. 0	2	EKG lead pads	3
No. 1	2	Three-way stopcock	2
No. 2	1	E-Z Heat hot packs	4
Infant McGill forceps	1	Stethoscope	1
Laryngoscope handle	1	1-mL and 3-mL syringe	3 each
Blades, Miller/Shaw #0,#1	1 each	ABG kit	3
Other equipment		Low-volume extension tubing	4
Benzoin applicators	6	Full set Mini-Med Tubing	1
Alcohol preps	4	Endotracheal tubes	
Adjustable wrench	1	2.5 mm	3
E-tank wrench	1	3.0 mm	3
Cable ties	10	3.5 mm	3
Scissors	1	4.0 mm	3
9-volt battery	1	4.5 mm	3
Assorted laryngoscope bulbs	4	Pedi-cap detector	2
Adjustable venturi	2	Istat Pack	1

ABG, arterial blood gas; EKG, electrocardiogram; Fr, French; MVB, manual ventilation bag; NCPAP, nasal continuous positive airway pressure; PEEP, positive end-expiratory pressure.

QUALITY ASSURANCE

Performance review of the transport program should be a continual process. All activities of the program should be reviewed periodically to ensure that standard operating procedures are being observed. These reviews are best conducted by people directly related to the program activities. Also, the medical care provided by the team should be scrutinized for adherence to protocols and quality assurance. For nonphysician teams, the medical director or a physician designate should conduct this level of review. In addition, to assure that every chart is reviewed and problems discovered in a timely fashion, peer review in the immediate post-transport period is valuable.

Quality assurance activities should be closely linked to education and research. Review of individual transport records can be an extremely valuable method of identify-

ing transport personnel in need of further education and training. The compilation of reviews and the monitoring of patient outcomes provide an assessment of the efficacy of existing protocols and procedures and may identify a need to alter program activities. In addition, new therapies and equipment can be evaluated using existing quality assurance techniques.

General guidelines for developing quality assurance programs have been published (48,49). Guidelines, specific for air transport, have been produced by the Association of Air Medical Services (50). The Commission on Accreditation of Medical Transport Systems (CAMTS) provides external quality assurance reviews for transport programs and allows programs to benchmark themselves against measurable standards (51). A number of states require CAMTS accreditation, and some states use CAMTS certification in lieu of state regulations (52).

TABLE 4-3
NEONATAL MEDICINE PACK

Drug	Amount
Isotonic saline vials, 20 mL	4
Heparin	1
Sodium chloride (2%)	1
Phenytoin	2
Naloxone	2
Epinephrine 1:1,000, 1 mL	1
Epinephrine 1:1,000, 30 mL	1
Ampicillin, 500 mg	1
Ampicillin, 250 mg	1
Gentamicin, 20 mg	1
Acyclovir	1
Cefotaxime, 1 g	1
Flumazenil	1
Calcium gluconate	1
Dobutamine	1
D$_{50}$W	1
Calcium chloride Bristoject	1
Atropine Bristoject	1
Survanta	2
Sterile water vials, 20 mL	4
Heparin lock flush	2
Dexamethasone	1
Furosemide	1
Artificial tears	1
Lidocaine 1%	1
Digoxin	1
Adenosine, 6 mg	2
Hydralazine, 20 mg	1
Clindamycin	1
Aminophylline	1
Dopamine	1
Pancuronium	1
Vecuronium	1
Amiodarone	2
Sodium bicarbonate	1
Lidocaine 2% Bristoject	1
Vitamin K, 1 mg/mL	1
Neonatal Narcotic Pack	
Morphine 2 mg/mL	2
Midazolam 5 mg/mL	1
Phenobarbital 130 mg/mL	1
Fentanyl 50 μg/mL	1
Lorazepam 2 mg/mL	1

D$_{50}$W, 50% dextrose water.

PSYCHOSOCIAL CONSIDERATIONS

Psychological Impact on the Family

It is impossible to eliminate the parental anxiety associated with neonatal transport; however, a few techniques exist that may help families in coping with this difficult situation. The transport team should provide the family with as much information as possible about the nature of their child's illness, the therapies and equipment that will be used, the NICU to which the infant will be transported, and the professionals who will provide care. A member of

the referring hospital staff should be in attendance during this discussion in preparation for dealing with questions that may arise after the departure of the transport team (53). This information should be provided both verbally and in written form. Many teams use brochures that describe their service, and provide relevant phone numbers and directions to the tertiary care center.

Parents should see their infant before departure from the referring hospital. The benefit of this interaction outweighs any delay in departure (54). This contact should be encouraged prior to the transport of even the most critically ill infant or when parents are reluctant to view their child. When possible, a photograph of the infant should be left with the family. On arrival in the receiving hospital, the transport team should call the family immediately to reassure them that their child has arrived safely. The transport team should alert the tertiary center staff to any unusual problems the parents might have in coping with their child's illness.

Relationships with Referring Hospital Personnel

Transporting a neonate from a community hospital to a tertiary center has the potential to either improve dramatically the relationship between institutions or to cause irreparable damage. Each transport represents an opportunity for success or failure. To ensure success, referring personnel must have easy access to and a quick response time from the transport team. Rapidity of response often is critical from a public relations standpoint, even when the infant's medical condition does not mandate speed.

Even the most responsive service will fail to satisfy personnel in the referring hospital if the team does not conduct itself appropriately. The team must understand the psychological milieu surrounding a transport. The event is often emotionally charged because of the acute nature of the infant's illness and feelings of inadequacy on the part of the referring hospital personnel. These feelings seem to arise even when excellent, comprehensive care is provided. Referring hospital personnel may be very sensitive to criticism, and any critique of care, unless requested, should be deferred until a later time. The team should seek information about the history and condition of the infant before their arrival, and they should ask for assistance from referral hospital personnel when practical. Members of the transport team should clearly state appreciation for the contribution made by the referring staff. The need for performing all procedures should be explained, this being particularly important when referring personnel have made the decision not to perform a procedure because of their lack of understanding of the transport environment. Nonphysician teams must avoid conflicts with referring physicians over the need for therapies or procedures. Any disagreements should be resolved through discussion between the referring physician and the consulting physician in the tertiary center.

TABLE 4-4
BACK TRANSPORT PACK

Equipment or Drug	Amount	Equipment or Drug	Amount
EQUIPMENT		Minimed full set	1
Istat Pack	1	Minimed half set	1
Lancets, sterile	5	Oximeter probes	2
Stethoscope	1	EKG electrodes	6
Syringes		Hot packs	
1 mL	3	Small	1
3 mL	3	Large	1
10 mL	1	Silver thermal hats	
20 mL	1	Small	1
60 mL	3	Large	1
Needles, 19 gauge	10	IV limb board	1
Bulb syringe	1	Intraosseous needle	1
Feeding tubes		BP cuffs (2,3,4,5)	1 each
5 French	1	Scissors	1
8 French	1	Hemostat	1
Butterfly needles		T-connector	2
23 gauge	2	Angiocath, 24 gauge	4
25 gauge	2	Safety pins	6
ET tubes, 2.5 through 5.0	2 each	Tape	2 rolls
Stylets	2	Benzoin	1
Laryngoscope and blades (Miller 0, 1)	1 each	Sterile gloves	
Face masks, assorted sizes	1 each	Size 6½	2
Face tent	1	Size 7½	2
Manual ventilation bag	1	Diapers	3
Nebulizer setup	1	Pacifiers	1
Venturi tubing	2	Oxygen tubing	2
Nasal cannula	2		
Alcohol and Betadine swabs	10 each	**MEDICATIONS**	
Thermometer	1	Isotonic saline	2
Suction catheters		Heparin flush	2
6 French	2	Sodium bicarbonate	2
8 French	2	Epinephrine 1:10,000 Bristoject	1
10 French	2	Atropine Bristoject	1
Yankauer suction	1	Sterile water	2
Three-way stopcock	2	$D_{10}W$, 500cc	1
IV tubing		D_5W, 100 cc	1
Low-volume extension	2	D_5/0.2 NaCl, 250 cc	1
Mini-volume extension	1	Normal saline, 250 cc	1

BP, blood pressure; cc, cubic centimeters; D_5/0.2 NaCl = dextrose 5% injection in 2% sodium chloride; D_5W, 5% dextrose in water; $D_{10}W$, 10% aqueous dextrose solution; EKG, electrocardiogram; ET, endotracheal; IV, intravenous.

LEGAL CONSIDERATIONS

Emergency medical services personnel may be held to a different standard of care while providing care at the scene of an accident or in a transport vehicle compared to performing the same tasks in the inpatient setting (55). Neonatal transport, however, is more closely associated with inpatient intensive care and less likely to be considered an emergency service (providing extraordinary care under adverse conditions). Therefore, neonatal transport personnel should assume that they have the same high risk of litigation as other perinatal caretakers.

Although there are few regulations and little case law defining the legal obligations of transport services, understanding the principles that are likely to govern legal decision making will help guide programs in establishing sound practices and limit risk of litigation (56). The principles of *respondeat superior* define the hospital as the party responsible for governing the protocols and procedures followed by its personnel (57). These principles appear to apply to mobile services as well as inpatient care. Therefore, the hospital that sponsors a transport program is responsible for selecting and training the personnel and defining their scope of practice. Logically, the medical director, as the medical professional delegated to ensure the quality of care, also is liable for the governance of the team. Team members assume personal liability only if they perform outside their enfranchised scope of practice.

Each transport program should construct a manual of operations clearly denoting its standard procedures. The method used for selecting, training, and certifying personnel should be documented. Similarly, protocols and procedures should be recorded and approved by the medical director. Activities of nonphysician personnel that exceed their usual scope of practice in the inpatient setting should be listed and approved by the respective governing bodies (e.g., Board of Nursing). All documentation should be kept on permanent file.

During the conduct of a transport, the team should adhere to established protocols and procedures (58) unless the patient's needs dictate an abridgement of usual standards. In this situation, advice from a consulting physician should be sought, and the recommendations of this physician should be carefully noted in the patient record.

Referring hospitals have both ethical and legal responsibilities to patients requiring interhospital transfer, with the latter responsibilities outlined primarily in the Consolidated Omnibus Budget Reconciliation Act (COBRA) of 1985 (59). This federal legislation assigns to the referring hospital the responsibility to adequately stabilize the patient prior to transport. The referring hospital also must establish an agreement with a hospital to receive the patient and must ensure that the receiving hospital is capable of providing for the predicted needs of the patient. Amendment of this act in 1989 added the requirement that referring hospitals make an effort to obtain written consent from parents of a minor patient prior to transport. Failure to comply with these requirements is considered medical abandonment.

Referring and receiving hospitals, and their personnel, have distinct responsibilities to patients at varying points in time during the conduct of a transport. There is no single point at which the responsibility shifts absolutely from referring to receiving hospital. From the time of a referral call to the arrival of the patient in the receiving hospital, there is a stepwise decline in the responsibility of the referring hospital (Fig. 4-3). Critical events that shift responsibility include:

- Arrival of the transport team in the referring hospital
- Assumption of direct patient care by the transport team
- Departure of the team and patient from the referring hospital
- Arrival in the receiving hospital (60)

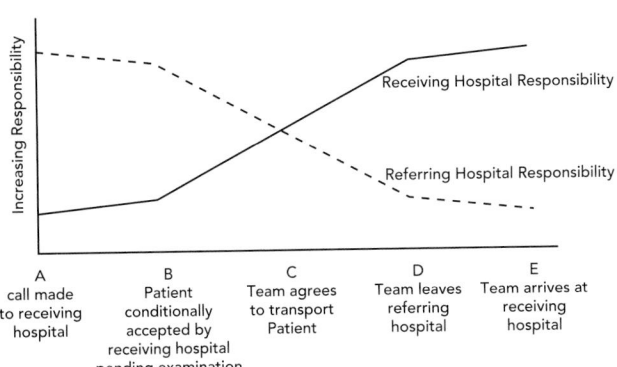

Figure 4-3 Changing levels of legal responsibility for patient care. (From Brimhall, DC. The Hospital Administrator's Perspective. In: MacDonald MG, ed., Miller MK, assoc. ed.. *Emergency transport of the perinatal patient.* Philadelphia: Little, Brown and Co, 1989: 148, with permission.)

The scope of nursing practice is usually established by two sets of regulations, the rules and regulations set forth by their employing hospital or agency and the nurse practice acts in the state in which they practice. Transport creates unique problems regarding nursing scope of practice because transport nurses often provide care in a hospital other than their sponsoring institution, and sometimes they may practice in a state other than the one in which they are licensed (60). Nurses in general are not permitted to practice under the supervision of a physician not associated with their employing hospital. Therefore, while providing care in the referral hospital and sharing responsibilities with the referring physician, a transport nurse must follow protocols and procedures established by the sponsoring institution, or receive verbal orders from the receiving hospital's MCO. In anticipation of problems during interstate transport, some adjacent states have established reciprocal relationships for licensure; however, this is not routine. Many transport teams circumvent this problem by "admitting" the patient to their home hospital at the time of first contact with the patient and thus team members are considered to be practicing in their licensed state.

Vendors who provide transportation for medical personnel and patients are governed by either state or federal legislation. The Emergency Medical Services Act of 1973 places the responsibility for the governance of ground transportation under the guidelines of state emergency medical service regulations. Air transportation services must comply with Part 135 of the Federal Aviation Administration regulations, which govern medical air operations.

BACK TRANSPORT

The return transport of convalescing infants to community hospitals before discharge home is referred to as back transport. Benefits of back transport include:

- Reserves tertiary center resources for critically ill patients, decreasing overcrowding in these units (61,62)
- Improves use of level I and level II center resources and helps prepare their personnel for the care of acutely ill patients
- Improves relationships between tertiary centers and their referral hospitals
- Familiarizes primary care physicians with infants before discharge home
- Improves family visitation and promotes family–infant bonding
- Reduces the total cost of medical care (63,64)

There are also potential disadvantages associated with back transport, including the following:

- Parental anxiety and loss of continuity of care caused by the change of caretakers
- Occasional requirement for readmission to the level III center (65)
- Lost opportunity by level III personnel to participate in convalescent care

■ Hazards and cost of transport
■ Lack of reimbursement by third party payers for the transport (64)

Back transport should be considered an option for all infants who no longer require the unique resources of the level III center and for whom the tertiary center is not the site of subsequent primary care (65).

REFERENCES

1. DeLee JB. Infant incubation, with the presentation of a new incubator and a description of the system at the Chicago Lying-In Hospital. *Chic Med Rec* 1902;22:22.
2. Butterfield LJ. Historical perspectives of neonatal transport. *Pediatr Clin North Am* 1993;40(2):221.
3. Losty MA, Orlofsky I, Wallace HM. A transport service for premature babies. *Am J Nurs* 1950;50:10.
4. Wallace HM, Losty MA, Baumgartner L. Report of two years experience in the transportation of premature infants in New York City. *Pediatrics* 1952;22:439.
5. Pettett G, Merenstein GB, Battaglia FC, et al. An analysis of air transport results in the sick newborn infant: Part I: the transport team. *Pediatrics* 1975;55(6):774.
6. Cifuentes J, Bronstein J, Phibbs CS, et al. Mortality in low birth weight infants according to level of neonatal care at hospital of birth. *Pediatrics* 2002;109(5):745.
7. Hohlagschwandtner M, Husslein P, Klebermass K. Perinatal mortality and morbidity: comparison between maternal transport, neonatal transport and inpatient antenatal treatment. *Arch Gynecol Obstet* 2001;265:113.
8. Richardson DK, Reed K, Cutler JC, et al. Perinatal regionalization versus hospital competition: the Hartford example. *Pediatrics* 1995;96(3):417.
9. Bose CL. Organization and administration of a perinatal transport service. In: MacDonald MG, Miller MK, eds. *Emergency transport of the perinatal patient*. Boston: Little, Brown and Co, 1989:43.
10. Hood JL, Cross A, Hulka B, et al. Effectiveness of the neonatal transport team. *Crit Care Med* 1983;11(6):419.
11. Chance GW, Matthew JD, Gash J, et al. Neonatal transport: a controlled study of skilled assistance. *J Pediatr* 1978;93(4):662.
12. American Academy of Pediatrics, Committee on Fetus and Newborn, and American College of Obstetricians and Gynecologists, Committee on Obstetric Practice. Guidelines for perinatal care, 5th ed. Evanston, IL: American Academy of Pediatrics and American College of Obstetricians and Gynecologists, 2002:58.
13. Brimhall D. Developing administrative support for the transport system. In: McCloskey K, Orr R, eds. *Pediatric transport medicine*. St. Louis, MO: CV Mosby, 1995:56.
14. Mitchell A, Watts J, Whyte R, et al. Evaluation of graduating neonatal nurse practitioners. *Pediatrics* 1991;88(4):789.
15. Karlowicz MG, McMurray JL. Comparison of neonatal nurse practitioners' and pediatric residents' care of the extremely-low-birth-weight infants. *Arch Peds Pediatr Adolesc Med* 2000;154(11):1123.
16. Thompson TR. Neonatal transport nurses: an analysis of their role in the transport of newborn infants. *Pediatrics* 1980;65(5):887.
17. Aylott M. Expanding the role of the neonatal transport nurse: nurse-led teams. *Brit J Nurs* 1997;6(14):800.
18. Cook LJ, Kattwinkel J. A prospective study of nurse-supervised versus physician-supervised neonatal transports. *JOGN Nurs* 1983;12(6):371.
19. American Academy of Pediatrics, Task Force on Interhospital Transport. *Guidelines for air and ground transport of neonatal and pediatric patients*. Elk Grove Village, IL: American Academy of Pediatrics, 1999:37.
20. Conn AKT, Bowen CY. The communications network for perinatal transport. In: MacDonald MG, Miller MK, eds. *Emergency transport of the perinatal patient*. Boston: Little, Brown and Co, 1989:93.
21. Perlstein PH, Edwards NK, Sutherland JM. Neonatal hot line telephone network. *Pediatrics* 1979;64(4):419.
22. Bostick JS, Hsiao HS, Lawson EE. A minicomputer-based perinatal/neonatal telecommunications network. *Pediatrics* 1983;71(2):272.
23. Risemberg HM. Financing a perinatal transport program in the United States. In: MacDonald MG, Miller MK, eds. *Emergency transport in the perinatal patient*. Boston: Little, Brown and Co, 1989:85.
24. Bose CL. The transport environment. In: MacDonald MG, Miller MK, eds. *Emergency transport of the perinatal patient*. Boston: Little, Brown and Co, 1989:195.
25. Philbin MK, Gray L. Changing levels of quiet in an intensive care nursery. *J Perinatol* 2002;22(6):455.
26. Kellman N. Noise in the intensive care nursery. *Neonatal Netw* 2002;21(1):35.
27. Robertson A, Cooper-Peel C, Vos P. Peak noise distribution in the neonatal intensive care nursery. *J Perinatol* 1998;18(5):361.
28. Shenai JP. Sound levels for neonates in transit. *J Pediatr* 1977;90(5):811.
29. Campbell AN, Lightstone AD, Smith JM, et al. Mechanical vibration and sound levels experienced in neonatal transport. *Am J Dis Child* 1984;138:967.
30. Gadeke R, Doring B, Keller R, et al. The noise level in a children's hospital and the wake-up threshold in infants. *Acta Paediatr Scand* 1969;58:164.
31. Blackburn S. Environmental impact of the NICU on developmental outcomes. *J Pediatr Nurs* 1998 13(5):279.
32. Shenai JP, Johnson GE, Varney RV. Mechanical vibration in neonatal transport. *Pediatrics* 1981;68(1):55.
33. MacNab A, Chen Y, Gagnon F, et al. Vibration and noise in pediatric emergency transport vehicles: a potential cause of morbidity? *Aviat Space Environ Med* 1995;66(3):212.
34. Floyd WN, Broderson AB, Goodno JF. Effect of whole-body vibration on peripheral nerve conduction time in the rhesus monkey. *Aerospace Med* 1973;44(3):281.
35. Clark JG, Williams JD, Hood WB, et al. Initial cardiovascular response to low frequency whole body vibration in humans and animals. *Aerospace Med* 1967;38(5):464.
36. Ando H, Ishitake T, Miyazaki Y, et al. The mechanism of a human reaction to vibration stress by palmar sweating in relation to autonomic nerve tone. *Internat Arch Occup Environ Health* 2000;73(1):41.
37. Adey WR, Winters WD, Kado RT, et al. EEG in simulated stresses of space flight with special reference to problems of vibration. *ElectroencephalogrElectroenceph Clin Neurophysiol* 1963;15:305.
38. Graybiel A, Knepton J. Sopite syndrome: a sometimes sole manifestation of motion sickness. *Aviationt Space Environ Med* 1976;47:873.
39. Lawson BD, Mead AM. The sopite syndrome revisited: drowsiness and mood changes during real or apparent motion. *Acta Astronauticat* 1998;43(3–6):181.
40. Wright MS, Bose CL, Stiles AD. The incidence and effects of motion sickness among medical attendants during transport. *J Emerg Med* 1995;13(1):15.
41. Patient compartment illumination. *Federal specifications for ambulance KKK-A-1822B*. Washington, DC: National Automotive Center, General Services Administration, 1985. Para 3.8.5.1.
42. American Academy of Pediatrics, Committee on Fetus and Newborn, and American College of Obstetricians and Gynecologists, Committee on Obstetric Practice. *Guidelines for perinatal care*, 5th ed. Evanston, IL: American Academy of Pediatrics and American College of Obstetricians and Gynecologists, 2002:45.
43. Kinsella JP, Griebel J, Schmidt JM, et al. Use of inhaled nitric oxide during interhospital transport of newborns with hypoxemic respiratory failure. *Pediatrics* 2002;109(1):158.
44. Schneider C, Gomez M, Lee R. Evaluation of ground ambulance, rotor-wing, and fixed-wing aircraft services. *Crit Care Clin* 1992;8(3):533.
45. Brink LW, Neuman B, Wynn J. Air transport. *Pediatr Clin North Am* 1993;40(2):439.
46. King BR, Woodward GA. Pediatric critical care transport—the safety of the journey: a five-year review of vehicular collisions involving pediatric and neonatal transport teams. *Prehosp Emerg Care* 2002;6(4):449.
47. DeLorenzo RA. Military and civilian emergency aeromedical services: common goals and different approaches. *Aviation Space Environ Med* 1997;68(1):56.
48. Council on Medical Service. Guidelines for quality assurance. *JAMA* 1988;259(17):2572.
49. Joint Commission on the Accreditation of Hospitals and Health Organizations. *Examples of monitoring and evaluation in emergency services*. Chicago: JCAHHO, 1988:13.

50. Eastes L, Jacobson J, eds. *Quality assurance in air medical transport.* Orem, UT: WordPerfect Publishers, 1990.
51. *Accreditation standards of the commission on accreditation of medical transport systems,* 3rd ed. Anderson, SC: Commission on Accredition of Medical Transport Systems, 1997.
52. Frazier E. How many state EMS agencies require CAMTS accreditation for air ambulance services. *Air Med J* 2001;20(1):8.
53. McBurney B. The role of the community hospital nurse in supporting parents of transported infants. *Neonatal Network* 1988; 6:60.
54. MacNab AJ, Gagnon F, George S, et al. The cost of family-oriented communication before air medical interfacility transport. *Air Med J* 2001;20(4):20.
55. Reimer-Brady JM. Legal issues related to stabilization and transport of the critically ill neonate. *J Perinat Neonatal Nurs* 1996; 10(3):62.
56. Ginzburg HM. Legal issues in medical transport. In: MacDonald MG, Miller MK, eds. *Emergency transport of the perinatal patient.* Boston: Little, Brown and Co, 1989:152.
57. Tonsic v Wagner, 458 Pa. 246; 329 A 2d 497;1974.
58. American Academy of Pediatrics, Task Force on Interhospital Transport. *Guidelines for air and ground transport of neonatal and pediatric patients.* Elk Grove Village, IL: American Academy of Pediatrics, 1999:16.
59. Ross M, Hayes C. Consolidated Omnibus Budget Reconciliation Act of 1985. *Soc Secur Bull* 1986;49(8):22.
60. Brimhall DC. The hospital administrator's perspective. In: MacDonald MG, Miller MK, eds. *Emergency transport of the perinatal patient.* Boston: Little, Brown and Co, 1989:147.
61. Jung AL, Bose CL. Back transport of neonates: improved efficiency of tertiary nursery bed utilization. *Pediatrics* 1983;71:918.
62. Zarif MA, Rest J, Vidyassagar D. Early retransfer: a method of optimal bed utilization of NICU beds. *Crit Care Med* 1979;7:327.
63. Bose CL, LaPine TR, Jung AL. Neonatal back transport: cost effectiveness. *Med Care* 1985;23(1):14.
64. Phibbs CS, Mortensen L. Back transporting infants from neonatal intensive care units to community hospitals for recovery care: effect on total hospital charges. *Pediatrics* 1992;90(1Pt1):22.
65. Lynch TM, Jung AL, Bose CL. Neonatal back transport: clinical outcomes. *Pediatrics* 1988;82(6):845.

Telehealth in Neonatology

Sarah C. Muttitt   *Mary M. K. Seshia*   *Liz Loewen*

Health care is facing many challenges and changes with increasing pressure to improve access and quality while reducing the administrative and financial burden of providing care. There is growing expectation that technology has a key role to play in meeting these demands. Telehealth, defined as the use of information and communications technology (ICT) to deliver health services, expertise, and information over barriers of distance, geography, time, and culture, fulfills this role (1). Telehealth can support services within the whole spectrum of health care including diagnosis, treatment, and prevention of disease, continuing education of health professionals and consumers, and research and evaluation. When well-integrated into routine clinical practice, telehealth can improve the efficiency and cost effectiveness of the health care system by moving people and information virtually rather than physically (1). Although not new, telehealth has experienced rapid expansion over the past decade and is being utilized in a growing number of medical specialties including dermatology, oncology, radiology, surgery, cardiology, mental health, and home health care. While telehealth may not have reached the volume and maturity required for large-scale randomized studies, the value of telehealth has been well accepted by consumers and health care providers alike (1).

Telehealth implementation addresses three major issues: access to health care services; retention, recruitment, and support of rural physicians and other health care providers; and potential cost savings to the health care system and/or patients and their families. In order to access specialty care, residents of rural areas are often forced to travel long distances at significant cost, inconvenience and, in some cases, aggravation of underlying medical conditions. Although some tertiary care centers provide itinerant specialty clinics, these services may not be available where and when a patient requires specialist advice. Physician travel for itinerant clinics also has associated risks and

costs, including the loss of valuable time while traveling between clinics. Telehealth has the potential to provide access to a broader range of comprehensive primary, secondary, and tertiary health care services, more timely intervention, earlier repatriation, and improved continuity of care for rural patients. Physicians and health care providers in rural areas have limited direct access to peers, specialists, education, and opportunities to participate in health care administration or professional association activities. This sense of professional and social isolation often contributes to clinicians leaving positions prematurely and the inability to recruit skilled practitioners, leaving rural communities largely underserviced. Access to education and peer support through telehealth may impact retention and recruitment and allow health care providers in rural settings to work to the full potential of their scope of practice as well as provide more complex care closer to home.

Although telehealth is primarily driven by the demand for more equitable access to health care for rural and remote residents, much attention has been given to the telehealth "business case." Cost avoidance and cost savings are constantly sought to offset the substantial costs of telehealth implementation and operations. Although there are cost savings associated with a reduced number of unnecessary medical transports, earlier patient discharge to community hospitals or home, and decreased education and administrative travel, the longer-term savings associated with more timely access to care resulting in less consumption of health care resources and improved health outcomes have yet to be measured (1–3). The ability of telehealth to contribute to greater efficiencies within the system may offer the opportunity to redirect any savings towards improved patient services. Even if telehealth does not result in a reduction in total health expenditures, improved access to quality health care services should be of high importance to patients, providers, and health care funders (1).

THE HISTORY OF TELEHEALTH

Health care at a distance, or telehealth, has been practiced for decades using less sophisticated communications technologies than we currently associate with telehealth. The National Aeronautics and Space Agency (NASA) played an important role in the early development of telehealth. The remote monitoring of crew, spacecraft, and environmental health has been an integral part of NASA operations. Similarly, the United States (U.S.) military has been actively involved in telehealth research and applications as a means of bringing medical expertise to those injured in battle with less risk of injury to health care personnel. In the 1960s, the Nebraska Psychiatric Institute became one of the first facilities in the United States to develop a two-way link via microwave technology to provide education and consultations between specialists and general practitioners. NASA's efforts at enhancing satellite communications provided the opportunity to pilot telehealth in more remote locations such as Alaska in the early 1970s (4). Satellite technology also facilitated the development of the Telemedicine Centre at Memorial University of Newfoundland (MUN) in 1977. Using simple, low-cost audio-conferencing technology, the MUN program linked hospitals, community colleges, university campuses, high schools, town halls, and education agencies throughout the province for educational programs and transmission of medical data (5). In the 1980s, there was a flurry of telehealth activity in North America as well as around the world, with new projects in Australia, New Zealand, the United Kingdom, France, and Norway. Early projects were largely focused on the technical feasibility of telehealth and often were developed around a single application and single clinical "champion." Because of the high capital costs of these projects, they were also extremely dependent on grant funding. Many came to end when funding expired or the clinical champion moved on to other areas of research interest.

In the late 1980s and early 1990s, telehealth technology became more robust and less expensive, making telehealth a more viable alternative for health care service delivery. The past decade has seen rapid expansion of telehealth sites and applications. The Telemedicine Information Exchange currently lists more than 160 telehealth programs internationally (6). A better understanding of the human factors associated with telehealth success has allowed improved planning, deployment, and management of telehealth programs. However, the majority of telehealth activity worldwide still remains grant funded or hospital supported with consequent vulnerability to annual funding cycles. Today's projects focus on assessing sustainability. It is becoming apparent that telehealth solutions have to be integrated within the traditional healthcare system to be sustainable. With careful attention to cost-effectiveness and quality services, telehealth is destined to become a standard component of health service delivery.

TECHNOLOGY

There are two main types of communications in telehealth. Asynchronous, or store-and-forward, involves the capture and later transmission of data or images for dissemination or interpretation. Teleradiology, the sending of radiographs, computed tomography (CT) scans, or other digital scans, is the most common store-and-forward application of telehealth in use today, and is often integrated into larger picture archiving and communication systems (PACS). Pathology and dermatology are other specialties that typically use store-and-forward technology for remote diagnosis. Synchronous, or real time, implies the transmission of information instantly and is primarily associated with the use of videoconferencing to support face-to-face consultation between a patient in one location and a provider in another. Almost all medical specialties have found an application for the use of videoconferencing technology and with the addition of appropriate peripheral medical devices, such as stethoscopes, otoscopes, and examination cameras, a comprehensive examination can be conducted remotely. Some telehealth applications use a combination of store-and-forward and videoconferencing technologies to allow both the review of still images and interactive consultation with peers and patients. In all cases, the clinical requirements must drive the technical solution. The price and performance of telehealth technology has improved dramatically over recent years and in many cases, off-the-shelf hardware now provides the necessary functionality at much lower cost than systems specifically designed for telehealth. All equipment should comply with accepted technical standards to ensure quality, flexibility, and compatibility between systems.

In addition to end points, telehealth requires a telecommunications network to facilitate the exchange of information. Although telecommunications infrastructure in urban settings has developed remarkably over the past decade, the primary focus of telehealth has been to serve rural and remote populations where connectivity continues to be a considerable challenge. Requirements for bandwidth (communication channel capacity) vary depending on the application. The higher the bandwidth, the more information can be sent in a measured time period. POTS (plain old telephone system) may be appropriate for transmitting low volumes of nonurgent X-ray images between two destinations for a teleradiology service. Larger volumes of images or a need for urgent interpretation would require a higher bandwidth solution. Similarly, higher bandwidth is required to support quality interactive videoconferencing for clinical applications. Although urban sites may be able to choose between a number of suitable solutions such as ISDN (Integrated Services Digital Network), DSL (digital subscriber lines), or high-speed cable, geographically remote communities may only have access to the necessary bandwidth through satellite or other high-cost wireless solutions. Telecommunications costs for rural education and health care networks in the United States are heavily subsidized through the Universal Service Fund, a fund generated through contributions from telecommunications companies. In Canada, the federal government continues to support the deployment of broadband to many rural, northern, and isolated communities through initiatives such as the Broadband for Rural and Northern Development and the National Satellite Initiatives. In some cases, sharing infrastructure costs with other sectors, such as education, justice, or industry, may improve the viability of telehealth in a small, remote community. The availability of low-cost telecommunications solutions is critical to the expansion and sustainability of telehealth in many of the neediest areas, including developing countries.

The advent of IP (Internet Protocol) videoconferencing is impacting the design and operations of telehealth networks everywhere. Traditional copper-based networks required dedicated connections so telehealth was often limited to a single site or "suite" within a health care facility. With line installation, monthly line rentals, and long-distance charges associated with each session, telecommunications costs often accounted for as much as 15% to 25% of total telehealth costs (2). With advances in digital video compression, composite audio and video signals can now be carried over typical IP network circuits either on a LAN (local area network) within a health center, across a broader WAN (wide area network), or private network. With nearly ubiquitous access, telehealth can be available on every physician's desktop, at the patient bedside, and throughout every hospital and primary health care facility—providing access wherever and whenever healthcare services are delivered. Although there is a fixed cost associated with an IP network, there is little or no additional cost associated with actual use. As a result, the actual per session cost for telehealth declines with increasing utilization. In addition to long-term cost savings, the convergence of voice, video, and data onto a single network will ultimately allow telehealth to interface with other health information, including PACS and electronic health records. Issues surrounding network quality, bandwidth requirements, and security continue to be refined but telehealth over IP networks is becoming an attractive option for many programs.

Choosing the right technology for telehealth is complicated in the face of declining equipment and telecommunications costs, inevitable capital depreciation, and rapid technical innovation. Clinical users of the equipment must be involved in purchasing decisions, as clinical and operational requirements will directly determine technical specifications; such involvement will also foster acceptance by the users. In general, a telehealth program should purchase the highest specification equipment available to meet user expectations at the lowest possible cost. Similarly, decisions regarding telecommunications infrastructure should be based on file size, immediacy, and volume of usage balanced by fiscal realities and whether or not funding or revenue streams can offset the associated capital and operating costs. Telehealth programs must also plan for equipment and network maintenance, support, and upgrading.

Vendor relationships are crucial to the success of telehealth programs. In addition to price and technical specifications, appropriate service level agreements should be instituted to ensure high-quality, reliable, and state-of-the art telehealth operations.

MEDICO-LEGAL AND REGULATORY ISSUES

The clinician's duty of care and clinical case responsibility in the telehealth setting adhere to the same principles found in face-to-face encounters. The ethical and quality standards of practice governing clinicians are not altered by the use of telehealth. Proper documentation, including written consent when applicable, should be maintained for all telehealth encounters. The advantage of telehealth is that it permits health care to be delivered anywhere, with no recognition of borders; however, this inherent distinction from traditional in-person care also raises new issues surrounding regulations and policy related to health care practice (7) (see also Chapter 8).

Licensing of health professionals is typically a jurisdictional responsibility. If physicians and patients are located in different provinces or states, it is important to determine whether the locus of accountability will be the patient site or provider site. If the service is deemed to occur at the patient site, the physician may be required to obtain appropriate licensing and credentialing as if practicing in person at that site. A number of policy options to overcome these licensing issues have been proposed including "universal" licensure, a special-purpose license for telehealth, and mutual agreements, but there is still a significant need to harmonize standards to support cross-jurisdictional telehealth activities (7).

The absence of policies regarding physician reimbursement for telehealth consultations has historically been a significant barrier to the widespread adoption of telehealth. Early telehealth initiatives were often pilot projects or clinical trials located at hospitals or universities, and physician reimbursement was not a major concern as most physicians treated their participation as a research initiative or were compensated through alternative payment arrangements (salary or capitation). However, as more practitioners incorporate telehealth into routine practice, compensation has become a pivotal issue. Although many insurance plans still require patients to be seen in person by a physician in order to bill, others have developed specific fee codes for telehealth services; however, these often have significant limitations related to geographic location, specific facilities, number and types of services, and professional category. Canada's publicly administered system is also inconsistent, with some provinces allowing direct reimbursement for telehealth services and others not. There is slow progress toward expanding telehealth reimbursement, but health care organizations should determine the policies in their jurisdiction regarding payment prior to implementing telehealth services.

All physicians engaging in telehealth consultations should verify with their insurance providers that telehealth is included within their malpractice insurance policies. To date, there has been very little litigation associated with telehealth, but there are some specific issues to be considered. Not all consultations are appropriate for telehealth. Providers must use their best clinical judgment to determine whether services can be safely and effectively provided by telehealth. In addition, a back-up process must be established to ensure that patients receive appropriate and timely care in the event of technical failure. Practitioners may require specialized training and expertise for telehealth and demonstrate acceptable technologic competence prior to providing telehealth services. Specific clinical protocols and guidelines may be necessary to ensure consistent, high-quality telehealth applications in some settings. At all times, telehealth services must adhere to basic quality assurance and professional standards of care (7).

Privacy of personal information related to the use of ICTs in health has been a developing issue over the last decade. Concerns over the use of technology to track everything from health care services to spending habits have spurred the development of policies to regulate the protection of individual privacy. Standards for maintaining the privacy of health information in a telehealth context do not differ from those in a face-to-face encounter; however, the introduction of technology adds privacy and security considerations (7). In addition to maintaining privacy through more traditional measures such as a private physical environment and organizational processes, delivery of telehealth requires attention to security of data during transmission and, in some cases, storage. Ensuring security in an ever-changing technologic environment requires a proactive and evolving approach (8). Ensuring confidentiality in a telehealth setting can be more challenging given the potential risks for interception, potential for a permanent video record, and additional people involved in each care session. This is compounded by the variety of equipment and complexity of transmitting images between two settings (9). As telehealth moves from single-room standalone applications to integration within direct patient care areas, such as the neonatal intensive care unit (NICU), the complexity of ensuring privacy increases.

THE ECONOMICS AND EVALUATION OF TELEHEALTH

The body of scientific literature related to the application of telehealth has been growing steadily over the last 30 years. A search for the keyword *telemedicine* on PubMed found only 24 references for the decade 1970 to 1979; this increased to 2,903 for 2000 to 2003. Several recent literature reviews have examined the current state of research knowledge related to telehealth, and most have determined that while telehealth shows promise, research and evaluation of telehealth is still maturing with few scientifically conclusive studies completed to date. The reviews completed to date have identified small numbers of studies which meet criteria for inclusion ranging from 7 for those requiring a randomized controlled trial to 50 when inclusion criteria were broadened to include any controlled design (10,11). The strongest studies examining clinical impacts have demonstrated support for telehomecare initiatives, management of chronic illness, psychiatry, dermatology, cardiology, teleradiology, transmission of digital images for neurosurgery consultation, and echocardiographic image transmission (10–14).

Most telehealth studies include some element of economic analysis. Whitten and colleagues (3) completed a systematic review of telemedicine cost effectiveness studies from 1966 to 2000 and found 612 articles that included some economic analysis, most of which were recorded as small-scale or short-term evaluations with less than ideal economic analysis and limited transferability. Only 55 included actual cost data, 24 of which met the requirements for a full review. Jennett and associates (1) identify more than 40 telehealth studies that found economic indicators (many of which are repeated from the Whitten study); however, again, most were rated as less than optimal analyses. Economic indicators for telehealth include costs related to travel and travel time for patients and providers; patient transport; equipment and telecommunications; shift of care from larger centers; and recruitment and retention related to access to continuing education.

While the reviews done to date have demonstrated the feasibility of telehealth, telehealth research has not yet included large-scale randomized studies (10). An additional challenge in the evaluation of telehealth is whether face-to-face care is, in fact, the gold standard against which any new service delivery method should be tested (10). As telehealth moves toward a more integrated model, evaluation approaches must also use an integrated and systemic approach rather than focusing on limited indicators to measure the impact of the technology. The potential for increased access to healthcare resulting from telehealth applications may have long-term systemic benefits not easily captured in a single study. A more recent review examining the socioeconomic impact of a variety of telehealth applications found benefits to patients, clinicians, and the health care system (1).

TELEHEALTH APPLICATIONS IN NEONATOLOGY

In 1970, regionalization of perinatal–neonatal care was advocated following the observation that neonatal mortality was highest in those hospitals delivering small numbers of infants compared with that of larger hospitals with neonatal referral units. Additionally since that time, the care of the sick neonate has become increasingly technologically dependent, providing further justification for regionalization of neonatal care. This has resulted in dislocation of families during complicated pregnancies, limited access to specialized resources for sick neonates, and difficulties in ensuring access to follow-up resources.

In this same time period, technologic advances have resulted in the ability to deliver health care effectively over distance. Those practicing neonatal–perinatal medicine need to harness this technology, incorporating it into daily care, to provide consultation (both emergent and elective) over distance, allow for televisitation by families, facilitate discharge from tertiary to secondary levels of care, and provide follow-up of high-risk newborns in their home communities, ideally within their home.

This section demonstrates how telehealth has been used effectively through the perinatal-neonatal continuum, both for the delivery of care and for education of health care providers.

Antepartum

Telehealth has been used successfully for a number of antepartum applications including genetic counseling and teleultrasound. In Queensland, Australia, a weekly connection, developed in 1997, allows maternal fetal medicine specialists to provide direction to a sonographer at the patient site while viewing the fetal ultrasound in real time. At the end of the consultation, the subspecialist counsels the parents on diagnosis, prognosis, and management and prepares a report for the referring physician. In addition to increasing patient access to the subspecialist, communication between the two hospitals is improved and knowledge transfer between health care providers is facilitated. A review of the program found only one missed fetal diagnosis out of 120 cases, and patients were highly satisfied with the consultative process. The real-time interaction is considered a key component of the success of this project (15,16).

Neonatal

Health care professionals caring for neonates know that even a low-risk pregnancy can result in a high-risk situation for the neonate in 2% to 4% of deliveries. Additionally, newborn infants who initially appear well can deteriorate rapidly, particularly from sepsis, respiratory problems, and congenital heart disease. Timely access to specialists in newborn care can be a problem for remote and isolated health facilities. In Manitoba, Canada, the provincial MBTelehealth Network supports a telehealth link between a tertiary NICU and a general hospital 760 kilometers north. Pediatricians at the remote site can consult the receiving NICU on an emergent basis for assistance with management and stabilization. In this integrated system, both the remote and receiving staff operate the equipment and only rely on technical support when problems are encountered. The equipment at the remote end is positioned to allow the NICU staff to see the newborn, cardiorespiratory monitor, and ventilator. The NICU health care professionals at the receiving site take over camera control from the remote site to ensure that the

remote staff members are not distracted from the care of the newborn. Image resolution is high—even the numbers on the side of the umbilical catheter can be read. The addition of the visual image of the baby to the usual telephone verbal description allows for improved assessment and advice on management (Fig. 5-1). The interaction between the neonatologist and referring physician provides a conduit for ongoing education in neonatal care; further, the "virtually present" neonatologist can talk the referring physician through procedures such as umbilical catheterization, which the referring physician may not have recently performed, enhancing that physician's confidence; and finally, but importantly, the parents are comforted by the ready availability of a specialist for their newborn. This link has also allowed parents and extended family to "visit" the neonate and participate in management decisions from the remote location in situations when they are unable to travel to the NICU. While technology is not going to replace the need for neonatal units, it does allow for improved access to care. In addition, if appropriate education is provided to those smaller referring facilities, earlier retrotransfer of newborns should occur, reducing family dislocation and costs. As telehealth networks expand and personnel realize both its potential and ease of use, this application will surely become more widespread.

Telecardiology

Digital echocardiography has enabled the transmission of echocardiograms from remote sites to pediatric cardiologists both by store-and-forward and real-time, synchronous transmission. Real-time transmission allows for continuous live contact between the cardiologist, sonographer, and other health professionals, and also family members at the remote site. Although this technology is used for all age groups, Finley (17) found that 51% of urgent examinations were for newborn infants. In addition to diagnosis, the utilization of interactive videoconferencing can support case conferencing and echocardiogram review between referring sites and remote surgical teams for infants being referred to a cardiac surgical center. Families can participate in this process, increasing their confidence in the care of their infant. With appropriate bandwidths, images can be of clinical quality. Ideally the sonographer at the remote end should have pediatric cardiology experience to ensure that more difficult diagnoses, such as total anomalous pulmonary venous return and coarctation of the aorta, are not missed (17–20). Although in many situations the neonate will still have to be transported to the tertiary center, with telecardiology, some transports can be avoided or undertaken more electively and more appropriate management decisions can be made.

Retinal Telephotoscreening

Retinopathy of prematurity (ROP) is a complication of surviving preterm low-birth-weight infants, with approxi-

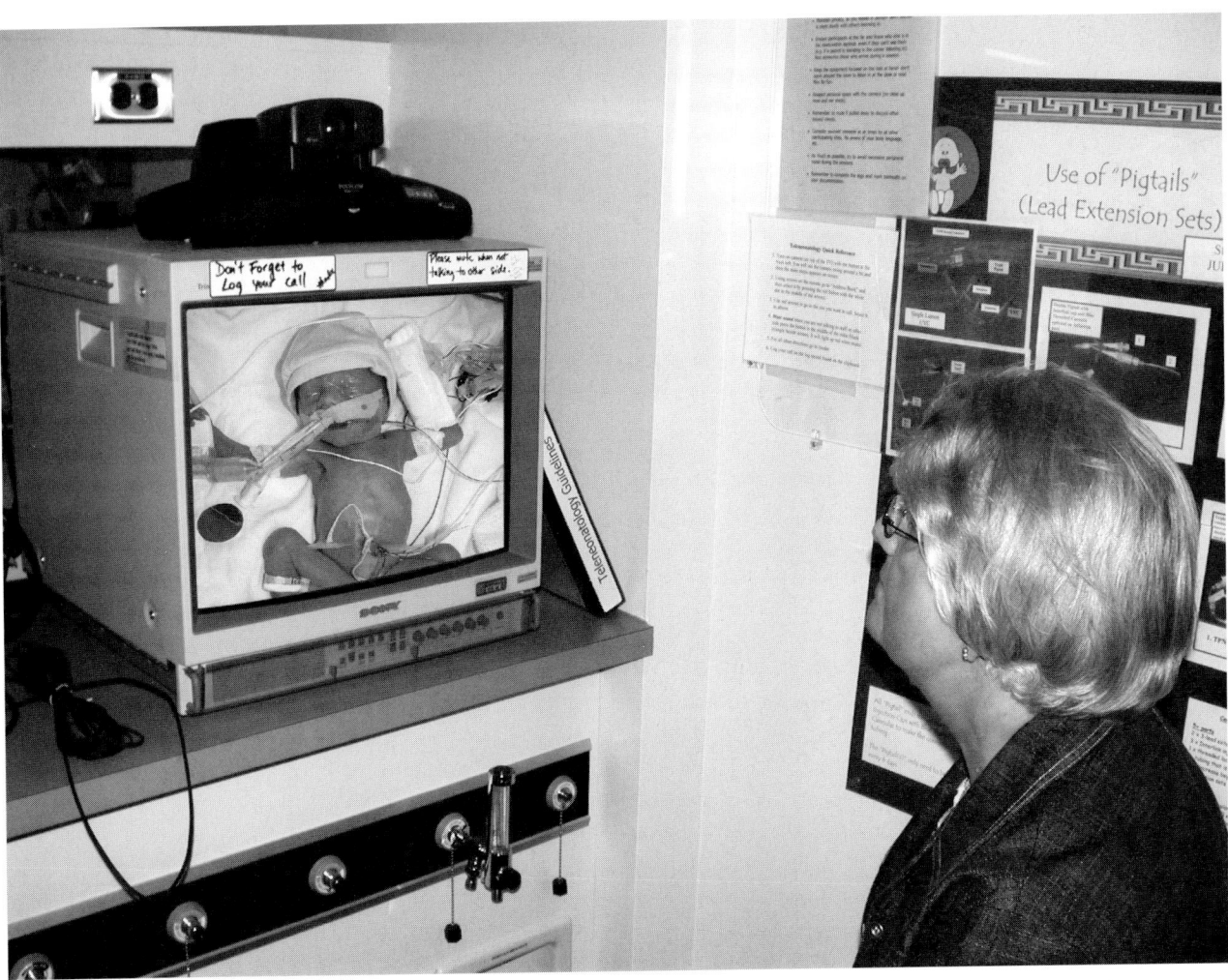

Figure 5-1   Videoconferencing between the neonatologist in the NICU and remote health care professionals following the delivery of this preterm infant.

mately 65% of infants <1,300g at birth and up to 80% of infants <1,000g developing ROP. These infants require frequent retinal screening once the disease is diagnosed to prevent blindness. The "gold standard" for screening is indirect ophthalmoscopy by a pediatric ophthalmologist with expertise in ROP management. Such subspecialists are few in number and with the geographical diversity of levels II and III NICUs, providing this service is challenging. Telehealth technology, using a digital retinal camera equipped with an ROP lens, is currently being investigated as an alternative method for retinal screening. The camera system provides an immediate wide-angle view of 120 degrees and also produces a real-time image on a computer monitor, which is then stored, uncompressed, on a digital videodisc (Figs. 5-2 and 5-3). Two recent studies concluded that the sensitivity was insufficient for recommendation as a screening tool for ROP (21,22). However Schwartz and associates (23) suggested that this telemedical strategy might be highly accurate when assessing whether a child's eye required the urgent attention of a physician capable of evaluating and managing threshold ROP. Ells (24) subsequently adopted a pragmatic approach; rather than using

this technology to differentiate between stages 1 and 2 ROP, she focused on whether this technology could identify those eyes that require treatment. In this approach, digital photography had a sensitivity of 100% and a specificity of 96% in detecting referral-warranted ROP. As the technology improves and more people become trained in its use, the use of digital retinal photography will become a useful adjunct to hospitals providing level II care; and growing premature infants at risk of ROP will be able to return to their home community rather than remaining in a center where there is access to a trained pediatric ophthalmologist.

Televisitation

Telehealth can promote a connection to the neonate's home setting both before and after neonatal discharge. Interactive videoconferencing can provide a link between the mother and her family. Gray and associates (25) have used a web-based solution designed to reduce the costs of care and at the same time provide enhanced medical, informational, and emotional support to families of very

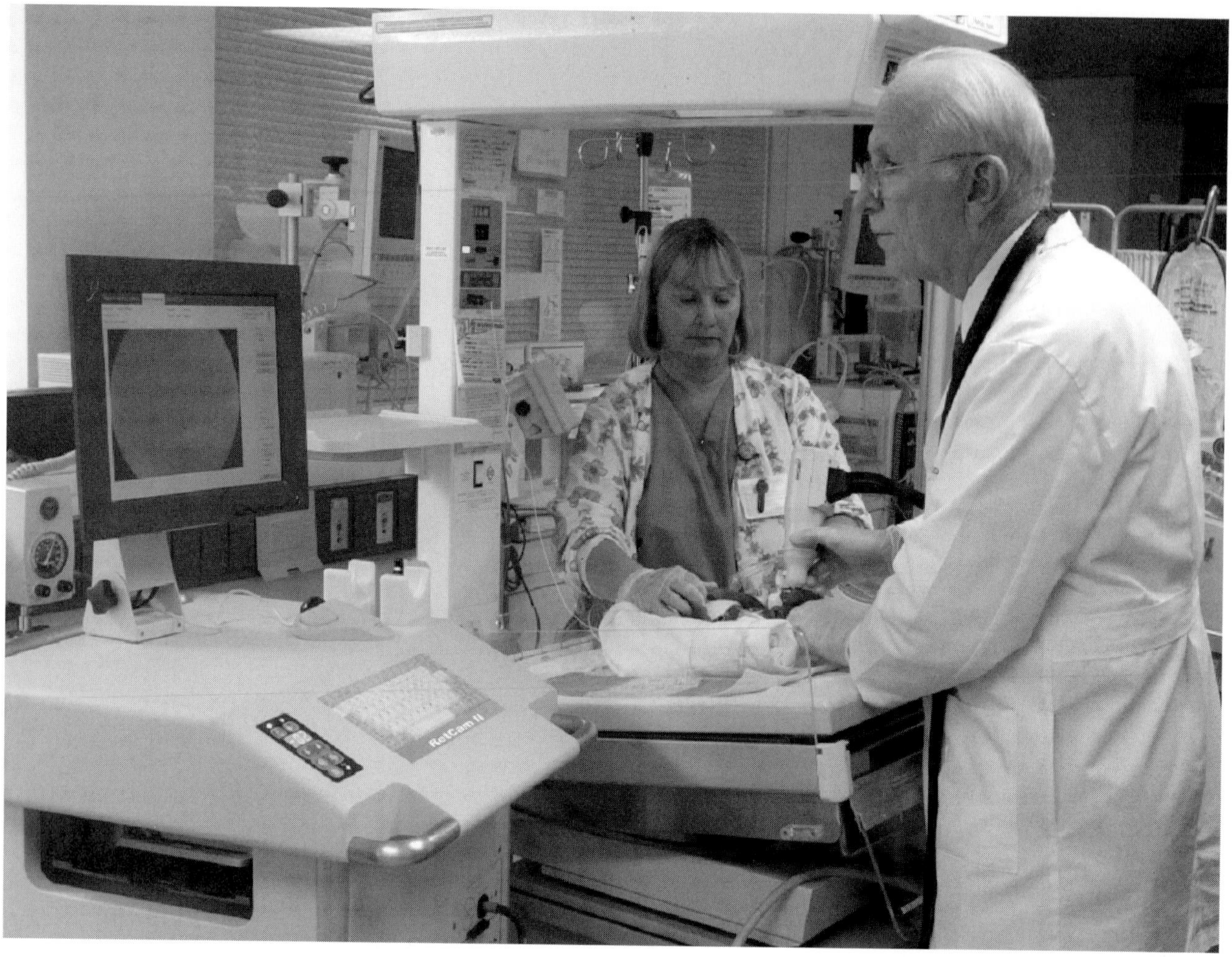

Figure 5-2 Retinal telephotoscreening taking place in the NICU using the RetCamII.

low-birth-weight infants in the NICU. Via the Internet, families can link to the NICU at any time to obtain information about their infant, as well as obtaining educational information and information on experiences of other families. Also incorporated, and perhaps the most exciting aspect for families, is the interactive videoconferencing that can occur. Parents can see their infant and receive information and support from staff at times when they cannot visit. In a small, randomized study of this technology, hospital stay was shorter and families experienced greater satisfaction with the care received. The system requires the installation of an easy-to-use computer in the home. Given that access to the Internet has been adopted more rapidly than any other technologic advance in history, the use of this technology as a means of delivering care can only expand.

Telehomecare

Telehomecare is a growing application with considerable potential to support neonatology. Telehomecare applications link patients from their home environment to hospital or community-based providers with ongoing monitoring of vital signs, and when indicated, videocon-

ferencing contact on a scheduled or urgent basis. Reviews of these applications in the non-neonatal population have demonstrated improved control of chronic conditions such as diabetes and chronic heart failure, along with high levels of patient satisfaction (1,12). Data such as blood

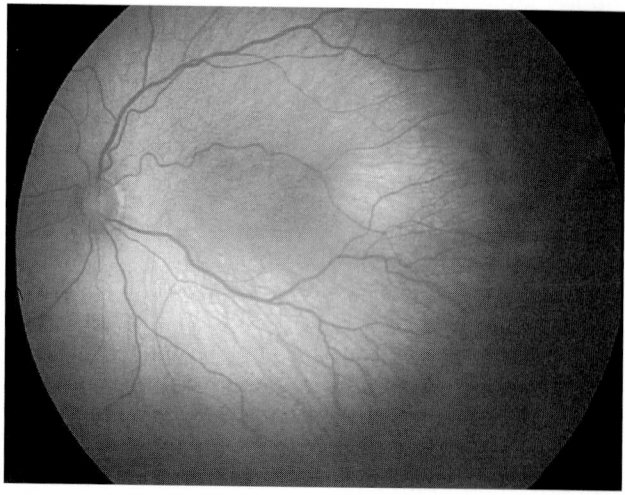

Figure 5-3 This image of an infant with ROP demonstrates the wide-field imaging capability of the RetCamII.

glucose, blood pressure, spirometry, or weight can be collected in the home by digital equipment and transmitted to a health care provider at a distance. Some applications include automated reminders about when to monitor and about opportunities to respond to specific questions to enhance the remote assessment and improve self-management. Access to assessment data on an ongoing basis allows providers to readily identify trends requiring intervention, and patients are motivated and reassured knowing their results are monitored routinely. Within the neonatal setting, telehomecare can be a support to parents following discharge, a time when families may feel inadequate and may be reluctant or have difficulty accessing care. Telehomecare may include regular vital sign monitoring as well as videoconferencing to assess color or respiratory status in conditions such as congenital heart disease or bronchopulmonary dysplasia.

Postdischarge telehealth applications can include improved access to a wide range of disciplines and support systems, including follow-up developmental assessments, feeding assessments, speech and language therapy, genetic counseling, and many others. For neonates with ongoing health issues, telehealth can also provide access to patient education and support for families in rural locations, who may not have regular access to other families supporting a newborn with a chronic condition. Telehealth can provide key support for neonates as they transition out of the institutional setting, and it may result in earlier discharge and improved patient outcomes.

Continuing Education

The education of healthcare professionals involved in newborn care is critical to maximizing telehealth's potential to improve neonatal care. Continuing education is challenging, particularly for professionals working at a site removed from a tertiary center. It is now recommended that all hospitals delivering newborns should have an individual certified in the Neonatal Resuscitation Program present at the delivery. In addition to initial certification, recertification is required every two years. Cronin and associates (26) have demonstrated that instruction via interactive videoconferencing, including the testing of practical skills, can be provided satisfactorily. Similarly, Loewen and associates (27) have demonstrated that the neonatal stabilization program, S.T.A.B.L.E.® (sugar, temperature, artificial breathing, blood pressure, lab work, and emotional support), can be delivered effectively. In a study of 56 health professionals randomized to receive the program either in person or by videoconferencing, both groups, with similar pretest scores, had a similar, but significant increase in their posttest scores.

In Canada, trans-Canada rounds have been established to allow neonatal fellows from across the country to interact and share information on unusual cases. These sessions are highly interactive and in addition to improving knowledge, have resulted in an element of friendly competitiveness.

PRACTICAL STEPS IN GETTING STARTED

As telehealth moves away from pilot projects to operational telehealth networks, there have been many lessons learned and some consensus on the critical factors for success. This background of experience has provided a framework for developing new telehealth services or programs.

Needs Assessment

Experience has proven that time and resources spent on a needs assessment will result in the ability to design systems that truly meet the user requirements. The needs assessment process includes obtaining information and ideas from many groups involved in the delivery of health services to determine the goals, objectives, and priorities for telehealth. The clinical needs identified will drive the goals of the telehealth program and system design. Engaging clinical staff early and promoting buy-in will ensure that clinical needs remain the primary focus of telehealth programs and will begin the change management process necessary to integrate telehealth into clinical workflow. A well-structured telehealth needs assessment will not only define the clinical direction of a potential telehealth application or network, but will identify strategies to resolve issues that could potentially add long delays and increased costs to telehealth implementation.

Readiness Assessment

Prior to telehealth investment, there is a clear need to determine the "telehealth readiness" of communities and organizations to reduce the risk of failure and losses in time, money, and effort. Although there is a fundamental requirement for sufficient bandwidth to support telehealth, non-technical organizational factors are equally important to successful telehealth implementation. The perception of need and the ability and willingness of users to adapt to the changes associated with the introduction of telehealth can have enormous impact on adoption and utilization. Telehealth success depends upon selecting communities, organizations, and programs that are aware of telehealth and its benefits, have a genuine need for and commitment to telehealth, and can provide or acquire the capacity to support and resource telehealth beyond implementation.

Telehealth Business Plan

To successfully deploy and evolve a telehealth program, it is important to develop a telehealth business plan. The business plan serves as a guide for the organization and as a communications tool for external stakeholders and funders. This plan should be generated in collaboration with a range of staff and be revisited frequently in response to changes in the environment. The plan should fully describe the telehealth opportunity, products, and services to be provided; organizational structure; operational and technical requirements; implementation plan; marketing and business development strategy; and financial analysis. There is increased pressure for telehealth programs to become viable commercial enterprises. Even in publicly funded health systems, telehealth is expected to show a return on investment realized through cost savings and improved health outcomes. The goal of the financial analysis is to define potential funding/revenue sources, expenses (capital and operating), and cost recovery, as well as to identify and mitigate financial risk. Projections should contain best-case, expected-case, and worst-case scenarios based upon a mix of alternative assumptions related to growth and use of the telehealth network, cost of operations, cost recovery, and sources of funding/revenue. Careful attention to longer-term sustainability is critical from the outset. Guidelines for developing a telehealth business plan can be found in several of the listed references (2,28).

Program Management

Successful telehealth initiatives are built upon a robust operational infrastructure that ensures efficient delivery of telehealth services on a daily basis. In addition to the obvious need for technical training and support for users, there are many other functions required for effective telehealth program management including scheduling, policy and standards development, workflow and process design, marketing and communications, research and evaluation, and financial management. Strategic clinical leadership is also essential to ensure buy-in of key clinical providers, validate clinical telehealth applications, and develop clinical policies and risk management strategies. Understanding these functions and the related skills and competencies will allow a telehealth program to implement an appropriate organizational structure and human resource plan to support operations. The optimal organizational model will also be determined by the degree of telehealth integration into existing organizational structures and functions.

Evaluation and Quality Assurance Plan

Evaluation and quality assurance are vital to ensuring quality telehealth activities. To date, telehealth evaluation has focused on technical accuracy and reliability, diagnostic quality and effectiveness, impact on clinical management, user satisfaction, and impact on service or program costs (9,10). There is still great need for standardization of evaluation tools, measures and key indicators to assess the impact of telehealth on cost, quality, and accessibility of care. An effective evaluation plan will provide evidence to funding agencies, health care administrators, providers, and patients and will significantly contribute to the strategic development and sustainability of a telehealth program.

Healthcare organizations, including telehealth programs, are adopting a focus on quality improvement in response to increased demands for accountability, height-ened consumer expectations, resource limitations, and fundamental changes in health service delivery models (29). Management tools such as the balanced scorecard are increasingly being adapted to the health care setting to guide ongoing evaluation and quality improvement initiatives and can be tailored to include telehealth and other ICTs (30–33). Regardless of the approach chosen, telehealth services should be continually monitored through a quality assurance process that allows rapid and responsive improvements to performance and the maintenance of quality practices. When possible, both evaluation and quality assurance processes should be aligned with broader program or organizational initiatives.

IMPLICATIONS FOR THE FUTURE

The introduction of advanced information and communications technology is inherently changing the way that medicine is practiced. With the introduction of health information systems, clinical decision support tools, and online learning, medical professionals are being provided the tools to support high-quality, evidence-based practice. Telehealth and the electronic health record allow access to health care services and information across sites, providers, and the continuum of care, removing the traditional organizational boundaries and building a foundation for integrated service delivery. These technologies are transforming the way that health care professionals and patients interact with the health care system. IP-based technologies will provide a convergence of data with images, video, and voice in a media-rich environment. Wireless network solutions will enable mobile access to the health care system and these supporting technologies.

Telehealth is about the relationships and processes that allow health care services to be delivered virtually—it is not just about technology. Limits to telehealth expansion have less to do with access to bandwidth and equipment costs than the human factors. Telehealth initiatives must have the necessary time and resources committed to address not only the technical solution but also the process redesign, and change management necessary to encourage more widespread adoption of telehealth. Unless those involved with telehealth programs develop their skill and expertise in these areas, the programs will run the risk of limited user acceptance and poor network use. With the relatively high cost of implementation and operations, low utilization threatens the sustainability of any telehealth program.

Neonatology has been accused of focusing on the "high tech." Telehealth is also viewed by some as yet another application of technology. Ultimately the fundamental purpose of both remains grounded in patient care and achieving the best possible outcomes for patients. Telehealth improves access to health care, which means access to specialist consultation for the neonate; improves access to education of health care professionals in the care of the neonate; and facilitates family involvement with their newborn infant over distance. Telehealth applications in neonatology can range from "low-tech" home care applications to high-end intensive care and wireless transport communications. For both, the ultimate goal of improved patient care remains. To achieve this goal, regardless of the technical solution chosen, the need for building user acceptance and confidence, as well as simplifying the telehealth process to support integration into the workplace, is essential.

REFERENCES

1. Jennett PA, Scott R, Hailey D, et al. *Socio-economic impact of telehealth: evidence now for health care in the future. Volume one: state of the science report.* Calgary, Alberta: Health Telematics Unit, University of Calgary, 2003.
2. Darkins AW, Cary MA. *Telemedicine and telehealth: principles, policies, performance and pitfalls.* New York: Springer Publishing Co., 2000.
3. Whitten PS, Mair FS, Haycox A, et al. Systematic review of cost-effectiveness studies of telemedicine interventions. *BMJ* 2002;324:1434–1437.
4. Brown N. A brief history of telemedicine. Updated June 03, 2004. Available at http://tie.telemed.org/articles/tmhistory.asp?www=t1&tree=telemed101/understand/. Accessed September 29, 2004.
5. Elford R. Telemedicine activities at Memorial University 1975-1997. November 28, 2002. Available at http://www.med.mun.ca/telemed/telehist/telemulti.htm. Accessed September 29, 2004.
6. TIE (telemedicine information exchange). Available at http://tie.telemed.org/. Accessed September 29, 2004.
7. Hasham S, Akalu R, Rossos PG. Medico-legal implications of telehealth in Canada. *Telehealth Law* 2003;4:9–20.
8. Blum JD. Telemedicine poses new challenges for the law. *Hlth Law Canada* 1999;20:115–126.
9. *National initiative for telehealth (NIFTE) framework of guidelines.* Ottawa, Ontario: NIFTE; 2003.
10. Currell R, Urquhart C, Wainwright P, et al. Telemedicine versus face to face patient care: effects on professional practice and health care outcomes. *Cochrane Database Syst Rev* 2000;2:CD002098.
11. Roine R, Ohinmaa A, Hailey D. Assessing telemedicine: a systematic review of the literature. *CMAJ* 2001;165:765–771.
12. Hersh WR, Helfand M, Wallace J, et al. Clinical outcomes resulting from telemedicine interventions: a systematic review. *BMC Med Inform Decis Mak* 2001;1:5.
13. Ohinmaa A, Hailey D, Roine R. *The assessment of telemedicine: general principals and a systematic review.* Alberta, Canada: Finish Office for Health Care Technology Assessment and Alberta Heritage Foundation for Medical Research, 1999.
14. Hersch W, Helfand M, Wallace J, et al. A systematic review of the efficacy of telemedicine for making diagnostic and management decisions. *J Telemed Telecare* 2002;8:197–209.
15. Chan FY, Soong B, Watson D, et al. Realtime fetal ultrasound by telemedicine in Queensland. A successful venture? *J Telemed Telecare* 2001;7 Suppl 2:7–11.
16. Soong B, Chan FY, Bloomfield S, et al. The fetal tele-ultrasound project in Queensland. *Aust Health Rev* 2002;25:67–73.
17. Finley JP, Sharratt GP, Nanton MA, et al. Paediatric echocardiography by telemedicine—nine years' experience. *J Telemed Telecare* 1997;3:200–204.
18. Casey FA. Telemedicine in paediatric cardiology. *Arch Dis Child* 1999;80:497–499.
19. Sable C. Digital echocardiography and telemedicine applications in pediatric cardiology. *Pediatr Cardiol* 2002;23:358–369.
20. Widmer S, Ghisla R, Ramelli GP, et al. Tele-echocardiography in paediatrics. *Eur J Pediatr* 2003;162:271–275.
21. Roth DB, Morales D, Feuer WJ, et al. Screening for retinopathy of prematurity employing the retcam 120: sensitivity and specificity. *Arch Ophthalmol* 2001;119:268–272.
22. Yen KG, Hess D, Burke B, et al. Telephotoscreening to detect retinopathy of prematurity: preliminary study of the optimum time to employ digital fundus camera imaging to detect ROP. *J AAPOS* 2002;6:64–70.
23. Schwartz SD, Harrison SA, Ferrone PJ, et al. Telemedical evaluation and management of retinopathy of prematurity using a fiberoptic digital fundus camera. *Ophthalmology* 2000;107:25–28.
24. Ells AL, Holmes JM, Astle WF, et al. Telemedicine approach to screening for severe retinopathy of prematurity: a pilot study. *Ophthalmology* 2003;110:2113–2117.
25. Gray JE, Safran C, Davis RB, et al. Baby CareLink: using the internet and telemedicine to improve care for high-risk infants. *Pediatrics* 2000;106:1318–1324.
26. Cronin C, Cheang S, Hlynka D, et al. Videoconferencing can be used to assess neonatal resuscitation skills. *Med Educ* 2001;35:1013–1023.
27. Loewen L, Seshia MM, Fraser Askin D, et al. Effective delivery of neonatal stabilization education using videoconferencing in Manitoba. *J Telemed Telecare* 2003;9:334–338.
28. Office for the advancement of telehealth. Available at http://telehealth.hrsa.gov/welcome.htm. Accessed September 29, 2004.
29. Harrigan M. Quest for quality in Canadian health care: continuous quality improvement. 2nd ed. Ottawa, Ontario: Minister of Public Works and Government Services Canada, 2000.
30. Baker GR, Pink GH. A balanced scorecard for Canadian hospitals. *Healthc Manage Forum* 1995;8:7–21.
31. Kaplan RS, Norton DP. *The balanced scorecard: translating strategy into action.* Boston, Mass: Harvard Business School Press, 1996.
32. Kaplan RS, Norton DP. *The strategy-focused organization: how balanced scorecard companies thrive in the new business environment.* Boston, Mass: Harvard Business School Press, 2001.
33. Castaneda-Mendez K, Mangan K, Lavery AM. The role and application of the balanced scorecard in healthcare quality management. *J Healthcare Qual* 1998;20:10–13.

Newborn Intensive Care Unit Design: Scientific and Practical Considerations

Robert D. White   Gilbert I. Martin   Judith Smith   Stanley N. Graven

DEVELOPING A MISSION STATEMENT

The first step in a successful newborn intensive care unit (NICU) design project is the development of a shared vision among NICU, hospital, and community leaders. The construction of a new unit or redesign of an existing facility should successfully address key problems in the region's current system of neonatal care. For an existing, stable unit wishing to modernize its facility, these problems may be primarily internal—the need for more space, current technology, and family support. For an entirely new facility, these issues will be predominantly external—who are the existing providers and what niche will this new unit most appropriately fill? A careful appraisal of medical care trends anticipated within the community over the next 20 years, especially with regard to obstetric and intensive care services, should precede any decision on a mission statement intended to guide NICU construction and operation. Whether a hospital is the only provider of NICU services in its area or one of several, it is crucial that it understand its niche and the responsibilities inherent to that role, so that appropriate physical facilities can be constructed to fulfill its mission.

A mission statement that might provide a framework for many NICUs is as follows:

The Newborn Intensive Care Unit will provide a state-of-the-art, integrated, family-centered approach to neonatal care. This interdisciplinary program will strive to give patients, families, and payers high quality and compassionate care through the provision of:

- Care that honors the racial, ethnic, cultural, religious, and socioeconomic diversity of family and staff
- Education, information, and emotional support
- Access to the most current effective therapies
- Integrated treatment plans emphasizing coordination throughout the continuum of care
- Encouragement of family support and involvement

When consensus is reached on a mission statement, specific goals and objectives can be defined that apply this mission to the local realities of demographics, care practices, and competition. Defining these goals will be the first step toward decisions on bed capacity, types of equipment needed, and changes in care practices. All of these can then be explored in depth by the teams described below. The goals and objectives should be measurable (e.g., survival and morbidity rates compared to regional and national standards, staff experience and turnover, parental satisfaction ratings, cost per patient day) and realistic, so that the overall value of the project can be ascertained at the time cost projections are available, and on an ongoing basis after construction is complete.

CREATING THE TEAMS

Once a decision has been made to proceed with the development of either a new or a renovated NICU, it is important to form specialized teams with well-defined goals. In many hospitals, several persons will serve on two or more teams. Each team should have access to the several excellent reference materials available to assist in the design of an NICU (1–6).

The Strategic Planning Team

The strategic planning team will continue to develop the vision and goals that led to the decision to pursue new construction. It should include, at a minimum, an administrator, a neonatologist, and a nursing director. This group will be responsible for reviewing utilization and demographic information (available from state and local planning and health agencies, the insurance industry, and the Census Bureau) in order to define the NICU's service area and appropriate number of beds. Some general guidelines in this area include estimates that 5% to 12% of all newborns will need intensive care at the time of birth, and 1% to 2% will need ventilator care. Total NICU days for a defined region will approximate 1.25 patient-days per live birth—if a region has 10,000 live births per year, it will generate approximately 13,000 NICU patient days, or an average census of 35 babies, with an average length of stay of 20 to 25 days. These numbers will be influenced considerably by the level of care provided by a particular NICU, referral and back transport patterns, admission and discharge criteria, and competing NICUs serving the same region. Because of fluctuations in census, a unit should have sufficient bed positions to care for 40% to 50% more babies than the average census calculations, so a region with 10,000 deliveries per year will need 50 to 55 NICU beds. Many areas currently exceed this number by a sizable proportion because of serving a particularly high-risk population, or because of inefficiencies inherent in multiple NICUs serving a single region.

The strategic planning team also should make some basic calculations regarding staffing patterns, if this is to be a new service for the hospital. Depending on patient mix, overall staffing patterns may require 4 to 6 nurses and 2 support staff (inclusive of nursing administration, respiratory therapy, developmental therapy, social work, ward clerk, and housekeeping staff) for every 10 babies. A unit with an average census of 20 babies, for example, would require 8 to 12 nurses on each shift, or 40 to 65 full-time equivalents (FTEs), with an additional 20 to 25 FTEs for support staff. One neonatologist is needed for each 6 to 8 babies (average census); this is one area, among several, where units with an average census of less than 20 infants encounter certain inefficiencies because of their size. On the other hand, large units (more than 40 beds or so) can be difficult to design and manage efficiently because of the space requirements. Some hospitals have addressed this issue by dividing their NICU into intensive care and continuing care, or step-down areas. Some units will also need to plan staffing for transport team or nurse practitioner coverage. Six to 7 full-time positions are required for 24-hour coverage of each position for these services. A transport team with 2 nurses and a respiratory therapist, for example, would require at least 12 nurses and 6 therapists to provide full-time, in-house coverage.

Next, the strategic planning team also will need to assess the impact of the new or renovated NICU on other hospital departments, especially obstetric, maintenance, and supply services. When these issues are clear, the team will proceed to interview and engage an architect. The timing of this step is important—the architectural firm should be involved before any design decisions are made, but after the strategic planning team has articulated a clear set of goals for the process. Several architectural firms can be asked to make formal presentations of their general concepts for the project, as well as present examples of other projects that they have designed. The architectural firm chosen should have complete engineering and interior design specialists on staff, as well as an equipment representative and a neonatal nurse planner. The entire architectural team should be familiar with the latest trends in NICU design and the scientific principles behind the design process. Once chosen, the architectural group and the strategic planning team can then develop a timetable for planning and construction of the new facility.

The Financial Planning Team

This group is composed of the hospital's chief financial and operational officers, nursing management, and any other individuals representing areas of the hospital whose budgets will be significantly affected by the new construction. Consultants, such as those helpful in the equipment selection process (see Equipment Selection section), also may be asked to join the team. The one-time costs for the project will include architectural fees, the physical plant, and new equipment. Ongoing costs may include increased staffing for direct patient care, housekeeping, and maintenance functions. These costs should be clearly identified early in the planning sequence, with the assistance of the care practices team (see The Care Practices Team section). This team should continue to meet intermittently throughout the planning process, because some unanticipated expenses often surface as the design takes shape.

The Care Practices Team

This is the largest group, and it represents caregivers in the NICU. At a minimum, the following disciplines should participate: neonatology, nursing management and staff, respiratory therapy, social work, pharmacy, laboratory, radiology, infection control, nutrition, housekeeping, and parents. Depending on local care practices, surgery, obstetrics, and clinical research may be appropriate additions to this list. As each individual provides information on his or her own specialty to enhance care for babies, families, and staff, the team should be encouraged to look beyond existing practices and view the new construction as an opportunity to change the way things are done. In particular, most NICUs will need to reevaluate their care practices with respect to parental access and developmentally supportive care, which may have been severely restricted under their previous NICU design. They should consider environmental design features that will provide the most optimal living conditions for babies, working conditions for staff, and integration of families, and they should begin to address some of the conflicts inherent in these ideals. As a team, this group can then identify general space, equipment, staffing, and maintenance and cleaning requirements, which can be reported to the financial and design teams for determination of feasibility.

The Design Team

When the strategic planning, financial planning, and care practice teams have agreed on the general scope of the project, including goals, approximate size and cost, major changes in care practices, and an architectural firm, the design team can begin its work. Members of this team should include the architectural group, the hospital's project manager, neonatology, nursing, respiratory therapy, parents, and the equipment consultant. After creating a functional plan that addresses all the needs identified by the care practices team, this group should visit new or updated NICUs to get additional ideas, learn how to avoid pitfalls, and solicit suggestions on their functional plan. This team then will meet regularly over several months as blueprints are developed to reconcile all these concepts into a working unit. Detailed minutes should be kept and reviewed at the beginning of each meeting.

SITE VISITS

Touring other NICUs can be a valuable investment for many reasons, whether planning for a renovation or new construction. Visits provide a firsthand look at design features that are and are not working for others. The benefits can include a better plan, fewer change orders, and a smoother transition because the planning team gained new ideas and a clearer understanding of the pros and cons of the proposed changes.

Careful planning will assure that site visits are productive. Start by identifying the objectives of the tours, areas of greatest interest, potential units to visit, and the best timing. The typical purpose of a site visit during the early stages of planning is to trigger ideas. Many NICU teams find it useful to tour other units during the stage when they have identified their vision, defined their care practices, and prepared a preliminary functional program. Others stagger their tours and see different units during various stages of planning. Waiting until the preparation of construction documents is underway is not usually the best timing for initial site visits, unless the objective is to clarify operational issues related to the selected design approach.

Two other essential components to be addressed are selecting the members of the tour group and funding the travel. Selecting tour team members should tie back to the objectives. Most units request a budget for site visits as part of the project funding. Some fortunate units have donors who help with the travel budget, and even include interested donors on the tour team, when appropriate. If a travel budget is not feasible, the next best strategy is virtual tours. In many cases, the NICUs or their architects have photos in hard copy, on Web sites, videos or other material

that could be viewed, and several of these are also available on a single Web site (6). A phone interview or written survey would be helpful to provide descriptive information for a virtual tour.

Tips for Planning a Site Visit

Performing the tasks below will enable the planning team to get maximum benefit from a site visit:

- Interview key people by telephone or in person before touring their unit.
- Obtain permission to photograph, videotape, or receive audiovisuals already available from public relations, architects, and other sources. If assigning photography to a team member, assure that he or she has the proper equipment and competence.
- Design a questionnaire that will be used consistently as a guide for all visits.
- Assign a person or people to key topics to assure all pertinent questions are answered before, during, or after the tour. Categorize questions by area of interest, and create the expectation that the responsible person will report on the findings.
- Determine how the information from the tour will be used and by whom.
- After the visit and in a timely manner, discuss and record general impressions of people who toured the facility.

Sample Questionnaire

A questionnaire should be developed to ensure that all needed information in relation to a site visit is captured and recorded. Segments of the questionnaire could be contact information, general statistics, and specific questions.

Contact Information

The contact information should include:

- Date of Visit
- Organization Name/Location
- Contact Names/Titles
- Phone Numbers/E-mail Addresses/Web Site
- Who attended from your organization

General Statistics

General statistics should include:

- Annual NICU volume (and birth volume, if relevant)
- Number of beds by level of care or other category
- Annual number of infant transports in and out
- Average length of stay (by level, if appropriate)
- Economic and cultural characteristics of population served
- Acuity of patients served (and information on how acuity is defined)
- Payer mix
- Date opened or renovated

Examples of Questions

The questions to ask at the site being visited should include, but not be limited to:

1. Describe the changes that resulted in the current services and facilities and the reasons driving the changes.
2. Were the objectives met? (How is success measured?)
3. What types of NICU health professionals practice at this hospital (number of neonatal nurse practitioners (NNPs), neonatologists, residents, etc.)?
4. What are the key staffing issues that were or need to be resolved?
5. What type of staffing education programss, orientation, budget, and amount of time were required to make changes to the current model?
6. How is each type of patient care room or area used?
7. Where and how are most procedures handled?
8. Describe communication systems among staff, between staff and families and others.
9. Describe special features of unit.
10. What was the biggest challenge related to this project?
11. What would be done differently based on the wisdom learned from the experience?
12. What were the benchmarks or other resources that were most helpful during the planning process?

Other Potential Topics for Questionnaire

Other topics that may be included on the site visit questionnaire are:

Family input
Visitation practices
Family space
Care practices
Admission process
Maintenance
Monitoring systems
Lighting
Sound control
Interior design
Storage
Communication Systems Security
Flow paths
Cleaning
Head walls
Staffing
Fundraising
Total project costs
Acceptance by staff/administration
Response by community/competitors
Ceiling/floor/wall/cabinet finishes patterns
Coordination with labor and delivery

One of the final planning steps is to determine how the information gained from the site visit will be shared with the stakeholders who could not participate directly in the tour. Good documentation of the visits and effective presentation of the information will provide maximum benefit from the activities.

SPECIFIC DESIGN ISSUES

Floor Space Requirements

NICUs have historically been undersized, with insufficient room for storage, parental access, and offices, even when accurate estimates are made for the number of babies to be cared for. Change has been incremental, as administrators, architects, and NICU staff gradually expand their horizons to accommodate new practices, particularly increased parental access.

Given this historical perspective and extrapolating from floor space requirements in adult and pediatric intensive care units (ICUs), it is likely that an NICU design should allow 600 gross square feet per bed to meet the needs of the babies, staff, and families. This figure includes office, storage, and support space as well as the patient care areas; gross square footage estimates also include space required for hallways, ductwork, restrooms, and the like. This figure is an average; teaching hospitals with active clinical research programs, for example, might require more than 600 gross square feet per bed, whereas a community NICU might require somewhat less. Any design that provides less than 500 gross square feet per bed will inevitably demand compromises and limit flexibility for the future, when parental access desires and lengths of stay (because of increasing survival of extremely low-birth-weight infants) may be even greater than they are today.

Previous estimates of floor space requirements often recommended square footage per bed position (e.g., 120 to 150 square feet per intensive care bed position), and most state codes still use this convention. If this method is used, an additional 30 square feet of storage space must be planned outside of the patient care area, as well as 24 cubic feet of cabinet storage at each bedside, at a minimum.

Location Within the Hospital

The NICU should be immediately adjacent to the high-risk delivery rooms whenever possible. There are few, if any, NICUs that are more than a few hundred feet from a high-risk delivery service that do not consider their location as the source of certain risks to optimal care. In some circumstances, especially very large hospital complexes or free-standing children's hospitals, this ideal may be impossible to achieve. In the former situation, a resuscitation area within the delivery room complex or in each delivery suite, always valuable, becomes crucial; in the latter case, all infants are accepted as transfers, and proximity to the ambulance entrance and heliport becomes particularly significant. When the NICU is on a different floor from the delivery suites, as often occurs in larger hospitals, controlled elevator access between these two areas is essential.

Many NICUs, particularly in small or medium-sized hospitals, share staff and responsibilities with the well-baby nursery or pediatric ICU. When these areas are contiguous, much of the support space (e.g., family lounge, staff lockers, equipment storage) can be shared, and the opportunities for staff to assist one another are enhanced.

Traffic patterns for infants who leave the NICU for procedures should be identified and private hallways created wherever possible, so that ill infants and their attendants do not need to use public areas.

Security Considerations

As family access to the NICU has become more prevalent, so have security considerations. Most NICUs now permit continuous access to families, so traffic in and out of the NICU is commonplace. Certain design features are necessary in this setting to protect babies and staff. First, the NICU should be designed with only a single public entrance. Other entrances and exits (e.g., to the delivery suite, the clean utility room, and the staff lockers) may be desirable, but these should be less apparent to the public (except as fire exits) and either within constant observation of the staff or equipped with alarms.

The public entrance to the NICU should be designed with the security of all major parties (babies, families, and staff) in mind. Families and staff need a secure locker area to store personal belongings. This area should be large enough to allow more than one family to enter or leave at a time and should be under constant observation. Electronic detection systems increasingly are being used in newborn nursery areas to prevent kidnapping; these are uncommon in NICU settings, but worthy of consideration if constant visual monitoring of all exits from the NICU is not feasible.

Fire exits should be carefully planned in the initial design, and clearly marked, as should the location of fire extinguishers. The fire marshal should be given the first draft of the design documents so that any problems can be corrected early.

Reception Area

In most NICUs, the reception area is part of or near the public entrance. This area also may encompass the family lounge and the ward clerk's workspace. The size and layout of this space is highly dependent on the size of the NICU and its *culture*, or typical practices.

The family lounge should always be large enough to accommodate at least two families (6–10 people) comfortably, with seating that is comfortable, but not conducive to overnight sleeping. Lockers for valuables, a coffee pot, a television set, reading material (including informational and educational literature for families of NICU babies), and a toy box for children are items found in many such areas; public restrooms and telephones should be nearby.

Families and the public should be able to immediately reach an NICU staff member from the reception area. In some larger units, the contact person might be a full-time ward clerk; in others, it might be a hot line or direct visual

contact into the patient care area. In any case, this function should be carefully thought out so that those who should be encouraged to enter (i.e., families) find themselves feeling welcomed, while others (e.g., curious individuals wandering through the hospital) are discouraged.

Direct Patient Care

As might be expected, the greatest design effort is spent creating the patient care area. The first and major decision to be made is the extent to which individualized environments are desirable. The goal to provide each baby with a space that is not impinged upon by noise, bright lights, and commotion from an adjacent bed position, and that has enough space to accommodate staff, family, and bedside equipment and storage seems intuitive and is certainly the norm for adult ICUs; but this has not historically been the pattern for NICUs, for several reasons.

NICUs in the 1970s and 1980s were routinely designed as large, open wards. These permitted care of the largest number of babies in a given space and allowed direct visibility of each baby by the staff, and of staff members by one another. Babies (and staff) were not thought to be adversely affected by the noise and bright lighting that were the norm for such designs. New practices and equipment (as long as they did not require much additional space) could be incorporated easily into this design, and highly variable census patterns also could be accommodated more easily than in the older premature nursery design of several smaller rooms. Parents were allowed, or expected, to visit for only short periods, so very little space at the bedside was allotted to them.

In recent years, many of these assumptions have changed. Direct, continuous observation of most babies no longer is considered necessary, thanks to improved monitoring systems (especially noninvasive oximetry and blood pressure monitoring), and certainly is no longer practiced except for the sickest babies, even in units where it is still physically possible. Babies clearly are affected by excessive, noxious levels of light and noise, and their response to these environmental hazards varies with their gestational age and medical condition. Extensive adult studies in workplace settings also have established that staff needs and responses can be quite different from those of babies (7). Perhaps, most dramatically, family expectations have changed. Many families now want continuous access to their babies and want to be able to stay at the bedside—without interfering with the ability of staff to care for their baby—in any but the most extraordinary circumstances.

Designing an NICU that takes these newer realities into consideration requires establishing a local philosophy on individualized environments. In some units, private or semiprivate rooms for at least some of the infants will be considered desirable and feasible; in others, space, staffing, or philosophical considerations will lead the design team in a different direction. Often, a combination of "pods" (one, two, or four beds), with a larger room for recovering neonates, has been the design of choice. In any NICU, however, the need for each baby to be protected as much as possible from the noise, light, and activity generated at other bed positions and the differing needs of babies from staff need to be discussed and integrated into the design process at the outset (8).

Certain principles can be established for all direct patient care area plans, regardless of whether a single large room, multiple smaller rooms, or private rooms are chosen as the model. First, each bed position must have sufficient space for families to stay for extended periods without interfering with staff duties. Second, each bed position must have individualized lighting, data entry, and communications systems. Third, traffic patterns must be well planned, with sufficient aisle widths to accommodate diagnostic equipment and personnel; generally, this requires aisles of at least 5 feet in width. Nursing functions should be separated from the bedside whenever possible. For babies, the NICU is perhaps ideally visualized as a bedroom for a sick infant; for staff, it is a workplace, where both work-related and social communication occurs. These concepts are often in conflict, yet the NICU design must accommodate both to the greatest extent possible. Therefore, the design team should (again, within the local culture and practices) separate those nursing functions that do not involve direct patient care (e.g., most charting, giving reports, receiving and making most phone calls) from the bedside to the greatest extent possible, especially if those activities require different lighting levels or create noise that would disturb the baby. This is done by providing adequate space for these functions away from the bedside, yet sufficiently proximate to allow appropriate response to the unpredictable needs of the baby. Finally, in any plan that uses modules or individual rooms, staffing patterns should be considered. In general, enough babies should be clustered together to justify staffing with at least three nurses. Designing smaller clusters creates significant staffing issues during those times when at least one nurse must leave the area.

After these considerations are adequately debated and decided, the general layout of the patient care area can proceed. Each bed position can be identified, as well as nursing work areas (charting, medication preparation, etc.), sinks, and traffic flow patterns. At this point, an infectious disease specialist also should be consulted, to assure that the design is conducive to good infection control practices. This individual also will be interested in airflow considerations and in floor, wall, and ceiling finishes (discussed below). Proximity to other important support areas also will begin to take shape at this stage (specific design features for each of these areas are discussed in the next section).

The design team then can spend considerable time planning the layout of a typical bed position. Perhaps most important in this regard is the headwall, including monitoring and communication systems. Construction of a full-size mockup of an individual bed position, complete with

headwall, monitors, and communications systems is well worth the effort and expense to be sure the ergonomics of the design have been adequately considered. Many members of the design team will be unable to fully visualize the layout from a blueprint, and it would be rare that a new NICU would resemble an existing design closely enough to bypass this step. Most NICUs will want to include one or more special care areas for isolation, treatment rooms, parent rooming in, and breast-feeding. In most units, some of these functions can be combined, and many will choose to eliminate one or more of these because of local practice patterns. The need for each should be carefully considered in new designs, however, and if not served by a dedicated space, at least clearly accommodated at some appropriate location in the NICU.

General Support Space

Clean utility, soiled utility, and general storage are functions that each require a dedicated space; in some units, a satellite pharmacy and clinical laboratory are also given designated areas. The layout of these rooms is straightforward; errors in design usually are made by allowing too little space or placing these rooms in an inconvenient position away from the direct patient care area. Ideally, these areas also should be accessible from an outside corridor so that restocking can take place without unnecessary traffic through the NICU, but this must be designed in accordance with security precautions (discussed previously). Storage areas should have a generous supply of electrical outlets and shelving so that battery-powered devices can be recharged. Additional specific considerations are outlined in each state's code documents and in several published guidelines (1–3).

Staff Support Space

As noted previously, some charting space, especially for the nursing and respiratory therapy staff, needs to be allocated within the direct patient care area. Additional space, especially for physician and nurse practitioner charting and discussion, should be provided adjacent to the patient care area, so that the noise and activity generated there does not impinge on the babies' bedsides. The communications systems (phone, computer terminal, printer) that link the NICU with the hospital laboratory, pharmacy, and central supply generally will be situated in this area as well, which will benefit from being centrally located.

The staff lounge and locker room should be adjacent to the NICU, with restroom facilities integral or nearby. The lounge should be large enough to accommodate at least one third of all NICU staff (nurses, therapists, physicians, and other support staff) at one time and be accessible to the NICU by phone or intercom.

Several disciplines should have office space immediately adjacent to the NICU, including social work, medical and nursing administration, and developmental and respiratory therapy. When parent support or research staff are actively involved in a unit's activities, they also will need nearby office space. On-call rooms and a conference room should be situated within this complex, with phone and computer links, including digital x-ray transmission, and restrooms with showers.

Family Support Space

In addition to generous provision of space at the bedside and in the family lounge, parents need space to stay overnight, to meet in private with staff to discuss their baby or to grieve, and to breast-feed. Again, depending on the size of the NICU and its local practices, some of these functions can be combined, but none can be ignored.

Rooming in, even with critically ill patients, is provided (indeed, encouraged) in most areas of a typical hospital, except for the NICU, where this practice usually is limited to those infants close to discharge. We are unaware of any documented factors, other than tradition, that justify the exclusion of parents from rooming in with NICU patients from immediately after birth, however, and suggest that future designs should anticipate that this practice will become more prevalent as families come to request and expect this opportunity. To be sure, many families will not choose or will be unable to room in with their ill newborn, so an ideal design need not anticipate that all babies will need space for rooming in at all times, but it should allow most parents who desire this privilege the opportunity to do so. Experience in NICUs that permit unlimited rooming in indicates that up to 50% of babies may have a family member staying overnight at a given time.

Breast-feeding of premature or ill infants is poorly accommodated in many existing NICUs because of space and privacy considerations. Mothers should be able to breast-feed babies at the bedside without compromising their privacy or being asked to wait until the baby is stable enough to be transferred to an area where these problems do not exist. Alternatives in this regard include private rooms for those babies whose mothers plan to room in and/or breast-feed, or moveable partitions. Breast-feeding rooms are also a good alternative for babies who are healthy enough to be moved and can be utilized by mothers who need to use a breast pump. These rooms should be designed with most of the capabilities of a headwall (e.g., oxygen, suction, monitor, electrical outlets, and direct communication to the NICU staff), yet be as much like home as possible.

Room for parent education and counseling should be available within the NICU complex. This is particularly important when private discussions need to occur with families of critically ill infants.

The location and content of signs are often overlooked when planning an NICU. Some thought should be given to traffic patterns for families and the public from the hospital entrance(s) and how signage will be used to direct them clearly to the NICU. Information on signs should be phrased warmly, in a way that will make families feel welcome, rather than sternly, in a way that could make them feel like outsiders and intruders.

Lighting

Planning appropriate lighting for the NICU requires consideration of the disparate needs of both the babies and staff. In general, babies need very little light, but exposure to moderate levels of illumination during part of the day may help establish circadian rhythmicity.

Staff need moderate levels of illumination at the bedside to evaluate babies and to perform charting and manual tasks. At times, intense levels of illumination are necessary to perform procedures and for phototherapy of hyperbilirubinemia. It is doubtful that babies need natural lighting, but studies of adult office workers and hospital patients document the benefit of windows for staff and families (9).

Consideration of these disparate needs should lead the design team to plan a multilevel lighting scheme. At the bedside, a low level of indirect ambient lighting (200 to 300 lux [20 to 30 foot-candles]) is desirable, so the baby is not exposed to a continuous or direct bright light source. Task lighting, both for the bed surface and the nursing work surface(s), should be highly focused (framed), and rheostatically controlled, so that only the amount of light needed is provided, and only to the specific location desired. This may require multiple light sources at the bedside. The ideal task light would be adjustable to an infinite variety of positions, yet be able to recess fully into the wall or ceiling. It would have a beam of adjustable width and intensity and be free of shadowing effects.

At nursing work areas and traffic circulation areas elsewhere in the patient care area, moderate lighting levels (300 to 1,000 lux) are suitable. The light sources used should avoid glare, especially on work surfaces and computer terminals, and should have multiple switches or rheostatic controls to allow flexibility in lighting levels. A single master switch may be useful, however, if a darkened room is desired for transillumination. All fixtures should have filters or shields that block ultraviolet radiation and minimize the risk to babies and staff if a bulb should shatter.

Provision of natural lighting is highly dependent on the NICU locale. Ideally, each room where adults spend several hours at a time would have a window with an attractive view, allowing the eye to escape and orient to external conditions. In the northern hemisphere, windows that face north are optimal, because they will not transmit glare or heat gain. Windows facing other directions should be appropriately shaded, either with an external overhang or with internal louvers. If the ability to completely darken the room is desired, internal (within a triple-glazed window unit) electrically operated louvers are essential. Because even well-insulated external windows allow some heat gain or loss, these should be situated several feet away from any baby's bed position.

Noise Abatement

The initial design issue in making an NICU as quiet as possible is to eliminate or reduce as many sources of background noise as possible. Some NICUs are situated in noisy communities, which requires extra insulation in the external walls to minimize the impingement of outside sounds into the NICU. Airflow through the heating and cooling ducts also can produce considerable background noise in an NICU, but this can be reduced through appropriate sizing and baffling of the ducts. These issues must be addressed in the design process, because it is prohibitively expensive to correct a poor design after construction begins.

Traffic patterns also play a role in determining the level of noise to which babies and staff are exposed. To the greatest extent possible, traffic flow should be designed so that an echocardiogram, ultrasound, x-ray, or electroencephalographic technician can get to each baby's bedside as directly as possible, without wheeling the equipment past several other bed positions. As noted previously, support areas should be designed so that restocking functions can be accomplished without creating unnecessary bedside traffic.

Noise production also should be a prime consideration in design of the monitoring and communication systems and in the selection of equipment. Whenever possible, equipment should be selected with a noise criterion rating of less than 40. Based on available data for sound levels that do not interfere with newborn sleep or adult conversation, overall background noise levels in the NICU should be maintained below 55 decibels on the A-weighted slow response scale, with peak levels not in excess of 70 dB (10).

Once all unnecessary sources of sound are minimized, the next design consideration is the abatement of unavoidable sound such as voices, equipment noise, and anything that might disturb a sleeping baby. Here, there is no substitute for adequate space, and another cogent argument for individualized environments becomes apparent. Increasing the distance between beds will diminish noise transfer from one baby's bedside to another, as will higher ceilings, especially those that are angled to reflect sound laterally rather than back to the bedside. Obviously, floor, wall, and ceiling materials are crucial in this regard (see the next section, *Surface Finishes*).

Finally, care practices should be evaluated as part of the design process to see whether many sources of noise produced by the staff can be diminished or eliminated. Radios, pagers, rounds, and reports are examples of care practices that may create considerable noise at the bedside, and that can be modified or eliminated.

Surface Finishes

In the past, selection of surface finishes was given little attention in NICU design, which focused primarily on integration of the newest technology. The choice of wall, ceiling, and floor finishes is important, however, for reasons of aesthetics, noise abatement, and infection control.

Perhaps the most controversial design issue in this regard is the choice between carpet and hard flooring. Hard flooring (usually a vinyl composite) is easily cleaned, durable, and provides little resistance to wheeled equipment. Carpeting provides noise abatement and may be more attractive and more comfortable to those who are on their feet for several hours a day. The differences between these two choices have started to blur in recent years, as carpet has become more durable and cleanable, and hard flooring has become more resilient and sound absorbent. It seems clear that vinyl or rubber flooring is the ideal for isolation, procedure, and clean and soiled utility areas and around sinks. Carpeting may be desirable for other areas; the direct patient care area is where this question remains most controversial. Carpet, however, has a significantly higher replacement factor and the hospital administration must demonstrate a commitment to the greater maintenance required to keep it clean.

Wall finishes increasingly include quilts or soft sculpture to provide aesthetic and sound-absorbent qualities. Extensive use of highly durable railings or moldings is necessary throughout the NICU, as walls are easily damaged by portable equipment.

Ceiling materials should be designated with a noise reduction coefficient (NRC) of at least 0.90. Many states are now allowing the use of certain types of nonfriable acoustical ceiling tile that helps with noise abatement. The method of cleaning the ceiling and changing lights should be considered in the design process so that this can be accomplished with minimal disruption to patient care.

Infection Control Considerations

As noted previously, an infection control practitioner will be an important member of the design team during the discussion of the layout of the NICU and the choice of surface finishes. In addition, they will be helpful in discussing air quality issues in design of the heating and cooling system. They also will be very interested in the location and design of hand washing areas.

Sinks should be readily accessible throughout the NICU, within a few steps of any bedside. They should be large and deep, so that a full surgical scrub can be performed with minimal splatter, and the walls and floor surrounding them should be covered with easily cleanable surfaces. Porcelain sinks generally are more attractive and quieter in use than stainless steel. Faucets should operate hands-free; and soap, hand-drying supplies, and large trash receptacles should be easily accessible. These should be designed to avoid cross-contamination, to be easily cleanable, and to minimize noise production. At least some sinks should be provided for children and individuals with handicaps. Signage above each sink should contain written and pictorial hand-washing instructions. A convenient space for waterless hand-cleaning solutions should also be available at each bedside.

Headwalls

The area surrounding the baby's bedside, containing service outlets, shelving, and bedside storage, is commonly referred to as the "headwall." It is the focal point for creating a self-contained workstation at each bedside. This area must be easily adaptable to changes in census and acuity and to future changes in care practices. It must support and provide easy access to necessary equipment and supplies, as well as to the baby. The headwall design also should contain a comfortable working area for the staff and provide space for the family to personalize the baby's surroundings. There are several vendors that supply headwall systems, or these can be built on site, using either moveable or fixed-rail systems that can be customized for local equipment and practices.

A complete headwall system might include the following items and capabilities:

- Dimmer (rheostat)-controlled task lighting
- Three oxygen ports
- Three compressed air ports
- Three vacuum ports
- Twenty to 30 electrical outlets
- Telephone jack
- Computer terminal jack

Consideration also should be given to allowing space for future needs.

All electrical, vacuum, and gas outlets need to be simultaneously and conveniently accessible, that is, usage of one outlet cannot obstruct other outlets, even when equipment contains oversized plugs. Some electrical outlets should provide normal power, whereas others should be on emergency power, because either system could be temporarily incapacitated.

A fixed or moveable shelf to contain monitoring equipment should be located as near to eye level as possible and within easy reach. A countertop should be provided as a work surface, with at least 24 cubic feet of cabinet space below to hold supplies. Raceways within this cabinetry to hold wiring and gas lines can minimize the danger and unattractiveness of a clutter of cords, but should be easily accessible for repairs or modifications. Support beams should be placed to avoid visual obstruction or access problems. A ledge at the base of the headwall will prevent moveable equipment, such as incubators or warmers, from damaging the wall.

Heating and Cooling Systems

Heating, ventilation, and air conditioning (HVAC) is perhaps the most mundane segment of NICU design, and the one in which most members of the design team feel they have the least expertise; yet it is important to consider for several reasons. We have previously discussed the contribution HVAC makes to background noise in the NICU, a problem that is amenable to some design considerations. The number of air changes per hour needs to be specified for the patient care area in general, and for the isolation and procedure areas in particular; minimums usually are dictated by state code. In the case of the isolation area(s) and soiled utility room, a negative air pressure design, with 100% of the air exhausted to the outside, is imperative. In all cases, a high-efficiency filtering system is needed to remove particulate matter from the air.

Control of temperature and humidity is particularly important when designing the HVAC system for an NICU. The system should be able to maintain ambient temperature in the NICU between 72 and 78 degrees Fahrenheit throughout the year, even at the extremes of outside temperatures for that particular locale. A relative humidity of 30% to 60% should be maintained as well, again, even at local extremes externally. Maintaining temperature and humidity within these guidelines will minimize heat and water loss for the babies and discomfort for the staff.

Delivery of airflow into the unit requires considerable forethought. Return ducts should be situated near the floor so that particulate matter is not carried upward. Supply ducts should be located where drafts will not be a problem and should be generous in number, so that high-velocity air flow is avoided. Placement of supply ducts near external walls and windows should be carefully planned to avoid condensation and to minimize convective heat loss or gain to the babies nearby. The fresh air intake into the hospital HVAC system should be planned carefully to avoid areas that will contain exhaust fumes from vehicles, nearby buildings, or from the hospital itself.

Communication Systems

Communication systems comprise, perhaps, the segment of NICU design that requires the greatest anticipation of future developments. It is likely that communication patterns among NICU staff, and between the NICU and other support areas of the hospital (e.g., laboratory, radiology, and pharmacy), will change dramatically in the next decade. Likewise, information transfer among infant monitoring devices, the staff, and the medical record will accelerate rapidly in the same time frame. Because unit design and construction typically take several years, lack of foresight in this area can be inconvenient at best and often quite expensive.

Those planning an NICU should anticipate digital transfer of virtually all information. It is likely that the entire medical record will be computerized, and work areas within the patient care area should be designed accordingly, with adequate space to add terminals. Ergonomics and lighting should be considered, so that staff can work at these terminals with minimal strain. Monitoring systems will be interfaced with all the equipment supporting the baby, such as the incubator, ventilator, and intravenous pumps, and then with the patient chart. This will allow the obvious benefit of making data acquisition faster and more accurate, and it will provide new alternatives for patient alarm systems. At present, most NICUs depend on audible alarms to alert staff that a baby needs attention; but, in the future, these alarms can be transmitted digitally to the staff via headsets, pagers, or other devices that will not add to the noise of the unit.

Telephone and intercom systems also will change drastically with newer technology. Much of the noise generated in the NICU is because of these devices, but alternatives already exist, such as wireless headsets, which allow communication to occur very efficiently without adding to noise levels. These systems also will facilitate communication among staff in the multiple room arrangement used in most NICUs currently being constructed. Because using these systems requires a considerable adjustment in the local culture of the NICU, the design process should include discussion with end users so that the system chosen will address their needs and concerns.

Maintenance Issues

Many NICU designs that looked good in the blueprint stage have required major revisions soon after construction because maintenance issues were not considered adequately. The choice of carpeting, lighting systems, HVAC design, computer devices, and bedside equipment should not be finalized until maintenance problems are identified fully with those who will be responsible for their upkeep. Many of these devices or systems cost more to maintain than to buy, so the economic perspective also should be considered carefully over the anticipated 15- to 20-year lifespan of the NICU, as well as the extent to which routine or unanticipated maintenance will interfere with patient care.

Designing for Renovations

Unless the pace of change slows dramatically, all NICUs will be faced with the desire to upgrade their facility every few years. Many of the suggestions (listed previously) are practical to implement without a major building program (e.g., reduced ambient lighting; some noise control measures; better, more welcoming signage). Others can be accomplished through a renovation-in-place project (e.g., adding carpeting, wall hangings, and acoustical tile; providing more rooming-in space for families), but some will be impossible without new construction and significant increases in available floor space. In the course of a new construction project, it will be impossible to anticipate all the changes that might occur in neonatal care and technology over the next 20 years, but a couple of general principles should be kept in mind.

First, there is no substitute for adequate space. The square footage needed for state-of-the-art NICU care has increased relentlessly, yet is still less per patient than that allotted to pediatric or adult ICUs in virtually all hospitals. Most NICU new construction projects completed in the last 20 years have been forced to accept reductions in floor space from the ideal for fiscal considerations, which often proved to be short sighted, as renovations were required only a few years later. It is hard to imagine new developments that would reduce the floor space requirements for NICUs, but it is easy to suggest those that might increase them, such as increased parental access and continued development of new technology to improve monitoring, diagnosis, and thereby survival and outcome of extremely low-birth-weight infants.

Second, we are in the midst of a dramatic transition from the NICU as a high-tech, sterile (in every sense of the word) environment, to one that resembles a baby's bedroom, with all the implications that carries for parental access. This does not mean technology will disappear, or that many bedsides will not continue to resemble an operating room setup. It does suggest that this latter situation should be the exception, and that NICU design teams will need to consider the norm to be an area where each baby is surrounded by its family and a nurturing environment.

EQUIPMENT SELECTION

Equipment selection is an integral part of the planning process, whether for renovation or new construction. It is important to recognize that equipment features change rapidly and that, with the advance of technology, specific plans for space allocation and cost must be easily modifiable. Categories of equipment that will need to be specified include:

- Environmental (incubators, radiant warmers)
- Life support (ventilators, extracorporeal membrane oxygenation, nitric oxide systems)
- Monitors
- Diagnostic (x-ray, ultrasound, electronic scales)
- Treatment (infusion pumps, phototherapy, suction, chest percussion)
- Communications (telephone, computer terminals, printers)
- General support (breast milk, pharmacy refrigerators)

All users, as well as consultants familiar with the process of equipment inventory, planning, procurement, and installation, and with maintenance of the equipment, should be part of the planning team.

The first step of the equipment selection process involves preparing a list of all fixed and portable equipment that will be needed. Next, existing equipment should be evaluated to determine which items can be used in the newly constructed NICU. At this point, dimensions and general space and equipment-mounting requirements should be transmitted to the design team so that design of the patient care and storage areas can proceed while decisions are being made regarding purchase of new equipment.

The choice and procurement of new equipment is itself a several-step process. After deciding exactly what equipment will be needed and the budget available, the selection team should become familiar with options available in the market. If a considerable amount of new equipment is anticipated, it is wise to organize an exhibitors' day where all the major vendors can demonstrate their products to the largest number of staff possible. Alternatively, most large medical and nursing conferences have displays by the major vendors.

When evaluating a new product, considerations should include ease of use, durability, ease of maintenance, the ability to interface easily with computer and monitor systems, hazards such as noise and electromagnetic radiation, size and portability, ability to upgrade, and cost. After all this information is gathered, the equipment consultant should organize it into a report that can be given to all interested parties (users, maintenance, and procurement staff) for comment. Procurement then can proceed with a request for bids, and a final purchasing decision can be made when these are available. A delivery schedule should be developed in coordination with the design and construction teams so that equipment will arrive in sufficient time to be assembled, tested, and installed before the NICU opens, but not so far in advance that upgrades and modifications in the technology occur while the equipment is sitting in storage.

After selecting the equipment, the financial planning team will need to consider decisions regarding purchase versus lease and service contracts on each item. Although many hospitals have standing policies for such decisions, certain factors may still be worth reviewing. If a piece of equipment is a newer model of an item from a manufacturer with which the hospital has had considerable experience, the biomedical maintenance department may feel quite comfortable with assuming the responsibility for repair without the benefit of a service contract, and purchase of the item usually will be less expensive than leasing in the long run (although the chief financial officer should confirm this based on the specific terms offered). However, if the piece of equipment is an entirely new device and only one or two are being acquired, lease or purchase with a service contract has considerable value in that repairs will be made by experienced technicians, and faulty equipment may be replaced more readily. In either case, the hospital should have a very clear understanding of how quickly service will be available, and whether replacement items will be immediately available if repairs cannot be made promptly, especially if the equipment is crucial to the management of a critically ill child. These commitments should be obtained in writing, and their reliability confirmed by calling other units currently using similar equipment from each manufacturer.

Before installation occurs, the equipment consultant should review architectural, mechanical, electrical, and plumbing drawings to ensure that all specifications are current and compatible with the equipment that has been selected. There is nothing more frustrating than trying to install a piece of equipment that does not fit or has inadequate electrical or plumbing support. There are also many human dynamics that are crucial to this process, and the equipment consultant must be able to work with each of the specialists involved and organize a process that will be well structured and successfully implemented. Again, the construction of a full-sized, functional mockup of a patient care area should be considered as part of this process before final approval of the blueprints.

REVIEW AND APPROVAL PROCESS

After several months of planning, the architects will review the completed plans with the design team for final comment and approval. The hospital administration will be asked to sign off on a series of construction documents before submitting them to contractors for bids. Although it is common knowledge to architects and construction managers, many members of the design team may be unaware that changes after this time usually are expensive and sometimes impossible. A design that has considerable flexibility built in will become an obvious benefit, so that interim changes in care practices or equipment can be accommodated easily. When bids on the project are received, however, some major changes may still be required, because financial projections by the architects are, of necessity in such one-of-a-kind projects, only rough estimates. Sometimes compromises are fairly straightforward, such as:

- If aisles were generously sized, a reduction in all aisle widths by 1 foot might save tens of thousands of dollars.
- Bed positions might be reduced in number or size.
- Offices and conference areas might be reduced in size, shared with adjacent units, or redesigned as flexible-use spaces.

The mission statement developed at the beginning of the planning process provides an important point of reference here. If compromises appear to be required that would make accomplishing that mission and the accompanying goals and objectives difficult or impossible, it may be more appropriate to revise the budget rather than the design or (particularly in areas that already have high-quality neonatal providers) to reconsider the project's feasibility altogether.

Before finalizing the blueprints, the design team should spend one more session exploring all the possible sources of unanticipated problems. Any device or system that could break or malfunction should be reevaluated to see if a change in the design would minimize the impact of such an event. For example, is there anything in, or attached to, the ceiling that could break or come loose and fall on a baby? Is there any wiring, plumbing, or ductwork hidden in a wall for which access might be very difficult or disruptive? Is there any passageway that might be obstructed by a piece of equipment just when a resuscitation became necessary? Architects cannot anticipate all of these events, which usually are not discussed in the planning process, and staff have difficulty visualizing the impact of such events from looking at blueprints, so this process usually is best done with several members of each discipline committed to brainstorming together for several hours. This is another reason visits to other NICUs can be particularly valuable to one who is as interested in the flaws as well as the positive features of the design.

After a bid is accepted (a process that, like the choice of an architect, should be based not only on cost but on the extent and quality of the contractor's previous experience), a meeting should be held with the contractor and members of all the planning teams to be sure the construction team has "caught the vision" so carefully thought out over the previous months. Far from being simply contractors, the construction team can offer many helpful suggestions along the way if they understand the planning teams desires, especially with regard to specifics such as easily accessible wiring, minimizing noise generation from HVAC and plumbing supplies, and so forth. Walkthroughs should be performed regularly throughout the construction process, as multiple fine-tuning issues that were not anticipated in advance undoubtedly will occur. Any resulting changes from the architectural drawings should be documented carefully on "as is" drawings, so that future renovations are not hampered by unpleasant surprises.

HUMAN DYNAMICS CRUCIAL TO A SUCCESSFUL MOVE

In renovation projects, construction often must proceed in stages, while patient care continues to be provided in the existing unit. With either new construction or renovation, the implementation of new equipment and care practices can be both exciting and stressful, and it is not unusual for turnover of staff to increase around the time of the move. There are two contrasting strategies that have been used to ease the transition to a new unit. One school of thought suggests that introducing new equipment and practices to the greatest extent possible before the move is valuable to minimize the culture shock of transition. An alternative strategy is based on the concept that acceptance of new practices is most successful when undertaken wholesale, especially if some issues that are anxiety provoking (e.g., increased access for families) are balanced by others about which the staff will be excited (more space, better equipment). In practice, the transition period requires belief of both philosophies, because some changes may not be possible until the new unit is built (e.g., rooming in for parents), whereas others will be desirable to implement as soon as possible (e.g., a new ventilator).

Certainly the most important strategy in this regard is to integrate the staff as fully as possible into the planning, design, and construction process. The staff must understand and buy into the conceptual changes intended by the mission statement and around which the design process proceeded. Attendance at committee meetings and posting blueprints are helpful in this regard, especially if comments are encouraged and used. Additionally, working with a full-scale mockup of a patient care area and occasional visits to the construction site are very helpful to those who have difficulty visualizing two-dimensional renderings.

CHANGE-IN-PLACE

The final step of any NICU construction is a commitment to "change-in-place." We are just beginning to understand the biological effects of the environment on premature infants, especially the positive and negative effects of light, sound, touch, movement, and smell at each gestation stage. Likewise, a better recognition of the role of parents and staff in the care and nurture of their babies will lead to improved care practices, and technological improvements are sure to continue. Each of these trends will influence our concept of the optimal NICU design and should be incorporated to the greatest extent possible on an ongoing basis within an existing structure, rather than waiting until new construction again becomes feasible. An agreement by all members of the planning process that the NICU will be considered a work in progress, rather than a finished edifice, will enhance the readiness of all disciplines to implement change when the need becomes apparent and will drive the design teams to build in as much flexibility as possible.

REFERENCES

1. Gilstrap LC, Oh W, eds. *Guidelines for perinatal care*, 5th ed. Elk Grove Village, IL: American Academy of Pediatrics, 2002.
2. Recommended standards for newborn ICU design. *J Perinatol* 2003;23:S3–S21.
3. American Institute of Architects Academy of Architecture for Health. *Guidelines for design and construction of hospital and health care facilities.* Washington, DC: The American Institute of Architects, 2001.
4. White RD (ed). The sensory environment of the MCU: scientific and design-related aspects. *Clin Perinatol* 2004;31:199–393.
5. White RD. Enhanced neonatal intensive care design: a physiological approach. *J Perinatol* 1996;16:381–384.
6. Pediatrix University, NICU Design Center Section. Available online at http://www.natalu.com.
7. Bullough J, Rea MS. Lighting for neonatal intensive care units: some critical information for design. *Lighting Res Technol* 1996; 28:189.
8. White RD. Individual rooms in the NICU—an evolving concept. *J Perinatol* 2003;23:S22–S24.
9. Rea MS, ed. *The IESNA lighting handbook*, 9th ed. New York: Illuminating Engineering Society of North America, 2000.
10. Philbin K, Graven S, Robertson A. The influence of auditory experience on the fetus, newborn, and preterm infant: report of the sound study group of the national resource center. *J Perinatol* 2000;20:S1–S142.

Organization of Care and Quality in the NICU

Richard Powers   Carolyn Houska Lund

Providing current, research-based care to critically ill newborns requires the collaboration of highly skilled, dedicated, and motivated caregivers from a variety of disciplines. Professional nurses, physicians, respiratory therapists, social workers, developmental care specialists, pharmacists, clinical dieticians, and occupational and physical therapists have roles to play in planning, implementing, and evaluating care for infants and their families in the neonatal intensive care unit (NICU). This chapter includes a brief review of the basic organization and components of the NICU. An in-depth discussion of quality improvement is presented, including the systems to monitor and improve the quality of care in the NICU. These systems involve all professional disciplines and are integral in providing care to high-risk infants.

ORGANIZATION OF CARE

The organization of care in the NICU includes the medical staff working in collaboration with nursing and other departments in the care of patients in the NICU. Decisions about delivery of care, unit philosophy, and future directions are best made through this collaborative process rather than by any one department or discipline.

However, most NICUs are organized structurally and financially around the nursing component. The organization and functioning of a NICU is dependent on nursing leadership that can provide knowledgeable support and nursing input for the following functions: strategic planning, budget development and implementation, staff development, education, quality assurance and improvement, interdepartmental collaboration, and clinical standards development.

Nursing leadership is provided by nurses with advanced education, training, and experience in the following roles: nurse manager, clinical nurse specialist (CNS), neonatal nurse practitioner (NNP), nurse educator, transport or extracorporeal membrane oxygenation (ECMO) coordinator, and case manager. Depending on the size and complexity of the NICU, some of these roles may be combined.

Caregivers who work in the NICU require emotional support because of the high stress and sensitive nature of their work with critically ill infants and families. The nursing leadership group actively seeks out situations that are stressful to staff and provides support to staff through stress debriefing and staff case conferences. Referrals to hospital ethics committees and appropriate professionals such as psychologists, psychiatric nurse liaisons, chaplains, and employee assistance programs should be made early to assist staff when needed.

Nurse Manager

The nurse manager has overall responsibility for the day-to-day operation of the NICU and for coordinating and collaborating with the medical staff, other department directors, and nursing managers from other units. The manager is usually expected to plan and implement both capital and operations budgets. Further, the manager works with the nursing leadership team to ensure that education, ongoing development, and competency of the nursing staff are attained. The nursing leadership group, in collaboration with the medical team and ancillary disciplines, is also responsible for assuring that the quality of care delivered in the NICU is safe and appropriate, meets regulatory standards, and demonstrates a commitment to ongoing quality improvement.

Although the nurse manager and nursing leadership group are accountable for the care delivered in the NICU, the staff nurses are the keystones of care delivery. Therefore, facilitating staff participation at every level of decision making is critical to the success of any unit operations. In some units, this collaboration may be formalized through a system of shared governance in which staff nurses are empowered to govern many aspects of unit operations. However, even in more traditional organizational structures, participation by staff is critical to the successful operation of the unit.

Advanced-practice Nurses

The CNS is an advanced practice nurse at the master's degree level. In a nonline position in the nursing structure, the CNS generally has no direct authority over other staff. The CNS role involves direct clinical care, consultation to nursing staff and other professionals, and education of staff and parents. Research is a component of the CNS role, and this is accomplished by keeping abreast of current research applicable to neonatal care, implementing research-based practices, supporting and facilitating research efforts in the NICU, and participating in research studies as primary investigator or co-investigator. Maintaining quality of care is another aspect of CNS practice; monitoring care practices, identifying problems, and participating in the NICU multidisciplinary practice committee are essential aspects of the CNS role and its effective implementation in the NICU (1).

Many units use the CNS in case management functions. Case management, a model of care delivery, focuses on multidisciplinary care throughout hospitalization to achieve desired patient outcomes in an expected time frame and with efficient use of resources (2,3). Within this model, the CNS follows a caseload of patients throughout their lengths of stay in the NICU, consulting with nursing staff, physicians, and other team members about the patients' expected courses and any variations that occur. The CNS coordinates the interdisciplinary model through weekly interdisciplinary rounds to discuss medical and social aspects of care for each infant in the NICU and identify needed interventions, procedures, or family communication. The CNS may identify a need for individual patient care conferences during which medical staff, nurses, and specialty consultants discuss a complicated patient and establish reasonable goals with evaluation criteria.

The NNP has formal education and certification in the medical management of high-risk newborns. NNPs generally carry a caseload of neonatal patients with consultation, collaboration, and supervision from a neonatologist. With extensive knowledge of physiology, pathophysiology, and pharmacology, the NNP functions both independently and interdependently with physicians in the assessment, diagnosis, and implementation of specific medical practices and procedures. Other responsibilities may include delivery room resuscitation, stabilization and transport either within the hospital or to other facilities, education, consultation, and research at varying levels (1,4,5). In addition to advanced-practice nurses, other nursing roles include neonatal clinical educators, outreach educators, transport nurses, discharge planners, nursing shift coordinators, and ECMO specialists.

The role of the charge nurse in the NICU is an important leadership position in the daily operations of the unit. Charge nurses may be nurse managers, shift coordinators, or experienced staff nurses responsible for the smooth functioning of the unit during each shift in a 24-hour day. Among their responsibilities are evaluating the number and level of acuity of all infants to determine the number of nursing and support staff required, and communicating the assignments of patients and staff. Charge nurses also arrange incoming and outgoing transports and may, in some settings, attend high-risk deliveries. They are often the "extra pair of hands" needed during emergency situations or special procedures, are consulted by other nurses in problem situations and conflict resolution, and become involved in crisis intervention with families. Astute assessment and problem-solving skills, along with excellent communication abilities, are necessary in the successful implementation of the charge nurse role and the daily running of the NICU.

Staff nurses help families in their adaptation to and resolution of crisis by providing consistency in the delivery of daily nursing care. Infants are regularly assigned to a nurse or a group of nurses on admission or shortly thereafter, and consistent care is delivered by this primary nurse or primary team throughout the hospital course.

Primary nurses provide direct patient care, organize and write individual care plans, and collaborate with the neonatologist, social worker, and advanced-practice nurse to facilitate the smooth transition of the infant throughout the hospital stay and discharge from the NICU. They have extensive knowledge about the individual responses of patients for whom they care on a daily basis and are invaluable to the neonatologist and other team members. Primary nursing care lends itself well to the developmental care that is specific in both assessment and interventions aimed at the individual needs and unique characteristics of neonatal patients.

Primary nursing is highly valued by families of infants in the NICU. Seeing the same person caring for their infant is comforting and establishes trust during this period of crisis and disequilibrium for families. Families often share their feelings and reactions with someone they have come to know and trust; this is often the primary nurse.

Other essential roles are necessary for the safe and effective functioning of the NICU. Respiratory specialists provide expertise in the NICU in areas of pulmonary care and assisted ventilation. Clinical dieticians consult regularly for both parenteral and enteral nutrition issues. Pharmacists assist regarding the safe and appropriate use of the multitude of medications administered in the NICU, as well as monitoring for adverse drug reactions and side effects. Developmental specialists, along with occupational and physical therapists, are responsible for the integration of developmentally appropriate interventions for specific infants, as well as educating other team members about developmental care and assisting in environmental modifications which can improve patient comfort and possibly even outcomes. Social workers assist in crisis intervention and provide psychosocial assessment and emotional support as they advocate for the wide range of families that encounter the NICU experience. In culturally diverse settings, translators are indispensable in the NICU to ensure that information is accurately provided to families.

Family-centered Care

The initial phase of hospitalization for high-risk infants results in significant disequilibrium for families. The expected outcome of their pregnancy has been changed from a healthy, full-term newborn to a premature newborn or a newborn with significant medical or surgical problems. With prenatal detection of problems, as well as perinatal care for premature labor, the families may have some idea of the situation they are facing. Yet, many have not faced a crisis of such importance and may need help in developing coping skills, understanding complicated medical information, and learning how to be an advocate for their infant. Nurses use therapeutic communication, crisis intervention, and supportive techniques to assist families during this time (6).

Because many families may have additional social risk factors, including language or cultural differences, poverty, chronic illness, or substance abuse, knowledge about the impact of these factors on coping with crises and parenting is needed. The importance of early intervention cannot be emphasized strongly enough, and interventions by neonatal nurses along with NICU social workers and neonatologists can have considerable positive effects for high-risk families during this time of disequilibrium.

Family-centered care is both a philosophy and approach to care that can enhance the potential of families to cope with the crisis and experience a positive outcome. Principles for family-centered neonatal care include open and honest communication in both medical and ethical considerations, providing in-depth medical information in terms that are meaningful, and accessibility to other parents who have had infants in similar circumstances. Information is provided to families early if neonatal problems are diagnosed prenatally. Parents are allowed to make decisions for their infants about aggressive treatments once they are fully informed with adequate medical knowledge. Additional areas addressed in family-centered care are alleviation of pain, ensuring an appropriate environment, providing safe and effective treatments, and policies and programs that promote parenting skills and maximum involvement of families with their infants in the NICU (7–9). Key elements of family-centered care are outlined in Table 7-1.

Parent and family education are necessary throughout the hospitalization in the NICU. Initially parents need information about their infant's medical condition and what the prognosis is, as well as an introduction to the NICU personnel they encounter ("who does what"). Pamphlets and booklets about premature infants or specific disease conditions may be helpful. There are also several books written by parents or NICU professionals that contain detailed information, illustrations, and accounts of other parents' reactions to the experience in the NICU (10,11). The Internet is another source of information for parents. Each unit should wisely evaluate which resources on the Internet contain the most up-to-date, factual, nonbiased information about specific conditions and post these resources for parents to access if they wish. Although written information is valuable, it is not a substitution for conferences and verbal interchange with parents. These conferences are focused on what the professional staff expects that the family needs to hear, what the parents are concerned about, and the parents' feelings and reactions to what is happening to them and their infant. Nurses can help parents become involved in the physical care of their

TABLE 7-1
THE KEY ELEMENTS OF FAMILY-CENTERED CARE

Incorporating into policy and practice the recognition that the family is the constant in a child's life while the service systems and support personnel within those systems fluctuate.
Facilitating family/professional collaboration at all levels of hospital, home, and community care:
    Care of an individual child
    Program development, implementation, evaluation, and evolution
    Policy formation
Exchanging complete and unbiased information between families and professionals in a supportive manner at all times.
Incorporating into policy and practice the recognition and honoring of cultural diversity, strengths, and individuality within and across all families, including ethnic, racial, spiritual, social, economic, educational, and geographic diversity.
Recognizing and respecting different methods of coping and implementing comprehensive policies and programs that provide developmental, educational, emotional, environmental, and financial supports to meet the diverse needs of families.
Encouraging and facilitating family-to-family support and networking.
Ensuring that hospital, home, and community service and support systems for children needing specialized health and developmental care and their families are flexible, accessible, and comprehensive in responding to diverse family-identified needs.
Appreciating families as families and children as children, recognizing that they possess a wide range of strengths, concerns, emotions, and aspirations beyond their need for specialized health and developmental services and support.

(Reprinted from Shelton T, Stepanek JS. Family-centered care for children needing specialized health and development services. Bethesda: Association for the Care of Children's Health, 1994, with permission.)

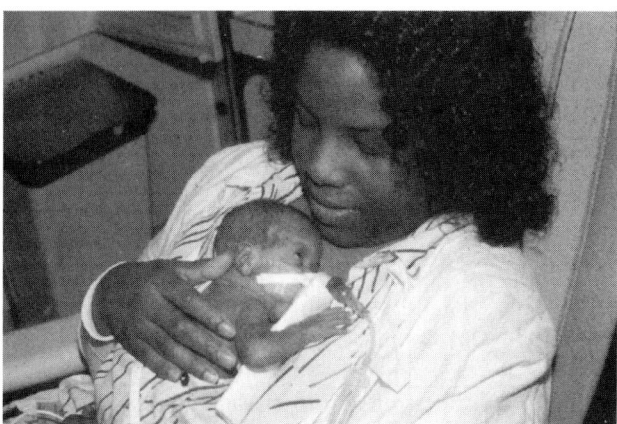

Figure 7-1 Photo of a mother holding her ventilated preemie skin to skin.

infant by showing them the things they can do such as comfort measures, bathing, skin or mouth care, changing diapers, taking the temperature, holding as soon as their infant is stable on the ventilator or oxygen (Fig. 7-1), and providing breast milk.

Discharge teaching is an important aspect of family-centered care. This includes well-baby care with knowledge about specific patterns of feeding, sleeping, urination, stooling, breathing, skin care, and appropriate use of infant car seats. Teaching about medication administration, including the purpose, method of administration, side effects, and where to obtain the medications, is essential. Special needs are described and skills taught, including gavage or gastrostomy feeding, oxygen administration, ostomy care, tracheostomy care, cardiorespiratory monitoring, and others. Different disease processes or conditions are identified for parents, such as bronchopulmonary dysplasia, short-bowel syndrome, and hydrocephalus, and symptoms are identified for parents so they can assess and seek medical care appropriately after the infant is home (12,13).

QUALITY IN THE NEONATAL INTENSIVE CARE UNIT

The many disciplines and personnel described above provide the structure around the delivery of care in the NICU. However, to move beyond day-to-day care delivery and improve the quality of care, a sound knowledge base in quality improvement theory and practice is essential.

Background of Quality Improvement

Over the past decades, medicine has witnessed a rapid expansion of knowledge and technology. This expansion has occurred in parallel with financial pressures brought on by inexorable increases in per capita costs of health care and limitations in financial resources available to the

health care system. These forces are especially applicable to intensive care subspecialties such as neonatology on which a significant amount of research and technology is focused and for which delivery of care can be extremely costly.

Research in the form of randomized controlled trials (RCTs) has become the "gold standard" for evaluating the efficacy of health care interventions. In 1966, about 100 articles were published annually in all fields of medicine from RCTs; by 1995, more than 10,000 were published (14). More than 3,000 articles about neonatology RCTs have been published alone (15).

In the face of this avalanche of information on clinical efficacy and rapid infusion of technology driven by the computer and pharmaceutical industries, health care workers and institutions have major challenges before them. Individuals in health care organizations need to efficiently evaluate new interventions and adopt the most compelling ones in a timely manner to provide optimal patient care and avoid preventable complications. It is through the principles of quality improvement, along with organizational adaptability, that continuous integration of research, technology, and improved patient care outcomes is accomplished.

Quality of care is defined by the Institute of Medicine as "the degree to which health services for individuals and populations increase the likelihood of desired health outcomes and are consistent with current professional knowledge" (16). This definition, first proposed in 1990, has become widely accepted and is still considered the best definition of health care quality today. The concept of "health services for individuals and populations" is especially important in neonatology where evaluation is often determined by population data such as infant and neonatal mortality rates or the incidence of neurological deficits among a specific subgroup such as extremely low-birth-weight survivors.

The definition also emphasizes that quality care "increases the likelihood" of beneficial outcomes, a reminder that quality is not merely the achievement of positive outcomes. Poor outcomes occur despite excellent care because diseases vary in severity and can defeat even the best efforts. Conversely, patients may do well despite poor quality of care. Assessing quality thus requires attention to both processes and outcomes of care. The last part of the definition of quality, "consistent with current knowledge" highlights the dynamic and evolving body of knowledge available to health care professionals and the need to revise and update measures of quality as new interventions become standards of care.

Problems in quality of health care can be classified in three categories: underuse, overuse, and misuse (14). Underuse is the failure to provide a health care service when it would have produced a favorable outcome. For example, failure to provide surfactant in a timely manner after the delivery of an extremely low-birth-weight infant with respiratory distress syndrome would indicate underuse. Overuse occurs when a health care service is provided despite the fact that its potential for harm exceeds its possible benefit.

The widespread use of postnatal steroids for chronic lung disease popular in the 1990s is an example of overuse in neonatology. Misuse occurs when a preventable complication arises during administration of an appropriately selected treatment. Misuse includes many of the common medical errors that occur during hospitalization or other health care encounters. Medical errors have been extensively discussed (17,18), driving numerous initiatives by the United States (U.S.) government and regulatory agencies aimed at understanding the human and systems factors that contribute to the errors. External reporting systems that collect information on adverse events and errors are important in the reduction of future errors by alerting practitioners to new hazards, using the experience of individual hospitals using new methods to prevent errors, and revealing trends that require attention (19). In neonatology, medical errors have been collated and classified as part of an anonymous error-reporting project in conjunction with the NIC/Q Quality Improvement Collaborative of the Vermont Oxford Network (Table 7-2) (20).

Regulatory agencies, in conjunction with federal and state governments, have traditionally been charged with the task of motivating health care professionals and organizations to maintain and improve quality. The Joint Commission on Accreditation of Healthcare Organizations, formed in 1951, initially developed standards for hospitals and evaluated compliance to these standards, hypothesizing that compliance with these standards would correlate with quality care and positive outcomes for patients in hospitals. In accreditation, quality is evaluated by monitoring adherence to accepted standards and measuring outcomes. Standards used by accreditation organizations are derived from a variety of sources, including government (via regulatory agencies at both the federal and state levels), as well as professional and community-based, standards of practice.

Regulation is for the most part successful in establishing minimal standards of performance and is an important means of protecting the public from egregiously poor providers. It has, however, numerous limitations. Standards are difficult to enforce uniformly, and regulation tends to be inflexible with difficulty in adapting quickly as knowledge changes. Regulation also fails to stimulate organizations to integrate new technologies or developments and does not motivate them to continuously improve. Continuous quality improvement (CQI) can supplement the deficiencies of regulation alone, while providing an impetus for individuals and organizations to strive for the highest quality of care.

Continuous Quality Improvement

CQI emerges from the industrial sector as an effective system to reduce errors in production. It motivates good performers to excel, emphasizes identification of potentially successful change opportunities, and facilitates change implementation throughout all levels of the organization. CQI provides the framework for organizations to keep abreast of current knowledge and innovations, identify appropriate changes, and implement them in a timely manner. There are three components to CQI: measurement, benchmarking, and collaboration.

Measurement

The first and most basic element of CQI is the acquisition of data. Data acquisition drives information, which in turn drives action. Over the past 25 years, numerous systems of quality measurement have been developed, encompassing the areas of outcomes, processes, and patient satisfaction.

Outcome measures represent the most objective and often the most meaningful data for health care organizations. When applied to populations, outcome measures provide essential feedback to leaders charged with resource allocation, managers charged with developing successful and efficient organizations, and individual health care providers.

Due to variability in disease severity among patients from different socioeconomic and cultural backgrounds, as well as differences in the type of patients cared for in highly specialized tertiary centers compared to community health facilities, data based on outcomes alone can be inaccurate or misleading. Process measures are also important in evaluating overall quality. Measures of process are needed to determine that accepted standards of care are being met regardless of good or bad outcomes.

TABLE 7-2

CLASSIFICATION OF MEDICAL ERRORS IN NEONATOLOGY (20)

Error Classification	Percent of Errors
Wrong medication/dose/schedule/infusion rate	53.4%
Error in performance of operation, procedure or test	12%
Patient misidentification	7.8%
Error in administration or method of using a treatment	7%
Error or delay in diagnosis	4.7%
Equipment failure	2.3%
Failure of communication	1.3%
Other system failure	6.7%

TABLE 7-3
TYPICAL QUALITY IMPROVEMENT MEASURES

Process measures
Intrapartum antibiotics for mothers with positive group B strep
  cultures
Intrapartum antibiotics for mothers with group B strep risk factors
Antenatal steroid use
Admission temperature
Postnatal steroid use
Surfactant administration
Incidence of hypocarbia (PaCO$_2$ <30)

Outcome measures
Mean 1-minute and 5-minute Apgar scores
Survival rate
Length of stay
Incidence of chronic lung disease
Incidence retinopathy of prematurity
Incidence of intraventricular hemorrhage
Nosocomial infection rate

Patient satisfaction measures[a]
Comfort of facilities
Appearance of room
Nurses' attitudes toward requests
Facilities for family information provided
Doctor's concern for questions/worries

[a] From Press, Ganey Associates, Inc., South Bend, IN. 2002

A third category of measurement in assessing quality of care is patient and family satisfaction. This is the result of applying traditional marketing techniques to the health care industry, and it has accompanied the adoption of CQI principles from industry to health care. It is also a natural result of a larger movement throughout health care that recognizes the autonomy and accountability of the patient and family. As the health care community expands its expectations that patients and their families take on a larger part of the responsibility to maintain their own health and wellness, the feedback obtained from patients and families regarding their interaction with the health care system is crucial. Table 7-3 shows examples of neonatology quality measures in the three areas of outcomes, processes, and patient satisfaction.

Benchmarking: Use of Comparative Databases

The second step in the process of CQI is benchmarking of outcomes. Opportunities for benchmarking are numerous, thanks to the recognition in the past 15 years of the contribution it brings to CQI. A number of regional, national, and international databases have been organized in neonatology, providing benchmarking opportunities through voluntary participation and confidential reporting of individual center outcomes.

One of the first neonatology databases, and currently the largest, is the Vermont Oxford Neonatal (VON) Network. Started in 1990 with 36 hospitals, this network has grown to 380 centers (21,22). The network includes data on more than 25,000 very low-birth-weight (<1,500 g;

VLBW) infants each year, more than 50% of all VLBW infants born in the United States annually.

In the VON Network, centers report outcomes, including survival and lengths of stay for all VLBW infants admitted to the NICU. They also report incidence of chronic lung disease and complications, including nosocomial infection, pneumothorax, necrotizing enterocolitis, intraventricular hemorrhage, retinopathy of prematurity, and other conditions. All participating centers receive a confidential annual report showing their performance compared with the database as a whole. Each center can see how they rank with all other centers, and with centers that are grouped in similar categories by number and type of NICU admissions. In the VON Network, all of the variables are reported in aggregate form showing the mean incidence rate and highest and lowest quartile of each measure. The mortality rate and length of stay for each center is also adjusted for patient acuity.

Other databases have been formed at regional and national levels. The National Institute of Child Health and Development Neonatal Research Network provides a venue for participating institutions to submit outcome measures; their aggregate data has been published to serve as a reference for other centers to compare their performances. These include general survival and complication rates in VLBW infants (23,24) and rates of neurological abnormalities (25). The Canadian Neonatal Network has published reports tracking overall outcomes and complications in infants of all gestational ages (26–28). Other national networks include the Scottish Neonatal Consultants and Nurses Collaborative Study Group, New South Wales Neonatal Intensive Care Unit Study Group, and Paulista Collaborative Group on Neonatal Care in Brazil (29–31).

Variability in Neonatal Intensive Care Unit Outcomes

Variability in neonatal outcomes becomes apparent when data from multiple newborn intensive care units is analyzed in comparative databases. The VON data describing the first full year of the collaborative in 1990 showed a number of differences in outcomes among VLBW infants in the 36 reporting centers. These included the incidence of respiratory distress syndrome, pneumothorax, chronic lung disease, patent ductus arteriosus, nosocomial infection, intraventricular hemorrhage, and retinopathy of prematurity (22). The annual VON reports provide the distribution of outcomes among centers by ranking the data and calculating the 25th and 75th percentiles for mean incidence of the given outcome from each center. Percentile ranking of mean values from individual centers represents a simple and effective means of illustrating one center's ranking among the entire sample of participants. Table 7-4 shows the 2001 data from the VON database, illustrating this methodology for selected outcomes (32).

Investigators also report variation in outcomes as part of multicenter prospective interventional trials or retrospectively as multicenter independent research. Brodie and

TABLE 7-4

OUTCOMES AND INTERVENTIONS (VERMONT OXFORD NETWORK 2001, 32)

Outcome/Intervention	Percent	Interquartile Range (25th, 75th Percentile)
Respiratory distress syndrome	72	63,82
Pneumothorax	6	3,7
Oxygen use	90	86,96
Nasal CPAP use	60	60,73
Ventilation	71	63,80
Chronic lung disease	29	17,36
Patent ductus arteriosus	33	22,40
Necrotizing enterocolitis	6	2,8
Nosocomial infection	21	12,26
Intraventricular hemorrhage		
Grade 3	4	2,6
Grade 4	5	2,7
Retinopathy of prematurity		
Stage 3	10	5,13
Stage 4	1	0,0

CPAP, continuous positive air pressure.

associates (33) studied nosocomial bloodstream infections in VLBW infants in 6 NICUs in the Boston area from 1994 to 1996; mean incidence of infections was 19.1% for the whole group, but varied from 8.5% to 42% among the 6 units. After adjusting for patient- and treatment-related variables, significant variation persisted. Variations in blood transfusions among 6 perinatal centers in Massachusetts and Rhode Island were studied, showing a mean total transfused volume ranging from 95.5 mL/kg (highest) to 35.0 mL/kg (lowest) (34). Avery and associates (35) described the variability in incidence of chronic lung disease among 8 units surveyed. Later, an in-depth review of the practices related to respiratory support for infants with respiratory distress syndrome was undertaken at the 8 centers, triggering the study and dissemination of a number of innovations in respiratory care practices from the unit reporting the best outcome.

Wide variation in outcomes among centers is often found when centers participate in comparative outcome studies. Even when the data has been adjusted for confounding risk factors, marked variability still exists in many cases. Explanations for this persistent variation include differences in case mix, data quality, and case finding. However, the final and most important factor is often variation in effectiveness of clinical practice.

It can be extremely useful and important for units to recognize how clinical effectiveness contributes to variability, especially in areas where the outcomes for the unit are in the lowest quartile. One of the major benefits of participating in the comparative analyses of outcome measures lies in the understanding that changing clinical care practices truly can influence their outcomes. In most cases, individual units find outcomes in the lowest quartile for only a few variables of the data set, with the majority

falling within the interquartile range (25th–75th percentile) or even exceeding the 75th percentile. The lowest quartile outcomes provide target areas to which focused improvement efforts can be directed. Furthermore, centers in the database that report better outcomes can be used as resources to identify practices that may benefit centers in the lowest quartile.

Identification of benchmark data through concurrent measurement among centers represents only one model for benchmarking. Published data can also be used as a benchmark when concurrent data is not available. It is important to review the methodology and data definitions in the published benchmark paper to allow for consistency in data acquisition before any extrinsic comparison can be made. An example is the nosocomial infection rates published by the National Nosocomial Infection Surveillance project of the Centers for Disease Control which is used by many NICUs to analyze their infection prevalence (36).

Collaboration

The concept of institutions collaborating with each other for the purpose of improving overall quality of care is novel, yet essential, in successfully and efficiently changing health care. Comparative databases with institutions prospectively reporting outcomes to identify opportunities for improvement are an example of how collaboration can benefit organizations. Collaboration is equally important for implementing practices that enable institutions to adopt new technology and bring about improved methods of delivering care.

Collaboration among different and sometimes competing companies is found in industries outside of health care. For example, in the semiconductor manufacturing industry corporations must maintain the pace of technologic research and development to compete. Yet 10 of the largest U.S. semiconductor manufacturers, including Intel, Motorola, Advanced Micro Devices, and Texas Instruments, joined forces in the mid-1990s to form a company called Semanteck to foster mutual information and advancement (Austin, TX) (37).

This motivation to achieve common improvement goals among different organizations has led to the formation of numerous quality improvement collaboratives in health care. A number of factors serve as incentives to collaboration. First is the substantial gap that exists between current knowledge and the actual provision of care. Second, collaboration among institutions can accelerate the infusion of existing knowledge into practice by providing insight into how the centers with the best outcomes were able to implement systems that yielded these results. Despite abundant literature describing practices that should or should not be done, little is written about specific activities that facilitate implementing desired practices (37). Dialogue between units, as well as visits involving a multidisciplinary team from one unit to another, provides an exchange of ideas and solutions to clinical problems.

The Institute of Healthcare Improvement Breakthrough Series is an example of large collaboratives working to accomplish common aims, including reducing cesarean section rates, improving asthma care, reducing adverse drug events and others (38–40). The NIC/Q Collaboratives on Quality Improvement in Neonatology, organized by the VON, have identified the goal of improving neonatal outcomes in chronic lung disease, nosocomial infection, nutrition and other areas (22). The California Perinatal Quality Care Collaborative is a regional collaborative with the goal of improving perinatal care in California. It involves more than 100 NICUs throughout the state and brings, in addition to health care providers, representatives from state certification agencies and various business groups into the process. Through this diverse collaboration, goals with a broader definition of quality are identified.

During the collaborative process, the decision to adopt new interventions or evaluate existing practices is often encountered. A critical review of the available evidence supporting new interventions and clinical practices is essential. With the pace of development of new drugs and technology, the consistent and systematic evaluation of evidence supporting new interventions becomes a priority.

Evidence-based Medicine

Evidence-based medicine is defined as "the conscientious, explicit, and judicious use of current best evidence in making decisions about the care of individual patients" (41). In the context of continuous quality improvement, the definition is expanded beyond the individual patient to decisions regarding institutional guidelines and policies in the care of multiple patients with similar diagnoses. In both applications, the principles are the same: an answerable clinical question is formulated, the best evidence is located, and the evidence is critically appraised. These steps are essential whether answering a question regarding treatment for a VLBW infant with a patent ductus arteriosus or creating a policy for management of all VLBW admissions who develop the diagnosis of patent ductus arteriosus.

Randomized Controlled Trials

Randomized controlled trials (RCTs) represent the highest level of evidence and are the foundation for establishing effectiveness of interventions. The methodology of RCTs is geared to minimize selection bias by the random allocation of study subjects at the time of enrollment. This unique characteristic of the RCT establishes it as the basis for traditional statistical comparisons in both clinical and basic science research. Sound scientific methodology must also address other potential biases that can impact validity of the results. These include performance bias, or nonuniform exposure to the intervention; exclusion bias, or incomplete follow-up in obtaining postintervention data; and assessment bias, or inaccurate measurement of outcomes.

Metanalyses

Although RCTs are considered the best single methodology to evaluate an intervention, there are sometimes more than one RCT for a given intervention. RCTs can be combined using the technique of quantitative systematic review, or metanalysis. Pooling results of similar RCTs can increase the statistical power lacking in multiple small RCTs or provide more support for decision making when conflicting results are reported in separate studies on the same treatment. The techniques used in performing metanalysis are rigorous. The methodology of metanalysis has been formally outlined and includes 5 stages: (a) specify the objectives of the review, (b) identify and select studies, (c) assess validity, (d) combine results of independent studies, and (e) make inferences (15).

Objectives of the review must be clearly and succinctly stated at the outset, with a principle objective and often secondary objectives given. The strategy for identifying and selecting studies must also be clearly stated in the review. This addresses one of the most challenging issues in any search and analysis of available literature, publication bias. Publication bias refers to the tendency for investigators to preferentially submit studies with positive results and the tendency for editors to preferentially select studies with positive results for publication. Klassen and associates (42) report that only 59% of abstracts presented at meeting of the Society for Pediatric Research between 1992 and 1995 were subsequently published. Abstracts were more likely to be published as a full study if they reported good news about newer therapies. To document their rigor in minimizing publication bias, authors of metanalyses must include a prospectively designed search protocol, a comprehensive and explicit search strategy, and strict criteria for inclusion and exclusion of studies.

Validity of each study in the metanalysis must be determined independently, based on each study's merits and exclusion of bias in all areas. Results of multiple studies are usually combined based on their principle outcomes or measures of treatment effect. These are typically expressed using relative estimators, the relative risk or odds ratio, and absolute estimators, event rate difference or risk difference. Derived from the estimators are the relative risk reduction, computed as (1 – relative risk), and the number needed to treat, computed as (1/risk difference). For continuous outcome data measurements, the effect of treatment is measured as the mean difference. These outcomes are determined for individual trials in the metanalysis, and then computed for the entire systematic review using statistical methodology that weights each trial based on its population size. The statistical significance of a treatment effect is determined when the confidence interval of the combined estimate for relative risk or odds ratio does not include 1, or when the confidence interval for the risk difference or weighted mean difference does not include 0.

Estimates of treatment effect or lack of effect are much stronger in metanalyses in which there is less heterogeneity. Heterogeneity refers to the observation of large differences in point estimates among the included studies. The ability to make inferences from a metanalysis depends on the methodologic quality of the primary trials on which the review was based, degree of consistency of results among the trials contributing to the review, and degree of confidence that the search for all trials relevant to the review was comprehensive (15).

The quality of a metanalysis is dependent upon the rigor of the methodology applied by its authors. The process of metanalysis has its critics; attempts at pooling results from various studies not only incorporates the biases of the primary studies, but may add additional bias attributable to study selection and heterogeneity of the selected studies (43). In addition, pooling data from small studies not adequately powered cannot answer questions about the potential side effects of new therapies, as compared to larger RCTs.

Evidence-Grading Systems

Although RCTs and metanalyses of RCTs represent the best sources of evidence, such high-quality evidence is not always available. Multiple systems for grading the strength of evidence have evolved that account for sources other than RCTs. The majority of grading systems place the most value on inferences from a systematic review of RCTs, with evidence from an individual RCT second, followed by evidence from well-designed trials without randomization, evidence from nonexperimental studies and, finally, opinions of respected authorities or reports of expert committees (44). Sources that may not meet the gold standard of an RCT are nevertheless important when this gold standard is either not yet achieved or is not achievable. Numerous systems have been developed to rate the strength of evidence, targeting evidence from metanalyses down to the opinion of experts (45). Table 7-5 shows a summary of 2 typical evidence-grading systems (46,47).

Despite the obvious value of evidence provided by RCT and metanalyses, examples of other forms of validation can be found in collaborative processes. The Vermont Oxford Quality Improvement Collaborative for Neonatology reported that one of the most fundamental components in reducing nosocomial infection in the NICU observed

---

TABLE 7-5
EVIDENCE-GRADING SYSTEMS (45)

Grade	Description
	Agency for Healthcare Research and Quality (45)
I.	Metanalysis of multiple well-designed controlled studies
II.	At least one well-designed experimental study
III.	Well-designed, quasi-experimental studies, such as nonrandomized controlled, single-group, pro-post cohort, time series, or matched case-controlled studies
IV.	Well-designed, non-experimental studies, such as comparative and correlational descriptive and case studies.
V.	Case reports and clinical examples
	Canadian Task Force on the Periodic Health Examination (46,47)
I.	Metanalysis of multiple well-designed controlled studies
II-1.	Evidence obtained from well designed controlled trials without randomization
II-2.	Evidence obtained from well-designed cohort or case-control analytic studies, preferably from more than 1 center or research group
II-3.	Evidence obtained from multiple time series with or without intervention
III.	Opinions of respected authorities, based on clinical experience, descriptive studies or reports of expert committees

(Adapted from The periodic health examination. Canadian Task Force on the Periodic Health Examination. *CMAS* 1979;121:1193–1254; Strom KL. Quality improvement interventions: what works? *J Healthc Qual* 2001;23:4–14, with permission.)

consistently in "best-performing" units was staff account-ability for nosocomial infections (48). Implementation of this valuable insight was critical for collaborative partici-pants desiring to reduce infections in their individual units. Although not meeting the usual criteria for high-grade evidence since it has not been formally studied sci-entifically, this form of observational data nevertheless represents an important category of evidence, i.e. evidence gained from collaborative benchmarking.

In addition to determining the efficacy of a certain intervention, disease prevalence, complication rates, finan-cial impact of treatment versus the disease itself, and cost of implementation of the policy are all critical issues before implementation of evidence-based treatments. Many of the questions can be answered by a critical sys-tematic review of available studies. Decisions to implement an intervention for a population of patients should be thor-oughly researched and analyzed to account for case mix, variation over time, availability of subspecialty resources, and baseline complication rate. Although only somewhat relevant in an individual treatment decision, financial cost-effectiveness and feasibility are vital issues to be addressed in adopting policies on a unit-, institution-, or system-wide basis. Especially when financial and staff resources are lim-ited, the implementation of one costly intervention could preclude the implementation of other interventions with more impact for a greater number of patients.

As critical analysis of research and benchmarking allows an organization to identify specific processes to improve, the actual incorporation of change into the organization requires an approach unique to each separate organiza-tion. Implementation of change requires individual com-mitment and open mindedness, a multidisciplinary group culture that embraces new ideas, and an institutional envi-ronment established by the management structure that encourages new ideas.

Organizational Change and Unit Culture

Each organization has a culture that is unique, represent-ing the individuals and relationships that make up that organization. As Baker points out, "teams and organiza-tions that attempt to implement quality improvement often identify organizational culture as an important bar-rier to or facilitator of success" (49).

Change, and an organization's readiness for change, has been the topic of numerous treatises in the field of indus-trial psychology. Although the traditional view of change management is that change begins at the top of an organi-zation pyramid, recent views emphasize that change must occur at all levels within the organization, especially on an individual level (50). O'Connor and Fiol (51) describe 3 elements: energizers or motivators that compel people to take action, impediments to change, and action steps needed for change to occur. Examples of energizers include objectives, benefits, and negative consequences. Barriers to change include apathy, errors, disturbed relationships, lost power, status, and money. Action steps are the steps taken

to overcome barriers and resistance to change. It is impor-tant in CQI to understand common obstacles and the unique interrelationships that characterize different orga-nizations in their quests for providing the same quality of care (51).

Tools for Quality Improvement

Fundamental to CQI is the use of improvement teams working together to solve problems or improve processes in which they are key players. In this approach, a process needing revision is analyzed using a series of tools, with multiple group discussions among the team, progressing through specific phases of analysis. This "diagnostic jour-ney" progresses through description, cause-effect analysis, elaboration of potential improvements, and prioritization of these improvements based on research and study. The end result is the identification and implementation of 1 or 2 improvements that will have the most constructive impact on the related process.

One of the tools used in this process is flowcharting, which allows teams to depict the sequence of activities that make up the process. As teams chart the sequence of activities in a process, they often identify problem areas that become potential opportunities for improvement. Subsequent analy-ses using another tool, the cause-effect diagram, allow the team to attribute causes to the problem areas in the process being studied. Causes are classified in generic categories, which include personnel, equipment, supplies, informa-tion, methods, measurement, and environment. The deter-mination of causes often requires analysis and chart review, with group discussion and consensus determining the likelihood of a cause-effect relationship. After group consensus and further study using a Pareto analysis (based on the "80-20" rule, ascribing 20% of the causes to account for 80% of the problems), the next step is to elaborate on the relationship between potential problems identified and their relative effect on the global process under review. The goal in this stage is to identify the relationship between factors identified with the adverse outcome of the process under review, as well as to systematically describe those factors which have the most potential to favorably influence the process under review.

Traditional CQI incorporates several tools for data col-lection and analysis. Data are essential in establishing the baseline activity or outcome of a process, ascertaining the relative role of various potential interventions, and mea-suring the process to document the desired improvement. Examples of data collection tools include simple check sheets, data sheets, interviews, and surveys. Analysis of the data is often performed using bar charts, histograms, line graphs, and scatter diagrams. Another important and more sophisticated tool useful in this stage is the process control chart (52,53) in which data is plotted over time; analyzing variation in the data allows the distinction of special-cause variation from common-cause variation. This distinguishes variation caused by the influence of extrinsic factors from normal variation intrinsic to the process itself.

The sequence described represents traditional CQI, which has evolved over time and led to important improvements in industry and health care. However, due to the demands placed on modern health care organizations to implement numerous changes over much shorter time periods, the traditional model may not be best, as it may be tedious, be unnecessarily time consuming, and tie up precious resources when used every time a change is needed.

Rapid-Cycle Continuous Quality Improvement

Most organizations are looking for results at a pace that meets objectives in a more timely manner than traditional CQI. The impetus for getting results more efficiently has led to the development of a new approach called "rapid-cycle CQI." Rather than merely speeding up the discrete stages of traditional CQI, rapid-cycle CQI represents a completely different approach. Rapid-cycle CQI is a system of parallel processes as compared to traditional CQI, a system composed of multiple sequential processes performed in series. Originally designed by Nolan, Langley, and colleagues (54,55), rapid-cycle CQI involves the identification of changes chosen as goals by an organization; introduction of change concepts in small cycles, or tests of change; and measurement of the effects of the change.

Rapid-cycle CQI has several basic prerequisites. Organizations with smaller, less hierarchical leadership structures are best suited for this methodology. The use of smaller sample size in initial assessment is another important element as it allows for more rapid feedback regarding the success or failure of a test of change. Rapid-cycle CQI also works best when potential solutions or successful change concepts are readily available through prior applications in other settings. For more complex, interdepartmental problems, other problem-solving methods, including traditional CQI teams, may be more effective.

The process of rapid-cycle CQI begins with the question. "What are we trying to accomplish?" The answer to this question constitutes the aim statement, the starting point in applying rapid-cycle CQI. Next is establishment of the measurement necessary to answer the question, "How will we know that a change is an improvement?" Measurement is key to any methodology of CQI, and it is especially key to rapid cycle because each small test of change is evaluated by measurement. The progression toward the final outcome requires successive or simultaneous cycles depending on measurement to provide the appropriate feedback regarding the value of the change concept being evaluated. Change concepts can be based on evidence in the literature, models of practice identified in benchmark centers, ideas generated during brainstorm sessions by teams within units, or modifications based on the result of previous tests of change.

Although not unique to the rapid-cycle CQI model, Plan-Do-Study-Act (PDSA) cycles are important elements of the process. The small tests of change are set in place with PDSA cycles. This involves the systematic planning of a specific adaptation of the change concept followed by the

unit making the adaptation. The unit staff then studies its effects through measurement, and finally acts on the outcome of the cycle, either deciding to continue with a further adaptation in another cycle, or determining that the aim has been achieved and concluding the process. The concept of building knowledge through PDSA cycles has a long history with roots that can be traced to the British philosopher John Dewey (56), and it has been adapted by Shewhart (57) and Deming (58) to the science of quality management. Figure 7-2 shows the flow diagram used in rapid-cycle CQI.

Plsek (56) points out numerous examples of successful applications of rapid-cycle CQI. These include 2 teams in the Breakthrough Series Collaborative sponsored by the Institute for Healthcare Improvement. One team, from the Mayo Family Medicine Clinic, identified the following change concepts: build capacity for routine assessment of patient outcomes, reduce unintended variation in care, streamline the process of care, and build information system capacity. By implementing these concepts through a series of small-scale cycles of change, the Mayo team reduced hospitalization in asthma patients by 47% and reduced emergency visits by 22% (39). In another example from the Breakthrough Series, a second team implemented a series of 3 change concepts and decreased readmission to the intensive care unit from 15.6% to 9.8% (40).

The Vermont Oxford NIC/Q 2000 collaborative for quality improvement in neonatology brought together

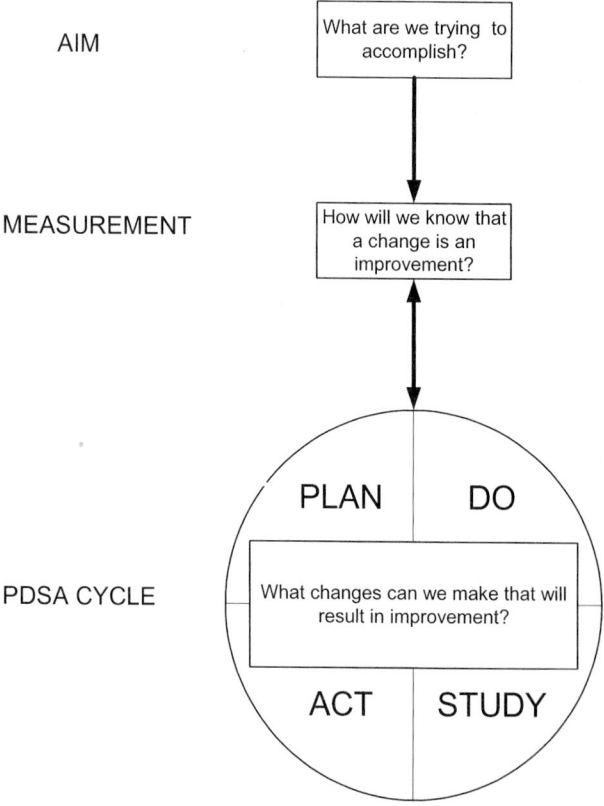

Figure 7-2 Flow diagram of rapid-cycle CQI. (From Plsek PE. Quality improvement methods in clinical medicine. *Pediatrics* 1999;103:203–214, with permission.)

teams from 34 participating centers, and provided education, content experts, and resources to facilitate the identification of change concepts in several clinical areas and the application of rapid-cycle CQI principles. One of the focus groups of the collaborative identified and prioritized 3 change concepts for reducing nosocomial infection in the NICU: improved hand hygiene, attention to the care of deep line connections, and standardized diagnosis of coagulase-negative staphylococcal sepsis. They were able to demonstrate a reduction in coagulase-negative staphylococcal sepsis from 25% to 16% (59).

In rapid-cycle quality improvement, pace is important. Successful application has been shown to depend on running small tests of change, short PDSA cycles, rather than running longer ones over an extended period of time. Each cycle provides the feedback forming the bases of learning and giving information on which to base further cycles of change. Efficiency of measurement is also critical for successful application of rapid cycle CQI. Teams have found that measurement within each cycle must be objective and sufficient enough to draw conclusions about the effect of the change concept. This often does not require the use of statistical techniques that would be very difficult given the sample sizes chosen for rapid cycle tests of change. Although not a requirement of many organizations successful at implementing widespread changes, statistical testing may be reserved for comparison of performance measures after large projects are completed, such as the examples of reduced hospitalization rates and nosocomial infection rates cited above.

CONCLUSION

The delivery of care in the NICU is a complex process involving numerous disciplines and personnel. The day-to-day management is important to the overall organization and keeps operations in motion. However, to continually improve practice and reduce medical errors, a system of continuous quality improvement is needed. The integration of comparative databases and benchmarking, evidence-based medicine principles, along with rapid-cycle processes that are compatible with concepts such as unit culture and change cycles, will help an individual unit to maintain quality in the face of technologic advances and organizational change.

REFERENCES

1. Stafford M, Appleyard JA. Clinical nurse specialists and nurse practitioners: who are they, what do they do, and what challenges do they face? In: McCloskey J, Grace HK, eds. *Current issues in nursing*. St. Louis: Mosby-Year Book, 1994.
2. Elizondo A. Nursing case management in the neonatal intensive care unit. Part 1: pioneering new territory. *Neonatal Netw* 1994;13:9–12.
3. Strong AG. Case management and the CNS. *Clin Nurse Specialist* 1992;6:64.
4. Farah AL, Bieda A, Shiao SY. The history of the neonatal nurse practitioner in the United States. *Neonatal Netw* 1996;15:11–21.
5. Buus-Frank ME, Conner-Bronson J, Mullaney D, et al. Evaluation of the neonatal nurse practitioner role: the next frontier. *Neonatal Netw* 1996;15:31–40.
6. Kenner C. Caring for the NICU parent. *J Perinat Neonatal Nurs* 1990;4:78–87.
7. Harrison H. The principles for family-centered neonatal care. *Pediatrics* 1993;92:643–650.
8. Johnson BH, Jeppson ES, Redburn L. *Caring for children and families: guidelines for hospitals*, 1st ed. Bethesda: Association for the Care of Children's Health, 1992.
9. Stepanek JS. *Moving beyond the medical/technical: analysis and discussion of psychosocial practices in pediatric hospitals*, 1st ed. Bethesda: Association for the Care of Children's Health, 1995.
10. Zaichkin J. *Newborn intensive care: what every parent needs to know*. 2nd ed. Petaluma, CA: NICU INK Book, 2002.
11. Linden DW, Paroli ET, Doron MW. *Preemies: the essential guide for parents of premature babies*. New York: Pocket Books, 2000.
12. Kenner C, Bagwell GA, Torok LS. Assessment and management in the transition to home. In: Kenner C, Lott JW, eds. *Comprehensive neonatal nursing: a physiologic perspective*, 3rd ed. St. Louis: WB Saunders Co., 2003.
13. Durfor SL, Murphy-Ratcliff M. Home- and community-based care. In: Kenner C, Lott JW, eds. *Comprehensive neonatal nursing: a physiologic perspective*, 3rd ed. St. Louis: WB Saunders Co., 2003.
14. Chassin MR, Galvin RW. The urgent need to improve health care quality. Institute of Medicine National Roundtable on Health Care Quality. *JAMA* 1998;280:1000–1005.
15. Sinclair JC, Bracken MB, Horbar JD, et al. Introduction to neonatal systematic reviews. *Pediatrics* 1997;100:892–895.
16. Lohr KN, ed. *Medicare: a strategy for quality assurance*. Washington, DC: National Academy Press, 1990.
17. Institute of Medicine. *Crossing the quality chasm: a new health system for the 21st century*. Washington, DC: National Academy Press, 2001.
18. Institute of Medicine. *To err Is human: building a safer health system*. Washington, DC: National Academy Press, 1999.
19. Leape LL. Reporting of adverse events. *N Engl J Med* 2002;347:1633–1638.
20. Suresh G, Horbar J, Plsek P, et al. Voluntary anonymous reporting of medical errors for neonatal intensive care. *Pediatric Res* 2003;53:426A.
21. The Vermont-Oxford Trials Network: very low birth weight outcomes for 1990. Investigators of the Vermont-Oxford Trials Network Database Project. *Pediatrics* 1993;91:540–545.
22. Horbar JD, Plsek PE, Leahy K. NIC/Q 2000: establishing habits for improvement in neonatal intensive care units. *Pediatrics* 2003;111:e397–e410.
23. Donovan EF, Ehrenkranz RA, Shankaran S, et al. Outcomes of very low birth weight twins cared for in the National Institute of Child Health and Human Development Neonatal Research Network's intensive care units. *Am J Obstet Gynecol* 1998;179:742–749.
24. Lemons JA, Bauer CR, Oh W, et al. Very low birth weight outcomes of the National Institute of Child health and human development neonatal research network, January 1995 through December 1996. NICHD Neonatal Research Network. *Pediatrics* 2001;107:E1.
25. Vohr BR, Wright LL, Dusick AM, et al. Neurodevelopmental and functional outcomes of extremely low birth weight infants in the National Institute of Child Health and Human Development Neonatal Research Network, 1993–1994. *Pediatrics* 2000;105:1216–1226.
26. Fernandez CV, Rees EP. Pain management in Canadian level 3 neonatal intensive care units. *CMAJ* 1994;150:499–504.
27. Lee SK, McMillan DD, Ohlsson A, et al. Variations in practice and outcomes in the Canadian NICU network: 1996–1997. *Pediatrics* 2000;106:1070–1079.
28. Sankaran K, Chien LY, Walker R, et al. Variations in mortality rates among Canadian neonatal intensive care units. *CMAJ* 2002;166:173–178.
29. Risk adjusted and population based studies of the outcome for high risk infants in Scotland and Australia. International Neonatal Network, Scottish Neonatal Consultants, Nurses Collaborative Study Group. *Arch Dis Child Fetal Neonatal Ed* 2000;82:F118–F123.
30. Sutton L, Bajuk B. Population-based study of infants born at less than 28 weeks' gestation in New South Wales, Australia, in 1992-3. New South Wales Neonatal Intensive Care Unit Study Group. *Paediatr Perinat Epidemiol* 1999;13:288–301.

31. Zullini MT, Bonati M, Sanvito E. Survival at nine neonatal intensive care units in Sao Paulo, Brazil. Paulista Collaborative Group on Neonatal Care. *Rev Panam Salud Publica* 1997;2:303–309.

32. Horbar JD, Carpenter JH, Burlington, VT: Vermont Oxford Network, 2002.

33. Brodie SB, Sands KE, Gray JE, et al. Occurrence of nosocomial bloodstream infections in six neonatal intensive care units. *Pediatr Infect Dis J* 2000;19:56–65.

34. Bednarek FJ, Weisberger S, Richardson DK, et al. Variations in blood transfusions among newborn intensive care units. SNAP II Study Group. *J Pediatr* 1998;133:601–607.

35. Avery ME, Tooley WH, Keller JB, et al. Is chronic lung disease in low birth weight infants preventable? A survey of eight centers. *Pediatrics* 1987;79:26–30.

36. National Nosocomial Infections Surveillance (NNIS) System report, data summary from January 1992–June 2001, issued August 2001. *Am J Infect Control* 2001;29:404–421.

37. Kilo CM. Improving care through collaboration. *Pediatrics* 1999;103:384–393.

38. Nolan TW, Schall MW, Roessner J. *Reducing delays and waiting times throughout the healthcare system.* Boston: Institute for Healthcare Improvement, 1996.

39. Weiss KB, Mendoza G, Schall MW, et al. *Improving asthma care in children and adults.* Boston: Institute for Healthcare Improvement, 1997.

40. Rainey TG, Kabcenell A, Berwick DM, et al. *Reducing costs and improving outcomes in adult intensive care.* Boston: Institute for Healthcare Improvement, 1996.

41. Sackett DL, Rosenberg WM, Gray JA, et al. Evidence based medicine: what it is and what it isn't. *BMJ* 1996;312:71–72.

42. Klassen TP, Wiebe N, Russell K, et al. Abstracts of randomized controlled trials presented at the society for pediatric research meeting: an example of publication bias. *Arch Pediatr Adolesc Med* 2002;156:474–479.

43. Soll RF, Andruscavage L. The principles and practice of evidence-based neonatology. *Pediatrics* 1999;103(1 Suppl E):215–224.

44. Muir Gray JA. *Evidence-based health care: how to make health policy and management decisions.* New York and London: Churchill Livingstone, 1997.

45. West S, King V, Carey T, et al. *Systems to rate the strength of scientific evidence.* Rockville, MD: Agency for Healthcare Research and Quality, 2002.

46. The periodic health examination. Canadian Task Force on the Periodic Health Examination. *Can Med Assoc J* 1979;121:1193–1254.

47. Strom KL. Quality improvement interventions: what works? *J Healthc Qual* 2001;23:4–14.

48. Kilbride HW, Powers R, Wirtschafter DD, et al. Evaluation and development of potentially better practices to prevent neonatal nosocomial bacteremia. *Pediatrics* 2003;111:e504–e518.

49. Baker GR, King H, MacDonald JL, et al. Using organizational assessment surveys for improvement in neonatal intensive care. *Pediatrics* 2003;111:e419–e425.

50. Baker GR, King H, MacDonald JL, et al. Using organizational assessment surveys for improvement in neonatal intensive care. *Pediatrics* 2003;111:e419.

51. O'Connor E, Fiol CM. In: Lowery JE, ed. *Culture shift: a leader's guide to managing change in health care.* Chicago: American Hospital Publishing, Inc., 1997:39–.

52. Plsek PE. Tutorial: introduction to control charts. *Qual Manag Health Care* 1992;1:65–74.

53. Carey RG, Lloyd RC. *Measuring quality improvement in healthcare: a guide to statistical process control applications.* New York: Quality Resources, 1995.

54. Langley GJ, Nolan KM, Norman CL, et al. *The improvement guide: a practical approach to enhancing organizational performance.* San Francisco: Jossey-Bass, 1996.

55. Nolan TW, Schall MW, Roessner J. *Reducing delays and waiting times throughout the healthcare system.* Boston: Institute for Healthcare Improvement, 1996.

56. Plsek PE. Quality improvement methods in clinical medicine. *Pediatrics* 1999;103:203–214.

57. Shewhart WA. *Economic control of quality of manufactured product.* New York: Van Nostrand, 1931.

58. Deming WE. *Out of the crisis.* Cambridge, MA: MIT Press, 1986.

59. Kilbride HW, Wirtschafter DD, Powers RJ, et al. Implementation of evidence-based potentially better practices to decrease nosocomial infections. *Pediatrics* 2003;111:e519–e533.

8

Law, Quality Assurance and Risk Management in the Practice of Neonatology

Harold M. Ginzburg   Mhairi G. MacDonald

BASIC LEGAL AND REGULATORY CONCEPTS

A brief historical overview of the transition from the past to present will help explain some of the current legal and social difficulties within the practice of medicine.

Health care professionals have always been subject to punishment should their medical skills or judgment fall below a community standard. Reports from the Middle Ages in England indicate that compensation was paid when patients were injured. In other nations during the Middle Ages the health care provider, if found responsible for poor medical care, was deformed in the same manner as the injury that he caused. Physicians were not motivated to treat patients with complicated illnesses unless the patient and his or her extended family clearly understood that treatment would be palliative. Although litigation has replaced amputation in modem western societies, health care providers and institutions still practice under the specter of retribution and public criticism.

Prior to the middle of the 20th century members of the healing profession functioned as an integral part of their local community. Since the 1940s there has been a progressive separation of health care providers from the communities they serve; this process has been accelerated by the advent of highly subspecialized and expensive intensive care. Neonatologists function in a crisis environment with little or no prior knowledge of their patients' family unit.

Isolation of patients from health care providers, except in times of crisis, can lead to poor or limited communication and unrealistic expectations. The family expects success.

Litigation may be initiated when negligence has occurred or is perceived to have occurred. A lack of good communication skills and empathy can be as self destructive as a faulty knowledge base, performing unacceptably, or functioning in an impaired manner. Thorough knowledge and understanding of one's medical subspecialty is insufficient to prevent involvement in malpractice litigation. Impersonal institutional and individual behaviors often precipitate a lawsuit. The failure to communicate and document patient and health care system interactions may place a health care system or provider in an untenable position when his or her actions are reviewed in an arbitration, mediation, or courtroom environment.

Health care providers are never able to succeed all the time. Sometimes the nature and extent of the disease is too severe, sometimes the course of treatment is too risky or aggressive to be tolerated by the patient, and sometimes errors of skill and judgment are made. Relatively recently the medical community and their legal advisors have come to the realization that explaining to a patient and family what went wrong in language that they can understand is not only the right thing to do but also appears to decrease the incidence of litigation (1,2). As part of its accreditation process, the Joint Commission on Accreditation of Healthcare Organizations (JCAHO) now requires health care organizations to disclose unanticipated injuries to the affected patients, investigate their root causes, and take action to prevent their recurrence (3).

Responsibility and Liability

The mundane aspects of medical care and treatment, such as scheduling of appointments, documentation of procedures, and understanding of the federal, state, and local guidelines, procedures, policies, regulations, and laws, are frequently the basis for confrontations between members of the medical and legal professions.

The vast majority of medical education pertains to understanding basic sciences and providing clinical services. Little formal attention is given to the myriad of governmental policies, procedures, and regulations that control all aspects of health care delivery.

Medical care is a contract between the health care professional and the patient. In almost all instances, if the patient is unable, because of age or illness, to render informed educated consent, then others must provide such consent. Thus, as a patient is examined or interviewed, law and medicine become intertwined.

The basic legal considerations relating the care and treatment of any patient, and particularly, a neonate, flow from the following four concepts:

1. The duty to act. When does the health care professional–patient or health care facility–patient relationship commence?
2. Knowledge and application of hospital policies and local, state, and federal mandates. What resources are available to facilitate information transfer to health care facilities and service providers?
3. Responsibility and accountability of the health care provider (individual or organization) to provide adequate care and treatment. Who is responsible for the decisions made in the provision of health care? Who monitors the quality of the services provided? Who ensures that the services provided are consistent with hospital policies and local, state, and federal mandates?
4. Information transfer to patients and their families or guardians. Who obtains educated informed consent, in what manner, and with what documentation? Who is responsible for providing ongoing medical information to the families or guardians of neonates and ensuring that the information, and the implications of the information, is understood? State and federal legislation, such as the Health Insurance Portability and Account-ability Act of 1996 (HIPAA) (4), do not set standards for the manner in which a clinician may or should communicate with a patient, family member or significant other.

Defensive Medicine

Defensive medicine has become a medical term of art. However, it can connote a thoughtful systematic approach to health care rather than the excessive ordering of investigatory studies because of anticipatory fear of litigation for malpractice. Medical malpractice lawsuits are based on the principle of negligence. Negligence implies some wrongful act of commission or omission (5). The essence of negligence is unreasonableness.

Due Care

Due care is simply reasonable conduct (6). In order for negligence to be demonstrated in a courtroom, the injured person/plaintiff must demonstrate that (a) there was a legal duty owed to him; (b) there was a breach of that duty (a deviation from the accepted standard of care); (c) as a result of the duty and the breach thereof, damages or an injury occurred; and (d) the damages or injury can be determined to have been caused by, or shown to have flowed from, the care or lack of care provided by the health care provider and/or organization responsible for the environment in which the health care was provided.

Quality assurance and risk management aspects of medical care are relatively recent innovations designed to improve patient care and outcome; they are discussed in greater detail in the second section of this chapter. Quality assurance activities accept the legal and medical position that a health care provider owes a duty to the patient to provide reasonable medical care, consistent with available resources. There are inherent, irreducible risks in the delivery of medical care and treatment, and quality assurance and risk management assessments are designed to identify and limit the risks. There are always risks in a medical intervention, and there are always risks in not rendering a medical intervention. The balance of relative risks needs to be understood by both the health care provider and the patient and/or parent/guardian.

The Duty to Act

The duty to act is determined when the health care professional– or organization–patient relationship commences (7). A "duty" is a legal and ethical responsibility. There is no legal duty under most circumstances for a health care provider or institution to accept a patient for care unless they hold themselves out as providing emergency care or they are required to do so by law, regulation, or contract. If a medical center, hospital, or physician represents itself to the public as a source of emergency medical care and the community has come to expect such care, then a patient cannot be arbitrarily denied such services (8). Once a health care service is initiated, a health care provider/institution–patient relationship exists, a duty is created, and there is then a legal and moral obligation not to abandon the patient. Further, the care that is being provided must be adequate under the circumstances. A moral and legal obligation attaches, which precludes abandonment or "dumping" of the patient (9). A referring hospital transferring an infant to another institution for further care is not perceived as abandoning the patient, as long as the reason for transfer is medical and not financial. The senior medical person responsible for the transport, whether stationed at a hospital or directly providing patient care during transport, is deemed to be supervising the health care until the transport team transfers care to the clinical staff at the receiving referral medical facility. The transport team's legal and ethical duty to the patient exceeds that of other parties, such as the referring or referral hospital.

The complexity of health care responsibility and liability increased rapidly during the 20th century. Public health care facilities have existed since the Middle Ages. Commencing in the 13th century, the Hotel Dieu in Paris provided indigent care for many centuries. In the United States, city, municipal, state, and federal public hospitals provided care for those unable to obtain it elsewhere, and the physicians and hospitals were not held liable for the outcome of care that was provided free of charge. The doctrine of charitable immunity protected hospitals from legal liability if medical negligence occurred within their boundaries. However, an individual's inability to pay for medical care no longer affects his or her ability to demand and receive services that are commensurate with those provided to patients who pay for their care directly or through third-party payment systems. Thus, providing care to patients who are unable to pay no longer protects a health care provider or medical institution from liability for negligence or malpractice. Physicians, other health providers, suppliers, and manufacturers of equipment, medical devices, and medicines can now all be sued for negligence and be held individually or jointly liable for their own actions, those that they supervise, and those that are performed by members of their health care team.

Licensure; Interstate-International Practice

In the United States, health care providers (physicians, nurses, emergency medical technicians, etc.) may be licensed in more than one state. They must be licensed in the state in which they maintain their primary office or place of employment. The authorities in most, but not all, states are not concerned about whether a health care provider who enters the state solely to transport a patient to another health care facility is licensed in that state; however, they are concerned that the individuals involved in the transport are competent to perform their job.

An individual who enters a state, regardless of the reason, will be subject to that state's laws. If a driver is involved in an accident, he or she is subject to the laws of the state in which the accident occurred, not to those of the state that issued the driving license; this legal principal also applies to medical transport vehicle operators (10). Failure to obtain informed consent may result in litigation in the state in which it was inadequately obtained or in the state to which the patient was transferred.

Patients and their guardians may initiate medical malpractice litigation in the state in which they reside, the state in which the alleged negligence occurred, the state in which the hospital is located, or the state in which the physician resides. If the patient/plaintiff can show that his or her residence is in a different state from that of the defendant/hospital and defendant/health care provider, then the plaintiff can commence the litigation in a federal court because the matter involves diversity of jurisdiction, i.e., opposing parties are located in two or more states. The defendant can request that the matter be removed to the federal court system for a similar reason (11). Most plaintiffs prefer state courts, especially if the defendant is from a different state. Some state courts are known for their large awards to plaintiffs, whereas others are known to be more sympathetic to defendants/health care providers.

Telemedicine

Recent advances in telephone-linked care (TLC) or "telemedicine" (see also Chapter 5) have initiated new questions regarding the practice of medicine across state lines (12). TLC has been applied as a supplement to direct patient care, to monitor patient progress, and as a service expander for specialized medical expertise and technology (e.g., the interpretation of neonatal radiologic or cardiologic films and tracings). Landwehr and associates (13) demonstrated the feasibility of telesonography for the interpretation of fetal anatomic scans from a remote location. Lewis and Moir (14) in Scotland and Landquist (15) in Finland demonstrated that telemedicine is an international technology.

TLC has been practiced for more than 30 years (in its simplest form, it includes giving advice over the telephone). In 1996 the U.S. Congress passed the Telecommunications Reform Act, which required a study of patient safety, efficacy, and the quality of services (16). The neonatologist has the opportunity to engage in "telehealth," which includes consultation, transportation, and interpretation of radiographic, cardiologic, and other data, as well as professional education, community health education, public health, and administration of health services. The American Medical Association and American Telemedicine Association have urged medical specialty societies to develop appropriate practice standards. Managed care organizations have begun to embrace telemedicine. Louisiana, in 1995, became the first state to enact legislation dealing with telemedicine reimbursement (17) that specifies a certain reimbursement rate for physicians at the originating site and includes language prohibiting insurance carriers from discriminating against telemedicine as a medium for delivering health care services.

California in 1996 (18), Oklahoma in 1997 (19), Texas in 1997 (20), and Kentucky in 2000 (21) have also passed telemedicine legislation. However, at the present time, issues relating to cross-state licensure are perceived to be potential barriers to the expansion of telemedicine, especially now that reimbursement is possible. States license physicians and other health care providers within their boundaries, but the federal government has the authority to prepare national licensure standards as they relate to national programs such as Medicaid and Medicare. In the future, there may be alternative approaches to licensure (22). Regardless of the end result of the issues surrounding telemedicine, neonatologists increasingly cross state and international boundaries and need to appreciate that the laws of political jurisdictions other than their home state may significantly impact the manner in which they practice.

The U.S. Food and Drug Administration (FDA) has become involved in telehealth activities on the Internet.

Over the past few years, some Web sites have offered illegal drugs or prescription drugs based on questionnaires rather than a face-to-face examination by a licensed health care practitioner. Some offshore sites offer prescription drugs without any prescription or medical consultation. The FDA works with the U.S. National Association of Boards of Pharmacy, which created a program in 1999 called Verified Internet Pharmacy Practice Sites to provide the consumer with the ability to verify the safety of medications being sold over the Internet (23). A number of U.S. federal and state regulatory agencies are working together to address health-related consumer problems on the Internet. They include state health authorities, FDA, Justice Department, and Federal Trade Commission. The Federal Trade Commission plays a key oversight and enforcement role in Internet commerce.

Medical Torts and Contracts

The legal system is divided into two broad areas. Civil litigation is based on the need to correct or remedy a wrong between one individual (corporation or partnership) and another. Criminal prosecution is instituted to correct a wrong against the community. In a civil litigation matter (or case), the plaintiff is the party bringing the lawsuit and alleging the wrong; the lawsuit is filed against the party (defendant) who is accused of causing the damage. In a criminal prosecution, the plaintiff is the government (local, state, federal) alleging that the community has been harmed by the action or inaction of a party (also known as the defendant).

Civil matters resulting in litigation generally are either contract disputes or torts. A contract dispute occurs when two or more parties have entered into an agreement and one or more parties believe that the terms and conditions of the agreement, either an oral or written contract, have not been met. It is important to appreciate that, in a court; most oral contracts have the same weight as written contracts.

A personal tort is an injury to a person or his or her reputation or feelings that directly results from a violation of a duty owed to the plaintiff (in medical malpractice cases, this is usually the patient) and produces damage. The remedy in any civil matter, after the nature and extent of the damages have been proved to the court (a judge with or without a jury), is determined by a preponderance of the evidence (more than 50.01%). Thus, to a medical degree of certainty means that it is more likely than not, and it is that standard upon which there are usually monetary damages awarded if the matter is found in favor of the plaintiff. In most instances in the United States, each side pays for its own legal services, regardless of the outcome of the case.

Battery

Battery is a tort; it is an intentional and volitional act without consent which results in touching that causes harm (e.g., the touching of a patient's body without consent). A technical battery can occur when there is no actual harm but touching occurred without consent. Patient care, even with a beneficial outcome but without informed consent, may be considered battery.

Plaintiffs may sue for an injury that occurred as a result of negligence or a tort (physical or mental harm), or both. Because the criminal court usually will not award monetary damages to the victim of a crime and because the standard of proof for conviction is "beyond a reasonable doubt" (quantitatively, this can be conceptualized as at least 95% certain), plaintiffs usually prefer to sue for injuries from a tort in civil court. In civil litigation, monetary damages may be awarded, and if the injury was determined to be egregious, punitive damages also can be assessed against the defendant. The standard of proof in civil litigation is the "preponderance of the evidence" or the "more likely than not" standard; it is a "superiority of weight" test that requires that for the plaintiff to be successful, 50.01% of the evidence must weigh in his or her favor (24). Thus, the preponderance of the evidence rule is a threshold test (25). In general, either the plaintiff proves that the damages were more likely to have been caused by the defendant agent than by any other source and is; therefore, entitled to full compensation, or he or she fails to meet the burden of proof and is entitled to nothing (26).

Professional Negligence

Negligence is "conduct, and not a state of mind" (27), "involves an unreasonably great risk of causing damage" (27) and is "conduct which falls below the standard established by the law for the protection of others against unreasonable risk of harm" (28,29).

Professional negligence, or medical malpractice, is a special instance of negligence. The medical profession is held to a specific minimum level of performance based on the possession, or claim of possession, of "special knowledge or skills" that have been accrued through specialized education and training.

Ely and associates (30) found that when family physicians recalled memorable errors, the majority fell into the following categories: physician distracters (hurried or overburdened), process of care factors (premature closure of the diagnostic process), patient-related factors (misleading normal results), and physician factors (lack of knowledge, inadequately aggressive patient management). Understanding the common causes of errors alerts the practitioner to situations when errors are most likely to occur.

The Elements of a Malpractice Case

To establish a *prima facie* medical malpractice case (one that still appears obvious after reviewing the medical evidence), the patient/plaintiff must demonstrate (Fig. 8-1): that (a) there is a duty on the part of the defendant/health care provider and/or defendant/health care facility to the patient/plaintiff, (b) the defendant failed to conform his or her conduct to the requisite standard of care required by the relationship, and (c) an injury to that patient/plaintiff resulted from that failure (31).

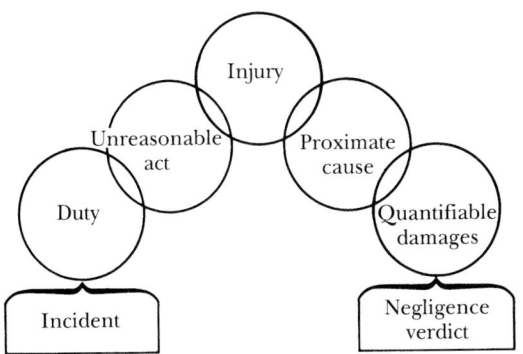

Figure 8-1   The elements of negligence. There must be an unbroken chain for successful litigation. If any link is not proved, the plaintiff will lose the case. (From Ginzburg HM. Legal issues in patient transport. In: MacDonald MG, ed.. *Emergency transport of the perinatal patient.* Philadelphia: Little, Brown and Company, 1989:163, with permission.)

Generally, in order for the plaintiff to establish a claim of medical malpractice, the plaintiff must establish by medical expert testimony (a) what the applicable standard of care is, (b) how the defendant breached or violated that standard of care, and (c) that the breach or violation (also referred to as the negligence) was the proximate cause of the injury.

A medical malpractice action can only proceed if the court determines that there is a genuine issue of material fact and if damages are quantifiable (e.g., the future costs of treatment, economic lost value of productive activities, etc.).

The most difficult element to prove is whether or not the standard of care was adequate. The plaintiff usually must provide expert witnesses to establish what a prudent health care provider in similar circumstances might have done. A "conspiracy of silence" may have existed in prior years in the United States, but today there are many "experts" willing to testify anywhere about anything. However, in Japan and other nations, it is difficult to find a local or even national expert to testify in medical malpractice cases (32).

More than 100 years ago in Massachusetts, it was held that a physician in a small town was bound to have only the skill that physicians of ordinary ability and skill in similar localities possessed. The court believed that a small-town physician should not be expected to have the skill of surgeons practicing a specialty in a large city (33). It was also held that a physician was required to use only ordinary skill and diligence, the average of that possessed by the profession as a body, and not by the thoroughly educated (34). However, a physician is now not excused for failing to keep himself or herself informed of medical progress. State requirements for continuing education and the effects of telemedicine consultations and educational programs essentially have removed clinicians' ability to say that they are too busy or so geographically inaccessible as to be precluded from keeping current with new treatments and new understanding of the illnesses that affect their patients.

Courts admit medical evidence based upon rules of evidence. In 1993, the U.S. Supreme Court in *Daubert v Merrill Dow Pharmaceuticals, Inc.* ruled that the Federal Rules of Evidence standards for acceptance of evidence would be used (35). This was an attempt to remove junk science from distracting the jury. The court held that scientific (medical) evidence had to be grounded in relevant scientific principles. The four criteria the court established are: (a) whether the theory or technique has been tested; (b) whether the theory or technique has been subjected to peer review and publication; (c) the known or potential rate of error of the method used and the existence and maintenance of standards controlling the technique's operation; and (d) whether the theory or method has been generally accepted by the scientific community. Thus, publication in a peer-reviewed or peer-refereed journal was not the only qualification for acceptance of evidence in a courtroom. The district (trial) court judges have the latitude to permit or exclude experts, based on the perceived scientific merit of the information they intend to provide to the court and, thus, to the jury. The fundamental issue for a clinician is not an understanding of the rules of evidence and the workings of the civil justice system but practicing medicine and acting in a professional manner, as documented in a patient's medical record.

Many states have medical peer-review panels in place. In these states, before a medical malpractice case may be heard in a court, the facts of the case are presented to the review panel on behalf of both the plaintiff and defendant. The medical facts often are buttressed by the opinions of retained medical experts for both sides. In some states the medical review panel is comprised of attorneys and physicians; in other states the medical review panel is chaired by an attorney and comprised of physicians in the same or similar medical specialty as the physician being accused of having committed malpractice. Even when there is a finding for the defendant by the medical review panel, the plaintiff may continue litigation in the local court. However, the findings of the medical review panel are admissible on behalf of either the plaintiffs or defendants.

Res ipsa loquitur

There are circumstances in which no expert witness is required to corroborate the findings of negligence. The doctrine of *res ipsa loquitur* essentially means that the thing speaks for itself. Under such circumstances, the negligence is inferred from the act itself, i.e., proof from circumstantial evidence. In the classic case *Ybarra v Spangard*, a patient was well prior to being anesthetized for an appendectomy, and when he woke up he had an injury to his arm (36). Clearly, he could not determine how his arm was injured; the operating room and recovery room staff either could not or would not explain the etiology of the injury. The court found for the injured plaintiff without the introduction of any expert witnesses because (a) the plaintiff had not done anything that in any way could have contributed to the injury, (b) the injury could not have occurred unless someone was negligent, and (c) the instrumentalities (hospital staff and physicians) that allegedly caused the injury were at all times under the control of the defendant hospital.

Informed Consent

Informed consent requires that sound, reasonable, comprehensible, and relevant information be provided by a health care professional to a competent individual (patient or guardian) for the purpose of eliciting a voluntary and educated decision by that patient (or guardian) about the advisability of permitting one course of clinical action as opposed to another (28). Physicians and other health care providers are held to have a fiduciary duty to their patients. Such a duty exists when one individual relies on another because of the unequal possession of information. The failure to obtain proper informed consent may result in the defendant/physician or defendant/hospital being sued for battery in some states or for negligence in others.

According to the battery theory, the defendant is to be held liable if any deliberate (not careless or accidental) action resulted in physical contact. The contact must have occurred under circumstances in which the plaintiff/patient did not provide either express or implied permission and the defendant/health care provider knew or should have known that the action was unauthorized. If the scope of consent obtained from the patient is exceeded, a claim of battery is proper. The plaintiff in *Mohr v Williams* consented to have surgery performed on her right ear (37). During the procedure, the surgeon determined that the right ear was not sufficiently diseased to require surgery, but the *left* ear required surgery. Because the patient was already anesthetized, the surgeon performed the operation. The operation was a success, but the patient successfully sued for battery. The court held that there was no informed consent for an operation to the left ear. Thus, it is not necessary for injury to occur for damages to be awarded; demonstration that there was unauthorized touching is sufficient. In this instance, the court found that there was no medical emergency that would have threatened the plaintiff/patient if the surgery had not immediately commenced. If there were evidence of a medical emergency, the court's decision might have been significantly different.

Failure to specifically identify the risks that accompany a surgical procedure also can result in a successful claim of battery. In *Canterbury v Spence*, the plaintiff/patient successfully proved that he was not informed of the risks attendant to the surgical procedure and that had he known them he would not have given permission (38). The court held that the physician has a duty to disclose all reasonable risks of a surgical procedure, and because he failed to perform that duty, the court held him liable for damages to the patient. The court noted that the concept of informed consent might be more appropriately replaced with the concept of educated consent. The court also articulated an objective standard that could be used in legal cases involving informed consent. This objective standard is based on

what a reasonable person in circumstances similar to that of the patient would have decided if he or she had been provided with an adequate amount of information. Therefore, the central issue in a medical battery is whether an educated, effective, or valid consent was given for the procedure that actually was performed.

A physician is not required to disclose every possible risk to a patient for fear of being guilty of battery (39). The court in *Cooper v Roberts* held that "[t]he physician is bound to disclose only those risks which a reasonable man would consider material to his decision whether or not to undergo treatment" (40). Thus, the court stated that such a standard creates no unreasonable burden for the physician. However, the physician must disclose risks that are material and feasible alternatives that are available. The information should be provided in a language and manner that reflects the emotional and educational status of the patient or, when the patient is a neonate, the parents. In *Davis v Wyeth*, the court held that any medical complication or risk that has a probability of greater than 1:1,000 should be included in the informed consent (41).

When a therapeutic procedure is for the benefit of a minor, the decision to proceed usually belongs to the parent or legal guardian. The failure of the parent to consent to blood transfusions (even if the refusal is based on sincere religious convictions) or other now routine procedures for a small child that are clearly medically indicated and required for the maintenance of life can be overridden by the physician and/or hospital petitioning the court for the appointment of a temporary legal guardian (42).

The unavailability of a parent in a life-threatening circumstance should not preclude therapeutic action. Just as informed consent is imputed to an unconscious accident victim who has a life-threatening condition that requires surgery, such rational behavior can be imputed to the absent parent in the case of a sick neonate. However, in such circumstances if time permits, detailed documentation and consultation with the hospital administration is recommended.

Informed consent in neonatal/perinatal medicine is not an empty gesture to reduce liability, but rather an interaction with the physician that helps parents to become full partners in decision making. Informed consent documents are intended to support decision makers in their choices, rather than to merely have them ratify decisions already made (43). Informed consent documents need to be routinely reviewed to determine that the reading level required to understand them is consistent with the educational and cultural experiences of those being asked to read, understand, and sign the forms (44).

The informed consent process can be extremely complex, with several legal "gray areas." For example, are maternal rights any more definitive in making critical decisions for a fetus or neonate than paternal rights? Conflicts can arise even when the putative or alleged father is not the legal spouse of the mother. Emergency hearings in front of local judges may be required to resolve conflicting opinions, especially when the decision of one parent may lead, to a medical degree of certainty (more likely than not), to the death of the infant.

It is one of the ironies of the law, in most states, that an unwed teenage mother has the ultimate legal responsibility for the care of her child, unless the court is petitioned to appoint an alternative guardian. In many states the live birth of a child, regardless of the age of the mother, results in the mother being declared an emancipated minor. In contrast, a non-pregnant teenager, living at home and attending school, does not have the legal right to make decisions about many aspects of her own medical care.

The disclosure of risks in the informed consent process tends to underscore a parent's sense of helplessness and to portray the physician as somewhat helpless as well. The powerlessness of the parents and their wish that the physician be omnipotent creates unrealistic expectations for the outcomes of procedures and treatment. Gutheil and associates (45) suggest that the physician acknowledge the parent's wish for certainty and substitute the mystical with a physician-parent alliance in which uncertainty is accepted.

Advanced Care Planning

Decision making in life and death situations is not easy. Advanced care planning efforts initially evolved in the care of the elderly (46). Advanced care planning, or contingency medical care planning, is no longer generally reserved for adults. The American Academy of Pediatrics Committee of Bioethics developed a policy statement about parental permission and informed consent (47). A distinction is made in this public policy statement and in case law in the United States between emergency medical treatment, life support efforts, and elective surgical procedures, such as circumcision or removing a kidney from one child to aid a sibling (48,49). Neonates need others to make decisions about their treatment and viability. Their treatment in a neonatal intensive care unit (NICU) is also never a series of leisurely scheduled elective procedures. There must be a designated person to whom the health care providers relate and who is held to render decisions about treatment. When potential conflicts in decision making are recognized, a conference among the concerned individuals, with representation from the hospital administration, may be a worthwhile endeavor to clarify who actually has the final decision-making authority. There may be times in the treatment of a patient when one person has to render an immediate decision, even if that decision is not a consensus. Decision-making issues are often confounded when the mother of the neonate is an adolescent herself and not wed to the father.

While all 50 states in the United States and the District of Columbia have passed legislation on advance directives, reinforcing the fact that adherence to such directives is mandatory rather than optional continues to be problematic (46). The majority of states do place restrictions on proxy decision making. If identification of the responsible party for decision making is not clear or keeps shifting, legal consultation, initiated by the health care providers, is

recommended. Most jurisdictions have the ability to hold emergency judicial proceedings when an impasse has been reached and a medical decision must be made before irreversible damage or death to the patient occurs (42).

Medical Records

As evidenced by HIPAA (4) and state regulations, medical records are legal documents. Medical and hospital records are designed to be a contemporaneous record of the available clinical information and medical and other decisions that flow from the clinical information and interactions with the patient's significant others. Records provide an opportunity for adequate documentation. Documentation is the key to management of patients, and it is the key to protecting physicians against malpractice litigation, especially in the instances in which the patients have difficult and complex clinical presentations. The course of treatment and meeting or failing to meet therapeutic goals should be noted in the hospital chart. Treatment options, including the option of no treatment when pertinent, should be explained to the patient's family and, if necessary, others potentially involved in the decision-making process; these interactions should be documented in the patient's chart. The patient's family's understanding, or lack thereof, of the various treatment options also should be noted, especially if there are divergent views among family members. Ultimately one family member or guardian has to be acknowledged by the family and health care providers as the decision maker. Identifying such an individual in the medical record will facilitate treatment decisions and posthospital treatment care and management. Such documentation may preclude the need for judicial intervention.

Adequate medical records will document that the risks of a given procedure have been shared with the patient's decision makers. A record that indicates that specific known adverse side effects, or rare but serious untoward events, were discussed with a patient's family members or guardians helps protect the clinician should one of these untoward events actually occur. No medical procedure is risk free, and although families may be informed of the relative risks of the various procedures and pharmacologic interventions, the stress of the moment may shorten their attention span, concentration, and recall. For example, prescriptions at the time of discharge are often for a limited period of time, with follow-up care being provided in either a hospital outpatient, clinic, or private clinical environment. Prescriptions must be written clearly, identifying the patient, date, dose, dose schedule, and route of administration. The parent or guardian to whom the prescription is provided needs to understand why the medication is being prescribed, adverse side effects, therapeutic effects of the medication, and consequences to the infant if the medication is not provided. Medical record documentation, including discharge instructions and prescriptions, at least provide a contemporaneous record of what information actually was provided.

Medical records provide the basis for reimbursement of the costs for patient care and treatment. The severity of a condition, justification for laboratory and other investigations, need for consultations, and manner in which the consultative advice is incorporated into patient care should be present within a patient's medical record. In the spring of 1998 the U.S. Justice Department announced the hiring of 250 Federal Bureau of Investigation (FBI) agents for the purpose of investigating Medicare and Medicaid fraud. The U.S. federal government continues to pay increasing attention to the issue of fraudulent billing for health care services whether the care is provided directly or via telemedicine. The FBI estimates that 10% of the money paid out for health care services under the Medicaid program is the result of fraudulent billing (50). Not all the money paid for fraudulent services is recovered. However, in 2002, $1.6 billion was collected in connection with health care fraud cases and matters (51). The absence of consistent, comprehensive reimbursement policies is frequently cited as one of the most serious obstacles to total integration of telemedicine into health care practice. This lack of an overall telemedicine reimbursement policy reflects the multiplicity of payment sources and policies within the current U.S. health care system.

Adequate documentation facilitates medical audit, permits those who prepare invoices for reimbursement or payment to justify the categories or International Classification of Diseases codes placed on the universal billing forms (sometimes identified as HCFA-1500 forms), and prevents errors that may result in the appearance of fraud (52).

Medical Confidentiality of Oral and Handwritten Communications

The Hippocratic oath states, in part, "Whatever, in connection with my professional practice or not in connection with it, I see or hear, in the life of men, which ought not to be spoken of abroad, I will not divulge, as reckoning that all should be kept secret" (53). This oath, taken by many physicians upon graduating from medical school, has been codified by state and federal law. The confidentiality of the information obtained by the physician is considered to be "privileged" (54). The privilege, however, belongs to the patient or his or her guardian; it does not belong to the physician or other health care provider. A court may order a health care provider to breach medical confidentiality; legislation may require it.

As the delivery of medical care becomes more complex, individuals not generally thought of as direct health care providers are requiring access to confidential medical information. The legitimate needs, for example, of physical therapists, occupational therapists, hospital administrative personnel, and medical insurance personnel may appear to conflict with the principle that medical information is confidential and should be restricted only to physicians. The ethical basis for confidentiality derives from the concept that assurance of confidentiality encourages patients

to seek the medical care that they require and to be candid with their health care providers. The legal basis for confidentiality is derived from statutes, which have been enacted in essentially all states within the United States.

There is significant variation among the states as to what classes of health care providers (doctors, nurses, social workers, etc.) can assert that they cannot share medical information provided to them without the patient's express permission or a court order directing them to do so.

Legislatures create state disease-reporting requirements that require medical confidentiality to be breached as historically the courts have found that the state has a compelling need to protect its citizens from certain infectious diseases (55). Certain behaviors, such as dangerousness, also have resulted in reporting requirements that compel a health care professional to notify authorities when a patient has made an explicit threat against a known individual (56) or even an unknown but identifiable group of individuals (57). Dangerous behaviors include spousal and child abuse.

Medical records also are protected by state and federal legislation. The U.S. Public Health Service Act provides for the explicit protection of medical records dealing with treatment for drug (58) and alcohol abuse (59). However, even the contents of substance abuse treatment records may be released "to medical personnel to the extent necessary to meet a *bonafide* medical emergency" (60,61). If release of the medical records is authorized by a court order, then appropriate safeguards need to be put into place to preclude unauthorized disclosure.

The courts recognize that they must balance the public interest and the need for disclosure against injury to the patient, physician–patient relationship, and treatment services (4,62,63).

"A hospital medical record is the property of the hospital, but it is kept for the benefit of the patient, the physician, and the hospital" (53). A patient's medical record is preserved to document events in a contemporaneous manner for later use. Later use includes further medical care and treatment, documentation for financial payment by third-party payers, and defense of medical malpractice claims.

The medical record librarian becomes the custodian of the medical records. The American Association of Medical Record Librarians has a code that is similar to the Hippocratic Oath taken by physicians. Hospital policies and procedures, consistent with state and federal statutes and regulations, prevent a medical record from being released without either a patient release or court order. Under certain defined circumstances, medical records can be admitted as evidence in a court of law. They can be authenticated as business records. They also can be used to refresh a doctor's memory and document his or her actions.

The American Hospital Association, JCAHO, and other health care professional organizations have asserted that a patient's medical records are to be protected from unauthorized and unnecessary access. Their positions are generally consistent with current HIPAA regulations and state regulations. Hematology, blood chemistry, urinalyses, and radiographic, sonographic, and electrodiagnostic findings are all considered a part of a patient's authorization or court order. Third-party payers, as a condition of their insuring the patient, almost invariably are given access to patient medical records, as are state and federal auditors.

The privilege of medical confidentiality does not extend to third parties present who are not part of the health care being delivered. That is, police officers present during an evaluation or treatment cannot be prevented from sharing with other law enforcement personnel or the courts any information that they obtained under such circumstances. When an individual engages in litigation in which his or her physical or mental status is an issue, that individual cannot assert the privilege to prevent unfavorable information from reaching the ear of the court. Thus, in a lawsuit for malpractice, the patient/plaintiff has waived his or her right to medical confidentiality of any oral, written, or electronic communication concerning his or her medical history, diagnosis, treatment, or prognosis. Medical confidentiality statutes were and are designed to protect a patient's privacy and to encourage treatment for conditions that may bear social or other stigmas. The laws were not made to give the moving party, the patient/plaintiff in a medical malpractice case, an unfair advantage by allowing the individual to select only those records considered testimony favorable to his or her case. A medical record cannot be used as both a sword and a shield.

In 1991 the Institute of Medicine (IOM) advocated the adoption of the computer-based patient record as standard medical practice in the United States (64). A computer-based record is perceived as a continuous chronological history of a patient's medical care. The medical care record can be linked to various aids, including reminders and alerts to clinicians and clinical decision-making instruments. However, a computer-based record increases access to a patient's record and increases the array of data maintained in a single record (65). The more information compressed into an easily accessible single location, the greater the precautions needed to prevent misuse. As Annas (66) notes, in a setting of private practice, medical information that identifies a patient is supposed to be transferred from physician to physician only with the patient's written informed consent. In contrast, he explains, within a medical institution, information is generally passed around on a perceived, usually self-designated, "need to know basis" without first obtaining a patient's informed consent. Individuals who receive their medical care through managed care facilities and integrated health care delivery systems that have multiple treatment sites and use computer-based patient records can anticipate that the traditional standards of medical confidentiality will be diminished. Even a minor error, such as dialing an incorrect fax number and sending an electronic report to an unintended recipient, can result in damage to the patient and ultimately cost to the individual who authorized the report to be transmitted in error.

A release of medical information request can be general or rather specific, depending on the clinical and social circumstances, needs of the treating health care providers, and instructions of the patient or guardian. In general, medical information is released upon written instruction; however, oral instructions frequently are sufficient or necessary. This may be the case in a medical emergency. Documentation of oral permission for release of medical information is recommended.

Health Insurance Portability and Accountability Act of 1996

The HIPAA, Public Law 104-191 (4), is concerned in general about the written word and not oral communications, especially those provided in an ongoing manner in the course of clinical treatment.

HIPAA set national standards for the protection of health information, as applied to the three types of covered entities: (a) health plans—an individual or group plan that provides or pays the cost of medical care that includes the diagnosis, cure, mitigation, treatment, or prevention of disease; health plans include private entities and government organizations such as Medicaid, Medicare, and the Veterans Health Administration; (b) health care clearinghouses—a public or private entity, including a billing service or community health information system that processes medical, financial, or other data; and (c) health care providers who conduct certain health care business transactions electronically. Health care providers such as physicians, hospitals, and clinics are covered entities if they transmit health information in electronic form in connection with a transaction for which a HIPAA standard has been adopted by the Department of Health and Human Services (DHHS).

The compliance date has passed; for larger entities it was April 14, 2003, for smaller entities it was April 14, 2004. If HIPAA is more stringent than a state's law, it governs; if the state law is more stringent than HIPAA, the state law governs. Generally, "covered entities" are required to comply with both HIPAA and state law whenever possible. HIPAA preempts any contrary provision of state law, including state law provisions that require written records rather than electronic ones. State law, however, is not preempted in the following circumstances: regulation of insurance or health plans; prevention of fraud and abuse; reporting on health care system operations and costs; regulations concerning controlled substances; when a state law requires the reporting of disease or injury; child abuse, birth, or death; public health surveillance, investigation, or intervention; or when a provision of state law is more stringent than the requirements of HIPAA.

As with every issue of conflict between state and federal laws, there are exceptions. Exceptions mean health care lawyers need to be consulted when a clinician is unsure as to his or her course of action with regard to HIPAA and state confidentiality laws. There are other federal laws that may be relevant to parental conduct, such as the federal

Drug and Alcohol Confidentiality Regulations (58) which govern the release of medical records that contain information about drug and alcohol use, and the terrorism provisions of HIPAA which allow access to medical records if matters of national security may be involved.

HIPAA was designed to protect patients' medical records and their confidentiality. Other laws have existed to do this. The U.S. Congress believed, in consultation with many patient advocates, health care providers, and other commentators, that more than 1,000 additional pages of laws and regulations were required. If HIPAA serves to demonstrate two basic principles that health care professionals have long recognized, it is that first, medicine is no longer a one-on-one relationship and second, medicine has evolved with all its disciplines, providers, and equipment to be a major economic force and component of every industrialized nation.

HIPAA has forced health care professionals to better communicate with patients and their relatives. More ironically, 9-11 and the potential for future terrorist activities, has demanded that the health care professions better communicate with potential patients, the general public, politicians, and the media. Risk communication has been transformed from an arcane technique used by military and emergency preparedness personnel to a staple of daily communication. The basic principles of risk communication are simple and totally applicable to the practice of medicine, especially neonatology: Tell what you know—clearly, succinctly, and in a manner that every sixth grader can understand. Tell what you do not know clearly, succinctly, and in a manner that every sixth grader can understand. Do not guess—information has to be data driven. It is better to say we do not know now, and when we do, we will share it with you rather than to provide incorrect information initially because incorrect information causes credibility to suffer, believability to suffer, cooperation to suffer, and ultimately there is more confusion, anxiety, and poorer outcomes. Communication issues are discussed further in the second section of this chapter.

HIPAA delegates to local health departments the task of collecting vital statistics that include birth, death, and marriage information. These documents generally are protected to some degree. Autopsy reports usually are not released beyond the treating physician and/or coroner/medical examiner, unless there is authorization to do so. Civil or criminal courts can order the contents of an autopsy revealed if it would assist a party in asserting his or her civil claim, criminal prosecution, or defense from prosecution.

Legal Issues Specific to Managed Care

Although the incidence of malpractice litigation against health professionals has increased exponentially in the U.S. since the 1970s (67), it is not a recent phenomenon. Documented medical professional liability cases date to 1374, when a surgeon in England was sued for negligent treatment of a wound (68). However, a hybrid of lawsuits

against health care providers, focusing on managed care issues, is new (69,70). Profit is the bottom line in today's health care system (71). Managed care developed in response to a perception on the part of both government and society in general that there were unnecessary medical procedures being performed with an associated overutilization of medical resources and services, and an unrestrained lack of uniformity of cost in health care. Managed care filled a vacuum; it was developed and marketed because of a perceived need to control by those who paid costs (the employers) and those who managed health care dollars (health care insurance companies). Health care providers did little to inform their constituencies of the potential problems associated with managed care.

Managed care may be defined as "any entity capable of negotiating to deliver health care to a group of recipients at a predetermined rate on a per capita basis" (71). The American Association of Health Plans claims that 150 million Americans were enrolled in health maintenance organizations (HMOs) or other managed care entities in 1995 (72). Almost 75% of those who receive health insurance through their employers are covered by some type of managed care plan (73).

Managed care has become "big business," with the administrative costs and profit deriving in major part from cost savings and efficiencies (74). The focus of the decision maker to authorize or perform a service or procedure or order a medication now has an aspect of a real or perceived profit motive: There has been considerable media coverage of managed care programs that firmly control costs to the detriment of those paying premiums and expecting the best services available. In many cases, unqualified personnel are placed in a position of second-guessing and overruling physician decision-making responsibilities and obligations. Delays in receiving permission for expensive procedures or outright denials for critical but costly procedures occur. In some instances, so-called "gag" orders had been inserted in physicians' contracts, which effectively prohibited physicians from disclosing expensive, and potentially more effective, alternative treatments to their patients (71). However, in February 1997 President Clinton requested that the DHHS send a letter to all state Medicaid directors informing them that "gag rules" are prohibited for Medicaid HMOs. He also supported national legislation to ban "gag rules" for all managed care organizations within the United States. Approximately half the states in the United States have enacted or introduced their own laws regulating "gag rule" provisions in medical care policies. In *Moore v Regents of the University of California*, the California Supreme Court held that the concept of informed consent is broad enough to include the physicians' duty to inform their patients that they have an economic interest which might affect that physician's professional judgment (75).

Although managed care attempts to reduce costs by creating economies of scale and coordinating care among health care providers and resources, they also attempt to reduce costs by eliminating unnecessary care, as they define it. In some instances, a managed care program's criteria for emergency or extensive and expensive care may conflict with those held by the physician. The physician's contract may have a provision in which a percentage of fees are paid only if utilization goals are met. The physician's contract also may have a capitation provision, which means that the physician is provided a fixed amount regardless of the level of service provided to each patient. In the latter circumstances, the physicians essentially become coinsurers and may have a perceived conflict of interest in the manner and degree to which they provide services to their patients.

The most unique feature of an HMO is that an enrolled patient pays a prepaid, fixed fee for medical services. This is in contrast to "fee for services" in which the patient pays a separate fee for each service rendered by the independent physician. Preferred provider organizations (PPOs) differ from HMOs in that a PPO is an organized group of health care providers offering their services at a discount. Services are provided on a predetermined fee-for-service basis. Members may choose physicians regardless of whether they are in the members' plan but receive "discounts" only from physicians within the plan. PPO physicians have relatively minimal financial incentive to limit services, and physicians practicing under such an arrangement would appear to have greater control of their practice and potential liability.

The HMO may contract directly with physicians and pay them a salary (staff model), or they may contract with a group of physicians. The physician group may or may not devote a majority of its time to serving the needs of a specific HMO. It may offer a mixture of financial arrangements to its patients, including fee for service. The HMO may contract with an individual practice association (IPA), usually a partnership or corporation of physicians, to provide health care services to the HMO membership. The IPA then contracts with its physicians to provide services to the HMO. The fundamental difference between the IPA and the staff and group physician arrangements is that IPA physicians usually work in their own facilities, use their own equipment, and keep their own records. The HMO pays the IPA a capitation fee (a specific amount per enrollee or subscriber); the IPA pays the treating physicians on a fee-for-services basis (76).

Physicians and their managed care carriers are being sued jointly. Allegations of malpractice now are joined with allegations of bad faith, and contract theories of liability are being added to the more traditional negligence/medical malpractice theories of liability (69,70,77). Under the doctrine of *respondeat superior*, HMOs have been found responsible for the alleged negligence of their employee—physicians (78). The doctrine of *respondeat superior* states that an employer is vicariously liable for negligence of an employee acting within the scope of his or her employment (79). The doctrine does not apply if the negligent party is a true independent contractor (80). The distinction between an employee and an independent contractor is control or independence; that is, an employee is subject to the immediate direction and control of the employer, and independent contractors use their own judgment and are not subject to direct control. In some instances, an HMO can be held vicariously liable for the negligence of a consultant requested by the HMO's physician (81). This issue may be decided on the wording in the promotional material provided to subscribers. A managed care contract can increase a physician's obligations to a patient; the contract cannot decrease or even limit the physician's obligations and legal liability to the patient. When a physician employed by an HMO makes a treatment decision, that treatment decision has financial consequences to the HMO (69). In a malpractice suit, there are now assertions that the HMO-paid physician's treatment decisions were economically motivated rather than being made in the best interests of the patient (69). Before a physician accepts a contractual obligation, whether it is the product of an employment contract with a hospital, group practice, HMO, or other form of managed or prepaid care program, it is strongly suggested that the physician seek legal advice regarding the terms of the contract and the consequences of those terms.

Regardless of the employment status of the health care provider, the hospital has an obligation to oversee the quality of patient care and services (82). Ultimately, however, the courts have held that it is the physician's responsibility to uphold good medical practice in the face of improper or incorrect cost-containment procedures put forth by HMOs or other managed care organizations. The California Court of Appeals has held that, "while we recognize, realistically, that cost consciousness has become a permanent feature of the health care system, it is essential that cost limitation programs are not permitted to corrupt medical judgment" (83). That court found for the plaintiff because the physician did not protest the health insurer's determination that a prolonged hospitalization for his patient was not necessary, with severe negative consequences for the patient (83).

The Employee Retirement Income Security Act of 1974 (ERISA) (84) "supersedes any and all state laws insofar as they may now or hereafter relate to any employee benefit" (85). In *Shea v Esensten*, a federal court found that ERISA requires HMOs to disclose to their enrollees the compensation agreement between the HMO and its physicians (86). That is, there is an affirmative duty by the HMOs to inform their subscribers of any financial incentives that the health care providers may receive as they manage their patients' care. These financial "incentives must be disclosed and the failure to do so is a breach of ERISA's fiduciary duties" (86). Physicians who have challenged managed care decisions about patient care have been removed from the HMO panels. Suits for reinstatement on the grounds that they were removed from the panel without good cause and in violation of public policy and the implied covenant of good faith and fair dealing traditionally read into contracts have had mixed results (87,88). Just as medicine has evolved significantly during the past several decades, so too has the law. Both will continue to change, and their progress, conflicts, and resolutions will be documented in the media, professional journals, legislature, and courts.

Physician Liability Arising from Nonphysician Providers

Liability exposure arising from the use of nonphysician providers (NPPs) (e.g., neonatal nurse practitioner, clinical nurse specialist, physician assistant) is relatively new. It can be assumed, however, that as NPPs increase their roles, there will be a concomitant increase in malpractice allegations against NPPs and the physicians working with them, based upon the fact that the NPP is acting as an agent for the physician.

To the extent that NPPs exercise control over their professional activities, they will be held responsible for their negligent acts. Under the old "captain of the ship" (*respondeat superior*) doctrine, the physician was presumed to be responsible for the activities of all the NPPs working with the physician. Contemporary courts have moved away from this theory and have placed responsibility on those professionals exercising control. However, this does not eliminate the liability risk for the supervising physician.

Potential areas of risk for neonatologists working with NPPs and methods for reducing risk are listed in Table 8-1.

The National Practitioner Data Bank

Some malpractice insurance carriers retain the right to settle lawsuits independent of the wishes or sentiments of the health care provider. The federally mandated and operated National Practitioner Data Bank contains information, available to hospitals and individuals, and lists settled medical malpractice claims (89). General medical malpractice carriers may not always be knowledgeable regarding the specific nuances of specialty practice.

Health professionals should do more than comparison shop the price of a malpractice policy. They need to determine the financial soundness of the malpractice carrier and their own rights to control settlement and to determine the sophistication and knowledge of the legal representation provided by their insurance carrier.

TABLE 8-1

LIABILITY RISK AND RISK REDUCTION FOR NEONATOLOGISTS WORKING WITH NONPHYSICIAN PROVIDERS

Areas of Risk	Risk Reduction

■ Inadequate supervision by physician
■ NPPs working beyond their scope
■ Parent unhappy about access to their newborn's physician
■ Physician viewed as "deep pocket" by plaintiff's bar
■ Apparent physician delay in seeing critical patient
	■ Check NPP credentials before hiring and maintain documentation
	■ Establish, and review at least annually, written policies, protocols, and procedures for:
	  • patient examination
	  • treatment
	  • delegation
	  • supervision
	  • patient's/parent's right of access to physician
	■ Instruct NPP to adhere as closely as possible to patient care protocols, using physician input when significant deviation may be required; the rationale for deviations should be documented
	■ Document completion of skills inventory check
	■ Document current competency and establish a quality monitoring system
	■ Educate other staff about the role and limits of the NPP
	■ Understand and keep current regarding statutory requirements for NPPs
	■ Use name tags to identify the professional status of the NPP
	■ Introduce NPP to parents and explain role
	■ Review NPP's charts on a regular basis and cosign orders in a timely fashion
	■ Establish protocol for physician to see patient and parents at set intervals
	■ Obtain adequate liability insurance for NPP; physician's liability insurer should be informed that they are supervising NPPs
	■ Ensure that NPP complies with hospital credentialing requirements and has sufficient time allotted for continuing professional education; require that copies of licensure renewal and certification of continuing education are kept on file
	■ Inform physicians covering call of NPP's role

QUALITY ASSURANCE, PERFORMANCE IMPROVEMENT, AND RISK MANAGEMENT

The process of quality monitoring and improvement (QMI) is also discussed in Chapter 7. This part of the chapter emphasizes how QMI and risk management are closely interwoven and how both monitoring systems are used to improve patient care.

The Growth of Risk Management

In the United States, risk management programs grew out of changes in the medical malpractice insurance market (insurance became more difficult and more expensive to obtain) as malpractice claims accelerated in the 1970s (67). As the cost of liability insurance increased, the establishment of risk management programs made health care facilities more attractive to insurance underwriters. When institutions formed their own self-insurance trust funds, risk management programs provided some assurances to hospital board members that the financial liability of the institution would be limited to the greatest extent possible by their own risk managers. Depending upon the size and complexity of the health care institution involved, there may be one set of professionals who provide risk management guidance relative to standards of care and a second set of professionals under the leadership of a compliance officer who assure compliance with the requirements of regulatory bodies. Ensuring compliance requires a thorough knowledge of applicable standards and a commitment of time specifically directed towards understanding compliance and related issues. In smaller institutions the compliance officer and risk manager may be the same individual.

Basic Elements of a Compliance Program

A compliance program is a set of procedures within a medical practice or other health care facility which are designed to ensure adherence to laws and regulations associated with either federal or privately insured health care programs and thereby to prevent or reduce improper conduct. Although the size (e.g., number of employees) and type of practice or organization determines in large part the extent and formality of its compliance program, even small, private, neonatology practices are expected to implement one. Compliance programs establish and communicate standards of conduct; provide channels of communication to inform employees of rights, benefits, and obligations, and to answer questions; enforce standards through the consistent application of disciplinary measures; and require ongoing auditing and monitoring to ensure that identified errors are corrected and future similar occurrences are prevented.

The rapid rise in health care costs in the United States during the past three decades has prompted a significant increase in governmental scrutiny. The results of government audits have created a dramatic change in public opinion regarding the level of waste, fraud, and abuse in the health care system. This has led to the passage of legislation that creates a trust fund for investigations and expands governmental prosecutorial powers and also has markedly increased penalties for noncompliance. For instance, a claim for payment for medical services to Medicaid or Medicare which is deemed to be "fraudulent" under the False Claims Act (90) requires payment of three times the amount of the overpayment plus a mandatory $5,000 to $10,000 fine per claim. And since each individual service billed for is a claim under the definitions used in the statute, penalties can become enormous. On the other hand, "erroneous" claims (i.e., those resulting from innocent errors) require only the return of the amount of the overpayment. Fraudulent claims result from three circumstances: (a) actual knowledge that the claim is false, (b) reckless disregard of the truth or falsity of the claim, or (c) deliberate ignorance of the truth or falsity of the information. To mitigate the potential and corresponding penalties for noncompliance, voluntary compliance programs have become commonplace and necessary in the health care world. The voluntary compliance programs recommended for health care providers are designed to detect and/or prevent illegal activity through self policing.

Providers meeting the requirements of an effective compliance program, listed below, demonstrate their commitment to creating an environment in which payment claims are accurate; fraudulent behavior does not occur; improper practices are prevented, detected, or rectified; wrongdoing is reduced; administrative liability is mitigated; and the mental state of reckless disregard is negated. Although all compliance programs do not need to be alike and the degree to which each element needs to be addressed varies among practice types, compliance programs should address the following seven basic elements (91):

> establish written standards of conduct, policies, and procedures
> designate a compliance officer or contact
> provide mandatory training and education
> create and publish accessible lines of communication
> audit and monitor compliance with guidelines
> enforce through clear disciplinary guidelines
> respond to violations and take corrective action

Although neonatal practitioners are not expected to be experts in law or regulation, they need to have a good working knowledge of relevant legal and regulatory requirements that relate directly to their duties and responsibilities. Regulations often are complex, ambiguous, and sometimes silent on key issues. Whenever in doubt about a legal or administrative issue, it is important for the practice or practitioner to consult with an expert before proceeding. The list of areas of law/regulation which the practitioner should understand includes, but is not limited to, the following (91):

> billing and coding
> patients' rights
> health care antifraud and antiabuse laws

Medicare/Medicaid antikickback statutes

conflicts of interest

harassment in the workplace

environmental protection laws (e.g., disposal of hazardous material and medical waste)

health and safety programs and Occupational, Safety, and Health Administration regulations

HIPAA regulations

receipt and giving of gifts, gratuities, and other business courtesies

credentialing requirements, including sanction screening

insider information and securities laws

patent, copyright, and intellectual property laws

record retention requirements

professional standards of care

Stark legislation (e.g., physician antireferral statues)

the Privacy Act

Establishing a Risk Management Program

Health care errors rarely are due solely to a mistake made by an individual; they are usually an indication of failure of a health care system. System issues are referred by risk managers to staff trained in quality improvement and to the hospital administration, and vice versa. An effective QMI program works in close cooperation with the risk management team, with the ultimate aim being the improved care and safety of patients and lowered liability exposure. The importance of monitoring all aspects of a health care system in the prevention of medical errors was emphasized by the IOM in their 1999 report (92) on the nature and extent of medical errors in the practice of medicine.

Risk Reduction as It Relates to Quality Monitoring and Improvement and Risk Management

Risk is the possibility of harm, the uncertainty of danger, and the probability of loss. The essence of a QMI program and of risk management lies in maximizing the areas in which there is some control over the outcome while minimizing the areas in which there is absolutely no control over the outcome. The existence of risk does not imply that there are always alternatives. The terms QMI and risk management are used to describe a process of examining any potential alternatives and thereby influencing, in a positive manner, the level of risk to which patients, health care providers, and institutions are exposed. An outcome of managing risk is the identification of a level of harm or danger that is the irreducible minimum. However, QMI and risk management differ in the order of priority of their primary goals. In the health care setting, harm or danger expressed in human terms pertains to the safety of patients, visitors, and employees, and to health care delivery practices; however, harm or loss can also be expressed in financial terms, such as losses in settlements, jury verdicts, legal expenses, and payment of increased insurance premiums.

QMI is the term used for the process in which the primary expected reduction is expressed in human terms; risk management is the term used when the primary expected reduction in risk is expressed in financial terms. Risk reduction is achieved using a process that involves investigating, evaluating, planning, organizing, and implementing procedures. The resulting benefit of risk reduction is improved quality and understanding of patient care and also preservation of the financial resources necessary to provide optimal patient care when there are fewer claims made and fewer lawsuits brought against the health care providers (93,94). Financial and psychological benefits also are realized when malpractice cases are dismissed or settled for reduced amounts, based on the strength of the defense.

The level of risk exposure in the health care environment is inversely proportional to the control maintained by the health care service providers. Total control is not possible in the face of complex disease processes and complex care and treatment managed in complex patient care delivery systems. In the critical care environment, a risk reduction program must be established that anticipates, identifies, and responds to risk. When it is possible in the process of delivering care to patients, fail-safe systems are established to prevent errors from affecting the patient.

The elements of a risk reduction program also reflect the health care organization's attempt to define, describe, and impute liability within the organizational structure. Functional definitions of health care executives and their roles and responsibilities for supervising and administering health care activities enable the health care providers to identify chains of management decision making and accountability. Health care providers need to understand who supervises each administrative component of a health care facility so that complaints, comments, and recommendations reach those who are in a position to respond affirmatively. The chain of responsibility for developing, implementing, supporting, monitoring, and evaluating a risk reduction program reflects multidisciplinary health and management skills and activities. It must be recognized that a risk reduction program is both a proactive (preventing potential incidents from occurring) and reactive (responding to an incident or seminal event and preventing future similar incidents) system of intervention to protect the patient, institution, and clinician. Although assignment of responsibility does occur in either a proactive or reactive risk assessment, responsibility is not to be perceived as the same as negligence. For example, there is no negligence in a situation in which a physician orders a specific dose of medication, the nurse responsible administers the proper dosage, and there is a resultant catastrophic effect on the patient. In many instances, either the risk was known and shared with the parents or the adverse consequences could not reasonably have been foreseeable.

Risk reduction programs strive to reduce risk to the greatest extent possible and to manage the remaining risk. Quality improvement committees, safety committees, and specialized subcommittees provide the administrative and management structures to review the various aspects of clinical care and support and to provide constructive guidance and assistance. The outcome of this effort is improved quality of care within the context of the goals of the health care team and the patient's family.

From the perspective of risk management, risk financing involves the financial arrangement (insurance) made for the payment of losses that inevitably do occur. The liability insurance program may be coordinated by the risk management department. The risk manager notifies the insurance carrier of reportable events, claims, and lawsuits. Members of the health care team have a shared responsibility to report adverse events, contribute to the data that will track these events, and alert the malpractice insurance carrier to potential financial loss. The risk manager may select defense counsel and assist counsel in the defense of the institution and/or health care providers. In addition to contributing to the quality of patient care, the risk manager, under the direction of counsel, contributes to the quality of the defense of the health care provider in a claim or suit (94,95). Conflicts of interest between the institution and health care provider need to be identified and addressed as soon as possible. Separate counsel for the medical institution or group practice and medical practitioners may be required when there are divergent institutional and personal interests. For instance, one party may wish to settle their portion of the case while the other named party or parties may wish to litigate the allegations against them.

From the QMI perspective, adequate risk financing, malpractice insurance, requires the acknowledgment that reducing the risk to patients and staff in the health care system never means totally eliminating it. There will always remain some minimal risk for an untoward event. Hence, malpractice insurance is needed to cover the cost of defending the claims and the cost of paying any judgment, should the defense efforts prove unsuccessful.

To achieve the goals of risk management, the following activities must take place:

Systematic and continuous investigation of risk exposures. Risk managers must be made aware of potential and actual exposures (adverse events) as they occur and of system changes that may affect patient and staff potential exposure to risk. To achieve this level of awareness, it is necessary for risk managers to establish a communication network that provides real-time feedback. The risk manager utilizes the knowledge, impressions, and experience of the health care team to investigate events that have occurred and to identify events that might occur in the future. Methods of communication to risk managers include incident reports, risk management presence on committees, and ready accessibility by electronic means.

Evaluation of risk loss exposure. An examination of the nature, frequency, severity of risk, and potential impact on the patient/organization detects patterns in recurrent events, which can be used to predict their recurrence. For example, if medication errors

are observed to occur just before a change of shift, examination of the human dynamics that contribute to these errors and breaking the pattern can lead to correction of an error-producing systems flaw. Administration and clinical staff are called upon to identify potential risk areas for evaluation.

Planning and organization of appropriate risk avoidance and prevention techniques to efficiently minimize loss to the organization. Currently in the United States, order, stability, and consistency are not the hallmarks of a successful health care organization. Risk management demands the establishment of an information-gathering network, which identifies emerging organizational changes. Areas of risk can be identified as projects are developed. The monitoring of system changes after implementation is used to detect any negative impact on patient care. Recommendations can then be made to adjust system changes. Anticipation is one of the most important considerations. Identifying pertinent questions regarding the level of risk for potential adverse events and those who should be involved in evaluating a system helps the direct clinical service providers avoid some significant errors (96).

Implementation of risk reduction. Good clinical staff are flexible, innovative, and creative; thus, there is constantly the potential for an adverse event to emerge from new technology or treatment modalities. Simplifying the organization or health care practices to gain control is not a realistic goal in today's complex health systems. By using reporting and communication connections within and outside the organization and analyzing data from the investigation of adverse events, areas of greatest risk can be identified. The information about potential risk is communicated to committees or individuals who then put in place mechanisms to reduce the risk to the patient and institution. That the risk cannot be controlled completely should also be communicated, particularly to the patient's family.

The Risk Management Plan

Risk management activities are outlined in a program description. Such a document provides clear and concise information about the risk management program, which is available to all those within the institution.

Staff Education

Personnel involved in QMI or risk management must recognize that they are educators. Every committee meeting, exchange with a staff member, or participation in orientation is an opportunity to dispel misinformation and increase understanding of the risk management process.

The fundamentals of risk management are not highlighted in medical and nursing schools but are necessary to prepare future health care providers for dealing with risk issues that arise in the clinical setting. The development of a risk management curriculum gives structure to educational efforts and provides a framework to cover essential topics, ranging from the orientation of new employees, staff physicians, and residents to seminars for advanced practitioners, department chairpersons, and administrators.

As an outcome of a core curriculum in risk management, all individuals in health care should be able to:

define risk

know the basics of how to set up a risk reduction study, including definitions of area of risk to be studied and sentinel events

describe what a risk manager does and why

understand what events need to be communicated to risk managers

recognize that if a facility, treatment, or system is replaced, the replacement must be monitored until proven to decrease risk

describe how to access risk managers for reporting and receiving information

describe what relationship risk managers have with professional liability insurers

Grupp-Phelan and associates (97) reported that pediatric residents were named in 26% of malpractice suits. All health care providers, including nurses, nurse practitioners, residents, house staff, and ancillary staff such as respiratory therapists and clinical nutritionists, should know what kind of process a risk management investigation will follow (Fig. 8-2).

Health care professionals should avoid making editorial comments in patient records and should not keep personal notes about clinical events. Objective clinical impressions belong in a patient's medical record. Physicians, nurses, and other health care professionals should understand that investigations take time and that the findings may be very different from the initial views of the staff. Speculation about the causes of adverse events or discussions of the events outside the peer-review/quality improvement areas should be discouraged.

With an understanding of the fundamentals of risk reduction/management, the health care provider can move on to identify systems and processes in his or her care that can be examined for safety and effectiveness. The risk manager analyzes the frequency or severity of adverse events or unexpected outcomes and the findings during the course of discovery in lawsuits, and then identifies topics that can be presented in an advanced risk reduction curriculum. These include: retroactive peer review (e.g., clinicopathologic review, regular review of perinatal or neonatal patient care statistics), documentation, communication, supervision, monitoring and assessment, coordination of care, medication administration, system fail-

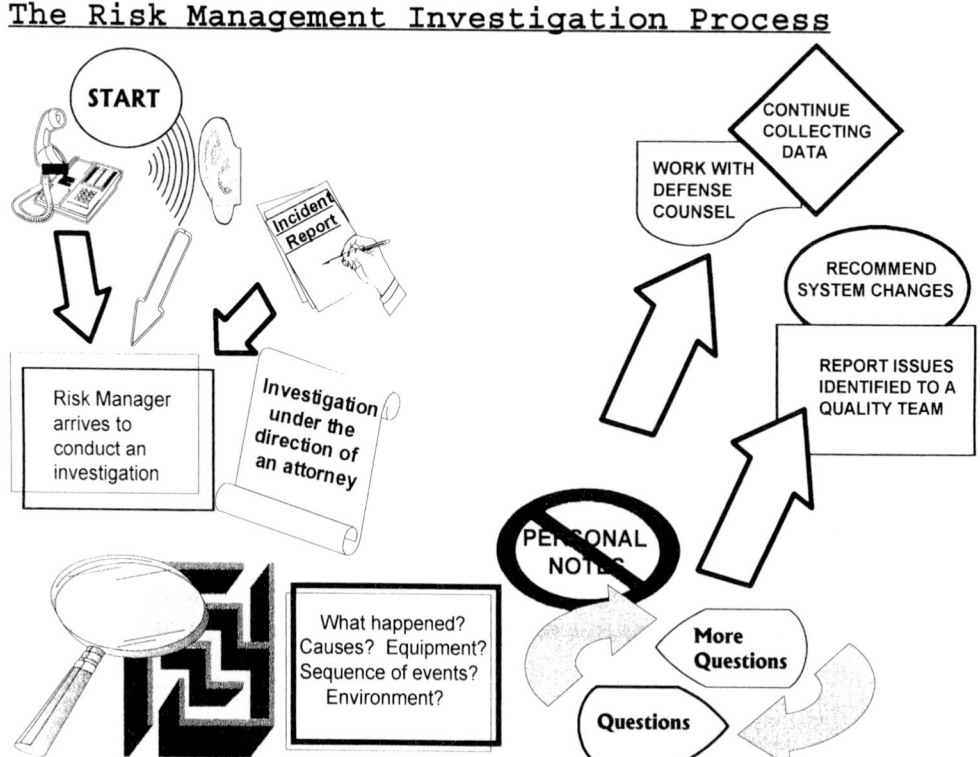

Figure 8-2 The risk management investigation process begins with the receipt of notice that an adverse event has occurred. An attorney directs some investigations in jurisdictions where the risk management activities are not protected from discovery in litigation. The personal notes of health care providers are not protected from discovery. After many rounds of questions, opportunities for improvement are reported to quality improvement councils. In a separate activity, the results of investigation directed by the defense attorney are sent to him or her.

ure(s) and human error, and changes in local, state, or national regulations or laws.

Adverse Events

Adverse sentinel events were defined by the JCAHO in 1996 as unexpected occurrences involving death or serious physical or psychologic injury or risk thereof. The term "sentinel" is used because the event should sound a warning that requires immediate attention. A root cause analysis is recommended by the JCAHO as the format for an intensive assessment to reduce the variation and prevent the event in the future. This type of analysis addresses these questions: what happened, why did it happen, and what processes were involved when it happened? The analysis can be used to piece together the reasons why a mistake or complication occurred. If the system worked previously, what elements have changed to produce the potential for error (98)?

In some instances, it is not possible to sort out the exact sequence of events. Interruptions in the system of care delivery that are identified should be repaired or redesigned to prevent further breakdowns. Because serious occurrences do not occur very often, it is necessary to optimize the lessons learned from each event, including an application of those potential events that did not occur. Adverse, unexpected, or poor patient outcomes do not necessarily indicate that a mistake has been made. It is important not to make this assumption within the health care team, nor to accuse or place blame. When there is an unexpected outcome, the risk manager is called upon to perform the process of identifying the possible contributing factors.

Receiving an incident report and investigating problems that have occurred or potentially might occur is viewed by the risk manager as an opportunity for improvement in the system of care delivery. This positive outlook may not be shared by the staff. The stigma of punishment or retaliation in relation to incident reports exists and is a deterrent to obtaining the information on which to base a recommendation for change and improvement in health care delivery.

Accountability versus Blame

System and practice patterns are the focus of a risk management investigation. Investigations may reveal systems and patterns that do not provide sufficient or effective safety checks to prevent human error or miscommunication. In addition to identifying the flaw in systems or processes that potentiate mistakes, adverse event investigations studied in the aggregate identify the types of patients most likely to be affected. Andrews and associates (99) found that more patients with a serious illness had an initial adverse event, and that the likelihood of an adverse event increased 6% for each additional hospital day. The analysis of event databases provides the health care team with information that they can use to modify practice or alert other practitioners, thereby improving care and reducing the likelihood of lawsuits.

Reported predictors of the outcome of pediatric litigation include severity of resulting disability (100), defensibility of the case (101), and parental anger (102) (often exacerbated by a perception that communication with health care providers was less than satisfactory). The importance of patient or parental anger was demonstrated by Andrews and associates (99), who found that of 1,047 patents with serious injury, 17.7% experienced serious adverse events that led to longer hospital stays, but only in 1% to 2% of these adverse events was a legal claim made for compensation.

Pichert and associates (102) studied 43 closed claims, covering 8 years, involving children. A significant portion of the claims were associated with high-risk medical conditions (37%) and problems associated with intravenous therapies, central lines, and catheters (21%). In 9% of the claims physicians relied on faulty information, and in 19% the parent(s) became particularly enraged by an injury.

Conventional wisdom holds the view that human beings are intrinsically unreliable. From this it follows that when something goes wrong, someone must have erred. It is assumed that mistakes such as these are the result of inattention, carelessness, and negligence. The remedies invoked to prevent further lapses include finding the culprit, assigning blame, and acting to correct future misdeeds. The truth is that the errors people make often are traceable to extrinsic factors that predispose an individual to fail. Whenever human error is suspected, it is a sound policy to trace the error to its root cause(s). To assign blame to an individual who makes an error is no assurance that the same error will not be made again by that individual or another (103).

The health care provider should not assume that he or she or another member of the team is responsible or liable for an unexpected outcome. Frequently the first impression regarding the cause of poor patient outcomes is significantly different from the cause(s) recorded at the conclusion of an investigation. There is also a possibility that a cause may never be found. There should be no speculation by those directly or peripherally involved as to the cause or etiology of the event. A defensive position in response to the family's accusations should be avoided, as should the assignation of blame to other disciplines, departments, and/or systems.

The analysis of a single event and analysis of event trends provide the health care team with information that they can use to modify practice or alert other practitioners, thereby improving care and reducing the likelihood of repeated errors.

Communication

Risk communication includes those techniques for disseminating information that may be complex and include elements of uncertainty as to diagnosis, treatment, and prognosis. Chess and associates (104) note that some common myths often interfere with the development and implementation of effective risk communication. The manner in which the information is provided (the style and process of information delivery) is just as important as the content of the message. Treatment options need to be provided, including the option of no treatment. Confrontation should be avoided. Questioning should be encouraged and not perceived to be a challenge to a clinician's knowledge, treatment interventions, or plans. Neonatal intensive care units are highly emotionally charged environments, both for the parents and concerned family members and health care providers.

Communication with Parents and Guardians

Many factors that lead to medical malpractice lawsuits are perceptual and qualitative in nature. In many cases, lawsuits are not the result of malpractice, but are instituted because the patient or patient's family feels that information was withheld from them or that they were not told the truth. Effective communication skills used in data collection, developing relationships, and dealing with parents' emotions help to prevent anger and possible malpractice litigation (105).

The perception by the family of the competency of the physicians, nurses, and other health care team members is drawn from their interactions with them. Ideally, contact with the family inspires trust, confidence, and openness. Positive contact with the family of a neonate is based upon the fundamentals of communication: body language that conveys attention to the family and infant, taking time to answer questions, asking for input from the family regarding their impressions of the baby's progress, and speaking in terms that can be understood by the family. These basic clinical and social skills represent the foundation of defensive medicine techniques. It is important to convey the message that team members taking care of the infant are communicating with each other, are fully aware of the treatment plan, and are coordinated in their approach to the care of the infant. Judgments and preconceived opinions about the family should be avoided, regardless of their lifestyle or behavior toward the health care team. A study by Cuttini and associates (106) concluded that parents generally are satisfied with the information received, although some complain about the style of communication and especially the need to ask repeatedly in order to be informed. The latter complaint may be more common in teaching hospitals because of the greater complexity of the health care hierarchy produced by the presence of medical students, interns, residents, and attending physicians, who may change every month. No matter how large the team caring for a neonate, the attending physician should be known to the parents and guardians and readily accessible to all salient parties.

Those who provide health care need to understand the manner in which they communicate to parents and other concerned parties. Health care providers must communicate in a manner which is linguistically, contextually, and culturally appropriate. The reluctance of many health care providers to convey the limitations as well as the achievements of the health care can significantly increase the family's distress when negative changes in their infant's condition occur. When the neonate or infant is not doing well, that is the critical time for more communication and more interaction with parents and significant others, not less. A decrease in communication at a critical juncture can and will damage the health care team's credibility. Training in risk communication, in conveying negative information, is essential.

Covello and Allen (107) identify seven cardinal rules of risk communication. Though these rules are designed for individuals who have to deal with the general public, they generally can be adapted to a hospital setting (91):

Accept and involve the family or guardian as a partner. Information is to be shared; concerns may not always be eliminated.

Present the plan or course of action that may even include alternative plans.

Listen to the concerns being stated. A concerned individual cares more about trust, credibility, competence, and empathy than cold statistics and complex details.

Be honest, frank, and open. Recognize that once trust and credibility are lost, they are almost impossible to regain.

Different health care providers may have different opinions; different family members may express different concerns. This is to be expected. Open and frequent communication minimize doubt and distrust. A single spokesperson, or a limited number of spokespersons, should be designated to minimize the diversity of opinions being provided.

Concerned parties are more interested in risks, simplicity of explanations, and the danger to the patient. The focus of the discussion needs to be on the patient, not on the health care provider.

Clear communication in a language and vocabulary understood by all parties needs to occur. Communication should be accompanied by compassion.

For the family of a critically ill neonate, the distinction is unclear between a bad outcome due to disease progression and unfortunate circumstances/errors/negligence. Anxiety over the uncertainty inherent in the care of the seriously ill may evoke feelings of helplessness. Outcomes that are expected by the physician but not clearly conveyed to the family may be a shock for the family. The nonoccurrence of expected outcomes leaves the parents feeling that a mistake has been made. Families who experience disappointments in clinical outcomes may take out their grief and despair on the health care provider. The provider may be unprepared for the parents' anger and distrust. Appearing uncertain, handling questions improperly, apologizing for oneself or the team, not knowing the available information, not involving the family in the decision-making process, not establishing rapport, appearing disorganized, and providing the wrong information (such as discussing the wrong patient) can all lead to a breakdown in communication.

Acknowledgment of hostility is acceptable; this indicates that the health care provider recognizes the reality of the situation. Anxiety undercuts confidence, concentration, and momentum. Listen to what others have to say, even if you disagree with them; recognize expressions of frustration. State conclusions and then provide supporting data. Above all, do not lie.

If an adverse event occurs, the honest, sincere, and compassionate response of the health care team to the family will reduce the family's view that there is a need to bring a lawsuit. Without burdening the family with personal feelings of inadequacy, regret, or vague misgivings, it is helpful to show concern and to express empathy regarding the patient outcome. Silverman (108) offers insight into how parents of infants blinded by retrolental fibroplasia (RLF) (retinopathy of prematurity) view the health professional who fails to convey appropriate concern:

> As compared with conversations with RLF-blind young adults, discussions with parents, singly and in groups, were much more difficult for me (and for them). Most of the parents were still bitterly angry at the medical profession, but not for the reason I imagined. They understood and accepted the fact of limited knowledge at the time their children were born. Most were convinced that physicians had rendered excellent care and had used supplemental oxygen liberally in well-meant efforts to improve the chances of the small babies for intact survival. But, almost without exception, parents recalled (with rancor) that once the diagnosis of RLF was made, a chill in relationships developed. At the very time when they needed support and advice, their physicians became distant and defensive, the parents recalled. Most blamed their doctors for failing to maintain interest and concern, not for the failure of clairvoyance! The parents said it was anger at personal, not professional, behavior of physicians which prompted many of the RLF legal suits charging malpractice which burgeoned in this country.

A member of the health care team should be designated as the primary communicator to share with the family the treatment plans that have been formulated in response to the adverse event. At the request of the family, extended family and other support may be included in family conferences and discussions of the causes or possible causes of the event. Maintenance of a coordinated and ongoing communication with the family may be difficult in the face of the family's anger and despair. However, the goal of the health care team must remain the support and treatment of the patient and family.

Communication with and within the Health Care Team

From the significant number of dangerous errors that occur in the intensive care unit, Donchin and associates (109) found many were attributed to problems of communication between physicians and nurses. They suggest that studying the weak points of communication in a unit may reduce errors, and that errors should not be considered an incurable disease but rather a preventable phenomenon.

Clear oral communication is vital in a NICU; the medical record alone cannot be relied upon to adequately convey urgent information between members of a health care team.

The medical record should be designed to achieve clear communication with and among the members of the health care team. Clinical information is focused on the patient and family, and it derives from repeated assessments, analyses, judgments, and actions aimed at achieving specific goals. Documentation in the patient record allows ongoing evaluation of patient progress and review of the clinical management plan. The individual contributions of the members of the health care team are recorded and used by other team members as a basis for planning each new step in patient care. This documentation of the exchange of information among the team and the recording of the outcome of each team member's analysis of the information also helps to support the team's choices and judgments. Documenting patient care, contemporaneous with the events, provides the clinical picture that will be used in the defense of the care provided should an adverse event occur. If the clinical record has the appearance of being a battleground for warring or defensive factions of the team, the record will reflect a lack of team cohesion and direction that is difficult to defend. The record should contain the facts of the event, assessments of the patient, the decision-making processes, and the interventions undertaken.

Any documentation of an abnormality in the medical record should be accompanied by the reassuring factors that support the overall interpretation of the clinical findings. All factors that explain decisions made in the face of abnormal finding(s) should be recorded. In fact, documentation of reassuring factors should accompany the recording of abnormal factors (110).

It is very important not to draw conclusions or relate events to outcomes that are speculative in nature. Avoid placing an inappropriate medical diagnosis as a label to clinical findings. The members of the team will erroneously draw upon speculative causal relationships and refer to them further in the record as an absolute. Applying an outcome, diagnosis, or finding from incomplete data does not lessen the impact of such a premature diagnosis during the course of either treatment or litigation. Concluding, for example, based on insufficient data that the encephalopathy found on a computerized tomographic scan is hypoxic encephalopathy and that the hypoxic encephalopathy is related to a specific hypotensive episode serves no meaningful clinical purpose and may lay the foundation for an accusation of medical negligence on those purported to be responsible for causing or failing to detect that specific hypotensive episode when the abnormal finding may not be secondary to hypoxic encephalopathy in the first place.

Imposition of unsubstantiated diagnoses is a frequent occurrence during follow-up care of high-risk infants and children. Recognizing that the medical records of infants discharged from an NICU may be voluminous, if a diagnosis cannot be confirmed by review of records, it should not be made in a follow-up summary.

TABLE 8-2
STEPS IN THE CONSULTATION PROCESS

- Identify when it is appropriate to obtain consultation
- Choose the type of consultant (sequencing of a variety of consultants)
- Share the purpose of the consultation with the family
- Decide what information is necessary to provide to the consultant, including the purpose of the consultation and provide as a written consultation request
- Arrange a formal consultation or designate this responsibility to a specific individual
- Give a time frame within which the consultation is to be done
- Agree with the consultant on how the consultation will be reported and who will discuss the findings with the family/parent(s)
- Share the outcome of the consultation with the family
- Tell the family what will be done with the resulting information
- Document in the medical record the reasons for requesting a consultation, discussions with the family, and plan of treatment, including the reasons why the recommendations of the consultant will or will not be followed

---

Clinical findings, if possible, are best graded using numeric values. Modifiers, such as the words "extreme," "severe," or "massive" do not provide objective information and will feed into the drama of a courtroom presentation. Contributors to the evaluation and care of the patient must avoid inflammatory language, markings, or punctuation that attempt to draw attention to the writer and imply that the team may be inattentive to the remarks otherwise.

It is possible that an infant's condition is changing so rapidly that thorough, contemporaneous notes in the medical record cannot be made. Although "not documented, not done" (111) is a well-known legal motto, there is much that occurs that cannot be documented in the patient record at the time of a critical event. It is often hindsight that focuses the care provider on events not recorded in contemporaneous records. A decision must be made as to whether an addendum to the medical record would contribute to patient care, or whether the additional information relates to system issues and should be conveyed to the risk manager by completing an incident report. An incident report is a confidential document that provides a means to communicate system issues. References to the completion of the incident report or discussions with the risk manager are not appropriate for, and should not appear in, the medical record (110). An incident report relates to an adverse event; the patient's record reflects care and treatment delivered, the patient's response, and the further plan of care.

When additional information, identified after an adverse event, is necessary to the care of the patient, communication of this information is achieved in an addendum to the medical record. Such entries must include the date and time that they were written. Under no circumstances should an attempt be made to make this entry appear contemporaneous with the adverse event. The addendum must be placed sequentially in the medical record in the next available space, not on a separate page, and never inserted into the text of previous entries. The purpose of an addendum is not to provide a defense or to make excuses.

Communication with Consultants

The "curbside" consultation between colleagues is a thing of the past. This type of consultation tends to be documented poorly, if at all, and can lead to damaging finger pointing in a court of law. Guidelines for the consultation process are shown in Table 8-2.

When a consultant is contacted for a specific patient with a formal request for evaluation and/or management, both the primary physician and consultant should interact in such a way as to limit unnecessary risk for both (111).

CONCLUSIONS

Almost coincident with publication of the fifth edition of this textbook (at the end of 1999), the IOM published their landmark report on the quality of health care in America (92). The reported finding that between 44,000 and 98,000 patient deaths per year are due to medical errors placed this as the eighth leading cause of death in the United States. In their report, the IOM estimated that at least 50% of these errors were preventable and challenged the health care system to reduce medical errors by 50% in the next 5 years. A further report entitled *Crossing the Quality Chasm: A New Health System for the Twenty-First Century* was published 2 years later in 2001 by the IOM (112) in which they listed six redesigned imperatives for the health care system in the United States:

redesign of the care process
use of information technologies
knowledge and skills management
development of effective teams
coordination of care
use of performance and outcome measurements

As the sixth edition of this textbook goes to press, there is abundant evidence that the IOM challenge has been noted and that the mouth of the quality chasm has been explored. There is little evidence however, at the 5-year anniversary of the IOM challenge that construction of a sound bridge across the quality chasm has progressed beyond the sinking of pylons.

REFERENCES

1. Witman AB, Park DM, Hardin SB. How do patients want physicians to handle mistakes? A survey of internal medicine patients in an academic setting. *Arch Intern Med* 1996;156:2565–2569.
2. Gallagher TH, Waterman AD, Ebers AG, et al. Patients' and physicians' attitudes regarding the disclosure of medical errors. *JAMA* 2003;289:1001–1007.
3. *Setting the Standard.* Oakbrook Terrace, Ill: Joint Commission on Accreditation of Healthcare Organizations (JCAHO) 2003.
4. *Eckert v Long Island R.R.,* 43 NY 502 (1871).

5. *Kambat v St. Francis Hospital*, 89 NY2d 489, 678 NE2d 456, NYS2d 844 (1997).
7. Keeton WP, Dobbs DB, Keeton RE. *Prosser and Keeton on the law of torts*. 5th ed. Eagan, Minn: West Group, 1984:356.
8. Mancini MR, Gale AT. *Emergency care and the law*. Rockville: Aspen Systems Corp., 1981:50.
9. Frew SA, Roush WR, LaGreca K. COBRA: implications for emergency medicine. *Ann Emerg Med* 1988;17:835–837.
10. *Hess v Paulowski*, 279 US 352 (1927).
11. Diversity of Citizenship; amount in controversy; costs, 28 USC §1332.
12. Friedman RH, Stollerman JE, Mahoney DM, et al. The virtual visit: using telecommunications technology to take care of patients. *J Am Med Inform Assoc* 1997;4:413–425.
13. Landwehr JB Jr, Zador IE, Wolfe HM, et al. Telemedicine and fetal ultrasonography: assessment of technical performance and clinical feasibility. *Am J Obstet Gynecol* 1997;177:846–848.
14. Lewis M, Moir AT. Medical telematics and telemedicine; an agenda for research evaluation in Scotland. *Health Bull (Edinb)* 1995;53:129–137.
15. Landquist A. Finland is a leading country when it comes to telemedicine. *Lakartidningen* l996;93:7–8.
16. Telecommunications Reform Act, S. 652, 104th Cong. §§ 709 (1996).
17. S. 773, 1995 Reg. Sess. (La. 1995).
18. Cal. Assembly 1665 (1996).
19. S. 48 (Okla. 1997).
20. H.R. 2033 (Tex. 1997).
21. H.R. 177 (Ky. 2000).
22. Telemedicine Report to Congress, January 31, 1997. Legal Issues, Licensure and Telemedicine. Available at: http://www.ntia.doc.gov/reports/telemed/.
23. Available at: http://www.napb.net/vipps/intro.asp.
24. *Jackson v Johns-Manville Sales Corp.*, 727 F2d 506,516 (5th Cir 1984).
25. McCormick C. *McCormick on evidence*, 2nd ed. St. Paul: West Publishing Co., 1972:§ 339.
26. Morgan E. *Basic problems of evidence*, 4th ed. Philadelphia: Joint Committee on Continuing Legal Education, 1963:24.
27. Terry HT. Negligence. *Harv Law Rev* 1915;29:40.
28. *Zebarth v Swedish Hospital Medical Center*, 81 Wash 2d 12,499 (P2d 1 1972).
29. Second Restatement of Torts, Section 282.
30. Ely JW, Levinson W, Elder EC, et al. Perceived causes of family physicians' errors. *J Fam Pract* 1995;40:337–344.
31. *Oelling v Rao*, 593 NE2d 189 (1992).
32. Available at: http://www.japantimes.co.jp/cgi_bin/getarticle.p15?ed20020705a1.htm. Accessed October 28, 2004.
33. *Small v Howard*, 128 Mass 131 (1880).
34. *Peck v Hurchinson*, 88 Iowa 320,55 NW 511.
35. *Daubert v Merrill Dow Pharmaceuticals, Inc.* 509 US 579 (1993).
36. *Ybarra v Spangard*, 25 Cal App 2d 486, 154 P2d 687 (1944).
37. *Mohr v Williams*, 104 NW 12, 5 Ct (1905).
38. *Canterbury v Spence*, 464 F2d 772 (DC Cit 1972), cert denied, 409 US 1064 (1972).
39. *Getchell v Mansfield*, 260 Or 174,489 P2d 953 (1971).
40. *Cooper v Roberts*, 286 A2d 647,650 (1971).
41. *Davis v Wyeth Laboratories, Inc.*, 399 F2d 121 (9th Cit 1968).
42. Application of President & Directors of Georgetown College, 331 F2d 1000 (DC Cir), cert denied, 377 US 978 (1964).
43. King NM. Transparency in neonatal intensive care. *Hastings Cent Rep* 1992;22:18–25.
44. Paasche-Orlow MK, Taylor HA, Brancati FL. Readability standards for informed-consent forms as compared with actual readability. *N Engl J Med* 2003;348:721–726.
45. Gutheil TG, Bursztajn H, Brodsky A. Malpractice prevention through the sharing of uncertainty. Informed consent and the therapeutic alliance. *N Engl J Med* 1984;311:49–51.
46. Gillick MR, Advance care planning. *N Engl J Med* 2004;350:7–8.
47. Committee on Bioethics, American Academy of Pediatrics. Informed consent, parental permission, and assent in pediatric practice. *Pediatrics* 1995;95:314–317.
48. *Little v Little*, 576 SW2d 493 (1979).
49. In Re Richardson, 284 So2d 185 (1973).
50. Medicaid fraud—a multibillion-dollar crime. Available at: http://www.newsmax.com/archives/articles/2002/12/30/170723.shtml.
51. U.S. Dept of Health and Human Services and U.S. Dept of Justice Health Care Fraud and Abuse Control Program. *Annual Report For FY 2002*. Washington, DC: U.S. Government Printing Office, 2003.
52. Federal crackdown puts risk managers in hot seat [Editorial]. *Health Care Risk Management* 1997;19:49.
53. Hayt E, Hayt LR, Groeschel AH. *Law of hospital, physician, and patient*, 2nd ed. New York: Hospital Textbook Co., 1952:637.
54. Beck JC. *Confidentiality versus the duty to protect: foreseeable harm in the practice of psychiatry*. Washington, DC: American Psychiatric Press, 1990.
55. *Reisner v Regents of the University of California* 31 Cal App 4th 1195,37 CalRptr2d518 (1995).
56. *Tarasoff v Regents of University of California*, 108 Cal Rptr 878 (Cal App 1973), superseded by *Tarasoff v Regents of University of California*, 13 Cal 3d 177, 118 Cal Rptr 129,529 P2d 553 (1974), subsequent op on on reh *Tarasoff v Regents of University of California*, 17 Cal 3d 425, 131 Cal Rptr 14,551 P2d 334 (1976).
57. *Lipari v Sears Roebuck & Co.*, 497 F Supp 185 (D Neb 1980).
58. 42 USC §290ee-3.
59. 42 USC §290dd-3.
60. 42 USC §290ee-3(b)(2)(A).
61. 42 USC §290dd-31(b)(2)(A).
62. 42 USC §290ee-3(tb)(2)(C).
63. 42 USC §290dd-3(b)(2)(C).
64. Dick RS, Steen EB, eds. *The computer-based patient record: an essential technology for health care*. Washington, DC: National Academy Press, 1991.
65. Woodward B. The computer-based patient record and confidentiality. *N Engl J Med* 1995;333:1419–1422.
66. Annas GJ. *The rights of patients: the basic ACLU guide to patient rights*, 2nd ed. Carbondale: Southern Illinois University Press, 1989:178.
67. Basalmo RR, Brown MD. Risk management. In: Sanbar SS, Gibofsky A, Firestone MH, eds. *Legal medicine*, 3rd ed. St. Louis: Mosby-Year Book, Inc., 1995:237.
68. Kramer C. Medical Malpractice 5 (1976), citing History of Reported Medical Professional Liability Cases, 30 Temple LQ 367 (1957).
69. *Pegram v Herdrich*, 530 US 211 (2000), 154 F3d 362, reversed.
70. Aetna Health Inc. v Davila, 542 US (2004), 307 F3d 298, reversed and remanded.
71. Malone TW, Thaler DH. Managed health care: a plaintiff's perspective. *Tort Insur Law J* 1996;32:123–153.
72. Clifford RA. Physician's liability in a managed care environment. *Health Lawyer* 1997;10:5.
73. Bodenheimer T. The HMO backlash—righteous or reactionary? *N Engl J Med* 1996;335:1601–1604.
74. Blum JL, ed. Monograph 5, achieving quality care: the role of the law. Health Law Section of the American Bar Association, Loyola University, Chicago, June 1997.
75. *Moore v Regents of the University of California*, 793 P2d 479, 51 Cal 2d 120 (1990).
76. Kanute M. Evolving theories of malpractice liability in HMOs. *Loy Univ Chic Law Rev* 1989;20:841–873.
77. *Fox v Health Net*, Civ No 21962 (Riverside County Super Ct, Cal 1993).
78. *Sloan v Metropolitan Health Council*, 516 NE2d 1104 (Ind Ct App 1987).
79. Restatement (second) of Agency paragraph sign 216, 1958.
80. Restatement (second) of Agency paragraph sign 250, 1958.
81. *Schleier v Kaiser Foundation Health Plan of the Mid-Atlantic States, Inc.*, 876 F2d 174 (DC Cir 1989).
82. *Darling v Charleston Community Memorial Hospital*, 211 NE2d 253 (1965), cert denied, 383 US 946 (1966).
83. *Wickline v State*, 192 Cal App 3d 1630, 239 Cal Rptr 810 (1986).
84. 29 USC Sections 1001–1461.
85. 29 USC Section 1144(a).
86. *Shea v Esensten*, 107 F3d 625 (8th Cir 1997).
87. *Harper v Healthsource New Hampshire*, 674 A2d 962 (NH 1996).
88. *Texas Medical Association v Aetna Life Insurance Co.*, 80 F3d 153 (5th Cir 1996).
89. 42 USCA 11131–11137 (West Supp 1995).
90. American Academy of Pediatrics Section on Perinatal Pediatrics, Committee on Practice Management. Understanding a practice venue: guidelines and suggestions regarding the non-clinical aspects of neonatology. *J Perinatol* 2002;22(Suppl 1):S1–S76.

91. Kohn LT, Corrigan JM, Donaldson MS, eds. *To err is human: building a safer health system.* Washington, DC: National Academy Press, 2000.

92. Fortescue EB, Kaushal R, Landrigan CP, et al. Prioritizing strategies for preventing medication errors and adverse drug events in pediatric inpatients. *Pediatrics* 2003;111:722–729.

93. Bernstein PL. *Against the gods: the remarkable story of risk.* New York: Wiley and Sons, 1996:197.

94. Morlock LL, Malitz FE. Do hospital risk management programs make a difference?: relationships between risk management program activities and hospital malpractice claims experience. *Law Contemp Probl* 1991;54:1–22.

95. Acerbo-Avalone N, Kremer K. Medical malpractice claims investigation: a step-by-step approach. Gaithersburg, MD: Aspen Publishers, 1997:xv.

96. Stelovich S. Framework for handling adverse events. *Forum* 2002;22:8–9.

97. Grupp-Phelan J, Reynolds S, Lingl LL. Professional liability of residents in a children's hospital. *Arch Pediatr Adolesc Med* 1996;150:87–90.

98. *Conducting a root cause analysis in response to a sentinel event.* Oakbrook Terrace, Ill: Joint Commission on Accreditation of Healthcare Organizations (JCAHO), 1996.

99. Andrews LB, Stocking C, Krizek T, et al. An alternative strategy for studying adverse events in medical care. *Lancet* 1997;349:309–313.

100. Brennan TA, Sox CM, Burstin HR. Relation between negligent adverse events and the outcomes of medical-malpractice litigation. *N Engl J Med* 1996;335:1963–1967.

101. Taragin MI, Willett LR, Wilczek AP, et al. The influence of standard of care and severity of injury on the resolution of malpractice claims. *Ann Intern Med* 1992;117:780–784.

102. Pichert JW, Hickson GB, Bledsoe S, et al. Understanding the etiology of serious medical events involving children: implications for pediatricians and their risk managers. *Pediatr Ann* 1997;26:160–172.

103. Van Cott H. Human errors: their causes and reduction. In: Bogner MS, ed. *Human error in medicine.* Hillsdale, NJ: Lawrence Erlbaum Associates, 1994:153.

104. Chess C, Hance BJ, Sandman PM. Improving dialogue with communities: a short guide to government risk communication. New Jersey Department of Environmental Protection, 1988.

105. Levison W. Doctor-patient communication and medical malpractice: implications for pediatricians. *Pediatr Ann* 1997;26:186–193.

106. Cuttini M, Romito P, Del Santo M, et al. Communication in the neonatal intensive therapy unit: the opinions of parents and of medical personnel compared. *Pediatr Med Chir* 1994;16:325–329.

107. Covello VT, Allen FW. *Seven cardinal rules of risk communication.* Washington, DC: U.S. Environmental Protection Agency, Office of Policy Analysis, 1988.

108. Silverman WA. *Retrolental fibroplasia: a modern parable.* New York: Grune and Stratton, Inc., 1980:83.

109. Donchin Y, Gopher D, Olin M, et al. A look into the nature and causes of human errors in the intensive care unit. *Crit Care Med* 1995;23:294–300.

110. Chilton JH, Shimmel TR. Inappropriate word choice in the labor and delivery and newborn medical record. In: Donn SM, Fisher CW, eds. *Risk management techniques in perinatal and neonatal practice,* 1996:603.

111. Hartline JV Smith CG. Risk management in medical consultation. In: Donn SM, Fisher CW, eds. *Risk management techniques in perinatal and neonatal practice.* Armonk, NY: Futura Publishing, 1996:617.

112. Committee on Quality of Health Care in America. Crossing the quality chasm: a new health system for the 21st century. Washington, DC: National Academy Press, 2001.

The Vulnerable Neonate and the Neonatal Intensive Care Environment

9

Penny Glass

Environmental factors in the neonatal intensive care unit (NICU) have major implications for the care of the sick newborn infant. Advances in medical technology during the last 3 decades are credited with dramatic reductions in mortality, with a 50% survival rate for newborns weighing 1,500 g in 1970 to a 50% survival rate for those weighing less than 700 g by 2000. Morbidity among survivors, however, is a problem of increasing proportions. Whereas the rate of major morbidity has remained fairly stable, around 10%, this focus on major morbidity has overlooked the much larger number of children born prematurely who have learning disabilities at school age. Broad evidence implicates the environment in the NICU as a factor in neonatal morbidity. Abnormal sensory input can be a source of potentially overwhelming stress and, at a sensitive period during development, can modify the developing brain. The NICU environment, therefore, assumes a crucial role in the care of the sick newborn infant.

Preterm birth is the most common single risk factor for developmental problems in childhood, and learning disability is the most pervasive developmental problem. This is a catch-all term, but includes children of low, average, or otherwise normal intelligence who have deficits in language, visual perception, or visuomotor integration; deficiencies in attention span, hyperactivity; or social immaturity. Such children require either special services to function in a regular classroom or placement in a special class. Reports of school-age children who were of very-low-birth-weight indicate that as many as half have learning disabilities (1–8). Such deficits may originate from overt damage to the brain or from a more general disturbance in brain organization.

Throughout infancy, both behavioral and neurologic differences exist between full-term and preterm infants, even when matched for conceptional age. The latter often exhibits manifestations of altered brain organization, including disrupted sleep, difficult temperament, both hyperresponsivity and hyporesponsivity to sensory input, prolonged attention to redundant information, inattention to novel stimuli, and poor quality of motor function (9–15). These precursors of learning problems in school are not fully explained by either the severity of illness among the preterm infants or by later conditions in the home environment (10).

The sensory environment in the NICU is different in virtually every respect, both from the environment of a fetus *in utero* and from that of a full-term newborn at home. The NICU experience also contains frequent aversive procedures, excess handling, disturbance of rest, noxious oral medications, noise, and bright light. These conditions are sources of stress and anomalous sensory stimulation, both of which may affect morbidity.

The immediate effects of stress are autonomic instability, apnea/bradycardia, vasoconstriction, and decreased gastric motility. Cortisol, adrenaline, and catecholamines are secreted during stress as part of an intricate hypothalamic–pituitary–adrenocortical system (16,17). High levels of these hormones interfere with tissue healing. Noxious stimuli disrupt sleep and can have biological consequences for the neonate. Even medical complications commonly associated with prematurity per se, such as bronchopulmonary dysplasia and necrotizing enterocolitis, may be, in part, stress-related diseases (18).

Sensory input is essential during maturation. Most of the cortex is part of one of the sensory systems. Abnormal experiences, both depriving and overstimulating, can modify the developing brain. The most vulnerable period occurs during rapid brain growth and neuronal differentiation

(19,20). The timing of these events for the human fetus corresponds to 28 to 40 weeks of gestation (21). It is assumed that, for the fetus, the optimal sensory environment is experienced within the womb. One of the most striking aspects of this environment is the bidirectional contingency between mother and fetus.

The potential impact of the anomalous NICU environment on the vulnerable newborn infant has raised unabated concerns for more than 2 decades (22–28). A more optimal NICU environment might reduce iatrogenic morbidity and improve the outcome of sick neonates; however, the parameters are not yet well defined. This chapter summarizes the maturation of each sensory system during late fetal development, with particular reference to evidence for the prenatal onset of function, compares the intrauterine and NICU sensory experience, and critiques techniques of developmental intervention.

NEONATAL SENSORY SYSTEMS: DEVELOPMENT, DISORDERS, ENVIRONMENT, AND INTERVENTION

Maturation of all the sensory systems begins during the latter part of embryogenesis; however, the process is neither unitary nor fixed. Within each system some reciprocity between structure and function probably exists. To some extent, sensory input drives maturation (29). In addition, the rate of maturation of each sensory system varies, with the onset of function generally in the following order: tactile, vestibular, gustatory–olfactory, auditory, and visual (30). These sensory systems also are interrelated in a hierarchical manner—stimulation of early maturing senses (e.g., tactile, vestibular) has a positive influence on development of later-maturing ones (e.g., visual) (31). Recent research also indicates that untimely stimulation within this sequence (e.g., visual) may disrupt the normal maturational process of another sensory system (e.g., auditory) (Philbin MK. *personal communication*, 1998.).

This hierarchical organization and integration of sensory function is well supported and bolsters two guiding principles for developmental intervention in the NICU:

1. Stimulation of the senses should begin with the most mature.
2. The optimal form of stimulation for initial postnatal development resembles the sources naturally available to the fetus and infant—those that come from the mother.

Tactile System

The cutaneous system includes sensation of pressure, pain, and temperature. Only pressure is discussed here; pain is discussed in Chapter 57. Receptors in the skin respond to pressure and then transmit impulses to the spinal cord through the dorsal root, ascending in the posterior tract and terminating in the gray matter of the cord. At this point, connecting fibers decussate and continue in the ventral spinothalamic tract to the medulla and the thalamus, terminating in the postcentral gyrus of the cortex. Representation here is somatotopic and contralateral to the stimulated side. Increased stimulation to an area of the body or loss of a limb can alter the pattern of representation in the somatosensory cortex.

Development

Like the vestibular system, the tactile sense develops early in fetal life and is thought to play a particularly pervasive role in the early development of the organism. Receptor cells are present in the perioral region in the fetus by 8 weeks of gestation and spread to all skin and mucosal surfaces by 20 weeks. The cortical pathway is intact by 20 to 24 weeks of gestation, and some myelin is already present. Response to tactile stimulation has been observed by ultrasound as early as 8 weeks of conceptional age (32). Response to stroking in the lip region occurs first, followed by a response to stimulation of the palms. Most of the body is sensitive to touch by 15 weeks (33).

Tactile threshold is very low in the preterm infant. It is more related to postconceptional age (PCA) than to natal age but increases by term. Infants younger than 30 weeks PCA respond by an unequivocal leg withdrawal to pressure of a 0.50-g von Frey hair applied to the plantar surface of the foot compared to 1.7-g pressure by 38 weeks PCA (34). A qualitative shift occurs around 32 weeks PCA. Infants less than 32 weeks PCA respond to repeated stimulation with sensitization and a diffuse behavioral response. In contrast, infants after this age show habituation to the same stimuli.

Classic studies by Harlow and Harlow (35) demonstrated the profound importance of contact comfort for normal development. In a parallel fashion, even preterm infants will seek and maintain contact with a physical object within their incubator and even more so if the tactile source contains rhythmic stimulation (36). These findings provide strong support for intervention in the tactile modality.

Disturbances

Tactile hypersensitivity, or tactile defensive behavior, is contained in clinical reports of children with developmental delay, many of whom were born preterm. It also is seen in infants and children who otherwise appear normal. The behavior frequently is said to be a manifestation of sensory integration deficit and thought to have its origins in the prenatal or perinatal period. It appears as an infant's overreaction to touch, generally the hands or oral–facial regions. With oral hypersensitivity, the infant may withdraw, gag, or retch when touched, even around the outside of the mouth. Some infants are intolerant of food with texture and resist transition from liquids or very smooth puree. Infants also may be hypersensitive to touch on their extremities, with prolonged palmar–mental reflex, exaggerated hand and toe grasp, or leg withdrawal. An extreme case was a 2-month-old (corrected age) infant who, when supine, arched his buttocks off the table surface in response to his legs being grasped. Additional manifestations of tactile sensitivity may appear as an intolerance for grasping toys or handling play materials of certain textures. In another extreme example, a 1-year-old infant would gag when his hand was placed in dry macaroni. Some children are intolerant of normal clothing and even may avoid body contact. Such aversion adversely affects parent–infant bonding. The link between early tactile disturbances and learning disabilities at school age is unlikely to be a causal one, but may be related to a similar mechanism of brain dysfunction.

Intrauterine Experience

The fetus is housed in a thermoneutral, fluid-filled space that is a source of cutaneous input throughout the body surface. Fetal movement provides tactile self-stimulation. Perhaps even more important, fetal movement often evokes a contingent maternal response. As term approaches and the intrauterine space becomes more constraining, the normal posture of flexion evokes hand-to-mouth, skin-to-skin, and body-on-body tactile feedback. The effect is progressive throughout gestation.

After a normal term birth, a ventral-to-ventral position is preferred by both mother and infant, with touch followed by slow stroking (37). Traditionally, the infant is then swaddled and held. As before birth, human proximity produces contingent touch.

Touch And Handling in the Neonatal Intensive Care Unit

After premature birth, tactile input is radically altered. The extrauterine fetus is frequently nursed naked, with the exception of maybe a diaper and a hat. The surface of the mattress generally is unyielding. She or he is exposed to air currents, cold stress, tape, instruments, handling by caregivers, and painful stimuli. Pressure is not uniform.

The type and frequency of tactile stimulation imposed on a preterm newborn in the NICU would be overwhelming even for a healthy adult. During a 2-week period, a sick neonate may be handled by more than 10 different nurses, in addition to physicians, occupational or physical therapists, laboratory and x-ray technicians, and, finally, the parents (38).

Handling occurs more often among the sickest infants, typically is related to procedures, generally is disturbing, and often is painful. In spite of wide attention in the literature to the consequences of excess handling in the NICU, the amount had not decreased from 1976 to 1990, even among the more severely ill infants (39). On the average, sick preterm newborns are handled more than 150 times per day, with less than 10 minutes of consecutive uninterrupted rest (26). Disturbance of sleep has biologic and immunologic consequences (40,41). Secretion of cortisol and adrenaline normally is inhibited during sleep. Growth hormone, which is released during quiet sleep, increases protein synthesis and mobilization of free fatty acids for energy use. Thus, sleep facilitates healing.

Excess handling has other significant physiologic consequences for the sick neonate. Blood pressure changes, alterations in cerebral blood flow, and episodes of oxygen desaturation are associated with noxious procedures, handling, or crying (42–46). Fluctuations in blood pressure may contribute to intracranial hemorrhage in the unstable preterm infant (47). Importantly, when caretakers monitor the infant's level of oxygenation during procedures, the severity of hypoxemic episodes can be reduced significantly (42).

In addition to the hemodynamic impact of obviously noxious procedures described earlier, more benign manipulations, such as those that occur during neurodevelopmental assessment, also may adversely affect the preterm infant (25,46). Decreased plasma growth hormone has been reported after administration of the Brazelton Neonatal Behavioral Assessment Scale to preterm infants at 36 weeks PCA (48). Even at the time of discharge, the evaluation was associated with elevated cortisol levels (17,49). It is not clear whether these effects were from the neurodevelopmental assessment or from the stress associated with crying, which normally occurs during administration of the Neonatal Behavioral Assessment Scale. Thus, handling could be stressful even for stable preterm infants.

Tactile Intervention in the Neonatal Intensive Care Unit

The two general approaches to tactile intervention in the NICU provide either reduction of general handling or provision of planned touch experiences. Touch may be pressure alone or may include stroking. The neonates may be acutely ill or medically stable. These distinctions are important.

As part of an individualized approach to developmental care for acutely ill preterm infants, Als and colleagues (50) provided "minimal handling" and clustering of routine procedures, as well as positive tactile input and containment from bunting, rolls, positioning, and the like. Short- and long-term outcomes were improved for her intervention group compared to a nonintervention group. This technique has had a major impact on developmental intervention as a whole. Although it is not possible to isolate which aspect of this multimodal approach was effective, a significant change was made in the role of the nurse/caregiver.

More specific to the tactile modality, Jay (51) evaluated the effects of planned, gentle, touch for 12-minute periods four times a day for acutely ill preterm infants. This intervention, which consisted of hands-on contact but not stroking or manipulating, was associated with a lower fraction of inspired oxygen (FIO_2) after 5 days compared to a similar nonintervention group.

In apparent contrast, Field and colleagues (52) and Scafidi and colleagues (53) initiated a touch intervention that differed from that of Jay (51) and Als and colleagues (50) in several important respects. The infants were recruited when "stable and growing" rather than during an acute period.

The treatment provided three 15-minute periods a day of massage (i.e., stroking and passive limb movement) for a 10-day treatment period. The massaged infants showed a greater weight gain, even though the groups did not differ in formula intake. These early effects on growth are thought to be mediated by induction of catecholamine release (48). The massaged infants also spent more time awake, showed better performance on the Brazelton neonatal assessment, were discharged to home 6 days sooner, and had better performance on developmental assessment at 8 months past term.

Although overall effects of the tactile intervention have been positive, the response of individual infants is variable and deserves attention. For example, an increase in periods of oxygen desaturation during parent touch, compared to baseline, has been reported (54). A number of infants have responded with apnea and bradycardia to the type of intervention described by Field and colleagues (52) and Scafidi and colleagues (53). This physiologic response may occur after the intervention. It is not clear whether the intervention itself was excessive or whether the abrupt shift after the cessation of tactile input led to an unexpected physiologic response. Individual differences exist among caregivers that also affect the infants' responses to the stimulation. Finally, the distinction between touch, stroking, and massage is probably important.

All of these issues advise against standardized protocols of stroking or massage for all preterm infants. When any form of tactile and kinesthetic intervention is applied, the caregiver should continue to monitor the infant's physiologic and behavioral responses before onset, during, and after the cessation of the intervention. Consistency of contact across caregivers would help.

Soft swaddling or clothing may provide tactile input in a more sustained fashion than periodic hands-on contact. Arguments that this obscures the view of the infant and interferes with temperature regulation by servocontrol simply argue against servocontrol rather than against covers. Clothing or swaddling actually could dampen the fluctuations in temperature that occur during incubator care and inhibit exaggerated movement or agitation, which in itself may be stabilizing. Creative swaddling with crisscrossed strips and Velcro could allow for more visualization of the infant. The use of swaddling in the NICU is necessary if the parent is to retain that option at home as a means of calming and supporting sleep. Swaddling is difficult to initiate after a period of not being swaddled.

Thus, the amount and type of stimulation are important and change with acuity, maturation, and the response of the infant. Parents need specific guidance and modeling from the beginning. The general order of tactile intervention might be:

- *If acutely ill*—minimal handling, containment (e.g., swaddling, rolls), and gentle touch (e.g., warm hand) without stroking
- *When medically stable*—holding, rocking gently, stroking, contining to swaddle

Minimal handling protocols have a definite place in the NICU, but not as the end point. It also is important during the hospital stay to help the infant develop increased tolerance for social contact and gentle handling, especially as discharge approaches. Systematic desensitization may even be necessary in cases of chronically ill infants.

Nonnutritive Sucking

Nonnutritive sucking is an important oral–tactile intervention that supports both feeding and early behavioral regulation. It represents an early endogenous rhythm and a manifestation of sensorimotor integration (55). As such, it is reported in the fetus (56) and observed in the preterm newborn before 28 weeks of gestation. The number of sucks per burst increases with maturation, whereas the duration of burst is fairly stable across ages.

Nonnutritive sucking experience may facilitate important physiologic and behavioral mechanisms and potentially reduce cost of care. Infants provided with nonnutritive sucking during gavage feeding showed significantly improved gastrointestinal transit time, greater suck pressure, more sucks per burst, and fewer sporadic sucks. They initiated bottle-feeding earlier, showed better weight gain, and thereby had shorter hospital stays (57,58). Having a pacifier continuously available, however, may not be beneficial and may, in fact, encourage inappropriate sucking patterns, particularly in the chronically ill neonate.

Nonnutritive sucking also acts as a behavioral organizer or facilitator. It has been shown to decrease motor activity and increase quiet states in stable preterm infants (59). It dampens an infant's behavioral response after a painful procedure such as circumcision or heelstick (60,61), although it does not appear to dampen the cortisol response (17). It is noteworthy that sucking on a pacifier before the onset of repeated painful procedures, such as heelsticks, may be inappropriate, because aversive conditioning to the pacifier could occur.

Nipples used for nonnutritive sucking abound, varying in size, configuration, consistency, and utility. A feeding nipple is not designed for nonnutritive sucking and is inappropriate. It readily collapses; the infant experiences little resistance to his or her suck and may loll the device. Gauze inserted in the nipple may absorb oral secretions and breed bacteria. In larger infants, the nipple is unsafe because of possible aspiration. A variety of commercially available pacifiers should be available in any NICU to suit the individual needs of each infant. Some neonates who are hypersensitive to touch in the perioral region often respond positively to contact (and perhaps smell) from their own hands.

Vestibular System

The vestibular system, situated in the nonauditory labyrinth of the inner ear, responds to movement as well as directional changes in gravity. The three fluid-filled semicircular canals, one for each major plane of the body, lie at right angles to each other. The ampulla, located at the end of each canal, contains hair fibers in a sac, or cupula. Motion of the body or head causes pressure changes that move the cupula, which stimulates the hair cells and transmits an impulse along the vestibular portion of the eighth cranial nerve to the vestibular nuclei of the medulla. The vestibular organs consist of the utricle and saccule, which respond to changes of head position involving linear motion. The macula, a thickening in the wall of the utricle and saccule, contains hair cells sensitive to the position of the head. Impulses from the macula transmit along the vestibular nerve to the medulla and cerebellum. From there, information is transmitted to motor fibers going to the neck, eye, trunk, and limb muscles. There are no connections to the cortex (63). Vestibular stimulation affects level of alertness. Slow, rhythmic, continuous movement induces sleep. Periodic or higher amplitude swing increases arousal.

Development

Initial vestibular development is concurrent with auditory development, emanating from the same otocyst early in gestation. The three semicircular canals begin to form before 8 weeks of gestation, reaching morphologic maturity by 14 weeks, and full size by week 20 (29). The vestibular sacs probably develop at the same time. Response to vestibular stimulation has been observed by 25 weeks of gestation (33). The traditional vertex presentation of the fetus at term gestation is thought to occur from fetal activity in response to vestibular input.

Disturbances

Considerable research with animals has demonstrated the importance of both tactile and vestibular input (35,63). Lack of normal vestibular stimulation in the developing organism is thought to affect general neurobehavioral organization (31). Children who were born preterm are reported to have deficits in balance at preschool age (8), but this is not necessarily a vestibular problem.

Intrauterine Experience

The fetus experiences both contingent and noncontingent vestibular stimulation that varies during gestation. From the beginning of embryonic life, the fluid environment of the womb provides periodic oscillations and movements that emanate from normal movements of the mother as well as activity of the fetus itself. Reports by mothers of fetal movement occur around 16 weeks. After 28 weeks of gestation, there is a decrease in the relative amount of amniotic fluid, and, thus, the movement of the fetus becomes partially constrained by the more limited physical space. Vestibular experience is then less contingent on self-activation and more related to normal maternal activity and position change, which often occurs in response to fetal activity. In general, maternal activity level slows as parturition approaches.

After birth, the infant is held normally. Movement is slow from maternal breathing and shifting. Change of position is gradual, even by experienced parents. Vestibular stimulation is used to affect state—moving to upright or laying down increases arousal; monotonous side-to-side rocking and walking in the form of parental pacing reduce the level of arousal.

Vestibular Experience in the Neonatal Intensive Care Unit

Vestibular stimulation after preterm birth is limited to efficient manipulation or turning of the neonate by the caregiver. It clearly lacks any of the temporal qualities or contingencies that the maternal environment may have provided. Spontaneous limb movement generally is diffuse, often unrestricted, and typically disorganizing in its effect.

Intervention in the Neonatal Intensive Care Unit

Like the tactile sense, the early development of the vestibular system provides a theoretical basis for primary intervention with preterm neonates. More than 3 decades ago, Neal (64) demonstrated that daily rocking facilitated the development of preterm infants. Subsequent research simulated the intrauterine environment and provided compensatory vestibular stimulation. An oscillating waterbed was devised, which moved with the rhythm of maternal respirations but with an amplitude of less than 2.5 mm at the surface of the unoccupied waterbed. The safety of this paradigm, as well as efficacy in reduction in apnea of prematurity, has been well demonstrated (65). In addition, the infants on waterbeds demonstrated more organized sleep state and motor behavior, decreased irritability, enhanced visual alertness, and improved somatic growth (65–68).

Difficulty in nursing sick infants on an oscillating surface may have precluded more widespread adoption of the waterbed. An infant's own movement also can induce more than optimal movement of the surface, as, for example, an infant with gastroesophageal reflux; however, some babies still are likely to benefit. At the least, it would seem prudent to provide a trial on a waterbed for a nonventilated infant with apnea of prematurity, before introduction of pharmacologic intervention.

Other sources of vestibular stimulation, such as rocking chairs, swings, and hammocks, have not been investigated formally. Rocking chairs probably belong in any nursery. Swings are questionable, given the excessive upright position of the baby and the standard rate of oscillation (i.e., too fast). A crib has been devised that provides controlled motion similar to a woman walking; the duration of motion may be individually controlled and proportionally reduced over time (69), but the rate of oscillation appears too rapid for a preterm infant. The device appears to be effective in modulating fussiness in full-term infants and is used with preterm infants. The infants are well swaddled and further contained on each side by rolls.

Positioning

The physical position of an infant is part of the NICU tactile–vestibular experience. Nursing sick preterm infants routinely has been with the infant in the supine position and exposed, which may simplify management but may not be advantageous for the infant. Prone positioning in the NICU has been strongly supported physiologically. The current NICU dilemma is that the prone sleep position is contrary to the recommendation by the American Academy of Pediatrics (AAP), which now supports supine positioning because epidemiologic data associate supine positioning with a lower rate of sudden infant death syndrome. The optimal position of the infant needs to address anatomic and physiologic consequences. Positioning for optimal care in the NICU needs to take account of the AAP recommendation before the infant is ready for discharge to home.

Yu (70) demonstrated that gastric emptying was facilitated in either the prone or right lateral position compared to the supine or left lateral position. This was particularly significant for the sick preterm who already showed a delay in gastric emptying. The prone position, compared to supine, is associated with more quiet sleep and less active sleep or crying. Quiet sleep, in turn, is associated with improved lung volume, more stable respiration, less apnea, and improved PAO$_2$ (71,72). Finally, the prone position compared to supine is associated with a higher PAO$_2$ among healthy preterm infants and, even more significantly, in those with respiratory distress syndrome (72,73). The evidence suggests that, when possible, the sick infant should be nursed in a prone or right lateral position.

Parents of preterm infants often complain that their baby's feet turn out. In fact, the legs more often are externally rotated at the hip. Grenier (74) described hip deformities seen on x-ray of preterm infants after prolonged nursing in a frog-leg position. The bulk of the diaper in extremely preterm infants exacerbates the problem. Winging of the scapula also is frequent in the preterm infant. Proper support of the trunk and limbs in the prone or supine position lessens this extreme rotation and may diminish orthopedic or neuromuscular complications.

In the prone position, placing the infant on a small folded strip from shoulder to hip, could allow more physiologic flexion and adduction. In side lying, it may be easier to position the infant in soft flexion. Gentle containment of the limbs usually can be managed with strips of soft cloth across the upper arm and thigh. Some movement should be allowed within a controlled range. A posture of physiologic flexion and adduction in the supine position requires swad-

dling. Maintenance of postures can be facilitated by nesting the infant in soft rolls, but the rolls must not reach above the level of the shoulder. Rolls placed at the buttocks don't allow for adequate leg/hip extension. Each posture should facilitate the infant bringing hands to mouth.

For older, more medically stable preterm infants, infant seats are used as an alternative to continuous lying in bed. The infant should be swaddled and nested, the angle probably no greater than 30 degrees, and the length of time should be limited. Oxygen desaturation has been reported in stable preterm infants placed in car seats.

Kangaroo Care

Kangaroo care is a technique that evolved primarily in South America (75). Traditionally, the infant is clad only in a diaper and placed under the mother's clothing between her breasts, remaining there according to the mother's comfort, and feeding on demand. The technique provides fairly sustained multimodal stimulation: tactile, vestibular, proprioceptive, olfactory, and auditory. It appears to be safe for larger preterm infants or those who are medically stable. Temperature regulation in the infant does not appear to be a problem, but needs to be carefully monitored on an individual basis. It seems to have the greatest benefit in terms of facilitating and maintaining lactation and enhancing maternal sense of competency for these infants. The studies, however, are of insufficient sample size to evaluate whether morbidity, such as intracranial hemorrhage, is increased. More data are needed among medically stable infants before kangaroo care should be attempted prior to 32 weeks conceptional age or with infants requiring mechanical ventilation. The increased tactile stimulation and additional handling easily could be overly stressful for the immature or sick infant.

Chemical Senses

The chemoreceptors include taste and olfaction. Taste receptors are in the taste buds, which are located primarily in the papillae of the tongue but also are found on the soft palate and epiglottis (29,76). Taste stimuli (i.e., sweet, sour, bitter, salt) transmit to the brainstem with a primary branch to the hypothalamus. Cortical regions are involved in learned taste preferences. The olfactory receptors are located in the lining of the olfactory epithelium in the posterior portion of the nasal passage. The afferent pathway has no cortical projection area, but is direct to the limbic system. Olfaction plays an important part in gustatory experiences. Olfaction also is an integral part of infant attachment to the caregiver and may even be mutual (77).

Development of Taste

The chemoreceptors are well developed within the first trimester (29,76). Taste buds appear around 8 to 9 weeks of gestation. The receptors are present at least by week 16 of gestation, and increase by term to adult levels. During the second half of gestation, morphologic changes occur that continue after term. Taste receptors are functional before birth. Injection of distinct tastes into the amniotic fluid of pregnant women between 34 and 39 weeks of gestation alter fetal swallowing behavior, which increases with the sweeter taste and decreases with bitter taste (29).

Taste discrimination has been measured by differential consumption, autonomic responses, and the presence of characteristic facial expressions. Plain water evokes an aversive response, which may be a biologically based protective mechanism. Taste is sufficiently sensitive at term to detect a 0.1 mol/L-concentration of NaCl in water (78). Full-term neonates, even anencephalic infants, demonstrate differential behavioral responses to sweet, bitter, sour, and salt (79). In a behavior described as "savoring," normal newborns discriminate between different concentrations of sucrose and even among various sugars (78). Preterm infants (30 to 36 weeks of gestation) show stronger sucking in response to glucose, compared to plain water, and characteristic behavioral expressions in response to sour or bitter solutions (80). Behavioral response to formula, or breast milk, administered to the tip of the tongue has been documented in preterm infants prior to 28 weeks of gestation (Zorc L. unpublished doctoral dissertation, 2000).

Stimulation of taste receptors has important implications for early feeding and behavioral regulation. Smotherman and Robinson (81) hypothesized that tastes of milk activate a centrally mediated endogeneous opioid system in newborn term infants, consistent with that shown in the animal model. This would suggest that, in normal development, the mechanism to support early feeding extends beyond maintenance of chemical or caloric balance and becomes "feeding to thrive."

Development Of Olfaction

The human olfactory system is composed of four anatomically distinct but integrated subsystems:

1. The main olfactory
2. The vomeronasal
3. The terminal
4. The trigeminal

Each of these differentiates very early in gestation and is nearly mature prior to term birth (29,82). Epithelia of the main olfactory system are evident around 5 weeks in the apical part of the nasal cavities. Nerve fibers and cells form the olfactory nerve, which links the epithelium to the main olfactory bulbs and then to the ventral wall of the forebrain. The vomeronasal system consists of bipolar sensory cells in the lower nasal septum, with axons terminating in the accessory olfactory bulb. The terminal system is comprised of free nerve endings in the anterior part of the nasal septum. The nerve endings of the trigeminal system, which originates from cranial nerve V, are diffusely distributed in the nasal cavity. The trigeminal system, although activated by touch, may be the earliest functioning chemoreceptor.

No information exists about the functional onset of human olfaction, but it is presumed to be present prenatally, having been demonstrated in a rat model. Rat fetuses exposed to citral in the amniotic fluid will selectively attach postnatally to a nipple of the same scent (83).

Human prenatal olfactory function is inferred from the sophistication present by term, including behavioral discrimination, preference, and conditioning to olfactory stimuli. For example, 1-week-old infants will reliably turn their heads away from a noxious smell (84). In response to a series of pleasant or aversive odors, infants less than 12 hours old will exhibit different facial expressions that are discriminable by adults (79). Infants younger than 1 week of age reliably prefer the odor of their mother's breast pad to the breast pad of another mother (85). Neonates who were given a period of familiarization to a novel odor subsequently demonstrated a preference for that odor, whereas infants exposed to it for the first time did not (77). Finally, classical conditioning to a novel olfactory stimulus has been demonstrated empirically within the first 48 hours after term birth (86). Given ten 30-second pairings of citrus odor with stroking, neonates the following day showed increased activity and head turning in the presence of the citrus but not to a novel odor. By 28 to 32 weeks gestation, the majority of preterm infants show reliable behavioral response to olfactory input (82).

Disorders

Feeding disorders are reported commonly among preterm infants, particularly those with chronic lung disease. The infant may even respond aversively to the introduction of food in the mouth. The cause generally is attributed to frequent stressful procedures around the mouth as well as poor coordination of suck and swallow. However, marked alteration of the orogustatory environment occurs by nature in a preterm birth. Feeding disorders also are common among neonates who have sustained brain damage. No studies have attempted to identify whether deficits in taste or smell are present in infants with feeding disorders. Certainly in adults, loss of the sense of smell radically affects eating habits.

Intrauterine Experience

The amniotic fluid is a complex solution of suspended particulate and dissolved odorants that changes in chemical composition during maturation of the fetal chemosensory system (29,82,87). Even as early as 18 weeks gestation, more than 120 compounds have been identified in single amniotic fluid samples. The mother contributes to the chemical variation through hormones and even the types of food consumed. The fetus contributes to the chemical status through urination, oral mucosa, and lung secretions. More directly, fetal respiratory movements, sucking, and swallowing cause pulsatile displacement of the amniotic fluid in contact with the chemoreceptors to probably affect adaptation by the receptor cells (82). A link has been proposed between the intrauterine orogustatory experience and the selective behavioral preference of the newborn to breast milk.

Experience In The Neonatal Intensive Care Unit

The environment in the NICU has not been described previously in terms of gustatory or olfactory content, but it clearly is not well adapted here. The necessary restriction of oral feeding in sick or extremely premature neonates is a marked alteration of the fetal orogustatory environment. The chemical composition of initial feedings (breast milk or formula) is different from amniotic fluid or colostrum. Common changes in formula composition (brand), concentration (dilute or hypercaloric), and temperature (too cool) introduce unwanted variability. The addition of noxious oral medications and electrolyte supplements to breast milk or formula typically activate a gag response in the newborn. Negative experiences temporally associated with feeding can lead to aversive conditioning. Finally, in contrast to the healthy full-term neonate, preterm infants in the NICU lack a stable olfactory source that would be provided by sustained body contact of a consistent caretaker.

Intervention in the Neonatal Intensive Care Unit

Stimulation of both smell and taste has significant implications for enhancing care in the NICU. A period of familiarization with the odor of breast milk or formula, before the oral introduction of food, can facilitate acquisition of oral feeding skills (77). For a medically fragile infant, the mother's breast pad can be placed nearby. From another standpoint, familiarization to the odor of medications before ingestion could make the medication less aversive by the process of habituation. Obviously, like breast milk from the source, bottle-feeding ideally should be at body temperature rather than the typical room temperature.

Small tastes of formula or breast milk before the introduction of the nipple may foster behavioral organization and facilitate the onset of feeding (87). Most babies who are restricted from oral feeds can safely tolerate a small drop of breast milk or formula on the lips or tongue tip. The limited research available suggests that gut priming in the extremely preterm or sick full-term infant probably should not bypass the mouth entirely. Based on the animal model, surfactant and colostrum may have unsuspected roles in initiation of human feeding (81).

Another important implication of orogustatory stimulation is the effect of oral feeding on activation of the endogenous opioid system, which raises the threshold to noxious tactile stimuli in the fetal rat model and human newborn infants (88), although it is no longer elicited in the human infant after 6 weeks of age (89). Sucrose solution has been applied to the tip of the tongue to decrease the pain response to a heelstick procedure or even to circumcision in healthy term infants (88,90). However, repeated use of this pathway to modulate pain in the neonatal period is currently unwarranted since it may have negative repercussions given the link to feeding behavior.

Auditory System

The auditory system is composed of both peripheral and central components (91–93). Sound waves are conducted through the auditory canal and physically displace the tympanic membrane. Movement of the membrane is amplified by the ossicles in the middle ear and transmitted to the oval window. This action displaces fluid in the cochlea. A mechanical disturbance differentially displaces hair cells at a specific place on the basilar membrane of the cochlea, as a function of both frequency and intensity of the sound. The hair cells are organized tonotopically, so that those that respond to high-frequency sounds are near the oval window and those that respond to low-frequency sounds are at the apex of the cochlea. The complex neural impulse thus generated proceeds to the auditory cortex via the cochlear nucleus, superior olivary nucleus, inferior colliculus, and medial geniculate body. The primary cortical reception area is the Heschl gyrus in the temporal region. Approximately 60% of the nerve fibers from each ear transmit to the contralateral hemisphere. The tonotopic organization is repeated in the cortical structures. The initial development of the central component of the auditory system is independent of peripheral maturation; however, once the auditory pathway is complete, the absence of auditory stimulation would cause cortical neuronal degeneration (93).

Development

Development of the auditory system begins around 3 to 6 weeks of gestation (93,94). By 25 weeks gestation all the major structures of the ear are essentially in place, although the adult dimensions of the external auditory canal, tympanic membrane, and middle ear cavity will not be attained until 1 year after birth. The ossicles have evolved from a thickening of mesenchymal tissue and are already of adult proportions, although residual mesenchyme may diminish auditory thresholds. The cochlear nucleus has reached adult proportions and differentiated sufficiently to be functional by this time, although microscopically the cochlea still is not mature even at term. The hair cells are fully present and in a process of differentiation. The frequency-specific place on the basilar membrane is shifting systematically during this period of development (93). The afferent pathway from the cochlea to the auditory cortex is complete, and even myelination of the auditory pathway is present.

With regard to function, both cortical auditory-evoked responses and brainstem auditory-evoked responses can be elicited by 25 to 28 weeks (95,96). Wave morphology is different from the full-term infant's, and the latency is prolonged. A blink response to vibroacoustic stimulation has been obtained in human fetuses of 24 to 25 weeks of gestational age. A more complex behavioral response to sound occurs at least by 28 weeks, but readily fatigues. The maximum rate of electrophysiologic change occurs in the cortical auditory-evoked response and brainstem auditory-evoked response between 28 and 34 weeks of gestation. Orienting behavior to soft sound can be elicited by this time.

Maturation of the fetal auditory system is marked by an increase in spectral sensitivity, in both lower and higher frequencies, and a decrease in auditory threshold (91–93). The range of auditory sensitivity initially is fairly restricted: from 500 to 1,000 Hz in the third trimester compared to around 500 to 4,000 Hz at term and an adult range of 30 to 20,000 Hz. Changes in auditory threshold are related to maturation of both peripheral and central components. Auditory thresholds in a preterm infant at 25 weeks of gestation have been obtained with a 65-dB stimulus compared to 25 dB at term.

Evidence for a functional auditory system in the fetus is strong. Specific anatomic sites are present in the cortex that are responsible for processing complex sounds, such as language. A biological predisposition to respond to the specific acoustic patterns of speech is present in full-term neonates. For example, they have lower thresholds for sound within the most important range for speech perception (i.e., 500 to 3,000 Hz) (97). Within this frequency range, they respond differently to speech and nonspeech stimuli. There are even hemispheric differences in auditory-evoked potentials that support this language sensitivity (98). Finally, healthy full-term neonates demonstrate a preference for sound they were exposed to *in utero*. Research shows that 2- to 4-day-old neonates prefer their mother's voice compared to another female voice and prefer a recording of a story read by their mother prenatally to a recording of a story read by their mother that was not read to them prenatally (99–103).

Deficits

Preterm infants are at increased risk for sensorineural hearing loss and developmental language disorders (20). Language disorders may be receptive or expressive dysfunctions. Receptive language disorders often are referred to as auditory processing deficits. These deficits primarily include phonemic-based disorders that involve discrimination between speech sounds, such as *ba* versus *pa*, short-term memory deficits, and difficulty in interpreting the meaning of words implied by grammatical structure. Expressive language problems may include disorders of speech (as in articulation or fluency), word-finding difficulty, and deficient or disordered sentence structure (grammar). Language disorders result from direct damage to central structures or can be incidental to more general brain dysfunction. They occur in children with normal hearing thresholds and otherwise normal intelligence. They occur

more commonly among children who were born preterm (104).

Intrauterine Experience

Development of the auditory system during fetal life occurs within a uterine environment that contains rhythmic, structured, and patterned sound emanating predominantly from the mother. Internal sounds include maternal respirations, borborygmi, placental and heart rhythms, and the like. Maternal speech transmits both externally and internally. Prosody (i.e., intonation, rhythm, stress) is probably the most salient aspect of speech available to the fetus. The intensity of internally recorded sound within the amniotic fluid is approximately 70 to 85 dB, with a predominance of low frequency (Fig. 9-1) (105). External sound also is transmitted to the fetus, but is attenuated by the time it reaches the intrauterine cavity, more so at higher frequencies (i.e., 70 dB at 4000 Hz) than lower frequencies (i.e., 20 dB at 50 Hz) (106). Given these considerations, the fetus probably is minimally exposed to frequencies above 1,000 dB (107). The available frequencies *in utero* also parallel cochlear development (100).

The auditory environment in the womb likely provides the most appropriate substrate for normal development of the sensory system, but defining the acoustic properties of

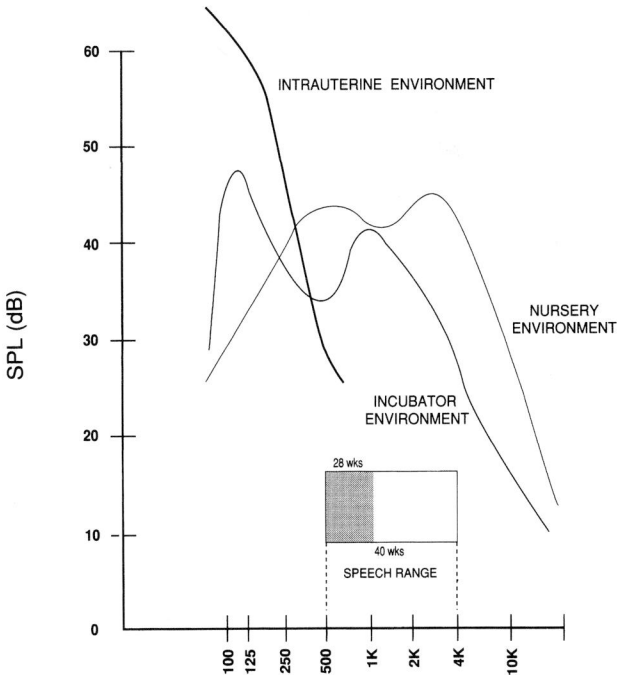

Figure 9-1 Comparison of the frequency-specific auditory environment of the fetus *in utero* and the preterm infant in the neonatal intensive care unit. SPL, sound pressure level. (From Walker D, Grimwade J, Wood C. Intrauterine noise: a component of the fetal environment. *Am J Obstet Gynecol* 1970;109:91, with permission; and Otho Boone, *personal communication*, December 1992, with permission.)

the sound actually transmitted to the inner ear of the fetus is problematic. The fluid-filled womb would alter the conductive property of the middle ear; however, data on this are unavailable. The best guess generally is that fetal hearing is limited to bone conduction. Hearing thresholds are elevated in the prematurely born infant, but no unequivocal data are available on the actual hearing thresholds of the fetus *in utero*.

After a normal, full-term birth, the auditory environment is quiet by contrast. This may serve to increase the salience of the human voice. Early speech directed to the neonate is subdued and generally contingent on the infant's response.

Neonatal Intensive Care Unit Environment

The acoustic environment in the NICU differs from the intrauterine environment in peak intensity, spectral characteristics, and pattern (Fig. 9-1). Ambient noise is generated by motors, fans, ventilator equipment, personnel, telephones, alarms, hand-washing areas, trash lids, pagers, intercoms, and carts, to name a few. The intensity of background noise is around 50 to 60 dB and, therefore, not louder than *in utero*, although episodic bursts of higher intensity (i.e. less than 100 dB) occur. It would appear (Fig. 9-1) that speech input for the neonate is selectively masked by the NICU auditory environment.

The auditory environment is different for babies nursed in open beds versus those nursed in incubators. To some degree, the incubator may partially attenuate high-frequency room noise (Fig. 9-1), but produces its own background noise level for the baby within (i.e., 50 to 70 dB). In addition, the infant in an incubator may be subjected to the closing of porthole doors, an object being placed on the top surface, or rapping on the incubator to stimulate an infant who is apneic or bradycardic, which may peak at more than 100 dB.

Effect of the Neonatal Intensive Care Unit Environment

Exposure to aberrant noise levels in the NICU may cause sensorineural damage, induce stress, and contribute to language or auditory processing disorders in the preterm neonate. Schulte and colleagues (20) reported nearly 12% hearing loss in a followup of preterm infants. Damage to the outer hair cells of the cochlea of neonatal guinea pigs has been reported after exposure to noise of similar intensities and frequencies found in the NICU (108). These researchers found no correlation between hearing loss and duration of exposure to incubator noise, but did report an association between hearing loss and a measure of severity of illness. Although not stated, more severely ill neonates may be exposed to increased NICU noise compared to healthy preterm infants. In other research, the combination of noise and ototoxic drugs commonly given to sick preterm infants (e.g., aminoglycosides, diuretics) was found to have a potentiating effect on hearing loss

(109–111). The data further suggest that the immature cochlea may be more susceptible to damage than the mature one. Increased susceptibility is coincident with the final stages of anatomic development and differentiation of the cochlea (111). Given these data, incubator manufacturers have lessened the noise level emitted by the incubator motor, but limits on the environmental source of noise in the NICU itself are few.

In addition to possible sensory nerve damage, loud noise could have physiologic consequences in the newborn preterm infant in the form of stress, leading to alterations in corticosteroid levels and autonomic changes. Decreases in oxygen saturation, increases in intracranial pressure, and peripheral vasoconstriction are reported in preterm infants after exposure to sudden noise (112). Finally, sleep is disrupted by intermittent noise in the NICU.

Abnormal auditory environmental conditions could contribute to language problems in preterm children. Normal auditory habituation patterns were impaired in chicks reared in an NICU-sound environment (113). Delayed cortical auditory-evoked responses among healthy preterm infants have been reported, in addition to deficits in brainstem response to linguistic stimuli (104,114). The NICU environment, like the fetal environment, has an important role in the normal development of the auditory system.

Intervention in the Neonatal Intensive Care Unit

Auditory intervention in the NICU includes efforts both to reduce ambient noise and to induce patterned auditory input. Personnel in the NICU generally have made focused efforts to lower the level of noise in the environment. Quiet times during each shift are prevailing, and radios are less constant. Evidence would suggest the value of caring for the smallest and sickest preterm infants inside an incubator, as a shield against environmental noise. The steady incubator noise may induce sleep in the preterm infant (115). At some point, however, the continuous white noise in the incubator masks more socially relevant auditory stimuli. Prolonged housing in this environment becomes disadvantageous at some point, but the timing is unknown.

Another approach to decreasing the level of ambient noise reaching the infant is by occluding the infant's ears. Zahr and de Traversay (116), using a within-subjects design, found increased quiet sleep and fewer state changes during the two observation periods. Caution here is warranted. Auditory input could be particularly critical for hearing-impaired infants. Preterm infants' auditory thresholds generally are not tested until near the time of discharge. Thus, if attenuation is practiced, the safer device would model that provided by the womb, where higher frequencies are selectively attenuated. Without a more selective approach, speech sounds also would be dampened. The strategy is, therefore, potentially harmful. On the other hand, short-term occlusion might be appropriate during a brief, acute phase of illness. Research is needed, with both short- and long-term consequences carefully evaluated, including speech stimuli and hearing thresholds as outcome measures.

Auditory stimulation, as a single modality, has been studied in the preterm infant. Schmidt and colleagues (115) reported that auditory stimulation, in the form of a heartbeat, lengthened the duration of the first quiet sleep period. Quiet sleep is a more stabilized state that reflects central nervous system maturity. Some NICUs have urged using sound as a protective window for the infant—when music is played, the infant will not be disturbed. This approach responds to the potential for conditioning in the preterm infant. Soothing sound is soft, simple, repetitive, and harmonic, with a limited dynamic range. Nonetheless, speech and nonspeech stimuli differentially stimulate the cerebral hemispheres (98). Availability of speech sounds may be more critical. In one of the earliest studies, Katz (117) reported using auditory stimulation in the form of recorded maternal speech, played to healthy preterm infants of 28 to 32 weeks of gestation, until each reached 36 weeks PCA. Compared to controls, the intervention group showed better neuromotor development and improved auditory and visual responses. This study highlights once more that the effects of an intervention may not be limited to the stimulated sense. Even so, exposure to recorded speech lacks the essential reciprocal nature of normal communication.

Visual System

The visual system is the most extensively studied sensory system; therefore, the mechanisms are better understood. The eye is like a window to the brain, as it contains two thirds of the afferent nerve fibers in the central nervous system. Light energy is transmitted through the cornea, pupil, lens, and optic media to the retina. There it bypasses the retinal blood vessels, a layer of ganglion cells, and a layer of bipolar cells before it finally reaches the outer segments of the photoreceptors (i.e., rods and cones). Light is absorbed by the photoreceptors in a photochemical response that converts the radiant energy to an electrical impulse. The amount of light energy necessary to stimulate a single photoreceptor cell is extremely small—one quantum (118). In the absence of a light stimulus, retinal firing still occurs in the form of a tonic discharge. Some processing occurs even at the level of the retina (118). From the photoreceptors, the impulse travels to the ganglion cells, the optic nerve, and through the lateral geniculate nucleus to the occipital cortex. Fibers from the medial portion of each retina decussate, whereas those from the lateral half do not. Thus, information from either the left or right visual field will fall on the contralateral portion of each retina and be transmitted to the same hemisphere of the brain. Representation in the cortex is topographic, but upside down and reversed.

Development

The eye is an outgrowth of the brain from the early embryonic stage. By 24 weeks of gestation, gross anatomic structures are in place and the visual pathway is complete. As shown in Table 9-1, the visual system is undergoing extensive maturation and differentiation between 24 and 40 weeks of gestation. Corresponding functional visual responses have been elicited in the preterm infant (10,119–125).

As early as 24 to 28 weeks of gestation, a visual-evoked response to bright light can be obtained, but it consists of a

TABLE 9-1
MATURATION OF THE FETAL EYE IN THE THIRD TRIMESTER

Fetal Eye Components	26–28 Weeks of Gestation	30–32 Weeks of Gestation	34–36 Weeks of Gestation
Eyelid	Fused early in development, now reopens.	Less translucent.	
Pupil	Tunica vasculosa lentis. begins to atrophy. No reflex present.	Fully atrophied by end of period. Sluggish reflex.	Few remnants. Complete reflex.
Lens	Second of four-layer nucleus forming.	Second layer complete, third begins.	
Media	Cloudy. Hyaloid system begins. to regress.	Clears. Hyaloid almost disappeared.	Some remnants may still be present.
Retina	Rod differentiation begins. Vascularization just beginning.	Complete except for fovea, cone differentiation begins. Nasal portion nearly complete.	Cone number in fovea increases. Temporal region nearly fully vascularized.
Visual cortex	Rapid dendritic growth and differentiation.	Marked development of dendritic spines and synapses.	Morphologically now similar to full term.

long-latency negative wave that readily fatigues. A behavioral response to bright light consists of lid tightening, but the response also fatigues quickly. The refractive error is approximately −5 diopters (D). The optic media is cloudy.

Important functional changes occur around 32 weeks of gestation. The morphology of the visual-evoked response becomes more complex with the addition of a positive wave, and the latency decreases. The pupillary reflex is more efficient. A bright light will cause immediate lid closure, and the response sustains. The optic media has often cleared. The eyes may open spontaneously, and the infant may even briefly fixate. This has been described as the beginning of "attention" (119). Attention as such may be best elicited with a large, high-contrast form held closer to the eyes than would be necessary at term, but under similar conditions of low illumination (i.e., 5 foot-candles [ft-c]).

By 36 weeks, the visual-evoked response resembles that of a full-term infant, but the latency is still longer for the preterm infant and remains so. Spontaneous eye opening, even *in utero*, has been observed on ultrasound. Although alertness still is less sustained than at term, the preterm infant now shows a spontaneous orientation toward a soft light and can track an object horizontally and vertically. Additionally, the infant prefers a patterned to a nonpatterned surface, in a manner similar to a full-term infant. The refractive error is near zero.

Relative to the other sensory systems, the visual system is the least mature by term birth, with considerable development continuing over the next 6 months (126). Having less dense optic media and less macular pigmentation than an adult, the eye of the newborn infant transmits more short-wavelength light by a factor of four (78). Newborns are photophobic; thus, visual attention is facilitated under low illumination (i.e., approximately 5 ft-c). Acuity estimates are in the range of 20/200 Snellen equivalents. The refractive error is normally slightly hyperopic (i.e., +1 D).

The newborn can attend to form, object, and face. Specifically, he or she can fixate a high-contrast form (i.e., a 1/16-inch wide line at a distance of 1 foot) and can show preference for patterns along dimensions of brightness and complexity. She or he will track a bright object horizontally across midline and vertically. Attention to the human face by a neonate can be explained as a predisposition to respond to contrast (e.g., eyes, open mouth) or to edge (e.g., hairline), to slow movement (e.g., nodding), and to contingent stimulation (e.g., adult's voice). In any event, this behavior is powerfully adaptive.

Deficits

It generally is agreed that the visual system of the preterm infant is particularly susceptible to insult. The most well-known visual problem is retinopathy of prematurity (ROP), which is a proliferative vascular disease of multifactorial origin. ROP has been linked to oxygen toxicity, but it occurs in preterm infants with cyanotic heart disease who have never been hyperoxic. ROP is most strongly associated with degree of immaturity of the retina (127–130). Visual disorders—

thicker lenses, poorer visual acuity, higher incidence of astigmatism, high myopia, strabismus, anisometropia, and color deficits (blue–yellow)—other than ROP are more common among children born prematurely (131–133). For example, among a sample of 5-year-old, low-birth-weight children, 35% lacked stereopsis and 25% had less than 20/20 corrected acuity in both eyes (132). Risk for visual disorders is inversely related to gestational age.

In addition to these visual problems, the preterm infant also has difficulty processing visual information at a more cognitive level. Performance on tests of visual attention, visual pattern discrimination, visual recognition memory, and visuomotor integration repeatedly indicates particular vulnerability for the preterm infant (9,12,13,134,135).

Intrauterine Environment

The womb generally is dark, but under certain conditions light can transmit to the fetus. A behavioral response by a fetus to light has been described (136). Transmission through all the tissue is limited to small amounts of red, or long-wavelength, light. Probably only 2% of incident light reaches the uterus (D. Sliney, *personal communication*, June 1992). In later pregnancy, the head of the human fetus is in the vertex position, the neck is flexed, and the face is posterior, thereby diminishing exposure. It is unlikely that light exposure is a necessary condition for the fetus, or that periodic exposure to low levels of long-wavelength light is harmful. Aspects of the light–dark cycle that reach the fetus probably are mediated more by maternal sources such as rest–activity cycles and hormones than by light directly.

After birth, ambient light increases markedly, although typically the room is kept dim and cycled with dark to some extent. A prolonged wake period linked to catecholamine release occurs during this transition to extrauterine life. In dim light, the newborn is more likely to open his or her eyes.

Neonatal Intensive Care Unit Environment

Modern intensive care nurseries are brightly lit environments with ambient light in excess of standard office lighting for adults (Fig. 9-2). The general range reported has been 30 to 150 ft-c, with peaks of more than 1,500 ft-c from sunlight (137,138). The intensity of ambient illumination for any individual infant is determined by the location of the crib in a room; the number of overhead light units; the size, location, and compass direction of windows; the season of the year; and even the prevailing weather conditions (i.e., sunny versus hazy). The duration of exposure generally is 24 hours a day over the length of hospital stay, which is a function of degree of immaturity and medical complications. Thus, light exposure is greater for those most vulnerable to visual problems.

In addition to ambient light, preterm infants routinely are exposed to supplementary sources, such as a bili light, heat lamp, and indirect ophthalmoscope. The standard double-bank phototherapy unit produces 300 to 400 ft-c

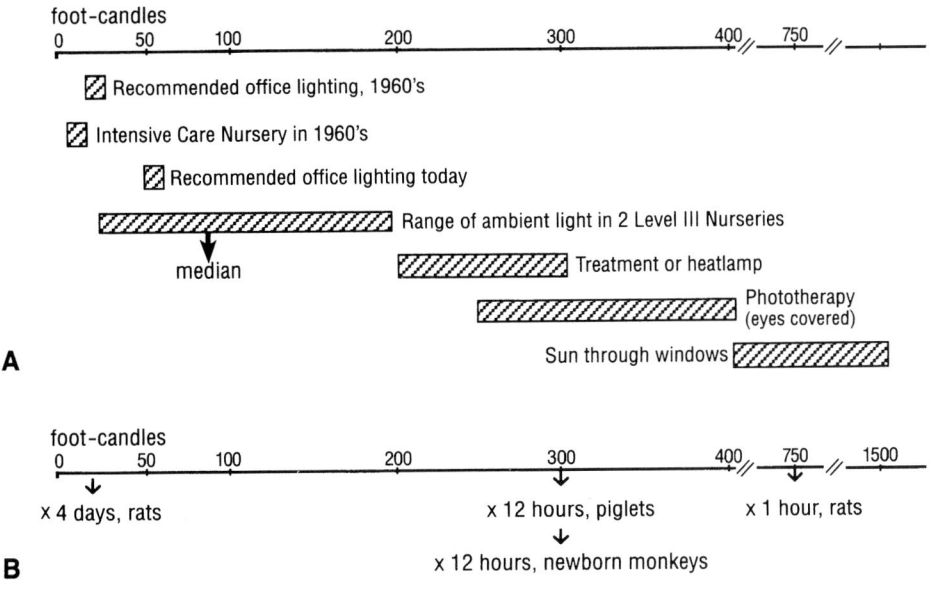

Figure 9-2   A: Levels of light exposure in the intensive care nursery. **B:** Light exposure and retinal damage in animals. (From Glass P, Avery GB, Subramanian KN, et al. Effect of bright light in the hospital nursery on the incidence of retinopathy of prematurity. *N Engl J Med* 1985;313:401, with permission.)

of illumination. The mini bili light has an intense beam, estimated at more than 10,000 ft-c. Infants' eyes are routinely patched under phototherapy; however, in some cases the eye pads are inadequate or may slip off. A commonly used heat lamp produces an intensity of more than 300 ft-c at an infant's face. Exposure time varies, but typically is longer for younger and sicker infants. The eyes of infants typically are not covered during procedures.

Finally, an indirect ophthalmoscope is used for the routine eye examinations to rule out ROP. Exposure for 2 minutes, which is the approximate time of retinal examination, at maximum power has been estimated as equivalent to exposure at 2,000 ft-c for 3 hours (139). Extra precautions for protecting the infant's dilated eyes from ambient or supplementary sources of light before and after the eye examination are not routine. For the smallest infants, the addition of a heat lamp during the examination often is necessary to maintain the baby's temperature.

Phototoxicity in Animals

Animals exposed to similar levels of light have sustained damage to their photoreceptors, pigment epithelium, and choroid (139,140). Phototoxicity is a consequence of a photochemical effect, but may be exacerbated by heat. The effectiveness of light in producing retinal damage is proportional to its efficiency in bleaching rhodopsin. A level of 100 ft-c bleaches rhodopsin to 80% in approximately 10 minutes. Continuous illumination is more potent than cyclic, but intermittent exposure may be cumulative.

Factors that enhance photochemical damage to the animal retina strikingly parallel the perinatal course of the preterm infant (137). Retinal damage in animals is facilitated by maintenance of the animal in constant dark

before light exposure, an increase in body temperature, conditions of hyperoxia, hypoxia, or ischemia, and retinal disease. Finally, light and oxygen may have a synergistic adverse effect on ROP (141). In spite of all these considerations, safety standards have not yet been determined.

Photobiological Effects of Light in the Neonatal Intensive Care Unit

Mounting data indicate that light has potent biological effects that are not considered routinely in standard NICU care. An association between light and ROP was first suggested by Terry (142) in 1946. Potential mechanisms to account for phototoxicity as one of the contributing factors in ROP have been proposed and are consistent with the oxygen toxicity hypotheses: damage to endothelial cells, alteration of normal retinal metabolism, disruption of the normal regenerative process of the retina, and generation of free radicals (137,141,143–146).

There is no evidence that light is a necessary condition for ROP or that maintaining a preterm infant in the dark will completely prevent it. Seiberth and colleagues (147) found no difference in incidence of ROP for preterm infants (birth weight less than 1,250 g) who had opaque eye patches day and night from birth to 35 weeks of gestation compared to an unpatched control group. The daytime ambient light levels were already low (30 to 40 lux, or approximately 3 to 5 ft-c), and the control group had cycled lighting at night.

Three converging lines of evidence lend empirical support to an association between light and ROP. In a prospective but nonrandomized study, preterm infants for whom the light levels were reduced for the duration of their hospital stay had a lower incidence of ROP compared to a similar group of preterm infants exposed to standard bright levels of nursery light (148). The same effect was found in both NICUs studied. Similar findings were reported by Hommura and colleagues (149). Reynolds and colleagues (150) reported no difference in incidence of ROP for preterm infants who wore light-reducing goggles compared to infants who did not; however, the goggles were discontinued at 31 weeks of gestation. In a separate study, increased ROP was identified in the region of the retina that is more exposed to light—specifically, more in the regions around 3 o'clock and 9 o'clock compared to the superior and inferior regions (151). In addition, preterm infants with a higher degree of retinal pigment are less likely to develop ROP than infants with less retinal pigment (152,153). Retinal pigment is protective against phototoxicity.

Photobiological effects are not limited to the retina. Elevated room light or phototherapy may cause degradation of riboflavin and vitamin A, which are common components of total parenteral nutrition (154). Solutions containing these vitamins may be covered at the source, but tubing often is not shielded. Light in the visible spectrum penetrates the skin and thereby may alter more than the bilirubin concentration in the blood. Riboflavin levels were reduced *in vivo* in infants undergoing phototherapy (155). Thrombocytopenia (i.e., platelets less than $150,000/mm^3$) was more than tripled among preterm infants exposed to phototherapy light (156). *In vitro* experiments demonstrated inhibition in the normal constriction of immature lamb ductal rings exposed to ambient laboratory light (157). Subsequently, Rosenfeld and colleagues (158) found a significant reduction in the occurrence of patent ductus arteriosus among preterm infants whose chests were shielded from exposure to phototherapy light.

Light and Behavior

Bright light in an infant's face is a source of stress (159). Even routine ambient light level affects sleep and wake states in preterm infants. Lower ambient light is associated with significantly less active rapid eye movement sleep and significantly more quiet sleep among preterm infants at 35 to 36 weeks PCA (160). Rapid eye movement is a more destabilized state, with greater fluctuations of oxygen saturation and more frequent occurrence of apnea and bradycardia. Lower ambient light also is associated with increased eye opening and awake periods. Light level influences an infant's response to sound. Under bright light, an infant shows an aversive response to a tone, whereas under a dim light the same tone elicits an orienting response (161). Dimming the light has a quieting effect on caregivers, who are apt to behave as though someone were sleeping.

Intervention in the Neonatal Intensive Care Unit

The optimal level of NICU lighting has not been determined; however, no study supports the safety of current bright light levels. Therefore, it would be prudent to limit

ambient nursery light to necessary levels and shield the infant's eyes and chest from ambient as well as supplementary sources. Shading does not mean occluding. Evidence does not suggest that infants' eyes should be patched beyond what is necessary for phototherapy. Prolonged patching may be detrimental, both in terms of stimulus deprivation and possible effects on corneal growth.

Opportunities for spontaneous eye opening under dim (i.e., 5 ft-c) or dark conditions should be provided. Visual attention is more likely to occur under low light levels. Animal studies suggest that dim–dark cycling may be beneficial for regeneration after retinal damage.

A day–night cycling regimen in the intermediate care nursery before hospital discharge affects behavior (162). Infants in the cycled nursery showed improved sleep patterns both in the hospital and after discharge, spent less time feeding, and gained more weight; however, light, noise, and handling all were reduced at night in the experimental unit. That does not negate the effect, but the necessity of entrainment of preterm infants to light–dark cycles is not supported. Rest–activity cycles may be more potent. Biological rhythms are much more complex (163,164).

The question then becomes whether to provide patterned visual stimulation. An infant's ability to respond to a level of stimulation does not necessarily mean that he or she should be stimulated at that level. For example, infants are more likely to respond to a louder sound, yet no one would recommend higher-intensity noise just because the baby hears it better. Likewise, babies attend more to high-contrast black-and-white stimuli than to pastel, but that does not necessarily mean that the baby should be stimulated with the stronger visual pattern either. Prolonged or obligatory visual attention is not a preferred behavior. Given that the visual system is the least mature, the most parsimonious approach would be to provide stimulation of the other senses first. Then the most appropriate visual stimulus to begin with is probably the human face, which bears no resemblance to strong black-and-white patterns.

GENERAL PRINCIPLES

A central issue in developmental intervention is whether to conceptualize the preterm infant as an extrauterine fetus and, therefore, attempt to reproduce the intrauterine environment, or whether by dint of being born, the system now requires other forms of stimulation to foster the unique development of the preterm infant. To some extent this is a nonissue; abrupt change to extrauterine life in altricial species almost always has been modulated by the mother. The aversive conditions found in the NICU would not be conducive to development for even the healthiest full-term infant. Further research is not necessary to determine whether excess handling, noise, and bright light ought to be reduced. The NICU environment is a potential source of stress and overt damage to the preterm brain. Research is needed to establish safety limits, rather than to study whether or not aversive conditions do harm.

Sensory deprivation also can affect development. Research still is necessary to determine the optimal type, timing, duration, and level of stimuli; however, basic guiding principles for developmental intervention do exist:

- Preterm infants are not a homogeneous group. Thus, determining the appropriate level of stimulation is based on an understanding of developmental neurophysiology and evaluation of an individual infant's medical status, neurologic maturation, physiologic stability, and social and physical needs.
- Sensory development is not a simple unitary process. The hierarchical organization and integration of function among the sensory systems provides the conceptual framework for developmental intervention. Thus, intervention should begin with the most mature system, should support the normal maturational process, and should not attempt to accelerate development.
- The model of optimal stimulation for early development lies in the sources naturally available to the fetus and infant (i.e., the mother). The optimal NICU model thus would begin with the intrauterine conditions, then parallel and extend the transition period that occurs immediately after a normal term birth.

A general algorithm therefore seems possible:

- Provide, for any infant, protective care, minimal handling, undisturbed rest, dim, and quiet. Provide for stabilization of autonomic, state, and motor processes through positioning and containment. Model supportive touch.
- Consider the role of olfaction and early bonding. Include positive taste experiences.
- If the infant is sufficiently mature (32 weeks gestation) and medically stable, introduce graded tactile–vestibular and auditory input. Introduce familiar forms of stimulation at lower intensity first and only if no major medical changes are occurring simultaneously. Other than a parent's face, wait for visual stimulation. Avoid any attempt to "accelerate" development.
- Monitor and modify the approach as the infant matures.

Decreasing aversive conditions, such as bright light, noise, and handling in the NICU, and enhancing comfort through touch, holding, positioning, and containment, benefit the infant and communicate directly to parents.

ACKNOWLEDGMENTS

I thank Cara Coffman and Susan Lydick for substantial contributions to a previous version of this chapter, and R.D. Walk, my mentor.

REFERENCES

1. Hack M, Breslau N, Weissman B, et al. Effect of very-low-birthweight and subnormal head size on cognitive abilities at school age. *N Engl J Med* 1991;325:231.
2. Hack M, Fanaroff AA. Outcomes of children of extremely low birthweight and gestational age in the 1990s. *Semin Neonatol* 2000;5:89–106.
3. McCormick MC, Gortmaker SL, Sobol AM. Very-low-birth-weight children: behavior problems and school difficulty in a national sample. *J Pediatr* 1990;117:687.
4. Klein N, Hack M, Gallaher J, et al. Preschool performance of children with normal intelligence who were very-low-birth-weight infants. *Pediatrics* 1985;75:531.
5. Ross G, Lipper EG, Auld PAM. Educational status and school-related abilities of very-low-birth-weight premature children. *Pediatrics* 1991;88:1125.
6. Taylor HG, Klein N, Minich NM, et al. Middle-school-age outcomes in children with very low birthweight. *Child Dev* 2000; 71(6):1495.
7. Volpe JJ. Cognitive deficits in premature infants. *N Engl J Med* 1991;325:276.
8. Sostek AM. Prematurity as well as IVH influence development outcome at five years. In: Friedman S, Sigman M, eds. *The psychological development of low birth weight children*. New York: Academic Press, 1992:259.
9. Kopp C, Sigman M, Parmelee A, et al. Neurological organization and visual fixation in infants at 40 weeks conceptional age. *Dev Psychobiol* 1975;8:165.
10. Parmelee AH, Sigman M. Development of visual behavior and neurological organization in pre-term and full-term infants. In: *Minnesota symposium on child psychology*, vol. 10. Minnesota: University of Minnesota Press, 1976:119.
11. Sostek AM, Quinn PO, Davitt MX. Behavior, development and neurologic status of premature and full term infants with varying medical complications. In: Field TM, Sostek A, Goldberg S, et al, eds. *Infants born at risk*. New York: Spectrum, 1979:281.
12. Caron A, Caron R. Processing of relational information as an index of infant risk. In: Friedman S, Sigman M, eds. *Preterm birth and psychological development*. New York: Academic Press, 1981: 219.
13. Rose SA. Enhancing visual recognition memory in preterm infants. *Dev Psychol* 1980;16:85.
14. Garcia-Coll C. Behavioral responsivity in preterm infants. *Clin Perinatol* 1990;17:113.
15. Sigman M. Early development of preterm and fullterm infants: exploratory behavior in eight-month olds. *Child Dev* 1976;47: 606.
16. Gunnar M, Hertsgaard L, Larson M, et al. Cortisol and behavioral responses to repeated stressors in the human newborn. *Dev Psychobiol* 1991;24:487.
17. Gunnar MR. Reactivity of the hypothalmic-pituitary-adrenocortical system to stressors in normal infants and children. *Pediatrics* 1992;90:491.
18. Gorski PA. Developmental intervention during neonatal hospitalization. *Pediatr Clin North Am* 1991;38:1469.
19. Weisel TN, Hubel DH. Single cell response in striate cortex of kittens deprived of vision in one eye. *J Neurophysiol* 1963;26:1003.
20. Schulte FJ, Stennert E, Wulbrand H, et al. The ontogeny of sensory perception in preterm infants. *Eur J Pediatr* 1977;126:211.
21. Dobbing J. Later development of the brain and its vulnerability. In: Davis JA, Dobbing J, eds. *Scientific foundations of paediatrics*. London: Heinemann, 1974:565.
22. Field T. Supplemental stimulation of preterm infants. *Early Hum Dev* 1980;4:301.
23. Cornell EH, Gottfried AW. Intervention with premature human infants. *Child Dev* 1976;47:32.
24. Lawson KR, Daum C, Turkewitz G. Environmental characteristics of the neonatal intensive care unit. *Child Dev* 1977;48:1633.
25. Gorski PA. Premature infant behavioral and physiological responses to caregiving interventions in the intensive care nursery. In: Call JD, Galenson E, Tyson RL, eds. *Frontiers of infant psychiatry*. New York: Basic Books, 1983:256.
26. Korones S. Iatrogenic problems in intensive care. In: Moore TD, ed. *Report of the sixty-ninth Ross conference on pediatric research*. Columbus, OH: Ross Laboratories, 1976:94.
27. Korner AF. Preventive intervention with high-risk newborns: theoretical, conceptual, and methodological perspectives. In: Osofsky JD, ed. *Handbook of infant development*, 2nd ed. New York: John Wiley and Sons, 1987:1006.
28. Avery GB, Glass P. The gentle nursery: developmental intervention in the NICU. *J Perinatol* 1989;9:204.

29. Bradley RM, Mistretta CM. Fetal sensory receptors. *Physiol Rev* 1975;55:352.
30. Gottlieb G. The psychobiological approach to developmental issues. In: Mussen PH, ed. *Handbook of child psychology*, vol. II, 2nd ed. New York: John Wiley and Sons, 1983:1.
31. Turkewitz G, Kenny PA. The role of developmental limitations of sensory input on sensory/perceptual organization. *J Dev Behav Pediatr* 1985;6:302.
32. Humphrey T. Correlation between appearance of human fetal reflexes and development of the nervous system. *Prog Brain Res* 1964;4:93.
33. Hooker D. *The prenatal origin of behavior*. New York: Hafner, 1969.
34. Fitzgerald M, Shaw A, MacIntosh N. Postnatal development of the cutaneous flexor reflex: comparative study of preterm infants and newborn rat pups. *Dev Med Child Neurol* 1988;30:520.
35. Harlow H, Harlow M. The effects of rearing conditions on behavior. *Bull Menninger Clin* 1962;26:213.
36. Thoman EB, Ingersoll EW, Acebo C. Premature infants seek rhythmic stimulation, and the experience facilitates neurobehavioral development. *J Dev Behav Pediatr* 1991;12:11.
37. Klaus MH, Kennell JH. *Maternal–infant bonding*. St. Louis: CV Mosby, 1976.
38. Tribotti SJ. Effects of gentle touch on the premature infant. In: Gunzenhauser N, ed. *Advances in touch: new implications in human development*. Skillman, NJ: Johnson & Johnson Consumer Products, 1990:80.
39. Eyler FD, Woods NS, Behnke M, et al. Changes over a decade: adult-infant interaction in the NICU, 1992 *(unpublished manuscript)*.
40. Adam K, Oswald I. Sleep helps healing. *BMJ* 1984;289:1400.
41. Sassin JF, Parker DC, Mace JW, et al. Human growth hormone release: relation to slow-wave sleep and sleep-waking cycles. *Science* 1969;165:513.
42. Long JG, Philip AGS, Lucey JF. Excessive handling as a cause of hypoxemia. *Pediatrics* 1980;65:203.
43. Murdoch DR, Darlow BA. Handling during neonatal intensive care. *Arch Dis Child* 1984;59:957.
44. Peabody JL, Lewis K. Consequences of newborn intensive care. In: Gottfried AW, Gaiter JL, eds. *Infant stress under intensive care: environmental neonatology*. Baltimore: University Park Press, 1985:201.
45. Perlman JM, Volpe JJ. Suctioning in the preterm infant: effects on cerebral blood flow velocity, intracranial pressure, and arterial blood pressure. *Pediatrics* 1983;72:329.
46. Speidel BD. Adverse effects of routine procedures on preterm infants. *Lancet* 1978;2:864.
47. Volpe JJ. Intraventricular hemorrhage and brain injury in the premature infant: diagnosis, prognosis, and prevention. *Clin Perinatol* 1989;16:387.
48. Schanberg S, Field T. Maternal deprivation and supplemental stimulation. In: Field T, McCabe P, Schneiderman N, eds. *Stress and coping across development*. Hillsdale, NJ: Erlbaum, 1988:3.
49. Kuhn CM, Schanberg SM, Field T, et al. Tactile-kinesthetic stimulation effects on sympathetic and adrenocortical function in preterm infants. *J Pediatr* 1991;119:434.
50. Als H, Lawhon G, Brown E, et al. Individualized behavioral and environmental care for the very-low-birth-weight preterm infant at high risk for bronchopulmonary dysplasia: neonatal intensive care unit and developmental outcome. *Pediatrics* 1986;78:1123.
51. Jay S. *The effects of gentle human touch on mechanically ventilated very short gestation infants*. Ph.D. Thesis, University of Pittsburgh, Pittsburgh, PA, 1982.
52. Field TM, Schanberg SM, Scafidi F, et al. Tactile/kinesthetic stimulation effects on preterm neonates. *Pediatrics* 1986;77:654.
53. Scafidi FA, Field TM, Schanberg SM, et al. Massage stimulates growth in preterm infants: a replication. *Infant Behav Dev* 1990;13:167.
54. Harrison LL, Leeper JD, Yoon M. Effects of early parent touch on preterm infants' heart rates and arterial oxygen saturation levels. *J Adv Nurs* 1990;15:877.
55. Hack M, Estabecek M, Robertson S. Development of sucking rhythm in preterm infants. *Early Hum Dev* 1985;11:133.
56. Birnholz J, Stephens J, Faria M. Fetal movement patterns: a possible means of defining neurologic developmental milestones in utero. *AJR* 1978;130:537.
57. Bernbaum JC, Pereira GR, Watkins JB, et al. Nonnutritive sucking during gavage feeding enhances growth and maturation in premature infants. *Pediatrics* 1983;71:41.
58. Field T, Ignatoff E, Stringer S, et al. Nonnutritive sucking during tube feedings: effects on preterm neonates in an intensive care unit. *Pediatrics* 1982;70:381.
59. Woodson R, Hamilton C. Effects of nonnutritive sucking on heart rate in pre-term infants. *Dev Psychobiol* 1988;21(3):207–213.
60. Dixon S, Syder J, Holve R, et al. Behavioral effects of circumcision with and without anesthesia. *J Dev Behav Pediatr* 1984;5:246.
61. Field T, Goldson E. Pacifying effects of nonnutritive sucking on term and preterm neonates during heelstick procedures. *Pediatrics* 1984;74:1012.
62. Geldard FA. *The human senses*. New York: John Wiley and Sons, 1967.
63. Mason WA. Wanting and knowing: a biological perspective on maternal deprivation. In: Thoman EB, ed. *Origins of infant's social response*. Hillsdale, NJ: Erlbaum, 1979:225.
64. Neal MV. Vestibular stimulation and developmental behavior of the small premature infant. *Nurs Res Rep* 1968;3:1.
65. Korner AF. The use of waterbeds in the care of preterm infants. *J Perinatol* 1986;6:142.
66. Cordero L, Clark DL, Schott L. Effects of vestibular stimulation on sleep states in premature infants. *Am J Perinatol* 1986;3:319.
67. Kramer LI, Pierpont ME. Rocking waterbeds and auditory stimuli to enhance growth of preterm infants. *J Pediatr* 1976;88:297.
68. Pelletier JM, Short MA, Nelson DL. Immediate effects of waterbed flotation on approach and avoidance behaviors of premature infants. In: Ottenbacher KJ, Short-DeGraff MA, eds. *Vestibular processing dysfunction in children*. Binghamton, NY: Haworth Press, 1985:81.
69. Gatts JD, Fernbach SA, Wallace HD, Singra TS. Reducing crying and irritability in neonates using a continuous controlled learning environment. *J Perinatol* 1995;15(3):215–221.
70. Yu VYH. Effect of body position on gastric emptying in the neonate. *Arch Dis Child* 1975;50:500.
71. Henderson-Smart DJ, Read DJ. Depression of intercostal and abdominal muscle activity and vulnerability to asphyxia during active sleep in the newborn. In: Guilleminault C, Dement W, eds. *Sleep apnea syndromes*. New York: Alan R. Liss, 1978:93.
72. Martin RJ, Herrell N, Rubin D, et al. Effect of supine and prone positions on arterial oxygen tension in the preterm infant. *Pediatrics* 1979;63:528.
73. Wagaman MJ, Shutack JG, Moomijian AS, et al. The effects of different body positions on pulmonary function in neonates recovering from respiratory disease. *Pediatr Res* 1978;12:571(abstract).
74. Grenier A. Prévention des déformations précoces de hanche chez les nouveau-nés à cerveau lésé: maladie de Little sans ciseaux? *Ann Pediatr (Paris)* 1988;35:423.
75. Anderson GC. Current knowledge about skin–skin (kangaroo) care for preterm infants. *J Perinatol* 1991;11:216.
76. Mistretta CM, Bradley RM. Development of the sense of taste. In: Blass EM, ed. *Handbook of behavioral neurobiology*. Vol. 8: *Developmental psychobiology and developmental neurobiology*. New York: Plenum Press, 1986:205.
77. Porter RH, Balogh RD, Makin JW. Olfactory influences on mother–infant interaction. In: Rovee-Collier C, Lipsitt LP, eds. *Advances in infancy research*. Camden, NJ: Ablex, 1988:39.
78. Werner JS, Lipsitt LP. The infancy of human sensory systems. In: Gollin ES, ed. *Developmental plasticity: behavioral and biological aspects of variations in development*. New York: Academic Press, 1981:35.
79. Steiner JE. Human facial expressions in response to taste and smell stimulation. *Adv Child Dev Behav* 1979;13:257.
80. Tatzer E, Schubert MT, Timischl W, et al. Discrimination of taste and preference for sweet in premature babies. *Early Hum Dev* 1985;12:23.
81. Smotherman WP, Robinson SR. Milk as the proximal mechanism for behavioral change in the newborn. *Acta Paediatr Suppl* 1994;397:64.
82. Schaal B, Orgeur P, Rognon C. Odor Sensing in the human fetus: Anatomical, functional, and chemoecological bases. In: Lecanuet J-P, Fifer WP, Krasnegor NA, et al., eds. *Fetal development: A psychobiological perspective*. Hillsdale, NJ: Erlbaum, 1995:205.
83. Pedersen PE, Greer CA, Shepherd GM. Early development of olfactory function. In: Blass EM, ed. *Handbook of behavioral neurobiology*. Vol. 8: *Developmental psychobiology and developmental neurobiology*. New York: Plenum Press, 1986:163.

84. Rieser J, Yonas A, Wikner K. Radial localization of odors by human newborns. *Child Dev* 1976;47:856.

85. Macfarlane JA. Olfaction in the development of social preferences in the human neonate. In: *Parent–infant interaction:* Ciba Foundation Symposium 33. Amsterdam: Elsevier, 1975:103.

86. Sullivan RM, Taborsky-Barba S, Mendoza R, et al. Olfactory classical conditioning in neonates. *Pediatrics* 1991;87:511.

87. Smotherman WP, Robinson SR. Dimensions of fetal investigation. In: Smotherman WP, Robinson SR, eds. *Behavior of the fetus.* Caldwell, NJ: Telford, 1988:19.

88. Blass EM, Hoffmeyer LB. Sucrose as an analgesic for newborn infants. *Pediatrics* 1991;87:215.

89. Barr RG, Quek VS, Cousineau D, et al. Effects of intra-oral sucrose on crying, mouthing and hand-mouth contact in newborn and six-week-old infants. *Dev Med Child Neurol* 1994;36:608.

90. Blass EM, Shah A. Pain-reducing properties of sucrose in human newborns. *Chem Senses* 1995;20:29.

91. Aslin RN, Pisoni DB, Jusczyk PW. Auditory development and speech perception in infancy. In: Mussen PH, ed. *Handbook of child psychology*, vol. II, 2nd ed. New York: John Wiley and Sons, 1983:573.

92. Hecox K. Electrophysiological correlates of human auditory development. In: Cohen LB, Salapatek P, eds. *Infant perception: from sensation to cognition. Perception of space, speech, and sound,* vol. II. New York: Academic Press, 1975:151.

93. Rubel EW. Auditory system development. In: Gottlieb G, Krasnegor N, eds. *Measurement of audition and vision in the first year of postnatal life: a methodological overview.* Camden, NJ: Ablex, 1985:53.

94. Parmelee HP, Sigman MD. Perinatal brain development and behavior. In: Mussen PH, ed. *Handbook of child psychology*, vol. II, 2nd ed. New York: John Wiley and Sons, 1983:95.

95. Birnholz JC, Benacerraf BR. The development of human fetal hearing. *Science* 1983;222:516.

96. Querleu D, Renard X, Boutteville C, et al. Hearing by the human fetus? *Semin Perinatol* 1989;13:409.

97. Berg, KM, Smith M. Behavioral thresholds for tones during infancy. *J Exp Child Psychol* 1983;35:409.

98. Molfese D, Freeman R, Palermo D. Ontogeny of brain lateralization for speech and non-speech stimuli. *Brain Lang* 1975;2:356.

99. Fifer W, Moon C. Psychobiology of newborn auditory preferences. *Semin Perinatol* 1989;13:430.

100. Fifer WP, Moon C. Auditory experience in the fetus. In: Smotherman WP, Robinson SR, eds. *Behavior of the fetus.* Caldwell, NJ: Telford, 1988:175.

101. DeCasper AJ, Fifer WP. Of human bonding: newborns prefer their mothers' voices. *Science* 1980;208:1174.

102. DeCasper AJ, Spence MJ. Prenatal maternal speech influences on newborn's perception of speech sounds. *Infant Behav Dev* 1986; 9:133.

103. Spence M, DeCasper A. Newborns prefer a familiar story over an unfamiliar one. *Infant Behav Dev* 1987;10:133.

104. Kurtzberg D, Stapells DR, Wallace IF. Event-related potential assessment of auditory system integrity: implications for language development. In: Vietze PM, Vaughan HG, eds. *Early identification of infants with developmental disabilities.* Philadelphia: Grune & Stratton, 1988:160.

105. Gerherdt K. Characteristics of the fetal sheep sound environment. *Semin Perinatol* 1989;13:362.

106. Armitage SE, Baldwin BA, Vince MA. The fetal sound of sheep. *Science* 1980;208:1174.

107. Walker D, Grimwade J, Wood C. Intrauterine noise: a component of the fetal environment. *Am J Obstet Gynecol* 1970;109:91.

108. Douek E, Dodson HC, Bannister LH, et al. Effects of incubator noise on the cochlea of the newborn. *Lancet* 1976;2:1110.

109. Falk SA. Combined effects of noise and ototoxic drug. *Environ Health Perspect* 1972;2:5.

110. Walton JP, Hendricks-Munoz K. Profile and stability of sensorineural hearing loss in persistent pulmonary hypertension of the newborn. *J Speech Hear Res* 1991;34:1362.

111. Carlier E, Pujol R. Supra-normal sensitivity to ototoxic antibiotic of the developing rat cochlea. *Arch Otorhinolaryngol* 1980;226: 129.

112. Long JG, Lucey JF, Philip AGS. Noise and hypoxemia in the intensive care nursery. *Pediatrics* 1980;65:143.

113. Philbin MK, Ballweg DD, Gray L. The effect of an intensive care unit sound environment on the development of habituation in healthy avian neonates. *Dev Psychobiol* 1994;27:11.

114. Salamy A, Mendelson T, Tooley WH, et al. Differential development of brainstem potentials in healthy and high-risk infants. *Science* 1980;210:553.

115. Schmidt K, Rose SA, Bridger WH. Effect of heartbeat sound on the cardiac and behavioral responsiveness to tactual stimulation in sleeping preterm infants. *Dev Psychol* 1980;16:175.

116. Zahr LK, de Traversay J. Premature infant responses to noise reduction by earmuffs: effects on behavioral and physiologic measures. *J Perinatol* 1995;15:448.

117. Katz V. Auditory stimulation and developmental behavior of the premature infant. *Nurs Res* 1971;20:196.

118. Gregory RL. *Eye and brain: the psychology of seeing,* 4th ed. Princeton, NJ: Princeton University Press, 1990.

119. Hack M, Mostow A, Miranda S. Development of attention in preterm infants. *Pediatrics* 1976;58:669.

120. Dreyfus-Brisac C. Neurophysiological studies in human premature and fullterm newborns. *Biol Psychiatry* 1975;10:485.

121. Mann I. *Development of the human eye.* New York: Grune & Stratton, 1964.

122. Purpura DP. Morphogenesis of visual cortex in the preterm infant. In: Brazier MAB, ed. *Growth and development of the brain: nutritional, genetic, and environmental factors. International Brain Research Organization monograph series.* New York: Raven Press, 1975:1.

123. Dubowitz LM, Dubowitz V, Morante A, et al. Visual function in the preterm and fullterm newborn infant. *Dev Med Child Neurol* 1980;22:465.

124. Miranda SB. Visual abilities and pattern preferences of premature infants and full-term neonates. *J Exp Child Psychol* 1970;10: 189.

125. Senecal J, Defawe G, Roussey M, et al. Le comportement visuel du premature. *Arch Fr Pediatr* 1979;36:454.

126. Abramov I, Gordon J, Hendrickson A, et al. Light and the developing visual system. In: Marshall J, ed. *Vision and visual dysfunction.* Boca Raton, FL: CRC Press, 1991.

127. James L, Lanman J. History of oxygen therapy and retrolental fibroplasia. *Pediatrics* 1976;57:590.

128. Lucey J, Dangman B. A reexamination of the role of oxygen in retrolental fibroplasia. *Pediatrics* 1984;73:82.

129. Johns KJ, Johns JA, Feman SS, et al. Reinopathy of prematurity in infants with cyanotic congenital heart disease. *Am J Dis Child* 1991;145:200.

130. Inder TE, Clemett, RS, Austin NC, et al. High iron status in very-low-birth-weight infants is associated with an increased risk of retinopathy of prematurity. *J Pediatr* 1997;131:541.

131. Fledelius T. Prematurity and the eye. *Acta Ophthalmol* 1976; 128:3.

132. Hoyt C. Long-term visual effects of short-term binocular occlusion of at-risk neonates. *Arch Ophthalmol* 1980;98:1967.

133. Dobson V, Quinn GE, Abramov I, et al. Color vision measured with pseudoisochromatic plates at five-and-a-half-years in eyes of children from the CRYO-ROP study. *Invest Ophthalmol Vis Sci* 1996;37:2467.

134. Sigman M, Parmelee A. Visual preferences of four month old premature and fullterm infants. *Child Dev* 1974;45:959.

135. Siegel L. The prediction of possible learning disabilities in preterm and fullterm children. In: Field T, Sostek A, eds. *Infants born at risk: physiological, perceptual, and cognitive processes.* New York: Grune & Stratton, 1983:295.

136. Brazelton TB, Field TM. Introduction. In: Gunzenhauser N, ed. *Advances in touch: new implications in human development.* Skillman, NJ: Johnson & Johnson Consumer Products, 1990:xiii.

137. Glass P. Light and the developing retina. *Doc Ophthalmol* 1990;74:195.

138. Landry RJ, Scheidt PC, Hammond RW. Ambient light and phototherapy conditions of eight neonatal care units: a summary report. *Pediatrics* 1985;75:434.

139. Lanum J. The damaging effects of light on the retina: empirical findings, theoretical and practical implications. *Surv Ophthalmol* 1978;22:221.

140. Williams TP, Baker BN, eds. *The effects of constant light on visual processes.* New York: Plenum Press, 1980.

141. Ham WT, Mueller HA, Ruffolo JJ. Mechanisms underlying the production of photochemical lesions in the mammalian retina. *Curr Eye Res* 1984;3:165.

142. Terry L. Retrolental fibroplasia. *J Pediatr* 1946;29:770.

143. Dorey CK, Delori FC, Akeo K. Growth of cultured RPE and endothelial cells is inhibited by blue light but not green or red light. *Curr Eye Res* 1990;9:549.

144. Riley PA, Slater TF. Pathogenesis of retrolental fibroplasia. *Lancet* 1969;2:265.

145. Stefansson E, Wolbarsht ML, Landers MB. In vivo O_2 consumption in rhesus monkeys in light and dark. *Exp Eye Res* 1983;37:251.

146. Zuckerman R, Weiter JJ. Oxygen transport in the bullfrog retina. *Exp Eye Res* 1980;30:117.

147. Seiberth V, Linderkamp O, Knorz MC, et al. A controlled clinical trial of light and retinopathy of prematurity. *Am J Ophthalmol* 1994;118:492.

148. Glass P, Avery GB, Subramanian KN, et al. Effect of bright light in the hospital nursery on the incidence of retinopathy of prematurity. *N Engl J Med* 1985;313:401.

149. Hommura S, Usuki Y, Takei K, et al. Ophthalmic care of very low birthweight infants, report 4: clinical studies of the influence of light on the incidence of ROP. *Nippon Ganka Gakkai Zasshi* 1988;92:456.

150. Reynolds JD, Hardy RJ, Kennedy KA, et al. Lack of efficacy of light reduction in preventing retinopathy of prematurity. *N Engl J Med* 1998;338:1572.

151. Fielder AR, Robinson J, Shaw DE, et al. Light and retinopathy of prematurity: does retinal location offer a clue? *Pediatrics* 1992;89:648.

152. Monos T, Rosen SD, Karplus M, et al. Fundus pigmentation in retinopathy of prematurity. *Pediatrics* 1996;97:343.

153. Schaffer D, Palmer E, Plotsky D, et al, on behalf of the CRYO-ROP Cooperative Group. Prognostic factors in the natural course of retinopathy of prematurity. *Ophthalmology* 1993;100:230.

154. Bhatia J, Mims L, Roesel R. The effect of phototherapy on amino acid solutions containing multivitamins. *J Pediatr* 1980;96:284.

155. Sisson T. Advances in phototherapy of neonatal hyperbilirubinemia. In: Helene C, Charlier M, Montenay-Garestier T, et al, eds. *Trends in photobiology.* New York: Plenum Press, 1982:339.

156. Maurer H, Fratkin M, McWilliams N, et al. Effects of phototherapy on platelet counts in low-birthweight infants and on platelet production and life span in rabbits. *Pediatrics* 1976;57:506.

157. Clyman RI, Rudolph AM. Patent ductus arteriosus: a new light on an old problem. *Pediatr Res* 1978;12:92.

158. Rosenfeld W, Sadhev S, Brunot V, et al. Phototherapy effect on the incidence of patent ductus arteriosus in premature infants: prevention with chest shielding. *Pediatrics* 1986;78:10.

159. Shogan MG, Schumann LL. The effect of environmental lighting on the oxygen saturation of preterm infants in the NICU. *Neonat Netw* 1993;12:7.

160. Glass P, Sostek A. *Sleep organization in preterm infants: the effect of nursery illumination.* Presented at the International Conference of Infancy Studies (poster session), New York, April 21, 1984.

161. Haith MM. *Rules that babies look by.* Hillsdale, NJ: Erlbaum, 1980.

162. Mann NP, Haddow R, Stokes L, et al. Effect of night and day on preterm infants in a newborn nursery: randomised trial. *BMJ* 1986;293:1265.

163. Glotzbach SF, Rowlett EA, Edgar DM, et al. Light variability in the modern neonatal nursery: chronobiologic issues. *Med Hypotheses* 1993;41(3):217–224.

164. Mirmiran M, Kok JH. Circadian rhythms in early human development. *Early Hum Dev* 1991;26:121.

The Fetal Patient

Prenatal Diagnosis in the Molecular Age—Indications, Procedures, and Laboratory Techniques

10

Arie Drugan   *Nelson B. Isada*   *Mark I. Evans*

The modern era of molecular and biochemical genetics commenced with the observations of Sir Archibald Garrod at the beginning of the twentieth century. He proposed that four diseases—namely, alkaptonuria, albinism, cystinuria, and pentosuria—resulted from inherited disorders of chemical metabolism. He also suggested that these disorders, which he called "inborn errors of metabolism," represented only a small fraction of every human's "chemical individuality" that had gone awry (1).

Advances in biochemistry have confirmed Garrod's concepts by characterizing the structural protein abnormality or enzymatic defect of many disorders. Other advances in molecular genetics have allowed precise identification of the defect in the deoxyribonucleic acid (DNA) message, sometimes before the protein defect itself is known (2). This knowledge has direct and immediate applications in the field of prenatal diagnosis (3). This chapter discusses gene organization; mutations and polymorphism analysis; molecular diagnostic techniques; DNA cloning; an approach to disorders diagnosable by molecular genetics; biochemical disorders not amenable to DNA technology or better studied by protein chemistry techniques; and carrier screening.

GENE ORGANIZATION

The Watson-Crick double-helix model of DNA organization is well known (4). DNA conveys information encoded by a series of four nucleotides—adenine (A), thymine (T), cytosine (C), and guanine (G)—that are connected sequentially on two strands. The two strands complement each other, with nucleotide base pairs (bp) being formed by hydrogen bonding between adenine–thymine and guanine–cytosine. Eukaryotic DNA is located in the nucleus and organized into structures called chromosomes. During interphase, chromosomes are not visible by light microscopy. They can be observed only when the genetic content has doubled and the chromosomes condense before mitosis. Chromosomal material is organized into euchromatin and heterochromatin. Euchromatin is vigorously transcribed into ribonucleic acid (RNA). Heterochromatin is relatively inactive. An example of heterochromatin is the inactivated X chromosome.

An unexpected discovery made in the 1970s was that some regions of the eukaryotic chromosome do not code for any known protein (5). Specifically, these noncoding regions (*introns*), were noted to be interspersed within coding regions (*exons*) (6,7). Exons carry information to direct the assembly of amino acids into a protein, whereas introns do not. Messenger RNA (mRNA) acts as an intermediate molecule to convey information encoded in the DNA by a process called *translation*. Posttranslational modification of mRNA takes place such that introns are removed and exons are joined together before amino acid sequences are formed. After additional biochemical modifications, the mRNA passes out of the nucleus into the cytoplasm, where protein-synthesizing organelles are located.

Approximately 60% of the human genome is comprised of regions of unique nucleotide sequences that presumably code for proteins (8). It is estimated that there are 50,000 to 100,000 expressed genes and proteins active in humans; however, expressed genes comprise less than 10% of total genomic DNA. A significant portion of the human genome, perhaps approximately 40%, contains repetitive DNA sequences (9). Various terms are used for the different classes of repetitive DNA sequences found in humans. Highly repetitive sequences are found in the chromosome region adjacent to the centromere. These are simple sequences that are repeated thousands of times, are present in more than 10^4 copies, and comprise approximately 20% of the genome.

Other repetitive, simple sequences are several hundred base pairs long, and are separated easily by centrifuging slightly fragmented DNA through a cesium chloride density gradient. DNA separated by this process is called *satellite DNA*, because the centrifuged DNA forms a main band and several satellite bands above and below the main band. In humans, four satellite bands comprise approximately 6% of the total DNA, each band representing tandem repeat sequences. Blocks of satellite DNA are readily localized by in situ hybridization to regions around the centromeres of metaphase chromosomes. Satellite DNA should not be confused with satellites, a cytogenetic term referring to the segment of an acrocentric chromosome distal to short arm and separated by a constriction.

Other classes of repetitive DNA include *moderately repetitive DNA*, which is gene size in length, repeated from 10 to 1,000 times, and comprises approximately 20% of genome (i.e., one-half of the 40% that is repetitive DNA); *tandem repeat sequences*, which are stretches of DNA in which a short nucleotide sequence is repeated 20 to 100 times, the exact number varying from person to person; *alphoid DNA*, which is a chromosome-specific, repeated, monomeric 170-bp unit located in centromeric regions; and *Alu sequences*, which are highly repetitive 300-bp sequences that are not clustered around centromeres, but are more evenly distributed throughout the genome and interspersed within longer stretches of unique or moderately repetitive DNA. Most contain a single cleavage site near the middle for the restriction enzyme Alu I, derived from the bacterium *Arthrobacter luteus* (see *Restriction Fragment Length Polymorphism Analysis* below). Almost 1 million *Alu* sequences are present in the human genome, accounting for 3% to 6% of the total DNA. Each individual human has a unique amount of repetitive DNA. This genetic fingerprint is used for paternity testing and forensic analysis.

A discovery involving repeat sequences demonstrates an association between changes in length of triplet repeats and human disease. A significant increase in length of the normal sequence of three repeated nucleotides is associated with marked tendency to clinical morbidity. This was first described in the fragile X syndrome, a common form of heritable male mental retardation, where a polymorphic sequence of -CGG- repeats on the X chromosome is increased from a mean of 29 repeats to more than 200 repeats in affected males. Triplet expansion of -GCT- is

associated with congenital myotonic dystrophy. Triplet expansion of -CAG- is found in spinal-bulbar muscular atrophy, spinocerebellar ataxia, and Huntington disease (10–12).

Regulation of gene expression occurs at many levels. Substrate concentrations both enhance and repress specific enzymes, especially in bacteria. In eukaryotes and prokaryotes, a region separate from a given gene but still involved in regulation of expression is called *promoter*; it binds RNA polymerase and initiates transcription. Similar functional areas have been found that bind a large group of transcription factors. In eukaryotes, such an area or box contains a common or consensus nucleotide sequence, CAAT, and is called a *CAAT box*. A conserved area associated with RNA polymerase positioning contains repeated sequences of the nucleotides thymine and adenine and is called a *TATA box*.

Extranuclear DNA found in mitochondria (mtDNA) is inherited independently of nuclear DNA, is 16.5 kb in length, contains no introns, and is organized as a double-stranded circle. mtDNA is subject to a relatively high rate of mutation compared to nuclear DNA and is inherited maternally, the paternal spermatic mitochondria being excluded from the oocyte at the time of fertilization. A variety of neonatal and pediatric disorders, predominantly neuromuscular, are associated with mtDNA deletions (13–15).

ELEMENTS OF MOLECULAR GENETICS

The deciphering of DNA structure and the genetic code has advanced understanding of the molecular basis of genetic disease. Alterations in DNA sequence may affect a gene structure or function, and may result in an altered gene product that may (or may not) be expressed as genetic disease. An alteration in the sequence of nucleotides within a gene is termed a mutation.

Many types of mutations can affect a gene. The DNA within a gene contains information for the final sequence of a protein and signals for the correct expression and processing of mRNA. If the actual coding region is altered, then the resultant protein may be changed. These alterations can be in the form of deletions that may be many kilobases in length or as small as a single base, inversions or translocations that produce no net nucleotide changes but potential or actual protein changes, or single-base substitution. Even a change at the junction of a coding and noncoding region can result in abnormal mRNA formation. Defects in the promoter region may result in too little or too much expression of mRNA, which will be reflected in abnormal protein synthesis. A deletion of all or part of the gene will almost always result in the disruption of normal gene expression.

Two examples of molecular pathology can be seen in Ashkenazi Jews (16). In the severe infantile type of Tay-Sachs disease, a mutation at an exon–intron splice site in the α-subunit has been identified (i.e., G to C transversion); another mutation is a four-base insertion in exon 11 of the α-subunit causing a frameshift mutation and marked reduction in mRNA (17,18). Another example is the F508 mutation, the most common (approximately 70%) mutation causing cystic fibrosis (CF) in people of northern European ancestry (19–21). The remaining 30% of CF cases in people of northern European ancestry are caused by a heterogeneous assortment of other mutations (i.e., W1282X). Commercial testing is available and can detect more than 90% of mutations in the northern European population (22). However, other ethnic groups carry their own particular repertoire of mutations and detection rate may be as low as 50% (23).

A variety of approaches have been used to detect mutations. Optimally, determination of DNA structure and sequence, followed by elucidation of gene structure and organization in the normal allele, are completed before beginning a search for specific defects. However, only 5% to 10% of clinically significant mutations are a result of gross alterations in gene structure that are detectable by Southern blot analysis of genomic DNA, leaving unknown the remaining 90% to 95%. The problem is compounded by normal variation in the nucleotide sequence (polymorphism). Thus, when variations from the normal sequence are found, additional analysis is required before these changes can be construed as being a disease-causing mutation.

Because DNA is present in each cell nucleus, any nucleated cell theoretically is suitable for DNA analysis, regardless of whether the gene in question is being transcribed and expressed. Thus, leukocytes, amniocytes, and chorionic villi all are candidate cells for DNA analysis, using Restriction Fragment Length Polymorphism (RFLP). Other methods also used for DNA diagnosis include Southern blot, oligonucleotide probes, and polymerase chain reaction (PCR). Northern blotting is used for RNA analysis.

RFLP analysis uses bacterial enzymes that recognize and cleave DNA at specific sites. Presumably, these enzymes evolved as a defense mechanism against hostile, invading DNA, as might occur with bacteriophages. Because these cleavage sites are quite specific, that is, are restricted to specific palindromic sequences 4 to 10 nucleotides in length, these enzymes are called *restriction endonucleases*. When these enzymes are added to eukaryotic DNA, the resultant mixture contains a variety of DNA fragments of different sizes, which can be separated by gel electrophoresis and transferred for analysis by Southern blotting. Each enzyme cuts an individual's DNA according to the positions of the cleavage sites, with every person having his or her own unique pattern of cleaved DNA fragments. Thus, people are polymorphic for the resulting lengths of DNA fragments. Many of these recognition-site polymorphisms are neutral and represent normal inherited variability. These characteristics have given rise to the term *restriction fragment length polymorphisms*, which refers to the polymorphic patterns observed in specific nucleotide sequences that are cleaved by bacterial restriction enzymes (Fig. 10-1). The resultant mixture of DNA fragments can be separated and further characterized by gel electrophoresis, Southern blotting, and oligonucleotide probes (24). DNA alterations that

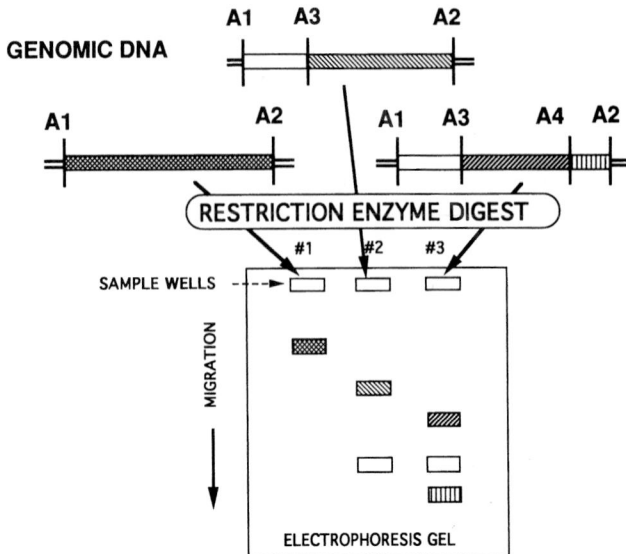

Figure 10-1 Restriction fragment length polymorphisms. Lane 1, A1, and A2 present; lane 2, A1–A3 present; lane 3, A1–A4 present; A1–A5, hypothetical polymorphisms.

affect an RFLP site either by creating a new site for endonuclease cleavage or eliminating a previously existing one can be detected on Southern blot as a result of changes in the size of the DNA fragment associated with this site (25). If, by chance, either a mutation or normal sequence corresponds to an RFLP site, this situation can be exploited for allele identification by using linkage analysis.

An initial use of such mapping involved the Huntington disease locus (26). Another early application was for prenatal identification of the sickle-cell mutation in the β chain of hemoglobin (27,28). For example, the restriction enzyme Dde I, derived from the bacterium *Desulfovibrio desulfuricans aestuarii*, recognizes the nucleotide sequence -CTNAG- (where N indicates that any nucleotide may occupy that position) that occurs within the hemoglobin A (-CTGAG-) and hemoglobin C (-CTAAG-) gene, but not within hemoglobin S (-CTGTG-). In hemoglobin S, the nucleotide thymine is substituted for adenine, which is not recognized by Dde I and thus is not cleaved by Dde I. This results in a much larger RFLP fragment that can be recognized on Southern blot. Initially, this technology used unamplified DNA and Southern blot transfer. Target gene sequences can now be preamplified a million-fold by PCR (see next page) and then cut by restriction endonucleases, which greatly facilitates target sequence recognition. This approach is potentially useful in prenatal diagnosis, particularly when the quantity of clinical material is limited.

When the precise nucleotide mutations of the abnormal gene causing the disease are unknown, linkage analysis is a very powerful technique that can be used for diagnosis by association of the diseased gene to a known gene or polymorphic site (29). This implies that the closer together two genetic traits are on a chromosome, the more likely they are to segregate together during meiosis and the less likely crossing-over occurs between them. When genes are in such close proximity that crossing-over rarely occurs, such as for hemophilia A and color blindness, the two sites are said to be linked (30). Any polymorphism that is linked with the trait of interest is termed informative. Unfortunately, family studies are not always informative, because linked molecular or clinical polymorphisms are not always present.

The likelihood that two given traits are linked can be described mathematically by the *logarithm of the odds* (LOD) score, developed in 1955 by Morton (31). It can be derived from recombination observed between clinical or biochemical traits from pedigree analysis, or from molecular polymorphisms (32). The probability of recombination during meiosis between two loci is quantified by the *recombination fraction* (i.e., theta or q), the maximum being 0.5. The LOD score is derived from various values of q. Viewed simplistically, the higher the LOD score, the higher the likelihood of linkage. Because this number is used on a logarithmic scale, each integer increase reflects a tenfold increase in likelihood of linkage. Thus, a LOD score of 4 suggests that there is linkage between two polymorphisms, the odds of random association being 10,000:1. A LOD score of zero suggests there is no linkage and that the two traits are on different chromosomes or are far apart on the same chromosome. Tight linkage indicates little or no recombination and suggests an actual physical proximity of two polymorphisms, measured in physical map distances, with the common unit of genetic distance reported as centimorgans (cM). Linkage disequilibrium describes closely linked genes that occur more frequently than would be expected from random distribution, suggesting nonrandom mating or some survival advantage from natural selection. Examples of linkage disequilibrium include the carrier states for sickle cell disease and thalassemia, where those affected have increased resistance to certain types of malarial infections.

Other methods used for DNA analysis include Southern blot, oligonucleotide probes, and PCR. Northern blot is used for RNA analysis. Southern blot is a standard method for DNA analysis in both the clinical and basic science settings. In the Southern blot technique, named after Edwin Southern, double-stranded DNA is digested by a restriction endonuclease chosen because of its ability to detect a DNA polymorphism (33). After endonuclease digestion, the resulting DNA fragments are separated using gel electrophoresis. The DNA in the gel is denatured to generate single-stranded DNA molecules. DNA fragments are transferred from the gel to nylon filter paper (blotting), and specific filter-bound DNA fragments then can be detected by hybridization. A radiolabeled DNA or RNA probe is used that has sequence homology to the DNA fragment of interest, usually 200 to 2,000 bases long. Subsequent autoradiography produces a radiographic film with banding patterns that indicate the hybridization locations on the filter that reflect the fragment sizes of the DNA sequences homologous to that particular probe (Fig. 10-2).

Allele-specific oligonucleotide hybridization has proven to be a valuable technique that measures the specific binding of short (18 to 20), labeled oligonucleotide probes, that match exactly either the wild-type) normal (or the

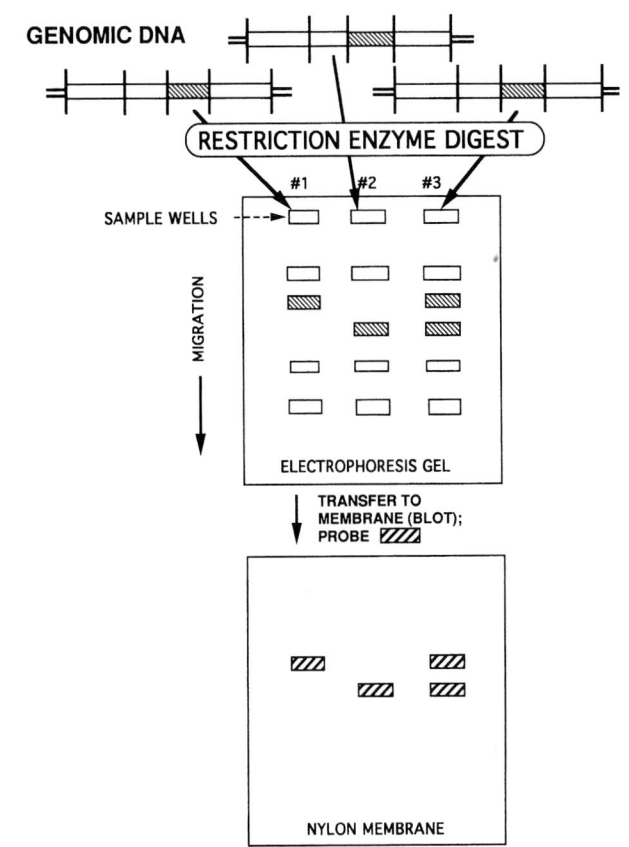

Figure 10-2 Southern blot for a hypothetical autosomal recessive disorder. Lane 1, unaffected; lane 2, affected; lane 3, carrier.

mutant DNA sequence, under stringent washing conditions. Only the probes that exactly complement the immobilized DNA will remain bound and thus generate a signal seen on autoradiography. Conner (34) originally described this technique for the detection of sickle cell β-globin allele. This technique greatly facilitates the evaluation of genetic disorders in which the gene has to be screened for numerous mutations such as thalassemia, Tay-Sachs, Gaucher, or CF.

PCR has revolutionized the field of molecular genetics (35,36). It's discoverer, Kary Mullis, won the Nobel Prize in Chemistry in 1993. This procedure allows *in vitro* amplification of minute amounts of DNA to generate sufficient quantities of signal to make detection by more traditional methods possible. PCR makes use of Taq I, a relatively heat-stable bacterial enzyme derived from *Thermus aquaticus*, a thermoacidophilic bacterium. If the target nucleotide sequence is known, a specific set of oligonucleotides, called *primers*, can be synthesized to encompass the target sequence. The target DNA, oligonucleotide primers, Taq I polymerase, and free nucleotides are placed in solution. This reaction mixture is further heated to allow already denatured DNA to anneal with the oligonucleotides, between which the polymerase synthesizes complementary strands (Fig. 10-3). Repeated cycles of heating and cooling result in cyclic primer sequence synthesis, leading to annealing and amplification of the target sequence, because

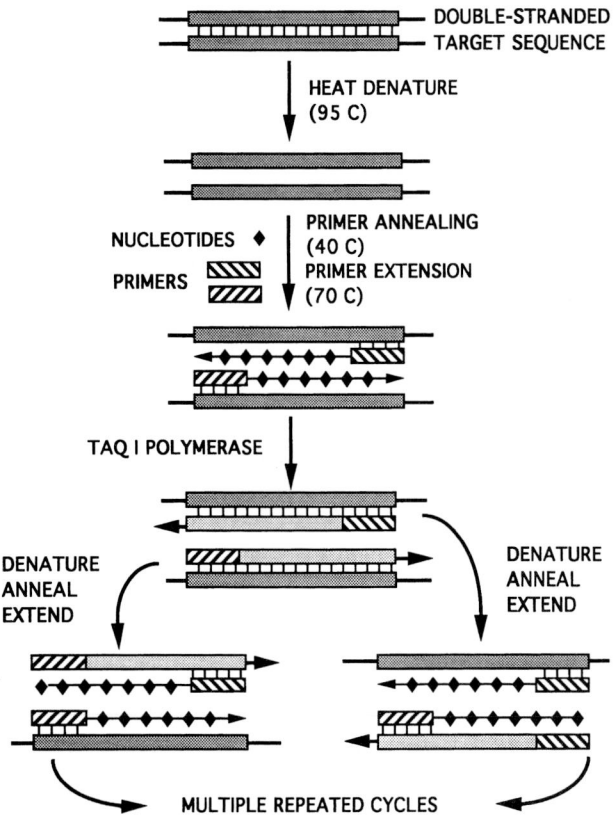

DOUBLE-STRANDED
TARGET SEQUENCE

HEAT DENATURE
(95 C)

NUCLEOTIDES ◆   PRIMER ANNEALING
(40 C)

PRIMERS ▨   PRIMER EXTENSION
(70 C)

TAQ I POLYMERASE

DENATURE
ANNEAL
EXTEND

DENATURE
ANNEAL
EXTEND

MULTIPLE REPEATED CYCLES

Figure 10-3 Polymerase chain reaction.

each set of DNA strands gives rise to two additional sets of sequence templates in each cycle of the reaction. This process can be automated to allow 20 to 30 cycles, which can produce more than a million-fold duplication of the target sequence within hours. Modifications of this process can be performed to allow:

- Analysis of RNA.
- Analysis of multiple DNA areas (multiplex PCR). This technique allows detection of more than 97% of deletions in Duchenne muscular dystrophy and all those of patients at risk for Becker muscular dystrophy (37).
- Selective amplification of one strand instead of both (i.e., asymmetric PCR).
- Simultaneous use of one primer set within another to increase specificity (i.e., nested PCR).
- Simultaneous use of two different primer sets, one of which selects for a normal sequence and the other for a mutant sequence (i.e., competitive oligonucleotide priming).
- Simultaneous use of a known amount of a second, easily identified target DNA to measure the amount of original DNA (i.e., semiquantitative PCR).

Many technical difficulties must be addressed to eliminate both false-positive and false-negative PCR results. Problems with reagent or reactant contamination can lead to false-positive results and require that appropriate control methods be performed simultaneously to verify positive PCR results. Other problems, such as primer instead of target

amplification and nonspecific amplification, must be recognized and avoided.

Northern blotting is used for RNA analysis. This requires prompt specimen processing and committed laboratory reagents and instruments because of ubiquitous ribonucleases, present even on finger surfaces. The general principles of the technique are similar to those for Southern blotting. Examination of the size and amount of a mRNA transcript is a useful initial step in evaluating the expression of mutated genes in cells or tissues. Fibroblasts and lymphocytes are good sources of mRNA. Hepatic or muscle tissue is also useful, if available. Placental tissue can be used if maternal cell contamination can be avoided. Of the cell's total RNA, only 1% to 2% is mRNA, which is highly unstable at room temperature because of tissue RNA-ases. The remainder of the RNA is mainly ribosomal RNA (rRNA) and transfer RNA (tRNA). Once isolated, the mRNA is denatured, separated by agarose gel electrophoresis, transferred to a membrane filter, and analyzed by hybridization of a specific fluorescent or radiolabeled probe.

For most diseases studied at the molecular level, 5% to 10% of patients have no detectable mRNA for the gene product in question; 10% to 20% have reduced but detectable amounts of normal mRNA; and approximately 5% have some alteration in mRNA size. The approximately 50% remaining have normal amounts of normal-size mRNA. Given this information, it is possible to deduce the general type of mutation at the DNA level, such as large or total gene deletions, which are suggested by a total absence of mRNA. Mutations in promoter regions are suggested by reduced amounts of normal mRNA. Mutations at exon–intron junctions are suggested by changes in mRNA size—normal–size mRNA but abnormal function of protein hints at point mutations.

In some instances, the quantity of RNA is insufficient to be detected in the previously mentioned methods. In these cases, reverse transcriptase PCR methodology permits identification and isolation of small quantities of mRNA and thereby analyze genes in a more fastidious manner. Grompe et al. (38) were unable to detect by Northern analysis the mRNA in an ornithine transcarbamylase-deficient patient. Nonetheless, the mRNA was isolated and successfully amplified (after synthesis of a single-stranded complementary DNA [cDNA] by using the RNA-directed DNA polymerase, reverse transcriptase), and the mutation responsible for the disease was identified. This technique also allows isolation of the shorter cDNA fragments corresponding to the coding region of the gene of interest. As in Menkes' ("kinky hair") disease, a neurodegenerative disorder associated with a disturbance of copper metabolism, exon splicing is the characteristic result of the splice-junction mutations seen in this rather large gene (39). By using reverse transcriptase PCR, one can discern which exons are lacking by the size of fragment seen on agarose gel or by sequence analysis.

The basic steps in the study of a gene start with the isolation of a DNA molecule complementary to its mRNA, called cDNA, that contains only exonic sequences. The first step in cDNA cloning is the isolation of mRNA from a particular cell or tissue that contains a significant amount of the desired mRNA. A retroviral enzyme, reverse transcriptase, is used to synthesize cDNA from the mRNA. Because the cell or tissue mRNA contains transcripts of many genes, the resultant pool of cDNA will be heterogeneous and must be sorted out. The cDNA strands are inserted into a vector to form a cDNA library. A second type of chromosome library is composed of fragments of native genomic DNA and contains introns and other noncoding regions. Vectors include viruses that can replicate within bacteria, such as bacteriophage lambda, or autonomous, self-replicating, circular DNA molecules found in bacteria, called *plasmids*. Another vector that combines properties of plasmids and bacteriophage lambda are called *cosmids*. Cosmids are plasmid vectors into which larger fragments of DNA can be cloned. The term *cosmid* is derived from the presence of internal cohesive end sites (cos) that have been inserted into a plasmid. Cos are nucleotide sequences from bacteriophage lambda between which DNA sequences are normally expressed as capsule proteins. In cosmids, these sequences can be replaced with other nucleotide sequences, which then can be expressed and concentrated *in vitro*.

An alternative approach to cDNA cloning uses mRNA itself instead of cDNA. Using mRNA is advantageous because the mRNA pool, although heterogeneous, is not nearly so complex as a corresponding pool of genomic DNA fragments that contains a mixture of introns, nonexpressed genes, and DNA from noncoding regions. Methods of cDNA cloning to detect the presence of a specific cDNA segment include screening a cDNA library with synthetic oligonucleotide probes and screening a bacteriophage lambda library with antibodies directed against the protein of interest. Using the first approach, a set of radiolabeled oligonucleotide probes is synthesized with sequences complementary to those predicted for the mRNA from the amino acid sequence found in the protein. These oligonucleotides are used to probe a cDNA library that contains bacterial colonies infected with bacteriophage lambda. With the second approach, antibodies against the protein of interest are used to detect a corresponding protein expressed by cDNA inserted into bacteriophage lambda.

cDNA for many genes have been cloned using these approaches. Nucleotide sequencing is the first step in the analysis of a cDNA. With this information, the investigator can identify potential sites of restriction endonuclease cleavage, can compare the deduced amino acid sequence with that of the protein of interest, and can identify regions of homology with other proteins, which may suggest evolutionary relationships and previously unrecognized functions. In addition to providing nucleotide and amino acid sequence information, these cDNA can be used as hybridization probes to characterize and quantitate corresponding mRNA in cells and tissues from patients with a variety of diseases.

The process by which DNA analysis leads to an identifiable protein abnormality was previously called "*reverse genetics*"; it is now called "*positional cloning*" (40,41). Several hundred genes associated with human disease have been identified. In some diseases, such as Cystic Fibrosis, the triple-nucleotide/single-amino-acid deletion in the CFTR protein has been recognized. For other diseases, the gene and protein are better characterized, such as for neurofibromatosis type 1 (42). For most human diseases, however, the genes and the defect in protein synthesis have yet to be defined.

PRENATAL DIAGNOSIS

Whether by cytogenetic, biochemical, or molecular methods, prenatal diagnosis of an affected fetus requires obtaining either fetal tissue (i.e., blood) or other tissue for analysis that is representative of the fetus (e.g., amniocytes or placenta). Invasive procedures for prenatal diagnosis of fetal disease are available throughout gestation, from the first trimester onward. Even earlier, assisted reproduction technologies (ART) enable diagnosis (or exclusion) of several disorders on the 4- to 8-cell embryo before implantation.

Invasive procedures for diagnosis in pregnancy of fetal genetic disorders have been available for almost four decades, since the introduction of techniques for culturing and karyotyping of amniotic fluid fibroblasts in the mid-1960s (43). The first diagnosis of a fetal chromosome anomaly by amniocentesis (44) was followed shortly by the diagnosis of an enzyme deficiency in amniotic fluid cells (45). Thereafter, collaborative studies established the safety and accuracy of midtrimester amniocentesis, so that this technique became a routine part of prenatal care in high-risk patients and the gold standard against which other procedures for prenatal diagnosis are compared (46,47).

Despite its proven efficacy, a major disadvantage of amniocentesis is the availability of results late in the second trimester, generally 18 to 20 weeks of gestation. The emotional and physical implications of termination of pregnancy this late in gestation are obvious. Improvement in ultrasonography machinery and increasing expertise in ultrasound-guided procedures enabled physicians in the late 1980s to attempt prenatal diagnosis in the first trimester, introducing chorionic villus sampling (CVS) and early amniocentesis. These technical developments are backed and reinforced by increasing preference on the part of patients for first trimester prenatal diagnosis (48). Chorionic villus sampling is usually performed between 11 and 13 weeks of gestation so that results are available by the end of the first trimester. The accuracy and safety of CVS are quite comparable to those of mid trimester amniocentesis (49,50) and the early results allow patients privacy in reproductive decisions and an earlier and safer termination of pregnancy if so opted. An alternative to CVS was offered by early amniocentesis performed between 10 and 14 weeks of gestation, but this technique has been largely abandoned (51).

Over the years, a change in the pattern of indications for prenatal diagnosis has been observed. The most common

TABLE 10-1
INDICATIONS FOR PRENATAL DIAGNOSIS

Increased risk of chromosome anomalies
    Advanced maternal age
    Previous offspring with chromosome anomalies
    Parental balanced translocation or inversion
    Ultrasonogram diagnosis of fetal malformations or anomalies
    Abnormal biochemical screening in maternal serum
Previous offspring with neural tube defect
Parents carriers of a mendelian genetic trait
    Molecular DNA diagnosis (e.g., cystic fibrosis, sickle cell anemia
       and fragile X syndrome)
    Enzymatic activity in villi or amniocytes (e.g., Tay-Sachs and
       Refsum disease)
    Precursor levels in cell free amniotic fluid (e.g., 17-hydoxycortico-
       steroids progesterone in congenital adrenal hyperplasia;
       7-dehydrocholesterol in Smith-Lemli-Opitz syndrome)

indication for genetic counseling and prenatal diagnosis is the need to evaluate the karyotype of the fetus, this being indicated in more than 70% of cases of advanced maternal age (defined as 35 years or older at birth). Other "classical" indications to evaluate fetal karyotype include a previous, affected offspring and a balanced structural rearrangement of parental chromosomes, the latter being clinically evident as recurrent pregnancy loss (Table 10-1). In recent years, increased use of biochemical serum screening and of ultrasonographic screening for fetal chromosome anomalies have caused more young patients, previously considered to be at low risk for fetal aneuploidy, to opt for invasive prenatal testing. The combination of "double," "triple," or "quadruple" serum screening (α-fetoprotein [AFP], human chorionic gonadotropin [hCG], and unconjugated estriol [uE3], with or without inhibin A) and

maternal age will select for prenatal testing a sub-group of patients among whom 65% to 75% of chromosomally abnormal conceptions will be contained. Using a risk cut-off for fetal aneuploidy equal to that of age 35 years, some 5% of young pregnant patients will have a positive screening test, and 1 in 50 amniocenteses performed for this indication will diagnose a chromosomally abnormal conception (52). In the second trimester, sonographic markers for fetal chromosome anomalies are observed in 3% to 5% of pregnancies (53) (Table 10-2) and are another indication for fetal karyotyping. The most worrisome of these findings are abnormalities of fetal neck, indicating the need for evaluation of fetal chromosomes even in association with normal biochemical serum screening in young patients (54).

The most effective screening test for Down syndrome is probably the integrated test, based on estimation of the nuchal translucency on ultrasonography, hCG, and pregnancy-associated plasma protein A (PAPP-A) in the first trimester, combined with AFP, HCG, estriol, and inhibin A in the second trimester of pregnancy. The integrated risk assessment is reported to have a 94% detection rate and a 5% false-positive rate (55). The results of biochemical or ultrasonography screening also can be used to modify the risk of aneuploidy in the population previously considered at risk, reducing the number of invasive diagnostic procedures in patients of advanced maternal age by more than half (56,57). Furthermore, "at-risk" patients who previously declined amniocentesis may be influenced to accept invasive prenatal diagnosis following a positive screen result (57). However, a major problem of this "integrated" approach is that results obtained in the first trimester are withheld from the patient, and the advantages of first trimester diagnosis are lost.

The need for rapid karyotyping may arise when fetal anomalies are suspected near the statutory limit for termi-

TABLE 10-2
RELATIVE RISK FOR ANEUPLOIDY ASSOCIATED WITH ISOLATED SONOGRAPHIC MARKERS

Sonographic Marker	Prevalence	Relative Risk*
Choroid plexus cysts	1.25%	× 9[†]
Nuchal Thickening or hygroma	4%–5%	
>4 mm		× 18
>5 mm		× 28
>6 mm		× 36
Left ventricular echogenic focus	5%	× 4
Hyperechoic bowel	0.6%–0.8%	× 14–16
Pyelectasis	2%	× 3.3–3.9
Fetal biometry		
Short CRL	7%	× 3
Short Femur Length	4%–5%	× 2.7
Short Humerus	4%–5%	× 4.1
Short Femur and Humerus	2.4%	× 11.5

* Risk for trisomy 21 as calculated in relation to maternal age alone or in combination with biochemical screening.
† Risk specific for trisomy 18 and possibly trisomy 21.

nation of affected pregnancies, that is, after an abnormal result on biochemical or ultrasonography evaluation. In those cases, the diagnostic options are "late" CVS (58) or cordocentesis and karyotyping of fetal blood lymphocytes. Other tests that may be performed on blood obtained by cordocentesis include hematologic parameters, acid–base balance, and immunologic status of the fetus (59).

Birth of a child with an inherited genetic disorder caused by malfunction in a single gene implies a 25% to 50% risk of recurrence in subsequent gestations, depending on the specific mode of inheritance of that disease. This risk and the associated genetic burden of the disease may be considered so high that many couples will opt to avoid further reproduction unless prenatal diagnosis is available. Fetal karyotype is uninformative in these cases. Prenatal diagnosis of mendelian disease is performed using biochemical or molecular techniques on fetal or placental tissue. Biochemical assays include assessment of gene products such as enzymes, receptors, and transport proteins, and metabolites such as amino acids, organic acids, vitamins, and hormones. When the underlying biochemical defect is known and is expressed in accessible fetal tissue or cells, prenatal diagnosis can be achieved by enzyme analysis of material obtained by CVS, amniocentesis, or cordocentesis. Because variability caused by different mutations and different genomic backgrounds exists among families, additional testing of leukocytes or cultured skin fibroblasts from presumably unaffected parents and siblings can provide valuable information. In addition to the benefit in interpretation of prenatal results, such studies may provide a reliable means for identification of other carriers among members of the extended family.

Prenatal diagnosis is now available for many inherited metabolic disorders. For an autosomal recessive disease, biochemical assays can be used should discriminate among homozygous affected, heterozygous unaffected, and homozygous normal fetuses. Assays for detection of autosomal dominant diseases, such as some of the porphyrias, usually are capable of identifying affected homozygotes, but sometimes fail to differentiate conclusively affected heterozygotes from unaffected fetuses. Heterozygote detection in X-linked disorders is difficult because of the random X inactivation occurring in every pregnancy with a female fetus. Depending on the ratio of an active mutant X to the normal X in tissues involved in the pathogenesis of the disease, a female heterozygous for an X-linked disorder may be clinically normal, or may have mild or even severe disease manifestations (60). To complicate matters further, measured enzymatic activities also vary depending on the ratio of mutant to normal X chromosomes that are active in the analyzed specimen—chorionic villi, for example. Occasionally, the activity levels in chorionic villi will not correlate with clinical expression. Males, conversely, have only one X chromosome and are either hemizygous affected with deficient enzyme activity or hemizygous normal with activity in the normal range. Thus, prenatal biochemical assessment of X-linked disorders is less complicated if the fetus is male.

The use of direct and cultured fetal specimens for prenatal evaluation of metabolic disorders ideally requires the availability of normal control preparations. Except for trophoblasts and amniotic fluid cells that can be maintained in culture, availability of fresh controls is often a problem, and in most instances long-term frozen controls with partial loss of activity must be used. There are other potential pitfalls that seem specific for each of these tissue, cell, and fluid types. All samples should be analyzed as soon as possible, except those requiring initial tissue culture. Chorionic villi, fetal tissue biopsies, cell pellets, amniotic fluid supernatant, and fetal serum or plasma that are not used for tissue culture can be kept frozen and shipped on dry ice. Cell and tissue cultures, however, should be shipped at room temperature. Whenever possible, appropriate controls matched by gestational age should accompany the samples to be analyzed. Extraction and analysis of labile enzymes is especially difficult, because test results are very sensitive with respect to the duration of homogenization or sonication. Using fresh chorionic villi or amniocytes or freshly harvested trophoblasts helps preserve the activity of such labile enzymes (61).

Fetal liver and muscle biopsy should be considered only in the absence of other alternatives, because the risk for pregnancy loss associated with these invasive procedures is significantly higher. Fetal muscle biopsy has been used in rare cases of Duchenne muscular dystrophy (DMD), when molecular analysis of trophoblasts, amniocytes, or fetal leukocytes is nondiagnostic and family studies are uninformative. An *in utero* fetal muscle biopsy can be performed in the middle of the second trimester to assess dystrophin levels in myoblasts by *in situ* hybridization (62). Absence of dystrophin suggests an affected fetus.

Fetal liver biopsy also can be performed for certain rare enzyme deficiencies. For example, in one type of glycogenosis, glucose-6-phosphatase is decreased; this enzyme is expressed only in fetal liver and kidney. In the absence of direct DNA techniques, the only option available for prenatal diagnosis is fetal liver biopsy in which glucose-6-phosphatase activity can be measured. Fetal liver biopsy also is applicable in rare cases of ornithine transcarbamylase deficiency where family studies are uninformative and known deletions cannot be detected (63). In the future, it is probable that most of these procedures will be considered obsolete, and prenatal diagnosis of most genetic disorders will be performed by molecular analysis, including some mitochondrial disorders that may be amenable to prenatal diagnosis (64).

Prenatal Diagnosis in the First Trimester

Chorionic Villus Sampling

The first attempts at first trimester prenatal diagnosis were made in the early 1970s for fetal gender determination. Prenatal diagnosis did not gain popularity in the Western world until 1983, when laboratory techniques to obtain adequate karyotypes from chorionic villi were developed by Simoni and Brambati in Milan (65). They also reported the first diagnosis of trisomy 21 by the direct method (66). Over the years, the quality of chromosome preparation from CVS material has improved considerably, approaching the banding quality obtained from amniocytes or blood karyotypes (67). The clinical procedure also has been refined, with the use of real-time ultrasonographic guidance and malleable catheters for villi aspiration.

Two types of cells are observed in chorionic villi. The outer layer consists of cytotrophoblast, which divide spontaneously, and is used for direct evaluation of metaphases. The inner mesenchymal core is used to initiate long-term cultures and is usually considered as more representative of fetal karyotype. Fetal karyotype is obtained from direct analysis, from long-term culture, or from both in 99.6% of successful sampling of villi (67). Results of direct analysis are equivocal in 0.5% to 2% of cases, but questions raised usually are resolved by long-term CVS or amniotic cell cultures (68). Most commonly, an abnormal direct result that proves to be normal on long-term culture will not be confirmed in karyotypes obtained from amniocytes or fetal lymphocytes. The unusual situation is a normal direct result followed by an abnormal result in long-term culture, with the abnormality being confirmed in fetal tissue in one-half of cases (67). Maternal cell contamination has been observed in 1.9% of long-term cultures, but usually is not observed in direct preparations and does not contribute to diagnostic error in any case (68).

Chromosomal mosaicism in CVS material affects 1.2% to 2.5% of cases (average 1.3%), and is more common in direct preparations than in long-term culture (69). Mosaicism was restricted to extraembryonic tissue in 70% to 80% of cases. Despite mosaicism being confined to the placenta, followup of these cases documented a significantly elevated fetal loss rate (7.5% to 16.7%), mostly in the second and third trimesters, suggesting that such placental mosaicism is not entirely benign (70,71). Intrauterine growth restriction (IUGR) also appears to be more common in this situation (72). Mosaic trisomy 3 is one of the most common types of mosaicism observed in placental cells (69). An adverse impact on pregnancy outcome seems to be most common in association with confined placental mosaicism of chromosomes 13, 16, and 22 (73).

The diagnosis of mosaicism in CVS presents difficulties in genetic counseling because it implies uncertainty with respect to fetal phenotype and genotype. Using both direct preparation and long-term culture might increase the accuracy of diagnosis by CVS. When further evaluation is needed, level II ultrasonography and amniocentesis is generally adequate for followup. The use of early amniocentesis in these cases may allow earlier clarification of fetal karyotype without a significant increase in procedure related fetal loss rate (71). In our experience, however, the frequency of mosaicism in amniotic fluid cultures is not significantly different from that observed in CVS (0.35% vs. 0.56%, respectively) (74). Cordocentesis may also be used in such cases to verify mosaicism in fetal blood (75). Even if fetal blood karyotype is normal,

however, there still remains a small chance that mosaicism is confined to specific fetal tissues, as observed in trisomy 20 mosaicism.

CVS can be offered to almost every patient who needs prenatal diagnosis in the first trimester. The most common indication for CVS is evaluation of fetal karyotype, which is indicated for patients with advanced maternal age (70% to 80% of cases), a previous child with chromosome anomalies, or a parent carrier of a balanced translocation or inversion. "Mendelian" genetic disease can be diagnosed in at-risk cases by enzyme level analysis in fresh or cultured villi (i.e., disorders such as Tay-Sachs disease or the mucopolysaccharidoses) (76). However, it is crucial to obtain for analysis chorionic villi that are only of fetal origin, with maternal cells either completely absent or extremely rare. For most biochemical prenatal tests in the first trimester, the recommended practice is to use fresh chorionic villi for preliminary evaluation followed by subsequent analysis of cultured trophoblast for confirmation of the diagnosis. One exception is with nonketotic hyperglycinemia (NKH). Although the glycine-to-serine ratio in amniotic fluid is elevated in this disease, there is a significant overlap with normal values. The potential for prenatal diagnosis of this disorder would rely exclusively on the results obtained in fresh chorionic villi, because the glycine cleavage system is not expressed in amniotic fluid cells or trophoblasts, but is detectable in fresh tissue (77). When the enzyme in question is very labile (e.g., sialidase), or when its normal activity in chorionic villi is extremely low, as for α-iduronidase, the use of frozen controls may cause false-negative diagnoses. Specific problems also may be encountered because of different distribution of enzymes and isozymes (78). The characteristic presence of high levels of arylsulfatase C activity in chorionic villi hampers the differential detection of arylsulfatase A in metachromatic leukodystrophy and arylsulfatase B in mucopolysaccharidosis VI.

Chorionic villus sampling is particularly suitable for prenatal molecular diagnosis of "mendelian" genetic disease. The amount of DNA obtained from even a few villi is much larger than that contained from 40 mL of amniotic fluid. The molecular techniques described throughout this chapter and in a large number of other sources have particular application to CVS material.

Technical Aspects of Chorionic Villus Sampling

CVS procedures are commonly performed between 11 and 13 weeks of gestation by the transcervical, transabdominal, or transvaginal route (Fig. 10-4). After 13 weeks, the procedure is best performed using a transabdominal approach (69,79). Fetal viability and gestational age must always be confirmed before the procedure. Placental location will usually dictate which approach to employ. Transcervical CVS is used when the placenta is low lying, whereas fundal placentas are most commonly an indication for transabdominal needle aspiration of the villi. Transcervical or transvaginal CVS should be avoided in patients who have an active vaginal or cervical infection (e.g., herpes); the transabdominal approach also should be

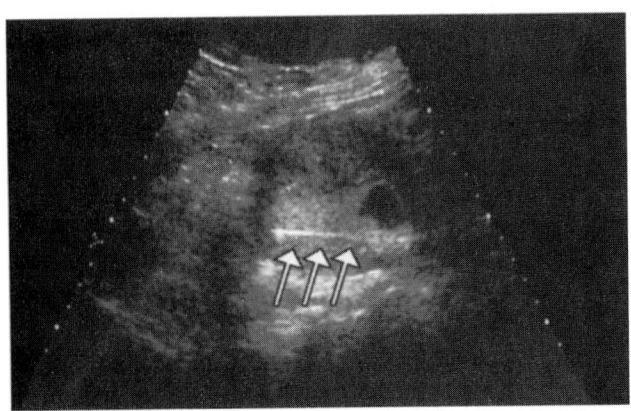

Figure 10-4 In transcervical chorionic villus sampling (CVS), the CVS catheter (*arrows*) is guided through the cervical canal and into the placenta.

avoided in patients who have an interposed bowel or marked uterine retroversion (68). In those cases, the procedure can be performed transvaginally with a needle guided by transabdominal or transvaginal ultrasonography (80).

Despite the preference of some American and European centers to use the transabdominal approach for CVS (81,82), our experience is that transabdominal sample size usually is lower than that obtained transcervically (83). Proficiency in both types of procedures is necessary, however. Tailoring the type of procedure to placental location is expected to reduce complication rates after CVS (83,84). It appears also that transabdominal CVS is more suitable for testing multifetal pregnancies and can be applied before fetal reduction (85). After the procedure, fetal heart activity should be verified by ultrasonography. Maternal vaginal bleeding should also be assessed.

The safety of CVS must be judged in view of the natural pregnancy loss rate in the first trimester. It is estimated that 3% to 5% of pregnancies are miscarried after documentation of fetal heart beats on ultrasound at 8 to 11 weeks of gestation; the likelihood of spontaneous abortion also increases with age (86). Both the Canadian and the American collaborative studies documented an excess loss of pregnancy rate in the CVS group of 0.6% to 0.8%, which was not significantly different than the loss rate in the amniocentesis group (48,49). Fundal placental location, three catheter insertions, and obtaining small amounts of villi are significantly associated with pregnancy loss after CVS. These factors may reflect technical difficulty during the procedure (68).

Concerns over an increased risk of limb reduction defects (LRDs) following CVS were raised in the early 1990s (87,88). Evaluation of more than 135,000 cases from experienced centers worldwide reveals that the incidence of LRD or of any other defect is identical to that of the background risk in this population (89). Furthermore, closer assessment of cases of LRD reported after CVS has shown that several patients had unaccounted for familial factors (90).

Because some of these cases were reported with CVS procedures done earlier than the recommended gestational age, it is advisable to postpone CVS until 10 weeks of gesta-

tion are completed. However, there are special circumstances under which earlier CVS may be appropriate. In populations at high risk for genetic disorders there is commonly a tendency for diagnosis as early in gestation as possible. For example, in Orthodox Judaism, abortions are permitted, but only until 40 days past conception (i.e., 54 days after the last menstrual period or 8 weeks). CVS in these patients has been performed at 7 weeks to get answers "in time" (91). The ethics of using a procedure with known higher risks to meet the theological needs of patients is a fascinating subject that is beyond scope of this chapter.

Another concern regarding CVS is the potential for fetomaternal transfusion. Transiently rising maternal serum AFP levels after CVS, suggest some transfer of fetal blood into maternal circulation, this being in correlation with sample size (92). The calculated mean volume of transfused fetal blood was 5.4 mL. Others have reported the volume of fetomaternal transfusion after CVS to reach 21% of fetoplacental blood volume (69). Thus, Rhesus (Rh) immunoprophylaxis (anti-D 300 μg) should be administered to Rh-negative patients. Prior Rh isoimmunization should be considered a relative contraindication to CVS.

Early Amniocentesis

Early amniocentesis refers to aspiration of amniotic fluid less than 15 weeks from the last menstrual period. The procedure is technically similar to later amniocentesis procedures; using continuous ultrasonography guidance and aseptic technique, a 22-gauge needle is inserted into a pocket of fluid, and about 1 mL of fluid per week of gestation is aspirated into a 20-mL syringe.

With improving ultrasonography technology and increasing experience with ultrasonography-guided needle manipulations, early amniocentesis late in the first trimester appeared, in the early to mid 1990s, to be an attractive alternative to CVS. However, women who had early genetic amniocentesis were more likely to have more postprocedure amniotic fluid leakage (2.9% vs. 0.2%), vaginal bleeding (1.9% vs. 0.2%), or fetal loss (2.2% vs. 0.2%) than were women undergoing amniocentesis at 16 to 19 weeks (93). Moreover, in approximately 5% of early procedures, aspiration of fluid can be hampered by tenting of membranes; rotating the needle or the use of a stylet longer than the needle allows the procedure to succeed in these situation (51,94).

The total unintentional loss rate after early amniocentesis is estimated as 1.4% to 4.2% (93,95). It appears that the principal determinant of total fetal loss after any procedure is gestational age. There seems to be a trend in all series toward increased loss rates after amniocentesis performed at 11 or 12 weeks of gestation (96–98).

Early amniocentesis has a lower rate of pseudomosaicism and maternal cell contamination than that observed in CVS analysis. Culture failure rates of early amniocytes have been reported as 0.32% to 1.6% (95,96,99,100). In our experience, culture failure rate is 1 in 700 after midtrimester amniocentesis, but approximately 1% after early procedures (nearly 5% when amniocentesis was performed before 12 weeks of gestation). It also should be noted that failure of culture at amniocentesis has been reported more commonly in association with fetal chromosome anomalies (97). The mean culture time may also be somewhat longer after early amniocentesis than after midtrimester procedures (98).

AFP peaks in amniotic fluid at 12 to 13 weeks of gestation and then gradually decline, similar to fetal serum (99). Analysis of AFP and acetylcholinesterase (AChE) in early amniotic fluid specimens may permit the diagnosis of fetal structural anomalies. High amniotic fluid AFP levels have been observed with fetal neural tube defects (NTDs) or omphalocele even in these early samples (100), and low amniotic fluid AFP values accompanied some conceptions diagnosed as aneuploid, as seen in samples of amniotic fluid obtained at midtrimester. The interpretation of AChE results in early amniotic fluid specimens is more complex. Acetyl cholinesterase usually is analyzed on gel electrophoresis as a bimodal result, either positive or negative. In early amniotic fluid samples, a faint, inconclusive band is frequently observed, this being associated with fetal anomalies only in a minority of cases (101). A normal sonogram in this situation is also reassuring in regard to fetal neural or abdominal wall defects, but a higher rate of adverse outcomes has been reported in these pregnancies (102).

First-Trimester Prenatal Diagnosis: Chorionic Villus Sampling or Early Amniocentesis?

A prospective, randomized evaluation of CVS and first trimester amniocentesis suggests that the two techniques are comparable in terms of accuracy and successful results (103). It is apparent also that the two procedures are equally efficient in providing a sample for evaluation (CVS 99.3%, early amniocentesis [EA] 100%) and in giving a nonmosaic cytogenetic result (CVS 97.5%, EA 97.9%) (104). Spontaneous pregnancy loss after early amniocentesis is, however, significantly higher than after CVS (4.9% vs. 2.1%, respectively). Similar results were concluded from analysis of the Cochrane database: more spontaneous miscarriages (relative risk [RR] 1.92, confidence interval [CI] 1.14 to 3.23) and more cases of neonatal talipes were observed in the EA group (105). Concerns have also been raised that removal of amniotic fluid so early in gestation may affect fetal lung development and function (106). Moreover, results of EA are available about 4 weeks later than after CVS. Thus, in cases that are diagnosed as abnormal, one advantage of first trimester CVS (that patients can have a less traumatic and less risky termination of pregnancy) is lost when early amniocentesis is employed.

Our opinion is that CVS *is* the diagnostic procedure of choice before 14 weeks of gestation for karyotyping, enzymatic, and DNA molecular analysis. Conversely, EA (after 12 gestational weeks) may be preferable in certain biochemical disorders and in situations in which CVS may not truly represent fetal tissue (i.e., contamination with maternal cells or with tissue from a twin pregnancy with fused placenta).

Prenatal Diagnosis in the Second and Third Trimesters

Midtrimester Amniocentesis

Midtrimester amniocentesis is the oldest, most commonly performed procedure for prenatal diagnosis. It also is considered the gold standard to which other procedures for prenatal diagnosis are compared. Indications for genetic amniocentesis include increased risk for metabolic disorders, for chromosome anomalies or for structural anomalies that may be associated with elevated AFP (see Table 10-1).

Some metabolic genetic disorders may be diagnosed by measurement of precursor levels in cell-free fluid or by enzyme activity in cultured amniocytes. Elevated concentrations of amino acids and organic acids in amniotic fluid serve as preliminary indications for several inherited disorders, such as amino and organic acidopathies or urea cycle defects.

Amniotic fluid supernatants should be divided into multiple vials to avoid the loss of activity that occurs with repeated freezing and thawing. Determinations of amniotic fluid concentrations of specific metabolites, as well as enzymes and other proteins, usually serve as supporting evidence in prenatal diagnoses. The variability in enzyme activities or in the levels of other proteins and metabolites frequently observed in cultured amniotic fluid cells and trophoblasts can be minimized by a careful choice of control cells. Preferably, the final diagnosis should rely on molecular analysis of specific mutations or on demonstration of the underlying biochemical defect in fetal cells or tissue (measuring the actual gene products responsible for the metabolic block).

In the cytogenetics laboratory, amniocytes are removed from amniotic fluid by centrifugation and cultured in flasks or on cover glasses to grow in monolayers. Dividing cells are arrested in metaphase, when chromosomes are maximally condensed, using agents such as Colchimide that prevent spindle formation. The cells are then harvested and placed in hypotonic saline, which causes intracellular swelling and better spreading of the chromosomes during slide preparation. After fixation, the chromosomes are stained with Giemsa or quinacrine for microscopic analysis. The use of triple gas incubators, specific growth media (e.g., Chang) that enhance cellular proliferation, and *in situ* culture on cover glass have shortened considerably the sampling–harvesting interval; in most laboratories, the results are available within 1 to 2 weeks. Additional improvement is obtained by computerized cytoanalyzers that expedite recognition of metaphase spreads and obviate the need for darkroom and photography.

Cytogenetic analysis of amniotic fluid cells reflects fetal status accurately in more than 99% of cases, but mosaicism sometimes may confuse the interpretation of results. In our experience, the frequency of results needing further investigation is similar in cultures from amniocentesis and from CVS (74). Differentiation between cytogenetic abnormalities that truly reflect fetal chromosome aberrations from those that are the result of laboratory artifacts may be difficult. One or more hypermodal cells that are limited to one colony or one culture flask are identified in 2% to 3% of all amniocytes cultures and are usually associated with a normal phenotype (107). True fetal mosaicism should be considered when hypermodal cells are identified in different culture flasks or in separate colonies in the same culture flask. The frequency of hypermodal cells in one or more colonies from the same flask is 0.7%. Hypermodal cells with the same abnormality originating from multiple culture flasks are observed in 0.2% of amniotic cultures (108). Even in the latter situation, however, the abnormality in culture may not represent true fetal mosaicism, as observed by Gosden and colleagues (75). Fetal blood sampling for karyotype should help to avoid termination of pregnancy of some normal fetuses in these cases.

The use of fluorescence *in situ* hybridization (FISH) is a valuable adjunct to standard cytogenetics (109). With this technique, fluorescent probes identify chromosome-specific repetitive DNA, unique sequence regions, or site-specific cosmids in uncultured cells. Fetal cells obtained at the time of amniocentesis or chorionic villus sampling can be analyzed with commercially available probes for chromosomes 21, 18, 13, X, and Y, the result being available in 24 hours. In addition, FISH analysis can be used to identify microdeletions that cannot be observed with standard cytogenetics, that is, microdeletions that may be found in Prader–Willi, Angelman, Williams, DiGeorge/velocardiofacial or Smith–Magenis syndromes (110). It must be emphasized that FISH is still an adjunct to standard cytogenetics and does not detect or identify some cases of mosaicism, translocations, marker chromosomes, or other rare aneuploidies; standard cytogenetics must still be performed. FISH is properly used on patients for whom rapid diagnosis is essential, for example, those with abnormalities seen on ultrasonography, or who are suspicious either at term or at the cusp of their legal options for termination, or who have had multifetal pregnancies prior to reduction. We have found it to be very reliable and efficient in allowing rapid diagnosis (111).

Technical Aspects of Amniocentesis

Genetic counseling is a prerequisite to amniocentesis as well as to any other procedure for invasive prenatal diagnosis (112). Pedigree information obtained during the counseling session will allow a more accurate ascertainment of genetic risks in patients referred for other indication (e.g., advanced maternal age or abnormal serum screening). Only experienced physicians trained in the procedure should perform amniocentesis. In general, a detailed ultrasonographic examination is performed to evaluate gestational age, placental location, and amount of amniotic fluid, and to exclude fetal anomalies. After sterile preparation of the skin, a draped sterile ultrasonography transducer is used to locate a suitable pocket of fluid. Then, under continuous ultrasonographic guidance, a 20- to 22-

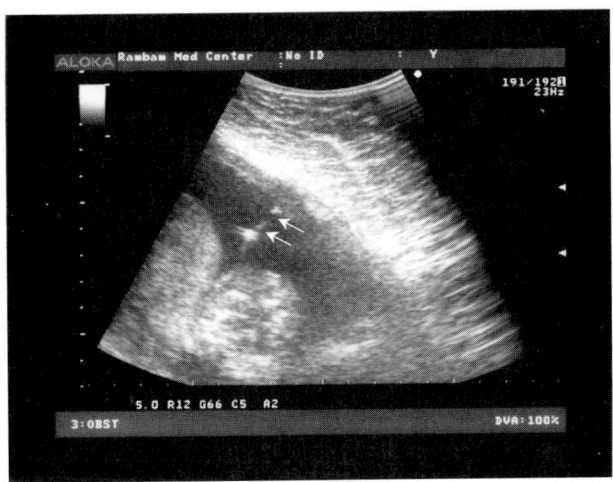

Figure 10-5 In amniocentesis, the needle (*arrows*) is inserted through the uterine wall and into the amniotic cavity.

gauge, 3.5-inch-long spinal needle is inserted in a single, smooth motion into the pocket of fluid. When the needle, which is visualized on ultrasonography as a bright spot (Fig. 10-5), is placed satisfactorily into the pocket of amniotic fluid, the stylet is removed. Twelve to 20 mL (depending on the laboratory) of amniotic fluid are then gently aspirated, transferred into sterile tubes, and transported at room temperature to the laboratory for processing.

The risk of Rh isosensitization in Rh-negative women with Rh-positive fetuses has been estimated to increase by 1% after amniocentesis (113). Thus, the patient's blood type and antibody status should be known before amniocentesis, and unsensitized Rh-negative women should receive Rh immunoprophylaxis after the procedure.

Amniocentesis is a safe procedure in experienced hands. The procedure-related pregnancy loss rate is 0.2% to 0.5% over and above the spontaneous loss rate at 16 weeks of gestation (the latter is estimated at 2% to 3%) (114). Pregnancy loss rates seem to be associated with the number of failed needle insertions at the same session and with vaginal bleeding after amniocentesis. Within reason, gestational age at the time of amniocentesis, volume of fluid removed, and amniocentesis repeated at a different session after a failed attempt do not seem to correlate with increased risk of pregnancy loss. Transplacental amniocentesis does not appear to increase the rate of fetal loss (115) provided the umbilical cord is avoided. However, the risk of Rh isosensitization is apparently increased by transplacental passage of the needle. With ultrasonography-guided amniocentesis, fetal injury by the needle should be very rare.

Leakage of amniotic fluid is a relatively frequent complication, affecting approximately 1% to 2% of patients after amniocentesis, but it usually is of minor long-term consequence; in most cases, it resolves with bed rest for 48 to 72 hours (116). Even patients with complete absence of fluid after amniocentesis may reaccumulate amniotic fluid and go on to have normal outcomes. Thus, as long as there is no evidence of infection, expectant management (for at least several days) seems prudent. Prolonged amniotic fluid leakage, however, may lead to severe oligohydramnios, which can result in fetal pressure deformities (e.g., arthrogryposis) and in pulmonary hypoplasia (117).

The risk of severe amnionitis endangering maternal health appears to be very low, around 0.1% (114). However, injury to maternal bowel or blood vessels and rare cases of mortality have also been reported (118).

"Late" Chorionic Villus Sampling

The technique of transabdominal CVS also has been applied successfully in the second and third trimesters. Nicolaides and associates first reported six successful human placental biopsies at 14 to 37 weeks of gestation, and suggested that CVS should not be confined to the first trimester (119). Chieri and Aldini performed transabdominal placental biopsy and amniocentesis in 220 patients at midtrimester; 210 of the procedures were indicated for advanced maternal age (120). A sample adequate for analysis (>2 mg of cleaned villi) was obtained in 90.9% of cases. The success rate was 94% with an anterior or fundal placenta, and 83.8% with a posterior placental location. In the latter situation, the approach to the placenta was transamniotic. Cytogenetic results were obtained in 95% of samples. No discrepancy could be found between cytogenetic results obtained in villi or in amniotic fluid, and when fetal anomalies were observed on CVS, they were acted on without waiting for corroboration from the amniotic fluid culture (120). Several studies since (121,122) have documented a sampling and diagnostic success rate of 98% to 99%, with a very low rate (0.3% to 1.8%) of procedure-related pregnancy loss, even with oligohydramnion.

The collaborative results of 2,058 late CVS procedures performed at 24 centers were reported by Holzgreve and colleagues (58). A fetal karyotype was obtained in 96% of procedures. The frequency of abnormal chromosome results was 21% when fetal anomalies were observed on ultrasound, and 6.2% with normal ultrasonographic findings. The pregnancy loss rate, excluding terminations, was 10.3% in the group with abnormal ultrasonography findings, and 2.3% in the normal ultrasonography group. Holzgreve and associates further presented their own data on 301 CVS procedures in the second and third trimester, 225 (74.7%) of which were performed for abnormal ultrasonography scans (123). Fetal karyotype was obtained in 99% of cases. The rate of chromosome anomalies was 20% in the group with abnormal ultrasonographic scans, and increased to 38% when the ultrasonography findings included abnormalities of amniotic fluid volume.

It was apparent from these studies that despite the decrease in mitotic index with placental aging, direct results could be obtained even with small amounts of placental tissue. The quality of karyotypes obtained from analysis of second and third trimester samples was similar to that obtained in the first trimester (124). Moreover, the risk of maternal cell contamination in late CVS samples actually may be lower than that observed in the first trimester because of less direct contact between villi and decidua at

later gestational age (125). Consequently, placental biopsies in the second and third trimesters are technically feasible procedures for prenatal diagnosis, with results apparently as accurate as those of amniocentesis and probably associated with a smaller risk of pregnancy loss than percutaneous umbilical blood sampling. The major advantage of late CVS is the possibility of obtaining rapid results in situations where such information is needed for decisions about pregnancy termination or fetal therapy. Such situations include the ultrasonography diagnosis of fetal anomalies late in the second trimester, close to the legal limit in gestational age after which termination of pregnancy is no longer possible. Late CVS also offers a distinct advantage over cordocentesis in cases complicated by oligohydramnion. Prenatal availability of fetal karyotype in pregnancies complicated by severe IUGR or fetal anomalies may influence the mode of delivery, the management of intrapartum fetal distress, which is a common phenomenon in fetuses with chromosome anomalies, or the decision for surgical intervention within the first few hours after birth.

Cordocentesis

Freda and Adamson originally attempted to access the vascular system of the fetus for treatment of Rh isoimmunization by hysterotomy and fetal exposure (126). This method soon was abandoned because of the unacceptably high risk for the mother and fetus. Subsequently, the development of fiberoptics allowed the introduction of fetoscopy to visualize and sample vessels on the chorionic plate or the umbilical cord (127). Although the risk of maternal compromise with this method was relatively small, the residual high rate of pregnancy loss associated with fetoscopy (up to 11.3%) was considered a major disadvantage (128).

Daffos introduced ultrasonography-guided percutaneous umbilical blood sampling (PUBS) in 1983 for the diagnosis of fetal infections (129). The procedure gained rapid and wide acceptance. In experienced hands, the risk of fetal loss is relatively small, between 1% to 2.3%, although numbers as high as 5.4% have been reported (130,131). Other complications, usually associated with excessive needle manipulations, include hematoma of the umbilical cord and placental abruption, chorioamnionitis (0.6%), and preterm delivery (9%) (131). Fetal exsanguination from the puncture site is a relatively rare complication but has been reported (132). Maternal complications are negligible, although one case of life-threatening amnionitis has been reported (133). It appears that the risks are higher when the mother is obese, the placenta is posterior, and the sampling is performed relatively early in gestation (i.e., before 19 weeks) (130).

Table 10-3 lists the indications for cordocentesis. With the development of better molecular tests, the use of cordocentesis has dramatically decreased over the last 10 years. Parental counseling before cordocentesis should include the risk of that pregnancy being affected by the conditions considered and the yield of information obtained through fetal blood sampling in such a situation. The risk and

TABLE 10-3
INDICATIONS FOR CORDOCENTESIS

Prenatal diagnosis of inherited blood disorders
 Hemoglobinopathies (e.g., homozygous thalassemia, sickle-cell disease)
 Coagulopathies (e.g., hemophillia A and B, von Willebrand disease)
Prenatal diagnosis of metabolic disorders
Fetal Infections
 Toxoplasmosis: specific IgM or DNA hybridization
 Rubella: specific IgM
 Cytomegalovirus: specific IgM and blood cultures
 Varicella zoster virus: specific IgM
 Human parvovirus (B19): viral DNA
 Human immunodeficiency virus: specific IgM
Rapid fetal karyotyping
 Late booking or failed amniocentesis
 Suspected fetal mosaicism on amniocentesis
 Abnormal maternal serum screening
 Ultrasound diagnosis of fetal malformations
Evaluation of the small-for-gestational-age fetus
 Acid–base status
 Oxygenation
Assessment and treatment of fetal anemia
Diagnosis and treatment of fetal thrombocytopenia

Adapted from ref. 104.

potential complications of the procedure itself also should be discussed. Before cordocentesis, a detailed ultrasonography examination should evaluate gestational age, placental location, and fetal anomalies. Fetal blood can be obtained by puncture of the fetal heart, the intrahepatic part of the umbilical vein, or by puncture of an umbilical vessel close to its placental insertion, the latter being by far the most common site for cordocentesis. When the placenta is located on the anterior or lateral wall of the uterus, the needle is introduced through the placenta into the umbilical cord (Fig. 10-6). In cases with a posterior placenta, the needle is introduced through the amniotic fluid and the cord is punctured close to its placental insertion. Different guidance techniques (i.e., fixed-needle guides vs. freehand), needles of lengths varying from 8 to 15 cm, gauges varying from 20 g to 27 g, and differing patient preparation protocols are used by various centers. Nicolaides and colleagues advocate an outpatient setting in the ultrasonography department, without need for maternal fasting, sedation, tocolytics, antibiotics, or fetal paralysis for the procedure (134).

Molecular diagnoses are now available for many of the mutations resulting in thalassemia, sickle cell disease, and hemophilia A and B, enabling diagnosis in the first trimester by CVS, with blood sampling performed only in noninformative cases or in cases with ambiguous results. Cordocentesis is, however, necessary for the diagnosis and management of congenital alloimmune thrombocytopenia (135). In alloimmune thrombocytopenia, cordocentesis allows the determination of fetal platelet phenotype and count. A low fetal platelet count in this

situation can be treated by weekly infusion of platelets until delivery (136).

In Rh isoimmunization, fetal blood sampling is performed for immediate confirmation of fetal antigenic status, obviating the need for further intervention in the Rh-negative fetus. If the fetus is Rh-positive, cordocentesis enables a more accurate assessment of fetal anemia and an immediate rise in fetal erythrocyte count on correction by intravascular transfusion. From case-control studies, it appears that at all gestational ages and at all levels of disease severity, intravascular correction of fetal anemia is more efficient and less risky to the mother and fetus than the intraperitoneal approach (137). Moreover, in cases with cardiac decompensation in which the fetus may be compromised by the volume overload needed to correct the severe anemia, better results were obtained by intravascular exchange transfusion (138). It should be noted, however, that cordocentesis might enhance maternal sensitization more than does amniocentesis, especially if blood sampling is performed by a transplacental approach (139). Rh immunoprophylaxis should be offered to all Rh-negative, nonsensitized patients with an Rh-positive fetus undergoing cordocentesis.

The diagnosis of fetal infection is based commonly on the demonstration of the agent-specific immunoglobulin (Ig) M in fetal blood, because the large molecule IgM does not cross the placenta. Fetal blood sampling should be scheduled to allow enough time from initial exposure for IgM to appear after immunocompetence develops in the fetus. For first trimester exposures, the best time for cordocentesis is probably after 20 weeks' gestation. In a few specific cases, *in utero* treatment also is available. Thus, after toxoplasmosis infection in the mother, and demonstration of IgM specific for toxoplasmosis in fetal blood, antibiotic treatment with spiramycin reduced significantly the risk of congenital toxoplasmosis, as well as the risk of late sequelae (140). Cordocentesis has also

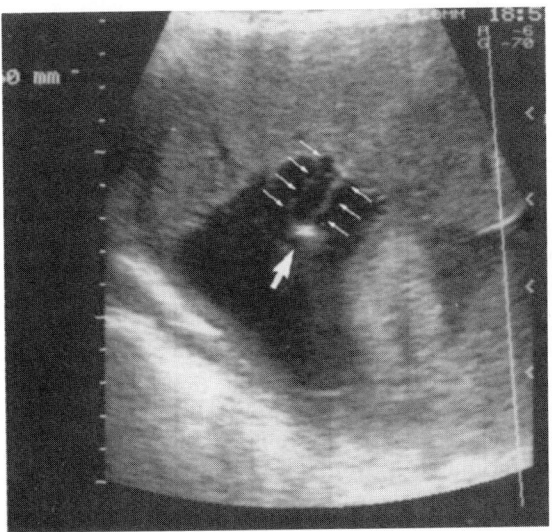

Figure 10-6 In cordocentesis, the umbilical cord insertion in the placenta (*small arrows*) must be located. The needle tip (*bright spot*) is placed in the umbilical vein (*large arrow*).

been used for repeated blood transfusions *in utero* to hydropic fetuses with hemolytic anemia caused by parvovirus B19 infection (141).

Severe, early onset IUGR commonly is associated with fetal chromosome anomalies. Cordocentesis allows for rapid fetal karyotyping, which can be available within 48 to 72 hours. Other abnormalities observed in blood samples from IUGR fetuses with normal chromosomes include hypoxemia, hypercapnia, lactic acidemia, leukopenia, thrombocytopenia, and disturbed carbohydrate, lipid, and protein metabolism (142). A statistically significant correlation was reported between increased umbilical systolic-to-diastolic ratio (>3.5) and fetal hypoxia and acidemia in cord blood (143), these relationships being even more pronounced with absent or reversed diastolic flow. Thus, when a fetus is severely growth restricted, fetal pressure of oxygen (PO_2) and pH may provide additional and crucial information to the biophysical score and umbilical blood flow studies, allowing us to decide between the risk of premature delivery and the risk of leaving the fetus to grow in a hostile intrauterine environment.

Preimplantation Genetic Diagnosis

Preimplantation genetic diagnosis (PGD) was developed for patients at high risk of transmitting an inherited disease to their offspring who, for whatever reason, do not want to have even a first trimester abortion. Patients have to go through *in vitro* fertilization (IVF) procedures to produce preimplantation embryos *in vitro*. One or two cells are biopsied from the cleavage-stage embryos, at the 6- to 8-cell stage (day 3 of development), and single-cell diagnosis with PCR or FISH is performed to determine which embryos are free of the genetic disease. This technique has been applied for a wide variety of disorders, including Tay-Sachs disease (144), β-thalassemia (145), cystic fibrosis (146), aneuploidy (147), and Marfan syndrome (148). Overall obstetric outcome appears normal (149).

Because only normal embryos are transferred to the uterus, PGD virtually eliminates the need for termination of an affected pregnancy. However, most centers still recommend that prenatal diagnosis be done, as errors have been made.

PGD appears to be the perfect solution for those couples who are at high risk of transmitting genetic diseases. However, for a multitude of reasons, relatively few centers worldwide offer the procedure, and fewer than 3,000 cycles have been performed in more than 10 years (150).

Single–Cell Diagnosis

Because it is difficult to karyotype single blastomeres, FISH has been used to analyze chromosomes in embryos. Several studies have shown that human embryos exhibit a high level of chromosome abnormalities, mainly mosaicism and chaotic chromosome makeup (151,152). Mosaic embryos can lead to problems in terms of certain PGD diagnoses because the blastomere biopsied may not be representative of the rest of the embryo; in some circumstances, this can be minimized by analyzing two independent blastomeres for PGD (152,153).

The most widespread application of FISH in prenatal diagnosis is for the rapid detection (1 to 2 working days) of the common numerical chromosome abnormalities using chromosome-specific probes applied to single blastomeres or to interphase cells from amniocentesis and chorionic villi samples (154,155). Most commonly, probes specific for chromosomes 13, 18, 21, X, and Y are used because, depending on the indications for invasive tests, numerical abnormalities involving these chromosomes account for 70% to 95% of the chromosome aberrations identified prenatally (154–156). The usefulness of interphase FISH in prenatal diagnosis and the test performance characteristics were recently assessed (156). The detection rate was nearly 100%, with a false-positive rate of only 0.003% and a false-negative rate of 0.024%. FISH results are now commonly acted on if, for example, a common trisomy is found, without waiting for the examination of a complete karyotype.

The diagnostic capability of interphase FISH is obviously limited by the choice of probe used; structural chromosome aberrations and numerical chromosome abnormalities other than those tested for will be missed. In addition, the incomplete hybridization of FISH probes or a reduction in signal size because of heteromorphism (154,157) may lead to false-negative prenatal FISH results. In cases of ambiguous FISH results, however, full karyotype should remain the gold standard.

FISH has also been used for the PGD of structural chromosome abnormalities (158,159). This has only been possible in recent years, as probes for the acrocentric chromosomes and specific locus probes were only recently developed. PGD of robertsonian translocations is a good example; minimum dual-color FISH with one probe for each chromosome is possible, but three-color FISH, with two probes for different areas of the most important chromosome, is better (160). PGD for reciprocal translocations is more difficult because specific probes for the region in question are required.

Another limiting factor in PGD for chromosome abnormalities is the high incidence of abnormalities, including mosaicism, seen in preimplantation embryos (160). For some translocations, 70% to 100% of embryos may be abnormal, consistent with the high reproduction failure of such couples. PGD offers these couples a potential major advantage in only transferring a chromosomally balanced embryo.

The techniques developed for PGD have also been applied to aneuploidy screening for patients going through IVF procedures (PGD-AS) (161,162). PGD-AS was initially performed for women of older reproductive age (older than age 35 years), with recurrent IVF failure (more than three attempts with no pregnancy) and after recurrent miscarriages when the couple have normal karyotypes (150). Several reports of an increased pregnancy rate have been published (161–163), but a randomized controlled clinical trial has not been performed.

Comparative genomic hybridization (164,165) has also now been successfully applied in PGD-AS, with one normal live birth (165). Because the time required for comparative genomic hybridization is 72 hours, embryos have to be frozen as they cannot be kept in culture for that length of time.

Whether by cytogenetics, biochemical, or molecular methods, prenatal diagnosis of an affected fetus requires obtaining for analysis either fetal tissue (i.e., blastomeres or blood) or other tissue that is representative of the fetus (e.g., amniocytes or placenta). Invasive procedures for prenatal diagnosis of fetal disease are available throughout gestation, from the first trimester onward. Assisted reproductive technologies have allowed preimplantation diagnosis (or exclusion) of several disorders. Despite its limitations, as the technology for genetics and assisted reproductive technologies improve, we believe there will be dramatic increases in the use of this modality.

REFERENCES

1. Garrod AE. The Croonian lectures. *Lancet* 1908;2:1.
2. Caskey CT. Disease diagnosis by recombinant DNA methods. *Science* 1987;236:1223–1229.
3. King CR. Prenatal diagnosis of genetic disease with molecular genetic technology. *Obstet Gynecol Surv* 1988;43:493–508.
4. Watson JD, Crick FHC. Molecular structure of nucleic acids: a structure for deoxyribose nucleic acid. *Nature* 1953;171:737–738.
5. Berget SM, Moore C, Sharp PA. Spliced RNA segments at the 5[T407]8-terminus of late adenovirus 2 in RNA. Proc *Natl Acad Sci U S A* 1977;74:3171–3175.
6. Gilbert W. Why genes in pieces? *Nature* 1978;271:501.
7. Gilbert W. Genes-in-pieces revisited. *Science* 1985;228:823–824.
8. Cooper DN, Smith BA, Cooke HJ, et al. An estimate of unique DNA sequence heterozygosity in the human genome. *Hum Genet* 1985;69:201–208.
9. Miller DA, Choi YC, Miller OJ. Chromosome localization of highly repetitive human DNAs and amplified ribosomal DNA with restriction enzymes. *Science* 1983;219:395–397.
10. Caskey CT, Pizzun A, Ying-Hui Fu, et al. Triplet repeat mutations in human disease. *Science* 1992;256:784–789.
11. Richards RI, Sutherland GR. Heritable unstable DNA sequences. *Nat Genet* 1992;1:7–9.
12. ACMG/ASHG Statement. Laboratory guidelines for Huntington disease genetic testing. *Am J Hum Genet* 1998;62:1243.
13. Poulton J, Marchington DR. Segregation of mitochondrial DNA (mtDNA) in human oocytes and in animal models of mtDNA disease: clinical implications. *Reproduction* 2002;123:751–755.
14. Smeitink J, van den Heuvel L, diMauro S. The genetics and pathology of oxidative phosphorylation. *Nature* 2001;2:342–352.
15. DiMauro S, Andreu AL. Mutations in mtDNA: are we scraping the bottom of the barrel? *Brain Pathol* 2000;10:431–441.
16. Petersen GM, Rotter JI, Cantor RM, et al. The Tay-Sachs disease gene in North American Jewish populations: geographic variation and origin. *Am J Hum Genet* 1983;35:1258–1269.
17. Myerowitz R, Costigan C. The major defect in Ashkenazi Jews with Tay-Sachs disease is an insertion in the gene for the alpha-chain for beta-hexosaminidase. *J Biol Chem* 1988;263:18587–18589.
18. Ohno K, Suzuki K. A splicing defect due to an exon–intron junctional mutation results in abnormal beta-hexosaminidase X-chain in RNAs in Ashkenazi Jewish patients with Tay-Sachs disease. *Biochem Biophys Res Commun* 1988;153:463–469.
19. Cutting GR, Kasch LM, Rosenstein BJ, et al. Two cystic fibrosis patients with mild pulmonary disease and nonsense mutations in each CFTR gene. *N Engl J Med* 1990;323:1685–1689.
20. Cutting GR, Kasch LM, Rosenstein BJ, et al. A cluster of cystic fibrosis mutations in the first nucleotide-binding fold of the cystic fibrosis conductance regulator protein. *Nature* 1990;346: 366–369.
21. Kerem E, Corez M, Kerem BS, et al. The relationship between genotype and phenotype in cystic fibrosis: analysis of the most common mutation (delta F508). *N Engl J Med* 1990;323: 1517–1522.
22. Stern RC. The diagnosis of cystic fibrosis. *N Engl J Med* 1997;336:487–491.
23. Kerem B, Chiba-Falek O, Kerem E. Cystic fibrosis in Jews: frequency and mutation distribution. *Genet Test* 1997;1:35–39.
24. Antonarakis SE, Phillips JA III, Kazazian HH Jr. Genetic diseases: diagnosis by restriction endonuclease analysis. *J Pediatr* 1982;100:845–856.
25. Gusella JF. DNA polymorphism and human disease. *Annu Rev Biochem* 1986;55:831–854.
26. Gusella JF, Wexler NS, Conneally PM, et al. A polymorphic DNA marker genetically linked to Huntington disease. *Nature* 1983;306:234–238.
27. Antonarakis SE, Kazazian HH Jr, Orkin SH. DNA polymorphism and molecular pathology of the human globin gene clusters. *Hum Genet* 1985;60:1–14.
28. Embury SH, Scharf SJ, Saiki RK et al: Rapid prenatal diagnosis of sickle cell anemia by a new method of DNA analysis. *N Engl J Med* 1987;316:656–661.
29. Smith CAB. The development of human linkage analysis. *Ann Hum Genet* 1986;50:293–296.
30. Haldane JBS, Smith CAB. A new estimate of the linkage between the genes for color-blindness and hemophilia in man. *Ann Genet* 1947;14:10.
31. Morton NE. Sequential tests for the detection of linkage. *Am J Hum Genet* 1955;7:277–310.
32. Risch N. Genetic linkage: interpreting LOD scores. *Science* 1992;255:803–804.
33. Southern EM. Detection of specific sequences among DNA fragments separated by electrophoresis. *J Mol Biol* 1975;98:503–517.
34. Conner BJ, Reyes AA, Morin C, et al. Detection of sickle cell beta S-globin allele by hybridization with synthetic oligonucleotides. *Proc Natl Acad Sci U S A* 1983;80:278–282.
35. Ehrlich HA, Gelfand D, Sninsky JJ. Recent advances in the polymerase chain reaction. *Science* 1991;252:1643–1651.
36. Saiki RK, Gelfand DH, Stoffel S, et al. Primer-directed enzymatic amplification of DNA with a thermostable DNA polymerase. *Science* 1988;239:487–491.
37. Beggs AH, Koenig M, Boyce FM, et al. Detection of 98% of DMD/BMD gene deletions by polymerase chain reaction. *Hum Genet* 1990;86:45–48.
38. Grompe M, Muzny DM, Caskey CT. Scanning detection of mutations in human ornithine transcarbamoylase by chemical mismatch cleavage. Proc *Natl Acad Sci U S A* 1989;86:5888–5892.
39. Das S, Levinson B, Shitney S, et al. Diverse mutations in patients with Menkes disease often lead to exon skipping. *Am J Hum Genet* 1994;55:883–889.
40. Collins FS. Positional cloning: let's not call it reverse anymore. *Nat Genet* 1992;1:3–6.
41. Ruddle FH. The William Allan Memorial Award address: reverse genetics and beyond. *Am J Hum Genet* 1984;36:944–953.
42. Xu G, O'Connell P, Viskochil D, et al. The neurofibromatosis type 1 gene encodes a protein related to GAP. *Cell* 1990;62: 599–608.
43. Steel MW, Breg WR. Chromosome analysis of human amniotic fluid cells. *Lancet* 1966;1:383–387.
44. Jacobson JB, Barter RH. Intrauterine diagnosis and management of genetic defects. *Am J Obstet Gynecol* 1967;99:795–801.
45. Nadler HL. Antenatal detection of hereditary disorders. *Pediatrics* 1968;42:912–918.
46. Medical Research Council. *Diagnosis of genetic disease by amniocentesis during second trimester of pregnancy.* Ottawa, Ontario: Author, 1977.
47. National Institute of Child Health and Human Development Amniocentesis Registry. *The safety and accuracy of midtrimester amniocentesis.* DHEW publication no (NIH) 78–190. Washington, DC: United States Department of Health, Education and Welfare, 1978.
48. Evans MI, Drugan A, Koppitch FC, et al. Genetic diagnosis in the first trimester: the norm for the 90s. *Am J Obstet Gynecol* 1989;160:1332–1336.
49. Canadian Collaborative CVS–Amniocentesis Clinical Trial Group. Multicenter randomized clinical trial of chorionic villus sampling and amniocentesis. *Lancet* 1989;1:1–18.

50. Rhoads GG, Jackson LG, Schlesselman SE, et al. The safety and efficacy of chorionic villus sampling for early prenatal diagnosis of cytogenetic abnormalities. *N Engl J Med* 1989;320:609–617.
51. Hanson FW, Happ RL, Tennant FR, et al. Ultrasonography-guided early amniocentesis in singleton pregnancies. *Am J Obstet Gynecol* 1990;162:1376–1381.
52. Drugan A, Reichler A, Bronshtein M, et al. Abnormal biochemical serum screening versus second trimester ultrasound-detected minor anomalies as predictors of aneuploidy in low-risk patients. *Fetal Diagn Ther* 1996;11(5):301–305.
53. Drugan A, Johnson MP, Evans MI. Ultrasound screening for fetal chromosome anomalies. *Am J Med Genet* 2000;90:98–107.
54. Zimmer EZ, Drugan A, Ofir C, et al. Ultrasound anomalies of the fetal neck: implications for the risk of aneuploidy and structural anomalies. *Prenat Diagn* 1997;17:1055–1058.
55. Wald NJ, Hackshaw AK. Advances in antenatal screening for Down's syndrome. *Baillieres Clin Obstet Gynaecol* 2000;14:563–580.
56. Haddow JE, Palomaki GE, Knight GJ, et al. Reducing the need for amniocentesis in women 35 years of age or older with serum markers for screening. *N Engl J Med* 1994;330:1114–1118.
57. Beekhuis JR, De Wolf BT, Mantingh A, et al. The influence of serum screening on the amniocentesis rate in women of advanced maternal age. *Prenat Diagn* 1994;14:199–202.
58. Holzgreve W, Miny P, Schloo R, et al. "Late CVS" international registry: compilation of data from 24 centers. *Prenat Diagn* 1990;10:159–167.
59. Hoskins IA. Cordocentesis in isoimmunization and fetal physiologic measurement, infection and karyotyping. *Curr Opin Obstet Gynecol* 1991;3:266–271.
60. Puck JM, Willard HF. X inactivation in females with X-linked disease [Editorial]. *N Engl J Med* 1998;338:325–328.
61. Ben-Yoseph Y, Evans MI, Bottoms SF, et al. Lysosomal enzyme activities in fresh and frozen chorionic villi and in cultured trophoblasts. *Clin Chim Acta* 1986;161:307–313.
62. Evans MI, Krivchenia EL, Johnson MP, et al. In utero fetal muscle biopsy alters diagnosis and carrier risks in Duchenne and Becker muscular dystrophy. *Fetal Diagn Ther* 1995;10(2):71–75.
63. Holzgreve W, Golbus MS. Prenatal diagnosis of ornithine transcarbamylase deficiency utilizing fetal liver biopsy. *Am J Hum Genet* 1984;320–328.
64. Faivre L, Cormier-Daire V, Chretien D, et al. Determination of enzyme activities for prenatal diagnosis of respiratory chain deficiency. *Prenat Diagn* 2000;20:732–737.
65. Simoni G, Brambati B, Danesino C, et al. Efficient direct chromosome analyses and enzyme determinations from chorionic villi samples in the first trimester of pregnancy. *Hum Genet* 1983;63:349–357.
66. Brambati B, Simoni G. Letter to the editor. *Lancet* 1989;1:586.
67. Ledbetter DH, Martin AO, Verlinsky Y, et al. Cytogenetic results of chorionic villus sampling: high success rate and diagnostic accuracy in the United States collaborative study. *Am J Obstet Gynecol* 1990;162:495–501.
68. Simpson JL. Chorionic villus sampling. *Semin Perinatol* 1990;14:446–455.
69. McGowan KD, Blackemore KJ. Amniocentesis and chorionic villus sampling. *Curr Opin Obstet Gynecol* 1991;3:221–229.
70. Johnson A, Wapner RJ, Davis GH, et al. Mosaicism in chorionic villus sampling: an association with poor perinatal outcome. *Obstet Gynecol* 1990;75:573–577.
71. Sundberg K, Lundsteen C, Philip J. Early filtration amniocentesis for further investigation of mosaicism diagnosed by chorionic villus sampling. *Prenat Diagn* 1996;16:1121–1127.
72. Kalousek DK, Dill FJ. Chromosomal mosaicism confined to the placenta in human conceptions. *Science* 1983;221:665–667.
73. Leschot NJ, Schuring Blum GH, Van Prooijen-Knegt AC, et al. The outcome of pregnancies with confined placental chromosome mosaicism in cytotrophoblast cells. *Prenat Diagn* 1996;16:705–712.
74. Wright DJ, Brindley BA, Koppitch FC, et al. Interpretation of chorionic villus sampling laboratory results is just as reliable as amniocentesis. *Obstet Gynecol* 1989;74:739–744.
75. Gosden C, Rodeck CH, Nicolaides KH. Fetal blood sampling in the investigation of chromosome mosaicism in amniotic fluid cell culture. *Lancet* 1988;1:613–617.
76. Evans MI, Moore C, Kolodny E, et al. Lysosomal enzymes in chorionic villi, cultured amniocytes, and cultured skin fibroblasts. *Clin Chim Acta* 1986;157:109–113.
77. Hayasaka K, Tada K, Fueki N, et al. Feasibility of prenatal diagnosis of nonketotic hyperglycinemia: existence of the glycine cleavage system in placenta. *J Pediatr* 1987;110:124–126.
78. Giles L, Cooper A, Fowler B, et al. Aryl sulphatase isozymes of chorionic villi: implications for prenatal diagnosis. *Prenat Diagn* 1987;245–252.
79. Podobnick M, Ciglar S, Singer Z, et al. Transabdominal chorionic villus sampling in the second and third trimesters of high risk pregnancies. *Prenat Diagn* 1997;17:125–133.
80. Sidransky E, Black SH, Soenksen DM, et al. Transvaginal chorionic villus sampling. *Prenat Diagn* 1990;10:583–586.
81. Brambati B, Oldrini A, Lanzani A. Transabdominal villus sampling: a free hand ultrasound guided technique. *Am J Obstet Gynecol* 1987;157:134–137.
82. Smidt-Jensen S, Hahnemann N. Transabdominal fine needle biopsy from chorionic villi in the first trimester. *Prenat Diagn* 1984;4:163–169.
83. Evans MI, Quigg MH, Koppitch FC, et al. First trimester prenatal diagnosis. In: Evans MI, Fletcher JC, Dixler AO, et al, eds. *Fetal diagnosis and therapy: science, ethics and the law.* Philadelphia: JB Lippincott, 1989:17.
84. Brambati B, Lanzani A, Tului L. Transabdominal and transcervical chorionic villus sampling: efficiency and risk evaluation of 2411 cases. *Am J Med Genet* 1990;35:160–164.
85. Eddleman KA, Stone JL, Lynch L, et al. Chorionic villus sampling before multifetal pregnancy reduction. *Am J Obstet Gynecol* 2000;185:772–774.
86. Simpson JL. Incidence and timing of pregnancy losses: relevance to evaluating safety of early prenatal diagnosis. *Am J Med Genet* 1990;35:165–173.
87. Firth HV, Boyd PA, Chamberlain P, et al. Severe limb abnormalities after chorionic villus sampling at 56–66 days' gestation. *Lancet* 1991;337:762–763.
88. Burton BK, Schulz CJ, Burd LI. Limb anomalies associated with chorionic villus sampling. *Obstet Gynecol* 1992;79:726–730.
89. Kuliev A, Jackson L, Froster U, et al: Chorionic villus sampling safety. Report of World Health Organization/EURO meeting. *Am J Obstet Gynecol* 1996;174:807–811.
90. Schloo R, Miny P, Holzgreve W, et al. Distal limb deficiency following chorionic villus sampling? *Am J Med Genet* 1992;42:404–413.
91. Wapner RJ, Evans MI, Davis G, et al: Procedural risks versus theology: chorionic villus sampling for Orthodox Jews at less than 8 weeks' gestation. *Am J Obstet Gynecol* 2002;186(6):1133–1136.
92. Shulman LP, Meyers CM, Simpson JL, et al. Fetomaternal transfusion depends on amount of chorionic villi aspirated but not on method of chorionic villus sampling. *Am J Obstet Gynecol* 1990;162:1185–1188.
93. Brumfield CG, Lin S, Conner W, et al. Pregnancy outcome following genetic amniocentesis at 11–14 versus 16–19 weeks' gestation. *Obstet Gynecol* 1996;88:114–118.
94. Dombrowsky MP, Isada NB, Johnson MP, et al. Modified stylet technique for tenting of amniotic membranes. *Obstet Gynecol* 1996;87:455–456.
95. Stripparo I, Buscaglia M, Longatii L, et al. Genetic amniocentesis: 505 cases performed before the sixteenth week of gestation. *Prenat Diagn* 1990;10:359–364.
96. Elejalde BR, de Elejalde MM, Acuna JM, et al. Prospective study of amniocentesis performed between weeks 9 and 16 of gestation: its feasibility, risks, complications and use in early genetic amniocentesis. *Am J Med Genet* 1990;35:188–196.
97. Reid R, Sepuvelda W, Kyle PM, et al. Amniotic fluid culture failure: clinical significance and association with aneuploidy. *Obstet Gynecol* 1996;87:588–592.
98. Diaz Vega M, De La Cueva P, Leal C, et al. Early amniocentesis at 10-12 weeks gestation. *Prenat Diagn* 1996;16:307–312.
99. Drugan A, Syner FN, Greb A, et al. Amniotic fluid alpha-fetoprotein and acetylcholinesterase in early genetic amniocentesis. *Obstet Gynecol* 1988;72:35–38.
100. Crandall BF, Chua C. Detecting neural tube defects by amniocentesis between 11 and 15 weeks' gestation. *Prenat Diagn* 1995;15:339–343.

101. Drugan A, Syner FN, Belsky RL, et al. Amniotic fluid acetylcholinesterase: implications of an inconclusive result. *Am J Obstet Gynecol* 1988;159:469–474.

102. Brown CL, Colden KA, Hume RF, et al: Faint and positive amniotic fluid acetylcholinesterase with a normal sonogram. *Am J Obstet Gynecol* 1996;175:1000–1003.

103. Byrne D, Marks K, Azar G, et al. Randomized study of early amniocentesis versus chorionic villus sampling: a technical and cytogenetic comparison of 650 patients. *Ultrasound Obstet Gynecol* 1991;1:235–240.

104. Nicolaides KH, Brizot ML, Patel F, et al. Comparison of chorionic villus sampling and early amniocentesis for karyotyping in 1492 singleton pregnancies. *Fetal Diagn Ther* 1996;11:9–15.

105. Alfirevic Z. Early amniocentesis versus transabdominal CVS for prenatal diagnosis *Cochrane Database Syst Rev* 2000;(2):CD000077.

106. Yuksel B, Greenough A, Naik S, et al. Perinatal lung function and invasive antenatal procedures. *Thorax* 1997;52:181–184.

107. Simpson JL. Amniocentesis: what it can tell you and what it can't. *Contemp Obstet Gynecol* 1988;31:33–35.

108. Hsu LYF, Kaffe S, Perlis ET. Trisomy 20 mosaicism in prenatal diagnosis: a review and update. *Prenat Diagn* 1987;7:581–596.

109. Schwartz S. Efficacy and applicability of interphase fluorescent *in situ* hybridization for prenatal diagnosis [Invited Editorial]. *Am J Hum Genet* 1993;52:851–853.

110. Ligon AH, Beaudet AL, Sheffer LG. Simultaneous multilocus FISH analysis for detection of microdeletions in the diagnostic evaluation of developmental delay and mental retardation. *Am J Hum Genet* 1997;61:51–59.

111. Evans MI, Henry GP, Miller WA, et al. International collaborative assessment of 146,000 prenatal karyotypes: expected limitations if only chromosome specific probes and fluorescent in situ hybridization are used. *Hum Reprod* 2000;15(1):228–230.

112. Cohn GM, Gould M, Miller RC, et al. The importance of genetic counseling before amniocentesis. *J Perinatol* 1996;16:352–357.

113. Murray JC, Karp LE, Williamson RA, et al. Rh isoimmunization as related to amniocentesis. *Am J Hum Genet* 1983;16:527–534.

114. Drugan A, Johnson MP, Evans MI. Amniocentesis. In: Evans MI, ed. *Reproductive risks and prenatal diagnosis.* Norwalk, CT: Appleton & Lange, 1992:191.

115. Bombard AT, Power JF, Carter S, et al. Procedure related fetal losses in transplacental versus nontransplacental genetic amniocentesis. *Am J Obstet Gynecol* 1995;172:868–872.

116. Crane JP, Rohland BM. Clinical significance of amniotic fluid leakage after genetic amniocentesis. *Prenat Diagn* 1986;6:25–31.

117. Nimrod C, Varela-Gittings F, Machin G, et al. The effect of very prolonged membrane rupture on fetal development. *Am J Obstet Gynecol* 1984;148:540–543.

118. Chervenak JL, Kardon NB. Advancing maternal age: the actual risks. *Female Patient* 1991;16(11):17–24.

119. Nicolaides KH, Soothill PH, Rodeck CH, et al. Prenatal diagnosis: why confine chorionic villus (placental) biopsy to the first trimester? *Lancet* 1986;1:543–544.

120. Chieri PR, Aldini AJR. Feasibility of placental biopsy in the second trimester for fetal diagnosis. *Am J Obstet Gynecol* 1989;160:581–583.

121. Ko TM, Tseng LH, Hwa HL, et al. Prenatal diagnosis by transabdominal chorionic villus sampling in the second and third trimesters. *Arch Gynecol Obstet* 1995;256:193–197.

122. Podobnik M, Ciglar S, Singer Z, et al. Transabdominal chorionic villus sampling in the second and third trimesters of high-risk pregnancies. *Prenat Diagn* 1997;17:125–133.

123. Holzgreve W, Miny P, Gerlach B, et al. Benefits of placental biopsies for rapid karyotyping in the second and third trimesters (late chorionic villus sampling) in high risk pregnancies. *Am J Obstet Gynecol* 1990;162:1188–1192.

124. Smidt-Jensen S, Lundsteen C, Lind AM, et al. Transabdominal chorionic villus sampling in the second and third trimester of pregnancy: chromosome quality, reporting time and fetomaternal bleeding. *Prenat Diagn* 1993;13:957–969.

125. Ganshirt-Ahlert D, Pohlschmidt M, Gal A, et al. Transabdominal placental biopsy in the second and third trimester of pregnancy: what is the risk of maternal contamination in DNA diagnosis? *Obstet Gynecol* 1990;75:320–323.

126. Freda VJ, Adamson KJ. Exchange transfusion *in utero. Am J Obstet Gynecol* 1964;89:817–821.

127. Rodeck CH, Cambell S. Umbilical cord insertion as source of pure fetal blood for prenatal diagnosis. *Lancet* 1979;1:1244–1245.

128. Ward RHT, Modell B, Fairweather DVI. Obstetric outcome and problems of midtrimester fetal blood sampling for antenatal diagnosis. *Br J Obstet Gynaecol* 1981;88:1073–1080.

129. Daffos F, Cappella-Pavlovsky M, Forestier F. Fetal blood sampling via the umbilical cord using a needle guided by ultrasound: report of 66 cases. *Prenat Diagn* 1983;3:271–277.

130. Buscaglia M, Ghisoni L, Bellotti M, et al. Percutaneous umbilical blood sampling: indication changes and procedure loss rates in a nine years' experience. *Fetal Diagn Ther* 1996;11:106–113.

131. Bernaschek G, Yildiz A, Kolankaya A, et al. Complications of cordocentesis in high risk pregnancies: effects on fetal loss and premature deliveries. *Prenat Diagn* 1995;15:995–1000.

132. Seligman SP, Young BK. Tachycardia as the sole fetal heart rate abnormality after funipuncture. *Obstet Gynecol* 1996;87:833–834.

133. Wilkins I, Mezrow G, Lynch L, et al. Amnionitis and life threatening respiratory distress after percutaneous umbilical blood sampling. *Am J Obstet Gynecol* 1989;160:427–428.

134. Nicolaides KH, Soothill PW, Rodeck CH, et al. Ultrasound guided sampling of umbilical cord and placental blood to access fetal well being. *Lancet* 1986;1:1065–1067.

135. Bussel JB, Berkowitz RL, McFarland JG, et al. Antenatal treatment of neonatal thrombocytopenia. *N Engl J Med* 1988;319:1374–1378.

136. Murphy MF, Pullon HWH, Metcalfe P, et al. Management of fetal allo-immune thrombocytopenia by weekly in utero platelet transfusions. *Vox Sang* 1990;58:45–49.

137. Harman CR, Bowman JM, Manning FA, et al. Intrauterine transfusion: intraperitoneal versus intravascular approach: a case control comparison. *Am J Obstet Gynecol* 1990;162:1053–1059.

138. Poissonier MH, Brossard Y, Demedeiros N, et al. Two hundred intrauterine exchange transfusions in severe blood incompatibilities. *Am J Obstet Gynecol* 1989;161:709–713.

139. Weiner CP, Grant S, Hudson J, et al. Effect of diagnostic and therapeutic cordocentesis on maternal serum alpha-fetoprotein concentration. *Am J Obstet Gynecol* 1989;161:706–708.

140. Daffos F, Forestier F, Capella-Pavlovsky M, et al. Prenatal management of 746 pregnancies at risk for congenital toxoplasmosis. *N Engl J Med* 1988;318:271–275.

141. Peters MT, Nicolaides KH. Cordocentesis for the diagnosis and treatment of human fetal parvovirus infection. *Obstet Gynecol* 1990;75:501–504.

142. Weiner CP. The relationship between the umbilical artery systolic/diastolic ratio and umbilical blood gas measurements in specimens obtained by cordocentesis. *Am J Obstet Gynecol* 1990;162:1198–1202.

143. Ribbert LSM, Sniders RJM, Nicolaides KH, et al. Relationship of fetal biophysical profile and blood gas values at cordocentesis in severely growth retarded fetuses. *Am J Obstet Gynecol* 1990;163:569–571.

144. Gibbons WE, Gitlin SA, Lansendorf SE, et al. Preimplantation genetic diagnosis for Tay-Sachs disease: successful pregnancy after pre-embryo biopsy and gene amplification by polymerase chain reaction. *Fertil Steril* 1995;63(4):723–728.

145. Ray PF, Kaeda JS, Bingham J, et al. Preimplantation genetic diagnosis of β-thalassaemia major. *Lancet* 1996;347:1696.

146. Strom CM, Verlinsky Y, Milayeva-Rechitsky S, et al. Preconception genetic diagnosis for cystic fibrosis by polar body removal and DNA analysis. *Lancet* 1995;336:306–307.

147. Verlinsky Y, Cieslak J, Friedine M, et al. Pregnancies following preconception diagnosis of common aneuploidies by fluorescence *in situ* hybridization. *Hum Reprod* 1995;10:1923–1927.

148. Harton GL, Tsipouras P, Sisson ME, et al. Preimplantation genetic testing for Marfan's syndrome. *Mol Hum Reprod* 1996;2(9):713–715.

149. Soussis I, Harper JC, Handyside AH, et al. Obstetric outcome of pregnancies resulting from embryos biopsied for pre-implantation diagnosis of inherited disease. *Br J Obstet Gynaecol* 1996;103:784–788.

150. ESHRE PGD Consortium Steering Committee. ESHRE Pre-implantation Genetic Diagnosis (PGD) Consortium: data collection III (May 2001). *Hum Reprod* 2000;17:233–246.

151. Harper JC, Coonen E, Handyside AH, et al. Mosaicism of autosomes and sex chromosomes in morphologically normal, monospermic pre-implantation human embryos. *Prenat Diagn* 1995;15:41–49.

152. Delhanty JDA, Harper JC, Ao A, et al. Multicolor FISH detects frequent chromosomal mosaicism and chaotic division in normal

pre-implantation embryos from fertile patients. *Hum Genet* 1997;99:755–760.

153. De Vos A, Van Steireghem A. Aspects of biopsy procedures prior to pre-implantation genetic diagnosis. *Prenat Diagn* 2001: 21:767–780.

154. Tepperberg J, Pettenati MJ, Rao PN, et al. Prenatal diagnosis using interphase fluorescence *in situ* hybridization (FISH): 2-year multi-center retrospective study and review of the literature. *Prenat Diagn* 2001;21:293–301.

155. Cheong Leung W, Chitayat D, Deaward G, et al. Role of amniotic fluid interphase fluorescence in situ hybridization (FISH) analysis in patient management. *Prenat Diagn* 2001;21:327–332.

156. Evans MI, Henry GP, Miller WA, et al. International collaborative assessment of 146,000 prenatal karyotypes expected limitations if only chromosome-specific probes and fluorescent *in situ* hybridization are used. *Hum Reprod* 1999;14:1213–1216.

157. Weremowicz S, Sandstrom DJ, Morton CC, et al. Fluorescence in situ hybridization (FISH) for rapid detection of aneuploidy: experience with 911 prenatal cases. *Prenat Diagn* 2001; 21:262–269.

158. Fridstrom M, Ahrlund-Richter L, Iwarsson E, et al. Clinical outcome of treatment cycles using PGD for structural chromosomal abnormalities. *Prenat Diagn* 2001;21:781–781.

159. Munne S, Sandalinas M, Escudero T, et al. Outcome of pre-implantation genetic diagnosis of translocations. *Fertil Steril* 2000;73:1209–1218.

160. Munne S, Magli C, Cohen J, et al. Positive outcomes after pre-implantation diagnosis of aneuploidy in human embryos. *Hum Reprod* 1999;14:2191–2199.

161. Magli MC, Sandalinas M, Escudero T, et al. Double locus analysis chromosome 21 for pre-implantation genetic diagnosis a of aneuploidy. *Prenat Diagn* 2001;21:1080–1085.

162. Conn CH, Harper JC, Winston RML, et al. Infertile couples with robertsonian translocations: pre-implantation genetic analysis of embryos reveals chaotic cleavage divisions. *Hum Genet* 1998;102:117–123.

163. Verlinsky Y, Cieslak J, Ivakhnenko V, et al. Preimplantation diagnosis of common aneuploidies by the first- and second-polar body FISH analysis. *J Assist Reprod Genet* 1998; 15:285–289.

164. Vouliare L, Slater J, Williamson R, et al. Chromosome analysis of blastomeres from human embryos by using CGH. *Hum Genet* 2000;105:210–217.

165. Wilton L, Williamson R, McBain J, et al. Birth of a healthy infant after pre-implantation confirmation of euploidy by comparative genomic hybridization. *N Engl J Med* 2001;345:1537–1541.

Feto-Maternal Interactions: Placental Physiology, the In Utero Environment, and Fetal Determinants of Adult Disease

11

Gabriella Pridjian

The human placenta has become a highly evolved, sophisticated interface between mother and fetus. As the gatekeeper for maternofetal interactions, its functions are diverse and essential. The *in utero* environment not only influences fetal and newborn growth and development, but possibly the development of adult disease.

HUMAN PLACENTATION

Based on the modified classification of Grosser, which separates placentas by the number of layers interfacing the maternal and fetal circulations, the human placenta is hemomonochorial, with only the syncytiotrophoblast, fetal connective tissue, and fetal capillary endothelium forming the barrier between the two circulations (Fig. 11-1) (1). The human placenta, with this most intimate interface, is similar to that of the guinea pig and the monkey. Placentation in other animals is different, and there is great variation in mammalian placentation. For example, the ovine placenta is epitheliochorial and almost impermeable to diffusional transfer of the ketone body β-hydroxybutyrate, but human placenta is permeable to this ketone body, which has been implicated with the fetal distress accompanying diabetic ketoacidosis (2). The human placenta is discoid and made up of 8 to 10 cotyledons. Fetal blood is supplied to the placenta by two umbilical arteries and drained by one umbilical vein. On the fetal surface of the placenta, the umbilical arteries, crossing over fetal veins, decrease in caliber and increase in divisions as they travel toward the placental edges and dive deeply into the placental disc to supply individual cotyledons. Within the substance of the placenta, the caliber of the arteries decreases until only fetal capillaries exist at the level of the terminal villi. The fetal capillaries are dilated, providing a broad surface area for maternofetal transfer. The maternal blood supply to the placenta originates from the uterine artery, which divides into spiral arteries and percolates through the intervillous space, bathing the terminal villi.

PLACENTAL TRANSFER

The fetus depends almost exclusively on the placenta for nutritional, respiratory, and excretory functions. The placenta, growing steadily as gestation progresses, parallels fetal growth. Studies of placental growth and physiology in disease states suggest that placental growth and size are determined by the fetus and modulated by maternal factors. Normal placental-to-fetal weight ratios are approximately 1:6. As the placenta grows, villous processes increase in number as fetal vasculature expands, and by the third trimester, a large surface area is available to the maternal and fetal circulations.

Most placental transport is transcellular. Although the placenta often is thought of as a "separating membrane," it is actually a series of membranes. The most efficient areas for maternofetal exchange are the epithelial plates, which consist of thinly stretched, attenuated villous tissue separating maternal blood in the intervillous space from fetal

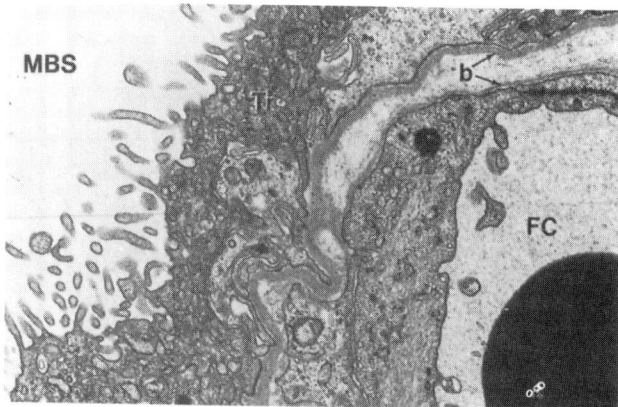

Figure 11-1 Electron micrograph of the placental barrier of the human hemomonochorial full-term placenta. Notice the numerous endocytotic vesicles in various stages of formation located on the maternal-side brush border membrane of the syncytiotrophoblast. b, basement membrane; FC, fetal capillary; MBS, maternal blood space or intervillous space; Tr, syncytiotrophoblast with microvillous brush border membrane. Bar = 0.5 mm. (From Thornberg KL, Faber JJ. *Placental physiology.* New York: Raven Press, 1983:19, with permission.)

blood in the fetal sinusoids. To cross epithelial plates from the maternal to the fetal side, a substance must traverse:

- The brush border membrane of the syncytiotrophoblast
- The cellular plasma of this cell
- The basement membrane of the syncytiotrophoblast
- The maternal side of the fetal capillary endothelial cell
- The fetal side of the same endothelial cell

The microvillous brush border membrane of the syncytiotrophoblast appears to be the membrane most involved in regulation of transport, especially of active or carrier mediated transport. Certain diffusible substances traverse the trophoblast and endothelial cell intact for release on the fetal side, some substances may be partially or completely metabolized by the placenta, and others may be involved in intricate transport systems (Fig. 11-2).

Simple Diffusion

Many nutrients, metabolites, and excretory products cross the placenta by diffusion. Diffusion of substances in the placenta depends on multiple factors, as summarized in Table 11-1.

The amount of a nutrient delivered to the placenta is directly proportional to its concentration in the maternal bloodstream, which depends on nutritional intake and gastrointestinal absorption. Famine, maternal gastrointestinal diseases that interfere with absorption, or maternal pulmonary diseases that interfere with alveolar exchange may significantly affect blood concentrations and the transfer and accrual of fetal fuels. A lack of fetal fuels produces fetal and placental growth restriction. Abnormalities in maternal homeostatic mechanisms may produce either an insufficiency or an abundance of nutrients. For example, in poorly controlled diabetes, maternal hyperglycemia, hyperaminoacidemia, and hypertriglyceridemia allow

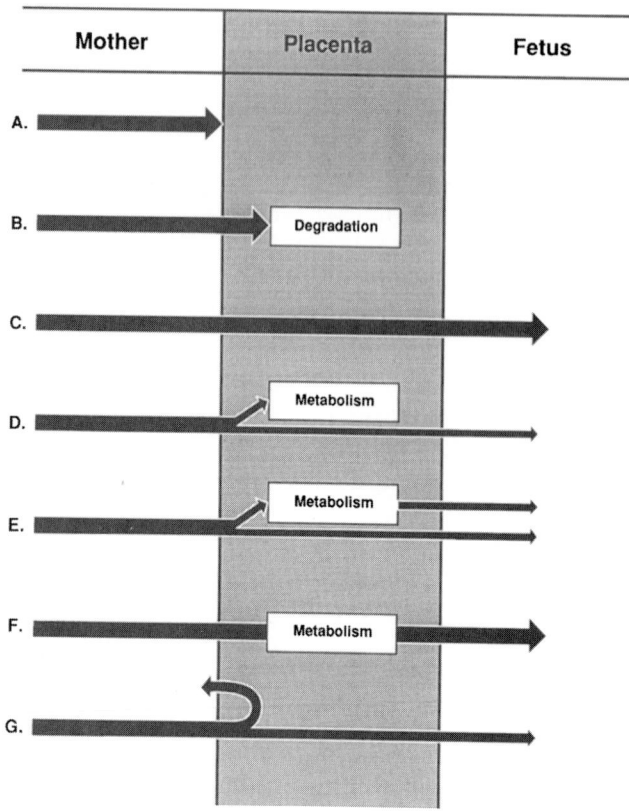

Figure 11-2 Patterns of maternofetal transport. **A:** Minimal or no placental uptake and no fetal transfer (e.g., succinylcholine, highly charged quaternary ammonium compounds). **B:** Placental uptake, degradation, and no fetal transfer (e.g., insulin). **C:** Placental uptake and transfer predominantly unmodified to the fetus (e.g., β-hydroxybutyrate, bilirubin). **D:** Placental uptake, partial use, and transfer to the fetus (e.g., oxygen, glucose, amino acids, free fatty acids). **E:** Uptake, partial metabolism, and transfer to the fetus (e.g., cyclosporine). **F:** Uptake, modification, and transfer to the fetus (e.g., 25-hydroxyvitamin D_3, of which most undergoes 1_α-hydroxylation in the placenta to form 1,25-dihydroxyvitamin D_3). **G:** Carrier-coupled uptake with release of the ligand to the fetal side and regeneration of the carrier on the maternal side (e.g., transferrin–iron complex).

unrestrained nutrient delivery to the fetus with excessive growth of fetal organs, body fat, and the placenta (3).

Delivery of a nutrient to the placenta is directly proportional to blood flow in the intervillous space. Maternal blood volume gradually increases to 30% to 40% higher than prepregnancy volume, with 40% directed to the uterus and placenta. Maternal cardiac disease with lower cardiac output may result in fetal and placental growth restriction. Even in healthy women, maternal position influences blood flow to the uterus. Normal pregnant women have an 18% lower cardiac output in the standing position compared with lying on their sides, perhaps explaining why women who stand at work throughout their pregnancy have newborns of lower birth-weight.

Fetal factors influencing diffusion are those that affect nutrient delivery to the fetal side of the placenta. The concentration of a substance in the umbilical artery depends on the amount of prior placental transfer, absorption from swallowed amniotic fluid, and fetal metabolism. Fetal blood flow to the uterus depends on fetal cardiac output

TABLE 11-1
FACTORS AFFECTING THE PLACENTAL TRANSFER OF A DIFFUSIBLE SUBSTANCE

Maternal Factors	Placental Factors	Fetal Factor
Amount Delivered to the Intervillous Space	**Transfer Physiology**	**Amount Delivered to the Fetal Capillaries**
Blood concentration	Area of diffusing membrane(s)	Blood concentration
Exogenous and endogenous supplies	Diffusion resistance	Fetal metabolic production or gastrointestinal absorption
Homeostatic mechanisms	Characteristics of transferred material (size, charge, polarity, shape)	Prior placental transfer
Arteriovenous mixing in the intervillous space	Characteristics of membrane (physiochemical composition, fluidity)	Flow rate in the fetal capillaries
Flow rate in intervillous space	Diffusion pressure across each placental cell membrane	Hemodynamic factors in fetus
Hemodynamic factors in mother	Maternofetal concentration gradients	Local circulatory factors
Local circulatory factors	Placental cellular production or use	Shunting
Shunting	Maternofetal blood flow characteristics; intervillous flow	

and placental vascular tone. Normally, fetal vessels on the chorionic plate are maximally dilated, providing the least resistance to flow.

Numerous placental factors influence diffusion. Overall, transfer is governed by the quantity of epithelial plates, which are specialized regions of enhanced diffusion where the interhemal barrier is less than a few micrometers. The human placenta has an intervillous pool flow system in which fetal capillaries in terminal villi are bathed in a maternal blood reservoir continuously filled by arteries and drained by veins (Fig. 11-3). Concurrent and countercurrent flows exist in areas of uneven distribution of flow (i.e., shunting), where a portion of the villus is well supplied by maternal blood but poorly supplied by fetal blood; in other areas, the opposite occurs.

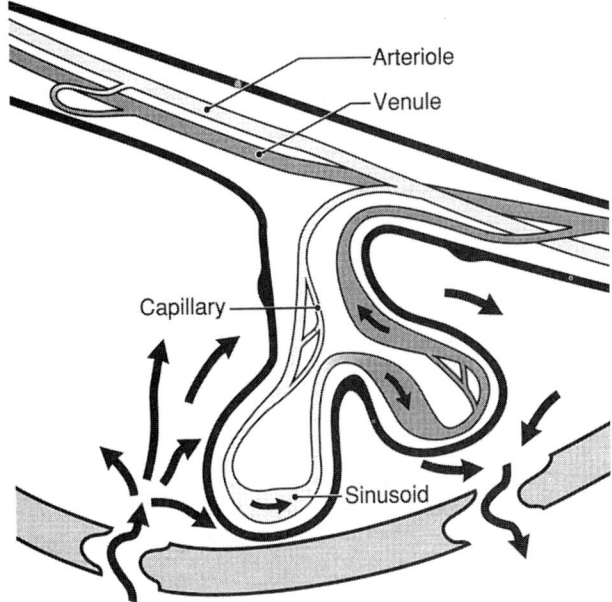

Figure 11-3 Areas of concurrent and countercurrent flow exist in the intervillous pool flow system of the human placenta.

Stereochemical characteristics of a substance are major factors in transferability. Small, compact, nonpolar, lipophilic substances are transferred most efficiently. The placenta is relatively impermeable to large, polar molecules that do not have specific transport systems or carrier proteins or are unable to take advantage of an analogous transport system to aid in their transfer. For example, α-fetoprotein (AFP), a 70-kd fetal protein, does not transfer to the maternal side in appreciable amounts despite large quantities in fetal blood. Maternal AFP is derived from transplacental transfer from fetal blood and transmembrane (i.e., chorioamnion) transfer from amniotic fluid. The fetal blood AFP level at 17 weeks of gestation is approximately 3 mg/mL when the maternal blood level is approximately 0.1 mg/mL, resulting in a fetomaternal gradient of approximately 30,000:1. The low level of fetomaternal transplacental transfer allows detection of elevated maternal serum levels from transmembrane (i.e., amniochorion) transfer of abnormally high amniotic fluid AFP, which provides the basis of maternal serum AFP screening for neural tube defects. False–positive elevations of maternal serum AFP (i.e., high maternal serum value with a structurally normal fetus) suggest placental microabruptions, or loss of integrity of the maternofetal barrier, and forecast a higher rate of fetal morbidity.

Membrane characteristics regulate transport. The fluidity of the membrane, determined by the degree and character of membrane-incorporated phospholipids, influences transfer of certain substances. Diseases, such as diabetes, may influence membrane fluidity (4).

The major driving force in favor of transfer by diffusion is the concentration gradient across the placenta; the resistance to diffusion is dictated by the nature of the molecule. The principles of diffusion of molecules that are generally applicable to biological membranes hold true in the placenta, although specifics remain to be defined. Availability of a substance for diffusional transfer across the placenta is not always related to blood levels of that substance, because many metabolites, nutrients, and drugs that are poorly water-soluble are protein bound.

Although proteins aid in delivery of these substances to the placenta, they may actually hinder transfer of the substances. It is the free, unbound—or soluble—fraction of a substance that is available for transfer. Conversely, high-affinity carrier proteins on the receiving side of the placenta drive diffusional transfer to their side by decreasing a ligand's free fraction and increasing its maternofetal gradient. Oxygen, for example, is 98% bound to hemoglobin. It is the transplacental difference in the partial pressure of dissolved oxygen (PO_2) that determines the diffusion pressure. The more oxygen-avid fetal hemoglobin counterbalances the resistance to transfer from the maternal circulation. The O_2 content (i.e., dissolved and hemoglobin-bound O_2) of the blood on each side of the placental membrane is determined principally by different affinities of maternal and fetal hemoglobin for oxygen. In humans, the fetal oxyhemoglobin dissociation curve is displaced leftward of the maternal curve, facilitating a much greater uptake of oxygen by fetal blood at the placental capillary level than would be possible otherwise (see Appendix B). At any given PO_2, a much higher O_2 content is achieved in fetal blood than in maternal blood. The O_2 content in the umbilical vein (14.5 mL/dL) is as high as that of the uterine artery (15.8 mL/dL), despite an umbilical venous PO_2 of only 27 mm Hg (Table 11-2). Relatively high fetal blood O_2 content confers on the fetus the ability to deliver sufficient oxygen to peripheral tissue despite low PO_2. Low PO_2 may be essential to fetal physiologic adaptation to maintain high pulmonary vascular resistance and to keep the ductus arteriosus open.

The excretion of bilirubin provides an example of fetomaternal interaction using specific permeability properties of the placenta to accomplish a given objective (5). Before birth, elimination of bilirubin from the fetus is by diffusional transfer through the placenta to the mother. The placenta is extremely permeable to unconjugated bilirubin but relatively impermeable to bilirubin glucuronide (i.e., conjugated bilirubin). In the fetus, because of minimal bilirubin glucuronyltransferase, hepatic conjugation of bilirubin is suppressed. Because fetal bilirubin is predominantly unconjugated and highly lipid soluble, it diffuses freely from the fetal to the maternal side. After transfer to the mother, it is efficiently conjugated and excreted (Fig. 11-4).

Facilitated Diffusion

Most substances cross the placenta by simple diffusion. Maternal glucose, the principal substrate for oxidative metabolism in the fetus, is a water-soluble, polar molecule that crosses the placenta by facilitated diffusion, which is a gradient-dependent, receptor-mediated, saturable process. In the human placenta, preferential transfer of D-glucose (over L-glucose) exists. Transfer stereospecificity implies a carrier-mediated process that provides the fetus with the appropriate isomer for metabolism. The presence of glucose transporter genes in the placenta, which code for glucose transporter proteins, confirms indirect experimental evidence for the existence of a membrane-bound D-glucose carrier protein (6,7). Under physiologic and pathologic human conditions, the carrier protein for glucose is not saturated, and the amount transferred to the fetus is directly related to the amount supplied to the placenta (8).

Active Transport

To provide appropriate fuels for fetal growth, specific energy-requiring transport mechanisms in the microvillous surface aid in transfer of substances that are not readily lipid soluble and are required in large amounts by the fetus.

Most amino acids cross the placenta by an active transport mechanism (9,10,11). Active amino acid uptake has two major purposes: transfer to the fetus and placental production of peptide hormones.

Transfer from maternal to fetal circulation is especially important for the essential amino acids required for fetal growth, including the essential adult amino acids histidine, isoleucine, leucine, lysine, methionine, phenylalanine, threonine, tryptophan, and valine; and the proposed fetal essential amino acids cysteine, tyrosine, histidine, and taurine. Early in development, before maturation of fetal metabolic systems, all amino acids are essential to the fetus. Fetal amino acid levels are 1.5- to 5-fold higher than maternal levels, confirming a transport process against a concentration gradient.

Placental transfer of amino acids is stereospecific, with the natural l-form preferred. Transport of amino acids by animal cells is mediated by specific carrier systems that have overlapping substrate reactivities. In human villous

TABLE 11-2
NORMAL OXYGEN VALUES IN MATERNAL AND FETAL BLOOD

Oxygen Measurements	Uterine Artery	Uterine Vein	Umbilical Vein	Umbilical Artery
PO_2 (torr)	95	40	27	15
Hemoglobin O_2 saturation (%)	98	76	68	30
O_2 content (mL/dL)	15.8	12.2	14.5	6.4
Hemoglobin (g/dL)	12.0	12.0	16.0	16.0

From Longo L. Disorders of placental transfer. In: Assali NS, ed. *Pathophysiology of gestation.* New York: Academic Press, 1972;2:11, with permission.

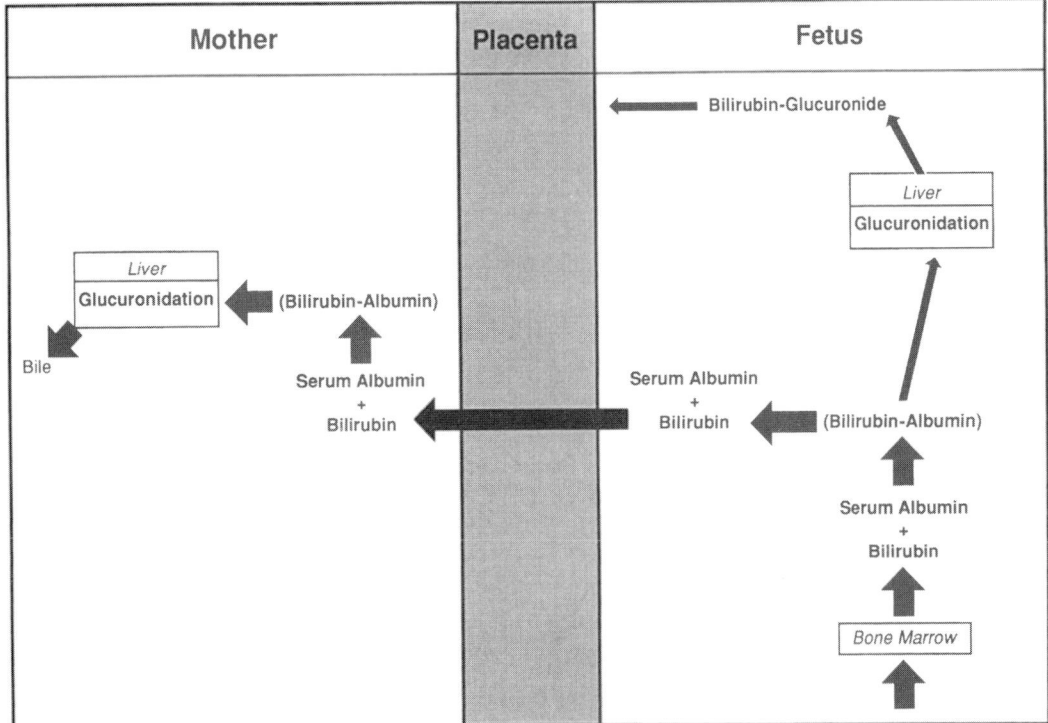

Figure 11-4   Antepartum excretion of bilirubin. Fetal bilirubin is transferred from fetal serum albumin through the placenta to maternal serum. It then is conjugated with glucuronic acid by the maternal liver and excreted into the bile. Fetal glucuronidation is suppressed. The placenta is relatively impermeable to the glucuronide.

tissue fragments, three carrier systems exist for neutral amino acids (12). System A is sodium dependent, reversible at low pH, and most reactive with amino acids that have short, polar, or linear side chains (e.g., alanine, glycine). System L is sodium independent and most reactive with large, apolar, branched-chain, and aromatic amino acids (e.g., leucine, isoleucine, tyrosine, tryptophan, valine, phenylalanine, methionine, glutamine). The ASC system is sodium dependent and is involved in transport of alanine, serine, and cysteine (ASC). Evidence suggests that a B system exists in placenta for taurine transport (13). Taurine, although produced by the maternal liver from cysteine and methionine, is essential for fetal neurologic development but is not produced by the fetus.

Certain drugs cross the placenta by active transport. Zidovudine, used for treating HIV, has been found in the perfused human placental model to cross from the maternal to the fetal side by energy-dependent transport (14). Because zidovudine is a thymidine analog, it may take advantage of placental thymidine transport systems. Zidovudine levels are higher in cord blood than in maternal blood, suggesting transport against a concentration gradient and an active transport mechanism. Maternal administration of zidovudine and other antiretroviral agents has become accepted therapy in HIV-positive mothers for prevention of vertical transmission to the fetus. In a collaborative, prospective study of pregnant, HIV-seropositive women, zidovudine administered orally

in the prenatal period and intravenously during labor was shown to decrease the vertical transmission to the fetus from 25.5% to 8.3% (15).

Receptor-Mediated Endocytosis

Although many large protein molecules cross the placenta by pinocytosis in extremely small quantities, specific receptor-mediated processes expedite transfer of certain larger substances that are required by the fetus. The receptor-rich microvillous brush border of the syncytiotrophoblast and the numerous coated micropinocytotic vesicles found just beneath it provide anatomic evidence for receptor-mediated endocytosis (16). The receptors involved in this process, found on the surface of the syncytiotrophoblast, are thought to extend through the glycocalyx layer of the cell membrane and bind to the protein clathrin to form a membrane complex. After the ligands are bound to their receptors, aggregation and internalization occur to form a cytoplasmic-coated vesicle (Fig. 11-5). Destiny of the contents of the vesicles depends on the ligand.

Maternal immunoglobulin (Ig) molecules are transferred to the fetus by receptor-mediated endocytosis. IgG subclasses 1 and 3 and IgA are known to cross the placenta. Once internalized, the intact Ig molecules within the vesicles are delivered from the cytoplasm of syncytiotrophoblast through the capillary endothelial cell and into the fetal circulation (17,18). Antenatal fetal transfer of maternal IgG antibodies may interfere with antibody-based

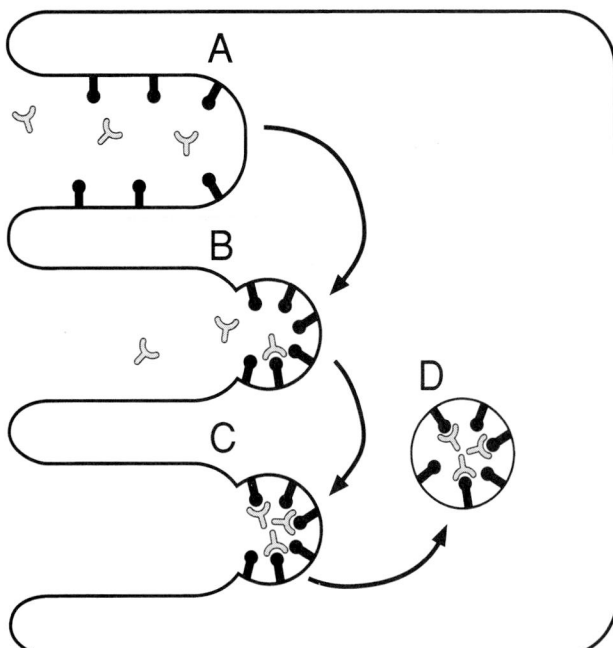

Figure 11-5 Receptor-mediated endocytosis. The placental syncytiotrophoblast with the microvillous maternal border (Fig. 11-1) has **(A)** specific receptors, located in the microvillous projections **(B)** clustering in intervening pits on exposure to specific ligand in the maternal blood stream. Endocytosis occurs. **C:** The receptor–ligand complexes and associated cell wall invert to form **(D)** an endocytic vesicle that is internalized. The destiny of the vesicle depends on the ligand.

diagnostic testing in the fetus, necessitating analysis of the fetal-specific IgM antibody. Developmentally, the transfer of maternal IgG to the fetus is probably protective and beneficial, but this transfer backfires in some situations, such as immune fetal hydrops (i.e., erythroblastosis fetalis) and alloimmune fetal thrombocytopenia. By receptor-mediated endocytosis, anti-D or another blood group antibody crosses the placenta to cause fetal hemolytic anemia, and anti-Pl^{A1} crosses the placenta to cause fetal thrombocytopenia (19).

Transfer of transferrin–iron complex into the placental syncytiotrophoblast occurs through receptor-mediated endocytosis. Brush border membrane transferrin-specific receptors on the maternal side of the syncytiotrophoblast bind transferrin–iron complex, and aggregate and internalize it to form vesicles of transferrin–iron complexes. In the cytoplasm, the complexes dissociate to form apotransferrin and ferrous iron. Apotransferrin is recycled to the maternal circulation, and ferrous iron is stored transiently as ferritin and released to the fetal circulation to be made into a complex with fetal transferrin. No maternal transferrin or placental ferritin is transferred to the fetus (20). Maternofetal iron transport is independent of maternal levels.

Uptake of low-density lipoprotein (LDL) cholesterol from maternal blood for progesterone synthesis by the placental trophoblast is accomplished through receptor-mediated endocytosis. Specific receptors that have a high affinity for LDL but not for high-density lipoprotein (HDL) are located on the microvillous brush border of the syncy-

tiotrophoblast. LDL binds to its receptor and is actively internalized. Within the cytoplasm, LDL vesicles fuse with lysosomes, where enzyme hydrolysis of cholesterol esters releases cholesterol for mitochondrial synthesis of progesterone.

Other Mechanisms of Transfer

A variety of other mechanisms of transfer probably are functional in the human placenta. Large protein molecules may cross the placental membranes by a slow, non–receptor-mediated process of pinocytosis. Ions may cross placental membranes with the aid of ion pumps. Evidence suggests that small molecules and ions may cross through intercellular channels.

PLACENTAL METABOLISM

The placenta is a highly metabolic organ. Oxygen is consumed at a rate of 10 mL/min per kg, representing the amount of maternal oxygen needed to supply the placenta and fetus for metabolic functions. Approximately 20% of placental oxygen uptake is used by the placenta; the remainder diffuses to the fetus. Glucose, the principle metabolic carbon source of the placenta, is converted to lactate or is oxidized to CO_2. Placental tissue requires energy for maintenance of active transfer systems, hormone production, and substrate metabolism.

PLACENTA AS AN ENDOCRINE ORGAN

It is the placenta that maintains the maternal milieu most favorable for pregnancy by elaboration of large amounts of steroid and peptide hormones, which are required to maintain the fetoplacental unit. Generally, placentally produced steroid hormones, but not peptide hormones, cross to the fetal side.

Human Chorionic Gonadotropin

Sensitive techniques demonstrate that the secretion of human chorionic gonadotropin (hCG) begins during implantation, when the cytotrophoblast differentiates into the syncytiotrophoblast. Although the messenger RNA for hCG can be found in the cytotrophoblast, this cell is thought not to be the origin of this peptide hormone, but only gains the ability to secrete hCG after it differentiates into a syncytiotrophoblast. The maternal plasma hCG level rises after implantation, peaks by 10 menstrual weeks of pregnancy, and declines to a nadir in the second trimester, after which levels remain low (Fig. 11-6).

The only well-established role of hCG is continued stimulation of the ovarian corpus luteum to produce 17-hydroxyprogesterone for maintenance of pregnancy. Although placental production of progesterone occurs early in gestation, the transition to placental autonomy from the ovary occurs

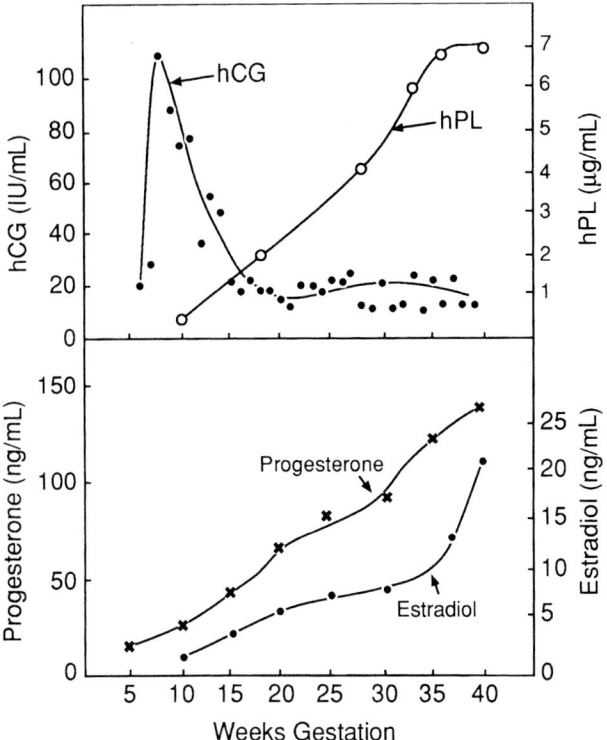

Figure 11-6 Maternal blood levels of the major hormones produced by the placenta throughout pregnancy. (From Ashitaka Y, Nishimura R, Takemori M, et al. Production and secretion of hCG and hCG subunits by trophoblastic tissue. In: Segal S, ed. *Chorionic gonadotropins*. New York: Plenum Press, 1980:151; Selenkow HA, Varma K, Younger D, et al. Patterns of serum immunoreactive human placental lactogen and chorionic gonadotropin in diabetic pregnancy. *Diabetes* 1971;20:696; and Speroff L, Glass RH, Kase NG. *Clinical gynecologic endocrinology and infertility*, 4th ed. Baltimore: Williams & Wilkins, 1989, with permission.)

between 10 and 12 menstrual weeks. Before this transition, loss of the corpus luteum results in loss of the pregnancy, unless exogenous progesterone is administered. Primary control of trophoblastic hCG production has not been determined, but hormonal modulation is apparent (21). Proposed roles for hCG include the immunologic protection of the trophoblast and regulation of placental progesterone production. Falling levels of hCG before 10 menstrual weeks heralds pregnancy loss and is associated with miscarriage or ectopic gestation. Higher-than-normal hCG levels are seen with multiple gestations, hydatidiform mole, choriocarcinoma, fetal triploidy when associated with molar changes of the placenta, and Down syndrome (22).

Human Placental Lactogen

Human placental lactogen (hPL) is a single-chain polypeptide that has approximately 85% similarity to human growth hormone. The quantity of hPL synthesized by the placental syncytiotrophoblast parallels placental mass, reaching its peak at term and falling dramatically after delivery of the placenta.

Functionally, hPL can be considered a fetal growth hormone, because it maintains the maternal metabolic milieu

optimal for delivery of nutrients to the fetus. Despite its name, hPL has not been demonstrated conclusively to exert a lactogenic effect in humans. The physiologic role of hPL appears to be in shifting the pattern of maternal energy metabolism during pregnancy from carbohydrate to one that depends on fat. The hormone promotes adipolysis and increases free fatty acid availability for maternal metabolism, saving glucose and amino acids for transfer to the fetus. Free fatty acids do not cross the placenta as readily as amino acids and glucose.

Human placental lactogen has antiinsulin effects thought to be mediated by the elevated free fatty acids, which promote peripheral tissue resistance to insulin. The subsequent increased pancreatic production of insulin leads to down regulation of peripheral insulin receptors.

Maternal blood levels of hPL correlate with placental function. It was once thought that low hPL levels could predict pregnancies with deteriorating placental function and those with fetal compromise (23). Unfortunately, hPL levels are not as clinically useful as other methods. Similarly, elevated maternal hPL levels were thought to be predictive of gestational diabetes or outcome in preexisting diabetes, but large biological variations in maternal levels preclude its use in prediction or diagnosis. There are no clinical applications for hPL levels at this time.

Estrogen

Estrogen production by the syncytiotrophoblast requires an elaborate concerted effort by the mother, fetus, and placenta (Fig. 11-7). Because there is no activity of 17-hydroxylase and 17,20-desmolase in the human placenta, estrogen precursors must be obtained from the fetal adrenal gland. The placenta produces three major estrogens—estradiol (E2), estriol (E3), and estrone (E1)—which are secreted predominantly into the maternal circulation. Maternal estrogen levels increase with gestational age.

Little is known about the specific functions of estrogen during pregnancy. Estrogens effect many general changes in the mother to prepare for and maintain pregnancy. The uterine myometrium responds exquisitely with increased protein synthesis and cellular hypertrophy. Estrogens cause vascular relaxation and increased blood flow to the uterus. Uterine contractility is increased by estrogens, supporting a role in the onset of parturition. Placental sulfatase deficiency, an X-linked fetal disorder, is associated with low estrogen levels. Except for dysfunctional labor, women with these fetuses have normal pregnancies.

A specific role for estrogens in the fetus has not been determined. The fetal liver can metabolize E3 to estetrol (E4), which binds to fetal estrogen receptors but has no estrogenic activity, protecting fetal tissue from massive amounts of free estrogen.

Progesterone

The placental syncytiotrophoblast produces progesterone from maternally derived LDL cholesterol (Fig. 11-8). Fetal

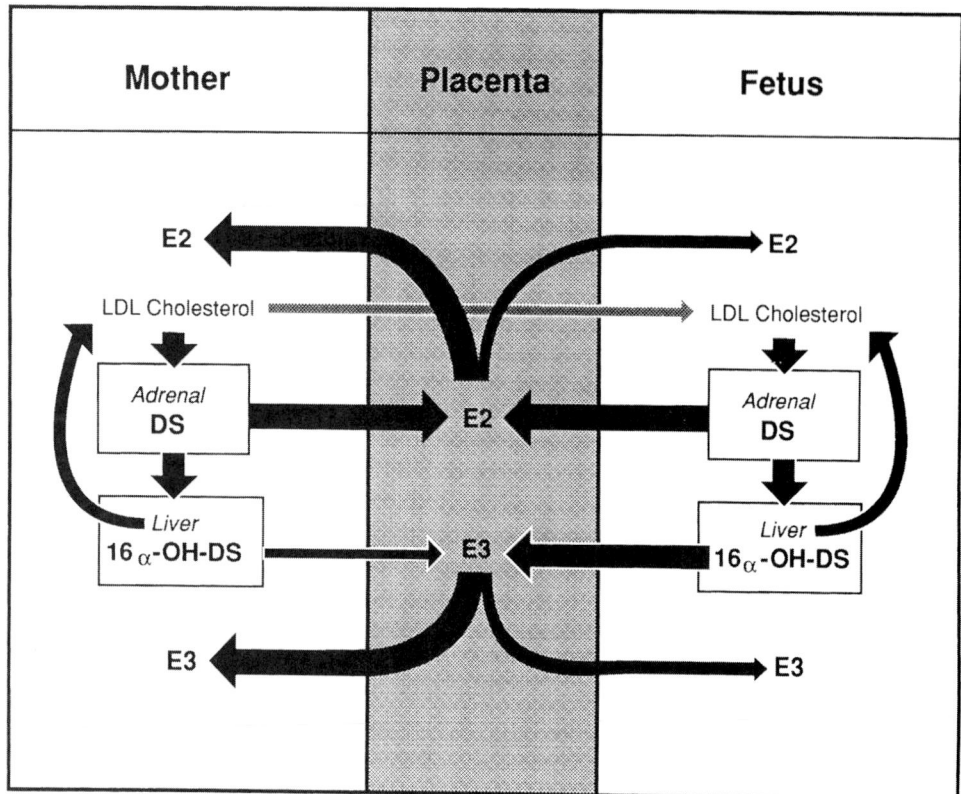

Figure 11-7 Placental estrogen synthesis from fetal and maternal precursors. After 20 weeks of gestation, the fetal compartment supplies most steroid precursors for placental estrogen production. The fetal adrenal uses low-density lipoprotein cholesterol, produced by the fetal liver or transferred from the maternal compartment, to synthesize dehydroepiandrosterone sulfate (DS). DS is converted to 16_α-OH-DS in the fetal liver. DS and 16_α-OH-DS undergo placental metabolism to estradiol (E2) and estriol (E3), respectively, which are released predominantly on the maternal side.

contribution to progesterone synthesis is minimal. Maternal progesterone levels increase with gestational age. The major role of progesterone is to maintain the pregnancy. Early production of progesterone is by the ovarian corpus luteum. After a transition period of shared function between 6 and 12 weeks of gestation, the placenta becomes the dominant producer of progesterone, and the pregnancy continues even if the corpus luteum is removed. Low levels of progesterone may be associated with first-trimester pregnancy loss.

The most important role of progesterone may be that of principal substrate for fetal adrenal gland production of glucocorticoids and mineralocorticoids. Progesterone may have a role in parturition and in suppressing the maternal immunologic response to fetal antigens.

AMNIOTIC FLUID

Formation and circulation of the amniotic fluid reflect intimate and dynamic maternal and fetal interactions. Amniotic fluid is ultimately derived from maternal water. Very early in pregnancy, amniotic fluid is cellular transudate with the same tonicity, but lower protein content, as maternal plasma. By at least 8 gestational weeks, when the maternal and fetal blood circulations are well established, most amniotic fluid water is thought to be derived from maternal plasma water by direct transfer from the maternal circulation to fetal capillaries in response to osmotic and hydrostatic forces. Once circulating in the fetus, water is filtered and excreted by the urinary system into the amniotic cavity. By 8 gestational weeks, the urethra is patent, and the fetal kidneys begin to form urine; by 10 to 11 weeks, a fetal bladder can be seen ultrasonographically. Concurrently, the fetus begins to swallow. Swallowed amniotic fluid is

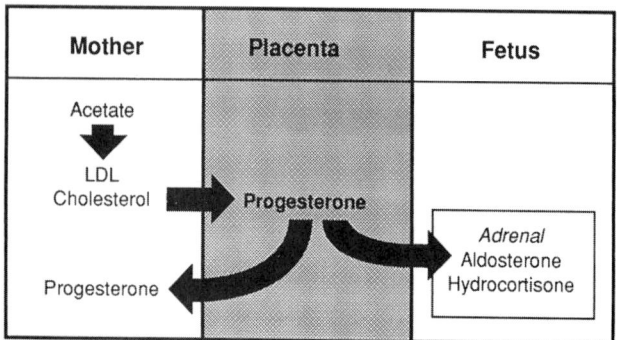

Figure 11-8 Placental progesterone synthesis depends only on maternal precursors.

reabsorbed into the fetal circulation to be reexcreted by the kidneys or transferred across the placenta to the mother. By the end of the first trimester, the amniotic fluid circulation has been established. Before fetal skin keratinization at 22 weeks, additional water transfer can occur directly through the highly permeable fetal skin.

The content of amniotic fluid changes over gestation. The early electrolyte content is similar to that of extracellular fluid. As the kidneys become functional, fetal urine electrolytes and excretory products become major components. As gestation progresses, the fetal kidneys mature and are better able to retain electrolytes and produce more dilute urine. At 20 weeks, the sodium content of amniotic fluid is 136 mEq/L and the osmolality is 276 mOsm/L; at 40 weeks, the sodium content is 124 mEq/L and the osmolality is 258 mOsm/L.

Amniotic fluid contains excretory products of the fetus and maternal products that can diffuse directly across the fetal membranes from the maternal compartment. In addition to electrolytes and proteins, amniotic fluid contains carbohydrates, amino acids, urea, creatinine, lactate, pyruvate, lipids, enzymes, hormones, and various other metabolites reflective of the fetal milieu. Their presence and the presence of desquamated fetal cells allow diagnosis of many fetal abnormalities by biochemical and genetic analysis of amniotic fluid. Amniotic fluid also contains fetal pulmonary fluid. The usefulness of the lecithin to sphingomyelin ratio in predicting maturity of the fetal lungs has its basis in contributions from this fluid. In fetal sheep, there is constant outpouring of pulmonary fluid into the trachea (24).

Although the range of normal amounts of amniotic fluid varies and depends on gestational age, abnormal volumes often herald fetal structural or growth abnormality. Maternal factors can affect amniotic fluid volume. Maternal plasma volume correlates with amniotic fluid volume. In hypovolemic mothers, expansion of plasma volume with albumin increases amniotic fluid volume (25). Maternal use of diuretics may influence amniotic fluid volume indirectly by decreasing maternal intravascular volume and directly by increasing fetal micturition after transplacental passage.

FETAL MEMBRANES

The fetal amnion and chorion, although simple in anatomic design, are intricately involved in fetomaternal interactions. The thin, avascular layer of epithelial cells that makes up the amnion arises from fetal ectodermal cells, and the chorion, several layers thick, arises from extraembryonic somatic mesoderm and a trophoblast layer. The trophoblast layer in the area of the chorion, which is destined to be the fetal surface of the term placenta, undergoes rapid proliferation and branching into villi. By 8 menstrual weeks, the trophoblast layer of the remaining chorion becomes compressed, attenuated, and microscopic. These microscopic cells are intimately intermingled with the

outermost maternal layer, the decidua or gestational endometrium, to allow paracrine interaction of these cells.

Paracrine interactions of the fetal chorionic cells with maternal decidual cells may be involved in the control of maternal production of prolactin and amniotic fluid volume regulation. Transport studies with tritiated water suggest that the net transport of water by the chorioamnion with adherent decidua is greatest in the fetomaternal direction, suggesting a net outflow of water from the amniotic fluid compartment to maternal circulation (26). Lower osmolality in the amniotic fluid compartment favors movement of water from the amniotic cavity to the maternal compartment.

The cells of the amnion, rich in esterified arachidonic acid, are active in prostaglandin metabolism and are at least indirectly involved in cervical ripening and the onset or maintenance of labor. Initiation of human labor may involve autocrine and paracrine mechanisms within the fetal membranes and possibly maternal decidua, resulting in amnion cell production of prostaglandin E2 (PGE2), a potent cervical-ripening and uterotonic agent (27). Although amnion cell production of PGE2 has been associated with initiation and maintenance of labor, control of its production is less well understood. Various inflammatory cytokines, in particular, tumor necrosis factor α interleukin-1α, interleukin-1β, interleukin-6, and interleukin-8, play a role affecting the common pathway of amnion cell production of PGE2 and subsequent labor (28–31).

UMBILICAL CORD

The umbilical cord contains one fetal vein and two fetal arteries, which are supported and protected by Wharton jelly, a gel-like connective tissue composed of a ground substance of open-chain polysaccharides in a network of collagen and microfibrils (32). Externally, the cord is covered by amnionic epithelium, but there is no chorionic epithelium. The length of the umbilical cord ranges from 30 to 100 cm (mean 55 cm) with reported extremes from 0 to 155 cm. Fetuses with no umbilical cords have a severe, fatal abdominal wall defect because of failure of formation of the body stalk. The association of a short cord with a low IQ raises the question of whether the length of the cord is determined by fetal movement mediated by antenatal neurologic function. Fetuses with long cords are more likely to have cord entanglement. Short cords are more likely to stretch and avulse during descent of the fetus, resulting in signs of fetal distress during expulsion or hemorrhage at birth.

The normal umbilical cord increases in circumference with gestation until term, when the average circumference is 3.8 cm (33). Although excessive Wharton jelly (i.e., thick cords) has not been associated with fetal abnormalities, lack of this connective tissue has. Thin cords frequently are seen with growth-retarded fetuses and may be associated with cord strictures, umbilical vessel rupture, or thrombi (34). Thin cords are more likely to allow symptomatic external compression, stretch, or occlusion of umbilical vessels. Resolution of umbilical venous bleeding after percutaneous umbilical blood sampling is facilitated by Wharton jelly surrounding the vessel.

PLACENTAL PHYSIOLOGY IN DISEASE STATES

Preeclampsia and Hypertensive Disorders of Pregnancy

Preeclampsia, a hypertensive disease unique to pregnancy, has its genesis in the placenta. It is more common in women with multiple gestations (i.e., multiple placentas) and molar pregnancies (i.e., excessive trophoblastic tissue), and it abates after delivery of the placenta (35). Altered placentation may be responsible for maternal vasospasm, the basic physiologic abnormality in preeclampsia (36). Vascular constriction in most maternal organs results in hypoperfusion of the uterus and placenta, making the fetus at risk for intrauterine growth restriction, placental abruption, and fetal death.

Placentas of preeclamptic women have a significantly lower total volume and volume of parenchymal and villous surface area than placentas of normal controls (37). There is a greater proportion of centrally located, infarcted areas because of poor intervillous maternal circulation. Histologically, cellular degenerative changes are found (38). An abundance of syncytial budding is common in histologic sections and teased preparations of villi. Budding, or knotting of the placental syncytiotrophoblast, consists of bunching of the cytoplasm of these cells with aggregation of nuclei, a histologic finding suggestive of perfusional compromise.

The maternal vascular response to placentation is inadequate in women who develop preeclampsia (39). Normally during implantation, cytotrophoblasts, or early placental cells, invade the lumen of the uterine spiral arterioles, anchor to the vessel wall, and cause dilatation of the arterioles to allow adequate perfusion of the placenta and, ultimately, the fetus. There is evidence of a "vascular transformation" of the cytotrophoblasts that invade the spiral arterioles manifested by at least modulation of adhesion molecules (40). In preeclampsia there is a loss of the normal modulation of adhesion molecules and an incomplete vascular invasion by the cytotrophoblasts (41). Some spiral arteries show absence of physiologic changes throughout the entire length, suggesting a complete lack of invasion by trophoblasts (Fig. 11-9).

Certain spiral arterioles at the implantation site undergo acute atherosis. Initially, fibrinoid degeneration and mural thrombosis of decidual vessels occurs. The vessel wall then becomes replaced by fibrin, and the intima is replaced by cholesterol-laden macrophages. Eventually, fibrinoid necrosis and total obstruction of the lumen lead to loss of maternal blood flow, which is likely responsible for placental infarcts (42).

There are no microscopic or macroscopic placental changes that are pathognomonic for preeclampsia. The pathologic changes in placentas of preeclamptic women suggest the disease is indistinguishable from that of women with lupus anticoagulant syndrome, signifying a shared physiology. In the lupus anticoagulant syndrome, autoimmune antiphospholipid antibodies, detectable in the maternal bloodstream, are associated with maternal arterial and venous thrombosis, recurrent miscarriage, early onset preeclampsia, placental and fetal growth restriction, and fetal death. Placentas from these women, whether or not they show signs of overt preeclampsia, have infarctions, fibrosis, a decrease in vasculosyncytial membranes, and an increase in syncytial knots (43).

Preeclampsia is a disease resulting from abnormal maternoplacental interaction, and its cause is unknown. More recently, preeclampsia has been considered a syndrome with various etiologies leading to a final common

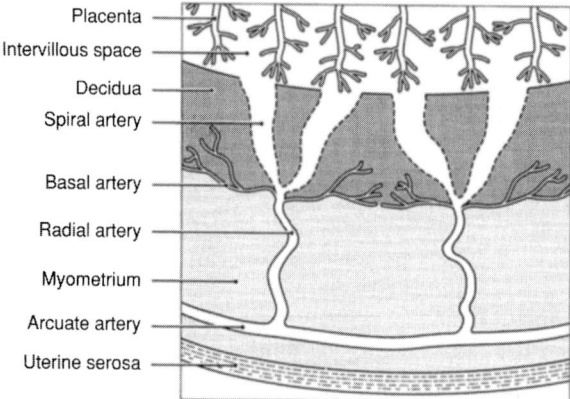
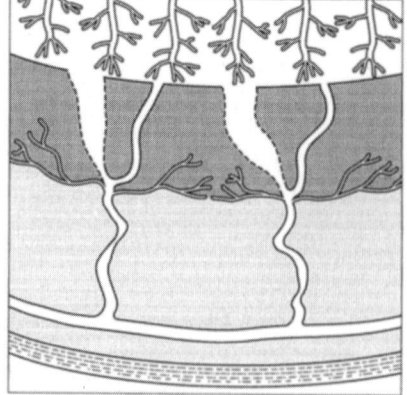

Placenta
Intervillous space
Decidua
Spiral artery
Basal artery
Radial artery
Myometrium
Arcuate artery
Uterine serosa

Figure 11-9 Maternal blood supply to the placenta in normal pregnancy **(left)** and preeclampsia **(right)**. Notice the lack of normal physiologic dilation of radial arteries and of some decidual segments of spiral arteries in preeclampsia. (From Khong TY, De Wolf F, Robertson, WB, et al. Inadequate maternal vascular response to placentation in pregnancies complicated by preeclampsia and by small for gestational age infants. *Br J Obstet Gynaecol* 1986;93:1049, with permission.)

constellation of signs and symptoms, hypertension, proteinuria, and edema. One of the more attractive pathogenetic mechanisms of preeclampsia is that of an immune-mediated disease, supported by similarities with the lupus anticoagulant syndrome. However, in preeclampsia, neither the exact antigenic stimulus nor the antibody response has been defined, although the former probably is derived from trophoblasts.

Preeclampsia may be caused by placental production of a circulating humoral factor, perhaps immunologic, which affects prostaglandin homeostasis. Prostaglandins are involved in normal vasodilation of pregnancy. Prostacyclin (PGI$_2$), because of its potent effect in relaxing vascular smooth muscle and lowering systemic arterial pressure, is thought to be most involved. Prostacyclin is produced in vascular endothelial cells and is thought to exert its effect on vascular smooth muscle in a paracrine fashion. It is an inhibitor of platelet aggregation and of uterine contractility. The combined effects of this prostaglandin prevent maternal hypertension, prevent platelet aggregation, and promote uteroplacental blood flow. Thromboxane, produced predominantly by platelets, is a powerful vasoconstrictor, stimulator of platelet aggregation, and stimulator of uterine contractility, favoring maternal hypertension, decreased utero- placental blood flow, and intrauterine growth restriction.

Abnormal prostaglandin homeostasis has been found in preeclampsia (44). Excessive placental production of thromboxane and insufficient production of PGI$_2$ result in an abnormally high ratio of thromboxane to PGI$_2$. Prostacyclin production is decreased in umbilical arteries, placental veins, and uterine vessels. Thromboxane production is increased in placental tissue and in circulating platelets from preeclamptic women with infants who are small for gestational age (45).

Compared with normal placentas, placental findings in women with chronic or essential hypertension vary from lower total volume, lower parenchymal tissue, and infarcts to normal volumes and large, villous surface areas. Findings differ with various degrees of severity of disease and lack of differentiation between chronic hypertension and chronic hypertension with superimposed preeclampsia.

Diabetes

Just as the infant of a diabetic mother can be macrosomic, growth restricted, or normally grown, the diabetic placenta can have various findings. Some investigators associate these findings with severity of maternal diabetes, especially the duration and complications of the disease, and others associate them with the degree of glycemic control.

Placentas of diabetic mothers without significant vascular disease (i.e., White's classes A–D) differ from normal by having more parenchymal and villous tissue, a higher cellular content, and a larger surface area of exchange between mother and fetus in terms of peripheral villous and capillary surface areas and intervillous space volume (46,47,48). These larger placentas are able to adequately support growth of large fetuses. Placentas of diabetic mothers with appropriate-for-gestational-age newborns are morphologically closer to control, nondiabetic placentas. It is the placentas of macrosomic infants that are heavier, predominantly because of a significant accumulation of nonparenchymal and parenchymal tissue. These placentas have retarded maturation of surface areas of terminal villi. Grossly, they appear large, thick, and plethoric. Microscopically, focal immaturity (i.e., dysmaturity) and villous edema are found.

The excessive growth and dysmaturity of these placentas suggest an accelerated growth process or a loss of the normal growth process that occurs in placentas of healthy women. Because the placenta is essentially a fetal organ, which is different from other fetal organs only in that it is subject to more direct maternal modulation, it is not surprising that macrosomic fetuses have large placentas. The major mechanism for organ enlargement, or macrosomia, in the fetus of a diabetic mother involves anabolic metabolism of excess glucose and its deposition as glycogen and fat. The placenta of a macrosomic infant of a diabetic mother has neither excessive fat nor glycogen, suggesting a different mechanism by which the fetus (or mother) increases placental size and surface areas of terminal villi to maintain fetal nutrition (the size of the placenta and quality and topography of the transfer surface regulate nutrient availability to the fetus).

Placental cells respond to maternally or fetally produced hormones directly by alterations in growth and indirectly by elaboration of certain substances that control their own growth. Insulin and its associated family of growth-promoting peptide hormones, such as insulin-like growth factor I (IGF-I) and insulin-like growth factor II (IGF-II), have been implicated in excessive placental growth of the diabetic placenta.

Insulin receptors have been localized to the apical brush border of the syncytiotrophoblast (bathed in maternal blood) (49). Maternal insulin binds to these receptors, is internalized, and eventually degraded by this cell. Investigators using the *in vitro* perfused human placental cotyledon model have shown that placental-facilitated uptake and metabolism of glucose do not appear to be regulated by insulin (50). The lack of insulin regulation of glucose transport in the intact placenta correlates with glucose transporter genes in placenta, *GLUT1* and *GLUT3*, both thought to code for insulin-unresponsive glucose transporter proteins. Why then is there active insulin uptake by the placental syncytiotrophoblast? Insulin, more likely fetal but possibly maternal, may have growth-promoting activity in the placenta and thereby affect placental size.

The placental trophoblast microvillous brush border membrane contains specific heterotetrameric IGF-I receptors that have been found in trophoblasts as early as 6 weeks of gestation (51). This somatomedin has been measured in placental explant cultures and placental fibroblast culture fluid and is thought to be involved in control of placental growth (52). Maternal serum IGF-I levels and the ratio of cord serum IGF-I to its binding protein correlate with birth-weight (53). Cord serum IGF-II levels are 50%

higher in infants of diabetic mothers than in those of non-diabetic mothers. Because fetal macrosomia in diabetic pregnancies cannot always be prevented, despite excellent maternal blood glucose control, attention has been turned to excessive placental transfer of fetal fuels other than glucose. Some investigators suggest a greater diffusional transfer of free fatty acids in diabetic pregnancies, probably related to greater maternal availability (e.g., maternal hyperlipidemia in diabetic pregnancies) and greater placental transfer surface (54). Excessive placental transfer of insulin-secretagogue amino acids (e.g., arginine) also may be responsible for fetal hyperinsulinemia and macrosomia.

Placentas of diabetic women with vascular complications (e.g., nephropathy, retinopathy, heart disease, White's class F, R, or H) frequently have infarcts and are associated with growth-retarded fetuses. The weights of the placentas of these diabetic women are lower than normal gestational age-matched placentas. There have been no specific placental findings to explain the higher stillborn rate in macrosomic fetuses of diabetic mothers.

Erythroblastosis

Erythroblastosis fetalis, or hemolytic disease of the newborn, is a condition in which specific IgG antibodies formed by the mother against erythrocyte antigens of the fetus cross the placenta by receptor-mediated endocytosis and coat fetal erythrocytes, causing splenic sequestration, intravascular hemolysis, anemia, and unconjugated hyperbilirubinemia. Unconjugated bilirubin is transported easily to the maternal side, conjugated, and excreted by the mother. Anemia stimulates fetal hematopoiesis, especially in the liver and spleen, resulting in release of immature erythrocyte precursors into fetal blood. Severe fetal anemia causes fetal and placental hydrops, and often hypoproteinemia and thrombocytopenia. The placenta of newborns with erythroblastosis fetalis is pale and enlarged, displaying villous immaturity, edema, and an increase in Hofbauer cells (i.e., macrophages). Erythrocyte precursors are found in the vascular spaces. The severity of placental changes parallels the severity of fetal disease. There is ultrasonographic evidence of reversal of placental thickening and edema as fetal hydrops improves with treatment.

Placental changes are secondary to the disease process and do not contribute to its formation. Hydropic placentas from fetuses with erythroblastosis fetalis are indistinguishable from those with other causes. In placentas of newborns with erythroblastosis fetalis, compensatory placental hematopoiesis, specifically in the villous stroma, is suggested because numerous erythrocyte precursors are found packed in fetal villous sinusoids mimicking *de novo* erythrocyte synthesis in the placenta. No specific erythrocyte synthesis occurs in the placenta.

Hydropic placentas produce elevated titers of hCG. Serum levels of this hormone are significantly higher than normal in women with hydropic fetuses and placentas (55). It is unclear whether this is because of overproduction of the hormone or normal production by larger pla-

cental cell mass. Other placental hormones, including hPL, are found in elevated quantities in serum of women with hydropic placentas.

Preeclampsia occurs frequently in mothers with fetal and placental hydrops. Reversal of preeclamptic signs and symptoms has been observed after fetal and placental hydrops resolved spontaneously or was reversed by fetal transfusion (56). Because hydropic placentas release greater amounts of placental hormones into the maternal circulation, this finding gives credence to a humoral placental product theory as the cause of preeclampsia.

Twin-to-Twin Transfusion Syndrome

Abnormal placental physiology because of congenital placental vascular malformations in monozygotic twins is the basis of twin-to-twin transfusion syndrome.

Although dizygotic twinning always involves separate placentas and membranes (i.e., diamnionic dichorionic), monozygotic twinning results in separation ranging from complete separation of the placentas and membranes (i.e., diamnionic dichorionic) to shared placentas and chorion (i.e., diamnionic monochorionic), to shared placentas, chorion, and amniotic cavity (i.e., monoamnionic monochorionic), to shared fetal tissues (i.e., monoamnionic conjoined).

Twin-to-twin transfusion syndrome is a disease of monochorionic twins. Extraembryonic somatic mesoderm lining the extraembryonic cavity of the developing embryo gives rise to the chorion and to the mesenchymal core of the placental villus and associated fetal vessels. Monozygotic twins who share chorions (i.e., monochorionic) also share fetal circulations by vascular connections. Fetal vascular anastomoses almost never are found on placentas of dichorionic twins, but they are usually found on those of monochorionic twins (57).

In monochorionic twin placentas, the normal 1:1 ratio between the artery supplying and the vein draining a cotyledon is lost. Haphazard vascular patterns exist (Fig. 11-10).

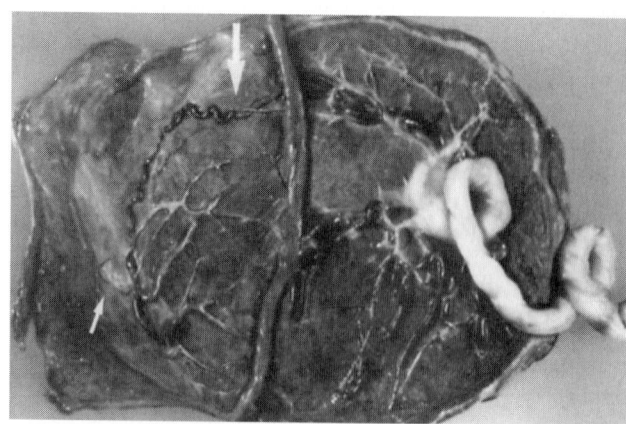

Figure 11-10 Diamnionic, monochorionic twin placenta, with the intervening amnion rolled in the center. Notice the haphazard vascularization (*large arrow*). The velamentous cord insertion (*small arrow*) of the smaller twin of this discordant pair is not an unusual finding in monochorionic twins.

Certain cotyledons are supplied from a single or anasto-motic artery from both twins and are drained by one or two veins. Others are supplied by an artery of one fetus and drained by a vein of the other. Drainage by the vein of the opposite fetus may not be obvious when capillaries join the venous system in a neighboring cotyledon before surfacing as a contralateral fetal vessel. An intertwin arteriovenous shunt should be suspected when an artery diving into a cotyledon is not accompanied by an adjacent emerging vein.

The most common fetal vascular anastomosis on the surface of the placenta is artery to artery, occurring in two thirds of monochorionic placentas (58). Vein-to-vein anastomoses are the least common, occurring in only 1 of 20 monochorionic placentas. Arteriovenous anastomosis, or arterial supply with contralateral fetal venous drainage of a cotyledon, which occurs in approximately two thirds of monochorionic placentas, is thought to be the most common placental lesion leading to inequality of blood flow and twin transfusion syndrome. Placental injection studies using contrast have been performed to ascertain vascular anastomosis, but injection studies only demonstrate the presence of anastomosis and do not establish overall inequality of flow.

In twin-to-twin transfusion syndrome, blood from the donor twin flows to the recipient twin through intertwin placental vascular connections. Remaining anastomoses are insufficient to allow return of the lost blood volume, and an imbalance of blood flow exists. The donor twin becomes hypovolemic, anemic, malnourished, and growth restricted; and responds with oliguria (i.e., oligohydramnios) and, in severe cases, anuria (i.e., ahydramnios). The recipient twin becomes hypervolemic and plethoric, develops cardiomegaly and polyuria (i.e., polyhydramnios), and, if severe, develops cardiac failure and hydrops fetalis. Grossly, the placental portion of the donor twin is anemic, pale, and usually smaller than that of the receiving twin. If hydrops has not yet occurred, the recipient twin's placental portion is red, thick, and congested. After hydrops ensues, the placenta becomes pale from villous edema. Microscopically, anemia and villous immaturity are found in the donor's placental portion and polycythemia and congestion in that of the recipient.

Despite the high frequency of cross-placental vascular anastomoses in monochorionic placentas, the incidence of clinically evident twin-to-twin transfusion syndrome in monochorionic twin pairs is only 5% to 10%. In some twin pairs, intertwin vascular connections may produce a chronic twin transfusion syndrome in which the larger twin responds with cardiac hyperplasia and hypertrophy (59). Cardiac hyperplasia may be compensatory, and certain sets of monochorionic twins may withstand the vascular inequalities throughout gestation (i.e., subclinical twin-to-twin transfusion syndrome). In others, the pumping capabilities of the enlarged heart are exceeded, and cardiac failure occurs. It is tempting to speculate that as the heart enlarges and fails, delicate pressure–flow characteristics in the placental vasculature are disrupted, exacerbating shunting to the recipient twin.

Twin-to-twin transfusion syndrome is a condition that begins early in embryonic vascular development. Benirschke (60) described the youngest example, a pair of aborted twin embryos measuring 7 and 8 cm (10 weeks of gestation) in which the heart of the donor twin was half the size of that of the recipient. Intertwin vascular distribution established early in the embryonic period may control intertwin placental mass distribution. Inequality in placental mass distribution may have an early, direct effect on fetal growth, causing significant growth restriction in one fetus. Antenatal ultrasonographic evaluation of placentation in the first trimester, or of the number of layers in intervening membranes in the latter trimesters, has allowed diagnosis of chorionicity with high sensitivity and positive predictive value (61). The obstetrician can confirm chorionicity and assess placental vascular patterns immediately after delivery of the twin placenta and should impart this information to the pediatrician.

Some antenatal treatment approaches for twin transfusion syndrome attempt to reverse the abnormal placental physiology. Selective termination of one fetus, usually the donor, prevents further transfusion to the recipient. This treatment introduces risks to the living twin from passage of emboli from the dead twin through anastomotic channels (i.e., twin embolization syndrome). Serial amniocentesis to decompress the polyhydramniotic sac of the recipient twin has reversed twin-to-twin transfusion syndrome in a few cases (62). Loss of amniotic fluid pressure on a large placental vascular anastomosis allows changes in fetal blood flow. After amniotic fluid decompression of severe polyhydramnios, ultrasonographically observed placentas appear thickened and less stretched. Fetoscopic laser occlusion of placental vessels, reported by De Lia and colleagues (63), may prove to be the most logical therapy, because treatment is directed at the cause of the problem. At the time of delivery, the placenta is two discs, separated by an area of infarcted cotyledons previously supplied by the coagulated vessels.

Acute transplacental fetus-to-fetus bleeding can occur in monochorionic twins and is distinct from twin transfusion syndrome. Acute fetus-to-fetus bleeding occurs in placentas with medium- or large-caliber vascular anastomosis when loss of established pressure–flow relations occurs. For example, the death of one twin of a monochorionic pair may allow large shifts of blood from the living twin to the deceased twin. Shifts may be sufficient to cause anemia and hydrops fetalis in the surviving twin. If the deceased twin was the growth-retarded donor of a twin-to-twin transfusion pair, paradoxical plethora of the donor twin may occur.

Acute transplacental fetal bleeding may occur at the time of labor. For example, during the uterine contractions, umbilical cord compression may occur to a sufficient degree that it diminishes umbilical venous return but not arterial perfusion. The resulting higher resistance in the placental venous system of the cord-compressed twin favors return of blood to the co-twin. Acute intraplacental fetal bleeding may occur after delivery of the first fetus. Loss of established placental pressure–flow relations after clamping of the umbilical cord favors intraplacental pooling of the second twin's blood through anastomoses, resulting in hypovolemia. Acute transplacental fetal bleeding can create disparate newborn hematocrits that do not reflect hematocrit levels during fetal life.

THE *IN UTERO* ENVIRONMENT AND FETAL DETERMINANTS OF ADULT DISEASE

The *in utero* environment has an overwhelming impact upon birth-weight and newborn disorders. Constriction of the uterine cavity because of leiomyomata (fibroid tumors), uterine anomalies, or lack of amniotic fluid may lead to deformation abnormalities such as club feet (64). Persistent, severe oligohydramnios, particularly in the second and third trimesters may lead to Potter sequence (65). Certain metabolic abnormalities of the mother causing an abnormal metabolic uterine milieu, such as uncontrolled diabetes (66) or uncontrolled phenylketonuria (67), may lead to congenital malformations, mental retardation, and growth abnormalities. Additionally, each fetus has a certain genetic predisposition to various disorders the development of which can be influenced by the *in utero* environment. For example, *in utero* positioning or abnormalities of labor may be associated with cranial synostosis in predisposed individuals (68).

Recently, the concept of the *in utero* environment influencing development of adult disease has become popular. This "fetal origins of adult disease" hypothesis says that human development is controlled not only by a combination of predetermined genes, but the effect on the fetus of the many variables of pregnancy.

The epidemiologic associations to support *in utero* programming and the fetal origins hypothesis were initially published in 1989 (69). The majority of the abnormal fetal origin hypotheses relate to poor fetal growth. Generally, investigators in these initial studies noted that outliers of normal birth-weight, either very large or more often very small newborns, had an increased risk for coronary artery disease, hypertension, and type 2 diabetes. This concept in humans has credibility from animal studies (70,71). The fetal origins hypothesis suggests, specifically, that lack of availability or use of fetal fuels *in utero* can program an individual's risk for chronic disease later in life.

Intrauterine fetal growth restriction is not only heterogeneous in etiology, but often multifactorial. The extensive placental and maternal physiologies discussed earlier in this chapter apply. Overall, the availability, delivery, and utilization of nutrients influence the growth of the fetus. Some of these influences can be modified such as promotion of adequate nutrition, cessation of smoking, and optimization of cardiac output to the uterus and placenta. Many other etiologies of growth restriction in newborns are evasive and lack both therapeutic and preventative prenatal measures.

BIRTH-WEIGHT AND CORONARY HEART DISEASE

Epidemiologic investigators have found an association of either low- or high-birth-weight with a higher risk of coronary heart disease later in life (72,73). The majority of the supporting data come from British epidemiologists evaluating birth records in three regions of Britain, specifically Hertfordshire, Sheffield, and Preston.

In a study of men born in Sheffield from 1907 to 1924 (74), death because of cardiovascular disease evaluated by standardized mortality ratios, fell in the birth-weight categories greater than 2,495 g. The standardized mortality ratio for cardiovascular disease fell from 119 in men who weighed 2,495 g (5.5 pounds) or less at birth to 74 in men who weighed more than 3,856 g (8.5 pounds). A significant fall was seen also in premature cardiovascular deaths and was associated as well with smaller head circumference and lower ponderal index. Notably in the study, men of low-birth-weight with large placentas (highest placenta-to-birth-weight ratio) had the highest rate of mortality from cardiovascular disease. Additionally, the risk appeared to be associated more with those who were low-birth-weight newborns who experienced catch-up growth later in life (75).

The association of low-birth-weight and higher incidence of cardiovascular disease has also been seen in other areas of the world. In an Uppsala study of nearly 15,000 Swedish men born between 1915 and 1929, a 1,000-g increase in birth-weight correlated with a 0.77 reduction in the rate of coronary artery disease (76).

The association of low-birth-weight and mortality from coronary artery disease appears to be stronger for men than women, but still significant in the latter. In Nurse's Health Study, performed in the United States, 70,297 women who completed questionnaires from 1976 to 1992 were assessed. An inverse relationship between birth-weight and cardiovascular disease and stroke was noted in these women (73).

Risk factors for coronary artery disease, specifically abnormalities of cholesterol metabolism and the coagulation system, were also linked to low-birth-weight, especially head-sparing growth restriction. In an English cohort study from Sheffield, a reduction in abdominal circumference and body length at birth predicted higher serum low-density lipoprotein cholesterol and plasma fibrinogen levels in adult life. It was postulated that the small abdominal circumference reflected impaired liver growth and "reprogramming" of liver metabolism (77). In a somewhat similar British study of newborn size and corresponding adult lipid profile, men and women who had smaller abdominal circumferences at birth were found to have higher serum levels of total and low density lipoprotein cholesterol and apolipoprotein B. The association was independent of social class, adult body weight, cigarette use, or alcohol use (78).

Higher birth-weights have also been associated with a higher risk of adult onset disease, but the association has not been as strong. Men born with large abdominal circumferences (presumed large liver as well) were also noted to have an increased risk for coronary heart disease (79).

BIRTH-WEIGHT AND HYPERTENSION

Birth-weight was associated with adult hypertension at least as early as 1985 by Wadsworth and investigators (80), who studied more than 5,000 36-year-old men and noted that, in addition to adult weight, newborn weight was also statistically related to blood pressure elevation. Law and colleagues (81) studied a national sample of British children and men and women in various age categories. At all age categories beyond the newborn period, men and women who had lower birth-weights developed a higher blood pressure in adulthood. Investigators in the Nurses' Health Study evaluated women at 30 to 55 years of age and found that their birth-weight (by recollection) was inversely proportional to blood pressure in adult life (82).

Barker and associates (83) studied adult blood pressure of 327 men and women 46 to 54 years of age in relation to the placental weight and the newborn parameters of length, ponderal index, and head circumference. Even in this small cohort, there was a strong trend of higher blood pressure in adult life with lower birth-weight. Those newborns with high placental weights were also at higher risk for development of hypertension later in life.

The association of low-birth-weight with a higher risk of hypertension in adulthood has not been found in all studies. Birth-weight has been found in at least one study (84) to have a nearly negligible influence upon adult hypertension when compared to the effect of adult body mass index. In that study, birth-weight accounted for only 5% of the risk of adult hypertension when compared to adult body mass index, which accounted for 12% of the risk.

BIRTH-WEIGHT AND DIABETES

Hales and coworkers (85) evaluated fasting plasma glucose, insulin, proinsulin, and 32/33 split proinsulin concentrations, as well as glucose levels after a 75 g glucose challenge, in 468 men in a British cohort born and raised in Hertfordshire. Men of lower birth-weight had the highest rate of glucose intolerance and diabetes. The association was independent of adult body mass at the time of the study. A higher level of 32/33 split proinsulin was also related to low-birth-weight and interpreted as representation of pancreatic β-cell dysfunction. In this cohort, hypertension in adulthood was also associated with impaired glucose tolerance in adulthood. Low-birth-weight has also been associated with a higher risk of syndrome X (type 2 diabetes, hypertension, and hyperlipidemia) in adult life (86).

In a British study of forty 21-year-old men, glucose intolerance after a 75 g glucose challenge was associated with lower birth-weight independent of gestational age at birth and adult body mass, height, and social class (87). In a different study, ponderal index at birth was indirectly correlated with insulin resistance in late adulthood as measured by the rate of drop of glucose concentration after injection of insulin (88). Thinner newborns had greater glucose intolerance in adulthood. The authors remarked that thinness at birth and thinness in adult life had opposing effects. Insulin resistance and glucose intolerance increased with a low-birth-weight, but decreased with high adult weight.

Huxley and colleagues (89), as well as others (90), question the fetal origins of adult disease hypothesis. They conducted a meta-analysis of 55 studies and concluded that the association of at least low fetal weight and an increased risk of high blood pressure in adulthood is at best weak. They believe that the strength of this association was primarily because of random error, selective emphasis of particular results, and inappropriate adjustments for adult weight and confounding factors.

Current epidemiologic data regarding fetal origins, fetal programming, and intrauterine effects on development of adult disease need further evaluation to confirm both association and causation. Both genetic and environmental factors affect fetal growth. For example, women with hypertension (and at risk for coronary artery disease later in life) are more likely to have growth-restricted newborns because of their hypertension during the pregnancy. These growth-restricted newborns are genetically at higher risk of developing hypertension and thus coronary heart disease irrespective of intrauterine conditions. Confounding variables need further evaluation. It remains to be seen if a newborn's small size alone is a risk factor for adult-onset disease. Nonetheless, it is exciting to think that efforts to promote a healthy pregnancy and optimize normal fetal growth may decrease development of certain common and widespread adult disorders.

REFERENCES

1. Ramsey EM. *The placenta: human and animal.* New York: Praeger, 1982:9.
2. Pridjian G, Moawad AH, Whitington PF. Handling of beta-hydroxybutyrate in the human placenta. In: *Scientific program and abstracts.* St Louis, MO: Society for Gynecologic Investigation, 1990:230(abst).
3. Lind T, Aspillaga M. Metabolic changes during normal and diabetic pregnancies. In: Reece EA, Coustan DR, eds. *Diabetes mellitus in pregnancy: principles and practice.* New York: Churchill Livingstone, 1988:75.
4. Neufeld ND, Corbo L. Increased fetal insulin receptors and changes in membrane fluidity and lipid composition. *Am J Physiol* 1982;243:E246.
5. Dancis J. Aspects of bilirubin metabolism before and after birth. *Pediatrics* 1959;24:980.
6. Kayano T, Fukumoto H, Eddy RL, et al. Evidence for a family of human glucose transporter-like proteins. *J Biol Chem* 1988;263:15245.
7. Tadakoro C, Yoshimoto Y, Sakata M, et al. Localization of human placental glucose transporter 1 during pregnancy. An immunohistochemical study. *Histol Histopathol* 1996;11:673.
8. Johnson LW, Smith CH. Monosaccharide transport across microvillous membrane of human placenta. *Am J Physiol* 1980;238:C160.
9. Yudelivech DL, Sweiry JH. Transport of amino acids in the placenta. *Biochim Biophys Acta* 1985;822:169.

10. Miller RK, Berndt WO. Characterization of neutral amino acid accumulation by human term placental slices. *Am J Physiol* 1974; 227:1236.

11. Schneider H, Mohlen KH, Dancis J. Transfer of amino acids across the in vitro perfused human placenta. *Pediatr Res* 1979;13:236.

12. Enders RH, Judd RM, Donohue TM, et al. Placental amino acid uptake. III. Transport systems for neutral amino acids. *Am J Physiol* 1976;230:706.

13. Hibbard JU, Pridjian G, Whitington PF, et al. Taurine transport in the in vitro perfused human placenta. *Pediatr Res* 1990;27:80.

14. Fortunato SJ, Bawdon RE, Swan KF, et al. Transfer of azidothymidine (AZT) across the in vitro perfused human placenta. In: *Scientific program and abstracts*. San Diego, CA: Society for Gynecologic Investigation, 1989:82(abst).

15. Connor EM, Sperlin RS, Gelber R, et al. Reduction of maternal–infant transmission of human immunodeficiency virus type 1 with zidovudine treatment. *N Engl J Med* 1994;331:1173.

16. Ockleford CD, Whyte A. Differentiated regions of human placental cell surface associated with the exchange of materials between maternal and fetal blood. The structure, distribution, ultrastructural cytochemistry and biochemical composition of coated vesicles. *J Cell Sci* 1977;25:293.

17. McNabb T, Koh TY, Dorrington KJ, et al. Structure and function of immunoglobulin domains V. Binding of immunoglobulin G and fragments to placental membrane preparations. *J Immunol* 1976; 117:182.

18. Niezgodka M, Mikulska J, Ugorski M, et al. Human placental membrane receptor for IgG-1. Studies on the properties and solubilization of the receptor. *Mol Immunol* 1981;18:163.

19. Bussel JB, Zabusky MR, Berkowitz RL, et al. Fetal alloimmune thrombocytopenia. *N Engl J Med* 1997;337:22.

20. Okuyama T, Tawada MD, Furuya H, et al. The role of transferrin and ferritin in the fetal-maternal-placental unit. *Am J Obstet Gynecol* 1985;152:344.

21. Ringler GE, Kallen CB, Strauss JF. Regulation of human trophoblast function by glucocorticoids: dexamethasone promotes increased secretion of chorionic gonadotropin. *Endocrinology* 1989;124:1625.

22. Eldar-Geva T, Hochberg A, deGroot N, et al. High maternal serum chorionic gonadotropin level in Downs' syndrome pregnancies is caused by elevation of both subunits messenger ribonucleic acid level in trophoblasts. *J Clin Endocrinol Metab* 1995;80:3528.

23. Cohen M, Haour F, Dumont M, et al. Prognostic value of human chorionic somatomammotropin plasma levels in diabetic patients. *Am J Obstet Gynecol* 1973;115:202.

24. Adams FH, Fujiwara T. Surfactant in fetal lab tracheal fluid. *J Pediatr* 1963;63:537.

25. Goodlin RC, Anderson JC, Gallagher TF. Relationship between amniotic fluid volume and maternal plasma volume expansion. *Am J Obstet Gynecol* 1983;146:505.

26. McCoshen JA. Associations between prolactin, prostaglandin E2 and fetal membrane function in human gestation. In: Mitchell BF, ed. *The physiology and biochemistry of human fetal membranes.* Ithaca, NY: Perinatology Press, 1988:117.

27. Okazaki T, Casey ML, Okita JR, et al. Initiation of human parturition, XII. Biosynthesis and metabolism of prostaglandins in human fetal membranes and uterine decidua. *Am J Obstet Gynecol* 1981;139:373.

28. Romero R, Brody DT, Oyarzun E, et al. Infection and labor III. Interleukin-1: a signal for the onset of parturition. *Am J Obstet Gynecol* 1989;160:1117.

29. Keelan JA, Sato T, Mitchell MD. Interleukin (IL)-6 and IL-8 by human amnion: regulation by cytokines, growth factors, glucocorticoids, phorbol esters, and bacterial lipopolysaccharide. *Biol Reprod* 1997;57:1438.

30. Romero R, Avila C, Santhanam U, et al. Amniotic fluid interleukin 6 in preterm labor: association with infection. *J Clin Invest* 1990;85:1392.

31. Goldberg RL, Hauth JC, Andrews WW. Intrauterine infection and preterm delivery. *N Engl J Med* 2000;342:1500.

32. Benirschke K, Kaufmann P. *Pathology of the human placenta,* 2nd ed. New York: Springer-Verlag, 1990:182.

33. Silver RK, Dooley SL, Tamura RK, et al. Umbilical cord size and amniotic fluid volume in prolonged pregnancy. *Am J Obstet Gynecol* 1987;157:716.

34. Robertson RD, Rubinstein LM, Wolfson WL, et al. Constriction of the umbilical cord as a cause of fetal demise following midtrimester amniocentesis. *J Reprod Med* 1981;26:325.

35. Pridjian G, Puschett JB. Preeclampsia part I: clinical and pathophysiologic considerations. *Obstet Gynecol Surv* 2002;57:598.

36. Pridjian G, Puschett JB. Preeclampsia part II: experimental and genetic considerations. *Obstet Gynecol Surv* 2002;57:619.

37. Boyd PA, Scott A. Quantitative structural studies on human placentas associated with preeclampsia, essential hypertension and intrauterine growth retardation. *Br J Obstet Gynaecol* 1985; 92(7):714–721.

38. Cibils LA. The placenta and newborn infant in hypertensive conditions. *Am J Obstet Gynecol* 1974;118:256.

39. Khong TY, De Wolf F, Robertson, WB, et al. Inadequate maternal vascular response to placentation in pregnancies complicated by preeclampsia and by small for gestational age infants. *Br J Obstet Gynaecol* 1986;93:1049.

40. Damsky CH, Fitzgerald ML, Fisher SJ. Distribution patterns of extracellular matrix components and adhesion receptors are intricately modulated during first trimester cytotrophoblast differentiation along the invasive pathway, in vivo. *J Clin Invest* 1992;89: 210.

41. Zhou Y, Damsky CH, Fisher SJ. Preeclampsia is associated with failure of human cytotrophoblasts to mimic a vascular adhesion phenotype. Once cause of defective endovascular invasion in this syndrome? *J Clin Invest* 1997;99:2152.

42. Zeek PM, Assali NS. Vascular changes in the decidua associated with eclamptogenic toxemia of pregnancy. *Am J Clin Pathol* 1950;20:1099.

43. Out HJ, Kooijman CD, Bruinse HW, et al. Histopathological findings in placentae from patients with intrauterine fetal death and antiphospholipid antibodies. *Eur J Obstet Gynecol Reprod Biol* 1991;41:179.

44. Walsh SW. Preeclampsia: an imbalance in placental prostacyclin and thromboxane production. *Am J Obstet Gynecol* 1985;152:335.

45. Wallenburg HC, Rotmans N. Enhanced reactivity of the platelet thromboxane pathway in normotensive and hypertensive pregnancies with insufficient fetal growth. *Am J Obstet Gynecol* 1982;144:523.

46. Teasdale F. Histomorphometry of the placenta of the diabetic woman. Class A diabetes mellitus. *Placenta* 1981;2:241.

47. Teasdale F. Histomorphometry of the human placenta in class B diabetes mellitus. *Placenta* 1983;4:1.

48. Teasdale F. Histomorphometry of the human placenta in class C diabetes mellitus. *Placenta* 1985;6:69.

49. Deal CL, Guyda HJ. Insulin receptors of human term placental cells and choriocarcinoma (JEG-3) cells: characteristics and regulation. *Endocrinology* 1983;112:1512.

50. Challier JC, Hauguel S, Desmaizieres V. Effect of insulin on glucose uptake and metabolism in the human placenta. *J Clin Endocrinol Metab* 1986;62:803.

51. Grizzard JD, D'Ercole AJ, Wilkins JR, et al. Affinity-labeled somatomedin-C receptors and binding proteins from the human fetus. *J Clin Endocrinol Metab* 1984;58:535.

52. Fant M, Monro H, Moses AC. An autocrine/paracrine role for insulin-like growth factors in the regulation of human placental growth. *J Clin Endocrinol Metab* 1986;63:499.

53. Hall K, Hansson U, Lundin G, et al. Serum levels of somatomedins and somatomedin-binding protein in pregnant women with type I or gestational diabetes and their infants. *J Clin Endocrinol Metab* 1986;63:1300.

54. Thomas CR. Placental transfer of non-esterified fatty acids in normal and diabetic pregnancy. *Biol Neonate* 1987;51:94.

55. Hatjis CG. Nonimmunologic fetal hydrops associated with hyperreactio luteinalis. *Obstet Gynecol* 1985;65[Suppl]:11S–13S.

56. Pryde PG, Nugent CE, Pridjian G, et al. Spontaneous resolution of nonimmune hydrops fetalis secondary to parvovirus B19 infection. *Obstet Gynecol* 1992;79:869.

57. Robertson EG, Neer KJ. Placental injection studies in twin gestation. *Am J Obstet Gynecol* 1983;147:170.

58. Benirschke K, Kaufmann P. *Pathology of the human placenta,* 2nd ed. New York: Springer-Verlag, 1990:658.

59. Pridjian G, Nugent CE, Barr M. Twin gestation: influence of placentation on fetal growth. *Am J Obstet Gynecol* 1991;165:1394.

60. Benirschke K. Prenatal cardiovascular adaptation, comparative pathophysiology of circulatory disturbances. In: Bloor CM, ed. *Advances in experimental medicine and biology.* New York: Plenum Press, 1972:3.

61. D'Alton ME, Dudley DK. The ultrasonographic prediction of chorionicity in twin gestation. *Am J Obstet Gynecol* 1989;160:557.

62. Elliott JP, Urig MA, Clewell WH. Aggressive therapeutic amniocentesis for treatment of twin-twin transfusion syndrome. *Obstet Gynecol* 1991;77:537.

63. De Lia JE, Cruikshank DP, Keye WR. Fetoscopic neodymium:YAG laser occlusion of placental vessels in severe twin-twin transfusion syndrome. *Obstet Gynecol* 1990;75:1046.

64. Christianson C, Huff D, McPherson E. Limb deformations in oligohydramnios sequence: effects of gestational age and duration of oligohydramnios *Am J Medical Genetics.* 1999;86:430.

65. Curry CJ, Jensen K, Holland J, et al. The Potter sequence: a clinical analysis of 80 cases. *Am J Med Genet* 1984;19:679.

66. Simpson JL, Elias S, Martin AO, et al. Diabetes in pregnancy, Northwestern University series (1977–1981). I. Prospective study of anomalies in offspring of mothers with diabetes mellitus. *Am J Obstet Gynecol* 1983;146:263.

67. Rouse B, Azen C, Koch R, et al. Maternal Phenylketonuria Collaborative Study (MPKUCS) offspring: facial anomalies, malformations, and early neurological sequelae. *Am J Med Genet* 1997;69:89.

68. Shahinian HK, Jackle R, Suh Rh, et al. Obstetrical factors governing the etiopathogenesis of lambdoid synostosis. *Am J Perinatol* 1998;15:281.

69. Barker DH, Winter PD, Osmond C, et al. Weight in infancy and death from ischaemic heart disease. *Lancet* 1989;2:577.

70. Koukkou E, Ghosh P, Lowy C, et al. Offspring of normal and diabetic rats fed saturated fat in pregnancy demonstrate vascular dysfunction. *Circulation* 1998;98:2899.

71. Vickers MH, Ikenasio BA, Breier BH. Adult growth hormone treatment reduces hypertension and obesity induced by an adverse prenatal environment. *J of Endocrinology* 2002;175:615.

72. Barker DJP, Osmond C. Infant mortality, childhood nutrition, and ischaemic heart disease in England and Wales. *Lancet* 1986;1:1077.

73. Rich-Edwards J, Stampfer M, Manson J, et al. Birth weight and risk of cardiovascular disease in a cohort of women followed up since 1976. *BMS* 1997;315:396–400.

74. Barker DJ. Osmond C, Simmonds SJ, et al. The relation of small head circumference and thinness at birth to death from cardiovascular disease in adult life. *BMJ* 1993;306:422.

75. Barker DJ, Eriksson JG, Forsen T, et al. Fetal origins of adult disease: strength of effects and biological basis. *Int J Epidemiol* 2002;31:1235.

76. Leon DA, Lithell HO, Vg D, et al. Reduced fetal growth rate and increased risk of death from ischaemic heart disease: cohort study of 15, 000 Swedish men and women born 1915–29. *BMJ* 1998;317:241.

77. Roseboom TJ, van der Meulen JH, Ravelli AC, et al. Plasma fibrinogen and factor VII concentrations in adults after prenatal exposure to famine. *Br J Haematol* 2000;111:112–117.

78. Barker DJ, Martyn CN, Hales, et al. Growth in utero and serum cholesterol concentrations in adult life. *BMJ* 1993;307:1524.

79. Barker DJP, Martyn CN, Osmond C, et al. Abnormal liver growth in utero and death from coronary heart disease. *BMJ* 1995;310:703.

80. Wadsworth ME, Cripps HA, Midwinter RE, et al. Blood pressure in a national birth cohort at the age of 36 related to social and familial factors, smoking and body mass. *BMJ* 1985;291:1534.

81. Law CM, de Swiet M, Osmond C, et al. Initiation of hypertension in utero and its amplification throughout life. *BMJ* 1993;306:24.

82. Curham GC, Chertow GM, Willett WC, et al. Birth weight and adult hypertension and obesity in women. *Circulation* 1996;94:1310.

83. Barker DJ, Godfrey KM, Osmond, et al. The relation of fetal length, ponderal index and head circumference to blood pressure and the risk of hypertension in adult life. *Paediatr Perinat Epidemiol* 1992;6:35.

84. Holland FJ, Stark O, Ades AE, et al. Birth weight and body mass index in childhood, adolescence, and adulthood as predictors of blood pressure at age 36. *J Epidemiol Commun H* 1993;47(6):432–435.

85. Hales CN, Barker DJ, Clark PM, et al. Fetal and infant growth and impaired glucose tolerance at age 64. *BMJ* 1991;303:1474.

86. Barker DJ, Hales CN, Fall CH, et al. Type 2 (non-insulin-dependent) diabetes mellitus, hypertension and hyperlipidemia (syndrome X): relation to reduced fetal growth. 1993;36:62.

87. Robinson S, Walton RJ, Clark PM, et al. The relation of fetal growth to plasma glucose in young men. *Diabetologia* 1992;35:444.

88. Phillips DI, Barker DJ, Hales CN, et al. Thinness at birth and insulin resistance in adult life. *Diabetologia* 1994;37:150.

89. Huxley R, Neil A, Collins R. Unraveling the fetal origins hypothesis: is there really an inverse association between birthweight and subsequent blood pressure? *Lancet* 2002;360:659–665.

90. Williams S, Poulton R. Birth size, growth, and blood pressure between the ages of 7 and 26 years: failure to support the fetal origins hypothesis. *Am J Epidemiol* 2002;155:849.

Fetal Imaging: Ultrasound and Magnetic Resonance Imaging

12

Dorothy I. Bulas

Advances in high-resolution sonographic imaging and rapid sequencing magnetic resonance imaging (MRI) have provided exquisite detail regarding the fetus and intrauterine environment. The ability to assess the health of the fetus and identify anomalies has changed the practice of both obstetrics and neonatology. By identifying the fetus with anomalies or at risk for intrauterine compromise, management can be guided by appropriate specialists with resultant improved outcome.

ASSESSMENT OF FETAL AGE, GROWTH, AND MATURITY

Accurate assessment of fetal age is crucial for perinatal management. Overestimating the age of a fetus can result in the delivery of a premature infant, whereas underestimating the age of a growth-retarded fetus can result in a fetal death.

Fetal age can be determined based on obstetric history and clinical data, but estimations can be inaccurate in up to 40% of patients (1). The use of ultrasound provides a method of significantly improving the accuracy of gestational age determination. Measurements used to assess age have been chosen on the basis of their relationship with gestational age and ease in obtaining these measurements and reproducibility. The fetal biparietal diameter (BPD) measurement was the first measurement used because the cranium was the most easily visualized body part (2). There are many tables and nomograms that describe the normal growth of various fetal organs. Most predictions of gestational age are based on the 50th percentile measurement with a wide range of normal values. At the various gestational ages, each fetal dimension differs in how easily

and reliably it can be measured. Thus, a combination of measurements is superior to a single measurement, with computer software that permits instantaneous calculation of fetal age and weight estimates and plotting growth curves. Functional studies of the fetus, such as breathing patterns, can also aid in the determination of gestational age.

DETERMINING FETAL AGE

First-Trimester Assessment

In the first trimester, fetal imaging using a transabdominal approach is often difficult because the uterus is low within the maternal pelvis and may be obscured by overlying gas. Transvaginal ultrasound transducers greatly improve fetal visualization in early pregnancy. The probe is placed into the maternal vagina in close proximity to the uterus and fetus. High-resolution fetal images can thus be obtained for accurate assessment of fetal morphology. By use of transvaginal scanning, a gestational sac can be seen by 5 weeks menstrual age, and fetal heart activity by 6 weeks menstrual age. With abdominal scanning, these findings are first identified reliably a week later, at 6 and 7 weeks, respectively.

Crown–rump length is the most accurate dimension for assessing gestational age in the first trimester, with a 95% confidence interval of ±2 to 3.5 days (3). Measurement of the gestational sac diameter can also be used to estimate age, although it is not as accurate as a result of variability in the shape of the sac. Fetal biparietal diameter and abdominal circumference are also relatively good predictors of menstrual age in the first trimester (4).

TABLE 12-1

RELATIONSHIPS AMONG SELECTED FETAL INDICES AS MEASURED BY ULTRASOUND AND GESTATIONAL AGE AS DETERMINED BY MENSTRUAL WEEKS

Menstrual Age (wk)	Biparietal Diameter (cm)	Head Circumference (cm)	Abdominal Circumference (cm)	Femur Length (cm)
12	2	7.1	5.6	0.8
13	2.3	8.4	6.9	1.1
14	2.7	9.8	8.1	1.5
15	3	11.1	9.3	1.8
16	3.3	12.4	10.5	2.1
17	3.7	13.7	11.7	2.4
18	4	15	12.9	2.7
19	4.3	16.3	14.1	3
20	4.6	17.5	15.2	3.3
21	5	18.7	16.4	3.6
22	5.3	19.9	17.5	3.9
23	5.6	21	18.6	4.2
24	5.8	22.1	19.7	4.4
25	6.1	23.2	20.8	4.7
26	6.4	24.2	21.9	4.9
27	6.7	25.2	22.9	5.2
28	7	26.2	24	5.4
29	7.2	27.1	25	5.6
30	7.5	28	26	5.8
31	7.7	28.9	27	6.1
32	7.9	29.7	28	6.3
33	8.2	30.4	29	6.5
34	8.4	31.2	30	6.6
35	8.6	31.8	30.9	6.8
36	8.8	32.5	31.8	7
37	9	33.1	32.7	7.2
38	9.1	33.6	33.6	7.3
39	9.3	34.1	34.5	7.5
40	9.5	34.5	35.4	7.6

From Hadlock FP, Deter RL, Harrist RB. Computer assisted analysis of fetal age using multiple fetal growth parameters. *J Clin Ultrasound* 1983;11:313, with permission.

Second- and Third-Trimester Assessment

After 12 weeks of gestation, the crown–rump length is difficult to obtain accurately. In the second and third trimesters, the main parameters of fetal age are the BPD, head circumference, abdominal circumference, and femoral length (Table 12-1).

The fetal BPD is quick, reliable, and easy to obtain. It measures the transverse diameter of the upper midbrain at the level of the thalamic nuclei and cavum septum pellucidum from the external surface of one proximal parietal bone to the inner surface of the contralateral parietal bone (Fig. 12-1) (5). The earlier the gestational age the greater the predictive accuracy of this measurement.

Inaccuracies in measurements of the BPD may result from improper selection of the measurement plane (6). In late pregnancy, the fetal head may be too low in the pelvis to measure. Cranial molding, either from fetal position or oligohydramnios, may result in BPD measurements that do not accurately reflect true gestational age (Fig. 12-2).

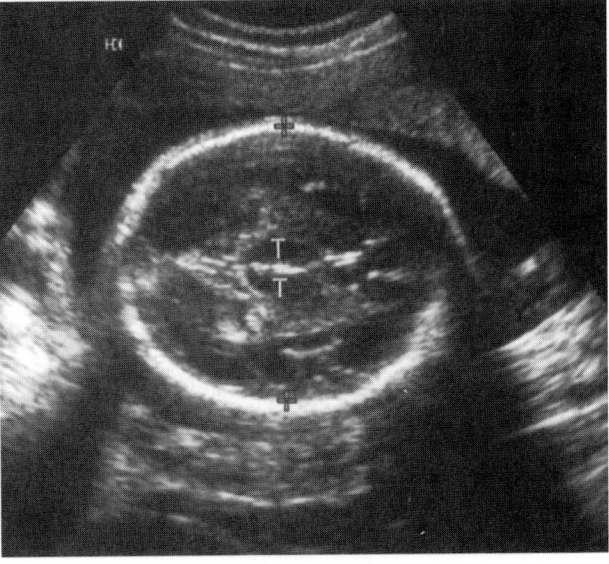

Figure 12-1 Fetal biparietal diameter (BPD). Axial scan of the head at the standardized level for BPD measurement shows the thalami.

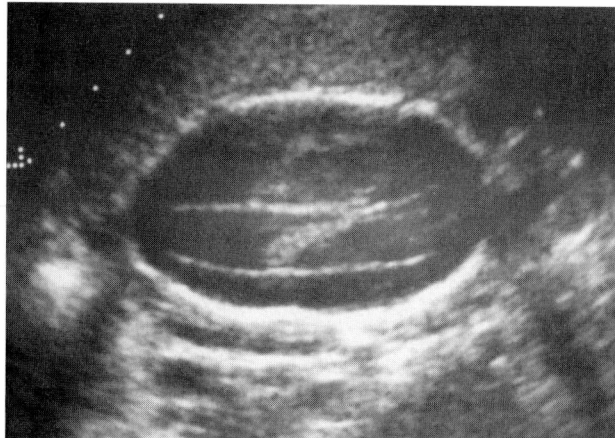

Figure 12-2 Transverse image of the brain of a 23-week fetus with severe oligohydramnios demonstrates a narrow and elongated skull. Cephalic index was abnormally low.

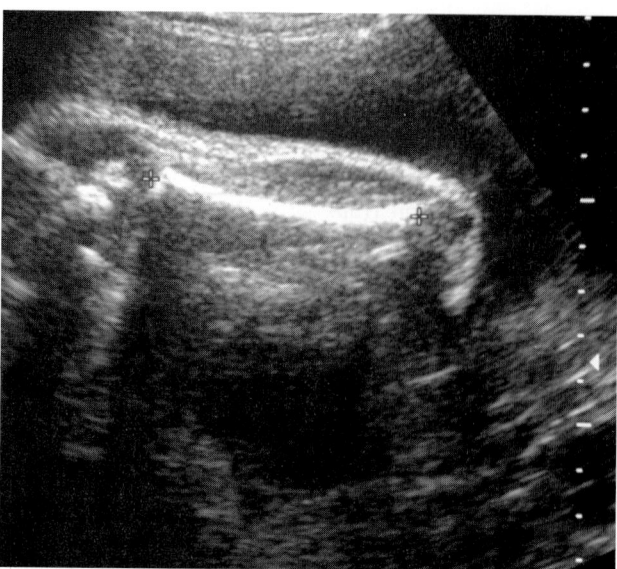

Figure 12-3 Longitudinal scan of the fetal thigh demonstrates a femur length of 3.5 cm consistent with a 21-week gestation. Measurement is from the greater trochanter to the distal end of the femur.

The cephalic index, which measures the relationship between the short and long axes of the fetal head, should be measured if the head shape appears abnormal. If this index is below 70 or above 86, the biparietal diameter should not be used in the age and weight estimates (7). The accuracy of BPD measurements decreases with advancing gestational age. In the second trimester, a BPD measurement carries a predictive accuracy of ±7 days, whereas in the late third trimester it carries a predictive accuracy of ±3 weeks (7). Serial measurements of BPD can improve the predictive accuracy (8). The fetal head circumference is obtained from the same axial image used for the BPD. This measurement is more accurate than the BPD in the third trimester, as it is less affected by shape (7).

The measurement of the fetal abdominal circumference is made from an axial image of the abdomen at the level of the portal vein. The circumference of the head is typically larger than the abdominal circumference up to 34 weeks of gestation, and the abdomen becomes larger thereafter. In the presence of intrauterine growth retardation (IUGR), head size tends to be preserved compared to abdominal size altering the head circumference to abdominal circumference ratio.

Femur length is defined as the distance between the greater trochanter and the distal end of the femur (Fig. 12-3) (9). Gestational age prediction from femur length is subject to error either from measurement difficulties caused by difficulty in visualizing the ends of the bone or from biological variation. The predictive accuracy of femur length ranges from ±1 week at 12 weeks of gestation to ±3 weeks at 36 weeks of gestation (10).

Estimation of fetal age is best accomplished using a composite assessment of multiple fetal measurements. A combination of head size (BPD or head circumference), femur length, and abdominal circumference is most commonly used. Estimates have an error of ±1.46 weeks between 24 and 30 weeks of gestation and increase to 2.3 weeks at 36 weeks of gestation (11). Individual measurements should not be used for assessing gestational age when they are affected by a pathological process; for exam-

ple, head measurements in a hydrocephalic fetus or long bone measurements in the fetus with a bone dysplasia. After 22 weeks, age-independent fetal body ratios are useful in identifying asymmetric measurements. If the cephalic index is normal, the ratio of femur length to BPD can be measured, with normal results ranging between 71 and 87. The ratio of femur length to abdominal circumference should range between 20 and 24 (12).

FETAL WEIGHT ESTIMATES

It would be helpful in the assessment of fetal age, growth, and maturity if an accurate, reproducible method of determining fetal weight were available. Ultrasonographic estimates of fetal weight have been derived from single measurements such as BPD or abdominal circumference (13) and by a combination of measurements such as abdominal circumference and BPD (14). All ultrasonographic methods for fetal weight estimations, however, contain inherent error. Measurement of abdominal circumference yields an average error of 18% (13). The BPD and abdominal circumference yield a similar error (20%) (15). The absolute estimated error decreases as birth weight decreases.

The use of multiple parameters, especially head, abdomen, and femur measurements, provides the most accurate measurement of fetal weight. However, it is still not accurate in extremely low or high birth weight fetuses. Because fetal weight estimates remain imprecise, estimation of fetal age based solely on estimates of fetal weight should not be used. Incremental fetal weight change can be determined with serial ultrasounds and is one way of detecting abnormal fetal growth (10). In the future, three-dimensional fetal MRI reconstruction and volume estimates may improve the accuracy of fetal weight determination (16).

ASSESSMENT OF FETAL GROWTH

Fetal growth abnormalities are often associated with increased risk of perinatal morbidity and mortality. The rate of growth in the normal fetus varies with gestational age, with an increasing exponential curve in the first trimester, a linear curve in the second and most of the third trimester, and a decreasing exponential curve after 36 weeks of gestation (17). Serial ultrasonographic measurements can be plotted to evaluate fetal growth and may include weight estimates derived from a combination of these variables.

Intrauterine Growth Retardation

The infant whose birth weight is below the tenth percentile for gestational age is considered small for gestational age (SGA). The population of SGA infants whose weight falls below the tenth percentile is heterogeneous. Normal but small fetuses represent up to 60% of the SGA group, fetuses with congenital anomalies account for up to 15%, and fetuses with true IUGR account for 25% (18). Management varies among these groups. The normal but small fetus is not at increased risk and does not require intervention. The small fetus with true growth restriction may be at high morbidity or mortality risk and may require immediate intervention. The small infant with congenital abnormalities may or may not require intervention. It can be difficult determining which group an SGA fetus falls into, particularly when the true gestational age is unknown.

Ultrasound's ability to identify the truly IUGR fetus is variable and is most successful when the disease state is severe. A slowing of the rate of head and femur growth is apparent with severe IUGR (19,20) but is more difficult to identify when the retardation is mild or early. Growth-adjusted sonographic age determination based on BPD or abdominal circumference (6,20) uses serial ultrasonographic measurements. This method assumes that fetal growth should remain within a narrow percentile band and that deviation from this may be an early sign of growth disorders (21). Because of the inherent errors, serial estimation of fetal weight identifies only the most severe growth disturbances. Asymmetric growth suggests IUGR. Abnormal ratios of head circumference to abdominal circumference, as a result of loss of liver mass with normal head growth, can be seen in severe IUGR but may not be present in milder cases (22).

Secondary signs aid in assessing the presence and severity of IUGR. Oligohydramnios often develops during episodes of uteroplacental insufficiency, most likely because of decreased fetal urine production and pulmonary fluid during episodes of fetal hypoxemia (23). Amniotic fluid volume may be assessed subjectively or by the semiquantitative method of measuring the vertical diameter of the largest visible pocket of amniotic fluid. The amniotic fluid index (AFI) is calculated by adding the vertical depths of the largest pocket in each of four equal uterine quadrants (24). Oligohydramnios has been defined by the absence of identifiable amniotic fluid pockets or when the maximum vertical pocket measures less than 2 cm in two perpendicular planes or when the amniotic fluid index measures less than 5 cm. Oligohydramnios as defined by any one of the methods is predictive of increased peripartum morbidity and mortality (24–26). Milder cases of IUGR, however, may not be associated with oligohydramnios (27).

Assessing fetal condition using the biophysical profile score (BPS) or Doppler velocity ratios of the umbilical artery and/or fetal middle cerebral artery are additional useful adjuncts in the diagnosis of IUGR (see Doppler Assessment of Blood Velocities in Umbilical and Fetal Vessels) (28). If a fetus who is being followed for IUGR has no signs of asphyxial compromise, continued observation rather than intervention may be reasonable.

Macrosomia

The infant whose birth weight is above the 90th percentile for gestational age is labeled large for dates (LGA) or macrosomic. This group of large infants is heterogeneous, composed of normal but large infants and infants with abnormally increased growth. Macrosomia is usually associated with maternal glucose abnormalities. Macrosomia may lead to obstetric complications such as shoulder dystocia, although maternal diabetes may cause neonatal complications such as hypoglycemia, polycythemia, and cardiac abnormalities (29). Detection of macrosomia sonographically includes serial assessment of growth and the relationship of the variables. The ratio of abdominal circumference to head circumference is particularly useful in identifying an enlarging abdomen indicative of excessive weight gain. Other measurements have been proposed to aid in the diagnosis of macrosomia, including soft tissue thickness of the humerus or femur and cheek-to-cheek diameter (30).

Fetal Maturity

The sonographic assessment of fetal maturity is useful in the optimal timing of perinatal management. The perinatologist must maintain a balance between the risk of fetal death and the risk of neonatal death based on an estimate of whether a fetus has reached an age and weight at which lung maturity is possible. Fetal age and weight determinations, evaluation of placental architecture, and the biophysical profile have been used to assess fetal maturity. Studies on elective deliveries based on BPD, or weight estimates based on BPD and abdominal circumference, have shown good results (31–33). The grading of placental maturity sonographically, however, has not been shown to be as accurate in assessing lung maturity as examination of the amniotic fluid (34).

FETAL ANATOMY

Congenital anomalies are present in 2% to 5% of newborns and account for 20% to 30% of perinatal deaths (35). High-resolution ultrasonography has produced significant

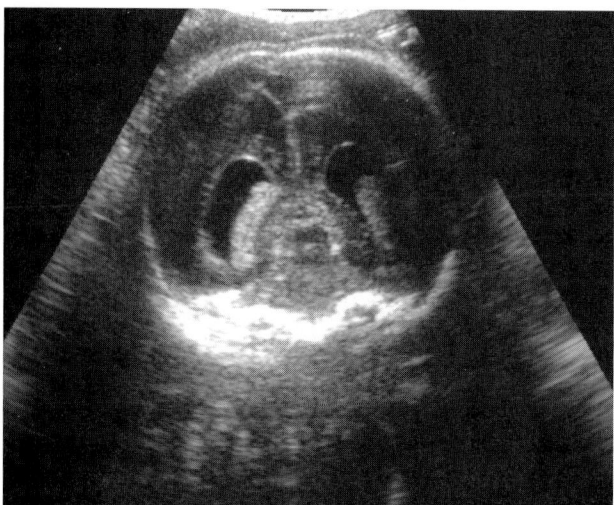

Figure 12-4 Transvaginal scan of the fetal brain in the coronal plane clearly demonstrates mild dilatation of both occipital horns.

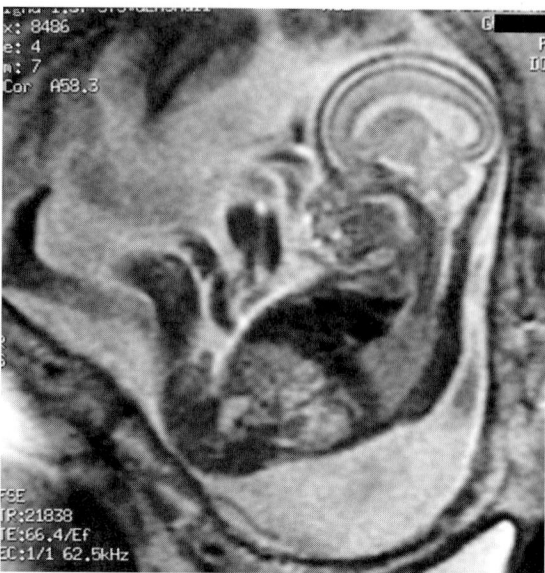

Figure 12-5 Large field of view T2 weighted sagittal image demonstrates the brain, chest, abdomen, and leg of a 20 week fetus.

changes in the diagnosis and management of these anomalies, including the potential for therapeutic intervention. Factors to be considered in the counseling of these cases include gestational age, effect on maternal outcome, and neonatal prognosis with or without therapy. Amniocentesis should be considered in cases at risk for a chromosomal anomaly.

Ultrasound is the initial imaging modality of choice for the assessment of the fetus as it is safe, inexpensive, and easily performed. A comprehensive sonographic review includes a survey of the fetus, followed by evaluation of amniotic fluid volume, cord structure, and the placenta. A functional review of the fetus including hand clenching and swallowing is informative. Because some anomalies may not become evident until later in gestation (such as progressive hydrocephalus, congenital diaphragmatic hernia), follow-up evaluation of the fetus at risk is important. Transvaginal sonography and three-dimensional sonographic imaging have provided a means of improved visualization of fetal anomalies, particularly of the face and brain (Fig. 12-4).

Fetal Magnetic Resonance Imaging

Factors such as fetal lie, maternal obesity, and oligohydramnios may interfere with the sonographic evaluation of fetus. MRI is an alternative modality to evaluate the fetus as it uses no ionizing radiation, has excellent tissue contrast, large field of view and multiplanar capabilities (Fig. 12-5) (36,37). The development of faster scanning techniques now allow studies to be performed without sedation in the second trimester with superior contrast, and without significant motion artifact.

Although there currently is no evidence that the use of clinical MRI produces deleterious effects on human embryos, the safety of MRI during pregnancy has not been definitively demonstrated (37,38). While there has been concern that prolonged exposure to electromagnetic radia-

tion may be linked to deleterious effects on embryogenesis, animal studies on embryos have so far demonstrated no growth abnormalities (40,41). Limited follow-up studies on children exposed to fetal MRI also have not demonstrated developmental abnormalities (40,42,43). Due to the possibility of unknown effects, MRI currently is used as a complementary study only when ultrasound results are inadequate for diagnosis or when MR imaging is expected to provide important additional information.

With advances in the diagnosis and treatment of fetal abnormalities there is an increasing need for precise depiction of abnormalities. Fetal MRI not only confirms the presence of lesions noted by ultrasound, but also can demonstrate additional subtle anomalies. This information helps appropriate specialists, including the neonatologist, counsel families when difficult decisions must be made regarding early and potentially invasive intervention and allows for optimal delivery planning.

Fetal Central Nervous System Abnormalities

Fetal central nervous system (CNS) abnormalities may be detected in the first trimester in severe cases such as anencephaly. The most favorable time to evaluate the fetal neural axis, however, is 18 to 24 weeks of gestation, when resolution is sufficient to identify most structures including the spine. Abnormal measurements of BPD and head circumference may be the first suggestion of a CNS abnormality. Structural evaluation includes the shape and size of the head, ventricles, and posterior fossa and an evaluation of the spine. If a CNS anomaly is identified, careful evaluation for other anomalies, especially of the face, heart, and kidneys, follows.

The ventricular diameter normally measures less than 10 mm throughout the second and third trimesters

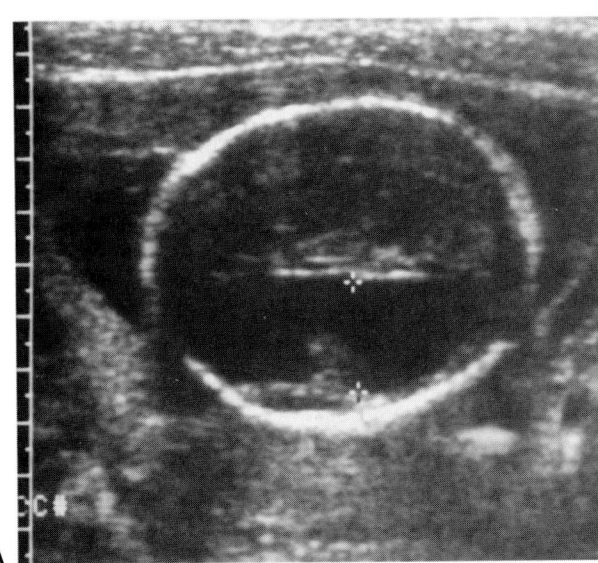 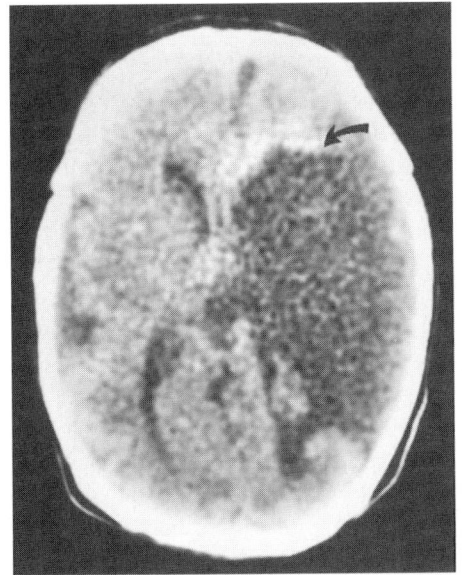

Figure 12-6 **A:** Axial sonogram of the brain at 29 weeks of gestation demonstrates unilateral dilatation of the left lateral ventricle (cursers). **B:** Follow-up CT scan at birth confirms the finding of left hemispheric porencephaly (arrow).

(44,45). Other criteria of ventriculomegaly include separation of choroid plexus from the medial ventricular wall. If the diagnosis of ventriculomegaly is established, a search for its etiology should be made. A differential diagnosis ranges from cerebral atrophy (hydranencephaly, porencephaly) (Fig. 12-6), dysgenesis (holoprosencephaly, agenesis of the corpus callosum), to true hydrocephalus.

There are significant limitations in the sonographic evaluation of the fetal brain as a result of refraction artifact from the skull and low sensitivity to cortical malformations. MRI better defines anomalies of the posterior fossa, corpus callosum, and developing gray and white matter. Three planes of the brain can be obtained with excellent delineation of the extraaxial spaces (Fig. 12-7). Sulcal and gyral development can be assessed allowing for estimation of brain maturity (Fig. 12-8) (46–48).

Hydrocephalus

Hydrocephalus can be caused by an increased rate of cerebrospinal fluid (CSF) formation as in choroid plexus papilloma, decreased resorption of CSF after hemorrhage, or obstruction of CSF flow as a result of tumor or aqueductal stenosis (49). In many cases, the etiology of hydrocephalus remains unknown. Up to 85% of cases are associated with other neurological, cardiac, renal, gastrointestinal (GI), or skeletal anomalies. Up to 10% are associated with chromosomal abnormalities (50). Fetuses with other anatomic or chromosomal abnormalities have a grim prognosis for long-term development. When ventriculomegaly is mild, and no associated abnormalities are identified, outcome is less severe. Up to 20% of these cases, however, may demonstrate neurological abnormalities later in life (51–53).

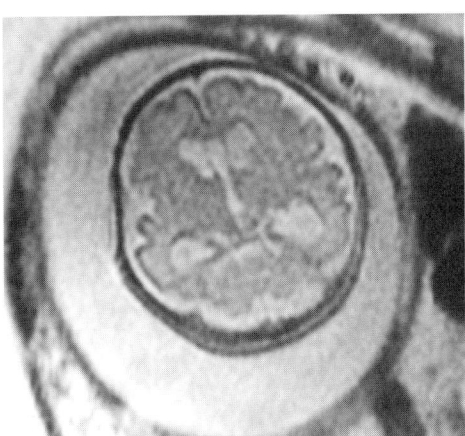

Figure 12-7 Coronal T2 weighted image through the brain of a 25 week fetus with aqueductal stenosis demonstrates moderate lateral and third ventricular dilatation.

Figure 12-8 Oblique T2 weighted image through the brain of a 32 week fetus with trisomy 21 demonstrates moderate ventriculomegaly with a more mature sulcation pattern.

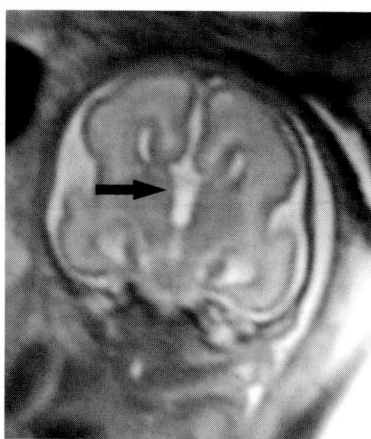

Figure 12-9 Coronal T2 weighted image through the brain of 19 week gestation demonstrates agenesis of the corpus callosum and high riding third ventricle.

MRI is useful in confirming the presence of ventriculomegaly, and can assess symmetry of ventricular size and contour. Irregularity of the ventricular wall and adjacent parenchymal abnormalities may indicate post inflammatory and destructive changes. Atrophy, hemorrhages, or masses may be identified (48). Identifying the etiology for ventriculomegaly, however, may still be difficult as subtle gyral abnormalities and parenchymal changes may be impossible to detect by MRI in the second trimester.

Multiplanar views are particularly useful in the evaluation of the corpus callosum, which develops between 8 to 17 weeks gestation (Fig. 12-9). When severe, holoprosencephaly can be identified by ultrasound; less severe semilobar and lobar types are more difficult to diagnose even by MRI.

The posterior fossa and brain stem are well delineated by MRI and can help differentiate Dandy Walker malformation for posterior fossa arachnoid cysts or mega cisterna magna (Fig 12-10).

Vascular CNS anomalies including vein of Galen aneurysms are well demonstrated by MRI. Hemorrhage and or encephalomalacia suggests a poorer prognosis and is better demonstrated by MRI.

Neural Tube Defects

The most common condition leading to ventriculomegaly is spina bifida. Evaluation of the fetal spine and cerebellum allows prenatal identification of over 95% of fetuses with meningomyeloceles. Screening programs using maternal serum α-fetoprotein identify pregnancies at risk for neural tube or ventral wall defects. Sonographic findings of meningomyelocele include splaying of pedicles, presence of a cystic collection posterior to the fetal spine with absent skin covering, and scoliosis. Because of the difficulty in identifying small spinal defects prenatally, the association of cranial abnormalities is useful in evaluating cases at risk. The Arnold-Chiari malformation, which often accompanies spina bifida, results in the herniation of the cerebellum through the foramen magnum into the upper cervical spinal canal. Cranial sonographic findings of this malformation include frontal bone scalloping (lemon sign), abnormal curvature of the cerebellum (banana sign), and obliteration of the cisterna magna (54,55). MRI is useful in the confirmation of Chiari malformations, with amount of tonsillar herniation measured (46).

Cranial defects involving brain (encephalocele) or meninges (meningocele) may present with ventriculomegaly (Fig 12-11). Typically on ultrasonography there is a posterior paracranial mass that is cystic or solid. It is important to identify a true skull defect because the diagnosis can be confused with scalp edema, cystic hygroma, or scalp hemangiomas, which carry a better prognosis (56). MRI is particularly useful in identifying intracranial anomalies associated with encephaloceles. Because encephalocele is a feature of other syndromes including Meckel-Gruber, additional anomalies should be excluded (57).

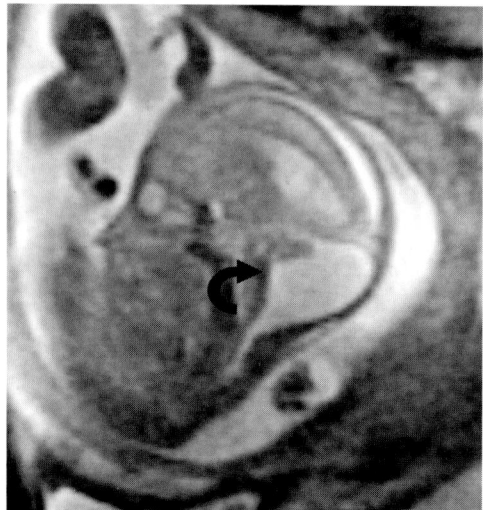

Figure 12-10 Sagittal T2 weighted image of a 22 week gestation demonstrates a Dandy Walker cyst with absent inferior vermis.

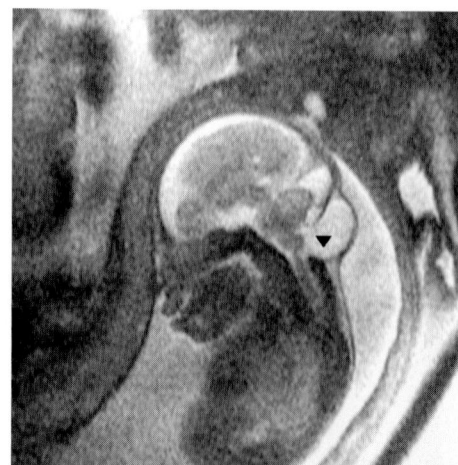

Figure 12-11 Sagitta T2 weighted image of a 24 week fetus demonstrates an occipital meningocele with microcephaly and sulcation anomalies.

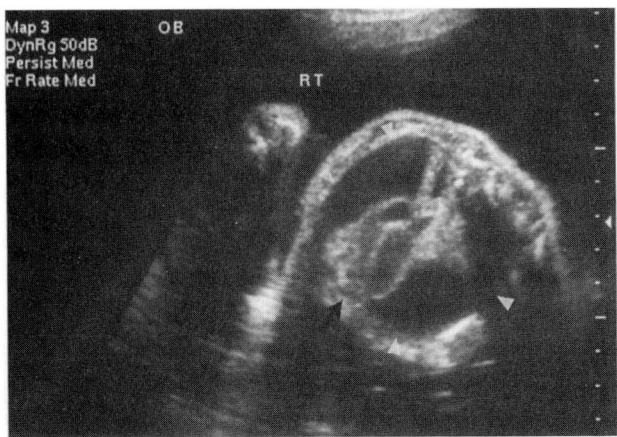

Figure 12-12 Transverse image through the chest of a 25-week fetus demonstrates bilateral large pleural effusions (white arrowheads). The heart (black arrow) is slightly deviated to the right.

Fetal Chest Abnormalities

Many major intrathoracic structures can be identified sonographically by the second trimester. A small chest circumference suggests pulmonary hypoplasia in the presence of oligohydramnios or skeletal dysplasia (58). Pleural effusions appear as fluid collections surrounding collapsed echogenic lung (Fig. 12-12). Effusions may be primary in chylothorax or secondary in nonimmune hydrops. In the presence of effusions, prognosis is variable, with 15% mortality if an effusion is isolated but up to 95% mortality if it is associated with severe hydrops (59,60).

The normal fetal mediastinum lies in the center of the chest, anterior to the spine, with the cardiac interventricular septum forming a 45-degree angle with the midline. Deviation of this axis or shift of the heart suggests a mass effect or cardiac pathology.

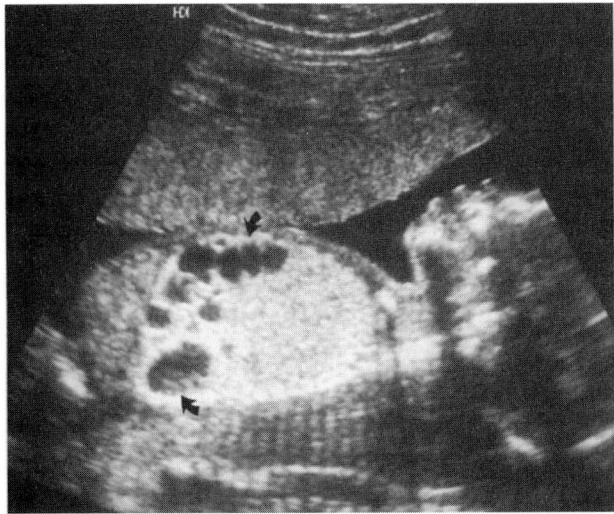

Figure 12-13 Cystic adenomatoid malformation. Sagittal image of the left fetal chest at 26 weeks of gestation demonstrates multiple cysts (arrows) within the left hemithorax dispersed between unusually echogenic lung parenchyma.

Fetal lung parenchyma should be homogeneously echogenic. If it is heterogenous and/or there is shift of midline structures, a chest mass is likely. Sonographic findings will vary depending on the type of chest mass. Cystic adenomatoid malformations (CCAM) type 1 are the most common and appear as a single or multiple macrocysts. Type 2 CCAM contain small cysts less than 1 cm in size and are often associated with other anomalies. Type 3 CCAM contain multiple microcysts that appear sonographically as a homogeneously echogenic mass (Fig. 12-13) (61,62). Sequestrations are intralobar or extralobar masses of pulmonary tissue that lack a tracheobronchial communication and have a vascular supply from the aorta. They present as a solid or mixed solid and cystic mass in the inferior portion of the chest (63). Up to 25% have a CCAM component that may be cystic. With color Doppler, a vessel can often be seen coursing from the aorta to feed the mass, confirming the diagnosis. Bronchogenic cysts typically present as a simple mediastinal or lower lobe cyst without a feeding vessel (64).

MRI is particularly valuable in the evaluation of fetal thorax. Fetal lungs are homogeneously intermediate in signal and clearly delineated from mediastinal structures, liver, and bowel (64,65). Cystic lung masses are typically higher in signal as a result of the high fluid content and can be separated from normal surrounding lung parenchyma (Fig. 12-14a and b) (67,68).

Prognosis depends on the size of the intrathoracic mass because marked lung compression during fetal development leads to hypoplastic lungs. Polyhydramnios, ascites, and hydrops are likely secondary to compression of the esophagus and vena cava and correlate with poor outcome (61). Type 3 CCAM tend to have the worst prognosis. The prenatal placement of shunts in cysts or pleura has resulted in some success in lung reexpansion (68). Spontaneous resolution of pleural effusions and pulmonary masses in utero has been reported (Fig. 12-13) (60–62). Prenatal therapy is reserved for those cases at highest risk for poor outcome (e.g., hydrops) (61,69–71). A fetus with a lung mass has an excellent prognosis if there is no hydrops and only minimal pulmonary hypoplasia (71).

Fetal neck masses such as cystic teratomas and lymphangiomas can occlude the airway resulting in hypoxic brain injury or death on delivery. The prenatal detection of a neck mass allows for the planning of a more controlled delivery such as Exutero Intrapartum Treatment (EXIT) procedure to establish an airway (72,73). Fetal MRI is particularly useful in providing additional detailed anatomic information in three planes of the larynx and trachea which are not visualized sonographically (72,73).

Congenital Diaphragmatic Hernia

When a fetal thoracic mass is identified, the differential diagnosis includes congenital diaphragmatic hernia. This defect results from incomplete fusion of the pleuroperitoneal membranes during the seventh week of gestation. Passage of bowel and liver may occur into the thorax at any

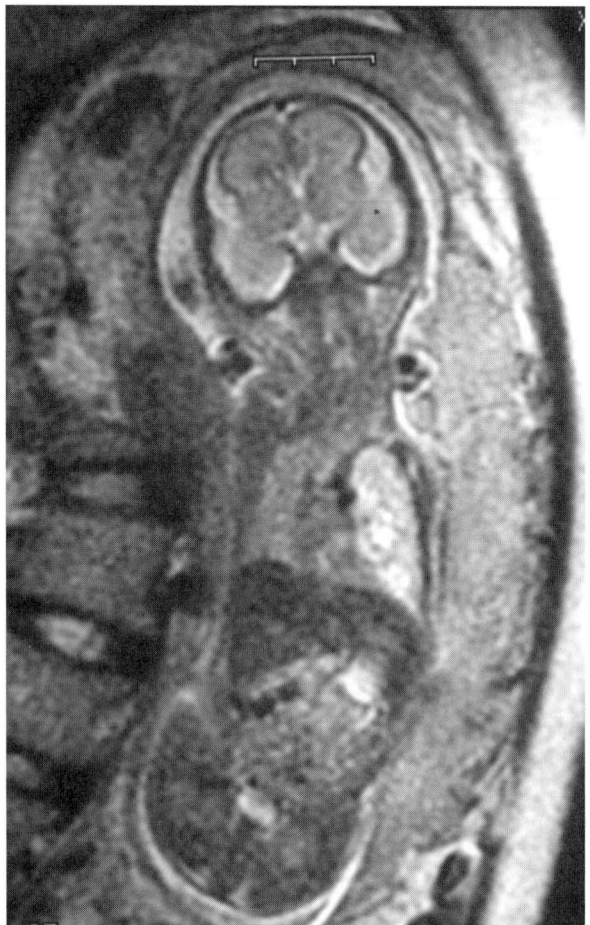

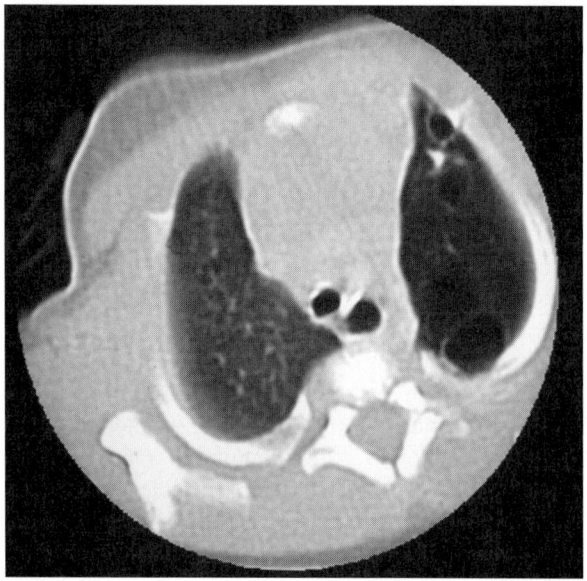

Figure 12-14 A. Coronal T2 weighted image of a fetal chest at 22 weeks gestation demonstrates multiple high signal cysts occupying the left hemithorax. **B.** Axial CT of the chest following delivery demonstrates multiple air filled cysts in the left upper lobe compatible with a cystic adenomatoid malformation.

time during pregnancy. Sonographic findings include contralateral mediastinal shift and fluid-filled loops of bowel within the chest that mimic pulmonary "cystic" masses (Fig. 12-15). Findings specific to congenital diaphragmatic

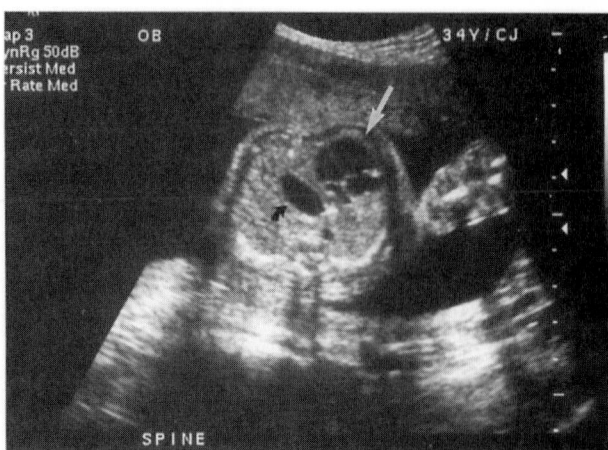

Figure 12-15 Congenital diaphragmatic hernia. Transverse sonographic image through the chest of a 23-week fetus demonstrates the heart (white arrow) to be shifted to the right by a herniated fluid-filled stomach (black arrow).

hernia (CDH) include absence of an intraabdominal stomach bubble or loops of bowel within the chest. Doppler flow studies demonstrating mesenteric vessels extending into the hemithorax confirm the diagnosis. Bowing of the umbilical portion of the portal vein suggests liver herniation. Associated anomalies often present include cardiac, genitourinary, CNS, and GI. Other conditions associated with congenital diaphragmatic hernia are Fryns' syndrome with nuchal thickening and limb anomalies and Pallister Killian syndrome (74).

Further evaluation includes fetal chromosomal analysis and fetal echocardiograms. Fetal MRI is particularly useful in differentiating a CCAM from a CDH. MRI can assess how much residual lung parenchyma remains expanded, and determine the amount of liver and bowel that has herniated into the thorax (Fig. 12-16) (36). Serial sonograms every 2 to 4 weeks are important as up to 75% of cases develop polyhydramnios, and all are at risk for IUGR (75). The mortality rate for infants with diaphragmatic hernia is variable. Cases with multiple anomalies are likely to be lethal. Less clear is whether sonographic findings such as marked mediastinal shift, IUGR, hydrops, and polyhydramnios predict uniformly poor outcome (75,76). Ratios of right lung area to head circumference and the presence of liver in the chest appear most useful in identifying which cases carry the poorest prognosis (77,78).

Congenital Heart Disease

Congenital heart disease is one of the most commonly recognized birth defects with a reported frequency of 0.8%. Any woman with a risk factor for a cardiac anomaly should undergo a detailed ultrasound examination of the fetal heart. Risk factors include nonimmune hydrops, suspected abnormality by screening sonogram, teratogen exposure, parental or sibling heart defect, aneuploidy, extracardiac anomalies, maternal diabetes, and fetal arrhythmia (80).

Detailed cardiac evaluation is difficult before 18 weeks of gestation. Examination includes visualization of the

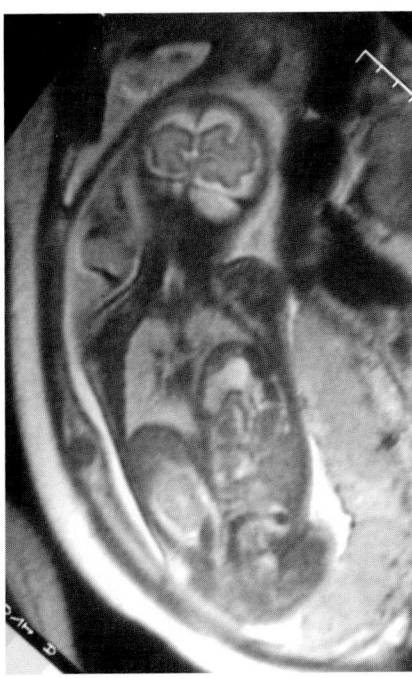

Figure 12-16 Congenital diaphragmatic hernia. Coronal T2 weighted image of a chest at 32 weeks gestation demonstrates herniation of stomach, bowel, and spleen into the left hemithorax. There is minimal deviation of mediastinal structures with the right lung and left upper lobes expanded.

four chambers and outflow tracts. A dedicated fetal echocardiogram requires additional cross-sectional views to demonstrate fetal heart integrity. M-mode echocardiography measures chamber size, wall thickness, and wall motion and facilitates cardiac rhythm assessment. Pulsed Doppler and color flow Doppler are useful to define blood flow. Sensitivity in detecting anomalies is dependent on fetal position, maternal size, and amniotic fluid volume and equipment and expertise. Ventricular septal defects, anomalous pulmonary venous return, and aortic or pulmonic stenosis are especially difficult to diagnose. Ott, in 1995, reported a 14% sensitivity for detection of congenital heart disease in a low-risk population compared with a 63% sensitivity in the high-risk group (81). Heart disease diagnosed prenatally is often severe and associated with a poor long-term prognosis with chromosomal or extracardiac structural defects often present (82).

Fetal Gastrointestinal Tract

The ultrasound appearance of fetal bowel varies, with significant overlap between normal and abnormal patterns (83). The stomach is first visualized at 13 to 16 weeks of gestation. If it is not identified by 16 weeks, especially in the presence of polyhydramnios, an abnormality such as esophageal atresia or congenital diaphragmatic hernia should be suspected (84). The esophagus is typically collapsed and not visualized by ultrasound scans (US), but the absence of a fluid-filled stomach and presence of polyhydramnios and a dilated proximal pouch are findings suggestive of esophageal atresia. In cases of tracheo-

esophageal fistula, 70% have a fluid-filled stomach, with polyhydramnios developing in only 60% of cases. Thus, sonographic detection of tracheoesophageal fistula (TEF) in unlikely (85). TEF may be detected by MRI if a proximal dilated esophageal pouch is noted and the distal esophagus is not visualized (86).

When an enlarged fluid-filled duodenum and stomach are identified, duodenal obstruction is present. Duodenal atresia is the most common cause, but the differential diagnosis includes annular pancreas, or duodenal stenosis. Up to 30% of fetuses with isolated duodenal atresia have trisomy 21, so chromosome analysis and fetal echocardiography are indicated. Serial sonograms will indicate development of polyhydramnios or IUGR.

In a normal fetus, small bowel is only occasionally visualized, and loops measuring over 7 mm in diameter are considered abnormal and suggestive of obstruction (87) (Fig. 12-17). Differential diagnosis includes a duplication cyst, mesenteric cyst, ovarian cyst, and hydroureter. Polyhydramnios is not always present and depends on the site of obstruction. Because a fetus with a large bowel obstruction or anal atresia typically does not develop polyhydramnios or dilated bowel, these entities are less readily diagnosed in utero. At times, bowel obstruction is associated with perforation and meconium spilling into the peritoneum, otherwise known as meconium peritonitis. Sonographic findings include fetal ascites, peritoneal calcifications, and meconium pseudocysts (88). The most common cause of small bowel obstruction is atresia felt to be secondary to an in utero vascular infarct. Fifteen percent of infants with cystic fibrosis present with meconium ileus and sonographic findings similar to those of bowel atresia. Echogenic bowel, meconium peritonitis, and pseudocyst formation occur in both meconium ileus and isolated bowel atresia. Echogenic bowel has also been associated with cytomegalovirus (CMV) and with chromosomal abnormalities such as trisomy 21 (89). Amniocentesis allows for karyotyping, CMV cultures, and analysis of amniocytes for the common cystic fibrosis (CF) mutations. In cases of suspected bowel abnormalities, serial sonograms will detect new onset of polyhydramnios and meconium peritonitis.

Fetal bowel is well visualized by MRI. Meconium is low signal on T2w and high signal on T1w. Proximal bowel loops are high signal on T2w and low on T1w. MR can provide additional information regarding level of obstruction. Anal atresia, typically missed by US may be identified by MRI (90).

Ventral Abdominal Wall Defects

The most common abdominal wall defects identified sonographically include omphalocele and gastroschisis (91). Through maternal serum alpha-fetoprotein screening, these defects can be diagnosed early in pregnancy. Omphaloceles result from failure of intestines to return to the abdomen during the tenth week of gestation with herniation of bowel or liver into the umbilical cord. A

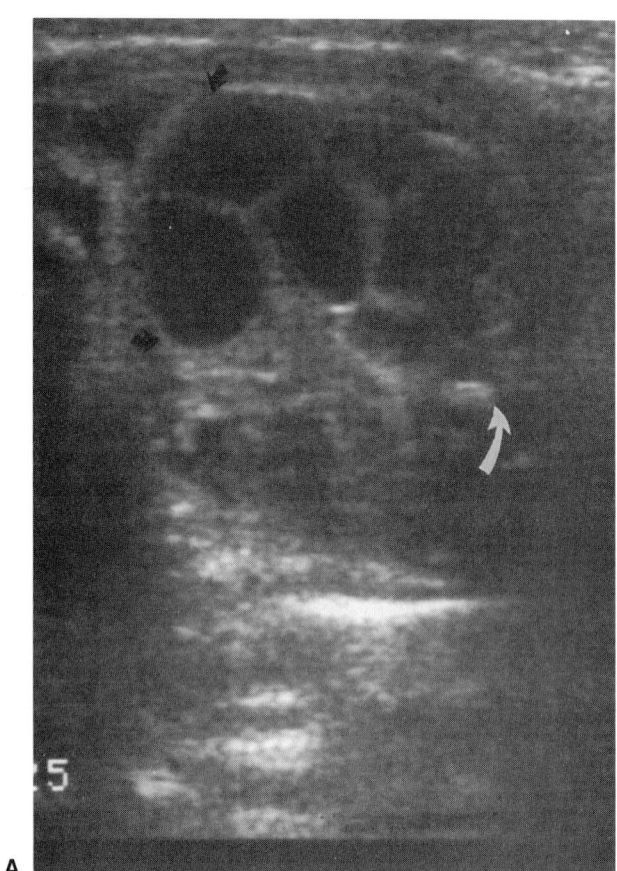
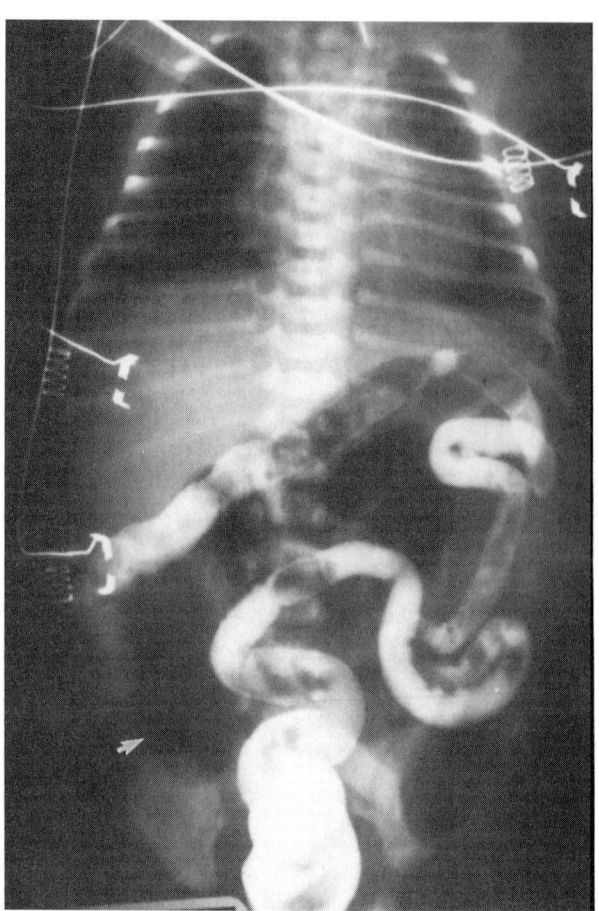

Figure 12-17 **A:** Transverse image of a 33-week gestation fetal abdomen demonstrates multiple dilated loops of bowel (black arrowheads). Echogenic focus (white arrow) is consistent with a peritoneal calcification. **B:** Following delivery at term, a water-soluble enema demonstrates a normal-caliber colon with dilated air-filled small bowel loops (arrow). Jejunal atresia was found at surgery.

surrounding peritoneal membrane is present, and the cord insertion is central (Figs. 12-18, 12-19). Gastroschisis, on the other hand, is a paraumbilical defect located to the right of the umbilicus and is a full-thickness abdominal wall defect without a covering membrane. It is important

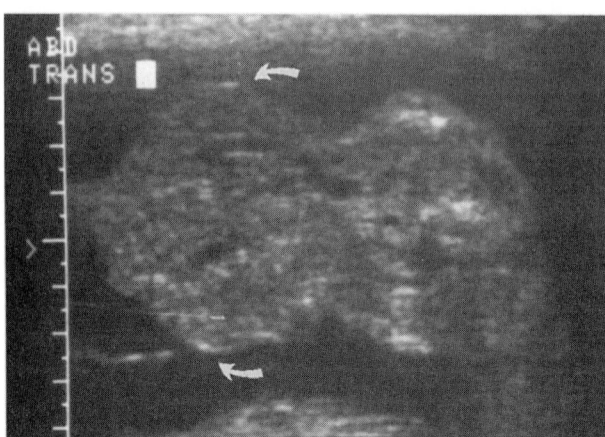

Figure 12-18 Omphalocele. Transverse sonographic image at the level of the umbilical cord insertion demonstrates a large outpouching (arrows) with a covering membrane containing liver and bowel.

to distinguish between the two entities for associated diagnosis and prognosis. Gastroschisis is classically an isolated entity felt to be caused by a vascular event and is not associated with chromosomal anomalies but is complicated by bowel fibrosis (92).

Omphaloceles, although not as likely to have bowel fibrosis, are more at risk for associated chromosomal abnormalities (30%–50%) and syndromes such as Beckwith-Wiedemann syndrome (macroglossia, organomegaly) and pentalogy of Cantrell (ectopia cordis) (93).

Normal fetal bowel migrates into the base of the cord by 12 menstrual weeks. Thus, the sonographic diagnosis of abdominal wall defects should be made only with caution before the second trimester. Chromosomal analysis and fetal echocardiography should be offered, and consultation with a pediatric surgeon is helpful. Serial sonograms will diagnose the development of polyhydramnios and IUGR (94,95).

Genitourinary Tract

Many asymptomatic genitourinary abnormalities are now being identified prenatally by sonography. Most renal lesions that are identified are cystic or obstructive. Increased detection and earlier diagnosis aid in minimizing

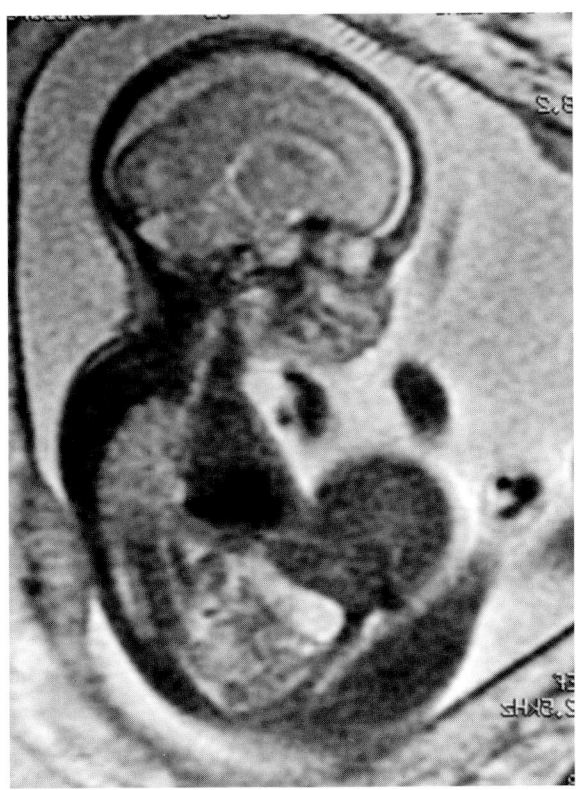

Figure 12-19 Omphalocele. Sagittal T2 weighted imaged demonstrates liver outpouching at the level of the cord insertion.

the risk of further renal damage after birth. Detection of the fetus with irreversible or lethal renal disease also assists in obstetric and perinatal management. Renal anomalies that can be diagnosed prenatally include renal agenesis, dilated obstructed or nonobstructed collecting systems, renal cystic disease, and tumors. It is estimated that 1 in 1,000 fetuses have a renal anomaly (96,97). In a series of 17,000 women screened prospectively at 16 to 18 weeks, renal anomalies were identified in 313 cases, 55 of which were significant. Upper tract dilation was the most common finding (298 cases), but it was transient in two-thirds of these cases. Obstruction was noted in 23 infants on follow-up, with 15 of these requiring surgery. Eight infants had unilateral multicystic kidney disease, and three had posterior urethral valves (98). Mortality after prenatal identification of fetal uropathy ranges from 20% to 50%.

A systematic approach to urinary tract abnormalities includes an assessment of amniotic fluid, characterization of the urinary tract abnormality, and a search for additional abnormalities. The kidneys contribute little amniotic fluid until 16 weeks of gestation, making it difficult to assess renal function before the second trimester. The presence of oligohydramnios secondary to a urinary abnormality carries a poor prognosis. Rarely, polyhydramnios may be present in a fetus with a mesoblastic nephroma, incomplete ureteropelvic junction (UPJ) obstruction, or associated cranial or GI abnormalities.

Fetal kidneys can be visualized as early as 14 weeks of gestation. Standard renal measurements include length [age in weeks = fetal kidney length (mm)], AP diameter, and renal circumference to abdominal circumference ratio (0.27–0.33). If a fetal renal pelvis is dilated and fluid-filled, one must determine if it is physiological, obstructive, secondary to reflux, or simply nonobstructive megacystis. In most cases, if the pelvic diameter measures less than 1 cm, the finding is nonpathological. When the pelvic diameter measures over 1 cm, the ratio of pelvic diameter to renal diameter measures greater than 0.5, or caliectasis or hydroureter is present, a pathological process is likely (99).

Obstructive Uropathy

The most common cause of fetal pyelectasis is UPJ obstruction (98). Differential includes extrarenal pelvis, vesicoureteral reflux, or a multicystic dysplastic kidney. When bilateral, the severity of obstruction is usually asymmetric. Rarely, dysplasia, urinoma, or urine ascites develops. MRI is helpful in defining anatomy of complex renal anomalies such as bladder extrophy and cloacal anomalies (100). If associated nonrenal anomalies are identified, chromosome analysis is indicated. The frequency of follow-up sonograms depends on whether both kidneys are involved and the severity of obstruction. Outcome is variable, with 10% increasing in dilation, 50% remaining stable, and 40% improving (101). Prophylactic antibiotics should be provided to the infant after delivery, until work up, including renal scans can document whether the dilatation is truly obstructive.

Bladder Outlet Obstruction

If hydroureter and pyelectasis are bilateral, the differential diagnosis includes urethral obstruction, bilateral reflux, or bilateral megacystis. In the male fetus, the differential also includes posterior urethral valves and prune belly syndrome. Accurate diagnosis of posterior valves includes the finding of a dilated, thick bladder with keyhole posterior urethral expansion, dilated tortuous ureters, and caliectasis. Fetal MRI may aid in the assessment of ureteral and urethral dilatation particularly if oligohydramnios is present. Urinary ascites may be present (Fig. 12-20). Findings that suggest a poor outcome include dysplastic echogenic renal parenchyma and oligohydramnios (102). If fetal bladder aspirate demonstrates elevated fetal urine electrolytes and elevated osmolarity, a poor outcome is also suggested.

Frequent sonograms will detect progressive oligohydramnios and IUGR. If severe oligohydramnios is present, up to 95% die from pulmonary hypoplasia. Those who survive require an emergency voiding cystourethrogram to confirm the diagnosis and valvuloplasty or cystostomy to relieve the obstruction. Up to 40% of survivors may develop renal failure at a later date.

Cystic Renal Disease

Cystic changes of the fetal kidneys may be secondary to hereditary diseases (autosomal recessive infantile polycystic

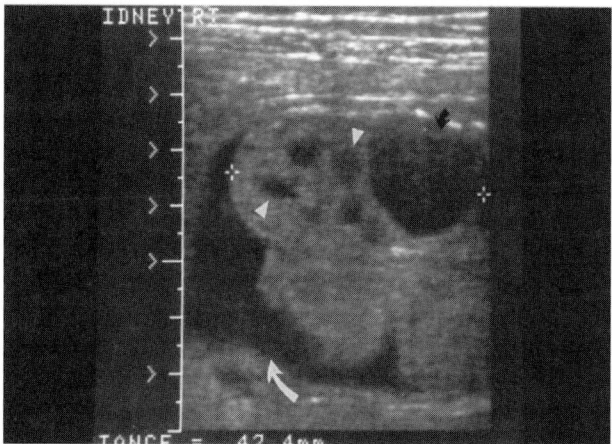

Figure 12-20 Longitudinal image of a right kidney in a 23-week gestation male fetus with posterior urethral valves demonstrates a kidney with a large upper pole cortical cyst (black arrow), caliectasis (arrowheads), and urinary ascites (white arrow).

kidneys), dysmorphology (multicystic dysplastic kidney disease), or severe obstruction (Potter type II). Differentiating the various diagnoses, at times, may be difficult. When renal cystic disease is identified, the most important factors to evaluate are amniotic fluid volume and whether one or both kidneys are affected. If the cysts are unilateral and amniotic fluid is normal, prognosis typically is good.

Multicystic dysplastic kidneys are felt to be an early error in development of mesonephric blastema or early obstructive uropathy. Up to 75% of multicystic dysplastic kidneys are associated with other renal abnormalities in the contralateral kidney, especially UPJ obstruction and vesicoureteral reflux. Sonographically, multiple cysts are identified in various sizes that do not connect to a renal pelvis. No normal renal parenchymal tissue is seen. Following delivery, the diagnosis is confirmed by renal radionuclide scan, and vesicoureteral reflux is excluded by voiding cystourethrogram.

Autosomal recessive infantile polycystic kidneys typically present with bilateral large echogenic kidneys with a large abdominal circumference. If severe oligohydramnios develops, outcome is poor because of pulmonary hypoplasia (Fig. 12-21).

Skeletal Dysplasia

Skeletal dysplasias include a heterogeneous group of over 160 disorders. The prevalence is 2.4 per 10,000 births (103). Up to one-fourth of affected infants are stillborn, with another one-third dying by 1 week of age. The most common lethal dysplasias include thanatophoric dysplasia, osteogenesis imperfecta type II, and achondrogenesis. The most common nonlethal skeletal dysplasia is achondroplasia (104).

Prenatally, a systematic approach is needed to analyze skeletal anomalies. Long bones should be evaluated for size, shape, bowing, and symmetry. Shortening of the extremities can involve the proximal segment (rhizomelic), midsegment (mesomelic), distal segment (acromelic), or the entire limb (micromelic). Fractures appear as bones that are irreg-

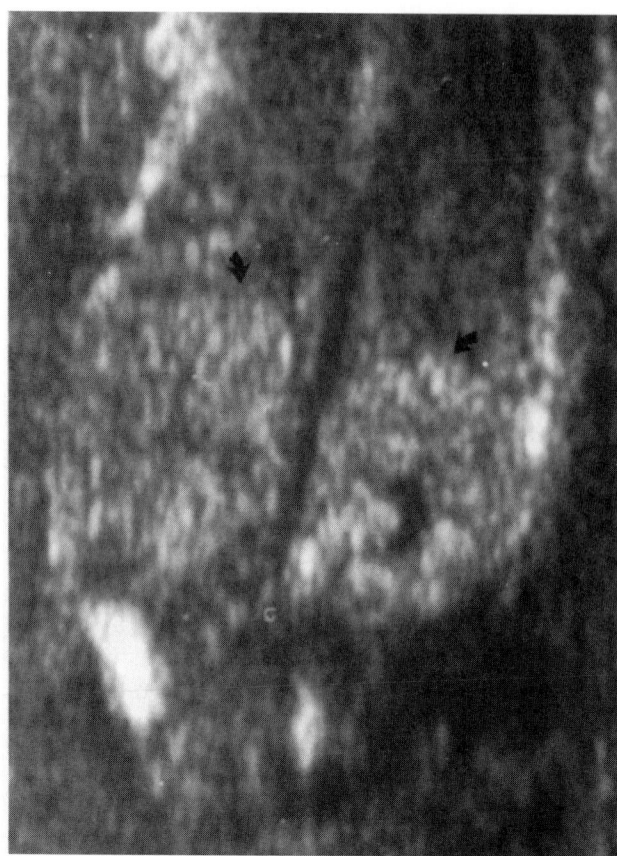

Figure 12-21 Infantile polycystic kidney disease. Coronal image of a 24-week fetus demonstrates bilateral enlarged echogenic kidneys (arrows). Severe oligohydramnios is present.

ular, angled, or bowed sonographically (Fig. 12-22). The skull should be evaluated for frontal bossing or cloverleaf deformity. Decreased skull echogenicity may be noted with osteogenesis imperfecta and hypophosphatasia. Hypertelorism, micrognathia, and abnormally shaped ears may be identified. Hands and feet should be evaluated for polydactyly, missing digits, or equinovarus deformities. The presence of hemivertebrae, scoliosis, and platyspondyly should be explored. Although short ribs may be difficult to recognize sonographically, the thoracic circumference can be measured and compared to normal values for gestational age. If gestational age is unknown, the ratio of thoracic to abdominal circumference can be used. A small thorax suggests a poor prognosis because chest restriction results in pulmonary hypoplasia and, at times, hydrops. Additional findings such as cleft lip, cardiac, and renal anomalies help narrow the differential diagnosis.

When there is a positive family history of a skeletal dysplasia, accurate prenatal diagnosis is possible. When a skeletal abnormality is noted incidentally, a precise diagnosis is more difficult. Fetal radiographs help confirm a diagnosis if fractures or joint calcifications are identified. Additional biochemical testing or karyotyping is useful. Because dysplasias may progress with time (e.g., achondroplasia and osteogenesis imperfecta), serial sonograms are useful for assessment of skeletal growth in cases at risk

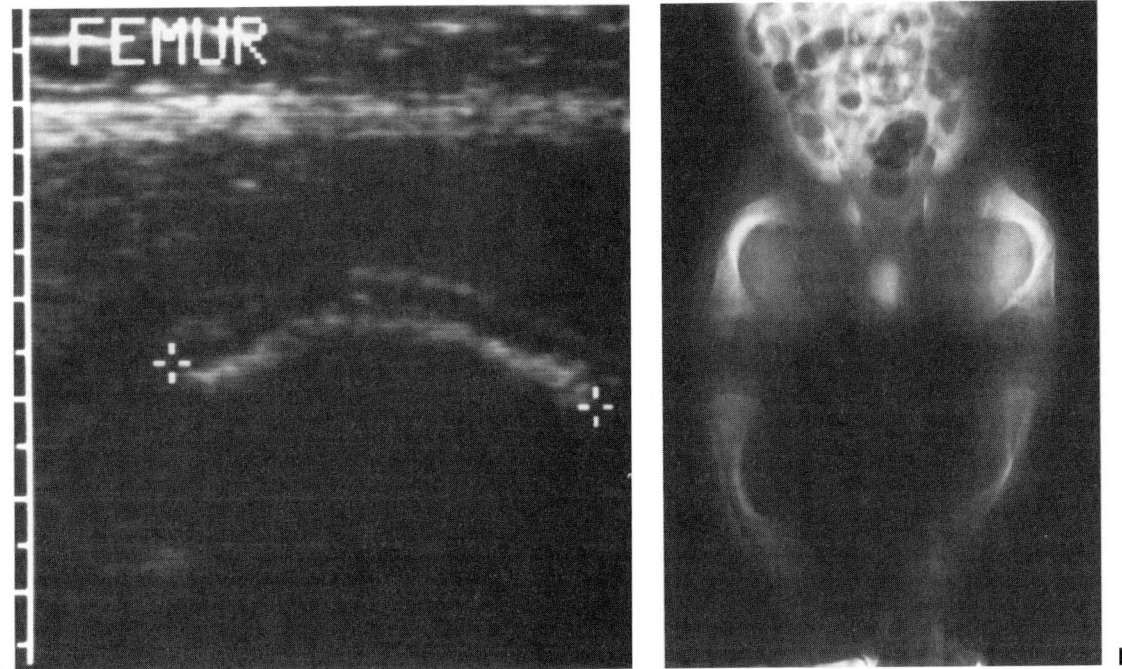

Figure 12-22 Osteogenesis imperfecta type III. **A:** Longitudinal image of a fetal thigh at 38 weeks of gestation demonstrates a short, bowed femur (cursors). **B:** Radiograph after delivery confirms the presence of short bowed femurs, tibia, and fibula bilaterally.

(105). The potential development of polyhydramnios and/or hydrops should also be noted. Differentiating intrauterine growth retardation or constitutional short stature from a true dysplasia is more difficult in the third trimester. Assessment of fetal well-being including the biophysical profile and umbilical arterial flow patterns aids in establishing the correct diagnosis.

DETECTION OF FETAL ASPHYXIA

Fetal asphyxia is a common cause of fetal injury or death. Fetal asphyxia is a spectrum of conditions ranging from transient episodes of hypoxemia to sustained hypoxemia with resultant metabolic acidosis. There are diverse signs of asphyxia with multiple organs potentially affected and a wide range in severity, duration, and chronicity. When asphyxia develops, the fetus redistributes cardiac output from nonvital organs (lung, kidney, skeleton) to vital organs (brain, adrenals, and myocardium. This protective redistribution is reflexive, resulting from hypoxemic or acidemic stimulation of aortic body chemoreceptors (23). When sustained, redistribution can be profound. Diminished amniotic fluid production develops as a result of decreased urine production. Oligohydramnios further endangers the fetus because the umbilical cord is more at risk for compression, especially during uterine contractions. Cerebral asphyxia results in alterations in biophysical activities and responses. It is unclear whether increasing degrees of hypoxemia cause progressive loss of a biophysical function or if all functions are lost simultaneously. Fetal

breathing has been noted to disappear early, whereas fetal movements disappear only with more severe disease (106,107).

Identification of an asphyxiated fetus is important because emergency delivery may improve outcome. Acute fetal asphyxia is rare except in cases of cord prolapse or placental abruption. These obstetric complications can be recognized sonographically and suggest appropriate intervention (108). Unfortunately, most asphyxiated fetuses exhibit both subacute and chronic signs of asphyxia. The fetus suffering from uteroplacental insufficiency typically has intermittent hypoxemic episodes induced during episodes of uterine contraction. Between these periods, the fetus can be normally oxygenated or demonstrate minimal compensated hypoxemia. Signs of hypoxemia thus depend on the duration, progression, and frequency of hypoxemic episodes.

The biophysical signs of asphyxia may be acute, such as loss of breathing movements and heart rate reactivity, or they may be chronic, such as oligohydramnios. Biophysical responses will change during hypoxemic episodes. Experiments in fetal lambs have demonstrated a decrease in fetal breathing and gross movements during hypoxemia (109,110). Fetal muscle tone and heart rate response to movement (i.e., accelerations) also decrease during hypoxemia (111). Maternal depressant medication and fetal cerebral anomalies can alter fetal biophysical activities, so these causes should be excluded. Ultrasound findings of chronic effects of intermittent hypoxemia include intrauterine growth retardation. Oligohydramnios should be considered a sign of fetal asphyxia unless renal abnormalities or premature rupture of membranes is identified (22).

Fetal Biophysical Profile

Monitoring fetal activity and its responses has altered the practice of perinatology (112,113). Any fetus at risk for uteroplacental insufficiency is a candidate for fetal evaluation in the third trimester. The first electronic fetal heart rate evaluation developed was the contraction stress test (CST), which relies on the fetal heart rate response to uterine contractions. The test records the fetal heart response as contractions are induced with oxytocin. If no fetal decelerations are recorded, uteroplacental function is considered normal. Disadvantages include the need to administer oxytocin intravenously and the length of the examination (average time of 90 minutes) (114).

The nonstress test (NST) evaluates fetal heart rate acceleration in response to fetal movement. As with a negative CST, a reactive NST is predictive of intrauterine survival for approximately 7 days subsequent to the test. This test has become popular because it requires relatively little time, cost, and technical skill (115). Reproducibility of NST interpretation, however, is problematic (116). Past acute asphyxial events are not excluded solely with a NST, and nonreactive patterns may exist for benign reasons.

The differentiation of the normal from the compromised fetus may be most accurate when several fetal and environmental parameters are evaluated together. Manning proposed the combined use of five ultrasound-monitored fetal variables to assess risk of asphyxia to reduce both false-positive and false-negative results. These include fetal breathing movements, gross body movements, tone, amniotic fluid volume, and heart rate reactivity (117). Each variable is evaluated according to tested criteria, and they are assigned scores of 2 when normal and 0 when abnormal (Table 12-2). Observation of each variable is continued until normal criteria are met or 30 minutes of continuous observation has been completed. The total score, termed the biophysical profile score (BPS), is an accurate method of differentiating if a fetus is normal or compromised (Table 12-3). Manning et al. reported that in a series of over 19,000 pregnancies, there was a false-normal test rate of approximately one per 1,000, with more that 97% of pregnancies tested having normal test results (118). Clinical studies from other centers have reported similar results with this method (119). In a follow up study, Manning and associates reported on 493 fetuses in which BPS were performed just before umbilical venous blood pH values were obtained via cordocentesis. A BPS of zero was associated with significant fetal acidemia, whereas scores of 8 or greater were associated with a normal pH 120). A score of 6 was a poor predictor of abnormal outcome, but a decrease from a score of 2 to 4 to a score of zero was an accurate predictor of abnormal outcome. In a similar study, for each of the four acute variables of the BPS, a substantial difference in mean umbilical venous pH was noted for the normal and abnormal results (121). Manning and associates prospectively studied the incidence of cerebral palsy in 22,336 high-risk pregnancies managed with serial BPS compared with 30,224 low-risk pregnancies that did not receive antepartum testing. Cerebral palsy (CP) diagnosed by 3 years of age was significantly associated with a low BPS. Incidence of CP was 0.8 per 1,000 when the BPS score was normal (10/10) and 250 per 1,000 when the BPS was very abnormal (0/10) (122).

Because the BPS is labor intensive, abbreviated screening tests have been evaluated. When normal, the four ultrasound monitored variables appear equal to that achieved by the addition of the NST component. The NST should be performed when one or more variables are abnormal

TABLE 12-2

BIOPHYSICAL PROFILE SCORING: TECHNIQUE AND INTERPRETATION

Biophysical Variable	Normal (score 2)	Abnormal (score 0)
FBMs	At least one episode of FBM of at least 30-sec duration in a 30-min observation period	Absent FBM or no episode of ≥ 30 sec in 30 min
Gross body movement	At least three discrete body or limb movements in 30 min (episodes of active continuous movement are considered a single movement)	Two or fewer episodes of body or limb movements in 30 min
Fetal tone	At least one episode of active extension with return to flexion of fetal limb(s) or trunk; opening and closing of hand considered normal tone	Either slow extension with return to partial flexion or movement of limb in full extension or absent fetal movement
Reactive FHR	At least two episodes in 30 min of FHR acceleration of ≥ 15 bpm of at least 15-sec duration associated with fetal movement	Less than two episodes of acceleration of FHR or acceleration of < 15 bpm in 30 min
Qualitative AFV	At least one pocket of AF that measures at least 2 cm in tow perpendicular planes	Either no AF pockets or a pocket < 2 cm in two perpendicular planes

AF, amniotic fluid; AFV, amniotic fluid volume; bpm, beats per minute; FBM, fetal breathing movement; FHR, fetal heart rate.
From Manning FA, Morrison I, Lange IR, et al. Fetal assessment based on fetal biophysical profile scoring: experience in 12,620 referred high risk pregnancies. I. Perinatal mortality by frequency and etiology. *Am J Obstet Gynecol* 1985;151:343, with permission.

TABLE 12-3

BIOPHYSICAL PROFILE SCORING: MANAGEMENT PROTOCOL

Score	Interpretation	Management
10	Normal infant, low risk for chronic asphyxia and patients over 42 weeks of gestation	-Repeat testing at weekly intervals; repeat twice weekly in diabetics
8	Normal infant, low risk for chronic asphyxia- diabetics and patients over 42 weeks of gestation;	-Repeat testing at weekly intervals; repeat testing twice weekly in oligohydramnios is an indication for delivery
6	Suspicion of chronic asphyxia	Repeat testing in 4–6 hours; deliver if oligohydramnios present
4	Suspicion of chronic asphyxia -weeks of gestation and L/Sª <2, repeat test in 24 hrs;	-If past 36 weeks of gestation and favorable, deliver; if less than 36 repeat score £4, deliver
0–2	Strong suspicion of chronic asphyxia regardless of gestational age	-Extend testing time to 120 min; if persistent score £4, deliver

ª L/S, lecithin–sphingomyelin ratio.
From Manning FA, Morrison I, Lange IR, et al. Fetal assessment based on fetal biophysical profile scoring: experience in 12,620 referred high risk pregnancies. I. Perinatal mortality by frequency and etiology. *Am J Obstet Gynecol* 1985;151:343, with permission.

(123). Provided amniotic fluid volume is normal, a BPS of 8 to 10 by whatever combination can be considered normal. All equivocal or abnormal BPS results should be based on a complete assessment including a NST (124).

Biophysical evaluation should be performed in patients with recognized high-risk factors. It allows for accurate differentiation of the normal fetus from the compromised one, information crucial in the timing of intervention. The variables used in the fetal BPS were selected because of ease and rapidity of measurement. Additional variables such as swallowing, fine hand movement, rapid-eye-movement state, peristalsis of fetal gut, urine output, and umbilical vessel flow rates may be found to add to the more precise evaluation of the fetal condition (125).

DOPPLER ASSESSMENT OF BLOOD VELOCITIES IN UMBILICAL AND FETAL VESSELS

Doppler ultrasound velocimetry can provide the clinician with important information on the hemodynamics of various vascular regions. Flow waveforms provide important information 12 through 40 weeks gestation from maternal vessels, placental circulation, and fetal systemic vessels. Gestational age-related reference values have been established for maternal uterine and arcuate artery, umbilical artery, fetal descending aorta, and fetal cerebral, renal, and femoral arteries (126). Values are obtained by directing an ultrasound beam toward a vessel and recording the frequency shift (Doppler effect) in the returning echoes. The Doppler shift principle states that echoes returning from moving structures are altered in frequency, and the amount of shift is directly proportional to the velocity of the moving structure. The frequencies of echoes returning from blood moving toward the transducer are increased, whereas the frequencies of echoes returning from blood moving away from the transducer are decreased. This method may not accurately measure velocity, but it does accurately evaluate the relative resistance to flow (127). The frequency spectrum can be analyzed by comparing the systolic to diastolic flow velocities. There are several different ratios for measurement of flow impedance. These include the difference between peak systolic and diastolic flow velocity over the mean flow velocity (pulsatility index), the difference between peak systolic and diastolic flow over the peak systolic flow (resistive index), and the ratio of the peak systolic to diastolic flow (S/D ratio). All indices are independent of the angle of insonation.

Measurement of flow velocity waveforms in the uterine artery, which depicts maternal vascular effects of the invading placenta, has been shown to be a method for early recognition of the pregnancy at risk for preeclampsia and IUGR (128,129). Uterine arterial remodeling occurs following successful placentation. Prepregnancy, uterine arteries show high resistance, elastic recoil with early diastolic notches and low diastolic flow. Successful placental invasion removes intimal muscle with increasing diastolic flow and loss of elasticity (130). Indices decrease as term approaches, with diastolic velocity increasing with advancing gestation. Fetal growth retardation has been reported when indices increase or notching in the waveform at end-systole develops at 22–24 weeks gestation (130,131). Uterine flow velocity waveforms are useful in predicting the frequency and severity of preeclampsia and intrauterine growth retardation (128–131). A major clinical obstetric application has been in the measurement of umbilical arterial flow using the S/D ratio (Fig. 12-23). In a normal pregnancy, the placental resistance declines slowly with advancing gestational age. The umbilical artery peak systolic flow velocity gradually decreases although diastolic flow velocity increases. Thus, the umbilical artery S/D ratio declines with advancing gestational age and should be less than 3 after 30 weeks of gestation (132). In growth-retarded fetuses and fetuses developing intrauterine distress, the umbilical artery blood velocity waveform changes as placental vascular resistance increases.

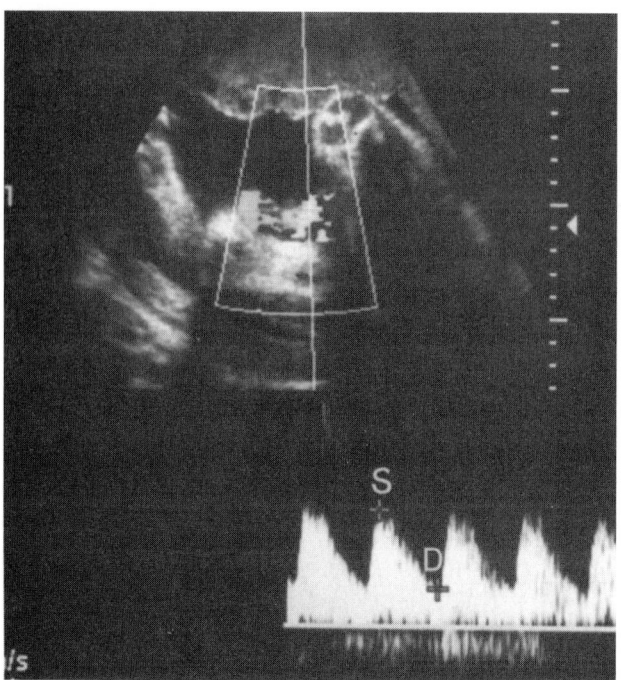

Figure 12-23   Umbilical artery velocimetry. S, systolic velocity; D, diastolic velocity. Note S/D ratio of approximately 3.

Abnormalities are progressive with reduction, loss, and finally reversal of diastolic flow. Absent or reversed end-diastolic flow (AREDV) is associated with a high risk of morbidity and mortality. Studies have compared the prediction of fetal acidosis by Doppler and cord blood gases. A statistically significant correlation has been found between an increased umbilical S/D ratio and fetal hypoxia particularly when diastolic blood flow is absent or reversed (133). In the preselected population of high-risk pregnancies, this method has a high predictive value regarding diagnosing fetal compromise and can be used for monitoring fetal health (128,134,135). If an abnormal umbilical velocimetry is identified in an SGA fetus, fetal heart rate variability should be tested. Fetuses that remain normal after a non-stress test have a low morbidity and can be closely followed (136,137).

Applied as a screening test in an unselected pregnant population, umbilical velocimetry has currently not been found to be cost-effective (138). A significant change in indices does not develop until more than 60% of the terminal placental arteries are obliterated (129). On the other hand, in preselected populations of high-risk pregnancies, Doppler of the umbilical artery has a high predictive value regarding diagnosing fetal compromise (135). These abnormal Doppler velocities are associated with higher mortality and morbidity in the neonatal period. Long term follow-up studies have shown an association between the abnormal intrauterine umbilical and fetal blood flow and subsequent postnatal neurodevelopmental impairment including mental retardation and severe motor impairment (139–141).

Absent diastolic flow velocity of the umbilical artery has been noted in up to 25% of fetuses with anomalies, typically

trisomy 13 or 18 (136). Because abnormal velocimetry may indicate a chronic fetal abnormality and not acute distress, delivery should not be undertaken based on umbilical artery Doppler velocimetry alone (130,137). In the fetus with IUGR and equivocal umbilical blood flow studies, Doppler studies of fetal systemic vessels can be useful.

The fetus with an abnormal umbilical artery velocimetry will redistribute blood flow detectable as vasodilation of the main arteries of the fetus including the heart and brain (23). Measurable fetal flow velocities include the middle cerebral, descending aorta, renal arteries and ductus venosus (142,143). These measures provide a means of assessing the distribution of fetal blood flow and can be useful in assessing the fetal cardiovascular adaptive responses to chronic hypoxemia. Doppler studies of the fetal circulation in intrauterine growth retardation and hypoxia have demonstrated a compensatory redistribution of arterial blood flow with increased flow to the brain and myocardium with decreased flow to the periphery (144,145). Redistribution of cardiac output reflects rising placenta resistance and results in "brain sparing" when cerebrovascular dilatation occurs (130).

Doppler waveforms of the middle cerebral artery (MCA) can be obtained at the level of the circle of Willis with a high degree of reproducibility. Normally, the MCA impedance decreases with advanced gestational age but remains higher than that of the umbilical artery (144). Fetal brain sparing during hypoxia is characterized by increase in diastolic and mean blood flow velocity in the MCA. If vasodilation of the MCA is lost, the fetus will begin to enter the acidotic stage. At term, evidence of fetal hemodynamic redistribution may exist in the presence of normal umbilical artery indices, so ratios such as the MCA/uric acid (UA) ratio can be useful. Normal cerebral to placental resistance ratio (CPR) is typically greater than 1 (146–148).

In the compromised IUGR fetus, precordial veins can illustrate fetal cardiac function. Which venous waveforms provide the best data are still being investigated (130,131). The ductus venosus regulates venous control, is a conduit of right atrial retrograde pulse waves, and is responsive to changes in oxygenation. In fetuses compromised by anemia or hypoxia, changes in pulsatile venous flow are being evaluated (130,131,18–49,150). When umbilical artery flow becomes abnormal, further evaluation of the fetal systemic Doppler may improve analysis of fetal distress. Doppler studies of fetal intracranial arteries and ductus venosus may thus result in improved timing of intervention to minimize morbidity (145–149).

SUMMARY

Ultrasonography has profoundly influenced the practice of perinatal medicine. Doppler and fetal MRI have also become useful adjuncts in the evaluation of the fetus. The ability to distinguish the normal from abnormal pregnancy has many applications. Serious complications such as developmental anomalies, intrauterine asphyxia, and growth abnormalities are now identified with greater frequency and accuracy as a result of these advances. Recognition of high-risk conditions such as placental abruption and cord prolapse and more chronic conditions such as intrauterine asphyxia allow for optimal preventive care. The improved accuracy in identifying fetal anomalies by ultrasound and MRI has increased the potential for prenatal intervention and optimizing the care and delivery of the fetus.

REFERENCES

1. Dewhurst CJ, Beasley JM, Campbell S. Assessment of fetal maturity and dysmaturity. *Obstet Gynecol* 1972;113:141.
2. Donald I. Ultrasound in obstetrics. *Br Med Bull* 1968;24:71.
3. Silva PD, Mahairas G, Schaper AM, et al. Early crown–rump length a good predictor of gestational age. *J Reprod Med* 1990;35:641.
4. Selbing A. Gestation age and U.S. measurement of gestational sac, CRL, and BPD during the first 15 weeks of pregnancy. *Acta Obstet Gynecol Scand* 1982;61:233.
5. Campbell S, Newman GB. Growth of the fetal biparietal diameter during normal pregnancy. *Br J Obstet Gynaecol* 1971;78:513.
6. Sabbagha RE, Hughey M. Standardization of sonar cephalometry and gestational age. *Obstet Gynecol* 1978;52:402.
7. Hadlock FP, Deter RL, Carpenter RL, et al. The effect of head shape on the accuracy of BPD I estimating fetal gestational age. *AJR Am J Roentgenol* 1981;137:83.
8. Sabbagha RE, Turner JH, Rockette H, et al. Sonar BPD and fetal age: definition of the relationship. *Obstet Gynecol* 1974;43:7.
9. Queenan JT, O'Brien GD, Campbell S. Ultrasound measurement of fetal limb bones. *Am J Obstet Gynecol* 1980;138:297.
10. Hadlock FP, Deter RL, Harrist RB. Computer assisted analysis of fetal age using multiple fetal growth parameters. *J Clin Ultrasound* 1983;11:313.
11. Deter RL, Harrist RB, Birnholz JC, et al. Evaluation of fetal dating studies. In: Hedlock F, Deter RL, eds. *Qualitative obstetrical ultrasonography.* New York: John Wiley & Sons, 1986:33.
12. Hadlock FP, Deter RL, Harrist RB, et al. A date independent predictor of IUGR:FL/AC ratio. *Am J Roentgenol* 1983;141:979.
13. Campbell S, Wilkin D. Ultrasound measurement of fetal abdominal circumference in the estimation of fetal weight. *Br J Obstet Gynaecol* 1975;82:689.
14. Warsof SL, Gohari P, Berkowitz RL, et al. The estimation of fetal weight by computer assisted analysis. *Am J Obstet Gynecol* 1977;128:881.
15. Shepard MJ, Richards VA, Berkowitz RL, et al. An evaluation of two equations for predicting fetal weight by ultrasound. *Am J Obstet Gynecol* 1982;142:47.
16. Kubik-Huch RA, Wildermuth S, Cettuzzi L, et al. Fetus and uteroplacental unit fast MRI and 3D volumetry feasibility study. *Radiology* 2001;219:567.
17. Deter RL, Harrist RB, Hadlock FP, et al. Longitudinal studies of fetal growth with the use of dynamic image ultrasonography. *Am J Obstet Gynecol* 1982;143:545.
18. Morrison I. Perinatal Mortality. *Semin Perinatol* 1985;9:144.
19. O'Brien GD, Queenan JT. Ultrasound fetal femur length in relation to intrauterine growth retardation. *Am J Obstet Gynecol* 1982;144:33.
20. Tamura RK, Sabbagha RE. Percentile ranks of sonar fetal abdominal circumference measurements. *Am J Obstet Gynecol* 1980;138:475.
21. Sabbagha RE. Intrauterine growth retardation: antenatal diagnosis by ultrasound. *Obstet Gynecol* 1978;52:252.
22. Wladimiroff JW, Bloemsma CA, Wallenburg HCS. Ultrasound assessment of fetal head and body sizes in relation to normal and retarded fetal growth. *Am J Obstet Gynecol* 1978;131:857.
23. Cohn HE, Sacks EJ, Heyman MA, et al. Cardiovascular responses to hypoxemia and acidemia in fetal lambs. *Am J Obstet Gynecol* 1974;120:817.
24. Phelan JP, Smith CV, Broussard P, et al. Amniotic fluid volume assessment with the four quadrant technique at 36–42 weeks gestation. *J Reprod Med* 1987;32:540.
25. Manning FA, Hill LM, Platt LD. Qualitative amniotic fluid volume determination by ultrasound: antepartum detection of intrauterine growth retardation. *Am J Obstet Gynecol* 1981;1139:254.
26. Marks AD, Divon MY. Longitudinal study of the amniotic fluid index in postdated pregnancy. *Obstet Gynecol* 1992;79:229.
27. Chamberlain PF, Manning FA, Morrison I, et al. Ultrasound evaluation of amniotic fluid volume: I. The significance of marginal and decreased amniotic fluid volume to perinatal outcome. *Am J Obstet Gynecol* 1984;150:245.
28. Manning FA, Morrison I, Lange IR, et al. Fetal assessment based on fetal biophysical profile scoring: experience in 12,620 referred high risk pregnancies: I. Perinatal mortality by frequency and etiology. *Am J Obstet Gynecol* 1985;151:343.
29. Boulet LS, Alexander GR, Salihu HM et al. Macorsomic births in the United States: Determinants, outcomes, and proposed grades of risk. *Am J Obstet Gynecol* 2003;188:137.
30. Petrikovsky B, Gelertner N, Oleschuk C. Fetal abdominal fat line: can macrosomia be diagnosed. *Am J Gynecol* 1996;174:428.
31. Goldstein P, Gershenson D, Hobbins JC. Fetal biparietal diameter as a predictor of mature L/S ratio. *Obstet Gynecol* 1976;438:667.
32. Strassner HT, Plat LD, Whittle M, et al. Amniotic fluid phosphatidylglycerol and real-time ultrasonic cephalometry. *Am J Obstet Gynecol* 1979;135:804.
33. Golde SH, Platt LD. The use of ultrasound in the diagnosis of fetal lung maturity. *Clin Obstet Gynecol* 1984;27:391.
34. Harman CR, Manning FA, Stearns E, et al. The correlation of ultrasonic placental grading and fetal pulmonic maturity in five hundred and sixty-three pregnancies. *Am J Obstet Gynecol* 1982;143:941.
35. Lee K, Khoshnood B, Chen L, et al. Infant mortality from congenital malformations in the United States 1970-1997. *Obstet Gynecol* 2001;98:620.
36. Hubbarb AM, Adzick NS, Crombleholme TM, et al. Leftsided congenital diaphragmatic hernia: value of prenatal MR imaging in preparation for fetal surgery. *Radiology* 1997;203:636.
37. Levine D, Barnes PD, Madsen JR, et al. Fetal central nervous system anomalies: MR imaging augments sonographic diagnosis. *Radiology* 1997;204:635.
38. Yip YP, Capriotti C, Tlagala, et al. Effects of MR exposure at 1.5 T on early embryonic development of the chick. *J Magn Reson Imaging* 1994;4:742.
39. Gu Y, Hasegawa T, Yamamato Y, et al. The combined efects of MRI and Xrays on ICR mouse embryos during organogenesis. *J Radiat Res* 2001;42:265.
40. Ginsberg JS, Hirsh J, Rainbow AJ, et al. Risks to the fetus of radiologic procedures uses in the diagnosis of maternal venous thromboembolic disease. *Thromb Haemost* 1989;61:189–196.
41. Okazaki R, Ootsuyama A, Uchida S, et al. Effects of a 4.7 T statid magnetic field on fetal development in ICR mice. *J Radiat Res* 2001;42:273.
42. Baker PN, Johnson IR, Harvey PR, et al. A three year follow up children imaged in utero with echoplanar magnetic resonance. *Am J Obstet Gynecol* 1994;170:32.
43. Mevissen M, Buntenkotter S, Loscher W. Effect of static and time varying magnetic field on reproduction and fetal development in rats. *Teratology* 1994;50:229–237.
44. Siedler DE, Filly RA. Relative growth of the higher brain structures. *J Ultrasound Med* 1987;6:573.
45. Pretorius D, Davis K, Manco-Johnson M, et al. Clinical course of fetal hydrocephalus: 40 cases. *ANJR Am J Neuroradiol* 1985;6:23.
46. Bilaniuk LT. MRI of the fetal brain. *Semin Roentgenol* 1999;32:48–61.
47. Girard N, Raybaud C, Ponset M. In vivo MR study of brain maturation in normal fetuses. *AJNR Am J Neuroradiol* 1995;16: 407-413.
48. Levine D, Barnes PD. Cortical maturation in normal and abnormal fetuses as assessed with prenatal MR imaging *Radiology* 1999;210:751–758.
49. Drugan A, Kraus B, Canady A, et al. The natural history of prenatally diagnosed cerebral ventriculomegaly. *JAMA* 1989;261:1785.
50. Chervenak FA, Berkowitz RL, Tortora M, et al. The management of fetal hydrocephalus. *Am J Obstet Gynecol* 1985;151:933.
51. Brown IM, Bannister CM, Rimmer S, et al. The outcome for infants diagnosed prenatally as having cerebral ventriculomegaly. *J Matern Fetal Neonatal Med* 1995;5:13.

52. Patel MD, Filly AL, Hersh DR, et al. Isolated mild fetal cerebral ventriculomegaly: Clinical course and outcome. *Radiology* 192:759:1994.

53. Levitsky DB, Mack LA, Nyberg DA, et al. Fetal aqueductal stenosis diagnosed sonographically: How grave is the prognosis? *Am J Roentgenol* 1995;164:725.

54. Benaceraff BR, Stryker J, Frigoletto FD. Abnormal US appearance of the cerebellum (banana sign). Indirect sign of spina bifida. *Radiology* 1989;171:151.

55. Van de Hof MC, Nicolaides KH, Campbell J, et al. Evaluation of the lemon and banana signs in one hundred thirty fetuses with open spina bifida. *Am J Obstet Gynecol* 1990;162:322.

56. Bulas DI, Johnson D, Allen J, et al. Fetal hemangioma. Sonographic and color flow Doppler findings. *J Ultrasound Med* 1992;11:499.

57. Benson JT, Dillard RG, Burton BK. Open spina bifida: does c-section delivery improve prognosis? *Obstet Gynecol* 1988;71:532.

58. Songster GS, Gray DL, Crane JP. Prenatal prediction of lethal pulmonary hypoplasia using US fetal chest circumference. *Obstet Gynecol* 1989;73:261.

59. Estroff JA, Parak R, Frigoletto FD, et al. The natural history of isolated fetal hydrothorax. *Ultrasound Obstet Gynecol* 1992;2:162.

60. Lein JM, Colmorgen GHC, Gehret JF, et al. Spontaneous resolution of fetal pleural effusion diagnosed during the second trimester. *J Clin Ultrasound* 1990;18:54.

61. Adzick NS, Harrison MR, Glick PL, et al. Fetal cystic adenomatoid malformation: prenatal diagnosis and natural history. *J Pediatr Surg* 1985;20:483.

62. Saltzman DH, Adzick NS, Benacerraf BR. Fetal cystic adenomatoid malformation of the lung: apparent improvement in utero. *Obstet Gynecol* 1988;71:1000.

63. Benya EC, Bulas DI, Selby DM, et al. Cystic sonographic appearance of extralobar pulmonary sequestration. *Pediatr Radiol* 1993;23:605.

64. Albright EB, Crane JP, Shackelford GD. Prenatal diagnosis of a bronchogenic cyst. *J Ultrasound Med* 1988;7:91.

65. Coakley FV, Lopoo JB, Ying LU, et al. Normal and hypoplastic fetal lungs: volumetric assessment with prenatal single shot rapid acquisition with relaxation enhancement MRI. *Radiology* 2000;216:107.

66. Duncan KR, Gowland PA, Moore RJ, et al. Assessment of fetal lung growth in utero with echoplanar MR imaging. *Radiology* 1999;210:197.

67. Hubbard AM, Cromplehome TM. Anomalies and malformation affecting the fetal neonatal chest. *Semin Roentgenol* 1998;33:117.

68. Hubbard AM. Magnetic resonance imaging of fetal thoracic abnormalities. *Top Magn Reson Imaging* 2001;12:18.

69. Blott M, Nicolaides KH, Greenough A. Pleuroamniotic shunting for decompression of fetal pleural effusions. *Obstet Gynecol* 1988;71:798.

70. Bromley B, Parad R, Estroff JA, et al. Fetal lung masses: prenatal course and outcome. *J Ultrasound Med* 1995;14:927.

71. Songster GS, Gray DL, Crane JP. Prenatal prediction of lethal pulmonary hypoplasia using US fetal chest circumference. *Obstet Gynecol* 1989;73:261.

72. Hubbard AM, Crombleholme TM, Adzick NS. Prenatal MRI Evaluation of Giant Neck Masses in Preparation for the Fetal EXIT procedure. *Am J Perinatol* 1998;15:253.

73. Kathary N, Bulas D, Newman K, et al. Fetal MRI evaluation of cervical neck masses. *Pediatr Rad* 2001;31:72774.

74. Bulas DI, Saal HM, Fonda J, et al. Cystic hygroma and CDH: early prenatal evaluation of Fryns syndrome. *Prenat Diag* 1992;12:867.

75. Adzick NS, Harrison MR, Glick PR. Diaphragmatic hernia in the fetus: prenatal diagnosis and outcome in 94 cases. *J Pediatr Surg* 1985;20:357.

76. Wilson JM, Fauza DO, Lund DP, et al. Antenatal diagnosis of isolated CDH is not an indicator of outcome. *J Pediatr Surg* 1994;29:815.

77. Metkus AP, Filly RA, Stringer MD, et al. Sonographic predictors of survival in fetal diaphragmatic hernia. *J Pediatr Surg* 1996;31:148.

78. Harrison MR. The fetus with a diaphragmatic hernia: pathophysiology, natural history and surgical management. In Harrison MR, Bolvus MS, Filly RA, eds. *The unborn patient*, 2nd ed. Philadelphia: WB Saunders, 1990:295.

79. VanderWall KJ, Skarsgard ED, Filly RA, et al. Fetendoclip: a fetal endoscopic tracheal clip procedure in a human fetus. *J Pediatr Surg* 1997;32:970.

80. Perone N. A practical guide to fetal echocardiography. *Contemp Obstet Gynecol* 1988;1:55.

81. Ott WJ. The accuracy of antenatal fetal echocardiography screening in high and low risk patients. *Am J Obstet Gynecol* 1995;172:1741.

82. Crawford DC, Chita SK, Allan LD. Prenatal detection of congenital heart disease: factors affecting obstetric management and survival. *Am J Obstet Gynecol* 1988;159:352.

83. Hertzberg BS. Sonography of the fetal gastrointestinal tract: anatomic variants, diagnostic pitfalls and abnormalities. *Am J Roentgenol* 1994;162:1175.

84. McKenna KM, Goldstein RB, Stringer MD. Small or absent fetal stomach: prognostic significance. *Radiology* 1995;197:729.

85. Pretorius DH, Drose JA, Dennis MA, et al. Tracheoesophageal fistula in utero: twenty-two cases. *J Ultrasound Med* 1986;6:509.

86. Langer JC, Hussain H, Khan A, et al. Prenatal diagnosis of esophageal atresia using MRI. *J Pediatr Surg* 2001;36:804.

87. Nyberg DA, Mack LA, Patten RM, et al. Fetal bowel, normal sonographic findings. *J Ultrasound Med* 1987;6:257.

88. Foster MA, Nyberg DA, Mahony BS, et al. Meconium peritonitis prenatal sonographic findings and their clinical significance. *Radiology* 1987;165:661.

89. Nyberg DA, Dubinsky TJ, Resta RG, et al. Echogenic fetal bowel during the second trimester: clinical importance. *Radiology* 1993;188:527.

90. Benachi A, Sonig P, Jounnic JM, et al. Detemination of the anatomical location of an antenatal intestinal occlusion by magnetic resonance imaging. *Ultrasound Obstet Gynecol* 2001;18:164–165.

91. Hertzberg BS, Bowie JD. Fetal gastrointestinal abnormalities. *Radiol Clin North Am* 1990;28:101.

92. Babcock CJ, Hedrick MH, Goldstein RB, et al. Gastroschisis: can sonography of the fetal bowel accurately predict postnatal outcome. *J Ultrasound Med* 1993;13:701.

93. Nicolaides KH, Snifders RJM, Cheng HH, et al. Fetal gastrointestinal and abdominal wall defects: associated malformation and chromosomal abnormalities. *Fetal Diagn Ther* 1992;7:102.

94. Chescheir NC, Azizkhan RG, Seeds JW, et al. Counseling and care for the pregnancy complicated by gastroschisis. *Am J Perinatol* 1991;8:323.

95. Fitzsimmons J, Nyberg DA, Cey DR, et al. Perinatal management of gastroschisis. *Obstet Gynecol* 1988;71:910.

96. Estes J, Harrison M. Fetal Obstructive Uropathy. *Semin Pediatr Surg* 1993;2:129.

97. Cusick E, Didier F, Droulle P, et al. Mortality after an antenatal diagnosis of fetal uropathy. *J Pediatr Surg* 1995;30:463.

98. Gunn TR, Moral JD, Pease P. Antenatal diagnosis of urinary tract abnormalities by ultrasonography after 28 weeks: incidence and outcome. *Am J Obstet Gynecol* 1995;172:479.

99. Fernbach SK, Maizels M, Conway JJ. Ultrasound grading of hydronephrosis; introduction to the system used by the Society for Fetal Urology. *Pediatr Radiol* 1993;23:478.

100. Hubbard A, Harty M, Ruchelli E, et al. Prenatal MRI of the fetal urinary tract: normal and abnormal anatomy with US and pathological correlation. *Radiology* 1998;209:259.

101. King LR, Hatcher PA. Natural history of fetal and neonatal hydronephrosis. *Pediatr Urol* 1990;35:433.

102. Hutton KE, Thomas DF, Arthur RJ, et al. Prenatally detected posterior urethral valves: is gestational age at detection a predictor of outcome? *J Urol* 1994;152:698.

103. Camera G, Mastroiacovo P. Birth prevalence of skeletal dysplasia in the Italian multicentric monitoring system for birth defects. In: Papadatos CJ, Bartsocas CCS, eds. *Skeletal dysplasias*. New York: Alan R Liss, 1982:441.

104. Clark RN. Congenital dysplasias and dwarfism. *Pediatr Rev* 1990;12:149.

105. Bulas DI, Stern HJ, Rosenbaum KN, et al. Variable prenatal appearance of osteogenesis imperfecta. *J Ultrasound Med* 1994;13:419.

106. Vintzileos AM, Rippert LSM, Sniders RJM, Nicolaides KH, et al. Relationship of fetal biophysical profile score and blood gas values in severely growth retarded fetuses. *Am J Obstet Gynecol* 1990;163:569.

107. Manning FA, Platt LD. Maternal hypoxemia and fetal breathing movement. *Obstet Gynecol* 1979;53:758.

108. Lange IR, Manning FA, Morrison I, et al. Cord prolapse: is antenatal diagnosis possible? *Am J Obstet Gynecol* 1985;151:1083.

109. Boddy K, Dawes GS. Fetal breathing. *Br Med Bull* 1976;31:3.
110. Natale R, Clewlow F, Dawes GS. Measurement of fetal forelimb movements in the lamb in utero. *Am J Obstet Gynecol* 1981; 140:545.
111. Brown R, Patrick J. The non-stress test: how long is enough? *Am J Obstet Gynecol* 1981;141:646.
112. Manning FA. Dynamic ultrasound based fetal assessment: the fetal biophysical profile score. *Clinical Obstet Gynecol* 1995; 3826:44.
113. William K. Amniotic fluid assessment. *Obstet Gynecol Surv* 1993;46:795.
114. Ray M, Freeman R, Pine S, et al. Clinical experience with oxytocin challenge test. *Am J Obstet Gynecol* 1972;114:1.
115. Freeman RK. The use of oxytocin challenge test for antepartum clinical evaluation of uteroplacental respiratory function. *Am J Obstet Gynecol* 1975;121:481.
116. Hage ML. Interpretation of nonstress tests. *Am J Obstet Gynecol* 1985;153:490.
117. Manning FA, Platt LD, Sipos L. Antepartum fetal evaluation: development of a fetal biophysical profile score. *Am J Obstet Gynecol* 1980;136:787.
118. Manning FA, Morrison I, Harman CR, et al. Fetal assesment based on fetal biophysical prophile score. Experience with 19,221 referred high risk pregnancies. *Am J Obstet Gynecol* 1987;157:880.
119. Baskett TF, Gray JH, Prewett ST, et al. Antepartum fetal assessment using a fetal biophysical profile score. *Am J Obstet Gynecol* 1983;148:630.
120. Manning FA, Snijder R, Harman CR, et al. Fetal BPS correlation with antepartum umbilical venous pH. *Am J Obstet Gynecol* 1993;169:755.
121. Vintzileos AM, Gaffney SE, Salinger LM, et al. The relationship between fetal biophysical profile and cord pH in patients undergoing C section. *Obstet Gynecol* 1987;70:196.
122. Manning FA, Harman C, Menticoglou S. Fetal BPS and cerebral palsy at age 3 years. *Am J Obstet Gynecol* 1996;174:319.
123. Manning FA, Harman CR, Lange IR, et al. Modified fetal BPS by selective use of the NST. *Am J Obstet Gynecol* 1987;156:709.
124. Manning FA. Dynamic ultrasound based fetal assessment: the fetal biophysical profile score. *Clin Obstet Gynecol* 1995;38:26.
125. Marsal K. Rational use of Doppler ultrasound in perinatal medicine. *J Perinat Med* 1994;22:463.
126. Johnson T. Maternal perception and Doppler detection of fetal movement. *Clin Perinatol* 1994;21:765.
127. Gill RW. Measurement of blood flow by ultrasound accuracy and source of error. *Ultrasound Med Biol* 1985;11:625.
128. Fleischer A, Schumlman H, Farmakides G. Uterine artery Doppler velocimetry in pregnant women with hypertension. *Am J Obstet Gynecol* 1986;154:806.
129. Thompson RS, Trudinger BJ. Doppler waveform pulsatility index and resistance pressure and flow in the unbilical placental circulation. *Ultasound Med Biol* 1990;16:449.
130. Harman C, Baschet A. Comprehensive assessment of fetal wellbeing: which Doppler tests should be performed? *Curr Opin Obstet Gynecol* 2003;15:147.
131. Detti L, Akiyama M, Mari G. Doppler blood flow in obstetrics. *Curr Opin Obstet Gynecol* 2002;14:587.
132. Giles WB, Trudinger BJ, Cook CM. Umbilical artery velocity time waveforms in pregnancy. *J Ultrasound Med* 1982;1:9.
133. Okamura K, Watanabe T, Ando J, et al. Blood gas profiles of fetuses with abnormal Doppler flow in the umbilical artery. *Am J Perinatol* 1996;13:297.
134. Weiner CP. The relationship between umbilical artery S/D ratio and umbilical blood gas measurements in specimens obtained by cordocentesis. *Am J Obstet Gynecol* 1990;162:1198.
135. Westergaard HB, Langhoff-Roos J, Lingman G, et al. A critical appraisal of the use of umbilical artery Doppler ultrasound in high risk pregnancies; use of metaanalyses in evidence based obstetrics. *Ultrasound Obstet Gynecol* 2001;17:46.
136. Rochelson B, Schulman H, Farmakides G, et al. The significance of absent end diastolic velocity in umbilical artery velocity waveforms. *Am J Obstet Gynecol* 1987;156:1213.
137. Giles W. Clinical use of Doppler US in pregnancy. Information from six randomised trials. *Fetal Diagn Ther* 1993;8:247.
138. Bricker L, Neilson JP. Routine Doppler ultrasound in pregnancy. *Cochrane Database Syst Rev* 2;2003.
139. Vossbeck S, de Camargo OD, Grab D, et al. Neonatal and neurodevelopmental outcome in infants born before 30 weeks of gestation with absent or reversed end diastolic flow velocities in the umbilical artery. *Eur J Pediatr* 2001;160:128.
140. Wienerroither H, Steiner H, Tomaselli J, et al. Intrauterine blood flow and long term intellectual neurologic and social development. *Obstet Gynecol* 2001;97:449.
141. Kurschera J, Tomaselli J, Urlesberger B, et al. Absent or reversed end-diatolic blood flow in the umbilical artery and abnormal Doppler cerebroplacental ratio-cognitive, neurological, and somatic development at 3-6 years. *Early Hum Dev* 2002;29:47.
142. Wladimiroff JW, Wijingaard JAGW, Degani S. Cerebral and umbilical blood flow velocity waveforms in normal and growth retarded pregnancies. *Obstet Gynecol* 1987;69:705.
143. Veille JC, Kanaan C. Duplex Doppler ultrasonographic evaluation of the fetal lamb artery in normal and abnormal fetuses. *Am J Obstet Gynecol* 1989;161:1502.
144. Dubiel M, Gudmundsson S, Gunnarson G, et al. Middle cerebral artery velocimetry as a predictor of hypoxemia in fetuses with increased resistance to blood flow in the umbilical artery. *Early Hum Dev* 1997;47:177.
145. Donofreio MT, Bremer YA, Schieken RM, et al. Autoregulation of Cerebral Blood Flow in Fetuses with Congenital Heart Disease: the brain sparing effect. *Pediatr Cardiol* 2003;28.
146. Harrington K, Carpenter RG, Nguyen M, et al. Changes observed in Doppler studies of the fetal circulation in pregnancies complicated by preeclampsia or SGA baby. *Ultrasound Obstet Gynecol* 1995;6:19.
147. Devine PA, Bracero LA, Lyskiewicz A, et al. Middle cerebral to umbilical artery Doppler ratio in post date pregnancies. *Obstet Gynecol* 1994;84:856.
148. Zimmermann P, Alback T, Koskinen J, et al. Doppler flow velocimetry of the umbilical artery, uteroplacental artery and fetal MCA in prolonged pregnancy. *Ultrasound Obstet Gynecol* 1995;5:189.
149. Hecher K, Campbell S, Doyle P, et al. Assessment of fetal compromise by Doppler ultrasound investigation of the fetal circulation. *Circulation* 1995;91:129.
150. Galan HL, Ferrazzi E, Hobbins JC. Intrauterine growth restriction: biometric and Doppler assessment. *Prenatal Diagn* 2002; 22:331.

Fetal Therapy

13

Mark I. Evans   Mark P. Johnson   Alan W. Flake
Yuval Yaron   Michael R. Harrison

Over the past three decades, physicians from multiple specialties have developed numerous methods for the diagnosis of structural and physiological fetal abnormalities (1,2). When they are severe or lethal, pregnancy termination is viewed by many as a reasonable consideration. For couples in countries that permit its availability and in cultures in which the fetus does not have more rights than the mother, a variable portion of patients chose this option (3,4). With more moderate fetal anomalies, obstetrical care can be modified to optimize outcomes and prevent secondary complications. In some instances, prenatal treatments of the underlying problem have become possible. In general, structural malformations are more logically approached with surgery, although metabolic disorders may benefit from pharmacological or genetic therapies (2).

Fetal therapy has evolved into four major areas: open surgical approaches, "closed" endoscopic surgical approaches, pharmacological therapy, and stem cell/gene therapy. Advances in the field have been characterized by alternating exuberance at spectacular successes, but also periods of intense frustration at technical challenges to be overcome to bring new approaches on line. "Moving goal posts" have also been a common problem, secondary to improvements in ancillary care that keep raising the bar to show intervention as having a positive benefit to risk ratio.

Even after four decades since the first transfusions by Lilley, the single most misunderstood and continuous issue about fetal therapy continues to be "why before and not after birth." There is no one single answer; rather there are multiple disorder-specific considerations. If something cannot be treated safely postnatally, then there is generally justification for prenatal intervention. However, for many conditions profound and irreparable damage occurs before birth, making fetal intervention the best or sometimes only way to ameliorate the damage. Some procedures have been quite rare. Others are more common. The expectation is that with improvements and increasing utilization of prenatal diagnosis, more women will choose to consider the opportunities to treat fetuses before birth.

SURGICAL THERAPY

In Utero "Closed" Fetal Surgery

The most successful *in utero* fetal surgery has been for the evaluation and treatment of obstructive uropathy (5,6). Lower urinary tract obstruction (LUTO) is a heterogeneous entity that affects 1:500—8,000 newborn males (5–8). Posterior urethral valves or urethral atresias are the most common causes, although stenosis of the urethral meatus, anterior urethral valves, ectopic insertion of a ureter and tumors of the bladder have also been observed. Massive distention of the bladder can be seen with compensatory hypertrophy and hyperplasia of the smooth muscle within the bladder wall. Loss of compliance and elasticity, and poor postnatal function generally require post natal surgical reconstruction (9). Elevated intravesicular pressures prevent urine inflow from the ureters, eventually distortion of the ureterovesical angles contributes to reflux hydronephrosis (5–7). Progressive pyelectasis and calyectasis compress the delicate renal parenchyma within the encasing serosal capsule, leading to functional abnormalities within the medullary and eventually the cortical regions (5–10). Focal compressive hypoxia likely contributes to the progressive fibrosis and perturbations in tubular function resulting in urinary hypertonicity. Obstructive processes can eventually lead to type IV cystic dysplasia and renal insufficiency (8–9).

The effects extend beyond the genitourinary tract. Progressive oligo/anhydramnios leads to compressive deformations as seen in Potter sequence, including extremity contractures, facial dysmorphology, and disruptions of abdominal wall musculature, as in prune belly. Absence of normal amniotic fluid volume profoundly impedes pulmonary growth and development. Constant compressive pressure on the fetal thorax leads to restriction of expansion of the chest through normal physiological "breathing movements." Babies born with LUTO mostly die because of pulmonary complications. They do not live long enough to die of renal failure.

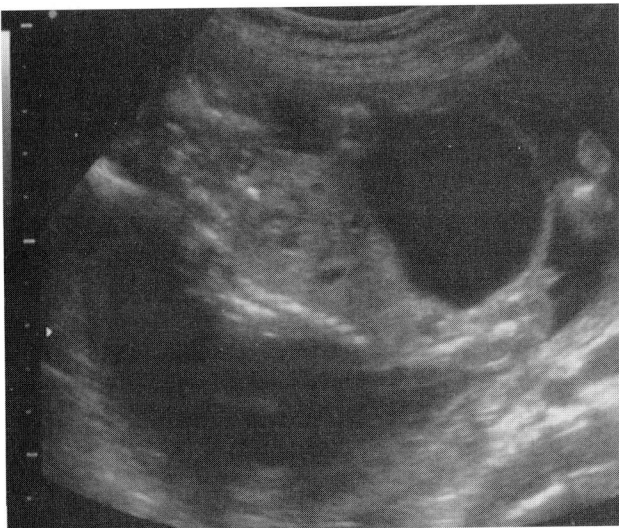

Figure 13-1 Oligohydramnios and dilated bladder in a fetus at 17 weeks with good electrolytes.

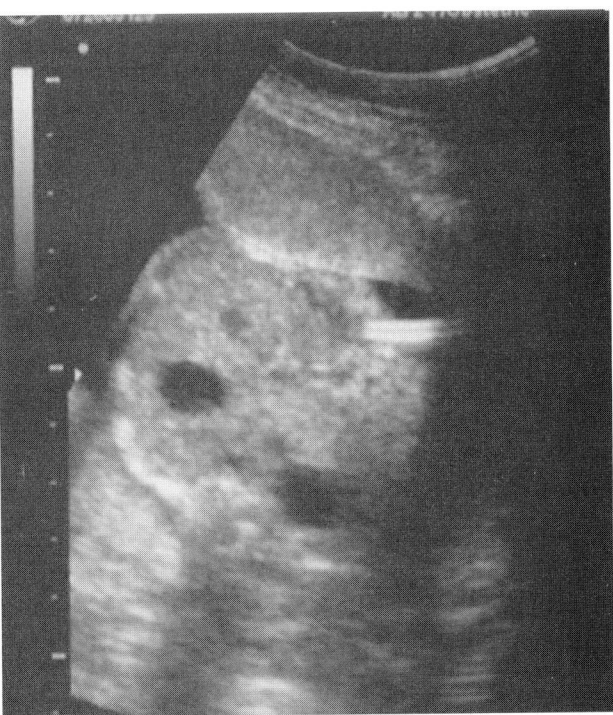

Figure 13-2 Vesicoamniotic shunt with the proximal portion lying within the fetal bladder although the distal portion lies within the amniotic fluid space allowing diversionary draining of urine into the appropriate space.

Sonographic findings in LUTO include dilated and thickened walls of the bladder, hydronephrosis, and oligohydramnios (Fig. 13-1). Urethral strictures or atresia, urethral agenesis, megalourethra, ureteral reflux, and cloacal anomalies may be present and have a very similar appearance on ultrasound. The typical "keyhole sign" of proximal urethral dilation is secondary to urethral obstruction present in posterior urethral valves or atresia. However, the precise diagnosis can only be made after birth (9).

The prenatal evaluation and management of fetuses with the sonographic findings of LUTO require multiple steps (5–8). Ruling out other congenital anomalies such as cardiac and neural tube defects is necessary before intervention can be considered.

Karyotyping is essential to confirm a normal male chromosomal status. Most are isolated problems, but the incidence of aneuploidy is higher than the general population. Female fetuses, however, almost always have more complex syndromes of cloacal malformations and do not benefit from *in utero* shunt therapy. Because of the presence of oligo/anhydramnios, we commonly obtain karyotypes by transabdominal chorionic villus sampling, which gives reliable results within several days during which the remainder of the prenatal evaluation is underway. Fluorescence in situ hybridization is now commonly used to get rapid status of chromosomes 13, 18, 21, X & Y (11, 12).

Essential to the prenatal workup is the evaluation of underlying renal status in the fetus. Over the past 15 years, a multicomponent approach has developed for the analysis of fetal urine that evaluates proximal tubular and possible glomerular status using sodium, chloride, osmolality, calcium, β-2 microglobulin, albumin, and total protein concentrations (6,8). It has been shown to be significantly improved by sequential samplings at 48- to 72-hour intervals to be useful approach. The degree of impaired renal function and damage with the extent of urinary hypertonicity and proteinuria can then be directly correlated.

The ability to counsel patients about the renal status of their fetus and the long-term prognosis has been dramatically improved as a result.

Vesicoamniotic catheter shunts bypass the urethral obstruction diverting the urine into the amniotic space to allow appropriate drainage of the upper urinary tract and prevention of pulmonary hypoplasia and physical deformations (Fig. 13-2). In fetuses with isolated LUTO, a normal male karyotype, and progressively improving urinary profile that meet threshold parameters (Table 13-1), intervention has been very successful in salvaging fetuses using percutaneous vesicoamniotic shunt therapy.

Subsequent experience in humans has been widely variable and appears to be related to the extent of prenatal evaluation prior to shunt placement, and the etiology of obstruction. Freedman and associates found that prune

TABLE 13-1

UPPER THRESHOLD VALUES FOR SELECTING FETUSES THAT MIGHT BENEFIT FROM PRENATAL INTERVENTION FOR URINARY OBSTRUCTION

Sodium	<100 mg/dl
Chloride	<90 mg/dl
Osmolality	<190 mOsm/L
Calcium	<8 mg/dl
β-2 microglobulin	<6 mg/L
Total protein	<40 mg/dl

belly infants, without complete urethral obstructions have very good renal outcomes following vesicoamniotic shunt therapy (9). They also found significant improvement in survival and renal function in infants with posterior urethral valves treated by shunting. However, many such children develop mild-to-moderate renal insufficiency at birth and several of these have progressed to renal failure, requiring dialysis, and transplantation. The worst prognosis appears to be for those with urethral atresia. There have been survivors, including some with urethral atresia, following early shunt intervention. Animal studies have indicated that early onset, complete obstructions result in more severe renal damage than later onset or partial obstructions. Such data emphasizes the necessity of early diagnosis, evaluation, and intervention to achieve the best outcomes in such cases.

 Data from our experience over the past 15 years suggest that patients having bladder shunts had a 91% survival, but that long-term renal function was not guaranteed. Just under half had "normal renal function," and about a quarter had mild impairments. The experience depended largely on the exact etiology of the disorder with posterior urethral value having the best outcomes and urethral atresia the worst. Our experience suggests that close pediatric urological/renal function assessment is essential to maximize outcomes. The Paris group has found, consistent with our experience, that about 25% of children had serious, long-term renal impairments and about 15% actually developed end-stage renal disease requiring transplant (10).

Although vesicoamniotic shunting has certainly improved survival and renal function in cases of early obstructive uropathy, complications of this procedure remain unacceptably high. We found in the eighties and nineties that in 40% of our cases, the shunts became physically displaced into the amniotic or intraperitoneal space, or have become blocked causing loss of drainage function and necessitating replacement. On balance, intervention for LUTO has clearly saved fetuses, who would otherwise have surely died. Many have normal to moderately impaired renal function. A carefully balanced approach in counseling is required for patients to determine what is right for them.

Other Shunt Procedures

Shunting was attempted for obstructive hydrocephalus, in the late 1970s (13). The results were almost uniformly dismal. Most of the patients operated on were, in retrospect, very poor candidates for intervention. Many had multisystem syndromic disorders, including aneuploidy, and hopeless congenital anomalies such as holoprosencephaly.

Ventriculoamniotic shunts were abandoned the early eighties. However, with a better understanding of the poor natural history of the anomaly, and improved, more accurate diagnostic techniques, there may eventually be some limited applications for prenatal neurological shunting. It may eventually be useful in cases of early onset, isolated, progressive obstructive hydrocephaly.

The other use of percutaneously placed shunts has been for thoracic abnormalities (14,15). The macrocystic form of congenital cystic adenomatoid malformation (CCAM) can present with a very large intrathoracic mass with a dominant macrocyst which causes cardiac and mediastinal shifts. Potential hemodynamic changes can result along with pulmonary compression and risk of lung hypoplasia. Such dominant cysts can be approached using pleuroamniotic shunts to chronically drain these structures, reducing their volume, and diminishing their space occupying effects within the thoracic cavity.

Isolated pleural effusions can enlarge, causing hemodynamic changes and onset of generalized hydrops and pulmonary compression. The mass interferes with normal lung development increasing the risk of hypoplasia. Small, unilateral effusions generally do not warrant intervention, but cannot be ignored as they have the potential for rapid progression (15).

As with all fetal interventions, prenatal evaluation prior to intervention is critical for appropriate case selection. Seemingly isolated effusions may be associated with cardiac malformations, aneuploidy, anemia, or an infectious process. Thoracoamniotic shunting is effective in carefully evaluated cases when the risk of pulmonary hypoplasia from large effusions early in gestation is present, or early signs of progressive hydrops (unilateral or bilateral effusion, skin or scalp edema, ascites, pericardial effusion) appear. Fetal anemia, per se, is not an indication for thoracoamniotic effusion shunting. Hydropic changes will usually resolve with timely fetal transfusion therapy. By the time the fetus develops significant ascites, the prognosis even with successful shunt intervention, diminishes considerably (15). However, several cases with suddenly progressive pleural effusions and onset of generalized hydrops have been treated with complete resolution of all hydropic complications and normal postnatal infants.

Open Surgery

Open fetal surgery has been performed for a limited number of indications for nearly two decades (3). There are appropriate concerns for maternal risks, rigorous selection criteria, and somewhat frustrating results. There has been continuing innovation and development of instruments and techniques, motivated by the clinical necessity to improve the safety of open fetal surgery for both the fetus and the mother, which have turned the field upside down in many instances.

Congenital Diaphragmatic Hernia

The surgical approach to congenital diaphragmatic hernia (CDH) has evolved considerably since the first attempted CDH repair in 1986 and the first success in 1989 (16–18). Definitive repair of CDH by reduction of viscera from the chest, diaphragmatic patch placement, and abdominal silo construction (to reduce intraabdominal pressure) satisfied the desire for a single step approach but had unacceptable

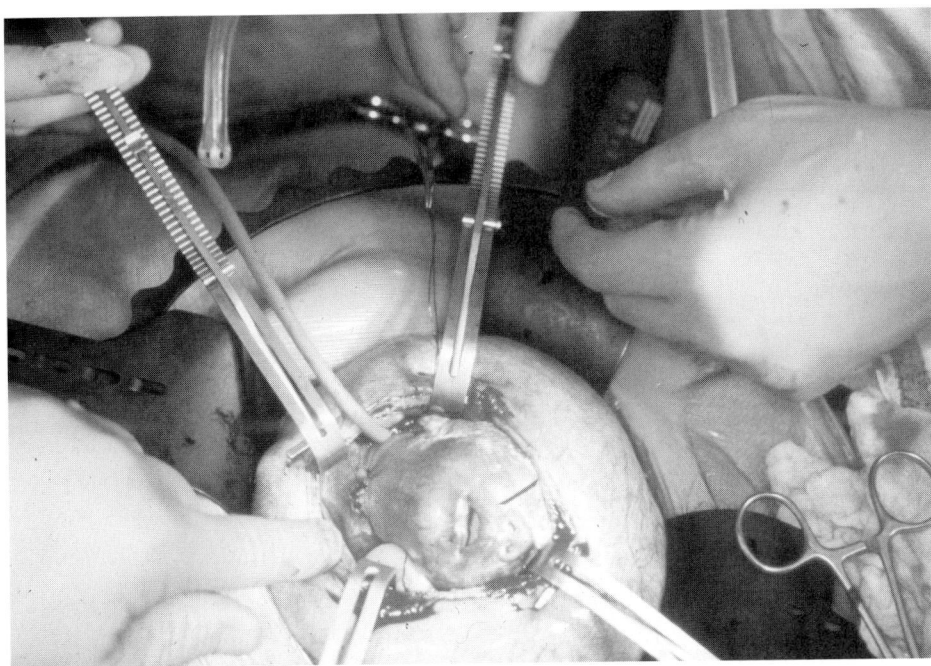

Figure 13-3 Surgical isolation of the fetal trachea prior to placement of hemoclips in a tracheal occlusion procedure for congenital diaphragmatic hernia.

mortality, particularly after a clinical trial showed that open fetal repair was no better than postnatal repair when the liver was herniated into the chest (19,20). The definitive repair was then abandoned and *in utero* tracheal occlusion took its place (Fig. 13-3) (20–26).

Tracheal occlusion produces increased lung size through accumulation of pulmonary secretions. The herniated viscera are reduced from the chest and therefore decrease the risk for lung hypoplasia. The technique of achieving reliable, complete and reversible tracheal occlusion has evolved. Initially, it could only be accomplished by open fetal surgery and fetal neck dissection (taking care to avoid the recurrent laryngeal nerves) and placement of occlusive hemoclips. Then, a fetoscopic technique was developed to accomplish the same neck dissection and tracheal clip (the Fetendo Clip Procedure) (24). While successful, it proved difficult, with a significant learning curve. Attempts to simplify the procedure by developing an appropriate polymer to use as a tracheal plug inserted through the fetal mouth have been generally unsuccessful. Unless there was complete occlusion, the pulmonary secretions would leak, thereby defeating the purpose of the plug. Finally, a relatively simple technique was developed in which a fetoscope passed through a single port is advanced into the fetal trachea (fetal bronchoscopy) and a detachable silicone balloon is inflated to occlude the trachea.

CDH has a prototype of rapid changes in technology, further clouding any simple attempts to understand the role for fetal surgery. With increasing sophistication of the surgical approach and concomitant improvements in neonatal care using extracorporeal membrane oxygenation, it was impossible to accurately determine the relative benefits of each approach without a prospective, randomized comparison that held all other details constant. Thus, after much debate, a randomized trial of surgery for CDH vs. optimal postnatal care was funded by National Institute of Child Health and Human Development (NICHD) (21). The principal component of the trial was that patients in the postnatal care arm (control group) would receive the same neonatal care by the same center as the surgical arm.

It was originally expected that patients having the surgery would have a survival rate of about 70%. The best data on controls showed survivals of about 35%. The surgically treated patients achieved the expected survival rate. However, by having the controls cared for at the same tertiary specialty centers as the surgical group, survival in the controls was essentially the same as the surgical group. Therefore, the trial was stopped prematurely. Such data show dramatically the principle of "the moving target" and how our use of technology must continually adapt to changing conditions (27).

Congenital Cystic Adenomatoid Malformation

CCAM is a space occupying congenital cystic lesion of the lung. Hydrops evolves by causing mediastinal shift which compromises venous return to the heart. When fetuses with CCAM develop hydrops, the fetal mortality approaches 100% (Fig. 13-4) (28–30). Fetal resection of CCAM can reverse hydrops and has improved survival dramatically (17). The fetal operation is performed by exposure of the arm and chest wall on the side of the lesion through the maternal hysterotomy. A large muscle sparing thoracotomy is performed through the midthorax of the fetus and the lobe containing the CCAM is isolated. The attachments of

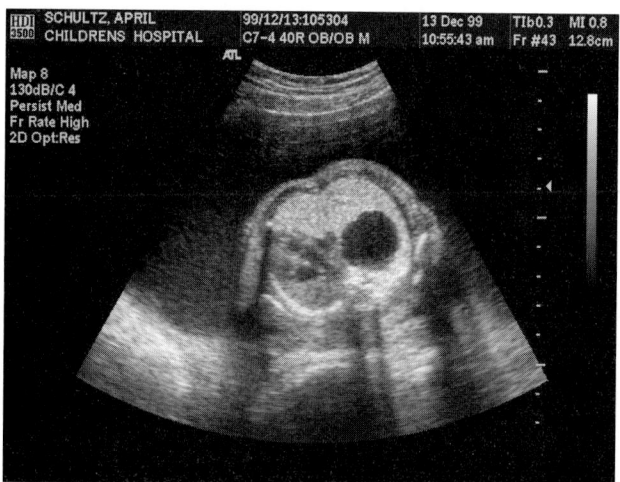

Figure 13-4 Microcystic congenital cystic adenomatous malformation (microcystic) with beginnings of hydrops.

the lobe to adjacent lung tissue are bluntly divided and the lobar hilum is divided by use of a stapler or a bulk ligature. During the remainder of the pregnancy, the remaining normal lung shows compensatory growth to fill the space left following removal of the mass.

Sacrococcygeal Teratoma

Fetal sacrococcygeal teratoma (SCT) arises from the presacral space, which may grow to massive proportions and in some fetuses induces high output congestive heart failure from tumor vascular steal. Fetal SCT with high output physiology and associated placentomegaly or hydrops uniformly results in fetal demise (Fig. 13-5) (31,32). The pathophysiological rationale for fetal surgery is to ligate the vascular connections to the tumor, remove the vascular shunt, and reverse the high output physiology. The fetal operation is performed by exteriorization of the fetal buttocks with attached tumor *(31)*. The head, torso, and lower extremities of the fetus are kept *in utero* if at all possible. Since the tumor can sometimes be larger than the fetus, significant loss of uterine volume occurs, and the uterus may contract increasing the risk for placental abruption, placental dysfunction because of compression, or postoperative preterm labor. Once exteriorized, the anus is identified, and the fetal skin is incised posterior to the anorectal sphincter complex to avoid injury to the continence mechanism. A tourniquet is then applied at the base of the tumor and brought down gradually as the tumor is finger fractured down to its vascular pedicle. The vascular pedicle is then ligated or stapled depending on the width of the pedicle. The entire fetal procedure can be performed in less than 15 minutes with minimal blood loss. Because of the increase in afterload following ligation of the low resistance tumor circuit, the fetal hemodynamic status must be monitored by fetal echocardiography during and in the immediate period following the ligation.

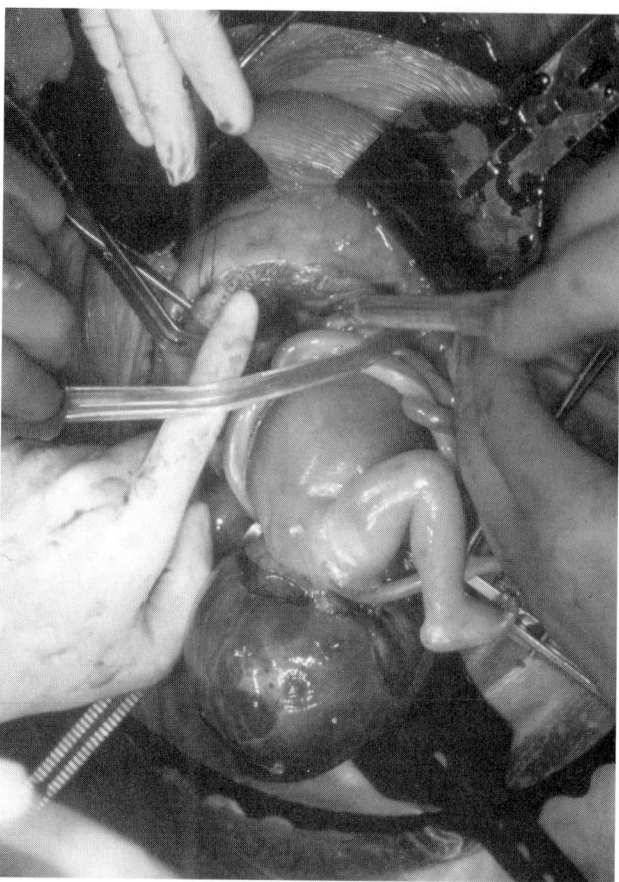

Figure 13-5 Sacrococcygeal teratoma in a fetus.

Neural Tube Defects

Neural tube defects (NTDs) result from abnormal closure of the neural tube which normally occurs between the third and fourth week of gestational age. The etiology is complex, with both genetic and environmental factors involved. There are historical data in humans suggesting increased NTD frequencies in subjects with poor dietary histories or with intestinal bypasses. Analysis of recurrence patterns within families and of twin-twin concordance data provides evidence of a genetic influence in nonsyndromal cases. However, factors such as socioeconomic status, geographic area, occupational exposure, and maternal use of antiepileptic drugs are also associated with variations in the incidence of NTDs (33). In 1980, Smithells and associates suggested that vitamin supplementation containing 0.36 mg folate could reduce the frequency of NTD recurrence by sevenfold (33–35). For almost a decade, there has been a great deal of controversy regarding the benefit of folate supplementation for the prevention of NTDs3 (36–39). In 1991, a randomized double-blinded trial designed by the Medical Research Council Vitamin Study Research Group demonstrated that preconceptual folate reduces the risk of recurrence in high risk patients (40). Subsequently, it was shown that preparations containing folate and other vitamins also reduce the occurrence of first time NTDs (41). In response to these findings, guidelines were issued calling for consumption of 4.0 mg/day folic acid by women with a prior child affected with an NTD, for at least 1 month prior to conception through the first 3 months of pregnancy. Additionally, 0.4 mg/day folic acid is recommended to all women planning a pregnancy to be taken preconceptually. The data on NTD recurrence prevention is now very well established, and has become routine practice for high-risk cases. As of January 1998, the United States Food and Drug Administration have mandated that breads and grains be supplemented with folic acid. The impact of food fortification with folic acid on NTDs birth prevalence during the years 1990–1999 was evaluated by assessing birth certificate reports before and after mandatory fortification (42). It was found that the birth prevalence of NTDs reported decreased by 19%. It is important to note that the continuing decline in NTDs rates are estimated to be as a result of the introduction and increased utilization of prenatal diagnosis in addition to the recommendation for multivitamin use in women of childbearing age and the population-wide increases in blood folate levels because food fortification was mandated (43). Recently, Evans and associates have shown a 32% drop in high maternal serum alpha-fetoprotein (MSAFP) values in the United States comparing 2000 values versus 1997 before the introduction of folic acid supplementation (44).

Folate plays a central part in embryonic and fetal development because of its role in nucleic acid synthesis mandatory for the widespread cell division that takes place during embryogenesis. Folate deficiency can occur because of low dietary folate intake or because of increased metabolic requirement as seen in particular genetic alterations such as the polymorphism of the thermolabile enzyme methyltetrahydrofolate reductase (MTHRF). However, evidence regarding its role in NTD is unsupported, except in certain populations, suggesting that these variants are not large contributors to the etiology of NTDs (45,46). Additional candidate genes other than MTHFR may be responsible for an increased risk for NTDs (47). It has recently been reported that methionine synthase polymorphisms are associated with increased risk for NTDs, that is not influenced by maternal preconception folic acid intake at doses of 0.4 mg/day (48). Other candidate genes include the mitochondrial membrane transporter gene UCP2 (49). Despite previous studies suggesting zinc deficiency to play a role in the etiology of NTDs (50,51), further studies were inconclusive (52,53). Because methionine deficiency may be involved in NTDs, it may be beneficial in NTD risk reduction (54). Preconception folic acid intake as a sole vitamin or as multivitamin supplementation reduces the risk of recurrence and first time NTDs.

Babies with meningomyeloceles have impaired lower motor function, loss of bowel, and bladder control. A significant percentage develop obstructive hydrocephalus, which requires ventriculoperitoneal shunting (55,56). Experience from the 1970s and 1980s showed that babies with meningomyelocele delivered atraumatically by cesarean section had a better level of motor function for the given level of anatomic defect, than those babies delivered through the vaginal canal (55). Such data suggest that compression and trauma to the cord in the delivery process can have permanent long-term sequelae to motor function. In theory, trauma to the spinal cord *in utero*, either from banging into the uterine wall or the toxic effects of the amniotic fluid in the third trimester, could be detrimental to the function of the spinal cord. Traditional dogma held that the pathogenesis of meningomyelocele was that an abnormally developed spinal cord, which did not engender the proper development of the bony spinal column, may not be the whole story. It is possible that the primary defect is in the bony spinal column, which exposes a presumptively undamaged spinal cord. The cord is then damaged by the toxic affects of amniotic fluid and trauma from the uterine environment and repeated contact with the uterine wall. Thus, the rationale for attempts to cover and protect the spinal cord in utero, to minimize the sequelae (57).

Three groups (58–60) have done most of the work in this area and have attempted to repair meningomyeloceles in utero, both as an open surgical procedure, and endoscopically, with the stated attempt to reduce long-term morbidity and mortality. The principal benefit of the surgery is likely secondary, i.e., a significant reduction in the number of babies requiring ventriculoperitoneal shunting for obstructive hydrocephalus (58,61). There is still much controversy surrounding the data (54). A randomized, prospective trial comparing fetal to postnatal neurosurgical closure began in 2003 but will take several years to be completed. A major milestone of this trial has been the agreement among the participating centers not to perform any cases outside the trial, and other centers around the country have agreed not to start programs until the trial is completed.

The Ex Utero Intrapartum Therapy Procedure

The ex utero intrapartum therapy procedure (EXIT) procedure is a modified cesarean delivery and may be applied to deliver fetuses after fetal surgical procedures such as tracheal ligation, or for fetuses with difficult airway problems such as massive cervical teratomas or cystic hygromas (62,63). The most important component of the EXIT procedure is maintenance of uteroplacental perfusion until the fetal airway is secured and ventilation is established. In direct contrast to cesarean section in which uterine contraction for hemostasis is encouraged, uterine relaxation is maintained by deep general anesthesia. The fetal manipulations are then performed with maternal support via the placenta. Clips can be removed, chest masses removed, bronchoscopy performed, and stable airway access established in otherwise very difficult circumstances with this approach. Once the fetus is ready for transport to the nursery or adjacent operating suite following these preliminary steps, the cord is clamped, cut and the cesarean delivery completed.

ENDOCRINE DISORDERS

Adrenal Disorders

Congenital Adrenal Hyperplasia

Congenital adrenal hyperplasia is actually not a single disorder but a group of autosomal recessive metabolic disorders, characterized by enzymatic defects in the steroidogenic pathway (64). A compensatory increase in adrenocorticotropic hormone secretion leads to overproduction of the steroid precursors in the adrenal cortex resulting in adrenal hyperplasia. Excess precursors often are converted to androgens that may result in virilization of female fetuses. The phenotype is determined by the severity of the cortisol deficiency and the nature of the steroid precursors which accumulate proximal to the enzymatic block. The most common abnormality, responsible for greater than 90% of patients with congenital adrenal hyperplasia (CAH) is caused by a deficiency of the 21-hydroxylase (21-OH) enzyme. Other, less common causes for CAH, include deficiencies in 11β-hydroxylase, 17β-hydroxylase, and 3α-hydroxysteroid-dehydrogenase. Reduced 21-OH activity results in accumulation of 17-hydroxyprogesterone (17-OHP) as a result of its decreased conversion to 11-deoxy-corticosterone. Excess 17-OHP is then converted via androstenedione to androgens, the levels of which increase by as much as several hundred-fold (Fig. 13-6). The excess androgens cause virilization of the undifferentiated female external genitalia. The degree of virilization may vary from mild clitoral hypertrophy to complete formation of a phal-lus and scrotum. In contrast, genital development in male fetuses is normal. The excess androgens cause postnatal virilization in both genders and may manifest in precocious puberty (64).

The "classical" form of CAH involves a severe enzyme deficiency or even a complete block of enzymatic activity, which is associated in two-thirds to three-fourths with salt-loss that may be life-threatening. The classical form is easy to recognize in female newborns but may be overlooked in males, which may present at a later stage with severe dehydration and even demise. The "nonclassical" attenuated form of 21-OH deficiency results in partial blockade of the enzymatic activity and is usually clinically apparent as simple virilization in women only later in life. It is estimated to occur in about 3.5% in Ashkenazi Jews and about 2% in Hispanics (65). In the late seventies and early eighties, diagnosis of CAH was made on amniocentesis by the finding of elevated levels of 17-OHP in the supernatant. In the eighties, with the development of chorionic villus sampling (CVS) linkage based molecular diagnosis in the first trimester became available, because the gene for 21-OH was found to be linked to the human leukocyte antigen (HLA) complex on chromosome 6 (66). The gene for 21-OH (CYP21B) was later mapped, allowing direct mutation analysis in informative families (67).

It has been known for two decades that the fetal adrenal gland can be pharmacologically suppressed by maternal replacement doses of dexamethasone (68). Suppression can prevent masculinization of affected female fetuses in couples who are carriers of classical CAH. Evans, and associates were first to administer dexamethasone to a carrier

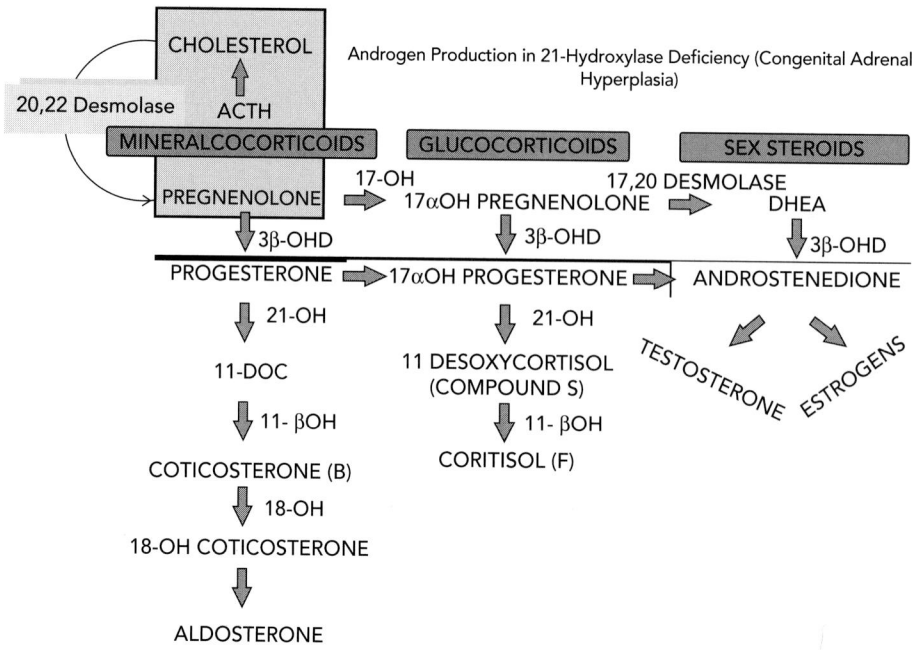

Figure 13-6 STEROIDOGENIC PATHWAY—Pathway of conversion from Cholesterol to Cortisol is vulnerable to enzymatic errors. Blockage at 21 hydroxylase leads to over production of 17 hydroxyprogesterone which ultimately leads to excess androgens that produce masculinization of the external genitalia.

mother beginning at 10 weeks of gestation in an attempt to prevent masculinization *(68)*. Serial maternal estriol and cortisol levels indicated that adrenal gland suppression had been achieved. The female fetus was born at 39 weeks gestation with normal external genitalia. A similar approach was employed successfully by Forrest and New (69,70). Differentiation of the external genitalia begins at about 7 weeks of gestation. Thus for a carrier couple, pharmacological therapy has to be initiated prior to diagnosis. Direct deoxyribonucleic acid (DNA) diagnosis or linkage studies are then performed by CVS in the first trimester and therapy is continued only if the fetus is found to be an affected female. Detailed inclusion criteria for treatment have been issued by the European Society for Pediatric Endocrinology and Wilkins Pediatric Endocrine Society (71).

Thyroid Disorders

Hyperthyroidism

Neonatal hyperthyroidism is rare with an incidence of 1:4,000 to 1:40,000/live births (72). Fetal thyrotoxic goiter is usually secondary to maternal autoimmune disease, most commonly, Graves' disease or Hashimoto's thyroiditis. As many as 12% of infants of mothers with a known history of Graves' disease are affected with neonatal thyrotoxicosis, which may occur even if the mother is euthyroid (73). The underlying mechanism is the transplacental passage of maternal IgG antibodies. In this case the antibodies, known as TSAb, are predominantly directed against the thyroid-stimulating hormone (TSH) receptor. Often in these cases, the fetal goiter is first diagnosed on ultrasound in patients with elevated thyroid stimulating antibodies. In some cases, fetal goiters are incidentally detected on routine ultrasonography. Others may be discovered in patients referred for scan because of polyhydramnios. Untreated fetal hyperthyroidism may be associated with a mortality rate of 12%–25% as a result of high-output cardiac failure (73).

Once the diagnosis of fetal hyperthyroidism is confirmed, fetal treatment should be initiated. Authors have attempted treating fetal hyperthyroidism with maternally administered antithyroid drugs. Porreco has reported maternal treatment of fetal thyrotoxicosis with propylthiouracil (PTU), which lead to a good outcome (74). The initial dose used was 100 mg p.o. three times a day, which was later decreased to 50 mg p.o. three times a day. A favorable outcome was shown using maternal methimazole to treat fetal hyperthyroidism in a patient who could not tolerate PTU (75). Hatjis also treated fetal goiterous hyperthyroidism with a maternal dose of 300 mg PTU (75). This patient however, required supplemental Synthroid to remain euthyroid. There was good fetal outcome in this case as well.

Hypothyroidism

Congenital hypothyroidism is relatively rare affecting about 1:3,000 to 1:4,000 infants (76). About 85% of the cases are the result of thyroid dysgenesis, a heterogeneous group of developmental defects characterized by inadequate amount of thyroid tissue. Congenital hypothyroidism is only rarely associated with errors of thyroid hormone synthesis, TSH insensitivity, or absence of the pituitary gland. Fetal hypothyroidism may not necessarily manifest in a goiter before birth because maternal thyroid hormones may cross the placenta. Congenital hypothyroidism presenting with a goiter can be found in only about 10%–15% of cases (77).

Fetal goiterous hypothyroidism is usually secondary to maternal exposure to thyrostatic agents such as PTU, radioactive I131, or iodide exposure used to treat maternal hyperthyroidism (78). Maternal ingestion of amiodarone or lithium may also cause hypothyroidism in the fetus. Finally, fetal hypothyroidism may follow transplacental passage of maternal blocking antibodies (known as TBIAb or TBII). Rarely it may be a result of rare defects in fetal thyroid hormone biosynthesis (72).

An enlarged fetal goiter may cause esophageal obstruction, polyhydramnios, leading to preterm delivery or premature rupture of membranes. Rarely, a goiter may even lead to high-output heart failure (78). A large fetal goiter can also cause extension of the fetal neck leading to dystocia. The effects of the fetal hypothyroidism itself may be devastating. Without treatment, postnatal growth delay and severe mental retardation may ensue. Even with immediate diagnosis and treatment at birth, long-term follow-up of children with congenital hypothyroidism has demonstrated that they have lower scores on perceptual-motor, visuospatial, and language tests (79).

In suspicious cases, an extensive maternal and family history should be obtained. In patients with a positive history, maternal thyroid hormone levels, and blocking immunoglobulin levels should be measured. Additionally, all women with a history of any thyroid disease (both hypothyroidism and hyperthyroidism) are advised to have monthly fetal ultrasound scans to screen for fetal goiter, polyhydramnios, or fetal tachycardia (79).

Occasionally, fetal goiterous hypothyroidism may be identified by a routine ultrasound performed as a result of increased uterine size caused by polyhydramnios secondary to esophageal obstruction and impaired swallowing. Sometimes, a fetal goiter may incidentally be discovered on a routine scan. Before the advent of cordocentesis, amniotic fluid levels of TSH and free thyroxine were used as potential indicators of fetal thyroid function. However, these proved to be inconsistent *(80)*. With cordocentesis, fetal thyroid status can be directly and accurately evaluated; fetal response to therapy can therefore be reliably measured using available appropriate nomograms for fetal serum levels of free T4, total T4, free T3, total T3, and TSH (81,82). In utero treatment was initially suggested by Van Herle and associates using i.m. injection of levothyroxine sodium (83). Subsequent studies however, have indicated that intraamniotic (IA) administration of thyroxine may be superior and can lead to resolution of the polyhydramnios as well. The dose of the injected drug may be refined using the fetal thyroid profile in the amniotic fluid and the thyroid size *(84)*. The doses commonly used for treatment range from 200–500 mg IA every week (23). With this regimen, fetal goiters have been shown to regress, the hyperextension of the fetal head have been shown to resolve and fetal and newborn TSH levels have normalized (84).

INBORN ERRORS OF METABOLISM

Methylmalonic Acidemia

The methylmalonic acidemias (MMA) are a group of autosomal recessive enzyme-deficiency diseases. Some cases are caused by mutations in the gene encoding methylmalonyl-coenzyme-A mutase. Others are a result of a defect that reduces the biosynthesis of adenosylcobalamin from vitamin B12. The disease has a wide clinical spectrum ranging from a benign condition to a fatal neonatal disease characterized by severe metabolic acidosis, developmental delay and biochemical abnormalities that include methylmalonic aciduria, long chain ketonuria, and intermittent hyperglycinemia. Neurological abnormalities may result from diminution of myelin content and of ganglioside N-acetylneuraminic acid in the cerebrum (85). Patients with defects in adenosylcobalamin biosynthesis may respond to administration of large doses of B12, which may enhance the amount of active holoenzyme (mutase apoenzyme plus adenosylcobalamin).

Ampola and associates first attempted prenatal diagnosis and treatment of a B12-responsive variant of MMA (86). Their patient previously had a child who died of severe MMA. In the subsequent pregnancy, amniocentesis at 19 weeks revealed an elevated methylmalonic acid level. Cultured amniocytes also demonstrated defective propionate oxidation and undetectable levels of adenosylcobalamin. When adenosylcobalamin was added, normal succinate oxidation and methylmalonyl-coenzyme-A mutase activity were noted, confirming that the fetus also suffered from MMA. Late in the pregnancy, cyanocobalamin (10 mg/day) was orally administered to the mother, only marginally altering maternal serum B12 level. They noted a slight reduction of maternal urinary methylmalonic acid excretion that remained several-fold above normal. At 34 weeks gestation, 5 mg of cyanocobalamin per day was administered intramuscularly. The maternal serum B12, level then rose gradually to more than sixfold above normal and was accompanied by a progressive decrease in urinary methylmalonic acid excretion. Maternal urinary methylmalonate was only slightly above the normal range when delivery occurred at 41 weeks. Amniotic fluid methylmalonic acid concentrations were three times the normal mean at 19 menstrual weeks and four times the normal mean at term, despite prenatal treatment. Postnatally, the diagnosis of methylmalonic acidemia was confirmed. The infant suffered no acute neonatal complications and had an extremely high serum B12 level. Long-term postnatal management involved protein restriction but continuous B12 treatment was not required.

It is not clear whether *in utero* treatment actually resulted in an improved outcome but it is likely that correction of the biochemical abnormality in the fetus had some beneficial effect on fetal development. In a cohort of 8 children with MMA, Andersson and associates described congenital malformations, probably caused by prenatally abnormal cyanocobalamin metabolism (87). Growth was significantly improved in most cases after initiation of therapy postnatally and in one case microcephaly resolved. However, developmental delay of variable severity was always present regardless of treatment onset. These data suggest that prenatal therapy of MMA may be effective and perhaps ameliorate some of the prenatal effects. Evans and associates have documented the changing dose requirements necessary over the course of pregnancy to maintain adequate levels of B12. They sequentially followed maternal plasma and urine levels in a prenatal treated pregnancy (88).

Multiple Carboxylase Deficiency

Biotin-responsive multiple carboxylase deficiency is an inborn error of metabolism caused by diminished activity of the mitochondrial biotin-dependent enzymes (pyruvate carboxylase, propionyl-coenzyme-A carboxylase and 3-methylcrotonyl-coenzyme-A carboxylase). The condition may arise from mutations in the holocarboxylase synthetase gene (HCS) or the biotinidase gene (89–93). Affected patients present with dermatitis, severe metabolic acidosis, and a characteristic pattern of organic acid excretion. Normal metabolism can be restored toward normal levels by biotin supplementation. Prenatal diagnosis is based on the demonstration of elevated levels of typical organic acids (3-hydroxyisovalerate, methylcitrate) in the amniotic fluid or in the chorionic villi. However, the existence of a mild form of HCS deficiency can complicate prenatal diagnosis as organic acids level in amniotic fluid might be normal (94). Therefore, prenatal diagnosis must be performed by enzyme assay in cultured fetal cells in biotin-restricted medium.

Roth and colleagues treated a fetus whose two previous siblings died of multiple carboxylase deficiency (95). The mother was first seen at 34 weeks gestation and prenatal diagnosis was not performed. Oral administration was begun at a dose of 10 mg/day of biotin. There were no apparent untoward effects. Maternal urinary biotin excretion increased by 100. Nonidentical twins were delivered at term. Cord blood and urinary organic acid profiles were normal, and cord blood biotin concentrations were 4–7 times greater than normal. The neonatal course for both twins was unremarkable. Subsequent study of the cultured fibroblasts of both twins indicated that the cells of one twin had complete deficiency of carboxylase activities. This was later confirmed by genetic studies. Other cases of such treatment were also reported (94,96,97).

Smith-Lemli-Optiz Syndrome

Smith-Lemli-Optiz syndrome (SLOS) is an autosomal recessive disorder characterized by multiple anomalies, dysmorphic features, growth and mental retardation. Males with SLOS frequently have ambiguous genitalia (98). The severe form is associated with a high rate of neonatal mortality (99). SLOS is estimated to occur in 1:20,000–40,000 live births with an estimated carrier frequency of 1:70 (100,101). SLOS is caused by an inborn error of cholesterol biosynthesis as a result of a deficiency of the enzyme dehydrocholesterol-Δ7 reductase leading to reduced cholesterol levels and elevated 7- and 8- dehydrocholesterol levels (7-DHC and 8-DHC respectively) in all body fluids and tissues including amniotic fluid and chorionic villi (100,102–104). The diagnosis is based on elevated levels of 7-DHC (100–1,000 times the normal value). Clinical manifestations correlate with cholesterol levels. Prenatal diagnosis of SLOS has been available since 1994 by either amniocentesis or chorionic villus sampling (105–107).

Since the identification of the cholesterol metabolic defect in SLOS, a treatment protocol has been attempted providing exogenous cholesterol. This form of therapy has now been provided to many patients with SLOS for the past several years in many centers in the United States and internationally (108–110), with the goal of raising cholesterol levels and decrease the precursors, 7-DHC and 8-DHC. It has been shown that dietary cholesterol supplementation can restore a normal growth pattern in children and adolescents with SLOS, alleviate behavioral abnormalities, and improve general health (108–110). Since significant development of the central nervous system and myelination occurs prior to birth it is reasonable to assume that providing cholesterol to the fetus, as early as possible would result in the most clinical benefit. However, providing cholesterol to the mother is of no use because cholesterol does not cross the placenta well in the second trimester and there is lack of evidence that it crosses the placenta in the third trimester. It is impractical to inject cholesterol into the amniotic fluid because it would precipitate. However, cholesterol can be given to the fetus by giving fresh frozen plasma in the form of low-density lipoprotein-cholesterol. A group at Tufts University has attempted treatment antenatally in several affected fetuses. In cases in which treatment was started late in pregnancy, the results were inconclusive. Although few descriptions of fetal therapy for SLOS exist, the latest report of antenatal treatment comes from that same group of investigators (111). Therapy was begun at 34 weeks of gestation and resulted in increased fetal cholesterol levels and red blood cell mean corpuscular volume with subtle improvement in fetal growth. However, no significant change in 7-DHC and 8-DHC levels was observed, further emphasizing the inconclusiveness of that treatment.

Galactosemia

Galactosemia is an autosomal recessive disorder caused by decreased activity of galactose-1-phosphate uridyltransferase (GALT). Clinical manifestations include cataracts, growth deficiency, and ovarian failure. Clinical symptoms appear in the neonatal period and can be largely ameliorated by elimination of galactose from the diet. Cellular damage in galactosemia is thought to be mediated by accumulation of galactose-1-phosphate intracellularly and of galactitol in the lens. Several disease-causing mutations in the GALT gene have been reported in classical galactosemia (112). Galactosemia can also be diagnosed prenatally by biochemical studies of cultured amniocytes and chorionic villi.

There are suggestions that even the early postnatal treatment of galactosemic individuals with a low galactose diet may not be sufficient to ensure normal development. Some have speculated that prenatal damage to galactosemic fetuses could contribute to subsequent abnormal neurological development and to lens cataract formation. Furthermore, it has been recognized that female galactosemics, even when treated from birth with galactose deprivation, have a high frequency of primary or secondary amenorrhea because of ovarian failure. This is because oocytes have already been damaged irreversibly long before birth (113,114). There also may be some subtle abnormalities of male gonadal function as well. Thus, galactose restriction during pregnancy may be beneficial in affected fetuses. In humans, ovarian meiosis begins at 12 weeks and ovarian damage may occur prior to prenatal diagnosis. Thus, anticipatory treatment in pregnancies at risk for having a galactosemic fetus might best be initiated very early in gestation or even preconceptually. There are no studies that adequately assess the impact of prenatal administration of a low-galactose diet to galactosemic infants. Nevertheless, prenatal galactose restriction is probably desirable in galactosemia and should be harmless.

PRENATAL HEMATOPOIETIC STEM CELL TRANSPLANTATION

The engraftment and clonal proliferation of a relatively small number of normal hematopoietic stem cells (HSCs) can sustain normal hematopoiesis for a lifetime. This observation provides the compelling rationale for bone marrow transplantation (BMT) and is now supported by thousands of long-term survivors of BMT who otherwise would have succumbed to lethal hematological disease (115,116). Realization of the full potential of BMT, however, continues to be limited by a critical shortage of immunologically compatible donor cells, the inability to control the recipient or donor immune response, and the requirement for recipient myeloablation to achieve engraftment. The price of HLA mismatch remains high: the greater the mismatch, the higher the incidence of graft failure, graft-versus-host disease (GVHD), and delayed immunological reconstitution. Current methods of myeloablation have high morbidity and mortality. In combination, these problems remain prohibitive for most patients who might benefit from BMT. A theoretically attractive alternative, which potentially can address many of the limitations of

BMT, is *in utero* transplantation of HSC. This approach is potentially applicable to any congenital hematopoietic disease that can be diagnosed prenatally and can be cured or improved by engraftment of normal HSCs.

Rationale for *In Utero* Transplantation

The rationale for *in utero* transplantation is to take advantage of the window of opportunity created by normal ontogeny of hematopoietic cell lines. There is a period, prior to population of the bone marrow and prior to thymic processing of self-antigen, when the fetus theoretically should be receptive to engraftment of foreign HSC without rejection and without the need for myeloablation. In the human fetus, the ideal window would appear to be prior to 14 weeks' gestation, before release of differentiated T lymphocytes into the circulation and although the bone marrow is just beginning to develop sites for hematopoiesis (117). It certainly may extend beyond that in immunodeficiency states, particularly when T-cell development is abnormal. During this time, presentation of foreign antigen by thymic dendritic cells theoretically should result in clonal deletion of reactive T cells during the negative selection phase of thymic processing. Recent advances in prenatal diagnosis have made possible the diagnosis of a large number of congenital hematological diseases during the first trimester. Technical advances in fetal intervention make transplantation feasible by 12 to 14 weeks' gestation. The ontological window of opportunity falls well within these diagnostic and technical constraints, making application of this approach a realistic possibility.

Because of the unique fetal environment, prenatal HSC transplantation could theoretically avoid many of the current limitations of postnatal BMT. There would be no requirement for HLA matching, resulting in expansion of the donor pool. Transplanted cells would not be rejected, and space would be available in the bone marrow, eliminating the need for toxic immunosuppressive and myeloablative drugs. The mother's uterus may ultimately prove to be the ultimate sterile isolation chamber, eliminating the high risk and costly 2 to 4 months of isolation required after postnatal BMT and prior to immunological reconstitution. Finally, prenatal transplantation would preempt the clinical manifestations of the disease, avoiding the recurrent infections, multiple transfusions, growth delay, and other complications that cause immeasurable suffering for the patient and often compromise postnatal treatment.

Source of Donor Cells

Identifying the best source of donor cells may ultimately prove to be the most critical factor for the success of engraftment. The most obvious advantage of the use of fetal hematopoietic stem cells is the minimal number of mature T cells in fetal liver-derived populations prior to 14 weeks' gestation. This alleviates any concern about GVHD and avoids the necessity of T cell depletion processes, which can negatively impact potential engraftment (115–119).

Although there may be important homing, proliferative, and developmental advantages to the use of fetal cells, there are practical and ethical advantages to the use of cord blood or postnatal HSC sources. Legitimate ethical concerns regarding the use of fetal tissue for transplantation must be addressed by the medical and lay community. Fetal tissue obtained by the usual methods at the time of elective abortion has a high degree of microbial contamination (120). The transplantation of transmissible viral, fungal, or bacterial disease could have disastrous consequences for the recipient fetus or mother. Although the fetal liver is a rich source of HSC, small size limits total cell yield, and current technology does not yet allow undifferentiated expansion of donor cells. In contrast, the use of adult-derived cells would allow a renewable, relatively infection-free, ethically acceptable source of donor cells. Tolerance induction by the in utero transplantation of highly purified adult bone marrow HSC from a living related donor, followed by a single or multiple postnatal "booster" injections offers an intriguing approach in situations in which postnatal BMT is necessary but an HLA-matched donor is not available (121–123).

Diseases Amenable to Prenatal Treatment

Generally speaking, any disease that can be diagnosed early in gestation, which is improved by BMT, and for which postnatal treatment is not entirely satisfactory, is a target disease. Some diseases, however, are far more likely to benefit from prenatal transplantation than others. The list can be divided into three general categories: hemoglobinopathies, immunodeficiency disorders, and inborn errors of metabolism. Each of the diseases has unique considerations for treatment, and in fact each disease may respond differently (Table 13-2). Issues such as availability of engraftment sites within the bone marrow at time of transplantation, and capacity of a needed enzyme to cross the blood–brain barrier at a particular gestational age need to be considered. Of particular relevance to the prenatal approach, in which experimental levels of engraftment have been relatively low, is the observation that in many of the target diseases, engrafted normal cells would be predicted to have a significant survival advantage over diseased cells. This would have the clinical effect of amplification of the level of engraftment in the peripheral circulation. Additionally, even with minimal levels of engraftment, specific tolerance for donor antigen should be induced, allowing additional cells from the same donor to be given to the tolerant recipient after birth.

Hemoglobinopathies

The sickle cell anemia and thalassemia syndromes make up the largest patient groups potentially treatable by prenatal stem cell transplantation (122–125). Both groups can be diagnosed within the first trimester. Both have been cured by postnatal BMT, but BMT is not recommended routinely because of its prohibitive morbidity and mortality,

TABLE 13-2
POTENTIAL CANDIDATES FOR IN UTERO STEM CELL FETAL THERAPY

Hematopoietic Disorders
Disorders affecting lymphocytes
  SCID (sex linked)
  SCID (adenosine deaminase deficiency)
  Ommen syndrome
  Agammaglobinemia
  Bare Lymphocyte syndrome
Disorders affecting granulocytes
  Chronic granulomatous disease
  Infantile agranulocytosis
  Neutrophil membrane GP-180
  Lazy leukocyte syndrome
Disorders affecting erythrocytes
  Sickle cell disease
  α-Thalassemia
  β-Thalassemia
  Hereditary spherocytosis
  Fanconi anemia
Mannosidosis
  α-Mannosidosis
  β-Thalassemia
Mucolipidoses
  Gaucher disease
  Metachromatic leukodystrophy
  Krabbe disease
  Niemann-Pick disease
  β-Glucoronidase deficiency
  Fabry disease
  Adrenal leukodystrophy
Mucopolysaccharidoses

MPS I	(Hurler Disease)
MPS II	(Hunter Disease)
MPS IIIB	(Sanfilippo B)
MPS IV	(Morquio)
MPS VI	(Maroteaux-Lamy)

and the relative success of modern medical management. In both diseases the success of BMT is indirectly related to the morbidity of the disease, that is, the younger the patient, the fewer transfusions received, and the less organ compromise from iron overload, the better the results. With both diseases the primary questions relevant to prenatal transplantation are: (a) what levels of normal peripheral cell expression are necessary to alleviate clinical disease, and (b) can adequate levels of donor cell engraftment be achieved by in utero HSC transplantation? At present only indirect evidence exists to answer these questions.

In sickle cell disease (SCD) the pathophysiology is directly related to the concentration of hemoglobin S (HbS) within red cells, which results in marked rheological abnormality, including hyperviscosity, cellular adherence, and sickling, with a result of vaso-occlusion and tissue ischemia. In examining the in vitro relationships between hematocrit (HCT) and viscosity using mixtures of sickle and normal red blood cells (RBCs), Schmalzer observed that the primary determinant of viscosity is the sickle HCT (fraction of RBCs that contain HbS) (126). Adverse effects of HCT on viscosity were seen at a sickle HCT level in the low twenties. Oxygen delivery, as gauged by the maximal point on the HCT vs. viscosity curve, was markedly improved by exchanging normal for sickle RBCs (even when the total HCT was held constant). The clinical correlate of this in vitro information presently is chronic exchange transfusion therapy with its inherent discomfort and potential complications. However, prenatal transplantation of normal hematopoietic stem cells was thought to offer a solution to this problem. Normal cells were expected to have a developmental advantage over HbS cells such that overall production of Hb-normal RBCs may exceed that of HbS cells. This could potentially decrease the overall HbS fraction, reducing the risk of hyperviscosity and vaso-occlusive/ischemic complications. However, experimental data have not yet born this out.

The clinical manifestations of thalassemia are secondary to hypoxia related to severe anemia and ineffective erythropoiesis. It is now standard therapy to transfuse patients with thalassemia major chronically from an early age, which suppresses endogenous erythropoiesis and maintains oxygen delivery. When instituted at an early age this effectively prevents the bone marrow expansion and secondary bony changes, and the hemodynamic and cardiac manifestations of the disease. The necessary normal hemoglobin (Hb) level required is controversial, but good results have been achieved with maintenance of an Hb of 9 g/dL.

Although these levels of normal Hb are higher than have been achieved experimentally (30% donor Hb is maximal), there would be a significant survival advantage of normal cells in both diseases. In SCD, erythrocytes have a circulating half-life of 10 to 20 days (normal half-life = 120 days) prior to destruction. In thalassemia, most cells (80%) never leave the bone marrow and also have shortened survival in the periphery. Therefore, engraftment of even a relatively small number of normal stem cells could result in significantly increased levels of peripheral donor cell expression. The problem, however, is creating spaces in the bone marrow for engraftment, which is an unsolved dilemma.

Immunodeficiency Diseases

These represent an extremely heterogeneous group of diseases, which differ in their likelihood of cure by their capacity to develop hematopoietic chimerism (115,116). Once again, the most likely to benefit from even low levels of donor cell engraftment are those diseases in which a survival advantage exists for normal cells. The best example of this situation is severe combined immunodeficiency syndrome (SCID). Several different molecular causes of SCID have been identified, with approximately two-thirds of cases being of X-linked recessive inheritance (X-SCID). The genetic basis of X-SCID has been defined recently (127) as a mutation of the gene encoding the common -Y chain (-γ c), which is a common component of several members of the cytokine receptor superfamily, including those for interleukin-2 (IL-2), IL-4, IL-7, IL-9, IL-15, and possibly IL-13. Children affected with X-SCID have simultaneous disruption of multiple cytokine systems, resulting in a block in thymic T-cell development and diminished T-cell response. B cells, although present in normal or even increased numbers, are dysfunctional, either secondary to the lack of helper T-cell function or an intrinsic defect in B-cell maturation. Another form of SCID is secondary to adenosine deaminase (ADA) deficiency. Clinical experience with HLA-matched sibling bone marrow, fetal liver or thymus transplantation generally has been successful without myeloablative therapy, suggesting that the lymphoid progeny of relatively few engrafted normal HSC have a selective growth advantage in vivo over genetically defective cells (128). The competitive advantage of normal cell populations in X-SCID is best supported by the discovery of skewed cross-inactivation in female carriers (129). Only T cells containing the normal X chromosome were found to be present in the circulation of recipients. Evidence that ADA production confers a survival advantage derives from the early experience with gene therapy for ADA deficiency SCID. ADA-gene-corrected autologous T cells have persisted for prolonged periods despite discontinuation of the T-cell infusions (130). Transfer of ADA-gene-corrected cells versus uncorrected cells from the same SCID patient into immunodeficient beige, nude, x-linked (BNX) mouse results in survival of the corrected cells and death of the uncorrected cells, confirming a survival advantage for ADA-producing cells even when there is normal ADA production in the surrounding environment. Unfortunately, other diseases such as chronic granulomatous disease would not be expected to provide a competitive advantage for donor cells. Nevertheless, in all these conditions even a partial engraftment and expression of normal cell phenotype might at least partially ameliorate the clinical manifestations of the disease and should result in donor-specific tolerance for later transplantation. If higher levels of engraftment are needed, further HSC transplants from the same donor could be performed after birth without fear of rejection.

Flake and associates reported the successful treatment of a fetus with X-SCID in a family in which a previously afflicted child died at 7 months of age (131). Diagnosis by chorionic villous sampling at 12 weeks in the second pregnancy showed another affected male. For this couple, abortion was not an option. After lengthy informed consent, paternal bone marrow was harvested, T cells depleted, and enriched stem cell populations injected intraperitoneally into the fetus beginning about 16 weeks of gestation. Subsequent injections were performed at 17 and 18 weeks. The baby presently shows a split chimerism with all of his T cells being his father's and the majority of B cells being his own. He has achieved developmentally normal milestones and immune progress through 8 years of age (123). Other cases have been recently tried using less T cell-depleted populations resulting in higher T cell concentrations that have ended in fetal demise (117,132–134).

Inborn Errors of Metabolism

An even more heterogeneous group of diseases, inborn errors of metabolism, can be caused by a deficiency of a specific lysosomal hydrolase, which results in the accumulation of substrates such as mucopolysaccharide, glycogen, or sphingolipid. Depending on the specific enzyme abnormality and the compounds that accumulate, certain patterns of tissue damage and organ failure occur (116). These include central nervous system (CNS) deterioration, growth failure, dysostosis multiplex and joint abnormalities, hepatosplenomegaly, myocardial or cardiac disease, upper airway obstruction, pulmonary infiltration, corneal clouding, and hearing loss. The potential efficacy of prenatal HSC transplantation for the treatment of these diseases must be considered on an individual disease basis. The purpose of BMT in these diseases is to provide HSC-derived mononuclear cells that can repopulate various organs in the body, including the liver (Kupffer cells), skin (Langerhans' cells), lung (alveolar macrophages), spleen (macrophages), lymph nodes, tonsils, and the brain (microglia). Patients who have been corrected by postnatal BMT, such as Gaucher's disease or Maroteaux-Lamy syndrome (minimal CNS involvement), are reasonable candidates for prenatal treatment. In many cases postnatal BMT has corrected the peripheral manifestations of the disease and has arrested the neurological deterioration. However, postnatal BMT has not reversed neurological injury that is present in such disorders as metachromatic leukodystrophy and Hurler's disease (115,116). In these cases the neurological injury may begin well before birth. Postnatal maturation of the blood–brain barrier restricts access to the CNS of transplanted cells or the deficient enzyme. These considerations suggest that prenatal treatment may be beneficial and offer the possibility for a cure. The primary unanswered question is whether donor HSC-derived microglial elements would populate the CNS, providing the necessary metabolic correction inside the blood-brain barrier.

To date, the only definitively successful transplants have been for SCID (115,116). All others have either failed to take or were afflicted with graft versus host disease. Much more work needs to be done to determine the optimal dosing, timing, and specific protocols for different conditions.

As reviewed recently by Shields and associates (116), as of 2002 there have been 39 published cases of in utero stem cell transplants. Since the first successful case performed in 1995, only immunodeficiency cases continued to be successful. Of 14 cases of α and β-thalassemia, none have been successful. Three sickle cell, 3 Rh isoimmunization, and 7 storage disease cases have likewise been unsuccessful (116). Of 12 immunodeficiency cases, 6 have shown at least split chimerism or "alive and well." The dosages used, timing, fresh vs. frozen tissue, and methods of evaluation before and after transplantation have been widely varied. While no definitive conclusions are possible at this time, it is clear that our lack of understanding of the mechanics or development of immunocompetency are persuasive. Until a better understanding of the processes obtained, better theories on treatment to achieve better outcomes may be limited.

CONCLUSION

There are an increasing number of congenital and genetic abnormalities for which in utero treatment is possible, and are in some cases, relatively routine now. Advances in therapies have progressed at different paces for different disorders, but there is great hope and enthusiasm that progress will continue to expand the number of disorders for which therapy can be effective (60).

REFERENCES

1. *Reproductive Risks and Prenatal Diagnosis.* Norwalk, CT: Appleton & Lange, 1992.
2. Harrison MR, Evans MI, Adzick NS, et al. The Unborn Patient. Philadelphia: WB Saunders, 2000.
3. Pryde PG, Isada NB, Hallak M, et al. Determinants of parental decision to abort or continue after non-aneuploid ultrasound-detected fetal abnormalities. *Obstet Gynecol* 1992;80(1)1:52–56.
4. Evans MI, Sobiecki MA, Krivchenia EL, et al. Parental decisions to terminate/continue following abnormal cytogenetic prenatal diagnosis: "what" is still more important than "when". *Am J Med Genet* 1996;61(4):353–355.
5. Johnson MP, Flake AW, Quintero RA, et al. *Invasive outpatient procedures in reproductive medicine.* New York: Raven Press, 1997.
6. Evans MI, Sacks AJ, Johnson MP, et al. Sequential invasive assessment of fetal renal function and the intrauterine treatment of fetal obstructive uropathies. *Obstet Gynecol* 1991;77(4):545–550.
7. Wilson RD, Johnson MP. Prenatal ultrasound guided percutaneous shunts for obstructive uropathy and thoracic disease. *Semin Pediatr Surg* 2003;12(3):182–189.
8. Johnson MP, Corsi P, Bradfield W, et al. Sequential urinalysis improves evaluation of fetal renal function in obstructive uropathy. *Am J Obstet Gynecol* 1995;173(1):59–65.
9. Freedman AL, Bukowski TP, Smith CA, et al. Fetal therapy for obstructive uropathy: diagnosis specific outcomes [corrected]. *J Urol* 1996;156(2 Pt 2):720–723, discussion 723–724.
10. Dommergues M, Meuller F. Experience of 100 Obstructive Uropathies. International Fetal Medicine and Surgery Society Meeting, 2003.
11. Feldman B, Aviram-Goldring A, Evans MI. Interphase FISH for prenatal diagnosis of common aneuploidies. *Methods Mol Biol* 2002;204:219–241.
12. Evans MI, Henry GP, Miller WA, et al. International, collaborative assessment of 146,000 prenatal karyotypes: expected limitations if only chromosome-specific probes and fluorescent in-situ hybridization are used. *Hum Reprod* 1999;14(5):1213–1216.
13. Drugan A, Krause B, Canady A, et al. The natural history of prenatally diagnosed cerebral ventriculomegaly. *JAMA* 1989; 261(12):1785–1788.
14. Ahmad FK, Sherman SJ, Hagglund KH, et al. Isolated unilateral fetal pleural effusion: the role of sonographic surveillance and in utero therapy. *Fetal Diagn Ther* 1996;11(6):383–389.
15. Nicolaides KH, Azar GB. Thoraco-amniotic shunting. *Fetal Diagn Ther* 1990;5:153–164.
16. Adzick NS, Harrison MR, Flake AW, et al. Automatic uterine stapling devices in fetal surgery: experience in a primate model. *Surgical Forum* 1985;34:479.
17. Jennings RW, Adzick NS, Longaker MT, et al. Radiotelemetric fetal monitoring during and after open fetal operation. *Surg Gynecol Obstet* 1993;176(1):59–64.
18. Harrison MR, Adzick NS, Longaker MT, et al. Successful repair in utero of a fetal diaphragmatic hernia after removal of herniated viscera from the left thorax. *N Engl J Med* 1990;322(22): 1582–1584.
19. Harrison MR, Adzick NS, Flake AW, et al. Correction of congenital diaphragmatic hernia in utero. VI. Hard-earned lessons. *J Pediatr Surg* 1993;28(10):1411–1417, discussion 1417–1418.
20. Harrison MR, Keller RL, Hawgood SB, et al. A randomized trial of fetal endoscopic tracheal occlusion for severe fetal congenital diaphragmatic hernia. *N Engl J Med* 2003;349(20):1916–1924.
21. Harrison MR, Sydorak RM, Farrell JA, et al. Fetoscopic temporary tracheal occlusion for congenital diaphragmatic hernia: prelude to a randomized, controlled trial. *J Pediatr Surg* 2003;38(7): 1012–1020.
22. Heerema AE, Rabban JT, Sydorak RM, et al. Lung pathology in patients with congenital diaphragmatic hernia treated with fetal surgical intervention, including tracheal occlusion. *Pediatr Dev Pathol* 2003;6(6):536–546.
23. Sydorak RM, Harrison MR. Congenital diaphragmatic hernia: advances in prenatal therapy. *Clin Perinatol* 2003;30(3):465–479.
24. Danzer E, Sydorak RM, Harrison MR, et al. Minimal access fetal surgery. *Eur J Obstet Gynecol Reprod Biol* 2003;108(1):3–13.
25. Evans MI, Harrison MR, Flake AW, et al. Fetal therapy. *Best Pract Res Clin Obstet Gynaecol* 2002;16(5):671–683.
26. Paek BW, Coakley FV, Lu Y, et al. Congenital diaphragmatic hernia: prenatal evaluation with MR lung volumetry—preliminary experience. *Radiology* 2001;220(1):63–67.
27. Wenstrom KD. Fetal surgery for congenital diaphragmatic hernia. *N Engl J Med* 2003;349(20):1887–1888.
28. Adzick NS, Kitano Y. Fetal surgery for lung lesions, congenital diaphragmatic hernia, and sacrococcygeal teratoma. *Semin Pediatr Surg* 2003;12(3):154–167.
29. Adzick NS, Harrison MR, Crombleholme TM, et al. Fetal lung lesions: management and outcome. *Am J Obstet Gynecol* 1998; 179(4):884–889.
30. Crombleholme TM, Coleman B, Hedrick H, et al. Cystic adenomatoid malformation volume ratio predicts outcome in prenatally diagnosed cystic adenomatoid malformation of the lung. *J Pediatr Surg* 2002;37(3):331–338.
31. Holterman AX, Filiatrault D, Lallier M, et al. The natural history of sacrococcygeal teratomas diagnosed through routine obstetric sonogram: a single institution experience. *J Pediatr Surg* 1998;33(6):899–903.
32. Paek BW, Vaezy S, Fujimoto V, et al. Tissue ablation using high-intensity focused ultrasound in the fetal sheep model: potential for fetal treatment. *Am J Obstet Gynecol* 2003;189(3)(Sep): 702–705.
33. Lemire RJ. Neural tube defects. *JAMA* 1988;259(4):558–562.
34. Frey L, Hauser WA. Epidemiology of neural tube defects. *Epilepsia* 2003;44[Suppl 3]:4–13.
35. Smithells RW, Sheppard S, Schorah CJ, et al. Possible prevention of neural-tube defects by periconceptional vitamin supplementation. *Lancet* 1980;1(8164):339–340.
36. Smithells RW, Nevin NC, Seller MJ, et al. Further experience of vitamin supplementation for prevention of neural tube defect recurrences. *Lancet* 1983;1(8332):1027–1031.
37. Younis JS, Granat M. Insufficient transplacental digoxin transfer in severe hydrops fetalis. *Am J Obstet Gynecol* 1987;157(5): 1268–1269.
38. Mills JL, Rhoads GG, Simpson JL, et al. The absence of a relation between the periconceptional use of vitamins and neural-tube defects. National Institute of Child Health and Human Development Neural Tube Defects Study Group. *N Engl J Med* 1989;321(7):430–435.
39. Mulinare J, Cordero JF, Erickson JD, et al. Periconceptional use of multivitamins and the occurrence of neural tube defects. *JAMA* 1988;260(21):3141–3145.
40. Prevention of neural tube defects: results of the Medical Research Council Vitamin Study. MRC Vitamin Study Research Group. *Lancet* 1991;338(8760):131–137.
41. Czeizel AE, Dudas I. Prevention of the first occurrence of neural-tube defects by periconceptional vitamin supplementation. *N Engl J Med* 1992;327(26):1832–1835.
42. Honein MA, Paulozzi LJ, Mathews TJ, et al. Impact of folic acid fortification of the US. food supply on the occurrence of neural tube defects. *JAMA* 2001;285(23):2981–2986.
43. Olney RS, Mulinare J. Trends in neural tube defect prevalence, folic acid fortification, and vitamin supplement use. *Semin Perinatol* 2002;26(4):277–285.
44. Evans MI, Llurba E, Landsberger EJ, et al. Impact of folic acid fortification in the United States: markedly diminished high maternal serum alpha-fetoprotein values. *Obstet Gynecol* 2004; 103(3):474–479.
45. Parle-McDermott A, Mills JL, Kirke PN, et al. Analysis of the MTHFR 1298A → C and 677C → T polymorphisms as risk factors for neural tube defects. *J Hum Genet* 2003;48(4):190–193.

46. Finnell RH, Shaw GM, Lammer EJ, et al. Does prenatal screening for 5,10-methylenetetrahydrofolate reductase (MTHFR) mutations in high-risk neural tube defect pregnancies make sense? *Genet Test* 2002;6(1):47–52.

47. Rampersaud E, Melvin EC, Siegel D, et al. Updated investigations of the role of methylenetetrahydrofolate reductase in human neural tube defects. *Clin Genet* 2003;63(3):210–214.

48. Zhu H, Wicker NJ, Shaw GM, et al. Homocysteine remethylation enzyme polymorphisms and increased risks for neural tube defects. *Mol Genet Metab* 2003;78(3):216–221.

49. Volcik KA, Shaw GM, Zhu H, et al. Risk factors for neural tube defects: associations between uncoupling protein 2 polymorphisms and spina bifida. *Birth Defects Res Part A Clin Mol Teratol* 2003;67(3):158–161.

50. Sever LE. Zinc deficiency in man. *Lancet* 1973;1(7808):887.

51. McMichael AJ, Dreosti IE, Gibson GT, et al. A prospective study of serial maternal serum zinc levels and pregnancy outcome. *Early Hum Dev* 1982;7(1):59–69.

52. Stoll C, Dott B, Alembik Y, et al. Maternal trace elements, vitamin B12, vitamin A, folic acid, and fetal malformations. *Reprod Toxicol* 1999;13(1):53–57.

53. Hambidge M, Hackshaw A, Wald N. Neural tube defects and serum zinc. *Br J Obstet Gynaecol* 1993;100(8):746–749.

54. Shoob HD, Sargent RG, Thompson SJ, et al. Dietary methionine is involved in the etiology of neural tube defect-affected pregnancies in humans. *J Nutr* 2001;131(10):2653–2658.

55. Adzick NS, Walsh DS. Myelomeningocele: prenatal diagnosis, pathophysiology and management. *Semin Pediatr Surg* 2003; 12(3):168–174.

56. Evans ML, Holzgreve W, Johnson MP, et al. Fetal cell testing: societal and ethical speculations. *Ann N Y Acad Sci* 1994;731: 257–261.

57. Meuli M, Meuli-Simmen C, Hutchins GM, et al. In utero surgery rescues neurological function at birth in sheep with spina bifida. *Nat Med* 1995;1(4):342–347.

58. Bruner JP, Tulipan N, Paschall RL, et al. Fetal surgery for myelomeningocele and the incidence of shunt-dependent hydrocephalus. *JAMA* 1999;282(19):1819–1825.

59. Sutton LN, Adzick NS, Bilaniuk LT, et al. Improvement in hindbrain herniation demonstrated by serial fetal magnetic resonance imaging following fetal surgery for myelomeningocele. *JAMA* 1999;282(19):1826–1831.

60. Tulipan N, Hernanz-Schulman M, Bruner JP. Reduced hindbrain herniation after intrauterine myelomeningocele repair: a report of four cases. *Pediatr Neurosurg* 1998;29(5):274–278.

61. Johnson MP, Sutton LN, Rintoul N, et al. Fetal myelomeningocele repair: short-term clinical outcomes. *Am J Obstet Gynecol* 2003;189(2):482–487.

62. Liechty KW, Crombleholme TM, Flake AW, et al. Intrapartum airway management for giant fetal neck masses: the EXIT (ex utero intrapartum treatment) procedure. *Am J Obstet Gynecol* 1997;177(4):870–874.

63. Hedrick HL. Ex utero intrapartum therapy. *Semin Pediatr Surg* 2003;12(3):190–195.

64. MacLaughlin DT, Donahoe PK. Sex determination and differentiation. *N Engl J Med* 2004;350(4):367–378.

65. Speiser PW, Dupont B, Rubinstein P, et al. High frequency of nonclassical steroid 21-hydroxylase deficiency. *Am J Hum Genet* 1985;37(4):650–667.

66. Dupont B, Oberfield SE, Smithwick EM, et al. Close genetic linkage between HLA and congenital adrenal hyperplasia (21-hydroxylase deficiency). *Lancet* 1977;2(8052–82–8053):1309–1312.

67. White PC, Grossberger D, Onufer BJ, et al. Two genes encoding steroid 21-hydroxylase are located near the genes encoding the fourth component of complement in man. *Proc Natl Acad Sci U S A* 1985;82(4):1089–1093.

68. Evans MI, Chrousos GP, Mann DW, et al. Pharmacologic suppression of the fetal adrenal gland in utero. Attempted prevention of abnormal external genital masculinization in suspected congenital adrenal hyperplasia. *JAMA* 1985;253(7):1015–1020.

69. Forrest M, David M. Prenatal treatment of congenital adrenal hyperplasia due to 21-hydroxylase deficiency. Paper presented at 7th International Congress of Endocrinology 1984; Quebec, Canada.

70. New MI, Carlson A, Obeid J, et al. Prenatal diagnosis for congenital adrenal hyperplasia in 532 pregnancies. *J Clin Endocrinol Metab* 2001;86(12):5651–5657.

71. Clayton PE, Miller WL, Oberfield SE, et al. Consensus statement on 21-hydroxylase deficiency from the European Society for Paediatric Endocrinology and the Lawson Wilkins Pediatric Endocrine Society. *Horm Res* 2002;58(4):188–195.

72. Fisher DA, Klein AH. Thyroid development and disorders of thyroid function in the newborn. *N Engl J Med* 1981;304(12):702–712.

73. Bruinse HW, Vermeulen-Meiners C, Wit JM. Fetal treatment for thyrotoxicosis in non-thyrotoxic pregnant women. *Fetal Ther* 1988;3(3):152–157.

74. Porreco RP, Bloch CA. Fetal blood sampling in the management of intrauterine thyrotoxicosis. *Obstet Gynecol* 1990;76(3 Pt 2): 509–512.

75. Hatjis CG. Diagnosis and successful treatment of fetal goitrous hyperthyroidism caused by maternal Graves disease. *Obstet Gynecol* 1993;81(5 Pt 2):837–839.

76. Fisher DA. Neonatal thyroid disease of women with autoimmune thyroid disease. *Thyroid Today* 1986;9:1–7.

77. Volumenie JL, Polak M, Guibourdenche J, et al. Management of fetal thyroid goitres: a report of 11 cases in a single perinatal unit. *Prenat Diagn* 2000;20(10):799–806.

78. Morine M, Takeda T, Minekawa R, et al. Antenatal diagnosis and treatment of a case of fetal goitrous hypothyroidism associated with high-output cardiac failure. *Ultrasound Obstet Gynecol* 2002;19(5):506–509.

79. Rovet J, Ehrlich R, Sorbara D. Intellectual outcome in children with fetal hypothyroidism. *J Pediatr* 1987;110(5):700–704.

80. Sack J, Fisher DA, Hobel CJ, et al. Thyroxine in human amniotic fluid. *J Pediatr* 1975;87(3):364–368.

81. Thorpe-Beeston JG, Nicolaides KH, McGregor AM. Fetal thyroid function. *Thyroid* 1992;2(3):207–217.

82. Ballabio M, Nicolini U, Jowett T, et al. Maturation of thyroid function in normal human foetuses. *Clin Endocrinol (Oxf)* 1989;31(5):565–571.

83. Van Herle AJ, Young RT, Fisher DA, et al. Intra-uterine treatment of a hypothyroid fetus. *J Clin Endocrinol Metab* 1975;40(3):474–477.

84. Gruner C, Kollert A, Wildt L, et al. Intrauterine treatment of fetal goitrous hypothyroidism controlled by determination of thyroid-stimulating hormone in fetal serum. A case report and review of the literature. *Fetal Diagn Ther* 2001;16(1):47–51.

85. Brusque A, Rotta L, Pettenuzzo LF, et al. Chronic postnatal administration of methylmalonic acid provokes a decrease of myelin content and ganglioside N-acetylneuraminic acid concentration in cerebrum of young rats. *Braz J Med Biol Res* 2001;34(2):227–231.

86. Ampola MG, Mahoney MJ, Nakamura E, et al. Prenatal therapy of a patient with vitamin-B12-responsive methylmalonic acidemia. *N Engl J Med* 1975;293(7):313–317.

87. Andersson HC, Marble M, Shapira E. Long-term outcome in treated combined methylmalonic acidemia and homocystinemia. *Genet Med* 1999;1(4):146–150.

88. Evans MI, Duquette DA, Rinaldo P, et al. Modulation of B12 dosage and response in fetal treatment of methylmalonic aciduria (MMA): titration of treatment dose to serum and urine MMA. *Fetal Diagn Ther* 1997;12(1):21–23.

89. Leon-Del-Rio A, Leclerc D, Akerman B, et al. Isolation of a cDNA encoding human holocarboxylase synthetase by functional complementation of a biotin auxotroph of Escherichia coli. *Proc Natl Acad Sci U S A* 1995;92(10):4626–4630.

90. Suzuki Y, Aoki Y, Ishida Y, et al. Isolation and characterization of mutations in the human holocarboxylase synthetase cDNA. *Nat Genet* 1994;8(2):122–128.

91. Aoki Y, Suzuki Y, Sakamoto O, et al. Molecular analysis of holocarboxylase synthetase deficiency: a missense mutation and a single base deletion are predominant in Japanese patients. *Biochim Biophys Acta* 1995;1272(3):168–174.

92. Dupuis L, Leon-Del-Rio A, Leclerc D, et al. Clustering of mutations in the biotin-binding region of holocarboxylase synthetase in biotin-responsive multiple carboxylase deficiency. *Hum Mol Genet* 1996;5(7):1011–1016.

93. Pomponio RJ, Hymes J, Reynolds TR, et al. Mutations in the human biotinidase gene that cause profound biotinidase deficiency in symptomatic children: molecular, biochemical, and clinical analysis. *Pediatr Res* 1997;42(6):840–848.

94. Suormala T, Fowler B, Jakobs C, et al. Late-onset holocarboxylase synthetase-deficiency: pre- and post-natal diagnosis and

evaluation of effectiveness of antenatal biotin therapy. *Eur J Pediatr* 1998;157(7):570–575.

95. Roth KS, Yang W, Allan L, et al. Prenatal administration of biotin in biotin responsive multiple carboxylase deficiency. *Pediatr Res* 1982;16(2):126–129.

96. Packman S, Cowan MJ, Golbus MS, et al. Prenatal treatment of biotin responsive multiple carboxylase deficiency. *Lancet* 1982; 1(8287):1435–1438.

97. Thuy LP, Jurecki E, Nemzer L, et al. Prenatal diagnosis of holocarboxylase synthetase deficiency by assay of the enzyme in chorionic villus material followed by prenatal treatment. *Clin Chim Acta* 1 999;284(1):59–68.

98. Smith DW, Lemli L, Opitz JM. A Newly Recognized Syndrome of Multiple Congenital Anomalies. *J Pediatr* 1964;64:210–217.

99. Curry CJ, Carey JC, Holland JS, et al. Smith-Lemli-Opitz syndrome-type II: multiple congenital anomalies with male pseudohermaphroditism and frequent early lethality. *Am J Med Genet* 1987;26(1):45–57.

100. Opitz JM. RSH/SLO ("Smith-Lemli-Opitz") syndrome: historical, genetic, and developmental considerations. *Am J Med Genet* 1994;50(4):344–346.

101. Kelley RI. A new face for an old syndrome. *Am J Med Genet* 1997;68(3):251–256.

102. Kelley RI. Diagnosis of Smith-Lemli-Opitz syndrome by gas chromatography/mass spectrometry of 7-dehydrocholesterol in plasma, amniotic fluid and cultured skin fibroblasts. *Clin Chim Acta* 1995;236(1):45–58.

103. Tint GS, Irons M, Elias ER, et al. Defective cholesterol biosynthesis associated with the Smith-Lemli-Opitz syndrome. *N Engl J Med* 1994;330(2):107–113.

104. Waterham HR, Wijburg FA, Hennekam RC, et al. Smith-Lemli-Opitz syndrome is caused by mutations in the 7-dehydrocholesterol reductase gene. *Am J Hum Genet* 1998;63(2):329–338.

105. Johnson JA, Aughton DJ, Comstock CH, et al. Prenatal diagnosis of Smith-Lemli-Opitz syndrome, type II. *Am J Med Genet* 1994;49(2):240–243.

106. Hobbins JC, Jones OW, Gottesfeld S, et al. Transvaginal ultrasonography and transabdominal embryoscopy in the first-trimester diagnosis of Smith-Lemli-Opitz syndrome, type II. *Am J Obstet Gynecol* 1994;171(2):546–549.

107. Sharp P, Haan E, Fletcher JM, et al. First-trimester diagnosis of Smith-Lemli-Opitz syndrome. *Prenat Diagn* 1997;17(4):355–361.

108. Irons M, Elias ER, Tint GS, et al. Abnormal cholesterol metabolism in the Smith-Lemli-Opitz syndrome: report of clinical and biochemical findings in four patients and treatment in one patient. *Am J Med Genet* 1994;50(4):347–352.

109. Irons M, Elias ER, Abuelo D, et al. Treatment of Smith-Lemli-Opitz syndrome: results of a multicenter trial. *Am J Med Genet* 1997;68(3):311–314.

110. Nowaczyk MJ, Whelan DT, Heshka TW, et al. Smith-Lemli-Opitz syndrome: a treatable inherited error of metabolism causing mental retardation. *CMAJ* 1999;161(2):165–170.

111. Irons MB, Nores J, Stewart TL, et al. Antenatal therapy of Smith-Lemli-Opitz syndrome. *Fetal Diagn Ther* 1999;14(3):133–137.

112. Elsas LJ. Prenatal diagnosis of galactose-1-phosphate uridyltransferase (GALT)-deficient galactosemia. *Prenat Diagn* 2001; 21(4):302–303.

113. Chen YT, Mattison DR, Feigenbaum L, et al. Reduction in oocyte number following prenatal exposure to a diet high in galactose. *Science* 1981;214(4525):1145–1147.

114. Bandyopadhyay S, Chakrabarti J, Banerjee S, et al. Prenatal exposure to high galactose adversely affects initial gonadal pool of germ cells in rats. *Hum Reprod* 2003;18(2):276–282.

115. Flake AW. Stem cell and genetic therapies for the fetus. *Semin Pediatr Surg* 2003;12(3):202–208.

116. Shields LE, Lindton B, Andrews RG, et al. Fetal hematopoietic stem cell transplantation: a challenge for the twenty-first century. *J Hematother Stem Cell Res* 2002;11(4):617–631.

117. Flake AW, Zanjani ED. In utero hematopoietic stem cell transplantation: ontogenic opportunities and biologic barriers. *Blood* 1999;94(7):2179–2191.

118. Liechty KW, MacKenzie TC, Shaaban AF, et al. Human mesenchymal stem cells engraft and demonstrate site-specific differentiation after in utero transplantation in sheep. *Nat Med* 2000;6(11):1282–1286.

119. Guidos CJ, Danska JS, Fathman CG, et al. T cell receptor-mediated negative selection of autoreactive T lymphocyte precursors occurs after commitment to the CD4 or CD8 lineages. *J Exp Med* 1990;172(3):835–845.

120. Touraine JL, Raudrant D, Laplace S. Transplantation of hemopoietic cells from the fetal liver to treat patients with congenital diseases postnatally or prenatally. *Transplant Proc* 1997;29(1-21-2): 712-713.

121. Flake AW, Zanjani ED. In utero hematopoietic stem cell transplantation. A status report. *JAMA* 1997;278(11):932–937.

122. Hayward A, Ambruso D, Battaglia F, et al. Microchimerism and tolerance following intrauterine transplantation and transfusion for alpha-thalassemia-1. *Fetal Diagn Ther* 1998;13(1):8–14.

123. Flake AW, Zanjani ED. Treatment of severe combined immunodeficiency. *N Engl J Med* 1999;341(4):291–292.

124. Westgren M, Ringden O, Eik-Nes S, et al. Lack of evidence of permanent engraftment after in utero fetal stem cell transplantation in congenital hemoglobinopathies. *Transplantation* 1996;61(8): 1176–1179.

125. Touraine JL, Raudrant D, Royo C, et al. In utero transplantation of hemopoietic stem cells in humans. *Transplant Proc* 1991;23(1 Pt 2):1706–1708.

126. Schmalzer EA, Lee JO, Brown AK, et al. Viscosity of mixtures of sickle and normal red cells at varying hematocrit levels. Implications for transfusion. *Transfusion* 1987;27(3):228–233.

127. Noguchi M, Yi H, Rosenblatt HM, et al. Interleukin-2 receptor gamma chain mutation results in X-linked severe combined immunodeficiency in humans. *Cell* 1993;73(1):147–157.

128. Buckley RH, Schiff SE, Schiff RI, et al. Haploidentical bone marrow stem cell transplantation in human severe combined immunodeficiency. *Semin Hematol* 1993;30(4)[Suppl 4]:92–101, discussion 102–104.

129. Puck JM, Stewart CC, Nussbaum RL. Maximum-likelihood analysis of human T-cell X chromosome inactivation patterns: normal women versus carriers of X-linked severe combined immunodeficiency. *Am J Hum Genet* 1992;50(4):742–748.

130. Slavin S, Naparstek E, Ziegler M, et al. Clinical application of intrauterine bone marrow transplantation for treatment of genetic diseases–feasibility studies. *Bone Marrow Transplant* 1992;9[Suppl 1]:189–190.

131. Flake AW, Roncarolo MG, Puck JM, et al. Treatment of X-linked severe combined immunodeficiency by in utero transplantation of paternal bone marrow. *N Engl J Med* 1996;335(24): 1806–10.

132. Bambach BJ, Moser HW, Blakemore K, et al. Engraftment following in utero bone marrow transplantation for globoid cell leukodystrophy. *Bone Marrow Transplant* 1997;19(4)1:399–402.

133. Peranteau WH, Hayashi S, Kim HB, et al. In utero hematopoietic cell transplantation: what are the important questions? *Fetal Diagn Ther* 2004;19(1):9–12.

134. Porta F, Mazzolari E, Zucca S, et al. Prenatal transplant in a fetus affected by Omenn Syndrome. *Bone Marrow Transplant* 2000; 25(Suppl):S43.

The Impact of Maternal Illness on the Neonate

Helain J. Landy

Progress in obstetric and neonatal care has directly contributed to improvements in neonatal outcome. The infant mortality rate (deaths in the first year of life per 1,000 live births), an established indicator of a nation's health status and well-being, has declined exponentially in the twentieth century with a drop of 46% since 1980 (1,2). The infant mortality rate, directly related to birth weight, has declined in spite of the increase in the percentage of low-birth-weight infants (2). These encouraging data largely reflect neonatal and pediatric advances in combination with regionalization of perinatal services and delivery of high-risk mothers in tertiary centers (2–5).

The mother's well-being during pregnancy has direct relevance for the newborn. Potential complications such as preterm delivery, growth disturbances (intrauterine growth restriction [IUGR] or macrosomia), congenital malformations, or chronic maternal illness may be important factors. This chapter discusses the impact of maternal illness on fetal development and well-being.

PRETERM DELIVERY

Preterm delivery is responsible for the majority of neonatal deaths and a major proportion of perinatal morbidity; in 1999, for the first time, prematurity constituted the leading cause of infant deaths in the first month of life (5,6). Approximately 11% of all deliveries in the United States occur prior to term (7) and these children are at higher risks of lifelong problems, including cerebral palsy, deafness, blindness, learning disabilities, and developmental delay (8). Encouraging data reveal increasingly effective care for pregnant women and neonates. This translates into a better prognosis for preterm infants, including increased survival rates (greater than 80%, compared with 74% in 1988) without an associated increase in morbidity (9).

Despite intense research efforts and technological advances, data demonstrate a steady rise in the preterm delivery rate in the United States over the past 20 years. In 1981, the preterm delivery rate was 9.4% and rose to 10.6% in 1990 (2). Recent data show a minor drop in the preterm birth rate from 11.8% in 1999 to 11.6% in 2000 (the latest year for which information exists); this represents the first such decline since 1992 (2). Compared with other industrialized nations, the United States ranks poorly (2,10). A number of confounding variables may explain these facts. These include a racial disparity regarding persistently higher mortality statistics for black infants, a lack of agreement in the diagnosis of preterm labor, an overlap in the characteristics of actual and threatened preterm labor, controversies over the effectiveness of available screening techniques and therapies for preterm labor, and varying dosages and administration of tocolytic medications (2).

Preterm Labor and Premature Rupture of Membranes

A significant proportion of spontaneous preterm deliveries result from preterm labor and premature rupture of the membranes (PROM). Approximately 70% of preterm births may be associated with clinical evidence of ruptured membranes or underlying maternal, obstetric, or fetal conditions (Table 14-1) (10–13).

Predisposing factors for preterm labor remain largely unknown. Epidemiologic studies consistently report an association with nonwhite race (African American relative risk [RR] = 3.3), lower socioeconomic status (RR = 1.83–2.65), low prepregnancy weight (odds ratio [OR] = 2.72), and maternal age younger than 17 years or older than 40 years (RR = 1.47–1.95) (14). Lack of prenatal care is strongly associated with higher rates of preterm delivery, low birth weight, and maternal and infant mortality (15). Other particularly important risk factors include maternal history of preterm birth, especially during the second trimester, with or without rupture of membranes, and vaginal bleeding in at least two trimesters (14,16–18). Prostaglandins, thought to be

TABLE 14-1
UNDERLYING CONDITIONS ASSOCIATED WITH PRETERM BIRTH[a]

Maternal Conditions	Fetal Conditions
Anatomic conditions	Fetal growth restriction
Uterine malformations	Multiple gestation
Unicornuate or bicornuate uterus	Fetal anomaly
Myomas	Fetal death
Cervical incompetence	
Placenta previa or abruption	
Ruptured membranes	
Medical conditions	
Systemic medical or obstetric illness	
Trauma	
Exogenous substance use	
Tobacco	
Cocaine	
Maternal *in utero* exposure to diethylstilbestrol (DES)	
Infection (subclinical or clinical)	
Urogenital tract	
Amniotic cavity	
Systemic	

[a] From Singh GK, Yu SM. Infant mortality in the United States: trends, differentials, and projections, 1950 through 2010. *Am J Public Health* 1995;85:957–964; Amon E, Anderson GD, Sibai BM, et al. Factors responsible for a preterm delivery of the immature newborn infant (less than or equal to 1000 gm). *Am J Obstet Gynecol* 1987;156:1143–1148; Meis PJ, Ernest JM, Moore ML. Causes of low birth weight births in public and private patients. *Am J Obstet Gynecol* 1987;156:1165–1168; and Tucker JM, Goldenberg RL, Davis RO, et al. Etiologies of preterm birth in an indigent population: is prevention a logical expectation? *Obstet Gynecol* 1991;77:343–347.

important mediators in the onset of labor at term, may have a role in preterm labor; in the absence of intrauterine infection, however, the data are not convincing (19).

Although PROM occurs in only 3% of pregnancies before term (20), it is associated with 20% to 50% of preterm deliveries (21) and represents the foremost predisposing factor for admissions to neonatal intensive care units (22). The pathophysiology underlying PROM appears to be multifactorial; evidence suggests that inflammatory weakening of the membranes or choriodecidual infection may be involved, especially at early gestational ages (20,23). Some clinical characteristics seen with PROM are also common to cases with preterm labor (e.g., lower socioeconomic status, young maternal age, sexually transmitted diseases, cigarette smoking, and vaginal bleeding) (20). Many studies suggest an association between bacterial vaginosis, a relatively common condition in which the normally predominant lactobacilli are overgrown by anaerobes and other peroxide-producing bacteria, and complications of premature birth, preterm labor, and PROM (14,24–26); however, conflicting data exist (27).

In most patients, spontaneous labor begins after the membranes rupture. The latency period, defined as the time between membrane rupture and onset of contractions, is shorter in patients close to term. More than half of preterm

patients will be in labor within 24 hours of ruptured membranes, and 50% to 60% will deliver within 1 week despite conservative management (7,20,28,29). PROM remote from viability is associated with significant rates of maternal and fetal morbidity and low rates of neonatal survival (7,8,19,29). Neonatal respiratory distress syndrome (RDS) is the most common complication at all gestational ages (7–8). Fetal demise resulting from intrauterine infection, umbilical cord compression, or placental abruption occurs in approximately 1% of cases of PROM at 30 to 36 weeks of gestation and up to 21.7% of cases of PROM in the midtrimester (7,8). Prolonged oligohydramnios can also be associated with fetal pulmonary hypoplasia, limb-positioning deformities, and abnormal facies (e.g., low-set ears and epicanthal folds) (19,30).

Pharmacologic tocolysis, employed in an attempt to prevent progression of preterm labor, is implemented most often before 34 weeks of gestation. The various agents used in pharmacologic tocolysis, which are administered orally, subcutaneously, or parenterally, can have potentially serious maternal and/or fetal side effects (Table 14-2) (31). Despite the widespread use and evaluation of tocolysis over the past 20 years, data fail to demonstrate benefits of tocolysis in terms of medical costs, improvements in neonatal survival, or improvements in other long-term outcome parameters (31). The major benefit of tocolysis is its ability to provide short-term pregnancy prolongation in order that corticosteroids can be administered (31).

Corticosteroids, which are given between 24 and 34 weeks of gestation to patients who are at risk for preterm delivery, are used to induce fetal pulmonary maturity. The recommended protocol includes a single course of betamethasone (12 mg intramuscularly [i.m.]) given in 2 doses 24 hours apart) or dexamethasone (6 mg i.m. given in 4 doses every 12 hours). Optimal benefit is seen within 24 hours and through 7 days after administration (32,33). A recent meta-analysis evaluating multiple randomized studies confirmed the decreased incidence and severity of neonatal RDS with antenatal administration of corticosteroids (34). Additional neonatal benefits include reductions in rates of intraventricular hemorrhage and death, even with treatment of less than 24 hours' duration and in gestations earlier than 30 to 32 weeks with ruptured membranes (33). Long-term data of infants exposed *in utero* to a single course of corticosteroids failed to demonstrate any significant adverse effects on physical development, growth, cognitive or motor skills, or early school performance (31).

The use of antibiotic therapy, particularly aimed at treating bacterial vaginosis, group B streptococcus, and other genital tract organisms, has been studied widely in recent years. Initially shown to decrease rates of preterm delivery, preterm labor, and neonatal sepsis in some studies, the data show mixed results (31,35–37). Routine antibiotic administration is not recommended if used only in an attempt at prevention of preterm delivery (31). While conservatively managing preterm PROM remote from term, however, aggressive antibiotic therapy with erythromycin and ampicillin or amoxicillin prolongs pregnancy and

TABLE 14-2

POTENTIAL COMPLICATIONS OF VARIOUS TOCOLYTIC AGENTS[a]

Agent	Side Effects
Magnesium sulfate	*Maternal:* Decreased respiratory, cardiovascular, and renal function; contraindicated in myasthenia gravis *Fetal:* Alterations in fetal heart rate patterns
Betamimetic agents (e.g., ritodrine, terbutaline)	*Maternal:* Pulmonary edema; myocardial ischemia or infarction (rare); hypotension; hyperglycemia; hypokalemia *Fetal:* Alterations in fetal heart rate patterns
Prostaglandin synthetase inhibitors (e.g., indomethacin, sulindac)	*Maternal:* Gastrointestinal bleeding *Fetal:* Constriction of ductus arteriosus; reversible, dose-dependent oligohydramnios from decreased fetal urinary output; pulmonary hypertension seen with prolonged use (rare)
Calcium channel blockers (e.g., nifedipine)	Well tolerated

[a] From Goldenberg RL. The management of preterm labor. *Obstet Gynecol* 2002;100:1020–1037.

decreases major neonatal morbidity (e.g., RDS, early sepsis, severe intraventricular hemorrhage, severe necrotizing enterocolitis) (20,38,39).

Screening for Preterm Delivery

Because a woman's past obstetric history may be important for subsequent pregnancies, several risk-scoring systems have been developed. The most widely applied system was devised by Papiernik and modified by Creasy (40). Application of these systems to various populations in the United States, however, has been disappointing (41), and applicability to nulliparae has not been accepted. A 1996 study of almost 3,000 gravidas that attempted to develop a risk-assessment system for predicting spontaneous preterm delivery by using clinical information at 23 to 24 weeks of gestation was similarly disappointing (18). A recent study demonstrated the utility of the preterm labor index, a clinical tool to assess the likelihood of overall preterm delivery and delivery within 1 week (42). The preterm labor index, originally proposed in 1973, combines four clinical parameters (uterine contractions, PROM, vaginal bleeding, and cervical dilation) and is comparable to newer biochemical markers for predicting preterm delivery (42,43). Its utility across populations remains to be studied.

Other screening tools have been proposed to help identify the pregnancy at risk for preterm delivery, including home uterine activity monitoring, screening for fetal fibronectin in vaginal secretions, cervical examination, and screening for genital tract colonization and/or infection.

Home Uterine Activity Monitoring

The working premise behind home uterine activity monitoring (HUAM) is that uterine contractions may increase in frequency in the 24 hours before the development of preterm labor (14,44). The use of HUAM involves tocody-

namometric recording of uterine contractions combined with interpretation and daily telephone contact by health care providers to try to detect early preterm labor. Oral tocolysis often is used in conjunction with HUAM. Data from many randomized studies evaluating the efficacy of HUAM are conflicting and the quality of supportive evidence is limited by study designs (14,31,45–47). Its use in clinical practice is widespread in spite of the lack of endorsement by the U.S. Preventive Services Task Force (46) and the American College of Obstetricians and Gynecologists (ACOG) (14).

Fetal Fibronectin

Fetal fibronectin (fFN), a protein produced by the fetal membranes, most likely functions to bind the placenta and membranes to the decidua. Disruption of this normal interface, as with preterm labor or PROM, allows leakage of fibronectin into cervicovaginal secretions. In normal pregnancy it is rarely present after 20 weeks of gestation, and it has been found to be of value in predicting preterm delivery (48–50). Positive tests for fFN can be seen in women with bacterial vaginosis or subsequent maternal and fetal infections (48,51). The most useful aspect of the fFN assay is its negative predictive value: Less than 1% of women with questionable preterm labor will deliver within the next 2 weeks with a negative test for fFN compared with approximately 20% of women with a positive test (31). At this time, however, its use as a routine screening test for the general obstetric population has not been endorsed by the ACOG Committee on Obstetric Practice (52).

Cervical Examination

The value of routine digital cervical examination in otherwise uncomplicated pregnancies is controversial. Asymptomatic cervical dilation may be a normal anatomic variant, and may represent the earliest sign of impending preterm delivery, implying cervical incompetence or undiagnosed preterm labor (53–55). Sonographic cervical examination is superior to digital assessment of cervical dilation, length, and effacement, and confirms the association of cervical shortening with preterm delivery (56–60). Predictive sonographic findings for increased risks of preterm delivery include cervical shortening (generally described as less than 2.5 to 3 cm), funneling or ballooning of membranes at the level of the internal os, and cervical dilation (57,60,61). Currently, routine use of sonographic cervical length in the prediction of preterm delivery is not recommended because of the lack of proven treatments affecting outcome (14). Combining transvaginal sonography with other biochemical markers, such as fFN, may prove more predictive, however (14,62).

Genital Tract Screening

Routine screening for various infections (e.g., syphilis, hepatitis B, and rubella) is recommended early in pregnancy. Additional testing for other sexually transmitted disorders, however, is left to the discretion of the practitioner based on the patient's history and physical examination (63). Infections with *Neisseria gonorrhoeae, Trichomonas vaginalis, Chlamydia trachomatis,* and group B streptococci, as well as urinary tract infections, asymptomatic bacteriuria, and bacterial vaginosis, are associated with premature delivery (64–66). Some investigators recommend more aggressive screening and treatment for these conditions during gestation, as well as in women contemplating pregnancy (65). Recently adopted guidelines from the Centers for Disease Control and Prevention in conjunction with ACOG and the American Academy of Pediatrics recommend the routine screening for group B streptococcus colonization in late pregnancy and antibiotic treatment for carriers in labor (67). This strategy reflects attempts to prevent early onset neonatal disease rather than impact on rates of prematurity (31,67).

MATERNAL NUTRITION

Recognition of the importance of proper nutrition during pregnancy has varied over the years. Earlier in this century, restrictions in maternal diet were implemented to lessen fetal growth in order to decrease the rates of preeclampsia and labor complications (68). Fetal growth, which is determined by complex interactions of environmental, genetic, and physiologic factors, is influenced by both maternal prepregnancy body mass index and pregnancy weight gain. Whereas low birth weight and IUGR are seen in infants of underweight mothers and mothers with poor weight gain, macrosomia is common in infants of overweight mothers and mothers with excessive weight gain (68–70). Current weight-gain recommendations for singleton pregnancies are 25–35 pounds for normal weight gravidas, 28–40 pounds for underweight gravidas, and 15–25 pounds for overweight gravidas; in twin gestations, ideal weight gain is 35–45 pounds (71). Recent epidemiologic evidence suggests an independent association between maternal obesity and fetal neural tube defects and other malformations (72), as well as increased maternal risks of diabetes mellitus, preeclampsia, and cesarean delivery (73).

Although it is common for multivitamins to be prescribed to pregnant women in the United States, a balanced diet with appropriate weight gain should supply the required vitamins and make supplementation unnecessary. In certain conditions, however, specific recommendations are warranted. There are relatively few food sources high in vitamin D, for example; in the United States, its major source is vitamin D-fortified milk (74). Vitamin D synthesis in the skin depends on ultraviolet light skin exposure; however, there is generally insufficient exposure in winter, especially at higher latitudes (74). Vitamin D deficiency in pregnant women varies based on the patient's racial and ethnic background as well as dietary customs; a fairly high prevalence has been reported among Indian and Pakistani women living in Britain (74). Maternal deficiency of vitamin D may be seen with neonatal hypocalcemia and tetany. If supplementation is to be administered, 400 to 500 IU doses daily have been reported as safe and adequate; excessive supplementation can result in calcium hyperabsorption, hypercalcemia, and calcification of soft tissues (74).

Vitamin supplementation of vitamin B_{12} and zinc are indicated for strict vegetarians; additional folic acid is suggested for women taking anticonvulsant medications, carrying multiple gestations, or with hemoglobinopathies. To prevent anemia, iron supplementation in the second and third trimesters is recommended (74). In contrast, excessive vitamin A, in daily doses of at least 25,000 to 50,000 IU, is teratogenic, producing malformations similar to those seen with maternal exposure to 13-*cis*-retinoic acid (Accutane) (75).

High-dose folic acid supplementation (4 mg/day) reduces the risk of a subsequent neural tube defect in women with a prior affected infant (76), and such doses, beginning 1 month before conception and continuing through the first 3 months of pregnancy, are advocated (77). Further studies led to the Centers for Disease Control and Prevention statement that all women of child-bearing age in the United States who are capable of becoming pregnant should consume 0.4 mg of folic acid daily (78). Beginning January 1998, the U.S. Food and Drug Administration ordered folic acid fortification of bread, flour, and other grain foods to help prevent these birth defects (79).

MATERNAL ILLNESSES

Hypertension

Hypertension complicates 5% to 8% of pregnancies and constitutes a major cause of maternal and perinatal morbidity and mortality (80–82). Potential fetal and neonatal complications associated with chronic hypertension include prematurity, increased overall perinatal morbidity, IUGR, and fetal death (80–82). Several studies document that the risk of perinatal mortality is increased two to four times if the mother is hypertensive compared with the general obstetric population (83). Maternal complications include superimposed preeclampsia, placental abruption, cesarean delivery, and potentially life-threatening complications such as pulmonary edema, hypertensive en-cephalopathy, retinopathy, cerebral hemorrhage, and acute renal failure (80–85). Low-risk patients have mild essential hypertension and no organ involvement; those with severe hypertension or superimposed preeclampsia are considered to be at high risk. The risks of significant complications are especially increased in patients with uncontrolled severe hypertension and underlying renal or cardiac disease prior to or early in gestation (82).

Classification and terminology of the different subdivisions of the hypertensive disorders in pregnancy is confusing. A recent recommendation by the National High Blood Pressure Education Program Working Group replaces the term "pregnancy-induced hypertension" with "gestational hypertension" to describe situations in which elevated blood pressure without proteinuria develops after 20 weeks of gestation and blood pressure levels return to normal postpartum (80,85). Up to 25% of women with gestational hypertension will develop proteinuria or preeclampsia; with severe chronic hypertension, this rate can approach 50% (84). Proteinuria is classified by at least 0.3 g of protein in a 24-hour urine specimen, which usually corresponds to 1+ or greater on a urine dipstick evaluation (83).

Preeclampsia is defined as hypertension with proteinuria in addition to other possible symptoms of headache, edema, visual disturbances, and epigastric pain; laboratory abnormalities may involve hemolysis, elevated liver enzymes, and low platelet count (known by the acronym HELLP). HELLP syndrome can occur in up to 20% of women with severe preeclampsia and may have a variety of clinical presentations (86). In past years, the diagnosis of preeclampsia included specific blood pressure elevations above the patient's baseline blood pressure; these clinical parameters have not been found to be a reasonable prognostic indicator of outcome (85). Eclampsia involves the development of seizures and/or coma, which represents central nervous system involvement, in a preeclamptic patient. Severe preeclampsia can be defined by the criteria listed in Table 14-3 (80,85). Thrombocytopenia (platelet count below 100,000/mL) is the most consistent finding in patients with preeclampsia (87). Table 14-4 outlines the risk factors for the development of preeclampsia (80,85).

The precise pathophysiologic factors involved in preeclampsia have been difficult to elucidate. Trophoblastic invasion by the placenta appears to be important because the severity of hypertension appears to be related to the degree of trophoblastic invasion (80,88). Vascular changes, specifically vasospasm, seem responsible for many of the serious clinical manifestations (e.g., hypertension and diminished renal function). Earlier investigations demonstrated support for the involvement of vasospasm in the etiology of preeclampsia. Specifically, the failure of the blunted pressor response to angiotensin II present in normal pregnancy is not seen in preeclampsia (89), and a progressive sensitivity to the pressor effects of infused angiotensin can be demonstrated after 18 weeks in patients destined to become preeclamptic (90). Other factors may involve an imbalance in the production of prostacyclin, a potent vasodilator, relative to levels of thromboxane, a vasoconstrictor, and alterations in the synthesis of nitric oxide and/or endothelin 1 (85).

TABLE 14-3
CLINICAL MANIFESTATIONS OF SEVERE PREGNANCY-INDUCED HYPERTENSION[a]

- Systolic blood pressure ≥160 mm Hg or diastolic blood pressure ≥110 mm Hg on two occasions at least 6 hours apart with the patient at bed rest
- Proteinuria ≥5 g in a 24-hour collection or ≥3+ on two random urine samples collected at least 4 hours apart
- Oliguria (<500 mL in 24 hours)
- Cerebral or visual disturbances
- Pulmonary edema
- Right upper quadrant or epigastric pain
- Hepatocellular dysfunction
- Thrombocytopenia
- Intrauterine growth restriction

[a] From National High Blood Pressure Education Program Working Group on high blood pressure in pregnancy. *Am J Obstet Gynecol* 2000;183(1):S1–S22; and Sibai BM, Lindheimer M, Hauth J, et al. Risk factors for preeclampsia, abruptio placentae, and adverse neonatal outcomes among women with chronic hypertension. *N Engl J Med* 1998;339:667–671.

TABLE 14-4
RISK FACTORS ASSOCIATED WITH THE DEVELOPMENT OF PREECLAMPSIA[a]

- Nulliparity
- Age >35 years
- African American race
- Family history of preeclampsia
- Prior history of preeclampsia
- Chronic hypertension
- Chronic renal disease
- Obesity
- Vascular and connective tissue disease
- Antiphospholipid syndrome
- Thrombophilia
- Pregestational diabetes mellitus
- Multiple gestation
- Gestational trophoblastic disease
- Fetal hydrops

[a] From National High Blood Pressure Education Program Working Group on high blood pressure in pregnancy. *Am J Obstet Gynecol* 2000;183(1):S1–S22; and Sibai BM, Lindheimer M, Hauth J, et al. Risk factors for preeclampsia, abruptio placentae, and adverse neonatal outcomes among women with chronic hypertension. *N Engl J Med* 1998;339:667–671.

Some fetal effects of preeclampsia reflect vasospasm with regard to placental perfusion. A decrease in uteroplacental perfusion may result in abruption, IUGR, oligohydramnios, or nonreassuring fetal status demonstrated on antepartum testing. Placental abruption, which occurs in fewer than 2% of patients with chronic hypertension, can be twice as high in those with superimposed preeclampsia (82,83). In 1990, Burrows and Andrews (91) found that neonatal thrombocytopenia occurred in more infants of hypertensive than in those born to normotensive mothers (9.2% compared with 2.2%).

Prematurity significantly contributes to the increased rates of perinatal morbidity and mortality associated with preeclampsia. Conservative management, recommended in a tertiary care setting or in consultation with a maternal–fetal medicine subspecialist, may be attempted for women with severe preeclampsia remote from term (80,82). Delivery remains the only definitive treatment, and ultimately may be required (92,93). In cases managed conservatively, patients are hospitalized; bed rest with frequent clinical and laboratory assessments and corticosteroids are administered to enhance fetal pulmonary maturity. Magnesium sulfate, an agent long recognized for its anticonvulsant effects, is often administered (85). Although phenytoin sulfate may be used, magnesium sulfate is the preferred drug (94,95). Blood pressure control is achieved with the use of antihypertensive agents such as labetalol, hydralazine, or nifedipine (80–82). A protocol of high-dose corticosteroid administration stabilizes both clinical and laboratory parameters in patients with HELLP syndrome before term (96,97).

Several different antihypertensive agents are used during pregnancy. α-Methyldopa is frequently used because it is a safe, effective agent that has been studied extensively. Newer antihypertensive drugs that are safe in pregnancy include beta-blockers, labetalol (a combination alpha- and beta-blocker), and calcium channel blockers such as nifedipine. There is concern about using diuretics during pregnancy because of an accompanying plasma volume reduction (83). The National High Blood Pressure Education Program Working Group on High Blood Pressure in Pregnancy suggests that diuretics can be used safely except in situations in which there is already evidence of diminished uteroplacental function (80,81). Angiotensin-converting enzyme (ACE) inhibitors, commonly used in young, nonpregnant adults, are both teratogenic and fetotoxic if administered during gestation. Skull defects (hypoplastic calvaria and encephalocele) and in utero renal failure leading to oligohydramnios, pulmonary hypoplasia, long-standing neonatal anuria, and fetal or neonatal death have been reported (98–100). In women using an ACE inhibitor, antihypertensive medication is changed to another agent once pregnancy is confirmed.

Over the years, prevention of preeclampsia has been attempted. Initially, a beneficial effect was demonstrated in high-risk groups that were given low-dose aspirin (60 to 80 mg daily), but subsequent studies have been conflicting and a similar effect was not found in low-risk women (101–104). Similarly, other studies have obtained disappointing results in evaluating supplementation with calcium, magnesium, zinc, fish oil, or use of different antihypertensive medication (103). More recently, evaluation of the uteroplacental circulation via transvaginal Doppler sonography at 12 to 16 weeks suggests an association with abnormal waveforms and increased risks of developing preeclampsia later in gestation (103–107). Further study is ongoing.

Diabetes Mellitus

Diabetes mellitus complicates nearly 4% of pregnancies (108,109). The disease is classified based on the requirement for insulin therapy into type 1 (insulin-dependent) or type 2 (non–insulin-dependent) diabetes. The White classification system for diabetes in pregnancy, developed in 1949, is based on age of onset and duration of disease, as well as disease progression with respect to vascular complications (110). With continued improvements in glucose control, assessment of fetal well-being, and neonatal management, the White classification is no longer as helpful as it once was in the management of the pregnant diabetic (111). Instead, the distinction can be made between diabetes that preceded a woman's pregnancy (pregestational diabetes) and diabetes first recognized during pregnancy (gestational diabetes).

Fetuses of diabetic mothers may have growth disturbances at both ends of the spectrum: IUGR and macrosomia. IUGR, fetal growth less than or equal to the 10th percentile for gestational age, is not an infrequent finding in pregnancies of women with vascular complications of pregestational diabetes. In diabetic pregnancies, IUGR often results from uteroplacental insufficiency, usually associated with maternal hypertension, although fetuses with congenital anomalies also may exhibit signs of IUGR.

Infants of mothers with both pregestational and gestational diabetes are at risk for macrosomia, which refers to fetal growth beyond a specific weight regardless of gestational age, usually above 4,000 g or 4,500 g (112). With the development of a new national reference for fetal growth based on data from over 3.8 million births (113), clinicians can distinguish between macrosomia and large-for-gestational-age (above the 90th percentile for a given gestational age) (112,113). Several large studies support the continued use of 4,500 g as a value above which a fetus should be considered to be macrosomic (112,114–117). The antenatal sonographic diagnosis of macrosomia remains inaccurate, especially in diabetics (118–120). In women with normal glucose tolerance, 2% of infants weighed more than 4,500 g compared with 6% of women with untreated borderline gestational diabetes (112,121). Even in the absence of gestational diabetes, however, higher infant weights are associated with higher maternal glucose levels (112,122,123). In patients with untreated gestational diabetes, up to 20% of infants may be macrosomic (112,124).

Macrosomia is accompanied by the additional risks of prolonged labor, fracture of the clavicle, birth trauma from shoulder dystocia, and instrumented or cesarean deliveries (125–129). Shoulder dystocia occurs in only 1.4% of all vaginal deliveries (130). Among deliveries of diabetic mothers, however, shoulder dystocia occurs two to six times more frequently than in the nondiabetic population (120,129,131). The complication has been reported to occur in 20% to 50% of infants of diabetic mothers with birth weights above 4,500 g (114–117,120). Brachial plexus injury is the most serious complication resulting from shoulder dystocia. Fortunately, it is rare, occurring in approximately 0.05% to 0.19% of vaginal deliveries (112,120), but that risk is increased 18- to 21-fold among vaginally delivered infants weighing more than 4,500 g (114,120,132–135). The majority of cases of brachial plexus injury resolve within 1 year (136,137), yet permanent injury is more commonly seen among infants with birth weights greater than 4,500 g (138). Important information for the practicing clinician to remember is that most cases of shoulder dystocia and brachial plexus injuries occur among infants who are not macrosomic (135). Clavicular fracture, which usually resolves without any permanent effect, can be seen in 0.3% to 0.7% of all deliveries (134,139,140), and its occurrence is increased up to ten times in the macrosomic infant (134).

Polyhydramnios, defined as excessive amniotic fluid, is not an unusual finding in diabetic pregnancies. A four-quadrant sonographic assessment of the amniotic fluid index (AFI) defines polyhydramnios as an AFI greater than the 95th percentile for gestational age (141). In diabetic pregnancies, the etiology is not clear, although fetal malformations or poor glucose control may be related. When polyhydramnios complicates maternal diabetes, higher rates of perinatal morbidity and mortality are reported (142).

Pregestational Diabetes Mellitus

Estimates from 1999 indicate that approximately 10,000 women in the United States with pregestational diabetes delivered live births (143). Pregnancies of women with pregestational diabetes are at significant risk for both spontaneous abortion and fetal anomalies (144–150), the latter representing the major cause of perinatal mortality in this group of patients (144,149,150). The frequency of congenital anomalies in infants of diabetic mothers occurs at two to three times the rate in the nondiabetic population (151). These malformations, which occur before 7 weeks of gestation, commonly include open neural tube defects, congenital heart defects, and the caudal regression syndrome (144,151,152).

Hyperglycemia is responsible for the increased risks of both fetal malformations and spontaneous abortion seen in diabetics (146–148,149). Poor glycemic control, combined with derangements in amino acid and lipid concentrations, is believed to underlie the development of fetal malformations (147,153). Hypertrophic cardiomyopathy, which can cause cardiomegaly and congestive heart failure, may result from elevated maternal glucose levels throughout pregnancy (154,155). A patient's degree of hyperglycemia can be assessed by the level of glycosylated hemoglobin (hemoglobin A$_{1c}$), a retrospective marker of glucose control (153). Intensive glycemic control in the periods before conception and organogenesis can lower the frequency of congenital anomalies in infants of diabetic mothers (144,156,157).

In the past, a major source of perinatal mortality among diabetic pregnancies was fetal demise, often unexplained and sudden. Among well-controlled diabetics, stillbirth is an uncommon event (144). With diabetic ketoacidosis, however, perinatal mortality rates may be as high as 50% to 90% (158). Fetal blood sampling has confirmed that these previously designated unexplained stillbirths result from hyperglycemia, metabolic disturbances, polycythemia, and acidemia (159,160). Efforts to prevent fetal demise at the Joslin Clinic in the 1960s resulted in the strategy of scheduled preterm deliveries. Even though reductions in the number of stillbirths occurred, neonatal deaths from RDS were prevalent, predominantly as a result of errors in estimates of gestational age (161). Although older data from the 1980s suggested a delay in fetal pulmonary maturation in diabetic pregnancies (162–164) more recent studies have disproved this assumption, especially in patients with good glucose control (165–168). Other complications seen in women with pregestational diabetes mellitus, especially those with end-organ dysfunction from long-standing vascular disease, include preterm delivery and preeclampsia (85).

In the immediate neonatal period, infants of diabetic mothers are at higher risks for a number of metabolic irregularities. Hypoglycemia may occur from a rapid decline in neonatal glucose levels after delivery. This results from a combination of removal of the continued placental source of glucose and fetal islet cell hyperplasia from chronic maternal hyperglycemia. Close maternal glucose control during labor with continuous insulin and glucose infusions can lessen the development of neonatal hypoglycemia (169). Other neonatal metabolic derangements include hypercalcemia, polycythemia, and hyperbilirubinemia (160,170,171).

Gestational Diabetes Mellitus

In the United States, gestational diabetes mellitus (GDM) is diagnosed by at least two abnormal values on a 3-hour 100-g oral glucose tolerance test subsequent to an elevated 1-hour 50-g glucose challenge test (108). GDM occurs in 2% to 5% of pregnancies but comprises the majority of cases of diabetes in pregnancy (108). Recent estimates suggest rising prevalence rates as a result of increased detection following the 1980s' recommendations for universal screening (172,173). In women with GDM, the risk of developing diabetes mellitus 20 years later is approximately 50% (174).

For most patients with GDM, glucose levels may be controlled with dietary therapy alone. Insulin therapy is suggested when fasting glucose levels exceed 95 mg/dL, 1-hour postprandial values exceed 130 to 140 mg/dL, or 2-hour postprandial value exceed 120 mg/dL (108). Regular exercise may help with glucose regulation in this group of patients (108). One randomized trial found similar results among patients with GDM comparing use of insulin versus glyburide, a second-generation sulfonylurea, although additional study is needed (175). In general, infants of mothers with GDM are at risk for macrosomia, operative and cesarean deliveries, birth trauma (including fracture of the clavicle, shoulder dystocia, and brachial plexus injury), fetal death, and neonatal hyperglycemia and/or hyperbilirubinemia (108,112). Patients diagnosed with GDM early in pregnancy and in whom glucose levels require intensive therapy with diet and insulin behave much like those with pregestational diabetes; these patients has a higher risk of fetal malformations and stillbirth than do patients with mild GDM (111). Postpartum recommendations for women diagnosed with GDM during pregnancy include evaluation of glucose status using a 75-g glucose tolerance test (108).

Fetal Assessment

Several tools are used to assess fetal well-being in diabetic and in other high-risk pregnancies. Obstetric ultrasonography can be of value in determining early fetal viability and in screening for various anomalies. Fetal echocardiography is employed generally after 20 weeks' gestation to evaluate fetal cardiac structure. In the third trimester, sonography can assess fetal growth and aid in the diagnosis of macrosomia, polyhydramnios, or septal hypertrophy. An ongoing sense of fetal well-being can be obtained through maternal perception of fetal movement counts. Serial fetal biophysical testing (e.g., nonstress tests and biophysical profiles) is usually implemented by 32 weeks in most insulin-dependent diabetics; pregnancies with well-controlled gestational diabetes, considered to be at low risk for fetal demise, may not require testing except in the presence of other obstetric factors (161).

Autoimmune Disorders

A number of disorders that involve circulating autoantibodies and/or deposition of immune complexes may have direct effects on pregnancy. These include the rheumatologic or connective tissue diseases and conditions associated with circulating antiphospholipid antibodies.

Rheumatologic Disorders

Rheumatologic disorders are chronic inflammatory diseases usually affecting the connective tissues and joints. The most common disorders occurring in young women include systemic lupus erythematosus, rheumatoid arthritis, scleroderma, and Sjögren's syndrome.

Systemic Lupus Erythematosus

Systemic lupus erythematosus (SLE) is the most common connective tissue disorder seen among reproductive-age women. Its various clinical presentations include polyarthritis, skin manifestations, Raynaud phenomenon, and nephri-

tis; laboratory abnormalities such as anemia, leukopenia, thrombocytopenia, and the presence of autoantibodies are common. The disease is characterized by remissions and exacerbations. Patients with SLE have a high prevalence of fetal wastage: spontaneous abortion, IUGR, preterm delivery, stillbirth, and perinatal death (176–181). A majority of the pregnancy losses result from fetal death in the second and third trimesters (182). Many lupus patients have pregnancies with high rates of preterm and term PROM (183). Fetal survival is higher when the disease is in remission (176,177,181–184). Other predictors of fetal wastage include active nephritis, hypertension, and circulating antiphospholipid antibodies (e.g., lupus anticoagulant or anticardiolipin antibodies), the latter likely the most important factor associated with pregnancy loss (176,177,179–182,184,185).

Despite older data that supported the opinion of disease exacerbation in lupus patients during pregnancy, most authorities now agree that pregnancy has no effect on disease progression (176,186,187). Treatment with corticosteroids is standard (178–180,185,188). Salicylates and other nonsteroidal antiinflammatory agents (e.g., paracetamol) are commonly used, although high doses are discouraged (188–191). Azathioprine, an immunosuppressive that has been used predominantly in renal transplantation patients (188,192–194), and antimalarial agents are used widely in SLE patients and considered to be safe during pregnancy (179,188,195–198). In some cases, plasmapheresis has been performed (199,200).

Infants of mothers with SLE are at risk for the neonatal lupus syndrome. This constellation of findings consists of abnormalities in the heart and skin or development of clinical features of SLE and occurs from transplacental passage of maternal antibodies (201). Congenital complete heart block is the most frequently seen heart abnormality (202), occurring in fewer than three percent of infants at risk (189). The pathophysiology involves deposition of immunoglobulin, specifically circulating IgG autoantibodies directed against ribosomal nucleoprotein antigens (anti-Ro or SSA and, to a lesser extent, anti-La or SSB antibodies) in fetal cardiac tissue (201,203). Anti-Ro (SSA) and anti-La (SSB) antibodies are detectable in 40% to 50% of SLE patients (181,202). Most cases of congenital complete heart block occur in fetuses whose mothers do not have overt clinical SLE (204). Many studies, however, indicate that the majority of mothers with affected children have detectable anti-Ro (SSA) antibodies (201,202). Heart block in the absence of structural defects has been documented as early as 16 weeks of gestation (205).

The presenting finding of congenital heart block is fetal dysrhythmia; sonography may reveal a pericardial effusion or hydrops resulting from either congestive failure or an immune mechanism (myocarditis) (203,206–208). Maternal treatment with dexamethasone and/or plasmapheresis, used to lower circulating antibody levels and to minimize inflammatory injury, has had some success in reversing fetal heart block and improving fetal cardiac contractility (207–210). Resolution of ascites has been reported with corticosteroid use (209). The technique of *in utero* cardiac pacing, demonstrated to be technically feasible in a hydropic 24-week fetus with heart block (211), may be a future option in severe cases. After birth, heart block is usually permanent; intermittent and incomplete cases, as well as unusual late presentations, have been described (201,212–214). Cardiac pacemaking is instituted for those infants that survive; however, mortality rates are high (12% to 28%) (201,215). Coexistent cardiac anomalies among infants with congenital heart block are common (214,216).

The skin is the other major organ system involved in the neonatal lupus syndrome. Cutaneous lesions are frequently widespread macular rashes, although a butterfly rash and discoid lesions are found occasionally (181,201). These histologically inflammatory lesions generally appear within the first few weeks of life and disappear spontaneously within 6 months, coexistent with the clearance of maternal autoantibodies from the neonatal circulation (181,201). Hematologic manifestations, such as anemia and thrombocytopenia, glomerulonephritis, hepatosplenomegaly, and neurologic symptoms, are unusual (201,202).

Rheumatoid Arthritis

Rheumatoid arthritis (RA) is the most common inflammatory joint disease, affecting approximately 1% of the population in North America and complicating approximately 1 in 1,000 to 2,000 pregnancies (217). The disorder affects women three times as often as men, with a peak incidence between the fourth and sixth decades of life (217). There is a familial preponderance associated with the tissue antigen HLA-DR4 (217). RA is characterized by chronic polyarthritis and inflammatory synovitis, usually of the peripheral joints, resulting in bone and cartilage destruction and joint deformities. Other clinical manifestations include anorexia, weakness, fatigue, and vague musculoskeletal complaints. The diagnosis is made based on specific criteria outlined by the American Rheumatism Association (218). Despite much study, it is not known why the symptoms of RA are ameliorated during pregnancy; studies evaluating cortisol levels and sex hormone concentrations have not provided any solid answers (219,220). In contrast to SLE, perinatal morbidity and mortality are not increased in patients with RA (220).

The major therapies for RA are acetylsalicylic acid (aspirin) and nonsteroidal antiinflammatory agents; concerns for adverse fetal and/or neonatal effects (such as impaired hemostasis, premature closure of the fetal ductus arteriosus, prolonged gestation, and long labor) have been largely theoretical (188,219). Gold therapy, which lowers the levels of rheumatoid factor, has been used for many years; antimalarial agents are also administered (188,219). Although D-penicillamine has been used, some reports have shown connective tissue defects similar to Ehlers-Danlos syndrome in children with antenatal exposure (221).

Scleroderma

Scleroderma is an autoimmune connective-tissue disorder that occurs at least five times more frequently in women of childbearing age than in men, affecting the skin, gastrointestinal tract, especially the esophagus, lungs, and kidneys (222). The typical remissions and exacerbations of the disease make it difficult to assess the effect of pregnancy. According to a 1989 report on 94 cases of scleroderma in pregnancy and a review of the literature, pregnancy had either no effect on the disease or was associated with exacerbations (223). A retrospective case control study of 48 women revealed an association with first trimester pregnancy loss in those patients with long-standing diffuse scleroderma and a 29% prematurity rate (222). Fetal mortality may be as high as 20% and the development of neonatal scleroderma has been described.

Sjögren Syndrome

This rare autoimmune disorder, also known as keratoconjunctivitis sicca or sicca syndrome, involves lymphocytic infiltration of the salivary and lacrimal glands resulting in loss of saliva and tears. Sjögren syndrome is both clinically and immunologically related to SLE. Many circulating autoantibodies are present, as well as anti-Ro (SSA) and anti-La (SSB) antibodies. Approximately 50% of patients with Sjögren syndrome have rheumatoid arthritis (224). Pregnancy complications of fetal loss and congenital heart block have been reported (225).

Antiphospholipid Antibodies and the Antiphospholipid Syndrome

Circulating antiphospholipid antibodies and the antiphospholipid syndrome (APS) are associated with clinical complications such as adverse pregnancy outcomes, autoimmune thrombocytopenia, and thrombosis (226). These antibodies are directed against negatively charged phospholipids present on cell membranes, notably platelets and endothelial cells (227). The most common antiphospholipid antibodies are the lupus anticoagulant and anticardiolipin antibodies. The lupus anticoagulant was originally described as a circulating anticoagulant identified in two patients with SLE (228). It is paradoxically named, however, for the anticoagulant activity is seen *in vitro*, whereas it acts is as a potent thrombotic agent *in vivo*.

Antiphospholipid antibodies may be found in the normal population, but they are more frequently detected in patients with SLE (229,230). Diagnosis of the APS involves both clinical and laboratory parameters: moderately high levels of the antiphospholipid antibodies (lupus anticoagulant and/or anticardiolipin antibodies) plus one clinical parameter (thrombosis, autoimmune thrombocytopenia, or pregnancy loss) (226,231–233). Potential pregnancy complications include those listed in Table 14-5 (226,227,234). The most striking adverse fetal outcomes associated with APS are fetal death and IUGR. Pregnancy loss may be the only clinical marker associated with the presence of antiphospholipid antibodies, however. A 1994 study demonstrated a very high rate of development of thrombotic complications after the identification of these antibodies, even

TABLE 14-5

PREGNANCY COMPLICATIONS SEEN IN ASSOCIATION WITH ANTIPHOSPHOLIPID ANTIBODIES[a]

- Fetal loss, including recurrent embryonic loss or fetal death after 10 weeks
- Intrauterine growth restriction
- Placental infarction
- Preterm birth
- Early onset severe preeclampsia
- Nonreassuring fetal heart rate patterns
- Unusual postpartum syndrome (e.g., cardiopulmonary disease, fever, hemolytic uremic syndrome)

[a] From American College of Obstetricians and Gynecologists. *Antiphospholipid syndrome. ACOG Educational Bulletin 244.* Washington, DC: ACOG, 1998; Branch DW. Antiphospholipid syndrome: laboratory concerns, fetal loss, and pregnancy management. *Semin Perinatol* 1991;15:230–237; and Kniaz D, Eisenberg GM, Elrad H, et al. Postpartum hemolytic uremic syndrome associated with antiphospholipid antibodies. A case report and review of the literature. *Am J Nephrol* 1992;12:126–133.

in asymptomatic individuals (235). Other unusual reported complications include fetal or neonatal thrombosis resulting from transplacental passage of maternal antibodies (236,237) and fetal effects of therapy.

Initial treatment of the APS involved use of low-dose aspirin (75 mg) and corticosteroids (238,239); successful pregnancy outcomes were reported by many investigators worldwide using similar regimens (227). Oropharyngeal candidiasis, gestational diabetes, osteoporosis, and PROM are some of the complications seen with corticosteroid use (227,240–242). An alternative regimen consisting of low-dose aspirin and heparin currently is the preferred therapy (226,240,243,244). Potential problems associated with heparin include thrombocytopenia and heparin-induced osteoporosis, although these complications are fewer with administration of low-molecular-weight heparin (243, 245). Intravenous immunoglobulin also has been used (246,247). In spite of aggressive treatment, however, successful pregnancy outcomes are not guaranteed.

Thyroid Disorders

The second most common endocrine disorder in women of reproductive age consists of disorders of thyroid metabolism (248). Pregnancy significantly affects thyroid physiology. Normal pregnancy is characterized by hypermetabolic effects that resemble the clinical findings of hyperthyroidism. Although some thyroid function tests may be altered during pregnancy, largely by hyperestrogenemia and the resulting increase in thyroid-binding globulin, levels of free-circulating hormone (T_4 and T_3) and thyroid-stimulating hormone (TSH) are unchanged. Moreover, several obstetric conditions, notably hyperemesis gravidarum or gestational trophoblastic disease, may cause abnormalities in thyroid function. These principles must be understood when making the diagnosis of thyroid disease during pregnancy.

Hyperthyroidism

Approximately 1 in 2,000 pregnancies will be complicated by thyrotoxicosis; the condition that results from excessive production of thyroid hormone. Most cases of hyperthyroidism are due to Graves disease, an autoimmune disorder characterized by production of thyroid-stimulating immunoglobulin (TSI) and thyroid-stimulating hormone-binding inhibitory immunoglobulin (TBII), both of which act on TSH production (248–250). Graves disease accounts for 95% of hyperthyroidism during pregnancy, affecting 1% of American women (249,250). Other causes of hyperthyroidism include excess TSH production, gestational trophoblast tumors, toxic multinodular goiter, subacute thyroiditis, overactive thyroid adenoma, and extrathyroid source of thyroid hormone (248). Poorly controlled or untreated hyperthyroidism during pregnancy is associated with greater risks of severe preeclampsia, congestive heart failure, and preterm delivery (248). The most serious consequence of uncontrolled thyrotoxicosis, thyroid storm, presents with exaggerated features of thyrotoxicosis including fever, altered mental status, vomiting, diarrhea, and cardiac dysfunction manifested by arrhythmia and heart failure (248). Usually, this rare condition is triggered by a precipitating event such as infection, trauma, or delivery; though the diagnosis can be difficult to make, treatment of the underlying condition is critical (248).

Medical treatment of hyperthyroidism involves blocking thyroid hormone production and controlling the peripheral clinical symptoms. Propylthiouracil (PTU) and methimazole, which block production of thyroid hormone, are safe in pregnancy (251). Both agents cross the placenta, but methimazole has been associated with a scalp disorder known as aplasia cutis (252). Peripheral manifestations such as tachycardia are controlled with beta-blockers, notably propranolol, widely used during pregnancy. In difficult cases, thyroidectomy may be performed during pregnancy after medical control of thyrotoxicosis has been achieved. Iodides may be used for short periods in preparation for thyroidectomy or for management of thyroid storm.

Most fetal morbidity and mortality develop from uncontrolled maternal hyperthyroidism. Prolonged iodide exposure after 10 to 12 weeks of gestation may result in fetal hypothyroidism and goiter (248,250). Fetal thyrotoxicosis, which results from transplacental passage of TSI (253), has been reported in approximately 1% of infants of mothers with Graves disease and is associated with fetal death (248,254–256). Fetal blood sampling has been helpful in measuring fetal thyroid status (255,256).

Hypothyroidism

Overt hypothyroidism rarely complicates pregnancy, although retrospective studies show high rates of stillbirths, low-birth-weight infants, medically indicated preterm delivery, preeclampsia, and abruption in women with inadequately treated hypothyroidism (248). In many cases, hypothyroidism develops after thyroidectomy or radioiodine therapy; other causes of hypothyroidism include Hashimoto thyroiditis, carcinoma, or insufficient thyroid replacement (248,250). Replacement therapy with thyroxine is recommended for these patients and TSH levels are used to guide therapeutic dosages. Replacement doses of thyroxine may need to be increased during pregnancy (257). Neonatal hypothyroidism needs to be excluded if maternal antenatal treatment involved radioactive iodine; however, because congenital hypothyroidism is a difficult diagnosis, screening for all infants is routine (248,258).

Perinatal Infections

Any infection occurring during pregnancy has the potential for causing infectious or teratogenic complications in the fetus, some with devastating effects. The two important routes for fetal infection are hematogenous via the placenta and ascending via the vagina and cervix, the latter usually occurring intrapartum. The effect of an infectious agent on fetal growth and development depends on, among other things, the type of organism, the infectious load, timing in gestation, and potential organ systems affected. Many different organisms have been implicated in causing fetal infection; Table 14-6 lists some of the important perinatal viral infections (259–265), and Table 14-7 lists some of the important perinatal nonviral infections (259–261, 266– 268).

Treatment of many perinatal infections either does not exist, as in cases with viruses, or may not prevent congenital infection, as with syphilis. Consequently, efforts to minimize the effect on the neonate focus primarily on prevention. Examples include cesarean delivery in cases of active maternal genital herpes infection, thereby decreasing the risk of intrapartum ascending infection, neonatal administration of the hepatitis B vaccine, or administration of prophylactic eyedrops to newborns to prevent gonococcal ophthalmia neonatorum. Attempts at preventing early onset neonatal disease from group B streptococcus have resulted in guidelines from the Centers for Disease Control and Prevention, adopted by ACOG, for universal third-trimester screening and administration of intrapartum antibiotics to carriers (266). There is much work to be done, however, in devising strategies to prevent other perinatally transmitted illnesses such as congenital cytomegalovirus infection or human immunodeficiency virus that may have damaging effects on a significant number of children annually.

Thromboembolic Disorders

The risk of venous thromboembolism is five times greater during pregnancy than in the nonpregnant population, with an absolute risk of 0.5 to 3.0 per 1,000 women (269). The most constant predisposing factor for thromboembolic disease during pregnancy is venous stasis, although other factors include prolonged bed rest, operative vaginal or cesarean delivery, sepsis, hemorrhage, multiparity, and

advanced maternal age (269,270). Although older reports demonstrated the greatest risk for development of thromboembolism during the third trimester and the immediate postpartum period, newer reports raise concerns that older studies may have been skewed by the practices of common operative deliveries, delaying postpartum ambulation, and suppression of lactation with oral estrogen (269–271). Newer data suggest not only equal frequencies in all trimesters but that antepartum events may occur at least as often as those postpartum (269,271).

Maternal thromboembolism may result from an underlying inherited coagulopathy (also known as thrombophilia). Most of these autosomally dominant disorders result in deficiencies of antithrombin III, protein C and protein S, or activated protein C resistance because of the factor V Leiden mutation (269,271–276). Other inherited thrombophilias include the prothrombin G20210A mutation, 4G/4G mutation in plasminogen activator inhibitor 1 (PAI-1) gene, and the thermolabile variant of methylenetetrahydrofolate reductase (C677T MTHFR), the latter resulting in hyperhomocysteinemia (269,272–274). Individuals with inherited coagulopathies have significantly increased risks of thromboembolism as well as pregnancy complications such as stillbirth, IUGR, and severe preeclampsia (269,271–276). The APS may also cause thromboembolic events (226,269,271).

The clinical diagnosis of deep vein thrombosis during gestation is imprecise. Noninvasive tests, such as impedance plethysmography or real-time Doppler sonography, accurate in nonpregnant patients, may be difficult to interpret during pregnancy; the data they provide as initial tests, however, may be useful (269,270). Duplex ultrasound venography has been the standard in diagnosing deep venous thromboembolism (277). For both pregnant and nonpregnant patients suspected of having a pulmonary embolism, the ventilation–perfusion (V/Q) scan is the recommended study (278). In recent years the utility of spiral computed tomography (CT) has been demonstrated (279). With a 90% sensitivity and 90% specificity, some authors recommend replacing the V/Q scan with the spiral CT scan, although studies in pregnancy are lacking (269).

Treatment for acute deep vein thrombosis or pulmonary embolism during pregnancy involves 5 to 10 days of intravenous heparin followed by subcutaneous heparin in doses to achieve full-dose anticoagulation for a minimum of 3 months (269–271). Antepartum prophylactic heparin therapy is indicated in patients with a previous thrombotic event (269,271). The preferred anticoagulant during pregnancy is heparin because it does not cross the placenta (280); the newer low-molecular-weight heparins are safe in pregnancy (269,281). Warfarin is avoided because of associated fetal malformations: first-trimester exposure may produce an embryopathy involving stippled epiphyses, nasal and limb hypoplasia, and hypertelorism (269,282,283), and second- or third-trimester exposure is associated with central nervous system abnormalities (284). Warfarin may be used postpartum in women who are breast-feeding (271).

TABLE 14-6

SOME PERINATAL VIRAL INFECTIONS[a]

Virus	Type of Virus	Route of Transmission	Time of Critical Exposure	Potential Severe Fetal or Neonatal Effect(s)
Cytomegalovirus (CMV)	Double-stranded DNA herpesvirus	Transplacental more than ascending; also breast-feeding	Gestational age not critical; primary infection more severe than recurrent	*Fetus*: IUGR, nonimmune hydrops, hepatosplenomegaly, chorioretinitis, microcephaly, cerebral calcifications, microophthalmia, hydrocephaly. *Newborn*: jaundice, petechiae, LBW, hepatosplenomegaly, thrombocytopenia
Rubella	RNA virus	Transplacental	First trimester	Congenital heart disease, purpura, cataracts, retinopathy, IUGR, microcephaly
Herpes simplex virus (HSV)	Double-stranded DNA virus	Ascending intrapartum	Intrapartum	Microcephaly, seizures, mental retardation, mircoophthalmia, retinal dysplasia, meningitis, chorioretinitis (HSV-2 more important than HSV-1)
Varicella zoster	DNA herpesvirus	Transplacental	*Congenital varicella* if <20 weeks; *neonatal varicella* if 5 days before or 2 days after delivery	*Congenital varicella*: limb hypoplasia, cutaneous scars, chorioretinitis, cortical atrophy, microcephaly; *Neonatal varicella* if contracted peripartum
Parvovirus B-19	Single-stranded DNA virus	Transplacental	Severe effects seen with exposure before 20 weeks	Low risk for fetal morbidity; possibly spontaneous abortion, hydrops (from aplastic anemia, myocarditis or chronic hepatitis) and/or stillbirth
Human immuno-deficiency virus (HIV)	Retrovirus	Transplacental; ascending intrapartum; breast-feeding	Any	Neonatal acquired immunodeficiency syndrome (AIDS)
Hepatitis B	DNA virus	85%–95% ascending intrapartum; rest transplacental during acute hepatitis or postnatal via breast-feeding and close contact		Postnatal chronic hepatitis, cirrhosis, hepatocellular carcinoma

DNA, deoxyribonucleic acid; IUGR, intrauterine growth restriction; LBW, low birth weight; RNA, ribonucleic acid.
[a] From Bale JF. Congenital infections. *Neurol Clin* 2002;20:1039–1060; Duff P. Maternal and Perinatal infection. In: Gabbe SG, Niebyl JR, Simpson JL, eds. *Obstetrics—normal and problem pregnancies*, 4th ed. New York: Churchill-Livingstone 2002:293–1348; American College of Obstetricians and Gynecologists. *Perinatal viral and parasitic infections. ACOG Practice Bulletin 20*. Washington, DC: ACOG, 2000; American College of Obstetricians and Gynecologists. *Viral hepatitis in pregnancy. ACOG Educational Bulletin 248*. Washington, DC: ACOG, 1998; American College of Obstetricians and Gynecologists. *Perinatal herpes simplex virus infections. ACOG Technical Bulletin 122*. Washington, DC: ACOG, 1988; American College of Obstetricians and Gynecologists. *Human immunodeficiency virus infections in pregnancy. ACOG Educational Bulletin 232*. Washington, DC: ACOG, 1997; and Kotler DP. Human immunodeficiency virus and pregnancy. *Gastroenterol Clin North Am* 2003;32:437–448, ix.

Renal Disorders

Mild renal dysfunction typically has little, if any, effect on pregnancy outcome; however, adverse pregnancy events are well described in women with moderate to severe renal insufficiency (e.g., serum creatinine >1.4 mg/dL) (285–287). These pregnancies are especially risky: maternal complications include anemia, vascular accidents, placental abruption, chronic hypertension, pregnancy-induced hypertension, preeclampsia, proteinuria, and worsening renal function; perinatal complications such as IUGR, stillbirth, prematurity, polyhydramnios, and midtrimester pregnancy loss are not unusual (285,287,288).

Dialysis may be used during pregnancies complicated by renal insufficiency. More literature is available for hemodialysis than for continuous ambulatory peritoneal dialysis (289–293). Pregnancy success rates in dialysis patients are at most 52% (290), and outcomes generally are more promising for women in whom dialysis has been initiated during pregnancy compared to patients already on dialysis before

TABLE 14-7

SOME NONVIRAL PERINATAL INFECTIONS[a]

Organism (Disease)	Type of Organism	Route of Transmission	Time of Critical Exposure	Potential Severe Fetal or Neonatal Effect(s)
Neisseria gonorrhoeae (gonorrhea)	Gram-negative diplococcus	Ascending	Intrapartum	Ophthalmia neonatorum
Group B streptococcus	Gram-positive bacteria	Ascending	Intrapartum	Early onset neonatal infection: sepsis, meningitis, pneumonia
Treponema pallidum (syphilis)	Spirochete	Transplacental	Any trimester but worse risk in first and second trimesters	Hepatosplenomegaly, osteitis, hemolytic anemia, thrombocytopenia, pneumonia, hydrops, cutaneous or mucous membrane lesions, hepatitis, stillbirth
Toxoplasma gondii (toxoplasmosis)	Intracellular parasite	Transplacental	More likely transmitted during the third trimester but more severe infection with earlier infection	Stillbirth, hydrocephalus, microcephaly, periventricular calcifications, hepatosplenomegaly, ascites; neonate with seizures, chorioretinitis leading to blindness, fever, rash, hearing loss, mental retardation

[a] From Bale JF. Congenital infections. *Neurol Clin* 2002;20:1039–1060; Duff P. Maternal and Perinatal Infection. In: Gabbe SG, Niebyl JR, Simpson JL, eds. *Obstetrics—normal and problem pregnancies*, 4th ed. New York: Churchill-Livingstone 2002:293–1348; American College of Obstetricians and Gynecologists. *Perinatal viral and parasitic infections. ACOG Practice Bulletin 20*. Washington, DC: ACOG, 2000; American College of Obstetricians and Gynecologists. *Viral hepatitis in pregnancy. ACOG Educational Bulletin 248*. Washington, DC: ACOG, 1998; American College of Obstetricians and Gynecologists. *Prevention of early-onset group B streptococcal disease in newborns. ACOG Committee Opinion 279*. Washington, DC: ACOG, 2002; Ray JG. Lues-lues: maternal and fetal considerations of syphilis. *Obstet Gynecol Surv* 1995;50:845–850; Ricci JM, Fojaco RM, O'Sullivan MJ. Congenital syphilis: the University of Miami/Jackson Memorial Medical Center experience, 1986–1988. *Obstet Gynecol* 1989;74:687–693.

conception (289,291). Complications associated with peritoneal dialysis in pregnancy include preterm labor (289) and acute peritonitis (291,294). Hemodialysis involves intermittent and often significant fluid shifts, which may be accompanied by hypotension, electrolyte imbalances, and preterm labor (288). In one reported case, in spite of efforts to eliminate major fluid shifts and changes in arterial pressure in a patient at 32 weeks gestation, uterine artery Doppler studies showed a significant increase after hemodialysis; redistribution of flow away from the uteroplacental vascular bed during hemodialysis was postulated (288).

Pregnancy is no longer an unusual event among women of childbearing age with functioning renal transplants, occurring in approximately 1 of 20 to 50 women (193,295). More than 7,000 pregnancies have been reported in renal transplant recipients (296). Overall, these pregnancies have low success rates, although repeated successful pregnancies have been reported (297,298). Hypertension before or during early pregnancy is associated with adverse perinatal events (295). Typically, pregnancy results in increased renal function, which transiently declines in late pregnancy. As many as 15% of patients with kidney disease may experience permanent renal impairment (298). High rates of preterm delivery, IUGR, hypertension and/or preeclampsia, and stillbirth are reported (193,295,296,298). The risk of graft rejection, however, is not influenced by pregnancy (193). Cyclosporine A, a potent anti–T-cell immunosuppressive agent, has replaced older regimens of azathioprine and steroids in preventing graft rejection (299). Cyclosporine has been used successfully during pregnancy without evidence of teratogenicity (299–301).

Heart Disease

Maternal cardiac disease may be accompanied by significant maternal and perinatal morbidity and mortality. Although the etiology of cardiac disease has changed in the past 30 years, with congenital heart disease now more common than rheumatic heart disease, the underlying pathophysiology remains the same. Functional status before or early in pregnancy is an important prognostic indicator of maternal and fetal outcome. A helpful and commonly used system for assessing cardiac function is the New York Heart Association classification (Table 14-8) (302,303). Better prognoses are expected during pregnancy for women with functional classes I and II than for those with classes III or IV. Gravidae with severe functional limitations account for 75% of the maternal deaths (304).

Preconception counseling is critical in this group of patients. The added cardiovascular demands of pregnancy may be associated with cardiac deterioration: more than 40% of women with heart disease will develop pulmonary edema for the first time during the third trimester (302,305). Maternal risks vary with the individual cardiac

TABLE 14-8

THE NEW YORK HEART ASSOCIATION (NYHA) FUNCTIONAL CLASSIFICATION OF HEART DISEASE[a]

Class	Symptoms
Class I	Asymptomatic
Class II	Symptoms with greater than normal activity
Class III	Symptoms with normal activity
Class IV	Symptoms at rest

[a] From American College of Obstetricians and Gynecologists. *Cardiac disease in pregnancy. ACOG Technical Bulletin 168*. Washington, DC: ACOG, 1992; Criteria Committee of the New York Heart Association. *Nomenclature and criteria for diagnosis of diseases of the heart and great vessels*, 8th ed. Boston: Little Brown, 1979.

lesion, several specific defects being associated with especially high risks of maternal mortality (Table 14-9) (302, 303,306).

Fetal risks include premature delivery, IUGR, and still-birth, especially with maternal cyanotic heart disease (302,307). A 2% to 5% incidence of fetal cardiac anomalies

has been suggested in women with congenital heart disease, although with specific lesions, the risk may be as high as 26% (302,306,308). Most of the drugs used in the treatment of cardiac disease are well tolerated and rarely associated with significant fetal problems (e.g., beta-blockers, calcium channel blockers, digitalis, and heparin) (304,306). Newer agents have not been well studied during pregnancy.

Cardiac surgery should be delayed until after completion of pregnancy if possible. If it is required, however, surgery during the second trimester is preferable (306). Maternal and perinatal mortality varies with the type of procedure. For example, in mitral valve commissurotomy, the cardiovascular procedure that has been performed the most during pregnancy, maternal mortality is under 3% and perinatal mortality is less than 10%; in contrast, with open-heart surgery, although maternal mortality is not significantly higher, fetal loss may be as high as 20% (306).

Myocardial infarction (MI) rarely occurs during pregnancy; the incidence is estimated at 1 in 10,000 pregnancies (309). Cases show a preponderance during the third trimester and in multiparous women older than age 33 years (310), with the majority of MIs located in the anterior wall (310,311). Maternal mortality ranges from 19% to 37%

TABLE 14-9

THE EFFECTS OF SOME MATERNAL CONGENITAL HEART LESIONS DURING PREGNANCY[a]

Cardiac Lesion	Specific Information
Aortic insufficiency	Well tolerated
Aortic stenosis	Valve diameter must decrease to ≤1/3 for hemodynamic significance; increased risk of angina, MI, syncope, or sudden death with severe disease because CO is fixed and may not be able to compensate; frequently associated with ischemic heart disease; most critical time is at pregnancy termination or delivery; PA catheterization may be most useful in labor
Ebstein anomaly	Right-to-left shunt ± pulmonary HTN; association with thromboembolism, CHF, arrhythmias; 25% of patients have Wolf-Parkinson-White syndrome and increased risk for tachyarrhythmias
Eisenmenger syndrome	Pulmonary HTN with left-to-right shunt; grave prognosis; maternal mortality 30% to 50%; high association with thromboembolism; therapeutic termination is recommended
Marfan syndrome	Autosomal dominant; aortic dissection or aortic or splenic artery aneurysm or rupture associated with worse outcomes; 50% mortality seen with aortic root diameter >40 mm
Mitral insufficiency	Well tolerated; CHF rare; pulmonary edema more likely with preeclampsia because of increase in afterload; because of increased risk of atrial enlargement and fibrillation, prophylactic digitalis recommended in severe disease
Mitral stenosis	Tachycardia may result in fall in CO and BP; fluid balance crucial; most critical time is immediately postpartum; hemodynamic monitoring is recommended
Mitral valve prolapse	Common; mostly asymptomatic; chest pain or palpitations possible; responds to beta-blockers
Tetralogy of Fallot	VSD, overriding aorta, RVH, and pulmonary stenosis; patients are cyanotic; maternal mortality 4% to 15% in uncorrected patients; corrected cases fairly good outcome
Tricuspid or pulmonic valve disease	Well tolerated

BP, blood pressure; CHF, congestive heart failure; CO, cardiac output; HTN, hypertension; MI, myocardial infarction; PA, pulmonary artery; RVH, right ventricular hypertrophy; VSD, ventricular septal defect.
[a] From American College of Obstetricians and Gynecologists. *Cardiac disease in pregnancy. ACOG Technical Bulletin 168*. Washington, DC: ACOG, 1992; Criteria Committee of the New York Heart Association. *Nomenclature and criteria for diagnosis of diseases of the heart and great vessels*, 8th ed. Boston: Little Brown, 1979.

(310–312). Fetal mortality is similarly high, most resulting from maternal death (310–312). Given that electrocardiography can be nondiagnostic in 50% of pregnant women with an acute MI, the use of cardiac troponin I levels has been found to be reliable in making an accurate diagnosis (309). Acute coronary artery angioplasty recently was successful during pregnancy (313,314). Treatment with thrombolytic agents for maternal myocardial infarction has been reported during the second trimester, although the fetal risk of such therapy has not been established (315). Some patients have had successful subsequent pregnancies (316,317).

Successful pregnancies have been reported in women who have undergone heart transplantation (304,318–322). Reported cases include four patients who initially received their allograft because of peripartum cardiomyopathy from an earlier pregnancy (322). Maternal hypertension, preeclampsia, and jaundice, as well as fetal IUGR, are common (322). Immunosuppression issues are the same as those discussed for patients with renal transplants.

Cancer

Cancer develops in approximately 1 of 1,000 pregnancies. The most common invasive carcinoma originates in the cervix, affecting one of 2,200 pregnancies (323,324). Almost 3% of all cervical cancers are diagnosed during pregnancy (325). The second most common site for malignancy during pregnancy is the breast, with cancer estimated to occur once in every 1,360 to 3,200 pregnancies (326). Other frequently seen neoplasias include vulvar, ovarian, and colorectal carcinoma, as well as leukemia, Hodgkin disease, and melanoma. Stage for stage, comparing diagnoses in nonpregnant women with those in pregnant women, carcinoma identified during pregnancy may be more advanced. Currently, this is thought to reflect a delay in diagnosis, possibly because of the physiologic changes of pregnancy, and not necessarily because the cancer is more aggressive during the pregnant state (327). It has never been substantiated that pregnancy termination alters cancer progression (327). Metastasis to the fetus or placenta has been reported in fewer than 70 cases, mostly involving the breast, cervix, leukemia, lymphoma, melanoma, and thyroid (328).

Decisions regarding the management of malignancies during pregnancy are difficult and involve risk assessment for both mother and fetus. The difficulty of these decisions is compounded by the timing in gestation. In general, first-trimester treatment risks spontaneous abortion or fetal malformation, and early third-trimester therapy places the pregnancy at risk for preterm labor. Surgery can be performed at any time, although it is preferred during the second trimester. Radiation or chemotherapy exposure in the first trimester may affect organogenesis, resulting in either pregnancy loss or fetal structural defects (329–331).

Radiation exposure just prior to and immediately after implantation poses the greatest risk of spontaneous abortion (330). Animal studies demonstrate an "all-or-nothing"

effect because at this early point in development, the few embryonic cells are not yet differentiated; therefore, the embryo either dies or develops normally (330). During the first 3 weeks of gestation, radiation exposure of at least 250 rads (2.5 cGy) poses the greatest risk for miscarriage (332). Exposure to more than 50 rads (0.5 cGy) is more commonly associated with development of severe malformations (333); however, congenital anomalies are unusual in embryos exposed to more than 5-rads (0.05 cGy) (332). Some malformations associated with radiation exposure during weeks 3 through 10 include microcephaly, low birth weight, mental retardation, cataracts, retinal degeneration, and skeletal abnormalities (332,333). Radiation exposure between 11 and 20 weeks of gestation is not commonly associated with fetal malformations (327,330). Pregnancy termination has been suggested when fetal exposure is greater than 10 rads (0.1 cGy) (334). In cases in which local irradiation is used to treat malignancies of the pelvis, spontaneous abortion or fetal demise usually occurs (325).

Use of cytotoxic chemotherapy is generally avoided in the first trimester, although data vary for different agents (325,329). Exposure beyond the first trimester has not been found to be associated with increased risks of congenital anomalies (325,331). Long-term developmental data are lacking, however. In treating patients with chemotherapeutic agents, recognition of the physiologic changes of pregnancy may alter the efficacy, toxicity, and/or dosage regimens.

SUMMARY

Many maternal conditions have relevance for a developing pregnancy. Counseling pregnant women with underlying medical disorders must encompass the effects of the illness on the pregnancy, the effects of the pregnancy on the condition, as well as potential complications of therapeutic interventions, and the risks of possible premature delivery. Statistics indicating reductions in neonatal mortality rates are encouraging; however, there is much yet to be learned in perinatology in order to impact on the unacceptably high rates of premature deliveries and to improve the health of women before and during pregnancy.

REFERENCES

1. Guyer B, Freedman MA, Strobino DM, et al. Annual summary of vital statistics: trends in the health of Americans during the 20th century. *Pediatrics* 2000;106:1307–1317.
2. Arias E, MacDorman MF, Strobino DM, et al. Annual summary of vital statistics—2002. *Pediatrics* 2003;112:1215–1230.
3. McCormick MC, Shapiro S, Starfield BH. The regionalization of perinatal services: summary of the evaluation of a national demonstration program. *JAMA* 1985;253:799–804.
4. Yeast JD, Poskin M, Stockbauer JW, et al. Changing patterns in regionalization of perinatal care and the impact on neonatal mortality. *Am J Obstet Gynecol* 1998;178:131–135.
5. Hein HA, Lofgren MA. The changing pattern of neonatal mortality in a regionalized system of perinatal care: a current update. *Pediatrics* 1999;104:1064–1069.

6. Wilcox A, Skjærven R, Buekens P, et al. Birth weight and perinatal mortality. A comparison of the United States and Norway. *JAMA* 1995;273:709–711.
7. American College of Obstetricians and Gynecologists. *Premature rupture of membranes. ACOG practice bulletin 1.* Washington, DC: ACOG, 1998.
8. Mercer BM, Lewis R. Preterm labor and preterm premature rupture of the membranes. Diagnosis and management. *Clin Infect Dis* 1997;11:177–201.
9. Stevenson DK, Wright LL, Lemons JA, et al. Very low birth weight outcomes of the National Institute of Child Health and Human Development Neonatal Research Network, January 1993 through December 1994. *Am J Obstet Gynecol* 1998;179:1632–1639.
10. Singh GK, Yu SM. Infant mortality in the United States: trends, differentials, and projections, 1950 through 2010. *Am J Public Health* 1995;85:957–964.
11. Amon E, Anderson GD, Sibai BM, et al. Factors responsible for a preterm delivery of the immature newborn infant (less than or equal to 1000 gm). *Am J Obstet Gynecol* 1987;156:1143–1148.
12. Meis PJ, Ernest JM, Moore ML. Causes of low birth weight births in public and private patients. *Am J Obstet Gynecol* 1987;156:1165–1168.
13. Tucker JM, Goldenberg RL, Davis RO, et al. Etiologies of preterm birth in an indigent population: is prevention a logical expectation? *Obstet Gynecol* 1991;77:343–347.
14. American College of Obstetricians and Gynecologists. *Assessment of risk factors for preterm birth. ACOG practice bulletin 31.* Washington, DC: ACOG, 2001.
15. Centers for Disease Control and Prevention. State-specific trends among women who did not receive prenatal care—United States 1980–1992. *MMWR Morb Mortal Wkly Rep* 1994;43:939–942.
16. Harger JH, Hsing AW, Tuomala RE, et al. Risk factors for preterm premature rupture of fetal membranes: a multicenter case-control study. *Am J Obstet Gynecol* 1990;163:130–137.
17. Kristensen J, Langhoff-Roos J, Kristensen FB. Implications of idiopathic preterm delivery for previous and subsequent pregnancies. *Obstet Gynecol* 1995;86:800–804.
18. Mercer BM, Goldenberg RL, Das A, et al. The preterm prediction study: a clinical risk assessment system. *Am J Obstet Gynecol* 1996;174:1885–1895.
19. Romero R, Brody DT, Oyarzun E, et al. Infection and labor. III. Interleukin-1: a signal for the onset of parturition. *Am J Obstet Gynecol* 1989;160:1117–1123.
20. Mercer BM. Preterm premature rupture of the membranes. *Obstet Gynecol* 2003:101:178–193.
21. Lee T, Carpenter MW, Heber WW, et al. Preterm premature rupture of membranes: risks of recurrent complications in the next pregnancy among a population-based sample of gravid women. *Am J Obstet Gynecol* 2003;188:209–213.
22. Kaltreider DF, Kohl S. Epidemiology of preterm delivery. *Clin Obstet Gynecol* 1980;23:17–31.
23. Bendon RW, Faye-Peterson O, Pavlova Z, et al. Fetal membrane histology in preterm premature rupture of membranes: comparison to controls, and between antibiotic and placebo treatment. The National Institute of Child Health and Human Development Maternal Fetal Medicine Units Network. *Pediatr Dev Pathol* 1999;2:552–558.
24. Cauci S, Hitti J, Noonan C, et al. Vaginal hydrolytic enzymes, immunoglobulin A against Gardnerella vaginalis toxin, and risk of early preterm birth among women in preterm labor with bacterial vaginosis or intermediate flora. *Am J Obstet Gynecol* 2002;187:877–881.
25. Hillier SL, Nugent RP, Eschenbach DA, et al. Association between bacterial vaginosis and preterm delivery of a low-birth-weight infant. *N Engl J Med* 1995;333:1737–1742.
26. Goldenberg RL, Iams JD, Mercer BM, et al. The preterm prediction study: the value of new vs. standard risk factors in predicting early and all spontaneous preterm births. NICHD MFMU Network. *Am J Public Health* 1998;88:233–238.
27. Carey JC, Klebanoff MA, Hauth JC, et al. Metronidazole to prevent preterm delivery in pregnant women with asymptomatic bacterial vaginosis. National Institute of Child Health and Human Development Network of Maternal-Fetal Medicine Units. *N Engl J Med* 2000;342:534–540.
28. Hauth JC, Gilstrap LC, Hankins GD, et al. Term maternal and neonatal complications of acute chorioamnionitis. *Obstet Gynecol* 1985;66:59–62.
29. Wilson JC, Levy DL, Wilds PL. Premature rupture of membranes prior to term: consequences of nonintervention. *Obstet Gynecol* 1982;60:601–606.
30. McIntosh N, Harrison A. Prolonged premature rupture of membranes in the preterm infant: a 7 year study. *Eur J Obstet Gynecol Reprod Biol* 1994;57:1–6.
31. Goldenberg RL. The management of preterm labor. *Obstet Gynecol* 2002:100:1020–1037.
32. Wright LL. National Institutes of Health (NIH) Consensus Development Conference. Effect of corticosteroids for fetal maturation on perinatal outcomes. Consensus Development Conference, February 28–March 2, 1994, Bethesda, MD. *Am J Obstet Gynecol* 1995:173:246–252.
33. National Institutes of Health Consensus Development Panel. Antenatal corticosteroids revisited: repeat courses-national institutes of health consensus development conference statement, August 17–18, 2000. *Obstet Gynecol* 2001;98:144–150.
34. Crowley P. Prophylactic corticosteroids for preterm birth. *Cochrane Database Syst Rev* 2000;2:CD000065.
35. Svare J, Langhoff-Roos J, Anderson LF, et al. Ampicillin-metronidazole treatment in idiopathic preterm labour: a randomised controlled multicentre trial. *Br J Obstet Gynaecol* 1997;104:892–897.
36. Norman K, Pattinson RC, de Souza J, et al. Ampicillin and metronidazole treatment in preterm labour: a multicentre, randomised controlled trial. *Br J Obstet Gynaecol* 1994;101:404–408.
37. King J, Flenady V. Antibiotics for preterm labour with intact membranes. *Cochrane Database Syst Rev* 2000;2:CD000246.
38. Mercer B, Miodovnik M, Thurnau G, et al. Antibiotic therapy for reduction of infant morbidity after preterm premature rupture of the membranes: a randomized controlled trial. *JAMA* 1997;278:989–995.
39. Kenyon SL, Taylor DJ, Tarnow-Mordi W, et al. Broad spectrum antibiotics for preterm, prelabor rupture of fetal membranes: the ORACLE I randomized trial. *Lancet* 2001;357:979–988.
40. Creasy RK, Gummer BA, Liggins GC. System for predicting spontaneous preterm birth. *Obstet Gynecol* 1980;55:692–695.
41. Main DM, Richardson DK, Hadley CB, et al. Controlled trial of a preterm labor detection program: efficacy and costs. *Obstet Gynecol* 1989;74:873–877.
42. Sakai M, Sasaki Y, Yamagishi N, et al. The preterm labor index and fetal fibronectin for prediction of preterm delivery with intact membranes. *Obstet Gynecol* 2003;101:123–128.
43. Baumgarten K, Gruber W. Tocolyseindex. In: Dudenhausen JW, Saling E, eds. *Perinatale medizin.* Stuttgart: Georg Thieme Verlag, 1974:197–199.
44. Katz M, Newman RB, Gill PJ. Assessment of uterine activity in ambulatory patients at high risk of preterm labor and delivery. *Am J Obstet Gynecol* 1986;154:44–47.
45. US Preventive Services Task Force. Home uterine activity monitoring for preterm labor. Policy statement. *JAMA* 1993;270:369–370.
46. US Preventive Services Task Force. Home uterine activity monitoring for preterm labor. Review article. *JAMA* 1993;270:371–376.
47. Iams JD, Newman RB, Thom EA, et al. The National Institute of Child Health and Human Development Network of Maternal–Fetal Medicine Units. Frequency of uterine contractions and the risk of spontaneous preterm delivery. *N Engl J Med* 2002;346:250–255.
48. Goldenberg RL, Mercer BM, Meis PJ, et al. The preterm prediction study: fetal fibronectin testing and spontaneous preterm birth. National Institute of Child Health and Human Development Maternal–Fetal Medicine Units Network. *Obstet Gynecol* 1996;87:643–648.
49. Peaceman AM, Andrews WW, Thorp JM, et al. Fetal fibronectin as a predictor of preterm birth in patients with symptoms: a multicenter trial. *Am J Obstet Gynecol* 1997;177:13–18.
50. Goldenberg RL, Mercer BM, Iams JD, et al. The preterm prediction study: patterns of cervicovaginal fetal fibronectin as predictors of spontaneous preterm delivery. National Institute of Child Health and Human Development Maternal–Fetal Medicine Units Network. *Am J Obstet Gynecol* 1997;177:8–12.
51. Goldenberg RL, Thom E, Moawad AH, et al. The preterm prediction study: fetal fibronectin, bacterial vaginosis, and peripartum infection. National Institute of Child Health and Human Development Maternal–Fetal Medicine Units Network. *Obstet Gynecol* 1996;87:656–660.

52. American College of Obstetricians and Gynecologists. *Fetal fibronectin preterm labor risk test. ACOG committee opinion 187.* Washington, DC: ACOG, 1997.

53. Amon E. Premature labor. In: Reece EA, Hobbins JC, Mahoney MJ, Petrie RH, eds. *Medicine of the fetus and mother.* Philadelphia: JB Lippincott, 1992:1404–1429.

54. Papiernik E, Bouyer J, Collin D. Precocious cervical ripening and preterm labor. *Obstet Gynecol* 1986;67:238–242.

55. Buekens P, Alexander S, Boutsen M, et al. Randomised controlled trial of routine cervical examinations in pregnancy. European Community Collaborative Study Group on Prenatal Screening. *Lancet* 1994;344:841–844.

56. Gomez R, Galasso M, Romero R, et al. Ultrasonographic examination of the uterine cervix is better than cervical digital examination as a predictor of the likelihood of premature delivery in patients with preterm labor and intact membranes. *Am J Obstet Gynecol* 1994;171:956–964.

57. Berghella V, Tolosa jE, Kuhlman K, et al. Cervical ultrasonography compared with manual examination as a predictor of preterm delivery. *Am J Obstet Gynecol* 1997;177:723–730.

58. Iams JD, Goldenberg RL, Meis PJ, et al. The length of the cervix and the risk of spontaneous premature delivery. National Institute of Child Health and Human Development Maternal–Fetal Medicine Units Network. *N Engl J Med* 1996;334:567–572.

59. Iams JD, Paraskos J, Landon MB, et al. Cervical sonography in preterm labor. *Obstet Gynecol* 1994;84:40–46.

60. Okitsu O, Mimura T, Nakayama T, et al. Early prediction of preterm delivery by transvaginal ultrasonography. *Ultrasound Obstet Gynecol* 1992;2:402–409.

61. Quinn MJ. Vaginal ultrasound and cervical cerclage: a prospective study. *Ultrasound Obstet Gynecol* 1992;2:410–416.

62. Iams JD, Goldenberg RL, Mercer BN, et al. The Preterm Prediction Study: recurrence risk of spontaneous preterm birth. National Institute of Child Health and Human Development Maternal–Fetal Medicine Units Network. *Am J Obstet Gynecol* 1998;178:1035–1040.

63. *Guidelines for perinatal care,* 4th ed. Elk Grove Village, IL: American Academy of Pediatrics; and Washington, DC: American College of Obstetricians and Gynecologists, 1997:75–76.

64. Gravett MG, Nelson HP, DeRouen T, et al. Independent association of bacterial vaginosis and *Chlamydia trachomatis* infection with adverse pregnancy outcome. *JAMA* 1986;256:1899–1903.

65. McGregor JA, French JI, Parker R, et al. Prevention of premature birth by screening and treatment for common genital tract infections: results of a prospective controlled evaluation. *Am J Obstet Gynecol* 1995;173:157–167.

66. Regan JA, Klebanoff MA, Nugent RP, et al. Colonization with group B streptococci in pregnancy and adverse outcome. VIP Study Group. *Am J Obstet Gynecol* 1996;174:1354–1360.

67. Centers for Disease Control and Prevention. Prevention of perinatal group B streptococcal disease: a public health perspective. *MMWR Morb Mortal Wkly Rep* 1996;45:1–24.

68. Abrams B, Pickett KE. Maternal nutrition. In: Creasy RK, Resnik R, eds. *Maternal–fetal medicine,* 4th ed. Philadelphia: WB Saunders, 1999:122–131.

69. American College of Obstetricians and Gynecologists. *Nutrition during pregnancy. ACOG technical bulletin 179.* Washington, DC: ACOG, 1993.

70. Johnson JWC, Longmate JA, Frentzen B. Excessive maternal weight and pregnancy outcome. *Am J Obstet Gynecol* 1992;167:353–372.

71. Institute of Medicine, Food and Nutrition Board, Committee on Nutritional Status During Pregnancy and Lactation, Subcommittee on Dietary Intake and Nutrient Supplements During Pregnancy and Subcommittee on Nutritional Status and Weight Gain During Pregnancy. *Nutrition during pregnancy. Part I. Weight gain.* Washington, DC: National Academies Press, 1990.

72. Castro LC, Avina RL. Maternal obesity and pregnancy outcomes. *Curr Opin Obstet Gynecol* 2002;14:601–606.

73. Lu GC, Rouse DJ, DuBard M, et al. The effect of the increasing prevalence of maternal obesity on perinatal morbidity. *Am J Obstet Gynecol* 2001;185:845–849.

74. Institute of Medicine, Food and Nutrition Board, Committee on Nutritional Status During Pregnancy and Lactation, Subcommittee on Dietary Intake and Nutrient Supplements During Pregnancy and Subcommittee on Nutritional Status and Weight Gain During

Pregnancy. *Nutrition during pregnancy. Part II. Nutrient supplements.* Washington, DC: National Academies Press, 1990.

75. American College of Obstetricians and Gynecologists. *Vitamin A supplementation during pregnancy. ACOG committee opinion 112.* Washington, DC: ACOG, 1992.

76. Medical Research Council Vitamin Study Research Group. Prevention of neural tube defects: results of the Medical Research Council vitamin study. *Lancet* 1991;338:131–137.

77. Centers for Disease Control and Prevention. Use of folic acid for prevention of spina bifida and other neural tube defects—1983–1991. *MMWR Morb Mortal Wkly Rep* 1991;40:513–516.

78. Centers for Disease Control and Prevention. Recommendations for the use of folic acid to reduce the number of cases of spina bifida and other neural tube defects. *MMWR Morb Mortal Wkly Rep* 1992;41:1–7.

79. Survey alert. Fortified pasta coming. *Obstet Gynecol Surv* 1997;52:191.

80. National High Blood Pressure Education Program Working Group on high blood pressure in pregnancy. *Am J Obstet Gynecol* 2000;183(1):S1–S22.

81. American College of Obstetricians and Gynecologists. *Chronic hypertension in pregnancy. ACOG practice bulletin 29.* Washington, DC: ACOG, 2001.

82. Sibai BM. Chronic hypertension in pregnancy. *Obstet Gynecol* 2002;100:369–377.

83. Livingston JC, Sibai BM. Chronic hypertension in pregnancy. *Obstet Gynecol Clin North Am* 2001;28:447–464.

84. Sibai BM, Lindheimer M, Hauth J, et al. Risk factors for preeclampsia, abruptio placentae, and adverse neonatal outcomes among women with chronic hypertension. *N Engl J Med* 1998;339:667–671.

85. American College of Obstetricians and Gynecologists. *Diagnosis and management of preeclampsia and eclampsia. ACOG practice bulletin 33.* Washington, DC: ACOG, 2002.

86. Martin JN, Blake PG, Perry KG, et al. The natural history of HELLP syndrome: patterns of disease progression and regression. *Am J Obstet Gynecol* 1991;164:1500–1513.

87. Leduc L, Wheeler JM, Kirshon B, et al. Coagulation profile in severe preeclampsia. *Obstet Gynecol* 1992;79:14–18.

88. Madazli R, Budak E, Calay Z, et al. Correlation between placental bed biopsy findings, vascular cell adhesion molecule and fibronectin levels in pre-eclampsia. *BJOG* 2000;107:514–518.

89. Talledo OE, Chesley LC, Zuspan FP. Renin-angiotensin in normal and toxemic pregnancies. III. Differential sensitivity to angiotensin II and norepinephrine in toxemia of pregnancy. *Am J Obstet Gynecol* 1968;100:218–222.

90. Gant NF, Daley GL, Chand S, et al. A study of angiotensin II pressor response throughout primigravid pregnancy. *J Clin Invest* 1973;52:2682–2689.

91. Burrows RF, Andrew M. Neonatal thrombocytopenia in the hypertensive disorders of pregnancy. *Obstet Gynecol* 1990;76:234–238.

92. Schiff E, Friedman SA, Sibai BM. Conservative management of severe preeclampsia remote from term. *Obstet Gynecol* 1994;84:626–630.

93. Sibai BM, Mercer BM, Schiff E, et al. Aggressive versus expectant management of severe preeclampsia at 28 to 32 weeks gestation: a randomized controlled trial. *Am J Obstet Gynecol* 1994;171:818–822.

94. The Eclampsia Trial Collaborative Group. Which anticonvulsant for women with eclampsia? Evidence from the Collaborative Eclampsia Trial. *Lancet* 1995;345:1455–1463.

95. Lucas MJ, Leveno KJ, Cunningham FG. A comparison of magnesium sulfate with phenytoin for the prevention of eclampsia. *N Engl J Med* 1995;333:201–205.

96. Magann EF, Bass D, Chauhan SP, et al. Antepartum corticosteroids: disease stabilization in patients with the syndrome of hemolysis, elevated liver enzymes, and low platelets (HELLP). *Am J Obstet Gynecol* 1994;171:1148–1153.

97. O'Brien JM, Milligan DA, Barton JR. Impact of high-dose corticosteroid therapy for patients with HELLP (hemolysis, elevated liver enzymes, and low platelet count) syndrome. *Am J Obstet Gynecol* 2000;183:921–924.

98. Barr M, Cohen MM. ACE inhibitor fetopathy and hypocalvaria: the kidney–skull connection. *Teratology* 1991;44:485–495.

99. Hanssens M, Keirse MJ, Vankelecom F, et al. Fetal and neonatal effects of treatment with angiotensin-converting enzyme inhibitors in pregnancy. *Obstet Gynecol* 1991;78:128–135.

100. Piper JM, Ray WA, Rosa FW. Pregnancy outcome following exposure to angiotensin-converting enzyme inhibitors. *Obstet Gynecol* 1992;80:429–432.
101. CLASP (Collaborative Low-Dose Aspirin Study in Pregnancy) Collaborative Group. CLASP: a randomised trial of low-dose aspirin for the prevention and treatment of pre-eclampsia among 9364 pregnant women. *Lancet* 1994;343:619–629.
102. Heyborne KD. Preeclampsia prevention: lessons from the low-dose aspirin therapy trials. *Am J Obstet Gynecol* 2000;183:523–528.
103. Sibai BM. Prevention of preeclampsia: a big disappointment. *Am J Obstet Gynecol* 1998;179:1275–1278.
104. Caritis S, Sibai B, Hauth J, et al. Low-dose aspirin to prevent preeclampsia in women at high risk. National Institute of Child Health and Human Development Network of Maternal–Fetal Medicine Units. *N Engl J Med* 1998;338:701–705.
105. Harrington K, Carpenter RG, Goldfrad C, et al. Transvaginal Doppler ultrasound of the uteroplacental circulation in the early prediction of pre-eclampsia and intrauterine growth retardation. *Br J Obstet Gynaecol* 1997;104:674–681.
106. Harrington K, Goldfrad C, Carpenter RG, et al. Transvaginal uterine and umbilical artery Doppler examination of 12–16 weeks and the subsequent development of pre-eclampsia and intrauterine growth retardation. *Ultrasound Obstet Gynecol* 1997;9:94–100.
107. Bower SJ, Harrington KF, Schuchter K, et al. Prediction of pre-eclampsia by abnormal uterine Doppler ultrasound and modification by aspirin. *Br J Obstet Gynaecol* 1996;103:625–629.
108. American College of Obstetricians and Gynecologists. *Gestational diabetes. ACOG practice bulletin 30*. Washington, DC: ACOG, 2001.
109. Report of the Expert Committee on the Diagnosis and Classification of Diabetes Mellitus. American Diabetes Association. Expert Committee on the Diagnosis and Classification of Diabetes Mellitus. *Diabetes Care* 2001;4[Suppl 1]:S5–S20.
110. White P. Pregnancy complicating diabetes. *Am J Med* 1949;7:609–616.
111. Lucas MJ. Diabetes complicating pregnancy. *Obstet Gynecol Clin North Am* 2001;28:513–536.
112. American College of Obstetricians and Gynecologists. *Fetal macrosomia. ACOG practice bulletin 22*. Washington, DC: ACOG, 2000.
113. Alexander GR, Himes JH, Kaufman RB, et al. A United States national reference for fetal growth. *Obstet Gynecol* 1996;87:163–168.
114. Menticoglou SM, Manning FA, Morrison I, et al. Must macrosomic fetuses be delivered by a cesarean section? A review of outcome for 786 babies ≥4,500 g. *Aust N Z J Obstet Gynaecol* 1992;32:100–103.
115. Lipscomb KR, Gregory K, Shaw K. The outcome of macrosomic infants weighing at least 4500 grams: Los Angeles county + University of Southern California experience. *Obstet Gynecol* 1995;85:558–564.
116. Bérard J, Dufour P, Vinatier D, et al. Fetal macrosomia: risk factors and outcome. A study of the outcome concerning 100 cases >4500 g. *Eur J Obstet Gynecol Reprod Biol* 1998;77:51–59.
117. Nesbitt TS, Gilbert WM, Herrchen B. Shoulder dystocia and associated risk factors with macrosomic infants born in California. *Am J Obstet Gynecol* 1998;179:476–480.
118. Johnstone FD, Prescott RJ, Steel JM, et al. Clinical and ultrasound prediction of macrosomia in diabetic pregnancy. *Br J Obstet Gynaecol* 1996;103:747–754.
119. Sandmire HF. Whither ultrasonic prediction of fetal macrosomia? *Obstet Gynecol* 1993;82:860–862.
120. Acker DB, Sachs BP, Friedman EA. Risk factors for shoulder dystocia. *Obstet Gynecol* 1985;66:762–768.
121. Naylor CD, Sermer M, Chen E, et al. Cesarean delivery in relation to birth weight and gestational glucose tolerance: pathophysiology or practice style? Toronto Trihospital Gestational Diabetes Investigators. *JAMA* 1996;275:1165–1170.
122. Verma A, Mitchell BF, Demianczuk N, et al. Relationship between plasma glucose levels in glucose-intolerant women and newborn macrosomia. *J Matern Fetal Med* 1997;6:187–193.
123. Sermer M, Naylor CD, Gare DJ, et al. Impact of increasing carbohydrate intolerance on maternal-fetal outcomes in 3637 women without gestational diabetes. The Toronto Tri-Hospital Gestational Diabetes Project. *Am J Obstet Gynecol* 1995;173:146–156.
124. Adams KM, Li H, Nelson RL, et al. Sequelae of unrecognized gestational diabetes. *Am J Obstet Gynecol* 1998;178:1321–1332.
125. Gross, TL, Sokol RJ, Williams T, et al. Shoulder dystocia: a fetal–physician risk. *Am J Obstet Gynecol* 1987;156:1408–1418.
126. Keller JD, Lopez-Zeno JA, Dooley SL, et al. Shoulder dystocia and birth trauma in gestational diabetes: a five-year experience. *Am J Obstet Gynecol* 1991;165:928–930.
127. Meshari AA, DeSilva S, Rahman I. Fetal macrosomia-maternal risks and fetal outcome. *Int J Gynecol Obstet* 1990;32:215–222.
128. Sacks DA. Fetal macrosomia and gestational diabetes: what's the problem? *Obstet Gynecol* 1993;81:775–781.
129. Bahar AM. Risk factors and fetal outcome in cases of shoulder dystocia compared with normal deliveries of a similar birthweight. *Br J Obstet Gynaecol* 1996;103:868–872.
130. Nocon JJ, McKenzie DK, Thomas LJ, et al. Shoulder dystocia: an analysis of risks and obstetric maneuvers. *Am J Obstet Gynecol* 1993;168:1732–1739.
131. Langer O, Berkus MD, Huff RW, et al. Shoulder dystocia: should the fetus weighing greater than or equal to 4000 grams be delivered by cesarean section? *Am J Obstet Gynecol* 1991;165:831–837.
132. McFarland LV, Raskin M, Daling JR, et al. Erb/Duchenne's palsy: a consequence of fetal macrosomia and method of delivery. *Obstet Gynecol* 1986;68:784–788.
133. Ecker JL, Greenberg JA, Norwitz ER, et al. Birth weight as a predictor of brachial plexus injury. *Obstet Gynecol* 1997;89:643–647.
134. Perlow JH, Wigton T, Hart J, et al. Birth trauma. A five-year review of incidence and associated perinatal factors. *J Reprod Med* 1996;41:754–760.
135. Bryant DR, Leonardi MR, Landwehr JB, et al. Limited usefulness of fetal weight in predicting neonatal brachial plexus injury. *Am J Obstet Gynecol* 1998;179:686–689.
136. Gordon M, Rich H, Deutschberger J, et al. The immediate and long-term outcome of obstetric birth trauma. I. Brachial plexus paralysis. *Am J Obstet Gynecol* 1973;117:51–56.
137. Hardy AE. Birth injuries of the brachial plexus: incidence and prognosis. *J Bone Joint Surg [Br]* 1981;63-B:98–101.
138. Kolderup LB, Laros RK, Musci TJ. Incidence of persistent birth injury in macrosomic infants: association with mode of delivery. *Am J Obstet Gynecol* 1997;177:37–41.
139. Oppenheim WL, Davis A, Growdon WA, et al. Clavicle fractures in the newborn. *Clin Orthop* 1990;250:176–180.
140. Chez RA, Carlan S, Greenberg SL, et al. Fractured clavicle is an unavoidable event. *Am J Obstet Gynecol* 1994;171:797–798.
141. Moore TK, Cayle JE. The amniotic fluid index in normal pregnancy. *Am J Obstet Gynecol* 1990;162:1168–1173.
142. Desmedt EJ, Henry OA, Beischer NA. Polyhydramnios and associated maternal and fetal complications in singleton pregnancies. *Br J Obstet Gynaecol* 1990;97:1115–1122.
143. Ventura SJ, Martin JA, Curtin SC, et al. *Births: final data for 1999. National vital statistics reports*, vol. 49, no. 1. Hyattsville, MD: National Center for Health Statistics, 2001.
144. Pregnancy outcomes in the Diabetes Control and Complications Trial. *Am J Obstet Gynecol* 1996;174:1343–1353.
145. Mills JL, Simpson JL, Driscoll SG, et al. Incidence of spontaneous abortion among normal women and insulin-dependent diabetic women whose pregnancies were identified within 21 days of conception. *N Engl J Med* 1988;319:1617–1623.
146. Dicker D, Feldberg D, Samuel N, et al. Spontaneous abortion in patients with insulin-dependent diabetes mellitus: the effect of preconceptional diabetic control. *Am J Obstet Gynecol* 1988;158:1161–1164.
147. Miller E, Hare JW, Cloherty JP, et al. Elevated maternal hemoglobin A_{1c} in early pregnancy and major congenital anomalies in infants of diabetic mothers. *N Engl J Med* 1981;304:1331–1334.
148. Miodovnik M, Mimouni F, Siddiqi TA, et al. Periconceptional metabolic status and risk for spontaneous abortion in insulin-dependent diabetic pregnancies. *Am J Perinatol* 1988;4:368–373.
149. Cousins L. Congenital anomalies among infants of diabetic mothers. Etiology, prevention, diagnosis. *Am J Obstet Gynecol* 1983;147:333–338.
150. Gabbe SG. Congenital malformations in infants of diabetic mothers. *Obstet Gynecol Surv* 1977;32:125–132.
151. Mills JL. Malformations in infants of diabetic mothers. *Teratology* 1982;25:385–394.
152. Mills J, Baker L, Goldman AS. Malformations in infants of diabetic mothers occur before the seventh gestational week. Implications for treatment. *Diabetes* 1979;28:292–293.

153. Leslie RDG, Pyke DA, John PN, et al. Hemoglobin A1 in diabetic pregnancy. *Lancet* 1978;2:958–959.

154. Reller MD, Kaplan S. Hypertrophic cardiomyopathy in infants of diabetic mothers: an update. *Am J Perinatol* 1988;5:353–358.

155. Veille J-C, Sivakoff M, Hanson R, et al. Interventricular septal thickness in fetuses of diabetic mothers. *Obstet Gynecol* 1992; 79:51–54.

156. Kitzmiller JL, Gavin LA, Gin GD, et al. Preconception care of diabetes. Glycemic control prevents congenital anomalies. *JAMA* 1991;265:731–736.

157. Lucas MJ, Leveno KJ, Williams ML, et al. Early pregnancy glycosylated hemoglobin, severity of diabetes, and fetal malformations. *Am J Obstet Gynecol* 1989;161:426–431.

158. Coustan DR. Perinatal mortality and morbidity. In: Reece EA, Coustan DR, eds. *Diabetes mellitus in pregnancy,* 2nd ed. New York: Churchill Livingstone, 1995:361–367.

159. Richey SD, Sandstad JS, Leveno KJ. Observations concerning unexplained fetal demise in pregnancy complicated by diabetes mellitus. *J Matern Fetal Med* 1995;4:169–172.

160. Salvesan DR, Brudenell MJ, Nicolaides KH. Fetal polycythemia and thrombocytopenia in pregnancies complicated by maternal diabetes mellitus. *Am J Obstet Gynecol* 1992;166:1287–1293.

161. Landon MB, Gabbe SG. Fetal surveillance and timing of delivery in pregnancy complicated by diabetes mellitus. *Obstet Gynecol Clin North Am* 1996;23:109–123.

162. Bourbon JR, Farrell PM. Fetal lung development in the diabetic pregnancy. *Pediatr Res* 1985;19:253–267.

163. Ojomo EO, Coustan DR. Absence of evidence of pulmonary maturity at amniocentesis in term infants of diabetic mothers. *Am J Obstet Gynecol* 1990;163:954–957.

164. Cruz AC, Buhi WC, Birk SA, et al. Respiratory distress syndrome with mature lecithin/sphingomyelin ratios: diabetes mellitus and low Apgar scores. *Am J Obstet Gynecol* 1976;126:78–82.

165. Curet LB, Olson RW, Schneider JM, et al. Effect of diabetes mellitus on amniotic fluid lecithin/sphingomyelin ratio and respiratory distress syndrome. *Am J Obstet Gynecol* 1979;135:10–13.

166. Fadel HE, Saad SA, Davis H, et al. Fetal lung maturity in diabetic pregnancies: relation among amniotic fluid insulin, prolactin, and lecithin. *Am J Obstet Gynecol* 1988;159:457–463.

167. Piper JM, Langer O. Does maternal diabetes delay fetal pulmonary maturity? *Am J Obstet Gynecol* 1993;168:783–786.

168. Parker CR Jr, Hauth JC, Hankins GD, et al. Endocrine maturation and lung function in premature neonates of women with diabetes. *Am J Obstet Gynecol* 1989;160:657–662.

169. Landon MB, Catalano PM, Gabbe SG. Diabetes Mellitus. In: Gabbe SG, ed. *Obstetrics—normal and problem pregnancies,* 4th ed. Orlando, FL: Churchill Livingstone, 2002:1105–1106.

170. Peevy KJ, Landaw SA, Gross SJ. Hyperbilirubinemia in infants of diabetic mothers. *Pediatrics* 1980;66:417–419.

171. Widness JA, Cowett RM, Coustan DR, et al. Neonatal morbidities in infants of mothers with glucose intolerance in pregnancy. *Diabetes* 1985;34[Suppl 2]:61–65.

172. Report of the Expert Committee on the Diagnosis and Classification of Diabetes Mellitus. *Diabetes Care* 1997;20: 1183–1197.

173. Metzger BE, Coustan DR. The Organizing Committee. Summary and recommendations of the Fourth International Workshop-Conference on Gestational Diabetes Mellitus. *Diabetes Care* 1998;21:B161–B167.

174. O'Sullivan JB. Body weight and subsequent diabetes mellitus. *JAMA* 1982;248:949–952.

175. Langer O, Conway DL, Berkus MD, et al. A comparison of glyburide and insulin in women with gestational diabetes mellitus. *N Engl J Med* 2000;343:1134–1138.

176. Petri M. Hopkins Lupus Pregnancy Center: 1987 to 1996. *Rheum Dis Clin North Am* 1997;23:1–13.

177. Mascola MA, Repke JT. Obstetric management of the high-risk lupus pregnancy. *Rheum Dis Clin North Am* 1997;23:119–132.

178. Le Huong D, Wechsler B, Vauthier-Brouzes D, et al. Outcome of planned pregnancies in systemic lupus erythematosus: a prospective study on 62 pregnancies. *Br J Rheumatol* 1997;36:772–777.

179. Lima F, Buchanan NM, Khamashta MA, et al. Obstetric outcome in systemic lupus erythematosus. *Semin Arthritis Rheum* 1995;25: 184–192.

180. Mintz G, Niz J, Gutierrez G, et al. Prospective study of pregnancy in systemic lupus erythematosus. Results of a multidisciplinary approach. *J Rheumatol* 1986;13:732–739.

181. Out HJ, Derksen RH, Christiaens GC. Systemic lupus erythematosus and pregnancy. *Obstet Gynecol Surv* 1989;44:585–591.

182. Faussett MF, Branch DW. Autoimmunity and pregnancy loss. *Semin Reprod Med* 2000;18:379–392.

183. Johnson MJ, Petri M, Witter FR, et al. Evaluation of preterm delivery in a systemic lupus erythematosus pregnancy clinic. *Obstet Gynecol* 1995;86:396–399.

184. Font J, Lopez-Soto A, Cervera R, et al. Antibodies to thromboplastin in systemic lupus erythematosus: isotype distribution and clinical significance in a series of 92 patients. *Thromb Res* 1997;86:37–48.

185. Ogasawara M, Aoki K, Hayashi Y. A prospective study on pregnancy risk of antiphospholipid antibodies in association with systemic lupus erythematosus. *J Reprod Immunol* 1995;28: 159–164.

186. Lockshin MD. Pregnancy does not cause systemic lupus erythematosus to worsen. *Arthritis Rheum* 1989;32:665–670.

187. Lockshin MD, Reinitz E, Druzin ML, et al. Lupus pregnancy. Case-control prospective study demonstrating absence of lupus exacerbation during or after pregnancy. *Am J Med* 1984;77:893–898.

188. Ramsey-Goldman R, Schilling E. Immunosuppressive drug use during pregnancy. *Rheum Dis Clin North Am* 1997;23:149–167.

189. Meehan RT, Dorsey JK. Pregnancy among patients with systemic lupus erythematosus receiving immunosuppressive therapy. *J Rheumatol* 1987;14:252–258.

190. Lockshin MD. Pregnancy associated with systemic lupus erythematosus. *Semin Perinatol* 1990;14:130–138.

191. Stuart MJ, Gross SJ, Elrad H, et al. Effects of acetylsalicylic-acid ingestion on maternal and neonatal hemostasis. *N Engl J Med* 1982;307:909–912.

192. Alstead EM, Ritchie JK, Lennard-Jones JE, et al. Safety of azathioprine in pregnancy in inflammatory bowel disease. *Gastroenterology* 1990;99:443–446.

193. Davison JM. Dialysis, transplantation, and pregnancy. *Am J Kidney Dis* 1991;17:127–134.

194. Pilarski LM, Yacyshyn BR, Lazarovits AI. Analysis of peripheral blood lymphocyte populations and immune function from children exposed to cyclosporine or to azathioprine in utero. *Transplantation* 1994;57:133–144.

195. Khamashta MA, Buchanan NM, Hughes GR. The use of hydroxychloroquine in lupus pregnancy: the British experience. *Lupus* 1996;5[Suppl 1]:S65–S66.

196. Parke A, West B. Hydroxychloroquine in pregnant patients with systemic lupus erythematosus. *J Rheumatol* 1996;23:1715–1718.

197. Parke AL, Rothfield NF. Antimalarial drugs in pregnancy—the North American experience. *Lupus* 1996;5[Suppl 1]:S67–S69.

198. Phillips-Howard PA, Wood D. The safety of antimalarial drugs in pregnancy. *Drug Saf* 1996;14:131–145.

199. Shumak KH, Rock GA. Therapeutic plasma exchange. *N Engl J Med* 1984;310:762–771.

200. Wei N, Klippel JH, Huston DP, et al. Randomised trial of plasma exchange in mild systemic lupus erythematosus. *Lancet* 1983;1:17–22.

201. Tseng C-E, Buyon JP. Neonatal lupus syndromes. *Rheum Dis Clin North Am* 1997;23:31–54.

202. Watson RM, Lane AT, Barnett NK, et al. Neonatal lupus erythematosus. A clinical, serological and immunogenetic study with review of the literature. *Medicine (Baltimore)* 1984;63: 362–378.

203. Olah KS, Gee H. Fetal heart block associated with maternal anti-Ro (SSA) antibody-current management. A review. *Br J Obstet Gynaecol* 1991;98:751–755.

204. Reichlin M, Friday K, Harley JB. Complete congenital heart block followed by anti-Ro-SS-A in adult life. Studies of an informative family. *Am J Med* 1988;84:339–344.

205. Buyon JP, Waltuck J, Kleinman C, et al. *In utero* identification and therapy of congenital heart block. *Lupus* 1995;4:116–121.

206. Richards DS, Wagman AJ, Cabaniss ML. Ascites not due to congestive heart failure in a fetus with lupus-induced heart block. *Obstet Gynecol* 1990;76:957–959.

207. Copel JA, Buyon JP, Kleinman CS. Successful in utero therapy of fetal heart block. *Am J Obstet Gynecol* 1995;173:1384–1390.

208. Copel JA. Management of fetal cardiac arrhythmias. *Obstet Gynecol Clin North Am* 1997;24:201–211.

209. Watson WJ, Katz VL. Steroid therapy for hydrops associated with antibody-mediated congenital heart block. *Am J Obstet Gynecol* 1991;165:553–554.

210. Herreman G, Galezewski N. Maternal connective tissue disease and congenital heart block [Letter]. *N Engl J Med* 1985;312:1328–1329.

211. Walkinshaw SA, Welch CR, McCormack J, et al. *In utero* pacing for fetal congenital heart block. *Fetal Diagn Ther* 1994;9:183–185.

212. McCarron DP, Hellmann DB, Traill TA, et al. Neonatal lupus erythematosus syndrome: late detection of isolated heart block. *J Rheumatol* 1993;103:1212–1214.

213. Reed BR, Lee LA, Harmon C, et al. Autoantibodies to SS-A/Ro in infants with congenital heart block. *J Pediatr* 1983;103:889–891.

214. Eronen M, Sirèn MK, Ekblad H, et al. Short- and long-term outcome of children with congenital complete heart block diagnosed *in utero* or as a newborn. *Pediatrics* 2000;106:86–91.

215. Rider LG, Buyon JP, Rutledge J, et al. Treatment of neonatal lupus: case report and review of the literature. *J Rheumatol* 1993;20:1208–1211.

216. Davison MB, Radford DJ. Fetal and neonatal congenital complete heart block. *Med J Aust* 1989;150:192–198.

217. Dedhia HV, DiBartolomeo A. Rheumatoid arthritis. *Crit Care Clin* 2002;18:841–854, ix.

218. Arnett FC, Edworthy SM, Bloch DA, et al. The American Rheumatism Association 1987 revised criteria for the classification of rheumatoid arthritis. *Arthritis Rheum* 1988;31:315–324.

219. Nelson JL, Ostensen M. Pregnancy and rheumatoid arthritis. *Rheum Dis Clin North Am* 1997;23:195–212.

220. Johnson MJ Obstetric complications and rheumatic disease. *Rheum Dis Clin North Am* 1997;23:169–182.

221. Buchanan WW, Needs CJ, Brooks PM. Rheumatic diseases: the arthropathies. In: Gleicher N, ed. *Principles and practice of medical therapy in pregnancy*, 3rd ed. Norwalk: Appleton & Lange, 1998:538–545.

222. Steen VD. Pregnancy in women with systemic sclerosis. *Obstet Gynecol* 1999;94:15–20.

223. Maymon R, Fejgin M. Scleroderma in pregnancy. *Obstet Gynecol Surv* 1989;44:530–534.

224. Belilos E, Carsons S. Rheumatologic disorders in women. *Med Clin North Am* 1998;82:77–101.

225. Julkunen H, Kaaja R, Kurki P, et al. Fetal outcome in women with primary Sjögren's syndrome. A retrospective case-control study. *Clin Exp Rheumatol* 1995;13:65–71.

226. American College of Obstetricians and Gynecologists. *Antiphospholipid syndrome. ACOG educational bulletin 244.* Washington, DC: ACOG, 1998.

227. Branch DW. Antiphospholipid syndrome: laboratory concerns, fetal loss, and pregnancy management. *Semin Perinatol* 1991;15:230–237.

228. Conley CL, Hartmann RD. A hemorrhagic disorder caused by circulating anticoagulant in patients with disseminated lupus erythematosus. *J Clin Invest* 1952;31:621–622.

229. Love PE, Santoro SA. Antiphospholipid antibodies: anticardiolipin and the lupus anticoagulant in systemic lupus erythematosus (SLE) and in non-SLE disorders. Prevalence and clinical significance. *Ann Intern Med* 1990;112:682–698.

230. Ninomiya C, Taniguchi O, Kato T, et al. Distribution and clinical significance of lupus anticoagulant and anticardiolipin antibody in 349 patients with systemic lupus erythematosus. *Intern Med* 1992;31:194–199.

231. Harris EN. Syndrome of the black swan. *Br J Rheumatol* 1987;26:324–326.

232. Hughes GRV, Harris EN, Gharavi AE. The anticardiolipin syndrome. *J Rheumatol* 1986;13:486–489.

233. Lockshin MD. Antiphospholipid antibody. Babies, blood clots, biology. *JAMA* 1997;277:1549–1551.

234. Kniaz D, Eisenberg GM, Elrad H, et al. Postpartum hemolytic uremic syndrome associated with antiphospholipid antibodies. A case report and review of the literature. *Am J Nephrol* 1992;12:126–133.

235. Silver RM, Draper ML, Scott JR, et al. Clinical consequences of antiphospholipid antibodies: an historic cohort study. *Obstet Gynecol* 1994;83:372–377.

236. Sheridan-Pereira M, Porreco RP, Hays T, et al. Neonatal aortic thrombosis associated with the lupus anticoagulant. *Obstet Gynecol* 1988;71:1016–1018.

237. Silver RK, MacGregor SN, Pasternak JF, et al. Fetal stroke associated with elevated maternal anticardiolipin antibodies. *Obstet Gynecol* 1992;80:497–499.

238. Lubbe WF, Butler WS, Palmer SJ, et al. Fetal survival after prednisone suppression of maternal lupus-anticoagulant. *Lancet* 1983;1(8338):1361–1363.

239. Lubbe WF, Liggins GC. Lupus anticoagulant and pregnancy. *Am J Obstet Gynecol* 1985;153:322–327.

240. Cowchock FS, Reece EA, Balaban D, et al. Repeated fetal losses associated with antiphospholipid antibodies: a collaborative randomized trial comparing prednisone with low-dose heparin treatment. *Am J Obstet Gynecol* 1992;166:1318–1323.

241. Landy HJ, Isada NB, McGinnis J, et al. The effect of chronic steroid therapy on glucose tolerance in pregnancy. *Am J Obstet Gynecol* 1988;159:612–615.

242. Landy HJ, Kessler C, Kelly WK, et al. Obstetric performance in patients with the lupus anticoagulant and/or anticardiolipin antibodies. *Am J Perinatol* 1992;9:146–151.

243. Kutteh WH. Antiphospholipid antibody-associated recurrent pregnancy loss: treatment with heparin and low-dose aspirin is superior to low-dose aspirin alone. *Am J Obstet Gynecol* 1996;174:1584–1589.

244. Rosove MH, Tabsh K, Wasserstrum N, et al. Heparin therapy for pregnant women with lupus anticoagulant or anticardiolipin antibodies. *Obstet Gynecol* 1990;75:630–634.

245. Nelson-Piercy C, Letsky EA, de Swiet M. Low-molecular-weight heparin for obstetric thromboprophylaxis: experience of sixty-nine pregnancies in sixty-one women at high risk. *Am J Obstet Gynecol* 1997;176:1062–1068.

246. Branch DW, Peaceman AM, Druzin M, et al. A multicenter, placebo-controlled pilot study of intravenous immune globulin treatment of antiphospholipid syndrome during pregnancy. The Pregnancy Loss Study Group. *Am J Obstet Gynecol* 2000;18:122–127.

247. Branch DW, Porter TF, Paidas MJ, et al. Obstetric uses of intravenous immunoglobulin: successes, failures, and promises. *J Allergy Clin Immunol* 2001;108:S133–S138.

248. American College of Obstetricians and Gynecologists. *Thyroid disease in pregnancy. ACOG practice bulletin 244.* Washington, DC: ACOG, 2002.

249. Mestman JH, Goodwin TM, Montoro MM. Thyroid disorders of pregnancy. *Endocrinol Metab Clin North Am* 1995;24:41–71.

250. Mazzaferri EL. Evaluation and management of common thyroid disorders in women. *Am J Obstet Gynecol* 1997;176:507–514.

251. Wing DA, Millar LK, Koonings PP, et al. A comparison of propylthiouracil versus methimazole in the treatment of hyperthyroidism in pregnancy. *Am J Obstet Gynecol* 1994;170:90–95.

252. Van Dijke CP, Heydendael RJ, De Kleine MJ. Methimazole, carbimazole and congenital skin defects. *Ann Intern Med* 1987;106:60–61.

253. Matsuura N, Konishi J, Fujieda K, et al. TSH-receptor antibodies in mothers with Graves' disease and outcome in their offspring. *Lancet* 1988;1:14–17.

254. Houck JA, Davis RE, Sharma HM. Thyroid-stimulating immunoglobulin as a cause of recurrent intrauterine fetal death. *Obstet Gynecol* 1988;71:1018–1019.

255. Wenstrom KD, Weiner CP, Williamson RA, et al. Prenatal diagnosis of fetal hyperthyroidism using funipuncture. *Obstet Gynecol* 1990;76:513–517.

256. Porreco RP, Bloch CA. Fetal blood sampling in the management of intrauterine thyrotoxicosis. *Obstet Gynecol* 1990;76:509–512.

257. Toft AD. Drug therapy: thyroxine therapy. *N Engl J Med* 1994;154:785–787.

258. American Academy of Pediatrics AAP Section on Endocrinology and Committee on Genetics, and American Thyroid Association Committee on Public Health: newborn screening for congenital hypothyroidism: recommended guidelines. *Pediatrics* 1993;91:1203–1209.

259. Bale JF. Congenital infections. *Neurol Clin* 2002;20:1039–1060.

260. Duff P. Maternal and Perinatal Infection. In: Gabbe SG, Niebyl JR, Simpson JL, eds. *Obstetrics—normal and problem pregnancies*, 4th ed. New York: Churchill-Livingstone, 2002:293–1348.

261. American College of Obstetricians and Gynecologists. *Perinatal viral and parasitic infections. ACOG practice bulletin 20.* Washington, DC: ACOG, 2000.

262. American College of Obstetricians and Gynecologists. *Viral hepatitis in pregnancy. ACOG educational bulletin 248.* Washington, DC: ACOG, 1998.

263. American College of Obstetricians and Gynecologists. *Perinatal herpes simplex virus infections. ACOG technical bulletin 122.* Washington, DC: ACOG, 1988.

264. American College of Obstetricians and Gynecologists. *Human immunodeficiency virus infections in pregnancy. ACOG educational bulletin 232.* Washington, DC: ACOG, 1997.

265. Kotler DP. Human immunodeficiency virus and pregnancy. *Gastroenterol Clin North Am* 2003;32:437–448, ix.

266. American College of Obstetricians and Gynecologists. *Prevention of early-onset Group B streptococcal disease in newborns. ACOG committee opinion 279.* Washington, DC: ACOG, 2002.

267. Ray JG. Lues-lues: maternal and fetal considerations of syphilis. *Obstet Gynecol Surv* 1995;50:845–850.

268. Ricci JM, Fojaco RM, O'Sullivan MJ. Congenital syphilis: the University of Miami/Jackson Memorial Medical Center experience, 1986–1988. *Obstet Gynecol* 1989;74:687–693.

269. American College of Obstetricians and Gynecologists. *Thromboembolism in pregnancy. ACOG practice bulletin 19.* Washington, DC: ACOG, 2000.

270. Toglia MR, Weg JG. Venous thromboembolism during pregnancy. *N Engl J Med* 1996;335:108–114.

271. Barbour LA, Pickard J. Controversies in thromboembolic disease during pregnancy: a critical review. *Obstet Gynecol* 1995;86:621–633.

272. Lockwood CJ. Inherited thrombophilias in pregnant patients: detection and treatment paradigm. *Obstet Gynecol* 2002;99:333–341.

273. Lockwood CJ. Heritable coagulopathies in pregnancy. *Obstet Gynecol Surv* 1999;54:754–765.

274. den Heijer M, Koster T, Blom HJ, et al. Hyperhomocysteinemia as a risk factor for deep-vein thrombosis. *N Engl J Med* 1996;334:759–762.

275. Dizon-Townson DS, Nelson LM, Jang H, et al. The incidence of factor V Leiden mutation in an obstetric population and its relationship to deep vein thrombosis. *Am J Obstet Gynecol* 1997;176:883–886.

276. Rouse DJ, Goldenberg RL, Wenstrom KD. Antenatal screening for factor V Leiden mutation: a critical appraisal. *Obstet Gynecol* 1997;90:848–851.

277. Weinmann EE, Salzman EW. Deep-vein thrombosis. *N Engl J Med* 1994;331:1630–1641.

278. The PIOPED Investigators. Value of the ventilation/perfusion scan in acute pulmonary embolism: results of the Prospective Investigation of Pulmonary Embolism Diagnosis (PIOPED). *JAMA* 1990;263:2753–2759.

279. Powell T, Müller NL. Imaging of acute pulmonary thromboembolism: should spiral computed tomography replace the ventilation-perfusion scan? *Clin Chest Med* 2003;24:29–38.

280. Ginsberg JS, Hirsh J. Use of antithrombotic agents during pregnancy. *Chest* 1995;108[Suppl 4]:305S–311S.

281. American College of Obstetricians and Gynecologists. *Prevention of deep vein thrombosis and pulmonary embolism. ACOG practice bulletin 21.* Washington, DC: ACOG, 2000.

282. Hall JG, Pauli RM, Wilson KM. Maternal and fetal sequelae of anticoagulation during pregnancy. *Am J Med* 1980;68:122–140.

283. Wong V, Cheng CH, Chan KC. Fetal and neonatal outcome of exposure to anticoagulants during pregnancy. *Am J Med Genet* 1993;45:17–21.

284. Stevenson RE, Burton OM, Ferlauto GJ, et al. Hazards of oral anticoagulants during pregnancy. *JAMA* 1980;243:1549–1551.

285. Cunningham FG, Cox SM, Harstad TW, et al. Chronic renal disease and pregnancy outcome. *Am J Obstet Gynecol* 1990;163:453–459.

286. Hou SH, Grossman SD, Madias NE. Pregnancy in women with renal disease and moderate renal insufficiency. *Am J Med* 1985;78:185–194.

287. Jones DC, Hayslett JP. Outcome of pregnancy in women with moderate or severe renal insufficiency. *N Engl J Med* 1996;335:226–232.

288. Krakow D, Castro LC, Schwieger J. Effect of hemodialysis on uterine and umbilical artery Doppler flow velocity waveforms. *Am J Obstet Gynecol* 1994;170:1386–1388.

289. Elliott JP, O'Keeffe DF, Schon DA, et al. Dialysis in pregnancy: a critical review. *Obstet Gynecol Surv* 1992;46:319–324.

290. Hou SH. Pregnancy in women on haemodialysis and peritoneal dialysis. *Ballieres Clin Obstet Gynaecol* 1994;8:481–500.

291. Jakobi P, Ohel G, Szylman P, et al. Continuous ambulatory peritoneal dialysis as the primary approach in the management of

292. Nageotte MP, Grundy HO. Pregnancy outcome in women requiring chronic hemodialysis. *Obstet Gynecol* 1988;72:456–459.

293. Yasin SY, Beydoun SN. Hemodialysis in pregnancy. *Obstet Gynecol Surv* 1988;43:655–668.

294. Tison A, Lozowy C, Benjamin A, et al. Successful pregnancy complicated by peritonitis in a 35-year old CAPD patient. *Perit Dial Int* 1996;16[Suppl 1]:S489–S491.

295. Sturgiss SN, Davison JM. Perinatal outcome in renal allograft recipients: prognostic significance of hypertension and renal function before and during pregnancy. *Obstet Gynecol* 1991;78:573–577.

296. Cohen D, Galbraith C. General health management and long-term care of the renal transplant recipient. *Am J Kidney Dis* 2001;38[Suppl 6]:S10–S24.

297. Ehrich JH, Loirat C, Davison JM, et al. Repeated successful pregnancies after kidney transplantation in 102 women (report by the EDTA registry). *Nephrol Dial Transplant* 1996;11:1314–1317.

298. Davison JM. Renal transplantation and pregnancy. *Am J Kidney Dis* 1987;9:374–380.

299. Burrows DA, O'Neil TJ, Sorrells TL. Successful twin pregnancy after renal transplant maintained on cyclosporine A immunosuppression. *Obstet Gynecol* 1988;72:459–461.

300. Gaughan WJ, Moritz MJ, Radomski JS, et al. National Transplantation Pregnancy Registry: report on outcomes in cyclosporine-treated female kidney transplant recipients with an interval from transplant to pregnancy of greater than five years. *Am J Kidney Dis* 1996;28:266–269.

301. Olshan AF, Mattison DR, Zwanenburg TS. International Commission for Protection Against Environmental Mutagens and Carcinogens. Cyclosporine A: review of genotoxicity and potential for adverse human reproductive and developmental effects. Report of a Working Group on the genotoxicity of cyclosporine A, August 18, 1993. *Mutat Res* 1994;317:163–173.

302. American College of Obstetricians and Gynecologists. *Cardiac disease in pregnancy. ACOG technical bulletin 168.* Washington, DC: ACOG, 1992.

303. Criteria Committee of the New York Heart Association. *Nomenclature and criteria for diagnosis of diseases of the heart and great vessels,* 8th ed. Boston: Little Brown, 1979.

304. Gei AF, Hankins GDV. Cardiac disease and pregnancy. *Obstet Gynecol Clin North Am* 2001;28:465–512.

305. Szekely P, Turner R, Snaith L. Pregnancy and the changing pattern of rheumatic heart disease. *Br Heart J* 1973;35:1293–1303.

306. McAnulty JH, Morton MJ, Ueland K. The heart and pregnancy. *Curr Probl Cardiol* 1988;9:589–660.

307. Patton DE, Lee W, Cotton DB, et al. Cyanotic maternal heart disease in pregnancy. *Obstet Gynecol Surv* 1990;45:594–600.

308. Whittemore R, Hobbins JC, Engle MA. Pregnancy and its outcome in women with and without surgical treatment of congenital heart disease. *Am J Cardiol* 1982;50:641–651.

309. Shade GH, Ross G, Bever FN, et al. Troponin I in the diagnosis of acute myocardial infarction in pregnancy, labor, and post partum. *Am J Obstet Gynecol* 2002;187:1719–1720.

310. Roth A, Elkayam U. Acute myocardial infarction associated with pregnancy. *Ann Intern Med* 1996;125:751–762.

311. Badui E, Enciso R. Acute myocardial infarction during pregnancy and puerperium: a review. *Angiology* 1996;47:739–756.

312. Hankins GDV, Wendel GD, Leveno KJ, et al. Myocardial infarction during pregnancy: a review. *Obstet Gynecol* 1985;65:139–146.

313. Ascarelli MH, Grider AR, Hsu HW. Acute myocardial infarction during pregnancy managed with immediate percutaneous transluminal coronary angioplasty. *Obstet Gynecol* 1996;88:655–657.

314. Eikman FM. Acute coronary artery angioplasty during pregnancy. *Cathet Cardiovasc Diagn* 1996;38:369–372.

315. Schumacher B, Belfort MA, Card RJ. Successful treatment of acute myocardial infarction during pregnancy with tissue plasminogen activator. *Am J Obstet Gynecol* 1997;176:716–719.

316. Dufour P, Berard J, Vinatier D, et al. Pregnancy after myocardial infarction and a coronary artery bypass graft. *Arch Gynecol Obstet* 1997;259:209–213.

317. Frenkel Y, Barkai G, Reisin L, et al. Pregnancy after myocardial infarction: are we playing safe? *Obstet Gynecol* 1991;77:822–825.

318. Baxi LV, Rho RB. Pregnancy after cardiac transplantation. *Am J Obstet Gynecol* 1993;169:33–34.

319. Key TC, Resnik R, Dittrich HC, et al. Successful pregnancy after cardiac transplantation. *Am J Obstet Gynecol* 1989;160:367–371.

320. Kirk EP. Organ transplantation and pregnancy: a case report and review. *Am J Obstet Gynecol* 1991;164:1629–1634.

321. Löwenstein BR, Vain NW, Perrone SV, et al. Successful pregnancy and vaginal delivery after heart transplantation. *Am J Obstet Gynecol* 1988;158:589–590.

322. Scott JR, Wagoner LE, Olsen SL, et al. Pregnancy in heart transplant recipients: management and outcome. *Obstet Gynecol* 1993;82:324–327.

323. Antonelli NM, Dotters DJ, Katz VL, et al. Cancer in pregnancy: a review of the literature. Part I. *Obstet Gynecol Surv* 1996;125–134.

324. Hacker NF, Berek JS, Lagasse LD, et al. Carcinoma of the cervix associated with pregnancy. *Obstet Gynecol* 1982;59:735–746.

325. Berman ML, DiSaia PJ, Brewster WR. Pelvic malignancies, gestational trophoblastic neoplasia, and nonpelvic malignancies. In: Creasy RK, Resnik R, eds. *Maternal–fetal medicine*, 4th ed. Philadelphia: WB Saunders, 1999:1128–1150.

326. Donegan WL. Breast cancer and pregnancy. *Obstet Gynecol* 1977;50:244–252.

327. Schwartz PE. Cancer in pregnancy. In: Reece EA, Hobbins JC, Mahoney MJ, Petrie RH, eds. *Medicine of the fetus and mother.* Philadelphia: JB Lippincott, 1992:1257–1281.

328. Dildy GA, Moise KJ, Carpenter RJ, et al. Maternal malignancy metastatic to the products of conception: a review. *Obstet Gynecol Surv* 1989;44:535–540.

329. Buekers TE, Lallas TA. Chemotherapy in pregnancy. *Obstet Gynecol Clin North Am* 1998;25:323–329.

330. Mayr NA, Wen BC, Saw CB. Radiation therapy during pregnancy. *Obstet Gynecol Clin North Am* 1998;25:301–321.

331. Sweet DL, Kinzie J. Consequences of radiotherapy and antineoplastic therapy for the fetus. *J Reprod Med* 1976;17:241–246.

332. Debakan A. Abnormalities in children exposed to x-irradiation during various stages of gestation: tentative timetable of radiation injury to the human fetus. Part I. *J Nucl Med* 1968;9:471–477.

333. Brent RC. The effect of embryonic and fetal exposure to x-ray, microwaves, and ultrasound: counseling the pregnant and nonpregnant patient about these risks. *Semin Oncol* 1989;16:347–368.

334. Orr JW Jr, Shingleton HM. Cancer in pregnancy. *Curr Prob Cancer* 1983;8:1–50.

The Effects of Maternal Drugs on the Developing Fetus

15

David A. Beckman   *Lynda B. Fawcett*   *Robert L. Brent*

Every conception has a risk of ending in abortion or serious congenital anomaly (Tables 15-1, 15-2). Furthermore it is axiomatic that every drug administered or taken by a pregnant woman presents the mother and fetus with both risks and benefits. The controversies in this field are primarily related to the nature and magnitude of the risks for these drugs.

Abortion and birth defects have some common etiologies, but in many instances the causes of these two areas of adverse reproductive outcome are divergent. Most human teratogens affect the embryo during a relatively narrow period of early embryonic development (18–40 days for major malformations excluding genital malformations and cleft palate which have longer periods of sensitivity). However, there are a few teratogens and many fetotoxic agents that have deleterious effects during the second and even the third trimester.

In this chapter, we evaluate the data concerning the potential risks of selected prescribed and self-administered drugs in human pregnancy. The evaluations were made after a review of the available clinical, epidemiological and experimental data and an analysis based on reproducibility, consistency and biological plausibility. Only key references or reviews are cited which will guide the reader to additional relevant literature.

CHARACTERIZATION OF ADVERSE REPRODUCTIVE OUTCOMES

Spontaneous Abortion

The definition of spontaneous abortion is based on the stage of embryonic development when viability was not possible outside the uterus. This stage is presently considered to be 20 weeks or less of gestation and a fetal weight of less than 500 grams, although these criteria are not universally accepted.

The frequency of spontaneous abortion varies with the stage of gestation (Table 15-2): more than 80% of abortions occur in the first trimester and there is a steady decline in the risk of abortion as pregnancy progresses. Therefore it is essential that epidemiological studies into the cause of abortion compare control and "exposed" populations with the same mean stage and range of abortion. Two pregnant populations with a 2-week difference in mean stage of pregnancy will have a different background incidence of abortion. Abortion in human populations include the following causes (Table 15-3):

Chromosomal Abnormalities

The earlier the abortion, the higher the proportion of chromosomal abnormalities (1,2). Approximately 53% of spontaneous abortions in the first trimester are as a result of chromosomal abnormalities, 36% are as a result of chromosomal abnormalities in the second trimester and only 5% of stillbirths in the third trimester are as a result of chromosomal abnormalities. Over 95% of abortuses with chromosomal abnormalities were as a result of autosomal trisomy, double trisomy, monosomy, triploidy or tetraploidy (3,4). Most chromosomal abnormalities are not the cause of repetitive abortion, although in about 4% of couples with two or more spontaneous abortions, a normal-appearing parent could be a carrier for a balanced translocation or may be a mosaic with abnormal cells in the germ cell line. Environmental exposures during pregnancy cannot account for any of these abortions because most aneuploidies result from meiotic nondisjunction during gametogenesis before conception.

TABLE 15-1

FREQUENCY OF REPRODUCTIVE RISKS IN THE HUMAN

Reproductive Risk	Frequency
Immunologically and clinically diagnosed spontaneous abortions per 10^6 conceptions	350,000
Clinically recognized spontaneous abortions per 10^6 pregnancies	150,000
Genetic diseases per 10^6 births	110,000
Multifactorial or polygenic (genetic-environmental interactions)	90,000
Dominantly inherited disease	10,000
Autosomal and sex-linked genetic disease	1,200
Cytogenetic (chromosomal abnormalities)	5,000
New mutations	3,000
Major congenital malformations per 10^6 births	30,000
Prematurity per 10^6 births	40,000
Fetal growth retardation per 10^6 births	30,000
Stillbirths per 10^6 pregnancies (>20 wks)	20,900

Modified from Brent RL. Environmental factors: miscellaneous. In: Brent RL, Harris ML, eds. *Prevention of embryonic fetal and perinatal disease.* Bethesda: DHEW (NIH), 1976:211–218, with permission.

Abortions With Normal Chromosomes (Euploidy)

Hertig (1) and many other investigators reported the occurrence of malformed or blighted embryos as a cause of abortion. These embryonic losses may occur later in the first trimester and have been shown to have normal karyotypes (3). The etiology of these abortions are manifold and include the following:

Genetic Abnormalities

Dominant mutations (lethals), polygenic genetic abnormalities, and recessive disease may rarely account for repetitive abortion but in most instances they will occur sporadically. A review of gene knockouts and mutations in mice suggests that embryonic death resulted from disrupting basic cellular functions, vascular circulation, hematopoiesis or nutritional supply from the mother rather than affecting embryonic organ systems (5).

Maternal Diabetes

Type I (insulin dependent) diabetes mellitus with poor metabolic control increases the risk of abortion and still births but there is no increased risk with good metabolic control.

Maternal Hyper- and Hypothyroidism

Abnormal thyroid function is rare in patients with recurrent abortion.

Corpus Luteum or Placental Progesterone Deficiency (Luteal Phase Deficiency)

It is controversial whether low hormone levels after implantation result from impending abortion or are the cause of the abortion.

Maternal Infection

Infections of the genital tract could be responsible for abortion but it is not easy to document causality. The data

TABLE 15-2

ESTIMATED OUTCOME OF 100 PREGNANCIES VERSUS TIME FROM CONCEPTION

Time from Conception	Percent Survival to Term	Last Time for Induction of Selected Malformations[a]
Preimplantation		
0–6 days	25	
Postimplantation		
7–13 days	55	
14–20 days	73	
3–5 wk	79.5	22–23 days; cyclopia; sirenomelia, microtia
		26 days; anencephaly
		28 days; meningomyelocele
		34 days; transposition of great vessels
6–9 wk	90	36 days; cleft lip,
		6 wk; diaphragmatic hernia, rectal atresia, ventricular septal defect, syndactyly
		9 wk; cleft palate
10–13 wk	92	10 wk; omphalocele
14–17 wk	96.26	12 wk; hypospadias
18–21 wk	97.56	
22–25 wk	98.39	
26–29 wk	98.69	
30–33 wk	98.98	
34–37 wk	99.26	
38+ wk	99.32	38+ wk; central nervous system (CNS) cell depletion

[a] Modified from Schardein JL, ed. *Chemically induced birth defects.* New York: Marcel Dekker, 1993.

TABLE 15-3
ETIOLOGY OF SPONTANEOUS ABORTION IN THE HUMAN

Chromosomal Abnormalities
  Chromosomal abnormalities from either the maternal or
    paternal gonadocytes account for 50%–70% of abortions
Abortions with Normal Chromosomes (Euploidy)
  Genetic abnormalities: dominant mutations (lethal), polygenic
    genetic abnormalities, recessive disease from either the
    maternal, paternal, or both parents gonadocytes.
  Severe maternal disease states: diabetes, hypothyroidism,
    hepatitis, collagen diseases, untreated hyperthyroidism,
    severe malnutrition
  Corpus luteum or placental progesterone deficiency (luteal
    phase deficiency)
  Maternal infection which results in fetal infection: *Treponema*
    pallidum, *Plasmodium falciparum*, *Toxoplasma gondii*, herpes
    simplex virus, parvovirus B19, or cytomegalovirus
  Antiphospholipid antibodies: lupus anticoagulant, anticardiolipin
    antibodies
  Maternal-fetal histocompatibility
  Overmature gametes
  Mechanical or physical problems: uterine abnormalities, multiple
    pregnancies, very rarely trauma
  Cervical incompetence
  Abnormal placentation: hypoplastic trophoblast, circumvallate
    implantation
  Embryos and fetuses with severe malformations or growth
    retardation

suggesting that infection with *Chlamydia trachomatis*, *Borrelia burgdorferi*, *Mycoplasma hominis*, *Listeria monocytogenes*, and *Ureaplasma urealyticum* result in abortion are not conclusive. In contrast, maternal disease resulting in fetal infection with *Treponema pallidum*, *Plasmodium falciparum*, *Toxoplasma gondii*, herpes simplex virus, parvovirus B19, or cytomegalovirus has the potential to cause stillbirth or spontaneous abortion.

Severe, Debilitating Maternal Diseases

Hepatitis, collagen diseases, untreated hyperthyroidism, Wilson's disease or severe malnutrition can lead to abortion.

Antiphospholipid Antibodies

Lupus anticoagulant and anticardiolipin antibodies predispose women to recurrent abortion in both first and second trimesters as a result of vascular disruption in the placenta.

Maternal-Fetal Histocompatibility

It is suggested that embryonic loss increases if the mother and fetus are more histocompatible at the human leukocyte antigen (HLA) locus, resulting in the failure to develop maternal blocking antibodies against paternal antigens.

Overmature Gametes

Either the ovum or sperm could age because insemination occurred a few days prior to ovulation or ovulation occurred prior to insemination. The magnitude of this risk factor as a cause of spontaneous abortion is not known

and some investigators are skeptical that this phenomenon is clinically significant.

Mechanical or Physical Problems Related to Uterine Abnormalities, Multiple Pregnancies or Trauma

A hostile intrauterine environment can result from submucosal or intramural myomas, adhesions (Asherman's syndrome), multiple embryos or abnormalities of the uterus (bifid uterus, infantile uterus). Uterine trauma from a direct blow or penetrating injury may rarely be responsible for an abortion and if this type of injury occurs it would be more likely to result in a still birth at midgestation or later.

Cervical Incompetence

Cervical incompetence is more likely to result in second trimester than first trimester abortions.

Abnormal Placentation

Hypoplastic trophoblast and circumvallate implantation increase the risk of fetal loss.

Some Environmental Teratogens and Reproductive Toxins

Severe malformations or growth retardation implantation increase the risk of fetal loss.

Congenital Malformations

The etiology of congenital malformations can be divided into three categories: unknown, genetic, and environmental (Table 15-4). The etiology of 65%–75% of human malformations is unknown. A significant proportion of congenital malformations of unknown etiology is likely to have an important genetic component. Malformations with an increased recurrence risk, such as cleft lip and palate, anencephaly, spina bifida, certain congenital heart diseases, pyloric stenosis, hypospadias, inguinal hernia, talipes equinovarus, and congenital dislocation of the hip, fit in the category of multifactorial disease and in the category of polygenic inherited disease (6). The multifactorial/threshold hypothesis postulates the modulation of a continuum of genetic characteristics by intrinsic and extrinsic (environmental) factors (6). Although the modulating factors are not known, they probably include: placental blood flow, placental transport, site of implantation, maternal disease states, maternal malnutrition, infections, drugs, chemicals, and spontaneous errors of development.

Spontaneous errors of development may account for some of the malformations that occur without apparent abnormalities of the genome or environmental influence. We postulate that there is some probability for error during embryonic development based on the fact that embryonic development is such a complicated process. It is estimated that 75% of all conceptions are lost before term; 50% within the first 3 weeks of development (1,2). The World Health Organization estimated that 15% of all clinically recognizable pregnancies end in a spontaneous abortion, 50%–60% of which are as a result of chromosomal abnormalities

TABLE 15-4
ETIOLOGY OF HUMAN CONGENITAL MALFORMATIONS OBSERVED DURING THE FIRST YEAR OF LIFE

Suspected Cause	Percent of Total
Unknown	65–75
Polygenic	
Multifactorial (gene-environment interactions)	
Spontaneous errors of development	
Synergistic interactions of teratogens	
Genetic	15–25
Autosomal and sex-linked inherited genetic disease	
Cytogenetic (chromosomal abnormalities)	
New mutations	
Environmental	10
Maternal conditions: alcoholism; diabetes; endocrinopathies; phenylketonuria; smoking and nicotine; starvation; nutritional deficits	4
Infectious agents: rubella, toxoplasmosis, syphilis, herpes simplex, cytomegalovirus, varicella-zoster, Venezuelan equine encephalitis, parvovirus B19	3
Mechanical problems (deformations): Amniotic band constrictions; umbilical cord constraint; disparity in uterine size and uterine contents	1–2
Chemicals, drugs, high dose ionizing radiation, hyperthermia	<1

Modified from Brent RL. Environmental factors: miscellaneous. In: Brent RL, Harris ML, eds. *Prevention of embryonic fetal and perinatal disease.* Bethesda: DHEW (NIH), 1976:211–218; Brent RL. Definition of a teratogen and the relationship of teratogenicity to carcinogenicity [Editorial]. Teratology 1986;34:359–360.

(4,7,8). Finally, 3%–6% of offspring are malformed, which represents the background risk for human maldevelopment. This means that, as a conservative estimate, 1,176 clinically recognized pregnancies will result in approximately 176 miscarriages and 30 to 60 of the infants will have congenital anomalies in the remaining 1,000 live births. The true incidence of pregnancy loss is much higher because undocumented pregnancies are not included in this risk estimate.

Based on his review of the literature, Wilson (9) provided a format of theoretical teratogenic mechanisms: mutation; chromosomal aberrations; mitotic interference; altered nucleic acid synthesis and function; lack of precursors, substrates, or coenzymes for biosynthesis; altered energy sources; enzyme inhibition; osmolar imbalance, alterations in fluid pressures, viscosities, and osmotic pressures; and altered membrane characteristics. We suggest a revised list of mechanisms for teratogenesis (Table 15-5).

Even though an agent can produce one or more of these pathological processes, exposure to such an agent does not guarantee that maldevelopment will occur. Furthermore, it is likely that a drug, chemical or other agent can have more than one effect on the pregnant woman and the developing conceptus and therefore the nature of the drug or its

TABLE 15-5
MECHANISMS OF TERATOGENESIS

1. Cell death or mitotic delay beyond the recuperative capacity of the embryo or fetus.
2. Inhibition of cell migration, differentiation and cell communication.
3. Interference with histogenesis by processes such as cell depletion, necrosis, calcification, or scarring.
4. Biologic and pharmacological receptor-mediated developmental effects.
5. Metabolic inhibition or nutritional deficiencies.
6. Physical constraint, vascular disruption, inflammatory lesions, amniotic band syndrome.

biochemical or pharmacological effects will not in themselves predict a teratogenic effect in the human. In fact, the discovery of human teratogens has come primarily from human epidemiological studies. Animal studies and in vitro studies can be very helpful in determining the mechanism of teratogenesis and the pharmacokinetics related to teratogenesis (10). However, even if one understands the pathological effects of an agent, one cannot predict the teratogenic risk of an exposure without taking into consideration the developmental stage, the magnitude of the exposure and the reparability of the embryo.

Various maternal viral, bacterial, and parasitic infections are known to cause maldevelopment in humans including cytomegalovirus, fetal herpes virus infections (type 1 or 2), parvovirus B19 (erythema infectiosum), rubella virus, congenital syphilis (*Treponema pallidum*), *T. gondii* infection, varicella-zoster virus, and venezuelan equine encephalitis (11). The incidence of serum antibody to human immunodeficiency virus (HIV) in pregnant women is increasing from the 1991 estimate of 1.5 per 1,000 women delivering in the United States (12); the incidence is as high as 31% in pregnant women in some African cities (13). Several studies support the conclusion that asymptomatic HIV pregnancies are not associated with an increased risk of congenital malformations, low birth weight or abortion (14–17). It is likely that sexually transmitted diseases, opportunistic maternal infections, and symptomatic HIV pregnancies may increase the risk of low birth weight and morbidity in noninfected offspring.

The lethal or developmental effects of infectious agents are the result of mitotic inhibition, direct cytotoxicity or necrosis. Repair processes may result in metaplasia, scarring or calcification, which causes further damage by interfering with histogenesis. Infectious agents appear to be exceptions to some of the principles of teratogenesis because the relevance of dose and time of exposure cannot be demonstrated as readily for replicating teratogenic agents. Transplacental transmission of an infectious agent does not necessarily result in congenital malformations, growth retardation, or lethality.

Vascular disruption is a rare event associated with intrauterine death and a wide range of structural anomalies, including cerebral infarctions, certain types of visceral and urinary tract malformations, congenital limb amputations of the nonsymmetrical type; and orofacial malformations such as mandibular hypoplasia, cleft palate, and Moebius syndrome, which vary too widely to constitute a recognized syndrome. Some anomalies associated with twin pregnancies can be explained by vascular disruption resulting from placental anastomoses in shared placenta of monozygotic twins, anastomoses in a small percentage of dichorionic placentas in the case of dizygotic twins, or death of one twin resulting in emboli, intravascular coagulation and altered fetal hemodynamics in the co-twin (18,19). Vascular disruption may also result from physical trauma causing chorion bleeding, such as chorionic villous sampling, and exposure to some developmental toxicants, such as cocaine and misoprostol. Although uterine bleeding during the first trimester may result in fetal anomalies, the malformations associated with vascular disruption can also occur later in gestation. This topic is discussed in greater detail below with specific drugs.

Adverse Effects Produced Later in Pregnancy

The fetal period is characterized by histogenesis involving cell growth, differentiation, and migration. Drugs that produce permanent cell depletion, vascular disruption, necrosis, specific tissue or organ pathology, physiological decompensation, or severe growth retardation have the potential to cause deleterious effects throughout gestation. Sensitivity of the fetus for induction of mental retardation and microcephaly is greatest at the end of the first and the beginning of the second trimester. Other permanent neurological effects can be induced in the second and third trimesters.

The classic example of a drug that presents little risk to the developing embryo during organogenesis but can affect the near-term fetus if high doses are used is aspirin. It is possible that other antiinflammatory drugs present a similar risk.

FACTORS THAT AFFECT SUSCEPTIBILITY TO THE DELETERIOUS EFFECTS OF DRUGS

A basic tenet of environmentally produced embryo- and fetotoxicity is the effects of teratogenic or abortigenic milieu which have certain characteristics in common and follow certain basic principles. These principles determine the quantitative and qualitative aspects of developmental toxicity (Table 15-6).

Stage of Development

The induction of developmental toxicity by environmental agents usually results in a spectrum of morphological anomalies or intrauterine death, which varies in incidence depending on stage of exposure and dose. The developmental period at which an exposure occurs will determine which structures are most susceptible to the deleterious effects of the drug or chemical and to what extent the embryo can repair the damage. The period of sensitivity may be narrow or broad, depending on the environmental agent and the malformation in question. Limb defects, produced by thalidomide,

TABLE 15-6
FACTORS THAT INFLUENCE SUSCEPTIBILITY TO DEVELOPMENTAL TOXICANTS

Stage of development: The developmental period at which an exposure occurs will determine which structures are most susceptible to the adverse effects of chemicals and drugs and to what extent the embryo can repair the damage.
Magnitude of the exposure: Both the severity and incidence of toxic effects increase with dose.
Threshold phenomena: The threshold dose is the dose below which the incidence of death, malformation, growth retardation, or functional deficit is not statistically greater than that of nonexposed subjects.
Pharmacokinetics and metabolism: The physiologic changes in the pregnant woman and during fetal development and the bioconversion of compounds can significantly influence the developmental toxicity of drugs and chemicals by affecting absorption, body distribution, active metabolites, and excretion.
Maternal diseases: A maternal disease may increase the risk of fetal anomalies or abortion with or without exposure to a chemical or drug.
Placental transport: Most drugs and chemicals cross the placenta. The rate and extent to which a drug or chemical crosses the placenta are influenced by molecular weight, lipid solubility, polarity or degree of ionization, plasma protein binding, receptor mediation, placental blood flow, pH gradient between the maternal and fetal serum and tissues, and placental metabolism of the chemical or drug.
Genotype: The maternal and fetal genotypes may result in differences in cell sensitivity, placental transport, absorption, metabolism, receptor binding and distribution of an agent, and account for some variations in toxic effects among individual subjects and species.

have a very short period of susceptibility (Table 15-7) although microcephaly produced by radiation has a long period of susceptibility. Our knowledge of the susceptible stage of the embryo to various environmental influences is continually expanding and is vital to evaluating the significance of individual exposures or epidemiological studies.

During the first period of embryonic development, from fertilization through the early postimplantation stage, the embryo is most sensitive to the embryolethal effects of drugs and chemicals. Surviving embryos have malformation rates similar to the controls not because malformations cannot be produced at this stage but because significant cell loss or chromosome abnormalities at theses stages have a high likelihood of killing the embryo. Because of the omnipotentiality of early embryonic cells, surviving embryos have a much greater ability to have normal developmental potential. Wilson and Brent (20) demonstrated that the all-or-none phenomenon, or marked resistance to teratogens, disappears over a period of a few hours in the rat during early organogenesis utilizing ionizing X-irradiation as the experimental teratogen. The term all-or-none phenomenon has been misinterpreted by some investigators to indicate that malformations cannot be produced at this stage. On the contrary, it is likely that certain drugs, chemicals, or other insults during this stage of development can result in malformed offspring, but the nature of embryonic development

TABLE 15-7
DEVELOPMENTAL STAGE SENSITIVITY TO THALIDOMIDE-INDUCED LIMB REDUCTION DEFECTS IN THE HUMAN

Days from Conception for Induction of Defects	Limb Reduction Defects
21–26	Thumb aplasia
22–23	Microtia
23–34	Hip dislocation
24–29	Amelia, upper limbs
24–33	Phocomelia, upper limbs
25–31	Preaxial aplasia, upper limbs
27–31	Amelia, lower limbs
28–33	Preaxial aplasia, lower limbs; phocomelia, lower limbs; femoral hypoplasia; girdle hypoplasia
30–36	Triphalangeal thumb

Modified from Brent RL, Holmes LB. Clinical and basic science lessons from the thalidomide tragedy: what have we learned about the causes of limb defects? Teratology 1988;38:241–251, with permission.

at this stage will still reflect the basic characteristic of the all-or-none phenomenon which is a propensity for embryo lethality rather than surviving malformed embryos.

The period of organogenesis (from day 18 through about day 40 of postconception in the human), is the period of greatest sensitivity to teratogenic insults and the period when most gross anatomic malformations can be induced. Most environmentally produced major malformations occur before the 36th day of gestation in the human. The exceptions are malformations of the genito-urinary system, the palate, the brain or deformations as a result of problems of constraint, disruption or destruction. Severe growth retardation in the whole embryo or fetus may also result in permanent deleterious effects in many organs or tissues.

The fetal period is characterized by histogenesis involving cell growth, differentiation, and migration. Teratogenic agents that produce permanent cell depletion, vascular disruption, necrosis, specific tissue or organ pathology, physiological decompensation, and/or severe growth retardation have the potential to cause deleterious effects throughout gestation. Additionally, sensitivity of the fetus for induction of mental retardation and microcephaly is greatest at the end of the first and the beginning of the second trimester. Other permanent neurological effects can be induced in the second and third trimesters. Effects such as cell depletion or functional abnormalities, not readily apparent at birth, may give rise to changes in behavior or fertility which are apparent only later in life. The approximate last gestational day on which certain malformations may be induced in the human is presented in Table 15-2.

Magnitude of the Exposure

The dose-response relationship is extremely important when comparing effects among different species because usage of mg/kg doses are, at most, rough approximations. Dose equivalence among species can only be accomplished

by performing pharmacokinetic studies, metabolic studies, and dose-response investigations in the human and the species being studied. Furthermore, the response should be interpreted in a biologically sound manner. One example is that a substance given in large enough amounts to cause maternal toxicity is likely to also have deleterious effects on the embryo such as death, growth retardation, or retarded development. Another example is that because the steroid receptors that are necessary for naturally occurring and synthetic progestin action are absent from nonreproductive tissues early in development, the evidence is against the involvement of progesterone or its synthetic analogues in nongenital teratogenesis (21,22).

An especially anxiety-provoking concept is that the interaction of two or more drugs or chemicals may potentiate their developmental effects. Although this is an extremely difficult hypothesis to test in the human, it is an especially important consideration because multichemical or multitherapeutic exposures are common. Fraser (23) warns that the actual existence of a threshold phenomenon when nonteratogenic doses of two teratogens are combined could easily be misinterpreted as potentiation or synergism. Potentiation or synergism should be invoked only when exposure to two or more drugs is just below their thresholds for toxicity.

Several considerations affect the interpretation of dose-response relationships:

Active metabolites: Metabolites may be the proximate teratogen rather than the administered chemical, i.e., the metabolites phosphoramide mustard and acrolein may produce maldevelopment resulting from exposure to cyclophosphamide (24).

Duration of exposure: A chronic exposure to a prescribed drug can contribute to an increased teratogenic risk, e.g., anticonvulsant therapy; in contrast an acute exposure to the same drug may present little or no teratogenic risk.

Fat-solubility: Fat-soluble substances such as polychlorinated biphenyls (25) can produce fetal maldevelopment for an extended period after the last ingestion or exposure in a woman because they have an unusually long half life.

Threshold Phenomena

The threshold dose is the dosage below which the incidence of death, malformation, growth retardation, or functional deficit is not statistically greater than that of controls. The threshold level of exposure is usually from less than one to three orders of magnitude below the teratogenic or embryopathic dose for drugs and chemicals that kill or malform half the embryos. A teratogenic agent therefore has a no-effect dose as compared to mutagens or carcinogens, which have a stochastic dose response curve. Threshold phenomena are compared to stochastic phenomena in Table 15-8. The severity and incidence of malformations produced by every exogenous teratogenic agent that has been appropriately tested have exhibited threshold phenomena during organogenesis (9).

TABLE 15-8

STOCHASTIC AND THRESHOLD DOSE-RESPONSE RELATIONSHIPS OF DISEASES PRODUCED
BY ENVIRONMENTAL AGENTS

Relationship	Pathology	Site	Diseases	Risk	Definition
Stochastic phenomena	Damage to a single cell may result in disease	deoxyribonucleic acid DNA	Cancer, mutation	Some risk exists at all dosages; at low exposures the risk is below the spontaneous risk	Incidence of disease increases but severity and nature of the disease remain the same
Threshold phenomena	Multicelluar injury	High variation in etiology, affecting many cell and organ processes	Malformation, growth retardation, death, chemical toxicity, etc.	No increased risk below the threshold dose	Both severity and incidence of the disease increase with dose

Modified from Brent RL. Definition of a teratogen and the relationship of teratogenicity to carcinogenicity [Editorial]. Teratology 1986;34:359–360, with permission.

Pharmacokinetics and Metabolism

The physiological alterations in pregnancy and the bioconversion of compounds can significantly influence the teratogenic effects of drugs and chemicals by affecting absorption, body distribution, active form(s), and excretion of the compound. Physiological alterations in the mother during pregnancy which affect the pharmacokinetics of drugs include the following: decreased gastrointestinal motility and increased intestinal transit time may delay absorption of drugs absorbed in the small intestine as a result of increased stomach retention but enhance absorption of slowly absorbed drugs; decreased plasma albumin concentration, which alters the kinetics of compound normally bound to albumin; increased plasma and extracellular fluid volumes that affect concentration-dependent transfer of compounds; renal elimination, which is generally increased but is influenced by body position during late pregnancy; inhibition of metabolic inactivation in the liver late in pregnancy; and variations in uterine blood flow, although little is known about how this affects transfer across the placenta (26–28).

The fetus also undergoes physiological alterations, which affect the pharmacokinetics of drugs (28): the amount and distribution of fat varies with development and affects the distribution of lipid-soluble drugs; the fetal circulation contains a higher concentration of unbound drug largely because the plasma fetal proteins are lower in concentration than in the adult and may lower drug affinity; the functional development of pharmacological receptors is likely to proceed at different rates in the various tissues; and i.v. drugs excreted by the fetal kidneys may be recycled by swallowing of amniotic fluid.

The role the placenta plays in drug pharmacokinetics, reviewed by Juchau and Rettie (29) and Miller (25), involves transport [discussed in detail in the section Placental Transport; the presence of receptors sites for a number of endogenous and xenobiotic compounds (β-adrenergic, glucocorticoid, epidermal growth factor, IgG-Fc, insulin, low-density lipoproteins, opiates, somatomedin, testosterone, transcobalamin II, transferrin, folate, retinoid)] (25); and the bioconversion of xenobiotics. Bioconversion of xenobiotics

has been shown to be important in the teratogenic activity of several xenobiotics. There is strong evidence that reactive metabolites of cyclophosphamide, 2-acetylaminofluorene, and nitroheterocycles (niridazole) are the proximal teratogens (30). There is also experimental evidence that suggests that other chemicals undergo conversion to intermediates that have deleterious effects on embryonic development including phenytoin, procarbazine, rifampicin, diethylstilbestrol, some benzhydrylpiperazine antihistamines, adriamycin, testosterone, benzo(a)pyrene, methoxyethanol, caffeine, and paraquat (29,30).

The major site of bioconversion of chemicals in vivo is likely to be the maternal liver. Placental P450-dependent monooxygenation of xenobiotics will occur at low rates unless induced by such compounds as those found in tobacco smoke (29). However, the fetus also develops functional P450 oxidative isozymes capable of converting proteratogens to active metabolites.

Maternal Disease

Maternal disease states such as diabetes mellitus, epilepsy, phenylketonuria, and endocrinopathies are associated with adverse effects on the fetus. In some cases, it may be difficult to determine whether a maternal disease or the treatment for the disease plays a role in the etiology of malformations associated with the treatment for that disease during pregnancy. For example, the genetic and environmental milieu, which cause epilepsy may also contribute to the maldevelopment associated with exposure to diphenylhydantoin (31).

The role of maternal malnutrition is an important area for investigation because it may be a contributing factor to many teratogenic milieu. A series of investigations provided evidence suggesting that folic acid supplementation could reduce the incidence of recurrence of neural tube defects in the human (32–35). It was later shown convincingly that periconceptional supplementation with folic acid, 4 mg/day, reduces the risk of recurrence of neural tube defects in subsequent siblings of children with neural tube defects (36). Furthermore, low-dose folic acid supplementation, 0.8 mg/day, was reported to decrease the incidence of neural tube defects in a population not at increased risk for these defects (37). Although folate supplementation reduces the incidence of neural tube defects, folate supplementation will not prevent all neural tube defects and it is not known whether folic acid supplementation corrects an undefined metabolic defect or a nutritional deficiency.

Placental Transport

The exchange between the mammalian embryo and the maternal organism is controlled by the placenta which includes the chorioplacenta, the yolk sac placenta and the paraplacental chorion. The placenta varies in structure and function among species and for each stage of gestation. As an example, the rodent yolk sac placenta continues to function as an organ of transport for a much greater part of gestation than in the human. Thus differences in placental function and structure may affect our ability to apply teratogenic data developed in one species directly to other species, including the human (38). As pharmacokinetic techniques and the actual measurement of metabolic products in the embryo become more sophisticated, the appropriateness of utilizing animal data to project human effects may improve.

Historically a placental barrier was thought to exist, which prevented harmful substances from reaching the embryo. It is now clear that there is no "placental barrier" per se. The fact is that most drugs and chemicals cross the placenta. It will be a rare substance that will cross the placental barrier in one species and be unable to reach the fetus in another (39). No such chemical exists except for selected proteins whose actions are species-specific.

Even before there were chemical techniques to demonstrate the presence of drugs or chemicals in the embryo there was clear evidence that they had reached the fetus because of clinical manifestations of the drugs: anticoagulants such as warfarin can affect the clotting of fetal blood; many drugs can affect the fetal cardiac rate; changes in the fetal electroencephalogram (EEG) can be demonstrated as a result of the many drugs that affect the central nervous system (CNS); and newborns may exhibit withdrawal symptoms from drugs taken by their mothers, either medications or substances of abuse such as alcohol or opiates.

These observations demonstrate clinically significant placental transport of drugs only in the latter portion of gestation and may not be a means of evaluating embryonic exposure during early organogenesis.

Those factors which determine the ability of a drug or chemical to cross the placenta and reach the embryo include: molecular weight, lipid affinity or solubility, polarity or degree of ionization, protein binding, and receptor mediation. Compounds with low molecular weight, lipid affinity, nonpolarity, and without protein-binding properties will cross the placenta with ease and rapidity. As an example, ethyl alcohol is a chemical which reaches the embryo rapidly and in concentrations equal to or greater than the level in the mother.

High molecular weight compounds like heparin, 20,000 daltons, do not readily cross the placenta and therefore heparin is used to replace warfarin-like compounds during pregnancy for the treatment of hypercoagulation conditions. Rose Bengal does not cross the placenta. In general, compounds with molecular weights of 1,000 or greater do not readily cross the placenta, although 600 dalton compounds usually do; most drugs are 250–400 daltons and cross the placenta (40).

In addition to the particular properties of the drug or chemical, three other conditions affect the quantitative aspect of placental transport: (a) placental blood flow, (b) the pH gradient between the maternal and fetal serum and tissues, and (c) placental metabolism of the chemical or drug. The biotransformation properties of the placenta and/or maternal organism are important because a number of chemicals or drugs are not teratogenic in their original form.

The most important concept regarding placental transport of teratogens must be reemphasized. An agent is teratogenic because it affects the embryo directly or indirectly by its ability to produce a toxic effect in the embryo or extraembryonic membranes at exposures which are attained in the human being, not because it crosses the placenta per se.

Genotype

The genetic constitution of an organism is an important factor in the susceptibility of a species to a drug or chemical. More than 30 disorders of increased sensitivity to drug toxicity or effects have been reported in the human as a result of an inherited trait (41). The effect of a drug or chemical depends on both the maternal and fetal genotypes and may result in differences in cell sensitivity, placental transport, absorption, metabolism (activation, inactivation, active metabolites), receptor binding, and distribution of an agent. This accounts for some variations in teratogenic effects among species and in individual subjects.

Estimating the Developmental Risks of Drugs During Human Pregnancy

Evaluation of Data Available for the Human

Although chemicals and drugs can be evaluated for fetotoxic potential by utilizing *in vivo* animal studies and *in vitro* systems, it should be recognized that these testing procedures are only one component in the process of evaluating the potential teratogenic risk of drugs and chemicals in the human. The evaluation of the teratogenicity of drugs and chemicals should include, when possible, (a) data obtained from human epidemiological studies, (b) secular trend data in humans, (c) animal developmental toxicity studies, (d) the dose-response relationship for developmental toxicity and the relationship to the human pharmacokinetic equivalent dose in the animal studies, and (e) considerations of biological plausibility (Table 15-9) (42,43). This method is of greatest value when utilized for

TABLE 15-9

EVIDENCE FOR POTENTIAL DEVELOPMENTAL TOXICITY IN THE HUMAN

Epidemiological studies: Epidemiological studies consistently demonstrate an increased incidence of pregnancy loss or of a particular spectrum of fetal effects in exposed human populations.

Secular trend data: Secular trends demonstrate a relationship between the incidence of pregnancy loss or a particular fetal effect and the changing exposures in human populations. The percent of the population exposed must be large for this analysis.

Animal developmental toxicity studies: An animal model mimics the human developmental effect at clinically comparable exposures. Since mimicry may occur in only one animal species, if it occurs at all, it would not necessarily be observed during an initial developmental toxicology study. Developmental toxicity studies are therefore indicative of a potential hazard in general rather than the potential for a specific adverse effect on the fetus.

Dose-response relationship: Developmental toxicity in the human increases with dose and the developmental toxicity in animals occurs at a dose that is pharmacokinetically equivalent to the human dose.

Biological plausibility: The mechanisms of developmental toxicity are understood or the results are biologically plausible.

Modified from Brent RL. Method of evaluating alleged human teratogens [Editorial]. *Teratology* 1978;17:83; Brent RL. Definition of a teratogen and the relationship of teratogenicity to carcinogenicity [Editorial]. Teratology 1986;34:359–360, with permission.

the evaluation of chemicals and drugs that have been in use for some time or for evaluating new drugs that have a similar mechanism of action, structure, pharmacology and purpose similar to other, extensively studied agents. The ability to establish a causal relationship between an environmental agent and abortigenic effect is more difficult, for the following reasons:

1. Abortion is a very frequent reproductive event and therefore the incidence can vary considerably between different populations of women. Differences in the abortion incidence between two populations in a single study may be as a result of chance alone.
2. There are multiple causes of abortion and most epidemiological studies dealing with abortion make no attempt to determine the etiology of the abortions. Since most abortions are as a result of preconceptual or periconceptual events, it is extremely difficult to match patients in case control studies and it would be necessary to have large increases in a particular etiological category of environmentally induced abortion to demonstrate a statistically significant increase in the incidence of spontaneous abortion in an "exposed" population of pregnant women.
3. Confounding factors appear to be more significant in abortion studies than in birth defect studies (cocaine, smoking, alcohol, syphilis, narcotics, caffeine). This fur-

ther decreases the possibility that the agent being studied has a direct abortigenic effect.

4. The incidence of therapeutic abortions is difficult to estimate or control for in most epidemiological studies (44,45).

One of the advantages of reproductive effects is that there is frequently, but not always, concordance of effects involving more than one parameter (growth, malformations, abortion, stillbirth, prematurity, etc.). Isolated abortion studies that do not study the totality of reproductive effects are at a serious disadvantage, because spurious or nonetiological results may be misinterpreted as being causally related to a drug or environmental toxicant.

Some investigators and regulatory agencies divide drugs and chemicals into developmentally toxic and nontoxic compounds. In reality, potential developmental toxicity can be evaluated only if one considers, as a minimum, the agent, the dose, the species and the stage of gestation. Working definitions for developmental toxicity in the human are suggested in Table 15-10.

Potential human teratogens and abortifacients comprise a large group of drugs because they include all drugs and chemicals that can produce embryotoxic and fetotoxic effects at some exposure. Since these exposures are not utilized or attained in the human, they represent no or minimal risks to the human embryo.

Misconceptions in Evaluating Developmental Toxicity in the Human

Misconceptions have lead to confusion regarding the potential effects of even proven teratogens. Examples of erroneous concepts include: if an agent can produce one

TABLE 15-10

DEFINITIONS OF POTENTIAL FOR DEVELOPMENTAL TOXICITY IN THE HUMAN

Developmental toxicant: An agent or milieu that has been demonstrated to produce permanent alterations or death in the embryo or fetus following intrauterine exposures that usually occur or are attainable in the human.

Potential for developmental toxicity: An agent or milieu that has not been demonstrated to produce permanent alterations or death in the embryo or fetus following intrauterine exposures that usually occur or are attainable in the human, but can affect the embryo or fetus if the exposure is raised substantially above the usual exposure. Most chemicals and drugs have the potential for interrupting a pregnancy or inducing developmental defects if the exposure is increased sufficiently.

Little or no potential for developmental toxicity: An agent or milieu that has been demonstrated to produce no embryo- or fetotoxicity at any attainable dose in the human. In contrast, an environmental agent may be so toxic that it has no developmental toxicity in the human because it kills the mother before or at the same dose that it begins to have adverse effects on the embryo.

Modified from Brent RL. Method of evaluating alleged human teratogens [Editorial]. *Teratology* 1978;17:83, with permission.

type of malformation, it can produce any malformation; an agent presents a risk at any dose, once it can be proven to be teratogenic; and an agent that is teratogenic is likely to be abortigenic.

These concepts are incorrect. The data clearly indicate that proven teratogens do not have the ability to produce every birth defect. Many teratogens can be identified on the basis of the malformations that are produced. Thus, the concept of the syndrome is probably more appropriate in clinical teratology than any other area of clinical medicine. Some symptoms or signs appear in many teratogenic syndromes, such as growth retardation or mental retardation, and therefore are not very discriminating. On the other hand, rare or specific effects, such as deafness, retinitis, or a pattern of cerebral calcifications, may point to a specific teratogen. It is also true that there is substantial overlap in malformation syndromes which may not always be separable. Environmentally produced birth defects may be confused with genetically determined malformations. Using thalidomide as an example, a patient with bilateral radial aplasia and a ventricular septal defect may have the Holt Oram syndrome or the thalidomide syndrome. It may or may not be possible to make a diagnosis with absolute certainty, even if one has a history of thalidomide ingestion during pregnancy. It is possible, however, to refute the suggestion that thalidomide was responsible for congenital malformations in an individual by the nature of the limb malformation.

The specificity of some teratogens can sometimes point to the mechanism or site of action. For instance, the predominant central nervous system effects of methyl mercury are understood when one realizes the propensity for organic mercury to be stored in lipid.

Epidemiologists sometimes use poor judgment when grouping malformations. As an example, limb reduction defects are frequently studied regarding their association with environmental teratogens but, in some studies, limb defects that are clearly related to problems of organogenesis are lumped with congenital amputations even though it is very unlikely that any agent will be responsible for both types of malformations. It is clear that epidemiological studies could be markedly improved if there was more input from clinical teratologists in planning and performing the studies.

Case control studies concerning spontaneous abortion may contain serious errors unless the populations being studied are similar regarding the stage of pregnancy when abortion occurred. This study design diminishes the possibility that the abortion rate will differ on the basis of the selection process and not the drug or environmental agent being studied. Unfortunately most epidemiological studies dealing with drug or environmentally induced abortion do not attempt to determine the etiology of the abortion.

Potential Embryo- and Fetotoxicity of Selected Prescribed and Self-administered Drugs

We evaluated the literature concerning selected drugs that cause or are suggested to cause deleterious effects during pregnancy in the human. The data included human epidemiological studies, secular trend data in humans where appropriate, and animal developmental toxicity studies. In our analysis we considered the dose-response relationship of teratogenicity, the relationship to the human pharmacokinetic equivalent dose in the animal studies and biological plausibility (Table 15-9) (42,43). Table 15-11 focuses on these drugs, listing their potential adverse effects in the human. Although these drugs account for a small percentage of all malformations and abortions, they are important because these exposures may be preventable.

Alcohol

Adverse effects in offspring from excessive alcohol consumption during pregnancy were recognized more than 200 years ago (46). It was Jones and associates (47) however, who defined the fetal alcohol syndrome (FAS) in children with intrauterine growth retardation, microcephaly, mental retardation, maxillary hypoplasia, flat philtrum, thin upper lip, and reduction in the width of palpebral fissures. Cardiac abnormalities were also seen. Many of the children of alcoholic mothers had FAS and all of the affected children evidenced developmental delay (47,48).

A period of greatest susceptibility is not clearly established but the risk for adverse effects increases with increased consumption and binge drinking early in pregnancy may be associated with an increased risk of alcohol-related effects (49). The risk of decreased brain growth and differentiation that results from high alcohol consumption is greater during the second and third trimester. Chronic consumption of 6 oz of alcohol per day constitutes a high risk although the FAS is not likely when the mother consumes fewer than two drinks (equivalent to 1 oz of alcohol) per day (50). Reduction of alcohol consumption or cessation of drinking early in pregnancy will reduce the incidence and severity of alcohol-related effects (49,51–53) but may not entirely eliminate the risk of some degree of physical or behavioral impairment. The human syndrome is likely to involve the direct effects of alcohol and the indirect effects of genetic susceptibility and poor nutrition. Alcoholism can have maternally deleterious effects on intermediary metabolism and nutrition, especially if alcoholic cirrhosis is present, which can contribute to an adverse milieu for the developing embryo.

Although alcoholic mothers frequently smoke and consume other drugs, there is little doubt from the human and animal data that alcohol ingestion alone can have a disastrous effect on the developing embryo or fetus. The reported incidence of FAS varies widely in different studies but appears to be approximately 6% in offspring of women who drink heavily during pregnancy (51). Fetal alcohol syndrome may be the most commonly recognized cause of environmentally induced mental deficiency; there are at least several hundred children born each year with full FAS and probably many more with subtler fetal alcohol effects (50,54).

TABLE 15-11

EFFECTS AND ESTIMATED RISKS OF SELECTED PRESCRIBED AND SELF-ADMINISTERED DRUGS HUMAN PREGNANCY

Selected Drugs	Reported Effects or Associations and Estimated Risks	Comments[a]
Alcohol	Fetal alcohol syndrome: intrauterine growth retardation, maxillary hypoplasia, reduction in width of palpebral fissures, characteristic but not diagnostic facial features, microcephaly, mental retardation. An increase in spontaneous abortion has been reported but since mothers who abuse alcohol during pregnancy have multiple other risk factors, it is difficult to determine whether this is a direct effect on the embryo. Consumption of 6 oz of alcohol or more per day constitutes a high risk but it is likely that detrimental effects can occur at lower exposures.	Quality of available information: good to excellent. Direct cytotoxic effects of ethanol and indirect effects of alcoholism. While a threshold teratogenic dose is likely it will vary in individuals because of a multiplicity of factors.
Aminopterin, methotrexate	Microcephaly, hydrocephaly, cleft palate, meningomyelocele, intrauterine growth retardation, abnormal cranial ossification, reduction in derivatives of first branchial arch, mental retardation, postnatal growth retardation. Aminopterin can induce abortion within its therapeutic range; it is used for this purpose to eliminate ectopic embryos. Risk from therapeutic doses is unknown but appears to be moderate to high.	Quality of available information: good. Anticancer, antimetabolic agents; folic acid antagonists that inhibit dihydrofolate reductase, resulting in cell death.
Androgens	Masculinization of female embryo: clitoromegaly with or without fusion of labia minora. Nongenital malformations are not a reported risk. Androgen exposures which result in masculinization have little potential for inducing abortion. Based on animal studies, behavioral masculinization of the female human will be rare.	Quality of available information: good. Effects are dose and stage dependent; stimulates growth and differentiation of sex steroid receptor-containing tissue.
Angiotensin-converting enzyme (ACE) inhibitors	The therapeutic use of ACE inhibitors has neither a teratogenic effect nor an abortigenic effect in the first trimester. Since this group of drugs does not interfere with organogenesis, they can be used in a woman of reproductive age; if the woman becomes pregnant, therapy can be changed during the first trimester without an increase in the risk of teratogenesis. Later in gestation these drugs can result in fetal and neonatal death, oligohydramnios, pulmonary hypoplasia, neonatal anuria, intrauterine growth retardation, and skull hypoplasia. Risk is dependent on dose and length of exposure.	Quality of available information: good. Antihypertensive agents; adverse fetal effects are related to severe fetal hypotension over a long period fo time during the second or third trimester.
Antibiotics	*Streptomycin:* Streptomycin and a group of ototoxic drugs can affect the eighth nerve and interfere with hearing; it is a relatively low-risk phenomenon. There are not enough data to estimate the abortigenic potential of streptomycin. Because the deleterious effect of streptomycin is limited to the eighth nerve, it is unlikely to affect the incidence of abortion.	Quality of available information: fair to good. Long duration maternal therapy during pregnancy is associated with hearing deficiency in offspring.
	Tetracycline: Bone staining and tooth staining can occur with therapeutic doses. Persistent high doses can cause hypoplastic tooth enamel. No other congenital malformations are at increased risk. The usual therapeutic doses present no increased risk of abortion to the embryo or fetus.	Quality of available information: good. Effects seen only if exposure is late in the first or during second or third trimester, since tetracyclines have to interact with calcified tissue.
	Penicillin G benzathine used for the treatment of syphilis produces no adverse fetal effects in the usual therapeutic regimens:	These antibiotics are used in late pregnancy for the treatment of sexually transmitted diseases.
	Ceftriaxone and doxycycline used for the treatment of gonorrhea produces no adverse fetal effects in the usual therapeutic regimens.	
	Erythromycin base or stearate used for the treatment of Chlamydia involves a possible increased risk of cholestatic hepatitis in the usual therapeutic regimens.	
Antihypertensive (excluding ACE inhibitors)	*Clonidine:* a direct alpha adrenergic agonist that appears to be relatively safe during pregnancy but there are few available data.	
	Hydralazine: a vasodilator often used in combination with methyldopa and is considered to be safe.	
	Methyldopa: a centrally acting adrenergic antagonist and currently the safest antihypertensive drug available for use during pregnancy with no reported adverse effects on the fetus or on mental and physical development.	

TABLE 15-11
(continued)

Selected Drugs	Reported Effects or Associations and Estimated Risks	Comments[a]
	Nifedipine: a calcium channel blocker whose potential for adverse effects with its long term use in the treatment of hypertension is unknown. *Propranolo:* a β-blocker whose prolonged use may increase the risk of intrauterine growth retardation.	
Antituberculosis therapy	Drugs prescribed for the treatment of tuberculosis include aminoglycosides, ethambutol, isoniazid, rifampin, and ethionamide. The ototoxic effects of streptomycin (discussed above) are the only proven adverse effects of these drugs on the fetus. Therapeutic exposures to other tuberculostatic drugs appear to represent a very small risk of teratogenesis and even less risk of abortion.	
Aspirin	No increased risk for malformations or abortion low dose regimen (60–150 mg per day). Aspirin should be discontinued 1 week before anticipated delivery to reduce the risk for maternal or neonatal bleeding.	Used for treatment of preeclamspia, idiopathic placental insufficiency, systemic lupus erythematosus, increased platelet aggregation
Benzodiazepines	Benzodiazepines appear to have minimal or no increased risk of malformations at therapeutic ranges; higher exposures may increase the risk. The risk for abortion is unknown. *Chlordiazepoxide* (Librium), appears to have a minimal risk for congenital anomalies and no increased risk for abortion at therapeutic doses. Higher exposures are likely to increase the risk of adverse effects on the fetus but the magnitude of the increase is not known. *Diazepam* (Valium): third trimester exposure can reversibly affect the fetus and neonate there is minimal increased risk of congenital malformations and no demonstrated increased risk of abortions from therapeutic exposures. *Meprobamate:* weakly associated with a variety of congenital malformations but the data are not sufficient to confirm or rule out a small increase risk of malformations due to exposures early in pregnancy.	The benzodiazepines are widely used as tranquilizers during pregnancy.
Caffeine	Caffeine is teratogenic in rodent species with doses of 150 mg/kg. There is no convincing data that moderate or usual exposures (300 mg per day or less) present a measurable risk in the human for any malformation or group of malformations. On the other hand, excessive caffeine consumption (exceeding 300 mg per day) during pregnancy is associated with growth retardation and embryonic loss.	Quality of available information: fair to good. Behavioral effects have been reported and appear to be transient or temporary; more information is needed concerning the population with higher exposures.
Carbamazepine	Minor craniofacial defects (upslanting palpebral fissures, epicanthal folds, short nose with long philtrum), fingernail hypoplasia, and developmental delay. Teratogenic risk is not known but likely to be significant for minor defects. There are too few data to determine whether carbamazapine presents an increased risk for abortion. Since embryos with multiple malformations are more likely to abort, it would appear that carbamazepine presents little risk because an increase in these types of malformations has not been reported.	Quality of available information: fair to good. Anticonvulsant; little is known concerning mechanism. Epilepsy may itself contribute to an increased risk for fetal anomalies.
Cocaine	Preterm delivery; fetal loss; placental abruption; intrauterine growth retardation; microcephaly; neurobehavioral abnormalities; vascular disruptive phenomena resulting in limb amputation, cerebral infarctions and certain types of visceral and urinary tract malformations. There are few data to indicate that cocaine increases the risk of first trimester abortion. The low but increased risk of vascular disruptive phenomena due to vascular compromise of the pregnant uterus would more likely result in midgestation abortion or stillbirth. It is possible that higher doses could result in early abortion. Risk for deleterious effects on fetal outcome is significant; risk for major disruptive effects is low, but can occur in the latter portion of the first trimester as well as the second and third trimesters.	Quality of available information: fair to good. Cocaine causes a complex pattern of cardiovascular effects due to its local anesthetic and sympathomimetic activities in the mother. Fetopathology is likely to be due to decreased uterine blood flow and fetal vascular effects. Because of the mechanism of cocaine teratogenicity, a well-defined cocaine syndrome is not likely. Poor nutrition accompanies drug abuse and multiple drug abuse is common.

(continued)

TABLE 15-11
(continued)

Selected Drugs	Reported Effects or Associations and Estimated Risks	Comments[a]
Coumarin derivatives	Nasal hypoplasia; stippling of secondary epiphysis; intrauterine growth retardation; anomalies of eyes, hands, neck; variable central nervous system anatomical defects (absent corpus callosum, hydrocephalus, asymmetrical brain hypoplasia). Risk from exposure 10% to 25% during 8th to 14th week of gestation. There is also an increased risk of pregnancy loss. There is a risk to the mother and fetus from bleeding at the time of labor and delivery.	Quality of available information: good. Anticoagulant; bleeding is an unlikely explanation for effects produced in the first trimester. CNS defects may occur anytime during second and third trimester and may be related to bleeding.
Cyclophosphamide	Growth retardation, ectrodactyly, syndactyly, cardiovascular anomalies, and other minor anomalies. Teratogenic risk appears to be increased but the magnitude of the risk is uncertain. Almost all chemotherapeutic agents have the potential for inducing abortion. This risk is dose-related; at the lowest therapeutic doses the risk is small.	Quality of available information: fair. Anticancer, alkylating agent; requires cytochrome P450 mono-oxydase activation; interacts with DNA, resulting in cell death.
Diethylstilbestrol (DES)	Clear cell adenocarcinoma of the vagina occurs in about 1:1,000 to 10,000 females who were exposed *in utero*. Vaginal adenosis occurs in about 75% of females exposed in utero before the 9th week of pregnancy. Anomalies of the uterus and cervix may play a role in decreased fertility and an increased incidence of prematurity although the majority of women exposed to DES *in utero* can conceive and deliver normal babies. *In utero* exposure to DES increased the incidence of genitourinary lesions and infertility in males. DES can interfere with zygote survival, but it does not interfere with embryonic survival when given in its usual dosage after implantation. Offspring who were exposed to DES *in utero* have an increased risk for delivering permaturely, but do not appear to be at increased risk for first trimester abortion.	Quality of available information: fair to good. Synthetic estrogen; stimulates estrogen receptor-containing tissue, may cause misplaced genital tissue which has a greater propensity to develop cancer.
Digoxin	No adverse fetal effects reported with usual therapeutic regimens.	Used for treatment of fetal dysrhythmia.
Diphenylhydantoin	Hydantoin syndrome: microcephaly, mental retardation, cleft lip/palate, hypoplastic nails and distal phalanges; characteristic, but not diagnostic facial features. Associations documented only with chronic exposure. Wide variation in reported risk of malformations but appears to be no greater than 10%. The few epidemiological data indicate a small risk of abortion for therapeutic exposures for the treatment of epilepsy. For short term treatment, i.e., prophylactic therapy for a head injury, there is no appreciable risk.	Quality of available information: fair to good. Anticonvulsant; direct effect on cell membranes, folate, and vitamin K metabolism. Metabolic intermediate (epoxide) has been suggested as the teratogenic agent.
Glucocorticoids	*Dexamethasone, Betamethasone, Dexamethasone, Hydrocortisone, Methylprednisone:* Glucocorticoids have not been shown to be teratogenic but chronic glucocorticoid therapy may result in prematurity and intrauterine growth retardation.	Glucocorticoids are used late in pregnancy to reduce respiratory distress in premature infants and to treat congenital adrenal hyperplasia. They are also used in the treatment of rheumatic diseases, other acute and chronic inflammatory diseases, and organ transplantation.
Indomethacin	Can prolong labor and may predispose neonate to necrotizing enterocolitis when used as a tocolytic.	Used for the prevention or reduction of intraventricular hemorrhage in premature infant and for treatment of polyhydramnious.
Lithium carbonate	Although animal studies have demonstrated a clear teratogenic risk, the effect in humans is uncertain. Early reports indicated an increased incidence of Ebstein's anomaly, other heart and great vessel defects, but as more studies are reported the strength of this association has diminished. Lithium levels within the therapeutic range (< 1.2 mg%) do not increase the risk of abortion.	Quality of available information: fair to good. Antidepressant; mechanism has not been defined.
Methylene blue	Hemolytic anemia and jaundice in neonatal period after exposure late in pregnancy. There may be a small risk for intestinal atresia but this is not yet clear. No indication of increased risk of abortion.	Quality of available information: poor to fair. Used to mark amniotic cavity during amniocentesis.

TABLE 15-11
(continued)

Selected Drugs	Reported Effects or Associations and Estimated Risks	Comments[a]
Misoprostol	Misoprostol is a synthetic prostaglandin analog that has been used by millions of women for illegal abortion. A low incidence of vascular disruptive phenomenon, such as limb reduction defects and Mobius syndrome, has been reported.	Quality of available information: Fair Classical animal teratology studies would not be helpful in discovering these effects, because vascular disruptive effects occur after the period of early organogenesis.
Oxazolidine-2,4-diones (trimethadione, paramethadione)	Fetal trimethadione syndrome: V-shaped eye brows, low-set ears with anteriorly folded helix, high-arched palate, irregular teeth, CNS anomalies, severe developmental delay. Wide variation in reported risk. Characteristic facial features are documented only with chronic exposure. The abortifacient potential has not been adequately studied, but appears to be minimal.	Quality of available information: good to excellent. Anticonvulsants; affects cell membrane permeability. Actual mechanism of action has not been determined.
D-Penicillamine	Cutis laxa, hyperflexibility of joints. Condition appears to be reversible and the risk is low. There are no human data on the risk of abortion.	Quality of available information: fair to good. Copper chelating agent; produces copper deficiency inhibiting collagen synthesis and maturation.
Phenobarbitol	No adverse fetal effects reported for usual therapeutic regimens.	May be used for the prevention or reduction of intraventricular hemorrhage in premature infant.
Progestins	Masculinization of female embryo exposed to high doses of some testosterone-derived progestins and may interact with progesterone receptors in the liver and brain later in gestation. The dose of progestins present in modern oral contraceptives presents no masculinization or feminization risks. All progestins present no risk for nongenital malformations. Many synthetic progestins and natural progesterone have been used to treat luteal phase deficiency, embryos implanted via in-vitro fertilization (IVF) threatened abortion or bleeding in pregnancy with variable results. Conversely, synthetic progestins that interfere with progesterone function may cause early pregnancy loss; RU-486 is presently used specifically for this purpose.	Quality of available information: good. Stimulates or interferes with sex steroid receptor-containing tissue.
Retinoids, systemic (isotretinoin, etrentinate)	Increased risk of CNS, cardio-aortic, ear, and clefting defects. Microtia, anotia, thymic aplasia and other branchial arch, aortic arch abnormalities and certain congenital heart malformations. Exposed embryos are at greater risk for abortion. This is plausible since many of the malformations, such as neural tube defects, are associated with an increased risk of abortion.	Quality of available information: fair. Used in treatment of chronic dermatoses. Retinoids can cause direct cytotoxicity and alter programmed cell death; affect many cell types but neural crest cells are particularly sensitive.
Retinoids, topical (tretinoin)	Epidemiological studies, animal studies and absorption studies in humans do not suggest a teratogenic risk. Regardless of the risks associated with systemically administered retinoids, topical retinoids present little or no risk for intrauterine growth retardation, teratogenesis or abortion because they are minimally absorbed and only a small percentage of skin is exposed.	Quality of available information: poor. Topical administration of tretinoin in animals in therapeutic doses is not teratogenic, although massive exposures can produce maternal toxicity and reproductive effects. More importantly, topical administration in humans results in non-measurable blood levels.
Rh immune globulin	No adverse fetal effects have been associated with Rh-Ig prophylaxis against Rh immunization.	
Smoking and nicotine	Placental lesions; intrauterine growth retardation; increased postnatal morbidity and mortality. While there have been some studies reporting increases in anatomical malformations, most studies do not report an association. There is no syndrome associated with maternal smoking. Maternal or placental complications can result in fetal death. Exposures to nicotine and tobacco smoke are a significant risk for pregnancy loss in the first and second trimester.	Quality of available information: good to excellent. While tobacco smoke contains many components, nicotine can result in vascular spasm vasculitis which has resulted in a higher incidence of placental pathology.

(continued)

TABLE 15-11
(continued)

Selected Drugs	Reported Effects or Associations and Estimated Risks	Comments[a]
Thalidomide	Limb reduction defects (preaxial preferential effects, phocomelia), facial hemangioma, esophageal or duodenal atresia, anomalies of external ears, eyes, kidneys, and heart, increased incidence of neonatal and infant mortality. The thalidomide syndrome, while characteristic and recognizable, can be mimicked by some genetic diseases. Although there are fewer data pertaining to its abortigenic potential, there appears to be an increased risk of abortion.	Quality of available information: good to excellent. Sedative–hypnotic agent. The etiology of thalidomide teratogenesis has not been definitively determined.
Thyroid: iodides, antithyroid drugs (thioamides)	Fetal hypothyroidism or goiter with variable neurologic and aural damage. Maternal hypothyroidism is associated with an increase in infertility and abortion. Maternal intake of 12 mg of iodide per day or more increases the risk of fetal goiter. Thioamides may cause fetal goiter but dose can be adjusted to minimize this effect.	Quality of available information: good. Fetopathic effect of iodides and antithyroid drugs involves metabolic block, decreased thyroid hormone synthesis and gland development.
Tocolytics	There are no reports of adverse fetal outcome resulting from exposure to therapeutic doses of terbutaline, ritodrine, or magnesium sulfate.	
Toluene	Intrauterine growth retardation; craniofacial anomalies; microcephaly. It is likely that high exposures from abuse or intoxication increase the risk of teratogenesis and abortion. Occupational exposures should present no increase in the teratogenic or abortigenic risk. The magnitude of the increased risk for teratogenesis and abortion in abusers is not known because the exposure in abusers is too variable.	Quality of available information: poor to fair. Neurotoxicity is produced in adults who abuse toluene; a similar effect may occur in the fetus.
Valproic acid	Malformations are primarily neural tube defects and facial dysmorphology. The facial characteristics associated with this drug are not diagnostic. Small head size and developmental delay have been reported with high doses. The risk for spina bifida is about 1% but the risk for facial dysmorphology may be greater. Because therapeutic exposures increase the incidence of neural tube defects, one would expect a slight increase in the incidence of abortion.	Quality of available information: good. Anticonvulsant; little is known about the teratogenic action of valproic acid.
Vitamins	*Biotin:* No adverse fetal effects for the usual therapeutic regimen

Cyanocobalamin: No adverse fetal effects for the usual therapeutic regimen.
Folic acid: The efficacy of folic acid supplementation for reducing the risk of neural tube defect recurrence may be limited to a select portion of the population. There are no adverse fetal effects for the usual therapeutic regimen.
Vitamin A: The same malformations that have been reported with the retinoids have been reported with very high doses of vitamin A (retinol). Exposures below 10,000 IU. present no risk to the fetus. Vitamin A in its recommended dose presents no increased risk for abortion.
Vitamin D: Large doses given in vitamin D prophylaxis are possibly involved in the etiology of supravalvular aortic stenosis, elfin faces, and mental retardation. There is no data on the abortigenic effect of vitamin D. | Used for treatment of multiple carboxylase deficiency
Used for treatment of vitamin B$_{12}$-responsive methylmalonic acidemia
Used for reduction in recurrence of neural tube defects

Quality of available information: good. High concentrations of retinoic acid are cytotoxic; it may interact with DNA to delay differentiation and/or inhibit protein synthesis.
Quality of available information: poor. Mechanism is likely to involve a disruption of cell calcium regulation with excessive doses. |

Modified from Friedman JM, Prolifka JE. Teratogenic effects of drugs (TERIS) 2nd ed. Baltimore: Johns Hopkins University Press, 2000.

Aminopterin and Methotrexate

Aminopterin and methotrexate (methylaminopterin) are folic acid antagonists that inhibit dihydrofolate reductase, resulting in cell death during the S phase of the cell cycle (55). Aminopterin-induced therapeutic abortions have resulted in malformations (hydrocephalus, cleft palate, meningomyelocele and growth retardation) in some of the abortuses (56–58). Three case reports of children exposed to aminopterin *in utero* included observations of growth retardation, abnormal cranial ossification, high-arched palate, and reduction in derivatives of the first branchial arch (59). The pattern of malformations associated with exposure to either compound has been referred to as the fetal aminopterin/methotrexate syndrome (60). Key features of this pattern of malformations include prenatal growth deficiency, abnormal cranial ossification, micrognathia, small low set ears, and limb abnormalities. There have also been three case reports to date of severe developmental delay in children with methotrexate syndrome (61–63). Methotrexate is used therapeutically as an abortifacient, treatment of rheumatoid arthritis and other autoimmune disorders, and as an antineoplastic agent. Skalko and Gold demonstrated a threshold effect and a dose-dependent increase in malformations in mice exposed to methotrexate in utero (64). Although malformations were induced in rats at doses exceeding those used in humans (65), smaller doses than those used in humans have resulted in malformation in rabbits (66). Analysis of human data indicate a critical period of exposure to methotrexate from 6–8 weeks from conception at a dose above 10 mg per week for the development of aminopterin/methotrexate syndrome (67). The risk of adverse effects as a result of aminopterin in the usual therapeutic range is not know precisely but appears to be moderate to high (58).

Androgens

Masculinization of the external genitalia of the female has been reported following in utero exposure to large doses of testosterone, methyltestosterone, and testosterone enanthate (68–70). The masculinization is characterized by clitoromegaly with or without fusion of the labia minora and no indication of nongenital malformations. Affected females experience normal secondary sexual development at puberty (71).

Many animal models show the masculinizing effects of androgens. Well-known studies were performed by Greene and coworkers in the rat, Raynaud in the mouse, Bruner and Witschi in the hamster, Jost in the rabbit, and Wells and Van Wagenen in the monkey (72–76). These studies demonstrated the masculinization of the urogenital sinus, its derivatives, and the external genitalia, although there was little effect on the mullerian ducts, and ovarian inversion did not occur. Based on experimental animal studies of altered sexually dimorphic behavior in female guinea pigs, rats and monkeys (77–82), behavioral masculinization of the female as a result of prenatal exposure to androgens in the human will be rare. The available literature indicates that the effects of androgens on the fetus are dependent on the dose and stage of development during which exposure occurred.

Angiotensin Converting Enzyme Inhibitors

The first angiotensin converting enzyme (ACE) inhibitor, captopril, was introduced in 1981 for the treatment of severe refractory hypertension. Since then the number of ACE inhibitors has increased and now includes enalapril, lisinopril, quinapril, perindopril, fosinopril, ramipril, and cilazapril (83). Their relative effectiveness, combined with a paucity of side effects as compared to other antihypertensives, have made these drugs extremely popular for the treatment of all types of hypertension and congestive heart failure and diabetic nephropathy.

ACE inhibitors are competitive inhibitors of ACE, a carboxypeptidase that forms an integral part of the renin angiotensin system (83). ACE catalyses the conversion of angiotensin I to angiotensin II, one of the most potent vasoconstrictors known. It is the same enzyme as kininase II, and also catalyses the breakdown of bradykinin. A vasodilatory peptide itself, bradykinin stimulates the release of other vasodilatory substances including prostaglandins and endothelium derived relaxation factor (84). Both mechanisms of action contribute to the decrease in blood pressure resulting from ACE inhibition (85).

Although they are considered relatively safe for the treatment of hypertension, the use of ACE inhibitors during pregnancy has been associated with adverse fetal outcomes in both humans and experimental animals. The first case of adverse fetal outcome in humans was reported in 1981 (86). In that report, treatment with captopril began on the 26th week of gestation, oligohydramnios was detected 2 weeks later, and a cesarean section was performed the following week. The child was anuric and hypotensive and died on day 7. The kidneys and bladder were morphologically normal but hemorrhagic foci were found in the renal cortex and medulla. Numerous cases of severe and often lethal adverse fetal effects associated with ACE inhibitor use during pregnancy have since been reported (87–89). The most consistent findings have been associated with a disruption of fetal renal function resulting in oligohydramnios and neonatal anuria accompanied by severe hypotension (87,89). Intrauterine growth retardation, pulmonary hypoplasia, hypocalvaria, persistent patent ductus arteriosis, and renal tubular dysgenesis have also been reported (89–91). Some of these effects may also result from the condition for which ACE inhibitors were prescribed (87). These effects have been associated with ACE inhibitor treatment only during the second and third trimester. There are no reports of adverse fetal outcome associated with ACE inhibitor use during the first trimester (89,91). As ACE inhibitors do not appear to affect organogenesis in either humans or in animal studies, it is not a classical teratogen. For this reason Pryde and associates (89) have proposed the term ACE inhibitor fetopathy to describe the characteristic syndrome that results from ACE inhibitor use during pregnancy.

The majority of adverse fetal effects associated with ACE inhibitor use during pregnancy result from the direct therapeutic action of ACE inhibitors on the fetus. ACE inhibitors readily cross the placenta in which they inhibit fetal ACE activity (89,92). The decreased renal blood flow caused by vasodilation of renal efferent arterioles results in a loss of glomerular filtration pressure leading to fetal anuria and oligohydramnios (92,93). This in turn may result in other adverse fetal outcomes, such as pulmonary hypoplasia. Fetal urine production and tubular function does not begin until approximately 9–12 weeks of gestation and probably explains the lack of adverse fetal effects when ACE inhibitor treatment is discontinued in the first trimester. Renal dysplasia, in particular a lack of renal proximal tubule differentiation, has also been noted in some effected fetuses (90,93,94).

Exposure to ACE inhibitors during pregnancy has also resulted in several cases of hypocalvaria, an ossification defect of the membranous bones of the skull that leaves the fetal brain inadequately protected (89,90). Although the pathogenesis is still unknown, inadequate perfusion of developing bone as a result of fetal hypotension combined with pressure from uterine muscles as a result of oligohydramnios may explain this defect (90,91). It has also been suggested that ACE inhibitors may affect ossification by acting on osteoblast-derived growth factors (90).

Despite consistent reports of adverse ace inhibitor fetopathy, there are no controlled studies available to assess the risks associated with the use of ACE inhibitors during pregnancy. Because there is no reported incidence of adverse fetal effects as a result of ACE inhibitor use during the first trimester of pregnancy, there is no contraindication to ACE inhibitors in women of reproductive age. If the woman becomes pregnant therapy is then changed to an alternative antihypertensive that represents less risk to the fetus.

Antibiotics

The incidence of intraamniotic infection is about 1% of all pregnancies but 3%–40% of women with ruptured membranes for 24 hours or more (95). Intraamniotic infection is associated with increased morbidity in the newborn including pneumonia, and sepsis. There is also a significant increase in perinatal mortality associated with intraamniotic infection although this is in part related to prematurity.

Increased neonatal mortality and morbidity, especially from group B streptococcal infection, can be largely prevented by intrapartum chemoprophylaxis. Neonatal sepsis is also significantly reduced if mothers receive intrapartum antibiotics. With few exceptions (such as streptomycin) acute exposure to antibiotics in usual therapeutic doses poses little significant risk to the fetus, especially in comparison to the potentially devastating effects of neonatal sepsis.

Aminoglycosides

This class of antimicrobials includes gentamicin, tobramycin, streptomycin and kanamycin. The only drug in this category with confirmed developmental toxicity is streptomycin. Based on case reports, there appears to be a small increased risk of sensorineural deafness in offspring of women treated with streptomycin for tuberculosis during pregnancy (96,97). Other congenital anomalies have not been associated with in utero exposure to streptomycin in the human (98). Because of the risk for ototoxicity, streptomycin should not be given during pregnancy. However, other aminoglycosides, such as kanamycin, appears to have minimal risk of causing similar adverse effects (99,100).

Anti-Tuberculosis Therapy

Drugs prescribed for the treatment of tuberculosis include aminoglycosides, ethambutol, isoniazid, rifampin, and ethionamide. The ototoxic effects of streptomycin are the only proven adverse effects of these drugs on the fetus. Neither ethambutol nor rifampin have been associated with an increase in the incidence of growth retardation, premature birth or malformations (96,97,101,102).

Early reports did not associate therapeutic exposures to isoniazid with an increased risk of malformations (96,97) but there is an unconfirmed association with CNS dysfunction (103,104). There was one attempted suicide involving 50 tablets of isoniazid per day during the 12th week that resulted in a stillbirth with arthrogryposis multiplex congenita syndrome (105). Isoniazid may have small increased risk for adverse effects on the CNS but there is no apparent increase in risk for congenital malformations or abortions with therapeutic exposures. Only one report associated ethionamide with an increased risk of teratogenic effects (106). However, this association is tenuous and not supported by other case reports (107).

As a general observation, the antituberculosis drugs produce adverse effects on the fetus of experimental animals in greater doses than those equivalent to therapeutic exposures and not in all species. Embryotoxicity can be demonstrated for streptomycin in the mouse, kanamycin in the guinea pig, isoniazid in the rat, rifampin in the rat, and ethionamide in the rabbit (108–110). While this does not eliminate the possibility of adverse effects on the fetus following exposure to the other prescribed tuberculostatic medications discussed, therapeutic exposures appear to represent a very small risk of teratogenesis and even less risk of abortion.

Cephalosporins

Cephalosporins are frequently prescribed during pregnancy. Examples include cephalexin (Keflex), cefixime (Suprax), and cefaclor (Ceclor). Although generally considered safe for use in pregnancy, epidemiological studies examining the effects of this class of antibiotics on the developing fetus are scarce. However, available data indicate that, although a small risk cannot be completely excluded, a high risk of congenital anomalies resulting from in utero exposure in the first trimester is unlikely (111).

Macrolides

This category includes erythromycin, azithromycin, and clarithromycin (Biaxin). Erythromycin does not readily cross the placenta and is generally considered safe for use in pregnancy. There is less available data on azithromycin and clarithromycin however existing data indicate that any potential risk is minimal. As is the case with other sexually transmitted diseases, chlamydia infection is on the increase. The infant most likely acquires chlamydial infection during parturition at an incidence of approximately 50%. Erythromycin is an effective prenatal treatment.

Metronidazole

Metronidazole (Flagyl) is used most frequently to treat trichomoniasis, various other protozoan and anaerobic bacterial infections, and to help prevent preterm labor. Administration is given orally, rectally and parenterally. Vaginal absorption occurs readily but plasma levels achieved are much lower than those achieved by other routes. There are a large number of studies examining the risk of exposure during pregnancy to the developing fetus. Epidemiological studies, and the majority of animal studies have not revealed an increased risk of congenital anomalies with exposure during the first trimester (112–117), or when used to prevent preterm labor in the third trimester (118,119). Based on these studies therapeutic use of metronidazole during pregnancy is generally considered safe. Although some bacterial test systems indicated mutagenicity, there is no evidence for increased chromosomal abnormalities in human cells (120–122).

Penicillin

The most frequently prescribed drugs in this category include penicillin, ampicillin, and amoxicillin. Newer agents may also contain an agent to enhance effectiveness against resistant microbials such as the use of amoxicillin with clavulanic acid (Augmentin). There are no adverse fetal effects reported for any penicillins. Among other uses penicillin is used in pregnancy to treat Treponema pallidum in pregnant women.

Quinolones

Fluoroquinolones (ciprofloxacin, norfloxacin, ofloxacin), are used to treat urinary infections. Reports of use in early pregnancy have not revealed any teratogenic or developmental risk (123–130). Studies in immature dogs and rodents revealed a potential for arthropathy and cartilage erosion (131). Musculoskeletal dysfunction was not noted in a multicenter prospective controlled study of 200 women exposed to fluoroquinolones during pregnancy (124). Effects on cartilage and bone would be unlikely in the first trimester and there are few studies addressing long term effects with late pregnancy exposure. Based on available evidence quinolone antibiotics do not appear to pose a risk to the fetus at therapeutic doses however more studies are needed to address the potential for osteotoxicity in the neonate and juvenile.

Sulfonamides

Sulfonamides are usually combined with other antibiotics, such as in trimethoprim-sulfamethoxazole (Bactrim). Due to the possibility of jaundice in the newborn, sulfonamides should not be used during the last trimester of pregnancy, or during nursing. Trimethoprim is a folate

metabolism antagonist and thus has potential for adverse embryonic and fetal effects (see Trimethoprim below).

Tetracyclines

This class of antibiotics includes tetracycline and doxycycline. Tetracycline crosses the placenta but is not concentrated by the fetus. Tetracyclines complex with calcium and the organic matrix of newly forming bone without altering the crystalline structure of hydroxyapatite (132). Although tetracycline has been shown to discolor teeth without affecting the likelihood of developing carries (133,134), very high doses may depress skeletal bone growth. No congenital malformations of any other organ system have been associated with antenatal tetracycline exposures (98). Several case reports of limb reduction defects in human embryos exposed to tetracycline are not supported by epidemiological studies or animals studies. Therapeutic doses of tetracycline are associated with no or minimal increased risk of congenital malformations but they are likely to result in some degree of dental staining, which does not appear to have a deleterious effect on the offspring.

Untreated Neisseria gonorrhoeae can lead to serious consequences for the infected woman. Treatment with ceftriaxone plus doxycycline has no reported adverse effects on the fetus.

Trimethoprim

Trimethoprim is an inhibitor of microbial dihydrofolate reductase, and is usually combined with a sulfonamide for treatment of urinary tract infections. Early studies did not report an association between exposure to trimethoprim during pregnancy and congenital anomalies (135–138). However, more recent studies using much larger study populations have reported increases in the incidence of neural tube defects, orofacial clefts and cardiovascular defects among infants exposed to trimethoprim during the first three months of pregnancy (139–142). Use of a vitamin supplement containing folic acid during treatment resulted in a reduced risk in these studies.

Trimethoprim was not teratogenic in rodents using less than 10 times the human therapeutic dose for treatment of urinary tract infections, and caused malformations and intrauterine death at high doses (>16 times therapeutic doses) (143–145). The relevance of these findings to human risk at therapeutic doses is unclear.

Due to the potential for adverse effects on folate metabolism in the pregnant woman and fetus, trimethoprim should be avoided during pregnancy.

Antihypertensives (Excluding Angiotensin Converting Enzyme Inhibitors)

Clonidine

Clonidine exerts its hypotensive effect by a direct alpha adrenergic agonistic action in the CNS. It is used to treat hypertension and may also be given epidurally with epidural anesthesia. It appears to be relatively safe during pregnancy but there are few available data regarding effects of exposure during the first trimester of pregnancy. When used during labor with epidural anesthesia there are reports of a small but increased frequency of fetal bradycardia (146,147) and, even less commonly, transient neonatal hypotension (148,149).

Hydralazine

Hydralazine is a vasodilator often used in combination with methyldopa for the treatment of preexisting hypertension in pregnancy and is considered to be safe. Although there is one report of fetal thrombocytopenia (150), over 120 normal pregnancies have been reported (151). Additionally there have been reports of an increased frequency of fetal distress in neonates born to women treated with hydralazine near term (152–154).

Methyldopa

Methyldopa is currently the safest antihypertensive drug available for use during pregnancy (155). Methyldopa is a centrally acting adrenergic antagonist with no reported adverse effects on the fetus or on mental and physical development.

Nifedipine

Nifedipine is a calcium channel blocker used for the treatment of preterm labor with no reported adverse effects. The potential for adverse effects with its long term use in the treatment of hypertension is unknown.

Propranolol

Propranolol is a β-blocker useful in treating preexisting hypertension during pregnancy. There have been no reports of associations with use in the first trimester and congenital anomalies (156). However, prolonged use may cause intrauterine growth retardation (157–163). Moreover, there have been several reports of difficulties in perinatal adaptation associated with maternal treatment late in pregnancy and shortly prior to delivery including apnea and respiratory distress (159,160,164–166).

Aspirin

Aspirin acts principally by inhibiting prostaglandin synthesis by irreversibly acetylating and inactivating fatty acid cyclooxygenase. Low-dose aspirin (60–150 mg per day) is used clinically in the prevention or treatment of a variety of conditions that affect maternal and fetal health. For instance, aspirin is used for the treatment of systemic lupus erythematosus, antiphospholipid syndrome, and preeclampsia.

Of obvious concern is the potential for increased fetal and maternal bleeding associated with low-dose aspirin use near the time of delivery or higher doses used to treat preterm labor. Jankowski and associates reported a study involving 25 women threatened with premature delivery who were given 3.6 g of oral aspirin per day for 4 successive days within 10 days prior to delivery (167). They and others have found no adverse effect on maternal bleeding at delivery, fetal hemorrhage, or circulatory disorders.

There is some evidence that aspirin combined with dipyridamole may prevent or ameliorate intrauterine growth retardation associated with idiopathic uteroplacental insufficiency. Fetal growth was also improved with aspirin (150 mg per day) alone in fetuses with high, but not extreme, umbilical artery systolic/diastolic ratio. Third trimester exposure to low daily doses of aspirin were not associated with adverse fetal outcome in these studies (168,169).

High fetal losses are associated with lupus anticoagulant antibodies, anticardiolipin antibodies and systemic lupus erythematosus. Surviving fetuses experience an increased incidence of growth retardation, fetal distress, and preterm delivery. Low-dose aspirin (60–80 mg per day) in combination with prednisone (20–80 mg per day) improves pregnancy outcome and greatly reduces thrombosis (170).

Case reports suggest that 75 to 300 mg of aspirin per day in combination with dipyridamole might reduce the risk of late fetal loss in patients with arterial thromboembolism, thrombotic thrombocytopenia purpura, and idiopathic or essential thrombocythemia (170).

Although doubts concerning the safety of aspirin during pregnancy have been expressed, aspirin use during the first trimester is not associated with an increased teratogenic risk (171). Third trimester exposure to 80 mg per day or less are not associated with an early constriction of the ductus arteriosus (172). Much larger doses of aspirin during the third trimester have been associated with an increased length of gestation, duration of labor, frequency of postmaturity and blood loss at delivery (173) and justify careful fetal surveillance.

Benzodiazepines

The benzodiazepines, such as chlordiazepoxide (Librium), diazepam (Valium), xanax, and meprobamate, are widely used as tranquilizers during pregnancy and, therefore, it is not surprising that they have been associated with congenital malformations in some publications.

Chlordiazepoxide was associated with various anomalies after exposure during early pregnancy but no syndrome was identified (98,174). Other studies were inconclusive or found no association (175–177). Chlordiazepoxide appears to have a minimal risk for congenital anomalies and no increased risk for abortion at therapeutic doses. Higher exposures are likely to increase the risk of adverse effects on the fetus but the magnitude of the increase is not known.

Some studies reported an association between diazepam and increased incidence of congenital malformations

(177). However, a follow-up study found no associations (178). The majority of studies of fetal outcome following *in utero* exposure to diazepam are negative (112,175–180). Behavior alterations have been reported in infants exposed to benzodiazepines, mostly diazepam (181), but this observation must be confirmed and the long-term developmental outcome evaluated before it can be appropriately interpreted. Although third trimester exposure to diazepam can reversibly affect the fetus and neonate (182) there is minimal increased risk of congenital malformations and no demonstrated increased risk of abortions from therapeutic exposures.

Meprobamate has been weakly associated with a variety of congenital malformations (183,184). Other studies found no associations (98,176). Because of inconsistencies, the data are not sufficient to confirm or rule out a small increase risk of malformations as a result of exposures early in pregnancy.

Benzodiazepines appear to have minimal increased risk of malformations at therapeutic ranges; higher exposures may increase the risk. The risk for abortion is unknown but given the widespread use of these drugs, it is unlikely that a significant abortigenic effect would have gone unnoticed.

Caffeine

Caffeine is a methylated xanthine, which acts as a CNS stimulant. It is contained in many beverages including coffee, tea, and colas, and chocolate. Caffeine is also present in many over-the-counter medications, such as cold and allergy tablets, analgesics, diuretics, and stimulants; the latter lead to relatively minimal population intakes. Caffeine containing food and beverages are consumed in large quantities by most of the human populations of the world. The per capita consumption of caffeine from all sources is estimated to be about 200 mg/day, or about 3 to 7 mg/kg per day (185). Consumption of caffeinated beverages during pregnancy is quite common and is estimated to be approximately 144 mg per day (186).

Current evidence, does not appear to implicate the usual exposure of caffeine as a human teratogen, however, associations between maternal coffee drinking during pregnancy and miscarriage or poor fetal growth have been reported in epidemiological studies (187–191). In many instances these associations are largely attributable to confounding effects of maternal cigarette smoking or other factors. Some of these studies (192) have serious methodological limitations. If maternal consumption of caffeine-containing beverages in conventional amounts during pregnancy does have an association with the rate of miscarriage or fetal growth retardation, the effect appears to be relatively small.

In other studies no association has been found between caffeine consumption during pregnancy and congenital defects (98,193,194). For instance, Rosenberg and associates analyzed six selected birth defects in relation to maternal ingestion of more than 8 mg/kg per day of tea, coffee, or cola (195). The defects were inguinal hernia, cleft lip/cleft palate, cardiac defects, pyloric stenosis, cleft palate (isolated) and neural tube fusion defects. None of the point estimates of relative risk was significantly greater than unity, suggesting that caffeine was not a major teratogen, at least for the defects evaluated.

Interpretation of the available information pertaining to the animal and human studies regarding the teratogenicity of caffeine leads us to conclude that the usual exposure of caffeine does not present a measurable risk in the human for any one malformation or group of malformations. There is a clear indication that the consumer must ingest a substantial amount of caffeine to have an effect on the developing embryo or fetus; total consumption of 300 mg/day may be a safe upper daily limit. Most reviewers and investigators concluded that there is a threshold, below which caffeine does not exert a detrimental effect, and the usual human consumption falls in this nontoxic range. The quantity of caffeine consumed in an average cup of coffee, about 1.4 to 2.1 mg/kg (196), is believed to be below the amount that induces congenital defects in animals. Quantities of caffeine in tea and soft drinks would be even less.

Carbamazepine

Although epidemiological and case report studies have not yielded consistent results, exposure to carbamazepine has been associated with minor craniofacial defects, fingernail hypoplasia, developmental delay (197,198), reduced birthweight, length and head circumference (199) and neural tube defects (200). Confounding the issue is the possibility that epilepsy itself may increase the risk for malformations (201). However, an attempted suicide involving carbamazepine produced blood levels of 27–28 µg/mL (the therapeutic range is 8–12 µg/mL) during what was estimated to be 3–4 weeks postconception (202). The fetus was later determined to have myeloschisis with carbamazepine the only known exogenous risk factor. This suggests that carbamazepine has the potential to produce neural tube defects at about two- to three-fold the therapeutic level. It appears that the risk for minor defects is significant but the risk for all teratogenic effects is not known. The risk for abortion is also not known but appears to be small.

Cocaine

Cocaine (benzoylmethylecgonine) is one of the most commonly used illicit drugs by women of reproductive age. Reported estimates for cocaine use during pregnancy range from 3% to 17%, the highest rates occurring in inner city populations (203). Because of its widespread use during pregnancy and the growing cost of caring for cocaine exposed neonates, there has been increasing concern over the risks associated with prenatal cocaine use to maternal and fetal health. Yet despite numerous clinical studies linking prenatal cocaine use with a variety of adverse maternal and fetal effects, methodological limitations in these studies have made it difficult to establish a causal relationship between these alleged effects and maternal cocaine use. Not only are the timing, frequency and dose of cocaine use hard to determine, but adverse effects as a result of low socioeconomic status, poor nutrition, multiple drug use, infections, and a lack of prenatal care are difficult to dissociate from effects as a result of cocaine use alone (203). As such the issue of how much risk to the fetus is associated with cocaine use during pregnancy is unresolved. Nonetheless a growing body of literature supports the concept that cocaine is a developmental toxicant. Adverse effects attributed to prenatal cocaine exposure include a higher incidence of spontaneous abortion, placental abruption, still birth, prematurity, low birth weight, growth retardation, decreased head circumference, intracerebral hemorrhage, congenital defects, neurobehavioral abnormalities, and a possible association with increased risk of sudden infant death syndrome (SIDS) (203,204). These effects are reduced but not eliminated in mothers receiving appropriate prenatal care. Like other developmental toxins, outcome is dependent on dose and time of use.

The majority of adverse effects associated with cocaine use during pregnancy appear to be as a result of high levels of cocaine abuse in later stages of gestation rather than in the first trimester or organogenesis (205). Moderate usage of cocaine only in the first trimester does not appear to result in adverse fetal outcome and may not pose an increased risk to the fetus (206).

Adverse fetal outcomes associated with maternal cocaine use are thought to primarily result from the vasoconstrictive effects of cocaine on both the maternal and fetal vasculature (205). Vasoconstriction of the uterine arteries, which are normally fully dilated during pregnancy, may compromise fetal growth and development. Studies in animals have confirmed that cocaine reduces uterine artery and placental blood flow leading to reduced oxygen and nutrient supply to the fetus (207). Fetal cardiovascular effects resulting from uterine vasoconstriction include hypertension, tachycardia, hypoxia and an increase in cerebral blood flow (207,208). Cocaine also crosses the placenta in which it has a direct effect on the fetal vasculature flow (207). Fetal hypertension combined with increased cerebral blood flow may result in intracerebral hemorrhage or infarction, which has been reported to occur in cocaine exposed fetuses in both human and animal studies (209–211).

Disruption of uterine and fetal vasculature may also lead to a variety of congenital anomalies that have been associated with cocaine abuse. A significant association between cocaine use and an increased incidence of genitourinary tract malformations has been found (209,211,212). Other defects reported include limb reduction defects, nonduodenal intestinal atresia, cardiac anomalies, hypospadias, prune belly syndrome as a result of urethral obstruction, hydronephrosis and crossed renal ectopia (208,209,211). Two cases of limb-body wall complex have also been

reported (213) With the exception of genitourinary tract malformations, the sample size in these clinical studies has not been sufficient to determine a statistically significant relationship between cocaine use and these congenital anomalies (214).

Coumarin Derivatives

Nasal hypoplasia following exposure to several drugs, including warfarin, during pregnancy was reported by DiSaia (215). Kerber and associates (216) were the first to suggest warfarin as the teratogenic agent. Coumarin anticoagulants have since been associated with nasal hypoplasia, calcific stippling of the secondary epiphysis, and CNS abnormalities. Warfarin embryopathy has been described and an overview of the difficulties in relating a congenital malformation to an environmental cause and has been published (217,218). There is an estimated 10% risk for affected infants following exposure during the period from the eighth through the fourteenth week of pregnancy, although this risk has been reported to be much lower in some series, and other factors besides dose and gestational stage seem to play a role (218). Low-dose warfarin (5 mg/day or less) throughout pregnancy did not result in any adverse effects in 20 offspring (219).

Coumarin inhibits the formation of carboxyglutamyl residues from glutamyl residues, decreasing the ability of proteins to bind calcium. The inhibition of calcium binding by proteins during embryonic/fetal development, especially during a critical period of ossification, could explain the nasal hypoplasia, stippled calcification, and skeletal abnormalities of warfarin embryopathy (218). Microscopic bleeding does not seem to be responsible for these problems early in development (217).

One case report was unique in that the time of exposure to warfarin was between 8 and 12 weeks of gestation, and the infant presented Dandy-Walker malformation, eye defects, and agenesis of the corpus callosum (220). This case report is the clearest evidence for a direct effect of warfarin on the developing CNS rather than an effect mediated by hemorrhage, because the exposure is well defined and occurs before the appearance of vitamin K-dependent clotting factors. Further supportive evidence for a direct pathogenic role of warfarin is the report of an infant with an inherited deficiency of multiple vitamin K-dependent coagulation factors whose congenital anomalies were similar to warfarin syndrome without exposure to warfarin (221). The risk of stillbirths and spontaneous abortions is increased in pregnant women treated with warfarin but the risk may be less if the exposure is in the last half of pregnancy. The risk of adverse effects as a result of hemorrhaging increases later in gestation.

Cyclophosphamide

Cyclophosphamide, a widely used antineoplastic agent, is also used in severe rheumatic disease. Cyclophosphamide is likely to be teratogenic in the human but the magnitude of the teratogenic risk is uncertain. The reported defects include growth retardation, ectrodactyly, syndactyly, cardiovascular anomalies, and other minor anomalies (222–224). Ten normal pregnancies have been reported after cyclophosphamide exposure (225).

The mechanism of cyclophosphamide teratogenesis was reviewed by Mirkes (24): cytochrome P-450 monooxygenases convert cyclophosphamide to 4-hydroxycyclophosphamide, which in turn breaks down to phosphoramide mustard and acrolein. Phosphoramide mustard may produce teratogenic effects by interacting with cellular DNA in an as yet undefined manner although acrolein acts in a different manner, possibly by affecting sulfhydryl linkages in proteins (226). Tissue sensitivity to phosphoramide mustard and acrolein is thought to be related to such processes as detoxification and cellular repair.

Diethylstilbestrol

The first abnormality reported following exposure to diethylstilbestrol (DES) during the first trimester was clitoromegaly in female newborns (227). Herbst and associates (228,229) and Greenwald and associates (230) later reported an association of vaginal adenocarcinoma in female offspring following first trimester exposures. DES is the only drug with proven transplacental carcinogenic action in the human. Almost all of the cancers occurred after 14 years of age and only in those exposed before the 18th week of gestation. There is a 75 percent risk for vaginal adenosis for exposures occurring before the ninth week of pregnancy; the risk of developing adenocarcinoma is about 1:1,000 to 1:10,000 (231). While the incidence of vaginal adenosis was related to the amount of DES administered, the incidence of vaginal carcinoma does not appear to be related to the maternal dose.

Although there does not appear to be an adverse effect on menstrual cycle functioning or on the rate of conception, the anatomic abnormalities of the uterus and cervix induced by intrauterine exposure to DES, including T-shaped uterus, transverse fibrous ridges and uterine hypoplasia, cause the increased incidence of ectopic pregnancies, spontaneous abortions and premature delivery in pregnancies of women exposed to DES *in utero* (232–235).

There have been reports that males exposed to DES *in utero* exhibited genital lesions and abnormal spermatozoa (236,237). Other studies reported no increase in the risk for the male for genitourinary abnormalities or infertility (238). An association between *in utero* exposure to DES and testicular cancer in male offspring has been suggested but the data are not conclusive (238,239). The controversial nature of the effects of DES exposure on the male may be attributable to study design or, more likely, to the fact that dose levels varied greatly according to different regimens: exposures during the first half of pregnancies varied from 1.5 to 150 mg per day with total doses from 135 mg to 18 g (231).

DES is a potent nonsteroidal estrogen and, as in the case of steroidal estrogens, must interact with the receptor proteins present only in estrogen-responsive tissues before exerting its effects by stimulating ribonucleic acid (RNA), protein, and DNA synthesis. The carcinogenic effect of DES is most likely indirect: DES exposure results in the presence of columnar epithelium in the vagina, and this misplaced tissue may have a greater susceptibility to developing the adenocarcinoma, much as teratomas and other misplaced tissues are more susceptible to malignant degeneration.

Digoxin

Digoxin is used to correct fetal tachyarrhythmias with no substantiated adverse fetal effects (240). However, the possibility of any adverse side effects must be balanced with the fetal prognosis if the dysrhythmia persists or is likely to lead to fetal cardiac failure.

Diphenylhydantoin

Hanson and Smith (241) characterized the fetal hydantoin syndrome in infants whose mothers were treated for epilepsy with hydantoin anticonvulsants. Chronic exposure to diphenylhydantoin has been suggested to present a maximum of 10% risk for the full syndrome and a maximum of 30% risk for some anomalies (242–245). Although cleft lip and palate, congenital heart disease, and microcephaly have been reported, hypoplasias of the nails and distal phalanges are possibly more common malformations in the exposed fetuses (246,247). Hanson and associates noted that, although the hydantoin syndrome is observed in 11% of the subjects in their study, three times that number exhibit mental deficits (31,248). Prospective studies demonstrate a much lower frequency of effects, and some do not demonstrate any effect; thus, the overall prospective risk may be much lower for the classically reported effects.

Factors associated with epilepsy may contribute to the etiology of these malformations (249). Based on the United States Collaborative Perinatal Project and a large Finnish registry, the incidence of malformations was 10.5% when the mother was epileptic, 8.3% when the father was epileptic and 6.4% when neither parent was affected (250).

Cleft lip and palate, skeletal anomalies, and cardiac defects have been produced in rabbits (31,251) mice (252–255), and rats (256,257), and the malformation rate was dose-dependent (253,258).

Glucocorticoids

Glucocorticoids (dexamethasone, betamethasone, hydrocortisone, methylprednisone) are effective in reducing the incidence of respiratory distress syndrome in premature newborns by inducing early lung maturation as first hypothesized by Liggins (259). Endogenous glucocorticoids mediate normal pulmonary maturation. Exogenous glucocorticoids are used to stimulate the production of surfactant. The adverse fetal effects observed in experimental animals exposed to pharmacological doses are not seen in humans at therapeutic levels (260–262).

Dexamethasone is used to suppress the fetal adrenal gland in cases of congenital adrenal hyperplasia (263). 21-Hydroxylase deficiency impairs the conversion of cholesterol to cortisol and results in excess 17-hydroxyprogesterone which in turn results in excess levels of androgens. The masculinization of female fetuses with congenital adrenal hyperplasia varies from clitoral hypertrophy to formation of a phallus. Maternal replacement doses of dexamethasone suppress both the maternal and fetal adrenal glands and prevent masculinization in most patients (264).

Glucocorticoids are also used in the treatment of rheumatic diseases, other acute and chronic inflammatory diseases, and organ transplantation. Although some studies have reported increased frequency of perinatal death, prematurity and intrauterine growth retardation with chronic therapy, women in these studies typically had severe autoimmune or other diseases, or history of fetal loss requiring treatment, thus these findings cannot be attributed to the glucocorticoid therapy itself (223,265–271). Dexamethasone poses minimal or no teratogenic risk at therapeutic doses in humans and the benefits of glucocorticoid treatment, particularly dexamethasone, for prevention of masculinization as a result of congenital adrenal hyperplasia, and betamethasone for the prevention of the respiratory distress syndrome in premature infants, and potentially other complications arising from prematurity are clear (272–276).

Indomethacin

Oral administration of the prostaglandin synthetase inhibitor, Indomethacin, is a prostaglandin synthetase inhibitor that is used as an analgesic, an antiinflammatory, and an antipyretic agent. Indomethacin is also effective in the treatment of polyhydramnios that is either idiopathic or related to maternal diabetes mellitus. Administration of indomethacin during the first trimester has not been shown to increase the frequency of congenital malformations (112). Late in pregnancy maternal administration of indomethacin may cause oligohydramnios, constriction of the ductus arteriosus (prostaglandins are necessary to maintain the patency of the fetal ductus arteriosus), fetal hydrops and persistent pulmonary hypertension in the newborn, potentially serious side effects of indomethacin that warrant careful fetal and neonatal surveillance (277–280). The risk for premature closure of the ductus arteriosus increases with treatment after 32 weeks (281–283). Indomethacin may also be used to prevent preterm labor or intraventricular hemorrhage; however its efficacy when used for this purpose is controversial. Indomethacin may also predispose the neonate to necrotizing enterocolitis when used as a tocolytic (284,285).

Lithium Carbonate

Lithium carbonate, widely used for treatment of manic-depressive disorders, was first associated with human congenital malformations in 1970 (286,287). The malformations described include heart and large-vessel anomalies, Epstein's anomaly, neural tube defects, talipes, microtia, and thyroid abnormalities (288–290). Lithium readily crosses the placenta (291), and appears to be a human teratogen at therapeutic dosages but it presents a small risk. Although early reports suggested a strong association of prenatal lithium exposure with cardiac defects, in particular Epstein's anomaly, more recent evidence from controlled epidemiological studies suggests that the risk for malformations is much lower than initially thought (292,293). The results of a retrospective study suggest that lithium may also increase the risk for premature delivery (294), but again the magnitude of the risk is likely to be small. Only one follow-up study has been published examining long-term effects of lithium on early development. In this study children exposed prenatally to lithium with no congenital abnormalities at birth did not show any signs of developmental delay at 7.3 years follow-up (295). Fetal toxicity has been associated with late gestational maternal lithium use with and without obvious maternal toxicity. One reported side effect is nephrogenic diabetes insipidus (296–298) and associated polyhydramnios which may increase the likelihood of premature labor (294,297). Transient toxic effects have also been reported in neonates exposed late in pregnancy. These include hypothyroidism, lethargy, hypostomia, cardiac murmur, renal toxicity, persistent fetal circulation and diabetes insipidus (299–302). To prevent lithium intoxication in the neonate the lithium dosage of the patient should be adjusted to avoid high serum levels in the second and third trimester (293).

Lithium can induce abnormal development in several laboratory animals, but the mechanisms of the teratogenic action of lithium is not known (303–305). The neurotropic activity of lithium suggests that CNS malformations may result from cell membrane disturbances which affect neural tube closure (306).

Because of the value of lithium carbonate for treating manic-depressive psychosis, the risk associated with psychiatric relapse on removing the drug may be more important clinically than the teratogenic risk. Moreover, the risk of alternative pharmacological agents for treatment of bipolar disorder may exceed the risk from lithium carbonate (307).

Methylene Blue

Methylene blue has been used clinically for a variety of purposes including the identification of anatomic structures, the treatment of methemoglobinemia, and to mark the amniotic cavity during amniocentesis. Use of methylene blue in late gestation to detect rupture of fetal membranes has been associated with adverse fetal effects including hyperbilirubinemia, hemolytic anemia and staining of the skin (308–311). There is currently not enough data to determine whether respiratory distress in these infants may also result from late gestation methylene blue exposure (312).

There have been several reports of an increased prevalence of small intestinal atresia in twins with intraamniotic exposure to methylene blue. Twinning itself results in an increased prevalence of intestinal atresia, increasing from approximately 2 to 2.5 per 10,000 in singletons to 5 to 7.3 per 10,000 amongst twins (313). However, in twins exposed to midgestational amniocentesis in which methylene blue was used to mark the amniotic cavity the prevalence of small intestinal atresia has been reported as high as 9.6% (314). The strongest evidence indicating that methylene blue is a teratogen is a retrospective study from Amsterdam. In this study methylene blue was injected into one amniotic cavity of 86 twin pregnancies undergoing midgestation amniocentesis. Jejunal atresia occurred in 17 infants, each from different pregnancies (314). In 15 of these cases it was possible to determine which twin was exposed to methylene blue, and in each case the twin exposed to methylene blue had jejunal atresia. Based on this evidence and several other reports there appears to be a significant risk of small intestinal atresia associated with exposure to methylene blue during midgestation amniocentesis (311,313,315–319). Intraamniotic exposure to methylene blue has not been associated with any other malformation (312). Whether midgestation exposure to methylene blue increases the incidence of fetal death has not been clearly established (320,321). In rats, intraamniotic injection of methylene blue increased fetal loss (322).

Misoprostol

Misoprostol is a synthetic prostaglandin E1 methyl analogue used for the prevention of gastric ulcers induced by nonsteroidal antiinflammatory drugs. It has known, but not very effective, abortifacient properties. Gonzalez and associates (323) recently reported seven newborns with vascular disruptive phenomena (limb reduction defects, Moebius syndrome) whose mothers used misoprostol early in pregnancy in an attempt to induce abortion. Although there is evidence that misoprostol is used illegally by thousands of pregnant Brazilian women as an abortifacient (324–326), controlled cohort or case control epidemiological studies of the fetal outcome of failed abortions are not available. Although the data available are not conclusive, the uterine bleeding produced by misoprostol and type of malformations produced suggest a vascular disruption mechanism for misoprostol induced teratogenesis.

If one is looking for vascular disruption, it will more likely be produced later in gestation. Therefore, classical animal teratology experiments will not detect the vascular disruptive effect of drugs or chemicals unless they are exposed beyond the period of early organogenesis (327). Furthermore, it has become clear that if an agent produces vascular disruption, it is a rare event and therefore large populations would need to be studied before the effect may be discovered (328).

Previous case reports are also of little assistance. Collins and Mahoney (329) reported an infant with hydrocephalus and attenuated digital phalanges after exposure intravaginally to 15-methyl F2alpha prostaglandin five weeks after conception. Schuler and associates (330) reported that 29% of women who used misoprostol in Brazil as an abortifacient failed to abort. Seventeen children who failed to abort were observed to have no malformations. Wood and associates (331) reported an infant exposed to oxytocin and prostaglandin E2 for the purpose of termination to have hydrocephaly and growth retardation. Schonhofer (332) and Fonesca and associates (333) reported five Brazilian infants with defects of the skull and overlying scalp who were exposed to misoprostol in utero. These case reports indicate the low risk of misoprostol exposure and the possibility that some of the features reported may or may not be as a result of misoprostol (334). It is too early to know the extent of the effects of misoprostol, but it is biologically plausible that they should include all of the features of vascular disruption.

Oxazolidine-2,4-diones (Trimethadione, Paramethadione)

Trimethadione and paramethadione are antiepileptic oxazolidine-2,4-diones that distribute uniformly throughout body tissues and exert their effects by means of the action of their metabolites. These drugs affect cell membrane permeability and vitamin K-dependent clotting factors, but their primary mode of action is unknown.

Zackai and associates (335) described the fetal trimethadione syndrome characterized by developmental delay, V-shaped eyebrows, low-set ears with anteriorly folded helix, high arched palate and irregular teeth. Clinical observations of these and other associated findings, such as cardiovascular, genitourinary and gastrointestinal anomalies, have been reviewed (335–338). The incidence of miscarriage, stillbirth and infant death was also increased. There are wide variations in reported risk, with estimates as high as 80% for major or minor defects. Because the number of exposures is small, the actual risk could vary considerably from these figures. Although there are variations in incidences reported amongst studies, the risk of malformation or other adverse fetal effects is considered high, therefore the drug should not be used in pregnant women.

D-Penicillamine

D-Penicillamine has been used in the treatment of rheumatoid arthritis and cystinuria. D-Penicillamine is a copper chelator and copper deficiency appears to be the mechanism for teratogenicity (339). Exposure to D-penicillamine can induce a connective tissue defect including generalized cutis laxa, hyperflexibility of the joints, varicosities and impaired wound healing (340–342). The exposure must be long enough to induce a copper deficiency sufficient to inhibit collagen synthesis and maturation. However, the condition appears to be reversible and the risk is low, 5% or less.

Phenobarbital

Phenobarbital is used as a sedative and anticonvulsant. Risk of congenital anomalies is unlikely with occasional exposure to phenobarbital in therapeutic doses during pregnancy. Use of phenobarbital for long term treatment of seizure disorders such as epilepsy may be associated with a small to minimal risk of increase in congenital malformations such as cleft palate and congenital heart defects (177,250,343–347). Some of these effects may relate directly to the disease being treated itself, rather than to phenobarbital (348). The risk appears to be greater in cases in which phenobarbital was combined with other drugs such as phenytoin (344,346,349–351). Some studies report no increased risk for congenital anomalies with use of phenobarbital for treatment of epilepsy. However, other studies report an increased incidence of minor congenital anomalies with phenobarbital monotherapy with a characteristic pattern of minor dysmorphic features, termed the "fetal anticonvulsant syndrome" including nail and midface hypoplasia and depressed nasal bridge (345, 352–354).

In two prospective, studies of patients in high risk groups for neonatal intraventricular hemorrhage, intravenous phenobarbital administered antenatally resulted in a significant reduction in the incidence of severe cases of intraventricular hemorrhage by increasing cerebral vascular resistance (355). Phenobarbital reduces peak arterial blood pressure, thereby reducing the risk for intraventricular hemorrhage, one of the leading complications of the very low birth-weight preterm infant (356). Initiation of intravenous phenobarbital in the early neonatal period is probably too late to derive the potential benefits of this therapy.

Progestins

It is often overlooked that, although various progestins utilized therapeutically as progestational agents act by means of similar receptors, their potential androgenic effects can differ markedly. This point is critical to the evaluation of the virilizing effects of these compounds in the human. It has been shown, for example, that the pharmacokinetic parameters that estimate steroid bioavailability and metabolism show great variability among subjects and between steroids conveniently grouped together, such as "progestins" (357). One must assume that these differences in bioavailability and metabolism reflect differences in the biological activity of these steroids in humans.

In contrast to progesterone and 17α-hydroxyprogesterone caproate, high doses of some of the synthetic progestins have been reported to cause virilizing effects in humans. Exposure during the first trimester to large doses of 17α-ethinyltestosterone has been associated with masculinization of the external genitalia of female fetuses (358). Similar associations result from exposure to large doses of 17α-ethinyl-19-nortestosterone (norethindrone) (358) and 17α-ethinyl-17-OH-5(10)estren-3-one (Enovid-R)

(68). The synthetic progestins, like progesterone, can influence only those tissues with the appropriate steroid receptors. The preparations with androgenic properties may cause abnormalities in the genital development of females only if present in sufficient amounts during critical periods of development. In 1959, Grumbach and associates (68) pointed out that labioscrotal fusion could be produced with large doses if the fetuses were exposed before the thirteenth week of pregnancy, whereas clitoromegaly could be produced after this period, illustrating that a specific form of maldevelopment can be induced only when the embryonic tissues are in a susceptible stage of development.

The World Health Organization (359) reported that there is a suspicion that combined oral contraceptives or progestogens may be weakly teratogenic but that the magnitude of the relative risk is small. In a large retrospective study, Heinonen and associates (360) reported a positive association between cardiovascular defects and in utero exposure to female sex hormones. A revaluation of some of the base data by Wiseman and Dodds-Smith, (361) however, did not support the reported association. Another retrospective study conducted by Ferencz and associates (188) did not find a positive association between female sex hormone therapy and congenital heart defects. Although neither study disproved the positive association reported by Heinonen and associates (360) their findings made the association less likely.

Epidemiological studies have reported an association between exposures to female sex hormones, oral contraceptives or progestogens, and congenital neural tube defects (362) and limb defects (363). Further studies and reevaluations have not supported either of these associations (9,21,22).

Further support for the absence of a nongenital effect of progestins comes from (a) a negative correlation between sex hormone usage during pregnancy and malformations, (b) no increased incidence in malformations following progesterone therapy to maintain pregnancy, and (c) no increased incidence in malformations following first trimester exposure to progestogens (mostly medroxyprogesterone) administered to pregnant women who had signs of bleeding. The Food and Drug Administration has recognized that the evidence does not support an increased risk of limb reduction defects, congenital heat disease, or neural tube defects following exposure to oral contraceptives or progestins (364).

It is generally accepted that the actions of steroid hormones are mediated by specific steroid (365) and therefore only those tissues with the specific receptors can be affected by steroid hormones.

Retinoids, Systemic Administration (Isotretinoin, Etretinate)

Vitamin A congeners, including retinol, retinal, all-trans-retinoic acid (tretinoin) and 13-cis-retinoic acid (isotretinoin), are all teratogenic in numerous species. Both isotretinoin (Accutane, Roche Laboratories), marketed for treating severe acne, and etretinate (Tigason, Sautier Laboratories), marketed for treating psoriasis, contained warnings by the manufacturers against exposure during pregnancy. Unfortunately, exposures occurred. Analyses of the resulting malformations have been reviewed (366,367). Human malformations include CNS, cardioaortic, microtia, clefting defects and, more controversially, limb defects. Isotretinoin has a serum half-life of 10 to 12 hours; there is no apparent risk to the fetus if maternal use is terminated before conception (368). However, the risk for malformations and subnormal results on standard intelligence tests is high for offspring of women who were treated with therapeutic doses of isotretinoin in the first 60 days after conception (369).

Etretinate exposure during the first 60 days of pregnancy is associated with a high risk of malformations. Etretinate persists in the body for up to 2 years (370,371). Whether the lower concentrations of etretinate remaining in the mother's circulation over these extended periods increases the risk of malformations is not known but, if there is an increased risk, it is likely to be low.

Experimental evidence suggests that endogenous retinoic acid may act as a natural morphogen. Exogenous retinoids act either directly, resulting in cytotoxicity, or via receptor-mediated pathways to interact with DNA and alter programmed cell death (372,373). It is likely that different specificities of retinoid binding proteins (374) account for the variations in placental transfer. Although retinoids can influence many types of cells, Lammer (366) emphasized that neuroectodermally derived cells of the rhomben-cephalon are particularly sensitive and that the resulting neural crest cell abnormality differs from that resulting in oculoauriculo-vertebral dysplasia or Goldenhar syndrome. The susceptibility of specific cell types to the effects of the retinoids may be determined by the intracellular concentration of cellular retinoic binding protein (366).

Retinoids, Topical Administration (Tretinoin)

There have been a number of case reports of congenital malformations occurring in the offspring of mothers who used topical tretinoin during their pregnancy. The United States Food and Drug Administration received adverse reaction reports involving approximately seventeen infants who were born from mothers who used topical tretinoin during pregnancy, with a higher than expected representation of holoprosencephaly (Rosa, F., personal communication). While there has not been an abundance of epidemiological studies involving topical tretinoin, there are three reports. Using Michigan Medicaid data, the incidence of birth defects in 147 pregnancies exposed to topical tretinoin was compared to the incidence of birth defects in 104,092 nonexposed; the relative risk was 0.8 in the exposed population (Rosa, F., personal communication). A relative risk of 0.7 for birth defects was determined in 215 pregnancies exposed to topical tretinoin as compared with 430 nonexposed mothers in data from Group Health of Puget Sound (375). De Wals and associates (376) evaluated the association of the occurrence of holoprosen-

cephaly with topical tretinoin exposure. Among 502,189 births there were 31 infants with holoprosencephaly. Eight patients had an abnormal karyotype and 16 had a normal karyotype. None of the patients with a normal karyotype were exposed to topical tretinoin during pregnancy.

Since all teratogens that have been appropriately studied have a no-effect dose, it would be paramount that topical administration of a known teratogen such as tretinoin must be absorbed and produce teratogenic concentrations in the blood. At conventional doses, the blood levels from topical administration are far below the teratogenic dose. It would appear that prudent use of this topical medication presents no risk to the embryo, because there would be no teratogenic exposure. The pharmacokinetics, animal studies and human studies support this conclusion.

Rh Immune Globulin

After exposure to Rh(D)-positive red cells, usually resulting from a fetal transplacental hemorrhage that occurs to some degree in 75% of pregnancies, (377) the Rh(D)-negative mother becomes Rh immunized. Rh immunization during a previous pregnancy results in brain damage of various degree or death in an Rh(D)-positive newborn in approximately 50% of cases (377). Once maternal Rh immunization has developed, it cannot be treated effectively, but it can be prevented by antenatal prophylaxis with 300 ug of RhIg at 28 weeks' gestation (377). No adverse fetal effects to immunoprophylaxis have been reported.

Smoking and Nicotine

Approximately 30% of all women of childbearing age smoke, and about 25% of all women will continue to smoke after they become pregnant (378). The evidence in humans indicates that smoking affects the fetus directly in a dose-related manner and probably involves more than one component of smoke (379). Placental lesions and fetal growth retardation have been consistently reported in epidemiological studies involving pregnant women who smoke cigarettes (380–382). Fetal death is 20%–80% higher among women who smoked cigarettes although pregnant (382). However, despite suggestions that smoking during pregnancy may increase the risk of limb anomalies, there is no proven relationship between smoking and specific malformations or malformations in general (383–385). Because of the large number of pregnant women who smoke and the documented effects of smoking on the fetus, one can conclude that smoking presents a significant risk to the fetus for growth retardation and abortion.

Thalidomide

Lenz and Knapp (386) were the first to associate thalidomide exposure during pregnancy with limb reduction defects and other features of the thalidomide syndrome. Limb defects resulted from exposure limited to a 2-week period from the 22nd to the 36th days postconception:

exposures from the 27th to the 30th days most often affected only the arm, whereas exposures from the 30th to the 33rd days resulted in both leg and arm abnormalities (387,388). Although there was no association of mental retardation, brain malformations, or cleft palate, other abnormalities included facial hemangioma, microtia, esophageal or duodenal atresia, deafness, and anomalies of the eyes, kidneys, heart, and external ears and increased incidence of miscarriages and neonatal mortality (386,387,389,390). A high proportion, about 20%, of the fetuses exposed during the critical period were affected. The current use of thalidomide in Brazil for the treatment of leprosy has resulted in more recent cases of embryopathy including at least 29 children born with thalidomide syndrome (391,392). Although the mechanism of teratogenic action for thalidomide is not yet defined, the subject has been critically reviewed by Stephens (393).

Thyroid: Iodides, Antithyroid Drugs (Thioamides)

There are several case reports of congenital goiter as a result of *in utero* exposures to iodide-containing drugs (394). Maternal intake of as low as 12 mg per day may result in fetal goiter (394). Iodinated diagnostic x-ray contrast agents used for amniofetography have been reported to affect fetal thyroid function adversely (395).

Thioamides are antithyroid drugs used to treat fetal thyrotoxicosis. Fetal thyrotoxicosis is induced by thyroid-stimulating immunoglobulins produced in euthyroid or hypothyroid women. The adverse fetal effects, e.g., craniosynostosis, intellectual impairment and increased mortality, are caused by excess fetal thyroid hormone production. The thioamides block thyroid hormone synthesis by inhibiting the oxidation of iodide or iodotyrosyl. Unlike other thioamides, propylthiouracil also inhibits the peripheral deiodination of thyroxine to triiodothyronine. All thioamides are associated with a significant risk of fetal goiter and teratogenesis (290). However, in the case of propylthiouracil, the fetal goiter can be reduced with intraamniotic injections of thyroxine (396) which also prevents other abnormalities caused by inhibition of fetal thyroid function.

Tocolytics

Fetal distress can result from uterine hypertonus, umbilical cord compression, premature rupture of the fetal membranes, oligohydramnios, placental abruption, and uteroplacental insufficiency. In some cases of severe fetal hypoxemia or acidosis, prompt delivery may be recommended. However, if immediate surgery is not feasible, tocolytics may help to reduce fetal distress until delivery is possible.

In cases of hypoxemia as a result of reduced blood flow to the fetus, inhibiting uterine activity should increase the delivery of oxygen to the fetus by increasing uterine and intervillous perfusion. In addition to inhibiting uterine activity, β-adrenergic agonists both increase maternal cardiac output and dilate uterine vessels resulting in a further increase in placental perfusion.

Ritodrine, a β2-adrenergic receptor agonist, may be administered as an intravenous bolus for acute fetal distress (397). Ritodrine's mechanism of action leads to a reduction in the intracellular calcium available for smooth muscle contraction.

Terbutaline sulfate, a nonspecific beta-adrenergic agonist, is associated with a higher incidence of cardiovascular side effects than ritodrine with prolonged use.

When the use of β-adrenergic agonists is contraindicated in cases of intraamniotic infection, uncontrolled maternal thyroid disease, diabetes mellitus, and cardiovascular disease, magnesium sulfate may be used as a tocolytic agent. Although its mechanism of action is unknown, it results in an uncoupling of the actin-myosin interaction in smooth muscle (398). An advantage of magnesium sulfate tocolysis is the absence of cardiovascular side effects.

The data concerning the fetal effects of tocolytic agents are restricted to case reports, but, there are no reports of adverse fetal outcome resulting from exposure to therapeutic doses of terbutaline (399), ritodrine (400), or magnesium sulfate (401).

Toluene

Although occupational exposure to toluene has not been associated with congenital malformations in offspring, there are case reports of malformations resulting from the abuse of toluene. The first description of an infant with features similar to FAS born to a chronic abuser of toluene appeared in 1979 (402). This case and 22 additional cases have been described in detail (403). Thirty-nine percent of the toluene-exposed infants were born prematurely and 9% died in the perinatal period. In the surviving infants, 52% exhibited growth deficiency, 67% were microcephalic, and 80% exhibited developmental delay. Craniofacial features similar to those in the FAS were observed in 89%. An increased incidence of prematurity, perinatal death, growth and developmental delay and phenotypic features similar to FAS were reported in 35 pregnancies of 15 toluene abusers (404). Pearson and associates (403) suggest that the clinical and experimental data can be interpreted to imply that alcohol and toluene may have a common mechanism of facial teratogenesis. Toluene appears to have the potential for developmental toxicity in the human but the magnitude of the risk is minimal for usual occupational exposures, although it may be moderate to high in inhalation abusers.

Tranquilizers

The minor tranquilizers as a group are probably the most frequently prescribed therapeutic agents. Within this group, the propanediol carbonates and the benzodiazepines, the two most widely used classes, have been associated with teratogenic effects (290). The strongest association has been between diazepam and cleft lip with or without cleft palate but even this association is not likely to be causal (405). Since these drugs are widely used, even a small increased risk would be expected to result in more reported adverse effects than has been the case. Continued surveillance is warranted because so many pregnancies are exposed to these drugs.

Valproic Acid

Valproic acid (dipropylacetic acid) is used for the treatment of various types of epilepsy. Dalens and associates (406), were the first to report the association of valproic acid and congenital malformations in the human. Although other reports followed, Robert and colleagues (407) described the associated malformations, consisting primarily of neural tube defects, and their incidence in detail. The neural tube defect observed is usually spina bifida in the lumbar or sacral region and increased risk appears to be correlated with higher serum levels (350,408). Other anomalies include postnatal growth retardation, microcephaly, midface hypoplasia, micrognathia and epicanthal folds. Therapeutic dosages during pregnancy present a teratogenic risk for spina bifida of about 1% (409) but the risk for facial dysmorphology may be greater. Valproic acid crosses the human placenta (410) but the fetal serum concentrations are not known.

Vitamins

Biotin

Biotin-responsive multiple carboxylase deficiency is an inborn error of metabolism in which there is a severe reduction in the activities of the mitochondrial biotin-dependent carboxylase enzymes. Affected individuals exhibit dermatitis, severe metabolic acidosis and a characteristic pattern of organic acid excretion. Metabolism in these patients is restored to normal levels by biotin supplementation. Prenatal administration of 10 mg per day of oral biotin initiated during the third trimester prevented neonatal complications with no adverse fetal effects (390).

Vitamin A

Case reports have associated congenital defects in humans with massive vitamin A ingestion during pregnancy (411). Although effects similar to those produced by vitamin A congeners, namely CNS, cardioaortic, microtia and clefting defects (see discussion of Retinoids above), may be predicted, no pattern of anomalies has emerged. Another fourteen infants of women who ingested high doses of vitamin A (25,000 IU or more) during pregnancy had no congenital anomalies, although three additional pregnancies ended in miscarriage (412).

A review of literature concerning retinoids and birth defects entitled "Recommendations for Vitamin A Use During Pregnancy" was published by the Teratology Society (411). Supplementation of 8,000 IU vitamin A per day should be the maximum during pregnancy and high

dosages (25,000 IU or more) are not recommended. Beta-carotene as a source of vitamin A is likely to be associated with a smaller risk than an equivalent dose of vitamin A as retinol (411).

Vitamin B12

Ampola and associates (413) were the first to report prenatal treatment of a vitamin-responsive inborn error of metabolism. Their report involved a fetus with a vitamin B12-responsive variant of methylmalonic acidemia, a metabolic disease involving a functional deficiency in the coenzymatically active form of vitamin B12. Oral cyanocobalamin, 10 mg per day, initiated at 32 weeks gestation resulted in only a slight increase in maternal serum B12 level. Oral therapy was therefore stopped at 34 weeks' gestation and 5 mg per day of intravenous cyanocobalamin was initiated. This regimen produced a progressive increase in maternal serum B12 and a decrease in urinary methylmalonic acid excretion. The infant had no acute neonatal complications after delivery at 41 weeks.

Vitamin D

There have been no large-scale studies examining the effects of ingestion of large doses of vitamin D during pregnancy. In several small studies no increased risk of malformations was seen in offspring of women who took large doses of vitamin D during pregnancy (414,415). There have been some reports that huge doses of vitamin D administered for rickets prophylaxis in pregnant women resulted in a marked increased incidence of a syndrome consisting of supravalvular aortic stenosis, elfin facies, and mental retardation similar to Williams syndrome in the human (416,417). However, more recent studies have demonstrated that Williams syndrome is caused by a gene deletion in most cases (418,419). Animal studies and additional clinical reports suggest that the teratogenic risk of therapeutic doses of vitamin D is none to minimal.

ACKNOWLEDGMENTS

The authors thank Yvonne Edney for her secretarial assistance.

REFERENCES

1. Hertig AT. The overall problem in man. In: K. Benirschke, ed. *Comparative Aspects of Reproductive Failure.* Berlin: Springer-Verlag, 1967:11–41.
2. Robert CJ, Lowe CR. Where have all the conceptions gone? *Lancet* 1975;1:498–499.
3. Kajii T, Ferrier A, Niikawa N, et al. Anatomic and chromosomal anomalies in 639 spontaneous abortions. *Hum Genet* 1980; 55:87.
4. Simpson JL. Genes, chromosomes and reproductive failure. *Fertil Steril* 1980;33:116–778.
5. Copp AJ. Death before birth: clues from gene knockouts and mutations. *Trends Genet* 1995;11.
6. Fraser FC. The multifactorial/threshold concept-uses and misuses. *Teratology* 1976;14:762–770.

7. World Health Organization. *Spontaneous and induced abortion.* World Health Organization: Geneva, 1970.
8. Boue J, Boue A, Lazar P. Retrospective and prospective epidemiological studies of 1,500 karyotyped spontaneous abortions. *Teratology* 1975;12:11–26.
9. Wilson JG. *Environment and birth defects.* New York: Academic Press, 1973.
10. Brent RL. Predicting teratogenic and reproductive risks in humans from exposure to various environmental agents using in vitro techniques and in vivo animal studies. *Congenit Anom Kyoto* 1988;28[Suppl]:S41–S55.
11. Sever JL. Infections in pregnancy: highlights from the collaborative perinatal project. *Teratology* 1982;25.
12. Gwinn M, Pappaioanou M, George JR, et al. Prevalence of HIV infection in childbearing women in the United States. *JAMA* 1991;265.
13. Braddick MR, Kreiss JK, Embree JE, et al. Impact of maternal HIV infection on obstetrical and early neonatal outcome. *AIDS* 1990;4.
14. Blanche S, Rouzioux C, Moscato MLG, et al. A prospective study of infants born to women seropositive for human immunodeficiency virus type 1. *N Engl J Med* 1989;320.
15. Embree JE, Braddick MR, Datta P, et al. Lack of correlation of maternal human immunodeficiency virus infection with neonatal malformations. *Pediatr Infect Dis J* 1989;8.
16. European Collaborative Study. Mother-to-child transmission of HIV infection. *Lancet* 1988;II.
17. Qazi QH, Sheikh TM, Fikrig S, et al. Lack of evidence for craniofacial dysmorphism in perinatal human immunodeficiency virus infection. *J Pediatrics* 1988;112.
18. Van Allen MI. Structural anomalies resulting from vascular disruption. *Pediatr Clin N Am* 1992;39:255–277.
19. Van Allen MI JS-B, Dixon J, et al. Construction bands and limb reduction defects in two newborns with fetal ultrasound evidence for vascular disruption. *Am J Med Genet* 1992;44.
20. Wilson JG, Brent RL, Jordan HC. Differentiation as a determinant of the reaction of rat embryo to x-irradiation. *Proc Soc Exp Biol Med* 1953;82.
21. Briggs MH, Briggs M. Sex hormone exposure during pregnancy and malformations. In: Briggs MH, Corbin A, eds. *Advances in steroid biochemistry and pharmacology.* London: Academic Press, 1979:51–89.
22. Wilson JG, Brent RL. Are female sex hormones teratogenic? *Am J Obstet Gynecol* 1981;114:567–580.
23. Fraser FC. Interactions and multiple causes. In: Wilson JG, Fraser FC, eds. *Handbook of teratology.* New York: Plenum Press, 1977:445–463.
24. Mirkes PE. Cyclophosphamide teratogenesis: a review. *Teratog Carcinog Mutagen* 1985;5:75–88.
25. Miller RK. Placental transfer and function: the interface for drugs and chemicals in the conceptus. In: Fabro S, Scialli AR, eds. *Drug and chemical action in pregnancy: pharmacologic and toxicologic principles.* New York: Marcel Dekker, 1986:123–152.
26. Jackson MJ. Drug absorption. In: Fabro S, Scialli AR, eds. *Drug and chemical action in pregnancy: pharmacologic and toxicologic Principles.* New York and Basel: Marcel Dekker, 1986:15–36.
27. Mattison DR. Physiologic variations in pharmacokintics during pregnancy. In: Fabro S, Scialli AR, eds. *Drug and Chemical Action in Pregnancy: pharmacologic and toxicologic principles.* New York: Marcel Dekker 1986:37–102.
28. Sonawane BR, Yaffe SJ. Physiologic disposition of drugs in the fetus and newborn. In: Fabro S, Scialli AR, eds. *Drug and chemical action in pregnancy: pharmacologic and toxicologic principles.* New York and Basel: Marcel Dekker, 1986:103–121.
29. Juchau MR, Rettie AE. The metabolic role of the placenta. In: Fabro S, Scialli AR, eds. *Drug and chemical action in pregnancy: pharmacologic and toxicologic principles.* New York and Basel: Marcel Dekker, 1989:153–169.
30. Juchau MR. Bioactivation in chemical teratogenesis. *Ann Rev Pharmacol Toxicol* 1989;29.
31. Hanson JW. Teratogen Update: fetal hydantoin effects. *Teratology* 1986;33:349–353.
32. Laurence KM, James N, Miller MH, et al. Double-blind randomized controlled trial of folate treatment before conception to prevent recurrence of neural tube defects. *Br Med J* 1981;282:1509–1511.

33. Smithells RW, Seller MJ, Nevin NC, et al. Further experience of vitamin supplementation for prevention of neural tube defect recurrences. *Lancet* 1983;1:1027–1031.
34. Smithells RW, Shepard S, Schorah CJ, et al. Apparent prevention of neural tube defects by periconceptional vitamin supplementation. *Arch Dis Child* 1981;56:911.
35. Smithells RW, Sheppard S, Wild J, et al. Prevention of neural tube defect recurrences in Yorkshire: final report. *Lancet* 1989;2:498–499.
36. Medical Research Council. Prevention of neural tube defects: results of the Medical Research Council Vitamin Study. *Lancet* 1991;338:131–137.
37. Cziezel AE, Dudas I. Prevention of the first occurrence of neural-tube defects by periconceptional vitamin supplementation. *N Engl J Med* 1992;327.
38. Brent RL. Environmental factors: miscellaneous. In: Brent RL, Harris MI, eds. *Prevention of embryonic fetal and perinatal disease.* Bethesda: DHEW(NIH), 1976:211–218.
39. Brent RL. Drugs and pregnancy: are the insert warnings too dire? *Contemp Ob/Gyn* 1976;20:42–49.
40. Mirkin BI. Maternal and fetal distribution of drugs in pregnancy. *Clin Pharmacol Ther* 1973;14:643–647.
41. McKusick VA. *Mendalian inheritance in man: catalogs of autosomal dominant, autosomal recessive, and X-linked phenotypes.* Baltimore: Johns Hopkins University Press, 1988.
42. Brent RL. Method of evaluating alleged human teratogens [Editorial]. *Teratology* 1978;17:83.
43. Brent RL. Definition of a teratogen and the relationship of teratogenicity to carcinogenicity [Editorial]. *Teratology* 1986;34:359–360.
44. Susser E. Spontaneous abortion and induced abortion: an adjustment for the presence of induced abortion when estimating the rate of spontaneous abortion from cross-sectional studies. *Am J Epidemiol* 1983;117:305–308.
45. Olsen J. Calculating the risk ratios for spontaneous abortions: the problem of induced abortion. *Int J Epidemiol* 1984;13:347–350.
46. Warner RH, Rosett HL. The effects of drinking on offspring: an historical survey of the American and British literature. *J Stud Alcohol* 1975;36:1395.
47. Jones KL, Smith DW, Streissguth AP, et al. Outcome in offspring of chronic alcoholic women. *Lancet* 1974;1:1076–1078.
48. Streissguth AP, Grant TM, Barr HM, et al. Cocaine and the use of alcohol and other drugs during pregnancy. *Am J Obstet Gynecol* 1991;164:1239–1243.
49. Streissguth AP, Sampson PD, Marr HM. Neurobehavioral dose-response effects of prenatal alcohol exposure in humans from infancy to adulthood. *Ann NY Acad Sci* 1989;562:145–158.
50. Streissguth AP, Landesman-Dwyer C, Martin JC, et al. Teratogenic effect of alcohol in humans and laboratory animals. *Science* 1980;209:353–361.
51. Day NL, Richardson GA. Prenatal alcohol exposure: a continuum of effects. *Semin Perinatol* 1991;15:271–279.
52. Autti-Ramo I, Granstrom M-L. The effect of intrauterine alcohol exposure of various durations on early cognitive development. *Neuropediatrics* 1991;22:203–210.
53. Autti-Ramo I, Granstrom M-L. The psychomotor development during the first year of life of infants exposed to intrauterine alcohol of various durations. Fetal alcohol exposure and development. *Neuropediatrics* 1991;22:59–64.
54. Clarren SK, Smith DW. The fetal alcohol syndrome. *N Engl J Med* 1978;298:1063–1067.
55. Skipper HT, Schabel FM Jr. Quantitative and cytokinetic studies in experimental tumor models. In: Holland JF, Frei E III, eds. *Cancer medicine.* Philadelphia: Lea and Bebieger, 1973:629–650.
56. Thiersch JB. Therapeutic abortions with a folic acid (4-amino PGA). *Am J Obstet Gynecol* 1952;63:1298–1304.
57. Goetsch C. An evaluation of amniopterin as an abortifacient. *Am J Obstet Gynecol* 1962;83:1474–1477.
58. Warkany J. Aminopterin and methotrexate: folic acid deficiency. *Teratology* 1978;17:353–358.
59. Warkany J, Beautry PH, Horstein S. Attempted abortion with amniopterin (4-aminopteroylglutamic acid). *Am J Dis Child* 1959;97:274–281.
60. Jones KL. Fetal amniopterin/methotrexate syndrome. In: Jones KL, ed. *Smith's Recognizable patterns of human malformation.* Philadelphia: WB Saunders, 1997:570–571.

61. Del Campo M, Kosaki K, Bennett FC, et al. Developmental delay in fetal aminopterin/methotrexate syndrome. *Teratology* 1999;60:10–12.

62. Bawle EV, Conard JV, Weiss L. Adult and two children with fetal methotrexate syndrome. *Teratology* 1998;57:51–55.

63. Shaw EB, Steinbach HL. Amniopterin-induced fetal malformation: survival of infant after attempted abortion. *Am J Dis Child* 1968;115:477–482.

64. Skalko RG, Gold MP. Teratogenicity of methotrexate in mice. *Teratology* 1974;9:159–164.

65. Baranov VS. Characteristics of the teratogenic effect of aminopterin compared to that of other teratogenic agents. *Bull Exp Biol Med* 1966;61:77–81.

66. Goeringer GC, DeSesso JM. Developmental toxicity in rabbits of the antifolate aminopterin and its amelioration by leucovorin. *Teratology* 1990;41:560–561.

67. Feldkamp M, Carey JC. Clinical teratology counseling and consultation case report: low dose methotrexate exposure in the early weeks of pregnancy. *Teratology* 1993;47:533–539.

68. Grumbach MM, Conte FA. Disorders of sex differentiation. In: Williams RH, ed. *Textbook of endocrinology*. Philadelphia: WB Saunders, 1981:422–514.

69. Moncrieff A. Nonadrenal female pseudohermaphroditism associated with hormone administration in pregnancy. *Lancet* 1958; 2:267.

70. Hoffman F, Overzier C, Uhde G. Zur frage der hormonalen erzengung fotaler zwittenbildugen beim menschen. *Geburtshilfe Frauerheikd* 1955;15:1061–1070.

71. Reschini E, Giustina G, D'Alberton A, et al. Female pseudohermaphroditism due to maternal androgen administration: 25-year follow-up. *Lancet* 1985;1:1226.

72. Greene RR, Burrill MW, Ivy AC. Experimental intersexuality: the effect of antenatal androgens on sexual development of female rats. *Am J Anat* 1939;65:415–469.

73. Raynaud A. Observations dur de development normal des ebauches de la glande mammaire des foetus maleset femelle de souris. *Ann Endocrinol* 1947;8:349–359.

74. Brunner JA, Witschi E. Testosterone-induced modifications of sexual development in female hamsters. *Am J Anat* 1946;79:293–320.

75. Jost A. Problems of fetal endocrinology: the gonadal and hypophyseal hormones. *Recent Prog Horm Res* 1953;8:379–418.

76. Wells, LJ, Van Wagenen G. Androgen induced female pseudohermaphroditism in the monkey (macaca mulatta) anatomy of the reproductive organs. *Carnegie Institute Contrib Embryol* 1954;35:93–106.

77. Dohler KD, Hancke JL, Srivastava SS, et al. Participation of estrogens in female sexual differentiation of the brain: neuroanatomical, neuroendocrine and behavioral evidence. *Prog Brain Res* 1984;6:99–117.

78. Goy RW, Bercovitch FB, McBrair MC. Behavioral masculinization is independent of genital masculinization in prenatally androgenized female rhesus macaques. *Horm Behav* 1988;22:552–571.

79. Goy RW, Bridson WE, Young WC. Period of maximal susceptibility of the prenatal female guinea pig to masculinizing actions of the testosterone propionate. *J Comp Physiol Psychol* 1964;57:166–174.

80. Hoepfner BA, Ward IL. Prenatal and neonatal androgen exposure interact to affect sexual differentiation in female rats. *Behav Neurosci* 1988;102:61–65.

81. Huffman L, Hendricks SE. Prenatally injected testosterone propionate and sexual behavior of female rats. *Physiol Behav* 1981;26:773–778.

82. Phoenix CH, Goy RW, Gerall AA, et al. Organizing action of prenatally administered testosterone propionate on the tissues mediating mating behavior in the female guinea pig. *Endocrinology* 1959;65:369–382.

83. Maxwell SRJ, Kendall MJ. ACE inhibition in the 1900s. *Br J Clin Pract* 1993;47:30–37.

84. German J, Kowal A, Ehlers KH. Trimethadione and human teratogenesis. *Teratology* 1970;3:349–362.

85. Gavras I, Gavras H. Ace inhibitors: a decade of clinical experience. *Hosp Pract (Off Ed)* 1993;28:117–127.

86. Guignard JP, Burgener F, Calame A. Persistent anuria in neonate: a side effect of captopril. *Int J Pediatr Nephrol* 1981;2:133.

87. Hanssens M, Keirse MJNC, Vankelecom F, et al. Fetal and neonatal effects of treatment with angiotensin-converting enzyme inhibitors in pregnancy. *Obstet Gynecol* 1991;79:128–135.

88. Piper JM, Ray WA, Rosa FW. Pregnancy outcome following exposure to angiotensin converting enzyme inhibitors. *Obstet Gynecol* 1992;80:429–432.

89. Pryde PG, Sedman AB, Nugent CE, et al. Angiotensin-converting enzyme inhibitor fetopathy. *J Am Soc Nephrol* 1993;3:1575–1582.

90. Barr M Jr, Cohen MM Jr. ACE inhibitor fetopathy and hypocalvaria: the kidney-skull connection. *Teratology* 1991;44:485–495.

91. Brent RL, Beckman DA. Angiotensin-converting enzyme inhibitors, an embryopathic class of drugs with unique properties: information for clinical teratology counselors. *Teratology* 1991;43:543.

92. Guignard JP. Effect of drugs on the immature kidney. *Adv Nephrol Necker Hosp* 1993;22:193–211.

93. Martin RA, Jones KL, Mendoza A, et al. Effect of ACE inhibition in the fetal kidney: decreased renal blood flow. *Teratology* 1992;46:317–321.

94. Cunniff C, Jones K, Phillipson J, et al. Oligohydramnios sequence and renal tubular malformation associated with maternal enalapril use. *Am J Obstet Gynecol* 1990;162:187–189.

95. Cox SM, Williams ML, Leveno KJ. The natural history of preterm ruptured membranes: what to expect of expectant management. *Obstet Gynecol* 1988;71:558–562.

96. Snider DE, Layde PM, Johnson MW, et al. Treatment of turberculosis during pregnancy. *Am Rev Respir Dis* 1980;122:65–79.

97. Warkany J. Antituberculosis drugs. *Teratology* 1979;20:133–138.

98. Heinonen OP, Slone D, Shapiro S, eds. Birth Defects and Drugs in Pregnancy. Littleton: Publishing Sciences Group, 1977.

99. Jones HG. Intrauterine toxicity: a case report and review of literature. *J Natl Med Assoc* 1973;65:201–203.

100. Nishimura H, Tanimura T, eds. *Clinical aspects of the teratogenicity of drugs.* New York: American Elsevier, Excerpta Medica, 1976.

101. Bobrowitz ID. Ethambutol in pregnancy. *Chest* 1974;66:20–24.

102. Lewit T, Nebel L, Terracina S, et al. Ethambutol in pregnancy: observations on embryogenesis. *Chest* 1974;66:25–26.

103. Monnet P, Kalb JC, Pujol M. Harmful effects of isoniazid on the fetus and infants. *Lyon Med* 1967;218:431–455.

104. Varpela E. On the effect exerted by the first line turberculosis medicines on the fetus. *Acta Tuberc Pneumol Scand* 1964;35:53–69.

105. Lenke RR, Turkel SB, Monsen R. Severe fetal deformities associated with ingestion of excessive isoniazid in early pregnancy. *Acta Obstet Gynecol Scand* 1985;64:281–282.

106. Potworowska M, Sianoz-Ecka E, Szufladowicz R. Treatment with ethionamide in pregnancy. *Gruzlica* 1966;34:341–347.

107. Zierski M. Effects of ethionamide on the development of the human fetus. Gruzlica 1966;34:349–352.

108. Dluzniewski A, Gastol-Lewinska L. The search for teratogenic activity of some tuberculostatic drugs. *Diss Pharm Pharmacol* 1971;23:383–392.

109. Nakamoto Y, Otani H, Tanaka O. Effects of aminoglycosides administered to pregnant mice on postnatal development of inner ear in their offspring. *Teratology* 1985;2:604–605.

110. Steen JSM, Stainton-Eldis DM. Rifampicin in pregnancy. *Lancet* 1977;2:604–605.

111. Friedman JM, Prolifka JE. Teratogenic effects of drugs (TERIS) 2nd ed. Baltimore: Johns Hopkins University Press, 2000.

112. Aselton P, Jick H, Milunsky A, et al. First-trimester drug use and congenital disorders. *Obstet Gynecol* 1985;65:451–455.

113. Burtin P, Taddio A, Ariburnu O, et al. Safety of metronidazole in pregnancy: a meta analysis. *Am J Obstet Gynecol* 1995;172:525–529.

114. Caro-Paton T, Carvajal A, Martin de Diego I, et al. Is metronidazole teratogenic? A meta analysis. *Br J Clin Pharmacol* 1997;44:179–182.

115. Morgan I. Metronidazole treatment in pregnancy. *Int J Gynaecol Obstet* 1978;15:501–502.

116. Piper J, Mitchel E, Ray W. Prenatal use of metronidazole and birth defects: no association. *Obstet Gynecol* 1993;82:348–352.

117. Rosa F, Baum C, Shaw M. Pregnancy outcomes after first trimester vaginitis drug therapy. *Obstet Gynecol* 1987;69:751–755.

118. Svare J JL-R, Anderson L, et al. Ampicillin-metronidazole treatment in idiopathic preterm labor: a randomized controlled multicentre trial. *Br J Obstet Gynaecol* 1997;104:892–897.

119. Norman K, Pattinson R, de Souza J, et al. Ampicillin and metronidazole treatment in preterm labor: a multicentre, randomized controlled trial. *Br J Obstet Gynaecol* 1995;102:267–268.

120. Dobias L, Cerna M, Rossner P, et al. Genotoxicity and carcinogenicity of metronidazole. *Mutat Res* 1994;317:177–194.

121. Roe F. Toxicologic evaluation of metronidazole with partucular reference to carcinogenic, mutagenic, and teratogenic potential. *Surgery* 1983;93:158–164.
122. Roe F. Safety of nitroimidizoles. *Scand J Infect Dis* 1985;[Suppl 46]:72–81.
123. Schaefer C, Amoura-Elefant E, Vial T, et al. Pregnancy outcome after prenatal quinolone exposure. Evaluation of a case registry of the European Network of Teratology Information Services. *Eur J Obstet Gynecol Reprod Biol* 1996;69:83–89.
124. Loebstein R, Addis A, Ho E, et al. Pregnanacy outcome following gestational exposure to fluoroquinolones: a multicenter prospective controlled study. *Antimicrob Agents Chemother* 1998;42:1336–1339.
125. Berkovitch M, Pastuszak A, Gazarian M, et al. Safety of the new quinolones in pregnancy. *Obstet Gynecol* 1994;84:535–538.
126. Koren G. Use of the new quinolones in pregnancy. *Can Fam Physician* 1996;42:1097–1099.
127. Pagnini G, Pelagalli GV, Di Carlo F. Effect of nalidixic acid on the chick embryo and on pregnancy and embryonic development in rabbits and rats. *Atti Soc Ital Sci Vet* 1971;25:137–140.
128. Sato T, Kaneko Y, Saegusa T, et al. Reproduction studies of cinoxacin in rats. *Chemotherapy* 1980;28[Suppl 4]:484–507.
129. Sato T, Kobayashi F. Teratological study on cinoxacin in rabbits. *Chemotherapy* 1980;28 [Suppl 4]:508–515.
130. Murray EDS. Nalidixic acid in pregnancy. *Br Med J* 1981;282:224.
131. Ingham B, Brentnall DW, Dale EA, et al. Arthropathy induced by antibacterial fused N-alkyl-4-pyridone-3-carboxylic acids. *Toxicol Lett* 1977;6:21–26.
132. Cohlan SQ, Bevelander G, Tiamsic T. Growth inhibition of prematures receiving tetracycline: clinical and laboratory investigation. *Am J Dis Child* 1963;105:453–461.
133. Baden E. Environmental pathology of the teeth. In: Gorlin RJ, Goldman HM, eds. *Thomas' oral pathology*. St Louis: Mosby, 1970:189–191.
134. Rebich T, Kumar J, Brustman B. Dental caries and tetracycline-stained dentition in an American-Indian population. *J Dent Res* 1985;64:462–464.
135. Colley DP, Kay J, Gibson GT. A study of the use in pregnancy of co-trimozazole and sulfamethizole. *Aust J Pharm* 1982;63:570–575.
136. Bailey RR. Single-dose antibacterial treatment for bacteriuria in pregnancy. *Drugs* 1984;27:183–186.
137. Williams JD, Brumfitt W, Condie AP, et al. The treatment of bacteriuria in pregnant women with sulphamethoxazole and trimethoprim. *Postgrad Med J* 1969;45[Suppl]:71–76.
138. Bailey RR, Bishop V, Peddie PA. Comparison of single dose with a 5-day course of co-trimoxazole for asymptomatic (covert) bacteriuria of pregnancy. *Aust NZ J Obstet Gynaecol* 1983;23:139–141.
139. Hernandez-Diaz S, Mitchell AA. Folic acid antagonists during pregnancy and risk of birth defects. *N Engl J Med* 2001;344:934–935.
140. Hernandez-Diaz S, Werler MM, Walker AM, et al. Folic acid antagonists during pregnancy and the risk of birth defects. *N Engl J Med* 2000;343:1608–1614.
141. Hernandez-Diaz S, Werler MM, Walker AM, et al. Neural tube defects in relation to use of folic acid antagonists during pregnancy. *Am J Epidemiol* 2001;153:961–968.
142. Cziezel AE, Rockenbauer M, Sorensen HT, et al. The teratogenic risk of trimethoprim-sulfonamides: a population based case control study. *Reprod Toxicol* 2001;15:637–646.
143. Elmazar MMA, Nau H. Trimethoprim potentiates valproic acid-induced neural tube defects (NTDs) in mice. *Reprod Toxicol* 1993;7:249–254.
144. Kreutz R. Investigation on the influence of trimethoprim at the intrauterine development of the rat. *Anat Anz* 1981;149.
145. Udall V. Toxicology of sulphonamide-trimethoprim combinations. *Postgrad Med J* 1969;45[Suppl]:42–45.
146. Chassard D, Mathon L, Dailler F, et al. Extradural clonidine combined with sufentanil and 0.0625% bupivacaine for analgesia in labour. *Br J Anaesth* 1996;77:458–462.
147. Cigarini I, Kaba A, Bonnet F, et al. Epidural clonidine combined with bupivicaine for analgesia in labor. Effects on mother and neonate. *Reg Anesth* 1995;20:113–120.
148. Boutroy MJ, Gisonna CR, Legagner M. Clonidine: placental transfer and neonatal adaptation. *Early Hum Dev* 1988;17:275–286.
149. Horvath JS, Phippard A, Korda A, et al. Clonidine hydrochloride-a safe and effective antihypertensive agent in pregnancy. *Obstet Gynecol* 1985;66:634–638.
150. Widerlov E, Karlman I, Storsater J. Hydralazine-induced neonatal thrombocytopenia [Letter]. *N Engl J Med* 1980;301:1235.
151. Bott-Kanner G, Schweitzer A, Reisner SH, et al. Propranolol and hydralazine in the management of essential hypertension in pregnancy. *Br J Obstet Gynaecol* 1980;87:110–114.
152. Derham RJ, Robinson J. Severe preeclampsia: is vasodilation therapy with hydralazine dangerous for the preterm fetus? *Am J Perinatol* 1990;7:239–244.
153. Kirshon B, Wasserstrum N, Cotton DB. Should continuous hydralazine infusions be utilized in severe pregnancy-induced hypertension? *Am J Perinatol* 1991;8:206–208.
154. Spinnato JA, Sibai BM, Anderson GD. Fetal distress after hydralazine therapy for severe pregnanacy-induced hypertension. *South Med J* 1986;79:559–562.
155. NHBPEP. Working Group Report on High Blood Pressure in Pregnancy, Public Health Service. In: National Institutes of Health publication, no. 91–2039. Bethesda, MD: NIH, 1991, p. 38.
156. Cziezel AE. Teratogenicity of ergotomine. *J Med Genet* 1989;26:69–70.
157. Eliahou HE, Silverberg DS, Reisen E. Propranolol for the treatment of hypertension in pregnancy. *Br J Obstet Gynaecol* 1978;85:431–436.
158. Lieberman BA, Stirrat GM, Cohen SL, et al. The possible adverse effect of propranolol on the fetus in pregnancies complictaed by severe hypertension. *Br J Obstet Gynaecol* 1978;85:678–683.
159. Oakley GD, McGarry K, Limb DG, et al. Management of pregnancy in patients with hypertrophic cardiomyopathy. *Br Med J* 1979;1:1749–1750.
160. Pruyn SC, Phelan JP, Buchanan GC. Long-term propranolol therapy in pregnancy: maternal and fetal outcome. *Am J Obstet Gynecol* 1979;135:485–489.
161. Redmond GP. Propranolol and fetal growth retardation. *Semin Perinatol* 1982;6:142–147.
162. Paran E, Holzberg G, Mazor M, et al. Beta-adrenergic blocking agents in the treatment of pregnancy-induced hypertension. *Int J Clin Pharmacol Ther* 1995;33:119–123.
163. Witter FR, King TM, Blake DA. Adverse effects of cardiovascular drug therapy on the fetus and neonate. *Obstet Gynecol* 1981;58:100S–105S.
164. Tunstall ME. The effect of propranolol on the onset of breathing at birth. *Br J Anaesth* 1969;41:792.
165. Habib A, McCarthy JS. Effects on the neonate of propranolol administered during pregnancy. *J Pediatr* 1977;91:808–811.
166. Rubin PC. Beta blockers in pregnancy. *N Engl J Med* 1981;305:1323–1326.
167. Jankowski A, Skublicki S, Wichlinski LM, et al. Clinical pharmacokinetic investigations of acetylsalicylic acid in cases of imminent premature delivery. *J Clin Hosp Pharm* 1985;10:361.
168. Trudinger BJ, Cook CM, Giles WB, et al. Low-dose aspirin in pregnancy. *Lancet* 1989;1:410.
169. Wallenburg HC, Rotmans N. Prevention of recurrent idiopathic fetal growth retardation by low-dose aspirin and dipyridamole. *Am J Obstet Gynecol* 1987;157:1230.
170. Barton JR, Sibai BM. Low-dose aspirin to improve perinatal outcome. *Clin Obstet Gynecol* 1991;34:251.
171. Werler MM, Mitchell A, Shapiro S. The relation of aspirin use during the first trimester of pregnancy to congenital cardiac defects. *N Engl J Med* 1989;321:1639.
172. McParland P, Pearce JM, Chamberlain GVP. Doppler ultrasound and aspirin in recognition and prevention of pregnancy-induced hypertension. *Lancet* 1990;335:1552.
173. Lewis RB, Schulman JD. Influence of acetylsalicylic acid, an inhibitor of prostaglandin synthesis, on the duration of human gestation and labour. *Lancet* 1973;2:1159.
174. Kullander S, Kallen B. A prospective study of drugs and pregnancy. *Acta Obstet Gynecol Scand* 1976;55:25–33.
175. Czeizel A. Lack of evidence of teratogenicity of benzodiazepine drugs in Hungary. *Reprod Toxicol* 1988;1:183–188.
176. Hartz SC, Heinonen OP, Shapiro S, et al. Antenal exposure to meprobamate and chloridiazepoxide in relation to malformations, mental development, and childhood mortality. *N Engl J Med* 1975;292:726–728.

177. Rothman K, Fuyler D, Goldblatt A, et al. Exogenous hormones and other drug exposures of children with congenital heart disease. *Am J Epidemiol* 1979;109:433–439.
178. Zierler S, Rothman KJ. Congenital heart disease in relation to maternal use of Bendectin and other drugs in early pregnancy. *N Engl J Med* 1985;313:347–352.
179. Safra MJ, Oakley GP. Association between cleft lip with or without cleft palate and prenatal exposure to diazepam. *Lancet* 1975;2:478–479.
180. Tikkanen J, Heinonen OP. Risk factors for conal malformations of the heart. *Eur J Epidemiol* 1992;8:48–57.
181. Laegried L, Hagberg G, Lundberg A. Neurodevelopment in late infancy after prenatal exposure to benzodiazepines—a prospective study. *Neuropediatrics* 1992;23:60–67.
182. Rementeria JL, Bhatt K. Withdrawal symptoms in neonates from intrauterine exposure to diazepam. *J Pediatr* 1977;90:123–126.
183. Milkovich L, van den Berg BJ. Effects of prenatal meprobamate and chlordiazepoxide hydrochloride on human embryonic and fetal development. *N Engl J Med* 1974;291:1268–1271.
184. Saxen I. Association between oral clefts and drugs taken during pregnancy. *Int J Epidemiol* 1975;4:37–44.
185. Barone JJ, Roberts H. Human consumption of caffeine. In: Dewes PB, ed. *Caffeine.* New York: Springer-Verlag, 1984:59–73.
186. Morris MB, Weinstein L. Caffeine and the fetus—is trouble brewing? *Am J Obstet Gynecol* 1981;140:607–610.
187. Beaulac-Baillargeon L, Desrosiers C. Caffeine-cigarette interaction on fetal growth. *Am J Obstet Gynecol* 1987;157:1236–1240.
188. Ferencz C, Matanoski GM, Wilson PD, et al. Maternal hormone therapy and congenital heart disease. *Teratology* 1980;21:225–239.
189. Srisuphan W, Bracken MB. Caffeine-consumption during pregnancy and association with late spontaneous abortion. *Am J Obstet Gynecol* 1986;154:14–20.
190. Watkinson B, Fried PA. Maternal caffeine use before, during and after pregnancy and effects upon offspring. *Neurobehav Toxicol Teratol* 1985;7:9–17.
191. Wilcox AJ, Weinberg CR, Baird DD. Risk factors for early pregnancy loss. *Epidemiology* 1990;1:382–385.
192. Berger A. Effects of caffeine consumption on pregnancy outcome—a review. *J Reprod Med* 1988;33:945–956.
193. Kurppa K, Holmberg PC, Kuosma E, et al. Coffee consumption during pregnancy and selected congenital malformations: a nationwide case-control study. *Am J Public Health* 1983;73:1397–1399.
194. van't Hoff W. Caffeine in pregnancy. *Lancet* 1982;1:1020.
195. Rosenberg L, Mitchell AA, Shapiro S, et al. Selected birth defects in relation to caffeine-containing beverages. *JAMA* 1982;247:1429–1432.
196. Felts JH. Coffee arabica. *N C Med J* 1981;42:281.
197. Jones KL, Lacro RV, Johnson KA, et al. Pattern of malformations in the children of women treated with carbamazepine during pregnancy. *N Engl J Med* 1989;320:1661–1666.
198. Nielsen M, Froscher W. Finger and toenail hypoplasia after carbamazepine monotherapy in late pregnancy. *Neuropediatrics* 1985;16:167–168.
199. Bertolini R, Kallen B, Mastroiacovo P, etal. Anticonvulsant drugs in monotherapy: effect on the fetus. *Eur J Epidemiol* 1987;3:164–167.
200. Rosa FW. Spina bifida in infants of women treated with carbamazapine during pregnancy. *N Engl J Med* 1991;10:674–677.
201. Janz D. Antiepileptic drugs and pregnancy: alered utilization patterns and teratogenesis. *Epilepsia* 1982;23:S53-S63.
202. Little BB, Santos-Ramos R, Newell JF, et al. Megadose carbamazapine during the period of neural tube closure. *Obstet Gynecol* 1993;82:705–708.
203. Slutsker L. Risk associated with cocaine use during pregnancy. *Obstet Gynecol* 1992;79:778–779.
204. Young SL, Vosper HJ, Phillips SA. Cocaine: its effects on maternal and child health. *Pharmacotherapy* 1992;12:2–17.
205. Jones KL. Developmental pathogenesis of defects associated with prenatal cocaine exposure: fetal vascular disruption. *Clin Perinatol* 1991;18:139–146.
206. Koren G, Graham K. Cocaine in pregnancy: analysis of fetal risk. *Vet Hum Toxicol* 1992;34:263–264.
207. Woods JR, Plessinger MA. Maternal-fetal cardiovascular system: a target of cocaine. *NIDA Res Monogr* 1991;108:7–27.
208. Plessinger MA, Woods JR. Maternal, placental, and fetal pathophysiology of cocaine exposure during pregnancy. *Clin Obstet Gynecol* 1993;36:267–278.
209. Chasnoff IJ, Chisum GM, Kaplan WE. Maternal cocaine use and genitourinary tract malformations. *Teratology* 1988;37:201–204.
210. Dogra VS, Menon PA, Poblete J, et al. Neurosonographic imaging of small for gestational age neonates exposed and not exposed to cocaine and cytomegalovirus. *J Clin Ultrasound* 1994;22:93–102.
211. Hoyme EH, Jones KL, Dixon SD. Prenatal cocaine exposure and prenatal vascular disruption. *Pediatrics* 1990;85:743.
212. Chavez GF, Mulinare J, Cordero JF. Maternal cocaine use during early pregnancy as a risk factor for congenital urogenital anomalies. *JAMA* 1989;262:795–798.
213. Viscarello RR, Ferguson DD, Nores J, et al. Limb-body wall complex associated with cocaine abuse: further evidence of cocaine's teratogenicity. *Obstet Gynecol* 1992;80:523–526.
214. Lutiger BK, Graham K, Einarson TR, et al. Relationship between gestational cocaine use and pregnancy outcome: a meta analysis. *Teratology* 1991;44:405–414.
215. DiSaia PJ. Pregnancy and delivery of a patient with a Starr-Edwards mitral valve prosthesis: report of a case. *Obstet Gynecol* 1966;29:469–472.
216. Kerber IJ, Warr OS, Richardson C. Pregnancy in a patient with prosthetic mitral valve. *JAMA* 1968;203:223–225.
217. Barr M, Burdi AR. Warfarin-associated embryopathy in a 17-week abortus. *Teratology* 1976;14:129–134.
218. Hall JG, Pauli RM, Wilson RM. Maternal and fetal sequelae of anticoagulation during pregnancy. *Am J Med* 1980;68:122–140.
219. Cotrufo M, deLuca TSL, Calabro R, et al. Coumarin anticoagulation during pregnancy in patients with mechanical valve prostheses. *Eur J Cardiothorac Surg* 1991;5:300–305.
220. Kaplan LC. Congenital Dandy Walker malformation associated with first trimester warfarin: a case report and literature review. *Teratology* 1985;32:333–337.
221. Pauli RM, Lian JB, Mosher DF. Association of congenital deficiency of multiple vitamin K-dependent coagulation factors and the phenotype of the warfarin embryopathy: clues to the mechanism of coumarin derivatives. *Am J Hum Genet* 1987;41:566–583.
222. Greenberg LH, Tanaka KR. Congenital anomalies probably induced by cyclophosphamide. *JAMA* 1964;188:423–426.
223. Scott JR. Fetal growth retardation associated with maternal administration of immunosuppressive drugs. *Am J Obstet Gynecol* 1977;128:668–676.
224. Toledo TM, Harper RC, Moser RH. Fetal effects during cyclophosphamide and irradiation therapy. *Ann Intern Med* 1971;74:87–91.
225. Blatt J, Mulvihill JJ, Ziegler JL, et al. Pregnancy outcome following cancer chemotherapy. *Am J Med* 1980;69:828–832.
226. Hales BF. Effects of phosphoramide mustard and acrolein, cytotoxic metabolites of cyclophosphamide, on mouse limb development in vitro. *Teratology* 1989;40:11–20.
227. Bongiovanni AM, DiGeorge AM, Grumbach MM. Masculinization of the female infant associated with estrogenic therapy alone during gestation: four cases. *J Clin Endocrinol Metab* 1959;19:1004–1011.
228. Herbst AL, Ulfelder H, Poskanzer DC. Adenocarcinoma of the vagina: association of maternal stilbestrol therapy with tumor appearance in young women. *N Engl J Med* 1971;284:878–881.
229. Herbst AL, Kurman RJ, Scully RE, et al. Clear-cell adenocarcinoma of the genital tract in young females. *N Engl J Med* 1972;287:1259–1264.
230. Greenwald P, Barlow JJ, Nasca PC, et al. Vaginal cancer after maternal treatment with synthetic estrogens. *N Engl J Med* 1971;285:390–392.
231. Herbst AL, Robboy SJ, Scully RE, et al. Clear-cell adenocarcinoma of the vagina and cervix in girls: analysis of 170 registry cases. *Am J Obstet Gynecol* 1974;119:713–724.
232. Barnes AB, Colton T, Gundersen J, et al. Fertility and outcome of pregnancy in women exposed in utero to diethylstilbestrol. *N Engl J Med* 1980;302:609–613.
233. Berger MJ, Goldstein DP. Impaired reproductive performance in DES-exposed women. *Obstet Gynecol* 1980;55:25–27.
234. Herbst AL, Hubby MM, Blough RR, et al. A comparison of pregnancy experience in DES-exposed and DES-unexposed daughters. *J Reprod Med* 1980;24:62–69.
235. Linn S, Liberman E, Schoenbaum SC, et al. Adverse outcome of pregnancy in women exposed to diethylstilbestrol in utero. *J Reprod Med* 1988;33:3–7.

236. Gill WB, Schumacher GFB, Bibbo M, et al. Association of diethylstilbestrol exposure in utero with cryptorchidism, testicular hypoplasia and semen abnormalities. *J Urol* 1979;122:36–39.

237. Shy KK, Stenchever MA, Karp LE, et al. Genital tract examinations and zona-free hamster egg penetration tests from men exposed in utero to diethylstilbestrol. *Fertil Steril* 1984;42:772–778.

238. Vessey MP. Epidemiological studies of the effects of diethylstilbestrol. *IARC Sci Publ* 1989;96:335–348.

239. Gershman ST, Stolley PD. A case-control study of testicular cancer using Connecticut tumour registry data. 1988;17:738–742.

240. Pinsky WW, Rayburn WF, Evans MI. Phamacologic therapy for fetal arythmias. *Clin Obstet Gynecol* 1991;34:304–309.

241. Hanson JW, Smith DW. The fetal hydantoin syndrome. *J Pediatr* 1975;87:285–290.

242. Speidel BD, Meadow SR. Maternal epilepsy and abnormalities of the fetus and newborn. *Lancet* 1972;2:839–843.

243. Frederick J. Epilepsy and pregnancy: a report from Oxford record linkage study. *Br Med J* 1973;2:442–448.

244. Monson RR, Rosenberg L, Hartz SC, et al. Diphenylhydantoin and selected malformations. *N Engl J Med* 1973;289:1049.

245. Albengres E, Tillement JP. Phenytoin in pregnancy: a review of the reported risks. *Biol Res Pregnancy Perinatol* 1983;4:71–74.

246. Barr M, Pozanski AK, Shmickel RD. Digital hypoplasia and anticonvulsants during gestation, a teratogenic syndrome. *J Pediatr* 1974;4:254–256.

247. Hill RM, Verland WM, Horning MG, et al. Infants exposed in utero to antiepileptic drugs. *Am J Dis Child* 1974;127:645–653.

248. Hanson JW, Myrianthopoulos NC, Harvey MAS, et al. Risks to the offspring of women treated with hydantoin anticonvulsants, with emphasis on the fetal hydantoin syndrome. *J Pediatr* 1976;89:662–668.

249. Keneko S. Antiepileptic drug therapy and reproductive consequences: functional and morphological effects. *Reprod Toxicol* 1991;5:179–198.

250. Shapiro S, Slone D, Hartz SC, et al. Anticonvulsants and parental epilepsy in the development of birth defects. *Lancet* 1976;1:272–275.

251. McClain RM, Langhoff L. Teratogenicity of diphenylhydantoin in the New Zealand White rabbit. *Teratology* 1980;21:371–379.

252. Collins MD, Fradkin R, Scott WI. Induction of postaxial forelimb ectrodactyly with anticonvulsant agents in A/J mice. *Teratology* 1990;41:61–70.

253. Finnell RH, Abbott LC, Taylor SM. The fetal hydantoin syndrome: answers from a mouse model. *Reprod Toxicol* 1989;3:127–133.

254. Elshave J. Cleft palate in the offspring of female mice treated with phenytoin. *Lancet* 1969;2:1074.

255. Harbinson RD, Becker BA. Relation of dosage and time of administration of diphenylhydantoin to its teratogenic effect in mice. *Teratology* 1969;2:305–312.

256. Rowland JF, Binkerd PE, Hendrickx AG. Developmental toxicity and pharmacokinetics of oral and intravenous phenytoin in the rat. *Reprod Toxicol* 1990;4:191–202.

257. Zengel AE, Keith DA, Tassinari MS. Prenatal exposure to phenytoin and its effect on postnatal growth and craniofacial proportion in the rat. *J Craniofac Genet Dev Biol* 1989;9:147–160.

258. Finnell RH. Phenytoin-induced teratogenesis: a mouse model. *Science* 1981;211:483–484.

259. Liggins GC, Howie RN. A controlled trial of antepartum glucocorticoid treatment for prevention of the respiratory distress syndrome in premature infants. *Pediatrics* 1972;50:515–525.

260. Collaborative Group on Antenatal Steroid Therapy. Effect of antenatal dexamethasone administration in the prevention of respiratory distress syndrome. *Am J Obstet Gynecol* 1981;141:276–287.

261. Cziezel AE, Rockenbauer M. Population based case-control study of teratogenic potential of corticosteroids. *Teratology* 1997;56:335–340.

262. Liu D-L, Zhou Z-L. Enhancement of fetal lung maturity by intraamniotic instillation of dexamethasone. *Clin Med J* 1985;98:915–918.

263. Chrousos GP, Evans MI, Loriaux DL, et al. Prenatal therapy in congenital adrenal hyperplasia. Attempted prevention of abnormal external genital masculinization by pharmacologic suppression of the fetal adrenal gland in utero. *Ann N Y Acad Sci* 1985;458:156–164.

264. Pang S. Congenital adrenal hypoplasia. *Endocrinol Metab Clin North Am* 1997;26:853–891.

265. Bar J, Fisch B, Wittenberg C, et al. Prednisone dosage and pregnancy outcome in renal allograft recipeints. *Nephrol Dial Transplant* 1997;12:760–763.

266. Kallen B. Drug treatment of rheumatic diseases during pregnancy: the teratogenicity of antirheumatic drugs-what is the evidence? *Scand J Rheumatol* Suppl 107:114–124.

267. Kwak J, Gilman-Sachs A, Beaman K, et al. Reproductive outcome in women with recurrent spontaneous abortion of alloimmune and autoimmune causes: preconception versus postconception treatment. *Am J Obstet Gynecol* 1992;166:1787–1798.

268. Laskin C, Bombardier C, Hannah M, et al. Predisone and aspirin in women with autoantibodies and unexplained fetal loss. *N Engl J Med* 1997;337:148–153.

269. Le Thi Huong D, Wechsler B, Vauthier-Brouzes D, et al. Outcome of planned pregnancies in systemic lupus erythematosis: a prospective study on 62 pregnancies. *Br J Rheumatol* 1997;36:772–777.

270. Cowchuck FS, Reece EA, Balaban D, et al. Repeated fetal losses associated with antiphopholipid antibodies: a collaborative randomized trial comparing prednisone with low-dose heparin treatment. *Am J Obstet Gynecol* 1992;166:1318–1323.

271. Reinisch JM, Simon NG. Prenatal exposure to prednisone in humans and animals retards intrauterine growth. *Science* 1978;202:436–438.

272. Higgins R, Mendelsohn A, DeFeo M, et al. Antenatal dexamethasone and decreased severity of retinopathy of prematurity. *Arch Opthalmol* 1998;116:601–605.

273. Leylek O, Ergur A, Senocak F, et al. Prophylaxis of the occurrence of hyperbilirubinemia in relation to maternal oxytocin infusion with steroid treatment. *Gynecol Obstet Invest* 1998;46:164–168.

274. Spinello A, Capuzzo E, Ometto A, et al. Value of antenatal corticosteroid therapy in preterm birth. *Early Hum Dev* 1995;42:37–47.

275. Silver R, Vyskocil C, Solomon S, et al. Randomized trial of antenatal dexamethasone in surfactant-treated infants delivered before 30 weeks gestation. *Obstet Gynecol* 1996;87:683–691.

276. Ward RA, Pharmacologic enhancement of fetal lung maturation. *Clin Perinatol* 1994;21:523–542.

277. Moise KJ. Indomethacin therapy in the treatment of symptomatic polyhydramnios. *Clin Obstet Gynecol* 1991;24:310.

278. Bessinger,R, Niebyl J, Keyes W, et al. Randomized comparative trial of indomethacin and ritodrine for the long-term treatment of preterm labor. *Am J Obstet Gynecol* 1991;164:981–988.

279. Bivens H, Newman R, Fyfe D, et al. Randomized trial of oral indomethacin and terbutaline sulfate for the long-term supression of preterm labor. *Am J Obstet Gynecol* 1993;169:1065–1070.

280. Mohen D, Newnham J, D'Orsonga L. Indomethacin for the treatment of polyhydramnios: a case of constriction of the ductus arteriosus. *Aust N Z J Obstet Gynaecol* 1992;32:243–246.

281. Eronen M. The hemodynamic effects of antenatal indomethacin and a beta-sympathomimetic agent of the fetus and the newborn: a randomized study. *Pediatr Res* 1993;33:615–619.

282. Moise KJ. Effect of advancing gestational age on the frequency of fetal ductal constriction in association with maternal indomethacin use. *Am J Obstet Gynecol* 1993;168:1350–1353.

283. Norton M. Teratogen update: fetal effects of indomethacin administration during pregnancy. Teratology 1997;56: 282–292.

284. Fejgin MD, Delpino ML, Bidiwala KS. Isolated small bowel perforation following intrauterine treatment with indomethacin administration. *Am J Perinatol* 1994;11:295–296.

285. Major CA, Lewis DF, Harding JA, et al. Tocolysis with indomethacin increases in incidence of necrotizing enerocolitis in the low-birth-weight neonate. *Am J Obstet Gynecol* 1994;170:102–106.

286. Lewis WH, Suris OR. Treatment with lithium carbonate: results in 35 cases. *Tex Med* 1970;66:58–63.

287. Vacaflor L, Lehmann HE, Ban TA. Side effects and teratogenicity of lithium carbonate treatment. *J Clin Pharmacol* 1970;10:387–389.

288. Frankenberg RR, Lipinski JF. Congenital malformations. *N Engl J Med* 1983;309:311–312.

289. Warkany J. Teratogen Update: lithium. *Teratology* 1988;38:593–596.

290. Schardein JL, ed. *Chemically induced birth defects.* New York: Marcel Dekker, 1993.

291. Rane A, Tomson G, Bjarke B. Effects of maternal lithium therapy in a newborn infant. *J Pediatr* 1974;93:296–297.
292. Jacobson SJ, Jones K, Johnson K, et al. Prospective multicentre study of pregnancy outcome after lithium exposure during first trimester. *Lancet* 1992;339:530–533.
293. Cohen LS, Friedman JM, Jefferson JW, et al. A reevaluation of risk of in utero exposure to lithium. *JAMA* 1994;271:146–150.
294. Troyer WA, Pereira G, Lannon RA, et al. Association of maternal lithium exposure and premature delivery. *J Perinatol* 1993;13:123–127.
295. Schou M. What happened later to the lithium babies? A follow-up study of children born without malformations. *Acta Psychiatr Scand* 1976;54:193–197.
296. Holtzman EJ, Ausiello DA. Nephrogenic diabetes insipidus: causes revealed. *Hosp Pract* 1994;29:89–93,97–98,103–104.
297. Krause S, Ebbsen F, Lange AP. Polyhydramnios with maternal lithium treatment. *Obstet Gynecol* 1990;75:504–506.
298. Lam SS, Kjellstrand C. Emergency treatment of lithium-induced diabetes insipidus with non-steroidal anti-inflammatory drugs. *Renal Failure* 1997;19:183–188.
299. Nars PW, Girad J. Lithium carbonate intake during pregnancy leading to a large goiter in a premature infant. *Am J Dis Child* 1977;131:123–127.
300. Filtenborg JA. Persistent pulmonary hypertension after lithium intoxication in the newborn. *Eur J Pediatr* 1982;138:321–323.
301. Morrell P, Sutherland GR, Buamah PK, et al. Lithium toxicity in the neonate. *Arch Dis Child* 1983;58:539–541.
302. Wilson N, Forfar JD, Godman MJ. Atrial flutter in the newborn resulting from lithium ingestion. *Arch Dis Child* 1983;58:538–539.
303. Weinstein MR, Goldfield M. Cardiovascular malformations with lithium use during pregnancy. *Am J Psychiatry* 1975;132:529–531.
304. Hansen DK, Walker RC, Grafton TF. Effect of lithium carbonate on mouse and rat embryos in vitro. *Teratology* 1990;41:155–160.
305. Klug S, Collins M, Nagao T, et al. Effect of lithium on rat embryos in culture: growth, development, compartmental distribution and lack of protective effect of inositol. *Arch Toxicol* 1992;66:719–728.
306. Jurand A. Teratogenic activity of lithium carbonate: an experimental update. *Teratology* 1988;38:101–111.
307. Llewellyn A, Stowe ZN, Strader JR. The use of lithium and management of women with bipolar disorder during pregnancy and lactation. *J Clin Psychiatry* 1998;59:57–64.
308. Cowett RM, Hakanson DO, Kocon RW, et al. Untoward neonatal effect of intraamniotic administration of methylene blue. *Obstet Gynecol* 1976;48:745–755.
309. Serota FT, Bernbaum JC, Schwartz E. The methylene blue baby. *Lancet* 1979;2:1142–1143.
310. Crooks J. Haemolytic jaundice in a neonate after intra-amniotic injection of methylene blue. *Arch Dis Child* 1982;57:872–886.
311. Dolk H. Methylene blue and atresia or stenosis of ileum and jejunum. *Lancet* 1991;338:1021–1022.
312. Cragan JD. Teratogen Update: methylene blue. *Teratology* 1999;60:42–48.
313. Cragen JD, Martin L, Waters et al. Increased risk of small intestinal atresia among twins in the United States. *Arch Pediatr Adolesc Med* 1994;148:733–739.
314. van der Pol JG, Wolf H, Boer K, et al. Jejunal atresia related to the use of methylene blue in genetic amniocentesis in twins. *Br J Obstet Gynecol* 1992;99:141–143.
315. Moorman-Voestermans CGM, Heig HA, Vos A. Jejunal atresia in twins. *J Pediatr Surg* 1990;25:638–639.
316. Moorman-Voestermans CGM, Heij HA, Vos A. Letter to the Editor. *J Pediatr Surg* 1992;27:133.
317. Nicolini U, Monni G. Intestinal obstruction in babies exposed in utero to methylene blue. *Lancet* 1990;336:1258–1259.
318. Cragen JD, Martin L, Khoury MJ, et al. Dye use during amniocentesis and birth defects [Letter]. *Lancet* 1993;341:1352–1353.
319. Gluer S. Intestinal atresia following intraamniotic use of dyes. *Eur J Pediatr Surg* 1995;5:240–242.
320. Kidd SA, Lancaster PA, Anderson JC, et al. Fetal death after exposure to methylene blue dye during mid-trimester amniocentesis. *Prenat Diagn* 1996;16:39–47.
321. Kidd SA, Lancaster PA, Anderson JC, et al. A cohort study of pregnancy outcome after amniocentesis in twin pregnancy. *Paediatr Perinat Epidemiol* 1997;11:200–213.
322. Piersma AH, Verhoet A, DeLiefde A, et al. Embryotoxicity of methylene blue in the rat. *Teratology* 1991;43:458–459.
323. Gonzalez CH, Vargas FR, Perez ABA, et al. Limb deficiency with or without Moebius sequence in seven Brazilian children associated with misoprotol use in the first trimester of pregnancy. *Am J Med Genet* 1993;46:59–64.
324. Coelho HLL, Misago C, Fonsecam WVC, et al. Selling abortifacients over the counter in pharmacies in Fortaleza, Brazil. *Lancet* 1991;338:247.
325. Costa SH, Vessey MP. Misoprostol and illegal abortion in Rio de Janeiro, Brazil. *Lancet* 1993;341:1258–1261.
326. Luna-Coelho HL, Teixeria AC, Santos AP, et al. Misoprostol and illegal abortion in Fortaleza, Brazil. *Lancet* 1993;341:1261–1263.
327. Brent RL. Relationship between uterine vascular clamping, vascular disruption, and cocaine teratogenicity [Editorial]. *Teratology* 1990;41:757–760.
328. NICHD Workshop. CVS and limb reduction defects. *Teratology* 1993;48:7–13.
329. Collins FS, Mahoney MJ. Hydrocephalus and abnormal digits after failed first trimester prostaglandin abortion attempt. *J Pediatr* 1983;102:620–621.
330. Schuler LS, Ashto PW, Sanseverino MT. Teratogenicity of misoprostol. *Lancet* 1992;339:437.
331. Woods JR, Plessinger MA, Clark KE. Effect on cocaine on uterine blood flow and fetal oxygenation. *JAMA* 1987;257:957–961.
332. Schonhofer PS. Brazil: misuse of misoprostol as a abortifacient may induce malformations. *Lancet* 1991;337:1534.
333. Fonseca W, Alencar AJC, Mota FSB, et al. Misoprostol and congenital malformations. *Lancet* 1991;336:56.
334. Castilla EE, Orioli IM. Teratogenicity of misoprostol: data from the Latin-American collaborative study of congenital malformations (ECLAMC). *Am J Med Genet* 1994;51:161–162.
335. Zackai EH, Melmen WJ, Neiderer B, et al. The fetal trimethadione syndrome. *J Pediatr* 1975;87:280–284.
336. Cohen MM. Syndromology—an updated conceptual overview. VII. Aspects of teratogenesis. *Int J Oral Maxillofac Surg* 1990;19:26–32.
337. Feldman GL, Weaver DD, Lovrien EW. The fetal trimethadione syndrome. *Am J Dis Child* 1977;131:1389–1392.
338. Smith ES, Dafoe CS, Miller JR, et al. An epidemiological study of congenital reduction deformities of the limbs. *Br J Prev Soc Med* 1977;31:39–41.
339. Keen CL, Mark-Savage P, Lonnerdal B, et al. Teratogenesis and low copper status resulting from D-penicillamine in rats. *Teratology* 1982;26:163–165.
340. Harpey J-P, Jaudon M-C, Clavel J-P, et al. Cutix laxa and low serum zinc after antenatal exposure to penicillamine. *Lancet* 1983;2:858.
341. Linares A, Zarranz JJ, Rodriguez-Alarcon J, et al. Reversible cutix laxa due to maternal D-penicillamine treatment. *Lancet* 1979; 2:43.
342. Solomon L, Abrams G, Dinner M, et al. Neonatal abnormalities associated with D-pencillamine treatment during pregnancy. *N Engl J Med* 1977;296:54–55.
343. Greenberg G, Inman W, Weatherall J, et al. Maternal drug histories and congenital abnormalities. *Br Med J* 1977;2:853–856.
344. Nakane Y, Okuma T, Takahashi R, et al. Multi-institutional study on the teratogenicity and fetal toxicity of antieplieptic drugs: a report of a collaborative study group in Japan. *Epilepsia* 1980; 21:663.
345. Robert E, Lofkvist E, Mauguiere F, et al. Evaluation of drug therapy and teratogenic risk in a Rhone-Alps district population of pregnant epileptic women. *Eur Neurol* 1986;25:436–443.
346. Dansky L, Finnell R. Parental epilepsy, anticonvulsant drugs, and reproductive outcome: epidemiologic and experimental findings spanning three decades; 2, Human studies. *Reprod Toxicol* 1991; 5:301–335.
347. Waters C, Belai Y, Gott P, et al. Outcomes of pregnancy associated with antiepileptic drugs. *Arch Neurol* 1994;51:250–253.
348. Kelly T. Teratogenicity of anticonvulsant drugs I: Review of the literature. *Am J Med Genet* 1984;19:413–434.
349. Dravet C, Julian C, Legras C, et al. Epilepsy, antiepileptic drugs, and malformations in children of women with epilepsy: a French prospective cohort study. *Neurology* 1992;42:75–82.
350. Lindhout D, Meinardi H, Meijer JWA, et al. Antiepileptic drugs and teratogenesis in two consecutive cohorts: changes in prescription policy paralleled by changes in pattern of malformations. *Neurology* 1992;42:94–110.

351. Tanganelli P, Regesta G. Epilepsy, pregnancy, and major birth anomalies: an Italian prospective controlled study. *Neurology* 1992;42:89–93.
352. Seip M. Growth retardation, dysmorphic facies and minor malformations following massive exposure to phenobarbitone in utero. *Acta Paediatr Scand* 1976;65:617–621.
353. Jones K, Johnson K, Chamber C. Pregnancy outcome in women treated with phenobarbitol monotherapy. *Teratology* 1992;45:452–453.
354. Koch S, Losche G, Jager-Roman E, et al. Major and minor birth malformations and antiepileptic drugs. *Neurology* 1992;42:83–88.
355. Morales WJ. Antenatal therapy to minimize neonatal intraventricular hemorrhage. *Clin Obstet Gynecol* 1991;34:328–335.
356. Morales WJ. Effect of intraventricular hemorrhage on the one-year mental and neurologic handicaps of the very low birth weight infant. *Obstet Gynecol* 1987;70:111–114.
357. Fotherby K. A new look at progestins. *Clin Obstet Gynecol* 1984;11:701–722.
358. Wilkins L. Masculinization due to orally given progestins. *JAMA* 1960;172:1028–1032.
359. World Health Organization. The effect of female sex hormones on fetal development and infant health. Geneva: World Health Organization, 1981.
360. Heinonen OP, Slone D, Monson RR, et al. Cardiovascular birth defects and antenatal exposure to female sex hormones. *N Engl J Med* 1977;296:67–70.
361. Wiseman RA, Dodds-Smith IC. Cardiovascular birth defects and antenatal exposure to female sex hormones: a reevaluation of some base data. *Teratology* 1984;30:359–370.
362. Gal I. Risks and benefits of the use of hormonal pregnancy test tablets. *Nature* 1972;240:241–242.
363. Janerich DT, Piper JM, Glebatis DM. Oral contraceptives and congenital limb reduction defects. *N Engl J Med* 1974;291:697–700.
364. Brent RL. The magnitude of the problem of congenital malformations. In: Marois M, ed. *Prevention of physical and mental congenital defect part a basic and medical Science, education and future strategies.* New York: Alan R. Liss, 1985:55–68.
365. O'Malley BW, Schrader DT. The receptors of steroid hormones. *Sci Am* 1976;234:32–43.
366. Lammer EJ. Developmental toxicity of synthetic retinoids in humans. *Prog Clin Biol Res* 1988;281:193–202.
367. Rosa FW. Teratogen Update: penicillamine. *Teratology* 1986;33:127–131.
368. Dai WS, Hsu M, Itri LM. Safety of pregnancy after discontinuation of isotretinoin. *Arch Dermatol* 1989;125:362–365.
369. Dai WS, LaBraico JM, Stern RS. Epidemiology of isotretinoin exposure during pregnancy. *J Am Acad Dermatol* 1992;26:599–606.
370. DiGiovanna JJ, Zech LA, Ruddel ME, et al. Etretinate: persistent serum levels of a potent teratogen. *Clin Res* 1984;32:579A.
371. Rinck G, Gollnick H, Organos CE. Duration of contraception after etretinate. *Lancet* 1989;1:845–846.
372. Alles AJ, Sulik KK. Retinoic-acid-induced limb-reduction defects: perturbation of zones of programmed cell death as a pathogenetic mechanism. *Teratology* 1989;40:163–171.
373. Yasuda Y, Konishi H, Kihara T, et al. Developmental anomalies induced by all-trans-retinoic acid in fetal mice: II. Induction of abnormal neuroepithelium. *Teratology* 1987;35:355–366.
374. Ong DE, Chytil F. Changes in levels of cellular retinol-and retinoic-acid-binding proteins of liver and lung during perinatal development rat. *Proc Natl Acad Sci U S A* 1976;73:3976–3978.
375. Jick SS, Terris BZ, Jick H. First trimester topical tretinoin and congenital disorders. *Lancet* 1993;341:1181–1182.
376. DeWals P, Bloch D, Calabro A, et al. Association between holoprosencephaly and exposure to topical retinoids: results of the EUROCAT survey. *Paediatr Perinat Epidemiol* 1991;5:445–447.
377. Bowman JM. Antenatal suppression of Rh alloimmunization. *Clin Obstet Gynecol* 1991;34:296–303.
378. Prager K, Malin H, Speigler D, et al. Smoking and drinking behavior before and during pregnancy of married mothers of liveborn and stillborn infants. *Public Health Rep* 1984;99:117–127.
379. Naeye RL. Effects of maternal cigarette smoking on the fetus and placenta. *Br J Obstet Gynaecol* 1979;85:732–737.
380. Chattingius S. Does age potentiate the smoking-related risk of fetal growth retardation? *Early Hum Dev* 1989;20:203–211.
381. Hjortdal JO, Hjortdal VE, Foldspang A. Tobacco smoking and fetal growth: a review. *Scand J Soc Med* 1989;45:1–22.
382. Stillman RJ, Rosenberg MJ, Sachs BP. Smoking and reproduction. *Fertil Steril* 1986;46:545–566.
383. Erickson JD. Risk factors for birth defects: data from the Atlanta defects case-control study. *Teratology* 1991;43:41–51.
384. Tikkanen J, Heinonen OP. Maternal exposure to chemical and physical factors during pregnancy and cardiovascular malformations in the offspring. *Teratology* 1991;43:591–600.
385. Werler MM, Pober BR, Holmes LB. Smoking and pregnancy. *Teratology* 1985;32:473–481.
386. Lenz W, Knapp K. Thalidomide embryopathy. *Arch Environ Health* 1962;5:100–105.
387. Brent RL, Holmes LB. Clinical and basic science lessons from the thalidomide tragedy: what have we learned about the causes of limb defects? *Teratology* 1988;38:241–251.
388. Lenz W. A short history of thalidomide embryopathy. *Teratology* 1988;38:203–215.
389. Kida M. *Thalidomide embryopathy in Japan.* Kodansha, Tokyo: 1987.
390. Ruffing L. Evaluation of thalidomide children. *Birth Defects Orig Artic Ser* 1977;13:287–300.
391. Cutler J. Thalidomide revisted. *Lancet* 1994;343:795–796.
392. Jones GRN. Thalidomide: 35 years on and still deforming. *Lancet* 1994;343:1041.
393. Stephens TD. Proposed mechanisms of action in thalidomide embryopathy. *Teratology* 1988;38:229–239.
394. Carswell F, Kerr MM, Hutchinson JH. Congenital goiter and hypothyroidism produced by maternal ingestion of iodides. *Lancet* 1970;1:1241–1243.
395. Rodesch F, Camus M, Ermans AM, et al. Adverse effect of amniofetography on fetal thyroid function. *Am J Obstet Gynecol* 1976;126:723–726.
396. Clewell WP. In utero treatment of thyrotoxicosis. In: Evans MI, et al, eds. *Fetal diagnosis and therapy: science, ethics, and the law.* Philadelphia: JB Lippincott, 1984:124.
397. Smith CV. Reversing acute intrapartum fetal distress using tocolytic drugs. *Clin Obstet Gynecol* 1991;34:353–359.
398. Caritis SN, Darby MJ, Chan L. Pharmacologic treatment of preterm labor. *Clin Obstet Gynecol* 1988;31:635–651.
399. Egarter CH, Husslein PW, Rayburn WF. Uterine hyperstimulation after low-dose prostagladin E2 therapy: tocolytic treatment in 181 cases. *Am J Obstet Gynecol* 1990;163:794–796.
400. Mendez-Bauer C, Shekarloo A, Cook V, et al. Treatment of acute intrapartum fetal distress by beta 2-symphatomimetics. *Am J Obstet Gynecol* 1987;148:104–106.
401. Reece EA, Chervenak FA, Romero R, et al. Magnesium sulfate in the management of acute intrapartum fetal distress. *Am J Obstet Gynecol* 1984;148:104–106.
402. Toutant C, Lippman S. Fetal solvents syndrome. *Lancet* 1979;1:1356.
403. Pearson MA, Hoyme HE, Seaver LH, et al. Toluene embryopathy: delineation of the phenotype and comparison with fetal alcohol syndrome. *Pediatrics* 1994;93:211–215.
404. Arnold GL, Kirby RS, Langendoerfer S, et al. Toluene embryopathy: clinical delineation and developmental follow-up. *Pediatrics* 1994;93:216–220.
405. Safra MJ, Oakley GP. Valium: an oral cleft teratogen? *Cleft Palate J* 1976;13:198–200.
406. Dalens B, Raynaud E-J, Gaulme J. Teratogenicity of valproic acid. *J Pediatr* 1980;97:332–333.
407. Robert E. Valproic acid as a human teratogen. *Congenit Anom Kyoto* 1988;28:S71-S80.
408. Omtzigt JGC, Nau H, Los FJ, et al. The disposition of valproate and its metabolites in the late first trimester and early second trimester of pregnancy in maternal serum, urine and amniotic fluid: effect of dose, co-medication, and the presence of spina bifida. *Eur J Clin Pharmacol* 1992;43:381–388.
409. Lammer EJ, Sever LE, Oakley GP. Valproic acid. *Teratology* 1987;35:465–473.
410. Dickinson RG, Hapland RC, Lynn RK, et al. Transmission of valproic acid across the placenta: half-lives of the drug in mother and baby. *J Pediatr* 1979;94:832–835.
411. Teratology Society. Teratology Society position paper: recommendation for vitamin A use during pregnancy. *Teratology* 1987;35:269–275.
412. Zuber C, Librizzi RJ, Vogt BI. Outcomes of pregnancies exposed to high doses of vitamin A. *Teratology* 1987;35:42A.

413. Ampola MG, Mahoney MJ, Nakamura E, et al. Prenatal therapy of a patient with vitamin B responsive methylmalonic acidemia. *N Engl J Med* 1975;293:313–317.

414. Goodenday L, Gordon G. No risk from vitamin D in pregnancy. *Ann Intern Med* 1971;75:807–808.

415. O'Brien J, Rosenwasser S, Feingold M, et al. Prenatal exposure to milk with excessive vitamin D supplementation. *Teratology* 1993;47:387.

416. Friedman WF. Vitamin D and the supravalvular aortic stenosis syndrome. In: Woollam DHM, ed. *Advances in teratology.* New York: Academic Press, 1968:83–96.

417. Garcia RE, Friedman WF, Kaback MM, et al. Idiopathic hypercalcemia and supravalvular stenosis: documentation of a new syndrome. *N Engl J Med* 1964;271:117–120.

418. Ewart A, Morris C, Atkinson D. Hemizygosity at the elastin locus in a developmental disorder, Williams syndrome. *Nature Genet* 1993;5:11–16.

419. Mari A, Amati F, Mingarelli R. Analysis of the elastin gene in 60 patients with clinical diagnosis of Williams syndrome. *Hum Genet* 1995;96:444–448.

Obstetric Anesthesia and Analgesia: Effects on the Fetus and Newborn

16

Judith Littleford

Many drugs and various techniques have been used to provide anesthesia and analgesia for surgery during pregnancy, for labor and delivery, and for breastfeeding. The following quote, which refers to the first administration of inhalational analgesia in childbirth, is as relevant to the practice of obstetric anesthesia today as it was in 1847, "It will be necessary *to ascertain anesthesia's precise effect*, both *upon the action of the uterus* and *on the* assistant *abdominal muscles*; its influence, if any, *upon the child*; whether it has the tendency to hemorrhage *or other complications*" (1). Between the mid-1800s and 1950s, descriptive reports of the presumed effect of maternally administered medication on the fetus and newborn appeared sporadically in the literature. Two developments eventually encouraged physicians to acknowledge the potential problems associated with placental transmission of anesthetic drugs:

1. Recognition that morphine, a popular ingredient of patent medicines, was addictive, and that signs of withdrawal could be identified in the fetus (violent fetal movements and/or sudden fetal death) when the mother's heavy opioid use was decreased.
2. Confirmation of the structure and dynamic function of the placenta and demonstration of the presence of chloroform in the umbilical blood of neonates.

In 1952 the pioneering work of anesthesiologist Virginia Apgar converted an intangible phenomenon, the clinical condition of a newly born baby, into a formally defined measurement (2). Thereafter, the well-being of the infant became a major criterion for evaluation of the obstetric and anesthetic management of pregnant women.

This chapter introduces the neonatal practitioner to the clinical aspects of obstetric anesthesia and analgesia and examines their effects on the fetus and newborn.

EVALUATION OF WELL-BEING

Several methods of evaluation have been adopted into common usage as anesthesiologists attempt to separate out the fetal/neonatal effects of their interventions from concomitant medical and nursing management, and from the influence of preexisting maternal conditions.

The Apgar Score

The Apgar score is a convenient method of reporting the status of the newborn and the effectiveness of resuscitation. It rates each of five physical signs traditionally used by anesthesiologists to monitor a patient's condition: heart rate, respiratory effort, muscle tone, reflex irritability, and color. Apgar demonstrated that her score was sufficiently sensitive to detect differences among newborns whose mothers had received spinal versus general anesthesia (GA) for cesarean section (2).

Elements of the score are partly dependent on the physiologic maturity of the infant. Likewise, neonatal conditions such as bradyarrhythmias affect heart rate, while infection, neuromuscular conditions, and certain medications affect respiratory effort and tone. Additional information is required to interpret Apgar scores meaningfully in infants receiving ongoing resuscitation.

Wider application has resulted in incorrect use of the Apgar score to evaluate infant morbidity/mortality and to predict the occurrence of intrapartum events and long-term disability. Apgar scores at 1 and 5 minutes correlate poorly with both cause and neurologic outcome. A joint statement from the American Academy of Pediatrics (AAP) and American College of Obstetricians and Gynecologists emphasizes the appropriate use of the Apgar Score (3).

When used as originally intended, the Apgar score remains a valuable tool to assess the condition of the infant at birth (4), but it is not specific for the effects of anesthesia on the newborn.

Umbilical Cord Blood Gas Analysis

Cord blood gas analysis is the gold standard for assessing fetal acid-base status and uteroplacental function at birth. Umbilical artery pH, base excess, and pCO_2 reflect fetal and immediate neonatal condition whereas umbilical vein values reflect maternal acid-base status and placental function.

"Normal" values vary depending on the definition of normality and the influence of factors (e.g., altitude, parity, breech vaginal delivery, and duration of labor) on the population studied (5). Helwig and associates (6) retrospectively examined the records of 15,000 vigorous newborns with a 5-minute Apgar score of >7. Median umbilical artery values, with the 2.5th percentile value in parentheses, were pH 7.26 (7.10) and base excess −4 mmol/L (−11 mmol/L). The means ± 2 standard deviations were similar. The generally accepted lower limit of normal umbilical artery pH extends to 7.10 and base excess to −12 mmol/L (5,7).

Values for pH, pCO_2, and base excess also vary with differences in sampling technique. Preanalytical error can be introduced if the cord is not clamped immediately, there is an excess quantity of heparin in relation to the amount of blood collected, air is present in the syringe, or the sample is kept at room temperature for longer than 15 minutes (8).

The supply of oxygen and the removal of volatile (CO_2) and fixed (e.g., lactate) acids by the placenta for excretion by the maternal lungs and kidneys, respectively, allow the fetus to maintain acid-base balance within a narrow range. Interruption of these processes can lead to acidemia in the fetus. In general, respiratory acidosis alone is not associated with newborn complications; rather, it reflects a sudden decrease in uteroplacental or umbilical perfusion such as placental abruption or cord prolapse immediately preceding delivery. Base excess values have greater usefulness than pH values because base excess does not change significantly with respiratory acidosis and demonstrates linear, rather than logarithmic, correlation to the degree of metabolic acidosis. Umbilic artery base excess is the most direct measure of fetal metabolic acidosis. Human and animal studies have confirmed normal values before and during labor and rates of base excess change in relation to events causing fetal hypoxemia (maternal hypoxemia, umbilical cord occlusion, and reduced uterine blood flow) (7).

The process of normal labor and delivery without anesthetic intervention stresses the fetus such that mild acidosis develops in almost all labors (9). Reynolds and associates (10) recently completed a metanalysis comparing epidural with systemic opioid analgesia to determine the effect of these anesthetic interventions on acid-base status at birth. They concluded that epidural analgesia was associated with an improvement in base excess, suggesting that placental exchange is well preserved in association with this technique.

While umbilical artery pH, base excess, and pCO_2 are considered sensitive and objective indicators of fetal hypoxia during labor, the results represent a "snapshot" of fetal status and depict the mixed effluent of all fetal tissues. Cord gases do not distinguish between primary fetal pathologic conditions, fetal effects of maternal conditions (e.g., acid-base disorders), or the influence of inadequate placental blood flow. They also do not indicate in which direction the condition of the fetus is moving, or at what rate, nor do they reflect events that occurred remote from delivery.

Fetal Scalp Blood Gas Analysis

This method is advocated to improve the specificity of fetal heart rate monitoring (11) but has not been used by anesthesiologists to measure the fetal effects of their interventions.

Evaluation of Newborn Neurobehavior

Brazelton, Scanlon, and Amiel-Tison assessed the effect of anesthetic medications on the neurobehavior of term, healthy newborns (12–14). Their belief was that central nervous system depression from drugs administered to the mother during labor and delivery could be distinguished from effects associated with perinatal asphyxia and trauma at birth. Several review articles have described these tests in detail and compared the Brazelton Neonatal Behavioral Assessment Scale (NBAS) (12) and Early Neonatal Neurobehavioral Scale (ENNS) (13) to the Neurologic and Adaptive Capacity Score (NACS) (14).

Researchers in obstetric anesthesia have tended to favor the NACS. It emphasizes muscle tone, avoids aversive stimuli, can be completed quickly, and is considered easier to learn than the NBAS and ENNS. The 20-item instrument is organized into two scales, adaptive capacity and neurologic assessment. The latter is further divided into four subscales, passive tone, active tone, primary reflexes, and general neurologic status assessment. A systematic review of the literature regarding use of NACS in obstetric anesthesia research concluded that reliability and validity evaluations of the tool were lacking, and it was unclear whether NACS could detect the existence of subtle neurobehavioral effects (15). The topic was the subject of an editorial that examined the widespread acceptance of this test notwithstanding the criticism that surrounded its initial publication (16). Subsequently, it has been determined that NACS has poor reliability when used to detect the effects of intrapartum drugs and other interventions on the neonate (17).

The NBAS is a much more detailed examination that may be more sensitive to environmental influences on behavior and reflect more accurately the capabilities of the neonate (18). Early studies involving concentrated epidural solutions tended to show that babies delivered to medicated mothers were less alert, had poorer muscle tone, and had difficulty habituating to repeated stimuli. This finding is much less likely to occur with modern obstetric analgesia (19), where emphasis is placed on administering the lowest effective dose of medication or combination of medications needed to achieve the desired maternal effect and reduce the likelihood of adverse influences on the fetus/newborn.

Electronic Fetal Monitoring

Electronic fetal monitoring, one technique in the overall strategy of intrapartum fetal surveillance (20,21), aims to improve outcomes by identifying fetuses with hypoxic acidemia at a point when the process is still completely reversible by intrauterine resuscitation or expedited delivery. The fetal heart rate (FHR), including variability, accelerations, and decelerations, if any occur, is recorded electronically on a paper trace. A reactive (normal or reassuring) cardiotocogram (CTG) is defined by the presence of accelerations. Baseline FHR normally ranges between 110 and 160 beats per minute. Reduced variability and the presence of decelerations are abnormal findings.

A systematic review of studies comparing the efficacy and safety of routine continuous electronic fetal monitoring versus intermittent auscultation (IA) of the FHR reveals the former to be associated with a significantly higher rate of cesarean and operative vaginal delivery (22). In the antecedent Cochrane review of this same topic, the incidence of GA to facilitate obstetric intervention was also increased. This aspect of management was not examined in the current review. The only significant benefit of the use of routine, continuous fetal monitoring was in the reduction of neonatal seizures; otherwise, neither IA nor continuous monitoring has been shown to decrease morbidity or mortality (22).

Difficulty in the visual interpretation of CTG patterns during labor can result in unnecessary operative intervention, while some significant changes go unrecognized. Computerized CTG systems, which do not rely on observer reading of the FHR tracing, are more accurate and reliable. Evaluation of the FHR pattern is given online continuously, and warnings are displayed if there is signal loss, reduction in fetal movements, or an abnormally flat or decelerative trace (23). Retrospective analysis of several thousand records enabled investigators to conclude that the most reliable single parameter of fetal condition was variability (short- and long-term). Absence of accelerations, presence of decelerations, decrease in the number of movements, and changes in baseline FHR all occurred occasionally in normal fetuses (24).

Recently, automatic ST segment and T-wave analysis of the fetal electrocardiogram (recorded continuously from the fetal scalp electrode used for FHR measurement) has been combined with conventional CTG. Elevation or depression of the ST segment occurs when the fetus is exposed to a hypoxic stress. When CTG is accompanied by computerized analysis of the ST segment, the number of operative deliveries for the indication of "fetal distress" can be reduced without jeopardizing fetal outcome (24). This

technique of fetal surveillance improves the practitioner's ability to identify cases of significant fetal hypoxia necessitating obstetric intervention, thus reducing the risk of an umbilical cord arterial metabolic acidosis at birth (25).

Anesthesiologists have used continuous fetal CTG recordings to evaluate the effect of maternal analgesia on FHR and variability. Solt and associates (26) demonstrated that intrapartum intravenous (IV) administration of meperidine (pethidine) 50 mg and promethazine 25 mg resulted in decreased variability and fewer accelerations on computerized CTG for the duration of their 40-minute recording. It is unclear whether the effect can be attributed to one of the two drugs or the combination, although this is a typical fetal response to systemic maternal opioid administration.

A randomized study was conducted to examine the effect of continuous epidural anesthesia with or without narcotic on intrapartum FHR characteristics as measured by computer analysis. The narcotic epidural consisted of an initial bolus of 10–12 mL 0.125% bupivacaine with fentanyl 50 μg, followed by continuous bupivacaine 0.125% with fentanyl 1.7 μg/mL infusion. The nonnarcotic epidural was initiated with a bolus of 10–12 mL bupivacaine 0.25% and followed by a bupivacaine 0.125% infusion. Investigators found no difference in pre- and postepidural baseline FHR, accelerations, or variability between the groups (27). These solutions are considerably less concentrated than those used 10–20 years ago and are in keeping with modern obstetric anesthesia practice, which aims to reduce motor block by using dilute local anesthetic (LA) plus narcotic epidural solution combinations.

In a double-blind randomized study of bolus epidural opioid effect on FHR variability, butorphanol 2 mg, fentanyl 50 μg, sufentanil 15 μg, or saline in combination with bupivacaine 0.25% did not change FHR short- or long-term variability (28).

FHR decreases in response to compression of the fetal head during passage through the birth canal and in response to umbilical cord compression or reduced uterine blood flow secondary to maternal hypotension or prolonged uterine contraction. This bradycardia is vagally mediated.

Biophysical Profile Score

This ultrasound-based method combines measures of acute biophysical variables, fetal breathing, heart rate accelerations, gross body movements, and fetal tone with amniotic fluid volume (29). The first four variables reflect acute fetal condition, whereas the last variable reflects chronic fetal condition. The observation period lasts 30 minutes because fetuses are known to sleep for intervals lasting approximately 30 minutes. When normal (≥8 out of a possible 10), the biophysical profile score (BPS) is a direct, reliable, and accurate measure of normal tissue oxygenation. A normal score is never associated with an abnormal fetal pH. Scores ≤6/10 during routine antepartum evaluation indicate the amount of oxygen delivered to target organs is insufficient to maintain function. The lower the score, the greater the likelihood that central acidemia is present (30).

Placental transfer to the fetus of maternally administered intramuscular (i.m.) narcotic medication (diamorphine 10 mg or morphine 10 or 15 mg administered with dimenhydrinate) resulted in transiently reduced fetal activity and, consequently, a lower BPS for the duration of the drug effect (31,32). A small dose of IV fentanyl (50 μg) given in early labor was associated with abolishment of fetal breathing at 10 minutes postdosing, fewer body movements, and reduced variability (33). The effect lasted approximately 30 minutes, in keeping with the pharmacodynamic profile of fentanyl. This should be taken into account when fentanyl is administered close to the time of delivery. In this study, none of the neonates required resuscitation, and all had umbilical artery pH values >7.2.

Fetal Pulse Oximetry

Fetal oxygen saturation monitoring by pulse oximetry (SpO$_2$) is poised to become the most significant advance for intrapartum fetal assessment in recent years. It relies on established, noninvasive technology and is based on the following assumptions: fetal well-being is dependent on perfusion of vital organs with oxygenated blood; SpO$_2$ correlates with saturation as measured by blood gas analysis; and a critical threshold for SpO$_2$ exists, above which the fetus will be nonacidemic and below which, acid-base decompensation may occur (34).

Based on animal and human data, fetal SpO$_2$ values ≥30% can be considered reassuring, whereas SpO$_2$ values <30% may be associated with acidosis. Low SpO$_2$ values warrant further assessment if they persist for periods of >2 minutes and necessitate intervention (intrauterine resuscitation or expedited delivery) if they persist for >10 minutes (34,35). The predictive value of intrapartum fetal SpO$_2$ compares favorably with fetal scalp blood analysis (36). The former has the advantage of being a continuous monitoring technique.

The United States Food and Drug Administration approved the Nellcor N-400/FS14 fetal pulse oximeter for clinical use in 2000 as an adjunct to electronic fetal monitoring in the presence of a nonreassuring tracing (Fig. 16-1). At present, this technology is limited to singleton, term fetuses in the vertex position.

Results of studies designed to investigate the effects on fetal oxygen saturation of administering epidurals to healthy parturients are beginning to appear in the literature. Neither an initial epidural bolus of 15 mL of ropivacaine 0.1% with sufentanil 10 μg or intermittent repeat plain ropivacaine boluses affected SpO$_2$ in healthy fetuses (37). In a study designed to account for the possible influence of maternal position, diastolic blood pressure, and preexisting FHR pattern, SpO$_2$ values were not affected by boluses of dilute epidural infusion solutions but did decrease with bolus administration of more concentrated LA at epidural insertion or top-up (38). Other than to

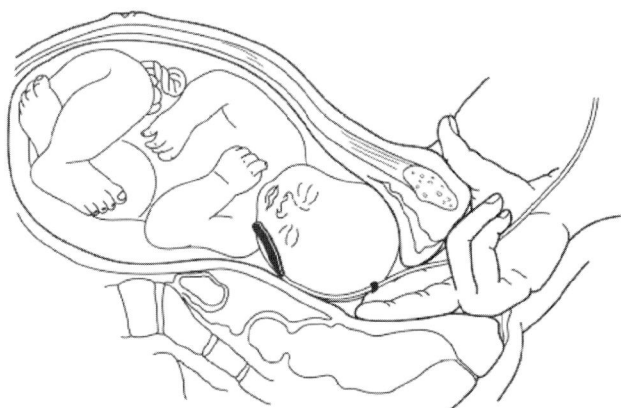

Figure 16-1 Oxifirst Fetal Pulse Oximetry. Reprinted with permission from TycoHealthcare. Copyright 2000 Mallinckrodt, Inc. All rights reserved.

comment on the variety of combinations and strengths of analgesic agents, details of the epidural solutions were not contained in the report. Further clinical trials are needed to assess and characterize the effect of all types of anesthetic intervention on fetal SpO$_2$ during normal and abnormal labor, in addition to various maternal conditions associated with fetal compromise (e.g., pregnancy-induced hypertension).

Fetal Doppler

Flow velocity waveforms from maternal vessels (uterine arteries), placental circulation (umbilical arteries), and fetal systemic vessels (e.g., middle cerebral artery), collectively known as Doppler evaluation, provide prognostic and diagnostic detail about placentation and fetal adaptation (39).

Regulation of the circulation is a complex fetal behavior, influenced by gestational age and the maternal environment. Under normal circumstances, the reduction in sympathetic tone created by epidural analgesia does not affect Doppler flow characteristics of either the uterine or umbilical artery vessels because the spiral arterioles are maximally dilated and the fetoplacental circulation is stable and tolerant of environmental changes. However, epidural analgesia has been shown to improve uteroplacental perfusion and effectively reduce maternal blood pressure in laboring patients with pregnancy-induced hypertension (40). This offers potential benefits for both the fetus and mother: when uteroplacental perfusion improves, fetal oxygenation and acid-base balance improve, and when blood pressure is restored to normal levels, the risk of vascular accidents and organ damage is reduced.

Static Charge-Sensitive Bed

A new method for long-term monitoring of respiration, heart rate, cardiac function, and body movements in newborn infants was presented in 1984, and possible clinical applications were discussed (41). The technology has been used to evaluate neonatal sleep states following unmedicated vaginal delivery or elective cesarean section delivery under spinal anesthesia (42) and, in combination with SpO_2 and ECG recording, to examine the influence on the newborn baby of maternal fentanyl analgesia in labor (43).

In the first study, mode of delivery did not affect sleep state distribution during the first day of life (42). Vaginally born neonates had fewer body movements and more episodes of SpO_2 <95% in the first 24 hours after birth. This result surprised the investigators since babies born by cesarean section are known to develop respiratory problems more often than infants who are delivered vaginally. In the second study, fentanyl (50 μg of IV bolus q5min until pain relief, then fentanyl patient-controlled analgesia) was compared with paracervical block (10 mL of bupivacaine 0.25%) in a prospective, randomized fashion. The trial was interrupted after enrolment of the twelfth healthy, term newborn because there was a significant decrease in SpO_2 to 59% in one of the babies. Interestingly, the SpO_2 improved with naloxone administration even though later analysis showed the concentration of fentanyl in the umbilical vein to be below the detection limit of the assay. Intrapartum electronic fetal monitoring did not reveal any difference in variability or heart rate between groups. As well, Apgar scores and analyses of umbilical artery pH were similar. The SpO_2 values were lower and the percentage of minimum SpO_2 values between 81% and 90% were more prevalent in the fentanyl group. The static charge-sensitive bed (SCSB) method proved sensitive enough to detect lower heart rates and less quiet sleep in the fentanyl group, suggesting a salutary effect of the opioid on delivery stress (43).

Summary

The nature of the association of anesthetic medications and interventions is complex and can be confounded by a myriad of factors. As yet, there is no one test that clearly separates effects on the fetus/newborn, if any, of maternally administered medication during labor and delivery, although newer technologies show some promise.

PAIN MANAGEMENT

For most women, childbirth is likely one of the most painful events in their lifetimes. There are both physiologic and psychologic aspects to pain and its management (44).

Labor pain evokes a generalized neuroendocrine stress response that has widespread physiologic effects on the parturient and fetus (45). The neuroendocrine model, presented in Figure 16-2, examines the potential detrimental consequences of untreated pain. The sequelae of hyperventilation, secretion of stress-related hormones, and increased oxygen consumption can be prevented, obtunded, or abolished by central neuraxial blockade (epidural or spinal anesthesia).

Research in humans supports elements of this model (46), but studies are not necessarily designed to consider the effects of simultaneously occurring care practices on these same physiologic responses. "This critique is needed because it is somewhat counterintuitive that the procreative physiologic process of labor and birth would by nature have detrimental effects on a healthy mother and fetus" (47). An example of a concurrent care practice is the administration of isotonic "sport drinks" versus water only during labor (48). Sports drinks were shown to prevent the development of maternal ketosis without increasing gastric volume, although there was no difference between the groups in neonatal outcome.

Labor Pain: Implications for the Fetus

Neural pathways and neurochemical systems involved in pain perception are functional from mid-gestation and are well developed by the third trimester (49,50). Gitau and associates (51) conducted a parallel study of the fetal and maternal hormonal responses to fetal blood transfusion. They confirmed that the fetus mounts a hypothalamic-pituitary-adrenal response to transfusion via the intrahepatic vein, which involves piercing the fetal trunk, but not to transfusion in the umbilical vein at the placental cord insertion, which has no sensory innervation. The rise in fetal cortisol and endorphin occurred independently of the maternal reaction. Pretreatment of the fetus with fentanyl for this same procedure attenuated the rise in β-endorphin (52).

Hormonal stress responses do not provide a direct index of pain. While it is true that a rise in cortisol and endorphin is seen as a consequence of painful stimuli in children, other nonpainful situations (e.g., exercise) are also associated with an increase in the levels of these hormones. Nonetheless, editorial review of Fisk's fentanyl pretreatment study suggests that fetal analgesia should be given during invasive *in utero* procedures (53).

At present, there is no literature on fetal "pain" during labor or delivery.

Labor and Delivery Pain: Implications for the Mother

Visceral pain predominates during the first stage of labor. Nociceptive information arising from uterine contractions, distention of the lower uterine segment, and cervical dilation is relayed in C afferent fibers to the dorsal horn of the spinal cord at the T10 to L1 levels. As labor progresses, a mixture of visceral and somatic (A-delta fibers) pain results from traction on the pelvic floor structures surrounding the vaginal vault, and eventually from distention and stretch of the vagina and perineum (L2-S1). Delivery pain (Stage II) is somatic in nature and transmitted along the pudendal nerve (S2-4). Synaptic input at the dorsal horn, mediated by neurotransmitters and chemicals (e.g., excitatory amino acids), is relayed via the spinothalamic tract to higher centers including the reticular formation, hypothalamus, and limbic system. Dorsal horn neurons also initiate segmental spinal reflexes. Descending spinal tracts, endogenous opioids, and other inhibitory systems modulate

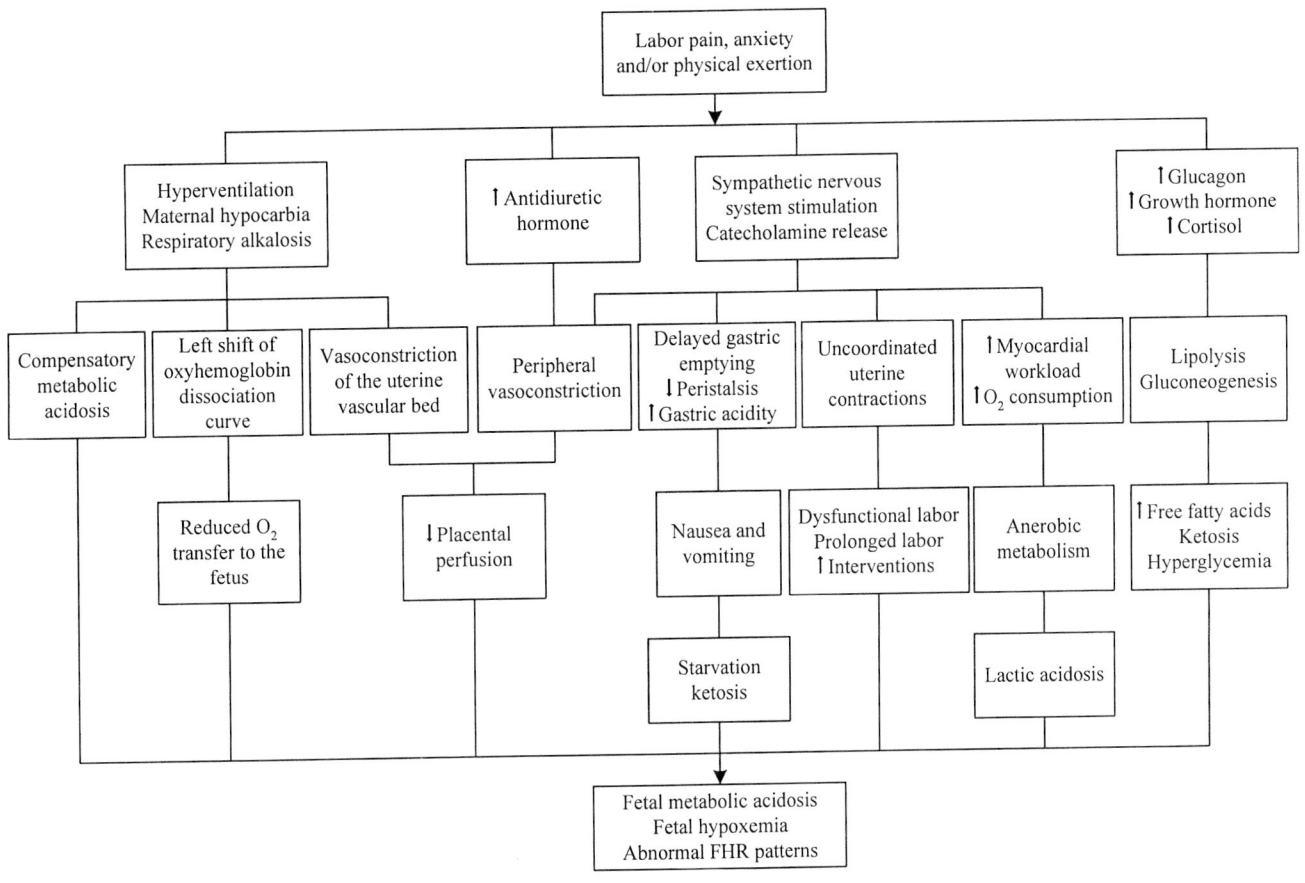

Figure 16-2   Potential adverse effects of untreated maternal pain on the fetus. (Modified from Brownridge P, Cohen SE, Ward ME. Neural blockade for obstetrics and gynecologic surgery. In: Cousins MJ, Bridenbaugh PO, eds. *Neural blockade in clinical anesthesia and management of pain*, 3rd ed. Philadelphia: Lippincott Williams & Wilkins, 1998:557–604, with permission.)

nociception centrally in the spinal cord. The neural mechanism of labor shares features with other forms of acute pain (54).

To view labor pain only as a neuroendocrine, sensory experience is limiting and undermines the complexity of this phenomenon (47). Pain is just one component of the totality of the labor and birth experience. Assisting women to cope with the affective or distress components of labor and birth in a supportive environment has been shown to reduce the need for pain-relieving drugs, decrease the incidence of operative delivery, result in higher Apgar scores, and improve breastfeeding success (44,55).

Practice guidelines, including a section devoted to specific analgesia techniques, have been developed to enhance the quality of anesthetic care for obstetric patients (56). For the obstetrician, analgesia options are outlined in a practice bulletin that was written to facilitate communication with patients and anesthesia and neonatology colleagues (57).

The management of pain and anxiety in labor is a worthwhile goal whether the techniques used are nonpharmacologic, pharmacologic, or include a combination of both. The choice depends on patient preferences, medical status of the mother and fetus, progress of labor, and resources available at the facility for pain management and treatment of potential complications.

ANALGESIC TECHNIQUES FOR LABOR: EFFECTS ON THE FETUS AND NEWBORN

Analgesia refers to pain relief without loss of consciousness. Regional analgesia denotes partial sensory blockade in a specific area of the body, with or without partial motor blockade. The term neuraxial analgesia pertains to the administration of pain-relieving medications using caudal, spinal, and/or epidural techniques.

Not all methods of pain relief are available or desirable in all centers, and certain methods are more popular in different parts of the world (58).

Nonpharmacologic Methods

Proponents of nonpharmacologic methods claim that these methods reduce requirements for analgesia during the first stage of labor. This does not necessarily imply that women who use these techniques have less pain, rather that they are able to cope with labor using less analgesia.

In a systematic review of comfort measures, Simkin and O'Hara (59) commented on five methods scientifically evaluated for their effectiveness in reducing indicators of labor pain. This review also mentioned pain-related outcomes such as obstetric interventions and duration of labor. *Continuous labor support* was associated with a decrease in duration of labor, requests for analgesia, rates of instrumental and cesarean deliveries, and occurrence of lower Apgar scores. The use of *baths* offered temporary pain relief and was considered safe provided water temperatures were maintained at or below maternal body temperature and that immersion duration was controlled. Perinatal morbidity and mortality did not increase, even if membranes were ruptured. The authors concluded that there had been insufficient study to provide clear conclusions regarding *touch/massage*, although emotional and physical relief was demonstrated with this intervention. *Intradermal water blocks* were effective in reducing severe back pain, and one randomized study reported a decrease in cesarean deliveries. Lastly, *maternal movement and positioning* was reported to impact pain relief in labor and impact several variables related to fetal and neonatal well-being. In this systematic review, no trials compared a policy of freedom to move spontaneously with a policy of restriction to a bed for outcomes such as comfort, labor progress, or fetal welfare. Mechanisms by which dystocia may be prevented or corrected through the use of maternal positioning have been discussed elsewhere (60).

Systemic Opioids

From the maternal perspective, efficacy and incidence of side effects with systemic opioid analgesia is largely dose- rather than drug-dependent. There is little evidence to suggest one agent is intrinsically superior. Most often, the choice is based on institutional tradition or personal preference.

Opioids may affect the fetus directly as a result of placental transfer and/or indirectly, for example, by altering maternal minute ventilation or uterine tone. As a group, these low-molecular-weight drugs are lipid-soluble weak bases (61) that readily cross the placenta. This implies that maternal to fetal concentration gradients are important; only free, not protein-bound, drug is available for transfer. The amount of "free" drug delivered to the placenta depends on placental blood flow and the degree of maternal protein binding. The amount of drug available to the fetus depends on the degree of placental uptake, metabolism, and clearance (62). In single-dose drug studies, key factors influencing umbilical vein/maternal drug ratio are lipid solubility and transit time through the placental bed. In multidrug dosing (e.g., patient-controlled narcotic analgesia [PCA] delivery systems), key factors influencing fetal

drug levels are the degree of ionization and degree of fetal protein binding (Fig. 16-3).

Fetal pH is lower than maternal pH; consequently, the fraction of opioid (and other basic drugs) existing in the ionized state is higher in the fetus than in the mother. Ionization results in drug trapping. The degree of ionization depends on the drug's pKa; the effect is greater for meperidine (pKa ~8.5) than morphine (pKa ~8.0), and more significant when the fetus is acidotic. This is a simplistic, albeit true, application of opioid pharmacokinetics, a complex, difficult to predict, and incompletely evaluated topic.

All opioids have the potential to decrease baseline FHR and reduce variability, making interpretation of fetal CTG recordings potentially problematic. It has been documented from observational studies that parenteral narcotics can be associated with neonatal respiratory depression, decreased neonatal alertness, inhibition of sucking, and delay in effective feeding. When evidence related to the use of parenteral opioids for labor pain relief was subjected to a systematic review (63), it was noted that none of the studies was sufficiently powered to address the primary outcome measure of neonatal resuscitation, a measure of safety. Intramuscular opioid was compared to placebo, different i.m. opioid, same i.m. opioid but different dose, and same opioid given intravenously; IV opioid was compared to different IV opioid and same IV opioid but different modes of administration. There was insufficient pooled information to draw conclusions regarding any of the secondary outcome measures, including fetal distress administration of naloxone, Apgar score <7 at 5 minutes, baby death, admission to a special care setting, feeding problems, and problems with mother-baby interaction.

The concept of genetic imprinting at birth for opiate or amphetamine addiction in later life has been associated with systemically administered pain-relieving labor medications (narcotics, barbiturates, or nitrous oxide) (63). The original studies that led to this conclusion were criticized regarding the matching of controls and the imprinting hypothesis proposed to explain the finding (64). Although a more recent study of drug-abusing subjects confirmed the phenomenon, these results will be considered controversial until there is more confirmatory evidence.

Meperidine is the most commonly used opioid for labor analgesia worldwide. It has been shown that, as the time increases from administration of single-dose, i.m. meperidine 1.5 mg/kg during labor to delivery of the baby, so too does the level of meperidine in the fetus (65). Maximum fetal concentrations reach a plateau between 1 and 5 hours after dosing; therefore, babies born within 1 to

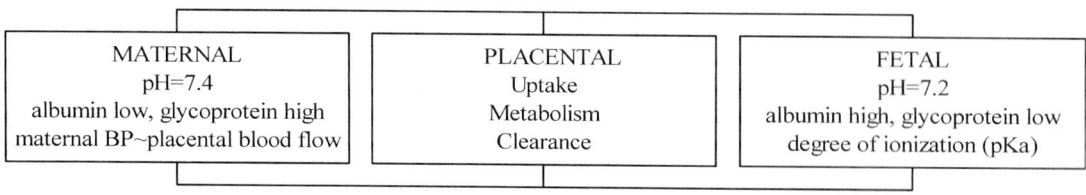

Figure 16-3   Factors influencing fetal drug levels with PCA narcotic administration.

5 hours after meperidine is given to the mother have the greatest chance of narcotic-induced depression. In contrast to single-dose studies, multiple doses of meperidine administered over many hours lead to accumulation of meperidine's metabolite, normeperidine, in the mother and fetus (66). Half-lives of 17–25 hours for this metabolite are common in the mother, whereas the half-life exceeds 60 hours in the fetus/newborn. Normeperidine is associated with respiratory depression, not reversible by naloxone, and seizures. Because of concerns about meperidine, research has focused on the newer, shorter-acting opioids with no active metabolites as alternatives.

Fentanyl has been available clinically for more than 20 years. It offers prompt analgesia coupled with a short duration of action and no active metabolites. Both maternal and fetal drug levels decline in a parallel fashion following a single dose of the drug (67). In the first report of its administration to laboring patients, fentanyl (50 to 100 µg IV q1h) was compared with meperidine (25 to 50 mg IV q2–3hr) (68). More mothers were nauseated and sedated and more babies required naloxone in the meperidine group.

Sufentanil is the most lipid soluble (octanol:water partition coefficient 1778) of the commonly used opioids (61). This feature should enhance placental transfer after a single dose, but transfer is impeded by the extent of maternal plasma protein binding (α1-acid glycoprotein) and uptake by the placenta. Sufentanil concentration in the fetus rises slowly, reaching a plateau between 45 and 80 minutes postadministration (69). It is a useful maternal analgesic for pain relief during second stage, when fetal delivery is imminent (<45 minutes).

Remifentanil is a novel, ultra-short-acting opioid. It has the most rapid onset of peak effect ($\sim$1 minute), shortest context-sensitive half time ($\sim$3–5 minutes), and greatest clearance (40 mL/kg/min) of the commonly used opioids (61). Although the maternal cardiovascular and side effect profiles are similar to other fentanyl congeners, remifentanil is chemically distinct because of its ester linkages. This ester structure renders it susceptible to hydrolysis by red cell- and tissue-nonspecific esterases, resulting in rapid metabolism. Remifentanil concentration decreases by 50% within 3 to 5 minutes of stopping drug administration, regardless of the duration of the infusion (61).

Labor pain occurs at intervals and increases in intensity over time. Rapid recovery between contractions and after delivery is desirable. Therefore, the most effective means of administering remifentanil to the laboring patient, taking advantage of the drug's characteristics, is via PCA with a background infusion. Bolus dose, lockout time, and rate of infusion can be titrated (70). The drug rapidly crosses the placenta and is quickly metabolized by fetal esterases (71). Maternal oxygen desaturation and sedation and reduced FHR variability have been observed (72). Newborns exposed to remifentanil *in utero* up until the time of delivery have been vigorous. There have been no reports of lower Apgar scores, unacceptable umbilical cord gas analyses, or respiratory depression necessitating naloxone use. (70,71,73)

Naloxone is used to reverse respiratory depression in narcotic-exposed newborns. It is contraindicated for infants of narcotic-dependent mothers, as administration may precipitate acute withdrawal and seizures. Naloxone has never been shown to reduce the need for assisted mechanical ventilation or reduce admission rates to special-care nurseries (74). No studies have evaluated the effect of naloxone on time to spontaneous effective respiration or long-term outcome. Naloxone use in adults has been associated with reports of hypertension, pulmonary edema, arrhythmias, and cardiac arrest (61).

Agonist-Antagonist Opioids

Nalbuphine is commonly used as a systemic analgesic during labor. Reports of severe perinatal cardiovascular and respiratory depression prompted Nicolle and associates (75) to carry out a study designed to delineate placental transfer and disposition of nalbuphine in the neonate. The estimated half-life was 4.1 hours (versus 0.9 hour in infants and 2 hours in adults). Given that the liver extensively metabolizes nalbuphine, the authors speculated that the slower neonatal plasma disappearance rate compared to the infant or adult could be due in part to immature hepatic function or bypass of the liver via the ductus venosus. All 28 babies had 5-minute Apgar scores of 10. Fifty-four percent of the FHR tracings showed reduced variability lasting 10–35 minutes after maternal injection.

One potential use for this class of drugs is in the treatment of opiate-dependent pregnant women. Babies born to mothers on a buprenorphine maintenance program showed little or no clinically measurable neonatal abstinence syndrome in contrast to findings with methadone, morphine, or heroin maintenance programs (76).

Nitrous Oxide

Nitrous oxide (N_2O) is an odorless inhalational agent that exerts weak but prompt analgesic activity. It is a relatively insoluble gas at room temperature, and therefore equilibrates rapidly between the alveoli, blood, and brain. To be fully effective, inhalation needs to be timed with contractions such that the patient begins to breathe the gas about 10 to 15 seconds in advance of the next contraction. This synchronizes the peak effect of N_2O with the zenith of pain, assuming the average contraction lasts 60 seconds and peaks at the midpoint. N_2O is combined with oxygen in a 50:50 mixture for obstetric use and is self-administered by the patient through a specialized breathing circuit equipped with a demand valve. The negative pressure generated at the onset of inspiration opens the valve, which remains open during inspiration and closes when the patient begins to exhale. Inhalation analgesia with N_2O during labor and delivery by itself, as a coanalgesic, or as a temporizing measure pending other forms of pain relief is less common in the United States than in other developed countries.

Any patient at risk of vitamin B12 deficiency (e.g., pernicious anemia or vegetarian) should not use N_2O as it irreversibly oxidizes vitamin B12, reducing the activity of methionine synthetase (necessary for myelin formation) and other B12-dependent enzymes. Many countries have set maximal environmental limits for N_2O, which necessitates the use of ventilation systems that allow exhaled gas to be scavenged.

N_2O readily crosses the placenta. The maternal-fetal concentration ratio reaches 0.8 within 15 minutes of continuous inhalation. It has no effect on uterine contractions or FHR. It is not metabolized and is eliminated quickly and entirely by the lungs with the onset of respiration at birth. This is true whether the mother inhales N_2O for 5 minutes or 5 hours. N_2O does not affect Apgar scores or sucking behavior (77).

Paracervical Block

This peripheral block provides a therapeutic alternative for first-stage labor pain when central neuraxial blockade is contraindicated or unavailable. The technique involves transvaginal injection of LA on either side of the cervix to interrupt pain transmission at the level of the uterine and cervical plexuses (located at the base of the broad ligament). Paracervical block (PCB) is relatively easy to perform and, when effective, it provides good to excellent analgesia that lasts 1–2 hours.

Since the introduction of PCB in the 1940s, reports of serious adverse sequelae, including injection of LA directly into the uterine arteries or fetal head, fetal death, and profound bradycardia, have resulted in modification of the injection technique and changes to the concentration and type of LA used. There are statements cautioning against employing this block in situations of uteroplacental insufficiency or nonreassuring FHR tracings.

Overall, in current practice the incidence of fetal bradycardia postblock is about 15% (78), with the onset beginning 2 to 10 minutes after injection and the bradycardia lasting 15 to 30 minutes. The exact etiology is unknown; however, a recent investigation comparing epidural with PCB using Doppler flow velocity waveforms of the maternal femoral and uterine arteries, and umbilical and fetal middle cerebral arteries has shed some light on this phenomenon (79). PCB was associated with a small but significant increase in uterine artery impedance, indicating uterine artery vasoconstriction. In this study, Apgar scores and umbilical arterial and venous pH determinations were within the normal range in both groups.

Neuraxial Analgesia

Spinal, epidural, and combined spinal-epidural (CSE) techniques are commonplace for managing childbirth pain. They are used to administer opioids, LAs, and other pain-modulating adjuvants. Collectively, these methods are considered the most effective forms of pain relief available to laboring women.

Although spinal anesthesia has been in use since 1899, spinal analgesia only became a viable possibility in the 1970s following the discovery of specific opioid receptors in the brain and spinal cord. From a practical standpoint, however, it was not an option for laboring women at that time for two reasons: there was an unacceptably high incidence of postspinal headache (also known as postdural puncture headache) in the young female population; and a single injection technique could not be relied upon to provide analgesia for more than 1 to 2 hours. The advantage of having an epidural catheter in place, either for subsequent bolus dosing or for continuous infusion, is the provision of uninterrupted analgesia between placement of the catheter and delivery of the baby.

The (re-)introduction of fine-gauge, pencil-point, atraumatic (noncutting) spinal needles in the late 1980s fostered a renewed interest in subarachnoid (intrathecal) injection (80). With the advent of CSE equipment and "needle-through-needle" technique, single-level subarachnoid injection, followed immediately by epidural catheter placement at the same site, became possible (81). The CSE procedure has become synonymous with subarachnoid injection of opioid (± a small dose of LA) and simultaneous initiation of a low-dose epidural infusion. The perceived advantages of CSE compared with more traditional methods continue to be debated, along with the consequences of routine dural puncture (81–83).

Epidural catheter analgesia alone has been popular for many years. Depending on the choice of agents used, it provides superior pain relief during the first and second stages of labor and can be extended, if necessary, for cesarean section, instrumented vaginal delivery, manual placental removal, or episiotomy repair.

Neuraxial Opioids

Opioids injected into the lumbar intrathecal space distribute between nerve tissue and cerebrospinal fluid (CSF) on the basis of their partition coefficients (lipid solubility). Opioids injected into the epidural space first diffuse across the dura to reach the subarachnoid space, and then behave as their intrathecal counterparts. Morphine, the least lipid soluble of the commonly used opioids, diffuses slowly from the CSF into the substantia gelatinosa of the dorsal horn to activate opioid receptors. This accounts for its delayed onset and prolonged duration of action. Morphine also spreads rostrally, moving by bulk flow with CSF to reach vasomotor, respiratory, and vomiting centers in the brainstem. In contrast, the highly lipophilic fentanyl and sufentanil penetrate nerve tissue quickly. They have a faster onset of activity coupled with a shorter duration of action. Remifentanil is not approved for use in the intrathecal space because it contains a glycine preservative.

All opioids have some minor intrinsic LA properties, but these effects are marked with meperidine (61), allowing it to be used as the sole agent, even for cesarean section, in the rare event of amide LA allergy. Intrathecal meperidine produces significant sympathetic and motor blockade as well as typical opioid side effects such as pruritus. It has little value as an adjunct to regional analgesia for labor.

The purported advantages of using opioid drugs alone to induce neuraxial analgesia for labor include:

1. Preservation of motor function, sustaining the ability to ambulate during first stage and to push during second stage
2. Avoidance of LA-induced sympathectomy which can be associated with undesirable cardiovascular sequelae such as hypotension
3. Reduction in the systemic side effects of opioids themselves, given the receptor-specific route and minute amount of drug needed to exert an effect. Less total opioid means less chance of drug transfer to the fetus and fewer unpleasant maternal side effects such as nausea, vomiting, pruritus, urinary retention, and sedation.

Fetal bradycardia may develop following administration of intrathecal opioid, although its occurrence can follow any type of effective labor analgesia (84). While technique-specific etiologies can occur (e.g., maternal hypotension or fetal LA toxicity), uterine hypertonus as the mechanism inciting the transient but profound drop in heart rate was first reported in 1994 (85). This topic has been the subject of study (86) and systematic review (87).

Pain relief can affect uterine function. Hunter (88) reported in 1962 that bilateral lumbar sympathetic block for first-stage labor pain caused abnormal uterine contraction patterns to normalize and previously normal patterns to become hyperactive. Although there is likely more than one mechanism, the etiology is thought to be related to a change in the balance of circulating catecholamines occurring with the advent of analgesia, favoring α- over β-activation of smooth muscle receptors (46,89). Uterine muscle tone and vascular resistance increase as a result of the contraction-inducing norepinephrine influence predominating over the contraction-relaxing epinephrine effect. FHR decreases because of a reduction in uteroplacental blood flow. The effect may be more pronounced in the face of oxytocin stimulation.

From an anesthetic perspective, any block that includes segments T10 to T12 (uterine afferent pain fibers enter the spinal cord at the T10-L1 level) will affect efferent nerves to the adrenal medulla (46). There is a temporal relationship between the speed of onset of labor pain relief and the appearance, if any, of bradycardia. It occurs faster with spinal analgesia (<10 minutes) and more slowly with epidural analgesia (15 to 30 minutes) (84). However, as Van de Velde and associates (86) point out, speed of onset of labor pain relief cannot be the only factor at work. Nonreassuring FHR tracings did not occur after CSE using a mixture of bupivacaine and sufentanil (1.5 μg) when compared to a larger dose of intrathecal sufentanil (7.5 μg) alone, despite equally fast pain relief. Metanalysis performed during a well-conducted systematic review of this topic revealed a significant increase in the risk of fetal bradycardia due to intrathecal opioid (odds ratio 1.8, 95% confidence interval 1.0 to 3.1) (87).

The clinical implications are not obvious because the occurrence of FHR changes in response to labor analgesia has not prompted an increase in the rate of interventional delivery (87). The hypertonus usually lasts less than 10 minutes and can be relieved by administration of a nitric oxide donor such as nitroglycerin (50 to 100 μg IV), or a β2 agonist such as terbutaline (125 to 250 μg IV), in cases of prolonged fetal bradycardia. The observed changes in FHR have not correlated with observable clinical differences in neonatal outcome, including Apgar scores, cord pH, prevalence of cord pH < 7.15, or admission rate to a neonatal intensive care unit (86).

Despite the utility of opioids as neuraxial agents during labor, their use without LAs is confined to early labor; by themselves, they do not provide adequate relief as labor progresses and pain intensifies (81,90).

Neuraxial Local Anesthetics

LAs exert their effect by penetrating the epineurium and neural cell membrane in the lipid-soluble (un-ionized) base form to reach the axoplasm. Cellular integrity and metabolism are unaffected. Once inside the cell, the molecules revert to ionized and un-ionized forms in equilibrium. The charged form blocks sodium channels, thereby disrupting sodium conductance and preventing depolarization. This interaction between LA and channel is reversible and ends when the concentration of LA falls below a critical minimum level.

There are several factors that influence the choice of LA agent and concentration employed for epidural or caudal analgesia. These include the delivery system used (intermittent bolus, continuous infusion, or patient-controlled epidural bolus ± background infusion), desired speed of onset, nature of the pain, progress of labor, degree of motor block tolerable for the patient and anesthesiologist, local practice and experience, and cost. In general, when LA is used alone, concentrated solutions are required to afford pain relief. Since block density is dose dependent, the more concentrated the solution used, the greater the degree of motor block expected; this has been implicated in pelvic muscle relaxation-induced fetal malposition, maternal inability to push, and need for instrumental delivery (91). In a recent metanalysis comparing randomized clinical trials of techniques using epidural LA alone with intrathecal opioid alone (92), the authors were unable to find sufficient information to comment on either similarities or differences in maternal and fetal outcomes. This study was accompanied by an insightful editorial that will assist readers to critically interpret the results of this and other systematic reviews and metanalyses (93).

LAs alone are not normally used for spinal analgesia, and use of the caudal technique for pain relief in labor is uncommon.

Combining Opioids, Local Anesthetics, and Pain-Relieving Adjuvants

When spinal, epidural, and CSE techniques involve combinations of pain-modulating drugs (sodium channel-blocking agents, opioid-receptor agonists, α-adrenergic agonists, and/or acetylcholinesterase inhibitors) acting by different mechanisms, there is potential to afford analgesia with minimal motor blockade and other relevant side effects (19,83,94). Lower doses of individual agents in combination often result in at least additive and, at times, synergistic analgesic effect.

Labor Epidurals and Outcome

An erudite and interesting historical review of anesthesia for childbirth by Caton and associates (95) provides the foundation for a discussion of the controversies and unresolved issues surrounding the influence of epidural analgesia on maternal outcomes that affect the fetus and newborn.

There have been five systematic reviews (63,96–99) comparing epidural to nonepidural analgesia methods. All focused in some manner on the clinical dilemma of balancing the alleviation of maternal pain with the possible increase in side effects and/or adverse outcomes for the mother and baby. The search strategies, choice of inclusion and exclusion criteria, assessment of individual trial validity, primary and secondary outcomes, and approach to the synthesis of information differed. Commentary about two of the reviews that were conducted in parallel is thought provoking (100).

The following is a simplified summary of the information provided by the reviews:

1. Epidural solution concentration and technique varied tremendously over the 38-year timespan covered. As a result, there were some qualitative differences in the effects of treatment (heterogeneity).
2. All reviewers concluded that there was insufficient evidence to support an increased incidence of cesarean section with the use of epidural analgesia.
3. Data on babies were scanty, apart from gross measures such as Apgar scores and results of umbilical cord blood gas analysis. Some issues remained unproven; e.g., the suggestion that "epidural analgesia is associated with less naloxone use and higher one-minute Apgar scores." No consistent picture emerged about the incidence of neonatal adverse effects associated with epidural. There was little evidence regarding the effects of epidural on fetal physiologic mechanisms.
4. Epidural analgesia was associated with (not necessarily a causal relationship):
   i. longer second-stage labor (approximately 14 minutes)
   ii. more fetal malposition (occiput posterior), possibly due to failure to rotate or because laboring with a fetus in this position results in more pain, which brings about the request for epidural analgesia
   iii. higher rate of instrumental vaginal deliveries
   iv. maternal fever
   v. increased use of oxytocin augmentation. This serves as an example of the "association versus causation" debate (101). Active labor management protocols,

including the routine use of oxytocin, may simply be associated with a higher demand for epidurals.

Halpern and associates noted (96) that the quality of the clinical trials included in their review improved with time; all trials after 1995 reported outcomes with patients grouped by intent to treat. Analysis conducted in this way (i.e., by groups to which patients were randomized) is vital because women who choose epidurals differ demographically from those who choose other methods of labor analgesia. The former are more likely to be nulliparous, be admitted to the hospital earlier in labor with higher fetal head positions, have slower rates of cervical dilation, bear heavier babies, and need oxytocin augmentation more frequently. All of these factors and degree of maternal pain independently predict the need for cesarean delivery for dystocia ("failure to progress" or prolonged labor) (102).

In the five reviews cited above, the nonepidural analgesia "control methods" primarily consisted of i.m. or IV administration of opioids. More recently, continuous infusion epidural has been compared to CSE (103) and patient-controlled epidural analgesia (104). These publications serve to highlight epidural technique modifications, such as choice of drug, dosage (volume and concentration), and method of administration, that have taken place over time.

Obstetric management practices have an important role to play in terms of the progress and outcome of labor (91). For instance, the presence of an epidural block may sometimes decrease the obstetrician's threshold for performing instrument-assisted deliveries, as well as for allowing instrument-assisted delivery for the purpose of teaching residents. Active management of labor (routine oxytocin augmentation and/or artificial rupture of membranes), delayed pushing in second stage, and promotion of ambulation have all been suggested as methods to reduce obstetric intervention and increase the number of spontaneous vaginal births (94).

Instrumental Vaginal Delivery

Attempts at operative vaginal delivery (vacuum extraction or forceps) put the baby at risk of injury, including hemorrhagic morbidities such as subgaleal hematoma and cerebral hemorrhage (105). Forceps use is also associated with facial nerve and brachial plexus injury (106). In a study comparing use of forceps and vacuum extractors, babies delivered by vacuum extraction showed a higher incidence of cephalohematomas, although need for resuscitation at birth, admission to a neonatal intensive care unit, and neonatal death rate were not different (107).

Epidural analgesia has been associated with a higher rate of operative vaginal deliveries (96–99). Recently, the "Comparative Obstetric Mobile Epidural Trial" (COMET) study group (108) showed that there was a decreased incidence of instrumental vaginal delivery when lower doses of medication (CSE, low-dose LA plus opioid infusion) were used in labor compared to conventional doses of LA (bupivacaine 0.25%). The presumed mechanism is the preservation of motor tone and bearing-down reflex. Mild neonatal depression necessitating neonatal resuscitation was more common among babies whose mothers were in low-dose LA plus opioid epidural infusion group, most likely due to the cumulative effect of the opioid over time. Neither the Apgar scores at 5 minutes nor the rates of admission to a neonatal intensive care unit differed between groups.

Newer methods of epidural analgesia offer the best chance of spontaneous delivery with satisfactory pain control (109).

Delayed Pushing

The "Pushing Early or Pushing Late with Epidural" (PEO-PLE) study, a multicenter, randomized, controlled trial, compared conventional early pushing commencing at full cervical dilation with pushing late, ≥2 hours after full dilation. Operative delivery was reduced with delayed pushing; however, umbilical arterial pH <7.10 occurred more frequently among babies whose mothers were in the delayed pushing group. The two groups had similar rates of neonatal morbidity, including asphyxia. Protocols advocating delayed pushing result in longer second stages and increased incidences of maternal fever (110).

Maternal Fever

Mothers who choose epidural are more likely to develop a fever during labor (111). The link between epidural analgesia, maternal fever, and the purported increase in neonatal septic work-ups is less clear (111–114); the concern is that babies are more likely to be treated with antibiotics since it is not currently possible to distinguish between maternal fever from infectious and noninfectious causes during labor. Many investigators believe the association of an epidural with fever is probably attributable to noninfectious causes, e.g., altered thermoregulation resulting from epidural analgesia. Neonates born to mothers who receive epidural analgesia do not have an increased risk of sepsis (91,111).

Breastfeeding

A succinct and thorough review of this topic concludes that intrapartum epidural analgesia does not adversely affect a baby's or mother's ability to breastfeed (115). The most critical factors for breastfeeding success are support of and education for the mother.

SURGERY DURING PREGNANCY

Urgent surgery during pregnancy requires modification of anesthetic and surgical approaches to address the safety of the mother and her fetus (116–118). Anesthetic considerations include:

1. Management of maternal risk factors resulting from physiologic adaptation to the demands of a growing fetus and ongoing support of the placental unit

2. Maintenance of the pregnant state
3. Optimization of uteroplacental perfusion and fetal oxygenation, and maintenance of a stable intrauterine environment
4. Attention to the direct and indirect actions of maternally administered medications on fetal well-being

The choice of anesthetic technique is guided by maternal indications, taking into account the site and nature of surgery. Efforts are made to reduce fetal drug exposure and, with reassurance, allay maternal anxiety. When possible, regional techniques are preferred because managing the airway of a pregnant patient poses unique challenges. Edema, weight gain, and increased breast size make intubation of the trachea technically difficult. Decline in functional residual capacity coupled with increased oxygen consumption predisposes the mother to rapid desaturation during induction of GA. Lower esophageal sphincter laxity leads to reflux of stomach contents, increasing the risk of aspiration once protective airway reflexes are abolished. Most abdominal procedures, however, require GA to provide sufficient muscle relaxation to facilitate surgical exposure.

Approximately 2% of pregnant women require surgery during pregnancy (117). The procedure may be directly related (e.g., cervical cerclage), indirectly related (e.g., ovarian cystectomy), or unrelated (e.g., appendectomy) to pregnancy. Semielective procedures should be delayed until the second trimester. Surgery at this time avoids the vulnerable period of organogenesis (approximately 15- to 60-day gestation) and technical difficulties of maneuvering around a large, gravid uterus or managing the maternal airway in an advanced stage of pregnancy. Special techniques, including laparoscopy, cardiopulmonary bypass, transplantation, and induced hypothermia have all been performed safely during pregnancy (116).

Premature labor represents the greatest risk to the fetus in the perioperative period. Neonatal mortality in the developed world is approximately 50% at 25 weeks, dropping to about 10% at 30 weeks (119). Postponing surgery during this period of rapid fetal maturation should weigh the advantages to the fetus against the hazards that delay poses to the mother. There is no evidence to suggest that any anesthetic agent, dose, or technique influences the risk of preterm labor (117). Rather, it is more likely to be related to the surgery itself, manipulation of the uterus, or the underlying condition of the mother (e.g., infection). The more advanced the pregnancy, the greater the probability of uterine irritability. Certain medications can be used as part of the anesthetic technique to promote uterine quiescence (e.g., magnesium sulfate, inhalational anesthetic agents, or β2 agonists), and surgical strategies can be employed to avoid handling the uterus. IV, sublingual, or transcutaneous administration of nitroglycerin is usually reserved for uterine relaxation during brief procedures or to manage refractory uterine activity (120).

The decision to monitor the fetus during surgery necessitates that someone be available for ongoing interpretation of fetal well-being and that there be a plan for intervention should fetal distress be diagnosed or suspected. Indicators of fetal distress are often indistinct because technical limitations at various gestational ages eclipse data acquisition, and FHR variability is reduced or eliminated by certain anesthetic drugs. Intervention may include delivery, reassessment of anesthetic depth, or a more aggressive approach to maximize uterine blood flow, tocolysis, and/or maternal oxygenation (116). If delivery of the fetus is planned to occur at the same time as surgery, a coordinated team approach involving anesthesia, obstetrics, surgery, nursing, respiratory therapy, and neonatology is vital.

The well-being of the fetus is dependent on the adequacy of the maternal blood supply to the placenta, which is mainly derived from the uterine arteries (121). Uterine artery blood flow increases during pregnancy and approaches 500 to 800 mL/min (10% to 15% of maternal cardiac output) at term. The uterine vascular bed is a low-resistance system, not capable of further dilatation and devoid of autoregulation. Therefore, placental blood flow varies directly with net perfusion pressure (uterine artery pressure − uterine venous pressure) across the intervillous space and inversely with uterine vascular resistance. When faced with maternal hypotension, to preserve uteroplacental perfusion in a "pressure-passive" system, a more aggressive approach to management (rapid fluid loading, vasopressor therapy, Trendelenburg and left lateral positioning) is required compared to strategies for the nonpregnant patient (118). Hypotension may be due to many different etiologies but commonly results from aortocaval compression in the supine position, general or high spinal anesthesia, or hemorrhage. Bleeding from the uterine vessels can be very brisk and can quickly lead to life-threatening hemorrhage. Left lateral decubitus positioning prevents aortocaval compression in the second and third trimesters. This can be accomplished by having the mother lie on her left side or by elevating the right hip with a wedge, as illustrated in Figure 16-4. Maintaining homeostasis in the intrauterine environment also requires attention to maternal oxygenation, temperature, and acid-base balance (respiratory and metabolic).

Most anesthetic agents are not known to be teratogens. When evaluating the possibility of teratogenicity from maternally administered anesthetic medications, points to be considered include (116,122):

1. The incidence of congenital anomalies in the developed world is 3%.
2. Human teratogenicity studies are impossible to perform for ethical reasons.
3. Extrapolation from animal studies may not be valid.
4. Hypoxemia and hypotension cause physiologic derangement that may be teratogenic.

Drugs that are usually avoided during anesthesia for long surgical procedures in early pregnancy include N_2O and benzodiazepines. N_2O is avoided because it causes oxidation of vitamin B12, rendering it incapable of functioning as a cofactor for methionine synthetase, an enzyme necessary for DNA synthesis in humans. Benzodiazepines are avoided because epidemiologic studies have shown a link to the development of congenital inguinal hernia (122).

Postoperative pain management may include plexus blocks or epidurals, when appropriate, to limit fetal exposure to drugs. Opioids and acetaminophen are used widely. Prolonged use of nonsteroidal antiinflammatory drugs (NSAIDs) is avoided due to concerns about premature constriction of the ductus arteriosus and development of oligohydramnios.

Fetal Surgery

Fetal surgery is defined as "the performance of procedures on the fetus or placenta designed to alter the natural history of a fetal disease that is diagnosed *in utero*" (123). Surgery can vary from minimally invasive percutaneous procedures, facilitated by local, spinal, or epidural anesthesia, to direct fetal operations following a hysterotomy incision. The latter requires maternal GA and attention to the possibility of inflicting pain on the fetus (124). Anesthetic considerations are identical to those for nonobstetric surgery during pregnancy. Once again, care needs to be

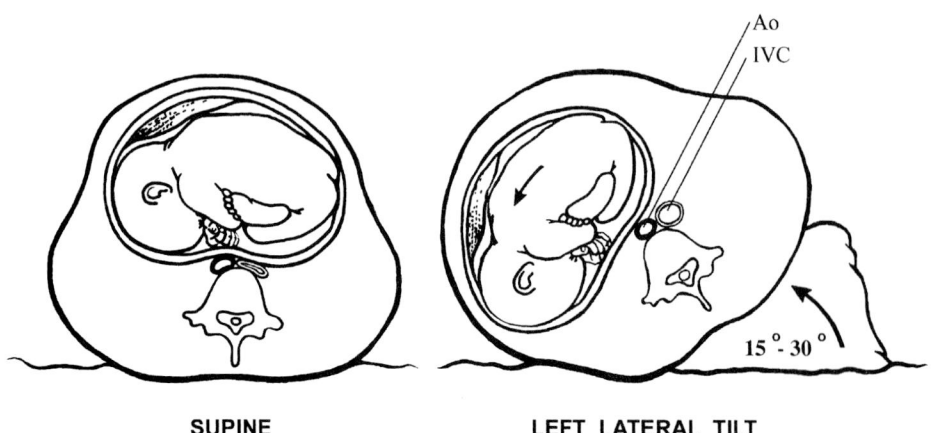

SUPINE   **LEFT LATERAL TILT**

Figure 16-4 Left lateral tilt to relieve aortocaval compression.

provided to two patients simultaneously, although the fetus is the primary patient in these circumstances.

Fetal sedation by placental transfer of maternally administered medication is not reliable and does not ensure an anesthetized or immobile fetus. Given enough time and subject to their individual solubilities, inhalation anesthetic agents used for maternal GA and uterine relaxation equilibrate in fetal tissues. Deep maternal inhalation anesthesia may result in progressive fetal acidosis by an uncertain mechanism. Fetal blood pressure, heart rate, oxygen saturation, and base excess can decrease due to direct impairment of fetal myocardial contractility, redistribution of fetal blood flow, or changes in uterine perfusion. Fetal distress and response to maneuvers can be recognized and managed by measuring heart rate, blood pressure, and umbilical blood flow, and by monitoring pH, pCO_2, pO_2, base deficit, glucose, and electrolytes. Vascular access facilitates this and the administration of fluid, blood products, and/or drugs (125).

Additional fetal anesthesia can be provided by direct i.m. or intravascular (via the umbilical vein) administration of opioids and neuromuscular blocking agents. Pancuronium is often chosen for fetal paralysis because of its long duration and vagolytic properties, which help elevate the FHR and maintain cardiac output. Fentanyl, in relatively large doses (12.5 to 25 μg/kg estimated fetal weight), attenuates the autonomic and hormonal stress response during potentially painful procedures (52,125). In the face of intense uterine tocolysis, maintenance of maternal blood pressure may require concomitant vasopressor therapy.

The ex utero intrapartum treatment (EXIT) procedure was developed for fetuses that have a predictably compromised airway, either because of prior *in utero* surgery (e.g., to treat congenital diaphragmatic hernia) or due to an obstructing mass, such as cystic hygroma or thyroid goiter. Delivery occurs by planned cesarean section with an anesthetic approach that maintains uterine relaxation. A hysterotomy incision is made with a device that limits uterine bleeding, and the fetus is partially delivered through the incision. The surgeon performs laryngoscopy or tracheotomy and secures the airway (endotracheal tube or tracheotomy tube) while the fetus is still attached to the umbilical cord and maintained on uteroplacental perfusion. Attention is paid to avoiding fetal hypothermia. The fetal lungs are expanded and surfactant administered if the infant is premature. The cord is then clamped and the remainder of the cesarean section proceeds as usual. Fetal well-being and operating conditions have been maintained for up to 2 hours during EXIT procedures (123,125).

Whether the fetus feels pain, and from what gestational age, has been the subject of vigorous debate (124,126,127). Prior to 22 weeks, the fetus does not have the neuroanatomic pathways in place to feel pain; between 22 and 26 weeks, thalamocortical fibers, considered to be crucial for nociception, are forming; and after 26 weeks, the fetus has the necessary neurologic development to feel pain. Investigators have used surrogate end points, including fetal "reflex" movement away from and biochemical stress response to noxious stimuli in an attempt to define markers of pain. Hormonal and circulatory stress responses to invasive procedures are observed by 20 weeks (49–53). Further definition of the neuroanatomic and neurophysiologic maturation of sensory pathways involved in pain transmission in the human fetus may provide more direct information about the fetal pain experience.

RESUSCITATION ISSUES DURING PREGNANCY

Intrauterine Resuscitation of the Compromised Fetus

The term "fetal distress" is used to identify a state of progressive fetal asphyxia with hypoxia and acidosis, which, if not corrected, results in decompensation and permanent organ damage. It is diagnosed or suspected when characteristically "abnormal" features emerge in one or more of the tests used to evaluate fetal well-being.

Intrauterine resuscitation consists of a series of maneuvers designed to reverse treatable causes of fetal asphyxia, restore fetal oxygenation, and correct fetal acidosis. These maneuvers are fundamental to the practice of obstetric anesthesia and are summarized, using an evidence-based template, by Thurlow and Kinsella (128). The circumstances surrounding the onset of fetal distress direct the order of application and determine which aspects of intrauterine resuscitation are appropriate for a particular patient. The goals and measures are:

1. Increase blood flow to the placenta
   i. treat maternal hypotension aggressively by administering a nonglucose-containing crystalloid/colloid IV fluid bolus, stopping the epidural infusion, and giving vasopressor therapy
   ii. alleviate aortocaval compression by changing the mother's position until an improvement in FHR occurs (left lateral, followed by right lateral, and finally knee chest position)
   iii. reverse uterine artery vasoconstriction induced by hypocapnia from maternal hyperventilation by managing pain and providing verbal reassurance
2. Relax uterine muscle
   i. stop oxytocin infusion
   ii. administer a tocolytic such as 50 to 100 μg of IV nitroglycerin
3. Increase fetal oxygenation
   i. administer 100% oxygen to the mother by face mask
   ii. relieve umbilical cord compression by changing the mother's position or, if oligohydramnios is present, consider amnioinfusion
4. Rule out umbilical cord prolapse or, if present, provide manual elevation of the presenting part per vagina, maintaining warmth and moisture for the cord until emergent delivery
5. Confirm fetal asphyxia by an alternate test
6. Prepare for emergent delivery

Maternal Cardiac Arrest

The management of cardiac arrest in pregnancy is outlined in the *Guidelines 2000 for Cardiopulmonary Resuscitation and Emergency Cardiovascular Care* (129). Acute cardiac life support protocols are modified in pregnancy, but the standard adult algorithms for medication, intubation, and defibrillation still apply.

The key to resuscitation of the fetus is resuscitation of the mother. Relief of aortocaval compression is paramount. Chest compressions are performed higher on the sternum to adjust for the shift of abdominal contents toward the head. Consideration of arrest etiologies unique to pregnancy (e.g., amniotic fluid embolism) and diagnoses exacerbated by the physiologic changes of pregnancy (e.g., peripartum cardiomyopathy) is important if response to resuscitative efforts is lacking. All medication infusions such as magnesium sulfate, oxytocin, or epidural are discontinued and early intubation is encouraged to reduce the risk of aspiration. Fetal surveillance monitors (e.g., scalp electrode lead) must be discontinued prior to defibrillation. The decision to perform open-chest cardiac massage or emergent cesarean section should occur earlier rather than later if circulation is not restored by usual measures. Perimortem cesarean section has the highest chance of improving outcome for both mother and baby when uterine size is >20 weeks (some would say >24 weeks) and delivery occurs within 5 minutes of the onset of the arrest (130).

Perimortem Cesarean Section

Perimortem cesarean section refers to emergent operative delivery of the fetus through a midline, classical uterine incision in situations in which the mother is moribund or pulseless and is being actively resuscitated. Emptying the uterine cavity increases maternal cardiac output (contraction of the myometrium results in autotransfusion of blood previously directed to the uterus and improved preload secondary to relief of inferior vena cava compression) and lung volume and makes it easier to perform effective chest compressions.

Accurate data regarding the incidence and outcome of this procedure for the mother or neonate are difficult to obtain. For example, the British Confidential Enquiry does not report deliveries during which the mother has been successfully resuscitated (131). There have been several case reports of expedient cesarean delivery during which both mother and baby have survived fully intact. Perimortem cesarean section is an established part of the resuscitation process in near-term pregnant women (129). In the largest series to date, Katz and associates (132) reviewed the literature from 1900 to 1985 for papers in which time from cardiopulmonary arrest to delivery was listed. Most fetal survivors were delivered within 5 minutes. The general consensus is that the likelihood of perimortem cesarean section resulting in a living and neurologically normal baby is related to the interval between onset of maternal cardiac arrest and delivery. Also, the chances of normal survival are good following delivery if the fetus lives past the first few days (131). For this technique to be an option, it must be considered in the context of immediately available staff and equipment to perform the cesarean section, and staff and equipment to conduct the neonatal resuscitation.

ANESTHETIC TECHNIQUES FOR CESAREAN SECTION: EFFECTS ON THE FETUS AND NEWBORN

General Anesthesia

GA is a reversible state characterized by loss of consciousness and lack of pain with or without skeletal muscle relaxation. Going to "sleep", staying "asleep", and "waking up" are known as induction, maintenance, and emergence. The state of GA is achieved through the use of drugs administered in a specific order, namely, induction agents (possibly including narcotics), neuromuscular blockers, inhalation agents, analgesics, and reversal agents.

Given enough time, all medication administered to the mother crosses the placenta and enters the umbilical vein, so gauging drug administration during the induction and maintenance phases of GA is important. An important factor affecting neonatal outcome is the elapsed time between the induction of anesthesia and clamping of the umbilical cord, as this represents the time of fetal exposure to maternally administered medication. A second factor is the time from uterine incision to delivery of the baby. A long incision-to-delivery time is associated with an increased incidence of fetal acidosis, presumably caused by uteroplacental vasoconstriction. If possible, induction-to-clamp time should be <10 minutes and uterine incision-to-delivery time <3 minutes (133).

The three determinants of placental transfer of drugs to the fetus include the physical-chemical properties of the drug, characteristics of the maternal, placental, and fetal circulations, and placental anatomy and physiology. Fetal and neonatal pharmacologic effects of anesthetic agents given to the mother during a cesarean section conducted under GA depend on the amount of drug reaching the fetus. Estimating this is not an easy task.

There are difficulties associated with human *in vivo* studies of placental transfer during pregnancy (134). The fetoplacental unit is inaccessible *in situ*, and there are ethical considerations in conjunction with maternal and fetal safety. *In vivo* studies are most commonly performed at birth by collecting maternal venous and umbilical cord arterial and venous blood samples. It is difficult to draw conclusions based on one set of measurements. Likewise, the applicability of animal placentas as models for the human placenta is limited because the structure and function of the placenta is species specific. Many studies of anesthetic pharmacology to date have been conducted using animal models. The alternative is to use a human *ex vivo* placental perfusion model. Ala-Kokko and associates

(134) make a strong case for the human placental perfusion model as the best method available for studying transplacental passage of drugs.

It will take time to study anesthesia drugs using this methodology. The conclusions reached in most of the studies cited in the following discussion derive from animal and *in vivo* blood sampling data.

The standard method by which anesthesia is induced for cesarean section is rapid sequence induction. The process consists of giving 100% oxygen by mask, IV administration of an induction agent ± narcotic and neuromuscular-blocking drug followed by application of cricoid pressure and intubation of the trachea. The induction agents used to initiate GA include sodium thiopental, methohexital, ketamine, propofol, and midazolam. Ketamine is usually reserved for situations involving maternal hemodynamic instability because it preserves sympathetic outflow. The others have been studied and compared (135–137). Midazolam and propofol have been associated with longer induction times, a lighter plane of maternal anesthesia (as measured by electroencephalogram), and lower Apgar scores. Both sodium thiopental and methohexital are highly lipid soluble. They share pharmacokinetic properties with thiamylal, another barbiturate that peaks in umbilical arterial plasma at 3 to 5 minutes and declines rapidly until 11 minutes (133,137). Induction to umbilical cord clamp times of approximately 10 minutes coincide with declining fetal levels of these agents and therefore little neonatal depression.

Neuromuscular-blocking drugs share a structural similarity, a quaternary ammonium ion, which slows but does not eliminate transfer of these drugs across the placenta (133). Succinylcholine is the only depolarizing drug available for clinical use. In the normal parturient, it is degraded so rapidly by plasma cholinesterase that virtually none reaches the fetus, whereas the percentage of nondepolarizing neuromuscular-blocking drug (e.g., rocuronium, pancuronium, and atracurium) that crosses the placenta ranges from 7% to 22%, depending on the drug. The literature is vague with respect to effects on the neonate. However, in the setting of high-dose nondepolarizing neuromuscular blockade (e.g., EXIT procedures), it may be necessary to support neonatal ventilation for a period of time or to administer reversal agents.

Inhalation anesthetics (not including N_2O) are also known as volatile agents. Halothane, enflurane, isoflurane, and the newer desflurane and sevoflurane are examples of drugs used to maintain anesthesia during cesarean section. Achieving adequate depth of inhaled anesthesia depends on how quickly partial pressures of a particular volatile agent equilibrate in alveolar, blood, and brain compartments. The less soluble the agent, the faster a deep plane of anesthesia is attained. Desflurane and sevoflurane are much less soluble than the other agents so theoretically they would be expected to cross the placenta and equilibrate in fetal tissues more rapidly than their more soluble counterparts, potentially resulting in a more depressed neonate. Equally expected, however, once the newborn

establishes ventilation, is that the lungs more quickly would excrete ("blow off") these relatively insoluble drugs. Desflurane is more pungent and irritating to the airway and may result in laryngospasm. This should be considered when suctioning the neonate whose mother has received desflurane (133). When compared with isoflurane 0.5%, sevoflurane 1% (equianesthetic concentration) was found to produce similar maternal and neonatal results (138). Cord blood gases and Apgar scores were equivalent. Desflurane in a subanesthetic dose (3%), mixed with N_2O-O_2, was considered safe and effective for cesarean section in healthy parturients when compared to enflurane 0.6%. Higher doses of desflurane delayed time to sustained respiration in the newborn (139).

Administration of GA to a parturient is demanding and dissimilar in terms of the drugs and techniques used to achieve the same state in an elective surgical patient. With the exception of a planned, elective cesarean section, circumstances surrounding labor and delivery are difficult to control. Consequently, the obstetric patient rarely comes to the operating room in optimal condition. Combine this with the effect on the parturient of the physiologic changes of pregnancy, add in the fact that mother and baby have unrelated anesthetic needs, and even a healthy woman becomes a high anesthetic risk.

Complications of GA for cesarean section remain the leading cause of anesthesia-related mortality. The case fatality ratio for GA versus regional anesthesia (RA) during obstetric delivery for the period 1991 to 1996 was 6.7:1 (140). In parturients who die from complications of GA, airway problems (failed intubation or aspiration) represent the most frequent cause of death (141). The incidence of failed intubation in obstetric patients is 1:250 to 1:280 compared with 1:2,230 for provision of GA in the main operating room (140,141); thus, the anesthesiologist working in the labor and delivery suite is seven times more likely to encounter failed intubation. The use of GA for cesarean section is declining in favor of RA techniques (142,143), prompting concern over the number of opportunities remaining for trainees to learn, and anesthesiologists to maintain, their obstetric airway management skills (144).

GA continues to be indicated in certain situations including, but not limited to, expedited delivery, technically impossible or failed RA, coagulopathy, cardiovascular instability, anticipated hemorrhage, tethered spinal cord, and patient preference.

Regional Anesthesia

RA is the loss of all sensation, motor function, and reflex activity in a specific area of the body. The surgical conduct of cesarean section under RA requires a sensory block to the fourth to sixth thoracic dermatome levels (T4–T6). Although the incision is most commonly in the lower abdomen, traction on the peritoneum ± uterine exteriorization can cause discomfort unless the area extending from mid-thoracic to sacral levels is blocked. Either an epidural or spinal approach will suffice, but larger doses of

LA and opioid medications are required than when the same techniques are used to provide analgesia in labor. As a result, the fetus/neonate may be affected directly by placental transfer of LAs and opioids, or indirectly by sympathetic blockade, with resultant alterations in uteroplacental perfusion (133).

LA toxicity manifests systemically as a progressive continuum of symptoms beginning with tongue numbness and tinnitus, moving to visual disturbance and muscle twitching, and finally escalating into convulsions, coma, arrhythmias, and respiratory arrest. Toxic LA levels are most often produced by inadvertent IV injection; however, toxicity can result through absorption from the epidural space, particularly given the large dose of LA required to produce T4 blockade. The search for LAs with low "toxic" profiles has led to four modern-day agents: lidocaine, bupivacaine, ropivacaine, and levobupivacaine (145,146). Lidocaine is subject to tachyphylaxis and is often mixed with low-dose epinephrine to delay its otherwise rapid absorption from the epidural space. Its toxicity profile includes central nervous rather than cardiac hyperactivity. Bupivacaine is marketed as a racemic mixture. In the 1970s and early 1980s epidural anesthesia with higher concentrations of this drug was associated with lethal ventricular arrhythmias and cardiovascular collapse. It became apparent that the R-enantiomer was responsible. Bupivacaine is still in widespread use today, but much smaller doses are employed for labor analgesia and it is not commonly used in the epidural space to provide anesthesia for cesarean section. Ropivacaine and levobupivacaine are single enantiomer (L-form) LAs. Evidence from a variety of experiments in several species supports a reduction in toxicity (145,146).

Labor epidural analgesia can be extended and made denser if the parturient is delivered by cesarean section. Under normal maternal and fetal conditions, skillfully conducted GA and RA are almost equivalent with respect to neonatal well-being (147,148). Nevertheless, given the risks to the mother and the association of lower Apgar scores with GA, RA for elective, and sometimes emergent, cesarean section is preferred (19,142,149,150). A compromised fetus may even benefit from anticipatory maternal epidural catheter placement in labor when there is a high risk of cesarean section (151) or primary epidural or spinal anesthesia for elective cesarean section (150,152). RA results in less neonatal exposure to drugs (especially when the spinal technique is used), allows the mother and her partner to participate in the birth of their baby, and provides better maternal postoperative pain relief (143).

For all the advantages of spinal anesthesia such as simplicity of technique, rapid onset, reduced risk of systemic toxicity, density of anesthetic block, and postoperative pain relief afforded by neuraxial morphine, the potential for hypotension with this technique poses the greatest threat to the mother and fetus (19). The incidence of hypotension is similar between epidural and spinal anesthesia but occurs earlier and more rapidly with the spinal approach. Hypotension results from temporary sympathectomy, an inevitable but undesirable component of

mid-thoracic blockade. Reduced preload (increased venous capacitance and pooling of blood volume in the splanchnic bed and lower extremities) and reduced afterload (decreased systemic vascular resistance) lower maternal mean arterial pressure (MAP), leading to nausea, lightheadedness and dysphoria, and reduced uteroplacental perfusion. When maternal MAP is maintained, maternal symptoms are averted and uteroplacental perfusion improves.

In their epidemiologic study of 5,806 cesarean deliveries, Mueller and associates (153) concluded that fetal acidemia was significantly increased after spinal anesthesia and maternal arterial hypotension was by far the most common problem encountered. The prevalence of fetal acidemia with RA for cesarean section has been confirmed in another study (150). However, isolated acidemia does not correlate with Apgar scores and is a poor indicator of outcome. Low umbilical artery pH reflects both the respiratory and metabolic components of acidosis, whereas base excess reflects only the metabolic component. It is base excess that correlates with neonatal outcome, values more negative than -12 mmol/L having an association with moderate to severe newborn encephalopathy (7). However, prevention of hypotension is advantageous to minimize any influence on neonatal acid-base status.

The routine measures used to maintain uteroplacental perfusion include left lateral tilt position, lower leg compressive stockings, and IV fluid loading (121,154). Vasopressor therapy is reserved for the treatment of hypotension. Prophylactic use of ephedrine in one study (155) and therapeutic use in another (150) possibly contributed to fetal acidemia. Likewise, ephedrine use was associated with lower umbilical arterial pH values when compared with phenylephrine in a systematic review (156). The literature is replete with debate regarding which vasopressor, a mixed αβ agonist (e.g., ephedrine) or a pure α agonist (e.g., phenylephrine), would be more appropriate for the management of hypotension during spinal anesthesia for cesarean delivery (157–160). The controversy revolves around the etiology of fetal acidemia: Is it due to the metabolic effects of β-stimulation in the fetus or insufficient maintenance of uteroplacental perfusion by failure to reclaim sequestered blood from the splanchnic bed to augment preload? Regardless, the choice of vasopressor drug is perhaps less important than the avoidance of hypotension (161).

Fetal Effects of Maternal Oxygen Administration

Providing supplemental oxygen to the parturient during cesarean section is common clinically, whether the procedure is elective, urgent, or emergent (162). This practice has been justified by the belief that raising the oxygen reserve of the mother is universally beneficial for the fetus. Since the advent of SpO$_2$, patients who may benefit from oxygen therapy are more easily identified and clinicians can be more selective about administering oxygen therapeutically. For example, SpO_2 readings obtained during elective cesarean section conducted under spinal anesthesia showed that maternal saturation was well maintained on room air, and administration of 35% oxygen by facemask failed to significantly change umbilical vein pH or partial pressure of oxygen (163). This finding was further substantiated in a study by Cogliano and associates (164).

Oxygen given to the mother does not increase fetal oxygenation to the same extent because of usage during intermediary placental metabolism. In comparison, neonatal oxygen therapy has the potential to raise newborn PaO_2 substantially. There is a growing body of clinical and experimental evidence that seems to indicate that the practice of routine supplemental oxygen during neonatal resuscitation may be injurious (165–167).

Oxidative stress is implicated as a common underlying mechanism in several neonatal conditions, including necrotizing enterocolitis, retinopathy of prematurity, periventricular leukomalacia, and chronic lung disease (168,179). It occurs when free radical generation exceeds the body's antioxidant defense mechanisms, and it is not exclusive to newborns; free radicals and antioxidants also play a role in adult diseases (170,171). The interest in free radicals as harbingers of disease prompted investigators to explore potential fetal effects of giving oxygen to mothers. Accordingly, the process of routine oxygen supplementation for healthy parturients undergoing elective cesarean delivery with RA has been questioned. (172).

Free radicals have a brief lifespan, making their detection difficult. Therefore, studies investigating oxidative stress usually measure surrogate markers, namely products of the attack by free radicals on lipids, proteins, and nucleotides. This methodology was used to examine the effect on the newborn of administering air or oxygen-enriched air to parturients undergoing elective cesarean section (173). There was a clear difference between groups, with greater free radical activity in the babies born to mothers breathing oxygen-enriched air. The main site of free radical generation was the placenta, as evidenced by the higher concentration of free radicals in the umbilical vein compared to the artery. As Backe and Lyons point out, "at present, we have no means of linking free radical formation with neonatal outcome following elective cesarean section. . . . . in a low-risk situation such as [this], a favorable outcome is unlikely to be influenced by maternal hyperoxia" (174). "The significance of [the Khaw and associates study] relates to the use of high inspired maternal oxygen fractions ($\geq$60%) for the delivery of compromised and premature [babies]." There are no published trials addressing maternal oxygen therapy for fetal distress (175).

POSTPARTUM PAIN MANAGEMENT

The genesis of postpartum pain is multifactorial. Postsurgical etiologies include episiotomy, manual placenta removal, postpartum tubal ligation, and/or visceral/incisional pain following cesarean delivery. For some women, cramping originating from uterine involution or localized pain resulting from perineal tears can result in distressing discomfort. The mother may suffer a postspinal headache as a complication of regional analgesia or anesthesia. Any method that reduces the magnitude of these painful experiences is desirable. This section is limited to pharmacologic therapy and its implications for the breastfeeding mother.

The goal of a pain management regimen is to prevent or control pain to a degree that is acceptable to the patient while facilitating activities of daily living and promoting quality of life. There are additional challenges for treating pain in women who have just given birth. New mothers are motivated to ambulate early and care for their babies, which requires them to be clear-headed and to experience minimal side effects from analgesics. Concern that postpartum analgesia could have implications for the baby may make the mother hesitant to take an analgesic, and therefore suffer unnecessarily. Breastfeeding calls for use of analgesic agents that are transferred minimally into breast milk and have little effect on the neonate (176).

The current trend is to use a balanced, multimodal approach (177,178). Additive or synergistic analgesic effects, with fewer side effects, have been demonstrated by combining agents with different mechanisms of action in smaller doses than would be required if the individual agents were used alone. This concept has become so important that, as part of the accreditation process, health care organizations are surveyed regarding pain assessment and management, looking for treatment initiatives that include a multimodal approach (179).

The act of breastfeeding results in milk production, secretion, let-down, and increased breast blood flow. Therefore, the timing of breastfeeding relative to drug administration influences the amount of drug that appears in the breast milk. Drug exposure can be minimized if the mother takes medication immediately after nursing or just before the baby is due to have a lengthy sleep, and uses short-acting medications. The neonatal dose of most medications obtained through breastfeeding is 1% to 2% of the maternal dose (122).

Breast milk content also affects the extent of drug transfer from maternal plasma. For instance, lipid-soluble drugs are less likely to accumulate in colostrum, which contains little fat. Colostrum has the same pH as maternal plasma, which is advantageous as far as narcotics are concerned. These weak bases are not sequestered in colostrum via ion trapping and therefore do not accumulate. Colostrum morphine concentrations have been measured during the first 48 hours of postcesarean IV patient-controlled analgesia (180). The milk-to-maternal plasma ratio for morphine was <1. Morphine was seen in very small concentrations in less than half of the milk samples. The authors concluded that the amount of drug likely to be transferred to the breastfed neonate was negligible. Only small amounts of colostrum are secreted during the first few postpartum days (10 to 120 mL/day) so newborn exposure from volume is limited. Ultimately, the concentration of drug in the baby's plasma is more important than the concentration of the drug in colostrum or breast milk. This depends on absorption across the gastrointestinal tract, volume of distribution, and extent of metabolism and excretion in the newborn. Little is known about the bioavailability of analgesics and their metabolites because of ethical issues involved in repeated blood sampling from babies.

Postcesarean section pain peaks on the second day after surgery (181), and analgesic usage begins to decline. Milk composition continues to change over the first 10 days after birth. There is a gradual increase in fat and lactose content and a reduction in protein and pH. By day 10 postpartum, factors such as high lipid solubility, low molecular weight, minimal protein binding, and the un-ionized state facilitate secretion of medications into mature breast milk (182). Women who breastfeed and require GA for surgery are usually counseled to feed their baby before the surgery and temporarily interrupt feeding postoperatively by wasting the first milk sample (express with a breast pump and discard). After that, if the mother feels well enough and there are no surgical contraindications, she is encouraged to resume feeding. Most anesthetics are rapidly cleared from the mother; some authors argue that no portion of human milk need be wasted (182).

Postdelivery analgesia should be tailored to match the changing severity of pain over time; as well, prompt recognition and treatment of side effects help to optimize pain management. Epidural or intrathecal morphine is commonly administered when neuraxial blockade is used for delivery. The analgesic effect following a single neuraxial dose can last up to 18 to 24 hours; however, in keeping with the multimodal approach, fixed regimen or "on-request" analgesics such as NSAIDs or acetaminophen (paracetamol) are usually prescribed concomitantly.

Mild analgesics (acetaminophen and NSAIDs) provide background pain relief to which opioids and/or adjuvant analgesics can be added (178,183). Fixed-dose combinations (e.g., acetaminophen plus codeine) have established efficacy and safety. They are widely used for postpartum pain management (184). Individual titration of opioids is essential. Different routes of administration, including oral, IV, and patient-controlled IV or patient-controlled epidural infusion should be available. A significant reduction in postpartum narcotic use can be achieved through implementation of a self-medication program (185). The AAP published a statement on drug transfer into human milk and possible effects on the infant or on lactation to assist prescribing practices (186). The AAP considers acetaminophen, most NSAIDs, and morphine compatible with breastfeeding.

CONCLUSION

The ideal analgesia/anesthesia for labor and delivery would meet the following criteria (82):

1. Provide fast, effective, and continuous pain relief while maintaining the parturient's ability to move and ambu-

late throughout labor, and to push during vaginal delivery
2. Not interfere with the progress of labor and possibly improve the course of a dysfunctional labor
3. Be technically straightforward and devoid of unacceptable side effects, complications, or risks
4. Not imperil the fetus *in utero*
5. Provide satisfactory conditions for delivery
6. Permit early mother-baby interaction
7. Have no short- or long-term impact on neonatal outcome

Not unexpectedly, no single technique of analgesia or anesthesia meets all of these criteria. The challenge for the anesthesiologist is to balance the needs of the mother and fetus while being flexible enough to modify or change the approach as circumstances dictate.

ACKNOWLEDGEMENT

My thanks to the staff at the Neil John Maclean Health Sciences Library, University of Manitoba; to online search system developers everywhere for helping to simplify the process of identifying and retrieving journal articles; to the inventors of systematic reviews and metanalyses; and to Mr. Hiscoke, my grade 7 science teacher, for introducing me to the thesaurus.

REFERENCES

1. Caton D. The history of obstetric anesthesia. In: Chestnut DH, ed. *Obstetric Anesthesia, Principles and Practice*, 2nd ed. New York: Mosby, 1999:1–13.
2. Apgar V. A proposal for a new method of evaluation of the newborn infant. *Curr Res Anesth Analg* 1953;32:260–267.
3. Committee on Fetus and Newborn, American Academy of Pediatrics, and Committee on Obstetric Practice, American College of Obstetricians and Gynecologists. Use and abuse of the Apgar score. *Pediatrics* 1996;98:141–142.
4. Papile LA. The Apgar score in the 21st century. *N Engl J Med* 2001;344:519–520.
5. Thorp JA, Rushing RS. Umbilical cord blood gas analysis. *Obstet Gynecol Clin North Am* 1999;26:695–709.
6. Helwig JT, Parer JT, Kilpatrick SJ, et al. Umbilical cord blood acid-base state: what is normal? *Am J Obstet Gynecol* 1996;174:1807–1812.
7. Ross MG, Gala R. Use of umbilical artery base excess: Algorithm for the timing of hypoxic injury. *Am J Obstet Gynecol* 2002;187:1–9.
8. National Committee for Clinical Laboratory Standards. Blood gas preanalytical considerations: specimen collection, calibration and controls (approved guideline C27-A). Wayne, PA: NCCLS; 1993.
9. Yoon BH, Kim SW. The effect of labor on the normal values of umbilical blood acid-base status. *Acta Obstet Gynecol Scand* 1994;73:555–561.
10. Reynolds F, Sharma SK, Seed PT. Analgesia in labour and fetal acid-base balance: a meta-analysis comparing epidural with systemic opioid analgesia. *BJOG* 2002;109:1344–1353.
11. Greene KR. Scalp blood gas analysis. *Obstet Gynecol Clin North Am* 1999;26:641–656.
12. Als H, Tronick E, Lester BM, et al. The Brazelton Neonatal Behavioral Assessment Scale (BNBAS). *J Abnorm Child Psychol* 1977;5:215–231.
13. Scanlon JW, Brown WU Jr, Weiss JB, et al. Neurobehavioral responses of newborn infants after maternal epidural anesthesia. *Anesthesiology* 1974;40:121–128.

14. Amiel-Tison C, Barrier G, Shnider SM, et al. A new neurologic and adaptive capacity scoring system for evaluating obstetric medications in full-term newborns. *Anesthesiology* 1982;56:340–350.
15. Brockhurst NJ, Littleford JA, Halpern SH. The neurologic and adaptive capacity score: A systematic review of its use in obstetric anesthesia research. *Anesthesiology* 2000;92:237–246.
16. Camann W, Brazelton TB. Use and abuse of neonatal neurobehavioral testing. *Anesthesiology* 2000;92:3–5.
17. Halpern SH, Littleford JA, Brockhurst NJ. The neurologic and adaptive capacity score is not a reliable method of newborn evaluation. *Anesthesiology* 2001;94:958–962.
18. Sepkoski CM, Lester BM, Ostheimer GW, et al. The effects of maternal epidural anesthesia on neonatal behavior during the first month. *Dev Med Child Neurol* 1992;34:1072–1080.
19. Richardson MG. Regional anesthesia for obstetrics. *Anesthesiol Clin North America* 2000;18:383–406.
20. Liston R, Crane J. Fetal health surveillance in labour, Part 1. SOGC Clinical Practice Guidelines No. 112, March 2002. Available at: http://www.sogc.org/SOGCnet/sogc_docs/common/guide/library_e.shtml#obstetrics Accessed May 6, 2003.
21. Liston R, Crane J. Fetal health surveillance in labour, Part 2. SOGC Clinical Practice Guidelines No. 112, April 2002. Available at: http://www.sogc.org/SOGCnet/sogc_docs/common/guide/library_e.shtml#obstetrics Accessed May 6, 2003.
22. Thacker SB, Stroup D, Chang M. Continuous electronic heart rate monitoring for fetal assessment during labor. *Cochrane Database Syst Rev* 2001;2:CD000063.
23. Dawes G, Meir YJ, Mandruzzato GP. Computerized evaluation of fetal heart-rate patterns. *J Perinat Med* 1994;22:491–499.
24. Neilson JP, Mistry RT. Fetal electrocardiogram plus heart rate recording for fetal monitoring during labour. (*Cochrane Database Syst Rev* 2000;2:CD000116.
25. Norén H, Ameer-Wåhlin I, Hagberg H, et al. Fetal electrocardiography in labor and neonatal outcome: data from the Swedish randomized controlled trial on intrapartum fetal monitoring. *Am J Obstet Gynecol* 2003;188:183–192.
26. Solt I, Ganadry S, Weiner Z. The effect of meperidine and promethazine on fetal heart rate indices during the active phase of labor. *Isr Med Assoc J* 2002;4:178–180.
27. Hoffman CT 3rd, Guzman ER, Richardson MJ, et al. Effects of narcotic and non-narcotic continuous epidural anesthesia on intrapartum fetal heart rate tracings as measured by computer analysis. *J Matern Fetal Med* 1997;6:200–205.
28. St Amant MS, Koffel B, Malinow AM. The effects of epidural opioids on fetal heart rate variability when coadministered with 0.25% bupivacaine for labor analgesia. *Am J Perinatol* 1998;15:351–356.
29. Manning FA. Fetal biophysical profile: a critical appraisal. *Clin Obstet Gynecol* 2002;45:975–985.
30. Manning FA, Snijders R, Harman CR, et al. Fetal biophysical profile score. VI. Correlation with antepartum umbilical venous fetal pH. *Am J Obstet Gynecol* 1993;169:755–763.
31. Farrell T, Owen P, Harrold A. Fetal movements following intrapartum maternal opiate administration. *Clin Exp Obstet Gynecol* 1996;23:144–146.
32. Kopecky EA, Ryan ML, Barrett JF, et al. Fetal response to maternally administered morphine. *Am J Obstet Gynecol* 2000;183:424–430.
33. Smith CV, Rayburn WF, Allen KV, et al. Influence of intravenous fentanyl on fetal biophysical parameters during labor. *J Matern Fetal Med* 1996;5:89–92
34. Dildy GA. Fetal pulse oximetry: current issues. *J Perinat Med* 2001;29:5–13.
35. East CE, Colditz PB, Begg LM, et al. Update on intrapartum fetal pulse oximetry. *Aust N Z J Obstet Gynaecol* 2002;42:119–124.
36. Carbonne B, Langer B, Goffinet F, et al. Multicenter study on the clinical value of fetal pulse oximetry. II. Compared predictive values of pulse oximetry and fetal blood analysis. *Am J Obstet Gynecol* 1997;177:593–598.
37. Paternoster DM, Micaglio M, Tambuscio B, et al. The effects of epidural analgesia and uterine contractions on fetal oxygen saturation during the first stage of labour. *Int J Obstet Anesth* 2001;10:103–107.
38. East CE, Colditz PB. Effect of maternal epidural analgesia on fetal intrapartum oxygen saturation. *Am J Perinatol* 2002;19:119–126.
39. Harman CR, Baschat AA. Comprehensive assessment of fetal wellbeing: which Doppler tests should be performed? *Curr Opin Obstet Gynecol* 2003;15:147–157.
40. Ramos-Santos E, Devoe LD, Wakefield ML, et al. The effects of epidural anesthesia on the Doppler velocimetry of umbilical and uterine arteries in normal and hypertensive patients during active term labor. *Obstet Gynecol* 1991;77:20–26.
41. Erkinjuntti M, Vaahtoranta K, Alihanka J, et al. Use of the SCSB method for monitoring of respiration, body movements and ballistocardiogram in infants. *Early Hum Dev* 1984;9:119–126.
42. Nikkola EM, Kirjavainen TT, Ekblad UU, et al. Postnatal adaptation after caesarean section or vaginal delivery, studied with the static-charge-sensitive bed. *Acta Paediatr* 2002;91:927–933.
43. Nikkola EM, Jahnukainen TJ, Ekblad UU, et al. Neonatal monitoring after maternal fentanyl analgesia in labor. *J Clin Monit Comput* 2000;16:597–608.
44. May AE, Elton CD. The effects of pain and its management on mother and fetus. *Baillieres Clin Obstet Gynaecol* 1998;12:423–441.
45. Brownridge P. The nature and consequences of childbirth pain. *Eur J Obstet Gynecol Reprod Biol* 1995;59 Suppl:S9–S15.
46. Neumark J, Hammerle AF, Biegelmayer C. Effects of epidural analgesia on plasma catecholamines and cortisol in parturition. *Acta Anaesthesiol Scand* 1985;29:555–559.
47. Lowe NK. The nature of labor pain. *Am J Obstet Gynecol* 2002;186(5 Suppl):S16–S24.
48. Kubli M, Scrutton MJ, Seed PT, et al. An evaluation of isotonic "sport drinks" during labor. *Anesth Analg* 2002;94:404–408.
49. Bhutta AT, Garg S, Rovnaghi CR. Fetal response to intra-uterine needling: is it pain? Does it matter? *Pediatr Res* 2002;51:2.
50. Glover V, Fisk NM. Fetal pain: implications for research and practice. *Br J Obstet Gynaecol* 1999;106:881–886.
51. Gitau R, Fisk NM, Teixeira JM, et al. Fetal hypothalamic-pituitary-adrenal stress responses to invasive procedures are independent of maternal responses. *J Clin Endocrinol Metab* 2001;86:104–109.
52. Fisk NM, Gitau R, Teixeira JM. Effect of direct fetal opioid analgesia on fetal hormonal and hemodynamic stress response to intrauterine needling. *Anesthesiology* 2001;95:828–835.
53. Anand KJ, Maze M. Fetuses, fentanyl, and the stress response: signals from the beginnings of pain? *Anesthesiology* 2001;95:823–825.
54. Rowlands S, Permezel M. Physiology of pain in labour. *Baillieres Clin Obstet Gynaecol* 1998;12:347–362.
55. Kitzinger S. Natural childbirth is inappropriate in a modern world. *Int J Obstet Anesth* 2002;11:30–32.
56. American Society of Anesthesiologists Task Force on Obstetrical Anesthesia. Practice guidelines for obstetrical anesthesia: a report. *Anesthesiology* 1999;90:600–611.
57. American College of Obstetrics and Gynecology. Obstetric analgesia and anesthesia. Number 36, July 2002. *Int J Gynaecol Obstet* 2002;78:321–335.
58. Marmor TR, Krol DM. Labor pain management in the United States: understanding patterns and the issue of choice. *Am J Obstet Gynecol* 2002;186(5 Suppl):S173–S180.
59. Simkin PP, O'Hara M. Nonpharmacologic relief of pain during labor: systematic reviews of five methods. *Am J Obstet Gynecol* 2002;186:S131–S159.
60. Fenwick L, Simkin P. Maternal positioning to prevent or alleviate dystocia in labor. *Clin Obstet Gynecol* 1987;30:83–89.
61. Bailey PL, Egan TD, Stanley TH. Intravenous opioid anesthetics. In: Miller RD, ed. *Anesthesia*. 5th ed. Philadelphia: Churchill Livingstone, 2000:273–376.
62. Ala-kokko T, Vähäkangas K, Pelkonen O. Placental function and principles of drug transfer. *Acta Anaesthesiol Scand* 1993;37 (S100):47–49.
63. Bricker L, Lavender T. Parenteral opioids for labor pain relief: a systematic review. *Am J Obstet Gynecol* 2002;186(5 Suppl):S94–S109.
64. Irestedt L. Current status of nitrous oxide for obstetric pain relief. *Acta Anaesthesiol Scand* 1994;38:771–772.
65. Tomson G, Garle RI, Thalme B, et al. Maternal kinetics and transplacental passage of pethidine during labour. *Br J Clin Pharmacol* 1982;13:653–659.
66. Kuhnert BR, Kuhnert PM, Philipson EH, et al. Disposition of meperidine and normeperidine following multiple doses during labor. II. Fetus and neonate. *Am J Obstet Gynecol* 1985;151:410–415.

67. Craft JB Jr, Coaldrake LA, Bolan JC, et al. Placental passage and uterine effects of fentanyl. *Anesth Analg* 1983;62:894–898.

68. Rayburn WF, Smith CV, Parriott JE, et al. Randomized comparison of meperidine and fentanyl during labor. *Obstet Gynecol* 1989;74:604–606.

69. Krishna BR, Zakowski MI, Grant GJ. Sufentanil transfer in the human placenta during in vitro perfusion. *Can J Anaesth* 1997;44:996–1001.

70. Saunders TA, Glass PS. A trial of labor for remifentanil. *Anesth Analg* 2002;94:771–773.

71. Kan RE, Hughes SC, Rosen MA, et al. Intravenous remifentanil: placental transfer, maternal and neonatal effects. *Anesthesiology* 1998;88:1467–1474.

72. Volmanen P, Akural EI, Raudaskoski T, et al. Remifentanil in obstetric analgesia: a dose-finding study. *Anesth Analg* 2002; 94:913–917.

73. Blair JM, Hill DA, Fee JP. Patient-controlled analgesia for labour using remifentanil: a feasibility study. *Br J Anaesth* 2001;87:415–420.

74. McGuire W, Fowlie PW. Naloxone for narcotic-exposed newborn infants. *Cochrane Database Syst Rev* 2002;4:CD003483.

75. Nicolle E, Devillier P, Delanoy B, et al. Therapeutic monitoring of nalbuphine: transplacental transfer and estimated pharmacokinetics in the neonate. *Eur J Clin Pharmacol* 1996;49:485–489.

76. Schindler SD, Eder H, Ortner R, et al. Neonatal outcome following buprenorphine maintenance during conception and throughout pregnancy. *Addiction* 2003;98:103–110.

77. Rosen MA. Nitrous oxide for relief of labor pain: a systematic review. *Am J Obstet Gynecol* 2002;186(5 Suppl):S110–S126.

78. Rosen MA. Paracervical block for labor analgesia: a brief historic review. *Am J Obstet Gynecol* 2002;186(5 Suppl):S127–S130.

79. Manninen T, Aantaa R, Salonen M, et al. A comparison of the hemodynamic effects of paracervical block and epidural anesthesia for labor analgesia. *Acta Anaesthesiol Scand* 2000;44:441–445.

80. Morgan P. Spinal anaesthesia in obstetrics. *Can J Anaesth* 1995;42:1145–1163.

81. Birnbach DJ, Ojea LS. Combined spinal-epidural (CSE) for labor and delivery. *Int Anesthesiol Clin* 2002;40:27–48.

82. Landau R. Combined spinal-epidural analgesia for labor: breakthrough or unjustified invasion? *Semin Perinatol* 2002;26:109–121.

83. Thallon A, Shennan A. Epidural and spinal analgesia and labour. *Curr Opin Obstet Gynecol* 2001;13:583–587.

84. Norris MC. Intrathecal opioids and fetal bradycardia: is there a link? *Int J Obstet Anesth* 2000;9:264–269.

85. Clarke VT, Smiley RM, Finster M. Uterine hyperactivity after intrathecal injection of fentanyl for analgesia during labor: a cause of fetal bradycardia? *Anesthesiology* 1994;81:1083.

86. Van de Velde M, Vercauteren M, Vandermeersch E. Fetal heart rate abnormalities after regional analgesia for labor pain: the effect of intrathecal opioids. *Reg Anesth Pain Med* 2001;26:257–262.

87. Mardirosoff C, Dumont L, Boulvan M, et al. Fetal bradycardia due to intrathecal opioids for labour analgesia: a systematic review. *BJOG* 2002;109:274–281.

88. Hunter CA Jr. Uterine motility studies during labor. Observations on bilateral sympathetic nerve block in the normal and abnormal first stage of labor. *Am J Obstet Gynecol* 1963;85:681–686.

89. Segal S, Csavoy AN, Datta S. The tocolytic effect of catecholamines in the gravid rat uterus. *Anesth Analg* 1998;87:864–869.

90. Connelly NR, Parker RK, Vallurupalli V, et al. Comparison of epidural fentanyl versus epidural sufentanil for analgesia in ambulatory patients in early labor. *Anesth Analg* 2000; 91:374–378.

91. Eltzschig HK, Lieberman ES, Camann WR. Regional anesthesia and analgesia for labor and delivery. *N Engl J Med* 2003;348:319–332.

92. Bucklin BA, Chestnut DH, Hawkins JL. Intrathecal opioids versus epidural local anesthetics for labor analgesia: a meta-analysis. *Reg Anesth Pain Med* 2002;27:23–30.

93. Halpern S. Why meta-analysis? *Reg Anesth Pain Med* 2002; 27:3–5.

94. Mayberry LJ, Clemmens D, De A. Epidural analgesia side effects, co-interventions, and care of women during childbirth: a systematic review. *Am J Obstet Gynecol* 2002;186(Suppl 5):S81–S93.

95. Caton D. Frölich MA. Euliano TY. Anesthesia for childbirth: controversy and change. *Am J Obstet Gynecol* 2002;186(Suppl 5): S25–S30.

96. Halpern SH, Leighton BL, Ohlsson A, et al. Effect of epidural vs parenteral opioid analgesia on the progress of labor: a meta-analysis. *JAMA* 1998;280:2105–2110.

97. Howell CJ. Epidural versus non-epidural analgesia for pain relief in labour. *Cochrane Database Syst Rev* 2000;2:CD000331.

98. Leighton BL, Halpern SH. The effects of epidural analgesia on labor, maternal, and neonatal outcomes: a systematic review. *Am J Obstet Gynecol* 2002;186(Suppl 5):S69–S77.

99. Lieberman E, O'Donoghue C. Unintended effects of epidural analgesia during labor: a systematic review. *Am J Obstet Gynecol* 2002;186(Suppl 5):S31–S68.

100. Thacker SB, Stroup DF. Methods and interpretation in systematic reviews: commentary on two parallel reviews of epidural analgesia during labor. *Am J Obstet Gynecol* 2002;186(Suppl 5):S78–S80.

101. Breen TW. Databases and obstetric anesthesia research: opportunity and limitations. *Int J Obstet Anesth* 2003;12:1–3.

102. Segal BS, Birnbach DJ. Epidurals and cesarean deliveries: a new look at an old problem. *Anesth Analg* 2000;90:775-777.

103. Norris M, Fogel ST, Conway-Long C. Combined spinal-epidural versus epidural labor analgesia. *Anesthesiology* 2001;95:913–920.

104. van der Vyver M, Halpern S, Joseph G. Patient-controlled epidural analgesia versus continuous infusion for labour analgesia: a meta-analysis. *Br J Anaesth* 2002;89:459–465.

105. Benedetti TJ. Birth injury and method of delivery. *N Engl J Med* 1999;341:1758–1759.

106. Towner D, Castro MA, Eby-Wilkens E, et al. Effect of mode of delivery in nulliparous women on neonatal intracranial injury. *N Engl J Med* 1999;341:1709–1714.

107. Weerasekera DS, Premaratne S. A randomised prospective trial of the obstetric forceps versus vacuum extraction using defined criteria. *J Obstet Gynaecol* 2002;22:344–345.

108. Comparative Obstetric Mobile Epidural Trial (COMET) Study Group UK. Effect of low-dose mobile versus traditional epidural techniques on mode of delivery: a randomised controlled trial. *Lancet* 2001;358:19–23.

109. Thornton JG, Capogna G. Reducing likelihood of instrumental delivery with epidural anaesthesia. *Lancet* 2001;358:2.

110. Fraser WD, Marcoux S, Krauss I, et al. Multicenter, randomized, controlled trial of delayed pushing for nulliparous women in the second stage of labor with continuous epidural analgesia. The PEOPLE (Pushing Early or Pushing Late with Epidural) Study Group. *Am J Obstet Gynecol* 2000;182:1165–1172.

111. Viscomi CM, Manullang T. Maternal fever, neonatal sepsis evaluation, and epidural labor analgesia. *Reg Anesth Pain Med* 2000;25:549–553.

112. Kaul B, Vallejo M, Ramanathan S, et al. Epidural labor analgesia and neonatal sepsis evaluation rate: a quality improvement study. *Anesth Analg* 2001;93:986–990.

113. Goetzl L, Cohen A, Frigoletto F Jr, et al. Maternal epidural use and neonatal sepsis evaluation in afebrile mothers. *Pediatrics* 2001;108:1099–1102.

114. Camann W. Intrapartum epidural analgesia and neonatal sepsis evaluations: a casual or causal association? *Anesthesiology* 1999;90:1250–1252.

115. Gaiser R. Neonatal effects of labor analgesia. *Int Anesthesiol Clin* 2002;40:49–65.

116. Goodman S. Anesthesia for nonobstetric surgery in the pregnant patient. *Semin Perinatol* 2002;26:136–145.

117. Beilin Y. Anesthesia for nonobstetric surgery during pregnancy. *Mt Sinai J Med* 1998;65:265–270.

118. Yarnell RW. Emergency surgery during pregnancy. Winterlude 1995. Available at: http://www.anesthesia.org/winterlude/wl95/wl95_6.html. Accessed May 5, 2003.

119. Goldenberg RL. The management of preterm labor. *Obstet Gynecol* 2002;100:1020–1037.

120. Dufour P, Vinatier D, Puech F. The use of intravenous nitroglycerin for cervico-uterine relaxation: a review of the literature. *Arch Gynecol Obstet* 1997;261:1–7.

121. Alahuhta S, Jouppila P. How to maintain uteroplacental perfusion during obstetric anaesthesia. *Acta Anaesthesiol Scand Suppl* 1997;110:106–108.

122. Rathmell JP, Viscomi CM, Ashburn MA. Management of nonobstetric pain during pregnancy and lactation. *Anesth Analg* 1997;85:1074–1087.

123. Cauldwell CB. Anesthesia for fetal surgery. *Anesthesiol Clin North America* 2002;20:211–226.

124. Smith RP, Gitau R, Glover V, et al. Pain and stress in the human fetus. *Eur J Obstet Gynecol Reprod Biol* 2000;92:161–165.

125. Rosen MA. Anesthesia for fetal procedures and surgery. *Yonsei Med J* 2001;42:669–680.

126. Report of the MRC expert group on fetal pain. August 28, 2001. Available at: http://www.mrc.ac.uk/pdf-fetal.pdf. Accessed May 5, 2003.

127. van Lingen RA, Simons SH, Anderson BJ, et al. The effects of analgesia in the vulnerable infant during the perinatal period. *Clin Perinatol* 2002;29:511–534.

128. Thurlow JA, Kinsella SM. Intrauterine resuscitation: active management of fetal distress. *Int J Obstet Anesth* 2002;11:105–116.

129. American Heart Association in collaboration with the International Liaison Committee on Resuscitation. Guidelines 2000 for cardiopulmonary resuscitation and emergency cardiovascular care. Part 8: advanced challenges in resuscitation: section 3: special challenges in ECC. *Circulation* 2000;102(8 Suppl):I229–I252.

130. Johnson MD, Luppi CJ, Over DC. Cardiopulmonary resuscitation. In: Gambling DR, Douglas MJ, eds. *Obstetric anesthesia and uncommon disorders*. Philadelphia: WB Saunders, 1997:51–74.

131. Whitten M, Irvine LM. Postmortem and perimortem caesarean section: what are the indications? *J R Soc Med* 2000;93:6–.

132. Katz VL, Dotters DJ, Droegemueller W. Perimortem cesarean delivery. *Obstet Gynecol* 1986;68:571–576.

133. D'Alessio JG, Ramanathan J. Effects of maternal anesthesia in the neonate. *Semin Perinatol* 1998;22:350–362.

134. Ala-kokko T, Myllynen P, Vähäkangas K. Ex vivo perfusion of the human placental cotyledon: implications for anesthetic pharmacology. *Int J Obstet Anesth* 2000;9:26–38.

135. Celleno D, Capogna G, Emanuelli M, et al. Which induction drug for cesarean section? A comparison of thiopental sodium, propofol, and midazolam. *J Clin Anesth* 1993;5:284–288.

136. Sánchez-Alcaraz A, Quintana MB, Laguarda M. Placental transfer and neonatal effects of propofol in caesarean section. *J Clin Pharm Ther* 1998;23:19–23.

137. Herman NL, Li AT, Van Decar TK, et al. Transfer of methohexital across the perfused human placenta. *J Clin Anesth* 2000;12:25–30.

138. Gambling DR, Sharma SK, White PF, et al. Use of sevoflurane during elective cesarean birth: a comparison with isoflurane and spinal anesthesia. *Anesth Analg* 1995;81:90–95.

139. Abboud TK, Zhu J, Richardson M, et al. Desflurane: a new volatile anesthetic for cesarean section. Maternal and neonatal effects. *Acta Anaesthesiol Scand* 1995;39:723–726.

140. Hawkins JL. Maternal mortality: anesthetic implications. *Int Anesthesiol Clin* 2002;40:1–11.

141. Hawthorne L, Wilson R, Lyons G, et al. Failed intubation revisited: 17-yr experience in a teaching maternity unit. *Br J Anaesth* 1996;76:680–684.

142. Tsen LC, Pitner R, Camann WR. General anesthesia for cesarean section at a tertiary care hospital 1990-1995: indications and implications. *Int J Obstet Anesth* 1998;7:147–152.

143. Reynolds F. The drive for regional anaesthesia for elective cesarean section has gone too far. *Int J Obstet Anesth* 2002;11:292–295.

144. Cooper G. The drive for regional anaesthesia for elective cesarean section has gone too far. *Int J Obstet Anesth* 2002;11:289–292.

145. Drysdale SM, Muir H. New techniques and drugs for epidural labor analgesia. *Semin Perinatol* 2002;26:99–108.

146. Lyons G, Reynolds F. Toxicity and safety of epidural local anaesthetics. *Int J Obstet Anesth* 2001;10:259–262.

147. Kavak ZN, Başgül A, Ceyhan N. Short-term outcome of newborn infants: spinal versus general anesthesia for elective cesarean section. A prospective randomized study. *Eur J Obstet Gynecol Reprod Biol* 2001;100:50–54.

148. Dick WF. Anaesthesia for caesarean section (epidural and general): effects on the neonate. *Eur J Obstet Gynecol Reprod Biol* 1995;59 Suppl:S61–S67.

149. Kolatat T, Somboonnanonda A, Lertakyamanee J, et al. Effects of general and regional anesthesia on the neonate (a prospective, randomized trial). *J Med Assoc Thai* 1999;82:40–45.

150. Ratcliffe FM, Evans JM. Neonatal wellbeing after elective caesarean delivery with general, spinal, and epidural anaesthesia. *Eur J Anaesthesiol* 1993;10:175–181.

151. Stuart KA, Krakauer H, Schone E, et al. Labor epidurals improve outcomes for babies of mothers at high risk for unscheduled cesarean section. *J Perinatol* 2001;21:178–185.

152. Levy BT, Dawson JD, Toth PP, et al. Predictors of neonatal resuscitation, low Apgar scores, and umbilical artery pH among growth-restricted neonates. *Obstet Gynecol* 1998;91:909–916.

153. Mueller MD, Brühwiler H, Schüpfer GK, et al. Higher rate of fetal acidemia after regional anesthesia for elective cesarean delivery. *Obstet Gynecol* 1997;90:131–134.

154. Emmett RS, Cyna AM, Simmons SW. Techniques for preventing hypotension during spinal anaesthesia for caesarean section. *Cochrane Database Syst Rev* 2001;3:CD002251.

155. Shearer VE, Ramin SM, Wallace DH, et al. Fetal effects of prophylactic ephedrine and maternal hypotension during regional anaesthesia for cesarean section. *J Matern Fetal Med* 1996;5:79–84.

156. Lee A, Ngan Kee WD, Gin T. A quantitative, systematic review of randomized controlled trials of ephedrine versus phenylephrine for the management of hypotension during spinal anesthesia for cesarean delivery. *Anesth Analg* 2002;94:920–926.

157. Ngan Kee WD. Obstetric neuraxial anaesthesia: which vasopressor should we be using? *Int J Obstet Anesth* 2003;12:55–56.

158. Harrop-Griffiths W. Ephedrine is the vasopressor of choice for obstetric regional anaesthesia. *Int J Obstet Anaesthesia* 2002;11:275–278.

159. Thomas DG. Ephedrine is the vasopressor of choice for obstetric regional anaesthesia. *International J Obstet Anesthesia* 2002;11:278–281.

160. Cooper DW, Carpenter M, Mowbray P, et al. Fetal and maternal effects of phenylephrine and ephedrine during spinal anesthesia for cesarean delivery. *Anesthesiology* 2002;97:1582–1590.

161. Wright PM, Iftikhar M, Fitzpatrick KT, et al. Vasopressor therapy for hypotension during epidural anesthesia for cesarean section: effects on maternal and fetal flow velocity ratios. *Anesth Analg* 1992;75:56–63.

162. Jordan, MJ. Women undergoing caesarean section under regional anesthesia should routinely receive supplementary oxygen. *Int J Obstet Anesth* 2002;11:282–285.

163. Kelly MC, Fitzpatrick KT, Hill DA. Respiratory effects of spinal anaesthesia for caesarean section. *Anaesthesia* 1996;51:1120–1122.

164. Cogliano MS, Graham AC, Clark VA. Supplementary oxygen administration for elective caesarean section under spinal anaesthesia. *Anaesthesia* 2002;57:66–69.

165. Saugstad OD, Rootwelt T, Aalen O. Resuscitation of asphyxiated newborn infants with room air or oxygen: an international controlled trial: the Resair 2 study. *Pediatrics* 1998;102:e1. Available at: http://www.pediatrics.org/cgi/content/full/102/1/e1. Accessed May 6, 2003.

166. Saugstad OD. Update on oxygen radical disease in neonatology. *Curr Opin Obstet Gynecol* 2001;13:147–153.

167. Saugstad OD. Is oxygen more toxic than currently believed? *Pediatrics* 2001;108:1203–1205.

168. Vento M, Asensi M, Sastre J, et al. Resuscitation with room air instead of 100% oxygen prevents oxidative stress in moderately asphyxiated term neonates. *Pediatrics* 2001;107:642–647.

169. Perlman J. Resuscitation—air versus 100% oxygen. *Pediatrics* 2002; 109:347–349.

170. Halliwell B. Free radicals, antioxidants, and human disease: curiosity, cause, or consequence? *Lancet* 1994;344:721–724.

171. Vendemiale G, Grattagliano I, Altomare E. An update on the role of free radicals and antioxidant defense in human disease. *Int J Clin Lab Res* 1999;29:49–55.

172. Hill D. Women undergoing caesarean section under regional anaesthesia should routinely receive supplementary oxygen. *Int J Obstet Anesth* 2002;11:285–288.

173. Khaw KS, Wang CC, Ngan Kee WD, et al. Effects of high inspired oxygen fraction during elective caesarean section under spinal anaesthesia on maternal and fetal oxygenation and lipid peroxidation. *Br J Anaesth* 2002;88:18–23.

174. Backe SK, Lyons G. Oxygen and elective Caesarean section. *Br J Anaesth* 2002;88:4–5.

175. Fawole B, Hofmeyr GJ. Maternal oxygen administration for fetal distress. *Cochrane Database Syst Rev* 2003;4:CD000136.

176. Halpern SH, Walsh VL. Multimodal therapy for post-cesarean delivery pain. *Reg Anesth Pain Med* 2001;26:298–300.

177. Jin F, Chung F. Multimodal analgesia for postoperative pain control. *J Clin Anesth* 2001;13:524–539.

178. Dahl V, Raeder JC. Non-opioid postoperative analgesia. *Acta Anaesthesiol Scand* 2000;44:1191–1203.

179. Gordon DB, Pellino TA, Miaskowski C. A 10-year review of quality improvement monitoring in pain management: recommendations for standardized outcome measures. *Pain Manag Nurs* 2002;3:116–130.

180. Baka N, Bayoumeu F, Boutroy MJ, et al. Colostrum morphine concentrations during postcesarean intravenous patient-controlled analgesia. *Anesth Analg* 2002;94:184–187.

181. Angle PJ, Halpern SH, Leighton BL, et al. A randomized controlled trial examining the effect of naproxen on analgesia during the second day after cesarean delivery. *Anesth Analg* 2002;95:741–745.

182. Spigset O. Anaesthetic agents and excretion in breast milk. *Acta Anaesthesiol Scand* 1994;38:94–103.

183. Windle ML, Booker LA, Rayburn WF. Postpartum pain after vaginal delivery. A review of comparative analgesic trials. *J Reprod Med* 1989;34:891–895.

184. Peter EA, Janssen PA, Grange CS, et al. Ibuprofen versus acetaminophen with codeine for the relief of perineal pain after childbirth: a randomized controlled trial. *CMAJ* 2001;165:1203–1209.

185. Greene JF, Kuiper O, Morosky M, et al. A postpartum self-medication program: effect on narcotic use. *J Womens Health Gend Based Med* 1999;8:1073–1076.

186. American Academy of Pediatrics Committee on Drugs. The transfer of drugs and other chemicals into human breast milk. *Pediatrics* 2001;108:776–789.

Transition and Stabilization

17

Cardiorespiratory Adjustments at Birth

Ruben E. Alvaro   *Henrique Rigatto*

Respiratory physiologists and physicians have long been interested in the respiratory and cardiovascular events that occur at birth. However, apart from occasional references to the pulmonary circulation, the fetal circulation only received serious consideration in the middle of the twentieth century, when it was recognized that dramatic changes in blood flow through the lungs occurred after birth.

The first detailed description of circulation in the mammalian fetus was provided by Harvey in 1628 (1). Although he correctly described blood flow from the inferior vena cava through the foramen ovale, he thought that the blood had to enter the pulmonary veins before returning to the left atrium. He was also perplexed by how the fetus survives *in utero* without the aid of respiration. The answer to the last question came in 1799, when Scheel noted light red blood in the umbilical vein and dark red blood in the umbilical artery in the fetal sheep, as well as darkening of that color when the pregnant ewe was asphyxiated (2). However, it was Zweifel, in 1876, who categorically stated that the placenta was the lung of the fetus, describing the presence of oxyhemoglobin in the umbilical blood before any breathing had occurred (3).

The conventional belief during the nineteenth century was that the fetal pulmonary blood flow progressively increased over gestation and that it was relatively higher in the fetus than after birth (4,5). It was not until the first part of the twentieth century that the right ventricular pressure was demonstrated to fall and pulmonary blood flow to increase after the establishment of breathing (6,7). It was only 50 years ago that Dawes and colleagues (8) demonstrated by direct measurements in fetal lambs that pulmonary blood flow increased when the lungs were ventilated with air. Over these past 50 years, the developmental changes in the pulmonary circulation and in its responses to stresses of hypoxia, and increases in pulmonary arterial pressure and blood flow, have become subjects of intense investigation (9).

It is well known now that during fetal life the placenta and not the lungs serves as the organ for gas exchange. Because of this, the normal fetal circulatory pattern is arranged very differently from that observed after birth and is quite satisfactory for survival in the womb. The placental circulation is in a parallel arrangement; that is, it receives blood from the descending aorta and drains blood to the systemic venous circulation. To accomplish this, the fetal circulation depends on a series of intra- and extracardiac shunts that allows the oxygenated blood to flow from the placenta to the systemic organs and for the deoxygenated blood to return to the placenta. This blood flow distribution allows the delivery of blood with the highest oxygen content (from the placenta) to the heart and brain and blood with lower oxygen content to the lower body and placenta. Because the lungs are not required for gas exchange, pulmonary blood flow is low (approximately 10% of the combined ventricular output), yet adequate for lung growth and development. Unique only to fetal life, the blood exiting the lungs has a lower saturation than does blood entering the pulmonary circulation, and although the lungs do not participate in gas exchange *in utero*, they are metabolically active, secreting liquid into the potential air spaces and synthesizing surfactant, a substance that is vital to achieve adequate ventilation at birth. The fetal lungs are also physically active in that they simulate breathing movements.

The transition from the placenta to the lungs at birth is accomplished by three main cardiopulmonary processes: (a) onset of breathing, resulting in lung expansion with concomitant decrease in pulmonary vascular resistance and increase pulmonary blood flow; (b) increase in blood oxygen content that further decreases pulmonary vascular resistance; and (c) loss of the placental circulation with resultant increase in systemic vascular resistance leading to the closure of the fetal cardiovascular shunts and transition from fetal to neonatal circulation. Thus, to establish the lungs as the site of gas exchange after birth, significant changes in the cardiac and pulmonary circulation as well as the initiation of pulmonary ventilation must occur. Many abnormal maternal, placental and fetal conditions may interfere with this physiologic transition and compromise the newborn infant.

The establishment of effective pulmonary ventilation at birth requires that the lungs develop to a stage where the alveoli can be inflated to provide adequate gas exchange. It also requires the lowering of the pulmonary vascular resistance to allow for the increase in pulmonary blood flow to accommodate the entire cardiac output. The successful transition also requires that the lung liquid volume be removed from the alveolar spaces and that surfactant material be secreted into the acinus to allow for satisfactory physical expansion of the lungs after the initial postnatal breaths. Adequate neurologic drive to generate and maintain spontaneous continuous breathing is essential to maintain ventilation postnatally.

The change to pulmonary ventilation at birth increases pulmonary venous oxygenation that serves to suppress active vasoconstriction of pulmonary vessels. The result is a tenfold increase in pulmonary blood flow and a rapid decrease in pulmonary vascular resistance. The removal of the placenta after constriction of the umbilical vessels in response to increased oxygenation, contributes to a rise in systemic vascular resistance. The decline in pulmonary vascular resistance below systemic values contributes to the closure of the foramen ovale and ductus arteriosus, establishing the adult circulatory patterns.

This chapter reviews some of the most important cardiorespiratory adjustments that occur at the time of delivery allowing the fetus to achieve a successful extrauterine transition.

PULMONARY ADAPTATION

Fetal Lung Fluid

During fetal life, the internal volume of the lungs is maintained by the secretion of liquid into the pulmonary lumen. This liquid expansion of potential air spaces is essential for the growth and the development of normal lung structure before birth, which, in turn, may influence lung function after birth (10).

The fluid in the fetal lung was for many years assumed to be aspirated amniotic fluid as a result of fetal breathing movements (11). In 1941, Potter and Bohlender (12) observed alveolar fluid in two human fetuses with malformations of the respiratory tract which blocked the entrance of amniotic fluid, thus establishing that the lung fluid was secreted, not inhaled. Experiments performed in other species confirmed that fetal pulmonary fluid was indeed generated within the lungs (13–15).

We know now that the fetal lung fluid is neither a mere ultrafiltrate of plasma nor aspirated amniotic fluid. Compared to plasma this lung fluid is rich in chloride and potassium, is significantly lower in bicarbonate and has similar sodium concentration. It is also quite different from amniotic fluid having much higher osmolality, Na^+ and Cl^- concentrations, and significantly lower K^+, protein and urea concentration (Table 17-1) (10,16–18). This distinctive composition of the lung liquid changes very little during gestation (17,19). The high Cl^- and the low protein content characteristics of the lung fluid result from active Cl^- secretion and tight junctions between epithelial cells respectively.

It is not known exactly when this secretory activity begins, but already during the glandular stage of lung development, at about 3 months of gestation, the lung epithelium actively secretes fluid (20,21). By this time the epithelium has developed tight junctions, which are evident by morphologic examination and also by the low protein concentration present in the lung liquid in relationship to the plasma. In fetal lambs, the volume of lung liquid increases from about 5 mL/kg of body weight at midgestation (18) to about 30 to 50 mL/kg at term (18,22–25). The secretion rate increases from about 2 mL/ kg body weight at midgestation (18) to about 5 mL/kg at term (26,27). More recently, Pfister and associates (28) demonstrated that the lung liquid volume exhibited a plateau level in the near-term fetal sheep before it began to decline toward birth. They also observed that the rate of lung liquid secretion declined in two linear phases that commenced earlier than the changes in lung liquid volume (28). In fetal lambs, the amount of lung liquid in relation to lung weight remains

TABLE 17-1

COMPOSITION OF LUNG LUMINAL LIQUID, AMNIOTIC LIQUID, AND PLASMA OF FETAL LAMBS

	Lung Liquid	Amniotic Liquid	Plasma
pH	6.27 ± 0.01	7.07 ± 0.22	7.34 ± 0.04
Osmolality	300 ± 6	257 ± 14	291 ± 8
Na^+ (mEq/L)	150 ± 1	113 ± 6	150 ± 1
Cl^- (mEq/L)	157 ± 4	87 ± 5	107 ± 1
HCO_3^- (mEq/L)	3 ± 1	19 ± 3	24 ± 1
Protein (g/dL)	0.03 ± 0.01	0.1 ± 0.1	4.1 ± 0.3

Values are mean ± SEM (standard error of mean) and are taken from the work of Adamson et al., Adams et al., and Humphreys et al.

relatively constant at approximately 90% through much of the pregnancy (29,30). The lung liquid secretion decreases with increased luminal hydrostatic pressure induced by a prolonged obstruction of the fetal trachea and increases when luminal pressure falls below amniotic fluid pressure and when fetal breathing movements are abolished (24).

This liquid secreted by the fetal lungs flows intermittently up the trachea with fetal breathing movements. Some of this fluid is swallowed and the remainder contributes directly to the formation of amniotic fluid production, accounting for approximately 25% to 50% of the amniotic fluid turnover in the sheep fetus, with the rest being formed by the fetal urine (10). The mechanism by which amniotic fluid is not aspirated into the lungs was demonstrated by Brown and associates (31) in 1983, when they showed that the larynx acts as a one-way valve allowing only liquid outflow under normal circumstances. The continuous secretion of liquid by the lungs confronted with a flow impediment produced by the larynx and the amniotic fluid pressure creates a small but important positive intrapulmonary pressure, which is essential for normal growth and for the structural and biochemical maturation of the developing lung (10,29,31,32). Thus, in fetal sheep, unimpeded leakage of tracheal liquid decreases lung size by arresting pulmonary tissue growth, whereas prolonged obstruction of tracheal outflow leads to lung hyperplasia (32,33). Nardo and associates (34) showed that lung hypoplasia in fetal sheep can be considerably improved by short-term obstruction at the tracheal level. Conversely, pulmonary hypoplasia in humans can be observed in pathologic conditions such as diaphragmatic hernia, pleural effusion, or severe oligohydramnios (Potter syndrome) as a result of the compression of the fetal lungs and the decrease in their internal volume (35,36).

Congenital high airway obstruction syndrome (CHAOS) is a clinical condition caused by complete or near-complete obstruction of the fetal airway that results in elevated intratracheal pressure, distention of the tracheobronchial tree, and lung hyperplasia. The enlarged lungs may cause cardiac and caval compression leading to *in utero* heart failure manifested by ascites, hydrops fetalis, and placentomegaly (37,38).

The production of fetal lung liquid depends on a system of active ion transport across the alveolar type II cells of the pulmonary epithelium (10,39,40). Olver and Strang (41) demonstrated that lung liquid secretion is coupled with active transport of Cl^- toward the pulmonary lumen, generating an electrical potential difference of -5 mV (lumen negative). This chloride secretion generates an osmotic gradient that causes liquid to flow from the microcirculation through the interstitium into the potential air spaces. This chloride secretion occurs through chloride channels in the apical membrane (alveolar side) and depends largely on chloride influx at a bumetanide-sensitive Na^+-K^+-$2Cl^-$ (NKCC) cotransporter system in the basolateral membrane (interstitial side) (42). Thus, Cl^- enters the cell on a cotransporter linked with K^+ and Na^+ down the electrochemical potential gradient for Na^+ generated by Na^+-K^+-adenosine triphos-

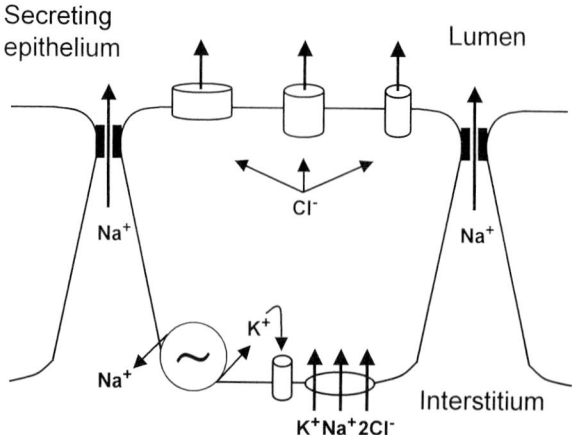

Figure 17-1 Lung liquid secretion. The present model for chloride secretion emphasizes the central role of basolateral Na-K-ATPase in maintaining high intracellular K^- and low NA^+ concentrations. Na^- re-enters the cell down its electrochemical gradient via the Na/K/2CL cotransporter on the basolateral membrane. K^+ may leave the cell through basolateral channels. The high intracellular Cl^- concentration and the negative intracellular membrane potential facilitate the rise of the Cl^- concentration to tally its electrochemical equilibrium. A further rise in intracellular Cl^- concentration will lead to opening of the apical Cl^- channels and flow of this anion into the lung lumen. Na^+ and water will follow Cl^- through a paracellular route. (Adapted from O'Brodovich HM. Immature epithelial Na^+ channel expression is one of the pathogenetic mechanisms leading to human neonatal respiratory distress syndrome. *Proc Assoc Am Physicians* 1996;108:345–355.)

phatase (ATPase) in the basolateral membrane of the cell. Consequently, Cl^- concentration increases inside the cell above its equilibrium potential, which provides an electrochemical gradient for Cl^- exit across the luminal membrane of the epithelial cell through Cl^- permeant ion channels (Fig. 17-1) (10). Addition of the loop diuretic bumetanide or furosemide (specific NKCC inhibitors) into the fetal lung liquid decreases fluid secretion by decreasing Cl^- entry into the epithelial cell through the basolateral membrane.

Clearance of Fluid at Birth

To allow adequate postnatal gas exchange, pulmonary fluid, which is essential to fetal lung development, must be rapidly removed at birth in order (43–45). Thus the transition from intra- to extrauterine life requires the effective clearance of lung liquid to support air breathing and the conversion of the pulmonary epithelium in the distal air spaces from fluid secretion to fluid absorption. Disruption of this process has been implicated in several disease states, including transient tachypnea of the newborn (TTN) and hyaline membrane disease (44,46–48). Preterm delivery and cesarean section without prior labor result in excessive retention of lung fluid and may contribute to respiratory compromise in the newborn infant (47,49–53).

A complete understanding of the mechanisms by which fetal lungs are able to clear themselves of fluid is still lacking. It is clear now that the traditional explanations for fluid reabsorption which relied on Starling forces, lymphatic uptake and vaginal squeeze at the time of birth, can only account for a very small fraction of the lung fluid clearance (54). More recently, several studies have strongly suggested that the primary mechanism of lung liquid reabsorption is the change in ion transport induced by catecholamines during labor (10,31,44,55–57). Although the mechanisms responsible for lung liquid clearance at birth develop gradually during the last part of pregnancy, the removal of lung liquid and the switch from fluid secretion to fluid absorption, triggered by events at birth, are probably quite rapid because in the human the functional residual capacity of the lungs rises to a near normal value of 25 to 30 mL/kg within 15 minutes after normal delivery (58).

Although there is disagreement about whether clearance begins prior to labor, or occurs entirely within labor, it is now clear that the vast bulk (>75%) of this liquid leaves the lung some time before normal term birth (59). In studies done in full-term fetal sheep, Pfister and associates (28) showed that the lung liquid volume began a gradual decline well before the onset of labor and it was mainly a result of a decrease in the secretion rate rather than active reabsorption. They also showed that this gradual decline was followed by a much more rapid decline within labor that was mainly a result of active reabsorption of fluid driven by active Na^+ transport through the pulmonary epithelium. This last process is stimulated by the catecholamine surge that occurs just before the onset of labor (31). Other authors, however, suggest that lung liquid volume continues to rise until the day before labor (24,25,60).

As explained in the previous section, chloride secretion across the distal lung epithelium results in the production of lung liquid which is necessary for proper lung development in fetal life. In contrast, sodium absorption allows for fluid reabsorption and is critical for efficient oxygenation in the newborn.

The movement of sodium across the pulmonary epithelium from the alveolar lumen to the interstitium with subsequent absorption into the vasculature can be considered a two-step process. In the first step, sodium passively enters the apical membrane of the alveolar type II cell through amiloride-sensitive epithelial Na^+ channels (ENaCs). Thus, intraluminal instillation of amiloride delays lung fluid clearance in fetal life (61–67) and induces severe respiratory distress and a persistence of fetal lung fluid postnatally (68). In the second step, sodium is actively pumped out of the cell into the interstitium through the basolateral membrane by the ouabain inhibitable Na^+-K^+-ATPase. Thus, Na^+-K^+-ATPase pump inhibition with ouabain consistently reduces liquid clearance in various species (62,66,69–72). To equilibrate the osmotic pressure, generated by the movement of Na^+, water diffuses from the alveolar to the interstitial space either through specific water channels (aquaporins) or through the paracellular junctions (Fig. 17-2) (44,73,74). Although recent data demonstrate that aquaporin-4 messenger RNA (mRNA) in the perinatal epithelium is developmentally regulated and peaks at birth (74,75) there is no evidence that these channels regulate fluid clearance (Fig. 17-2) (10,44,55,72,73,76–78). The mechanisms of Na^+ absorption through the pulmonary epithelium have been con-

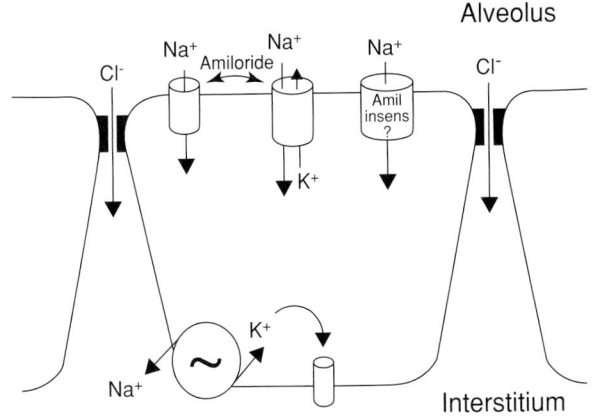

Figure 17-2 Lung liquid absorption. At birth, to offset Cl^- secretion Na^+ channels on the epithelial cell are activated, establishing conduit for the osmotically active Na^+ ion. Basolateral membrane Na^+-K^+-ATPase generates the gradient for apical Na^+ entry into the epithelial cell and switches the distal lung epithelium from a secreting to an absorbing organ. The net movement of Na^+ to the basolateral direction induces a parallel movement of Cl^- and fluid through the paracellular route or the transcellular pathway, using specific water channels, that is, aquaporins. Amil insens, amiloride insesitivity. (Adapted from O'Brodovich HM. Immature epithelial Na^+ channel expression is one of the pathogenetic mechanisms leading to human neonatal respiratory distress syndrome. *Proc Assoc Am Physicians* 1996;108:345–355.)

firmed by isolation and culture of fetal alveolar type II cells (68,79–82).

The gene for the amiloride-sensitive epithelial sodium channel has been cloned; it consists of three homologous subunits called α-, β-, and γ-ENaC. The α subunit is a prerequisite unit for any channel activity. The expression of the three subunits is necessary for maximum ion transport (83). The α-ENaC (84) and the β- and γ-ENaC subunits (85) were detected in early midtrimester on the apical domain of human airway cells suggesting that sodium absorption might begin significantly before birth, even if secretion is still dominant. The three subunits increased sharply around the time of birth, were highest shortly after birth, and declined in parallel with endogenous plasma epinephrine concentration during the first week of life. The importance of the ENaC was confirmed by studies showing that α-ENaC knockout mice were unable to clear lung liquid from the alveolar spaces after birth resulting in death from respiratory failure (86). Mice with β- or γ-ENaC null mutations had delayed liquid clearance but had near-normal lung water content 12 hours after birth (86,87).

It is well known now that net alveolar fluid clearance occurs at a rapid rate late in gestation and that this clearance is driven by elevations of endogenous epinephrine. The critical link between β-adrenergic stimulation and lung fluid clearance was made in 1978 by Walters and Olver who found that intravenously infused epinephrine caused rapid absorption of lung fluid in near-term fetal lambs and that this response could be inhibited by prior treatment with propanolol (88). The intravenous epinephrine caused an immediate and reversible increase in luminal electronegativity by stimulating the active transport of Na^+ out of the lung lumen (55). In the absence of adrenergic stimulation the amiloride-sensitive Na^+ channels remain closed (secretory state). Thus, the opened or closed state of the Na^+ channels determines whether the fetal lungs, at any particular time, are secretory or reabsorptive (10). The epinephrine stimulation of amiloride-sensitive alveolar fluid clearance is mediated by cyclic adenosine monophosphate (cAMP) and Ca^{2+} likely acting as a intracellular second messenger (89,90).

The induced reabsorption with epinephrine increases strikingly with advancing gestational age and can be induced by pretreatment of fetal sheep with the combination of corticosteroids and triiodothyronine (91). These two hormones are required to switch the effect of β-adrenergic stimulation from net chloride and liquid secretion to net sodium and liquid absorption (30,56,57,92,93). Consistent with *in vivo* observations, α-ENaC mRNA is increased by glucocorticoids in the primary cultures of alveolar type II cells FDLE, while the expression of β- and γ-ENaC mRNA is unaffected by glucocorticoid (94).

Another factor that appears to be particularly important in the switch of transepithelial liquid flow from secretion to absorption is the sharp increase in alveolar pressure of oxygen (P_AO_2) that occurs at birth. It was recently shown that fetal PO_2 favored the development of fluid filled cyst-like structures while the rise of PO_2 to postnatal levels reduced fluid in the cysts (95). The effect of oxygen seems to be the result of an increase in Na^+-K^+-ATPase activity and the response is also enhanced by glucocorticoids and thyroid hormones. Thus, at birth, epinephrine, oxygen, glucocorticoid and thyroid hormones interact to produce a permanent switch from secretion to absorption in the distal epithelium.

Although the switch from Cl^- secretion to sodium absorption is the critical mechanism for lung fluid clearance at the time of delivery, other passive factors play a role in clearing the residual liquid present in potential air spaces at birth. The first is transient and peaks early and relates to enlarged transepithelial pores produced by spontaneous ventilation (22,29,47,51). Thus air inflation, by passive reabsorption down the transpulmonary pressure gradient associated with ventilation, shifts residual liquid from the lung lumen into the interstitium around distensible perivascular spaces of large pulmonary blood vessels and airways. These perivascular cuffs progressively diminish in size as the fluid is removed by small pulmonary blood vessels and lymphatics. Bland and associates (96,97) showed that the pulmonary circulation absorbs most of the residual liquid present in potential air spaces at birth and that elevated left atrial pressure or reduction of plasma protein concentration slows the rate of liquid clearance in mature animals. Although there is a small and transient increase in lymph flow after postnatal breathing begins, the amount of excess liquid drained postnatally by pulmonary lymphatics is only approximately 11% of the residual liquid in the lungs at birth (98). The second mechanism is the transvascular protein gradient that facilitates the movement of fluid from the essentially protein-free lung fluid into the interstitium, followed by passage of liquid into the bloodstream.

RESPIRATORY ADAPTATION

Fetal Breathing

The discovery of fetal breathing in the late 1960s immediately stimulated interest in the factors that control breathing *in utero* (99–101). Although of unknown purpose, because no gas exchange is involved, fetal breathing may represent preparation *in utero* for a vital function important in life. Shortly after its discovery, the Oxford group (102) showed that, although fetal breathing was influenced by fetal behavior, occurring essentially in rapid eye movement (REM) sleep, it was clearly regulated by other chemical factors, such as carbon dioxide and oxygen concentration. Subsequent work confirmed and expanded these findings by recording the electrical activity of the diaphragm and clearly demonstrating the central origin of the respiratory output in utero (103–107). Using ultrasonographic technology, breathing movements were also identified in the human fetus, being present approximately 40% of the time during late pregnancy, a figure similar to that in sheep (108–111).

The discovery of fetal breathing not only stimulated the development of the area of fetal assessment but it also brought a new dimension to the events occurring at birth. What has been traditionally called "the initiation of breathing at birth" must now be called "the establishment of continuous breathing at birth." Breathing begins long before birth. The question is not what determines the appearance of breathing at birth, but what makes it continuous. From another angle, what makes fetal breathing episodic in late gestation and present only during low-voltage electrocortical activity? The answer to this question remains unknown.

Fetal breathing in sheep is mostly continuous in early gestation (90 to 115 days) but becomes episodic in late gestation, primarily occurring during periods of low-voltage electrocortical activity (99,101,107,112,113). During high-voltage electrocortical activity there is no established breathing present, but occasional breaths may surface after episodic, generalized, tonic muscular discharges associated with body movements (Fig. 17-3) (107). During low-voltage electrocortical activity, breathing is irregular, the diaphragmatic electromyelogram (EMG) being characterized by an abrupt beginning and end. The physiologic mechanism responsible for the occurrence of fetal breathing only during low-voltage electrocortical activity is unknown.

Modulation of Fetal Breathing by CO_2, O_2, and Neurochemicals

Many studies clearly show that the fetal breathing apparatus is capable of responding well to chemical stimuli and other agents known to modify breathing postnatally. Thus it

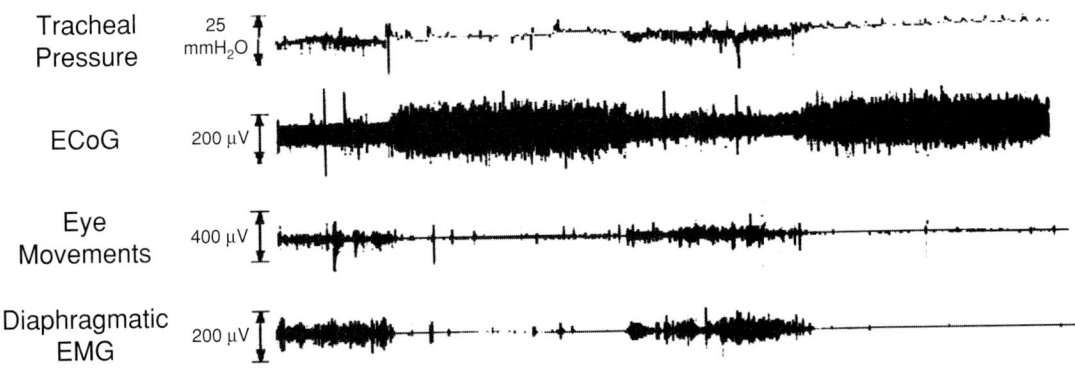

Figure 17-3 Fetal breathing in a fetal lamb at 134 days of gestation. The deflections in tracheal pressure and diaphragmatic activity occur during periods of raid eye movement (REM) in low-voltage electrocortical activity only. In high-voltage electrocortical activity (quiet sleep) breathing is absent. (From Rigatto H. Regulation of fetal breathing. *Reprod Fertil Dev* 1996;8:23–33, with permission.)

became clear that the fetus responds to an increase in arterial carbon dioxide pressure ($PaCO_2$) with an increase in breathing (102,108,114–118). The increased breathing activity is prolonged into the transitional high voltage electrocochleography but does not continue into the established (Fig. 17-4) (118). There is much evidence suggesting that the actions of CO_2 are central.

Administration of low oxygen to the fetus by having the ewe breathe hypoxic mixtures abolished fetal breathing; this was associated with a decrease in body movements and in the amplitude of the ECoG (102,119,120). Transection of the brain at the upper level of the pons prevents the inhibitory action of hypoxia and induces continuous breathing. Conversely, increase in arterial PO_2 to levels above 200 mm Hg through the administration of 100% O_2 to the fetus via an endotracheal tube stimulated breathing and induced continuous breathing in 35% of the experiments in fetal sheep (121). These findings suggest that low partial tension of O_2 in the fetus at rest may be a normal mechanism inhibiting breathing *in utero*.

A comprehensive review of the effects of various neurochemicals agents on fetal breathing has been published (122). In general, fetal breathing is inhibited by muscimol (123), a γ-aminobutyric (GABA) agonist, pentobarbiton (124), and diazepam (125) acting at the $GABA_A$

receptor complex (126). Other endogenous inhibitors include adenosine, prostaglandin E_2 (PGE_2) (see next subsection), and endorphins, which may be present at high levels in the fetal circulation. Agents that stimulate fetal breathing movements include prostaglandin inhibitors such as indomethacin, meclofenamate, morphine, caffeine, pilocarpine, and 5-hydroxy-L-tryptophan (5-HTP). Fetal breathing is inhibited by maternal hypoglycemia whereas it is stimulated after maternal meals and hyperglycemia.

Establishment of Continuous Breathing at Birth

The traditional view has been that labor and delivery produce a transient fetal asphyxia that stimulates the peripheral chemoreceptors to induce the first breath. Breathing would then be maintained through the input of other stimuli, such as cold or touch (127,128). More recent observations have questioned this general view. First, the denervation of the carotid and aortic chemoreceptors does not alter fetal breathing or the initiation of continuous breathing at birth (Fig. 17-5) (129,130). Second, continuous breathing can be established *in utero*, with manifestations of arousal, by raising fetal PO_2 and occluding the

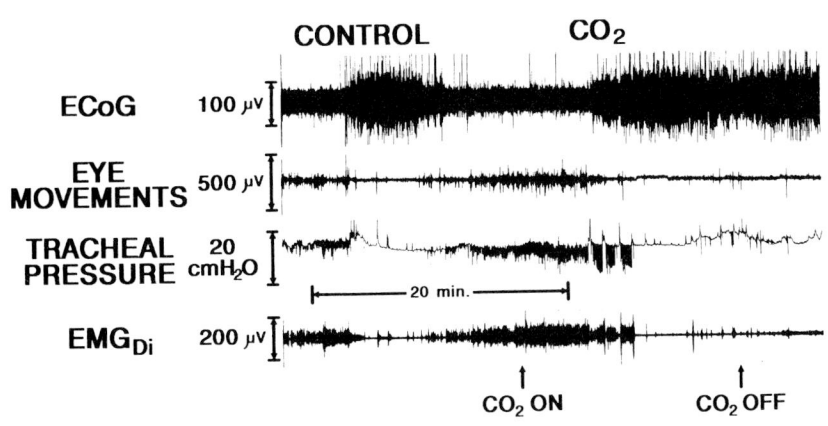

Figure 17-4 Fetal breathing during control and during CO_2 rebreathing. Note the increase in tracheal pressure and diaphragmatic activity during CO_2 rebreathing. Fetal breathing was prolonged into the transitional low- to high-voltage ECoG, but stopped in established high-voltage ECoG. (From Rigatto H. Regulation of fetal breathing. *Reprod Fertil Dev* 1996;8:23–33, with permission.)

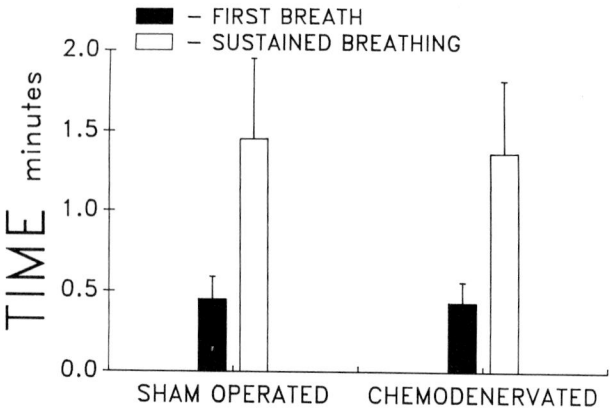

Figure 17-5 Delay in minutes from opening of the window to (■) the appearance of the first breath and to (□) sustained breathing. There were no significant differences between the sham-operated and the chemodenervated groups. (From Rigatto H. Regulation of fetal breathing. *Reprod Fertil Dev* 1996;8:23–33, with permission.)

uli, such as cold, once thought to be important for the establishment of continuous breathing at birth.

Thus, the physiologic mechanism responsible for the inhibition of fetal breathing and the establishment of continuous breathing at birth remains unknown. It has been debated whether the key factors in inducing these changes are intrinsic to the fetal brain or are in the placenta. Because placental separation at birth is associated with the onset of continuous breathing, we, together with others, have hypothesized that placental factors might be responsible for the inhibition of fetal breathing (131–135). This line of thinking is based on the assumption that the release of a factor by the placenta into the fetal circulation prevents fetal breathing from being continuous, with inhibition during high-voltage ECoG, and present only during periods of reticular activation as it occurs during low-voltage ECoG. In the absence of this factor from the placenta at birth, after cord clamping, the state-related inhibition observed during high-voltage ECoG is insufficient to disrupt continuous breathing. Teleologically, it is interesting that nature may have delegated to the placenta the important role of providing the fetus with gas exchange and nutrients and it is conceivable that it may also have endowed the placenta with some form of chemoreceptor

umbilical cord (Fig. 17-6) (121). These observations during administration of high O_2 or cord occlusion suggest that the fetus can be made to resemble a neonate *in utero* without the transient hypoxemia to stimulate the peripheral chemoreceptors and without any of the sensory stim-

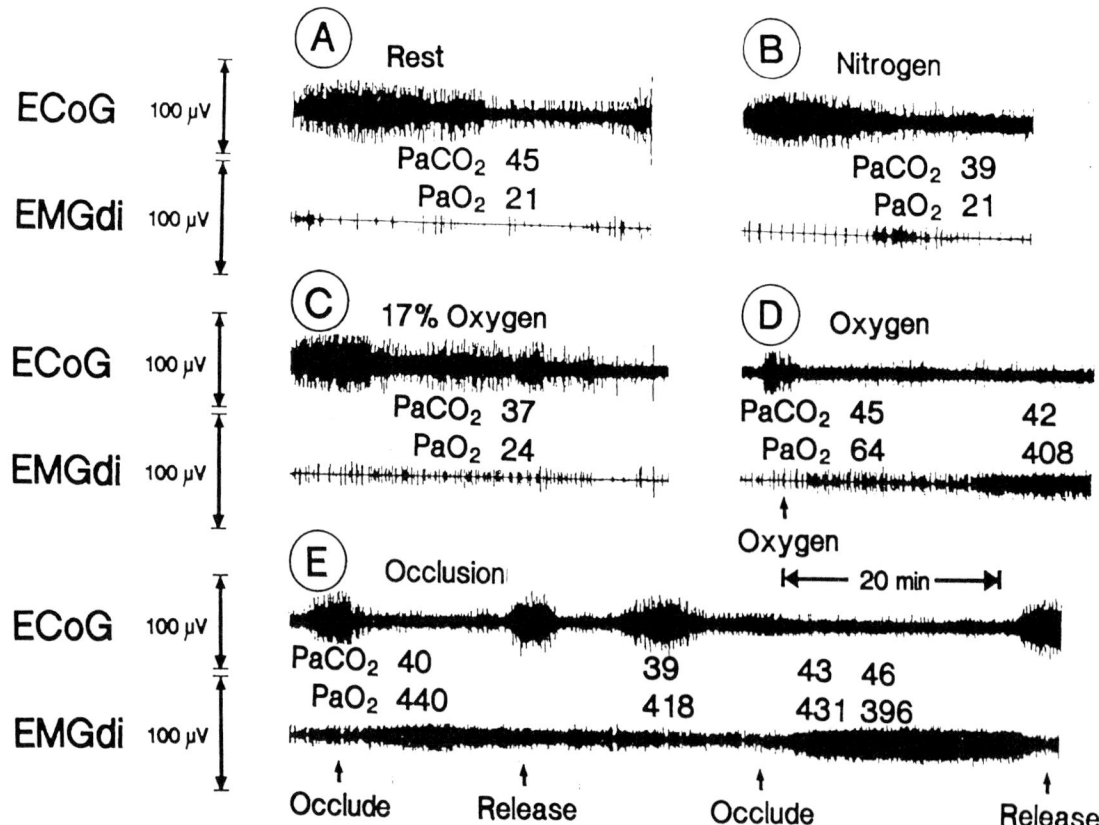

Figure 17-6 Representative tracing showing the effect of fetal fraction of inspired oxygen (FiO_2) on fetal breathing and electrocortical activity. **A**: Control cycle showing little breathing in fetus in early labor at 143 days of gestation. **B**: Lung distention (mean airway pressure 30 cm H_2O) and inspired N_2 does not affect baseline tracing. **C**: Seventeen percent O_2 also does not alter breathing. **D**: One hundred percent O_2 induces continuous breathing. **E**: Occlusion on two occasions induces more forceful breathing than that observed with O_2 alone. Note that continuous breathing was elicited despite preventing the rise of $PaCO_2$ by ventilating the fetus with high-frequency ventilation (15 Hz, stroke = 7 cm H_2O). ECoG, electrocochleography; EMGdi, electromyogram of the diaphragm. (From Rigatto H. Regulation of fetal breathing. *Reprod Fertil Dev* 1996;8:23–33, with permission.)

activity regulating fetal breathing and behavior by the secretion of chemical substances into the fetal circulation.

More direct evidence for a placental role has been present since Dawes (127) and Harned and Ferreiro (128) showed that only after clamping the umbilical cord does the newborn lamb start breathing and behaving like a neonate. Subsequently, Adamson and associates (133) induced breathing in the fetus with umbilical cord occlusion and supply of O_2 via an endotracheal catheter. On release of the cord, breathing ceased immediately, before any change in blood gases or pH, suggesting that a factor from the placenta might be involved. In our laboratory, we were able to induce continuous breathing and wakefulness in fetal sheep by occluding the umbilical cord, as long as we provided a gas exchange area for the fetus via an endotracheal tube (132,136–138). These experiments suggest the origin in the placenta of a compound that inhibits fetal breathing and fetal activity.

In trying to prove the hypothesis that a factor is released by the placenta, we injected the fetal sheep with a placental extract (juice of cotyledons acutely dissected, sliced, and immersed in Krebs solution) after continuous breathing was induced by cord occlusion (Fig. 17-7) (132). In all experiments the placental extract decreased or abolished breathing. The infusion of the placental extract into the fetal circulation also inhibited spontaneous fetal breathing present during low-voltage electrocortical activity without inducing significant changes in blood gas tensions, pH, heart rate, and blood pressure (139). This factor appeared specific to the placenta because the breathing response was absent with extracts from other tissues, such as liver, muscle, or blood. We have demonstrated that this factor in the placental extract is likely a prostaglandin, because treatment of the extract with indomethacin/acetylsalicylic acid (ASA), which significantly reduced the concentration of prostaglandins, eliminated the activity of the extract (Fig. 17-8) (140).

Indirect evidence that placental prostaglandins, especially PGE_2, are the mediators responsible for the inhibition of

breathing in fetal life has been provided by Kitterman and associates (141) and Wallen and associates (142) who showed that infusion of PGE_2 into the circulation of the fetal sheep induced a prompt and complete cessation of breathing movements. In addition, the incidence of fetal breathing movements was inversely correlated with both the PGE_2 dose and the mean PGE_2 concentration. Conversely, intravenous infusion of prostaglandin synthetase inhibitors, such as indomethacin or meclofenamate, induces continuous breathing for many hours in the fetus (141,143,144). Thus, the rate of placental prostaglandin production, plays a significant role in setting the level of fetal breathing activity by producing a sleep-related inhibition in the fetal brainstem.

It is unlikely, however, that prostaglandins are involved in the inhibition of fetal breathing observed during hypoxia, because this inhibition persists after the administration of prostaglandin inhibitors. Several studies show that adenosine is the likely mediator of the respiratory depression observed during hypoxia because intravascular administration of adenosine inhibits fetal breathing and eye movements (145) and the infusion of adenosine receptor antagonists blunts this inhibition (145,146). Also, brain disruptions that eliminate hypoxic inhibition of breathing also abolish the depressant effects of adenosine (147). Koos and associates (148) have shown that hypoxia inhibits fetal breathing through activation of central adenosine receptors, specially the A(2A) subtype.

Mechanics of the First Postnatal Breaths

Although the neural and chemical control mechanisms responsible for establishment of continuous breathing at birth are not completely understood, the mechanical processes responsible for inflating the lungs at birth are in some detail accepted.

It is well known that a sufficient force (opening pressure) must be generated across the lungs with the first inspiration to overcome the viscosity of the fluid in the

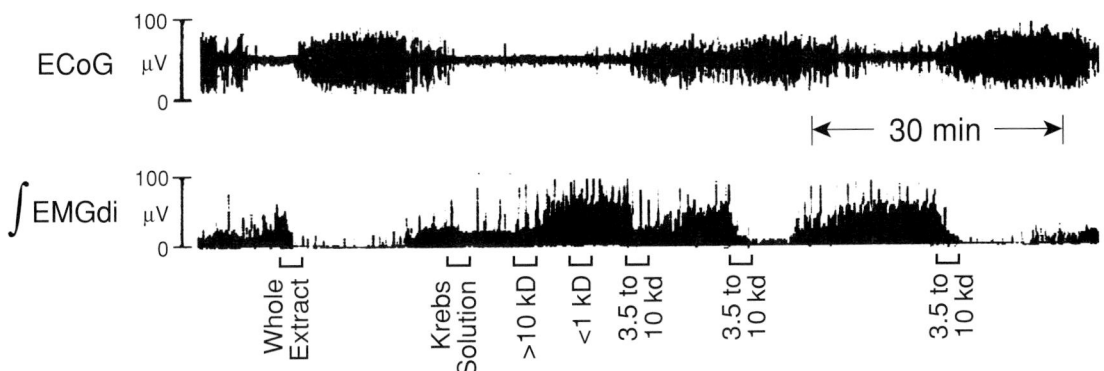

Figure 17-7 Representative tracing showing the effects of different placental infusates on fetal breathing and ECoG. The whole placental extract and the subfraction 3–5 to 10 kDa decreased or abolished breathing in all cases, and when given in low-voltage ECoG, this was associated with a switch to high voltage. No significant effects were seen with infusates having molecular mass greater than 10 kDa or less than 1 kDa. ECoG, electrocochleography; EMGdi, electromyogram of the diaphragm. (From Rigatto H. Regulation of fetal breathing. *Reprod Fertil Dev* 1996;8:23–33, with permission.)

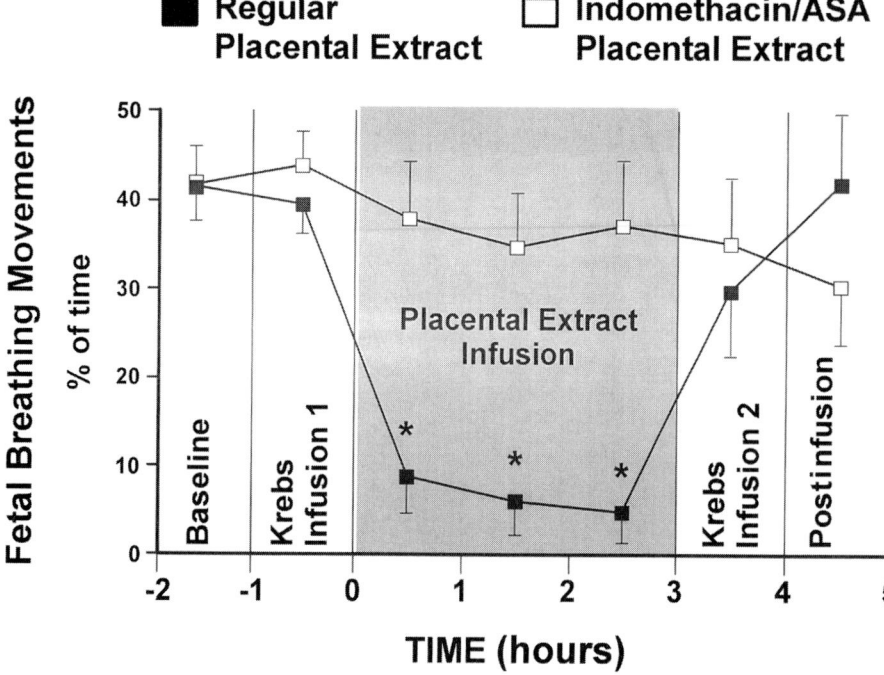

Figure 17-8 Incidence of fetal breathing movements during the infusion of placental extracts. The regular placental extracts (■) induced a profound inhibition of fetal breathing that progressively recovered upon discontinuation of the infusions. This effect disappeared when the extracts were treated with indomethacin/acetylsalicylic acid (ASA) (□). Values are mean ± standard error (SE). * p. <0.05.

airways, as well as the forces of surface tension and tissue resistance (149). As we described in the subsection "Clearance of Fluid at Birth" in preparation for lung ventilation at birth, the volume of pulmonary fluid in the fetus decreases during late gestation, especially during initiation of labor, as a result of reduction in the rate of secretion and an increase in reabsorption of fluid in response to catecholamines. Pfister and associates (28) found large negative intrapulmonary pressure in fetal sheep during labor, which implied that the lung volume was less than functional residual capacity. The findings of a negative intrapulmonary pressure near the end of labor may in part explain reports that the first inspiration in human infants does not require diaphragmatic contraction. The elastic recoil of the chest wall after delivery would tend to rebound to the resting position causing a small passive inspiration of air.

Although most of the lung fluid is reabsorbed during labor and delivery, a small but significant amount of fluid is still present in the lungs at the time the newborn infant is ready to take the first postnatal breath. A pressure of about 60 cm H_2O is required to make this fluid flow through the airways with the first inspiration (150). However, a much higher opening pressure would be needed to overcome the high surface tension forces if the airways were not partially distended with this fluid (Fig. 17-9) (151). According to the Laplace equation for a cylinder state, the pressure required to overcome surface tension is directly proportional to the surface tension and indirectly proportional to the radius of curvature (P = t/r). If the airways were not partially distended by liquid, the opening pressure in the terminal airway would be very large because of the small radius of curvature. Thus, the normal fluid content of the lung at birth facilitates the first breath by lowering the opening pressure, and ensuring a more homogeneous filling of the lung with air. A significant reduction in the volume of fetal pul-

monary fluid, as seen sometimes in postterm deliveries, may not be beneficial at birth. First, greater pressures would be required to inflate the air sacs in fluid-free lungs, and second, the distribution of inspired air during the first breath may not be as uniform. Faridy (151) showed that the highest opening pressure is seen in fluid-free lungs and the lowest in lungs containing fluid of approximately 25% of maximum lung volume.

The opening pressure of the lungs at birth also depends on the compliance of the alveolar tissue and the surface forces at air–fluid interface. During labor and birth, a massive release of surfactant in pulmonary fluid facilitates lung opening by lowering the opening pressure through the decrease in surface forces and the improvement of lung compliance (151–154). Thus, as seen in Fig. 17-10, the first postnatal breath (I) begins with no air volume in the lungs

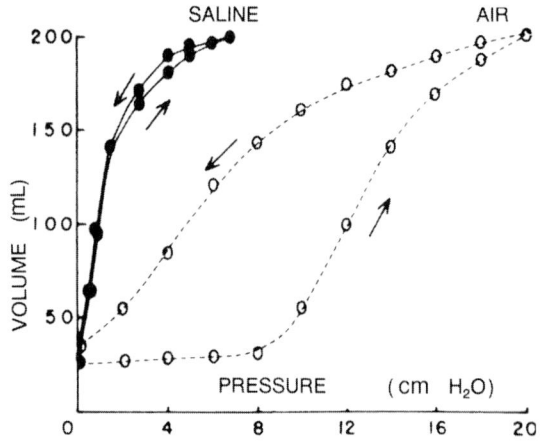

Figure 17-9 Pressure–volume curves after air versus liquid expansion of the lung. (From Radford EP. In: Remington JW, ed. *Tissue elasticity*. Washington, DC: American Physiological Society, 1957, with permission.)

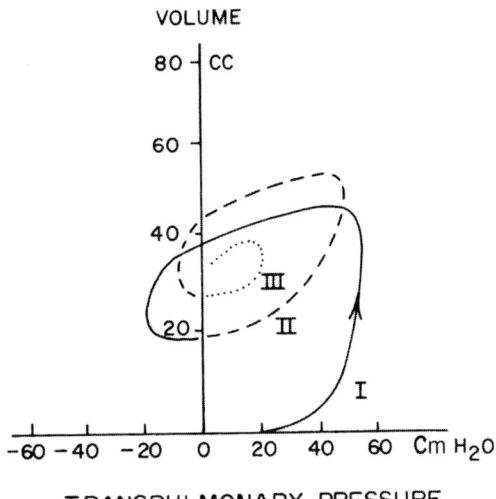

VOLUME

TRANSPULMONARY PRESSURE

Figure 17-10 Pressure–volume curves of the first three extrauterine breaths. (From Smith CA, Nelson NM. *Physiology of the newborn infant*, 4th ed. Springfield, IL: Charles C. Thomas, 1976:125, with permission.)

and no transpulmonary pressure gradient. As the chest wall expands, the transpulmonary pressure increases until it overcomes the surface tension of small airways and alveoli. At this point, actively inspired air begins to enter the lungs and, according to the Laplace equation, as the radius increases, the distending pressure required to open up those units decreases.

Although the first inspiratory effort is extremely important for lung opening, the creation of functional residual capacity (FRC) at the end of the first expiratory effort is essential for the normal pulmonary adaptation at birth. It is obvious that if all the air that entered the lung were to leave the lung, every breath would necessarily resemble the first breath (155). This FRC can only be created if the pulmonary surfactant is present allowing for the stabilization of the peripheral air spaces. The near-zero surface tension and the bubble formation produced by surfactant allows for retention of large volumes of air at the end of the first expiration. When surfactant is deficient, the consequences are a tendency to airlessness with each expiration and the application of high inspiratory pressures to maintain respiration. This leads to the marked retractions so commonly associated with atelectasis and hyaline membrane disease (HMD) as seen in preterm infants with surfactant deficiency.

Mortola and associates (156) showed that in healthy term infants born by cesarean section, the amount of air exhaled after the first breath was less than the inhaled volume representing the formation of the FRC. This FRC continued to rise after the first breath in a very irregular fashion from a mean of about 10 mL/kg at birth to 30 mL/kg by the second day of life (157). The first breaths are actively exhaled by the high negative transpulmonary pressures (see Fig. 17-10). These expiratory breaths are also associated with interruptions in the expiratory flow ("braking of the expiration"), likely as a result of closure in the

pharyngeal/laryngeal region, as indicated by the radiographic studies of Bosma and associates (158). The resulting positive pressure in the airway generated by this respiratory pattern would not only facilitate liquid absorption, but it would also improve air retention at the end of expiration, as well as increase lung compliance. Boon and associates (159) showed that the formation of FRC in asphyxiated neonates born by cesarean section was associated with a stepwise increase in tidal volume presumably indicating that the physical characteristics of the lungs had changed sufficiently to allow the lungs to remain inflated. Although vaginally delivered infants have not been extensively studied, it is likely that they require similar pressures for the first inflation as cesarean-delivered infants. In both vaginal- and cesarean-delivered infants, the major sources of resistance to inflation (surface forces caused by air–liquid interface and the frictional forces caused by the movement of the column of liquid in the airway) may be very similar and yield comparable inspiratory volume and FRC of the first breath (156).

CIRCULATORY ADAPTATION

Fetal Circulation

A combination of preferential flow and streaming through structural shunts in the liver (ductus venosus) and heart (foramen ovale and ductus arteriosus), allows the highest oxygen content blood coming from the placenta to be delivered to the heart, brain, and upper torso (Fig. 17-11). This relative parallel flow contrasts with the flow in series and without shunts of the adult circulation. Thus, the volume of blood in the fetal heart ventricles is not equal. In fact, the right ventricle ejects approximately two-thirds of total fetal cardiac output (300 mL/kg per minute), whereas the left ventricle ejects only a little more than one third (150 mL/kg per minute) (160).

Placenta blood is delivered to the fetus through the umbilical vein. Approximately 50% of this umbilical blood flow passes through the ductus venosus directly into the inferior vena cava and mixes with the systemic venous drainage from the lower body. The other 50% of the umbilical blood flow joins the hepatic portal venous system and passes through the hepatic vasculature (161). Preferential streaming allows the well-oxygenated blood derived from the ductus venosus to travel through the dorsal and leftward wall of the inferior vena cava (162). A tissue flap called the *eustachian valve*, located at the junction of the inferior vena cava and right atrium, serves to direct the highly oxygenated blood from the ductus venosus across the foramen ovale into the left atrium and then the left ventricle and ascending aorta (162–164). The less-oxygenated anterior stream (mainly blood from the lower body and the hepatic circulation) joins the oxygen-poor blood from the superior vena cava (which drains the head and upper body) and the coronary sinus (which delivers venous return from the myocardium) at the right atrium,

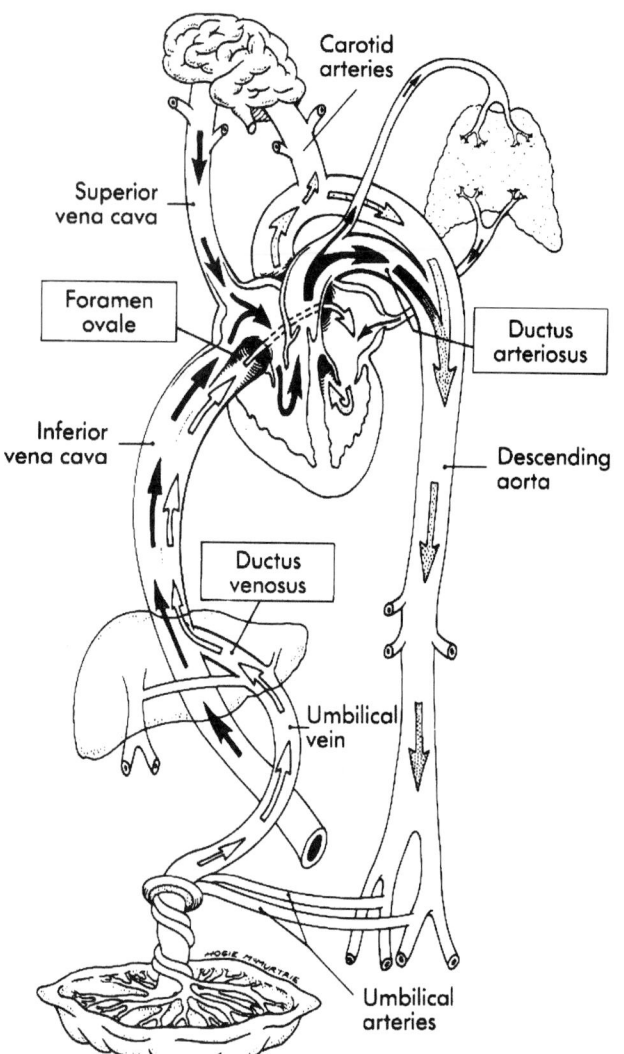

Figure 17-11   Fetal blood circulation. (From Bloom RS. Delivery room resuscitation of the newborn. In: Fanaroff AA, Martin RJ, eds. *Neonatal and perinatal medicine: diseases of the fetus and infant,* 5th ed. St. Louis: Mosby-Yearbook, 1992:302, with permission.)

directing the blood through the tricuspid valve into the right ventricle (Fig. 17-11).

Because the placenta is responsible for gas exchange *in utero,* very little blood flow is sent to the lungs. The pulmonary circulation is a high-resistance, low-flow circuit that receives less than 10% of the ventricular output. Instead of entering the pulmonary arteries, most of the right ventricular blood is diverted away from the lungs through the widely patent ductus arteriosus to the descending aorta, reaching the placenta for oxygenation through the umbilical arteries.

The well-oxygenated blood coming across the foramen ovale joins the small amount of blood returning from the lungs via the pulmonary veins in the left atrium and traverses the mitral valve into the left ventricle. This blood is then ejected across the aortic valve into the ascending aorta bringing well-oxygenated blood to the myocardium, brain, head, and upper torso (see Fig. 17-11).

Regulation of Fetal Pulmonary Vascular Resistance

There is a close association between pulmonary arterial development and airway development. As gestation progresses, synchronization of airway and vessel branching occurs, suggesting they may be regulated by common mediators or exchange messenger molecules (165,166). The embryonic endothelial channels later acquire a smooth-muscle layer and thus the ability to regulate vascular tone and blood flow.

During early gestation, pulmonary blood flow is limited by the paucity of pulmonary vessels. However, although the number of small blood vessels per unit of lung volume increases tenfold during the last trimester, pulmonary blood flow remains low because of a high pulmonary vascular resistance (Fig. 17-12). In addition to the mechanical compression of pulmonary vessels by the fluid-filled, atelectatic lungs and the lack of rhythmic distention, this high-resistance low-flow state is probably maintained in part by vasoconstriction because the fetal pulmonary vascular bed responds readily to vasodilators.

Sympathetic tone does not appear to be responsible for the high pulmonary vascular resistance of the fetus,

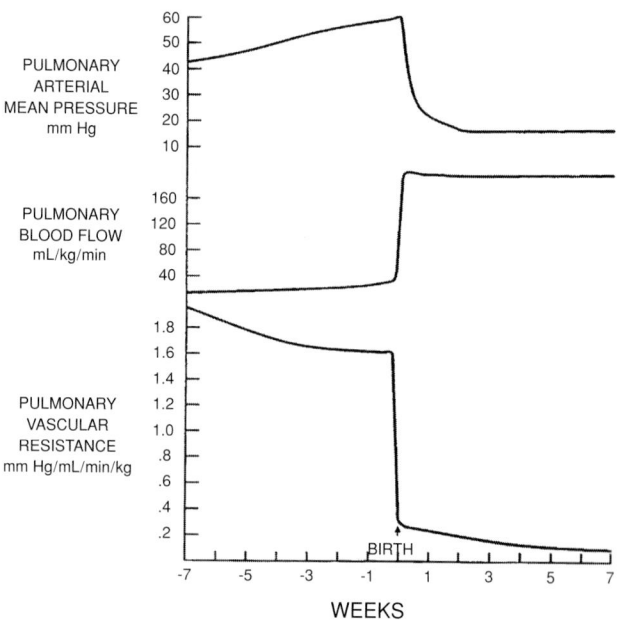

Figure 17-12   Representative changes in the pulmonary hemodynamics during transition from the late-term fetal circulation to the neonatal circulation. P pulmonary vascular resistance (PVR) decreases progressively during later gestation as a consequence of lung growth and increased cross-sectional area for flow. PVR decreases dramatically at birth as a consequence of the vasodilating effect of lung aeration. PVR continues to fall more gradually over the first 6 to 8 weeks of life. Pulmonary blood flow remains at relatively low levels during fetal growth, then increases abruptly with lung expansion and the rapid fall in PVR. Mean pulmonary artery pressure falls rapidly immediately after birth because the pulmonary vasodilation causes PVR to fall more than pulmonary blood flow increases. (Adapted from Rudolph AM. Fetal circulation and cardiovascular adjustment after birth. In: Rudolph AM, Hoffman JIE, Rudolph CD, eds. *Rudolph's pediatrics,* 19th ed. Norwalk, CT: Appleton & Lange, 1991:1309–1313, with permission.)

because neither sympathectomy nor α-adrenergic blockade decreases the resistance (167–169). Although arachidonic acid and its cyclooxygenase products, prostaglandin $F_{2\alpha}$ and thromboxane A_2 are vasoconstrictors in the fetal and newborn lung, their blockade does not decrease vascular resistance (170–172).

The discovery that the effects of some vasodilators agents, such as acetylcholine, bradykinin, and histamine, were dependent on release of an endothelium-derived relaxing factor (EDRF), later shown to be nitric oxide (NO) (173,174), led to the exploration of its possible role in the perinatal decrease in pulmonary vascular resistance. Nitric oxide, an inorganic, gaseous free radical discovered in the late 1980s, is produced by the endothelial cells from the terminal nitrogen of L-arginine by nitric oxide synthase (NOS). NOS can be stimulated by pharmacologic agents such as acetylcholine or bradykinin, and by birth, shear stress, and oxygen. Nitric oxide activates soluble guanylate cyclase, which produces smooth-muscle relaxation by activation of protein kinase C (Fig. 17-13) (175). Hydrolysis of cyclic guanosine monophosphate (cGMP) is accomplished by phosphodiesterases that control the intensity and duration of cGMP signal transduction (176). In fetal

life, NO production is also stimulated by activation of adenosine triphosphate (ATP)-dependent K^+ channels. A maturational increase in NO-mediated relaxation has been documented during the late fetal and early postnatal period, which parallels the dramatic fall in pulmonary vascular resistance at birth (177–181). In fetal lambs, inhibiting NO synthesis increases resting pulmonary vascular resistance and inhibits the ventilation-induced fall in pulmonary vascular resistance. Increased oxygen tension increases both basal and stimulated NO release and inhibition of NO blocks virtually the entire increase in fetal pulmonary blood flow caused by hyperbaric oxygenation without ventilation (182–184). Shear stress resulting from increased pulmonary blood flow and rhythmic distention of the lung without changing oxygen tension also induces endothelial NOS gene expression and contributes to pulmonary vasodilatation at birth (185,186).

Endothelin-1 (ET-1), a 21-amino acid peptide also produced by vascular endothelial cells, has potent vasoactive activities (187). Although ET-1 appears to play an important and active role in mediating pulmonary vascular resistance, *in vivo* studies indicate that the effects of exogenous endothelin are complex and depend on the site, develop-

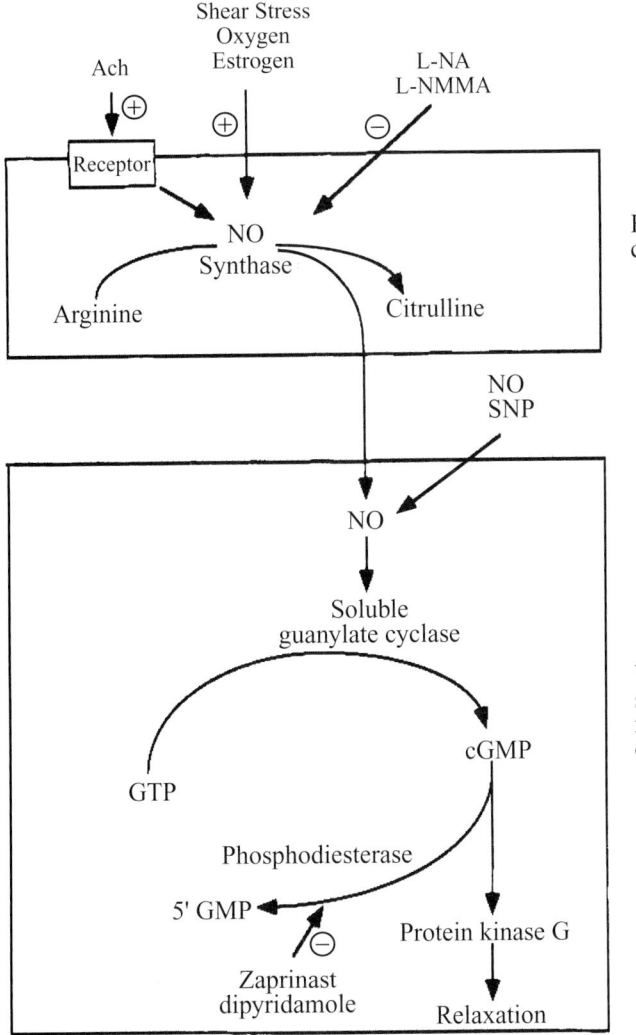

Figure 17-13 The proposed mechanism of synthesis and action of nitric oxide. Nitric oxide (NO) is produced in the endothelium from the terminal guanido nitrogen of L-arginine by NO synthase. NO synthase can be stimulated by pharmacologic agents such as acetylcholine (Ach) or bradykinin, and by birth, shear stress, and oxygen. Endothelial production of NO can be blocked by arginine analogues that have modifications of the guanido nitrogen of the molecule. Nitric oxide activates soluble guanylate cyclase, increases cyclic guanosine monophosphate (cGMP) concentrations in vascular smooth muscle, and initiates the cascade resulting in smooth-muscle relaxation. The magnitude and duration of the effect of cGMP is controlled by its inactivation by specific phosphodiesterases. GMP, guanosine monophosphate; GTP, guanosine triphosphate; L-NA, nitro-L-arginine; L-NMMA, N^G-mono-methyl-L-arginine. (From Lakshminrusimha S, Steinhorn R. Pulmonary vascular biology during neonatal transition. *Clin Perinatol* 1999;26(3):601–619, with permission.)

mental age, and tone of the vascular bed (188–190). Consequently, exogenous ET-1 predominantly vasodilates the fetal and newborn pulmonary circulations by acting on the ET_B receptors located on the endothelial cells but causes vasoconstriction in the adult pulmonary circulation by acting on the ET_A receptors located in the smooth muscle cells (191,192). Increasing data also suggest that endogenous NO and ET-1 participate in the regulation of each other through an autocrine feedback loop. Thus, ET-1 stimulates the release of NO, and NO inhibits the ET-1 system (193,194).

The low oxygen tension in fetal life is a physiologic stimulus for the pulmonary vasculature to be constricted. This hypoxic pulmonary vasoconstriction develops over the period of gestation when the cross-sectional area of the vascular bed is increasing rapidly. Decreasing oxygen tension in the fetus at 103 days of gestation does not increase pulmonary vascular resistance, but in the 132- to 138-day fetus it doubles the resistance. Conversely, increasing oxygen tension before 100 days of gestation does not decrease pulmonary vascular resistance, but by 135 days it decreases resistance markedly and increases pulmonary blood flow to normal newborn levels. Its mechanism of action may be in part through regulation of activity and gene expression of voltage-gated K^+ channels (195), nitric oxide synthase and/or endothelin (196,197).

Unlike the mature pulmonary circulation, the fetal pulmonary vasculature appears to regulate flow through a myogenic response. The fetal pulmonary vasculature exhibits a time-limited vasodilation in response to dilating stimuli, including shear stress, oxygen, and many pharmacologic vasodilators, with return to the constricted resting state despite continued exposure to the vasodilating stimulus. This unique mechanism limits pulmonary blood flow and preserves placental perfusion and gas exchange.

Transition to Extrauterine Circulation

At birth, a number of complex events must take place so that the fetal circulation that depends on the placenta for gas exchange and intracardiac and extracardiac shunts to deliver oxygenated blood to the heart and brain, switches to the neonatal circulation in which the gas exchange is transferred to the lungs and the fetal shunts are eliminated. A rapid and sustained decrease in pulmonary vascular resistance during the first breaths facilitate this adaptation. Although this normal pulmonary vascular transition occurs spontaneously and quickly in most neonates, failure of the pulmonary circulation to undergo this changes results in persistent pulmonary hypertension of the newborn (PPHN). This condition, which carries significant morbidity and mortality, develops when the pulmonary vascular resistance fails to decrease adequately during the transition to extrauterine life. Altered intrauterine environment producing structural changes in the pulmonary circulation or hypoxemia, acidosis and/or hypercarbia secondary to meconium aspiration, surfactant deficiency, or pneumonia at birth abnormally constricts the transitional pulmonary circulation. In this condition, right-to-left shunts at the atrial and ductus arteriosus

levels continue secondary to the high pulmonary vascular resistance, producing significant hypoxemia, which, in turn, causes an increase in pulmonary vasoconstriction. Thus, two major hemodynamic events must occur at delivery to allow for a normal transition from fetal to neonatal circulation.

Pulmonary Vasodilatation

At birth, pulmonary arterial blood flow increases eight- to tenfold and pulmonary vascular resistance (PVR) decreases by 50% within the first 24 hours, as the lung assumes the function of gas exchange (Fig. 17-14) (198–202). This decrease in PVR is brought about by active vasodilation which is regulated by a complex and incompletely understood interaction among metabolic, hormonal, and mechanical factors, triggered by a number of birth-related stimuli. Three main factors contribute to the increase in pulmonary blood flow during this transition: (a) ventilation of the lungs, (b) increased oxygenation, and (c) hemodynamic forces such as increased shear stress. The effects of these factors on pulmonary circulation at birth appears to be mediated primarily by the release of NO from the vascular endothelium which results in smooth muscle relaxation via activation of the intracellular cGMP-dependent protein kinase (203). The initial partial increase in pulmonary vasodilation may be independent of oxygenation and may be caused by physical expansion of the lungs and the production of prostaglandins (204). The next component is maximal pulmonary vasodilation associated with oxygenation, which may be mainly caused by NO synthesis. The increased shear forces related to the rise in pulmonary blood flow may stimulate endothelial cells to produce NO, which helps maintain pulmonary vasodilation (Fig. 17-14).

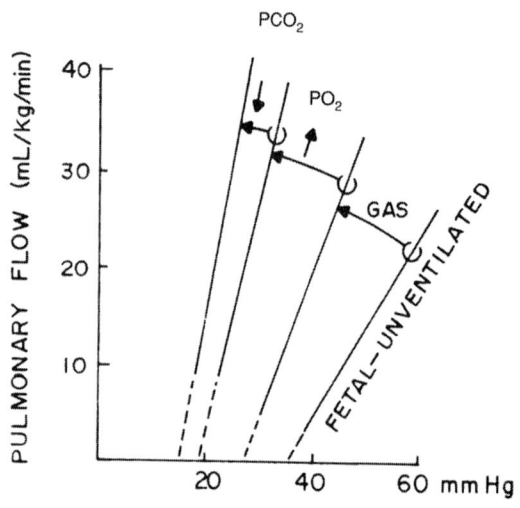

Figure 17-14 Pulmonary vascular conductance increases with the onset of ventilation. Separate curves depict the contributions of gaseous inflation, increased PO_2, and decreased PCO_2. (Adapted from Strang LB. The lungs at birth. *Arch Dis Child* 1965;40:575, with permission.)

Ventilation of the Lungs

It has long been known that the initiation of rhythmic breathing causes vasodilation, even in the absence of increase in oxygen tension (see Fig. 17-14) (8,199). However, physical expansion of the lungs alone produces only partial increase in pulmonary blood flow and a decrease in PVR. A small proportion of this relates to the mechanical distention of the lungs and the establishment of an air–liquid interface, as alveolar fluid is replaced by gas, which increases vessel radius by exerting a negative dilating pressure on the small pulmonary arteries and veins (205,206). Ventilation of the lung also releases vasoactive substances such as prostacyclin (PGI_2) from vessel walls, which increases pulmonary blood flow and decreases PVR (207). Cyclooxygenase inhibition, which blocks PGI_2 production, prevents the normal decrease in PVR with lung expansion, but not the changes that occur with oxygenation (207–210). Other prostaglandins, such as PGD_2 and histamine released by the mast cells during lung expansion, may also contribute to the initial postnatal pulmonary vasodilation (211). NOS and K_{ca} channel inhibition also blunt ventilation-induced pulmonary vasodilatation (212,213).

Increased Oxygenation

Oxygen is a potent stimulus for pulmonary vasodilation. Even in the absence of ventilation, increased oxygen tension reduces PVR. Ventilation plus increased oxygen tension produces complete pulmonary vasodilation and both are particularly crucial in the normal transition to postnatal circulation and pulmonary gas exchange (see Fig. 17-14) (199). Although the mechanisms of oxygen-induced pulmonary vasodilation are not completely understood, several factors appear to contribute to this response. It is known that K^+ channels are the major regulators of resting membrane potential in pulmonary arterial smooth muscle cells and that hypoxia decreases K^+ current by repressing K^+ channel gene expression (214,215). Gosche and associates (216) have found that $K_{voltage}$ but not K_{ca} or K_{ATP} channel activation contributes to the oxygen-induced vasodilation in isolated third-generation pulmonary arterioles from term fetal rats. Whether K^+ channels function as sensors of, or effectors for, oxygen-induced changes in pulmonary vascular tone is unknown. Thus, changes in K^+ channel activity may occur via a direct effect of oxygen tension on the K^+ channel (217) or, alternatively, K^+ channels may open in response to changes in the concentration of a second messenger substance like NO (218,219). Many studies show that the effect of oxygen on perinatal pulmonary circulation appears to be mediated primarily by the effects of NO on K^+ channels in arterial smooth muscle cells either directly or through a cGMP-sensitive kinase (220–223). Endothelium-derived nitric oxide modulates pulmonary vascular tone under basal conditions in the fetus and during transition of the pulmonary circulation at birth. Several studies show that the *in utero* increase in pulmonary blood flow observed in response to either ventilation with oxygen or maternal hyperbaric oxygen exposure can be markedly attenuated with inhibition of NO synthe-

sis (219). It has also been shown that the maturational rise in NO production seen from late gestation to 4 weeks postnatally is modulated by oxygen. Thus, the sudden increase in oxygen tension that occurs at birth appears to enhance NO synthesis and NOS inhibition blunts the oxygen-induced decrease in PVR. Although it is assumed that oxygen may act directly on endothelial cells to increase NO production, it is possible that it stimulates release of another agent, such as bradykinin, calcitonin gene-related peptide, or adrenomedullin, which, in turn, stimulates NO production (224,225).

Oxygen could also increase plasma and red blood cell ATP, which releases NO from endothelial cells and is a potent fetal pulmonary vasodilator (226). It is known that the release of NO from cultured human vascular endothelial cells is stimulated by ATP and that the inhibition of NOS by N-nitro-L-arginine attenuates the vasodilation caused by ATP and its metabolites in the fetal circulation. Konduri and associates (227) suggested that an increase in oxidative phosphorylation and a release of ATP can also mediate the endothelium-dependent pulmonary vasodilation that occurs in response to oxygen exposure.

Other studies show that NO release and pulmonary vasorelaxation can also be mediated by endothelial α_2-adrenoreceptors activation (228–230). Magnenant and associates suggested that α_2-adrenoreceptors are involved in the control of basal pulmonary vascular tone and in the pulmonary vasodilator effect of norepinephrine during fetal life through activation of the NO-dependent pulmonary vasodilation (231).

Recent studies also support the hypothesis that hypoxia causes ET_A-mediated inhibition of a K^+ channels, which leads to vessel depolarization and calcium influx, resulting in vasoconstriction (232–235). Goirand and associates (236) showed that ET_A receptor blockade opposes hypoxic pulmonary vasoconstriction in the rat isolated perfused lung through the suppression of the inhibition of K^+ channels by endogenous ET-1. Thus, the increase in oxygen, together with the perinatal decrease in ET_A receptor message, probably contributes also to decreased hypoxic pulmonary vasoconstriction observed at birth.

Increased Shear Stress

Partial or complete compression of the ductus arteriosus *in utero* increases pulmonary blood flow and causes a progressive fall in pulmonary vascular resistance in response to flow- or shear stress-induced pulmonary vasodilation (237,238). The initial increase in pulmonary blood flow that occurs with lung expansion and oxygenation at birth raises shear stress in the pulmonary vascular endothelium, causing further pulmonary vasodilation (239). This blood flow-dependent pulmonary vasodilation is mainly caused by nitric oxide, which is produced by an increase in shear stress of vascular endothelium (240–242). The released of NO from arterial and venous endothelial cells contributes to the maintenance of the physiologically low basal pulmonary vascular tone. Stepwise elevations in flow increased exhaled NO and nonselective inhibition of NOS completely blocks the shear stress-induced pulmonary vasodilation (240,242). This NO shear stress-induced vasodilation is mediated by activation of both voltage- and Ca^{2+}-dependent K^+ channels (241–244). Ralevic and associates (245) showed that vascular endothelial cells also release ATP when they are exposed to shear stress. Inhibition of receptors for ATP attenuates the pulmonary vasodilation that occurs in response to stepwise increases in flow (246).

Loss of the Placental Circulation and Closure of the Fetal Shunts

At birth, the umbilical circulation is abolished as the vascular smooth muscle of the umbilical cord go into spasm in response to the abrupt longitudinal stretching and the increased oxygenation (247). The removal of the low-resistance bed of the placenta produces much of the increase in systemic vascular resistance at birth. Without umbilical venous flow, the ductus venosus receives little blood flow and a passive, as well as active, constriction begins. Complete closure of the ductus venosus usually occurs by the end of the first week of life. The reasons for closure of the foramen ovale after birth are twofold. First, the occlusion of the umbilical cord decreases the volume of blood flowing up the inferior vena cava decreasing the right–left atrial pressure difference. Second, the increase in pulmonary venous return to the left atrium in response to the marked increase in pulmonary blood flow increases left atrial pressure. The reverse pressure difference across the foramen ovale pushes the foramen ovale flap against the atrial septum, closing the shunt. The foramen ovale remains patent, with no flow through it for weeks or months. The closure of the third fetal shunt, the ductus arteriosus, depends predominantly on the net balance between vasodilators, mainly oxygen, prostaglandins, and other vasoactive substances (248,249). Increased oxygen tension is known to be a potent stimulant of ductal smooth muscle constriction after birth (249). Prostaglandins, mainly PGE_2, are major mediators of ductal relaxation pre- and postnatally. The rapid fall in circulating prostaglandins at birth, caused by increased lung metabolism (from increased pulmonary blood flow) and the loss of placental prostaglandins, facilitates the constrictive effects of oxygen on the ductal tissue. Although functional closure of the ductus arteriosus occurs in the first 72 hours of life (250), permanent or anatomical closure takes several days and weeks and is achieved by endothelial destruction, subintimal proliferation, and connective-tissue formation (251). When the ductus arteriosus fails to close or reopens in the first days of life, as is frequently observed in small preterm infants, a significant left-to-right shunt may occur. The incidence of reopening is inversely related to birth weight. The closure of the patent ductus arteriosus effectively separates the pulmonary and systemic circulations and establishes the normal postnatal circulatory pattern.

CONCLUSION

The transition from fetal to neonatal life represents one of the most dynamic and difficult periods in human life cycle. Dramatic neurohormonal, metabolic, and cardiorespiratory adjustments must occur over hours to days around the time of delivery to insure the smooth and successful transition to extrauterine life. These changes are invoked by a variety of processes, including perinatal surges in hormones, labor, delivery, gaseous ventilation and oxygenation of the lungs, cord occlusion, and decrease in environmental temperature. Intensive research over the last century has significantly improved our understanding of the normal development of the cardiorespiratory system that allows the fetus to rapidly and efficiently adapt to air breathing at birth. This transitional period is characterized by removal of the lung liquid volume from the alveolar spaces and by the secretion of surfactant material into the acinus for satisfactory physical expansion of the lungs after the initial postnatal breaths. To maintain adequate ventilation and oxygenation the newborn infant must also switch from intermittent fetal breathing to continuous breathing at birth, a process that it is still not completely understood. The switch from placental to pulmonary gas exchange also requires the elimination of the fetal shunts and a rapid and sustained decrease in pulmonary vascular resistance to allow a significant increase in pulmonary blood flow. Thus, the circulation changes from one characterized by a relatively low combined ventricular output, right ventricular dominance, and pulmonary vasoconstriction, to a circulation in series with a high cardiac output equally divided between the two ventricles, and a greatly dilated pulmonary vascular bed. Many factors can disrupt this physiologic process causing significant morbidity and mortality.

REFERENCES

1. Harvey W. *Exercitatio anatomica de motu cordis et sanguinis in animalibus*. London: 1628. Surrey, England, 1847. Barnes WR, translator.
2. Scheel P. Comentatio de Liquoris amnii aspiras arteriae foetuum humanorum natura et usu. HFNIAE, 1799:86.
3. Zweifel P. Die Respiration des Fötus. *Arch Gynakol* 1876;9:291.
4. Bichat X. *Anatomie générale, àppliqueé à la physiologie et à la médecine*. Paris: Brosson, Gabon, 1801.
5. Kilian HF. *Ueber den Kreislauf des Blutes im Kinde, welches noch nicht geathmet hat*. Karlsruhe: Muller, 1826.
6. Hamilton WF, Woodbury RA, Woods EB. The relation between systemic and pulmonary blood pressures in the fetus. *Am J Physiol* 1937;119:206–212.
7. Barclay AE, Barcroft J, Barron DH, et al. A radiographic demonstration of the circulation through the heart in the adult and in the foetus, and the identification of the ductus arteriosus. *Br J Radiol* 1939;12:505.
8. Dawes GS, Mott JC, Widdicombe JG, et al. Changes in the lungs of the newborn lamb. *J Physiol* 1953;121:141–162.
9. Rudolph AM. In: Weir IK, Archer SL, Reeves JT, eds. The development of concepts of the ontogeny of the pulmonary circulation. Armonk, NY: Futura Publishing, 1999;3–18.
10. Strang LB. Fetal lung liquid: secretion and reabsorption. *Physiol Rev* 1991;71:991–1016.
11. Preyer W. *Specielle Physiologic des Embryo*. Leipzig: Greeben Verlag (L. Fernau), 1885:149.

12. Potter EL, Bohlender GP. Intrauterine respiration in relation to development of the fetal lung. *Am J Obstet Gynecol* 1941;42:14–22.

13. Jost A, Policard A. Contribution experimental a l'etude du development prenatal du poumon chez le lapin. *Arch Anat Microsc* 1948;37:323–332.

14. Reynolds SRM. A source of amniotic fluid in the lamb nasopharyngeal and buccal cavities. *Nature* 1953;175:307.

15. Dawes GS, Mott JC, Widdicombe JG. The foetal circulation in the lamb. *J Physiol* 1954;126(3):563–587.

16. Adams, FH, Moss AJ, Fagan L. The tracheal fluid in the fetal lamb. *Biol Neonate* 1963;5:151–158.

17. Adamson TM, Boyd RDH, Platt HS, et al. Composition of alveolar liquid in the fetal lamb. *J Physiol* 1969;204:159–168.

18. Olver RE, Schneeberger EE, Walters DV. Epithelial solute permeability, ion transport and tight junction morphology in the developing lung of the fetal lamb. *J Physiol* 1981;315:395–412.

19. Mescher EJ, Platzker ACG, Ballard PL, et al. Ontogeny of tracheal fluid, pulmonary surfactant, and plasma corticoids in the fetal lamb. *J Appl Physiol* 1975;39:1017–1021.

20. Burri PH. Fetal and postnatal development of the lung. *Annu Rev Physiol* 1984;46:617–628.

21. Adamson IYR. Development of lung structure. In: Crystal RG, West JB, Barnes PJ, Cherniack NS, Weibel ER, eds. *The lung: scientific foundations*. New York: Raven Press, 1991:663–670.

22. Humphreys PW, Normand ICS, Reynolds EOR, et al. Pulmonary lymph flow and the uptake of liquid from the lungs of the lamb at the start of breathing. *J Physiol* 1967;193:1–29.

23. Normand ICS, Olver RE, Reynolds OR, et al. Permeability of lung capillaries and alveoli to non-electrolytes in the fetal lamb. *J Physiol* 1971;219:303–330.

24. Harding R, Hooper S. Regulation of lung expansion and lung growth before birth. *J Appl Physiol* 1996;81:809–224.

25. Hooper SB, Harding R. Fetal lung liquid; a major determinant of the growth and functional development of the fetal lung. *Clin Exp Pharmacol Physiol* 1995;22:235–247.

26. Mescher EJ, Platzker ACG, Ballard PL, et al. Ontogeny of tracheal fluid, pulmonary surfactant, and plasma corticoids in the fetal lamb. *J Appl Physiol* 1975;39:1017–1021.

27. Adamson TM, Brodecky V, Lambert TF, et al. Lung liquid production and composition in the 'in utero' foetal lamb. *Aust J Exp Biol Med Sci* 1975;53:65–75.

28. Pfister RE, Ramsden CA, Neil HL, et al. Volume and secretion rate of lung liquid in the final days of gestation and labour in the fetal sheep. *J Physiol* 2001;535;3:889–899.

29. Orzalesi MM, Motoyama EK, Jacobson HN, et al. The development of the lungs of lambs. *Pediatrics* 1965;35:373–381.

30. Walters DV. Fetal lung liquid: secretion and absorption. In: Hanson MA, Spencer JAD, Rodeck CH, Walters D, eds. *Fetus and neonate: physiology and clinical application*, vol. 2: breathing. Cambridge: Cambridge University Press, 1994:43–62.

31. Brown MJ, Olver RE, Ramsden CA, et al. Effects of adrenaline and of spontaneous labour on the secretion and absorption of lung liquid in the fetal lamb. *J Physiol* 1983;344:137–152.

32. Alcorn D, Adamson TM, Lambert TF, et al. Morphological effects of chronic tracheal ligation and drainage in the fetal lamb lung. *J Anat* 1977;123:649–660.

33. Fewell JE, Johnson P. Upper airway dynamics during breathing and during apnea in fetal lambs. *J Physiol* 1983;339:495–504.

34. Nardo I, Hopper SB, Harding R. Lung hypoplasia can be reversed by short-term obstruction of the trachea in fetal sheep. *Pediatr Res* 1995;38:690–696.

35. Scurry JP, Adamson TM, Cussen LJ. Fetal lung growth in laryngeal atresia and tracheal agenesis. *Aust Paediatr J* 1989;25:47–51.

36. Souza P, O'Brodovich H, Post M. Lung fluid restriction affects growth, but not airway branching of embryonic rat lung. *Int J Dev Biol* 1995;39:629–637.

37. Crombleholme TM, Albanese CT. The fetus with airway obstruction. In: Harrison MR, Evans MI, Adzick NS, et al., eds. *The unborn patient: the art and science of fetal therapy*, 3rd ed. Philadelphia: WB Saunders, 2001:357–371.

38. Lim F, Crombleholme M, Hedrick HL, et al. Congenital high airway obstruction syndrome: natural history and management. *J Pediatr Surg* 2003;38:940–945.

39. Matalon S. Mechanisms and regulation of ion transport in adult mammalian alveolar type II pneumocytes. *Am J Physiol* 1991;261:C727–C738.

40. Saumon G, Basset G. Electrolyte and fluid transport across the mature alveolar epithelium. *J Appl Physiol* 1993;74:1–15.

41. Olver RE, Strang LB. Ion fluxes across the pulmonary epithelium and the secretion of the lung liquor in the fetal lamb. *J Physiol* 1974;241:327–357.

42. Frizzell RA, Field M, Schultz SG. Sodium-coupled chloride transport by epithelial tissues. *Am J Physiol* 1979;236:FI–F8.

43. Bland RD, Nielson DW. Developmental changes in lung epithelial ion transport and liquid movement. *Annu Rev Physiol* 1992;54:373–394.

44. O'Brodovich HM. Immature epithelial Na$^+$ channel expression is one of the pathogenetic mechanisms leading to human neonatal respiratory distress syndrome. *Proc Assoc Am Physicians* 1996;108:345–355.

45. Adams FH, Yanagisawa M, Kuzela D, et al. The disappearance of fetal lung fluid following birth. *J Pediatr* 1971;78:837–843.

46. O'Brodovich HM, Hannam V. Exogenous surfactant rapidly increases PaO$_2$ in mature rabbits with lungs that contain large amounts of saline. *Am Rev Respir Dis* 1993;147:1087–1090.

47. Egan EA, Dillon WP, Zorn S. Fetal lung liquid absorption and alveolar epithelial solute permeability in surfactant deficient, breathing fetal lambs. *Pediatr Res* 1984;18:566–570.

48. Barker PM, Gowen CW, Lawson EE, Knowles MR. Decreased sodium ion absorption across nasal epithelium of very premature infants with respiratory distress syndrome. *J Pediatr* 1997;130:373–377.

49. Aherne W, Dawkins MJR. The removal of fluid from the pulmonary airways after birth in the rabbit, and the effect on this of prematurity and pre-natal hypoxia. *Biol Neonate* 1964;7:214.

50. Bland RD, Carlton DP, Scheerer RG, et al. Lung fluid balance in lambs before and after premature birth. *J Clin Invest* 1989;84;568–576.

51. Bland RD, McMillan DD, Bressack MA, et al. Clearance of liquid from lungs of newborn rabbits. *J Appl Physiol* 1980;49:171–177.

52. Sundell HW, Brighman KL, Harris TR, et al. Lung water and vascular permeability-surface area in newborn lambs delivered by cesarean section compared with the 3–5 day old lamb and adult sheep. *J Dev Physiol* 1980;2:191–204.

53. Sundell HW, Harris TR, Cannon JR, et al. Lung water and vascular permeability-surface area in premature newborn lambs with hyaline membrane disease. *Circ Res* 1987;60:923–932.

54. Jain L. Alveolar fluid clearance in developing lungs and its role in neonatal transition. *Clin Perinatol* 1999;26(3):585–599.

55. Olver RE, Ramsden CA, Strang LB, et al. The role of amiloride-blockable sodium transport in adrenaline-induced lung liquor reabsorption in the fetal lamb. *J Physiol* 1986;376:321–340.

56. Walters DV, Ramsden CA, Olver RE. Dibutyryl cAMP induces a gestation-dependent absorption of fetal lung liquid. *J Appl Physiol* 1990;68:2054–2059.

57. Chapman DL, Carlton DP, Cummings JJ, et al. Intrapulmonary terbutaline and aminophylline decrease lung liquid in fetal lambs. *Pediatr Res* 1991;29:357–361.

58. Barker PM, Olver RE. Clearance of lung liquid during the perinatal period. *J Appl Physiol* 2002;93:1542–1548.

59. Berger PJ, Kyriakides MA, Smolich JJ, et al. Massive decline in lung liquid before vaginal delivery at term in the fetal lamb. *Am J Obstet Gynecol* 1998;178:223–227.

60. Lines A, Hopper SB, Harding R. Lung liquid production rates and volumes do not decrease before labour in healthy fetal sheep. *J Appl Physiol* 1997;82:927–932.

61. Crandall ED, Heming TH, Palombo RL, et al. Effect of terbutaline on sodium transport in isolated perfused rat lung. *J Appl Physiol* 1986;60:289–294.

62. Basset G, Crone C, Saumon G. Significance of active ion transport in transalveolar water absorption: a study on isolated rat lung. *J Physiol* 1987;384:311–324.

63. Berthiaume Y, Boraddus VC, Gropper MA, et al. Alveolar liquid and protein clearance from normal dog lungs. *J Appl Physiol* 1988;65:585–593.

64. O'Brodovich H, Hanman V, Seear M, et al. Amiloride impairs lung liquid clearance in newborn guinea pigs. *J Appl Physiol* 1990;68:1758–1762.

65. Smedira N, Gates L, Hastings R, et al. Alveolar and lung liquid clearance in anesthetized rabbits. *J Appl Physiol* 1991;70:1827–1835.

66. Sakuma T, Okaniwa G, Nakada T, et al. Alveolar fluid clearance in the resected human lung. *Am J Respir Crit Care Med* 1994;150:305–310.

67. Yue G, Matalon S. Mechanisms and sequelae of increased alveolar fluid clearance in hyperoxic rats. *Am J Physiol Lung Cell Mol Physiol* 1997;272:L407–L412.

68. O'Brodovich H, Hannam V, Rafii B. Sodium channel but neither Na$^+$-H$^+$ nor Na-glucose symport inhibitors slow neonatal lung water clearance. *Am J Respir Cell Mol Biol* 1991;5:377–384.

69. Sakuma T, Pittet JF, Jayr C, et al. Alveolar liquid and protein clearance in the absence of blood flow or ventilation in sheep. *J Appl Physiol* 1993;74:176–185.

70. Jayr C, Garat C, Meignan M, et al. Alveolar liquid and protein clearance in anesthetized ventilated rats. *J Appl Physiol* 1994;76:2636–2642.

71. Icard P, Saumon G. Alveolar sodium and liquid transport in mice. *Am J Physiol Lung Cell Mol Physiol* 1999;277:L1232–L1238.

72. Matthay MA, Folkesson HG, Clerici C. Lung epithelial fluid transport and the resolution of pulmonary edema. *Physiol Rev* 2002;82:569–600.

73. Walters DV. Fetal lung liquid: secretion and absorption. In: Hanson MA, Spencer JAD, Rodeck CH, et al., eds. *Fetus and neonate: physiology and clinical application.* vol. 2: *breathing.* Cambridge: Cambridge University Press, 1994:43–62.

74. Umenishi F, Carter EP, Yang B, et al. Sharp increase in rat lung water channel expression in the perinatal period. *Am J Respir Cell Mol Biol* 1996;15:673–679.

75. Ruddy MK, Drazen JM, Pitkanen OM, et al. Aquaporin-4 is expressed in rat fetal distal lung epithelial cells (FDLE) where it may function in Na$^+$ mediated water reabsorption during the perinatal period. *Am J Respir Crit Care Med* 1996;153:A2321(abst).

76. Fyfe GK, Kemp PJ, Cragoe EJ Jr, et al. Conductive cation transport in apical membrane vesicles prepared from fetal lung. *Biochim Biophys Acta* 1994;1224:355–364.

77. Matthay MA, Folkesson HG, Verkman AS. Salt and water transport across alveolar and distal airway epithelium in the adult lung. *Am J Physiol Lung Cell Mol Physiol* 1996;270:L487–L503.

78. Ma T, Fukuda N, Song Y, et al. Lung fluid transport in aquaporin-5 knockout mice. *J Clin Invest* 2000;105:93–100.

79. Cott GR. Modulation of bioelectric properties across alveolar type II cells by substratum. *Am J Physiol* 1989;257:C678–C688.

80. Orser BA, Bertlik M, Fedorko L, et al. Cation selective channel in fetal alveolar type II epithelium. *Biochim Biophys Acta* 1991;1094:19–26.

81. Rao AK, Cott GR. Ontogeny of ion transport across fetal pulmonary epithelial cells in monolayer culture. *Am J Physiol* 1991;261:L178–L187.

82. Barker PM, Boucher RC, Yankaskas JR. Bioelectric properties of cultured monolayers from epithelium of distal human fetal lung. *Am J Physiol* 1995;268:1270–1277.

83. Canessa CM, Schild L, Buell G, et al. Amiloride-sensitive epithelial Na$^+$ channel is made of three homologous subunits. *Nature* 1994;367:412–413.

84. Smith DE, Otulakowski G, Yeger H, et al. Epithelial Na(+) channel (ENaC) expression in the developing normal and abnormal human perinatal lung. *Am J Respir Crit Care Med* 2000;161:1322–1231.

85. Gaillard D, Hinnrasky J, Coscoy S, et al. Early expression of β- and γ-subunits of epithelial sodium channel during human airway development. *Am J Physiol Lung Cell Mol Physiol* 2000;278:L177–L184.

86. Hummler E, Barker P, Gatzy J, et al. Early death due to defective neonatal lung liquid clearance in αENaC-deficient mice. *Nat Genet* 1996;12:325–328.

87. Barker PM, Nguyen MS, Gatzy JT, et al. Role of γ-ENaC subunit in lung liquid clearance and electrolyte balance in newborn mice. Insights into perinatal adaptation and pseudohypoaldosteronism. *J Clin Invest* 1998;102:1634–1640.

88. Walters DV, Olver RE. The role of catecholamines in lung liquid absorption at birth. *Pediatr Res* 1978;12:239–242.

89. Niisato N, Ito Y, Marunaka Y. cAMP stimulates Na$^+$ transport in rat fetal pneumocyte: involvement of a PTK- but not a PKA-dependent pathway. *Am J Physiol Lung Cell Mol Physiol* 1999;277:L727–L736.

90. Norlin, Andreas, Folkensson Hans G. Ca^{2+}-dependent stimulation of alveolar fluid clearance in near-term fetal guinea pigs. *Am J Physiol Lung Cell Mol Physiol* 2002;282:L642–L649.

91. Brown MJ, Olver RE, Ramsden CA, et al. Effects of adrenaline and spontaneous labour on the secretion and absorption of lung liquid in the fetal lamb. *J Physiol* 1983;344:137–142.

92. Krochmal-Mokrzan EM, Barker PM, Gatzy JT. Effects of hormones on potential difference and liquid balance across

93. explants from proximal and distal fetal rate lung. *J Physiol* 1993;463:647–665.

93. Cott GR, Rao AK. Hydrocortisone promotes the maturation of the Na$^+$ dependent ion transport across the fetal pulmonary epithelium. *Am J Respir Cell Mol Biol* 1993;9:166–171.

94. Tehepichev S, Ueda J, Canessa C, et al. Lung epithelial Na channel subunits are differentially regulated during development and by steroids. *Am J Physiol* 1995;269:C805–C812.

95. Barker PM, Gatzy JT. Effects of gas composition on liquid secretion by explants of distal lung of fetal rat in submersion culture. *Am J Physiol Lung Cell Mol Physiol* 1993;265:L512.

96. Raj JU, Bland RD. Lung luminal liquid clearance in newborn lambs. Effect of pulmonary microvascular pressure elevation. *Am Rev Respir Dis* 1986;134:305.

97. Cummings JJ, Carlton DP, Poulain FR, et al. Hypoproteinemia slows lung liquid clearance in young lambs. *J Appl Physiol* 1993;74:153–160.

98. Bland RD, Hansen TN, Haberkern CM, et al. Lung fluid balance in lambs before and after birth. *J Appl Physiol* 1982;53:992–1004.

99. Dawes GS, Fox HE, Leduc BM, et al. Respiratory movements and paradoxical sleep in the fetal lamb. *J Physiol* 1970;210:47P.

100. Merlet C, Hoerter J, Devilleneuve C, et al. Mise en evidence de mouvements respiratoires chez le foetus d'agneau au cours du dernier mois de la gestation. *C R Acad Sci Ser D* 1970;270:2462–2464.

101. Dawes GS, Fox HE, Leduc MB, et al. Respiratory movements and rapid eye movement sleep in the fetal lamb. *J Physiol* 1972;220:119–143.

102. Boddy K, Dawes GS, Fisher R, et al. Fetal respiratory movements, electrocortical and cardiovascular responses to hypoxaemia and hypercapnia in sheep. *J Physiol* 1974;243:599–618.

103. Maloney JE, Adamson TM, Brodecky V, et al. Modification of respiratory center output in the unanesthetized fetal sheep "in utero." *J Appl Physiol* 1975;39:552–558.

104. Maloney JE, Bowes G, Wilkinson M. "Fetal breathing" and the development of patterns of respiration before birth. *Sleep* 1980;3:299–306.

105. Ioffe S, Jansen AH, Russell BJ, et al. Respiratory response to somatic stimulation in fetal lambs during sleep and wakefulness. *Pfluegers Arch* 1980;388:143–148.

106. Ioffe S, Jansen AH, Russell BJ, et al. Sleep, wakefulness and the monosynaptic reflex in fetal and newborn lambs. *Pfluegers Arch* 1980;388:149–157.

107. Rigatto H, Moore M, Cates D. Fetal breathing and behavior measured through a double-wall Plexiglas window in sheep. *J Appl Physiol* 1986;61:160–164.

108. Boddy K, Dawes GS. Fetal breathing. *Br Med Bull* 1975;31:3–7.

109. Dawes GS, Fox HE, Leduc MB, et al. Respiratory movements and rapid eye movement sleep in the fetal lamb. *J Physiol* 1972;220:119–143.

110. Patrick J, Campbell K, Carmichael L, et al. A definition of human fetal apnea and the distribution of fetal apneic intervals during the last ten weeks of pregnancy. *Am J Obstet Gynecol* 1980;136:471–477.

111. Patrick J, Campbell K, Carmichael L, et al. Patterns of human fetal breathing during the last 10 weeks of pregnancy. *Obstet Gynecol* 1980;56:24–30.

112. Dawes GS. Breathing before birth in animals and man. *N Engl J Med* 1974;290:557–559.

113. Kitterman JA, Liggins GC, Clements JA, Tooley WH. Stimulation of breathing movements in fetal sheep by inhibitors of prostaglandin synthesis. *J Dev Physiol* 1979;1:453–466.

114. Dawes GS, Gardner WN, Johnston BM, et al. Effects of hypercapnia on tracheal pressure, diaphragm and intercostal electromyograms in unanesthetized fetal lambs. *J Physiol* 1982;326:461–474.

115. Jansen AH, Ioffe S, Russell BJ, et al. Influence of sleep state on the response to hypercapnia in fetal lambs. *Respir Physiol* 1982;48:125–142.

116. Moss IR, Scarpelli EM. Generation and regulation of breathing in utero: fetal CO_2 response test. *J Appl Physiol* 1979;47:527–531.

117. Rigatto H. A new window on the chronic fetal sheep model. In: Nathanielsz PW, ed. *Animal models in fetal medicine.* Ithaca, NY: Perinatology Press, 1984:57–67.

118. Rigatto H, Hasan SU, Jansen A, et al. The effect of total peripheral chemodenervation on fetal breathing and on the establishment

of breathing at birth in sheep. In: Jones CT, ed. *Fetal and neonatal development*. Ithaca, NY: Perinatology Press, 1988:613–621.

119. Clewlow F, Dawes GS, Johnston BM, et al. Changes in breathing, electrocortical and muscle activity in unanesthetized fetal lambs with age. *J Physiol* 1983;341:463–476.

120. Koos BJ, Sameshima H, Power GG. Fetal breathing, sleep state, and cardiovascular responses to graded hypoxia in sheep. *J Appl Physiol* 1987;62:1033–1039.

121. Baier RJ, Hasan SU, Cates DB, et al. Effects of various concentrations of O_2 and umbilical cord occlusion on fetal breathing and behavior. *J Appl Physiol* 1990;68:1597–1604.

122. Moss IR, Inman JG. Neurochemicals and respiratory control during development. *J Appl Physiol* 1989;67:1–13.

123. Johnston BM, Gluckman PD. GABA mediated inhibition of breathing in the late gestation sheep fetus. *J Dev Physiol* 1983;5:353–360.

124. Boddy K, Dawes GS, Fisher R, et al. The effects of pentobarbitone and pethidine on foetal breathing movements in sheep. *Br J Pharmacol* 1976;57:311–317.

125. Piercy WN, Day MA, Nims AH, et al. Alteration of ovine fetal respiratory-like activity by diazepam, caffeine and doxapram. *Am J Obstet Gynecol* 1977;127:43–49.

126. Paul SM, Maraugos PJ, Skolnick P. The benzodiazepine-GABA-chloride ionophore receptor complex: common site of minor tranquilizer action. *Biol Psychol* 1981;16:213–229.

127. Dawes GS. The establishment of pulmonary respiration. In: *Foetal and neonatal physiology*. Chicago: Year Book, 1968:125–159.

128. Harned H, Ferreiro J. Initiation of breathing by cold stimulation: effects of change in ambient temperature on respiratory activity of the full-term fetal lambs. *J Pediatr* 1973;88:663–669.

129. Jansen AH, Ioffe S, Russell BJ, et al. Effect of carotid chemoreceptor denervation on breathing in utero and after birth. *J Appl Physiol* 1981;51:630–633.

130. Rigatto H, Lee D, Davi M, et al. Effect of increased arterial CO_2 on fetal breathing and behavior in sheep. *J Appl Physiol* 1988; 64:982–987.

131. Alvaro R, Weintraub Z, Alvarez J, et al. The effects of 21 or 30% O_2 plus umbilical cord occlusion on fetal breathing and behavior. *J Dev Physiol* 1992;18:237–242.

132. Alvaro R, deAlmeida V, Al-Alaiyan S, et al. A placental extract inhibits breathing induced by umbilical cord occlusion in fetal sheep. *J Dev Physiol* 1993;19:23–28.

133. Adamson SL, Richardson BS, Homan J. Initiation of pulmonary gas exchange by fetal sheep *in utero*. *J Appl Physiol* 1987;62: 989–998.

134. Adamson SL, Kuiper IM, Olson DM. Umbilical cord occlusion stimulates breathing independent of blood gases and pH. *J Appl Physiol* 1991;70:1796–1809.

135. Thorburn GD. The placenta and the control of fetal breathing movements. *Reprod Fertil Dev* 1995;7:577–594.

136. Alvarez JE, Baier RJ, Fajardo CA, et al. The effect of 10% O_2 on the continuous breathing induced by O_2 or O_2 plus cord occlusion in the fetal sheep. *J Dev Physiol* 1992;17:227–232.

137. Baier, RJ, Fajardo CA, Alvarez J, et al. The effects of gestational age and labour on the breathing and behavior response to oxygen and umbilical cord occlusion in the fetal sheep. *J Dev Physiol* 1992;18:93–98.

138. Baier, RJ, Hasan SU, Cates DB, et al. Hyperoxemia profoundly alters breathing pattern and arouses the fetal sheep. *J Dev Physiol* 1992;18:143–150.

139. Alvaro RE, Robertson M, Lemke R, et al. Effects of a prolonged infusion of a placental extract on breathing and electrocortical activity in the fetal sheep. *Pediatr Res* 1997;41:300A.

140. Alvaro RE, Hasan S, Chemtob S, et al. The inhibition of breathing observed with a placental extract in fetal sheep is due to prostaglandin. *Pediatr Res* 2002;51:332A.

141. Kitterman J, Liggins GC, Fewell JE, et al. Inhibition of breathing movements in fetal sheep by prostaglandins. *J Appl Physiol* 1983;54:687–692.

142. Wallen LD, Mural DT, Clyman RI, et al. Regulation of breathing movements in fetal sheep by prostaglandin E_2. *J Appl Physiol* 1986;60:526–531.

143. Koos BJ. Central stimulation of breathing movements in fetal lambs by prostaglandin synthetase inhibitors. *J Physiol* 1985;362: 455–456.

144. Kitterman J. Arachidonic acid metabolites and control of breathing in the fetus and newborn. *Semin Perinatol* 1987;11:43–52.

145. Koos BJ, Maeda T. Fetal breathing, sleep state and cardiovascular response to adenosine in sheep. *J Appl Physiol* 1990;68:489–495.

146. Bissonette JM, Hohimer AR, Knopps SJ. The effect of centrally administered adenosine on fetal breathing movements. *Respir Physiol* 1991;84:273–285.

147. Koos BJ, Maeda T, Jan C. Adenosine A_1 and A_{2A} receptors modulate sleep state and breathing in fetal sheep. *J Appl Physiol* 2001;91:343–350.

148. Koos BJ, Phil D, Takatsugu M, et al. Adenosine A_{2A} receptors mediate hypoxic inhibition of fetal breathing in sheep. *Am J Obstet Gynecol* 2002;186:663–668.

149. Chernick V. Mechanics of the first inspiration. *Semin Perinatol* 1977;1:4:347–355.

150. Agostoni E, Talietti A, Agostoni AF, et al. Mechanical aspects of the first breath. *J Appl Physiol* 1958;13:344.

151. Faridy EE. Air opening pressure in fluid filled lungs. *Resp Physiol* 1987;68:279–291.

152. Faridy EE. Fetal lung development in surgically induced prolonged gestation. *Resp Physiol* 1981;45:153–166.

153. Faridy EE. Air opening pressure in fetal lungs. *Resp Physiol* 1987;68:293–300.

154. Lowson EE, Brown ER, Torday DL, et al. The effect of epinephrine on tracheal fluid flow and surfactant efflux in fetal sheep. *Am Rev Respir Dis* 1978;118:1–23.

155. Avery ME, Mead J. Surface properties in relation to atelectasis and hyaline membrane disease. *Am J Dis Child* 1959;97:517.

156. Mortola JP, Fisher JT, Smith JB, et al. Onset of respiration in infants delivered by cesarean section. *J Appl Physiol* 1982;52(3): 716–724.

157. Polgar G, Weng TR. The functional development of the respiratory system. *Am Rev Respir Dis* 1979;120:625–695.

158. Bosma JF, Lind J, Gentz N. Motions of the pharynx associated with the initial aeration of the lungs of the newborn. *Acta Paediatr Scand* 1959;48[Suppl 117]:117–122.

159. Boon AW, Milner AD, Hopkin IE. Lung expansion, tidal exchange, and formation of the functional residual capacity during resuscitation of asphyxiated neonates. *J Pediatr* 1979;95(6): 1031–1036.

160. Heymann MA, Creasy RK, Rudolph AM. Quantitation of blood flow patterns in the foetal lamb *in utero*. In: *Proceedings of the Sir Joseph Barcroft centenary symposium: foetal and neonatal physiology*. Cambridge: Cambridge University Press, 1973.

161. Edelstone DI, Rudolph AM, Heymann MA. Liver and ductus venosus blood flows in fetal lambs in utero. *Circ Res* 1978;42: 426.

162. Edelstone DI, Rudolph AM. Preferential streaming of ductus venosus blood to the brain and heart in fetal lambs. *Am J Physiol* 1979;237:1172–1174.

163. Berhman RE, Lees MH, Peterson EN, et al. Distribution of the circulation in the normal and asphyxiated fetal primate. *Am J Obstet Gynecol* 1970;108:957.

164. Reuss ML, Rudolph AM, Heymann MA. Selective distribution of microspheres injected into the umbilical veins and inferior venae cavae of fetal sheep. *Am J Obstet Gynecol* 1981;141:427.

165. Hislop A, Reid L. Intrapulmonary arterial development during fetal life: branching pattern and structure. *J Anat* 1972;113:35–48.

166. Hislop A, Reid L. Formation of the pulmonary vasculature. In: Hodson WA, ed. *Lung biology in health and disease: development of the lung*. New York: Marcel Dekker, 1977:37–86.

167. Colebatch H, Dawes G, Goodwin J, et al. The nervous control of the circulation in the foetal and newly expanded lungs of the lamb. *J Physiol* 1965;178:544–562.

168. Barrett C, Heymann M, Rudolph A. Alpha and beta adrenergic receptor activity in fetal sheep. *Am J Obstet Gynecol* 1972;112: 1114–1121.

169. Rudolph A, Heymann M, Lewis A. Physiology and pharmacology of the pulmonary circulation in the fetus and newborn. In: Hodson WA, ed. *Lung biology in health and disease: development of the lung*. New York: Marcel Dekker, 1977:497–523.

170. Clozel M, Clyman R, Soifer S, et al. Thromboxane is not responsible for the high pulmonary vascular resistance in fetal lambs. *Pediatr Res* 1985;19:1254–1257.

171. Tod M, Cassin S. Thromboxane synthase inhibition and perinatal pulmonary response to arachidonic acid. *J Appl Physiol* 1985;58:710–716.

172. Velvis H, Moore P, Heymann M. Prostaglandin inhibition prevents the fall in pulmonary vascular resistance as a result of

rhythmic distension of the lungs in fetal lambs. *Pediatr Res* 1991;30:62–68.

173. Furchgott RF, Zawadzki JV. The obligatory role of endothelial cell in the relaxation of arterial smooth muscle by acetylcholine. *Nature* 1980;288:373–376.

174. Ignarro LJ, Byrns RE, Buga GM, et al. Endothelium-derived relaxing factor from pulmonary artery and vein possesses pharmacologic and chemical properties identical to those of nitric oxide radical. *Circ Res* 1987;61:866–879.

175. Warner T, Mitchell J, Sheng H, et al. Effects of cyclic GMP on smooth muscle relaxation. In: Murad F, ed. *Advances in pharmacology.* San Diego, CA: Academic Press, 1984;26:171–194.

176. Thompson W. Cyclic nucleotide phosphodiesterases: pharmacology, biochemistry and function. *Pharmacol Ther* 1991;51:13–33.

177. Perreault T, De Marte JM. Maturational changes in endothelium-derived relaxation in newborn piglet pulmonary circulation. *Am J Physiol* 1993;264:H302.

178. Steinhorn RH, Morin FC III, Gugino SF, et al. Developmental differences in endothelium-dependent responses in isolated ovine pulmonary arteries and veins. *Am J Physiol* 1993;264: H2162–H2167.

179. Shaul PW, Farrar MA, Magness RR. Pulmonary endothelial nitric oxide production is developmentally regulated in the fetus and newborn. *Am J Physiol* 1993;265:H1056–H1063.

180. North AJ, Star RA, Brannon TS, et al. Nitric oxide synthase type I and type III gene expression are developmentally regulated in rat lung. *Am J Physiol* 1994;266:L635–L641.

181. Bloch KD, Filippov G, Sanchez LS, et al. Pulmonary soluble guanylate cyclase, a nitric oxide receptor, is increased during the perinatal period. *Am J Physiol* 1997;272:L400–L406.

182. Moore P, Velvis H, Fineman JR, et al. EDRF inhibition attenuates the increase in pulmonary blood flow due to O₂ ventilation in fetal lambs. *J Appl Physiol* 1992;73:2151–2157.

183. McQueston JA, Cornfield DN, McMurtry IF, et al. Effects of oxygen and exogenous L-arginine on EDRF activity in fetal pulmonary circulation. *Am J Physiol* 1993;264:H865–H871.

184. Tiktinsky MH, Morin FC III. Increasing oxygen tension dilates fetal pulmonary circulation via endothelium-derived relaxing factor. *Am J Physiol Heart Circ Physiol* 1993;265:H376–H380.

185. Abman SH, Chatfield BA, Hall SL, et al. Role of endothelium-derived relaxing factor during transition of pulmonary circulation at birth. *Am J Physiol* 1990;259:H1921–H1927.

186. Cornfield DN, Reeve HL, Tolarova S, et al. Oxygen causes fetal pulmonary vasodilation through activation of a calcium-dependent potassium channel. *Proc Natl Acad Sci USA* 1996;93: 8089–8094.

187. Yangisawa M, Kurihara H, Kimura S, et al. A novel potent vasoconstrictor peptide produced by vascular endothelial cells. *Nature* 1998;332:411–415.

188. Chatfield BA, McMurtry IF, Hall SL, et al. Hemodynamic effects of endothelin-1 on ovine fetal pulmonary circulation. *Am J Physiol* 1991;261:R182–R187.

189. Hislop AA, Zhao YD, Springall DR, et al. Postnatal changes in endothelin-1 binding in porcine pulmonary vessels and airways. *Am J Respir Cell Mol Biol* 1995;12:557–566.

190. Wong J, Vanderford PA, Fineman JR, et al. Developmental effects of endothelin-1 on the pulmonary circulation in sheep. *Pediatr Res* 1994;36:394–401.

191. Arai H, Hori S, Aramori I, et al. Cloning and expression of a cDNA encoding an endothelin receptor. *Nature* 1990;348:730–732.

192. Sakurai T, Yanagisawa M, Takuwa Y, et al. Cloning of a cDNA encoding a non-isopeptide-selective subtype of the endothelin receptor. *Nature* 1990;348:732–735.

193. Boulanger C, Luscher TF. Release of endothelin from the porcine aorta. Inhibition by endothelium-derived nitric oxide. *J Clin Invest* 1990;85:587–590.

194. Luscher TF, Yang Z, Tschudi M, et al. Interaction between endothelin-1 and endothelium-derived relaxing factor in human arteries and veins. *Circ Res* 1990;66:1088–1094.

195. Gosch JR. Oxygen dilation in fetal pulmonary arterioles: role of K⁺ channels. *J Surg Res* 2001;97:159–163.

196. Weir EK, Archer SL. The mechanism of acute hypoxic pulmonary vasoconstriction: the tale of two channels *FASEB J* 1995;9: 183–189.

197. Sham JS, Crenshaw EB Jr, Deng LH, et al. Effects of hypoxia in porcine pulmonary arterial myocytes: roles of K(V) channel and endothelin-1. *Am J Physiol* 2000;279:L262–L272.

198. Dawes GS, Mott JC. Vacular tone of the foetal lung. *J Physiol* 1962;164:465–477.

199. Cassin S, Dawes GS, Ross BB. Pulmonary blood flow and vascular resistance in immature foetal lambs. *J Physiol* 1964;171:80–89.

200. Emmanouilides GC, Moss AJ, Duffie ER, et al. Pulmonary arterial pressure changes in human newborn infants from birth to 3 days of age. *J Pediatr* 1964;65:327–333.

201. Heymann MA, Soifer SJ. Control of fetal and neonatal pulmonary circulation. In: Weir EK, Reeves JT, eds., *Pulmonary vascular physiology and pathophysiology.* New York: Marcel Dekker, 1989:33–50.

202. Heymann MA. Control of the pulmonary circulation in the fetus and during the transitional period to air breathing. *Eur J Obstet Gynecol Reprod Biol* 1999;84:127–132.

203. Raj U, Shimoda L. Oxygen-dependent signaling in pulmonary vascular smooth muscle. *Am J Physiol Lung Cell Mol Physiol* 2002;283:L671–L677.

204. Heymann MA. Control of the pulmonary circulation in the fetus and during the transitional period to air breathing. *Eur J Obstet Gynecol Reprod Biol* 1999;84:127–132.

205. Enhorning G, Adams FH, Norman A. Effect of lung expansion on the fetal lamb circulation. *Acta Paediatr Scand* 1996;55:441–451.

206. Gilbert RD, Hessler JR, Eitzman DV, et al. Site of pulmonary vascular resistance in fetal goats. *J Appl Physiol* 1972;32:47–53.

207. Leffler C, Hessler J, Green R. Mechanism of stimulation of pulmonary prostacyclin synthesis at birth. *Prostaglandin* 1984;28: 877–887.

208. Leffler CW, Hessler JR, Green RS. The onset of breathing stimulates pulmonary vascular prostacyclin synthesis. *Pediatr Res* 1984;18:938–942.

209. Leffler CW, Tyler T, Cassin S. Effect of indomethacin on pulmonary vascular response to ventilation of fetal goats. *Am J Physiol* 1978;234:H346–H351.

210. Leffler CW, Hessler JR, Terragno NA. Ventilation-induced release of prostaglandin-like material from fetal lungs. *Am J Physiol* 1980;238:H282–H286.

211. Soifer SJ, Morin FC III, Kaslow DC, et al. The developmental effects of prostaglandin D₂ on the pulmonary and systemic circulations in the newborn lamb. *J Dev Physiol* 1983;5:237–250.

212. Cornfield DN, Resnik ER, Herron JM, et al. Pulmonary vascular K⁺ channel expression and vasoreactivity in a model of congenital heart disease. *Am J Physiol Lung Cell Mol Physiol* 2002;283: L1210–L1219.

213. Tristani-Firouzi M, Martin E, Tolarova S, et al. Ventilation-induced pulmonary vasodilation at birth is modulated by potassium channel activity. *Am J Physiol* 1996;271:H2353–H2359.

214. Archer SL, Huang JMC, Hampl V, et al. Nitric oxide and cGMP cause vasorelaxation by activation of a charybdotoxin-sensitive K channel by cGMP-dependent protein kinase. *Proc Natl Acad Sci U S A* 1994;91:7583–7587.

215. Cornfield DN, Reeve HL, Toarova S, et al. Oxygen causes fetal pulmonary vasodilation through activation of a calcium-dependent potassium channel. *Proc Natl Acad Sci U S A* 1996;93:8089.

216. Gosche JR. Oxygen dilation in fetal pulmonary arterioles: role of K(⁺) channels. *J Surg Res* 2001;97(2):159–163.

217. Hulme JT, Coppock EA, Felipe A, et al. Oxygen sensitivity of cloned voltage-gated K⁺ channels expressed in the pulmonary vasculature. *Cir Res* 1999;85:489.

218. Abman SH, Chatfield BA, Hall SL, et al. Role of endothelium derived relaxing factor during transition of pulmonary circulation at birth. *Am J Physiol* 1990;259;H1921–H1927.

219. Tiktinshy MH, Morin FC 3rd. Increasing oxygen tension dilates fetal pulmonary circulation via endothelium-derived relaxing factor. *Am J Physiol* 1993;265(1 Pt 2):H376–H380.

220. Bolotina VM, Najibi S, Palacino JJ, et al. Nitric oxide directly activates calcium-dependent potassium channels in vascular smooth muscle. *Nature* 1994;368:850–853.

221. Robertson BE, Schubert R, Hescheler J, et al. cGMP dependent protein kinase activates Ca-activated K channels in cerebral artery smooth muscle cells. *Am J Physiol* 1993;265:1993:C299–C303.

222. Archer SL, Huang JMC, Hampl V, et al. Nitric oxide and cGMP cause vasorelaxation by activation of a charybdotoxin-sensitive K channel by cGMP-dependent protein kinase. *Proc Natl Acad Sci U S A* 1994;91:7583–7587.

223. Saqueton CB, Miller RB, Porter VA, et al. NO causes perinatal pulmonary vasodilation through K⁺-channels activation and intracellular Ca²⁺ release. *Am J Physiol* 1999;276:L925–L932.

224. De Vroomen M, Takahashi Y, Roman C, et al. Calcitonin gene-related peptide increases pulmonary blood flow in fetal sheep. *Am J Physiol* 1998;274:H277–H282.

225. Godecke A, Decking U, Ding Z, et al. Coronary hemodynamics in endothelial NO synthase knockout mice. *Circ Res* 1998;82:186–194.

226. Konduri G, Woodard L. Selective pulmonary vasodilation by low-dose infusion of adenosine triphosphate in newborn lambs. *J Pediatr* 1991;199:94–102.

227. Konduri GG, Mattei J. Role of oxidative phosphorylation and ATP release in mediating birth-related pulmonary vasodilation in fetal lambs. *Am J Physiol Heart Circ Physiol* 2002;283:H1600–H1608.

228. Pepke-Zaba J, Higenbottam TW, Dinh-Xuan AT, et al. Alpha-adrenergic stimulation of porcine pulmonary arteries. *Eur J Pharmacol* 1993;235:169–175.

229. MacLean MR, McCulloch KM, McGrath JC. Influences of the endothelium and hypoxia on α_2-adrenoceptor-mediated responses in the rabbit isolated pulmonary artery. *Br J Pharmacol* 1993;108:155–161.

230. Miller VM, Vanhoutte PM. Endothelial α_2-adrenoceptors in canine pulmonary and systemic blood vessels. *Eur J Pharmacol* 1985;118:123–129.

231. Magnenant E, Jaillard S, Deruelle P, et al. Role of the alpha$_2$-adrenoceptors on the pulmonary circulation in the ovine fetus. *Pediatr Res* 2003;54:1–8.

232. Shimoda LA, Sylvester JT, Sham JS. Inhibition of voltage-aged K$^+$ current in rat intrapulmonary arterial myocytes by endothelin-1. *Am J Physiol* 1998;274:L842–L853.

233. Barman SA. Pulmonary vasoreactivity to endothelin-1 at elevated vascular tone is modulated by potassium channels. *J Appl Physiol* 1996;80:91–98.

234. Li H, Elton TS, Chen YF, et al. Increased endothelin receptor gene expression in hypoxic rat lung. *Am J Physiol* 1994;266:L553–L560.

235. Peng W, Michael JR, Hoidal JR, et al. ET-1 modulates K$_{ca}$-channel activity and arterial tension in normoxic and hypoxic human pulmonary vasculature. *Am J Physiol* 1998;275:L729–L739.

236. Goirand F, Bardou M, Guerard P, et al. ET$_A$, mixed ET$_A$/ET$_B$ receptor antagonists, and protein kinase C inhibitor prevent acute hypoxic pulmonary vasoconstriction: influence of potassium channels. *J Cardiovas Pharmacol* 2003;41:117–125.

237. Adman SH, Accurso FJ. Acute effects of partial compression of ductus arteriosus on fetal pulmonary circulation. *Am J Physiol* 1989;257:H626–H634.

238. Abman SH, Chatfield BA, Hall SL, et al. Role of endothelium-derived relaxing factor during transition of pulmonary circulation at birth. *Am J Physiol* 1990;259:H1921–H1927.

239. Heymann MA. Control of the pulmonary circulation in the fetus and during the transitional period to air breathing. *Eur J Obstet Gynecol Reprod Biol* 1999:84(2):127–132.

240. Rairigh RL, Storme L, Parker TA, et al. Inducible NO synthase inhibition attenuates shear stress-induced pulmonary vasodilation in the ovine fetus. *Am J Physiol* 1999;276:L513–L521.

241. Cornfield DN, Chatfield BA, McQueston JA, et al. Effects of birth-related stimuli on L-arginine-dependent pulmonary vasodilation in ovine fetus. *Am J Physiol* 1992;262:H1474–H1481.

242. Ogasa T, Nakano H, Ide H, et al. Flow-mediated release of nitric oxide in isolated, perfused rabbit lungs. *J Appl Physiol* 2001;91(1):363–370.

243. Storme L, Rairigh RL, Parker TA, et al. K$^+$-channel blockade inhibits shear stress-induced pulmonary vasodilation in the ovine fetus. *Am J Physiol* 1999;276:L220–L228.

244. Cooke JP, Rossitch E Jr, Andon NA, et al. Flow activates an endothelial potassium channel to release an endogenous nitrovasodilator. *J Clin Invest* 1991;88:1663–1671.

245. Ralevic V, Milner P, Kirkpatrick KA, et al. Flow-induced release of adenosine 5'-triphosphate from endothelial cells of the rat mesenteric arterial bed. *Experientia* 1992;48:31–34.

246. Hassessian H, Bodin P, Burnstock G. Blockade by glibenclamide of the flow-evoked endothelial release of ATP that contributes to vasodilation in the pulmonary vascular bed of the rat. *Br J Pharmacol* 1993;109:466–472.

247. Nelson N. Physiology of transition. In: Avery GB, Fletcher MA, Fletcher MA, MacDonald MG, eds. *Neonatology: pathophysiology and management of the newborn*, 4th ed. Philadelphia: JB Lippincott, 1994:223–247.

248. Starling MB, Elliott RB. The effects of prostaglandins, prostaglandin inhibitors, and oxygen on the closure of the ductus arteriosus, pulmonary arteries and umbilical vessels *in vitro*. *Prostaglandins* 1974;8(3):187–203.

249. Sharpe GL, Larsson KS. Studies on closure of the ductus arteriosus. X. *In vivo* effect of prostaglandin. *Prostaglandins* 1975;9(5):703–719.

250. Lim MK, Hanretty K, Houston AB. Intermittent ductal patency in healthy newborn infants: demonstration by colour Doppler flow mapping. *Arch Dis Child* 1992;67:1218.

251. Hammerman C. Patent ductus arteriosus: clinical relevance of prostaglandins and prostaglandin inhibitors in PDA pathophysiology and treatment. *Clin Perinatol* 1995;22(2):457–470.

Delivery Room Management

Virender K. Rehan   *Roderic H. Phibbs*

Although more than 90% of neonates undergo smooth feto/neonatal transition, of the 10% who require some resuscitative assistance during delivery, a small minority requires extensive resuscitative efforts (1,2). More importantly, because the need for resuscitation can come as a complete surprise, at every delivery there should be at least one person whose primary responsibility is the management of the newly born and who is capable of initiating resuscitation. Either this person or someone else who is immediately available should be skilled in all aspects of neonatal resuscitation. However, if the need for resuscitation is anticipated, additional skilled personnel should be called on before delivery. Furthermore, because many high-risk deliveries occur in nonteaching and smaller hospitals, all personnel involved in delivery room care of the newborn should be trained adequately in all aspects of neonatal resuscitation. All necessary resuscitation equipment should be checked and in working order before each delivery.

There is a high risk of asphyxia, defined as a combination of hypoxemia, hypercapnia, and acidosis, during labor, delivery, and in the first minutes after birth. This is because the newborn infant must successfully inflate his or her lungs and make adaptations to the circulation immediately after birth. Failure of either to occur leads to asphyxia. The key changes during feto/neonatal transition are the establishment of effective ventilation and perfusion of the lungs to raise partial pressure of arterial oxygen (PaO_2) from the normal low levels of the fetus to the normal, relatively higher level of the neonate, together with the shutting down of the fetal circulatory pathways, which include the right-to-left shunts through the foramen ovale and the ductus arteriosus. Skillful resuscitation of infants with impaired transition can prevent brain damage and minimize subsequent morbidity and mortality. An understanding of the physiologic changes in the respiratory and circulatory systems that occur normally as the newborn infant adapts to extrauterine life is essential for a rational and effective approach to resuscitation.

RESPIRATORY ADAPTATION

At birth, the lungs must transition rapidly to become the site for gas exchange or else hypoxia and cyanosis (see Color Plate) will rapidly develop. For the lungs to exchange gas adequately after birth, the airways and the alveoli must be cleared of fetal lung fluid, and an increase in pulmonary blood flow must occur. *In utero*, fetal pulmonary vascular resistance is high and the fetal systemic vascular resistance is low; most of the cardiac output is shunted away from the lungs and is directed to the placenta where fetoplacental gas exchange occurs. Within minutes of delivery, the newborn's pulmonary vascular resistance may decrease eight- to tenfold, causing a corresponding increase in neonatal pulmonary blood flow. Effective transition requires that the lung fluid be expelled or quickly absorbed to allow effective gas exchange. In fact, the decrease in lung fluid begins during labor (3). As a consequence of increased catecholamine levels, during labor, there is also an increase in lymphatic drainage. The absence of these physiologic events accounts for the increased incidence of transient tachypnea of the newborn after a cesarean section without labor. The first breath must generate a high transpulmonary pressure to overcome the viscosity of the lung fluid and the intraalveolar surface tension. It also helps to drive the alveolar fluid across the alveolar epithelium. Lung expansion and aeration also stimulate surfactant release with the resultant establishment of an air–fluid interface and development of functional residual capacity (FRC) (4). Normally, 80% to 90% of FRC is established within the first hour of birth in the term neonate with spontaneous respirations.

CIRCULATORY ADAPTATION

At birth, the clamping of the umbilical cord increases the systemic vascular resistance with a resultant increase in left ventricular and aortic pressures. Lung aeration and subsequent gas exchange result in increased PaO_2 and pH, which result in pulmonary vasodilation. These physiologic changes increase flow of blood to the left atrium via the pulmonary veins, so that left atrial pressure exceeds right atrial pressure, resulting in functional closure of foramen ovale. When pulmonary vascular resistance decreases to a level lower than the systemic vascular resistance, the ductus arteriosus closes functionally. As a result of the cessation of umbilical venous return, clamping of the umbilical cord also leads to the closure of the ductus venosus.

Asphyxia has the potential to set in motion a series of responses that can not only impair the normal feto/neonatal transition, but may, in fact, reverse this process and lead to the persistence of the fetal circulatory state. Hypoxia keeps the ductus arteriosus open and causes pulmonary vasoconstriction leading to right-to-left flow across the ductus. Tissue hypoxia causes metabolic acidosis worsening the pulmonary vasoconstriction. The pulmonary hypertension leads to tricuspid insufficiency, raising right atrial pressure, which leads to right-to-left shunting of blood through the foramen ovale, causing further tissue hypoxia. However, in the majority of instances, with timely and appropriate resuscitation, the changes leading to a persistent fetal circulation like state can be reversed quickly.

PATHOPHYSIOLOGY OF INTRAPARTUM ASPHYXIA AND RESUSCITATION

Asphyxia occurs when the organ of gas exchange fails. When this happens, arterial carbon dioxide partial pressure ($PaCO_2$) rises, and PaO_2 and pH fall. Despite the low PaO_2, tissues continue to consume O_2, although at a lower rate in some organs. When the PaO_2 is very low, anaerobic metabolism sets in, producing large quantities of metabolic acids. These are buffered partly by the bicarbonate in the blood (5).

The human infant is particularly vulnerable to asphyxia in the perinatal period. During normal labor, transient hypoxemia occurs with uterine contractions, but the healthy fetus tolerates this well. There are five basic events that lead to asphyxia during labor and delivery:

1. Interruption of umbilical blood flow (e.g., cord compression);
2. Failure of gas exchange across the placenta (e.g., placental abruption);
3. Inadequate perfusion of the maternal side of the placenta (e.g., severe maternal hypotension);
4. An otherwise compromised fetus who cannot further tolerate the transient, intermittent hypoxia of normal labor (e.g., the anemic or growth-retarded fetus); and
5. Failure to inflate the lungs and complete the changes in ventilation and lung perfusion that must occur at birth. This failure may occur because of airway obstruction, excessive fluid in the lungs, or weak respiratory effort. Alternatively, it may occur as a result of fetal asphyxia from one of the other four events, because fetal asphyxia

often results in an infant who is acidotic and apneic at birth.

The umbilical cord blood pH, partial pressure of oxygen (PO_2), partial pressure of carbon dioxide (PCO_2), and calculated base excess are standard measures of fetal asphyxia (6–8). With fetal acidosis, the pH can vary over a wide range. Consequently, it is important to remember that pH is a logarithmic function of hydrogen ion concentration. A decrease of 0.3 pH units from 7.40 to 7.10 indicates only a 40 nmol/L increase in hydrogen ion (i.e., from 40 to 80 nmol), whereas a 0.3 decrease from 7.10 to 6.80 indicates an increase of 80 nmol/L (i.e., from 80 to 160 nmol). The gradient in blood gas tensions between umbilical artery and vein gives some indication of placental perfusion at the time of birth. The slower the flow of fetal blood through the placenta, the more complete the equilibration of gas tensions between fetal and maternal blood. For example, an arterial PO_2 of 25 mm Hg with a venous PO_2 of 32 mm Hg suggests good placental blood flow. An arterial PO_2 of 12 mm Hg with a venous PO_2 of 45 mm Hg suggests very slow flow. Metabolic acidosis suggests asphyxia, although some of the increased lactic acid in the blood may be a result of reduced uptake of lactate by the asphyxiated liver rather than increased lactate production from anaerobic metabolism (6,9). If asphyxia occurred just before birth, there may be lactic acid in the tissues that has not yet reached the central circulation. This will be detected only by blood gas measurements a few minutes after birth. If the fetus was asphyxiated an hour before delivery and recovered, that event may not be reflected in the umbilical cord blood gases at birth. Other indicators of asphyxia include plasma hypoxanthine, which increases because of lack of aerobic metabolism, plasma erythropoietin, which increases in response to fetal hypoxia, increased plasma levels of several lipid mediators, such as platelet-activating factor, and increased cerebrospinal fluid levels of several proinflammatory cytokines such as interleukin (IL)-1β, IL-6, and IL-8 (10–12).

Asphyxia in the fetus or newborn infant (including a preterm infant) is a progressive and reversible process. The speed and extent of progression are highly variable. Sudden, severe asphyxia can be lethal in less than 10 minutes. Mild asphyxia may progressively worsen over 30 minutes or more. Repeated episodes of brief, mild asphyxia may reverse spontaneously but produce a cumulative effect of progressive asphyxia. In the early stages, asphyxia usually reverses spontaneously if its cause is removed. Once asphyxia is severe, spontaneous reversal is unlikely because of the circulatory and neurologic changes that accompany it. Other sources provide a more detailed review of these phenomena (13,14).

Figure 18-1 schematically represents the sequence of pathophysiologic changes that accompany asphyxia. Although there are some quantitative differences between the changes that occur in the fetus and those in the newborn infant, the scheme generally applies to both. It is useful to consider the changes in both fetus and newborn infant together, because many cases of neonatal asphyxia

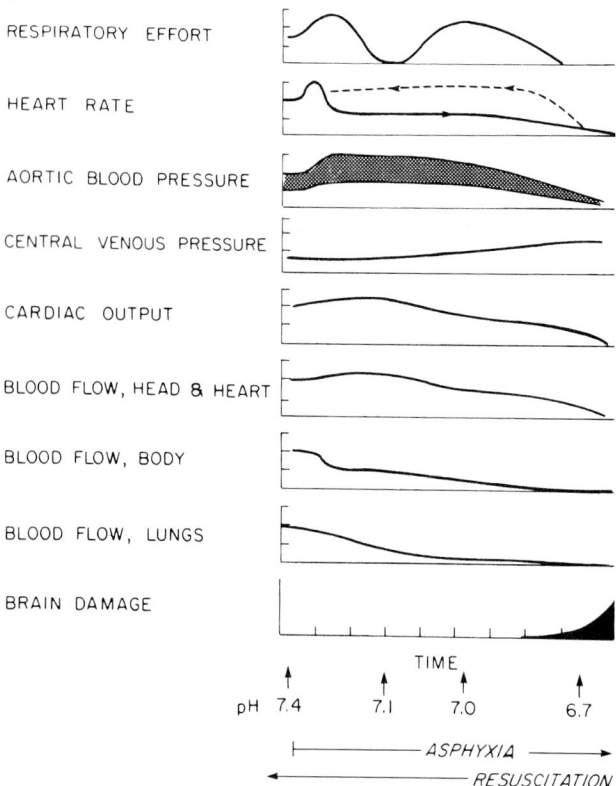

RESPIRATORY EFFORT

HEART RATE

AORTIC BLOOD PRESSURE

CENTRAL VENOUS PRESSURE

CARDIAC OUTPUT

BLOOD FLOW, HEAD & HEART

BLOOD FLOW, BODY

BLOOD FLOW, LUNGS

BRAIN DAMAGE

TIME

pH   7.4   7.1   7.0   6.7

ASPHYXIA

RESUSCITATION

Figure 18-1 The sequence of cardiopulmonary changes with asphyxia and resuscitation. If there is complete interruption of respiratory gas exchange, the entire process of asphyxia could occur in about 10 minutes. It could take much longer with an asphyxiating process that only partly interrupts gas exchange or one that does so completely but only for repeated brief periods. With resuscitation, the process reverses, beginning at the point to which the asphyxia has proceeded. (Adapted from Dawes G. *Fetal and Neonatal Physiology.* Chicago: Year-Book, 1968, with permission.)

begin in the fetus and continue after birth. Cardiac output is maintained early in asphyxia, but its distribution changes radically. Selective regional vasoconstriction reduces blood flow to less vital organs and tissues such as gut, kidneys, muscle, and skin (15). Blood flow to the brain and myocardium increases, thereby maintaining adequate oxygen delivery despite reduced oxygen content of the arterial blood. Other organs and tissues must depend on increased oxygen extraction to maintain oxygen consumption (16,17). Pulmonary blood flow is low in the fetus. It is decreased further by hypoxia and acidosis (18). As a consequence of these adaptations, fetal oxygen consumption decreases (19).

Early in asphyxia, newborns make vigorous attempts to inflate their lungs. If successful, the lungs become adequately ventilated and perfused, but the mere presence of gasping does not ensure that this will happen. As asphyxia becomes more severe, the respiratory center is depressed, and the chances of an infant spontaneously establishing effective ventilation and pulmonary perfusion diminish.

If asphyxia progresses to the severe stage, oxygen delivery to the brain and heart decreases. The myocardium then uses its stored reserve of glycogen for energy. Eventually, the glycogen reserve is consumed and the myocardium is

exposed simultaneously to progressively lower values of PO_2 and pH. The combined effects of hypoxia and acidosis lead to decreased myocardial function and decreased blood flow to the vital organs (20,21). Brain injury begins late during this phase (13,14).

This sequence of cardiovascular events is manifested by changes in heart rate and aortic and central venous pressures (see Fig. 18-1), all of which are measured easily in the newborn immediately after birth. The early bradycardia and hypertension are caused by the reflexes that shunt blood away from nonvital organs. Early in asphyxia, central venous (i.e., right atrial) pressure may rise slightly, owing to pulmonary hypertension and constriction of systemic capacitance vessels. As the myocardium fails, central venous pressure rises further, aortic pressure decreases, and heart rate is reduced further.

The initial adaptations of the systemic circulation to asphyxia are mediated by various physiologic reflexes (22). There also are major hormonal responses to asphyxia, including elevations in plasma corticotrophin, glucocorticoids, catecholamines, arginine vasopressin, renin, and atrial natriuretic factor, and a decrease in insulin (23,24). Some of these are important in maintaining the circulatory adaptations to asphyxia. Catecholamines, which come mainly from the adrenal medulla, maintain myocardial function in the presence of asphyxia, thereby increasing survival (25,26). Arginine vasopressin helps maintain the hypertension, bradycardia, and redistribution of systemic flow (27). Increased hepatic glycogenolysis helps maintain plasma glucose concentrations (9).

The physiology of resuscitation is essentially a reversal of the pathophysiology of asphyxia. In Fig. 18-1, which illustrates both processes, asphyxia proceeds from left to right, and resuscitation from right to left. It is crucial to determine where the infant is in this sequence of pathophysiologic events when resuscitation is started. If asphyxia has proceeded to myocardial failure, resuscitation must include restoration of cardiac output as well as establishment of effective ventilation and perfusion of the lungs. Generally, myocardial failure does not occur until both pH and PaO_2 are extremely low, approximately 6.9 and 20 mm Hg, respectively. Cardiac output is reestablished through rapid correction of the severe hypoxia and acidosis. Until this is done, output must be maintained by cardiac massage. As soon as pH is raised to approximately 7.1 and PaO_2 to 50 mm Hg, the myocardium responds rapidly, heart rate rises, aortic pressures rise, and pulse pressure widens, whereas central venous pressure falls. These changes indicate that cardiac massage can be stopped. At this point, the infant may be hypertensive because the vasoconstriction in nonvital organs is still present. This vasoconstriction is relieved only by continued adequate oxygenation and correction of acidosis. Pressures then will fall toward normal. The vasoconstriction also is manifested by intense pallor of the skin. As the vasoconstriction is relieved, the skin becomes pink and well perfused, with rapid capillary refilling (i.e., less than 2 seconds) when blanched by pressure. As peripheral flow improves, lactic acid sequestered in these tissues enters the central circulation and a large base deficit, which may have been corrected earlier, now reappears.

If asphyxia is only moderately severe, resuscitation begins in the middle of the sequence depicted in Fig. 18-1. There is hypertension, indicating that the myocardium has not yet failed. Effective ventilation of the lungs with a high oxygen concentration may correct acidosis by lowering the $PaCO_2$, oxygenating the blood, and adequately dilating the pulmonary vascular bed. If significant acidosis persists after alleviation of the hypercarbia, alkali might be needed to correct the metabolic component of the acidosis, relieve pulmonary vasoconstriction, and establish good pulmonary perfusion. Generally, raising pH to 7.25 is sufficient for this purpose, but there are some important exceptions (discussed below) in which a higher pH is needed to dilate the pulmonary vascular bed.

When the effects of asphyxia are alleviated, spontaneous respiratory efforts return. The duration between the onset of resuscitation and reappearance of spontaneous respiratory efforts is directly proportional to the amount of brain injury that has occurred (13).

Onset of spontaneous respiratory efforts is not necessarily an indication to withdraw assisted ventilation. Often, there is residual atelectasis and the infant does not have strong, regular respiratory efforts. $PaCO_2$ may be normal, and PaO_2 may rise to a high level with assisted ventilation. But when assisted ventilation is withdrawn, effective ventilation may decrease and the whole process of asphyxia recurs. Therefore, assisted ventilation and supplemental oxygen should be only gradually withdrawn.

The blood volume of the asphyxiated infant may be abnormal. Asphyxia during labor usually shifts blood from the placenta to the fetus. There are certain situations, however, in which the infant's blood volume may be reduced. The most obvious of these is hemorrhage from the fetoplacental unit, which is manifested by vaginal bleeding. Three other conditions that shift blood volume from the fetus to the placenta are compression of the umbilical cord, in which umbilical venous flow is reduced selectively more than arterial flow; severe hypotension in the mother; and asphyxia occurring only at the end of labor (28).

Initially, it may be difficult to determine whether or not blood volume is adequate in the asphyxiated newborn. There are two reasons for this. First, many of the circulatory responses to asphyxia are similar to those associated with loss of blood volume. Either asphyxia or hypovolemia may cause bradycardia, metabolic acidosis, poor peripheral perfusion indicated by pallor and slow capillary filling, and a large difference between core and skin temperature. A low aortic pressure could be a result of either the end stage of asphyxia or to shock. Only changes in central venous pressure are in the opposite direction, and even here the coexistence of the two processes can have offsetting effects. Second, the circulatory changes during asphyxia and resuscitation may determine the adequacy or inadequacy of the circulating blood volume. If an infant is moderately asphyxiated and has systemic and pulmonary vasoconstriction (see

Fig. 18-1, *center*) and a small blood volume, aortic and central venous pressures will be nearly normal. Administration of a blood volume expander at this point would only overload the circulation. The effects of volume expansion would be even worse if the asphyxia were more severe and myocardial failure were present. Correction of asphyxia (see Fig. 18-1, going from right to left) relieves the vasoconstriction of resistance and capacitance vessels, and the small blood volume now becomes inadequate to support the circulation. Reperfusion of asphyxic and ischemic tissues also increases loss of intravascular water from these capillary beds, leading to edema and reduced plasma volume.

During recovery from asphyxia, several metabolic abnormalities appear. There may be hypoglycemia caused by depletion of carbohydrate reserves during the asphyxia. Hypoglycemia must be prevented because it can cause myocardial failure in a heart recently subjected to asphyxia (29). Hyperglycemia caused by excessive glucose administration similarly is dangerous during asphyxia because it worsens the acidosis by increasing lactic acid production (30). Hypocalcemia also develops, possibly as a result of increased calcitonin release during asphyxia (31), and can lead to myocardial failure.

Hyperkalemia occurs during asphyxia, when, in the process of buffering acidosis, H^+ enters the erythrocytes and K^+ is displaced from them. Although this increases plasma K^+ while the patient is asphyxiated, total body K^+ decreases as some of the K^+ is excreted by the kidney. On relief of asphyxia, the buffering processes are reversed and K^+ leaves the plasma and reenters the erythrocytes, leading to hypokalemia.

HIGH-RISK PREGNANCIES

Certain situations during pregnancy, labor, or delivery carry an increased risk of intrapartum asphyxia. If these high-risk deliveries are identified before birth, their progress during labor and delivery should be closely monitored and resuscitation can be initiated at birth. Tables 18-1 and 18-2 list some of the factors that alert the physician to a high-risk delivery. Optimal management of these cases requires good communication between the obstetrician, anesthesiologist, and pediatrician.

RESUSCITATION OF THE ASPHYXIATED INFANT

If a severely asphyxiated infant is expected, a resuscitation team must be present at delivery. In the majority of instances, good communication between the obstetrician and pediatrician will provide timely notice of the impending delivery of an asphyxiated infant. The actual extent of resuscitation needed can be determined only after someone with considerable clinical experience evaluates the infant's condition. It is helpful to assign the responsibility of each member of the resuscitation team before delivery.

TABLE 18-1

SOME FACTORS THAT PLACE THE NEWBORN AT HIGH RISK FOR ASPHYXIA

Maternal Conditions	Labor and Delivery Conditions	Fetal Conditions
Diabetes mellitus	Forceps delivery other than low-elective or vacuum-extraction delivery	Premature delivery
		Postmature delivery
Preeclampsia, hypertension, chronic renal disease	Breech or other abnormal presentation and delivery	Acidosis determined by fetal scalp capillary blood
Anemia (i.e., hemoglobin <10 g/dL)	Cephalopelvic disproportion: shoulder dystocia, prolonged second stage	Abnormal heart rate pattern or dysrhythmia
Blood type or group alloimmunization	Cesarean section	Meconium-stained amniotic fluid
Abruptio placentae, placenta previa, or other antepartum hemorrhage	Prolapsed umbilical cord	Oligohydramnios
		Polyhydramnios
Narcotic, barbiturate, tranquilizer, psychedelic drug use or alcohol intoxication	Cord compression (e.g., nuchal cord, cord knot, compression by aftercoming head in breech delivery)	Decreased rate of growth: uterine size or fetal size determined by ultrasonography
History of previous perinatal loss	Maternal hypotension or hemorrhage	
Prolonged rupture of membranes		Macrosomia
Lupus		Immaturity of pulmonary surfactant system
		Fetal malformations determined by sonography
Maternal heart disease		Hydrops fetalis
Maternal fever or other evidence of amnionitis		Low biophysical profile
Abnormal umbilical artery		
Doppler velocity		Multiple birth; in particular, discordant, stuck, or monamniotic

The following is an example of outlining the responsibilities of each member of the resuscitation team.

Member A:

1. Assess infant.
2. Manage airway and intubate the trachea, if needed.
3. Provide positive-pressure ventilation.
4. Secure endotracheal tube (ET).

Member B:

1. Listen for heart rate and, if needed, give cardiac massage.
2. Auscultate chest to be sure ET is in proper position and gas exchange is good.

TABLE 18-2

FETAL HEART RATE PATTERNS ASSOCIATED WITH FETAL AND NEONATAL DISTRESS

Heart Rate Pattern	Fetal or Neonatal Problems
Severe (i.e., <80 beats/min), sustained bradycardia, with loss of variability	Fetal hemorrhage, fetal asphyxia
Sustained tachycardia, uncomplicated by other abnormal patterns	Infection, often with apnea
Late decelerations with loss of variability	Asphyxia
Severe, recurrent variable decelerations, with loss of variability	Asphyxia and possible hypovolemia
Sinusoidal	Severe anemia with asphyxia

3. Catheterize umbilical vessel or vessels and maintain patency of catheters.
4. Measure intravascular pressures, assess perfusion, sample blood for pH, PO_2, and PCO_2, and draw blood cultures.
5. Administer fluids and drugs.
6. Continue assessment of infant.

Member C:

1. Blot baby dry; apply electrocardiograph (ECG) monitor leads, radiant monitor servocontrol, and transcutaneous oxygen sensor.
2. Keep timed, written record of resuscitation and vital signs and assign the Apgar scores at 1 and 5 minutes and every 5 minutes thereafter until the score is 7 or greater; time and record the rate and volume of infusions such as alkali and blood volume expanders.
3. Assist member A by providing ET suction, adjusting the fraction of oxygen inspired (FiO_2), and helping to secure ET.
4. Help member B by providing medications and blood volume expanders in sterile syringes; B is working in a sterile field early in resuscitation.
5. Monitor baby's temperature and capillary blood glucose.

Resuscitation Equipment and Supplies for Optimal Resuscitation (Modified from Reference 1)

All resuscitation equipment (listed below) should be checked before each delivery and should be fully operational.

Resuscitation table with heat source
Suction equipment
Bulb syringe

Mechanical suction and tubing

Suction catheters: 5 Fr, 6 Fr, 8 Fr, 10 Fr, and 12 Fr

8 Fr feeding tube and 20 mL syringe

Meconium aspirator

Bag and mask equipment

Neonatal resuscitation bag with a pressure-release valve or pressure manometer (the bag must be capable of delivering 90% to 100% oxygen)

Face masks, newborn and premature sizes (cushioned-rim masks preferred)

Oxygen source with flowmeter (flow rate up to 10 L/min) and tubing

Intubation equipment

Laryngoscope with straight blades: No. 00 (very-low-birth-weight infant); No. 0 (preterm infant); and No. 1 (term infant)

Endotracheal tubes, 2.5-, 3.0-, 3.5-, 4.0-mm internal diameter (ID)

Stylet (optional)

Scissors

Tape or securing device for ET

Alcohol sponges

CO_2 detector (optional)

Laryngeal mask airway (optional)

Medications

- Epinephrine 1:10,000 (0.1 mg/mL)-3-mL or 10-mL ampules
- Isotonic crystalloid (normal saline or Ringer lactate) for volume expansion: 100 or 250 mL
- Sodium bicarbonate 4.2% (5 mEq/10 mL)-10-mL ampules
- Naloxone hydrochloride 0.4 mg/mL-1-mL ampules or 1.0 mg/mL-2-mL ampules
- Dextrose 10%, 250 mL
- Normal saline for flushes

Feeding tube, 5 Fr (optional)

Umbilical vessel catheterization supplies

Sterile gloves

Scalpel or scissors

Povidone-iodine solution

Umbilical tape

Umbilical catheters, 3.5 Fr, 5 Fr

Three-way stopcock

Syringes: 1, 3, 5, 10, 20, and 50 mL

Needles: 25, 21, and 18 gauge, or puncture device for needleless system

Miscellaneous

- Gloves and appropriate personal protection
- Radiant warmer or other heat source
- Firm, padded resuscitation surface
- Clock (timer optional)
- Warmed linens
- Stethoscope (neonatal head preferred)
- Tape: $1/2$ or $3/4$ inch
- Cardiac monitor and electrode or pulse oximeter and probe

- Oropharyngeal airways (0, 00, 000 sizes or 30-, 40-, and 50-mm lengths)
- Arterial and venous pressure monitor with waveform displays; transducers can be connected to the catheters beforehand so that aortic pressure is displayed as soon as the umbilical artery catheter is inserted, and the venous waveform can be used to localize the catheter tip in the thoracic inferior vena cava (32)
- Indirect blood pressure monitor
- Tube thoracostomy tray with instruments and catheters from 10 to 14 Fr
- Blood gas electrodes with a trained operator of the blood gas machines close enough to the resuscitation area so that results are available in less than 5 minutes

In selected situations (see the section "Special Problems"), it is useful to have present in the delivery room a unit of whole blood or packed erythrocytes that have been cross-matched against the mother; this blood can be kept in a cold pack and returned to the blood bank if not used.

Clinical Assessment of Severity of Asphyxia

The Apgar score was the first attempt at a systematic assessment of birth asphyxia (6,33). There is a loose correlation between low Apgar scores and umbilical cord blood gases. However, some infants with severe acidosis have normal Apgar scores, and some with normal blood gases and pH have very low scores (34,35). Maternal anesthetics, sedatives, maternal drugs, fetal sepsis, and central nervous system pathologic conditions can lower the Apgar score; extremely premature infants often have low scores without any other evidence of asphyxia (36,37). Regardless of the cause, an Apgar score that remains low calls for action. The clinical significance of the Apgar score increases with time. Scoring should continue every 5 minutes until the score increases to 7 or above. The length of time it takes to reach a score of 7 is a rough indication of severity of asphyxia. Umbilical cord blood gases, discussed previously, are useful measures of fetal asphyxia, but this information will not be available until a few minutes after birth, and resuscitation must be started before that. Thus, their main value is in guiding subsequent management of the infant.

It is important to point out that the term *perinatal asphyxia* should be used with caution because an inaccurate use of this term may have medicolegal ramifications. It should be reserved in the clinical context of damaging hypoxemia and metabolic acidosis. A neonate who suffers from hypoxemia proximate to delivery that is severe enough to result in hypoxic encephalopathy will show other evidence of hypoxic damage, including severe metabolic or mixed acidemia (pH <7.00) on an umbilical cord arterial sample; persistence of an Apgar score of 0 to 3 for longer than 5 minutes; neonatal neurologic sequelae, for example, seizures, coma, hypotonia; and evidence of multiorgan system dysfunction. However, because neonatal neurologic problems may be attributed to factors other than those involving labor and delivery, the term *neonatal depression* should be used when cause is uncertain.

The following resuscitation approach is based mostly on the recommendations of the American Academy of Pediatrics and the American Heart Association for neonatal resuscitation (1). However, it must be pointed out that most of these recommendations are based on anecdotal experience and a review of the available literature, but have not been rigorously tested. It is expected that in the future some of these recommendations will undergo close scrutiny and possible change.

Initial Steps in Resuscitation

Initial assessment, performed within a few seconds of delivery, dictates the extent of resuscitation needed. Initial assessment includes determining whether or not the infant is breathing, if there is good muscle tone, if the color is pink, and whether the infant looks term or preterm. If the infant is term, vigorous, without any known risk factors, and born through clear amniotic fluid, the infant need not be separated from the mother to receive initial care. Thermal care can be given by putting the infant on the mother's chest (direct skin-to-skin contact), drying the infant, and covering the infant with dry linen. If the infant is apneic, gasping, has decreased muscle tone, or is cyanotic, immediate resuscitation is needed. Place the infant under a radiant warmer; quickly towel dry the baby; open the airway by laying the infant in the sniffing position; suction the mouth first and then the nose; provide tactile stimulation (by gently slapping or flicking the soles of the feet or by gently rubbing the back); and, if necessary, give oxygen. In the majority of instances, with these initial steps, the infant will start breathing adequately and demonstrate a color change to pinkish. If the infant starts breathing adequately, but continues to have central cyanosis, provide free-flow 100% oxygen. However, if the infant does not start breathing adequately or has a heart rate of less than 100 beats per minute, positive pressure ventilation (PPV) should be instituted immediately. The entire process up to this point should not take more than 20 to 30 seconds.

Positive Pressure Ventilation

Ensuring adequate ventilation is the single most important step in the cardiopulmonary resuscitation of the compromised newborn infant (38). Indications for initiating PPV include (a) apnea or gasping breaths; (b) heart rate of less than 100 beats per minute (bpm); and (c) persistent central cyanosis despite the provision of free-flow 100% oxygen. Initial PPV can be provided by either a flow-inflating bag (also called an anesthesia bag) or a self-inflating bag. Each type has its own advantages and disadvantages, and the resuscitator should be familiar with the type of bag used in his or her institution. If PPV is needed for a term infant, provide bag-and-mask ventilation at a rate of 40 to 60 breaths per minute with initial pressures of as high as 30 to

40 cm H_2O. Subsequently, however, one should ventilate with the lowest pressures required to produce a gentle chest rise. Begin ventilation by slowly applying a pressure of 20 to 30 cm H_2O. Maintain this inflating pressure for 1 to 2 seconds, then ventilate at a rate of 40 to 60 breaths per minute, using an inflation time of 0.3 to 0.5 seconds and enough pressure to provide a visible rise of the upper portion of the chest. Repeat the application of the initial inflating pressure pattern three to four times over the first 2 minutes. These prolonged breaths inflate regions of the lungs that were gasless and create necessary FRC (39). Figure 18-2 illustrates this process. Care must be taken to avoid rapid inflation or overdistension of the lungs.

It is important to realize that infants respond to initial lung inflation by eliciting a variety of physiologic responses. The infant may respond by the "rejection response," in which the infant responds to PPV with a positive intraesophageal pressure to resist the inflation, that is, the infant actively resists attempts to inflate the lungs by generating an active exhalation. This response acts to not only reduce lung inflation, but also may cause high transient inflation pressures. Another response is "Head's paradoxical response" in which the neonate responds to PPV with an inspiratory effort, causing a negative intraesophageal pressure. This inspiratory effort, with the resultant negative pressure produces a fall in inflation pressures but results in a transient increase in tidal volume. Of course, the neonate may demonstrate no response to the inflation attempt, that is, not generating any change in intraesophageal pressure during the positive pressure inflation, and passive inflation subsequently results. It is important to recognize that these physiologic responses to positive pressure inflation in the delivery room may cause large variability in the tidal volume and intrapulmonary pressures, despite constant delivery of inflation pressure.

The very premature infant with a very small lung volume and a surfactant-deficient lung presents special problems for initial ventilation that are discussed later (see section "Special Problem"). Whether low tidal volume ventilation starting in the delivery room, in an attempt to avoid lung injury and hypocapnia in premature infants, can be safely delivered, and whether it is as efficacious as normal tidal volume ventilation remains to be seen.

In the majority of instances, provision of appropriate PPV is followed by an increase in heart rate, improvement in color, and spontaneous breathing. Rate and pressures of PPV should be gradually reduced before deciding to see if the infant will tolerate its discontinuation. Free-flow oxygen may be continued as long as necessary to keep the infant pink. Some of the factors determining the success of PPV using a bag and mask include choosing the correct size mask, proper positioning of the infant, achieving tight seal between the face and the mask, and using adequate inspiratory pressure. If despite correct bag-and-mask PPV the infant fails to improve or continues to deteriorate, consider beginning chest compressions and bag-and-endotracheal-tube ventilation.

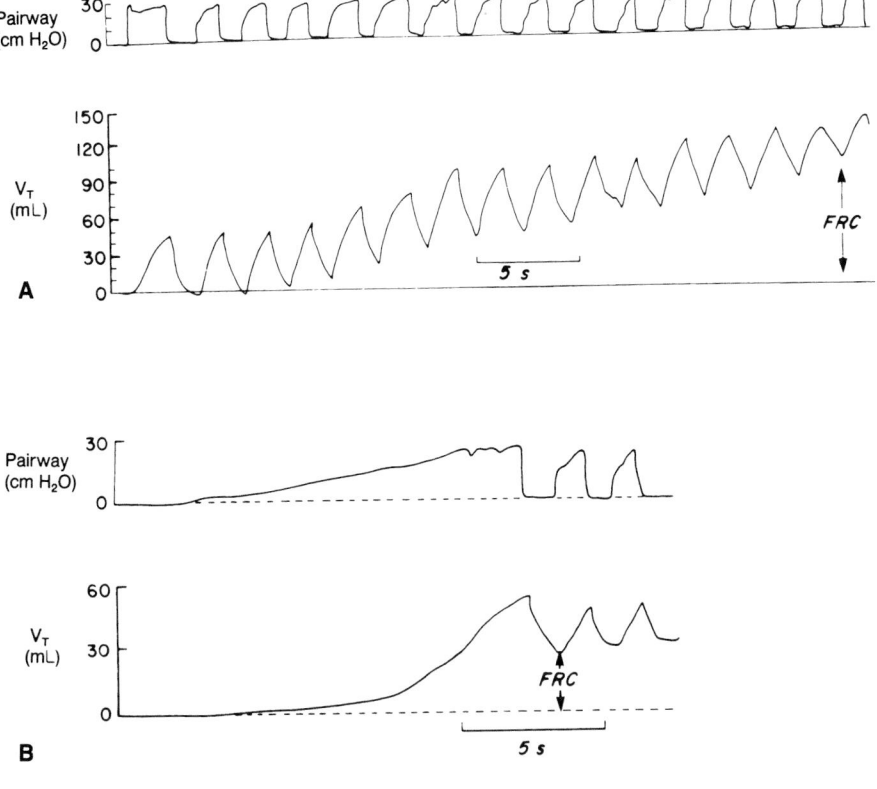

Figure 18-2 Initial inflation of the lungs by assisted ventilation in two asphyxiated infants. **A**: An inflation pressure of 30 cm H_2O is applied repeatedly for 1 to 2 seconds. For the first several breaths, the volume entering and leaving the lungs is the same. Then the volume out is slightly less than the volume in for several breaths, and this trapped gas begins to form the functional residual capacity (FRC). **B**: The first inflation is with a pressure that is increased slowly up to 30 cm H_2O over 8 seconds and held at that pressure for 2 seconds. During exhalation, less gas leaves than what entered; therefore, some FRC has been generated with the first breath. P_{air}, pressure applied to the airway; V_T, tidal volume. (Adapted from Boon AW, Milner AD, Hopkin IE. Lung expansion, tidal exhange, and formation of the functional residual capacity during resuscitation of asphyxiated neonates. *J Pediatr* 1979;95: 1031; and Vyas H, Milner AD, Hopkin IE, et al. Physiologic responses to prolonged and slow-rise inflation in the resuscitation of the asphyxiated newborn infant. *J Pediatr* 1981:99:635.)

Chest Compressions

Chest compressions are infrequently needed during neonatal resuscitation. However, infants who have a heart rate of less than 60 bpm, despite 30 seconds of effective PPV, need immediate chest compressions (Fig. 18-3) Chest compressions can be provided by either the thumb technique or the two-finger technique, the thumb technique being preferred. Chest compressions are performed by placing thumbs or finger on the sternum immediately above the xiphoid and compressing at a rate of 90 per minute with an accompanying breath rate of 30 per minute (chest-compressions-to-ventilation ratio = 3:1). To provide effective chest compressions, one should ensure that the depth of compressions is one-third the depth of the chest, thumbs or fingers remain in contact with the chest at all times, the duration of the downward stroke of the compression is shorter than that of the release, compressions are well coordinated with ventilation, and there is adequate chest movement during ventilation. Continue chest compressions until the heart rate is greater than 60 bpm

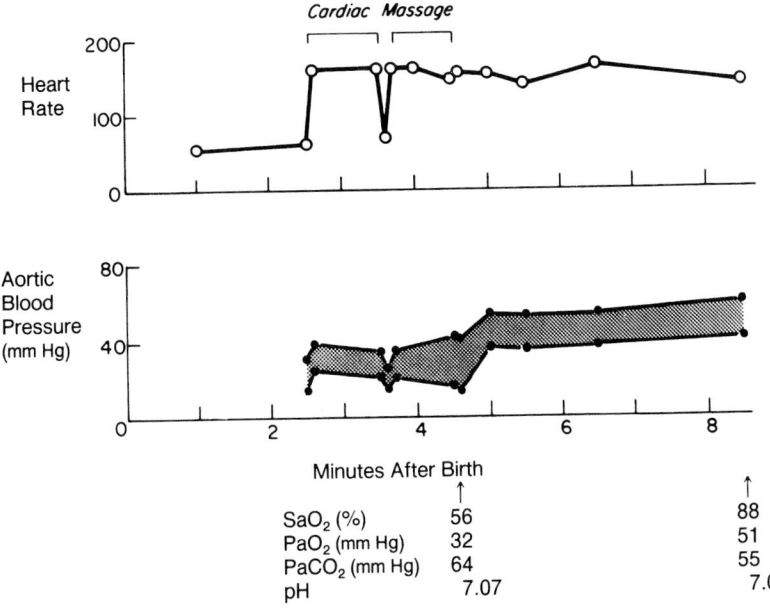

Figure 18-3 Resuscitation and cardiac massage were performed on a 2.1-kg infant who was delivered by cesarean section because of signs of fetal asphyxia at 34 weeks of gestation. The infant was intubated and ventilated with 60% oxygen beginning 30 seconds after birth. An electrocardiogram was begun at 1 minute, and at 2.5 minutes an umbilical artery catheter connected to a pressure transducer and a recorder was passed into the descending aorta. Note persistent bradycardia despite assisted ventilation and low aortic pressure with narrow phasic pressure. Cardiac massage raised heart rate and pressure. When briefly discontinued after 1 minute, pressure and heart rate fell. After another minute of massage and assisted ventilation, good cardiac output had returned. This was manifested by a sustained higher heart rate and higher blood pressure with wider phasic pressure when massage was discontinued a second time 5 minutes after birth. By 8.5 minutes, the infant was still acidotic, but there was adequate oxygenation and aortic pressure continued to rise. $PaCO_2$, arterial carbon dioxide partial pressure; PaO_2, arterial oxygen partial pressure; SaO_2, saturation of arterial blood hemoglobin with oxygen.

and ventilate until heart rate is greater than 100 bpm, at which point the infant's own respiratory effort is assessed for adequacy. Ventilation can then be discontinued if heart rate remains above 100 bpm and the infant continues to breathe spontaneously. However, if the heart rate remains below 60 bpm despite effective chest compressions and ventilation, ET intubation (if it has not been already done) and administration of medications may be needed. However, it is important to realize that the most important reason for continued bradycardia during resuscitation is failure to establish effective postnatal ventilation rather than perinatal asphyxia. Therefore, it important to make every effort to optimize ventilation before chest compressions and medication administration are considered.

Endotracheal Intubation

Endotracheal intubation is probably the most difficult step in neonatal resuscitation and the one that requires constant practice to maintain sharp skills in this technique. Someone experienced in endotracheal intubation should be available to assist at every delivery. Therefore, if the resuscitator is not comfortable with endotracheal intubation, he/she should focus on providing effective ventilation via bag and mask until somebody experienced in endotracheal intubation arrives. Indications for endotracheal intubation include (a) to suction meconium; (b) to improve ventilation when bag-and-mask ventilation is ineffective; (c) to coordinate ventilation and chest compressions; (d) to administer medications such as epinephrine; (e) when prolonged ventilation is needed, for example, extreme prematurity; (f) to administer surfactant; and (g) when congenital diaphragmatic hernia is suspected (probably the only absolute indication for endotracheal intubation).

The correct size laryngoscope blade is No. 1 for a term and No. 0 for a preterm infant. For a very-low-birth-weight (VLBW) infant, a size 00 blade may be used. The ET should be of uniform internal diameter as tubes with shoulders may obstruct the line of vision during insertion and are more likely to cause trauma to the vocal cords. The choice of ET is based on the infant's weight or gestational age: for infants weighing less than 1000 g (<28 weeks' gestational age), use a 2.5-mm internal diameter (ID) tube; for infants weighing 1000 to 2000 g (28 to 34 weeks' gestational age), use a 3.0-mm ID tube; for infants weighing 2000 to 3000 g (34 to 38 weeks' gestational age), use a 3.5-mm ID; and for larger infants, a 3.5- to 4.0-mm ID tube may be used. To minimize the risk of vocal cord trauma and the subsequent development of laryngeal stenosis, one should make sure that the inserted ET is not too tight a fit in the larynx. In general, gas should leak from the space between the ET and the trachea when 15 to 30 cm H_2O pressure is applied to the airway. Cutting the tube at the 13- to 15-cm mark prior to insertion makes it easier to handle during the procedure, decreases the chances of inserting the tube too far, and decreases the resistance to airflow. The use of a stylet during ET insertion is optional. If a stylet is used to stiffen the

ET, it should be ensured that its tip is approximately 0.5 cm above from the tip of the tube and does not protrude from the end or the side hole of the ET. In addition, the stylet should be well secured so that it does not advance farther into the ET during intubation. If the stylet extends beyond the tip of the ET, it could traumatize the airway.

For intubation, stabilize the infant's head in the sniffing position, slide the laryngoscope into the mouth and advance it gently beyond the base of the tongue, lift the blade, and look for landmarks, suctioning if necessary. Once the vocal cords are visualized (as an inverted letter V [Λ] within the glottis), insert the ET gently until the vocal cord guide is at the level of the vocal cords. Application of downward pressure on the cricoid may facilitate intubation. Preoxygenating the infant before attempting intubation, delivering free-flow oxygen during intubation, and limiting actual intubation attempts to no longer than approximately 20 seconds minimizes hypoxia associated with intubation. If intubation is unsuccessful in 20 seconds, ventilate the infant by bag and mask for at least 1 minute before again attempting intubation. Other complications of intubation include apnea and bradycardia; contusion or laceration of the tongue, gums, or airway; perforation of the trachea or esophagus; infection; and pneumothorax. With all these complications possible, intubate gently.

If the ET is inserted to aspirate meconium, immediately connect a meconium aspirator and apply suction as the tube is gradually withdrawn. Repeat the procedure as necessary until little additional meconium is suctioned or until the infant's heart rate indicates that PPV is required. If the ET is inserted to ventilate the infant, after insertion, immediately ensure that the ET is in the trachea by observing the chest rise with each breath, listening for good breath sounds with each breath, the absence of breath sounds over the stomach, and observing vapor condensation on the inside of the tube during exhalation. If there is still any doubt whether the tube is in the esophagus or trachea, a color change on a CO_2 detector attached to the ET may be helpful. However, be aware that extremely premature infants and infants with very poor cardiac output may exhale insufficient CO_2 to be detected reliably by CO_2 detectors. Correct placement of the ET within the trachea is guided by the lip-to-tip distance in centimeters (6 + the infant's body weight in kilograms), which places the ET tip midway between the vocal cords and the carina. Correct placement is further suggested by listening to equal air entry on both sides of chest, in the axillae. If the breath sounds are louder on the right side of chest, the ET is likely to be in the right main stem bronchus and should be slowly pulled back until equal breath sounds are heard over both sides of chest before it is taped in place. If the ET is to be left in place beyond initial resuscitation, final confirmation of appropriate placement should be made through a chest radiograph.

Medications

More than 99% of infants requiring resuscitation improve with timely and skillful implementation of initial steps of resuscitation and establishment of effective ventilation. Only a small fraction of infants require medications during resuscitation (2). Each delivery area should have a chart displaying the appropriate dosages and concentrations of all medications used in neonatal resuscitation. All medications needed for resuscitation can be administered via the ET or via an umbilical venous or an arterial catheter.

Epinephrine is usually the first drug administered during resuscitation. It is indicated when the heart rate remains less than 60 bpm after 30 seconds of adequate PPV and another 30 seconds of chest compressions and PPV. It is administered either via an ET or umbilical vein (40). Administration via the umbilical route is probably more effective, but is often delayed because of the time required to establish an umbilical venous access. Therefore, during neonatal resuscitation, administration via an ET is generally the most rapidly accessible and practical route for epinephrine administration. The recommended dose is 0.1 to 0.3 mL/kg of a 1:10,000 solution, given rapidly. In addition to its β_1 effect on the heart, it also has a peripheral α_1 effect that results in peripheral vasoconstriction and increased blood flow to the heart and brain. The heart rate should increase promptly after epinephrine has been administered; if it does not, epinephrine can be repeated every 3 to 5 minutes. Epinephrine should not be given before establishing adequate ventilation, because in the absence of available oxygen it may cause myocardial damage by increasing the workload and oxygen consumption of the heart muscle. One area of controversy is the use of high-dose epinephrine during neonatal resuscitation. Because of the theoretical risks of higher doses coupled with lack of any human data proving its added advantage, higher doses are not currently recommended for neonatal resuscitation.

If the infant looks pale and there is evidence of blood loss, administration of a volume expander is indicated. Although it is most commonly given through the umbilical vein, the intraosseous route can be used (41). The recommended solution for treating hypovolemia during neonatal resuscitation is an isotonic crystalloid solution (normal saline or Ringer lactate at 10 mL/kg). Whether albumin can be given safely in this situation, and whether it is as effective as normal saline is not known. O-negative blood crossmatched with the mother's blood (if available) can be transfused. This should be prepared before delivery if low fetal blood volume is suspected antenatally. A volume expander can be repeated if the infant shows minimum improvement after the first dose and evidence of hypovolemia persists (persistent pallor despite adequate oxygenation, weak pulses, and poor response to adequate resuscitation). Although hypovolemia should be corrected fairly quickly, there is concern that too rapid infusion of the volume expander may result in intracranial hemorrhage, especially in the preterm infant. Therefore, each infusion should be given over 5 to 10 minutes.

The use of sodium bicarbonate ($NaHCO_3$) during resuscitation is controversial. The current recommendation is to use $NaHCO_3$ if the infant has undergone all other steps of resuscitation appropriately and has failed to respond. Although there is a lack of data documenting its benefit, if the pH is less than 7.05 as a consequence of a mixed acidosis, or the base deficit is 15 mEq/L or more, correction of the metabolic component of the acidosis with an infusion of NaHCO3 may be helpful. The immediate objectives are twofold: to reverse the myocardial failure and low cardiac output that occurs from acute metabolic, but not respiratory, acidosis (22,42,43); and to relieve the intense pulmonary vasoconstriction that occurs with severe acidosis, particularly in full-term infants (19,44,45). The degree of pulmonary vasoconstriction is approximately the same for metabolic and respiratory acidosis (46). The recommended dose is 2 mEq/kg [4 mL/kg of 4.2% solution, osmolarity = 900 mOsm/L]) given slowly (no faster than 1 mEq/kg per minute). Some studies suggest that there is an association between rapid infusions of large volumes of concentrated $NaHCO_3$ and intracranial hemorrhage in preterm infants. The hemorrhages might be caused by transient hypernatremia from too rapid an infusion, by an acute rise in $PaCO_2$ from inadequate ventilation during the $NaHCO_3$ infusion, which would cause cerebral vasodilation, or by the asphyxia for which the $NaHCO_3$ was given. However, infusion of $NaHCO_3$ into the inferior vena cava at the rate of 1 mEq/kg per minute, for a total dose of up to 5 mEq/kg, causes only a slight transient increase in the arterial sodium concentration.

The ability of $NaHCO_3$ buffer to raise pH depends on the ability of the lungs to eliminate the CO_2 produced by the buffering process, as determined by the following equation:

$$H^+ + NaHCO_3 \leftrightarrow Na^+ + H_2CO_3 \leftrightarrow H_2O + CO_2$$

Consequently, $NaHCO_3$ should not be given unless ventilation is adequate and $PaCO_2$ is low, normal, or declining toward normal. Continue ventilation during bicarbonate therapy to eliminate the excess CO_2 produced. CO_2 is highly diffusible, so even if ventilation is adequate, some of the CO_2 produced by buffering could enter cells and transiently increase acidosis. The implications of this intracellular acidosis following sodium bicarbonate infusion are not known, and remain to be studied.

Tris(hydroxymethyl)-aminomethane (THAM acetate), although generally not used during resuscitation, may also be helpful in correcting metabolic acidosis. It has the dual advantage of reducing $PaCO_2$ and buffering metabolic acid. It is most useful for treating infants with severe mixed metabolic and respiratory acidosis and for situations of severe asphyxia with suspected extreme acidosis in which blood gas measurements are not available. It may cause respiratory depression, and so should be used only in situations in which ventilation already is assisted. Also it may cause hypoglycemia. Further, it should not be used in patients who are anuric or uremic. An earlier preparation was very hyperosmolar, highly alkaline and tended to cause sclerosis of blood vessels. These problems have been corrected by the use of the 0.3 mol/L preparation (can be used without dilution), which also is adjusted to pH 8.6. Figure 18-4 illustrates correction of a severe mixed acidosis.

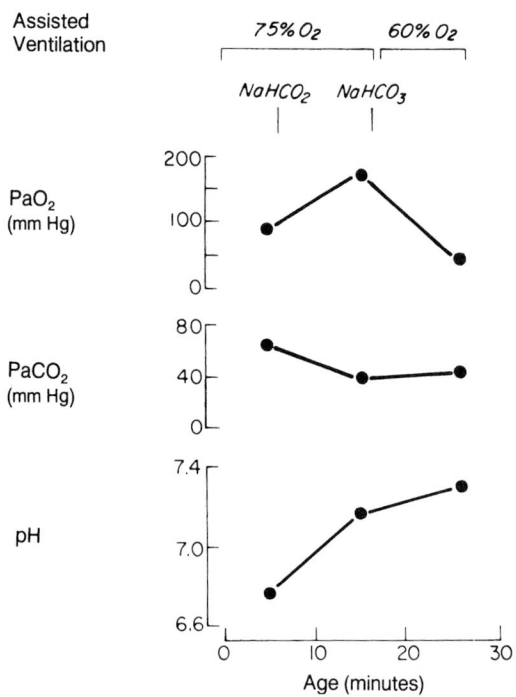

Assisted Ventilation

75% O₂   60% O₂

NaHCO₂   NaHCO₃

PaO₂ (mm Hg)

PaCO₂ (mm Hg)

pH

Age (minutes)

Figure 18-4 The sequence of events following the onset of ventilation. (From Smith CA, Nelson NM. Physiology of the newborn infant. 4th ed. Springfield, IL: Charles C. Thomas, 1976:131.)

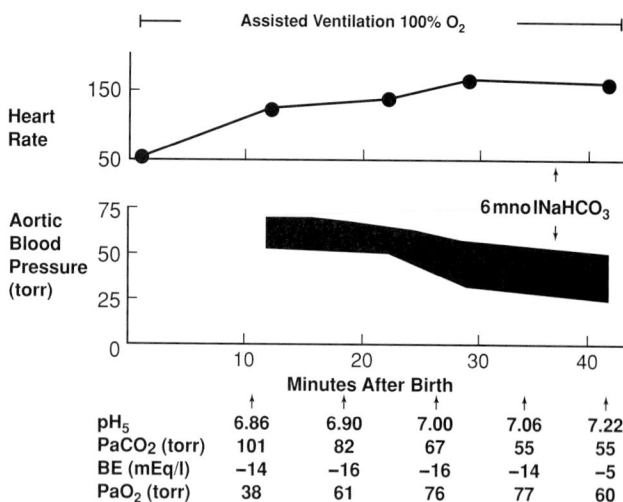

Assisted Ventilation 100% O₂

Heart Rate

Aortic Blood Pressure (torr)

6 mmol NaHCO₃

Minutes After Birth

pH₅	6.86	6.90	7.00	7.06	7.22
PaCO₂ (torr)	101	82	67	55	55
BE (mEq/l)	−14	−16	−16	−14	−5
PaO₂ (torr)	38	61	76	77	60

Figure 18-5 Changes occurred in heart rate, aortic blood pressure, and arterial blood gas tensions during the first 45 minutes after birth of a 1.2-kg premature infant with severe asphyxia complicated by bilateral pleural effusions. The child's trachea was intubated immediately after birth, and he was manually ventilated with 100% oxygen throughout this time. Note the severe mixed acidosis in the first blood gas measurement at 11 minutes after birth. Administration of NaHCO3 at this point would have been inappropriate and ineffective because assisted ventilation had not yet achieved adequate elimination of CO₂. NaH CO₃ was given only after adequate CO₂ elimination was achieved. Note that there was no rise in the arterial carbon dioxide partial pressure (PaCO₂) after this, indicating that all the CO₂ produced during the buffering process was eliminated, and the only change was a reduction in base deficit form -14 to -5 mEq/L, which raised the pH from 7.06 to 7.22. Note the high initial aortic pressure, which was due to the vasoconstriction of asphyxia, indicating that myocardial failure had not yet developed. As asphyxia was relieved, aortic pressure fell to normal. (BE, base excess; PaO₂, arterial oxygen partial pressure.)

Figure 18-5 shows how the cardiovascular effects of an infusion of alkali differ depending upon the severity of the asphyxia.

If the infant's respiratory depression is suspected to be caused by maternal narcotics (e.g., morphine, meperidine, or butorphanol tartrate), administered within 4 hours prior to delivery, administration of naloxone hydrochloride (Narcan), a narcotic antagonist should quickly reverse the respiratory depression. However, prompt and adequate ventilatory support should always precede the administration of naloxone and should be continued until the infant is breathing normally. As the duration of action of narcotics often exceeds that of naloxone, continued close observation is necessary and repeated doses of naloxone may be required. Because naloxone can precipitate an acute withdrawal reaction, it should not be given to the infant of a mother who is suspected of being addicted to narcotics or is on methadone maintenance. The recommended dose of naloxone hydrochloride is 0.1 mg/kg (1.0 mg/mL solution). It should be given preferably endotracheally or intravenously; however, intramuscular and subcutaneous routes are also acceptable, although they have a delayed onset of action.

Infants who have had severe asphyxia and who do not respond promptly to adequate resuscitation are likely to have myocardial depression with decreased cardiac output and hypotension. These infants may respond to dopamine starting at 5 μg/kg per minute and increasing to 15 to 20 μg/ kg per minute, as needed. Rarely, dobutamine might need to be added (starting at 5 μg/kg per minute and increasing

to 15 to 20 μg/kg per minute). During vigorous resuscitation it is useful to monitor heart rate and oxygen saturation electronically and have ECG electrodes applied.

Umbilical Vessel Catheterization

Catheterization of umbilical vessels is invaluable during neonatal resuscitation. The umbilical vein is readily accessible in the newborn and can be quickly catheterized. It is most often used for the administration of medications and volume expanders. For these purposes, the catheter should be inserted only 3 to 5 cm, or until free flow of blood is established, to avoid placing the tip in the portal circulation. The umbilical artery can be catheterized to obtain blood for arterial blood gas and other samples as well as to monitor blood pressure. The umbilical arterial catheter can be connected to a precalibrated pressure transducer, so that blood pressure can be monitored continuously. Alternatively, it can be connected to the transducer ahead of time and the blood pressure displayed as soon as the catheter is passed into the aorta. This also reduces the risk of accidentally injecting air bubbles through the catheter into the infant's circulation while the catheter is being connected to the transducer.

It is important to obtain quickly a measurement of pH and $PaCO_2$ to determine that ventilation is neither inadequate nor excessive and to detect metabolic acidosis. Although a venous blood gas analysis is not as representative as an arterial one, it will suffice as an initial measurement to detect severe acidosis and to determine whether or not $PaCO_2$ is near the normal range. Venous $PaCO_2$ is about 6 mm Hg higher and pH is about 0.03 units lower than in arterial blood (32).

Other aspects of infant's care that need to be closely followed are discussed in the following sections.

Hematology

Consumption of coagulation factors may complicate severe asphyxia. This is almost always a transient process rather than continuing disseminated intravascular coagulation. Thrombocytopenia is the most consistent finding. In extreme cases, clinical bleeding occurs and requires replacement of platelets and plasma clotting factors. Other hematologic changes include a transient rise in the number of granulocytes, including immature forms, and in erythroid precursors in the peripheral blood. These can rise to very high levels and could be misleading when considering diagnoses such as infection and hemolytic anemia. If the changes are secondary to asphyxia, however, they will disappear in a day or so.

Glucose

When hypoxia and acidosis have been relieved, begin a continuous infusion of 10% dextrose in water at 3 mL/kg per hour to maintain a normal concentration of blood glucose. This provides 5 mg of glucose per kg per minute. Begin screening for hyperglycemia and hypoglycemia with repeated testing of capillary blood. Hypoglycemia can be corrected by a bolus infusion of 10% dextrose (2 mL/kg over 2 to 3 minutes) and by temporarily increasing the infusion rate to 5 mL/kg per hour (8.4 mg/kg per minute), which is sufficient in all but the most extreme cases of asphyxia-induced hypoglycemia. Rapid infusions of more concentrated solutions of dextrose can be dangerous because of their hyperosmolarity and their tendency to produce serious vascular injury.

Fluid and Electrolytes

Asphyxia causes renal ischemia, which may persist after birth and resuscitation (47). Many asphyxiated infants are oliguric for the first day of life and have a rising serum creatinine (48,49). Very high serum creatinine concentrations in the first days of life, however, are not caused by renal failure but are caused by tissue necrosis after severe asphyxia. When urine output increases, there is transient hematuria and polyuria. With extreme asphyxia, corticomedullary hemorrhagic necrosis occurs and the renal failure is more severe. As renal function returns, sodium, potassium, and chloride can be added to parenteral fluids.

As acidosis is corrected, extracellular potassium shifts back into cells and postasphyxial infants with good renal function may become hypokalemic. The usual maintenance amounts of electrolytes may be adequate to maintain serum electrolyte concentrations, but in many cases renal losses of electrolytes are very high during this diuresis, so it will be necessary to administer higher concentrations of electrolytes. When planning sodium requirements, consider the sodium given as $NaHCO_3$ during resuscitation and the NaCl in catheter-flush solutions. Infants who are asphyxiated often become hypocalcemic by the first day after birth (31). Serum ionized calcium should be measured and supplemental calcium given as needed.

Gastrointestinal Function

During asphyxia, blood flow to the small and large bowel is reduced. *Severe* asphyxia may cause serious ischemic injury to these organs and gastrointestinal blood flow may remain abnormal for up to 3 days after delivery and resuscitation (47). Because of this, it may be advisable to continue intravenous fluids and delay enteral feedings for several days. Occasionally, acute necrotizing enterocolitis occurs when severely asphyxiated infants are fed in the first day or two after birth. This is particularly important in infants who also have suffered hypovolemic shock, because shock severely compromises intestinal blood flow.

Central Nervous System

Severe asphyxia can lead to hypoxic ischemic encephalopathy. Because the homeostatic responses to asphyxia tend to preserve oxygen delivery to the brain at the expense of other organs, asphyxial encephalopathy tends to occur in infants with evidence of multiorgan injury (47,49). However, there are situations in which encephalopathy appears in isolation. A significant portion of the damage to the brain is reperfusion injury, which occurs some time after recovery from asphyxia (50,51). This interval raises the potential for treatment that could prevent this portion of the injury. Several forms of therapy that might provide such neuroprotection are under investigation, but none has been shown to be effective (50). However, there are some lessons from these studies that are applicable to clinical care. Many studies point to hypocarbia as a contributor to neurologic injury (50,52). Closely monitoring $PaCO_2$ and adjusting ventilation to avoid hypocarbia has been discussed previously. There is much conflicting information about the beneficial versus the harmful effects of hyperglycemia in the asphyxiated infant. So it seems prudent to keep the blood glucose concentration in the physiologic range. Recent experimental studies have shown that moderate cerebral hypothermia initiated as soon as possible in the latent phase, before the onset of secondary injury, and continued for 48 hours or more, is associated with potent, long-lasting neuroprotection. There are several recently published and ongoing randomized clinical trials to test the safety and efficacy of whole-body hypothermia and selective head cooling (53,54). Current data suggest that whole-body cooling is feasible in term neonates, with no life-threatening adverse events, but improvements are needed to maintain stable hypothermia for prolonged periods, and its impact on long-term outcome remains to be seen (55).

DISCONTINUATION OF RESUSCITATION

Discontinuation of resuscitation in an infant with cardiorespiratory arrest should be strongly considered, and may be appropriate, if despite all the steps of resuscitation, heartbeat remains absent after 15 minutes. Current data support the position that after 10 minutes of asystole, a newborn infant is very unlikely to survive, and if it survives, is likely to have severe neurologic compromise (1,56–58). Of course, parents should have a major role in determining the care of their newly born infant and the extent of resuscitation offered. Based on the data at hand, every effort should be made to plan the resuscitation approach before delivery, with the provision that the plan may change according to the infant's condition at delivery and the infant's response to resuscitative efforts.

Situations When Noninitiation of Resuscitation is Reasonable

In recent years there has been considerable debate over the concept of the lower limit of viability and other circumstances when noninitiation of resuscitation can be recommended. Although there are still no clear answers to such a sensitive subject, noninitiation of treatment may be appropriate for infants with confirmed gestation of less than 23 weeks or a birthweight of less than 400 g, anencephaly, or confirmed trisomy 13 or 18. Present data support the position that despite resuscitation these infants are very unlikely to survive, or if they do survive, it will be with severe disability. However, in situations of uncertain prognosis, including uncertain gestational age (antenatal prediction of gestational age is variable; see Chapter 11), resuscitation options may include a trial of resuscitation, noninitiation, or discontinuation of resuscitation following assessment of the infant. If after initial assessment, there is still any doubt, full resuscitation and continuation of life support can allow time to obtain more complete clinical information and the family's viewpoint, and will allow for counseling to the family regarding continuation versus withdrawal of support. Then, if agreed on, withdrawal of support may be appropriate. In general, it is a bad idea to decide initially not to resuscitate and then, many minutes later, change the decision to aggressively resuscitate.

Continuing Supportive Care After Resuscitation

After adequate ventilation and circulation have been established, the infant may still be at risk for deterioration. Consequently, continuing close monitoring of heart rate, respiratory rate, blood pressure, arterial oxygen saturation, blood gas analysis, blood glucose, and the administered oxygen concentration may be indicated.

Monitoring Respiratory Status

During this time, the infant should be closely monitored for complications of assisted ventilation. The ET may be dislodged from the trachea and advance into the esophagus. Alternatively, the tube may advance into the right main bronchial stem, leading to nonventilation of the entire left lung and the upper lobe of the right lung. This is the most common serious complication of endotracheal intubation. Clinical suspicion may need to be confirmed by a repeat chest radiograph. Examine the abdomen for distension that may elevate the diaphragm and interfere with ventilation. This usually is a consequence of assisted ventilation via a face mask and can be relieved by an orogastric tube.

Following successful resuscitation, pulmonary function may change rapidly, leading to several complications. First, PaO_2 will rise as ventilation and perfusion become better matched and may reach levels that are dangerously high in the very premature infant. Hyperoxia is better managed initially by reducing the inspired oxygen concentration rather than by withdrawing ventilatory assistance. Second, improved ventilation may lead to acute hypocarbia, which will reduce cerebral and myocardial blood flow (59–61). Correct the hypocarbia by reducing the rate of assisted ventilation and inspiratory pressure. Figure 18-6 illustrates these changes. Third, as lung compliance increases, the ventilatory pressure that was appropriate initially will become excessive. If the excess pressure is mild, the result will be hyperventilation and hypocarbia. If it is extreme, however, there will be tamponade of the pulmonary circulation and right-to-left shunting of blood at the atrial and ductal levels and low systemic blood flow. This phenomenon is manifested by a low aortic pressure, wide fluctuations in blood pressure in phase with the positive-pressure ventilation, and arterial hypoxemia. This situation can be detected by briefly disconnecting the ET from the ventilation system. Aortic pressure will rise within 5 seconds. If this occurs, restart ventilation using lower airway pressures. The hypoxia caused by the shunting of blood from right to left will decrease quickly as the lungs are ventilated with lower pressures.

Tension pneumothorax may occur during spontaneous or assisted ventilation of any infant. A tension pneumothorax of small or moderate size may restrict ventilation and cause hypoxia and hypercarbia. Pneumothorax must be suspected whenever PaO_2 decreases despite a ventilation system that is functioning properly. Sometimes the diagnosis of pneumothorax is difficult to make by physical examination alone. Breath sounds may be unequal bilaterally, but often they are equal. The upper portion of the affected side of the chest tends to lag behind the unaffected side during inflation of the lungs. Transillumination with a cold fiberoptic light may cause the affected side to glow brightly; however, the absence of this sign does not rule out pneumothorax, particularly in the larger infant with a

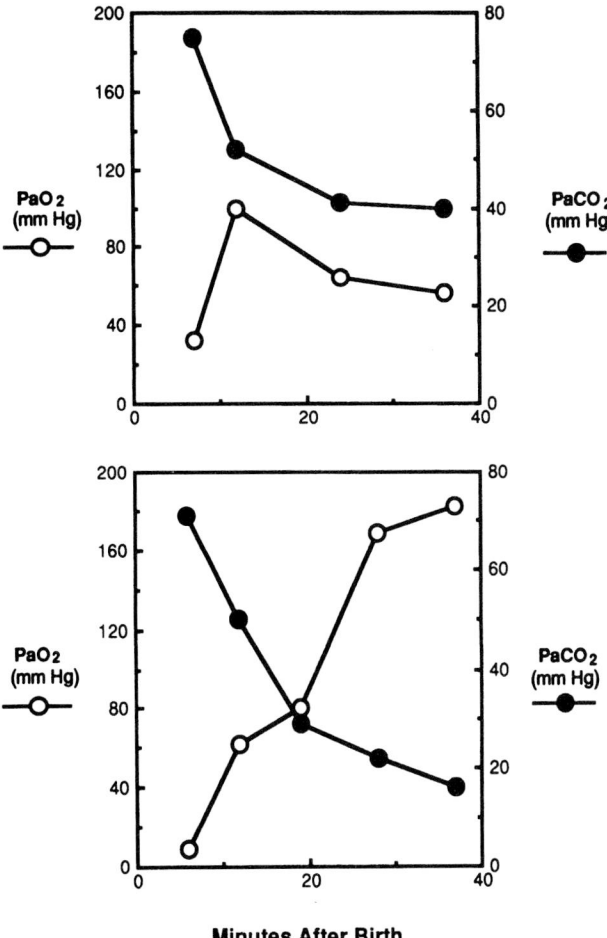

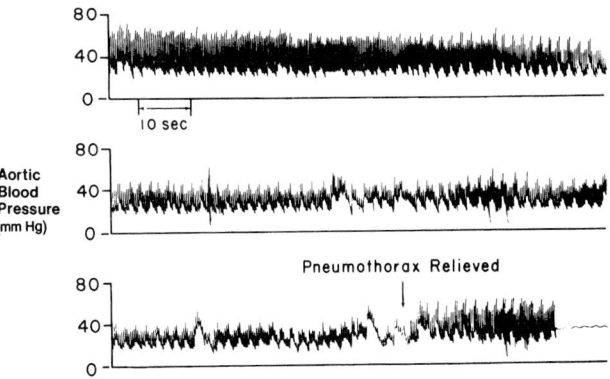

Figure 18-7 Aortic blood pressure of a premature, 1.5-kg infant at 32 gestational weeks of age during development of a tension pneumothorax. This is a continuous tracing at 2 hours of age. Because the patient's condition was rapidly worsening, as shown by hypotension, a narrow pulse pressure, and rapidly worsening, as shown hypotension, a narrow pulse pressure, and rapidly increasing cyanosis despite assisted ventilation with 100% oxygen, thoracentesis of the right pleural cavity was done (*arrow*) before radiologic confirmation of the pneumothorax was obtained. About 50 mL of air escaped when the pleural cavity was opened. The patient's color improved, and blood pressure promptly returned to normal.

Minutes After Birth

Figure 18-6 Changes in arterial blood gas tensions occurred during the resuscitation of two very-low-birth-weight infants. Each was intubated immediately after birth, and in each the umbilical artery was catheterized before 10 minutes after birth to allow frequent measurements of blood gasses. Both were hypoxic and hypercarbic at the first measurements at 6 and 7 minutes after birth. As ventilation and oxygenation improved, ventilation pressures, rates, and inspired oxygen concentration were reduced. In the baby in the *upper panel*, this led to normal blood gas tensions. In the baby in the *lower panel*, adjustments were made too slowly, leading to hyperoxia and extreme hypocarbia. $PaCO_2$, arterial carbon dioxide partial pressure; PaO_2, arterial oxygen partial pressure.

thicker chest wall. The diagnosis of pneumothorax can be made best by a chest radiograph, but this often is difficult to obtain quickly in the resuscitation area. The arterial and central venous pressures may not change with small pneumothoraces. If hypoxia and hypercarbia become severe, it may be necessary to perform a diagnostic thoracentesis with a small-gauge angiocatheter and syringe before there is time to obtain a radiograph. The situation changes when a pneumothorax is large and under tension. Venous return to the heart and cardiac output may fall precipitously to extremely low levels. If blood pressure, PaO_2, and $PaCO_2$ are being measured, this critical situation will be diagnosed easily because the onset of hypoxia and hypercarbia will be accompanied by severe hypotension rather than the hypertension of asphyxia (see Fig. 18-1) (62). This situation warrants intervention, which is as urgent as in cardiac arrest. One cannot wait for a confirmatory radiograph.

Figure 18-7 illustrates the diagnosis and successful treatment of such a case. Satisfactory decompression of a tension pneumothorax usually requires insertion of a thoracostomy tube and continuous suction applied to the tube through an underwater suction system. Aspiration with a needle and syringe usually gives only very brief relief. While assembling equipment for decompression of the pneumothorax, however, insert a 22-gauge Angiocath connected to a three-way stopcock and a 30-mL syringe. This is a convenient and relatively safe method for temporary decompression of the pneumothorax.

Pulmonary function will improve rapidly in many infants as compliance improves with absorption of lung water. Pulmonary perfusion will increase in response to a rising pH and PaO_2. On the other hand, if ischemia has caused more severe asphyxia with lung injury, there may be continued respiratory distress that is indistinguishable from early hyaline membrane disease. This will require continued ventilatory assistance. Unlike hyaline membrane disease, however, this form of respiratory failure usually begins to improve within a few hours after birth (63), whereas hyaline membrane disease as a result of immaturity of the surfactant system worsens over the first day after birth. When a fetus with immature lungs has suffered significant intrapartum asphyxia, the ensuing hyaline membrane disease generally will be more severe (64). Figure 18-8 illustrates these divergent courses of respiratory distress.

Infants with early onset hyaline membrane disease should be given exogenous surfactant as soon as the condition is apparent and the ET is in proper position with its tip above the carina. Early treatment with surfactant is more effective than treatment that has been delayed several hours (65). At this early stage in the infant's course, it often is impossible to distinguish between hyaline membrane

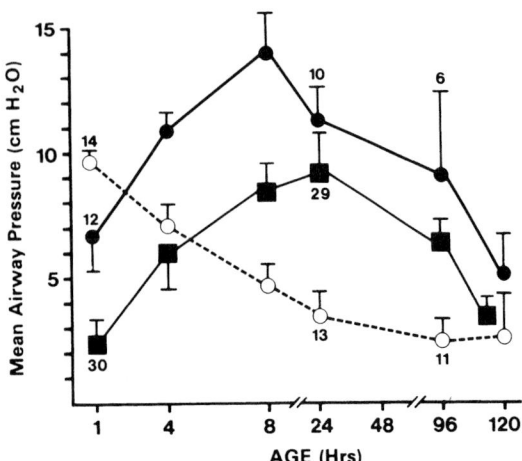

Figure 18-8 The course of respiratory distress is characterized by changes in mean airway pressure in three groups of infants: those with severe perinatal asphyxia but no hyaline membrane disease; those with perinatal asphyxia plus hyaline membrane disease; and those with no perinatal asphyxia but hyaline membrane disease. In both groups with hyaline membrane disease, the disease worsens, as indicated by the increased mean airway pressure required over the first 24 hours. Those who also had asphyxia had more severe disease. Those with severe asphyxia but no hyaline membrane disease had a completely different course, with progressive improvement over the first 24 hours of life. ○, No respiratory distress syndrome—severe acidosis; ●, respiratory distress syndrome—severe acidosis; ■, respiratory distress syndrome—mild or no acidosis. (From Thibeault DW, Hall FK, Sheehan MB, et al. Postasphyxial lung disease in newborn infants with severe perinatal acidosis. *Am J Obstet Gynecol* 1984;150:393.)

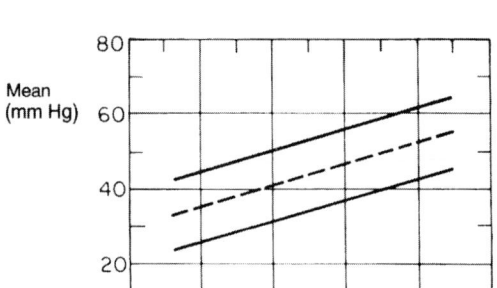

Figure 18-9 Mean aortic blood pressure was obtained from an umbilical artery catheter. The *dashed line* is the average blood pressure at each birth weight, and the *solid lines* are the 95% confidence limits of this relationship. Blood pressure values below the lower confidence line are hypotensive. (From Versmold HT, Kitterman JA, Phibbs RH, et al. Aortic blood pressure during the first twelve hours of life in infants with birth weights 610–4220 grams. *Pediatrics* 1981;67:607).

disease, postasphyxial respiratory distress, and congenital pneumonia. This is not a reason to withhold surfactant treatment, because it has virtually no adverse effects (under proper monitoring) and may be of some benefit in some infants with other pulmonary diseases (66,67).

Monitoring Circulatory Status

Asphyxia disrupts the newborn's ability to compensate for the loss of large amount of blood volume (68). However, most asphyxiated infants have a normal or greater-than-normal blood volume; only a few have a low blood volume (28). Consequently, hypovolemic shock does not develop in most asphyxiated infants. Of the few infants in whom hypovolemic shock develops in the first hours after birth, however, almost all have had intrapartum asphyxia (69). Blood volume expansion is essential for the infant who is in hypovolemic shock, but may be harmful for the asphyxiated infant who has a normal blood volume.

Because some circulatory changes caused by asphyxia may either mimic or mask hypovolemic shock, it is impossible to identify those infants who need blood volume expansion until resuscitation has produced adequate oxygenation of arterial blood and a normal $PaCO_2$. Acute hypocarbia causes systemic hypotension, and severe overventilation may reduce systemic blood flow (see above). Neither of these states requires blood volume expansion.

Signs that suggest an inadequate blood volume include low aortic pressure and a narrow and abnormal aortic wave-

form (Figs. 18-9 and 18-10), falling hematocrit, persistent metabolic acidosis, low central venous PO_2 (i.e., <30 mm Hg) after correction of arterial hypoxia, cold extremities, and delayed (i.e., >3 seconds) filling of capillaries in the skin after they have been blanched under pressure, provided that core temperature is normal. Tachycardia often is absent in the early stages of severe shock and may be present from too many other causes to be a reliably useful sign (70,71).

If some findings suggest shock but the diagnosis is uncertain it is useful to directly monitor the central venous pressure through the umbilical venous catheter with the tip positioned in the inferior vena cava or right atrium (32). Central venous pressure may be low or normal during hypovolemic shock, but it will be high with circulatory tamponade from excessive PPV, tension pneumothorax, or postasphyxial myocardiopathy. The findings of low or normal central venous pressure in combination with signs of

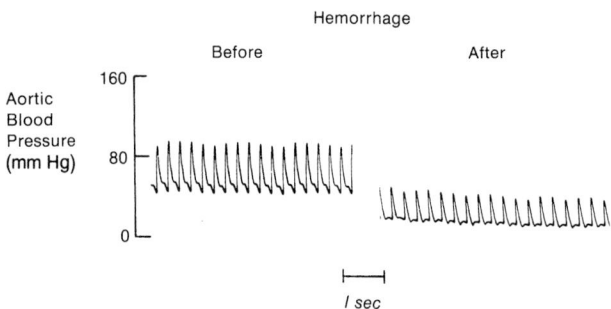

Figure 18-10 Changes in aortic blood pressure during rapid hemorrhage in a newborn lamb. Blood pressure falls and pulse pressure (i.e., systolic minus diastolic) narrows. Note the difference in waveform before and after hemorrhage. Before the hemorrhage, pressure continues to decrease after the dicrotic notch, indicating continued systemic flow during diastole. This disappears after hemorrhage, indicating little or no systemic flow during diastole. Heart rate has not yet increased but will do so later.

poor systemic perfusion support a trial of volume expansion. Low central venous oxygen content is a very sensitive, but nonspecific, indicator of increased oxygen extraction in the microcirculation in response to inadequate oxygen delivery from any cause. It is one of the earliest changes during hypovolemic shock (72).

Hypovolemic shock is best treated with repeated small infusions of whole blood that has been crossmatched against the mother before delivery and is available in the resuscitation area at birth. Group O Rh-negative blood given to newborns without crossmatching against the mother's serum occasionally has produced fatal transfusion reactions caused by incompatibility in minor blood groups and should not be used. If only packed erythrocytes are available, give equal volumes of cells and a plasma substitute, such as isotonic saline. If no erythrocytes are available, use normal saline for initial resuscitation, then give packed cells as soon as they are available. However, this is less effective than giving blood initially. The objective of therapy is prompt restoration of adequate tissue perfusion. This must be done rapidly enough to avoid the cumulatively harmful effects of prolonged underperfusion of tissues. The latter can lead to the secondary effects of shock, including increased capillary permeability and pulmonary disease, which make therapy more difficult. Excessive speed in volume replacement is also dangerous, however. Some vascular beds, such as that of the brain, vasodilate in response to

systemic hypotension. If treatment produces an abrupt rise in systemic pressure, there is not enough time for the vasculature to partially constrict, and as a result the higher pressure is transmitted to the capillaries, where it may cause capillary injury, edema, or hemorrhage. In some instances, with the initial correction of hypovolemia, systemic vasoconstriction is relieved, and pressure falls again, requiring further volume expansion provided other signs of poor perfusion persist. Occasionally, when there has been massive hemorrhage, volume may have to be replaced more rapidly. In such a case, monitor aortic pressure continuously to avoid abrupt rises in pressures. Figure 18-11 shows the course of successful treatment during the first hour of life in an infant who lost approximately 50% of his blood volume during delivery and also suffered asphyxia. Figure 18-12 shows the course in an infant in whom hypovolemia did not become evident until assisted ventilation relieved asphyxia and unmasked hypovolemia.

Transient myocardial failure of 1 to 2 days of duration can occur after asphyxia (29,73). The resulting circulatory failure is differentiated from that caused by hypovolemic shock by an elevated central venous pressure. Postasphyxial cardiomyopathy responds to a continuous infusion of dopamine with improved systemic perfusion and decreased central venous pressure. Start with a dose of 5 μg/kg per minute and increase the dose as needed to obtain adequate systemic perfusion pressures. If possible, correct hypoxia and acidosis to improve myocardial function before starting dopamine. If pulmonary vasoconstriction and hypertension coexist with systemic hypotension caused by myocardial failure, venous-to-arterial shunting of blood through the foramen ovale and ductus arteriosus often occurs. This leads

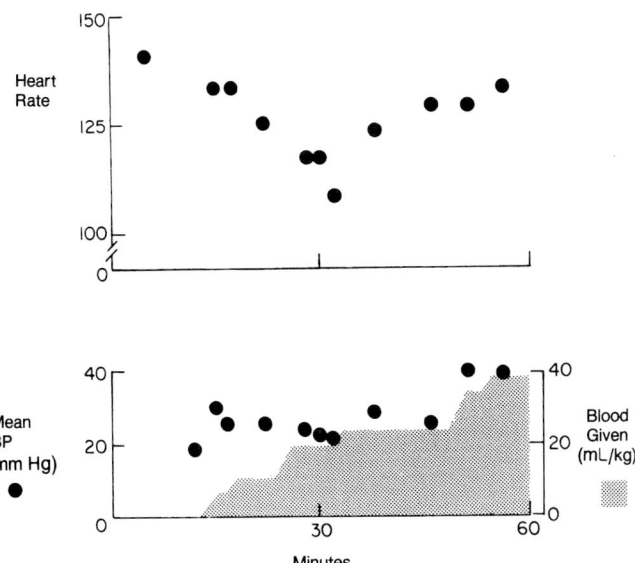

Figure 18-11 Heart rate, aortic blood pressure, and blood volume replacement were monitored during the first hour after birth in a 2.8-kg infant who suffered massive blood loss when the anteriorly placed placenta was incised deeply at cesarean section delivery. The shaded area shows the cumulative volume of whole blood given expressed as mL/kg body weight. The final volume, which produced a normal aortic blood pressure and relieved signs of poor perfusion, was 40 mL/kg: approximately one-half the total blood volume for a normal newborn infant. The blood was given as a series of small transfusions guided by the changes in blood pressure. Note that the heart rate is not elevated at first, despite the extreme hypotension, and that subsequently heart rate does not consistently change in the opposite direction of blood pressure changes.

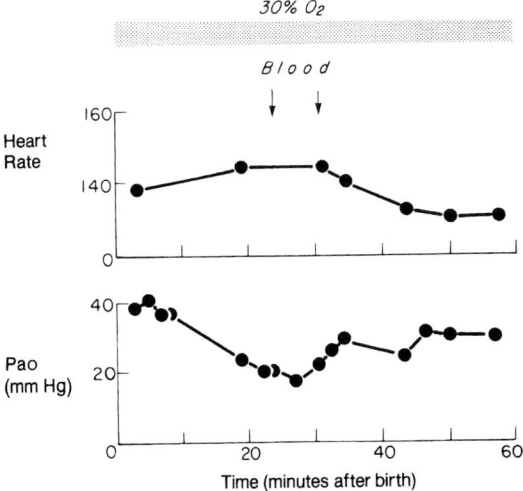

Figure 18-12 Heart rate, aortic blood pressure (Pao), and therapy were monitored during the first hour after the birth of a 1.5-kg second twin delivered by cesarean section. There had been a large abruption of the placenta. Initially, the infant was hypoxic and acidotic, and aortic pressure was normal. As blood gas tensions normalized, aortic pressure fell and the infant continued to appear pale and poorly perfused. This probably is an example of the intense vasoconstriction of asphyxia keeping blood pressure at a normal level despite a subnormal blood volume. Relief of the asphyxia allowed sufficient vasodilation to unmask the hypovolemia.

to additional systemic hypoxemia and worsening metabolic acidosis. When correcting acidosis in this situation, it is important to avoid hyperventilation, because hypocarbia constricts the coronary circulation and causes systemic hypotension (60,61). Some infants of poorly controlled diabetic mothers have a particularly severe form of cardiomyopathy. The antecedents of this cardiomyopathy are asphyxia plus hypoglycemia plus hypocalcemia, and all of these must be corrected to improve myocardial performance.

Additional Measures

These may include treatment of hypoglycemia, suspected infection, or seizures. Complete documentation of all observations, resuscitative actions, and timings of these actions is absolutely essential not only for good clinical care but also for medicolegal purposes. Postresuscitation may also be the first time to meet the family in situations where there has not been the opportunity to meet the family before delivery. The family should be informed about the infant's condition at the earliest opportunity, the resuscitative measures that have been taken, why they were necessary, and, in fact, parents should be encouraged to interact with the newly born as soon as possible.

SPECIAL PROBLEMS

Meconium-Stained Amniotic Fluid

Meconium staining of amniotic fluid occurs in 10% to 15% of all deliveries (74,75). Mature fetuses pass meconium in response to various stimuli, including asphyxia. Meconium staining diminishes with decreasing gestational age and is rare before 34 weeks of gestation, whereas it is quite common in postmature fetuses. The proportion of infants admitted to the neonatal intensive care unit (NICU) is several-fold higher among infants born through meconium-stained amniotic fluid (MSAF) than in those born through clear amniotic fluid (76,77). Furthermore, meconium-stained infants are 100-fold more likely to develop substantial respiratory distress than those born through clear amniotic fluid (78). Meconium can be aspirated into the airway by gasping, which may occur *in utero* in response to a variety of stimuli, including hypoxia, or, by inhalation after delivery. Aspiration of meconium can cause pulmonary disease both by plugging of the airways or by producing a chemical pneumonitis. Clinical pulmonary disease is more likely if meconium staining occurs before the second stage of labor, if meconium-stained fluid is thick with particulate matter, if infant is depressed at delivery, and if there is meconium below the vocal cords (76). However, a significant proportion of infants with meconium aspiration syndrome (MAS) are born through thin consistency meconium staining of amniotic fluid or are vigorous at birth (79,80).

In many instances, infants with meconium aspiration demonstrate symptoms immediately after birth. However, sometimes, infants are clinically well at birth and manifest symptoms of MAS during the first few hours after birth.

Severe disease nonetheless can develop in infants with this more gradual onset of symptoms. Pulmonary air leaks are ten times more likely to develop in infants with meconium aspiration than in infants without meconium staining; this air leak often occurs during resuscitation. Infants with meconium aspiration are at a great risk of developing hypoxemia, acidosis, hypercapnia, and the resultant persistent pulmonary hypertension of the newborn (PPHN). Approximately one-third of infants with MAS have PPHN, and two-thirds of infants with PPHN are associated with MAS (78,81).

When MSAF is identified before delivery, personnel trained in all aspects of neonatal resuscitation must be present in the delivery room. On delivery of the head, the infant's nasopharynx and nares be should be suctioned with a catheter or a bulb syringe before delivering the shoulders. Previous recommendations included that after suctioning at the perineum, suctioning via ET intubation should immediately follow if the amniotic fluid is stained with thick meconium versus thin meconium, irrespective of infant's general condition. However, no study documents the efficacy of this approach. In fact, a multicenter, prospective, randomized, controlled trial demonstrated that, regardless of the consistency of meconium, there was no increase in the incidence of respiratory distress or MAS when vigorous infants were not intubated and suctioned following delivery (80). Consequently, present recommendations include ET intubation and suctioning soon after delivery only if the infant is *nonvigorous*, that is, if the infant has depressed respirations, depressed muscle tone, and/or heart rate less than 100 bpm. To avoid initiation of breathing, vigorous stimulation and drying should be delayed until intubation and suctioning are performed in these infants. Endotracheal intubation and suctioning should be repeated until little additional meconium can be recovered or until the infant has significant bradycardia and requires positive pressure ventilation or chest compressions. Therefore, during endotracheal suctioning, a second person should monitor heart rate continuously. Furthermore, to avoid hypoxemia, free-flow oxygen should be provided throughout the suctioning procedure. Other procedures to prevent meconium aspiration such as squeezing baby's chest, chest physiotherapy, or inserting a finger in baby's mouth, which are sometimes performed, have not been rigorously tested and may actually be harmful. These procedures are not recommended, and should be strongly discouraged.

Preterm Infants

Preterm (<37 weeks' gestation) infants constitute a special group because of the special needs and problems encountered in the resuscitation of these infants. As a group premature infants make up the largest proportion of infants requiring resuscitation after delivery. The majority of infants born at less than 28 weeks' gestation require some degree of resuscitation. The immature respiratory system in these infants makes it extremely hard for them to spontaneously achieve adequate lung inflation and create an adequate FRC. As lung inflation stimulates surfactant release from the type II alveolar cells, the majority of extremely premature infants do require some ventilatory assistance beginning in the delivery room. Further, there is a large body of evidence suggesting that the pathogenesis of bronchopulmonary dysplasia begins during the first few minutes of life, with aggressive ventilation that results in volutrauma and hypocapnia (82). Therefore, initial ventilation requires special attention in the extremely preterm infant with a small lung volume and surfactant deficiency. Ventilating such lungs with very large tidal volumes even for a very brief period can do serious lung damage. In premature lambs, as few as five sustained inflations of 35 to 40 mL/kg leads to the release of proinflammatory cytokines and gross histopathologic changes (83). The large inflating breaths recommended earlier in this chapter for resuscitation of larger infants may not be appropriate for extremely premature infants. Therefore, it has been suggested that a gentler and noninvasive mode of supporting ventilation, that is, starting continuous positive airway pressure (CPAP) in the delivery room may be an effective strategy to prevent the development of bronchopulmonary dysplasia (84). However, there are no convincing data as yet to support this notion. Whether low-tidal-volume ventilation starting in the delivery room, in an attempt to avoid lung injury and hypocapnia in premature infants, could be safely delivered and whether it is as efficacious as normal-tidal-volume ventilation remains to be seen. As pulmonary function improves and these smallest infants are weaned from assisted ventilation, it is important to remember that many of them cannot maintain an adequate FRC, even in the absence of lung disease, and progressive atelectasis will gradually develop unless end-expiratory distending pressure is applied to their lungs.

As with the prevention of volutrauma, special emphasis should also be given to prevent oxygen-induced lung injury by providing the lowest level of oxygen supplementation that maintains adequate delivery of oxygen to tissues. This requires not only keeping vigilance on the oxygen concentration provided but also optimizing cardiac output and hemoglobin concentration. Continuous monitoring of oxygen saturation starting in the delivery room is likely to reduce overall oxygen exposure (85). Further, recent data suggest that resuscitation with 100% oxygen may generate oxygen free radicals that may cause tissue damage, particularly to the brain. Some clinical studies suggest that resuscitation with room air may be both effective and possibly even safer than with 100% oxygen, but no large, randomized, controlled trial has tested the efficacy of using room air versus 100% oxygen for resuscitation (86–89). Such a trial is eagerly awaited, but until then, the recommendation is to continue to use 100% oxygen for resuscitation. However, if supplemental oxygen is unavailable, and PPV is indicated, use of room air may be acceptable.

Although clinical trials have proven that surfactant therapy is effective in improving the clinical outcome of premature newborns, it is unclear whether preventive (prophylactic or delivery room administration) or therapeutic (selective or rescue administration) strategy is better. A recent meta-analysis suggests that prophylactic surfactant administration to premature infants judged to be at risk for developing respiratory distress syndrome, compared to selective use of surfactant in infants with established respiratory distress syndrome (RDS), improves clinical outcome (90). However, it remains unclear as to exactly which criteria should be used to judge "at risk" infants who require prophylactic surfactant administration. A reasonable approach is to administer surfactant to the infant delivered at less than 28 weeks' gestation born to a mother who did not receive antenatal steroids. The disadvantages of this approach include that the infant has to be intubated and a significant number of infants may not develop RDS, and would receive surfactant unnecessarily. As more and more infants are being treated with CPAP in the delivery room, it has been speculated that transient intubation of the infant solely for the purpose of surfactant administration and continuation of CPAP may a more cost-effective way of managing RDS in preterm infants (91).

Because of the relatively larger surface area-to-body mass ratio, thin permeable skin, decreased amount of subcutaneous fat, and diminished metabolic response to cold stress, premature infants are at great risk of developing hypothermia. Hypothermia, especially in extremely preterm infants, may result in adverse outcomes; therefore, during the delivery of premature infants, especially those of 28 weeks or less of gestation, preventing heat loss should be a top priority. One should take all the necessary steps to reduce heat loss, even if these infants do not initially appear to require resuscitation. The radiant heat required to maintain normal body temperature during resuscitation evaporates water from the infant's skin. This can produce very high insensible water losses from very premature infants. Once the ET and the umbilical catheter are in place and secured and other emergency procedures are completed, cover the infant with a clear plastic wrap to reduce insensible water loss. One study suggests that wrapping premature infants in polyethylene immediately after delivery prevents heat loss (92). This practice needs to be further evaluated to determine its potential value in changing the outcome of extremely preterm infants.

Furthermore, preterm infants have a very fragile network of capillaries in the germinal matrix of their brains and, therefore, are at high risk of developing intraventricular bleeds and lifelong neurodevelopmental problems. Both periventricular leukomalacia and intraventricular hemorrhage are linked to birth asphyxia, need for resuscitation, hemodynamic instability, early significant hypocarbia, and metabolic acidosis (93). To avoid the rupture blood vessels in the germinal matrix, preterm infants should be handled very gently, and too rapid administration of blood and volume expanders should be avoided.

Newborn with Airway Compromise

The management of a newborn with a compromised airway can be challenging and requires careful identification of the source of the airway obstruction. In mild situations, appropriate positioning of the infant's head and neck or provision of short-term positive pressure ventilation is all that may be needed. However, in infants with severe airway obstruction or with multiple problems, laryngeal airway, intubation (either oral or nasal) requiring fiberoptic endoscopy, or emergent tracheostomy may be required. If the problem is known prenatally, it may require a team approach involving the obstetrician, neonatologist, anesthesiologist, and otolaryngologist. In some situations, an *ex utero* intrapartum tracheloplasty (EXIT) following a planned cesarean section in which the maternal–fetal placental circulation can be prolonged for several minutes following delivery can be lifesaving. Laryngeal mask airway may be a useful temporizing device until a more definitive intervention for the compromised airway can be arranged. It is particularly helpful when tracheal visualization is impaired because of glossoptosis, macroglossia, hypoplastic mandible, or cervical immobility. However, its use requires considerable practice (94).

Newborn with a Surgical Condition

The general principles of stabilization for any infant also apply to an infant requiring surgical intervention during the initial care. These include establishment of airway patency and adequate ventilation, effective circulation, correct fluid and electrolyte balance, paying careful attention to thermoregulation, and providing appropriate antibiotic coverage. However, specific early management will depend on the underlying surgical condition. In infants with gastroschisis or omphalocele, avoidance of both direct and ischemic trauma to the eviscerated viscera by appropriate infant positioning, keeping up with the infant's excessive fluid and heat losses from the exposed viscera, and preventing infection of the exposed abdominal contents are the biggest challenges. In an infant with a suspected diaphragmatic hernia, the greatest emphasis during the initial management should be on avoiding bag and mask ventilation and immediate endotracheal intubation. Insert an orogastric tube into the stomach and aspirate its contents immediately. This reduces the risk of regurgitation and aspiration, which can occur despite the presence of an ET. This also prevents the compression on the already hypoplastic lungs in these patients. If the diagnosis is not known prenatally, a scaphoid abdomen and difficulty in achieving adequate ventilation suggest a diaphragmatic hernia. Furthermore, because invariably there is accompanying pulmonary hypertension, strategies such as sedation, paralysis, correction of acidosis, avoidance of systemic hypotension, and selective pulmonary vasodilation might be required from the outset.

Hydrops

Resuscitation and delivery room management of a newborn with hydrops fetalis pose a unique set of problems for the neonatologist. Usually, the diagnosis is known before delivery. Every effort should be made to establish the cause of hydrops before delivery to help with preparations for resuscitation at delivery. With improvements in prenatal care, hydrops because of Rh alloimmunization has considerably decreased and now hydrops because of nonimmune causes is much more frequent. More personnel are needed for resuscitation of infants with hydrops than for a routine resuscitation. Have whole blood or packed erythrocytes crossmatched against the mother in the resuscitation area, even if the hydrops is not caused by Rh disease or other alloimmune hemolysis, because many infants with nonimmune hydrops are also anemic at birth. In addition to the usual supplies for resuscitation, supplies needed for a partial exchange transfusion, thoracentesis, and paracentesis, plus tubes required for diagnostic studies must be on hand. Two umbilical vessel catheters should be connected to pressure transducers and a recorder with one channel calibrated for arterial pressures and the other for venous pressure. Blood should be obtained from the umbilical cord at birth to measure hematocrit or hemoglobin immediately.

An ultrasonography examination should be done just before delivery to assess for the presence and size of pleural effusions and ascites. On many occasions, drainage of large pleural effusions and ascites may be needed before delivery to facilitate delivery as well as to facilitate postnatal gas exchange (95). Similarly, postnatal drainage of pleural effusions and ascites is often required in the delivery room (96). Lung inflation and ventilation often are difficult in hydropic infants because the lungs are compressed by the diaphragm, which is elevated by ascites and by large pleural effusions. There is also low compliance because of excessive lung water. Resuscitation usually requires immediate endotracheal intubation and ventilation with oxygen at high pressures. If paracentesis needs to be performed because of abdominal distension due to ascites, it should be performed in the flank region to avoid puncturing a potentially large liver or spleen. Remove just enough fluid so that the abdomen becomes soft and the diaphragm moves easily upon inflation. If ventilation remains difficult and there are pleural effusions, these should be reduced to allow ventilation. Even after fluid is removed from the abdomen and chest, many of these infants continue to require high pressures to provide adequate ventilation because of excess lung water, surfactant deficiency, and in some cases of long-standing hydrops, pulmonary hypoplasia.

While the infant is being ventilated and the effusions are being reduced, catheterize the umbilical vein and artery and measure venous and arterial pressures, blood gas tensions and pH to assess the state of circulation. Anemia compromises tissue oxygenation, and anemic hydropic infants usually do not respond well to resuscitative measures until the hematocrit is at least 30% to 35% (97). Transfused blood is virtually 100% hemoglobin A, which transports oxygen much more efficiently after birth than hemoglobin F. How the anemia is corrected depends on the state of the circulation. Most infants with hydrops caused by alloimmune disease have low or normal blood volumes (98). The blood volume of infants with nonimmune hydrops of various causes is unpredictable. If intravascular pressures indicate that blood volume is adequate, do a partial exchange transfusion and keep the blood volume constant. If there is evidence of hypovolemia, infuse more blood than is withdrawn until the intravascular pressures are normal. Alternately, infuse a bolus of packed erythrocytes, as is done for the treatment of hypovolemic shock. In most cases, evidence of hypovolemia does not appear until asphyxia is relieved (97). The most common scenario is a partial exchange transfusion that keeps blood volume constant while raising the hematocrit, and then repeated small infusions of packed erythrocytes or fresh-frozen plasma to support the circulation. Fresh-frozen plasma may partially correct the coagulation defects that are often present in these infants (99). Most infants with alloimmune hydrops have very low concentrations of serum albumin and a low plasma oncotic pressure (97,100). About one-half of those with nonimmune hydrops are also hypoalbuminemic. There is no evidence, however, that albumin infusion or correction of hypoproteinemia is beneficial (96). Moreover, there is concern that giving albumin and fresh frozen plasma to these infants during resuscitation may raise plasma oncotic pressure enough to draw excessive volumes of fluid into the circulation and worsen pulmonary edema. If this occurs, appropriate adjustments to ventilatory support are needed. Pulmonary vasoconstriction is particularly common in infants with hydrops (96,101). Anticipate and promptly correct metabolic derangements such as acidosis and hypoglycemia. Surfactant deficiency and hypoplastic lungs may be associated with hydrops, and are managed accordingly. Therefore, if pulmonary perfusion does not improve during resuscitation, correction of metabolic acidosis may be required. After resuscitation is complete, there usually is pulmonary disease that requires assisted ventilation. This may be transient respiratory distress, hyaline membrane disease, pulmonary hypoplasia, or some combination of these.

Multiple Births

The three features of multiple births that complicate delivery room management are the following:

1. Increased incidence of preterm labor and delivery. This affects management only by increasing the number of personnel needed for resuscitation. The risk of intrapartum asphyxia is somewhat increased in the second-born twin.
2. Increased incidence of congenital anomalies in monozygotic multiple births.
3. Increased risk of intrauterine growth retardation because the placenta may be unevenly shared among the fetuses. This results in the usual problems associated with intrauterine growth retardation, for example, intrapartum asphyxia, polycythemia, hypoglycemia, and pulmonary hemorrhage (see Chapter 11). Twin-to-twin syndrome with the most severe form being "stuck twin syndrome."

The twin-to-twin transfusion syndrome, which occurs in at least 5% of multiple pregnancies, results from vascular anastomosis between the circulations of monozygotic twins, primarily with a monochorionic placenta. Both the degree of transfusion from one fetus to the other and the time course are quite variable and determine the clinical presentation at birth. Transfusion may have been relatively recent or may have begun in the second trimester and been long-standing at the time of birth. If the transfusion is primarily in one direction, the donor twin becomes anemic and the recipient twin polycythemic. With ongoing transfusion, the recipient grows normally while the donor becomes progressively smaller for gestational age. As the process becomes more severe, polyhydramnios develops in the recipient fetus and oligohydramnios in the donor. Ultimately, either twin may become hydropic, one from volume overload and the other from anemia. In severe cases, the donor twin may die (102).

When twins suffering from this syndrome are delivered, management during resuscitation can be extremely complicated. Findings in the mother should lead to close ultrasonographic surveillance of the fetuses and prenatal recognition of the unidirectional twin-to-twin syndrome. The polycythemic infant might need to have his or her hematocrit reduced. Management of the anemic donor is less straightforward. Recent blood loss requires the same management as in any other hypovolemic infant (see above). More often, the anemia is prolonged and severe, so the donor circulation may be compromised and may not tolerate blood volume expansion. In this situation, proper therapy is partial exchange transfusion with packed cells to raise the hematocrit to a normal level. Both arterial and central venous pressures should be monitored beginning immediately after birth to assess the circulatory status and make the correct adjustments in both hematocrit and intravascular volume. Rapidly measure hematocrit or hemoglobin in each twin and begin appropriate therapy.

In monochorionic twins, the vascular anastomoses may be multidirectional, so that the direction of flow is determined at least in part by the difference in circulatory resistance between the twins. Such twin-to-twin transfusions are not diagnosed so easily, nor are the hemoglobin measurements necessarily different at birth even when the blood volumes are.

The "stuck twin syndrome" is a poorly understood phenomenon in monochorionic twins. There is discordant growth with oligohydramnios in the growth restricted fetus and polyhydramnios in the appropriate-for-gestational-age fetus. The growth-restricted fetus becomes impacted into a small volume within the uterus. Lung growth is often restricted, which leads to pulmonary hypoplasia that is lethal, if severe. If mild, it requires positive-pressure ventilation at high pressures and rates. In some cases, there is marked myocardial dysfunction in one or both twins, which can be detected antenatally by echocardiography. Preparations for delivery are the same as for any other severe twin-to-twin transfusion syndrome.

Birth Injury

Severe birth injury and intrapartum asphyxia often occur together. The main problem for delivery room management in these infants is significant hemorrhage from the traumatized tissues, which complicates the resuscitation. The blood loss almost always is internal and, therefore, not immediately evident. Moderate blood loss can occur in fractured limbs or into the perineum in a difficult breech delivery. Sites for major blood loss include intracranial, mediastinal, and intraabdominal (e.g., ruptured spleen, hepatic subcapsular hematoma). A subgaleal hematoma can produce a massive loss of blood volume because of the extremely large potential space. Any of these hematomas can contain several hundred milliliters of blood and are particularly dangerous because they can consume large quantities of coagulation factors and lead to generalized bleeding that perpetuates the hypovolemia. In severe cases, only early and aggressive therapy can bring the situation under control. Treatment includes replacement of the lost blood volume and erythrocyte mass and, if there is depletion of clotting factors, treatment with fresh-frozen plasma, platelets, and, occasionally, cryoprecipitate.

Early detection of internal hemorrhage from birth trauma is crucial. Abdominal distention and discoloration suggest intraabdominal bleeding, which may need to be verified by abdominal ultrasonography, computed tomographic scanning, magnetic resonance imaging, or needle aspiration. Control of intraabdominal bleeding may require surgery. Intracranial hemorrhage sufficient to cause hypovolemia usually is manifested by a bulging fontanelle and can be confirmed by ultrasonography. Small intracranial hemorrhages also may cause circulatory instability through their effects on the autonomic nervous system. A mediastinal hematoma does not declare itself by the physical signs, but a chest radiograph often suggests its presence when the mediastinum is widened. If suspected, it can be diagnosed quickly by an ultrasonographic examination of the mediastinum. Early swelling of the back of the neck from a subgaleal hematoma may be hard to recognize, but an expanding subgaleal hemorrhage pushes the ears laterally and forward. This often is the earliest sign of this condition. Subgaleal hemorrhage, too, can be confirmed by ultrasonography.

Overall, remarkable progress has been made since the first publication of the neonatal resuscitation guidelines by the American Academy of Pediatrics and American Heart Association in 1985. However, many recommendations for neonatal resuscitation still are based on accepted practice rather than research data. Many of these are being questioned, and are now being rigorously tested. Undoubtedly, based on the analysis of new data, novel recommendations will emerge. Fortunately, with skillful intervention, resuscitation of a newborn infant is usually successful, in contrast to resuscitation attempts in an older child or an adult.

ACKNOWLEDGMENTS

We are extremely grateful to Nik Phou for his help in the preparation of the manuscript, and to M. Vasudeva Kamath, MD, MPH, for helpful suggestions.

REFERENCES

1. Kattwinkel J, ed. American Academy of Pediatrics/American Heart Association: Textbook of Neonatal Resusitation, 4th ed. Elk grove village, IL, American Academy of Pediatrics, American Heart Association, 2000.
2. Perlman JM, Risser R. Cardiopulmonary resuscitation in the delivery room. *Arch Pediatr Adolesc Med* 1995;149:20–25.
3. Brown MJ, Oliver RE, Ramsden CA, et al. Effects of adrenaline and spontaneous labour on the secretion and absorption of lung fluid in the fetal lamb. *J Physiol* 1983;344:137–152.
4. Wirtz HR, Dobbs LG. The effects of mechanical forces on lung function. *Respir Physiol* 2000;119:1–17.
5. Torrance S, Wittnich C. The effect of varying arterial oxygen tension on neonatal acid-base balance. *Pediatr Res* 1992;31: 112–116.
6. James LS, Weisbrot IM, Prince CE, et al. The acid-base status of human infants in relation to birth asphyxia and onset of respiration. *J Pediatr* 1958;52:379–394.
7. Yeomans ER, Hauth JC, Gilstrap LC, et al. Umbilical cord pH, PCO$_2$, and bicarbonate following uncomplicated term vaginal deliveries. *Am J Obstet Gynecol* 1985;151:798–800.
8. Goodwin TM, Belai I, Hernandez P, et al. Asphyxial complications in the term newborn with severe acidemia. *Am J Obstet Gynecol* 1992;167:1506–1512.
9. Rudolph CD, Roman C, Rudolph AM. Effect of acute umbilical cord compression on hepatic carbohydrate metabolism in the fetal lamb. *Pediatr Res* 1989;25:228–233.
10. Sapirstein A, Bonventre JV. Phospholipases A$_2$ in ischemic and toxic brain injury. *Neurochem Res* 2000;25:745–753.
11. Savman K, Blennow M, Gustafson K, et al. Cytokine response in cerebrospinal fluid after birth asphyxia. *Pediatr Res* 1998;43: 746–751.
12. Ruth V, Fyhrquist F, Clemons G, et al. Cord plasma vasopressin, erythropoietin, and hypoxanthine as indices of asphyxia at birth. *Pediatr Res* 1988;24:490–494.
13. Dawes G. *Fetal and neonatal physiology.* Chicago: Year Book, 1968.
14. Volpe JJ. *Neurology of the newborn,* 4th ed. Philadelphia: WB Saunders, 2001.
15. Cohn HE, Sacks EJ, Heymann MA, et al. Cardiovascular responses to hypokalemia and acidemia in fetal lambs. *Am J Obstet Gynecol* 1974;120:817–824.
16. Fisher DJ. Increased regional myocardial blood flows and oxygen deliveries during hypoxemia in lambs. *Pediatr Res* 1984;18:602–606.
17. Boyle DW, Hirst K, Zerbe GO, et al. Fetal hind limb oxygen consumption and blood flow during acute graded hypoxia. *Pediatr Res* 1990;28:94–100.
18. Rudolph AM, Yuan S. Response of the pulmonary vasculature of hypoxia and H$^+$ ion concentration changes. *J Clin Invest* 1966;45:339–411.
19. Parer JT. The effect of acute maternal hypoxia on fetal oxygenation and the umbilical circulation in the sheep. *Eur J Obstet Gynecol Reprod Biol* 1980;10:125–136.
20. Fisher DJ. Acidemia reduces cardiac output and left ventricular contractility in conscious lambs. *J Dev Physiol* 1986;8: 23–31.
21. Lewinsky R, Szware R, Benson L, et al. The effects of hypoxic acidemia on left ventricular end-diastolic pressure elastance in fetal sheep. *Pediatr Res* 1993;34:38–43.
22. Itskovitz J, LaGamma EF, Bristow J, et al. Cardiovascular responses to hypoxemia in sinoaortic-denervated fetal sheep. *Pediatr Res* 1991;30:381–385.
23. Jones CT, Roebuck MM, Walker DW, et al. The role of the adrenal medulla and peripheral sympathetic nerves in the physiological responses of the fetal sheep to hypoxia. *J Dev Physiol* 1988; 10:17–36.
24. Cheung CY, Brace RA. Fetal hypoxia elevates plasma atrial natriuretic factor concentration. *Am J Obstet Gynecol* 1988;159:1263–1268.
25. Fisher DJ. β-Adrenergic influence on increased myocardial oxygen consumption during hypoxemia in awake newborn lambs. *Pediatr Res* 1989;25:585–590.
26. Slotkin TA, Seidler FJ. Adrenomedullary catecholamine release in the fetus and newborn: secretory mechanisms and their role in stress and survival. *J Dev Physiol* 1988;10:1–16.

27. Perez R, Espinoza M, Riquelme R, et al. Arginine vasopressin mediates cardiovascular responses to hypoxia in fetal sheep. *Am J Physiol* 1989;256:R1011–1018.

28. Linderkamp O, Versmold HT, Messow-Zahn K, et al. The effects of intrapartum and intrauterine asphyxia on placental transfusion in premature and full-term infants. *Eur J Pediatr* 1978; 127:91–99.

29. Bucciarelli RL, Nelson RM, Egan EA, et al. Transient tricuspid insufficiency of the newborn: a form of myocardial dysfunction in stressed newborn. *Pediatrics* 1977;59:330–337.

30. D'Alecy LG, Lundy EF, Barton KJ, et al. Dextrose containing intravenous fluid impairs outcome and increases death after eight minutes of cardiac arrest and resuscitation in dogs. *Surgery* 1986;100:505–511.

31. Venkataraman PS, Tsang RC, Chen IW, et al. Pathogenesis of early neonatal hypocalcemia; studies of serum gastrin and plasma glucagon. *J Pediatr* 1987;110:599–603.

32. Kitterman JA, Phibbs RH, Tooley WH. Catheterization of umbilical vessels in newborn infants. *Pediatr Clin North Am* 1970; 17:895–912.

33. Apgar V. A proposal for a new method of evaluation of the newborn infant. *Curr Res Anesth Analg* 1953;32:260–267.

34. Sykes GS, Molloy PM, Johnson P, et al. Do Apgar scores indicate asphyxia? *Lancet* 1982;1:494–496.

35. Marrin M, Paes BA. Birth asphyxia: does the Apgar score have diagnostic value? *Obstet Gynecol* 1988;72:120–123.

36. Meyer BA, Dickinson JE, Chambers C, et al. The effect of fetal sepsis on umbilical cord blood gases. *Am J Obstet Gynecol* 1992;166:612–617.

37. Catlin EA, Carpenter MW, Brann BS, et al. The Apgar score revisited: influence of gestational age. *J Pediatr* 1986;109:865–868.

38. Milner A. The importance of ventilation to effective resuscitation in the term and preterm infant. *Semin Neonatol* 2001;6:219–224.

39. Vyas H, Milner AD, Hopkin IE, et al. Physiologic responses to prolonged and slow-rise inflation in the resuscitation of the asphyxiated newborn infant. *J Pediatr* 1981;99:635–639.

40. Lindemann R. Resuscitation of the newborn with endotracheal administration of epinephrine. *Acta Paediatr Scand* 1984;73: 210–212.

41. Ellemunter H, Simma B, Trawoger R, et al. Intraosseous lines in preterm and full term neonates. *Arch Dis Child Fetal Neonatal Ed* 1999;80:F74–F75.

42. Downing SE, Talner NS, Gardner TH. Influences of hypoxemia and acidemia on left ventricular function. *Am J Physiol* 1966; 210:1327–1334.

43. Effron MB, Guarnieri T, Frederiksen JW, et al. Effect of *tris* (hydroxymethyl) aminomethane on ischemic myocardium. *Am J Physiol* 1978;235:H167–H174.

44. Lewis AB, Heymann MA, Rudolph AM. Gestational changes in pulmonary vascular responses in fetal lambs *in utero*. *Circ Res* 1976;39:536–541.

45. Schreiber MD, Heymann MA, Soifer SJ. Increased arterial pH, not decreased PaCO$_2$, attenuates hypoxia-induced pulmonary vasoconstriction in newborn lambs. *Pediatr Res* 1986;20:113–117.

46. Wiklund L, Oquist L, Skoog G, et al. Clinical buffering of metabolic acidosis: problems and a solution. *Resuscitation* 1985;12:279–293.

47. Akinbi H, Abbasi S, Hilpert PL, et al. Gastrointestinal and renal blood flow velocity profile in neonates with birth asphyxia. *J Pediatr* 1994;125:625–627.

48. Martin-Ancel A, Garcia Alix A, Gaya F, et al. Multiple organ involvement in perinatal asphyxia. *J Pediatr* 1995;127:786–793.

49. Perlman JM, Tack ED. Renal injury in the asphyxiated newborn infant: relationship to neurologic outcome. *J Pediatr* 1988;113: 875–879.

50. Vannucci RC, Perlman J. Interventions for perinatal hypoxic-ischemic encephalopathy. *Pediatrics* 1997;100:1004–1014.

51. Fellman V, Raivio KO. Reperfusion injury as the mechanism of the brain damage after perinatal asphyxia. *Pediatr Res* 1997; 41:599–606.

52. Vannucci RC, Brucklacher RM, Vannucci SJ. Effect of carbon dioxide on cerebral metabolism during hypoxic-ischemia in the immature rat. *Pediatr Res* 1997;42:24–29.

53. Gunn AJ. Cerebral hypothermia for prevention of brain injury following perinatal asphyxia. *Curr Opin Pediatr* 2000;12(2): 111–115.

54. Shankaran S, Laptook A, Wright LL, et al. Whole body hypothermia for neonatal encephalopathy: animal observations as a basis

for a randomized controlled pilot study in term infants. *Pediatrics* 2002;110:377–385.

55. Debillon T, Daoud P, Durand P, et al. Whole-body cooling after perinatal asphyxia: a pilot study in term neonates. *Dev Med Child Neurol* 2003;45:17–23.

56. Davis DJ. How aggressive should delivery room cardiopulmonary resuscitation be for extremely low birth weight neonates? *Pediatrics* 1993;92:447–450.

57. Jain L, Ferre C, Vidyasagar D, et al. Cardiopulmonary resuscitation of apparently stillborn infants: survival and long-term outcome. *J Pediatr* 1991;118:778–782.

58. Casalaz DM, Marlow N, Speidel BD. Outcome of resuscitation following unexpected apparent stillbirth. *Arch Dis Child Fetal Neonatal Ed* 1998;78:F112–F115.

59. Patel J, Marks K, Roberts I, et al. Measurement of cerebral blood flow in infants using near infrared spectroscopy with indocyanine green. *Pediatr Res* 1998;43:34–39.

60. Kruyswijk H, Jansen BH, Muller EJ. Hyperventilation-induced coronary artery spasm. *Am Heart J* 1986;112:613–615.

61. Case RB, Felix A, Wachter M, et al. Relative effect of CO$_2$ on canine coronary vascular resistance. *Circ Res* 1978;42:410–418.

62. Ogata ES, Kitterman JA, Gregory GA, et al. Pneumothorax in the respiratory distress syndrome: incidence and effect on vital signs, blood gases, and pH. *Pediatrics* 1976;58:177–183.

63. Desmond MM, Kay JL, Megarity AL. The phases of transitional distress occurring in neonates in association with pro-longed postnatal umbilical cord pulsations. *J Pediatr* 1959;55:131–151.

64. Thibeault DW, Hall FK, Sheehan MB, et al. Post-asphyxial lung disease in newborn infants with severe perinatal acidosis. *Am J Obstet Gynecol* 1984;150:393–393.

65. The OSIRIS Collaborative Group. Early versus delayed neonatal administration of a synthetic surfactant—the judgment of OSIRIS. *Lancet* 1992;340:1363–1369.

66. Segerer H, Stevens P, Schadow B, et al. Surfactant substitution in ventilated very low birth weight infants: factors related to response types. *Pediatr Res* 1991;30(6):591–596.

67. Robertson B. New targets for surfactant replacement therapy: experimental and clinical aspects. *Arch Dis Child Fetal Neonatal Ed* 1996;75:F1–F3.

68. Simbruner G, Rudolph AM. Relationship between peripheral blood flow and blood temperatures in lambs during hypoxemia and hemorrhage. *Biol Neonate* 1982;42(1–2):31–38.

69. Paxon CL Jr. Neonatal shock in the first postnatal day. *Am J Dis Child* 1978;132:509–514.

70. Sola A, Spitzer AR, Morin FC, et al. Effects of arterial carbon dioxide tension on the newborn lamb's cardiovascular responses to rapid hemorrhage. *Pediatr Res* 1983;17:70–76.

71. Meyers RL, Paulick RP, Rudolph CD, et al. Cardiovascular responses to acute, severe hemorrhage in fetal sheep. *J Dev Physiol* 1991;15:189–197.

72. Weil MH, Rackow EC, Trevino R, et al. Difference in acid-base state between venous and arterial blood during cardiopulmonary resuscitation. *N Engl J Med* 1986;315:153–156.

73. Walther FJ, Siassi B, Ramadan NA, et al. Cardiac output in newborn infants with transient myocardial dysfunction. *J Pediatr* 1985;107:781–785.

74. Gregory GA, Gooding C, Phibbs RH, et al. Meconium aspiration in infants: a prospective study. *J Pediatr* 1974;85:848–852.

75. Wiswell TE, Tuggle JM, Turner BS. Meconium aspiration syndrome: have we made a difference? *Pediatrics* 1990;85: 715–721.

76. Anyaegbunam A, Fleischer A, Whitty J, et al. Association between umbilical artery cord pH, five-minute Apgar scores and neonatal outcome. *Gynecol Obstet Invest* 1991;32:220–223.

77. Nathan L, Leveno KJ, Carmody TJ, et al. Meconium: a 1990's perspective on an old obstetric hazard. *Obstet Gynecol* 1994; 83:329–332.

78. Fleischer A, Anyaegbunam A, Guidetti D, et al. A persistent clinical problem: profile of the term infant with significant respiratory complications. *Obstet Gynecol* 1992;79:185–190.

79. Cleary GM, Wiswell TE. Meconium-stained amniotic fluid and the meconium aspiration syndrome: an update. *Pediatr Clin North Am* 1998;45:511–529.

80. Wiswell TE, Gannon CM, Jacob J, et al. Delivery room management of the apparently vigorous meconium-stained neonate: results of the multicenter, international collaborative trial. *Pediatrics* 2000;105:1–7.

81. Abu-Osba YK. Treatment of persistent pulmonary hypertension of the newborn: update. *Arch Dis Child* 1991;66:74–77.

82. Auten RL, Vozzelli M, Clark RH. Volutrauma. What is it, and how do we avoid it? *Clin Perinatol* 2001;28:505–515.

83. Bjorklund LJ, Ingimarsson J, Curstedt T, et al. Manual ventilation with a few large breaths at birth compromises the therapeutic effect of subsequent surfactant replacement in immature lambs. *Pediatr Res* 1997;42:348–355.

84. Narendran V, Donovan EF, Hoath SB, et al. Early bubble CPAP and outcomes in ELBW preterm infants. *J Perinatol* 2003; 23:195–199.

85. Kopotic RJ, Lindner W. Assessing high-risk infants in the delivery room with pulse oximetry. *Anesth Analg* 2002;94:S31–S36.

86. Saugstad OD, Rootwelt T, Aalen O. Resuscitation of asphyxiated newborn infants with room air or oxygen: an international controlled trial: the Resair 2 study. *Pediatrics* 1998;102:e1.

87. Vento M, Asensi M, Sastre J, et al. Resuscitation with room air instead of 100% oxygen prevents oxidative stress in moderately asphyxiated term neonates. *Pediatrics* 2001;107:642–647.

88. Vento M, Asensi M, Sastre J, et al. Six years of experience with the use of room air for the resuscitation of asphyxiated newly born term infants. *Biol Neonate* 2001;79:261–267.

89. Saugstad OD, Ramji S, Irani SF, et al. Resuscitation of newborn infants with 21% or 100% oxygen: follow-up at 18 to 24 months. *Pediatrics* 2003;112:296–300.

90. Soll RF, Morley CJ. Prophylactic versus selective use of surfactant in preventing morbidity and mortality in preterm infants. *Cochrane Database Syst Rev* 2001;2:CD000510.

91. D'Angio CT, Khalak R, Stevens TP, et al. Intratracheal surfactant administration by transient intubation in infants 29–35 weeks gestation with RDS requiring CPAP decreases the likelihood of later mechanical ventilation: a randomized controlled trial. *Pediatr Res* 2003;53:A2088.

92. Vohra S, Frent G, Campbell V, et al. Effect of polyethylene skin wrapping on heat loss in very low birth weight infants at delivery: a randomized trial. *J Pediatr* 1999;134:547–551.

93. Ozdemir A, Brown MA, Morgan WJ. Markers and mediators of inflammation in neonatal lung disease. *Pediatr Pulmonol* 1997;23:292–306.

94. Lopez-Gil M, Brimacombe J, Cebrian J, et al. Laryngeal mask airway in pediatric practice: a prospective study of skill acquisition by anesthesia residents. *Anesthesiology* 1996;84:807–811.

95. Holzgreve W, Holzgreve B, Curry CJ. Nonimmune hydrops fetalis: diagnosis and Management. *Semi Perinatol* 1985;9:52–67.

96. Carlton DP, McGillivray BC, Schreiber MD. Nonimmune hydrops fetalis: a multidisciplinary approach. *Clin Perinatol* 1989;16:839–851.

97. Phibbs RH, Johnson P, Kitterman JA, et al. Cardiorespiratory status of erythroblastotic newborn infants: III. Intravascular pressures during the first hours of life. *Pediatrics* 1976;58:484–493.

98. Phibbs RH, Johnson P, Tooley WH. Cardiorespiratory status of erythroblastotic newborn infants: II. Blood volume hematocrit and serum albumin concentrations in relation to hydrops fetalis. *Pediatrics* 1974;53:13–23.

99. Hey E, Jones P. Coagulation failure in babies with rhesus isoimmunization. *Br J Haematol* 1979;42:441–454.

100. Baum JD, Harris D. Colloid osmotic pressure in erythroblastosis fetalis. *Br Med J* 1972;1:601–603.

101. Phibbs RH, Johnson P, Kitterman JA, et al. Cardiorespiratory status of erythroblastotic infants: I. Relationship of gestational age, severity of hemolytic disease and birth asphyxia to idiopathic respiratory distress syndrome and survival. *Pediatrics* 1972; 49:5–14.

102. Rehan VK, Menticoglou SM. Mechanism of visceral damage in fetofetal transfusion syndrome. *Arch Dis Child Fetal Neonatal Ed* 1995;73:F48–F50.

Physical Assessment and Classification

Michael Narvey   Mary Ann Fletcher

The approach to the newborn examination differs in several ways from that of the adult patient. It is imperative that one seizes opportunities as they arise, rather than force an unwilling infant to an assessment based on the examiner's preferred order. Such forcing often culminates in the infant crying, which although informative may render a complete examination impossible at that time. Instead, during a quiet moment, one may appreciate the heart sounds or the clarity of breath sounds. Similarly during an awake, active period, simple observation may yield a plethora of information regarding the neurologic status of the infant. In the acutely ill infant, delaying the complete examination until such time that the infant may be handled safely is prudent. Inspection, palpation, percussion, and auscultation are all important tools for examination at any age and are incorporated into the neonatal assessment. It is important to provide a thorough systematic assessment of the newborn, but flexibility must be inherent in the approach.

Antenatal ultrasound screening and more recently the evaluation of fetal abnormalities by MRI have provided physicians with the capability of preparing for the delivery of newborns with anticipated problems. For example, antenatal discovery of congenital diaphragmatic hernia allows planned delivery in a tertiary care hospital with neonatal staff present at delivery. Despite improvements in triaging of deliveries, the physical examination at birth remains a critical tool in the management of all newborns. In the above example, assessment of vital signs, work of breathing, color, and the presence of other anomalies at birth determine subsequent management, not just the diagnosis itself. In other cases, significant anomalies may be present but their impact on the newborn not appreciated until examination after birth.

Physical assessment in neonates serves to determine anatomic normality for the first time in a new life and the state of health in someone unable to describe their symptoms. A challenge is to determine which findings will be transient or are merely variations of normal and which are markers of major malformations or syndromes. Most of the clinical descriptions of specific syndromes are made of findings that become typical only after there has been sufficient growth and maturation. An example is the subtlety or absence of obvious findings in aborted fetuses or extremely premature infants with Down syndrome.

Because many of the physical signs of early disease also present as part of the normal physiologic changes occurring at birth or in the newborn period, differentiating the markers of subtle illness from transitional variations is a particular challenge in neonatal physical diagnosis. Additionally, there are unique findings that appear quite dramatic but carry little medical significance. Once the examiner has determined that findings represent a disease process, he or she then has to decide just how sick that infant is, or is likely to become. To that end, there have been devised a number of acuity of illness scores that range from the very simple to complex systems that include physiologic monitoring and laboratory values (1–5). The primary advantage of such scoring systems is in forcing a systematic and quantitative assessment that can be compared among observers and over time. Such scores have been used as indicators of mortality risk (5).

The first neonatal examination occurs immediately after birth in the assigning of Apgar scores at 1 and 5 minutes of age and every 5 minutes thereafter until the total is above 7. The scores summarize encapsulated assessments of the cardiopulmonary and neurologic systems after inspection for color, heart rate, respiratory efforts, tone, and muscle activity and assigning a value of 0, 1, or 2 for each of the five observations. Also part of this first examination is inspection for designation of gender and a cursory inspection for major anomalies. Any obvious abnormality merits more immediate evaluation, but the definitive examination in healthy infants should take place after initial transition and the first bath.

The first complete examination ordinarily occurs within the first 24 hours after birth, but if any portion of an assessment is deferred or abnormal at that time reexamination prior to discharge is warranted. For infants discharged before 48 hours after delivery, an examination should take place within 48 hours of discharge by a health professional competent in newborn assessment (6).

During the first outpatient visit, the physician should fully reevaluate the infant, especially those systems not as easily assessed immediately after birth, e.g., the eyes, and those that undergo the greatest changes during transition, e.g., the cardiovascular and hepatobiliary systems. The areas emphasized with subsequent well-baby examinations include neuromuscular and sensory development, the heart, and the hips, as well as parameters of growth including head circumference, length, and weight.

This chapter is a brief discussion of the steps for assessing the newborn infant and interpreting some of the findings. A thorough textbook on how to perform and interpret the physical examination in neonates is available (7).

NEWBORN HISTORY

It is tempting to start the physical examination of neonates before reviewing the history and available laboratory information of the mother. If a newborn is critically ill, the clinician should initiate therapy for stabilization after a cursory examination and before obtaining the complete history, but too much delay can lead to missed or partial diagnoses. Historic information is just as important for neonates as for any other patient. Even if it is more practical to examine an apparently healthy newborn before obtaining the history, a complete evaluation includes all available information. Knowledge of certain historic details may increase one's vigilance for signs of drug withdrawal in a baby born to a drug abuser, for instance. A key part is the mother's pregnancy history as well as her prior medical and social history. Other essential elements include general family history, postnatal history, and information about the placental examination.

Maternal history includes the mother's age, gravidity, parity, time and type of previous fetal losses, general fertility issues, and premature births and their outcomes; maternal illness before or during pregnancy; extent and location of prenatal care; results of any prenatal laboratory tests, especially those for hepatitis, human immunodeficiency virus (HIV), and sexually transmitted diseases; labor and delivery history including duration, assessments of fetal well-being, anesthesia, and route of delivery, drug, alcohol, and tobacco use; prescription and nonprescription medication use; and her vocation. The general family history includes current or significant past medical illnesses in other family members, including siblings; physical traits or appearance, including birth weights of other siblings; consanguinity; social information, educational levels, and vocations; and ethnic or racial background. Helpful information about the newborn period of siblings includes suc-cess in breast-feeding, infections, congenital anomalies, genetic conditions, jaundice, and other concerns. To include the postnatal course as part of the newborn history, the clinician should review events surrounding the birth and response to resuscitation, vital signs, feeding, eliminations, and behavior. If there were any complications or requirement for anything other than routine care, this information is a key part of the total neonatal history.

Placental Information

Often more overlooked than history in evaluating neonates is information about the placenta and the clues it provides about the gestational history. Several features of the placenta and cord can be readily assessed on gross examination by anyone at the time of delivery. The placenta should be examined for size, odor, color, and the number and character of fetal membranes. In the last trimester the ratio of fresh placental weight to infant weight is normally 1:6. There should be a uniform thickness and density throughout. Depressions and adherent clots or changes in firmness on the maternal surface suggest abruption or infarction. The placenta is essentially odorless except for a slight odor of fresh blood. Malodor may indicate the presence of infection although this is controversial.

The color of the fetal surface changes with gestational age (GA), but pallor or plethora suggest aberrations in fetal blood volume or hemoglobin level. Elevated bilirubin in the amniotic fluid stains the placenta bright yellow. Meconium will discolor the fetal surface greenish-brown but so too can old blood. If either meconium passage or bleeding occurred more than 1 day prior to delivery, it can be difficult to differentiate the two by gross examination.

The fetal surface should be examined for cloudiness of fetal membranes, which suggests an inflammatory reaction but not necessarily due to infection. Nodules on the amnion indicate prolonged, extreme oligohydramnios. Fetal pulmonary hypoplasia is highly probable in this setting and is a key finding in renal agenesis. Their presence suggests futility if resuscitation is underway.

In multiple gestations with a single placenta, the dividing membranes should be assessed. Membranes can be teased apart and counted: four layers indicate dichorionic placentation and two layers indicate a monochorionic placenta. With a dichorionic placenta or completely separate placentas and same gender twins, one cannot say if they are identical or fraternal from the placental examination. Monochorionicity has traditionally been viewed as pathognomonic for identical twins; however, a recent report refutes this assertion (8). Just as monozygotic twins can have separate placentas, dizygotic twins can have tightly fused placentas that appear to be one mass. If there are any remnants of vessels seen in translucent dividing membranes held to a light, there are four membrane layers. If there is only a transparent membrane with no chorionic remnants, it is likely to contain only amnion.

GESTATIONAL AGE ASSESSMENT

For standard reporting of reproductive health statistics and as a prerequisite to determining normality, all infants should be classified by GA and birth weight (6). Ultrasonography has improved the accuracy of pregnancy dating, but discrepancies in dates, physical appearance, or size require further evaluation. If there has been no prenatal care, physical assessment remains the primary clinical determinant of GA.

GA is noted in completed weeks after the onset of the last menstrual period (LMP). For example, a fetus who is 37 weeks and 2 days is in its 38th week of gestation. A term infant is any infant whose birth occurs from the beginning of the first day of week 38 through the end of the last day of week 42 after the onset of the LMP (i.e., 260 to 294 days of gestation). A preterm infant is one born before 37 completed weeks or at 36 weeks and 6 days (259 days) or less. A postterm infant is one whose birth occurs from the beginning of the first day of week 43 (i.e., after 294 days or at 42 weeks and 1 day or more). Correct classification of GA has assumed great importance when discussing the outcome of preterm infants. GAs should never be *rounded up*. For example, a preterm infant of 24 weeks and 6 days should be considered and classified as 24, not 25 weeks. Classifying infants born at term, preterm, or postterm helps to establish the level of risk for neonatal morbidity and long-term developmental problems. The terms premature and postmature often are used clinically to connote physical or physiologic findings not always correlating with GA. Postdates is an obstetric term meaning a pregnancy that has continued to any time after the expected date of confinement but is not necessarily postterm.

Assessment Techniques

Estimation of GA by physical examination is possible because there is a predictable pattern of physical changes that occur throughout gestation. The most popular score for GA assessment was originally developed in part by Saint-Anne-Dargassies (9), Amiel-Tison (10), and Dubowitz and associates (11). These systems have been applied to infants with GAs of 22 to 27 weeks despite the fact that no infants below 28 weeks were included in their development. In these very premature infants, the GA was consistently overestimated by up to 2 weeks when compared to reliable ultrasound dates. Conversely, in postterm pregnancies they tended to underestimate the age of postterm infants (12). A further modification by Ballard and associates (13), which included infants with GAs ≥26 weeks, purportedly improved reliability. However, even in infant cohorts of <1,500 g and <2,500 g, the Ballard score similarly yielded a 1- to 2-week error, being greatest at lower birth weights (14–17). A final modification produced the New Ballard Score (NBS), which claimed to improve the accuracy of age assessment to within 1 week (Fig. 19-1) (18). The strength of this study was inclusion of infants ≥20 weeks, designed to improve accuracy because of larger

numbers of extremely premature infants. However a recent study in 24- to 27-week premature infants refuted these findings, showing persistent miscalculation by up to 2 weeks (19). Some have attributed the tendency to overestimate true GA to accelerated neurologic maturity (14,18). It is likely that factors contributing to preterm birth cause stress in the developing fetus and bring about faster neurologic maturation compared to unstressed fetuses in continuing pregnancies. Using last menstrual period (LMP) or early ultrasound as the gold standard, some studies show a closer correlation between physical criteria alone and GA compared to neurologic or total Ballard score. In a multicenter study, infants who were small for their GA had consistent overestimation of their GA. (14).

Due to the inaccuracy of the NBS in extreme prematurity, one must continue to use maternal LMP and early ultrasound as the gold standard for determining GA (see Chapter 12). This becomes imperative when deciding aggressiveness of support in an infant born at 22 to 23 weeks by dates. Despite the aforementioned concerns, the NBS remains the best method available to estimate GA in the presence of uncertain dates.

Other methods for GA assessment have emerged over the years. Prior to gestation of 27 weeks, the cornea is too hazy to permit examination of intraocular structures. The vessels in the anterior vascular capsule of the lens mature in a predictable enough pattern in the last trimester to allow determination of GA with a 2-week margin of error in infants at 28 to 34 weeks of gestation. (20) The exam must be performed within the first 24 to 48 hours of life as the vessels atrophy rapidly after this time. It may prove useful when a neurologic abnormality and uncertain dates render the NBS inadequate. As well, it has been validated in infants who are small for GA, which compromises the accuracy of the NBS (21).

One final technique is the use of changes in skin reflectance during fetal development to determine GA of infants at 24 to 42 weeks of gestation (22). A reflectance spectrophotometer at a wavelength of 837 nm obtains a measurement of skin reflectance independent of melanin, yielding an estimate of GA unaltered by skin color. Initially considered for use in black infants who were thought to be more neurologically mature at birth than other ethnic groups, the requirement for special equipment and discovery that GA assessment tools were not influenced by racial differences likely prevented widespread use of this technique (23).

Accurate estimation of GA requires experience and consideration of the infant's history and overall condition at the time of scoring; for example, maternal medications or drugs and the infant's fetal position or sleep state affect the neuromuscular response in a normal infant. Significant hypertonia or hypotonia is particularly powerful in affecting the neuromotor scores but does not affect the physical maturity score. Examination as soon as possible after initial stabilization or by 12 hours increases the accuracy in gestations shorter than 28 weeks (18). The use of NBS is particularly

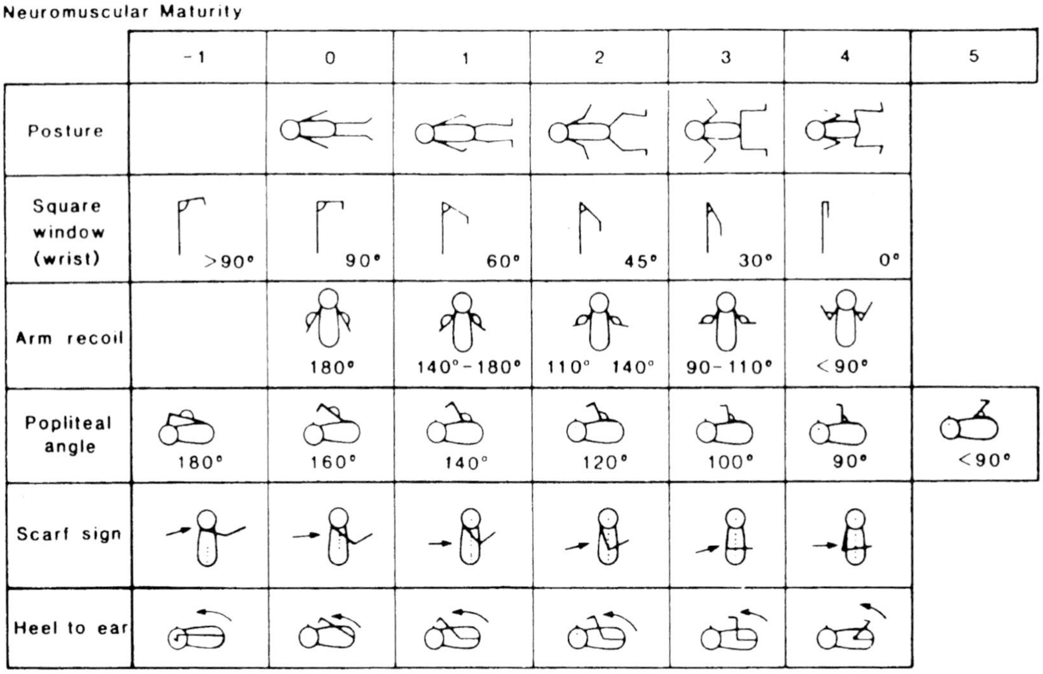

Neuromuscular Maturity

	-1	0	1	2	3	4	5
Posture							
Square window (wrist)	>90°	90°	60°	45°	30°	0°	
Arm recoil		180°	140°-180°	110° 140°	90-110°	<90°	
Popliteal angle	180°	160°	140°	120°	100°	90°	<90°
Scarf sign							
Heel to ear							

Physical Maturity

Skin	sticky friable transparent	gelatinous red, translucent	smooth pink, visible veins	superficial peeling &/or rash. few veins	cracking pale areas rare veins	parchment deep cracking no vessels	leathery cracked wrinkled
Lanugo	none	sparse	abundant	thinning	bald areas	mostly bald	
Plantar surface	heel-toe 40-50mm: -1 <40mm: -2	>50 mm no crease	faint red marks	anterior transverse crease only	creases anterior 2/3	creases over entire sole	
Breast	imperceptible	barely perceptible	flat areola no bud	stippled areola 1-2 mm bud	raised areola 3-4 mm bud	full areola 5-10 mm bud	
Eye/ear	lids fused loosely: -1 tightly: -2	lids open pinna flat stays folded	slightly curved pinna; soft; slow recoil	well-curved pinna; soft but ready recoil	formed & firm instant recoil	thick cartilage ear stiff	
Genitals, male	scrotum flat, smooth	scrotum empty faint rugae	testes in upper canal rare rugae	testes descending few rugae	testes down good rugae	testes pendulous deep rugae	
Genitals, female	clitoris prominent labia flat	prominent clitoris small labia minora	prominent clitoris enlarging minora	majora & minora equally prominent	majora large minora small	majora covers clitoris & minora	

Maturity Rating

Score	Weeks
-10	20
-5	22
0	24
5	26
10	28
15	30
20	32
25	34
30	36
35	38
40	40
45	42
50	44

Figure 19-1   Assessment of maturity by the expanded Ballard score (18).

attractive for neonates who are immature and instrumented because it does not require lifting the infant. Although described here separately from other components of the examination, the steps for assessing GA can be done as part of the general physical examination and can provide information for the neurologic evaluation. The neurologic examination of infants during the first year continues to use a number of these assessment elements (24,25).

Neuromuscular Maturity

The resting posture is that observed with the infant in a quiet unrestrained environment. Tone increases in a caudocephalad direction to a pattern of full flexion at term (Fig. 19-1).

The square window is assessed by flexing the wrist and measuring the minimal angle between the palm and flexor surface of the forearm. This angle decreases with advancing

GA. Conditions of marked intrauterine compression, such as severe oligohydramnios, increase wrist flexion. As an extremely premature newborn advances through corrected GA, he or she will not continue to develop as much wrist flexion after birth as the infant would have had he or she stayed *in utero*.

The scarf sign indicative of shoulder and superior axial tone is assessed by pulling the hand across the chest to encircle the neck as a scarf and observing the position of the elbow in relation to the midline. There is decreased range and a higher score if there is marked obesity, chest wall edema, an abnormally shortened humerus, or shoulder girdle hypertonicity. Brachial plexus injury or generalized hypotonia produces a spuriously low score.

With the infant supine and head midline, arm recoil is assessed by first flexing the elbow and holding the arm against the forearm for 2 to 5 seconds. The elbow is then fully extended and released with observation of how quickly and fully the infant resumes a flexed posture. Assessing recoil should not be done as part of testing arm traction or with forceful extension because other responses may interfere with a normal reaction. Any pathology affecting the motor strength or tone of the arm will decrease this score.

To determine the popliteal angle, one should first flex the hips with the thighs alongside the abdomen rather than over the front. With the hips held in flexion and the pelvis flat, the knee is then extended as far as possible to estimate the popliteal angle. If an infant was in frank breech presentation with legs extended, the popliteal angles would be greater than expected for age.

In the heel-to-ear maneuver, the legs are held together and pressed as far as possible toward the ears without lifting the pelvis from the table. The angle made by an arc from the back of the heel to the table decreases with maturity.

Physical Maturity

Skin in the most premature infants is gelatinous and almost transparent, allowing the abdominal vessels to be visible. It becomes opaque with maturity as it thickens and keratinizes, eventually shedding the lubricating vernix after it dries and cracks.

Lanugo, which is the fine hair evenly distributed over the body, first emerges at 19 to 20 weeks, but for a few weeks after initial emergence it is not readily apparent. Maximally apparent at 27 to 28 weeks, lanugo sheds first from the areas of greatest contact. Lanugo is distinct from the more pigmented body hair that may be quite prominent in infants of medium to dark complexion.

Assessment of the plantar surface includes measuring the foot because its length reliably corresponds to early GA. With normal muscle activity and uterine compression, creases develop in the sole, progressing from the toes toward the heel. Inappropriate sole creasing is seen in infants with serious neuromotor deficit in the lower extremities (e.g., decreased creasing or only deep vertical creasing) or with oligohydramnios (e.g., increased creasing).

The breast develops with an increase in color, stippling of the areola, and increase in the size of the breast tissue. Although the volume of the breast somewhat depends on fetal nutrition and fat deposition, areolar development with increasing GA is more consistent and independent of these factors.

Ear cartilage becomes firmer with gestation if there is no continuous, extrinsic pressure and the auricular muscles have normal anatomy and activity. Concurrently, as gestation advances, the number of ear folds increase as well. Unfusing of the eyelids can occur over several weeks, and a fused condition by itself is not a sign of extreme, nonviable immaturity. Opening starts by 22 weeks; complete unfusing is evident by at latest 28 weeks (18).

Maturity of the external genitalia is one of the more reliable individual indicators of GA (18). Due to timed descent in the third trimester, testicular progress through the canal into the scrotum is a GA marker. The testes are usually palpable high in the scrotum at 36 weeks and fully descended by 40 weeks. For the scrotum to develop fully into a pendulous, rugose, term appearance, testicular descent must occur at some time, even if the sac is empty at the time of birth.

The appearance of term female genitalia depends on fat deposition and is abnormally immature in a poorly nourished infant. The clitoris approaches term size well before 38 weeks so it is disproportionately large in premature females (26,27). The appearance of a pigmented vertical line, the linea nigra, above the pubis toward the umbilicus suggests a GA of at least 36 weeks.

Influences on Age Assessment Results

If there is a discrepancy between expected and achieved scores, factors that influence the demonstrated findings should be sought before assigning GA.

Resting posture reflects progressive flexion into the position assumed when a term fetus occupies virtually all available intrauterine space and is no longer in a freely floating state. To minimize the volume occupied, this flexion logically progresses in a caudal to cephalic sequence. Compression from oligohydramnios accelerates flexion; it gives an artificially advanced estimate of maturity. Conversely, poor fetal motor activity over a long period spuriously decreases estimated age. Fetuses with markedly decreased motor activity and polyhydramnios have decreased plantar and palmar horizontal creasing and inappropriately immature posturing. Any condition affecting the position or activity of the lower extremities, such as frank breech presentation with hyperextended knees or myelomeningocele with paresis leads to an aberrantly lowered neuromotor score. Similarly, an infant who is hypotonic from illness or sedation has less flexion than normal for true GA.

GROWTH

Measurement Techniques

Infants weighing less than 2,500 g are low birth weight (LBW) regardless of GA; very low birth weight (VLBW) refers to a weight less than 1,500 g, and extremely low birth weight (ELBW) indicates an infant weighing less than 1,000 g. Classification by these weight groups helps establish the level of risk for neonatal and long-term morbidity and mortality, particularly when the weight classification is coupled with an accurate GA (28).

Of all measurements, crown-heel length is the most subject to variability, because it depends on achieving full extension of an infant who is more naturally in flexion. This measurement is performed with the infant supine, neck neutral, leg fully extended, and ankle flexed to 90 degrees. If there is deviation from an expected norm, the first step in evaluation is to remeasure the infant for confirmation. Although not part of routine practice, a measuring board definitely improves accuracy.

When anomalies of the lower extremities make crown-heel length implausible, the crown-rump measurement may still be feasible. Crown-rump length is measured with the infant supine and the hips flexed 90 degrees. Congenital dwarfism may be classified as those with a short trunk, short legs, or both. These subtypes can be readily differentiated by the crown-rump to total length ratio. From 27 to 41 weeks of gestation the value is fairly consistent at 0.665 ± 0.027 (29). The ratio is normal if a condition causes proportional reductions in length of the upper and lower body; increased if the legs are shortened to a greater degree; and decreased if the trunk is foreshortened. Standards for separate lengths of upper and lower limbs are available (30,31).

The head circumference is the largest dimension around the head obtained with a tape placed snugly above the ears. This is the occipital frontal circumference (OFC). Head circumference undergoes a marked increase during the last trimester, averaging 25 cm at 28 weeks and 35 cm at term (32). The average head circumference is 0.5 cm greater in male compared with female neonates (33). Due to greater reliability of repeated measurements, paper rather than reusable cloth tape measures should be used (34). Minor changes in head circumference occur during the first week after birth as scalp edema and molding resolve. The molding seen after prolonged breech positioning can lead to an OFC that is as much as 2 cm higher than it will be after molding resolves.

The OFC predictably falls on the same percentile curve as the length. If the OFC differs from length by more than one quartile, the cause should be sought because head size in part reflects brain growth. The most frequent reason for a head percentile to exceed that of length is familial. In this situation the head circumference follows a persistently higher but consistent growth curve. In contrast, pathologic macrocephaly tends to cross to higher percentile curves as it progresses. A decreased rate of head growth, manifested by a flat curve or by dropping to a lower percentile, may indicate poor brain growth, atrophy, or premature suture fusion (craniosynostosis [CS]). As OFC may be normal in some forms of CS, the head width index (maximal biparietal diameter divided by the OFC) and head length index (glabella to occipital prominence divided by the OFC) may be more informative (35). For example, a patient with

scaphocephaly secondary to sagittal suture closure may have a normal OFC but have an abnormally small width index and excessive length index. Normal ranges for these indices are available (35). The fetal head circumference exceeds the abdominal circumference until 32 weeks. Between 32 and 36 weeks, the two circumferences are equivalent, and after 36 weeks the abdominal circumference normally is greater.

Interpretation of Growth Parameters

Interpretation of growth parameters requires plotting the measurements on percentile charts constructed from a similar race and environmental population. If birth weight falls between the 10th and 90th percentiles for a given GA, the infant is appropriate for gestational age (AGA); if less than the 10th percentile, the infant is small for gestational age (SGA); and if above the 90th percentile, the infant is large for gestational age (LGA). Some literature cites the 3rd and 97th percentiles as outer limits, but for most clinical purposes this broader range underselects for some at-risk infants, particularly in the lower sizes. Accuracy in GA assessment is critical in determining if a weight is appropriate. AGA infants born at term are at lowest risk for problems associated with neonatal mortality and morbidity (28).

Infants are considered symmetric if the three parameters of weight, length, and head circumference fall on the same curve. The infant is asymmetric if the parameters are on different curves, usually with the weight on a curve lower than those of the head circumference or length. If an infant has either a slowing of intrauterine growth rate documented by serial fetal sonography or a presumed slowing by very low weight for length measurements, he or she is classified as having intrauterine growth retardation (IUGR). All infants who fall below the 10th percentile for weight are both SGA and IUGR. Infants above the 10th percentile are AGA but may be IUGR if they did not achieve their expected growth potential. An infant who demonstrates a deceleration in growth from the 50th to the 20th percentile during the last trimester due to maternal hypertension is such an example.

Infants who are SGA, IUGR, or LGA are at risk for perinatal and long-term problems. Several of the problems encountered by LGA infants include the following:

Iatrogenic prematurity due to overestimation of GA by late size estimates
Increased requirement for delivery by cesarean section
Pulmonary hypertension
Shoulder dystocia
Birth injuries

Ecchymoses
   Local fat necrosis associated with forceps applications
   Cephalohematoma, skull fracture
   Brachial plexus injuries
   Paralysis of diaphragm
   Fracture of clavicle or humerus

Polycythemia
    Jaundice
    Hyperviscosity syndrome
    Seizures
    Renal vein thrombosis

Increased total blood volume
Poor feeding
Hypoglycemia

EXAMINATION

Examination Conditions

A routine neonatal examination, normally 5 to 10 minutes, should take place in a quiet, warm environment. The room's light should be bright enough to detect skin markings and color but not so bright as to discourage open eyes. When an infant is ill, attention to optimizing the environment and recognizing the potential effect of noxious nursery surroundings on his or her state is fundamental.

Even healthy infants do not tolerate handling in extended examinations. The sicker or more immature they are, the less they tolerate manipulation and environmental assaults. For all examinations, the prime consideration must be that no harm should come by the process. In routine care situations, having one or both parents present during an examination allows discussion about physical findings and offers the opportunity to point out behaviors that can help them better understand their infant. They can address directly any questions about history or therapy at that time as well.

General Assessment

The specifics of neonatal examination are discussed in the following sections. Some systems that are discussed in more detail in other chapters are given less emphasis in this chapter than they would merit in an actual examination.

Inspection

Inspection begins before making any physical contact and from enough of a distance to encompass the infant as a whole. An immediate assessment of wellness can come from simply noting the state, color, respiratory effort, posture, and spontaneous activity. Even simple observations of spontaneous movement patterns can suggest future neurologic deficits or well-being (36).

State

Important indicators of infant well-being are the states or levels of arousal the infant achieves throughout the examination and throughout the day as described by the parents or nursing staff. One categorization of states listed here was originally defined by Prechtl and Beintema (37).

Modifications have been made but are not clinically important for general assessments (38–41).

    Deep sleep
    Light sleep
    Awake, light peripheral movements
    Awake, large movements, not crying
    Awake, crying

During examination, a healthy infant should demonstrate several levels of arousal. The most useful states for assessing an infant are those of light sleep and quiet awake so irritating maneuvers are held until the conclusion of the assessment. What it takes to assist an infant in moving from one state to another or how well he or she does it without assistance is noteworthy. Because the deep sleep that follows a recent feeding may give an appearance of lethargy on arousal, knowing the feeding history and pattern is prerequisite to determining aptness of state.

Newborns spend nearly two-thirds of each day in sleep (42). Each 24-hour period involves cycling between periods of active sleep (AS) and quiet sleep (QS). These periods are also known as rapid eye movement (REM) and non-REM sleep, respectively. During AS, infants demonstrate phasic limb movements, eye movements, and irregular respirations. Breathing is typically rapid and shallow interspersed between periods of more regular respiration (43). In comparison, QS is characterized by regular respirations and the absence of eye and limb movements. As GA increases, the proportion of time spent in QS increases (44). Stress during the perinatal period may alter the proportion of time spent between AS and QS as firstborns and infants born after cesarean section spend more time in AS than babies from subsequent pregnancies or vaginal deliveries (42).

Quieting an infant may require anything from simply stopping the handling to holding and talking to him or her. The amount of time spent in unstimulated crying is normally limited in the first 24 hours but may increase significantly each day thereafter. Excessive crying that requires more than routine consoling, particularly if there are no intervals of quiet alert states, indicates abnormal irritability, but other causes include a proper response to pain or to a cold environment (45,46).

Color

Color assessment includes judging perfusion and skin color for the presence of cyanosis, (see color plate) jaundice, pallor, plethora, or any unusual pigmentation.

Respiratory Effort

The degree of respiratory effort is a primary indicator of how distressed or comfortable a newborn infant is, even if the cause of distress is not pulmonic. The examiner can observe the respiratory rate, depth of excursions, use of accessory muscles with retractions or nasal flare, any emitted sounds (e.g., grunting or wheezing), and crying pattern. Understanding the infant's pattern of respiratory

TABLE 19-1

PATTERNS OF NEONATAL RESPIRATORY EFFORT[a]

Conditions	Pattern Observed
Distal airway or lung parenchyma	Intercostal retractions, sternal retractions, flaring, tachypnea, grunts, increased work in breathing
Upper airway obstruction	Suprasternal retraction, subcostal retractions
Cardiac pattern	Tachypnea without effort, infant is quiet but not somnolent
Neurodepression	Poor effort compared with physiologic need, apnea
Metabolic acidosis of sepsis	Tachypnea, apnea, lethargy, whining, minimal retractions

[a] Early in disease process before patterns merge with multiple system involvement.

effort can suggest a specific illness and direct the examination. As the severity of a condition increases, these distinctions may be lost (Table 19-1).

Posture

The normal resting postures at different GAs are shown in Fig. 19-1. While observing neck position, the examiner looks for symmetry between the sides and compares the upper and lower extremities. If there is lateral asymmetry and the head is turned to one side, there may be an asymmetric tonic neck reflex with the extremities on the mental side in extension and those on the occipital side in flexion. In that case, the head should be turned to the opposite side to verify that the asymmetry reverses.

If the fetal presentation is nonvertex or unknown or there is asymmetry or deformation, it is helpful to assist the infant in assuming a position reflecting his or her intrauterine attitude. The physician can fold the extremities into the fetal position by applying moderate pressure to a relaxed infant's feet while gently shaking the infant's legs and by directing the arms toward the thorax through gentle pressure on the elbows.

Spontaneous Activity

The examiner should observe what the infant does in light sleep and awake states. Does the infant stretch, move all extremities equally, open and close hands, root and start sucking when something touches his or her face, and yawn with great facial expression, or does the infant lie quietly and move only in response to stimulation?

Premature infants spend more time sleeping but should have spontaneous activity and resting postures commensurate with their GA (47). Because they habituate and become disorganized and stressed quickly on handling, inspection before contact in a benign environment is important.

Vital Signs

Temperature

It is unusual for neonates to develop fevers except in response to increased environmental temperature. If an

infant's skin temperature is above 38°C and remains elevated after the environment returns to normal, a rectal temperature should be obtained. Unless the temperature has been elevated for a prolonged time, the rectal temperature is less likely to be affected by environment, and evaluation for infectious or neurologic causes is indicated (48). Recurrent or profound hypothermia also requires additional evaluation.

In a warm environment, overbundling may cause temperature elevation into the febrile range (49). The infant's postural response to hyperthermia is arm and leg extension, decreased spontaneous activity, and increased sleep duration in order to maximally dissipate heat. Conversely, hypothermic infants assume a flexed posture to conserve heat. During the first week of life, only 30% of infants born at less than 30 weeks are capable of limb extension, but by 2 weeks this number increases to 87% (50). As such, premature infants in the first week of life and hypotonic or myopathic infants are most at risk for temperature instability because they are less capable of altering position to aid heat dissipation or conservation.

Term infants in the first day of life sweat in response to overheating, but not as efficiently as in a child or adult (51). Infants less than 36 weeks, in comparison, are incapable of sweating on the first day but do so by 2 weeks of age (52). Furthermore, the minimal temperatures required to induce sweating are higher in preterm than in term infants. The first site capable of sweating is the forehead with recruitment of other sites happening in a caudal direction. Visible sweating at rest or on feeding in an afebrile infant is abnormal and may indicate distress, typically from cardiac disease.

Respiratory Rate and Heart Rate

The respiratory rate is obtained by looking at the upper abdomen for a full minute. As soon as an infant is touched, the respiratory rate and depth change. The normal respiratory rate is 30 to 60 inspirations per minute in a term infant, with lower rates occurring after the period of cardiopulmonary transition. When awake, some normal infants breathe shallowly and rapidly but are able to slow sufficiently to feed well.

The heart rate is 110 to 160 beats per minute (bpm) in healthy term infants, but it may vary significantly during deep sleep or active awake states. Preterm infants have resting heart rates at the higher end of the normal range. Tachycardia, with a rate persistently greater than 160 bpm, may be a sign of many conditions, including central nervous system (CNS) irritability, congestive heart failure, sepsis, anemia, fever, or hyperthyroidism. Conversely, low resting heart rates may be observed following mild perinatal asphyxia.

Blood Pressure

Measuring blood pressure is not a routine part of vital signs in most newborn nurseries but is used for infants requiring special care and for evaluating coarctation of the aorta. There are wide variations of normal at different GAs (53–56). The Committee on Fetus and Newborn of the American Academy of Pediatrics states that hypertension should be diagnosed only after three separate measurements (57).

The range of normal blood pressure in neonates depends on the method used for assessment and GA (see Appendix C-1 for blood pressure values). The values obtained by the blanching and flush methods are mean pressures and are lower than those registered by direct intravascular or Doppler monitoring. The flush method for obtaining mean pressure is easier in an active infant and requires only a sphygmomanometer (58). The Doppler methods, although providing diastolic and systolic pressures, require electronic equipment and a quieter patient. Two important elements for obtaining accurate blood pressure are a quiet infant and a properly sized cuff with a width two-thirds the length of the upper arm.

Facies

Assessment of facies includes looking for symmetry, size, shape, and the relations of all parts of the face and how the infant holds or uses them. A seemingly unusual facial appearance dictates analyzing the individual components to decide if the constellation represents malformation, deformation, a syndrome, or merely familial appearance.

Head and Neck

Inspection of the head includes assessment of the shape and size relative to the rest of the body, face distribution and character of the hair, and the underlying scalp.

Head circumference was discussed previously. Even when the OFC is normal, it is important to notice if the size of the head seems appropriate for the size of the face. The shape of the cranial vault reflects interaction of internal forces (i.e., brain anatomy, volume, intracranial pressure) against external forces (i.e., intrauterine and extrauterine molding, suture mobility). Normal intrauterine molding for a vertex presentation leads to a narrowed biparietal diameter and a maximal occipitomental dimension. After breech presentation, there may be marked accentuation of the occipitofrontal dimension with parietal flattening, an occipital shelf, and apparent frontal prominence. This normal breech shape requires differentiation from the abnormal occipital prominence found in posterior fossa masses (e.g., Dandy-Walker malformation), frontal prominence due to increased cranial volume, or the boat-shaped scaphocephaly from synostosis of the sagittal suture. Normal molding resolves within a few weeks, but other aberrations progress. Pathologic conditions that prevent normal molding of the fetal head should be suspected in infants who failed to engage in vertex and descend in labor. These conditions are unusual but important to detect as early as possible.

Unusual head shapes are found in approximately 10% of newborns with the most common abnormality being posterior or lateral plagiocephaly (i.e., flattening) (59). Associated risk factors are primiparity, assisted delivery, prolonged labor, and twin pregnancies (59). Right-sided flattening occurs more often than left due to the more common left occiput anterior descent during birth. It has been postulated that plagiocephaly present at birth may contribute to the development of positional plagiocephaly in infancy. Initiatives to decrease the incidence of sudden infant death syndrome through supine sleep positioning may accentuate plagiocephaly, as the infants may lay on the side of the preexisting flattening (59). Plagiocephaly and torticollis often coexist; occipital flattening with contralateral frontal prominence dictates determining range of motion for the neck. The infant's head should turn as far as the shoulder in both directions; farther if it is premature. Frontooccipital plagiocephaly may be manifested by a unilateral epicanthal fold or asymmetric positioning of the ears (60). To fully assess position, the ears should be viewed *en face* and from the top of the head.

Hair and Scalp

The hair is inspected for color, texture, distribution, and directional patterns. Although hair color may change, there should be racial concordance. For example, reddish or blond hair in a dark-skinned infant may indicate albinism. The hair color should also be fairly uniform. Random patches of white hair are familial or sporadic and inconsequential, but white forelocks with other pigment defects and anomalies are associated with deafness and retardation (61). The texture of hair at birth is relatively fine. Most of the conditions associated with abnormal textures or fragility appear some time later. With immaturity, the hair is even finer and more sparse.

The hairline may vary at the frontal margin, and normal but hirsute infants have hair well down the forehead but without synophrys (i.e., eyebrows which have grown together). The posterior hairline has a more consistent limitation, so that hair roots well below the neck creases, particularly at the lateral margins, suggest syndromes associated with short or webbed necks. Although neonatal hair initially appears quite disheveled, its growth direction normally is consistent.

In 97.5% of newborns, there is a single parietal hair whorl, located in or just to the right of the midline approximately 80% of the time (62). Nearly 90% of these whorls have a clockwise rotation. More than two, an isolated frontal or a significantly abnormally positioned whorl may be a sign of abnormal development of underlying structures. Due to hair kinkiness, whorls are identified in only 10% of black infants. Consequently, the absence of a whorl should not trigger unnecessary investigations of the CNS in this population. It is unusual for hair to be strongly upswept at the neck or forehead at birth. If there is extreme hair unruliness with multiple directions of growth, particularly with unusual facies, microcephaly, or SGA, there may be poor brain growth of early fetal onset (63). Unruliness is typical but not diagnostic of a number of genetic syndromes, including Cornelia de Lange and Down syndromes.

Superficial ecchymoses and abrasions of the scalp are common after vaginal deliveries, especially after extraction by forceps or vacuum. Incision sites for fetal scalp electrodes or blood sampling should be small and inconsequential, although some are deep enough to require closure. A small defect of the scalp, cutis aplasia, that appears coincidentally at a potential monitoring spot may be confused with an electrode lesion because it sometimes appears ecchymotic or blistered. Telangiectatic or staining lesions appear over the scalp, neck, and face, ranging from the superficial and transient flammeus nevus or stork bite to the more intense, permanent port wine stain. Scalp nodules less than 3 cm in size and covered by a port wine stain are not benign. This lesion, encircled by a long thick whorl of hair is known as the "hair collar sign." All of these nodules contain a small encephalocele and thus neuroimaging is indicated (64).

An unusual finding is scalp rugae along with a normal scalp hair pattern. The skull beneath the rugae has collapsed during fetal development and portends a very poor neurologic outcome (65).

Transillumination of the skull may detect large fluid collections, but the method has been supplanted by more precise diagnostic techniques. Transillumination remains an important adjunct to examining the chest, abdomen, and genitalia for fluid or air accumulations.

Palpation of the Head

Palpation detects motility and firmness of adjacent bones, size of the sutures, and bony or dermal defects. There are six bony plates to the cranial vault; one frontal, two parietal, two temporal, and one occipital. Normally at birth, these bones are separated by suture lines of which there are also six: metopic, sagittal, and paired coronal and lambdoid (Fig. 19-2). Depending on the extent and direction of molding, there is variable overlap in the sagittal, coronal, or lambdoid sutures. With CS, the fused sutures do not move freely when alternate sides are pressed. Primary CS implies that the suture fusion is present at birth whereas secondary CS occurs when poor brain growth culminates in premature closure of the sutures. This is an important distinction because while the neurologic outcome for primary CS is often normal, that of secondary CS is almost invariably poor. If secondary CS is present, one should evaluate the infant for other signs of thyrotoxicosis and exclude it as a cause (66). Sutures that are overlapping but not fused feel like a mountain cliff, with a drop-off from the overriding bone to the lower bone. Sutures that are fused feel more like a mountain range, with equal build-up on both sides. Growth of the skull plates is perpendicular to the suture lines. If the sutures fuse prematurely, growth is impaired, giving rise to the various forms of CS (Fig. 19-3). Isolated CS occurs in 0.6 of 1,000 live births, in a 2 to 3:1 male to female ratio, with affected sutures found to be metopic in 50%, sagittal in 28%, coronal in 16.5%, and lambdoid in 5.5% (67).

Any suture, particularly the metopic, may be normally widened in the absence of increased intracranial pressure;

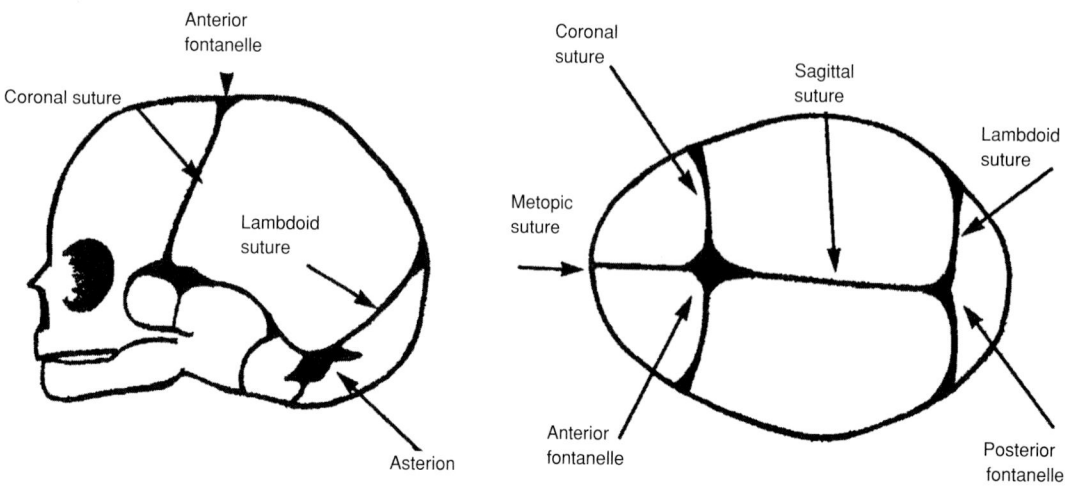

Figure 19-2 Lateral and sagittal views of the cranial sutures. (From full reference citation, with permission).

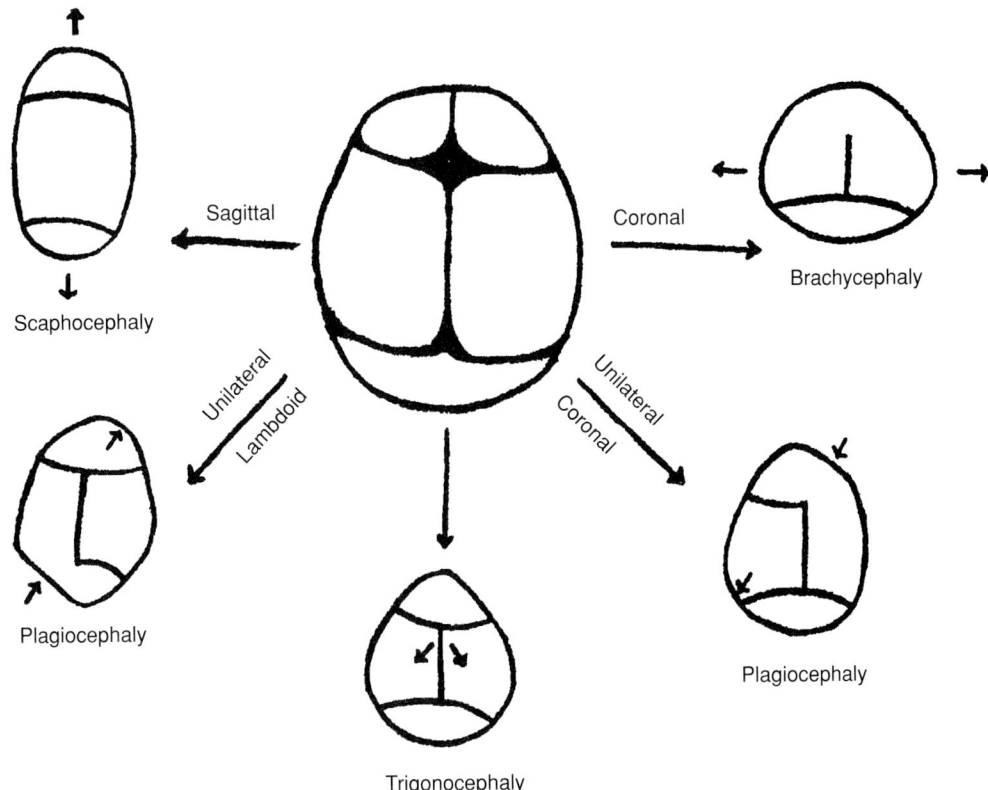

Scaphocephaly

Sagittal

Coronal

Brachycephaly

Unilateral Lambdoid

Unilateral Coronal

Plagiocephaly

Trigonocephaly

Plagiocephaly

Figure 19-3 The various forms of craniosynostosis displaying lack of growth perpendicular to the prematurely fused suture line. (From full reference citation, with permission.

the exception is a wide lambdoid suture, which ordinarily indicates increased pressure. Palpation of the bones adjacent to the sagittal suture may reveal a give and return similar to that felt when pressing on an aluminum can. These softer areas, indicating craniotabes, occur most often in premature infants or term gestations if the fetal head was compressed against the maternal bony pelvis for several weeks. Physiologic craniotabes resolves within a few weeks after birth (68). Pathologic craniotabes occurs in syphilis and rickets but may not be evident from these associations in the early neonatal period.

The fontanelles vary in size between and within race and by GA (69–72). There is little clinical application for measurements in otherwise normal infants because head growth can occur despite apparently closed fontanelles. Regardless of size, a pulsatile bulging fontanelle is a strong indicator of raised intracranial pressure. The rate of fontanelle closure is independent of gender, growth parameters, and bone age (71,73,74). Infants with a closed posterior fontanelle at birth have smaller anterior fontanelles, and those with smaller anterior fontanelles also have smaller head circumferences (72). Although aberrantly large fontanelles are seen in genetic syndromes and metabolic or endocrine diseases, they are not pathognomonic.

There are several other palpable findings on the head unique to the neonatal period. The most frequent, caput succedaneum, presents at birth with pitting edema and initially is most prominent over the presenting area. It repre-

sents fluid accumulation within and under the scalp. Although a caput initially may be limited to overlying a single bone, it will shift to dependent regions and be more apparent in crossing sutures.

Cephalohematoma is less common and rarely is present immediately upon delivery. Any nonfluctuant swelling that is palpable in the delivery suite is more likely a caput. Typically a cephalohematoma develops after delivery and expands during the first few hours as blood accumulates between the surface of a calvarial bone and its pericranial membrane (75). The cephalohematoma is rounded and discrete with boundaries limited by suture lines. There may be pitting edema if a caput overlies a cephalohematoma, but an isolated cephalohematoma feels fluctuant. Because of periosteal reflection at the margins, there is often a false sensation of underlying bony depression. The blood contained in a cephalohematoma may take several weeks to resorb and prolong neonatal jaundice. Any resolving cephalohematoma that begins to increase in size and becomes erythematous should be aspirated to rule out infection. Unless there are neurologic indicators, radiographs to look for the occasional underlying skull fracture are not indicated.

The least frequent scalp injury is a subgaleal hematoma, which may feel crepitant with less pitting and more discoloration than found in caput succedaneum. Because there is little anatomic restriction to accumulation of fluid under the aponeurosis, large amounts may redistribute and deplete total body volumes in massive subgaleal hemorrhage (76). Cephalohematomas and subgaleal hematomas occur most often after vacuum or difficult forceps extractions but may develop spontaneously even in cesarean or unassisted vaginal deliveries (77). If a subgaleal hematoma is suspected, observation for tracking of the swelling towards the nape of the neck and bluish discoloration will confirm the diagnosis. Serial measurements of OFC should be made in the first 24 hours in all cases of suspected subgaleal hemorrhage; an increasing OFC will allow for early identification and treatment of hypovolemia.

A thorough examination of the head includes auscultating for bruits over the temporal arteries and anterior fontanelle, particularly if there are conditions involving high-output cardiac failure or neuropathology.

The neck should be extended for maximal exposure to look for branchial clefts or cysts anywhere from the ear along the anterior border of the sternocleidomastoid. The isthmus of a normal thyroid is just palpable in the sternal notch on neck extension; midline enlargements rarely represent a goiter. Other congenital neck masses include cystic hygroma, lymphangioma, and cervical teratoma (78). A teratoma will usually be found in the anterior midline with extension to the right, which differs from the more exclusively midline goiter (79). Any mass may produce feeding difficulties, torticollis, and respiratory distress if airway compression is present. Finally, a firm mass in the belly of the sternocleidomastoid is a fibroma, which may cause torticollis. If present, the head tilt is to the involved side with the chin pointing away from the involved muscle.

Eyes

Examining the eyes of a neonate requires patience and a cooperative infant. Stimulating sucking or taking the infant from a supine to an upright position and rocking gently back and forth may encourage spontaneous eye opening in dim light; however, if the infant is crying inconsolably, delaying the examination is prudent. It is inadvisable to pry the infant's eyes open as doing so will usually elicit crying and result in tighter eye closure.

The emphasis of the neonatal eye examination is on the structure and appearance of the eye and its surroundings rather than assessment of visual acuity or extraocular muscles. The examination may proceed from anterior to posterior structures: eyebrows, eyelids, eyelashes, eye socket, conjunctiva, sclera, cornea, iris, and pupils.

The eyebrows are examined for symmetry and synophrys. Synophrys may raise suspicion that the infant has a syndrome such as Cornelia de Lange or others. Do the eyelids rise and fall symmetrically? Failure of one side to elevate may indicate a congenital ptosis, which may be due to several causes. A miotic pupil on the ipsilateral side suggests the presence of congenital Horner's syndrome. Absent eyelashes may be a clue to a disorder of the ectoderm and should prompt further evaluation.

Additional observations include determining the relative size, shape, and position of the eye in its socket and demonstrating if the infant appears to have vision by reacting to light. One looks for symmetry and observes whether the eyes seem to fit their sockets; they should sit neither too deeply nor too far forward. The size and shape of the socket needs to be related to the size and shape of the surrounding skull. Marked molding with depression of the forehead may make normal eyes appear to sit too far forward unless their position relative to the cheeks is considered. Standard measurements for the eyes are available (80).

Subconjunctival hemorrhages may be present following vaginal delivery. These are transient, disappearing after a few days, and related to increased intravascular pressure during delivery.

Tearing or persistent eye crusting after the first 2 days calls for evaluation for glaucoma, infection, corneal abrasion, mass lesions with obstruction of the nasolacrimal duct, or absence of the puncta. The signs of congenital glaucoma that may be noticed during the neonatal examination include photophobia, excessive tearing, cloudy cornea, or eyes that appear large (81).

The pupillary response to light requires a relatively dark room with only a moderately bright beam to avoid stimulating reflex eye closure. The pupil diameter decreases toward term as its response to light increases. Pupil reaction occurs consistently only after 32 weeks but may develop as early as 28 weeks of gestation. Pupillary reaction and size are not affected by the presence of intraventricular hemorrhage as had been previously thought (82). Pupils of term infants are anomalously dilated if their diameter is larger than 5.4 mm or anomalously constricted if smaller than 1.8 mm (83). The pupils may appear discrepant in size (anisocoria) but if more than 1 mm in diameter different, a cause should be sought (84).

Iris color is poorly defined at birth. The iris should form a continuous circle without interruptions or unusual stretching or banding. In infants less than 28 weeks of gestation, corneal cloudiness permits only a cursory inspection of the iris and pupils.

A thorough fundoscopic examination with mydriasis is not routine, but there should be an attempt to detect cloudiness, masses, or large hemorrhages. Assessment of vision is best with an alert, quiet infant, but a startle in response to a bright light flash through closed lids even with the infant asleep indicates intact optic pathways. The corneal edema normally present in the first 2 days after birth may prevent an accurate detection of a red reflex or visualization of the fundus without mydriasis. This is especially problematic in darkly pigmented eyes. The red reflex is best visualized using a direct ophthalmoscope with the widest beam of light possible, held 30 cm from the infant such that both eyes are within the field of light (85). An abnormal red reflex indicates an ocular abnormality anywhere from the cornea to the retina and warrants an urgent ophthalmologic assessment to determine its exact location.

Ears

Each ear is examined for shape, size, position, presence of a canal, and any extraneous tags or pits. The ear canal should be examined, especially in the presence of an auricular abnormality. However, the presence of vernix and debris from birth may obscure visualization of the tympanic membrane until after the first few days of life. The shape of the external ear is determined in part by intrauterine forces and by the activity of extrinsic and intrinsic auricular muscles. Abnormal formation may be a sign of neuromuscular weakness or abnormalities in auricular muscles (86,87). This is quite uncommon, with a recent estimate of 0.011% having a malformed auricle at birth (86). The length of the ear roughly approximates the vertical distance from the arch of the brow to the bottom of the nose. Ear length measurements at different GAs are available (88). Posteriorly rotated or low-set ears occur when cephalad migration and anterior rotation fail to complete. Molding or deformation from the birth process may also yield an abnormal position, but this will resolve after a few days. The position at term should be similar on both sides, with at least 30% of the pinna above a line extended between the medial canthi (89). Because a line extended between the medial and lateral canthi on one eye reflects variable slanting of the eye, it is better to use a more consistently positioned marker such as the two medial canthi.

A behavioral reaction to a standardized sound excludes only gross bilateral deficits, but it should be elicited in all neonates. Assessment of hearing by brainstem-evoked potential or otoacoustic emission is specifically indicated in infants at risk for hearing deficits, particularly those with anomalies of the head and neck, a family history of childhood deafness, very low birth weight, severe asphyxia, fetal infection, meningitis, severe jaundice, and intracranial hemorrhage. Even though congenitally acquired hearing deficits may result from anomalies, infections, or other perinatal conditions, loss may not develop for months or be detectable until behavioral audiometry is feasible. Early detection of hearing deficits may improve with the institution of universal hearing screening, which is becoming standard in many institutions worldwide.

Nose

The nose is assessed for shape, size, patency, presence of swelling over the nasolacrimal duct, size of the philtrum, and definition of the nasolabial folds. It should appear appropriately sized for the face when viewed laterally and *en face*.

Nasal deformation with asymmetry of the nares and apparent deviation occurs as part of facial compression and molding. The triangular cartilage rarely may be dislocated during delivery causing septal deviation, which is best treated by surgical relocation during the first week. With depression of the tip of the nose, a dislocated septum appears even more angled within the nares but a normal septum merely compresses. After release, a dislocated septum does not return to upright nor can it be readily molded into a normal shape (90).

Nasal patency is assessed by free passage of a small catheter through both nares and into the stomach. Air flow is detected by holding a strand of thread in front of each nostril and observing fluttering with breathing.

Congenital obstruction of the nasolacrimal duct occurs in approximately 20% of newborns, 95% of whom are symptomatic within the first month of life (91). Common signs are a large tear meniscus at the lower lid, tearing without stimulation, dried mucoid residue after a nap, or a discharge during waking. A distally obstructed nasolacrimal duct is diagnosed by pressing the finger over the lacrimal sac and sliding it along the course of the duct toward the eye to express material from the puncta. Dacryocystocele is a dilation of the lacrimal drainage system due to obstruction at both ends and filling of the enclosed space. Dacryocystoceles are observed at birth as immobile, tense, sometimes blue-gray cystic swellings no more than 1 cm in length located just below the medial canthal tendon (92).

Mouth and Throat

The shape of the mouth is a marker of fetal position and neuromotor activity. For the mouth to develop properly, there must be muscle activity of the tongue against an intact hard palate. If there is a large palatal defect so the tongue does not meet superior resistance, the mandible is more receded and small. If the hard palate is intact but the tongue inactive, the hard palate may have a high arch or have prominent lateral palatine ridges.

The more common oral findings have counterparts in neonatal dermatology and are benign (Table 19-2). The mouth should be observed with the infant at rest and crying. The shape and size of the mouth is best determined by looking at the mandible and how well it fits the maxilla. It should open at equal angles bilaterally. If the head was tilted *in utero* for an extended period just before delivery, there may be mandibular deviation causing the jaw to open at an angle. This deformation resolves spontaneously, but significant oral asymmetry causes difficulty in breast-feeding on one side compared to the other. Asymmetry on crying occurs with facial nerve paresis, in which the nasolabial folds are asymmetric, or with absence of the depressor anguli oris muscle, in which the folds are symmetric (93, 94). The side with the absent muscle feels thinner.

The tongue, buccal surface, palate, uvula, and back of the mouth should be visualized. The gums and hard palate are best assessed by palpating with a gloved finger while the strengths of the suck and gag reflex also are assessed. A bifid uvula should alert one to the presence of a submucous cleft palate.

Oral cysts in various locations may be present in up to 80% of newborns (95). One to six pairs of small benign midline cysts known as "Epstein pearls" may be present at the junction of the hard and soft palates. Other cysts may be found along the maxillary or mandibular alveolar ridges or on the buccal surfaces. These cysts are benign and often

TABLE 19-2
NEONATAL ORAL FINDINGS

Finding	White (%)	Nonwhite (%)	Comments
Palatal cysts (e.g., Bohn nodules, Epstein pearls)	73–85	65–79	Yellow-white elevated cysts 1 mm in diameter; nests of epithelial cells in the midpalatal raphe at the fusion points of the soft and hard palates
Alveolar or gingival cysts	54	40	Appear similar to palatal cysts
Alveolar lymphangioma	0	4	Blue-domed, fluid-filled cysts in posterior regions; no more than one per quadrant; may cause discomfort during feeding if cysts are large
Alveolar eruption of cysts with or without teeth	<0.1	<0.1	Clear, fluid-filled cysts; mandibular central incisor; rates range from 1:2,500 in Hong Kong to 1:3,392 in Canada
Leukoedema	11	43	Filmy, white hue of mucosa, nonblanching; of no significance compared with thrush
Median alveolar notch	16	26	Reduces when teeth erupt or persists as notch between central incisors
Ankyloglossia	~2	~2	Male to female ratio of 3:1; lingual frenum prevents protrusion of tongue, extends to papillated surface of tongue, or causes fissure in tip
Commissural lip pits	1	3	Blind-ended pits at corners of mouth; autosomally dominant; associated with preauricular pits; medial pits more syndromic
Thrush			Adherent white plaques on tongue and buccal and palatal surfaces; will scrape off; caused by *Candida* sp.
Bifid uvula	<1	<1	Associated with submucous cleft palate
Ranula	≪1	≪1	Cyst of sublingual salivary gland
Epulis	≪1	≪1	Large, pedunculated cyst of incisor region

Data from refs. 120–125.

resolve by 3 months of age. Epstein pearls are always found in the midline except when there is a submucous cleft, in which case they appear as paired cysts along either side of the median raphe (95).

Natal teeth, often in pairs, may be found most commonly along the mandibular alveolar ridge. These fairly mobile teeth are present in 1:2,000 to 3,000 live births and are often removed due to concerns of aspiration (96). Despite the probable low risk of aspiration, removal should be considered due to ulceration of the ventral surface of the tongue, which may occur if they are retained (97).

A prominent tight frenulum (ankyloglossia or "tongue tie") has been cited as causing poor latch and nipple pain during breast-feeding. While prophylactic frenuloplasty cannot be advocated, it may be considered for the infant with severe persistent feeding problems or nipple pain unresponsive to usual therapeutic interventions (98).

Other abnormalities involving the tongue include one that is too large, preventing mouth closure, and tongue protrusion because of low oral-facial tone or small oral cavity.

Skin and Lymph Nodes

The skin is assessed for general color, presence of any extra markings or rashes, texture, turgor, edema or areas of induration, thickness of underlying fat, and maturity. Icterus progresses in a cephalocaudal pattern and is best appreciated in natural light. Detection may be improved by gently blanching the skin to remove the blood from the dermal capillaries. Levels requiring phototherapy are seldom attained if icterus is not present past the nipple line (99).

The distribution and types of pigmentation should also be noted. Areas of hypo- or hyperpigmentation such as café au lait spots are important to document as they may be associated with neurologic disorders.

A common finding is the presence of a line of demarcation with pallor above and deep erythema in the dependent area below (harlequin color change). Another frequent skin pattern is marbling of the extremities from vasoconstriction (cutis marmorata) occurring when the infant undergoes hypothermic stress.

If any mark on the skin is to be considered to be a "birth mark," there is rarely an infant born without several. In view of the many variations of normal and the important signs of other diseases or syndromes that are manifested on the skin, understanding the common physical findings of the neonatal skin is fundamental.

Lymph nodes are palpable in more than one-third of all neonates, most commonly in the inguinal region and independent of perinatal history. These nodes, from 3 to 12 mm in diameter, tend to persist (100). A benign node commonly palpable in the femoral triangle serves as a reliable landmark for finding the femoral pulse adjacent to it.

The most frequent, abnormal congenital lymphatic masses are cystic hygroma or cystic lymphangiomas, which are soft, compressible, and often poorly defined masses in almost any part of the body, but commonly in the head, neck, abdomen, and axilla. If markedly distended, the hygroma may transilluminate. Ultrasonography reveals their cystic anatomy. A discussion on the congenital abnormalities of the lymphatic system is available (101).

Chest and Abdomen

Size and Symmetry

In term neonates, the chest circumference is 1 to 2 cm less than the head circumference; it is relatively smaller with lower GA. The thorax is normally symmetric and wider than its anteroposterior dimension. The ribs are compliant, and their shape is easily impacted by external and internal form. Compression from the infant's own arm or a twin's body part may lead to marked asymmetry in thoracic shape and pattern on inspiration. By encouraging the infant to assume the fetal position, the cause of a chest deformation may become apparent.

The abdomen is mildly protuberant compared with the chest. It should be softly rounded, with a diameter slightly greater above than below the umbilicus. The abdominothoracic relation is reversed in diaphragmatic defects, with herniation of abdominal contents into the thorax leaving a scaphoid abdomen. Diastasis recti, a separation between the rectus abdominus muscles, is a normal finding during the newborn exam. Supraumbilical fullness is increased in the presence of duodenal atresia with gastric distension or hepatomegaly, and infraumbilical fullness is increased with distension of the urinary bladder or in severe cases of IUGR with an abnormally small liver. Any significant abdominal visceral enlargement causes distension, as does forced depression of the diaphragm.

Retractions

Mild subcostal and intercostal retractions are common even in healthy neonates because of their compliant chest walls. Suprasternal retractions, indicating proximal airway resistance, are normally less pronounced; supraclavicular retractions are never normal. In conditions notable for loss of lung volume and poor compliance, respiratory movements may become paradoxical (i.e., seesaw) with a collapse of the chest wall on inspiration as the abdominal wall expands. With air trapping and increased thoracic volume, there is an increase in the anteroposterior dimension and abdominal distension as the diaphragm is pushed down.

Because the diaphragm is the primary muscle of breathing with little contribution by accessory muscles, quiet breathing is abdominal, with only mild but equal subcostal retractions. The umbilical stump moves caudally in the midline with each contraction of the diaphragm. In the absence of abdominal abnormalities, any lateral deviation of the umbilicus with inspiration suggests a diaphragmatic paresis with the deviation toward the nonfunctioning side

(102). This belly dancer sign is lost during mechanical ventilation. Albeit rare, neonatal diaphragmatic paresis occurs most often with brachial plexus injuries, and it should be considered if an arm is weak.

Auscultation of Breath Sounds

Neonatal lung sounds are relatively more bronchial than vesicular because of better transmission of large airway sounds across a small chest. Changes in the pitch of bronchial sounds from one side to the other or between regions most likely represent main stem or conducting bronchial narrowing. The coarse crackle of a distal airway opening is particularly common in neonates in whom there is a natural tendency in many conditions for microatelectasis. If heard at the end of inspiration, adventitial sounds represent more distal disease compared with those in beginning inspiration, which usually represent conducting airway secretions. A characteristic sound of crushing styrofoam or walking on dry snow signals pulmonary interstitial emphysema.

Locating abnormal sounds requires listening carefully bilaterally. Breath sounds should be symmetric when auscultating right and left corresponding regions of the chest. If they are not, air leaks or fluid collections or consolidations may be present and the cause should be identified. If bowel sounds are heard, the examiner should differentiate direct transmission from herniated contents or referred abdominal sounds.

If there is stridor or wheezing, auscultation of the nose or throat may reveal a site of extrathoracic obstruction. Because there must be sufficient air flow to cause stridor or wheezing in the first place, stimulating the infant may accentuate an obstruction. If an endotracheal tube is in place and an air leak is present, a whistling sound corresponding to ventilator breaths may be evident in the periphery of the lung fields but is loudest over the upper trachea or outside the mouth.

Clavicles

Clavicular fracture is the most common form of birth trauma. If carefully sought by radiographs or repeated examinations, clavicular fractures are found in at least 1.7% to 2.9% of term deliveries and more frequently on the right side (103). These fractures most commonly occur in pregnancies complicated by macrosomia, shoulder dystocia, or operative vaginal delivery. Most clavicular fractures are asymptomatic and are incidental findings on a chest radiographs. When symptomatic, the most frequent findings are swelling from hematoma, crepitations, asymmetrical bone contour, and crying with passive movement. There may be an associated brachial plexus injury or pseudoparesis, with poor movement in the affected arm and an asymmetric Moro reflex. As well, an infant may not be willing to breast-feed on one side because of discomfort with positioning. Standing at the foot of the infant, the examiner feels each clavicle, compares ease of outlining the distinct borders of the bones, and assesses tenderness, swelling, or crepitation. Finally, the clavicles may be hypoplastic or absent as in cleidocraniodysostosis. If they are absent, the shoulders may be made almost to touch in the anterior midline.

Nipples

The breasts of term infants vary in diameter from 0.5 cm to several centimeters, with clinically insignificant differences between genders. The internipple distance varies with GA and body weight, but its relation to chest circumference is more constant. If the internipple distance divided by the chest circumference is greater than 0.28 cm, the space is more than 2 standard deviations above the mean regardless of body size (104). Larger breasts, influenced by maternal hormones, may secrete a thin, milky substance (i.e., "witches' milk") for a few days or weeks. Although the degree of enlargement may not be the same in both breasts, they should never be hot, red, or notably tender. Unless there are specific signs of inflammation, enlarged breasts should be left alone.

Supernumerary nipples occur in 1.2% to 1.6% of darkly pigmented infants but are more unusual in lightly pigmented infants. These supernumerary nipples, seen in the milk line below and lateral to the true breast, are rudimentary, occasionally only distinguishable because of the presence of a small pigmented mark or dimple. Speculation that infants with supernumerary nipples have a higher incidence of renal and urinary tract malformations has been refuted (105).

Umbilicus

The umbilicus normally is positioned approximately halfway between the xiphoid and pubis. A caudally placed insertion occurs in conditions of caudal regression or underdeveloped lower body segment. The neonatal appearance of the umbilicus does not indicate what the adult appearance will be because most are relatively protuberant with redundant skin.

The umbilical cord is assessed for appearance, length and diameter, number of vessels, and insertion site. The cord is a uniform ivory color ranging in length from 30 to 100 cm; a shorter cord suggests decreased fetal movement and a reason for fetal distress, failed descent, or avulsion. Deep green staining of the cord is a sign of prior fetal distress reflecting the passage of meconium at least several hours prior to delivery. Superficial staining reflects very recent passage of meconium. Longer cords are more likely to result in fetal entanglement or prolapse. At term, the cord diameter is an average of 1.5 cm and is relatively uniform throughout its length, without strictures. If the base of the umbilical cord itself is especially broad or remains fluctuant after vascular pulsations have stopped, there may be a herniation of abdominal contents into the cord.

At birth, the presence of two arteries and a single vein should be identified. Single umbilical arteries occur in approximately 1% of pregnancies with nearly 10% of iden-

tified cases having another congenital malformation. A thin cord with a paucity of Wharton's jelly is present in neonates with IUGR and may be compressed more easily by fetal parts. As the cord dries, it should remain odorless. The base should not appear red or indurated. After the cord falls off, the umbilicus should be examined for granuloma or continued leakage through a patent urachus.

Palpation of Abdomen

The infant tolerates palpation of the abdomen best when the organs are brought to the examining hand rather than the fingertips pushing into the abdomen and probing for the organs. Standing at the right side of the infant, with the left hand lifting the legs and raising the pelvis slightly off the mattress to relax the abdominal muscles, the examiner can keep the right hand flat and use the fingerpads rather than fingertips to palpate the abdominal organs. Palpation should start below the umbilicus on both sides and proceed toward the diaphragm. In some instances, it is helpful to palpate the abdomen with the infant in the decubitus or prone position, allowing the contents to fall toward the hand rather than being pushed away (106). Palpation of the abdomen in ill neonates increases centrally measured blood pressure by as much as 25% above baseline (107). The liver is normally palpable 3.0 ± 0.7 cm below the costal margin in the midclavicular line and across the midline as a left lobe that is distinguishable from the spleen, which is felt more laterally (108). Finding a left lobe larger than the right may reflect situs inversus. A liver edge that is palpable greater than 4.4 cm below the costal margin is indicative of hepatomegaly although hyperinflated lungs may falsely give this impression (108). Assessing the liver span in this circumstance will provide a better assessment of liver size (109). By 34 weeks, the normal liver span, determined by percussing the upper and lower margins, is at least 6 cm in the midclavicular line (110). An exception to this is infants who are SGA in whom the span may be up to 1 cm less (110). An effective technique to outline the margins of the liver or any solid abdominal mass is to scratch lightly across the skin surface while auscultating with the diaphragm of the stethoscope held over the mass. The pitch elevates when the stroking overlies the solid mass or liver.

The normal edge of the liver is thin and soft, and the hepatic surface is smooth. A full or firm edge commonly represents a marked increase in total blood volume, increased extramedullary hematopoiesis, chronic infection, early cirrhosis, or an infiltrative process. Hepatomegaly is a late and inconsistent finding in cardiac failure. Cardiac pulsations in the liver occur in right-sided obstructive cardiac lesions, but these hepatic pulsations should be differentiated from a normally transmitted cardiac impulse or respiratory excursions. In the first 24 to 48 hours after birth, the liver often decreases markedly in size, probably reflecting redistribution of circulating blood volume.

Although the spleen is often not palpable in the newborn period, an attempt should be made to palpate it. Beginning in the right lower quadrant, one gently palpates with the right hand in a direction cephalad and to the left side of the abdomen until the fingers come to rest under the left subcostal margin. Successful palpation may be achieved by placing the left hand under the left posterior subcostal margin and applying gentle anterior pressure to bring the spleen forward. If this maneuver is not fruitful, then positioning in the right lateral decubitus may displace the spleen in an anteriomedial direction, allowing for easier palpation.

The kidneys are palpable if the abdomen is soft, and they are moderately firm and rounded. It is often easier to palpate the right kidney as it is displaced more caudally than the left by the liver. An enlarged ureter simulates a filled segment of large bowel, although it is less mobile. A fullness in the lower abdomen may be a distended bladder in an infant with infrequent voiding.

An infant reveals abdominal tenderness by a grimace, cry, or drawing up of the legs on light palpation. True guarding is unusual. Rebound tenderness is difficult to detect, and infants with significant peritoneal disease are often too obtunded to show a reliable response. The presence of localized edema or discoloration of the abdominal wall is an important indicator of intraperitoneal disease. An unusual exception is ecchymosis caused by leaking of an umbilical vessel or urine edema from a patent urachus leaking into the subcutaneous space above the peritoneum. In either case, the dramatic findings are limited to the abdominal wall below the umbilicus. A thin abdominal wall allows transillumination of fluid- or gas-filled masses to outline their position and size. Meconium-filled bowel loops do not transilluminate, but stomach or bowel distended with air, hydronephrotic kidneys, or a distended bladder will. A transillumination pattern that shifts with patient rotation suggests free air.

Auscultation of the abdomen includes listening for pitch and activity of bowel sounds and for bruits. Infants normally have relatively inactive bowel sounds on their first day of life or if they are extremely premature and not fed for several days or weeks. Even in infants with clinical ileus, bowel sounds tend to persist to some extent; however, a true absence of bowel sounds is always significant. Detecting changes in the pattern of bowel sounds is more helpful than the findings of a single examination. Auscultation may reveal the presence of a bruit over the liver, indicating an arteriovenous fistula, or over the kidneys in the presence of renal artery stenosis.

Cardiovascular System

The changes that occur in the cardiovascular system during the neonatal period complicate the cardiac examination until the pulmonary and systemic pressures reverse their fetal associations, all communications have closed, and the left ventricle becomes predominant. The role for most clinicians in the newborn examination is not to determine precisely what the cardiac anatomy is but to rule out cardiac disease as part of a routine newborn examination, and in a symptomatic infant, to determine if the cause of the symptoms is cardiac.

The physician must determine the urgency of the condition by asking some basic questions. Is this a cardiac disease that could be fatal if not immediately diagnosed and treated (e.g., ductal-dependent lesions, cyanotic heart disease)? Is its presence aggravating or relieving other conditions (e.g., patent ductus arteriosus [PDA] in the presence of lung disease or pulmonary hypertension)? Is this something that requires following the patient and potential future intervention but is not emergent and should not interfere with newborn and parental adjustment (e.g., mild pulmonic stenosis or a small septal defect)?

Palpation of the chest may be informative in several ways. The position of the point of maximal impulse (PMI) may be displaced downward and laterally from its common location in the fourth or fifth intercostal space in the midclavicular line. This finding suggests cardiac enlargement, which should be followed by palpation at the lower edge of the xiphoid. A strong impulse in this location is indicative of significant right ventricular enlargement, which could reflect right-sided or biventricular enlargement as the cause of PMI displacement. Additional information obtained from palpation may be parasternal heaves, another sign of ventricular enlargement, or thrills in the presence of significant murmurs.

Careful auscultation of the chest will reveal two heart sounds with an occasional splitting of the second heart sound due to changes in pulmonary blood flow with normal respiration. This split may be difficult to appreciate, however, in infants with heart rates in the upper range of normal or in those with frank tachycardia. In addition to examining the heart sounds, it is important to palpate the strength of the peripheral pulses, taking special note of the intensity of the femoral pulse relative to the brachial pulse. The femoral pulse is located just lateral to the femoral triangle beneath the inguinal ligament. The typical radial-femoral delay observed in older children with coarctation of the aorta is difficult, if not impossible, to appreciate in the setting of such rapid heart rates. It is critical, therefore, to establish the strength of the femoral pulses and if weak or not palpable, urgent echocardiographic examination is required. Bounding peripheral pulses are indicative of a *run-off* situation, such as a PDA with marked left to right shunt or less commonly an arterio-venous malformation.

Murmurs persisting after the first 12 hours are likely to reflect structural abnormalities even though they may not be hemodynamically significant. In one study of infants referred to the cardiology department for murmurs between 12 hours and 14 days, 84% had identifiable lesions, with ventricular septal defects (39%), pulmonic stenosis (15%), and PDA (15%) most common (111). The remaining 16% had normal hearts with innocent murmurs due to tricuspid regurgitation or peripheral pulmonic stenosis. Very commonly a systolic murmur from a closing PDA will be present in the first 24 to 48 hours of life. The key to diagnosing this murmur is serial examinations to confirm that in fact the murmur has disappeared. Whether or not echocardiac evaluation is warranted requires clinical judgment if there is no option for reexamination in a timely manner. It is important to remember that infants with the most serious forms of congenital heart disease may have no murmur but often will have other clues in the cardiac examination.

Evaluation of the cardiovascular system begins in the delivery room with assessment of the Apgar scores and includes evaluation of heart rate, color, and respiratory effort. Frequently, a line of demarcation is observed, with the head, right arm, and right side of the chest pink and the rest of the infant pale or cyanotic until there is functional closure of the ductus. With vigorous crying, its disappearance indicates an appropriate drop in pulmonary vascular resistance and transductal shunting. Another reassuring milestone in cardiac transition often noticed at the first bath by nursing staff is a brief but bright red flush over the entire body and extremities. This blush, reminiscent of cooked lobster, is distinguishable from the darker, ruddy, plethoric color of polycythemia, which is accentuated in the mucous membranes and less so on the palms and soles and is more persistent. The blush is not seen in infants with cyanotic cardiac disease. Specific points to be considered in the cardiac examination are outlined in Table 19-3.

Genitourinary System

In the delivery room, one of the first documented observations of the neonate is assignment of gender. Genital abnormalities are relatively uncommon but cause significant stress to new parents, and so it is important to distinguish the variations of normal from pathologic malformations. It is always urgent to start an appropriate evaluation of gender if it is in question.

The male infant should be examined by stretching the penis for an expected penile length at term of at least 2.5 cm. Although previously unrecognized, a recent study has indicated that there may be racial differences in the size of infant genitalia. As such, infants having measurements at the extremes of the standard length curves should be compared to others from their racial background if this information is available (112). The presence of chordee prevents complete stretching, but a twisted median raphe is of no significance. In obese infants, the shaft may be retracted and covered by suprapubic fat, appearing to be too small unless it is stretched. The observation of the presence of erectile tissue essentially eliminates true micropenis as a consideration. The meatal opening should be located although completely retracting the foreskin is unnecessary. Any significant glandular hypospadias generally is accompanied by incomplete foreskin and therefore is readily apparent on simple inspection. Fortunately, the newborn frequently provides opportunities to observe the origin, direction, and force of his stream on urination.

The presence of both testes deep in the scrotal sac indicates term gestation. If a testicle is not felt within the sac or canal, use a lubricated finger to sweep from the anterior iliac crest along the canal while palpating the scrotum. The volume of the testes should be estimated. Table 19-4 summarizes the normal values. If the scrotum or a testis is distended but soft and nontender, transillumination may reveal a

hydrocele. Deep discoloration suggests hematoma or torsion and a need for immediate surgical evaluation, but superficial scrotal cyanosis (see color plate) may represent benign ecchymosis after breech presentation. Only in rare instances will a salvageable testicle be found as most often it is a remote vascular insult and was resorbed before birth ("vanishing testicle"). Hydrocele of the cord, a harbinger of inguinal hernia, is not so likely to transilluminate but is easily felt.

The female genitalia should be inspected for size and location of the labia, clitoris, meatus, vaginal opening, and the relations of the posterior fourchette to the anus (Table 19-4). Virtually all female newborns have redundant hymenal tissue. Hymens tend be annular with a smooth or fimbriated edge and a central or ventrally displaced opening. Tags of tissue may extend from 1 to 15 mm beyond the rim of the hymen and occur in at least 13% of female neonates. These tags disappear within a few weeks. A complete review of hymenal variations in newborns is available (113). An imperforate hymen can present with a hydrometrocolpos, a build-up of mucoid or bloody secretions causing a mass protruding from the vagina, which usually resolves with spontaneous rupture or regression but can enlarge significantly and cause urinary obstruction or apparent discomfort. Assessment for virilization in the female is difficult because there are varying degrees of clitoral hypertrophy and labioscrotal fusion. With clitoral size realized by 27 weeks of gestation but with little deposition of fat in the labia, there is particular confusion about clitoral hypertrophy in premature infants. As gestation progresses, the labia majora enlarge and by term should completely cover the labia minora. Masculinization causes posterior fusion of the labioscrotal folds independent of clitoral hypertrophy. The distance of the anus from the posterior fourchette varies by GA and body size, but its relation relative to other genital landmarks is more constant (Table 19-4). Measurements are made with the hips flexed and the infant relaxed so that the perineum does not bulge. It is important in both genders to identify a normally positioned anus. Anterior displacement of the anus, while not problematic in the early months of life, frequently causes significant constipation after the stools become more formed.

Musculoskeletal System

Examination of the spine includes observation for abnormal curving and cutaneous manifestations of underlying deformities such as sacral agenesis or spina bifida. A pilonidal sinus is suspected if the bottom of a sacral pit is not visible or there is moisture in an otherwise dry area. Long tufts of hair, an overlying hemangioma, or pigmented nevus potentially indicate a tethered cord unless well below the origin of the cauda equina. A palpable mass usually indicates a lipoma if covered by normal skin that moves with it. A sacrococcygeal teratoma tends to be a fixed mass just lateral to midline, and spinal dysraphism presents as a midline mass, most frequently without full skin coverage. One assesses the extremities for symmetry, size and length, range

TABLE 19-3
NEONATAL CARDIAC EXAMINATION

Finding	Key Location	Points to Consider
Color	Over entire surface except presenting part; inside oral mucous membranes	Peripheral cyanosis may include area around mouth but not inside mucous membranes Prominent venous-capillary plexus around mouth and eyes simulates cyanosis Acrocyanosis of extremities reverses with warming Mild cyanosis may appear as pallor or mottling Infant with PDA run-off looks washed out, particularly in the feet
Respiratory pattern	Lateral view of chest and abdomen Alae nasi	Most often have respiratory rate within normal range May be cyanotic but tachypneic without distress (e.g., retractions, labored breathing) unless there is pulmonary edema or severe acidosis
Heart rate rhythm	PMI	Resting rate 120–130 bpm (range 100–150); higher second to fourth weeks and in premature infants Most premature beats are transient and benign
Precordial bulge	Thorax compared side to side and to the abdomen	Thoracic asymmetry indicates bulge with AVM, tricuspid regurgitation (i.e., Ebstein anomaly), tetralogy with absent PV, intrauterine arrhythmia, or myocardopathy Most commonly, asymmetry indicates pneumothorax, diaphragmatic hernia, atelectasis, or lobar emphysema
PMI	Left parasternal area	Visible until 4–6 h of life during transition; beyond 12 h, associated with volume overload lesions (e.g., AP shunt, transposition, or outflow obstruction) Normally more visible in premature infants but increases with PDA Abnormal to have PMI beyond 1–2 cm left of LSB at less than 1 wk of age Right sided indicates dextrocardia versus shift due to intrathoracic pressures Absence of increased impulse with cyanosis indicates pulmonary atresia, tetralogy, and or tricuspid atresia Increase with cyanosis indicates transposition Thrill: gross insufficiency of AV valve, severe pulmonary stenosis, absent PV
BP	Right arm and leg	Pressure in lower extremities is equal to or minimally higher than pressure in upper extremities in the first week Pressures are preserved by ductal flow in the presence of severe left-sided obstructive disease Norms vary by gestational and chronologic age and method
Pulses	Right and left brachial and simultaneous femoral and right brachial	Look for equality of intensity and timing, synchronicity, slope of impulse curve, no delay in peak between preductal and postductal pulses Easily seen axillary pulses suggest run-off or wide pulse pressure
Pulse pressure	Systolic minus diastolic BP	25–30 cm of H_2O in term; 15–25 cm of H_2O in preterm Narrow indicates myocardial failure, vasoconstriction, and or vascular collapse Widened indicates AV malformation, truncus arteriosus, AP window, and or PDA; may not be widened until pulmonary vascular resistance has dropped
S_1	Upper LSB Lower LSB	Usually single and relatively accentuated; audible split indicates Ebstein anomaly or slow heart rate; decreased with CHF, prolonged AV conduction Increased accentuation with increased flow across AV valve indicates PDA, MI, VSD, TAPVR, AVM, and or tetralogy
S_2	Upper LSB	Two components should be heard by 6–12 h of age Single sound indicates aortic atresia, pulmonary atresia, truncus arteriosus, and or transposition of great arteries Wide split indicates pulmonary stenosis, Ebstein anomaly, TAPVR, tetralogy, and or occasionally left-to-right atrial shunts Loud sounds indicate systemic or pulmonary hypertension
S_3 and S_4	Base or apex	S_3 indicates increased atrioventricular valve flow, PDA, and or CHF S_4 indicates severe myocardial disease with diminished LV compliance
Click	Lower LSB	Benign first several hours; abnormal after transition Dilation of great vessel indicates truncus arteriosus, tetralogy of Fallot, left- or right-sided ventricular outflow obstructions
Murmur	Precordium, back, under both axilla	Many serious cardiac malformations do not have their classic murmurs in early neonatal period but will have some combination of signs suggesting pathology; absence of murmur does not preclude presence of serious malformation (e.g., transposition, TAPVR) At least 60% of infants have murmurs during the first 48 h of life; PDA, peripheral pulmonary stenosis, and or tricuspid regurgitation may be indicated Quiet is necessary to auscultate murmurs; may need to disconnect the infant from the ventilator for a few beats Persistent murmurs first heard right after birth indicate ventricular outflow obstruction; most often pulmonic stenosis

(continued)

TABLE 19-3

NEONATAL CARDIAC EXAMINATION (*continued*)

Finding	Key Location	Points to Consider
Venous pulse	Jugular vein, liver	Jugular a and v waves in sleeping infant In presence of cyanosis, pulsating liver suggests RA or RV obstruction
Abdomen	Liver (left and right)	Span greater than 5.5 cm at term; late sign of CHF, presence of left-sided or central liver suggests likely cardiac anomaly
Edema	Presacrum, eyelids, legs and feet; Chest: hydrops	Causes are more often noncardiac except when associated with abnormalities of renal blood flow (e.g., left-sided obstruction of severe hydrops associated with myocardiopathy, such as severe anemia)

AP, aortopulmonary; AV, atrioventricular; AVM, arteriovenous malformation; BP, blood pressure; bpm, beats per minute; CHF, congestive heart failure; LA, left atrium; LSB, left sternal border; LV, left ventricle; MI, mitral insufficiency; PDA, patent ductus arteriosus; PMI, point of maximal impulse; PV, pulmonary valve; RA, right atrium; RV, right ventricle; S_1, first heart sound; S_2, second heart sound; S_3, third heart sound; S_4, fourth heart sound; TAPVR, total anomalous pulmonary venous return; VSD, ventricular septal defect.
From refs. 85 and 86.

of active and passive motion, and obvious deformity. The length of the upper extremities should allow the fingers to reach to the upper thighs on extension. The muscles are not well defined but should not feel atrophic or fibrotic.

Hand examination consists of observing its activity and appearance, including the nails, joints, and palmar creases. The creases of the fifth digit should be parallel. If there is shortening of the mid phalanx, the nonparallel creases mark a radial deviation, clinodactyly. Any curve less than 10 to 15 degrees is normal. The thumb should reach just beyond the base of the index finger. Extra digits that are postaxial or on the ulnar side are most often equivalent to skin tags and of no significance; they may be familial, most often in families of color. Extra digits on the preaxial or radial side are often enough associated with hematologic and cardiac abnormalities to warrant further evaluation, regardless of racial background.

The neonate's hips require assessment with each visit because dislocations may not be detectable on every examination. If the femur freely dislocates, it may appear to jerk spontaneously when the infant extends or flexes his or her hip. The legs should be symmetric in length on extension and with the knees flexed as the feet rest on the bed. If they are unequal, suggesting dislocation of the shorter leg (i.e.,

Galeazzi sign), the next maneuver is to attempt reduction on the shorter side while stabilizing the pelvis (i.e., Ortolani maneuver). With the hip and knee flexed, the thigh is grasped with the third finger over the greater trochanter and the thumb near the lesser trochanter. The other hand stabilizes the pelvis. As the thigh is abducted, gentle pressure applied to the greater trochanter reduces the dislocated femoral head into the acetabulum with a clunking sensation. The commonly felt, benign clicks are distinct from the pathologic clunks, which often are seen as much as they are felt when the femoral head jerks into place. If the legs are of equal length or if they rest in full abduction, the first maneuver is to attempt to dislocate the head (i.e., Barlow maneuver). With the hip and knee flexed, the thigh is grasped and adducted to 15 degrees beyond midline while applying downward pressure. If the hip dislocates on the maneuver, the Ortolani maneuver should then reduce it. If the hip rides to the edge but not out of the acetabulum during the Barlow maneuver, it is subluxable. Even if dislocation is undetectable, there may be telescoping with free movement of the femur up and down, indicating some degree of instability. The Ortolani maneuver may be negative if a teratologic hip dysplasia cannot be reduced. Unless both hips are involved, discrepancy

TABLE 19-4

NEWBORN GENITALIA

	Parameter	Normal Range	Abnormal Range
Penis	Length	3.5 cm ± 1 cm	<2.5 cm
	Width	0.9–1.2 cm	
Testis	Volume	1–2 cm	
Anus			
Location, male	Anus to scrotum/coccyx to scrotum	0.58 ± 0.06 cm	<0.46 cm
Location, female	Anus to fourchette/coccyx to fourchette	0.44 ± 0.05 cm	<0.34 cm
Size	Diameter	7 mm + (1.3 × weight in kg)	
Masculinization (i.e., labioscrotal fusion)	Anus to fourchette/anus to clitoris	<0.5 cm	>0.5 cm

[a] From refs. 87 and 88.

TABLE 19-5
NEONATAL NEUROLOGIC EVALUATION

Test	Technique	Normal for Term	Deviant for Term
Resting posture	Observe unswaddled infant without contact in quiet awake, quiet active, or light sleep states	Moderate flexion of 4 limbs, held off bed Equal side-to-side and upper-to-lower if head is in midline Extension of neck in face presentation or legs in breech presentation	Constant tight flexion Full extension, flaccid or forced Knees abducted to bed (i.e., frog leg) Elbows flexed with dorsum of hands on bed Tight, persistent fisting ATNR persistent ≥30 seconds Strong lateral preference
State	Deep sleep Light sleep Awake, light peripheral movements Awake, large movements, not crying Awake, crying	Moves from one to the other with appropriate stimuli Self calms Modulated cry with expression	Is difficult to move from one to the other Stays too alert or cries without physical reason Does not come to fully awake state Weak or monotonous cry
Motor activity	Observe throughout physical examination	Appropriate for state of alertness Symmetric, fairly smooth Expressive face with yawn or cry	Bicycling, swatting without stimulus Asymmetric, weak Jittery while sucking Flat facial expression
Phasic (i.e., passive) tone: resistance to movement	Measure resistance to extension (limb recoil) Scarf, heel to ear	Response appropriate for gestational age	Resists too much or too little Asymmetry
Tendon reflexes	Test patellar reflex with head midline	Patellar reflex only one reliably present at birth	Sustained clonus
Postural (i.e., active) tone: resistance to gravity			
Traction response	Pull to sitting while grasping infant's hands	Infant pulls back with flexion at elbows, knees, and ankles Head comes with body with minimal lag and falls forward when sitting is obtained	Asymmetry in pulling back No resistance Full head lag Pull to stand instead Head does not fall forward as infant goes past upright
Upright suspension	Suspend infant facing examiner with both hands in axillae	Infant supports himself then yields slowly Holds head erect, flexes hips, knees, and ankles Eyes open	Infant falls through immediately Legs extend Eyes fail to open Infant fails to relax and fall through after 1 min
Ventral suspension	Hold infant under chest and suspend in prone position Galant: stroke adjacent to spine Landau: stroke caudocephalad along spine	Flexes arms, extends neck, holds back straight Curves toward side of stimulus Extends back, lifts head and pelvis, micturates	Hangs limply or excessively rigidly Asymmetric incurving Weak or absent response
Positive support	Hold infant to support trunk with feet touching firm, flat surface	Infant extends hips to bear his or her own weight and relaxes after 1 min	Infant fails to bear weight or extends too much or too long
Integrated reflexes Moro reflex	Hold infant in supine position; support head and neck with hand; allow head to drop while still supporting it	Spreading: arms abduct, extend; hands open Hugging: arms adduct and flex; hands close	Unequal laterality Absence of spread Asymmetry Exaggeration with disorganization in state
Tonic neck reflex	Infant in supine, neutral position; turn head to one side; repeat opposite side;	Mental extension, occipital flexion primarily of arms; does not remain in position for >30 seconds	Exaggerated response and stays in position >30 seconds
Withdrawal reflex	Painful stimulus to one foot	Withdrawal of stimulated foot; variable extension of opposite leg	Absence of flexion in stimulated leg

ATNR, asymmetric tonic neck reflex.

TABLE 19-6
ASSESSMENT OF CRANIAL NERVES

Cranial Nerve	Assessment	Pitfalls
I	Withdrawal or grimace to strong odor (e.g., peppermint, oil of cloves)	Rarely tested clinically; rapid habituation
II	Behavioral response to light (i.e., blinking fixing, follwing, turning to light source); searching nystagmus	Room too bright; infant too deeply asleep; overstimulation of other senses
III, IV, VI	Ocular movement, doll's eyes, oculovestibular response, pupil size, gemini red reflex	Should not force eyes to open; ocular alignment usually poor in neonates; light for pupil response causes eye closing
VII	Facial muscle tone at rest and during crying	Poor mouth opening due to absence of depressor anguli oris muscle
V, VII, XII	Sucking strength, rooting reflex	Gestational age dependent; infant should be hungry
VIII auditory a portion	Behavioral response to horn (i.e., blinking widened eyes); quieting to voice	Room too loud; difficult to distinguish unilateral loss; rapid habituation
IX, X	Swallowing with normal gag	Irritated throat after suctioning
VII, IX	Facial expression to strong flavor	Rapid habituation
XII	Tongue fasciculation, thrust, ability to shape around nipple	Macroglossiaa

in leg length and inability to abduct fully to the affected side should be present.

Nervous System

Neurologic evaluation begins with the initial observations made on approaching the infant and continues as the infant is positioned and stimulated for the remainder of the routine physical examination. As discussed earlier, assessing GA includes many of the steps also used to evaluate motor tone and symmetry. Much can be learned about the neurologic state just by observing what the infant does on his or her own; little more is needed unless the observations indicate abnormality or there are particular risk factors. Subtle differences in tone or use require more specific evaluation.

A neonate with facial asymmetry while crying and who has a flattened or absent nasolabial fold has a facial palsy. These are most often acquired during forceps delivery and have an incidence of 1.8 per 1,000 deliveries. More than 90% are expected to recover in the first few years of life (114).

Infants display patterns of spontaneous muscular activity referred to as general movements. In the first three months they are typically writhing of slow to moderate speed and small amplitude (115). There appears to be a correlation between abnormal general movements and later development of cerebral palsy (116,117).

These abnormalities are characterized as those confined to one or few body parts (poor repertoire), involving simultaneous contraction of all limb and trunk muscles (cramped-synchronized), or are chaotic with large amplitude. The most worrisome are the "cramped-synchronized" as they have been most closely linked to the later development of cerebral palsy (117).

The most common peripheral nerve injury associated with vaginal delivery is a brachial plexus injury. Injuries may be incurred secondary to traction on an arm during birth. The upper roots, C-5 and C-6, are most commonly damaged, leaving the infant with a prone adducted arm at his or her side. It is generally advised that infants undergo operative repair if function is not recovered by 3 months of age (114).

Fortunately quite rare, spinal cord injury initially may be confused with bilateral brachial plexus injury if it occurs below C-5. Careful exam, however, will disclose paresis or paralysis in the lower extremities as well. Lesions above this level are likely to incapacitate the diaphragm and present with apnea or severe respiratory distress and may also be complicated by cardiovascular instability (114).

Jitteriness, characterized by rhythmic tremors of equal amplitude around a fixed axis in an extremity or the jaw, may occur in 41% to 44% of healthy newborns in the first hours of life and thus deserves special comment (118). It occurs more often if the infant is awake, after a startle, or after crying. Accompanying symptoms of CNS irritation, hypertonicity, and low-threshold startle may also be present. Jitteriness is distinguishable from clonic seizure activity because of its more rapid rate and its cessation either by pressure or by stimulating sucking; it is most often a physiologic activity. If it fails to cease during sucking, it may be a sign of hypoglycemia, hypocalcemia, or drug withdrawal (118). Jitteriness may persist in some infants for many months with the infants having more severe accompanying CNS symptoms having longer persistence (119).

The basics of the neonatal neurologic examination include assessment of state; spontaneous muscle activity for assessing amount, quality, and strength; passive and active muscle tone; and functioning of the cranial nerves. The steps are described in Tables 19-5 and 19-6.

REFERENCES

1. Silverman WA, Andersen DH. A controlled clinical trial of effects of water mist on obstructive respiratory signs, death rate and necropsy findings among premature infants. *Pediatrics* 1956;17:1–10.
2. Morley CJ, Thornton AJ, Cole TJ, et al. Baby Check: a scoring system to grade the severity of acute systemic illness in babies under 6 months old. *Arch Dis Child* 1991;66:100–105.
3. Gray JE, Richardson DK, McCormick MC, et al. Neonatal therapeutic intervention scoring system: a therapy-based severity-of-illness index. *Pediatrics* 1992;90:561–567.
4. Richardson DK, Gray JE, McCormick MC, et al. Score for Neonatal Acute Physiology: a physiologic severity index for neonatal intensive care. *Pediatrics* 1993;91:617–623.
5. Richardson DK, Corcoran JD, Escobar GJ, et al. SNAP-II and SNAPPE-II: simplified newborn illness severity and mortality risk scores. *J Pediatr* 2001;138:92–100.
6. American Academy of Pediatrics and the American College of Obstetricians and Gynecologists. *Guidelines for perinatal care*, 5th ed. Elk Grove Village, Ill and Washington, DC: AAP and ACOG, 2002.
7. Fletcher MA. *Physical diagnosis in neonatology*. Philadelphia: Lippincott-Raven Publishers, 1998.
8. Souter VL, Kapur RP, Nyholt DR, et al. A report of dizygous monochorionic twins. *New Engl J Med* 2003;349:154–158.
9. Saint-Anne-Dargassies S. *Neurological development in the full-term and premature neonate*, 1st ed. Amsterdam: Elsevier, 1977.
10. Amiel-Tison C. Neurological evaluation of the maturity of newborn infants. *Arch Dis Child* 1968;43:89–93.
11. Dubowitz LM, Dubowitz V, Goldberg C. Clinical assessment of gestational age in the newborn infant. *J Pediatr* 1970;77:1–10.
12. Alexander GR, de Caunes F, Hulsey TC, et al. Validity of postnatal assessments of gestational age: a comparison of the method of Ballard et al. and early ultrasonography. *Am J Obstet Gynecol* 1992;166:891–895.
13. Ballard JL, Novak KK, Driver M. A simplified score for assessment of fetal maturation of newly born infants. *J Pediatr* 1979;95:769–774.
14. Constantine NA, Kraemer HC, Kendall-Tackett KA, et al. Use of physical and neurologic observations in assessment of GA in low birth weight infants. *J Pediatr* 1987;110:921–928.
15. Sanders M, Allen M, Alexander GR, et al. Gestational age assessment in preterm neonates weighing less than 1500 grams. *Pediatrics* 1991;88:542–546.
16. Alexander GR, de Caunes F, Hulsey TC, et al. Validity of postnatal assessment of gestational age: a comparison of the method of Ballard et al. and early ultrasonography. *Am J Obstet Gynecol* 1992;166:891–895.
17. Wariyar U, Tin W, Hey E. Gestational assessment assessed. *Arch Dis Child* 1997;77:F216–F220.
18. Ballard JL, Khoury JC, Wedig K, et al. New Ballard score, expanded to include extremely premature infants. *J Pediatr* 1991;119:417–423.
19. Donovan EF, Tyson JE, Ehrenkranz RA, et al. Inaccuracy of Ballard scores before 28 weeks' gestation. *J Pediatr* 1998;135:147–152.
20. Hittner HM, Hirsch NJ, Rudolph AJ. Assessment of gestational age by examination of the anterior vascular capsule of the lens. *J Pediatr* 1977;91:455–458.
21. Hittner HM, Gorman WA, Rudolph AJ. Examination of the anterior vascular capsule of the lens: II. assessment of gestational age in infants small for gestational age. *J Pediatr Ophthalmol Strabismus* 1981;18:52–54.
22. Lynn CJ, Saidi IS, Oelberg DG, et al. Gestational age correlates with skin reflectance in newborn infants of 24–42 weeks gestation. *Biol Neonate* 1993;64:69–75.
23. Stevens-Simon C, Cullinan J, Stinson S, et al. Effects of race on the validity of clinical estimates of gestational age. *J Pediatr* 1989;115:1000–1002.
24. Ellison P. The infant neurological examination. *Adv Dev Behav Pediatr* 1990;9:75.
25. Amiel-Tison C, Grenier A. *Neurological assessment during the first year of life*, 1st ed. New York: Oxford University Press, 1986.
26. Litwin A, Aitkin I, Merlob P. Clitoral length assessment in newborn infants of 30 to 41 weeks gestational age. *Eur J Obstet Gynecol Reprod Biol* 1991;38:209–212.
27. Oberfield SE, Mondok A, Shahrivar F, et al. Clitoral size in full-term infants. *Am J Perinatol* 1989;6:453–454.
28. Wilcox AJ, Russell IT. Birthweight and perinatal mortality: II. on weight-specific mortality. *Int J Epidemiol* 1983;12:319–325.
29. Merlob P, Sivan Y, Reisner SH. Ratio of crown-rump distance to total length in preterm and term infants. *J Med Genet* 1986;23:338–340.
30. Sivan Y, Merlob P, Reisner SH. Upper limb standards in newborns. *Am J Dis Child* 1983;137:829–832.
31. Merlob P, Sivan Y, Reisner SH. Lower limb standard in newborns. *Am J Dis Child* 1984;138:140–142.
32. Amiel-Tison C, Gosselin J, Infante-Rivard C. Head growth and cranial assessment at neurological examination in infancy. *Dev Med Child Neurol* 2002;44:643–648.
33. Raymond GV, Holmes LB. Head circumference standards in neonates. *J Child Neurol* 1994;9:63–66.
34. Sutter K, Engstrom JL, Johnson TS. Reliability of head circumference measurements in preterm infants. *Pediatr Nurs* 1997;23:485–490.
35. Sivan Y, Merlob P, Reisner SH. Head measurements in newborn infants. *J Craniofac Genet Dev Biol* 1984;4:259–263.
36. Prechtl HF, Einspieler C, Cioni G, et al. An early marker for neurological deficits after perinatal brain lesions. *Lancet* 1997;349:1361–1363.
37. Prechtl HF, Beintema D. *The neurologic examination of the full-term newborn infant. Clinics in developmental medicine*, vol. 12. London: SIMP Heinemann, 1964.
38. Brazelton TB. *Neonatal behavioral assessment scale*, 2nd ed. *Clinics in developmental medicine*, vol. 88. Philadelphia: JB Lippincott, 1984.
39. Lester BM, Boukydis CF, McGrath M, et al. Behavioral and psychophysiologic assessment of the preterm infant. *Clin Perinatol* 1990;17:155–171.
40. Thoman EB. Sleeping and waking states in infants: a functional perspective. *Neurosci Biobehav Rev* 1990;14:93–107.
41. Haddad GG, Jeng HJ, Lai TL, et al. Determination of sleep state in infants using respiratory variability. *Pediatr Res* 1987;21:556–562.
42. Sadeh A, Dark I, Vohr BR. Newborns' sleep-wake patterns: the role of maternal delivery and infant factors. *Early Hum Dev* 1996;44:113–126.
43. Hathorn MK. The rate and depth of breathing in new-born infants in different sleep states. *J Physiol* 1974;243:101–113.
44. Stern E, Parmelee AH, Akiyama Y, et al. Sleep cycle characteristics in infants. *Pediatrics* 1969;43:65–70.
45. Poole SR. The infant with acute, unexplained, excessive crying. *Pediatrics* 1991;88:450–455.
46. Heine RG, Jaquiery A, Lubitz L, et al. Role of gastro-oesophageal reflux in infant irritability. *Arch Dis Child* 1995;73:121–125.
47. Als H, Lester BM, Tronick EC, et al. Manual for the assessment of preterm infants' behavior (APIB). In: Fitzgerald HE, Lester BM, Yogman MW, eds. *Theory and research in behavioral pediatrics*, vol. 1. New York: Plenum Press, 1982:65–132.
48. Grover G, Berkowitz CD, Lewis RJ, et al. The effects of bundling on infant temperature. *Pediatrics* 1994;94:669–673.
49. Cheng TL, Partridge JC. Effect of bundling and high environmental temperature on neonatal body temperature. *Pediatrics* 1993;92:238–240.
50. Harpin VA, Chellappah G, Rutter N. Responses of the newborn infant to overheating. *Biol Neonate* 1983;44:65–75.
51. Rutter N, Hull D. Response of term babies to a warm environment. *Arch Dis Child* 1979;54:178–183.
52. Harpin VA, Rutter N. Sweating in preterm babies. *J Pediatr* 1982;100:614–619.
53. Hegyi T, Carbone MT, Anwar M, et al. Blood pressure ranges in premature infants. I. The first hours of life. *J Pediatr* 1994;124:627–633.
54. Park MK, Lee DH. Normative arm and calf blood pressure values in the newborn. *Pediatrics* 1989;83:240–243.
55. Perry EH, Bada HS, Ray JD, et al. Blood pressure increases, birth weight-dependent stability boundary, and intraventricular hemorrhage. *Pediatrics* 1990;85:727–732.
56. Engle WD. Blood pressure in the very low birth weight neonate. *Early Hum Dev* 2001;62:97–130.
57. American Academy of Pediatrics Committee on Fetus and Newborn. Routine evaluation of blood pressure, hematocrit, and glucose in newborns. *Pediatrics* 1993;92:474–476.
58. Goldring D, Wohltmann HJ. Flush method for blood pressure determinations in newborn infants. *J Pediatr* 1952;40:285–289.

59. Peitsch WK, Keefer CH, LaBrie RA, et al. Incidence of cranial asymmetry in healthy newborns. *Pediatrics* 2002;110:e72.

60. Jones MD. Unilateral epicanthal fold: diagnostic significance. *J Pediatr* 1986;108:702–704.

61. Jones KL, ed. *Smith's recognizable patterns of human malformation,* 4th ed. Philadelphia: WB Saunders, 1988.

62. Samlaska CP, James WD, Sperling LC. Scalp whorls. *J Am Acad Dermatol* 1989;21:553–556.

63. Smith DW, Greely MJ. Unruly scalp hair in infancy: its nature and relevance to problems of brain morphogenesis. *Pediatrics* 1978; 61:783–785.

64. Drolet BA, Clowrey L Jr, McTigue MK, et al. The hair collar sign; marker for cranial dysraphism. *Pediatrics* 1995;96: 309–313.

65. Corona-Rivera JR, Corona-Rivera E, Romero-Velarde E, et al. Report and review of the fetal brain disruption sequence. *Eur J Pediatr* 2001;160:664–667.

66. Johnsonbaugh RE, Bryan RN, Hierlwimmer R, et al. Premature craniosynostosis: a common complication of juvenile thyrotoxicosis. *J Pediatr* 1978:93:188–191.

67. Shuper A, Merlob P, Grunebaum M, et al. The incidence of isolated craniosynostosis in the newborn infant. *Am J Dis Child* 1985;139:85–86.

68. Graham JM Jr, Smith DW. Parietal craniotabes in the neonate: its origin and significance. *J Pediatr* 1979;95:114–116.

69. Popich GA, Smith DW. Fontanels: range of normal size. *J Pediatr* 1972;80:749–752.

70. Faix RG. Fontanelle size in black and white term newborn infants. *J Pediatr* 1982;100:304–306.

71. Duc G, Largo RH. Anterior fontanel: size and closure in term and preterm infants. *Pediatrics* 1986;78:904–908.

72. Adeyemo AA, Omotade OO. Variations in fontanelle size with gestational age. *Early Hum Dev* 1999;54:207–214.

73. Lloyd FA, Finkelstein SI. Normal head growth in infant with nonidentifiable anterior fontanel. *J Pediatr* 1975;87:490–494.

74. Kataria S, Frutiger AD, Lanford B, et al. Anterior fontanelle closure in healthy term infants. *Infant Behav Dev* 1988;11:229.

75. Potter EL, Craig JM. *Pathology of the fetus and the infant,* 3rd ed. Chicago: Year Book Medical Publishers, 1975.

76. Benaron D. Subgaleal hematoma causing hypovolemic shock during delivery after failed vacuum extraction: a case report. *J Perinatol* 1993;13:228–231.

77. Govaert P, Vanhaesebrouck P, De Praeter C, et al. Vacuum extraction, bone injury and neonatal subgaleal bleeding. *Eur J Pediatr* 1992;151:532–535.

78. Gundry SR, Wesley JR, Klein MD, et al. Cervical teratomas in the newborn. *J Pediatr Surg* 1983;18:382–386.

79. Carr MM, Thorner P, Phillips JH. Congenital teratomas of the head and neck. *J Otolaryngol* 1997;26:246–252.

80. Sivan Y, Merlob P, Reisner H. Eye measurements in preterm and term newborn infants. *J Craniofac Genet Dev Biol* 1982;2:239–242.

81. Crouch ER Jr, Crouch ER. Pediatric vision screening: why? when? how? *Contemp Pediatr* 1991;8:9–30.

82. Isenberg SJ, Vazquez M. Are the pupils of premature infants affected by intraventricular hemorrhage? *J Child Neurol* 1994;9: 440–442.

83. Isenberg SJ. Clinical application of the pupil examination in neonates. *J Pediatr* 1991;118:650–652.

84. Roarty JD, Keltner JL. Normal pupil size and anisocoria in newborn infants. *Arch Ophthalmol* 1990;108:94–95.

85. Goldbloom RB, ed. *Pediatric clinical skills,* 2nd ed. New York: Churchill Livingstone, 1997.

86. Smith DW, Takashima H. Ear muscles and ear form. *Birth Defects Orig Artic Ser* 1980;16:299–302.

87. Zerin M, Van Allen MI, Smith DW. Intrinsic auricular muscles and auricular form. *Pediatrics* 1982;69:91–93.

88. Ruder RO, Graham JM Jr. Evaluation and treatment of the deformed and malformed auricle. *Clin Pediatr (Phila)* 1996;35: 461–465.

89. Sivan Y, Merlob P, Reisner SH. Assessment of ear length and low set ears in newborn infants. *J Med Genet* 1983;20:213–215.

90. Silverman SH, Leibow SG. Dislocation of the triangular cartilage of the nasal septum. *J Pediatr* 1975;87:456–458.

91. MacEwen CJ, Young JD. Epiphora during the first year of life. *Eye* 1991;5:596–600.

92. Ogawa GS, Gonnering RS. Congenital nasolacrimal duct obstruction. *J Pediatr* 1991;119:12–17.

93. Levin SE, Silverman NH, Milner S. Hypoplasia or absence of the depressor anguli oris muscle and congenital abnormalities, with special reference to the cardiofacial syndrome. *S Afr Med J* 1982;61:227–231.

94. Miller M, Hall JG. Familial asymmetric crying facies. Its occurrence secondary to hypoplasia of the anguli oris depressor muscles. *Am J Dis Child* 1979;133:743–746.

95. Richard BM, Qiu CX, Ferguson MW. Neonatal palatal cysts and their morphology in cleft lip and palate. *Br J Plast Surg* 2000;53:555–558.

96. Hayes PA. Hamartomas, eruption cyst, natal tooth and Epstein pearls in a newborn. *ASDC J Dent Child* 2000;67:365–368.

97. Zhu J, King D. Natal and neonatal teeth. *ASDC J Dent Child* 1995;62:123–128.

98. Ballard JL, Auer CE, Khoury JC. Ankyloglossia: assessment, incidence, and effect of frenuloplasty on the breastfeeding dyad. *Pediatrics* 2002;110:e63.

99. Moyer VA, Ahn C, Sneed S. Accuracy of clinical judgment in neonatal jaundice. *Arch Pediatr Adolesc Med* 2000;154:391–394.

100. Bamji M, Stone RK, Kaul A, et al. Palpable lymph nodes in healthy newborns and infants. *Pediatrics* 1986;78:573–575.

101. Hilliard RI, McKendry JB, Phillips MJ. Congenital abnormalities of the lymphatic system: a new clinical classification. *Pediatrics* 1990;86:988–994.

102. Nichols MM. Shifting umbilicus in neonatal phrenic palsy (the belly dancer's sign). *Clin Pediatr (Phila)* 1976;15:342–343.

103. Joseph PR, Rosenfeld W. Clavicular fractures in neonates. *Am J Dis Child* 1990;144:165–167.

104. Hassan A, Karna P, Dolanski EA. Intermamillary indices in premature infants. *Am J Perinatol* 1988;5:54–56.

105. Grotto I, Browner-Elhanan K, Mimouni D, et al. Occurrence of supernumerary nipples in children with kidney and urinary tract malformations. *Pediatr Dermatol* 2001;18:291–294.

106. Senquiz AL. Use of decubitus position for finding the "olive" of pyloric stenosis. *Pediatrics* 1991;87:266.

107. Sinkin RA, Phillips BL, Adelman RD. Elevation in systemic blood pressure in the neonate during abdominal examination. *Pediatrics* 1985;76:970–972.

108. Ashkenazi S, Mimouni F, Merlob P, et al. Size of liver edge in full-term, healthy infants. *Am J Dis Child* 1984;138:377–378.

109. Reiff MI, Osborn LM. Clinical estimation of liver size in newborn infants. *Pediatrics* 1983;71:46–48.

110. Brion L, Avni FA. Clinical estimation of liver size in newborn infants. *Pediatrics* 1985;75:127–128.

111. Du ZD, Roquin N, Barak M. Clinical and echocardiographic evaluation of neonates with heart murmurs. *Acta Paediatr* 1997;86: 752–756.

112. Phillip M, De Boer C, Pilpel D, et al. Clitoral and penile sizes of full term newborns in two different ethnic groups. *J Pediatr Endocrinol Metab* 1996;9:175–179.

113. Berenson A, Heger A, Andrews S. Appearance of the hymen in newborns. *Pediatrics* 1991;87:458–465.

114. Medlock MD, Hanigan WC. Neurologic birth trauma. Intracranial, spinal cord, and brachial plexus injury. *Clin Perinatol* 1997;24: 845–857.

115. Einspieler C, Prechtl HF, Ferrari F. The qualitative assessment of general movements in the preterm, term and young infants—review of the methodology. *Early Hum Dev* 1997;50:47–60.

116. Prechtl HF, Einspieler C, Cioni G, et al. An early marker for neurological deficits after perinatal brain lesions. *Lancet* 1997;349: 1361–1363.

117. Ferrari F, Cioni G, Einspieler C, et al. Cramped synchronized general movements in preterm infants as an early marker for cerebral palsy. *Arch Pediatr Adolesc Med* 2002;156:460–470.

118. Linder N, Moser AM, Asli I, et al. Suckling stimulation test for neonatal tremor. *Arch Dis Child* 1989;64:44–46.

119. Kramer U, Nevo Y, Harel S. Jittery babies: a short-term follow-up. *Brain and Dev* 1994;16:112–114.

120. Jorgenson RJ, Shapiro SD, Salinas CF, Levin LS. Intraoral findings and anomalies in neonates. *Pediatrics* 1982;69:577.

121. Levin LS, Jorgenson RJ, Jarvey BA. Lymphangiomas of the alveolar ridge in neonates. *Pediatrics* 1976;58:88.

122. Fromm A. Epstein's Pearls, Bohn's nodules and inclusion-cysts of the oral cavity. *J Dent Child* 1967;34:275.

123. King NM, Lee AMP. Prematurely erupted teeth in newborn infants. *J Pediatr* 1989;114:807.

124. Leung AKC. Natal teeth. *Am J Dis Child* 1986;140:249.

General Care

Ian Laing

This chapter describes the general care of the well infant and discusses how a pediatrician may meet the needs of the majority of families whose infants do not require admission to a neonatal unit.

No pediatrician should act independently of midwives, neonatal nurses, obstetricians, fetal medicine specialists, radiologists, geneticists, and practitioners of many other disciplines. The pediatrician should be a member of a multidisciplinary group that meets weekly to discuss the anticipated antenatal problems and to provide an audit of outcomes from the previous months.

There are four phases of care:

- Antenatal
- Intrapartum
- Neonatal
- Postdischarge

ANTENATAL

The past 20 years have seen a revolution in the general public's expectations regarding the standard of care received and the quality and extent of information provided. Midwives and obstetricians are not the only professionals responsible for providing this care and information. The pediatrician must work with these other professionals to ensure the clarity and accuracy of information provided antenatally to mothers and their partners. The team must also grapple with the legal and ethical aspects of "informed consent." Wherever possible, all professionals should strive toward evidence-based medicine. The concept of risk is not yet well understood by the general population.

Information

The developed world has now emerged from the days when underinformed patients conveyed their decisions to professionals. The patient–professional partnership is now crucial. Information should be given to mother and partner as fully as possible, in verbal and written form. Such information should maintain perspective, while being spoken or written in language that the patient can understand.

Risk

Today our communities strive toward "natural" childbirth, emphasizing that birth should ideally be a normal physiologic phenomenon for a healthy woman and fetus. Nevertheless, even the healthiest pregnancy carries a small risk of maternal mortality and a significant risk of morbidity. For the fetus and neonate the risks are much higher: The perinatal mortality is usually between 6 and 10 deaths per 1,000 total deliveries in the developed world. The anticipated risk may change. New possibilities may emerge unexpectedly. Unforeseen emergencies occur without time to discuss them completely. Furthermore, some pregnancies may appear to cause initial concern, and such worries may resolve as the pregnancy progresses. The clinician must address the question of whether the mother should be told of all possibilities, even those that may occur once in 500 events. In striving to do so, there is a chance that all perspective may be lost for the patient. A value judgment must be taken in each individual case. This risk, however great or small, is communicated to mother and a plan is chosen accordingly. Written information should capture the idea that the plan may have to change in light of forthcoming events.

Because labor is usually a tiring process for the mother, it is not an ideal time to discuss options that could be better addressed beforehand. Mode of feeding, vitamin K prophylaxis, and immunization schedules are examples of subjects that should be explored in depth before the mother enters labor.

Informed Consent

In theory, there should be "fully informed consent at all times." This is an important goal, but it is not entirely achievable. Pregnancy, labor, delivery, and the neonatal period are all times when unexpected events may arise. Anticipating them all is impossible and would be detrimental to the perspective that a woman and her partner require. Fully informed consent can be aimed at exploring all likely events and their outcomes, test findings, including the implications of false-positive and false-negative results, and the concept of changing risk. These goals are commendable, very time-consuming, and potentially bewildering, even for educated parents. Compromises therefore must be embraced. Professionals should obtain written informed consent where possible, and those who administer, manage, and finance the health program must recognize that the informed consent procedure is time-consuming and requires increased staff resources.

Infant Feeding Information

There is great variation throughout the world in rates of breast-feeding. This variation is largely cultural in origin. Some parts of the developed world, including Europe, the United States, and Canada, have low rates of breast-feeding and physicians are required to provide mothers with clear information about the proven advantages of breast-feeding. Advantages include lower prevalence of maternal breast cancer, lower incidence of infant infections (1) (including necrotizing enterocolitis), lower prevalence of obesity in childhood (2), and lower incidence of sudden infant death syndrome (SIDS) (3,4). Breast-feeding may also provide some protection against allergic disease in childhood.

Vitamin K Information

Hemorrhagic disease of the newborn (HDN) can cause significant neonatal morbidity and mortality. It may present in the early days of neonatal life as bleeding from the umbilicus, skin, or as intestinal hemorrhage. Late-onset HDN may cause intracranial bleeding, with consequent death or brain damage. Infants who are breast-feeding or born of mothers taking anticonvulsants are at particular risk (5). Because of these hazards, all parents should be advised to choose vitamin K prophylaxis for their newborn infants. One intramuscular dose of vitamin K can prevent almost all episodes of HDN. This is a simple and reliable method of prophylaxis. Some reports suggest that there is an increased incidence of childhood malignancy after intramuscular vitamin K prophylaxis, whereas other studies fail to confirm this.

Oral prophylaxis may be given on days 1, 8, and 28, and is effective at dramatically reducing the incidence of HDN (6). Oral prophylaxis requires a motivated parent to remember to administer the second and third dose, or else

an efficient community support program must be in place to ensure that the infant is similarly protected.

Written information should be available for all parents to examine the evidence, and professionals should be available to discuss the issues and provide parents with a recommendation. Anxieties expressed in the literature, whether justified or not, should not lead parents to reject vitamin K prophylaxis altogether. HDN is a potentially lethal condition.

Immunization Information

Throughout the world there are differences in immunization programs. These depend on varying risks of disease in different parts of the planet, availability of vaccines and ability to refrigerate them, and community education programs. Preterm infants should be immunized at the same postnatal age as their term counterparts. Provided the infant is clinically well, the timing of immunization should be unaffected by gestation. Table 20-1 shows an example of recommended immunization schedules in the developed world. Because each country has its own schedule, the pediatrician should check both the local and current recommendations.

INTRAPARTUM

Ideally the pediatrician attending the delivery of a newborn infant has full information available. The reality is often different. An urgent call to a labor suite is followed gradually by an unfolding history. The pediatrician relies on close observation of the neonate to guide emergency care while the history is gathered.

Information from case records should include the following:

■ *Maternal health:* Diseases prior to and during the pregnancy are documented; these include diabetes mellitus and positive human immunodeficiency virus (HIV) status. In addition, there should be an account of diseases associated with the pregnancy, such as pregnancy-induced hypertension and gestational diabetes.
■ *Prescribed drugs during pregnancy:* Some therapeutic drugs may have significant effects on the fetus and neonate (see Chapter 15).

TABLE 20-1

IMMUNIZATION SCHEDULE

Age (Months After Delivery)	Immunization
At birth	BCG (high risk) Hep B (mother carrier)
2	Dip Tet Pertuss Polio HIB MenC
3	Dip Tet Pertuss Polio HIB MenC
4	Dip Tet Pertuss Polio HIB MenC

BCG, Bacille Calmette-Guérin (tuberculosis); Dip, diphtheria; HIB, *Haemophilus influenzae* B; MenC, meningococcal C; Pertuss, pertussis; Tet, tetanus.

- *Drug abuse:* A mother may be a chronic drug abuser. Frequently this involves a cocktail of drugs, only some of which are known by professionals. The chronic drug abuser may be a caring mother with feelings of guilt and sincere intentions of creating a healthy environment for the new baby. The mother however, may have a chaotic lifestyle, and there might also be coincident malnutrition, heavy smoking, alcoholism, and positive HIV status.
- *Fetal growth and apparent well-being, including all tests of fetal assessment:* These may involve fetal ultrasonography scans for structural anomalies and nuchal translucency. Data from amniocentesis or chorionic villus sampling may be available. Doppler studies of uterine arteries may have been used to predict preeclampsia and fetal growth retardation. Umbilical arterial Doppler studies may have predicted placental damage and vascular occlusion. Doppler studies of fetal arteries and veins can also be used to assess fetal hypoxemia. Biophysical profile scoring involves cardiotocography, amniotic fluid volume, and three dynamic ultrasonography variables (fetal movement, fetal breathing, and fetal tone). Chapter 12 includes a detailed discussion of these techniques.
- *Gestation:* It is important to know the best estimate of gestation and how this was calculated. An ultrasonography examination in the first trimester is accurate to within ±2 to 3.5 days. The mother's history of the first day of the last menstrual period may be helpful but is not always available. Remember too that a mother may experience a menstrual period even after conception has taken place, and in these circumstances an early ultrasonography scan may correctly declare that the pregnancy is 4 weeks further advanced than the mother's history would suggest.
- *Date and time of rupture of membranes:* The definition of prolonged rupture of the amniotic membranes is not consistent and is variously described as 12, 18, 24, 48, and 72 hours. It is associated with chorioamnionitis and an increased risk of fetal and neonatal infection.
- *Events during labor:* Assessment of fetal well-being including cardiotocography, passage of meconium, maternal pyrexia, and the results of any fetal scalp pH measurements may guide the resuscitation. The combination of profound fetal acidosis and neonatal apnea requires the presence of an experienced pediatric team that can begin immediate assisted ventilation.
- *Mode of delivery:* Resuscitation of the infant in the room where mother has labored allows the pediatrician to learn firsthand about the ease or difficulty of delivery. Forceps or ventouse (vacuum) deliveries may account for local trauma observed.

NEONATAL

Chapter 18 describes resuscitation of the neonate in detail.

The transformation from fetus to neonate is a remarkable one. The placenta, which until this point has been the provider of food and oxygen and the remover of fetal waste products, is clamped off and the neonate must immediately adapt to take responsibility for these functions. Collapsed, liquid-filled lungs become inflated within seconds, and the capillaries and lymphatics drain most of the pulmonary fluid in a few hours. The fetal partial pressure of arterial oxygen (PaO_2) changes from 32 mm Hg to 80 mm Hg in minutes and achieves 100 mm Hg in a few days. Approximately 95% of infants establish spontaneous respiration by 1 minute after delivery and thereafter become pink and vigorous spontaneously. The purpose of resuscitation is to intervene when these natural processes are disturbed pathologically. Dr. Virginia Apgar's scoring system for assessment of the neonate at 1 and 5 minutes is still used widely today, but the pediatrician should concentrate on assisting the infant to achieve a heart rate greater than 100 per minute and active, crying respirations. In the absence of congenital abnormalities, central pinkness is soon achieved thereafter.

General Principles of Resuscitation

The following principles are guides to the general care of the newborn in the early minutes of life:

- Resuscitation in the delivery room can be readily described to parents while it is happening. Parents fear silences.
- Identification anklets or wristbands are important, but not at the expense of causing a tiny infant to become cold.
- The loudly crying baby never needs to be intubated or to be given bag-and-mask insufflation. Enrichment of the inspired gas may be required but never under positive pressure. The infant is more efficient than the clinician.
- Do not ever sound frustrated or critical of colleagues during resuscitations. Such sentiments result in a breakdown of essential teamwork and sap the confidence of parents.

Meconium

The contents of the fetal bowel may have been passed prematurely and may have been inhaled during asphyxial gasping prior to delivery. Meconium is a chemical irritant to the lungs as well as a marker of fetal distress. In 9% to 11% of deliveries, meconium is present. The caregiver should thoroughly suction any meconium from the mouth and nares with the head on the perineum. Whether or not meconium should be aspirated from the newborn's oropharynx is controversial (7); the current author is in favor of this practice, but recognizes that more data are required to support or refute this maneuver. It is clear that those infants who are vigorous do not require invasive care. Those who are in poor condition should be intubated and any inhaled meconium aspirated from the trachea.

Cord Clamping

Data are currently being gathered about the ideal time of cord clamping and whether the infant should be held for a few seconds below the placenta in order to receive a gravitational transfusion (8). Consequences of receiving too much blood volume are fluid overload, polycythemia, and (later) hyperbilirubinemia. Until the data from research studies are complete, it may be reasonable to allow a 15-second delay to achieve a modest blood transfusion. Because delayed clamping of the cord increases the infant's blood volume, it may be advantageous in extreme preterm infants to ensure an adequate intravascular volume, and perhaps to decrease the necessity for subsequent blood transfusion. There is no place for "stripping" of the cord by "milking" the blood from placenta to baby. The cord should initially be clamped several centimeters from the umbilicus and then be cut (9). Then the cord should be clamped 1 or 2 cm from the umbilicus using a disposable clamp, and cut with sterile scissors distal to the clamp. The cord clamp can be safely removed during the second day of life, at which time the cord should be inspected to insure that there is no residual hemorrhage.

Drying

The neonate is delivered covered in amniotic fluid that immediately extracts latent heat by evaporation from the infant's body. Consequently, most infants should be thoroughly dried with warm towels.

Temperature Control

Newborn infants lose heat by four physical mechanisms: evaporation, conduction, convection, and radiation. Evaporation is at its most important in the early seconds of life when the newborn is covered in amniotic fluid. Conduction in general contributes little to heat loss because the infant is in contact with warm garments of low conductivity. Convection losses become important when a child is exposed to drafts, and most especially when a child is being nursed naked on an open radiant warmer. Radiant heat loss occurs to cold surrounding objects, that is, the incubator wall in a cool room. Recognition of these physical principles allows heat loss to be minimized by early drying, warm clothing, freedom from drafts, and ensuring that incubators are double-walled with warm gas between the walls. Physical examination, weighing, and bathing of the infant should always be carried out in a warm environment. The neonatal unit and postnatal wards should audit the incidence of neonatal hypothermia and identify the sources of baby cooling. The areas or procedures at fault should be corrected and the quality of care surveyed prospectively.

Identification

Before leaving the delivery room, every infant should be identified by the fixing of a wristband and anklet; the parent(s) should witness the bands being attached. In addition, many institutions now routinely do footprinting, handprinting, and fingerprinting, although it is not yet clear that this is reliable and worthwhile (10).

Security

Because of sporadic baby abductions in maternity units, each unit should have a written policy to protect the infants. Both antenatally and postnatally, parents should be given instructions to maximize the safety of the infant. Parents and staff must verify the identity of anyone requesting to remove the baby from the room. Parents should be encouraged, when in any doubt, to summon another member of the staff to check the identification of the person asking to take the child.

Bonding

The early minutes and hours of a child's life are important times for establishing a close bond between mother and infant. After the majority of deliveries it should be possible to put the infant immediately to the maternal breast for close physical contact even if the mother does not intend to breast-feed.

Control of Infection

Even today infection is one of the major causes of mortality and morbidity in newborn infants. Gowning does not decrease bacterial colonization of the baby nor the incidence of neonatal sepsis (11). The maternity service, in all its departments, must have high-quality handwashing facilities. The troughs should be large with elbow-operated, knee-operated, or automatic taps that produce warm water. Soap must be plentiful. Alcohol rubs should be readily available wherever infants are cared for. Staff should be free of all clothes and jewelry from elbows to fingertips. Each institution should have regular (at least annual) education sessions for staff, and a culture of nonthreatening criticism by peers should be ever-present. All staff on entering a nursery must wash their hands and forearms with an antiseptic (e.g., chlorhexidine or hexachlorophene). Before and after touching each baby, staff should douse hands and forearms in at least 5 mL of alcohol rub or thoroughly wash their hands (12).

Eye Prophylaxis

Throughout the developed world there is great variation in the use of eye prophylaxis. Each individual community should make a risk assessment depending on the incidence of identified *Chlamydia* and gonococcal infections. Erythromycin 0.5% and tetracycline 1% are effective antibiotics against sensitive gonococci, but penicillinase-producing gonococci are increasing in numbers and are best prevented with silver nitrate 1% (13).

If prophylaxis is to be given, the ointments should be instilled within the first hour of life into the lower conjunctival sac. The lids are then gently massaged. It is difficult to produce effective prophylaxis against *Chlamydia*. If conjunctivitis is identified, scrapings of the tarsal conjunctiva should be sent to the laboratory to identify typical cytoplasmic inclusion bodies. Treatment with combined oral and topical erythromycin has the advantage of eradication of nasopharyngeal carriage of *Chlamydia*. Equally, if the mother is known to have gonococcal disease, prophylaxis with ointments is insufficient for the infant, who should be fully treated with parenteral antibiotics (13).

General Concepts of Clinical Examination

Chapter 19 describes the details of clinical examination. The purpose of newborn clinical examination is to identify the child who is unwell and the child who has an evident congenital abnormality. Reassurance is given, along with an opportunity for parents to ask questions of the examining doctor. There is no universally accepted ideal time for carrying out the examination. The pediatrician cannot exclude all congenital abnormalities but rather is highlighting those that can be identified at that time. On day 1 the systolic murmur of ventricular septal defect is not yet manifest. On day 4 the infant may seem well yet may perish on day 5 from aortic atresia as the ductus arteriosus closes. Congenital metabolic diseases may occasionally take weeks, months, or even years to be symptomatic. It should be made clear in writing to parents that the examination is a description of the child's condition on a particular day and time, and that a normal examination does not guarantee that the neonate is perfect in every respect.

Birth weight and head circumference should be accurately measured. This is documented as a baseline for any further consultations, which may arise, and also to contribute to epidemiological data for the population.

Screening Tests

The developed world has the opportunity to use bloodspot screening for conditions not readily identifiable by other means. These diseases screened for vary from country to country and even from region to region. In the United Kingdom, the national universal newborn screening program for phenylketonuria was introduced in 1969, and the program for congenital hypothyroidism was introduced in 1981. Galactosemia, tyrosinemia, and maple syrup urine disease have been screened for in the past but have been discontinued. Cystic fibrosis and anonymous testing for HIV-positive blood are screened for in some regions, and there are plans to screen for sickle cell disorders in the future.

The screening may be done in the hospital, or the midwife or public health nurse may do it during a home visit. The baby's heel is pricked, and four "bloodspots" are collected on a filter paper (the "Guthrie" card). Each country must decide whether they have the time to obtain fully informed written consent from a parent in every case. Some authorities recognize that making written consent compulsory may have the undesirable side effect of reducing uptake of the screening program, with consequent detriment to the individual children with undetected disease. Written information should be provided to parents both antenatally and postnatally. There should also be high-quality verbal communication with all mothers on the subject of newborn bloodspot screening. Pediatricians caring for newborns must be acquainted with their local newborn screening program, not only for the diseases being screened but also for the timing and implementation of the screening and the procedure to be followed for questionable and abnormal results.

Fluids and Growth

Of all infants, 95% are observed to pass urine in the first 24 hours of life (14). The 5% who have dry diapers have probably voided during labor or in the labor suite. Failure to pass urine in 48 hours should trigger careful examination and investigation.

Meconium is usually passed in the first day of life. Failure to do so should prompt the clinician to ask whether meconium was passed prior to or during labor. If failure to pass meconium is confirmed, careful examination should exclude anorectal atresia. Abdominal examination should ensure that there is no evidence of distention. Hirschsprung's disease and meconium ileus may both present with delayed passage of meconium, and the child should be evaluated for these conditions. The infant should be observed until there is reliable documentation of the passage of meconium (14).

Meconium is a dark green viscous substance consisting of bile-stained intestinal secretions, intestinal debris, and cells. It is usually observed more than once per day for the first 3 days of life. After approximately 3 days of milk feedings, the meconium appears mixed with milk stool ("changing stool") and in 2 more days there are well-established yellow milk stools. Delay in appearance of milk stools should trigger the clinician to question the adequacy of oral feedings. Passage of stool in the neonatal period varies in frequency and consistency. Breast-fed infants typically pass stool several times daily, and the laxity is occasionally confused with diarrhea. The stool frequency of formula-fed infants is usually less, and the stool is of a firmer consistency, occasionally confused with constipation (Table 20-2).

Breast-feeding

Breast-feeding should be actively promoted in all societies. Whenever possible the infant is put directly to the breast at delivery. This maintains baby's temperature, promotes bonding, and allows early suckling, which in turn stimulates prolactin production by the anterior pituitary, resulting in milk production in the maternal breast. Nipple stimulation also promotes oxytocin release by the posterior pituitary gland. Oxytocin leads to contraction of the myoepithelial cells in the breast, and this causes the lactiferous sinuses to release milk ("the let-down reflex"). For the first 3 days mother produces colostrum, which is high in protein, immunoglobulins, hormones, and white cells. These probably have a role in protecting the infant against infection. Initially the volumes of fluid produced are low,

TABLE 20-2
FREQUENCY OF VOIDING AND STOOLING IN THE EARLY DAYS OF LIFE

	Days 1–2	Days 3–4	Day 5 Onward
Passage of urine	2 or more	3 or more	5 or more heavy diapers
Passage of stool	1 or more meconium	2 or more changing stool, brownish green	2 or more yellow

and the infant must break down stored glycogen to maintain blood glucose concentrations.

After the first 3 days, mother reports that her "milk has come in". The clear colostrum is now replaced by creamy-colored breast milk, rich in fat. The exact composition of breast milk varies from mother to mother, and the hindmilk, that which is produced later in the feed, is richer in fat and calories. Once the mother and infant have established satisfactory breast-feeding, almost all of the milk taken is in the first 10 minutes; any suckling thereafter is for social purposes. Suckling for too long, such as greater than 20 minutes, might exhaust both mother and baby and can result in trauma to the nipple with consequent interference with pleasurable breast-feeding.

Pediatricians tend to delegate the instruction and encouragement of breast-feeding to midwives and nurses. Although it is highly probable that these professionals give the best advice to mothers, pediatricians should possess a working knowledge of the mechanics of breast-feeding and the most common associated problems. Infants who fail to breast-feed may develop hypernatremic dehydration, a condition that can be fatal or cause major morbidity. For a detailed review of this lethal and underrecognized condition, see reference 15.

All staff should be familiar with the following principles of breast-feeding:

- Mother and baby should be relaxed and comfortable.
- No artificial teats (soothers, dummies) should be used.
- No artificial milks should be given unless medically indicated.
- Babies are commonly "sleepy" in the first 24 hours but may demand feeds every 2 to 3 hours thereafter.
- After the full fatty milk has been established on day 3 or 4, infants settle with demand feeds every 3 to 4 hours.
- Babies should suckle often, especially in the early days of life.
- Successful breast-feeding involves a wide-mouthed approach of the baby, the tongue underneath the nipple, the chin pressed into the breast tissue, and the nose high.
- Sucking should be powerful and rhythmic with pause periods for breath while the child remains latched on.
- If mothers are separated from their infants out of necessity, they should be shown how to manually express breast milk manually.

- Posseting and small vomits are common, but all bile-stained vomiting should be considered pathologic until proven otherwise.
- Term babies lose up to 10% of their birth weight and then should show a growth velocity thereafter of approximately 150 to 200 g per week. If there is any doubt about the adequacy of breast-feeding, accurate weighing can be a simple and helpful intervention.
- There is no place for "test weighing," a procedure whereby a baby is weighed before and after a feed.

Despite these important written recommendations, there is no substitute for an experienced breast-feeding counselor sitting with mother during the early feeds, optimizing mother's position, baby's position, observing latching onto the breast, ensuring that the tongue is able to milk the ducts, and noting that milk supply is adequate and that the infant successfully receives the nutrition required. Every neonatal unit and postnatal ward should possess a copy of the WHO/UNICEF recommendations on "The 10 Steps to Successful Breast-feeding" (16).

Bottle-feeding

If a mother has made an informed decision to bottle-feed her infant, there is no reason why a small formula feed should not be offered in the early minutes or hours of life. Some professionals prefer to offer a water feed first (17), but in healthy newborn infants with no history of polyhydramnios, it is not clear that this is required. Glucose feeds should not be offered, on the grounds that inhalation of glucose can cause a severe chemical pneumonitis. Newborns may take 15 to 30 mL of formula every 3 to 4 hours in the first day, rising to 90 mL feeds 4 to 5 times a day by day 5 (18). A healthy infant can establish demand feeds in the early days of life.

Poor Feeding

Poor breast-feeding is common. Poor bottle-feeding is not. The infant who is thought to be feeding poorly at the breast should be seen by an experienced professional to ensure that there is no underlying serious structural or systemic problem. Never forget infection. If the child is thought to be well, then the most important therapeutic measure is the prolonged patient attentions of a member of staff who is an expert on teaching breast-feeding.

Primigravid mothers often experience difficulties in achieving good breast-feeding, but even mothers who have breast-fed before may require further encouragement and assistance. They might say, "I have breast-fed other babies before, but I have never breast-fed that baby."

Poor bottle-feeding is much simpler to approach. The milk is available and the intake is readily measured. Again, however, structural and systemic problems should be considered, because the baby with meningitis may feed neither at the breast nor at the bottle. If there is thought to be no underlying pathology, the technique of feeding should be observed. Is the teat (nipple) adequate to allow milk flow? How is the mother holding the infant and bottle? Is the child lethargic, indicating some disease process? Is the child irritable and frustrated, indicating some mechanical difficulty in obtaining the milk desired?

Posseting

Posseting refers to the recurrent production of mouthfuls of milk from a recently fed, satisfied child. This is normal and perhaps universal. The experienced clinician must provide reassurance to the parent on the basis of a careful history and observation of the phenomenon. Adequate weight gain strongly implies that the infant is thriving. In the first few days, when weight loss is the norm, a healthy eager child who produces mouthfuls of milk is unlikely to be concealing a serious disease.

Vomiting

Vomiting is the production of larger amounts of emesis than mere mouthfuls. The occasional episode is common, even in the healthy infant, but this symptom should always be taken seriously. The vomiting infant who is otherwise clinically well and gaining weight at a normal rate is being overfed: there is no other logical explanation. This simple principle can be very reassuring to parents. The infant who is vomiting and failing to gain weight adequately has a problem that must be taken very seriously. The differential diagnosis is large (see Chapter 40). The following general principles may be helpful to the pediatrician.

- Establish the timing and quality of the vomiting. Huge projectile vomits may indicate pyloric stenosis (note that this is more common in 4 to 8 weeks of life and in boys, but it has been described in newborns and in females). Meningitis may also present as projectile vomiting. *Warning:* Both pyloric stenosis and meningitis may present in more subtle ways.
- Always observe a feed and try to establish whether it is accomplished satisfactorily. Mechanical problems, such as cleft palate, may present as vomiting during the feed itself.
- Any child who looks unwell and is vomiting may be septic. Other possibilities include metabolic disease.
- A full clinical examination is required for any newborn presenting with vomiting. Abdominal palpation may

reveal the tenderness and guarding associated with necrotizing enterocolitis. Tachypnea may point to infection or metabolic disease, triggering a full infection screen, often including lumbar puncture, and preliminary investigations for underlying metabolic conditions.

Common Neonatal Problems

Potential neonatal problems include cold and hypoglycemia.

Cold

Delivery suites that are designed for maternal comfort may be at inadequate temperatures for the infant. The neonate is limited in compensatory mechanisms, including shivering and vasoconstriction. An acute cold insult may cause the infant to become hypoglycemic and apneic. Chronic cold injury may result in failure to thrive (19).

Hypoglycemia

Over the years neonatal hypoglycemia has been defined in a multitude of ways. An infant may be said to be hypoglycemic when the blood glucose concentration is less than 2.6 mmol/L (20). Indications for testing blood glucose concentration include growth retardation, jitteriness, lethargy, cold injury, suspected infection, asphyxia, and if the infant is born of a mother with diabetes mellitus. When present, the predisposing condition should be treated. Meanwhile, a strategy must be adopted that will return the plasma glucose to normal levels promptly. This may require the establishment of an intravenous infusion of glucose. There is no "evidence-based" level for such treatment, but if the blood glucose is less than 1.7 mmol/L consideration should be given to the use of intravenous therapy. If the baby is systemically well, it is usually possible to avoid admission to a neonatal unit. Increasing the frequency of oral feeds, hand expression of breast milk, and supplementation with proprietary milk may keep the infant by mother's side. Asymptomatic hypoglycemia warrants careful observation, and the need for intervention is carefully assessed.

Skin Appearance

Chapter 55 addresses this topic in detail. The most common skin appearances that cause parental anxiety are capillary hemangioma; dry, cracked skin; an inflamed perineum; and a maculopapular rash.

Capillary hemangioma ("stork's beak mark"), is seen most frequently at the bregma and the nape of the neck. This red or pink capillary nevus blanches on pressure and fades over the early months of life, being most prominent during crying.

Dry, cracked skin is common particularly in postmature infants. Weeping and erythema should lead the clinician to further pursuit of a diagnosis.

Inflamed perineum, is usually caused by one of two events: ammoniacal dermatitis and candida. Ammoni-acal dermatitis tends to show itself as acute erythema on areas of skin exposed to the diaper. Candida is similar except that the abnormality also invades the perineal crease including the groins and often produces satellite lesions over the suprapubic area. This finding should trigger the search for thrush in the mouth; especially on the buccal mucosa.

In the early days of life a maculopapular rash is commonly seen. The papules are typically pale in the center and surrounded by a halo of erythema. In the well child, this is almost certainly erythema toxicum, which is an entirely benign self-resolving appearance requiring only reassurance. In its most flamboyant form, even experienced neonatologists may wish to culture any weeping area to ensure that the infant does not have staphylococcal dermatitis.

The Clicky Hip

In the absence of a screening program, the incidence of developmental dysplasia of the hip (DDH) would be approximately 1 in 1,000 infants delivered (21).

Chapter 19 describes how to examine an infant for DDH. Only after examining many hundreds of neonatal hips can the clinician be confident of differentiating between a lax dislocatable hip and one that is stable. The dislocatable hip provides a "clunk" in the examiner's hands. A "click" is frequently felt and can be differentiated because it is not associated with a movement of the femoral head at the acetabular lip. Indeed the source of the click is often tendon movement at the knees. Where there is doubt, the clinician should not hesitate to refer the child for an orthopedic opinion. It is much better to have a click confirmed than to miss DDH. The American Academy of Pediatrics has produced an extensive review of this subject as well as clinical practice guidelines (22,23). Primary screening of all newborn infants with ultrasonography examination of the hips is unlikely to be helpful (24). Ultrasonography may, however, be a useful adjunct in studying the hips of infants suspected to have DDH on clinical examination.

The Systolic Murmur

The population of babies with systolic murmurs changes according to the discharge policy of the hospital. If infants are discharged home in the early hours of life, there has frequently not been time for the common systolic murmurs to be heard, because the pulmonary arterial pressures are still similar to aortic pressures, and therefore shunts are small in volume. Thus the ductus arteriosus and ventricular septal defect (VSD) are probably inaudible on day 1. The VSD may first present at the community pediatrician's office when the second examination takes place.

Murmurs have been found in 1% to 2% of babies undergoing routine newborn examination (25), but less than half of these are caused by congenital malformations (26). Furthermore, of babies found to have congenital cardiac malformations, fewer than half have a murmur heard

in the newborn period (27). What should the clinician do in the hospital when a systolic murmur is heard? It is a council of perfection that all parents should be told the diagnosis before discharge home. Currently this ideal may not be achievable because of lack of local expertise in echocardiography. In practice, the pediatrician must be satisfied that the child is well, in no distress, with a normal oxygen saturation in room air and with no cardiac failure. Careful auscultation may lead to a probable diagnosis based on the character, position, and transmissibility of the murmur. Even the most experienced pediatrician should avoid being dogmatic about the complete diagnosis: the typical murmur of VSD may be the only evidence of tetralogy of Fallot, and parents will rightly feel aggrieved by being told that this is a small hole in the inner heart wall that should close off by itself. An electrocardiogram is carried out, and, provided this is normal, the family is provisionally reassured and an appointment is made for early review when the ductus arteriosus might be expected to have closed. On review, persistence of a murmur requires early referral to a pediatric cardiologist for a definitive opinion including echocardiography.

Jaundice

Jaundice is a yellow pigmentation of the skin and sclera, and is manifest to some degree in two thirds of babies in the first week of life (28). Most jaundiced babies are normal (29). The differential diagnosis and treatment of neonatal jaundice are described in Chapter 35. Each jaundiced infant should be carefully examined to exclude infection. The pediatrician should also inquire about mother and infant blood groups and the result of the Coombs (direct antiglobulin) test. In a child established on milk feeds, test a sample of urine for reducing substances: the finding of a nonglucose sugar may indicate a diagnosis of galactosemia. If the child is well, however, the majority of infants manifest jaundice as a transient phenomenon that is more common in breast-feeding babies (30). This is often a result of lower volumes of milk swallowed in early breast-feeding, and the difference is largely eliminated by encouraging the mother to feed her infant every 2 to 3 hours (31). Jaundice should never be a reason for changing a baby from breast-feeding to bottle-feeding. Transcutan-eous bilirubin monitoring is a useful, noninvasive technique that can help identify a population of babies who require to be tested by plasma bilirubin levels. Each perinatal unit should have clear protocols for initiation of phototherapy, a therapy whose main purpose is to avoid exchange transfusion, which, in turn, is intended to avoid bilirubin encephalopathy.

Cryptorchidism

At birth approximately 2% of males exhibit failure of descent of one or both testes. Most of these will descend in the next four months of life, perhaps because of a postnatal surge of testosterone. It is true that cryptorchidism is associated with decreased fertility and increased malignancy, but it is not yet clear that orchidopexy is preventive. Nevertheless, pediatric surgeons may wish to operate when the child is around 1 year of age.

SPECIFIC CONGENITAL INFECTIONS

Syphilis

Syphilis is again beginning to show itself as a significant pathogen worldwide, and consequently congenital syphilis is a resurgent problem. Adequate treatment of the mother prior to 18 weeks gestation almost always protects the fetus. If the mother is untreated, there is up to a 70% chance that the newborn will be infected. There may be fetal loss or hydrops. A surviving newborn infant may present with anemia, hepatosplenomegaly, and pneumonia.

The subject of screening is a vexed one, and each community may reasonably develop a program based on the incidence of congenital syphilis and its anticipated occurrence in years to come.

The Centers for Disease Control and Prevention (CDC) (32) recommends that

Pregnant women should be screened early in pregnancy. . . . In areas of high syphilis prevalence, or in patients at high risk, screening should be repeated in the third trimester and again at delivery. . . . An infant should not be released from the hospital until the serologic status of its mother is known.

Diagnosis in the mother is based on the visualization of *Treponema pallidum* by dark ground microscopy or complement fixation (Wasserman) or flocculation tests (Kahn, Venereal Disease Research Laboratory [VDRL]). The *T. pallidum* immobilization test (TPI) and the direct fluorescent treponema antibody absorption (FTA-Abs) immunoglobulin (Ig) M test are more specific. The obstetrician and pediatrician should work closely with the microbiology laboratory to ensure that the results are correctly interpreted. Such interpretation may vary based on the mother's treatment or partial treatment during pregnancy.

Evaluation of the infant includes the following measures (32):

- Complete physical examination
- Serologic test for syphilis (the same test performed on the mother so that titers can be compared)
- Lumbar puncture for analysis of cells, protein, and VDRL
- Long-bone radiographs

The evaluation and treatment of maternal and congenital syphilis are complicated and should always be managed by a multidisciplinary team.

Hepatitis B

The mother who tests positive for hepatitis B surface antigen (HBsAg-positive) can transmit hepatitis B virus (HBV) perinatally to her newborn. In up to 90% of newborns, the immune response to infection is incomplete and a chronic infective carrier state occurs. The disease in the newborn may present as a very wide spectrum from apparent normality to severe, fatal hepatitis. Perinatally infected infants are at particular risk of becoming chronic carriers, and, even if free of chronic hepatitis, they are at increased risk of developing later cirrhosis or hepatocellular carcinoma. Because immunoprophylaxis against HBV initiated at birth is 98% to 99% effective in preventing virus acquisition by the infant, identification of HBsAg-positive pregnant women is essential (33). In the developed world each country must make decisions about a screening program based on prevalence of hepatitis B, incidence of congenital disease, and the resources available to tackle this major problem. In the United States and Canada, confining testing to high-risk women (e.g., Asian or African race, intravenous drug abuse, multiple sexual partners) may miss 50% of those who are HBsAg-positive; therefore, "prenatal HBsAg testing of all pregnant women is recommended. . ." (33).

Treatment of the infant whose mother is HBsAg-positive or hepatitis B e antigen (HBeAg)-positive or who has had acute hepatitis during pregnancy consists of immediate, thorough bathing; administration of 0.5 mL of hepatitis B immunoglobulin (HBIg) intramuscularly within 12 hours of birth; and the first dose of hepatitis B vaccine (0.5 mL) intramuscularly, concurrently with HBIg but at a different site.

Additional doses of vaccine are given at 1 and 6 months of age (33).

Babies born to mothers who are HBsAg-positive and anti-HBeAg-positive should have hepatitis B vaccine but not HBIg. When in doubt, the pediatrician must always consult with a virologist expert in perinatal disease.

Note that no special isolation is necessary. Although HBV is found in breast milk, breast-fed infants, even if they are not receiving immunoprophylaxis, are not at increased risk of acquiring HBV infection, and breast-feeding therefore is allowed. In the United States, infants born to known HBsAg-positive women should receive HBIg and the recommended 3 doses of vaccine, but there is no need to delay the initiation of breast-feeding until after the infant is immunized (33).

In some countries a hepatitis B immunization series is recommended for all infants, including those of HBsAg-negative mothers. National guidelines must be consulted and local programs adapted to the community need. This requires the input of an expert multidisciplinary team.

Recently, because of concerns about thiomersal, which is an organic compound containing mercury, thimerosal-free hepatitis B vaccines have been developed.

Human Immunodeficiency Virus (HIV)

Human immunodeficiency virus (HIV) is a retrovirus that can cause meningitis and encephalopathy. Vertical transmission may occur transplacentally, and also acutely during labor. Such transmission occurs in 13% to 45% of cases, but this risk

---

can be reduced by zidovudine and perhaps by cesarean section delivery. Approximately one-third of infected children will become symptomatic in the first year of life.

Maternal antibodies are transferred passively to the infant and are detectable for 15 to 18 months; therefore, HIV culture and identification of HIV proviral deoxyribonucleic acid (DNA) by means of the polymerase chain reaction (PCR) are the preferred diagnostic tests for the newborn. Because false-negative results are common within the first month of life, retesting at 4 to 6 months is recommended. All exposed infants need comprehensive follow up, preferably by a pediatrician with a particular expertise in HIV infection and its profound effects on families.

There are documented cases of infants acquiring HIV infection through breast-feeding. The American Academy of Pediatricians (AAP) recommendation states, "In the United States, where safe alternative sources of feeding are readily available and affordable, HIV-infected women should be counseled not to breastfeed their infants. . ." (34). This recommendation is now widely adopted throughout the developed world. No special isolation for mother or infant is necessary as long as universal precautions are followed.

POST-DISCHARGE

Car Safety

Car safety ideally should be planned before delivery of the infant. Staff should be aware of the regulations of the national car safety authorities to ensure that the guidelines available in the perinatal service are compatible with the law and are up to date.

The following principles are important:

- The child car seat should be suitable for the weight and size of the child.
- The seat should have a United Nations "E" mark, a British standards "kitemark," or a European "e" mark.
- The parent fitting the car seat should ensure that the adult seat belt passes through all the correct guides.
- If the adult seat has an airbag in front of it, do not fit a rear-facing child restraint.
- It should be possible to fit an adult hand between the child's chest and the restraining harness.

Timing and Planning

Throughout the developed world there is great variation in the timing of discharge home. It should be dictated primarily by the well-being of the infant and of the mother. Mothers with other children at home may be anxious to achieve early discharge, perhaps within hours of delivery. In the United Kingdom this is exemplified by the DoMInO (Domiciliary Midwife In and Out) scheme, where a mother is cared for antenatally, intrapartum and postpartum by the same midwife or team of midwives. No matter what the program available, the professionals should ensure that mother and baby are healthy and that they have been adequately prepared for life in the community.

A checklist should be completed and signed by parents and professionals prior to discharge. The checklist should include at least the following items:

- Parents are able to care for their infant independently.
- Feeding is satisfactory and will be further supported in the community.
- If the child is bottle-feeding, parents demonstrate ability to sterilize bottles and teats.
- Parents have been given information on choking, crying, frequency and consistency of passage of stool.
- Parents given advice on baby's day and night clothing, outdoor clothing, and how to assess baby's temperature.
- Parents given verbal and written information about prevention of sudden infant death syndrome.
- Audiologic screening has been performed (where this is available).
- Arrangements for follow up are clear, whether this is domiciliary visiting, at the practitioner's office in the community, or by return to a hospital clinic.
- Parents have discussed car seat safety and have a car seat that meets the national safety requirements.
- Parents have demonstrated satisfactory knowledge of elementary cardiopulmonary resuscitation.
- Parents possess any drug prescriptions and have demonstrated ability to administer drugs to the baby.
- Parents possess a written record of any immunizations given and have clear written plans for future immunizations.

It is also important that the discharge plan for mother and infant be individualized. Factors that may alter the plan include baby's birth weight, any illnesses or congenital abnormalities present, parents' wishes and confidence, educational attainment of the parents, staff knowledge of parents' lifestyle and support available, whether the home is urban or rural, and whether transportation is readily available. Special planning is required to support an adolescent mother and her infant: the responsibility of care must be clear, and robust systems should be put into place to allow the teenage mother to return to school whenever this is practical.

The hospital should communicate clearly with the team responsible for care of the family in the community to ensure that continuity of care is seamless.

REFERENCES

1. Howie PW, Forsyth JS, Ogston SA, et al. Protective effect of breast-feeding against infection. *BMJ* 1990;300:11–16.
2. Gillman MW, Rifas-Shiman SL, Camargo CA Jr, et al. Risk of overweight among adolescents who were breast-fed as infants. *JAMA* 2001;285:2461–2467.
3. Alm B, Wennergren G, Norvenius SG, et al. Breastfeeding and the sudden infant death syndrome in Scandinavia, 1992–1995. *Arch Dis Child* 2002;86(6):400–402.
4. McVea KL, Turner PD, Peppler DK. The role of breast feeding in sudden infant death syndrome. *J Hum Lact* 2000;16(1):13–20.

5. Lane PA, Hathaway WE. Vitamin K in infancy. *J Pediatr* 1985; 106:351–359.

6. AAP Committee on Fetus and Newborn and ACOG Committee on Obstetrics: Maternal and fetal medicine. Postpartum and follow-up care. In: Freeman RK, Poland RL, eds. *Guidelines for perinatal care*, 3rd ed. Elk Grove Village, IL: American Academy of Pediatrics and American College of Obstetricians and Gynecologists, 1992:91.

7. Wiswell TE, Gannon CM, Jacob J, et al. Delivery room management of the apparently vigorous meconium-stained neonate: results of the multicenter, international collaborative trial. *Pediatrics* 2000;105:1–7.

8. Mercer JS. Current best evidence: a review of the literature on umbilical cord clamping. *J Midwifery Womens Health* 2001;46: 402–414.

9. Cunningham FG, MacDonald PC, Gant NF. *Williams Obstetrics*, 18th ed. Norwalk, CT: Appleton & Lange, 1989:307.

10. Thompson JE, Clark DA, Salisbury B, et al. Footprinting the newborn infant: not cost effective. *J Pediatr* 1981;99:797–798.

11. Birenbaum HJ, Glorioso L, Rosenberger C, et al. Gowning on a postpartum ward fails to decrease colonization in the newborn infant. *Am J Dis Child* 1990;144:1031–1033.

12. Hudome SM, Fisher MC. Nosocomial infections in the neonatal intensive care unit. *Curr Opin Infect Dis* 2001;14(3):303–307.

13. Committee on Infectious Diseases, American Academy of Pediatrics. Prevention of neonatal ophthalmia. In: Peter G, Lepow ML, McCracken GH Jr, et al., eds. *Report of the committee on infectious diseases*, 22nd ed. Elk Grove Village, IL: American Academy of Pediatrics, 1991:546.

14. Clark DA. Times of first void and first stool in 500 newborns. *Pediatrics* 1977;60:457–459.

15. Laing IA, Wong CM. Hypernatraemia in the first few days: is the incidence rising? *Arch Dis Child Fetal Neonatal Ed* 2002;87:F158–F162.

16. World Health Organization. *Protecting, promoting and supporting breast feeding: the special role of maternity services (a joint WHO/UNICEF statement)*. Geneva: World Health Organization, 1989.

17. Olson M. The benign effects on rabbits' lungs of the aspiration of water compared with 5% glucose or milk. *Pediatrics* 1970;46: 538–547..

18. Driscoll JM Jr. Routine and special care. In: Fanaroff AA, Martin RJ, eds. *Neonatal-perinatal medicine*, 4th ed. St. Louis: CV Mosby, 1987:441.

19. Oliver TK Jr. Temperature regulation and heat production in the newborn. *Pediatr Clin North Am* 1965;12:765–799.

20. Lucas A, Morley R, Cole TJ. Adverse neurodevelopmental outcome of moderate neonatal hypoglycaemia. *BMJ* 1988;297:1304–1308.

21. Leck I. Congenital dislocation of the hip. In: Wald N, Leck I, eds. *Antenatal and neonatal screening*. Oxford: Oxford University Press; 2000.

22. Committee on Quality Improvement and Subcommittee on Developmental Dysplasia of the Hip. Clinical practice guideline: early detection of developmental dysplasia of the hip. *Pediatrics* 2000;105:896–905.

23. Lehmann HP, Hinton R, Morello P, et al. Developmental dysplasia of the hip practice guideline: technical report. Committee on Quality Improvement, and Subcommittee on Developmental Dysplasia of the Hip. *Pediatrics* 2000;105:e57.

24. Gardiner HM, Dunn PM. Controlled trial of immediate splinting versus ultrasonographic surveillance in congenitally dislocatable hips. *Lancet* 1990;336:1553–1556.

25. Arlettaz R, Archer N, Wilkinson AR. Natural history of innocent heart murmurs in newborn babies: controlled echocardiographic study. *Arch Dis Child* 1998;78:F166–F170.

26. Ainsworth SB, Wyllie JP, Wren C. Prevalence and significance of cardiac murmurs in neonates. *Arch Dis Child* 1999;80:F43–F45.

27. Wren C, Richmond S, Donaldson L. Presentation of congenital heart disease in infancy: implications for routine examination. *Arch Dis Child* 1999;80:F49–F53.

28. Maisels MJ, Newman TB. Jaundice in the healthy full-term infant: time for reevaluation. In: Klaus MH, Fanaroff AA, eds. *1990 Yearbook of neonatal and perinatal medicine*. St. Louis: Mosby Year Book, 1990:iv.

29. Newman TB, Maisels MJ. Does hyperbilirubinemia damage the brain of healthy full-term infants? *Clin Perinatol* 1990; 17:331–358.

30. Schneider AP II. Breast milk jaundice in the newborn. *JAMA* 1986;255:3270.

31. Yamauchi Y, Yamanouchi I. Breast-feeding frequency during the first 24 hours after birth in full-term neonates. *Pediatrics* 1990;86:171–175.

32. Centers for Disease Control and Prevention. 1989 Sexually transmitted diseases treatment guidelines. *MMWR Morb Mortal Wkly Rep* 1989;38:9.

33. Committee on Infectious Diseases, American Academy of Pediatrics. Hepatitis B. In: Peter G, Lepow ML, McCracken GH Jr, et al, eds. *Report of the committee on infectious diseases*, 22nd ed. Elk Grove Village, IL: American Academy of Pediatrics, 1991; 238 .

34. Committee on Infectious Diseases, American Academy of Pediatrics. AIDS and HIV infections. In: Peter G, Lepow ML, McCracken GH Jr, et al, eds. *Report of the committee on infectious diseases*, 22nd ed. Elk Grove Village, IL: American Academy of Pediatrics, 1991:115.

Fluid and Electrolyte Management

Edward F. Bell   William Oh

Infants who are born prematurely or who are critically ill cannot regulate their own intake of fluids and nutrients. Moreover, enteral feeding is often limited by feeding intolerance or medical problems that preclude or limit use of the gastrointestinal tract for feeding. In other cases, the infant presents with disordered fluid and electrolyte balance as a primary result of an underlying illness. In all of these situations, water and electrolytes must be provided by prescription of the health provider. Prescribing the correct amounts of water and electrolytes helps to assure the infant's healthy recovery.

The goal of fluid and electrolyte management is to replace losses of water and electrolytes so as to maintain normal balance of these essential substances during growth and recovery from disease. A subsidiary aim in the first days of life is to allow successful transition from the aquatic environment of the uterus into the arid extrauterine milieu. The principles of fluid and electrolyte management in the neonatal period are similar to those established for older children, except for some variations and specific features of body composition, insensible water loss (IWL), renal function, and neuroendocrine control of fluid and electrolyte balance.

To manage fluid therapy of newborns appropriately, the clinician should understand the normal physiologic mechanisms that govern water and electrolyte balance and the variations in these mechanisms that can occur in sick or premature infants. The clinician should develop a systematic approach to the estimation of fluid and electrolyte requirements for correction of deficits and replacement of ongoing losses, both normal and abnormal. Finally, the results of fluid and electrolyte management must be carefully monitored so that the intakes of water and electrolytes can be adjusted as needed.

BODY COMPOSITION OF THE FETUS AND NEWBORN INFANT

Changes in Body Water During Growth

The total body water (TBW) is divided into two major compartments, intracellular (ICW) and extracellular (ECW). The ECW is further divided into the interstitial water and the plasma volume, which is the intravascular component of the ECW (Fig. 21-1).

In the early stages of fetal development, a large part of the body consists of water (1). It has been estimated that TBW is 94% of the body weight during the third month of fetal life. As gestation progresses, the TBW per kilogram declines. By 24 weeks the TBW is approximately 86%, and by term it is about 78% of body weight (Fig. 21-2). There also are characteristic changes in the partition of body water between ECW and ICW during development. ECW decreases from 59% of body weight at 24 weeks of gestation to about 44% at term, and ICW increases from 27% to 34% of body weight during the same period (Table 21-1) (1–6). Infants born prematurely thus have higher TBW and ECW per kilogram than their term counterparts (7–9), and small-for-gestational-age infants have higher TBW per kilogram than do appropriate-for-gestational-age infants (9).

After birth, TBW per kilogram of body weight continues to fall, due primarily to contraction of the ECW (2,7,8, 10–13). This mobilization of extracellular fluid occurs in conjunction with the improvement in renal function that takes place following birth (14,15), which is thought to occur as a result of increasing glomerular filtration rate and perhaps, too, as a result of increasing levels of the epithelial transport proteins involved in renal tubular function (16). It has also been suggested that atrial natriuretic peptide

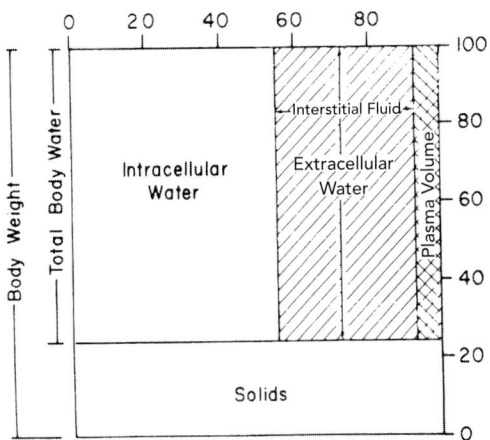

Figure 21-1 Distribution of body water in a term newborn infant.

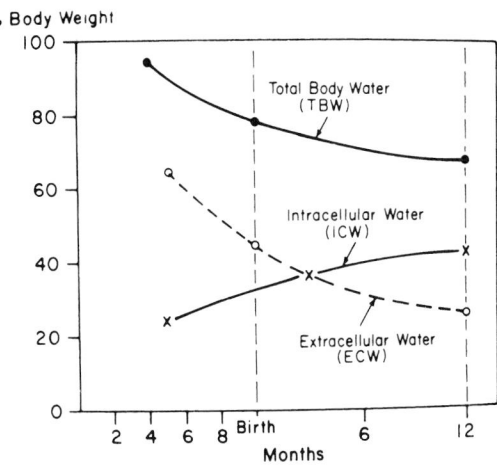

Figure 21-2 Changes in body water during gestation and infancy. (Adapted from Friis-Hansen B. Changes in body water compartments during growth. *Acta Paediatr* 1957;46(Suppl 110):1–68., with permission.)

plays a role in the postnatal contraction of the ECW (13). Various studies have shown an increase, decrease, or no change in the ICW after birth. ICW probably increases roughly in proportion to body weight in the first weeks of postnatal life (2,7,8,17). Thereafter, ICW increases faster than body weight and exceeds ECW by 3 months of age (Fig. 21-2) (1,2). These postnatal changes in body water and its partition between ECW and ICW are influenced by the intake of water and electrolytes (11,18). Failure to allow the normal postnatal contraction of ECW in premature infants may increase the risk of significant patent ductus arteriosus (PDA) (19), necrotizing enterocolitis (NEC) (20–22), and bronchopulmonary dysplasia (BPD) (23,24).

Solute Distribution in Body Fluids

The major cation in the blood plasma is sodium (Fig. 21-3). Potassium, calcium, and magnesium constitute the bal-

ance of the cation fraction. The primary anion is chloride, with protein, bicarbonate, and some undetermined anions constituting the balance of the anions. The interstitial fluid (i.e., nonplasma ECW) has a solute composition that is similar to plasma except that its protein content is lower. The ICW contains potassium and magnesium as its primary cations, and phosphate, both organic and inorganic, is the major anion, with bicarbonate contributing a smaller fraction.

The electrolyte composition of the body fluids of the newborn infant is largely determined by gestational age. Premature infants contain more sodium and chloride per kilogram of body weight than term infants (3–5) because of their larger ECW (Table 21-1). Total body potassium content largely reflects ICW and is similar or slightly lower

TABLE 21-1
CHANGES IN BODY WATER AND ELECTROLYTE COMPOSITION DURING INTRAUTERINE AND EARLY POSTNATAL LIFE

	Gestational Age (Weeks)					
Component	24	28	32	36	40	1 to 4 Weeks After Term Birth
Total body water (%)	86	84	82	80	78	74
Extracellular water (%)	59	56	52	48	44	41
Intracellular water (%)	27	28	30	32	34	33
Sodium (mEq/kg)	99	91	85	80	77	73
Potassium (mEq/kg)	40	41	40	41	41	42
Chloride (mEq/kg)	70	67	62	56	51	48

Data from Friis-Hansen B. Changes in body water compartments during growth. *Acta Paediatr* 1957;6 (Suppl 110):1–68; Friis-Hansen B. Body water compartments in children: changes during growth and related changes in body composition. *Pediatrics* 1961;28:169–181; Ziegler EE, O'Donnell AM, Nelson SE, et al. Body composition of the reference fetus. *Growth* 1976;40:329–341; Forbes JB, Perley A. Estimation of total body sodium by isotopic dilution. II. Studies on infants and children: an example of a constant differential growth ratio. *J Clin Invest* 1951;30:566–574; Cheek DB. Observations on total body chloride in children. *Pediatrics* 1954;14:5–10; Romahn A, Burmeister W. [Body composition during the first two years of life: analysis with the potassium 40 method]. *Klin Pädiatr* 1977;189:321–327.

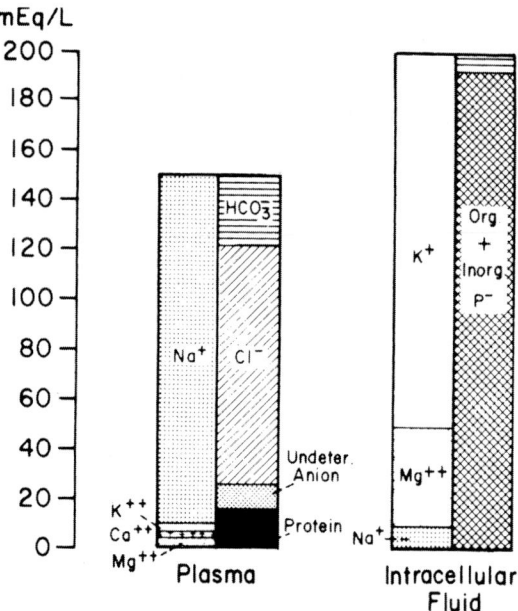

Figure 21-3 Ion distribution in the blood plasma, which represents extracellular fluid, and in the intracellular fluid compartment.

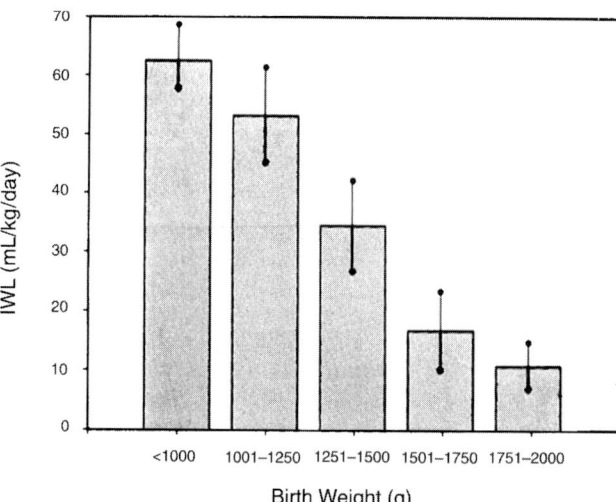

Figure 21-4 Relation between insensible water loss (IWL) and birth weight of 5-day-old (mean) infants in incubators. (Data from Wu PY, Hodgman JE. Insensible water loss in preterm infants: changes with postnatal development and non-ionizing radiant energy. *Pediatrics* 1974;54:704–712, as redrawn in Shaffer SG, Weismann DN. Fluid requirements in the preterm infant. *Clin Perinatol* 1992;19: 233–250, with permission.)

per kilogram of body weight in premature infants than at term (3,6). These concepts are important in the management of fluid and electrolyte therapy for newborn infants.

In the fetus, fluid and electrolyte balance depends on maternal homeostasis and placental exchange. Thus, fluid and electrolyte status at birth is influenced by the maternal fluid and electrolyte management in labor (25–28).

INSENSIBLE WATER LOSS

The loss of water by evaporation from the skin and respiratory tract is known as insensible water loss (IWL). About 30%

of IWL normally occurs through the respiratory tract as moisture in expired gas (29–31), with the remaining 70% lost through the skin. IWL can be expressed in reference to body surface area (m^2) or weight (kg). IWL depends more on surface area than weight, but it is commonly expressed per kilogram because weight is more easily determined than area.

A number of factors are known to influence IWL in a predictable manner (Table 21-2) (29–60). When expressed per kilogram of body weight, IWL is inversely proportional to birth weight and gestational age (Figs. 21-4 and 21-5) (32,33,35). In other words, smaller, more immature infants have larger IWL per kilogram (Table 21-3). The

TABLE 21-2
FACTORS AFFECTING INSENSIBLE WATER LOSS IN NEWBORN INFANTS

Factor	Effect on Insensible Water Loss (IWL)
Level of maturity (32,33,35–37)	Inversely proportional to birth weight and gestational age (Fig. 21-4)
Respiratory distress (hyperpnea) (38)	Respiratory IWL increases with rising minute ventilation when dry air is being breathed
Environmental temperature above neutral thermal zone (29,39,40)	Increased in proportion to increment in temperature
Elevated body temperature (29,39)	Increased by up to 300%
Skin breakdown or injury	Increased by uncertain magnitude
Congenital skin defect (e.g., gastroschisis, omphalocele, neural tube defect)	Increased by uncertain magnitude until surgically corrected
Radiant warmer (33,41–45)	Increased by about 50%
Phototherapy (43,46,47)	Increased by about 50%
Motor activity and crying (29,49,50)	Increased by up to 70%
High ambient or inspired humidity (29,31)	Reduced by 30% when ambient vapor pressure is increased by 200%
Plastic heat shield (32,44,52)	Reduced by 30% to 70%
Plastic blanket (52–54) or chamber (54,55)	Reduced by 30% to 70%
Semipermeable membrane (56–58)	Reduced by 50%
Topical agents (59,60)	Reduced by 50%

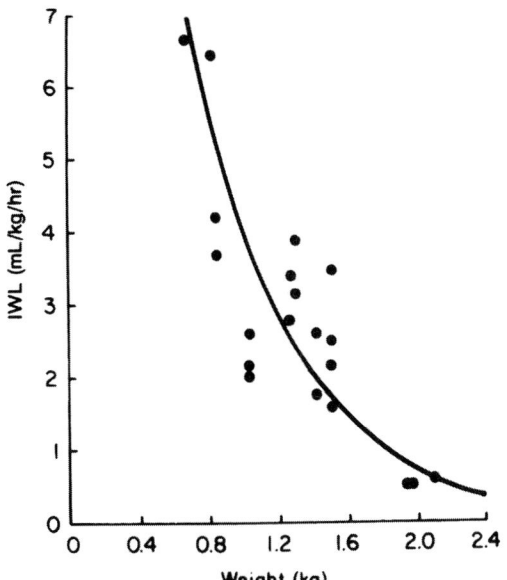

Figure 21-5 Insensible water loss (IWL) as a function of birth weight in premature infants nursed under radiant warmers. (Adapted from Costarino AT, Baumgart. Controversies in fluid and electrolyte therapy for the premature infant. *Clin Perinatol* 1988; 15:863–878, with permission.)

same is true if IWL is expressed per square meter of body surface (36,37). Therefore, although the greater IWL of smaller premature infants is partly due to the increased ratio of surface area (skin and respiratory tract) to body weight, it also is thought to be related to their thinner skin, greater skin blood flow, larger body water per kilogram of body weight, and higher respiratory rate. Because skin permeability to water varies inversely with gestational age, the degree of immaturity is an important determinant of cutaneous IWL independent of birth weight.

Factors That Increase Insensible Water Loss

An increase in minute ventilation increases the respiratory IWL (38) as long as the water vapor pressure is less in the

inspired than in the expired gas. Increased minute ventilation may occur in infants with cardiac disease, pulmonary dysfunction, or metabolic acidosis.

Environmental temperature above the neutral thermal zone increases IWL in proportion to the increment in temperature (29,39,40). This effect can occur even without a rise in body temperature. In contrast, a subneutral environmental temperature is not associated with reduced IWL, although metabolic heat production is increased (40). Increased body temperature, whether caused by fever or environmental overheating, elevates IWL (29,39).

Skin breakdown or injury disrupts the barrier against cutaneous evaporation and raises IWL. Skin trauma from thermal, chemical, or mechanical injury is common among critically ill, small, premature infants. Such injury may result from removal of tape and adherent monitoring devices or from prolonged skin exposure to disinfectant solutions. IWL also is increased in conjunction with the skin manifestations of essential fatty acid deficiency, a potential problem in infants receiving fat-free parenteral nutrition. Congenital skin defects, such as those seen in gastroschisis, omphalocele, and neural tube defects, are associated with increased IWL until surgically corrected.

Use of nonionizing radiant energy, in the form of either a radiant warmer or phototherapy, has been shown to increase IWL by about 50% (33,41–48). For infants in incubators with controlled air temperature, the increase in IWL with overhead phototherapy is most likely a result of increased body temperature because of the warmer incubator walls (46). For infants in incubators operated to control skin temperature, the rise in IWL with phototherapy can be explained by the lower absolute humidity resulting from the reduced air temperature that accompanies the warming of the incubator walls by the phototherapy. The impact on IWL of phototherapy delivered by fiberoptic blankets or pads is not known but is probably negligible unless the blanket produces a warmer or moister microenvironment around the infant. Investigators using direct measurements of transepidermal and respiratory water loss have obtained

TABLE 21-3

AVERAGE INSENSIBLE WATER LOSS[a] OF PREMATURE INFANTS IN INCUBATORS

Age (d)	Birth Weight Range (kg)					
	0.50–0.75	0.75–1.00	1.00–1.25	1.25–1.50	1.50–1.75	1.75–2.00
0–7	100[a]	65	55	40	20	15
7–14	80	60	50	40	30	20

[a] Insensible water loss (mL/kg/day).
Data from Wu PY, Hodgman JE. Insensible water loss in preterm infants: changes with postnatal development and non-ionizing radiant energy. *Pediatrics* 1974;54:704–712; Okken A, Jonxis JH, Rispens P, et al. Insensible water loss and metabolic rate in low birthweight newborn infants. *Pediatr Res* 1979;13:1072–1075; Hammarlund K, Sedin G. Transepidermal water loss in newborn infants. III. Relation to gestational age. *Acta Paediatr Scand* 1979;68:795–801.

TABLE 21-4

RELATIVE AND ABSOLUTE HUMIDITY AS RELATED TO INSENSIBLE WATER LOSS IN INCUBATORS AND UNDER RADIANT WARMERS

Measurement	Incubator	Radiant Warmer
Air temperature (°C)	35.0	27.6
Saturation pressure (mm Hg)	42.1	27.7
Relative humidity (%)	31.4	39.0
Absolute humidity (mm Hg)	13.2	10.8
Insensible water loss (mL/kg/hour)	2.37	3.40

Data from Bell EF, Weinstein MR, Oh W. Heat balance in premature infants: comparative effects of convectively heated incubator and radiant warmer, with and without plastic heat shield. *J Pediatr* 1980;96: 460–465.

conflicting results regarding the effect of overhead phototherapy on IWL. One group (47) found an increase in transepidermal water loss with phototherapy, but another did not (61,62).

If an infant's IWL is measured at the same skin temperature under a radiant warmer and in an incubator, the IWL is higher (by about 50%) under the radiant warmer. IWL is higher because absolute humidity (water vapor pressure) is lower under the radiant warmer than in the incubator (44). This may be true even if relative humidity is higher under the radiant warmer (43,44) because the lower air temperature with the radiant warmer means that the saturation pressure of water vapor is considerably lower than in the incubator (Table 21-4). This finding has been confirmed using direct measurements of transepidermal water loss (45). It is now understood that the higher IWL with radiant warmers arises from the lower ambient water vapor pressure and not from higher air velocity or a direct effect of nonionizing radiation on the skin. The same phenomenon explains the effect of phototherapy on IWL of infants in incubators operated by skin temperature servocontrol. The effects on IWL of radiant warmers and phototherapy are additive; the IWL with the combination is approximately twice as large as in an incubator without phototherapy (43,48).

Increased motor activity and crying increase IWL by up to 70% (29,49,50). This effect may be partly due to elevated minute ventilation.

Factors That Reduce Insensible Water Loss

Increasing the humidity or water vapor pressure of inspired gas reduces respiratory IWL. The inspired humidity is raised by humidifying the air-oxygen mixture delivered to a head hood or directly to the infant's upper airway (e.g., via nasal cannula, face mask, or endotracheal tube) if respiratory support is required. If the temperature and water content of the inspired and expired gas are the same, the respiratory IWL will be entirely eliminated (51). Increasing ambient humidity, for example in an incubator, reduces

total IWL, but respiratory IWL is decreased more than cutaneous IWL (29); a threefold increase in ambient water vapor pressure, from an average of 7 to 25 mm Hg, resulted in a 30% reduction in total IWL. Increasing ambient humidity is facilitated by the design of certain recent models of incubators. The use of incubator humidification systems should not be overlooked as a way of reducing IWL.

Plexiglas heat shields are effective in reducing the IWL of small premature infants in incubators (32,44), especially if the ends are at least partially enclosed to decrease air movement near the skin. Plexiglas heat shields are not effective for infants under radiant warmers (44,52) because Plexiglas is opaque to the infrared energy produced by the radiant heaters. Thin barriers of saran and other materials reduce IWL of infants under radiant warmers while allowing the infrared heat to reach the skin (52). These heat shields presumably reduce IWL by limiting air movement and raising water vapor pressure near the infant's body surface.

Thin plastic blankets have been found to reduce IWL by 30% to 70% for infants under radiant warmers and in incubators (52–54). Chambers made of thin plastic material also reduce IWL by a similar amount (54,55). Semipermeable membranes (56–58) and waterproof topical agents (59,60) reduce IWL from the covered areas by an average of approximately 50%.

Knowledge of these factors that affect IWL is essential for estimating the water intake required by newborn infants and for making appropriate adjustments in water intake with changes in care. Of all infants, premature and critically ill infants are the ones whose IWL is most significantly influenced by these factors. This is especially true for the extremely premature infant, of whom more are surviving each year. However, these are exactly the infants for whom precise maintenance of fluid and electrolyte balance is most important and for whom the margin of error is smallest.

NEUROENDOCRINE CONTROL OF FLUID AND ELECTROLYTE BALANCE

The pituitary gland, adrenal cortex, parathyroid glands, and heart are the major organs producing hormones involved in the regulation of water and electrolyte balance in the body. The basic mechanisms by which the antidiuretic hormone, arginine vasopressin (AVP), is produced and secreted by the posterior pituitary gland appear to be intact in newborn infants (63–65), even in those who are born prematurely (66). It is not clear at what age precise quantitative hypothalamic control of AVP production is established. However, it is known that even in the first week of life, breast-fed term infants release AVP in response to a 10% loss of body weight (65).

Aldosterone is the most potent mineralocorticoid produced and secreted by the adrenal cortex. Its synthesis is regulated by the renin-angiotensin system, adrenocorticotropic hormone, and plasma concentrations of sodium and potassium. These mechanisms appear to be intact in newborn infants, even those born prematurely (67–71). Increased sodium loss in the urine of premature infants in the presence of high plasma concentrations of aldosterone and elevated urinary aldosterone excretion suggests that the renal tubule is less responsive in premature than in term infants (69,70). Under conditions of low sodium intake, however, the high plasma aldosterone concentrations found in sick newborn infants seems to promote increased sodium reabsorption in the distal nephron (71).

Calcium concentration in the blood of newborn infants is regulated by the balance between parathyroid hormone (PTH), which is produced by the parathyroid glands, and calcitonin, which is produced in the thyroid. Serum PTH concentration is low at birth and rises slowly during the first few days, both in term and premature infants (72–74). The same pattern has been observed with serum calcitonin concentrations, low at birth and rising thereafter (73,74). Intravenous calcium infusion to large premature and term infants caused elevation of serum calcitonin and a corresponding fall in serum PTH (75). These data together indicate that the hormonal regulation of calcium metabolism is basically intact in newborn infants, even those born prematurely.

Atrial natriuretic factor (ANF) is present in the fetal heart early during development (76). In the human fetus, cardiac atrial levels of ANF increase during gestation and, by the beginning of the third trimester, exceed adult human levels; during the same period, fetal ventricular ANF levels decrease (77). Plasma ANF levels rise after birth, peaking at the time of maximal postnatal diuresis, usually 48 to 72 hours, and then returning to levels below those at birth (78–80). ANF secretion is stimulated by volume loading (81), and ANF levels correlate with atrial size (82). ANF in turn stimulates diuresis and natriuresis and seems to play an important role in the regulation of extracellular fluid volume in newborn infants (82–84). However, studies of the effects of sodium supplementation on ANF levels and sodium excretion (83) indicate that premature infants are less responsive to ANF than are adults.

RENAL FUNCTION IN RELATION TO FLUID AND ELECTROLYTE THERAPY

Most aspects of renal function are incompletely developed at birth, especially in premature infants (15,58–90). Both glomerular and tubular functions increase with gestational age at birth (15,85–87,90) and with postnatal age (15,87–89). This development seems to depend most directly on postmenstrual age (gestational age at birth plus postnatal age) and occurs at approximately the same rate, regardless of whether the infant has been born or is *in utero* (86,87,89).

In spite of the immaturity of some aspects of renal tubular function at birth, the tubules seem to respond to AVP from the first day of life, even in small premature infants (66). However, the maximal urine concentration of prema-

ture infants, typically 600 mOsm/L, is less than that of term newborn infants (800 mOsm/L) or adults (1200 mOsm/L) (91,92). Both term and premature infants can excrete urine with osmolarity as low as 50 mOsm/L when challenged with an acute water load (92–95). Although they can produce dilute urine, newborn infants cannot excrete a water load as rapidly as adults can (93).

The limitations in renal function in premature infants contribute to the problems of fluid and electrolyte regulation in various disease states. The glomerular and tubular functions of premature infants allow them to handle some physiologic variations in water and electrolyte load, but imbalance readily occurs when estimations of the water and electrolyte needs are misjudged, particularly in the case of extremely premature infants.

PRINCIPLES OF FLUID AND ELECTROLYTE THERAPY

As in older children, three steps should be followed in the management of infants with fluid and electrolyte disorders:

1. Estimate the deficits of fluid and electrolytes.
2. Calculate the amounts of fluid and electrolytes required for replacement of deficits, maintenance, and replacement of ongoing abnormal losses.
3. Institute a system of monitoring the response to therapy.

Estimation of Fluid and Electrolyte Deficits

Fluid Deficit

The body water deficit can be estimated by the degree of dehydration. If serial body weight measurements are available, the acute weight loss is considered to represent the water deficit. During the first week of life, however, weight loss of up to 15% occurs normally as a result of contraction of extracellular water and tissue catabolism. Even those small premature infants who can be enterally fed lose an average of 10% of their body weight during the first 5 days of life (96). Among premature infants who must be nourished intravenously, it is not uncommon to observe weight loss of 15% or more without evidence of circulatory or renal insufficiency resulting from dehydration (97). The precise amount of weight loss desired during the first week of life has not been established because of a lack of reliable physiologic data. In general, smaller infants tend to lose larger fractions of their weight following birth (97). For small premature infants, a weight loss of 2% to 3% per day is a reasonable target in the first week of life. Efforts to completely prevent postnatal weight loss risk overhydration and problems with symptomatic PDA (19). Beyond the first week of life, acute weight loss should be considered to indicate nonphysiologic dehydration, and the calculated deficit of water should be replaced.

If serial body weight data are not available, urine volume and concentration and physical signs can be used to estimate the degree of dehydration. Infants with 5% isotonic (i.e., serum sodium concentration of 130 to 150 mEq/L) dehydration have dry mucous membranes, subnormal tear production with crying, flat or slightly sunken anterior fontanel (when quiet in the upright position), and oliguria. Infants with 10% isotonic dehydration have dry mucous membranes, absent tears, sunken eyes and fontanel, cool extremities, poor skin turgor, and oliguria. Infants with 15% isotonic dehydration have the aforementioned signs as well as signs of shock, such as hypotension, tachycardia, weak pulses, mottled skin, and altered sensorium. Infants with hypertonic dehydration (i.e., serum sodium concentration above 150 mEq/L) have less severe symptoms than infants with isotonic dehydration who have lost the same fraction of body water; the intravascular volume is preserved better with hypernatremia than with isotonic dehydration. However, infants with hypotonic dehydration (i.e., serum sodium below 130 mEq/) may have more severe symptoms with the same degree of dehydration.

The usual clinical signs of dehydration are more difficult to evaluate in small premature infants. Their skin and mucous membranes may appear dry because of thermal or mechanical injury, particularly in infants kept under radiant warmers. In addition, skin turgor is harder to judge because of the lack of subcutaneous fat.

Electrolyte Deficits

The nature and extent of electrolyte disturbances often can be determined by history and physical examination and by measurement of electrolyte concentrations in serum. Based on serum sodium concentration, electrolyte disturbances are divided into isotonic, hypertonic, and hypotonic abnormalities. The type of electrolyte disorder seen in a clinical situation depends on the cause of fluid and electrolyte abnormality. For example, severe acute diarrhea usually leads to isotonic dehydration. High IWL, such as

may occur in small premature infants under radiant warmers, may result in hypernatremic dehydration. Inadequate replacement of salt losses from diarrhea may produce hypotonic dehydration. Although it may be possible to anticipate the type of electrolyte disorder accompanying dehydration in some situations, confirmation must be made by measurement of serum electrolyte concentrations.

Calculation of Fluid and Electrolyte Requirements

After replacement of any fluid and electrolyte deficits, the requirements of newborn infants for water and electrolytes are determined by the rates of loss of these substances from the body by various routes and by the net amounts retained by body tissues during changes in body weight and composition. Knowledge of the usual rates of loss and of expected changes in body weight and composition in the first postnatal days and during subsequent growth helps to estimate water and electrolyte requirements. These estimates are then used to guide the management of fluid and electrolyte therapy.

Replacement of Fluid and Electrolyte Deficits

The deficit of fluid is calculated from the estimated degree of dehydration determined from measured body weight loss or by clinical examination. The rate and composition of initial fluid replacement depend on the severity of dehydration. As a rule, dehydration of acute onset and short duration requires more rapid correction. An exception to this rule is the case of hypertonic dehydration, in which rapid expansion of body water may cause brain swelling and convulsions.

The deficit of electrolytes is calculated as the difference between total body solute expected before dehydration and that observed in the dehydrated state (Table 21-5). It is common to replace half the water deficit over the first 8 hours and the other half over the next 16 hours. The

TABLE 21-5
CALCULATION OF SODIUM DEFICIT

Type of Dehydration	Serum Sodium Concentration (mEq/L)	Calculation of Total Solute Deficit (mOsm/kg)[a]	Solute Deficit (mOsm/kg)	Sodium Deficit (mEq/kg)[b]
Isotonic (10%)	140	$(0.7 \times 280) - (0.6 \times 280)$	28	14
Hypertonic (10%)	153	$(0.7 \times 280) - (0.6 \times 306)$	12	6
Hypotonic (10%)	127	$(0.7 \times 280) - (0.6 \times 254)$	44	22

[a] Total solute deficit = $(TBW_e \times solute_e) - (TBW_o \times solute_o)$, where subscripts e and o indicate expected and observed, respectively. $TBW_e = 0.7$ L/kg; $TBW_o = 0.7 - 0.1 = 0.6$ L/kg; $solute_e = 140 \times 2 = 280$ mOsm/L, assuming total solute concentration in body water is twice the sodium concentration in serum; $solute_o$ = observed serum sodium $\times 2$.
[b] Total solute deficit is assumed to be half sodium. Although the serum (and ECW) has lost this amount of sodium, only half this amount has been lost to the environment; the other half has been lost into the cells in exchange for potassium, which in turn has been lost from the body. In practice, therefore, only half the amount listed as "sodium deficit" should be replaced as sodium, and the other half should be given as potassium. TBW, total body water. ECW, extracellular water.

sodium deficit is replaced over 24 hours; more rapid replacement is not necessary and may risk overcorrection. If the potassium deficit is large, one should replace it over a longer period (i.e., 48 to 72 hours) to allow ascertainment of adequate renal function and to avoid the possible cardiac effects associated with rapid potassium infusion. Initiation of potassium replacement is best deferred until urine flow is established.

Maintenance Fluid and Electrolytes

IWL, urine, fecal water, and water retained in new tissues during growth are the four components that one must consider in estimating the daily maintenance water requirement. Fecal water loss is approximately 5 to 10 mL/kg/day (98,99). The water retained for growth is about 10 mL/kg/day, assuming a weight gain of 10 to 20 g/kg/day, 60% to 70% of which is water (3). In the first week of life, fecal water loss is small and no water is deposited in new tissues because growth has not yet begun. In fact, water is lost from body tissues during the period of physiologic extracellular dehydration. After growth begins, replacement of fecal and growth water may require up to 20 g/kg/day, but this amount is small compared with the insensible and urine water losses, the two major routes of water loss that must be considered in estimating the water intake required to maintain the desired water balance.

A small portion of the water used to replace these normal losses is derived from the oxidation of metabolic fuels (i.e., carbohydrate, protein, and fat). This water of oxidation consists of about 0.60 mL/g of carbohydrate oxidized, 0.43 mL/g protein, and 1.07 mL/g fat (100). A newborn infant usually produces 5 to 10 mL/kg/day as water of oxidation. This amount is small enough to be neglected in most calculations but, for practical purposes, can be considered to offset the normal fecal water loss of 5 to 10 mL/kg/day.

For a term infant under basal conditions, IWL is approximately 20 mL/kg/day (29). Urine volume depends on the excess of water intake over losses by other routes (i.e., IWL, feces, growth), and urine concentration is determined by the urine volume and renal solute load. The range of urinary water loss within which the infant's immature kidneys can safely excrete the total renal solute load is determined by the limits of urine concentration (volume = solute load/urine concentration) (101). A renal solute load of 15 to 30 mOsm/kg/day would require urine volume of 50 to 100 mL/kg/day to maintain an average urine concentration of 300 mOsm/L. This urine concentration is near the middle of the range of urine osmolarity that can be produced by the neonate's kidneys, and it allows a margin of safety for over- or underestimation of other water requirements.

In the first days of life, a term infant receiving intravenous fluid and electrolytes would need to excrete about 15 mOsm/kg/day, assuming that both endogenous solute production and tissue deposition of solute are negligible. The urine volume of 50 mL/kg/day plus the IWL of 20 mL/kg/day yield a total maintenance water requirement of 70 mL/kg/day; this assumes growth and fecal water to be small enough to be offset by the water of oxidation. If one allows for a negative water balance of 10 mL/kg/day, the true water requirement at birth is about 60 mL/kg/day. With increasing postnatal age and enteral feedings, the renal solute load and fecal water loss increase, and water is deposited in new tissues as growth begins. By the second week of life, a growing term infant needs 120 to 150 mL/kg/day.

In premature infants, the maintenance water requirement is larger because of higher IWL (33,35). Therefore, the IWL component of maintenance water should be increased with decreasing birth weight or gestation. During the first days of life, the renal solute load is less because little exogenous solute is provided. If sodium chloride is administered at a rate of 2 mEq/kg/day (4 mOsm/kg/day) and a solute load of 8 mOsm/kg/day resulting from tissue catabolism is assumed to be excreted (102), a urine volume of only 40 mL/kg/day is required to excrete this solute with a urine concentration of 300 mOsm/L. Thus, a small premature infant requires about 80 mL/kg/day on day 1 (60 IWL + 40 urine −20 for negative balance). The water requirement for this same infant would be about 150 mL/kg/day in the second or third week (55 IWL + 85 urine + 10 feces + 10 growth − 10 oxidation). Very premature (less than 26 weeks of gestation) infants in the first week of life may have considerably higher IWL, raising the total water requirement to 200 or 300 mL/kg/day or even higher, especially if maintained in dry air. The minimum water intake of premature infants is also higher than that of term infants because of premature infant's slightly lower urinary concentrating capacity (91,92). However, the aforementioned urine volumes (40 to 100 mL/kg/day) were selected to avoid taxing this limit of concentration and so are not influenced by this effect of immaturity.

The allowance for IWL should be increased by about 50% for infants under radiant warmers (33,41–44) or receiving overhead phototherapy (33,46). If both are used, the allowance for IWL should be increased by approximately 100% (43). The effect of fiberoptic phototherapy blankets or pads on IWL is not known but is probably less than that of overhead phototherapy. The IWL of infants in incubators also is increased if body or environmental temperature is too high (29,39,40). The IWL can be reduced by increasing the ambient or inspired humidity (29,31) or by using certain types of heat shields (32,44,52), plastic blankets (52–54) or chambers (54,55), semipermeable membranes (56–58), or waterproof topical agents such as paraffin (59,60) (Table 21-2).

The infant's maintenance requirements of sodium, potassium, and chloride can be estimated by adding the dermal, urinary, and fecal losses to the amounts retained in the body tissues during growth. The estimated requirements for sodium, potassium, and chloride are each between 2 and 4 mEq/kg/day (103,104). Small premature infants may require additional sodium because of increased urinary excretion (105–107), especially during the second and third weeks of life. The magnitude of urinary sodium excretion is inversely proportional to gestational age (Fig. 21-6) (85).

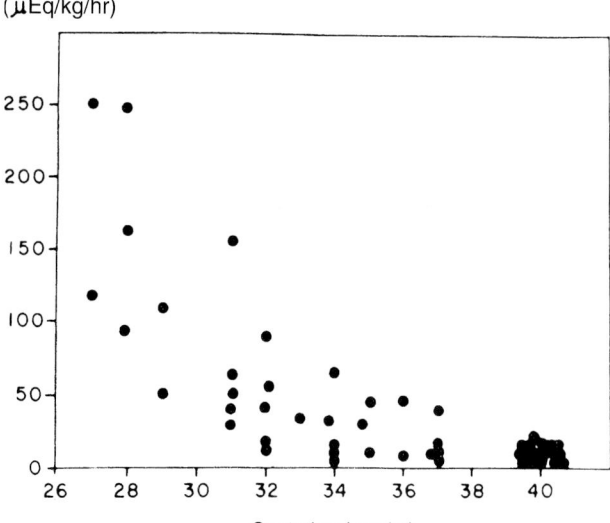

(μEq/kg/hr)

Figure 21-6 Urinary sodium excretion in infants from 27 to 40 weeks of gestation. (From Siegel SR, Oh W. Renal function as a marker of human fetal maturation. *Acta Paediatr* Scand 1976;65: 481–485, with permission.)

Ongoing Abnormal Losses of Fluid and Electrolytes

Ongoing abnormal losses must be replaced along with correction of established deficits and provision of maintenance fluid and electrolytes. Abnormal losses may occur with vomiting or diarrhea, ileostomy output, or removal by aspiration of gastrointestinal, pleural, peritoneal, or cerebrospinal fluid. The amount of extra water required can be determined by carefully measuring the volume lost. The additional amounts of electrolytes required can be estimated by measuring their concentrations in an aliquot of fluid (Table 21-6).

Example of Fluid and Electrolyte Calculation

Consider a 3-kg infant who presents with 10% isotonic dehydration (i.e., serum sodium = 140 mEq/L). In the first 24 hours of therapy, the infant should be given 27 mEq of sodium chloride in 600 mL of water as a dextrose solution (Table 21-7). If the potassium deficit is to be corrected over 72 hours, 13 mEq of potassium chloride (21/3 + 6) should be given during the first 24 hours. This fluid could then be ordered as dextrose solution with 45 mEq NaCl/L and 20 mEq KCl/L to be infused at 25 mL/hour. If the infant also has significant metabolic acidosis, some or all of the sodium could be given as sodium bicarbonate or sodium acetate.

The initial glucose concentration is determined by the estimated water requirement and the desired glucose intake, which is usually 5 to 8 mg/kg/minute. Smaller, more premature infants, because they require more water and may tolerate less glucose, are usually begun on solutions containing lower concentrations of glucose (e.g., 5 g/dL); larger term or near-term infants require higher glucose concentrations (e.g., 10 g/dL).

The fluid and electrolyte requirements of very small premature infants vary widely and are difficult to predict. Therefore, close monitoring of the fluid and electrolyte balance of these infants is especially important so that any imbalance can be detected as soon as possible.

Monitoring the Effectiveness of Fluid and Electrolyte Therapy

During the course of parenteral fluid therapy, detailed and organized data collection is necessary for monitoring the adequacy of fluid and electrolyte intake. Data that should be collected and recorded regularly at designated intervals include water and electrolyte intake by all routes, measurable output of water, body weight change, and serum electrolyte concentrations; in addition, clinical assessment should be made for the presence of dehydration, edema, or acute water overload. A calibrated infusion pump should be used to assure accurate administration of prescribed parenteral fluids. Accurate measurement of urine volume is difficult in small infants. It is possible to collect urine from male infants by placing the penis into a collecting vessel that is taped to the abdomen. Urine is then aspirated from the vessel with a catheter and syringe. Urine volume can also be estimated by comparison of the weights of dry and wet diapers, provided the diaper is weighed soon enough to avoid evaporation of the urine.

Inadequate fluid may be administered if the fluid maintenance requirement is underestimated or if a preexisting

TABLE 21-6
ELECTROLYTE CONTENT OF BODY FLUIDS

Fluid Source	Sodium (mEq/L)	Potassium (mEq/L)	Chloride (mEq/L)
Stomach	20–80	5–20	100–150
Small intestine	100–140	5–15	90–120
Bile	120–140	5–15	90–120
Ileostomy	45–135	3–15	20–120
Diarrheal stool	10–90	10–80	10–110
Cerebrospinal fluid	130–150	2–5	110–130

TABLE 21-7

CALCULATION OF FLUID AND ELECTROLYTE INTAKE FOR A 3-KG INFANT WITH 10% ISOTONIC DEHYDRATION

	Water (mL)	Sodium (mEq)	Potassium (mEq)
Deficit	300[a]	21[b]	21[b,c]
Maintenance	300[d]	6	6
Ongoing losses	0	0	0
Total	600	27	27[c]
Total/kg	200	9	9[c]

[a] Water deficit: 0.10×3 kg.
[b] Electrolyte deficits calculated as in Table 21-5 (14 mEq/kg $\times$ 3 kg divided between sodium and potassium).
[c] Potassium deficit should be replaced slowly over 48 to 72 hours.
[d] Maintenance water requirement assumed to be 100 mL/kg/day.

deficit or ongoing loss is neglected or underestimated. Insufficient water intake leads to reduced urine volume and increased urine concentration, and if these compensatory measures are inadequate, water is mobilized from body stores to provide for obligatory insensible loss and to allow solute excretion. This results in weight loss, clinical signs of dehydration, metabolic acidosis, and hemoconcentration. As serum osmolarity rises, neurologic sequelae of hypertonicity may occur. In severe cases, untreated dehydration may lead to decreased circulating blood volume, acute renal failure, and finally to death from cardiovascular collapse.

Excessive water intake leads to increased excretion of dilute urine. If these compensatory mechanisms are overtaxed, water will be retained in the body, resulting in edema and weight gain. Rapid overhydration may produce congestive heart failure and pulmonary edema, particularly in ill infants with cardiopulmonary disorders. Even gradual daily administration of excess water (i.e., volumes larger than can be readily eliminated by the kidneys) may increase the risk of heart failure from PDA in premature infants (19).

If appropriate fluid therapy is being provided, body weight should be stable or slowly increasing after the first week of life, and there should be no evidence of dehydration or fluid overload. During the first week of life, loss of as much as 15% of body weight is considered normal, provided urine output is adequate and there is no acidosis or evidence of dehydration. This "physiologic" weight loss is at least partly the result of postnatal contraction of the extracellular water volume. Efforts to prevent this weight loss are ill advised and may lead to fluid overload, edema, and significant PDA. Plotting daily weights on a standard postnatal growth chart (97) may help in detecting excessive weight loss or inappropriate weight gain.

Routine measurement of serum electrolyte concentrations is the best way to monitor the body's electrolyte status and the adequacy or excess of electrolyte intake. It is not necessary to add sodium to the parenterally administered fluid during the first 24 hours of life; in fact, starting sodium on the day of birth may delay the physiologic contraction of the extracellular water compartment (108,109).

On the other hand, adding some sodium as bicarbonate or acetate facilitates the use of permissive hypercapnia to reduce lung trauma while still maintaining acceptable arterial pH. In any case, it is advisable to determine the serum electrolyte concentrations soon after birth in infants who require parenteral fluids; if the mother received sodium-free fluid during labor, the infant may be hyponatremic (25–28) and require immediate addition of sodium to the prescribed fluid. If not required earlier, sodium in the form of sodium chloride or sodium acetate should be administered at a dose of 2 to 4 mEq/kg/day beginning on the second day of life. Use of the acetate salt helps to correct the metabolic acidosis sometimes seen in young premature infants as a result of renal immaturity; it also helps the kidneys in buffering the respiratory acidosis resulting from permissive hypercapnia.

During the first week of life, infants are usually in negative sodium balance as a result of the mobilization of sodium along with water from the extracellular compartment. This negative balance should be allowed as long as the serum sodium concentration remains normal. In the second and third weeks of life, small premature infants may require more sodium to replace the large amounts that are lost in the urine (105–107). It is important to understand that most cases of hyponatremia or hypernatremia result from excessive or inadequate intake of water.

Potassium supplementation (2 mEq/kg/day) may be started after the infant urinates unless the serum potassium concentration is elevated. In most infants, potassium should be added to the infused fluids by the second day. In very small, critically ill premature infants, however, it is wise to wait until the serum potassium concentration falls below 4 mEq/L before administering potassium; these infants are at increased risk of hyperkalemia due to catabolism and release of potassium from cells in combination with decreased renal potassium excretion (110–114). Another mechanism proposed for the hyperkalemia often seen in extremely premature infants is the movement of potassium from cells to the extracellular compartment as a result of decreased sodium-potassium-ATPase activity in erythrocytes (115).

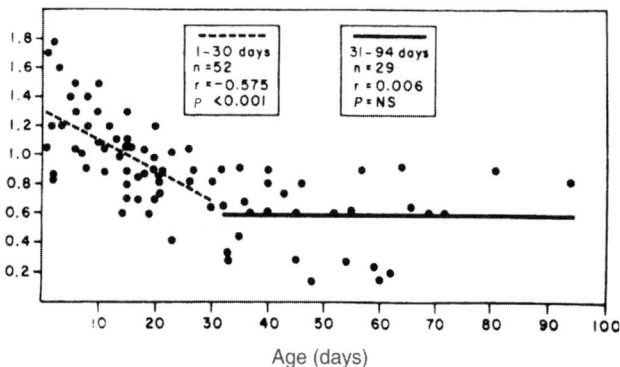

Figure 21-7 Plasma creatinine levels of premature infants during the first 3 months of life. (From Stonestreet BS, Oh W. Plasma creatinine levels in low-birth-weight infants during the first three months of life. *Pediatrics* 1978;61:788–789, with permission.)

Hyperkalemia is the most common life-threatening electrolyte disturbance in newborn infants. If an elevated serum potassium level is reported by the laboratory, it should not be attributed to *in vitro* hemolysis without verification of the result with another blood sample obtained with good technique to minimize hemolysis. If the serum potassium concentration is higher than 6 mEq/L, only potassium-free fluids should be administered. If the serum potassium concentration is above 7 mEq/L, rectal administration of sodium polystyrene sulfonate (Kayexalate) or another potassium-binding resin should be considered. Binding resins, if used, should be given carefully to limit the risk of colonic necrosis and perforation (116–118). If a cardiac arrhythmia occurs in the presence of hyperkalemia, calcium, bicarbonate, and insulin with glucose should be given to force potassium into body cells. In small premature infants, hyperkalemic arrhythmias include sinus bradycardia—especially if it occurs without hypoxia—and ventricular tachycardia.

Blood urea nitrogen and serum or plasma creatinine levels (Fig. 21-7) (119) are useful for assessing renal function, although the urea nitrogen may also be elevated with dehydration.

ACID–BASE BALANCE

The physiologic buffer system—primarily bicarbonate and its weak acid counterpart carbonic acid—and the renal and respiratory compensatory systems are the major mechanisms responsible for the maintenance of normal acid–base equilibrium in the body fluids. Changes in the hydrogen ion concentration in body fluids are governed by the Henderson-Hasselbach equation:

$$pH = 6.1 + \log([HCO_3^-]/[H_2CO_3])$$

in which 6.1 is the pK or dissociation constant for carbonic acid (120) and $[H_2CO_3]$ is the concentration of carbonic acid. It can be seen from this equation that increase or decrease in the bicarbonate (HCO_3^-) concentration results in *metabolic alkalosis* or *metabolic acidosis*, respectively.

Because H_2CO_3 is interchangeably linked to the partial pressure of carbon dioxide (PCO_2) under the influence of carbonic anhydrase, any alteration in PCO_2 in body fluid also alters pH. Thus, hyperventilation, by reducing PCO_2, produces *respiratory alkalosis*, and hypoventilation, by increasing PCO_2, causes *respiratory acidosis*.

Metabolic alkalosis occurs with pyloric stenosis because persistent vomiting results in the loss of hydrochloric acid and thus produces a relative excess of bicarbonate. Metabolic acidosis is most commonly seen as a consequence of lactic acid accumulation from anaerobic metabolism in hypoxic infants. Respiratory alkalosis may occur in an infant who is hyperventilated with a mechanical ventilator. Respiratory acidosis occurs as a result of hypercapnia in infants with respiratory distress syndrome or other pulmonary disease.

In all types of acid–base disturbance, compensation by the lungs or kidneys occurs to restore the pH toward 7.4. Metabolic acid–base disorders are corrected by change in ventilation, and respiratory disorders are compensated for by change in renal bicarbonate excretion. If the compensation is adequate to correct the pH to normal, the acid–base disturbance is said to be compensated. For example, if an infant with respiratory distress syndrome has a pH of 7.38, PCO_2 of 32 torr, bicarbonate concentration of 18 mEq/L, and base excess of −5 mEq/L, the acid–base status is called *compensated metabolic acidosis*. If the same infant has a pH of 7.38, PCO_2 of 50 torr, bicarbonate concentration of 29 mEq/L, and base excess of +3 mEq/L, the acid–base status is *compensated respiratory acidosis*.

FLUID AND ELECTROLYTE PROBLEMS ASSOCIATED WITH SPECIFIC CLINICAL CONDITIONS

Extreme Prematurity

Infants born at gestational ages younger than 26 weeks present special problems in fluid and electrolyte management. These infants have large IWL (36,37), in some cases more than 200 mL/kg/day if the infant is nursed under a radiant warmer. The large IWL of extremely premature infants results from their meager skin barrier to evaporation and their large ratio of surface area to body weight. The average water requirement for an infant with birth weight between 500 and 750 grams in the first week of life is estimated to be about 170 mL/kg/day if the infant is in an incubator with low ambient humidity and without phototherapy and perhaps 150 mL/kg/day if moderate humidity is added to the incubator. The requirement would be 210 to 220 mL/kg/day if a radiant warmer or overhead phototherapy is used and 250 to 270 mL/kg/day if both radiant warmer and photo therapy are used (121). In the first week of life, the water requirement may be even higher in infants born after only 22 or 23 weeks of gestation. In these extremely premature infants, the cutaneous IWL and consequently the total water requirement decrease toward the end of the first week of life, as the stratum corneum matures and becomes less permeable to water.

Extremely premature infants, unless hyponatremic from maternal hypotonicity (25–28), should initially be started on electrolyte-free solutions of glucose (5 g/dL) in water or solutions that provide sodium in a dose of 2 to 3 mEq/kg/day as sodium acetate or sodium bicarbonate. The latter bases compensate for respiratory acidosis while allowing hypercapnia with the goal of minimizing lung trauma. Administering some or all of the maintenance sodium as sodium acetate or sodium bicarbonate also serves to mitigate the metabolic acidosis present in many extremely premature infants as a result of renal immaturity and transient renal tubular acidosis. If sodium is not begun initially, it should be added by the second day, provided the serum sodium concentration is below 145 mEq/L.

Hyperkalemia is a very common problem in extremely premature infants during the first week of life. This potentially dangerous condition results from potassium release from catabolized cells in the presence of immature distal renal tubular function (110,112,113). Hyperkalemia is exacerbated if dehydration and oliguria occur as a result of inadequate water intake. No potassium should be given to extremely premature infants until the serum potassium concentration falls below 4 mEq/L. If the serum potassium concentration exceeds 7 mEq/L, rectal administration of a potassium-binding resin should be considered.

Respiratory Distress Syndrome and Bronchopulmonary Dysplasia

The renal function of infants with respiratory distress syndrome (RDS) is similar to that of infants of the same gestational age without respiratory distress, provided their cardiorespiratory status is not significantly compromised (122–124). If infants with RDS become hypoxic and acidotic, however, they may have decreased glomerular filtration, reduced renal blood flow, and lower renal bicarbonate threshold (123–126). It has been observed that clinical improvement in infants with RDS is accompanied by an increase in urine volume that occurs on the second and third days of life (127) and, at the same time, by a rise in circulating levels of atrial natriuretic peptide (13). It is not clear whether this diuresis causes or is caused by the improving pulmonary function, or whether each enhances the other. These associated events may, in fact, be causally unrelated because this is the time when all infants, especially premature infants, are in negative water balance (128,129) and experience contraction of the extracellular water.

In addition to any changes in renal function that may occur with pulmonary dysfunction resulting from severe RDS, positive-pressure ventilation may also cause water retention through effects on renal function. Positive-pressure ventilation can impair water and sodium excretion by mechanisms that are not well defined but probably include increased aldosterone secretion (130) and increased production of antidiuretic hormone (131,132). It is also possible for impaired filtration and solute excretion

to result from decreased aortic pressure and renal perfusion if excessive mean airway pressure is used during ventilatory support. Infants with RDS and other pulmonary disorders may have increased secretion of antidiuretic hormone, especially if they develop pneumothorax (64,133,134). When carefully used, positive-pressure ventilation, either conventional or high-frequency ventilation, does not impair diuresis or cause water retention (135).

PDA is a problem that affects premature infants; those with RDS are more likely to develop cardiorespiratory signs related to PDA than those without RDS. Infants receiving carefully limited intake of water are less likely to develop significant PDA (19,21,22).

RDS is commonly associated with a combined respiratory and metabolic acidosis resulting from hypercapnia and lactic acidemia. In severe RDS, when the acidosis is primarily respiratory, assisted ventilation should be instituted. If the acidosis is primarily metabolic, the underlying cause should be identified and corrected; if this cannot be done, sodium bicarbonate may be given to correct the acidosis. There is little evidence to support the routine use of bicarbonate in infants with RDS (21,136–138). Therefore, the current approach is to treat only significant metabolic acidosis, generally if the pH is below 7.25. When bicarbonate is used, the dose should be calculated from the following equation:

$$\text{NaHCO}_3 \text{ dose} = (\text{base deficit})(\text{body weight})(0.5 \text{ L/kg})$$

The 0.5 value in the equation is the volume of distribution (i.e., bicarbonate space), which is confined mostly to the extracellular fluid compartment (Fig. 21-3). There is some disagreement regarding the true bicarbonate space; the reported values range from 0.3 to 0.6 L/kg. The 0.5 value in the preceding equation applies to term infants; 0.6 L/kg is a more appropriate value for premature infants because of their larger volume of extracellular water (1).

The calculated bicarbonate dose should be diluted to a concentration of 0.5 mEq/mL and given intravenously at a rate no faster than 1 mEq/kg/minute. A slow infusion over 30 to 60 minutes is preferable, especially for premature infants, because it may reduce the risk of rapid osmolar changes in the intravascular and interstitial fluid compartments (139), which have been associated with intracranial hemorrhage in infants receiving bicarbonate infusions (140).

Infants with RDS or BPD are sometimes treated with dexamethasone or other corticosteroid hormones in an attempt to ameliorate the severity of their lung disease. During dexamethasone therapy, infants may have impaired glucose tolerance, growth failure, and elevated blood urea nitrogen resulting from the catabolic effects of dexamethasone (141–143). Dexamethasone also perturbs the balance of phosphorus and potassium by increasing urinary excretion of these elements (144).

Perinatal Asphyxia

Infants with hypoxia or ischemia of the brain and kidneys during the perinatal period may suffer brain or kidney injury. Increased secretion of AVP often accompanies hypoxic encephalopathy (64,145,146). Moreover, acute renal failure may result from renal ischemia in these infants (147,148). Both conditions cause oliguria and therefore decrease the need for exogenous water. After birth asphyxia, it is advisable to restrict water intake in anticipation of possible increased AVP secretion (also known as inappropriate antidiuretic hormone secretion) or acute renal failure. During the first 24 hours of life, the water intake for asphyxiated infants should be limited to IWL plus urine output minus about 20 mL/kg/day to allow for some physiologic contraction of the extracellular water volume. If urine production is normal by the third postnatal day, water intake can be restored to a normal level.

During the oliguric phase of acute renal failure, potassium should not be administered unless the serum potassium concentration is less than 3.5 mEq/L. With acute renal failure resulting from hypoxia or ischemia, the initial period of oliguria may be followed by a diuretic phase with polyuria. If urine output increases and body weight falls below the expected level (i.e., the weight before fluid retention began), the intake of water must be increased to prevent dehydration. This diuretic phase may be accompanied by large losses of sodium and other electrolytes, which must be replaced. Replacement of the urinary sodium losses is facilitated by measuring the volume and sodium concentration in an aliquot of urine from a timed collection.

Central Nervous System Injury

Infants with brain injury from other causes, such as intracranial hemorrhage or central nervous system infection, may also have oliguria and water retention because of inappropriately increased secretion of AVP (64,145).

Sepsis and Necrotizing Enterocolitis

Systematic reviews of randomized clinical trials of varying fluid intake in premature infants have identified overhydration as a risk factor in the pathogenesis of NEC (20–22). Infants with septicemia who also have meningitis may develop inappropriate AVP secretion, reducing their water requirement. Infants with septicemia or NEC may also develop shock from endotoxin production or from hypovolemia due to loss of intravascular water and protein to the interstitial and peritoneal spaces or to the intestinal lumen, or from frank hemorrhage resulting from thrombocytopenia, disseminated intravascular coagulopathy, or intestinal injury. In infants with shock, it is essential to replace lost water and solutes in the form of blood products or other solute-containing fluids. Even if properly treated, septic shock may cause renal injury, which then further complicates fluid and electrolyte management.

Pyloric Stenosis

With pyloric stenosis, water, electrolytes, and hydrogen ions are lost from the stomach as a result of repeated vomiting of gastric contents. Infants with severe vomiting caused by pyloric stenosis have elevated intracellular concentrations of sodium and decreased concentrations of potassium. Infants with pyloric stenosis are likely to be dehydrated and may have hypochloremic metabolic alkalosis and hypokalemia. The alkalosis may cause lethargy, hypoventilation, and, in severe cases, tetany.

Parenteral fluid therapy consists of replacing the deficits of water, potassium, and chloride. The chloride should initially be given as sodium chloride. Potassium chloride should be added after adequate urination has been established. Specific treatment of the metabolic alkalosis with acidic agents is not necessary. In most cases, control of vomiting, correction of dehydration, and replacement of chloride and potassium deficits will restore the blood acid–base status to normal.

Abdominal Wall Defects

Infants born with abdominal wall defects (gastroschisis or omphalocele) have increased IWL from the exposed viscera and require extra water prior to surgical repair. This is especially true of infants with gastroschisis because there is no membrane covering the extruding organs. Once the abdominal wall has been closed, evaporative water loss is no longer increased, although there may still be abnormal loss of water into the peritoneal cavity or interstitial fluid compartment.

Diarrhea

The principles of parenteral fluid therapy of diarrheal dehydration in the newborn infant are similar to those applied to older infants and children. Because of their limited renal concentrating ability, newborn infants are quicker to develop severe dehydration, hypovolemia, and cardiovascular collapse. Therefore, rapid establishment of intravenous access for vascular expansion is of the utmost importance in newborn infants with moderate to severe dehydration from diarrhea. After stabilization, fluid and electrolyte deficits should be estimated as described earlier in this chapter. Water and electrolytes should be given to correct established deficits, meet maintenance requirements, and counteract ongoing losses.

Metabolic acidosis is a frequent finding in diarrheal dehydration. During initial volume reexpansion, preexisting acidosis may worsen as the body bicarbonate is further diluted with bicarbonate-free replacement fluids. Prerenal azotemia is common with diarrheal dehydration. It usually corrects spontaneously within several days as the infant is rehydrated.

Oral fluids and feeding should be withheld during recovery from diarrheal dehydration. Oral rehydration has been used successfully in older children with diarrhea, but there has been less experience with this technique in newborn infants (149). For this reason, oral rehydration is not recommended for newborn infants in areas where adequate personnel and supplies are available to maintain parenteral infusions. However, oral rehydration provides an important alternate therapy when intravenous therapy is not feasible for economic or technical reasons. The appropriate period of fasting for diarrhea depends on the severity and duration of the diarrheal episode. As a rule, a more severe, protracted bout requires a longer period of fasting. How long diarrheal stools persist following the onset of fasting also helps to determine the duration of fasting. Reintroduction of oral fluids should be carried out with extreme care. Aggressive refeeding may precipitate a recurrence of diarrhea or even protracted chronic diarrhea and malabsorption with consequent growth failure.

Fluid and Electrolyte Management of Neonatal Surgical Patients

If a condition that requires surgery (e.g., pyloric stenosis) results in dehydration and electrolyte or acid–base disturbance, the infant should be restored as close as possible to normal fluid, electrolyte, and acid–base status before surgery. Otherwise, the risks of anesthesia and surgery might be increased by dehydration, acidosis, alkalosis, or abnormal serum potassium concentration.

During surgery, the prescribed fluid and electrolyte therapy should be continued with the same fluid composition and rate of infusion unless additional intraoperative losses require replacement. The anesthesiologist and surgeons should be apprised of the plan for parenteral fluid therapy to avoid errors resulting from lack of communication. The operative losses of fluid and blood should be recorded and replaced either during surgery or shortly thereafter.

During the initial postoperative period, some infants have reduced urine output as a result of fluid loss from the vascular compartment or increased secretion of AVP. Therefore, the fluid provided for maintenance may need to be reduced during the immediate postoperative period. However, this reduction may be offset by the extra fluid required to replace abnormal operative and postoperative losses. A system of careful monitoring of fluid and electrolyte balance is essential in the surgical patient, as in other ill newborn infants.

TECHNICAL ASPECTS OF PARENTERAL FLUID THERAPY

Blood Sampling

Sampling of capillary blood by heel puncture is a safe and commonly used technique in newborn infants. Automated, spring-loaded lancets provide a safe and simple way to create an incision of standardized length and depth. Capillary blood is adequate for determination of serum electrolyte and blood urea nitrogen concentrations because most of these values agree closely with venous samples. Serum potassium concentration is slightly higher when obtained by heel puncture, but the difference is min-

imized if the blood flows freely from the puncture wound so that little squeezing is required. Blood flow can be enhanced by prior warming of the foot. Because the amount of blood that can be obtained by heel puncture is limited, the neonatology service should be supported by a laboratory in close proximity to the nurseries that is capable of performing the required analyses on blood samples of small volume. Such laboratory support is also crucial to minimize blood transfusions, which are necessitated in part by phlebotomy blood losses (150).

Blood samples for blood gas and acid–base determination can also be obtained by heel puncture. Their reliability is enhanced by warming the skin to 44°C, which reduces the arterial-capillary differences in blood gases and pH; however, oxygen pressure (PO_2) measurements on samples obtained by heel puncture tend to underestimate true arterial PO_2, especially in the hyperoxic range. Sufficient information for clinical management can usually be obtained by using capillary acid–base and PCO_2 values in conjunction with oxygen saturation values determined by continuous pulse oximetry. However, indwelling umbilical or radial artery catheters often are used in infants who are extremely ill and require continuous blood pressure monitoring or high levels of oxygen and ventilatory support. Because indwelling arterial catheters are associated with serious thromboembolic complications, they should be removed as soon as possible. For occasional sampling of arterial blood, direct puncture and aspiration from a peripheral artery can be used. This procedure is fairly safe in skilled hands but can cause serious complications, such as arterial obstruction or nerve injury.

Intravenous Fluid Infusion

Short catheters inserted into peripheral veins in a limb or the scalp can be used for infusion of water, electrolytes, and nutrient solutions. Hypertonic and vasoconstrictive solutions should be infused with caution into peripheral veins. Peripheral infusion of solutions containing dextrose in concentrations higher than 12.5 g/dL is generally contraindicated. Central venous access, if available, is preferred for such infusions. Shaving scalp hair to expose veins is distressing to many parents; the scalp should be used only if extremity sites have been exhausted and only after the procedure has been discussed with the parents. Intravenous sites must be carefully inspected on each nursing shift for evidence of infection at the insertion site or for extravasation of infusate that might injure subcutaneous tissues.

Long catheters of silicone elastomer or other materials can be inserted percutaneously so that the tip lies centrally in a large vein within the abdomen or chest. These catheters can be used for long-term intravenous access with lower risks of infection and thrombosis than occur with surgically inserted central vein catheters. Serious complications are rare with percutaneous central vein catheters. However, infectious complications are an ever-present threat. In addition, life-threatening complications, such as pleural effusion and cardiac tamponade, are possible (151).

Venous cutdown for vascular access is seldom necessary if skilled personnel are available to insert and maintain standard intravenous catheters. Surgical cutdown for venous access risks local infection or septicemia and permanent venous obstruction. Moreover, catheters inserted by cutdown usually do not last as long in newborn infants as they do in older children and adults. For these reasons, venous cutdown should be avoided in newborns whenever possible.

A catheter in the umbilical vein with its tip in the inferior vena cava may be used for infusion of fluid, electrolytes, and nutrients during the first few days, until potential infection can be treated and percutaneous central vein access can be established if needed. Umbilical vein catheters ordinarily should be removed within a few days of birth because of the risks of infection, portal phlebitis, and liver damage. Umbilical vein catheters can also be used for central venous pressure monitoring and exchange transfusions. Except in unusual circumstances, an umbilical vein catheter should be removed by the end of the first week of life, when the risks of infection and thrombosis probably surpass the advantages of continued catheter use.

With any route of parenteral fluid administration to newborn infants, it is essential to use infusion pumps that can be precisely regulated and can deliver fluids at an absolutely steady rate, even when very low flow rates are used. A fluctuating infusion rate may cause erratic delivery of water, glucose and other nutrients, or drugs.

REFERENCES

1. Friis-Hansen B. Changes in body water compartments during growth. *Acta Paediatr* 1957;46(Suppl 110):1–68.
2. Friis-Hansen B. Body water compartments in children: changes during growth and related changes in body composition. *Pediatrics* 1961;28:169–181.
3. Ziegler EE, O'Donnell AM, Nelson SE, et al. Body composition of the reference fetus. *Growth* 1976;40:329–341.
4. Forbes GB, Perley A. Estimation of total body sodium by isotopic dilution. II. Studies on infants and children: an example of a constant differential growth ratio. *J Clin Invest* 1951;30:566–574.
5. Cheek DB. Observations on total body chloride in children. *Pediatrics* 1954;14:5–10.
6. Romahn A, Burmeister W. [Body composition during the first two years of life: analysis with the potassium 40 method]. *Klin Pädiatr* 1977;189:321–327.
7. Shaffer SG, Bradt SK, Hall RT. Postnatal changes in total body water and extracellular volume in the preterm infant with respiratory distress syndrome. *J Pediatr* 1986;109:509–514.
8. Bauer K, Bovermann G, Roithmaier A, et al. Body composition, nutrition, and fluid balance during the first two weeks of life in preterm neonates weighing less than 1500 grams. *J Pediatr* 1991;118:615–620.
9. Hartnoll G, Bétrémieux P, Modi N. Body water content of extremely preterm infants at birth. *Arch Dis Child Fetal Neonatal Ed* 2000;83:F56–F59.
10. Cheek DB, Maddison TG, Malinek M, et al. Further observations on the corrected bromide space of the neonate and investigation of water and electrolyte status in infants born of diabetic mothers. *Pediatrics* 1961;28:861–869.
11. Kagan BM, Stanincova V, Felix NS, et al. Body composition of premature infants: relation to nutrition. *Am J Clin Nutr* 1972; 25:1153–1164.
12. Heimler R, Doumas BT, Jendrzejczak BM, et al. Relationship between nutrition, weight change, and fluid compartments in preterm infants during the first week of life. *J Pediatr* 1993;122:110–114.
13. Modi N, Bétrémieux P, Midgley J, et al. Postnatal weight loss and contraction of the extracellular compartment is triggered by atrial natriuretic peptide. *Early Hum Dev* 2000;59:201–208.
14. Oh W, Oh MA, Lind J. Renal function and blood volume in newborn infant related to placental transfusion. *Acta Paediatr Scand* 1966;55:197–210.
15. Aperia A, Broberger O, Elinder G, et al. Postnatal development of renal function in pre-term and full-term infants. *Acta Paediatr Scand* 1981;70:183–187.
16. Horster M. Embryonic epithelial membrane transporters. *Am J Physiol Renal Physiol* 2000;279:F982–F996.
17. Cassady G, Milstead RR. Antipyrine space studies and cell water estimates in infants of low birth weight. *Pediatr Res* 1971;5:673–682.
18. Stonestreet BS, Bell EF, Warburton D, et al. Renal response in low-birth-weight neonates. Results of prolonged intake of two different amounts of fluid and sodium. *Am J Dis Child* 1983;137:215–219.
19. Bell EF, Warburton D, Stonestreet BS, et al. Effect of fluid administration on the development of symptomatic patent ductus arteriosus and congestive heart failure in premature infants. *N Engl J Med* 1980;302:598–604.
20. Bell EF, Warburton D, Stonestreet BS, et al. High-volume fluid intake predisposes premature infants to necrotising enterocolitis. *Lancet* 1979;2:90.
21. Bell EF. Fluid therapy. In: Sinclair JC, Bracken MB, eds. *Effective care of the newborn infant.* Oxford: Oxford University Press, 1992:59–72.
22. Bell EF, Acarregui MJ. Restricted versus liberal water intake for preventing morbidity and mortality in preterm infants. *Cochrane Database Syst Rev* 2001;2:CD000503.
23. Brown ER, Stark A, Sosenko I, et al. Bronchopulmonary dysplasia: possible relationship to pulmonary edema. *J Pediatr* 1978; 92:982–984.
24. Van Marter LJ, Leviton A, Allred EN, et al. Hydration during the first days of life and the risk of bronchopulmonary dysplasia in low birth weight infants. *J Pediatr* 1990;116:942–949.
25. Battaglia F, Prystowsky H, Smisson C, et al. Fetal blood studies. XIII. The effect of the administration of fluids intravenously to mothers upon the concentrations of water and electrolytes in plasma of human fetuses. *Pediatrics* 1960;25:2–10.
26. Tarnow-Mordi WO, Shaw JC, Liu D, et al. Iatrogenic hyponatraemia of the newborn due to maternal fluid overload: a prospective study. *Br Med J* 1981;283:639–642.
27. Grylack LJ, Chu SS, Scanlon JW. Use of intravenous fluids before cesarean section: effects on perinatal glucose, insulin, and sodium homeostasis. *Obstet Gynecol* 1984;63:654–658.
28. Zimmer EZ, Goldstein I, Feldman E, et al. Maternal and newborn levels of glucose, sodium and osmolality after preloading with three intravenous solutions during elective cesarean sections. *Eur J Obstet Gynecol Reprod Biol* 1986;23:61–65.
29. Hey EN, Katz G. Evaporative water loss in the new-born baby. *J Physiol* 1969;200:605–619.
30. Sulyok E, Jéquier E, Prod'hom LS. Respiratory contribution to the thermal balance of the newborn infant under various ambient conditions. *Pediatrics* 1973;51:641–650.
31. Sosulski R, Polin RA, Baumgart S. Respiratory water loss and heat balance in intubated infants receiving humidified air. *J Pediatr* 1983;103:307–310.
32. Fanaroff AA, Wald M, Gruber HS, et al. Insensible water loss in low birth weight infants. *Pediatrics* 1972;50:236–245.
33. Wu PY, Hodgman JE. Insensible water loss in preterm infants: changes with postnatal development and non-ionizing radiant energy. *Pediatrics* 1974;54:704–712.
34. Shaffer SG, Weismann DN. Fluid requirements in the preterm infant. *Clin Perinatol* 1992;19:233–250.
35. Okken A, Jonxis JH, Rispens P, et al. Insensible water loss and metabolic rate in low birthweight newborn infants. *Pediatr Res* 1979;13:1072–1075.
36. Hammarlund K, Sedin G. Transepidermal water loss in newborn infants. III. Relation to gestational age. Acta Paediatr *Scand* 1979;68:795–801.
37. Costarino AT, Baumgart. Controversies in fluid and electrolyte therapy for the premature infant. *Clin Perinatol* 1988;15:863–878.

38. Hooper JM, Evans IW, Stapleton T. Resting pulmonary water loss in the newborn infant. *Pediatrics* 1954;13:206–210.
39. Rutter N, Hull D. Response of term babies to a warm environment. *Arch Dis Child* 1979;54:178–183.
40. Bell EF, Gray JC, Weinstein MR, et al. The effects of thermal environment on heat balance and insensible water loss in low-birth-weight infants. *J Pediatr* 1980;96:452–459.
41. Williams PR, Oh W. Effects of radiant warmer on insensible water loss in newborn infants. *Am J Dis Child* 1974;128:511–514.
42. Jones RW, Rochefort MJ, Baum JD. Increased insensible water loss in newborn infants nursed under radiant heaters. *Br Med J* 1976;2:1347–1350.
43. Bell EF, Neidich GA, Cashore WJ, et al. Combined effect of radiant warmer and phototherapy on insensible water loss in low-birth-weight infants. *J Pediatr* 1979;94:810–813.
44. Bell EF, Weinstein MR, Oh W. Heat balance in premature infants: comparative effects of convectively heated incubator and radiant warmer, with and without plastic heat shield. *J Pediatr* 1980; 96:460–465.
45. Kjartansson S, Arsan S, Hammarlund K, et al. Water loss from the skin of term and preterm infants nursed under a radiant heater. *Pediatr Res* 1995;37:233–238.
46. Oh W, Karecki H. Phototherapy and insensible water loss in the newborn infant. *Am J Dis Child* 1972;124:230–232.
47. Grünhagen DJ, de Boer MG, de Beaufort AJ, et al. Transepidermal water loss during halogen spotlight phototherapy in preterm infants. *Pediatr Res* 2002;51:402–405.
48. Engle WD, Baumgart S, Schwartz JG, et al. Insensible water loss in the critically ill neonate. Combined effct of radiant-warmer power and phototherapy. *Am J Dis Child* 1981;135:516–520.
49. Day R. Respiratory metabolism in infancy and in childhood: XXVII. Regulation of body temperature of premature infants. *Am J Dis Child* 1943;65:376–398.
50. Zweymüller E, Preining O. The insensible water loss of the newborn infant. *Acta Paediatr Scand* 1970;205(Suppl):1–29.
51. O'Brien D, Hansen JDL, Smith CA. Effect of supersaturated atmospheres on insensible water loss in the newborn infant. *Pediatrics* 1954;13:126–132.
52. Baumgart S, Fox WW, Polin RA. Physiologic implications of two different heat shields for infants under radiant warmers. *J Pediatr* 1982;100:787–790.
53. Marks KH, Friedman Z, Maisels MJ. A simple device for reducing insensible water loss in low-birth-weight infants. *Pediatrics* 1977;60:223–226.
54. Baumgart S, Engle WD, Fox WW, et al. Effect of heat shielding on convective and evaporative heat losses and on radiant heat transfer in the premature infant. *J Pediatr* 1981;99:948–956.
55. Fitch CW, Korones SB. Heat shield reduces water loss. *Arch Dis Child* 1984;59:886–888.
56. Knauth A, Gordin M, McNelis W, et al. Semipermeable polyurethane membrane as an artificial skin for the premature neonate. *Pediatrics* 1989;83:945–950.
57. Vernon HJ, Lane AT, Wischerath LJ, et al. Semipermeable dressing and transepidermal water loss in premature infants. *Pediatrics* 1990;86:357–362.
58. Mancini AJ, Sookdeo-Drost S, Madison KC, et al. Semipermeable dressings improve epidermal barrier function in premature infants. *Pediatr Res* 1994;36:306–314.
59. Rutter N, Hull D. Reduction of skin water loss in the newborn. I. Effect of applying topical agents. *Arch Dis Child* 1981;56:669–672.
60. Nopper AJ, Horii KA, Sookdeo-Drost S, et al. Topical ointment therapy benefits premature infants. *J Pediatr* 1996;128:660–669.
61. Kjartansson S, Hammarlund K, Sedin G. Insensible water loss from the skin during phototherapy in term and preterm infants. *Acta Paediatr* 1992;81:764–768.
62. Kjartansson S, Hammarlund K, Riesenfeld T, et al. Respiratory water loss and oxygen consumption in newborn infants during phototherapy. *Acta Paediatr* 1992;81:769–773.
63. Leung AK, McArthur RG, McMillan DD, et al. Circulating antidiuretic hormone during labour and in the newborn. *Acta Paediatr Scand* 1980;69:505–510.
64. Wiriyathian S, Rosenfeld CR, Arant BS Jr, et al. Urinary arginine vasopressin: pattern of excretion in the neonatal period. *Pediatr Res* 1986;20:103–108.
65. Marchini G, Stock S. Thirst and vasopressin secretion counteract dehydration in newborn infants. *J Pediatr* 1997;130:736–739.
66. Rees L, Brook CGD, Shaw JC, et al. Hyponatraemia in the first week of life in preterm infants. Part I. Arginine vasopressin secretion. *Arch Dis Child* 1984;59:414–422.
67. Siegel SR, Fisher DA, Oh W. Serum aldosterone concentrations related to sodium balance in the newborn infant. *Pediatrics* 1974;53:410–413.
68. Dillon MJ, Rajani KB, Shah V, et al. Renin and aldosterone response in human newborns to acute change in blood volume. *Arch Dis Child* 1978;53:461–467.
69. Aperia A, Broberger O, Herin P, et al. Sodium excretion in relation to sodium intake and aldosterone excretion in newborn pre-term and full-term infants. *Acta Paediatr Scand* 1979;68: 813–817.
70. Sulyok E, Németh M, Tényi I, et al. Postnatal development of renin-angiotensin-aldosterone system, RAAS, in relation to electrolyte balance in premature infants. *Pediatr Res* 1979;13:817–820.
71. Kojima T, Fukuda Y, Hirata Y, et al. Effects of aldosterone and atrial natriuretic peptide on water and electrolyte homeostasis of sick neonates. *Pediatr Res* 1989;25:591–594.
72. David L, Anast CS. Calcium metabolism in newborn infants. The interrelationship of parathyroid function and calcium, magnesium, and phosphorus metabolism in normal, "sick," and hypocalcemic infants. *J Clin Invest* 1974;54:287–296.
73. David L, Salle B, Chopard P, et al. Studies on circulating immunoreactive calcitonin in low birth weight infants during the first 48 hours of life. *Helv Paediatr Acta* 1977;32:39–48.
74. Hillman LS, Rojanasathit S, Slatopolsky E, et al. Serial measurements of serum calcium, magnesium, parathyroid hormone, calcitonin, and 25-hydroxy-vitamin D in premature and term infants during the first week of life. *Pediatr Res* 1977;11:739–744.
75. David L, Salle BL, Putet G, et al. Serum immunoreactive calcitonin in low birth weight infants. Description of early changes; effect of intravenous calcium infusion; relationships with early changes in serum calcium, phosphorus, magnesium, parathyroid hormone, and gastrin levels. *Pediatr Res* 1981;15:803–808.
76. Smith FG, Sato T, Varille VA, et al. Atrial natriuretic factor during fetal and postnatal life: a review. *J Dev Physiol* 1989;12:55–62.
77. Mercadier JJ, Zongazo MA, Wisnewsky C, et al. Atrial natriuretic factor messenger ribonucleic acid and peptide in the human heart during ontogenic development. *Biochem Biophys Res Commun* 1989;159:777–782.
78. Shaffer SG, Geer PG, Goetz KL. Elevated atrial natriuretic factor in neonates with respiratory distress syndrome. *J Pediatr* 1986;109:1028–1033.
79. Liechty EA, Johnson MD, Myerberg DZ, et al. Daily sequential changes in plasma atrial natriuretic factor concentrations in mechanically ventilated low-birth-weight infants. Effect of surfactant replacement. *Biol Neonate* 1989;55:244–250.
80. Rozycki HJ, Baumgart S. Atrial natriuretic factor and postnatal diuresis in respiratory distress syndrome. *Arch Dis Child* 1991;66:43–47.
81. Robillard JE, Weiner C. Atrial natriuretic factor in the human fetus: effect of volume expansion. *J Pediatr* 1988;113:552–555.
82. Bierd TM, Kattwinkel J, Chevalier RL, et al. Interrelationship of atrial natriuretic peptide, atrial volume, and renal function in premature infants. *J Pediatr* 1990;116:753–759.
83. Tulassay T, Rascher W, Seyberth HW, et al. Role of atrial natriuretic peptide in sodium homeostasis in premature infants. *J Pediatr* 1986;109:1023–1027.
84. Kojima T, Hirata Y, Fukuda Y, et al. Plasma atrial natriuretic peptide and spontaneous diuresis in sick neonates. *Arch Dis Child* 1987;62:667–670.
85. Siegel SR, Oh W. Renal function as a marker of human fetal maturation. *Acta Paediatr Scand* 1976;65:481–485.
86. Leake RD, Trygstad CW, Oh W. Inulin clearance in the newborn infant: relationship to gestational and postnatal age. *Pediatr Res* 1976;10:759–762.
87. Arant BS Jr. Developmental patterns of renal functional maturation compared in the human neonate. *J Pediatr* 1978;92:705–712.
88. Ross B, Cowett RM, Oh W. Renal functions of low birth weight infants during the first two months of life. *Pediatr Res* 1977;11: 1162–1164.
89. Wilkins BH. Renal function in sick very low birthweight infants: 1. Glomerular filtration rate. *Arch Dis Child* 1992;67: 1140–1145.
90. Wilkins BH. Renal function in sick very low birthweight infants: 2. Urea and creatinine excretion. *Arch Dis Child* 1992;67:1146–1153.

91. Hansen JD, Smith CA. Effects of withholding fluid in the immediate postnatal period. *Pediatrics* 1953;12:99–113.
92. Calcagno PL, Rubin MI, Weintraub DH. Studies on the renal concentrating and diluting mechanisms in the premature infant. *J Clin Invest* 1954;33:91–96.
93. McCance RA, Naylor NJ, Widdowson EM. The response of infants to a large dose of water. *Arch Dis Child* 1954;29:104–109.
94. Leake RD, Zakauddin S, Trygstad CW, et al. The effects of large volume intravenous fluid infusion on neonatal renal function. *J Pediatr* 1976;89:968–972.
95. Aperia A, Herin P, Lundin S, et al. Regulation of renal water excretion in newborn full-term infants. *Acta Paediatr Scand* 1984;73:717–721.
96. Brosius KK, Ritter DA, Kenny JD. Postnatal growth curve of the infant with extremely low birth weight who was fed enterally. *Pediatrics* 1984;74:778–782.
97. Shaffer SG, Quimiro CL, Anderson JV, et al. Postnatal weight changes in low birth weight infants. *Pediatrics* 1987;79:702–705.
98. Lemoh JN, Brooke OG. Frequency and weight of normal stools in infancy. *Arch Dis Child* 1979;54:719–720.
99. Patrick CH, Pittard WB. Stool water loss in very-low-birth-weight neonates. *Clin Pediatr (Phila)* 1988;27:144–146.
100. Williams GS, Klenk EL, Winters RW. Acute renal failure in pediatrics. In: Winters RW, ed. *The body fluids in pediatrics, medical, surgical, and neonatal disorders of acid-base status, hydration, and oxygenation.* Boston: Little, Brown and Company, 1973:523–557.
101. Gamble JL, Butler AM. Measurement of the renal water requirement. *Trans Assoc Am Phys* 1944;58:157–161.
102. Sinclair JC, Driscoll JM Jr, Heird WC, et al. Supportive management of the sick neonate. Parenteral calories, water, and electrolytes. *Pediatr Clin North Am* 1970;17:863–893.
103. Ziegler EE. Feeding the low birth weight infant. In: Gellis SS, Kagan BM, eds. *Current pediatric therapy,* 13th ed. Philadelphia: WB Saunders, 1990:713–716.
104. American Academy of Pediatrics Committee on Nutrition. Nutritional needs of the preterm infant. In: Kleinman RE, ed. *Pediatric nutrition handbook,* 5th ed. Elk Grove Village, Ill: American Academy of Pediatrics, 2004:23–54.
105. Roy RN, Chance GW, Radde IC, et al. Late hyponatremia in very low birthweight infants (<1.3 kilograms). *Pediatr Res* 1976;10:526–531.
106. Engelke SC, Shah BL, Vasan U, et al. Sodium balance in very low-birth-weight infants. *J Pediatr* 1978;93:837–841.
107. Al-Dahhan J, Haycock GB, Chantler C, et al. Sodium homeostasis in term and preterm neonates. I. Renal aspects. *Arch Dis Child* 1983;58:335–342.
108. Costarino AT Jr, Gruskay JA, Corcoran L, et al. Sodium restriction versus daily maintenance replacement in very low birth weight premature neonates: a randomized, blind therapeutic trial. *J Pediatr* 1992;120:99–106.
109. Hartnoll G, Bétrémieux P, Modi N. Randomized controlled trial of postnatal sodium supplementation on body composition in 25 to 30 week gestational age infants. *Arch Dis Child Fetal Neonatal Ed* 2000;82:F24–F28.
110. Gruskay J, Costarino AT, Polin RA, et al. Nonoliguric hyperkalemia in the premature infant weighing less than 1000 grams. *J Pediatr* 1988;113:381–386.
111. Brion LP, Schwartz GJ, Campbell D, et al. Early hyperkalaemia in very low birthweight infants in the absence of oliguria. *Arch Dis Child* 1989;64:270–272.
112. Shaffer SG, Kilbride HW, Hayen LK, et al. Hyperkalemia in very low birth weight infants. *J Pediatr* 1992;121:275–279.
113. Sato K, Kondo T, Iwao H, et al. Internal potassium shift in premature infants: cause of nonoliguric hyperkalemia. *J Pediatr* 1995;126:109–113.
114. Lorenz JM, Kleinman LI, Markarian K. Potassium metabolism in extremely low birth weight infants in the first week of life. *J Pediatr* 1997;131:81–86.
115. Stefano JL, Norman ME, Morales MC, et al. Decreased erythrocyte Na$^+$,K$^+$-ATPase activity associated with cellular potassium loss in extremely low birth weight infants with nonoliguric hyperkalemia. *J Pediatr* 1993;122:276–284.
116. Milley JR, Jung AL. Hematochezia associated with the use of hypertonic sodium polystyrene sulfonate enemas in premature infants. *J Perinatol* 1995;15:139–142.
117. Bennett LN, Myers TF, Lambert GH. Cecal perforation associated with sodium polystyrene sulfonate-sorbitol enemas in a 650 gram infant with hyperkalemia. *Am J Perinatol* 1996;13:167–170.
118. Grammatikopoulos T, Greenough A, Pallidis C, et al. Benefits and risks of calcium resonium therapy in hyperkalaemic preterm infants. *Acta Paediatr* 2003;92:118–120.
119. Stonestreet BS, Oh W. Plasma creatinine levels in low-birth-weight infants during the first three months of life. *Pediatrics* 1978;61:788–789.
120. Karlowicz MG, Simmons MA, Brusilow SW, et al. Carbonic acid dissociation constant (pK1) in critically ill newborns. *Pediatr Res* 1984;18:1287–1289.
121. Bell EF. Nutritional support. In: Goldsmith JP, Karotkin EH, eds. *Assisted ventilation of the neonate,* 4th ed. Philadelphia: WB Saunders, 2003:416–428.
122. Siegel SR, Fisher DA, Oh W. Renal function and serum aldosterone levels in infants with respiratory distress syndrome. *J Pediatr* 1973;83:854–858.
123. Broberger U, Aperia A. Renal function in idiopathic respiratory distress syndrome. *Acta Paediatr Scand* 1978;67:313–319.
124. Tulassay T, Ritvay J, Bors Z, et al. Alterations in creatinine clearance during respiratory distress syndrome. *Biol Neonate* 1979;35:258–263.
125. Torrado A, Guignard JP, Prod'hom LS, et al. Hypoxaemia and renal function in newborns with respiratory distress syndrome (RDS). *Helv Paediatr Acta* 1974;29:399–405.
126. Guignard JP, Torrado A, Mazouni SM, et al. Renal function in respiratory distress syndrome. *J Pediatr* 1976;88:845–850.
127. Langman CB, Engle WD, Baumgart S, et al. The diuretic phase of respiratory distress syndrome and its relationship to oxygenation. *J Pediatr* 1981;98:462–466.
128. Bidiwala KS, Lorenz JM, Kleinman LI. Renal function correlates of postnatal diuresis in preterm infants. *Pediatrics* 1988;82:50–58.
129. Lorenz JM, Kleinman LI, Ahmed G, et al. Phases of fluid and electrolyte homeostasis in the extremely low birth weight infant. *Pediatrics* 1995;96:484–489.
130. Cox JR, Davies-Jones GA, Leonard PJ, et al. The effect of positive pressure respiration on urinary aldosterone excretion. *Clin Sci* 1963;24:1–5.
131. Bark H, LeRoith D, Nyska M, et al. Elevations in plasma ADH levels during PEEP ventilation in the dog: mechanisms involved. *Am J Physiol* 1980;239:E474–E481.
132. Hemmer M, Viquerat CE, Suter PM, et al. Urinary antidiuretic hormone excretion during mechanical ventilation and weaning in man. *Anesthesiology* 1980;52:395–400.
133. Paxson CL Jr, Stoerner JW, Denson SE, et al. Syndrome of inappropriate antidiuretic hormone secretion in neonates with pneumothorax or atelectasis. *J Pediatr* 1977;91:459–463.
134. Stern P, LaRochelle FT Jr, Little GA. Vasopressin and pneumothorax in the neonate. *Pediatrics* 1981;68:499–503.
135. Bauer K, Buschkamp S, Marcinkowski M, et al. Postnatal changes of extracellular volume, atrial natriuretic factor, and diuresis in a randomized controlled trial of high-frequency oscillatory ventilation versus intermittent positive-pressure ventilation in premature infants <30 weeks gestation. *Crit Care Med* 2000;28:2064–2068.
136. Sinclair JC, Engel K, Silverman WA. Early correction of hypoxemia and acidemia in infants of low birth weight: a controlled trial of oxygen breathing, rapid alkali infusion, and assisted ventilation. *Pediatrics* 1968;42:565–589.
137. Hobel CJ, Oh W, Hyvarinen MA, et al. Early versus late treatment of neonatal acidosis in low-birth-weight infants: relation to respiratory distress syndrome. *J Pediatr* 1972;81:1178–1187.
138. Corbet AJ, Adams JM, Kenny JD, et al. Controlled trial of bicarbonate therapy in high-risk premature newborn infants. *J Pediatr* 1977;91:771–776.
139. Siegel SR, Phelps DL, Leake RD, et al. The effects of rapid infusion of hypertonic sodium bicarbonate in infants with respiratory distress. *Pediatrics* 1973;51:651–654.
140. Simmons MA, Adcock EW 3rd, Bard H, et al. Hypernatremia and intracranial hemorrhage in neonates. *N Engl J Med* 1974;291:6–10.
141. Brownlee KG, Ng PC, Henderson MJ, et al. Catabolic effect of dexamethasone in the preterm baby. *Arch Dis Child* 1992;67:1–4.
142. Williams AF, Jones M. Dexamethasone increases plasma amino acid concentrations in bronchopulmonary dysplasia. *Arch Dis Child* 1992;67:5–9.

143. Van Goudoever JB, Wattimena JD, Carnielli VP, et al. Effect of dexamethasone on protein metabolism in infants with bronchopulmonary dysplasia. *J Pediatr* 1994;124:112–118.

144. Schanler RJ, Shulman RJ, Prestridge LL. Parenteral nutrient needs of very low birth weight infants. *J Pediatr* 1994;125:961–968.

145. Moylan FMB, Herrin JT, Krishnamoorthy K, et al. Inappropriate antidiuretic hormone secretion in premature infants with cerebral injury. *Am J Dis Child* 1978;132:399–402.

146. Speer ME, Gorman WA, Kaplan SL, et al. Elevation of plasma concentrations of arginine vasopressin following perinatal asphyxia. *Acta Paediatr Scand* 1984;73:610–614.

147. Dauber IM, Krauss AN, Symchych PS, et al. Renal failure following perinatal anoxia. *J Pediatr* 1976;88:851–855.

148. Anand SK, Northway JD, Crussi FG. Acute renal failure in newborn infants. *J Pediatr* 1978;92:985–988.

149. Pizarro D, Posada G, Mata L, et al. Oral rehydration of neonates with dehydrating diarrhoeas. *Lancet* 1979;2:1209–1210.

150. Widness JA, Seward VJ, Kromer IJ, et al. Changing patterns of red blood cell transfusion in very low birth weight infants. *J Pediatr* 1996;129:680–687.

151. Beardsall K, White DK, Pinto EM, et al. Pericardial effusion and cardiac tamponade as complications of neonatal long lines: are they really a problem? *Arch Dis Child Fetal Neonatal Ed* 2003;88:F292–F295.

Nutrition

22

Michael K. Georgieff

The provision of nutrition to term and preterm newborn infants remains one of the most important aspects of neonatal care. With increasing survival rates among sick newborns, the nourishment of full-term and preterm infants has assumed an increasingly greater role in the neonatal intensive care unit in the past 25 years. Great strides have been made in understanding neonatal nutritional physiology and pathophysiology in these years, allowing physicians to more precisely estimate the nutritional needs of the infants in their care. Knowledge of newborn infants' nutritional requirements and of their neurological, gastrointestinal, and metabolic capabilities is a prerequisite to informed decision making about nutritional therapy in the nursery. It is also important to understand the tools available for assessment of neonatal nutritional status to judge the success or failure of nutritional therapies.

The goal of nutritional therapy in the term neonate is to ensure a successful growth transition from the fetal to the postnatal period. In the preterm infant, the goal has been to continue the process of intrauterine growth in what is now an extrauterine environment until 40 weeks postconception and to foster catch-up growth and nutrient accretion in the postdischarge period. Until lately, the goal for the growing preterm infant has been to match the third trimester intrauterine rates of weight gain, linear growth, and brain growth. Even if these rates are successfully attained, the body composition of the preterm infant raised in an extrauterine environment nevertheless remains remarkably different than that of the same postconceptional-age infant who has remained in utero (1,2). Current efforts are aimed at understanding the metabolic processes that determine the body composition of the preterm infant. Additionally, the preterm infant is still likely to be well below the standard gestational growth curves at discharge (3) because of nutrient deficits that have accrued during the prolonged period of neonatal illness (4). The effect of illness on neonatal metabolism and nutritional requirements is being recognized (5). Conditions such as bronchopulmonary dysplasia (BPD), congestive heart failure (CHF), acute respiratory distress, intrauterine growth retardation, and sepsis (and their treatments) have negative effects on neonatal energy, protein, and mineral and vitamin requirements. These conditions may also affect the digestive and absorptive capacities of the neonate.

This chapter reviews the nutritional requirements, digestive capabilities, and expected growth of term and preterm infants. These factors will be addressed in the context of the three time phases of neonatal nutritional development: transition, premie growth, and postdischarge. The chapter also provides an overview of various nutrient delivery systems, both enteral and parenteral. Finally, the chapter covers techniques of nutritional assessment and offers suggestions for appropriate monitoring of neonatal nutritional status.

NUTRITIONAL CAPABILITIES OF THE NEWBORN INFANT

The ability to suck and swallow a meal in a coordinated fashion and then process those nutrients for utilization by the body may be one of the most complex developmental tasks facing the newborn infant (6). Success depends on a certain amount of neurological, digestive, absorptive and metabolic maturity. The term infant is quite mature in these respects. However, the preterm infant's physiology is progressively more immature as a function of decreased gestational age.

Neurological Maturity

The neurologically intact term infant is able to suck and swallow in a coordinated fashion within minutes of birth (7). In the preterm infant, the sucking reflex is strong at the limit of viability (23 weeks) and likely prior to that age (8). However, the ability to coordinate the suck reflex with swallowing to ensure that food is propelled into the gastrointestinal tract rather than the airway matures at approximately 34 weeks gestation (9). To a great extent, this coordinated suck and swallow reflex appears to be postconceptional-age mediated; that is, it does not appear that "practice" can stimulate the infant to become more mature at an earlier postconceptional age. Nevertheless, the age at which the infant matures varies widely, and some preterm infants are able to suck and swallow in a coordinated manner by 32 weeks postconception.

Motility in the gastrointestinal tract is also dependent on neurological maturation (10). For example, the esophagus shows a very discoordinated pattern of peristalsis at 24 weeks gestation, with weak peristaltic waves beginning sporadically and propagating either rostrally or caudally (11). By term, the pattern has matured into a coordinated pattern that propels food downward to the stomach (12). The lower esophageal sphincter of the very preterm infant is tenuous and provides little barrier to gastroesophageal reflux (GER). GER disease in the preterm infant can be associated with apnea and bradycardia, aspiration syndromes, and feeding intolerance. At term, although GER remains demonstrable in most infants, it is generally not the potentially life-threatening problem seen at earlier gestational ages.

The stomach also undergoes maturation during the third trimester. The preterm infant's stomach does not coordinately "wring" the stomach from antrum to pylorus, frequently being subject to periods of antiperistalsis, which in turn promotes GER disease (13). Additionally, pyloric function is different in the preterm compared to the term infant. Gastric emptying is longer in the preterm infant, although stomach volume is smaller (14). The small stomach capacity frequently results in the need to feed small volumes to preterm infants on a more frequent schedule. The prolonged gastric emptying time, however, causes retention of the food in the stomach and subsequent obtainment of "preaspirates" prior to the next feeding. Since the presence of preaspirates may also signify an ileus associated with more severe diseases such as necrotizing enterocolitis (NEC), feedings are often discontinued with this sign.

The maturation of small intestinal motility has been extensively studied by Berseth and her colleagues (15–18). They have demonstrated an orderly progression of peristaltic frequency, amplitude, and duration with increasing gestational age. They have also demonstrated a two-hour periodicity to peristalsis in very preterm infants (18). This finding may influence decisions about feeding schedules. The lack of a coordinated motility pattern in the very preterm infant makes it more likely that they will present with signs of feeding intolerance, usually marked by abdominal distention. When compared to adults, neonates retain food in their small intestine for proportionately longer periods and in their colon for shorter periods. The newborn's ability to modulate stool water and electrolyte content is immature compared to adults.

In summary, multiple neuromaturational factors work against the preterm infant's ability to enterally feed as successfully as the term infant (9). These immaturities have an impact on feeding management, as will be discussed in a later section.

Digestive and Absorptive Capabilities

The newborn infant does not have the capability to digest and absorb nutrients from a complex diet (9). Fortunately,

the term human infant has a ready source of nutrition in the form of human milk (7). Human milk is remarkably adapted to fit the digestive capacities of the term newborn and to meet the infant's nutritional needs for at least the first 6 months of life (7). Recent studies have also shown the nutritional value of feeding human milk to preterm infants; however, for infants weighing more than 1,500 g, human milk needs to be fortified (19).

The functional immaturities of the gastrointestinal, hepatic, and renal systems in the newborn have an impact on the delivery of all classes of nutrients: macronutrients, minerals, trace elements, and vitamins.

Protein

Protein digestion begins in the stomach with the action of pepsin on the intact protein (20). Pepsin is activated by acid hydrolysis of its precursor molecule, pepsinogen. The newborn is capable of creating an acidic stomach environment by 1 week of age (21); thus, pepsin activation is thought to be intact. Dietary protein is then acted upon by pancreatic peptidases released into the duodenum. These enzymes include trypsin, chymotrypsin, carboxypeptidases A and B, and elastase, and are amino acid selective with respect to cleavage sites, resulting in peptides of relatively small length. The peptides are subsequently cleaved once more by peptidases located in the intestinal mucosal cells, absorbed as amino acids or dipeptides, and transported to the liver. Protein digestion and absorption in adults is very efficient; up to 95% of a protein load can be fully digested. Although term and preterm infants have relatively low concentrations of chymotrypsin, the carboxypeptidases, and elastase (22), they nevertheless achieve more than 80% protein digestion.

Fat

The efficiency of fat digestion in the neonate has been a controversial topic. Data from the 1970s and 1980s suggested that fat is the most poorly digested macronutrient in the neonate (23). Whereas adults will absorb close to 95% of a fat meal and term infants absorb 85% to 90%, early studies indicated that preterm infants absorb as little as 50%, depending on the type of fat presented to them (24). The perceived functional immaturity of fat digestion in the preterm infant led to modification of fat blends in the formulas used in preterm infants.

Fat digestion in the neonate begins in the stomach with the action of a lipase secreted in the mouth (lingual lipase) or by the gastric mucosa (gastric lipase) (25). The two lipases are identical, function ideally at acid pH, work primarily on medium-chain triglycerides (MCT), and do not require bile salts. Hamosh has estimated that this enzyme may be responsible for up to 50% of fat digestion in the newborn (26). Infants fed human milk have the additional benefit of a lipase secreted into the milk by the mother (27). This lipase is found in all carnivores (but not herbivores) and functions more like pancreatic or intestinal lipases found in adults. It works primarily on long-chain triglycerides at a neutral pH, as is found in the intestine, and requires bile salts. This lipase may be responsible for the digestion of up to 20% of dietary fat (28). These two lipases are referred to as the "compensatory lipases" of the newborn and function in place of pancreatic and intestinal lipases seen in more mature humans (29).

Long-chain fatty acids are dependent on bile salts for proper micellization and uptake into the intestinal lymphatics. From there, the micelles are carried to the venous system via the thoracic duct, ultimately destined for the liver. Medium-chain fatty acids do not require micellization and can be directly absorbed into the blood stream. The bile acid, and hence bile salt, pools of the preterm newborn are low, thus restricting the fat-absorption capacity of the infant. Prenatal administration of glucocorticoids to the mother can mature the fetal bile salt pool in the preterm infant less than 34 weeks gestation to the level of the term infant (30). Without such priming, however, the preterm infant has significant impairment of fat absorption (including fat-soluble vitamins) prior to 34 weeks gestation. The fat blend in preterm infant formulas designed for infants less than 34 weeks gestation has been significantly modified to optimize fat absorption. These formulas contain a higher percentage of MCT and higher vitamin A, D, and E levels than formulas manufactured for term infants.

Carbohydrate

Like fats, carbohydrates can present a significant digestive challenge. The neonate has a limited ability to digest complex carbohydrates because of relatively small amounts of pancreatic amylase (31). Thus, beikost in the form of cereal rarely makes up a significant portion of the infant's diet until after 4 months of age. The term and preterm newborn readily uses glucose, which can be delivered either parenterally or enterally. Intestinal glucose uptake is seen as early as ten weeks gestation, long before the fetus is viable (32). However, provision of all carbohydrate calories as glucose would result in the neonatal gut being exposed to a hyperosmolar solution with a high potential for mucosal damage.

The primary carbohydrate found in mammalian milk is the disaccharide lactose. Like other disaccharides (sucrose, maltose, isomaltose), enzymatic cleavage by a disaccharidase must occur before the monosaccharides can be absorbed. In the case of lactose, glucose and galactose are produced by the action of lactase. The disaccharidases sucrase and maltase appear very early in gestation and appear to be inducible enzymes (33). In contrast, lactase begins to appear at 24 weeks gestation and rises in concentration very slowly until term. It does not appear to be a particularly inducible enzyme (34). The preterm infant is thus functionally somewhat lactose intolerant and will have typical symptoms of gas formation, diarrhea, and acidic stools characteristic of lactose malabsorption when fed high doses of lactose. Positive hydrogen breath tests

have been documented in preterm infants following lactose challenges (35).

Preterm infant formulas have lower lactose contents than term formulas for this reason. Up to 60% of carbohydrate calories in preterm infant formulas are derived from linear glucose polymers, which produce a lower osmolar load than the equivalent number of individual glucose molecules. The enzyme required to digest glucose polymers (glucoamylase) is present from 24 weeks gestation (36). The lower lactose content is also present in the premature discharge formulas, although it is likely that the preterm infant is fully mature with respect to lactose absorption at the time of discharge (37).

NUTRIENT REQUIREMENTS FOR TERM AND PRETERM INFANTS

Estimation of nutrient requirements is an inexact process, particularly when the goal is unclear. To date, the goal has been to achieve the same growth rates and body composition as the "reference" infant; the healthy breastfed infant serves as the "gold standard" for the term infant. Nevertheless, it is clear that breastfed babies have different growth rates and body compositions than formula-fed infants (38). Human milk composition varies greatly among mothers, and the length of time that it remains sufficient for all the nutrient needs of the infant is not uniform. Breastfed infants may have lower iron stores (39) and be at greater risk for vitamin D deficiency than formula-fed infants (40).

Determining the ideal growth for the infant born before term is far more problematic. Indeed, the ideal growth rate and body composition of the "healthy" preterm infant remain unknown and are likely to be different from his or her gestationally age-matched fetal counterpart. Until recently, the daily and weekly accretion rates of various nutrients in the preterm infant have been modeled on in utero accretion rates of these nutrients in gestationally age-matched fetuses. The "reference fetus" described by Widdowson and again by Ziegler has served as the benchmark by which neonatal nutritionists judge fetal growth and body composition (2,41). Nevertheless, energy requirements are likely to be different in a 28-week-gestational-age newborn exposed to the thermal stresses of extrauterine life than in a 28-week fetus comfortably surrounded by amniotic fluid.

The rates of weight gain, linear growth, and head growth between the ages of 24 and 36 weeks gestation can be calculated from the standard growth curves generated from infants born prematurely (42,43). It must be recognized that the data used to generate these plots are necessarily cross-sectional and thus need smoothing to create the resemblance of a curve. Additionally, since premature birth is an abnormal event and up to 30% of very-low-birth-weight (VLBW) infants are small for dates (most likely as a result of the pregnancy failing over time), the reliability of newborn data to assess the growth velocity of healthy fetuses is suspect. Nevertheless, these curves are used extensively as guideposts for neonatal growth of the preterm infant. On average, these curves predict that the preterm infant should gain 10 to 15 g/kg body weight each day, grow 0.75 to 1.0 cm per week linearly, and demonstrate 0.75 cm per week of head growth. These values had been utilized to calculate the energy and protein needs of the preterm infant until recently. More accurate ultrasonographic techniques have been used to measure fetal growth in healthy pregnancies. These studies suggest that the rate of weight gain is closer to 18 to 20 g/kg body weight per day (44).

The nutrient requirements of term and preterm infants can be calculated based on fetal reference figures, balance studies, serum nutrient values, or a combination of these.

Energy Requirements

Energy requirements must take into account the amount and caloric density of the solution ingested, the route of administration (enteral versus parenteral), the amount lost in stool or urine, and the energy requirements in the body (e.g., basal metabolic rate, cost of growth, energy cost of food processing by the body) (45). Many of these are now measurable, and reasonable estimates of energy requirements to maintain optimal growth velocities can be made for both term and preterm infants.

Energy is predominantly derived from carbohydrates and fat in the diet, which provide 4 and 9 kcal/g, respectively. The infant fed human milk receives calories predominantly from fat (46), whereas the formula-fed infant receives calories more evenly distributed between fat and carbohydrate (47). The calories derived from these sources are used first to maintain the total energy need of the infant, which consists of the basal metabolic rate, the thermic effect of feeding, and physical activity. Energy intake beyond this baseline is stored and recorded as weight gain. Protein is not normally utilized as an energy source, unless the total energy intake is less than the total energy expenditure of the infant. In those cases, certain amino acids can be deaminated and shunted into the gluconeogenic pathways to provide approximately 4 kcal/g of protein (48).

Energy requirements can be affected by numerous factors, including the route of delivery and the disease state. Energy requirements are lower when infants are fed parenterally as opposed to enterally because no energy is excreted in the stool. Thus, the term infant who normally requires 100 kcal/kg/day enterally may be fed 90 kcal/kg/day parenterally. Diseases that increase energy needs include CHF (49), BPD (50), acute respiratory disease (51), and overwhelming sepsis (52). Diseases that decrease energy needs include hypoxic-ischemic encephalopathy and degenerative neurological conditions in which there is paucity of physical movement.

Term Infants

Healthy breastfed term infants show adequate growth on as little as 85 to 100 kcal/kg body weight per day during the first four months of life (53). Formula-fed infants have higher energy requirements (100–110 kcal/kg), most likely as a result of a lower efficiency of digestion and absorption of fat (54). The presence of a lipase in human milk increases the digestibility of its fats.

Preterm Infants

Preterm infants have higher energy requirements than term infants because of a higher resting energy expenditure and greater stool losses as a result of immature absorptive capacities (55,56) (Appendix J-1). Whereas the resting energy expenditure of the term infant is 45 to 50 kcal/kg/day, the preterm infant less than 34 weeks gestation consumes 50 to 60 kcal/kg/day (55,56). Stool losses vary between 10% and 40% of intake, depending on the diet. For example, a diet in which the carbohydrate is 100% lactose and the fats are predominantly long-chain triglycerides will promote more stool losses because of the low levels of lactase and the small bile salt pools in the premature infant. Replacement of up to 50% of the lactose with glucose polymers and between 10% and 40% of the fat with medium-chain triglycerides (MCT) appears to reduce malabsorption to approximately 10% (57). The preterm infant will need an additional 50 to 60 kcal/kg/day beyond the daily energy expenditure and the loss of energy in the stool to maintain growth along the intrauterine growth curve (10 to 15 g/kg/day). Thus, barring any excess needs from diseases that increase oxygen consumption or from malabsorption, the preterm infant will gain weight adequately on approximately 120 kcal/kg/day. Assuming that 2.5 kcal are needed to achieve 1 gram of weight gain, this upward adjustment of expected weight gain would require feeding an additional 10 to 15 kcal/kg body weight per day to the preterm infant. Thus, it is likely that energy intake on the order of 130 to 135 kcal/kg/day is a more reasonable target for the premature infant than the previous recommended intake of 120 kcal/kg/day (57).

Energy Sources

Carbohydrates

Newborn infants are highly dependent on a source of glucose for normal brain metabolism (58). The primary source of glucose in the term infant is lactose in human milk and cow-milk formulas. Soy-based formulas provide glucose from the metabolism of dietary sucrose or glucose polymers. Preterm infants also receive glucose, initially as dextrose in parenteral solutions, but subsequently enterally from lactose or glucose polymers. Galactose is also important to the newborn, as it is needed for glycogen storage (59). The newborn infant typically utilizes between 4 and 8 mg/kg/minute of glucose (60). This figure is commonly used as the glucose infusion rate for parenteral nutrition. Because of their low glycogen stores and poorer gluconeogenic capacities, preterm infants are more prone to hypoglycemia than term infants (61). Higher rates of glucose delivery (up to 15 mg/kg/minute) may be required in growth-retarded infants and in infants of diabetic mothers to maintain normal glucose concentrations.

Intravenous dextrose infusion rates up to 12.5 mg/kg/minute are commonly used in preterm infants to promote catch-up weight gain. Beyond this rate, a cost/benefit analysis must be made. Although faster rates of weight gain can be achieved on higher glucose infusion rates (especially if the serum glucose is controlled with exogenous insulin infusion) (62), a higher metabolic rate and a shift in the respiratory quotient will also occur. Thus, a higher oxygen consumption rate coupled with proportionately more carbon dioxide generated by the cells may significantly affect serum carbon dioxide and ventilatory requirements. In one study, infants who received glucose and insulin remained on the respirator an average of 13 days longer than their counterparts given lower glucose infusion rates (63). Moreover, the increased "growth rates" demonstrated with high glucose infusion rates are as a result of fatty weight gain, without any increase in linear or brain growth (62). The overall metabolic cost of glucose infusion rates > 12.5 mg/kg/minute must be weighed against the benefit of increased rates of nonlean weight gain.

Fats

Lipids constitute the other major energy source for neonates. Certain fatty acids, such as linoleic (omega-6, 18:2) and linolenic (omega-3, 18:3), are essential in the diet, and their absence will produce deficiency syndromes characterized by growth failure and skin rash (64). Although the full syndrome is rare, lower essential fatty acid concentrations are seen within one week of discontinuing lipid intake. Infants receiving parenteral nutrition or on a fat-restricted enteral diet require 0.5 mg/kg/day of an intravenous fat blend containing these fatty acids at least three times per week to prevent deficiency. The American Academy of Pediatrics (AAP) has recommended that 3% of total energy intake in infants should be in the form of linoleic acid (65).

Daily fat intake varies greatly based on the method of delivery (enteral vs. parenteral) and the dietary source (human milk vs. formula). Enterally fed term infants consume approximately 5 to 6 g/kg/day of fat, whereas parenterally fed infants rarely receive greater than 4 g/kg/day, largely because of concerns about toxicity. Infants receiving human milk (especially human milk expressed by mothers who have delivered preterm) may receive up to 7 g/kg/day.

Infants fed human milk receive a unique blend of fats that has not been precisely replicated in infant formulas. Cow-milk fat is generally not well tolerated by newborn infants, forcing formula manufacturers to use vegetable oils as substitutes. The spectrum of fatty acids found in palm, palm-olein, corn, and coconut oils are distinctly different from human-milk fats.

The role of omega fatty acids such as docosahexaenoic acid (DHA) and arachidonic acid (ARA) in the infant diet continues to be a subject of intense research (57,66). These fatty acids are products of an elongation pathway from linoleic acid and are important in cell membrane structure, in cell-signaling cascades and in myelination (67). The synthetic pathways may be immature in preterm infants, and for some undetermined period of time after birth in term infants (68). Sources of these fatty acids include the placenta and human milk. In contrast, cow-milk fat and vegetable oil do not contain these compounds. A number of studies addressed whether these particular fatty acids are essential in the preterm and term infant (69–72). Because the preterm infant may be less capable of synthesizing the compounds and would have received them in utero, the European Society for Pediatric Gastroenterology and Nutrition has recommended that a source of these fatty acids be added to preterm infant formula (73). Evidence of their efficacy includes studies that demonstrate better visual acuity, more mature electroretinograms, and short-term gains in general neurodevelopment (74–76). Studies of the longer-term growth and developmental outcomes of infants who have been supplemented with these fatty acids are in their early stages but suggest continued positive effects on the visual system at one year of age (77). It remains unclear whether potential early neurodevelopmental gains are sustained beyond the first year (78). A review assessing the role of long-chain polyunsaturated fatty acid (LC-PUFA) supplementation on neurodevelopment concluded that the studies remain too underpowered to support a positive long-term effect (79). The lack of a consistent effect may be as a result of suboptimal dosing of the compounds. Additionally, any time a single component of human milk can be isolated and added to cow-milk-based infant formula, an important consideration is whether the component exerts its nutritional effect individually or in consort with other compounds (80).

The Food and Drug Administration (FDA) in the United States has recently approved a fungal source of DHA and ARA and its incorporation into infant formula under a provision termed "Generally Recognized as Safe" (GRAS). This designation confirms that the FDA has no questions of the manufacturers regarding the safety of the source and stability of these compounds when used in the intended matrix (e.g., infant formula). The GRAS designation is used to indicate that the ingredient in question has been in the food chain of humans and, based on prior usage or experimental evidence reviewed by an expert scientific panel, poses no safety concern. The GRAS determination does not assess efficacy claims; indeed, claims of efficacy for a new ingredient added to infant formula would be subjected to a more thorough examination process by the FDA, not unlike that required of new drugs. The major formula manufacturers in the United States have now added DHA and ARA to their term, preterm hospital, and preterm discharge formulas without making efficacy claims. The formulas appear to be as safe as formulas without added DHA and ARA. It is likely that formulas without the added fats will be phased out over time.

Carnitine is another compound involved in fat metabolism in the neonate. Although carnitine deficiency is rare in the enterally fed infant because of high levels in human milk and supplementation of formulas, it remains a concern in infants receiving long-term exclusive parenteral nutrition in which carnitine has not been supplemented (81). Carnitine supplements can be added to total parenteral nutrition (TPN), and this is recommended in infants who receive TPN for greater than 3 weeks (82).

Protein Requirements

Protein requirements in humans are determined by a number of factors including protein quality and quantity, the amount of energy delivered, and the protein nutritional status of the subject (20). The latter is influenced by the degree of previous malnutrition, by the rate of catch-up growth, and potentially by inflammatory processes. The sick newborn infant is exposed to many of these influences. Additionally, they have a high basal requirement for protein accretion based on in utero nitrogen accretion rates (2,41). Adequate energy intake is important to promote optimal protein utilization, with a nonprotein calorie-to-gram nitrogen ratio of 200:1 considered ideal. Overall protein intake in the neonate is ultimately limited to about 4 to 4.5 g/kg/day because of the inability of the immature kidney to excrete titratable acid, blood urea nitrogen (BUN), and ammonium ion (83). The renal excretion limitations are proportional to the degree of prematurity.

Protein requirements, in general, and branched-chain amino acid needs, in particular, are increased in adults with physiological instability as a result of septic or surgical illness (84). Recently, the possibility that similar changes might occur in sick neonates has been preliminarily investigated (51,52,85). Neither acute respiratory disease nor sepsis nor surgical ligation of the patent ductus arteriosus (PDA) results in increased protein requirements (51,52,85). At this time, increasing protein delivery routinely on the basis of illness or physiological instability is not recommended. Conversely, practitioners frequently limit nutrient delivery during illness out of concern that high loads may be metabolically taxing. Recent studies demonstrate that up to 3 g of protein/kg body weight can be administered daily to sick preterm infants beginning in the first 24 hours after birth (86).

Term Infants

The full-term breastfed infant grows adequately and maintains normal serum and somatic i.e., muscle protein status on as little as 1.5 g/kg/day of protein. Although the protein content is low (1.1%), the quality of human milk protein is excellent because the spectrum of amino acids provides a unique "match" for the amino acid needs of the newborn. The protein content is predominantly lactalbumin, as opposed to casein, which makes for smaller curds and easier digestibility. Additionally, human milk is replete with nondietary nitrogen sources including nucleotides, which may enhance the immune system (87); immunoglobulins and other antimicrobial factors, which help protect the gut epithelium (88,89); growth factors, which stimulate intestinal growth (90); and enzymes (e.g., lipases), which aid digestion.

The term infant fed a cow-milk or soy-based infant formula requires a greater protein delivery rate, most likely to compensate for the less-than-ideal protein quality. Thus, the infant on cow-milk formula typically requires 2.14 g/kg/day and the infant on soy formula up to 2.7 g/kg/day of protein (47). Cow-milk protein is predominantly casein, although a number of cow-milk-based formulas are modified to be whey predominant. The soy formulas also promote adequate growth of lean body mass. However, these formulas contain a smaller percentage of available nitrogen as essential or semi-essential amino acids (91).

Protein can also be delivered to the term infant by way of protein hydrolysate or individual amino acid formulas. These formulas are specifically designed to decrease the exposure of the infant to potentially antigenic cow- or soy-milk proteins. By hydrolyzing the cow-milk-based protein such that greater than 90% of the proteins have a molecular weight of 1,250 Daltons or less, allergic disease as a result of cow-milk allergy can be treated or potentially prophylaxed. These formulas provide approximately 2.8 g/kg/day of protein at an energy delivery of 100 kcal/kg/day.

Preterm infants

Recommendations for protein intake in preterm infants follow many of the same parameters as in term infants. However, the needs of the preterm infant appear to be greater than the term infant. Early studies suggested that the most rapid weight gain and most efficient energy utilization was achieved with protein intakes of 3 to 5 g/kg/day (92,93). Kashyap and associates refined these goals when they demonstrated that weight gain and nitrogen retention were greatest in healthy 32-week-gestational-age infants fed 3.9 g/kg/day of protein (94). They also attempted to define the optimal energy-to-protein ratio which promoted growth, finding that approximately 30 kcal were necessary for each gram of protein delivered. In a later study by the same group, Schulze and associates proposed that preterm infants tolerate 3.6 g/kg/day of protein with an energy intake of at least 120 kcal/kg/day (95). Heird has emphasized that increasing protein delivery requires increased energy delivery, and vice versa (96). His conclusions include:

- The low-birth-weight (LBW) infant who can take feeds soon after birth requires a protein intake of at least 2.8 g/kg/day.
- Infants who do not receive protein in the first few days of life lose at least 1% of their endogenous protein stores daily. (These findings are consistent with research stating that preterm neonates were in better nutritional status if amino acids were added to dextrose solutions in the first days of life [97].)
- Infants with delayed protein intake subsequently require higher protein intakes to correct for early losses.

Denne has used stable isotopes of nitrogen to study the protein requirements and distribution (synthesis versus breakdown) in extremely-low-birth-weight (ELBW) infants (98). His calculations indicate that an average daily intake of 3.2 g/kg of protein is necessary to counter the negative nitrogen balance of neonatal illness and to match the expected in utero protein accretion rate. Ziegler's data in stable, growing premature infants also confirms that enteral protein delivery less than 3.5 g/kg/day results in suboptimal growth (99).

Besides total protein delivery, recent studies have considered which amino acids may limit protein accretion in the preterm infant. The terms "essential" and "nonessential" amino acids have been replaced in the neonatal lexicon by "indispensable" or "limiting" and "dispensable" (100) because they are more descriptive of the effects of amino acids on protein metabolism. Threonine and lysine are clearly indispensable because they cannot be synthesized de novo from products of carbon intermediary metabolism. Heird suggests that these two amino acids may currently be the limiting amino acids in TPN solutions.

Finally, illnesses or medications that increase protein turnover or muscle breakdown will have an influence on protein delivery. Van Goudoever and associates demonstrated that the steroids used for the treatment of BPD cause negative nitrogen balance by increasing the rate of protein breakdown but have little effect on protein synthesis (101).

Many preterm infants receive protein initially as part of a regimen of parenteral nutrition. Intravenous amino acid solutions have advanced to the point of being specifically formulated for preterm infants. These amino acid solutions are designed to normalize the plasma amino acid profile of the healthy infant, promoting levels similar to those of a one-month-old breastfed infant (102). Anderson and associates demonstrated that dextrose solutions with amino acids given early in life promote better nutritional status than dextrose solutions without protein (97). Denne et al. have shown that newborn preterm infants respond to parenteral nutrition with an acute increase in protein synthesis and a decrease in proteolysis (103). Thus, it appears that amino acid delivery in the first days of life is critical.

The recommended amount of amino acids to be delivered and the rate of advancement remain to be determined, and are influenced by the infant's condition. Based on the estimates of protein loss by Heird and associates (96), it is prudent to begin amino acids on day one. The BUN and acid-base status of the infant must be followed. Older studies in sick neonates suggest that 1.5 g/kg/day of amino acids on day two would achieve neutral nitrogen balance (51). However, more recent data from Thureen and associates indicate that preterm infants can be safely started on 3.0 g/kg/day on day one (86). Ultimately, the goal is to deliver between 3.0 and 4.0 g/kg/day of parenteral amino acids. Some newborn intensive care units carry stock solutions of dextrose with added protein to be started upon admission to the nursery before parenteral nutrition from the pharmacy can be ordered and obtained. The amount of protein is designed to deliver 2 g/kg/day when the fluid solution is prescribed at 75 cc/kg/day.

Preterm infants who begin enteral feeds in the first days after birth will be relatively protein restricted because they are typically given human milk or low amounts of preterm infant formula. Although human milk from mothers delivering preterm is initially higher in protein (Table 22-1) compared to term human milk (104–106), the content is still relatively low and the infant will likely receive low volumes. Fortification with a human milk fortifier addresses this low protein issue. Preterm infant formula has a high concentration of protein (3.1 to 3.6 g/120 kcal), but it is unlikely that the infant will achieve that type of delivery in the first week. With the trend toward increased protein delivery to the preterm infant, Ziegler and others have stressed the importance of supplying adequate energy intake (99,107).

TABLE 22-1
NUTRIENT AND MINERAL CONTENT OF PRETERM MILK

Element[a]	Days 3–7	Day 21	Days 29–42	Days 57–98
Protein (g/dL)	3.24 ± 0.31	1.83 ± 0.14	1.31–1.81 ± 0.12	1.8 ± 0.07
Lactose (g/dL)	5.96 ± 0.2	6.49 ± 0.21		
Fat (g/dL)	1.63 ± 0.23	3.68 ± 0.4		
Energy (kcal/dL)	51.4 ± 2.4	65.6 ± 4.3		
Sodium (mEq/dL)	2.66 ± 0.3	1.3 ± 0.18	0.76 ± 0.09	0.55 ± 0.05
Chloride (mEq/dL)	3.16 ± 0.3	1.7–0.17		
Potassium (mEq/dL)	1.74 ± 0.07	1.63–0.09	1.1 ± 0.1	1.1 ± −0.1
Calcium (mg/dL)	20.3–26.3 ± 1.7	20.4 ± 1.5	24.6–26.2 ± 2.2	31.5 ± 1.3
Phosphorous (mg/dL)	9.5–14.6 ± 0.7	14.9 ± 1.3	13.3 ± 0.3	
Magnesium (mg/dL)	2.8 ± .1	2.4 ± 0.1	4.9 ± 0.1	

[a] From Gross SJ, David RJ, Bauman L, et al. Nutritional composition of milk produced by mothers delivering preterm. *J Pediatr* 1980;96:641–644; Schanler RJ, Oh W. Composition of breast milk obtained from mothers of premature infants as compared with breast milk obtained from donors. *J Pediatr* 1980;96:679–681; Feeley RM, Eitenmiller RR, Jones JB, et al. Calcium, phosphorus and magnesium contents of human milk during early lactation. *J Pediatr Gastroenterol Nutr* 1983;2:262–267, with permission.

Mineral And Element Requirements

Mineral requirements in newborns are influenced by the immature status of the kidney, prematurity, and medications that affect mineral metabolism (108). In general, preterm infants require higher amounts of minerals than term infants. The daily needs of some minerals (e.g., sodium, potassium chloride) are determined by measuring serum levels, although others (e.g., calcium, phosphorus) are estimated from in utero accretion rates (2,41). A more comprehensive discussion of these needs can be found in other chapters in this volume (e.g., Fluid/Electrolyte, Bone Mineralization) and in other sources (109). The following discussion focuses on selected minerals, comparing requirements in the preterm infant to the term infant and emphasizing the effects of diseases and their treatments on mineral status.

Sodium, Potassium, and Chloride

The typical term infant requires 1 to 3 mEq/kg/day of sodium (108). Breastfed infants have a lower sodium intake than formula-fed infants, although formula manufacturers have reduced the sodium content of cow-milk formula to levels comparable to human milk. Preterm infants have higher sodium requirements and may become hyponatremic on human milk (19,110). Baseline sodium requirements range from 2 to 4 mEq/kg day in the preterm infant. The higher sodium requirement with lower gestational age is due predominantly to the immaturity of the proximal renal tubule in the small preterm infant. Treatment of these infants with salt-wasting diuretics, e.g., furosemide, hydrochlorothiazide may increase the needs to 10 to 13 mEq/kg/day.

Potassium requirements in the term infant generally range between 1 and 2 mEq/kg/day. Because potassium is also reabsorbed at the proximal tubule, the preterm infant needs 2 to 4 mEq/kg/day (110). Diuretics such as furosemide, metolazone, and hydrochlorothiazide can increase requirements to 8 mEq/kg/day.

Sodium and potassium are provided in human milk and infant formulas to satisfy the daily requirement for the normal infant. However, excessive demands from prior or ongoing losses may require supplementation. Supplements are typically in the form of chloride salts (NaCl or KCl) and are dosed based on calculations of maintenance requirements plus deficits. Depending on the acid-base status of the infant receiving parenteral nutrition, sodium and potassium can be added as chloride or as acetate.

Calcium, Magnesium, and Phosphorus

The term infant who has not experienced intrauterine growth retardation has well-mineralized bones. Analysis of the reference fetus demonstrated that the average fetus accretes 80% to 90% of its calcium during the last trimester (2). If there has been no interruption of the process, the average term infant will grow well and remain well mineralized on a diet that provides approximately 40 to 60 mg/kg/day of calcium and 20 to 30 mg/kg/day of phosphorus. Human milk is an excellent source for this rate of delivery. Infant formulas have higher concentrations of calcium than human milk, but there is little evidence that term infants who are formula fed are better mineralized.

LBW infants (intrauterine growth retarded or preterm) have significantly lower calcium and phosphorus content than term, appropriate-for-dates infants. Daily enteral calcium and phosphorus requirements in the preterm infant are estimated at 120 to 230 and 60 to 140 mg/kg/day, respectively (111). This rate of daily accretion can only be achieved enterally. The two minerals become insoluble in typical TPN solutions when added at concentrations that would provide more than 60 mg/kg/day of calcium and 30 mg/kg/day of phosphorus (at typical fluid delivery of 150 cc/kg/day). Human milk is relatively low in calcium and phosphorus and thus must be supplemented with a fortifier to achieve adequate mineralization in the less than 1,500 g infant (112). Preterm infant formula contains enough calcium and phosphorus to deliver the recommended daily amount and some excess to begin to replace previously acquired deficits. This is important because most preterm infants do not tolerate full enteral feedings immediately after birth. Preterm infants will invariably need intakes greater than the projected daily in utero requirement to avoid becoming osteopenic since parenteral nutrition results in negative calcium and phosphorus balance (4). Because serum calcium levels will always be maintained at the expense of the bone, following calcium levels as a way of monitoring status is not useful. Instead, indicators of bone activity (serum alkaline phosphatase) or urinary phosphorus excretion are used to monitor long-term calcium status.

As with calcium, the rates of magnesium accretion *in utero* are high during the third trimester. Thus, the magnesium requirement for infants born preterm are greater than those for term infants. Human milk and preterm infant formula appear to support normal magnesium levels. Magnesium delivery in parenteral nutrition is titrated based on serum magnesium levels, which should be monitored. The daily enteral magnesium intake should be 10 to 26 mg/kg/day (57) although the advisable parenteral intake should be 4.3 to 7.2 mg/kg/day (111).

Iron

The majority of total body iron found in the term infant is accreted during the third trimester. The fetus maintains a constant total body iron content of 75 mg/kg during the last trimester, increasing from 35 to 40 mg at 24 weeks gestation to 225 mg at term (113). Preterm delivery results in disruption of this process, and premature infants are therefore born with lower iron stores than term infants. Small-for-dates infants are frequently born with low iron stores, presumably because of decreased placental iron transport (114). Infants of diabetic mothers are born with low stores because much of the fetal iron is in the expanded red cell mass (114). These infants also appear to be low in total body iron, most likely as a result of altered transport of iron by the diabetic placenta, such that the increased iron need of the infants of diabetic mothers exceeds the placental transport capacity (116,117).

Term Infants

The appropriate-for-dates newborn infant has sufficient iron stores to last four to six months; the small-for-dates infant has closer to a 2-month supply (118,119). In the absence of adequate dietary iron, these stores are mobilized for hemoglobin synthesis in the rapidly expanding blood volume of the growing infant. An adequate source of iron generally maintains iron stores until the infant begins to obtain iron from other dietary sources in the second 6 months of life. The estimated daily iron requirement for the term infant is 1 mg/kg/day (118,119).

The major source of iron for the healthy, term infant is dietary, either through human milk or infant formula fortified with iron (119). Although human milk has a low iron content (0.3 mg/L) compared to either iron-fortified infant formula (10–12 mg/L) or "low-iron" formula (4.5 mg/L), the iron is much more bioavailable as a result of proteins such as lactoferrin (120). Greater than 50% of the iron in human milk is absorbed, compared to only 4% to 12% of formula iron (121). The rate of iron deficiency in breastfed infants before six months is relatively low, although few methodologically sound studies have been performed (122). After 6 months, iron deficiency rates of 20% to 30% have been recorded in breastfed infants (123), although it has been unclear whether the infants in these studies were exclusively breastfed. Innis and associates showed an iron-deficiency anemia rate of 15% in 8-month-old breastfed infants (124). Given this, it may be wise to screen the breastfed infant's iron status at 6 months.

The FDA defines "low-iron formulas" as those containing less than 6.7 mg/L. Prior to changes in the iron content of "low-iron formula" at the end of the millennium, the rate of iron deficiency in infants fed exclusively a low-iron formula containing less than 2 mg/L was unacceptably high, with rates between 28% and 38% (123). This compares with a rate of less than 5% in infants fed iron-fortified formula (12 mg/L) during the first 6 months of life. Indeed, the introduction of iron fortification of formulas in the early 1970s represents one of the most effective public health campaigns in this country. Recent studies indicate that infants fed formulas containing either 4 or 7 mg/L remain iron sufficient (125). No advantage in iron status is conferred to infants consuming formulas containing 8 as compared to 12 mg/L (126). Low-iron formulas have been reconstituted during the last 4 years such that they all contain at least 4 mg of iron/L, thus meeting the AAP recommendations (119). They continue to carry the designation "low iron" because of the FDA standard.

Low-iron formula continues to account for 9% to 30% of elective, e.g., non WIC formula sales. The reasons appear to involve the unfounded perception that iron in formula causes gastrointestinal symptoms such as colic, diarrhea, constipation, and GER. Double-blind studies have failed to support these claims (127,128).

Preterm Infants

The preterm infant that is not growth retarded begins extrauterine life with the same iron stores per kilogram body weight as the term infant (approximately 12 mg/kg). However, the preterm infant is exposed to several stressors that perturb iron balance, with the result that by the time of hospital discharge, the infant may be iron deficient (129,130) or iron overloaded (131,132). The range of iron status of the preterm infant at 40 weeks postconception appears to be far wider than the term infant, although systematic studies are lacking.

The preterm infant frequently goes into negative iron balance because of blood lost during phlebotomy although sick, coupled with a rapid growth rate (and expansion of the red cell mass) during the convalescent period. In the past, phlebotomy losses were replaced by red cell transfusions, but criteria for transfusion have become more stringent because of concerns of exposure to infectious agents (133). Recombinant human erythropoietin has been used to stimulate endogenous red cell production in place of red cell transfusion, and produces additional negative stress on neonatal iron balance (134). Since 3.4 mg of iron are necessary to synthesize 1 g of hemoglobin, the therapeutic use of recombinant erythropoietin significantly taxes the already low iron stores of the preterm infant. Because of these factors, the daily enteral iron requirement for the preterm infant who does not receive recombinant erythropoietin is 2 to 4 mg/kg/day, with the greater requirement for the more preterm infant (108). Infants who receive recombinant erythropoietin require at least 6 mg/kg/day of iron (108).

The issue of when to begin iron supplementation in the preterm infant is controversial. Iron is necessary for normal growth and development of all tissues, including the brain. A rich literature supports the hypothesis that early iron deficiency results in neurodevelopmental sequelae at the time of the deficiency and persists well after iron has been repleted (135). Iron deficiency in infants as young as 6 months of age slows nerve conduction (136), a finding that persists even after repletion of iron (137). Nevertheless, iron is also a very potent oxidant stressor since it catalyzes the Fenton reaction to produce reactive oxygen species. Since preterm infants have immature antioxidant systems, there is concern that free iron (i.e., in excess of the total iron-binding capacity) can exacerbate diseases that may be related etiologically to oxidative stress, including BPD, necrotizing enterocolitis, neuronal injury, and retinopathy of prematurity (ROP) (137,138,139,140,141). Although definitive studies on the role of iron in these diseases of prematurity have not been performed, it is clear that infants who are multiply transfused with packed red blood cells and those who receive parenteral iron are at risk for having free circulating iron and increased markers of oxidative stress

TABLE 22-2
RECOMMENDED MICROMINERAL INTAKES FOR PRETERM INFANTS[d]

	Transitional Period (0–14 days)		Stable/Postdischarge Periods	
	Enteral (μg/kg/day)	Parenteral (μg/kg/day)	Enteral (μg/kg/day)	Parenteral (μg/kg/day)
Zn	500–800	150	1,000[a]	400
Cu	120	0, ≤20[b]	120–150	20[b]
Se	1.3	0, ≤1.3	1.3–3.0	1.5–2.0
Cr	0.05	0, ≤0.05	0.1–0.5	0.05–0.2
Mo	0.3	0	0.3	0.25[c]
Mn	0.75	0, ≤0.75[b]	0.75–7.5	1.0[b]
I	11–27	0, ≤1.0	30–60	1.0

[a] Postdischarge supplement of 0.5 mg/kg/day for infants fed human milk.
[b] Should be withheld when hepatic cholestasis is present.
[c] For long-term total parenteral nutrition only.
[d] From Reifen RM, Zlotkin SH. Microminerals. In: Tsang RC, Lucas A, Vauy R, et al., eds. Nutritional needs of the preterm infant. Baltimore: Williams & Wilkins, 1993:195–207; Greene H, Hambridge K, Schanler R, et al. Guidelines for the use of vitamins, trace elements, calcium, magnesium, and phosphorus in infants and children receiving total parenteral nutrition: report of the Subcommittee on Pediatric Parenteral Nutrient Requirements from the Committee on Clinical Practice Issues of the American Society for Clinical Nutrition. *Am J Clin Nutr* 1988;48:1324–1342, with permission.

(131,132,142). Because of these concerns, parenteral iron should be used very sparingly. Since infants are born with adequate iron stores, there is no need to begin iron supplementation in a sick, nongrowing preterm infant. Therefore, enteral iron supplementation should not be started before two weeks postnatal age (108,138). Conversely, delaying iron supplementation until after two months confers a very high risk of iron deficiency in the postdischarge period (129).

Generally, human milk should be used whenever possible in preterm infants. However, because of the low iron content of human milk and the rapid growth rate of these infants, iron supplementation is highly recommended. Additionally, those who receive recombinant human erythropoietin should be supplemented earlier with iron sulfate to have an adequate erythropoietic response. It is clear that iron must be available to see a sustained erythropoietic response with recombinant erythropoietin treatment (143). Preterm infant formulas are iron fortified and should provide adequate amounts to the larger preterm infant. However, preterm infants less than 30 weeks gestation may well need enteral iron supplementation in addition to their preterm formula to bring their total dose closer to 4 mg/kg/day.

Trace Elements

Ten trace elements are nutritionally essential for the human: zinc, copper, selenium, chromium, manganese, molybdenum, cobalt, fluoride, iodine, and iron (144). Zlotkin and associates have written an excellent review of trace element requirements in newborns (144). Most trace elements are accreted during the last trimester. Thus, the term infant is fully replete and needs modest dietary intake of these elements. Both human milk and infant formula ensure adequate intakes. The preterm infant or the term infant on prolonged TPN would rapidly go into negative balance of any of these elements if not provided with an exogenous source. While on TPN, infants should receive neonatal trace elements (Table 22-2). Preterm infant formulas and preterm human milk appear to supply adequate amounts of trace elements to the enterally fed premature infant (145).

Selenium is a potent antioxidant. Preterm infants have lower selenium stores than term infants (146), and this has been proposed as an etiology for diseases such as BPD and ROP (147). Studies linking selenium insufficiency with these diseases have not been persuasive (148), but the general consensus is that selenium status should be supported in the preterm infant (149). Selenium is not found in commercially available products and must be added separately to TPN at the rate of 2 μg/kg/day (149). Iodine is not added to TPN, but adequate amounts of iodine are absorbed through the infant's skin from iodine solutions applied topically (144). Nevertheless, a dose of 1 μg/kg/day has been recommended for infants who are on TPN for more than 6 weeks (149).

Vitamins

Vitamin requirements in newborn infants can be most easily conceptualized by considering water- and fat-soluble vitamins separately. An extensive review of all of the vitamins and their deficiencies is beyond the scope of this chapter and the reader is referred to sources dedicated to this subject (150). This section will deal primarily with vitamins that are of particular relevance to neonates and to those with a specific risk for deficiency.

Water-Soluble Vitamins

Term newborns are rarely deficient of water-soluble vitamins in the B group (150). As with all humans, neonates need a daily source of vitamin C and folate. These are provided in adequate concentrations in human milk, infant formulas and multivitamin preparations added to parenteral nutrition. The AAP has stated that term breastfed infants do not need supplemental water-soluble vitamins during the first six months unless there are extenuating circumstances (7). Preterm infants also do not appear to need supplemental water-soluble vitamins once they are taking an adequate amount of formula or fortified human milk. The minimum amount of enteral feeds needed to maintain vitamin sufficiency varies among the formulas and the human milk fortifiers available. Infants receiving Enfamil Premature Formula or human milk fortified with Enfamil Human Milk Fortifier need no vitamin supplementation if their intake exceeds 150 mL/day. Those receiving Similac Special Care Formula or human milk fortified with Natural Care must exceed 300 mL/day to remain vitamin sufficient (151).

Fat-Soluble Vitamins

Fat-soluble vitamin deficiencies are also rarely a problem for term, healthy newborns fed human milk or infant formula. Nevertheless, certain groups of infants are at risk for vitamin D deficiency (150). These include breastfed infants whose mothers are vitamin D deficient as a result of their diet (vegan) or whose mothers completely protect their own skin from sunlight. Their infants must also be exposed to less than 30 minutes of sunlight per day to be at greatest risk. Most reports of rickets in breastfed infants in these circumstances have been in far-northern climates, although in the United States the problem has been seen as far south as San Diego and North Carolina (152,153). The AAP has recently recommended that all infants receive 200 IU of vitamin D daily. For infants consuming less than 500 mL of infant formula per day (including all breastfed infants), the least expensive and easiest way to achieve this goal is through a tri-vitamin preparation.

Virtually all infants receive vitamin K in the delivery room to prevent hemorrhagic disease of the newborn. The prevalence of this condition is very low, but the neurological consequences are so disastrous and preventable that the current recommendation is to continue to give vitamin K at birth. Once a gut flora has been established in the first 2 postnatal days, vitamin K deficiency is exceedingly rare (154). However, infants who receive broad-spectrum antibiotics, which markedly reduce the intestinal flora, should be supplemented with vitamin K at least twice per week (154).

Whereas infants are not wholly dependent on dietary sources for vitamin D (it can be synthesized de novo from sterol precursors by 1 week of age) and vitamin K (supplied by gut bacteria), vitamins E and A must be provided in the diet. The term infant who consumes human milk or infant formula receives an adequate amount of each, assuming that there are no impediments to fat absorption,

such as cystic fibrosis or short bowel syndrome. In infants with those conditions, a water-soluble A and E preparation should be utilized and serum levels monitored.

There are significant issues with fat-soluble vitamins, particularly vitamins A and E, in preterm infants less than 34 weeks gestation because of their relatively poor digestion of fats. As with term infants, vitamin K and, most likely, vitamin D are not a major problem, although preterm infant formulas are supplemented with more vitamin D than are term formulas. Even the most premature infants are capable of synthesizing the active vitamin D metabolite by one week of age (155).

Vitamin A deficiency in growing mammals results in significant tissue fibrosis, particularly of the lung and liver. In 1925, Wolbach and Howe noted that lambs born to vitamin A-deficient mothers had significant lung disease that, in retrospect, bears remarkable similarity to BPD (156). These animals had squamous metaplasia, loss of cilia, and loss of ciliary motility. Several investigators have noted that preterm infants have low vitamin A levels and hepatic stores (157). Moreover, preterm infants with respiratory distress syndrome who had low cord-blood vitamin A concentrations are more likely to develop BPD (158). Additionally, both prenatal and postnatal steroid administration increased serum vitamin A levels in preterm infants although preventing and treating BPD, respectively (159, 160). Two small but well-controlled studies assessed whether prophylactically administering 2,000 IU of vitamin A intramuscularly every other day from birth in <1500 g infants prevented BPD. Shenai and associates found a significant reduction of BPD in their treated infants, from 85% to 45%, with a concomitant rise in serum vitamin A levels (161). The serum retinol levels of placebo-treated infants remained abnormally low (<20 µg/dL). In contrast, Pearson et al., utilizing the same protocol, found no difference in BPD between the vitamin A- and placebo-treated groups (46% vs. 44%) despite a significant rise in serum retinol concentrations in the treated group (162). Of note was that retinol levels remained above 20 µg/dL in the placebo group. The unifying conclusion of these two studies is that vitamin A deficiency, as seen in the control group of Shenai and associates is indeed a risk factor for BPD, but not all infants less than 1,500 g are vitamin A deficient in the first month of life. Further supplementation of infants with adequate vitamin A status does not appear to further reduce the risk of BPD according to Pearson's data (162). More recently, the National Institute of Child Health and Human Development network addressed this issue in a multi-center, randomized trial (163). There was a small but statistically significant reduction in the rate of BPD in the vitamin A-treated group. The data were not analyzed as a function of initial serum retinol concentration. At this time, treatment with vitamin A for all infants at risk for BPD is not unreasonable. The risks are relatively small, but include three-time-weekly intramuscular injections for 4 weeks in infants with little muscle mass and the relatively remote possibility of vitamin A toxicity. Vitamin A levels should be followed weekly to monitor for toxicity and efficacy since the early studies suggest the greatest benefit occurs in infants with low initial vitamin A levels. Another approach is to check vitamin A levels in preterm infants at risk for BPD at birth and treat only those with low serum concentrations, realizing that serum concentrations are not the most reliable measure of tissue vitamin A status.

Ever since Oski and associates reported on hemolytic anemia caused by vitamin E deficiency, studies have assessed vitamin E sufficiency in the context of oxidative stress (164). Clearly, phospholipid membranes are at high risk for oxidative stresses; and if not adequately protected by circulating antioxidants such as vitamin E, selenium and superoxide dismutase will be damaged, with subsequent cell death. Thus, it was hoped that vitamin E supplementation of the preterm infant who has an immature antioxidant system might prevent or ameliorate established BPD or ROP. Studies along those lines have been a disappointment; after initial reports that vitamin E supplementation at birth prevented BPD (165–168), subsequent studies have not been able to duplicate the effect (168). Similarly, a meta-analysis of trials of vitamin E supplementation to prevent the occurrence or progression of ROP has not shown a significant effect (169). Moreover, high vitamin E levels following supplementation appear to increase the risk of sepsis and NEC (170).

Preterm infant formulas are supplemented with vitamins E and A. For most infants fed the preterm infant formula with higher vitamin E and A concentrations, serum levels remain in the normal range. However, routine assessment of these levels in the high-risk infant less than 1,500 g may be prudent, since it is likely that the deficiency state is not advantageous to the growing infant. The consensus panel recommendations for daily vitamin intake via parenteral nutrition were published in 1993 (171) and were adapted from a special report of the subcommittee on pediatric parenteral nutrient requirements (149).

The Effect Of Neonatal Illness on Nutritional Requirements

Most studies of neonatal nutritional requirements have dealt with defining the needs of the healthy growing term or preterm infant. Nevertheless, adults and older children who are ill undergo profound changes in metabolism based on the type and degree of illness (172,173). Cerra and associates have investigated the independent effects of surgery, trauma, and sepsis on adult metabolism and have found consistent changes in protein-energy requirements (173). Each incident increases cellular oxygen consumption and promotes more negative nitrogen balance; sepsis has the most profound effects. Cytokines such as tumor necrosis factor (TNF-alpha), interleukin-6 (IL-6) and interleukin-1 (IL-1) appear to be important mediators of the response (174). These are elevated in preterm and term infants with sepsis (175). The adult studies suggest that energy and amino acid delivery must be significantly modified in sick patients. In particular, these patients appear to require higher energy delivery and more protein to remain in neutral or positive nitrogen balance. Special amino acid solutions that are rich in branched-chain amino acids are utilized to support nitrogen balance (176). Fewer studies have assessed these issues in preterm and term newborns. Nevertheless, some of the metabolic effects of acute lung disease, chronic lung disease, CHF, and sepsis have been studied (5). The conclusions of these studies support the concept that simply supplying the nutrients normally required by the healthy newborn will not be sufficient for infants with these illnesses.

Overall Approach Based on Stage of Illness in Preterm Infants

In 1995, the Canadian Pediatric Society proposed a novel approach to neonatal nutrition, primarily designed for premature infants but adaptable for term infants (177). This approach acknowledged that nutritional needs of premature infants change based on the phase of their illnesses. The initial "transition" phase is characterized as the time of neonatal illness and physiological instability. Although defined as the first ten postnatal days, the timing is flexible based on the duration of neonatal illness. The sick premature infant is likely to be relatively insulin resistant and to have increased circulating counter-regulatory (gluconeogenic) hormones, including cortisol and glucagon. Vasopressor therapy with dopamine, dobutamine, or epinephrine may have effects similar to the endogenous hormones. These factors, combined with the release of cytokines during illness (177), place the infant in a catabolic rather than anabolic state. Under such circumstances, growth factors are down-regulated (178) and growth is unlikely. Premature infants typically show weight loss and lack of head growth during their period of illness. The nutritional strategy for this first phase is incompletely defined. Principles gleaned from the adult critical care literature would suggest that energy delivery should at least meet resting energy expenditure to prevent further glycogen, muscle, and fat breakdown for gluconeogenesis. Once resting energy expenditure has been met in the stable, growing infant (approximately 60 kcal/kg/d), excess calories are channeled for growth, with a cost of about 2.5 calories per gram of weight gain. However, in the insulin-resistant sick infant with down-regulated growth factors, these extra calories are likely to increase the cellular metabolic rate, generating more carbon dioxide but not resulting in growth. Carbohydrates, with their respiratory quotient of 1.0, are more likely than fat to create more carbon dioxide. The source of nutrition is usually parenteral with minimal enteral or trophic feedings. Administration of protein appears to be beneficial during this period to reduce the degree of negative nitrogen balance. Recent data of Thureen and associates demonstrating the safety and efficacy of 3 grams of protein/kg body weight on day one supports this concept (86). The use of specialized protein blends to replace particular amino acids lost during illness has not yet been studied extensively.

The in-hospital growth period is characterized by physiological stability and an anabolic state. The goal during this period is to match intrauterine growth rates and mineral accretion. For the preterm infants less than 34 weeks postconception, nutrient delivery should be adjusted to take into account digestive and absorptive immaturities. Fortification of preterm human milk and the use of premature infant formulas typically address these issues.

Preterm infants in the postdischarge phase are also anabolic and growing. Compared to the term infant, their physiology is characterized by a mature absorptive and digestive system. Unlike the term infant, however, these infants have accrued large energy, protein, and mineral deficits (3,4), and their growth is frequently below the 5th percentile for their age adjusted for prematurity. Premature infant discharge formula and fortification/supplementation of human milk after hospital discharge are indicated. The premature infant discharge formulas have increased energy, protein, calcium, phosphorus, iron, vitamin A, and vitamin D compared to term infant formulas. Infants on these formulas have more rapid catch-up growth and mineralization than premature infants-fed term formula (179).

In summary, a tri-phasic system seeks to customize nutritional delivery for the preterm infant based on physiology and nutrient needs. Future directions may include better definition of specific nutrient needs (e.g., amino acids, growth factors) for each phase and the development of noninflammatory formulas to be delivered enterally during transition or periods of medical instability.

Specific Disease Effects on Nutrient Needs

Whether acute lung disease, such as hyaline membrane disease, increases the oxygen consumption of the infant in direct proportion to the degree of respiratory illness remains debated (51,86,98). Unlike in adults, however, nitrogen balance in newborns appears to be unaffected by respiratory illness. The mean protein requirement to maintain neutral nitrogen balance during respiratory disease is 1.5 to 2.0 g/kg/day. Severe respiratory illness is associated with a higher incidence of hypocalcemia and hypoglycemia. There appears to be no indication to increase protein delivery beyond what would normally be given.

BPD increases the resting energy expenditure by up to 30% (50), and infants with BPD will require energy intakes up to 150 kcal/kg/day to grow adequately. Much of the growth failure in BPD occurs in the first month, after which the rate of weight gain can be quite similar (although at a lower percentile) to infants without BPD (180). Protein requirements have not been extensively studied in infants with BPD, but those who are treated with steroids have increased muscle breakdown and a more negative nitrogen balance (101). Clearly, malnutrition plays an important role in the genesis of the disease and the rate of recovery (181). Sodium and potassium requirements are increased in infants with BPD treated with salt-wasting diuretics, occasionally requiring supplementation. Calcium balance is more tenuous as a result of more prolonged periods of parenteral nutrition, renal cal-

cium wasting as a result of calciuric diuretics (furosemide), and bone demineralization as a result of corticosteroid therapy. A relationship between vitamin A deficiency and BPD has been documented (161,163); thus, it is important to monitor and support vitamin A status in infants with BPD.

CHF has a profound effect on resting energy expenditure equal to that of BPD. Infants with CHF as a result of structural heart disease may require up to 150 kcal/kg/day on the basis of both an increased metabolic rate and malabsorption as a result of intestinal edema. The protein requirement of infants with CHF has not been studied, although it is clear many fail to thrive and have reduced muscle mass. It is prudent to increase the protein delivery commensurate with the increase in energy delivery, maintaining a 25 to 30 kcal:g protein ratio. Diuretics used to treat CHF cause the same sodium, potassium, and calcium deficiencies seen in infants with chronic lung disease. Furthermore, the use of citrated blood products to replace losses perioperatively can cause profound hypocalcemia. Persistent cyanosis (See color plate) causes an additional nutritional stress by increasing the infant's need for iron. Since many of these infants have secondary polycythemia, there must be enough iron in the diet to support augmented erythropoiesis. Failure of a cyanotic infant to maintain an elevated hemoglobin may be as a result of iron deficiency, which can be screened for with a ferritin concentration and by assessing the red cell indices for microcytosis.

The effect of sepsis on neonatal nutritional status has not been well evaluated. Infants rarely present with the overwhelming multi-system organ failure that adults routinely have with sepsis. This may be as a result of an incomplete cytokine response. Septic infants have increased TNF and IL-6 levels, but their levels are not nearly as high as in adults (52). Furthermore, neonatal sepsis does not result in a profoundly negative nitrogen balance. Sepsis does increase oxygen consumption—although this appears to be a nonspecific response to illness, as it is seen in other nonseptic states. It appears that sepsis increases energy but not protein needs in the neonate.

NUTRIENT DELIVERY

Almost all term infants and many preterm infants more than 33 weeks gestation will feed orally on demand immediately after birth. Breastfed infants should be offered the breast within 30 minutes of delivery. However, ill term infants and preterm infants who are not physiologically mature or who are unstable will require alternate forms of nutrient delivery. The first decision revolves around whether the infant is stable enough to be fed enterally or if parenteral nutrition is indicated. If long-term parenteral nutrition is anticipated, decisions will need to be made whether a central catheter should be placed or whether the nutrients should be given through a peripheral vein. If the infant is to be enterally gavage fed, the practitioner has multiple options with respect to where the gavage tube is placed, whether it remains indwelling or is replaced after each feed, and whether the feedings are by continuous drip or bolus.

Parenteral Nutrition

Indications

Parenteral nutrition is indicated in all infants in which enteral nutrition is contraindicated or delivers less than 75% of total protein and energy requirements. Although parenteral nutrition has become a more refined nutritional tool with fewer complications over the past decade, the enteral route remains the preferred way to nourish babies. For all practical purposes, infants on ventilators in the acute stage of their diseases are rarely enterally fed nutritionally meaningful amounts. It is also not appropriate to simply provide these infants with a dextrose and electrolyte solution. Anderson et al. demonstrated that the addition of amino acids to dextrose solutions shortly after birth improves the nutritional status of infants (97). Earlier initiation of parenteral nutrition was one factor associated with higher weight, length, and OFC percentiles at discharge and better long-term developmental outcome (182). Therefore, it is appropriate to begin parenteral nutrition for infants within 24 hours of birth. The trend in the past five years has been to begin feedings earlier in preterm infants to promote ongoing maturity of the intestinal tract, to avoid villous atrophy as a result of disuse, and to kindle gut hormone activity (183). Thus, infants who still require moderate respiratory support will receive "trophic" feeds, but these feedings are hypocaloric, and parenteral nutrition is indicated in these infants.

Absolute indications for parenteral nutrition include surgical lesions such as omphalocele, gastroschisis, intestinal tract atresias (e.g., tracheoesophageal atresia, duodenal atresia, ileal atresia), meconium peritonitis, diaphragmatic hernia, short bowel syndrome, and Hirschsprung's disease. Medical indications include NEC (or feeding intolerance), meconium ileus, ileus as a result of generalized illness, infants on extracorporeal membrane oxygen (ECMO) therapy, and preterm infants on slowly advancing feedings.

Routes of Delivery

The decision whether to supply parenteral nutrition centrally or peripherally requires weighing the benefits versus the risks. Parenteral nutrition administered through a central line allows for greater energy delivery because solutions with dextrose concentrations more than 12.5% can be administered. Dextrose concentrations of that magnitude and calcium infusions are poorly tolerated by peripheral veins and carry a high rate of venous sclerosis (184). Skin sloughs are likely to occur if the solution extravasates from the vein. For the same reasons, many intensive care nurseries will not allow or will limit the amount of calcium to be run through a peripheral venous line. This practice is sound, but effectively limits the amount of calcium

and phosphorus that can be delivered to an infant who is already at great risk for osteopenia.

The risks of central TPN relate primarily to the risk of central venous line placement and maintenance. Umbilical venous catheters placed at birth have traditionally been used as the primary central catheter, but the incidence of venous thromboses is high (185). Clots can be detected as early as 24 hours after catheter placement. The clots are frequently infected with Staphylococcus epidermidis, which has become the most common pathogen isolated in the ELBW infant after seven days of age (186). Equally concerning is the high rate of Candida septicemia seen with high dextrose delivery and high serum concentrations (187).

One risk of peripheral TPN is undernutrition. The infant receiving maximal concentrations of dextrose (D12.5%), amino acids (3.0 g/kg/day), and intravenous fat (3.5 g/kg/day) at an average fluid rate of 150 cc/kg/day will receive approximately 95 nonprotein kcal/kg/day. Although this amount of intake meets the daily resting energy expenditure of the premature infant (65 kcal/kg/day), there are insufficient "extra" calories to sustain weight gain at 15 to 18 g/kg/day. Thus, long-term peripheral TPN will result in preterm infants slowly falling away from the growth curve. Calcium delivery will also be constrained, either because of an absolute contraindication (in some nurseries) or because of osmolarity issues. Each day on peripheral TPN results in a larger deficit calcium balance and a higher risk of osteopenia of prematurity.

Infants who are not expected to tolerate oral feedings within a week of starting parenteral nutrition should have a central line placed and be maintained on central parenteral nutrition. The choice of venous access also involves weighing the risks and benefits. Surgical placement of an anchored catheter (e.g., Broviak) is a riskier procedure than placement of a peripherally inserted central catheter (PICC). However, it is likely that the Broviak, placed under sterile operating room conditions, will last longer. Additionally, the choice of lines (single lumen vs. double lumen, differences in gauges) is greater with surgically placed lines, and frequently blood can be drawn from one of the ports for laboratory monitoring. Conversely, the PICC lines are easily placed in the unit, can be as small as 27 gauge, and are silastic (which are less prone to clotting and infection). Their disadvantage is that they generally cannot be used for blood drawing. In our unit we try to remove all umbilical venous catheters after the infant has been stabilized following delivery room resuscitation and attempt to place a percutaneously inserted central catheters (PICC) line within the first 24 to 48 hours if the infant is expected to be on parenteral nutrition. Because of the low incidence of infection with these lines, we typically do not use peripheral parenteral nutrition.

Maintaining patency of the lines is important for the success of parenteral nutrition. Most centers use heparin in TPN solutions to keep central lines patent and reduce the formation of a fibrin sheath around the catheters. These fibrin sheaths are most likely to be the site of infectious agents. In order to maintain patency, our unit utilizes the following protocol for PICC lines: for flow rates more than 7 cc/hour, no heparin is used; for flow between 2 and 7 cc/hr, 0.25 U of heparin/cc is added; for flow rates more than 2 cc/hour, 0.5 U of heparin/cc is added. We do not "heparin-lock" our PICC lines and run them with a minimum rate of 0.5 cc/hour with 1 U heparin/cc of solution. We do heparin-lock surgically placed lines, administering 10 Units of heparin in 1 cc of solution, given every 12 hours.

Catheter occlusions are usually treated with removal of the line because so many of the clots are infected. Nevertheless, catheter occlusions that occur without signs of sepsis (e.g., if the line was inadvertently shut off) can be treated with urokinase (5000 U/mL). The amount of urokinase solution should approximate the internal volume of the catheter (0.2 to 0.5 mL). After instillation, the solution should be allowed to dwell in the catheter for 30 minutes. If two attempts at clearing the line fail or if a positive blood culture has been obtained from the clotted line, the catheter should be removed (188).

Nutritional Management

Parenteral nutrition should be started within 24 hours of delivery, since dextrose solutions alone cannot meet the resting energy requirements or the protein requirements of the neonate.

Dextrose delivery should typically begin between 4 and 6 mg/kg/minute and be advanced as tolerated. Extremely preterm infants are frequently glucose intolerant because of relative insulin hypoactivity and poor peripheral glucose utilization. Although their energy needs are higher because of higher basal metabolic rates and higher brain–liver weight ratios, they frequently develop hyperglycemia and glycosuria. These are serious complications that must be treated immediately. Persistent glycosuria will result in a large free-water diuresis, intravascular dehydration, hypernatremia, and azotemia. Persistent hyperglycemia is a significant risk factor for fungal infection. Dextrose delivery can be slowly advanced based on how well the infant tolerates this. Typically we do not administer more than 12.5 g/kg/day because of the significant effect on the respiratory quotient. However, others have advocated rates up to 20 g/kg/day, aided by the administration of insulin to maintain normoglycemia (62). As stated earlier, I do not advocate this approach because the weight gain is predominantly fat rather than lean body mass, and the metabolic cost of fat synthesis from glucose is high in terms of both oxygen consumption and carbon dioxide production. On the other hand, insulin is very useful in treating the hyperglycemia seen in ELBW infants in the first week of life, in which glucose intolerance may necessitate decreasing dextrose delivery to unacceptably low rates (<4 mg/kg/minute).

Protein in the form of amino acid solutions designed for newborns should be administered within the first 24 hours. There are few contraindications to early protein delivery, and there is evidence that amino acid solutions

improve nitrogen balance (52,86,97,98,189). At energy intakes above resting energy expenditure (65 kcal/kg/day), the main determinant of positive nitrogen balance is the nitrogen intake (190). The goal is to achieve in utero nitrogen accretion rates although compensating for nitrogen losses as a result of illness. This appears to be possible with amino acid delivery rates of 2.7 to 4.0 g/kg/day (86,98,191). Although protein requirements may be higher as a result of prior malnutrition, to diseases that increase nitrogen turnover, or to catch-up growth, it is rarely practical to give more than 4.0 g/kg/day of parenteral amino acids because of increasing BUN concentrations. Recent studies demonstrate that administration of amino acids is safe for all infants on day one to two. Most infants can be safely started on at least 2 g/kg/day and advanced by 1 g/kg/day to a maximum of 4.0 g/kg/day, thus ensuring that they will be on full protein delivery within 48 hours. Very unstable preterm infants and those with renal insufficiency as a result of indomethacin administration, surgery, a patent ductus arteriosus, or shock may need to be advanced more slowly. Monitoring the BUN allows the practitioner to decide on a daily basis whether the protein delivery can increase. A rising BUN is an indication that the infant is not clearing nitrogen waste and that the rate of amino acid infusion should not be increased. Initially, when amino acid solutions intended for adults were given to infants, significant complications occurred because these solutions did not meet their metabolic needs. In the mid-1980s, improved solutions were introduced that added the semi-essential amino acids taurine, water-soluble tyrosine, and L-cysteine. Potentially toxic amino acids such as phenylalanine and glycine were reduced. These newer solutions promote a more normal serum amino acid profile (103), better nitrogen retention and weight gain (190–193), and lower rates of cholestasis (194). The lower rates of cholestasis may be as a result of the addition of taurine, which may also be important in neuronal development (194–196). Nevertheless, the neonatal parenteral amino acid solutions are not perfectly formulated, and investigations continue to determine whether threonine, lysine, and glutamine are limiting amino acids (100). There is no evidence that specialized solutions such as HepatAmine, BranchAmine or NephrAmine are indicated in newborns and the spectrum of amino acids found in them may dangerously imbalance an infant's serum amino acid profile.

Intravenous fats provide a low-volume source of calories and shift cellular metabolism toward less carbon dioxide production, perhaps improving the respiratory load of the infant. They can be utilized within the first three days of life and are important in preventing essential fatty acid deficiency (197). Close monitoring of serum triglyceride levels is important during intravenous fat therapy. Intravenous fat solutions can be started at a delivery rate of 1 g/kg/day and advanced to a maximum of 4 g/kg/day. Total fat calories should be less than 60% of the diet and typically are in the 30% to 40% range. Like amino acids, intravenous fats can be advanced by 1 g/kg/day if tolerated. Since fat incorporation into cells is dependent on insulin, fat intolerance in

VLBW infants is more likely to be manifested by hyper-triglyceridemia or, interestingly, hyperglycemia, requiring a slower rate of advancement (0.5 g/kg/day) or interruption of fat delivery. Infants with birth weights less than 1,250 g and gestational ages less than 30 weeks may need to have their fat dose held at 1 g/kg/day until their hyperbilirubinemia begins to resolve. This group of infants seems to be at greatest risk for intravenous lipids exacerbating hyperbilirubinemia (see TPN complications). Fat emulsions are predominantly 20% solutions and are generally infused over no fewer than 16 hours to allow for metabolic clearing. It is important both to run them separately from other solutions, so as not to disturb the stability of the emulsion, and to cover the solution from light, to decrease breakdown. The solutions can be joined with the amino-acid-containing solution with a Y-connector near the infusion point on the infant.

Since infants initially undergo a free-water diuresis before a salt diuresis, sodium needs remain low until after day three of life (198). Thereafter, sodium and potassium requirements increase rapidly and serum concentrations should be monitored at least daily although infants are on intravenous solutions. Table 22-3 lists the approximate electrolyte requirements for premature infants in the face of no extraneous losses, such as those incurred by renal failure or diuretic therapy. However, requirements may approach 10 mEq/kg/day for each if there are excessive urinary losses. Chloride is the usual anion for both sodium and potassium; however, these cations also can be given as acetates, allowing for fine tuning of acid–base balance. Amino acid solutions have an inherent chloride and acetate load (e.g., TrophAmine contains 1 mEq of acetate for every gram of amino acid).

Calcium and phosphorus are the most difficult minerals to maintain in positive balance in the preterm infant because of the large requirements for adequate mineralization, excessive losses as a result of calciuric diuretics and steroids, and the limited solubility of these nutrients in TPN (199). A calcium-to-phosphorus ratio of 1.7:2.0 appears to be optimal for mineralization (200). Because of solubility

issues, calcium concentrations more than 16.6 mEq/L with a concomitant phosphorus concentration of 8.3 mM are rarely obtained. In an infant receiving 150 cc/kg/day, these values are equivalent to a calcium delivery of 50 mg/kg/day and a phosphorus delivery of 25 mg/kg/day—far less than the *in utero* accretion rate. Strategies to increase calcium retention and bone mineralization have been largely unsuccessful, but have included infusing calcium in one line and phosphorus in another and alternate infusions of higher doses of the two minerals (201,202). Monitoring of serum phosphorus and calcium levels is important. Infants are prone to hypocalcemia in the first 72 hours as a result of transient hypoparathyroidism and to hypophosphatemia. Both calcium and phosphorus should be added early during TPN therapy. Calcium delivery without phosphorus delivery should be avoided because of the likelihood of hypophosphatemia. This complication tends to occur in the first 72 to 96 hours because of the focus on the diagnosis and treatment of neonatal hypocalcemia. More acidic TPN solutions appear less likely to cause calcium-phosphorous precipitation (203,204).

Infants on TPN receive 0.2 mL/kg body weight of a neonatal trace element solution that supplies 0.02 mg/kg of copper, 0.3 mg/kg of zinc, 5 µg/kg of manganese, and 0.17 µg/kg of chromium. This supplement should be added with initiation of TPN and given daily. Selenium should be added after 2 weeks of TPN (149). Although we do not routinely measure zinc, copper, chromium, manganese, or selenium levels in infants on TPN, the practitioner should be aware that preterm infants in particular have low stores of these trace elements and that deficiencies have been described (205–207). Water- and fat-soluble vitamins are added as a pediatric multi-vitamin solution to match the recommended parenteral dosing guidelines (149,171). This supplement should be added at initiation of TPN and given daily.

Complications of TPN

Administration of parenteral nutrition remains an inexact science. Because it is not the normal mode of nutritional delivery, it is not surprising that complications occur. For the most part, complications can be divided into those associated with catheters and those related to the nutrients themselves. As discussed above, centrally placed catheters are prone to thrombosis and infection. Thrombi can occur in the right atrium or in the veins. Clotting in the superior vena cava is of particular concern. Superior vena cava syndrome with or without hydrocephalus can result. Occasionally, back pressure from the clot on the thoracic duct will cause a chylothorax. Additionally, nonseptic complications such as skin sloughs can occur. Erosion of catheters through vessels or cardiac walls has caused pleural effusions, pericardial effusions, and endothelial damage. Improper technique of catheter insertion can result in pneumothorax or nerve injuries, although improper handling of fluids can result in air or fat embolisms. It is important for all personnel involved in parenteral nutrition

TABLE 22-3

DAILY REQUIREMENTS OF TOTAL PARENTERAL NUTRITION

Nutrient	Requirement
Protein	2.5–3.5 g/kg
Fat emulsion	2–4 g/kg (max 3.5 g/kg in infants <2.5 kg)
Calories	90–110 kcal/kg or as needed
H20	125–150 mL/kg or as needed
Na	3–4 mEq/kg
K	2–3 mEq/kg
Ca	50–100 mg/kg, depending on size of infant
P	1–1.5 mM/kg
Mg	0.5–1 mEq/kg
Multivitamins (e.g., MVI Pediatric)	10 mL (40%/kg/d)

therapy, including nurses, pharmacists, and physicians, to be aware of the complications and the techniques to avoid them.

Intravenous lipids have been associated with hypoxia, pulmonary hypertension, hyperbilirubinemia, and infection (208). Infants with respiratory disease have minimally lower PaO_2 values when given intravenous lipids, most likely because lipids can uncouple hypoxic vasoconstriction (209). Normally, to optimize ventilation/perfusion matching, the pulmonary vasculature supplying a poorly oxygenated alveolar area will constrict. This effect is reduced by the infusion of lipids, most likely moderated by serotonin. Similarly, higher pulmonary arterial pressures are seen in neonatal lambs infused with pharmacological doses of lipids (6 mg/kg over 1–4 hours) (210). Finally, trials that have assessed whether early administration of intravenous lipids causes chronic lung disease (211,212) have had mixed results. Overall, given the profound and early onset of growth failure in infants with severe lung disease, it seems prudent to start small amounts of lipids early in life.

Free fatty acids can displace bilirubin from albumin-binding sites, prompting some practitioners to limit the dose of lipids to very small preterm infants. A study of infants weighing 670 to 3360 g demonstrated adequate albumin binding of bilirubin and no effect on serum bilirubin levels (213,214). There are no reports of fat emulsions increasing the incidence of kernicterus. Theoretically, chylomicrons can be taken up by the reticuloendothelial system and interfere with fighting infection. Fat emulsions are also good media for fungi, including *Candida albicans* and *Malassezia furfur* (215). Whether these risks clinically outweigh the benefits of higher energy intake for small preterm infants has not been studied. At this time it is likely that intravenous lipids improve the survival of infants through better growth.

Parenteral amino acids also are associated with toxicity. Excessive amino acid delivery will lead to increased serum BUN and ammonia levels as a result of the newborn infant's relatively immature renal and hepatic status. Parenteral amino acids also have been associated with cholestasis, although the mechanism remains unknown (216). Infants at greatest risk are those who receive TPN for more than 3 weeks, those with intestinal disease, particularly NEC, those with sepsis, and those who remain NPO. Small amounts of trophic feeds reduce the prevalence of cholestasis, most likely by stimulating bile flow via cholecystokinin. Reduced bile flow from prolonged TPN is frequently associated with gallstones. In rare cases, prolonged TPN with no enteral intake will lead to cirrhosis.

Aluminum toxicity is worth considering in infants who have been on TPN for more than 3 weeks. The largest contamination comes from the calcium and phosphorus salts that are added (217). The risk to the neonate is two-fold. Aluminum accumulates in the bones of infants on TPN in which it is avidly taken up because of underlying osteopenia of prematurity (218). Of greater concern is the possibility that aluminum will cross the blood–brain barrier and

induce an acute or chronic encephalopathy, as has been described in adult patients (219). Reduced renal capacity for excreting aluminum appears to be a necessary setting for this to occur, but it is not unusual for preterm infants to have a significant measure of renal insufficiency after treatment with indomethacin (220). Some have proposed that aluminum toxicity may be a factor in the poorer neurodevelopment of preterm infants. Since the body has no need for aluminum, manufacturers are being pressured to reduce the aluminum content of their solutions (221).

Monitoring TPN Efficacy and Toxicity

Administering TPN is an inexact science still in the process of evolution. Matching nutrient delivery to the infant's needs presupposes knowledge of how a particular disease or its treatment affects the infant's metabolism and, therefore, nutritional requirements. Careful monitoring of growth is indicated for any infant on TPN or partial parenteral nutrition. Weight should be measured daily and length and head circumference weekly. Standards have been published for arm muscle area and arm fat area for preterm and term infants, and these areas can be measured using a tape measure and skin caliper (180,222). Protein status can be assessed in two ways: somatic protein deposition (arm muscle area) and serum protein synthesis (serum albumin and prealbumin). The former provides a longitudinal view of protein accretion, although the latter reflects a more rapidly turned-over pool of protein. Assessment of serum concentrations of proteins with short half-lives such as prealbumin has been shown to reflect recent protein intake and to predict future weight gain (223). Prealbumin, also known as transthyretin, has a half-life of 1.9 days and can be measured once or twice per week to yield useful nutritional information. If the serum concentration remains stable or increases, one can expect that the infant is in reasonable nitrogen balance and will gain weight subsequently (224). A decrease of more than 10% from the previous measurement suggests relative protein-energy malnutrition and the need for a higher intake. Like most rapidly turned-over proteins, prealbumin acts as an acute-phase reactant and will rise rapidly with stress, infection, and glucocorticosteroid administration, rendering it useless as a nutritional marker. Serum albumin, which has a half-life of 21 days, can be monitored every two to four weeks.

It is important to monitor infants on parenteral nutrition because of the toxicities associated with its administration. Table 22-4 provides guidelines for nutritional monitoring of infants on TPN. At the least, infants on TPN should have a set of electrolytes and a serum glucose checked daily. Serum glucose concentrations more than 110 mg/dL are an indication not to increase the glucose infusion rate; concentrations more than 150 mg/dL are an indication to reduce the rate. Serum triglyceride concentrations should be checked at least twice per week, or more frequently if the infant is showing signs of lipid intolerance. ELBW infants and infants with sepsis are especially

TABLE 22-4
SUGGESTED MONITORING FOR TOTAL PARENTERAL NUTRITION

Variable	First Week	Later
Growth		
Weight	Daily	Daily
Length and head circumference	Weekly	Weekly
Chemistry		
Na, K, Cl, CO_2	Daily until stable	Daily
Glucose (Chemstrip bG)	Daily	Daily
Triglycerides	With each increase in IL	Twice weekly when stable
Ca (ionized Ca is most accurate)	Daily until stable	Weekly
P	Initially	Twice weekly for first week, then weekly
Albumin	Initially	Monthly
Prealbumin	Initially	Weekly (biweekly) in infants < 1000 g
Alkaline phosphatase	Initially	Weekly
Bilirubin	Initially	Every 4 wk or PRN
Mg	Initially	Weekly
Ammonia	As needed	As needed
Gamma GT	Initially	Weekly
Alanine aminotransferase	As needed	Monthly
Amino acids	As needed	Monthly
Zinc		Monthly
Serum osmolarity	Initially	Weekly
Vitamin A (if infant is < 1,300 g)	Weekly	Weekly while supplemented
Hematology		
Complete blood count	Initially	At least weekly
Type and screen	Initially	
Urinalysis		
Sugar	Each void	Each shift
Protein	Each void	Each shift
Specific gravity	Each void	Each shift

prone to hypertriglyceridemia, even if they have tolerated intravenous fat previously. Methylxanthines and glucocorticosteroids increase the likelihood of both glucose and fat intolerance in preterm infants. A triglyceride level more than 150 mg/dL measured with the infant off lipid infusion is an indicator of impending intolerance and lipid doses should not be increased. A triglyceride concentration more than 200 mg/dL is considered a sign of intolerance and the lipid dose should be decreased. Since persistent hypertriglyceridemia represents a risk to the pulmonary system, daily serum triglyceride levels should be monitored in the infant who exhibits intolerance.

Calcium status must be monitored carefully in the first days of postnatal life because hypocalcemia is commonly seen in ill newborns. Preterm infants, growth-retarded infants, and infants of diabetic mothers appear particularly prone to hypocalcemia. Infants receiving large amounts of citrated blood products, such as those who are postoperative, who are on ECMO or who have disseminated intravascular coagulopathy, will require large amounts of calcium. Similarly, maintenance of normophosphatemia is important for normal metabolism. Therefore, serum calcium, phosphorus, and magnesium should be monitored daily in the first week of life, or until stable, and then weekly thereafter (Table 22-4).

Bone mineralization is problematic for the preterm infant on long-term parenteral nutrition; therefore, close monitoring is indicated. Unfortunately, this can be quite difficult. Although osteopenia of prematurity is predominantly as a result of deficient intakes of calcium and phosphorus, the serum levels of these minerals will be maintained at the expense of the bones. Thus, serial measurements of calcium and phosphorus are not useful in monitoring this complication. Serum alkaline phosphatase is an indirect measure of osteopenia because its level will increase with the bone remodeling that takes place to supply the serum calcium pool. The level should be monitored weekly, particularly in preterm and growth-retarded infants. The level may be difficult to interpret, since the alkaline phosphatase will rise with cholestatic liver disease (a complication of parenteral nutrition itself) and with intestinal injury (such as NEC). Fractionating the alkaline phosphatase level into its bone and nonbone components can be done, but may take weeks depending on whether the laboratory has the capability to perform the fractionation. As with monitoring of the prealbumin concentration, the most important aspect of the alkaline phosphatase to follow is the trend. Rising alkaline phosphatase levels generally mean aggressive bone remodeling and an increased risk of osteopenia.

Strategies to increase calcium and phosphorus delivery should be considered.

The incidence and severity of hepatic toxicity from parenteral nutrition has been on the decline with the introduction of more specialized neonatal amino acid solutions. The toxicity is typically cholestatic in nature, with an initial rise in serum bile acids followed by an increase in the direct bilirubin, alkaline phosphatase, and gamma glutamyl transferase. Transaminase elevations are seen only in very severe cases. The liver toxicity was initially thought to be as a result of intravenous lipids (fatty liver), but has now quite conclusively been associated with amino acid solutions. Although these solutions have been refined (192,193), the problem persists and its cause is unknown. Total and direct bilirubin concentrations will typically be monitored in all newborns in the first week of life. Infants on prolonged TPN should have direct bilirubin measured weekly. If it is elevated, the remaining liver function tests should be assayed and followed weekly.

Trace minerals are rarely deficient in infants on TPN because of supplementation. Nevertheless, the importance of maintaining normal zinc status for growth and protein utilization (225) makes it wise to monitor the serum zinc concentration monthly, particularly if the infant is not growing adequately or has physical signs of zinc deficiency.

With the exception of vitamins E and A, vitamin status generally need not be checked in infants on TPN. Most vitamin assays are cumbersome and are a poor reflection of total body load. Serum vitamin E and A levels also do not necessarily reflect total body stores. Nevertheless, the association of low serum retinol (circulating vitamin A) levels with an increased risk for BPD in the VLBW infant suggests that monitoring may be appropriate (161,163). An initial measurement in all infants less than 1500 g with respiratory disease should indicate the degree of risk. Infants with levels less than 20 µg/dL should be supplemented and their levels followed weekly. The methodologies for assaying vitamin A (high performance liquid chromatography or fluorometry) are the same as for vitamin E and the values for both can be done simultaneously. As with vitamin A, it is important to keep vitamin E concentrations in the normal range, as an insufficient concentration has been associated with anemia (164) and perhaps ROP (165), although toxic levels increase the risk of sepsis and NEC (170).

Enteral Nutrition

Oral Feeding

The goal for virtually all infants prior to discharge from the hospital is full oral feedings, preferably by breast. Oral feedings come naturally to infants born at term, but can be a significant task for those born at less than 34 weeks gestation, those with significant central nervous system disease, and those with anatomical abnormalities that prevent oral feedings.

Oral feedings should be initiated within half an hour of birth by placing the infant to the mother's breast. Infants who are breastfed will have a different sucking motion than those who are bottle fed. Thus, it is important that artificial nipples (and probably pacifiers) not be introduced as the infant is establishing breastfeeding (7). The oral pattern associated with breastfeeding is typically well established within two weeks, although a substantial number of infants who are then supplemented with bottles will demonstrate nipple confusion and may give up on breastfeeding. The healthy breastfed infant has no need for supplemental water, juice, or formula (7). Breastfeeding can be supported in the delivery hospital by training all of the staff to encourage mothers to breast-feed and to provide the necessary environment to promote breastfeeding. This includes allowing the mother to nurse within half an hour of delivery, having the infant room with the mother, and having the mother learn the cues of her infant's hunger. Hospitals can contribute by eliminating policies about supplementing breastfed babies and by supplying charts that assess the infant's feeding and hydration status (7).

Oral feedings can be more problematic for the healthy premature infant. These infants rarely show any interest in oral feeding until approximately 32 weeks gestation and rarely have a mature, safe feeding pattern until 34 weeks gestation (9). Coordination of sucking, swallowing, and breathing is most difficult; the issue is predominantly one of inappropriate swallow-respiration interface rather than suck-swallow interaction (226). There is little evidence that "practice" helps the gestationally immature infant to feed orally sooner. Nevertheless, Meier has reported that breast-fed premature infants have longer periods of sucking with fewer obstructive apnea and desaturation spells than comparably sized bottle-fed infants (227). This may relate to the more metered rate of milk flow. It is important to note that preterm infants are frequently exposed to pacifiers to stimulate nonnutritive sucking, which improves gastric motility and likely increases the flow of important gastrointestinal hormones (228–230). It is unclear whether this nonnutritive sucking at an earlier postconceptional age affects the success of breastfeeding at 34 weeks gestation.

A strong case can be made for feeding breast milk to the preterm infant, either by gavage tube or by breastfeeding, because of its superior performance with respect to immune status and neurodevelopment, among other advantages (19,227,231). In order to successfully breast-feed the premature infant, the mother needs to be available to begin the process as the infant nears 33 weeks gestation. Before that point, it is important that she maintain her milk supply. The intensive care nursery can help by providing a place to nurse, an electric breast pump, storage containers, and a freezer for storing the milk. An organized program with an informed leader is quite useful in timing the introduction of actual breastfeeding and in overseeing the progress made by the individual infant. With such a program, more than 60% of preterm infants whose mothers desire to nurse can successfully breast-feed at the time of discharge.

Preterm infants who are bottle fed also require close observation as they transition from gavage to nipple feeds. There is an energy cost to bottle feeding. Gavage feedings require between 4% and 17% less energy to process, and excessive oral feedings may tire an infant and reduce weight gain velocity (232,233). Typically, attempts at bottling should begin around 33 weeks' gestation with one feeding per day. If the infant shows no interest or has significant obstructive apnea, it may be prudent to wait several days before attempting again. The frequency of feedings can be increased as the infant shows more aptitude. Once the infant has advanced to full oral feedings, it is important to see whether weight gain can be maintained on an ad libitum on-demand schedule prior to discharge. Consistency in feeding personnel can improve the infant's performance, and in the best of all worlds, having the mother give most of the feedings is ideal. Adopting a cue-based feeding program, in which personnel pay attention to the feeding cues exhibited by the infant, may reduce the number of episodes in which the infant refuses to feed because of fatigue and aversion.

Oral aversion is a significant problem in infants who have been NPO or on ventilators for long periods of time. Symptoms include aversive behaviors such as tongue-thrusting, head-turning, pooling of milk in the mouth, and occasionally breath-holding apneic spells. A barium swallowing study with fluoroscopy can help identify whether the problem is anatomical, or is as a result of discoordination, immaturity, or neurological pathology. For infants with severe cases, the worst course is to force oral feedings. The involvement of an occupational or speech therapist can be invaluable in desensitizing the oral area.

Gavage Feeding

Gavage feedings are indicated for infants who can be fed enterally but not orally. For the most part, this approach is used in premature infants who are neurologically immature and the full expectation is that they will feed orally. Infants who will not be candidates for oral feeds either because of anatomical or neurological conditions can have gastrostomy tubes placed. Gavage feedings are most frequently accomplished by placing a naso- or orogastric tube and bolusing feedings intermittently. Some practitioners prefer to place an indwelling transpyloric tube to reduce aspirates and to ensure nutrient delivery. Infants can receive feeds by continuous drip and by bolus.

Oro- or nasogastric tube feedings can be initiated using a soft silastic 5-French or 8-French catheter. The tube is most commonly placed into the stomach prior to a feeding and the contents of the stomach aspirated to ensure there are no residuals from the previous feeding. The feeding is allowed to run in by gravity, although in some infants with very slow gastric emptying the feeding can be titrated in over one hour. The tube is typically withdrawn rapidly after the feeding, although there is some increased risk of the infant vomiting in response to this stimulus. A long-term indwelling catheter can be placed, but this type of catheter may lose flexibility over time and increase the risk of stomach perforation.

Gastric gavage feedings can be given on a schedule between every one and four hours. Typically, smaller infants do not tolerate excessive stomach distention with large-volume feedings and may exhibit respiratory compromise. They may need to be fed small amounts on a more frequent schedule. Infants less than 1,000 g can be fed on a bolus schedule of every one to two hours or with continuous-drip feedings. This approach may reduce oxygen consumption and total energy expenditure, and potentially contribute to faster rates of weight gain. Infants may be fed on this schedule until 1,250 to 1,500 g, after which every-3-hour feeds are more appropriate. Nevertheless, larger infants who are not tolerating bolus feedings, those who remain on ventilators, or those with severe apnea and bradycardia may require drip feedings. Term infants who require gavage feedings may do best on an every-four-hour schedule.

Tube placement and maintenance may cause significant problems in the infant. Tubes can be malpositioned in the airway instead of in the stomach. With the placement of any new tube it is important to document its position by auscultation and by checking the pH of aspirated stomach contents. Placement of the tube can cause significant vagal stimulation that results in apnea or bradycardia. The presence of an indwelling tube can cause apnea and bradycardia either by excessive vagal stimulation or, more commonly, by upper airway obstruction. Although nasogastric tubes are more stable, they appear to cause more problems with airway obstruction. Gastric and esophageal perforations are rare but must be considered if there is a significant change in the infant's behavior or physical exam.

Gavage feedings can also be given through a transpyloric tube. The advantages of this type of feeding include ensured nutrient delivery and a smaller chance of GER and aspiration pneumonia. There are significant mechanical and nutritional disadvantages to this approach. The mechanical problems include the difficulty of placing the tube, although this becomes easier with practice. In order to place the tube, the infant is turned with his or her right side down and the tube is inserted into the stomach with small amounts of injected air. As the infant remains in the right-side-down position, the tube has a reasonable chance of advancing through the pylorus into the duodenum. The tube has reached the duodenum when bile-stained fluid is returned or when the pH of the aspirated fluid changes from acidic (pH 3) to alkaline (pH 5–7). Infants on histamine-2 blocking agents cannot be assessed in this way. The procedure can also be done in the radiology suite under fluoroscopy with a weighted tube. The position of the tube is confirmed on x-ray. Frequently, the tip of the tube will curl back on itself or simply move back into the stomach, and the process will need to be repeated. Although rare, the most devastating complication of transpyloric feedings is intestinal perforation and peritonitis.

Transpyloric feedings also pose significant nutritional risks (233–235). Bypassing the stomach decreases fat digestion and absorption, since up to 50% of fat processing takes place in the stomach by the lingual and gastric lipase enzymes. Additionally, secretion of gut hormones such as cholecystokinin and gastrin are dependent in part on stomach distention by a meal. Potassium accretion may

TABLE 22-5

ORAL FEEDING SCHEDULE FOR THE LOW-BIRTH-WEIGHT INFANT

Time	Substance[a]	≤1,000 g		1,001–1,5000 g		1,501–2,000 g		> 2000 g	
		Amount	Frequency	Amount	Frequency	Amount	Frequency	Amount	Frequency
First feeding	Full-strength human milk or 1/4 strength formula	1–2 mL/kg	1–2 h or continuous drip	1–3 mL/kg	2 h	3–4 mL/kg	2–3 h	10 mL/kg (full strength)	3 h
Subsequent feedings, 12–72 h	Formula or full-strength human milk	Increase 1 mL every other feeding to maximum of 5 mL	2 h	Increase 1 mL every other feeding to maximum of 20 mL	2 h	Increase 2 mL every other feeding to maximum of 15 mL	2–3 h	Increase 5 mL every other feeding to maximum of 20 mL	3 h
Final feeding schedule, 150 mL/kg	Full-strength formula or human milk	10–15 mL	2 h	20–28 mL	2–3 h	28–37 mL	3 h	37–50 mL, then *ad libitum*	3–4 h
Total time to full feeds		10–14 d or more for infants <705 g		7–10 d		5–7 d		3–5 d	

[a] Supplemental intravenous fluids should be given to fulfill requirements of 140–160 mL/kg and caloric requirements of 90–130 cal/kg.

be impaired. Bacterial colonization of the normally sterile intestine may be a significant risk since the normal mechanism by which the stomach acid kills bacteria has been bypassed.

Initiation of gavage feedings through any of the tubes mentioned above requires a careful assessment of the infant. The stable infant more than 1500 g birth weight can typically be fed within hours of birth, although if the infant is less than 35 weeks gestation it is prudent to advance the strength and volume of feedings in a proscribed manner. Table 22-5 provides a sample of feeding schedules in stable infants based on birth weight. Advancement at a rate of 20 cc/kg body weight per day appears to be safe as long as the infant shows no signs of feeding intolerance. Interestingly, a meta-analysis of randomized or quasi-randomized trials of rapid versus slow rates of advancement revealed that more rapid rates were associated with a shorter time to regain birth weight and to achieve full enteral feedings without an increase in morbidity (236). Infants with birth weights more than 1,500 g can be started on every-3-hour feedings; infants between 1,000 and 1,500 g on every-two-hour feedings; and infants less than 1,000 g on every-one-hour, two-hour, or continuous-drip feedings. It must be remembered that although low-volume feedings are better tolerated from a respiratory standpoint, the gastric emptying time of the preterm infant is often between 60 and 90 minutes. Therefore, it is likely that gastric aspirates will be present in an infant fed every hour or by continuous drip. In the infant fed every two hours or less frequently, gastric aspirates should be less than 2 cc/kg body weight. Aspirates greater than that amount may be indicative of an ileus as a result of feeding intolerance or impending NEC. A thorough evaluation including an abdominal examination is indicated before resuming feedings. The availability and

ease of administration of parenteral nutrition makes a strong argument for being conservative with feeding advancement in preterm infants.

Trophic Feeds

Slow advancement of feedings is recommended in an infant who has been ill and likely had an ileus. The trend in the last ten years has been to start with trophic feeds in infants who in the past would otherwise have remained NPO. Trophic feedings are defined as continuous-drip feedings at 1 cc/hour or less. Studies of VLBW infants begun on trophic feedings in the first week of life have shown a lower incidence of feeding intolerance and NEC, a more mature gastrointestinal tract, and a shorter duration of time to regain birth weight (237–241). Animal studies demonstrate that early feedings prevent involution of the gut villi and loss of intestinal enzymes normally seen as few as three days after beginning intravenous feedings (242). Trophic feedings can be considered more as "oral medication" than as true feedings because little is gained nutritionally from them. Trophic feedings have not been studied in infants less than 800 g birth weight, and it is unclear whether the benefits, if any, of early feedings in these infants would outweigh the risks. Most practitioners agree that these infants should not receive feedings although they are unstable. However, mechanical ventilation or the presence of an umbilical arterial catheter per se is not absolute contraindication to initiating feedings.

WHAT TO FEED NEWBORN INFANTS

What one decides to feed infants is dependent on understanding the developmental physiology of the newborn gastrointestinal tract, the requirements of the infant for normal growth and body composition, and the available mechanisms of nutrient delivery. It is not surprising that term infants will thrive on different amounts and types of foods than will preterm infants, and that allowances in both groups must be made for the effect of illness on nutrient requirements.

Term Infants

Human Milk

Human milk is species-specific food for human beings (7). As such, it represents the best choice of food for the newborn infant. Substitute feedings, usually made from an animal-milk base, have been available for hundreds of years and have been highly refined in the past century. Nevertheless, no manufactured food can match the content of human milk for several reasons. Human milk is delivered fresh and has no "shelf life." This simple property allows live cells, growth factors, enzymes, and immune factors to remain intact and active. Formulas, which are designed to have a shelf life of one to two years (depending on the type of formulation), do not incorporate most of these factors because they would be unstable and would degrade over time. The factors found in human milk are thought to be responsible for many of its immunological and developmental advantages. Human milk is always at the correct temperature and requires no sterilization.

Approximately 69% of women in the United States elect to breast-feed their infants (243). This figure has remained relatively stable during the past five years and represents a rise from the nadir of 40% in the 1950s. It falls short of the goal of 75% set by the Healthy People 2000 initiative sponsored by the National Institutes of Health and endorsed by the AAP (7). The obstacles to improving the rate of initiation of breastfeeding include physician apathy or misinformation (244), insufficient prenatal breastfeeding education (245), and the lack of a perception of breastfeeding as culturally normal (246). By 6 months of age, only 33% of infants are breastfed even though human milk is nutritionally sufficient for infants through the first six months (243). This figure falls far short of the Healthy People 2000 goal of 50%. The decrement is due primarily to failure to maintain a milk supply in the first days after birth and discontinuation of breastfeeding upon the mother's return to work, typically at 6 or 12 weeks postpartum. The former relates to hospital and office practices that encourage formula feeding or are, at best, ambivalent to breastfeeding. For example, early hospital discharges combined with lack of timely routine follow-up care and postpartum health visits contribute to this early loss (247,248). The late dropout relates to the fact that many mothers work and many workplaces are not equipped to support the mother to maintain her milk supply (249–251). The AAP reaffirmed its support of breastfeeding and provided recommendations to improve the initiation and retention rates (7).

There are few absolute contraindications to breastfeeding. Infants with galactosemia should not be breastfed (252), nor should infants whose mothers are using illegal drugs (253). Mothers with active tuberculosis and mothers in first world countries who have human immunodeficiency virus (HIV) should also not breast-feed (254,255). Mothers who are taking certain medications (e.g., amethopterin, bromocriptine, cimetidine, clemastine, cyclophosphamide, ergotamine, gold salts, methimazole, phenindione, thiouracil) should not breast-feed. Complete lists of maternal medications that contraindicate breastfeeding are available (256,257). Temporary disorders, such as maternal mastitis or engorgement, are not contraindications to breastfeeding.

Human milk is nutritionally complete for most term infants for the first 6 months of life. Its primary carbohydrate is lactose. The protein content is low (1.1%) but the amino acid spectrum is well matched for the human infants' needs, and the predominance of lactalbumin ensures a low curd tension. The fat content of human milk is high and may approach 55% of total calories. The fat blend is unique and has been difficult to imitate in formula. In particular, the presence of certain omega fatty acids (DHA and ARA) may be important for optimal retinal and neurological development (258). Human milk is relatively low in sodium and osmolality. Not surprisingly, gastric emptying is rapid with human milk, making it ideal for infants with slow gastrointestinal motility as a result of illness. Human milk is relatively low in iron content but high in iron bioavailablity. The vast majority of term infants exclusively fed human milk will remain iron sufficient, although their stores at 6 months may be lower than infants fed iron-supplemented formula (124). Human milk may have a low-vitamin D content, particularly in women consuming a diet low in vitamin D and having low exposure to sunshine. Their infants are at risk of developing rickets if they too are not exposed to sunshine or given a vitamin D supplement. The AAP now recommends that all breastfed infants receive 200 IU of vitamin D daily.

Epidemiological studies provide evidence for the advantages of human milk over formulas, including better immune status, fewer infections (259–262), greater psychological benefits, more rapid neurodevelopment (263), protection from chronic childhood diseases (264–266), protection for the mother from certain diseases (267,268), and a lower rate of allergic disease (269,270). The reader is referred to the AAP statement on breastfeeding for a more complete review of these benefits (7).

Infant Formula

Many women choose formula feeding instead of breastfeeding for their infants. Infant formulas promote excellent growth and development when used as an alternative to breastfeeding. They should be given for the first year (271). Formula manufacturers are continuously attempting to improve their products, with the goal of matching human milk composition or performance. Most infant formulas are cow-milk based and are formulated at 20 calories per ounce. Alternatives include soy-based formula and elemental formulas.

Carbohydrates provide approximately 40% to 45% of the calories in formula. The most commonly used cow-milk-based formulas contain lactose as the primary carbohydrate, whereas the soy formulas contain either sucrose or glucose polymers.

The protein in formula provides approximately 10% of the total calories. Cow-milk protein is casein predominant, which is reported to have a higher curd tension than whey. Formula manufacturers have increasingly processed the cow-milk protein to make the formulas whey predominant with the whey-to-casein ratio approaching 60:40. The ratio in human milk is 70:30 (19). One formula in the United States has hydrolyzed the whey. Soy formulas contain soy proteins, which also support normal linear growth and muscle accretion. The protein content of soy formulas is higher than that of cow-milk formula. Soy formulas contain phytic acid, which may bind divalent cations (Ca, Mg) in the formula. For this reason, the calcium content of soy formulas is greater than that of cow-milk formulas. Both bone mineralization and linear bone growth in term infants fed soy formulas appear to be adequate.

Fat constitutes 40% to 55% of calories in infant formula and is usually a blend of vegetable oils, such as corn, coconut, soy, or palm-olein. Vegetable oils are added to cow-milk-based formulas because babies do not tolerate butterfat well. The fat blends are generally well tolerated, although infants will malabsorb up to 1 g/kg/day of ingested fat in the first 10 days of life (272). This malabsorption is lower than what is observed with whole milk (2 g/kg/day) or evaporated milk (1 to 2 g/kg/day). Recent research has focused on whether LC-PUFAs, such as DHA and ARA, are essential in the diets of newborns. Human milk contains these fatty acids whereas cow milk does not. Newborn infants have a relatively limited ability to synthesize these fats at birth, although the rates of maturation of the enzymatic pathways (elongation and desaturation) in the postnatal period are only now being elucidated. The content of DHA in human milk decreases rapidly after 44 weeks postconception, yet infants maintain adequate DHA levels, suggesting that the synthetic process is intact near that age (273). Addition of DHA to term infant formula has yielded mixed results with respect to growth and neurodevelopment (69,70,72,77). Those studies that have shown a positive effect on early retinal development or neurodevelopment have failed to demonstrate long-term or permanent benefits. From a safety standpoint, the FDA has determined that it has no questions whether the addition of LC-PUFAs derived from fungal sources are GRAS (generally recognized as safe), as claimed by the manufacturer. Based on this safety designation, major formula manufacturers in the United States have added DHA and ARA to their term infant formulas, although formula without the added PUFAs remain available.

Substantial alterations need to be made to whole cow milk to create a formula that a newborn infant will tolerate and thrive on. Whole cow milk is highly osmolar, low in calcium, high in phosphorus, low in vitamins A and D, and very low in bioavailable iron. Significant adjusting of all of these nutrients, in addition to the protein and fat manipulations, is necessary before an infant formula is safe for newborns.

Soy formulas are indicated for infants with galactosemia or lactase deficiency, infants whose mothers choose a vegetarian diet for their family, and infants with documented IgE-mediated allergy to cow-milk protein (274). On the other hand, there is no evidence that soy formula prevents atopic disease. Soy formulas do not relieve colic and are not indicated for premature infants (see below).

Elemental and casein hydrolysate formulas continue to make up a larger part of the infant formula market despite their very high cost and poor taste. Their main use has been in the treatment and prevention of allergy because 90% of the protein fragments are less than 1250 Daltons molecular weight. These low molecular weight fragments are less antigenic than cow-milk protein. In spite of this, anaphylaxis to these formulas has been reported (275,276). Additionally, the rate of true cow-milk protein allergy in newborns is less than 3%. Whey hydrolysate formulas are similar in cost to standard term infant formulas but are not as finely hydrolyzed as the casein hydrolysates and thus may present more of an antigenic challenge. Their ability to prevent and treat cow-milk allergy is debatable. All hydrolysate formulas promote adequate growth and nitrogen retention. Hydrolysates are not indicated for refeeding infants after gastroenteritis or for treating colic. They are more osmolar than standard cow-milk or soy formulas and thus possess a potential risk to the intestinal epithelium, particularly in the preterm infant.

Preterm Infants

Human Milk

Extensive research has assessed the adequacy and desirability of human milk feedings in the preterm infant. The reader is referred to a recent review of the subject (19). This research is predicated on the argument that human milk is the ideal food for the term neonate and that the immunological, gastrointestinal trophic, and psychological aspects are even more relevant to the preterm infant. When beginning human milk feedings in the preterm neonate, one must ask whether human milk is a good match for the preterm infant's nutritional requirements.

Mothers who deliver preterm produce a milk that has a higher protein content, higher caloric density, higher calcium content, and higher sodium content than milk from mothers who deliver at term (103–106). To a certain extent these higher concentrations match the increased needs for these nutrients in preterm infants. The composition of preterm human milk changes during the first month postnatally and becomes more like term human milk thereafter. Table 22-1 demonstrates the change in content of preterm human milk in the first months of life.

Human milk provides multiple nutritional advantages for the LBW infant (19). The carbohydrate composition is predominantly lactose, but also includes oligosaccharides that are important for intestinal host defenses (277). These oligosaccharides may play a role in protecting the human-milk-fed premature infant from NEC (19).

The fat blend of preterm human milk is unique and allows up to 95% absorption of dietary fat. This is due in part to the presence of lipases in human milk, but also apparently as a result of the fat blend. Preterm human milk also has detectable concentrations of omega-3 and omega-6 fatty acids. These fatty acids, particularly DHA, are important constituents of phospholipid membranes in the brain (278) and are normally delivered transplacentally. They are not found in cow milk, but are currently added to preterm infant formula in the United States. They do not appear to be readily synthesized by the preterm infant from linoleic and linolenic acid precursors and are thus considered by some to be semi-essential. Studies of infants who receive a source of these fatty acids either from human milk or in preterm infant formula suggest better visual acuity (71,74,279). Studies of long-term developmental outcome continue to determine whether any early advantages fade over time.

The protein content of human milk is predominantly whey, as opposed to the casein predominance of whole cow milk. Although preterm infant formulas are whey predominant, there are important differences in the proteins that make up the whey. The main human milk whey protein is alpha-lactalbumin, as opposed to β-lactalbumin in cow milk. Additionally, only human milk has significant concentrations of important proteins involved in host defense, such as lactoferrin and secretory IgA, in the whey fraction. These proteins may contribute to the observed protective effect that human milk has on the occurrence of NEC. There is evidence that these proteins act at a local (280) and systemic (281) level. Their effects may be in combination with a more benign fecal flora (282). Human milk contains multiple growth factors (19), including erythropoietin (283) and epidermal growth factor (284).

In spite of these advantages, feeding human milk to preterm infants poses several nutritional problems, particularly for the infant less than 1500 g. Preterm infants fed unsupplemented human milk have slow growth rates and higher rates of hyponatremia and osteopenia (285–289). These findings suggest that despite the altered content of preterm human milk, there is still not enough energy, protein, calcium, phosphorus and sodium to sustain adequate growth and bone mineralization. There is concern that some of the energy loss occurs when fat separates from human milk (290) and adheres to delivery tubing and storage containers.

Rather than abandon human-milk feedings, the solutions to these nutritional inadequacies include preventing losses by using short tubing lengths and employing a syringe and pump, maintaining the syringe upright (19).

Most importantly, human milk delivered to all infants less than 1,500 g should be fortified with commercial products that increase the caloric, protein, sodium, and calcium density of the milk (19). Two preformulated powder products are currently available. Each promotes better growth and bone mineralization than unsupplemented preterm human milk when fortified to a presumed caloric density of 24 kcal/ounce.

There is great variability in the milk expressed by mothers delivering preterm. Therefore, monitoring of nutritional status is critically important in preterm infants fed fortified human milk. In particular, growth rates, serum sodium concentrations, and bone mineralization status (serum alkaline phosphatase concentration, urinary excretion of phosphorus) must be assessed with regularity in these infants. Inadequate weight gain (<15 g/kg/day consistently over one week) can be treated by giving the infant more hind milk in the diet (19). Persistent increases in serum alkaline phosphatase concentrations despite fortification may necessitate adding some feedings of preterm infant formula.

Care must be taken in handling human milk to protect its important nutritional and immunological advantages. Fresh human milk is best, but is often impractical, particularly if the mother lives out of town. Fresh milk can be kept refrigerated up to 24 hours, but must then be frozen. Although live cells are destroyed by deep freezing (291), proteins remain largely intact. Suboptimal freezing results in fat breakdown. Rewarming frozen human milk can be dangerous as microwaving heats milk unevenly and can cause esophageal or gastric burns (292). It is more prudent to thaw an aliquot of milk for the entire shift or day and dispense it once it has been warmed in a water bath.

Initiating, advancing, and maintaining human milk feedings in the preterm infant who cannot take oral feeds can be accomplished in many ways. Unlike preterm infant formula, human milk does not need to be diluted since gastric aspirates are less of a problem with human milk because of better gastric emptying.

Preterm Infant Formulas

The development of formulas specifically designed for the preterm infant represented an important advancement in the nutrition of these infants. Prior to the introduction of these formulas in the late 1970s through mid-1980s, preterm infants were fed various formulations intended for infants with very different intestinal maturity, nutrient assimilation capability, and nutritional requirements. The science that went into developing preterm infant formulas carefully measured the nutrient needs of the preterm infant (described above) and the digestive and absorptive capabilities. When these two factors were considered together, a unique formulation for preterm infants evolved. For the most part, the preterm infant formulas are designed with the physiology of the less than 34 week gestational age infant in mind. Infants more than or equal to 34 weeks whose mothers choose not to breast-feed can be started on term infant formulas. If they show signs of intolerance (usually diarrhea, excessive gas, abdominal distention), relative lactase insufficiency as a result of immature intestinal development should be suspected, and a preterm formula can be used.

Two preterm infant formulas are available in the United States, and their nutritional constituents are remarkably similar. The carbohydrate source for both is a combination of lactose and glucose polymers. The lactose content is reduced compared to term infant formulas because of the relatively lower lactase concentration found in the preterm intestine. Glucose polymers are easily digested and are low-osmolar.

The protein source is cow milk that has been made whey predominant. The concentration of protein is quite high, delivering up to 3.6 g/kg/day when the formula is fed at a typical volume of 150 cc/kg/day. This high rate of delivery is designed to match the intrauterine accretion of nitrogen and follows the guidelines established by Heird and associates (96). Protein intakes at this rate maintain reasonable muscle mass accretion and support normal serum albumin and prealbumin concentrations.

As in term formulas, the fat blend is derived from vegetable oils. However, preterm infant formulas contain between 10% and 50% of the fat content as MCT. The necessity of MCT remains controversial (57). Addition of MCT was stimulated by the finding that lingual and gastric lipases are particularly effective at hydrolyzing fatty acids of this length and because long-chain fatty acids require an adequate bile salt pool for absorption. As discussed previously, preterm infants have low bile salt pools, which contributes to their higher fat malabsorption rate. Excessive MCT are not indicated, as they are poorly utilized for fat storage. They are an excellent source of energy, with the excess being excreted in the form of dicarboxylic acids (293). As a result of the GRAS determination of LC-PUFAs in infant formula, manufacturers of preterm infant formula are now adding DHA and ARA to their products.

The sodium and potassium contents of preterm infant formulas are higher than term formulas to compensate for renal tubular immaturity. Levels of trace elements are likewise higher. The preterm infant formulas contain the most calcium and phosphorus of any formula available. The current formulations, when fed at a volume of 150 cc/kg/day, will provide approximately 225 mg/kg/day of calcium and 110 mg/kg/day of phosphorus. This is well in excess of intrauterine accretion rates, allowing these formulas to be utilized to provide catch-up bone mineralization for those infants who have been on prolonged parenteral nutrition or dilute formulas. In spite of this high content, most premature infants less than 1,500 g have evidence of osteopenia of prematurity at the time of discharge. The bones of VLBW infants are frequently demineralized at discharge (294). Preterm infant formulas have recently been supplemented with iron in recognition of the fact that preterm infants are born with low iron stores compared to term infants, and that a rapid expansion of the red cell mass when catch-up growth ensues places a large stress on maintaining iron balance.

The preterm infant formulas are replete with water- and fat-soluble vitamins. Both formulations have higher vitamin D, E, and A concentrations compared to term formulas because of the poor fat absorption in preterm infants and the concern about the consequences of deficiency states in the infants. Studies assessing vitamin A and E levels in preterm infants fed the preterm infant formula with higher vitamin A and E concentrations demonstrated that additional supplementation with vitamins is not necessary once the infant is consuming at least 150 cc. Infants on the product that has a lower concentration may need additional supplementation. In either case, serum vitamin A and E levels should be followed weekly in preterm infants less than 1,500 g birth weight.

Techniques for the initiation, advancement, and maintenance of preterm infant formula feedings vary widely. The formula manufacturers have recommended initiating feedings with dilute (12 kcal/ounce) formula. Most infants will be on parenteral nutrition although their feedings are advanced. Although opinions vary greatly regarding whether formula volume or strength should be increased first, one should keep in mind that 1 cc of fully advanced peripheral parenteral nutrition (D12.5%, 3.0 g/kg/day of amino acids, 3.5 g/kg/day of lipids) is equivalent to approximately three-quarter-strength formula. Thus, volume-for-volume substitution of TPN with half-strength formula will dilute the caloric delivery to the infant, although substitution with full-strength formula will advance caloric intake.

Other Formulas

Although a large number of other formulas have been used for preterm infants, none are specifically designed to meet the nutritional needs of these infants. Any potential advantage of these formulas must be weighed against some fairly serious side effects. For example, soy formulas were used extensively in the late 1970s and early 1980s for preterm infants because they do not contain lactose and because of the concern that the preterm infant's intestine was particularly permeable to translocation of antigenic milk proteins (295). However, calcium absorption from soy formulas is very poor because the phytates in soy bind divalent cations. The incidence of osteopenia and rickets in preterm infants who are fed soy formulas is too high to justify recommending these products for this population (296).

Similarly, the possibility of using elemental or casein hydrolysate formulas for preterm infants has been suggested. The attractiveness of these formulas stems from their more elemental nature, thus presenting less of a digestive challenge to the immature preterm intestine. Unfortunately, these formulas are a poor nutritional match for the preterm infant from a fat-soluble vitamin and mineral standpoint. The vitamin E and A contents of the hydrolysates are one-quarter to one-half that of premature infant formula. The significantly lower vitamin D levels, lower calcium levels, and poor calcium-to-phosphorus ratio (1.4:1) place the preterm infant at high risk for osteopenia of prematurity. Finally, the osmolarity of these formulas ranges from 290 to 330 mOsm/L at 20 kcal/ounce, 25% higher than the preterm infant formulas, which have osmolarities of 210 to 220 mOsm/L at 20 kcal/ounce and 250 to 270 mOsm/L at 24 kcal/ounce. Hyperosmolarity is associated with a higher risk of NEC in preterm infants. As currently formulated, elemental or casein hydrolysate formulas are not recommended for routine use in preterm infants.

Preterm Discharge Formulas

Follow-up formulas for preterm infants have recently been introduced. Prior to their introduction, the preterm infant was usually switched to a formula designed for term infants prior to discharge from the hospital. This made sense from a digestive standpoint because most intestinal capacities are similar to term by 34 weeks postconception and preterm infants rarely leave the hospital prior to that age. Nevertheless, this practice did not take into account the large deficits in muscle stores, fat stores, and bone mineralization that occur in many of these infants (3,4), nor did they take into account the high rates of growth in preterm infants in the first year. Follow-up formulas represent a hybrid between preterm and term infant formulas. The ones marketed in the United States are powders designed to be diluted to 22 cal/ounce, but able to be prepared at various concentrations. At the 22-kcal/ounce concentration, they have a 50% higher calcium and vitamin D content than cow-milk-based formula for term infants (297). The carbohydrate content is a blend of lactose and glucose polymers, and the fat blends contain MCT oil in a manner similar to preterm infant formulas. There is less vitamin A and less sodium than in preterm infant formulas, but more vitamin A and D than in term formulas. The recommendation has been to give these formulas for at least the first six months postdischarge, although the manufacturers state that the formulas are safe for the entire first postnatal year. These formulas promote better growth rates and mineral status than does term formula in the preterm infant at follow-up (179). This is an important concept because of the large nutritional deficits that are accrued by the preterm infant in the neonatal intensive care unit (NICU) and the association between poor in-hospital growth and neurodevelopmental disability (182,298). The protein-energy deficit at hospital discharge at 25 grams of protein and 1000 kcal per kg of body weight (e.g., 50 grams of protein and 2000 kcal of energy for the average 2 kg premature infant at discharge) (4).

An alternative approach has been to continue to feed the discharged patient premature infant formula (299). Two problems arise with this solution: the formulas are not available commercially, and the improved fat digestive capacity of the infant after 34 weeks postconception raises the possibility of excessive vitamin A absorption. Moreover, the preterm infant formulas were designed for the special physiology of the less than 1,500 g, less than 34 week-postconceptional age infant.

NUTRITIONAL MONITORING

Any plan to nourish newborn infants should include plans for monitoring the nutritional status. For the healthy term infant, periodic plotting of the infant's weight, length, and head circumference on a standard growth curve is sufficient (Appendix I). The assessment of these parameters at birth provides a metric of the quality of fetal growth and also provides a starting point for postnatal monitoring. Small-for-dates infants should be assessed for signs and symptoms of intrauterine growth retardation. Signs of intrauterine wasting include small weight-for-length and midarm circumference:head circumference ratio (300,301), and may be seen in many small-for-dates infants and some appropriate-for-dates infants. It is important to plot newborns on a population-appropriate growth curve. For example, the growth curves published by Lubchenco in the 1960s are widely used, but were generated from a predominantly inner-city population born at high altitude (43) (Appendix D and I). Both factors tend to be associated with less intrauterine growth. It would not be appropriate to plot an infant of Scandinavian heritage (in which birth weights are on average 11 oz higher than in the United States [302,303]) born at sea level on the Lubchenco curves as it would overestimate the rate of macrosomia. The current debate is whether breastfed infants should be plotted on their own unique curve rather than on one generated from a mixed or formula-fed population (53).

Similarly, appropriate curves must be used to judge the growth and nutritional health of preterm infants. The IHDP growth curves (Infant Health and Development Program, Ross Laboratories) have separate charts for VLBW and LBW infants and for boys and girls (304) (Appendix I). These curves can be used for the first two postnatal years. The weight gain velocity of the VLBW infant is not as rapid as the LBW infant or the term infant, and little catch-up growth occurs in the first year after discharge (305). Catch-up growth has been reported to occur during late childhood (306).

The importance of monitoring protein-energy status in the hospitalized newborn cannot be overemphasized. It is state of the art for NICUs with substantial numbers of nutritionally at-risk infants to have nutrition support services that review the infants' status at least weekly and provide nutritional recommendations. Ideally, these nutrition support teams should include a registered dietician, a doctor of pharmacy, and a physician. All should have a background or additional training in neonatal nutritional principles. Studies support the positive effect of such teams on nutritional status of the infants at discharge (182).

Daily weights and weekly length and head circumference measurements should be routinely performed and charted. The effect of manipulating protein-energy delivery should be reflected with delays in the rate of weight gain. Interpretation of protein-energy status from weight measurements can be complicated by fluid retention or dehydration. Length measurements are the least reliable because of the difficulty in obtaining reproducible numbers. Assessments of energy requirements can also be made by indirect calorimetry to estimate resting energy expenditure. These measurements require special equipment and provide only a brief (usually 20 min) glimpse into energy utilization. The daily energy expenditure is extrapolated from the short-term measurement with the potential errors introduced by the extrapolation. Stable isotope techniques such as double-labeled water are the province of research institutions and are not used for clinical monitoring. Similarly, dual photon absorptiometry x-ray (DEXA) has been used in research studies to assess fat and lean body mass. A more practical assessment of the infant's relative fat status can be achieved with skinfold measurements and calculation of the arm fat area (180).

Protein status can be assessed by measurements of somatic or serum proteins or the serum BUN and creatinine concentrations in the absence of renal disease. The BUN will reflect recent nitrogen intake although the creatinine will index muscle mass. Low values are valid screening markers of poor protein status. Somatic protein status is best reflected in measurements of peripheral muscles, usually in the arm. The arm muscle area is calculated from the arm circumference and the skinfold thickness (307). The somatic muscle pool turns over relatively slowly and serial measurements, like those of length, do not provide acute information with respect to recent nutritional manipulations. Serum proteins have various half-lives and thus give differential time information. Serum prealbumin (transthyretin) concentrations reflect recent protein intake and predict subsequent weight gain velocity (224). The half-life of the protein is 1.9 days; therefore, a weekly assessment of the serum prealbumin is useful. Serum albumin has a half-life of 10 to 21 days, can be used as a marker of chronic protein status, and can be assessed monthly if needed. It is not very responsive to recent manipulations in protein delivery. Serum transferrin concentrations, used extensively in older children and adults because of its half-life of 10 days, is not useful in premature infants either for assessing recent intake or for predicting weight gain (308). It likely reflects a combination of iron and protein status and thus can be difficult to interpret. Nitrogen balance, urinary excretion of 3-methyl histidine, and stable isotope assessments using N-15 glycine or H-3 leucine are research tools that assess protein status.

Rapidly changing glucose, mineral, and electrolyte status is best monitored with serum levels. Sodium and potassium levels should be followed in infants on who are on TPN or are receiving diuretics. Similarly, infants on TPN should have their serum glucose concentrations monitored. In the first days after birth, sick infants should have serum calcium, magnesium, and phosphorus levels assessed.

Chronic calcium and bone mineralization status should not be monitored solely with serum calcium and phosphorus levels because they will usually be in the normal to low-normal range. The serum alkaline phosphatase concentration is an indirect measurement of bone mineralization since it is closely tied to rapid bone turnover. An infant who is becoming osteopenic will have more rapid bone turnover and will have a higher alkaline phosphatase

level. It should be expected that any growing premature infant will have relatively higher levels than a term infant, but a rapidly rising weekly alkaline phosphatase level is often indicative of active osteopenia. X-ray changes demonstrating demineralization are late findings and indicate that the bones are at least 33% demineralized. An elevated urinary excretion of phosphorus is also found during osteopenia of prematurity (309). DEXA can also be used to assess bone mineralization, but is used primarily in the research setting (310).

In general, it is unnecessary to routinely monitor trace element or vitamin status in the healthy, growing premature infant (See Appendix J-2 for nutrients in commercially available foods). However, higher risk infants should be monitored periodically, depending on the micronutrient in question and the disease state of the infant. Infants less than 1,500 g who are at high risk for BPD should have a vitamin A level measured at birth and should be treated with supplemental vitamin A if the level is less than 20 μg/dL (161,162). Concomitant vitamin E measurements can also be obtained. Weekly vitamin A and E levels should be followed in infants treated for deficiency.

The recent introduction of recombinant human erythropoietin has made monitoring of iron status an important consideration in the preterm infant. The iron status of the premature infant can fluctuate widely; infants who are multiply transfused have extremely high ferritin concentrations (311). Conversely, the meager iron stores of those who receive few or no transfusions will be rapidly consumed by erythropoiesis. Those treated with recombinant erythropoietin experience a decrease in their ferritin levels (134). They are likely to need iron supplementation earlier than premature infants who have been transfused. Currently, reference values for ferritin, serum iron, and transferrin concentrations in newborn infants have not been generated. Since iron has a narrow therapeutic-to-toxic ratio, better norms for assessing iron status in preterm infants are needed. At this time, it may be prudent to assay the serum ferritin concentration at one month of age to assess iron stores.

REFERENCES

1. Reichman B, Chessex P, Putet G, et al. Diet, fat accretion and growth in premature infants. *N Engl J Med* 1981;305:1495–1500.
2. Ziegler EE, O'Donnell AM, Nelson SE, et al. Body composition of the reference fetus. *Growth* 1976;40:239–241.
3. Lemons JA, Bauer CR, Oh W, et al. Very low birth weight outcomes of the National Institute of Child Health and Human Development neonatal research network, January 1995 through December 1996. *Pediatrics* 2001;107:E1.
4. Cooke RJ, Griffin IJ, McCormick K, et al. Feeding preterm infants after hospital discharge: effect of dietary manipulation on nutrient intake and growth. *Pediatr Res* 1998;43:355–360.
5. Wahlig TM, Georgieff MK. The effects of illness on neonatal metabolism and nutritional management. *Clin Perinatol* 1995;22:77–96.
6. Mathew OP. Science of bottle feeding. *J Pediatr* 1991;119:511–519.
7. American Academy of Pediatrics Work Group on Breastfeeding. Breastfeeding and the use of human milk. *Pediatrics* 1997;100:1035–1039.

8. Pritchard JA. Fetal swallowing and amniotic fluid volume. *Obstet Gynecol* 1966;28:606–610.

9. Montgomery RK, Mulberg AW, Grand RJ. Development of the human gastrointestinal tract: twenty years of progress. *Gastroenterology* 1999;116:702–731.

10. Wood JD. Intrinsic neural control of intestinal motility. *Annu Rev Physiol* 1981;43:33–51.

11. Gryboski JD. The swallowing mechanisms of the neonate: I. Esophageal and gastric motility. *Pediatrics* 1965;35:445–449.

12. Broussard DL. Gastrointestinal motility in the neonate. *Clin Perinatol* 1995;22:37–59.

13. Ittmann PI, Amarnath R, Berseth CL. Maturation of antroduodenal motor activity in preterm and term infants. *Dig Dis Sci* 1992;37:14–19.

14. Siegel M, Lebenthal E, Krantz B. Effect of caloric density on gastric emptying in premature infants. *J Pediatr* 1984;104:118–122.

15. Berseth CL. Gestational evolution of small intestine motility in preterm and term infants. *J Pediatr* 1989;115:646–651.

16. Berseth CL. Neonatal small intestinal motility: Motor responses to feeding in term and preterm infants. *J Pediatr* 1990;117:777–782.

17. Al-Tawil Y, Klee G, Berseth CL. Extrinsic neural regulation of antroduodenal motor activity in preterm infants. *Dig Dis Sci* 2002;47:26567–26563.

18. Berseth CL. Feeding methods for the preterm infant. *Semin Neonatol* 2001;6:417–424.

19. Schanler RJ. The use of human milk for premature infants. *Pediatr Clin North Am* 2001;48:207–219.

20. Sunshine P. Digestion and absorption of proteins. In: Bloom RS, Sinclair JC, Warshaw JB, eds. *Selected aspects of perinatal gastroenterology.* Evansville: Mead Johnson, 1977;(11)17–21.

21. Euler AR, Byrne WJ, Cousins LM, et al. Increased serum gastrin concentrations and gastric acid hyposecretion in the immediate newborn period. *Gastroenterology* 1977;72:1271–1273.

22. Hadorn B, Zoppi G, Schmerling DH. Quantitative assessment of exocrine pancreatic function in infants and children. *J Pediatr* 1968;73:39–50.

23. Watkins JB. Mechanisms of fat absorption and the development of gastrointestinal function. *Pediatr Clin North Am* 1975;22:721–730.

24. Balistreri WF. Anatomical and biochemical ontogeny of the gastrointestinal tract and liver. In: Tsang RC, Nichols B, eds. *Nutrition during infancy,* 1st ed. Philadelphia: Hanley & Belfus, 1988:33–55.

25. Hamosh M. Fat digestion in the newborn: role of lingual lipase and preduodenal digestion. *Pediatr Res* 1979;13:615–622.

26. Hamosh M. Lingual and breast milk lipases. *Adv Pediatr* 1982;29:33–67.

27. Jensen RG, Jensen GL. Specialty lipids for infant nutrition: I. Milks and formulas. *J Pediatr Gastroenterol Nutr* 1992;15:232–245.

28. Hernell O, Olvecrona T. Human milk lipases. II. Bile salt stimulated lipase. *Biochim Biophys Acta* 1974;369:234–244.

29. Hamosh M, Bitman J, Wood DL, et al. Lipids in milk and the first steps in their digestion. *Pediatrics* 1985;75[Suppl]:146–150.

30. Watkins JB, Szczepanik P, Gould JB, et al. Bile salt metabolism in the human premature infant. *Gastroenterology* 1975;69:706–713.

31. Lifschitz CH. Carbohydrate needs in preterm and term newborn infants. In: Tsang RC, Nichols B, eds. *Nutrition during infancy,* 1st ed. Philadelphia: Hanley & Belfus, 1988:122–140.

32. Koldovsky O. *Development of the functions of the small intestine in mammals and man.* Basel, Switzerland: S Basel and AG Karger, 1969:168–189.

33. Gray GM. Carbohydrate absorption and malabsorption. In: Johnson LR, ed. *Physiology of the gastrointestinal tracts.* New York: Raven Press 1981:1063–1081.

34. Auricchio S, Rubino A, Murset G. Intestinal glycosidase activities in the human embryo, fetus and newborn. *Pediatrics* 1965;35:944–949.

35. MacLean WC Jr, Fink BB. Lactose malabsorption by premature infants: magnitude and clinical significance. *J Pediatr* 1980;97:383–388.

36. Lebenthal E, Lee PC. Glycoamylase and disaccharidase activities in normal subjects and in patients with mucosal injury of the small intestine. *J Pediatr* 1980;97:389–394.

37. Georgieff MK. Taking a rational approach to the use of infant formulas. *Contemp Pediatrics* 2001;18:112–130.

38. Salmenpera L, Perheentupa J, Siimes MA. Exclusively breast-fed healthy infants grow slower than reference infants. *Pediatr Res* 1985;19:307–312.

39. Duncan B, Schifman RB, Corrigan JJ Jr, et al. Iron and the exclusively breast-fed infant from birth to six months. *J Pediatr Gastroenterol Nutr* 1985;4:421–425.

40. Wright AL, Holberg CJ, Taussig LM, et al. Relationship of infant feeding to recurrent wheezing at age 6 years. *Arch Pediatr Adolesc Med* 1995;149:758–763.

41. Widdowson EM, Spray CM. Chemical development in utero. *Arch Dis Child* 1951;26:205–214.

42. Babson SG, Benda GI. Growth graphs for the clinical assessment of infants of varying gestational age. *J Pediatr* 1976;89:814–820.

43. Lubchenco L, Hansman C, Boyd E. Intrauterine growth in length and head circumference as estimated from live births at gestational ages from 26 to 42 weeks of gestation. *Pediatrics* 1966;37:403–408.

44. Alexander GR, Himes JH, Kaufman RB, et al. A United States national reference for fetal growth. *Obstet Gynecol* 1996;87:163–168.

45. Butte NF. Meeting energy needs. In: Tsang RC, Zlotkin SH, Nichols B, et al, eds. *Nutrition during infancy,* 2nd ed. Cincinnati: Digipub 1997:57–82.

46. Hamosh M. Lipid metabolism in premature infants. *Biol Neonat* 1987;50[Suppl 1]:50–64.

47. Ross Pediatrics. *Composition of feedings for infants and young children.* Ross Ready Reference. Columbus, Ohio: Ross Products Division, Abbott Laboratories, 1996.

48. Motil KJ. Meeting protein needs. In: Tsang RC, Zlotkin SH, Nichols B, et al, eds. *Nutrition during infancy,* 2nd ed. Cincinnati: Digipub 1997:83–104.

49. Stocker FP, Wilkoff W, Mietinen OS, et al. Oxygen consumption in infants with heart disease. *J Pediatr* 1972;80:43–51.

50. Weinstein MR, Oh W. Oxygen consumption in infants with bronchopulmonary dysplasia. *J Pediatr* 1981;99:958–961.

51. Wahlig TM, Gatto CW, Boros SJ. Metabolic response of preterm infants to variable degrees of respiratory illness. *J Pediatr* 1994;124:283–288.

52. Mrozek JD, Georgieff MK, Blazar BR, et al. Neonatal sepsis: effect on protein and energy metabolism. *Pediatr Res* 1997;41:237A.

53. Heinig MJ, Nommsen LA, Peerson JM, et al. Energy and protein intakes of breast-fed and formula-fed infants during the first year of life and their association with growth velocity. The DARLING study. *Am J Clin Nutr* 1993;58:152–161.

54. Butte NF, Wong WW, Ferlic L, et al. Energy expenditure and deposition of breast-fed and formula-fed infants during early infancy. *Pediatr Res* 1990;28:631–640.

55. Whyte RK, Campbell D, Stanhope R, et al. Energy balance in low birth weight infants fed formula of high or low medium chain triglyceride content. *J Pediatr* 1986;108:964–971.

56. Sauer PJJ, Dane HF, Visser HKA. Longitudinal studies on metabolic rate, heat loss, and energy cost of growth in low birth weight infants. *Pediatr Res* 1984;18:254–259.

57. Klein CJ. Nutrient requirements for preterm infant formulas. *J Nutr* 2002;132:1395S–1577S.

58. Hay WW Jr. Fetal and neonatal glucose homeostasis and their relation to small for gestation age infants. *Semin Perinatol* 1984;8:101–116.

59. Kliegman RM, Morton S. Sequential intrahepatic metabolic effects of enteric galactose alimentation in newborn rats. *Pediatr Res* 1988;24:302–307.

60. DiGiacomo JE. Carbohydrates: metabolism and disorders. In: Hay WW Jr, ed. *Neonatal nutrition and metabolism.* St. Louis: Mosby 1991:93–109.

61. Lilien LD, Pildes RS, Srinivasan G, et al. Treatment of neonatal hypoglycemia with mini-bolus and intravenous glucose infusions. *J Pediatr* 1980;97:295–298.

62. Collins JW Jr, Hoppe M, Brow K, et al. A controlled trial of insulin infusion and parenteral nutrition in extremely low birth weight infants with glucose intolerance. *J Pediatr* 1991;118:921–927.

63. Binder ND, Rasschko PK, Benda GI, et al. Insulin infusion with parenteral nutrition in extremely low birth weight infants with hyperglycemia. *J Pediatr* 1989;114:273–280.

64. Burr GO, Burr MM. A new deficiency disease produced by rigid exclusion of fat from the diet. *J Biol Chem* 1929;82:345–367.

65. American Academy of Pediatrics, Committee on Nutrition. Nutritional needs of low birth weight infants. *Pediatrics* 1985;75: 976–986.

66. Lucas A. Long-chain polyunsaturated fatty acids, infant feeding and cognitive development. In: Dobbing J, ed. *Developing brain and behaviour: the role of lipids in infant formula.* San Diego: Academic Press 1997:3–36.

67. Innis SM. Essential fatty acids in growth and development. *Prog Lipid Res* 1991;30:39–103.

68. Innis SM. Polyunsaturated fatty acid nutrition in infants born at term. In: Dobbing J, ed. *Developing brain and behaviour: the role of lipids in infant formula.* San Diego: Academic Press 1997: 103–140.

69. Carson SE, Werkman SH, Tolley EA. Effect of long-chain n-3 fatty acid supplementation on visual acuity and growth of preterm infants with and without bronchopulmonary dysplasia. *Am J Clin Nutr* 1996;63:687–697.

70. Carlson SE, Werkman SH, Peeples JM, et al. Arachidonic acid status correlates with first year growth in preterm infants. *Proc Natl Acad Sci U S A* 1993;90:1073–1077.

71. O'Connor DL, Hall R, Adamkin D, et al. Growth and development in preterm infants fed long-chain polyunsaturated fatty acids: a prospective, randomized controlled trial. *Pediatrics* 2001;108:359–371.

72. Auestad N, Halter R, Hall R, et al. Growth and development in term infants fed long-chain polyunsaturated fatty acids: a double-masked randomized, parallel, prospective multi-variate study. *Pediatrics* 2001;108:372–381.

73. European Society of Paediatric Gastroenterology and Nutrition (ESPGAN). Nutrition and feeding of preterm infants. *Acta Paediatr Scand* 1987;336[Suppl]:1–14.

74. Uauy RD, Birch DG, Birch EE, et al. Effect of dietary omega-3 fatty acids on retinal function of very-low-birth-weight neonates. *Pediatr Res* 1990;28:485–492.

75. Birch EE, Birch DG, Hoffman DR, et al. Dietary essential fatty acid supply and visual acuity development. *Invest Ophthalmol Vis Sci* 1992;33:3242–3253.

76. Hoffman DR, Birch EE, Castaneda YS, et al. Visual function in breast-fed term infants weaned to formula with or without long-chain polyunsaturates at 4 to 6 months: a randomized clinical trial. *J Pediatr* 2003;142:669–677.

77. Jensen CL, Heird WC. Lipids with an emphasis on long-chain polyunsaturated fatty acids. *Clin Perinatol* 2002;29:261–281.

78. Lucas A, Stafford M, Morley R, et al. Efficacy and safety of long-chain polyunsaturated fatty acid supplementation of infant-formula milk: a randomised trial. *Lancet* 1999;354:1948–1954.

79. Wroble M, Mash C, Williams L, et al. Should long chain polyunsaturated fatty acids be added to infant formula to promote development? *J Appl Dev Psychol* 2002;23:99–112.

80. MacLean WC Jr, Benson JD. Theory into practice: the incorporation of new knowledge into infant formula. *Semin Perinatol* 1989;13:104–111.

81. Penn D, Schmidt-Sommerfeld E, Wolf H. Carnitine deficiency in premature infants receiving total parenteral nutrition. *Early Hum Dev* 1980;4:23–34.

82. Helms RA, Whitington PF, Mauer EC, et al. Enhanced lipid utilization in infants receiving oral L-carnitine during long-term parenteral nutrition. *J Pediatr* 1986;109:984–988.

83. Lorenz JM, Kleinman LI. Otogeny of the Kidney. In: Tsang RC, Nichols B, eds. *Nutrition during infancy.* Philadelphia: Hanley & Belfus 1988:58–80.

84. Ziegler TR, Gatzen C, Wilmore DW. Strategies for attenuating protein-catabolic responses in the critically ill. *Annu Rev Med* 1994;45:459–480.

85. Keshen TH, Jaksic T, Jahoor F. Measurement of the protein metabolic response to surgical stress in extremely low birthweight neonates. *Pediatric Res* 1997;41:234A.

86. Thureen PJ, Melara D, Fennessey PV, et al. Effectof low versus high intravenous amino acid intake on very low birth weight infants in the early neonatal period. *Pediatr Res* 2003;53:24–32.

87. Carver JD, Pimentel B, Cox WI, et al. Dietary nucleotide effects upon immune function in infants. *Pediatrics* 1991;88:359–363.

88. Goldman AS, Garza C, Nichold B, et al. Effect of prematurity on the immunologic system in human milk. *J Pediatr* 1982;101: 901–905.

89. Mestecky J, Blair C, Ogry PL et al. Immunology of milk and the neonate. *Adv Exp Med Biol* 1990;310:1–177.

90. Uauy R, Stringel G, Thomas R, et al. Effect of dietary nucleosides on growth and maturation of the developing gut in the rat. *J Pediatr Gastroenterol Nutr* 1990;10:497–503.

91. Graham GG, Placko RP, Morales E, et al. Dietary protein quality in infants and children. *Am J Dis Child* 1970;120:419–423.

92. Davidson M, Levine SZ, Bauer CH, et al. Feeding studies in low-birth-weight infants. I. Relationships of dietary protein, fat, and electrolytes to rates of weight gain, clinical courses, and serum chemical concentrations. *J Pediatr* 1967;70:695–713.

93. Kagan BM, Stanincova V, Felix NS, et al. Body composition of premature infants: relation to nutrition. *Am J Clin Nutr* 1972;25: 1153–1164.

94. Kashyap S, Schulze KF, Forsyth MS, et al. Growth, nutrient retention, and metabolic response in low birth weight infants fed varying intakes of protein and energy. *J Pediatr* 1988;113: 713–721.

95. Schulze KF, Stefanski M, Masterson J, et al. Energy expenditure, energy balance and composition of weight gain in low birth weight infants fed diets of different protein and energy content. *J Pediatr* 1987;110:753–759.

96. Heird WC, Kashyap S, Gomez MR. Protein intake and energy requirements of the infant. *Semin Perinatol* 1991;15:438–448.

97. Anderson TL, Muttart C, Bieber MA, et al. A controlled trial of glucose vs. glucose and amino acids in premature infants. *J Pediatr* 1979;94:947–951.

98. Denne SC. Protein and energy requirements in preterm infants. *Semin Neonatol* 2001;6:377–382.

99. Ziegler EE, Thureen PJ, Carlson SJ. Aggressive nutrition of the very low birthweight infant. *Clin Perinatol* 2002;39:225–244.

100. Uauy R, Greene HL, Heird WC. Conditional nutrients. In: Tsang RC, Lucas A, Uauy R, et al, eds. *Nutritional needs of the preterm infant.* Baltimore: Williams & Wilkins, 1993:267–280.

101. van Goudoeveer JB, Wattimena JDL, Carnielli VP, et al. Effect of dexamethasone on protein metabolism in infants with bronchopulmonary dysplasia. *J Pediatr* 1994;124:112–118.

102. Wu PY, Edwards NB, Storm MC. Plasma amino acid pattern in normal term breast-fed infants. *J Pediatr* 1986;109:347–349.

103. Clark SC, Karn CA, Ahlrichs JA, et al. Acute changes in leucine and phenylalanine kinetics produced by parenteral nutrition in premature infants. *Pediatr Res* 1997;41:568–574.

104. Gross SJ, David RJ, Bauman L, et al. Nutritional composition of milk produced by mothers delivering preterm. *J Pediatr* 1980;96: 641–644.

105. Schanler RJ, Oh W. Composition of breast milk obtained from mothers of premature infants as compared with breast milk obtained from donors. *J Pediatr* 1980;96:679–681.

106. Feeley RM, Eitenmiller RR, Jones JB, et al. Calcium, phosphorus and magnesium contents of human milk during early lactation. *J Pediatr Gastroenterol Nutr* 1983;2:262–267.

107. Kashyap S, Towers HM, Sahni R, et al. Effects of quality of energy on substrate oxidation in enterally fed, low-birth-weight infants. *Am J Clin Nutr* 2001;74:374–380.

108. American Academy of Pediatrics. Nutritional needs of preterm infants. In: Kleinman R, ed. *Pediatric nutrition handbook,* 4th ed. Elk Grove Village, IL: AAP, 1998:55–79.

109. *Vitamin and mineral requirements in preterm infants.* Tsang RC, ed. New York: Marcel Dekker, 1985:1–212.

110. Holliday MA. Requirements for sodium chloride and potassium and their interrelation with water requirement. In: Tsang RC, Nichols B, eds. *Nutrition during infancy.* Philadelphia: Hanley & Belfus 1988:160–191.

111. Koo WWK, Tsang RC. Calcium, magnesium, phosphorus and vitamin D. In: Tsang RC, Lucas A, Uauy R, et al, eds. *Nutritional needs of the preterm infant.* Baltimore: Williams & Wilkins 1993:135–156.

112. Schanler RJ, Garza C. Improved mineral balance in very low birth weight infants fed fortified human milk. *J Pediatr* 1987; 112:452–456.

113. Oski FA. The hematologic aspects of the maternal-fetal relationship. In: Oski FA, Naiman JL, eds. *Hematologic problems in the newborn,* 3rd ed. Philadelphia: WB Saunders, 1982:32–61.

114. Chockalingam UM, Murphy E, Ophoven JC, et al. Cord transferrin and ferritin levels in newborn infants at risk for prenatal uteroplacental insufficiency and chronic hypoxia. *J Pediatr* 1987;111:283–286.

115. Georgieff MK, Landon MB, Mills MM, et al. Abnormal iron distribution in infants of diabetic mothers: spectrum and maternal antecedents. *J Pediatr* 1990;117:455–461.

116. Petry CD, Eaton MA, Wobken JD, et al. Placental transferrin receptor localization and binding characteristics in diabetic pregnancies characterized by increased fetal iron demand. *Am J Physiol* 1994;E507-E514.

117. Georgieff MK, Petry CD, Mills MM, et al. Increased N-glycosylation and reduced transferrin binding capacity of transferrin receptor isolated from placentas of diabetic mothers. *Placenta* 1997;18:563-568.

118. American Academy of Pediatrics. Iron deficiency. In: Kleinman R, ed. *Pediatric nutrition handbook*, 4th ed. Elk Grove Village, IL: AAP, 1998:233-246.

119. Committee on Nutrition, American Academy of Pediatrics. Iron fortification of infant formulas. *Pediatrics* 1999;104:119-123.

120. Siimes MA, Vuori E, Kuitunen P. Breast milk iron: a declining concentration during the course of lactation. *Acta Paediatr Scand* 1979;68:29-31.

121. Lonnerdal B. Iron in human milk and cow's milk—effects of binding ligands on bioavailability. In: Lonnerdal B, ed. *Iron metabolism in infants*. Boca Raton, FL: CRC Press, 1990:87-103.

122. Pisacane A, De Vizia B, Valiante A, et al. Iron status in breast-fed infants. *J Pediatr* 1995;127:429-431.

123. Pizarro F, Yip R, Dallman PR, et al. Iron status with different infant feeding regimens: relevance to screening and prevention of iron deficiency. *J Pediatr* 1991;118:687-692.

124. Innis SM, Nelson CM, Wadsworth LD, et al. Incidence of iron-deficiency anaemia and depleted iron stores among nine-month-old infants in Vancouver, Canada. *Can J Pub Health* 1997;88:80-84.

125. Lonnerdal B, Hernell O. Iron, zinc, copper and selenium status of breast-fed infants and infants fed trace element fortified milk-based infant formula. *Acta Paediatr* 1994;83:367-373.

126. Foman SJ, Ziegler EE, Serfass RE, et al. Erythrocyte incorporation of iron is similar in infants fed formulas fortified with 12 mg/L or 8 mg/L of iron. *J Nutr* 1997;127:83-88.

127. Oski FA. Iron-fortified formulas and gastrointestinal symptoms in infants: a controlled study. *Pediatrics* 1980;66:168-170.

128. Nelson SE, Ziegler EE, Copeland AM, et al. Lack of adverse reactions to iron-fortified formula. *Pediatrics* 1988;81:360-364.

129. Hall RT, Wheeler RE, Benson J, et al. Feeding iron-fortified premature formula during initial hospitalization to infants less than 1800 grams birth weight. *Pediatrics* 1993;92:409-414.

130. Winzerling JJ, Kling PJ. Iron deficient erythropoiesis in premature infants measured by blood zinc protoporphyrin/heme. *J Pediatr* 2001;139:134-136.

131. Cooke RW, Drury JA, Yoxall CW, et al. Blood transfusion and chronic lung disease in preterm infants. *Eur J Pediatr* 1997;156:47-50.

132. Inder TE, Clemett RS, Austin NC, et al. High iron status in very low birth weight infants is associated with an increased risk of retinopathy of prematurity. *J Pediatr* 1997;131:541-544.

133. Widness JA, SewardVJ, Kromer IJ, et al. Changing patterns of red blood cell transfusion in very low birth weight infants. *J Pediatr* 1996;129:680-687.

134. Shannon K, Keith J, Mentzer W, et al. Recombinant human erythropoietin stimulates erythropoiesis and reduces erythrocyte transfusions in very low birth weight preterm infants. *Pediatrics* 1995;95:1-8.

135. Lozoff B, Jimenez E, Hagen J, et al. Poorer behavioral and developmental outcome more than 10 years after treatment for iron deficiency in infancy. *Pediatrics* 2000;105:E51.

136. Roncagliolo M, Garrido M, Walter T, et al. Evidence of altered central nervous system development in infants with iron deficiency anemia at 6 mo: delayed maturation of auditory brainstem responses. *Am J Clin Nutr* 1998;68:683-690.

137. Algarin C, Peirano P, Garrido M, et al. Iron deficiency anemia in infancy: long-lasting effects on auditory and visual system functioning. *Pediatr Res* 2003;53:217-223.

138. Berger HM, Mumby S, Gutteridge JM. Ferrous ions detected in iron-overloaded cord blood plasma from preterm and term babies: implications for oxidative stress. *Free Radic Res* 1995;22:555-559.

139. Chockalingam U, Murphy E, Ophoven JC, et al. The influence of gestational age, size for dates and prenatal steroids on cord transferrin in newborn infants. *J Pediatr Gastroenterol Nutr* 1987;6:276-280.

140. Jansson LT. Iron, oxygen stress and the preterm infant. In: Lonnerdal B, ed. *Iron metabolism in infants*. Boca Raton, FL: CRC Press, 1990:73-85.

141. Buonocore G, Perrone S, Longini M, et al. Non protein bound iron as early predictive marker of neonatal brain damage. *Brain* 2003;126:1224-1230.

142. Pollak A, Hayde M, Hayn M, et al. Effect of intravenous iron supplementation on erythropoiesis in erythropoietin treated premature infants. *Pediatrics* 2001;107:78-85.

143. Peters C, Georgieff MK, DeAlarcon P, et al. The effect of chronic erythropoietin administration on iron in newborn lambs. *Biol Neonate* 1996;70:218-228.

144. Zlotkin SH, Atkinson S, Lockitch G. Trace elements in nutrition for premature infants. *Clin Perinatol* 1995;22:223-240.

145. Reifen RM, Zlotkin SH. Microminerals. In: Tsang RC, Lucas A, Uauy R, et al, eds. *Nutritional needs of the preterm infant*. Baltimore: Williams & Wilkins, 1993:195-207.

146. Bayliss PA, Buchanan BE, Hancock RGV, et al. Tissue selenium accretion in premature and full-term human infants and children. *Biol Trace Elem Res* 1985;7:755-759.

147. Sinkin RA, Phelps DL. New strategies for the prevention of bronchopulmonary dysplasia. *Clin Perinatol* 1987;14:599-620.

148. Lipsky CL, Spear ML. Recent advances in parenteral nutrition. *Clin Perinatol* 1995;22:141-155.

149. Greene H, Hambridge K, Schanler R, et al. Guidelines for the use of vitamins, trace elements, calcium, magnesium, and phosphorus in infants and children receiving total parenteral nutrition: report of the Subcommittee on Pediatric Parenteral Nutrient Requirements from the Committee on Clinical Practice Issues of the American Society for Clinical Nutrition. *Am J Clin Nutr* 1988;48:1324-1342.

150. American Academy of Pediatrics. Vitamins. In: Kleinman R, ed. *Pediatric nutrition handbook*, 4th ed. Elk Grove Village, IL: AAP, 1998:267-281.

151. Pereira GR. Nutritional care of the extremely premature infant. *Clin Perinatol* 1995;22:61-75.

152. Feldman KW, Marcuse EK, Springer DA. Nutritional rickets. *Am Fam Physician* 1990;42:1311-1318.

153. Kreiter SR, Schwartz RP, Kirkman NH Jr, et al. Nutritional rickets in African-American breast-fed infants. *J Pediatr* 2000;137:153-157.

154. Riedel BD, Greene HL. Vitamins. In: Hay WW Jr, ed. *Neonatal nutrition and metabolism*. St. Louis: Mosby, 1991:143-170.

155. Hillman L, Hoff N, Salmons SJ, et al. Mineral homeostasis in very premature infants: serial evaluation of serum 25 hydroxy vitamin D, serum minerals and bone mineralization. *J Pediatr* 1985;106:970-980.

156. Wolbach SB, Howe PR. Tissue changes following deprivation of fat-soluble vitamin A. *J Exp Med* 1925;42:753-777.

157. Shenai JP, Stahlman MT, Chytil F. Vitamin A delivery from parenteral alimentation solutions. *J Pediatr* 1981;99:661-663.

158. Shenai JP, Chytil F, Stahlman MT. Vitamin A status of neonates with bronchopulmonary dysplasia. *Pediatr Res* 1985;19:185-188.

159. Georgieff MK, Chockalingam UM, Sasanow SR, et al. The effect of antenatal betamethasone on cord blood concentrations of retinol-binding protein, transthyretin, transferrin, retinol and vitamin E. *J Pediatr Gastroenterol Nutr* 1988;7:713-717.

160. Georgieff MK, Mammel MC, Mills MM, et al. Effect of postnatal steroid administration on serum vitamin A concentrations in newborn infants with respiratory compromise. *J Pediatr* 1989;114:301-304.

161. Shenai JP, Kennedy KA, Chytil F, et al. Clinical trial of vitamin A supplementation in infants susceptible to bronchopulmonary dysplasia. *J Pediatr* 1987;111:269-277.

162. Pearson E, Bose C, Snidow T, et al. Trial of vitamin A supplementation in very low birth weight infants at risk for bronchopulmonary dysplasia. *J Pediatr* 1992;121:420-427.

163. Tyson JE, Wright LL, Oh W, et al. Vitamin A supplementation for extremely-low-birth-weight infants. National Institute of Child Health and Human Development Neonatal Research Network. *N Engl J Med* 1999;340:1962-1968.

164. Oski FA, Barnes LA. Vitamin E deficiency: a previously unrecognized cause of hemolytic anemia in the premature. *J Pediatr* 1967;70:211-220.

165. Johnson L, Schaffer D, Boggs TR. The premature infant, vitamin E deficiency and retrolental fibroplasia. *Am J Clin Nutr* 1974;27:1158-1173.

166. Hittner HM, Godio LB, Rudolph AJ, et al. Retrolental fibroplasia: efficacy of vitamin E in a double-blind clinical study of preterm infants. *N Engl J Med* 1981;305:1365-1371.

167. Hittner HM, Godio LB, Speer ME, et al. Retrolental fibroplasia: further clinical evidence and ultrastructural support for efficacy of vitamin E in the preterm infant. *Pediatrics* 1983;71: 423–432.

168. Phelps DL, Rosenbaum AL, Isenberg SJ, et al. Tocopherol efficacy and safety for preventing retinopathy of prematurity: a randomized, controlled, double-masked trial. *Pediatrics* 1987;79: 489–500.

169. Phelps DL. Retinopathy of prematurity. *Curr Probl Pediatr* 1992; 22:349–371.

170. Johnson L, Bowen FW, Abbasi S, et al. Relationship of prolonged pharmacologic serum levels of vitamin E to incidence of sepsis and necrotizing enterocolitis in infants with birth weights of 1500 grams or less. *Pediatrics* 1985;75:619–638.

171. Heird WC, Gomez MR. Parenteral Nutrition. In: Tsang RC, Lucas A, Uauy R, et al, eds. *Nutritional needs of the preterm infant.* Baltimore: Williams & Wilkins 1993:225–242.

172. Steinhorn DM, Green TP. Severity of illness correlates with alterations in energy metabolism in the pediatric intensive care unit. *Crit Care Med* 1991;19:1503–1509.

173. Cerra FB, Siegel JH, Coleman B, et al. Septic autocannibalism: a failure of exogenous nutritional support. *Ann Surg* 1980;192: 570–580.

174. Fleck A. Acute phase response: implications for nutrition and recovery. *Nutrition* 1988;4:109–116.

175. Harris MC, Costarino AT, Sullivan JS, et al. Cytokine elevations in critically ill infants with sepsis and necrotizing enterocolitis. *J Pediatr* 1994;124:105–111.

176. Maldonato J, Gil A, Faus MJ, et al. Differences in the serum amino acid pattern of injured and infected children promoted by two parenteral nutrition solutions. *JPEN* 1989;13:41–46.

177. Canadian Paediatric Society and Nutrition Committee. Nutrient needs and feeding of premature infants. *CMAJ* 1995;152: 1765–1785.

178. Priego T, Ibanez de Caceres I, Martin AI, et al. Glucocorticoids are not necessary for the inhibitory effect of endotoxic shock on serum IGF-I and hepatic IGF-I mRNA. *J Endocrinol* 2002;172: 449–456.

179. Carver JD, Wu PY, Hall RT, et al. Growth of preterm infants fed nutrient-enriched or term formula after hospital discharge. *Pediatrics* 2001;107:683–689.

180. deRegnier R-AO, Guilbert TW, Mills MM, et al. Growth failure and altered body composition are established by one month of age in infants with bronchopulmonary dysplasia. *J Nutr* 1996;126:168–175.

181. Frank L, Sosenko IRS. Undernutrition as a major contributing factor in the pathogenesis of bronchopulmonary dysplasia. *Am Rev Respir Dis* 1988;138:725–729.

182. Georgieff MK, Mills MM, Lindeke L, et al. Changes in nutritional management and outcome of very-low-birth-weight infants. *Am J Dis Child* 1989;143:82–85.

183. Berseth CL. Minimal enteral feedings. *Clin Perinatol* 1995;22: 195–205.

184. Roberts JR. Cutaneous and subcutaneous complications of calcium infusions. *JACEP* 1977;6:16–20.

185. Hruszkewycz V, Holtrop PC, Batton DG, et al. Complications associated with central venous catheters inserted in critically ill neonates. *Infect Control Hosp Epidemiol* 1991;12:544–548.

186. Polin RA, St. Geme JW 3rd. Neonatal sepsis. *Adv Pediatr Infect Dis* 1992;7:25–61.

187. Rowen JL, Atkins JT, Levy ML, et al. Invasive fungal dermatitis in the less than or equal to 1000 gram neonate. *Pediatrics* 1995;95:682–687.

188. Duffy LF, Kerzner B, Gebus V, et al. Treatment of central venous catheter occlusions with hydrochloric acid. *J Pediatr* 1989;114: 1002–1004.

189. Kashyap S. Nutritional management of the extremely-low-birth-weight infant. In: Cowett RM, Hay W, eds. *The micropremie: the next frontier.* Report of the 99th Ross Conference on Pediatric Research, 1990:115–119.

190. Zlotkin SH, Bryan MH, Anderson GH. Intravenous nitrogen and energy intakes required to duplicate in utero nitrogen accretion in prematurely born human infants. *J Pediatr* 1981;99:115–120.

191. Helms RA, Christensen ML, Mauer EC, et al. Comparison of a pediatric versus standard amino acid formulation in preterm neonates requiring parenteral nutrition. *J Pediatr* 1987;110: 466–470.

192. Helms RA, Johnson MR, Christenson ML, et al. Evaluation of two pediatric amino acid formulations (abst). *JPEN* 1988;12:4.

193. Heird WC, Dell RB, Helms RA, et al. Amino acid mixture designed to maintain normal plasma amino acid patterns in infants and children requiring parenteral nutrition. *Pediatrics* 1987;80:401–408.

194. Hayes KC, Carey RE, Schmidt SY. Retinal degeneration associated with taurine deficiency in the cat. *Science* 1975;188:949–951.

195. Guertin F, Roy CC, Lepage G, et al. Effect of taurine on parenteral nutrition-associated cholestasis. *JPEN* 1991;15:247–251.

196. Tyson JE, Lasky R, Flood D, et al. Randomized trial of taurine supplementation for infants <1,300 gram birth weight: effect on auditory brainstem-evoked responses. *Pediatrics* 1989;83:406–415.

197. White HB, Turner AC, Miller RC. Blood lipid alterations in infants receiving intravenous fat-free alimentation. *J Pediatr* 1973;83:305–313.

198. Costarino AT, Baumgart S. Modern fluid and electrolyte management of the critically ill premature infant. *Pediatr Clin North Am* 1986;33:153–178.

199. Dunham B, Marcuard S, Khazanie PG, et al. The solubility of calcium and phosphorus in neonatal parenteral nutrition solutions. *JPEN* 1991;15:608–611.

200. Pelegano JF, Rowe JC, Carey DE, et al. Effect of calcium/phosphorus ratio on mineral retention in parenterally fed premature infants. *JPEN* 1991;12:351–355.

201. Hoehn GJ, Carey DE, Raye JR, et al. Alternate-day infusion of calcium and phosphate in very low birth weight infants: wasting of the infused mineral. *JPEN* 1987;6:752–757.

202. Kimura S, Nose O, Seino Y, et al. Effects of alternate and simultaneous administration of calcium and phosphorus on calcium metabolism in children receiving total parenteral nutrition. *JPEN* 1986;10:513–516.

203. Fitzgerald KA, MacKay MW. Calcium and phosphate solubility in neonatal parenteral nutrient solutions containing Trophamine. *Am J Hosp Pharm* 1986;43:88–93.

204. Schmidt GL, Baumgartner TG, Fischlschweiger W, et al. Cost containment using cysteine HCl acidification to increase calcium/ phosphate solubility in hyperalimentation solutions. *JPEN* 1986;10:203–207.

205. Thorp JW, Boeckx RL, Robbins S, et al. A prospective study of infant zinc nutrition during intensive care. *Am J Clin Nutr* 1981;34:1056–1060.

206. Heller RM, Kirchner SG, O'Neill JA, et al. Skeletal changes of copper deficiency in infants receiving prolonged total parenteral nutrition. *J Pediatr* 1978;92:947–949.

207. Lane HW, Barroso AO, Englert D, et al. Selenium status of seven chronic intravenous hyperalimentation patients. *JPEN* 1982;6: 426–431.

208. Stahl GE, Spear ML, Hamosh M. Intravenous administration of lipid emulsions to premature infants. *Clin Perinatol* 1986;13: 133–162.

209. Hageman JR, McCullough K, Gora P, et al. Intralipid alterations in pulmonary prostaglandin metabolism and gas exchange. *Crit Care Med* 1983;11:794–798.

210. McKeen CR, Brigham KL, Bowers RE, et al. Pulmonary vascular effects of fat emulsion infusion in unanesthetized sheep. Prevention by indomethacin. *J Clin Invest* 1978;61:1291–1297.

211. Hammerman C, Aramburo MJ. Decreased lipid intake reduces morbidity in sick premature neonates. *J Pediatr* 1988;113: 1083–1088.

212. Gilbertson N, Kovar IZ, Cox, DJ, et al. Introduction of intravenous lipid administration on the first day of life in the very low birth weight neonate. *J Pediatr* 1991;119:615–623.

213. Eggert LD, Rusho WJ, MacKay MW, et al. Calcium and phosphorus compatibility in parenteral nutrition solutions for neonates. *Am J Hosp Pharm* 1982;39:49–53.

214. Adamkin DH, Radmacher PG, Klingbeil RL. Use of intravenous lipid and hyperbilirubinemia in the first week. *JPEN* 1992;14: 135–139.

215. Aschner JL, Punsalang A, Maniscalco WM, et al. Percutaneous central venous catheter colonization with Malassezia furfur: incidence and clinical significance. *Pediatrics* 1987;80:535–539.

216. Merritt RJ. Cholestasis associated with total parenteral nutrition. *JPEN* 1986;5:9–22.

217. Koo WWK, Kaplan LA, Horn J, et al. Aluminum in parenteral solutions—sources and possible alternatives. *JPEN* 1986;10: 591–595.

218. Koo WWK, Kaplan LA, Bendon R, et al. Response to aluminum in parenteral nutrition during infancy. *J Pediatr* 1986;109:877–883.
219. Alfrey AC. Aluminum. *Adv Clin Chem* 1983;23:69–91.
220. Sedman AB, Klein GL, Merritt RJ, et al. Evidence of aluminum loading in infants receiving intravenous therapy. *N Engl J Med* 1985;312:1337–1343.
221. ASCN/A.SPEN. Working Group on Standards for Aluminum Content of Parenteral Nutrition Solutions. Parenteral drug products containing aluminium as an ingredient or a contaminant: response to food and drug administration notice of intent and request for information. *JPEN* 1991;15:194–198.
222. Sann L, Durand M, Picard J, et al. Arm fat and muscle areas in infancy. *Arch Dis Child* 1988;63:256–260.
223. Georgieff MK, Sasanow SR, Pereira GR. Serum transthyretin levels and protein intake as predictors of weight gain velocity in premature infants. *J Pediatr Gastroenterol Nutr* 1987;6:775–779.
224. Georgieff MK, Sasanow SR, Mammel MC, et al. Cord prealbumin values in newborn infants: effect of prenatal steroids, pulmonary maturity and size for dates. *J Pediatr* 1986;108:972–976.
225. Vallee BL, Galdes A. The metallobiochemistry of zinc enzymes. *Adv Enzymol Relat Areas Mol Biol* 1984;56:283–430.
226. Lau C, Smith EO, Schanler RJ. Coordination of suck-swallow and swallow respiration in preterm infants. *Acta Paediatr* 2003;92:721–727.
227. Meier P. Bottle and breastfeeding effects on transcutaneous oxygen pressure and temperature in preterm infants. *Nurs Res* 1988;37:36–41.
228. Lucas A, Morley R, Cole TJ, et al. A randomised multicentre study of human milk versus formula and later development in preterm infants. *Arch Dis Child Fetal Neonatal Ed* 1994;70:F141-F146.
229. Bernbaum JC, Pereira GR, Watkins JB, et al. Nonnutritive sucking during gavage feeding enhances growth and maturation in premature infants. *Pediatrics* 1983;71:41–45.
230. Field T, Ignatoff E, Stringer S, et al. Nonnutritive sucking during tube feedings: effects on preterm neonates in an intensive care unit. *Pediatrics* 1982;70:381–384.
231. Widstrom AM, Marchini G, Matthieson AS, et al. Nonnutritive sucking in tube-fed preterm infants: effects on gastric motility and gastric contents of Somatostatin. *J Pediatr Gastroenterol Nutr* 1988;7:517–523.
232. Toce SS, Keenan WJ. Enteral feeding in very-low-birth-weight infants. *Am J Dis Child* 1987;141:436–444.
233. Roy RN, Pillnitz RP, Hamilton JR, et al. Impaired assimilation of nasojejunal feeds in healthy low-birth-weight newborn infants. *J Pediatr* 1977;90:431–434.
234. Wells DH, Zachman RD. Nasojejunal feeds in low-birth-weight infants. *J Pediatr* 1975;87:276–279.
235. Challacombe D. Bacterial microflora in infants receiving nasojejunal tube feeding [Letter]. *J Pediatr* 1974;85:113.
236. Kennedy KA, Tyson JE, Chamnanvankij S. Rapid versus slow rate of advancement of feedings for promoting growth and preventing necrotizing enterocolitis in parenterally fed low-birth-weight infants. *Cochrane Database Syst Rev* 2000;2:CD001241.
237. Lucas A, Bloom SR, Aynsley-Green A. Gut hormones and "minimal enteral feeding." *Acta Paediatr Scand* 1986;75:719–723.
238. Slagle TA, Gross SJ. Effect of early low-volume enteral substrate on subsequent feeding tolerance in the very low birth weight infants. *J Pediatr* 1988;113:526–531.
239. Dunn L, Hulman S, Weiner J, et al. Beneficial effects of early hypocaloric enteral feeding on neonatal gastrointestinal function: preliminary report of a randomized trial. *J Pediatr* 1988;112:622–629.
240. Meetze W, Valentine C, Sacks J, et al. Effects of gastrointestinal (GI) priming prior to full enteral nutrition in very low birth weight (VLBW) infants. *Pediatr Res* 1990;27:287A(abst).
241. Neu J, Valentine C, Mietze W. Scientifically-based strategies for nutrition of the high-risk low birth weight infant. *Eur J Pediatr* 1990;150:2–13.
242. Hughes CA, Dowling RH. Speed of onset of adaptive mucosal hypoplasia and hypofunction in the intestine of parenterally fed rats. *Clin Sci* 1980;59:317–327.
243. Ryan AS, Wenjun Z, Acosta A. Breastfeeding continues to increase into the new millennium. *Pediatrics* 2002;110:1103–1109.
244. Freed GL, Clark SJ, Sorenson J, et al. National assessment of physicians' breast-feeding knowledge, attitudes, training, and experience. *JAMA* 1995;273:472–476.
245. World Health Organization. *Protecting, promoting and supporting breast-ceeding: the special role of maternity services.* Geneva, Switzerland: WHO, 1989.
246. Spisak S, Gross SS. *Second Followup Report: the Surgeon General's Workshop on Breastfeeding and Human Lactation.* Washington, DC: National Center for Education in Maternal and Child Health, 1991.
247. Braveman P, Egerter S, Pearl M, et al. Problems associated with early discharge of newborn infants. *Pediatrics* 1995;96:716–726.
248. Williams LR, Cooper MK. Nurse-managed postpartum home care. *J Obstet Gynecol Neonatal Nurs* 1993;22:25–31.
249. Gielen AC, Faden RR, O'Campo P, et al. Maternal employment during the early postpartum period: effects on initiation and continuation of breast-feeding. *Pediatrics* 1991;87:298–305.
250. Frederick IB , Auerback KG. Maternal-infant separation and breast-feeding: the return to work or school. *J Reprod Med* 1985;30:523–526.
251. Spisak S, Gross SS. *Second Followup Report: the Surgeon General's Workshop on Breastfeeding and Human Lactation.* Washington, DC: National Center for Education in Maternal and Child Health, 1991.
252. Wilson MH. Feeding the healthy child. In: Oski FA, DeAngelis CD, Feigin RD, et al, eds. *Principles and practice of pediatrics.* Philadelphia: JB Lippincott, 1990:553–572.
253. Rohr FJ, Levy HL, Shih VE. Inborn errors of metabolism. In: Walker WA, Watkins JB, eds. *Nutrition in pediatrics.* Boston: Little, Brown, 1983:412–422.
254. American Academy of Pediatrics, Committee on Drugs. The transfer of drugs and other chemicals into human milk. *Pediatrics* 1994;93:137–150.
255. American Academy of Pediatrics, Committee on Pediatric AIDS. Human milk, breastfeeding, and transmission of human immunodeficiency virus in the United States. *Pediatrics* 1995;96:977–979.
256. Centers for Disease Control and Prevention. Recommendation for assisting in the prevention of perinatal transmission of human T-lymphotropic virus type III/lymphadenopathy-associated virus and acquired immunideficiency syndrome. *MMWR* 1985;34:721–723.
257. Briggs GG, Freeman RK, Yaffe SJ. Drugs in Pregnancy and Lactation. Baltimore: Williams & Wilkins, 1990.
258. Uauy-Dagach R, Mena P. Nutritional role of Omega-3 fatty acids during the perinatal period. *Clin Perinatol* 1995;22:157–175.
259. Kovar MG, Serdula MK, Marks JS, et al. Review of the epidemiologic evidence for an association between infant feeding and infant health. *Pediatrics* 1984;74:615–638.
260. Frank AL, Taber LH, Glezen WP, et al. Breast-feeding and respiratory virus infection. *Pediatrics* 1982;70:239–245.
261. Saarinen UM. Prolonged breast feeding as prophylaxis for recurrent otitis media. *Acta Paediatr Scand* 1982;71:567–571.
262. Lucas A, Cole TJ. Breast milk and neonatal necrotising enterocolitis. *Lancet* 1990;336:1519–1523.
263. Mortensen EL, Michaelsen KF, Sanders SA, et al. The association between duration of breastfeeding and adult intelligence. *JAMA* 2002;287:2365–2371.
264. Mayer EJ, Hamman RF, Gay EC, et al. Reduced risk of IDDM among breast-fed children. *Diabetes* 1988;37:1625–1632.
265. Koletzko S, Sherman P, Corey M, et al. Role of infant feeding practices in development of Crohn's disease in childhood. *Br Med J* 1989;298:1617–1618.
266. Davis MK, Savitz DA, Graubard BI. Infant feeding and childhood cancer. *Lancet* 1988;2:365–368.
267. Rosenblatt KA, Thomas DB. Lactation and the risk of epithelial ovarian cancer. WHO Collaborative Study of Neoplasia and Steroid Contraceptives. *Int J Epidemiol* 1993;22:192–197.
268. Newcomb PA, Storer BE, Longnecker MP, et al. Lactation and a reduced risk of premenopausal breast cancer. *N Engl J Med* 1994;330:8–87.
269. Saarinen UM, Kajosaari M. Breastfeeding as prophylaxis against atopic disease: prospective follow-up study until 17 years old. *Lancet* 1995;346:1065–1069.
270. Lucas A, Brooke OG, Morley R, et al. Early diet of preterm infants and development of allergic or atopic disease: randomised prospective study. *Br Med J* 1990;300:837–840.
271. American Academy of Pediatrics. *Pediatric nutrition handbook,* 4th ed. Kleinman RE, ed. Elk Grove Village, IL: AAP, 1998:29–42.

272. Fomon SJ, Ziegler EE, Thomas LN, et al. Excretion of fat by normal full-term infants fed various milks and formulas. *Am J Clin Nutr* 1970;23:1299–1313.

273. Henderson TR, Hamosh M, Hayman L. Serum long chain polyunsaturated fatty acids (LC-PUFA) are adequate in full term breast fed infants in spite of low milk LC-PUFA after >3 months lactation. *Pediatr Res* 1996;39:311A.

274. American Academy of Pediatrics, Committee on Nutrition. Soy protein formulas. Recommendations for use in infant feeding. *Pediatrics* 1983;72:359–363.

275. Saylor JD, Bahna SL. Anaphylaxis to casein hydrolysate formula. *J Pediatr* 1991;118:71–74.

276. Ellis MH, Short JA, Heiner DC. Anaphylaxis after ingestion of a recently introduced hydrolyzed whey protein formula. *J Pediatr* 1991;118:74–77.

277. Schanler RJ. Human milk for preterm infants: Nutritional and immune factors. *Semin Perinatol* 1989;13:69–77.

278. Uauy R, Hoffman DR. Essential fatty acid requirements for normal eye and brain development. *Semin Perinatol* 1991;15:449–455.

279. Carlson SE, Werkman SH, Rhodes PG, et al. Visual-acuity development in healthy preterm infants: effect of marine-oil supplementation. *Am J Clin Nutr* 1993;58:35–42.

280. Kleinman RE, Walker WA. The enteromammary immune system. *Dig Dis Sci* 1979;24:876–882.

281. Hutchens TW, Henry JF, Yip T-T, et al. Origin of intact lactoferrin and its DNA-binding fragments found in the urine of human milk-fed preterm infants. Evaluation by stable isotope enrichment. *Pediatr Res* 1991;29:243–250.

282. Balmer SE, Wharton BA. Diet and faecal flora in the newborn: breast milk and infant formula. *Arch Dis Child* 1989;64:1672–1677.

283. Kling PJ. Roles of erythropoietin in human milk. *Acta Paediatr* 2002;91[Suppl]:31–35.

284. Dvorak B, Fituch CC, Williams CS, et al. Increased epidermal growth factor levels in human milk of extremely premature infants. *Pediatr Res* 2003;54:15–19.

285. Atkinson SA, Bryan MH, Anderson GH. Human milk feeding in premature infants: protein, fat and carbohydrate balances in the first 2 weeks of life. *J Pediatr* 1981;99:617–624.

286. Roy RN, Chance GW, Radde IC, et al. Late hyponatremia in very low birth weight infants (<1.3 kilograms). *Pediatr Res* 1976;10:526–531.

287. Schanler RJ. Calcium and phosphorus absorption and retention in preterm infants. *J Exp Med* 1991;2:24–29.

288. Schanler RJ, Oh W. Nitrogen and mineral balance in preterm infants fed human milk or formula. *JPEN* 1985;4:214–219.

289. Ziegler EE, O'Donnell AM, Nelson SE, et al. Body composition of the reference fetus. *Growth* 1976;40:329–341.

290. Stocks RJ, Davies DP, Allen F, et al. Loss of breast milk nutrients during tube feeding. *Arch Dis Child* 1985;60:164–166.

291. Williams FH, Pittard WB 3rd. Human milk banking: Practical concerns for feeding premature infants. *J Am Diet Assoc* 1981;74(5):565–568.

292. Puczynski M, Rademaker D, Gatson RL. Burn injury related to improper use of microwave ovens. *Pediatrics* 1983;72:714–715.

293. Henderson MJ, Dear PRF. Dicarboxylic aciduria and medium chain triglyceride supplemented milk. *Arch Dis Child* 1986;61:610–611.

294. Koo WW, Tsang RC. Mineral requirements of low-birth-weight infants. *J Am Col Nutr* 1991;10:474–486.

295. Lake AM, Walker WA. Neonatal necrotizing enterocolitis: a disease of altered host defense. *Clin Gastroenterol* 1977;6:463–480.

296. Hillman LS, Hoff N, Martin LA, et al. Osteopenia, hypocalcemia, and low 25-hydroxyvitamin D (25-CHD) serum concentration with use of soy formula. *Pediatr Res* 1979;13:A448(abst).

297. Georgieff MK. Taking a rational approach to the use of infant formulas. *Contemp Pediatrics* 2001;18:112–130.

298. Georgieff MK, Hoffman JS, Pereira GR, et al. The effect of neonatal caloric deprivation on head growth and one-year developmental status in preterm infants. *J Pediatr* 1985;107:581–587.

299. Cooke RJ, Griffin I, Wells J, et al. Formula feeding preterm infants after hospital discharge: 2. Effects on body composition. *Pediatr Res* 1996;39:306A.

300. Miller HC, Hassanien K. Diagnosis of impaired fetal growth in newborn infants. *Pediatrics* 1971;48:511–522.

301. Georgieff MK, Sasanow SR, Chockalingam UM, et al. A comparison of the mid-arm cirumference/head circumference ratio and ponderal index for the evaluation of newborn infants after abnormal intrauterine growth. *Acta Paediatr Scand* 1988;77:214–219.

302. Bjerkedal T, Bakketeig L, Lehmann DH. Percentiles of birthweights of single live births at different gestational periods. *Acta Paediatr Scand* 1973;62:449–457.

303. Sterky G. Swedish standard curves for intra-uterine growth. *Pediatrics* 1970;46:7–8.

304. Casey PH, Kraemer HC, Berbaum J, et al. Growth status and growth rates of a varied sample of low birth weight, preterm infants: a longitudinal cohort from birth to three years of age. *J Pediatr* 1991;119:599–604.

305. Georgieff MK, Mills MM, Zempel CE, et al. Catch-up growth, muscle and fat accretion, and body proportionality of infants one year after newborn intensive care. *J Pediatr* 1989;114:288–292.

306. Hack M, Weissman B, Borawski-Clark E. Catch-up growth during childhood among very-low-birth-weight children. *Arch Pediatr Adolesc Med* 1996;150:1122–1129.

307. Gurney JM, Jelliffee D. Arm anthropometry in nutritional assessment: normogram for rapid calculation of muscle circumference and cross-sectional muscle and fat areas. *Am J Clin Nutr* 1973;26:912–915.

308. Georgieff MK, Amarnath UM, Murphy EL, et al. Serum transferrin levels in the longitudinal assessment of protein energy status in preterm infants. *J Pediatr Gastroenterol Nutr* 1989;8:234–239.

309. Shenai JP, Jhaveri BM, Reynolds JW, et al. Nutritional balance studies in very-low-birth-weight infants: role of soy formula. *Pediatrics* 1981;67:631–637.

310. Koo WW. Laboratory assessment of nutritional bone disease in infants. *Clin Biochem* 1996;29:429–438.

311. Inder TE, Clemett RS, Austin NC, et al. High iron status in very low birth weight infants is associated with an increased risk of retinopathy of prematurity. *J Pediatr* 1997;131:541–544.

Breastfeeding and the Use of Human Milk in the Neonatal Intensive Care Unit

Kathleen A. Marinelli   Kathy Hamelin

OVERVIEW

Over the past two decades, as advances in technology have markedly improved our success in neonatal medicine, we have concomitantly recognized that nutrition is the cornerstone of the care we provide to sick and preterm neonates. The introduction and refinement of total parenteral nutrition, and the development of specialty premature enteral formulas have paralleled these improved outcomes. Over this same time period, there has also been an increasing awareness by both the general public and the medical community of the short- and long-term advantages of both human milk and breastfeeding. Based on a rapidly increasing body of research, there is no question that human milk is uniquely superior to other forms of nutrition for infants. The most recent American Academy of Pediatrics (AAP) policy statement on the use of human milk reminds us that the breastfed infant is the reference or normative model against which all alternative feeding methods must be measured regarding growth, health, development, and other short- and long-term outcomes (1). This position is endorsed and echoed by the American College of Obstetrics and Gynecology (2), the American Academy of Family Physicians (3), the American Dietetic Association (4), and the Canadian Pediatric Society (5). The evidence for the advantages of human milk to not only babies, but mothers, families and society in such diverse areas as health, nutrition, development, and immunology, with psychological, social, economic, and environmental impact (1–4) is so compelling that the U. S. government has made the support

and promotion of breastfeeding a national public health priority. With the release of the Surgeon General's HHS *Blueprint for Action on Breastfeeding* (6) and the United States Breastfeeding Committee's *Breastfeeding in the United States: A National Agenda* (7) the federal government has embraced the Healthy People 2010 breastfeeding goals of 75% initiation, 50% breastfeeding at 6 months, and 25% breastfeeding at 1 year (8). The June 2004 launching of a 3 year, $40 million National Breastfeeding Awareness Campaign by the U.S. Department of Health and Human Services, Office of Women's Health, with the tag line "Babies were born to be breastfed" exclusively for 6 months, is clear indication of the commitment to breastfeeding promotion and support (9). Produced in conjunction with the Ad Council, whose previous credits include "Only you can prevent forest fires," "A mind is a terrible thing to waste," and "Friends don't let friends drive drunk," these Public Service Announcements will target the general market, particularly first time parents, and the African American community, as rates of breastfeeding are lowest among this population (10).

In the ideal scenario, a discussion of breastfeeding generally conjures up a Madonna-like picture of a robust, healthy term newborn, eagerly latched and nursing well with a mother who has had an uncomplicated delivery and is supported and empowered by her ability to continue to nourish her baby. However, the reality of the neonatal intensive care unit (NICU) is often in stark contrast to this. Are the uncertainty, the stress, the technology, the constantly changing and critical nature of our patients and our environment incompatible with the concept of breast-feeding? On the contrary, for these most vulnerable of our patients and their families, the exponentially increasing body of research supports that both the provision of human milk and breastfeeding are not only as important as they are in the full term population, but in fact may be more critical to the ultimate health and developmental outcome of these sick and premature babies. The AAP policy statement specifically recommends human milk as the preferred feeding not only for healthy term infants, but for sick and premature infants as well (1).

It is incumbent on us as practitioners to have the knowledge and the expertise to promote and successfully support lactation in the NICU population. Unfortunately, most of us received a cursory education on lactation, if at all, during medical school, residency and fellowship training. The same is true of nursing, nurse practitioner and physician assistant training. This is evidenced by the lack of physician knowledge of and confidence in the subject (11–13), the variable and non-evidence-based information present in current general pediatric textbooks (14) and the paucity of neonatal textbooks that even include it. This chapter presents our current knowledge of the unique benefits of the use of human milk in a preterm and sick NICU population, supporting an evidence-based rationale for its important role in our therapeutic regimen. It will also detail the challenges to the provision of human milk, including the decision to express human milk and breastfeed, initiating and maintaining lactation with a breast pump, breast milk supply, the use of donor human milk, the developmental progression toward breastfeeding, the use of alternative feeding methods, and supporting breastfeeding in the NICU and after discharge.

BACKGROUND

Prior to the advent of NICUs and the technology that has made them possible, most premature infants did not survive. Those that were developmentally and physiologically mature enough did so if they could be kept warm, and nourished. The source of that nourishment was human milk. It would then not be an unreasonable leap of faith to say, that until this past century, the survival of premature infants was in large part dependent on the provision of human milk. As early as 1907, Pierre Budin, at L'Hôpital Maternité in Paris, encouraged mothers of premature infants to breastfeed to improve survival (15). Julius Hess, who in Chicago began the first continuously operating center for premature infants in the United States, wrote in 1922 "by far the best results are obtained in the premature infant weighing less than 1500 grams when it is fed human milk" (16). He advocated that human milk was the choice for feeding premature infants, with artificial milk a poor substitute, resulting in increased mortality. It is astounding that at that time there was even positive discussion about the survival of very low birth weight babies, let alone the association of improved survival with human milk feedings!

So why are we just now "re-discovering" the value of human milk in the neonatal unit? In 1947 Gordon showed that premature infants fed two different formulas based on bovine milk gained weight faster than infants who were fed human milk (17). It had also been previously shown that human milk did not support bone mineralization in premature infants unless supplemented with calcium and phosphorus (18). Based on studies like these, the use of human milk was abandoned in the United States for formulas that provided higher protein and mineral intakes. Although the latter was an important observation that needs to be considered today, what was not realized at the time, was how much was lost to obtain this gain.

INCIDENCE OF BREASTFEEDING OR PROVISION OF HUMAN MILK

Until very recently (19,20), the only on-going large-scale source of breastfeeding data in the United States has been the Ross Laboratories Mothers Survey (21,22), which was developed in 1954 and is periodically updated. Ross Products is a division of Abbott Laboratories, a manufacturer of infant formulas. Surveys are mailed to large numbers of mothers who have given birth within the previous year. Included among concerns of using this data to define breastfeeding rates and goals in the United States are low response rates (average 28% per month since 1997) (21), inability to determine exclusivity of breastfeeding, no differentiation between breastfeeding and breast milk feeding, and conflict of interest in a formula company monitoring breastfeeding rates. Although the population of NICU babies or premature babies per se are not analyzed, data is reported on the subset of babies with birth weights less than 2,500 grams, which would combine both premature babies and small for gestational age term babies. For 1990 the in-hospital breastfeeding rates in this weight category are given as 36.5% (compared to overall population breastfeeding rate of 51.5%) with steady increases to 62.7% (compared to overall increase to 69.5%) in 2001 (21,22). In comparison, recently published data from the Centers for Disease Control and Prevention (CDC), using questions added to the National Immunization Survey for the third quarter of 2001, showed a similar overall U.S. initiation of 65.1% (95% CI: 59.5%–70.7%) (19). The CDC has also looked at breastfeeding in 10 states using the Pregnancy Risk Assessment and Monitoring System (PRAMS). For 1993 they report 57% overall initiation, with 40.3% for babies less than 2500 grams, and 49.4% for babies admitted to the NICU. This improved in 1998 to 67.5% overall initiation, 57.9% low birth weight initiation, and 64.3% NICU initiation (20). These data, although less commercially biased, are still difficult to interpret and compare to other studies as a result of inconsistency of definitions. The definition of initiation of breastfeeding varies between studies, and often includes any attempt at putting a baby to breast or initiating lactation with a breast pump in the first several days of life or during the initial hospitalization. It also does not indicate whether other liquids are given at that time.

These same reports have tried to look at duration of breastfeeding by surveying for any breastfeeding activity later in the first year of life. The Ross Mothers Surveys report continued breastfeeding at 6 months in babies less than 2,500 grams birth-weight increasing from 9.5% in 1990 to 22.1% in 2001 (with concomitant changes in the entire population of 17.6% to 32.5%) (21,22). This data looked at babies with "any breastfeeding"; including only breastfed, breast milk/breastfeeding mixed with formula feedings (no quantification determined), and only occasional breast milk/breastfeeding (again no quantification). For 2001 they added the category of "exclusive" breastfeeding, reporting for all infants in-hospital as 46.3%, falling to 17.2% at 6 months; for babies less than 2,500 grams, 27.1% in-hospital falling to 8.4% at 6 months (21). Exclusive was defined as "fed only human milk; no supplemental formula and/or cow's milk." No information on solid foods or other non-formula supplements (e.g., water, juices) fed to infants were collected (21). The PRAMS study looked at "predominant" breastfeeding at 10 weeks postpartum and showed decreases between 1993 to 1998 of 58.5% to 57.9% in the entire population, 47.9% to 45.1% in the low birth weight subgroup, and 55.1% to 47.3% in the NICU subgroup (20). When duration data is given, it has historically been *any* breastfeeding or breast milk consumption, with no differentiation made for whether other liquids or solids are ingested and in what quantities. This issue was addressed in 1988 by the Interagency Group for Action on Breastfeeding, who developed a set of definitions to standardize terminology. In the system they describe, full breastfeeding is distinguished from partial breastfeeding, with full subdivided into categories of exclusive and almost-exclusive breastfeeding, and partial differentiated into three levels (23). The hope was that consistent widespread implementation of these definitions would assist researchers and agencies to describe, interpret and compare breastfeeding practices accurately. Clearly, this has not occurred.

In March 2004, the Breastfeeding Committee for Canada issued a document on breastfeeding definitions. They used work previously done in this area, including the definitions from the Interagency Group for Action on Breastfeeding, to develop definitions in an algorithmic format that will facilitate data collection that is consistent, and can be used to compare breastfeeding practices between Canadian provinces and territories (Table 23-1) (24). These definitions are well thought out, and clearly delineate the amount of human milk vs. other liquids that are being consumed. The one thing they do not do, however, is to separate out *breast milk feedings* from *breastfeeding*.

When attempting to elucidate trends in breastfeeding and human milk consumption specifically in a NICU population, one can examine a number of reports from individual NICUs. For example, in one author's NICU (KM), breastfeeding rates have been tracked over a 15-year period. During this time, breast-feeding promotion and support has been

TABLE 23-1
BREASTFEEDING DEFINITIONS

Definition	Description
Exclusive Breast milk	No food or liquid other than breast milk, not even water, is given to the infant from birth by the mother, health care provider, or family member/supporter
Total breast milk	No food or liquid other than breast milk, not even water, is given to the infant from birth by the mother, health care provider, or family member/supporter during the past 7 days
Predominant breast milk	Breast milk, given by the mother, health care provider, or family member/supporter plus 1 or a maximum of 2 feeds of any food or liquid including nonhuman milk, during the past 7 days
Partial breast milk	Breast milk, given by the mother, health care provider, or family member/supporter plus 3 or more feeds of any food or liquid including nonhuman milk, during the past 7 days
No breast milk	The infant/child receives no breast milk

Breast milk includes breastfeeding, expressed breast milk or donor milk and undiluted drops or syrups consisting of vitamins, mineral supplements or medicines.
From The Breastfeeding Committee for Canada Breastfeeding Definitions, March 2004, with permission.

greatly increased (which will be detailed later in this chapter). In the entire NICU population, only 20.2% of babies received any human milk (either by breastfeeding or alternative feeding method) in 1989, which steadily increased to 70.8% in 2002. Continuing to receive any human milk at discharge increased from 5.9% to 55.9% of all NICU discharges over this same time period. Even more striking is the data for the population less than 1,500 grams: initiation increased from 10.6% to 82.6% with continued provision of any human milk at discharge from 1.6% to 38.2% (25).

Although the numbers vary, overall trends show an increase in initiation and continuation of breastfeeding activity over the past decade, with significantly fewer babies in low birth weight or NICU categories than healthy, full term babies breastfeeding at any time point. Single institutional reports from the United States and Canada have substantiated that NICU breastfeeding rates are lower than in their equivalent well-baby populations (26–29), with rapid attrition over the course of the hospitalization and after discharge (29–33). Factors often associated with continued lactation in this population are mothers who are older, married, of Caucasian race, with more than a high school education, a good social support system and having babies with increasing birth weight (27,30,33–35). An interesting recent multicenter study by Powers and associates used an administrative database to look at breastfeeding in 42,891 neonates admitted to 124 NICUs from January 1999 to December 2000 (36). They show that 50% of neonates discharged home from

NICUs are not receiving human milk, and they confirm that greater birth weight, older gestational age, white race, increasing maternal age, and married parents are associated with increased likelihood of receipt of at least some human milk at discharge. Of note, they also showed that site of care is a significant independent factor associated with human milk use. This raises questions regarding site differences that are more or less likely to promote successful breastfeeding in an intensive care setting.

It is also important to note that these trends in North American NICUs are not necessarily replicated in other parts of the world. As early as the 1980s, reports from European (37–39), Brazilian (40), and Australian (41) units demonstrate breastfeeding initiation rates, duration, and eventual exclusivity in premature babies that are equal to or higher than those we currently see in our term healthy population! Importantly, these countries have breastfeeding cultures, in which breastfeeding in the term healthy population is the norm, with close to 100% initiation.

ADVANTAGES OF HUMAN MILK FOR PREMATURE AND COMPROMISED BABIES

Human milk is a living, changing fluid. It contains over 200 known components, including live lymphocytes, macrophages, neutophils; immunoglobulins, complement, and other host defense factors; lactoferrin; enzymes and hormones such as corticosteroids, erythropoietin, and insulin to name a few, in addition to its nutrients. There are complex interactions between these components, which likely enhance and contribute to their functions. It is ever-changing, from the beginning to the end of a feeding session, throughout the course of the day, and over the course of lactation. It can never be replicated, no matter how much advertising to the contrary is implied. Adding a "new" component to artificial formula that is present in human milk does not in any way guarantee that its function or performance will be identical. Human milk has changed and adapted over the course of human evolution to provide exactly what human infants need. It differs from the milk of other mammalian species, including bovines, which have concomitantly evolved to provide what the young of each of those species require to optimally grow and mature.

Accepting that human milk is the species-specific gold standard in nutrition for human babies, the outcomes associated with its use are then the norm to which other forms of nutrition are compared. That being the case, instead of a discussion of the "benefits of breastfeeding" as has been our habit, it is more accurate to look at the "risks of artificial feeding." There is a large evidence-based body of literature detailing improved health and developmental outcomes of human milk-fed term babies and their mothers, over artificially fed babies, which have been well reviewed elsewhere (1–4,42–46). The economic savings to families, health care payers, employers, and society have also been

TABLE 23-2
SUMMARY OF THE DISADVANTAGES OF NOT BREASTFEEDING

Infant/Child:
  Increased incidence/severity of:
    Diarrheal diseases
    Respiratory infections
    Otitis media
    Urinary tract infections
    Infant botulism
    Sudden infant death
      syndrome
    Sepsis
    Meningitis
    Allergic diseases
    Type 1 Diabetes mellitus
    Celiac disease
    Some childhood cancers
      (leukemias, lymphomas)
    Inflammatory bowel disease
Mother:
  Increased potential risk for:
    Postpartum blood loss
    Anemia
    Premenopausal breast
      cancer
    Ovarian cancer
    Osteoporosis
Inability to take advantage of
  Lactational Amenorrhea
  Method (LAM) of family
  planning

Economic:
  Families:
    Cost of formula
    Increased sick child visits
    Increased medication use
      and costs
    Lost wages for sick child
      care
  Employers:
    Employee absence for sick
      child care
    Reduced productivity
    Potential for higher health
      insurance rates
  Payers:
    Increased physician
      fees
    Increased emergency room
      fees
    Laboratories/x-rays fees
    Increased prescriptions
    Hospitalization costs
  Society:
    Use of natural resources in
      production of artificial
      feedings
    Environmental costs of
      production and wastes
      generated

studied. Table 23-2 summarizes these disadvantages of using artificial formulas.

There is every reason to assume that these same advantages of human milk to term, healthy babies also apply to preterm and sick neonates. Additionally, there is increasing research-based evidence of both short- and long-term positive effects on prematurity-related conditions, including nutrition, gastrointestinal (GI) function, host defense, neurodevelopment, and physiological well-being.

Nutritional Advantages

Both the AAP (1) and the Canadian Paediatric Society (5) strongly recommend that breast milk is not only the preferred nutrition for healthy term infants, but for all infants, including premature and sick newborns, with rare exceptions (1). For an excellent in-depth examination of this topic please see Chapter 22. The reader is also referred to a recent review article of the use of human milk for premature infants (47).

There are several points that are worth reiterating here. Preterm milk is different than term milk (Table 23-3). Notably, preterm milk has higher concentrations of protein, fatty acids, sodium, and chloride (48,49), which interestingly, are all components required in higher amounts by babies born early. This phenomenon was initially attributed to lower milk volumes produced by mothers of preterm babies, thus causing a concentrating effect on these nutrients.

TABLE 23-3
COMPARISON OF PRETERM TO TERM HUMAN MILK

Increased in Preterm Milk	Unchanged in Preterm Milk
Total nitrogen	Volume
Protein nitrogen	Calories
Long-chain fatty acids	Lactose (?less)
Medium-chain fatty acids	Fat
Short-chain fatty acids	Linolenic acid
Sodium	Potassium
Chloride	Calcium
Magnesium (?)	Phosphorous
Iron	Copper
	Zinc
	Osmolality
	Vitamin B1–12

Lawrence KA, Lawrence RM. eds. Reprinted with permission from Breastfeeding. A Guide for the Medical Profession, 1999:445.

However, contrary to this theory, other components of preterm milk are present in the same concentrations as in term milk. It has subsequently been shown that preterm milk has similar volumes as term milk, so this is a true occurrence. Some have speculated that this is a maternal adaptation to the delivery of her premature baby, although others suggest that these differences are the end result of the interruption in maturation of the mammary gland during pregnancy. In a recent study looking at total nitrogen, fat, lactose and carbohydrate concentrations, gestational age at birth (GA) was inversely related to carbohydrate concentration; postmenstrual age (PMA; an indicator of autonomous developmental processes not affected by the moment of birth) was not related to milk composition; although postnatal age (PNA) was related to a decrease in total nitrogen and an increase in lactose concentration. This data was interpreted to indicate that PNA strongly influences the development of the composition of very preterm human milk, GA affects carbohydrate content with a negligible effect on the nutritional value of the milk, although PMA has no effect (50).

The higher concentration of nutrients in preterm human milk all decrease to approximately term milk levels over the course of the first postnatal month, regardless of the gestational age of the baby at delivery, although the premature baby's increased needs continue until approximately term corrected gestational age. With the advantage the earlier higher concentrations, particularly of protein and electrolytes, that premature milk afforded no longer being present, we are often required to fortify human milk for the smallest babies. Babies less than 1,500 grams have been shown to require fortification with more calories, protein, calcium, phosphorus, sodium chloride and some vitamins to preclude poor growth rates, hyponatremia, hypochloremia, and osteopenia (47). Larger, more mature babies thrive on mother's milk alone. Because human milk content differs not only over the course of lactation, but during the course of a feed or milk expression session, at different times of the day, and for those babies requiring feeding by alternative methods, by the method used, it is critical to monitor these very low birth weight babies for growth rates, serum sodium levels, and bone mineralization status (see Chapter 22).

Protein

Human milk protein is 80% whey, as opposed to bovine milk protein, which is 80% casein. The whey in human milk, α-lactalbumin, is much more easily digested than bovine whey, which is β-lactalbumin, an important factor to consider for premature babies with immature gut function. Additionally, human milk protein also includes nucleotides, secretory immunoglobin A (sIgA) and other immunoglobulins, and an enzyme, lysozyme, all of which are thought to aid in host defense; growth factors that stimulate gut growth and maturation; a variety of hormones; and enzymes (e.g., mammary amylase, lipases) that enhance the immature intestinal tract's ability to digest nutrients. The amino acid taurine, which serves many functions in the newborn including bile acid conjugation, osmoregulation, neurotransmission, and as an antioxidant and a growth factor, is present in high concentrations in human milk and is almost absent in bovine milk. Hence, it is added to artificial feedings. Unlike bovine milk, human milk is also low in phenylalanine and tryrosine, which the premature and newborn infant are poorly equipped to metabolize. For these reasons among others, human milk protein composition is well-adapted to the needs of premature babies (see Chapter 22) (51).

Lipids

Human milk lipids have sparked the greatest interest in milk components recently, with the increasing body of literature on the positive neuro-developmental effects of the long-chain polyunsaturated fatty acids (LC-PUFA's), in particular docosahexaenoic acid (DHA) and arachidonic acid (AA). They are found in phospholipids in the brain, retina and red blood cell membranes. These LC-PUFA's are not readily synthesized by preterm babies, and are normally delivered via the placenta. They occur naturally in human milk, but are not found in bovine milk. For premature babies, they must be delivered via an external source, in this case easily by human milk. Because of studies that show improved neuro-developmental outcome and visual function in breastfed preterm babies and in formula-fed preterm babies supplemented with exogenous sources of LC-PUFA's, DHA and AA have now been added commercially to most term and preterm infant formulas. Of concern is that these additives are of plant origin and are structurally different than human LC-PUFA's (see Neurodevelopmental Advantages).

Human milk lipids are an easily digested source of energy, in part as a result of their composition and in part as a result of their packaging with lipases in the milk, providing approximately 50% of the calories. Additionally they provide cholesterol, which is an essential component of membranes. Human milk-fed babies show significantly higher plasma cholesterol levels than formula-fed babies (52). Although one might then expect them to have higher cholesterol levels than formula-fed babies as adults, the opposite has been found to be true (53). Additionally, coronary artery disease has been shown to be less frequent in persons up to 20 years of age who were initially breast-fed (54). It has been postulated that this early exogenous exposure to cholesterol, a necessary nutrient, keeps endogenous cholesterol production down-regulated, thus resulting in lower cholesterol levels in adult life. The mechanisms remain to be elucidated.

Carbohydrates

The disaccharide lactose is the predominant carbohydrate in human milk. It is a ready source of energy, and is broken down by the enzyme lactase, located in the brush border of the intestinal mucosa, to galactose and glucose, necessary for energy supply to the rapidly growing brain. Lactase activity is low in premature babies, but is readily inducible by exposure to lactose, enabling them to absorb more than 90% from human milk. The remaining unabsorbed lactose contributes to softer stool consistency, and colonization of the gut by nonpathogenic fecal flora. It also enhances calcium absorption, critical to preventing nutritional rickets in prematures. Oligosaccharides, present in human milk as well, act in host defense by preventing bacterial attachment to intestinal mucosa, thus serving a protective role for the relatively immunocompromised preterm infant.

Energy

Several previous studies have suggested that human milk-fed term (55,56) and preterm (57,58) infants have lower sleeping energy expenditure compared with formula-fed infants. A recent randomized, cross-over study of gavage-fed preterm babies showed significantly lower energy expenditure in the human milk fed babies at prefeeding, during feeding, and postfeeding measurements (59). With the vast difference in composition of the nutrients and other factors between human and artificial milk, it is not possible to say what causes this difference, but it is an intriguing difference that remains to be investigated.

Gastrointestinal Advantages

In addition to the species specificity and superior digestibility of the nutrients in human milk for premature babies, human milk also favorably affects the function and maturation of the GI tract. It has been shown *in vivo* to decrease intestinal permeability in preterm infants when compared to preterm formula (60). Several studies have found that human milk promotes more rapid gastric emptying than artificial formula (61,62), with one revealing that on average, human milk emptied twice as fast as formula (62). This has implications for clinical practice.

Delayed gastric emptying, which generally presents clinically as measured gastric residuals or vomiting, prevents advancement of enteral nutrition. Babies who cannot reach full enteral feeds require longer periods of parenteral nutrition, with the concomitant risks inherent in both prolonged intravenous catheter usage (e.g., infection, thrombosis, chemical infiltrates) and prolonged intravenous nutrition (e.g., mineral or electrolyte imbalance, hepatic damage). Any of these can impact length of stay, which in turn has economic and social/family implications, all of which are important to consider in the therapeutic plan in our NICUs today. In fact, other studies suggesting that human milk is better tolerated by the GI tract of premature babies than formula have looked at the marker "time to full feeds." Several have shown that infants fed human milk achieve full enteral feeds significantly faster than those fed artificial formulas (63,64). This would also be expected to have a positive impact on length of stay.

Another related finding is the induction of lactase activity by feedings. Lactase, the enzyme responsible for the digestion of lactose, is present in the fetal intestine early in gestation, but the greatest increase occurs during the third trimester. Hence, premature babies are lactase-deficient at birth. In one study, lactase activity was induced in preterm babies (26–30 weeks gestation) by the initiation of enteral feeds. Of greatest significance, the highest levels of enzyme activity were seen with the introduction of "early" feeds (4 days old) as opposed to "standard" feeds (15 days old) and in human milk-fed vs. formula-fed babies (65). There was also an inverse correlation between lactase activity at 28 days, and the time to achieve full enteral feeds. It appears that the level of lactase activity may be a marker of intestinal maturity, with human milk use being directly related to the progression of that maturity.

There are a large number of "bioactive components" in human milk that are not present in formulas. They variously provide antiinflammatory effects or protection from infectious agents; or are hormones and growth factors that influence development; or are immune function modulators (66). This is an active area of research with many questions remaining to be answered. At least a few of these factors have activity suggesting they may be involved in GI maturation, growth and motility (67). Epidermal growth factor (EGF) is a major growth-promoting cytokine that stimulates proliferation of intestinal mucosa and epithelium and strengthens the mucosal barrier to antigens (68,69). In an animal model, EGF isolated from human milk has been shown to facilitate gut healing after induced injury (69). Other factors identified in human milk, known as human growth factors I, II and III and insulin-like growth factor, have been shown to have growth-promoting functions, including stimulation of deoxyribonucleic acid (DNA) synthesis and cellular proliferation. *In vivo* studies in animal species have shown remarkable increases in the mass of intestinal mucosa after feedings with colostrum, which contains these factors, but not after feedings with artificial milk (70,71). It is intriguing to postulate that factors such as these in human milk may be important to the maturation and development of the premature GI tract, as well as being important to intestinal repair after damage as a result of disease processes such as necrotizing enterocolitis.

Host Defense Advantages

One of the single most extraordinary advantages of the use of human milk over formula in the preterm and NICU patient is the effect on host defense and infections. This reason alone is enough to make the use of human milk the gold standard in this population. The myriad of hormones, factors, cytokines, proteins, enzymes, nucleotides, antioxidants, immunoglobulins, and live, functioning leukocytes contained within human milk (72), their interactions and the milieu in which they effect action, is not and cannot ever be duplicated in an artificial milk. And our knowledge is just beginning to scratch the surface.

One can think of human milk as not only the perfect form of nutrition, but also as "baby's first immunization." One type of immunization is the passive transfer of antibody. Examples include the use of intravenous immune globulin, tetanus immune globulin, rabies immune globulin, or respiratory syncytial immune globulin. The immunoglobulins represented in a mother's milk are a history of many of the infectious agents she has been exposed to, and developed antibody to, during her lifetime. By transferring these antibodies to her baby through her milk, she is then in effect "immunizing" her baby against those organisms. This process is a continuum from the one begun in utero by the passage of maternal antibody across the placenta. Taking this one step further is the concept of the enteromammary immune system, first proposed in 1979 by Kleinman and Walker (73) (Fig. 23-1). In this schema, antigen presented to the maternal mouth and gut is brought into proximity of lymphoid follicles in the maternal GI tract. The antigen's presence commits maternal lymphoblasts to specific IgA production against that antigen. These lymphoblasts migrate via the mesenteric nodes and the thoracic duct into the systemic circulation, in which they find their way into the active mammary tissue. There these cells manufacture sIgA, which is secreted into the milk. When the infant ingests the milk, the immunoglobulin present functions in the infant's gut as protection against that specific pathogen. Most sIgA is not absorbed in the infant's intestine, but rather plays an active role in mucosal defense. Although intact immunoglobulin has been found in infant urine, signifying some systemic absorption, most survives intact in the GI tract, and is excreted into the feces. The environment of the neonatal intensive care unit is full of potentially pathogenic organisms. What makes this concept of the enteromammary immune system even more appealing is that during skin to skin (kangaroo) care, a neonate is held by the mother at her chest, and is touched, kissed, and caressed. The mother exposes herself to any potential pathogens to which her baby has also been in contact. Through the enteromam-

mary immune system, she makes antibody to those particular organisms, and then in subsequent feedings, she passes that antibody to her baby, to help protect him/her. Imagine—individually prepared immunizations to help protect each different baby in the NICU!

Similarly to our previous discussion of concentrations of specific nutrients, many of these immune modulators are in higher concentration in preterm milk than term milk, helping to compensate for the premature baby's immature immune function (Table 23-4). When major factors were quantified and compared between colostrum of mothers delivering both prematurely (28–36 weeks) and at term (38–40 weeks), mean concentrations of IgA, lysozyme, lactoferrin, and absolute counts of total cells, macrophages, lymphocytes, and neutrophils were found to be significantly higher in the preterm colostrum (74). The degree of prematurity did not influence the antiinfective levels in the colostrum. However, the total cells and macrophages were significantly higher in the colostrum of mothers delivering at 28–32 weeks of gestation compared to 33–36 weeks gestation ($p < 0.05$) (74). These differences make the use of early colostrum and human milk critical in the care of premature and sick babies, both as prevention and also possibly in treatment of infectious disease.

Another likely factor in improved immune defense with the use of human milk is the affect on fecal flora. The normal flora of the intestines of a breastfed infant is predominantly the gram positive bacteria *Lactobacillus bifidus*. Non-human milk-fed babies are colonized with many more types of bacteria, most of which are the potentially pathogenic gram negative bacteria. With establishment of *Lactobacillus* as the predominant bacteria inhabiting the premature infant's GI tract, the likelihood of a serious or life-threatening gram negative infection would be expected to decrease.

It has long been known that breastfed babies are at decreased risk of a number of infectious diseases—respiratory infections, otitis media, gastroenteritis, and diarrhea—and are at decreased risk of mortality. These protections accrue in a dose-dependent fashion—i.e., the more breast milk a baby receives, statistically the better protected they are. Although much of the earlier work was done in Third-World countries, and commonly held beliefs are that breastfeeding does not make a difference in industrialized nations like the United States, there are now many studies that show significant impact in these populations as well (75–78). There has even been a study looking at breastfeeding and the risk of postneonatal deaths in the United States which shows promoting breastfeeding has the potential to save or delay about 720 postneonatal deaths each year (79)! It is probably fair to assume that babies admitted to NICUs, once attaining term corrected gestational age and discharged to home, will accrue similar advantages from breast milk/breastfeeding as their healthier term counterparts in these studies. But even more importantly for our population, an increasing body of research has been done looking at the effects of a diet of

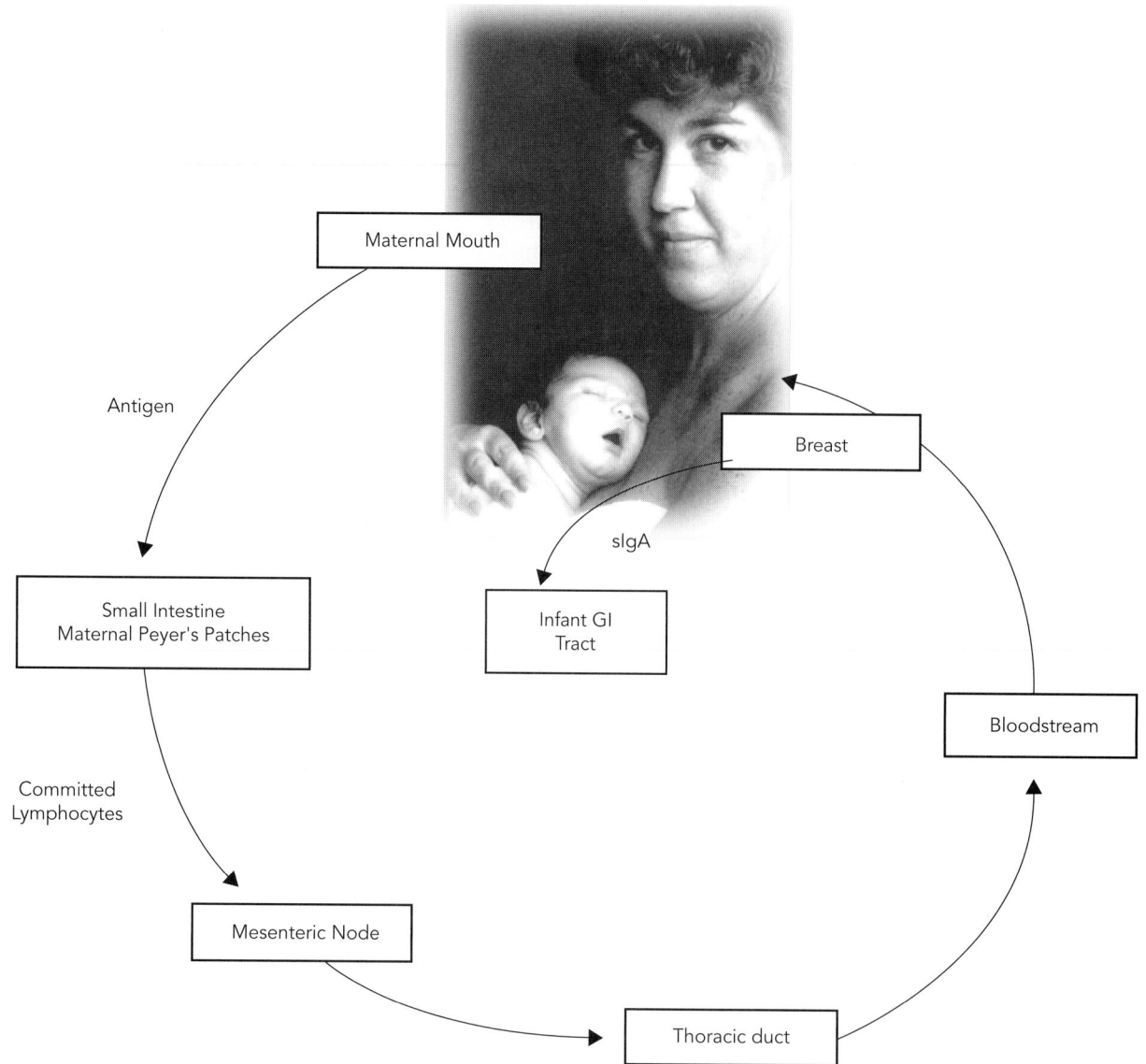

Figure 23-1 The Enteromammary Immune System. Adapted from Kleinman RE, Walker, WA. The enteromammary immune system: an important new concept in breast milk host defense. *Dig Dis Sci* 1979;24:880.

human milk compared to preterm formula in premature and low birth weight babies, with respect to clinical infections. The data is clear—premature babies fed human milk are at significantly less risk of serious diseases, including necrotizing enterocolitis, urinary tract infections, sepsis, and meningitis.

As early as 1971, a report from Sweden showed a protective effect of breastfeeding against sepsis in the newborn (80). Then in 1980, Narayanan and her group in India reported that even partial use of human milk (81), and subsequently exclusive use (82) could significantly decrease the incidence of infection in a premature and low birth weight population. In the first study, infants fed human milk supplemented with formula had a 6% incidence of sepsis, compared to a 21% incidence in those fed formula alone (81). In the second, in 62 infants studied, no sepsis occurred in those infants receiving human milk exclusively,

although six episodes occurred in those fed formula (82). A further study by this group looked at the dose-response effect of human milk in the prevention of infection (83). Infections noted were sepsis, diarrhea, pneumonia, meningitis, conjunctivitis, pyoderma, thrush, and upper respiratory infections. The strongest effect was noted in those babies fed exclusive human milk, followed by partial feedings of human milk. In a United States study, a decrease in blood culture proven sepsis was seen in those infants fed their own mothers' milk compared to those fed formula (27% vs. 58%, $p < 0.05$) (63) More recently in another U.S. neonatal unit, El-Mohandes and associates showed a significantly decreased incidence of sepsis, in each of three time periods through the first 38 days of life, for infants admitted to the NICU who received human milk vs. formula (odds ratio for sepsis in human milk-fed infants was 0.4, 95% confidence limits, 0.15 to 0.95, $p = 0.04$) (84).

TABLE 23-4

COMPARISON OF ANTIINFECTIVE PROPERTIES OF PRETERM AND TERM MOTHER'S COLOSTRUM

	Preterm Colostrum	Term Colostrum
Total protein (g/L)	0.43 ± 1.3	0.31 ± 0.05*
IgA (mg/g protein)	310.5 ± 70	168.2 ± 21*
IgG (mg/g protein)	7.6 ± 3.9	8.4 ± 1
IgM (mg/g protein)	39.6 ± 23	36.1 ± 16
Lysozyme (mg/g protein)	1.5 ± 0.5	1.1 ± 0.3*
Lactoferrin (mg/g protein)	165 ± 37	102 ± 25*
Total cells/ ml3	6794 ± 1946	3064 ± 424*
Macrophages	4041 ± 1420	1597 ± 303*
Lymphocytes	1850 ± 543	954 ± 143*
Neutrophils	842 ± 404	512 ± 178**

$* p < 0.001; ** p < 0.005$
Modified from Mathur NB, Dwarkadas AM, Sharma VK, et al. Anti-infective factors in preterm human colostrum. *Acta Paediatr Scand* 1990;79:1039–1044.

Hylander and colleagues published an elegant study in 1998 in which they looked at 212 VLBW infants born at Georgetown University Medical Center (85). They not only looked at incidence of infection among these babies in relationship to their type of feeding, but they also controlled for confounding factors. Infection was documented as clinical signs of sepsis along with positive cultures for pathogenic organisms from one or more of the following sites: blood, spinal fluid, urine, stool, pleural fluid, nasopharyngeal, intravascular catheter, umbilicus, eye, or surgical wound. Additionally, pneumonia (by chest radiograph) and necrotizing enterocolitis (Bell's classification) were included. Human milk feeding was defined as receiving any human milk, with supplemental formula feedings when milk was not available. Formula-fed babies received only formula. They found that the incidence of infection (human milk 29.3% vs. formula 47.2%) and sepsis/meningitis (human milk 19.5% vs. formula 32.6%) dif-

fered significantly by type of feeding (Fig. 23-2). Human milk was independently correlated with a reduced odds ratio of infection (OR = 0.43, 95% CI, 0.23–0.81), controlling for gestational age, 5-minute APGAR score, days on mechanical ventilation, and days without enteral feeds. Human milk feeding was also independently correlated with a reduced odds ratio of sepsis/meningitis (OR = 0.47, 95% CI 0.23–0.95), controlling for gestational age, mechanical ventilation days, and days without enteral feeds. And remember, the human milk-fed babies were supplemented with formula, so if they had been exclusively breastfed, one wonders if the difference would have been even more remarkable?

In 1999, Schanler and his colleagues showed that in a group of premature infants between 26 to 30 weeks gestation, those fed predominantly fortified human milk were discharged earlier (73 ± 19 vs. 88 ± 47 days) and had lower incidence of necrotizing enterocolitis (NEC) and late-onset sepsis than infants fed preterm formula (86). This data on NEC confirms a previous study by Lucas and Cole (87), who showed that in a cohort of 926 infants with birthweights below 1850 grams, formula fed babies were six to ten times more likely to develop NEC than those fed human milk exclusively; and three times more likely than babies who received a combination of human milk and formula supplements. Once again, this data shows a dose-response effect of human milk. While reviewing the data on NEC it is also important to point out that in addition to these significant clinical decreases in incidence of NEC, there are also concomitant significant savings in economic costs. This is an enormous issue to us as practitioners, to the health care system as a whole, and certainly to the individual families we care for. A reduction in the cases of NEC would engender significant savings in medical charges, and length of stay (LOS). Bisquera and associates (88) showed that infants with surgical NEC exceeded LOS by 60 days over matched controls, and medical NEC by 22 days over

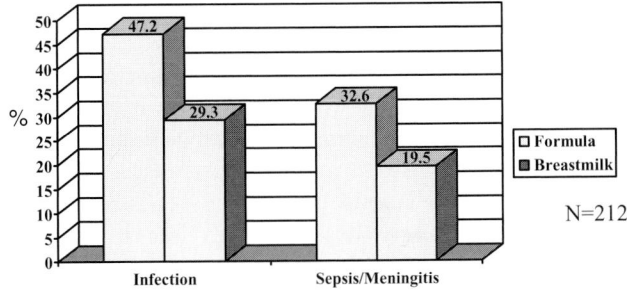

Figure 23-2 The incidence of all infections and of significant infections (sepsis/meningitis) in VLBW babies in formula vs. breast milk-fed groups, is significantly different even when controlling for confounding factors. Infection OR = 0.43; 95% CI 0.23–0.81; sepsis/meningitis OR = 0.47; 95% CI 0.23–9.95) n = 212. From Hylander MA, Strobino DM, Dhanireddy R. Human milk feedings and infection among very low birth weight infants. *Pediatrics* 1998;102:e38.

controls. Based on LOS, the estimated total hospital charges per baby for surgical NEC averaged $186,200 more and medical NEC $73,700 more than controls. This translated into yearly additional hospital charges at their institution for NEC of $6.5 million, or $216,666 per survivor! When parents' time and wages and prevention of premature deaths are also considered, the total savings in the United States alone are more than $3 billion if only 75% of preterm infants received human milk feedings and their incidence of NEC decreased from 7% to 1% (89)! The significance of these statistics cannot be ignored.

Just as the etiology of NEC is not completely understood, and is certainly multi-factorial, so the mechanism underlying the protection against NEC afforded by breast milk is also not completely understood, and most likely multi-factorial. One study showed a decreased prevalence of NEC in premature infants who were given enteral doses of a serum-derived IgA-IgG product, with IgA predominance, similarly to that found in human milk (90). This leads one to postulate that the immunoglobulins, in particular IgA, present in human milk have a role to play in NEC prevention. It is also known that platelet-activating factor (PAF) is one of the inflammatory mediators that is known to be higher in babies with NEC, and that in experimental models, it causes bowel necrosis similar to that seen in NEC, when injected intravenously. PAF is rapidly broken down by PAF acetylhydrolase, which has been shown to be not only present in human milk, but to be approximately 5-fold higher in preterm than in term milk (91). This may yet be another mechanism by which breast milk is protective. Additionally we have previously discussed the predominance of nonpathogenic fecal flora in breastfed infants. Could this not be another protective mechanism? There are certainly many other biologically active substances in human milk that may ultimately be found to have a role in the prevention of NEC.

It is unclear how much human milk is needed to see these effects. In the previously discussed Hylander study (85), the human milk-fed group also received supplements of formula and still showed significant benefit. Narayanan (83) showed a dose-response in that exclusive human milk was more protective than partial, which was still more protective than no human milk. And Lucas and Cole showed that in NEC, partial human milk feeding was protective, but less so than exclusive human milk feedings (87). Furman and colleagues, looking at 119 VLBW babies, identified a daily threshold amount of at least 50 ml/kg/day of maternal milk through week 4 of life as needed to decrease rates of sepsis in this group (92). These data are convincing that by providing human milk, we do make a difference in these serious morbidities in even the tiniest of our patients. And it certainly appears that there is a dose-response relationship. That being the case, with all the potential morbidities that our patients face, and the costs both economically and emotionally for these families and society, it is without a doubt worth our efforts to make human milk the gold standard in neonatal intensive care for these reasons alone. It has also been shown that

upper respiratory symptoms are reduced for those low birth weight babies through seven months corrected age who continue to receive human milk after discharge from the NICU (93). Although not significant, a trend appears to exist for otitis media, bronchiolitis, and gastroenteritis as well. More studies with larger cohorts are needed to confirm these data.

Neurodevelopmental Advantages

Much press has been given to recent work that shows improved cognitive development in babies who receive human milk. In 1988 Morley and associates showed an 8-point cognitive advantage using the Bayley Scales of Infant Development for 771 infants with birth weights less than 1850 grams (94). After controlling for demographic and perinatal factors, a 4.3-point advantage still remained. When this cohort was followed up at 7.5 to 8 years of age, infants who had received human milk by tube (rather than breastfeeding) continued to show an 8.3-point IQ advantage (over half a standard deviation) even after adjustments were made for difference in mother's education and social class (95). They also showed a dose response relationship between the proportion of human milk in the diet and subsequent IQ. In a second randomized prospective study, these same researchers compared premature infants who received mature donor human milk with those who received premature formula as their early enteral nutrition. These diets were compared as sole enteral feeds or as supplemental feeding to their own mother's expressed milk. No differences in outcome were seen at 18 months between the two diet groups, despite the low nutrient content of mature donor milk in relation to preterm formula. Additionally, when they compared the infants from this study fed solely on mature donor milk with infants from a previous study fed solely standard term formula, the infants fed the mature donor milk had higher developmental scores, again supporting the positive role of human milk on cognitive development (96). Bier and colleagues have also looked at the effects of human milk on both cognitive and motor development. They found that in a cohort of 39 premature infants, those who received human milk had significantly higher motor scores at 3 and 12 months corrected ages than those fed formula. Additionally, when adjusting for oxygen requirement and maternal vocabulary scores, human milk-fed babies continued to show an advantage in both cognitive and motor scores at 12 months. There was also an association between the amount of human milk intake while in the special care nursery (dose response relationship!), and cognitive development at both 7 and 12 months corrected ages (97).

There has been one meta-analysis of controlled studies looking at the question of human milk and cognitive development (98). It demonstrated a 3.16-point higher score for cognitive development in human milk-fed babies compared with formula after adjustment for significant covariates. This difference was observed as early as 6 months and was sustained through 15 years of age, the last time of reliable measurement. Longer duration of breast-feeding was accompanied by greater differences in cognitive development (dose related response). Whereas normal weight infants showed a 2.66-point difference in IQ scores between breastfed and formula fed groups, the difference was even more remarkable, a 5.18-point difference, in low-birth-weight infants. The results of this meta-analysis suggest that not only does human milk contribute to higher neurodevelopment, but that the effect is even more striking in a much more high-risk population, the low-birth-weight infant.

Postulated to be responsible for at least a portion of these neurodevelopmental advantages of human milk is the presence of long-chain polyunsaturated fatty acids (LC-PUFAs), which until recently, were not present in formulas (Please see Chapter 22 for a more in-depth review). Docosahexaenoic acid (DHA), normally accounts for greater than one-third of the total fatty acids of the gray matter of the brain and the retina of the eye (99). Most of the prenatal accumulation of DHA in these tissues occurs in the third trimester—thus by definition, premature infants are deficient compared to their term counterparts. Animal studies have shown that deficiency of DHA in neural tissues during development leads to behavioral and retinal changes.

Other examples of the effects of human milk on neurological maturation have also been observed. Premature infants receiving human milk have been shown to have faster brainstem maturation than those on formula (100). Visual acuity and the development of retinopathy of prematurity have also been studied. A number of studies were performed before the routine addition of the LC-PUFAs to preterm formulas. In one, the researchers showed improved visual acuity of preterm infants up to four months of age in supplemented vs. nonsupplemented formulas (99). In another, improved retinal function was present in LC-PUFA sufficient VLBW neonates fed human milk or supplemented formula as compared to an unsupplemented formula group with lower LC-PUFA cell composition (101). Better visual evoked potentials and acuity in both preterm and term infants at 57 weeks postconception has been seen in those fed human milk as opposed to those fed formula (102). Additionally, another interesting study in which healthy term infants who breastfed to 4 or 6 months, and then were weaned, were randomly assigned to commercial formulas with or without DHA and arachidonic acid (ARA) supplements. At 1 year of age, the level of DHA as measured in the red blood cells was reduced by 50% from weaning level in the unsupplemented group, although there was an increase of 24% in the supplemented group (103). The conclusions drawn from this study were that the critical period during which a dietary supply of DHA and ARA can contribute to optimizing visual development in term infants extends through the first year of life. This supports the AAP recommendation that breastfeeding continue through the first year of life (1), and begs consideration then of the length of time

breastfeeding should be encouraged and supported for the baby born prematurely.

Physiological Advantages

Breastfeeding is widely assumed to be more stressful than bottle feeding for premature infants, an assumption that has led in many intensive care units to the introduction of bottle feedings as the first oral feeds, and postponing attempts at breastfeeding until babies "can prove themselves with the bottle." There are also often concerns for the small premature baby's ability to maintain temperature while breastfeeding, leading to "rules" restricting initiating breastfeeding until a certain weight is achieved. Additionally, there is the widely held belief that the "suck-swallow-breathe" mechanism is not mature until approximately 34 weeks gestation. Because of the fear that they will choke, desaturate and aspirate, this leads to more "rules" concerning not initiating oral feeds, including breastfeeding, until at least 34 weeks corrected gestational age. It is important to point out that there is no scientific evidence to back any of these statements. On the contrary, the exact opposite is the case as we will discuss. It is also important to understand that these policies, in addition to being unsupported scientifically, are also harmful in that they (a) preclude premature babies and their mothers from early breastfeeding experiences; (b) allow babies whose mothers want to breastfeed to learn to suck from a bottle, which then in many cases makes it hard for them to transfer to the breast at a latter time, as the sucking mechanisms are different; and (c) introduces breastfeeding so late in the hospital stay, that in addition to struggling to overcome what they have learned with an artificial nipple, the mother and baby are often discharged before they have had time to learn together and develop the confidence and skills necessary to allow successful breastfeeding in this population. It is important to re-emphasize our medical dictum in this circumstance: *Primum non nocere.*

Data does exist that enables us to develop breastfeeding policies that are physiologic, safe and supportive of breastfeeding. As early as the 1980s, Meier was publishing data concerning physiologic stability at breast compared to bottle-feeding. She was able to show that in babies less than 1,500 grams at the time of first feeding, different sucking mechanisms were employed for breast and bottle, with better coordination of suck-swallow-breathe during breastfeeding, particularly in the smaller less mature babies. Concomitantly, there are markedly different patterns of transcutaneous oxygen pressure (tcPO2) for the two methods of feeding. TcPO2 patterns suggest less ventilatory interruption during breastfeeding than during bottle-feeding with greater declines in tcPO2 during bottle-feeding than during breastfeeding over the course of a feeding session. Additionally, babies became significantly warmer during breastfeeding than during bottle-feeding (104–106). Similar studies done by Bier and colleagues in first VLBW (107), and then ELBW (108) babies showed they could tolerate beginning breast- and bottle feedings at the same postnatal age; that they were less likely to have oxygen desaturations to less than 90% during breastfeeding; and that they had lower intakes during breastfeeding. Given that there is no data supporting the safety of initiating bottles as first feeds, and that there is data to show that during breastfeeding premature babies are more physiologically stable, it would then seem reasonable, safe and scientifically sound to allow mothers to put their babies to nuzzle at breast and to begin early steps toward breastfeeding, once they are physiologically ready!

CHALLENGES TO THE PROVISION OF HUMAN MILK

The Decision to Express Human Milk and Breastfeed

Expressing human milk and subsequently breastfeeding a premature infant has been described as a contribution to the care of her infant that only the mother can make. This is a very powerful, tangible opportunity for these mothers. Additionally, this feeding choice has been considered the one aspect of natural caregiving that the mother does not have to forfeit when she delivers a sick or premature infant. In the past, the decision to provide expressed human milk for the premature infant was regarded as a matter of parental choice with professional responsibility limited to implementing the parent's decision. With increasing and irrefutable evidence that human milk supports the optimal health and nutrition of sick and premature infants, NICU care providers must actively encourage mothers to initiate lactation and provide milk to their infants, even if they do not plan to ultimately feed at the breast.

Parental decisions related to infant feeding must be based on informed choice. Emphasizing the importance of human milk to the health of the infant assists mothers in making an informed decision about feeding method. Health care providers should share research-based evidence about the superiority of human milk and the value of this intervention for the sick or premature infant. It is also important to communicate the maternal benefits of lactation to these mothers, both in terms of her immediate ability to be actively involved in the care of her baby, no matter how sick he or she is, and also in terms of the health benefits she will accrue (2,3). Optimally, this information should be discussed with the family as soon as the premature birth of their baby becomes a possibility. With the understanding that this is not always feasible, it must be discussed as soon after the infant's birth as realistic, so that milk expression can be initiated and colostrum expressed when the hormones of lactation are optimal. Even mothers who had indicated prior to the birth of their child that they desired to feed formula, are often more than willing to initiate milk expression to obtain colostrum for their babies when they understand all the advantages it confers. Written information should reinforce that early human milk is considered "medicine" that prevents infection in this vulnerable popula-

tion. Although staff may worry that this approach is coercive or may make mothers feel guilty about initial feeding plans, mothers who are educated to make an informed choice to provide human milk for their infant report they are thankful for the information that assisted them to support the health of their infant. It is important that families understand that a decision to initiate milk expression does not commit them to breastfeeding. They can decide to stop at any point along the continuum. This is very empowering to these women, who with the birth of a baby who requires intensive care, acutely feel the loss of normal maternal control. Research has demonstrated that structured education and support programs within NICUs are effective in increasing lactation initiation rates, often in mothers who had intended to formula feed (109–110). The positive breastfeeding outcomes of such programs clarify the critical role of health care providers in sharing the science of human milk with mothers so that they can make an informed choice related to infant feeding.

Initiating and Maintaining Lactation with a Breast Pump

Mothers who provide breast milk and eventually breastfeed their premature infants must develop their milk supply through manual or mechanical milk expression techniques. These techniques may be suboptimal compared to actually breastfeeding in stimulating and maintaining a full milk supply. As a result, compromised milk production is a well-documented constraint to extended breastfeeding in the premature mother-infant dyad. An understanding of the physiology of lactogenesis and the effects of various pumps and pumping styles on milk production is critical to understanding this issue and supporting mothers to establish and maintain optimal milk volumes.

The transition from pregnancy to lactation is called lactogenesis. The first half of pregnancy is characterized by growth and proliferation of the mammary ductal system; during the second half of pregnancy, secretory activity increases and the alveoli become distended by accumulating colostrum (111). The capacity of the mammary gland to secrete milk after approximately 16 weeks gestation is referred to as lactogenesis I. The onset of copious milk secretion 2 to 8 days after birth is called lactogenesis II. Triggered by a rapid drop in serum progesterone levels after the delivery of the placenta, lactogenesis II results in a rapid increase in milk volumes from 36 to 96 hours postpartum. Ongoing lactation is dependent on a delicate interplay of hormones and effective stimulation and emptying of the breast. Interference with these processes can delay and/or suppress milk production (112).

Prolactin and oxytocin are the predominant hormones of lactation. Prolactin, the milk-making hormone, is essential for both initiating and maintaining milk supply. As progesterone and estrogen levels abruptly drop after birth, the anterior pituitary gland is no longer inhibited by these hormones and releases pulsatile surges of prolactin in response to suckling at the breast. Frequent breastfeeding in early lactation stimulates the development of receptors to prolactin in the mammary glands and results in a faster increase in milk synthesis (113). The number of prolactin receptors increases in early breastfeeding and remains constant thereafter (114,115). Therefore, early breast stimulation during this critical period is a predictor of later milk production. Oxytocin is the hormone responsible for the removal of milk from the breast. Excreted by the posterior pituitary gland in response to suckling, oxytocin causes the myoepithelial cells surrounding the alveoli to contract and milk to be ejected into the ducts in which it is available to the newborn. The secretion of oxytocin is negatively affected by stress and pain. Therefore, the birth of a premature infant (often by cesarean delivery) and the subsequent stressors associated with this event can interfere with the milk ejection reflex or "let down" of milk from the breast.

After the first few days postpartum, lactation shifts from endocrine control (hormone driven) to autocrine control (driven by milk removal). Galactopoiesis (the maintenance of milk production) is driven by the quality and quantity of milk removal. As long as milk is being removed from the breasts, the alveolar cells will continue to make milk. This supply-demand phenomenon regulates milk production to match intake by the infant (112).

The birth of a premature infant can negatively influence milk production. If a mother has delivered very prematurely, mammary development may be poor because the mother may not have received the full component of pregnancy related hormones to prepare the breasts for lactation (116,117). Additionally, the close infant contact most frequently experienced by mothers following term delivery is limited or absent after premature delivery. As a result, the neurohormonal stimulus of the lactogenic hormones is impaired. An additional barrier to optimal milk expression is the fact that anxiety, fatigue and emotional stress, all powerful inhibitors of lactation, are experienced almost universally in mothers of premature infants (118). As a result, for mothers of premature infants, concerns related to milk production and transfer of adequate milk to the infant are primary reasons for discontinuing breastfeeding or providing supplements. Early, frequent and optimal stimulation of maternal milk supply must replace the natural breastfeeding process to ensure adequate milk production and duration of breastfeeding in this population.

Current research points to three factors that are independently associated with optimizing milk production in mothers who are pumping for a preterm baby. After controlling for maternal age, race, marital status and maternal education, factors significantly associated with ongoing milk supply and breastfeeding at term include initiating breast pumping before 6 hours postpartum, pumping more that 6 times a day, and skin-to-skin contact with the infant (119–121). An additional factor that optimizes ongoing milk production is expressing milk for an adequate duration of time to completely empty the breasts (120). The degree of breast emptying is a strong stimulus

TABLE 23-5
OPTIMAL INITIAL MILK EXPRESSION REGIME

Lactogenesis I—Establishing initial milk supply
- Begin milk expression as soon after birth as possible (optimally within 6 hours)
- Pump frequently (no less than 8 times in 24 hours)
- Pump at least once at night (between 1 AM and 4 AM)
- Use a full-sized (hospital grade) electric breast pump with the ability to pump both breasts simultaneously
- Increase pump suction until milk is flowing and comfort maintained
- Hold infant skin-to-skin prior to pumping if possible
- Use breast massage prior to and during milk expression
- Pump for 10 to 15 minutes and/or until all milk droplets cease flowing
- Maximize rest and minimize stress as much as possible

Lactogenesis II—Maintaining milk supply
- Continue with above regime
- To ensure breasts are emptied, do not pump a specific amount of time, but pump until milk stops flowing, for 2 to 3 minutes

for milk synthesis and may be even more important than the frequency of pumping. Clinical advice therefore should include early ($<$ 6 hours postpartum), frequent (8–10 times in 24 hours) and effective pumping to achieve milk volumes between 800 and 1000 ml per day by 2 weeks postpartum (112) (Table 23-5). This oversupply of milk provides a reserve against diminishing milk production later in lactation.

Mothers who initiate long-term milk expression require a hospital grade electric breast pump; the clinical challenge is ensuring that these pumps are available. Although hospital-grade electric pumps are available through pharmacies, lactation consultants and home health agencies, many mothers are unable to incur this expense. Support and advocacy from health care providers related to the necessity of this equipment for the health of the infant may assist with payment from third party payers. Although some researchers advocate simultaneous pumping as a significant predictor of eventual milk volumes (122,123), other studies have not supported the necessity of pumping both breasts simultaneously (119). However, simultaneous (double) pumping requires less time and effort than sequential (single) pumping; this difference may influence ultimate maternal commitment and ongoing willingness to continue pumping over time.

Human Milk Supply

Despite their best efforts, mothers of premature infants may experience persistent low milk volumes or milk production that decreases over time. Researchers have described a frequent phenomenon of a decreasing milk supply during the second month of pumping (124), which is very often seen by these authors. Because a breast pump does not mimic the physical contact and closeness of an infant during breastfeeding, suboptimal hormonal stimulation may play a role in decreasing milk supply. Little is known about the physiologic response of mechanical milk expression to milk production. Therefore strategies to manage low milk volumes in mothers of premature infants have focused on pharmacological and nonpharmacological enhancement of prolactin secretion (112,125–127).

Kangaroo Care, also called skin-to-skin Care, is an effective nonpharmacological method to enhance maternal milk production through skin-to-skin contact. This intimate contact stimulates the release of the hormones of lactation and positively influences maternal milk supply (128–129). Mothers who engage in Kangaroo Care frequently note feelings of milk-ejection and report pumping larger volumes immediately following holding their infants skin-to-skin. Hurst and colleagues report that mothers who held their infants in Kangaroo Care for 30 minutes per day had significantly greater milk volumes both early (2 weeks) and later (4 weeks) in the postpartum period (128). Breast massage has also been demonstrated to increase volumes of pumped milk. It is done similarly to a breast self-exam. Using the palmar surface of her three middle fingers, a mother starts close to the chest wall and slowly massages in a circular motion, moving toward the areola. Mothers should be instructed to palpate each breast after pumping and subsequently massage the firmer areas to promote complete breast emptying (117).

Ongoing clinical observation of pumped milk volumes will ensure timely intervention to prevent significantly inadequate milk production. Because most premature infants require a minimum of 500 mL per day at discharge, intervention to increase milk volumes should be put into place when milk volumes fall below this level (112). Nonpharmacological interventions to increase milk volumes include increasing pumping frequency and resuming and/or increasing pumping at night, pumping at the infant's bedside, or while holding a picture or an article of baby's clothing or bedding; alternatively pumping in a quiet, low-stress environment; and covering the milk collection bottles with a receiving blanket or towel while pumping (decreases anxiousness, stress hormones? It really works!). Pharmacological measures however should be considered if alternative strategies to increase milk volumes have been employed unsuccessfully for 7 days, milk supply is not fully established despite optimal breast stimulation, and/or milk supply has decreased significantly (by 50% or < 500 mL/day) after optimal initiation.

Pharmacological prolactin enhancers are another strategy to assist with increasing milk supply. Dopamine inhibitors such as Metoclopramide and Domperidone have been used to induce lactation in clinical situations with varying results (125,126,130). Both increase circulating prolactin levels and, with accompanying breast stimulation, are postulated to cause an increase in prolactin receptors and subsequent milk production (113). As a result, these medications are most effective in the early postpartum period when the breast tissue is sensitive to the formation of prolactin receptors. Companies that manufacture these drugs do not endorse their use as galactogogues, so they are used off-label for this purpose (Use of Galactogogues in Initiating or Augmenting Maternal Milk Supply, Appendix C-1). When other strategies to increase milk supply have been applied, however, pharmacological alternatives may be considered to optimize milk production and support ongoing breastfeeding.

THE USE OF MOTHER'S MILK IN NEONATAL INTENSIVE CARE

Guidelines for the collection and storage of human milk ensure optimal quality of human milk that is collected and fed to premature infants. Milk storage and handling are slightly different for the term healthy baby/infant compared to the hospitalized/sick/premature infant (131, 132). Collection technique, collection container and storage conditions play a role in maintaining the unique constituents of human milk and reducing bacterial colonization. Even with meticulous technique, no mother's milk is sterile. Attention to hand washing and cleaning of expression equipment, however, is extremely important in reducing colonization by pathogens other than normal skin flora. Mothers require instruction to ensure that anything coming in contact with the milk or the breasts be cleansed thoroughly prior to each pumping session. Each mother must have her own personal kit. Instructions should include washing all pump parts with hot soapy water after each pumping and sterilizing all equipment once a day. Most NICUs provide sterile hard plastic containers for the collection of human milk in the hospital and at home. These containers provide for the stability of water-soluble constituents and immunoglobulins. Plastic milk bags are not recommended for the collection of milk for hospitalized infants as a result of loss of milk constituents and chance of leakage and contamination during storage and handling. The temperature at which milk is stored determines the duration of storage. Fresh milk, considered optimal for premature infants, must be used or refrigerated, within one hour of expression. If the infant is not fed immediately, expressed milk can be safely kept in the refrigerator for 48 hours. If the milk will not be used within this time frame, it should be frozen. Milk that has been fortified with additives should be used with 24 hours, and should never be frozen (Appendix C-2).

All milk that is used for infant feeding should be stored in the hospital under controlled conditions. Environmental issues are an important aspect of quality control. This includes monitoring refrigerator/freezer temperatures, and routine cleaning and maintenance of storage units and milk preparation areas. All milk should be clearly identified with infant's name, medical record number and date and time of collection and kept in an environment that eliminates the potential for tampering (Appendix C-2).

Human milk, like blood, is a living fluid and should be handled as such. Proper handwashing and/or wearing gloves during preparation and administration prevents potential bacterial contamination. Stringent quality control standards, including a two-nurse check system of identification, minimize potential administration errors (Appendix C-2).

The Use of Donor Human Milk

No chapter on the use of human milk in the NICU is complete without a discussion of donor human milk and its uses. It is beyond the scope of this chapter to present this subject in great depth—for that the reader is referred to more comprehensive discussions (133–136).

If human milk is the perfect food nutritionally, immunologically and developmentally for the sick or premature infant, what happens when that milk is not available? What if the mother died in the postpartum period? What if the mother, despite her best efforts, is not providing adequate volumes to cover the baby's needs? What if the mother is HIV positive in North America? What if the mother was delivered prematurely because she had a diagnosis of breast cancer made during pregnancy, and she must now undergo chemotherapy? What if the mother, despite being optimally informed, decided not to provide breast milk, and now her baby has a severe allergic colitis and is not thriving on any of the expensive hypoallergenic formulas? What if . . . . ? Do these questions sound far-fetched? They are not. They have all occurred within recent memory in one intensive care unit. The answer has always been "provide formula"—or "keep changing formulas around until you find one that works." But is this the best answer? The World Health Organization (WHO) and the United Nations Children's Fund (UNICEF), in their 2003 *Global Strategy for Infant and Young Child Feeding*, recommend banked donor milk as the next option when mother's own milk is not available (137). Although the AAP fell short of endorsing the use of donor milk in its 1997 statement (1), the AAP's 2003 Red Book does contain a section on human milk banks and donor milk (138). The international physician breast-feeding organization, the Academy of Breastfeeding Medicine, supports donor human milk as the preferred human milk supplement in its published clinical protocol for supplementing healthy, term infants in the hospital (139). Many other countries in Europe and South America have donor milk banks and make extensive use of donor human milk.

In North America, the Human Milk Banking Association of North America (HMBANA) developed guidelines that are now mandatory for all member milk banks (140). They require thorough donor screening and testing (similar to that required for organ donors), pasteurization of all milk, and bacteriological quality control of all dispensed milk. The pasteurization process kills all known viruses (including CMV and HIV) and bacteria known to date. Most of the immunologic factors remain intact. IgA is reduced by 20% to 30%; lysozyme activity is only minimally affected; lactoferrin iron-binding capacity is reduced by as much as 60% (141). Even with these reductions, donor milk still has more immunoglobulin, lysozyme, and lactoferrin than formula! There is little effect of pasteurization on the long chain polyunsaturated fatty acids (141).

In 2002 the six milk banks belonging to HMBANA dispensed 501,100 ounces of milk, approximately half of which went to premature or ill NICU babies (when surveyed in 1994) (142).

The benefits of using donor milk are the same as have been discussed for mother's own milk. In fact, many of the studies from Europe on the prevention of NEC and neurodevelopmental outcomes were done using donor milk when own mother's milk was not available. In addition to prematurity and low or nonexistent maternal milk supply, other uses in the NICU include formula intolerance/allergy; short bowel syndrome; other issues of malabsorption such as gastroschisis; multiple births; recovery from NEC; supplementation of the hypoglycemic baby; and supplementation of the dehydrated, hyperbilirubinemic breastfed baby.

Donor milk requires a doctor's prescription. Although the milk is donated to the milk banks and not sold, there are processing fees charged to help defray the costs of donor screening and processing of the milk. That fee is currently approximately $3.50 an ounce plus shipping fees. In Canada, the use of donor milk is covered by the national health plan. In the United States, its coverage by insurance and health plans is variable. It often requires an extra effort by the physician to speak to the medical director of the health plan and educate him or her on the benefits of using donor milk. Although the cost may seem exorbitant, it has been estimated that for every $1 spent on donor milk, $11 to $37 in NICU costs are saved (136). Arnold calculated the cost of supplying donor human milk and fortifier to a hypothetical preterm infant as being $1350 (134). Using the previously discussed (86) estimated additional costs of surgical NEC averaging $186,200 more and medical NEC $73,700, the potential for preventing a case of NEC by the use of donor human milk seems more than economical! Most milk donated to milk banks comes from mothers who have delivered at term. However, they do receive milk from preterm mothers—mothers who have large milk supplies, and even mothers who have ultimately lost their baby, but donate their milk as part of working through the grieving process, to help another baby. Preterm and full term milk is processed separately. Donor preterm milk can be specifically requested, and if available, it will be shipped to you. It is shipped frozen overnight. It is worth having a policy in place for the timely transport of the milk from your receiving area to your unit, where it must be transferred to the freezer on arrival. For a sample donor human milk policy, please see Appendix C-3.

FORTIFICATION OF HUMAN MILK FOR VERY LOW BIRTH WEIGHT BABIES

There are many times when babies in the NICU do not show adequate growth and good weight gain. For babies who are receiving breast milk, there are a number of things that can be done. One of the most obvious, and most frequently overlooked, is increasing the volumes. As neonatologists, we have firmly entrenched in our minds that we cannot exceed

160 cc/kg/day. For some babies this is true—in particular those who are fluid restricted, on diuretics, or for those who do not tolerate advancing beyond that volume enterally. However as we also know, term babies, when allowed to feed ad libitum, often exceed 200 to 220 cc/kg/day. So it is worth remembering that at least in some of our population, we do not have to adhere to such tight fluid control. When we cannot advance volume any further, there are generally two ways to advance calories with breast milk: using hind milk and using commercial fortifiers.

Hind Milk

The fat content of human milk increases throughout the course of a feeding or a milk expression session. We can take advantage of that to provide higher caloric milk to a baby who is either receiving breast milk through an alternative feeding method or who is breastfeeding. Hind milk refers to the milk at the end of the feed that is higher in fat content; foremilk is the milk from the early part of the feed that is lower in fat. Because the fat changes along a continuum, this is in some ways an artificial construct, but one that is useful to this concept. For a mother to provide hind milk, she must be producing more than the baby's requirement in milk per day. Essentially it consists of having her pump off a specified volume of milk at the beginning of a session, change containers, and then continue to pump until she is "empty." If these containers are then compared, the foremilk will look thin and bluish (lower fat content) and the hind milk will look whiter and creamier. The decision regarding how much is foremilk and how much is hind milk is based on how much milk mother makes, and how much is needed for a feed. For example, if she generally pumps 4 ounces of milk total, and the baby receives 2 ounces at a feeding, we would have mom pump off approximately 1 ounce from each breast as her foremilk, and the remaining 2 ounces total as her hind milk. The containers need to remain separate and be labeled as foremilk and hind milk respectively. If a baby is receiving some or all of his/her nutrition at the breast, this method can still be used. Mother can express the initial one ounce from her breast, and then let the baby drain the breast to receive the higher fat content milk. This method has been used successfully in a developing country to improve growth when commercial fortifiers were not available (143). A word of caution—hind milk is only higher in fat and therefore calories. It does not provide the extra protein, vitamins or minerals that many of our babies need. These are provided by the commercial fortifiers. However, if a baby on fortified milk is not showing acceptable rate of weight gain, one can successfully use fortified hind milk (144).

Commercial Fortifiers

Either liquid or powdered commercially manufactured substances generally provide fortification. Powdered forti-

fiers add the additional nutrients without diluting out any of the substances in the human milk. Liquid fortifiers are added in equal volume to the human milk, thus diluting out its components by half. Traditionally, when a mother's milk production has equaled or exceeded her baby's requirements, powdered fortifier has been used. When her production has not met her baby's needs, liquid fortifier has been used in an attempt to "extend" her milk. There have recently been a number of reports of significant Enterobacter sakazakii infections in neonates, including sepsis, meningitis and necrotizing enterocolitis, with premature and sick babies being at highest risk (145–150). They are associated with the use of complete milk-based powdered infant formula products from a variety of manufacturers. Powdered milk-based infant formulas are not sterile; they are heat treated during processing, but unlike liquid formula products, not subjected to the high temperatures for sufficient time to make the product commercially sterile (145,151). Recommendations from the CDC included that "formula products should be selected based on nutritional needs; alternatives to powdered forms should be chosen when possible" (145). At the time of this writing, there have been no reports of infection following the use of powdered human milk fortifiers. However, based on these reports and the CDC recommendations for powdered "formula products," many NICUs are preferentially using the liquid fortifiers, unless there is a cogent reason for using the powdered.

The protein in these fortifiers, which is derived from cow's milk, is of concern to many neonatologists and nutritionists. One of the risks of artificial feedings compared to human milk is the development of allergic GI symptoms to the bovine protein they contain. The ideal fortification of milk for preterm babies could be obtained by a process known as lactoengineering, in which specific components are removed from either excess own mother's milk, or donor milk, and then added to the human milk feeding to increase those needed nutrients. Studies have shown babies fed own mother's milk fortified with human milk protein (152) or with human milk protein plus human milk fat (153) grow comparably to both intrauterine growth curves and to other premature babies who have been exclusively fed fortified preterm formulas. This is an expensive process, but is feasible, and has been under investigation in several European countries (154–156). The ideal may well become human milk proteins packaged with other components for use as fortifiers for preterm babies. In the meantime, for these very low birthweight babies, human milk with added fortification is the ideal nutrition available.

It is a widely held belief by staff at all levels in NICUs that the addition of commercial human milk fortifiers increases feeding intolerance; there is, however, no evidence for this. Numerous controlled clinical trials have shown no difference in signs of feeding intolerance, increased gastric residuals, bilious gastric residuals, abdominal distention, or blood in the stools when compared to human milk alone or preterm formulas (157–162).

There has also been concern that nutritional additives to human milk may in fact alter its complex system of anti-infective/host defense properties. In one clinical study fortified human milk has been shown to increase, but not to a significant degree, the incidence of necrotizing enterocolitis (5.8% compared with 2.2%, $p = 0.12$), and infections (suspected plus proven; 43% compared with 31%, $p = 0.04$) over human milk alone (163).

Laboratory research in this area has shown that fortification does not affect total IgA content (164,165), or inhibition to *E. coli*, although it does decrease lysozyme activity by 19%, which was not considered significant (164). When fortified human milk was evaluated under simulated nursery conditions, bacterial colony counts did not rise appreciably for the first 20 hours under refrigeration, but did increase approximately 10-fold in the following 4 hours under incubator conditions (165). More recently, Chan evaluated the effect of addition of powdered fortifiers to human milk on antibacterial activity. Human milk alone inhibited the growth of *E. coli*, *Staphylococcus aureus*, *Enterobacter sakazakii*, and Group B Streptococcus. Fortifier that contains iron, and iron alone, affected the antimicrobial activity of the milk, causing no zone of inhibition for any of these organisms (166). The fortifier containing no iron had similar inhibitory effects to human milk alone. It was postulated that the iron may have saturated the lactoferrin in the milk, thus decreasing its antibacterial activity. Another *in vitro* study looked at the effect of human milk fortifier added to human milk on the concentration of transforming growth factor-α (TGF-α). TGF-α is a gut peptide found in human milk that is believed to exert a maturational effect on the neonatal gut. They found that the addition of fortifier did not affect the whole milk or aqueous portion of TGF-α, but significantly decreased its concentration in the fat fraction, in addition to altering its molecular mass profile characteristics (167). Thus far, the data does not suggest a change in our current practice of fortification. Whether these laboratory findings are of clinical significance remains to be seen. But it is worth keeping in mind that the addition of exogenous substances to human milk, although our intent is good, may in fact be found later to alter and compromise the balance of nutrients, enzymes, hormones, immunological and other factors and thus their effects.

One final note on fortification—mothers of NICU babies are already dealing with many stresses, not the least of which are the circumstances that brought her and her baby to the NICU. We must always be very cautious when talking about "inadequate growth" and "fortification" with her. Remember—providing breast milk is the one thing only she can do for her baby. If we are careless when we broach these subjects, the message she will take away is that her milk is not adequate, and that her infant's slow growth relates to something she is not doing right. It is important to point out to her that her milk is the best possible nutrition for her baby, and helping the baby to fight infections, and that she is doing an excellent job providing it. The issue at this time is that her small baby has enormous nutritional needs, which can be met by using hind milk and/or commercial fortifiers. It is important as well to emphasize that this is a time-limited issue, and that as her baby grows, matures, and becomes healthier, her milk alone will provide all her baby needs.

Colostrum Oral Care

It is well known that sIgA is present in large quantities in premature colostrum (Table 23-4). Almost 75% of ingested IgA from human milk survives passage through the intestinal tract and is excreted in the feces (168). This immunoglobulin provides passive protection against antigens (including viruses and bacteria) crossing the immature, permeable mucosal barrier (169). As early as 1983, Narayanan and colleagues from India reported that small quantities of colostrum (10 cc three times a day) administered to low birth weight infants resulted in a significantly decreased incidence of infection compared to solely formula-fed controls (170). It is common practice in NICUs to provide oral care to babies who are not being orally fed—including the new, ventilated ELBW and VLBW infants, and those with significant cardiovascular instability. This is generally accomplished using sterile water applied to a cotton-tipped swab, or to a piece of gauze. In our unit, we have instituted a practice of "colostrum oral care" in which any baby who is not being enterally fed can be provided with oral care using mother's expressed colostrum instead of sterile water. The reasoning behind this is that knowing the sIgA is active in protecting the mucosal surfaces of these immunocompromised babies, by swabbing the oral cavity with colostrum, we are providing some of that protection to the oral mucosa and possibly the upper GI tract if any is swallowed. Additionally, it accomplishes another very important purpose. In the early days before a mother can hold a very small or sick baby, before the milk she is working so hard to express can be used for feeds, she is playing a vital role in the care of her infant. This procedure can be initiated within hours of birth, even in the most premature babies. NICU staff or parents dip a sterile swab in the colostrum container, and swab over the tongue and oral mucosa. The swab should not be dipped back into the container. This may be done as frequently as every 4 hours, generally in conjunction with hands-on care. Once minimal enteral feedings are begun, remaining colostrum should be used for those early feedings, and oral care continued according to standard routine.

THE DEVELOPMENTAL PROGRESSION TOWARD BREASTFEEDING

In hospital breastfeeding management, the process of establishing breastfeeding in the preterm population begins with the facilitation of frequent skin-to-skin contact

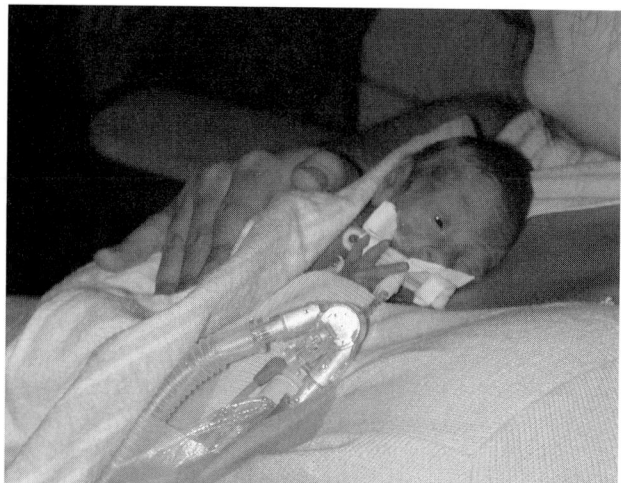

Figure 23-3 Mother and 600-gram 23-week infant engaging in skin-to-skin contact.

through Kangaroo (skin to skin) care (Fig. 23-3). Originally proposed by Rey and colleagues in Bogota Columbia (171), subsequent studies in developed nations illustrate that the practice is safe, beneficial and an essential component of high-quality neonatal intensive care (172–175). Kangaroo care has also been consistently associated with improved milk production, enhanced maternal breastfeeding competence and extended lactation (175–178). Mothers who provide skin-to-skin contact report that their infant makes rooting and sucking movements toward the nipple, note feelings of milk ejection and leaking, and often express larger amounts of milk immediately following a Kangaroo Care session (179–180). Kangaroo care provides the mother with the opportunity to become more confident in handling her small infant. Mothers who engage in Kangaroo Care report a sense of efficacy, increased self-esteem, and confidence in caring for their babies (181). Kangaroo care also provides the infant with frequent access to the breast, increases opportunity for nonnutritive sucking, and assists in the gradual transition to breastfeeding. It is the optimal position for an infant to receive gavage feedings prior to the establishment of breastfeeding and during supplemental feedings. Tornhage and colleagues report that infant plasma cholecystokinin levels increase when receiving nasogastric feedings during Kangaroo Care (182). This stimulates GI function and infant growth.

The transition from breast milk feedings to breastfeeding is critical. When successful breastfeeding is established in the hospital setting, breastfeeding is more likely to continue at home. However, the process of breastfeeding the premature infant can be challenging for the infant, the mother and the health care professional. The transition phase from providing expressed human milk to nutritive breastfeeding has not been extensively studied. Factors to consider in transitioning the premature infant from breast milk feedings to feeding at the breast include assessment of feeding readiness, optimizing opportunity for early breastfeeding, encouraging increased breastfeeding as the infant

nears discharge and ensuring post discharge support based on the individual needs of the mother and infant.

Assessment of feeding readiness is determined by the maturation of the infant, measured chronologically as corrected gestational age and influences the development of feeding skills. The bottle-feeding skill of the premature infant has been positively correlated with the development of sucking skills and is a function of maturation (183). The infant must be able to coordinate bursts of sucking interspersed with pauses for breathing to manage the bottle-feeding skills. This ability is variable but often occurs by about 34 weeks' gestational age.

Restrictions in breastfeeding policies for preterm infants are commonly based on studies of bottle-feeding, in which it has been established that infants with immature cardirespiratory control show less coordinated suck-swallow-breathe pattern, resulting in apnea, hypoxia, and bradycardia (184). However, at the breast the preterm infant coordinates sucking, swallowing, and breathing with minimal fluctuations in transcutaneous oxygen pressure (104,106), and as discussed earlier, is more physiologically stable.

There is no scientific evidence linking gestational age, growth/weight milestones, or the ability to drink from a bottle as evidence for breastfeeding readiness in a premature infant. Although maturation plays a role in the premature infant's ability to breastfeed, clinicians observe a wide range of variability related to breastfeeding readiness and competence among premature infants, with infants as young as 34 weeks gestation fully breastfeeding although some term infants take several weeks to effectively breastfeed. This suggests that the emergence of breastfeeding competence in preterm infants is a multifactorial process that is dependent on both infant and maternal factors. The role of experience and learning in acquiring breastfeeding skills has recently been investigated (185). Nyquist and colleagues suggest that the development of nutritive sucking is not solely maturational but a result of learning and extrinsic factors such as maternal-infant interaction and the frequency and time spent breastfeeding (185). The same investigators examined early oral behavior of preterm infants during breastfeeding via electromyographic study (186). Data provided evidence of early sucking competence during breastfeeding, with wide individual variations. The authors concluded that preterm infants are capable of suckling at the mother's breast at low maturational levels and that both maturation and experience play a role in breastfeeding success (186). With experience and maturation, preterm infants will demonstrate increasing competence in latching onto the breast and maintaining a latch. Over time, they will subsequently engage in more efficient suckling and demonstrate gradual increase in vigor, intake velocity and volume at the breast (187). Research also indicates that breastfeeding is less stressful for premature infants than bottle-feeding with less hypoxia, apnea, bradycardia, and oxygen desaturation experienced during breastfeeding than during bottle feeding (104). Therefore, when infant stability is

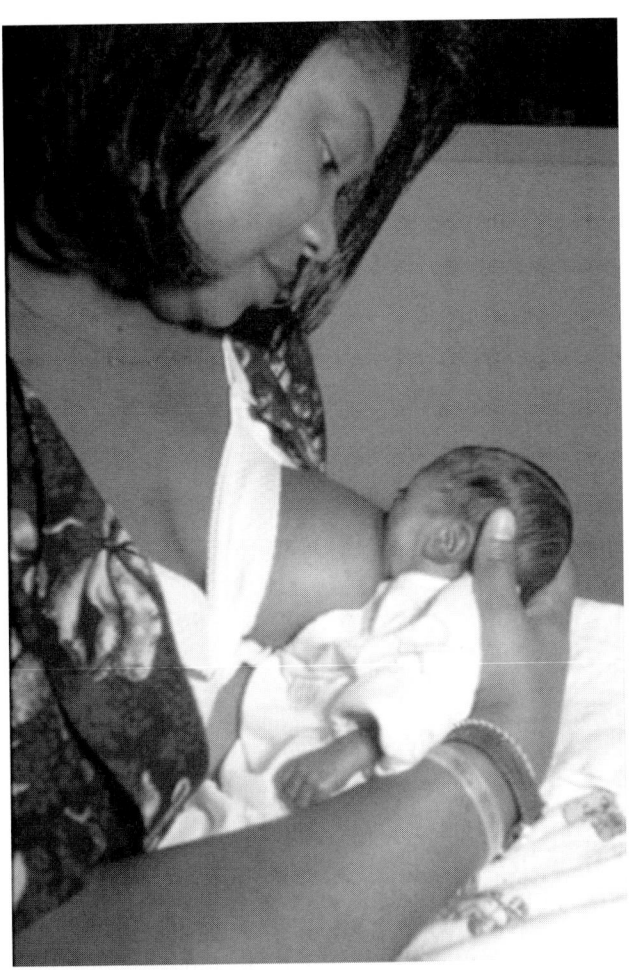

Figure 23-4   Premature infant at the breast.

attained, neonatal staff should encourage early and frequent opportunities to breastfeed.

Readiness criteria for early breastfeeding sessions include individual assessment of physiological stability during Kangaroo Care or holding, wakeful periods during feeding, rooting when hungry, and periods of nonnutritive sucking. The goal of early breastfeeding for a premature infant is to promote an enjoyable experience for both mother and baby although simultaneously teaching proper position and latch at the breast. Some oral feeding is possible at the breast between 28 to 30 weeks gestation; by 32 to 34 weeks gestation, some infants may be able to take a full breastfeed once or twice a day, while others may become proficient at breast; from 35 weeks onward, efficient breastfeeding that maintains growth is possible (Fig. 23-4).

Early breastfeeding sessions provide opportunity to introduce breastfeeding as the first oral feeding experience for the premature infant. These are in effect, practice sessions. Mothers do not feel the pressure to "make it work" because their baby's nutrition does not depend on their success. So they become comfortable handling the baby, and working on the skills of positioning and latching, while enjoying this process and the time spent with their baby. These sessions are also excellent times to give the baby a gavage feed, in effect teaching the baby as well.

time the baby becomes "imprinted" with "this is the position I am in, this is the taste and smell of my mother (and maybe even a little taste of the milk that can be expressed onto her nipple!), and this is the nice feeling I get when my stomach becomes full." During this early breastfeeding stage, mothers should be encouraged to put baby to the breast one to two times per day. Making the mother and baby as comfortable as possible is key. Chairs used for these postpartum women should be padded and give the mother good support with enough room to maneuver and provide support to the infant's body. The large reclining chairs used in geriatric wards or dialysis units make perfect breastfeeding or skin to skin chairs. Mothers often maintain better position if a small stool is used under their feet to raise their legs somewhat. Pillows may be necessary to help support her arms in correct position. The baby needs to be supported as well. Commercial breastfeeding pillows, made of hospital grade materials that can be wiped off with disinfectant between babies, are available and work well. They can be covered with a towel or receiving blanket for comfort. Alternatively, some come with removable, washable covers that can be changed between babies. In our experience they seem to work better than using bed pillows, which are another option. Neonatal staff should provide a constant presence to reassure the mother, point out the positive aspects of this early breastfeeding, ensure infant stability, and optimize the latch of the premature infant at the breast.

The premature infant has unique characteristics that may interfere with latch at the breast. These include low muscle tone, limited energy, and the propensity to fall asleep at the breast from fatigue rather than satiety (188). Compared to a full-term infant, physical characteristics include a proportionately larger head, weaker neck muscles, and a mouth that is smaller in relationship to the areola and breast. These characteristics require breastfeeding positions that assist in placing the infant's mouth over the areola. Failure to support the infant in this optimal position will result in inability to compress the lactiferous sinuses, decreased milk transfer and nipple trauma. Additionally, failure to provide adequate support for the premature infant at the breast can result in the baby slipping away from a good latch and tiring easily as a result of the additional effort expended during breastfeeding to try and stay latched. Mothers may become discourage because of some of these issues. It is important to reassure them that these are time-limited concerns. As the baby grows and develops, the hypotonia will improve. Early on for many of these dyads, the problem of "trying to fit a quarter-sized nipple into a dime-sized mouth" is a real problem. It is easy to point out to a frustrated mom, that although her nipple is not expected to grow any more, her baby's mouth will!

Effective techniques to assist the premature infant to latch vary and depend on the configuration of the breast and the strength and skill of the infant (188). Data from nonnutritive sucking and bottle-feeding reveal that the amount of suction that the premature infant generates

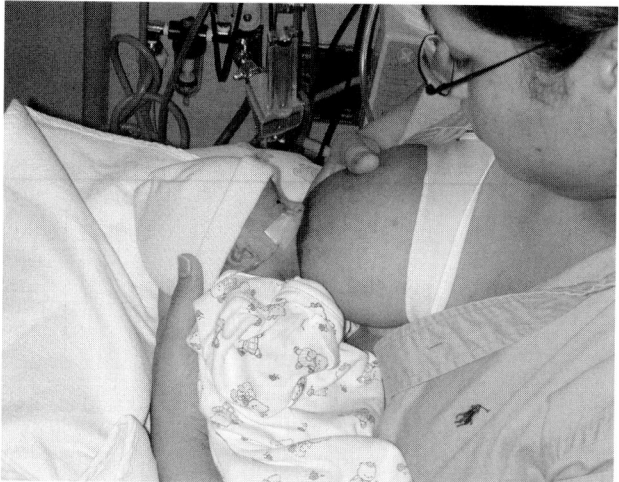

Figure 23-5 Cross-cradle position at the breast.

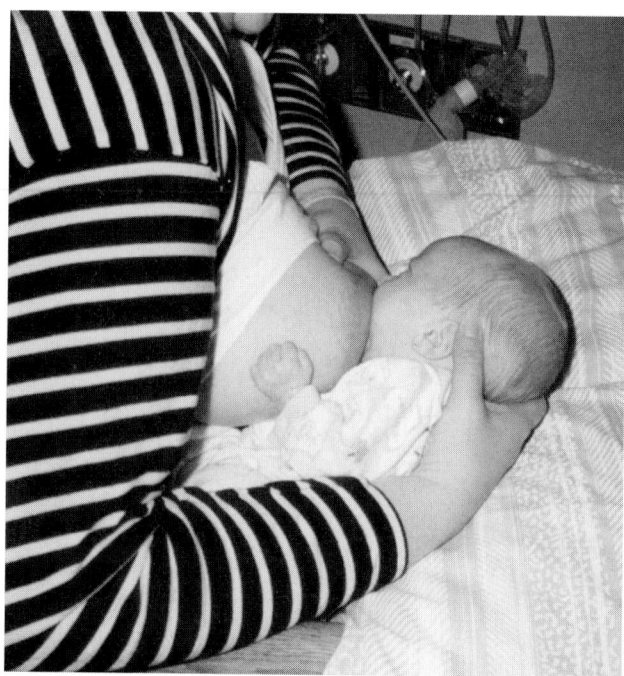

Figure 23-6 Football hold with a premature baby at breast, demonstrating compression of the breast to increase milk flow during the feed.

while at the breast is maturationally dependent (189). Because of this limitation, small premature infants need to be "placed" and "kept" on the nipple/areola, because limited suction inhibits their ability to bring and keep the nipple /areola in the correct position for milk extraction. Mothers of small premature infants require instruction to place and support the baby at the breast. This includes supporting the baby's head at the nape of the neck during latch and throughout breastfeeding. Additional head support assists weak neck musculature of the premature infant to maintain neck stability and prevents undirected head movement that can lead to airway collapse, apnea, and bradycardia (190). For some mothers with large breasts, it is helpful to roll a towel or blanket to place under the breast to hold it up, to make it easier for mom to see as she is placing the baby, and easier for the baby to stay latched because the breast is being supported. Supportive positions for breastfeeding the premature infant include the underarm/football hold or cross-cradle (across the lap) positions. These positions support the infant's head and torso, guide the infant to the nipple/areolar area, ensure optimal latch, and subsequently maintain the baby in a close flexed position throughout the feeding. To maintain the airway and to help in swallowing in the cross-cradle position, it is important to maintain the infant's body facing the mother, keeping the baby's ear, shoulder and hip in a straight line, and then flexing their legs around the mother's body (Fig. 23-5). In the football hold, care should be taken to ensure that the baby's neck is not overly flexed (Fig. 23-6). The typical breastfeeding Madonna hold, which most mothers have seen so will naturally try, in which the baby is held with her arm on the same side of her body as the breast she is feeding from, is not appropriate for premature or other low tone babies. The baby's head, which is supported in the crook of the mother's arm, tends to fall through, and is poorly supported for optimal feeding.

When optimal position is attained, the infant's head can be moved toward the breast, by the hand supporting the

neck and head. The mother's nipple can then be lightly brushed against the infant's mouth. The infant will spontaneously open his mouth when ready. The mother should then gently guide the infant onto the nipple/areolar area. The mother with everted, elongated nipples may find it easier to elicit a sucking response at the breast as her nipple will automatically stimulate the roof of the baby's mouth and elicit the sucking response. Mothers with flatter nipples may require additional assistance to achieve latch. This may include manipulating the nipple to make a "teat" which will then stimulate the infant suck reflex. It can be done by either having the mother use the electric pump briefly right before the feed to draw the nipple out, or by having the mother roll her nipple between her thumb and forefinger. This requires additional assistance from nursing staff or a lactation consultant during the first several breastfeeding sessions or until the infant has demonstrated effective latch.

It is important here to discuss the concept of "on-cue" feedings. In neonatal units, we are very entrenched in calculating, ordering, measuring and reporting the exact input and the intervals at which it must occur. It is critical to our care when our patients are very small or very sick. However, we need to learn to relax that somewhat as we begin to introduce feedings at breast. If the baby is due for an interval feeding at a specific time but is asleep, it often will prove fruitless to try to put the baby to breast at that time. However, an hour later, before the next feed is due, when the baby is awake and the mother is at the bedside, it is the right time to allow them to practice breastfeeding. If the baby takes nothing or if the baby actually ingests a few ccs, it really does not matter. But the dyad have had the perfect opportunity to learn—that is what matters. As the baby matures, bedside staff will often notice a pattern to their wakeful periods. It is not unusual for them to be at night. So a mother who comes in every afternoon to put the sleeping baby to breast may have gotten nowhere. But if she changes her pattern, and manages to come in at night when the baby is often active, their breastfeeding skills may take off and amaze everyone. From there, we often see the babies becoming more wakeful for feeds, so on-cue breastfeeding times can advance in number. If the baby is awake 2 hours after the last feed, and is giving feeding cues, it is perfectly reasonable to have her put the baby to breast again, even though it is "too early" based on our feeding orders. That is what the mother will do once she is home—that is what we must ultimately aim for before discharge.

Mothers must be taught indicators of milk transfer/ swallowing at the breast. This includes the soft "caw" sound of swallowing. This also includes the open-pause-close pattern of suckling during which the wide-open pause of the infant's mouth during breastfeeding indicates that the infant is swallowing a mouthful of milk. When evidence of milk transfer diminishes during a feed, switching breasts and using breast compression may increase volume of milk ingested. During breast compression, the mother uses her "free" hand, which has been supporting her breast, to grasp the breast in a C-hold (fingers on one side, thumb on the other) and when the baby is suckling, compresses her breast between her fingers to eject more milk (Fig. 23-6). This will often keep the baby interested and actively suckling. When bursts of these indicators are evident during breast-feeding, and accuracy of intake is important, intake at the breast can be estimated by the use of prefeeding and postfeeding weights (191,192). The difference between pre- and post-weights in grams equals the amount of milk transfered in cc's. Volume of intake at the breast can be extremely variable. It is, however, virtually impossible to estimate by observing the feed, even by experts in lactation. Most premature infants will experience marginal intake during early breastfeeding. However some infants can consume adequate quantities of milk during early breastfeeding because mothers have copious milk supply and it flows readily. Thus milk volume and ejection can compensate for a marginally effective suck in some small premature infants. Test weighing or prefeeding and postfeeding weights under identical conditions may be helpful in determining the ability of the infant to stimulate milk transfer, amount of supplements required, and maternal milk supply. The scale used must be an accurate electronic scale. "Under identical conditions" means the baby must be weighed immediately before and after the feeding session, with the same clothing, diaper, blankets, leads, tubes, and so on at both of these times. Using this data, instead of trying to guess how much supplementation must be given for that feed, the difference between the ordered feeding amount and the amount taken at breast can be calculated and given via gavage. Prefeeding and postfeeding weights may also provide an indicator of breastfeeding progress and therefore reassurance for mother and staff. Test weighing should be introduced when it appears that milk transfer is occurring or when discharge is imminent. This information can assist in tailoring ongoing breastfeeding support and discharge preparation.

ONGOING BREASTFEEDING SESSIONS

The Use of Alternative Feeding Methods

The goal of ongoing breastfeeding sessions is to support the infant to consume adequate volumes of milk from the breast in anticipation of discharge. Research indicates that premature infants are able to coordinate the suck, swallow and breathe pattern of breastfeeding before bottle-feeding (104). This data also illustrates that mean volumes of milk transfer/intake during early breastfeeding sessions is often minimal but that the range for intake at the breast is variable and may be quite high. Early breastfeeding sessions are almost always supplemented by gavage feedings, which optimize this early learning experience. Typically, other methods of supplemental and/or complemental feedings are initiated when the maturity, energy and ability of the infant to suckle increases. These include bottle-feeding, cup feeding, finger feeding, and feeding tube at the breast. Currently there is limited evidence to guide hospital practice related to transitioning the premature infant to the breast. Although protocols to eliminate or minimize bottle feeds have been published and used clinically (193), the majority have not been tested in randomized controlled trials. Hospital policies and practices related to the use of supplemental or complemental feedings however can potentially interfere with breastfeeding outcomes (194,195).

The majority of neonatal units introduce bottle-feeding as a supplementation method for the preterm infant who is not exclusively breastfed during neonatal hospitalization. The degree that bottle-feeding may interfere with the acquisition of breastfeeding skills is controversial. Most experts would agree that the oral dynamics of breastfeeding and bottle-feeding are significantly different (196,197). Breastfeeding is dependent on the massaging action of the tongue and jaw while bottle-feeding depends more on suction. Additionally, the characteristic of milk flow from the bottle is different from the flow of milk from the breast. A quicker flow that provides immediate reward for minimal sucking may be another factor in the preference of bottle over breastfeeding. Therefore the suckling pattern learned through bottle-feeding may result in infants resisting latching to the breast, refusing the breast, or having difficulty with latch-on (198,199). Research indicates that the use of artificial nipples interferes with breastfeeding success in term infants and that they may be detrimental in preterm infants as well (194,200,201). Consequently, for preterm infants whose supplementary feedings are provided by bottle, subsequent breastfeeding may be difficult. Alternative feeding methods that do not adversely affect breastfeeding duration in this population are highly desirable. This need, coupled with recommendations emerging from the 1991

WHO/UNICEF Baby Friendly Initiative (202,203) that no artificial nipples or pacifiers be used if breastfeeding is to be established, has resulted in an increased use of alternate feeding methods in neonatal units. Methods that may foster the transition of preterm infants to full breastfeeding include continued tube feeding, cup feeding, finger feeding, or a nursing supplementer tube (feeding tube device). A nipple shield may also be a consideration at this stage of breastfeeding. Currently there is no agreement on the best method of supplementing the preterm infant or the timing of transitioning the preterm infant to the breast. Supplementation method and timing are based on a combination of maternal and infant factors. Various levels of evidence support each strategy.

Until the preterm infant establishes a pattern of nutritive oral feeding, periodic gastric tube feedings are required. Although guidelines and protocols for gastric feeding differ, continuous nasogastric tube placement is the most common protocol and tube sizes include numbers 5, 6.5, and 8 French (204). Nasogastric feedings have been associated with negative impacts on breathing, sucking, irritation, and delayed transition to oral feeding. A prospective randomized trial evaluated the impact of an indwelling smaller bore feeding tube (3.4 French) during the transition to breastfeeding as an alternative to supplementation by bottle. Infants who received nasogastric supplementation were 4.5 times more likely to be partially and 9.4 times fully breastfeeding at discharge compared to the bottle-fed group (205). Method of supplementation continued to be predictive of long-term breastfeeding as well (205). Although there were risk and stressors associated with continued nasogastric feeding (greater numbers of apnea and bradycardia requiring stimulation) the authors suggest that this method can be used safely during hospitalization to support ongoing breastfeeding.

Cup feeding has been used primarily in full term infants as a short-term method of providing a supplement to a breastfeeding baby. Early reports suggested that cup feeding is a safe alternative method of supplementation for preterm infants 30 weeks gestational age and older (206). Breastfeeding rates were increased when cup feeding replaced bottle-feeding and replaced or supplemented tube feedings in this early study (206). More recently, the safety of cup feedings and bottle feedings were compared in a prospective randomized cross-over study of 56 infants ≤34 weeks at birth by Marinelli and colleagues (207). Results indicate that a 10-fold increase in desaturations occurs during bottle-feeding compared to cup feeding. Although volumes taken were lower and duration of feeds longer during cup feedings, the study supported the use of cup feeding as a safe alternative feeding method for premature infants learning to breast-feed (207). The mechanics and safety of cup feeding were also evaluated by Dowling and colleagues through observation of 18 cup feeding sessions by 8 preterm infants with a mean gestational age of 30.7 weeks (208). Data indicate that the infants remained physiologically stable during cup feeding but that low volume of intake may

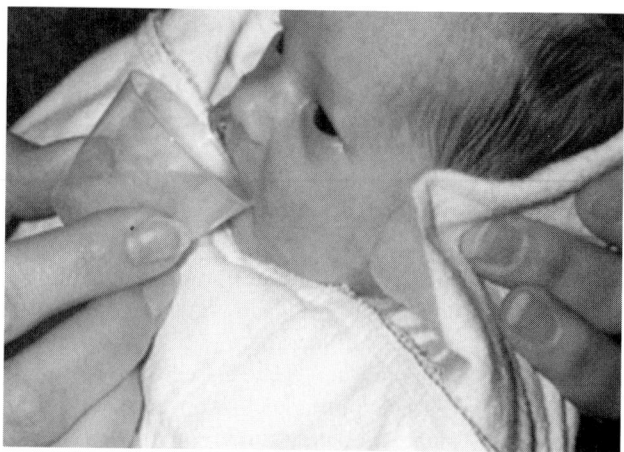

Figure 23-7 Cup feeding.

account for this stability and is also cause for concern (208). Spillage was a common occurrence during cup feeding, indicating that cup feeding may not be as easy for the infant or caregiver as previously described. Therefore, the efficacy and efficiency of cup feeding as an alternative method of supplementation is questioned and requires further study (208) (Fig. 23-7).

Finger feeding is another alternative feeding method that eliminates the need for bottle-feedings while the premature infant is learning to breastfeed and/or nearing discharge. Finger feeding is proposed as a method of feeding that assists with the development of appropriate tongue position and movements of sucking. Finger feeding is considered more similar to breastfeeding that bottle-feeding and can be used while the infant is learning to breastfeed, is too tired to breastfeed or when mother is not available (194). Little data exists to evaluate finger feeding as an alternative feeding method. Oddy and Glenn assessed the effectiveness of finger feedings in encouraging a breastfeeding-type suck and breastfeeding outcomes in preterm infants who required supplementation (209). Data was collected on rates of breastfeeding at discharge before and after this alternative feeding method was introduced. Results indicated higher rates of breastfeeding on discharge in preterm infants who were supplemented with finger feeding vs. bottle-feeding (209). One of the concerns with finger feeding is that it is introducing a hard surface into the baby's mouth, and may not ultimately fair any better than the use of artificial bottles with nipples. It is a tool that is used widely and successfully in "suck-training" babies with dysfunctional sucking mechanisms (210). Although further research is required to evaluate this strategy, finger feeding may provide an option to support breastfeeding learning in this population.

Alternative methods of transitioning the premature infant to the breast can be used when the mother is present; these include a nipple shield and a feeding tube device at the breast (supplemental nurser). Recent literature supports the use of a thin silicone nipple shield to assist the premature infant to latch when the infant cannot draw in enough nipple/areola, the areola is too puffy or the nipple

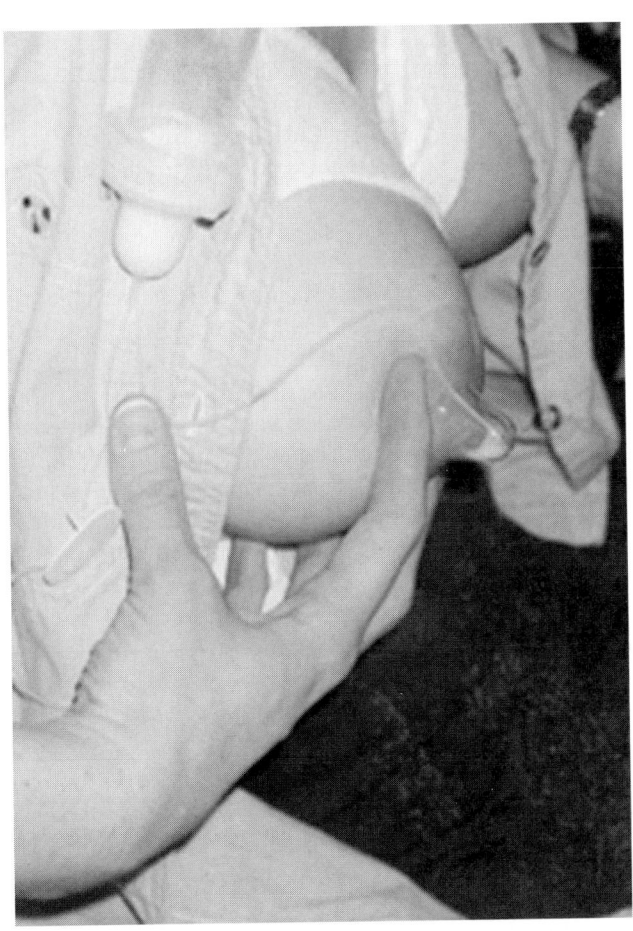

Figure 23-8 Silicone nipple shield with feeding tube device.

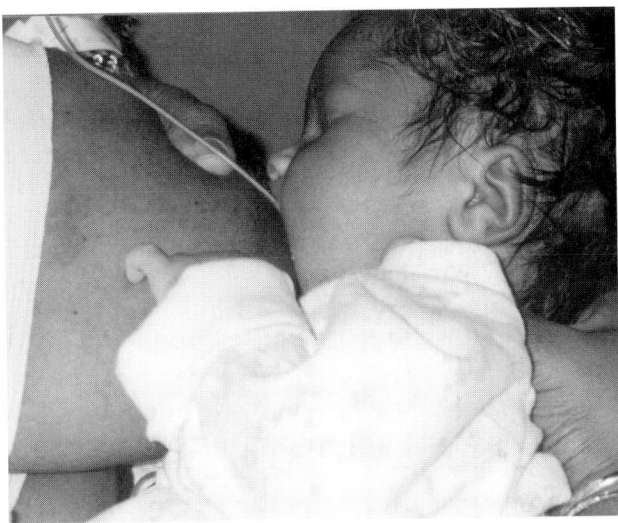

Figure 23-9 Feeding tube device at the breast.

is very large (211,212). Because the nipple shield is less pliable than the maternal nipple, it can stimulate a stronger sucking reflex. It has been hypothesized that the nipple shield functions to increase the effectiveness of infant suck by remaining in the correct position within the infant's mouth in the absence of strong suck pressures. A nipple shield maintains its shape when the infant pauses, keeping him/her on the breast with little effort, minimizing the tendency to slip off during feedings. Additionally, once the baby begins to suckle, negative pressure appears to be generated in the empty space between the nipple and the tip of the shield. These pressures have been postulated to compensate for the weaker suck of the infant, allowing milk to accumulate in the chamber, and thus making it more readily available (212). In these circumstances, the nipple shield may make it easier for the premature infant to maintain attachment to the breast and extract milk. As a result, temporary use of a nipple shield may increase both the duration of suckling and volume of milk consumed during breastfeeding (211,212) (Fig. 23-8). In the past, nipple shields were considered taboo in the lactation field. They were made of thick rubber, and mothers often developed decreasing milk supplies as a result of less sensory stimulation to the breast, ultimately leading to cessation of breastfeeding. The newer thin silicone nipple shields are less likely to precipitate these negative outcomes. Premature

infants who may benefit from the use of a thin silicone nipple shield include those with short inefficient bursts of sucking, limited energy and low suction at the breast, who fall asleep quickly at the breast, or whose mothers have flat or ill-defined nipples that make grasp and sustained latch difficult. A nipple shield is often well accepted by mothers because it allows the infant to feed at the breast with increased vigor, alert periods and intake at the breast (112,212).

Attempts should be made to wean the baby from the nipple shield prior to discharge. However, if the baby can only maintain total enteral intake with the shield, discharge home can be considered, but only if there is experienced lactation support available. The dyad must have close follow-up with intent to wean from the shield when the baby is able to suckle well without it. Additional research is required to continue to explore the use of a silicone nipple shield as a temporary milk transfer device for premature infants.

A feeding tube device at the breast (supplemental nurser) can be beneficial for a mother with a limited milk supply or for an infant who achieves a good latch but is unable to transfer adequate milk volumes (214). This device reinforces the position and latch of breastfeeding, provides for additional infant intake at the breast without supplementary time and energy expenditure, and increases maternal milk supply through optimal breast stimulation (Fig. 23-9). Mothers often feel initially awkward with placing the tube and then latching the baby, but with assistance from staff and a little practice, it will become much easier for her. The tube should be placed so that the tip is close to, but not at or past the end of the nipple. If that occurs, babies often figure out quickly how to use it like a straw instead of latching correctly! A feeding tube device can be placed inside a nipple shield to aid a baby with milk transfer, especially if the mother has low milk supply, or the baby has limited energy and needs help with efficiently transferring milk (Fig. 23-8).

It is important to recognize that the safety, efficacy and breastfeeding outcomes of all methods of supplementing the premature infant during the transition to full breast-feeding have not been studied systematically in controlled trials. Therefore, the method, timing and duration of supplementation should be based on individual assessment of the infant and mother and follow informed consent.

DISCHARGE PLANNING

Transition to cue-based full breastfeeding occurs over time with the majority of premature infants able to achieve this milestone by the time they are equivalent to term. This process is facilitated by increasing the frequency of breastfeeding as the infant's ability to transfer milk at the breast improves. Several protocols to facilitate this outcome are documented in the literature. All require ongoing assessment of breastfeeding adequacy and intervention as required.

Breastfeeding assessment should include regular visual assessment of the baby at the breast by staff with knowledge and experience in the care of breastfeeding families. Several "breastfeeding tools" are available to promote an objective assessment of latch, milk transfer and other attributes associated with optimal breastfeeding (215–220). The Preterm Infant Breastfeeding Behavior Scale specifically measures the maturational steps in breastfeeding progress and is useful in the clinical setting (220). Utilization of an objective breastfeeding assessment tool has the potential to identify early breastfeeding issues and assist staff to intervene in a timely and consistent manner. These tools are also excellent teaching tools for families which assist mothers in assessing progress toward successful breastfeeding.

As the infant matures, mothers should be given opportunity to breastfeed not only on cue, but ad libitum. Frequent on-demand or cue-based breastfeeding ad libitum provides information about the infant's energy level to engage in full breastfeeding, rate of growth with this plan, and assists with setting realistic goals for discharge preparation and feeding at home. Feeding options should be discussed with mothers and fathers to ensure they participate in and are fully informed about individualized breastfeeding plans. An individualized transition to home plan should be put into place for each mother-infant dyad based on the skills of the infant, the mother's milk production and the infant's caloric needs. Because the behavioral feeding cues of the preterm infant are less distinct than the full-term infant, mothers require time and learning to interpret correctly (185). The availability of a parent suite for overnight stays facilitates this learning, allowing maximal access to the infant and a trial of breastfeeding on cue. This opportunity can also provide valuable information related to maternal milk supply and the adequacy of infant intake at the breast. Prior to discharge, if the facilities are available, parents should be offered and encouraged to room-in with their baby for at least 24 hours. This is helpful in both trouble shooting any concerns or issues that arise, and for building parental confidence that they will be able to manage once home.

Many premature infants are otherwise ready for discharge before reaching term. Lack of maturity may continue to interfere with their ability to fully breastfeed. Other premature infants are discharged at term but have size and energy limitations that preclude full breastfeeding. Mothers therefore may need to modify their expectations about their infant's breastfeeding potential at discharge. All mothers require a detailed feeding plan at discharge that addresses the ongoing nutritional needs of the infant while supporting ongoing breastfeeding. This plan must support the mother's knowledge of expected feeding patterns, assessment of adequate intake, supplementation (method, frequency and amount) to ensure adequate intake, and the need for continued pumping to ensure full milk production until the baby is fully breastfed. It is optimal that this plan be not only developed collaboratively with the parents, but also given to them in written format to refer to once home. It must also be communicated to the primary care provider and the lactation expert who will be following and managing this dyad closely at home (Appendix C-4).

SUPPORTING BREASTFEEDING IN THE NEONATAL INTENSIVE CARE UNIT AND AFTER DISCHARGE

It is critical to have a "breastfeeding friendly" NICU to optimize a dyad's chances of successfully breastfeeding. One of the largest roadblocks to this is the inaccurate and inconsistent advice and assistance that is given to these mothers and families by the health care professionals (relatives and friends as well) they come into contact with. Much of that is based on knowledge deficits in lactation, attitudes and beliefs that influence what we say and how we present it, and personal factors such as age, education and own breastfeeding experiences (221,222). Additionally, nurses, who spend more time at the bedside than any other caregivers, are viewed by families as breastfeeding authorities, regardless of their knowledge or expertise. Although a number of studies have looked at the effect of education on caregiver attitudes on breastfeeding, one has examined this approach in the NICU. Siddell, Marinelli, and colleagues examined the change in breastfeeding knowledge and attitudes in their NICU staff after a structured mandatory 8-hour educational intervention (223). Nurses' breastfeeding knowledge and some attitudes improved significantly, with indication that other attitudes were changed as well. Although more study is necessary, it appears that the time and effort placed on educating a NICU staff so that advice and assistance can become more consistent, has the potential to make a difference.

The environment also must be breastfeeding friendly. Many mothers are very shy about breastfeeding openly, and their privacy must be respected. Because milk volume is often increased when a mother pumps at her baby's bedside, pumping is another activity that requires some privacy. Portable screens in sufficient numbers are an easy way to cordon off a small area. It is interesting to observe that once pumping and breastfeeding become the cultural norm in a given unit, it is not unusual to see mothers request the screens less. Having enough portable hospital-grade electric breast pumps, comfortable chairs for skin to skin and breastfeeding, breastfeeding pillows, and stools are equally as important. If space permits, small rooms in which mothers can rest between feeding sessions, express milk, or take their babies to as discharge nears are ideal, as are rooms for overnight/rooming-in.

Another major issue is the influence of the formula/drug companies on our NICU culture, and that of medicine as a whole. The giving out of free formula samples and discharge gift packs have been associated with decreased duration of breastfeeding in the less vulnerable well-baby population (224,225). The Baby–Friendly Hospital Initiative was designed by the United Nations Children's Fund (UNICEF) and the WHO as an intervention to increase breastfeeding rates (202,203). One of the issues it addresses is the negative influence of these products, and other informational materials provided by these companies for our patients—for example booklets on breastfeeding. Two recent U.S. studies, one in a NICU, have shown that these interventions can improve breastfeeding initiation rates (226,227). Instead of discharging a vulnerable breastfeeding NICU family with a discharge gift pack from a formula company, some units have put together their own packs with noncommercial information and supplies to support them.

The period immediately following discharge from the neonatal unit is a time of extreme vulnerability for mothers and may precipitate a breastfeeding crisis (188). Follow up care in the community is critical and must be arranged and provided prior to discharge home. Access to a telephone support number and referral to a lactation consultant or a breastfeeding clinic has been shown to increase the transition to home and support ongoing breastfeeding in this vulnerable group (Appendix C-4).

SPECIAL CIRCUMSTANCES

The Near-Term Infant

Infants born at 35 to 37 weeks gestation are considered near term. In the past, these small but physically stable infants were cared for in a special care nursery until close to 40 weeks gestation. Currently, most stable near-term infants are placed on the postpartum unit with their mothers and treated as though they are full-term. Many of these infants appear deceptively vigorous at first glance but have subtle immaturities that may compromise their outcomes. Clinical challenges in temperature control and glucose/metabolic stability are examples of this immaturity. Potential difficulties in establishing and maintaining breast feeding present an additional challenge in this population.

Common breastfeeding problems experienced by term infants and their mothers are magnified in infants who are born before term. These include the ability to latch to the breast, the incidence of jaundice, weight loss in the first few days to weeks of life, and the establishment of maternal milk supply. As a result, the near term infant is at risk of hypoglycemia, dehydration and slow growth/failure to thrive. Recent literature has reported an increased incidence of kernicterus among breastfed infants; this literature identifies breastfed infants born at less than 37 weeks gestation at increased risk for this devastating and preventable morbidity (228,229). These issues are more likely to occur in near term infants who are breastfeeding.

The predominant characteristic of the near term infant that interferes with breastfeeding is decreased stamina. This characteristic results in less effective suckling at the breast, decreased milk transfer and suboptimal breast stimulation. Additionally, the suck, swallow, breathe cycle of the near term infant may not be fully developed, further compromising intake at the breast. Poor muscle tone also contributes to fatigue and suboptimal breastfeeding. A common pattern among these infants is to latch and suckle for a short time and then pause to rest with subsequent difficulty resuming a nutritive sucking pattern. The inability of these infants to sustain a suck/swallow/breathe pattern limits milk transfer and contributes to insufficient intake at the breast. This scenario predisposes the near term infant to morbidity in the early newborn period (230).

The two basic principles in breastfeeding support of the near term infant are to ensure adequate infant nutrition and to assist with establishing and maintaining maternal milk supply. The near term infant requires adequate nutrition with minimal calorie/energy expenditure. Early frequent breastfeeding should be accompanied by assessment of latch and intake at the breast. Once lactogenesis II is established, measurement of intake at the breast with an electronic scale can provide information about the infant's ability to transfer milk effectively and maternal milk supply. The infant may need to be supplemented after breastfeeding with small quantities of expressed breast milk or formula. A full/generous milk supply assists the infant to receive adequate intake at the breast with minimal effort. Because the near term infant may not have the ability to optimally stimulate milk production, mothers should be encouraged to use a full-sized electric breast pump after breastfeeding to ensure early and ongoing milk supply. Discharge from the hospital must be accompanied by a discharge plan that is communicated to the family and care providers. Early and ongoing follow up is required to ensure infant health and nutrition and maternal health and milk supply. With continuing support, the majority of near term infants will transition to full breastfeeding at term.

Other infants who have decreased energy and potential for poor breastfeeding may also benefit from this approach. The NICU graduate may be discharged before term or at term but not displaying term characteristics. Infants born to diabetic mothers, term infants who have been ill at birth, and term infants with physical or neurological issues that interfere with energy or feeding may have compromised breastfeeding ability similar to the near term infant. Similar to the near term infant, these vulnerable infants should be carefully assessed for breastfeeding competency and supported until the transition to full breastfeeding is made. For more information see the Academy of Breastfeeding Medicine Protocol #10. Breastfeeding the Near-Term Infant at www.bfmed.org.

Hypoglycemia and the Breastfeeding Infant

It is important to briefly touch on the issue of hypoglycemia and the breastfeeding infant, from the standpoint of prevention and maintaining the breastfeeding relationship. The topics of metabolic adaptation to extra-uterine life, glucose homeostasis, and causes of hypoglycemia are well covered in other venues (231,233). As described by Williams (231) there are two principles to guide us in preventing hypoglycemia: (a) early and exclusive breastfeeding meets the nutritional requirements of healthy, full-term newborn infants; and (b) healthy full-term infants do not develop symptomatic hypoglycemia simply as a result of underfeeding. An excellent guide to the prevention and management of hypoglycemia is the Academy of Breastfeeding Medicine Clinical Protocol Number 1: Guidelines for Glucose Monitoring and Treatment of Hypoglycemia in the Breastfed Neonate (233). In brief, this is put into practice by putting babies skin to skin, which facilitates normal temperature and metabolic adaptation, to initiate breastfeeding within 30 to 60 minutes of delivery, and allowing them to room-in, and feed on cue as frequently as every 10 to 12 times in 24 hours or more. Given these tenants, there is no need to "routinely" monitor blood glucose levels in healthy, full-term breastfeeding infants (1,233). If hypoglycemia does develop, asymptomatic babies can continue to breastfeed frequently with careful follow-up and monitoring. If a need for intravenous glucose develops, once the baby is stable and able to feed, breastfeeding should resume as weaning from the i.v. glucose occurs.

Jaundice and the Breastfeeding Infant

It is beyond the scope of this chapter to cover this topic in detail. The reader is referred to in-depth articles on jaundice (234,235) that cover the pathophysiology and prevention of "lack of" breastfeeding jaundice. With increasing cases of kernicterus being reported, the importance of good management and frequent follow-up of breastfeeding babies, especially those who are feeding poorly, whose mothers have not developed a good milk supply, or who develop jaundice, cannot be over-stated. It is critical that when a breastfed baby needs intervention or is admitted to the hospital for treatment of dehydration or jaundice, that it be emphasized to the mother and the family that breastfeeding is not harmful or dangerous to the baby. This can not be emphasized enough. Mothers immediately get the message that they have done something wrong to cause

their child to have this problem. As often health care providers, in their explanations of the pathophysiology, lay blame on the failure of breastfeeding, mothers immediately assume enormous guilt. With that comes pressure from within themselves or their families to stop breastfeeding and begin formula feeding. It is critical that these mothers be supported to continue breastfeeding through this family crisis. That support in the hospital setting includes continuing breast-feeding; having a qualified person (lactation consultant, trained staff member) immediately evaluate and begin working on fixing the mother's milk supply and the baby's latch and transfer of milk, and allowing the mother to room-in with her baby. If supplements are needed, and the baby can latch, consider use of a feeding tube device at breast, so the mother will continue to stimulate her breasts to produce more milk, and her feedings can continue at breast. If milk supply is at issue, evaluate possible causes. Most commonly one finds a baby with a poor or inadequate latch; a mother with sore nipples; and a vicious cycle of less stimulation to the breasts resulting in inadequate milk supply. If the mother's nipples are significantly painful and traumatized because of poor latch, she may need a rest from breastfeeding. In either of these scenarios, it is critical that she be given the use of a hospital-grade electric pump in the hospital to use, and that she initiates frequent expression (see Table 23-5) to empty her breasts and increase her milk supply. The gentle support of this mother and her family are as important as the diagnosis and treatment of the dehydration and the jaundice.

CONTRAINDICATIONS TO BREAST FEEDING

There are surprisingly few contraindications to the provision of breast milk and breastfeeding. We will cover a few of the most important here (for a more in-depth review the reader is referred to 236–239).

Infections

Human Immunodeficiency Virus

The one clear infectious contraindication to breastfeeding, in developed countries, is maternal HIV (138,240). HIV can be transmitted through human milk, with rates varying from 5% to 20% depending on many contributing factors, and up to 29% when the infection is acquired just before or during the breastfeeding period (236). In developed countries in which sanitary affordable replacement feedings are readily available, women should be counseled strongly not to breastfeed. In developing countries in which safe and affordable substitutes are not readily available, and in which malnutrition and infectious diseases cause high infant and child mortality, breastfeeding remains the nutrition of choice. These recommendations will continue to be re-evaluated as more study is done on the specifics of the transmission of HIV and the possible affects of maternal and infant antiretroviral therapy.

Human T-Cell Lymphotrophic Virus

HTLV-1 and HTLV-2 are retroviruses similar to HIV. The virus is transmitted in human milk, so women with this infection are advised not to breastfeed. Recommendations in developed countries are the same as for HIV (138).

Hepatitis

The risk of transmission of Hepatitis A is rare, so breast-feeding is encouraged. Breastfeeding does not increase the risk of transmission of Hepatitis B. Babies born to mothers who are positive for hepatitis B should be treated according to recommended guidelines. There is no need to delay initiation of breastfeeding. Hepatitis C transmission via breast milk has not been documented. Mothers should be advised it is theoretically possible, but maternal hepatitis C is not a contraindication to breastfeeding (138).

Cytomegalovirus

Cytomegalovirus (CMV) maternal infection is a bit more complicated. It is a ubiquitous virus, and is transmitted via breast milk. Acquisition in healthy full-term infants does not result in clinical disease, leading to the term "natural vaccination" (241). Recent reports of transmission, thought to be through breast milk to premature infants, some of whom developed significant disease, have caused some concern (242). Some units use only frozen milk, which has been reported to kill the virus, in the smallest, most immunosuppressed babies. No authoritative guidelines have been issued.

MEDICATIONS AND DRUGS

The vast majority of medications are compatible with lactation. Many health care providers will tell a mother to stop breastfeeding when a medication is prescribed. This is rarely indicated, and it is always worth looking up the drug in a reliable source. If a drug is found to be contraindicated, it is almost always possible to find another that will be efficacious and is compatible with breastfeeding. Drugs that require cautious use when used in breastfeeding mothers of newborns or preterm infants include: sulfonamides (jaundice possible; do not use in G6PD deficiency); ergotamine and bromocriptine (reduce milk supply); pseudoephedrine and estrogens (may inhibit milk supply); meperidine (neonatal sedation reported); fluoxetine (tremulousness, colic, crying and hypotonia reported); angiotensin-converting enzyme inhibitors (may predispose to neonatal hypotension) and anticancer agents (239). Drugs of abuse—marijuana, cocaine, heroin, phencyclidine—are contraindicated in lactation. When in doubt—do not tell a mother to pump and dump or discontinue breastfeeding—go to a good source and

find out! Medications that are found in breast milk are shown in Appendix H-1a through H-1e.

Resources for Medication Use During Lactation

Publications

- American Academy of Pediatrics Committee on Drugs. The transfer of drugs and other chemicals into human milk. Pediatrics 2001; 108:776–789.
- Briggs GG, Freeman RK, Yaffe SJ. *Drugs in Pregnancy and Lactation: A Reference Guide to Fetal and Neonatal Risk.* 6th edition. Philadelphia: Lippincott Williams and Wilkins, 2002.
- Hale, Thomas W. *Medications and Mother's Milk.* 11th edition. Amarillo, TX: Pharmasoft Medical Publishing, 2004.
- Hale, Thomas W. *Clinical Therapy in Breastfeeding Patients.* 1st edition. Amarillo, TX: Pharmasoft Medical Publishing, 1999.
- Lawrence, Ruth A and Lawrence Robert M. *Breastfeeding: A Guide for the Medical Profession.* 6th edition. St. Louis: Mosby, 2005.

Telephone Consultation

- Lactation Study Center, University of Rochester: 1-585-275-0088
- Poison and Drug Control Centers: (Check your local poison control center for availability of drug information)

Internet

- Breastfeeding Pharmacology—Dr. Thomas Hale http://neonatal.ttuhsc.edu/lact/index.html

CONCLUSION

In today's high-tech world of neonatal intensive care, there is one relatively low tech intervention that we as neonatologists can give with just a little effort, understanding, and education—the gift of mother's milk. The research supports it. The cost/benefit ratio is very appealing. The advantages to our patients and their mothers and families are high. The drawbacks are very low. Promoting, encouraging, and supporting mothers to succeed is a very small price to pay. We just need to remember, and to embrace, that *all babies were born to be breastfed.*

Acknowledgment

With deep gratitude to Ms. Linda Kaczmarczyk, Pediatric Clinical Librarian at Connecticut Children's Medical Center, for her invaluable aid in preparing this chapter.

REFERENCES

1. American Academy of Pediatrics, Work Group on Breastfeeding. Breastfeeding and the use of human milk. *Pediatrics* 1997;100: 1035–1039.

2. Breastfeeding: maternal and infant aspects. ACOG Educational Bulletin 2000;258:1–16.
3. American Academy of Family Physicians. Breastfeeding (Position Paper). AAFP Policies on Health Issues. Available at http://www.aafp.org/x6633.xml. Last accessed 1/26/05.
4. Position of the American Dietetic Association: promotion of breastfeeding. J Am Diet Assoc 1997;97(6):662–666.
5. Nutrition Committee, Canadian Paediatric Society (CPS). Nutrient needs and feeding of premature infants. CMAJ 1991;144(11):1451–1454. Available at http://www.cps.ca/english/statements/N/n95-01.htm. Last accessed 1/26/05.
6. U.S. Department of Health and Human Services. HHS Blueprint for Action on Breastfeeding. Washington: U.S. Department of Health and Human Services; Office of Woman's Health; 2000.
7. United States Breastfeeding Committee. Breastfeeding in the United States: a national agenda. Rockville, MD: US Department of Health and Human Services, Heath Resources and Services Administration, Maternal and Child Health Bureau; 2001.
8. U.S. Department of Health and Human Services. Healthy People 2010: conference Edition—volumes I and II. Washington: Department of Health and Human Services, Public Health Service, Office for the Assistant Secretary for Health; 2000(Jan): 47–48. Available at http://www.healthypeople.gov/document/ Last accessed 1/26/05.
9. The National Women's Health Information Center. US Department of Health and Human Services. Available at http://www.4woman.gov/ Last accessed 1/26/05.
10. The Ad Council. Breastfeeding Awareness Campaign. Available at http://www.adcouncil.org/campaigns/breastfeeding/ Last accessed 1/26/05.
11. Freed GL, Clark SJ, Sorenson J, et al. National assessment of physician's breast-feeding knowledge, attitudes, training and experience. JAMA 1995;273(6):472–476.
12. Freed GL, Clark SJ, Curtis P, et al. Breast-feeding education and practice in family medicine. J Fam Pract 1995;40(3):263–269.
13. Williams EL, Hammer LD. Breastfeeding attitudes and knowledge of physicians-in-training. Am J Prev Med 1995;11:26–33.
14. Philipp BL, Merewood A, Gerendas E. Breastfeeding information in pediatric textbooks needs improvement. Academy of Breastfeeding Medicine News and Views 2002;8(3):27.
15. Budin P. The nursling: the feeding and hygiene of premature and full-term infants. London, UK: Caxton Publishing, 1907. Maloney WJ, translator.
16. Hess JH. Premature and congenitally diseased infants. Philadelphia: Lea and Febiger, 1922.
17. Gordon HH, Levine SZ, McNamara H. Feeding of premature infants. A comparison of human and cow's milk. Am J Dis Child 1947;73:442–452.
18. Benjamin MH, Gordon HH, Marples E. Calcium and phosphorus requirements of premature infants. Am J Dis Child 1943; 65:412–425.
19. Ruowei L, Zhao Z, Mokdad A, et al. Prevalence of breastfeeding in the United States: the 2001 National Immunization Survey. Pediatrics 2003;111:1198–1201.
20. Ahluwalia I, Morrow B, Hsia J, et al. Who is breast-feeding? Recent trends from the pregnancy risk assessment and monitoring system. J Pediatr 2003;142:486–491.
21. Ryan AS, Wenjun Z, Acosta A. Breastfeeding continues to increase into the new millennium. Pediatrics 2002;110: 1103–1109.
22. Ross Products Division. Breastfeeding trends through 2000. Available at http://ross.com/aboutross/Survey.pdf. Last accessed 1/26/05.
23. Labbok M, Krasovec K. Toward consistency in breastfeeding definitions. Stud Fam Plan 1990; 21:226.
24. Breastfeeding Committee for Canada. Breastfeeding Definitions and Data Collection Periods, March 2004. http://www.breastfeedingcanada.ca Date last accessed: 1/26/05
25. Marinelli K. Personal communication from Connecticut Children's Medical Center NICU database: 2004.
26. Erenkrantz RA, Ackerman BA, Mezger J, et al. Breast-feeding premature infants: incidence and success. Pediatr Res 1985;19: 199A(abst530).
27. Furman L, Minich NM, Hack M. Breastfeeding of very low birth weight infants. J Hum Lact 1998;14(1):29–34.
28. Hill PD, Ledbetter RJ, Kavanaugh KL. Breastfeeding patterns of low-birth-weight infants after hospital discharge. JOGN Nurs 1997;26(2):189–197.
29. Lefebvre FL, Ducharme M. Incidence and duration of lactation and lactational performance among mothers of low-birth-weight and term infants. CMAJ 1989;140:1159–1164.
30. Marinelli K, Page K, Burke G. Influence of NICU admission on choice and duration of breastfeeding in mothers of preterm infants. Academy of Breastfeeding Medicine News and Views 1998;4:23.
31. Hill PD, Ledbetter RJ, Kavanaugh KL. Breastfeeding patterns of low-birth-weight infants after hospital discharge. JOGN Nurs 1997;26:189–197.
32. Richards MT, Lang MD, McIntosh C, et al. Breastfeeding the VLBW infant: successful outcome and maternal expectations. Pediatr Res 1986;20:383A(abst1385).
33. Kaufman KJ, Hall LA. Influence of the social network on choice and duration of breast-feeding in mothers of preterm infants. Res Nurs Health 1989;12:149–159.
34. Killersreiter B, Grimmer I, Buhrer C, et al. Early cessation of breast milk feeding in very low birthweight infants. Early Hum Dev 2001;60:193–205.
35. Furman L, Minich N, Hack M. Correlates of lactation in mothers of very low birth weight infants. Pediatrics 2002;109(4):e57 Available at http://www.pediatrics.org/cgi/content/full/109/4/e57. Last accessed _____.
36. Powers NG, Bloom B, Peabody J, et al. Site of care influences breast milk feedings at NICU discharge. J Perinatol 2003;23: 10–13.
37. Meberg A, Willgraff S, Sande HA. High potential for breastfeeding among mothers giving birth to pre-term infants. Acta Paediatr Scand 1982;71:661–662.
38. Verronen P. Breast feeding of low birthweight infants. Acta Paediatr Scand 1985;74:495–499.
39. Hunkeler B, Aebi C, Minder CE, et al. Incidence and duration of breast-feeding of ill newborns. J Pediatr Gastroenterol Nutr 1994;18:37–40.
40. Barros FC, Victoria CG, Vaughn JP, et al. Birth weight and duration of breast-feeding: are the beneficial effects of human milk being over-estimated? Pediatrics 1986;78:656–661.
41. Yip E, Lee J, Sheehy Y. Breast-feeding in neonatal intensive care. J Paediatr Child Health 1996;32:296–298.
42. Heinig MJ. Host defense benefits of breastfeeding for the infant: effect of breastfeeding duration and exclusivity. Pediatr Clin North Am 2001;48(1):105–123.
43. Davis MK. Breastfeeding and chronic disease in childhood and adolescence. Pediatr Clin North Am 2001;48(1):125–141.
44. Reynolds A. Breastfeeding and brain development. Pediatr Clin North Am 2001;48(1):159–171.
45. Labbok MH. Effects of breastfeeding on the mother. Pediatr Clin North Am 2001;48(1):143–158.
46. Butte N. The role of breastfeeding in obesity. Pediatr Clin North Am 2001;48(1):189–198.
47. Schanler RJ. The use of human milk for premature infants. Pediatr Clin North Am 2001;48:207–219.
48. Gross SJ, David RJ, Bauman L, et al. Nutritional composition of milk produced by mothers delivering preterm. J Pediatr 1980;96: 641–644.
49. Hibberd CM, Brooke OG, Carter ND, et al. Variations in the composition of breast milk during the first five weeks of lactation: implications for the feeding of preterm infants. Arch Dis Child 1982;57:658–662.
50. Maas YGH, Gerritsen J, Hart AAM, et al. Development of macronutrient composition of very preterm human milk. Br J Nutr 1998; 80:35–40.
51. Lawrence RA, Lawrence RM. Breastfeeding: a guide for the medical profession. Philadelphia: Mosby, 1999.
52. Wagner V, Stockhausen JG. The effects of feeding human milk and adapted milk formulae on serum lipid and lipoprotein levels in young infants. Eur J Pediatr 1988;147:292–295.
53. Owen CG, Whincup PH, Odoki K, et al. Infant feeding and blood cholesterol: a study in adolescents and a systematic review. Pediatrics 2002;110:597–608.
54. Bergstrom E, Hernell O, Persson LA, et al. Serum lipid values in adolescents are related to family history, infant feeding and physical growth. Atherosclerosis 1995;117:1–13.
55. Butte NF, Wong WW, Ferlic L, et al. Energy expenditure and deposition of breast-fed and formula-fed infants during early infancy. Pediatr Res 1990;28:631–640.
56. Butte NF, Smith EO, Garza C. Energy utilization of breast-fed and formula-fed infants. Am J Clin Nutr 1990;51:350–358.

57. Putet G, Senterre J, Rigo J, et al. Nutrient balance, energy utilization and composition of weight gain in very-low-birth-weight infants fed pooled human milk or preterm formula. *J Pediatr* 1984;105:79–85.

58. Whyte RK, Haslam R, Vlainic C, et al. Energy balance and nitrogen balance in growing low birthweight infants fed human milk or formula. *Pediatr Res* 1983;17:891–898.

59. Lubetzky RL, Vaisman N, Mimouni FB, et al. Energy expenditure in human milk- versus formula-fed preterm infants. *J Pediatr* 2003;143:750–753.

60. Shulman RJ, Schanler RJ, Lau C, et al. Early feeding, antenatal glucocorticoids, and human milk decrease intestinal permeability in preterm infants. *Pediatr Res* 1998;44:519–523.

61. Cavell B. Gastric emptying in infants fed human milk or infant formula. *Acta Paediatr Scand* 1981;70:639–641.

62. Ewer AK, Durbin GM, Morgan MEI, et al. Gastric emptying in preterm infants. *Arch Dis Child* 1994;71:E24–E27.

63. Uraizee F, Gross S. Improved feeding tolerance and reduced incidence of sepsis in sick very low birthweight infants fed maternal milk. *Pediatr Res* 1989;25:298A.

64. Lucas A. AIDS and milk bank closures. *Lancet* 1987;1:1092–1093.

65. Shulman RJ, Schanler RJ, Lau C, et al. Early feeding, feeding tolerance, and lactase activity in preterm infants. *J Pediatr* 1998;133:645–649.

66. Hamosh M. Bioactive factors in human milk. *Pediatr Clin North Am* 2001;48:69–86.

67. Sheard NF, Walker WA. The role of breast milk in the development of the gastrointestinal tract. *Nutr Rev* 1988;46:1–8.

68. Carpenter G. Epidermal growth factor is a major growth-promoting agent in human milk. *Science* 1980;210:198–199.

69. Petschow BW, Carter DL, Hutton GD. Influence of orally administered epidermal growth factor on normal and damaged intestinal mucosa of rats. *J Pediatr Gastroenterol Nutr* 1993;17:49–57.

70. Heird WC, Schward SM, Hansen IH. Colostrum-induced enteric mucosal growth in beagle puppies. *Pediatr Res* 1984;18:512–515.

71. Widdowson EM, Colombo VE, Artavanis CA. Changes in the organs of pigs in response to feeding for the first 24 hours after birth. II. The digestive tract. *Biol Neonate* 1976;28:272.

72. Xanthou M, Bines J, Walker WA. Human milk and intestinal host defense in newborns: an update. *Adv Pediatr* 1995;42:171–208.

73. Kleinman RE, Walker WA. The enteromammary immune system. An important new concept in breast milk host defense. *Dig Dis Sci* 1979;24:876–882.

74. Mathur NB, Dwarkadas AM, Sharma VK, et al. Anti-infective factors in preterm human colostrum. *Acta Paediatr Scand* 1990;79:1039–1044.

75. Scariati PD, Grummer-Strawn LM, Fein SB. A longitudinal analysis of infant morbidity and the extent of breastfeeding in the United States. Pediatrics 1997;99(6)URL: Available at http://www.pedatrics.org/cgi/content/full/99/6/e5. Last accessed 1/26/05.

76. Bachrach VR, Schwarz E, Bachrach LR. Breastfeeding and the risk of hospitalization for respiratory disease in infancy. *Arch Dis Adolesc Med* 2003;157:237–243.

77. Dewey KG, Heinig MJ, Nommsen-Rivers LA. Differences in morbidity between breast-fed and formula-fed infants. *J Pediatr* 1995;126:696–702.

78. Duncan B, Ey J, Holberg CJ, et al. Exclusive breast-feeding for at least 4 months protects against otitis media. *Pediatrics* 1993;91:867–872.

79. Chen A, Rogan WJ. Breastfeeding and the risk of postneonatal death in the United States. Pediatrics 2004;113:e435-e439. Available at URL: http://www.pediatrics.org/cgi/content/full/113/5/e435. Last accessed 1/26/05.

80. Winberg J, Wessner G. Does breast milk protect against septicaemia in the newborn? *Lancet* 1971;1:1091–1094.

81. Narayanan I, Prakash K, Bala S, et al. Partial supplementation with breast-milk for prevention of infection in low-birth-weight infants. *Lancet* 1980;2:561–563.

82. Narayanan I, Prakash K, Gujral VV. The value of human milk in the prevention of infection in the high-risk low-birth-weight infant. *J Pediatr* 1981;99:496–498.

83. Narayanan I, Prakash K, Prabhakar AK, et al. A planned prospective evaluation of the anti-infective property of varying quantities of expressed human milk. *Acta Paediatr Scand* 1982;71:441–445.

84. El-Mohandes AE, Picard MB, Simmens SJ, et al. Use of human milk in the intensive care nursery decreases the incidence of nosocomial sepsis. *J Perinatol* 1997;17:130–134.

85. Hylander MA, Strobino DM, Dhanireddy R. Human milk feedings and infection among very low birth weight infants. Pediatrics 1998;102:e38. Available at http://www.pediatrics.org/cgi/cotent/full/102/3/e38; Accessed 1/26/05.

86. Schanler RJ, Shulman RJ, Lau C. Feeding strategies for premature infants: beneficial outcomes of feeding fortified human milk versus preterm formula. *Pediatrics* 1999;103:1150–1157.

87. Lucas A, Cole TJ. Breast milk and neonatal necrotising enterocolitis. *Lancet* 1990;336:1519–1523.

88. Bisquera JA, Cooper TR, Berseth CL. Impact of necrotizing enterocolits on length of stay and hospital charges in very low birth weight infants. *Pediatrics* 2002;109:423–428.

89. Weimer J. *The economic benefits of breastfeeding—a review and analysis.* Washington: Food and Rural Economic Research Service; U.S. Department of Agriculture; Food and Assistance Research report no 13; 2001.

90. Eibl MM, Wolf HM, Furnkranz, et al. Prevention of necrotizing enterocolitis in low-birth-weight infants by IgA-IgG feeding. *N Engl J Med* 1988;319:1–7.

91. Moya FR, Eguchi H, Zhao B, et al. Platelet-activating factor acetylhydrolase in term and preterm human milk: a preliminary report. *J Ped Gastroenterol Nutr* 1994;19:236–239.

92. Furman L, Taylor G, Minich N, Hack M. The effect of maternal milk on neonatal morbidity of very-low-birth-weight infants. *Arch Pediatr Adolesc Med* 2003;157:66–71.

93. Blaymore Bier JA, Oliver T, Ferguson A, et al. Human milk reduces outpatient upper respiratory symptoms in premature infants during their first year of life. *J Perinatol* 2002;22: 354–359.

94. Morley R, Cole TJ, Powell R, et al. Mother's choice to provide breast milk and developmental outcome. *Arch Dis Child* 1988;63:1382–1385.

95. Lucas A, Morley R, Cole TJ, et al. Breast milk and subsequent intelligence quotient in children born preterm. *Lancet* 1992;339:261–264.

96. Lucas A, Morley R, Cole TJ. A randomized multicentre study of human milk versus formula and later development in preterm infants. *Arch Dis Child* 1994;70:F141–F146.

97. Blaymore Bier JA, Oliver T, Ferguson AE, et al. Human milk improves cognitive and motor development of premature infants during infancy. *J Hum Lact* 2002;18:361–367.

98. Anderson JW, Johnstone BM, Remley DT. Breast-feeding and cognitive development: a meta-analysis. *Am J Clin Nutr* 1999;70:525–535.

99. Carlson SE, Werkman SH, Rhodes PG, et al. Visual-acuity development in healthy preterm infants: effect of marine-oil supplementation. *Am J Clin Nutr* 1993;58:35–42.

100. Amin SB, Merle KS, Orlando MS, et al. Brainstem maturation in premature infants as a function of enteral feeding type. *Pediatrics* 2000;106:318–322.

101. Uauy RD, Birch DG, Birch EE, et al. Effect of dietary omega-3 fatty acids on retinal function of very-low-birth-weight neonates. *Pediatr Res* 1990;28:485–492.

102. Birch E, Birch D, Hoffmann D, et al. Breast-feeding and optimal visual development. *J Pediatr Ophthalmol Strabismus* 1993;30:33–38.

103. Hoffman DR, Birch EE, Castaneda YS, et al. Visual function in breast-fed term infants weaned to formula with or without long-chain polyunsaturates at 4 to 6 months: a randomized clinical trial. *J Pediatr* 2003;142:669–677.

104. Meier P. Bottle- and breast-feeding; effects on transcutaneous oxygen pressure and temperature in preterm infants. *Nurs Res* 1988;37:36–41.

105. Meier P. Suck-breathe patterning during bottle and breastfeeding for preterm infants. In: David TJ, ed. *Major controversies in infant nutrition*, International Congress and Symposium, series 215. London: Royal Society of Medicine Press, 1996:9–20.

106. Meier P, Anderson GC. Responses of small preterm infants to bottle- and breast-feeding. *MCN Am J Matern Child Nurs* 1987;12:97–105.

107. Blaymore Bier J, Ferguson A, Anderson L, et al. Breast-feeding of very low birth weight infants. *J Pediatr* 1993;123:773–778.

108. Blaymore Bier JA, Ferguson AE, Morales Y, et al. Breastfeeding infants who were extremely low birth weight. Pediatrics 1997;100:e3.

109. Meier PP. Supporting lactation in mothers with very low birth weight infants. Pediatr Ann 2003;32:317–325.

110. Meier PP, Engstrom JL, Spanier-Mingolelli SR et al. Dose of own mothers' milk provided by low-income and non-low income mothers of very low birthweight infants (abstract). Pediatr Res 2000; 47:292A.

111. Russo J, Russo IH. Development of the human mammary gland. In: Neville MD, Daniel CE eds. *The mammary gland: development, regulation and function.* New York: Plenum Press, 1987:67–97

112. Riordan J. Anatomy and physiology of lactation. In: Riordan J, ed. *Breastfeeding and human lactation,* 3rd ed. Massachusetts: Jones and Bartlett, 2005.

113. deCarvalho M, Anderson DM, Giangreco A, et al. Frequency of milk expression and milk production by mothers of nonnursing premature neonates. *Am J Dis Child* 1985;139(5):483–485.

114. Hinds LA, Tyndale-Biscoe CH. Prolactin in the marsupial macropus engenii during the estrous cycle, pregnancy and lactation. *Biol Reprod* 1982;26:391–398.

115. Zuppa AA, Tornesello A, Papacci P, et al. Relationship between maternal parity, basal prolactin levels and neonatal breast milk intake. *Biol Neonate* 1988;53(3):144–147.

116. Ellis L, Picciano MF. Prolactin variants in term and preterm milk: altered structural characteristic, biological activity and immunoreactivity. *Endocr Regul* 1993;27:193–200.

117. Morton JA. Strategies to support extended breastfeeding of the premature infant. *Adv Neonatal Care* 2002;2(5):267–282.

118. Chatterton RT, Hill PD, Aldag JC, et al. Relation of plasma oxytocin and prolactin concentrations to milk production in mothers of preterm infants: influence of stress. *J Clin Endocrinol Metab* 2000;85(10):3661–3668.

119. Hill PD, Aldag JC, Chatterton RT. Effects of pumping style on milk production in mothers of non-nursing preterm infants. *J Hum Lact* 1999;15(3):209–216.

120. Hill PD, Aldag JC, Chatterton RT. Initiation and frequency of pumping and milk production in mothers of non-nursing preterm infants. *J Hum Lact* 2001;17(1):9–13.

121. Furman L, Minich N, Hack M. Correlates of lactation in mothers of very low birth weight infants. *Pediatrics* 2002;109(4):1–7.

122. Hill PD, Aldag JC, Chatterton RT. The effect of sequential and simultaneous breast pumping on milk volumes and prolactin levels: a pilot study. *J Hum Lact* 1996;12(3): 193–199.

123. Jones E, Dimmock PW, Spencer SA. A randomised controlled trial to compare methods of milk expression after preterm delivery. *Arch Dis Child Fetal Neonatal Ed* 2001;85(2): 91–95.

124. Hill PD, Brown LP, Harker TL. Initiation and frequency of breast expression in breastfeeding mothers of LBW and VLBW infants. *Nurs Res* 1995;44(6):352–355.

125. Budd SC, Erdman SH, Long DM, et al. Improved lactation with metoclopramide: a case report. *Clin Pediatr (Phila)* 1993;32(1): 53–57.

126. da Silva OP, Knoppert DC, Angelini MM, et al. Effect of domperidone on milk production in mothers of premature newborns: a randomized, double-blind, placebo-controlled trial. *CMAJ* 2001;164(1):17–21.

127. Emery MM. Galactogogues: drugs to induce lactation. J Hum Lact 1996;12(1):55–57.

128. Hurst NM, Valentine CJ, Renfro L, et al. Skin-to-skin holding in the neonatal intensive care unit influences maternal milk volume. *J Perinatol* 1997;17(3):213–217.

129. Bier JA, Ferguson AE, Morales Y, et al. Comparison of skin-to-skin contact with standard contact in low-birth-weight infants who are breast-fed. *Arch Pediatr Adolesc Med* 1996;150(12):1265–1269.

130. Ehrenkranz RA, Ackerman BA. Metoclopramide effect on faltering milk production by mothers of premature infants. *Pediatrics* 1986;78(4):614–620.

131. Williams-Arnold LD. *Human Milk Storage for Healthy Infants and Children.* Sandwich, MA, Health Education Associates Inc, 2000.

132. Arnold, LDW. *Recommendation for Collection, Storage and Handling of a Mother's Milk for Her Own Infant in the Hospital Setting.* 3rd edition. Denver, The Human Milk Banking Association of North America, 1999.

133. Arnold LDW. Using banked donor milk in clinical settings. In: Cadwell K, ed. *Reclaiming breastfeeding for the United States; protection, promotion and support.* Boston: Jones and Bartlett, 2002: 137–159.

134. Arnold LDW. The cost-effectiveness of using banked donor milk in the neonatal intensive care unit: prevention of necrotizing enterocolitis. *J Hum Lact* 2002;18:172–177.

135. Arnold LDW. Donor human milk banking. In: Riordan J, ed. *Breastfeeding and human lactation,* 3rd ed. Boston: Jones and Bartlett, 2005:409–431.

136. Wight NE. Donor milk for preterm infants. *J Perinatol* 2001;21: 249–254.

137. World Health Organization. *Global strategy for infant and young child feeding.* Geneva: WHO, 2003.

138. American Academy of Pediatrics. Human Milk. In: Red Book: 2003 Report of the Committee on Infectious Diseases, Pickering LK, Baker CJ, Overtorf GD, Prober CG, ed. 26th ed. Elk Grove Village, IL, American Academy of Pediatrics 2003:117–123.

139. Protocol Committee Academy of Breastfeeding Medicine. In: Cordes R, Howard CR, Powers N, et al, eds. *Clinical Protocol Number 3: Hospital guidelines for the use of supplementary feedings in the healthy term breastfed neonate.* Academy of Breastfeeding Medicine. 2002. Available at www.bfmed.org; accessed 1/26/05.

140. Human Milk Banking Association of North America (HMBANA). In: Tully M, ed. *Guidelines for the establishment and operation of a donor human milk bank.* Raleigh, NC: HMBANA, 2003.

141. Tully DB, Jones F, Tully MR. Donor milk: what's in it and what's not. *J Hum Lact* 2001;17:152–155.

142. Arnold LDW. How North American donor milk banks operate: results of a survey, part 2. *J Hum Lact* 1997;13:243–246.

143. Slusher T, Hampton R, Bode-Thomas F, et al. Promoting the exclusive feeding of own mother's milk through the use of hindmilk and increased maternal milk volume for hospitalized, low birth weight infants (< 1800 grams) in Nigeria: a feasibility study. *J Hum Lact* 2003;19:191–198.

144. Valentine CJ, Hurst NM, Schanler RJ. Hindmilk improves weight gain in low-birth-weight infants fed human milk. *J Pediatr Gastroenterol Nutr* 1994;18:474–477.

145. Centers for Disease Control and Prevention. Enterobacter sakazakii infections associated with the use of powdered infant formula—Tennessee, 2001. *MMWR Morb Mort Wkly Rep* 2002; 51:297–300.

146. Van Acker J, de Smet F, Muyldermans G, et al. Outbreak of necrotizing enterocolitis associated with enterobacter sakazakii in powdered milk formula. *J Clin Microbiol* 2001;39:293–297.

147. Weir E. Powdered infant formula and fatal infection with Enterobacter sakazakii. *CMAJ* 2002;166(12):1570.

148. Clark NC, Hill BC, O'Hara CM, et al. Epidemiologic typing of Enterobacter sakazakii in two neonatal nosocomial outbreaks. *Diagn Microbiol Infect Dis* 1990;13(6):467–472.

149. Simmons BP, Gelfand MS, Haas M, et al. Enterobacter sakazakii infections in neonates associated with intrinsic contamination of a powdered infant formula. *Infect Control Hosp Epidemiol* 1989;10(9):398–401.

150. Biering G, Karlsson S, Clark NC, et al. Three cases of neonatal meningitis caused by Enterobacter sakazakii in powdered milk. *J Clin Microbiol* 1989;27(9):2054–2056.

151. US Food and Drug Administration. Health professionals letter on Enterobacter sakazakii infections associated with use of powdered (dry) infant formulas in neonatal intensive care units. April 11, 2002; rev. October 10, 2002. Available at http://www.cfsan.fda.gov/~dms/inf-ltr3.html. Last accessed 1/26/05.

152. Ronnholm KAR, Perheentupa J, Siimes MA. Supplementation with human milk protein improves growth of small premature infants fed human milk. *Pediatrics* 1986;77:649–653.

153. Chappell JE, Clandinin MT, Kerney-Volpe C, et al. Fatty acid balance studies in premature infants fed human milk or formula: effect of calcium supplementation. *J Pediatr* 1986;102:439.

154. Michaelsen KF, Skafte L, Badsberg JH, et al. Variation in micronutrients in human bank milk: influencing factors and implications for human milk banking. *J Pediatr Gasrtoenter Nutr* 1990;11:229–239.

155. Voyer M, Senterre J, Rigo J, et al. Human milk lacto-engineering. *Acta Paediatr Scand* 1984;73:302–306.

156. Polberger S, Raiha NCR, Juvonen P, et al. Individualized protein fortification of human milk for preterm infants: composition of ultrafiltrated human milk protein and a bovine whey fortifier. *J Pediatr Gasrtoenter Nutr* 1999;29:332–338.

157. Lucas A, Fewtrell MS, Morley R, et al. Randomized outcome trial of human milk fortification and developmental outcome in preterm infants. *Am J Clin Nutr* 1996;64:142–151.

158. Schanler RJ, Schulman RJ, Lau C, et al. Feeding strategies for premature infants: randomized trial of gastrointestinal priming and tube-feeding method. *Pediatrics* 1999;103:434–439.

159. Reis BB, Hall RT, Schanler RJ, et al. Enhanced growth of preterm infants fed a new powdered human milk fortifier: a randomized control trial. *Pediatrics* 2000;106:581–588.

160. Ewer AK, Yu VYH. Gastric emptying in preterm infants: the effect of breast milk fortifier. *Acta Paediatr* 1996;85:1112–1115.

161. Sankaran K, Papageorgiou A, Ninan A, et al. A randomized, controlled evaluation of two commercially available human breast milk fortifiers in health preterm neonates. *J Am Diet Assoc* 1996;96:1145–1149.

162. Moody GJ, Schanler RJ, Lau C, et al. Feeding tolerance in premature infants fed fortified human milk. *J Pediatr Gastoenterol Nutr* 2000;30:408–412.

163. Lucas A, Fewtrell MS, Morley R, et al. Randomized outcome trial of human milk fortification and developmental outcome in preterm infants. *Am J Clin Nutr* 1996;64:142–151.

164. Quan R, Yang C, Rubinstein S, et al. The effect of nutritional additives on anti-infective factors in human milk. *Clin Pediatr* 1994;33:325–328.

165. Jocson MAL, Mason EO, Schanler RJ. The effects of nutrient fortification on varying storage conditions on host defense properties of human milk. *Pediatrics* 1997;100:240–243.

166. Chan GM. Effects of powdered human milk fortifiers on the antibacterial actions of human milk. *J Perinatol* 2002;23:620–623.

167. Lessaris KJ, Forsythe DW, Wagner CL. Effect of human milk fortifier on the immunodetection and molecular mass profile of transforming growth factor-alpha. *Biol Neonate* 2000;77:156–161.

168. Lawrence RM. Host resistance factors and immunologic significance of human milk. In: Lawrence RA, Lawrence RM, eds. *Breastfeeding: a guide for the medical profession*, 5th ed. New York: Mosby, 1999;172.

169. Walker WA. Antigen penetration across the immature gut: effect of immunologic and maturational factors in colostrum. In: Ogra PL, Dayton D, eds. *Immunology of breast milk*. New York: Raven Press, 1979.

170. Narayanan I, Prakash K, Verma RK, et al. Administration of colostrum for the prevention of infection in the low birth weight infant in a developing country. *J Trop Pediatr* 1983;29: 197–200.

171. Gomez HM, Sanabria ER, Marquette CM. The mother kangaroo programme. *International Child Health* 1992;3:55–56.

172. Cattaneo A, Davanzo R, the International Network for Kangaroo Mother Care, et al. Recommendations for the implementation of kangaroo mother care for low birth weight infants. *Acta Paediatrica* 1998;87:440–445.

173. Ludington SM, Ferreira CN, Goldstein MR. Kangaroo care with a ventilated preterm infant. *Acta Paediatrica* 1998;87:711–716.

174. Tornhage CJ, Stuge E, Lindberg T, et al. First week kangaroo care in sick very preterm infants. *Acta Paediatrica* 1999;88:1402–1404.

175. Whitelaw A, Heisterkamp G, Sleath K, et al. Skin to skin contact for very low birthweight infants and their mothers. *Arch Dis Child* 1998;63:1377–1381.

176. Charpak N, Ruiz-Pelaez JG, Figueroa de CZ, et al. A randomized, controlled trial of kangaroo mother care: results of follow-up at 1 year of corrected age. *Pediatrics* 2001;108:1072–1079.

177. Hurst NM, Valentine CJ, Renfro L, et al. Skin-to-skin holding in the neonatal intensive care unit influences milk volume. *J Perinatol* 1997;17:213–217.

178. Kirsten GF, Bergamn NJ, Hann FM. Kangaroo mother care in the nursery. *Ped Clin North Am* 2001;48:443–452.

179. Anderson GC. Current knowledge about skin-to-skin (kangaroo care) for preterm infants. *J Perinatol* 1991;11:216–226.

180. Hurst NM, Valentine CJ, Renfro L, et al. Skin-to-skin holding in the neonatal intensive care unit influences maternal milk volume. *J Perinatol* 1997;17(3):213–217.

181. Furman L, Kennell J. Breast milk and skin-to-skin kangaroo care for premature infants. Avoiding bonding failure. *Acta Paediatrica* 2000;89:1280–1283.

182. Tornhage CJ, Serenius F, Uvnas-Moberg K, et al. Plasma somatostatin and cholecystokinin levels in preterm infants during kangaroo care with and without tube-feeding. *J Pediatr Endocrinol Metab* 1998;11:645–651.

183. Lau C, Alaguagurusamy R, Schanler RJ, et al. Characterization of the developmental stage of sucking in preterm infants during bottle feeding. *Acta Paediatrica* 2000;89:846–852.

184. Daniels H, Devlieger H, Minami T, et al. Infant feeding and cardiorespiratory maturation. *Neuropediatrics* 1990;21:9–10.

185. Nyquist KH, Sjoden P, Ewald U. The development of preterm infants' breastfeeding behavior. *Early Hum Dev* 1999;55; 247–264.

186. Nyquist KH, Farnstrand C, Eeg-Olofsson KE, et al. Early oral behavior in preterm infants during breastfeeding: an electromoygraphic study. *Acta Pediatrica* 2001;90:658–663.

187. Martell M, Martinez G, Gonzalez M, et al. Suction pattern in preterm infants. *J Perinat Med* 1993;21:363–369.

188. Morton JA. The long road home: strategies to support extended breastfeeding of the premature infant. *Adv Neonatal Care* 2002;2(5):267–282.

189. Lau C, Sheena HR, Shulman RJ, et al. Oral feeding in low birth weight infants. *J Pediatr* 1997;130(4):561–569.

190. Neifert M, Seacat J. Practical aspects of breastfeeding the premature infant. Perinatology *Neonatology* 1988;12:24–30.

191. Meier PP, Lysakowski TY, Engstrom JL, et al. The accuracy of test weighing for preterm infants. J Pediatr Gastroent Nutr 1990; 10:62–65.

192. Meier PP, Engstrom JL, Crichton CL. A new scale for in-home test weighing for mothers of preterm and high risk infants. J Hum Lact 1994;10:163–168.

193. Stine MJ. Breastfeeding the premature newborn: A protocol without bottles. J Hum Lact 1990;6(4):167–170.

194. Newman J. Breastfeeding problems associated with early introduction of bottles and pacifiers. *J Hum Lact* 1990;6(2):59–63.

195. Walker M. Breastfeeding the premature infant. NAACOG's Clinical Issues in Perinatal and Women's health. *Nursing* 1992;3:620–633.

196. Woolridge MW. The anatomy of infant sucking. *Midwifery* 1986;2:164–171.

197. Righard L, Alade MO. Sucking technique and its effect on success of breastfeeding. *Birth* 1992;19:185–189.

198. Hill PD, Ledbetter RJ, Kavanaugh KL. Breastfeeding pattern of low-birth-weight infants after hospital discharge. *J Obstet Gynecol Neonatal Nurs* 1997;26:190–197.

199. Neifert M, Lawrence R, Seacat J. Nipple confusion: towards a formal definition. *J Pediatr* 1995;126:125–129.

200. Barros FC, Victora CG, Semer TC, et al. Use of pacifiers is associated with decreased breastfeeding duration. *Pediatrics* 1995;95: 497–499.

201. Righard L. Are breastfeeding problems related to incorrect breastfeeding technique and the use of bottles and pacifiers? *Birth* 1998;25:40–44.

202. World Health Organization. *Protecting, Promoting and Supporting Breastfeeding: The Special Role of Maternity Services.* Geneva, Switzerland: World Health Organization; 1989.

203. World Health Organization, Division of Child Health and Development. *Evidence for the Ten Steps to Successful Breastfeeding.* Geneva, Switzerland: World Health Organization; 1998.

204. Shiao PK, DiFiore TE. A survey of gastric tube practices in level 11 and level 111 nurseries. *Compr Pediatr Nurs* 19:209–220.

205. Kliethermes PA, Cross ML, Lanese MG, Johnson KM, Simon SD. Transitioning preterm infants with nasogastric tube supplementation: increased likelihood of breastfeeding. *JOGNN* 1999;28: 264–273.

206. Lang SL, Lawrence CJ, L'E Orme R. Cupfeeding: an alternative method of infant feeding. *Arch Dis Child* 1994;71:365–369.

207. Marinelli KA, Burke GS, Dodd VL. A comparison of the safety of cupfeedings and bottlefeedings in premature infants whose mothers intend to breastfeed. *J Perinatol* 2001;21(6):350–355.

208. Dowling DA, Meier PP, DiFiore JM, et al. Cup-feeding for preterm infants: mechanics and safety. *J Hum Lact* 2002;18(1): 13–20.

209. Oddy WH, Glenn K. Implementing the baby Friendly Hospital initiative: the role of finger feeding. *Breastfeeding Rev* 2003; 11(1):5–9.

210. Wolf LS, Glass RP. *Feeding and Swallowing Disorders in Infancy.* Therapy Skill Builders, San Antonio, TX; 1992.

211. Jones L, Spencer A. Establishing successful preterm breastfeeding. part 3. *Pract Midwife* 2002;5(6):18–19.

212. Meier PP, Brown LP, Hurst NM, et al. Nipple shields for preterm infants: effect on milk transfer and duration of breastfeeding. *J Hum Lact* 2000;16(2):106–114.

213. Hurst NM, Meier PP. Breastfeeding the preterm infant. In: Riordan J, ed. *Breastfeeding and Human Lactation.* 3rd ed. Massachusetts: Jones and Bartlett, 2005;395–376

214. Riordan J, Hoover K. Perinatal and intrapartum care. In: Riordan J, ed. *Breastfeeding and Human Lactation.* 3rd ed. Massachusetts. Jones and Bartlett, 2005:199.
215. Jensen D, Wallace S, Kelsay P. LATCH: a breastfeeding charting system and documentation tool. *J Obstet Gynecol Neonatal Nurs* 1994;23(1):27–32.
216. Mulford, C. The mother-baby assessment (MBA): an "Apgar Score" for breastfeeding. *J Hum Lact* 1992;8(2):79–82.
217. Shrago L, Bocar D. The infant's contribution to breastfeeding. *J Obstet Gynecol Neonatal Nurs* 1990;19(3):209–215.
218. Matthews MK. Developing an instrument to assess infant breastfeeding behavior in the early neonatal period. *Midwifery* 1988; 4:154–163.
219. Janke JR. Development of the breastfeeding attrition prediction tool. *Nurs Res* 1994;43(2):100–104.
220. Hedberg Nyquist K, Rubertsson C, Ewald U, et al. Development of the Preterm Infant Breastfeeding Behavior Scale (PIBBS): a study of nurse-mother agreement. *J Hum Lact* 1996;1:207–219.
221. Winikoff B, Laukaran V, Meyers D, Stone R. Dynamics of mother-infant feeding: mothers, professionals, and the institutional context in a large urban hospital. Pediatrics 1986; 77:357–365.
222. Bernaix L. Nurses' attitudes, subjective norms, and behavioral intentions toward support of breastfeeding mothers. J Hum Lact 2000;16:201–209.
223. Siddell E, Marinelli K, Froman R, Burke G. Evaluation of an educational intervention on Breastfeeding for NICU Nurses. J Hum Lact 2003;19(3):293–302.
224. Bergevin Y, Dougherty C, Kramer MS. Do infant formula samples shorten the duration of breastfeeding? Lancet 1983;1:1148–1153.
225. Frank DA, Wirtz SJ, Sorenson JR, Heeren T. Commercial discharge packs and breastfeeding counseling: effects on infant feeding practices in a randomized trial. Pediatrics 1987;80: 845–854.
226. Philipp BL, Merewood A, Miller LW, et al. Baby-Friendly Hospital Initiative improves breastfeeding initiation rates in a US hospital setting. Pediatrics 2001;108:677–681.
227. Merewood A, Phillip BL, Vchawala N, Vcimo S, The baby-friendly hospital initiative increases breastfeeding rates in a US neonatal intensive care unit. *J Hum Lact* 2003;19:166–171.
228. Maisels MJ, King E. Length of stay, jaundice and hospital readmission. *Pediatrics* 1998; 101:995–998.
229. Brown AK, Damus K, Kim MT, et. al. Factors relating to readmission of term and near-term neonates in the first two weeks of life. *J Perinatal Med* 1999; 27(4):263–275.
230. Wight NE, Breastfeeding the borderline (near-term) preterm infant. *Pediatr Ann* 2003;32(5):329–336.
231. Williams A. *Hypoglycemia of the newborn: review of the literature.* Geneva: World Health Organization, 1997;75:261–290. Download from: http://www.who.int/reproductive-health/docs/hypoglycae mia_newborn.htm
232. Eidelman AI. Hypoglycemia and the breastfed neonate. *Pediatr Clin North Am* 2001;48:377–387.
233. Protocol Committee Academy of Breastfeeding Medicine, Eidelman AI, Howard CR, et al. *Clinical protocol number 1: guidelines for glucose monitoring and treatment of hypoglycemia in breastfed neonate.* Academy of Breastfeeding Medicine. Available at http//www.bfmed.org/protos.html; accessed 1/26/05.
234. Gartner LM, Herschel M. Jaundice and breastfeeding. *Pediatr Clin North Am* 2001; 48:389–399.
235. Gartner LM, Herschel M. Jaundice and the breastfed baby. In: Riordan J, ed. *Breastfeeding and human lactation,* 3rd ed. Boston: Jones and Bartlett, 2005;311–321.
236. Lawrence RM, Lawrence RA. Given the benefits of breastfeeding, what contraindications exist? *Pediatr Clin North Am* 2001;48: 235–251.
237. Howard CR, Lawrence RA. Xenobiotics and breastfeeding. *Pediatr Clin North Am* 2001;48:485–504.
238. American Academy of Pediatrics. Committee on Drugs. The transfer of drugs and other chemicals into human milk. *Pediatrics* 2001;108:776–789.
239. Hale TW. Medications in breastfeeding mothers of preterm infants. *Pediatr Annu* 2003;32:337–347.
240. World Health Organization. *HIV and infant feeding: a review of HIV transmission through breastfeeding.* Publication WHO/FRH/ NUT 98.3, UNAIDS/98.5, UNICEF/PD/NUT/(J) 98.2 Geneva: WHO, 1998.
241. Stagno S, Reynolds DW, Pass RF, et al. Breast milk and the risk of cytomegalovirus infection. *N Engl J Med* 1980;302: 1073–1076.
242. Vochem M, Hamprecht K, Jahn G, et al. Transmission of cytomegalovirus to preterm infants through breast milk. *Pediatr Infect Dis J* 1998;17:53–58.

Thermal Regulation

Michael Friedman   Stephen Baumgart

A HISTORICAL PERSPECTIVE

Tarnier was an obstetrician in Paris who first applied modern concepts of incubation to human infants starting around 1830 (1,2). Tarnier's incubator, the couveuse, has been widely recognized as the first one designed specifically to care for premature babies. Tarnier and his student, Budin, studied premature human incubation into the next century, reporting almost doubled survival in infants born at less than 2 kg. In the United States, commercialization of Tarnier's and Budin's designs occurred, and the Rotch Incubator appeared at the Colombian Exposition in Chicago in 1893 (3–5). Thereafter, in 1933 Blackfan and Yaglou (6) provided humidity along with air warming within incubators, which improved the stability of infant temperature control. In the 1940s Chappel in Philadelphia added air isolation techniques to incubator care to prevent neonatal septic infections recognized to occur more frequently in humid environments (7,8). In 1958, Silverman and associates (9) challenged the need for humidity in incubators and used higher air temperatures than previously reported to care for an ever smaller premature population surviving with modern techniques.

Toward Defining the Optimal Thermal-Neutral Environment

In 1959 Cross and Hill from the United Kingdom described a metabolically neutral temperature for achieving the optimal environmental care of newborn animals and humans, suggesting that poor temperature maintenance resulted in increased metabolic rates of oxygen and substrate consumption (10–12) (Fig. 24-1). Physiologic responses to environmental temperature during incubation of premature newborn infants were investigated systematically in 1962 by Brück and coworkers (13,14) from Germany. In 1969 Hey and associates (15–17) from the United Kingdom defined the best operational incubator temperatures for preterm babies by describing an algorithm of air and wall temperatures, taking humidification and swaddling (insulation) into account as well. The Hey and Katz

nomograms for regulating incubators following preterm birth, growth, and maturation remain the benchmark standard for modern human incubation to date (Fig. 24-2).

THERMAL BALANCE AT THE BEGINNING OF LIFE

Fetal Thermal Regulation

The fetus generates heat during metabolism with cellular proliferation and differentiation, maintenance of intra- and extracellular ion gradients, and transport of nutrients and wastes across cell membranes. Cardiac and skeletal muscle work also generates heat *in utero* (18). Fetal ovine and human studies suggest that the rate of fetal heat production is about 33 to 47 cal/kg/minute (18,19). Fetal-maternal temperature gradients in mammals and humans have demonstrated that a difference in temperature of only 0.45°C to 0.50°C between the umbilic arterial and venous blood is sufficient to eliminate the majority of metabolic heat via the placental circulation (i.e., by forced convective transfer into the mother's uterine circulation) (20–22). Probably less than 10% to 20% of heat is dissipated from the fetal skin into the amniotic fluid (natural convection and conduction from the uterine wall). The mother additionally serves as a heat reservoir for the fetus, favoring the dissipation of heat as a byproduct of fetal metabolism. Fatal hyperthermia may occur with an elevation of maternal temperature or if the mother is unable to dissipate the excess heat produced during pregnancy. Therefore, pregnant women are advised to avoid prolonged hot baths and exertion on hot and humid days. Maternal fever should be treated aggressively with environmental cooling and with antipyretics and antibiotics when indicated.

Transition in the Delivery Suite

At birth, a newly born infant is immediately exposed to a wet and cold environment. Without intervention, rapid cooling by convection from the neonate's skin into the cold delivery room air (at least a 10.0°C drop) and by

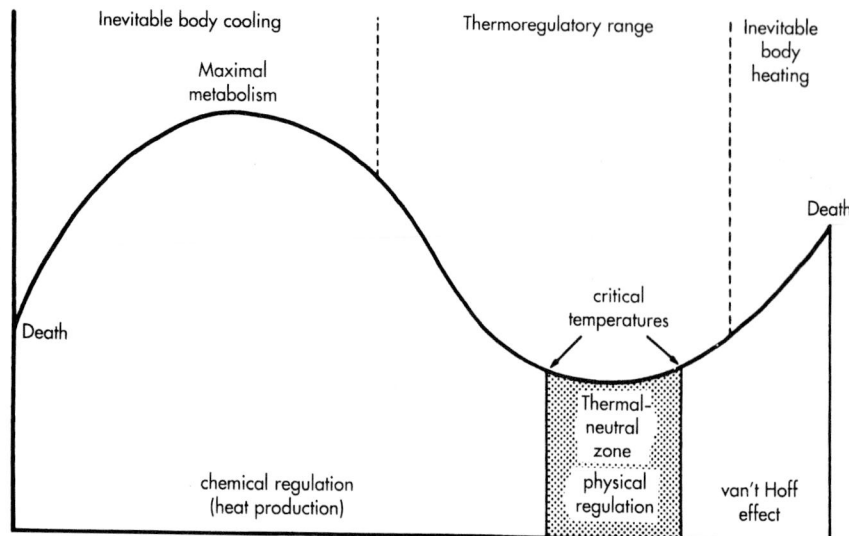

Figure 24-1 Basic concepts for defining neonatal thermal-neutral environmental temperature (horizontal axis) as the minimal observed metabolic rate (vertical axis, measured indirectly as oxygen consumption). The shaded region of this graph (the relatively narrow thermal-neutral zone) is bounded by upper and lower critical temperatures for nonmetabolic or physical regulation of normal body temperature (e.g., by vasoconstriction, vasodilatation, or changes in posture). Variation of environmental temperature outside this limited range results in a metabolic rate increase, in which infant core temperature may remain normal, but at the expense of increased metabolic expenditure (e.g., cold stress). Outside the thermal regulatory range of metabolic heat production, inevitable body cooling or heating results, with eventual death at environmental extremes. (From Baumgart S. Incubation of the human newborn infant. In: Pomerance JJ, Richardson CJ, eds. *Neonatology for the clinician.* Norwalk, Conn: Appleton & Lange, 1993:139–150, with permission.)

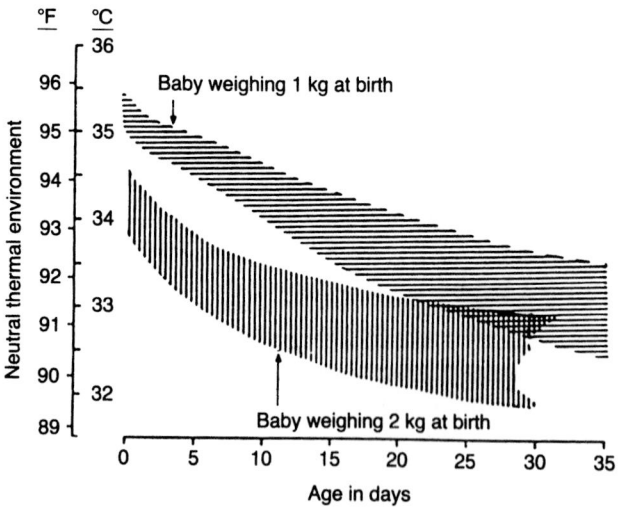

Figure 24-2 Range of temperatures needed to provide neutral environmental conditions for babies lying naked on an insulated mattress in draft-free surroundings (at about 50% relative humidity) with equal mean radiant wall temperature and air temperature. The top graph represents a 1-kg infant at birth and the bottom graph a 2-kg infant. Optimum temperature probably approximates the lower limit of each neutral range as defined here. Approximately 1°C should be added to these operative temperatures to derive the appropriate neutral air temperature for a single-walled incubator when room temperature is less than 27°C (80°F), and more should be added if room temperature is very much less than this. (From Hey EN, Katz G. The optimum thermal environment for naked babies. *Arch Dis Child* 1970;45:328–334, with permission.)

evaporation at a tremendous rate (0.58 kcal/mL of water loss) may result in a drop of the infant's body temperature at a rate of 0.2°C to 1.0°C/minute. Although fetal response to cold stress is relatively insensitive prenatally (22,23), increased infant activity (crying with agitated movement characteristic of cold exposure upon birth), vasoconstriction, and nonshivering thermogenesis (shivering is not active in the human newborn) occurs the instant the baby hits the cold air, mediated by the sympathetic nervous system (24). Triggered by temperature sensation of the skin, infant metabolic rate may increase by two- to threefold and thus maintain body temperature for a period of several hours in the term subject before thermogenic reserves of glycogen and brown fat become depleted.

Physiology of Neonatal Thermal Response

Brown fat is especially thermogenic in the term newborn, with large reserves located between the scapula, in the axillae and perithymic region, and in the paraspinal and perinephric areas. Penetrated extensively by blood vessels, which give it the brown appearance and which conduct heat generated into the central circulation, these adipocytes are laden with excess triglyceride stores and numerous mitochondria. With cold stress, the sympathetic surge acts directly upon cell surface receptors, which stimulate

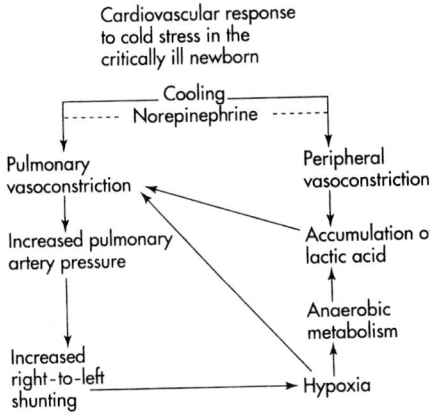

Figure 24-3 Immediate and potentially detrimental cardiovascular response to a sympathetic surge in norepinephrine released after birth upon exposure of the neonate's temperature-sensitive skin to a cold extrauterine environment (convection and evaporation). (From Baumgart S. Incubation of the human newborn infant. In: Pomerance JJ, Richardson CJ, eds. *Neonatology for the clinician.* Norwalk, Conn: Appleton & Lange, 1993:139–150, with permission.)

cyclic-AMP–mediated lipoprotein lipase. Thyroid hormone also surges at birth and augments this effect (5,25,26). β-Oxidation is uncoupled in brown adipocytes, however, resulting in triglyceride breakdown and resynthesis producing heat (27).

Preterm infants with immature thermogenic response and without metabolic substrate reserves deposited over the last trimester of pregnancy fare worse. As shown in Fig. 24-3, a sympathetic surge occurs at birth, with massive neurohumoral secretion of noradrenaline from paraaortic nodes and the fetal adrenal (28). Systemic and pulmonary vasoconstriction result, which may end in poor oxygen uptake and relative peripheral tissue hypoxia. Lactic acid production ensues, with demise ultimately occurring secondary to cold stress. Tarnier in the 1800s recognized this in Paris, where there was no central heating and poor home and hospital insulation.

Early Intervention

Drying infants in the delivery suite interrupts the process of evaporation, and bundling infants in cotton blankets to prevent exposure to cold air interrupts convective heat loss and provides insulation to retain the infant's metabolic heat. Placing infants at the mother's breast and cradled into her axillary fold engenders conductive heat transfer from the mother to the infant. Alternatively, and especially if early intervention is required to aid transition (e.g., suctioning or oxygen administration), the infant is dried first and then placed onto dry bedding under a radiant warmer while these procedures are performed. A convectively warmed incubator enclosure with air temperatures ranging from 35.0°C to 37.0°C and a variety of plastic swaddling heat shields have been advocated to prevent excessive cold exposure, especially during transition and hospital transport of premature infants (29–31).

Once in the nursery or mother's room, bundled infants may be placed into either an open bassinet or incubator (naked or bundled) and provided close monitoring of either axillary (preferred, 36.0°C to 36.5°C) or rectal (37°C to 37.5°C) temperatures through the first few hours of life. Slightly premature infants (32 to 35 weeks) or small-for-gestational-age babies may appear to have normal body temperature at the expense of metabolically generated heat (9). Glass and associates (32) demonstrated that premature infants nurtured in dry incubator environments of either 35.0°C (slightly cool) or 36.5°C in the first few days of life maintained a normal body temperature, but experienced more weight loss in the cooler environment.

Kangaroo Care

Skin-to-skin care, now termed kangaroo care, has been promoted for nurturing premature infants who are held naked between the mother's breasts as if in a kangaroo's pouch. The infant is in contact with the mother's warm skin and is close to the breast for unlimited feeding. Fathers also can provide thermal support in this way. Kangaroo care was first reported from Bogotá, Columbia, where use of conventional incubators was limited and mortality in nonincubated preterm births high. A large randomized trial from this country recently showed that infants less than or equal to 2.00 kg placed under kangaroo care shortly after birth for prolonged periods achieved transition safely and grew normally, had fewer nosocomial infections, and were discharged earlier, particularly at less than or equal to 1.80 kg (33). Significant reduction in early mortality also has been observed. During the 1980s the kangaroo technique was promoted for nurturance of nonmechanically ventilated, growing premature infants in Scandinavian and some other European countries. Randomized clinical trials also have demonstrated enhanced mother-infant attachment, greater maternal self-esteem, prolonged and enhanced lactation, increased infant alertness, and better weight gain (34). Physiologic studies have focused on demonstrating thermal-neutral metabolic response (minimal observed oxygen consumption) and temperature stability in stable growing premature babies during kangaroo care. Moreover, vital signs and oxygenation parameters were demonstrated to be more stable in preterm infants recovering from bronchopulmonary dysplasia, with absence of periodic breathing and reduced apnea and bradycardia. Behavioral studies demonstrate more homogenous sleep patterns, less irritability later in infancy, and more direct social eye contact with caregivers (35).

In the intensive care nursery, kangaroo care may be initiated even during mechanical ventilation with uncomplicated patients. Mothers are instructed to wear front-opening shirts, maintain careful hygiene without open sores or rashes, and avoid use of lotions, oils, or perfumes. Maximum skin surface area contact is desirable with a covering blanket to avoid outward convective and evaporative heat losses. Privacy and quiet must be provided by the nursery staff for periods of 0.5 to 1 hour initially, and careful temperature monitoring by surface thermistor or axillary thermometer should be performed at least every 15 minutes, along with cardiorespiratory and noninvasive oxygen monitoring when indicated. Temperature deviation of more than 0.5°C of normal skin temperature (36.5°C to 37.0°C) should result in termination of the session and return to incubator care. Periods up to 4 hours may be achieved. Mothers are encouraged to pump their breasts before and after sessions because milk production is enhanced. Parents are empowered with the care of their infants, and kangaroo care integrates the family into the neonatal intensive care team. Presently, no adverse reports have been published, and the use of kangaroo care in modern intensive care settings is on the rise.

CONVECTION-WARMED INCUBATORS

A modern incubator consists of an optically transparent, plastic hood (≥3 mm thick) covering the infant, with sidewall and hand-access ports. The infant lays on a bed platform, underneath which a tungsten element electronically heats the air. Air is forced over this element by a fan, circulating heated air within the hood. Temperature may be controlled thermostatically to regulate either the air or infant skin temperature (15,36).

Thermodynamics of Incubation

The physiology of mammalian (homeothermic) thermal regulation (37) may be summarized by the equation:

$$\dot{Q}_{metabolic} = \dot{Q}_{convection} + \dot{Q}_{conduction} + \dot{Q}_{evaporation} + \dot{Q}_{radiation} + \dot{Q}_{stored}$$

in which $\dot{Q}$ is the rate of either metabolic heat production (left side of the equation) or of heat loss and heat stored (right side of the equation), generally expressed in kcal/kg/hour or in W/m^2 ($J/sec/m^2$). By convention, heat production and heat losses (or storage) are expressed as positive values. When a mammal is successfully maintaining normal body temperature, heat storage is zero, otherwise body temperature either increases or decreases until a new thermal equilibrium is established at another temperature. Also, when an environmental heat loss becomes a heat gain (e.g., under a radiant warmer), the gain is expressed as a negative loss.

Convection

The rate of heat transferred from an infant's skin into the incubator environment depends in part on the insulation provided by the dermis and subcutaneous fascia (comprised primarily of white fat deposited late in gestation). Preterm babies have almost no fatty fascia and, therefore, are more vulnerable to heat loss through air (and skin blood flow) convection (37). Air convection is heat loss that takes place from the skin's surface into the surrounding environment and is summarized by the equation:

$$\dot{Q}_{convection} = k_1(T_{mean\ skin} - T_{air}) + k_2(T_{mean\ skin} - T_{air})V^n$$

in which two forms of skin-to-air convective heat loss occur, depending on the gradient between skin and air temperatures (ΔT), the complex geometry of surface area exposed and air thermal density k, and air movement velocity V^n (38). The first is natural convection, which results from the gradient of temperature between the skin surface and surrounding air (38,39). Natural convection cells form as warm air rises from the skin, conveying heat and body moisture away from the surface of the baby. Air thus warmed subsequently cools and falls back toward the baby, forming the convection cell. Such cells form over the curvature of the baby's exposed body surface area. An infant in flexion leaves less surface area exposed (38). An infant extended and flaccid is able to dissipate more heat. Posture may be a valuable observation in deciding the thermal comfort or discomfort of even a preterm infant.

The second form of convection is forced convective air movement, usually occurring at air velocities ≥0.27 m/sec. Forced convective heat loss is roughly proportional to an exponential power (n) of the velocity (V) of air movement. Within forced convection-warmed incubators, manufacturers strive to render still the air near the baby. Recent estimates of natural and forced-air convective heat loss from premature neonates nursed within incubators indicate success in this strategy because natural convection was the only major loss observed to occur (40). Heat also is lost to a lesser degree by respiratory convection and evaporation.

An example of different incubator convection designs affecting skin-to-air heat transfer is shown in Fig. 24-4,

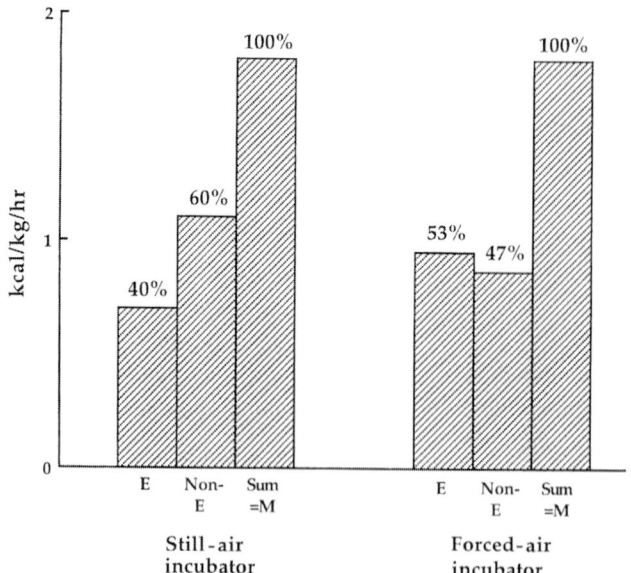

Figure 24-4 Partitional calorimetry performed for premature infants in two different types of convection-warmed incubators, natural and forced air. The rate of evaporative heat loss (E) is greater proportionally for babies nurtured in a conventional forced-air warmed environment than nonevaporative heat losses (non-E) from convection, conduction, and radiation. Heat balance is regulated by metabolic rate (M) and nonmetabolic mechanisms for thermal conservation (e.g., vasoconstriction). (Adapted from Okken A, Blijham C, Franz W, et al. Effects of forced convection of heated air on insensible water loss and heat loss in preterm infants in incubators. *J Pediatr* 1982;101:108–112, with permission.)

TABLE 24-1

CALCULATED BODY SURFACE AREA: BODY MASS RATIO FOR ADULTS, LOW-BIRTH-WEIGHT NEONATES, AND VERY-LOW-BIRTH-WEIGHT NEONATES

	Body Mass (kg)	BSA (m^2)	BSA/Mass (cm^2/kg)
Adult	70	1.73	250
LBW premature	1.5	0.13	870
LBW premature	1.0	0.10	1,000
VLBW	0.5	0.065	1,300

LBW, low birth weight; VLBW, very low birth weight. (Adapted from Costarino AT, Baumgart S. Neonatal water metabolism. In: Cowett RM, ed. *Principles of perinatal neonatal metabolism.* New York: Springer-Verlag, 1991:623, with permission.)

adapted from a study of partitional calorimetry performed by Okken and associates (41). The left incubator partition in this figure represents a natural convection-warmed incubator with no circulating fan. Air rose passively from heating elements underneath the baby's mattress to warm the interior of the incubator hood. The second partition on the right represents a more standard, fan-forced convection incubator as described previously. Nonevaporative heat loss in the passive device (non-E, the sum of convection, radiation, and conduction) was 60% compared to 47% in the forced convection-warmed incubator, whereas evaporative heat loss (E) was 13% higher in the forced convective environment. These authors attributed this increased evapora-

tive loss to disturbance by the incubator's fan of a microenvironment of humid air layered near the baby's skin.

Evaporation

The premature neonate loses large amounts of water (and, therefore, latent heat at 0.58 kcal/mL) through evaporation from the skin for several reasons (42–49). First and most important is the premature neonate's thin epidermis lacking keratin, which normally serves as a vapor barrier for older infants, children, and adults. Very immature skin is associated with reduced survival, and evaporative rates from infants less than 700 g may be likened to those of severe burn victims. Second, premature neonates lose excessive amounts of water and heat due to an increased body surface area:body mass ratio as demonstrated in Table 24-1 (50). The very-low-birth-weight premature infant of less than or equal to 500 grams exposes six times the area of the adult subject per kilogram of the largely water body mass. Third, the proportion of the extracellular water mass in the very-low-birth-weight infant, which is exposed to the external environment through the nonkeratinized epidermal layer, is significantly larger (51).

Hammerlund and Sedin (45) (Fig. 24-5) summarized the rate of transepidermal water loss in premature newborn infants nurtured in incubators throughout the first month of life at different gestational ages. This figure demonstrates that the newborn at 26 weeks of gestation may lose as much as 60 grams of water per m^2/hour (more than 180 mL/kg/day or 100 kcal/kg/day). Additional amounts of water may also be lost from upper airways during respiration of nonhumidified air in incubators.

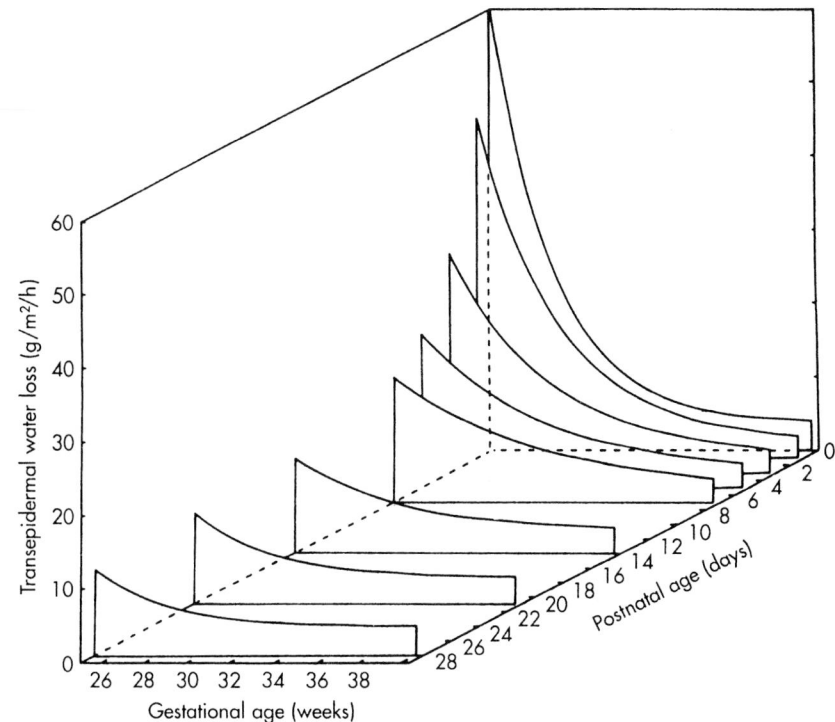

Figure 24-5 Transepidermal water evaporation from the skin of premature neonates of gestations ranging from 25 to 40 weeks, followed longitudinally from birth over the first month of life. Dehydration is most dangerous in the most immature babies less than 28 weeks of gestation in the first week of life before skin keratinization occurs. (From Sedin G, Hammarlund K, Nilsson GE, et al. Measurements of transepidermal water loss in newborn infants. *Clin Perinatol* 1985;12: 79–99, with permission.)

Incubator Humidification

Humidification inside modern incubators is accomplished by the evaporation of water from a reservoir located in the air path over the heating element beneath the incubator mattress (52). Earlier descriptions of humidification in incubators cited the use of nebulized mist to saturate the infant's environment ($\geq$80% to 90% relative humidity) (53,54). These latter techniques resulted in the proliferation of *Pseudomonas* infections and were rejected resoundingly by a number of reports (53–56). Unfortunately, abandoning all use of vapor (invisible humidification) based on infection risks encountered with particulate mists (visible humidification) has resulted in running incubator hoods completely "dry." Relative humidity levels inside dry incubators at 36°C to 36.5°C may drop to less than 10% to 15%, promoting large insensible water and latent heat losses (52). In response to these concerns, the American Academy of Pediatrics recommended only moderate use of air humidification 50% relative humidity in the vapor phase (i.e., gaseous), and not a particulate mist (liquid phase) (57). Put simply, if water circulating near an infant is visible, infection may be more likely.

A more recent reevaluation of incubator humidification was conducted by Harpin and Rutter (52) in 1985. Thirty-three infants less than 30 weeks of gestation and less than 2 weeks of age were nurtured in vapor-humidified incubators saturated at between 80% and 90% relative humidity. Two infants acquired *Pseudomonas* sepsis and one died. Twenty-nine babies of similar gestation and maturity were nurtured in dry incubators: one suffered an episode of *Pseudomonas* sepsis and died. Those who died with *Pseudomonas* infections did so after the study had ended after the first 2 weeks of life. The authors recommended that humidification be used routinely in the first 2 weeks of life to prevent evaporative losses and prevent skin desiccation. Humidification early in life may be prudent for incubation of the very-low-birth-weight infant, in whom heat and water losses are excessive and probably pathologic. Modern incubators now may be equipped with sophisticated solid-state temperature and humidity control devices to prevent condensation at higher relative humidity levels between 60% and 80%. Although verification is yet lacking, hopefully a reduced risk of infection will occur by maintaining humidity without visible condensation.

Conductive Heat Loss and Warming Mattresses

Conductive heat loss results from contact of a baby's body with the solid surface of a bed platform:

$$\dot{Q}_{conduction} = k(T_{core\ temp} - T_{mean\ skin})/D$$

in which k is contact surface area and the bed's heat conductivity constant, and (ΔT) represents the temperature gradient between the infant's body core (containing heat) and mean skin contact surface. D is the thickness of the bed's conducting material. In general, insulating foam rubber (about 2.5-cm thickness) and double cotton blanket batting results in negligible conductive heat loss by providing insulation from the metal or plastic bed table (i.e., reducing the value of k). Recently, however, incubator manufacturers and water mattress companies have provided evidence that exogenous heat application through carefully conducted bed surfaces maintained at less than or equal to 39°C to prevent burn injury to areas of skin contact may reduce environmental heat requirements from incubators or radiant warmers for very-low-birth-weight subjects (58,59). Moreover, application of warmed mattresses during extreme environmental conditions encountered in infant transports also may prove beneficial (59,60).

Radiant Heat Loss

Radiant heat loss is the least intuitive aspect of newborn incubation. Radiant heat loss occurs as a transfer of infrared electromagnetic energy virtually instantly from one warm body to another of lesser warmth:

$$\dot{Q}_{radiation} = (\beta)(\epsilon_1)(\epsilon_2)(T_{mean\ skin} - T_{walls})$$

in which a radiant heat transfer constant β (Stefan-Boltzmann), the physical emissivity of the infant's skin and incubator's plastic walls (ϵ_{skin}, ϵ_{walls}), the absolute temperature gradient (ΔT), and the infant's exposed surface area and posture determine the rate of radiant heat loss within incubators (37). In a single-walled incubator, heat transfers from the infant's skin (36.5°C to 37.0°C) to the mean temperature of the cooler walls of the incubator's plastic interior (approximately 28.0°C to 36.5°C). The incubator walls then reradiate heat to the nursery walls and windows, which are even cooler (18.0°C to 27.0°C). A massive heat sink is represented by the nursery walls, which may determine 60% of the operant environmental temperature perceived by the skin in room air conditions:

$$T_{operant\ environment} = 0.60(T_{walls}) - 0.40(T_{air})$$

Double-Walled Incubators

The importance of radiant heat transfer within incubators is demonstrated in Fig. 24-6 (40). Two incubators of different designs are compared. Partitional calorimetry for a single-walled incubator is shown on the left, whereas a double-walled incubator design is depicted on the right. The double-walled incubator constitutes a plastic chamber similar to the single-walled incubator with an additional inner wall suspended several centimeters interior to the outer wall of the incubator. Warmed air is circulated between these two incubator walls, warming both the outer and inner surfaces of the inner wall, as well as the inner surface of the outer wall of the incubator. The result is an elevated inner wall plastic temperature exposed to an infant's skin. Radiant heat loss to the inner wall of the incubator exposed to the infant's skin is significantly reduced. Convective heat loss is higher in the double-walled incubator because a cooler air temperature is

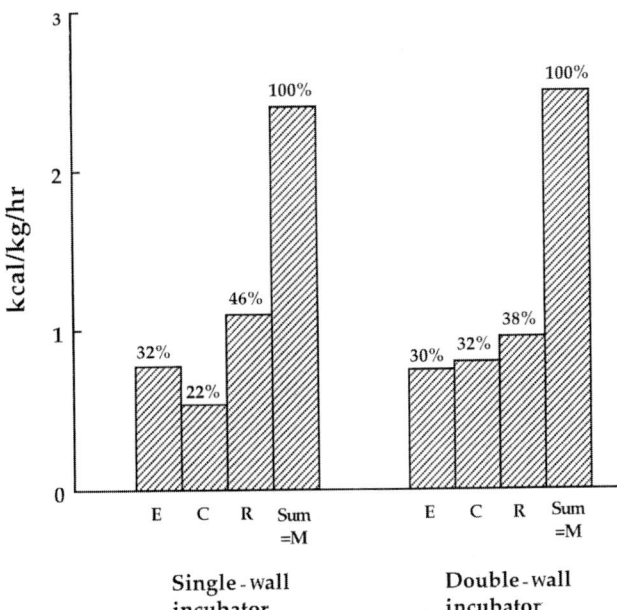

Figure 24-6 Partitional calorimetry performed for preterm infants at steady-state, thermal-neutral temperature in two forced-air, convection-warmed incubators, either with only a single wall between the infant and surrounding nursery's environmental air and wall temperatures, or with an inner wall (double-walled incubator) interposed between the infant and incubator's outer wall. Forced-air warming of both sides of the inner wall reduces radiant heat loss, resulting in lower servocontrolled incubator air temperature (higher infant convective heat loss). Evaporative loss was not altered by insertion of the double wall. (Adapted from Bell EF, Rios GR. A double-walled incubator alters the partition of body heat loss of premature infants. *Pediatr Res* 1983;17:135–140, with permission.)

required to maintain the infant when radiant heat loss is thus conserved. Because vapor pressure is constant, evaporative heat loss is the same in both incubator devices.

Skin Surface Servocontrol Temperature

As a result of the difficulties encountered in measuring and controlling the whole environment defined by all of the parameters described previously, Silverman and associates (36) proposed that any set of environmental conditions that rendered a normothermic skin surface temperature would provide a thermal-neutral environment. They defined a skin temperature servocontrol set point between 36.2°C to 36.5°C over the anterior abdominal wall for thermostatic control of incubator air temperature warming (with or without humidification, mattress warming, or radiant walls protection) to guarantee a minimal observed metabolic rate of oxygen consumption and, therefore, a thermal-neutral environment. Proportional response, servocontrolled skin temperature now has become the standard of care for regulating convection-warmed incubator heating over much of the world.

Servocontrolled Incubator Homeothermy

All incubator studies demonstrating a thermal-neutral environment under a variety of conditions evaluating air

temperature, convection, and humidity; incubator wall temperature; and nursery temperature were performed at steady-state conditions. Infant metabolic rates often were determined in noncritical subjects at rest. Such steady-state conditions are theoretical, however, in critically ill premature neonates in thermostatically servocontrolled incubators, subjected to the many variations encountered in the modern neonatal intensive care nursery. Hand ports and doors may be opened and closed several times a day for access to nursing and minor surgical procedures, as well as radiographic, ultrasound, and echocardiographic examinations. Incubators may be invaded as often as once an hour for delivery of intensive care. This can result in overshooting and undershooting of air temperature for as long as 1 hour after the door has been closed.

THE RADIANT WARMER BED

The radiant warmer bed is a variable-level, waist-high platform with a mattress surface (which may be either heated or may incorporate an electronic scale), upon which the critically ill newborn lies without an encumbering plastic enclosure. Suspended about 80 to 90 cm above this platform is a radiant heat source with an electrically heated metal alloy wire coiled within a quartz tube. A thermostatic skin servocontrol device regulates the radiant heat, which is distributed across near and far wavelengths of the infrared spectrum (Fig. 24-7). At full power, the sum of infrared

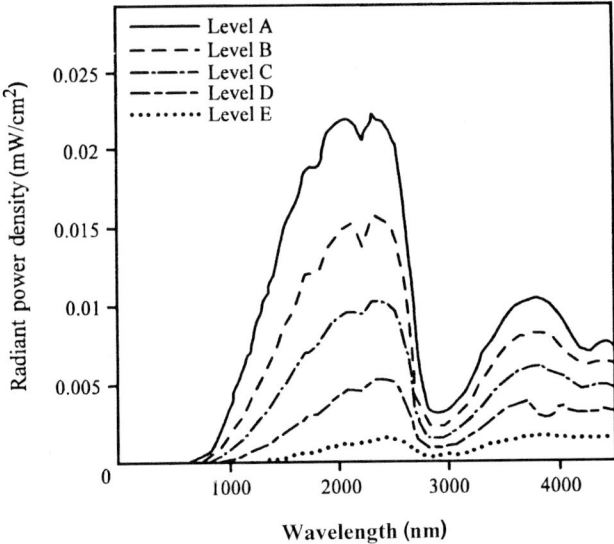

Figure 24-7 Spectral irradiance measured at bed level with increasing power from a radiant warmer's heating element. Note two peaks of energy indicating the wire element's emission (near infrared wavelength spectrum at the left) and the quartz containment tube's reemission of absorbed heat from the wire (far spectrum at the right). The notch in the near peak probably indicates infrared adsorption by water vapor. Integrated over the entire peak emissions, levels of near and far infrared exposure are felt to be safe for the developing skin and eyes. (From Baumgart S, Knauth A, Casey FX, et al. Infrared eye injury not due to radiant warmer use in premature neonates. *Am J Dis Child* 1993;147: 565–569, with permission.)

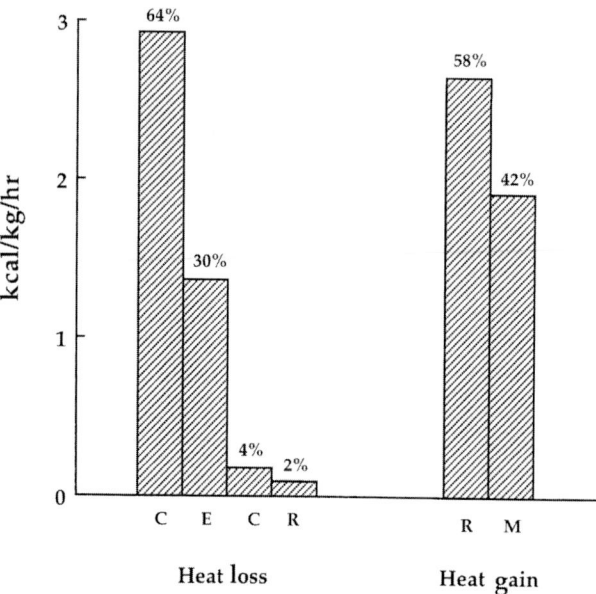

Figure 24-8 Partitional calorimetry for infants nurtured naked under radiant warmers servocontrolled to maintain anterior abdominal wall skin temperature at 36.5°C. Shown on the left are convective, evaporative, conductive, and radiant heat losses (from the infant's sides), and on the right are radiant heat gain (facing the warmer) and heat generated by the infant's metabolism. (Adapted from Baumgart S. Radiant heat loss versus radiant heat gain in premature neonates under radiant warmers. *Biol Neonate* 1990;57:10–20, with permission.)

irradiance is less than 100 mW/cm² of surface area on the bed platform. The heat delivered in the near portion of the infrared spectrum (less than 1,000 nm) is less than 10 mW/cm² of surface area irradiated. These levels of radiant exposure recently have been judged as biologically safe for the developing skin and eyes in the prematurely born newborn infant when exposed briefly. The servocontrolled warmer generally operates at about one-half this peak power, and radiant power density delivered at bed level usually is well below the 50 to 60 mW/cm² felt to be potentially deleterious at longer periods of exposure. The head, foot, and sides of the radiant warmer bed platform receive less radiant power and, therefore, less warming than is delivered to the center of the bed platform. Optimally, infants are positioned in the center of this device.

Figure 24-8 demonstrates experience with complete partitional calorimetry for critically ill premature infants nurtured under radiant warmers (61). Both radiant heat losses under a radiant warmer as well as heat gains are demonstrated. The effects of evaporation, convection, and conduction and of infant metabolic heat production are demonstrated for infants nurtured naked and supine under these devices. Heat loss comprised 64% toward convection to the surrounding cool air of the nursery's environment. The majority of convective heat loss occurred naturally, whereas a minor component was composed of forced convective air movement from doors opening and closing within the nursery, nursery personnel bustling near the bedside, as well as the cycling of heating and cooling vents

supplying the nursery's ambient air control. These turbulent convective air movements contributed to evaporative heat loss, which comprised 30% of total heat loss in this figure. Thermal equilibrium is maintained under a radiant warmer by replacement of heat losses through convection, evaporation, conduction, and radiation, by radiant heat gain directly from the warming element. Almost 58% of heat replacement is derived from the servocontrolled radiant warmer. Metabolic heat production M comprises 42% of the thermal balance and is overpowered by the radiant heating element.

Thermal-Neutral Radiant Warming

Le blanc (62) summarized a metanalysis comparing radiant warmers to convectively heated incubators. The thermal-neutral environment was defined for each warming device as the minimal observed metabolic rate of oxygen consumption (MOMR measured in oxygen consumption, $\dot{V}O_2$, in mL/kg/minute) when skin temperature was servocontrolled between 36.0°C and 36.5°C and at steady-state conditions. Eleven of 16 infants demonstrated slightly higher rates of oxygen consumption when nursed at similar temperatures under radiant warmers ($\dot{V}O_2$ 6.84 ± 0.37 [standard error of the mean] vs. 7.45 ± 0.44 mL/kg/minute), an increase of 8.8% in metabolic rate under radiant warmers.

A more recent metanalysis compiled by Flenady and Woodgate (63) again compared radiant warmers to incubators using MOMR to define the thermal-neutral environment. This review found that nursing under radiant warmers caused a statistically significant increase in insensible water loss and a nonsignificant trend toward higher oxygen consumption when compared to incubators. When a heat shield was added to the radiant warmer and compared to the incubator, there was a trend toward higher insensible water loss that was not statistically significant and there was no difference in oxygen consumption.

The assumptions involved in the calculation of MOMR are that the infant is (a) at rest and asleep, (b) postprandial at least 2 to 3 hours, and (c) at thermal-neutral temperature conditions. Typically premature infants demonstrate slightly higher oxygen consumptions than term infants, and small-for-gestational-age infants manifest oxygen consumptions slightly higher than premature and term infants. The minimum requirement for oxygen consumption in these studies demonstrates a metabolic rate of caloric expenditure of roughly 60 to 75 kcal/kg/day. Above this amount, 9 to 10 kcal/kg/day may be required for growth. However, intensive care conditions provided to critically ill neonates rarely approximate those of a growing premature baby at rest and at steady-state.

Figure 24-9 shows results of oxygen consumption measurements from studies conducted in an intensive care nursery in a 1.2-kg infant nurtured naked and supine under a radiant warmer while intubated endotracheally and receiving ventilatory support (64). During a 90-minute period of relatively mild cold stress (servocontrol skin temperature 35.5°C), oxygen consumption fluctuated

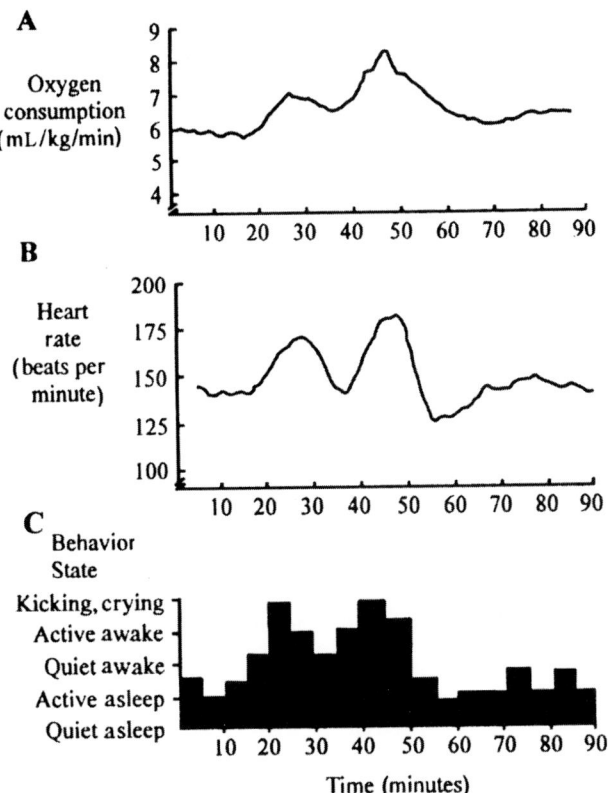

A
Oxygen consumption (mL/kg/min)

B
Heart rate (beats per minute)

C
Behavior State
Kicking, crying
Active awake
Quiet awake
Active asleep
Quiet asleep

Time (minutes)

Figure 24-9 Metabolic rate of oxygen consumption **(A)** parallels heart rate **(B)** and infant activity **(C)** with the performance of indirect calorimetry in a premature baby weighing approximately 1.2 kg. Variation with infant behavior is demonstrated in this relatively cool condition (servocontrol 35.5°C). (From Baumgart S. Partitioning of heat losses and gains in premature newborn infants under radiant warmers. *Pediatrics* 1985;75:89–99, with permission.)

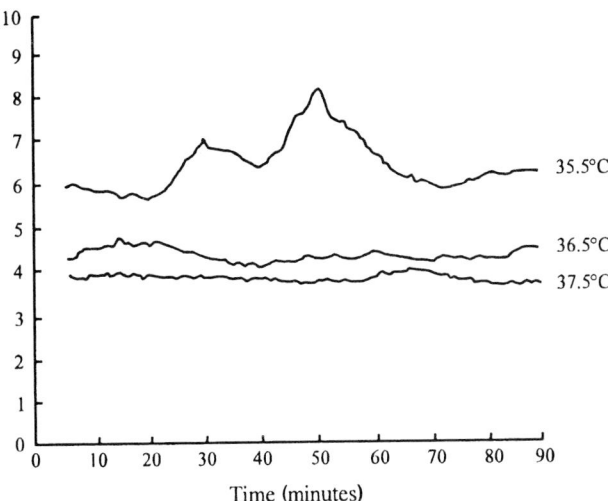

35.5°C
36.5°C
37.5°C

Time (minutes)

Figure 24-10 The metabolic rates of oxygen consumption from the same infant shown in Fig. 24-9 are compared at 35.5°C, 36.5°C, and 37.5°C servocontrol skin temperature. Behavioral activity is attenuated, and basal metabolism is significantly reduced at warmer temperatures. (From Malin SW, Baumgart S. Optimal thermal management for low birth weight infants nursed under high-power radiant warmers. *Pediatrics* 1987;79:47–54, with permission.)

36.5°C skin temperature set point represented optimal control under intensive care circumstances. Increasing anterior abdominal wall skin temperature above this point by 1°C resulted in no significant additional reduction in metabolic rate, and when servocontrolled to 37.5°C, the gradient for heat loss (from the infant's core to the skin) narrowed sufficiently for a number of them to become hyperthermic (38.2°C to 38.5°C). It is therefore recommended to avoid skin control temperatures above

between 5.5 and 8.5 mL/kg/minute, paralleled closely by the infant's heart rate and behavior. These observations of preterm infant behavior linked to metabolism are typical, even in critically ill infants. Criteria for determining MOMR suggest that oxygen consumption for this subject is 5.5 mL/kg/minute. However, the integrated sum of behavior over the entire study period reflects a higher rate of global metabolism. Such observations led Schulze and associates (65) to speculate that a thermal-neutral environment should be evaluated over periods considerably longer than 10 to 30 minutes of MOMR at steady state. Figure 24-10 shows oxygen consumption over three 90-minute periods for the same infant as shown in Fig. 24-9 at three different radiant warmer servocontrol skin temperatures—35.5°C, 36.5°C, and 37.5°C (66). From these studies over longer study periods, it seems clear that infant behavior may constitute a significant part of metabolic rate determination, affecting the thermal-neutral zone. Figure 24-11 shows 18 premature infants nurtured under radiant warmers demonstrating a thermal-neutral environmental temperature (between 36.2°C and 36.5°C servocontrolled anterior abdominal wall skin temperature) in which all infant behavior was incorporated (66). Approximately 7.2 mL/kg/minute VO₂ at the warmer's

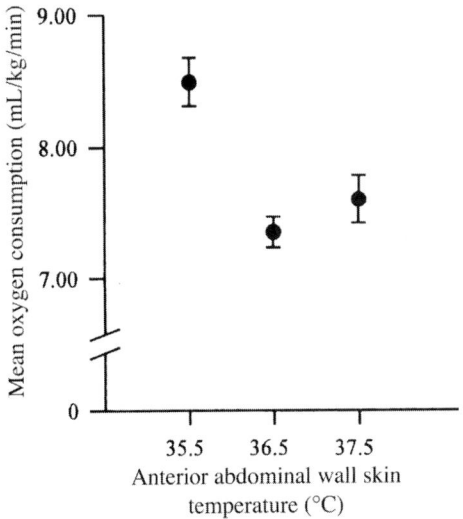

Mean oxygen consumption (mL/kg/min)

9.00

8.00

7.00

0

35.5   36.5   37.5
Anterior abdominal wall skin temperature (°C)

Figure 24-11 Significantly lower oxygen consumption is demonstrated at 36.5°C compared to 35.5°C servocontrol temperature for a series of 18 infants under radiant warmers. No additional significant reduction in oxygen consumption is achieved by increasing servocontrol temperature to 37.5°C, and several infants demonstrated deep rectal hyperthermia at 37.5°C. (From Malin SW, Baumgart S. Optimal thermal management for low birth weight infants nursed under high-power radiant warmers. *Pediatrics* 1987;79:47–54, with permission.)

36.7°C and 37.0°C for infants in the weight range studied (between 0.87 and 1.60 kg).

HEAT SHIELDING

Rigid, Plastic Heat Shields

A 1- to 2-mm thickness of plastic used as a miniature incubator hood and placed over infants on open radiant beds has been proposed by several authors. Yeh and associates (67) reported that insensible water loss was reduced by more than 25% for infants nurtured under a plastic hood. Bell and associates (68) failed to replicate any difference in water loss using a rigid plastic body hood under radiant warmers. The configuration of the plastic hoods used in each of these studies was different, in some cases permitting free air exchange at the open ends of the hood. Moreover, the interposition of radiantly opaque plastic between infant and the radiant element may have interfered with the delivery of radiant heat to the baby's skin (69). Disruption of the servocontrol mechanism by interposition of a radiant opaque plastic heat sink between the infant and the warmer seems to be a futile strategy.

Occlusive Plastic Blankets or Bags

A flexible plastic blanket made of saran seems more efficient than the body hood, particularly under a radiant warmer (Fig. 24-12) (39,70). Saran is thin, permitting free heat exchange without excessive evaporation (70). The flexible plastic blanket reduces the effect of forced convection, which disrupts the microenvironment of warm, humid air near the infant's skin (39). The reduction in both convective and evaporative heat losses is about 30% (70). Insensible water loss is diminished from about 2.0 to 1.2 mL/kg/hour. Oxygen consumption is reduced from 9.0 to 8.0 mL/kg/minute in this study. The net effect of saran blanket heat shielding under radiant warmers renders the environment more homeothermic, with lower power required to achieve thermal equilibrium, both from the radiant warmer and the baby's rate of metabolic heat production.

A polyethylene plastic body bag was proposed by Vohra and associates (71) for use during delivery room resuscitations in premature neonates. Significantly higher core temperatures and survival was reported for babies less than 28 weeks of gestation. A multicenter randomized trial of this device has been proposed by the authors.

Adverse effects with plastic blankets or bags have been cited. In extremely low-birth-weight infants, the immature skin may stick to the plastic, causing maceration. Moreover, if the servocontrol thermistor fails or becomes detached, serious hyperthermia may result and deaths have been reported. Nursing management of thermal care should prevent plastic from directly contacting the skin wherever possible. Infant core temperatures (axillary or rectal) should also be monitored frequently without relying on the skin servoprobe. Finally, infection control risk with plastic blankets/bags has not been adequately documented. With careful regard to these complications, however, these techniques are presently the most effective under radiant warmers for more consistent thermal-neutral temperature regulation.

EPIDERMAL BARRIER PROTECTION

Semiocclusive Artificial Skin

A novel strategy for thermal protection is covering the exposed surfaces of immature skin with semiocclusive polyurethane dressings (Tegaderm and Opsite) (72). In early studies using this technique, insensible water loss from days 1 to 4 of life was reduced by 30% to 50%. Upon careful removal of the artificial polyurethane dressing, skin moisture barrier development (keratinization) was consistent with development over the adjacent naked skin sites tested. A report by Porat and Brodsky (73) indicated that applying an adherent polyurethane layer over the entire torso and extremities early in very-low-birth-weight infants under 800 g improved fluid and electrolyte balance, reduced patent ductus arteriosus and intraventricular hemorrhage, as well as improved survival. Mancini and associates (74) found a similar result and reported a decrease in bacterial growth on skin guarded by a semipermeable dressing.

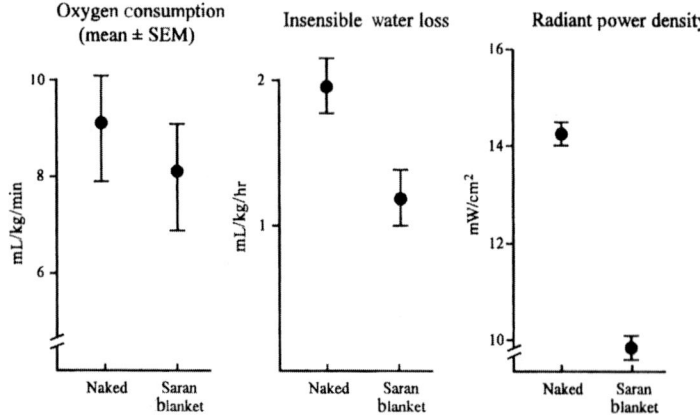

Figure 24-12 Comparison of radiant power density delivered (right), insensible water loss (middle), and oxygen consumption (left) in preterm neonates nurtured either naked or covered by a saran plastic blanket under radiant warmers. The blanket significantly reduced all three measurements in all babies tested, suggesting better environmental maintenance under saran. SEM, standard error of the mean. (From Baumgart S. Reduction of oxygen consumption, insensible water loss, and radiant heat demand with use of a plastic blanket for low-birth-weight infants under radiant warmers. *Pediatrics* 1984;74:1022–1028, with permission.)

Emollients and Aquaphor

Rutter and Hull (76) originally reviewed topical agents for reduction of transepidermal water loss. They found high water content creams ineffective in this regard, whereas paraffin produced a modest effect. Calculated evaporative rate was initially halved in preterm infants less than 30 weeks of gestation; however, this effect was transient, with return to a higher rate of water loss within 4 to 8 hours (75,76). Nopper and associates (77) conducted a randomized trial investigating barrier effects of a topical, petroleum-based, preservative-free ointment (Aquaphor) applied twice daily for 2 weeks to the skin of preterm infants. Transepidermal water loss was decreased by 67% initially compared to control infants and remained at 34% below controls after 4 to 6 hours. Dermatologic scores of skin integrity were improved in treated infants, and there was a decline in bacterial colonization of axillary skin, with a significantly lower incidence of positive blood and spinal fluid cultures. The authors also suggested better temperature control and fluid balance in treated subjects. Commentary by Rutter (76) on this work suggests, however, that temperature control may not benefit babies weighing less than 1 kg early after birth, and only high humidity incubators eliminate this problem in the smallest infants.

Aquaphor results early on were encouraging for improving skin care and reducing insensible water loss (77); however, the findings of a multicenter randomized trial are still awaiting publication (Vermont Oxford Network 2001) (78). One preliminary study, however, implies that bacterial infection may be more likely (79). Until complications of any shielding technique are better defined, nurses and doctors should remain cautious adopting them for routine care of extremely low-birth-weight patients.

HYBRID INCUBATOR/RADIANT WARMER DESIGN

One new incubator design recently marketed is the hybrid design. The accessibility of a radiant warmer is combined with the protection of an incubator enclosure. In the incubator mode, plastic walls surround the baby, and temperature is regulated by convection air warming. In the radiant warmer mode, these plastic walls are rotated down below the bed platform to facilitate handling with procedures. An overhead radiant heater switches on automatically to regulate servocontrolled skin temperature. No plastic is positioned between the infant and radiant warming element. Although expensive, these devices are an alternative to moving fragile infants requiring procedural interventions.

FEVER

Generally, fever may be defined as a core body temperature greater than 37.5°C. Depending on the limits chosen, approximately 1% to 2.5% of all newborns admitted to the normal nursery are febrile by rectal or axillary temperature (80). Although relatively more uncommon, the most life-threatening cause of fever in the neonate is bacterial sepsis. Fever, however, is an unreliable marker for infection in the newborn as less than 10% of all febrile neonates have culture-proven sepsis, and many more infected infants demonstrate normothermia or most commonly, hypothermia.

PHYSIOLOGIC CONTROL OF BODY TEMPERATURE

Central control of body temperature occurs at the level of the hypothalamus, where a set point temperature defines normothermia. When body temperature falls below this set point, the hypothalamus initiates heat conservation mechanisms that include peripheral vasoconstriction and nonshivering thermogenesis. If body temperature rises above the set point, heat dissipation mechanisms are activated; in the neonate, these consist mainly of peripheral vasodilation and to limited degree, sweating. It is thought that fever occurs when this set point is displaced to a higher level.

MECHANISMS PRODUCING NEONATAL FEVER

Bacterial and viral toxins, like endotoxins of bacterial membranes, are examples of exogenous pyrogens that can initiate an immunologic cascade resulting in fever (80). Exogenous pyrogens stimulate granulocytes and macro-phages to produce endogenous pyrogen (interleukin-1). Endogenous pyrogen then activates phospholipase A2, which ultimately results in the production of prosta-glandins. One of these prostaglandins, PGE2, is thought to be one of the mediators that raises the hypothalamic set point producing the fever seen with infection.

In addition, exposure to excess heat or insulation (excessive swaddling) can quickly increase core temperature of newborn infants due to their poor heat dissipation mechanisms, particularly the inability to effectively sweat. Such overheating commonly occurs when term babies are nursed in uncontrolled incubators or under radiant warmers. Temperature elevation may also occur with increased infant metabolic rate, as seen with skeletal muscle rigidity and status epilepticus. Another cause of temperature elevation is occasionally observed in well, breast-feeding newborn infants on the third to fourth day of life and is felt to result from dehydration due to insufficient maternal milk production. Finally, there are more recent reports of an increased incidence of maternal and neonatal fever when mothers receive epidural anesthesia (81).

REFERENCES

1. Cone TE. *History of the care and feeding of the premature infant*. Boston: Little, Brown & Co, 1985.
2. Berthod P. La couveuse et le gavage a la maternite de Paris [doctoral thesis]. Paris: G. Rougier, 1887.
3. Marx S. Incubation and incubators. *Am Med Surg Bull* 1896; 9:311–.
4. Rotch TM. Description of a new incubator. *Arch Pediatr* 1893;10: 661–665.
5. Swanson HE. Interrelations between thyroxin and adrenalin in the regulation of oxygen consumption in the albino rat. *Endocrinology* 1956;59:217–225.
6. Blackfan KD, Yaglou CP. The premature infant. a study of effects of atmospheric conditions on growth and on development. *Am J Dis Child* 1933;46:1175–1236.
7. Bolt RA. The mortalities of infancy. In: Abt I-A, ed. *Pediatrics*, 1st ed, Philadelphia: WB Saunders, 1923.
8. Mauriceau F. *Traite des maladies des femmes grosses et accouchees*. Paris: Chez l'Auteur, 1669:100–.
9. Silverman WA, Fertig JW, Berger AP. The influence of the thermal environment upon the survival of newly born premature infants. *Pediatrics* 1958;22:876–886.
10. Cross KW, Dawes GS, Mott JC. Anoxia, oxygen consumption and cardial output in new-born lambs and adult sheep. *J Physiol* 1959;146:316–343.
11. Hill JR, Rahimtulla KA. Heat balance and the metabolic rate of new-born babies in relation to environmental temperature, and the effect of age and of weight on basal metabolic rate. *J Physiol* 1965;180:239–265.
12. Hill JR. The oxygen consumption of new-born and adult mammals. Its dependence on the oxygen tension in the inspired air and on the environmental temperature. *J Physiol* 1959;149:346–373.
13. Brück K, Parmelee AH Jr, Brück M. Neutral temperature range and range of "thermal comfort" in premature infants. *Biol Neonate* 1962;4:32–51.
14. Brück K. Temperature regulation in the newborn infant. *Biol Neonate* 1961;3:65–119.
15. Hey EN, Katz G. The optimum thermal environment for naked babies. *Arch Dis Child* 1970;45:328–334.
16. Hey EN. The relation between environmental temperature and oxygen consumption in the new-born baby. *J Physiol* 1969;200: 589–603.
17. Hey E. Thermal neutrality. *Br Med Bull* 1975;31:69–74.
18. Power GG, Schroder H, Gilbert RD. Measurement of fetal heat production using differential calorimetry. *J Appl Physiol* 1984;57: 917–922.
19. Ryser G, Jequier E. Study by direct calorimetry of thermal balance on the first day of life. *Eur J Clin Invest* 1972;2:176–187.
20. Morishima HO, Yeh MN, Niemann WH, et al. Temperature gradient between fetus and mother as an index for assessing intrauterine fetal condition. *Am J Obstet Gynecol* 1977;129:443–448.
21. Power GG, Kawamura T, Dale PS, et al. Temperature responses following ventilation of the fetal sheep in utero. *J Dev Physiol* 1986;8:477–484.
22. Schroder H, Gilbert RD, Power GG. Computer model of fetal-maternal heat exchange in sheep. *J Appl Physiol* 1988;65:460–468.
23. Hodgkin DD, Gilbert RD, Power GG. In vivo brown fat response to hypothermia and norepinephrine in the ovine fetus. *J Dev Physiol* 1988;10:383–391.
24. Alexander G, Williams D. Shivering and non-shivering thermogenesis during summit metabolism in young lambs. *J Physiol* 1968;198:251–276.
25. Bray GA, Goodman HM. Studies on the early effects of thyroid hormones. *Endocrinology* 1965;76:323–328.
26. Klein AH, Reviczky A, Padbury JF. Thyroid hormones augment catecholamine-stimulated brown adipose tissue thermogenesis in the ovine fetus. *Endocrinology* 1984;114:1065–1069.
27. Silva JE, Larsen PR. Adrenergic activation of triiodothyronine production in brown adipose tissue. *Nature* 1983;305:712–713.
28. Baumgart S. Incubation of the human newborn infant. In: Pomerance JJ, Richardson CJ, eds. *Neonatology for the clinician*. Norwalk, Conn: Appleton & Lange, 1993:139–150.
29. Baum JD, Scopes JW. The silver swaddler. Device for preventing hypothermia in the newborn. *Lancet* 1968;1:672–673.
30. Besch NJ, Perlstein PH, Edwards NK, et al. The transparent baby bag. A shield against heat loss. *N Engl J Med* 1971;284:121–124.
31. Dahm LS, James LS. Newborn temperature and calculated heat loss in the delivery room. *Pediatrics* 1972;49:504–513.
32. Glass L, Silverman WA, Sinclair JC. Effect of the thermal environment on cold resistance and growth of small infants after the first week of life. *Pediatrics* 1968;41:1033–1046.
33. Charpak N, Ruiz-Pelaez JG, de Figueroa CZ, et al. Kangaroo mother versus traditional care for newborn infants ≤2000 grams: a randomized, controlled trial. *Pediatrics* 1997;100:682–688.
34. Bell RP, McGrath JM. Implementing a research-based kangaroo care program in the NICU. *Nurs Clin North Am* 1996;31:387–403.
35. Anderson GC. Current knowledge about skin-to-skin (kangaroo) care for preterm infants. *J Perinatol* 1991;11:216–226.
36. Silverman WA, Sinclair JC, Agate FJ Jr. The oxygen cost of minor changes in heat balance of small newborn infants. *Acta Paediatr Scand* 1966;55:294–300.
37. Sinclair JC. Metabolic rate and temperature control. In: Smith CA, Nelson NM, eds. *The physiology of the newborn infant*. Springfield, Ill: Thomas, 1976:354–415.
38. Wheldon AE, Rutter N. The heat balance of small babies nursed in incubators and under radiant warmers. *Early Hum Dev* 1982;6: 131–143.
39. Baumgart S, Engle WD, Fox WW, et al. Effect of heat shielding on convective and evaporative heat losses and on radiant heat transfer in the premature infant. *J Pediatr* 1981;99:948–956.
40. Bell EF, Rios GR. A double-walled incubator alters the partition of body heat loss of premature infants. *Pediatr Res* 1983;17:135–140.
41. Okken A, Blijham C, Franz W, et al. Effects of forced convection of heated air on insensible water loss and heat loss in preterm infants in incubators. *J Pediatr* 1982;101:108–112.
42. Baumgart S, Engle WD, Fox WW, et al. Radiant warmer power and body size as determinants of insensible water loss in the critically ill neonate. *Pediatr Res* 1981;15:1495–1499.
43. Baumgart S, Langman CB, Sosulski R, et al. Fluid, electrolyte, and glucose maintenance in the very low birthweight infant. *Clin Pediatr (Phila)* 1982;21:199–206.
44. Bell EF, Neidich GA, Cashore WJ, et al. Combined effect of radiant warmer and phototherapy on insensible water loss in low-birth-weight infants. *J Pediatr* 1979;94:810–813.
45. Hammarlund K, Sedin G, Stromberg B. Transepidermal water loss in newborn infants. VIII. Relation to gestational age and postnatal age in appropriate and small for gestational age infants. *Acta Paediatr Scand* 1983;72:721–728.
46. Hey EN, Katz G. Evaporative water loss in the new-born baby. *J Physiol* 1969;200:605–619.
47. Sedin G, Hammarlund K, Nilsson GE, et al. Measurements of transepidermal water loss in newborn infants. *Clin Perinatol* 1985;12:79–99.
48. Williams PR, Oh W. Effects of radiant warmer on insensible water loss in newborn infants. *Am J Dis Child* 1974;128:511–514.
49. Wu PY, Hodgman JE. Insensible water loss in preterm infants: changes with postnatal development and non-ionizing radiant energy. *Pediatrics* 1974;54:704–712.
50. Costarino AT, Baumgart S. Neonatal water metabolism. In: Cowett RM, ed. *Principles of perinatal–neonatal metabolism*. New York: Springer-Verlag, 2nd ed., 1998;1045–1075.
51. Costarino AT, Baumgart S. Modern fluid and electrolyte management of the critically ill premature infant. *Pediatr Clin North Am* 1986;33:1–53.
52. Harpin VA, Rutter N. Humidification of incubators. *Arch Dis Child* 1985;60:219–224.
53. Moffet HL, Allan D, Williams T. Survival and dissemination of bacteria in nebulizers and incubators. *Am J Dis Child* 1967;114: 13–20.
54. Moffet HL, Allan D. Colonization of infants exposed to bacterially contaminated mists. *Am J Dis Child* 1967;114:21–25.
55. Brown DG, Baublis J. Reservoirs of pseudomonas in an intensive care unit for newborn infants: mechanism of control. *J Pediatr* 1977;90:453–457.
56. Hoffman MA, Finberg L. Pseudomonas infections in infants associated with high-humidity environments. *J Pediatr* 1955;46: 626–630.
57. American Academy of Pediatrics and the American College of Obstetricians and Gynecologists. *Guidelines for perinatal care*, 2nd ed. Elk Grove Village, Ill and Washington, DC: AAP and ACOG, 2002:.

58. Topper WH, Stewart TP. Thermal support for the very-low-birth-weight infant: role of supplemental conductive heat. *J Pediatr* 1984;105:810–814.
59. Koch J. Physical properties of the thermal environment. In: Okken A, Koch J, eds. *Thermal regulation of sick and low birth weight neonates*. Berlin: Springer-Verlag, 1995:103.
60. Sedin G. Physics of neonatal heat transfer, routes of heat loss and heat gain. In: Okken A, Koch J, eds. *Thermal regulation of sick and low birth weight neonates*. Berlin: Springer-Verlag, 1995:21–.
61. Baumgart S. Radiant heat loss versus radiant heat gain in premature neonates under radiant warmers. *Biol Neonate* 1990;57:10–20.
62. Leblanc MH. Relative efficacy of radiant and convective heat in incubators in producing thermoneutrality for the premature. *Pediatr Res* 1984;18:425–428.
63. Flenady VJ, Woodgate PG. Radiant warmers versus incubators for regulating body temperature in newborn infants. *Cochrane Database Syst Rev* 2003;4:CD000435.
64. Baumgart S. Partitioning of heat losses and gains in premature newborn infants under radiant warmers. *Pediatrics* 1985;75:89–99.
65. Schulze K, Kairam R, Stefanski M, et al. Spontaneous variability in minute ventilation oxygen consumption and heart rate of low birth weight infants. *Pediatr Res* 1981;15:1111–1116.
66. Malin SW, Baumgart S. Optimal thermal management for low birth weight infants nursed under high-power radiant warmers. *Pediatrics* 1987;79:47–54.
67. Yeh TF, Amma P, Lilien LD, et al. Reduction of insensible water loss in premature infants under the radiant warmer. *J Pediatr* 1979;94:651–653.
68. Bell EF, Weinstein MR, Oh W. Heat balance in premature infants: comparative effects of convectively heated incubator and radiant warmer, with and without plastic heat shield. *J Pediatr* 1980;96:460–465.
69. Baumgart S, Fox WW, Polin RA. Physiologic implications of two different heat shields for infants under radiant warmers. *J Pediatr* 1982;100:787–790.
70. Baumgart S. Reduction of oxygen consumption, insensible water loss, and radiant heat demand with use of a plastic blanket for low-birth-weight infants under radiant warmers. *Pediatrics* 1984;74:1022–1028.
71. Vohra S, Frent G, Campbell V, et al. Effect of polyethylene occlusive skin wrapping on heat loss in very low birth weight infants at delivery: a randomized trial. *J Pediatr* 1999;134:547–551.
72. Knauth A, Gordin M, McNelis W, et al. Semipermeable polyurethane membrane as an artificial skin for the premature neonate. *Pediatrics* 1989;83:945–950.
73. Porat R, Brodsky N. Effect of Tegaderm use on outcome of extremely low birth weight (ELBW) infants. *Pediatr Res* 1993;33:231(A).
74. Mancini AJ, Sookdeo-Drost S, Madison KC, et al. Semipermeable dressings improve epidermal barrier function in premature infants. *Pediatr Res* 1994;36:306–314.
75. Rutter N, Hull D. Reduction of skin water loss in the newborn. I. Effect of applying topical agents. *Arch Dis Child* 1981;56:669–672.
76. Rutter N. Waterproofing our infants. *J Pediatr* 1997;130:333–334.
77. Nopper AJ, Horii KA, Sookdeo-Drost S, et al. Topical ointment therapy benefits premature infants. *J Pediatr* 1996;128:660–669.
78. Edwards WH, Conner JM, Soll RF for the Vermont Oxford Network. The effect of Aquaphor original emollient ointment on nosocomial sepsis rates and skin integrity in infants of birth weight 501 to 1000 grams. *Pediatr Res* 2001;49:388A (abstract).
79. Edwards WH, Conner JM, Soll RF. Vermont Oxford Network Neonatal Skin Care Study Group. The effect of prophylactic ointment therapy on nosocomial sepsis rates and skin integrity in infants with birth weights of 501–1000 g. *Pediatr* 2004; 113:1195–1203.
80. Craig WS. The early detection of pyrexia in the newborn. *Arch Dis Child* 1963;38:29–39.
81. Lieberman E, Lang JM, Frigoletto F Jr, et al. Epidural analgesia, intrapartum fever, and neonatal sepsis evaluation. *Pediatrics* 1997;99:415–419.

The Low-Birth-Weight Infant

IV

The Extremely Low-Birth-Weight Infant

Apostolos Papageorgiou   *Ermelinda Pelausa*   *Lajos Kovacs*

Tremendous progress in the survival of newborn infants has resulted in the need for population descriptors other than "premature" or "low birth weight." Such descriptors require subdivision by both gestational ages and birth weights to have meaningful diagnostic and prognostic value.

In the 1960s, the term "low birth weight" (LBW) defined all infants with a birth weight less than 2,500 g. With improved survival of infants born weighing less than 1,500 g in the 1970s and 1980s, the term "very low birth weight" (VLBW) was introduced to better express the problems and outcomes unique to this group of infants.

In the 1990s, it became clear that a new category was necessary to reflect the prevailing reality, namely, the large number of surviving infants born weighing less than 1,000 g. Thus, the term "extremely low birth weight" (ELBW) was added to identify these infants.

At the start of the millennium, we have witnessed the survival of a new cohort of infants who weigh less than 500 grams at birth, i.e., below the weight limit which the World Health Organization had designated for reporting live births. These infants, referred to by some authors as "fetal infants" or "micropremies," are rarely treated in our neonatal units but, nevertheless, reflect a new reality of modern Neonatology. Although their care showcases the tremendous clinical and technological progress achieved in recent years, their survival has also brought a substantial additional demand on human and financial resources, and major ethical dilemmas. Most of the fetal infants who do survive are small for gestational age (SGA) and, at this point in time, their long-term prognosis is not reassuring, which makes their neonatal intensive care unit (NICU) management a hotly contentious issue (1–3).

In recent years, few medical specialties have demonstrated as much progress and success as has neonatology. With regionalization of perinatal care, improved technology, and better understanding of their pathophysiology and specific needs, the survival of ELBW infants has

improved dramatically (4–12). In fact, in most well organized perinatal centers in North America and Europe, neonatal deaths are uncommon for infants with birth weights more than 1,000 g, in the absence of congenital anomalies. Recent reports demonstrate the improvement in overall perinatal and neonatal mortality and the increasing survival of VLBW and ELBW infants over time. Joseph and colleagues describe the reduction in infant mortality rates in Canada between the years 1985 to 1987 and 1992 to 1994, with the magnitude of reductions ranging from 14% (95% CI, 7–21) at 24 to 25 weeks gestation to 40% (95% CI, 31–47) at 28 to 31 weeks (13). Data in Table 25-1 reflect the progress as experienced in our own perinatal center over the last 15 years for infants born weighing less than 1,000 g. Our own perinatal mortality statistics at the Sir Mortimer B. Davis-Jewish General Hospital, a McGill University tertiary care perinatal referral center with near 4,000 deliveries per year and a catchment area of 12,000 deliveries, show a neonatal mortality consistently between 0.3 and 0.5 per 1,000 live births for infants weighing more than 1,000 g, including those who died from lethal congenital anomalies.

Thus, the care of VLBW infants, and particularly of ELBW infants, occupies an important part of the daily activities of all NICUs and contributes heavily to the cost of neonatal care (14–17).

As mortality has much decreased, concerns have been expressed regarding whether morbidity has followed the same rate of improvement (12,16,18–24). There is current evidence that for infants born weighing more than 750 g, the decline in morbidity is a significant one, although not parallel to mortality. However, for infants with birth weights less than 750 g, their long-term prognosis remains less favorable. Although the incidence of cerebral palsy and other physical impairments is relatively low, the incidence of later-appearing cerebral dysfunction is quite elevated, with requirement for additional resources to manage behavioral and school difficulties in later childhood.

TABLE 25-1

DECLINE IN MORTALITY BY BIRTHWEIGHT AT THE JEWISH GENERAL HOSPITAL, McGILL UNIVERSITY, FROM 1984 TO 2002

Birth Weight (g)	1984–1985		2001–2002		Percent Improvement
	Births	Mortality	Births	Mortality	
500–750	25	14 (56.0%)	41	18 (43.9%)	22
751–1,000	36	10 (27.8%)	40	4 (10.0%)	64
500–1,000	61	24 (39.3%)	81	22 (27.2%)	31

Major problems related to ELBW infants are listed in Table 25-2.

The aim of this chapter is to present a global approach to the care of ELBW infants, with emphasis on the problems and management issues particular to them. The reader is referred to the specific chapters in the textbook for a more comprehensive review of each problem.

Much of what is written in this chapter is based on our own experience in the management of ELBW infants, with appropriate reference to the most recent published data. We expect that our experience may be different from many in other parts of the world. It is important to appreciate that the Canadian health care system, which provides uni-

versal access to health care, emphasizes prevention and has a very successful antenatal referral policy, with the vast majority of VLBW infants being inborn. Table 25-3 indicates the number of infants weighing less than 1,500 g born in the five level III maternity hospitals in the province of Quebec in comparison with the number born in levels II and I (25). The success of the regionalization of perinatal care can be better appreciated by knowing the size of the province (approximately four times the size of France) and the weather conditions.

EPIDEMIOLOGY

Until recently, statistics on ELBW infants were analyzed exclusively by birth weight. Although this method offers the advantage of an objective measurement, it does not take into account the effect of gestational age (26). In other words, many infants born weighing less than 1,000 g are more mature than their birth weight may indicate, hence denoting the problems of intrauterine growth restriction (IUGR) superimposed on prematurity. The neonatal problems and long-term prognosis can be quite different for the more mature, SGA infant than for the less mature, appropriate for gestational age (AGA) infant of the same birth weight. The distinction between AGA and SGA infants born before 28 weeks of gestation became possible only in recent years, thanks to the introduction of early pregnancy ultrasonography. In Canada, and particularly in the Province

TABLE 25-2

MAJOR PROBLEMS IN EXTREMELY-LOW-BIRTH-WEIGHT INFANTS

Respiratory
  Respiratory distress syndrome
  Respiratory failure
  Apnea
  Air leaks
  Chronic lung disease
Cardiovascular
  Patent ductus arteriosus
Central nervous system
  Intraventricular hemorrhage
  Periventricular leukomalacia
  Seizures
Renal
  Electrolyte imbalance
  Acid–base disturbances
  Renal failure
Ophthalmologic
  Retinopathy of prematurity
  Strabismus
  Myopia
Gastrointestinal–nutritional
  Feeding intolerance
  Necrotizing enterocolitis
  Inguinal hernias
  Cholostatic jaundice
  Postnatal growth retardation
Immunologic
  Poor defense to infection

TABLE 25-3

LIVE BIRTHS ACCORDING TO THE LEVEL OF HOSPITAL CARE IN THE PROVINCE OF QUÉBEC, 1998

Level of Care	500–999 g		1,000–1,499 g	
	n = 244	%	n = 345	%
I	7	2.9	3	0.9
II	35	14.3	37	10.7
III	202	82.8	305	88.4

TABLE 25-4

IMPACT OF BIRTH WEIGHT ON OUTCOME IN THE CANADIAN COLLABORATIVE STUDY

Gestational Age	Weight (g)	Mortality
24 wk	<700	63.3%
n = 241	>700	37.2%
25 wk	<760	43.3%
n = 364	>760	35.9%

From SB Effer, unpublished data.

TABLE 25-5

IMPACT OF GESTATIONAL AGE ON SURVIVAL OF 533 INFANTS AGED 24 TO 25 WEEKS IN THE CANADIAN COLLABORATIVE STUDY

Gestational Age (d)	No. of N.B.	Neonatal Mortality (%)
168–171	125	55.2
172–176	177	47.4
177–181	171	34.5

From SB Effer et al., unpublished data.

of Quebec, systematic ultrasonography between 16 and 18 weeks of gestation has permitted not only the early detection, and the potential for termination of major congenital anomalies but, at the same time, it has provided a reasonably accurate dating of almost all pregnancies. Precise gestational age assignment, along with the birth weight of premature infants, has made it possible to relate specific problems, diagnoses and prognoses to the degree of immaturity, and to recognize the implications of IUGR at a very early gestational age (26). In our perinatal center, in the last 6 years, the incidence of IUGR, defined as a birth weight beyond two standard deviations (2SDs) below the mean for a given gestational age, has been 24.5% for infants born weighing less than 1,000 g (Table 25-4). It is hoped that as gestational age dating becomes universal and more accurate, the current method of reporting perinatal statistics based on birth weight will be complemented by the gestational age, thus reflecting both the degree of maturity and the degree of appropriateness of intrauterine growth. Hence, neonatal pathology and prognosis can be based on both gestational age and birth weight.

Although mortality rates of VLBW and ELBW infants are declining, the incidence of these births has not changed significantly. In the province of Quebec, the rate of live births for infants weighing 500 to 999 g has increased slightly from 0.3 in 1992 to 0.4% in 1998 and for those weighing 1,000 to 1,500 g from 0.4 to 0.5%. Similarly, the incidence of births less than 26 weeks increased from 0.1 to 0.2% and that of births between 26 and 28 weeks from 0.4 to 0.5% (25).

Factors that have long been recognized as being associated with prematurity include extremes of maternal age, socioeconomic status, low level of education, adverse social habits, maternal diseases, gynecologic infections and, more recently, multiple pregnancies secondary to *in vitro* fertilization (27).

Significant predictors for the survival of ELBW infants are older gestational age, heavier birth weight, female gender, African American race, singleton birth, and the absence of severe fetal growth restriction (28). The importance of birth weight for the survival of infants born at 24 and 25 weeks of gestation has been demonstrated clearly in a multicenter study of Canadian tertiary care centers (Table 25-5). In this particular study, all infants were

inborn, and the gestational ages were confirmed by early ultrasonography. Likewise, maturity by only a few days has been shown to add significant chances of survival, as shown in Table 25-6. Whether analysis is done by increments of 100 g or by increments of a few days, the impact of these two factors on the survival of ELBW infants is very important. Tables 25-4 and 25-7 indicate the survival rate of infants born weighing less than 1,000 g in our institution between 1995 and 2002, analyzed by weight and gestational age. In our experience, infants born before 27 weeks of gestation with a birth weight beyond 2SD below the mean are at a disadvantage compared to appropriate-for-gestational-age infants of the same gestational age in terms of acute and chronic problems, the most striking complication being the higher incidence of retinopathy of prematurity (ROP) (26).

In terms of global epidemiologic evaluation of outcomes for ELBW infants, many factors contribute to the inaccuracy of data. A number of countries, and particularly some developing ones, do not keep statistics for infants born before 28 weeks of gestation. In other countries,

TABLE 25-6

POPULATION PROFILE OF INFANTS WITH BW <1,000 g BORN IN 1995–2002, N = 369

Birth Weight (g)	Live Births # Infants	Survivors	
		# Infants	%
< 500	17	4	(23.5%)
500–750	151	87	(57.6%)
751–999	201	166	(82.6%)
500–999	352	253	(71.9%)
<1000	369	257	(69.6%)
Gestational age	26 ± 1.3 wks		
Birth weight	758 ± 142 g		
Apgar 1 min.	4.3 ± 2.2		
Apgar 5 min.	6.5 ± 1.9		
SGA rate	24.6%		
C/Section rate	47.7%		
Days in hospital	88 ± 36		
(for survivors)	mean, 1 s.d.		

TABLE 25-7

SURVIVAL RATE BY GESTATIONAL AGE OF 352 INBORN INFANTS WEIGHING 500–1,000 g AT THE SMBD-JEWISH GENERAL HOSPITAL, McGILL UNIVERSITY, FROM 1995 TO 2002

Gestational Age (wk)	Total Births	Survivors
< 23	10	2 (20.0%)
23–24	105	50 (47.6%)
25–26	129	98 (76.0%)
27–28	76	73 (96.1%)
29–30	25	23 (92.0%)
31–32	7	7 (100%)
All ages	352	253 (71.9%)

when death occurs rapidly in the first day of life, the death is not recorded as a neonatal death. Also, information originating from small private institutions may be inaccurate and difficult to control. National and regional data can also be seriously affected by the ratio of inborn to outborn infants and the number of extremely premature infants who are resuscitated. Indeed, great variations do exist in terms of intervention and resuscitation in the delivery room between institutions and countries, and they reflect not only differences in the capacity of some institutions to manage newborns near the limits of viability, but also differences in philosophy. Tables 25-4, 25-7 to 25-9 indicate the survival, management, and complications of infants weighing less than 1,000 g born in our center over a 8-year period (1995–2002).

TABLE 25-8

OUTCOME OF 352 INBORN INFANTS WEIGHING 500–1,000 g AT THE SMBD-JEWISH GENERAL HOSPITAL, McGILL UNIVERSITY, 1995–2002

	No. of Infants (n = 352)	%
Survived	253	71.9
Antenatal betamethasone	265	75.3
Cesarean section	168	47.7
Oxygen for at least 24h	318	90.3
Ventilation	296	84.1
Respiratory distress syndrome	239	67.9
Surfactant for respiratory distress syndrome	197/239	82.4
Drained pneumothorax	19	5.4
Pulmonary interstitial emphysema only	51	14.5
Intraventricular hemorrhage all grades	86	24.4
Grades III–IV	27	7.7
Patent ductus arteriosus	220	62.5
Surgical necrotizing enterocolitis	9	2.6
Apnea	249	70.7

TABLE 25-9

COMPLICATIONS AMONG 253 SURVIVORS 500–1,000 g AT THE SMBD-JEWISH GENERAL HOSPITAL, McGILL UNIVERSITY, FROM 1995–2002

	No. of Infants 253	%
Oxygen 28 d	161	63.6
Oxygen 36 wks PCA	79	31.2
Ventilation	193	76.3
IVH all grades	42	16.6
IVH grades III–IV	12	4.7
Periventricular leukomalacia	14	5.5
Ventriculomegaly	82	32.4
Retinopathy of prematurity all stages	159	62.8
≥ stage III	49	19.4
Threshold	15	5.9
Laser	15	5.9
Patent ductus arteriosus	162	64.0
Closure with indomethacin	135/162	83.3
Surgery	27/162	16.7
Sepsis	70	27.7
Surgical necrotizing enterocolitis	4	1.6
Home O_2	15	5.9
Days in hospital	88 ± 36	

PERINATAL MANAGEMENT

Prenatal

With the advent of routine early ultrasonography, the gestational age is fairly well established on admission to the Obstetrics unit for the vast majority of women presenting with premature labor, premature rupture of membranes or other problems diagnosed in the second trimester of pregnancy. Such patients need to be immediately placed in the charge of a specialist in high risk Obstetrics (Obstetrical Perinatologist or Specialist in Maternal Fetal Medicine) to coordinate the evaluation and management plans and to ensure appropriate communication and counseling. Based on the investigation for the causes of the problem at hand, the evaluation of the degree of cervical dilatation, the condition of the membranes, the presence or absence of chorioamnionitis and, if possible, the most recent evaluation of fetal well-being by bedside or formal ultrasonography, the Perinatologist can decide on the best course to be taken, such as an estimate of the likelihood of controlling labor with tocolysis to allow adequate time for antenatal corticosteroid therapy (7,29), often with consultation with their colleagues in neonatology.

The prospective parents should receive accurate information regarding all facets of the proposed management, including the possible need for cesarean delivery, and information regarding the subsequent management of the newborn infant, including the potential risks related to both the degree of prematurity and the therapeutic interventions that may be necessary to keep the infant alive.

Ideally, this information should be provided conjointly by both the obstetric perinatologist and the neonatologist and should be based not only on general statistical information, but also on the specific institutional experience with outcomes of newborn infants of similar gestational age. In our center, the attending neonatologist provides a written consultation on all patients admitted to the obstetric high-risk unit. We meet with the family, offer an extensive review of our experience with similar cases, and answer their questions regarding risks and outcomes. The father and mother are invited to visit the NICU and to familiarize themselves with the environment and the personnel. If the mother is not able to visit for medical reasons, we show her a book with pictures explaining each step of the baby's treatments, from the delivery room to the time of discharge.

The lowest gestational age at which resuscitation should be initiated has long been the subject of debate. Guidelines are available from both the American and the Canadian Fetus and Newborn Committees (30,31). Based on our experience, we offer an optimistic opinion in terms of survival and potential morbidity for pregnancies of 25 weeks' gestation and over. Between 24 and 25 weeks, although we underline that the chances of survival are quite good, we also emphasize the increased risk of potential complications, such as intraventricular hemorrhage (IVH), periventricular leukomalacia (PVL), retinopathy of prematurity (ROP), chronic lung disease (CLD), neurosensory impairments, and later school and behavioral difficulties. For pregnancies between 23 and 24 weeks of gestation, we describe the higher incidence of complications previously mentioned, and the lower survival rate; however we also mention the possibility of intact survival or survival with minimal handicaps. Finally, for pregnancies below 23 weeks of gestation, we do not recommend intervention. For parents who request full intervention, we strongly advise that resuscitation will be undertaken only if the newborn has at least the degree of maturity predicted by dates and/or ultrasonography, and if, in the judgment of the neonatologist present in the delivery room, the newborn has reasonable chances of responding to resuscitation. We always make it clear to the parents that initiation of resuscitation and subsequent treatments in the NICU do not preclude discontinuation of therapy if a major complication such as severe IVH is detected in the hours or days following birth. The presence of a staff neonatologist in the delivery room is an integral part of our protocol for the management of ELBW infants.

One of the most difficult questions that parents ask, and which our obstetric colleagues continuously debate, is the safest route of delivery in the presence of either a breech presentation or evidence of fetal distress (32). In our institution, based on our own results, we advise cesarean delivery in such situations as of 25 weeks' gestation. Between 24 and 25 weeks, we feel less inclined to recommend cesarean delivery, particularly in view of the fact that many may require a classical incision. The decision to proceed with such an intervention is taken with a clear

TABLE 25-10

CESAREAN SECTION RATE IN 352 INFANTS WEIGHING 500–1,000 g AT THE SMBD-JEWISH GENERAL HOSPITAL, McGILL UNIVERSITY, 1995–2002

GA by Wks	No. Deliveries	No. C/Sections	%
<23	10	0	0
23–24	105	31	29.5
25–26	129	71	55.0
27–28	76	39	51.3
29–30	25	20	80.0
31–32	7	7	100
All ages	352	168	47.7

understanding by the parents of all the medical implications for both the mother and the infant. Finally, at less than 24 weeks of gestation, cesarean delivery is performed strictly for maternal indications. Our incidence of cesarean section by gestational age is indicated in Table 25-10. It is obvious that a large number of cesarean deliveries, and particularly those between 22 and 24 weeks of gestation, are performed strictly for maternal indications, i.e., severe abruption, preeclampsia, etc.

Another difficult management situation relates to ruptured membranes between 18 and 22 weeks of gestation, resulting in severe oligohydramnios, with the inherent risk of lung underdevelopment (33–34). Serial ultrasound studies can evaluate the degree of reaccumulation of amniotic fluid and allow for a better-educated decision regarding whether continuation of pregnancy is advisable (35). However, in the vast majority of these cases, the outcome is very poor, and termination of pregnancy constitutes reasonable advice, particularly if rupture of membranes occurred before 20 weeks of gestation with poor reaccumulation of amniotic fluid. Amnioinfusion has been proposed and attempted as a means of overcoming the problem of chest compression, with limited success thus far (36).

Impending Delivery

The management of a patient with impending premature delivery should include the following: evaluation of gestational age by dates and/or early ultrasound, fetal size and position, condition of the fetal membranes, amniotic fluid volume, and evidence of chorioamnionitis and other obstetric complications such as bleeding, toxemia, and so on. Vaginorectal cultures for the detection of group B streptococcal colonization and initiation of therapy with penicillin are also in order (37). If culture results return negative, penicillin can be discontinued. In all patients from 24 weeks of gestation who are not infected and for whom there is no maternal indication for immediate delivery, such as massive bleeding, and in whom the cervix is dilated less than 5 cm, we propose tocolysis with magnesium sulfate and administration of betamethasone (29,38). Our experience over the years with the combination of tocolysis and betamethasone has been fully supported by the 1994 NIH Statement on Antenatal Use of Corticosteroids (39). For patients between 24 and 34 weeks' gestation, we administer two doses of 12 mg of betamethasone, 24 hours apart. Beyond 34 weeks, we use steroids only when an amniocentesis indicates lung immaturity. Multiple pregnancies are offered similar therapy (40). We also monitor body temperature and changes in leukocyte count, keeping in mind the possible transient leukocytosis after the administration of betamethasone.

If a patient has fever or demonstrates other signs of chorioamnionitis, broad-spectrum antibiotics are initiated. In the presence of ruptured membranes, a number of obstetricians use a combination of ampicillin and erythromycin in an attempt to temporarily stop labor and administer steroids (41–43). This seems a reasonable approach, because between 30% and 50% of premature births are believed to be precipitated by common genital tract infections.

Delivery Room Management

The successful management of the ELBW infant begins in the delivery room (Table 25-11). A well-organized and equipped delivery room and the presence of a competent team headed by an experienced neonatologist are essential ingredients to the proper reception of these very fragile newborns. The basic principle guiding successful management is directed toward prevention of any physiologic deviation from normality, such as hypothermia, acidosis, or hypoxia. At the same time, it is important that each

TABLE 25-11
THE FIRST 60 MINUTES OF LIFE

1. **Expert resuscitation in the delivery room.**
2. **Good thermoregulation.**
   a. Keep the infant warm and dry in the delivery room
   b. Provide high-humidity environment in the incubator
3. **Minimum handling and avoidance of brisk maneuvers.**
4. **Expert cardiorespiratory support.**
   a. Liberal use of nasopharyngeal CPAP.
   b. Intubation when indicated, avoiding excessive ventilatory pressures.
   c. Continuous monitoring of oxygenation with pulse oximetry.
   d. Monitoring of blood pressure. Prudent administration of volume expanders.
   e. Catheterization of umbilical vessels, when indicated.
   f. Close monitoring of blood gases, Hb, WBC + diff, blood glucose.
   g. Radiographic evaluation of lung pathology and position of catheters.
   h. Administration of surfactant, when indicated. Rapid adjustment of ventilatory support.
5. **Intravenous D$_{10}$W and antibiotics when indicated.**
6. **Parental information**

intervention during the resuscitation process be carefully adapted to the size and to the needs of the tiny infant. Brisk maneuvers, excessive positive pressure with bagging, or inappropriate administration of drugs and fluids may induce permanent central nervous system (CNS) or lung injuries.

It seems particularly inappropriate when high-risk mothers are referred to a tertiary care center for specialized perinatal care, to have their premature newborn infants cared for in the delivery room and during the critical first hours of their lives by unsupervised and inexperienced in-training personnel. Major decisions, such as whether to initiate resuscitation and for how long, often need to be made in extremely short periods of time and under heavy pressure for infants at the limit of viability. This can be done only by experienced personnel (44).

In our center, the birth of an ELBW infant is always attended by a neonatologist in addition to the pediatric house staff and a trained delivery room nurse. Appropriate equipment is used according to the American Heart Association and American Academy of Pediatrics (AAP) guidelines for neonatal resuscitation, with particular emphasis on temperature control i.e., radiant heater set at maximum temperature and prewarmed blankets (45).

During the initial steps of stabilization, the condition of the infant is rapidly assessed. After drying, positioning on warm blankets, and suctioning, most ELBW infants require immediate initiation of positive pressure ventilation with a bag and mask. Resuscitation is initiated using an inspired oxygen concentration of 100%, which is rapidly reduced as the infant's condition improves. Although concerns have recently been raised that such a practice may result in potential exposure to oxygen free radical species (46,47), the available data is limited to asphyxiated newborn infants at term, and there is currently insufficient evidence to support a change in practice. We found that, for ELBW infants, ventilation is more effective if performed at a higher ventilatory rate than for the term infant. We use anesthesia bags and ventilate at a rate of 60 to 80 breaths per minute, adjusting the pressure to provide adequate bilateral air entry and chest wall excursion. For extremely premature infants, intubation in the delivery room may rapidly follow.

With proper ventilation, in our experience, rarely will an infant require chest compressions or epinephrine. The prognosis of ELBW infants requiring this extent of resuscitation is very guarded, particularly if their birth weight is below 750 g. Fluid resuscitation is reserved only for those infants in which significant blood loss is suspected.

Even following optimal resuscitation, the Apgar scores of ELBW infants rarely exceed 6 or 7 in view of their decreased tone and reactivity, poor respiratory effort, and initially poor peripheral perfusion (48). The infant's heart rate is thus the best measure of the effectiveness of resuscitation efforts.

The topic of delivery room management would not be properly covered without mentioning the ethical dilemmas faced by the neonatologist when parental and medical opinions regarding resuscitation differ, or when an ELBW infant is severely asphyxiated and requires prolonged resuscitation. It is our view that reasonable parental opinions must be respected after full and honest discussion of the infant's chances of meaningful survival.

Admission to the Neonatal Intensive Care Unit

Expert management in the delivery room and during the first hours after admission to the NICU is of paramount importance to prevent immediate and long-term complications in the ELBW infant. It is well established that the majority of cerebral injuries occur around the time of delivery or in the immediate postnatal period. Acute changes in cerebral blood flow may predispose the very fragile network of periventricular vessels to rupture. Hence, it is essential to handle these very fragile infants with extreme care, avoiding unnecessary disturbances, and preventing, rather than correcting physiological deviations in acid–base balance, blood gases, blood pressure, or body temperature. Also, overly aggressive ventilation either in the delivery room or in the NICU may predispose to significant acute or chronic pulmonary problems such as hyperinflation and loss of elasticity of the alveoli, pulmonary interstitial emphysema, pneumothorax, and eventually CLD.

The vast majority of our ELBW infants who require assisted ventilation are intubated in the NICU. Only in exceptional situations, when the infant does not respond to bag and mask ventilation, is intubation performed in the delivery room. We use the nasotracheal route, and an endotracheal tube (ETT) of 2.5 mm for infants with a birth weight less than 1000 g. We believe that it is important to use a low-caliber ET tube to avoid subglottic trauma, strictures, and eventually stenosis. We have never had to perform a tracheostomy in an infant, and stridor has been very rare among our patients.

If the newborn infant is in distress, an umbilical arterial catheter is inserted. The arterial line is used exclusively for blood sampling. We favor the "high" position of the tip of the catheter, just above the level of the diaphragm. After each blood sampling, the catheter is flushed with a heparinized solution of 0.45% saline. In infants weighing less than 750 g, we also insert an umbilical venous line. We use the venous line to infuse fluids, thus avoiding excessive handling and disturbance to the newborn infant during the first 24 to 48 hours of life. The tip of the catheter is positioned at the junction of the inferior vena cava and the right atrium, hence avoiding the liver. This is important, particularly when infusing hypertonic solutions, such as sodium bicarbonate or calcium gluconate.

Blood is analyzed for glucose, electrolytes, blood gases, hemoglobin, and leukocytes. An intravenous with 10% dextrose is initiated at a rate of 65 to 85 mL/kg/d and the infant is placed in a high humidity closed incubator. Serum glucose levels are closely monitored, and the concentration of dextrose administered is adjusted accordingly. In very tiny babies, when more than ten percent of the baby's blood volume has been removed, we replace it with packed red cells. We use a single donor, collecting the blood in small packs, which may be used for up to several weeks (49). Donors are extensively screened for all viral illnesses. We encourage parents who wish to donate blood to their infants to do so, as long as they are of a compatible blood group and are free of viral and other infections. Very sick infants receive 1:1 nursing care until the condition is stabilized, at which point the ratio of nurse-to-baby becomes 1:2.

A percutaneous central venous catheter is usually inserted between the second and third day of life for intravenous alimentation (50,51). As portal of entry, we use the upper extremities of the infant, and we aim for the tip of the catheter to be in the superior vena cava, being careful to avoid intracardiac positioning, with its attendant risks of erosion into the pericardial space (52,53). In case of failure to properly position a central line, peripheral venous access is maintained using an extremity or scalp vein. Parenteral nutrition (TPN) is generally introduced within the first 24 hours of life. When the mother receives intravenous fluids during her labor, a baseline electrolytic profile of the newborn shortly after birth appears to be the proper way to follow subsequent changes. Electrolytes are repeated between 12 and 18 hours of age. During the first 72 hours, the body weight is recorded every 8 hours, and fluid intake is adjusted accordingly. The new incubators have incorporated scales, allowing recordings without excessive handling and disturbance of the newborn infant. One other major advantage of the new incubators is that they can provide a high level of humidity, hence substantially reducing the need for large volumes of fluid.

To establish prognostic criteria, it is important to obtain a cranial ultrasound in the first 24 hours of life (54,55). This ultrasound needs to be repeated at least one week later, or as often as necessary, depending on the pathology detected on admission or, if the infant's condition has deteriorated, suggesting CNS involvement. It is also important, before discharge from the hospital, to repeat the cranial ultrasound to evaluate the presence or absence of periventricular leukomalacia (PVL) (56). Ideally, this last ultrasound should be performed at 35 to 36 weeks of postmenstrual age.

Respiratory Support

The vast majority of infants with a birth weight less than 1,000 g will need some form of respiratory assistance to survive. For vigorous infants, nasal continuous positive airway pressure (CPAP) or recently, nasal ventilation, is the preferred mode of support (57). Some controversy surrounds the timing and criteria for the initiation of assisted ventilation. Likewise, controversy also exists regarding whether these tiny infants should receive prophylactic exogenous surfactant in the delivery room (58–62). We do not systematically intubate infants born weighing less than 1,000 g, and we do not administer surfactant unless the infant requires assisted ventilation and a minimum FiO_2 of 0.30.

The introduction of exogenous surfactant therapy has reduced significantly the mortality of all newborns suffering from respiratory failure secondary to respiratory distress syndrome (RDS), but its impact has been particularly important among the most premature infants (63–69). Administration of surfactant in these very tiny infants requires extra care, as rapid changes in lung compliance may not only damage the lungs by creating overinflation and overdistention, but also may predispose to acute changes in ductal circulation which, in turn, could lead to both cerebral and/or pulmonary hemorrhage. With rapid improvement in oxygenation, persistent hyperoxia also may be detrimental to the eyes. Hence, the administration of surfactant should be performed by an experienced person, under close monitoring of ventilatory parameters, and with rapid reduction of peak inspiratory pressures (PIP) and oxygen concentrations. If necessary, a second dose of surfactant may be administered as soon as 6 hours after the first. However, in our experience, if the response to the second dose is not satisfactory, it is highly unlikely that the condition will improve with additional administration of surfactant. In our center, 64% of the babies improved rapidly, requiring only a single dose of surfactant. Natural surfactant preparations are nowadays practically the only ones used (70).

Mechanical ventilation has dramatically improved the survival of infants weighing less than 1,000 g. In the 1970s, very few infants born weighing less than 1,000 g survived. In the early 1980s, survival of infants weighing 500 to 750 g varied from 3% to 25%, and that of infants weighing 750 to 1,000 g ranged from 30% to 70% (71). In initiating mechanical ventilation, it is imperative that minimal effective settings be used (72). Studies have shown that hyperventilation and overinflation of the lungs increase the loss of surface active phospholipids (73). Also, overinflation predisposes to air leaks and particularly to pulmonary interstitial emphysema (PIE). The latter is a serious complication in the tiny infant, and is a relatively frequent one. It is probably related to structural immaturity of the lungs, particularly to the relative lack of elastic tissue, which normally increases progressively throughout gestation (74). Also, the interstitium is larger in the more immature infant as a result of poor alveolization. Although drainage of a pneumothorax may lead to rapid improvement, management of PIE is far more complicated. As lung compliance is reduced, there is a need for increased PIPs to maintain adequate ventilation. This results in increased barotrauma to the small airways. Chorioamnionitis has been reported as a risk factor predisposing to PIE (75). The highest incidence of PIE in tiny infants has been observed when intrauterine pneumonia complicates the RDS. To overcome the problems related to PIE, a number of strategies have been devised. These include acceptance of higher levels of partial pressure of CO_2 (PCO_2) and lower levels of potential of hydrogen (pH), reduction of the positive end-expiratory pressure (PEEP) to between 2 and 3 cm water (H_2O), selective intubation of the contralateral lung, positioning the infant on the affected side, increasing the expiratory time,

and systemic corticosteroid therapy. The combination of the above strategies can occasionally produce quite spectacular recovery from this condition. However, high frequency oscillatory or JET ventilation is probably the most effective therapy (76,77).

A variety of ventilatory strategies have been promoted to maintain satisfactory ventilation and to reduce the risk of complications (78), such as high PIP–low rates, low PIP–high rates, variation in the I:E ratio, variations in the flow, permissive hypercapnia, tolerance of lower pH and, more recently, high-frequency oscillation and even ventilation via nasal prongs. In recent years, however, the general trend is to use the lowest possible PIP to achieve acceptable ventilation and oxygenation. Of course, the question is what is considered "acceptable"? Some neonatologists will tolerate a pH as low as 7.20 and a PCO_2 as high as 65 mm Hg. Most centers also aim for PaO_2 values between 50 and 70 mm Hg. Our own approach to the ventilation of tiny infants over the years has been to favor nasotracheal intubation with a 2.5-mm ET tube. Our PIPs rarely exceed 14 to 15 cm H_2O, and we set the PEEP at 5 cm H_2O, with initial rates of 65 to 75 per minute. We aim for arterial oxygen pressure (PaO_2) values between 45 and 50 mm Hg, which is enough to abolish production of lactic acid and, at the same time, remains relatively close to intrauterine values. Our pulse oximeters (79) are set to alarm at a lower limit of 80% and an upper limit of 93% for the first few weeks of life. We believe that this modest degree of oxygenation offers the advantage of reducing the need for administration of elevated oxygen concentrations, thus minimizing lung toxicity, and may help to avoid retinal damage. Our incidence of bronchopulmonary dysplasia (BPD) and ROP are shown in Table 25-9. We believe that by using the lowest possible PIP and initially, a relatively rapid respiratory rate, we reduce overdistention and barotrauma and minimize the risk of lung injury. Because, in RDS, there are compartments in the lung with relatively normal ventilation perfusion ratios and others with poor ventilation and adequate perfusion, it seems reasonable to attempt to improve ventilation of the poor ventilation perfusion (V-Q) compartment without overdistention of the normal V-Q compartment. Raising the ventilatory rate, which raises the mean airway pressure without changing the PIP, appears to accomplish this (80). We also have observed that with initially higher respiratory rates, the tiny infant very rapidly stops fighting the respirator, thus making the gas exchange smoother and possibly decreasing the incidence of air leaks. Relatively high respiratory rates also seem to be more physiologic for the very immature infant, as observed by Greenough and collaborators (81). For toilet of the airways, we use the Ballard closed suction circuit, thus avoiding disconnecting the infant from the ventilator (82). We suction sparingly during the first few days of life, when the volume of secretions is minimal. Analgesia/sedation is given for nonemergent intubation and for infants who remain agitated while on mechanical ventilation.

Most of our ventilated babies have their umbilical vessels cannulated for blood sampling and for fluid infusion.

As soon as the procedures of intubation and catheterization of the umbilical vessels are completed, we perform chest and abdominal radiography to assess the position of the ET tube and the umbilical catheters and, at the same time, to evaluate the severity of lung pathology. Fifteen minutes after the initiation of ventilation, we obtain an arterial blood gas and adjust the ventilatory parameters accordingly. We generally aim for a pH above 7.25 and a PCO_2 between 45 and 55 mm Hg, but when the PIPs are elevated or in the presence of PIE, we tolerate partial pressure of CO_2 (PCO_2) values up to 60 mm Hg as long as the pH is at least 7.20. Our ET tubes are sutured to the tape placed on the upper lip. We record the level at which sutures were placed on the ET tube, thus avoiding the need to repeat a chest radiograph to evaluate the tube position when reintubation is required. Actually, we take very few radiographs, and we rely extensively on clinical assessment, blood gases, and pulse oximetry. However, a chest radiograph should be taken if there are concerns about the position of the endotracheal tube or the development of any form of air leak.

Avery and associates (83) reported in 1987 that the incidence of BPD varied between neonatal units. The unit with the lowest incidence used CPAP much more frequently than did the other units. Epidemiologic data from 36 units in the Vermont-Oxford Trial Network also indicate large differences in the incidence of BPD, from 16% to 70% for infants weighing between 501 and 1,500 g (84). The incidence of BPD was lower in units allowing higher PCO_2 values. More evidence of the association of BPD and PCO_2 was provided by Kraybil and associates (85). More recently, Garland and associates (86) reported the highest incidence of BPD among infants with the lowest PCO_2 before the administration of surfactant.

The concept of permissive hypercapnia for patients requiring mechanical ventilation gives priority to the prevention or limitation of severe pulmonary hyperinflation over the maintenance of normal ventilation. The principle consists of allowing the PCO_2 to rise by minimizing ventilator pressures and tidal volume (87). Potential risks of high PCO_2 values include increased cerebral perfusion, increased retinal perfusion, increased pulmonary vascular resistance, and reduction of pH. Based on epidemiologic observations, it appears that respiratory acidosis, unlike metabolic acidosis, is not associated with poor neurologic outcomes. Vannucci and associates (88) demonstrated similar findings in animal studies involving rats.

Flow rate also can affect ventilation and increase airway injury. We generally use a flow rate between 3 and 5 L/min. Only when we need very high pressures, for instance, in the presence of pulmonary hemorrhage, do we allow the flow rate to exceed 5 L/min.

Several reports in the literature have expressed concern about potential side effects of low PCO_2 values (89). Graziani and associates (90) reported that, along with other factors, marked hypocarbia during the first 3 postnatal days was associated with increased risk of periventricular white matter injury in premature infants. The theoretical model of ischemic brain injury has been described by Wigglesworth and Pape (91). These authors hypothesize that cerebral blood flow could be decreased by several factors, including hypotension, hyperoxia, hypocarbia, and increased venous pressures. Concern also has been expressed in the literature about high-frequency ventilation, which may lead to low PCO_2 values as a result of effective alveolar ventilation (92). However, the data regarding the development of PVL among infants managed with these devices remain controversial. Most authors agree, however, that for hypocarbia to be dangerous for the brain, it has to reach levels below 30 mm Hg. Our policy is to avoid PCO_2 values below 40 mm Hg by first reducing PIP before reducing respiratory rates.

High frequency oscillatory ventilation (HFOV) has been used in recent years in an attempt to reduce the incidence of early ventilatory complications and to prevent bronchopulmonary dysplasia. Published reports are often contradictory and, so far, there is no clear evidence that HFOV offers an advantage over conventional ventilation (93,94). HFOV, however, offers an advantage when treating infants with PIE, pulmonary hypertension, or diaphragmatic hernias (95).

More recently, the effects of patient-triggered ventilation with volume-guarantee have been explored in the management of preterm infants (96). This novel technique calls for an automatic adjustment of the peak inspiratory pressure to ensure a minimum set mechanical tidal volume.

The timing of extubation of ELBW infants is very important, because they are prone to develop severe apnea, with the potential risk of cerebral injury. Nowadays, with early administration of surfactant and improvement in lung compliance, rapid extubation and placement on nasal CPAP or nasal ventilation is possible in the majority of ELBW infants. However, some extremely premature infants develop severe episodes of apnea and desaturation, requiring frequently reintubation. For this reason, for the tiniest infants, we often favor a more progressive weaning process by maintaining them for a few extra days at a very low PIP of 10 to 12 mmHg and rates of 15 to 25 per minute, although providing maximum intravenous and oral alimentation (97). When the infant is stronger and starting to gain weight, we administer caffeine and proceed directly to extubation. The infant then is placed on nasal CPAP. The CPAP is discontinued when, after periodic trials, the infant can maintain good oxygenation without significant apnea, bradycardia, and desaturations. If an infant on nasal CPAP shows signs of fatigue manifested by recurrent apnea and retention of CO_2, we try nasal ventilation prior to reintubation. In many circumstances, this approach provides the extra help that these tiny infants require to avoid reintubation (98,99).

Cardiovascular Support

By far, the major cardiovascular problem in ELBW infants is the presence of a patent ductus arteriosus (PDA). More than 50% of infants born weighing less than 1000 g will have a PDA diagnosed during the first few days of life (100,101). The onset of clinical manifestations of the PDA is related to the timing of improvement of the infant's respiratory status, which is associated with a decreasing pulmonary vascular resistance and a predominantly left-to-right shunt. The patency of the ductus arteriosus can be easily documented in the first hours of life, with the help of echocardiography. At this early stage of life, the shunt is either right-to-left or bidirectional, depending on the severity of the infant's respiratory condition. In our center, the incidence of clinically significant PDA requiring therapy has been around 65% of all infants weighing less than 1,000 g. The left-to-right ductal shunting can be diagnosed as early as in the first day of life in infants with RDS who improved following surfactant therapy (102). An active precordium, with bounding pulses and visible carotid pulse, will often precede auscultation of a murmur. If left untreated, the infant may develop left-sided heart failure and pulmonary edema or hemorrhagic pulmonary edema, with significant deterioration of the respiratory status. Significant left-to-right ductal shunting may cause decreased peripheral perfusion and oxygen delivery. ELBW infants with significant PDA are at risk for IVH, necrotizing enterocolitis (NEC), renal failure, CLD, and metabolic acidosis (103). The size of the ductus arteriosus, and the ratio of the left atrium to aortic root can be easily measured by echocardiography (104). We consider as significant a PDA of diameter greater than 1.5 mm and/or a ratio of left atrium to aortic root greater than 1.3 for ELBW infants.

The ductus arteriosus of the premature infant is less responsive to the vasoconstrictive effect of oxygen and is less likely to close spontaneously than that of term infants, especially in infants with RDS. The classic management of PDA first involves medical and supportive measures, i.e., fluid restriction, diuresis, distending airway pressure, transfusion of packed red blood cells to keep the hematocrit above 0.4. If these measures fail to close the ductus arteriosus, pharmacologic closure is possible with a cyclooxygenase inhibitor, namely indomethacin (105–107). In ELBW infants, because closure of the ductus arteriosus is unlikely to occur spontaneously, the infant is at risk for the short- and long-term complications mentioned previously. Hence, therapy with indomethacin has become standard practice for the majority of these infants. Different protocols of treatment have been proposed. We treat most infants with 0.2 mg/kg of indomethacin every 12 hours for three doses. For infants developing clinical and/or biochemical signs of renal failure, we subsequently use 0.1 mg/kg per dose (108). A reduction in fluid intake is advisable prior to administration of indomethacin. In our experience about 80% of the treated infants will respond with a functional closure of the ductus. However, about 30% of these may reopen, in which case, further indomethacin is administered. If the ductus arteriosus fails to close after three courses of indomethacin, or if indomethacin cannot be administered because of significant renal dysfunction on previous treatment, then surgical ligation is necessary. In the last 8 years, 16.7% of ELBW infants required surgical ligation of the ductus after repeated failures of pharmacologic therapy. The more premature the infant, and the greater the postnatal age at the time of treatment, the greater the failure of indomethacin (109). A group particularly resistant to indomethacin therapy is ELBW infants with severe IUGR (26). Suggested hypotheses for this high failure rate of indomethacin therapy among this group of infants include chronic hypoxia, altered levels of prostaglandin, and altered number or sensitivity of their receptors (110).

Contraindications to indomethacin therapy include renal failure, active bleeding, and thrombocytopenia. The presence of IVH does not appear to be an absolute contraindication to the use of indomethacin. Recent studies indicate that there is no progression of the severity of IVH after administration of indomethacin for PDA closure (111). Until additional data are available, it is prudent in the presence of IVH to verify the platelet count prior to the administration of indomethacin and to eliminate any bleeding diathesis.

The optimal timing of administration of indomethacin has been a matter of debate. Although early or prophylactic use of indomethacin may result in a higher initial PDA closure rate and in a reduction in the incidence of severe IVH, it does not appear to ultimately reduce the need for surgical PDA ligation, does not confer any long-term respiratory advantage, and does not change the rate of survival without neurosensory impairment at 18 months (112,113).

Another cyclooxygenase inhibitor that seems very promising is ibuprofen (114). It has the theoretical advantage over indomethacin that it may increase the range of blood pressure at which cerebral blood flow is autoregulated, but has little effect on cerebral blood flow during normotension (115,116). In a Phase I study carried out in our center, we observed a dramatic response in 12 ELBW infants treated with ibuprofen within 3 hours of birth (117). All twelve infants had their PDA permanently closed after three doses of ibuprofen. We also observed a significant trend in the reduction of IVH and practically no side effects. These findings have since been confirmed by other groups of investigators. The efficacy of ibuprofen for the treatment of PDA appears to be equivalent to that of indomethacin, with a lower likelihood of oliguria (118). Furthermore, in a series of patients evaluated by near-infrared spectroscopy and Doppler ultrasonography, ibuprofen therapy did not result in a significant reduction in cerebral perfusion and oxygen availability (119). One reported side effect of ibuprofen, namely the development of transient severe pulmonary hypertension and hypoxemia in a few infants treated within six hours of birth, may still require further evaluation (120).

Finally, in the presence of a clinically significant ductus that fails to respond to pharmacologic closure or in the presence of contraindications to the use of indomethacin, surgical ligation should not be delayed, as the presence of a continuous left-to-right shunt may contribute to ventilator and oxygen dependency with well-known consequences in terms of CLD.

Regarding early management of low blood pressure, with the exception of hypovolemic shock, when volume replacement is an urgent matter, we rarely use volume expanders and β-adrenergic drugs to maintain blood pressure. We pay particular attention to skin perfusion. As a rule of thumb, we aim for a mean blood pressure that is numerically slightly above the gestational age of the infant.

FLUIDS AND ELECTROLYTES

The management of fluids and electrolytes remains one of the most challenging aspects in the care of the ELBW infant. Knowledge of the body composition of these infants and better understanding of their renal function has helped to determine their requirements (121,122).

It is important to remember that the body of the ELBW infant is made up of 85 to 90% water, which is distributed as one-third intracellular water (ICW) and two-thirds extracellular water (ECW). Immediately following birth, glomerular filtration rate and fractional excretion of sodium (FENa) are low and urine output is minimal. This is followed by a diuretic phase, which results in a decrease in the ECW compartment. Furthermore, because of the large body surface area to body weight ratio and the underdeveloped epidermis of the ELBW infant, evaporative losses, if uncontrolled, may be of very significant magnitude, i.e., 5.7 mL/kg/h (123,124). Additionally, the immature kidney, having a limited concentrating ability (less than 700 mOsm), produces large amounts of diluted urine. Thus, without close control of fluid intake and the infant's environment, the infant is very vulnerable to dehydration and hypertonicity, which may predispose to IVH. One has to be also careful not to overload the infant with fluids, because this may have an impact on PDA, with possible congestive heart failure, pulmonary edema, worsening pulmonary function and CLD (125).

Shortly after admission, once the infant's respiratory status has stabilized and the need for ready access to the infant is not as essential, the infant is transferred from a radiant warmer to an incubator, maintaining 75 to 80% humidity for the first few days of life. This approach significantly reduces water and heat loss and allows limitation of fluid intake to between 65 and 85 mL/kg/d for the first day of life. Additionally, we monitor the infant's weight every 8 hours during the first days of life, and adjust fluid intake consequently. Under these described conditions, there is rarely a need to exceed an intake of 170 to 180 mL/kg/d even for infants with a birth weight less than 600 g.

Electrolyte abnormalities such as hypernatremia, hyponatremia, and hyperkalemia are frequently seen in ELBW infants. Hypernatremia is usually the result of severe insensible water loss, but can be secondary to the treatment of metabolic acidosis with large amounts of sodium bicarbonate. Hyponatremia (less than 130 mmol/L) is more frequently seen because of the high FENa during the diuretic phase. It may also be noted during the first day of life if the mother has received large amounts of hypotonic intra-venous fluids. Hyponatremia is also seen following therapy with indomethacin without prior proper reduction of fluid intake, and later on when diuretics are used for the treatment of CLD.

On admission, infants receive only a 10% dextrose solution in water. We monitor blood glucose and electrolytes closely and we test all urine for glucose. We subsequently adjust the intravenous dextrose according to the blood glucose values. Protein and lipid intake is generally initiated during the first 24 hours of life in the form of parenteral alimentation. We begin sodium supplementation only when its serum value is less than 140 mmol/L, which usually occurs between the second and third day of life.

Hyperkalemia (K+ greater than 7 mmol/L) is a severe acute problem in this ELBW group of infants, even in the absence of oliguria and potassium intake (126). A rapid rise in serum potassium may be seen during the first 24 hours of life, especially in the most immature infants. A few mechanisms have been proposed for this hyperkalemia, i.e., relative hypoaldosteronism, immaturity of the renal distal tubules, and internal potassium shift from the intracellular space to the extracellular space. Hyperkalemia is also more severe in infants with intraventricular or pulmonary hemorrhage, extensive bruising, or renal failure. It is prudent to obtain a baseline measurement of electrolytes following birth, particularly when the mother has received intravenous fluids. We routinely repeat the electrolytes every twelve to eighteen hours during the first couple days of life, or more frequently if indicated, especially for the smallest infants.

We treat hyperkalemia when it exceeds 7 mmol/L with insulin and sodium bicarbonate to allow an intracellular shift of potassium and calcium gluconate for stabilization of the myocardium. Potassium supplements are introduced only after the serum level has stabilized below 4.5 mmol/L.

We also monitor urine output, and use the urine specific gravity and osmolality as an additional guide to assess the renal function and hydration status of the infant. Typically, the urine pH of the ELBW infant is greater than 7 in the first few of days of life, then decreases as the tubular reabsorption of bicarbonate increases. Microscopic hematuria is consistently seen in the ELBW infant during the first few days after birth, regardless of the health status of the infant. Monitoring for the presence of glucose in the urine can be a good indicator of the carbohydrate homeostasis of the newborn infant. Some extremely premature infants have a low glucose renal tubular threshold and may be predisposed to osmotic diuresis.

Management of fluids in the ELBW infants is very much dependent on securing an intravenous line. Intravenous access may, at times, become very difficult, thus compromising fluid, electrolyte, and glucose homeostasis, thermoregulation, and physiologic stability as a result of the pain induced by multiple attempts to insert a venocath. The umbilical vessels usually provide an easy access route for the first days of life. Subsequently, small neonatal infusion needles (IMP Group International Inc.) are inserted in the scalp, or a venocath is inserted in one of the extremities. In our center, we favor the insertion of a percutaneous central venous catheter, which gives continuous venous access for as long as necessary (50). In our experience, this technique has not increased the incidence of infection when compared to peripheral catheters used for prolonged parenteral alimentation. (51)

The Skin of the Extremely Low Birth Weight Infant

The skin of an infant born at 23 to 26 weeks of gestation is extremely immature. Maturity of the epidermis is present at birth only in infants born after 32 weeks of gestation (127). Prior to this time, the epidermis is underdeveloped, especially the stratum corneum, predisposing to very high transepidermal water loss, and to the risk of trauma and percutaneous absorption of toxic agents. The skin also is permeable to gases, allowing for diffusion of oxygen and carbon dioxide. The tremendous transepidermal water loss of the ELBW infant predisposes to dehydration, electrolyte imbalance, and evaporative heat loss. Trauma to the skin may provide a portal of entry for infectious organisms. Fortunately, after birth, there is acceleration of epidermal maturation, such that, by 2 weeks of age, the skin of the premature infant almost resembles that of the term infant. Preservation of skin integrity and prevention of transepidermal water loss have been, and still are, areas of challenge in neonatology. Under a radiant warmer, water loss is extensive. Plastic shields have been used to decrease this loss, with variable success. When the infant is placed in an incubator, increasing the ambient humidity to 80% reduces total extracellular loss to a minimum. Initial studies using the topical ointment Aquaphor® had shown reduced losses for up to 6 hours following application, improved skin condition and decreased skin bacterial colonization, thus possibly reducing the risk of nosocomial infection (128). However, more recent studies indicate no advantage with this approach. (129)

Nutrition

Nutrition is an essential part of the care of the ELBW infant. These tiny infants are born with very low reserves of fat and carbohydrates, and they rapidly develop nutritional deficiencies in calcium, phosphorus, iron, trace minerals, and vitamins. Their endocrine and enzymatic capability is limited as a result of immaturity. Postnatally, they rapidly enter a catabolic state unless provided with sufficient nutrients. On the other hand, reversal of this catabolic state often is difficult because of limited feeding tolerance. The gastrointestinal (GI) tract is immature in terms of digestive pathways and motor function, increasing the risk of developing NEC.

The first goal of nutrition is to prevent catabolism. Usually, this will be achieved by providing a minimum of 50 kcal/kg/d. Growth will require additional caloric intake. Achieving steady growth is essential for the ELBW infant,

because the intrauterine growth velocity at 25 to 30 weeks' gestation is relatively higher than at term. If reasonable caloric intake cannot be provided, catch-up growth may never be achieved.

In the early days of life, satisfactory nutrition can never be achieved exclusively with milk. Parenteral nutrition provides the additional calories (130). In contrast to enteric nutrition, parenteral administration starting at 80 to 85 kcal/kg/d can provide the necessary calories for growth. When the infant no longer is receiving intravenous nutrition, 100 to 120 kcal/kg/d are needed to maintain growth. However, this level of caloric intake may not be sufficient in infants suffering from CLD and other high-energy–requiring conditions (131). Appropriate growth, if one wants to mimic intrauterine growth, should be a 2% daily increase in body weight, slowing to 1% near term.

Both parenteral nutrition and enteral nutrition are not without difficulties and complications in the ELBW infant. TPN requires intravenous access and, this can be associated with a variety of infections, with *Staphylococcus epidermidis* being the most common. The composition of TPN has been, and remains, an area of active research, especially regarding the composition of essential amino acids and fatty acids. Exclusive intravenous nutrition affects the mucosal lining of the GI tract, which is bypassed and eventually may lead to villus atrophy. TPN also requires regular metabolic monitoring for glucose, electrolytes, urea, lipids, and acid–base balance. Cholestatic jaundice is a frequent complication of TPN (132). In the vast majority of cases, this is a self-limited condition, the exact etiology of which is not completely understood, but appears to implicate both amino acids and lipids.

Enteral nutrition may consist of either breast milk or premature formulas. During fetal life, the fetus constantly swallows amniotic fluid, promoting intestinal development. Enteral feeding, even in small amounts, has been demonstrated to stimulate trophic factors and hormonal maturation of the GI tract, thus improving overall intestinal function and potentially improving feeding tolerance and preventing mucosal atrophy (133,134). Whether early introduction of feedings and stimulation of the GI tract could prevent or decrease the incidence of NEC has not yet been established.

The current standard for postnatal nutrition is to duplicate as much as possible in utero fetal growth rates (135). To achieve this goal, high intravenous amino acid and lipid intake are necessary. Recent studies indicate that more aggressive amino acid intakes up to 3 g/Kg/d from the first days of life not only are well tolerated, but they also suppress protein breakdown and provide increased protein accretion and synthesis. (136)

In our center, we start TPN from day one, as soon as the infant is metabolically stable, with 1 g/kg/d of amino acids, 1g/kg/d of lipids, and glucose according to tolerance. Calcium, phosphorus, vitamins, and trace minerals also are added. Sodium and potassium are added according to the electrolytic profile. The intake of amino acids and lipids is rapidly increased to a maximum of 3 to 3.5 g/kg/d. Lipids are restricted in the presence of severe indirect hyperbilirubinemia. We also adjust the amino acid intake according to urea, pH, and the degree of TPN-related cholestasis. Monitoring of urea, creatinine electrolytes, glucose, and bilirubin is performed daily for the first 3 to 4 days of life and then is reduced to twice a week. When the oral intake is half of the total caloric requirement, monitoring is performed only once a week. During the past 8 years, the mean duration of any amount of TPN administration among 253 survivors born weighing less than 1,000 g was 31.5 ± 15 days (median 28.5 days, range 9 to 121 days).

In terms of enteral nutrition, we attempt to introduce minimal feedings, starting in stable infants as early as 48 hours of life. In the vast majority, we use breast milk or, if necessary, a premature formula (68 kcal/100 mL). However, tolerance varies widely from one infant to the other. We encourage mothers to pump their own milk, which is used exclusively for their own babies. The progression of enteral feedings and the addition of a breast milk fortifier varies from one neonatal unit to the other. For the smallest infants, we increase the volume per feeding by 1 mL every 24 hours, up to 10 mL, and then by 1 mL every 12 hours. Generally, we add a fortifier to the breast milk, thus increasing its caloric content to 81 kcal/100 mL when oral intake is between one-quarter and one-half of the total daily intake. For those infants on premature formula, we also advance to a more calorie dense formulation (81 kcal/100 mL). Intolerance to milk feeds is not an infrequent occurrence. Tolerance of full enteral feeding, in our experience, usually is achieved between 20 and 30 days of life. In the 192 survivors mentioned previously, birth weight was regained at a mean of 12.2 ± 6.8 days (median 13 days, range 2 to 48 days). These data are comparable to that reported by Berry and associates (137).

Glucose, Calcium, and Phosphorus Homeostasis

Early hypoglycemia frequently is seen in this group of infants, because of poor glycogen reserves and the immaturity of the postnatal adaptive mechanism of endocrine and enzymatic control of glucose. In particular, ketogenesis and lipogenesis, which lead to the production of alternate fuels, are limited in very premature infants, making the infant more dependent on glucose (138,139). Hence, an infusion of dextrose at a rate of 8 to 10 mg/kg/min is necessary to maintain normoglycemia.

Hyperglycemia is a frequent and challenging complication, particularly in extremely immature infants of 23 to 24 weeks' gestation and in those with IUGR. This condition is usually the result of high glucose infusion rates, but may also occur because of incomplete suppression of hepatic glucose production in the presence of hyperglycemia, reflecting the immaturity of the regulatory mechanisms mentioned previously (140). Hyperglycemia poses the risk of osmotic diuresis, and thus of increased water loss, which eventually may have cerebral implications. Insulin can be used to control hyperglycemia. Although the exact mechanism of its action in the extremely premature infant is not completely clear, it is thought to work by decreasing hepatic production of glucose and increasing glucose utilization by peripheral tissues.

We monitor blood glucose within 1 hour of birth and as often as required, until stabilization. We also test all urine for glycosuria. We tolerate blood glucose values up to 8 or even 10 mmol/L, provided there is no glycosuria. If an insulin infusion is used, one must remember to preflush the tubing with the infusate, because insulin adheres to plastic and, unless the binding sites are saturated prior to infusion, a very erratic infusion of insulin may occur, making the interpretation of glucose values difficult (141,142). The sudden onset of glycosuria in a previously stable infant may be an early sign of infection. Hyperglycemia also is seen frequently with initiation of dexamethasone therapy for BPD (143). Because of the slow metabolic adaptation of the ELBW infant, rapid and significant changes in glucose intake should be avoided to prevent episodes of hypo- or hyperglycemia, which can become difficult to control. Finally, for the treatment of acute and severe hypoglycemia, a bolus of no more than 200 mg/kg of dextrose can be administered as needed, although, at the same time, increasing the concentration of the intravenous glucose infusion.

Additional calcium is necessary in ELBW infants both in the early days of life and later, when their limited calcium reserves are rapidly depleted during this period of rapid growth. However, it is important to appreciate that, because of the low serum albumin of the immature infant, total serum calcium rarely exceeds 1.75 mmol/L. Measurement of ionized calcium is, of course, the ideal way to evaluate hypocalcemia. Because hypocalcemia also can induce apnea, we always verify calcium levels after the first 24 hours of life. It is important to remember that metabolic acidosis can give falsely reassuring values of serum calcium, which decline rapidly with the improvement of acid–base balance. Mechanisms involved in the early manifestations of hypocalcemia include parathyroid dysfunction, renal immaturity, and calcitonin stimulation. Treatment of hypocalcemia consists of administering 500 mg/kg/d of calcium gluconate. As soon as we introduce TPN, 300 mg/kg/d of calcium gluconate is added daily to the solution, together with multivitamins. Because maternal milk has an inadequate mineral and vitamin content, we use a human milk fortifier and vitamins. In the presence of persistent hypocalcemia, it is important to verify the levels of magnesium. The daily recommended dose of Vitamin D in ELBW infants is between 800 and 1,000 IU. (144)

Acid–Base Balance

No other investigation is ordered more frequently in ELBW infants than measurements of acid–base balance. Both the respiratory and metabolic components need frequent adjustments. Acid–base homeostasis varies in relation to the degree of renal maturity. The renal threshold of bicarbonate can be as low as 15 mEq/L. Hence, in ELBW infants, there is often a need for additional buffering with sodium bicarbonate. The need for supplemental sodium bicarbonate also is frequent with high amounts of amino acids in the TPN. We initiate correction of the acid–base balance as soon as the base deficit exceeds 5 to 6 mEq/L. Because TPN contains calcium, the addition of sodium bicarbonate may induce precipitation. For this reason, we have elected to administer sodium bicarbonate via slow push of 0.5 mEq/kg every 2 to 6 hours, according to the severity of the metabolic acidosis, while evaluating the progress of correction and adjusting the frequency of administration accordingly. With this approach, we do not need to discontinue intravenous alimentation, nor do we need to start a second intravenous line. Sodium acetate added to the TPN as an additional buffer, is an alternative treatment to acidosis (145). The late metabolic acidosis of prematurity also is related to a combination of increased nitrogen load and low renal threshold.

Although acidosis is the main concern in the early days of life, later on, many of these tiny babies may develop a metabolic alkalosis as a result of the administration of diuretics, in combination with fluid restriction, as part of the management of CLD. On occasion, we have found it helpful to administer acetazolamide at a dosage of 2.5 mg/kg every 12 hours to overcome a significant metabolic alkalosis (pH more than 7.45).

Jaundice

Rarely will an infant weighing less than 1,000 g escape the need for phototherapy. Hepatic immaturity and reduced erythrocyte lifespan, blood group incompatibilities, extensive extravasation of blood, and increased enterohepatic circulation as a result of poor bowel motility all contribute to the fact that ELBW infants are very prone to develop jaundice. Because the serum bilirubin binding capacity is decreased in premature infants as a result of the lower serum albumin, the level at which toxicity for the brain and acoustic nerves may occur is much lower than that of the more mature infant. Guidelines for the initiation of phototherapy have been proposed in the past and have undergone frequent revisions. However, some basic principles are universally accepted and govern the management of jaundice. These include age of the baby in hours or days from birth, gestational age, presence of a hemolytic disorder, degree of bruising or other extravasation of blood, and level of serum albumin. We find it helpful in our decision to initiate or discontinue phototherapy to estimate the serum binding capacity from the level of serum albumin (146). Based on this principle, we have not seen a single case of kernicterus clinically or on autopsy material. Although we do not initiate phototherapy immediately after birth, we believe that relatively early phototherapy can decrease significantly the need for exchange transfusion, which incidentally is poorly tolerated in the very immature infant. We generally initiate phototherapy when the bilirubin level has reached 80 micromol/L in the first 24 hours of life, or if we note an increment of more than

40 micromol/L/d. When phototherapy is used, it is important to increase the fluid intake by 15% to 20% to avoid excessive insensible water loss. When the bilirubin level approaches the exchange transfusion level, it is important to avoid variations in acid–base balance, high levels of lipid infusion, hypothermia, and certain medications, which may compete with and displace bilirubin from albumin, thus precipitating kernicterus.

MAJOR MORBIDITIES OF THE EXTREMELY LOW-BIRTH-WEIGHT INFANT

Neurologic Disorders

The neurologic examination of the newborn infant is related to gestational age and is affected greatly by any disturbance in the CNS. The ELBW infant is typically hypotonic. The primitive reflexes are absent but brain stem function (corneal, gag, oculocephalic reflexes, facial grimacing, nasal tickle) can be tested. Neuronal migration usually is completed by 24 weeks of gestation, but synaptic development and myelinization are just beginning at this age.

Intraventricular Hemorrhage

IVH is a major morbidity for the ELBW infant, with serious potential sequelae in surviving infants, which include hemorrhagic periventricular infarction, posthemorrhagic hydrocephalus, seizures, PVL, and in the long-term, neurosensory and neurodevelopmental impairments. Despite modern advances, this remains a common problem, with an incidence of up to 44% of ELBW cohorts (147,148). Fortunately, the majority of ELBW infants develop less severe IVH (Grade I or II). There is evidence that the overall incidence of IVH may be declining in recent years (149). In a study of a large cohort of infants with birth weight of 500–1500 g from the National Institute of Child Health and Human Development (NICHD) Neonatal Network, Shankaran and associates (147) observed a significant decrease in severe intracranial hemorrhage (Grades III and IV) from 19% to 15% over a 3-year period. Significant variation in the rates of all grades of IVH has been observed between centers.

The degree of prematurity is a very strong predictor for IVH, with gestational age and birth weight inversely correlated with the incidence and severity of IVH. Thus, the smallest and youngest infants are at greatest risk for more severe IVH. Recent reports described the incidence of Grades III and IV IVH at 9% to 13% for ELBW infants, in contrast to 2% to 5% for infants with birth weights greater than 1,000 g. Severe IVH was found in 16% of infants with gestational age at birth less than 25 weeks, in contrast to about 1% to 2% in which gestation was greater than 25 weeks.

In our center, among 253 ELBW infants born between 1995 and 2002, we observed an overall incidence of 24.4%

for any IVH and 7.6% for severe IVH (Grades III and IV) (Table 25-8). It is important in assessing the incidence of IVH to know whether it is representative of the whole population born weighing less than 1,000 grams or only among survivors, in which the incidence of IVH would be much lower. Indeed, among our survivors, the incidence of IVH was 16.6% and for grades III and IV, 4.7% (Table 25-9).

The variations in the incidence of IVH could also be explained by the multifactorial pathogenesis proposed by Volpe (150,151), describing intravascular, vascular and extravascular factors, superimposed on the fragility of the germinal matrix and the limited cerebral blood flow autoregulation in ELBW infants.

We are particularly attentive to rapid stabilization, avoidance of hypo- and hyperoxia, and hypo- and hypercarbia, maintenance of normoglycemia, and control of the environment with the use of high humidity in the first few days of life to prevent excessive water loss, hypernatremia and hyperosmolarity. We attempt to maximize synchronization of the ventilator breaths to the infant's own respiratory efforts. We use the Ballard closed suction circuit, thus avoiding frequent disconnection of the infant from the ventilator. We avoid volume expanders, unless there is documented blood loss or significant hypotension. We favor early medical PDA closure. Finally, we minimize handling of the infant, with clustering of care or use of sedative/analgesics as warranted to decrease significant discomfort and pain. We also avoid significant apnea by initiating prompt supportive management, such as early nasal CPAP/ventilation, methylxanthines or mechanical ventilation, as necessary, and by rapid diagnosis and treatment of causative factors, such as infection, hypoglycemia, and hypocalcemia.

IVH may present acutely, leading to shock and death. It may be clinically silent or, more commonly, it may present with worsening cardiorespiratory instability. The time of occurrence of IVH has been well investigated and our experience is similar to published data. About 50% of bleeds occur during the first day of life, 25% during the second day, and 15% on the third day of life. (152). It is unusual for an infant to develop IVH after 7 days of life.

Ultrasonography is the most reliable and safest neuroimaging technique to diagnose IVH in premature infants (153). We obtain a cranial ultrasound in the first 24 hours of life. If no IVH is detected, the study is repeated 1 week later, or sooner if the infant suffers from any acute event in the interim. If pathology is present, ultrasonography may be repeated at intervals of 48 to 72 hours, until stabilization of the intracranial pathology and as clinically warranted to facilitate parental counseling and decisions for care.

The immediate management of IVH involves stabilization of the cardiovascular system, correction of any bleeding diathesis, and monitoring for hyperbilirubinemia and hyperkalemia. Careful neurologic examination and serial measurements of the head circumference along with serial cranial ultrasounds must be planned for the early detection and management of progressive posthemorrhagic

hydrocephalus. If there is rapid dilatation of the ventricles, neurosurgical intervention may be necessary for temporary or permanent drainage of the cerebrospinal fluid. We have not found repeated lumbar punctures to be effective as a temporizing technique to control progressive posthemorrhagic hydrocephalus.

Prognosis for mortality and long-term morbidity is related to the extent of the brain injury, hallmarked primarily by the extent of the bleed. Severe IVH with periventricular hemorrhagic ischemia in the ELBW cohort has a mortality of more than 50% and leads to progressive ventricular dilatation in 80% of infants. Many studies have confirmed the significant association between Grade IV IVH, periventricular leukomalacia and ventriculomegaly with cerebral palsy. One study gave an odds ratio (OR) of 15.4 (95% CI, 7.6–31.1) for a diagnosis of CP at 2 to 9 years of age in the presence of Grade IV IVH, PVL, or ventriculomegaly. Furthermore, Grade IV IVH and moderate to severe ventriculomegaly were strongly associated with the risk of mental retardation or neuropsychiatric disorders at 2 to 9 years, with the odds ratio ranging from 9.97 to 19.0 (154,155).

We believe that transport *in utero*, antenatal steroids, judicious obstetrical management, and expert delivery room stabilization and NICU care are important preventative measures against IVH. Pharmacologic strategies, specifically indomethacin administered within the first 12 hours of birth in ELBW infants, can reduce the incidence of severe IVH (112), but without significant long-term benefit at 18 months and hence is not current or recommended practice in our center (148). Further innovative research is needed to impact this serious complication for ELBW infants.

Periventricular Leukomalacia

PVL is the other significant injury of the developing premature brain, with an incidence estimated to range from 4% to 15%. In our center, PVL is uncommon, with an incidence of 5.5%. It is believed to be a consequence of hypoxic–ischemic events, leading to necrosis of the white matter (156). The most commonly affected areas are the white matter near the trigone of the lateral ventricles and around the Foramen of Monro. Although often diagnosed in association with IVH, PVL may also occur independently as an isolated lesion. Sometimes, the origin is clearly intrauterine. Chorioamnionitis is recognized as a risk factor for PVL (156). Postnatally acquired PVL is seen more frequently in male infants, in infants with severe RDS, in infants with septicemia, and in those with significant cardiovascular instability or apnea (156).

Cystic PVL among preterm infants is the single best predictor of adverse long-term neurologic outcomes (157). The frequency of cerebral palsy developing after cystic PVL has been reported to vary between 62 and 100%. (158). Its characteristic manifestation is a spastic paresis involving predominantly the lower extremities (spastic diplegia), and it is usually diagnosed in the first 2 years of life.

Although uncommon, severe disability with spastic quadriplegia, strabismus and impaired visual acuity, developmental delays, cognitive impairment, and seizures may be observed in early childhood.

The diagnosis of PVL is made primarily by cranial ultrasonography. When the lesions have occurred in utero, it is possible to make the diagnosis soon after birth, with the first or second studies. However, prenatally or postnatally acquired PVL is usually diagnosed by 3 to 6 weeks or later, as time is necessary to develop the cavitation of the injured periventricular white matter. This ultrasound, usually performed prior to discharge home, provides important prognostic information for the neurodevelopment of the infant, facilitating parental counseling and planning for long-term multidisciplinary follow-up.

Magnetic resonance imaging (MRI) may allow greater detection of white matter abnormalities than ultrasound. However, there have been insufficient follow-up studies to indicate whether the additional findings provide more information about neurodevelopmental prognosis. Therefore, the routine use of MRI and other techniques of neuroimaging for the detection of PVL and other brain injury in the ELBW is not yet a recommendation, and should be an avenue for future research. (155). Because of the later appearance of cystic lesions or residual ventricular dilatation secondary to involution of the periventricular white matter and resorption of the cysts, it is important to repeat the cranial ultrasound study between 36 and 40 weeks' postmenstrual age (155).

Seizures

Seizures are relatively rare in the ELBW infant, despite many potential risk factors, such as intracranial hemorrhage, hypoglycemia, and electrolyte disturbances. Compared to full-term infants, seizures in very premature infants are even more challenging to diagnose, due primarily to cortical immaturity coherent with the gestational age. Subtle, tonic or myoclonic seizures may be difficult to differentiate from the general uncoordinated movements, tremulousness and myoclonic jerks often seen in extremely premature infants. The etiologies of seizures in the ELBW infant, as for the term infant, include CNS pathology, metabolic derangements (e.g. hypoglycemia, hypocalcemia, severe hyponatremia), infection, and drug withdrawal.

The investigation and management of seizures is described comprehensively elsewhere. Suffice it to say that the electroencephalogram (EEG) can be difficult to interpret, because a conventional surface EEG may not detect the electrical activity of deeper cortical and subcortical structures. The treatment of seizures in ELBW infants involves correction of any metabolic derangements, appropriate antibiotic therapy for infection as warranted, and control of seizure activity to avoid brain injury as a result of alteration in cerebral energy metabolism. As for term infants, the prognosis in the face of neonatal seizures depends primarily on the underlying cause. However, the prognosis is generally worse for ELBW with seizures, compared to term infants. Our preference for medical control of seizures is with phenobarbital at a loading dose of 20 mg/kg, which can be increased by another 10 mg/kg if control is not achieved (maximum loading dose 30–40 mg/kg). If control is not achieved, phenytoin is added, at a loading dose of 15 mg/kg (maximum loading dose 30–40 mg/kg). Rarely, the use of sedative-hypnotic anticonvulsants, such as lorazepam (0.05–0.1 mg/kg/dose) or diazepam (0.1–0.2 mg/kg/dose), and rectal paraldehyde (0.3 ml/kg, diluted 1:2 in mineral oil) may be considered for resistant seizures. There should be proper attention to adverse effects of these agents on very premature infants, such as the potential exacerbation of jaundice secondary to bilirubin displacement from its albumin-binding site by the sodium benzoate in diazepam and the abnormal movements (muscle twitchiness, myoclonus) seen with lorazepam (159,160).

Hearing Impairment

ELBW infants are at increased risk for hearing impairment because of multisystemic illness and the frequent use of potentially ototoxic medications, such as aminoglycosides and diuretics. The estimated prevalence of hearing impairments in extremely immature (< 26 weeks gestation) survivors ranges from 1.7% to 3.8%. (161). In the TIPP study, the prevalence of hearing loss requiring amplification for surviving ELBW infants was 2% (20/876 infants). (162)

Reporting on the outcomes of VLBW infants at age 19 years, Ericson and Kallen found high rates of persistent hearing impairment, with the odds ratio for severe hearing loss being 2.5 (95% CI, 1.2–5.0) (163). In 1994, the Joint Committee on Infant Hearing issued a Position Statement recommending that all infants born with birth weight less than 1500 grams undergo auditory screening. (164). Early diagnosis of hearing loss and amplification with hearing aids as early as 6 months of age, together with speech therapy, are essential to reduce the progressive disability in speech and language development caused by hearing impairment. The tests commonly used to detect hearing loss in the ELBW include the evoked auditory brainstem responses (ABR) and otoacoustic emission (OAE). (165). In our unit, a hearing screen is obtained prior to discharge using the OAE, with a diagnostic ABR confirming abnormal screening results.

Hematologic Disorders

Anemia

Low iron stores, multiple blood tests, blood loss as a result of either organ hemorrhage or hemolysis, and rapid growth are some of the factors that make anemia a practically unavoidable hematologic complication for any ELBW infant. The ELBW infant usually has a hemoglobin concentration of 140 to 160 g/L at birth. Those who have suffered from IUGR may have a hemoglobin concentration as high as 200 g/L. Their blood volume is 85 to 90 mL/kg. However, these values can be affected by the extent of placental transfusion at delivery (166). We generally allow for a 10-second placental transfusion in ELBW infants not suffering from IUGR.

The need for transfusion of blood products is a source of anxiety for parents. Any measure that can decrease the frequency and severity of anemia should be implemented. These measures include limiting blood tests to those essential for appropriate management of the infant, use of microtechniques, and use of pulse oximetry and other transcutaneous devices to monitor partial pressure of oxygen (PO_2) and PCO_2.

Although the administration of erythropoietin with iron supplementation does not eliminate completely the need for blood transfusion, it can reduce the number of transfusions (167,168). The lack of universal use of erythropoietin is probably as a result of the fact that it is expensive and that, at least in sick infants, it does not eliminate the need for blood transfusions.

To decrease the risk of infection, one unit of packed red cells from a single, properly screened donor, divided into several small bags (satellite bags), could be used for the same infant for several weeks (169). We have found this approach useful and more reassuring to parents.

We also have implemented a protocol for direct blood donation from compatible parents (father or mother) who are cytomegalovirus, human immunodeficiency virus, and hepatitis B and C negative. Blood is irradiated prior to transfusion to avoid graft-vs.-host disease. However, preparation of such blood requires time. The issue of blood transfusion is discussed with the family, antenatally whenever possible, or soon after admission of the infant to the NICU, and the parental decision is documented in the chart.

Our guidelines for the management of anemia with blood transfusion in ELBW infants are as follows: (a) infants born with severe anemia and/or hypovolemic shock; (b) replacement of blood taken from an umbilical line in the first days of life for frequent blood monitoring and exceeding 10% of the baby's blood volume; (c) maintenance of hematocrit between 0.35 and 0.40 during the first week of life and between 0.30 and 0.35 during the second week; (d) maintenance of hematocrit greater than 0.35 in infants with PDA and in those still having severe lung disease in the second week of life; (e) in infants with CLD, we maintain the hematocrit between 0.30 and 0.35; (f) after the second week of life, the hemoglobin is allowed to decrease as long as the baby has no signs of symptomatic anemia such as poor feedings, high output cardiac failure, apnea, edema, failure to gain weight, tachycardia, and tachypnea. Finally, 4 to 6 mg/kg/d of elemental iron is commenced at 4 to 6 weeks of life.

When transfusion is necessary, it should be administered slowly, especially during the first weeks of life, when any acute change in blood volume may be translated into changes in cerebral blood flow, thus predisposing to IVH, and when there is cardiorespiratory instability. We usually transfuse a volume of 10 mL/kg of packed red blood cells, which may be repeated at 12 hours, according to the need. Furosemide 1 mg/kg can be given with transfusions.

Hemostasis and Bleeding Diathesis

Vitamin K and vitamin-K–dependent coagulation factors are present at low concentrations at birth (170). As a result, all of our ELBW infants receive 0.5 mg of vitamin K intramuscularly immediately after delivery. Additionally, parenteral nutrition is supplemented with vitamin K.

Conditions requiring immediate administration of additional vitamin K include hemorrhagic pulmonary edema, pulmonary or gastric hemorrhage, and disseminated intravascular coagulation. The management of these conditions often will require, additionally to vitamin K, administration of fresh frozen plasma, transfusion of platelets, and treatment of the underlying condition.

Thrombocytopenia (platelet count less than 100×10^9/L) is commonly observed in ELBW infants and, if severe enough, may put the infant at risk for IVH. Thrombocytopenia is more frequent in infants born to preeclamptic mothers and infants with IUGR (171). Accelerated platelet destruction is seen in infants with sepsis, indwelling catheters, or active bleeding, or following exchange transfusion. In practice we transfuse platelets to infants with a platelet count below 30 to 40×10^9/L. However, in case of active bleeding and a platelet count less than 60×10^9/L, transfusion of platelets should be considered.

Chronic Lung Disease

A large number of ELBW infants continue to require oxygen supplementation at one month of life, and many of them will remain oxygen dependent beyond 36 weeks of postmenstrual age. Both dates have been proposed in the literature to define CLD. It is also not rare to see a number of infants discharged on home oxygen programs. Up to 70% of infants weighing less than 1000 g have been reported to develop CLD, and an important number of survivors are discharged home on supplemental oxygen (172). Thus, for many ELBW infants, CLD seems practically unavoidable.

It is beyond the scope of this chapter to discuss the pathogenesis and pathophysiology of CLD, and we refer the reader to the appropriate chapter. Hence, we will limit our discussion to a few aspects of the problem that are more specific to the ELBW infant. CLD encompasses more than the classic BPD described by Northway and associates in 1969 (173). Over the years, we have observed two distinct groups of infants developing CLD (97). The first group consists of infants with severe RDS, who require early intubation and mechanical ventilation. In our center, close to 65% of these infants receive exogenous surfactant. This is followed by a rapid decrease in oxygen requirement and need for ventilatory support. By day 3 of life, the majority of these infants are breathing room air or require a minimal amount of supplemental oxygen. However, in most of these

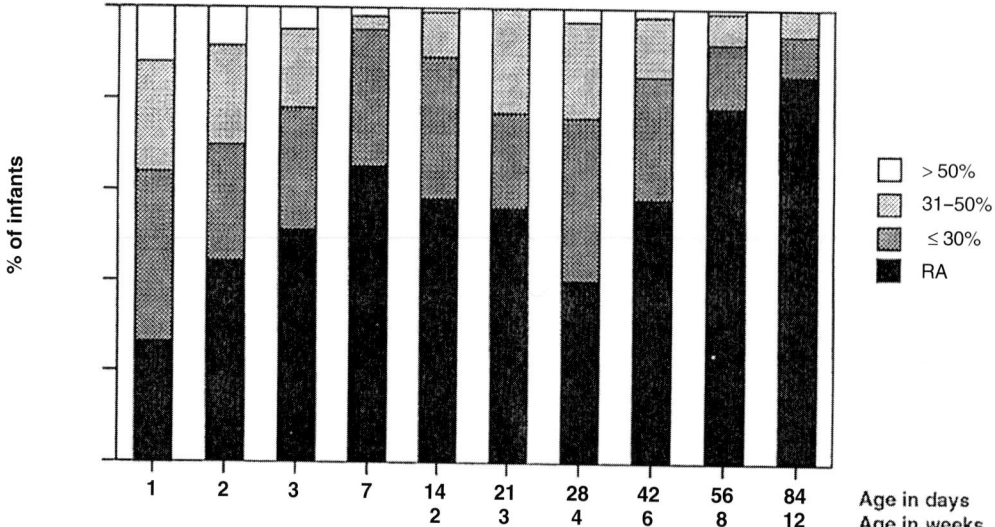

Figure 25-1 Variation in O$_2$ requirement in 120 survivors. RA, room air. 500–1000 g (1993–97).

infants, this improvement is transient, as ventilatory support and oxygen supplementation become necessary after 7 to 10 days of life, with eventual resolution of the respiratory problem over the ensuing weeks. The period of deterioration is usually accompanied by the presence of increased airway secretions, which require frequent toilet of the airways. The second group is composed of infants who had no initial lung pathology, and who required intubation for immaturity and/or apnea, but needed only minimal oxygen supplementation, if any. A number of these infants go on to develop clinical and radiological signs of CLD. They follow the same pattern of deterioration, and eventual improvement as the group with initial lung pathology. Fig. 25-1 indicates the bimodal fluctuation in oxygen requirement among 120 survivors of birth weight less than 1000 g in our center between 1993 and 1997.

In our population of ELBW survivors, 63.6% required oxygen supplementation at 28 days of age, and 31.2% at 36 weeks' postmenstrual age, with 5.9% of infants requiring supplemental oxygen after discharge home (Table 25-9).

The proposed management of the infant with CLD is based on a combination of the following interventions:

Respiratory support. Acceptance of a PCO$_2$ value up to 65 mm Hg, provided that the pH is at least around 7.25. Once the infant attains a postmenstrual age of 35 weeks, we aim for a steady oxygen saturation above 90% on pulse oximetry to prevent cor pulmonale. The hematocrit is generally kept above 0.35.

Prevention of fluid overload. Early closure of the PDA, fluid restriction to 120 to 130 mL/kg/d, or even less in some cases, administration of diuretics on a chronic basis, i.e., hydrochlorothiazide 1 mg/kg/dose and spironolactone 1 mg/kg/dose every 12 hours. Additional diuresis can be obtained with furosemide, when necessary.

Nutritional support. It has been increasingly recognized that infants with CLD require particular attention to nutri-

tional support. These infants may fail to thrive as a result of an increase in energy expenditure associated with an increased work of breathing, and their enteric intake may be suboptimal as a result of frequently associated feeding intolerance and gastroesophageal reflux. Lung growth and repair of damaged pulmonary tissue requires an adequate intake of all nutrients (174). We thus aim for an energy intake of 120 to 140 kcal/kg/d, encourage early initiation of enteral feeds, and use diuretics as needed to eliminate excess fluid.

Control of nosocomial infections. As ETT tubes frequently become colonized, it is important to periodically send secretions for culture and sensitivity to antibiotics. However, we do not treat the colonized infant if the condition remains stable, but rather monitor the infant carefully for clinical and laboratory signs compatible with infection. We may treat, however, infants colonized with ureaplasma, mycoplasma, or chlamydia with erythromycin if the respiratory status presents an unusual progression.

Control of inflammation. Because an inflammatory response seems to be an important mechanism leading to CLD, corticosteroids had been used extensively during the 1990s to decrease pulmonary edema, prevent inflammation, and increase surfactant and antioxidant production. Systemic dexamethasone had been the drug of choice, and various protocols were proposed in terms of onset and duration of treatment (175,176). Most infants responded favorably, with rapid extubation and a significant decrease in oxygen requirement. Initially, the side-effects of this therapy were believed to be limited to transient hypertension and hyperglycemia, an increased risk of infection, reversible hypertrophic cardiomyopathy, and a flattening of the growth curve.

With the onset of the new millennium, new data became available regarding the long-term outcomes of steroid-treated infants. Of note were some serious concerns that corticosteroid therapy may be independently associated with poor brain growth and with the development of cerebral palsy (177). This new information has resulted in a joint statement by the AAP and Canadian Pediatric Society, in which the routine use of systemic dexamethasone for the prevention or treatment of CLD in VLBW infants is no longer recommended (178). We currently limit the administration of systemic steroids to the most unstable ventilator-dependent infants with severe, life-threatening CLD, and the duration of therapy is limited to a three-day pulse of dexamethasone of 0.1 to 0.2 mg/kg/day, after parental consultation.

It remains to be clarified whether less potent systemic corticosteroids, such as hydrocortisone, administered at very low doses, may have a role to play in the future treatment of CLD (179). The same can be said of inhaled steroid preparations such as budesonide, the efficacy of which has likely been limited to date by inadequate methods of pulmonary delivery (180,181).

Bronchodilators. In infants with decreased air entry and wheezing, we have found that the administration of nebulized salbutamol at a dose of 1.25 mg diluted in 2.5mL physiologic saline solution, can be helpful (182). We have often observed that, immediately after a treatment, air entry improves and clearance of secretions becomes easier, particularly in combination with chest physiotherapy.

Home Oxygen Therapy

Despite maximum therapy, some infants remain dependent on supplemental oxygen beyond 40 weeks' postmenstrual age. In our center, such infants are evaluated and followed after discharge by a pediatric pulmonologist. The parents undergo specific training for home oxygen therapy. Prior to discharge, participation is organized with a multidisciplinary follow-up program, which include in its membership the pediatric pulmonologist, nutritionist and occupational therapist. For the years 1995 to 2002, the incidence of home oxygen therapy in our surviving ELBW infants was 5.9%. In comparison, the incidence of supplemental oxygen at discharge to home in the TIPP study was 18% to 20% (148).

Necrotizing Enterocolitis

NEC is the major GI disorder that selectively affects the sick premature infant. Its etiology is multifactorial and includes suspected predisposing factors such as intestinal immaturity, poor intestinal motility, hypoxemia, ischemia, PDA, umbilical catheter placement, IUGR, feeding practices, exchange transfusion, and systemic infections (183).

Antenatal administration of steroids appears to accelerate intestinal maturation and provides additional protection against NEC to the prematurely born infant (184). The incidence of NEC varies widely, from center to center, and is estimated at between 9% and 25% for ELBW infants (185). Our incidence of surgical NEC between 1995 and 2002 was 2.6% (Table 25-8). Variation in the incidence probably reflects differences in diagnostic criteria and clinical practices. Indeed, the successful reduction in the inci-

dence of NEC is related essentially to prevention, by avoiding all known predisposing factors and by intervening and interrupting the cascade of progression of the disease at the earliest signs, which many of us like to call "pre-NEC." These signs include increased gastric residuals, abdominal distension, cardiovascular instability, deterioration of skin perfusion, clusters of apneic spells, and unexplained glycosuria and lipemia. In the presence of these signs and depending on their severity, it is our practice either temporarily to discontinue feedings or to decrease the volume by 50% and reevaluate the situation in a few hours. In the presence of further abdominal distension, we do not hesitate to discontinue oral feeds and insert an orogastric catheter under continuous low suction. In the majority of cases of benign distension, the intestinal decompression reestablishes the intestinal vascular supply and, within 2 to 4 hours, the abdomen returns to normal. In an otherwise healthy looking and active infant, we do not necessarily initiate therapy with antibiotics unless there is blood in the stools or the abdominal radiograph demonstrates, besides dilated bowel loops, signs compatible with evolving NEC, such as pneumatosis intestinalis. In these cases, a septic workup is performed and antibiotics are begun immediately. Our initial treatment is a combination of gentamicin and ampicillin, to which clindamycin is added in case of additional deterioration, or when the presentation is that of overwhelming NEC. One of the most distressing situations in neonatology occurs when a previously stable premature infant, in whom milk intake has progressed well, suddenly develops fulminant abdominal distension accompanied by sepsis, profound metabolic acidosis, neutropenia, thrombocytopenia, and cardiovascular shock followed by rapid death. Fortunately, this dramatic clinical presentation is rare, as it is difficult to anticipate or to prevent, let alone to treat.

The management of NEC, besides antibiotics and orogastric suction, requires close monitoring of vital signs, frequent abdominal radiographs, with lateral views to visualize the possible presence of free air in the peritoneal cavity, correction of metabolic abnormalities, and cardiovascular support with volume expanders and vasopressors. Many infants with NEC may require assisted ventilation, as apnea frequently complicates the situation. TPN is also an integral part of the management of these infants. Persistent intractable metabolic acidosis, severe neutropenia and thrombocytopenia are ominous prognostic signs and usually reflect extensive intestinal necrosis.

For infants managed medically, the time of reintroduction of oral feeds is a critical one. We usually reinitiate enteric feeds after 7 to 14 days of therapy, depending on the rapidity of resolution of clinical and radiologic signs. The presence of bowel sounds, a stable condition, and a well-perfused infant without significant apnea are the basic requirements for starting oral feeds. We initially use an elemental formula and progress slowly to full enteric feeds over a period of 7 days or longer, as tolerated. For those infants on maternal milk, mother's own fresh milk is used. Post-NEC intestinal strictures are not unusual and can present several weeks after the initial episode, with milk intolerance, vomiting, and abdominal distension. Strictures may also be the result of subclinical injury of the intestine and can be seen in infants in whom the diagnosis of NEC was never made before.

In summary, much still needs to be learned about NEC, its prevention, and its management. In the meantime, every neonatal unit needs to develop its own philosophy and approach to reduce the risks of NEC. In our view, strategies that decrease the risk of NEC include antenatal administration of steroids, use of mother's own milk, early priming of the GI system with a very small volume of milk prior to the advancement of feedings, and, above all, careful observation of the infant's condition, with reduction or temporary discontinuation of feeds and intestinal decompression at the earliest suspicion.

Inguinal Hernias

Inguinal hernias occur frequently in ELBW infants, with a reported incidence between 14 and 30% (186,187). In our center, the incidence of inguinal hernia diagnosed prior to discharge home ranges from 10% to 15%. Predisposing factors are weakness of the abdominal musculature and tissues of the inguinal canal and increased intraabdominal pressure, especially in the presence of CLD. They can present as early as 2 weeks of age, often becoming very large and causing intermittent feeding intolerance, abdominal distension or bouts of crying and irritability. Surgical repair must be planned in consultation with a Pediatric Surgeon, preferably prior to discharge home where appropriate. Recurrence in the first year of life is a common observation.

Retinopathy of Prematurity

ROP remains a frequently diagnosed morbidity for ELBW infants and may result in significant visual impairment, ranging from correctible myopia and astigmatism to bilateral blindness. The incidence and severity of ROP is inversely proportional to birth weight and gestational age (188,189). Thus, as survival has increased, so has the number of surviving ELBW infants with severe ROP, particularly in infants born at the limits of viability at 23 and 24 weeks. Severe ROP is defined as unilateral or bilateral stage 4 or 5 disease or disease requiring laser or cryotherapy in at least one eye. Schmidt et al found an incidence of about 7% in a surviving ELBW cohort (162). However, blindness has become a rare outcome, with an estimated prevalence of 2% in ELBW survivors (162). The incidence and severity of ROP in our center is shown in Table 25-9.

The etiology and pathogenesis are complex and discussed in greater detail elsewhere in this book. Arterial oxygen tension remains a great risk factor, despite the introduction of noninvasive continuous O_2 monitors, such as pulse oximetry, and the presumed tighter control of the arterial pO_2. In addition to immaturity, we have recently reported that the combination of IUGR and severe prematurity further increases the risk of developing severe ROP (26).

Based on current knowledge of predisposing factors and years of careful observation, we have developed a policy of keeping stringent control of the PaO_2 below 50 mm Hg for all infants with birth weight less than 1,000 g in the first weeks of life. We have established guidelines for pulse oximetry, primarily based on gestational age and birth weight. Our long-standing practice to accept lower limits of arterial oxygen saturation (SaO_2) and to avoid brisk variations is in keeping with recent publications supporting the safety of this practice in an attempt to decrease the incidence of ROP (190). Furthermore, avoidance of swings from normoxemia to hyperoxemia and hypoxemia has been reported to decrease the incidence of ROP (191). For ELBW infants, the upper limit of SaO_2 is set at 93% and we try to avoid rapid fluctuations in PaO_2. We favor permissive hypercapnia, although we avoid prolonged hypercapnia, with values of pCO_2 greater than 55 mm Hg in the first weeks of life. We have a low tolerance of recurrent apnea associated with significant oxygen desaturation. In such cases, we do not hesitate to use respiratory support (nasal CPAP/ventilation; endotracheal ventilation) if the episodes are not readily controlled by respiratory stimulant medication, e.g. caffeine.

Early diagnosis and treatment of prethreshold and threshold ROP is required to preserve maximal visual acuity and prevent progression to blindness. This is achieved by expert serial ophthalmologic examinations as described by the joint statement of the AAP, the American Association of Pediatric Ophthalmology and Strabismus, and the Academy of Ophthalmology, such that all ELBW infants should be screened for ROP, with the first examination at 4 weeks of postnatal age or between 31 and 33 weeks postmenstrual age (192).

Like others, we have observed a few unpredicted cases of "rush" disease developing early, between 30 and 33 weeks, or progressing at later corrected gestational ages after a period of quiescence at stage 1 or 2. Consequently, in our center, we schedule the first ophthalmologic screen at 4 weeks after birth or at 30 weeks of postmenstrual age, whichever comes first. This practice is coherent with a recent publication by Subhani and associates (193), which recommended earlier screening in ELBW infants, beginning by 5 to 6 weeks of age using the postnatal age criterion and not waiting for the corrected postmenstrual age. Follow-up examinations are scheduled depending on the findings (e.g., degree of vascularization, zone and stage of retinal changes, tortuosity, plus disease) at intervals of 1 to 2 weeks. If the disease process seems to accelerate, examinations are performed twice a week. Infants with threshold and plus disease are candidates for laser therapy. In our center, 6% of ELBW underwent laser therapy in the past few years with satisfactory results.

Apnea of Prematurity

Apnea of prematurity is a feature of nearly all infants with a birth weight less than 1,000 g. Its incidence and frequency decrease with advancing gestational age, but at times it may be seen up to 42 weeks of postmenstrual age (194). In the ELBW population, it is a frequent indication for mechanical ventilation, thus exposing these infants to potential complications related to respiratory support.

Apnea usually is defined as a cessation of breathing for 20 seconds or more, or of a shorter duration if associated with cyanosis or bradycardia. Different patterns have been observed in premature infants: central apnea (absent breathing movements), obstructive apnea (breathing movements, but no airflow) or mixed apnea (central and obstructive) (195). ELBW infants are particularly prone to obstructive apnea, especially when in supine position with the neck in the midline, because of the weakness of the muscles of the oropharynx. Apnea as a result of obstruction of the lower airways also has been reported, suggesting immaturity of lung mechanics. The cessation of gas exchange during a significant apneic episode is manifested by hypoxemia and/or bradycardia. Recurrent episodes of apnea may affect neurodevelopmental outcome. Although it is difficult to relate frequency and severity of apnea to outcome, one can only stress the importance of monitoring these infants by pulse oximetry. Because apneic episodes can occur in premature infants as a result a variety of underlying diseases, investigation of other pathologic causes must be undertaken before diagnosing apnea of prematurity.

Patient management will depend on the severity and frequency of apneic episodes. Methylxanthines, which stimulate the respiratory center, are the most effective pharmacologic treatment for apnea of prematurity. Methylxanthines, aside from reducing the frequency of apneic pauses, have other actions that are equally important. They increase respiratory rate, tidal volume, and minute ventilation, and they decrease diaphragmatic fatigue. They also increase the sensitivity of the chemoreceptors to carbon dioxide and improve blood pressure and cardiac output (196–198). Treatment with either aminophylline or theophylline is effective but needs to be repeated two to four times per day. In our center, we treat apnea of prematurity with caffeine, which is the metabolite of theophylline (199). We found that caffeine has fewer GI side effects and causes less CNS irritability. It also has a much broader therapeutic index and achieves more stable plasma levels. In view of its long half-life, it only needs to be given once daily. We use caffeine base at a loading dose of 10 mg/kg, followed 24 hours later by a single daily dose of 2.5 mg/kg. Caffeine can be administered intravenously or orally. When given intravenously, the injection should be performed slowly, as it may otherwise be quite painful. We verify the serum level of caffeine in cases of intractable apnea or in the presence of clinical signs of toxicity. Caffeine is also the drug of choice when we start weaning an infant from the mechanical ventilator. The therapeutic range of serum caffeine levels is very broad, between 23 and 104 micromol/L, and the mean half-life is 102 hours.

If we cannot control apnea in a satisfactory manner with caffeine, we rapidly initiate nasal CPAP or nasal ventilation, which, in combination with caffeine, offers very good stabilization in the vast majority of cases. Finally, if apnea persists, we do not hesitate to intubate and ventilate such an infant with low pressures and rates. In infants with persisting apnea and desaturations after 40 weeks' postmenstrual age, we perform a respirogram prior to discharging them home on xanthines and a home monitoring program. It is important, before closing the discussion on apnea, to underline the fact that pharmacologic treatment of apnea should be considered only after proper investigation has eliminated any underlying condition requiring specific treatment, such as anemia, infection, or metabolic disorders.

Neonatal Infections

The ELBW infant is particularly vulnerable to bacterial, viral, and fungal infections. A significant number of premature labors are likely precipitated by infection. Chorioamnionitis is a frequent finding after a premature birth, particularly in the presence of prolonged rupture of membranes. As the clinical signs of infection are often nonspecific, the index of suspicion and the concern about the possibility of intrauterine infection should be very high in the presence of a premature birth. Hence, screening for infection should be an integral part of the evaluation of the ELBW infant. The diagnosis of neonatal infection can sometimes be difficult, as early neonatal infection often manifests with respiratory symptomatology, which is also the overwhelming pathology of prematurity. This is particularly true in the presence of group B streptococcal pneumonia, which is often indistinguishable clinically and radiologically from RDS (200). However, early appearance of recurrent apnea, poor perfusion, hypotension, and significant metabolic acidosis, often in the presence of an abnormal leukocyte count, are very strong elements in favor of infection.

In symptomatic infants, we obtain a skin surface culture, blood culture, and leukocyte count, and we initiate broad-spectrum antibiotic coverage with ampicillin and gentamicin. We do not routinely perform a lumbar puncture on admission. However, if the blood culture is positive or if there is clinical evidence of deterioration compatible with meningitis, then a lumbar puncture is performed. If the result suggests the presence of meningitis, we adjust the duration of therapy, antibiotic coverage and dosage accordingly. If the infant's condition improves rapidly, the blood culture is negative, and the acute phase reactants are normal, we discontinue antibiotics after 2 to 5 days.

Nosocomial infections are not rare among infants whose hospitalization can be as long as 3 to 4 months. Aside from the immaturity of the immune system, predisposing factors include ventilator care, intravenous alimentation via central or peripheral lines, and exposure to extensive handling. In recent years, *S. epidermidis* has emerged as the most common organism (201,202). However, in ventilated infants and in those with CLD, Pseudomonas, Klebsiella, and *S. aureus* are the predominant organisms found. Fungal infections are not rare and should be suspected in the presence of unexplained thrombocytopenia, hyperthermia (203), and clinical signs of progressive deterioration.

It is common practice to initiate intravenous therapy with vancomycin and a third-generation cephalosporin on suspicion of nosocomial sepsis, particularly when the infant is critically ill. One must, however, bear in mind that the widespread use of antibiotics in any neonatal intensive care unit may rapidly result in the development of drug-resistant bacterial strains (204–206). Another acceptable approach in more stable infants is to use a combination of cloxacillin and an aminoglycoside such as gentamicin, with subsequent adjustment of antibiotic therapy according to bacterial susceptibility testing results.

It is our policy not to treat colonization of ET tubes with antibiotics unless there are signs of pneumonia or systemic infection. In the absence of signs of infection, the vast majority of our ventilated infants are left without antibiotic coverage under close observation, with weekly monitoring of ETT colonization and sensitivity to antibiotics. This information can be used in case of clinical deterioration suggesting infection.

Concern has been expressed regarding the risk of infection in infants treated in incubators with high humidity. Our experience, using the new incubators providing up to 80 percent humidity, has generally been positive. However, after the first 48 hours of life, we do reduce the humidity level to 60% to 65%.

In the past, considerable effort was placed on measures believed to protect the newborn infant from nosocomial infections. These efforts included the restriction of visitors, and the use of gowns, gloves, masks, and hair nets. However, no studies have shown any evidence supporting these measures (207). In our unit, despite no longer using gowns for several years, we have not observed any change in the incidence of infection. We recommend gowning only when parents handle their babies in their arms or in cases requiring strict isolation. Parental visiting is unrestricted, and siblings are allowed to visit if they are healthy. In our view, the cornerstone of a relatively low incidence of nosocomial infection has been the enforcement of a very strict program of hand hygiene for both visitors and staff. In addition to routine hand-washing before and after patient contacts, an alcohol-based hand gel is also available at the bedside for unanticipated interventions (208).

Pain Control, Sensory Overload, and Developmental Care

During their NICU stay, preterm infants are exposed to external stimuli that are very different from those experienced by the fetus *in utero*: noise, lights, frequent disturbances, a nonliquid environment promoting different body movements and postures, and pain. Although neonatal pain was largely ignored in the past, it is now widely accepted that all newborns, including the ELBW, do experience pain. Furthermore, because ascending pain pathways are well developed by 24 weeks, but because descending pathways with endogenous opiates that may modulate incoming pain impulses are not present before 32 weeks, it is probable that the pain experienced by the very premature infant may actually be more intense. (209). Appropriate management of neonatal pain and stress is a very important aspect of modern neonatal care (210). Many nonpharmacologic strategies have been proposed to minimize the pain and stress experienced by infants for minor and major procedures, such as bundling, nonnutritive sucking, clustering of interventions and expertise in performing the procedures. Pharmacologic options include the use of opiate and nonopiate analgesics and local anesthetics. Topical anesthetics have not been fully evaluated for use in ELBW infants. Sedation and analgesia for elective intubation maintains physiologic stability for the neonate and facilitates the procedure for both the neonate and the operator (211). The safety of continuous opiate infusion early in life and for prolonged periods of time in very premature infants is still in the phase of evaluation (212). Although oral sucrose does attenuate the pain response for less invasive procedures such as heel sticks, i.v. insertion, and endotracheal suctioning, it remains unclear if there are adverse long-term effects secondary to repeated sucrose treatments of premature infants (213). Clearly, further research is required to better manage the stress and pain experienced by premature infants, to understand the long-term effects on the growth and development of the premature brain from episodes of stress and pain and exposure to exogenous opiates, and to demonstrate the long-term safety and utility of strategies to control neonatal stress and pain. Our efforts to reduce neonatal pain should succeed without inadvertent harm to the infants.

How the *ex utero* sensory input experienced by the premature infant affects the development of cerebral pathways and systems, including programmed cell death or apoptosis, is not known. These pathways are established after the period of neuronal migration, which is often completed around the 24th week of gestation. Unfortunately this time is often marked by clinical instability in the newborn very premature infant, e.g., from RDS, electrolyte disturbances, PDA, and limited energy and nutrient intakes, which may compound an adverse effect on the development of the premature brain.

These concerns have been the impetus for the wide implementation by most NICUs of global developmental care practices (e.g., control of light and noise, kangaroo care, massage and music therapy) and individualized developmental care (e.g. Newborn Individualized Developmental Care and Assessment Program [NIDCAP]) to minimize the stress, limit the sensory overload, and thereby optimize the health and neurodevelopment of each infant and facilitate parent-child bonding (214). Many studies have been published about developmental care, but because most have been limited by small samples, differing reported outcomes and other methodological problems, there continues to be controversy regarding the utility of these practices. Systematic reviews of the effectiveness of developmental care do confirm short-term benefits, such as improved growth outcomes, shorter duration of mechanical ventilation and oxygen supplementation, decreased length of stay and cost of hospitalization, and improved neurodevelopmental outcomes to 9 to 12 months corrected age, but not at 24 months; effects at older ages have not been reported (215,216).

In our nursery, the medical and nursing personnel have been sensitized to these issues over the years. The bedside nurse is responsible for implementing and maintaining the developmental care and comfort of the infant, with clustering of care to minimize external interventions and eliminate unnecessary disturbances, although promoting close parent-infant bonding. Particular attention is given to the parents' needs during hospitalization. Preparation for discharge involves the multi-disciplinary NICU and Neonatal Follow-Up teams, in collaboration with the family. Parents' group meetings are held regularly, allowing free discussion of common problems and concerns, and providing a ready support group.

Planning for Hospital Discharge

Preparing for hospital discharge is a momentous time for ELBW infants and their parents. This very much anticipated step is also fraught with emotional upheavals, with some parents pushing for early discharge and other parents clearly afraid to take their child home. It is the role of the NICU staff not only to judge the medical readiness of the infant for discharge, but also the readiness of the parents and family, and to support and educate the parents such that they are well prepared to take their infant home and that the discharge process is orderly. The AAP recently published guidelines for hospital discharge of high-risk infants (217). Discharge planning should be a multidisciplinary process with participation of the Neonatal Follow-Up team. The medical complications should be reviewed with the parents and plans for specific follow-up organized. Parents should be clear about who will be involved in their infant's care after they leave the NICU, who to call in emergencies, and should be taught about worrisome signs that should prompt assessment of their infant by a health care professional. Children with special needs, such as home oxygen therapy, will require even more planning, preparation and clear instructions for the parents. We plan the first Follow-Up Clinic visit within 1 to 2 weeks of discharge mainly to reassure parents that they are doing well, as we review the infant's weight gain, feeding problems, and check the hemoglobin for late anemia. Thus, transition from the NICU to home should be planned such that parents do not feel cut off from the security of the NICU, and such that they feel confident in their ability to safeguard and nurture their precious infant.

FOLLOW-UP OF THE EXTREMELY LOW BIRTH WEIGHT INFANT

The ultimate goal of neonatal intensive care for ELBW infants is to improve survival without impairment or dis-

ability attributable to the very premature birth. Fortunately, as survival has improved, follow-up studies have not shown an increase in the rates of neurodevelopmental delays or neurosensory impairments, such as cerebral palsy, blindness, deafness, or mental retardation (218–220). Although the majority of survivors do well, the improved survival rate translates to an increase in the absolute number of infants with neurodevelopmental and/or neurosensory problems and for whom long-term follow-up would be of benefit. Recent studies of outcomes of ELBW and VLBW infants at school age, adolescence and early adulthood reveal high rates of school difficulties, persistent neurosensory impairments, and health-related problems (221–224). Other studies describe the positive perceptions and values of these survivors and their families (225–230).

In 1993, Allen and associates reported the 36 month corrected age survival and morbidity rates for infants born between 22 and 25 weeks gestation (7). There were no survivors at 22 weeks, whereas 15%, 56%, and 80% of infants survived at 23, 24, and 25 weeks, respectively. Only 2% of those born at 23 weeks survived without severe intracranial abnormality. Intact survival was 21% at 24 weeks and 69% at 25 weeks. The authors concluded that aggressive resuscitation is warranted for infants born at 25 weeks or greater, but not for those born at 22 weeks or less. The Canadian Pediatric Society forwarded similar recommendations, with great deference to parental wishes at 23 and 24 weeks gestation (231). The Neonatal Resuscitation Program (NRP) emphasizes that the limit of viability is a moving target and up-to-date outcome data will assist in decision-making and care (232). An example of this is the change in the limit of viability in Japan, as stipulated in the Eugenic Protection Law, from 24 to 22 completed weeks of gestation. Nishida and associates reported that ELBW infants treated at the Tokyo Women's Medical College from 1984 to 2001 had a survival rate of 82%, with 50% survival for infants with birth weights of 400 to 499 grams (9/18 infants), 50% survival at 22 weeks gestation (3/6 infants) and low rates of neurosensory complications, such as cerebral palsy in 6.3% and mental retardation in 17.3%, at the 6-year follow-up (233).

There are many publications about the early neonatal outcomes based on birth weight, which encompass inborn, outborn, center-specific, and regional or population-based cohorts. With a regionalized perinatal program and population-based data from Australia, Yu described significant improvements in the survival of ELBW infants, increasing from 25% in 1979 to 56% by 1992 (234). Decreases in neurosensory deficits at 2 years of age were also observed, with severe disability reduced from 18 to 11%, severe cerebral palsy from 3 to 1%, blindness from 7 to 3% and deafness from 6 to 0.5%. The TIPP study described 1202 infants with birth weights of 500 to 999 grams. Survival to 18 months of age corrected for prematurity was 80%, with the following rates of neurosensory impairments: cerebral palsy 12%, severe cognitive delay 27%, hearing loss requiring amplification 2%, and bilateral blindness 2%. Death after a postmenstrual age of 36 weeks occurred in 4% of the sample (148). A review of the current literature by

Msall and associates provides a general summary of the rates of the major neurodevelopmental outcomes of ELBW infants in the first 2 to 3 years: cerebral palsy 9% to 26%, blindness 1% to 15%, deafness 1% to 9%, and cognitive disability 10% to 42% (235).

Early outcome data by gestational age is less encouraging. A regional study from Ontario, Canada, published in 1993, observed an absence of any handicap at 2 years of age in 50% of surviving infants born at 23 weeks, 41% of those born at 24 weeks, and 59% of those born at 25 weeks (6). In the same year, a regional study from Oxford, England reported moderate-to-severe functional handicaps at 4 years of age in 80% of surviving infants born at less than 25 weeks of age and in 66% of those born at 25 weeks (236). The large EPICure study described the outcomes of infants born at 25 or fewer completed weeks in the United Kingdom and Ireland in 1995 (237,238). This study added more fuel to the controversy regarding care of the extremely premature infants as they reported dismal survival and neurodevelopmental outcomes based on total births by gestational age, including stillbirths and cases not resuscitated in the delivery room. The outcomes of 283 surviving infants (92% follow-up rate) were described at a median age of 30 months: 49% had any disability, 23% had severe disability, and 18% had cerebral palsy.

Studies at school age consistently show significant difficulties for the ELBW population. Hack and Fanaroff (219) described the school-age outcomes in infants born weighing less than 750 grams, found that 56% of these extremely small infants required special education classes, and concluded that infants with birth weights less than 750 grams are expected to have significant problems with cognitive ability, psychomotor skills and academic achievements. Gross and associates (239) found that ELBW at 10 years did less well in school than term controls. They found that family factors, such as stable family units, were stronger predictors of school performance than were perinatal complications. This study illustrates the importance of variables other than prematurity and perinatal events on eventual cognitive outcome and also points to new directions for potential intervention to impact on behavior and learning for ELBW infants.

Studies of outcomes into early adulthood primarily describe VLBW cohorts. Consistent findings were persistence of chronic health problems and neurosensory impairments, smaller and lighter stature with an impact on physical work capacity, difficulties in educational attainment and lower IQ even in the absence of neurosensory impairment. (240,241) Bjerager and associates (228) describe the quality of life (QoL) at 18 to 20 years of age for VLBW cohort born in Copenhagen between 1971 and 1974 and found that VLBW subjects free of handicaps had a quality of life comparable to normal birth weight controls. Dinesen and associates (229) found that the VLBW cohort born in 1980 to 1982 achieved higher QoL scores in comparison to the VLBW cohort born in 1971 to 1974.

Mazurier and associates (242) described a Canadian ELBW cohort at 16 to 21 years of age. They found that ELBW subjects had a mean intelligence quotient (IQ) in the normal range (95 +/− 11) but lower than that of the control group (107 +/− 14), had significantly more school failures, and a lower rate of completion of secondary school education (61% vs. 87%).

Monset-Couchard (243) and associates reported on the mid- and long-term outcomes of 166 premature SGA, ELBW infants born in Paris, France. Language delays were observed at some stage in 31% of cases; behavioral disturbances in 42% (with 12% having severe problems); cerebral palsy in 2%; visual deficits increased to 68% with age; hearing losses after otitis media in 8%; 47% entered high school at their proper age and only 50% of the older individuals obtained their "baccalaureate" in their 19th/20th year.

The limited number of studies describing outcomes of ELBW and VLBW infants into adolescence and adulthood indicate that problems with health, education and adaptation may persist. It is unclear if the long-term outcomes of ELBW and VLBW individuals without neurosensory impairment, whether SGA or not, differ significantly from those of the normal-birth weight population. Furthermore, the current studies describe the outcomes of infants born in the 1970s and 1980s, prior to the current innovations in neonatal practices such as surfactant, alternative ventilation strategies, intensive nutrition and developmental care, and recent changes in obstetrical practices that may have a positive impact on neonatal outcomes, which include higher utilization of antenatal steroids, planned maternal transfers to tertiary care perinatal centers and intrapartum antibiotics. Whether the current ELBW and VLBW graduates have the same risks of long-term difficulties as their predecessors is not known. The importance of longitudinal follow-up of ELBW and VLBW infants and long-term follow-up studies cannot be overstated.

Our own longitudinal follow-up of infants born between 22 and 25 weeks of gestation is on-going. From April 1988 to March 1994, 110 infants born between 22 and 25 weeks gestation were admitted to our NICU. There were 58 survivors (survival rate 53%). In the first two years of life, problems with growth and general health were noted, with 56% requiring at least one rehospitalization for hernia repair, ear tubes, eye surgery, bronchiolitis-asthma or pneumonia. Reactive airway disease was seen in 59% and recurrent otitis media in 57%, with the need for hearing aid in 6%. The Griffiths Scales of Mental Development scores at a corrected age of 24 months were in the normal range (mean GQ 96 ± 4) and no infant scored in the mentally retarded range of less than 70. Outcomes at 5 years of age were available for 53 infants. For this cohort of 53 infants (91% follow-up rate), the mean gestational age was 24.9 ± 0.7 weeks and the mean birthweight was 715 ± 112 gms. There was a progressive improvement of their general health, as shown in Table 25-12. The rates of neurosensory impairments at 5 years of age were as follows: 5.2% had significant visual impairment, 5.5% required hearing aids and 9.4% were diagnosed with cerebral palsy (1 child had quadriplegia and 4 had monoplegia). Normal cognition was seen in 67%, with 12 children (23%) having mild deficits

TABLE 25-12

HEALTH IMPROVEMENT OVER 5-YEAR PERIOD AMONG 53 CHILDREN BORN BETWEEN 22–25 wks GA

	NICU Discharge to 2 Years	2–5 Years	Difference	p Value
Re-hospitalization	56%	10.5%	−44	0.01
Asthma	56%	31%	−25.5	0.04
Otitis media	53%	31%	−25	0.06

and 5 children (9%) having severe deficits. Behavioral difficulties such as hyperactivity and attention-deficit features were present in 28%, and speech delay in 37%. Overall, a higher incidence of deficits was present among SGA children compared to AGA (67% vs. 37%). Microcephaly (head circumference <5th centile) was found to be an important prognostic factor and was a predominant finding in SGA children (244).

The overall experience to date with ELBW infants allows us to come to the following conclusions:

(a) The vast majority of the surviving ELBW infants can hope for a very meaningful life.

(b) As survival of infants born less than 26 weeks has increased, there is an increase in the absolute numbers of ELBW infants who are healthy, and also of infants with long-term complications.

(c) A substantial number of ELBW infants will have physical, intellectual and behavioural impairments resulting in significant functional disability, which may persist into adolescence and adulthood.

(d) Because of the sequelae of extremely premature birth, it is important to have an organized, long-term Follow-Up Program as part of the postdischarge care of ELBW infants, to insure appropriate diagnosis and assist with therapy, resources and support to the child and family.

(e) Evidence of significant brain injury, such as Grade III or IV IVH, cystic PVL and ventricular dilatation, is an ominous predictor of future handicaps. Concomitant diagnosis of chronic lung disease at 36 weeks corrected age and severe retinopathy of prematurity increase the likelihood of neurodevelopmental problems. These provide important information to counsel the parents during care in the NICU and prior to discharge home.

One of the on-going challenges for Neonatal Follow-up of ELBW infants is to advocate for appropriate resource and service supports to these high-risk children and their families, and to insure longer-term follow-up, ideally into school entry.

In the past, the exceptional circumstances of birth at extreme prematurity offered no chance for survival. Although a very difficult road, fraught with major medical complications, parental stress and unanswerable ethical dilemmas, modern neonatal care for these extremely premature and ELBW infants has afforded many parents the opportunity to realize their hope of taking home a healthy infant with the potential for a good future.

FUTURE DIRECTIONS AND ETHICAL ISSUES

Although the birth weight barrier of 500 grams has been broken (2), the debate regarding the lower limit of viability remains open (30,31).

Early follow-up of infants born with a weight less than 500 grams is not very reassuring (1). It is obvious that beyond the heavy cost in human and financial resources in the NICU, these children will require extensive and careful long-term evaluation and support. Their performance at school age and as young adults is not yet clear.

However, it seems unlikely at this point that their management will cease. Therefore, it is our responsibility as neonatologists to provide short-and long-term accurate information to both parents and society, if we want to defend our interventions with credibility. We need to establish general and institutional guidelines and to address the ethical, financial and philosophical issues related to our interventions. Parental decisions need to be respected, but parents need also to be well informed of the potential risks. It is likely that with improved medical knowledge and technology, avoidance of major complications, and with better

TABLE 25-13

MEASUREMENT OF DEVELOPMENT AND COGNITIVE FUNCTION OVER TIME FOR INFANTS BORN BETWEEN 22–25 WEEKS GA

	Griffiths GQ 6 Mo	Griffiths GQ 12 Mo[a]	Griffiths GQ 24 Mo[a]	Stanford-Binet IQ 5 Years
Mean	103 ± 7	97 ± 7	96 ± 4	92 ± 5
Median	103	97	97	94
Range	78–115	80–121	78–115	70–110

[a] Age corrected for prematurity; Griffiths GQ: Griffiths Mental Development Scales General Quotient

nutrition, the outcome of all ELBW infants will improve. However, as we follow with great interest the future of these children born at the limit of viability, it is important to focus our attention on improving their management in our NICUs rather than on trying to break new barriers.

It is also evident that not all neonatologists, nor all NICUs, should undertake the treatment of ELBW infants. The management of these infants requires great expertise and ample resources. A critical mass is essential to maintain high medical and nursing standards. Ideally, only regional perinatal centers should be involved in the care of ELBW infants, and treatment should be undertaken only when adequate resources are available, without compromising the care of more mature infants having better chances of intact survival. Finally, the ultimate decision regarding the management and degree of intervention in the delivery room remains the responsibility of the neonatologist because, very often, there may not be time for multiple consultations and because, after all, the neonatologist is the person with the wider experience to make such decisions. However, it is also important that neonatologists involved in the care of the ELBW infant be sensitive to the wishes of the family and be objective in their presentation of information and interpretation of outcome data to the family. The neonatologist also should be prepared to advise parents when therapy has reached its limits, and should avoid heroic interventions when the expected outcome, based on current scientific knowledge, is definitely unfavorable. In our view, as we enter the new millennium, the moving target in the management of the ELBW infant should no longer be the gestational age or the birth weight, but rather the condition of the infant at birth, his or her potential to survive, the parents' desire, and our own honest evaluation of the capabilities, commitment, and resources of our own environment to provide lengthy support to the infant and to his or her family.

ACKNOWLEDGMENTS

We would like to express our profound gratitude to the NICU nursing personnel for many years of competent and devoted care of our ELBW infants. Our deep appreciation to Mrs. Judi Garon for her dedication and secretarial expertise.

REFERENCES

1. Rowan CA, Lucey JF, Shiono P, et al. Fetal infants: the fate of 4172 inborn infants with birth weights of 401–500 grams. The experience of the Vermont Oxford Network (1996–2000). *Pediatr Res* 2003;53:397A.
2. Fanaroff AA, Poole K, Duara S, et al. Micronates: 401–500 grams: the NICHD Neonatal Research Network Experience 1996–2001. *Pediatr Res* 2003;53:398A.
3. Whitelaw A, Yu VYH. Ethics of selective non treatment in extremely tiny babies. *Semin Neonatol* 1996;1:297.
4. Fanaroff AA, Wright LL, Stevenson DK, et al. Very low birth weight outcomes of the National Institute of Child Health and Human Development Neonatal Research Network, May 1995–December 1992. *Am J Obstet Gynecol* 1995;173:1423.
5. Tudhope D, Burns YR, Grey TA, et al. Changing patterns of survival and outcomes at four years of children who weighed 500–999 grams at birth. *J Pediatr Child Health* 1995;31:451.
6. Whyte HE, Fitzhardinge PM, Shennan AT, et al. Extreme immaturity: outcome of 568 pregnancies of 23–26 weeks gestation. *Obstet Gynecol* 1993;82:1.
7. Papageorgiou AN, Doray JL, Ardila R, et al. Reduction of mortality, morbidity and respiratory distress syndrome in infants weighing less than 1000 grams by treatment with betamethasone and ritodrine. *Pediatrics* 1989;83:493.
8. Piecuch RE, Leonard CA, Cooper BA, et al. Outcome of extremely low birth weight infants (500–999 grams) over a twelve year period. *Pediatrics* 1997;100:633.
9. Allen MC, Donohoe PK, Dusman AE. The limit of viability-neonatal outcome of infants born at 22–25 weeks gestation. *N Engl J Med* 1993;329:1597.
10. Synnes AR, Ling EWY, Whitfield MF, et al. Perinatal outcomes of a large cohort of extremely low gestational age infants (23–28 weeks gestation). *J Pediatr* 1994;125:925.
11. Ferrara TB, Hoekstra RE, Couser RJ, et al. Survival and follow-up of infants born at 23–26 weeks of gestational age (effects of surfactant therapy). *J Pediatr* 1994;124:119.
12. Kitchen WH, Doyle LW, Ford WG, et al. Changing two year outcome in infants weighing 500–999 grams at birth: a hospital study. *J Pediatr* 1991;118:938.
13. Joseph KS, Kramer MS, Allen AC, et al. Gestational age and birth weight-specific declines in infant mortality in Canada, 1985–1994. Fetal and Infant Health Study Group of the Canadian Perinatal Surveillance System. *Paediatr Perinat Epidemiol* 2000;14:332.
14. Pomerance JJ, Pomerance LJ, Gottlieb JA. Cost of caring for infants weighing 500–749 grams at birth. *Pediatr Res* 1993;4:231A.
15. McCormick MC, Bernabol JC, Eisenberg JM, et al. Cost incurred by parents of very low birth weight infants after the initial neonatal hospitalization. *Pediatrics* 1991;88:533.
16. Bennett-Britton S, Fitzhardinge PM, Asby S. Is intensive care justified for infants weighing less than 801 grams at birth? *J Pediatr* 1981;99:937.
17. Bohin S, Draper ES, Field I. Impact of extremely immature infants on neonatal services. *Arch Dis Child* 1996;74:F110.
18. Saigal S, Zsatmari P, Rosenbaum P, et al. Cognitive abilities and school performance of extremely low birth weight infants and matched term control children at eight years: regional study. *J Pediatr* 1991;118:751.
19. Harpe M, Taylor JG, Kline N, et al. School age outcomes of children with birth weights under 750 grams. *N Engl J Med* 1994;331:753.
20. Lahayne LA, Pine TR, Jackson C, et al. Outcome of infants weighing less than 800 grams at birth: 15 years experience. *Pediatrics* 1995;96:479.
21. Saigal S, Rosenbaum P, Hattersley B, et al. Decreased disability rate among 3-year old survivors weighing between 501 to 1000 gms at birth and born to residents of a geographically defined region from 1981 to 1984 compared with 1977 to 1980. *J Pediatr* 1989;114:839.
22. Halsey CR, Collin MF, Anderson CL. Extremely low birth weight children and their peers: a comparison of preschool performance. *Pediatrics* 1993;91:807.
23. Halsey CR, Collin MF, Anderson CL. Extremely low birth weight children and their peers: a comparison of school age outcomes. *Arch Pediatr Adolesc Med* 1996;150:790.
24. Zelkowitz P, Papageorgiou A, Zelazo P, et al. Behavioral adjustment of very low birth weight and normal birth weight children. *J Clin Child Psychol* 1995;24:21.
25. Comité d'Enquête sur la mortalité et morbidité périnatale, Rapport pour 1998. Collège des Médecins du Québec, 2002.
26. Bardin C, Zelkowitz P, Papageorgiou A. Comparison of outcomes of AGA and SGA infants born between 24 and 27 weeks gestation. *Pediatrics* 1997;100:1.
27. Vasa R, Vidyasagar D, Winegar A, et al. Perinatal factors influencing the outcome of 501 to 1000 gram newborns. *Clin Perinatol* 1986;13:267.
28. Ott WJ. Small for gestational age fetus and neonatal outcome: reevaluation of the relationship. *Am J Perinatol* 1995;12:396.
29. Crowley P, Chalmers I, Keirse MJ. The effects of corticosteroid administration before preterm delivery: an overview of evidence from controlled trials. *Br J Obstet Gynecol* 1990;97:11.

30. American Academy of Pediatrics—Committee on Fetus and Newborn, and American College of Obstetricians and Gynecologists—Committee on Obstetric Practice. Perinatal care at the threshold of viability. *Pediatrics* 1995;96:974.

31. Fetus and Newborn Committee, Canadian Pediatric Society—Maternal Fetal Medicine Committee, Society of Obstetricians and Gynecologists of Canada. Management of the woman with threatened birth of an infant of extremely low gestational age. *CMAJ* 1994;151:547.

32. Bottoms SF, Paul RH, Iams JD, et al. Obstetric determinants of neonatal survival: influence of willingness to perform cesarean delivery on survival of extremely low birth weight infants. *Am J Obstet Gynecol* 1997;176:960.

33. Thibeault DW, Beatty EC, Hall RT, et al. Neonatal pulmonary hypoplasia with premature rupture of fetal membranes and oligohydramnios. *J Pediatr* 1985;107:273.

34. Blott M, Greenough A. Neonatal outcome after prolonged rupture of the membranes starting in the second trimester. *Arch Dis Child* 1988;63:1146.

35. Nimrod C, Davies D, Iwaniski S, et al. Ultrasound prediction of pulmonary hypoplasia. *Obstet Gynecol* 1986;68:495.

36. Vergani P, Locatelli A, Strobelt N, et al. Amnioinfusion for prevention of pulmonary hypoplasia in second-trimester rupture of membranes. *Am J Perinatol* 1997;14:325.

37. Baker CJ. Group B Streptococcal infections. *Clin Perinatol* 1997;24:59.

38. Papageorgiou A, Desgranges MF, Masson M, et al. The antenatal use of betamethasone in the prevention of RDS: a controlled double-blind study. *Pediatrics* 1979;63:83.

39. National Institutes of Health. *Effects of corticosteroids for fetal maturation on perinatal outcomes.* Bethesda, MD: National Institutes of Health, 1994;12:1.

40. Ardila J, Le Guennec JC, Papageorgiou A. Influence of antenatal betamethasone and gender cohabitation on outcome of twin pregnancies 24–34 weeks gestation. *Semin Perinatol* 1994;18:15.

41. Mercer BM, Arheart KL. Antimicrobial therapy in expectant management of preterm premature rupture of the membranes. *Lancet* 1995;346:1271.

42. Hillier SL, Nugent RR, Eschenbach DA, et al. Association between bacterial vaginosis and preterm delivery of a low birth weight infant. *N Engl J Med* 1995;333:1737.

43. John C, Hauth MD, Robert L, et al. Reduced incidence of preterm delivery with metronidazole and erythromycin in women with bacterial vaginosis. *N Engl J Med* 1995;333:1732.

44. Bhat R, Zikos-Labropoulou E. Resuscitation and respiratory management of infants weighing less than 1000 grams. *Clin Perinatol* 1986;13:285.

45. Kattwinkel J, ed. *Textbook of neonatal resuscitation,* 4th ed. American Academy of Pediatrics and American Heart Association, 2000.

46. Vento M, Asensi M, Sastre J, et al. Resuscitation with room air instead of 100% oxygen prevents oxidative stress in moderately asphyxiated term neonates. *Pediatrics* 2001;107:642.

47. Saugstad OD, Rootwelt T, Aalen O. Resuscitation of asphyxiated newborn infants with room air or oxygen: an international controlled trial: the Resair 2 study. *Pediatrics* 1998;102:e1.

48. Hegyi T, Carbone T, Anwar M, et al. The Apgar score and its components in the preterm infant. *Pediatrics* 1998;107:77.

49. Strauss RG. AS-1 red cells for neonatal transfusions: a randomized trial assessing donor exposure and safety. *Transfusion* 1996;36:873.

50. Chathas MK, Paton JB, Fisher DE. Percutaneous central venous catheterization. *Am J Dis Child* 1990;144:1246.

51. Liossis G, Bardin C, Papageorgiou A. Comparison of risks from percutaneous central venous catheters and peripheral lines in infants of extremely low birth weight: a cohort controlled study of infants > 1000 g. *J Matern Fetal Neonatal Med* 2003;13:1.

52. Nowlen TT, Rosenthal GL, Johnson GL, et al. Pericardial effusion and tamponade in infants with central catheters. *Pediatrics* 2002;110:137.

53. Nadroo AM, Lin J, Green RS, et al. Death as a complication of peripherally inserted central catheters in neonates. *J Pediatr* 2001;138:599.

54. Pinto-Martin JA, Riolo S, Cnaan A, et al. Cranial ultrasound prediction of disabling and nondisabling cerebral palsy at age two in a low birth weight population. *Pediatrics* 1995;95:249.

55. Nwaesei CG, Pape KE, Martin DJ, et al. Periventricular infarction diagnosed by ultrasound: a postmortem correlation. *J Pediatr* 1984;105:106.

56. Rodriguez J, Claus D, Verellen G, Lyon G. Periventricular leukomalacia: ultrasonic and neuropathological correlations. *Dev Med Child Neurol* 1990;32:347.

57. Gittermann MK, Fusch C, Gittermann AR, et al. Early nasal continuous positive airway pressure treatment reduces the need for intubation in very low birth weight infants. *Eur J Pediatr* 1997;156.

58. Soll RF. Prophylactic synthetic surfactant for preventing morbidity and mortality in preterm infants (Cochrane Review). In: The Cochrane Library, Issue 4, 2004. Chichester, UK: John Wiley & Sons, Ltd.

59. Sagstad OD, Bevilacqua G, Katona M, et al. Surfactant therapy in the newborn. *Prenat Neonat Med* 2001;6:56.

60. Merritt TA, Hallman M, Berry C, et al. Randomized, placebo-controlled trial of human surfactant given at birth versus rescue administration in very low birth weight infants. *J Pediatrics* 1991;118:581.

61. Kendig JW, Notter RH, Cox C, et al. A comparison of surfactant as immediate prophylaxis and as rescue therapy in newborns of less than 30 weeks' gestation. *N Engl J Med* 1991;324:865.

62. Dunn MS, Shennan AT, Zayack D, et al. Bovine surfactant replacement therapy in neonates of less than 30 weeks' gestation: a randomized controlled trial of prophylaxis versus treatment. *Pediatrics* 1991;87:377.

63. Morley CJ. Surfactant treatment for premature babies: a review of clinical trials. *Arch Dis Child* 1991;66:445.

64. Merritt TA, Hallman M, Vaucher Y, et al. Impact of surfactant treatment in cost of neonatal intensive care. *J Perinatol* 1990;10:416.

65. Corbet A, Bucciarelli R, Zoldan S, et al. Decreased mortality rate among small premature infants treated at birth with a single dose of synthetic surfactant: a multicenter controlled trial. *J Pediatr* 1001;118:277.

66. Kwong M, Egan E, Nutter RH, et al. Double blind clinical trial of calf lung surfactant extract for the prevention of hyaline membrane disease in extremely premature infants. *Pediatrics* 1985;76:585.

67. Kovacs L, Bardin C, Rossignol M, et al. Reduction in mortality but not in chronic lung disease after surfactant therapy in infants < 1000 grams. *Pediatr Res* 1995;37:339A.

68. Ferrara TB, Hoekstra RE, Couser RJ. Effect of surfactant on outcome of infants with birth weight of 600–750 grams. *Pediatr Res* 1991;27:243A.

69. Horbar ID, Wright EC, Oustand L, et al. Decreasing mortality associated with the introduction of surfactant therapy: an observational study of neonates weighing 601–1300 grams at birth. *Pediatrics* 1993;92:191.

70. Vermont-Oxford Neonatal Network. A multicenter, randomized trial comparing synthetic surfactant with modified bovine surfactant extract in the treatment of neonatal respiratory distress syndrome. *Pediatrics* 1996;97:1.

71. Brans YW, Escobedo MB, Hayashi RH, et al. Perinatal mortality in a large perinatal center: five year review of 31,000 births. *Am J Obstet Gynecol* 1984;148:284.

72. Carlo WA, Stark AR, Wright LL, et al. Minimal ventilation to prevent Bronchopulmonary dysplasia in extremely low birth-weight infants. *J Pediatr* 2002;141:370.

73. Wyszogrodski I, Kyei-Aboagye K, Taeush HW, et al. Surfactant inactivation by hyperventilation: conservation by end-expiratory pressure. *J Appl Physiol* 1975;38:461.

74. Avery ME, Fletcher BD, Williams RG. *The lung and its disorders in the newborn infants.* Philadelphia: WB Saunders, 1981.

75. Heneghan MA, Sosulski R, Alarcon MB. Early pulmonary interstitial emphysema in the newborn: a grave prognostic sign. *Clin Pediatr* 1987;26:361.

76. Andreou A. One-sided high frequency oscillatory ventilation in the management of an acquired neonatal lobar emphysema: a case report and review. *J Perinatol* 2001;21:61.

77. Cotten M. The science of neonatal high-frequency ventilation. *Respir Care Clin N Am* 2001;7:611.

78. Goldsmith JP, Karotkin E. *Assisted ventilation of the neonate.* Philadelphia: WB Saunders, 1996:21.

79. Thilo EH, Andersen D, Wesserstein MC, et al. Saturation by pulse oximetry: comparison of the results obtained by instruments of different brands. *J Pediatr* 1993;122:620.

80. Heicher DA, Kasting DS, Harrod JR. Prospective clinical comparison of two methods for mechanical ventilation of neonates: rapid rate and short inspiratory time versus slow rate and long inspiratory time. *J Pediatr* 1981;98:957.

81. Greenough A, Greenall F, Gamsu H. Synchronous respiration: which ventilator rates are better? *Acta Paediatr Scand* 1987; 76:813.

82. Castling D, Greenough A, Giffin F. Neonatal endotracheal suction: comparison of open and closed suction techniques. *Br J Intens Care* 1995;5:218.

83. Avery ME, Tooley WH, Keller JB, et al. Is chronic lung disease in low birth weight infants preventable? A survey of eight centers. *Pediatrics* 1987;73:20.

84. Vermont-Oxford Network Database Project. Very low birth weight outcomes for 1990. *Pediatrics* 1993;91:540.

85. Kraybil EN, Runyan DK, Bose CL, et al. Risk factors for chronic lung disease in infants with birth weight of 751 to 1000 grams. *J Pediatr* 1989;115:115.

86. Garland JS, Buck RK, Allred EN, et al. Hypocarbia before surfactant therapy appears to increase the bronchopulmonary dysplasia risk in infants with respiratory distress syndrome. *Arch Ped Adolesc Med* 1995;149:617.

87. Feihl F, Perret C. Permissive hypercapnia. *Am J Respir Crit Care* 1994;150:1722.

88. Vannucci RC, Towfigh J, Heitjan DF, et al. Carbon dioxide protects the perinatal brain from hypoxic ischemic damage: an experimental study in the immature rat. *Pediatrics* 1995;95:868.

89. Fujimoto S, Togari H, Yamanuchi N, et al. Hypocarbia and cystic periventricular leukomalacia in premature infants. *Arch Dis Child* 1994;71:F107.

90. Graziani LJ,Spitzer AR, Mitchell DG, et al. Mechanical ventilation in preterm infants: neurosonographic and developmental studies. *Pediatrics* 1992;90:515.

91. Wigglesworth JS, Pape KE. An integrated model for hemorrhagic and ischaemic lesions in the newborn brain. *Early Hum Dev* 1978;2:179.

92. Wiswell TE, Graziani LS, Kornhauser MS, et al. Effects of hypocarbia on the development of cystic periventricular leukomalacia in premature infants treated with high frequency jet ventilation. *Pediatrics* 1996;98:918.

93. Courtney SE, Durand DJ, Asselin JM, et al. High- frequency oscillatory ventilation versus conventional mechanical ventilation for very low birth weight infants. *N Eng J Med* 2002;347:643.

94. Johnson AH, Peacock JL, Greennough A, et al. High-frequency oscillatory ventilation for prevention of chronic lung disease of prematurity. *N Eng J Med* 2002;347:633.

95. Priebe GP. High-frequency oscillatory ventilation in pediatric patients. *Respir Care Clin Am* 2001;7:633.

96. Herrera CM, Gerhardt T, Claure N, et al. Effects of volume-guaranteed synchronized intermittent mandatory ventilation in preterm infants recovering from respiratory failure. *Pediatrics* 2002;110:529.

97. Le Guennec JC, Rufai M, Papageorgiou A. Spectrum of oxygen dependency in surviving infants weighing 600 to 1000 grams: decreased incidence of severe chronic lung disease. *Am J Perinatol* 1993;10:292.

98. Barrington KJ, Bull D, Finer NN. Randomized trial of nasal synchronized intermittent mandatory ventilation compared with continuous positive airway pressure after extubation of very low birth weight infants. *Pediatrics* 2001;107:638.

99. DePaoli AG, Davis PG, Lemyre B. Nasal continuous airway pressure versus nasal intermittent positive ventilation for preterm neonates: a systematic review and meta-analysis. *Acta Paediatr* 2003;92:70.

100. Clyman RI. Medical treatment of patent ductus arteriosus in premature infants. In: Long WA, ed. *Fetal and neonatal cardiology*, Philadelphia: WB Saunders, 1990;682.

101. Gonzalez A, Ventura-Junca P. Incidence of clinically apparent ductus arteriosus in premature infants less than 2000 g. *Rev Chil Pediatr* 1991;62:354.

102. Hoekstra RE, Jackson JC, Myers TF, et al. Improved neonatal survival following multiple doses of bovine surfactant in very premature neonates at risk for respiratory distress syndrome. *Pediatrics* 1991;88:10.

103. Cotten RB, Stahlman MT, Kovar I, et al. Medical management of small preterm infants with symptomatic patent ductus arteriosus. *J Pediatr* 1978;92:467.

104. Mellander M, Larsson LE, Ekström-Jodal B, et al. Prediction of symptomatic patent ductus arteriosus in preterm infants using Doppler and M-mode echocardiography. *Acta Paediatr Scand* 1987;76:553.

105. Mahony L, Carnero V, Brett C, et al. Prophylactic indomethacin therapy for patent ductus arteriosus in very-low-birth-weight infants. *N Engl J Med* 1982;306:506.

106. Rennie JM, Doyle J, Cooke RW. Early administration of indomethacin to preterm infants. *Arch Dis Child* 1986;61:233.

107. Fowlie PW. Prophylactic indomethacin: systematic review and meta-analysis. *Arch Dis Child Fetal Neonatal Ed* 1996;74:F81.

108. Ment LR, Oh W, Ehrenkranz RA, et al. Low-dose indomethacin and prevention of intraventricular hemorrhage: a multicenter randomized trial. *Pediatrics* 1994;93:543.

109. Robie DK, Waltrip T, Garcia-Prats JA, et al. Is surgical ligation of a patent ductus arteriosus the preferred initial approach for the neonate with extremely low birth weight? *J Pediatr Surg* 1996; 31:1134.

110. Heymann MA. Prostaglandins and leukotrienes in the perinatal period. *Clin Perinatol* 1987;14:857.

111. Ment LR, Oh W, Ehrenkranz RA, et al. Low-dose indomethacin therapy and extension of intraventricular hemorrhage: a multi-center study. *J Pediatr* 1994;124:951.

112. Van Overmeire B, Van de Broek H, Van Laer P, et al. Early versus late indomethacin treatment for patent ductus arteriosus in premature infants with respiratory distress syndrome. *J Pediatr* 2001;138:205.

113. Schmidt B, Davis P, Moddemann D, et al. Long-term effects of indomethacin prophylaxis in extremely-low-birth-weight infants. *N Engl J Med* 2001;344:1966.

114. Mitchell JA, Akarasereenout P, Thiemermann C, et al. Selectivity of non-steroidal anti-inflammatory drugs as inhibitors of constitutive and inducible cyclo-oxygenase. *Proc Natl Acad Sci U S A* 1993;90:11693.

115. Mosca F, Bray M, Lattanzio M, et al. Comparative evaluation of the effects of indomethacin and ibuprofen on cerebral perfusion and oxygenation in preterm infants with patent ductus arteriosus. *J Pediatr* 1997;131:549.

116. Aranda JV, Varvarigou A, Beharry K, et al. Pharmacokinetics and protein binding of intravenous ibuprofen in the premature newborn infant. *Acta Paediatr* 1997;86:289.

117. Varvarigou A, Bardin CL, Beharry K, et al. Early ibuprofen administration to prevent patent ductus arteriosus in premature newborn infants. *JAMA* 1996;275:539.

118. Van Overmeire B. A comparison of ibuprofen and indomethacin for closure of patent ductus arteriosus. *N Engl J Med* 2000; 343:674.

119. Mosca F. Comparative evaluation of the effects of indomethacin and ibuprofen on cerebral perfusion and oxygenation in preterm infants with patent ductus arteriosus. *J Pediatr* 1997;131:549.

120. Gournay V, Savagner C, Thiriez G, et al. Pulmonary hypertension after ibuprofen prophylaxis in very preterm infants. *Lancet* 2002;359:1486.

121. Hellerstein S. Fluids and electrolytes: physiology. *Pediatr Rev* 1993;14:70.

122. Guignard JP, John EG. Renal function in the tiny, premature infant. *Clin Perinatol* 1986;13:377.

123. Shaffer SG, Bradt SK, Meade VM, et al. Extracellular fluid volume changes in very low birth weight infants during first 2 postnatal months. *J Pediatr* 1987;111:124.

124. Lorenz JM, Kleinman LI, Ahmed G, et al. Phases of fluid and electrolyte homeostasis in the extremely low birth weight infant. *Pediatrics* 1995;96:484.

125. Takahashi N, Hoshi J, Nishida H. Water balance, electrolytes and acid-base balance in extremely premature infants. *Acta Paediatr Jpn* 1994;36:250.

126. Sato K, Kondo T, Iwao H, et al. Internal potassium shift in premature infants: cause of nonoliguric hyperkalemia. *J Pediatr* 1995;126:109.

127. Rutter N. The immature skin. *Eur J Pediatr* 1996;155:18.

128. Nopper AJ, Horil KA, Sookdeo-Drost S, et al. Topical ointment therapy benefits premature infants. *J Pediatr* 1996;128:660.

129. Campbell JR. Systemic candidiasis in extremely low birth weight infants receiving topical petrolatum ointment for skin care: a case-control study. *Pediatrics* 2000;105:1041.

130. Heird LW, Gomez MR. Parenteral nutrition in low birth weight infants. *Annu Rev Nutr* 1996;16:471.

131. Yeh TF, McClenan DA, Ayahi OA, et al. Metabolic rate and energy balance in infants with bronchopulmonary dysplasia. *J Pediatr* 1989;114:448.

132. Merritt RJ. Cholestatic jaundice with total parenteral nutrition. *J Pediatr Gastroenterol Nutr* 1980;5:9.

133. Carver JD, Barness LA. Trophic factors for the gastrointestinal tract. *Clin Perinatol* 1996;23:265.

134. Berseth CL. Effect of early feeding on maturation of the preterm infant's small intestine. *J Pediatr* 1992;120:947.

135. American Academy of Pediatrics, Committee on Nutrition, 1998. Nutritional needs of preterm infants. In: Kleinman R, ed. *Pediatric nutrition handbook.* Elk Grove Village, IL: American Academy of Pediatrics, 55.

136. Thurreen PJ, Melara D, Fennessey PV, et al. Effect of low versus high intravenous aminoacid intake on very low birth weight infants in the early neonatal period. *Pediatr Res* 2003;53:24.

137. Berry MA, Conrod H, Usher RH. Growth of very premature infants fed intravenous hyperalimentation and calcium-supplemented formula. *Pediatrics* 1997;100;647.

138. Ogata E. Carbohydrate metabolism in the fetus and neonate and altered neonatal glucoregulation. *Pediatr Clin North Am* 1989; 33:25.

139. Pildes RS, Pyatis P. Hypoglycemia and hyperglycemia in tiny infants. *Clin Perinatol* 1986;13:351.

140. Pildes RS. Neonatal hyperglycemia. *J Pediatr* 1986;5:905.

141. Hewson M, Nawadra V, Oliver J, et al. Insulin infusion in the neonatal unit: delivery variation due to adsorption. *J Pediatr Child Health* 2000;36:216.

142. Fuloria M, Friedburg MA, DuRant RH, et al. Effect of flow rate and insulin priming on the recovery of insulin from microbore infusion tubing. *Pediatrics* 2000;105:915.

143. Ferrara TB, Couser RJ, Hoekstra RE. Side effects and long term follow-up of corticosteroid therapy in very low birth weight infants with bronchopulmonary dysplasia. *J Perinatol* 1990;10:137.

144. Salle BL, Delvin EE, Lapillone A, et al. Perinatal metabolism of vitamin D. *Am J Clin Nutr* 2000;71:1317S.

145. Peters O, Ryan S, Matthew L, et al. Randomized controlled trial of acetate in preterm neonates receiving parenteral nutrition. *Arch Dis Child Fetal Neonatal Ed* 1997;77:F12.

146. Odell GB, Storey GNB, Rosenberg LA. Studies in kernicterus: the staturation of serum protein bilirubin during neonatal life and its relationship to brain damage at 5 years. *J Pediatr* 1970;76:12.

147. Shankaran S, Bauer CR, Bain R, et al. Prenatal and perinatal risk and protective factors for neonatal intracranial hemorrhage. *Arch Pediatr Adolesc Med* 1996;150;491.

148. Schmidt B, Davis P, Moddemann D, et al. Long-term effects of indomethacin prophylaxis in extremely-low-birth-weight infants. *N Eng J Med* 2001;344:1966.

149. Batton DG, Holtrop P, DeWitte D, et al. Current gestational age-related incidence of major intraventricular hemorrhage. *J Pediatr* 1994;125:623.

150. Volpe JJ. Current concepts of brain injury in the premature infant. *Am J Radiol* 1989;153:243.

151. Volpe JJ. *Neurology of the newborn.* Philadelphia: WB Saunders, 1995.

152. Dolfin T, Skidmore MB, Fongk W, et al. Incidence, severity and timing of subependymal and intraventricular hemorrhages in preterm infants born in a perinatal unit as detected by serial real-time ultrasound. *Pediatrics* 1983;71:541.

153. Perlman JM, Rollins N. Surveillance protocol for the detection of intracranial abnormalities in premature neonates. *Arch Pediatr Adolesc Med* 2000;154:822.

154. Pinto-Martin JA, Whitaker AG, Feldman J, et al. Relationship of cranial ultrasound abnormalities in low-birth-weight infants to motor or cognitive performance at 2, 6 and 9 years. *Dev Med Child Neurol* 1999;41:826.

155. Ment L, Bada HS, Barnes P, et al. Practice Parameters: neuroimaging of the neonate: report of the Quality Standards Subcommittee of the American Academy of Neurology and the Practice Committee of the Child Neurology Society. *Neurology* 2002;58:1726.

156. Perlman JM, Risser R, Broyles RS. Bilateral cystic periventricular leukomalacia in premature infants: associated risk factors. *Pediatrics* 1996;97:822.

157. Levene MI. Cerebral ultrasound and neurologic impairment: telling the future. *Arch Dis Child* 1990;65:469.

158. Kuban KCK, Leviton A. Medical progress: cerebral palsy. *N Engl J Med* 1994;330:188.

159. Painter MJ, Alvin J. Neonatal Seizures. *Cur Treat Options Neurol* 1;3:237.

160. Sexson WR, Thigpen J, Stajich GV. Stereotypic movements after lorazepam administration in premature neonates: a series and review of the literature. *J Perinatol* 1995;15:146.

161. Lorenz JM, Wooliever DE, Jetton JR, et al. A qualitative review of mortality and developmental disability in extremely premature newborns. *Arch Pediatr Adolesc Med* 1998;152:425.

162. Schmidt B, Asztalos EV, Toberts RS, et al. Impact of bronchopulmonary dysplasia, brain injury and severe retinopathy of prematurity on the outcome of extremely low-birth-weight infants at 18 months. *JAMA* 2003;289:1124.

163. Ericson A, Kallen B. Very Low birthweight boys at the age of 19. *Arch Dis Child Fetal Neonatal Ed* 1998;78:F171.

164. Joint Committee on Infant Hearing 1994. Position statement. *Pediatrics* 1995;95:152.

165. Kennedy CR, Kim L, Dees DC, et al. Otoacoustic emission and auditory brain stem responses in the newborn. *Arch Dis Child* 1991;66:1124.

166. Berry MA, Conrod H, Usher RH. Growth of very premature infants fed intraveous hyperalimentation and calcium-supplemented formula. *Pediatrics* 1997;100:647.

167. Phibbs RH. Erythropoietin therapy for the extremely premature infant. *J Perinat Med* 1995;23:127.

168. Soubasi V, Kremenopoulos G, Diamandi E, et al. In which neonates does early recombinant human erythropoietin treament prevent anemia of prematurity? Results of a randomized controlled study. *Pediatr Res* 1993;34:675.

169. Strauss RG, Villhauer PJ, Cordle DG. A method to collect, store and issue multiple aliquots of packed red blood cells for neonatal transfusion. *Vox Sang* 1995;68:77.

170. Lane PA, Hathawy WE. Vitamin K in infancy. *J Pediatr* 1985; 106:351.

171. Burrows RF, Andrew M. Neonatal thrombocytopenia in hypertensive disorders of pregnancy. *Obstet Gynecol* 1990;76:234.

172. Hudak BB, Allen MC, Hudak ML, et al. Home oxygen therapy for chronic lung disease in extremely-low-birth-weight infants. *Am J Dis Child* 1989;143:357.

173. Northway WH Jr, Rosan RC, Porter DY. Pulmonary disease following respiratory therapy of hyaline-membrane disease. Bronchopulmonary dysplasia. *N Engl J Med* 1967;276:357.

174. Vaucher YE. Bronchopulmonary dysplasia: an enduring challenge. *Pediatr Rev* 2002;23:349.

175. Avery GB, Fletcher AB, Kaplan M, et al. Controlled trial of dexamethasone in respirator-dependent infants with bronchopulmonary dysplasia. *Pediatrics* 1985;75:106.

176. Cummings JJ, D'Eugenio DB, Gross SJ. A controlled trial of dexamethasone in preterm infants at high risk for bronchopulmonary dysplasia. *N Eng J Med* 1989;320:1505.

177. Shinwell ES. Early postnatal dexamethasone treatment and increased incidence of cerebral palsy. *Arch Dis Child Fetal Neonatal Ed* 2000;83:F177.

178. American Academy of Pediatrics, Committee on Fetus and Newborn and Canadian Paediatric Society, Fetus and Newborn Committee. Postnatal corticosteroids to treat or prevent chronic lung disease in preterm infants. *Pediatrics* 2002;109:330.

179. Watterberg KL, Gerdes JS, Gifford KL, et al. Prophylaxis against early adrenal insufficiency to prevent chronic lung disease in premature infants. *Pediatrics* 1999;104:1258.

180. Kovacs L, Davis GM, Faucher D, et al. Efficacy of sequential early systemic and inhaled corticosteroid therapy in the prevention of chronic lung disease of prematurity. *Acta Paediatr* 1998;87:792.

181. Shah V, Ohlsson A, Halliday HL, et al. Early administration of inhaled corticosteroids for preventing chronic lung disease in ventilated very low birth weight preterm neonates (Cochrane Review). *Cochrane Database Syst Rev* 2000;2:CD001969.

182. Kao LC, Warburton D, Platzker AC, et al. Effect of isoproterenol inhalation on airway resistance in chronic bronchopulmonary dysplasia. *Pediatrics* 1984;73:509.

183. Covert RF, Neu J, Elliot MJ, et al. Factors associated with age of onset of necrotizing enterocolitis. *Am J Perinatol* 1989;6:455.

184. Bauer CR, Morrison JC, Poole WK, et al. A decreased incidence of necrotizing enterocolitis after prenatal glucocorticoid therapy. *Pediatrics* 1984;73:682.

185. Mauy RD, Fanaroff AA, Korones SB, et al. Necrotizing enterocolitis in very low birth weight infants. Biodemographic and clinical correlates. *J Pediatr* 1991;119:630.

186. Uemura S, Woodward AA, Amerena R, et al. Early repair of inguinal hernia in premature babies. *Pediatr Surg Int* 1999;15:36.

187. Kumar VH, Clive J, Rosenkrantz TS, et al. Inguinal hernia in preterm infants (< or + 32-week gestation). *Pediatr Surg Int* 2002;18:147.

188. Ng YK, Fielder AR, Shaw DE, Levene M. Epidemiology of retinopathy of prematurity. *Lancet* 1988;2:1235.

189. Palmer EA, Flynn JT, Hardy RJ, et al. Incidence and early course of retinopathy of prematurity. The Cryotherapy for Retinopathy of Prematurity Cooperative Group. *Ophthalmology* 1991;98:1628.

190. Tin W, Milligan DWA, Pennefather P, et al. Pulse oximetry, severe retinopathy, and outcome at one year in babies of less than 28 weeks gestation. *Arch Dis Child Fetal Neonatal Ed* 2001; 84:F106.

191. Chow LC, Wright KW, Sola A. CSMC Oxygen Administration Study Group. Can changes in clinical practice decrease the incidence of severe retinopaty of prematurity in very low birth weight infants? *Pediatrics* 2003;111:139.

192. Fierson WM, Palmer EA, Biglan AW, et al. Screening examination of premature infants for retinopathy of prematurity. *Pediatrics* 1997;100:273.

193. Subhani M, Combs A, Weber P, et al. Screening guidelines for retinopathy of prematurity: the need for revision in extremely low birth weight infants. *Pediatrics* 2001;107:656.

194. Poets C, Samuels M, Southall DP. Epidemiology and pathophysiology of apnea of prematurity. *Biol Neonate* 1994;65;211.

195. Finer NN, Barrington KJ, Hayes BJ, et al. Obstructive mixed and central apnea in the neonate: physiologic correlates. *J Pediatr* 1992;121:943.

196. Davi M, Shankaran K, Simons KJ, et al. Physiologic changes induced by theophylline in the treatment of apnea in preterm infants. *J Pediatr* 1978;92:91.

197. Gerhardt T, McCarthy J, Bancalari E. Effect of aminophylline on respiratory center activity and metabolic rate with idiopathic apnea. *Pediatrics* 1979;63;537.

198. Fesslova V, Caccano ML, Salice P, et al. Assessment of cardiovascular effects of theophylline in premature newborns by means of echocardiography. *Acta Paediatr Scand* 1984;73:404.

199. Aranda JV, Turmen T, Davis J, et al. Effects of caffeine on control of breathing in infantile apnea. *J Pediatr* 1983;103:975.

200. Baker CJ. Group B streptococcal infections. *Clin Perinatol* 1997;24:59.

201. Rubin LG, Sanchez PJ, Siegel J, et al. Evaluation and treatment of neonates with suspected late-onset sepsis: a survey of neonatologists' practices. *Pediatrics* 2002;110:e42.

202. Stoll BJ, Hansen N, Fanaroff AA, et al. Late-onset sepsis in very low birth weight neonates: the experience of the NICHD Neonatal Research Network. *Pediatrics* 2002;110:285.

203. Makhoul IR, Kassis I, Smolkin T, et al. Review of 49 neonates with acquired fungal sepsis: further characterization. *Pediatrics* 2001;107:61.

204. Karlowicz MG, Buescher ES, Surka AE. Fulminant late-onset sepsis in a neonatal intensive care unit, 1988–1997, and the impact of avoiding empiric vancomycin therapy. *Pediatrics* 2000;106:1387.

205. Du B, Chen D, Liu D, et al. Restriction of third-generation cephalosporin use decreases infection-related mortality. *Crit Care Med* 2003;31:1088.

206. Bryan CS, John JF Jr, Pai MS, et al. Gentamicin vs cefotaxime for therapy of neonatal sepsis. Relationship to drug resistance. *Arch Pediatr Adolesc Med* 1985;139:1086.

207. Donowitz LG. Failure of the overgown to prevent nosocomial infection in a pediatric intensive care unit. *Pediatrics* 1986;77:35.

208. Harbarth S, Pittet D, Grady L, et al. Interventional study to evaluate the impact of an alcohol-based hand gel in improving hand hygiene compliance. *Pediatr Infect Dis J* 2002;21:489.

209. Anand KJ. Clinical importance of pain and stress in preterm neonates. *Biol Neonate* 1998;73:1.

210. Joint Statement of the CPS and AAP. Prevention and management of pain and stress in the neonate. *Paediatr Child Health* 2000;5:31.

211. DeBoer SL, Peterson LV. Sedation for nonemergent neonatal intubation. *Neonatal Netw* 2001;20:19.

212. Anand KJ, Barton BA, McIntosh N, et al. Analgesia and sedation in preterm neonates who require ventilatory support: results from the NOPAIN trial. Neonatal Outcome and Prolonged Analgesia in Neonates. *Arch Pediatr Adolesc Med* 1999;153:331.

213. Johnston CC, Filion F, Snider L, et al. Routine sucrose analgesia during the first week of life in neonates younger than 31 weeks' postconceptional age. *Pediatrics* 2002;110:523.

214. Als H, Lawhon G, Duffy FH, et al. Individualized developmental care for the very low birth weight preterm infant-medical and neuro-functional effects. *JAMA* 1994;272:853.

215. Symington A, Pinelli J. Developmental care for promoting development and preventing morbidity in preterm infants (Cochrane Review). In: The Cochrane Library, Issue 4, 2004. Chichester, UK: John Wiley & Sons, Ltd.

216. Jacobs SE, Sokol J, Ohlsson A. The Newborn Individualized Developmental Care and Assessment Program is not supported by meta-analyses of the data. *J Pediatr* 2002;140:699.

217. Committee on Fetus and Newborn, American Academy of Pediatrics. Hospital discharge of the high-risk neonate—proposed guidelines. *Pediatrics* 1998;102:411.

218. Lee KS, Kim BI, Khoshnood B, et al. Outcomes of very low birth weight infants in industrialized countries: 1947–1987. *Am J Epidemiol* 1995;141:1188.

219. Hack M, Fanaroff AA. Outcomes of children of extremely low birthweight and gestational age in the 1990s. *Semin Neonatol* 2000;5:89.

220. O'Shea TM, Klinepeter KL, Goldstein DJ, et al. Survival and developmental disability in infants with birth weights of 501 to 800 grams, born between 1979 and 1994. *Pediatrics* 1997;100:982.

221. Leonard CH, Piecuch RE. School age outcome in low birth weight preterm infants. *Semin Perinatol* 1997;21:240.

222. Hack M, Taylor HG, Klein N, et al. Functional limitations and special health care needs of 10- to 14-year-old children weight less than 750 grams at birth. *Pediatrics* 2000;106:554.

223. Hille ET, den Ouden AL, Saigal S, et al. Behavioural problems in children who weight 1000 g or less at birth in four countries. *Lancet* 2001;357:1641.

224. Saigal, S, Hoult L, Streiner D, et al. School difficulties at adolescence in a regional cohort of children who were extremely low birth weight. *Pediatrics* 2000;105:325.

225. Saigal S, Lambert M, Russ C, et al. Self-esteem of adolescents who were born prematurely. *Pediatrics* 2002;109:429.

226. Saigal S, Rosenbaum PL, Feeny D, et al. Parental Perspectives of the health status and health-related quality of life of teen-aged children who were extremely low birth weight and term controls. *Pediatrics* 2000;105:569.

227. Taylor HG, Klein N, Minich NM, et al. Long-term family outcomes for children with very low birth weights. *Arch Pediatr Adolesc Med* 2001;155:155.

228. Bjerager M, Steensberg J, Greisen G. Quality of life among young adults born with very low birthweights. *Acta Paediatr* 1995;84:1339.

229. Dinesen SJ, Greisen G. Quality of life in young adults with very low birth weight. *Arch Dis Child Fetal Neonatal Ed* 2001;85:F165.

230. Saigal S, Feeny D, Furlong W, et al. Comparison of the health-related quality of life of extremely low birth weight children and a reference group of children at age eight years. *J Pediatr* 1994; 125:418.

231. Canadian Pediatric Society Statement on Resuscitation Management of the woman with threatened birth of an infant of extremely low gestational age. A Joint Statement with the Society of Obstetricians and Gynaecologists of Canada and the Canadian Paediatric Society. *CMAJ* 1994;151:547.

232. Kattwinkel J, ed. *Textbook of neonatal resuscitation*, 4th ed. American Academy of Pediatrics and American Heart Association, 2000:7.

233. Nishida H. Marginally viable, fetal infants-who is too young or small to live: Japanese experience. Ross Special Conference. Hot Topics 2002 in Neonatology Syllabus, Dec 8–10, 2002, Washington DC.

234. Yu VYH. Developmental outcomes of extremely preterm infants. *Am J Perinat* 2000;17:57.

235. Msall ME, Tremont MR. Measuring functional outcomes after prematurity: developmental impact of very low birth weight and extremely low birth weight status on childhood disability. *Ment Retard Dev Disabil Res Rev* 2002;8:258.

236. Johnson A, Townshed P, Yudkin P, et al. Functional abilities at age 4 years of children born before 29 weeks of gestation. *Brit Med J* 1993;306:1715.

237. Costeloe K, Hennessy E, the Epicure Study Group, et al. The EPICURE Study: outcomes to discharge from hospital for infants born at the threshold of viability. *Pediatrics* 2000;104:659.

238. Wood NS, Marlow N, the EPICure Study Group, et al. Neurologic and Developmental Disability after Extremely Preterm Birth. *N Eng J Med* 2000;343:378.
239. Gross S, Mettelman BB, Dye TD, et al. Impact of family structure and stability on academic outcome in preterm children at 10 years of age. *J Pediatr* 2001;138:169.
240. Hack M, Flannery DJ, Schuchter M, et al. Outcomes in young adulthood for very-low-birth-weight infants. *N Eng J Med* 2002;346:149.
241. Ericson A, Kallen B. Very low birthweight boys at the age of 19. *Arch Dis Child Fetal Neonatal Ed* 1998;78:F171.

242. Mazurier E, Lefebvre F, Tessier R. Educational achievement and intelligence at 16–21 years of ex-prematures born at <1000 g. *Pediatr Res* 1999;45:25-A(abst).
243. Monset-Couchard M, de Bethmann O, Kastler B. Mid- and long-term outcome of 166 premature infants weighing less than 1000 g at birth, all small for age. *Biol Neonate* 2002;81: 244.
244. Piuze G, Bardin C, Papageorgiou A. Comparison of outcome at 5 years of age of SGA & AGA infants <28 weeks of gestation: a case control study. *Pediatr Res* 2001;49:334A.

Intrauterine Growth Restriction and the Small-For-Gestational-Age Infant

26

Marianne S. Anderson   William W. Hay

INTRODUCTION

Much of the interest in infants who are small for gestational age (SGA) at birth, and much of the impetus for studying intrauterine growth restriction (IUGR) that produces SGA infants, began with the observation by pediatricians and neonatologists that newborn infants who were classified according to birth weight as small, average, or large for gestational age (SGA, AGA, and LGA, respectively) showed specific morbidities and rates of death that were unique to each of these birth weight–gestational age classifications (1) (See Appendix D for intrauterine growth charts). SGA infants were recognized as having more frequent problems with perinatal depression ("asphyxia"), hypothermia, hypoglycemia, polycythemia, long-term deficits in growth, neurodevelopmental handicaps, and higher rates of fetal and neonatal mortality (2) (Fig. 26-1). Although there have been tremendous improvements in perinatal diagnosis and treatment, severe IUGR and the birth of markedly SGA infants continue to be frequent problems, and the perinatal morbidity and mortality rates of IUGR fetuses and SGA infants continue to exceed those of normal fetuses and infants.

DEFINITIONS

Small for Gestational Age

SGA infants are classically defined as having a birth weight that is more than two standard deviations below the mean or less than the 10th percentile of a population-specific birth weight vs. gestational age plot. Broader definitions include less than normal anthropometric indexes, such as length and head circumference, and marked differences between growth parameters, even when they are within the normal range. For example, an infant can be considered "relatively" SGA when its weight is at the 25th percentile, but its length and head circumference are at the 75th percentile. In this case, the weight/length ratio (or the Ponderal index = [weight (g)]/[length (cm)]3) is less than normal, indicating that growth rates of adipose tissue and skeletal muscle, the principal determinants of weight, were less than normal (Fig. 26-2) (3).

Intrauterine Growth Restriction

IUGR is defined as a rate of fetal growth that is less than normal for the population and for the growth potential of a specific infant. IUGR therefore produces infants who are SGA. SGA infants can be the result of normal but slower than average rates of fetal growth, such as those constitutionally small but not abnormal infants whose parents, siblings, and more distant relatives are small (4). SGA infants also can be the result of abnormally slow fetal growth that is caused by pathophysiologic conditions or diseases. Because growth is one of the essential features of the fetus, nearly any aberration of biologic activity in the fetus can lead to growth failure. Thus, small size at birth can be either a normal outcome or one that is a result of intrinsic or extrinsic factors that limit fetal growth potential.

Birth Weight Classification of Growth

Many terms are used to describe variations in fetal growth. For example, human newborns are classified as having normal birth weight (greater than 2,500 g), low birth weight (LBW, less than 2,500 g), very low birth weight (VLBW, less than 1,500 g), or extremely low birth weight (ELBW, less

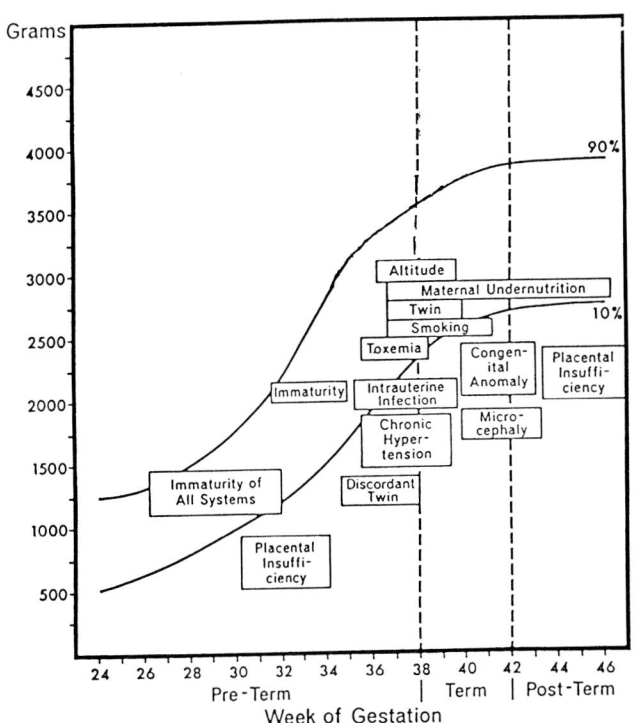

Figure 26-1 Morbidities specific to small-for-gestational-age infants. (Adapted from Lubchenco LO. The high risk infant. In: Schaffer AJ, Markowitz M, eds. *Major problems in clinical pediatrics*, volume XIV. Philadelphia: WB Saunders, 1976:6.)

than 1,000 g). Obviously, classification by weight alone says little about fetal growth rate, as most infants with less than normal birth weights are the result of a shorter than normal gestation, i.e., they are preterm. Similarly, classifying newborns as preterm or term on the basis of birth weight is erroneous, as infants with IUGR are smaller than normal at any gestational age.

Normal Variations and the Assessment of Fetal Growth

Normal fetal growth varies almost twofold. For example, mean birth weight for neonates born in New Guinea is 2,400 g (5), whereas normal birth weights in other populations can exceed 4,000 g (6). Such variations are related to genetic and environmental factors, the latter usually reflecting local diets (e.g., the relatively obese infants of Polynesian women who eat relatively large amounts of starchy foods in their normal diet). These and other normal anthropometric variations must be considered in relation to the diagnosis of IUGR in fetuses and SGA status of newborns.

Symmetric and Asymmetric Growth Restriction

SGA infants have been classified as having symmetric or asymmetric IUGR. Symmetric IUGR implies that brain and body growth both are limited. Asymmetric growth indicates that body growth is restricted to a much greater extent than head (and thus, brain) growth. In such cases, brain growth is considered "spared." Mechanisms that allow brain growth

to continue at a faster rate than adipose tissue and skeletal muscle are not completely known. Contributing factors may include an increased rate of cerebral blood flow relative to the umbilical and systemic circulations, which has been observed in some of these infants (7). In some experimental models, cerebral glucose transporter concentrations are preserved despite fetal hypoglycemia, indicating preservation of cerebral glucose uptake capacity (8). The most severely affected infants have marked reductions in both brain and body growth. Even moderately IUGR infants have growth restrictions of both brain and body, but to varying degrees that depend on the duration and severity of the insults that inhibit growth. Asymmetric and symmetric growth restriction are best thought of, therefore, as extreme examples (Fig. 26-3). Asymmetric fetal growth differentially affects organs other than the brain. As shown in Fig. 26-4, the heart also is larger for body weight in these infants, whereas the liver, probably representing glycogen deficit, and thymus, perhaps indicating a response to stress but also showing a potential for immunologic inadequacy, are smaller for body weight.

In general, factors intrinsic to the fetus cause symmetric growth restriction, whereas external factors cause asymmetric growth. Patterns of symmetric growth restriction develop early during fetal life, reflecting their intrinsic nature. Asymmetric patterns also can develop as early as the second trimester (9) and as much as 30% to 50% of extremely preterm neonates (less than 1,000 g) are SGA, probably reflecting pathology that produced growth restriction and led to preterm birth. Factors that limit the growth of both the fetal brain and body include chromosomal anomalies (e.g., particularly trisomy conditions), congenital infections (toxoplasmosis, rubella, cytomegalovirus), dwarf syndromes, some inborn errors of metabolism, and some drugs (10). The mechanisms by which these factors limit fetal growth are multifactorial.

Asymmetric growth restriction classically develops during the late second and third trimesters when fetal nutrients, particularly glucose and lipids, increasingly contribute to energy storage in the form of glycogen and fat (in both brown and white adipose tissue) (11). Slight reductions of energy substrate supply to the fetus limit fat and glycogen storage and the growth of skeletal muscle, but allow for continued bone and brain growth. More extreme limitations of energy substrates, for longer periods, affect both growth and energy storage. Timing is important; with decreased nutrient supply early in gestation, growth of all body organs is restricted, whereas decreased fetal nutrient supply later in gestation primarily restricts growth of glycogen content, adipose tissue, and skeletal muscle.

INTERPRETATION OF FETAL GROWTH CURVES

Growth Curves Based on Neonatal Measurements

Cross-sectional growth curves have been developed from anthropometric data in populations of infants born at

Colorado Intrauterine Growth Charts

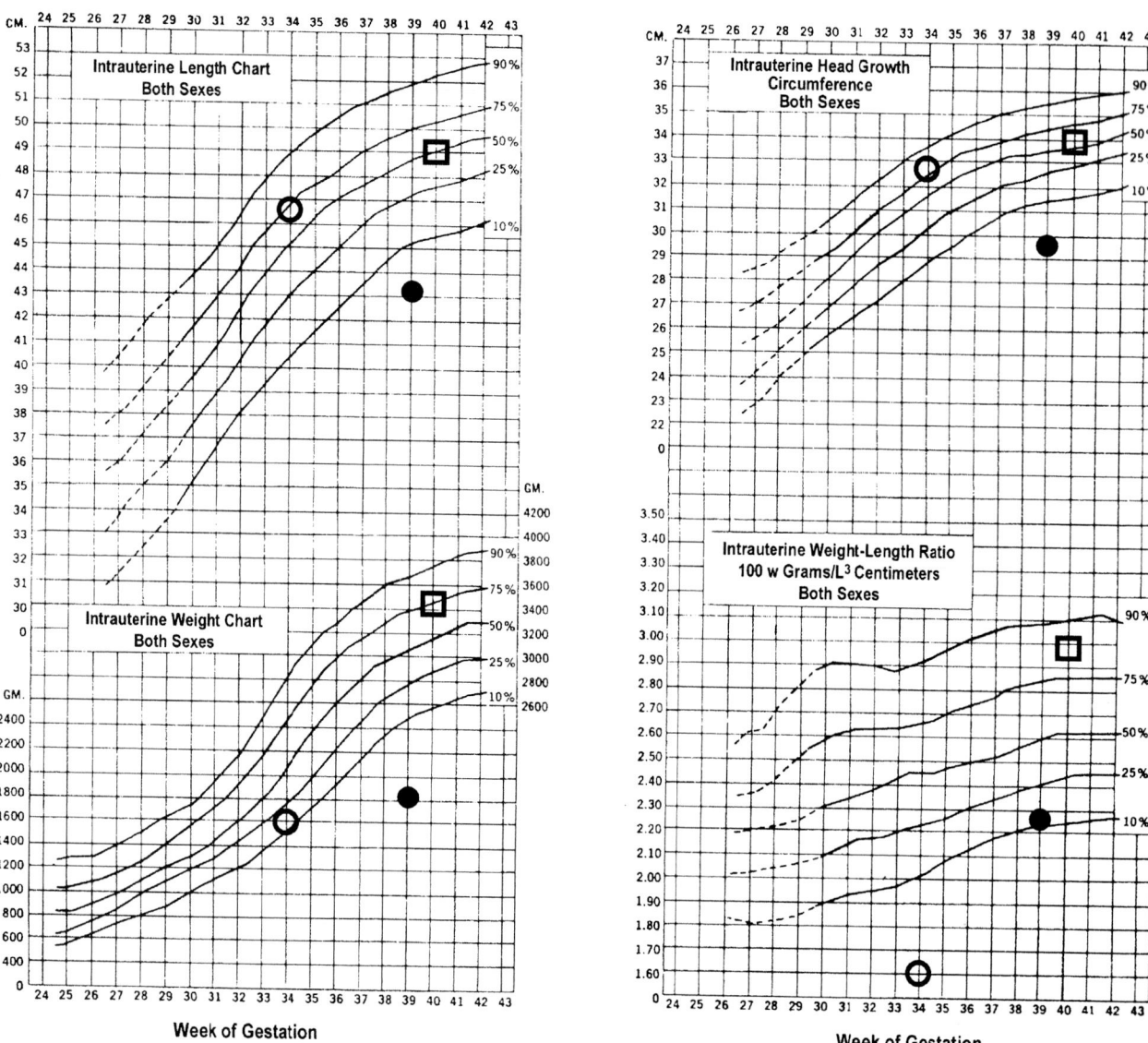

Figure 26-2   The Colorado Intrauterine Growth Charts, including symbols that define the anthropometric measurements for the three infants shown in Fig. 26-2. (O) Preterm infant at 34 weeks of gestation, showing asymmetry of weight (15th percentile) versus length and head circumference (75th percentile) and weight-to-length ratio (85th percentile); (•) severely but symmetrically small-for-gestational-age infant at 39 weeks, showing weight, length, head circumference, and weight-to-length ratio all about equally and markedly (<10th percentile); and (□) symmetric average-for-gestational-age infant at 40 weeks, showing weight, length, head circumference, and weight-to-length ratio about the 65th to 75th percentile. (Growth charts from Lubchenco LO, Hansman C, Boyd E. Intrauterine growth in length and head circumference as estimated from live births at gestational ages from 26 to 42 weeks. Pediatrics 1966;37:403 (ref. 13).

different gestational ages (12). Such curves have been used to demonstrate whether an infant's weight is within the normal range for a given gestational age and thus to estimate whether that infant's in utero growth was greater or less than normal. The normal range is defined as birth weights between the 10th and 90th percentile of the population-specific birth weight vs. gestational age relationship. Fetuses and neonates who are within the 10th and 90th percentiles for weight vs. gestational age are considered

AGA. Those who are less than the 10th percentile are considered SGA. Those who are greater than the 90th percentile are considered LGA. Other terms for SGA infants include light for dates and small for dates.

Most growth curves usually are confined to the third trimester. Each curve is based on local populations with variable composition of maternal age, parity, socioeconomic status, race, ethnic background, body size, degree of obesity or thinness, health, pregnancy-related problems, and nutrition,

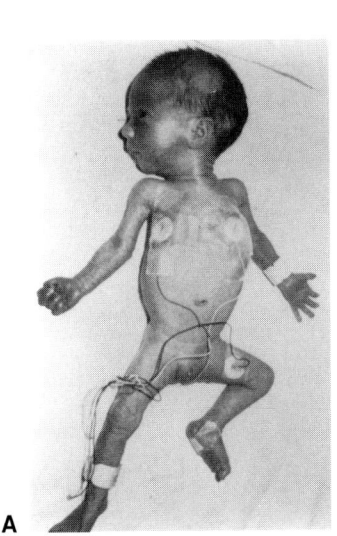
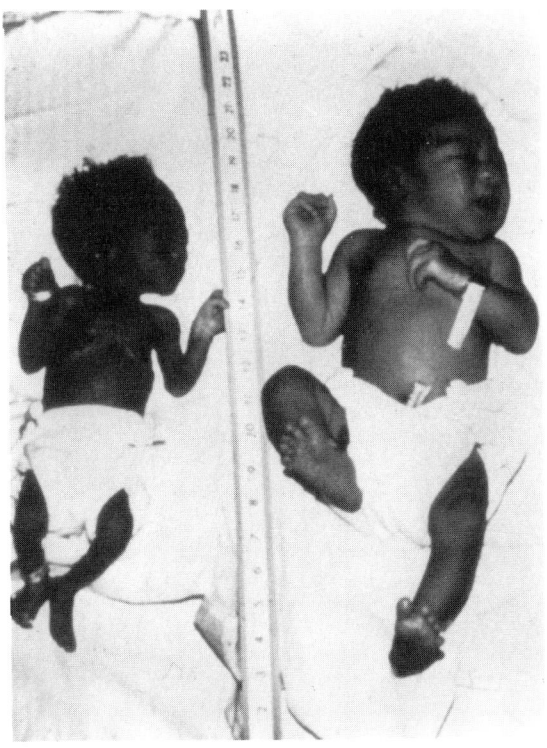

A

B

Figure 26-3 Preterm, small-for-gestational-age infant at 34 weeks of gestation **(left)**, severely small-for-gestational-age infant at 39 weeks **(middle)**, and average-for-gestational-age infant at 40 weeks **(right)**.

and the number of fetuses per mother, the number of infants included in the study, and by what methods and how accurately measurements of body size and gestational age were made. Estimating gestational age, in particular, has considerable error. Such error is derived from variability in dating conception because of maternal postimplantation bleeding and irregular menses, wide variability in the development physical features of maturation in the infant, and interobserver variability in assessing an infant's developmental stage. The growth curves shown in Fig. 26-2 are those of Lubchenco and colleagues (13) in Denver, Colorado, published in 1966. They are biased to slightly lower birth weights compared with many other growth curves, especially close to term, as a result of the unique mix of racial and ethnic groups in the population of babies who were born at Colorado General Hospital, Denver, Colorado, at the time the data were collected. Although the higher altitude of Denver (5,280 feet or ~1,600 m) has been considered a factor in the smaller birth weights shown in these curves, the independent effect of high altitude on restricting fetal growth is not clearly demonstrable at 1 mile (1.6 km). In fact, growth curves similar to those of Lubchenco et al. have been produced at sea level among lower socioeconomic groups with a high proportion of blacks and Hispanics in the population (Fig. 26-5).

Mathematical analyses of various fetal growth curves have been used to determine growth rates over relatively short gestational periods or at discrete gestational ages (12). For example, the data used in the Lubchenco growth curves (Figs. 26-2 and 26-5) can be approximated by a simple exponential function showing fetal weight increasing at about 15 g/day/kg. This rate will vary from the smallest to the largest infants. For a given weight percentile, however, there are only differences of 1% to 2% for this exponential function among different populations and studies.

Growth Curves Based on Fetal Measurements

Fetal growth curves also have been developed from serial ultrasound measurements of fetuses who subsequently were born at term in healthy condition and with normal

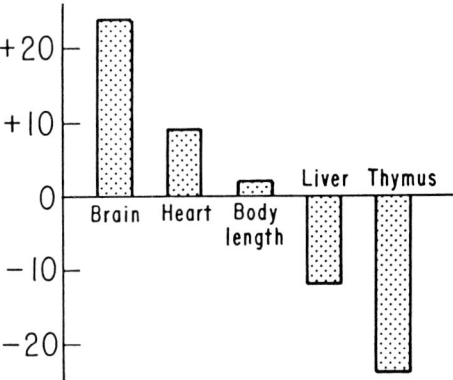

Figure 26-4 Body length and selective organ weight percent changes from normal preterm infants of similar birth weights in necropsy series of IUGR fetuses. (After Gruenwald P. Growth patterns in the normal and deprived fetus. In: Jonxis JHP, Visser HKA, Troelstra JA, eds. *Aspects of prematurity and dysmaturity.* Springfield: Charles C. Thomas, 1968:43.)

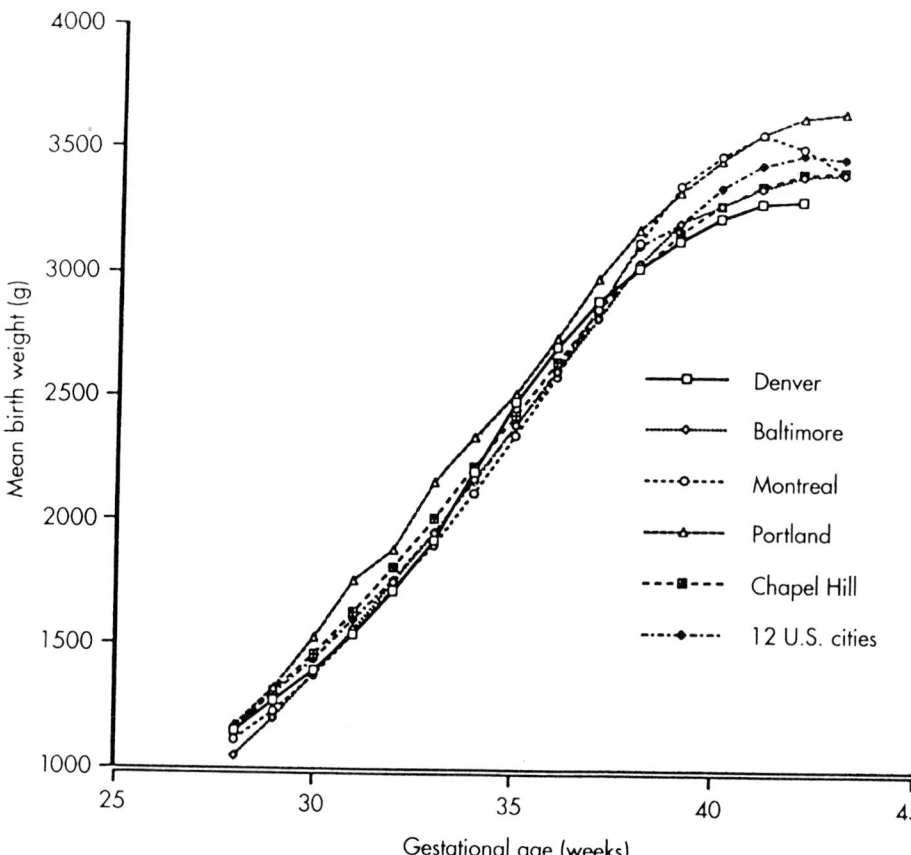

Figure 26-5 Birth weights by gestational age from six sources. (Adapted from Naeye R, Dixon J. Distortions in fetal growth standards. *Pediatr Res* 1978;12:987).

measurements, providing continuous rather than cross-sectional indexes of fetal growth. These curves can be better correlated with the expected fetal growth rate of a particular fetus than can cross-sectional, population-based growth curves. Serial ultrasound measurements of fetal growth also can more accurately determine how environmental factors, such as severe maternal illness and under nutrition, can inhibit fetal growth. Figure 26-6 shows an example of ultrasound data for fetal growth curves, including evidence for a particular fetus whose growth rate clearly was affected adversely by poor maternal health and beneficially by improved maternal nutrition. Further, fetal ultrasound-derived growth curves show less of the midgestational exponential increase in fetal growth rate that is typical of cross-sectional growth curves derived from neonatal measurements at different gestational ages. This observation strengthens the concept that, because preterm birth is not a normal outcome, one must be suspicious of growth parameters and growth curves derived from cross-sectional measurements of preterm infants assessed at birth. The intrauterine growth of these preterm infants probably was affected adversely by the same pathologic factors that led to their preterm birth. Thus, there probably is no ideal fetal growth curve derived from postbirth, cross-sectional measurements. Future growth curves to assess in utero growth of a specific newborn should be based instead on more thoroughly and accurately determined fetal growth parameters from ultrasound measurements in pregnancies with definitely known dates of conception and birth at term of normally grown and developed infants.

INTRAUTERINE GROWTH RESTRICTION AND PRETERM BIRTH

Most cases of fetal growth restriction represent only minimal growth delay and are natural, reproductively successful, although not perfect, adaptations to nutrient limitation. Most cases of IUGR, therefore, are not major causes of preterm delivery, and fetal growth rate and length of gestation usually are not related. In cases of severe IUGR, the pathophysiologic processes causing the IUGR also can lead to preterm labor and preterm delivery. Thus, IUGR frequently occurs with a variety of maternal conditions that are associated with preterm delivery (Table 26-1) (14–17).

Established maternal conditions that are associated with both IUGR and preterm delivery include very low maternal prepregnancy weight, prior preterm delivery, cigarette smoking, indirect effects of very young or advanced maternal age, and lower maternal socioeconomic status (14). Regarding race, African-American women who were born in the United States have a twofold greater incidence of both preterm birth and IUGR than do white women from the United States or African-American women who emigrated from Africa. Reasons for this are multifactorial and include nearly all of the generally associated risks

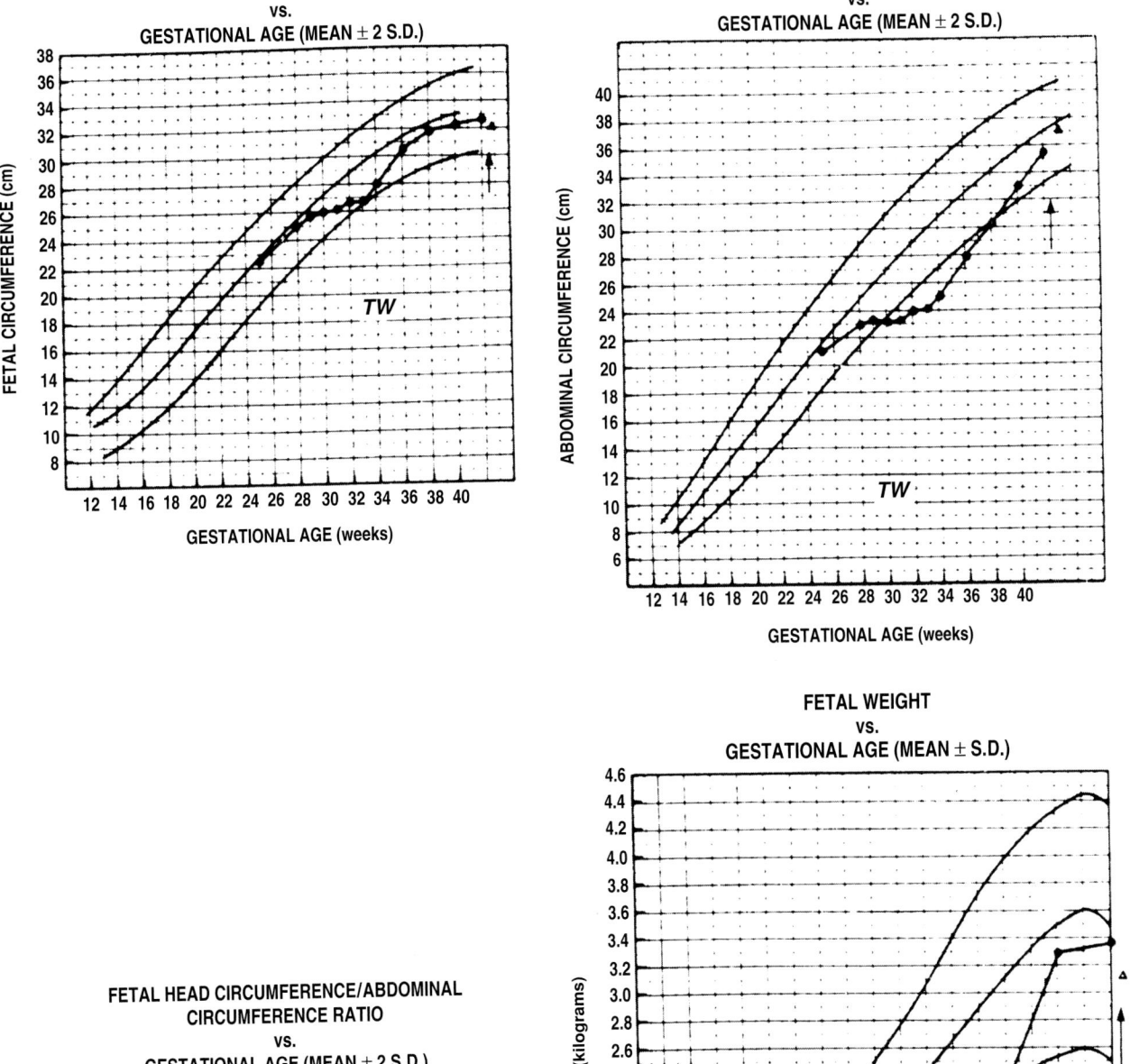

Figure 26-6 Serial fetal body measurements in a mother with severe ulcerative colitis. Note that fetal growth (—•—•—) begins to decrease markedly in mid-gestation but returns to normal following the initiation of central hyperalimentation at approximately 28–30 weeks. Solid lines represent the mean ± 2 S.D. of a reference population of human fetuses with normal fetal growth rates according to ultrasound measurements. Reproduced with permission from Creasy RK, Resnik R. Intrauterine growth retardation. In: Creasy RK, Resnik R, (Editors), Maternal-Fetal Medicine, Second Edition. Philadelphia: W.B. Saunders Co., 1989, p. 558.

TABLE 26-1

MATERNAL CONDITIONS ASSOCIATED WITH INTRAUTERINE GROWTH RESTRICTION AND PRETERM DELIVERY

Both very young and advanced maternal age
Maternal prepregnancy short stature and thinness
Poor maternal weight gain during the latter third of pregnancy
Maternal illness during pregnancy
Nulliparity
Failure to obtain normal medical care during pregnancy
Lower socioeconomic status
Black race (in the United States)
Multiple gestation
Uterine and placental anomalies
Polyhydramnios
Preeclampsia
Diabetes
Intrauterine infections
Cigarette smoking, cocaine use, and other substance abuse

and causes of IUGR and preterm delivery (15). Stretch-activated mechanisms probably induce preterm labor in cases of multiple gestation, uterine and placental space-occupying anomalies (e.g., fibroids), and polyhydramnios. Insufficient endometrial surface area for placental invasion and growth, plus abnormal placental perfusion, also combine to restrict nutrient delivery to the fetus, leading to IUGR. Poor placental growth and function limit placental supply of growth promoting hormones to the fetus, e.g., human placental lactogen (hPL), steroid hormones, and insulin-like growth factor-I (IGF-I) (18–20), and limit effective maternal–fetal nutrient exchange. In cases of polyhydramnios, IUGR often is related to the primary pathologic processes such as fetal infection, anemia, cardiac failure, and neuromuscular disorders. Intrauterine fetal infections can limit fetal growth by damaging the fetal brain and the neuroendocrine axis that support fetal growth via insulin-like growth factors (IGFs) and insulin. Intrauterine infections also can damage the fetal heart, leading to diminished cardiac output, poor placental perfusion, and inadequate nutrient substrate uptake. Fetal infections and ascending infections of the membranes from the vagina also are associated with preterm delivery. They probably do this by enhancing the fetal supply of prostaglandins, which causes fetal and uterine production of various cytokines that are associated with or cause the onset of labor (21). Chronic placental and fetal infections also limit placental perfusion, in some cases by inhibition of nitric oxide production, which leads to uteroplacental vasoconstriction, placental insufficiency, and IUGR (22). Preeclamptic women have poor endometrial vascular support for growth of the placenta, leading to placental growth failure, fetal nutrient deficit, and IUGR (23). Fetal hypoglycemia, hypoxemia, and acidosis usually are present in such cases of poor placental development and perfusion. These factors lead to increased production of prostaglandins and the activation of labor-promoting

cytokines, leading also to preterm delivery (24). Many of these cases are delivered preterm to protect the mother from eclampsia or the fetus from hypoxic–ischemic injury. Very young and very old women both produce IUGR infants who often are born prematurely. Nutritional, uterine, and vascular mechanisms may be common in these situations. Young still-growing adolescent girls appear less capable of mobilizing fat reserves in late pregnancy, apparently reserving them instead for their own continued development (25). Failure to mobilize such reserves can limit nutrient supply to the fetus and the rate of fetal growth (26). IUGR in cases of maternal smoking and substance abuse may be as a result of reduced placental blood flow, inhibition of uteroplacental vascular development, or direct fetal toxicity.

These examples illustrate that IUGR is commonly associated with conditions that also are related to preterm delivery. It is not surprising, therefore, and important to note, that IUGR is an increasingly common finding among infants born at earlier gestational ages. Whereas at term 10% of infants are classified as SGA, at less than 28 to 30 weeks gestational age, 30% to 40% of infants may be the result of IUGR (27).

FETAL GROWTH

The period of fetal growth is from the end of embryogenesis, at about the end of the first third of gestation, until term. During the embryonic period, growth occurs primarily by increased cell number (hyperplasia) (28). In the middle third of gestation, cell size also increases (hypertrophy), although the rate of cell division becomes stable. In the last third of gestation, the rate of cell division declines, although cell size continues to increase. Thus, insults that limit fetal growth in the embryonic period result in global reduction in fetal growth, whereas insults in the third part of gestation usually limit growth of fetal adipose tissue and skeletal muscle with less effect on the growth of other organs, especially the brain and heart (29).

GROWTH OF BODY COMPONENTS IN THE FETUS

Water

Fetal body water content, expressed as a fraction of body weight, decreases over gestation as a result of relative increases in protein and mineral accretion (Fig. 26-7) (30) and in humans because of the development of relatively large amounts of adipose tissue in the third trimester. Fetuses with marked IUGR and SGA neonates who have decreased body fat content have even lower fractional contents of body water. Extracellular water also decreases more than intracellular water as gestation advances, primarily because of increasing cell number and increasing cell size rather than the intracellular concentration of osmotic

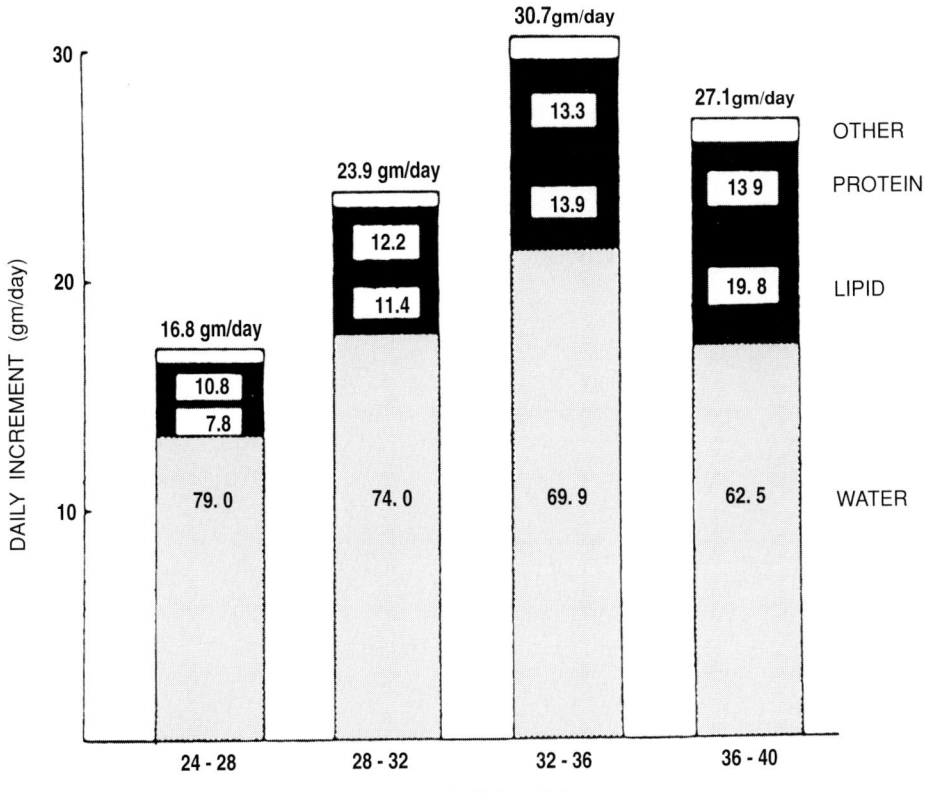

Figure 26-7 Composition of weight gain in normal human fetuses. From Ziegler EE, O'Donnell AM, Nelson SE, et al. Body composition of the reference fetus. *Growth* 1976;40:329.

substances. Measurements of extracellular space in SGA infants usually are normal for gestational age, as adipose tissue, skeletal muscle, and mineral accretion all are decreased to about the same extent (31).

Minerals

Fetal calcium content in SGA and AGA fetuses increases exponentially with a linear increase in length, because bone density, area, and circumference increase exponentially in

relation to linear growth (12). Accretion of other minerals varies more directly with body weight and according to the distribution of the minerals into extracellular (e.g., sodium) or intracellular (e.g., potassium) spaces (Table 26-2).

Nitrogen and Protein

There are very few chemical composition studies of normal human infants. Based on data from 15 studies accounting for 207 infants, Sparks has shown that nonfat dry weight and

TABLE 26-2

CHEMICAL COMPOSITION OF THE BODY OF THE DEVELOPING FETUS[a]

Body Weight (g)	Approximate Fetal Age (wk)	Per Kilogram Whole Body			Per Kilogram Fat-free Body									
		Water (g)	Fat (g)	Water (g)	N (g)	Ca (g)	P (g)	Mg (g)	Na (mEq)	K (mEq)	Cl (mEq)	Fe (mg)	Cu (mg)	Zn (mg)
30	13	900	5	906	10	3.0	2.0	0.10	20	40	81	—	—	—
100	15	890	5	894	10	3.0	2.0	0.10	100	40	70	50	—	—
200	17	885	5	889	14	4.0	3.0	0.15	100	40	70	50	3.5	18
500	23	880	6	885	14	4.4	3.0	0.20	100	44	66	56	3.5	18
1,000	26	860	10	869	14	6.1	3.4	0.22	90	44	66	65	3.5	18
1,500	31	847	23	867	17	6.8	3.8	0.24	85	44	66	68	3.8	18
2,000	33	810	50	853	20	7.9	4.3	0.24	85	44	63	84	4.2	18
2,500	35	776	74	838	21	9.0	4.8	0.25	85	48	56	95	4.3	18
3,000	38	727	120	826	21	9.5	5.3	0.27	90	49	55	95	4.5	18
3,500	40	686	160	816	21	10.2	5.8	0.27	95	51	54	95	4.8	18

[a] From Widdowson EM. Changes in body proportions and composition during growth. In: Davis JA, Dobbing J, eds. *Scientific foundations of paediatrics.* Philadelphia: WB Saunders, 1974:155, with permission.

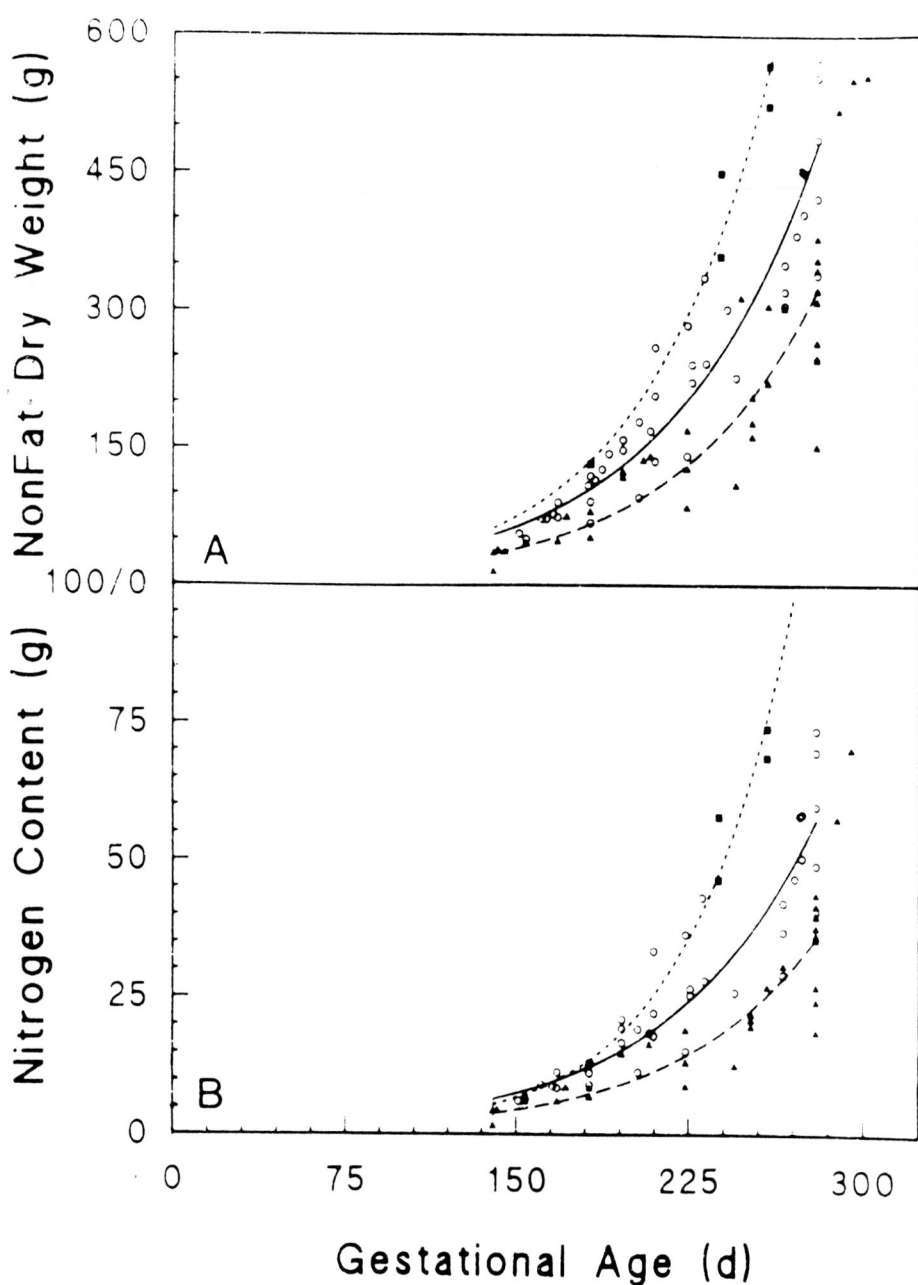

Figure 26-8 Nonfat dry weight **(A)** and nitrogen content **(B)** are plotted against gestational age for LGA (■, · · · ·), AGA (O, ——), and SGA (▲,- - - -) infants. Reproduced with permission from Sparks JW. Intrauterine growth and nutrition. In: Polin RA, Fox WW, (eds.), *Fetal and neonatal physiology.* Philadelphia: W. B. Saunders Co., 1992:184, with permission.

nitrogen content (predictors of protein content) have a linear relationship with fetal weight and an exponential relationship with gestational age (Fig. 26-8) (12,32). Table 26-3 shows nitrogen, protein, and selected amino acid composition and accretion rates for normal human fetuses. About 80% of fetal nitrogen content is found in protein; the rest is found in urea, ammonia, and free amino acids. The data for fetal protein content and accretion in Table 26-3 thus may be high, as they are based solely on nitrogen content.

Nitrogen and Protein Accretion in Small-for-Gestational-Age Infants

Among SGA infants, nitrogen and protein contents are reduced for body weight, primarily as a result of deficient production of muscle mass. In fact, they often are reduced below that of fat as a fraction of body weight (33).

Glycogen

Many tissues in the fetus, including brain, liver, lung, heart, and skeletal muscle, produce glycogen over the second half of gestation (34). Liver glycogen content, which increases with gestation (Fig. 26-9), is the most important store of carbohydrate for systemic glucose needs, because only the liver contains sufficient glucose-6-phosphatase for release of glucose into the circulation. Skeletal muscle glycogen content increases during late gestation and forms a ready source of glucose for glycolysis within the myocytes. Lung glycogen content decreases in late gestation with change in

TABLE 26-3

INCREMENTS PER DAY OF NUTRIENTS IN THE FETAL BODY AT SELECTED INTERVALS DURING GESTATION[a]

Fetal Age Range (wk) Weight Range (kg)	12–16 0.02–0.1	16–20 0.1–0.3	20–24 0.3–0.75	24–28 0.75–1.35	28–32 1.35–2.0	32–36 2.0–2.7	36–40 2.7–3.4
Increments of nitrogen (N) and protein in fetal body per 24h							
Total N	29	93	243	326	386	504	714
Protein (gm) (N = 6.25)	0.18	0.58	1.52	2.04	2.41	3.15	4.46
Increments of individual amino acids in fetal body (mg/d)							
ILE	6	26	53	71	82	109	148
LEU	13	43	111	151	174	231	330
LYS	13	41	107	145	167	222	313
MET	4	11	28	39	44	59	92
PHE	7	23	61	83	95	127	184
TYR	5	17	44	59	68	91	127
THR	7	23	61	83	95	127	184
VAL	8	27	70	94	109	145	210
ARG	14	43	114	154	177	236	340
HIS	5	15	39	53	61	81	112
ALA	13	41	107	145	167	222	319
ASP	17	52	136	183	211	281	392
GLU	23	74	195	263	303	403	568
GLY	21	68	177	240	276	367	513
PRO	15	48	125	168	194	258	300
SER	8	25	66	89	102	136	191

[a] From Widdowson EM. Chemical composition and nutritional needs of the fetus at different stages of gestation. In: Aebi H, Whitehead R, eds. *Maternal nutrition during pregnancy and lactation.* Berne: H. Huber, 1980:39–48, with permission.

cell type, leading to loss of glycogen-containing alveolar epithelium, development of type II pneumocytes, and onset of surfactant production. Cardiac glycogen concentration decreases with gestation, owing to cellular hypertrophy, but cardiac glycogen appears essential for postnatal cardiac energy metabolism and contractile function. Glycogen synthesis rates are low in human fetuses, about 2 mg/d/g of liver, accounting for less than 5% of fetal glucose utilization (35). Net synthesis, degradation, and accumulation rates of fetal glycogen are controlled by the functional states of two enzymes, glycogen synthase, which promotes glycogen formation, and glycogen phosphorylase, which promotes glycogen degradation (34,36,37). The total liver content of these two enzymes is relatively constant over gestation. Their functional states are regulated by hormone and substrate concentrations. For example, insulin acts synergistically with glucose to build hepatic glycogen stores, whereas close to term, cortisol, epinephrine, and glucagon develop the capacity to promote glycogenolysis and glucose release into the plasma.

Glycogen Deficiency in Small-for-Gestational-Age Infants

Glycogen content is markedly reduced in SGA infants, both in the liver and in the skeletal muscles (34). This is as a result of lower fetal plasma concentrations of glucose and insulin, which are the principal regulators of glycogen synthesis. If the SGA fetus also experiences repeated episodes of hypoxemia, epinephrine secretion in response will further deplete glycogen by activating glycogen phosphorylase and increasing glycogenolysis.

Adipose Tissue

At term, fetal fat content, expressed as a fraction of fetal weight, varies markedly among species (Fig. 26-10) (37). The fat content of newborns of almost all land mammals at term is 1% to 3%, which is considerably less than the 15% to 20% fat content of human term infants. Even in those species, such as the human, that take up fat from the placenta and deposit fat in fetal tissues, the rate of fetal fatty acid oxidation is presumed low. This condition occurs because plasma concentrations of fatty acids (and keto acid products, such as b-hydroxybutyrate and acetoacetate) are low, and because the carnitine palmityl transferase enzyme system is not sufficiently developed to deliver long-chain fatty acids to the respiration pathway inside the mitochondria. Fat accretion for the human fetus is shown in Fig. 26-11. Between 26 and 30 weeks of gestation, nonfat and fat components contribute equally to the carbon content of the fetal body (12,38). After that period, fat accumulation exceeds that of the nonfat components. By term, the deposition of fat accounts for more than 90% of the carbon accumulated by the fetus. The rate of fat accretion is approximately linear between 36 and 40 weeks of gestation, and, by the end of gestation, fat accretion ranges between 1.6 and 3.4 g/d/kg. At 28 weeks of gestation, it is slightly less and ranges between 1.0 and 1.8 g/d/kg.

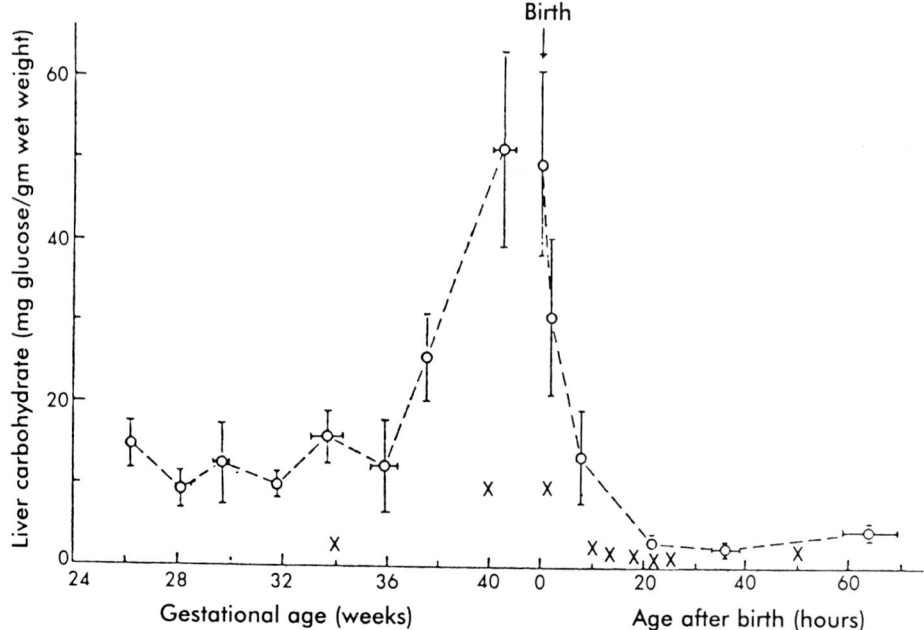

Figure 26-9 Liver glycogen content (as carbohydrate) in normal human fetuses and newborn infants with normal birth weights for gestational age (O - - - O, mean ± SEM) and infants of low birth weight for gestational age (X). From Shelley HJ, Neligan GA. Neonatal hypoglycaemia. *Br Med Bull* 1966;22:34, with permission.

Adipose Tissue Deficiency in Small-for-Gestational-Age Infants

By term, fat content in human fetuses with IUGR may be less than 10% of body weight (33). In these cases, the smaller placenta limits fetal fatty acid and triglyceride supply. Similarly, the smaller placenta decreases fetal glucose supply, which reduces glycerol production and triglyceride synthesis. Insulin deficiency, a result of decreased glucose and amino acid supply to the fetus, also limits fat synthesis. The insulin activation of peripheral lipoprotein lipase is thereby reduced, which normally is necessary to release fatty acids from circulating lipoproteins for

adipocyte uptake and triglyceride synthesis, and to decrease the normal insulin stimulation of fatty acid synthase within adipocytes.

Calories (Total Energy Storage)

The energy value of various tissue components is shown in Table 26-4. Fat has a high energy content, 9.5 kcal/g, and a very high carbon content, approximately 78%. Thus, differences in fetal fat concentration lead to large differences in calculated caloric accretion rates and carbon requirements of the fetal tissues for growth. The caloric concentration of nonfat dry weight is fairly consistent at different developmental stages, indicating that the ratio of protein to nonprotein substrates in the tissues is relatively constant (Table 26-5). Thus, caloric accretion rate of any fetus can be estimated from the growth curve of the fetus and the changing fat and water concentrations (38).

Caloric Accretion Deficiency in Small-for-Gestational-Age Infants

Growth of fat and nonfat (protein plus other) tissues is metabolically linked through energy supply that is used for protein synthesis and the production of anabolic hormones (39). These promote positive protein, fat, and carbohydrate growth. Thus, restriction of nutrient supply is likely to produce growth deficits of all tissues, not just fat. Indeed, growth restriction involves limitation of muscle growth and fat and glycogen (33). For example, chronic selective caloric (glucose) restriction in the experimental fetal sheep model leads to increased protein breakdown and lower rates of fetal growth and lipid content (40). Some growth curves, such as those shown in Figs. 26-8 and 26-11 from human

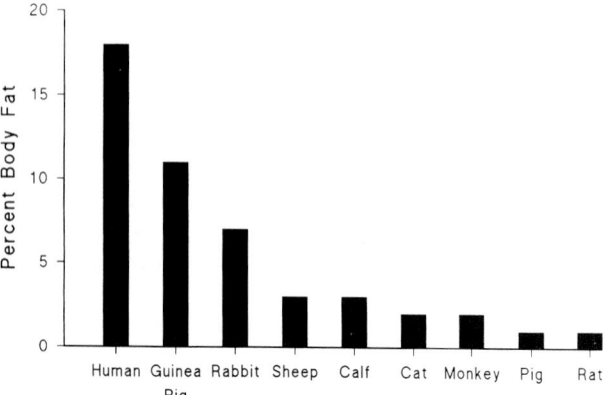

Figure 26-10 Fetal fat content at term as a percent of fetal body weight among species. Reproduced with permission from Hay WW Jr. Nutrition and development of the fetus: carbohydrate and lipid metabolism. In Walker WA, Watkins JB (Editors), *Nutrition in Pediatrics,* Second Edition. Hamilton: BC Decker, 1966, p. 376, with permission.

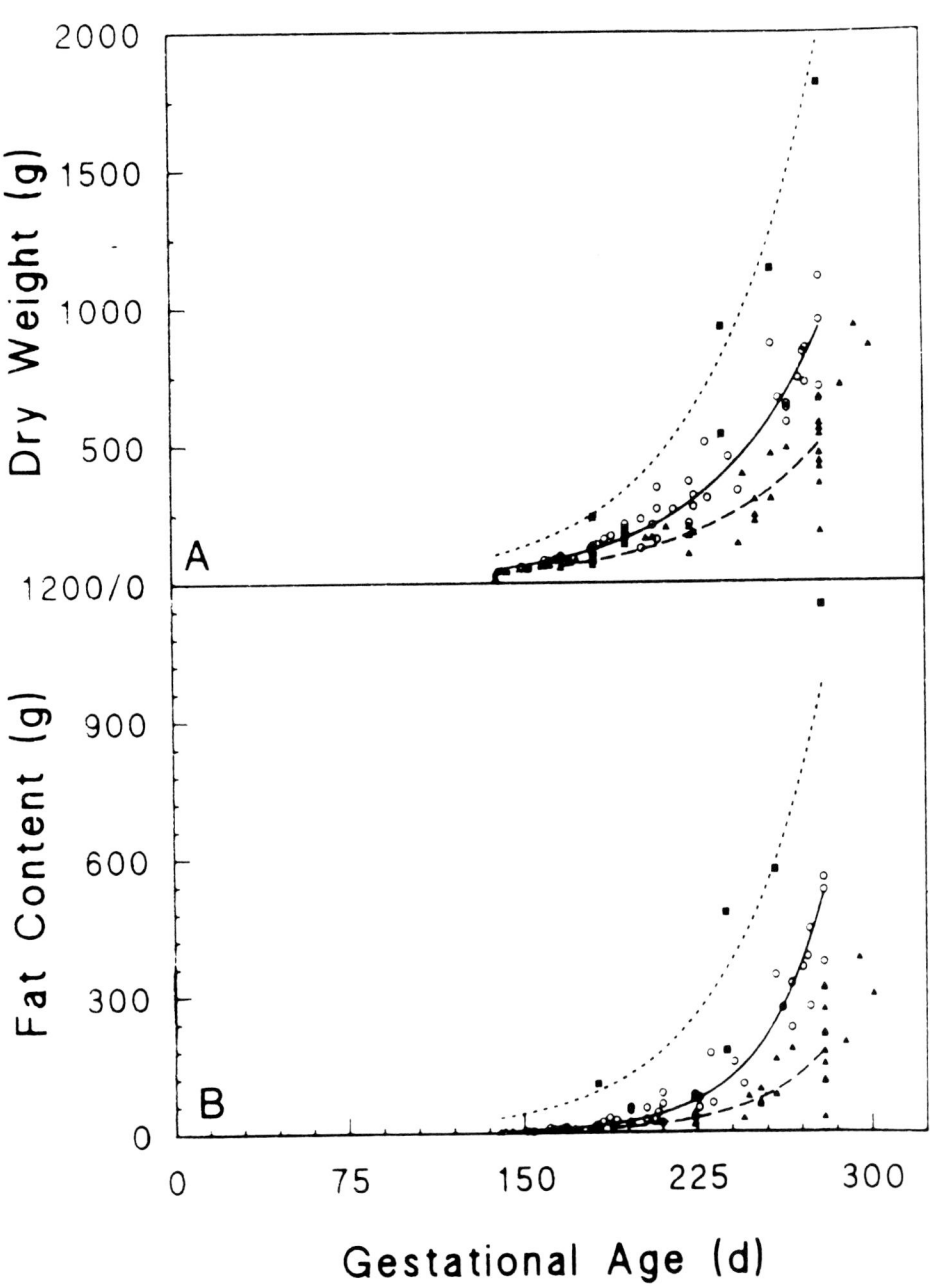

Figure 26-11 Dry weight **(A)** and fat content **(B)** plotted against gestational age in the same newborn human infants shown in Fig. 26-8 for LGA (■, · · · ·), AGA (O, ———), and SGA (▲, - - - -) infants. Reproduced with permission from Sparks JW. Intrauterine growth and nutrition. In: Polin RA, Fox WW, (eds.), *Fetal and neonatal physiology.* Philadelphia: W. B. Saunders Co., 1992:184, with permission.

infants born prematurely at different times over the last third of gestation, show a bias toward thinner SGA infants with less fat relative to nonfat weight and nitrogen content (32). These infants, however, were stillborn and may have suffered extensive wasting and IUGR. Other studies have shown that human SGA infants can be markedly deficient in muscle mass, even more than for fat (33,41).

REGULATION OF FETAL GROWTH

Fetal growth is regulated by maternal, placental, and fetal factors, representing a mix of genetic mechanisms and environmental influences through which genetic growth potential is expressed and modulated.

Epidemiologic Considerations

The major maternal risk factors for IUGR that vary among populations and among individuals within populations include small maternal size (height and prepregnancy weight) and low maternal weight gain during pregnancy. Low maternal body mass index (the degree of thinness or fatness, defined as [weight (kg)]/[height (cm)]2) is a major predicator of IUGR. This characteristic interacts with other risk factors, such as diet, smoking, illnesses, and so forth, to affect fetal growth, especially in thin women. For example, smoking has only half the impact on fetal growth in obese vs. thin women, and in black vs. white women (42). Low blood pressure has a detrimental impact on fetal growth, mostly in thin women (43). Moderate obesity,

TABLE 26-4
ENERGY VALUE OF HUMAN TISSUE COMPONENTS[b]

Tissue Component	Energy Value (kcal/g)[a]
H_2O	0
Fat	9.45
Nonfat dry weight	
Pig	4.0–4.6
Lamb	4.4–4.6
Guinea pig	4.6
Carbohydrate	4.15 (3.7–4.2)
Protein	5.65
In vivo catabolism	4.35

[a] 1 kcal = 4,190 J.
[b] From Battaglia FC, Meschia G. *An introduction to fetal physiology.* Orlando: Academic Press, 1986, with permission.

TABLE 26-6
FACTORS DETERMINING VARIANCE IN BIRTH WEIGHT[a,b]

	Percent of Total Variance
Fetal	
Genotype	16
Sex	2
Total	18
Maternal	
Genotype	20
Maternal environment	24
Maternal age	1
Parity	7
Total	52
Unknown	30

[a] From Penrose LS. Proceedings of the Ninth International Congress of Genetics, Part 1, 520, 1954, with permission.
[b] From Milner RDG, Gluckman PD. Regulation of intrauterine growth. In: Gluckman PD, Heymann MA, eds. Pediatrics & perinatology: the scientific basis, 2nd ed. London: Arnold, 1993:284, with permission.

therefore, protects against most growth-inhibiting risk factors except for black race and female gender. This pattern also holds for certain therapies. For example, zinc supplementation has a major impact on fetal growth in black women who have relatively low plasma zinc levels early in pregnancy, with all of the impact occurring in relatively thin women (44). Also, low-dose maternal aspirin treatment has been shown to improve fetal growth primarily in thin women (45).

Genetic Factors

Many genes contribute to fetal growth. Table 26-6 lists estimates of the quantitative contribution of fetal and parental factors to fetal growth and birth weight at term. Maternal genotype is more important than fetal genotype in the overall regulation of fetal growth. However, the paternal genotype is essential for trophoblast development, which secondarily regulates fetal growth by the provision of nutrients. More specific gene targeting studies have shown the importance of genomic imprinting on fetal growth. For example, normal fetal and placental growth in mice require that the

IGF-II gene be paternal and the IGF-II receptor gene be maternal, whereas maternal disomy producing IGF-II underexpression results in fetal dwarfism (39).

Nongenetic Maternal Factors

Under usual conditions, fetal growth follows its genetic potential, unless the mother is unusually small and limits fetal growth by a variety of factors considered collectively as "maternal constraint." Maternal constraint represents a relatively limited uterine size, including placental implantation surface area and uterine circulation, and thus the capacity to support placental growth and nutrient supply to the fetus. A clear example of maternal constraint is the reduced rate of fetal growth of multiple fetuses in a species—human—that optimally supports only one fetus (Fig. 26-12). Obviously, small fetuses of small parents do not reflect fetal growth restriction; in fact, their rates of growth are normal for their genome and for the size of the mother. Unless maternal constraint is particularly prominent, such fetuses would not grow faster or to a larger size if more nutrients were provided, although they might grow somewhat larger if the maternal uterine endometrial surface area, and thus placental implantation and growth area, were increased. The nongenetic, maternal nature of this effect has been demonstrated by embryo transfer and cross-breeding experiments (29). For example, a small-breed embryo transplanted into a large-breed uterus will grow larger than a small-breed embryo remaining in a small-breed uterus. Furthermore, partial reduction in fetal number in a polytocous species, such as the rat, produces greater than normal birth weights in the remaining offspring. Conversely, embryo transfer of a large-breed embryo into a small-breed uterus will result in a newborn that is smaller than in its natural large-breed environment. Such

TABLE 26-5
CALCULATION OF THE CALORIC DISTRIBUTION IN THE TERM HUMAN INFANT[a]

	Wet Weight	Fat	Nonfat Wet Weight	Nonfat Dry Weight
Weight (g)	3,450	386	3,064	511
Total calories (kcal)	5,950	3,650	2,300	2,300
Caloric concentration (kcal/g)	1.73	9.45	0.75	4.5

[a] Data from Ziegler EE, O'Donnell AM, Nelson SE, et al. Body composition of the reference fetus. *Growth* 1976;40:329, with permission.

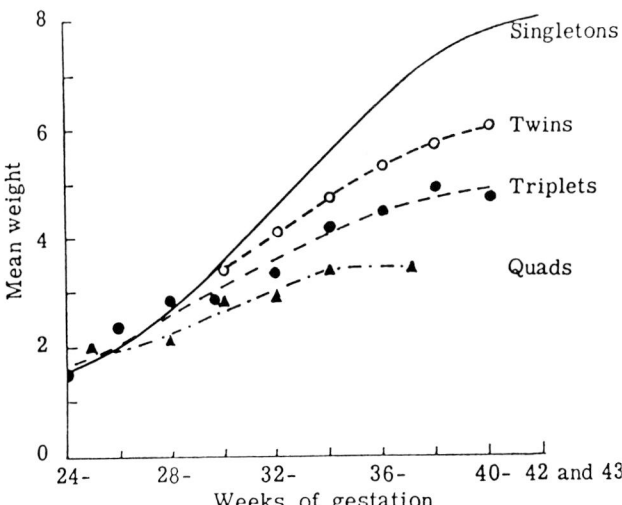

Figure 26-12   Mean birth weight of single and multiple human fetuses related to duration of gestation. Adapted from McKeown T, Record RG. Observation on foetal growth in multiple pregnancy in man. *J Endocrinol* 1952;8:386, with permission.

evidence supports the concept that fetal growth is normally constrained, and this constraint comes from the maternal environment, i.e., the size of the uterus.

Maternal Nutrition

The single most important environmental influence that affects fetal growth is the nutrition of the fetus. Normal variations in maternal nutrition, however, have relatively little impact on fetal growth and the severity of IUGR. This is because changes in maternal nutrition, unless extreme and prolonged, do not markedly alter maternal plasma concentrations of nutrient substrates or the rate of uterine blood flow, the principal determinants of nutrient substrate delivery and transport to the fetus by the placenta (46). Human epidemiologic data from conditions of prolonged starvation, and nutritional deprivation in experimental animals, indicate that severe limitations in maternal nutrition limit fetal growth only by 10% to 20%. Epidemiologic data from the Dutch during the Hunger Winter of 1944 showed an average reduction in fetal weight at term of 300 g (47), whereas birth weight at term was reduced by 500 g in women who suffered a more severe and prolonged famine in wartime Leningrad (48). Interestingly, second-generation daughters of women who suffered extreme nutritional deficit during gestation in turn tend to produce SGA infants who are 200 to 300 g less than normal at term with their first pregnancies (49). However, attempts to limit weight gain in pregnancy with a 1,200-kcal diet (50% of what is now recommended to prevent preeclampsia) increased the incidence of fetal growth restriction up to tenfold (50). Restrictions of calorie and protein intakes to less than 50% of normal for a considerable portion of gestation are needed before marked reductions in fetal growth are observed. Such

severe conditions often result in fetal loss before the impact of fetal growth rate in late gestation and fetal size at birth are manifested.

Attempts to increase fetal weight gain with maternal nutritional supplements have produced mixed results. Higher caloric feeding usually increases fetal adiposity, not growth of muscle mass or gain in length or head circumference. In contrast, high protein supplements tend to produce delayed fetal growth (51). Mechanisms responsible for this phenomenon are not known.

Maternal Chronic Diseases

Chronic hypertension, pregnancy-induced hypertension, and preeclampsia, like other vascular disorders including severe and long-standing diabetes mellitus and serious autoimmune disease associated with the lupus anticoagulant, have a common effect of limiting trophoblast invasion, placental growth and development, uteroplacental blood flow, and fetal oxygen and nutrient deficiency (52). Maternal cyanotic congenital heart disease can limit fetal oxygen supply, which can limit fetal growth (53). High-altitude hypoxia also can limit fetal growth (54), but usually this is only clinically significant for nonindigenous women who move to altitudes above 10,000 feet. Severe sickle cell crises can damage uterine vasculature, leading to placental growth and transport capacities (55).

Maternal Drugs

Specific effects of drugs on fetal growth (Table 26-7) are often difficult to sort out clinically, as many women who abuse drugs do so with many drugs taken intermittently, at different doses, and at different periods of fetal vulnerability. These women also frequently suffer from other disorders

TABLE 26-7

DRUGS ASSOCIATED WITH INTRAUTERINE GROWTH RESTRICTION

Amphetamines
Antimetabolites (e.g., aminopterin, busulfan, methotrexate)
Bromides
Cocaine
Ethanol
Heroin and other narcotics, such as morphine and methadone
Hydantoin
Isotretinoin
Metals such as mercury and lead
Phencyclidine
Polychlorinated biphenyls (PCBs)
Propranolol
Steroids
Tobacco (carbon monoxide, nicotine, thiocyante)
Toluene
Trimethadione
Warfarin

that could lead to poor fetal growth, such as poor nutrition, recurrent acute illnesses, and chronic diseases (56). Fetal growth restriction does appear to be a major part of the fetal alcohol syndrome. It is not clear when during gestation the specific effects of alcohol on fetal growth rate occur. Alcohol may exert its nonteratogenic effects by limiting placental-to-fetal amino acid transport (57). Cocaine probably exerts its primary effects on producing fetal growth restriction by causing uterine and perhaps umbilical vasoconstriction and reduced placental perfusion (58). The most consistent drug reducing fetal growth is cigarette smoking (41). Deficits of at least 300 g (about 10% of normal term weight) are not uncommon. A likely common mechanisms is the effect of nicotine, and of catecholamines released in response, to constrict the uterine and perhaps the umbilical vasculature, reducing placental perfusion. Carbon monoxide, cyanide, and other cellular toxins may limit oxygen transport to fetal tissues and cellular respiration.

Placenta

The size of the placenta and its directly related nutrient transport functions are the principal regulators of nutrient supply to the fetus and thus the rate of fetal growth (36). Nearly all cases of IUGR are associated with a smaller-than-normal placenta. Figure 26-13 shows a direct relationship between fetal weight and placental weight in

humans, demonstrating that LGA, AGA, and SGA infants are directly associated with LGA, AGA, and SGA placentas (59). Placental growth normally precedes fetal growth, and failure of placental growth is directly associated with decreased fetal growth. Variable limitations in placental nutrient transfer capacity modulate this primary effect of placental size on fetal growth. In some cases of experimentally reduced placental size, for example, fetal weight is not reduced proportionately (60). This indicates that either the capacity of the smaller placenta to transport nutrients to the fetus increases adaptively or the fetus develops increased capacity to grow. More characteristically, though, fetal growth fails first, or in direct relation to decreased nutrient supply. With primary fetal growth failure, placental growth can increase disproportionately, resulting in a larger than normal placental-to-fetal weight ratio for gestational age. This is characteristically seen under chronic hypoxic conditions of high altitude exposure or maternal anemia and has been seen in certain experimental situations of maternal undernutrition in early gestation (61). A variety of placental pathologic conditions are associated with IUGR (Table 26-8). In most of these cases, the placenta is simply smaller than normal. In many, there also is abnormal trophoblast development, including abnormal vascular growth in the trophoblast villi, frequently associated with limited uterine vascular perfusion of the intervillous spaces.

Placental and fetal growth both depend on an adequate supply of maternal blood to the placenta. IUGR is associated with inadequate development of the uteroplacental circulation, and radioisotope studies have demonstrated more than a twofold blood flow reduction in

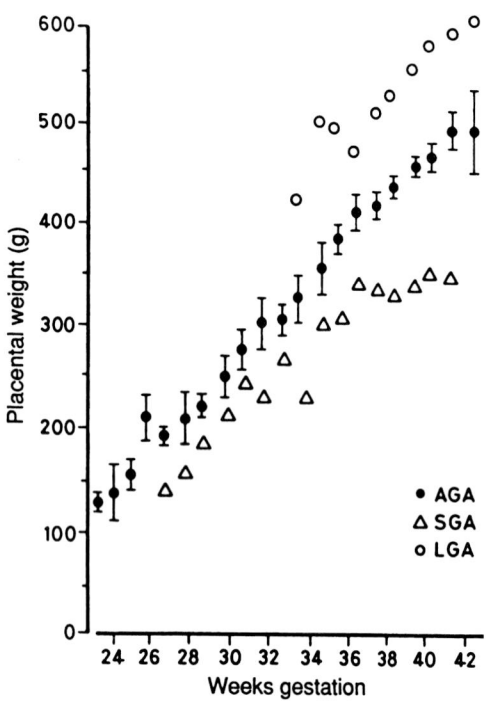

Figure 26-13 Mean placental weights for large-for-gestational-age (O), average-for-gestational-age (•), and small-for-gestational-age (Δ) human infants at each gestational age. ± SEM given for AGA infants alone. From Molteni RA, Stys SJ, Battaglia FC. Relationship of fetal and placental weight in human beings: fetal/placental weight ratios at various gestational ages and birth weight distributions. *J Reprod Med* 1978;21:327, with permission.

TABLE 26-8

PLACENTAL GROWTH DISORDERS THAT LEAD TO OR ARE ASSOCIATED WITH INTRAUTERINE GROWTH RESTRICTION

Abnormal umbilical vascular insertions (circumvallate, velamentous)
Abruption (chronic, partial)
Avascular villi
Decidual arteritis
Fibrinosis, atheromatous changes, cytotrophoblast hyperplasia, basement membrane thickening
Infectious villitis (as with TORCH infections)
Ischemic villous necrosis and umbilical vascular thromboses
Multiple gestation (limited endometrial surface area, vascular anastomoses)
Multiple infarcts
Partial molar pregnancy
Placenta previa
Single umbilical artery
Spiral artery vasculitis, failed or limited erosion into intervillous space
Syncytial knots
Tumors, including chorioangioma and hemangiomas

comparison with normal pregnancies (62). IUGR in the second half of gestation is due primarily to a failure of the normal villous vascular tree, mainly in the phase of non-branching angiogenesis, because terminal villi are critical for oxygen and nutrient transport to the fetus (63). This angiogenesis in turn depends on cytotrophoblast invasion of the uterus and its arterioles. Cytotrophoblast invasion is actually a differentiation process whereby the cells lose the ability to proliferate and modulate their expression of state-specific antigens. These antigens include members of the integrin family of cell–extracellular matrix receptors that are required for migration and invasion of the endometrium and decidua of the uterus (64). Preeclampsia, which is associated with IUGR, is characterized by shallow cytotrophoblast invasion (65). Abnormal cytotrophoblast differentiation also occurs, evidenced by the cells' inability to switch on their integrin repertoire (66). The same observations have been made on cultured normal cytotrophoblast cells in a hypoxic environment (67). These in vitro results indicate that whatever leads to hypoxia of the invading cytotrophoblast cells increases cytotrophoblast proliferation over differentiation and invasion, thus setting the stage for deficient placental development that can result in deficient nutrient and growth factor supply to the fetus, producing fetal growth restriction.

At more advanced stages of placental development, placental production of growth factors and growth regulating hormones develops, leading to significant autocrine regulation of placental growth and placental regulation of fetal growth processes. Human placental lactogen is synthesized and secreted by the syncytiotrophoblast cells of the placenta (68). Fetal growth-promoting actions of placental lactogen are mediated by stimulation of IGF production in the fetus and by increasing the availability of nutrients to fetal tissues (69). Obviously, placental growth failure and/or nutrient deficit to the placenta can result in decreased placental production of growth factors that then would lead to fetal growth failure.

FETAL NUTRIENT UPTAKE AND METABOLISM AND REGULATION OF FETAL GROWTH

In general, decreased rates of fetal growth represent an "adaptation" to inadequate nutrient supply. IUGR that results from decreased nutrient supply can be interpreted, therefore, as a successful, if not perfect, adaptation to maintain fetal survival. Fetal undernutrition also appears to affect rapidly growing fetuses more than slowly growing fetuses who may have been programmed to grow more slowly for genetic or embryonic and early fetal pathologic reasons (70). Reintroduction of nutrients can return fetal growth to normal in those fetuses whose rapid growth rate was decreased by undernutrition, but too rapid an introduction of nutrients has often caused fetal pathology,

including hyperlactatemia (70) and occasionally even acidosis and hypoxemia.

Glucose Uptake, Metabolism, and Regulation of Fetal Growth

Nearly all IUGR fetuses, whether studied experimentally in animal models or in women by cordocentesis (direct umbilical blood sampling), have relatively lower plasma glucose concentrations compared with normally grown fetuses (71,72). Fetal "hypoglycemia" has several consequences important to fetal adaptation and survival when maternal glucose supply is limited. First, relative fetal hypoglycemia is an important and natural compensatory mechanism that helps to maintain the maternal-to-fetal glucose concentration gradient and thus the transport of glucose across the placenta to the fetus (73). Despite this compensation, fetal hypoglycemia limits tissue glucose uptake directly by diminished mass action and indirectly by limiting fetal insulin secretion and thus the effect of insulin to promote tissue glucose uptake by skeletal muscle, heart, adipose tissue, and liver. Insulin also normally suppresses hepatic glucose production and release, and it acts as an anabolic hormone that increases net protein balance by inhibiting protein breakdown. Thus, a decrease in fetal plasma insulin concentration initially may allow fetal glucose production to take place, thereby providing glucose for both fetal and placental needs, but subsequently, combined with hypoglycemia, results in increased protein breakdown and decreased protein accretion (39,74,75).

Circulating concentrations and tissue-specific expression of growth factors such as IGF-I and IGF-II (see Fetal Amino Acid Metabolism) also are decreased during fetal hypoglycemia (76), which may contribute to increased fetal protein breakdown and decreased rates of fetal growth. Thus, fetal hypoglycemia in response to a decrease in maternal glucose supply acts to maintain fetal glucose supply, but it also leads to lower anabolic hormone concentrations, which limit the rate of fetal growth, thereby decreasing fetal nutrient needs.

Fetal Amino Acid Metabolism

The placenta contains a large variety of amino acid transporters, most of which use energy to actively concentrate amino acids in the trophoblast, which then diffuse into the fetal plasma, producing higher concentrations than in the maternal plasma (77). With small placentas, fetal amino acid supply is reduced, as are fetal amino acid concentrations, fetal protein synthesis, fetal protein and nitrogen balance, and, ultimately, fetal growth rate. Reduced energy supply to the placenta also reduces amino acid transport to the fetus. This is especially the case for oxygen deficit, either from primary hypoxemia or from reduced uteroplacental blood flow, and glucose deficit from chronic maternal and fetal hypoglycemia (78,79). Of course, hypoxemia and hypoglycemia could reduce fetal growth independently of reduced amino acid transport, for example, by limiting anabolic hormone and growth factor production or by decreasing energy supply, both of which are necessary to produce protein synthesis and to limit protein breakdown in fetal tissues.

The reason why amino acid and energy supplies are so important for fetal protein and nitrogen balance and for fetal growth is illustrated in Fig. 26-14. This figure shows results of experiments in fetal sheep over the second half of gestation, comparing fractional protein synthesis rates derived from tracer amino acid data and fractional body growth rates derived from carcass analysis data. The fractional rate of protein turnover per unit wet weight of fetus is several fold higher at 50% to 60% of term gestation (equivalent to about 20 to 24 weeks of human gestation). Such high rates of protein turnover require a much greater rate of amino acid supply and energy than at term, when fetal protein turnover rate is much lower. Indeed, in midgestation fetal sheep, glucose utilization rates per whole fetal weight and oxygen consumption rates per dry fetal weight are much higher in the early fetus than at term (80). These conditions result in a 50% higher rate of net protein accretion and fractional rate of fetal growth at midgestation than at term. Clearly, amino acid and energy deficits will affect the growth rate of the fetus at earlier stages of gestation, when fetal growth normally is very rapid much more than at term, when fetal growth rate is slower.

In the normally growing fetus, net protein synthesis exceeds net protein breakdown, resulting in net protein accretion. The mechanisms underlying the reduction in protein synthesis rate over gestation appear to be intrinsic to the fetus, and not to limitation of nutrient supply by the placenta. These mechanisms include changing proportions of the organs as fractions of body mass (Table 26-9).

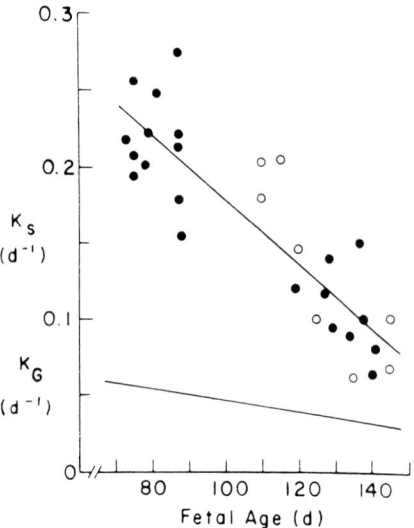

Figure 26-14 Fractional rate of protein synthesis (K_s) over gestation in fetal sheep studied with leucine (●) and lysine (O) radioactive tracers compared with the fractional rate of growth (K_G) in the lower portion of the figure (——). From ref. 77. Adapted from refs. 46 and 80; and from Meier PR, Peterson RG, Bonds DR, Meschia G, Battaglia FC. Rates of protein synthesis and turnover in fetal life. *Am J Physiol* 1981;240:E320.

TABLE 26-9

PERCENT CONTRIBUTION OF ORGANS AND TISSUES TO THE BODY WEIGHT OF HUMAN FETUSES AND NEWBORN INFANTS[a]

	Fetus (20–24 wk)	Full-term Infant
Skeletal muscle	25	25
Skin	13	15
Skeleton	22	18
Heart	0.6	0.5
Liver	4	5
Kidneys	0.7	1
Brain	13	13

[a] From Widdowson EM. Growth and composition of the fetus and newborn. In: Assali NS, ed. *Gestation*. New York: Academic Press, 1968:27, with permission.

Fetal Endocrine and Autocrine/Paracrine-Acting Growth Factor Effects on Fetal Growth

Table 26-10 lists those hormones whose deficiency results in a reduction in fetal growth supported by experimental evidence (81). These fetal hormones promote growth (and development) in utero by altering both the metabolism and gene expression of fetal tissues. These hormonal actions ensure that fetal growth rate is commensurate with nutrient supply.

Insulin

Insulin has direct mitogenic effects on cellular development and thus can regulate cell number. It also enhances glucose consumption by many cells, particularly in muscle, and limits protein breakdown (75). The latter effects are associated with reduced fetal growth when insulin concentration is low. This has been produced directly by experimental surgical (82) and chemical (83) ablation of the pancreas and/or the function of the pancreatic beta cells to secrete insulin, and has been observed clinically in infants who suffer pancreatic agenesis (84). Figure 26-15 shows reduced rates of growth in fetal sheep that underwent surgical pancreatectomy and a return to normal rates of growth with insulin replacement. Much of the growth reduction with hypoinsulinemia from pancreatectomy is caused by a release of insulin's normal inhibitory role on glucose production, resulting in fetal hyperglycemia, a secondary decrease in the maternal–fetal glucose concentration gradient, and thus a decrease in glucose transport to the fetus. Without this glucose, fetal growth decreases, as has been shown by a direct decrease in glucose uptake by the fetus following the production of chronic maternal hypoglycemia (85). Fetal amino acid uptake decreases under the same circumstances. Thus, insulin deficiency, directly and indirectly, results in a decrease in fetal nutrient supply. Initially, fetal protein breakdown results in fetal

TABLE 26-10

EFFECTS OF SPECIFIC ENDOCRINE DEFICIENCIES ON BODY WEIGHT AND CROWN–RUMP LENGTH, AND INDIVIDUAL TISSUES ADVERSELY AFFECTED BY TREATMENT IN SHEEP FETUSES DELIVERED NEAR TERM (>95% GESTATION)[a]

Endocrine Deficiency	Procedure	Gestational Age at Onset (d)	Body Weight	Crown-rump Length	Tissues with Specific Developmental Abnormalities
Insulin	Streptozotocin	70–85	↓50%	↓20%	None
	Pancreatectomy	115–120	↓30%	↓15%	None
Thyroid hormones	Thyroidectomy	80–96	↓30%	↓10%	Skeleton, skin, lungs, nervous system
		105–115	↓20%	↓10%	Skeleton, nervous system
Adrenal hormones	Adrenalectomy	110–120	↑10–15%	No change	Liver, lungs, gut, pituitary
Pituitary hormones	Hypophysectomy	70–79	↓30%	↓8%	Bones, liver, lungs, placenta
		105–110	↓20%	↓10%	Bones, liver, lungs, placenta, adrenal, gonads
		110–125	No change to ↓5%	No change	Bones, gonads, adrenal, liver
	Pituitary stalk section	108–112	↓15%	No change	Adrenals, other tissues?

[a] From Fowden AL. Endocrine regulation of fetal growth. In: Harding R, Genkin G, Grant A, eds. Progress in perinatal physiology. *Reprod Fertil Dev* 1995;7:50, with permission.

amino acid release for energy (via direct amino acid oxidation in the tricarboxylic [citric] acid cycle) and glucose production. Later on, the reduced rate of fetal growth during conditions of low insulin, glucose, and amino acid concentrations is sustained by increased protein breakdown (40); however, amino acids are used to maintain protein turnover rate and not for protein accretion, oxidation, or glucose production.

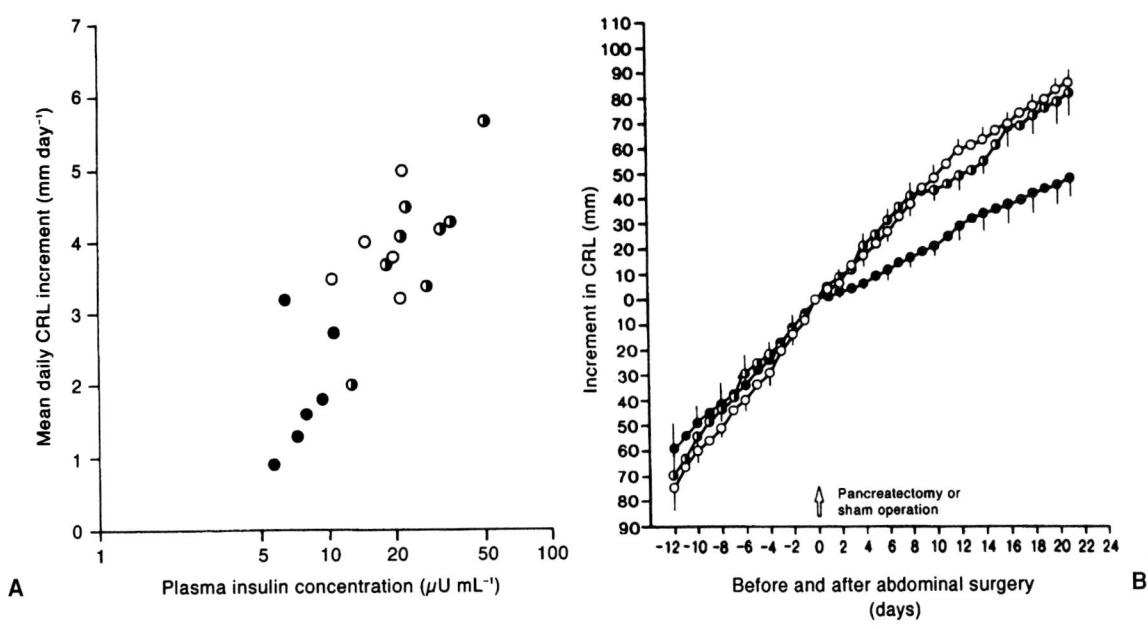

Figure 26-15 Relationship between growth and plasma insulin concentrations in the sheep fetus. **A:** Mean daily crown–rump length (CRL) increment with respect to plasma insulin concentration in individual sheep fetuses [sham operated (O); pancreatectomized (•); pancreatectomized and given insulin treatment (◑)]. **B:** Daily increment in CRL with respect to time before and after abdominal surgery in fetuses that were sham-operated (O), pancreatectomized (•), and given insulin treatment to restore normal insulin concentrations (◑). From Fowden AL. The role of insulin in prenatal growth. *J Dev Physiol* 1989;12:173; Fowden AL. Endocrine regulation of fetal growth. In: Harding R, Genkin G, Grant A, (eds.). *Progress in perinatal physiology. Reprod Fertil Dev* 1995;7:50, with permission.

Insulin-Like Growth Factor-I

IGF-I is positively regulated by glucose supply in the fetus. Infusion of IGF-I into fetal sheep decreases protein breakdown, especially when protein breakdown is increased by fasting-induced hypoglycemia. Metabolic effects of a decreased plasma concentration of IGF-I have not been studied, although, as for insulin, such effects might be difficult to separate from simultaneous changes in nutrient substrate supply and concentration. Thus, IGF-I probably can regulate metabolic processes that affect fetal protein balance and growth, but these have been difficult to measure.

Plasma IGF-I concentrations are positively related to fetal size at birth. A causative role for IGF-I has been shown by the production of transgenic models of mice that have shown that decreased expression of IGF-I results in markedly reduced rates of fetal growth. Other transgenic models with increased expression of IGF-I have been associated with increased brain growth (86,87), and this growth can be inhibited by overexpression of IGF binding protein-1 (IGFBP-1) (88). IGF-I stimulates an increase in oligodendrocytes and neuronal number, and neuronal outgrowth with increased dendritic arborization and axon terminal fields (89). Because IGF-I is decreased directly by reduced nutrient supply, particularly glucose, and IGFBP-1 is decreased under these circumstances, the smaller, more densely packed neuronal structure of the undernourished brain that is seen in some infants with severe IUGR may have been mediated by nutrient regulation of IGF-I and IGFBP-1 expression. Such developmental limitations might underlie the poorer neurodevelopmental outcome of severely SGA infants who have relative microcephaly.

Insulin-Like Growth Factor-II, Insulin-Like Growth Factor Binding Protein-2, Insulin-Like Growth Factor Binding Protein-3, and Vasoactive Intestinal Polypeptide

Although serum concentrations of IGF-II do not correlate with fetal size at birth in human infants, it has been shown conclusively that targeted mutation of the IGF-II gene reduces fetal size in mice (90,91). Furthermore, IGF-II is the predominant IGF expressed in the tissues of embryos and fetuses of all species. As with IGF-I and IGFBP-1, transgenic overexpression of IGF-II and IGFBP-2 shows that cellular growth is dependent on the balance between the binding protein and the IGF molecule itself. IGFBP-3 is the predominant IGF binding protein in several mammalian species including humans (92,93) and is reduced in cord blood of infants with IUGR (94). Vasoactive intestinal peptide (VIP) is another growth factor in the fetus that affects neuronal and whole body growth (95–97). Antagonists to VIP in pregnant mice produce smaller fetuses that are particularly microcephalic (98), with central nervous system neurons that show reduced mitosis and migration. These effects of VIP occur in the first half of gestation, coincident with transiently high VIP concentrations in the maternal plasma (99).

Thyroid Hormones

In all species, fetal thyroid hormone deficiency produces developmental abnormalities in certain tissues. When maternal thyroid hormones cannot compensate, as in the sheep, which does not transport maternal thyroid hormones to the fetus, fetal growth restriction develops, primarily reflecting deficient carcass growth (skin, bone, and muscle) (81). This growth restriction results from both hypoplasia (in muscle) and hypotrophy (in lung). More generally, fetal hypothyroidism decreases oxygen consumption and oxidation of glucose, thereby potentially decreasing fetal energy supply for growth. Hypothyroidism also can decrease circulating and tissue concentrations of IGF-I.

Glucocorticoids

Glucocorticoids do not have strong effects on fetal growth rate, but they are important in the maturation of many fetal enzymatic pathways (39). These include glycogen deposition, gluconeogenesis, fatty acid oxidation, induction of surfactant production and release, structural maturation of alveoli, structural maturation of the gastrointestinal tract, increased expression of digestive enzymes, increased adrenal function, switch from fetal to adult hemoglobin synthesis, and others. Many IUGR fetuses have increased cortisol concentrations that appear to result from intermittent hypoxic stress. This may account for much of the apparent increased maturation of IUGR fetuses, even when born preterm.

Growth Hormone

Growth hormone, which is the major hormonal regulator of postnatal growth, has no demonstrable effect on fetal growth (39,81).

ANTENATAL CARE OF THE INTRAUTERINE GROWTH-RESTRICTED FETUS

Diagnosis of Intrauterine Growth Restriction

Antenatal diagnosis of IUGR is difficult and often inaccurate. Despite careful attention to gestational dating by maternal history and early and serial fetal ultrasound evaluation, frequent maternal physical examinations, and repeated assessment of risks for IUGR, more than one-half of infants with IUGR may not be identified before birth (100).

Serial ultrasound evaluation of fetal growth rate and fetal body proportions and Doppler velocimetry of the uterine, placental, and fetal circulations are now the standard diagnostic approaches to determining the severity of IUGR. In particular, Doppler velocimetry has provided increasingly accurate prognostic evidence of worsening fetal condition and impending fetal death (101–106). Chronic fetal distress resulting from placental insufficiency, hypoxia, and ischemia (with or without acidosis) is associated with increased Doppler arterial waveform amplitudes that indicate increased vascular resistance and reduced systemic flow in the descending aorta and umbilical artery. Various ratios of systolic-to-diastolic flow velocity (amplitude) waveforms have been used, including the systolic-to-diastolic ratio, systolic-diastolic/systolic ratio (resistance index), and systolic-diastolic/mean ratio (pulsatility index). Ratios or indexes greater than two standard deviations from the mean are associated with IUGR, whereas reversed or absent diastolic waveforms represent severe fetal hypoxia and increased risk of fetal death. The most severely affected IUGR fetuses with the greatest risk of death demonstrate absent or reversed diastolic flow in systemic fetal arteries (104), along with increased umbilical venous pulsation and reversed flow in the abdominal vena cava. Interestingly, these same fetuses often have decreased cerebral (internal carotid artery) pulsatility index, indicating increased cerebral blood flow (105). This flow pattern has been interpreted as one way in which brain growth is spared, as body growth rate slows as a result of placental ischemia and/or placental growth failure. Doppler waveform abnormalities usually precede less specific signs of fetal distress, such as abnormal changes in fetal heart rate, spontaneously or in response to oxytocin challenge testing.

The fetus also should be examined by ultrasound for anatomic abnormalities that indicate congenital malformations, genetic syndromes, and deformations. Amniotic fluid index also is useful to identify oligohydramnios. The latter is a risk factor for congenital anomalies, severe IUGR with reduced urine production, pulmonary hypoplasia, variable decelerations from cord compression, and intrauterine fetal death in as many a 5% to 10% of affected fetuses.

Future Diagnosis and Treatment of Intrauterine Growth Restriction

Altered fetal growth rate, and pathophysiology associated with IUGR, usually develop insidiously, such that once these conditions are clinically obvious, injury has already taken place. It is important, therefore, to develop and apply diagnostic techniques to the fetus that would establish accurately even minimal changes in growth rate and physiologic function. Currently, Doppler ultrasound measurements of fetal cardiac output, systemic blood flow, and organ blood supply are close to achieving this goal, particularly with respect to the placental circulation (107). Other recent research trials have focused on quantifying placental transfer functions in pregnant women who are carrying a severely IUGR fetus. For example, women carrying an IUGR fetus can be given stable isotopes of nutrients normally transported across the placenta, such as glucose and selected amino acids, followed by timed cordocentesis to measure placental transfer characteristics of these substrate isotopes (108). This information can be compared with that from normal pregnancies with normal placental function and fetal growth rates.

It is also important that diagnostic techniques are developed to assess what damage is being done in the more extreme cases of IUGR. Current techniques include magnetic resonance imaging, Doppler measurements of blood flow to specific organs (107), cordocentesis (109–112), and neurologic and neuromuscular response to vibroacoustic stimulation (113). Based on such advances in fetal diagnosis, it soon may be possible to assess whether detected changes in fetal growth rate and measured fetal pathophysiology associated with IUGR are, in fact, as serious and indicative of future handicap as current postnatal follow-up studies have indicated.

Considerably more research is necessary to determine when and how damage to the fetus can be reversed or ameliorated. Some efforts have been made in animal models to improve maternal and fetal nutrition (114) and to enhance development by organ-specific hormone targeting (115). Examples of the latter include glucocorticoids that have been administered (such as betamethasone) to both the mother and the fetus to increase lung surfactant maturity (116), with additional potential benefits to the maturation of other fetal organs including the gut, heart, adrenals, and kidneys (115). Also, thyroid-releasing hormone has been administered along with corticosteroids to increase lung maturity, although currently there are mixed reports of its effectiveness (117). Continued work is necessary to assess brain development with such treatments, and long-term growth and development of all affected organs. More philosophically, it is important to consider whether it is wise to change normal developmental relationships among organs by using organ-specific hormone therapy; more information is needed to determine how altered patterns of organ development during fetal life are beneficial and how they may promote, or hinder, normal fetal development (118).

Antenatal Management

There are few, if any, proven treatments of IUGR. Bed rest and treatment of acute and chronic illnesses appear beneficial. Having the mother breathe supplemental oxygen improves fetal oxygenation, and in a few studies of severe IUGR fetuses with signs of chronic distress this has been associated with improved rates of fetal growth and reduced fetal aortic blood flow velocity (increased flow) (119). Trials of low-dose aspirin therapy, aimed primarily at treating preeclampsia, have not consistently improved fetal growth (120). Correction of maternal nutritional deficiencies also is useful, particularly when the mother is markedly undernourished. Maternal dietary zinc supplements have improved fetal growth when zinc deficiency was prominent. High protein intakes have not helped and, in fact, have been associated with worse IUGR and perinatal morbidity and mortality.

Fetal surveillance techniques should be instituted to determine whether the fetal condition is beginning to fail and if delivery would be more likely to result in a successful pregnancy outcome. Traditional fetal surveillance techniques have included fetal activity recordings, the oxytocin challenge test, which measures fetal heart rate changes after oxytocin-induced uterine contractions, and the nonstress test, which measures the acceleration and beat-to-beat variability of the fetal heart rate after spontaneous fetal movement. These tests, although still done, have been replaced by Doppler velocimetry and the biophysical profile, which combine analyses of fetal breathing movements, gross body movements, fetal heart rate, fetal heart rate reactivity to movement, and estimated amniotic fluid volume. The combined use of Doppler velocimetry and the biophysical profile has improved the antenatal management of IUGR (121,122). A low biophysical profile correlates with fetal hypoxia determined by absent or reversed diastolic flow in the umbilical artery and fetal blood gas and acid-base measurements obtained by cordocentesis, and with impending fetal demise.

Most obstetricians avoid labor when combined fetal surveillance techniques show severe fetal growth restriction and evidence of severe chronic distress (123,124), including absent or reversed diastolic flow in the fetal aorta, increased pulsations and/or reversed flow in the umbilical veins, and a low biophysical profile score. Fetuses with these conditions also usually have a nonreactive nonstress test result and a flat baseline fetal heart rate variability pattern. Such fetuses tolerate labor poorly and readily develop signs of acute distress. Saline amnioinfusion may be beneficial in the presence of oligohydramnios and an amniotic fluid index of less than 5 cm (125). Amnioinfusion to an index greater than 8 cm may decrease the incidence of meconium-stained fluid, variable decelerations in the fetal heart rate, end-stage bradycardia, and acute fetal acidosis. In all such severe cases the delivery should be coordinated with the neonatology service to provide prompt postnatal evaluation and care and to prepare for resuscitation of a depressed or asphyxiated neonate.

In the absence of repeated observations of severe or progressively worsening IUGR and signs of fetal distress, the moderately affected IUGR fetus should be left in utero, although providing good nutrition, perhaps bed rest, and optimal health care to the mother, and continuing fetal surveillance. Decisions to deliver these fetuses prematurely to prevent fetal death should be tempered by the difficulties of accurately diagnosing the worsening of fetal condition and successfully managing all potential neonatal problems of a preterm infant. Although lung maturity may be present, the many other problems associated with preterm delivery should add caution to a decision for early delivery, especially before 31 to 32 weeks of gestation.

CLINICAL EVALUATION AND TREATMENT OF THE SMALL-FOR-GESTATIONAL AGE INFANT

General Evaluation in the Delivery Room

SGA infants often present a variety of clinical problems immediately after birth in the delivery room. Because of their large surface area relative to body weight, SGA infants lose heat rapidly. To prevent hypothermia, they should be dried quickly and completely, placed under a radiant warmer, and protected from drafts with warmed blankets. Severely SGA infants who suffered marked oxygen and substrate deprivation in utero may have cardiopulmonary difficulties at birth. Closer to term they may pass meconium and present with meconium aspiration syndrome, signs of asphyxia, including hypoxemia, hypotension, mixed metabolic and respiratory acidosis, and persistent pulmonary hypertension. Immediately after birth, these infants need prompt and careful attention to their airway, breathing, and oxygen needs.

Brief Physical Examination in the Delivery Room

SGA infants have several characteristic features, even when those infants with obvious anomalies and syndromes and those born to mothers with severe illness or malnutrition are excluded (126–128). Severely SGA infants who had marked IUGR have relatively large heads for their undergrown trunks and extremities. The abdomen often appears shrunken or "scaphoid" and must be distinguished from infants with diaphragmatic hernias. The extremities appear scrawny with thin skinfolds, with evidence of decreased subcutaneous fat and skeletal muscle. The skin is loose and often rough, dry, and peeling. In term and postterm severely SGA infants, the fingernails may be long, and the hands and feet tend to look large for the size of the body. The face appears shrunken or "wizened." Cranial sutures may be widened or overriding, and the anterior fontanelle may be larger than expected, representing diminished membranous bone formation. The umbilical cord often is thinner than usual. When meconium has been passed in utero, the cord is yellow-green stained, as are the nails and skin.

Gestational Age Assessment of the Small-for-Gestational-Age Infant

Gestational age assessment based on physical criteria often is erroneous. Vernix caseosa frequently is reduced or absent as a result of diminished skin perfusion during periods of fetal distress or because of depressed synthesis of estriol, which normally enhances vernix production. In the absence of this protective covering, the skin is continuously exposed to amniotic fluid and will begin to desquamate. Sole creases appear more mature as a result of increased wrinkling from increased exposure to amniotic fluid. Breast tissue formation also depends on peripheral blood flow and estriol levels and will be reduced in SGA infants. The female external genitalia will appear less mature because of the absence of the perineal adipose tissue covering the labia. Ear cartilage also may be diminished. Specific organ maturity often continues at normal developmental rates despite diminished somatic growth in most IUGR infants. Cerebral cortical convolutions, renal glomeruli, and alveolar maturation all relate to gestational age and are not delayed with IUGR.

Neurologic Examination of the Small-for-Gestational-Age Infant

Neurologic examination for gestational age assessment may be little affected by IUGR. These infants often appear to have advanced neurologic maturity, although this observation is derived mostly from comparisons with infants of similar birth weight, not similar gestational age. Peripheral nerve conduction velocity and visual- or auditory-evoked responses correlate well with gestational age and are not impaired as a result of IUGR. These aspects of neurologic maturity are not sensitive to nutritional deprivation. Active and passive tone and posture are usually normal in SGA infants and are reliable guides to gestational age, assuming that infants with significant central nervous system and metabolic disorders are excluded.

Behavioral Observations

SGA infants demonstrate specific abnormal behaviors. They often have a "hyperalert" appearance and generally look "starved and hungry," and they often are described as being jittery and hypertonic, even without simultaneous hypoglycemia. They may be hyperexcitable, showing aberrations in tone from hypertonia to hypotonia and, in many cases, apathy. The Moro response is increased, with exaggerated extension and abduction of the arms, windmill motions, and prolongation of the tonic neck posture (129,130). When IUGR is particularly severe, SGA infants tend to show abnormal sleep cycles and a more consistent picture of diminished muscle tone, deep tendon and facial tactile reflexes, general physical activity, and excitability. These more severe changes indicate that functional central nervous system maturity is impaired, despite the presence of electrical neurologic maturity (131–133). Such severely SGA infants often appear floppy and develop exhaustion more easily after handling (134). The behavioral disorders occur even in the absence of significant central nervous system disease. The hypoexcitability indicates an adverse effect on polysynaptic reflex propagation and implies that central nervous system functional maturity does not necessarily proceed independently of the intrauterine events that result in IUGR.

Deferred Physical Examination to be Done in the Neonatal Intensive Care Unit

Careful evaluation is important as there is an increased incidence of severe malformation, chromosomal abnormality, and congenital infection among SGA infants (135,136). Dysmorphic features, "funny-looking facies," abnormal hands and feet, and the presence of palmar creases, in addition to gross anomalies, suggest congenital malformation syndromes, chromosomal defects, or teratogens. Ocular disorders, such as chorioretinitis, cataracts, glaucoma, and cloudy cornea, in addition to hepatosplenomegaly, jaundice, and a blueberry-muffin rash, suggest a congenital infection. Toxoplasmosis, other (syphilis, hepatitis, Zoster), rubella, cytomegalovirus, and herpes simplex (maternal infections) (TORCH) infections resulting in IUGR are unusual in the absence of other clinical signs of chronic congenital infection; however, screening cord blood for antibodies and antigens specific to certain infections (which can be augmented by polymerase chain reaction techniques), and a urine culture for cytomegalovirus may be indicated. Radiographic examination of the long bones, looking for possible anomalies and for the quality of mineralization, may be useful. Examination of the head with ultrasonography to establish the presence of congenital anatomic abnormalities or evidence of congenital infection also may be helpful in making a diagnosis.

CLINICAL PROBLEMS OF THE SMALL-FOR-GESTATIONAL-AGE NEONATE (TABLE 26-11)

Mortality

The consequences of small size for gestational age depend on the etiology, severity, and duration of growth restriction. There continues to be much debate on this subject. Previous studies have included heterogeneous groups of infants with respect to the degree and cause of IUGR, the degree of prematurity, and the severity of clinical problems in the early neonatal period. By now, many studies have been conducted over extended periods of changing perinatal management and increasing survival rates of smaller, more preterm infants, many of whom have been classified differently at different times and among different studies regarding their degree of IUGR. Some studies have indicated that the fetus responds to the "stress" of growth restriction with an acceleration of maturity, which ultimately is protective for the infant. Others have found no evidence of improved survival after perinatal stress, and SGA status has been shown to be an independent predictor of increased fetal, perinatal, and neonatal death (137). On balance, there is little evidence to support the concept of improved survival after perinatal stress in SGA infants, and the perinatal mortality rate for SGA infants with relatively severe IUGR is 5 to 20 times that of AGA infants of the same gestational age (136,137). Particularly when adjusted for maternal neonatal risk factors of IUGR, including birth weight percentile, gestational age at birth, maternal height, prepregnancy weight, gestational weight gain, race, and parity, a subgroup of SGA infants is defined that has consistently and markedly higher perinatal mortality and morbidity rates than normally grown infants (138).

Intrauterine Growth Restriction/Small-for-Gestational-Age Status vs. Preterm Birth, and Effects on Mortality and Morbidity

Preterm and growth-restricted infants have independent and overlapping problems. Constitutionally small infants are not likely to have increased risks of mortality or morbidity. As gestational age decreases, the problems of

TABLE 26-11
CLINICAL PROBLEMS OF THE SMALL-FOR-GESTATIONAL-AGE NEONATE

Problem	Pathogenesis/Pathophysiology	Prevention/Treatment
Intrauterine death	Chronic hypoxia	Antenatal surveillance
	Placental insufficiency	Fetal growth by ultrasound
	Growth failure	Biophysical profile
	Malformation	Doppler velocimetry
	Infection	Maternal treatment: ? bed rest, ?O$_2$
	Infarction/abruption	Delivery for severe/worsening fetal distress
	Preeclampsia	
Asphyxia	Acute hypoxia/abruption	Antepartum/intrapartum monitoring
	Chronic hypoxia	Adequate neonatal resuscitation
	Placental insufficiency/preeclampsia	
	Acidosis	
	Glycogen depletion	
Meconium aspiration definite, severe	Hypoxia	Resuscitation including tracheal suctioning for aspiration
Hypothermia	Cold stress	Protect against increased heat loss
	Hypoxia	Dry infant
	Hypoglycemia	Radiant warmer
	Decreased fat stores	Hat
	Decreased subcutaneous insulation	Thermoneutral environment
	Increased surface area	Nutritional support
	Catecholamine depletion	
Persistent pulmonary hypertension	Chronic hypoxia	Cardiovascular support
		Mechanical ventilation, Nitric oxide
Hypoglycemia	Decreased hepatic/muscle glycogen	Frequent measurement of blood glucose
	Decreased alternative energy sources	Early intravenous glucose support
	Heat loss	
	Hypoxia	
	Decreased gluconeogenesis	
	Decreased counterregulatory hormones	
	Increased insulin sensitivity	
Hyperglycemia	Low insulin secretion rate	Glucose monitoring
	Excessive glucose delivery	Glucose infusion <10 mg/min/kg
	Increased catecholamine and	Insulin administration glucagon effects
Polycythemia/hyperviscosity	Chronic hypoxia	Glucose, oxygen
	Maternal–fetal transfusion	Partial volume exchange transfusion
	Increased erythropoiesis	
Gastrointestinal perforation	Focal ischemia	Cautious enteral feeding
	Hypoperistalsis	
Acute renal failure	Hypoxia/ischemia	Cardiovascular support
Immunodeficiency	Malnutrition	Early, optimal nutrition
	Congenital infection	Specific antibiotic and immune therapy

prematurity have a larger role in the outcome of both SGA and AGA infants. In contrast, the more mature preterm or term infant may suffer more from the impact of growth restriction. When IUGR has been severe and prolonged, these infants have a higher perinatal mortality rate than their AGA peers. Intrauterine fetal death from chronic fetal hypoxia, immediate birth asphyxia, the multisystem disorders associated with asphyxia (hypoxic–ischemic encephalopathy, persistent fetal circulation, cardiomyopathy, meconium aspiration), and lethal congenital anomalies are the main contributing factors to the high mortality rate for IUGR fetuses and neonates. Most intrauterine fetal deaths occur between 38 and 42 weeks of gestation. Improved survival depends on achieving an optimal balance between the consequences of elective preterm delivery and the risks of continued IUGR.

Asphyxia

Perinatal asphyxia is an uncommon event in SGA infants, but it does occur at increased frequency in SGA infants and can complicate the immediate neonatal course of severe IUGR infants. SGA infants frequently do not tolerate labor and vaginal delivery, and signs of fetal distress are common. In such cases, the already stressed, chronically hypoxic infant is exposed to the acute stress of diminished blood flow during uterine contractions. Cord blood lactate concentrations are often increased despite overall normal cord blood pH. Preterm SGA infants are delivered by cesarean section twice as often as preterm AGA infants (136,139). SGA infants have an increased incidence of low Apgar scores at all gestational ages (136), and these infants frequently need resuscitation.

The acute fetal hypoxia, acidosis, and cerebral depression may result in fetal death or neonatal asphyxia. Severe IUGR results in a large proportion of stillborn infants. Myocardial infarction, amniotic fluid and meconium aspiration, and cerebral edema and necrosis often are noted at autopsy in these severely IUGR stillborn infants. An inadequate resuscitation at birth adds double jeopardy to the in utero insults. Sequelae of perinatal asphyxia include multiple organ system dysfunction that, in the more severe cases, includes hypoxic–ischemic encephalopathy, heart failure from hypoxia–ischemia and glycogen depletion, meconium aspiration syndrome, persistent pulmonary hypertension, gastrointestinal hypoperistalsis and ischemia- induced necrosis leading to focal perforation, and acute renal tubular necrosis and renal failure. However, surfactant-deficiency respiratory distress syndrome is not increased in more mature SGA infants closer to term, despite the increased incidence of other forms of respiratory distress. Hypocalcemia may occur following asphyxia in SGA infants, although this is uncommon unless there is excessive phosphate released from damaged cells by acidosis followed by correction with sodium bicarbonate.

Neonatal Metabolism

Hypoglycemia

Hypoglycemia is extremely common in SGA infants, increasing with the severity of IUGR (Fig. 26-16) (140–148). The risk of hypoglycemia is greatest during the first 3 days of life, but fasting hypoglycemia, with or without ketonemia, can occur repeatedly up to weeks after birth. Early hypoglycemia usually is as a result of diminished hepatic and skeletal muscle glycogen contents (145,147). Early hypoglycemia is aggravated by diminished alternative energy substrates, including reduced concentrations of fatty acids from the scant adipose tissue and decreased concentrations of lactate from the hypoglycemia. Hyperinsulinemia, increased sensitivity to insulin, or both may contribute to a greater incidence of hypoglycemia, although there are very few, if any, accurate measures of insulin sensitivity at different times and among different conditions in SGA infants to support such assumptions (142). SGA infants also demonstrate decreased gluconeogenesis (149), and resolution of persistent hypoglycemia is coincident with improved capacity for, and rates of, gluconeogenesis.

Deficient counterregulatory hormones also contribute to the pathogenesis of hypoglycemia in SGA infants (150). Catecholamine release is deficient in these neonates during periods of hypoglycemia. Although basal glucagon levels may be elevated, exogenous administration of glucagon fails to enhance glycemia because of the decreased hepatic glycogen stores.

Fasting hypoglycemia is now less common in SGA infants as conventional nutritional treatment now involves earlier enteral and intravenous feeding and a more liberal use of intravenous glucose (139). All SGA infants should

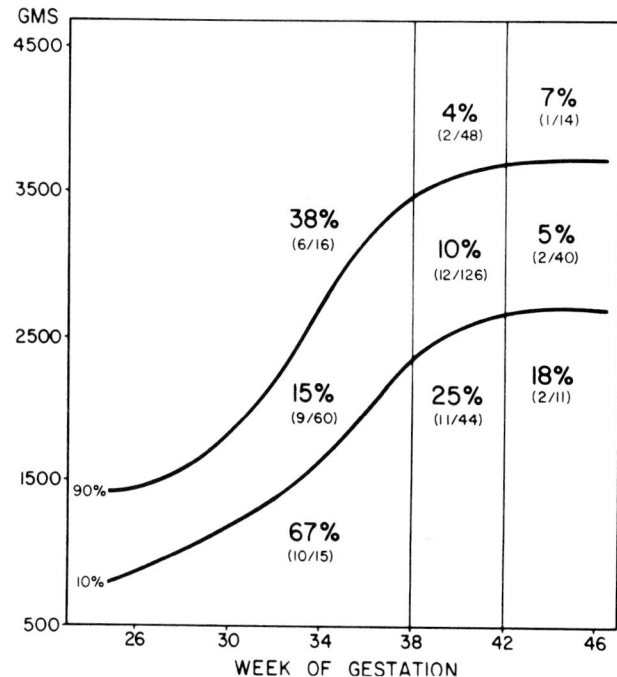

Figure 26-16 Incidence of hypoglycemia prior to first feeding (blood glucose less than 30 mg/dL) among large-for-gestational-age, average-for-gestational-age, and small-for-gestational-age (SGA) infants, demonstrating the much greater incidence of early hypoglycemia among SGA infants at all gestational ages. From Lubchenco LO, Bard H. Incidence of hypoglycemia in newborn infants classified by birth weight and gestational age. *Pediatrics* 1971;47:831, with permission.

have early and frequent measurements of blood or plasma glucose concentrations. Blood glucose concentrations should be kept at greater than 50 mg/dL. Early enteral feeding usually can prevent hypoglycemia. In less mature infants or those who have other clinical problems, intravenous glucose should be started at 4 to 8 mg/min/kg as soon after birth as possible—preferably by 30 minutes of age. This initial infusion rate should be adjusted in response to measurements of blood glucose concentration every 30 to 60 minutes until these values are consistently greater than 50 mg/dL. Less frequently repeated measurements should be continued until the infant is tolerating reasonably full enteral feedings. Infants with severe hypoglycemia (less than 20 mg/dL) that is persistent for more than 10 to 30 minutes, with coma and seizures, should be treated immediately with an intravenous "minibolus" of 10% dextrose in water at 200 mg/kg (2 mL/kg), followed by a glucose infusion of 10% dextrose in water at 4 to 8 mg/min/kg. Glucose concentrations should be measured at least every 30 minutes until concentrations are consistently above 45 mg/dL for blood or above 50 mg/dL plasma (or serum). Infants at greatest risk of having severe hypoglycemia are those who have been asphyxiated and those who are the thinnest according to the Ponderal index, representing those infants with the least amount of body glycogen content. Similarly, breast-fed twins who are not supplemented with a carbohydrate source are at risk, particularly the smaller twin, and they should be monitored carefully.

Hyperglycemia

Very preterm SGA infants have developmentally low insulin secretion rates and plasma insulin concentrations, which may underlie the relatively common problem of hyperglycemia in ELBW SGA infants (151). Unnecessarily high rates of glucose infusion (greater than 14 mg/min/kg) also contribute to this hyperglycemia (152). Higher concentrations of counterregulatory hormones, such as epinephrine, glucagon, and cortisol, also may contribute, although there is only limited evidence to support this commonly held assumption. In contrast, administration of insulin to even preterm SGA infants usually produces prompt decreases in glucose concentration, indicating at least normal and probably greater than normal insulin sensitivity (153).

Lipid Metabolism

SGA infants also have lower plasma free fatty acid levels than normally grown infants. Fasting blood glucose levels in SGA infants directly correlate with plasma free fatty acid and ketone body levels. Additionally, once fed, SGA infants have a deficient utilization of intravenous triglycerides. After the intravenous administration of triglyceride emulsion, SGA infants have high free fatty acid and triglyceride levels, but ketone body formation is attenuated (154,155). These observations indicate that the utilization and oxidation of free fatty acids and triglycerides are diminished in SGA neonates. Free fatty acid oxidation is important because it spares peripheral tissue use of glucose, whereas the hepatic oxidation of free fatty acids may contribute the reducing equivalents and energy required for hepatic gluconeogenesis. Deficient provision or oxidation of fatty acids may be partly responsible for the development of fasting hypoglycemia in these infants.

Energy Metabolism

When nursed in a neutral thermal environment, SGA infants demonstrate the usual decline of the respiratory quotient after birth, representing a shift toward free fatty acid oxidation. During the first 12 hours after birth, basal oxygen consumption may be diminished in SGA neonates. Similar observations have been recorded in utero among spontaneously SGA fetal lambs, indicating a deficiency of potentially oxidizable substrates in both situations. Supporting this hypothesis is the marked increment of oxygen consumption that occurs in well-fed SGA infants (156), similar to the increase in energy production after nutritional rehabilitation of infants with marasmic kwashiorkor. The increment of oxygen consumption after fetal or infantile malnutrition represents the energy cost of growth. Partly because of enhanced caloric intake, and because metabolic rate and oxygen consumption are related more to gestational age than birth weight, SGA infants have a higher oxygen consumption rate and a higher rate of total energy expenditure (primarily as a result of increased rest-

ing energy expenditure) than less mature neonates (155). This also reflects an increase in cell number relative to total mass and greater heat production in response to increased heat loss. Although some nutritional balance studies of preterm SGA infants have demonstrated an increase of fecal fat and protein loss, more recent studies indicate adequate digestion of nutrients and percent nutrient retention of metabolizable nutrient intake. Thus, these infants can achieve normal, and occasionally faster, rates of growth compared with preterm AGA infants.

Those SGA infants who, because of chromosomal or infectious insults early in gestation, cannot increase their growth rate do not demonstrate increased rates of oxygen consumption after appropriate caloric intake.

Amino Acid and Protein Metabolism

SGA infants are particularly deficient in muscle mass. Improving nutrition of skeletal muscle, and total body protein, is a priority in these infants. There is conflicting information from a limited number of studies, however, about how well SGA infants tolerate aggressive amino acid and protein nutrition. ELBW and VLBW SGA infants have higher rates of protein loss in stools, and of lipids (141), with 11% to 14% lower rates of absorption. This may be partly compensated for by higher intakes, which can normalize metabolizable protein intakes. Further, although growth rate may be increased in SGA infants by increased intake of protein and nonprotein calories, specific evidence for this comes largely from preterm infants, some of whom were AGA and some SGA (157). Also, animal studies show more limited pancreatic development and intestinal size in SGA offspring (158,159), which may limit feeding tolerance, protein digestion, and the production of insulin.

Some studies have shown that amino acid turnover rates are higher in SGA LBW infants (160), but other studies show no difference (161,162). SGA infants may be more energy efficient in protein synthesis (162). This could explain faster rates of growth in SGA vs. AGA infants of the same gestational age, who are fed the same diet (156,157). Thus, SGA infants possibly may tolerate higher protein intake, but the benefit of increased intake is not clear (157).

Nutritional Problems and Management

In fetal sheep that are acutely glucose deficient, amino acids are used for oxidation and for glucose production (163). With chronic glucose deficiency, protein breakdown remains increased and IUGR develops, but amino acids are not used for glucose production or oxidation more than normally (164). It is not clear if human infants born following similar patterns of IUGR and nutrient deficiency will have similar patterns of metabolism after birth, nor is it known what types and amounts of nutrients are best fed to such infants to restore normal metabolism and to reestablish normal rates of growth as quickly as possible. A rapid rate of glucose supply can lead to marked hyperglycemia, especially in the ELBW preterm SGA infant. On the other hand, amino acid intolerance is not exaggerated in SGA infants, despite some earlier evidence that amino acids are not used as readily for gluconeogenesis. If insulin and IGF-I are deficient in these infants, one would also expect lower anabolic rates until glucose and amino acid supplies and concentrations, and production rates of these growth factors, are restored. Similar issues may apply to lipid tolerance. Such considerations have prompted some reluctance to feed the SGA infant as aggressively as their deprived nutritional state would indicate, but large-scale, rigorous trials of different rates and amounts of nutrition to such infants have not been conducted. Such trials are needed to determine whether these infants will tolerate more aggressive feeding and whether this will result, safely, in improved nutritional rehabilitation, growth, and perhaps, neurodevelopmental outcome.

Temperature Regulation

Impaired placental function leading to ineffective heat elimination from the SGA fetus may result in a higher than normal temperature in the infant at birth (150,153). A normal increase in nonshivering thermogenesis is seen in these infants because brown fat is available (165,166). However, depletion of brown fat may occur more readily if exposure to cold is prolonged (167). In utero stress that depletes catecholamine stores can contribute to a failure of brown fat to produce heat. Compared with term infants, SGA infants have a narrow thermoneutral range. Heat production cannot match the rate of heat loss with continued cold stress. The rapid heat loss as a result of the large head-to-body ratio and increased surface area seen in all infants is exaggerated in the SGA infant. Heat is also lost more quickly through a thin layer of subcutaneous fat insulation (165,167). Because they are gestationally more mature than their preterm peers, SGA infants do have a more generous thermoneutral range for weight and are better able to maintain the increased metabolic rate necessary to increase heat production (168). Also, SGA infants of more than 30 weeks of gestation may have increased skin maturity and less evaporative heat loss than AGA infants of comparable weight (169), indicating that thermal neutral environments should be based on gestational age and not weight alone (170). Heat production may be impaired by concurrent conditions of hypoglycemia and hypoxia seen commonly in these patients. The normal response to cold involves increased muscular activity and catecholamine (norepinephrine) release. Central nervous system depression may prevent this normal response to cold (165).

During the first few hours of life, oxygen consumption and heat production may be less than anticipated as a result of decreased available substrate. Fewer fatty acids are available for oxidation. Later, as nutritional support is provided, the infant may have higher than expected oxygen consumption. Brain oxygen requirements are high, and in the SGA infant brain tissue represents a large proportion of body weight. Limited availability of glucose in utero limits metabolic rate. After delivery, as glucose substrate is provided, the brain increases its metabolic rate and oxygen consumption. Based on brain size, increased rates of oxygen consumption are appropriate in the SGA infant (171). It is critical, therefore, that the SGA infant be resuscitated and nursed in a thermoneutral environment. The newborn should be placed immediately under a radiant warmer and dried well. A prewarmed hat will minimize excessive heat loss from the head. A flexed posture decreases exposed surface area and may slow heat dissipation.

Current and future studies of the value of selective brain cooling of infants suffering perinatal hypoxic–ischemic encephalopathy may indicate an advantage for this unique approach in SGA infants as well.

Polycythemia–Hyperviscosity Syndrome

SGA infants manifest an increased incidence of polycythemia (172). Increased red blood cell volume is likely related to chronic in utero hypoxia leading to increased erythropoiesis (173,174). Maternal–fetal transfusion may occur chronically with fetal hypoxia or more acutely with episodes of fetal distress. Even when not polycythemic (venous hematocrit greater than 60), SGA infants have higher than normal hematocrit (174). Approximately half of all term SGA infants have a central hematocrit above 60% and about 17% of term SGA infants have a central hematocrit above 65% in contrast to only about 5% in AGA term infants (175,176). The plasma volume of SGA infants immediately after birth averages 52 mL/kg, as opposed to 43 mL/kg in AGA infants. Once equilibrated at 12 hours of life, the plasma volume becomes equivalent in the two groups. In addition to an enhanced plasma space, the circulating red blood cell mass is expanded.

Viscosity is directly related to venous hematocrit, and increased viscosity interferes with normal tissue perfusion. Although the incidence of hyperviscosity is about 5% in the general population, it is seen much more frequently (18%) in SGA infants (175). In these cases, polycythemia is the most likely etiology of hyperviscosity. Most polycythemic infants remain asymptomatic, but SGA infants are at greater risk of symptoms and clinical consequence (176). Interestingly, male SGA infants are at highest risk. Polycythemia contributes to hypoglycemia and hypoxia. Altered viscosity interferes with neonatal hemodynamics and results in abnormal postnatal cardiopulmonary and metabolic adaptation. There is also an increased risk of necrotizing enterocolitis. In addition to correcting hypoxia and hypoglycemia in these infants, partial volume exchange transfusion should be considered to lower hematocrit and minimize the risks of polycythemia and hyperviscosity.

Immune Function and Infectious Disease Risk

Immunologic function of SGA infants may be depressed at birth and may persist into childhood, as in older infants with postnatal onset of malnutrition (177). Deficiencies have been demonstrated in lymphocyte number and function, which include decreased spontaneous mitogenesis and reduced response to phytohemagglutinin. Similarly, these infants tend to have lower immunoglobulin levels during infancy and demonstrate an attenuated antibody response to oral polio vaccine.

Miscellaneous Problems

At birth, cord prealbumin and bone mineral content are low in term SGA infants (178). Calcium and iron stores may be low as a result of chronic decreased placental blood flow and insufficient nutrient supply. Significant hypocalcemia can occur after stressful birth complicated by acidosis. Thrombocytopenia, neutropenia, prolonged thrombin and partial thromboplastin times, and elevated fibrin degradation products are also problems among SGA infants (179–181). Sudden infant death syndrome may be more common after IUGR. Inguinal hernias also disproportionally follow preterm IUGR.

OUTCOMES AND LONG-TERM CONSEQUENCES OF SMALL-FOR-GESTATIONAL-AGE INFANTS

Hospitalization

At term, SGA infants are admitted more frequently to the intensive care unit and have longer hospital stays than their AGA counterparts. Even among term infants well enough to avoid neonatal intensive care unit admission as newborns, the incidence of readmission to hospital during the first year is significantly increased for SGA infants. Neurologic disorders and other morbidities requiring follow-up and hospitalization are more frequent among IUGR infants, occurring 5 to 10 times more often than among AGA infants. SGA infants also are more likely to be hospitalized for serious respiratory infections, especially if the mother smoked cigarettes at the time of conception and at other times.

Growth and Developmental Outcome

Most studies of normal and restricted fetal growth and development support the concept that critical windows of time are present in human development during which normal growth of certain tissues (e.g., fat, muscle, bone) or organs (pancreas, brain) must occur. Insults at such times limit growth and can program persistent, even lifelong failures in growth and development (182). In rats, for example, undernutrition at a vulnerable period of brain development permanently decreases brain size, brain cell number, normal behavioral development, learning, and memory (183,184). Permanent deficits may result if growth failure occurs during these critical periods (185).

SGA infants are a heterogeneous group of babies with the potential for a variety of outcomes. Some are small from genetic or familial causes and therefore may be expected to achieve their full growth potential and have normal neurodevelopment (186). Others have specific chromosomal errors or injury from infections, which are likely to result in severe and unrecoverable failure of growth and development. Most have a less defined reason for abnormal in utero growth. The infant with symmetric growth restriction may have little chance for postnatal catch-up growth after an early, global disruption of growth. However, a neonate who had normal growth in early gestation, but developed growth restriction from limited nutrient availability in later gestation later, has a reasonable potential for catch-up growth and normal development.

Studies of growth-restricted infants have been plagued by methodologic problems. Many early studies included all small infants without adequate distinction between those born at different gestational ages or those with limited familial or genetic growth potential. Infants with obvious chromosomal abnormalities and evidence of congenital infection also were included. Only relatively recently have studies of outcome of IUGR and SGA infants included in the study design the recognition that the etiology of small size at birth carries great prognostic value. More recent studies of this subject also have been limited by uncontrolled confounding factors. An infant's perinatal morbidity, including inborn or outborn (requiring transport) status, presence of abnormal umbilical artery waveforms (121), and a variety of neonatal complications, such as asphyxia, hypoglycemia, polycythemia, and cold stress, can impact on ultimate outcome (185–187). Multiple gestation and even birth order can influence future growth potential.

Socioeconomic status and environment are among the most important, but difficult to control for, variables affecting the growth and development of SGA infants. Several studies have attempted to differentiate between the influences of biologic and environmental variables (187, 188). There are strong associations between socioeconomic factors and the cognitive development and school performance of growth-restricted children.

Postnatal Physical Growth of Small-for-Gestational-Age Infants

Although measurements of weight, length (or height), and head circumference are standardized and reproducible, many authors have given more attention to one measurement over another or have been more concerned with a specific interrelationship of measurements, such as the Ponderal index (189). In general, SGA infants continue to be smaller and relatively underweight for age as they grow older, even through adolescence and early adulthood (Fig. 26-17). These infants more commonly have short stature as teenagers and young adults, indicating lifelong growth deficit.

Differences in patterns of early growth have been observed in SGA infants. Normal infants experience a period of rapid growth during the first 3 years of life. Adult size correlates with the individual growth curve after this time. Moderately affected SGA infants who had primarily a reduction in weight in the third trimester of gestation

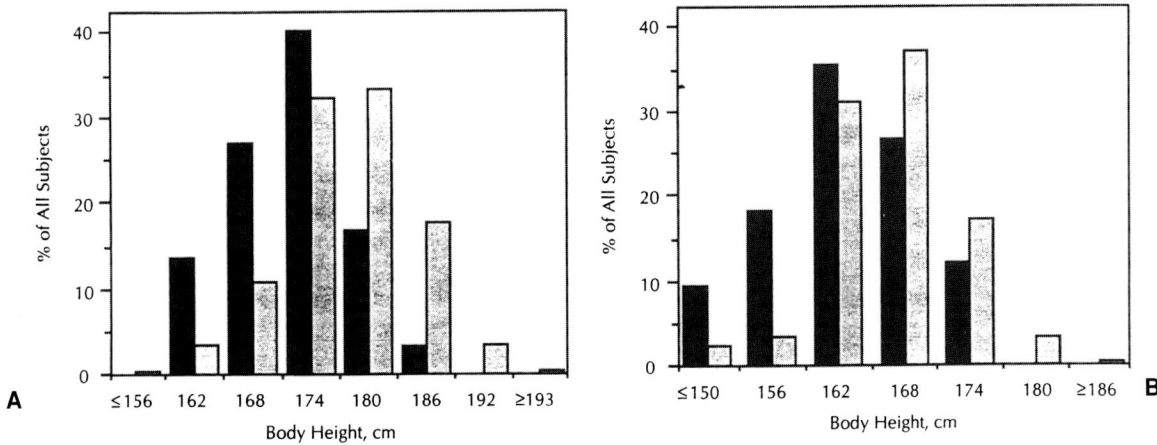

Figure 26-17 Distribution of height at age 17 years in 30 boys (**A**) and 34 girls (**B**) born small for gestational age (solid bars) and their peers who were born appropriate for gestational age (shaded bars). From Paz I, Seidman DS, Danon YL et al. Are children born small for gestational age at increased risk of short stature? *AM J Dis Child* 1993;147:337.

follow the same pattern of normal neonatal and infant growth, but tend to have an accelerated velocity of growth during the first 6 months (189). This catch-up growth occurs primarily from birth to 6 months of age, with some infants continuing an accelerated rate of growth for the first year. A few of these infants will achieve a normal growth percentile and thereafter have a growth rate similar to appropriately grown children (189,190). Head circumference parallels growth in length during catch-up and sustained growth periods. After the first year, no difference in the rate of growth has been noted (189,190).

Ultimate weight and height are less in SGA children when compared to their normal siblings (189,190). In one study of 4- to 6-year-old children (189), 45% of siblings were at or above the 50th percentile for weight and height, whereas only 12% of their SGA siblings achieved the 50th percentile. Interestingly, a subgroup of severely growth-restricted infants (less than 40% of expected birth weight) compared to less affected SGA peers showed no difference in weight or height at 6 months of age, adding concern for the growth outcome of even modest degrees of IUGR. Former SGA infants have been shown to have no delay in bone age, puberty, or sexual maturation at adolescence, although they were shorter, lighter, and had smaller heads. Muscle mass between the two groups was similar, but adipose tissue development was less in the SGA group (191).

Because head size correlates with brain size, volume, weight, and cellularity, head growth at the time of birth and the degree of catch-up growth thereafter are prognostic of future neurodevelopment. Deficient fetal head growth recognized by relative microcephaly at birth, whether at term or preterm, is felt to be a poor prognostic indicator, as it reflects the severity and duration of *in utero* growth failure. A lack of head sparing and small occipital-frontal circumference (OFC) is associated with poor neurologic and psychological outcome (192). Head size, if catch-up head growth has not occurred by 8 months of age, is a predictor

of lower intelligence test scores at 3 years of age (193). This correlation seems to be independent of environmental or other risks. Decreased head size when compared to siblings carries significant risks of deficient mental and motor function (188).

Postnatal Neurodevelopmental Outcome of Full-Term, Small-for-Gestational-Age Infants

Neurologic disorders and other morbidities are more frequent in SGA infants as a group, occurring 5 to 10 times more often than in AGA infants. However, in full-term, mild-to-moderately SGA infants who have normal brain growth, no hypoxic-ischemic injury, and good environmental support, IUGR may have little impact on behavior or mental ability in adolescence or adulthood (185,186, 192). There is no increased incidence of major handicap (189,191,193,194) and no increased risk of severe neurologic morbidity (192) in term infants born small for gestational age. Cerebral palsy is infrequent in this group (194). Routine neurologic examination is usually normal (191).

Although the absence of gross neurologic outcome in the term SGA infant is reassuring, evidence of minimal brain dysfunction among these children continues to be of concern. Many studies have revealed signs of minor brain damage, including hyperactivity, short attention span, learning problems, poor fine motor coordination, and hyperreflexia. An increased number of diffuse abnormalities are seen on electroencephalogram (194). In one study, 30% of term SGA children at 5 years of age had speech problems, which included a delayed onset of speech, immature vocabulary with persistent infantile articulation, and poor receptive and expressive abilities for age (194). In contrast, only 1.5% of the general population and about 5% of their siblings had speech difficulties.

Former term SGA infants more frequently have substandard school performance and display subtle neurologic and

TABLE 26-12

FETAL, NEONATAL/INFANCY, AND ADULT DISORDERS THAT MIGHT RESULT FROM FETAL PROGRAMMING AS A CONSEQUENCE OF FETAL UNDERNUTRITION AT DIFFERENT STATES OF GESTATION[a,b]

	Trimester of Pregnancy		
	First	**Second**	**Third**
Consequences	Low growth trajectory	Disturbed fetal–placental	Brain growth sustained, but not relationships body
Fetal adaptation	Down regulation of fetal growth	Insulin resistance	Growth factor(s) resistance/deficiency
Anthropometry	Symmetric	Mixed	Asymmetric
Infant growth	Reduced infant growth	Reduced infant growth	Catch-up growth possible
Adult life	Increased BP	Increased BP, NIDDM,	Increased BP, NIDDM, ischemic heart disease hypercholesterolemia, ischemic heart disease

[a] BP, blood pressure; NIDDM, noninsulin-dependent diabetes mellitus.
[b] From Barker D. *Mothers, babies, and diseases later in life*. London: BMJ Books, 1994, with permission.

behavioral problems despite a normal IQ. Sensori-motor abilities are frequently affected. Overall there is no correlation between the severity of growth restriction and learning deficit, although those with poor early brain growth in infancy have more problems (193). Measures of cognition at 4 to 6 years of age correlate well with testing at adolescence. This suggests that cognitive potential is reached early, with little change later. It seems likely that environmental and socioeconomic factors play a significant role in the learning deficiencies seen in these children (188).

At adolescence, trends toward lower test scores, especially in mathematics, and an increased incidence of learning disabilities have been noted (191,194). There also is a trend toward slower alternating movements on physical examination. Most believe, however, that the cognitive and academic differences in these children are small and do not significantly affect school performance or ultimate intellectual ability.

Postnatal Neurodevelopmental Outcome in Preterm, Small-for-Gestational-Age Infants

The prognosis for preterm SGA infants is less clear and is easily confounded by other problems of preterm birth. In general, subnormal intellectual outcomes are more common among preterm SGA infants than term SGA infants. Some authors have shown that those infants suffering the dual insults of preterm birth and growth restriction are at higher risk of neurodevelopmental deficit (195,196). Among extremely preterm infants, gestational age, and not growth status, has been the most significant predictor of intellectual outcome (197). By 3 years of age, social and environmental factors play an increasing role and may impact on development in either a positive or negative way (197). Socioeconomic status is independently associated with learning disabilities in these children (187).

When compared with their appropriately grown same-weight counterparts, SGA preterm infants have a lower incidence of major developmental handicaps and cerebral palsy. Specific motor deficits are more common in AGA infants (198,199). Minor neurologic abnormalities are more frequently observed in SGA infants (198). Diffuse cerebral damage as a result of hypoxia and decreased intrauterine blood flow, especially to the brain, probably accounts for the differences in expression of brain damage seen in preterm AGA and SGA children (200). Restricted growth for gestational age is associated with more cognitive disability in infants who were born preterm (199,201). The need for special education is higher and becomes apparent at an earlier age in these preterm SGA infants when they reach school age (200).

Possible Adult Disorders Resulting from Intrauterine Growth Restriction

Recent epidemiologic evidence indicates that obesity, insulin resistance, diabetes, and cardiovascular disease are more common among adults who were smaller than normal at birth and very likely SGA secondary to IUGR, particularly those who had a high placental-to-fetal-weight ratio (202). A variety of animal studies support this concept, including the greater incidence of obesity, glucose intolerance, plasma lipid abnormalities, and hypertension in offspring whose mothers were fed a low-protein diet during pregnancy (203–206). These examples indicate that certain adult pathologies may be unavoidable consequences of environmentally imposed conditions, such as severe and prolonged fetal undernutrition, which lead to fetal growth restriction to ensure fetal survival. These conditions may represent an example of "programming," in which an insult, when applied at a critical or sensitive stage in development, may result in a lasting, even lifelong, effect on the structure or function of the organism (183). IUGR, therefore, is increasingly seen as an adaptive physiologic process, even though it can produce adverse fetal, neonatal, and potentially adult consequences (Table 26-12) (207). Mechanisms responsible for these later-life morbidities in adults, who were growth restricted in utero, are not yet established. There is some evidence of diminished pancreatic growth and development, which might becomes manifest in later life as pancreatic insufficiency when the adult starts and then continues eating a diet rich in simple carbohydrates and lipids. Peripheral insulin resistance may develop in the same way, and hypertension in adulthood may be the result of altered adrenal development in response to IUGR.

REFERENCES

1. Lubchenco LO, Searls DT, Brazie JV. Neonatal mortality rate: relationship to birth weight and gestational age. *J Pediatr* 1972; 81:814.
2. Lubchenco LO. *The high risk infant.* Philadelphia: WB Saunders, 1976.
3. Chard T, Costeloe K, Leaf A. Evidence of growth retardation in neonates of apparently normal weight. *Eur J Obstet Gynecol Reprod Endocrinol* 1992;45:59.
4. Chard T, Yoong A, Macintosh M. The myth of fetal growth retardation at term. *Br J Obstet Gynaecol* 1993;100:1076.
5. Wark L, Malcolm LA. Growth and development of the Lumi child in the Sepik district of New Guinea. *Med J Aust* 1969;2:129.
6. Ashcroft MT, Buchanan IC, Lovell HG, et al. Growth of infants and preschool children in St. Christopher-Nevis-Anguilla West Indies. *Am J Clin Nutr* 1966;19:37.
7. Evans MI, Mukherjee AB, Schulman JD. Animal models of intrauterine growth retardation. *Obstet Gynecol Surv* 1983;38:183.
8. Simmons RA, Gounis AS, Bangalore SA, et al. Intrauterine growth retardation: fetal glucose transport is diminished in lung but spared in brain. *Pediatr Res* 1992;32:59.
9. Sabbagha RE. Intrauterine growth retardation. In: Sabbagha RE, ed. *Ultrasound applied to obstetrics and gynecology.* Philadelphia: JB Lippincott, 1987:112.
10. McGiven J, Pastor Angladi A. Regulatory and molecular aspects of mammalian amino acids transport. *Biochem J* 1993;299:321.
11. Hill RDG. Insulin as a growth factor. *Pediatr Res* 1985;19:879.
12. Sparks JW, Ross JR, Cetin I. Intrauterine growth and nutrition. In: Polin RA, Fox WW, eds. *Fetal and neonatal physiology,* 2nd ed. Philadelphia: WB Saunders, 1998:267.
13. Lubchenco LO, Hansman C, Boyd E. Intrauterine growth in length and head circumference as estimated from live births at gestational ages from 26 to 42 weeks. *Pediatrics* 1966;37:403.
14. Kramer MS. Intrauterine growth and gestational duration determinants. *Pediatrics* 1987;80:502.
15. Virgi SK, Cottington E. Risk factors associated with preterm deliveries among racial groups in a national sample of married mothers. *J Perinatol* 1991;8:347.
16. Klebanoff MA, Schulsinger C, Mednick BR, et al. Preterm and small-for-gestational-age birth across generations. *Am J Obstet Gynecol* 1997;176:521.
17. Abrams B, Newman V. Small-for-gestational-age birth: maternal predictors and comparison with risk factors of spontaneous preterm delivery in the same cohort. *Am J Obstet Gynecol* 1991;164:785.
18. Freemark M, Comer M. The role of placental lactogen in the regulation of fetal metabolism and growth. *J Pediatr Gastroenterol Nutr* 1989;8:281.
19. Lacroix MC, Devinov E, Servely JL, et al. Expression of the growth hormone gene in ovine placenta: detection and cellular localization of the protein. *Endocrinology* 1996;137:4886.
20. Gluckman PD. The endocrine regulation of fetal growth in late gestation—the role of insulin like growth factors. *J Clin Endocrinol Metab* 1995;80:1047.
21. Gibbs RS, Eschenbach DA. Use of antibiotics to prevent preterm birth. *Am J Obstet Gynecol* 1997;177:375.
22. Salas SP, Altermatt F, Campos M, et al. Effects of long-term nitric oxide synthesis inhibition on plasma volume expansion and fetal growth in the pregnant rat. *Hypertension* 1995;26:1019.
23. Krebs C, Macara LM, Leiser R, et al. Intrauterine growth restriction with absent end-diastolic flow velocity in the umbilical artery is associated with maldevelopment of the placental terminal villous tree. *Am J Obstet Gynecol* 1996;175:1534.
24. Nicolaides KH, Economides DL, Soothill PW. Blood gases, pH, and lactate in appropriate- and small-for-gestational-age fetuses. *Am J Obstet Gynecol* 1989;161:996.
25. Scholl TO, Hediger ML, Schall JO, et al. Maternal growth during pregnancy and the competition for nutrients. *Am J Clin Nutr* 1994;60:183.
26. Wallace JM, Aitken RP, Cheyne MA. Nutrient partitioning and fetal growth in rapidly growing adolescent ewes. *J Reprod Fertil* 1996;107:183.
27. Lucas A, Gore SM, Cole TJ, et al. A multicentre trial on feeding low birthweight infants: effects of diet on early growth. *Arch Dis Child* 1984;59:722.
28. Davis JA, Dobbing J. *Scientific foundations of paediatrics.* Philadelphia: WB Saunders, 1974.
29. Ounsted M, Ounsted C. On fetal growth rate. *Clinics in developmental medicine* no. 46. Philadelphia: JB Lippincott, 1973.
30. Ziegler EE, O'Donnell AM, Nelson SE, et al. Body composition of the reference fetus. *Growth* 1976;40:329.
31. Nimrod CA. The biology of normal and deviant fetal growth. In: Reece EA, Hobbins JC, Mahoney MJ, et al, eds. *Medicine of the fetus & mother.* Philadelphia: JB Lippincott, 1992:285.
32. Widdowson EM. Changes in body proportions and composition during growth. In: Davis JA, Dobbing J, eds. *Scientific foundations of paediatrics.* Philadelphia: WB Saunders, 1974:155.
33. Lapillonne A, Brailon P, Claris O, et al. Body composition in appropriate and in small for gestational age infants. *Acta Paediatr* 1997;86:196.
34. Shelley HJ. Glycogen reserves and their changes at birth. *Br Med Bull* 1961;17:137.
35. Philipps AF. Carbohydrate metabolism of the fetus. In: Polin RA, Fox WW, eds. *Fetal and neonatal physiology,* 2nd ed. Philadelphia: WB Saunders, 1998:560.
36. Hay WW Jr. Glucose metabolism in the fetal-placental unit. In: Cowett RM, ed. *Principles of perinatal-neonatal metabolism,* 2nd ed. New York: Springer-Verlag, 1998:337.
37. Hay WW Jr. Nutrition and development of the fetus: carbohydrate and lipid metabolism. In: Walker WA, Watkins JB, eds. *Nutrition in pediatrics,* 2nd ed. Hamilton: BC Decker, 1996:364.
38. Sparks JW, Girard J, Battaglia FC. An estimate of the caloric requirements of the human fetus. *Biol Neonate* 1980;38:113.
39. Milner RDG, Gluckman PD. Regulation of intrauterine growth. In: Gluckman PD, Heymann MA, eds. *Pediatrics & perinatology: the scientific basis,* 2nd ed. London: Arnold, 1993:284.
40. Carver TD, Quick AN Jr, Teng CC, et al. Leucine metabolism in chronically hypoglycemia, hypoinsulinemic growth restricted fetal sheep. *Am J Physiol* 1997;272:E107.
41. Yau K-IT, Chang M-H. Growth and body composition of preterm, small for gestational age infants at a postmenstrual age of 37–40 weeks. *Early Hum Dev* 1993;33:117.
42. Cliver SP, Goldenberg RL, Cutter GR, et al. The effect of cigarette smoking on neonatal anthropometric measurements. *Obstet Gynecol* 1995;85:635.
43. Goldenberg RL, Cliver SP, Cutter GR, et al. Blood pressure, growth retardation, and preterm delivery. *Int J Technol Assess Health Care* 1992;8:82.
44. Goldenberg RL, Tamura T, Neggers Y, et al. The effect of zinc supplementation on pregnancy outcome. *JAMA* 1995;274:463.
45. Goldenberg RL, Hauth JC, DuBard MD, et al. Fetal growth in women using low-dose aspirin for the prevention of preeclampsia: effect of maternal size. *J Matern Fetal Med* 1995;4:218.
46. Battaglia FC, Meschia G. *An introduction to fetal physiology.* Orlando: Academic Press, 1986.
47. Lumey LH. Decreased birthweights in infants after maternal in utero exposure to the Dutch famine of 1944–1945. *Paediatr Perinat Epidemiol* 1992;6:240.
48. Antonov AM. Children born during the siege of Leningrad in 1942. *J Pediatr* 1947;30:250.
49. Stein Z, Susser M, Rush D. Prenatal nutrition and birth weight: experiments and quasi-experiments in the past decade. *J Reprod Med* 1978;21:287.

50. Hickey CA, Cliver SP, Goldenberg RL, et al. Prenatal weight gain, term birth weight, and fetal growth retardation among high-risk multiparous black and white women. *Obstet Gynecol* 1993;81:529.

51. Rush D, Stein Z, Susser M. A randomized controlled trial of prenatal nutritional supplementation in New York City. *Pediatrics* 1980;68:683.

52. Sibai B, Anderson GD. Pregnancy outcome of intensive therapy in severe hypertension in first trimester. *Obstet Gynecol* 1986;67:517.

53. Novy MJ, Peterson EN, Metcalfe J. Respiratory characteristics of maternal and fetal blood in cyanotic congenital heart disease. *Am J Obstet Gynecol* 1968;100:821.

54. Lichty JA, Ting RY, Bruns PD, et al. Studies of babies born at high altitude. *Am J Dis Child* 1957;93:666.

55. Brown AK, Sleeper LA, Pegelow CH, et al. The influence of infant and maternal sickle cell disease on birth outcome and neonatal course. *Arch Pediatr Adolesc Med* 1994;148:1156.

56. Goldenberg RL, Davis RO, Nelson KG. Intrauterine growth retardation. In: Merkatz IR, Thompson JE, Mullen PD, et al, eds. *New perspectives on prenatal care.* New York: Elsevier, 1990:461.

57. Abel EL. Consumption of alcohol during pregnancy: a review of effects on growth and development of offspring. *Hum Biol* 1982;54:421.

58. Woods JR, Plessinger MA, Clark KE. Effect of cocaine on uterine blood flow and fetal oxygenation. *JAMA* 1986;257:957.

59. Molteni RA, Stys SJ, Battaglia FC. Relationship of fetal and placental weight in human beings: fetal/placental weight ratios at various gestational ages and birth weight distributions. *J Reprod Med* 1978;21:327.

60. Owens JA, Falconer J, Robinson JS. Effect of restriction of placental growth on fetal and utero-placental metabolism. *J Dev Physiol* 1987;9:225.

61. Beischer NA, Sivasamboo R, Vohra S, et al. Placental hypertrophy in severe pregnancy anaemia. *J Obstet Gynaecol Br Commonw* 1970;77:398.

62. Nylund L, Lunell NO, Lewander R, et al. Uteroplacental blood flow index in intrauterine growth retardation of fetal or maternal origin. *Br J Obstet Gynaecol* 1983;90:16.

63. Macara L, Kingdom JC, Kaufman P, et al. Structural analysis of placental terminal villi from growth-restricted pregnancies with abnormal umbilical artery Doppler waveforms. *Placenta* 1996;17:37.

64. Damsky CH, Fitzgerald ML, Fisher SJ. Distribution of extracellular matrix components and adhesion receptors are intricately modulated during first trimester cytotrophoblast differentiation along the invasive pathway, in vivo. *J Clin Invest* 1992;89:210.

65. Damsky CH, Librach C, Lim K-H, et al. Integrin switching regulates normal trophoblast invasion. *Development* 1994;120:3057.

66. Zhou Y, Damsky CH, Chiu K, et al. Preeclampsia is associated with abnormal expression of adhesion molecules by invasive cytotrophoblasts. *J Clin Invest* 1993;91:950.

67. Genbacev O, Joslin RJ, Damsky CH, et al. Hypoxia alters early gestation human cytotrophoblast differentiation/invasion in vitro and models the placental defects that occur in preeclampsia. *J Clin Invest* 1996;97:540.

68. Handwerger S. The physiology of placental lactogen in human pregnancy. *Endocr Rev* 1992;12:329.

69. Freemark M, Handwerger S. The role of placental lactogen in the regulation of fetal metabolism. *J Pediatr Gastroenterol Nutr* 1989;8:281.

70. Harding JE, Johnston BM. Nutrition and fetal growth. *Reprod Fertil Dev* 1995;7:539.

71. Thureen PJ, Trembler KA, Meschia G, et al. Placental glucose transport in heat induced fetal growth retardation. *Am J Physiol* 1992;263:R578.

72. Marconi AM, Cetin I, Davoli E, et al. An evaluation of fetal gluconeogenesis in intrauterine growth retarded pregnancies. *Metabolism* 1993;42:860.

73. Molina RD, Meschia G, Battaglia FC, et al. Gestational maturation of placental glucose transfer capacity in sheep. *Am J Physiol* 1991;61:R697.

74. Ross JC, Fennessey PV, Wilkening RB, et al. Placental transport and fetal utilization of leucine in a model of fetal growth retardation. *Am J Physiol* 1996;270:E491.

75. Milley JR. Effects of insulin on ovine fetal leucine kinetics and protein metabolism. *J Clin Invest* 1994;93:1616.

76. Townsend SF, Briggs KK, Carver TD, et al. Altered fetal liver and kidney insulin-like growth factor II mRNA in the sheep after chronic maternal glucose or nutrient deprivation. *Clin Res* 1992;40:91A.

77. Hay WW Jr. Fetal requirements and placental transfer of nitrogenous compounds. In: Polin RA, Fox WW, eds. *Fetal and neonatal physiology,* 2nd ed. Philadelphia: WB Saunders, 1998:619.

78. Milley JR. Ovine fetal leucine kinetics and protein metabolism during decreased oxygen availability. *Am J Physiol* 1998;274:E618.

79. Milley JR. Ovine fetal protein metabolism during decreased glucose delivery. *Am J Physiol* 1993;265:E525.

80. Bell AW, Kennaugh JM, Battaglia FC, et al. Metabolic and circulatory studies of the fetal lamb at mid gestation. *Am J Physiol* 1986;250:E538.

81. Fowden A. Endocrine regulation of fetal growth. *Reprod Fertil Dev* 1995;7:469.

82. Fowden AL, Hay WW Jr. The effects of pancreatectomy on the rates of glucose utilization, oxidation and production in the sheep fetus. *Q J Exp Physiol* 1988;73:973.

83. Hay WW Jr, Meznarich HK, Fowden AL. The effects of streptozotocin on rates of glucose utilization, oxidation and production in the sheep fetus. *Metabolism* 1988;38:30.

84. Sherwood WG, Chance GW, Hill DE. A new syndrome of pancreatic agenesis. The role of insulin and glucagon in cell and cell growth. *Pediatr Res* 1974;8:360.

85. Carver TD, Anderson SM, Aldoretta PW, et al. Glucose suppression of insulin secretion in chronically hyperglycemic fetal sheep. *Pediatr Res* 1995;38:754.

86. Mathews LS, Hammer RE, Behringer RR, et al. Growth enhancement of transgenic mice expressing human insulin-like growth factor I. *Endocrinology* 1988;123:2827.

87. Behringer RR, Lewin TM, Quaife CJ, et al. Expression of Insulin-like growth factor I stimulates normal somatic growth in growth hormone-deficient transgenic mice. *Endocrinology* 1990;127:1033.

88. D'Ercole AJ, Dai Z, Xing Y, et al. Brain growth retardation due to the expression of human insulin like growth factor binding protein 1 (IGFBP-1) in transgenic mice: an in vivo model for the analysis of IGF function in the brain. *Dev Brain Res* 1994;82:213.

89. Ye P, Carson J, D'Ercole AJ. In vivo actions of insulin-like growth factor-I (IGF-I) on brain myelination: studies of IGF-I and IGF binding protein-1 (IGFBP-1) transgenic mice. *J Neurosci* 1995;15:7344.

90. Delhanty PJD, Han VKM. The expression of insulin-like growth factor (IGF)-binding protein-2 and IGF-II genes in the tissues of the developing ovine fetus. *Endocrinology* 1993;132:41.

91. Wood TL, Rogler L, Streck RD, et al. Targeted disruption of IGFBP-2 gene. *Growth Regul* 1993;3:3.

92. Pintar JE, Wood TL, Streck RD, et al. Expression of IGF-II, the IGF-II/mannose-6-phosphate receptor and IGFBP-2 during rat embryogenesis. *Adv Exp Med Biol* 1991;293:325.

93. Wood TL, Streck RD, Pintar JE. Expression of the IGFBP-2 gene in post-implantation rat embryos. *Development* 1992;114:59.

94. Crystal RA, Giduice LC. Insulin-like growth factor binding protein (IGFBP) profiles in human fetal cord sera: ontogeny during gestation and differences in newborns with intrauterine growth retardation (IUGR) and large for gestational age (LGA) newborns. In: Spencer EM, ed. *Modern concepts of insulin-like growth factors.* New York: Elsevier, 1991:395.

95. Brenneman DE, Eiden LE. Vasoactive intestinal peptide and electrical activity influence neuronal survival. *Proc Natl Acad Sci U S A* 1986;83:1159.

96. Hill JM, Agoston DV, Gressens P, et al. Distribution of VIP mRNA and two distinct VIP binding sites in the developing brain; relation to ontogenic evens. *J Comp Neurol* 1994;342:186.

97. Gressens P, Hill JM, Gozes I, et al. Growth factor function of vasoactive intestinal peptide in whole cultured mouse embryos. *Nature* 1993;362:155.

98. Gressens P, Hill JM, Paindaveine B, et al. Severe microcephaly induced by blockade of vasoactive intestinal peptide function in the primitive neuroepithelium of the mouse. *J Clin Invest* 1994;94:2020.

99. Hill JM, McCune SK, Alvero RJ, et al. Maternal vasoactive intestinal peptide and the regulation of embryonic growth in the rodent. *J Clin Invest* 1996;97:202.

100. Kliegman RM. Intrauterine growth retardation. In: Fanaroff A, Martin R, eds. *Neonatal-perinatal medicine,* 6th ed. St. Louis: Mosby-Year Book, 1997:203.

101. Arduini D, Rizzo G, Romanini C. The development of abnormal heart rate patterns after absent end-diastolic velocity in umbilical artery: analysis of risk factors. *Am J Obstet Gyencol* 1993; 168:43.

102. Beattie RB, Whittle MJ. Doppler and fetal growth retardation. *Arch Dis Child* 1993;69:271.

103. Hitschold T, Weiss E, Beck T. Low target birthweight or growth retardation? Umbilical Doppler flow velocity waveforms and histometric analysis of fetoplacental vascular tree. *Am J Obstet Gynecol* 1993;168:1260.

104. Karsdorp VHM, vanVugt JMG, vanGeijn HP, et al. Clinical significance of absent or reversed end-diastolic velocity waveforms in umbilical artery. *Lancet* 1994;344:1664.

105. Noordam MJ, Heydanus R, Hop WC, et al. Doppler colour flow imaging of fetal intracerebral arteries and umbilical artery in the small for gestational age fetus. *Br J Obstet Gynaecol* 1994;101:504.

106. Valcamonico A, Danti L, Frusca T, et al. Absent end-diastolic velocity in umbilical artery: risk of neonatal morbidity and brain damage. *Am J Obstet Gynecol* 1994;170:796.

107. Marconi AM, Ferrazzi E, Cetin I, et al. *Umbilical velocimetry differentiates growth retarded fetuses at risk of acidemia.* Third Congress of the International Perinatal Doppler Society, Los Angeles, CA, 1990.

108. Cetin I, Marconi AM, Baggiani AM, et al. In vivo transplacental transport of 1-13C-glycine and 1-13C-leucine in human pregnancies. *Ital J Gastroenterol* 1992;24:8.

109. Marconi AM, Ferrazzi E, Cetin I, et al. Lactate metabolism in normal and growth retarded human fetuses. *Pediatr Res* 1990;28:652.

110. Pardi G, Cetin I, Marconi AM, et al. Diagnostic value of blood sampling in fetuses with growth retardation. *N Engl J Med* 1993;328:692.

111. Pardi G, Cetin I, Marconi AM, et al. Venous drainage of the human uterus: respiratory gas studies in normal and fetal growth-retarded pregnancies. *Am J Obstet Gynecol* 1992;166:699.

112. Pardi G, Cetin I, Marconi AM, et al. The role of fetal blood sampling in relation to fetal heart rate and Doppler velocimetry in growth retarded fetuses. *J Soc Gynecol Invest* 1993:220.

113. Richards DS. The fetal vibroacoustic stimulation test: an update. *Semin Perinatol* 1990;14:305.

114. Charlton V, Johengen M. Effects of intrauterine nutritional supplementation on fetal growth retardation. *Biol Neonate* 1985;48:125.

115. Padbury JF, Ervin MG, Polk DH. Extrapulmonary effects of antenatally administered steroids. *J Pediatr* 1996;128:167.

116. Liggins GC, Howie RN. A controlled trial of antepartum glucocorticoid treatment for the prevention of the respiratory distress syndrome in premature infants. *Pediatrics* 1972;50:515.

117. Ikegami M, Polk D, Tabor B, et al. Corticosteroid and thyrotropin-releasing hormone effects on preterm sheep lung function. *J Appl Physiol* 1991;70:2268.

118. Hay WW Jr, Catz CS, Grave GD, et al. Workshop summary: fetal growth: its regulation and disorders. *Pediatrics* 1997;99:585.

119. Battaglia FC, Battaglia C, Artini PG, et al. Maternal hyperoxygenation in the treatment of intrauterine growth retardation. *Am J Obstet Gynecol* 1992;167:430.

120. McFarland P, Pearce JM, Chamberlain GVP. Doppler ultrasound and aspirin in recognition and prevention of pregnancy-induced hypertension. *Lancet* 1990;335:1552.

121. McDonnell M, Serra-Serra V, Gaffney G, et al. Neonatal outcome after pregnancy complicated by abnormal velocity waveforms in the umbilical artery. *Arch Dis Child* 1994;70:F84.

122. Hobbins J. Morphometry of fetal growth. *Acta Paediatr Suppl* 1997;423:165.

123. Gaziano EP, Knox L, Ferrera B, et al. Is it time to reassess the risk for the growth-retarded fetus with normal Doppler velocimetry of the umbilical artery? *Am J Obstet Gynecol* 1994;170:1734.

124. Gazzolo D, Scopesi FA, Bruschettini PL, et al. Predictors of perinatal outcome in intrauterine growth retardation: a long-term study. *J Perinat Med* 1994;22:71.

125. Strong TH Jr, Hetzler G, Sarno AP, et al. Prophylactic intrapartum amnioinfusion: a randomized clinical trial. *Am J Obstet Gynecol* 1990;162:1370.

126. Morrison J, Olsen J. Weight-specific stillbirths and associated causes of death: an analysis of 765 stillbirths. *Am J Obstet Gynecol* 1985;152:975.

127. Yogman MW, Kraemer HC, Kindon D, et al. Identification of intrauterine growth retardation among low birth weight preterm infants. *J Pediatr* 1989;115:799.

128. Villar J, deOnis M, Kestler E, et al. The differential neonatal morbidity of the intrauterine growth retardation syndrome. *Am J Obstet Gynecol* 1990;163:151.

129. Frederickson WT, Brown JV. Gripping and moro responses: differences between small-for-gestational age and normal weight newborn. *Early Hum Dev* 1980;4:69.

130. Michaelis R, Schulte FS, Nolte R. Motor behavior of small for gestation age newborn infants. *J Pediatr* 1970;76:208.

131. Cruz Martinez A, Perez Conde MC, Ferrer MT. Motor conduction velocity and H-reflex in infancy and childhood. I: Study in newborns, twins and small-for-dates. *Electromyogr Clin Neurophysiol* 1977;17:493.

132. Moosa A, Dubowitz V. Assessment of gestational age in newborn infants: nerve conduction velocity vs maturity score. *Dev Med Child Neurol* 1972;14:290.

133. Schulte FJ, Michaelis R, Linke I, et al. Motor nerve conduction velocity in term, preterm and small-for-dates newborn infants. *Pediatrics* 1968;42:17.

134. Als H, Tronick E, Adamson L, et al. The behavior of the full-term but underweight newborn infant. *Dev Med Child Neurol* 1976;18:590.

135. Chiswick ML. Intrauterine growth retardation. *BMJ* 1985;291:845.

136. Wennergren M, Wennergren G, Vilbergasson G. Obstetric characteristics and neonatal performance in a four-year small for gestational age population. *Obstet Gynecol* 1988;72:615.

137. Piper JM, Xenakis EM-J, McFarland M, et al. Do growth-retarded premature infants have different rates of perinatal morbidity and mortality than appropriately grown premature infants? *Obstet Gynecol* 1996;87:169.

138. Sciscione AC, Gorman R, Callan NA. Adjustment of birth weight standards for maternal and infant characteristics improves the prediction of outcome in the small-for-gestational-age infant. *Am J Obstet Gynecol* 1996;175:544.

139. Hawdon JM, Platt MPW. Metabolic adaptation in small for gestational age infants. *Arch Dis Child* 1993;68:262.

140. Antunes JD, Geffner ME, Lippe BM, et al. Childhood hypoglycemia: differentiating hyperinsulinemic from nonhyperinsulinemic causes. *J Pediatr* 1990;116:105.

141. Chessex P, Reichman B, Verellen G, et al. Metabolic consequences of intrauterine growth retardation in very low birthweight infants. *Pediatr Res* 1984;18:709.

142. Collins J, Leonard JV. Hyperinsulinism in asphyxiated and small for dates infants with hypoglycemia. *Lancet* 1984;2:311.

143. Frazer T, Karl IE, Hillman LS, et al. Direct measurement of gluconeogenesis from [2,313C2] alanine in the human neonate. *Am J Physiol* 1981;240:615.

144. Haymond MW, Karl IE, Pagliana AS. Increased gluconeogenic substrates in the small for gestational age infant. *N Engl J Med* 1974;291:322.

145. Kliegman RM. Alterations of fasting glucose and fat metabolism in intrauterine growth-retarded newborn dogs. *Am J Physiol* 1989;256:E380.

146. LeDune M. Response to glucagon in small for dates hypoglycemic and nonhypoglycemic newborn infants. *Arch Dis Child* 1972;47:754.

147. Shelly HJ, Neligan GA. Neonatal hypoglycemia. *Br Med Bull* 1966;22:34.

148. Holtrop PC. The frequency of hypoglycemia in full-term large and small of gestational age newborns. *Am J Perinatol* 1993;10:150.

149. Williams PR, Fiser RH Jr, Sperling MA, et al. Effects of oral alanine feeding on blood glucose, plasma glucagon, and insulin concentrations in small for gestational age infants. *N Engl J Med* 1975;292:612.

150. Hawdon JM, Weddell A, Aynsley-Green A, et al. Hormonal and metabolic response to hypoglycemia in small for gestational age infants. *Arch Dis Child* 1993;68:269.

151. King RA, Smith RM, Dahlenberg GW. Long term postnatal development of insulin secretion in early premature neonates. *Early Hum Dev* 1986;13:285.

152. Cowett RM, Oh W, Pollak A, et al. Glucose disposal of low birth weight infants: steady state hyperglycemia produced by constant intravenous glucose infusion. *Pediatrics* 1979;63:389.

153. Hay WW Jr. Fetal and neonatal glucose homeostasis and their relation to the small for gestational age infant. *Semin Perinatol* 1984;8:101.

154. Bougneres PF, Castano L, Rocchiccioli F, et al. Medium-chain fatty acids increase glucose production in normal and low birth weight newborns. *Am J Physiol* 1989;256:E692.

155. Sabel K, Olegard R, Mellander M, et al. Interrelation between fatty acid oxidation and control of gluconeogenic substrates in small for gestational age (SGA) infants with hypoglycemic and with normoglycemia. *Acta Paediatr Scand* 1982;71:53.

156. Wahlig TM, Georgieff MK. The effect of illness on neonatal metabolism and nutritional management. *Clin Perinatol* 1995;22:77.

157. Hay WW Jr. Nutritional requirements of the extremel-low-birth-weight infant. In: Hay WW Jr, ed. *Neonatal nutrition and metabolism.* St. Louis: Mosby-Year Book, 1991:361.

158. De Prins FA, Van Assche FA. Intrauterine growth retardation and development of endocrine pancreas in the experimental rat. *Biol Neonate* 1981;1:16.

159. Lebenthal E, Nitzan M, Lee PC, et al. Effect of intrauterine growth retardation on the activities of fetal intestinal enzymes in rats. *Biol Neonate* 1981;39:14.

160. Pencharz PB, Masson M, Desgranges F, et al. Total-body protein turnover in human premature neonates: effects of birth weight, intrauterine nutritional status and diet. *Clin Sci* 1981;61:207.

161. Cauderay M, Schutz Y, Micheli JL, et al. Energy-nitrogen balances and protein turnover in small and appropriate for gestational age low birthweight infants. *Eur J Clin Nutr* 1988;42:125.

162. FAO/WHO/UNU. *Energy and protein requirements.* World Health Organization Technical Report Series. Report of a Joint Expert Consultation. 1985;724:1.

163. Van Veen LCP, Ten C, Hay WW Jr, et al. Leucine disposal and oxidation rates in the fetal lamb. *Metabolism* 1987;36:48.

164. Carver TD, Hay WW Jr. Uteroplacental glucose metabolism and oxygen consumption after long term hypoglycemic in pregnant sheep. *Am J Physiol* 1995;269:E299.

165. Sinclair J. Heat production and thermoregulation in the small for date infant. *Pediatr Clin North Am* 1970;17:147.

166. Bhakoo ON, Scopes JW. Minimal rates of oxygen consumption in small for dates babies during the first week of life. *Arch Dis Child* 1974;49:583.

167. Aherne W, Hull D. Brown adipose tissue and heat production in the newborn infant. *J Path Bact* 1966;91:223.

168. Silverman WA, Sinclair JC, Agate FJ Jr. Oxygen cost of minor variations in heat balance of small newborn infants. *Acta Paediatr Scand* 1966;55:294.

169. Hanmerlund K, Sedis G. Transepidermal water loss in newborn infants. IV. Small for gestational age infants. *Acta Paediatr Scand* 1980;69:377.

170. Klaus MH, Fanaroff AA, eds. *Care of the high-risk neonate,* 2nd ed. Philadelphia: WB Saunders, 1979.

171. Sinclair JC, Silverman WA. Intrauterine growth in active tissue mass of the human fetus, with particular reference to the undergrown baby. *Pediatrics* 1966;38:48.

172. Hakanson DO, Oh W. Hyperviscosity in the small-for-gestational age infant. *Biol Neonate* 1980;37:109.

173. Cassady G. Body composition in intrauterine growth retardation. *Pediatr Clin North Am* 1970;17:79.

174. Snijders RJM, Abbas A, Melby O, et al. Fetal plasma erythropoietin concentration in severe growth retardation. *Am J Obstet Gynecol* 1993;168:615.

175. Wirth FH, Goldberg KE, Lubchenco LO. Neonatal hyperviscosity. Incidence and effect of partial plasma exchange transfusion. *Pediatr Res* 1975;19:372(abst).

176. Humbert JR, Abelson H, Hathaway WE, et al. Polycythemia in small for gestational age infants. *J Pediatr* 1969;75:812.

177. Ferguson S. Prolonged impairment of cellular immunity in children with intrauterine growth retardation. *J Pediatr* 1978;93:52.

178. Minton S, Steichen JJ, Tsang RC. Decreased bone mineral content in small for gestational age infants compared with appropriate for gestational age infants: normal serum 25-hydroxyvitamin D and decreasing parathyroid hormone. *Pediatrics* 1983;71:383.

179. Meberg A. Hermatologic syndrome of growth-retarded infants. *Am J Dis Child* 1989;143:1260.

180. Mehta P, Vasa R, Neumann L, et al. Thrombocytopenia in the high-risk infant. *J Pediatr* 1980;97:791.

181. Perlman M, Dvilansky A. Blood coagulation status of small for dates and postmature infants. *Arch Dis Child* 1975;50:424.

182. Lucas A. *Programming by early nutrition in man.* In: Block GR, Whelan J, eds. The childhood environment and adult disease (CIBA Foundation Symposium 156). Chichester: Wiley, 1991:38.

183. Smart J. *Undernutrition, learning and memory: review of experimental studies.* In: Taylor TG, Jenkins NK, eds. Proceedings of XII International Congress of Nutrition. London: John Libbey, 1986:74.

184. Dobbing J. Nutritional growth restriction and the nervous system. In: Davison AN, Thompson RHS, eds. The *molecular bases of neuropathology.* London: Edward Arnold, 1981:221.

185. Hack M. Effects of intrauterine growth retardation on metal performance and behavior outcomes during adolescence and adulthood. *Eur J Clin Nutr* 1998;52:S65.

186. Spinillo A, Stronati M, Ometto A, et al. Infant neurodevelopmental outcome in pregnancies complicated by gestational hypertension and intra-uterine growth retardation. *J Perinat Med* 1993;21:195.

187. Low JA, Handley-Derry MH, Burke SO, et al. Association of intrauterine fetal growth retardation and learning deficits at age 9 to 11 years. *Am J Obstet Gynecol* 1992;167:1499.

188. Strauss RS, Dietz WH. Growth and development of term children born with low birth weight: effects of genetic and environmental factors. *J Pediatr* 1998;133:67.

189. Fitzhardinge PM, Steven EM. The small-for-date infant. I. Later growth patterns. *Pediatrics* 1972;49:671.

190. Behrman RE. Handicap in the preterm small-for-gestational age infant. *J Pediatr* 1979;94:779.

191. Westwood M, Kramer MS, Munz D, et al. Growth and development of full-term nonasphyxiated small-for-gestational-age newborns: follow-up through adolescence. *Pediatrics* 1983;71:376.

192. Berg AT. Indices of fetal growth retardation, perinatal hypoxia-related factors and childhood neurological morbidity. *Early Hum Dev* 1989;19:271.

193. Hack M, Breslau N, Weissman B, et al. Effect of very low birth weight and subnormal head size on cognitive abilities at school age. *N Engl J Med* 1991;325:231.

194. Fitzharding PM, Steven EM. The small-for-date infant. II. Neurologic and intellectual sequelae. *Pediatrics* 1972;50:50.

195. Pena IC, Teberg AJ, Finello KM. The premature small-for-gestational-age infant during the first year of life: comparison by birth weight and gestational age. *J Pediatr* 1988;113:1066.

196. Allen MC. Developmental outcome and follow up of the small for gestational age infant. *Semin Perinatol* 1984;8:123.

197. Sung I, Vohr B, Oh W. Growth and neurodevelopmental outcome of very low birth weight infants with intrauterine growth retardation: comparison with control subjects matched by birth weight and gestational age. *J Pediatr* 1993;123:618.

198. Veelken N, Stollhoff K, Claussen M. Development and perinatal risk factors of very low-birth-weight infants. Small versus appropriate for gestational age. *Neuropediatrics* 1992;23:102.

199. Hutton JL, Pharoah POD, Cooke RWI, et al. Differential effects of preterm birth and small gestational age on cognitive and motor development. *Arch Dis Child* 1997;76:F75.

200. Kok JH, den Ouden AL, Verloove-Vanhorick SP, et al. Outcome of very preterm small for gestational age infants: the first nine years of life. *Br J Obstet Gynaecol* 1998;105:162.

201. McCarton CM, Wallace IF, Divon M, et al. Cognitive and neurologic development of the premature, small for gestational age infant through age 6: comparison by birth weight and gestational age. *Pediatrics* 1996;98:1167.

202. Barker DJP. Fetal and infant origins of adult disease. *BMJ* 1993;301:1111.

203. Snoeck A, Remacle C, Reusens B, et al. Effect of a low protein diet during pregnancy on the fetal rat endocrine pancreas. *Biol Neonate* 1990;57:107.

204. Dahri S, Snoeck A, Reusesn B, et al. Islet function in offspring of mothers on a low protein diet during pregnancy. *Diabetes* 1991;40:115.

205. Dahri S, Cherif H, Reusens B, et al. Effect of an isolcaloric low protein diet during gestation in rat on in vitro insulin secretion by islets of the offspring. *Diabetologia* 1994;37:A80.

206. Rasschaert J, Reusens B, Dahri S, et al. Impaired activity of rat pancreatic islet mitochondrial glycerophosphate dehydrogenase in protein malnutrition. *Endocrinology* 1995;136:2631.

207. Hay WW Jr, Catz CS, Grave GD, et al. Workshop summary: fetal growth: its regulation and disorders. *Pediatrics* 1997;99:585.

Multiple Gestations

Mary E. Revenis   *Lauren A. Johnson-Robbins*

The incidence of twins, triplets, and higher-order multiple gestations now accounts for approximately 3% of all pregnancies in the United States. The products of multiple gestations comprise a disproportionate number of admissions to neonatal intensive care units and suffer greater morbidity than do singletons. In 2002 16% of all preterm deliveries in the United States were due to multifetal gestations (1). In addition to prematurity, the products of multiple gestations are susceptible to unique problems which may intensify as the numbers increase. A review of the major problems can help the clinician to anticipate the medical needs and prepare the parents for what lies ahead. Most of the issues about twins discussed in this chapter apply to all multiple gestations.

EPIDEMIOLOGY

The incidence of multiple gestations in the United States has increased dramatically during the past three decades as a result of the shift in maternal age distribution to older ages, as well as the increased use of fertility enhancement therapy. The number of births from twin deliveries and higher-order multiples rose respectively to 31.1 and 1.84 per 1,000 live births in 2002 (1). The actual rate of twin conceptions is much higher because early fetal loss with a vanishing twin is far more common than clinically recognized (2). In 1,000 pregnancies studied early with ultrasonography, Landy and associates (2) found a twin conception rate of 3.29%, with subsequent reduction to a single fetus in 21.2% of those pregnancies.

The incidence of naturally conceived higher-multiple births is mathematically described by the Hellin-Zeleny law, which states that if twins occur at a frequency of 1/N, triplets occur at a frequency of $(1/N)^2$, quadruplets at $(1/N)^3$, and so on. Because most epidemiologic studies exclude data on twins with no live-born member, they grossly underestimate the incidence of multiple gestations.

Natural monozygotic twinning occurs at a fairly constant rate of 3.5 per 1,000 live births, with limited variation among populations. The occurrence of monozygosity is not affected by environment, race, physical characteristics,

or fertility. The relatively new reproductive technology of zona manipulation enhances artificial reproductive technology success, but is also associated with a remarkable increase in monoamniotic twinning. Following zona manipulation, 17.3% of the resulting multiple gestations are monoamniotic. The zona may act as a container for the dividing cell mass, disruption of which may allow for monozygotic twinning (3).

In contrast, rates for dizygotic twins vary greatly among populations, from 1.3 per 1,000 live births in Japan to 49 per 1,000 live births in Nigeria (4). Other factors that influence the incidence of dizygotic twinning include a maternally transmitted familial tendency, race, nutrition, parity, advanced maternal age, coital frequency, and seasonality. Twins are found most often in black populations and least often in Asians. Taller, heavier women bear twins at a rate 25% to 30% higher than short, undernourished women (4). Parity is an independent risk factor, with multiparous women having a greater likelihood for multiple gestations (5). Advanced maternal age predisposes to dizygotic twinning, with peak incidence at 37 years of age (5). Coital frequency has a positive affect, with a high rate of twin conceptions within the first 3 months of marriage (6). Another factor is the effect of the climatic seasons. In the Northern hemisphere, most dizygotic births are autumnal, reflecting more multiple ovulations during the winter and spring months. The seasonality of multiple births does not coincide with the peak months of singleton births (7).

High circulating levels of follicle-stimulating hormone (FSH) and luteinizing hormone (LH) lead to the release of more than one ovum per menstrual cycle, making multizygotic conceptions more likely. Conception stimulants such as clomiphene citrate (Clomid, Serophene), which act by stimulating endogenous secretion of gonadotropins, raise the incidence of multiple gestations by 6.8% to 17%; exogenous gonadotropins such as menotropins (FSH and LH; Pergonal) or human chorionic gonadotropins (APL., Follutein, Pregnyl, Profasi HP) may increase the incidence as much as 18% to 53.5% (8). The women of the Nigerian Yoruba tribe, who have naturally elevated levels of FSH and LH, have a remarkably high rate of spontaneous, dizygotic twinning (1 in 20) (9). Martin and associates (10) examined another population and found that women with dizygotic twins have higher levels of FSH and estradiol than women bearing singletons. A phenomenon likely due to increased pituitary gonadotropin release is the twofold higher incidence of twin conceptions in the 2 months after the cessation of oral contraceptives (11). High FSH and LH levels probably account for the seasonal variation in twinning observed in many countries (12,13).

IMPACT OF REPRODUCTIVE TECHNOLOGY

The increasing use of ovulation-inducing drugs and assisted reproductive technology (ART; *in vitro* fertilization, gamete intrafallopian transfer, and zygote intrafallopian transfer) has contributed to the recent 65% increase in multiple-gestation births in the past two decades. In 2000 there were 99,629 ART procedures in the United States. Of the 35,025 infants born after these procedures, 53% were products of multifetal pregnancies (44% twins and 9% triplets and higher-order multiples) (14). It is estimated that the number of nonART fertility treatments (ovulation induction and intrauterine insemination) are comparable in number to the ART procedures and associated with even more triplet and higher-order multiple gestations. In 2000 only 18% of triplets were naturally conceived, with 40% a result of ART and estimated 40% due to ovulation induction (15). In addition to the expected increase in dizygotic twins following assisted reproduction, monozygotic twinning with its higher incidence of complications is also more frequent in multiple gestations following assisted reproduction with an incidence of 3.2%, eight times higher than for spontaneously conceived pregnancies (16).

The multiple births resulting from ART are the major factor responsible for the increase in preterm delivery to 12.1%, up 29% from 1981. The use of ART accounts for 3.5% of low-birth-weight (LBW) infants and 4.3 % of very-low-birth-weight infants in the United States because of absolute increases in multiple gestations and also because of higher rates of LBW among singleton infants conceived with this technology (17).

The number of embryos transferred during ART procedures is directly related to the risk of multiple gestations. The multiple rate increases from 33.9% with transfer of two embryos to 41.4%, 43.2%, and 46.5% with transfer of three, four, or five or more embryos, respectively. The rate of triplets increases from 0.8% with transfer of two embryos to 7.4%, 8.4%, and 10.7% with transfer of three, four, or five or more embryos (14).

Each cycle of ART is expensive and not often covered by insurance. An attempt to improve pregnancy success has encouraged transfer of multiple embryos during each procedure, especially for older women. As increasing the number of embryos transferred with ART increases the risk of multiple gestations and thus the risk of complications, the live birth rate is not always improved. For women less than

age 35, the live birth rate for each embryo transferred is higher when only two embryos are transferred (42%) than when three (39.7%), four (35.4%), or five or more (33%) embryos are transferred (14,18).

The increase in multiple gestations due to ART and nonART fertility procedures are associated with significant expenses due to increased need for perinatal surveillance and intervention, increased neonatal intensive care utilization, and long-term costs of care for chronic disabilities such as cerebral palsy. To reduce health care expenses, several European countries have passed regulations or guidelines addressing the number of embryos permitted to be transferred during ART procedures (19) or have agreed to pay the expense of ART cycles if a reduced number of embryos are transferred. In the United States, the progressively rising higher-order multiple birth rate finally decreased 9% from 193.5 per 100,000 live births in 1998 to 180.5 in 2000 (1), possibly indicating some moderation of the number of embryos transferred during ART procedures. There is ongoing debate as to whether regulations in the United States would be effective in reducing the numbers of multiple gestations following ART procedures and improving outcome at a lower cost.

ZYGOSITY

Zygosity is determined by the number of ova fertilized. Higher-order pregnancies may be monozygotic, dizygotic, or multizygotic. In 1955 Corner (20) postulated that monozygotic twins develop by splitting of the conceptus at any time from day 2 after conception through days 15 to 17. The timing of division determines whether monozygotic twins are dichorionic, monochorionic, or conjoined. Dizygotic or multizygotic gestations result if more than one ovum has undergone fertilization at the same coitus or even at different times or with different mates.

At birth, zygosity can be determined by gender differences or by direct placental examination. Other techniques include blood typing, dermatoglyphics, and chromosome banding (21,22). The most precise technique is DNA-variant restriction fragment length polymorphisms (23). Because monozygotic twins carry significantly higher risks of morbidity and mortality prenatally and postnatally, establishing the zygosity of all multiple gestations is clinically important. More effort is going into determining zygosity prenatally using ultrasonography or genetic identification techniques.

PLACENTATION

The placenta from a twin gestation can be monochorionic or dichorionic; if dichorionic, it can be fused or separated, making four types of placentation possible:

1. Diamniotic, dichorionic separate
2. Diamniotic, dichorionic fused

TABLE 27-1
ZYGOSITY DETERMINATION

Clinical Finding	Percentage of Total Deliveries	Zygosity
Different genders	35	Dizygotic
Monochorionic placenta	20	Monozygotic
Same gender and dichorionic placenta	45	8% of monozygotic and 37% of placenta dizygotic infants[a]

[a] Further differentiation can be obtained by genotyping.
From Cameron AH. The Birmingham twin survey. *Proc R Soc Med* 1968;61:229–234, with permission.

3. Diamniotic, monochorionic
4. Monoamniotic, monochorionic

All dizygotic twins have a diamniotic, dichorionic placenta; all monochorionic twins are monozygotic. Zygosity should be determined in the case of twins of the same gender if the placenta is not monochorionic, because these siblings may be monozygotic or dizygotic. Fusion of the placenta does not differentiate zygosity. Table 27-1 lists zygosity determination based on placental examination.

Benirschke (24) described how to determine chorionicity of a fused placenta based on examination of the dividing membranes. The amnion contains no blood vessels and is more transparent than the chorion, which contains fetal vessels and remnants of villous tissue. A monochorionic placenta is one in which the septum is composed of a thin, translucent amnion that can be easily separated and lifted from the chorionic plate. In a dichorionic placenta, the septum is thicker and more opaque. It does not separate as easily from the chorionic plate. Ultrasonography of the dividing membranes early in gestation is useful in some cases to determine the chorionicity, but it is not always technically feasible (25).

A monochorionic, monoamniotic placenta is formed by division of the embryonal disc at 7 to 13 days, which is after differentiation of the amnion. Only 1% to 2% of monozygotic twins are monoamniotic; the fetal mortality rate is as high as 50%, primarily due to twisting, knotting, or entanglement of the umbilical cords (26). Conjoined twins with their necessarily monoamniotic placenta result from the latest and incomplete splitting of the embryonic disc at days 13 to 15 of gestation. The monochorionic, diamniotic placenta with a dividing membrane consisting of two layers of amnion without an intervening chorion is formed at approximately 5 days of gestation. Dichorionic, diamniotic placentas are formed the earliest, within the first 3 days after conception.

ANTEPARTUM COMPLICATIONS

Many complications of pregnancy occur more frequently in multiple gestations. Preterm labor is the most frequent com-

plication, occurring in 20% to 50% of multiple gestations, most likely due to uterine overdistention. Pregnancy-induced hypertension, placenta previa, antenatal and intrapartum hemorrhage, hyperemesis gravidarum, and premature rupture of membranes all occur at a higher rate (27,28). Polyhydramnios, an almost expected complication of multiple gestations, is transient in pregnancies in which there are no other complications. If persistent, the polyhydramnios suggests abnormal fetal conditions, such as twin-to-twin transfusion syndrome (TTTS) or congenital anomalies (29).

ANTENATAL MANAGEMENT

Recommendations for managing multiple gestations are controversial. The only unquestioned aspect of management is the benefit of early diagnosis, facilitating referral to an appropriate facility for high-risk infants. Antenatal management includes the following components:

- Early diagnosis
- Nutritional intervention
- Cervical cerclage
- Prophylactic tocolysis
- Steroid stimulation of fetal lung maturity
- Therapeutic amniocentesis
- Multifetal reduction
- Bed rest

Bed rest beginning before 28 weeks is commonly advised to decrease perinatal mortality (30). The National Institutes of Health (NIH) Collaborative Study showed no significant effect of antenatal betamethasone therapy in inducing fetal lung maturity in twins, but it is important to note that a relatively small number of twins were enrolled in the study (31). The 1994 NIH Consensus Statement on antenatal corticosteroids recommends betamethasone for all fetuses between 24 and 34 weeks of gestation, including multiple gestations (32).

There are several approaches to limiting the complications seen in higher-order multiple gestation. The first is to limit the number of embryos transferred during *in vitro* fertilization to two. This results in a reduction in pre- and postnatal complications in the mother and infants without affecting the pregnancy or take-home baby rates (18). An alternative is the use of multifetal reduction. Reduction, most often to twins, is usually performed at 9 to 12 weeks of gestation via either the transvaginal or transabdominal route (33). Reduction of quadruplets to twins improves overall outcome, but studies on the effect of reduction of triplets to twins have had conflicting results (33). Infants who are the products of reduced twin gestations have an increased incidence of impaired fetal growth and a lower gestational age at delivery when compared with nonreduced twins (17). Selective termination is used during the second trimester in pregnancies in which one twin is discordant for a major genetic disease or anomaly (34).

LABOR AND DELIVERY

The total duration of labor in a twin gestation is similar to a singleton gestation, with some differences in the lengths of each stage. Friedman and Sachtelben (35) observed a shorter latent phase during twin labor but a longer active phase and second stage, probably due to dysfunctional labor in an overdistended uterus.

There are many potential complications associated with delivery of multiple gestations, including malpresentation, cord prolapse, cord entanglement, vasa previa, locked twins, and fetal distress. Locked twins occur most often if the chins interlock to prevent expulsion or extraction of the first twin. Locking occurs at a rate of 1 per 817 twin gestations, and uterine hypertonicity, monoamniotic twinning, fetal demise, and decreased amniotic fluid are all contributing factors (36).

The best method of delivery depends on the number of fetuses, presentation of the first fetus, and gestational age. Table 27-2 details the frequencies of each variation of presentation. If both twins are vertex, there is no evidence that cesarean section improves outcome (37). In vertex-nonvertex twin gestations longer than 32 weeks, vaginal delivery is recommended (38). Delivery of the nonvertex second twin can be by total breech extraction or external cephalic version under ultrasound guidance and epidural anesthesia (39). If the first twin is nonvertex, delivery is usually by cesarean section.

Mode of delivery of the preterm multiple gestation depends on many factors, only one of which is the fetal presentation. If premature twins present in a vertex-vertex pattern without other complications, vaginal delivery is attempted, whereas a cesarean section is recommended for all other combinations of presentation if the gestational age is less than 34 weeks (40). When these recommendations are followed, there is no effect of mode of delivery or birth order on the incidence of intracranial hemorrhage in very-low-birth-weight twins (41,42). Extremely low-birth-weight twins (less than 1,000 grams) have been shown to benefit from cesarean section, regardless of their positioning, with a reduction in postnatal mortality (43).

Delayed-interval delivery of multiple gestations is reported (44,45). Management typically involves the placement of a cervical cerclage, tocolysis, and antibiotic therapy following the delivery of the first fetus to delay the delivery of the remaining fetuses as long as fetal distress is not present. The duration of pregnancy extension is highly variable, with one series achieving a mean of prolongation of 49 days (45). Delayed delivery allows for fetal maturation through either antenatal steroid administration or increasing gestational age.

MORTALITY

The frequency of single fetal demise in multiple gestation is reported as 0.5% to 6.8%, although early ultrasonography suggests a much higher rate of early loss (2,46–48). The causes of antepartum death include cord accidents, vascular anastomoses with overwhelming blood volume shifts, and velamentous insertion of the umbilical cord. Velamentous insertion, which makes the cord more vulnerable to trauma from twisting and compression, is six to nine times more common with twin gestation and increases the risks for fetal distress and for vasa previa with fetal hemorrhage (49). Most intrauterine deaths in twins are associated with monochorionic placentation (46–48).

After the demise of a fetal twin, the surviving fetus is at increased risk for distress, abnormal presentation, or dystocia, and the mother is at risk for toxemia, chorioamnionitis, or disseminated intravascular coagulation. In dichorionic twins, if the cause of death is intrinsic only to that fetus, complications to the surviving co-twin are rare, except from spontaneous premature labor (48). When one twin dies after at least 15 weeks of gestation in diamniotic pregnancies, a fetus papyraceous develops. The fetus loses all water content, becomes compressed, and because of oligohydramnios, may be mistakenly identified on sonography as a stuck twin. A retained twin may be large enough to hinder labor mechanically, necessitating cesarean section (50). Before 15 weeks, the fetus is resorbed; this is called the vanishing twin phenomenon.

For most monochorionic twins, the death of one twin has little adverse effect on the surviving fetus (51). However, if vascular connections are present, the surviving twin is at risk for complications related to interfetal blood exchange, including disseminated intravascular coagulation. After the death of one twin, partial abruptio placentae, which separates further during labor, may cause asphyxia or demise of the other twin (47). Fetal transfusion syndrome may be related to many of the antepartum deaths complicating twin pregnancy (46–48,52).

Fetal mortality for twins 20 or more weeks gestation declined from 31.2 to 20.7 twin fetal deaths per 1,000 live twin births from 1981 to 1997 (53,54). This improvement is associated with an increased preterm birth rate and reductions of complications of the placenta, cord, and membranes, intrauterine hypoxia, and birth asphyxia, suggesting intensified obstetric management of prenatal care and earlier obstetric intervention. The mortality of multiple gestations higher than two is greater than for twins because of smaller fetal size and placental or cord compromise from competition for space (55).

TABLE 27-2
TWIN PRESENTATION

Delivery (A–B)[a]	Percentage of Total Deliveries
Vertex-vertex	42.5
Vertex-nonvertex	38.4
Nonvertex	19.1

[a] A, first-born twin; B, second-born twin. (From Young BK, Suidan, J, Antoine C, et al. Differences in twins: the importance of birth order. *Am J Obstet Gynecol* 1985;151:915–921, with permission.)

Multiple gestations account for 10% to 12% of perinatal deaths (1). Increased frequencies of prematurity, pre-eclampsia, hydramnios, placenta previa, abruptio placentae, and cord prolapse contribute to increased mortality. The perinatal mortality rate for triplet pregnancies is reported as 7% to 23% and is strongly related to gestational age at delivery (56).

Despite recent increased rates of preterm delivery of twins, infant mortality of twins has improved in the United States and Canada (53,54), with a decrease from 54 per 1,000 live births in 1983–1984, to 30 per 1,000 live births in 1996 (53) compared to a general infant mortality rate of 6.9 per 1,000 live births in 2000 (1).

TWIN-TO-TWIN TRANSFUSION SYNDROME

Interfetal blood exchange occurs almost exclusively in monochorionic twins with circulations shared through vascular anastomoses that are present in most monochorionic placentas. Only 5% to 18% of these communications are sufficiently imbalanced to produce TTTS, but the actual rate would be higher if all cases of early fetal death of one twin were identified (27,46,57). Placentas from twin pregnancies complicated by TTTS have been shown to have significantly fewer vascular anastomoses, which are more commonly deep than superficial in location, compared to monochorionic placentas in pregnancies not complicated by TTTS (58). Vascular anastomoses and TTTS are rare in fused dichorionic placentas of dizygotic or monozygotic twins (46,49,51,57).

Acute and chronic forms of TTTS have been described (59,60). The onset of symptoms depends on what type of vessels are in communication, with an unbalanced, arteriovenous anastomosis and unidirectional shunt leading to the earliest and most profound symptoms. If anastomoses are balanced (i.e., artery to artery, vein to vein), the onset and severity of symptoms depend on changes in perfusion pressures that may be temporary and vary throughout gestation or become problematic only after delivery or demise of one twin.

Chronic, unidirectional TTTS manifests at any time after 16 weeks and can occur when an arteriovenous anastomosis joins a high-pressure system with a low-pressure system. The donor twin becomes progressively anemic, hypovolemic, and growth retarded, with oligohydramnios, and is at risk for tissue hypoxia and acidosis from reduced perfusion (52,61). The recipient twin becomes polycythemic and hypervolemic, with polyhydramnios developing from increased urine production to relieve the circulatory volume overload. Disparities in the weight of the heart and other viscera and in the size of glomeruli and pulmonary and systemic arterioles have been reported (52). Both twins are at risk for ischemia, thromboembolism, disseminated intravascular coagulation, and death. In the donor twin, there is hypotension and poor tissue perfusion; in the recipient, there also is poor tissue perfusion from hyperviscosity and polycythemia. Although the net transfusion is in the direction of the recipient, thrombi can exchange freely in either direction through vascular anastomoses, resulting in infarcts or the death of either twin.

Manifestations of TTTS range in severity from mild differences in blood hematocrit to the extremes of anemia and polycythemia affecting the pair (62,63). In the most severe cases, the growth-retarded donor twin may die of chronic hypoxia; the recipient develops congestive heart failure and hydrops and may die. Premature rupture of membranes, preterm labor, and delivery of compromised, premature infants are the usual sequelae. The perinatal mortality is 70% or more (64,65). Prognosis is better if symptoms, diagnosis, and delivery occur at a later gestational age or if hydrops does not develop.

In rare cases, after death of one twin with TTTS, the polyhydramnios resolves and a healthy survivor is born at a later time. However, compromising volumes of blood may be lost from the survivor into the dead twin. Other morbidity results from the release of thrombogenic material from degenerating fetal tissues, resulting in disseminated intravascular coagulation, multiple infarcts, and tissue necrosis in the live twin (46). Possibly related to thromboembolic arterial occlusion, severe defects, such as porencephaly, multicystic encephalomalacia, renal cortical necrosis, infarcts of the spleen, cutis aplasia, small bowel atresia, colonic and appendiceal atresia with horseshoe kidney, hemifacial microsomia, and necrotic limb, have been observed in the survivor of monochorionic twins after one fetal demise (46,48,66–69). An increased incidence of these defects is not reported in dichorionic twin survivors after the death of a cotwin.

One suggested criterion for diagnosing chronic TTTS is a hemoglobin difference between twins of 5 g/dL or more. In itself, this is not sufficient to establish TTTS because large differences in hemoglobin concentration also can occur in separate, dichorionic placentas (70). Tan and associates (58) diagnosed TTTS if a birth weight difference of 20% and a hemoglobin difference of 5 g/dL or more was found. However, a birth weight difference of more than 20% occurs with similar frequency in monochorionic and dichorionic pregnancies. The smaller twin may have polycythemia, secondary to intrauterine growth retardation (70). Fetal transfusion studies using adult cells as markers indicate significant interfetal blood exchange sufficient to cause discordant growth, and amniotic fluid volumes occur far more often than differences in hemoglobin concentrations suggest (71). Because TTTS in all degrees is limited to monochorionic placentations, differentiating the type of placenta and detecting vascular anastomoses are important. Measurement of the difference in pulsatility index between fetuses by Doppler examination of umbilic arterial blood flow has been shown to be helpful in the diagnosis of TTTS even before the development of fetal hydrops (72).

Acardiac twinning (i.e., reversed arterial perfusion syndrome) is a rare but interesting variation of TTTS, occurring in 1% of monozygotic twins (73). The nonviable acardiac twin's survival depends on the existence of artery-to-artery and vein-to-vein anastomoses to the other twin (74). The structurally normal, pump twin provides the circulation for itself and for its abnormal, acardiac twin, permitting slow growth of the abnormal twin. This can be detected by pulsed and color Doppler flow studies demonstrating arterial blood flow perfusing the acardiac twin. The reversed direction of flow in the umbilical arteries of the acardiac twin (75) leads to unusual congenital anomalies. Often assuming an amorphous shape, the cephalic pole is affected most severely, because it is the region most distal to the retrograde perfusion. The closer and better perfused lower part of the body is relatively spared (74). The diagnosis of acardiac twinning can be suspected prenatally by absence or marked undergrowth of the heart, head, and trunk, and by increased body soft tissue (75,76) of the acardiac twin. Frequent complications include congestive heart failure of the pump twin developing between 22 and 30 weeks of gestation, with cardiomegaly, hepatomegaly, hydrops, intrauterine growth failure, maternal hydramnios, preterm delivery, malpresentation, and fetal distress (74,77). Increased right atrial enlargement, increased reverse flow in the inferior vena cava, reversed flow in the ductus venosus, and pulsatile flow in the umbilical vein are early indications of hemodynamic decompensation in the pump twin (34,64), which can guide timing of intervention. The mortality rate of the pump twin is 50% to 55%, primarily due to prematurity (74,77).

An acute form of TTTS occurs with rapid transfer of blood through large superficial artery-to-artery or vein-to-vein anastomoses during labor and delivery, resulting in a hypovolemic donor and a hypervolemic recipient with similar birth weights (59,60). The transfusion is from the first to the second twin during the delivery of the first twin. However, if the first cord clamping is delayed, blood from the undelivered twin can be transfused into the first infant. The potential for acute volume changes during labor and delivery of monochorionic twins contributes to their vulnerability, need for resuscitation, and volume management.

Antenatal management of the TTTS previously was limited to close observation and bed rest. Acute polyhydramnios, which often complicates TTTS, is managed with serial amniocenteses of enough amniotic fluid to lessen fetal symptoms (78). Digoxin has been used successfully to treat cardiac failure in a recipient twin (79). Endoscopic laser coagulation of connecting vessels is used in treating severe TTTS (64,65). When the death of both twins is anticipated, selective feticide or fetectomy of the donor twin may permit survival of the recipient twin (80). In some instances, decreasing the polyhydramnios seems to stop or ameliorate the interfetal transfusion dramatically. Serial amniocentesis of the recipient twin with polyhydramnios has a 50% to 60% survival rate with 25% neurologic complications, while endoscopic laser photocoagulation of the communicating vessels has a 52% to 70% survival with only 4% neurologic complications (34,64,65).

STUCK TWIN

The stuck twin phenomenon occurs in a diamniotic pregnancy if there is a relatively acute onset of severe disparity in amniotic volumes, with one growth-retarded twin in an oligohydramniotic sac compressed against the uterine wall. If the oligohydramnios is severe enough, this twin may suffer all the complications of prolonged compression, including pulmonary hypoplasia, abnormal facies, and orthopedic deformation. The other twin is in a distended, polyhydramniotic sac, adding to compression of the smaller twin (81).

The stuck twin phenomenon occurs to some degree in as many as 35% of monochorionic diamniotic twin pregnancies, and it can develop in dichorionic pregnancies (82). In monochorionic twins, the phenomenon may be related to TTTS. Other causes, regardless of placentation, include uteroplacental dysfunction, congenital infection, discordant aneuploidy, and structural malformations. Both twins are structurally normal in 95% of cases. Disparity in volumes of amniotic fluid can occur if one twin has structural anomalies that lead to polyhydramnios (e.g., neural tube defect, upper gastrointestinal obstruction, congenital heart disease) or oligohydramnios (e.g., ruptured amnion, urinary tract anomalies, growth retardation) (83). The onset is usually between 18 and 30 weeks of gestation (82). Premature labor, possibly related to uterine distention from polyhydramnios and to preterm rupture of membranes, develops in most cases. Without intervention to reverse the fetal compression and uterine overdistention, the chance of survival of both twins is less than 20% (84).

ASPHYXIA

Despite the clinical impression that the first-born twin does better than the second-born twin, there is no demonstrable increase in neonatal death in the second-born twin (37,85). Breech presentation is more frequent, and large placental abruptions are more common in second twins (85). Differences in the 1-minute Apgar score, umbilical venous pH, oxygen pressure, and partial carbon dioxide pressure favor the first-born twin, regardless of route of delivery, placentation, interval between twins, or presentation (86). The second-born twin has potentially greater risk for hypoxia and trauma, regardless of the route of delivery, suggesting physiologic changes after the birth of the first twin. Findings in the venous blood gases suggest compromised intervillous placental blood flow after delivery of the first twin as a major factor.

In triplet pregnancies, although preterm labor is the most frequent complication and most important factor in perinatal morbidity and mortality, the mode of delivery is also important. If delivery is by cesarean section, the third-born triplet has a higher 5-minute Apgar score, and the second- and third-born triplets have increased survival compared with triplets of vaginal delivery (87). If triplets are delivered by cesarean section, the three triplets have a similar acid-base status despite the finding of lower 1-minute Apgar scores for the third-born triplet (88). The influence of birth order on acid–base status becomes significant during vaginal births if there is a longer time *in utero* after delivery of the first triplet. Triplets of more than 34 weeks of gestation and with birth weights greater than 2,000 g for each fetus tolerate vaginal delivery more successfully than smaller triplets (87).

GROWTH

Examination of fetuses between 8 and 21 weeks of gestation show similar weight-to-length ratios for singleton and twin fetuses (89). Birth weights of live-born twins up to 30 weeks of gestation are slightly smaller but similar to singletons of the same gestational age, indicating that the growth rate is similar in twins and singletons until 30 weeks of gestation (Table 27-3) (90–92). After 30 weeks, the singleton fetus has accelerated, exponential growth, and twin fetuses have a more linear rate of growth (93). Triplet growth previously was reported to decline progressively after 27 weeks of gestation (64). More recent studies indicate that growth of individual triplets and triplet sets remains linear throughout the third trimester (94) (See Appendices E-1 and E-2).

Better growth in the third trimester for multiple gestations reflects the positive impact of more aggressive maternal nutritional and obstetric care management. In a prospective study of nutritional intervention, the incidence of preterm delivery, LBW, and very low birth weight was lowered by 30%, 25%, and 50%, respectively, compared with twin pregnancies without nutritional intervention, but the rates of intrauterine growth retardation were not affected (95). Singletons are more likely to have LBW if there had been more than one fetal heart on early ultrasonography, and twins are more likely to have LBW if there had been more than two fetal hearts (17), indicating a persistent effect of the prior multiple condition.

Multiple gestations account for 17% of intrauterine growth retardation, with higher mortality rates for affected infants, particularly for the growth-retarded twin if only one is affected (90,96). Monochorionic twins show greater degrees of intrapair variation in birth weight than dichorionic twins, and true intrauterine growth retardation occurs more often in monochorionic twins. The individual members of twin pairs frequently are discordant for the rate of growth due to TTTS, placental insufficiency, intrauterine crowding, or an unequal impact of maternal complications that impair growth, such as preeclampsia. Ultimately, the underlying factor in most instances is a limitation of intrauterine nutrition, which may be shared unequally by the fetuses.

The incidence of discordant fetal growth as measured by biparietal diameter increases significantly as gestation advances. It is important to differentiate discordant growth due to TTTS, in which both twins are at increased risk for morbidity and mortality often before the last trimester, from a twin gestation in which only one fetus shows growth retardation, which usually becomes evident during the last trimester. With discordant growth not due to TTTS, the prognosis for the growth-retarded fetus depends on the severity of the growth failure and its cause, and the prognosis for the normally growing fetus may not be compromised. During the postnatal period, the smaller of the discordant twins has an increased incidence of hypoglycemia and is more likely to have retarded growth and development during childhood (97,98).

CONGENITAL ANOMALIES

Monozygotic twins have an increased frequency of congenital anomalies compared with dizygotic twins or singletons (69). Monozygotic twins frequently are discordant for malformations or for the severity of a given malformation. Some structural defects are related to the monozygotic twinning process, such as conjoined twins or some amorphous twins. Early embryonic malformations and malformation complexes such as sirenomelia, holoprosencephaly, and anencephaly are increased in monozygotic twins, suggesting a common cause for monozygotic twinning and early malformation complexes. Structural defects that result from the disruption of previously normal tissues are associated with the exchange of circulation in monochorionic twins with vascular connections. Those defects in which a vascular disruptive cause has been suggested include central nervous system defects (e.g., microcephaly, porencephalic cysts, hydranencephaly), gastrointestinal defects (e.g., intestinal atresia), renal cortical necrosis, hemifacial microsomia, cutis aplasia, and terminal limb defects (67). Deformations due to crowding and constraint molding of the normal fetus *in utero* during late gestation are similar in type and frequency in dizygotic and monozygotic twins and include foot-positioning deformations. The products of multiple gestation resulting from the use of ART and nonART fertility enhancement procedures are not at higher risk for major congenital malformations compared to naturally conceived multiples. However, limited data show a

TABLE 27-3
BIRTH STATISTICS FOR MULTIPLE GESTATIONS

	Gestational Age (average in weeks)	Birth Weight (average in grams)
Twins[a]	37.1	2,390
Triplets[b]	33.0	1,720
Quadruplets[c]	31.4	1,482

[a] From Newton W, Keith L, Keith D. The Northwestern University multihospital twin study. IV. Duration of gestation according to fetal sex. *Am J Obstet Gynecol* 1984;149:655–658, with permission.
[b] From Sassoon DA, Castro LC, Davis JL, et al. Perinatal outcome in triplet versus twin gestations. *Obstet Gynecol* 1990;75:817–820, with permission.
[c] From Collins MS, Bleyl JA. Seventy-one quadruplet pregnancies: management and outcome. *Am J Obstet Gynecol* 1990;162:1384–1391, with permission.

slight but significant increase in the rate of spontaneous sex-chromosome anomalies (0.8%) (99) (aneuploidies and structural *de novo* autosomal aberrations) after intracytoplasmic sperm injection (which is used in cases of male infertility), compared to 0.2% in the general population. Most of the abnormalities are paternally transmitted, consistent with the higher incidence of chromosomal abnormalities in the sperm of men with infertility.

Conjoined twins represent a unique structural defect of monozygotic monoamnionic twins. The nonseparated parts of the otherwise normal twins remain fused throughout the remaining period of development (100). The incidence of conjoined twins is between 1 in 80,000 to 1 in 25,000 births, and 70% to 80% of these cases are female twins (101). Approximately 40% are joined at the chest (thoracopagus), 34% at the anterior abdominal wall (xiphopagus or omphalopagus), 18% at the buttocks (pygopagus), 6% at the ischium (ischiopagus), and 2% at the head (craniopagus). With ultrasonography, the diagnosis of conjoined twins can be established as early as week 12 of gestation (102). Forty percent of conjoined twins are stillborn, and an additional 35% survive only 1 day (103). Long-term survival with or without surgical separation depends on the anatomic site of attachment and the extent of shared organs (104).

NEONATAL DISORDERS

Prematurity

The preterm birth rate of twins in the United States increased from 40.9% of twin gestations in 1981 to 55% in 1997. This increase was related to more aggressive prenatal surveillance, an increase in labor induction, and an increase in first cesarean delivery (53). Canadian data similarly shows an increase in the preterm birth rate of twins, with a decline in stillbirth rates at and near term gestation (54). Despite increased rates of preterm delivery of twins, infant mortality of twins has improved in the United States and Canada (53,54). Ninety percent of triplets are born prematurely. In 2002, 12 % of twins, 36% of triplets, and 60% of quadruplets were born prior to 32 completed weeks of gestation (1).

Hyaline Membrane Disease

Twins are at increased risk of developing hyaline membrane disease due to the increase in preterm delivery. Both twins are usually affected by hyaline membrane disease. However, if only one twin is affected, it is usually the second-born twin, who had a lower Apgar score at 1 minute and a higher birth weight than the first-born twin (105). The greater risk to the second-born twin probably is related to birth asphyxia (105). Monozygotic twins more often are born prematurely and at an earlier gestational age than dizygotic twins, and they are more prone to develop hyaline membrane disease.

Necrotizing Enterocolitis

Unique risk factors for the development of necrotizing enterocolitis have not been identified for twins or higher multiple gestations, but as a group, they are at an increased risk due to the greater likelihood of prematurity and LBW. Comparisons of twins showed that the most significant factor in predicting the occurrence of necrotizing enterocolitis and need for surgical intervention was a lower 1-minute Apgar score for the affected twins, predominantly the second-born twin, compared with unaffected cotwins (106). Samm and associates (107) found that, in all their case pairs, it was the first-born twin who had developed necrotizing enterocolitis; in no case did only the second twin have necrotizing enterocolitis. In that study, the first-born infants were more stable, were fed sooner, and had feedings advanced more rapidly than the second-born twins, implicating feeding practices in the higher incidence of necrotizing enterocolitis for the first-born twin.

Infection

One early study reported an increased rate of early-onset group B streptococcal disease in LBW twins compared to LBW singletons (108). Subsequent large population-based studies failed to show an increased risk of early-onset group B streptococcal disease in multiple gestations independent of prematurity (109,110). If just one of a pair of twins is infected or colonized with group B *Streptococcus in utero*, it is most likely the twin positioned adjacent to the cervix, with the exposure due to ascending spread of group B *Streptococcus* through the membranes. Spread of infection through the vascular connections between monochorionic twins has not been documented, although it is theoretically possible. However, spread of group B *Streptococcus* from the amniotic fluid of an exposed twin to a co-twin may occur through intact dividing membranes (111).

The risk of neonatal listeriosis infection is increased with multiple gestations, to 2.8 and 21 times the risk for twin and triplet pregnancies, respectively, compared to singleton births (112). The risk is especially increased when maternal age is greater than 35 years. It is possible that the increased production of hormones or other inhibitors due to larger placental mass with multiple gestations versus singletons decreases immunity to *Listeria*. Discordance of infection is 66%, with the first-born twin at greater risk.

One study showed that multiple-birth preterm infants with bronchopulmonary dysplasia are at an increased risk of developing respiratory syncytial virus illness and pneumonia than are singletons matched for gestational age, and that if one member of a multiple gestation developed respiratory syncytial virus disease, usually the other member(s) did also. Other risk factors that contributed to this were the higher density of adults and children in the households of multiple gestations (113).

Sudden Infant Death Syndrome

Monozygotic and dizygotic twins are at some increased risk of sudden infant death syndrome (SIDS) compared with singletons, and this is especially true for LBW pairs (114). If the birth weights of the twins differ significantly, it is usually the smaller twin who dies of SIDS (114). For twins discordant for size, the risk of SIDS for the smaller of twins is greater than for LBW and premature singletons or other groups of infants at high risk for SIDS (114). It is unusual for the surviving cotwin also to die of SIDS.

POSTNEONATAL CARE AND FOLLOW-UP

In addition to the long-term impact of some of the perinatal conditions previously mentioned, twins and higher multiples continue to be at risk for medical, developmental, and social problems beyond those experienced by singletons born at similar gestational ages. A brief list of factors that should be considered in following these patients is included to assist the clinician in anticipating the problems, many of which can be lessened by preventive measures, such as the following:

Parental stress of child rearing (115,116)
Child abuse and neglect (116,117)
Intratwin favoritism (118)
Developmental delay (e.g., performance below chronologic age, especially in language and speech) (119)
Mental retardation (120,121)
Cerebral palsy (120,122), Growth delay (123,124)
Glucose intolerance (125)

REFERENCES

1. Martin JA, Hamilton BE, Sutton PD, et al. Births: final data for 2002. *National Vital Statistics Reports* 52(10). Hyattsville, MD: Centers for Disease Control and Prevention/National Center for Health Statistics, 2003.
2. Landy HJ, Weiner S, Corson SL, et al. The "vanishing twin": ultrasonographic assessment of fetal disappearance in the first trimester. *Am J Obstet Gynecol* 1986;155:14–19.
3. Slotnick RN, Ortega JE. Monoamniotic twinning and zona manipulation: a survey of U.S. IVF centers correlating zona manipulation procedures and high-risk twinning frequency. *J Assist Reprod Genet* 1996;13:381–385.
4. Nylander PP. Biosocial aspects of multiple births. *J Biosoc Sci Suppl* 1971;3:29–38.
5. Bulmer MG. The effect of parental age, parity and duration of marriage on the twinning rate. *Ann Hum Genet* 1959;23:454–458.
6. James WH. Dizygotic twinning, marital stage and status and coital rates. *Ann Hum Biol* 1981;8:371–378.
7. Picard R, Fraser D, Hagay ZJ, et al. Twinning in southern Israel. Seasonal variation and effects of ethnicity, maternal age and parity. *J Reprod Med* 1990;35:163–167.
8. Schenker JG, Yarkoni S, Granat M. Multiple pregnancies following induction of ovulation. *Fertil Steril* 1981;35:105–123.
9. Nylander PP. Serum levels of gonadotrophins in relation to multiple pregnancy in Nigeria. *J Obstet Gynaecol Br Commonw* 1973; 80:651–653.
10. Martin NG, Olsen ME, Theile H, et al. Pituitary-ovarian function in mothers who have had two sets of dizygotic twins. *Fertil Steril* 1984;41:878–880.
11. Bracken MB. Oral contraception and twinning: an epidemiologic study. *Am J Obstet Gynecol* 1979;133:432–434.
12. Timonen S, Carpen E. Multiple pregnancies and photoperiodicity. *Ann Chir Gynaecol Fenn* 1968;57:135–138.
13. Elwood JM. Maternal and environmental factors affecting twin births in Canadian cities. *Br J Obstet Gynaecol* 1978;85:351–358.
14. Wright VC, Schieve LA, Reynolds MA, et al. Assisted reproductive technology surveillance—United States, 2000. *MMWR Surveill Summ* 2003;52:1–16.
15. Contribution of assisted reproduction technology and ovulation-inducing drugs to triplet and higher-order multiple births—United States, 1980–1997. *MMWR Morb Mortal Wkly Rep* 2003; 49:535–538.
16. Wenstrom KD, Syrop CH, Hammitt DG, et al. Increased risk of monochorionic twinning associated with assisted reproduction. *Fertil Steril* 1993;60:510–514.
17. Schieve LA, Meikle SF, Ferre C, et. al. Low and very low birth weight in infants conceived with use of assisted reproductive technology. *N Engl J Med* 2002;346:731–737.
18. Templeton A, Morris JK. Reducing the risk of multiple births by transfer of two embryos after in vitro fertilization. *N Engl J Med* 1998;339:573–577.
19. Katz P, Nachtigall R, Showstack J. The economic impact of the assisted reproductive technologies. *Nat Cell Biol* 2002;4 Suppl:S29–S32.
20. Corner GW. The observed embryology of human single-ovum twins and other multiple births. *Am J Obstet Gynecol* 1955;70: 933–951.
21. Robertson JG. Blood grouping in twin pregnancy. *J Obstet Gynaecol Br Commonw* 1969;76:154–156.
22. McCracken AA, Daly PA, Zolnick MR, et al. Twins and Q-banded chromosome polymorphisms. *Hum Genet* 1978;45:253–258.
23. Hill AV, Jeffreys AJ. Use of minisatellite DNA probes for determination of twin zygosity at birth. *Lancet* 1985;2:1394–1395.
24. Benirschke K. Multiple pregnancy. In: Fox W, Polin R, eds. *Fetal and neonatal physiology*. Philadelphia: WB Saunders, 1998:115–123.
25. Robinson JN, Abuhamad AZ. Determining chorionicity and amnionicity in multiple pregnancies. *Contemp Ob/Gyn* 2002;6: 92–108.
26. Timmons JD, De Alvarez RR. Monoamniotic twin pregnancy. *Am J Obstet Gynecol* 1963;86:875–881.
27. Newton ER. Antepartum care in multiple gestation. *Semin Perinatol* 1986;10:19–29.
28. Polin JI, Frangipane WL. Current concepts in management of obstetrics problems for pediatricians. II. Modern concepts in the management of multiple gestation. *Pediatr Clin North Am* 1986;33:649–661.
29. Hashimoto B, Callen PW, Filly RA, et al. Ultrasound evaluation of polyhydramnios and twin pregnancy. *Am J Obstet Gynecol* 1986;154:1069–1072.
30. Gilstrap LC 3rd, Hauth JC, Hankins GD, et al. Twins: prophylactic hospitalization and ward rest at an early gestational age. *Obstet Gynecol* 1987;69:578–581.
31. Collaborative Group on Antenatal Steroid Therapy. Effect of antenatal dexamethasone administration on the prevention of respiratory distress syndrome. *Am J Obstet Gynecol* 1981;141: 276–287.
32. Effect of corticosteroids for fetal maturation on perinatal outcomes. *NIH Consens Sci Statements* 1994;12:1–24.
33. Bush M, Eddleman KA. Multifetal pregnancy reduction and selective termination. *Clin Perinatol* 2003;30:623–641.
34. Moldenhauer JS, Gillert A, Johnson A. Vascular occlusion in the management of complicated multifetal pregnancies. *Clin Perinatol* 2003;30:601–621.
35. Friedman EA, Sachtelben MR. The effect of uterine overdistention on labor I. Multiple pregnancy. *Obstet Gynecol* 1964;23: 164–172.
36. Cohen M, Kohl SG, Rosenthal AH. Fetal interlocking complicating twin gestation. *Am J Obstet Gynecol* 1965;91:407–412.
37. McCarthy BJ, Sachs BP, Layde PM, et al. The epidemiology of neonatal death in twins. *Am J Obstet Gynecol* 1981;141:252–256.
38. Adam C, Allen AC, Baskett TF. Twin delivery: influence of presentation and method of delivery on the second twin. *Am J Obstet Gynecol* 1991;165:23–27.
39. Chervenak FA. The controversy of mode of delivery in twins: the intrapartum management of twin gestation (part II). *Semin Perinatol* 1986;10:44–49.

40. Cetrulo CL. The controversy of mode of delivery in twins: the intrapartum management of twin gestation (part I). *Semin Perinatol* 1986;10:39–43.

41. Morales WJ, O'Brien WF, Knuppel RA, et al. The effect of mode of delivery on the risk of intraventricular hemorrhage in nondiscordant twin gestations under 1500 g. *Obstet Gynecol* 1989;73:107–110.

42. Pearlman SA, Batton DG. Effect of birth order on intraventricular hemorrhage in very low birth weight twins. *Obstet Gynecol* 1988; 71:358–360.

43. Zhang J, Bowes WA Jr, Grey TW, et al. Twin delivery and neonatal and infant mortality: a population-based study. *Obstet Gynecol* 1996;88:593–598.

44. Lavery JP, Austin RJ, Schaefer DS, et al. Asynchronous multiple birth. A report of five cases. *J Reprod Med* 1994;39:55–60.

45. Arias F. Delayed delivery of multifetal pregnancies with premature rupture of membranes in the second trimester. *Am J Obstet Gynecol* 1994;170:1233–1237.

46. Benirschke K. Twin placenta in perinatal mortality. *NY State J Med* 1961;61:1499–1508.

47. Litschgi M, Stucki D. [Course of twin pregnancies after foetal death in utero.] *Z Geburtshilfe Perinatol* 1980;184:227–230.

48. D'Alton ME, Newton ER, Cetrulo CI. Intrauterine fetal demise in multiple gestation. *Acta Genet Med Gemellol* 1984;34:43–49.

49. Benirschke K. Multiple gestation: incidence, etiology and inheritance. In: Creasy RK, Resnik R, eds. *Maternal-fetal medicine: principles and practice.* Philadelphia: WB Saunders, 1984:511–526.

50. Leppert PC, Wartel L, Lowman R. Fetus papyraceus causing dystocia: inability to detect blighted twin antenatally. *Obstet Gynecol* 1979;54:381–383.

51. Johnson SF, Driscoll SG. Twin placentation and its complications. *Semin Perinatol* 1986;10:9–13.

52. Naeye R. Human intrauterine parabiotic syndrome and its complications. *N Engl J Med* 1963;268:804–809.

53. Kogan MD, Alexander GR, Kotelchrch M, et. al. Trends in twin birth outcomes and prenatal care utilization in the United States, 1981-1997. *JAMA* 2000;284:335–341.

54. Joseph KS, Marcoux S, Ohlsson A, et al. Changes in stillbirth and infant mortality associated with increases in preterm birth among twins. *Pediatrics* 2001;108:1055–1061.

55. McKeown T, Record RG. Observations on foetal growth in multiple pregnancy in man. *J Endocrinol* 1952;8:386–401.

56. Egwuata VE. Triplet pregnancy: a review of 27 cases. *Int J Gynaecol Obstet* 1980;18:460–464.

57. Robertson EG, Neer KJ. Placental injection studies in twin gestation. *Am J Obstet Gynecol* 1983;147:170–174.

58. Tan KL, Tan R, Tan SH, et al. The twin transfusion syndrome. Clinical observations on 35 affected pairs. *Clin Pediatr (Phila)* 1979;18:111–114.

59. Bajoria R, Wigglesworth J, Fisk NM. Angioarchitecture of monochorionic placentas in relation to the twin-twin transfusion syndrome. *Am J Obstet Gynecol* 1995;172:856–863.

60. Klebe JG, Ingomar CJ. The fetoplacental circulation during parturition illustrated by the interfetal transfusion syndrome. *Pediatrics* 1972;49:112–116.

61. Dudley DK, D'Alton ME. Single fetal death in twin gestation. *Semin Perinatol* 1986;10:65–72.

62. Benirschke K, Driscoll SG. *The pathology of the human placenta.* New York: Springer-Verlag, 1967:87–.

63. In: Fox H. *Pathology of the placenta.* Philadelphia: WB Saunders, 1978:81–.

64. Quintero RA, Morales W. Operative fetoscopy: a new frontier in fetal medicine. *Contemp Ob/Gyn* 1999;44:45–68.

65. Quintero, RA. Twin-twin transfusion syndrome. *Clin Perinatol* 2003;30:591–600.

66. Galea P, Scott JM, Goel KM. Feto-fetal transfusion syndrome. *Arch Dis Child* 1982;57:781–783.

67. Hoyme HE, Higginbottom MC, Jones KL. Vascular etiology of disruptive structural defects in monozygotic twins. *Pediatrics* 1981;67:288–291.

68. Mannino FL, Jones KL, Benirschke D. Congenital skin defects and fetus papyraceus. *J Pediatr* 1977;91:559–564.

69. Schinzel AA, Smith DW, Miller JR. Monozygotic twinning and structural defects. *J Pediatr* 1979;95:921–930.

70. Danskin FH, Neilson JP. Twin-to-twin transfusion syndrome: what are appropriate diagnostic criteria? *Am J Obstet Gynecol* 1989;161:365–369.

71. Fisk NM, Borrell A, Hubinont C, et al. Fetofetal transfusion syndrome: do the neonatal criteria apply *in utero? Arch Dis Child* 1990;65:657–661.

72. Ohno Y, Ando H, Tanamura A, et al. The value of Doppler ultrasound in the diagnosis and management of twin-to-twin transfusion syndrome. *Arch Gynecol Obstet* 1994;255:37–42.

73. Napolitani FE, Schreiber I. The acardiac monster. A review of the world literature and presentation of 2 cases. *Am J Obstet Gynecol* 1960;80:582–589.

74. Van Allen MI, Smith DW, Shepard TH. Twin reversed arterial perfusion (TRAP) sequence: a study of 14 twin pregnancies with acardius. *Semin Perinatol* 1983;7:285–293.

75. Billah KL, Shah D, Odwin C. Ultrasonic diagnosis and management of acardius acephalus twin pregnancy. *J Med Ultrasound* 1984;8:108–113.

76. Stiller RJ, Romero R, Pace S, et al. Prenatal identification of twin reversed arterial perfusion syndrome in the first trimester. *Am J Obstet Gynecol* 1989;160:1194–1196.

77. Moore TR, Gale S, Benirschke K. Perinatal outcome of forty-nine pregnancies complicated by acardiac twinning. *Am J Obstet Gynecol* 1990;163:907–912.

78. Radestad A, Thomassen PA. Acute polyhydramnios in twin pregnancy. A retrospective study with special reference to therapeutic amniocentesis. *Acta Obstet Gynecol Scand* 1990;69:297–300.

79. De Lia J, Emery MG, Sheafor SA, et al. Twin transfusion syndrome: successful *in utero* treatment with digoxin. *Int J Gynaecol Obstet* 1985;23:197–201.

80. Wittman BK, Farquarson DF, Thomas WD, et al. The role of feticide in the management of severe twin transfusion syndrome. *Am J Obstet Gynecol* 1986;155:1023–1026.

81. Urig MA, Clewell WH, Elliott JP. Twin-twin transfusion syndrome. *Am J Obstet Gynecol* 1990;163:1522–1526.

82. Chescheir NC, Seeds JW. Polyhydramnios and oligohydramnios in twin gestations. *Obstet Gynecol* 1988;71:882–884.

83. Pretorius DH, Mahony BS. Twin gestations. In: Nyberg DA, Mahony BS, Pretorius DH, eds. *Diagnostic ultrasound of fetal anomalies.* Chicago: Year Book Medical, 1990:609–622.

84. Mahony BS, Petty CN, Nyberg DA, et al. The "stuck twin" phenomenon: ultrasonographic findings, pregnancy outcome, and management with serial amniocenteses. *Am J Obstet Gynecol* 1990;163:1513–1522.

85. Naeye RL, Tafari N, Judge D, et al. Twins: causes of perinatal death in 12 United States cities and one African city. *Am J Obstet Gynecol* 1978;131:267–272.

86. Young BK, Suidan J, Antoine C, et al. Differences in twins: the importance of birth order. *Am J Obstet Gynecol* 1985;151:915–921.

87. Deale CJ, Cronje HS. A review of 367 triplet pregnancies. *S Afr Med J* 1984;66:92–94.

88. Creinin M, MacGregor S, Socol M, et al. The Northwestern University triplet study. IV. Biochemical parameters. *Am J Obstet Gynecol* 1988;159:1140–1143.

89. Iffy L, Lavenhar MA, Jakobovits A, et al. The rate of early intrauterine growth in twin gestation. *Am J Obstet Gynecol* 1983; 146:970–972.

90. Hendricks CH. Twinning in relation to birth weight, mortality, and congenital anomalies. *Obstet Gynecol* 1966;27:47–53.

91. Naeye RL, Benirschke K, Hagstrom JW, et al. Intrauterine growth of twins as estimated from liveborn birth-weight data. *Pediatrics* 1966;37:409–416.

92. Wilson RS. Twins: measures of birth size at different gestational ages. *Ann Hum Biol* 1974;1:57–64.

93. Arbuckle TE, Sherman GJ. An analysis of birth weight by gestational age in Canada. *CMAJ* 1989;140:157–160.

94. Jones JS, Newman RB, Miller MC. Cross-sectional analysis of triplet birth weight. *Am J Obstet Gynecol* 1991;164:135–140.

95. Dubois S, Dougherty C, Duquette MP, et al. Twin pregnancy: the impact of the Higgins Nutrition Intervention Program on maternal and neonatal outcomes. *Am J Clin Nutr* 1991;53:1397–1403.

96. Powers WF. Twin pregnancy, complications and treatment. *Obstet Gynecol* 1973;42:795–808.

97. Reisner SH, Forbes AE, Cornblath M. The smaller of twins and hypoglycaemia. *Lancet* 1965;144:524–526.

98. Babson SG, Phillips DS. Growth and development of twins dissimilar in size at birth. *N Engl J Med* 1973;289:937–940.

99. Van Steirteghem A, Bonduelle, M, Liebaers I, et al. Children born after assisted reproductive technology. *Am J Perinatol* 2002;19: 59–65.

100. Benirschke K, Temple WW, Bloor CM. Conjoined twins: nosology and congenital malformations. *Birth Defects Orig Artic Ser* 1978;16:179–192.

101. Rudolph AJ, Michaels JP, Nichols BL. Obstetric management of conjoined twins. *Birth Defects Orig Artic Ser* 1967;3:28–.

102. Schmidt W, Heberling D, Kubli F. Antepartum ultrasonographic diagnosis of conjoined twins in early pregnancy. *Am J Obstet Gynecol* 1981;139:961–963.

103. Edmonds LD, Layde PM. Conjoined twins in the United States, 1970-1977. *Teratology* 1985;25:30–308.

104. Filler RM. Conjoined twins and their separation. *Semin Perinatol* 1986;10:82–91.

105. de la Torre Verduzco R, Rosario R, Rigatto H. Hyaline membrane disease in twins. A 7 year review with a study on zygosity. *Am J Obstet Gynecol* 1976;125:668–671.

106. Powell RW, Dyess DL, Luterman A, et al. Necrotizing enterocolitis in multiple-birth infants. *J Pediatr Surg* 1990;25:319–321.

107. Samm M, Curtis-Cohen M, Keller M, et al. Necrotizing enterocolitis in infants of multiple gestation. *Am J Dis Child* 1986;140:937–939.

108. Pass MA, Khare S, Dillon HC Jr. Twin pregnancies: incidence of group B streptococcal colonization and disease. *J Pediatr* 1980;97:635–637.

109. Schuchat A, Oxtoby M, Cochi S, et al. Population-based risk factors for neonatal group B streptococcal disease: results of a cohort study in metropolitan Atlanta. *J Infect Dis* 1990;162: 672–677.

110. Schuchat A, Deaver-Robinson K, Plikaytis BD, et al. Multistate case-control study of maternal risk factors for neonatal group B streptococcal disease. *Pediatr Infect Dis J* 1994;13:623–629.

111. Benirschke K. Routes and types of infection in the fetus and the newborn. *Am J Dis Child* 1960;99:714–721.

112. Mascola L, Ewert DP, Eller A. Listeriosis: a previously unreported medical complication in women with multiple gestations. *Am J Obstet Gynecol* 1994;170:1328–1332.

113. Simoes EA, King SJ, Lehr MV, et al. Preterm twins and triplets. A high-risk group for severe respiratory syncytial virus infection. *Am J Dis Child* 1993;147:303–306.

114. Beal S. Sudden infant death syndrome in twins. *Pediatrics* 1989;84:1038–1044.

115. Goshen-Gottstein ER. The mothering of twins, triplets and quadruplets. *Psychiatry* 1980;43:189–204.

116. Tanimura M, Matsui I, Kobayashi N. Child abuse of one of a pair of twins in Japan. *Lancet* 1990;336:1298–1299.

117. Groothuis JR, Altemeier WA, Rubarge JP, et al. Increased child abuse in families with twins. *Pediatrics* 1982;70:769–773.

118. Minde K, Corter C, Goldberg S, et al. Maternal preference between premature twins up to age four. *J Am Acad Child Adolesc Psychiatry* 1990;29:367–374.

119. Record RG, McKeown T, Edwards JH. An investigation of the difference in measured intelligence between twins and single births. *Ann Hum Genet* 1970;34:11–20.

120. Durkin MV, Kaveggia EG, Pendleton E, et al. Analysis of etiologic factors in cerebral palsy with severe mental retardation. I. Analysis of gestational, parturitional and neonatal data. *Eur J Pediatr* 1976;123:67–81.

121. Kragt H, Huisjes HJ, Touwen BC. Neurobiological morbidity in newborn twins. *Eur J Obstet Gynecol Reprod Biol* 1985;19: 75–79.

122. Petterson B, Nelson KB, Watson L, et. al. Twins, triplets and cerebral palsy in births in Western Australia in the 1980s. *BMJ* 1993;307:1239–1243.

123. Silva PA, Crosado B. The growth and development of twins compared with singletons at ages 9 and 11. *Aust Paediatr J* 1985;21: 265–267.

124. Morley R, Cole TJ, Powell R, et al. Growth and development in premature twins. *Arch Dis Child* 1989;64:1042–1045.

125. Jefferies CA, Hofman PL, Knoblauch H, et al. Insulin resistance in healthy prepubertal twins. *J Pediatr* 2004;144:608–613.

126. Cameron AH. The Birmingham twin survey. *Proc R Soc Med* 1968;61:229–234.

127. Newton W, Keith L, Keith D. The Northwestern University multi-hospital twin study. IV. Duration of gestation according to fetal sex. *Am J Obstet Gynecol* 1984;149:655–658.

128. Sassoon DA, Castro LC, Davis JL, et al. Perinatal outcome in triplet versus twin gestations. *Obstet Gynecol* 1990;75:817–820.

129. Collins MS, Bleyl JA. Seventy-one quadruplet pregnancies: management and outcome. *Am J Obstet Gynecol* 1990;162:1384–1391

The Newborn Infant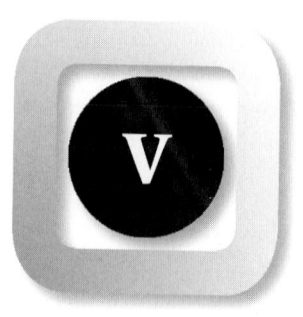

Control of Breathing: Development, Apnea of Prematurity, Apparent Life-Threatening Events, Sudden Infant Death Syndrome

28

Mark W. Thompson   *Carl E. Hunt*

The fetus makes breathing movements *in utero* and these movements change in character and frequency throughout gestation (1). This "maturation" of breathing control is likely critical to initiation of spontaneous, regular respiratory effort at birth and normal control of postnatal breathing. Studies in animals and preterm infants have explored the complexities of this maturational process, but an exact timeline has yet to be delineated. In this chapter, normal control of breathing will first be reviewed, the "end-state" of this maturational process will be described, genetic influences on control of breathing will be summarized, and then what is known about fetal breathing, the effects of sleep on fetal breathing, and the factors involved with establishing normal patterns of breathing at birth will be reviewed. Finally, we will review apnea of prematurity (AOP), how this disorder may shed light on the normal maturational process of breathing control, how to treat AOP, and the potential adverse clinical consequences.

NORMAL CONTROL OF BREATHING

The control and maintenance of normal breathing largely reside within the respiratory control centers of the bulbopontine region of the brainstem. Neurons within this area of the brain respond to multiple afferent inputs to modulate their own inherent rhythmicity and provide efferent output to the respiratory control muscles. Multiple afferent inputs induce modulation of the central respiratory center efferent outputs to the respiratory and airway muscles and lungs. These afferent inputs are "categorized" by the respiratory control center; some inputs cause an instantaneous response in the control center output, while others only act to "shape" the respiratory response, resulting in small changes in muscular output, tidal volume, and airway tone (2). Among these inputs are signals from central and peripheral chemoreceptors, pulmonary stretch receptors, and cortical and reticuloactivating system neurons. These afferent inputs and resultant efferent outputs of the central respiratory center are summarized in Fig. 28-1. Sleep state can also have a profound effect on respiratory pattern.

In the adult, these multiple afferent inputs act upon the neurons within the respiratory control center and provide a well-integrated response to perturbations in the system and characteristic respiratory patterns. For example, increased respiratory rate and depth will characteristically result from activation of central chemoreceptors in response to hypercarbia. In the newborn infant and especially in the preterm infant, however, these responses are less well-organized and apnea is a common result of a disorganized response to multiple nonintegrated afferent inputs.

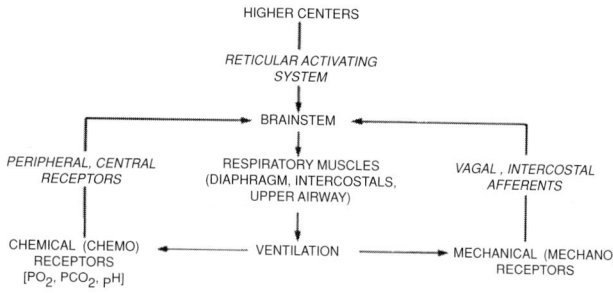

Figure 28-1 Major factors influencing respiratory control. PCO_2, carbon dioxide partial pressure; PO_2, oxygen pressure. (Reprinted from Martin RJ, Miller MJ, Carlo WA. Pathogenesis of apnea in preterm infants. *J Pediatr* 1986;109:733–741, with permission.)

Genetic Influences

Sequencing the approximately 25,000 genes in the human genome has resulted in fundamental changes in our understanding of the role of specific gene products in the pathophysiology of all diseases. Partly related to studies of sudden infant death syndrome (SIDS) pathophysiology, recent genetic studies of cardiorespiratory regulation linking specific genotypes to specific components of brainstem autonomic regulation are also relevant to understanding control of breathing and its developmental regulation in general and to understanding the pathophysiology of AOP and apparent life-threatening events (ALTE) in particular (3).

Neural control of breathing and sleep are closely integrated, and abnormalities in regulation of sleep and circadian rhythmicity can impair cardiorespiratory integration and arousal responsiveness from sleep (4). Circadian rhythmicity has been extensively studied in animals, and homologous counterparts of essential circadian clock genes isolated in *Drosophila* have been identified in mammals (3). Since the sleep-wake cycle is under control of the circadian clock, these circadian master genes, as well as other sleep-related genes, likely influence sleep regulation.

Targeted gene inactivation studies in animals have identified several genes involved with prenatal brainstem development of respiratory control including arousal responsiveness (3). During embryogenesis, the survival of specific cellular populations composing the respiratory neuronal network is regulated by neurotrophins, a multigene family of growth factors and receptors. Brain-derived neurotrophic factor (BDNF) is required for development of normal breathing behavior in mice, and newborn mice lacking functional BDNF exhibit ventilatory depression associated with apparent loss of peripheral chemoafferent input (5). Ventilation is depressed and hypoxic ventilatory drive is deficient or absent.

Krox-20, a homeobox gene important for mouse hindbrain morphogenesis, also appears to be required for normal development of the respiratory central pattern generator (6). *Krox-20*-null mutants exhibit an abnormally slow respiratory rhythm and increased incidence of respiratory pauses, and this respiratory depression can be further modulated by endogenous enkephalins. Inactivation of *Krox-20*

may result in the absence of a rhythm-promoting reticular neuron group localized in the caudal pons and could thus be a cause of life-threatening apnea (3).

Brainstem muscarinic cholinergic pathways are important in ventilatory responsiveness to carbon dioxide (CO_2) (3). The muscarinic system develops from the neural crest, and the *ret* proto-oncogene is important for this development. *Ret* knockout mice have a depressed ventilatory response to hypercarbia, implicating absence of the *ret* gene as a cause of impaired hypercarbic responsiveness. Diminished ventilatory responsiveness to hypercarbia has also been demonstrated in male newborn mice heterozygous for *Mash-1* (7). There is a molecular link between *ret* and *Mash-1*, and the latter is expressed in embryonic neurons in vagal neural crest derivatives and in brainstem locus coeruleus neurons, an area involved with arousal responsiveness.

Serotonergic receptors in the brainstem are critical components of respiratory drive, and abnormalities have been implicated as causal in SIDS (8). Review of the genetics of serotonin metabolism may be very pertinent to understanding important genetic risk factors for SIDS, and serotonin metabolism may be a model for multiple other genetically derived neurotransmitter systems important in maturation and development of control of breathing. Serotonin is a widespread neurotransmitter affecting breathing, cardiovascular control, temperature, and mood (3,9). Serotonin modulates activity of the circadian clock and appears to be the major neurotransmitter of nonrapid eye movement (nonREM), or quiet, sleep. Many genes are involved in the control of serotonin synthesis, storage, membrane uptake, and metabolism. The serotonin transporter gene is located on chromosome 17, and variations in the promoter region of the gene appear to have a role in serotonin membrane uptake and regulation (3,9). Several transporter polymorphisms have been described, including one in the promoter region; the long "L" allele increases effectiveness of the promoter and hence leads to reduced serotonin concentrations at nerve endings compared to the short "S" allele. The L/L genotype is associated with increased serotonin transporters on neuroimaging, and increased postmortem binding. Although no studies have been done in AOP or ALTE subjects, recent data in white, African-American, and Japanese infants indicate that SIDS victims are more likely than controls to have the "L" allele (9,10).

Fetal Breathing

Fetal sheep make regular breathing movements during REM sleep (11). Studies in animal models and human fetuses have demonstrated that there is a maturational progression in fetal breathing movements over gestation and that this respiratory pattern can be altered by a variety of pharmacologic and physiologic inputs.

In the human fetus, ultrasound evidence of fetal breathing movements was first noted with development of high-speed ultrasound in the mid-1970s. These fetal breathing movements have been characterized throughout gestation in response to maternal condition and as a potential indicator of overall fetal condition (12). From these studies, several characteristics of fetal breathing are evident. First, regardless of gestation, fetal breathing is not a continuous process. Significant periods of apnea, up to 122 minutes, are seen even in near-term fetuses (13). These periods of apnea are generally more frequent and of longer duration in younger gestational age fetuses (14), but significant respiratory pauses are still seen in presumed healthy near-term fetuses. Second, during periods of frequent respiratory motion, there are patterns of both regular and irregular breathing documented by chest/abdominal wall movements and by Doppler sonography assessing tracheal fluid flow (15). Third, there does appear to be a circadian rhythmicity to fetal breathing movements, with well-documented increases during certain periods of the day as compared to others (13). Fourth, maternal condition, particularly maternal glucose status, can have significant effects on fetal breathing frequency, with well-documented increases in fetal breathing frequency after maternal glucose loading following maternal fasting. This response to maternal glucose loading is not as pronounced when the mother is not fasting but rather ingesting normal meals during continuous 24-hour ultrasound monitoring (16). Fifth, fetal breathing does appear to be a potential measure of fetal well-being when used in conjunction with other ultrasound parameters. Several studies have documented diminished fetal breathing activity in association with poor fetal health, and this decreased activity, along with other measures of fetal well-being, can be helpful in guiding obstetric actions in terms of need for urgent delivery (17,18).

The fetal breathing pattern responds to a variety of pharmacologic and physiologic manipulations. Fetal breathing has been noted to increase three-fold if the mother inhales 5% CO_2 for 15 minutes (19). Maternal hyperoxia does not alter fetal breathing movements or pattern in near-term normally grown fetuses (20), but growth-restricted fetuses do exhibit an increase in respiratory rate with maternal hyperoxia (21). Tocolytics, indomethacin, and terbutaline increase fetal breathing movements almost two-fold when administered to women in preterm labor between 26 and 32 weeks of gestation (22). Despite the increased sensitivity of ultrasound to detect and characterize fetal breathing movements, almost all of the studies described have been observational in nature and have lacked characterization of several other very important fetal physiologic correlates, such as diaphragmatic electrical activity and sleep state. These human ultrasound studies have also not addressed the effects of pharmacologic and physiologic manipulation on fetal breathing in a controlled fashion. Animal studies, however, do augment the human ultrasound data and provide a clearer picture of the maturational development of breathing control.

Fetal breathing activity in sheep starts early in gestation, arises from centrally mediated stimuli, and occurs primarily during periods of low-voltage electrocortical activity (REM sleep) (11). REM sleep comprises about 40% of fetal life during the last trimester in sheep. Breathing does occur during periods of high-voltage electrocortical activity (quiet sleep), but there is no significant pattern to this breathing—it is only episodic in nature and generally occurs after tonic muscular discharges, i.e., body movements (23).

Additional insights have been obtained using chronically instrumented fetal lambs with direct visualization of fetal breathing and state at baseline and after physiologic manipulations (23). Fetal sheep do not show any periods of wakefulness as indicated by eye opening and purposeful movement of the head. The fetus alternates between REM sleep (low-voltage electrocortical activity) and quiet sleep (high-voltage electrocortical activity). Breathing movements, swallowing, licking, and other body movements occur almost exclusively during REM sleep. The fetus responds to an increase in arterial carbon dioxide pressure ($PaCO_2$) with an increase in breathing as determined by increases in tracheal pressure, breathing frequency, and integrated diaphragmatic activity, suggesting that both breathing rate and "tidal volume" increase in response to increasing hypercapnia (24–26). This breathing activity only occurs in REM sleep and during transitions to quiet sleep. Hypoxic levels of maternal oxygen abolish fetal breathing movements (27). These observations suggest that the relative low oxygen levels in the fetus at baseline contribute to the relative "lack" of fetal breathing movements throughout gestation and that the several-fold rise in oxygen partial pressure at birth is a contributing factor to the initiation of a regular respiratory pattern.

The use of pharmacologic agents in the fetal sheep model has also enhanced our understanding of fetal breathing. Indomethacin, pilocarpine, 5-hydroxytryptophan, and morphine all cause continuous breathing in both REM and quiet sleep. After these "breakthroughs" of breathing activity into quiet sleep, the intensity eventually diminished even when the fetus transitions back to REM sleep in association with decreasing drug levels (1,28).

In summary, animal experiments confirm that fetal breathing does occur. Under baseline conditions and non-pharmacologic manipulation (i.e., hypercarbia, hypoxia, hyperoxia), it occurs primarily during REM sleep (low-voltage electrocortical activity). The fetus does respond to central chemoreceptor input as evidenced by its response to hypercapnia. The fetal response to hypoxia appears to be centrally mediated and results in diminished normal neuronal activity and diminished or absent fetal breathing movements. The peripheral chemoreceptors may also be immature in the fetus and hence further contribute to absence of the "adult" response to hypoxia of an increase in respiratory rate and tidal volume.

Initiation of Breathing at Birth

Despite the enhanced understanding of fetal maturation of breathing control, the understanding remains incomplete regarding factors responsible for initiating and maintaining a regular pattern at birth. The traditional view is that mild fetal asphyxia during labor stimulates peripheral chemoreceptors leading to the first breath, and breathing is then maintained via input of other sensory stimuli, e.g., cold and touch. However, this view has been challenged by animal experiments showing that denervation of the carotid and aortic chemoreceptors does not alter fetal breathing or the initiation/continuation of breathing at birth (29). A stable respiratory pattern can also be initiated *in utero* with cord occlusion and hyperoxia, independent of $PaCO_2$. Postdelivery studies have also documented the importance of cooling in establishing a regular respiratory pattern and of CO_2 in maintaining that pattern (30). There are some data to suggest that a placentally derived factor inhibits fetal breathing and removal of this factor at birth then permits initiation of a regular respiratory pattern (1). This placental inhibitor "theory" is intriguing, but it does not explain the totality of response needed to initiate and maintain a normal respiratory pattern at birth; also, no candidate inhibitor has been suggested. Development and maintenance of respiration in the newborn is more likely due to a complex interaction of sensory stimuli and both central and peripheral chemoreceptor inputs (Fig. 28-1). The degree of maturation in the central respiratory centers also appears to be important since the responses to these stimuli in the term infant are more developed than in the preterm infant.

The Preterm Infant

The respiratory responses to hypercarbia are diminished in preterm infants less than 33 weeks' postconceptional age (PCA) (31), unrelated to any mechanical limitations in achieving adequate tidal volumes. The slope of the CO_2 response curve (Fig. 28-2) increases significantly between 29 to 32 and 33 to 36 weeks of gestation. The cause of this decreased sensitivity of central respiratory centers to CO_2 in preterm infants is related to central nervous system immaturity as indicated by decreased synaptic connections and incomplete dendritic arborization.

Preterm infants and full-term infants up to approximately 3 weeks postnatal age have a characteristic response to hypoxia that is quite different than in older infants. In contrast to the sustained hyperventilation in older infants, preterm infants have only a transient hyperventilation lasting

30 seconds to a minute. Subsequently, minute ventilation returns to baseline over several minutes and then progresses to ventilatory depression despite continued low inspired oxygen concentrations (1). The initial hyperventilatory response may be completely blunted in extremely premature infants (32). It is thought that this transient hyperventilation is in response to peripheral chemoreceptor input that is subsequently overridden by depression of central respiratory centers by hypoxia, and the hypoxic ventilatory depression is secondary to descending inhibition from the upper brainstem, midbrain, or higher structures (33,34).

Upper airway reflexes also may play a role in inhibiting respiration, particularly in preterm infants. Multiple sensory afferent fibers exist within the upper airways, and stimulation of these fibers by various mechanisms can result in abnormal respiratory responses. Responses to upper airway afferent fiber stimulation can change markedly with maturation. Newborn rabbits, for example, can exhibit irreversible, fatal apnea with stimulation of the nares. This response does not occur in mature animals (34). Negative pressure in the upper airways in human infants results in depressed ventilation, and isolated application of negative pressure to the upper airway in a rabbit model can result in diaphragmatic inhibition (35). This inhibition may contribute to the centrally mediated apnea (central apnea) occurring in mixed apneas initiated by obstructed breaths. As upper airway obstruction occurs, the infant makes respiratory efforts against this obstruction and the resulting increased negative pressure in the upper airway may result in reflex inhibition of diaphragmatic contraction. Due to a blunted response to hypercarbia and hypoxic ventilatory depression, less mature preterm infants with apnea may be less able to recover spontaneously and hence more likely to require active intervention by health care providers.

Laryngeal reflexes can also have significant effects on control of breathing. Apnea has been associated with overt regurgitation of gastric contents into the upper airway (36). Either regurgitation or reflux of the acidic contents of the stomach into the area of the larynx appears to stimulate chemoreceptors in the receptor-rich area of the larynx. This leads to an inhibitory afferent signal to the central respiratory centers. Animal studies have demonstrated that the area of the larynx is rich in chemoreceptors connecting with afferent fibers leading back to the brainstem. Stimulation of these chemoreceptors results in apnea in a lamb model (37,38).

Periodic Breathing

Periodic breathing is defined as a pattern of breathing alternating with respiratory pauses lasting through three cycles of breathing, with the pauses or apneic periods lasting at least 3 seconds (1,39). Periodic breathing is frequently seen in preterm infants and also in term neonates and young infants.

Periodic breathing appears to occur predominantly during REM sleep, but it also occurs during quiet sleep (32,40). During quiet sleep, periodic breathing is "regular" with consistent durations of the apneic and breathing periods,

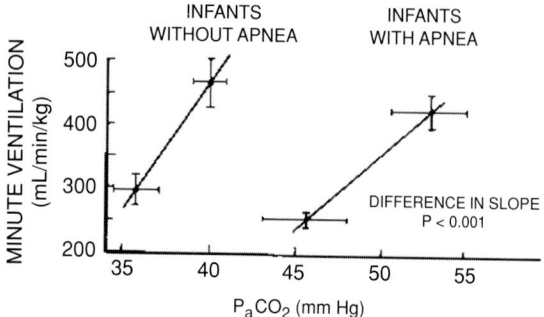

Figure 28-2 CO_2 response curves for preterm infants with and without apnea of prematurity. $PaCO_2$, arterial carbon dioxide pressure. (Reprinted from Gerhardt T, Bancalari E. Apnea of prematurity: I. Lung function and regulation of breathing. *Pediatrics* 1984; 74:58–62, with permission.)

while during REM sleep periodic breathing tends to be irregular with inconsistent durations of cycles of periodic breathing. These episodes of periodic breathing are reflective of immaturity of the respiratory control system. While initially thought to be a "benign" respiratory pattern, increasing evidence has indicated that periodic breathing can have pathologic consequences. Particularly in more immature preterm infants, minute ventilation can diminish significantly during episodes of periodic breathing, and oxygen saturations can decrease to hypoxemic levels in association with longer apnea durations and increased time spent in periodic breathing. Since more immature infants generally spend more time in sleep and more of this sleep time is characterized by periodic breathing, these infants can spend a significant amount of time with low oxygen saturations. These extreme degrees of periodic breathing likely reflect a greater general immaturity of the central respiratory control centers; the more "severe" the periodic breathing, the more likely an infant is to demonstrate overt clinical symptoms related to AOP.

It is very likely that both periodic breathing and AOP arise from the same pathophysiology, i.e., inability of the central respiratory control centers to adequately modulate multiple afferent inputs and resulting inhibitory outputs to the muscles of respiratory control. AOP may simply reflect a more severe variant of this dysmodulation. Not all studies have linked periodic breathing with more prolonged apneas (41), but preterm infants that demonstrate frequent intervals of periodic breathing also demonstrate an increased incidence of AOP and hence a general immaturity of the respiratory control system. While periodic breathing can thus be a normal respiratory pattern in both term and preterm infants, the higher the percent sleep time spent in periodic breathing and the greater the length of apnea during apneic periods, the more likely it is that these intervals represent a clinically significant immaturity of the central respiratory system associated with "pathologic" disturbances in central respiratory control.

The prevalence of periodic breathing is not precisely known since most studies have been based on convenience samples not necessarily representative of asymptomatic as well as symptomatic infants. Differing definitions for periodic breathing are an additional concern. In preterm infants less than 1,000 grams, many authors have reported the prevalence to be 100% (1,41). In term infants, the prevalence has been reported to be lower, but still as high as 80% (42,43). The high initial prevalence in both term and preterm neonates diminishes over time, most significantly in the first 6 to 8 weeks of life.

CLINICAL DISORDERS IN CONTROL OF BREATHING

Apnea

Apnea is defined as the cessation of breathing for longer than 20 seconds, or a shorter duration in the presence of

TABLE 28-1

ETIOLOGY OF APNEA IN PRETERM INFANTS

Cause	Comment
Idiopathic	Apnea of prematurity with immaturity of respiratory centers; modified by sleep state
Central Nervous System	Intracranial hemorrhage, seizures, depressant drugs, hypoxemia, hypothermia, hyperthermia
Respiratory	Pneumonia, obstructive airway lesions, Respiratory Distress Syndrome, laryngeal reflex, phrenic or vocal cord paralysis, pneumothorax, hypoxemia, hypercarbia, nasal occlusion caused by phototherapy eye patches, tracheal occlusion caused by neck flexion
Cardiovascular	Heart failure, hypotension, hypertension, hypovolemia, increased vagal tone
Gastrointestinal	Gastroesophageal reflux, abdominal distension, peritonitis
Infection	Pneumonia, sepsis, meningitis
Metabolic	Acidosis, hypoglycemia, hypocalcemia, hyponatremia, hypernatremia
Hematological	Anemia

Adapted from Hunt, CE. Apnea and sudden infant death syndrome in strategies in pediatric diagnosis and therapy. Editors: RM Kliegman. W.B. Saunders Co. Philadelphia, PA 1996.

pallor, cyanosis (See Color Plate), or bradycardia (44). There are multiple possible etiologic factors leading to symptomatic apnea in the preterm and full-term infant (Tables 28-1 and 28-2). The occurrence of apneic episodes thus requires clinical and laboratory assessments to rule out conditions requiring definitive treatment. There are no systematic prevalence data for symptomatic apnea in full-term infants, but most occurrences will have an identifiable medical cause (Table 28-2). In preterm infants less than 1,500 grams at birth, approximately 70% will have at least one clinically observed episode of symptomatic apnea while in the neonatal intensive care unit (NICU), and about 20% of these infants will have a specific medical cause (Table 28-1). The other 80% of preterm infants with symptomatic apnea do not have a specific medical cause and by exclusion are then diagnosed as having AOP, the most important and prevalent "disorder" of respiratory control occurring in preterm infants.

Apnea of Prematurity

Pathophysiology

The maturation of cardiorespiratory control and the clinical course of premature infants with AOP parallel each other and are consistent with the data reported in fetal animal studies. AOP is a direct consequence of immaturity of brainstem respiratory control centers. Both the presence

TABLE 28-2

ETIOLOGY OF APNEA AT BIRTH IN FULL TERM INFANTS

Cause	Comment
Intrapartum asphyxia	Hypoxemia, acidosis, brain stem depression
Placental transfer of CNS-depressant	Narcotics, magnesium sulfate, general anesthetics
Airway obstruction	Choanal atresia, macroglossia-mandibular hypoplasia (Pierre-Robin Sequence), tracheal web or stenosis, airway mass lesions
Neuromuscular disorders	Absent or uncoordinated sucking/swallowing, uncoordinated sucking and breathing, congenital myopathies or neuropathies
Trauma	Intracranial hemorrhage, spinal cord transaction, phrenic nerve palsy
Infection	Pneumonia, sepsis, meningitis
Central nervous system	Seizures, congenital central hypoventilation syndrome, Arnold-Chiari malformation, Dandy-Walker malformation

Adapted from Hunt, CE. Apnea and sudden infant death syndrome in strategies in pediatric diagnosis and therapy. Editors: RM Kliegman. W.B. Saunders Co. Philadelphia, PA 1996.

and severity progressively increase the lower the gestational age. This autonomic immaturity is not unique to respiratory control centers, however. Although there is no objective way to clinically quantify degree of immaturity for other brainstem autonomic control systems, brainstem auditory maturation can be quantified by serial measurements of brainstem conduction time from the auditory-evoked response (wave VI interval) (45). Both improved synaptic efficiency and myelination appear to be responsible for shortening of brainstem auditory conduction times with advancing gestational age. The brainstem auditory nuclei are located in close proximity to the cardiorespiratory centers, and there is a strong association between long brainstem conduction times for the auditory-evoked responses and clinical episodes of AOP. Since not all very-low-birth-weight preterm infants develop AOP and the severity varies even among affected infants of the same gestational age, other genetic and/or environmental risk factors are also likely to be important. Although no genetic, neurotransmitter, or neuropathologic studies have been performed in preterm infants with AOP, performance of such studies may be as informative in AOP as they appear to be in other control-of-breathing disorders.

Apneic episodes in AOP are subclassified as central, obstructive, or mixed (34,46). Figure 28-3 demonstrates the respiratory patterns during these events. Central apneas result from lack of respiratory effort. Obstructive apneas (obstructed breaths) are also central in origin but are related to absence of neuromuscular control of upper airway patency rather than absence of inspiratory diaphragmatic stimulation. Hence, obstructive apneas are characterized

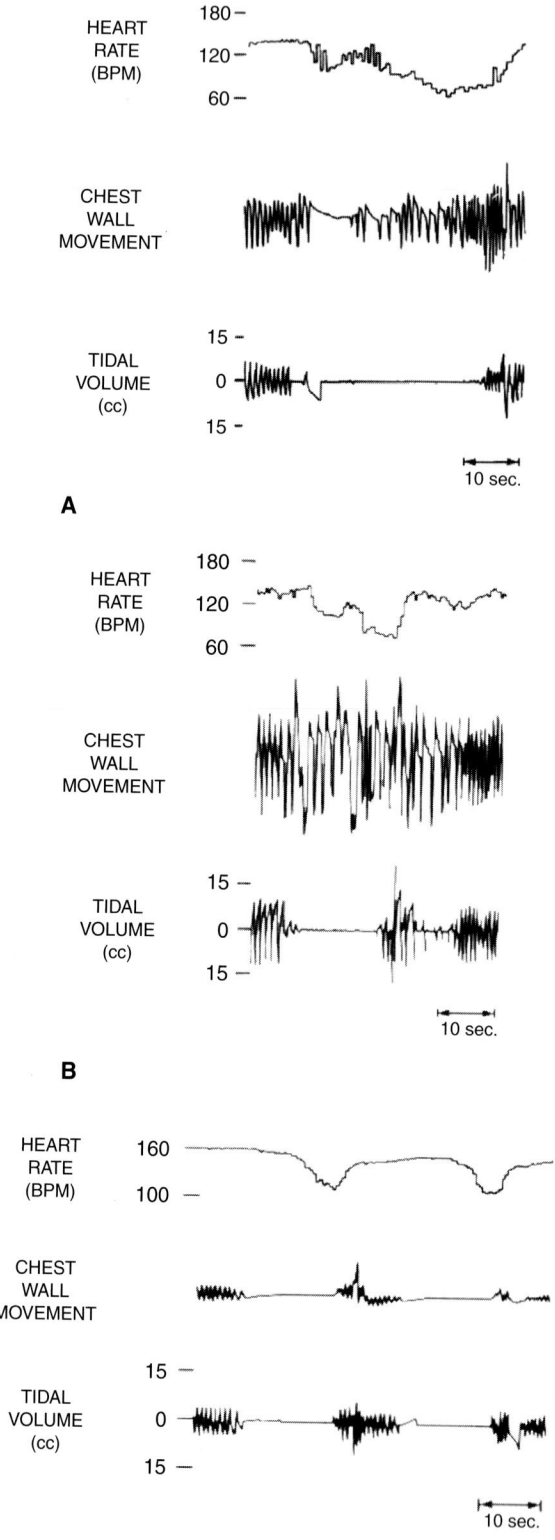

Figure 28-3 Examples of mixed, obstructive, and central apnea episodes occurring in apnea of prematurity. **A:** Mixed apnea. Obstructed breaths precede and follow a central respiratory pause. **B:** Obstructive apnea. Breathing efforts continue, although no nasal airflow occurs. **C:** Central apnea. Both nasal airflow and breathing efforts are absent. BPM, beats per minute. (Reprinted from Miller MJ, Martin RJ, Carlo WA. Diagnostic methods and clinical disorders in children. In Edelman NH, Santiago TV, eds. *Breathing disorders of sleep.* New York: Churchill Livingstone, 1986:157–180, with permission.)

by cessation of inspiratory air flow into the lungs despite persisting respiratory effort. Mixed apneas represent a combination of missed breaths (central apnea) and obstructed breaths. Mixed episodes of AOP can begin either with obstructed breaths or with central apnea, and there can be multiple alternations between obstructed breaths and central apnea within any single episode. In terms of relative frequency of each type, mixed apnea generally accounts for 53% to 71% of events, with obstructive apnea 12% to 20% and central apnea 10% to 25% (34). Preterm infants with AOP have significantly lower ventilatory responses to CO_2 than preterm infants matched for gestational age without AOP (31) (Fig. 28-2).

Incidence and Diagnosis

Threshold criteria for diagnosis have not been objectively defined and there is no established diagnostic test. Reported incidence data are therefore not based on any standardized criteria for diagnosis, but range from a low of less than 10% in preterm infants born at 34 weeks of gestation or more to approximately 60% at birth weights less than 1,500 grams and to a high of greater than 85% among infants born at less than 28 weeks of gestation (44,47,48). The first episodes can manifest themselves within the first 24 hours of life in spontaneously breathing infants without respiratory distress but are typically delayed in infants still receiving mechanical ventilatory support (49).

The identification of individual episodes of AOP is routinely based on detection of: a) central apnea lasting at least 20 seconds using standard impedance-based cardiorespiratory monitoring, b) bradycardia of less than 80 to 100 beats per minute (bpm) depending on gestational age, or c) arterial oxygen desaturation using a pulse oximeter (SpO_2). These symptoms are typically associated with clinically observed cyanosis. To be certain that monitor alarms are clinically significant, episodes initially detected by a monitor alarm need to be confirmed by visual observation (34,50). Since impedance-based cardiorespiratory monitors cannot detect obstructive apneas unless and until associated with bradycardia, however, episodes of AOP will not be detected by the monitor until central apnea has persisted long enough to trigger a monitor alarm or until the bradycardia threshold has been reached. Isolated respiratory pauses of less than 20 seconds without associated bradycardia or desaturation may not be of clinical significance and are not sufficient to justify a diagnosis of AOP. Periodic breathing is typically prominent in infants with AOP but is not sufficient for diagnosis in the absence of associated bradycardia and/or desaturation.

In infants with AOP, the periodic respiratory pauses associated with periodic breathing may be longer than in infants without AOP, and the total time spent in periodic breathing may be longer. Both of these factors contribute to the occurrence and severity of associated bradycardia and/or desaturation (39). Visually confirmed episodes of apnea with associated heart rate decelerations and desaturation are classified as symptomatic episodes. There is no

consensus-based threshold number of clinical episodes required for a "diagnosis" of AOP, but the minimum is at least one visually confirmed symptomatic episode unrelated to another medical cause (Table 28-1). The severity of AOP in individual patients and the threshold for initiating treatment are determined by the frequency and severity of subsequent clinically observed episodes. Although a multihour and multichannel recording that includes monitoring for both central and obstructive apneas, bradycardia, and desaturation might provide more objective threshold criteria for diagnosis and treatment, such recordings are not part of routine clinical care and no criteria have been established.

Treatment

Once other medical causes of apnea have been excluded (Table 28-1) and a diagnosis of AOP established, multiple treatment strategies are available. The first step is to ensure that borderline levels of baseline hypoxemia, anemia, hypocalcemia, and hypoglycemia have been corrected. Infants with intermittent hypoxemia due to episodes of AOP will be at increased risk for reduced tissue oxygen delivery (if they are also anemic) and for further exacerbation of AOP symptoms. Blood transfusions can be effective in reducing the severity of episodes (52–53), but some studies have not shown any correlation between degree of hypoxemia and degree of anemia (54–56). Some studies suggest that transfusion may be helpful in ameliorating symptoms of AOP only if the baseline hematocrit is less than 25 %. Clinicians should address the following questions when considering transfusion to improve symptoms related to AOP (57):

Are the symptoms related to AOP new in origin?
Has the severity of AOP increased as anemia has worsened?
Is the child receiving oxygen or other ventilatory support?
Has the heart rate increased?
Are other respiratory rhythm changes, such as periodic breathing, more prominent?

Affirmative answers to these questions increase the likelihood that a transfusion may improve clinical symptoms attributed to AOP.

The criteria for pharmacologic or ventilatory support vary among neonatologists, and there are no established clinical guidelines. Treatment is indicated, however, whenever clinical episodes are recurring, do not resolve spontaneously or in response to minimal stimulation, and are associated with bradycardia and intermittent hypoxemia. The first line of therapy is generally a methylxanthine, either caffeine or aminophylline.

Methylxanthines

Methylxanthines are central respiratory stimulants that increase CO_2 sensitivity and hence lead to improved tidal

TABLE 28-3

DOSING REGIMENS FOR INITIATING METHYLXANTHINE THERAPY (IV/po) FOR TREATMENT OF SYMPTOMATIC EPISODES IN PRETERM INFANTS WITH APNEA OF PREMATURITY

Drug	Loading	Maintenance
Aminophylline[a]	4 to 6 mg/kg	1 to 3 mg/kg every 8 to 12 hours
Caffeine[b]	10 to 20 mg/kg	2.5 to 4.0 mg/kg per day (base)
Caffeine Citrate[c]	20 to 40 mg/kg	5.0 to 8.0 mg/kg per day

[a] Start maintenance dose 8 to 12 hours after loading dose. If changing from IV to po aminophylline, increase dose by 20%. If changing to po theophylline, no change in dose is required.
[b] Start maintenance dose 24 hours after loading dose. Caffeine citrate may be given IV or po.
IV, intravenous; po, oral.

and minute volumes and blood gas values. Methylxanthines also increase diaphragmatic function, decrease muscle fatigue, and increase metabolic rate and catecholamine activity. These medications can be given by either oral or intravenous route. Both aminophylline and caffeine have been studied in placebo-controlled trials, and both have been shown to reduce the incidence of apnea (44,58–60). Table 28-3 reviews the recommended starting doses and dosing intervals for caffeine and aminophylline. The recommended therapeutic blood levels are 5 to 10 μg/mL for aminophylline and 8 to 20 μg/mL for caffeine. Methylxanthine side effects are secondary to catecholamine stimulation and include tachycardia, jitteriness, and irritability. Caffeine has a wider therapeutic index and side effects are uncommon at the recommended blood levels. There is consequently less need to check frequent blood levels. Direct comparisons of aminophylline and caffeine indicate similar efficacy at equivalent levels of central ventilatory stimulation. At equivalent degrees of central chemostimulation, however, side effects are less with caffeine than with aminophylline (61–63). Many neonatologists thus recommend caffeine as the preferred methylxanthine for treatment of AOP.

Regardless of which methylxanthine is chosen, most infants will have a significant reduction in central apnea events and hence in the severity of episodes. While individual studies measure efficacy in different ways, the number of clinical episodes was generally reduced by 50% to 90% (58–60,64–67). A Cochrane collaborative review found that both caffeine and aminophylline reduce the number of episodes of apnea and decrease the need for intermittent positive pressure ventilation (68).

The necessary duration of treatment with a methylxanthine is highly variable. AOP improves as brainstem respiratory control centers progressively mature, but there is considerable individual variation in the PCA at which maturation is sufficient to eliminate clinically documented episodes. By 32 to 36 weeks' PCA, most infants with AOP

can be weaned from treatment. Since there is no objective threshold to define resolution of AOP, neonatologists will usually use a combination of PCA, length of time since the last documented episode, and general clinical status to decide when to stop treatment. Once therapy is stopped, most physicians will continue to monitor an infant for a variable period of time (3 to 8 days) during drug "washout" before concluding that the infant is ready for discharge. Infants with recurrent clinical symptoms of bradycardia or cyanosis related to AOP will require reinstitution of medical treatment.

Continuous Positive Airway Pressure

Continuous positive airway pressure (CPAP), usually administered using nasal prongs (NCPAP), is also an effective treatment for AOP and is typically used when clinically significant episodes persist despite optimal methylxanthine therapy. At CPAP levels of 2- to 5-cm water, infants with AOP will have fewer episodes (69). This reduction is primarily related to significant reductions in episodes of obstructive and mixed apneas (Fig. 28-4) and has been attributed to splinting open of the upper airways by the positive airway pressure. CPAP levels of 2- to 5-cm water are generally sufficient to reduce upper airway resistance in sleeping premature infants and eliminate clinical symptoms of AOP related to mixed and obstructive apneas.

If NCPAP, in conjunction with a methylxanthine, is not sufficient to prevent recurring episodes associated with bradycardia and intermittent hypoxemia, some investigators have suggested using nasal intermittent positive pressure ventilation (70-72). Combined NCPAP and intermittent positive pressure ventilation may most likely be needed when episodes are related predominately to central apneas that are not being effectively eliminated by the NCPAP.

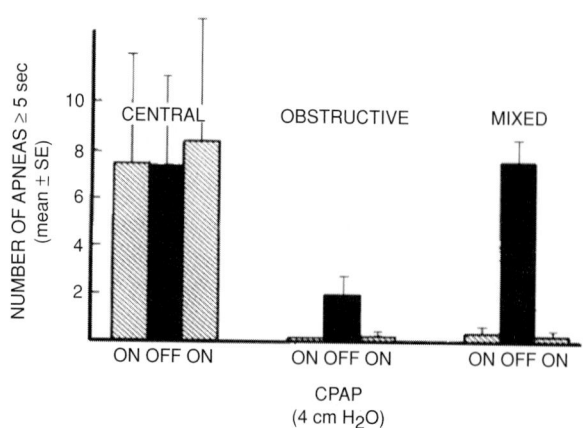

Figure 28-4 Effect of continuous positive airway pressure (CPAP) on a number of apneic episodes 10 seconds or longer in 10 infants with apnea of prematurity. Mixed and obstructive apnea decreased significantly during both periods of CPAP, with no evident effect on central apneas. (Reprinted from Miller MJ, Carlo WA, Martin RJ. Continuous positive airway pressure selectively reduces obstructive apnea in preterm infants. *J Pediatr* 1985;106: 91–94, with permission.)

Doxapram

Doxapram is an intravenous analeptic agent used in central hypoventilation syndrome and acute respiratory failure, and as a postoperative respiratory stimulant (44,73). Treatment with doxapram should be considered whenever methylxanthine therapy and NCPAP have been optimized but significant bradycardia and/or hypoxemia episodes persist. Its mechanism of action appears to be related to stimulation of carotid chemoreceptors at lower doses and to direct stimulation of central respiratory control neurons at higher doses. It is effective in diminishing the number of clinical episodes in small clinical trials and may be most effective when used in low doses in combination with low-dose methylxanthine treatment (74,75). The intravenous loading dose for doxapram is 2.5 to 3.0 mg/kg over 15 minutes followed by a continuous infusion of 1.0 mg/kg titrated to the lowest responsive dose (maximum dose 2.5 mg/kg/hour). At these low doses of doxapram used in AOP, significant side effects are uncommon but increased blood pressure and other side effects of catecholamine stimulation can occur, including lowering seizure threshold.

Intubation and Assisted Ventilation

If an infant is still having clinically significant episodes of bradycardia and/or cyanosis (See Color Plate) secondary to AOP despite optimal pharmacologic and noninvasive positive airway pressure, then endotracheal intubation and positive pressure ventilation is the treatment of last resort. It is infrequent that such invasive treatment is necessary, but no data as to frequency of need are available. Since intubation for treatment of AOP is uncommon, infants with AOP requiring intubation also need to be evaluated for intercurrent illnesses such as sepsis/meningitis and seizures.

Gastroesophageal Reflux

Significant controversy exists as to whether gastroesophageal reflux (GER) makes a significant contribution to episodes of AOP. Multiple studies indicate that stimulation of upper airway and especially laryngeal receptors leads to inhibitory influences on central respiratory centers and subsequent apnea. However, the preponderance of data from human studies indicates no causal link between GER and AOP (76–78). Some studies using intraluminal impedance techniques have shown a positive correlation between GER and AOP (79), but other studies using the same technique have not shown this correlation (78). GER and AOP may thus coexist in preterm infants and both may require treatment; however, in the absence of specific symptoms of GER, there is no evidence that treatment for GER will ameliorate symptoms of AOP.

Feeding-Related Symptoms

Both the establishment of adequate oral intake and resolution of any apneic or hypoxemic episodes related to persisting AOP are developmentally regulated. Just as resolution of AOP can be tracked by measuring maturation of brainstem auditory conduction using brainstem auditory-evoked responses, so can the attainment of coordinated oral feeding (45). Many infants will resolve their AOP and begin successful oral feeding at approximately the same time developmentally, but it is also possible that oral feedings may further aggravate episodes of AOP if the brainstem areas related to ventilatory control and oropharyngeal coordination are not sufficiently mature.

Feeding is a complex motor task that involves three coordinated steps: sucking, swallowing, and breathing. While full-term infants will breathe while sucking, the preterm infant has greater difficulty with this motor task. In addition, the preterm infant is very likely at the beginning of a feeding session to spend an exaggerated period of time in the initial sucking stage and not breath at all while in this stage. The full-term infant with no lung disease and a mature suck/swallow mechanism may have a brief period of mild desaturation during oral feeding, but rarely does this lead to bradycardia and apnea. The preterm infant with borderline respiratory status and an immature suck/swallow response, however, is more likely to hypoventilate while feeding due to immature suck/swallow pattern and response (80,81). If a preterm infant with AOP is demonstrating desaturations with feeding that are leading to bradycardia or apnea, decreased oral intake may be necessary pending further maturational development in oropharyngeal and ventilatory control as related to AOP. In addition to continuing methylxanthine treatment, additional therapeutic intervention may be as simple as providing oxygen immediately prior to and during the feeding (80).

Natural History: Implications for Discharge Planning and Home Care

Most preterm infants with AOP progressively improve with increasing PCA and are clinically normal without treatment by 34 to 36 weeks' PCA. Even after apparent resolution of AOP symptoms, however, symptoms can recur under well-defined conditions. Infection with respiratory syncytial virus (RSV) places infants at risk for apneic episodes, and apnea can be the presenting sign of an RSV infection (82,83). It is unclear why RSV places premature infants at risk for recurrent episodes of apnea, but RSV may alter laryngeal chemoreceptor sensitivity. With recovery from the RSV infection, the apnea episodes also resolve.

Exposure to general anesthesia also places premature infants at risk for recurrent apneic events (84). This is particularly true when inhalational anesthetic agents are used. Apnea-related symptoms can be related to anemia, especially at hematocrit levels below 30% (85). Unrelated to anemia, the incidence of apnea-related symptoms after discharge from the recovery room may be as high as 5% at 48 to 50 weeks' PCA and does not decrease to less than 1% until 54 to 56 weeks' PCA (84). Most clinically significant episodes, however, occur at less than 44 weeks' PCA, which is very consistent with Collaborative Home Infant Monitoring Evaluation (CHIME) data (46). Premature infants below these PCA limits, especially at lower hematocrit levels, thus need to receive adequate monitoring postoperatively to prevent life-threatening events.

Persisting or recurring symptoms at home associated with a prior history of AOP in former premature infants has become an issue of increasing clinical importance. At least in part related to discharge at younger PCAs, a significant minority of AOP patients have persisting symptomatic episodes related to apnea, bradycardia, cyanosis, or a combination thereof, when otherwise ready for discharge. In the CHIME study, for example, 17% of 443 infants less than 1,750 grams and 34 weeks or less of gestational age at birth were still symptomatic at the time of discharge home and 29% of these 443 infants were discharged with a methylxanthine (46).

Numerous studies have attempted to establish the minimum number of symptom-free hospital days without treatment required to ensure that symptoms would not recur after discharge home. Based on retrospective chart reviews in otherwise healthy preterm infants 1,500 grams or less and 32 weeks or less at birth and noting frequency of clinical episodes of apnea, bradycardia, and/or color change related to AOP, infants may be symptom-free for up to 8 days and still have another event (86). These investigators thus concluded that 8 symptom-free days were required to ensure resolution of AOP. In a different study based on monitor alarms, preterm infants with bedside monitor alarms had very infrequent apnea 20 seconds or more in duration when approaching discharge but had a higher frequency of desaturation and bradycardia with short apneas compared to preterm infants free of monitor alarms for at least 2 days (87). Among preterm infants with birth weights less than 1,250 grams, not having any clinically apparent episodes, and otherwise ready for discharge, 24-hour recordings of oxygen saturation, heart rate, respiratory impedance, and end-tidal CO_2 partial pressure revealed significant apnea in 91%, the majority of which were obstructive (88). Significant apnea was defined as apnea of longer than 12 seconds in association with a heart rate decrease of at least 10% or a decrease of at least 10 percentage points in oxygen saturation. Since there was no apparent correlation between severity of these predischarge recorded events and apparent life-threatening events or sudden unexpected death in the first 6 months of age, however, these data do not clarify whether one should delay discharge or prescribe home-based intervention for events detected only by overnight recording and not evident by bedside observation. In the absence of a clear standard of care in this regard, individual practice is highly variable. Some centers discharge preterm infants after as few as 3 days or as long as 5 to 7 days or more without a clinical event. There are no data to suggest that the relative risk of having an ALTE or dying of SIDS is any greater in infants discharged after just 3 days versus 5 to 7 or more days or that the relative risk is greater in infants in whom the event-free period is determined only by clinical observation versus overnight recordings.

The CHIME provides new insights regarding how long AOP-related events can persist after discharge home and the potential value of home-based memory monitor recordings in assessing risk for subsequent life-threatening or fatal events (46). The CHIME study was performed with a specially designed memory monitor utilizing respiratory inductance plethysmography to detect obstructed breaths as well as central apneas. Healthy full-term infants, premature infants, subsequent siblings of prior SIDS victims, and infants with a prior idiopathic ALTE were monitored until 6 months' postnatal age. The events stored for analysis included events exceeding conventional alarm thresholds (apnea of at least 20 seconds or heart rate less than 60 to 80 bpm for at least 5 seconds, depending on PCA) and extreme events (apnea of at least 30 seconds or heart rate less than 50 to 60 bpm for at least 5 seconds, depending on PCA).

Conventional events were common in all groups and at least one occurred in 41% of infants. Of those conventional events with apnea of at least 20 seconds, 50% included three or more obstructed breaths. Extreme events occurred in 10% of all infants. Among extreme events with apnea of at least 30 seconds, 70% included three or more obstructed breaths. In general, the degree of hypoxemia increased with increasing duration of apnea or bradycardia, and 25% of extreme events were associated with a decrease in oxygen saturation (SpO_2) of at least 10%. Compared to healthy term infants, preterm infants were more likely to have at least one extreme event, especially preterm infants younger than 34 weeks of gestation and with birth weights of less than 1,750 grams. Among these preterm groups, the relative risk of at least one extreme event was 18.0 in those who had persisting symptoms related to AOP within the last 5 days prior to NICU discharge and was 10.1 in those who had no clinical AOP-related events for at least 5 days before discharge. In these two groups, the risk of at least one extreme event and at least one conventional event remained higher than in the healthy term infants until approximately 43 weeks' PCA.

The CHIME study does not establish whether it is clinically important to detect conventional or extreme cardiorespiratory events by home memory monitoring. It is not known, for example, whether infants with a prior history of AOP are at greater risk for SIDS than gestational age-matched preterm infants without such a history, and the CHIME study was not designed to determine to what extent the presence and severity of extreme events in preterm infants after discharge home may be contributing to the greater prevalence of SIDS in preterm infants.

Neurodevelopmental Outcome

Most reports have found little evidence of any neurodevelopmental risk directly attributed to a history of AOP or ALTE (39,89). All of these AOP studies are limited due to nonstandardized criteria for diagnosis and for quantifying severity of apnea-related events in the NICU, and due to variable treatment strategies (89,90). Precisely measured predischarge apnea related to AOP, however, has been reported to be predictive of lower developmental indices at two years of age (91).

No outcome studies in preterm infants with AOP have considered the potential impact of cardiorespiratory events occurring at home during early infancy even though persistence beyond term gestation appears to be common, especially at lower birth weights (46,92). Using treatment with doxapram as a surrogate for severe AOP in preterm infants with birth weights of less than 1,250 grams, the duration of doxapram treatment and total dose received are significantly greater in children with isolated mental delay at 18 months compared to matched controls not receiving doxapram (93).

The CHIME study also provides some insights regarding risk for neurodevelopmental sequelae in infants with events documented using home memory monitoring (94). Among 256 infants (46% preterm) who used the home monitor and returned at 92 weeks' PCA for performance of the Bayley Scales of Infant Development-Revised (BSID-II), there was an inverse relationship between number of conventional events detected by home cardiorespiratory monitoring and neurodevelopmental outcome. This decrease in neurodevelopmental performance was observed both in full-term and preterm infants but was limited to the Mental Development Index (MDI). The adjusted difference in mean MDI scores with at least five events compared to no events was 5.6 points lower in full-term infants and 4.9 points lower in preterm infants. There was a trend toward a lower adjusted difference in mean Psychomotor Development Index scores with at least five events compared to no events in full-term infants ($P = 0.07$) but not in preterm infants. A dose effect is suggested by the tendency for mean BSID-II values with 1 to 4 events to be intermediate between 0 and at least 5 events. These findings are consistent with recent studies of sleep-disordered breathing in children showing diminished school performance several years later and in adults showing neuropsychologic deficits and gray matter loss by high-resolution magnetic resonance imaging in multiple sites (95–97). These CHIME data do not clarify, however, whether lower developmental performance at 1 year of age in preterm infants is caused by the events documented at home or whether the events and developmental delay are both the consequence of antecedent events in the NICU or antenatally. Since the findings in preterm infants are similar to those observed in full-term infants, however, the developmental outcomes appear at least in part attributable to the home-based events. It is unknown to what extent these developmental delays in preterm infants can be reduced or eliminated by improvements in hospital-based treatment of AOP or in home-based treatment of persisting events.

IDIOPATHIC APPARENT LIFE-THREATENING EVENTS

An ALTE is defined as a sudden, unexpected change in an infant that is frightening to the caregiver but does not lead to death or persistent collapse (98). Most patients are younger than 12 months and generally younger than 6 months of age. Episodes are characterized by some combination of apnea, color change, change in muscle tone, choking, and gagging (39). Approximately 40% to 50% of ALTE cannot be explained by the history and clinical evaluation and are hence classified as idiopathic. The percent of idiopathic cases is likely higher when symptoms are sleep related. Incidence rates for an ALTE vary from 0.5 to 10.0 per 1,000 live births; this 20-fold difference is likely related to different case definitions and methods of ascertainment. Most studies of ALTE do not include information about birth weight and gestational age, but the incidence in preterm infants has been estimated to be in the range of 8% to 10% (88). In the CHIME study, 30% of 152 infants with an idiopathic ALTE were 37 weeks of gestation or less at birth. Preterm infants thus are at increased risk for an idiopathic ALTE, but it is unknown to what extent this might be related to a prior history of AOP or to persisting symptoms of AOP.

Infants with an idiopathic ALTE are at increased risk for SIDS, but there is no consensus as to the magnitude of this risk or the extent to which prematurity or AOP might be a related factor. History of an idiopathic ALTE has been reported in 5% to 9% of SIDS victims (98,99). The risk of SIDS appears to increase with two or more idiopathic events, but no definitive incidence rates are available. In the CHIME study, the relative risk of having at least one extreme event was increased in preterm infants with a history of an idiopathic ALTE, but only until about 43 weeks' PCA (46).

Infants experiencing an idiopathic ALTE are candidates for home memory monitoring. In such patients, memory monitors can be useful in determining risk for, and timely identification of, recurrent life-threatening episodes, and perhaps useful in reducing the risk for neurodevelopmental sequelae from subsequent events (94). There are no data to indicate, however, that the risk for SIDS can be reduced by using a home monitor (100).

SUDDEN INFANT DEATH SYNDROME

SIDS is defined as the sudden death of an infant that is unexpected by history and unexplained by a thorough postmortem examination, which includes a complete autopsy, investigation of the scene of death, and review of the medical history (101). An autopsy is essential in all sudden and unexpected infant deaths because the history and scene investigation do not exclude all causes, including unsuspected congenital abnormalities and fatal child abuse. Comprising more than 7% of all infant mortality in the United States, SIDS was the third leading cause of infant mortality in 2000, ranked below congenital anomalies (21%) and disorders relating to short gestation/low birth weight (15%). About 2,650 infants died of SIDS in the United States in 1999, a rate of 0.67 in 1,000 live births; preliminary data suggest a lower rate for 2000 (102).

SIDS is the most common cause of postneonatal infant mortality in developed countries, generally accounting for 40% to 50% of infant deaths between 1 month and 1 year of age and about 20% of all deaths in infants discharged from a NICU. In full term infants, SIDS is rare before 1 month of age; the peak incidence occurs at 2 to 4 months of age, and 95% of all cases have occurred by 6 months of age. Compared to full-term infants, SIDS in preterm infants occurs at a younger PCA but older postnatal age (103).

Pathology

There is no autopsy finding pathognomonic of SIDS and no finding required for the diagnosis. There are, however, some common pathologic observations (104). Petechial hemorrhages are found in more than 90% of cases and may be more extensive than in other causes of infant mortality. Pulmonary edema is often present and may be substantial. Autopsy studies demonstrate structural evidence (tissue markers) indicative of preexisting, chronic low-grade asphyxia in nearly two-thirds of SIDS subjects (105). These tissue markers include persistence of adrenal brown fat, hepatic erythropoiesis, brainstem gliosis, and increased substance P. SIDS infants as a group have both prenatal and postnatal growth retardation, again consistent with prenatal and postnatal low-grade asphyxia. Vascular endothelial growth factor, which is upregulated by hypoxia, is elevated in cerebrospinal fluid of SIDS victims compared to control cases, confirming that SIDS is preceded by hypoxia and suggesting that it is prolonged hypoxia (106). The elevated levels of hypoxanthine in vitreous humor observed in SIDS infants further indicate a relatively long period of tissue hypoxia preceding death (105,107). Since adenosine, a precursor of hypoxanthine, is a respiratory inhibitor, these observations suggest that asphyxia from any cause could cause a secondary acceleration of adenosine monophosphate catabolism and adenosine accumulation and hence a vicious cycle leading to progressive hypoventilation and worsening asphyxia.

Brainstem structure and function have been a major focus of postmortem studies in SIDS victims. In addition to gliosis, findings include a persistent increase of dendritic spines and delayed maturation of synapses in the medullary respiratory centers, decrease of tyrosine hydroxylase immunoreactivity, and decreased catecholaminergic neurons in the brainstem (108). Significant decreases in serotonin receptor immunoreactivity in vagal medullary centers important in control of breathing have also been observed (109). Collectively, these results suggest that a maturational delay or malfunction related to cardiorespiratory autonomic regulation is one mechanism leading to SIDS.

The arcuate nucleus in the ventral medulla has been a particular focus for studies in SIDS victims. It is an integrative site for vital autonomic functions, including breathing and arousal, and is integrated with other regions that regulate arousal and autonomic chemosensory function. Quantitative three-dimensional anatomic studies indicate that a small subset of SIDS victims have hypoplasia of the arcuate nucleus, and histopathologic studies have observed bilateral, partial, and monolateral hypoplasia in as many as 57% of SIDS victims (110,111). Neurotransmitter studies of the arcuate nucleus have also identified receptor abnormalities in some SIDS victims that involve several receptor types relevant to autonomic control overall and to ventilatory and arousal responsiveness in particular. These deficits include significant decreases in binding to kainate, muscarinic cholinergic, and serotonergic receptors (8). Protein kinase C (PKC) and neuronal nitric oxide synthase (NOS) in the brainstem are critical components of respiratory drive, and abnormalities have been implicated as causal in SIDS (112). Prenatal cigarette smoke exposure is an important risk factor for SIDS, and decreased immunoreactivity to selected PKC and NOS isoforms have been observed in rats exposed prenatally to cigarette smoke.

Environmental Risk Factors

Numerous maternal and infant risk factors for SIDS have been identified (Table 28-4). Some of these risk factors may be surrogates for more fundamental factors (99). Some risk factors that are modifiable have been the successful focus of risk-reduction campaigns, resulting in

TABLE 28-4
ENVIRONMENTAL FACTORS ASSOCIATED WITH INCREASED RISK FOR SIDS

Maternal and antenatal risk factors
  Smoking
  Drug exposure (e.g., cocaine, heroin)
  Nutritional deficiency
  Inadequate prenatal care
  Low socioeconomic status
  Decreased age, education
  Single marital status
  Increased parity
  Shorter interpregnancy interval
  Intrauterine hypoxia
  Fetal growth retardation
Infant risk factors
  Age (peak 2–4 months)
  Male gender
  Race/ethnicity (e.g., African American and American Indian)
  Growth failure
  No pacifier (dummy)
  Prematurity
  Prone (and side) sleep position
  Recent (febrile) illness
  Smoking exposure (prenatal and postnatal)
  Soft sleeping surface, soft bedding
  Thermal stress/overheating
  Colder season, noncentral heating

Reprinted from Hunt CE, Hauk F: Sudden infant death syndrome, in Nelson textbook of pediatrics, 17th Edition, ed. by RE Behrman, RM Kliegman and HB Jenson, Philadelphia: W.B. Saunders Company 2003:1380, with permission.

TABLE 28-5
EPIDEMIOLOGICAL FACTORS ASSOCIATED WITH RISK FOR SIDS IN PRETERM INFANTS

Factor	Adjusted Odds Ratio
Birth weight	
500 to 999 g	3.1[a]
1000 to 1499 g	3.8[a]
1500 to 2499 g	2.5[a]
>2,499 g	1.0
Gestational age	
17 to 28 wks	2.9[a]
29 to 32 wks	2.8[a]
33 to 36 wks	1.8[a]
>36 wks	1.0
Race	
Non-Black	1.0
Black	1.7[a]
Gender	
Male	1.5[a]
Female	1.0
Maternal age	
<18 y	1.7[a]
18 to 35 y	1.0
>35 y	0.5[a]
Maternal education	
<12 y	1.7[a]
≥12 y	1.0
Pregnancies	
1	0.6[a]
2 to 3	1.0
>3	1.1[a]
Maternal smoking	
No	1.0
Yes	2.8[a]

[a]Statistically significant difference compared to reference group
SIDS, sudden infant death syndrome. Adapted from Malloy MH, Freeman DH Jr. Birth weight- and gestational age-specific sudden infant death syndrome mortality: United States, 1991 versus 1995. *Pediatrics* 2000;105:1227–1231, with permission.

TABLE 28-6
POSTCONCEPTIONAL AND POSTNATAL AGES (WEEKS) OF SIDS VICTIMS

Gestational Age	Postconceptional Age	Postnatal Age
24 to 28	44[a]	18[b]
29 to 32	45[a]	16[b]
33 to 36	47[a]	11
>36	50	11

[a] P < 0.05 compared to >36 weeks' gestational age
[b] P < 0.05 compared to the two older groups
Adapted from Malloy MH, Hoffman HI. Prematurity, SIDS, and age of death. *Pediatrics* 1995;96:464–471, with permission.

The odds ratio for SIDS in prone-sleeping infants in a metanalysis of case-control studies was 2.8 (95% confidence intervals [CI] 2.1–3.6) (99). The highest risk for SIDS may occur in infants usually placed nonprone but placed prone for last sleep ("unaccustomed prone") or found prone ("secondary prone"). Unaccustomed prone is more likely to occur in day care or other settings outside the home and highlights the importance of educating all infant caretakers about appropriate sleep positioning. As prone sleeping rates have declined following SIDS risk-reduction campaigns, side sleeping has also emerged as an independent risk factor for SIDS, with a relative risk of 2.0 compared to supine sleeping. The American Academy of Pediatrics has recommended since 1996 that supine sleeping be the preferred sleeping position for all infants (100), but they did not explicitly include preterm infants in this recommendation. As prone- and side-sleeping prevalence have decreased, unsafe sleeping practices, including soft sleep surfaces and soft bedding, have emerged as significant risk factors (99). Bed sharing has been implicated as another risk factor for SIDS, but studies have not classified risk for SIDS according to reason for bed sharing and have only partially adjusted for other pertinent risk factors such as breastfeeding.

Despite initial concern that supine sleeping would increase the risk for adverse events such as aspiration, vomiting, and trouble sleeping, studies have not identified any adverse consequences of supine sleeping compared to prone sleeping (115). No symptom or illness was increased among nonprone sleepers during the first 6 months of age, and some illnesses were less common, especially ear infections. Aspiration has not been observed to occur more frequently in infants sleeping supine, and infants sleeping supine do not appear to be at increased risk for episodes of apnea or cyanosis (See Color Plate).

Preterm infants were initially excluded from "back-to-sleep" campaigns. This exclusion was based on data from the NICU that ventilation and oxygenation, especially with persisting respiratory symptoms, were better when positioned prone compared to supine. When preterm infants are sufficiently mature and healthy to be discharged home without supplemental oxygen, however,

decreased SIDS rates (100). Preterm infants are approximately 3 to 6 times more likely to die of SIDS than full-term infants (100,103,113,114). The environmental risk factors associated with SIDS in preterm infants are not substantially different than those observed in full-term infants (Table 28-5), and there is an inverse relationship between risk for SIDS and birth weight/gestational age. The postnatal age of preterm infants dying of SIDS is 5 to 7 weeks later than that of full-term infants, and the PCA is 4 to 6 weeks earlier than that for full-term infants (Table 28-6).

In response to international back-to-sleep campaigns introduced in numerous countries in the 1990s, SIDS rates have declined by 50% or more as the prevalence of placing infants prone for sleep has decreased dramatically. These dramatic decreases in SIDS rates have generally not been associated with significant decreases in other risk behaviors. The 40% reduction in SIDS rates in the United States in 1992–1998 as prone prevalence decreased by approximately 50%, however, was associated with a 25% decrease in maternal reporting of smoking during pregnancy.

there is no clinically significant impairment in respiratory status when sleeping supine compared to prone. The American Academy of Pediatrics has therefore recommended since 2000 that all infants should sleep supine at home regardless of gestational age at birth (100), but adherence with this recommendation remains limited. Infants with birth weights of less than 1,500 grams are more likely to be placed to sleep in the prone position at home than infants with a birth weigh of 1,500 to 2,499 grams (26% versus 14%) even though risk for SIDS is greater at birth weights less than 1,500 grams compared to greater than 1,500 grams (113). Strategies are needed to reassure health care providers that the supine position for sleeping is as safe and effective in preterm as in full-term infants and to model safe sleeping practices in the NICU as the discharge planning process begins.

Maternal smoking during pregnancy has consistently been associated with increased risk of SIDS (99). The relative risk is in the range of 4.7 and represents one of the most significant modifiable risk factors following declines in prone sleeping. There appears to be a small independent effect of paternal smoking during pregnancy, but studies examining the influence of other household members have been inconsistent. Infants dying from SIDS tend to have higher concentrations of nicotine in their lungs than control infants, regardless of reported smoking exposure (116). Elimination of prenatal exposure to cigarette smoke could theoretically reduce the risk of SIDS by approximately 30% to 40% (117). It is difficult to assess the independent effect of postnatal exposure to cigarette smoke because smoking exposure during and after pregnancy are highly correlated, but studies do suggest that eliminating postnatal exposure to environmental cigarette smoke might further reduce risk for SIDS. In some studies of bed sharing as a risk factor for SIDS, this association has been linked with postnatal maternal smoking.

There are several potential mechanisms to explain why cigarette smoke exposure is a risk factor for SIDS. Maternal smoking can potentiate hyperplasia of pulmonary neuroendocrine cells, and dysfunction of these cells may contribute to the pathophysiology of SIDS (3). Both animal and clinical studies indicate decreased ventilatory and arousal responsiveness to hypoxia following fetal exposure to nicotine (118). The age-specific attenuation of hypoxic defenses following nicotine exposure suggests impaired brain catecholamine metabolism. *In vitro* studies suggest that smoking increases risk for SIDS due to greater susceptibility to viral and bacterial infections and enhanced bacterial binding after passive coating of mucosal surfaces with smoke components (119).

Most studies have not identified an association between SIDS and maternal alcohol use during or following pregnancy after adjusting for cigarette smoke exposure (99). A recent study, however, identified an increased frequency of binge drinking during pregnancy of 73% in mothers of SIDS victims compared to 45% in control mothers (120).

Maternal drug use during pregnancy is a risk factor for SIDS, with a two-fold increased risk of SIDS observed in the National Institute of Child Health and Human Development Cooperative Epidemiological Study after adjusting for birth weight, race, and age (121). Another study identified a seven-fold increased risk for SIDS among infants of substance-abusing mothers compared with drug-free mothers (122). Relative risks vary from 3.1 (CI 0.43–21.74) for phencyclidine and 6.9 (4.04–11.68) for cocaine to 15.1 (6.30–36.20) for opiates. The variable and sometimes conflicting results appear related at least in part to failure to control for confounding variables and sometimes to inadequate sample size.

No clear association has been identified between SIDS and specific viral or bacterial pathogens (99). It has been suggested that upper respiratory infections or other minor illnesses in conjunction with other factors, such as prone sleeping, may play a role in the pathogenesis of SIDS. Deficient inflammatory responsiveness to infection has also been hypothesized to be a mechanism for SIDS (3,119,123). Partial deletions in the *C4* gene may contribute to this apparent link between upper respiratory infection and SIDS. Mast cell degranulation has been reported in SIDS victims; this is consistent with an anaphylactic reaction to a bacterial toxin, and some family members of SIDS victims also have mast cell hyperreleasability and degranulation, suggesting a genetic component to risk for an anaphylactic reaction (124).

Gene-Environment Interactions

The actual risk for SIDS in individual infants is determined by complex interactions between genetic and environmental risk factors (3). There appears, for example, to be an interaction between prone/side sleep position and impaired ventilatory and arousal responsiveness. Face-down or nearly face-down sleeping does occasionally occur in prone-sleeping infants and can result in episodes of airway obstruction and asphyxia in healthy full-term infants (125). Healthy infants will arouse before such episodes became life threatening, but infants with insufficient arousal responsiveness to asphyxia would be at risk for sudden death. There may also be links between modifiable risk factors such as soft bedding, prone-sleep position, and thermal stress, and links between genetic risk factors such as ventilatory and arousal abnormalities and temperature or metabolic regulation deficits. The increased risk for SIDS associated with fetal and postnatal exposure to cigarette smoke also appears at least in part to depend on genetic risk factors (3).

There are substantial data indicating that both genetic and environmental factors contribute to an increased risk for death from most natural causes in siblings. The next-born siblings of first-born infants dying of any noninfectious cause, for example, are at significantly increased risk for infant death from the same cause, including complications of prematurity and SIDS (3). The relative risk is 9.1 for concordance of cause of recurrent death versus 1.6 for a discordant cause of death, and the relative risk for recurrence of each cause of infant death is similar for SIDS (5.4–5.8) and for each of the other causes (range 4.6–12.5). The risk

TABLE 28-7

PHYSIOLOGIC ABNORMALITIES THAT HAVE BEEN ASSOCIATED WITH SIDS

Deficient regulation of brainstem autonomic control, affecting
  Arousal/gasping
  Ventilatory responsiveness
  Respiratory pattern
  Heart rate
  Temperature
  Vagal tone
  Blood pressure
  Sleep/Circadian Rhythm
Metabolic (e.g.; fatty acid defects)
Abnormal inflammatory/immune response to infection
Prolonged QT syndrome

SIDS, sudden infant death syndrome.
Adapted from Hunt, CE, Hauck FR. Sudden infant death syndrome. In: Behrman RE, Kliegman RM, Jenson HB, eds. Nelson textbook of pediatrics, 17th ed. Philadelphia: Elsevier, 2004: 1380, with permission.

for recurrent infant mortality in subsequent siblings from the same cause as in the index sibling thus appears to be increased to a similar degree for both explained causes and for SIDS. These increased risks in SIDS families are consistent with genetic risk factors associated with brainstem abnormalities in autonomic control interacting with environmental risk factors.

Physiologic Studies

Physiologic studies have been performed in healthy infants during early infancy, a few of whom later died of SIDS (99). Physiologic studies have also been performed in infant groups at increased risk for SIDS, especially in infants having experienced an unexplained ALTE and in subsequent siblings of SIDS victims (Table 28-7). In the aggregate, these physiologic studies are indicative of a brainstem abnormality related to neuroregulation of cardiorespiratory control and other autonomic functions and are consistent with the autopsy findings in SIDS victims. The observed physiologic abnormalities include respiratory pattern, chemoreceptor sensitivity, control of heart and respiratory rate or variability, and asphyxic arousal responsiveness. A deficit in arousal responsiveness may be a necessary prerequisite for SIDS to occur but may be insufficient to cause SIDS in the absence of other genetic or environmental risk factors. Autoresuscitation (gasping) is a critical component of the asphyxic arousal response, and a failure of autoresuscitation in victims of SIDS may be the final and most devastating physiologic failure (126). Most full-term infants less than 9 weeks of age arouse in response to mild hypoxia, but only 10% to 15% of normal infants older than 9 weeks of age arouse (127). These data thus suggest that as full-term infants mature, their ability to arouse to mild/moderate hypoxic stimuli diminishes as they reach the age range of greatest risk for SIDS.

The ability to shorten Q-T interval as heart rate increases appears to be impaired in some SIDS victims, suggesting that such infants may be predisposed to ventricular arrhythmia (100). Infants studied physiologically and later dying of SIDS have higher heart rates in all sleep-waking states, diminished heart rate variability during wakefulness, and significantly lower heart rate variability at the respiratory frequency across all sleep-waking cycles. Even in early infancy, therefore, future SIDS victims differ in the extent to which cardiac and respiratory activity are coupled. No heart rate variability data are available in preterm infants with AOP compared to gestational age-matched infants without AOP or to full-term infants.

Part of the decreased heart rate variability and increased heart rate observed in infants who later die of SIDS may be related to decreased vagal tone. This decreased tone appears at least in part to be related to vagal neuropathy or to brainstem damage in areas responsible for parasympathetic cardiac control. Comparing heart rate power spectra before and after obstructive apneas in infants, future SIDS victims do not have the decreases in low-frequency to high-frequency power ratios observed in control infants (128). Some future SIDS victims thus have different autonomic responsiveness to obstructive apnea, perhaps indicating impaired autonomic nervous system control associated with higher vulnerability to external or endogenous stress factors and hence to reduced electrical stability of the heart.

Home cardiorespiratory monitors with memory capability have recorded the terminal events in some SIDS victims (129). These recordings, however, have not included SpO2 and do not permit identification of obstructed breaths due to reliance on transthoracic impedance for breath detection. In most instances, there has been sudden and rapid progression of severe bradycardia that is either unassociated with central apnea or appears to occur too soon to be explained by the central apnea. These observations are consistent with an abnormality in autonomic control of heart rate variability, or with obstructed breaths and associated bradycardia or hypoxemia.

Reducing Risk for Sudden Infant Death Syndrome

The international back-to-sleep campaigns have significantly reduced environmental risks for SIDS and have been associated with reductions in SIDS rates of 50% or more since the early 1990s. Despite the successes with risk reduction, however, there is no intervention that can be guaranteed to prevent SIDS in individual infants. Home electronic surveillance for apnea and bradycardia has been utilized for more than two decades, but no suitably designed prospective studies have been performed and hence no data exist to support a role for home cardiorespiratory monitors in preventing SIDS (130).

Limited data are available from the National Maternal and Infant Health Survey regarding extent of home monitor use in preterm and full-term SIDS victims and live controls (132). The prevalence estimates for monitor use for birth weights of 500 to 1,499, 1,500 to 2,499, and 2,500 grams or more were 20%, 3%, and 1% in African-American infants versus 44%, 9%, and 1% for other infants. In no instance was there a significant difference in prevalence of home monitor use in SIDS versus case controls, and in African-American infants with birth weights of 500 to 1,499 grams, the adjusted odds ratio for SIDS was significantly higher (3.9) with a home monitor. This higher odds ratio likely reflects a higher risk for SIDS in those infants monitored in this retrospective nonrandomized observational study.

Preventing extreme events such as observed in the CHIME study may be necessary if home monitors are to have any potential for reducing risk for SIDS (47). Even if prolonged apnea including obstructed breaths were not a primary autonomic abnormality contributing to risk for SIDS, home monitoring could still be potentially helpful if apnea of any type causing bradycardia or hypoxemia as part of the terminal event could be reliably detected sufficiently early to be amenable to intervention before the onset of life-threatening hypoxemia. However, this hypothesis remains untested and neither home electronic surveillance using current technology nor any other intervention can be recommended as a strategy to prevent SIDS. Despite absence of any proven prospective intervention to prevent SIDS, dramatic decreases in population-based risk can be achieved by eliminating modifiable risk factors associated with SIDS.

REFERENCES

1. Rigatto H. Maturation of breathing. *Clin Perinatol* 1992;19: 739–756.
2. Haddad G. Respiratory control in the newborn: comparative physiology and clinical disorders. In: Mathew OP, ed. *Respiratory control and disorders in the newborn.* New York: Marcel Dekker, 2003:1–13.
3. Hunt CE. Sudden infant death syndrome and other causes of infant mortality: diagnosis, mechanisms, and risk for recurrence in siblings. *Am J Respir Crit Care Med* 2001;164:346–357.
4. Kahn A, Franco P, Scaillet S, et al. Development of cardiopulmonary integration and the role of arousability from sleep. *Curr Opin Pulm Med* 1997;3:440–444.
5. Katz DM, Balkowiec A. New insights into the ontogeny of breathing from genetically engineered mice. *Curr Opin Pulm Med* 1997;3:433–439.
6. Fortin G, del Toro ED, Abadie V, et al. Genetic and developmental models for the neural control of breathing in vertebrates. *Respir Physiol* 2000;122:247–257.
7. Dauger S, Renolleau S, Vardon G, et al. Ventilatory responses to hypercapnia and hypoxia in Mash-1 heterozygous newborn and adult mice. *Pediatr Res* 1999;46:535–542.
8. Panigrahy A, Filiano J, Sleeper LA, et al. Decreased serotonergic receptor binding in rhombic lip-derived regions of the medulla oblongata in the sudden infant death syndrome. *J Neuropathol Exp Neurol* 2000;59:377–384.
9. Narita N, Narita M, Takashima S, et al. Serotonin transporter gene variation is a risk factor for sudden infant death syndrome in the Japanese population. *Pediatrics* 2001;107:690–692.
10. Weese-Mayer DE, Berry-Kravis EM, Maher BS, et al. Sudden infant death syndrome: association with a promoter polymorphism of the serotonin transporter gene. *Am J Med Genet* 2003;117A:268–274.
11. Dawes GS. Breathing before birth in animals and man. An essay in developmental medicine. *N Engl J Med* 1974;290:557–559.
12. Kaplan M. Fetal breathing movements. An update for the pediatrician. *Am J Dis Child* 1983;137:177–181.
13. Patrick J, Campbell K, Carmichael L, et al. A definition of human fetal apnea and the distribution of fetal apneic intervals during the last ten weeks of pregnancy. *Am J Obstet Gynecol* 1980;136:471–472.
14. Natale R, Nasello-Paterson C, Connors G. Patterns of fetal breathing activity in the human fetus at 24 to 28 weeks of gestation. *Am J Obstet Gynecol* 1988;158:317–321.
15. Kalache KD, Chaoui R, Marcks B, et al. Differentiation between human fetal breathing patterns by investigation of breathing-related tracheal fluid flow velocity using Doppler sonography. *Prenat Diagn* 2000;20:45–50.
16. Goodman JD. The effect of intravenous glucose on human fetal breathing measured by Doppler ultrasound. *Br J Obstet Gynaecol* 1980;87:1080–1083.
17. Trudinger BJ, Lewis PJ, Petit B. Fetal breathing patterns in intrauterine growth retardation. *Br J Obstet Gynaecol* 1979;86:432–436.
18. Manning FA, Platt LD. Fetal breathing movements: antepartum monitoring of fetal condition. *Clin Obstet Gynaecol* 1979;6: 335–349.
19. Ritchie JW, Lakhani K. Fetal breathing movements in response to maternal inhalation of 5% carbon dioxide. *Am J Obstet Gynecol* 1980;136:386–388.
20. Devoe LD, Abduljabbar H, Carmichael L, et al. The effects of maternal hyperoxia on fetal breathing movements in third-trimester pregnancies. *Am J Obstet Gynecol* 1984;148:790–794.
21. Bekedam DJ, Mulder EJ, Snijders RJ, et al. The effects of maternal hyperoxia on fetal breathing movements, body movements and hear rate variation in growth retarded fetuses. *Early Hum Dev* 1991;27:223–232.
22. Hallak M, Moise K Jr, Lira N, et al. The effect of tocolytic agents (indomethacin and terbutaline) on fetal breathing and body movements: a prospective, randomized, double-blind, placebo-controlled clinical trial. *Am J Obstet Gynecol* 1992;167: 1059–1063.
23. Rigatto H, Moore M, Cates D. Fetal breathing and behavior measured through a double-wall Plexiglas window in sheep. *J Appl Physiol* 1986;61:160–164.
24. Boddy K, Dawes GS. Fetal breathing. *Br Med Bull* 1975;31:3–7.
25. Dawes GS, Gardner WN, Johnston BM, et al. Effects of hypercapnia on tracheal pressure, diaphragm and intercostal electromyograms in unanaesthetized fetal lambs. *J Physiol* 1982;326:461–474.
26. Moss IR, Scarpelli EM. Generation and regulation of breathing in utero: fetal CO_2 response test. *J Appl Physiol* 1979;47:527–531.
27. Clewlow F, Dawes GS, Johnston BM, et al. Changes in breathing, electrocortical and muscle activity in unanaesthetized fetal lambs with age. *J Physiol* 1983;341:463–476.
28. Condorelli S, Scarpelli EM. Fetal breathing: induction in utero and effects of vagotomy and barbiturates. *J Pediatr* 1976;88:94–101.
29. Jansen AH, Ioffe S, Russell BJ, et al. Effect of carotid chemoreceptor denervation on breathing in utero and after birth. *J Appl Physiol* 1981;51:630–633.
30. Gluckman PD, Gunn TR, Johnston BM. The effect of cooling on breathing and shivering in unanaesthetized fetal lambs in utero. *J Physiol* 1983;343:495–506.
31. Gerhardt T, Bancalari E. Apnea of prematurity. II. Respiratory reflexes. *Pediatrics* 1984;74:63–66.
32. Alvaro R, Alvarez J, Kwiatkowski K, et al. Small preterm infants (less than or equal to 1500 g) have only a sustained decrease in ventilation in response to hypoxia. *Pediatr Res* 1992;32:403–406.
33. Gluckman PD, Johnston BM. Lesions in the upper lateral pons abolish the hypoxic depression of breathing in unanaesthetized fetal lambs in utero. *J Physiol* 1987;382:373–383.
34. Miller MJ, Martin RJ. Apnea of prematurity. *Clin Perinatol* 1992;19:789–808.
35. Thach BT, Schefft GL, Pickens DL, et al. Influence of upper airway negative pressure reflex on response to airway occlusion in sleeping infants. *J Appl Physiol* 1989;67:749–755.
36. Menon AP, Schefft GL, Thach BT. Frequency and significance of swallowing during prolonged apnea in infants. *Am Rev Respir Dis* 1984;130:969–973.
37. Lawson EE. Prolonged central respiratory inhibition following reflex-induced apnea. *J Appl Physiol* 1981;50:874–879.
38. Perkett EA, Vaughan RL. Evidence for a laryngeal chemoreflex in some human preterm infants. *Acta Paediatr Scand* 1982;71:969–972.

39. National Institutes of Health Consensus Development Conference on Infantile Apnea and Home Monitoring, Sept 29 to Oct 1, 1986. *Pediatrics* 1987;79:292–299.

40. Rigatto H. Breathing and sleep in preterm infants. In: Loughlin GM, Carroll JL, Marcus CL, eds. *Sleep and breathing in children. a developmental approach.* New York: Marcel Dekker, 2000:495–523.

41. Glotzbach SF, Baldwin RB, Lederer NE, et al. Periodic breathing in preterm infants: incidence and characteristics. *Pediatrics* 1989; 84:785–792.

42. Richards JM, Alexander JR, Shinebourne EA, et al. Sequential 22-hour profiles of breathing patterns and heart rate in 110 full-term infants during their first 6 months of life. *Pediatrics* 1984;74: 763–777.

43. Kelly DH, Stellwagen LM, Kaitz E, et al. Apnea and periodic breathing in normal full-term infants during the first twelve months. *Pediatr Pulmonol* 1985;1:215–219.

44. Hunt CE. Apnea and sudden infant death syndrome. In: Kliegman RM, Nieder ML, Super DM, eds. *Practical strategies in pediatric diagnosis and therapy.* Philadelphia: WB Saunders, 1996: 135–147.

45. Henderson-Smart DJ, Pettigrew AG, Campbell DJ. Clinical apnea and brain-stem neural function in preterm infants. *N Engl J Med* 1983;308:353–357.

46. Ramanathan R, Corwin MJ, Hunt CE, et al. Cardiorespiratory events recorded on home monitors. Comparison of healthy infants with those at increased risk for SIDS. *JAMA* 2001;285: 2199–2207.

47. Hunt CE. Sudden infant death syndrome. In: Spitzer AR, ed. *Intensive care of the fetus and neonate,* 2nd ed. St. Louis: Elsevier, 2005:.

48. Alden ER, Mandelkorn T, Woodrum DE, et al. Morbidity and mortality of infants weighing less than 1,000 grams in an intensive care nursery. *Pediatrics* 1972;50:40–49.

49. Carlo WA, Martin RJ, Versteegh FG, et al. The effect of respiratory distress syndrome on chest wall movements and respiratory pauses in preterm infants. *Am Rev Respir Dis* 1982;126:103–107.

50. Kattwinkel J, Nearman HS, Fanaroff AA, et al. Apnea of prematurity. Comparative therapeutic effects of cutaneous stimulation and nasal continuous positive airway pressure. *J Pediatr* 1975; 86:588–592.

51. Joshi A, Gerhardt T, Shandloff P, et al. Blood transfusion effect on the respiratory pattern of preterm infants. *Pediatrics* 1987;80: 79–84.

52. Ross MP, Christensen RD, Rothstein G, et al. A randomized trial to develop criteria for administering erythrocyte transfusions to anemic preterm infants 1 to 3 months of age. *J Perinatol* 1989;9: 246–253.

53. Sasidharan P, Heimler R. Transfusion-induced changes in the breathing pattern of healthy preterm anemic infants. *Pediatr Pulmonol* 1992;12:170–173.

54. Bifano EM, Smith F, Borer J. Relationship between determinants of oxygen delivery and respiratory abnormalities in preterm infants with anemia. *J Pediatr* 1992;120:292–206.

55. Keyes WG, Donohue PK, Spivak JL, et al. Assessing the need for transfusion of premature infants and role of hematocrit, clinical signs, and erythropoietin level. *Pediatrics* 1989;84:412–417.

56. Poets CF, Pauls U, Bohnhorst B. Effect of blood transfusion on apnoea, bradycardia and hypoxaemia in preterm infants. *Eur J Pediatr* 1997;156:311–316.

57. Lawson EE. Nonpharmacological management of idiopathic apnea of the premature infant. In: Mathew OP, ed. *Respiratory control and disorders in the newborn.* New York: Marcel Dekker, 2003:335–354.

58. Peliowski A, Finer NN. A blinded, randomized, placebo-controlled trial to compare theophylline and doxapram for the treatment of apnea of prematurity. *J Pediatr* 1990;116:648–653.

59. Aranda JV, Gorman W, Bergsteinsson H, et al. Efficacy of caffeine in treatment of apnea in the low-birth-weight infant. *J Pediatr* 1977;90:467–472.

60. Erenberg A, Leff RD, Haack DG, et al. Caffeine citrate for the treatment of apnea of prematurity: a double-blind, placebo-controlled study. *Pharmacotherapy* 2000;20:644–652.

61. Fuglsang G, Nielsen K, Kjaer NL, et al. The effect of caffeine compared with theophylline in the treatment of idiopathic apnea in premature infants. *Acta Paediatr Scand* 1989;78:786–788.

62. Bairam A, Boutroy MJ, Badonnel Y, et al. Theophylline versus caffeine: comparative effects in treatment of idiopathic apnea in the preterm infant. *J Pediatr* 1987;110:636–639.

63. Brouard C, Moriette G, Murat I, et al. Comparative efficacy of theophylline and caffeine in the treatment of idiopathic apnea in premature infants. *Am J Dis Child* 1985;139:698–700.

64. Sims ME, Yau G, Rambhatla S, et al. Limitations of theophylline in the treatment of apnea of prematurity. *Am J Dis Child* 1985; 139:567–570.

65. Murat I, Moriette G, Blin MC, et al. The efficacy of caffeine in the treatment of recurrent idiopathic apnea in premature infants. *J Pediatr* 1981;99:984–989.

66. Gupta JM, Mercer HP, Koo WW. Theophylline in treatment of apnoea of prematurity. *Aust Paediatr J* 1981;17:290–291.

67. Jones RA. Apnoea of immaturity. 1. A controlled trial of theophylline and face mask continuous positive airways pressure. *Arch Dis Child* 1982;57:761–765.

68. Henderson-Smart DJ, Subramaniam P, Davis PG. Continuous positive airway pressure versus theophylline for apnea in preterm infants. *Cochrane Database Syst Rev* 2001;4:CD001072.

69. Miller MJ, Carlo WA, Martin RJ. Continuous positive airway pressure selectively reduces obstructive apnea in preterm infants. *J Pediatr* 1985;106:91–94.

70. Khalaf MN, Brodsky N, Hurley J, et al. A prospective randomized, controlled trial comparing synchronized nasal intermittent positive pressure ventilation versus nasal continuous positive airway pressure as modes of extubation. *Pediatrics* 2001;108: 13–17.

71. Courtney SE, Pyon KH, Saslow JG, et al. Lung recruitment and breathing pattern during variable versus continuous flow nasal continuous positive airway pressure in premature infants: an evaluation of three devices. *Pediatrics* 2001;107:304–308.

72. Lemyre B, Davis PG, De Paoli AG. Nasal intermittent positive pressure ventilation (NIPPV) versus nasal continuous positive airway pressure (NCPAP) for apnea of prematurity. *Cochrane Database Syst Rev* 2000;3:CD002272.

73. Hunt CE, Inwood RJ, Shannon DC. Respiratory and nonrespiratory effects of doxapram in congenital central hypoventilation syndrome. *Am Rev Respir Dis* 1979;119:263–269.

74. Barrington KJ, Finer NN, Peters KL, et al. Physiologic effects of doxapram in idiopathic apnea of prematurity. *J Pediatr* 1986; 108:124–129.

75. Brion LP, Vega-Rich C, Reinersman G, et al. Low-dose doxapram for apnea unresponsive to aminophylline in very low birth-weight infants. *J Perinatol* 1991;11:359–364.

76. Arad-Cohen N, Cohen A, Tirosh E. The relationship between gastroesophageal reflux and apnea in infants. *J Pediatr* 2000;137: 321–326.

77. Kahn A, Rebuffat E, Sottiaux M, et al. Lack of temporal relation between acid reflux in the proximal oesophagus and cardiorespiratory events in sleeping infants. *Eur J Pediatr* 1992;151: 208–212.

78. Peter CS, Sprodowski N, Bohnhorst B, et al. Gastroesophageal reflux and apnea of prematurity: no temporal relationship. *Pediatrics* 2002;109:8–11.

79. Wenzl TG, Schenke S, Peschgens T, et al. Association of apnea and nonacid gastroesophageal reflux in infants: investigations with the intraluminal impedance technique. *Pediatr Pulmonol* 2001;31:144–149.

80. Mathew OP. Respiratory control during nipple feeding in preterm infants. *Pediatr Pulmonol* 1988;5:220–224.

81. Shivpuri CR, Martin RJ, Carlo WA, et al. Decreased ventilation in preterm infants during oral feeding. *J Pediatr* 1983;103:285–289.

82. Bruhn FW, Mokrohisky ST, McIntosh K. Apnea associated with respiratory syncytial virus infection in young infants. *J Pediatr* 1977;90:382–386.

83. Kneyber MC, Brandenburg AH, de Groot R, et al. Risk factors for respiratory syncytial virus associated apnoea. *Eur J Pediatr* 1998;157:331–335.

84. Cote CJ, Zaslavsky A, Downes JJ, et al. Postoperative apnea in former preterm infants after inguinal herniorrhaphy. A combined analysis. *Anesthesiology* 1995;82:809–822.

85. Welborn LG, Hannallah RS, Luban NL, et al. Anemia and postoperative apnea in former preterm infants. *Anesthesiology* 1991; 74:1003–1006.

86. Darnall RA, Kattwinkel J, Nattie C, et al. Margin of safety for discharge after apnea in preterm infants. *Pediatrics* 1997;100:795–801.

87. Di Fiore JM, Arko MK, Miller MJ, et al. Cardiorespiratory events in preterm infants referred for apnea monitoring studies. *Pediatrics* 2001;108:1304–1308.

88. Barrington KJ, Finer N, Li D. Predischarge respiratory recordings in very low birth weight newborn infants. *J Pediatr* 1996;129: 934–940.

89. Schmidt B. Methylxanthine therapy in premature infants: sound practice, disaster, or fruitless byway? *J Pediatr* 1999;135:526–528.

90. Martin RJ, Fanaroff AA. Neonatal apnea, bradycardia, or desaturation: does it matter? *J Pediatr* 1998;132:758–759.

91. Cheung PY, Barrington KJ, Finer NN, et al. Early childhood neurodevelopment in very low birth weight infants with predischarge apnea. *Pediatr Pulmonol* 1999;27:14–20.

92. Eichenwald EC, Aina A, Stark AR. Apnea frequently persists beyond term gestation in infants delivered at 24 to 28 weeks. *Pediatrics* 1997;100:354–359.

93. Sreenan C, Etches PC, Demianczuk N, et al. Isolated mental developmental delay in very low birth weight infants: association with prolonged doxapram therapy for apnea. *J Pediatr* 2001;139:832–837.

94. Hunt CE, Baird T, The Collaborative Home Infant Monitoring Evaluation (CHIME) Study Group, et al. Cardiorespiratory events detected by home memory monitoring and neurodevelopmental outcome at one year of age. *J Pediatr* 2004;145:465–471

95. Gozal D. Sleep-disordered breathing and school performance in children. *Pediatrics* 1998;102:616–620.

96. Macey PM, Henderson LA, Macey KE, et al. Brain morphology associated with obstructive sleep apnea. *Am J Respir Crit Care Med* 2002;166:1382–1387.

97. Kim HC, Young T, Matthews CG, et al. Sleep-disordered breathing and neuropsychological deficits. A population-based study. *Am J Respir Crit Care Med* 1997;156:1813–1819.

98. Samuels MP. Apparent life-threatening events: pathogenesis and management. In: Loughlin GM, Carroll JL, Marcus CL, eds. *Sleep and breathing in children: a developmental approach.* New York: Marcel Dekker, 2000:423–441.

99. Hunt CE, Hauck FR. Sudden Infant Syndrome. In: Behrman RE, Kliegman RM, Jenson HB, eds. *Nelson textbook of pediatrics,* 17th ed. Philadelphia: Elsevier, 2004:1380–1385.

100. American Academy of Pediatrics. Task Force on Infant Sleep Position and Sudden Infant Death Syndrome. Changing concepts of sudden infant death syndrome: implications for infant sleeping environment and sleep position. *Pediatrics* 2000;105: 650–656.

101. Willinger M, James LS, Catz C. Defining the sudden infant death syndrome (SIDS): deliberations of an expert panel convened by the National Institute of Child Health and Human Development. *Pediatr Pathol* 1991;11:677–684.

102. Hoyert DL, Freedman MA, Strobino DM, et al. Annual summary of vital statistics: 2000. *Pediatrics* 2001;108:1241–1255.

103. Malloy MH, Hoffman HJ. Prematurity, sudden infant death syndrome, and age of death. *Pediatrics* 1995;96:464–471.

104. Valdes-Dapena M. The sudden infant death syndrome: pathologic findings. *Clin Perinatol* 1992;19:701–716.

105. Naeye RL. Sudden infant death syndrome, is the confusion ending? *Mod Pathol* 1988;1:169–174.

106. Jones KL, Krous HF, Nadeau J, et al. Vascular endothelial growth factor in the cerebrospinal fluid of infants who died of sudden infant death syndrome: evidence for antecedent hypoxia. *Pediatrics* 2003;111:358–363.

107. Rognum TO, Saugstad OD. Hypoxanthine levels in vitreous humor: evidence of hypoxia in most infants who died of sudden infant death syndrome. *Pediatrics* 1991;87:306–310.

108. Obonai T, Yasuhara M, Nakamura T, et al. Catecholamine neurons alteration in the brainstem of sudden infant death syndrome victims. *Pediatrics* 1998;101:285–288.

109. Ozawa Y, Okado N. Alteration of serotonergic receptors in the brain stems of human patients with respiratory disorders. *Neuropediatrics* 2002;33:142–149.

110. Filiano JJ, Kinney HC. Arcuate nucleus hypoplasia in the sudden infant death syndrome. *J Neuropathol Exp Neurol* 1992;51:394–403.

111. Matturri L, Biondo B, Suarez-Mier MP, et al. Brain stem lesions in the sudden infant death syndrome: variability in the hypoplasia of the arcuate nucleus. *Acta Neuropathol (Berl)* 2002; 104:12–20.

112. Hasan SU, Simakajornboon N, MacKinnon Y, et al. Prenatal cigarette smoke exposure selectively alters protein kinase C and nitric oxide synthase expression within the neonatal rat brainstem. *Neurosci Lett* 2001;301:135–138.

113. Vernacchio L, Corwin MJ, Lesko SM, et al. Sleep position of low birth weight infants. *Pediatrics* 2003;111:633–640.

114. Malloy MH, Freeman DH Jr. Birth weight- and gestational age-specific sudden infant death syndrome mortality: United States, 1991 versus 1995. *Pediatrics* 2000;105:1227–1231.

115. Hunt CE, Lesko SM, Vezina RM, et al. Infant sleep position and associated health outcomes. *Arch Pediatr Adolesc Med* 2003;157: 469–474.

116. McMartin KI, Platt MS, Hackman R, et al. Lung tissue concentrations of nicotine in sudden infant death syndrome (SIDS). *J Pediatr* 2002;140:205–209.

117. Wisborg K, Kesmodel U, Henriksen TB, et al. A prospective study of smoking during pregnancy and SIDS. *Arch Dis Child* 2000;83: 203–206.

118. Froen JF, Akre H, Stray-Pedersen B, et al. Adverse effects of nicotine and interleukin-1beta on autoresuscitation after apnea in piglets: implications for sudden infant death syndrome. *Pediatrics* 2000;105:E52.

119. Gordon AE, El Ahmer OR, Chan R, et al. Why is smoking a risk factor for sudden infant death syndrome? *Child Care Health Dev* 2002;28(Suppl 1):23–25.

120. Iyasu S, Randall LL, Welty TK, et al. Risk factors for sudden infant death syndrome among northern plains Indians. *JAMA* 2002;288:2717–2723.

121. Hoffman HJ, Hillman LS. Epidemiology of the sudden infant death syndrome: maternal, neonatal, and postneonatal risk factors. *Clin Perinatol* 1992;19:717–737.

122. Ward SL, Bautista D, Chan L, et al. Sudden infant death syndrome in infants of substance-abusing mothers. *J Pediatr* 1990;117:876–881.

123. Blackwell CC, Weir DM, Busuttil A. Infection, inflammation and sleep: more pieces to the puzzle of sudden infant death syndrome (SIDS). *APMIS* 1999;107:455–473.

124. Gold Y, Goldberg A, Sivan Y. Hyper-releasability of mast cells in family members of infants with sudden infant death syndrome and apparent life-threatening events. *J Pediatr* 2000; 136:460–465.

125. Waters KA, Gonzalez A, Jean C, et al. Face-straight-down and face-near-straight-down positions in healthy, prone-sleeping infants. *J Pediatr* 1996;128:616–625.

126. Poets CF, Meny RG, Chobanian MR, et al. Gasping and other cardiorespiratory patterns during sudden infant deaths. *Pediatr Res* 1999;45:350–354.

127. Ward SL, Bautista DB, Keens TG. Hypoxic arousal responses in normal infants. *Pediatrics* 1992;89:860–864.

128. Franco P, Szliwowski H, Dramaix M, et al. Decreased autonomic responses to obstructive sleep events in future victims of sudden infant death syndrome. *Pediatr Res* 1999;46:33–39.

129. Meny RG, Carroll JL, Carbone MT, et al. Cardiorespiratory recordings from infants dying suddenly and unexpectedly at home. *Pediatrics* 1994;93:44–49.

130. American Academy of Pediatrics. Committee on Fetus and Newborn. Apnea, sudden infant death syndrome, and home monitoring. *Pediatrics* 2003;111:914–917.

131. Malloy MH, Hoffman HJ. Home apnea monitoring and sudden infant death syndrome. *Prev Med* 1996;25:645–649.

132. Martin RJ, Miller MJ, Carlo WA. Pathogenesis of apnea in preterm infants. *J Pediatr* 1986;109:733–741.

133. Gerhardt T, Bancalari E. Apnea of prematurity: I. Lung function and regulation of breathing. *Pediatrics* 1984;74:58–62.

134. Miller MJ, Martin RJ, Carlo WA. Diagnostic methods and clinical disorders in children. In Edelman NH, Santiago TV, eds. *Breathing disorders of sleep.* New York: Churchill Livingstone, 1986: 157–180.

Acute

29

Respiratory Disorders

Jeffrey A. Whitsett   *Ward R. Rice*   *Barbara B. Warner*
Susan E. Wert   *Gloria S. Pryhuber*

Successful adaptation to air breathing at the time of birth is the culmination of an orderly process of growth and differentiation of pulmonary cells, leading to alveolar and capillary surfaces capable of providing oxygen and eliminating carbon dioxide. Failure to achieve adequate gas exchange at birth represents a major cause of perinatal morbidity and mortality. This chapter reviews the common disorders of neonatal respiratory adaptation, including respiratory distress syndrome (RDS), pulmonary meconium aspiration syndrome (MAS), pulmonary hypertension, pneumonia, air leak, pulmonary hemorrhage, transient tachypnea of the newborn (TTN), and other causes of acute respiratory dysfunction in the perinatal period. The clinical manifestations and therapy of these disorders are discussed in the context of the morphologic, biochemical, and physiologic factors critical to normal pulmonary growth, maturation, and function in the newborn.

HUMAN LUNG DEVELOPMENT

Human lung development is normally divided into five distinct stages of organogenesis, which describe the histologic changes that the lung undergoes during morphogenesis and maturation of its structural elements (1,2). These five stages include the embryonic, pseudoglandular, canalicular, saccular, and alveolar stages of lung development. Human lung development is initiated during the early embryonic period of gestation (3–7 weeks postcoitum) as a small saccular outgrowth of the ventral foregut called the respiratory diverticulum. During the subsequent pseudoglandular stage of lung development (5–17 weeks postcoitum), formation of the conducting airways, i.e., the tracheobronchial tree, occurs by elongation and repetitive branching of the primitive bronchial tubules. Vascularization of the surrounding mesenchyme with formation of the air-blood barrier, i.e., the

alveolar-capillary membrane, occurs during the canalicular stage of lung development (16–26 weeks postcoitum). Cytodifferentiation of bronchiolar and alveolar epithelial cells is also initiated during this stage. Enlargement and expansion of the peripheral air spaces occurs during the saccular stage of lung development (24–38 weeks postcoitum), resulting in the formation of primitive sac-like alveoli and thick interalveolar septa. Formation of thin secondary alveolar septa and remodeling of the capillary bed occurs during the alveolar stage of lung development (36 weeks postcoitum to 8 years of age), giving rise to the mature alveolar organization of the adult lung (Fig. 29-1).

The human lung is a derivative of the primitive foregut endoderm and the surrounding splanchnic mesoderm. The primitive respiratory diverticulum appears at 3 weeks of gestation as an enlargement of the caudal end of the laryngotracheal sulcus located in the median pharyngeal groove, which is an outgrowth of the ventral wall of the primitive esophagus. During the fourth week of gestation, the respiratory diverticulum enlarges and subdivides into the left and right primary bronchi (see Fig. 29-1A,B). The primitive lung grows caudally, expanding into the mesenchyme surrounding the primitive foregut, although the trachea becomes separated from the esophagus by a band of mesenchymal tissue called the tracheoesophageal septum. Between 4 and 5 weeks of gestation, the left and right primary bronchi subdivide to produce secondary, or lobar, bronchi (see Fig. 29-1C,D). Further subdivision of lobar bronchi into tertiary or segmental bronchi occurs during the sixth week of gestation, with the lung taking on a lobulated appearance as the segmental buds are formed (see Fig. 29-1E,F). The developing respiratory tract is lined by endodermally derived epithelium that forms the conducting airways and alveoli. The surrounding mesoderm is composed of mesenchymal cells that will differentiate into connective tissue components,

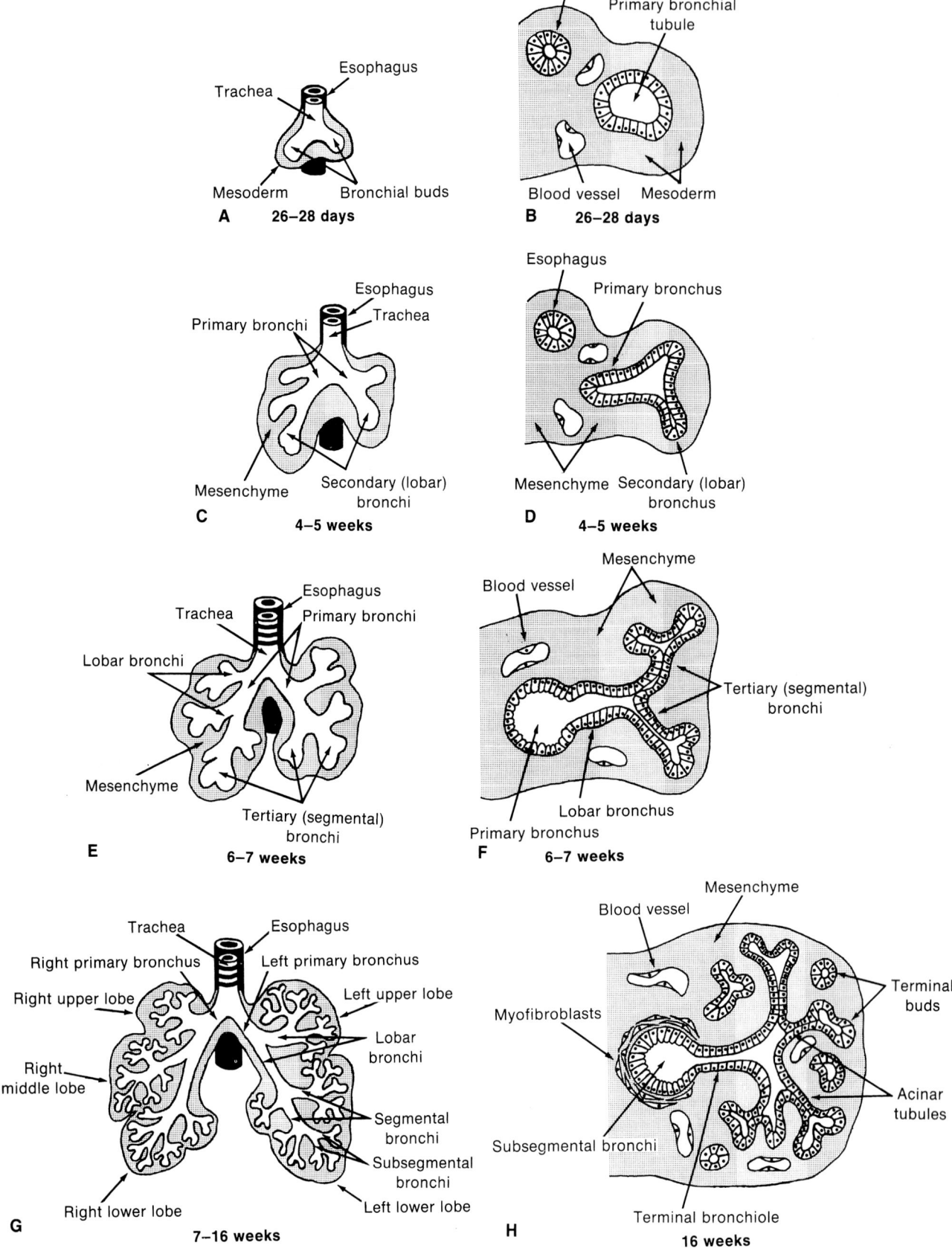

Figure 29-1 Lung development during the embryonic (A–F) and pseudoglandular (G,H) stages of organogenesis. The overall branching pattern of the primitive lung (left panels) results in the development of the bronchial tree. The histologic organization of the fetal lung becomes more complex as branching morphogenesis progresses through these stages (right panels).

including blood vessels, fibroblasts, smooth muscle cells, and cartilage.

Preacinar blood vessels first appear at the end of week 4. Pulmonary arteries arise from the sixth pair of aortic arches and grow into the mesenchyme, in which they accompany the developing airways, segmenting with each bronchial subdivision. Pulmonary veins develop as outgrowths of the left atrium of the heart and subdivide several times before connecting to the pulmonary vascular bed. Intraacinar vessels develop later, in parallel with alveolar formation.

The pseudoglandular stage of fetal lung development extends from about 5 to 17 weeks of gestation and is marked by the formation of the bronchial portion of the lung. This occurs through a process known as branching morphogenesis, during which the segmental tubules of the developing lung undergo repetitive lateral and terminal dichotomous branching to form the primitive bronchial tree (see Fig. 29-1G,H). By week 17 of gestation, the segmental bronchi have subdivided to produce approximately 23 generations of bronchial tubules ending in the terminal bronchioles. These bronchial tubules are lined initially by a pseudostratified columnar epithelium containing large pools of glycogen. A prominent basement membrane underlies the epithelium, and mesenchymal cells adjacent to these tubules differentiate into fibroblasts, which become organized in a circumferential orientation, perpendicular to the long axis of the tubules. As branching progresses, pseudostratified columnar epithelium is reduced to a tall columnar epithelium, especially in distal regions of the bronchial tree. During this period, cytodifferentiation of the airway epithelium occurs in a centrifugal direction with ciliated, nonciliated, goblet, neuroendocrine, and basal cells appearing first in the more proximal airways. Cartilage, smooth muscle cells, and mucous glands are also found in the trachea during the pseudoglandular stage of development and extend as far as the segmental bronchi.

The canalicular stage of fetal lung development extends from week 16 to 26 of gestation. By the end of week 16, the terminal bronchioles have divided into two or more respiratory bronchioles that have subdivided into small clusters of short acinar tubules and buds lined by cuboidal epithelium. These structures undergo further differentiation and maturation to become the adult respiratory unit, or pulmonary acinus, consisting of the alveolated respiratory bronchiole, alveolar ducts, and alveoli. Clusters of acinar tubules and buds continue to grow by lengthening, subdividing, and widening at the expense of the surrounding mesenchyme (Fig. 29-2A). This peripheral growth is accompanied by the formation of intraacinar capillaries, which align themselves around the air spaces, establishing contact with the overlying cuboidal epithelium. During this stage of lung development, type II epithelial cell differentiation occurs in acinar tubules with formation of intracellular multivesicular bodies and multilamellar bodies, the storage form of pulmonary surfactant phospholipids. Type I epithelial cell differentiation occurs in conjunction with development of the air-blood barrier, wherever

endothelial cells of the developing capillary system come into contact with the overlying epithelial cells.

During the saccular stage of fetal lung development, which extends from week 24 to 38 of gestation, the terminal clusters of acinar tubules and buds begin to dilate and expand into thin, smooth-walled, transitory ducts and saccules that later become the true alveolar ducts and alveoli of the adult (Fig. 29-2B). During this stage, there is a marked reduction in the amount of interstitial tissue. Intersaccular and interductal septa develop, which contain a delicate network of collagen fibers and the intraacinar capillary bed. Near the end of this stage, elastin is deposited in regions in which future interalveolar septa will form. Increasing amounts of tubular myelin, the secretory form of pulmonary surfactant, are seen in the air spaces.

The alveolar stage, which extends from 36 weeks of gestation to between 2 and 8 years of age, is the last stage of lung development and is marked by the formation of secondary alveolar septa, which partition the transitory ducts and saccules into true alveolar ducts and alveoli (Fig. 29-2C,D). This process of alveolarization greatly increases the surface area of the lung available for gas exchange. At the beginning of this period, the secondary interalveolar septa consist of short buds or projections of connective tissue that contain a double capillary network and interstitial cells that are actively synthesizing collagen and elastic fibers. By 5 months of age, these secondary interalveolar septa have lengthened and thinned, and now contain only a single capillary network. Although definitive alveoli can be found in the human lung by 36 weeks of gestation, 85 to 90% of all alveoli are formed within the first 6 months of life. Overall the number of alveoli increases by about six-fold between birth and adulthood, i.e., from an average of 50 million alveoli in the term lung to 300 million in the adult human lung. After the first 6 months of life, alveolar formation occurs at a slower pace until about 2 to 8 years of age, when further growth of the lung becomes proportional to growth of the body. The surface area available for gas exchange, and its diffusion capacity, increases linearly with body weight up to about 18 years of age. The conducting airways also increase in length and diameter, although airspace and capillary volume increase coordinately at the expense of interstitial volume.

DEVELOPMENTAL ANOMALIES

Each of these stages of lung development includes distinct changes in tissue organization and cellular differentiation that are important for subsequent growth and maturation of the lung. Structural and functional defects in lung development at birth can often be traced to arrested or aberrant development during one of these periods of organogenesis, often as a result of mutations in genes critical for patterning and growth of the lung, such as the GLI gene (Pallister Hall Syndrome), which is a component of the

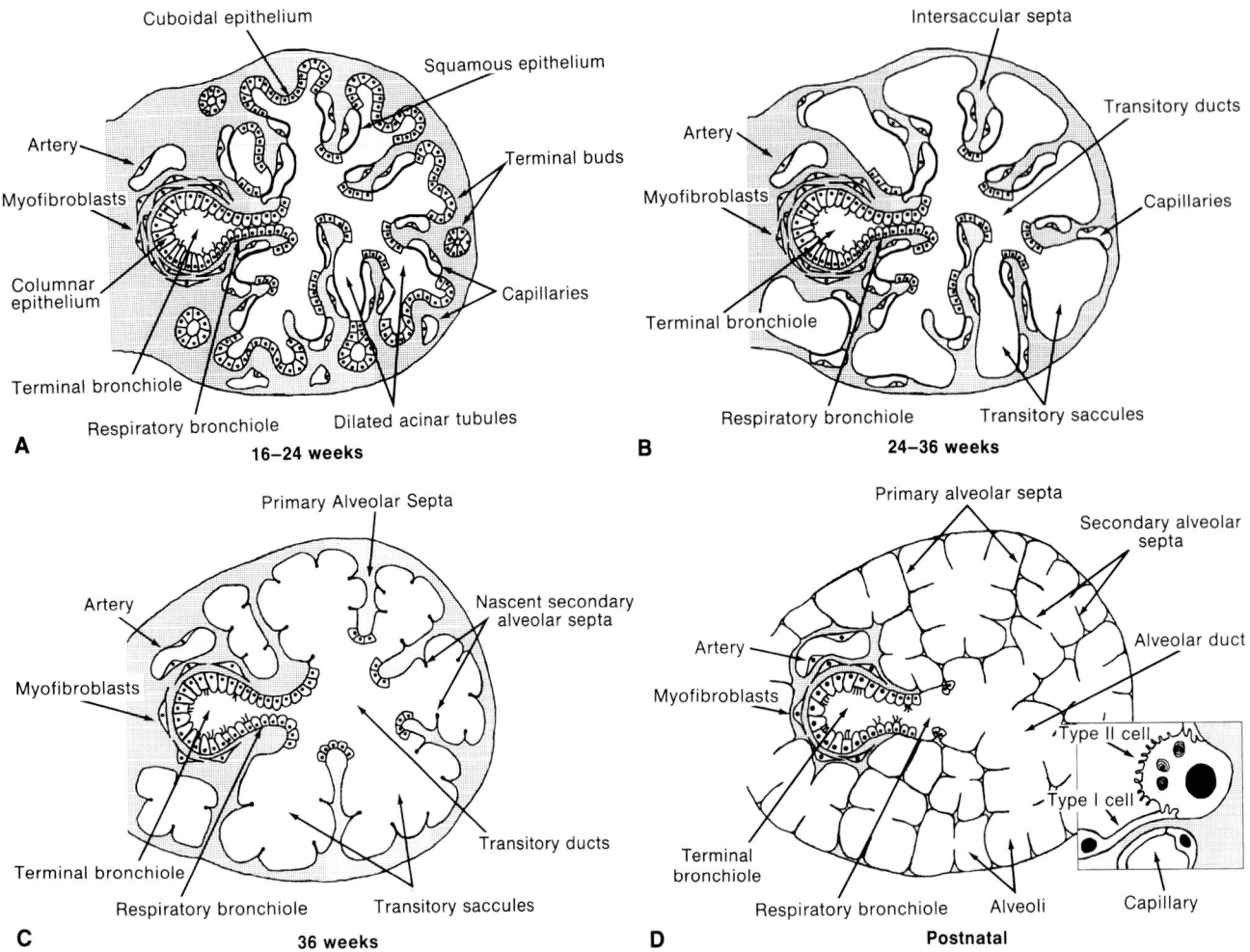

Figure 29-2 Lung development during the canalicular (A), saccular (B), and alveolar stages of organogenesis (C,D). Dramatic histologic changes in tissue organization occur during these periods. The adult alveolar epithelium is composed of squamous type I cells and cuboidal type II cells (inset).

Sonic Hedgehog signaling pathway, and the fibroblast growth factor receptor, FGFR2, gene (Pfeiffer's, Apert's, and Crouzon's syndromes). Developmental anomalies of the lung occur through defective division and differentiation of the lung bud, of the left or right bronchial bud or of the trachea and esophagus. Pulmonary agenesis, tracheal and bronchial malformations, tracheoesophageal fistulas, ectopic lobes, and bronchogenic and pulmonary cysts arise during the embryonic and pseudoglandular stages of lung development. Clinical disorders related to pulmonary hypoplasia, acinar dysplasia, alveolar capillary dysplasia, and respiratory insufficiency are associated with later periods of development. Pulmonary hypoplasia can be caused by a reduction of space within the pleural cavity, usually as a consequence of another primary developmental defect, such as congenital diaphragmatic hernia, or by a reduction in the amount of amniotic fluid following premature rupture of membranes or in association with renal dysgenesis Potter's syndrome. Respiratory distress syndrome and bronchopulmonary dysplasia are associated with premature birth at a time when biochemical functions (e.g., surfactant

production) and structural functions (e.g., elasticity) of the lung are still underdeveloped.

Hereditary-Genetic Causes of Acute Respiratory Failure in the Newborn

Mutations in the surfactant protein B and C genes are rare causes of acute respiratory failure in neonates (3,4). Hereditary SP-B deficiency causes respiratory distress, generally in full-term infants, within the first day of life. Respiratory failure progresses despite ventilatory support, surfactant replacement or ECMO, generally causing death from respiratory failure in the first months of life. Mutations in the SP-B gene are inherited as autosomal recessive traits, resulting in the lack of SP-B in the airways and severe surfactant dysfunction. Hereditary SP-B deficiency is a lethal disease, although some infants have been successfully treated with lung transplantation. The definitive diagnosis is made by genotyping. Mutations in the SP-C gene are generally inherited as autosomal-dominant, and cause both acute and chronic interstitial lung disease in newborns, infants, and adults. This disorder is associated with the lack of SP-C protein in alveolar lavage and with mutations in the proSP-C protein. The diagnosis of SP-C deficiency is made by genotyping. Mutations in a transport protein, ABCA3, also cause neonatal respiratory failure. Like hereditary SP-B deficiency, ABCA3 defects are inherited as autosomal recessive genes and cause respiratory failure that is refractory to ventilation and surfactant therapy (5).

THE SURFACTANT SYSTEM

The unique physical-chemical boundary between the alveolar gases and the highly solvated molecules at the apical surface of the respiratory epithelium generates a region of high surface tension produced by the unequal distribution of molecular forces among water molecules at an air-liquid interface. Surface-active material at this interface in the alveoli provides surface-tension-lowering activity that contributes to the remarkable pressure-volume associations characteristic of the lung. This surface-active material, called surfactant, has been subject to intense study in recent decades (6–8).

Deficiency or dysfunction of pulmonary surfactant plays a critical role in the pathogenesis of respiratory diseases in the newborn period. Pulmonary surfactant exists in a variety of physical forms when isolated from the alveolar wash of the lung. These physical forms include lamellated and

vesicular forms and highly organized tubular myelin. Tubular myelin is highly surface active and, although composed predominately of phospholipids, its unique structure depends on Ca2+ and lung surfactant proteins A (SP-A), B (SP-B), and D (SP-D). Tubular myelin represents the major extracellular pool of surfactant from which a lipid monolayered/multilayered film is generated to produce an interface between the hydrated cellular surfaces and alveolar gas (Fig. 29-3). Lamellated and vesicular forms of surfactant represent nascent or catabolic forms of surfactant material respectively; the latter is taken up by type II epithelial cells and recycled. Surfactant proteins A, B, C, and D play important roles in the organization and function of the surfactant complex regulating surfactant homeostasis. Alveolar surfactant concentrations are tightly controlled by a variety of mechanisms that modulate lipid and protein synthesis, storage, secretion, and recycling.

Composition of Surfactant

Pulmonary surfactant is composed primarily of the phospholipids phosphatidylcholine and phosphatidylglycerol (Fig. 29-4). These lipid molecules are enriched in dipalmitoyl acyl groups attached to a glycerol backbone that pack tightly and generate low surface pressures (Fig. 29-5). Rapid spreading and stability of pulmonary surfactant are achieved by the interactions of surfactant proteins and phospholipids. Surfactant is synthesized and secreted by

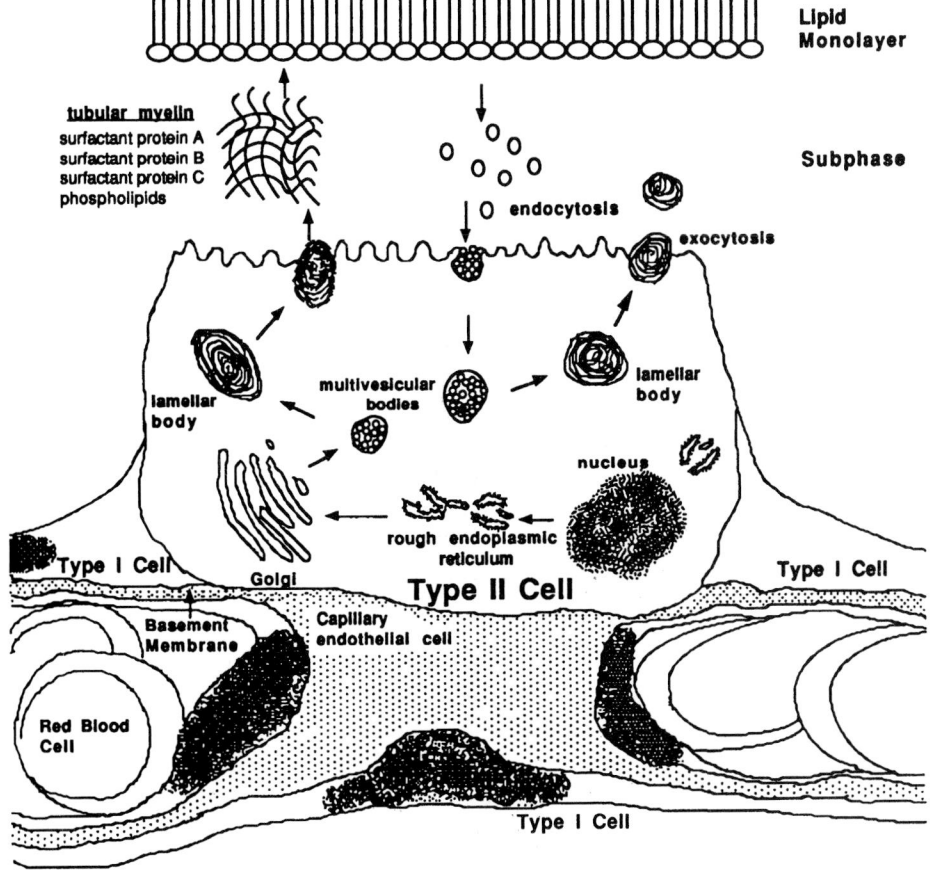

Figure 29-3 Surfactant phospholipids are synthesized in the endoplasmic reticulum, transported through the Golgi apparatus to multivesicular bodies, and ultimately packaged in lamellar bodies before secretion. After exocytosis of the lamellar bodies, surfactant phospholipids are organized into a complex lattice called tubular myelin phospholipid that provides material for a monolayer-multilayer at the air–fluid interface in the alveolus. Surfactant phospholipids and proteins are taken up by type II cells, probably transported by endosomal multivesicular bodies, and then catabolized or transported to lamellar bodies for recycling. A fraction of surfactant proteins and lipids are also catabolized by alveolar macrophages. Surfactant proteins are synthesized in polyribosomes and extensively modified in the endoplasmic reticulum, Golgi apparatus, and multivesicular bodies. Surfactant proteins are detected within lamellar bodies or in secretory vesicles closely associated with lamellar bodies before secretion into the alveolus.

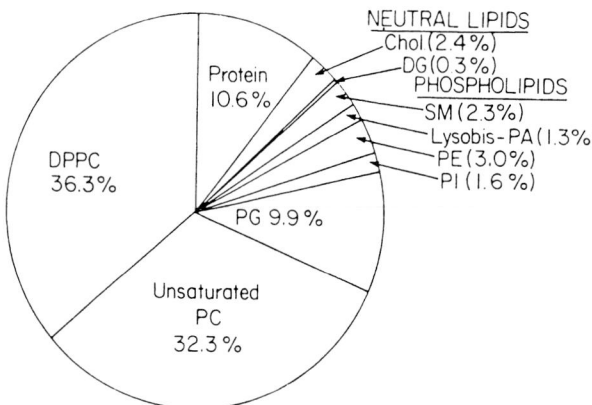

Figure 29-4 Pulmonary surfactant components are expressed as a percentage of the total weight. Chol, cholesterol; DG, diacylglycerol; DPPC, dipalmitoylphosphatidylcholine; PA, phosphatidic acid; PC, phosphatidylcholine; PE, phosphatidylethanolamine; PG, phosphatidylglycerol; PI, phosphatidylinositol; SM, sphingomyelin. Adapted from Possmayer F. Pulmonary surfactant. *Can J Biochem Cell Biol* 1984;62:1121, with permission.

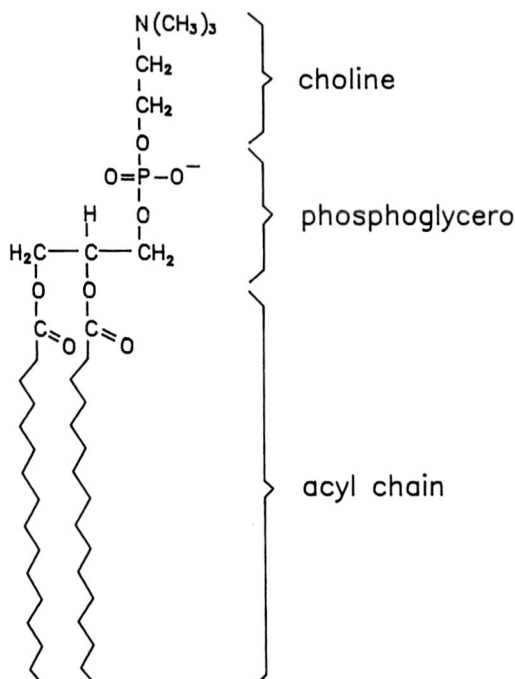

Figure 29-5 Dipalmitoylphosphatidylcholine (DPPC) is the most abundant phospholipid in pulmonary surfactant. The acyl chains of DPPC pack tightly to form the surfactant monolayer, reducing surface tension in the alveolus.

type II epithelial cells in the alveolus. Synthesis of phosphatidylcholine, surfactant proteins, and lamellar bodies, an intracellular storage form of pulmonary surfactant, increases with advancing gestation. Lamellar bodies are secreted into the lung liquid that contributes to the amniotic fluid. The measurement of amniotic fluid phosphatidylcholine, disaturated phosphatidylcholine, phosphatidylglycerol, or the surfactant proteins has provided useful biochemical markers that predict lung maturation and the adequacy of lung function at birth (e.g., lecithin-sphingomyelin [L-S] ratio and phosphatidylglycerol values). Surfactant function can be assessed by a variety of physical and physiologic tests that measure its ability to reduce surface tension at an air-liquid interface and to spread rapidly during dynamic compression and expansion. The Wilhelmy balance, Langmuir trough, pulsating bubble meter, and a variety of animal models have been used to assess the efficacy of surfactant and surfactant replacements.

Control of Surfactant Synthesis and Secretion

Synthesis of pulmonary surfactant is closely linked to the morphologic and biochemical differentiation of alveolar type II cells in the peripheral respiratory epithelium. Interactions between mesenchymal and epithelial cells, mediated by direct cell-cell contact or by paracrine factors, contribute to the differentiation process. Endocrine factors also modulate the differentiation of type II epithelial cells and the synthesis of surfactant components. In vivo and in vitro evidence supports the role of glucocorticoids in the modulation of morphologic differentiation and production of phospholipids and surfactant proteins by the lung.

Phospholipid Synthesis

Phosphatidylcholine is produced by type II epithelial cells using extracellular substrate and the glycogen stores that accumulate in the pretype II cells of the fetal lung. Metabolic pathways producing phosphatidylcholine depend on the production of phosphatidic acid and a glycerophosphate backbone (see Fig. 29-5); the latter is produced as an intermediate of the glycolytic pathway (9). The synthesis of phosphatidylcholine involves the deacylation of phosphatidic acid and its reaction with cytidine diphosphocholine (CDP-choline).

Disaturated forms of phosphatidylcholine may be formed de novo, using disaturated acyl precursors or by remodeling, i.e., salvage pathway, of phospholipids by deacylation and reacylation reactions. Production of CDP-choline is critical to phosphatidylcholine synthesis and is achieved by phosphorylation of choline and transfer to cytidine triphosphate in a reaction dependent on choline kinase and choline phosphate cytidylyltransferase. The activities of many of the enzymes in the synthetic pathway for phosphatidylcholine increase with advancing gestation in the lung, generally increasing in the last third of gestation (9,10).

Glucocorticoid Enhancement of Pulmonary Maturation

A variety of hormonal factors influence the rate of production of the enzymes controlling phosphatidylcholine synthesis in the developing lung (9,10). Glucocorticoids are the most clinically relevant and useful of these agents. Studies in fetal lambs and humans demonstrated that administration of glucocorticoid to the dam or mother resulted in precocious respiratory function in prematurely born offspring. The initial clinical studies of Liggins and Howie demonstrated that maternal administration of glucocorticoid decreased the incidence of respiratory distress in premature infants (11). Although the precise mechanisms by which glucocorticoids induce pulmonary maturation and lung function in premature infants have not been discerned, increased phosphatidylcholine synthesis and morphologic remodeling of the alveolar architecture, including the thinning of interstitial components of the fetal lung, are observed after glucocorticoid treatment. Glucocorticoids regulate several genes that are associated with the differentiation of the fetal lung, including the genes encoding enzymes involved in the synthesis of phosphatidylcholine and the surfactant proteins. The effects of glucocorticoid on lung cell differentiation are mediated in part by glucocorticoid receptors, which, when occupied by hormones, influence gene transcription and mRNA stability, altering the abundance of the proteins synthesized by pulmonary cells. Prenatal glucocorticoid therapy is useful in prevention of RDS in preterm infants.

Other Hormonal Influences

Thyroid hormones i.e., T3, T4, thyrotropin-releasing hormone (TRH), estrogens, prolactin, epidermal growth factor, β-adrenergic agents, and other agents that enhance cellular cAMP levels influence pulmonary maturation or biochemical indices of pulmonary maturation. Both T3 and T4 increase the synthesis of phospholipids in mammalian lung but do not readily cross the placenta.

Surfactant Secretion

Surfactant is stored within type II cells in large lipid-rich organelles called lamellar bodies. Secretion of lamellar bodies occurs by a process of exocytosis that is regulated by a number of physical and hormonal factors. Stretch, the mode of ventilation, and the labor process enhance surfactant secretion and extracellular surfactant pool sizes at birth. Catecholamines, purinoceptor agonists (e.g., adenosine triphosphate) that activate protein kinases, and Ca2+ ionophores enhance phospholipid secretion by type II cells *in vitro* (9). Hyperglycemia and hyperinsulinemia inhibit surfactant phospholipid secretion. Newly secreted surfactant enters the extracellular space and undergoes dramatic structural reorganization to form tubular myelin, a process dependent on SP-A, Ca2+, phospholipids, and SP-B. Phospholipids must move from tubular myelin to form monolayers and multilayers at the air-liquid interface, thereby reducing collapsing forces in the alveoli.

Surfactant Recycling and Catabolism

The process of inflation and deflation produces spent forms of surfactant phospholipids that are taken up by type II cells and reused or catabolized. Surfactant proteins B and C enhance the reuptake of phospholipids *in vitro*. Surfactant phospholipid is recycled. In the adult rabbit lung, the half-life of surfactant phospholipids is approximately 8 hours, and in newborn animals, the half-life is 3.5 days. The intracellular and extracellular pools of surfactant are generally larger in the newborn animal than in adults. A relatively small fraction of the alveolar surfactant pool is cleared by catabolism and alveolar macrophages, with most of the surfactant phospholipid recycled or catabolized by type II epithelial cells. Recent studies support an important role for granulocyte/macrophage-stimulating factors and their receptors in the mediation of surfactant clearance, acting primarily on the alveolar macrophage. Defects in granulocyte-macrophage cerebrospinal fluid (GM-CSF) signaling, caused by autoantibodies to GM-CSF or mutations in its receptor, cause alveolar macrophage dysfunction leading to marked lipid accumulation in the postnatal lung, in turn, causing the syndrome of pulmonary alveolar proteinosis. Exogenously administered surfactant is reused efficiently by adult and newborn lungs (12). The effects of surfactant replacement therapy are therefore related both to the direct surface-tension-lowering properties of surfactant introduced into the airway and to the recycling of the exogenously delivered phospholipids by type II cells.

The Role of Surfactant in Lung Disease

Quantitative and qualitative abnormalities of pulmonary surfactant contribute to the pathogenesis of lung disease in the newborn infant. In premature infants, deficiencies in surfactant production and secretion decrease intracellular and extracellular pools of surfactant, leading to alveolar surfactant insufficiency and atelectasis. Qualitative abnormalities of surfactant are also associated with many types of lung injury. Alveolar-capillary leak, hemorrhage, pulmonary edema, and alveolar cell injury fill the alveolus with proteinaceous material that inactivates surfactant. Serum and nonserum proteins, including albumin, fibrinogen, hemoglobin, and meconium, are potent inactivators of pulmonary surfactant in vivo and in vitro; SP-A, SP-B, and SP-C act synergistically to stabilize the surface properties of phospholipids in the presence of these inactivating proteins. Inhibitory factors associated with surfactant dysfunction in acute lung injury can be overcome by the administration of exogenous surfactants that contain the surfactant proteins.

Surfactant Replacement

The first successful surfactant replacement therapy in humans was reported by Fujiwara and colleagues in 1980 (13). Natural synthetic and semisynthetic surfactants have been successfully administered into the lungs of premature infants for treatment of RDS, for the treatment of meconium aspiration, and are being tested for therapy of other lung diseases. Surfactant replacement has become standard for prevention and treatment of RDS. Animal surfactant preparations containing phospholipids, SP-B, and SP-C (e.g., Survanta, Curosurf, Infasurf) and synthetic preparations composed primarily of phospholipids mixed with spreading agents (e.g., Exosurf) are in clinical use (7,8), although the animal based preparations are most widely used. The surfactant preparations containing surfactant proteins provide highly surface active material to the alveolus. Surfactant replacement also contributes to the pool size of surfactant phospholipids, providing substrate for surfactant synthesis by means of the recycling pathways.

RESPIRATORY DISTRESS SYNDROME

Respiratory distress syndrome, previously called hyaline membrane disease, is a common cause of morbidity and mortality associated with premature delivery. Respiratory distress syndrome is a developmental disorder rather than a disease process per se, and it is usually associated with premature birth. The incidence and severity of RDS generally increase with decreasing gestational age at birth and are usually worse in male infants. Infants of diabetic mothers with poor metabolic control and infants born after fetal asphyxia, maternofetal hemorrhage, or after pregnancies complicated by multiple births are at higher risk for RDS. Respiratory distress syndrome affects approximately 20,000 to 30,000 infants each year in the United States and complicates about 1% of pregnancies. Approximately 50% of the infants born between 26 and 28 weeks of gestation develop RDS, whereas fewer than 20% to 30% of premature infants at 30 to 31 weeks have the disorder.

Clinical Presentation

Infants with RDS present at birth or within several hours after birth with clinical signs of respiratory distress that include tachypnea, grunting, retractions, and cyanosis (See Color Plate) accompanied by increasing oxygen requirements. Physical findings include rales, poor air exchange, use of accessory muscles of breathing, nasal flaring, and abnormal patterns of respiration that may be complicated by apnea. Chest radiographs are characterized by atelectasis, air bronchograms, and diffuse reticular-granular infiltrates, often progressing to severe bilateral opacity characterized by the term "white-out" (Fig. 29-6). Radiographic patterns in RDS are variable and may not reflect the degree of respiratory compromise.

The infant attempts to maintain alveolar volume by prolonging and increasing expiratory pressures by breathing against a partially closed glottis, causing the grunting noise characteristic of RDS, but often seen in other respiratory disorders as well. Increasing oxygen requirements and the need for ventilatory support often occur rapidly in the first 24 hours of life and continue for several days thereafter. The clinical course depends on the severity of RDS and the size and maturity of the infant at birth. In uncomplicated RDS, typically seen in more mature infants, recovery occurs over several days, and infants generally no longer require oxygen or ventilatory support after the first week of life. The most premature infants are at greatest risk

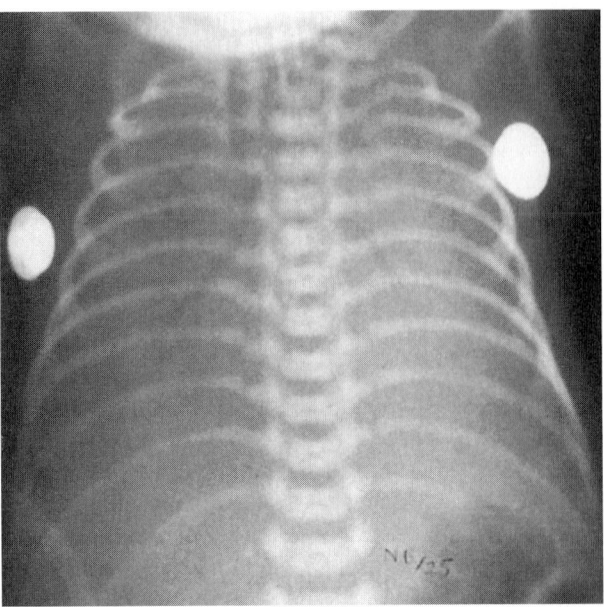

Figure 29-6 This premature infant presented with grunting, retractions, and cyanosis after delivery. The diffuse reticular–granular opacification, air bronchograms, and decreased lung volumes in the chest radiograph film indicate respiratory distress syndrome.

for severe RDS and frequently develop complications, including central nervous system (CNS) hemorrhage, patent ductus arteriosus (PDA), air leak, and infection, which contribute to prolonged requirements for oxygen and ventilatory support.

Pathology

Pathologic findings early in the course of RDS include atelectasis, pulmonary edema, pulmonary vascular congestion, pulmonary hemorrhage, and evidence of direct injury to the respiratory epithelium (Fig. 29-7). Epithelial cell injury is especially evident in the bronchiolar region of the lung. Histologic findings include the presence of hyaline membranes, the characteristic eosinophilic material derived from bronchial and bronchiolar injury to epithelial cells. Alveolar spaces are generally not inflated, and at autopsy, the lungs of infants with RDS are often airless on passive deflation. Leukocytic infiltration is not observed early in the course of RDS unless complicated by infection. Pulmonary edema, hemorrhage, and hemorrhagic edema are common pathologic features in RDS, especially if the clinical course is further complicated by PDA and congestive heart failure.

Pathophysiology

Avery and Mead first demonstrated the paucity of alveolar surfactant in the lungs of infants dying of RDS (14). Quantitative and qualitative abnormalities of the pulmonary surfactant system are critical to the pathogenesis of RDS in premature infants. Lack of pulmonary surfactant leads to progressive atelectasis, loss of functional residual

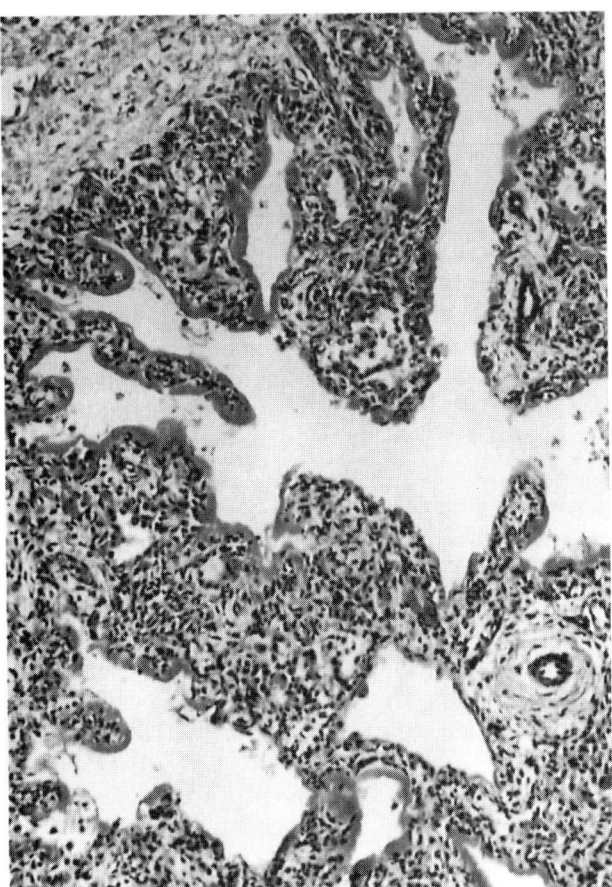

Figure 29-7 Dilated air spaces, hyaline membranes, and extensive atelectasis are seen throughout the lung of an infant born at 28 weeks of gestation with severe respiratory distress syndrome (Hematoxylin and eosin stain; original magnification × 250). (Courtesy of Edgar Ballard, Cincinnati Children's Hospital, Cincinnati, OH.)

capacity, alterations in ventilation-perfusion ratio, and uneven distribution of ventilation. The RDS is further complicated by the relatively weak respiratory muscles and the compliant chest wall of the premature infant, which impair alveolar ventilation. Diminished oxygenation, cyanosis (See Color Plate), and respiratory and metabolic acidosis contribute to increased pulmonary vascular resistance (PVR). Right-to-left shunting through the ductus arteriosus, foramen ovale, and intrapulmonary ventilation-perfusion mismatch further exacerbate hypoxemia.

Prevention

Although the incidence of premature birth in the United States (approximately 7%) has not changed significantly in recent decades, the incidence of severe RDS has decreased at each gestational age as advances in maternal care and strict attention to avoidance of asphyxia and infection at birth have become standard treatment. Careful fetal monitoring, treatment of underlying maternal disorders, determination of amniotic fluid lamellar body number or other biochemical indicators of fetal lung maturity, and administration of tocolytics and maternal glucocorticoids have

decreased the incidence of RDS. Although a single course of antenatal steroids improves lung function and reduces the risk of newborn death, current evidence from animal and clinical studies suggests that additional courses of steroids do not further improve lung function and are associated with risks of adverse consequences (15). Surfactant replacement can further decrease the incidence and severity of RDS. Rapid restoration of blood volume after hemorrhage and correction and avoidance of anemia, acidosis, and hypothermia improve the clinical outcomes in RDS as well. Positive-pressure ventilation and continuous positive airway pressure (CPAP) improve the course of severe RDS, but do not prevent the disease itself.

Treatment

Postnatal therapy of RDS begins with careful assessment and resuscitation. Adequate ventilation, oxygenation, circulation, and temperature must be assured before the infant is transferred from the delivery room to the appropriate site of care. Surfactant replacement therapy may be initiated at birth in infants at risk for RDS or thereafter, as symptoms of RDS are established and the diagnosis of RDS is confirmed. Ventilatory management of neonatal respiratory disorders has been reviewed and is detailed in Chapter 30 (16).

Adequacy of ventilation and oxygenation must be established as soon as possible to avoid pulmonary vasoconstriction, further ventilation-perfusion abnormalities, and atelectasis. Positive-pressure ventilation, CPAP, and oxygen therapy may be required at any time during the course of RDS and must be readily available to the infant. Close monitoring of pH, oxygen saturation, partial pressure of CO_2 (PCO_2), and partial pressure of oxygen (PO_2) by transcutaneous monitors and by arterial catheterization or sampling of arterialized capillary blood is critical in guiding mechanical ventilation and ambient oxygen requirements. Surfactant replacement therapy is provided through the endotracheal tube and is often used several times during the early course of RDS to maintain pulmonary function. Exogenous surfactants are given by intratracheal instillation of doses of approximately 100 to 150 mg of phospholipid per 1 kg of body weight. Animal-derived surfactants cause a more rapid improvement in oxygenation and lung compliance when compared to currently available synthetic surfactants (17).

Mild or moderate RDS can be managed by CPAP applied by mask, nasal cannula, nasal prongs, or endotracheal or nasopharyngeal tubes. In general, 3 to 6 cm of water (H_2O) pressure is applied to the infant's airway. Oxygenation and effort of breathing are usually rapidly improved by CPAP. Rapid fluctuations in blood gases may occur, requiring careful monitoring of PCO_2 and PO_2. As forced inspiratory oxygen requirements decrease during recovery, airway pressure is decreased, and the infant is weaned to head hood or nasal cannula oxygen. Apnea, inadequacy of ventilation, atelectasis, mucous plugging, hyperaeration, or air leak may complicate the care of infants with RDS.

Careful attention to the mechanical details of the application of CPAP or mechanical respirators is required. Mandatory ventilation should be instituted well in advance of respiratory failure and severe respiratory acidosis to avoid severe hypoxemia and atelectasis. Ventilation is maintained through an endotracheal tube, which can be placed nasally or orally, for delivery of oxygen and positive pressure. Pressure-cycled ventilators are most frequently used in the neonatal intensive care unit (NICU) and are controlled by setting positive inspiratory pressure, rate, inspiratory-expiratory times, and positive end-expiratory pressures (PEEP). Volume-cycled ventilators, in which fixed volumes are delivered to define the respiratory cycle, are used less frequently in the newborn. As in all respiratory therapy, critical attention to adequacy of ventilation, as assessed by PO_2, PCO_2, pH, and transcutaneous oxygen saturation, is required on an almost continual basis to adjust to the rapid changes in respiratory status occurring in these critically ill infants. Barotrauma and oxygen toxicity to the lung represent significant pulmonary complications in the therapy of RDS. Excesses in ventilation, peak or mean airway pressure, and oxygen therapy should be avoided. Because hyperoxia is associated with retrolental fibroplasia, a major cause of blindness in premature infants, arterial PO_2 must be carefully monitored, generally maintaining PO_2 between 50 to 80 mm Hg. Other forms of ventilation such as high-frequency or jet ventilators are often used in combination with exogenous surfactant for the treatment of RDS. These therapies are often considered for treatment of severely affected infants whose ventilation has not been adequately supported by conventional mandatory ventilation and surfactant therapy. Although some controlled trials indicate high frequency ventilation may reduce the risk of chronic lung disease in preterm infants, this mode of therapy may increase the usual adverse neurologic outcomes and should therefore be utilized with caution [18]. Nitric oxide (NO) has also been used successfully in the treatment of respiratory failure in term infants. However, for premature infants, there has been no clear demonstration of improvement in any clinically relevant outcome in the randomized trials conducted to date [19].

Complications

CNS hemorrhage, intraventricular hemorrhage (IVH), and PDA represent significant clinical problems affecting the care of infants with RDS. Patent ductus arteriosus and subsequent congestive heart failure and pulmonary edema further compromise respiratory function, decreasing pulmonary compliance and perhaps inactivating pulmonary surfactant. Prompt diagnosis and medical or surgical treatment of PDA are indicated during the treatment of RDS. Acute CNS hemorrhage is often associated with shock, pulmonary compromise, and pulmonary hemorrhage. Fluctuations in respiratory status may contribute to IVH and can be minimized by careful attention to respiratory care and by judicious use of sedation. Intravenous fluids

and administration of oral feedings must be adjusted carefully during acute and convalescent care of infants with RDS. Excessive fluid administration impairs pulmonary function and increases the risk of PDA.

MECONIUM ASPIRATION SYNDROME

Meconium-stained amniotic fluid (MSAF) occurs in approximately 12% of live births. The cause, pathophysiology, and treatment of MSAF and MAS have been recently reviewed [20].

Meconium first appears in the fetal ileum between 10 and 16 weeks of gestation as a viscous, green liquid composed of gastrointestinal secretions, cellular debris, bile and pancreatic juice, mucus, blood, lanugo, vernix and approximately 72% to 80% water. The dry weight composition consists primarily of mucopolysaccharides, with less protein and lipid. Although meconium appears in the intestine very early in gestation, MSAF rarely occurs before 38 weeks of gestation. Incidence of MSAF increases thereafter, and approximately 30% of newborns have MSAF if born after 42 weeks of gestation. The increased incidence of MSAF with advancing gestational age probably reflects the maturation of peristalsis in the fetal intestine. Motilin, an intestinal peptide that stimulates contraction of the intestinal muscle, is in lower concentrations in the intestine of premature vs. postterm infants. Umbilical cord motilin concentration is higher in infants who have passed meconium than in infants with clear amniotic fluid. Intestinal parasympathetic innervation and myelination also increase throughout gestation and may play a role in the increased incidence of passage of meconium in late gestation.

In utero passage of meconium is also associated with fetal asphyxia and decreased umbilical venous blood PO_2 (Fig. 29-8). Experimentally, intestinal ischemia produces a transient period of hyperperistalsis and relaxation of anal sphincter tone, leading to the passage of meconium. The fetal diving reflex, which shunts blood preferentially to the brain and heart and away from the visceral organs during hypoxia may enhance intestinal ischemia. The gasping respiratory efforts that accompany fetal asphyxia contribute to the actual entry of meconium into the respiratory tract, resulting in MAS.

Meconium in amniotic fluid is a hallmark of fetal compromise and demands critical evaluation of fetal well-being. However, most infants with MSAF do not have lower Activity, Pulse, Grimace, Appearance, and Respiration (APGAR) scores, more acidosis, or clinical illness than infants born with clear amniotic fluid. Fetal heart rate patterns do predict those infants at greatest risk of significant meconium aspiration syndrome and poor outcome. When normal fetal heart rate patterns are observed in cases of MSAF, the neonatal outcome is generally comparable to deliveries with clear amniotic fluid. In contrast, perinatal morbidity is increased in newborns with abnormal fetal heart rates and MSAF. Neonatal outcomes of

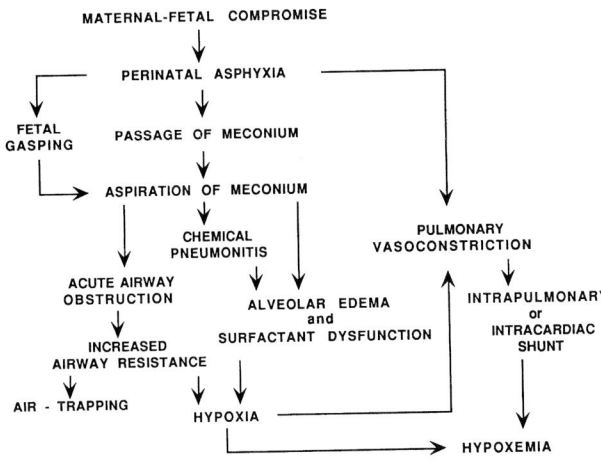

Figure 29-8 Pathogenesis of meconium aspiration syndrome.

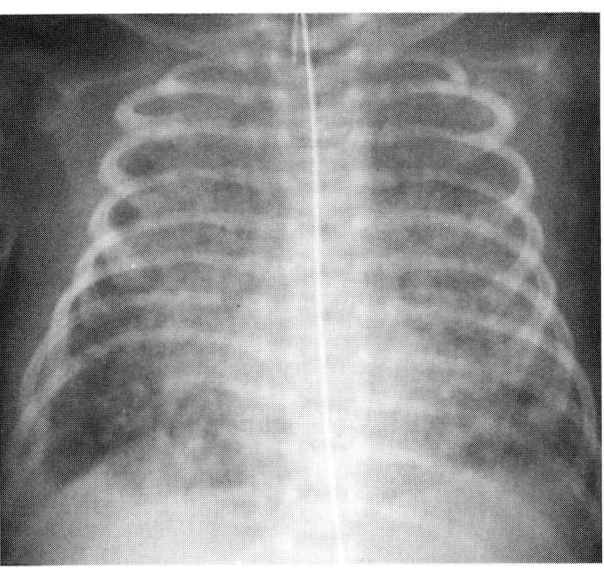

Figure 29-9 This full-term infant was born with fetal brady-cardia and thick meconium in the amniotic fluid. Cyanosis and respiratory distress were evident within minutes of delivery. The chest radiograph film demonstrates coarse, irregular infiltrates, hyperinflation (left and right diaphragms at ribs 10 to 11) and right pleural effusion indicative of meconium aspiration syndrome. Endotracheal and nasogastric tubes are in position.

deliveries complicated by MSAF associated with fetal tachycardia or decreased fetal heart rate variability are similar to those of nonmeconium-stained infants with similar abnormalities of fetal heart rate. Those babies with abnormal fetal tracings are at greatest risk for the meconium aspiration syndrome. However, in infants with a normal fetal heart rate pattern, MSAF generally carries a low risk for perinatal morbidity.

Clinical Presentation

Meconium found below the vocal cords defines MAS. MAS occurs in approximately 35% of live births with MSAF or in approximately 4% of all live births. Meconium aspiration syndrome describes a wide spectrum of respiratory disease, ranging from mild respiratory distress to severe disease and death despite mechanical ventilation. MAS typically presents as respiratory distress, tachypnea, prolonged expiratory phase and hypoxemia soon after birth in an infant heavily stained on the nails, hair, and umbilical cord with meconium or born through thick meconium. Infants with severe MAS often have an increased anterior–posterior dimension of the thorax, a "barrel" chest, secondary to obstructive airway disease. Persistent pulmonary hypertension is also frequently observed in infants with severe MAS. Less severe meconium aspiration, typically of nonparticulate meconium, may present with the appearance of a pneumonitis with mild increased work of breathing or peaceful tachypnea reaching a peak at one to three days and resolving slowly over the first week of life.

The chest radiographs of infants with MAS, especially when associated with thick particulate meconium, are heterogeneous and demonstrate coarse infiltrates, with widespread consolidation and areas of hyperaeration (Fig. 29-9). Pleural effusions are detected in approximately 30% of infants with MAS. There is an increased risk of pneumothorax or pneumomediastinum, which occur in approximately 25% of severely affected infants. Chest radiographs are abnormal in more than one-half of infants with meconium detected below the vocal cords, although

fewer than 50% of the infants with abnormal radiographs have significant respiratory distress. The severity of chest radiographic abnormalities may not correlate well with the severity of clinical disease.

Pathology

Postmortem examination of lungs from infants with severe MAS reveals meconium, vernix, fetal squamous cells and cellular debris in the air spaces from the airways to the alveoli. An inflammatory response with polymorphonuclear leukocytes, macrophages, and alveolar edema may be observed, but large quantities of meconium may be present without histologic signs of inflammation. Hyaline membrane formation, pulmonary hemorrhage, and necrosis of pulmonary microvasculature and parenchyma can occur. Platelet-rich microthrombi in small arterioles and increased muscularization of distal arterioles have been described in some infants dying of MAS.

Pathophysiology

The pulmonary abnormalities in MAS are related primarily to acute airway obstruction, decreased lung tissue compliance, and parenchymal lung damage (see Fig. 29-8). Instillation of meconium into adult rabbit and newborn dog tracheas causes acute mechanical obstruction of proximal and distal airways (21). A ball-valve mechanism producing partial airway obstruction contributes to air trapping, which results in increased anterior-posterior chest diameter, increased expiratory lung resistance, and increased functional residual capacity. Complete obstruction of small airways may result in regional atelectasis and ventilation-perfusion inequalities. Disruption of surfactant function by serum and nonserum proteins and fatty acids contributes to atelectasis, decreased compliance, and resulting hypoxia. Additionally, meconium may be toxic to pulmonary epithelial cells and may itself contain, and stimulate, the production of pro-inflammatory cytokines including IL-8 and TNF-α.

In more than one-half of the infants with severe MAS, pulmonary hypertension with right-to-left shunting contributes to the characteristically severe and sometimes refractory hypoxemia. Such clinical pulmonary hypertension correlates with increased muscularization of distal pulmonary vessels pathologically and, experimentally, with chronic intrauterine hypoxia. Perinatal asphyxia is a critical underlying factor in the pathogenesis of MAS, increasing the risks for pulmonary hypertension and meconium aspiration.

Prevention

Before the late 1970s, it was thought that aspiration of amniotic fluid and meconium occurred during the first few breaths after delivery. Therapy was aimed at preventing MAS at the time of delivery by DeLee suctioning of the nasopharynx before delivery of the shoulders and before the first breath and, after delivery, immediate intubation and suctioning of the trachea to limit aspiration of meconium from the oropharynx and trachea into the distal lung. Mortality from MAS was decreased when the trachea was suctioned immediately after birth (22). DeLee suctioning of the nasopharynx while the infant was at the perineum also decreased morbidity and mortality from MAS. However, meconium aspiration syndrome continues to occur in infants who are adequately suctioned in the delivery room. Aspiration of meconium or amniotic fluid in utero probably occurs in some infants with MAS, particularly in those with perinatal asphyxia. Generally, fetal lung fluid flows outward from the lungs into the amniotic sac. However, studies with radiopaque contrast and 51Cr-labeled erythrocytes injected into the amniotic sac demonstrated that some amniotic fluid enters the fetal lung even in the nonasphyxiated human fetus. Gasping associated with inhalation of amniotic fluid or meconium occurs in fetal lambs, rhesus monkeys, and humans in response to fetal asphyxia induced by compression of the umbilical cord or maternal aorta. Fetal gasping may be a critical factor in entry of meconium into the lung before birth. Antenatal diagnosis and treatment of fetal asphyxia is therefore critical for prevention of MAS. Amnioinfusion, the infusion of saline into the amniotic sac, decreases cord compression and dilutes meconium, potentially minimizing its toxicity after aspiration (23). Despite clinical studies supporting the use of intrapartum amnioinfusion to decrease the rate of emergency cesarean section and to decrease morbidity related to MAS, data regarding its efficacy have not supported its widespread use in MSAF.

Based on the findings that meconium aspiration may occur in utero, is occasionally accompanied by asphyxia,

and that the benefit of immediate intubation in the delivery room of infants with MSAF may be out-weighed by the risks of trauma to the airway, a more selective approach to intubation of neonates exposed to meconium in utero is now recommended (24). The oropharynx and nasopharynx of all meconium-exposed neonates should be cleared on delivery of the head by a wall-mounted DeLee suction device. Immediate tracheal intubation and suctioning is recommended only if the infant is depressed. The utilization of this type of protocol has decreased the need for emergent intubation by up to 40% without an increase in incidence or severity of meconium aspiration syndrome. Clearing the airway and establishing respiration and oxygenation remain however basic to the resuscitation of all infants.

Treatment

Postnatal therapy for MAS begins with continuous observation and monitoring of infants at risk. Vigorous treatment of nonrespiratory sequelae of neonatal asphyxia, including temperature instability, hypoglycemia, hypocalcemia, hypotension, and decreased cardiac function are critical to promoting the fetal-to-newborn physiologic transition. Attention also needs to be given to the potential effects of multi-organ hypoxemia and ischemia, including reduced renal function, reduced liver production of clotting factors, hypoalbuminemia, cerebral edema, and seizures. Pulmonary vasoconstriction is associated with MAS, and correction of hypoxemia and acidosis is indicated. Chest physiotherapy and suctioning of particulate meconium may be useful if there is airway obstruction and the infant maintains adequate oxygenation during such therapy. Exogenous surfactant has been used successfully for the treatment of meconium aspiration, decreasing air leak and the need for extracorporeal membrane oxygenation. Continuous monitoring of oxygenation by transcutaneous oxygen monitoring or pulse oximetry and assessment of PaO_2, $PaCO_2$, and pH should be used to guide the application of oxygen therapy and mechanical ventilation. The presence and severity of pulmonary hypertension should be evaluated by echocardiography in the hypoxemic infant with meconium aspiration syndrome. Broad-spectrum antibiotics are routinely used in the therapy of MAS in infants with abnormal radiographic findings and respiratory distress, although their efficacy in MAS is unproven. Treatment of acute MAS with glucocorticoids has not been beneficial.

Surfactant Treatment

Recent research suggests beneficial effects of surfactant replacement therapy, inhaled NO, and high-frequency oscillatory ventilation for MAS. Meconium instilled into canine or piglet lungs or mixed with surfactant in vitro inactivates surfactant function, decreasing lung compliance, lung volumes, and oxygenation. Surfactant inactivation can be overcome by addition of exogenous surfactant. Several studies suggest that surfactant therapy may decrease respiratory failure associated with MAS (25). Findlay and associates (26) determined that surfactant replacement (6 mL/kg, Survanta) improved oxygenation and reduced the incidence of air leaks and the severity of pulmonary morbidity when begun within 6 hours after birth. Response to the first dose was moderate. However, after the second and third doses, given 6 hours apart, improvements were documented in mean arterial-to-alveolar PO_2 ratio and in oxygenation index. Optimal dose, method, and timing of instillation of surfactant in MAS remain to be determined.

Ventilatory Support

Mechanical ventilation is required in up to 30% of infants with severe MAS and must be managed carefully. Although improvement in oxygenation was observed in patients with MAS treated with 4 to 7 cm H_2O PEEP, further studies to confirm the safety and efficacy of positive end-expiratory pressure in MAS are needed. Continuous positive airway pressure or PEEP may aggravate hyperinflation associated with MAS and should be used with caution. Pneumothorax or pneumomediastinum occur frequently during the course of MAS because of the ball-valve effect of meconium and may occur before the application of positive-pressure ventilation. Lengthening the expiratory time of the ventilatory cycle may minimize hyperinflation. Oscillation and high-frequency jet ventilation have been used in the treatment of MAS, but reports of their safety and efficacy in MAS are conflicting.

High-frequency oscillatory ventilation (HFOV) has been studied alone and in combination with INO as treatment for MAS. Kinsella and associates (27) found that the response rate of infants with MAS to HFOV plus INO was greater than the response rate to either HFOV or INO with conventional ventilation alone. Extracorporeal membrane oxygenation (ECMO) has been used successfully in rescue treatment of severe MAS refractory to conventional ventilatory therapy. As of June 2003, more than 6,300 neonates with MAS were registered as receiving ECMO in the Extracorporeal Life Support Organization (ELSO) database, with a 94% survival rate (28). Surfactant therapy during ECMO reduced the perfusion time required and the overall rate of complications after ECMO.

PERSISTENT PULMONARY HYPERTENSION OF THE NEWBORN

Gersony and colleagues (29) described hypoxemia in two infants with "persistent physiologic characteristics of the fetal circulation (PFC) in the absence of recognizable cardiac, pulmonary, hematologic, or central nervous system disease." Because the placenta is no longer present and the ductus arteriosus may or may not be patent, the term persistent pulmonary hypertension of the newborn (PPHN)

is now used to describe this disorder. The pathophysiology of PPHN is related to a failure to make the transition from high pulmonary vascular resistance (PVR) and low pulmonary blood flow, characteristic of the fetus, to the relatively low PVR and high pulmonary blood flow of the postnatal infant. The clinical syndrome of PPHN has been recently reviewed (30).

Pathophysiology

The pathophysiology of PPHN is best understood within the framework of the current knowledge of the transitional circulation. Normal transition occurs in four phases: the *in utero* phase, the immediate phase occurring in the first minutes after birth, the fast phase developing in the first 12 to 24 hours, and the final phase, which requires days or months to complete.

In Utero Circulation

The in utero phase is characterized by PVR that exceeds systemic vascular resistance, resulting in right atrial and ventricular pressures exceeding left atrial and ventricular pressures. As a result of this pressure differential, more than one-third of the oxygenated blood returning from the placenta through the inferior vena cava streams across the patent foramen ovale (PFO), is ejected from the left ventricle, and perfuses the head and neck vessels and the lower body. Venous blood returning through the superior vena cava preferentially flows into the right ventricle and main pulmonary artery. A small amount of this deoxygenated blood, comprising approximately 8% of the cardiac output and with a PO_2 less than 20 mm Hg, does perfuse the lungs, but because of elevated PVR, most is shunted across the PDA to mix with the blood in the aorta distal to the cervical and subclavian arteries. The lower body is therefore perfused with relatively less well oxygenated blood than the head and neck. Because of the large right-to-left shunt at the PFO and the PDA, blood bypasses the lungs in utero. Persistence of the elevated PVR after birth, without the benefit of placental oxygenation, results in the profound hypoxemia characteristic of PPHN. The mechanisms that maintain the fetal state of high PVR are under study. Pulmonary vasoconstriction induced by hypoxia, alterations in NO and arachidonic acid metabolism, and systemic acidosis probably contribute to physiologic abnormalities in PPHN.

Immediate Phase

The second stage of normal transition, the immediate phase, is accomplished in the first minute after birth when the fluid-filled fetal lungs are distended with air during the first breath. A rapid decrease in PVR occurs with the mechanical distention of the pulmonary vascular bed, allowing more oxygenated blood to perfuse the lungs. The entry of air into the alveoli improves the oxygenation of the pulmonary vascular bed, further decreasing PVR.

Fast Phase

The fast phase of the transitional circulation occurs for 12 to 24 hours after birth and accounts for the greatest reduction in PVR. The drop in PVR has been associated with the production of vasodilators, such as prostacyclin and endothelial-derived relaxing factor i.e., NO. Prostacyclin is produced in the neonatal lung in response to rhythmic distension of the lungs. Pretreatment of the fetal lamb with cyclooxygenase inhibitor decreased prostacyclin production and prevented the late fall in PVR. The role of cyclooxygenase and prostacyclin in the transitional circulation may have clinical implications. Persistent pulmonary hypertension of the newborn has been observed in infants of mothers receiving aspirin or nonsteroidal antiinflammatory agents that inhibit cyclooxygenase activity. However, prostacyclin induction at birth is transient, and it does not account for pulmonary vasodilation occurring in response to increasing oxygen tension. Likewise, indomethacin did not reverse decreased PVR caused by hyperbaric oxygen. The role of pulmonary production of potent vasodilatory leukotrienes, which also occurs during the initiation of ventilation, is unclear.

The pulmonary vasodilation and increase in pulmonary blood flow occurring in response to oxygenation can be virtually masked by inhibitors of the endothelial-derived relaxing factor, NO. NO is induced by oxygen, adenosine triphosphate (ATP), and sheer stress and is elevated in 1-day-old lamb pulmonary arteries and pulmonary veins in comparison to near-term fetuses and few-week-old lambs. NO causes vasodilation by inducing the guanylate cyclase enzyme. The resultant increase in cGMP in turn activates a kinase that decreases intracellular calcium, allowing smooth muscle cell relaxation. The vascular effects of NO are specific and localized because of its great affinity for hemoglobin, especially deoxyhemoglobin. Thus, INO can cause pulmonary vasodilation without systemic hypotension. Prostaglandin, PGI2 in particular, and NO are believed to be the principal agents responsible for the decrease in pulmonary vascular resistance in the fast phase of transition to air breathing.

Final Phase

The final phase of the neonatal pulmonary vascular transition involves remodeling of the pulmonary vascular musculature (31). In the normal fetal and term lung, fully muscularized, thick-walled preacinar arteries extend to the level of the terminal bronchioles. Intraacinar and alveolar wall arteries are not muscularized. Within days after delivery, medial wall thickness of preacinar vessels smaller than 250 mm in diameter decreases, and within months, medial wall thickness of vessels larger than 250 and smaller than 500 mm also decreases. Hypoxia at birth prevents the remodeling and regression of the smooth muscle of the preacinar bronchiolar arteries. In utero, or after birth, high-flow states and chronic hypoxia stimulate cells of the intraacinar and alveolar arteries to differentiate into smooth muscle and connective tissue, resulting in abnormally thickened and reactive arteriolar musculature. Distal extension of smooth muscle with increased numbers of adventitial fibroblasts and extracellular matrix has been described in pulmonary arteries of infants dying of severe MAS with PPHN.

Etiology

Persistent pulmonary hypertension of the newborn has a variety of causes that can be classified by the predominant abnormality involved (Table 29-1). Identification of the cause and subclass of PPHN is helpful in predicting severity and reversibility of PPHN in the neonate. Assessment of the clinical severity of PPHN helps determine the need for referral to nurseries with ECMO and NO capability.

Clinical Presentation

Clinically, PPHN presents as labile hypoxemia that is often disproportionate to the extent of pulmonary parenchymal disease. Infants with PPHN are commonly appropriate for gestational age and near term. The perinatal history frequently includes factors associated with perinatal asphyxia. Clinical symptoms include tachypnea, respiratory distress, and often rapidly progressive cyanosis (See Color Plate), particularly in response to stimulation of the infant. The cardiovascular examination may be normal or may reveal a right ventricular heave, closely split or single loud S2, and low-pitched systolic murmur of tricuspid regurgitation suggesting that pulmonary arterial pressure is equal to or greater than systemic arterial pressure. A gradient of 10 mm Hg between right arm and lower extremity oxygen pressures suggests right-to-left shunting at the ductus arteriosus and is consistent with, although not required for, the diagnosis of PPHN. PPHN may occur without differential oxygen saturations if the ductus arteriosus is closed and mixing of cyanotic and oxygenated blood is occurring within the lungs or at other intracardiac sites. Differential diagnosis of PPHN includes severe pulmonary parenchymal disease, such as severe MAS, RDS, pneumonia, or pulmonary hemorrhage, and congenital heart disease, such as transposition of the great arteries. Critical pulmonic stenosis, hypoplastic left ventricle, or severe coarctation should be considered in the differential diagnosis. Methods used to differentiate PPHN from pulmonary parenchymal disease or cardiac disease are outlined in Table 29-2.

The oxygenation of infants with severe pulmonary parenchymal disease without PPHN generally improves after treatment with oxygen or mechanical ventilation. Infants with PPHN often have little or no parenchymal lung disease. They are easily ventilated but remain hypoxic despite high fraction of inspiratory oxygen (FiO_2). Oxygenation will frequently improve markedly with improved ventilation and/or correction of metabolic acidosis in infants with PPHN. Cyanotic congenital heart disease (CCHD) is usually associated with fixed, structural mixing of venous and arterial blood. In infants with CCHD,

TABLE 29-1
CLASSIFICATION SYSTEM FOR PERSISTENT PULMONARY HYPERTENSION OF THE NEWBORN

Pathology	Associated Diseases	Proposed Mechanism	Prognosis
Functional vasoconstriction; normal pulmonary vascular development	Acute perinatal hypoxia Acute meconium aspiration Sepsis or pneumonia (especially group B streptococci) Respiratory distress syndrome Hypoventilation CNS depression[a] Hypothermia Hypoglycemia	Response to acute hypoxia, particularly in the presence of acidemia	Good; reversible
Fixed decreased diameter; abnormal extension and hypertrophy of distal pulmonary vascular smooth muscle	Placental insufficiency Prolonged gestation In utero closure of ductus arteriosus Aspirin Nonsteroidal antiinflammatory agents Single ventricle without pulmonic stenosis Chronic pulmonary venous hypertension TAPVR[a] Obstructive left-sided heart lesions Idiopathic diseases	Response to chronic hypoxia Excessive pulmonary blood flow in utero Elevated pulmonary venous pressure	Poor; fixed structural lesion
Decreased cross-sectional area of the pulmonary vascular bed	Space-occupying lesions Diaphragmatic hernia Lung dysgenesis Pleural effusions Congenital lung hypoplasia Potter syndrome Thoracic dystrophies	Hypoplasia of alveoli and associated vessels	Poor; fixed structural lesion
Functional obstruction to pulmonary blood flow	Polycythemia Hyperfibrinogenemia	Increased blood viscosity	Good, unless chronic

[a] CNS, central nervous system; TAPVR, total anomalous pulmonary venous return.

hypoxemia is generally unresponsive to increased exogenous oxygen, mechanical ventilation, hyperventilation, or alkalinization. Diagnosis of PPHN can be complicated by the coexistence of pulmonary hypertension, parenchymal lung disease, or CCHD. Echocardiography is useful in the diagnosis of structural heart disease and assessment of pulmonary hypertension in this clinical setting.

Therapy

Supportive medical management includes correction of underlying abnormalities that may include shock, polycythemia, hypoglycemia, hypothermia, diaphragmatic hernia, or CCHD. Metabolic acidosis and hypotension should be corrected.

Specific therapy for PPHN is aimed at increasing pulmonary blood flow, decreasing right-to-left shunting and reducing ventilation/perfusion (V/Q) mismatch. High ambient oxygen and mechanical ventilation are the pulmonary therapeutic interventions for treatment of PPHN. Ligation of the PDA is not useful, and it may be detrimental. Cardiac failure may occur after PDA ligation as the right ventricle fails in the face of high pulmonary resistance without the safety valve of the patent ductus. Shunting between the pulmonary and systemic circulations, such as through the ductus arteriosus or patent foramen ovale, depends on the relative pressures of each system. Therefore, optimal therapy decreases pulmonary artery pressure although increasing or not changing systemic arterial pressure and cardiac output.

Infants with severe PPHN are often sensitive to activity and agitation. Stimulation should be minimized during the care of these infants. Transcutaneous and intravascular monitoring equipment and temporal clustering of interventions reduce agitation. Muscle relaxants (e.g., pancuronium) and sedatives are frequently beneficial but should be used with caution. Paralysis may further compromise ventilation and may mask clinical signs of respiratory insufficiency. Sedatives should be chosen to minimize cardiovascular side effects such as systemic hypotension. Infants with PPHN, especially if asphyxiated or septic, frequently develop systemic hypotension and signs of cardiac failure. The hematocrit should be maintained at or above 45%, and volume expansion may be used to support the circulation. Elevated right heart pressure with increased PVR, poor venous return secondary to high intrathoracic pressures during mechanical ventilation, and predisposing asphyxia may contribute to myocardial dysfunction that may be responsive to dobutamine. Adrenergic pressors are commonly used for refractory hypotension but should be

TABLE 29-2
DIAGNOSTIC EVALUATION OF SEVERE NEONATAL HYPOXEMIA

Test	Method	Result[a]	Suggested Diagnosis
Hyperoxia	Expose to 100% FiO_2 for 5–10 min	PaO_2 increases to >100 mm Hg	Pulmonary parenchymal disease
		PaO_2 increases to <20 mm Hg	Persistent pulmonary hypertension or cyanotic congenital heart disease
Hyperventilation–hyperoxia	Mechanical ventilation with 100% FiO_2 and respiratory rate 100–150 breaths/min	PaO_2 increases to >100 mm Hg without hyperventilation	Pulmonary parenchymal disease
		PaO_2 increases at a critical PCO_2, often to <25 mm Hg	Persistent pulmonary hypertension
		No increase in PaO_2 despite hyperventilation	Cyanotic congenital heart disease or severe, fixed pulmonary hypertension
Simultaneous–preductal–postductal PO_2	Compare PO_2 of right arm or shoulder to that of lower abdomen or extremities	Preductal PO_2 ≥ 15 + postductal PO_2	Patent ductus arteriosus with right-to-left shunt
Echocardiography	M-mode	Increased RVPEP and RVET	Right ventricular systolic time interval ratio (RVSTI = RVPEP/RVET > 0.5) predicts PPHN
	Venous contrast injection	Simultaneously appears in PA and LA	Patent foramen ovale
	Two-dimensional echocardiography	Deviation of intraatrial septum to left; rule out congenital heart defect	Increased pulmonary arterial pressure
	Doppler	Failure of acceleration of systolic blood flow between large main pulmonary artery and small peripheral pulmonary artery	Suggests right-to-left PDA or intracardiac shunt

[a] LA, left atrium; PA, pulmonary artery; PDA, patent ductus arteriosus; PPHN, persistent pulmonary hypertension of the newborn; RVET, right ventricular ejection time; RVPEP, right ventricular ejection period.

used with caution, as they may contribute to pulmonary vasoconstriction. There is anecdotal evidence supporting efficacy of hydrocortisone, 10 mg/kg/dose, for the treatment of refractory hypotension in the newborn with PPHN and right-to-left intravascular shunt.

Respiratory and Metabolic Alkalosis

The often dramatic response of infants with PPHN to respiratory or metabolic alkalosis has lead to their use in the care of infants with severe PPHN, however the sometimes transient benefit of alkalosis must be balanced against the risk of secondary lung injury, neurologic compromise from hypocapnic alkalosis and cellular effects of infusion of hypertonic solutions. The degree of pulmonary parenchymal disease and risk of barotrauma may affect the clinical choice of inducing respiratory or metabolic alkalosis. Although it may be necessary to transiently raise arterial pH with increased ventilation and base to reverse severe pulmonary vasoconstriction, because of pulmonary and neurologic concerns, sustained hypocapnia and metabolic acidosis are not advocated. INO and normalization of acid–base and ventilatory status are preferred. Excessive mechanical ventilation with overdistension of the lung may increase right-to-left shunting. Pulmonary barotrauma

associated with aggressive ventilation should be avoided. Hypocarbic alkalosis, by shifting the hemoglobin–oxygen dissociation curve, may also compromise the release of oxygen at the tissue level. Hyperoxia and hypocarbia may adversely affect cerebral blood flow. When used, weaning from ventilation NO and oxygen must proceed with caution, because dramatic liability of PO_2 is often observed in infants with PPHN.

Nitric Oxide and High-Frequency Oscillatory Ventilation

Pharmacotherapy of PPHN was recently reviewed (32). Various vasodilators such as tolazoline and prostaglandins D2 and E1 have been studied for treatment of PPHN (32). At doses required to decrease PVR, these agents often cause undesirable systemic vasodilation and hypotension. Tolazoline was previously used for therapy for PPHN but has not been shown to improve outcome.

At low pharmacologic doses, <40 parts per million, INO specifically dilates the pulmonary vasculature. Avid binding to hemoglobin prevents INO from dilating systemic blood vessels. Additionally, INO preferentially vasodilates vessels of alveoli that are patent, thus improving V/Q matching. Other less specific vasodilators may increase blood flow to atelectatic alveoli, increasing V/Q mismatch. Inhaled NO combined with conventional ventilation increased oxygenation and decreased the oxygen index of approximately 30% of infants with PPHN. The likelihood of response to INO appeared inversely related to the severity of parenchymal disease (27). In patients with moderate PPHN, (alveolar-arterial oxygenation gradient, A-aDO2 = 500–599), 15% of those treated with INO, vs. 58% of controls, progressed to severe PPHN (33). Approximately 25% of PPHN infants failing to respond to INO responded to INO combined with HFOV, suggesting improved response to INO if ventilation strategies are optimized to recruit atelectatic alveoli. The combined use of exogenous surfactant, HFOV and INO to coordinately enhance alveolar recruitment and perfusion appears to provide at least additive if not synergistic effects, especially in RDS and meconium aspiration cases. A systematic review of twelve randomized controlled trials in term or near-full term infants with hypoxic respiratory failure, concluded that INO reduced the need for ECMO. Approximately 50% of infants demonstrated improved oxygenation with INO treatment, those with diaphragmatic hernia were least likely to respond (34). No adverse effects of INO were reported.

Extracorporeal Membrane Oxygenation

Extracorporeal membrane oxygenation has been useful for the treatment of severe PPHN refractory to medical management. The first newborn survivor of ECMO therapy was reported by Bartlett and colleagues in 1975 (35). In 1999, the National Registry of Neonatal ECMO, and in 2003, the International Summary data of the ELSO Registry reported an 80% survival rate for the infants with the primary diagnosis of PPHN who were treated with ECMO (28,36). Most of these infants met criteria for greater than 80% risk of mortality with conventional medical management. However, criteria used to determine risk of mortality vary from institution to institution and frequently are based on retrospective chart reviews, reflecting older methods of medical management. It is impossible to determine how these infants would have done with modern conventional therapy.

Long-Term Outcome

Most infants treated for PPHN have few residual respiratory symptoms, neurologic or developmental sequelae by 1 year of age (37). Of infants with more severe parenchymal disease, qualifying for INO or ECMO, approximately 25% have persistent BPD or recurrent reactive airway disease at 1 and 2 years of age. Of 133 children with moderately severe persistent PPHN, with oxygenation index of 24 ± 9 at study entry, randomized to receive INO or placebo, approximately 13% had major neurologic abnormalities, 30% had cognitive delays, and 19% had hearing loss (38). There was no difference between INO treated and control infants. Particularly, infants with severe MAS or congenital

diaphragmatic hernia and PPHN have an increased risk for chronic pulmonary sequelae (39). Continued oxygen therapy, bronchodilators, diuretics, and enhanced nutrition may be necessary to treat residual disease and establish adequate growth. Hearing, vision, and neurologic development should be followed closely in infants treated for PPHN, especially if severely asphyxiated. Approximately 25% of infants treated with INO or ECMO for PPHN remain below 5% for weight at 1 to 2 years of age. Approximately 10% to 12% are diagnosed with severe neurodevelopmental disability. The risk of neurologic, growth, and pulmonary sequelae is greatest in infants with PPHN secondary to congenital diaphragmatic hernia (39).

Pneumonia

Pneumonia remains a significant cause of morbidity and mortality for preterm and term infants. The incidence of pneumonia in NICU patients exceeds 10% (40), with mortality of perinatally acquired pneumonia varying between 4% and 20% (40,41). Pneumonia may be acquired transplacentally, during the birth process, or postnatally, and it is caused by a variety of pathogens, including viruses, bacteria, and fungi (Table 29-3). Unique environmental and host factors predispose the neonate to pulmonary infections. The increased susceptibility of neonates for pneumonia may be related to immaturity of mucociliary clearance, small size of the conducting airways, and lowered host defenses. Invasive procedures, such as tracheal intubation, barotrauma, and hyperoxic damage to the respiratory tract may further impair resistance to pneumonia. The nosocomial flora of the hospital nursery, whether derived from nursery equipment or the unwashed hands of caregivers, are important vectors of pathogenic organisms.

Transplacental Viral Pneumonias

Pneumonia acquired through the transplacental route is most commonly of viral origin. Rubella, varicella-zoster, cytomegalovirus (CMV), herpes simplex virus (HSV), and human immunodeficiency virus (HIV) are acquired by this route. Transplacentally acquired pneumonitis is also associated with adenoviral, enteroviral, and influenza viral infections. Viral pneumonia is usually part of a systemic illness, reflecting hematogenous spread from the mother. Severity and onset of respiratory symptoms varies from respiratory failure at delivery to chronic pneumonia evolving months after birth.

Fetal infection may result from a primary maternal infection acquired during pregnancy or from reactivation of a latent infection. *In utero* transmission of rubella occurs as a result of primary infection acquired during pregnancy. Transmission of varicella-zoster, HSV, and CMV occurs as a result of primary or recurrent maternal infection. The timing of maternal infection in relation to birth is often a critical factor in outcome. Congenital varicella typically develops when primary maternal chickenpox

TABLE 29-3

PRIMARY PATHOGENS OF NEONATAL PNEUMONIA

Vector	Viruses[a]	Bacteria	Other Agents
Transplacental	Rubella	L. monocytogenes	
	Varicella-zoster	M. tuberculosis	
	HIV	T. pallidium	
	CMV		
	HSV		
Perinatal	HSV	Group B streptococci	C. trachomatis
	CMV	Gram-negative enteric (i.e., E. coli, Klebsiella)	U. urealyticum
Postnatal	CMV	S. aureus	C. albicans
	HSV	P. aeruginosa	
	Community based (i.e., RSV, influenza, parainfluenza)	Flavobacterium	
		S. marcescens	

[a] HIV, human immunodeficiency virus; CMV, cytomegalovirus; HSV, herpes simplex virus; RSV, respiratory syncytial virus.

occurs within the 21 days preceding parturition. If maternal varicella occurs less than 5 days before birth, antepartum transfer of maternal antibody to the fetus is minimal, increasing the risk of systemic varicella infection in the neonate. Varicella pneumonia usually presents 2 to 4 days after the onset of the exanthem. Although varicella pneumonia is often self-limited, it can cause significant mortality and morbidity. Treatment with varicella-zoster immune globulin within 72 hours of birth improves clinical outcome in neonates exposed to varicella. Pneumonitis is not a common presentation in congenital CMV or herpes, but it is more common in perinatally acquired CMV and HSV. Pulmonary disease caused by transplacental transfer of the HIV virus generally presents after the neonatal period.

Transplacental Bacterial Pneumonias

Transplacental bacterial infections are less common causes of pneumonia. *Listeria monocytogenes*, *Mycobacterium tuberculosis*, and *Treponema palladium* are the most common organisms. Maternal listeriosis classically presents with a flu-like syndrome, with fever and chills occurring up to 2 weeks before delivery. Preterm labor and meconium staining of amniotic fluid, even in preterm infants, are common. Early onset listeriosis generally presents soon after birth with respiratory distress and pneumonia. Radiographic findings are nonspecific, consisting of peribronchial or widespread infiltrates. Congenital tuberculosis occurs most commonly in infants born to women with primary infections. Respiratory symptoms in neonatal tuberculosis typically present at 2 to 4 weeks of age. Transplacental transfer of *T. palladium* occurs most commonly during primary or secondary maternal infection, usually after 20 weeks of gestation. *Pneumonia alba* is relatively uncommon in congenital syphilis and refers to the pale, firm, and enlarged lungs seen at autopsy. Although the rate of congenital syphilis has declined from its peak in

1991, clinicians must remain aware of all manifestations of congenital syphilis.

Pneumonia Acquired in the Perinatal Period

Neonatal pneumonia is most commonly acquired during the process of labor and delivery. Infection occurs from organisms ascending from the genital tract after rupture of fetal membranes or acquired during passage of the infant through the birth canal. Respiratory symptoms are often present at delivery or have their onset in the first few days of life. Despite the abundance and heterogeneity of organisms in the genital tract, only a few commonly cause pneumonia. These organisms parallel pathogens causing early onset of sepsis.

In U.S. nurseries, group B Streptococcus (GBS) remains the most frequently identified organism causing neonatal pneumonia and sepsis (42). The second most common group of organisms to produce early onset sepsis or pneumonia are the gram-negative enteric bacilli: *Escherichia coli*, Klebsiella, Enterobacter, and Proteus species. For term infants, as the rate of GBS disease has declined with the introduction of intrapartum antibiotic prophylaxis, the rate of disease caused by other organisms has been relatively stable (42). In very low birth weight (VLBW) infants, as the rate of Group B streptococcal disease has declined, there has been an increase in *E. coli*, the majority of which is ampicillin resistant (42–44). Herpes simplex and CMV are the most common viral agents causing early onset pneumonia. Pneumonia caused by *Chlamydia trachomatis* usually begins at 2 to 8 weeks of age with upper respiratory tract symptoms, a staccato cough, and apnea. Antecedent conjunctival infection is common but not always observed. Interstitial pneumonitis and hyperinflation are associated with chlamydial pneumonia. *U. urealyticum* is a common inhabitant of the lower genital tract of women and is frequently associated with histologic evidence of chorioamnionitis. *U. urealyticum* is a cause of acute congenital pneumonia and has also been associated with chronic lung disease in infants.

Pneumonia Acquired in the Postnatal Period

Newborns exposed to respiratory equipment or humidified incubators are at risk for respiratory infection by Pseudomonas species, Flavobacterium, Klebsiella, or *Serratia marcescens*. Direct contamination by the hands of caretakers as a result of inadequate hand washing is associated with outbreaks of *Staphylococcus aureus* and gram-negative enteric organisms. Cytomegalovirus that is acquired postnatally through blood products or breast milk commonly presents as a pneumonitis. With advances in transfusion technology, acquisition through blood products is rare. Cytomegalovirus is shed intermittently in human milk, and can be transmitted to the infant. In term infants there is typically no resulting clinical illness. In preterm infants clinical symptoms have been reported, including development of systemic disease (45).

Neonatal HSV infection is most often associated with HSV type II. However, data from the National Institute of Allergy and Infectious Disease indicate that 27% of symptomatic neonatal HSV infections were caused by HSV type I (46). Postnatal infection from HSV generally occurs from orolabial, oropharyngeal, or breast lesions. Community-based respiratory pathogens, including respiratory syncytial virus, influenza, parainfluenza, and enteroviruses, occur in the nursery. Pneumonia resulting from epidemic outbreaks of various enteroviral agents, including echovirus 22 and coxsackievirus type B, is often associated with other clinical manifestation of enteroviral disease. Risk factors for nosocomial fungal infections include VLBW, prolonged antibiotic therapy, intubation, central line catheter placement, intravenous alimentation, and corticosteroids. Pneumonia caused by Candida albicans usually presents in the context of disseminated disease. Mycoplasma species may also cause pneumonia in the postnatal period.

Pathologic Findings

Three common histopathologic patterns have been associated with neonatal pneumonia: hyaline membrane formation, suppurative inflammation, and interstitial pneumonitis. Hyaline membrane formation is a nonspecific response seen in lung injury associated with surfactant deficiency, pneumonia, and oxygen therapy. Damage to the alveolar epithelium results in cell necrosis and leakage of cell and serum proteins into the alveolar space. Hyaline membranes in neonatal pneumonia are often observed after GBS infection, but they are also associated with fatal pneumonia caused by *H. influenzae*, gram-negative enteric organisms, and viral agents. Bacteria are commonly seen within the hyaline membranes (Fig. 29-10). Disruption of alveolar capillary permeability and cell injury results in leakage of proteins into the alveolus that further inactivate pulmonary surfactant, leading to atelectasis. The decreased compliance, atelectasis, and hypoxemia seen in pneumonia are often indistinguishable from findings in surfactant-deficient lungs in premature infants. The chest radiographic findings in RDS and neonatal pneumonia may be identical, although bronchopneumonia and pleural effusions are more common in GBS and other bacterial causes of neonatal pneumonia than in RDS.

Suppurative Pneumonia

Staphylococcus aureus, enteric bacilli such as *Klebsiella pneumoniae*, *E. coli*, and Pseudomonas species, and fungi can cause

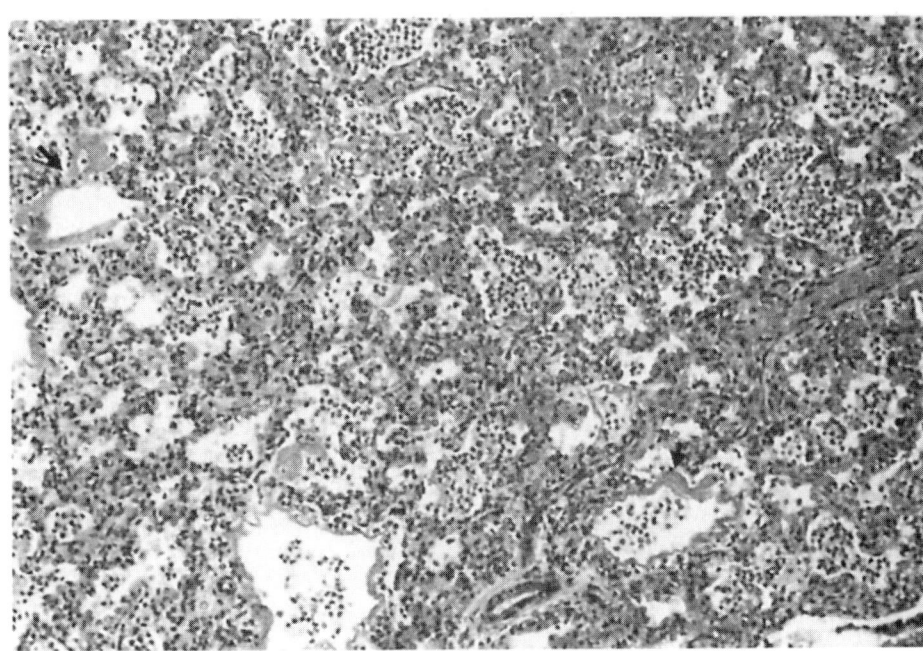

Figure 29-10 Acute neutrophilic response with atelectasis and hyaline membranes (arrows) are seen in lung tissue from a full-term infant who died at 2 days of age of group B streptococcal pneumonia. (Hematoxylin and eosin stain; original magnification × 200) (Courtesy of Edgar Ballard, Cincinnati Children's Hospital, Cincinnati, OH.)

suppurative pneumonia. An intense inflammatory response often occurs in the lungs during these bacterial infections. Necrosis of lung parenchyma, microabscess formation, and partial obstruction of terminal bronchioles results in thin-walled, air-filled pneumatoceles. Spontaneous rupture of these structures can produce pneumothorax. Microabscesses may consolidate into larger cavities or rupture to the pleural space, causing emphysema. Pneumonia may be focal or may consolidate to produce large confluent abscesses. Perfusion of consolidated lung tissue causes venous admixture and hypoxemia.

Interstitial Pneumonitis

Interstitial pneumonitis is typically caused by a virus and characterized by interstitial inflammation, edema, mononuclear infiltration, and septal hyperplasia. Alveolar spaces may remain uninvolved, but in severe cases, a serous exudate containing desquamated pneumocytes and macrophages may be associated with hyaline membrane formation. Septal wall necrosis may occur, adding a component of hemorrhage to the inflammatory exudate. Alveolar capillary block associated with the inflammation may impair respiratory function. CMV, HSV, varicella-zoster, rubella, HIV, enteroviruses, and the community-based pathogens, such as respiratory syncytial, influenza and parainfluenza viruses, are commonly associated with interstitial pneumonitis.

Group B Streptococcal Pneumonia

During the 1970s, GBS emerged as the predominant pathogen causing neonatal sepsis and pneumonia. Colonization rates in pregnant women, because that time, have remained relatively stable at 10% to 30% (41,47). Infants become infected by aspiration of contaminated amniotic fluid or acquisition during passage through the birth canal. Vertical transmission rates for untreated GBS is approximately 50% (46). Invasive disease is much less common, developing in 1% to 3% of colonized infants. Factors increasing the risk for infection include maternal group B streptococcal bacteria, prolonged rupture of membranes (>18 hours), maternal intrapartum temperature (>100.4), chorioamnionitis, and prematurity (41). Mortality from invasive disease has declined from 50% to approximately 4% secondary to advances in neonatal care in the 1990s (48).

Intrapartum chemoprophylaxis has been shown to be effective in preventing early onset of GBS disease. With the introduction of intrapartum antibiotic prophylaxis, the incidence of early onset disease has decreased by 70% from 18 cases per 1,000 live births to 0.5 cases per 1,000 live births (41,49). In 2002, the Center for Disease Control and Prevention recommended universal screening of all pregnant women at 35 to 37 weeks' gestation, and intrapartum antibiotics for all GBS colonized women (41).

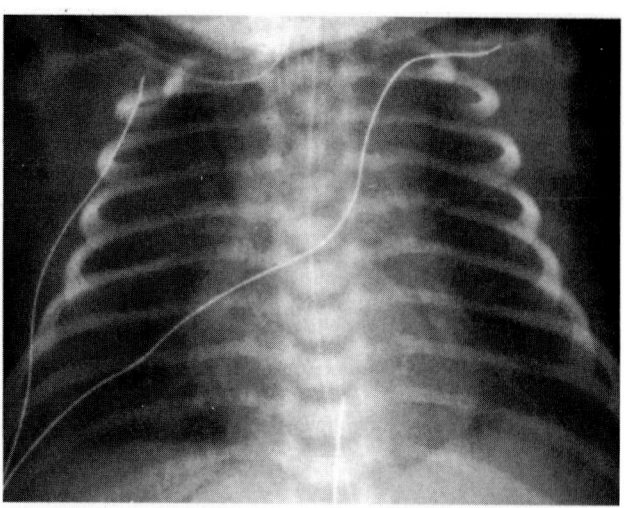

Figure 29-11 A full-term infant of an uncomplicated pregnancy developed respiratory distress, cyanosis, and periods of apnea within 6 hours of life. The blood culture and urine latex particle agglutination assay were positive for group B streptococci. Diffuse reticulogranular pattern, air bronchograms, and right pleural effusion without significant volume loss are consistent with common radiologic features of group B streptococcal pneumonia.

Early onset GBS disease presents within the first week of life. Septicemia (30%–40%), meningitis (20%–30%), and pneumonia (30%–40%) are the most common presentations. Exposure to intrapartum antibiotics has not changed the clinical presentation of illness with up to 95% of infants presenting within 24 hours and 90% of affected infants present with respiratory distress (49). Radiographic features of GBS infection may be indistinguishable from RDS, although pleural effusions may help differentiate GBS from RDS (Fig. 29-11). In two-thirds of affected infants, increased vascular markings or patchy infiltrates are observed on the initial chest radiographs. Respiratory distress in the absence of radiographic abnormalities may be associated with pulmonary vascular hypertension and hypoxemia. Late-onset GBS usually presents from 1 to 6 weeks after birth and is commonly associated with meningitis.

Respiratory failure in GBS pneumonia results from hyaline membrane formation, atelectasis, and pulmonary hypertension. Pulmonary hypertension is proposed to be mediated by high-molecular-weight polysaccharide exotoxin. In animals, infusion of GBS exotoxin results in an initial increase in pulmonary vascular pressures and fever, followed by a second phase characterized by granulocytopenia, granulocyte trapping in the lung, and increased pulmonary vascular permeability (50).

Isolation of GBS from cultures of blood, cerebrospinal fluid, or suppurative foci is diagnostic of GBS infection. Surface cultures of skin or mucous membranes are not useful because of the large number of infants colonized but not infected. Antimicrobial therapy is usually instituted before an organism is identified and consists of a penicillin and an aminoglycoside. After the organism is identified and meningitis is excluded, therapy can continue with penicillin alone at 200,000 U/kg/day, usually for 10 to 14 days. Extensive supportive care, including oxygen, mechanical ventilation, and cardiovascular support, may also be required in treating an overwhelming infection.

Herpes Simplex Pneumonia

The incidence of neonatal HSV is increasing in the United States, affecting 1,500 to 2,200 infants per year. Classification of HSV infection is based on the site and extent of involvement; HSV may be classified as a cutaneous infection; as encephalitic, with or without cutaneous infection; and as a disseminated infection. Mortality is highest among infants with disseminated disease. The mortality rate of infants with HSV pneumonitis is approximately 79% (46,51). Transmission of HSV infection to the neonate is most frequently related to direct contact with virus at delivery. Most women delivering infants with symptomatic HSV disease shed virus asymptomatically at delivery, and fewer than 20% of these women reported a history of previous infection (51). Whether the maternal infection is primary or recurrent is important in the pathogenesis of neonatal HSV infection. Infants of women with serologic evidence of a recent primary infection are more likely to develop disease than infants of women with recurrent herpes. Primary infections are associated with higher titers of viral shedding and with low levels of protective antibodies, placing the neonate at higher risk. Rupture of the amniotic sac for longer than 6 hours is associated with increased risk of neonatal HSV infection, although infection after cesarean section with intact membranes has also been reported.

Herpes simplex virus pneumonitis usually presents as part of a disseminated HSV infection. Many severely involved infants have no skin lesions. Infants typically develop signs of infection at 4 to 5 days of life. Fever, tachypnea, jaundice, and irritability, progressing to respiratory failure, shock, and disseminated intravascular coagulation are commonly seen. Diffuse interstitial pneumonitis and hemorrhagic pneumonitis are characteristic of HSV infection of the lung.

Diagnosis of HSV may be made by identification of HSV DNA through PCR or viral isolation by culture. Viral cultures should be obtained from skin lesions, cerebrospinal fluid, stool, urine, throat, nasopharynx, and conjunctiva. HSV deoxyribonucleic acid (DNA) may be identified in cerebrospinal fluid (CSF), aspirated skin vesicles, or blood. Hepatic dysfunction, neutropenia, bleeding diathesis, and interstitial pneumonitis are commonly associated with HSV but are not diagnostic. Serologic assays are not of clinical value, because they do not differentiate between antibodies to HSV types 1 and 2 or between maternal IgG and endogenously produced antibodies. Intranuclear inclusions and multinucleated giant cells observed in scrapings from cutaneous lesions are supportive but not diagnostic of HSV infection.

Early antiviral therapy decreases the progression from localized, cutaneous HSV infection to disseminated disease, and decreases the mortality from HSV infection. High-dose parental acyclovir is now widely used in treatment of HSV infection in the neonate and is currently considered the treatment of choice (52).

Transient Tachypnea of the Newborn

TTN was first described in 1966 by Avery and colleagues in a group of eight patients, seven of whom were delivered vaginally at or near term (53). All of the infants presented at or shortly after birth with grunting, retractions, and an increased respiratory rate. Respiratory rates of the original infants ranged from 80 to 140 breaths/min, and the symptoms persisted for 2 to 5 days. These infants could be differentiated from infants with other acute lung diseases by their clinical course and radiographic findings. Although the precise cause of TTN remains unknown, it was originally postulated that infants with TTN had reduced lung compliance because of delayed resorption of lung fluid at the time of birth. Many clinicians support the original proposal of Avery and colleagues that TTN results from distention of interstitial spaces by fluid, leading to alveolar air trapping and decreased lung compliance. Because the original description, others have postulated that TTN may result from mild immaturity of the surfactant system. Lack of phosphatidylglycerol in amniotic fluid samples obtained from infants with TTN supports the latter concept.

The incidence of TTN is approximately 11 per 1,000 live births. The risk factors for TTN include prematurity, maternal sedation, maternal fluid administration, maternal asthma, exposure to b-mimetic agents, and fetal asphyxia. Delivery by cesarean section also predisposes the term infant to TTN (54). Children with TTN as neonates are also more likely to develop asthma during ages zero to 4 (55).

Infants with TTN initially present with grunting, retractions, and increased respiratory rate. The symptoms of tachypnea may persist for several days, and most infants require less than 40% oxygen to maintain adequate systemic oxygenation. The radiographic findings in this disorder are ill defined but include increased central vascular markings, hyperaeration, evidence of interstitial and pleural fluid, prominent interlobar fissures, and cardiomegaly (Fig. 29-12). Furosemide has been utilized to treat TTN, but a recent meta-analysis failed to demonstrate any benefit of this therapy (56). Because TTN is self-limited, no specific therapy is indicated, although adequate ventilation and oxygenation must be maintained. Because the symptoms of TTN are nonspecific and consistent with neonatal sepsis or pneumonia, most infants with TTN are evaluated for infection and are treated with broad-spectrum antibiotics pending a definitive diagnosis.

Pulmonary Hemorrhage

Pulmonary hemorrhage in the newborn may vary from a focal, self-limited disorder to massive, lethal hemorrhage.

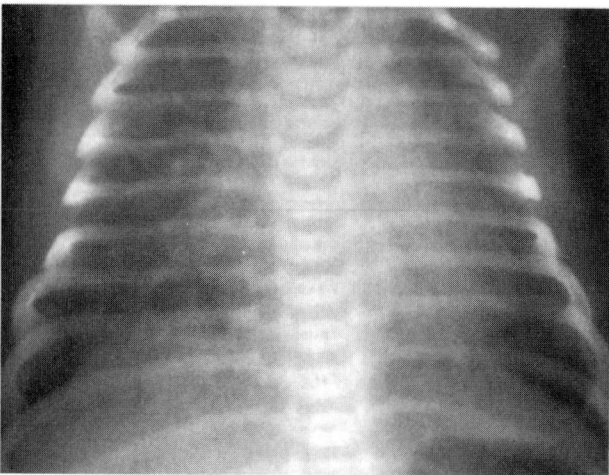

Figure 29-12 This full-term infant was born by cesarean section and developed tachypnea and grunting that resolved 48 hours after birth. Perihilar vascular densities, streaky opacities of interstitial edema, fluid in the interlobar fissures, small pleural effusions, and cardiomegaly are observed on the radiograph. These features are indicative of transient tachypnea of the newborn.

The incidence of pulmonary hemorrhage in the neonatal period ranges from 0.8 to 1.2 per 1,000 live births, although the incidence was 74% of all liveborn infants in one autopsy series of 70 newborns and is as high as 10% in babies less than 30 weeks gestation (57). Asphyxia, prematurity, intrauterine growth retardation, infection, hypothermia, oxygen therapy, severe Rh hemolytic disease, and coagulopathy are associated risk factors. In some studies, surfactant therapy has been associated with an increased incidence of pulmonary hemorrhage, although this remains controversial. Although disseminated intravascular coagulation may precede pulmonary hemorrhage, most infants with pulmonary hemorrhage do not have a coagulopathy. Pulmonary hemorrhage generally presents within the first week of life, and the mortality rate after pulmonary hemorrhage is estimated to be 75% to 90%. Although most infants who develop pulmonary hemorrhage have the predisposing factors of extreme prematurity and underlying asphyxia and stress, there are a few case reports describing previously healthy, term infants with pulmonary hemorrhage associated with an inborn error of the urea cycle and elevated blood ammonia.

Clinical Findings

The observation that the hematocrit of lung effluent in pulmonary hemorrhage is lower than the hematocrit of blood supports the concept that most of these infants have hemorrhagic pulmonary edema. Neonatal pulmonary hemorrhage is therefore thought to result from shock, hypoxia, and acidosis, which lead to left ventricular failure and increased pulmonary capillary pressure with subsequent hemorrhagic pulmonary edema. Chest radiographic findings in pulmonary hemorrhage depend on whether the hemorrhage is focal or massive. Because blood or hemor-

rhagic edema fluid has tissue density, hemorrhagic tissue appears opacified. It is often difficult to differentiate focal hemorrhage from atelectasis or pneumonia by chest radiographs. In the case of massive pulmonary hemorrhage, the lungs can be atelectatic and opacified. The clinical course of massive pulmonary hemorrhage usually involves rapid deterioration of ventilatory function. Affected infants develop progressive hypoxia and hypercarbia with resultant respiratory acidosis and may rapidly succumb to this disorder.

Treatment

Early detection and aggressive intervention improve the outcome of massive pulmonary hemorrhage, an otherwise lethal syndrome. Positive-pressure ventilation and oxygen are critical components of therapy. Blood volume and hematocrit should be vigorously restored and maintained with erythrocyte transfusions. Careful correction of hypotension, hypoxemia, and acidosis is also indicated. Coagulation abnormalities should be assessed and may be corrected with fresh-frozen plasma or appropriate clotting factors. Pressors and diuretics are indicated if congestive heart failure develops. Surfactant therapy has also been suggested as a useful adjunct in neonates with a clinically significant pulmonary hemorrhage.

AIR LEAKS

Air leaks include pneumothorax, pneumomediastinum, pneumopericardium, and pulmonary interstitial emphysema (PIE).

Pathophysiology

Pulmonary interstitial emphysema, pneumomediastinum, pneumothorax, and pneumopericardium are closely related clinical entities. Air leak begins with formation of PIE in which alveoli rupture into the perivascular and peribronchial spaces. Air may be trapped in the interstitium of the lung, leading to PIE, but it may also dissect into the mediastinum along the perivascular and peribronchial spaces, producing pneumomediastinum. Mediastinal air ruptures into the pleural space, producing pneumothorax, or into the pericardial space, producing pneumopericardium. In some instances, air can form blebs on the surface of the lung that rupture to produce pneumothorax. Rupture of the lung directly into the pleural space is thought to occur rarely.

Risk Factors

Air leaks occur in 1% to 2% of all newborn infants, but they are thought to cause symptoms in only 0.05% to 0.07%. Mechanical ventilation and CPAP are important risk factors contributing to air leak in infants with lung disease. Cystic adenomatoid malformation also predisposes infants to spontaneous pneumothorax. Summarizing data from 11 studies, Madansky found that air leak occurred in 12% of infants with RDS who were not on assisted ventilation, 11% of infants on CPAP, and 26% of infants on mechanical ventilation (58). The incidence of air leak in infants admitted to the NICU is approximately 2% to 8%, but it is higher if only low-birth-weight infants are considered. As of 1986, of infants weighing 500 to 999 g at birth who developed air leak, 35% had PIE, 20% had pneumothorax, 3% had pneumomediastinum, and 2% had pneumopericardium (58). Infants developing air leak are at higher risk of death, but the risk changes with postnatal age at the time of the air leak. Aspiration syndromes, including MAS, are frequently complicated by air leak.

Radiographic Evaluation

The chest radiographs of infants with PIE have been described as demonstrating a salt-and-pepper pattern in which the radiolucent interstitial air is juxtaposed to lung parenchyma (Fig. 29-13). Radiolucent air is present in the pleural space in a pneumothorax. Because chest radiographs of neonates are usually performed in the supine position, pleural air of a pneumothorax may accumulate in the anterior chest and may be visible only on a cross-table lateral or decubitus radiograph. In a tension pneumothorax, the lung and mediastinal organs may be displaced away from the side of the pneumothorax (Fig. 29-14). The thymus may be outlined in pneumomediastinum, seen on radiographs. Pneumopericardium results in a characteristic outline of the heart by radiolucent air.

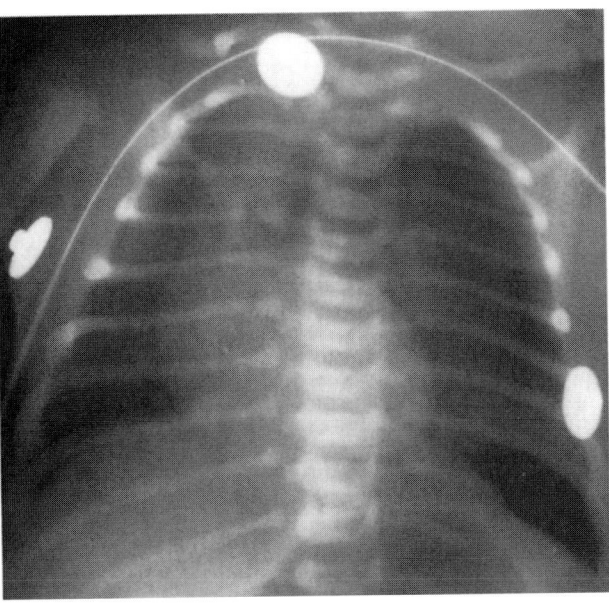

Figure 29-14 A full-term infant born by a difficult breech delivery presented shortly after birth with crepitus in the neck area, tachypnea, grunting, and retractions. An anteroposterior chest x-ray film demonstrates bilateral pneumothorax under tension on the left. The heart and mediastinum are compressed and shifted to the right. The left pleural air herniates across the midline. The left diaphragm is depressed and inverted. Subcutaneous emphysema is seen in the soft tissues of the neck.

Pulmonary Interstitial Emphysema

Pulmonary interstitial emphysema occurs most frequently in smaller infants being treated by mechanical ventilation for primary lung disease. In this clinical setting, PIE is associated with a mortality rate of more than 50%. Unilateral PIE can be managed by placing the infant with the affected side down for 24 to 48 hours. Selective bronchial intubation and high-frequency or jet ventilation have been used to treat unilateral PIE. Careful attention to peak and mean inspiratory pressures may be beneficial in preventing and treating PIE. High-frequency ventilation may be helpful. Bronchopulmonary dysplasia is a frequent sequel in infants surviving PIE.

Pneumothorax, Pneumomediastinum, and Pneumopericardium

Infants with pneumothorax often present with grunting, tachypnea, cyanosis (See Color Plate), and retractions. Accumulated air may collapse the lung or shift the mediastinum to the side opposite the air leak. A shift of the trachea or point of maximal impulse and decreased breath sounds on the affected side may be found on clinical examination. Pneumothoraces fall into two major groups: spontaneous pneumothorax in otherwise healthy, full-term infants, which most often occurs within minutes of birth, and pneumothorax in infants with significant pulmonary disease, which frequently occurs several days after birth, during therapy for pulmonary disease.

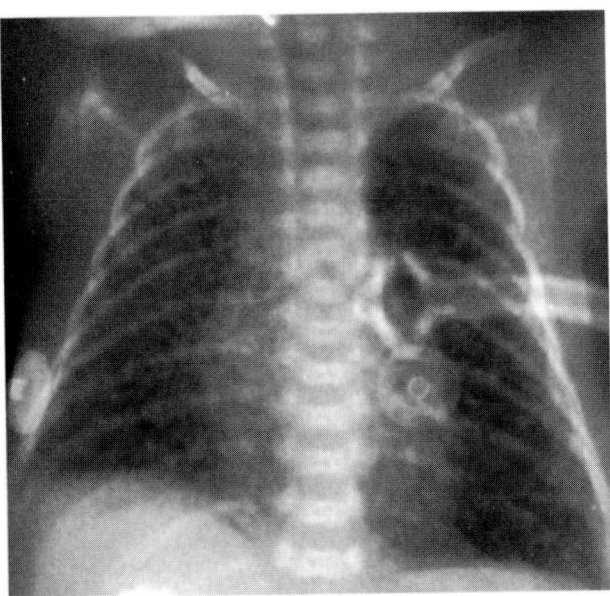

Figure 29-13 Chest x-ray film of pulmonary interstitial emphysema (PIE). A premature infant with severe respiratory distress syndrome requiring mechanical ventilation developed worsening respiratory acidosis and hypoxia refractory to increased ventilatory support. An anteroposterior chest x-ray film demonstrates a salt-and-pepper pattern resulting from radiolucent interstitial air surrounding compressed lung tissue. A left chest tube was placed to treat pneumothorax, a common complication of pulmonary interstitial emphysema.

Prompt recognition of air leak is essential for effective therapy. Unexpected changes in ventilatory requirements or status and abrupt fall in blood pressure, heart rate, respiratory rate, and PO2 may indicate an air leak. Transillumination of the thorax can be useful in the diagnosis of pneumothorax and the response to therapy. Treatment of tension pneumothorax requires immediate surgical drainage and placement of a chest tube. For treatment of pneumothorax that does not involve tension or cardiovascular compromise, inhalation of 100% oxygen, usually for 4 to 6 hours, can be used as a nitrogen washout method in term infants. Premature infants should not be treated with hyperoxia because they are at risk for retrolental fibroplasia. Pneumomediastinum and pneumopericardium that does not unduly stress the infant can also be managed with 100% oxygen therapy. Tension pneumopericardium is life threatening, must be drained surgically, and is associated with a high incidence of morbidity and mortality.

REFERENCES

1. Burri PH. Postnatal development and growth. In: Crystal RG, West JB, Barnes PJ, Cherniack NS, Weibel ER, eds. *The lung: scientific foundations.* New York: Raven Press, 1991:677.
2. Randell SH, Young SL. Structure of alveolar epithelial cells and the surface layer during development. In: Polin RA, Fox WW, eds. *Fetal and neonatal physiology.* Philadelphia: WB Saunders, 1992:962.
3. Nogee LM, Wert SE, Proffit SA, et al. Allelic heterogeneity in hereditary surfactant protein B (SP-B) deficiency. *Am J Respir Crit Care Med* 2000;161:973–981.
4. Nogee LM, Dunbar AE 3rd, Wert SE, et al. A mutation in the surfactant protein C gene associated with familial interstitial lung disease. *N Engl J Med* 2001;344:573–579.
5. Shulenin S, Nogee LM, Annilo T, et al. The *ABCA3* gene is frequently mutated in human newborns with fatal surfactant deficiency. *N Engl J Med* 2004;350:1296–1303.
6. Van Golde LM, Batenburg JJ, Robertson B. The pulmonary surfactant system: biochemical aspects and functional significance. *Physiol Rev* 1988;68:374–455.
7. Whitsett JA. RDS in the premature infant. In: Crystal RG, West JB, Barnes PJ, Cherniack NS, Weibel ER, eds. *The lung: scientific foundations.* New York: Raven Press, 1991:1723.
8. Shapiro DL, Notter RH. Surfactant replacement therapy. New York: Alan R Liss, 1989.
9. Rooney S. Regulation of surfactant associated phospholipid synthesis and secretion. In: Polin RA, Fox WW, eds. *Fetal and neonatal physiology.* Philadelphia: WB Saunders, 1992:986.
10. Ballard PL. Hormonal regulation of pulmonary surfactant. *Endocrinol Rev* 1989;10:165–181.
11. Liggins GC, Howie RN. A controlled trial of antepartum glucocorticoid treatment for prevention of the respiratory distress syndrome in premature infants. *Pediatrics* 1972;50:515–525.
12. Jobe A. Phospholipid metabolism and turnover. In: Polin RA, Fox WW, eds. *Fetal and neonatal physiology.* Philadelphia: WB Saunders, 1992:986.
13. Fujiwara T, Maeta H, Chida S, et al. Artificial surfactant therapy in hyaline membrane disease. *Lancet* 1980;1:55-59.
14. Avery ME, Mead J. Surface properties in relation to atelectasis and hyaline membrane disease. *Am J Dis Child* 1959;97:517–523.
15. Newnham JP, Moss TJ, Nitsos I, et al. Antenatal corticosteroids: the good, the bad and the unknown. *Curr Opin Obstet Gynecol* 2002;14:607–612.
16. Spitzer AR, Shaffer TH, Fox WW. Assisted ventilation: physiologic implications and application. In: RA Polin, WW Fox, eds. *Fetal and neonatal physiology.* Philadelphia: WB Saunders, 1991:894.
17. Suresh GK, Soll RF. Lung surfactants for neonatal respiratory distress syndrome: Animal-derived or synthetic agents? *Paediatr Drugs* 2002;4:485–492.
18. Henderson-Smart DJ, Bhuta T, Cools F, et al. Elective high frequency oscillatory ventilation versus conventional ventilation for acute pulmonary dysfunction in preterm infants. *Cochrane Database Syst Rev* 2003;1:CD000104.
19. Barrington KJ, Finer NN. Inhaled nitric oxide for respiratory failure in preterm infants. *Cochrane Database Syst Rev* 2001;4:CD000509.
20. Wiswell TE. Handling the meconium-stained infant. *Semin Neonatol* 2001;6:225–231.
21. Tran N, Lowe C, Sivieri EM, et al. Sequential effects of acute meconium obstruction on pulmonary function. *Pediatr Res* 1980;14:34–38.
22. Ting P, Brady JP. Tracheal suction in meconium aspiration. *Am J Obstet Gynecol* 1975;122:767–771.
23. Hofmeyr GJ. Amnioinfusion for meconium-stained liquor in labour. *Cochrane Database Syst Rev* 2002;1:CD000014.
24. Halliday HL. Endotracheal intubation at birth for preventing morbidity and mortality in vigorous, meconium-stained infants born at term. *Cochrane Database Syst Rev* 2001;1:CD000500.
25. Soll RF, Dargaville P. Surfactant for meconium aspiration syndrome in full term infants. *Cochrane Database Syst. Rev* 2000;2:CD002054.
26. Findlay RD, Taeusch HW, Walther FJ. Surfactant replacement therapy for meconium aspiration syndrome. *Pediatrics* 1996;97:48–52.
27. Kinsella JP, Truog WE, Walsh WF, et al. Randomized, multicenter trial of inhaled nitric oxide and high-frequency oscillatory ventilation in severe, persistent pulmonary hypertension of the newborn. *J Pediatr* 1997;131:55–62.
28. Extracorporeal Life Support Registry Report, International Summary. July, 2003.
29. Gersony W, Duc G, Sinclair J. "PFC" syndrome. *Circulation* 1969;40[Suppl III]:87.
30. Walsh MC, Stork EK. Persistent pulmonary hypertension of the newborn. Rational therapy based on pathophysiology. *Clin Perinatol* 2001;28:609–627.
31. Rabinowitz M. Structure and function of the pulmonary vascular bed: an update. *Cardiol Clin* 1989;7:227.
32. Weinberger B, Weiss K, Heck DE, et al. Pharmacologic therapy of persistent pulmonary hypertension of the newborn. *Pharmacol Ther* 2001;89:67–79.
33. Sadiq HF, Mantych G, Benawra RS, et al. Inhaled nitric oxide in the treatment of moderate persistent pulmonary hypertension of the newborn: A randomized controlled, multicenter trial. *J Perinatol* 2003;23:98–103.
34. Finer NN, Barrington KJ. Nitric oxide for respiratory failure in infants born at or near term. *Cochrane Database Syst Rev* 2001;4:CD000399.
35. Bartlett RH, Gazzaniga AB, Huxtable RF, et al. Extracorporeal circulation (ECMO) in neonatal respiratory failure. *J Thorac Cardiovasc Surg* 1977;74:826–823.
36. Rais-Bahrami K, Short BL. The current status of neonatal extracorporeal membrane oxygenation. *Semin Perinatol* 2000;24:406–417.
37. Ballard RA, Leonard CH. Developmental follow-up of infants with persistent pulmonary hypertension of the newborn. *Clin Perinatol* 1984;11:737–744.
38. Lipkin PH, Davidson D, Spivak L, et al. Neurodevelopmental and medical outcomes of persistent pulmonary hypertension in term newborns treated with nitric oxide. *J Pediatr* 2002;140:306–310.
39. Rosenberg AA, Kennaugh JM, Moreland SG, et al. Longitudinal follow-up of a cohort of newborn infants treated with inhaled nitric oxide in persistent pulmonary hypertension. *J Pediatr* 1997;131:70–75.
40. Gaynes RP, Edwards JR, Jarvis WR, et al. Nosocomial infections among neonates in high risk nurseries in the United States. National Nosocomial Infection's Surveillance System. *Pediatrics* 1996;98:357-361.
41. Schrag S, Gorwitz R, Fultz-Butts K, et al. Prevention of perinatal group B streptococcal disease. Revised guidelines from CDC. *MMWR Recomm Rep* 2002;51:1–22.
42. Hyde TB, Hilger TM, Reingold A, et al. Trends in incidence and antimicrobial resistance of early-onset sepsis: population-based surveillance in San Francisco and Atlanta. *Pediatrics* 2002;110:690–695.
43. Stoll BJ, Hansen N, Fanaroff AA, et al. Pathogens causing early-onset sepsis in very low birth weight infants. *N Engl J Med* 2002;347:240–247.

44. Schuchat A, Zywicki SS, Dinsmoor MJ, et al. Risk factors and opportunities for prevention of early-onset neonatal sepsis: a multicenter case-control study. *Pediatrics* 2000;105:21–26.
45. Hamprecht K, Maschmann J, Vochem M, et al. Epidemiology of transmission of cytomegalovirus from mother to preterm infant by breastfeeding. *Lancet* 2001;357:513–518.
46. Kimberlin DW, Lin CY, Jacobs RF, et al. Natural history of neonatal herpes simplex virus infection in the acyclovir era. *Pediatrics* 2001;108:223–229.
47. Hickman ME, Rench MA, Ferrieri P, et al. Changing epidemiology of group B streptococcal colonization. *Pediatrics* 1999;104: 203–209.
48. Schrag SJ, Zywicki S, Farley MM, et al. Group B streptococcal disease in the era of intrapartum antibiotic prophylaxis. *N Engl J Med* 2000;342:15–20.
49. Bromberger P, Lawrence JM, Braun D, et al. The influence of intrapartum antibiotics on the clinical spectrum of early-onset group B streptococcal infection in term infants. *Pediatrics* 2000; 106:244–250.
50. Rojas J, Stahlman M. The effect of group B *Streptococcus* and other organisms on the pulmonary vasculature. *Clin Perinatol* 1984;11: 591–599.
51. Whitley R, Arvin A, Prober C, et al. Predictors of morbidity and mortality in neonates with herpes simplex virus infections. The National Institute of Allergy and Infectious Diseases Collaborative Antiviral Study Group. *N Engl J Med* 1991;324:450–454.
52. Kimberlin DW, Lin CY, Jacobs RF, et al. Safety and efficiency of high dose intravenous acyclovir in the management of neonatal herpes simplex virus infection. *Pediatrics* 2001;108:230–238.
53. Avery ME, Gatewood OB, Brumley G. Transient tachypnea of newborn. Possible delayed resorption at birth. *Am J Dis Child* 1966;111:380–385.
54. Levine EM, Ghai V, Barton JJ, et al. Mode of delivery and risk of respiratory diseases in newborns. *Obstet Gynecol* 2001;97: 439–442.
55. Schaubel D, Johansen H, Dutta M, et al. Neonatal characteristics as risk factors for preschool asthma. *J Asthma* 1996;33:255–264.
56. Lewis V, Whitelaw A. Furosemide for transient tachypnea of the newborn. *Cochrane Database Syst Rev* 2002;1:CD003064.
57. Kluckow M, Evans N. Ductal shunting, high pulmonary blood flow, and pulmonary hemorrhage. *J Pediatr* 2000;137:68–72.
58. Madansky DL, Lawson EE, Chernick V, et al. Pneumothorax and other forms of pulmonary air leak in newborns. *Am Rev Respir Dis* 1979;120:729–737.

30

Bronchopulmonary Dysplasia

Jonathan M. Davis   *Warren N. Rosenfeld*

Bronchopulmonary dysplasia (BPD) is a chronic lung disease that develops in newborn infants treated with oxygen and positive-pressure mechanical ventilation for a primary lung disorder. The introduction of new treatment modalities (e.g., surfactant replacement therapy, high-frequency ventilation, extracorporeal membrane oxygenation, inhaled nitric oxide [INO]) has significantly improved the outcome for many critically ill premature and term infants. As a result, more infants are surviving the newborn period and developing BPD. Approximately 10,000 new cases of BPD occur each year in the United States and there is significant associated morbidity and mortality. There has been significant debate about the exact definition of BPD, further complicated because the specific nature of the disease has changed with the widespread use of surfactant and other therapeutic interventions. Although the current form of BPD appears to be much less severe than in the past, BPD is still an extremely important complication of neonatal intensive care (NICU) and the most common form of chronic lung disease in infants.

The modern history of BPD began with Northway's observations in 1967 (1). This study documented the clinical course, radiographic findings, and histopathologic lung changes in a group of infants who had received oxygen and ventilatory support for treatment of respiratory distress syndrome (RDS) and established the term BPD. Although Northway originally postulated that oxygen toxicity caused BPD, the exact mechanisms causing the lung injury are complex and are currently the subject of intense investigation. Treatment with positive-pressure ventilation appears to be a critical factor in the development of BPD, although factors such as oxygen toxicity, prematurity, genetic predisposition, infection and inflammation may also play important roles. Therapies for infants with BPD are directed toward improving the pathophysiologic abnormalities after they occur and include oxygen, mechanical ventilation, fluid restriction, and a variety of medications. Many different therapies can be used in these infants, often concurrently. The optimal treatment and prevention strategies have not been definitively established.

This chapter reviews the definition and incidence of BPD (also known as chronic lung disease in newborns), its pathogenesis, pathophysiologic changes, treatment strategies, and long-term outcome. Newly developed approaches for the prevention of BPD in high-risk infants are presented.

DEFINITION AND INCIDENCE

In the original description of BPD, Northway defined chronic lung changes in a group of premature neonates who survived mechanical ventilation for treatment of RDS (1). Northway's definition of BPD included radiologic, pathologic, and clinical criteria. BPD was divided into four developmental stages. The acute stages, I and II were indistinguishable from RDS and were seen in the first 10 days of life. Stages III and IV marked the transition to the chronic stages of this disease, with stage IV forming the basis for the definition of BPD. This stage described abnormalities that persisted beyond 1 month of age in patients who continued to require respiratory support (i.e., ventilation or oxygen supplementation). Chest radiographs demonstrated cyst formation and hyperexpansion alternating with areas of atelectasis.

As the care of neonates has become more sophisticated and smaller, sicker infants survived, the clinical and radiographic findings that define BPD have changed. Northway's original criteria depended heavily on a progression of radiographic changes, and clinical criteria were considered secondary. Further refinement was offered by Bancalari, whose criteria included ventilation for at least the first 3 days of life and respiratory symptoms (e.g., tachypnea, auscultatory rales, retractions) at 28 days of life, a need for supplemental oxygen to maintain a partial pressure (PaO_2) greater than 50 mm Hg and an abnormal chest radiograph at 28 days of life (2).

TABLE 30-1
DEFINITION OF BRONCHOPULMONARY DYSPLASIA: DIAGNOSTIC CRITERIA[a]

Gestational Age	<32 Wk	≥32 Wk
Time point of assessment	36 wk PMA or discharge to home, whichever comes first	>28 d but <56 d postnatal age or discharge home, whichever comes first
Treatment with oxygen >21% for at least 28 d **plus**		
Mild BPD	Breathing room air at 36 wk PMA or discharge, whichever comes first	56 d postnatal age or discharge, whichever comes first
Moderate BPD	Need for <30% oxygen at 36 wk PMA or discharge, whichever comes first	Need for <30% oxygen at 56 d postnatal age or discharge, whichever comes first
Severe BPD	Need for ≥30% oxygen and/or positive pressure, (PPV or NCPAP) at 36 wk PMA or discharge, whichever comes first	Need for ≥30% oxygen and/or positive pressure (PPV or NCPAP) at 56 d postnatal age or discharge, whichever comes first

Definition of abbreviations: BPD = bronchopulmonary dysplasia; NCPAP = nasal continuous positive airway pressure; PMA = postmenstrual age; PPV = positive-pressure ventilation.
[a] From Jobe AH, Bancalari E. Bronchopulmonary dysplasia. *Am J Respir Crit Care Med* 2001;163:1723, with permission.

Many infants who eventually develop chronic lung disease do not require prolonged mechanical ventilation, nor have significant radiographic abnormalities. Several studies have used less stringent criteria to define BPD such as simply the requirement for oxygen supplementation at 28 days of life (3,4). Shennan and associates questioned the large number of normal neonates who would be included by this criterion and suggested that the need for supplemental oxygen at 36 weeks postconceptual gestational age may be a more accurate predictor of ultimate pulmonary outcome (5). Other investigators have found that the most reliable method to definitively establish the diagnosis of BPD is the presence of chronic respiratory symptoms (e.g., asthma, repeated pulmonary infections) requiring treatment with bronchodilators or corticosteroids in the first year or two of life (6,7). Recently, a consensus conference convened by the National Institutes of Health suggested a new definition of BPD that incorporates many elements of previous definitions and attempts to categorize the severity of BPD (Table 30-1) (7). Ultimately, the definition of BPD will need to be validated with clinically important long-term endpoints in a prospective fashion.

The incidence of BPD depends on the definition used and the patient population studied. Several surfactant replacement trials have reported the incidence of BPD, defined as oxygen dependency at 28 days with appropriate radiographic findings, to be in the range of 11% to 63% and varying significantly by center (8–11). It appeared from these studies that the incidence of BPD decreased only slightly after surfactant therapy. However, the prevalence, or total number of infants with BPD, increased because of improved survival. Fenton and associates subsequently reported that exogenous surfactant had significantly improved the survival of many low-birth-weight infants in their geographically defined population and was actually associated with a marked increase in the incidence of BPD (12). BPD will continue to be an important problem for the neonatologist and pediatric pulmonologist in the future. Further study of the mechanisms involved in the lung injury process and the development of possible prevention strategies are urgently needed.

PATHOGENESIS

No single factor has been identified as the cause of BPD. Its origin is multifactorial and may depend on the nature of the injury, mechanisms of response, or the infant's inability to respond appropriately to the injury process (Fig. 30-1). Although Northway attributed the occurrence of BPD primarily to prolonged hyperoxia in infants with RDS, numerous other causes have been proposed.

Barotrauma/Volutrauma

Although the initial phases of lung injury in BPD are the result of the primary disease process (e.g., RDS), superimposed positive-pressure mechanical ventilation appears to

PATHOGENESIS OF BPD

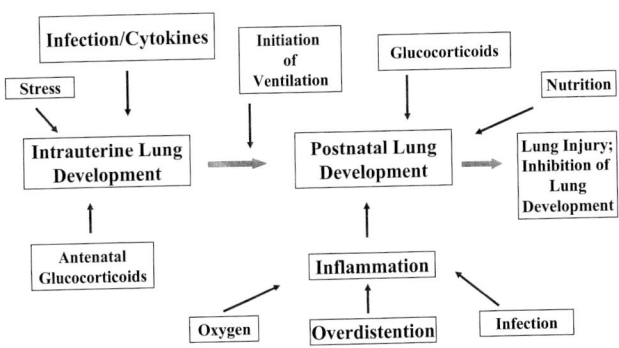

Figure 30-1 An overview of the pathogenesis of BPD showing prenatal and postnatal factors. Adapted from Jobe AH. The new BPD: an arrest of lung development. *Pediatr Res* 1999;46:641, with permission.

add to the lung injury and provoke a complex inflammatory cascade that ultimately leads to chronic lung disease. Barotrauma is the term generally used to describe the lung injury that occurs secondary to positive-pressure mechanical ventilation, although volutrauma from excessive tidal volume ventilation may be a more appropriate term to describe this lung injury process.

The role of barotrauma in BPD depends on several factors, including the structure of the tracheobronchial tree and the physiologic effects of surfactant deficiency. With surfactant deficiency, surface tension forces are elevated, aeration is unequal, and most terminal alveoli are largely collapsed. The pressure needed to distend these poorly compliant saccules is high and is transmitted to the terminal bronchioles and alveolar ducts. In the premature infant, these airways are highly compliant and subject to rupture. Gas then dissects into the interstitium and pleural space, resulting in the development of pulmonary interstitial emphysema (PIE) and pneumothorax. These complications are strongly associated with the development of BPD, suggesting that ventilator-induced lung injury is important in the pathogenesis (13,14).

Nilsson and colleagues have shown that even brief periods of positive-pressure ventilation cause bronchiolar epithelial damage in the lung, with the severity of the injury correlating with the amount of peak pressure used (15). Even with normal tidal volumes, ventilation of the immature or injured newborn lung results in nonuniform inflation and relative overdistension of ventilated segments, especially in the presence of low functional residual capacity (FRC) as a result of surfactant deficiency. Stretching of capillary endothelium and distal lung epithelium increases permeability to serum proteins that may further inhibit surfactant function, creating a vicious cycle that promotes lung injury.

The adverse effects of tidal volume breaths in lungs with low FRC can be ameliorated with better lung recruitment by application of higher positive end-expiratory pressure (PEEP). Experimental studies have shown that overdistension of the lung (not increased pressure) is responsible for lung injury in the surfactant-deficient lung (14). For example, strapping the chest wall to restrict overexpansion increases lung pressure but limits lung stretch, and ameliorates lung injury in animal models (16). Tremblay and associates have observed that mechanical ventilation with high tidal volumes and low PEEP markedly increases edema and cytokine production in the lung of rats (17). In this same model, lung injury increased cytokine release from the lungs into the systemic circulation, suggesting a potential mechanism linking multi-organ dysfunction and sepsis syndrome with lung injury. Improved survival of adults with acute respiratory distress syndrome (ARDS) has been found when employing a ventilator strategy that used low tidal volumes with high PEEP to recruit atelectatic lung regions and improve FRC (18).

Strategies to prevent lung injury have included changes in methods of ventilation. Even brief exposure to large tidal volume breaths during resuscitation shortly after birth can initiate early lung injury, which decreases the subsequent response to surfactant therapy (19). With the increased use of nasal continuous positive airway pressure (NCPAP), many preterm infants may be able to be managed without the need for endotracheal intubation and mechanical ventilation, which may lessen the risk for lung injury. Synchronized intermittent mechanical ventilation (SIMV) and high-frequency devices have also been extensively studied. Bernstein and associates reported that infants ($<1,000$ g) treated with SIMV developed less BPD than those receiving conventional ventilation (20). Several multicenter trials have demonstrated that high-frequency oscillatory ventilation (HFOV) or high frequency jet ventilation (HFJV) using high volume, alveolar recruitment strategies in conjunction with surfactant replacement therapy reduced complications of mechanical ventilation (PIE, pneumothorax) and lowered the incidence of BPD compared to conventional ventilation (21,22). However, these findings have not been consistently found in other trials. Regardless of the type of ventilation strategy used, it is important to avoid even brief periods of overdistension, because high tidal volumes and hypocarbia are associated with a greater risk for developing both BPD and neurologic injury (23,24). A retrospective study of 1,105 newborns born with birth weights about 2,000 g between 1984 to 1987 demonstrated a strong relationship between prolonged hypocapnia ($PaCO_2 < 35$ torr) and the development of cerebral palsy (CP) (24).

The use of surfactant replacement therapy has reduced some complications of mechanical ventilation. Surfactant permits more equal distribution of pressures and ventilation to all alveoli, prevents overdistension of distal air spaces and bronchioles, and stabilizes lung volume. A major benefit of surfactant therapy has been the ability to reduce airway pressures and the incidence of air leak, while maintaining a greater uniformity of lung recruitment. However, BPD continues to be an important problem despite the widespread use of exogenous surfactant and strategies to minimize lung injury from mechanical ventilation (e.g., permissive hypercapnia). Van Marter and associates recently studied 452 premature infants weighing 500 to 1,500 g at birth who were born at specific neonatal centers in either Boston or New York. They found that the incidence of BPD was significantly higher in Boston (22%) compared to New York (4%), even after adjusting for baseline risk factors, such as severity of prematurity (25). Using multivariate analyses to examine differences in specific respiratory care practices during the first week of life, most of the increased risk of BPD was associated with the early initiation of mechanical ventilation. Interestingly, the use of both exogenous surfactant and indomethacin increased the risk for BPD. This suggests that attempts to minimize the use of mechanical ventilation using nasal continuous positive airway pressure (NCPAP) (with or without exogenous surfactant) may actually lower the incidence and severity of BPD in high-risk infants. Ongoing multicenter trials of early NCPAP in premature infants are currently underway. BPD continues to be a serious problem, suggesting that barotrauma is only one of many factors involved in the pathogenesis of BPD.

Oxygen and Antioxidants

Under normal conditions, a delicate balance exists between the production of oxygen free radicals (also called reactive oxygen species) and the antioxidant defenses that protect cells in vivo. Free radicals are molecules with extra electrons in their outer ring and they are toxic to living tissues (Table 30-2). Oxygen has a unique molecular structure and is abundant within cells. It readily accepts free electrons generated by oxidative metabolism within the cell, producing free radicals. Increased free-radical production can occur under conditions of hyperoxia, reperfusion, or inflammation. Alternatively, free radicals can increase because of an inability to quench production because of inadequate antioxidant defenses. Damage caused by oxygen free radicals includes lipid peroxidation, mitochondrial injury, protein nitration and unraveling of nucleic acids.

The premature neonate may be more susceptible to free-radical damage because adequate concentrations of antioxidants may be absent at birth. Frank and associates documented the development of the antioxidant enzymes superoxide dismutase (SOD), catalase, and glutathione peroxidase in the lungs of rabbits during late gestation (Fig. 30-2) (26). The 150% increase in these enzymes during the last 15% of gestation parallels the maturation pattern of pulmonary surfactant. These developmental changes in the fetal lung allow proper ventilation by reducing surface tension and provide for the transition from the relative hypoxia of intrauterine development to the oxygen-rich extrauterine environment. Premature birth can occur before the normal upregulation of these antioxidant systems and other free radical scavengers (e.g. vitamin E, ascorbic acid, glutathione, and ceruloplasmin) and may result in an imbalance between oxidants and antioxidants and an increased risk for the development of BPD. Experimental animal models have shown that exposure to chronic hyper-

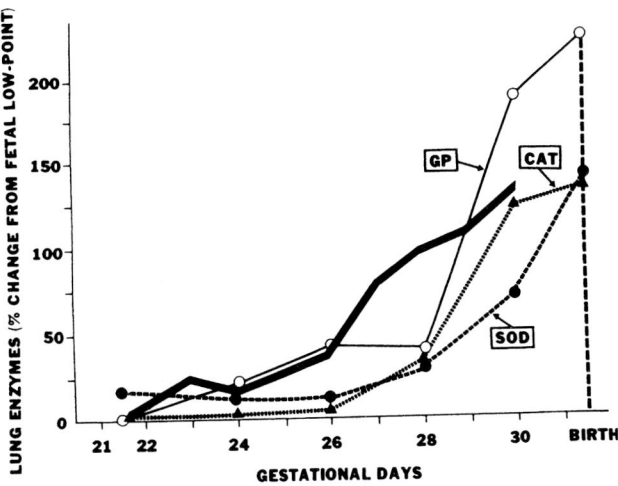

Figure 30-2 Developmental changes in antioxidant levels and activity during gestation. The increases in superoxide dismutase (SOD), catalase (CAT), and glutathione peroxidase (GP) late in gestation are similar to those seen for pulmonary surfactant (dark, thick line). From Frank L, Groseclose EE. Preparation for birth into an O_2-rich environment: the antioxidant enzymes in the developing rabbit lung. *Pediatr Res* 1984;18:240, with permission.

oxia can induce inflammation and lung injury that has many features seen in infants developing BPD. Both epithelial and endothelial cells are extremely susceptible to oxidant injury, leading to increased permeability edema and cell dysfunction. Hyperoxia also impairs mucociliary function, promotes inflammation and inactivates antiproteases, further complicating clinical outcome.

Clinical studies suggest that free radicals are involved in the pathogenesis of BPD. Plasma concentrations of allantoin, an oxidation byproduct of uric acid, has been shown to be significantly elevated in the first 48 hours of life in infants developing BPD compared to controls (27). Expired pentane and ethane have also been measured as indirect evidence of free radical-induced lipid peroxidation in the first week of life and found to be significantly elevated in neonates subsequently developing BPD (28). Varsila and colleagues analyzed proteins in tracheal aspirates in the first week of life and found evidence of protein oxidation (carbonyl formation) in infants developing BPD (29). Banks and associates found a fourfold increase in plasma 3-nitrotyrosine concentration in infants developing BPD compared to controls, indicating increased evidence of reactive nitrogen species (endogenous nitric oxide [NO] reacting with superoxide) modifying serum proteins (30). Of note, the multicenter STOP-retinopathy of prematurity (ROP) trial examined whether exposing premature infants to higher inspired oxygen concentrations would prevent the development of severe ROP. Although the effects of the increased oxygen were minimal on the eyes, exposed infants had a marked increase (55%) in the incidence of BPD and pulmonary infections (31).

Further evidence for the role of oxygen free radicals in lung injury comes from animal studies, which have shown that antioxidant supplementation with SOD and catalase reduces cell damage, increases survival, and prevents lung

TABLE 30-2
FREE RADICALS

Radical	Symbol[a]	Antioxidant
Superoxide anion	O_2^-	Superoxide dismutase, uric acid, vitamin E
Singlet oxygen	$^1O_2$	β-carotene, uric acid, vitamin E
Hydrogen peroxide	H_2O_2	Catalase, glutathione peroxidase, glutathione
Hydroxyl radical	OH•	Vitamins C and E
Peroxide radical	LOO•	Vitamins C and E
Hydroperoxyl radical	LOOH	Glutathione transferase, glutathione peroxidase

[a] L, lipid.

injury from prolonged hyperoxia and mechanical ventilation (32,33). Genetically engineered mice overexpressing SOD survive longer, whereas mice with disrupted SOD genes die more quickly in a hyperoxic environment compared to normal diploid controls (34,35). These studies all demonstrate that oxygen free radicals are intimately involved in the development of acute lung and chronic lung disease in newborn infants.

Inflammation

Marked inflammation in the lung appears to begin a cascade of destruction and abnormal repair that develops into BPD. The initial stimuli activating the inflammatory process in the lung may be oxygen free radicals, pulmonary barotrauma, infectious agents, or other stimuli that result in the attraction and activation of leukocytes. Inflammation appears to play an important role in the pathogenesis of BPD and allows many factors to be unified into a single cause of this disease. Inflammatory mediators and cellular responses have been found to be prominent in animal models of lung injury and in infants who develop BPD.

A sustained increase in the number of neutrophils that generate excessive oxygen free radicals in tracheal fluid samples distinguishes infants who develop BPD from those who recover spontaneously (36,37). Additionally, the presence of activated macrophages, high concentrations of lipid products, inactivated α-1-antitrypsin activity, and other markers of active inflammation are strongly linked with the development of BPD (38). Release of early response cytokines, such as tumor necrosis factor-α (TNF-α), interleukin-1β (IL-1β), interleukin-8 (IL-8), and transforming growth factor (TGF)-β by macrophages and the presence of soluble adhesion molecules (e.g., selectins) may impact other cells to release chemoattractants and recruit neutrophils which further amplify the inflammatory response (38–42). Elevated concentrations of pro-inflammatory cytokines (IL-6, IL-8) in conjunction with reduced antiinflammatory products, (IL-10) usually appear in tracheal aspirates within a few hours of life in infants subsequently developing BPD (40–42). All these agents recruit and activate leukocytes resulting in significant pulmonary damage, including breakdown of capillary endothelial integrity and leakage of macromolecules (e.g., albumin) into alveolar spaces. Albumin leakage and pulmonary edema are known to inhibit surfactant function and have been postulated to be important factors in the development of BPD (43).

The release of elastase and collagenase from activated neutrophils directly destroys the elastin and collagen framework of the lung. The breakdown products of collagen (hydroxyproline) and elastin (desmosine) have been recovered in the urine of infants who develop BPD (44). The major defense against the action of elastase activity is α1-proteinase inhibitor, which may be inactivated by oxygen radicals. Increased elastase activity accompanied by compromised antiproteinase function may enhance lung injury. This combination has been demonstrated in tracheal aspirates and serum of neonates who develop BPD (45–47).

As the acute cycle of injury continues with further production and accumulation of inflammatory mediators, significant injury to the lung can occur during a particularly critical period of rapid growth; six divisions from 24 to 40 weeks of gestation. It appears likely that this abnormal inflammatory process is primarily responsible for the acute and the chronic changes that occur in the lungs of infants with BPD. Watterberg and associates have demonstrated that extremely premature infants have evidence of adrenal insufficiency at birth with the lowest serum cortisol concentrations during the first week of life correlating with increased lung inflammation and adverse respiratory outcome (48). Pilot studies examining early treatment with low-dose hydrocortisone in extremely low birth weight (LBW) infants increased the likelihood of survival without BPD, a benefit that was particularly apparent in infants born to mothers with chorioamnionitis (49). The mechanisms of action may include suppression of lung inflammation with less inhibition of lung growth observed with higher doses of steroids or even beneficial effects of low dose hydrocortisone on lung development. These studies all clearly support the notion that this abnormal inflammatory process is primarily responsible for the acute and the chronic changes that occur in the lungs of infants with BPD.

Infection

Subclinical intrauterine infection and the ensuing inflammatory response have been clearly implicated in the etiology of preterm labor and premature rupture of membranes (50). Growing evidence indicates that prenatal infection and inflammation are major risk factors for the subsequent development of BPD. Although several investigators have found a lower incidence of RDS in preterm infants born to mothers with chorioamnionitis and funisitis (possibly as a result of an adaptive response to in utero stress), they also observed a significantly higher incidence of BPD in these same infants (51). This suggests that although intrauterine infection may accelerate lung maturation, the ensuing inflammatory response may also "prime the lung," causing lung injury, progressive inflammation and subsequent inhibition of lung growth. Subsequent exposure to hyperoxia and mechanical ventilation may further exacerbate the injury process in an already infected and/or inflamed lung.

Ureaplasma urealyticum has been recovered from cervical cultures of pregnant women and implicated as a possible cause of chorioamnionitis, prematurity, and BPD (52). Cassell and colleagues cultured tracheal aspirates and blood and found that BPD developed in 82% of infants (<1,000 g) colonized with Ureaplasma, compared with 41% of those with negative cultures (52). In contrast, other studies have found that although Ureaplasma was frequently detected (by culture or polymerase chain reaction) in many LBW infants, its presence was not associated with the development of BPD (53,54). It is possible that infection simply acts as a stimulus for the inflammatory response, with recruitment of leukocytes and the production of cytokines and oxygen free radicals, ultimately leading to the development of BPD. Normal defense mechanisms against infection can be compromised in the lungs of these chronically ventilated, premature infants. This makes them more susceptible to colonization and subsequent infection with a variety of infectious agents (e.g., virus, bacteria, fungi) that may affect the severity of BPD (55). Several large clinical studies have found a strong correlation between the presence of BPD and the development of late-onset sepsis, usually with organisms such as staphylococcus epidermidis (56,57). These infections are associated with increased morbidity, mortality, and length of hospital stay and appear to contribute to the severity of BPD.

Nutrition

The nutritional status of the critically ill premature infant may also be important in the development of BPD. Adequate calories and essential nutrients for growth may be lacking during a period of stress and growth; vital components for immunologic and antioxidant defenses may be inadequate; and the nutritional supplements provided may actually contribute to ongoing damage.

Premature infants have increased nutritional requirements because of increased metabolic needs and rapid growth requirements. If these increased energy needs are not met, the infant will develop a catabolic state, which most likely contributes to the pathogenesis of BPD. Inadequate nutrition could interfere with normal growth and maturation of the lung and may potentiate the deleterious effects of oxygen and barotrauma. Newborn rats with inadequate caloric intake have decreased lung weights, protein levels, and DNA content (58). These abnormalities were even greater in pups that were nutritionally deprived at birth and exposed to hyperoxia.

Antioxidant enzymes may play a vital role in the protection of the lung and the prevention of BPD. Many of these enzymes have trace elements (e.g., copper, zinc, selenium) that are an integral part of their structure. Deficiencies in these elements may compromise the premature infant's defenses and predispose the lung to further injury. The repair of elastin and collagen is limited in animals that are undernourished, and copper and zinc may be necessary for this repair (59). Although supplementation with these elements may provide protection to the lung and prevent hyperoxic lung injury, clinical trials using limited dosing strategies have not been able to demonstrate a beneficial effect in preventing BPD (60). Vitamin deficiency has been postulated to be important in the development of BPD. Although current nursery feeding and hyperalimentation regimens appear to provide adequate amounts of vitamin E for preterm infants, a relative decrease in the concentrations of other vitamins may be important in the pathogenesis of BPD. For example,

Vyas and colleagues reported significant decreases in levels of ascorbate (which can function as an antioxidant) in tracheal aspirate fluid from infants developing BPD compared to control infants, suggesting that supplementation with vitamin C might be beneficial (61). However, early supplementation with high dose "antioxidant" vitamins has been studied in preterm baboons and was not efficacious in preventing lung damage from prolonged hyperoxia (62).

Concentrations of vitamin A (retinol) may also be deficient in very LBW infants (63–65). This vitamin appears to be important in maintaining cell integrity and in tissue repair. Its deficiency has been associated with changes in the ciliated epithelium of the tracheobronchial tree (66). Hustead and associates demonstrated lower serum retinol levels in cord blood and at day 21 of life in infants who developed BPD (65). Similarly, Shenai and colleagues demonstrated lower plasma retinol concentrations in the first month of life in infants who subsequently developed BPD (67). Despite adequate supplementation, some infants remain vitamin A deficient, presumably from increased absorption of parenteral vitamin A into the tubing of the intravenous administration set or from higher nutritional requirements (68). A multicenter trial of vitamin A supplementation in premature infants at risk for developing BPD recently demonstrated that large doses of intramuscular vitamin A given three times per week was associated with a small (7%), but significant reduction in the incidence of BPD, suggesting that vitamin A deficiency is an important contributor to lung injury (69).

Large volumes of intravenous fluids are often administered to premature infants to provide adequate fluid requirements (from increased insensible water losses) and sufficient calories. Excessive fluid administration can be associated with the development of a patent ductus arteriosus and pulmonary edema, which can lead to an increase in oxygen and ventilator requirements and the subsequent risk of BPD (55,70). Early closure of the ductus, using indomethacin or surgical ligation, has been associated with improvements in pulmonary function, but these approaches have not affected the incidence of BPD (71).

Genetics

Numerous investigators have observed that neonates were more likely to develop BPD if there was a strong family history of atopy and asthma. Nickerson and Taussig found a positive family history of asthma in 77% of infants with RDS who subsequently developed BPD, compared with only 33% who did not (72). Bertrand evaluated the relationship of prematurity, RDS, and need for mechanical ventilation to a family history of airway hyperactivity (73). The severity of lung disease was directly related to the degree of prematurity and the duration of oxygen exposure. However, siblings and mothers of infants with the most significant lung disease had evidence of airway reactivity, suggesting that all three factors are involved in determining long-term outcome. When histocompatibility loci (HLA) were examined, Clark and associates found that only infants with HLA-A2 developed BPD, again suggesting that other underlying factors that are poorly understood may be important in the pathogenesis of BPD (74). More recently, Hagan reported that a family history of asthma is associated with an increase in the overall severity of BPD in premature infants but does not appear to be a causative factor (75).

PATHOPHYSIOLOGIC CHANGES

Infants with BPD demonstrate abnormal findings on clinical examination, chest radiograph, pulmonary function testing, echocardiogram, and morphologic examination of the lung. The severity of BPD is directly proportional to the degree of the pathophysiologic insult and can be assessed through all of these techniques. Determining the severity of BPD is complex and has been the subject of several workshops sponsored by the National Institutes of Health and many publications. Several scoring systems have been developed to address this important issue.

Clinical Assessment

A clinical scoring system to help evaluate the severity of BPD was developed by Toce and colleagues (76). Infants with BPD are tachypneic and may have intercostal and subcostal retractions. Accessory muscles may be used to assist with respiration. Infants can be hypoxic and hypercarbic and may grow poorly despite adequate caloric intake. The Toce system attempts to standardize clinical assessment, and a severity score can be assigned to each infant at 28 days of postnatal age and at 36 weeks postconceptual age. The clinical assessment should be adjusted if infants are receiving multiple medications for their BPD (e.g., diuretics, methylxanthines), NCPAP, or positive-pressure mechanical ventilation.

Radiographic Abnormalities

Northway and associates first described radiographic abnormalities characteristic of BPD in 1967 (1). A staging system was employed that documented the progression of the disease process through four distinct stages. The first stage was similar to uncomplicated RDS and occurred in the first few days of life. The BPD often progressed to pulmonary parenchymal opacities (stage II), a bubbly appearance (stage III), and then to an inhomogeneous appearance with marked hyperinflation, bleb formation, irregular fibrous streaks, and cardiomegaly (stage IV).

The radiographic progression of BPD is now seldom categorized by these four stages, so Edwards and colleagues redefined the radiologic changes (77). Their system is based on the four most prominent radiographic findings in BPD, including lung expansion, emphysema (including bleb formation), interstitial densities, and cardiovascular (CV) abnormalities (Table 30-3). More severe changes are associated with higher scores (maximum of 10). The occurrence of hyperinflation or interstitial abnormalities on chest radiograph appears to correlate with the development of airway obstruction later in life (78). Because the severity of BPD has continued to change so significantly over the past decade, Weinstein developed a new scoring system incorporating some of the more subtle radiographic signs that are often seen today in infants with BPD (Fig. 30-3) (79). The utility of these scoring systems remains to be demonstrated.

Computed tomography (CT) and magnetic resonance imaging (MRI) of the lung may provide more details of the structural disease in BPD, and can reveal significant abnormalities that are not readily apparent on chest radiographs (Fig. 30-4) (80). These findings can be important in determining ultimate pulmonary morbidity. CT scans often show regional heterogeneity, with regions of hyperinflation or "emphysema" and sparse arterial density alternating with relatively normal appearing regions. MRI of ventilated premature newborns may demonstrate striking regional variations in lung disease, with marked gravity-dependent

TABLE 30-3

ROENTGENOGRAPHIC SCORING SYSTEM FOR SEVERITY OF BRONCHOPULMONARY DYSPLASIA[b]

Variable	Score[a]		
	0	1	2
Cardiovascular abnormalities	None	Cardiomegaly	Gross cardiomegaly or RVH or enlarged MPA
Hyperexpansion (anterior plus posterior rib count)	≤14	14.5–16	≤16.5, or flattened hemidiaphragms
Emphysema	No focal areas	Scattered, small, abnormal lucencies	At least one large bleb or bulla
Fibrosis or interstitial abnormalities	None	Interstitial prominence; few abnormal, streaky densities	Dense fibrotic bands, many abnormal strands
Subjective	Mild	Moderate	Severe

[a] Rib counts intersecting level of the dome of the right hemidiaphragm. MPA, main pulmonary artery; RVH, right ventricular hypertrophy.
[b] From Edwards DK. Radiographic aspects of bronchopulmonary dysplasia. *J Pediatr* 1979;95:823, with permission.

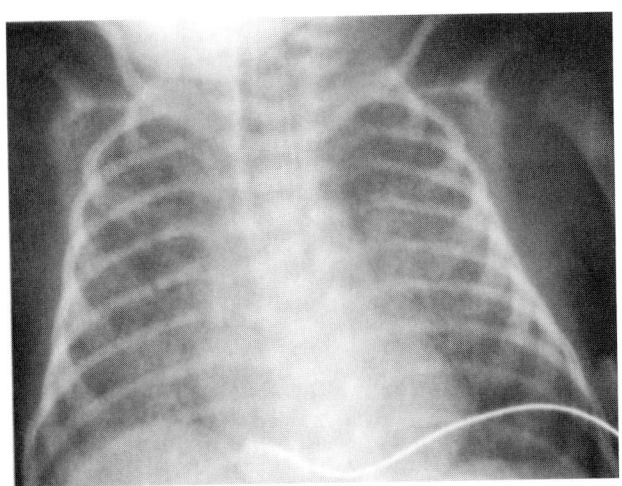

Figure 30-3 Typical chest radiograph of a 1-month-old infant with evolving bronchopulmonary dysplasia. The bilateral hazy appearance represents inflammatory exudate, edema, and atelectasis.

atelectasis and edema. More studies of the role of CT and MRI in BPD are needed to correlate structural and functional changes.

Cardiovascular Changes

In addition to adverse effects on airways and alveoli, acute lung injury also impairs growth, structure and function of the developing pulmonary circulation after premature birth (81). Endothelial cells have been shown to be particularly susceptible to oxidant injury and the media of small pulmonary arteries may also undergo smooth muscle cell proliferation (82). Structural changes in the lung vasculature contribute to high pulmonary vascular resistance (PVR) as a result of narrowing of the vessel diameter and decreased angiogenesis. In addition to these structural changes, the pulmonary circulation is further characterized by abnormal vasoreactivity, which also increases PVR (83). Overall, injury to the pulmonary circulation can lead to the development of pulmonary hypertension and cor pulmonale, which contributes significantly to the morbidity and mortality of severe BPD (84). Echocardiographic assessment is an extremely valuable tool in confirming these diagnoses.

In addition to pulmonary vascular disease and right ventricular hypertrophy, other CV abnormalities that are associated with BPD include left ventricular hypertrophy (LVH) and systemic hypertension. Steroid therapy can cause LVH, which tends to be transient and resolves when the drug is stopped. A high incidence of systemic hypertension can be seen in BPD, but its etiology remains obscure (85). Systemic hypertension may be mild, transient or severe and usually responds to pharmacologic therapy. On occasion, further evaluation of such infants may reveal significant renal vascular or urinary tract disease. Whether the high incidence of systemic hypertension in BPD reflects altered neurohumoral regulation, or increased catecholamines, angiotensin or antidiuretic hormone levels are still unknown.

Changes in Pulmonary Mechanics

The development of computerized pulmonary function systems has enabled more accurate measurements of pulmonary mechanics in newborn infants with BPD. Increased respiratory system resistance and bronchial hyperactivity can be demonstrated even during the first week of life in preterm neonates who subsequently develop BPD (86). These abnormalities are common in older infants with BPD and can cause dynamic airway collapse and expiratory flow limitation (Fig. 30-5) (87). Other abnormalities of lung function include increased dead

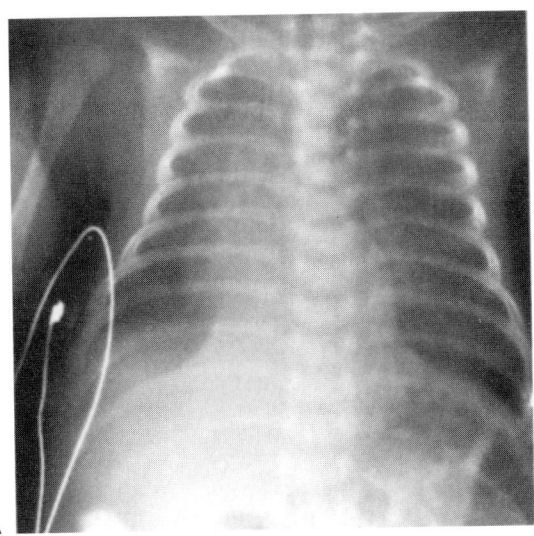
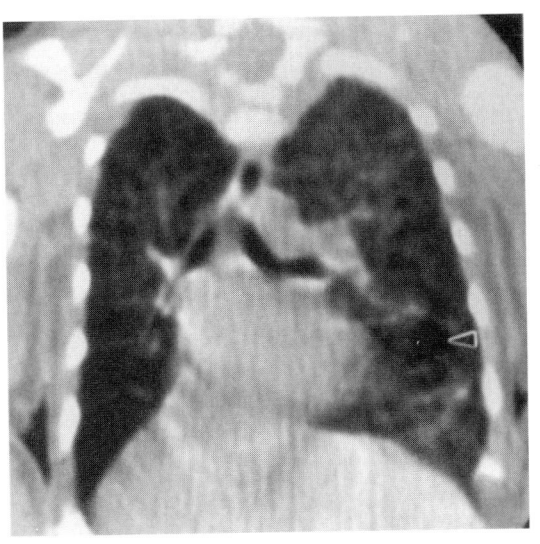

Figure 30-4 A: Chest radiograph of a 2-month-old infant with bronchopulmonary dysplasia, showing right-sided atelectasis and a shift of the mediastinum. The lung fields have a hazy appearance. B: Computed tomography scan on the same infant. The major bronchi and areas of atelectasis are apparent. Fibrotic changes and a bleb are seen on the left (arrow).

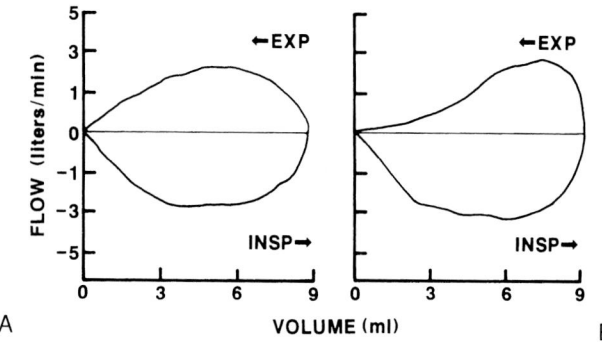

Figure 30-5 A: Normal flow–volume loop. B: Expiratory flow limitation as a result of dynamic collapse of small airways during expiration. INSP, inspiration; EXP, expiration.

space ventilation, decreased lung compliance, maldistribution of ventilation and abnormal ventilation-perfusion matching (88). Functional residual capacity (FRC) is often reduced early in the course as a result of atelectasis, but increases during the later stages of BPD as a result of gas trapping and hyperinflation. Increased respiratory rate with shallow breathing increases dead space ventilation that results from marked regional variability and decreased lung surface area. Nonuniform damage to the airways and distal lungs results in variable time constants for different areas of the lungs, altering the distribution of inspired gas to relatively poorly perfused lung segments and worsening ventilation-perfusion matching.

Two methods used to measure lung compliance include dynamic measurement and passive expiratory techniques after airway occlusion (89). Both methods show a reduction of lung compliance in infants with BPD. The decrease in lung compliance appears to correlate well with morphologic changes in the lung (e.g., atelectasis, edema, fibrosis). Compliance can be reduced because of increased resistance,

with frequency dependence of compliance, when infants are breathing rapidly (90). The use of pulmonary function testing to follow the progression of BPD and the response of the lung to various therapeutic interventions has become widespread, but care must be used in the interpretation of results because of inherent variability in the measurement and possible error from excessive chest wall distortion (91,92).

Pathologic Changes

Detailed morphometric studies have extensively characterized the lung pathology of infants dying with BPD (7,93–95). The pathology of BPD provides insights into the effects of acute lung injury and repair processes in the developing lung, and the impact of the timing of this injury. Pathologically, the original reports of BPD described a continuous process through distinct stages of the disease, originating with an acute exudative phase and progressing to a chronic proliferative phase of the disease (93). Older reports describe a gross cobblestone appearance of the lungs, representing alternating areas of atelectasis, marked scarring and regional hyperinflation. Typical histologic features of this BPD include marked airway changes, such as squamous metaplasia of large and small airways, increased peribronchial smooth muscle and fibrosis, chronic inflammation and airway edema, and hyperplasia of submucosal glands. Parenchymal disease is characterized by volume loss from atelectasis and alveolar septal fibrosis alternating with overdistension or emphysematous regions (Fig. 30-6). Mesenchymal thickening with increased cellularity and destruction of alveolar septae with alveolar hypoplasia is present, suggesting a marked reduction in surface area available for gas exchange. Growth of capillary beds is reduced and small pulmonary arteries have hypertensive structural

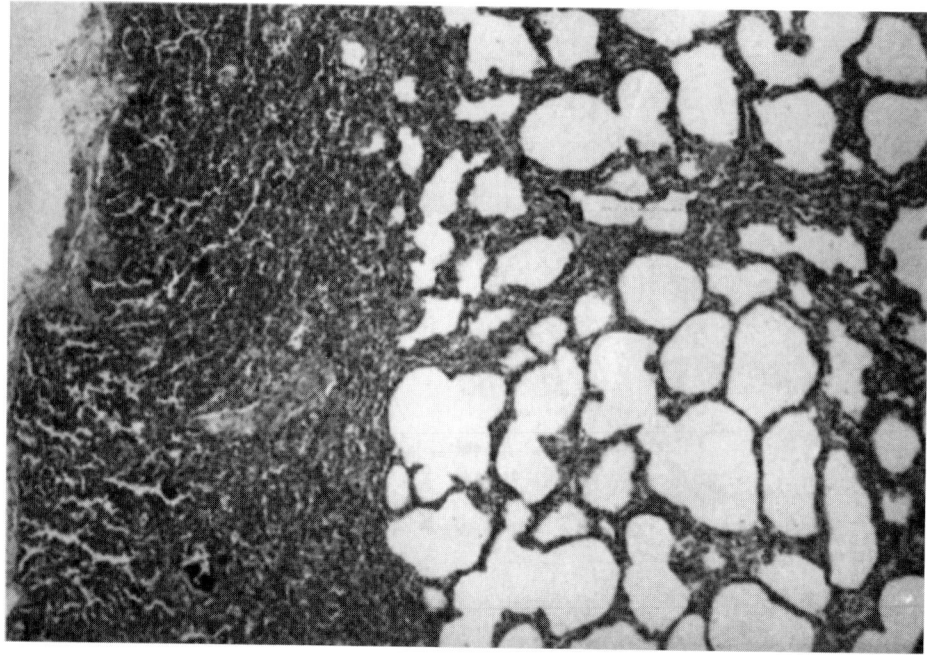

Figure 30-6 Light micrograph from a 1-year-old infant with bronchopulmonary dysplasia shows areas of atelectasis alternating with areas of hyperinflation (Original magnification times 4.).

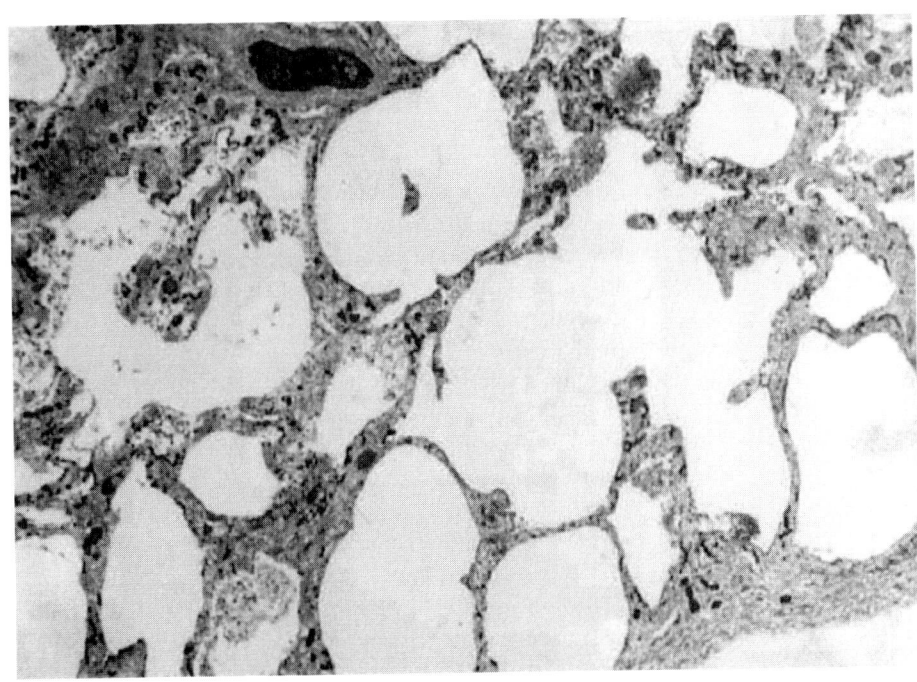

Figure 30-7 Lung histology from an infant dying in the postsurfactant era with the typical changes of the "new BPD," showing alveolar simplification and reduced septation (original magnification times four; provided by Dr. Steven Abman).

remodeling, which includes smooth muscle hyperplasia and distal extension of smooth muscle growth into vessels that are normally nonmuscular.

Although reductions in alveolar number were described in older infants dying with BPD, a pattern of "alveolar simplification" has become the most striking pathologic feature of the "new BPD" (Fig. 30-7) (7,94). In contrast with past reports, recent studies of infants dying with BPD describe fewer signs of airway injury and interstitial fibrosis, but emphasize persistent reductions of distal airspace and vascular growth (95). Decreased alveolarization and impaired growth of small pulmonary arteries results in decreased lung surface area for gas exchange, which has important functional implications regarding late cardiopulmonary sequelae (see above). In addition to changes in the distal lung, the pathology of BPD is further characterized by abnormal airway structure. The trachea and main bronchi of infants with BPD often reveal significant lesions, depending on the frequency and duration of endotracheal intubation. Grossly, mucosal edema or necrosis can be focal or diffuse. The earliest histologic changes include patchy loss of cilia from columnar epithelial cells, which can then become dysplastic or necrotic, resulting in breakdown of the epithelial lining and decreased pulmonary clearance of mucous and other material. Ulcerated areas may involve the mucosa or extend into the submucosa. Infiltration of inflammatory cells (neutrophils and lymphocytes) into these areas may be prominent. Goblet cells appear hyperplastic, suggesting greater capacity for increased mucous production that can mix with cellular debris. Granulation tissue often develops in the subglottis as a result of damaged from the endotracheal tube or more distally throughout the airway as a result of trauma from repeated suctioning. Significant narrowing of the trachea

and main bronchi secondary to injury can lead to subglottic stenosis, tracheal cysts and polyps, and related lesions. Tracheomalacia may often complicate the course of severe BPD and can appear as marked redundancy of the posterior wall of the trachea, as a result of chronic ventilation of the compliant premature airway.

MANAGEMENT

The current approach to infants with BPD is multidisciplinary and directed toward improving the complex pathophysiologic abnormalities that have been previously described. In addition to chronic respiratory disease, infants with BPD have significant growth, nutritional, neurodevelopmental, and CV problems. The severity of respiratory disease varies widely among infants with BPD. In its most severe presentation, children with BPD may require chronic ventilation or prolonged home oxygen therapy. Even infants who have successfully weaned off supplemental oxygen therapy have recurrent hospitalizations for lower respiratory exacerbations as a result of viral infections (respiratory syncytial virus and influenza), reactive airways disease, pulmonary hypertension or congestive heart failure. Additionally, persistent or recurrent respiratory exacerbations may also be as the result of structural lesions (e.g., tracheomalacia, subglottic stenosis, bronchomalacia), chronic aspiration (gastroesophageal reflux or swallowing dysfunction), or others. In addition to supplemental oxygen therapy, chronic treatment with bronchodilators, diuretics, corticosteroids, and nutritional supplements are commonly used as supportive therapy. Often, many of these therapies are used concurrently with the potential for significant side effects.

The major treatment approaches are described in the following sections.

Mechanical Ventilation

With established disease, patients with BPD who require prolonged ventilatory assistance generally require larger tidal volume breaths and a slower rate to enhance the distribution of gas as a result of heterogeneity of lung units. Ventilation of infants with severe BPD with fast rates and smaller tidal volumes increases dead space ventilation and may worsen gas exchange and increase gas trapping. Arterial blood gases should be optimally maintained with a pH of 7.25 to 7.40, PCO_2 of 45 to 55 mm Hg, and PO_2 of 55 to 70 mm Hg. The best method of assessing adequate oxygenation and ventilation is an arterial blood gas obtained from an indwelling arterial catheter when the infant is quiet. Intermittent arterial puncture may be accurate if obtained quickly or if local anesthesia is used, but may not be representative if the infant is awake and agitated. Capillary blood gases should not be used to make significant therapeutic decisions because of wide variability and poor correlation with arterial blood gases (especially in older infants who have already had multiple heel sticks for phlebotomy) (96). However, if samples are obtained properly (i.e., after adequate warming and without squeezing the heel or finger), the pH and PCO_2 may correlate with arterial values. The use of pulse oximetry can assist in ventilatory management and may reflect arterial values. End-tidal CO_2 measurements may not correlate well with arterial values in infants with significant ventilation–perfusion mismatch and chronic lung disease. As mentioned previously, hypocarbia and hyperventilation may increase the risk for BPD and should definitively be avoided (23,24).

Because oxygen appears to cause more significant lung damage than mechanical ventilation in animal models, sufficient mean airway pressure should be used to avoid atelectasis and maintain the fraction of inspired oxygen (FiO_2) at less than 0.5 (97). Inspired gas temperature should be maintained from 36.5°C to 37.5°C to ensure adequate humidity and minimize core temperature fluctuations and the progression of chronic lung disease (98). Weaning infants with BPD from mechanical ventilation is often difficult and should be done slowly. When peak inspiratory pressures have been reduced to approximately 15 to 20 cm H_2O and FiO_2 to less than 0.4 with acceptable blood gases, the ventilator rate (if using a conventional, time cycled ventilator) should be reduced slowly to allow the infant to gradually breathe more independently. This is essential because prolonged ventilation may be associated with atrophy of the muscle fibers of the diaphragm and increased diaphragmatic fatigue (99). When infants have been weaned to a ventilator rate of 10 to 20 breaths/min, elective extubation should be attempted. With synchronized mechanical ventilation, the infant is allowed to set his/her own inspiratory time and respiratory rate. Weaning infants from this type of ventilation involves reducing the

inspiratory pressure as previously described. Analysis of pulmonary mechanics before extubation may not be useful in determining optimal time of extubation because multiple factors (e.g., central inspiratory drive, diaphragmatic endurance, chest wall stability) may be important (100). Infants should not be weaned to continuous endotracheal tube positive airway pressure (CPAP) because increased airway resistance and work of breathing can cause fatigue, apnea, and carbon dioxide (CO_2) retention (101). The use of methylxanthines before extubation or NCPAP just after extubation may facilitate successful extubation (102,103). Higgins and colleagues demonstrated that infants weighing less than 1,000 g were almost four times as likely to be successfully extubated on the first attempt when NCPAP was used compared with an oxyhood (76% vs. 21%) (103). Chest physiotherapy and suctioning should be performed frequently to maintain a patent airway and prevent atelectasis.

Prolonged intubation and ventilation may be associated with the development of airway abnormalities (e.g., subglottic stenosis, tracheomalacia) (104). These should be considered in infants who rapidly and repeatedly fail attempts at extubation. A bronchoscopic evaluation should be performed in these infants or in any infant intubated for more than 2 to 3 months who continues to require prolonged ventilation. Surgical intervention (e.g., cricoid split, tracheostomy) should be performed if necessary.

Oxygen

In infants with BPD, chronic hypoxia results in pulmonary vasoconstriction, pulmonary hypertension, and the development of cor pulmonale. This contributes significantly to the morbidity and mortality of BPD. Elevated pulmonary artery pressures and pulmonary vascular resistance have been described in infants with BPD undergoing cardiac catheterization (83–85,105). Significant reductions in pulmonary pressures were found when oxygen was administered. Oxygen is now known to act as a pulmonary vasodilator by stimulating the production of endogenous NO (106). The NO diffuses into the vascular smooth muscle and stimulates the production of cyclic GMP (cGMP), which causes vasodilation by sequestering calcium. Ideally, PaO_2 should be maintained between 55 and 70 mm Hg in infants with BPD.

Pulse oximetry has become the most popular noninvasive method of neonatal oxygen monitoring. Pulse oximeters are most accurate when operating along the steep portion of the oxygen–hemoglobin dissociation curve and may be more reliable than measuring PaO_2 (107). Keeping the oxygen saturation (SaO_2) generally between 90% to 95% should exclude values of PaO_2 that are less than 45 mm Hg or greater than 100 mm Hg. Careful monitoring of oxygen status is essential because hypoxia can cause pulmonary hypertension, increased airway constriction, and growth failure. Repeated episodes of oxygen desaturation often develop in premature neonates with BPD during mechanical ventilation (108). This appears to be related to a decrease in central respiratory drive and alterations in pulmonary mechanics. Prone positioning (with careful monitoring) may increase SaO_2 and decrease the frequency of hypoxemic episodes (109).

Hyperoxia may worsen BPD or increase the risk of retinopathy of prematurity (110). The STOP-ROP trial examined the role of oxygen therapy in retinopathy of prematurity, and suggested that infants who were treated with supplemental oxygen to maintain oxygen saturations more than 95% had a higher risk for BPD than infants treated with supplemental oxygen that targeted lower saturations (31). However, interpretation of these data in the setting of preventing or treating infants with pulmonary hypertension are limited, because the targeted ranges for the low and high oxygen saturation groups fell between typical recommendations for oxygen therapy. Current recommendations for treatment of patients with BPD and pulmonary hypertension are to maintain oxygen saturations at 92% to 96%. Whether higher oxygen saturations increase lung injury remains unproven, but the adverse effects of hypoxemia are clear.

Oxygen can be administered through an endotracheal tube, hood, tent, or nasal cannula. Increased FiO_2 may be needed during periods of increased stress (e.g., during feedings). Oxygen should be withdrawn gradually and may be required for months. If oxygen-dependent infants can maintain an SaO_2 of more than or equal to 90% for at least 40 minutes in room air, then it appears that they can be successfully weaned from supplemental oxygen (111). Infants with BPD can be discharged from the neonatal intensive care unit and receive oxygen at home. The use of booster transfusions to increase oxygen-carrying capacity in oxygen-dependent infants with BPD is controversial. Alverson and associates demonstrated significant increases in oxygen content and systemic oxygen transport and decreases in oxygen consumption and oxygen use in infants with BPD after booster blood transfusion (112). However, hemoglobin levels did not appear to correlate well with systemic oxygen transport and did not predict which infants would benefit physiologically from transfusion. The need for multiple transfusions has been significantly reduced by minimizing phlebotomy and by using human recombinant erythropoietin therapy (113).

Nutrition

Because infants with BPD have increased metabolic demands, calories must be maximized to support tissue repair and growth. Enteral feedings with fortified breast milk or with premature formulas provide the best source of calories. Feedings should be given by intermittent or continuous gavage until the infant can be fed orally. Feedings can be concentrated to increase caloric density, or glucose polymers (e.g., polycose), protein supplements (ProMod) and medium-chain triglycerides (MCT) can be added to provide optimal calories although minimizing fluid intake. Infants may require 120 to 140 calories/kg of body weight each day to gain weight (10 to 30 g/day). If fluid restriction

interferes with the administration of adequate calories, a diuretic can be used to prevent fluid overload.

Intravenous nutrition should be started early (day 1–2 of life) to provide adequate sources of protein, fat, and carbohydrates. This may affect the ultimate outcome and severity of BPD, especially in the very-low-birth-weight infant. The early use of percutaneous silastic central catheters has greatly enhanced the ability to provide more optimal calories to LBW infants (114). Progressive increases in intravenous amino acid concentrations should optimally provide up to 3.5 g of protein per kilogram each day. The acid–base status of the infant should be monitored because acid loads may not be well tolerated. Intravenous lipids (20% suspension) should be administered as a continuous infusion over 20 to 24 hours. Up to 3 g of lipids per kilogram each day can be safely infused if serum triglyceride levels are closely followed. However, early administration of lipids may be associated with more severe BPD (115,116). Intravenous glucose is a good source of calories, but excessive loads (>4 mg/kg/min) may result in increased oxygen consumption, CO_2 production, and resting energy expenditures in infants with BPD (117). Adequate calcium and phosphorus intake is necessary, especially in infants receiving furosemide, to promote bone mineralization and prevent secondary hyperparathyroidism and rickets. Vitamins and trace metals should also be supplemented. Many premature infants are deficient in vitamin A, and adequate supplementation may promote tissue regeneration and growth in the lung and decrease the incidence and severity of BPD (66). Trace metals such as copper, zinc, and selenium are essential for the structure and function of antioxidant enzymes and should be provided.

Medications

Many different types of drug therapies are used, often concurrently, to improve the clinical status of infants with BPD. The exact dosages, efficacy, mechanisms of action, pharmacokinetics, and side effects have not been well established. National Institutes of Health (NIH)/FDA consensus panels are currently working to establish optimal treatment regimens for infants with BPD.

Diuretics

Furosemide (Lasix) is the treatment of choice for fluid overload in infants with BPD. It acts on the ascending loop of Henle and blocks chloride transport. Furosemide increases plasma oncotic pressure and lymphatic flow and decreases interstitial edema and pulmonary vascular resistance (118,119). Several studies have demonstrated that daily, alternate-day or even aerosolized furosemide improves clinical respiratory status and pulmonary mechanics and facilitates weaning from mechanical ventilation in infants with BPD (120–122). Side effects of furosemide are numerous and include volume depletion, contraction alkalosis, hyponatremia, hypokalemia, chloride depletion, renal calculi secondary to hypercalcinuria, nephrocalcinosis, cholelithiasis, osteopenia, and ototoxicity (118). Supplemental potassium chloride is usually needed to prevent electrolyte depletion and alkalosis, but sodium chloride supplements should be avoided if possible.

The thiazides affect renal tubular excretion of electrolytes, but they are less potent than furosemide (123). Potassium and bicarbonate excretion accompany the sodium and chloride excretion produced by the thiazides. For this reason, the thiazides are usually given in conjunction with spironolactone (Aldactone), which is a competitive inhibitor of aldosterone. Spironolactone is a relatively weak diuretic that causes increased sodium, chloride, and water excretion although sparing potassium. Although a few controlled trials examining the use of a thiazide diuretic and spironolactone in infants with moderate BPD demonstrated increased urine output and improvements in pulmonary mechanics, others could find no effect on gas exchange or pulmonary mechanics (124–126). Side effects of the combination of a thiazide with spironolactone include azotemia, hyperuricemia, hyponatremia, hyperkalemia or hypokalemia, hyperglycemia, hypercalcinuria, and hypomagnesemia (118). Overall, although it appears that short-term administration of diuretics may improve pulmonary mechanics in premature infants, there is limited data regarding the long-term benefits of these agents in reducing the need for ventilatory support, reducing the length of hospitalization or improving long-term clinical outcome (127). Longer-term studies establishing optimal treatment regimens in infants with evolving or established BPD are definitely needed. Diuretic dosing is shown in Table 30-4.

Bronchodilators

Albuterol is a specific β_2-agonist that has become the inhaled agent of choice in the treatment of reversible bronchospasm in infants with BPD. Albuterol aerosolization has been associated with acute improvements in pulmonary resistance and lung compliance secondary to bronchial smooth muscle relaxation (128). These changes in pulmonary mechanics returned to baseline by 4 hours after administration. Side effects are infrequent but can include tachycardia and hypertension. Tolerance may develop with prolonged usage.

Atropine is a competitive inhibitor of acetylcholine. In the lung, atropine decreases mucus secretion and transport in large airways and causes significant bronchial smooth muscle relaxation (129). Ipratropium bromide is a related muscarinic antagonist that is a much more potent bronchodilator than atropine and has significantly fewer side effects. In infants with BPD, ipratropium causes a significant improvement in pulmonary mechanics that is similar to that seen after treatment with albuterol (130). The combination of ipratropium and albuterol may be more effective than either agent alone (129,130). A selective β_2 agent should initially be used in older infants with BPD; ipratropium can be added if clinical improvement is not seen. Ipratropium can be used alone if significant side effects from albuterol occur.

The methylxanthines (e.g., caffeine, theophylline) are routinely used to increase respiratory drive and reduce the frequency of apnea in infants with apnea of prematurity (99). They are also used in the treatment of infants with BPD. Measurements of pulmonary mechanics in infants with BPD have shown that caffeine and

TABLE 30-4

COMMONLY USED MEDICATIONS FOR BRONCHOPULMONARY DYSPLASIA

Medication	Dosage[a]
Diuretics	
Furosemide	0.5–2.0 mg/kg/dose i.v or p.o. bid (qd in infants <31 weeks postconceptual age)
Chlorthiazide	5–20 mg/kg/dose i.v. or p.o. bid
Hydrochlorthiazide	1–2 mg/kg/dose p.o. bid
Spironolactone	1.5 mg/kg/dose p.o. bid
Inhaled agents	
Albuterol	0.02–0.04 mL/kg/dose of a 0.5% solution diluted to 1–2 mL with half-normal or normal saline q4–6h
Ipratropium bromide	0.025–0.08 mg/kg diluted to 1.5–2.5 mL in half-normal or normal saline q6h; doses up to 0.176 mg may be used
Systemic agents	
Aminophylline (i.v.), theophylline (p.o.)	LD 5 mg/kg; MD 2 mg/kg/dose q8–12h; serum levels of 5–15 mg/L
Caffeine citrate	LD 20 mg/kg; MD 5 mg/kg i.v. or p.o. q24h
Dexamethasone	0.1–0.2 mg/kg/day i.v. or p.o. divided q12h for 2–3 days, decrease by 50% for 2–3 days, then taper another 50% for 2–3 days and discontinue

[a] LD, loading dose; MD, maintenance dose.

theophylline can reduce pulmonary resistance and increase lung compliance, presumably through a direct bronchodilator action (131,132). These agents act as mild diuretics and improve skeletal muscle and diaphragmatic contractility. This is particularly important in chronically ventilated infants who may develop diaphragmatic atrophy and fatigue. Improved skeletal muscle contractility may stabilize the chest wall and improve functional residual capacity (133). These actions may facilitate successful weaning from mechanical ventilation. There may be a synergistic effect if theophylline and a diuretic are used concurrently (124).

The half-life of theophylline is 30 to 40 hours in newborns, and theophylline is metabolized primarily to caffeine in the liver and excreted in the urine. Adverse reactions include gastrointestinal (GI) (e.g., gastroesophageal reflux, diarrhea), central nervous system (e.g., agitation, seizures), CV (e.g., tachycardia, hypertension), and endocrine (e.g., hyperglycemia) disturbances (118). The half-life of caffeine may be as long as 100 hours. It is excreted unchanged in the urine. Side effects of caffeine are similar to those of theophylline, but are rarely encountered. Caffeine is a safer drug with a wider therapeutic index and fewer side effects than theophylline and may be a more appropriate adjunct in the treatment of apnea and BPD in preterm infants. Although all of these agents appear to improve lung mechanics in infants with BPD short-term, it is unclear whether prolonged therapy causes sustained clinical benefits. Older patients with BPD often have asthma, characterized by intermittent and reversible airways obstruction during acute respiratory exacerbations, and seem to be highly responsive to bronchodilator therapy.

Corticosteroids

Corticosteroids are synthesized by the adrenal cortex and are composed of mineralocorticoids, which affect fluid and electrolyte balance, and glucocorticoids, which affect the metabolism of many tissues and possess potent antiinflammatory properties (134). Dexamethasone is a synthetic corticosteroid that has been used in the prevention and treatment of BPD. Dexamethasone has multiple pharmacologic effects, although the down-regulation of the inflammatory cascade is thought to be primarily responsible for the improvements in pulmonary function in infants with severe BPD. Clinical studies have consistently shown that steroids acutely improve lung mechanics, gas exchange and reduce inflammatory cells and their products in tracheal samples of patients with BPD (135–137). Despite these studies, there have been multiple experimental and clinical studies that have raised concerns that excessive doses and prolonged use of corticosteroids can impair head growth, neurodevelopmental outcome, lung structure and long-term survival (138,139). Additionally, a recent multicenter study was halted prior to completion as a result of a high incidence of GI perforation (140). Steroids (e.g., dexamethasone) should be selectively used at lower doses and tapered appropriately over shorter durations (5–7 days) in ventilator dependent infants with severe, persistent lung disease. Discussions with the family regarding potential risks and benefits should occur prior to the initiation of treatment (139). The use of steroids should be delayed if possible until approximately one month of age. Other side effects include systemic hypertension, hyperglycemia, cardiac hypertrophy, poor somatic growth, sepsis, intestinal bleeding, and myocardial hypertrophy (141,142). Inhaled steroids have been studied, but the major effect was to decrease the perceived need for the use of systemic steroids (143). Recognition that some premature newborns may have adrenal insufficiency that could increase the risk for BPD prompted interest in the use of low dose cortisol replacement therapy (48). A randomized multicenter study was initiated to examine this question, but even this trial was recently halted as a result of excessive side effects in infants receiving low-dose hydrocortisone supplementation.

Physical Therapy

Physical therapy may help overcome various types of motor deficits (144). Infants with RDS and BPD are at increased risk for subsequent gross motor, fine motor, or cognitive developmental delays. To optimize ventilation, these infants use neck extension and accessory muscles. This produces abnormal posture of the neck, scapula, shoulder, and trunk. Efforts to reduce this abnormal posture and normalize tone should be provided in conjunction with a physical therapist. Infants are first positioned in a more neutral alignment. Strengthening of neck and trunk muscles follows this, although independent movements and exploration of the environment through infant stimulation techniques can be performed. A pacifier is used to facilitate and strengthen the suck reflex, especially when the infant is able to tolerate gavage feedings. When infants are fed orally, coordination of breathing, sucking, and swallowing may be difficult. Positioning the infants in natural flexion and using mandibular compression and cheek and upper palate stimulation may be helpful. Nasal oxygen is often necessary to assist the infant in feeding without tiring.

At the time of discharge, a comprehensive home therapy program is implemented. Nursing needs and home physical and occupational or speech therapy are ordered as necessary. Reevaluation at appropriate intervals is scheduled in a neonatal high-risk follow-up program, with emphasis on the possible need for an early intervention program. These treatment programs emphasize teaching parents specific handling, positioning, and stimulation techniques. Normalizing muscle tone and posture and stimulating desired patterns of movements are the goals of these therapies.

OUTCOME

Most neonates who develop BPD ultimately achieve normal lung function and thrive. However, this group of neonates is at higher risk of dying in the first year of life and developing significant long-term complications. During infancy, continued normal lung growth should result in slow improvement of pulmonary function and weaning from oxygen therapy. Later in childhood, other respiratory problems (e.g., reactive airway disease) and abnormal neurologic development are additional complications that may occur and require careful follow-up. Interpreting outcome studies has become more difficult as a result of the frequent introduction of new treatment modalities such as exogenous surfactant which has significantly influenced neonatal outcome.

Mortality

In Northway's original group of 32 infants, only 13 survived the first month of life (1). Nine (69%) of these survivors developed BPD and five died within the first year of life primarily of pulmonary hypertension and cor pulmonale. The remaining four infants with BPD had persistent respiratory abnormalities that resolved slowly over time. In sharp contrast to this 66% mortality rate, more recent studies have shown a significant improvement in mortality which has continued to fall with the changing epidemiology of BPD. Several surfactant replacement studies have demonstrated significantly improved survival, even in infants who develop BPD. Although Phibbs found a 32% incidence of BPD in his surfactant treatment and control groups, there were no deaths from BPD in the surfactant-treated group and only three deaths in the control group (145). Palta followed a cohort of 533 infants weighing less than 1500 grams who were born between 1988 and 1990 and survived until discharge (6). The incidence of BPD was 25% in this group. Only 9 patients (1.7%) died following hospital discharge, but it is unclear whether these deaths were related to the development of BPD. Twenty-one percent of all infants in this cohort had respiratory problems at 2 years corrected age, which correlated only weakly with a diagnosis of BPD at 36 weeks postconceptual age. In a more recent study from Finland, 211 survivors from the NICU weighing less than 1,000 grams were followed (146). Although 39% of neonates met criteria for a diagnosis of BPD, only one patient died as a result of causes associated with BPD (mortality 1.2%) and none died of sudden infant death syndrome (SIDS). More recent studies from the postsurfactant era suggest that BPD has generally become less severe than seen in the past and is associated with a better outcome if it does develop.

Cardiopulmonary Function

Although pulmonary function in most survivors with BPD improves over time with continued lung growth and permits normal activity, abnormalities detected by pulmonary function testing may remain. Follow-up studies of children with BPD have shown increased airway resistance and reactivity, decreased lung compliance, ventilation–perfusion mismatch, and blood gas abnormalities (e.g., increased PCO_2) that may continue into later years (147,148). These abnormalities appear to correlate extremely well with the presence of clinical respiratory symptoms such as wheezing. Although some authors have suggested that the pulmonary dysfunction is directly related to the development of BPD, others have demonstrated that many mechanically ventilated premature babies (with/without BPD) can have abnormal pulmonary function in later life. Blayney investigated patients with BPD at 7 and 10 years of age and found that although lung growth had occurred normally, residual volumes were increased and forced expiratory volumes and flow rates were reduced (149). Fifty percent of these children had a history of wheezing, suggesting airway hyperactivity. Significant improvement in pulmonary function occurred from years 7 through 10, indicating that pulmonary abnormalities from BPD persist well into childhood and continue to improve slowly over time. Filippone and colleagues reported similar results from a cohort of patients (<1250 grams at birth) with BPD who were followed up to 8–9 years of age (150). At 2 years of age, 66% had abnormalities on pulmonary function testing (diminished maximal flow at FRC). At school age only 16% reported any clinical difficulties, but abnormalities of pulmonary mechanics persisted with forced expiratory volume (FEV1) reduced to 76% of predicted and forced mid-expiratory flow (FEF) (25–75) to 63%. Hakulinen also found lower airway conductance and increased residual volumes in children who had BPD (151). The most significant abnormalities were found in children who had clinical respiratory symptoms, especially early in their childhood (<2 years of age). Although there was an increased need for hospitalization because of pulmonary problems for the first 2 years of life in children with BPD, by 6 to 9 years of age, none had evidence of wheezing or respiratory distress.

As the overall severity of BPD has decreased in recent years, so have the long-term clinical and cardiopulmonary sequelae. Baraldi and colleagues demonstrated progressive improvements in pulmonary function tests over the first 2 years of life, although evidence of airway dysfunction persisted (152). Mitchell and Teague studied premature infants with and without BPD at 6 to 9 years of age (153). They found reduced soluble gas transfer at rest and with exercise in children with BPD, explained by abnormal pulmonary architecture and/or right ventricular dysfunction affecting cardiac output. It appears that abnormal cardiopulmonary function is greatest in the first 2 years of life in infants with BPD. Survival beyond that age permits children to function at near normal capacity, although persistent abnormalities can be detected into adolescence.

Infection

Increased susceptibility to infection has been documented in infants with BPD. Respiratory syncytial virus (RSV) is a major pathogen that causes illness and the need for rehospitalization and mechanical ventilation in children with BPD. Infants are more susceptible to RSV infection because of impaired lung defenses secondary to damaged lung tissue (154,155). Monthly intramuscular injections of monoclonal antibodies (palivuzumab) have been shown to decrease the incidence and severity of RSV infection in high-risk premature infants by 55% (156). Indications for use include significantly premature infants who are home and less than 6 months of age during RSV season (November–December to March–April), infants under 2 years of age with BPD, or any preterm infant with BPD who has received supplemental oxygen in the previous 6 months. Other viruses such as rhinovirus and influenza, although not as common as RSV, may also be an important cause of lower respiratory tract disease in infants with BPD (157).

Growth and Neurologic Development

It is not surprising that the most critically ill and premature infants who develop BPD have an increased risk for growth failure and abnormal neurodevelopmental outcome. Infants with BPD have increased metabolic demands and caloric requirements and may grow poorly during infancy and childhood (158–160). Markestad observed that children with improving respiratory function exhibited faster catch-up growth, and those with continued respiratory problems failed to do so (161). Other studies have shown that a significant proportion of infants with BPD are consistently in the lower percentiles for height, weight, and head circumference (162). This is frequently found during the first 2 years of life, when respiratory symptoms and illness may be prominent (151). Huysman found that although infants with BPD increased in length, total body fat and free fat mass, growth was significantly less than term controls (163). Gregoire compared growth rates in extremely premature infants with and without BPD and found that significant differences existed at birth, but had resolved by 18 months corrected age (164).

Giacoia studied a group of preterm infants with BPD over the first 2 years of life and compared them to a group of age-matched premature infants and term controls (165). Both groups of premature infants had comparable growth rates and average mean standard scores for Wechsler IQ. However, all of the premature infants were significantly smaller than the term controls and had lower scores for performance and full-scale IQ. Singer found no difference in intelligence between infants with BPD and age-matched premature controls at 3 years of life, but motor function was significantly impaired (166). Hack and associates also followed a group of extremely premature infants who received exogenous surfactant at birth and found that BPD was among the most significant predictors of an abnormal motor developmental index (MDI) (odds ratio (OR 2.18) and neurologic abnormalities (OR 2.46) (167). Several more recent follow-up studies have confirmed that a diagnosis of BPD continues to be associated with a higher risk for abnormal neurodevelopmental outcome in premature infants (168,169). The relative contribution of BPD to poor outcome continues to be defined. However, infants developing BPD are often the smallest, sickest patients in the neonatal intensive care unit and consequently can develop

other conditions such as periventricular leukomalacia, intraventricular hemorrhage, retinopathy of prematurity and sepsis which also appear to be important variables in determining developmental outcome (168).

The introduction of surfactant replacement therapy has resulted in significantly improved survival and the development of less severe BPD. It is reassuring that follow-up studies have found that the number of children with significant neurodevelopmental handicaps has not increased despite the survival of an increased number of smaller, sicker infants who frequently develop BPD.

PREVENTION STRATEGIES

A multidisciplinary approach to the prevention of BPD in infants is needed. The use of antenatal steroids in mothers at high risk of delivering a premature infant may reduce the severity and incidence of BPD (170). The early use of NCPAP (with or without prior surfactant treatment) may eliminate the need for mechanical ventilation in some premature infants or facilitate successful extubation in others (103). Aggressive treatment of symptomatic patent ductus arteriosus with fluid restriction, diuretics, indomethacin (or possibly ibuprofen), or surgical closure may reduce the severity of BPD. Tidal volumes and inspired oxygen concentrations should be reduced as low as necessary to reduce hypocarbia, volutrauma, and oxygen toxicity. Using more aggressive lung recruitment strategies, such as more liberal PEEP, HFV or perhaps, prone positioning may also be beneficial. The early use of synchronized mechanical ventilation or high frequency ventilation (HFV) in newborn infants with significant RDS may reduce the severity and incidence of BPD (20–22). The combined use of HFV and surfactant replacement may prevent significant lung damage in premature and term infants with significant lung disease unresponsive to surfactant replacement and conventional mechanical ventilation (171,172). Further conclusive evidence of the beneficial effects of both synchronized ventilation and HFV in premature infants is needed.

Aggressive nutritional support is critical in helping to promote normal lung growth, maturation, and repair. It also protects the lung from the damaging effects of hyperoxia, infection, and barotraumas (173). Systemic supplementation with vitamin A in sufficient quantities to establish normal serum retinol concentrations has been reported to reduce the incidence of BPD, although the need to administer repeated doses through the intramuscular route over a prolonged period of time has limited the widespread use of this therapy.

Numerous studies have demonstrated that the early use of dexamethasone may reduce the incidence of BPD, presumably by treating cortisol deficiency and minimizing inflammation (138). However, early dexamethasone should not be used to prevent BPD because of significant concerns regarding increased mortality, side effects (e.g., GI perforation) and long-term sequelae (CP) (139,140). A

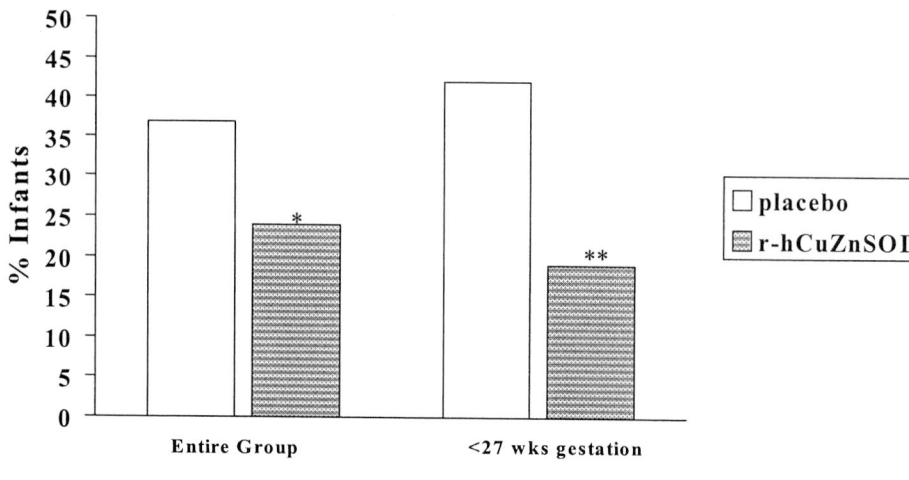

Asthma Medications

Figure 30-8 The use of asthma medications to treat significant respiratory illness in infants at 1–2 years of age from the multicenter trial of rhSOD in preterm infnats. The entire group is presented and a subset of infants <27 weeks gestation at birth. The open bars represent the percent of treated infants in the placebo group and the shaded bars the r-h CuZnSOD group (*$p = 0.05$; **$p < 0.01$). From Davis JM, Parad RB, Michele T, et al. Pulmonary outcome at 1 year corrected age in premature infants treated at birth with recombinant human CuZn superoxide dismutase. *Pediatrics* 2003;111: 469, with permission.

promising method for preventing the development of BPD appears to be prophylactic supplementation of human recombinant antioxidant enzymes. This seems to be a logical strategy in preventing BPD, because oxygen free radicals appear to play a major role in the pathogenesis of lung injury and premature infants are known to be relatively deficient in these enzymes at birth. Several animal studies have shown that prolonged exposure to high oxygen concentrations can cause severe lung damage and death, and administration of antioxidants can prevent many of these complications (174–181). Recombinant human CuZnSOD (rhSOD) has been administered prophylactically to the lung of premature infants at high risk for developing BPD. In preliminary studies in premature infants, the prophylactic use of both single and multiple intratracheal doses of rhSOD appeared to mitigate inflammatory changes and severe lung injury from oxygen and mechanical ventilation with no apparent associated toxicity (179,180). In animal studies, the rhSOD appeared to localize both in intracellu-

lar and extracellular compartments following intratracheal instillation with significant quantities of active protein present 48 hours after the dose is given (182). Multicenter trials using prophylactic, intratracheal rhSOD in premature infants at high-risk for developing BPD have recently been completed (181). Premature infants (birth weight 600–1,200 g) receiving intratracheal instillation of rhSOD at birth had significantly (44%) less episodes of respiratory illness (wheezing, asthma, pulmonary infections) severe enough to require treatment with bronchodilators or corticosteroids at a median of one year corrected age compared to placebo controls (Fig. 30-8). The largest effects were seen in infants less than 27 weeks gestation, with decreased episodes of respiratory illness accompanied by significant reductions (>50%) in emergency room visits and hospital readmissions (Fig. 30-9). This suggests that rhSOD did prevent long-term pulmonary injury from RDS in high-risk premature infants. Further therapeutic intervention trials are needed to ultimately develop a therapy that can prevent

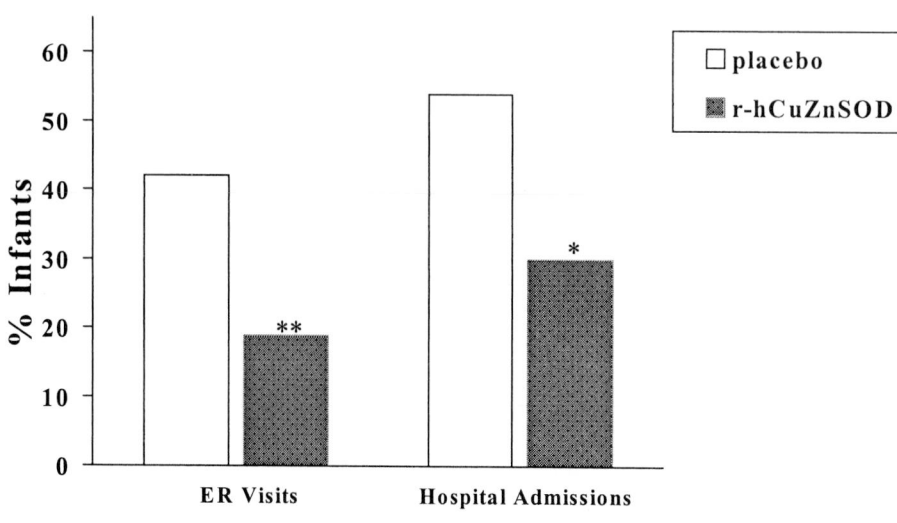

< 27 Weeks Gestation

Figure 30-9 The number of emergency room visits and hospital admissions (all causes) in a subset of infants <27 weeks gestation at birth who had received placebo (open bars) or rhSOD (shaded bars) (*$p = 0.05$; **$p = 0.01$). From Davis JM, Parad RB, Michele T, et al. Pulmonary outcome at 1 year corrected age in premature infants treated at birth with recombinant human CuZn superoxide dismutase. *Pediatrics* 2003;111:469, with permission.

or significantly ameliorate this important chronic lung disease.

Another area that is currently being investigated involves protecting the pulmonary vasculature from injury with inhaled NO (INO). INO may not only lower PVR and improve gas exchange, but may also enhance distal lung growth and improve long-term outcome. Extensive laboratory and clinical studies suggest that INO lowers PVR and improves oxygenation in patients with pulmonary hypertension, including premature infants with severe RDS and BPD (183,184). However, there are persistent concerns about potential toxicity and adverse effects of INO therapy in premature infants (185). Experimental data have suggested that INO therapy may be "lung protective" in several animal models, including premature lambs with RDS (186). Whether INO therapy has a potential role in the prevention of pulmonary vascular injury in premature newborns at risk for BPD is unknown. A multicenter clinical trial of low-dose INO therapy (5 ppm) was recently performed in severely ill premature newborns with RDS who had marked hypoxemia despite surfactant therapy (183). In this study, INO acutely improved PaO_2, but did not improve survival. Notably, there was no increase in the frequency or severity of intracranial hemorrhage or BPD, and the duration of mechanical ventilation was reduced. Based on these findings, a multicenter trial is now underway to determine whether early treatment with low dose INO therapy will prevent the early inflammatory changes that contribute to BPD, and protect the pulmonary circulation from injury during this critical time period.

REFERENCES

1. Northway WH Jr, Rosan RC, Porter DY. Pulmonary disease following respirator therapy of hyaline-membrane disease. *N Engl J Med* 1967;276:357.
2. Bancalari E, Abdenour GE, Feller R, et al. Bronchopulmonary dysplasia: clinical presentation. *J Pediatr* 1979;95:819.
3. Avery ME, Tooley WH, Keller JB, et al. Is chronic lung disease in low birth weight infants preventable? A survey of eight centers. *Pediatrics* 1987;79:26.
4. Sinkin RA, Cox C, Phelps DL. Predicting risk for bronchopulmonary dysplasia: selection criteria for clinical trials. *Pediatrics* 1990;86:728.
5. Shennan AT, Dunn MS, Ohlsson A, et al. Abnormal pulmonary outcomes in premature infants: prediction from oxygen requirement in the neonatal period. *Pediatrics* 1988;82:527.
6. Palta M, Sadek M, Barnet JH, et al. Evaluation of criteria for chronic lung disease in surviving very infants. Newborn Lung Project. *J Pediatr* 1998;132:57.
7. Jobe AH, Bancalari E. Bronchopulmonary Dysplasia. *Am J Resp Crit Care Med* 2001;163:1723.
8. Soll RF, Hoekstra RE, Fangman JJ, et al. Multicenter trial of single-dose modified bovine surfactant extract (Survanta) for prevention of respiratory distress syndrome. *Pediatrics* 1990;85:1092.
9. Bose C, Corbet A, Bose G, et al. Improved outcome at 28 days of age for very low birth weight infants treated with a single dose of a synthetic surfactant. *J Pediatr* 1990;117:947.
10. Liechty EA, Donovan E, Purohit D, et al. Reduction of neonatal mortality after multiple doses of bovine surfactant in low birth weight neonates with respiratory distress syndrome. *Pediatrics* 1991;88:19.
11. Long W, Thompson T, Sundell H, et al. Effects of two rescue doses of a synthetic surfactant on mortality rate and survival without bronchopulmonary dysplasia in 700- to 1350-gram infants with respiratory distress syndrome. The American Exosurf Neonatal Study Group I. *J Pediatr* 1991;118:595.
12. Fenton AC, Mason E, Clarke M, et al. Chronic lung disease following neonatal ventilation. Changing incidence in a geographically defined population. *Pediatr Pulmonol* 1996;21:24.
13. Dreyfus D, Saumon G. Should the lung be rested or recruited? *Am J Respir Crit Care Med* 1994;149:1066.
14. Dreyfuss DD, Saumon G. Ventilator induced lung injury: lessons from experimental studies. *Am J Respir Crit Care Med* 1998;157:294.
15. Nilsson R, Grossman G, Robertson B. Lung surfactant and the pathogenesis of neonatal bronchiolar lesions induced by artificial ventilation. *Pediatr Res* 1978;12:249.
16. Hernandez LA, Peevy KJ, Moise AA, et al. Chest wall restriction limits high airway pressure induced lung injury in young rabbits. *J Appl Physiol* 1989;66:2364.
17. Tremblay L, Valenza F, Ribeiro SP, et al. Injurious ventilatory strategies increase cytokines and c-fos m-RNA expression in an isolated rat lung model. *J Clin Invest* 1997;99:944.
18. Acute Respiratory Distress Syndrome Network. Ventilation with lower tidal volumes as compared with traditional tidal volumes for acute lung injury and the ARDS. *N Engl J Med* 2000;342:1301.
19. Bjorklund LJ, Ingimarsson J, Curstedt T, et al. Manual ventilation with a few large breaths at birth compromises the therapeutic effect of subsequent surfactant replacement in immature lungs. *Pediatr Res* 1997;42:348.
20. Bernstein G, Mannino FL, Heldt GP, et al. Randomized multicenter trial comparing synchronized and conventional intermittent mandatory ventilation in neonates. *J Pediatr* 1996;128:453.
21. Clark RH, Gerstmann DR, Null DM, et al. Prospective, randomized comparison of high-frequency oscillatory and conventional ventilation in respiratory distress syndrome. *Pediatrics* 1992;89:5.
22. Keszler M, Modanlou HD, Brudno DS, et al. Multicenter controlled clinical trial of high-frequency jet ventilation in preterm infants with uncomplicated respiratory distress syndrome. *Pediatrics* 1997;100:593.
23. Garland JS, Buck RK, Allred EN, et al. Hypocarbia before surfactant therapy appears to increase bronchopulmonary dysplasia risk in infants with respiratory distress syndrome. *Arch Pediatr Adolesc Med* 1995;149:617.
24. Collins MP, Lorenz JM, Jetton JR, et al. Hypocapnia and other ventilation-related risk factors for cerebral palsy in low birth weight infants. *Pediatr Res* 2001;50:712.
25. Van Marter LJ, Allred EN, Pagano M, et al. Do clinical markers of barotrauma and oxygen toxicity explain interhospital variation in rates of chronic lung disease? The Neonatology Committee for the Developmental Network. *Pediatrics* 2000;105:1194.
26. Frank L, Groseclose EE. Preparation for birth into an O_2-rich environment: the antioxidant enzymes in the developing rabbit lung. *Pediatr Res* 1984;18:240.
27. Ogihara T, Okamoto R, Kim HS, et al. New evidence for the involvement of oxygen radicals in triggering neonatal chronic lung disease. *Pediatr Res* 1996;39:117.
28. Pitkanen OM, Hallman M, Andersson SM. Correlation of free oxygen radical-induced lipid peroxidation with outcome in very low birth weight infants. *J Pediatr* 1990;116:760.
29. Varsila E, Pesonen E, Andersson S. Early protein oxidation in the neonatal lung is related to the development of chronic lung disease. *Acta Paediatr* 1995;84:1296.
30. Banks BA, Ischiropoulos H, McClelland M, et al. Plasma 3-nitrotyrosine is elevated in premature infants who develop bronchopulmonary dysplasia. *Pediatrics* 1998;101:870.
31. The STOP-ROP Multicenter Study Group. Supplemental therapeutic oxygen for prethreshold retinopathy of prematurity, a randomized, controlled trial. *Pediatrics* 2000;105:295.
32. Davis JM, Rosenfeld WN, Sanders RJ, et al. Prophylactic effects of recombinant human superoxide dismutase in neonatal lung injury. *J Appl Physiol* 1993;74:2234.
33. Padmanabhan RV, Gudapaty R, Liener IE, et al. Protection against pulmonary oxygen toxicity in rats by the intratracheal administration of liposome-encapsulated superoxide dismutase or catalase. *Am Rev Respir Dis* 1985;132:164.
34. Carlsson LM, Jonsson J, Edlun T, et al. Mice lacking extracellular superoxide dismutase are more sensitive to hyperoxia. *Proc Natl Acad Sci U S A* 1995;92:6264.

35. Wispe JR, Warner BB, Clark JC, et al. Human Mn-superoxide dismutase in pulmonary epithelial cells of transgenic mice confers protection from oxygen injury. *J Biol Chem* 1992;267:23937.
36. Brus F, van Oeveren W, Okken A, et al. Activation of circulating polymorphonuclear leukocytes in preterm infants with severe idiopathic respiratory distress syndrome. *Pediatr Res* 1996; 39:456.
37. Buss IH, Senthilmohan R, Darlow BA, et al. 3-Chlorotyrosine as a marker of protein damage by myeloperoxidase in tracheal aspirates from preterm infants: association with adverse respiratory outcome. *Pediatr Res* 2003;53:455.
38. Groneck P, Speer CP. Inflammatory mediators and bronchopulmonary dysplasia. *Arch Dis Child Fetal Neonatal Ed* 1995;73:F1.
39. Jones CA, Cayabyab RG, Kwong KY, et al. Undetectable interleukin (IL)-10 and persistent IL-8 expression early in hyaline membrane disease: a possible developmental basis for the predisposition to chronic lung inflammation in preterm newborns. *Pediatr Res* 1996;39:966.
40. Pierce MR, Bancalari E. The role of inflammation in the pathogenesis of bronchopulmonary dysplasia. *Pediatr Pulmonol* 1995; 19:371.
41. Munshi UK, Niu JO, Siddiq MM, et al. Elevation of interleukin-8 and interleukin-6 precedes the influx of neutrophils in tracheal aspirates from preterm infants who develop bronchopulmonary dysplasia. *Pediatr Pulmonol* 1997;24:331.
42. Ramsay PL, O'Brian SE, Hegemier S, et al. Early clinical markers for the development of bronchopulmonary dysplasia: soluble E-Selectin and ICAM-1. Pediatrics 1998;102:927.
43. Groneck P, Gotz-Speer B, Opperman M, et al. Association of pulmonary inflammation and increased microvascular permeability during the development of bronchopulmonary dysplasia: a sequential analysis of inflammatory mediators in respiratory fluids of high-risk neonates. *Pediatrics* 1994;93:712.
44. Alnahhas MH, Karathanasis P, Kriss VM, et al. Elevated laminin concentrations in lung secretions of preterm infants supported by mechanical ventilation are correlated with radiographic abnormalities. *J Pediatr* 1997;131:555.
45. Ossanna PJ, Test ST, Matheson NR, et al. Oxidative regulation of neutrophil elastase–alpha-1-proteinase inhibitor interactions. *J Clin Invest* 1986;77:1939.
46. Walti H, Tordet C, Gerbaut L, et al. Persistent elastase/proteinase inhibitor imbalance during prolonged ventilation of infants with bronchopulmonary dysplasia: evidence for the role of nosocomial infections. *Pediatr Res* 1989;26:351.
47. Stiskal JA, Dunn MS, Shennan AT, et al. alpha1-Proteinase inhibitor therapy for the prevention of chronic lung disease of prematurity: a randomized, controlled trial. *Pediatrics* 1998; 101:89.
48. Watterberg KL, Scott SM, Backstrom C, et al. Links between early adrenal function and respiratory outcome in preterm infants: airway inflammation and patent ductus arteriosus. *Pediatrics* 2000;105:320.
49. Watterberg KL, Gerdes JS, Gifford KL, et al. Prophylaxis against early adrenal insufficiency to prevent chronic lung disease in premature infants. *Pediatrics* 1999;104:1258.
50. Yoon BH, Romero R, Jun JK, et al. Amniotic fluid cytokines (interleukin-6, tumor necrosis factor-alpha, interleukin-1 beta, and interleukin-8) and the risk for the development of bronchopulmonary dysplasia. *Am J Obstet Gynecol* 1997;177:825.
51. Watterberg KL, Demers LM, Scott SM, et al. Chorioamnionitis and early lung inflammation in infants in whom bronchopulmonary dysplasia develops. *Pediatrics* 1996;97:210.
52. Cassell GH, Waites KB, Crouse DT, et al. Association of Ureaplasma urealyticum infection of the lower respiratory tract with chronic lung disease and death in very-low-birth-weight infants. *Lancet* 1988;2:240.
53. Da Silva O, Gregson D, Hammerberg O. Role of Ureaplasma urealyticum and Chlamydia trachomatis in development of bronchopulmonary dysplasia in very low birth weight infants. *Pediatr Infect Dis J* 1997;16:364.
54. Heggie AD, Jacobs MR, Butler VT, et al. Frequency and significance of isolation of Ureaplasma urealyticum and Mycoplasma hominis from cerebrospinal fluid and tracheal aspirate specimens from low birth weight infants. *J Pediatr* 1994;124:956.
55. Gonzalez A, Sosenko IRS, Chandar J, et al. Influence of infection or patent ductus arteriosus and chronic lung disease in premature infants weighing 1000 grams or less. *J Pediatr* 1996;128:470.
56. Stoll BJ, Fanaroff AA, Wright LL, et al. Late-onset sepsis in very low birth weight neonates: the experience of the NICHD network. *Pediatrics* 2002;110:285.
57. Makhoul IR, Sujov P, Smolkin T, et al. Epidemiological, clinical and microbiological characteristics of late-onset sepsis among very low birth weight infants in Israel: a national survey. *Pediatrics* 2002;109:134.
58. Frank L, Groseclose E. Oxygen toxicity in newborn rats: the adverse effects of undernutrition. *J Appl Physiol* 1982;53:1248.
59. O'Dell BL, Kilburn KH, McKenzie WN, et al. The lung of the copper-deficient rat: a model for developmental pulmonary emphysema. *Am J Pathol* 1978;91:413.
60. Darlow BA, Winterbourne CC, Inder TE,, et al. The effect of selenium supplementation on outcome in very low birth weight infants: A randomized controlled trial. *J Pediatr* 2000;136:473.
61. Vyas JR, Currie A, Dunster C, et al. Ascorbate acid concentration in airways lining fluid from infants who develop chronic lung disease of prematurity. *Eur J Pediatr* 2001;160:177.
62. Berger TM, Frei B, Rifai N, et al. Early high dose antioxidant vitamins do not prevent bronchopulmonary dysplasia in premature baboons exposed to prolonged hyperoxia: a pilot study. *Pediatr Res* 1998;43:719.
63. Shenai JP, Rush MG, Stahlman MT, et al. Plasma retinol-binding protein response to vitamin A administration in infants susceptible to bronchopulmonary dysplasia. *J Pediatr* 1990;116:607.
64. Darlow BA, Graham PJ. Vitamin A supplementation for preventing morbidity and mortality in very low birth weight infants. *Cochrane Database Syst Rev* 2002;4:CD00051.
65. Hustead VA, Gutcher GR, Anderson SA, et al. Relationship of vitamin A (retinol) status to lung disease in the preterm infants. *J Pediatr* 1984;105:610.
66. Anzano MA, Olson JA, Lamb AJ. Morphologic alterations in the trachea and the salivary gland following the induction of rapid synchronous vitamin A deficiency in rats. *Am J Pathol* 1980; 98:717.
67. Shenai JP. Vitamin A supplementation in very low birth weight neonates: rationale and evidence. *Pediatrics* 1999;104:1369.
68. Hartline JV, Zachman RD. Vitamin A delivery in total parenteral nutrition solution. *Pediatrics* 1976;58:448.
69. Tyson JE, Wright LL, Oh W, et al. Vitamin A supplementation for extremely-low-birth-weight infants. National Institute of Child Health and Human Development Neonatal Research Network. *New Engl J Med* 1999;340:1962.
70. Van Marter LJ, Leviton A, Allred EN, et al. Hydration during the first days of life and the risk of bronchopulmonary dysplasia in low birth weight infants. *J Pediatr* 1990;116:942.
71. Bancalari E, Sosenko I. Pathogenesis and prevention of neonatal chronic lung disease: recent developments. *Pediatr Pulmonol* 1990;8:109.
72. Nickerson BG, Taussig LM. Family history of asthma in infants with bronchopulmonary dysplasia. *Pediatrics* 1980;65:1140.
73. Bertrand JM, Riley SP, Popkin J, et al. The long-term pulmonary sequelae of prematurity: the role of familial airway hyperreactivity and the respiratory distress syndrome. *N Engl J Med* 1985; 312:742.
74. Clark DA, Pincus LG, Oliphant M, et al. HLA-A2 and chronic lung disease in neonates. *JAMA* 1982;248:1868.
75. Hagan R, Minutillo C, French N, et al. Neonatal chronic lung disease, oxygen dependency, and a family history of asthma. *Pediatr Pulmonol* 1995;20:277.
76. Toce SS, Farrell PM, Leavitt LA, et al. Clinical and radiographic scoring systems for assessing bronchopulmonary dysplasia. *Am J Dis Child* 1984;138:581.
77. Edwards DK. Radiographic aspects of bronchopulmonary dysplasia. *J Pediatr* 1979;95:823.
78. Mortensson W, Andreasson B, Lindroth M, et al. Potential of early chest roentgen examination in ventilator treated newborn infants to predict future lung function and disease. *Pediatr Radiol* 1989;20:41.
79. Weinstein MR, Peters ME, Sadek M, et al. A new radiographic scoring system for bronchopulmonary dysplasia. *Pediatr Pulmonol* 1994;18:284.
80. Oppenheim C, Mamou-Mani T, Sayegh N, et al. Bronchopulmonary dysplasia: value of CT in identifying pulmonary sequelae. *Am J Roentgenol* 1994;163:169.
81. Abman SH. Pulmonary hypertension in chronic lung disease of infancy. Pathogenesis, pathophysiology and treatment. In: Bland RD, Coalson JJ, eds. *Chronic lung disease of infancy.* New York: Marcel Dekker, 2000;619.
82. Jones R, Zapol WM, Reid LM. Oxygen toxicity and restructuring of pulmonary arteries: a morphometric study. *Am J Pathol* 1985; 121:212.

83. Abman SH, Wolfe RR, Accurso FJ, et al. Pulmonary vascular response to oxygen in infants with severe BPD. *Pediatrics* 1985; 75:80.

84. Abman SH, Sondheimer HS. Pulmonary circulation and cardiovascular sequelae of BPD. In: Weir EK, Archer SL, Reeves JT, eds. *Diagnosis and treatment of pulmonary hypertension.* Mt. Kisco: Futura Publishing, 1992:155.

85. Abman SH. Monitoring cardiovascular function in infants with chronic lung disease of prematurity. *Arch Dis Child Fetal Neonatal Ed* 2002;87:F15.

86. Lui K, Lloyd J, Ang E, et al. Early changes in respiratory compliance and resistance during the development of bronchopulmonary dysplasia in the era of surfactant therapy. *Pediatr Pulmonol* 2000;30:282.

87. Tepper RS, Morgan WJ, Cota K, et al. Expiratory flow limitation in infants with bronchopulmonary dysplasia. *J Pediatr* 1986; 109:1040.

88. Greenspan JS, DeGiulio PA, Bhutani VK. Airway reactivity as determined by a cold air challenge in infants with bronchopulmonary dysplasia. *J Pediatr* 1989;114:452.

89. McCann EM, Goldman SL, Brady JP. Pulmonary function testing in the sick newborn infant. *Pediatr Res* 1987;21:313.

90. Gerhardt T, Bancalari E. Lung function in bronchopulmonary dysplasia. In: Bancalari E, Stocker JT, eds. *Bronchopulmonary dysplasia.* Washington, DC: Hemisphere Publishing, 1988:182.

91. Nickerson BG, Durand DJ, Kao LC. Short-term variability of pulmonary function tests in infants with bronchopulmonary dysplasia. *Pediatr Pulmonol* 1989;6:36.

92. Hanrahan JP, Tager IB, Castile RG, et al. Pulmonary function measures in healthy infants. Variability and size correction. *Am Rev Respir Dis* 1990;141:1127.

93. Cherukupalli K, Larson JE, Rotschild A, et al. Biochemical, clinical, and morphologic studies on lungs of infants with bronchopulmonary dysplasia. *Pediatr Pulmonol* 1996;22:215.

94. Jobe AH. The new BPD: an arrest of lung development. *Pediatr Res* 1999;46:641.

95. Bhatt AJ, Pryhuber GS, Huyck H, et al. Disrupted pulmonary vasculature and decreased vascular endothelial growth factor, Flt-1, and TIE-2 in human infants dying with bronchopulmonary dysplasia. *Am J Respir Crit Care Med* 2001;164:1971.

96. Courtney SE, Weber KR, Breakie LA, et al. Capillary blood gases in the neonate. *Am J Dis Child* 1990;144:168.

97. Davis JM, Dickerson B, Metlay L, et al. Differential effects of oxygen and barotrauma on lung injury in the neonatal piglet. *Pediatr Pulmonol* 1991;10:157.

98. Tarnow-Mordi WO, Reid E, Griffiths P, et al. Low inspired gas temperature and respiratory complications in very low birth weight infants. *J Pediatr* 1989;114:438.

99. Aranda JV, Turmen T. Methylxanthines in apnea of prematurity. *Clin Perinatol* 1979;6:87.

100. Veness-Meehan KA, Richter S, Davis JM. Pulmonary function testing prior to extubation in infants with respiratory distress syndrome. *Pediatr Pulmonol* 1990;9:2.

101. Kim EH. Successful extubation of newborn infants without pre-extubation trial of continuous positive airway pressure. *J Perinatol* 1989;9:72.

102. Viscardi RM, Faix RG, Nicks JJ, et al. Efficacy of theophylline for prevention of post-extubation respiratory failure in very low birth weight infants. *J Pediatr* 1985;107:469.

103. Higgins RD, Richter SE, Davis JM. Nasal continuous positive airway pressure facilitates extubation of very low birth weight neonates. *Pediatrics* 1991;88:999.

104. Miller RW, Woo P, Kelman RK, et al. Tracheobronchial abnormalities in infants with bronchopulmonary dysplasia. *J Pediatr* 1987;111:779.

105. Goodman G, Perkin RM, Anas NG, et al. Pulmonary hypertension in infants with bronchopulmonary dysplasia. *J Pediatr* 1988;112:67.

106. Morin FC, Davis JM. Persistent pulmonary hypertension. In: Spitzer AR, ed. *Intensive care of the fetus and newborn.* St Louis: CV Mosby, 1996:506.

107. Ramanathan R, Durand M, Larrazabal C. Pulse oximetry in very low birth weight infants with acute and chronic lung disease. *Pediatrics* 1987;79:612.

108. Dimaguila MA, Di Fiore JM, Martin RJ, et al. Characteristics of hypoxemic episodes in very low birth weight infants on ventilatory support. *J Pediatr* 1997;130:577.

109. McEvoy C, Mendoza ME, Bowling S, et al. Prone positioning decreases episodes of hypoxemia in extremely low birth weight infants with chronic lung disease. *J Pediatr* 1997;130:305.

110. Higgins RD, Phelps DL. Oxygen-induced retinopathy: lack of adverse heparin effect. *Pediatr Res* 1990;27:580.

111. Simoes EAF, Rosenberg AA, King SJ, et al. Room air challenge: prediction for successful weaning of oxygen-dependent infants. *J Perinatol* 1997;17:125

112. Alverson DC, Isken VH, Cohen RS. Effect of booster transfusion on oxygen utilization in infants with bronchopulmonary dysplasia. *J Pediatr* 1988;113:722.

113. Messer J, Haddad J, Donato L, et al. Early treatment of premature infants with recombinant human erythropoietin. *Pediatrics* 1993;92:519.

114. Gilhooly J, Lindenberg J, Reynolds JW. Central venous silicone elastomer catheter placement by basilic vein cutdown in neonates. *Pediatrics* 1986;78:636.

115. Hammerman C, Aramburo MJ. Decreased lipid intake reduces morbidity in sick premature infants. *J Pediatr* 1988;113:1083.

116. Sosenko IR, Rodriguez-Pierce M, Bancalari E. Effect of early initiation of intravenous lipid administration on the incidence and severity of chronic lung disease in premature infants. *J Pediatr* 1993;123:975.

117. Yunis KA, Oh W. Effects of intravenous glucose loading on oxygen consumption, carbon dioxide production, and resting energy expenditure in infants with bronchopulmonary dysplasia. *J Pediatr* 1989;115:127.

118. Davis JM, Sinkin RA, Aranda JV. Drug therapy for bronchopulmonary dysplasia. *Pediatr Pulmonol* 1990;8:117.

119. Bland RD, McMillan DD, Bressack MA. Decreased pulmonary transvascular fluid filtration in awake newborn lambs after intravenous furosemide. *J Clin Invest* 1978;62:601.

120. Engelhardt B, Elliott S, Hazinski TA. Short- and long-term effects of furosemide on lung function in infants with bronchopulmonary dysplasia. *J Pediatr* 1986;109:1034.

121. Rush MG, Engelhardt B, Parker RA, et al. Double-blind, placebo-controlled trial of alternate-day furosemide therapy in infants with chronic bronchopulmonary dysplasia. *J Pediatr* 1990;117:112.

122. Brion LP, Primhak RA, Yong W. Aerosolized diuretics for preterm infants with (or developing) chronic lung disease. *Cochrane Database Syst Rev* 2001;2:CD001694.

123. Weiner IM, Mudge GH. Diuretics and other agents employed in the mobilization of edema fluid. In: Gilman AG, Goodman LS, Rall TW, et al, eds. *The pharmacological basis of therapeutics.* New York: Macmillan, 1985:887.

124. Kao LC, Durand DJ, McCrea RC, et al. Randomized trial of long-term diuretic therapy for infants with oxygen-dependent bronchopulmonary dysplasia. *J Pediatr* 1994;124:772.

125. Kao LC, Durand DJ, Phillips BL, et al. Oral theophylline and diuretics improve pulmonary mechanics in infants with bronchopulmonary dysplasia. *J Pediatr* 1987;111:439.

126. Engelhardt B, Blalock WA, DonLevy S, et al. Effect of spironolactone-hydrochlorothiazide on lung function in infants with chronic bronchopulmonary dysplasia. *J Pediatr* 1989;114:619.

127. Brion LP, Primhak RA, Ambrosio-Perez I. Diuretics acting on the distal renal tubule for preterm infants with (or developing) chronic lung disease. *Cochrane Database Syst Rev* 2002;1: CD001817.

128. Wilkie RA, Bryan MH. Effect of bronchodilators on airway resistance in ventilator-dependent neonates with chronic lung disease. *J Pediatr* 1987;111:278.

129. Weiner N. Atropine, scopolamine, and related antimuscarinic drugs. In: Gilman AG, Goodman LS, Rall TW, et al, eds. *The pharmacologic basis of therapeutics.* New York: Macmillan, 1985: 130.

130. Brundage KL, Mohsini KG, Froese AB, et al. Bronchodilator response to ipratropium bromide in infants with bronchopulmonary dysplasia. *Am Rev Respir Dis* 1990;142:1137.

131. Davis JM, Bhutani VK, Stefano JL, et al. Changes in pulmonary mechanics following caffeine administration in infants with bronchopulmonary dysplasia. Pediatr Pulmonol 1989;6:49.

132. Rooklin AR, Moomjian AS, Shutack JG, et al. Theophylline therapy in bronchopulmonary dysplasia. *J Pediatr* 1979;95:882.

133. Polgar G. Mechanical properties of the lung and chest wall. In: Thibeault DW, Gregory GA, eds. *Neonatal pulmonary care.* Norwalk: Appleton-Century-Crofts, 1986:49.

134. Haynes RC, Murad F. Adrenocorticotropic hormone; adrenocortical steroids and their synthetic analogs: inhibitors of adrenocortical steroid biosynthesis. In: Gilman AG, Goodman LS, Rall TW, et al, eds. *The pharmacological basis of therapeutics.* New York: Macmillan, 1985:1459.

135. Cummings JJ, D'Eugenio DB, Gross SJ. A controlled trial of dexamethasone in preterm infants at high risk for bronchopulmonary dysplasia. *N Engl J Med* 1989;320:1505.

136. Wang JY, Yeh TF, Lin YJ, et al. Early postnatal dexamethasone therapy may lessen lung inflammation in premature infants respiratory distress syndrome on mechanical ventilation. *Pediatr Pulmonol* 1997;23:193.

137. Yoder MC Jr, Chua R, Tepper R. Effect of dexamethasone on pulmonary inflammation and pulmonary function of ventilator-dependent infants with bronchopulmonary dysplasia. Am Rev Respir Dis 1991;143:1044.

138. Halliday HL, Ehrenkranz RA, Doyle LW. Early post-natal steroids for preventing chronic lung disease in preterm infants. *Cochrane Database Syst Rev* 2003;1:CD001146.

139. Postnatal corticosteroids to treat or prevent chronic lung disease in preterm infants. *Pediatrics* 2002;109:330.

140. Stark AR, Carlo WA, Tyson JE, et al. Adverse effects of early dexamethasone in extremely-low-birth-weight infants. NICHD neonatal research network. *N Engl J Med* 2001;344:95.

141. Marinelli KA, Burke GS, Herson VC. Effects of dexamethasone on blood pressure in premature infants with bronchopulmonary dysplasia. *J Pediatr* 1997;130:594.

142. Rizvi ZB, Aniol HS, Myers TF, et al. Effects of dexamethasone on the hypothalamic-pituitary-adrenal axis in preterm infants. *J Pediatr* 1992;120:961.

143. Cole CH, Colton T, Shah BL, et al. Early inhaled glucocorticoid therapy to prevent bronchopulmonary dysplasia. *N Engl J Med* 1999;340:1005.

144. Parker A. Expert handling. *Nurs Times* 1990;86:35.

145. Phibbs RH, Ballard RA, Clements JA, et al. Initial clinical trial of Exosurf, a protein-free synthetic surfactant, for the prophylaxis and early treatment of hyaline membrane disease. *Pediatrics* 1991;88:1.

146. Tommiska V, Heinonen K, Kero P, et al. A national two year follow up study of extremely low birthweight infants born in 1996–1997. *Arch Dis Child Fetal Neonatal Ed* 2003;88:F29.

147. Bader D, Ramos AD, Lew CD, et al. Childhood sequelae of infant lung disease: exercise and pulmonary function abnormalities after bronchopulmonary dysplasia. *J Pediatr* 1987;110:693.

148. Andreasson B, Lindroth M, Mortensson W, et al. Lung function eight years after neonatal ventilation. *Arch Dis Child* 1989;64:108.

149. Blayney M, Kerem E, Whyte H, et al. Bronchopulmonary dysplasia: improvement in lung function between 7 and 10 years of age. *J Pediatr* 1991;118:201.

150. Filippone M, Sartor M, Zacchello F, et al. Flow limitation in infants with bronchopulmonary dysplasia and respiratory function at school age. *Lancet* 2003;361:753.

151. Hakulinen AL, Heinonen K, Lansimies E, et al. Pulmonary function and respiratory morbidity in school-age children born prematurely and ventilated for neonatal respiratory insufficiency. *Pediatr Pulmonol* 1990;8:226.

152. Baraldi E, Filippone M, Trevisanuto D, et al. Pulmonary function until two years of life in infants with bronchopulmonary dysplasia. *Am J Respir Crit Care Med* 1997;155:149.

153. Mitchell SH, Teague WG. Reduced gas transfer at rest and during exercise in school-age survivors of bronchopulmonary dysplasia. *Am J Respir Crit Care Med* 1998;157:1406.

154. Weisman LE. Populations at risk for developing respiratory syncytial virus and risk factors for respiratory syncytial virus severity: infants with predisposing conditions. *Pediatr Infect Dis J* 2003; 22:S33-S37.

155. Groothuis JR, Gutierrez KM, Lauer BA. Respiratory syncytial virus infection in children with bronchopulmonary dysplasia. *Pediatrics* 1988;82:199.

156. The IMpact-RSV Study Group. Palivizumab, a humanized respiratory syncytial virus monoclonal antibody, reduces hospitalization from respiratory syncytial virus infection in high-risk infants. *Pediatrics* 1998;102:531.

157. Chidekel AS, Rosen CL, Bazzy AR. Rhinovirus infection associated with serious lower respiratory illness in patients with bronchopulmonary dysplasia. *Pediatr Infect Dis J* 1997;16:43.

158. Kalhan SC, Denne SC. Energy consumption in infants with bronchopulmonary dysplasia. *J Pediatr* 1990;116:662.

159. Kao LC, Durand DJ, Nickerson BG. Improving pulmonary function does not decrease oxygen consumption in infants with bronchopulmonary dysplasia. *J Pediatr* 1988;112:616.

160. Kurzner SI, Garg M, Bautista DB, et al. Growth failure in infants with bronchopulmonary dysplasia: nutrition and elevated resting metabolic expenditure. *Pediatrics* 1988;81:379.

161. Markestad T, Fitzhardinge PM. Growth and development in children recovering from bronchopulmonary dysplasia. *J Pediatr* 1981;98:597.

162. Yu VYH, Orgill AA, Lim SB, et al. Growth and development of very low birth weight infants recovering from bronchopulmonary dysplasia. *Arch Dis Child* 1983;58:791.

163. Huysman WA, de Ridder M, de Bruin NC, et al. Growth and body composition in preterm infants with bronchopulmonary dysplasia. *Arch Dis Child Fetal Neonatal Ed* 2003;88:F46.

164. Gregiore MC, Lefebvre F, Glorieux J. Health and developmental outcomes at 18 months in very preterm infants with bronchopulmonary dysplasia. *Pediatrics* 1998;101:856.

165. Giacoia GP, Venkataraman PS, West-Wilson KI, et al. Follow-up of school-age children with bronchopulmonary dysplasia. *J Pediatr* 1997;130:400.

166. Singer L, Yamashita T, Lilien L, et al. A longitudinal study of developmental outcome of infants with bronchopulmonary dysplasia and very low birth weight. *Pediatrics* 1997;100:987.

167. Hack M, Wilson-Costello D, Friedman H, et al. Neurodevelopment and predictors of outcomes of children with birth weights of less than 1,000 grams; 1992–1995. *Arch Pediatr Adolesc Med* 2000;154:725.

168. Schmidt B, Asztalos EV, Roberts RS, et al. Trial of Indomethacin Prophylaxis in Preterms (TIPP) Investigators. Impact of bronchopulmonary dysplasia, brain injury, and severe retinopathy on the outcome of extremely low-birth-weight infants at 18 months: results from the trial of indomethacin prophylaxis in preterms. *JAMA* 2003;289:1124.

169. Hanke C, Lohaus A, Gawrilow C, et al. Preschool development of very low birth weight children born 1994–1995. *Eur J Pediatr* 2003;162:159.

170. Van Marter LJ, Leviton A, Kuban KC, et al. Maternal glucocorticoid therapy and reduced risk of bronchopulmonary dysplasia. *Pediatrics* 1990;86:331.

171. Soll RF, Dargaville P. Surfactant for meconium aspiration syndrome in full term infants. *Cochrane Database Syst Rev* 2000;2: CD002054.

172. Davis JM, Richter SE, Kendig JW, et al. High frequency jet ventilation and surfactant treatment of newborns with severe respiratory failure. *Pediatr Pulmonol* 1992;13:108.

173. Frank L, Sosenko IR. Undernutrition as a major contributing factor in the pathogenesis of bronchopulmonary dysplasia. *Am Rev Respir Dis* 1988;138:725.

174. de Los Santos R, Seidenfeld JJ, Anzueto A, et al. One hundred percent oxygen lung injury in adult baboons. *Am Rev Respir Dis* 1987;136:657.

175. Jacobson JM, Michael JR, Jafri MH Jr, et al. Antioxidants and antioxidant enzymes protect against pulmonary oxygen toxicity in the rabbit. *J Appl Physiol* 1990;68:1252.

176. Tanswell AK, Freeman BA. Liposome-entrapped antioxidant enzymes prevent lethal O2 toxicity in the newborn rat. *J Appl Physiol* 1987;63:347.

177. Walther FJ, Gidding CE, Kuipers IM, et al. Prevention of oxygen toxicity with superoxide dismutase and catalase in premature lambs. *J Free Radic Biol Med* 1986;2:289.

178. Rosenfeld W, Evans H, Concepcion L, et al. Prevention of bronchopulmonary dysplasia by administration of bovine superoxide dismutase in preterm infants with respiratory distress syndrome. *J Pediatr* 1984;105:781.

179. Rosenfeld WN, Davis JM, Parton L, et al. Safety and pharmacokinetics of recombinant human superoxide dismutase administered intratracheally to premature neonates with respiratory distress syndrome. *Pediatrics* 1996;97:811.

180. Davis JM, Rosenfeld WN, Richter SE, et al. Safety and pharmacokinetics of multiple doses of recombinant human CuZn superoxide dismutase administered intratracheally to premature neonates with respiratory distress syndrome. *Pediatrics* 1997; 100:24.

181. Davis JM, Parad RB, Michele T, et al. Pulmonary outcome at 1 year corrected age in premature infants treated at birth with recombinant human CuZn superoxide dismutase. *Pediatrics* 2003;111:469.

182. Sahgal N, Davis JM, Robbins C, et al. Localization and activity of recombinant human CuZn superoxide dismutase after intratracheal administration. *Am J Physiol* 1996;271:L230

183. Kinsella JP, Walsh WF, Bose C, et al. Randomized controlled trial of inhaled nitric oxide in premature neonates with severe hypoxemic respiratory failure. *Lancet* 1999;354:1061.

184. Banks BA, Seri I, Ischiropoulos H, et al. Changes in oxygenation with inhaled nitric oxide in severe bronchopulmonary dysplasia. *Pediatrics* 1999;103:610.

185. Robbins CG, Davis JM, Merritt TA, et al. Combined effects of nitric oxide and hyperoxia on surfactant function and pulmonary inflammation. *Am J Physiol* 1995;269:L545.

185. Kinsella JP, Parker TA, Galan H, et al. Effects of inhaled NO on pulmonary edema and lung neutrophil accumulation in severe experimental HMD. *Pediatr Res* 1997;41:457.

Principles of Management of Respiratory Problems

William E. Truog　　**Sergio G. Golombek**

Although the principles of management of respiratory disorders are constant, the techniques of treatment have become more complex recently because of increasing and increasingly sophisticated technology. This complexity results from the incorporation into routine care of highly technical equipment and the necessity for skilled personnel—dedicated to the smooth functioning of life-sustaining devices. Knowledge of the pathophysiology of lung disorders and the maturational status of the lung is essential to applying the imperfect evidence derived from clinical trials and from experience to everyday use of assisted ventilation.

The goal of respiratory treatment is to provide tissue oxygenation and carbon dioxide (CO_2) removal in a safe and effective manner. Excessive oxygen delivered to the airways or to organs can be harmful. Excessive lung distention can result in stretching and tearing of the lung. Excessive alveolar ventilation with resultant respiratory alkalosis and hypocarbia can in a detrimental manner alter blood flow distribution and oxygen unloading. In contrast, respiratory and/or metabolic acidosis may constrict pulmonary blood vessels, thus affecting pulmonary blood flow and oxygen uptake. Attention to organ system dysfunction other than the lung must occur in parallel with respiratory management or the efforts directed to optimizing delivery of assisted ventilation will be useless. One of the most challenging aspects of ventilatory treatment is the dynamic way in which the ventilatory needs can change because of either the treatment applied or the progression of the underlying disease. This chapter reviews the indications, methods, and complications of respiratory management and available methods of assessment.

OXYGEN THERAPY

Optimal Level Of Oxygenation

Considerable debate has occurred about what constitutes an acceptable level of oxygen tension or hemoglobin saturation, especially in extremely preterm infants (1). The debate has focused on the contribution of excessive or of insufficient supplemental oxygen levels and hence levels of arterial pO_2 in the etiology of multiple disorders of prematurity. These disorders include central nervous system injuries, especially leukomalacia or hemorrhagic infarction; development or progression of retinopathy of prematurity (ROP); chronic lung disease of prematurity; and perhaps other disorders associated with excess level of reactive oxygen species (ROS).

Because of the direct relationship between elevated fraction of inspired oxygen (FiO_2) and arterial oxygen partial pressure (PaO_2) and the generation of ROS, it is reasonable that the arterial partial pressure of oxygen (PO_2) and/or oxyhemoglobin saturation be minimized to a level sufficient to allow adequate oxygen tissue delivery with satisfactory reserves. There are several practical limitations to this seemingly innocent idea. Cardiopulmonary status of extremely preterm babies is inherently unstable. There is intrinsic cyclicity to such physiologic events as cardiac output and to spontaneous respiration rate and depth, and the variable contribution of spontaneously generated respirations in addition to those associated with assisted respiration.

Hemoglobin concentration is subject to significant changes and the relative quantity of the various forms of hemoglobin can change rapidly over the first days and weeks (e.g., decreasing fetal hemoglobin and increasing adult hemoglobin). As this occurs, the relationship between partial pressure of oxygen tension and oxygen saturation can change in somewhat unpredictable ways in short periods of time. Relying on only one measurement exclusively (e.g., PaO_2 or pulse oximeter saturation [SpO_2]) either may mask or may exaggerate changes in the tissue oxygen delivery. Hemoglobin concentration is measured per mL or 100 mL of blood, but the actual blood volume, and hence total body hemoglobin concentration, can vary in sometimes unpredictable ways also.

The overall limitation in assessing tissue gas exchange is that all the elements of tissue oxygen delivery are not routinely assessed at bedside. For example, arterial blood pressure measurements, either by sphygmometry or by direct arterial measurement, do not measure cardiac output or oxygen tissue delivery. Clinicians have available only summary information, at best, of total body oxygen delivery and consumption. In fact the body might be considered as interdependent organs with individualized oxygen consumption. Satisfactory levels of oxygen delivery in one or most of these may not be satisfactory for a particularly high-consuming area, and interorgan changes and distribution of blood flow can have a marked impact on local oxygen tissue delivery and consumption and hence on the risk of organ-specific ischemic injury.

For babies treated with assisted ventilation, it is possible to manipulate arterial oxygen tension, perhaps at the cost of other kinds of injury, especially to the lung. The tradeoff between mean airway pressure and FiO_2 in the treatment of conditions associated with low end expiratory volume (e.g., respiratory distress syndrome or RDS) is one example of a difficult balancing act in clinical medicine. Central venous sampling or selective sampling of organ specific venous drainage would be crucial to optimizing the pressure FiO_2–dichotomy, but obtaining that information is impractical.

Two randomized studies (2,3) and one case series (4) demonstrated that maintaining pulse Doppler oximetry levels in a higher end of normal range in a group of babies with progressive ROP did not result in reduced progression of ROP, but was associated with borderline statistically and clinically significant increases in pulmonary problems. However, Schultz and associates (5) demonstrated that with oxygen saturation and FiO_2 maintained in a lower range of "normal," there appeared to be an elevated pulmonary vascular resistance (PVR) and subsequent VA/Q mismatch (Fig. 31-1). Should episodes of lower SpO_2 and higher PVR be exacerbated, then altered gas exchange with acute elevations in CO_2 and subsequent ill effects on cerebral circulation could develop. The interdependency of these variables has meant that at present it is difficult to recommend, based on clinically relevant outcomes, a proper oxygen level.

An arterial PaO_2 of 45 mm Hg results in a saturation of fetal hemoglobin (HbF) of approximately 90%. Maintaining the PaO_2 above 50 mm Hg should be sufficient for tissue oxygen needs but excessive levels are quickly achieved. Mitochondrial PO_2 is about 2 mm Hg.

The gap between the alveolar partial pressure of oxygen (PaO_2) and the PaO_2 indicates the magnitude of the arterial O2 gradient across the lungs and provides an indication of the magnitude of right-to-left shunting of blood. A simplification of the alveolar air equation provides an estimate of PaO_2 i.e., $PaO_2 = PiO_2 – PaCO_2$.

Because at sea level the barometric pressure, minus water vapor pressure, is approximately 700 mm Hg, the percent of inspired oxygen multiplied by 7 equals PiO_2 in mm Hg (e.g., 21% $\cong$ 147 mm Hg, 50% $\cong$ 350 mm Hg). Because $PaCO_2$ approximates $PaCO_2$ because of a usually small arterial–alveolar CO_2 gradient ($aADCO_2$), $PaCO_2$ can be substituted for $PACO_2$, and PAO_2 can be derived. For example, if an infant is breathing gas with FIO_2 of 0.6, with the measured PaO_2 of 70 mm Hg and the $PaCO_2$ of 40 mm Hg, the $PAO_2 = 420 - 40 = 380$ mm Hg, and the alveolar–arterial gradient for O_2 ($AaDO_2$) approximates 310 mm Hg. In an infant without either lung disease or a significant right-to-left cardiac shunt, the $AaDO_2$ should not exceed 25 mm Hg while breathing ambient air. Infants with severe RDS may have an $AaDO_2$ in excess of 500 mm Hg while breathing 100% oxygen.

Oxygen Delivery

Each gram of HbF binds 1.37 dL of oxygen. The full-term newborn with a hemoglobin (Hb) of 17 g/dL binds and transports 23 dL of oxygen per 100 dL of blood. Less than 2% of transported O_2 is carried as oxygen dissolved in plasma. Normal tissue oxygen consumption extracts 4 mL O_2/100 mL if oxygen consumption and cardiac output are normal. HbF binds oxygen with a greater affinity than adult HbA. The oxyhemoglobin saturation curve is nonlinear, and the P_{50}, the PaO_2 at which Hb is 50% saturated, increases with gestational age (Fig. 31-2). The higher the P_{50}, the greater the driving pressure for oxygen unloading. The curve gradually shifts to the right as hemoglobin A increases after birth. Several factors can adversely affect tissue oxygen delivery, including decreased cardiac output, maldistribution of cardiac output, arterial vasoconstriction, and shifts in the O_2 dissociation curve. Oxygen unloading in the tissues is increased with a shift to the right of the O_2 dissociation curve (i.e., decreased O_2 affinity of Hb) facilitated by a local decrease in pH, increase in $PaCO_2$, and increase in temperature. A shift to the right of the O_2 dissociation curve can result from transfusion of adult red blood cells. Oxygen uptake depends on adequate

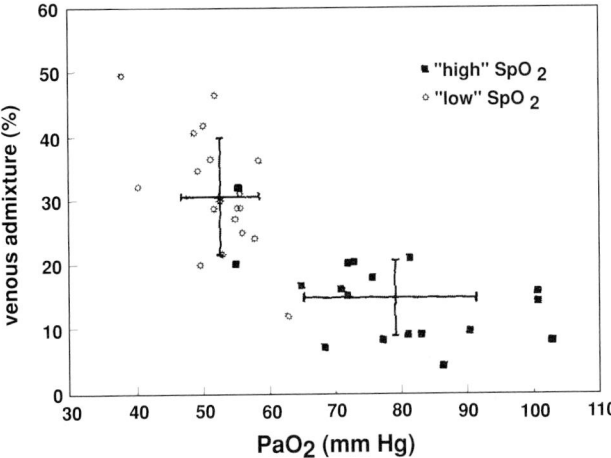

Figure 31-1 Relationship between venous admixture and PaO_2. From Schulze A, Whyte RK, Way RC, Sinclair JC. Effect of the arterial oxygenation level on cardiac output, oxygen extraction, and oxygen consumption in low birth weight infants receiving mechanical ventilation. J Pediatr 1995;126(5):777, with permission.

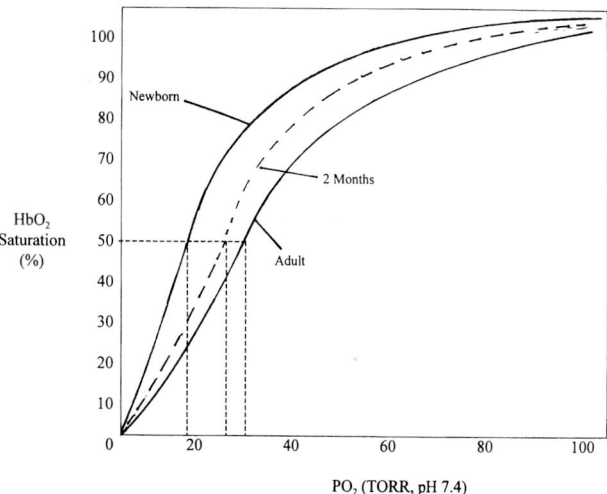

Figure 31-2 Oxygen equilibrium curves of hemoglobin at birth, 2 months of age, and adulthood. Note the increase in P_{50} with age.

alveolar ventilation ($\dot{V}_A$), an appropriate ventilation–perfusion match in the lungs, and absence of right-to-left shunting. Oxygen uptake or increased O_2 affinity of Hb (associated with a shift of the curve to the left) is enhanced by alkalosis, decreased temperature, decreased 2,3-diphosphoglycerate, and increased HbF.

Oxygen Administration

There are two methods by which to deliver supplemental oxygen to neonates: an oxygen hood with sufficient gas flow to prevent CO_2 retention and a nasal cannula or prongs. The concentration and the rate of flow are varied, and the precise amount of oxygen delivered to the lungs by nasal prongs is difficult to determine. This is because there may be dilution of inspired air through ill-fitting prongs or through an open mouth. Estimates of the effective FiO_2 have been based on patient's weight, gas flow rate, and concentration of oxygen blended in the blender (6). The O_2–air mixture should be warmed to the same temperature as the incubator air, which should be in the range of thermal neutrality (see Chapter 24).

ASSESSMENT OF GAS EXCHANGE

Clinical Assessment

The infant with respiratory problems may present with a wide spectrum of clinical findings. The infant's response depends on the degree of prematurity, lung and chest wall development, and maturation of respiratory control. The full-term infant may be able to increase the work of breathing to accomplish adequate gas exchange without treatment, including oxygen administration. The extremely premature infant will have a much weaker respiratory drive and inadequate muscular development and, thus, is less able to compensate for lung abnormalities. The classic

clinical signs of respiratory distress are helpful in the assessment of the mature newborn infant. Nasal flaring, grunting respirations, and tachypnea are almost always present. With progression of lung disease and decreased lung compliance, chest wall retractions become more marked. With increased work of breathing, retractions progress from sternal to subcostal, to intercostal, and then to a seesaw pattern of chest and abdominal wall movement. The full-term infant may increase respiratory rate above 100 per minute, with shallow respirations. This pattern is the most efficient way to increase gas exchange, with the least costly work of breathing. Expiratory grunting represents an effort to retard expiratory flow to increase end-expiratory pressure and maintain alveolar patency. It is unsafe to rely on color changes as an indication of oxygenation, as abnormalities in peripheral perfusion as a result of poor cardiac output, hypotension, or hypovolemia may be misleading. Similarly, infants with recurrent apnea will have intermittent deficiency in gas exchange. Auscultation assists in determining the quality of air entry in various parts of the lung and the presence of airway secretions or obstructions.

Measurement and Techniques

The measurement of blood gases and pH helps to confirm clinical impressions, and verifies the values obtained by pulse oximetry, transcutaneous electrodes, and end-tidal CO_2 monitoring. Most importantly, it helps to minimize the risks of hypoxia, hyperoxia, hypocapnia, hypercapnia, and metabolic acidosis.

Blood Gas Tension Measurements

Blood may be obtained by puncture of a peripheral artery, cannulation of a peripheral or umbilical artery, venous blood sampling, or capillary puncture. Venous and/or capillary blood values provide an approximation of arterial partial pressure of CO_2 (PCO_2) and pH but limited information about arterial oxygenation. The PCO_2 in venous blood is approximately 6 mm Hg higher and the pH is 0.03 lower than in arterial blood.

Peripheral arterial blood most often is sampled from the radial or posterior tibial arteries using a 23- or 25-gauge needle. Peripheral puncture is indicated when the anticipated number of samples will be small, or if arterial cannulation is unsuccessful. The painful nature of the procedure may result in altered breathing and a spurious result.

Cannulation

The choice of peripheral artery or umbilical artery catheterization usually is determined by the size of the infant, and the anticipated duration of the cannulation. The major advantage of a peripheral arterial catheter is the avoidance of umbilical cannulation and risk of thrombosis. A right radial arterial catheter has the unique advantage of sampling preductal PaO$_2$, which more accurately reflects retinal artery PO$_2$.

The need to insert a catheter into the umbilical artery should be based on the infant's maturation, postnatal age, and the type, severity, and expected duration of the illness. The high incidence of thrombus formation on the catheter tip, with its attendant risk of mural thrombus or emboli, must be weighed against the potential benefits to the infant. The tip of the umbilical catheter should rest in a low or high position to avoid the risk of occlusion, thrombosis, or direct infusion into a major branching artery. The distance to various levels within the aorta is estimated from the infant's shoulder to umbilicus distance and the chart of Dunn (Fig. 31-3) (7). The high location range is below the ductus arteriosus and above the takeoff of the celiac artery, with the tip resting between T5 and T10. At the lower site, the tip should be above the bifurcation of the aorta (L3 to L5) and below the takeoff of the renal and inferior mesenteric arteries. There appears to be a higher complication rate with catheters in the low position. The higher position allows greater leeway for catheter migration, although there is a greater risk of downstream embolization. A thoracoabdominal radiograph should be obtained immediately after catheter placement and before medications are infused. Once the catheter is in place, there is a risk of intraluminal clotting. Therefore, a continuous infusion is required, as is flushing of the line following blood sampling. Heparinization of fluid infusions is performed in many special care nurseries routinely. The umbilical arterial catheter fluids serve as a site of low grade hemolysis. Amino acid containing fluids can reduce this risk and supply some necessary protein constituents (8). A pressure strain gauge should be connected to the catheter, with alarm limits to indicate changes in blood pressure. Dampening of the pressure waveform indicates intraluminal or catheter tip narrowing or obstruction. The catheter should be removed once the infant has improved, the frequency of blood gas determinations has decreased to once or twice per day, and systemic arterial pressure monitoring no longer is essential.

The complications of umbilical artery catheterization are listed in (Table 31-1). The most frequent problem is peripheral vasospasm associated with blanching or patchy cyanosis (See Color Plate) of the distal leg, foot, or toes. If this does not improve with reflex vasodilation by warming of the contralateral leg, or worsens over the next 15 to 20 minutes, the catheter should be removed. Some thrombosis at the catheter tip is inevitable. Fortunately, the rate of complications from thrombus formation is relatively low.

Transcutaneous PO$_2$ and PCO$_2$

Transcutaneous PO$_2$ monitoring can be used selectively in conjunction with pulse oximetry. Most devices contain oxygen (O$_2$) and CO$_2$ electrodes. Noninvasive PO$_2$ measurements continue to be helpful in certain situations, particularly if transcutaneous PCO$_2$ also is obtained. Calibration before use and correlation with an arterial

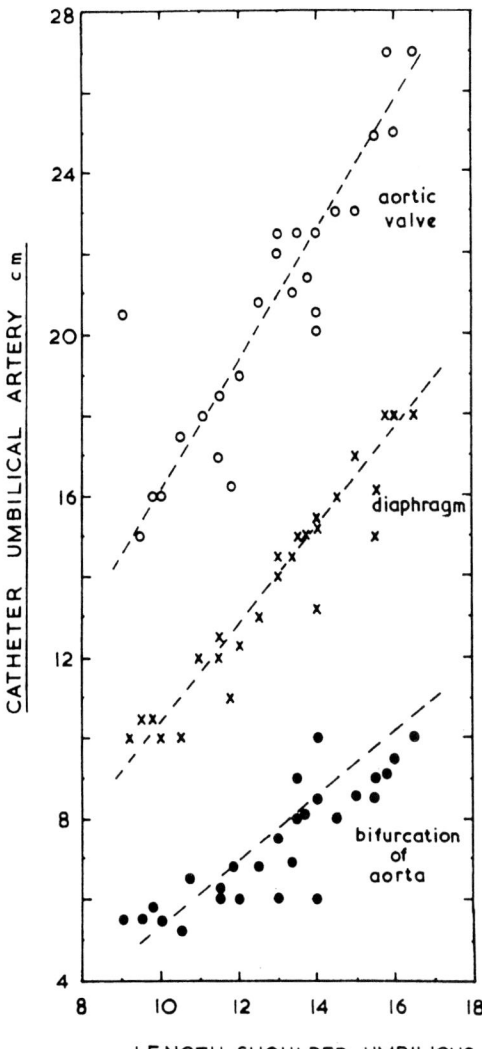

Figure 31-3 Relation between the shoulder-to-umbilicus measurement and the length of umbilical artery catheter needed to reach the aortic bifurcation, diaphragm, and aortic valve. From Dunn PM. Localization of the umbilical catheter by post-mortem measurement. Arch Dis Child 1966;41:69, with permission.

sample are necessary, but the need for subsequent blood samples should be reduced.

Arterial PO$_2$ and transcutaneous PO$_2$ are not identical. Differences can arise from local O$_2$ consumption by the skin or by the electrode itself, heating of the skin, O$_2$ diffusion time, and response time of the electrode (9). Skin blood flow may be affected by vasopressor medications, hypotension, and shock (10). Use of transcutaneous PO$_2$ can reduce the number of blood sampling procedures, particularly during a period when rapid changes in O$_2$ administration or mechanical ventilatory settings are taking place. Continuous monitoring for several hours also allows assessment of changes as a result of position, handling, suctioning, and feeding and for comparison with arterial oxygen saturation (SaO$_2$) monitoring. The risk of partial thickness burns precludes its use for longer than 5 hours at a single site on the body.

TABLE 31-1

COMPLICATIONS OF UMBILICAL CATHETERIZATION

Complication	Incidence	Comment
Limb ischemia	<20%	Assess Doppler arterial and venous flow from femoral region to dorsalis pedis; if reflex and unilateral, apply warmth to contralateral extremity; if persistent (>15 min), remove catheter
Thrombosis	<90%	Assess by aortic ultrasonography
Infection		Remove in presence of gram-positive blood culture if catheter was inserted more than 24 h previously; no relation to duration of catheter
Colonization	57%	
Sepsis	5%	
Blood loss	Rare	Connection to blood pressure transducer with alarm should prevent significant loss
Vascular perforation	Extremely rare	On removal, clamp for 5–10 min

Pulse Oximetry

Pulse oximetry provides a safe, accurate, and noninvasive adjunct to the assessment of tissue oxygenation (11,12). Oxygen saturation is determined by infrared spectrometry, utilizing two electrodes and a small cuff that can be placed around a hand, foot, or toe without requiring heating or calibration. One electrode contains two diodes that emit light at two wavelengths: red at 660 nm and infrared at 940 nm. The other electrode senses the light from both of these diodes that has not been absorbed by blood or tissue. The relative concentration of hemoglobin–oxygen (HbO_2) and deoxyhemoglobin determines the amount of transmitted light, because different forms of Hb have markedly different absorption characteristics. The ratio of the amount of light absorbed at each wavelength is used to calculate a SaO_2 value. The pulsed element of the apparatus allows the instrument to differentiate added arterial blood oxygenation and absorption from tissue, and it subtracts the amount contributed by nonpulsatile venous blood flow. With PO_2 values greater than 40 mm Hg, the saturation accurately reflects measurements of PO_2 obtained by catheter sample or by transcutaneous PO_2 (12).

A PaO_2 of 60 to 90 mm Hg results in a saturation value of 94% to 98% (see Fig. 31-2), and changes of 1% to 2% usually reflect a PaO_2 change of 6 to 12 mm Hg. The point of inflection at which the HbO_2 dissociation curve grows steep has considerable variability and depends on proportions of hemoglobin A, HbF, PCO_2, pH, and temperature. Generally, these variables are not so critical to the interpretation of the percent SaO_2 in arterial blood as they are to PaO_2. Below 40 mm Hg, the SaO_2 falls below 90%. Poor correlation with PaO_2 exists when the SaO_2 is above 96%, in which case the PaO_2 may be well above 100 mm Hg. In very low birth weight (VLBW) infants who require chronic oxygen administration and who are at risk for developing ROP, the upper limit of saturation should be reduced to 95% or less depending on local nursery policies. Inaccuracies may reflect improper placement, movement, or peripheral ischemia. Motion artifacts also produce invalid readings. However, these problems are less significant with newer pulse-Doppler devices.

Near-Infrared Spectroscopy

Utilization of the unique light-absorbing properties of Hb and HbO_2, as used in pulsed oximetry, has led to a sophisticated method of appraising tissue oxygenation by means of near-infrared spectroscopy. Near-infrared light penetrates the skin, bone, and various tissues and can be detected by electrodes placed on opposite sides of an infant's skull. This permits assessment of cerebral tissue O_2 and alterations in cerebral blood volume. Hb and cytochrome a and a_3 (cyt a, a_3) change their absorption characteristics according to the degree of oxygenation. The wavelength at which maximal absorption occurs is different for $HbO2$, deoxygenated Hb, total Hb, and reduced and oxygenated cyt a, a_3. The small cranial size of the infant weighing less than 1500 g makes cross-temple spectroscopy feasible. However, the technique has not gained widespread use in clinical neonatology.

End-Tidal CO_2 Monitoring

The concentration of CO_2 at the mouth or nose rises to reach a plateau at the end of each breath. This plateau reflects the alveolar CO_2 concentration under normal conditions, but may be inaccurate if there is marked ventilation–perfusion inequality or inhomogeneity of lung disease. Recent refinements to end-tidal CO_2 detection equipment permit in-line or "mainstream" infrared monitoring just proximal to the endotracheal tube (capnography), with a continuous display of the PCO_2 waveform. There is minimal dead space of the apparatus, and sampling accuracy has improved to compensate for the low expiratory flow rates characteristic of small premature infants. End-tidal CO_2 is less reliable in extremely small premature infants. Capnography is as accurate as capillary PCO_2 but is less precise than transcutaneous monitoring (13,14,15).

Hazards of High or Low Arterial CO_2

Identifying a safe range of PCO_2 has proven as difficult as for PaO_2. There are substantial risks to hypocarbia (Fig. 31-4)

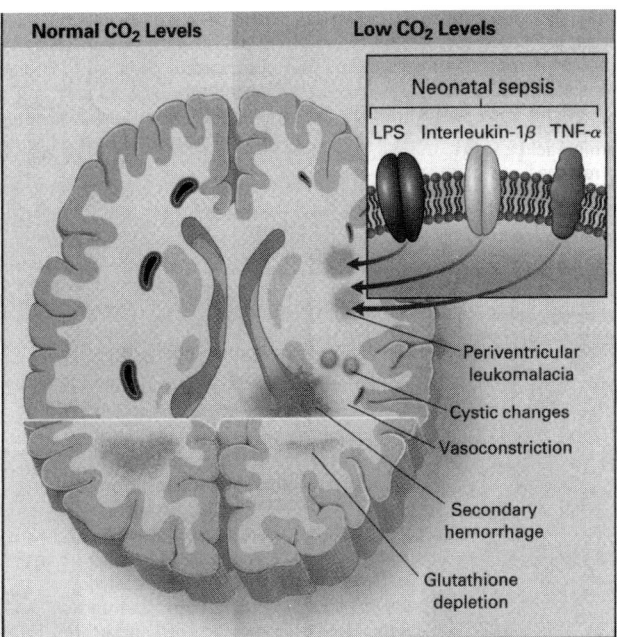

Figure 31-4 Effects of Hypocapnia on the Brain in Premature Infants. Hypocapnia has been implicated in the pathogenesis of neonatal white-matter injuries, including periventricular leukomalacia, resulting in intraventricular hemorrhage. At normal carbon dioxide levels (left-hand side of figure), cerebral blood flow is determined by local metabolic demand. Prolonged or severe hypocapnia includes severe cerebral vasoconstriction, resulting in brain ischemia, particularly in poorly perfused areas of the brain such as watershed areas (right-hand side of figure). This ischemia may initiate white-matter destruction in the brain of premature infants. Additionally, antioxidant depletion (caused by excitatory amino acids), lipopolysaccharide (LPS), and cytokines produced in response to sepsis, such as interleukin-1β and tumor necrosis factor α (TNF-α), potentiate the process. Finally, restoration of the normal partial pressure of arterial carbon dioxide can result in cerebral vasodilation, which may precipitate or contribute to intraventricular hemorrhage. From Laffey JG, Kavanagh BP. Hypocapnia. *N Engl J Med* 2002;347(1):43, with permission.

(16) (Table 31-2). Limiting the exposure time to hypocarbia may be important in presenting the development of cystic periventricular leukomalacia or decreasing the risk of CLD (17–19). There has been an increase in use of permissive hypercarbia, by which $PaCO_2$ levels of 50 to 60 mm Hg are sought and maintained. The rationale is to avoid high peak inspiratory pressure or to delay the onset of or to avoid assisted ventilation (20,21).

STRATEGIES FOR RESPIRATORY SUPPORT

Continuous Positive Airway Pressure

The application of end-expiratory pressure is intended to prevent alveoli and/or terminal airways from collapsing to airlessness. Continuous positive airway pressure (CPAP) may be applied during spontaneous breathing or as positive end-expiratory pressure (PEEP) during mechanical ventilation. This usually requires pressures between 4 to 6 cm H_2O for CPAP and 3 to 8 cm H_2O for PEEP.

TABLE 31-2

RISKS OF HYPOCARBIA AND HYPERCARBIA

Hypocarbia
- Overventilation increases risk for pulmonary injury
- Decreases cerebral perfusion, associated with ischemic white matter injury
- Increase in pH, interfering with tissue O_2 unloading

Hypercarbia
- Underventilation may increase areas of lung collapse and increase VA/Q mismatching necessitating higher F_1O_2
- May decrease pH elevating pulmonary vascular resistance and increase VA/Q mismatching
- Increases cerebral perfusion with associated risk of hemorrhagic infarctions

The physiologic effects of CPAP/PEEP may vary depending on the underlying pulmonary pathology, although the primary goal is to prevent alveolar collapse. Grunting respirations in infants with respiratory distress suggest laryngeal narrowing and increased resistance to expiratory flow to increase end-expiratory alveolar pressure. In the surfactant-deficient state, alveoli will collapse at end-expiration unless a minimum distending pressure is maintained. CPAP of 3 to 4 cm H_2O will prevent alveolar collapse but will not recruit atelectatic alveoli. Opening pressures of 12 to 15 cm H_2O are required to inflate collapsed alveoli. The infant will need to create a large distending airway pressure in the absence of CPAP. The shear forces from opening and closing of small airways may contribute to alveolar epithelial damage. Additionally, resultant abnormal distending forces on terminal or respiratory bronchioles will contribute to small airway injury. CPAP above physiologic levels of 3 to 4 cm H_2O may cause overinflation of some alveoli. Therefore, inflation and deflation may occur on the flatter portion of the pressure–volume curve and increase the work of breathing. CPAP theoretically could stimulate surfactant secretion. Maintenance of alveolar volume will reduce right-to-left shunting of blood through atelectatic alveoli, hence reducing oxygen needs.

Indications

The clinical indications for CPAP are varied. Initial use was directed at infants with RDS with the goal of avoiding or at least delaying intubation and mechanical ventilation. The gestational age, birth weight, and stage and severity of respiratory disease should be factored into the decision to initiate CPAP. If infants have severe lung disease, e.g., meconium aspiration, severe respiratory distress syndrome with FiO_2 needs >.6, or idiopathic pulmonary hypertension, more appropriate therapy would include assisted ventilation.

Infants <1,000 g birth weight are at considerable risk for developing chronic lung disease (CLD) and recurrent apneic episodes; therefore, they commonly are intubated and supported with mechanical ventilation as a result of their inability to sustain an adequate respiratory effort. They often develop an increasing oxygen need during the second week of life, associated with radiographic signs of CLD and attributed, in part, to assisted ventilation. CPAP may be beneficial in maintaining patency of extremely small terminal airways and prealveolar gas exchange units in these very immature infants. CPAP appears to be well tolerated by such infants over a period of many days. The increased enthusiasm for the use of CPAP is stimulated by the desire to minimize or prevent CLD. Because assisted ventilation is one putative factor in the etiology of CLD, the use of CPAP shortly after birth to avoid or minimize barotrauma has much appeal. Avoidance of endotracheal intubation should decrease the chances for tracheal injury, airway infection, abnormal mucociliary function, and over-inflation from excess ventilator pressure or volume.

Brief intubation and the administration of a single dose of surfactant followed by nasal CPAP has been advocated as another method of reducing the need for mechanical ventilation in infants with moderate RDS (22). Improvement in gas exchange has been demonstrated; however, more evidence of its efficacy in reducing the incidence or severity of CLD is required.

Recurrent Apnea

CPAP helps some infants with recurrent apnea of prematurity to sustain a more regular respiratory rate. The mechanism of its action is not well understood, although an increase in functional residual capacity (FRC) may alter the Hering–Breuer reflex or stabilize the thoracic cage, minimizing chest wall distortion and possibly altering inhibitory spinal cord reflexes (23). CPAP also helps to overcome obstructive apnea and decreases total respiratory system resistance (24,25).

Earlier methods of applying CPAP utilized an enclosed head box, face masks, and nasopharyngeal tubes. More recently, nasal prongs have been adapted to fit most infants. One device (the ALADDIN Infant Flow System, Hamilton Medical Inc., Reno, NV) appears to be well tolerated by both large and small infants. This apparatus maintains a constant flow of air by incorporating a double fluidic jet system within the apparatus. During inspiration, one jet maintains the flow to match the infant's inspiratory effort; during expiration, gas flow is reversed by a second jet to assist outflow while maintaining a constant minimum pressure. This system presumably does not add to the work of breathing and reduces the need to use high flow rates to compensate for air leak around the nasal prongs. A second system utilizes a variable depth water seal for the expiratory circuit to sustain continuous airway pressure (26). CPAP can also be applied utilizing constant flow ventilators.

Complications

CPAP may have adverse effects. Overinflation can result in increased work of breathing and decreased efficiency of gas exchange. Pneumothorax and pneumomediastinum may result from lung overdistension. Carbon dioxide retention may occur as a result of either increased dead space or ineffective ventilation of some alveoli. If the mean thoracic pressure is elevated with high levels of PEEP or CPAP, e.g., above 7 to 8 cm H20 in the absence of lung disease, cardiac output may be decreased because of impaired systemic and pulmonary venous return. The nasal prongs may cause irritation if the fit is not appropriate or the infant is active. Gastric distention may occur, making gastric feedings difficult, and often an indwelling or gastric tube is required for decompression.

Effectiveness

Does the use of CPAP decrease the need for assisted ventilation and does it prevent or ameliorate CLD in VLBW infants? Clinical trials conducted before the era of routine surfactant use and contemporary neonatal ventilation devices are now of limited relevance. Recent studies comparing the efficacy of conventional mechanical ventilation (CMV) to CPAP following the administration of surfactant found some differences in need for ventilation as an outcome although the number of infants studied was small (22,28).

CPAP is used to facilitate weaning from mechanical ventilation. Some infants, experiencing recurrent apneic episodes, appear to benefit (29), whereas infants evaluated in other studies have shown no benefit (30). Additional information is needed to confirm whether CPAP is an effective adjunct to successful extubation. The technique of nasal intermittent positive pressure ventilation (NIPPV) may gain widespread use if it can be shown to improve long-term outcome (31).

Assisted Mechanical Ventilation

Treatment with assisted ventilation is applied commonly to newborns across the neonatal birth weight spectrum (Fig. 31-5) (32). Illustrated is the rate of use of assisted ventilation, adjusted by birth weight, and the percent of all infants treated for more than or equal to 24 hours. Thirty-eight percent of treated infants were over 2,500 g birth weight in this survey, covering all California and New York State births for 1994–1995. Neonatologists must be expert in providing assisted ventilation across a 10-fold range of patient weight (0.5 kg–5.0 kg) and providing safe and effective assisted ventilation across a range of lung development from premature airways with preacinar gas exchange spaces to a virtually completely alveolarized organ. Thus, both size (patient and lung volume) and range of development are immense.

The Immature Lung

The immature lung presents a special hazard for the application of assisted ventilation. The application of positive pressure for the purpose of increasing ventilation and optimizing ventilation–perfusion ($\dot{V}A/\dot{Q}$) matching may injure

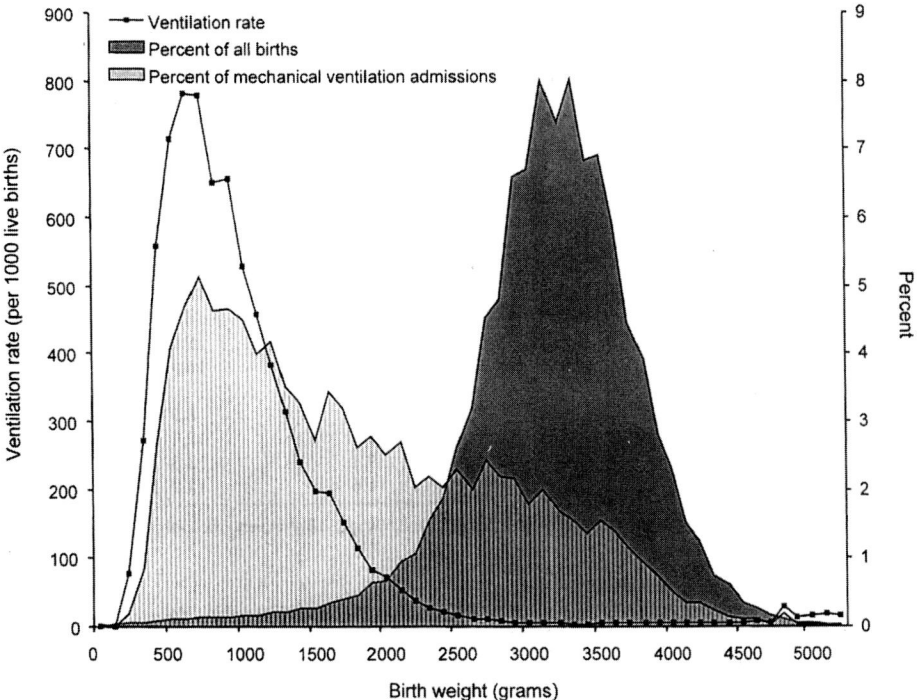

Figure 31-5   Distribution of total births and neonatal mechanical ventilation by birth weight. The primary y axis is the mechanical ventilation rate per 1000 live births within a given weight category. The secondary y axis is the percentage of all births and of all mechanical ventilation hospitalizations. Data are from New York and California for 1994. Higher mechanical ventilation rates are seen in smaller babies. However, because most babies are >2500 g, a large proportion of ventilated babies are of normal weight. From Angus DC, Linde-Zwirble WT, Clermont G, Griffin MF, Clark RH. Epidemiology of neonatal respiratory failure in the United States. Projections from California and New York. *Am J Respir Crit Care Med* 2001;164:1154, with permission.

epithelial and endothelial tissues. In the incompletely developed lungs, structures are less elastic and more vulnerable to barotrauma. Injury to the mesenchymal and epithelial tissues that later give rise to alveolar septation and vascular formation may be irreversible. Studies in adult animals have demonstrated that otherwise healthy lungs can suffer injury, which is reflected by increased airway fluid and deterioration of gas exchange, if inappropriate distending lung pressures are applied (33). The particular problems of providing assisted ventilation are illustrated in Fig. 31-6 (34). Relative immaturity of distal bronchioles and respiratory ducts, coupled with fluid-filled and collapsed alveoli, create a set of conditions leading to overdistention of some areas and underventilation of other areas, with resultant ineffective gas exchange. This uneven ventilation, coupled with injury produced by reactive oxygen species, contributes to the common problem of chronic lung disease of prematurity. The risk of its development is inversely correlated with birth weight.

Great strides have been made in understanding how the immature lung differs from a mature lung in phospholipid and surfactant-associated protein biosynthesis. However, there are factors other than surfactant biosynthesis that are unique to the immature lung and that increase the susceptibility to injury. These factors include, but are not limited to, incomplete development of the supportive net of collagen and elastin (35,36), incomplete development of the

capillary bed in the gas exchange areas (37), relative instability of the chest wall with reduced capacity to maintain expiratory lung volume at FRC, immaturity of the neural control producing sustained spontaneous respiratory effort, and probable immaturity of the metabolic functions of the pulmonary endothelium.

Respiratory failure ensues when spontaneous breathing efforts fail to produce adequate alveolar ventilation. In newborn infants, this may occur because of failure of adequate output from central nervous system respiratory centers, an overly compliant chest wall that increases the work of breathing, metabolic problems as a result of limited energy stores, or profoundly noncompliant lungs requiring more work and depleting available energy stores. Each of these may be an indication for assisted ventilation. In most neonatal respiratory disorders, these problems occur in combination, and the diagnosis of respiratory failure cannot be ascribed to any single cause.

Establishment of an Artificial Airway

Physiologic and Anatomic Airway Peculiarities

The newborn infant has distinct anatomic and physiologic characteristics of the airways and a strong preference for nasal breathing for the first few months of life (38). Nasal or nasopharyngeal obstruction because of secretions, mucosal

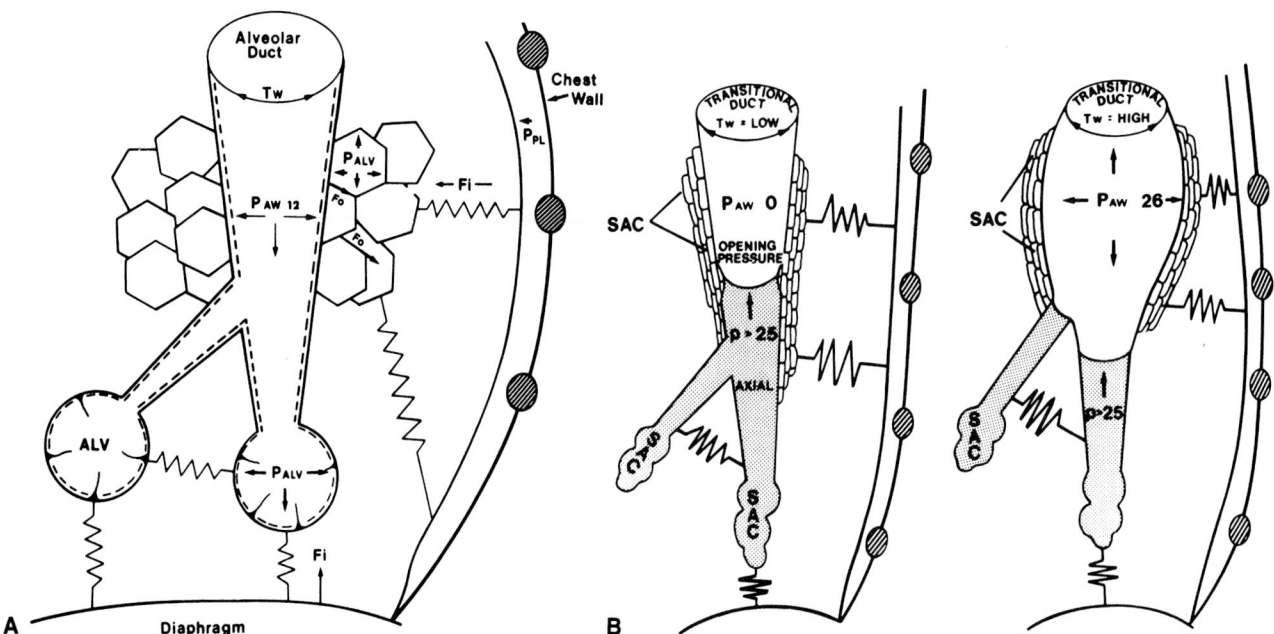

Figure 31-6 A: A mature alveolar duct and alveoli. Dotted line, surfactant; P_{ALV}, alveolar pressure; P_{AW}, airway pressure; P_{PL}, pleural pressure; Fi, tissue force (stretched springs) acting inward; Fo, tissue force directed outward; Tw, wall tension or recoil pressure. B: The end-expiratory airway pressure (P_{AW}) equals zero in an immature distal airway (left). The saccules (SAC) and airways contain fluid (shaded area). The axial airway is concave at the air–liquid interface as a result of the surface tension forces. The peripheral SACs are collapsed or fluid filled. The lax tissues are represented by relaxed springs. The inspiratory airway pressure (P_{AW}) is equal to 26 cm H_2O (right). The distended distal airway has a high wall tension (TW). The liquid front has been pushed peripherally, but the SACs are still not inflated. From Thibeault DW, Lang MJ. Mechanisms and pathobiologic effects of barotrauma. In: Merritt TA, Northway WH Jr, Boynton BR, eds. Bronchopulmonary dysplasia. *Contemporary issues in fetal neonatal medicine.* Boston: Blackwell Scientific Publishers, 1988:82, with permission.

injury, or congenital abnormalities may produce respiratory distress. Approximately one-half of the infant's airway resistance occurs in the nose, although the narrowness of the lower respiratory tract results in a total airway resistance approximately 15 times greater than that of an adult (39). Edema and inflammation can produce extremely high resistance to air flow in these narrow airways. During expiration, the airways become narrower, and resistance increases.

Endotracheal Intubation

Route

Orotracheal and nasotracheal intubation may be used for prolonged mechanical ventilation of term and premature infants. The principal advantage of the nasal route is the stabilization of the tube afforded by the close fit within the naris, but the nasal passages may limit the size of tube that can be used. Necrosis of the nasal septum or the alae nasi can occur if circulation is impaired because the tube is too large. Orotracheal intubation is more easily and quickly accomplished and is indicated for delivery room and emergency situations. It is the preferred route for prolonged mechanical ventilation.

The endotracheal tube should allow a small air leak between the tube and the glottis. A tube that fits too snugly within the trachea is likely to cause pressure necrosis of the

mucosa. If too large a leak is allowed, it may be difficult to achieve sufficient pressure for ventilation of noncompliant lungs. A tube with a 2.5-mm inner diameter usually fits infants weighing less than 1,000 g; a 3-mm tube fits those from 1,000 to 2,000 g; a 3.5-mm tube fits those from 2,000 to 3,000 g; and 3.5- to 4.0-mm tube fits larger infants.

Technique

Orotracheal intubation is a simple procedure that can be accomplished atraumatically within a few seconds. The necessary equipment consists of a straight-bladed laryngoscope, a suction catheter connected to a suction apparatus, an endotracheal tube of the appropriate size with an adapter for the bag or respirator, and an optical flexible Teflon introducer, bent to prevent its tip from protruding beyond the end of the endotracheal tube. The infant is ventilated with 100% oxygen by mask for a few breaths. A catheter to deliver oxygen can be taped to the laryngoscope blade to enhance oxygen delivery during intubation (40). The infant's neck is straightened without hyperextension by placing a small towel under the shoulders, and the head is steadied by an assistant. The laryngoscope is held in the left hand between the thumb and first two fingers. The heel of the hand is placed against the infant's left cheek to provide stability. The blade is introduced into the right side of the mouth, and the tongue is deflected to the left as the blade is advanced into the vallecula, anterior to the epiglottis. The laryngoscope is

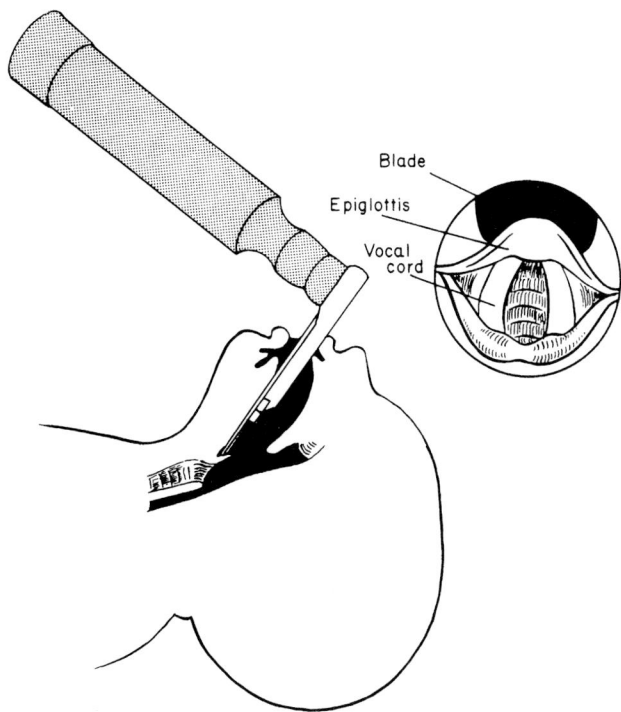

Figure 31-7 Laryngoscopy for endotracheal intubation.

TABLE 31-3	
DEPTH OF INSERTION OF AN OROTRACHEAL TUBE FROM THE LIPS OF A PREMATURE INFANT	
Infant Weight (kg)	**Depth of Insertion (cm)**
1.0	7
2.0	8
3.0	9
4.0	10

tion of an endotracheal tube, as determined by post-mortem and radiographic measurements, is related to body weight (43). Suggested depths of insertion for orotracheal intubation are given in (Table 31-3) (43,44).

Immediately after intubation, the position of the tube should be confirmed by inspection and auscultation. Identification of humidity in the tube or of CO_2—by a sensitive color detector—helps confirm endotracheal tube placement. Two common errors of tube placement are intubation of the esophagus and intubation of the right main-stem bronchus. The former should be suspected if insufflation through the tube produces abdominal distention with little chest expansion and if air movement is heard better over the stomach than over the chest. Breath sounds that are louder over the right chest than the left suggest that the tube is in the right main-stem bronchus. Auscultation, although helpful, is not reliable because breath sounds are well transmitted in a small chest. A chest radiograph should be obtained to confirm tube placement.

Care of Endotracheal Tubes

A tube in the trachea interferes with the physiologic mechanisms for clearance of respiratory secretions and may itself stimulate secretions. Meticulous care is needed to prevent accumulation and inspissation of secretions which can obstruct the tube. Routine changing of the tube is unnecessary and subjects the infant to the repeated risk of trauma to the larynx and interruption of ventilation. However, the most common reason for sudden deterioration of an otherwise stable ventilated infant is dislodgment or blockage of the tracheal tube. The volume and quality of secretions vary with the type of pulmonary disease and with the individual patient. Suction frequency may vary from once each hour to fewer than two or three times per day. Both "in-line" techniques and discontinuation of positive-pressure ventilation are used for suctioning of airway secretions. "In-line" techniques offer the advantage of no loss of distending pressure during the suctioning process. However, no formal comparisons of the safety of the two techniques have been conducted.

Another important aspect of the care of artificial airways is the provision of adequate humidification. The endotracheal tube bypasses the nasal and pharyngeal mucosa, which normally warms and humidifies inspired gases. If heat and humidity are not provided from an external

lifted rather than rotated so that the larynx is elevated and the glottis is brought into view (Fig. 31-7). The pharynx is suctioned if necessary. The endotracheal tube is introduced into the mouth to the right of the laryngoscope and gently guided into the glottis under direct vision.

The nasotracheal tube is inserted without an introducer through the naris and gently guided along the floor of the nose. The laryngoscope is placed in the mouth to the right of the orotracheal tube, and the tip of the nasotracheal tube is seen in the posterior pharynx. A Magill forceps is held in the right hand and introduced to the right of the laryngoscope. The nasotracheal tube is grasped a few millimeters back from its tip with the forceps, and the tip of the tube is elevated until it is almost at the glottis. It is helpful to have an assistant grasp the exterior end of the nasotracheal tube to assist in advancing it. The orotracheal tube is left in place until just before insertion of the nasotracheal tube in the glottis.

Pretreatment with pancuronium bromide and atropine may minimize heart rate and intracranial pressure changes associated with endotracheal intubation (41,42). Morphine and/or midazolam are commonly provided prior to intubation attempts to reduce agitation. Size and stability of the patient dictate the exact choice of adjunctive mediation use.

Positioning

The length of the trachea from the vocal cords to the carina varies from about 3.6 cm in the smallest premature infants to 6 cm in large, term infants. Optimal positioning for the tip of an endotracheal tube is in the middle of the trachea, in which it is least subject to dislodgment into the pharynx or displacement into a bronchus. The proper depth of inser-

source, drying of the lower airway mucosa, thickened secretions, and hypothermia may result. Inspired gases should be passed through a heated nebulizer with a constant readout temperature probe so that they are delivered to the airway already warmed to a range of 34°C to 36°C, and saturated. Inadequate humidification can contribute to airway injury (45).

Indications for Assisted Ventilation

The decision for initiation of assisted ventilation should be individualized for each baby. Factors to consider include underlying disease and its expected natural history, birth weight, gestational age, postnatal age, chest radiographic appearance, progression of clinical signs, serial arterial blood gas tension measurements, and pH measurements. The criteria indicating a need for mechanical ventilation are difficult to define, and there is lack of unanimity about a particular threshold for PaO_2, partial pressure of CO_2 ($PaCO_2$), or FiO_2. In general, the PaO_2 should be maintained at or above 50 mm Hg because of reasonable oxyhemoglobin saturation at this level, but the maximal level of inspired O_2 dictating intubation and application of assisted ventilation remains controversial. A trend of rising $PaCO_2$ with concomitant decrease in pH or onset of apnea indicates a need for mechanical assistance. After assisted ventilation is initiated, the generally accepted goals are to maintain the PaO_2 between 45 and 70 mm Hg, $PaCO_2$ at 45 and 60 mm Hg or less, and pH at 7.25 or more although minimizing PIP and FiO_2, and optimizing mean airway pressure (PAW[gas]) and PEEP. These general guidelines must be interpreted and often must be modified to provide optimal support for the individual patient.

Because acute lung disease is usually more severe and protracted in more immature infants, criteria for intervention for infants weighing less than 1,000 g differ from those for larger or older infants. For example, a 750 g infant with RDS has a high probability of developing apnea, fatigue, or both, and most of these infants require assisted ventilation even if the FiO_2 need is less than 40%. A 2,500 g, 36-week-old infant with RDS has greater muscular and caloric reserve and is able to sustain rapid ventilatory rates and higher respiratory work for several days without assistance. With a normal $PaCO_2$, inspired O_2 may be increased to between 80% and 90% before intubation in some infants. Infants of gestational age 35 to 39 weeks and older than 24 hours who develop respiratory failure with RDS may benefit from surfactant treatment (46).

Physiologic Considerations

An understanding of the effects of mechanical ventilation on the lungs requires knowledge of the interplay among thoracic mechanics, including pulmonary compliance and airway resistance, lung volumes, respiratory control mechanisms, and alveolar gas exchange.

Lung compliance change in lung volume per unit pressure change, in units of mL/cm H_2O depends on the elastic properties of the tissue, which are influenced by the lung volume

and abnormalities such as tissue inflammation and edema. Compliance is low if there is alveolar collapse or overdistention. Expansion from alveolar collapse requires inflation pressures of 12 to 20 cm H_2O in preterm infants with RDS to achieve tidal volumes of 3 to 5 ml/kg. The lungs of infants with RDS have areas of collapse and overexpansion, and there is nonuniformity of compliance. Other conditions, such as pneumothorax, lobar atelectasis or consolidation, and pulmonary edema, decrease compliance. The most relevant measure of compliance, specific compliance, is calculated by normalizing compliance by end-expiratory volume (EEV), the functional equivalent of FRC measured during positive pressure ventilation. Very low or high values for EEV will reduce compliance. Changes in compliance, EEV, and gas exchange are not concordant, at least not during RDS. This has limited the value of bedside measurements of compliance, particularly without concomitant measurements in EEV. Chest wall compliance usually is high and does not present a problem to mechanical ventilation.

Airway resistance (cm H_2O/L/s) is inversely related to the fourth power of the radius during laminar air flow. Airway resistance is high in infants, increasing with low lung volumes and with obstruction of the airway. High rates of air flow increase resistance by producing turbulence in the airways.

The rate at which lung areas inflate and deflate is determined by resistance and compliance. An increase in airway resistance increases the time required for air to reach the alveoli; a decrease in compliance results in less time required to reach equilibrium. The product of resistance and compliance is the pulmonary time constant. Changes in resistance or compliance can alter the pattern or distribution of ventilation, and recognition of the variations in the time constant (e.g., short with poor compliance, prolonged with increased airway resistance) helps determine respirator settings. Unfortunately, a single time constant does not exist for all lung areas during complex pulmonary disorders. Thus, all conventional positive-pressure ventilators produce areas of overinflation and underinflation of gas exchanging areas, each contributing to suboptimal gas exchange.

Because RDS should result in a short time constant, rapid inspiratory and expiratory respirator times are permissible, and mean airway pressure should be increased to improve oxygenation. With meconium aspiration or airway edema, the time constant is slower, and sufficient time for expiration is important to avoid gas trapping, overdistention of the lungs, and possible air leak. If the expiratory time (T_E) is shorter than the time constant of the lung for expiration, overdistention results. If the overall time constant for the lung is longer than the imposed ventilator inspiratory time (T_I), inadequate ventilation could result. Unequal time constants coexisting in different parts of the lung are most likely to occur if pulmonary abnormalities are unevenly distributed, as in pneumonia, meconium aspiration, pulmonary interstitial emphysema, pneumothorax, or CLD, in which case the optimal T_I or T_E becomes difficult to determine.

The circulatory effects of mechanically applied pressure to the alveoli are important. Normal breathing results in negative intrapleural pressure that enhances venous return and cardiac output. Positive-pressure breathing can impede venous return and may diminish cardiac output. Pressure during inspiration decreases the pulmonary capillary circulation as long as alveolar pressure exceeds capillary pressure and can affect total pulmonary blood flow and hence gas exchange.

Lung Volume Measurements During Mechanical Ventilation

Application of hot wire anemometry or pneumotachography to time-cycled pressure- limited ventilation systems allows measurement of inspiratory and expiratory tidal volumes, minute ventilation ($\dot{V}_E$), and air leak, the difference between tidal volumes measured during inspiration and expiration at any combination of ventilator settings. Tidal volume can be correlated with peak inspiratory pressure (PIP), inspiratory gas flow rate, T_I and PEEP. Knowledge of tidal volume from bedside measurements helps allow determination of the optimal PIP to achieve optimal tidal volume. For many clinical situations, this value is between 3 and 5 ml/kg. This knowledge allows minimizing PIP, which, if excessive, otherwise may induce or exacerbate the small airway injury of CLD. However, knowledge of tidal volume and V_E does not provide knowledge of distribution of inspired ventilation and of $\dot{V}_A/\dot{Q}$ matching. Distribution of tidal volume may vary with the associated PIP; low PIP can result in tidal volume distribution only to already overinflated lung regions, resulting in worsened $\dot{V}_A/\dot{Q}$ matching, development or exacerbation of high $\dot{V}_A/\dot{Q}$ areas, and worsening of CO2 retention, despite normal or elevated $\dot{V}_E$.

Many ventilators now have pulmonary graphic systems to monitor breath-by-breath pressure-volume and flow-volume loops. These graphics can be helpful in evaluating the extent of airway instability during inspiration and especially expiration. Pressure-volume curves may be helpful in detecting overdistention and/or air trapping or small airway obstruction. One limitation in the use of pulmonary graphics is the considerable breath-to-breath variability in the pattern exhibited, probably more than exists with assisted ventilation of adults. There is as yet no strong evidence suggesting that a clinically important outcome can be modified in neonates with reliance on interpretation of these patterns of airflow and pressure.

Automated bedside EEV measurements are now available. The devices utilize helium dilution methodology and early trials demonstrated safe use and reproducible measurements. Their use may allow a more individualized approach to application of PEEP in infants.

Investigation of New Forms of Assisted Ventilation

The gold standard approach to the introduction of new therapies in medicine is the performance of prospective,

definitive, randomized clinical trials (RCT) with predetermined clinically relevant primary outcomes. This approach has been followed belatedly but now enthusiastically in Neonatology. Part of the acceptance of the results of RCTs devolves from effective blinding of the treatment group assignment, and the widespread agreement that the control group received the best available therapy known at the time. When these principles are applied to trials testing new approaches in assisted ventilation, there are several obvious limitations.

It is difficult to conduct a blinded clinical study of two different types of assisted ventilation, especially if different ventilators are used. It is difficult to agree on what constitutes optimal standard of care to be used for the control group. This applies not only to the minutia of management of the ventilation device itself, but also to the ancillary supportive care. Even if agreement about standards of care is achieved, it is difficult to sustain adherence to these standards of care.

Contemporary ventilators designed for application to neonates are very complex devices. This complexity mandates a balance in the performance of clinical trials between the rigid prescriptions of ventilator management vs. the "field level" studies with greater tolerance for physician specific practices. The latter study design may have perhaps more applicability to broad populations, but runs the risk that center-to-center variance in approach and in outcome may be greater, potentially diluting the signal of interest. Although these issues are inherent in all prospective definitive trials, they are particularly acute when applied to testing modes of assisted ventilation in neonates.

Identifying a clinically relevant outcome can be difficult. Death is the obvious outcome of interest, but for most populations of neonates treated with assisted ventilation, it may be an insensitive marker and not informative for other important outcomes. Utilizing a surrogate marker for death (e.g., need for ECMO) has worked well for clinical trials of near term infants, but will not work well for babies ineligible for ECMO, (those less than 34 to 35 weeks gestation). For preterm infants, evidence of pulmonary injury (i.e., CLD) in combination with death is commonly used. However, even these outcomes pose problems because of the poorly understood pathogenesis of CLD and the role of factors other than assisted ventilation that contributes to its development and severity. Combined outcomes melded into one also have the problem that reduction in one part of the primary outcome (death) may increase the incidence of the adverse-associated outcome. Some studies testing different forms of assisted ventilation were plagued by the problem that to qualify for the study, infants first were treated with one form of assisted ventilation for a variable period before the application of different patterns of ventilation could be undertaken. More recent trials, especially those testing HFV (47,48,49), have largely avoided this problem. Some studies, even those purporting to show a benefit from an experimental form of ventilation, may demonstrate the benefit because the control patients demonstrated a higher than expected rate of adverse outcomes. Successful recruitment of sufficiently large populations in sufficiently short time and the ability to stratify them in a meaningful way can also prove to be difficult. This is increasingly true, given the role of economics in the decision regarding whether eligible patients for definitive clinical trials are moved from one center to another to participate in those trials (50).

Despite these limitations and others, advances have occurred in the application of assisted ventilation using randomized clinical trials. RCTs will remain valuable to better understand the limitations and strengths of the many different patterns of assisted ventilation.

Conventional Ventilation

Available Modes and Details of Use

Several manipulations of applied pressure allow for an increase in PaO_2. The physician decides whether to increase FiO_2 or $P_{AW}[gas]$ by considering the prior settings and balancing the possible harmful effects of increasing PAW[gas] against those of increasing FiO_2, recognizing that threshold limits are arbitrary. If the FiO_2 is approaching 1.0, and SpO_2 or PaO_2 are unacceptably low, then other options must be invoked. During time-cycled, pressure-limited ventilation, if PEEP is already 5 to 6 cm H_2O, the PIP or the T_I is increased. The use of PEEP helps to maintain patent small airways and prevent collapse to airlessness of those alveoli already open. Inspiratory pressures of >15 cm H_2O usually are required to open collapsed or fluid-filled acinar areas. A combination of an increase in the TI with 6 cm H_2O PEEP may be helpful during the initial phase of assisted ventilation for RDS. With subsequent opening of air spaces, the optimal TI may need to be decreased. The use of an end-inspiratory pause or plateau should improve the distribution of inspired gas if there are regional differences in airway resistance. However, if the alveolar pressure exceeds capillary pressure, there will be tamponade of the pulmonary circulation and development of high $\dot{V}_A/\dot{Q}$ areas.

Hypoxemia may persist during all combinations of ventilator settings in some conditions, and other underlying abnormalities should be suspected. The clinician should always consider the degree of air leak around the endotracheal tube when adjusting pressure and flow rates. Echocardiographic evaluation of the infant for coexisting pulmonary vascular hypertension or structural or functional heart disease is then indicated. Other management considerations are listed in Table 31-4.

If there is airway obstruction, as may occur with CLD or meconium aspiration, optimal ventilator settings may differ from those used for RDS. Because there is a relatively long time constant, the gas flow rate should not be too rapid, and there should be adequate time for expiration. One of the multiple available newer modes of assisted ventilation may then be useful.

TABLE 31-4
MANAGEMENT CONSIDERATIONS

- Utilize alternative mode of ventilation (e.g., HFV, SIMV, A/C, PRVC)
- Raise the hematocrit to 45–50% with packed erythrocyte transfusions
- Reposition baby into prone position if supine or into left or right lateral positions
- Use of sedation with or without paralysis; if infant is paralyzed, discontinue its use
- Change to a larger size endotracheal tube to diminish air leak
- Consider repeated doses of exogenous surfactant beyond 24 h of age
- Administer diuretics to change pulmonary fluid concentration
- Increase cardiac output and/or systemic blood pressure with agents
- Undertake trial of NO
- Consider use of corticosteroids

A/C, assist/control; HFV, high-frequency ventilation; IMV, intermittent mandatory ventilation; SIMV, synchronous intermittent mandatory ventilation; PRVC = pressure regulated volume control.

Patient-Triggered Ventilation

The goal of patient-triggered ventilation is to maximize the efficiency of spontaneous breathing efforts although minimizing the risk of insufficient ventilation or trauma to airways (51). All patterns of patient-triggered ventilation require a rapidly responding sensor and transducer that can detect the onset of spontaneous inspiratory effort and provide the mechanical initiation of machine-assisted ventilation during the early phase of the infant's inspiration. Currently used methods to signal the initiation of inspiratory effort are listed in Table 31-5. The current methodology allows transduction to be accomplished in as short a time as 30 to 50 ms, approximately one-tenth the duration of the inspiratory phase of a spontaneous respiratory cycle (Fig. 31-8) (52). The means by which this signal is provided and the addition of other subtle but potentially important changes in the capabilities of particular ventilators differentiate one type of conventional neonatal ventilator from another (53). A list of available modes and their theoretical advantages is found (Table 31-6).

Although it is not clear that modern means of patient-triggered ventilation have achieved their optimum, these methods have already gained widespread acceptance for three reasons. These include the clinical impression that infants are more comfortable and less distressed although being ventilated with patient-triggered ventilation; there may be at least modest improvements in pulmonary gas exchange (53) during patient-triggered ventilation; and there appears to be decreased need for sedation and muscle relaxation. Even with patient-triggered ventilation, it is important to recognize the pitfalls that may occur when the synchronized intermittent mandatory ventilation (SIMV) rates are too high or when the patient is allowed to breathe in the assist/control mode (Fig. 31-9) (53). With assist/control, hyperventilation may occur, especially if the sensor

TABLE 31-5

AVAILABLE MECHANISMS FOR DETECTING ONSET OF RESPIRATION

	Advantage	Disadvantage
Body movement measurement	No deadspace	Position-dependent
Transthoracic impedence	No deadspace	Position-dependent
Airway pressure sensors	Little deadspace	Speed
Airflow sensors		
Pneumotachygraphy	Sensitive	Added deadspace
Hotwire anaemometer	Sensitive	Too sensitive

for initiation of respiration is inappropriately sensitive and triggers ventilator breaths that are not associated with patient inspiratory effort. If the goal is to avoid breaths triggered late in inspiration or during expiration, then flow-triggering systems are less prone to auto triggering and have a shorter and more consistent response time than impedance-triggered systems (54). The "Pressure-Regulated Volume Control" mode available with the Siemens Series 300 ventilator has proven useful in correcting gas exchange problems in larger preterm infants or term infants. However, the set tidal volume is arbitrary because of loss of volume to the compliant breathing circuit leading to inaccuracy of its measurement (55). If end tidal CO_2 is measured with the ventilator, then a second measure of tidal volume (V_T) is made at the breathing tube, which may be more reflective of actual V_T. No definitive clinical trial of this variable flow mode of ventilation compared to conventional patterns of ventilation in the treatment of low-birth-weight (LBW) infants has been reported.

A limitation of many devices is that the individual breaths generated by the ventilator are monomorphic. Proportional assist ventilation may be one way to overcome

the problem and provide improved individualization of support. With proportional assist ventilation, the relationship between patient-induced inspiratory effort and ventilator response is interactive (56). During proportional assist ventilation the ventilator amplifies the patient's effort throughout the inspiratory phase of the cycle. With each spontaneously generated breath, the patient can individualize the machine-initiated tidal volume and flow patterns. Sensors monitor instantaneous flow rate and volume of gas from ventilator to patient; the applied pressure then changes according to the equation of motion. This system may allow for both greater patient comfort and reduction of peak airway pressure required to sustain ventilation, with less likelihood of over-ventilation compared to assist/control modes. (56). Another newer patient-interactive system is available with the Drager 8000 neonatal ventilator. The modality is called pressure-support ventilation with volume guarantee. The goal is to provide stable tidal volumes but with the capacity to alter inspiratory time and peak inflating pressure.

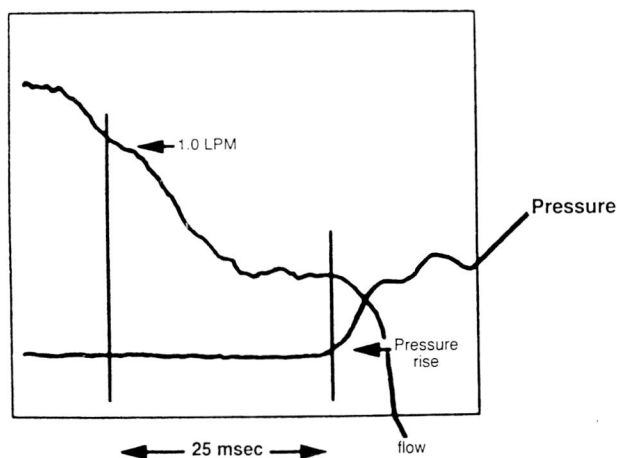

Figure 31-8 System response time, also known as trigger delay. The flow change trigger is set at 1.0 LPM. It took 25 ms from the time this threshold was reached (vertical line on the left) until there was a measurable rise in airway pressure (vertical line on the right). From Donn SM, Sinha SK. Controversies in patient-triggered ventilation. *Clin Perinatol* 1998;25:49, with permission.

TABLE 31-6

MODES OF ASSISTED VENTILATION VIA ENDOTRACHEAL TUBE

Modes	Theoretical Advantages
IMV	Pressure and time limited breaths
	Fresh gas flow allowing efforts at spontaneous breathing
SIMV	Synchronized, controllable number of assisted breaths
A/C	Every spontaneous breath assisted with a monomorphic wave form
PAV	Respiratory pressure is servo- controlled and is proportional to endogenous volume and flow
PSV	Inspiratory time and flow are variable but PIP is still fixed
PSV + VG	Time variable inspiration
	Constant flow
	Automatic attempt to deliver same tidal volume

IMV = Intermittent mandatory ventilation, SIMV = Synchronized intermittent mandatory ventilation, A/C = Assist/Control, PAV = Proportional assist ventilation, PSV = Pressure support ventilation, VG = Volume guarantee

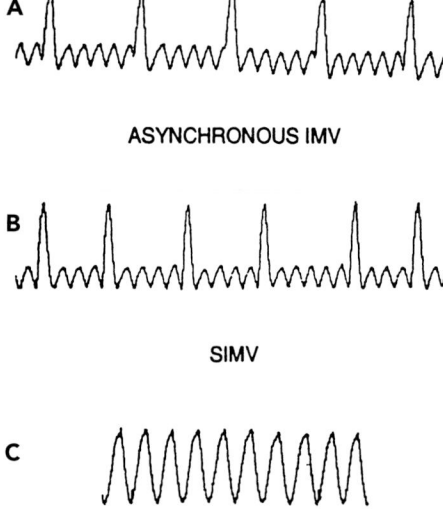

Figure 31-9 Tidal volume tracings (inspiration = upward) demonstrating three patterns of ventilator interaction with spontaneous breathing. In this illustration, tidal volume of spontaneous breaths is less than that of ventilator breaths. A: Asynchronous intermittent mandatory ventilation (IMV) with ventilator breaths delivered during spontaneous expiration. During IMV, ventilator breaths occur at a constant rate, with random timing with respect to spontaneous breaths. B: Synchronous intermittent mandatory ventilation (SIMV) with ventilator breaths delivered early in selected spontaneous inspirations. During SIMV, ventilator breaths occur more irregularly, but the ventilator delivers the set rate synchronously with spontaneous breaths. C: Assist/control mode, with ventilatory breaths delivered early in all spontaneous inspirations. The assist/control mode delivers ventilatory breaths synchronously with all spontaneous breaths and may lead to increased ventilation. From: Cleary JP, Bernstein G, Mannino FL, Heldt GP. Improved oxygenation during synchronized intermittent mandatory ventilation in neonates with respiratory distress syndrome: a randomized, crossover study. *J Pediatr* 1995;126:407, with permission.

No studies have been reported to date which measured a clinically important outcome after a significant duration of exposure to a patient interactive device compared to another similar device. One study did examine in a crossover design in infants with respiratory distress syndrome the effect of pressure-support ventilation plus volume guarantee, a volume targeted form of ventilation. Results of measurements of end expiratory volume and of minute ventilation are shown Figs. 31-10 and 31-11 (57). No obvious improvement could be detected in VE, a/A, or EEV when PCO_2 was controlled.

The ability to reduce assisted ventilatory support in a controlled manner with patient-interaction devices is improved compared to that with ventilator models available previously. Decremental changes in back-up rate, PIP and FiO_2 can be accomplished smoothly and cumulatively reduce the reliance on the "trial-and-error" approach to reduction in ventilatory support necessary with older generation devices. One established adjunctive therapy for VLBW infants is the use of methylxanthine therapy with discontinuation of assisted ventilation. Routine use of this medical therapy reduces the need for reintubation and reintroduction of assisted ventilation (58).

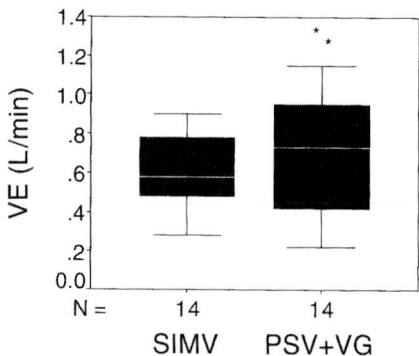

Figure 31-10 The relationship between the VE and the mode of ventilation (SIMV or PSV + VG). The difference between the two modes is significant (*p = 0.012). From Olsen SL, Thibeault DW, Truog WE. Crossover trial comparing pressure support with synchronized intermittent mandatory ventilation. *J Perinatol* 2002;22: 461, with permission.

Pressure-Regulation vs. Volume Guidance

It is helpful to think of current modes of conventional rate assisted ventilation as either pressure-controlled or volume targeted (59). The reintroduction of volume-controlled ventilation after unsuccessful use of this modality in the 1970s allows more choices after decades of pressure- and time-controlled neonatal ventilation. Some adjunctive features of volume-control ventilation include variable and limited Ti, decelerating inspiratory flow rates and patient-ventilator interaction. They can provide variable pressure support to maintain relatively constant minute ventilation. During pressure-controlled assisted breathing, there can also be pressure-support breaths—pressure once generated is constant during Ti but flow is decelerating. In summary, availability of many choices within the realm of conventional rate assisted ventilation allows greater individualization of assistance between patients and in the same patient during different stages of pulmonary insufficiency. However, definitive evidence of improvement in mortality or of decrease in clinically important morbidity with these new tools, compared to older modes of assisted ventilation, is lacking.

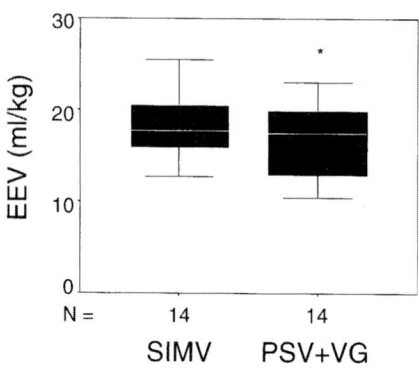

Figure 31-11 The relationship between the EEV and the model of ventilation (SIMV or PSV + VG). The difference between the two modes is significant (*P = 0.011). From Olsen SL, Thibeault DW, Truog WE. Crossover trial comparing pressure support with synchronized intermittent mandatory ventilation. *J Perinatol* 2002; 22:461, with permission.

High-Frequency Ventilation

Principles of Use

High-frequency ventilation (HFV) is defined as the use of small tidal volumes at supraphysiologic rates to provide oxygenation and ventilation. It generally refers to the use of rates above 150 breaths per minute. In some cases, V_T is less than the dead space. Thus, the mechanisms of high-frequency ventilation differ from the conventional combination of conduction and diffusion. This mode can still achieve adequate gas exchange. Many theoretical and experimental studies have demonstrated that a number of convective and diffuse mechanisms act in concert to affect gas transport during high-frequency ventilation (Fig. 31-12) (60). There is augmented mixing of gas in the airways, through increased energy of the gas molecules at high ventilator frequencies and high flows. The end result is that

fresh gas reaches the alveoli. Various patterns of high-frequency ventilation are illustrated in Fig. 31-13 (61).

The major advantage of high-frequency ventilation seems to be its potential to prevent some deleterious consequences of mechanical ventilation. When used in animal models with a strategy of optimizing lung inflation. High-frequency oscillatory ventilation (HFOV) improved gas exchange and lung mechanics, promoted uniform inflation, reduced air leak, and decreased the concentration of inflammatory mediators in the lung, as compared with conventional mechanical ventilation (62,63). Attempts have been made to differentiate high-frequency ventilators based on several ventilator-specific factors (Table 31-7) (61). The distinction among the types of high-frequency ventilators may be relevant to the appropriate matching of any one type of high-frequency ventilator to a particular part of the natural history of a neonatal pulmonary disorder.

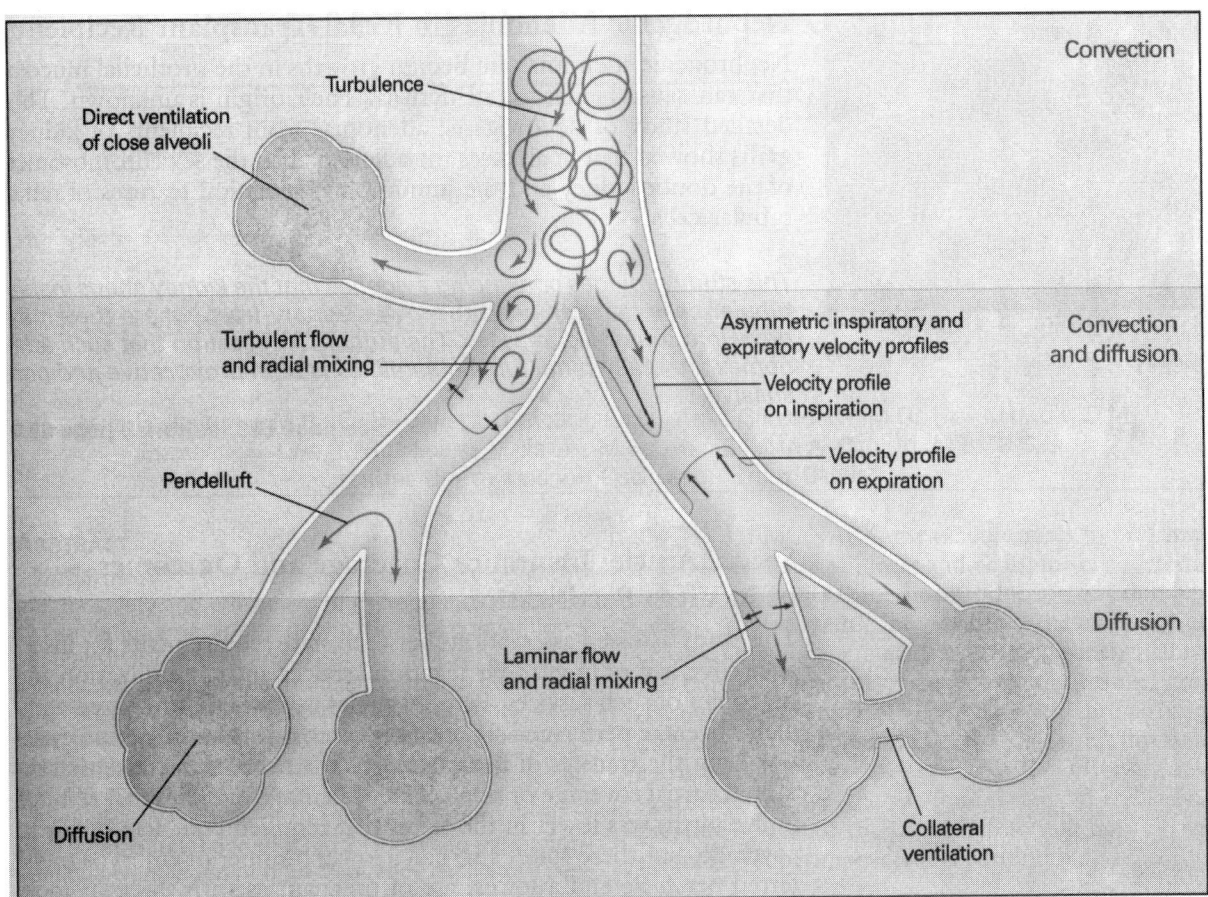

Figure 31-12 Gas-Transport Mechanisms During High-Frequency Ventilation. The major gas-transport mechanisms that are operative under physiologic conditions in each region (convection, convection and diffusion, and diffusion alone) are shown. There are seven potential mechanisms that can enhance gas transport during high-frequency ventilation: turbulence in the large airways, causing enhanced mixing; direct ventilation of close alveoli; turbulent flow with lateral convective mixing; pendelluft (asynchronous flow among alveoli as a result of asymmetries in airflow impedance); gas mixing as a result of velocity profiles that are axially asymmetric (leading to the streaming of "fresh" gas toward the alveoli along the inner wall of the airway and the streaming of "alveolar" gas away from the alveoli along the outer wall); laminar flow with lateral transport by diffusion (Taylor dispersion); and collateral ventilation through nonairway connections between neighboring alveoli. From Slutsky AS, Drazen JM. Perspective. Ventilation with small tidal volumes. *N Engl J Med* 2002; 347(9):630, with permission.

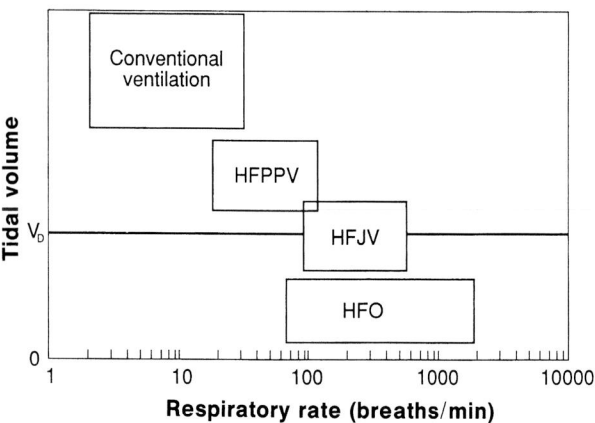

Figure 31-13 Respiratory rate vs. tidal volume. HFJV, high-frequency jet ventilation; HFO, high-frequency oscillation; HFPPV, high-frequency positive-pressure ventilation. From Slutsky AS. Nonconventional methods of ventilation. *Am Rev Respir Dis* 1988; 138:175, with permission.

Ventilation Devices and Their Indications

Three main types of high-frequency ventilators are used to treat neonates: high-frequency jet ventilators (HFJV), high-frequency flow interrupters (HFFI), and HFOV. These devices differ both in the way they generate HFV breaths and in the parameters that can be adjusted to control ventilation and oxygenation (Table 31-7).

High-Frequency Jet Ventilation

High-frequency jet ventilators are designed for the delivery of high-flow, short-duration pulses of pressurized gas directly into the upper airway through a specifically designed endo-tracheal tube lumen. These systems operate at rates of 150 to 600 breaths/min. Exhalation is passive. Effective tidal volumes are greater than the anatomic dead space. The ventilator is servocontrolled and operates to maintain a constant pressure at the endotracheal tube tip. The technique of high-frequency jet ventilation has been investigated to determine its efficacy in the management of VLBW infants to reduce mortality or the development of chronic lung disease in this population (64,65). Using chronic lung disease as a outcome variable is difficult in any study because of the multiple confounding factors that may develop (66).

The current status of jet ventilation as a primary mode of support for low-birth-weight infants is unclear. Keszler and associates (65) conducted a multicenter study in which 130 patients were enrolled. Half were treated with HFJV and half were treated with a continuation of conventional mechanical ventilation (nonsynchronized intermittent ventilation). Virtually all the infants had been treated with exogenous surfactant. Mortality and need for ventilatory support at 28 days of life were the same in the two groups, but there was a reduction from 40% to 20% for continuing respiratory support at 36 weeks postconceptional age among infants treated with high-frequency ventilation. This study also showed the HFJV was superior to tidal ventilation for preventing pulmonary interstitial emphysema. It is interesting to note that the 28-day BPD rate and the survival rate were comparable to that found 10 years earlier in a study comparing HFOV with conventional ventilation in infants without prior delivery of surfactant (67). These encouraging results are contrasted with another prospective randomized study in a comparable but smaller population of VLBW infants (68). In that study with HFJV there was an increased risk of adverse outcomes, defined as large intraventricular hemorrhage, periventricular leukomalacia, or

TABLE 31-7

HIGH-FREQUENCY VENTILATORS

	Flow Interruption	Jet Ventilator	Oscillatory Ventilators	
Commercially available device	Infant Star (Infrasonics, San Diego, CA)	Bunnell Life Pulse (Bunnell, Salt Lake City, UT	Sensormedics (Sensormedics, Anaheim, CA)	Draeger Babylog 8000 plus (Draeger Medical Inc, Telford, PA)
Indications	Failure of conventional ventilation in VLBW infants; PIE	PIE; intractable air leak; failure of conventional ventilation	Primary or rescue treatment of respiratory failure; prevention of ECMO	
Variables	Rate of conventional breaths; frequency of high-frequency	Variable inspiratory "on-time" rate of 240–600 beats/min	Rate; mean airway pressure; I—E ratio	Can be used as continuous flow, pressure limited, time cycled ventilator or as HFOV*, with flow and volume monitoring
Use with conventional ventilation	Yes	Yes	No	
Expiratory phase	Passive (?)	Passive	Active	Passive (conventional vent.)/active (HFOV)
Special precautions	>2 kg; no published trials	Sudden decrease in PCO$_2$; respiratory alkalosis	Sudden decrease in PCO$_2$; respiratory alkalosis	

* HFOV is not available in the USA

death. No difference in incidence of chronic lung disease was noted. The finding of leukomalacia had been previously associated with hypocarbia produced by treatment with HFJV during the first 3 days of life (68), although no cause-and-effect relationship could be established.

Hybrid Patterns of Ventilation

A hybrid device combining elements of jet and flow interruption to generate high-frequency ventilation, coupled with low-rate conventional ventilation, is available (Infrasonics, San Diego, CA). This device is operated at 10 to 15 Hz, with pauses in the high-frequency ventilator operation during the conventional breath inspiratory phase of ventilation. When operated in its mixed conventional and high-frequency mode, this device generates high-pressure, short, and nonvariable inspiratory flow with a variable shut-off phase, allowing passive lung deflation. One attractive feature is the minimal patient disturbance involved in changing from high-frequency to conventional forms of ventilation. No published study has demonstrated that this device offers any significant advantage as primary or rescue therapy compared to other types of high-frequency ventilation.

High-Frequency Oscillatory Ventilation

HFOV differs from the other two types by delivering smaller tidal volumes at higher rates and has an active expiratory phase. The Sensormedics 3100A high-frequency ventilator (Sensormedics, Anaheim, CA) has an additional feature of operating with an independently adjustable T_I. This device has been licensed for use for primary initial treatment of assisted ventilation and for alternative therapy in intractable respiratory failure unresponsive to conventional mechanical ventilation in neonates. The oscillating movement of the diaphragm causes active inspiratory and expiratory phases that drive the mixing of gas (Fig. 31-14). The amplitude of the pressure wave (measured as "delta pressure") is proportional to the tidal volume of the breath being delivered to the patient, and is adjusted to manipulate changes in ventilation. The mean airway pressure affects oxygenation, by changing the rate of gas flow into the circuit and the resistance to the gas flow out the expiratory side of the circuit (69).

Several prospective, randomized, controlled studies have been conducted using different types of HFOV (47–49,67,70–73) compared to conventional ventilation. The rationale for the postulated superiority of HFOV was that diminished distending pressures, combined with more adequate recruitment of and maintenance of lung volume, would be associated with fewer dysplastic cellular changes of the lung and less frequent or milder BPD. Cumulatively, these studies provide evidence that HFOV can be used safely and effectively in a wide variety of newborn infants, although its effectiveness as rescue therapy is still debated (74,75).

One question raised, but not answered, by clinical studies of HFOV is the potential benefit gained by its application at birth. Two studies using premature primate models of RDS demonstrated improved gas exchange if HFOV was used without any prior conventional mechanical ventilation (76,77). Jackson and associates (76) found decreased proteinaceous alveolar edema and improved gas exchange after 6 hours of HFOV applied from the first breath. However, all animals in both treatment groups had evidence of pulmonary cellular injury. The finding of both short-term benefit and concomitant cellular damage implies that HFOV used from birth could still be associated with significant lung injury. These findings are consistent with those of Solimano and associates (78), who showed that fluid and protein leaks in preterm lambs still occurred, although HFOV was applied from the first breath after delivery.

A possible second indication for high-frequency ventilation is to preclude the need for more invasive pulmonary support with extracorporeal membrane oxygenation (ECMO). Studies enrolling patients eligible for ECMO demonstrated that approximately one-half responded favorably to HFOV and did not need ECMO (79,80). Most babies responding to high-frequency ventilation were larger infants suffering from severe RDS. Other acute pulmonary disorders, such as meconium aspiration pneumonia with severe airway obstructive changes as shown by chest radiography, may not respond as well to oscillatory ventilation. Kinsella and associates (81) showed that the delivery of inhaled nitric oxide (INO), in association with HFOV, produced an improved outcome compared to either conventional ventilation with nitric oxide (NO) or HFOV alone. There was a reduced need for ECMO, especially in near-term infants with RDS or meconium aspiration syndrome (Fig. 31-15). The synergistic effect of these two treatment modalities may help reduce dependence on invasive ECMO support in this group of fragile term infants.

Two large contemporary trials comparing high-frequency oscillatory ventilation and conventional ventilation in preterm infants at high risk were done in the United Kingdom (49) and in the United States (48). The results of the study by Johnson and associates (49) (that enrolled infants with a gestational age of 23 to 28 weeks, assigned either to HFOV (n = 400) or to conventional ventilation

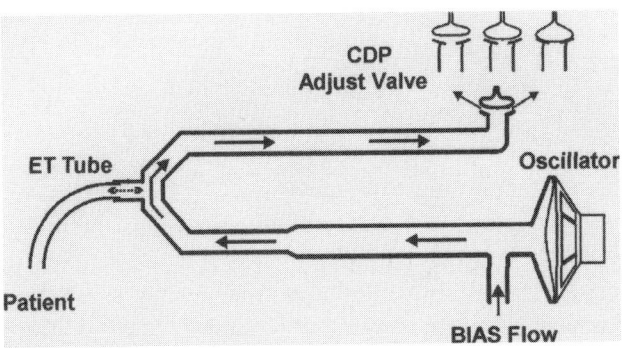

Figure 31-14 HFOV Principle.

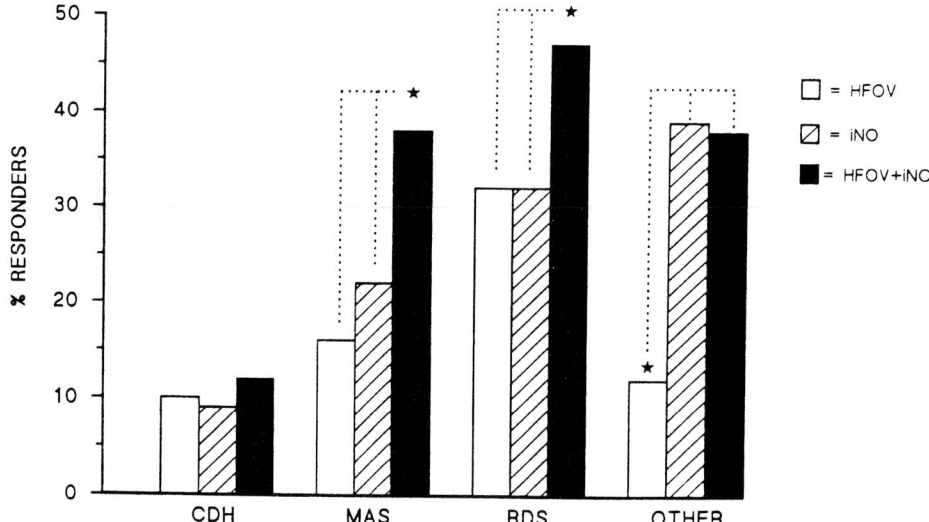

Figure 31-15 Percentage of patients responding to high-frequency oscillatory ventilation (HFOV); inhaled nitric oxide (INO); or combined HFOV plus INO by disease category. More patients with RDS or MAS responded to combination therapy with HFOV plus INO than to either treatment alone. Response to INO during conventional ventilation was more effective than response to HFOV in patients without significant lung disease ("other" category). Asterisk indicates $p < 0.05$. From Kinsella JP, Truog WE, Walsh WF, et al. Randomized, multicenter trial of INO and high-frequency oscillatory ventilation in severe, persistent pulmonary hypertension of the newborn. *J Pediatr* 1997;130:55, with permission.

($n = 397$)) were similar to those of a previous recent trial that also showed no difference between the modes of ventilation (47); the combined primary outcome, death or chronic lung disease (BPD), occurred in approximately two thirds of the infants, and similar proportions of infants in the two treatment groups survived without BPD. In contrast, Courtney and associates (48) found that in infants with birth weight of 601 to 1200 g, high-frequency oscillatory ventilation conferred a small but significant benefit in survival without bronchopulmonary dysplasia (56% vs. 47%; $p = 0.046$). Infants assigned to HFOV ($n = 234$) had a lower rate of pulmonary hemorrhage, a slightly higher rate of pulmonary interstitial emphysema, and were successfully extubated one week earlier compared to infants assigned to synchronized intermittent mandatory ventilation ($n = 250$). Neither trial showed an increased incidence of intracranial abnormalities or risk for air leak, two previously described complications (82,83).

There are differences between the designs of both trials that could explain the different results. However, the majority of available evidence suggests that in the usual clinical circumstances, the choice of the mode of ventilation does not affect the pulmonary outcome, which may be influenced more by prenatal risk factors, initial resuscitation, and other aspects of neonatal care (84).

Complications of Assisted Ventilation

Airway-Associated Problems

Acute and chronic complications of mechanical ventilation may develop in neonates. All patients with tracheal intubation demonstrate some degree of mucosal injury, usually squamous metaplasia or mucosal necrosis. In most infants, there seems to be spontaneous healing without significant sequelae. Hoarseness and stridor often occur after prolonged intubation but usually resolve in a few days. Persistent lesions, including laryngomalacia and subglottic stenosis, may develop in some patients occasionally requiring tracheostomy. Duration of intubation, pressure from oversized tubes, inadequate humidification, and airway pressure produced by the ventilator contribute to the development of laryngotracheal lesions.

The duration of intubation is dictated by the need for continued ventilatory support. In some infants requiring lengthy assisted ventilation tracheostomy may facilitate development of normal feeding patterns and social interaction and bypass already traumatized areas of the upper airway. However, infant tracheostomy itself is associated with a significant morbidity and mortality (85,86). Complications can include fatal loss of airway after accidental extrusion of the tube, paratracheal soft tissue infection, severe paratracheal air leak resulting in inadequate generation of PIP, and tracheal cartilage softening, making decannulation difficult. A bedside evaluation of the airway using flexible fiberoptic endoscopy can be helpful in assessing need for additional, more invasive procedures (87).

Pulmonary Air Leak Complications

Pulmonary air leak may occur as a complication of any of the life-threatening disorders of the newborn or as a result of their treatment. The air leak may take the form of pulmonary interstitial emphysema, pneumomediastinum, pneumoperitoneum, pneumopericardium, or pneumothorax. Pneumopericardium and pneumothorax occurring during positive-pressure ventilation require immediate treatment by evacuation of the free air.

Pneumothorax must be considered if there is abrupt worsening of the respiratory or circulatory status of an infant at risk. Unilateral hyperresonance, decreased breath sounds, a shift of the apical cardiac impulse, and skin mottling are useful clinical clues. High-intensity illumination may demonstrate the presence of a pneumothorax if the room can be adequately darkened. A definite diagnosis often can be made only by radiographic examination. The volume of the extrapulmonary air collection is not always a valid indication of tension. Interstitial emphysema, often a precursor of pneumothorax, causes the lung to remain partly expanded, even when intrapleural pressure is high. Bilateral pneumothorax may lead rapidly to death and must always be considered in cases of severe deterioration.

Pneumothorax in otherwise asymptomatic infants often resolves without therapy. However, marked mediastinal shift, coexisting pulmonary disease, or use of mechanical ventilation indicates a need for evacuation of the air. Aspiration with a syringe and needle may be done as an emergency procedure but is rarely adequate by itself and should be followed with tube thoracostomy.

Thoracostomy tubes should be sterile and made of nonreactive rubber or plastic. The wall thickness should be sufficient to prevent kinking, and the lumen should be large enough to prevent occlusion by exudate. The presence of at least two holes in the tube reduces the likelihood of occlusion by tissue. Polyvinylchloride feeding tubes or 8Fr (2.6 mm) to 10Fr (3.3 mm) catheters are suitable for thoracostomy use. The tube is inserted by grasping the tip with a clamp and pressing through a previously made incision through the pleura. The catheter is inserted after a skin incision has been made and can be Z-tracked over a rib for a better seal. Catheters with a trocar within the lumen often require considerable force to insert, and puncture of the lung and liver has been reported with their use.

The thoracostomy tube is connected to continuous suction at a negative pressure of 10 to 15 cm H_2O with an underwater seal. A chest radiograph should be obtained soon after thoracostomy. If the pneumothorax has not been evacuated, the infant should be repositioned and the tube stripped or, if necessary, a second tube should be inserted.

A thoracostomy tube is left in place until air ceases to bubble from the tube and until the risk of recurrent pneumothorax is reduced (i.e., until respiratory distress has subsided or mechanical ventilation is no longer required). The tube is then clamped. If there is neither clinical nor radiographic evidence of recurrent pneumothorax, the thoracostomy tube can be removed.

Liquid Ventilation

One experimental approach to reducing the lung injury associated with gas ventilation is liquid ventilation. Lung injury may be the result of abnormal inflation patterns produced because of elevated alveolar surface tension. Liquid inflation of the lungs with saline eliminates the alveolar gas–lung liquid interface with its tendency to induce collapse and perhaps injury. However, saline is too poor a carrier of oxygen to supply the body. Liquid perfluorocarbon solutions are able to dissolve large volumes of oxygen and carbon dioxide at 1 atm. Perfluorocarbon solutions have been used as carriers for O_2 and CO_2 in moribund human infants (88).

Two methods of liquid ventilation are being tested. The first is total liquid ventilation, which uses a completely perfluorocarbon-filled ventilator circuit, and a membrane oxygenator to prime the inspired liquid flow. The second is perfluorocarbon-assisted gas exchange, in which a portion of the lung volume, the EEV, is filled with perfluorocarbon liquids and the lungs are ventilated with a conventional infant mechanical ventilator. Liquid ventilation is an attractive form of pulmonary rescue therapy because the perfluorocarbons seem to be nontoxic and the technique is less invasive than ECMO. Definitive trials in neonates are yet to be reported.

MANAGEMENT IN THE INTENSIVE CARE SETTING

Management of respiratory problems requires specialized personnel working effectively as a team and specialized equipment. A physician skilled in neonatal intensive care techniques should be available within the unit at all times, and other specialists should be immediately accessible for consultation.

Nurses must be carefully trained in the techniques for the intensive care of infants. Necessary skills include application of ventilatory support equipment, recognition of equipment malfunction, airway management, assessment of ventilation, and use of monitoring equipment. Respiratory therapists are critical to the effective use of respiratory equipment. Maintenance and calibration of all oxygen administration and oxygen-measuring devices require the presence of a respiratory therapist within the hospital at all times.

Equipment needs for neonatal intensive care include wall sources of compressed air and oxygen, oxygen dilutors, heating and humidification devices, and oxygen-monitoring systems with alarms. Critically ill infants need continuous monitoring of temperature, respiratory rate, and heart rate by electrical devices with alarm systems. In the acute phase of illness, or if an umbilical or peripheral arterial catheter is in use, blood pressure monitoring and electrocardiographic display must be available.

The parents of severely ill infants need understanding and support. They experience feelings of anxiety, fear, guilt, and hostility. Most families are ill equipped for the unexpected emotional and financial burden imposed by the child's hospitalization. A social worker should be available exclusively to the neonatal intensive care unit to provide assistance to parents by delineating parental concerns and helping coordinate communication with the medical and nursing staff and other hospital personnel.

The physical design of the intensive care unit must facilitate the management of acute respiratory problems. Each patient area should be large enough to accommodate the necessary personnel and the enormous amount of equipment, without generating intolerable crowding. A small number of patients in each area of the nursery facilitates parental visits and alleviates the overall level of stress. The proliferation of monitors and alarms may result in monitor fatigue, with the risk that monitors are ignored. Although neonatology is often thought of as an acute care specialty, it more accurately is categorized as a chronic care specialty, because of the many days and weeks of specialized care that small, sick infants require. The physical design of intensive care units is catching up to that new reality.

Adequate attention paid to these ancillary features of intensive respiratory care of the newborn helps ensure the optimal outcome expected for critically ill infants.

REFERENCES

1. Tin W. Oxygen therapy: 50 years of uncertainty. *Pediatrics* 2002;110(3):615.
2. The STOP-ROP Multicenter Study Group. Supplemental therapeutic oxygen for prethreshold retinopathy of prematurity (STOP-ROP), a randomized, controlled trial. I. Primary outcomes. *Pediatrics* 2000;105:295.
3. Askie L, Henderson-Smart D, Irwig L, et al. The effect of differing oxygen saturation targeting ranges on long term growth and development of extremely preterm, oxygen dependent infants: the BOOST trial. *Pediatr Res* 2002;51:378(abst).
4. Chow LC, Wright KW, the CSMC Oxygen Administration Study Group, et al. Can changes in clinical practice decrease the incidence of severe retinopathy of prematurity in very low birth weight infants? *Pediatrics* 2003;111(2):339.
5. Schulze A, Whyte RK, Way RC, et al. Effect of the arterial oxygenation level on cardiac output, oxygen extraction, and oxygen consumption in low birth weight infants receiving mechanical ventilation. *J Pediatr* 1995;126(5):777.
6. Benaron DA, Benitz WE. Maximizing the stability of oxygen delivered via nasal cannula. *Arch Pediatr Adolesc Med* 1994;148(3):294.
7. Dunn PM. Localization of the umbilical catheter by post-mortem measurement. *Arch Dis Child* 1966;41:69.
8. Jackson JK, Biondo DJ, Kilbride H, et al. Can an alternative umbilical arterial catheter solution and flush regimen decrease iatrogenic hemolysis while enhancing nutrition? *Ped Res* 2002;51(4):373A.
9. Cassady G. Transcutaneous monitoring in the newborn infant. *J Pediatr* 1983;103:837.
10. Peabody JL, Gregory GA, Willis MM. Transcutaneous oxygen tension in sick infants. *Am Rev Respir Dis* 1978;118:83–87.
11. Hay WW Jr, Brockway J, Eyzaquirre M. Neonatal pulse oximetry: accuracy and reliability. *Pediatrics* 1989;83:717.
12. Hay WW, Thilo E, Curlander JB. Pulse oximetry in neonatal medicine. *Clin Perinatol* 1991;18:441.
13. Epstein MF, Cohen AR, Feldman HA, et al. Estimation of $PaCO_2$ by two noninvasive methods in the critically ill newborn infants. *J Pediatr* 1985;106:282.
14. McEvedy BAB, McLeod ME, Kirpalani H, et al. End-tidal carbon dioxide measurement in critically ill neonates: a comparison of sidestream and mainstream monitors. *Can J Anaesth* 1990;37:322.
15. Rozycki HJ, Sysyn GD, Marshall MK, et al. Mainstream end-tidal carbon dioxide monitoring in the neonatal intensive care unit. *Pediatrics* 1998;101(4 Pt 1):648.
16. Laffey JG, Kavanagh BP. Hypocapnia. *N Engl J Med* 2002;347(1):43.
17. Garland JS, Buck RK, Allred EN, et al. Hypocarbia before surfactant therapy appears to increase bronchopulmonary dysplasia

risk in infants with respiratory distress syndrome. *Arch Pediatr Adolesc Med* 1995;149:617.
18. Wiswell TE, Graziani LJ, Kornhauser MS, et al. Effects of hypocarbia on the development of cystic periventricular leukomalacia in premature infants treated with high-frequency jet ventilation. *Pediatrics* 1996;98:918.
19. Wyatt JS, Edwards AD, Cope M, et al. Response of cerebral blood volume to changes in arterial carbon dioxide tension in preterm and term infants. *Pediatr Res* 1991;29:553.
20. Kraybill EN, Runyan DK, Bose CL, et al. Risk factors for chronic lung disease in infants with birth weights of 751–1000 grams. *J Pediatr* 1989;115:115.
21. Poets CF, Sari B. Change in intubation rates and outcome of very low birthweight infants: a population-based study. *Pediatrics* 1996;98:24.
22. Verder H, Robertson B, Greisen G, et al. Surfactant therapy and nasal continuous positive airway pressure for newborns with respiratory distress syndrome. *N Engl J Med* 1994;331:1051.
23. Martin RJ, Nearman HS, Katona PG, et al. The effect of a low continuous positive pressure on the reflex control of respiration in preterm infants. *J Pediatr* 1977;90:976.
24. Miller MJ, Waldeman AC, Martin RJ. Continuous positive airway pressure selectively reduces obstructive apnea in preterm infants. *J Pediatr* 1985;106:91.
25. Miller MJ, DiFiore JM, Strohl KP, et al. Effects of nasal CPAP on supraglottic and total pulmonary resistance in preterm infants. *J Appl Physiol* 1990;56:141.
26. Narendran V, Donovan EF, Hoath SB, et al. Early bubble CPAP and outcomes in ELBW preterm infants. *J Perinatol* 2003;24:195.
27. So BH, Tamura M, Kamoshita S. Nasal continuous positive airway pressure following surfactant replacement for the treatment of neonatal respiratory distress syndrome. *Acta Paediatr* 1994;35:280.
28. So BH, Tamura M, Mishima J, et al. Application of nasal continuous positive airway pressure to early extubation in very low birth-weight infants. *Arch Dis Child* 1994;72:F191.
29. Annibale DJ, Halsey TC, Engstrom PC, et al. Randomized controlled trial of nasopharyngeal continuous positive airway pressure in the extubation of very low birthweight infants. *J Pediatr* 1994;124:455.
30. Tapia JL, Bancalari A, Gonzalez A, et al. Does continuous positive airway pressure (CPAP) during weaning from intermittent mandatory ventilation in very low birth weight infants have risks or benefits? A controlled trial. *Pediatr Pulmon* 1995;19:269.
31. Khalaf MN, Brodsky N, Hurley J, et al. A prospective randomized, controlled trial comparing synchronized nasal intermittent positive ventilation versus nasal continuous postive airway pressure as modes of extubation. *Pediatrics* 2001;108(1):13.
32. Angus DC, Linde-Zwirble WT, Clermont G, et al. Epidemiology of neonatal respiratory failure in the United States. Projections from California and New York. *Am J Respir Crit Care Med* 2001;164:1154.
33. Dreyfuss D, Saumon G. Ventilator-induced lung injury. *Am J Respir Crit Care Med* 1998;157:294.
34. Thibeault DW, Lang MJ. Mechanisms and pathobiologic effects of barotrauma. In: Merritt TA, Northway WH Jr, Boynton BR, eds. *Bronchopulmonary dysplasia. Contemporary issues in fetal nenoatal medicine.* Boston: Blackwell Scientific , 1988;82.
35. Thibeault DW, Mabry SM, Ekekezie II, et al. Lung elastic tissue maturation and perturbations during the evolution of chronic lung disease. *Pediatrics* 2000;106(6):1452.
36. Thibeault DW, Mabry SM, Ekekezie II, et al. Collagen scaffolding during development and its deformation with chronic lung disease. *Pediatrics* 2003;11:766–776.
37. Thibeault DW, Truog WE, Ekekezie II. Acinar arterial changes with chronic lung disease of prematurity in the surfactant era. *Pediatr Pulm* 2003;36:482–489.
38. Rodenstein DO, Perlmutter N, Stanescu DC. Infants are not obligatory nasal breathers. *Am Rev Respir Dis* 1985;131:343.
39. Polgar G, Kong GP. The nasal resistance of newborn infants. *J Pediatr* 1965;67:557.
40. Wung JT, Stark FI, Indyk L, et al. Oxygen supplementation during endotracheal intubation of the infant. *Pediatrics* 1977;59:1046.
41. Fanconi S, Duc G. Intratracheal suctioning in sick preterm infants: prevention of intracranial hypertension and cerebral hypoperfusion by muscle paralysis. *Pediatrics* 1987;79:538.
42. Kelly MA, Finer NN. Nasotracheal intubation in the neonate: physiologic responses and effects of atropine and pancuronium. *J Pediatr* 1984;105:303.

43. Tochen ML. Orotracheal intubation in the newborn infant: a method for determining depth of tube insertion. *J Pediatr* 1979; 95:1050.

44. Kohelet D, Goldberg A, Goldberg M. Depth of endotracheal tube placement in neonates. *J Pediatr* 1982;101:157.

45. Tarnow-Mordi WO, Reid E, Griffiths P, et al. Low inspired gas temperature and respiratory complications in very low birth weight infants. *J Pediatr* 1989;114:438.

46. Golombek S, Truog WE. Acute effects of exogenous surfactant treatment in near term infants with RDS. *J Invest Med* 1995;43:463.

47. Thome U, Kossel H, Lipowsky G, et al. Randomized comparison of high-frequency ventilation with high-rate intermittent positive pressure ventilation in preterm infants with respiratory failure. *J Pediatr* 1999;135:39.

48. Courtney SE, Durand DJ, the Neonatal Ventilation Study Group, et al. High-frequency oscillatory ventilation versus conventional mechanical ventilation for very-low-birth-weight infants. *N Engl J Med* 2002;347(9):643.

49. Johnson AH, Peacock JL, the United Kingdom Oscillation Study Group, et al. High-frequency oscillatory ventilation for the prevention of chronic lung disease of prematurity. *N Engl J Med* 2002;347(9):633.

50. Stark AR, Davidson D. Inhaled nitric oxide for persistent pulmonary hypertension of the newborn: implication and strategy for future "high-tech" neonatal clinical trials. *Pediatrics* 1995;96(6): 1147.

51. Amitay M, Etches PC, Finer NN, et al. Synchronous mechanical ventilation of the neonate with respiratory disease. *Crit Care Med* 1993;21:118.

52. Donn SM, Sinha SK. Controversies in patient-triggered ventilation. *Clin Perinatol* 1998;25(1):49.

53. Cleary JP, Bernstein G, Mannino FL, et al. Improved oxygenation during synchronized intermittent mandatory ventilation in neonates with respiratory distress syndrome: a randomized, crossover study. *J Pediatr* 1995;126(3):407.

54. Hummler HD, Gerhardt T, Gonzalez A, et al. Patient-triggered ventilation in neonates: comparison of a flow-and an impedance-triggered system. *Am J Respir Crit Care Med* 1996;154:1049.

55. Castle RA, Dunne CJ, Mok Q, et al. Accuracy of displayed values of tidal volume in the pediatric intensive care unit. *Crit Care Med* 2002;30(11):2566.

56. Younes M, Puddy A, Roberts D, et al. Proportional assist ventilation, a new approach to ventilatory support. *Am Rev Resp Dis* 1992;145:114.

57. Olsen SL, Thibeault DW, Truog WE. Crossover trial comparing pressure support with synchronized intermittent mandatory ventilation. *J Perinatol* 2002;22:461.

58. Henderson-Smart DJ, Davis PG. Prophylactic methylaxanthines for extubation in preterm infants. *Cochrane Database Syst Rev* 2002.

59. Sinha SK, Donn SM. Volume-controlled ventilation. Variations on a theme. *Clin Perinatol* 2001;28(3):547.

60. Slutsky AS, Drazen JM. Perspective. Ventilation with small tidal volumes. *N Engl J Med* 2002;347(9):630.

61. Slutsky AS. Nonconventional methods of ventilation. *Am Rev Respir Dis* 1988;138:175–183.

62. Meredith KS, deLemos RA, Coalson JJ, et al. Role of lung injury in the pathogenesis of hyaline membrane disease in premature baboons. *J Appl Physiol* 1989;66:2150.

63. Yoder BA, Siler-Khodr T, Winter VT, et al. High-frequency oscillatory ventilation: effects on lung function mechanics, and airway cytokines in the immature baboon model for neonatal chronic lung diseases. *Am J Respir Crit Care Med* 2000;162:1867.

64. Keszler M, Donn SM, Bucciarelli RL, et al. Multi-center controlled trial comparing high-frequency jet ventilation and conventional mechanical ventilation in newborn infants with pulmonary interstitial emphysema. *J Pediatr* 1991;119:85.

65. Keszler M, Madanlou HD, Brudno DS, et al. Multicenter controlled clinical trial of high-frequency jet ventilation in preterm infants with uncomplicated respiratory distress syndrome. *Pediatrics* 1997;100:593.

66. Bhuta T, Henderson-Smart DJ. Elective high frequency jet ventilation versus conventional ventilation for respiratory distress syndrome in preterm infants (Cochrane Review). In: *The Cochrane Library*, Issue 2, 2003. Oxford: Update Software.

67. The HIFI Study Group. High-frequency oscillatory ventilation compared with conventional ventilation in the treat-ment of respiratory failure in preterm infants. *N Engl J Med* 1989; 320:88.

68. Wiswell TE, Graziani LJ, Kornhauser MS, et al. High-frequency jet ventilation in the early management of respiratory distress syndrome is associated with a greater risk for adverse outcomes. *Pediatrics* 1996;98:1035.

69. Durand DJ, Asselin JM. Physiology of high-frequency ventilation. In: Polin R, Fox WJ, eds. *Fetal and neonatal physiology*, 2nd ed. Philadelphia: WB Saunders, 1998.

70. Clark RH, Gerstmann DR, Null DM Jr, et al. Prospective randomized comparison of high-frequency oscillatory and conventional ventilation in respiratory distress syndrome. *Pediatrics* 1992;89:5.

71. Gerstmann DR, Minton SD, Stoddard RA, et al. Results of the Provo multicenter surfactant high frequency oscillatory ventilation controlled trial. *Pediatrics* 1996;98:1044.

72. HIFO Study Group. Randomized study of high frequency oscillatory ventilation in infants with severe respiratory distress syndrome. *J Pediatr* 1993;122:609.

73. Ogawa Y, Miyaska K, Kawano T, et al. A multicenter randomized trial of high frequency oscillatory ventilation as compared with conventional mechanical ventilation in preterm infants with respiratory failure. *Early Hum Dev* 1993;32:1.

74. Bhuta T, Clark RH, Henderson-Smart DJ. Rescue high frequency oscillatory ventilation vs. conventional ventilation for infants with severe pulmonary dysfunction born at or near term (Cochrane Review). In: The *Cochrane Library*, Issue 2, 2003. Oxford: Update Software.

75. Bhuta T, Henderson-Smart DJ. Rescue high frequency oscillatory ventilation versus conventional ventilation for pulmonary dysfunction in preterm infants (Cochrane Review). In: *The Cochrane Library*, Issue 2, 2003. Oxford: Update Software.

76. Jackson JC, Truog WE, Standaert TA, et al. Effect of high-frequency ventilation on the development of alveolar edema in premature monkeys at risk for hyaline membrane disease. *Am Rev Respir Dis* 1991;143:865–871.

77. Meredith KS, de Lemos RA, Coalson JJ, et al. Role of lung injury in the pathogenesis of hyaline membrane disease in premature baboons. *J Appl Physiol* 1989;66:2150.

78. Solimano A, Bryan C, Jobe A, et al. Effects of high-frequency and conventional ventilation on the premature lamb lung. *J Appl Physiol* 1985;59:1571.

79. Carter MJM, Gerstmann DR, Clark MRH, et al. High-frequency oscillatory ventilation and extracorporeal membrane oxygenation for the treatment of acute neonatal respiratory failure. *Pediatrics* 1990;85:159.

80. Clark RH, Yoder BA, Sell MS. Prospective, randomized comparison of high-frequency oscillation and conventional ventilation in candidates for extracorporeal membrane oxygenation. *J Pediatr* 1994;124:447.

81. Kinsella JP, Truog WE, Walsh WF, et al. Randomized, multicenter trial of inhaled nitric oxide and high-frequency oscillatory ventilation in severe, persistent pulmonary hypertension of the newborn. *J Pediatr* 1997;130:55.

82. Moriette G, Paris-Llado J, Walti H, et al. Prospective randomized multicenter comparison of high-frequency ventilation and conventional ventilation in preterm infants of less than 30 weeks with respiratory distress syndrome. *Pediatrics* 2001;107:363.

83. Henderson-Smart DJ, Bhuta T, Cools F, et al. Elective high-frequency oscillatory ventilation versus conventional ventilation for acute pulmonary dysfunction in preterm infants (Cochrane Review). In: *The Cochrane Library*, Issue 3. Oxford: Update Software, 2001.

84. Stark AR. High-frequency oscillatory ventilation to prevent bronchopulmonary dysplasia: are we there yet? *N Engl J Med* 2002; 347(9):682–683.

85. Massie RJ, Robertson CF, Berkowitz RG. Long-term outcome of surgically treated acquired subglottic stenosis in infancy. *Pediatr Pulmonol* 2000;30(2):125–130.

86. Kremer B, Botos-Kremer AI, Eckel HE, et al. Indications, complications, and surgical techniques for pediatric tracheostomies—an update. *J Pediatr Surg* 2002;37(11):1556–1562.

87. Downing GJ, Kilbride HW. Evaluation of airway complications in high-risk preterm infants: application of flexible fiberoptic airway endoscopy. *Pediatrics* 1995;95:567.

88. Leach CL, Greenspan JS, Rubenstein SD, et al. Partial liquid ventilation with perflubron in premature infants with severe respiratory distress syndrome. *N Engl J Med* 1996;335:761.

Extracorporeal Membrane Oxygenation

Billie Lou Short

In 1944 Kolff and Berk observed that blood became oxygenated as it passed through cellophane chambers of their artificial kidney membrane (1). This historic observation led to the recognition by those involved in the fast-developing field of cardiopulmonary bypass that blood could be oxygenated through a semipermeable membrane lung. In the bubble and disk oxygenators used during the early 1950s for open-heart surgery, oxygen and blood were mixed directly. This mixing resulted in considerable damage to blood products and the potential for producing lethal fibrin emboli, making these systems unsuitable for prolonged clinical use (2). For this reason, and in light of Kolff and Berk's findings, attention was directed to the development of semipermeable membrane oxygenators that separated blood and oxygen, decreasing or eliminating the risks of the earlier oxygenators.

The first membrane lung, which used an ethylcellulose membrane, was described by Clowes in 1956 and was used successfully in open-heart surgery 1 year later (3). With this report began the study of prolonged cardiopulmonary bypass and potential application of extracorporeal membrane oxygenation (ECMO) as an artificial lung.

The 1960s witnessed intensive research on materials and techniques (2). Silicone polymers, available in thin sheets that enhanced gas transfer through membranes, began to be characterized and developed. The development of the Kolobow silicone membrane lung made the field of ECMO possible, and clinical trials, using prolonged bypass or ECMO as an artificial lung, began in the late 1960s (2,4–6).

The concept of an artificial placenta, a device capable of continuing *ex utero* the gas-exchange functions of the placenta, developed in parallel with that of an artificial lung. In 1961 Callaghan and colleagues began using animal models of respiratory distress syndrome of the newborn to test the efficacy of an extracorporeal oxygenation circuit as an artificial placenta (7). During the early 1960s investigators, including Rashkind, White, Dorson, and Avery, used

ECMO as an artificial placenta for premature infants (8–10). Although the infants died, this was an extremely important period for the development and refinement of the mechanical and surgical techniques that laid the foundation for the subsequent success of ECMO.

It was not until ECMO therapy was applied to the term infant through the pioneering work of Bartlett and colleagues that its full potential as a powerful therapy for infants in severe respiratory failure was recognized. In 1976 Bartlett and his associates reported the first neonatal ECMO survivor, a term infant with severe meconium aspiration syndrome (MAS) (11). During the next 10 years, neonatal ECMO was used to treat 99 term infants with respiratory failure in three centers in the United States and produced an overall survival rate of 65%. Since 1986, ECMO therapy has developed explosively, and more than 19,000 infants have been treated in more than 90 ECMO programs, with an overall survival rate of 77% (12). ECMO is also being used to support the cardiac patient postoperatively and the older child in respiratory failure. This chapter will only address the use of ECMO in the neonatal patient in respiratory failure.

The most common use for ECMO is in the term or near-term infant with failure to oxygenate as a result of MAS, idiopathic persistent pulmonary hypertension (PPHN), congenital diaphragmatic hernia (CDH), sepsis and pneumonia, or hyaline membrane disease. Although overall survival is 77% nationally, the best results are for the MAS (94%) and PPHN (79%) groups (Table 32-1). In the last 3 years, the survival rate for the MAS patient at Children's National Medical Center in Washington, DC has been 100%, PPHN 94%, and sepsis/pneumonia 100%. So although new therapies such as inhaled nitric oxide (iNO) and high frequency ventilation (HFV) may be delaying the initiation of ECMO, it does not appear that they have affected survival (13). As with Gill and associates, the time at Children's National Medical Center on ECMO has increased from 5 days to 8.9 days with the initiation

TABLE 32-1
RESULTS OF EXTRACORPOREAL OXYGENATION[a]

Diagnosis	Survival After Therapy (%)
Meconium aspiration syndrome	94
Persistent pulmonary hypertension	79
Sepsis and pneumonia	75
Respiratory distress syndrome	84
Congenital diaphragmatic hernia	53
Total	77

[a] From the Extracorporeal Life Support Neonatal Registry, July 2003, 19,061 patients.

of these additional therapies pre-ECMO. At Children's National Medical Center, a 34- to 36-week gestation infant with respiratory failure has not been placed on ECMO in the last 3 years due to therapies such as surfactant therapy and HFV. The survival rate for the CDH population requiring ECMO has not increased over time and remains between 50% to 60% nationally, perhaps because of the heterogeneity of this group of infants, who have various degrees of pulmonary hypoplasia and pulmonary hypertension (14,15). Only 30% to 40% of the CDH population require ECMO therapy, and those patients not requiring ECMO have a survival rate close to 100%. Therefore, with ECMO therapy, the overall survival rate for the CDH population as a whole has increased to more than 70% and in some centers has been reported to be as high as 80% (16,17). Most centers are now repairing the diaphragmatic defect in the critical CDH either on ECMO or immediately post-ECMO (14).

INDICATIONS

Among the most controversial aspects of ECMO therapy have been the clinical criteria used to determine its use (18–26). Because of the invasive nature of ECMO therapy and the potential risks associated with this therapy, the criteria are designed to select a population of infants who have an 80% or greater mortality risk with conventional therapy. Assumptions about the ability of ECMO to increase survival are valid only if the criteria are specific for each high-risk population. The ultimate test for the efficacy of ECMO, and the predictive value of ECMO criteria, is a prospective, randomized trial. Although two randomized trials have been completed, most centers have used historic controls to develop their criteria (18,19,24,26). In the prospective, randomized trial reported by O'Rourke and colleagues, a crossover design was used, which may have skewed the predictions of their criteria. The criteria used in O'Rourke's study, which were thought to predict a mortality over 80% based on retrospective data, predicted a mortality of only 40% when used prospectively (24). It is imperative that all centers continually evaluate their criteria, especially as less invasive therapies become available.

The United Kingdom collaborative randomized trial did not involve a crossover design and therefore represents a more ideal trial for ECMO therapy (27). Of the 185 patients enrolled in the study, 93 were allocated to ECMO therapy and 92 to conventional therapy, which included high-frequency ventilation and iNO therapy. Mortality was significantly different between the ECMO and conventional groups, 32% versus 59% ($P = 0.0005$). This benefit of ECMO was sustained when severe disability at 1 year of age was taken into account ($P = 0.002$). The CDH population in this study had the highest mortality rate, 82% in the ECMO group and 100% in the conventional group. Severity of illness was also a predictor, with mortality higher in the patients with an oxygen index (OI) of 60 or greater at the time of entry into the study, indicating that early transfer of these patients to an ECMO center is essential. The authors also noted that mortality was lower if the referring hospital was a teaching hospital.

The potential risks associated with ECMO therapy include those associated with ligation of the carotid artery (in venoarterial ECMO) and jugular vein, prolonged exposure to systemic heparinization, alterations in pulsatile blood flow patterns, exposure to potential toxins such as phthalate esters (i.e., plasticizer) from the circuit, and others yet to be determined (28,29). With its long-term outcome still unknown, use of ECMO should be limited to the term or near-term infant who has a 20% or less chance of survival with conventional therapy. Although criteria developed at other centers are available, they are based on the clinical management and patient populations in those centers and may not be valid when applied to patients in other institutions (19,20,24). What is considered maximal conventional therapy (e.g., hyperventilation) in one institution may not be used in others. Differences in patient populations, such as the percentage of patients who are inborn versus outborn, may significantly alter applicability of criteria from one center to another. All ECMO centers should attempt to develop criteria based on their own management techniques and patient population.

Several important inclusion criteria for ECMO are based on known complications of the procedure. These are listed in Table 32-2.

Age and Weight Limitations

The requirement for systemic heparinization of the ECMO patient places significant limitations on the population

TABLE 32-2
INCLUSION CRITERIA FOR EXTRACORPOREAL MEMBRANE OXYGENATION

Gestational age ≥34 weeks or birth weight ≥2,000 g
No uncontrolled bleeding complications
No major intracranial hemorrhage, e.g., not greater than grade II
Mechanical ventilation provided for 10 to 14 days
Reversible lung disease

that can be treated. Use of ECMO in the late 1960s and early 1970s in premature infants weighing less than 2,000 grams or younger than 34 weeks of gestation resulted in a significant mortality rate from intracranial hemorrhage (ICH) (30–32). This increased risk may be a result of the combination of systemic heparinization with a more direct effect of ECMO on the brain (33,34). Data from a review of the premature infant treated with ECMO by Hirschl and colleagues indicates that the ICH rate in the infant down to 32 weeks of gestation is lower than previously noted (35). Although the ICH rate is lower in infants at 32 to 33 weeks of gestation than in the earlier experience with this group, the rate is still close to 50%; thus, if one is considering ECMO therapy for this population, the information given to parents should appropriately address the high risk for ICH. A better understanding of the pathophysiology of the intracranial bleeds seen in the ECMO population may allow alteration of the risk for this complication and thus lower the gestational age cutoff in the future (33,34).

Hematologic Limitations

The requirement for systemic heparinization places the infant with a significant coagulopathy or with bleeding complications at extreme risk. All attempts should be made to correct any coagulopathy before instituting ECMO.

The septic infant is of particular concern because of the commonly associated coagulopathy. Although these infants are at an increased risk for bleeding complications on ECMO, correction of their coagulopathy and meticulous heparin management have resulted in successful treatment (36).

The necessity for heparinization during ECMO precludes the treatment of any infant with a major ICH. Infants with grade I to II intraventricular hemorrhages or small parenchymal hemorrhages can be treated if heparin management is monitored closely and activated clotting times (ACTs) are kept low (e.g., 160 to 180 seconds).

Prior Mechanical Ventilation

The limit of 10 to 14 days of assisted ventilation before ECMO therapy is imposed because of the probable development of chronic lung disease after aggressive assisted ventilation of this duration. ECMO is unable to reverse this disease process within a safe period. After 3 weeks of ECMO, the risks for complications related to the ECMO procedure itself, such as clot formation, nosocomial infections (e.g., neck wound infections), and mechanical failures (e.g., tubing ruptures), begin to increase. The maximal time that a neonatal patient can be kept on the ECMO circuit is unknown, but in view of the increasing risk of complications and usual lack of response beyond this time period, most centers limit time on the circuit to around 3 weeks. Infants with diseases, such as chronic lung disease, that do not improve in a short period should not be considered for ECMO unless there is a life-threatening

underlying disease state, such as acute pulmonary hypertension or sepsis/pneumonia, that can be rapidly reversed by ECMO.

Cardiopulmonary Disease

Candidates for ECMO must have reversible lung disease. Because of the cardiopulmonary support provided by this therapy, ECMO has allowed many infants thought to have irreversible lung disease to live. The diagnosis of irreversible lung disease has become progressively more difficult to make (14,37,38).

Significant cardiac disease must be ruled out before ECMO, but infants with severe reversible lung disease superimposed on congenital heart disease may be candidates for ECMO support before cardiac surgery.

Risk Assessment and Mortality Criteria

If the infant is failing maximal conventional therapy, ECMO should be considered. The next task is to predict which infants have a high mortality risk without ECMO.

Commonly used criteria (Table 32-3) are the alveolar–arterial oxygen gradient ($AaDO_2$), OI, and arterial partial pressure of oxygen (PaO_2) levels less than 50 mm Hg over a specific time period (19,20,23,39). The $AaDO_2$ can be calculated as follows:

$$AaDO_2 = P_B - 47 - PaCO_2 - PaO_2$$

when the fraction of inspired oxygen (FiO_2) is 1.00, P_B is the barometric pressure, 47 is the water vapor pressure, and $PaCO_2$ is the arterial carbon dioxide pressure. The OI can be calculated with the following equation:

$$OI = MAP \times FiO_2 \times 100/PaO_2$$

in which MAP is the mean airway pressure.

Deciding when to transfer an infant to an ECMO center is a difficult task. Most infants with disorders treated by ECMO improve without ECMO. Before the infant becomes too moribund for transport, the referring physician must attempt to determine which infants are at high risk for failing maximal conventional therapy. This is an enormous responsibility, which can be eased by early consultation

TABLE 32-3

NEONATAL EXTRACORPOREAL MEMBRANE OXYGENATION CRITERIA[a]

aaDO$_2$ 605–620 mm Hg[b] for 4 to 12 hr[b]
Oxygen index 35 to 60[b] for 0.5 to 6 hr[b]
PaO$_2$ 35 to 50[b] mm Hg for 2 to 12 hr[b]
pH <7.25 for 2 hr with hypotension
Acute deterioration PaO$_2$ <30 to 40 mm Hg

[a] Criteria used only after maximal therapy instituted; 50% of centers use more than one criterion.
AaDO$_2$, alveolar–arterial oxygen gradient; PaO$_2$, arterial partial pressure of oxygen.
[b] Represents the ranges used in various centers

with ECMO center personnel. Earlier studies by Boedy and associates (40) found that 12% of their ECMO referrals died before arrival of the transport team or during inter-hospital transport. Of importance, 32% of the deaths occurred in infants with CDH, indicating that early referral of these patients was warranted. This concern becomes even more important with the addition of therapies such as iNO. Centers providing iNO without ECMO capabilities need to have a close association with an ECMO center, so consultation can be obtained to determine when infants should be transported to the ECMO center (41,42).

The studies that are performed before transfer of a patient to an ECMO center include an echocardiogram to rule out heart disease; cranial ultrasound scan to rule out significant ICH; coagulation studies, including a partial thromboplastin time, prothrombin time, fibrinogen level, fibrin degradation products, and platelet count; calcium and electrolyte levels; leukocyte count with a differential analysis; and hemoglobin and hematocrit levels. These studies help the team at the ECMO center determine whether the patient should be considered for ECMO and if so, assist them in anticipating difficulties.

Once the patient is admitted to the ECMO center, it must be determined if the patient is an appropriate ECMO candidate. The ultrasound examination of the central nervous system (CNS) is repeated to ensure that an ICH did not occur during transport. The cardiac evaluation is repeated if there is any residual question about the possibility of cardiac disease. Doppler flow techniques are used to document the severity of pulmonary hypertension. This information can be used later if the infant does not wean from ECMO appropriately. Serum electrolyte and calcium levels; hemoglobin and hematocrit; clotting studies including fibrinogen level, fibrin degradation products, partial thromboplastin and prothrombin times; platelet count; and baseline ACT should be obtained on admission to detect abnormalities that require correction before ECMO.

Many ECMO candidates receive muscle relaxants before admission, making the neurologic status difficult to evaluate. It is imperative to obtain a complete perinatal history, including Apgar scores, resuscitation and seizure activity, and description of the neurologic status of the infant before paralysis. Infants who have sustained severe irreversible neurologic damage should not be considered for ECMO.

PROCEDURE

Venoarterial Method

Venoarterial (VA) ECMO involves the use of two catheters: the venous outflow catheter in the right internal jugular vein with the tip in the right atrium and the arterial return catheter in the right carotid artery with the tip at the junction with the aortic arch. Blood is removed through the jugular catheter by means of gravity drainage into a venous reservoir (Fig. 32-1). Blood is pulled out of the reservoir by

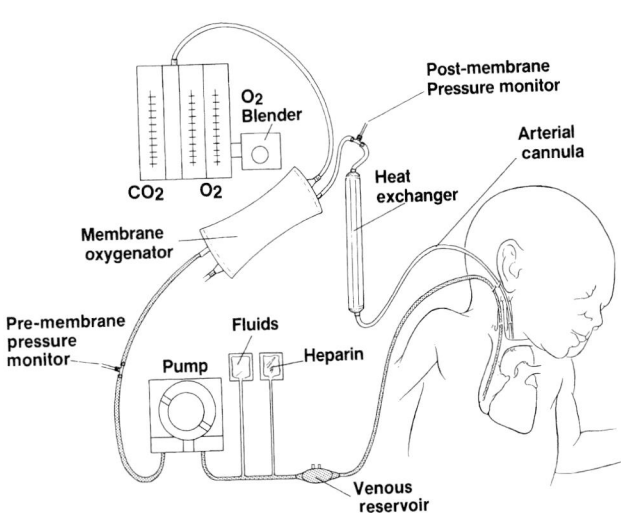

Figure 32-1 Components of the venoarterial extracorporeal membrane oxygenation circuit. (From Short BL. Physiology of extracorporeal membrane oxygenation (ECMO). In Polin RA, Fox WW, eds. *Fetal and neonatal physiology.* Philadelphia: WB Saunders, 1992:932, with permission.)

a roller occlusion pump and pushed through the membrane lung, where gas exchange occurs. Gas transfers across the silicone membrane lung into the blood because of pressure gradients, increasing the oxygen level and removing carbon dioxide (Fig. 32-2). Blood then enters the heat exchanger, where it is warmed to body temperature and returned to the infant through the arterial catheter.

This form of bypass provides pulmonary and cardiac support. Although most infants requiring ECMO have only a pulmonary disorder, some have cardiac dysfunction secondary to severe hypoxia and require the cardiac support that VA ECMO provides. Oxygenation is achieved by allowing the pump to support as much of the cardiac output as is needed to oxygenate the infant, usually 120 to 150 mL/kg/minute in the first few days.

It is easy to support and oxygenate with VA ECMO, and it remains the gold standard for ECMO therapy. However, ligation of the carotid artery, alteration of pulsatile arterial blood flow patterns, and the possibility that particles or air in the circuit may enter the cerebral or coronary circulation remain concerns.

Venovenous Method

Venovenous (VV) techniques for ECMO have been developed because of the concerns about carotid ligation. VV ECMO is currently achieved using a single double-lumen catheter placed through the internal jugular vein into the right atrium (Fig. 32-3) (43,44). This catheter has inflow and outflow ports that attach into the circuit. Because blood return and outflow happen in the right atrium, recirculation can occur, resulting in limited oxygenation with this technique (Fig. 32-4). Because the heart is the pump for VV ECMO, the use of this catheter depends on intact cardiac function (43,44). The advantages of this technique are the lack of necessity for ligation of the carotid artery,

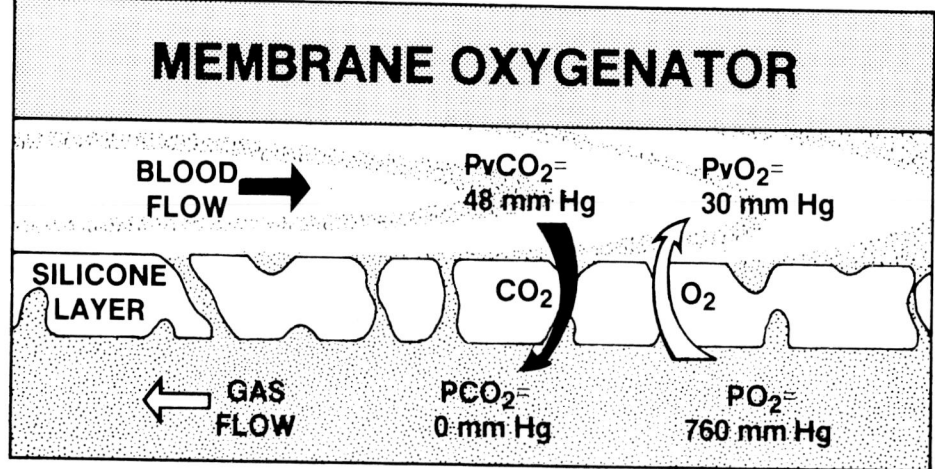

Figure 32-2 The silicone membrane lung promotes gas transfer across a gradient for oxygen and carbon dioxide. The pore size does not allow blood products to cross. PCO_2, carbon dioxide partial pressure; PO_2, oxygen pressure; $PvCO_2$, mixed venous carbon dioxide partial pressure; PvO_2, mixed venous oxygen partial pressure. (From Short BL. Physiology of extracorporeal membrane oxygenation (ECMO). In Polin RA, Fox WW, eds. *Fetal and neonatal physiology*. Philadelphia: WB Saunders, 1992:932, with permission.)

maintenance of normal pulsatile blood flow, and the theoretical advantage that particles entering the circuit enter the lungs rather than the cerebral or coronary circulation. Disadvantages are the lack of cardiac support and limited oxygenation.

EQUIPMENT AND SYSTEMS

Most equipment currently used for ECMO therapy is modified cardiopulmonary bypass equipment designed for short-term use. To ensure safe and effective use of the ECMO equipment, the limitations of each piece of equipment should be understood and considered before it is used for long-term bypass.

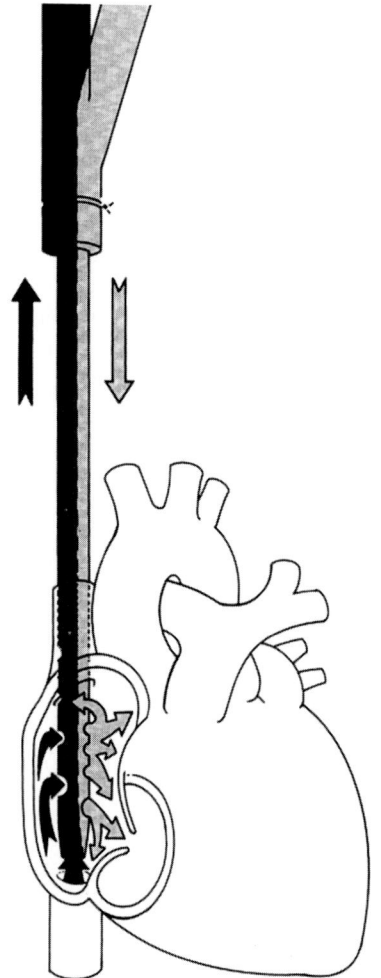

Figure 32-3 The inflow and outflow characteristics of the venovenous catheter in the right atrium. (From Short BL, O'Brien A, Poindexter C, eds. *CNMC ECMO training manual*. Washington, DC: Children's National Medical Center, 1993, with permission.)

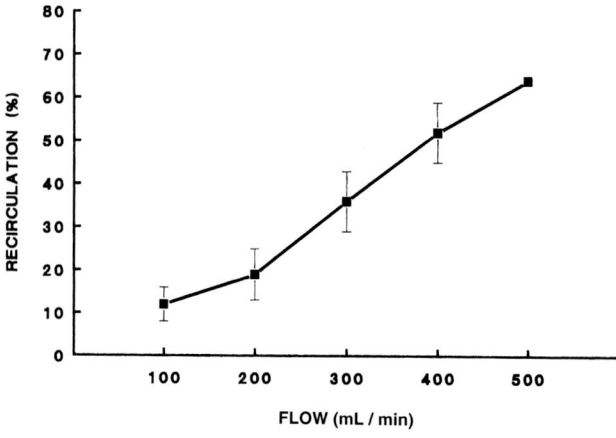

Figure 32-4 Recirculation occurs with the use of the venovenous extracorporeal membrane oxygenation catheter. Flows greater than 400 mL/min result in greater than 50% recirculation and decreased oxygenation. (From Anderson HL 3rd, Otsu T, Chapman RA, et al. Venovenous extracorporeal life support in neonates using a double lumen catheter. *ASAIO Trans* 1989;35: 650–653, with permission.)

TABLE 32-4

EQUIPMENT FOR NEONATAL EXTRACORPOREAL MEMBRANE OXYGENATION

Roller occlusion pump
Pump base
Venous return monitor or pressure monitoring module
Heating unit
Coagulation timer
Membrane mounting board
Oxygen blender
Carbon dioxide or carbogen tank
O_2 and CO_2 flowmeters
Inline temperature probes
Inline oxygen saturation monitor

There is no single ECMO machine. Each ECMO center must design an ECMO system by using equipment evaluated and designed to meet space and other specific requirements of their center. Bioengineering experts and cardiopulmonary perfusionists should be consulted in the design and evaluation of the ECMO system. The basic equipment needed for a complete system is listed in Table 32-4.

Space requirements and the possible need to transport the patient on ECMO should be taken into consideration in the design of an ECMO system (Figs. 32-1 and 32-5).

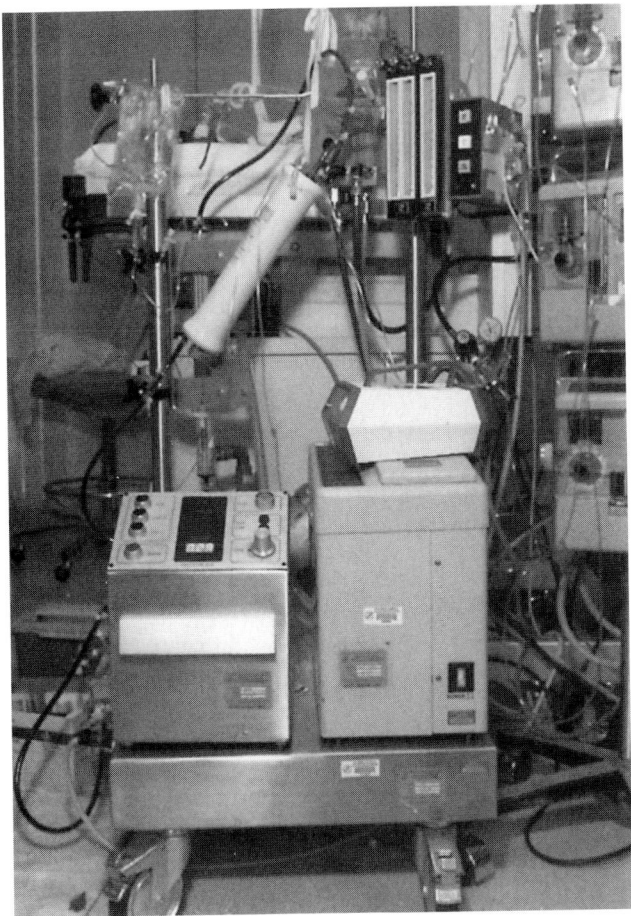

Figure 32-5 The extracorporeal membrane oxygenation system used at the Children's National Medical Center has a modular design.

The system should be on a cart or other movable base. The nondisposable equipment required includes a roller occlusion pump, water bath to maintain normothermic bypass temperatures, venous return monitor (VRM) or pressure monitoring system to insure adequate blood flow through the circuit, gas flow meters for CO_2 and O_2 delivery into the membrane lung, an inline venous saturation monitor, and membrane pressure monitors. Necessary disposable equipment includes the ECMO catheters (i.e., venous and arterial for VA ECMO; double-lumen venous for VV ECMO), tubing packs designed for the system, venous reservoir, heat exchanger, and membrane lung.

Those involved in providing ECMO therapy must know the potential complications related to each piece of equipment, especially the thrombogenic characteristics and flow dynamics. Several of these concepts are discussed in this chapter; however, additional information can be found elsewhere (45).

In VA ECMO, the venous catheter is the oxygenation catheter because the rate of blood flow through this catheter determines the percentage of the cardiac output that is supported by the ECMO pump. Oxygenation is determined by the percentage of cardiac output passing through the ECMO membrane (i.e., artificial lung) and bypassing the patient's lungs. If a small-gauge venous catheter is placed, minimal flow through the ECMO circuit occurs, and oxygenation may be compromised. Blood flow rates (Q) are directly proportional to the fourth power of the radius (r) of the tubing and inversely proportional to the length (L) of the tubing:

$$Q \propto r^4$$
$$Q \propto 1/L$$

To maximize flow into the circuit, a relatively short venous catheter with as large a lumen as possible is used.

The arterial catheter, which supplies return of flow from the circuit into the arch of the aorta, is the smallest-diameter component in the circuit and acts as the major resistance component in the circuit. A small arterial catheter may cause significant backpressure and lead to restricted blood flow, hemolysis, or eventual rupture of the circuit. Resistance to flow (R) depends on the dimensions and geometry of the tubing and the characteristics of the fluid used. Poiseuille's Law defines this concept by the following equation:

$$R = 8\eta L/\pi r^4$$

in which $8/\pi$ is the constant of proportionality, L (cm) is the length of the tubing, η is the coefficient of viscosity (i.e., Poise = dyne X sec/cm^2), and r (cm) is the radius of the tubing. The longer the tubing and the smaller the radius, the greater is the resistance. An 8-F (2.6-mm) catheter has much greater resistance than a 10-F (3.3-mm) catheter. A short, large-lumen catheter is ideal, but the size of catheter placed is limited by the diameter of the patient's carotid artery (46).

The double-lumen catheter used in VV ECMO has a small lumen for blood return, which produces a relatively high backpressure in the circuit. Kinking of this catheter significantly increases circuit pressures and must be diligently avoided.

The VRM is an electronic device that monitors the blood flow from the patient into the ECMO circuit (Fig. 32-1). Some systems do this through pressure monitoring instead of volume monitoring. The VRM functions as a servoregulator for the ECMO system and sounds an alarm and stops the pump if venous flow from the patient slows, ensuring that aortic blood input equals venous output. If a VRM system is not in place and venous return decreases without servoregulation, the roller pump continues to pump and causes the tubing to collapse, creating a negative pressure that pulls gas out of solution in the blood and air into the circuit at the connection points. The most common causes of loss of venous return are malplacement of the venous catheter (usually in the inferior vena cava), pneumothorax, or pneumopericardium; unrecognized bleeding (e.g., ICH, hemothorax); kinking of the venous catheter; or placing an anchoring suture too tightly around the catheter during cannulation.

The only membrane lung approved for long-term ECMO use in the United States is the silicone membrane lung made by Medtronics (Minneapolis, MN). The 0.8-m^2 membrane is most commonly used for neonates and can support oxygenation up to a blood flow rate of 1 L/min. CO_2 transfer is so efficient with this membrane that CO_2 must be added to the gases flowing into the membrane.

PATIENT MANAGEMENT

A team approach to the management of the ECMO patient is critical. Duties of the bedside nurse, respiratory therapist, and ECMO specialist should be clearly delineated to ensure efficient and effective care (47).

Daily Medical Management

Most neonatal patients, with the exception of those with CDH, require ECMO support for 7 to 8 days. During this period, the patient who was in respiratory failure and dying before ECMO shows evidence of reversal of disease, can be slowly weaned off ECMO to minimal ventilator settings, and can usually be extubated within 24 to 48 hours after coming off the ECMO circuit. The rapidity of recovery is remarkable, given the severity of the illness suffered by these infants before ECMO. For this level of recovery to occur in such a short time, many physiologic changes must take place rapidly, making daily care of the infant a fine art. Routine care must incorporate the fact that these infants are systemically heparinized, and tasks such as suctioning of the airway should be done with caution.

As the lungs improve, less blood flow is required to pass through the artificial lung, and the ECMO blood flow can be reduced. In the first few days, a blood flow rate of 120 to 150 mL/kg/min is required to oxygenate the infant (47). With improvement of the infant's lungs, arterial blood gases improve, and the ECMO blood flow can be decreased by 10 to 20 mL/min. The venous saturation of blood in the ECMO circuit can be monitored continuously, providing a representation of a mixed venous saturation level. However, this saturation is measured in blood from the right atrium, and right atrial blood saturation does not represent true mixed venous saturation if there are intracardiac shunts. Because most infants on ECMO develop left-to-right shunts, often occurring at the level of the foramen ovale, venous saturations must be interpreted in terms of other clinical signs. The following concepts must be understood:

$$C_VO_2 = CaO_2 - \dot{V}O_2/flow$$
$$\text{Oxygen content} = (Hb)(\% \text{ saturation})1.36 + 0.0031(PO_2)$$

in which C_VO_2 is venous oxygen content, CaO_2 is arterial oxygen content, $\dot{V}O_2$ is oxygen consumption, flow is cardiac output, Hb is hemoglobin, and PO_2 is oxygen pressure.

For venous oxygen saturation to represent a true indication of relative arterial oxygen content, several assumptions must be made: the cardiac output remains stable, hemoglobin concentrations remain stable, and metabolic rate of the patient does not change. Any one of these factors can cause a change in the venous saturation. Therefore, the patient should be carefully evaluated before this parameter is used alone to wean the ECMO flows. Obviously this parameter cannot be used in VV ECMO, where the venous saturation only represents recirculation. Patient arterial blood gases are needed to determine the pH and $PaCO_2$ status of the patient and membrane lung. If the arterial $PaCO_2$ of the membrane decreases below 35 mm Hg during VA ECMO, a decrease in respiratory rate may result because the brain detects the blood gas levels in blood from the membrane lung during VA ECMO. If the patient's respiratory rate falls, and he or she is on low bypass, the result is deterioration in blood gas status. The problem is corrected by increasing the CO_2 coming from the membrane to stimulate the infant to breathe. A high membrane PCO_2 may indicate membrane failure and is an emergency, and a normal membrane PCO_2 with an abnormal patient PCO_2 indicates a change in the patient's clinical condition such as development of pneumothorax or secondary pneumonia.

After being stabilized on ECMO, the infant is placed on lung-rest settings on the ventilator (e.g., FiO_2 = 0.21, peak inspiratory pressures [PIP] = 15 to 18 cm H_2O; peak end-expiratory pressures [PEEP] = 5 to 6 cm H_2O; rate = 10 to 15 breaths/min). It is typical for the lungs to appear opaque on chest radiographs during the first 1 to 3 days of ECMO (48–50). This is probably caused by the acute decrease in ventilatory settings, capillary leak, activation of complement as a result of interaction of blood products with the artificial surfaces in the circuit, and surfactant deficiency secondary to lung injury (51,52). Lotze and associates (53,54) showed that surfactant replacement therapy in infants on ECMO can decrease time on ECMO for all infants except those with CDH. A study conducted

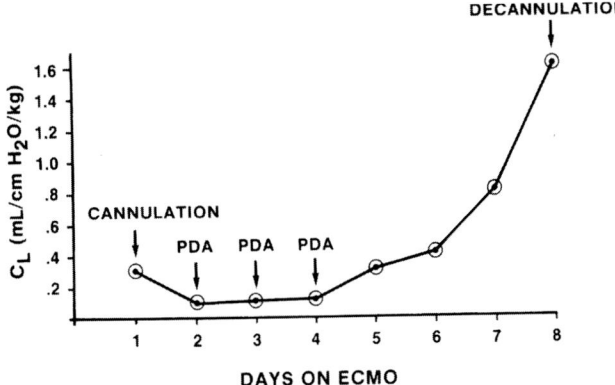

Figure 32-6 The typical lung compliance curve for an infant with meconium aspiration syndrome on extracorporeal membrane oxygenation (ECMO). Infants in this study were successfully taken off ECMO if a lung compliance (C_L) of 0.8 mL/cm H_2O/kg was attained. PDA, patent ductur arteriosus. (From Lotze A, Short BL, Taylor GA. Lung compliance as a measure of lung function in newborns with respiratory failure requiring extracorporeal membrane oxygenation. *Crit Care Med* 1987;15:226–229, with permission.)

using surfactant before ECMO revealed that a significant number of infants in the low-mortality group (OI 15 to 22) could be kept off ECMO with the use of surfactant (55). Lung compliance studies can help in predicting successful decannulation, especially in the infant who is borderline, and when a decision is being made about removing an infant from ECMO because of complications (49). A typical lung compliance curve is shown in Fig. 32-6. An old-fashioned but effective technique for assessing pulmonary improvement is to hand-ventilate the infant daily. When the chest moves easily with a peak pressure of 20 cm H_2O or less, the infant can successfully come off ECMO.

Heparin is administered continuously into the ECMO circuit to prevent clotting (47). Heparin management varies, depending on events before and during ECMO. Optimal heparin management can achieve the level of heparinization needed to decrease the risk for fibrin and clot formation in the circuit while minimizing the risk for bleeding complications in the patient. Because heparinization must be evaluated rapidly and at the bedside, most centers use the ACT (56). The ACT is determined in a system that uses activators, such as glass beads, to initiate the clotting cascade. The specimen is warmed to accelerate the clotting process. This test gives values of 80 to 120 seconds in a nonheparinized infant, compared with standard non-activated bleeding time values longer than 5 minutes (56,57).

The primary cause of death in the ECMO population is ICH (30,31,58). The risk factors associated with the development of an ICH include significant hypoxic or ischemic cerebral insult before ECMO, sepsis with coagulopathy, or gestational age less than 37 weeks. Initial heparin management is based on pretreatment risk factors (45).

Fibrin formation is related to flow rate; if there are low blood flow rates in the circuit, the heparin dose is increased to decrease the risk for clot formation. At the beginning of an ECMO run, blood flows are high, and the

ACTs can be maintained in a lower range. At the end of a run, the ACTs are increased, especially when the idling phase (i.e., 60 to 80 mL/min) is reached. When the blood flow rate in the circuit is below 150 mL/min, ACTs are increased to 200 to 220 seconds. Clinical factors that affect the ACT values are renal function (heparin excretion is directly proportional to urine output), transfusion of non-heparinized blood products or platelets, and a significant patent ductus arteriosus with a left-to-right shunt that may decrease renal blood flow.

Fluid requirements while on ECMO range from 80 to 120 mL/kg/day. Electrolyte requirements are significantly different from those before ECMO is started. Most infants require little sodium, usually 1 to 2 mEq/kg/day, and a large amount of potassium, usually 4 to 5 mEq/kg/day. The rationale for these requirements is unknown. Although renin levels increase on bypass, aldosterone levels decrease, and atrial natriuretic peptide levels do not change (59,60). Calcium requirements range from 40 to 50 mg/kg of elemental calcium per day.

Systemic hypertension is a common medical complication of ECMO (59–61). Hypertension (mean blood pressure greater than 65 mm Hg for more than 3 hours) can affect as many as 70% of these patients. Hypertension usually develops shortly after cannulation and is transient, but 1% to 5% of infants require long-term antihypertensive therapy. The risk of ICH is increased by hypertension (60). Although a subject of controversy, the hypertension may be related to an increase in serum renin levels (59,60). Fluid restriction and diuretic therapy may decrease the risk for prolonged hypertension.

As pulmonary vascular resistance decreases, it is common to develop a left-to-right shunt across the patent ductus arteriosus, resulting in oxygenation difficulty (62). Most of these shunts close with fluid restriction and diuretic therapy. Few patients require surgical intervention. Indomethacin should not be used in this population because it decreases platelet aggregation. After the shunt closes, an immediate increase in the patient's PaO_2 is observed.

Cardiac stun is an interesting complication of ECMO therapy that also occurs in patients on cardiopulmonary bypass (63). Cardiac stun occurs in infants with severe hypoxia or in infants in whom the tip of the arterial catheter is placed too close to the coronary arteries. This syndrome is characterized by a pulse pressure of 10 mm Hg or less on ECMO, with the patient's PaO_2 equal to or within 50 to 100 mm Hg of the pump PO_2 (e.g., a pump PO_2 of 400 mm Hg while on an FiO_2 of 1.00, with a patient PaO_2 between 300 and 350 mm Hg). The electrocardiographic pattern is normal, indicating that electrical conduction is normal, but cardiac output is markedly reduced. The pathophysiology is not understood (63,64). When data on infants with cardiac stun while on ECMO at the Children's National Medical Center were evaluated, there was a significant difference in pre-ECMO blood gases relative to infants who did not develop cardiac stun. Infants in stun were sicker before ECMO and had a higher incidence of death from ICH, indicating the marked hypoxic–ischemic insult suffered by these patients before ECMO. Treatment of cardiac stun consists of maintaining ECMO blood flow rates high enough to supply appropriate cardiac output. Afterload reduction does not improve cardiac function in this population (65). As stun resolves, the pulse pressure returns to normal, and the patient's PaO_2 no longer mirrors the pump PO_2.

Weaning from VA ECMO occurs slowly as the arterial blood gases and venous saturations improve. Idling flows, defined as flows at 10% of the cardiac output (i.e., 60 to 80 mL/minute) are continued for 6 to 8 hours, and if blood gases are normal during this period, most infants can be successfully taken off ECMO. A lung compliance measurement of at least 0.8 mL/cm H_2O/kg indicates that the infant can successfully come off ECMO (Fig. 32-6) (50). For patients on VV ECMO, the flows can be kept high and the membrane lung can be capped off, so no gas flow occurs. Monitoring blood gases for 2 to 4 hours will determine if the patient is ready to come off ECMO. Typical ventilator settings for infants after completing an ECMO course are FiO_2 of 0.30 to 0.40; rate of 30 to 40 breaths/minute; PIP of 18 to 20 cm H_2O; and PEEP of 5 to 6 cm H_2O.

Patient Care after Extracorporeal Membrane Oxygenation

A neuromuscular blocking agent with an intermediate half-life is used at decannulation to help the patient breathe spontaneously as soon as possible after coming off ECMO. By the end of the ECMO run, it is common for the ECMO patient to require high $PaCO_2$ levels (i.e., 45 to 55 mm Hg) to stimulate respiratory drive. Many of these infants have been receiving narcotics such as fentanyl and may need to be weaned slowly from this therapy to avoid withdrawal symptoms. PaO_2 levels of 60 to 70 mm Hg are accepted, and every effort is made to wean the patient from the ventilator. At Children's National Medical Center, the average time to extubation post ECMO is 23 hours. The CDH patient is an exception; these patients require slower weaning to ensure that pulmonary hypertension does not recur.

Hemoglobin, hematocrit, calcium, and electrolyte measurements should be obtained 6 to 8 hours after ECMO. These can then be monitored every 24 hours or as clinically indicated. The platelet count should be followed closely (i.e., values every 12 hours for 24 hours) because rebound thrombocytopenia may occur. Intravenous sodium is increased to 2 to 3 mEq/kg/day, and potassium supplementation is decreased to 1 to 2 mEq/kg/day.

After extubation, the infant usually requires oxygen therapy for another 5 to 7 days. Most ECMO infants feed poorly and may require feeding by tube for a few days. The cause of this problem is uncertain, but it is usually transient and does not indicate long-term developmental problems.

Because not all intracranial abnormalities are detected by ultrasound, a computed tomographic or magnetic reso-nance scan is recommended before discharge (66). A baseline hearing screen and neurologic assessment are also recommended before discharge. All infants should be followed in a neonatal high-risk follow-up program.

Outcome Data

Developmental outcome is encouraging, with most centers reporting that 60% to 70% of ECMO survivors are normal at 1 to 2 years of age (67–69). Risk factors associated with poor outcome include finding a severe abnormality on neuroimaging, chronic lung disease, prematurity, and group B streptococcal sepsis (67,70–72). When ECMO survivors were evaluated at 5 years of age though, Glass and associates (73) found that 37% were at risk for school failure; however, Rais-Bahrami and colleagues (74) found a similar risk in the population of "near-miss" ECMO patients, defined as those referred for ECMO but who improved without ECMO. Wagner and associates (75) followed the ECMO population studied in the Glass study into school and found that indeed, a high percentage had academic problems (37%). Therefore, although a great majority of post-ECMO patients are doing well, a thorough neuropsychologic evaluation prior to starting school should be considered to identify those children who may benefit from special education programs.

The need for carotid artery ligation for VA ECMO has caused concern that right-sided CNS lesions may result, but most studies have not shown this to be true (58,66,70,72). Analysis of the first 360 patients treated at Children's National Medical Center did not reveal lateralizing hemorrhagic or nonhemorrhagic abnormalities, but there was a high incidence of posterior fossa hemorrhage, raising the concern that jugular venous ligation might increase venous backpressure and the risk of hemorrhage (76). Data published by Taylor and Walker (77) showed that decreased sagittal sinus blood flow velocity is associated with ICH (70%) in the ECMO population. Whether this is cause or effect has yet to be determined. Also noted in this study was a marked decrease in sagittal sinus blood flow when the infant's head was turned to the left, obviously obstructing the left internal jugular vein when the right was ligated, resulting in obstruction of venous flow. The association of this with cerebral hemorrhage could not be determined because of the small number of patients, but it does address the need for keeping the infants head midline during the ECMO run. Because of this concern, many ECMO teams are now placing jugular bulb catheters in the right internal jugular vein, advanced up to the jugular bulb area, to drain the venous outflow from the brain into the venous side of the circuit, and thus reduce the potential obstruction caused by the venous catheter and ligation of the jugular vein.

The infant with CDH may have unique long-term problems, including significant gastroesophageal reflux and chronic lung disease (14,38). These infants require close follow-up in a multidisciplinary clinic to prevent problems such as failure to thrive and respiratory compromise.

SUMMARY

Care of the ECMO patient requires highly trained nurses, respiratory therapists, perfusionists, and physicians. The team must continually evaluate the treatment modalities and use the information to improve techniques and define the indications for ECMO therapy. Prior to the use of iNO, it was estimated that only 1,000 to 2,500 term infants required ECMO each year in the United States (78). That number is obviously going to be smaller since iNO has been shown to reduce the need for ECMO, making the need for tailoring the development and expansion of ECMO centers based on regional need even more important. Regionalization of ECMO programs can help to maintain cost control and optimize quality of care.

REFERENCES

1. Kolff WJ, Berk HT. Artificial kidney: a dialyzer with a great area. *Acta Med Scand* 1944;17:121–134.
2. Kenedi RM, Courtney JM, Gaylor JDS, et al, eds *Artificial organs.* Baltimore: University Park Press, 1976:87–88.
3. Clowes GHA Jr, Hopkins AL, Neville WE. An artificial lung dependent upon diffusion of oxygen and carbon dioxide through plastic membranes. *J Thorac Surg* 1956;32:630–637.
4. Kolobow T, Stool EW, Sacko KL, et al. Acute respiratory failure. Survival following ten days' support with a membrane lung. *J Thorac Cardiovasc Surg* 1975;69:947–953.
5. Zapol WM, Snider MT, Hil JD, et al. Extracorporeal membrane oxygenation in severe acute respiratory failure. A randomized prospective study. *JAMA* 1979;242:2193–2196.
6. Gille JP, Bagniewski AM. Ten years of use of extracorporeal membrane oxygenation (ECMO) in the treatment of acute respiratory insufficiency (ARI). *Trans Am Soc Artif Intern Organs* 1976;22:102–109.
7. Callaghan JC, de los Angeles J. Long-term extracorporeal circulation in the development of an artificial placenta for respiratory distress syndrome of the newborn. *Surg Forum* 1961;12:215–217.
8. Rashkind WJ, Freeman A, Klein D, et al. Evolution of a disposable plastic, low volume, pumpless oxygenator as a lung substitute. *J Pediatr* 1965;66:94–102.
9. White JJ, Andrews HG, Risemberg H, et al. Prolonged respiratory support in newborn infants with a membrane oxygenator. *Surgery* 1971;70:288–296.
10. Dorson W Jr, Baker E, Cohen ML, et al. A perfusion system for infants. *Trans Am Soc Artif Intern Organs* 1969;15:155–160.
11. Bartlett RH, Gazzaniga AB, Jefferies MR, et al. Extracorporeal membrane oxygenation (ECMO) cardiopulmonary support in infancy. *Trans Am Soc Artif Intern Organs* 1976;22:80–93.
12. Extracorporeal Life Support Organization quarterly report, July 2003.
13. Gill BS, Neville HL, Khan AM, et al. Delayed institution of extracorporeal membrane oxygenation is associated with increased mortality rate and prolonged hospital stay. *J Pediatr Surg* 2002;37:7–20.
14. Van Meurs K, Short BL. State-of-the-art management of congenital diaphragmatic hernia: a neonatologist's perspective. *Pediatr Rev* 1999;20:e79–e87.
15. Sanchez LS, O'Brien A, Anderson KD, et al. Best postductal PO_2 and PCO_2 do not predict outcome of CDH infants in extremis, stabilized with ECMO prior to surgical repair. *Pediatr Res* 1992;31:221A.
16. Boloker J, Bateman DA, Wung JT, et al. Congenital diaphragmatic hernia in 120 infants treated consecutively with permissive hypercapnea/spontaneous respiration/elective repair. *J Pediatr Surg* 2002;37:357–366.
17. Kays DW, Langham MR Jr, Ledbetter DJ, et al. Detrimental effects of standard medical therapy in congenital diaphragmatic hernia. *Ann Surg* 1999;230:340–348.
18. Bartlett RH, Roloff DW, Cornell RG, et al. Extracorporeal circulation in neonatal respiratory failure: a prospective randomized trial. *Pediatrics* 1985;76:479–487.
19. Beck R, Anderson KD, Pearson GD, et al. Criteria for extracorporeal membrane oxygenation in a population of infants with persistent pulmonary hypertension of the newborn. *J Pediatr Surg* 1986;21:297–302.
20. Cole CH, Jillson E, Kessler D. ECMO: regional evaluation of need and applicability of selection criteria. *Am J Dis Child* 1988;142:1320–1324.
21. Dworetz AR, Moya FR, Sabo B, et al. Survival of infants with persistent pulmonary hypertension without extracorporeal membrane oxygenation. *Pediatrics* 1989;84:1–6.
22. Krummel TM, Greenfield LJ, Kirkpatrick BV, et al. Alveolar–arterial oxygen gradients versus the neonatal pulmonary insufficiency index for prediction of mortality in ECMO candidates. *J Pediatr Surg* 1984;19:380–384.
23. Marsh TD, Wilkerson SA, Cook LN. Extracorporeal membrane oxygenation selection criteria: partial pressure of arterial oxygen versus alveolar–arterial oxygen gradient. *Pediatrics* 1988;82:162–166.
24. O'Rourke PP, Crone RK, Vacanti JP, et al. Extracorporeal membrane oxygenation and conventional medical therapy in neonates with persistent pulmonary hypertension of the newborn: a prospective randomized study. *Pediatrics* 1989;84:957–963.
25. Wung JT, James LS, Kilchevsky E, et al. Management of infants with severe respiratory failure and persistence of the fetal circulation, without hyperventilation. *Pediatrics* 1985;76:488–494.
26. Sacks H, Kupter S, Chalmero TC. Are uncontrolled clinical studies ever justified? *N Engl J Med* 1980;303:1059.
27. UK Collaborative ECMO Trial Group. UK collaborative randomised trial of neonatal extracorporeal membrane oxygenation. *Lancet* 1996;348:75–82.
28. Karle VA, Short BL, Martin GR, et al. Extracorporeal membrane oxygenation exposes infants to the plasticizer, di(2-ethylhexyl)-phthalate. *Crit Care Med* 1997;25:696–703.
29. Schneider B, Schena J, Truog R, et al. Exposure to di(2-ethylhexyl)phthalate in infants receiving extracorporeal membrane oxygenation. *N Engl J Med* 1989;320:1563.
30. Cilley RE, Zwischenberger JB, Andrews AF, et al. Intracranial hemorrhage during extracorporeal membrane oxygenation in neonates. *Pediatrics* 1986;78:699–704.
31. Revenis ME, Glass P, Short BL. Mortality and morbidity rates among lower birth weight infants (2000 to 2500 grams) treated with extracorporeal membrane oxygenation. *J Pediatr* 1992;121:452–458.
32. Toomasian JM, Snedecor SM, Cornell RG, et al. National experience with extracorporeal membrane oxygenation for newborn respiratory failure. Data from 715 cases. *ASAIO Trans* 1988;34:140–147.
33. Short BL, Walker LK, Bender KS, et al. Impairment of cerebral autoregulation during extracorporeal membrane oxygenation in newborn lambs. *Pediatr Res* 1993;33:289–904.
34. Short BL, Walker LK, Gleason CA, et al. Effects of extracorporeal membrane oxygenation on cerebral blood flow and cerebral oxygen metabolism in newborn sheep. *Pediatr Res* 1990;50:50–53.
35. Hirschl RB, Schumacher RE, Snedecor SN, et al. The efficacy of extracorporeal life support in premature and low birth weight newborns. *J Pediatr Surg* 1993;28:1336–1340.
36. McCune S, Short BL, Miller MK, et al. Extracorporeal membrane oxygenation therapy in neonates with septic shock. *J Pediatr Surg* 1990;25:479–482.
37. Newman KD, Anderson KD, Van Meurs K, et al. Extracorporeal membrane oxygenation and congenital diaphragmatic hernia: should any infant be excluded? *J Pediatr Surg* 1990;25:1048–1052.
38. Van Meurs KP, Newman KD, Anderson KD, et al. Effect of extracorporeal membrane oxygenation on survival of infants with congenital diaphragmatic hernia. *J Pediatr* 1990;117:954–960.
39. Ortiz RM, Cilley RE, Bartlett RH. Extracorporeal membrane oxygenation in pediatric respiratory failure. *Pediatr Clin North Am* 1987;34:39–46.
40. Boedy RF, Howell CG, Kanto WP Jr. Hidden mortality rate associated with extracorporeal membrane oxygenation. *J Pediatr* 1990;117:462–464.
41. American Academy of Pediatrics. Committee on Fetus and Newborn. Use of inhaled nitric oxide. *Pediatrics* 2000;106:344–345.

42. Clark RH. How do we safely use inhaled nitric oxide? *Pediatrics* 1999;104:296–297.

43. Anderson HL 3rd, Otsu T, Chapman RA, et al. Venovenous extracorporeal life support in neonates using a double lumen catheter. *ASAIO Trans* 1989;35:650–653.

44. Rais-Bahrami K, Walton DM, Sell JE, et al. Improved oxygenation with reduced recirculation during venovenous ECMO: comparison of two catheters. *Perfusion* 2002;17:415–419.

45. Short BL. Pre-ECMO considerations for neonatal patients. In: Arensman RM, Cornish D, eds. *Extracorporeal life support.* Cambridge, MA: Blackwell Scientific, 1993:156–174.

46. Van Meurs KP, Mikesell GT, Seale WR, et al. Maximum blood flow rates for arterial cannulae used in neonatal ECMO. *ASAIO Trans* 1990;36:M679–M681.

47. Short BL. Clinical management of the neonatal ECMO patient. In: Arensman RM, Cornish D, eds. *Extracorporeal life support.* Cambridge, MA: Blackwell Scientific, 1993:195–206.

48. Taylor GA, Short BL, Kriesmer P. Extracorporeal membrane oxygenation: radiographic appearance of the neonatal chest. *AJR Am J Roentgenol* 1986;146:1257–1260.

49. Lotze A, Short BL, Taylor GA. Lung compliance as a measure of lung function in newborns with respiratory failure requiring extracorporeal membrane oxygenation. *Crit Care Med* 1987;15: 226–229.

50. Keszler M, Subramanian KN, Smith YA, et al. Pulmonary management during extracorporeal membrane oxygenation. *Crit Care Med* 1989;17:495–500.

51. Lotze A, Whitsett JA, Kammerman LA, et al. Surfactant protein A concentrations in tracheal aspirate fluid from infants requiring extracorporeal membrane oxygenation. *J Pediatr* 1990;116:435–440.

52. Anderson JM, Kottke-Marchant K. Platelet interactions with biomaterials and artificial devices. In: Williams DF, ed. *Blood compatibility,* vol I. Boca Raton, FL: CRC Press, 1987:127–.

53. Lotze A, Knight GR, Martin GR, et al. Improved pulmonary outcome after exogenous surfactant therapy for respiratory failure in term infants requiring extracorporeal membrane oxygenation. *J Pediatr* 1993;122:261–268.

54. Lotze A, Knight GR, Anderson KD, et al. Surfactant (beractant) therapy for infants with congenital diaphragmatic hernia on ECMO: evidence of persistent surfactant deficiency. *J Pediatr Surg* 1994;29:407–412.

55. Lotze A, Mitchell BR, Bulas DI, et al. Multicenter study of surfactant (beractant) use in the treatment of term infants with severe respiratory failure. Survanta in Term Infants Study Group. *J Pediatr* 1998;132:40–47.

56. Hattersley PG. Activated coagulation time of whole blood. *JAMA* 1966;196:436–440.

57. Kay LA, ed. *Essentials of haemostasis and thrombosis,* 2nd ed. New York: Churchill-Livingstone, 1988.

58. Taylor GA, Short BL, Fitz CR. Imaging of cerebrovascular injury in infants treated with extracorporeal membrane oxygenation. *J Pediatr* 1989;114:635–639.

59. Marinelli KA, Short BL, Martin GR, et al. Extracorporeal membrane oxygenation: its effect on renin, aldosterone and natriuretic peptide. *Pediatr Res* 1989;25:241A.

60. Sell LL, Cullen ML, Lerner GR, et al. Hypertension during extracorporeal membrane oxygenation: cause, effect, and management. *Surgery* 1987;102:724–730.

61. Boedy RF, Goldberg AK, Howell CG Jr, et al. Incidence of hypertension in infants on extracorporeal membrane oxygenation. *J Pediatr Surg* 1990;25:258–261.

62. Martin GR, Short BL. Doppler echocardiographic evaluation of cardiac performance in infants on prolonged extracorporeal membrane oxygenation. *Am J Cardiol* 1988;62:929–934.

63. Martin GR, Short BL, Abbott C, et al. Cardiac stun in infants undergoing extracorporeal membrane oxygenation. *J Thorac Cardiovasc Surg* 1991;101:607–611.

64. Marban E. Myocardial stunning and hibernation. The physiology behind the colloquialisms. *Circulation* 1991;83:681–688.

65. Martin GR, Chauvin L, Short BL. Effects of hydralazine on cardiac performance in infants receiving extracorporeal membrane oxygenation. *J Pediatr* 1991;118:944–948.

66. Bulas DI, Taylor GA, O'Donnell RM, et al. Intracranial abnormalities in infants treated with extracorporeal membrane oxygenation: update on sonographic and CT findings. *Am J Neuroradiol* 1996; 17:287–294.

67. Glass P, Miller M, Short B. Morbidity for survivors of extracorporeal membrane oxygenation: neurodevelopmental outcome at 1 year of age. *Pediatrics* 1989;83:72–78.

68. Schumacher RE, Palmer TW, Roloff DW, et al. Follow-up of infants treated with extracorporeal membrane oxygenation for newborn respiratory failure. *Pediatrics* 1991;87:451–457.

69. Towne BH, Lott IT, Hicks DA, et al. Long-term follow-up of infants and children treated with extracorporeal membrane oxygenation (ECMO): a preliminary report. *J Pediatr Surg* 1985;20: 410–414.

70. Glass P, Bulas DI, Wagner AE, et al. Severity of brain injury following neonatal extracorporeal membrane oxygenation and outcome at age 5 years. *Dev Med Child Neurol* 1997;39:441–448.

71. Schumacher RE, Barks JDE, Johnston MV, et al. Right-sided brain lesions in infants following extracorporeal membrane oxygenation. *Pediatrics* 1988;82:155–161.

72. Bulas DI, Glass P, O'Donnell RM, et al. Neonates treated with ECMO: predictive value of early CT and US neuroimaging findings on short-term neurodevelopmental outcome. *Radiology* 1995; 195:407–412.

73. Glass P, Wagner AE, Papero PH, et al. Neurodevelopmental status at age five years of neonates treated with extracorporeal membrane oxygenation. *J Pediatr* 1995;127:447–457.

74. Rais-Bahrami K, Wagner AE, Coffman C, et al. Neurodevelopmental outcome in ECMO vs near-miss ECMO patients at 5 years of age. *Clin Pediatr (Phila)* 2000;39:145–152.

75. Wagner AE, Coffman CE, Short BL, et al. Neuropsychological outcome and educational adjustment to first grade of ECMO-treated neonates. *Pediatr Res* 1996;39(Suppl 2):283. (abstr.)

76. Bulas DI, Taylor GA, Fitz CR, et al. Posterior fossa intracranial hemorrhage in infants treated with extracorporeal membrane oxygenation: sonographic findings. *AJR Am J Roentgenol* 1991;156: 571–575.

77. Taylor GA, Walker LK. Intracranial venous system in newborns treated with extracorporeal membrane oxygenation: Doppler US evaluation after ligation of the right jugular vein. *Radiology* 1992; 183:453–456.

78. Rais-Bahrami K, Short BL. The current status of neonatal extracorporeal membrane oxygenation. *Semin Perinatol* 2000;24:406–417.

79. Short BL. Physiology of extracorporeal membrane oxygenation (ECMO). In: Polin RA, Fox WW, eds. *Fetal and neonatal physiology.* Philadelphia: WB Saunders, 1992:932.

Cardiac Disease

Michael F. Flanagan   *Scott B. Yeager*   *Steven N. Weindling*

INCIDENCE

The incidence of congenital heart disease detectable by routine clinical examination has been estimated to be 7.5 per 1,000 live births (1). The incidence of congenital heart anomalies in neonates seen with detailed echocardiographic examination is four- to 10-fold higher, with most of the difference being clinically insignificant ventricular septal defects (20–50 per 1,000) and nonstenotic bicommissural aortic valves (2). Severe forms of cardiac anomalies requiring cardiac catheterization or surgery, or resulting in death, occur in 2.5 to 3 infants per 1,000 births (2,3). Almost one-half of these are diagnosed during the first week of life. Additionally, moderately severe forms of cardiac anomalies occur in another 3 per 1,000 live births, and another 13 of 1,000 live births have a bicommissural aortic valve that may require care eventually (2). The distributions of congenital heart anomalies in newborns seen at a primary and a tertiary pediatric cardiac center are shown in Table 33-1.

INFANT MORTALITY

Before aggressive intervention, Mitchell found that 2.3 of 1,000 live births died with cardiac problems in infancy (1). Infant cardiac mortality in developed countries has progressively declined over the last several decades with better prenatal and postnatal recognition, and with the development and refinement of definitive interventions and periprocedural management. The infant cardiac fatality rate in the United States was 0.15 per 1,000 births in 2000, ranking tenth among leading causes of infant death (4). At high-volume surgical centers more commonly occurring cyanotic cardiac anomalies such as transposition of the great arteries and tetralogy of Fallot have surgical mortality rates of 1% to 5% or less. Complex anomalies with the highest risk have also had significant improvements in neonatal survival in developed countries. For example, surgical survival of neonates with hypoplastic left heart syndrome increased from 40% to 60% to 75% to 93% at specialized surgical centers (5), with overall mortality in infancy approximately twice this. Although surgical surgery outcomes are much

improved, including in babies with prematurity and multiple anomalies, prematurity and associated noncardiac anomalies still strongly influence the potential for salvaging infants with cardiac disease (Table 33-2) (4). In some situations, the mortality attributable to these problems is considerable.

LONG-TERM SURVIVAL

This chapter focuses on infancy; however, discussions with parents concerning their newborn with a cardiac anomaly often quickly, and appropriately, move to the length and quality of life anticipated in later childhood and adulthood. It is important that parents are accurately advised of likely and potential long-term outcomes with current therapies by cardiologists or other practitioners up-to-date with recent advances and outcome findings. In general, those with common acyanotic anomalies such as uncomplicated septal defects or pulmonary valve stenosis, and most of those with cyanotic anomalies such as simple transposition of the great arteries now can anticipate an essentially near-normal life after appropriate intervention. Even with many complicated anomalies, most can expect to survive to at least mid-adulthood, although long-term survival is highly dependent on the specific diagnosis, with the highest mortality now generally occurring in infancy (see Table 33-2). With few exceptions, a cardiac operation or catheter intervention can lengthen and improve the quality of life of a child with heart disease. Even when the nature of the long-term management is unclear, care has proceeded with the conviction that childhood survival often allows yet to be planned later interventions, resulting from future progress in the field, to provide even longer and better survival. The palliative shunt operations of 20 to 40 years ago unexpectedly produced candidates for later Fontan procedures. The central principle continues to be "where there is life, there is hope."

With reductions in mortality, and new generations of adults and older children with repaired and palliated cardiac anomalies, it has become evident that cardiac anomalies, and procedures utilized to treat them, sometimes have late residua and sequelae, including neurologic and cognitive morbidity not evident until preschool or school

TABLE 33-1
NEONATAL (FIRST MONTH) CARDIAC DIAGNOSTIC DISTRIBUTION[a]

	Percent
Ventricular septal defect	41
Atrial septal defect secundum	12
Valvar pulmonary stenosis	11
Coarctation of the aorta	6
Tetralogy of Fallot	5
Cardiomyopathy	4
Transposition of the great arteries	3
Endocardial cushion defects	3
Hypoplastic left heart syndrome	2
Aortic stenosis	2
Tricuspid atresia	1
Malposition	1
Total anomalous pulmonary venous connection	1
Truncus arteriosis	1
Aortic-Pulmonary window	1
Hemitruncus	<1
Interrupted Aortic Arch	<1
L-Transposition of the great arteries	<1
Tricuspid valve diseases	<1
Pulmonary atresia and intact interventricular septum	<1
Single ventricle	<1

[a] Based on 361 patients diagnosed by echocardiography by age 1 month at Childrens Hospital at Dartmouth. Neonates with patent ductus arteriosus, persistent fetal circulation, arrhythmia and normal heart exams are not included.

age (6–8), and arrhythmias and ventricular dysfunction developing in adolescence and adulthood. Most difficult, and not yet fully delineated have been the neurologic and cognitive morbidity. These abnormalities appear rarely with common septal and valvar malformations, and tend to be more frequent and severe with more complicated anomalies and repairs. Cardiac, neurologic and cognitive outcomes after repair of septal defects have appeared generally normal (8). Although most children with complex anomalies and procedures, such as hypoplastic left heart syndrome and operative circulatory arrest, have neurocognitive outcome within the normal range, on average, they have slower development, lower IQ scores, and higher rates of learning disabilities and special needs than normal. Moreover, a significant number have major impairments (8). The etiologies are complex, and include possible genetic issues, coexistent brain anomaly, potentially diminished cerebral blood flow or oxygenation in utero with some anomalies (e.g., hypoplastic left heart syndrome), pre- and/or peri-operative low cardiac output, cyanosis (See color plate), thrombo-embolism, or intracerebral hemorrhage, and operative use of hypothermic circulatory arrest (6–8). The possibility that brain injury or other injury may be acquired prenatally, pretreatment or in the process of treatment should be understood.

The goal is to provide a satisfying life through childhood and adulthood. The long-range future of patients undergoing intracardiac repair, arterial switch operations, staged multiple complex palliative operations, Fontan operations, or cardiac transplantation requires detailed discussion. The ramifications of treating a child who has major anomalies must be discussed with the parents in understandable language. The expected physical capabilities of the patient after treatment should be delineated. After the physician is confident that the parents thoroughly understand the known facts, he or she is free to express an opinion about what may be best for the child.

ETIOLOGY

Heart formation is a fantastic metamorphosis regulated by many sequences of genes. Given the remarkably complex orchestration of molecular and morphologic processes in formation of the heart, even small genetic and/or environmental changes in the control of these processes can have major, and variable, consequences. Truly, it is wonderful that development occurs and it does, as often as it does. Nevertheless, understandably, parents ask why their baby was born with a cardiac abnormality and whether it is likely to recur with a subsequent pregnancy.

Occasionally, children with isolated cardiac anomaly have a parent who has survived with cardiac anomaly, or another family member with a cardiac anomaly, but more often, there is no family history. However, an inheritable defect in a single gene (e.g., Marfan syndrome) or a chromosomal anomaly (e.g., trisomy) is identified in a significant minority of patients with cardiac malformations. More commonly there may be susceptibility from inherited or acquired mutations in two or more genes, perhaps with additional alterations in gene transcription or posttranscriptional processes from maternal-fetal folate metabolism, or fetal exposure to specific pharmacologic, biochemical, infectious and environmental factors that cumulatively surpass a threshold of liability (9). These result in pathogenetic changes in embryonic development, including defects in mesenchymal tissue migration (tetralogy of Fallot, truncus arteriosus, interrupted aortic arch, malalignment conal-septal ventricular septal defects, transposition of great arteries), extracellular matrix defects (endocardial cushion defects), abnormal cell death (muscular ventricular septal defect, Ebstein anomaly), targeted growth (anomalous pulmonary vein connection, single atrium), defective situs and cardiac looping (heterotaxy syndromes, L-transposition), and secondary effects from alterations in blood flow in the right heart (secundum atrial septal defect, pulmonary valve stenosis and atresia) or left heart (hypoplastic left heart syndrome, coarctation of aorta, aortic valve stenosis, patent ductus arteriosus) (9–12).

Approximately 13% of children with cardiac anomalies have chromosomal syndromes associated with cardiovascular malformation. Another approximately 8% to 13% of children have inheritable syndromes with associated cardiovascular abnormalities (11–13). The genes affected in many of these syndromes have been identified (9,14–16) (Table 33-3). The most common human mutations are in a critical 30 gene region of chromosome 22q11 involved in neural crest and cardiac development that cause DiGeorge

TABLE 33-2
INFANT (FIRST-YEAR) CARDIAC DIAGNOSTIC DISTRIBUTION AND MORTALITY

Diagnosis	Frequency (%)	Mortality (%)
Ventricular Septal Defect	31	0.7
Pulmonary Valve Stenosis	19	0.5
Atrial Septal defect	12	0.2
Aortic Valve Stenosis	8	4
Atrio-ventricular Canal Septal Defects	5	1.8
Coarctation of Aorta	4	3.5
D-Transposition of Great Arteries	4	1.0
Tetralogy of Fallot with pulmonary outflow stenosis	4	2.2
Malposition	3	9
Hypoplastic Left Heart Syndrome	2	22
Pulmonary Valve Atresia with Intact Ventricular Septum	2	4
Pulmonary Valve Atresia with Tetralogy of Fallot	1	11
Double Outlet Right Ventricle	0.9	6
Total anomalous pulmonary venous connection	0.8	7
Truncus arteriosis	0.7	5
Single Ventricle	0.7	<0.1
Tricuspid Atresia	0.5	<0.1
Interupted Aortic Arch	0.3	<0.1
Aortic-Pulmonary window	0.2	<0.1
Hemitruncus	0.1	<0.1
L-Transposition of Great Arteries	0.1	<0.1
Total	2.2	

Data is based on 5,182 infants diagnosed at Childrens Hospital, Boston between January 1,1998 and January 1,2002, and their overall mortality by age 1 year. Babies with patent ductus arteriosus and primary cardiomyopathy were not included. Mortality by age 1 year was significantly influenced by coexistent prematurity and noncardiac disease.

and velocardiofacial syndromes and associated conotruncal and aortic arch malformations (15). Other mutations in the genes encoding the extracellular matrix proteins fibrillin-1 and elastin are responsible, respectively, for Marfan and Williams syndrome. Genetic syndromes associated with abnormal cardiac development are generally associated with specific cardiac malformations, for instance Down syndrome and endocardial cushion defects, Williams syndrome and supravalvar aortic stenosis, DiGeorge syndrome and tetralogy of Fallot, truncus arteriosus, and interrupted aortic arch (Table 33-3). Recognition that a child has a syndrome associated with a cardiac anomaly, or vice versa, should prompt an investigation for possible associated anomalies (16–20).

Most children with cardiac malformations, even those with tetralogy of Fallot, have isolated cardiac anomalies, without generalized syndrome or other apparent abnormality. Many specific cardiac anomalies are rarely associated with a noncardiac syndrome, for example, transposition of the great arteries, and pulmonary atresia with intact ventricular septum (Table 33-4). Although the molecular biology of cardiovascular development is being unraveled, the specific genetic and/or environmental causes of isolated cardiac anomalies remain unknown in most individual cases (14,15,21). Mutations in 22q11 cause 20% to 30% of isolated conotruncal and aortic arch malformations. Other mutations are involved with at least some of the remainder

(15). For example, alterations in cardiac specific transcription factor control genes, or their function (e.g., NKX2.5, TBX5), sometimes in combination with genes that they control, are being identified in children with isolated cardiac anomalies (15).

Although the occurrence of cardiac malformation has been mostly constant year by year, and by location, there are exceptions. Biochemical and chance events during fetal development may play roles in causation of new genetic mutations and in transcriptional and posttranscriptional processes (9,14,15,22). For instance, the risk for development of conotruncal anomalies is significantly influenced by maternal-fetal intake and metabolism of folic acid and homocysteine (24–28). Although fetal exposure to specific pharmacologic, biochemical, infectious and environmental factors may increase the risk for developing a cardiac abnormality (Table 33-5) (9,29–31), these factors alone do not appear to explain most cases. In individual cases, it is usually difficult or impossible to identify specific extrinsic factors that may have modified the baby's genotype or genotypic expression.

A singular abnormality results in characteristic complex cardiac malformation by altering migration or function of embryonic primordial cells, such as in the neural crest or endocardial cushion, before formation of cardiac structures in the conotruncus or atrioventricular valves, respectively. Animal studies have demonstrated that embryonic

TABLE 33-3
CONGENITAL DISORDERS ASSOCIATED WITH CARDIAC DISEASE

Selected Disorders	Identified Gene(s)	Chromosome Location	% Heart Disease	Cardiovascular Anomalies
Autosomal Dominant				
Alagille Arteriohepatic dysplasia	Jagged 1	20p12	100	multiple PA stenosis and hypoplasia, PDA, ASD, VSD
Apert acrocephalosyndactyly	FGFR-2	10q26		VSD, hypoplastic PA
Beckwith-Wiedemann syndrome	BWS	11pter-p15.4	15 ?	HCM, ASD, VSD, TF, PDA
de Lange syndrome	CDL	3q26.3	30	VSD, ASD, PDA, AS, EFE
CATCH 22/ DiGeorge syndrome	DiGeorge chromosome region	22q11	>50	TF, interrupted Ao arch, truncus arteriosus, right Ao arch
Goldenhar hemifacial microsomaia	HFM	14q32	15	TF, VSD, PDA, COARC
Hereditary hemorrhagic telagiectasia Osler-Weber-Rendu	endoglin	9q34.1	100	pulmonary and systemic AVM, anuerysms, angiectasia
Holt-Oram Heart-hand syndrome	TBX5	12q24.1	100	ASD-2, VSD or PDA in 2/3, conduc. block, HLHS, TAPVC, truncus art.
Klippel-Feil syndrome	KFSL	8q22.2	May-70	VSD, dextrocardia
Marfan syndrome	fibrillin-1	15q21.1	up to 100 %	Ao anuerysm; AR, MR, TR & prolapse
Neurofibromatosis type I	NFI	17q11.2	rare	PS, COARC, renal artery stenosis
Noonan syndrome	NS 1	12q22-qter		PS/dysplasia, PDA, HCM, COARC
Rubinstein-Taybi Broad thumb-hallux syndrome	CREB binding protein	16p13.3	35	VSD, PDA, ASD, COARC, PS
Saethre-Chotzen syndrome	TWIST, FGFR-3&2	7p21,10q26	?	bicupid Ao valve, complex various, subvalvar AS
Shprintzen velocardiofacial syndrome	DiGeorge chromosome region	22q11	80	VSD, TF, right Ao arch, aberrant right subclavian artery
Treacher Collins syndrome	TCOF1	5q32-q33.1	10	ASD, VSD, PDA
Tuberous sclerosis	TSC1	9q34	30	rhabdomyomas, rarely Ao aneuerysm
Williams-Beuren syndrome	elastin	7q11.2	50–80	supravalvar AS, small aorta, stenoses LCA, multiple PAs, cerebral & renal arteries
Autosomal Recessive				
Carpenter acrocephalopolsndactyly type 2	?	?	33	PDA, PS, VSD, TF, TGA, ASD
Coffin-Siris fifth digit syndrome	?	7q32-q34	?	ASD, VSD, TF, PDA
Ellis van Creveld	EVC	4p16	50–60	single atrium, primum ASD, COARC, HLHS
Mucopolysaccharidosis type1 type 2	iduronidase iduronate 2-sulfatase	4p16.3 Xq28	>50	all types have valvular disease, coronary disease (type 2)
type 3D	GNS	12q14		

636

Syndrome	Gene/Etiology	Chromosome	Frequency (%)	Cardiac defects
type 6	arylsulfatase B	5q11-q13	2q32.3-q33.2	TF, COARC, pulmonary hypertension
Pierre Robin syndrome	?	?	20/100	VSD, PDA, ASD, TF, AV canal, COARC
Smith-Lemli-Opitz syndrome 1&2	SLOS	7q32.1	33	ASD, TF
Trombocytopenia absent radius	unknown	unknown		VSD, ASD, PDA
Zellweger cerebro-hepato-renal syndrome	multiple-peroxin-5,2,6,12	7q11.23		
Selected Chromosomal Disorders				
Trisomy 13 Patau syndrome		13	80	PDA, VSD, ASD, COARC, AS, PS
Trisomy 18 Edwards syndrome		18	90–100	VSD, polyvalvular, ASD, PDA
Trisomy 21 Down syndrome		21	40–50	AV canal, VSD, ASD1&2, PDA, TF
+8 Mosaicism		8	25	VSD, PDA, CoAo, PS
+9 Mosaicism		9	70	VSD, PDA, LSVC
XO Turners syndrome		X	>50	bicusp AV, COARC, Ao anuerysm, AS, VSD
4p- Wolfe syndrome		4p	33	VSD, ASD, COARC
5p- Cri-du-Chat syndrome		5p	20	VSD, PDA, ASD, PS
7q-		7q	20	
13q-		13q-	common	VSD, ASD, PDA, PS
18q-		18q	25	COARC, PA hypoplasia, HLHS, LSVS
ring 18		18	20	
10p trisomy		10p	30	AV canal, VSD, ToF
10q24 trisomy		10q24	50	TAPVC, TF
22+ Cat eye syndrome		22	40	Ao root enlargement, MR
Fragile X		x	50	
Syndromes with unknown etiology				
Asymmetric crying facies			44	VSD
CHARGE Association			65–75	TF, DORV, ASD, VSD, PDA, COARC, AV canal
VACTERL Association			10	VSD, ASD, TF
Nonrandom Associations				
cleft lip and palate			25	VSD, PDA, TGA, TF, SV
diaphramatic hernia			25	TF
lung agenesis			20	PDA, VSD, TF, TAPVC
omphalocele			20	TF, ASD
intestinal atresia			10	VSD
renal agenesis unilateral/bilateral			17/75	VSD

Abbreviations: Ao, aortic; AR, aortic regurgitation; AS, aortic stenosis; ASD, atrial septal defect; ASD-1, primum atrial septal defect; ASD-2, secundum atrial septal defect; AV, aortic valve; AV canal, atrioventricular canal defect; AVM, arteriovenous malformation; COARC, coarctation of the aorta; DORV, double-outlet right ventricle; EFE, endocardial fibroelastosis; HLHS, hypoplastic left heart syndrome; LCA, left coronary artery; LSVC, left superior vena cava; MR, mitral regurgitation; PAs, pulmonary arteries; PDA, patent ductus arteriosus; PS, pulmonary valve stenosis; TAPVC, totally anomalous pulmonary venous connection; TF, tetralogy of Fallot; TGA, transposition of great arteries; TR, tricuspid regurgitation; truncus art., truncus arteriosus; VSD, ventricular septal defect. References 9,12,16–20.

637

TABLE 33-4

INCIDENCE OF SEVERE ASSOCIATED NONCARDIAC ANOMALIES AMONG 2,220 INFANTS WITH HEART DISEASE

Diagnosis	Incidence (%)
Endocardial cushion defect	43
Patent ductus arteriosus	31
Ventricular septal defect	24
Malpositions	13
Tetralogy of Fallot	10
Coarctation of aorta	9
Pulmonary atresia with intact septum	1
D-Transposition of the great arteries	1

cervical neural crest cells migrate into the thorax and contribute to formation of the aortic arch and conotruncal outflow region of the heart. Blockage of the normal function of these embryonic neural crest cells results in aortic arch anomalies including aortic interruption; conotruncal abnormalities including tetralogy of Fallot, truncus arteriosus, and transposition; and ventricular inlet anomalies including tricuspid atresia and double-inlet single left ventricle (11,14). Cells in the embryonic endocardial tissue undergo a different developmental sequential process controlled by a large number of factors. Perturbation of specific steps in these embryonic cell process changes developmental sequences in characteristic ways and alters blood flow patterns affecting vascular growth downstream in characteristic ways (9–11). Because growth of specific cardiovascular structures is flow dependent, limitation of flow can cause additional hypoplasia of downstream structures (10,11). For example, a mildly stenotic bicommis-

TABLE 33-5

POSSIBLE TERATOGENS FOR CONGENITAL HEART DISEASE

Vitamin deficiency
  Folate deficiency[a]
Environmental agents
  High altitude,[a] trichloroethylene, irradiation
Drugs
  Ethanol,[a] folic acid antagonists (trimethoprim,[a] sulfasalazine,[a] triamterene,[a] timethadione,[a] phenytoin,[a] primidone,[a] phemobarbitol,[a] carbamazepine,[a] methotrexate)[a], valproic acid,[a] lithium,[a] thalidomide,[a] retinoic acid,[a] antineoplastic agents (?), coumadin,[a] amphetamine, cocaine
Metabolic factors
  Maternal diabetes,[a] maternal phenylketonuria,[a] homocysteine
Immune factors
  Maternal autoimmune disease with anti-Ra anti-LA antibodies
Infectious agents
  Rubella,[a] mumps (?), cytomegalovirus (?)

[a]It is generally accepted that these prenatal factors increase the risk for congenital heart disease.
From refs. 9,12,13,18,23–31,114.

sural aortic valve may decrease blood flow through the aortic isthmus and result in coarctation.

Certain cardiac anomalies are associated with prematurity or low birth weight. Because closure of the ventricular septum may be delayed until the first months of life, it is not surprising that there is a somewhat greater incidence of ventricular septal defect among premature infants. The increased incidence of patent ductus arteriosus in prematurely born infants can be viewed as the result of birth long before the programmed time for closure of the ductus. Hypoxemia of pulmonary origin also promotes ductal patency.

As with gross anatomic cardiac anomalies, specific causes of cardiac muscle diseases unknown until recently are being identified. Many of the hypertrophic and dilated cardiomyopathies previously known as idiopathic are now known to be caused by specific gene mutations and pathogenetic mechanisms (9,16,32–34). Most patients with isolated hypertrophic cardiomyopathy have newly acquired or autosomally dominant inherited mutations in the genes encoding sarcomeric contractile proteins, most commonly cardiac B-myosin heavy chain, cardiac myosin-binding protein C or troponin T2 (32,33). Isolated dilated cardiomyopathy has been associated to date with 19 genetic loci, involving contractile, cytoskeletal and other proteins, and identification of more is likely (9,16,33). Dilated and hypertrophic cardiomyopathies also occur in association with a large number of more generalized neuromuscular and metabolic disorders occurring from specific nuclear and mitochondrial genetic mutations (see Cardiomyopathy and Tables 33-16 and 33-17) (9,16,34).

Some specific arrhythmia syndromes are also caused by specific genetic mutations. These include patients with ventricular tachycardia associated with prolonged QT syndrome and arrhythmogenic right ventricular dysplasia and rare forms of Wolf–Parkinson–White syndrome with supraventricular tachycardia. Long QT syndrome results from mutations in genes encoding specific cardiac potassium and sodium ion channels that regulate repolarization (35); the ensuing prolongation of repolarization results in ventricular tachycardia.

FETAL CARDIOLOGY

Fetal Circulation

Extensive information about the circulatory physiology of the fetus and newborn has accumulated. The works of Barcroft (37), Dawes (38), Lind and associates (39), and Rudolph (40) should be consulted for details, but the central features are discussed here. The circulation before birth consists of parallel circuits (Fig. 33-1). Blood in the aorta may follow several routes to a capillary bed in the fetus or the placenta, back to the heart, passing through either ventricle, and out again to the aorta. The stream of newly oxygenated blood from the placenta passes through the umbilical vein, the ductus venosus, the inferior vena cava,

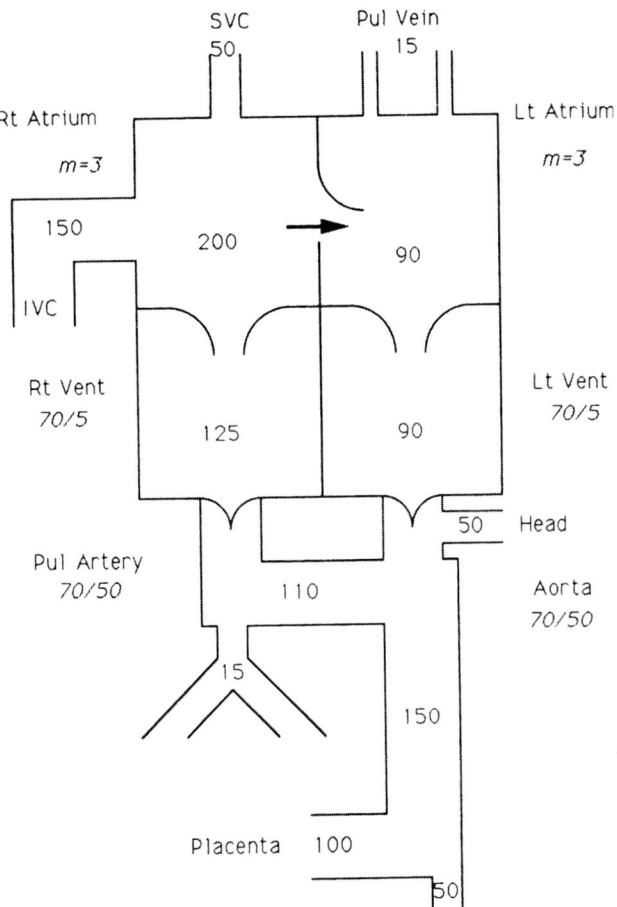

Figure 33-1 Fetal circulation is in parallel, and the amount of blood handled by the left and right ventricles is 125 and 90 mL, respectively. Only 40 mL passes through the aortic arch to the descending aorta, and only a small fraction passes through the lungs. The numbers inside the diagram represent relative blood flow (mL); the numbers in italics are pressure measurements. Modified from Rudolph AM. *Congenital diseases of the heart.* Chicago: Year Book, 1974, with permission.

and the right atrium. Unlike the circulation after birth, the streams of oxygenated and unoxygenated blood are not completely separated, although the more oxygenated blood from the inferior vena cava is mostly diverted through the foramen ovale into the left atrium. Consequently, blood from the left ventricle entering the ascending aorta and coronary and carotid circulations is somewhat higher in oxygen than that entering the descending aorta from the right ventricle by way of the ductus arteriosus.

The volume pumped by the right ventricle is normally about 55% of the combined output of both ventricles. Because both ventricles pump against the systemic resistance, the level of pressure in the two ventricles is comparable. The resistance to blood flow through the lungs is relatively great; only minimal flow through the lungs occurs *in utero*, and almost all of the right ventricular output into the pulmonary artery passes through the ductus arteriosus to the descending aorta. The parallel arrangement of the ventricles allows fetal survival despite a wide variety of cardiac lesions.

With total obstruction of either ventricle, the other ventricle assumes the entire cardiac output. Reversal of the pulmonary arterial and aortic streams of blood, as occurs in transposition of the great arteries, produces no deleterious effect on the fetus. Additionally, ductal or ascending aortic flow may reverse in the presence of severe semilunar valvar stenosis or atresia. Despite this remarkable ability to adapt, grow, and survive, the fetus is affected by limitations in myocardial contractility. Prolonged, severe pressure or volume loading of the heart or primary myocardial disease may result in congestive heart failure, manifested by hydrops fetalis. The interplay between the metabolic effects of congestion in the fetus and the possible compensatory role of the placenta is not understood. Because lesions that may be expected to cause gross intrauterine difficulty are tolerated surprisingly well, the postulate that the placenta helps compensate for the metabolic abnormalities resulting from congestive heart failure is tenable.

Circulatory Adjustments at Birth

Changes in the Source of Oxygenated Blood and in the Ductus Venosus and Ductus Arteriosus

With the first breath, the resistance to pulmonary blood flow drops sharply. The oxygen content of the left heart and systemic circulation rapidly reaches levels well above that of the fetal circulation. Oxygen saturation in the ascending aorta rises from about 65% in the fetus, to about 93% immediately after birth. The ductus venosus functionally closes, establishing the portal circulation as an independent loop between two capillary beds. With removal of the low-resistance placenta, systemic resistance increases. The relative fall in the pulmonary resistance and rise in the systemic resistance result in a transitory left-to-right shunt through the ductus arteriosus. In half of term babies the ductus is completely constricted by the end of the first day of life, and is normally becoming anatomically obliterated at about 10 days of age. Even among cyanotic newborns who are duct dependent, the ductus may inexorably close, often severing the infant's only source of pulmonary or systemic blood flow. The mechanisms causing closure of the ductus arteriosus are not completely understood but involve decreased prostaglandins and increased blood oxygen. Prostaglandin levels in the blood decrease at birth as a result of removal of their placental source of production from the circulation and increase in perfusion of the lungs, in which prostaglandins are metabolized.

Foramen Ovale

Functional closure of the foramen ovale occurs soon after birth, largely as a result of increased left atrial volume and pressure secondary to the increased pulmonary venous return, the ductal left-to-right shunt, and the developing differences in diastolic pressure of the two ventricles. Anatomic closure normally is delayed for months or years.

Among infants with cardiac defects, lesions with increased right atrial pressure favor indefinite patency of the foramen ovale (e.g., pulmonary stenosis), but abnormally increased left atrial pressure promotes early anatomic closure (e.g., ventricular septal defect). Before birth, the pulmonary arterioles are relatively muscular and constricted.

Pulmonary Vasculature

With the first breath, total pulmonary resistance falls rapidly because of the unkinking of the vessels with expansion of the lungs and because of the vasodilatory effect of inspired oxygen. The muscular constriction relaxes, and gradually, during the subsequent days and weeks, the muscular wall of the pulmonary arterioles thins. During the first weeks of life, the muscular arterioles retain a significant capacity for constriction. Pulmonary alveolar hypoxia normally produces an increase in pulmonary artery pressure at all ages, but in the young infant, the response is more profound and occurs more rapidly. Therefore, pulmonary hypertension equal to or greater than systemic pressure occurs commonly in neonates with severe respiratory disease.

Ventricular Work

Before birth, the two ventricles share in supplying systemic blood flow and placental flow, and after birth, the two ventricles sequentially and independently handle the entire cardiac output. At birth, the volume of blood to be pumped by the right ventricle decreases to the level of the systemic blood flow; right ventricular pressure falls as a result of the decrease in pulmonary resistance and closure of the ductus arteriosus. Although right ventricular work decreases, left ventricular work increases (Fig. 33-2). At birth, the left ventricle abruptly becomes the sole supplier of systemic blood flow, and the volume that it pumps is fractionally increased. The left-to-right shunt through the ductus arteriosus adds further volume work, and the elevated systemic resistance must be overcome. Although this is a stressful time for the left ventricle, the magnitude of these suddenly acquired burdens is not so great that detectable left ventricular difficulties are seen normally, but any impairment of myocardial function may be magnified as a consequence. Myocardial disease as a cause of symptoms is more common in the first days of life than at any other time during infancy; 25% of infants with myocardial disease presented in the first week of life (4).

Myocardial Function

Important changes occur in the fetus and neonate in many aspects of myocardial biochemistry and structure. These include myocyte size and number, microvascular structure, myocyte utilization of lactate and fatty acids, and anti-oxidant systems. Many structures and proteins involved in calcium handling within the myocyte, such as t-tubules, sarcoplasmic reticulum, Na+–Ca2+ exchange, Ca2+-ATPase, and phospholamban, have important developmental

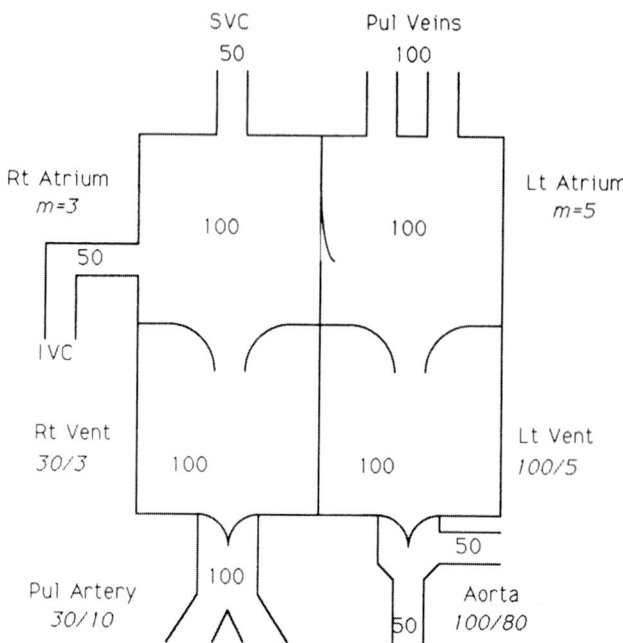

Figure 33-2 Mature circulation is in series, and the amount of blood carried by the two ventricles is approximately the same as before birth. The lungs carry an amount equivalent to the cardiac output, as does the ascending aorta. The numbers inside the diagram represent relative blood flow (mL); the numbers in italics are pressure measurements.

changes. These changes influence the effects on ventricular rhythm and function of normal development, prematurity, ischemia, cardioplegia, and various inborn errors of metabolism.

Fetal Echocardiography

High-resolution two-dimensional ultrasound evaluation of the fetal heart is a useful and accurate technique in the diagnosis and management of the fetus at risk for structural or functional cardiac abnormalities. Indications for prenatal echocardiography may include maternal, fetal, and genetic considerations (Table 33-6). The optimal time for performing fetal echocardiography is 18 to 24 weeks of gestation. At this age, the fetal heart is usually large enough for detailed anatomic evaluation, and the images are unimpaired by dense rib or spine calcification. There is also a relatively large volume of amniotic fluid that facilitates imaging from a variety of angles. For accurate diagnoses the examiner must be experienced in the technical aspects of fetal ultrasonography and knowledgeable in the anatomic patterns and physiologic consequences of congenital heart defects (46). Trans-vaginal ultrasound can provide diagnostic information as early as 10 to 12 weeks gestation, and may be useful when there is a high suspicion of major cardiac anomalies. Three dimensional echocardiography and magnetic resonance imaging has been applied to fetal cardiac evaluation and may improve diagnostic accuracy, although difficulty gating to the fetal heart rate has limited their utility to date.

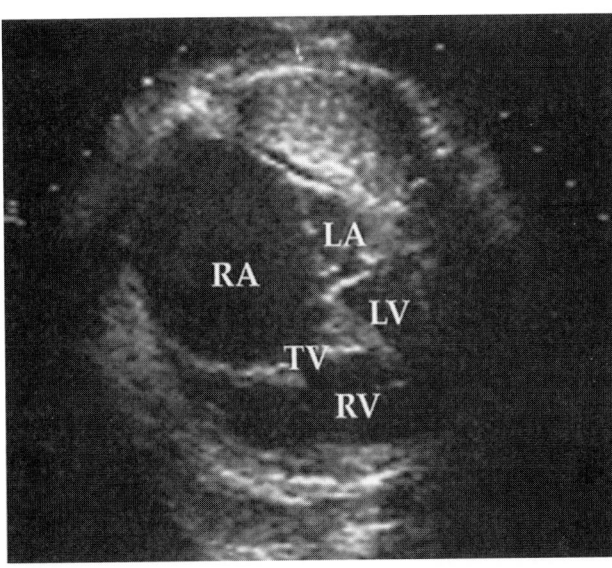

Figure 33-4   Echocardiographic cross-sectional views of the fetal chest in an infant with Ebstein anomaly of the tricuspid valve. The right atrium (RA) is markedly dilated and fills much of the thorax. The left atrium (LA) and left ventricle (LV) are of normal size but are dwarfed by the right-sided structures. The severely regurgitant tricuspid valve has apical displacement of the septal leaflet into the right ventricle (RV).

TABLE 33-6
INDICATIONS FOR FETAL ECHOCARDIOGRAPHY

Suspected cardiac malformation on general ultrasound
Other malformations noted on general ultrasound
Oligo- or polyhydramnios
Fetal dysrhythmia
Suspected or known chromosomal abnormality
Family history of congenital heart disease
Family history of chromosomal abnormality
Maternal diabetes
Maternal collagen vascular disease
Rubella exposure
Evidence of hydrops fetalis
Intrauterine growth retardation
Maternal drug exposure, including:
    Lithium
    Hormones
    Anticonvulsants
    Chemotherapy
    Alcohol

Cardiac Anatomy

Virtually all major cardiac malformations can be detected prenatally using high-resolution two-dimensional, real-time sector scanning by an experienced examiner. The details of systemic and pulmonary venous connections, arterial alignment, chamber size and orientation, and valve position and function can be determined (Fig. 33-3) and abnormal structures demonstrated (Figs. 33-4 and 33-5).

Cardiac Physiology

Color Doppler provides a quick and sensitive means of evaluating the function of atrioventricular and semilunar valves,

the direction of flow in fetal vessels, and the presence of normal and abnormal connections (Fig. 33-5). If abnormal flow is detected, it can be evaluated further using the quantitative capabilities of pulsed or continuous-wave Doppler.

Cardiac Function

A qualitative assessment of cardiac function is obtained by visual inspection of ventricular motion during real-time

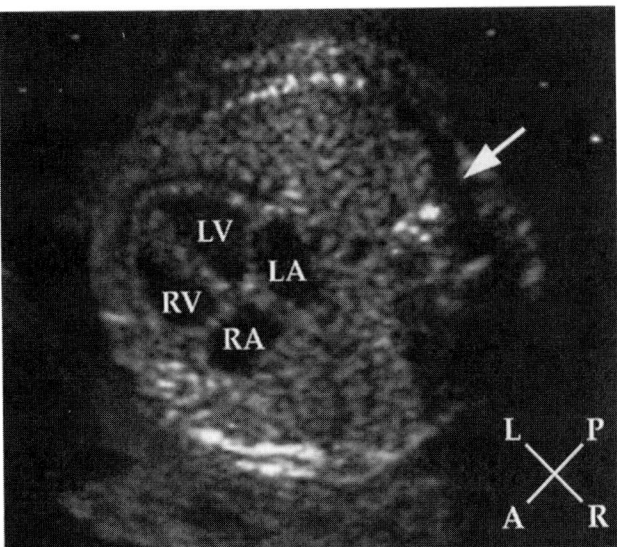

Figure 33-3   Echocardiogram of the normal fetal heart in a four-chamber view demonstrating the position of the heart and the cardiac chambers in a cross-section of the chest. A, anterior; L, left; LA, left atrium; LV, left ventricle; P, posterior; R, right; RA, right atrium; RV, right ventricle; arrow denotes the spine.

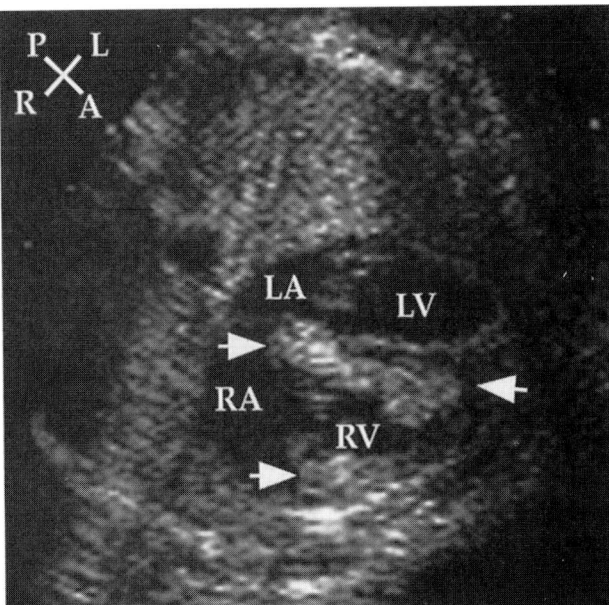

Figure 33-5   Echocardiographic cross-sectional view of a fetus with multiple intramyocardial rhabdomyomas (arrows). The infant was subsequently diagnosed with tuberous sclerosis. A, anterior; L, left; LA, left atrium; LV, left ventricle; P, posterior; R, right; RA, right atrium; RV, right ventricle.

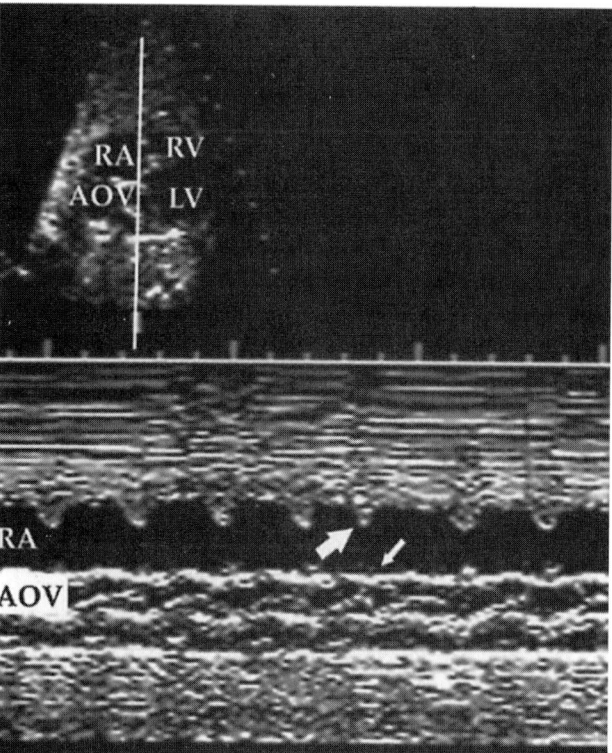

Figure 33-6 Echocardiogram of a fetus with a premature atrial beat. The upper left image is a two-dimensional view with a cursor (line) through the fetal right atrium (RA) and aortic valve (AOV), demonstrating the axis of the simultaneous M-mode echocardiogram seen in the lower panel. The M-mode tracing depicts the motion of the fetal right atrial wall and aortic valve in the cursor line over a time frame of 3 seconds. A series of normal atrial wall contractions are interrupted by a premature contraction (large arrow) followed by opening of the aortic valve (small arrow), demonstrating a premature atrial beat conducted to the ventricle. LV, left ventricle; RV, right ventricle.

sector scanning. When more quantitative information is desired, M-mode recording can provide precise dimensions and an accurate measure of ventricular shortening (Fig. 33-6). Doppler derived indices of cardiac function may also provide insight into fetal cardiac performance and three-dimensional imaging and fetal MRI may ultimately prove useful as well. Severe ventricular dysfunction may manifest as generalized hydrops fetalis, which is readily recognized by ultrasound as pleural and peritoneal fluid accumulation and cutaneous edema.

Arrhythmias

Tachyarrhythmias, bradyarrhythmias, and irregular cardiac rhythms are common reasons for referral for evaluation. Structural and functional abnormalities should be excluded, as described above. The mechanism of the rhythm disturbance can usually be elucidated by determining the timing of atrial and ventricular contraction using an M-mode (Fig. 33-6), two-dimensional and Doppler echocardiography, which simultaneously display atrial and ventricular wall and valve motions and flows. By this means, the timing and sequence of atrial and ventricular activation can be deduced. The most common rhythm disturbance is iso-

lated premature atrial contractions in a structurally normal heart or in association with an atrial septal aneurysm. Sustained tachyarrhythmia usually represents a reentrant or ectopic atrial tachycardia. These infants must be monitored closely for the development of congestive heart failure and hydrops fetalis, which would be an indication for induced delivery of the mature fetus or maternal antidysrhythmic therapy in the immature fetus. Sustained bradyarrhythmias may be secondary to heart block, nonconducted premature atrial contractions, or noncardiac sources of fetal distress. The mechanism can be inferred as described above and appropriate therapy initiated if indicated (see Arrhythmias).

FETAL CARDIAC INTERVENTION

Improvements in prenatal diagnostic techniques have led to renewed interest in fetal cardiac intervention. The restoration of more normal flow and pressure relationships in the developing heart may encourage normal or near normal growth and function, improving the postnatal outcomes and surgical and medical options. Exteriorization of the fetus and surgical intervention has been performed, but the inevitable development of premature labor remains a major obstacle to the development of fetal cardiac surgical techniques. Improvements in fetal imaging techniques are compatible with interventional catheterization methodology. The technical feasibility of aortic valve dilation in the fetus using new, low-profile coronary balloons and wires to dilate aortic valves in fetuses likely to acquire hypoplastic left heart syndrome without intervention has recently been demonstrated. Additionally, there has been some success in creating atrial communications in fetuses with premature closure of the foramen ovale in association with left sided obstruction. Attempts have also been made to re-establish communication between the right ventricle and pulmonary arteries in fetuses with valvar pulmonary atresia. Issues of patient selection, timing and outcome are only beginning to be addressed, and the clinical utility of prenatal interventions is yet to be determined.

PREMATURITY

The circulatory adjustments and myocardial biochemical changes at birth and in the neonatal period are modified in direct relation to the degree of prematurity. The muscular coat of the pulmonary arterioles develops late in gestation; the more premature the infant, the less muscular are the pulmonary arterioles at birth. The most notable consequence of this is that the difference between systemic and pulmonary resistance after birth is greater among premature than among normal infants. Shunting through a ductus arteriosus is often audible. Developmental biological factors in the ductus arteriosus and hypoxia, so common among premature infants, may be factors that contribute to the delay in closure of the ductus in premature infants. The propensity of the ductus to close at around 41 weeks after conception is clinically recognized. Developmental changes in myocardial structure and biochemistry may influence the function of the left ventricle in response to stress such as volume overload associated with the left-to-right shunt through a patent ductus arteriosus.

RECOGNITION OF CLINICAL FEATURES

Only a few infants are born in hospitals equipped for all eventualities. Infants with serious heart anomalies require transportation to a specialized pediatric cardiac center for detailed diagnostic assessment with echocardiography, and treatment that may include cardiac catheterization and/or surgery. Timely clinical recognition of the likely presence of a specific cardiac anomaly, that without intervention will result in serious deterioration of the baby's condition

(e.g., critical coarctation of the aorta, pulmonary valve atresia), is necessary for initiation of medical therapy to prevent and/or reverse clinical deterioration (e.g., administration of prostaglandin, inotropic agents, oxygen, and ventilation) and thereby provide the time and conditions necessary to transfer, evaluate, and treat the baby.

Initial evaluation includes assessment for cyanosis (See Color Plate) and of the infant's well-being, perfusion, pulses and blood pressure in the extremities, respiratory work and rate, precordial activity, second heart sound splitting, and murmur intensity, quality, pitch, and timing. Chest radiograph and electrocardiogram (ECG) remain cost- and time-efficient tests that aid in the initial evaluation of suspected congenital heart disease. Any one of these alone is rarely diagnostic. A number of lesions result in cyanosis; quite a number of lesions are also associated with loud murmurs; others are associated with little or no murmur; some cause shock (see Figs. 33-7 and 33-8). Others have chest

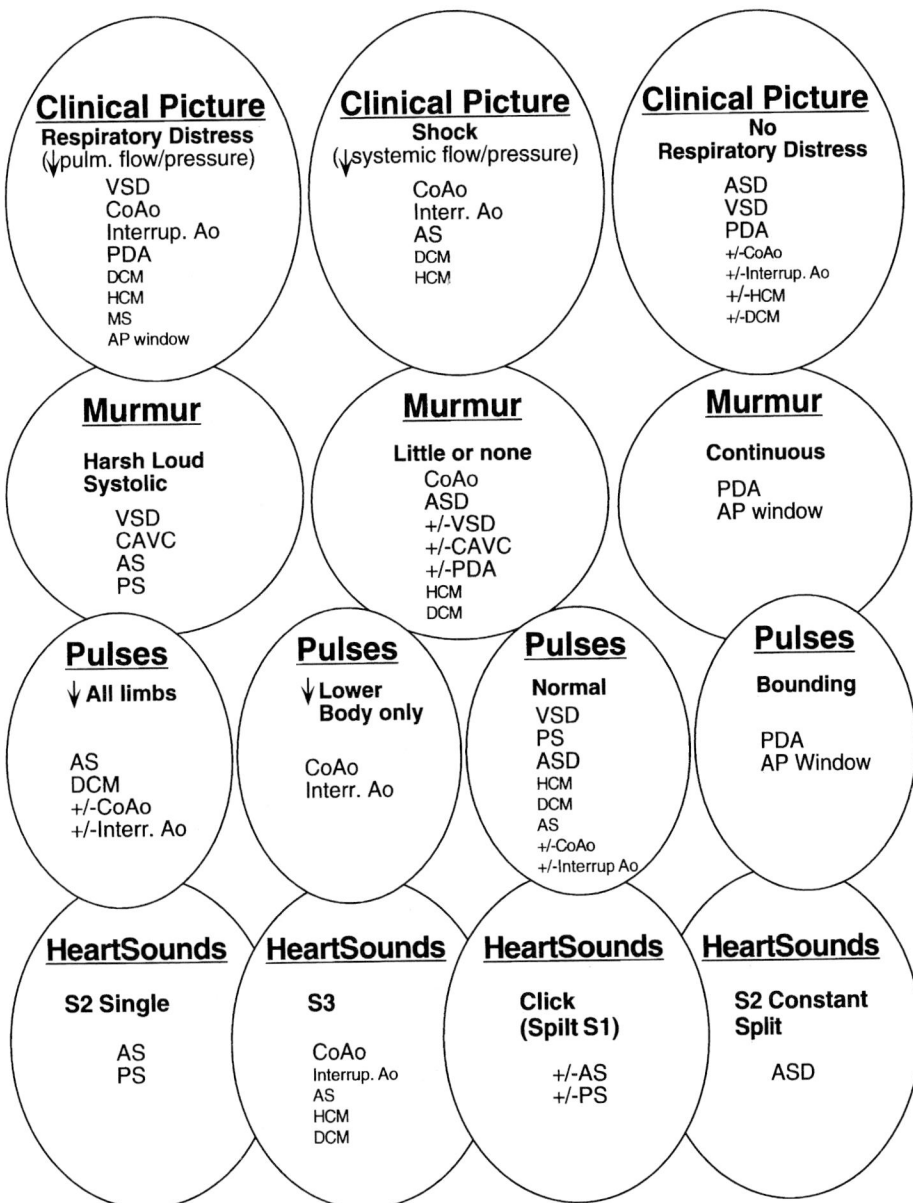

Figure 33-7 The differential diagnosis of cardiac exam findings in acyanotic neonates. Anomalies in larger print are more common. +/−, sometimes; up arrow, increased; down arrow, decreased; AP window, aorticopulmonary window; AS, aortic stenosis; ASD, atrial septal defect; CAVC, complete atrioventricular canal defect; CoAo, coarctation of the aorta; DCM, dilated cardiomyopathy; HCM, hypertrophic cardiomyopathy; Interrup. Ao, interrupted aortic arch; MS, mitral stenosis; PDA, patent ductus arteriosus; PS, pulmonary stenosis; VSD, ventricular septal defect.

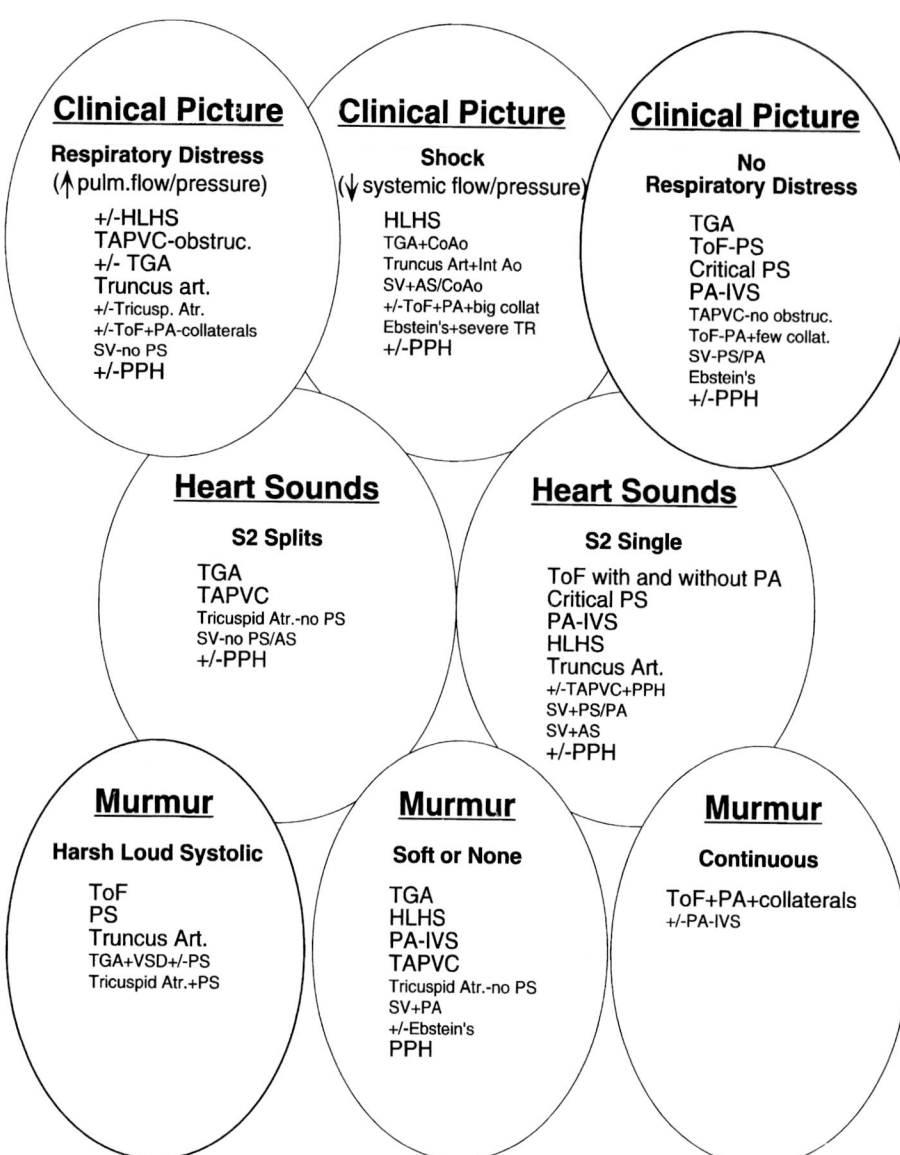

Figure 33-8 The differential diagnosis of cardiac exam findings in cyanotic neonates. +/−, sometimes; up arrow, increased; down arrow, decreased; AS, aortic stenosis; CoAo, coarctation of aorta; collat., systemic to pulmonary artery collateral vessels; Ebstein's, Ebstein anomaly of the tricuspid valve; HLHS, hypoplastic left heart syndrome; Int Ao, interrupted aorta; PA, pulmonary atresia; PA-IVS, pulmonary atresia with intact interventricular septum; PPH, persistent pulmonary hypertension syndrome; PS, pulmonary stenosis; SV, single ventricle; TAPVC, totally anomalous pulmonary venous connection; TGA, transposition of great arteries; ToF, tetralogy of Fallot; tricuspid atr., tricuspid atresia.

radiographs with increased pulmonary arterial or venous markings, others have diminished pulmonary vascular markings. Most have an undistinguished electrocardiogram at birth, although some have left axis deviation on electrocardiogram (see Figs. 33-9 and 33-10). Most cardiac anomalies vary in their characteristics at presentation. Furthermore, often it is not possible to determine with certainty if the second heart sound is split or not, or if the pulmonary vascular markings on chest radiograph are normal vs. increased or normal versus decreased. Clinical analysis requires weighting of the categories of evidence regarding its certainty and other possibilities. A classical diagnostic approach based on sequential analysis of data categories is limited by these types of weakness in the clinical information and is no stronger than the weakest link in the chain of information. However, interweaving of the findings provides a matrix of diagnostic information that remains intact even when one category of findings is weak. Overlapping possible anomalies suggested from history, physical examination, chest radiograph and electrocardiogram, as if with a series of Venn diagrams (see Figs. 33-7, 33-8, 33-9, and 33-10), provides information that allows a careful observer to quickly determine which anomaly, or which two or three possible anomalies, is likely present. Comparing the anomalies consistent with the clinical presentation with the anomalies consistent with the murmur findings, other physical exam findings, chest radiograph findings, and electrocardiographic findings, usually focuses the list of possible anomalies on one or two primary choices (see Fig. 33-11). This may provide an important advantage in the timely and efficient management of potentially life threatening anomalies. For example, the combination of cyanosis, soft or no murmur, single S2, chest radiograph with decreased pulmonary vascular markings and normal heart size, and electrocardiogram R axis of 50° suggests pulmonary atresia, which is an anomaly in which life depends on maintaining ductal patency (see Figs. 33-8 and 33-10). Two-dimensional echocardiogram should be obtained promptly if significant cardiac disease is suspected. This technique when done by personnel trained for evalua-

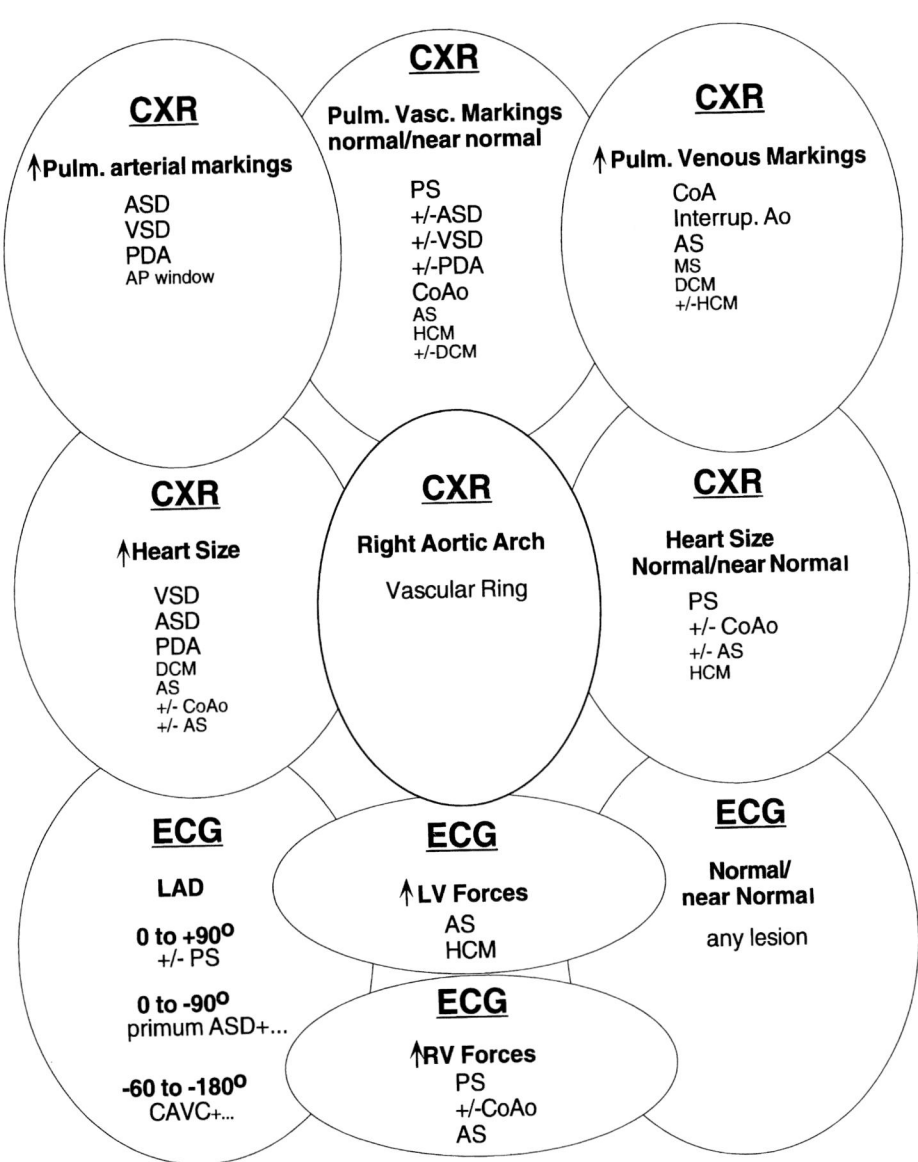

Figure 33-9 The differential diagnosis of chest radiographic and electrocardiographic findings in acyanotic neonates. Abbreviations, see Fig. 33-7; CXR, chest radiograph; LAD; left axis deviation; LV, left ventricle; Pulm. vasc. markings, pulmonary vascular markings; RV, right ventricle.

tion of congenital cardiac anomalies in neonates accurately demonstrates the anatomy, occasionally uncovering a potentially lethal lesion before symptoms. Appropriate initial management (e.g., infusion of PGE1 in a cyanotic infant suspected to have pulmonary atresia) need not await availability of echocardiography (see Fig. 33-12 and Management Procedures for Severe Cardiac Disease).

Age of Presentation

Most children with critical congenital cardiac anomaly develop symptoms within the first weeks of life (8). The age when infants develop cardiac symptoms is diagnostically useful. For instance, although ventricular septal defect is far more common (Table 33-2), transposition of the great arteries, coarctation of the aorta, and the hypoplastic left heart syndrome are the most common life-threatening anomalies presenting in the first days of life (see Table 33-7). Isolated ventricular septal defect is not associated with cyanosis, the associated murmur generally develops after several days or

more, and respiratory symptoms usually do not develop until after the first week of life. Among those whose problem is cyanosis, transposition of the great arteries is the leading cause through the third week of life; after that time, tetralogy of Fallot becomes the dominant cause of cyanosis. Among neonatal cardiac patients admitted because of respiratory symptoms, the hypoplastic left heart syndrome is the leading cause in the first week, complex coarctation leads in the second week, and thereafter, ventricular septal defect becomes the main cause (see Table 33-6).

Physical Examination

Respiratory Symptoms

Persistent tachypnea may be the first clue to heart disease or lung disease. Cardiac abnormalities with excessive pulmonary arterial flow or pulmonary venous hypertension cause pulmonary vascular engorgement, pulmonary edema, and decreased lung compliance that often result in

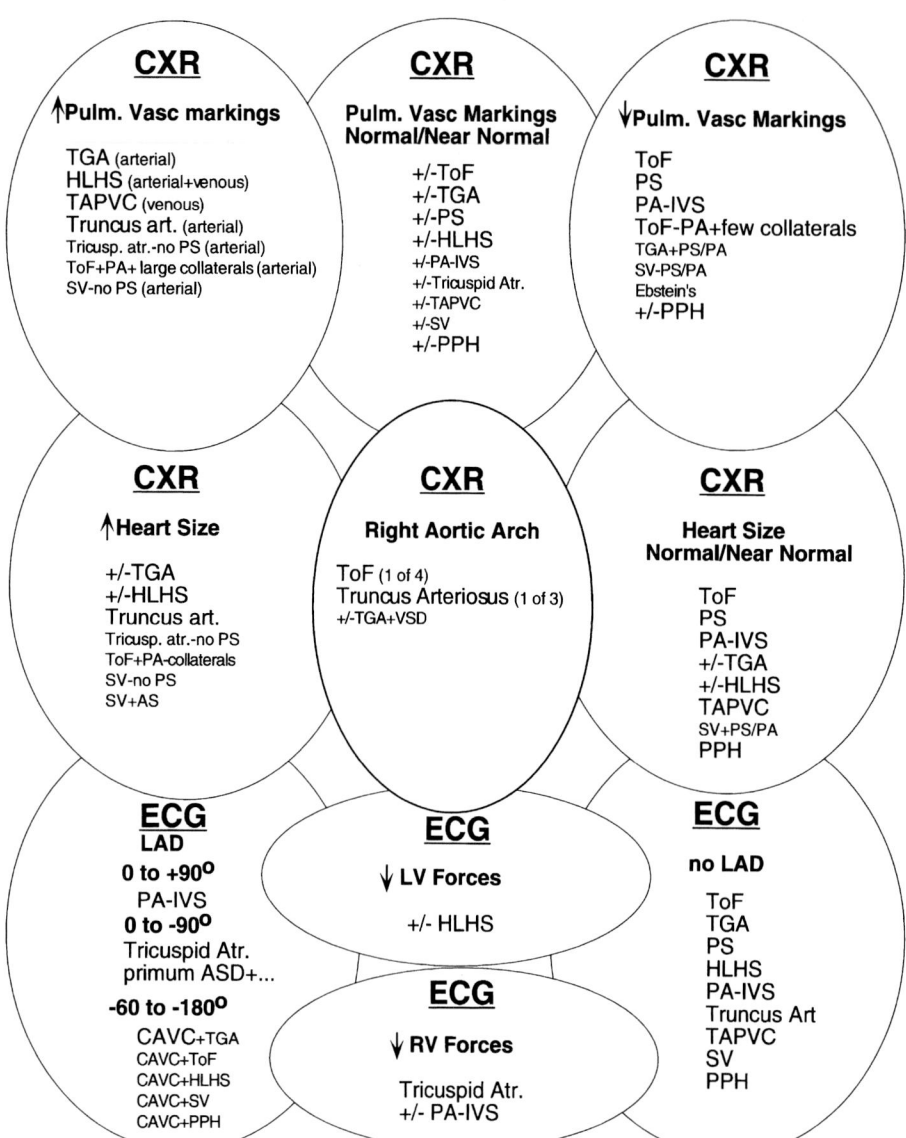

CXR

↑Pulm. Vasc markings

TGA (arterial)
HLHS (arterial+venous)
TAPVC (venous)
Truncus art. (arterial)
Tricusp. atr.-no PS (arterial)
ToF+PA+ large collaterals (arterial)
SV-no PS (arterial)

CXR

Pulm. Vasc Markings
Normal/Near Normal

+/-ToF
+/-TGA
+/-PS
+/-HLHS
+/-PA-IVS
+/-Tricuspid Atr.
+/-TAPVC
+/-SV
+/-PPH

CXR

↓Pulm. Vasc Markings

ToF
PS
PA-IVS
ToF-PA+few collaterals
TGA+PS/PA
SV-PS/PA
Ebstein's
+/-PPH

CXR

↑Heart Size

+/-TGA
+/-HLHS
Truncus art.
Tricusp. atr.-no PS
ToF+PA-collaterals
SV-no PS
SV+AS

CXR

Right Aortic Arch

ToF (1 of 4)
Truncus Arteriosus (1 of 3)
+/-TGA+VSD

CXR

Heart Size
Normal/Near Normal

ToF
PS
PA-IVS
+/-TGA
+/-HLHS
TAPVC
SV+PS/PA
PPH

ECG
LAD

0 to +90°
PA-IVS
0 to -90°
Tricuspid Atr.
primum ASD+...
-60 to -180°
CAVC+TGA
CAVC+ToF
CAVC+HLHS
CAVC+SV
CAVC+PPH

ECG

↓ LV Forces

+/- HLHS

ECG

↓ RV Forces

Tricuspid Atr.
+/- PA-IVS

ECG

no LAD

ToF
TGA
PS
HLHS
PA-IVS
Truncus Art
TAPVC
SV
PPH

Figure 33-10 The differential diagnosis of chest radiographic and electrocardiographic findings in cyanotic neonates. Abbreviations, see Figs. 33-8 and 33-9.

increased respiratory effort and rate. Cardiac anomalies with decreased pulmonary blood flow often have intense cyanosis that elicits a reflex "peaceful" tachypnea without respiratory distress. Experienced parents often observe that the affected baby had always breathed too fast. Persistent respiratory rates of 60 per minute or greater, often with minimally labored but persistently increased depth of respiration, commonly precede other findings and may presage clinical deterioration. A chest radiograph may differentiate cardiac from pulmonary disease.

Systemic Perfusion and Pressure

Decreased systemic cardiac output is an ominous sign that requires rapid assessment and rapid appropriate management for the infant to survive. There are many potential noncardiac causes, the most common being sepsis, and important cardiac causes (see Figs. 33-7 and 33-8). Signs of diminished systemic perfusion include poorly perfused, cool, and/or mottled skin, listlessness,

diminished peripheral pulse intensity, diminished systolic and pulse pressure, decreased urine output, and metabolic acidosis. Blood pressure should be measured in all four extremities in an infant who appears severely ill with these signs, particularly with coexistence of a murmur or cyanosis. Oscillometric devices can quickly and noninvasively measure blood pressure, although their correlation with centrally measured blood pressure declines in the presence of very low perfusion and pressure. It is very important to establish if the pulse amplitude and systolic blood pressure are diminished only in the postductal arterial distribution or throughout the body, that is, if the right arm systolic blood pressure is similar to or higher than that in the other extremities. Significant differential in the systolic blood pressure between the arms (usually right) and the legs (and umbilical artery) is diagnostic of an aortic obstruction. The additional presence of a murmur, gallop, hepatomegaly, or cyanosis further strongly suggests that a cardiac anomaly is causative of poor perfusion.

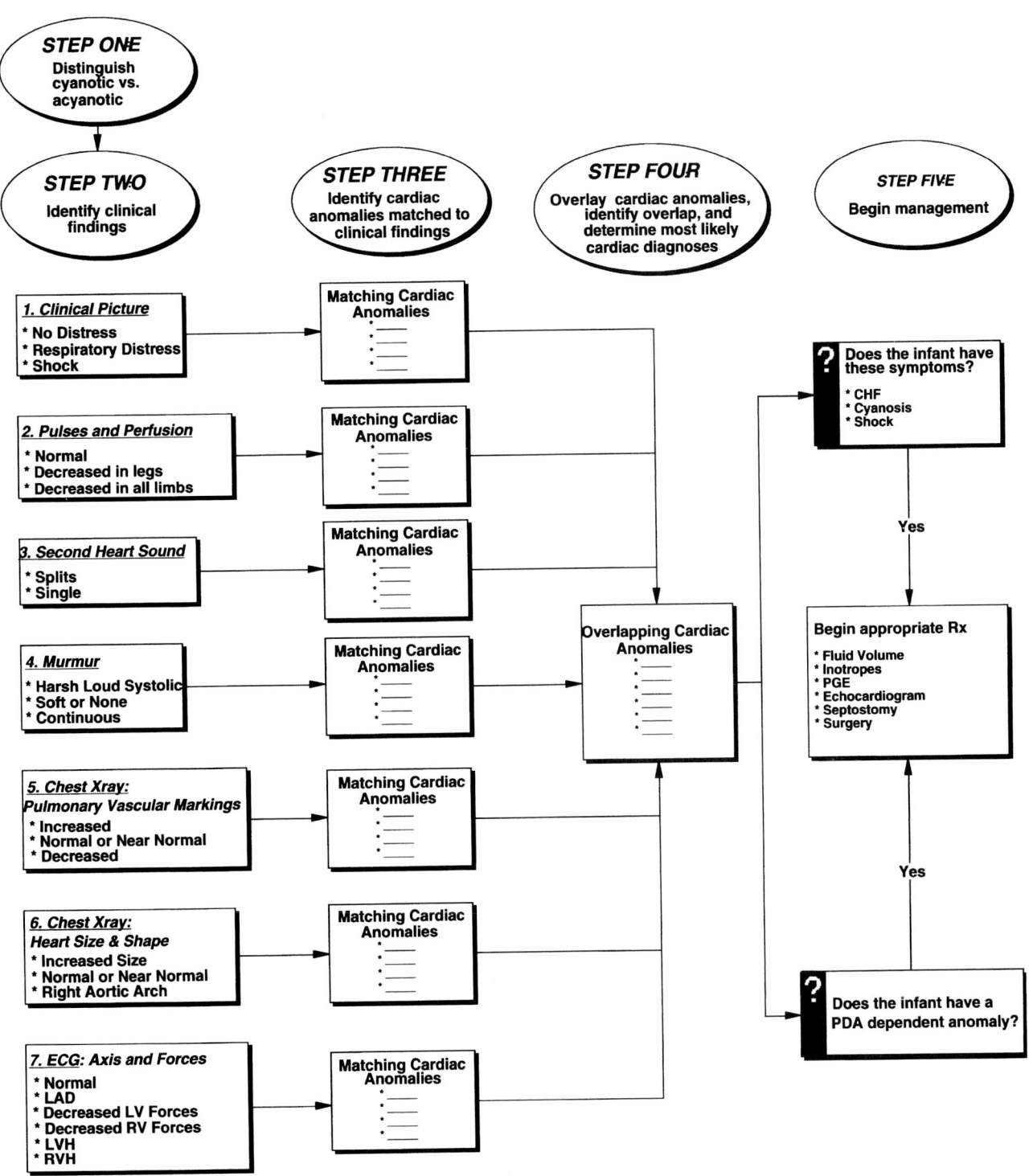

Figure 33-11 A process for diagnosing cardiac anomalies from findings on cardiac exam, chest radiograph, and electrocardiogram. ASAP, as soon as possible; c/w, consistent with; FiO₂, fractional percentage of inspired oxygen; PDA, patent ductus arteriosus.

Murmur

Hearing a murmur is the most common means of recognizing the presence of heart disease in an infant. Determining the diagnosis requires ascertaining the characteristics of the murmur. These include the history of the baby's age when the murmur was first audible and examination findings of murmur timing in systole versus diastole, loudness, pitch

and the association of a thrill. The murmurs of valvar regurgitation and stenosis are audible immediately after birth, and the murmurs of septal defects are usually delayed days to weeks, or as long as several months in the case of atrial septal defects. Diastolic murmurs are rare but indicative of cardiac pathology. A prominent continuous murmur in a cyanotic neonate, particularly in the back or axilla, is rare but is very characteristic of tetralogy of Fallot with

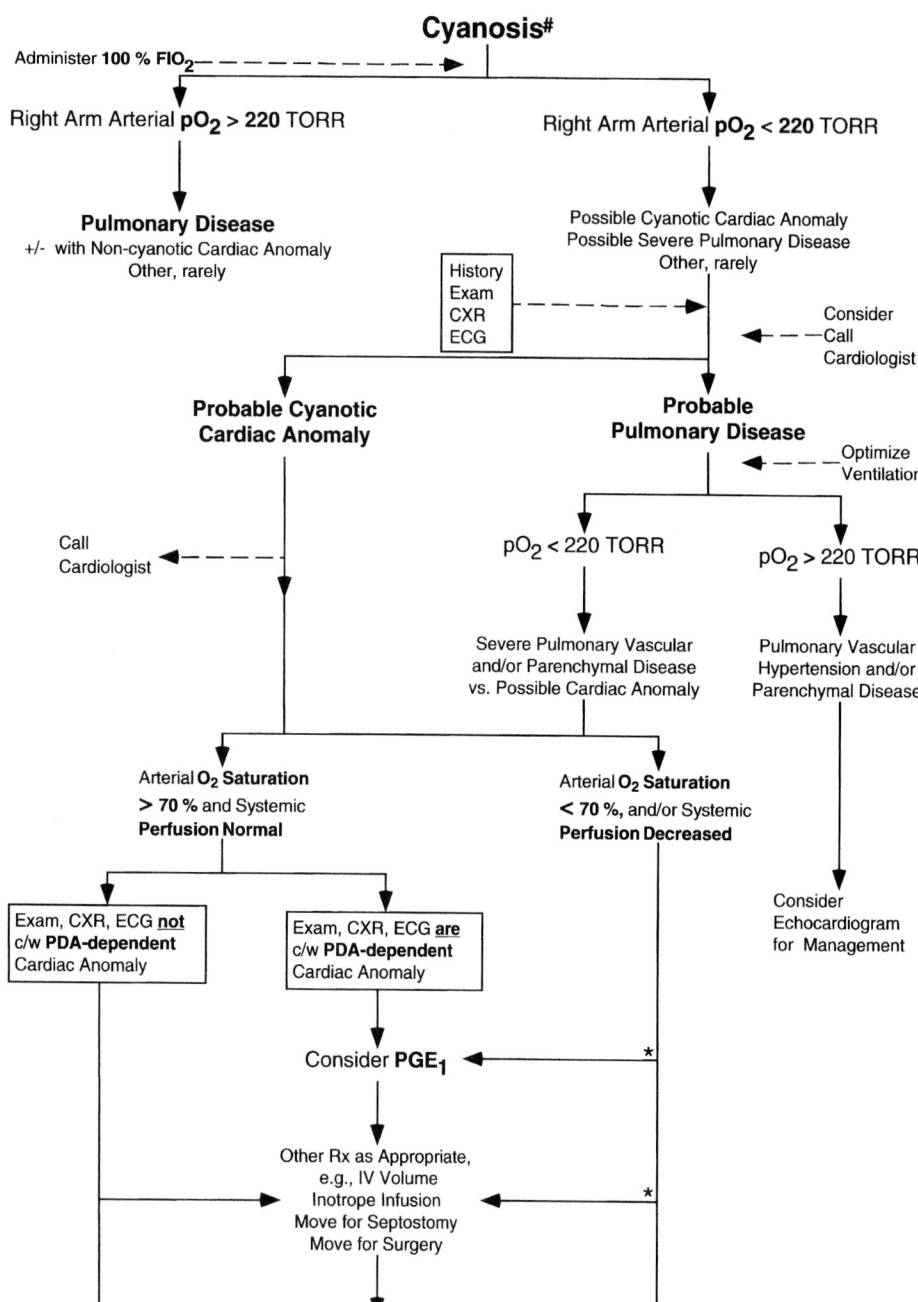

Figure 33-12 An approach to the diagnosis and management of cyanotic infants. #, cyanosis; see text for additional details of assessment of cyanosis; +/−, possibly; *, see text concerning management of specific anomalies; ASAP, as soom as possible; c/w, consistent with; FiO₂, fraction inspired oxygen; Rx, treatment.

pulmonary atresia and systemic-to-pulmonary-artery collateral vessels (the latter being the cause of the murmur). The loudness of a murmur, in combination with other findings, may suggest the likelihood of various anomalies but is often not proportional to the severity of the lesion. The absence of a murmur does not preclude serious heart disease. To the contrary, many life-threatening cardiac anomalies may be associated with little or no murmur. In a neonate with cyanosis and/or shock and suspected cardiac anomaly, the presence of little or no murmur provides a diagnostic clue (see Figs. 33-7 and 33-8). The pitch of a murmur is associated with the pressure gradient across the abnormality causing the murmur. Tiny ventricular septal defects develop a characteristic fairly high-pitched murmur

when the right ventricular pressure decreases to much less than the left ventricular pressure. Severe pulmonary or aortic stenosis can sometimes be distinguished from mild stenosis by a high-pitched harsh loud murmur and an associated thrill.

Heart Sounds

Auscultation of the heart sound splitting is the most difficult part of the cardiac examination in neonates because of the relatively rapid heart and respiratory rates in neonates. However, when abnormalities of the first and second heart sounds are strongly suspected or excluded, it provides important information. Detection of splitting of the heart

TABLE 33-7

TOP FIVE DIAGNOSES PRESENTING AT DIFFERENT AGES

Diagnosis	Percentage of Patients
Age on admission: 0–6 days (n = 537)	
D-Transposition of great arteries	19
Hypoplastic left ventricle	14
Tetralogy of Fallot	8
Coarctation of aorta	7
Ventricular septal defect	3
Others	49
Age on admission: 7–13 days (n = 195)	
Coarctation of aorta	16
Ventricular septal defect	14
Hypoplastic left ventricle	8
D-Transposition of great arteries	7
Tetralogy of Fallot	7
Others	48
Age on admission: 14–28 days (n = 177)	
Ventricular septal defect	16
Coarctation of aorta	12
Tetralogy of Fallot	7
D-Transposition of great arteries	7
Patent ductus arteriosus	5
Others	53

sounds requires practice and a minute or so of focused attention on just that sound, using a quality stethoscope, in a quieted baby. The absence of splitting may result from a heart rate too fast to discern splitting or a truly single-component sound. A split first heart sound in a neonate suggests a click. The second heart sound emanates from closure of the aortic and pulmonary valves. Determining that the second heart sound is split (i.e., has two components) suggests that both aortic and pulmonary valves are not severely abnormal; that is, it is against the presence of aortic or pulmonary valve atresia or severe stenosis. However, other serious anomalies with two semilunar valves may still be present, for example, simple transposition of the great arteries. A second heart sound that always appears single, particularly at heart rates not greater than 120 per minute, may be caused by relatively early pulmonary valve closure associated with elevation of pulmonary artery pressures comparable to aortic pressures, but it suggests that the pulmonary or aortic valve may be abnormal (as in pulmonary atresia or critical stenosis, hypoplastic left heart syndrome, truncus arteriosus). Although difficult to detect, constant splitting of the second heart sound, as opposed to the usual intermittent splitting, suggests a atrial septal defect.

Cyanosis

Much more threatening than a murmur is the presence of cyanosis. Cyanosis without pulmonary disease is almost invariably the result of a serious cardiac abnormality.

Cyanosis may result from poor mixing of separate parallel circulations (e.g., transposition of the great arteries, other anomalies with transposition physiology such as Taussig–Bing-type double-outlet right ventricle); restricted pulmonary blood flow and right-to-left shunting of un-oxygenated systemic venous blood to the systemic arterial circulation (e.g., tetralogy of Fallot, critical pulmonary stenosis, tricuspid atresia); or right-to-left shunting from intracardiac mixing with normal or increased pulmonary blood flow (e.g., total anomalous pulmonary venous connection without obstruction, truncus arteriosus, single ventricle without pulmonary stenosis, hypoplastic left heart syndrome). Especially in the first week of life, cyanosis may be the sole evidence of an important cardiac lesion. One-third of infants with potentially lethal congenital heart disease have cyanosis as their major symptom; another one-third have cyanosis associated with respiratory symptoms. Prompt cardiac evaluation of all cyanotic babies is mandatory because prompt infusion of prostaglandin endothelin (E1) to open the ductus arteriosus or catheter intervention to create an atrial septal defect may be necessary for survival, and most of the responsible lesions are amenable to surgery.

The clinical recognition of cyanosis is dependent on the amount of oxygen desaturation of arterial hemoglobin and therefore is influenced by the total blood hemoglobin concentration. An anemic infant may have severe arterial oxygen unsaturation without obvious cyanosis, and infants with polycythemia may appear cyanotic with near normal arterial oxygen levels. Hypothermic infants may seem blue; babies viewed in fluorescent lighting or in blue surroundings may make the estimation of cyanosis more difficult. Persistent cyanosis secondary to hypoglycemia or methemoglobinemia is rare. Cyanosis is particularly evident in the lips. Peri-oral or nail-bed cyanosis without lip cyanosis is usually not caused by cyanotic heart disease. When cyanosis is suspected, indirect assessment of arterial oxygen saturation by the transcutaneous method can provide a rapid noninvasive check.

Acute Lung Disease and Cardiac Disease

Rapid determination of the diagnosis and initiation of appropriate management is most pressing when the infant is dyspneic and cyanotic. A chest radiograph may suggest lung disease, particularly if the findings are asymmetric. In the presence of diffuse symmetric changes possibly compatible with pulmonary edema or increased vascular markings, caution is necessary, particularly in the full-term neonate. The differential diagnosis between primary lung disease and heart disease causing pulmonary edema (e.g., total anomalous pulmonary venous connection with obstruction) can be difficult. Persistent pulmonary arterial hypertension with right-to-left shunting may coexist with lung disease and cause severe cyanosis. Although carbon dioxide retention is usually prominent among babies with primary lung disease, some severely cyanotic infants with cardiac anomalies can have marked hypercarbia. It can also be difficult to differentiate cardiac anomalies with diminished pulmonary blood flow and little murmur (e.g., pulmonary valve atresia) from persistent pulmonary arterial hypertension without other, radiographically apparent, lung parenchymal disease. Although the absence of hypercarbia suggests cardiac disease, some severely cyanotic infants with pulmonary vascular disease have normal partial pressure of CO_2 (PCO_2) values.

The response of the arterial partial pressure of oxygen (PO_2) to administration of 100% oxygen, with the exceptions noted below, can differentiate cyanotic heart disease from lung disease. The infant who responds to breathing pure oxygen with a rise in arterial PO_2 to 220 mm Hg or more does not have cyanotic heart disease, and the infant who does not raise his preductal arterial PO_2 above 100 mm Hg is likely to have heart disease. Transcutaneous estimation of arterial oxygen saturation is not an accurate alternative because any arterial PO_2 greater than 70 mm Hg will result in arterial oxygen saturation greater than 95%. Because the hyperoxia test is inconclusive when the arterial PO_2 is between 100 and 220 mm Hg, these babies should be approached as possibly having cyanotic heart disease (see Fig. 33-12). The arterial PO_2 while the baby is breathing 100% oxygen may initially be most rapidly measured from an umbilical artery catheter positioned in the descending aorta. However, a low arterial PO_2 measured in the descending aorta may be from right-to-left shunting through a ductus arteriosus from coexisting persistent pulmonary hypertension. Comparison of the PO_2 measured in blood from the right radial artery with the PO_2 measured in blood from the umbilical arterial catheter may help to differentiate persistent pulmonary hypertension from cyanotic cardiac anomaly. The former may have a high PO_2 in the right radial artery. Simultaneous mechanical hyperventilation and administration of oxygen may decrease pulmonary resistance and increase pulmonary flow, increasing the PO_2 to greater than 220 mm Hg in the descending aortic and/or right radial arterial blood, allowing differentiation of lung disease or persistent pulmonary hypertension from cyanotic cardiac anomaly. Difficulties arise when pulmonary and cardiac pathology coexist. For example, in the baby with both lung and heart disease or those with coexistence of persistent pulmonary hypertension and predominant right-to-left shunting through the foramen ovale (see Chapters 29 and 32) or the baby with heart disease causing pulmonary venous hypertension and pulmonary edema, results may be confusing. Arterial PO_2 may not significantly increase in response to 100% oxygen with severe persistent pulmonary hypertension and predominant right-to-left shunting through the foramen ovale. If doubt persists, the physician can make the diagnosis with two-dimensional echocardiography (see Fig. 33-12).

Noncardiac Anomalies

It is useful to know the relative frequency of the cardiac diagnostic possibilities when there are associated noncardiac anomalies (see Tables 33-3 and 33-4) or prematurity.

Among premature infants, patent ductus arteriosus, coarctation of the aorta, and ventricular septal defect occur more often. Chromosomal abnormalities and congenital syndromes are also associated with lower birth weight cardiac malformations (e.g., Down syndrome).

DIAGNOSTIC TOOLS

Chest Radiography

Chest radiography is rarely diagnostic of specific cardiac lesions, but it is a relatively quick and relatively inexpensive method to identify lung disease and screen for suspected cardiac anomaly in symptomatic infants. Chest radiographs often appear normal or near normal in the first day or days of life with many cardiac anomalies, and may not be cost effective in asymptomatic infants with an isolated murmur (i.e., no cyanosis (See Color Plate) or congestive signs or symptoms). However, in cyanotic or symptomatic infants, the presence or absence of cardiomegaly, increased pulmonary arterial or venous markings, diminished pulmonary arterial markings, or right aortic arch provides important information regarding the presence of a cardiac anomaly (see Figs. 33-9 and 33-10). In combination with physical exam and electrocardiographic findings, chest radiographic findings may provide important information concerning the possible presence of specific cardiac anomalies that may aid in early management before an echocardiogram can be obtained. The heart size should be differentiated from the thymic shadow. Cardiomegaly is indicated by a cardiothoracic ratio greater then 0.6 in an anterior–posterior projection in the presence of an adequate inspiration. The aortic arch position can be assessed, even in the presence of a large overlying thymus, by deviation of the trachea to the opposite side. Associated noncardiac anomalies that provide clues to the cardiac diagnosis may be discovered by radiographic findings, for example, heterotaxy (asplenia syndrome, malrotation), absence of the thymus gland (DiGeorge syndrome), vertebral anomalies (VACTERL association), and abnormal sternal ossification (Down syndrome).

Electrocardiography

Electrocardiography can be useful in evaluation for cardiac anomaly and arrhythmogenic disorders and in particular for diagnosis and management of arrhythmia (see Arrhythmias). Electrocardiographic interpretation in neonates has several caveats. However, when placed within the context of other physical exam and radiographic findings, electrocardiographic findings can provide a timely advantage in diagnosis and management of suspected cardiac anomaly (see Figs. 33-9 and 33-10). Electrocardiography is also useful for timely recognition of life-threatening arrhythmogenic disorders, particularly within the context of other findings; for example family history and borderline prolonged QT interval (QTc).

TABLE 33-8
NORMAL MATURATIONAL ECG CHANGES

Age	Heart Rate* (beats per min)	R Axis* (+ degrees)	R Amplitude V1* (mm)	R Amplitude V6* (mm)	T Amplitude V1* (mm)
0–1 day	93–154 (123)	59–192 (135)	5–26	0–11	−30–+40
1–3 days	91–159 (123)	64–197 (134)	5–27	0–12	−41–+41
3–7 days	90–166 (129)	77–187 (132)	3–24	0.5–12	−45–+25
7–30 days	1–7–182 (149)	65–160 (110)	3–21.5	2.5–16	−10–−52
1–3 months	121–179 (150)	31–114 (75)	3–18.5	5–21	−12–−62

* 2–98th percentile (mean)
from ref 43,45

Interpretation of neonatal electrocardiograms requires knowledge of maturational changes in heart rate, and electrocardiographic intervals, axes, voltages and repolarization that occur normally during the first days and weeks of life (see Table 33-8 and Fig. 33-13) (43–45). Within the first days of life, there are significant changes in repolarization, including T axis and rate-corrected QTc, and changes in R and S wave amplitudes, that influence interpretation. Compared with a 1 year old, 1 day old babies normally have relatively fast heart rates (93–154, average 123/minute), relatively rightward R axis (60–195, average 123 degrees) and relative right ventricular hypertrophy (R in V1 5–16 mm) (44). During the first 4 days of life there is variability of the QTc, an evolution of changes in T wave polarity and

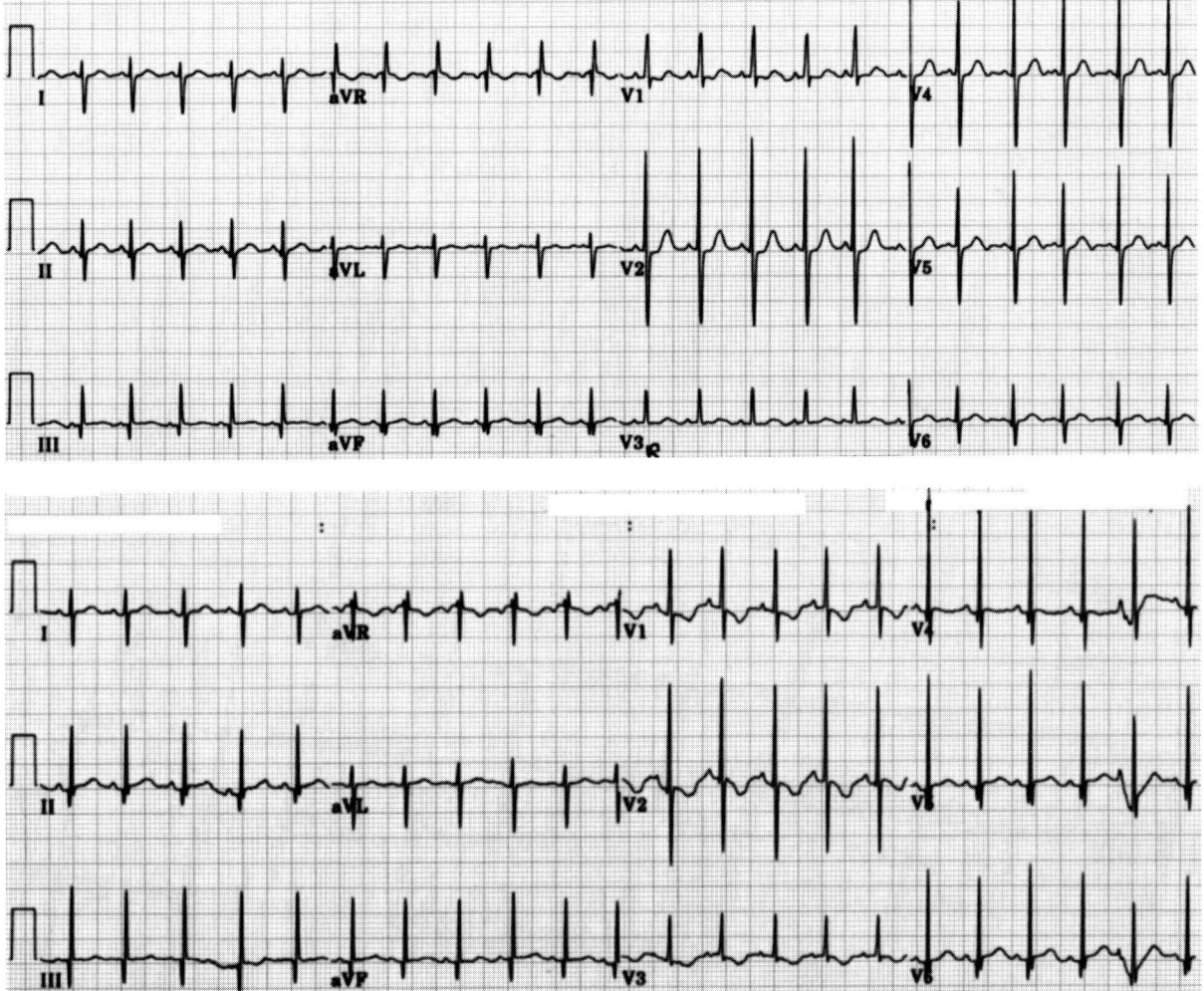

Figure 33-13 Electrocardiograms from healthy ½ day old (top) and 5 day old infants (lower) demonstrate normal neonatal repolarization changes. V1 T wave morphology chanbges from upright to inverted.

voltage (e.g., in V1 from upright to inverted), and nonspecific ST segment changes are common. QTc is 440 milliseconds or less in 97.5% of newborns, but can be much longer with electrolyte abnormality (e.g., hypocalcemia, hypokalemia), drug effect, brain injury and genetic prolonged QT syndromes. Premature neonates tend to have higher heart rates (141–160/min), slightly more leftward R axis 107–135 degrees), slightly less R amplitude in V3R (median 3 mm), slightly greater R amplitude in V6 (median 6–7 mm) and slightly longer QTc interval (411–412 ms) (46).

Ventricular hypertrophy in the electrocardiogram at birth is a consequence of the hemodynamic abnormalities imposed on the fetal circulation. The hemodynamic changes and the ventricular hypertrophy associated with various cardiac anomalies are often much different in the fetal circulation than postnatal. For example, neonates with coarctation, and other obstructive anomalies with less than normal blood flow volume through the fetal left ventricle and more than normal flow through the fetal right ventricle, often have right ventricular hypertrophy from increased fetal right ventricular workload. Furthermore, anomalies associated with systemic-level right ventricular hypertension later in infancy often have neonatal electrocardiographic right ventricular forces that are difficult to differentiate unambiguously from normal in the neonate. Therefore, the differential diagnosis of ventricular hypertrophy in the neonate is different from later in infancy (see Figs. 33-9 and 33-10). In term neonates electrocardiographic findings of right ventricular hypertrophy include R amplitude in V1 above the 98th percentile (44) (>26 mm in 1st week, >21 mm in 2nd to 4th week), presence of Q wave in V1, or persistence of upright T waves in V1 beyond age 1 week. Findings of left ventricular hypertrophy include elevated R amplitude in V6 (44) (>12 mm in 1st week, >16 mm in 2nd to 4th week) and deep Q wave in V6 (>4 mm), often accompanied by T wave flattening or inversion in V6.

Although most anomalies do not have R axis deviation at birth, when axis deviation is present the electrocardiogram can be very helpful in diagnosis (see Figs. 33-9 and 33-10). Left axis deviation in acyanotic newborns is most often associated with endocardial cushion anomaly (e.g., primum atrial septal defect, complete atrioventricular canal defect), although in cyanotic newborns left axis deviation occurs with tricuspid atresia and other cyanotic anomalies in combination with an endocardial cushion anomaly (e.g., tetralogy or double outlet right ventricle with complete atrioventricular canal defect).

Echocardiography

Examination of the heart by two-dimensional echocardiography with color Doppler ultrasound allows excellent analysis of the intracardiac anatomy in small infants. The equipment is portable and can be readily brought to the bedside of critically ill neonates thus avoiding transport elsewhere, interruption of ongoing care, or anesthesia. The examination in neonates requires no or little sedation. Neonates are particularly good candidates for echocardio-

graphic imaging because they are less active and have excellent echocardiographic imaging windows. Detailed segmental examination from sub-xiphoid, parasternal, apical, supra-sternal notch, and additional modified views as necessary delineates almost all relevant cardiac anatomy and anomalies in most neonates. The situs, ventricular relationship, great artery relationships, systemic and pulmonary venous cardiac connections, atrial and ventricular septum, valve structure, great artery anatomy and coronary origins can be accurately determined.

Doppler echocardiography demonstrates the direction and velocity of blood flow within the heart and vessels. Color Doppler visualizes valve regurgitation and blood flow in valvar and sub-valvar stenoses, patent ductus arteriosus, septal defects, abnormal coronary arteries, systemic venous anomalies, and arterio-venous malformation. Pulsed and continuous-wave Doppler techniques enable estimation of physiologic measurements such as the pressure gradient across stenotic valves, septal defects, and patent ductus arteriosus (see Fig. 33-14). When physiologic or pathologic tricuspid regurgitation is present, right ventricular peak systolic pressure may be estimated by Doppler measurement of the magnitude of the pressure gradient between the right ventricle and right atrium and the addition of the right atrial V-wave pressure, whether assumed or directly measured through an umbilical vein catheter (usually 3 to 10 mm Hg) (see Fig. 33-15). Right ventricular systolic pressure relative to left ventricular pressure can also be qualitatively assessed by the curvature of the interventricular septum. Contrast echocardiography with injection of agitated saline or albumin into intravenous or umbilical artery catheters can sometimes serve as a useful adjunct to color Doppler in detection of shunts.

The ventricular systolic performance, size, and wall thickness can be assessed. The shortening fraction of the left ventricular internal short-axis dimension is the most commonly used measurement to assess left ventricular systolic function in children. In the sick neonate right ventricular systolic pressure often is close to left ventricular systolic pressure, resulting in flattening of the ventricular septal curvature; such that shortening fraction may not be indicative of global systolic performance. When regional wall motion abnormalities are present, ventricular systolic performance is assessed by estimation or measurement of the relative change in ventricular volume with contraction, the ejection fraction. The shortening and ejection fractions measure left ventricular performance, which is a function of contractility, afterload, preload, and heart rate. Contractility can be independently assessed by measuring the relationship of end-systolic wall stress velocity to fiber shortening using directed M-mode echocardiography, indirect central pulse tracing, and phonocardiography. This technique is also impaired when right ventricular hypertension results in ventricular septal systole flattening.

Echocardiography has limitations. Because complete examination of cardiac anatomy in neonates is labor intensive and requires expensive additional technology, the cost is often nearly that of a computerized tomography

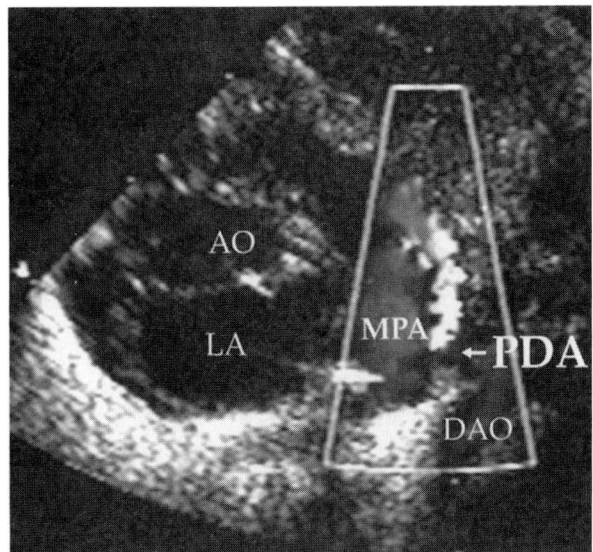

A

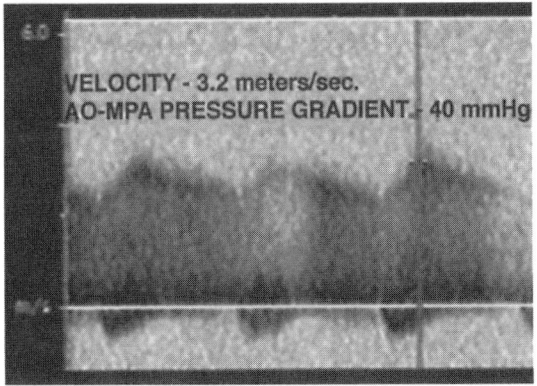

B

Figure 33-14 Echocardiographic parasagittal parasternal view of a patent ductus arteriosus. Doppler analysis demonstrates flow away from the transducer within the pulmonary artery and aortic isthmus and, in white, a jet of flow toward the transducer through the patent ductus arteriosus into the pulmonary artery. **B:** Quantification of the velocity of the flow jet through the ductus arteriosus with a continuous-wave Doppler technique and application of the Bernoulli principle allows the aortic-to-pulmonary-artery systolic pressure gradient to be measured. The pressure gradient by this technique is $4 \times$ (maximum instantaneous velocity)^2. The pulmonary artery peak systolic pressure can be estimated by the difference in the arterial systolic pressure and the pressure gradient across the ductus arteriosus. AO, aorta; DAO, descending aorta; LA, left atrium; MPA, main pulmonary artery; PDA, patent ductus arteriosus.

or magnetic resonance scans. The evaluation has often been unsatisfactory when performed in which the use of echocardiography to recognize heart disease in neonates is infrequent and echocardiographic transducers with frequencies appropriate for infants are not available. Training and performance standards for echocardiographic examination of congenital heart disease in fetuses and children have been disseminated (46). Cases of delayed transfer of babies because of erroneous diagnoses of inoperable congenital heart disease and erroneous impression that there is no significant lesion have been encountered. With limited experience in the diagnosis of congenital heart disease in neonates, it may be best to transport the infant to the nearest center for echocardiographic examination. If

personnel adequately trained in performing a complete study for congenital heart disease are available, it may be possible to send or transmit a tape of the examination for a second opinion.

Magnetic Resonance Imaging

Magnetic resonance imaging (MRI) can provide accurate assessment of intracardiac anatomy and function, and perhaps more importantly, can provide detailed images of intrathoracic structures, such as peripheral pulmonary arteries, systemic-to-pulmonary collateral vessels, and right ventricular function, that often are not adequately provided by echocardiography (see Coarctation, Fig. 33-35). Use of echocardiography and magnetic resonance imaging, in conjunction with the history and physical examination, enables precise diagnosis without resorting to diagnostic cardiac catheterization in most neonates.

DIAGNOSTIC CARDIAC CATHETERIZATION AND ANGIOGRAPHY

Anatomy

Catheterization is rarely used to learn the basic anatomy of the heart. The diagnostic information necessary for most cardiac surgical procedures in neonates is now obtained noninvasively by echocardiography. Diagnostic cardiac catheterization is used to provide specific data unavailable through echocardiography that are useful in planning management (47). What is the anatomy of the pulmonary arteries and systemic-to-pulmonary collaterals in the patient with tetralogy of Fallot and pulmonary atresia? (see Tetralogy, Fig. 33-22) Is catheter closure of the collaterals possible? What is the anatomy of the coronary arteries in the patient with pulmonary atresia and intact ventricular septum? (see Pulmonary Atresia, Fig. 33-26) What is the anatomy of the coronary arteries with tetralogy of Fallot or transposition in which abnormality is suspected and/or echocardiographic imaging is nondiagnostic? In selected patients with cardiomyopathy, light and electron microscopic analysis of ultrastructural anatomy and biochemical analysis of myocardium obtained by biopsy may provide a diagnosis. In many situations diagnostic catheterization may be safer or more useful after initial palliative surgery, such as in hypoplastic left heart syndrome or following shunt procedures in those with complex intracardiac anomalies and pulmonary atresia.

The decision to perform a cardiac catheterization should be guided by a careful assessment of the long-term benefits in management versus the risk of the procedure. Before catheterization the medical condition is optimized for the anomalies present and the rapidity with which catheterization may provide critical information to further stabilize the situation. Infants with a duct-dependent anomaly are best managed with an infusion of prostaglandin E1, begun before and continued throughout the

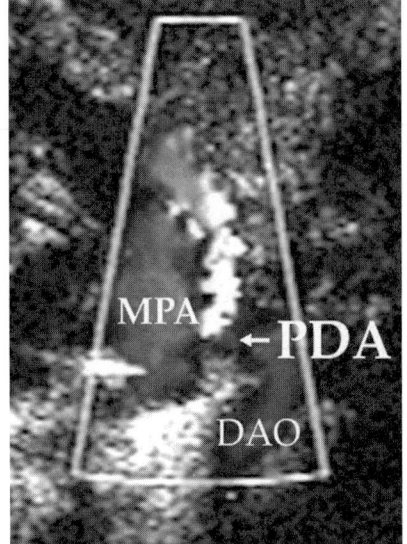
A

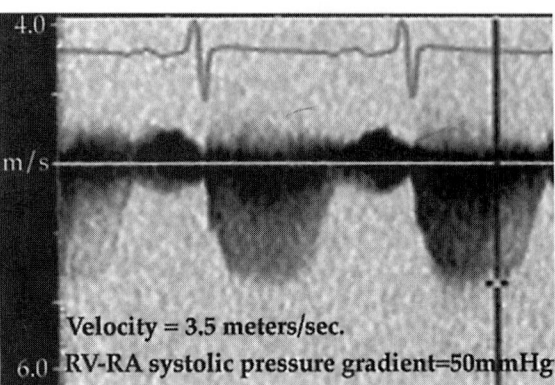
B

Figure 33-15 **A:** Echocardiographic apical four-chamber view in systole. Color Doppler analysis of the right heart demonstrates a jet of tricuspid regurgitation depicted by the blue flow jet (white arrow). **B:** Quantification of the velocity of the regurgitant jet by application of continuous-wave Doppler technique along the axis of the dotted line in the upper panel. Application of the measured triscuspid regurgitant velocity within the Bernoulli equation allows the right-ventricle-to-right-atrial peak pressure gradient to be measured and estimation of the right ventricular pressure (LA, left atrium; LV, left ventricle; RA, right atrium; RV, right ventricle; TR tricuspid regurgitation).

catheterization. The potential for procedural morbidity and mortality is greater in the sick newborn (47). Potential morbidity includes blood loss, hypothermia, metabolic and respiratory acidosis, arrhythmia, electrolyte imbalance, hypoglycemia, thrombosis of femoral arteries, and angiographic myocardial stains.

Hemodynamic Measurements

Hemodynamic data obtained by catheterization can now largely be deduced from noninvasive measurements of blood pressure, oxygen saturation, and echocardiographic Doppler measurements of pressure gradients. Direct measurement does not help preoperative neonatal surgical management of most anomalies. When catheterization is done primarily for delineation of anatomy, hemodynamic measurements can be readily obtained and can facilitate delineating the clinical status and management. Hemodynamic measurements are often used to guide interventional catheterization such as valvuloplasty. Sometimes, particularly postoperatively, information from implanted catheters is useful for management of sick babies in the intensive care unit. Catheters in the right atrium placed through an umbilical vein, systemic vein, or trans-thoracically in the operating room may be used to obtain central venous pressure and blood oxygen saturation. These data can be used to infer preload and adequacy of cardiac output and, in combination with blood pressure measurements, to infer relative afterload. Catheters in the pulmonary artery, placed trans-thoracically at surgery or trans-venously, can be used to measure left-to-right shunts and to measure pulmonary pressure to titrate pulmonary vasodilators.

The hemodynamic principals for these calculations are based on Ohm's law and the Fick principle (see Table 33-9) (47). The former, when applied to hemodynamics, is the pressure drop across a vascular bed equals the product of the flow and resistance across it. Therefore, the resistance equals the difference of the arterial and venous pressure divided by the flow. The flow can be calculated from the Fick principal, which is based on the premise that oxygen delivery to the body equals oxygen consumption by the body. Oxygen consumption is routinely measured in the catheterization laboratory and, in the intensive care unit, can be assumed to be 200 to 240 mL/min/m2 in neonates (48). Oxygen delivery is the product of flow and the arterial–venous oxygen content difference. Arterial and venous oxygen contents are calculated from the products of the measured blood oxygen saturations and blood hemoglobin concentration and the hemoglobin oxygen-carrying capacity (1.36 mL O_2/g hemoglobin). Systemic and pulmonary flow can be calculated as in Table 33-8. In those without a hemodynamic shunt, cardiac output can be measured by the thermodilution method.

MANAGEMENT PROCEDURES FOR SEVERE CARDIAC DISEASE

Preprocedure

An infant in difficulty in the first days of life because of heart disease has the potential for rapid deterioration. Too often, the baby looks as though he will survive but is near death hours later. The earlier symptoms appear, the faster deterioration can take place. By the time the infant has

TABLE 33-9

HEMODYNAMIC FORMULATIONS

O_2 consumption = O_2 delivery

$\qquad$ = Q × (arterial O_2 content − venous O_2 content)

Blood O_2 content (mL/L) = Hgb (g/dl) × 10 (dL/L) × 1.36 (ml O_2/g Hgb) × Hgb O_2 Sat.

Average neonate O_2 consumption = 200–220 mL/min/m^2

Q_s (L/min/m^2) = O_2 consumption/Hgb × 13.6 × (arterial O_2 Sat. − venous O_2 Sat.)

Q_p (L/min/m^2) = O_2 consumption/Hgb × 13.6 × (pulm. venous O_2 Sat. − pulm. arterial O_2 Sat.)

Q_p/Q_s = $\dfrac{\text{(arterial } O_2 \text{ Sat.} - \text{venous } O_2 \text{ Sat.)}}{}$

ΔP (mmHg) = Q × R (Woods units)

R_s = Q_s/(arterial mean pressure − RA mean pressure)

R_p = Q_p/(pulm. arterial mean pressure − LA mean pressure)

Q, cardiac output or blood flow; Hgb, blood hemoglobin concentration; Sat., saturation; Q_s, systemic flow or cardiac output; Q_p, pulmonary flow; ΔP, arterial mean pressure minus arterial atrial mean pressure; pulm., pulmonary; R, vascular resistance; R_s, systemic vascular resistance; R_p, pulmonary vascular resistance. From ref. 47.

reached 1 or 2 months of age, concern about sudden shifts in status is less warranted.

Infants who present with severe cyanosis (See Color Plate) in the first days to weeks of life may do so because right ventricular outflow is critically obstructed and adequate pulmonary blood flow is dependent on a closing ductus arteriosus, or because the great arteries are transposed and adequate mixing of the pulmonary and systemic circulations is decreasing as the ductus arteriosus constricts. Babies with congestive heart failure in the first week of life often have obstructed left ventricular or aortic outflow, with descending aortic flow supplied by a closing ductus arteriosus. In these babies, survival may depend on persistent patency of the ductus arteriosus; dependency should be suspected, and prostaglandin E1 therapy considered. If possible, echocardiography should be used to confirm a specific anatomic diagnosis, but this may not be available in many primary care facilities, and the infant's condition may not provide the time before starting treatments to transport to a facility in which echocardiography is available. If a duct-dependent anomaly is suspected from physical examination, ECG, and chest radiograph (e.g., pulmonary atresia, hypoplastic left heart syndrome), or if the condition of a baby with undiagnosed cardiac anomaly is significantly worsening so that arterial oxygen saturation is less than 70% (e.g., as in d-transposition of the great arteries or critical pulmonary stenosis) or there is severe congestive heart failure because of ductal closure (e.g., as in critical aortic stenosis or coarctation), prostaglandin E1 therapy should be initiated even if echocardiography is not available (see Fig. 33-12). The usual starting dose of 0.1 mg/kg/min can frequently be reduced to 0.05 to 0.02 mg/kg/min after stabilization. The occurrence of relatively common side effects, particularly central apnea, vasodilation with hypotension, and fever should be anticipated. Endotracheal intubation should be performed prior to transport in infants receiving prostaglandins, to reduce the risk should later-onset apnea occur.

Despite prostaglandin therapy, these critically ill infants may have low cardiac output that may respond to the cor-

rection of common metabolic perturbations including hypothermia, intravascular hypovolemia, hypocalcemia, and hypoglycemia, but frequently, inotropic support is needed (Tables 33-10 and 33-11). Measurement of pressure in a central venous catheter may guide fluid therapy and permit administration of concentrated infusions of dextrose, calcium, and vasoactive amines. After appropriate steps to correct contributing metabolic abnormalities, fluid can be given in 5- to 10-mL/kg doses until adequate response is achieved or circulatory congestion occurs. Infusion of dopamine or dobutamine (5 to 20 mg/kg/min) or amrinone, should be added to support pump function as needed. Higher doses or continuous infusion of epinephrine can be considered to support refractory neonates until surgical palliation can be achieved. Digitalis preparations are much less desirable for acute inotropic support of critically ill infants who have variable renal and hepatic functions and electrolyte status.

Hyperventilation should be avoided in babies with certain lesions in which the pulmonary and systemic circulations are in parallel, such as hypoplastic left heart syndrome. Hyperventilation and oxygen administration in these babies can drop pulmonary vascular resistance to low levels, resulting in runoff into the pulmonary vasculature, systemic hypotension, and very low systemic blood flow.

The acyanotic cardiac infant who develops symptoms of increased respiratory work and poor feeding after 2 to 4 weeks of life often has congestive heart failure from decreasing pulmonary vascular resistance and increasing left-to-right shunt. Treatment with digoxin, diuretics, and, in refractory cases, systemic vasodilators is often indicated (see Table 33-10). Rarely, these infants have left-sided obstructive lesions or myocardial disease (e.g., anomalous left coronary artery) that requires different treatment (see Therapeutic Catheterization).

Therapeutic Catheterization

Interventions now performed on neonates in the catheterization laboratory include balloon atrial septostomy by

TABLE 33-10
COMMON ORAL DRUGS FOR THE TREATMENT OF CONGESTIVE HEART FAILURE

Genetic Drug	Proprietary Name	Form	Dose	Action	Toxicity
Digoxin	Lanoxin	Elixir: 50 µg = 0.05 mg/mL	Digitalizing dose: Premature, 20 µg/kg Term, 30 µg/kg Initial dose, ½ In 6 h, ¼ In 12 h, ¼ Maintenance dose: Premature, 3–4 µg/kg/12 hr Term, 4–5 µg/kg/12 hr	Na–K ATPase inhibitor, increases contractility	Atrioventricular block (monitor ECG during loading), tachydysrhythmias, vomiting; use with caution in renal failure and myocarditis; decrease dose by one-half if used with quinidine
Furosemide	Lasix	Suspension: 10 mg/mL	1 mg/kg/12 hr PRN to 2.0 mg/kg/8 hr	Loop of Henle Cl-pump inhibition, diuretic	Hyponatremia, hypokalemia, hypochloremic alkalosis, nephrocalcinosis
Chlorothiazide	Diuril	Suspension: 10 mg/mL	10–15 mg/kg/12 hr	Blocks distal tubular Na reabsorption, diuretic	Hyponatremia, hypokalemia, hypochloremic alkalosis, hyperbilirubinemia, hyperuricemia, hyperglycemia
Spironolactone	Aldactone	Suspension: 5 mg/mL Tablet: 25 mg	1–3 mg/kg/d, ¼ tab– ½ tab, crushed, qod–qd	Blocks tubular aldosterone receptor, diuretic	Hyperkalemia
Captopril	Capoten	Tablet: 12.5 mg, 25 mg	Term, 0.1–1.0 mg/kg/8 hr Preterm, 0.05–0.2 mg/kg/8–12 hr	Angiotensin-converting enzyme inhibition, decreases afterload	Hypotension, azotemia, proteinuria, may cause hyperkalemia when given with spironolactone or potassium; use with caution in low dose in premature neonates

TABLE 33-11
INTRAVENOUS VASOACTIVE DRUGS

Drug	Dose (μg/kg/min)	Action	Preload	Systemic Resistance	Pulmonary Resistance	Contractility	Heart Rate	Use	Toxicity
Dopamine	2–5 5–20	D, β₁ D, β, α	+/-→ ↓	+/-→ ↓, ↑↑	0 ↑	↑ ↑↑	+/-↑ ↑↑	↑CO, ↑BP	Tachycardia, dysrhythmias, necrosis with extravasation, ↓renal blood flow at higher doses
Dobutamine	2–20	β₁, mild β₂, α	+/-→	→	→	↑↑	↑	↑CO	Tachycardia, dysrhythmias, necrosis with extravasation
Epinephrine	0.05–1.0	α, β₁, β₂	↓, ↑	↓, ↑↑	→, ↑	↑↑	↑↑↑	↑CO, ↑BP, ↑HR	Tachycardia, dysrhythmias, necrosis with extravasation, ↓renal blood flow
Isoproterenol	0.05–2.0	β₁, β₂	→	↓↓	→	↑↑↑	↑↑↑	↑CO, ↑HR	Marked tachycardia, dysrhythmias, hypotension when volume depleted
Amrinone	5–10 (load: 1.0 mg/kg)	Phosphodiesterase inhibition	↓	↓↓	↓, ↑↑	↑	0	↑CO	Thrombocytopenia, dysrhythmias
Nitroprusside	0.5–5	EDRF-like action	↓↓	↓↓↓	→	0	↑	↑CO, ↓BP	Hypotension, V/Q mismatch, thiocyanate toxicity
Nitroglycerin	1–5	EDRF-like action	↓↓↓	↓↓	→	0	↑	↑CO, ↓preload	Hypotension, V/Q mismatch, methemoglobinemia
Phenylephrine	0.5–4.0	α	↑	↑↑↑	↑	+/-↑	+/-↓	TF, cyanotic spells	Cardiac output, ↓renal blood flow

+/−, may or may not; ↓, decrease; ↑, increase; α, α-adrenergic; β, β-adrenergic; BP, blood pressure; CO, cardiac output; D, dopaminergic; EDRF, endothelial-derived relaxing factor; HR, heart rate; TF, tetralogy of Fallot; V/Q, pulmonary ventilation–perfusion ratio.

TABLE 33-12
DIFFERENTIAL DIAGNOSIS OF CYANOTIC HEART DISEASE

Diagnosis	Physical Examination	Radiographic Findings	Electrocardiographic Findings
Hypoplastic left heart syndrome	Single S$_2$, ↑ respiratory work, ↓ pulse amplitude, ↓ perfusion, +/− SRM	↑ Pulmonary arterial markings, cardiomegaly	↓ LV force usually, develops RAE, RAD, RVH
Transposition of great arteries (IVS, VSD)[a]	Split S$_2$, +/− murmur, +/− ↑ respiratory work (i.e., peaceful cyanosis)	↑ Pulmonary arterial markings, +/− cardiomegaly with narrow mediastinum (i.e., "egg on a string")	Develops RAE, RAD, RVH
Truncus arteriosus	Split S$_2$, multiple clicks, soft to loud SEM, +/− DRM, ↑ respiratory work	↑ Pulmonary arterial markings, cardiomegaly	Develops RAE, RAD, BVH
Total anomalous pulmonary venous connection	Narrow S$_2$ split, +/− murmur, ↑ respiratory work	↑ Pulmonary venous markings, ↑ diffuse interstitial markings	Develops RAE, RAD, RVH
Tricuspid atresia			Left axis deviation
Without PS	Split S$_2$, heave, SRM	↑ Pulmonary arterial markings, cardiomegaly	
With PS	Single S$_2$, SEM	↓ Pulmonary arterial markings, +/− cardiomegaly	
Tetralogy of Fallot			
With PS	Single S$_2$, SEM	+/− ↓ Pulmonary arterial markings, +/− boot–shaped heart	Develops RAE, RAD, RVH
With PA	Single S$_2$ continuous murmur, LSB back, axillae	↑, ↓ Pulmonary arterial markings and heart size	
Pulmonary stenosis (IVS or SV)	Single S$_2$, click, SEM	↓ Pulmonary arterial markings	In IVS QRS axis 0°–100°, develops RAE, RAD, RVH
Pulmonary atresia (IVS or SV)	Single S$_2$, soft SRM	↓ Pulmonary arterial markings	In IVS QRs axis 0–80°, ↓ RV forces, +/− develops Q waves
Persistent pulmonary hypertension	Narrow split or single S$_2$, ↑ S$_2$ loudness, +/− SRM	↓ Pulmonary arterial markings, +/− parenchymal infiltrates, +/− cardiomegaly	Develops RAE, RAD, RVH

[a] Single ventricle is usually associated with transposition of the great arteries, and in the absence of PS or PA, it presents similar to transposition with ventricular septal defects.

+/−, may or may not be present; ↓, decreased; ↑, increased; BVH, biventricular hypertrophy; DRM, diastolic regurgitant murmur; IVS, intact ventricular septum; LSB, left sternal border; LV, left ventricle; PA, pulmonary atresia; PS, pulmonary stenosis; RAD, right axis deviation; RAE, right atrial enlargement; RVH, right ventricle; RV, right ventricular hypertrophy; SEM, systolic ejection murmur; SRM, systolic regurgitant murmur; SV, single ventricle; VSD, ventricular septal defect.

Rashkind technique for transposition of the great arteries, creation of an atrial septal defect in mitral atresia or hypoplastic left heart syndrome with restrictive atrial communication using Brockenbrough atrial puncture and balloon dilation, pulmonary and aortic valvuloplasty, pulmonary artery angioplasty, angioplasty of discrete aortic coarctation with otherwise normal caliber aortic arch, and closure of systemic-to-pulmonary arterial collateral vessels (47,49–52). To perform a therapeutic procedure and to extract vital diagnostic information with the least danger to the patient requires vigilance against a multitude of treacherous pitfalls and acute sense of the clinical cost and benefit of each maneuver contemplated. The neonate undergoing study is ill, often critically ill, and may have a widely fluctuating physiologic state. Before catheterization the baby is medically stabilized as best possible as dictated by the baby's anomalies, condition, and the rapidity with which catheterization may be required to further stabilize the situation. Duct-dependent infants are managed with an infusion of prostaglandin E1 (53,54). Careful and constant attention to maintenance of proper thermal environment, minimization of blood loss, vascular access and hemostasis, anticoagulation, metabolic status, respiratory status, and catheter manipulation optimizes the outcome.

Surgery

Life threatening heart disease in neonates often requires surgery. Early recognition, safe transport to a cardiac center, accurate diagnosis, and an experienced surgical team are needed for success. Anesthesiologists familiar with the problems of neonatal cardiac patients and a well-equipped intensive care unit with trained personnel contribute to successful management of these babies. The postoperative care requires fine adjustment of blood volume, body temperature, fluid and electrolyte balance, oxygenation, ventilation, and hemodynamic measurements. Close cooperation between the cardiologists, intensivists, and surgeons responsible for the care of these infants is mandatory.

The timing of surgical intervention depends on the anatomic diagnosis and the relative outcome of surgery sooner or later. Single-stage repair should be used if possible when outcomes are at least equivalent to those for staged procedures to avoid the added jeopardy of performing and additional procedure before a definitive procedure is done. There is also increasing evidence that early repair results in improved cardiac status and neurologic function (12,55). For complex anomalies, particularly those with one functional ventricle, a staged approach is often required, with initial life-saving, palliative operation done in infancy, followed months or years later by additional reparative surgery.

CYANOTIC LESIONS

The differential diagnosis of cyanotic heart disease includes many disorders (Table 33-12). Lesions usually associated with decreased pulmonary flow include the tetralogy of Fallot, pulmonary stenosis, tricuspid atresia, pulmonary atresia with intact ventricular septum, and Ebstein disease. Cyanotic lesions usually associated with increased pulmonary vascular markings include d-transposition of the great arteries, hypoplastic left heart syndrome, total anomalous pulmonary veins, truncus arteriosus, and single ventricle.

Anomalies with Cyanosis Caused by Separate Transposed Systemic and Pulmonary Circulations

d-Transposition of the Great Arteries

With transposition of the great arteries, the aorta arises from the right ventricle and the pulmonary artery from the left ventricle. In the most common form, d-transposition, the aorta is anterior to and to the right of the pulmonary artery rather than in its normal rightward and posterior position.

Transposition of the great arteries is one of the most common congenital heart lesions presenting in the newborn period (see Tables 33-1 and 33-2), and is a frequent cause of death among un-operated neonates with congenital heart disease. The male–female ratio is 1.8:1, and the average birth weight is greater than that for other patients with congenital heart disease, although not for the general population. Transposition is associated with other cardiac abnormalities, including ventricular septal defect, patent ductus arteriosus, pulmonary valve stenosis, hypoplastic right ventricle, and coarctation.

Pathophysiology

The systemic and pulmonary circulations are normally in series with each other, but in complete transposition, the circulations are in parallel. Deoxygenated systemic venous blood returns to the right atrium, enters the right ventricle, and exits through the aorta. Maximally oxygenated pulmonary venous blood enters the left atrium and the left ventricle, and then returns to the pulmonary arteries and the lungs. Without some communication between the pulmonary and systemic circulations, survival is impossible; oxygenated blood cannot be delivered to the systemic circulation, nor can systemic venous blood be directed to the lung to become oxygenated. An atrial communication, ventricular defect, or patent ductus arteriosus, singly or in combination, may provide for mixing between the circulations (Fig. 33-16 and 33-17). The foramen ovale and ductus arteriosus, both normally patent in the fetus, usually close soon after birth. Infants with transposition and intact ventricular septum become extremely cyanotic within the first few hours or days after delivery, as closure of the foramen ovale and ductus arteriosus occurs and mixing between the circulations diminishes. The severe hypoxemia may lead to metabolic acidosis. Survival depends on prompt supportive medical care and reestablishment of patency of the ductus arteriosus and interatrial communication to improve mixing and oxygenation.

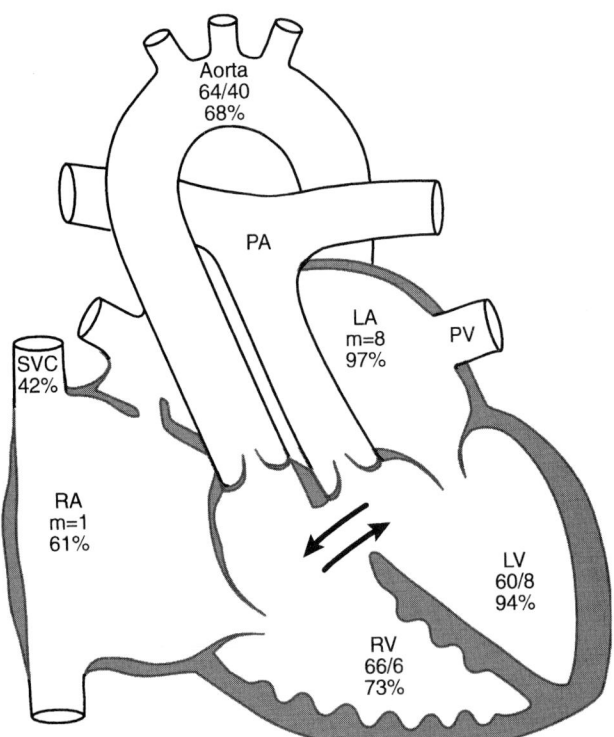

Figure 33-16 Diagram of the anatomy and physiology of transposition of the great arteries with a single membranous ventricular septal defect in a 1-month-old baby who had mild cyanosis and controlled congestive heart failure. There is equilibration of pressure between the ventricles and elevation of left-sided diastolic pressures. After balloon septostomy, the arterial saturation rose to 75%. The numbers below the chamber name are pressure measurements (mm Hg) determined at cardiac catheterization; the percentages indicate oxygen saturation. LA, left atrium; LV, left ventricle; PA, pulmonary artery; PV, pulmonary vein; RA, right atrium; RV, right ventricle; SVC, superior vena cava. Adapted from Mullins CE, Mayer DC. *Congenital heart disease: a diagramatic atlas.* New York: Alan R Liss, 1988, with permission.

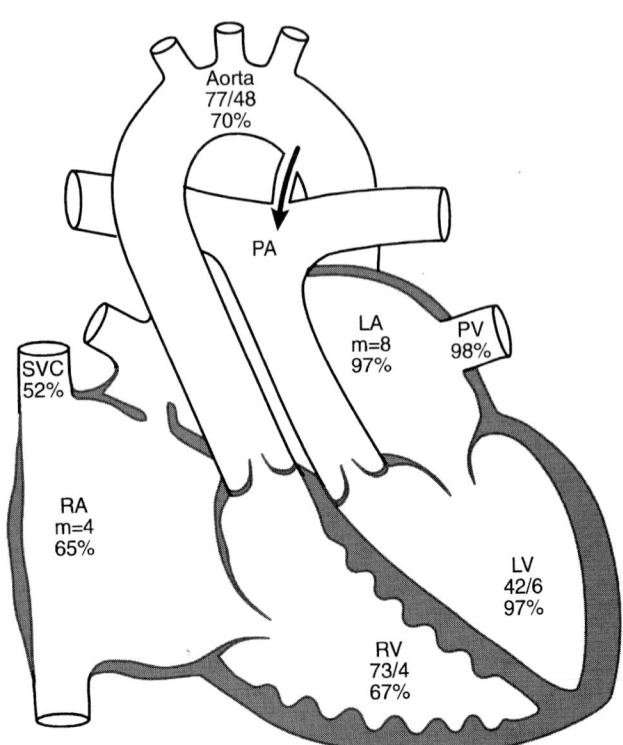

Figure 33-17 Diagram of the anatomy and physiology of transposition with intact ventricular septum in a 1-day-old girl who was cyanotic at birth. At catheterization, she had less than systemic pressure in the left (i.e., pulmonary) ventricle. The patent ductus arteriosus shunts blood into the pulmonary circuit, and the foramen ovale shunts an equal amount out of the pulmonary circuit. If this were not the case, relative blood volume would shift to one side of the circulation in a matter of minutes. If the ductus spontaneously closed, the infant's condition would become precarious. If the ductus were dilated with prostaglandins, the infant would become pinker but might experience respiratory difficulty because of excess pulmonary flow. The numbers below the chamber name are pressure measurements (mm Hg) determined at cardiac catheterization; the percentages indicate oxygen saturation. LA, left atrium; LV, left ventricle; PA, pulmonary artery; PV, pulmonary vein; RA, right atrium; RV, right ventricle; SVC, superior vena cava. Adapted from Mullins CE, Mayer DC. *Congenital heart disease: a diagramatic atlas.* New York: Alan R Liss, 1988, with permission.

Infants born with transposition and a large ventricular septal defect are less cyanotic because the ventricular defect allows mixing. These babies may not be recognized in the newborn period but appear in subsequent weeks with congestive failure. The combination of a large pulmonary flow, pulmonary hypertension, and elevation of left atrial pressure leads to the development of congestive heart failure (see Fig. 33-16) and later pulmonary vascular obstructive disease. Anatomic changes during the first few months of life may result in important hemodynamic changes. A large ventricular septal defect may spontaneously diminish in size or close, reducing mixing and increasing hypoxemia. Increasing pulmonary stenosis may decrease pulmonary flow and thereby increase cyanosis (See Color Plate) but improve congestive heart failure. Atrial septal defects created by balloon septostomy and those made by surgical septectomy may spontaneously diminish in size or close.

Clinical Findings

Infants with transposition of the great arteries and an intact ventricular septum develop marked cyanosis accompanied by mild tachypnea soon after birth. Often the infants, although tachypneic, do not seem distressed (i.e., peaceful cyanosis). The cardiac examination, chest radiograph, and ECG may otherwise be normal. The heart sounds are normal (i.e., the second heart sound splits), and there may be no significant murmur. Because the usual clinical findings, besides cyanosis, can be unremarkable, one of the most important diagnostic tests is the hyperoxia test. Failure of the arterial arterial oxygen pressure (PaO_2) (often <30 mm Hg in room air) to rise significantly after the inhalation of 100% oxygen for a 10-minute period is strong presumptive evidence for cyanotic heart disease, most commonly complete transposition.

The ECG may show some excessive right ventricular forces. On chest radiograph the heart and pulmonary vascularity may initially appear normal, although cardiac enlargement, a narrow mediastinum, and pulmonary plethora are frequently present or develop.

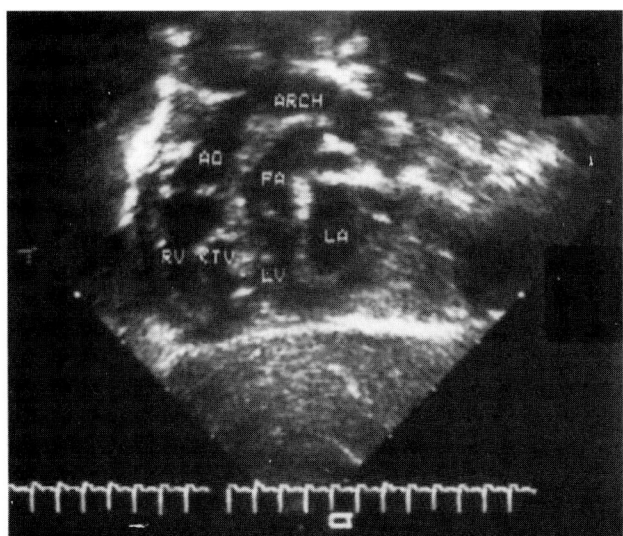

Figure 33-18 Echocardiographic subxiphoid view of a neonate with transposition of the great arteries. (AO aorta; ARCH, aortic arch; LA, left atrium; LV, left ventricle; PA, pulmonary artery; RV, right ventricle; TV, tricuspid valve.)

Subcostal echocardiography reveals the diagnosis. The great artery arising from the left ventricle has an abnormal course and then bifurcates into the right and left pulmonary artery. The right ventricle gives rise to a great artery that passes relatively straight superiorly to the posterior arching aorta (Fig. 33-18). Echocardiographic examination can also determine the patency of the foramen ovale and ductus arteriosus, the nature of associated anomalies, and the coronary anatomy relevant to the surgical arterial switch procedure.

Infants with transposition and a large ventricular septal defect usually present with congestive failure and mild cyanosis, between zero and 6 weeks of age. Poor weight gain, tachypnea, and excessive diaphoresis are common, and wheezing occurs in older infants. A loud systolic murmur is present maximally at the lower left sternal border, often associated with a mid-diastolic flow rumble. An S3 may produce a gallop rhythm. Rales may be audible in the lungs.

ECG reveals right axis deviation and right atrial and right ventricular hypertrophy. Infrequently, if the right ventricle is hypoplastic, right ventricular forces may be absent or reduced, and left ventricular hypertrophy is present. Chest radiograph characteristically shows considerable cardiomegaly and pulmonary plethora.

Echocardiographic examination should identify the location of the ventricular septal defect, its relation to the great arteries and the atrioventricular valves, and complex associated problems including straddling or abnormal tricuspid valve, hypoplastic right ventricle, valvar or sub-valvar pulmonary stenosis, coarctation of the aorta, juxtaposition of the atrial appendages, and anomalous systemic or pulmonary venous drainage.

Differential Diagnosis

Most infants with transposition and intact ventricular septum are readily recognized as cyanotic infants with little

respiratory distress and without significant murmur. Often a split second heart sound can be distinguished on exam, and chest radiograph demonstrates cardiomegaly and increased pulmonary flow, helping to distinguish transposition from other lesions with cyanosis and little murmur, pulmonary valve atresia with intact ventricular septum, and total anomalous pulmonary venous connection. Diagnosis of transposition of the great arteries can be complicated if other abnormalities, such as straddling tricuspid valve, hypoplastic right ventricle, coarctation of the aorta, or pulmonary stenosis, exist (see Table 33-12). Depending on the type and severity of the associated cardiac malformations, the clinical symptoms and findings in infants with complicated transposition of the great arteries may closely resemble those of almost any other cyanotic heart lesion.

The clinical picture in infants with transposition of the great arteries, ventricular septal defect, and pulmonary stenosis or atresia is virtually indistinguishable from that of tetralogy of Fallot or pulmonary atresia with a ventricular septal defect. If d-transposition of the great arteries is associated with a large ventricular septal defect and limited cyanosis, it is sometimes mistaken for other lesions with a large left-to-right shunt, such as a ventricular septal defect with normal aortic root or total anomalous pulmonary venous return without obstruction. The absence of cyanosis identifies the former, and echocardiography can differentiate all of these anomalies.

Treatment

In those with established or suspected transposition with intact ventricular septum, prostaglandin E1 is infused to open and maintain patency of the ductus arteriosus, to improve mixing and systemic oxygenation. Because prostaglandin E1 may cause apnea and vasodilation, support with mechanical ventilation, volume infusion, and sometimes inotropic agents may be required. Some babies also require a widely open atrial defect for adequate oxygenation, and most do better with one. Balloon atrial septostomy usually results in considerable clinical improvement in those sick from severe cyanosis, and some require it promptly for survival (see Fig. 33-19). The anatomy of the coronary arteries and associated lesions may also be established by catheterization. The type of surgical procedure employed depends on the associated cardiac defects. "Anatomic repair" with an arterial switch operation has been demonstrated to be the procedure of choice in neonates with uncomplicated transposition (56,57). The aorta and pulmonary arteries are transected, and the distal vessels are rejoined to provide normal physiologic connections. A button of proximal aortic tissue surrounding each coronary artery origin is cut, and both coronaries with the surrounding aortic button are moved from the native transposed aorta and attached to the neo-aorta. The ductus arteriosus is ligated, and the atrial septostomy is closed. Infants with transposition and isolated ventricular septal defect undergo arterial switch procedure and closure of the ventricular septal defect. Long-term outcome of arterial

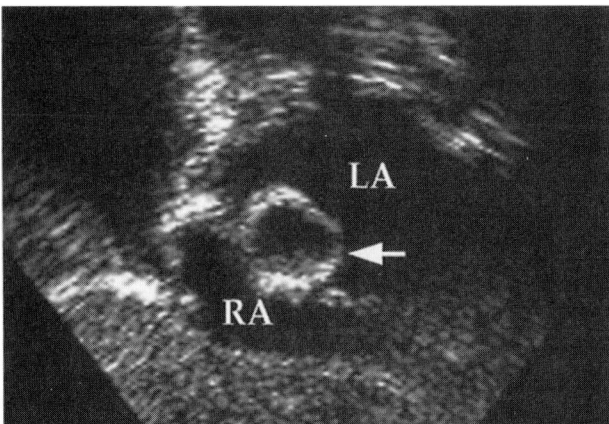

Figure 33-19   Echocardiographic subxiphoid view demonstrating a balloon septostomy catheter with the inflated balloon (arrow) being pulled from the left atrium (LA) to the right atrium (RA) through the foramen ovale. This septostomy technique is used in neonates with transposition of the great arteries to create an atrial septal defect to increase intracardiac mixing of fully and incompletely oxygenated blood, thereby improving systemic oxygenation.

switch procedure is not yet known but appears promising (58). Although a small number have difficulty with the coronary artery kinking, pulmonary artery compression, or anastomotic narrowing, the large majority do very well and lead essentially normal lives in childhood.

The additional presence of significant pulmonary or aortic valvar or sub-valvar stenosis can prohibit a straightforward arterial switch procedure. Severe pulmonary valve stenosis generally occurs with a large ventricular septal defect, and a Rastelli procedure or variation of it is done by placing a patch from the crest of the ventricular septum into the upper right ventricle to direct left ventricular blood to the transposed aorta and directing blood flow from the lower right ventricle to the pulmonary artery by interposition of a conduit (generally homograft) from a right ventriculotomy to the distal transected main pulmonary artery. The presence of native aortic valve stenosis can be dealt with by a modification of the Damus–Kaye–Stansel type in which left ventricular blood flow to the body is through anastomosis of the transected proximal main pulmonary artery to the ascending aorta, and pulmonary blood flow is through a conduit interposed between the right ventricle and distal main pulmonary artery. These procedures require revision of the surgically implanted conduits with growth and in the not infrequent occurrence of extrinsic compression. Without therapy, 95% of infants born with transpositions die within 1 year. With aggressive medical and surgical treatment, mortality is less than 5% to 10%.

Anomalies with Cyanosis from Decreased Pulmonary Blood Flow

Tetralogy of Fallot

The tetralogy of Fallot is characterized by a large ventricular septal defect and infundibular pulmonary stenosis or pul-

monary atresia. Both environmental factors and a number of genetic disorders are associated with tetralogy of Fallot. Many have microdeletions in a critical region of chromosome 22q11 (25,30). The primary anatomic pathologic abnormality appears to be anterior deviation of the upper part of the ventricular septum, known as the conal septum that separates the anterior pulmonary outflow of the right ventricle from the sub-aortic left ventricular outflow. This results in the sub-aortic anterior malalignment ventricular septal defect and in the right ventricular infundibulum being hypoplastic and narrow. There is often considerable valvar pulmonary stenosis, hypoplasia of the pulmonary arteries, right ventricular hypertrophy, a relatively large ascending aorta, and a right aortic arch (25%). In infants with pulmonary atresia, pulmonary perfusion occurs by way of a patent ductus arteriosus or by systemic-to-pulmonary arterial collateral vessels. Five percent of patients have abnormal coronary distribution that may influence surgical correction. Tetralogy is one of the most common cyanotic congenital heart lesions presenting in the newborn period (see Tables 33-1 and 33-2) and is occasionally (10%) associated with severe extra-cardiac malformations.

Pathophysiology

Depending on the severity of right ventricular outflow obstruction, there may be intracardiac left-to-right flow or right-to-left shunt and hypoxemia. Pressures equalize between the ventricles through the large septal defect. The peripheral arterial oxygen saturation depends on the amount of systemic venous admixture and the absolute pulmonary flow (Fig. 33-20). The extent of systemic venous admixture, that is, right-to-left shunting of systemic venous blood away from the pulmonary outflow through the ventricular septal defect to the aorta, is directly related to the severity of the pulmonary stenosis and inversely related to the systemic vascular resistance. The amount of pulmonary blood flow depends on the amount of antegrade flow through the right ventricle outflow and the existence of alternative sources of flow (through a ductus arteriosus or systemic-to-pulmonary arterial collateral vessels). For example, in pulmonary atresia with a ventricular septal defect, the entire right heart output passes right to left through the ventricular defect, and pulmonary flow is supplied by a ductus arteriosus or collateral vessels and is usually less than normal. Cyanosis is the result. If the newborn has large aortic-pulmonary collateral vessels perfusing the lung, pulmonary blood flow may be large; and the infant may be barely cyanotic and some have congestive heart failure.

The pulmonary outflow stenosis in tetralogy of Fallot is progressive. Clinically significant cyanosis is present at birth in 25%, by 1 year of age in 75%, and almost all have become cyanotic by 20 years of age. Infundibular hypoplasia and stenosis are progressive in both absolute and relative terms. Progression of the stenosis during the first 6 months of life is most often largely relative because of a lack of adequate infundibular expansion during rapid somatic growth and need for proportionately greater pulmonary flow (59).

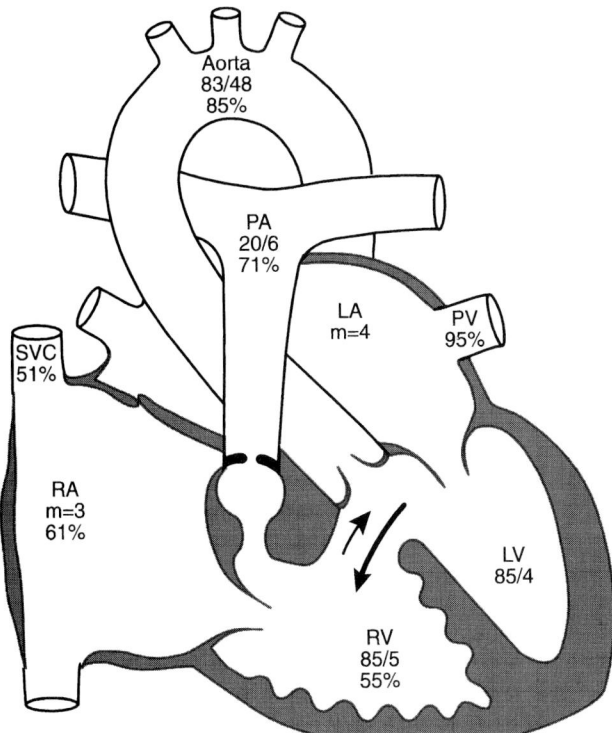

Figure 33-20 Diagram of the cardiac anatomy and physiology in a girl with mild cyanosis and a loud murmur audible at birth. She was found to have tetralogy of Fallot and was followed without medication prior to primary reparative surgery. The numbers below the chamber name are pressure measurements (mm Hg) determined at cardiac catheterization; the percentages indicate oxygen saturation. LA, left atrium; LV, left ventricle; PA, pulmonary artery; PV, pulmonary vein; RA, right atrium; RV, right ventricle; SVC, superior vena cava. (Adapted from Mullins CE, Mayer DC. *Congenital heart disease: a diagramatic atlas.* New York: Alan R Liss, 1988, with permission.)

With time, complete atresia can occur. A patent ductus arteriosus usually closes within the first week of life, resulting in severe and often sudden hypoxemia or cyanotic spells.

Hypoxemia of rapid onset is characteristic of a "tet" spell secondary to an infundibular spasm. This may be associated with an increased adrenergic contractile state, systemic vasodilation associated with a meal, warm bath, or certain types of anesthesia, or constriction of a ductus arteriosus. Hypoxemia may result in a fall in systemic vascular resistance, metabolic acidosis, hyperpnea, and further hypoxemia. Hyperventilatory compensation for the metabolic acidosis may be ineffective because of inadequate pulmonary blood flow. The self-aggravating cycle of increasing hypoxemia and metabolic acidosis can progress to unconsciousness and convulsions.

Clinical Findings

Cyanosis of various degree and mild tachypnea often develop soon after delivery. If hypoxemia becomes severe, the infant may become hypotonic, hypotensive, and bradycardic. "Tet" spells characterized by a sudden onset of irritability, hyperpnea, and increasing cyanosis may develop. Spells may end in a loss of consciousness, seizures, cerebral injury, hemiparesis, or death. The disappearance of a previ-

ously heard right ventricular outflow systolic murmur with increased cyanosis suggests a spell and constitutes an indication for immediate therapy.

The second heart sound is single. With typical tetralogy, systolic murmurs from the pulmonary stenosis and/or ventricular septal defect are at the left upper and mid sternal border, respectively. With pulmonary atresia, when the systolic murmur is absent; there may be a constant apical systolic ejection click and prominent continuous murmurs of a patent ductus arteriosus or aortic-pulmonary collaterals, audible at the base, in the axillae, and/or over the back. A patent ductus arteriosus usually does not cause a continuous murmur in the first months of life; therefore, the presence of murmurs with cyanosis and a single S2 in a neonate strongly suggests tetralogy of Fallot with pulmonary atresia. Delay in height, weight, and skeletal maturation is common, particularly when DiGeorge syndrome is present, but some infants flourish despite severe hypoxemia.

Some young infants with the anatomic but acyanotic tetralogy of Fallot experience congestive heart failure from left-to-right ventricular septal shunting, later develop increased pulmonary stenosis, recover from congestion, and become cyanotic. Congestive heart failure also sometimes occurs in infants with pulmonary atresia when numerous or very large aortic-pulmonary collaterals are present. Although sub-acute bacterial endocarditis and brain abscess are common in older children with tetralogy of Fallot, these complications are extremely rare in infancy. However, spontaneous cerebrovascular accidents are common, particularly in infants with severe hypoxemia and relative anemia (<6–8 g/dL of oxyhemoglobin).

Chest radiograph shows a normal-sized heart, sometimes with right ventricular enlargement resulting in an upturned apex and an absent or diminished main pulmonary artery segment (i.e., boot-shaped heart), diminution of the pulmonary vasculature, and, in 25%, the aorta arching to the right.

ECG demonstrates right axis deviation, right atrial enlargement, and right ventricular hypertrophy, which at birth is often difficult to differentiate from normally prominent right ventricular forces.

Echocardiographic examination shows anterior and leftward deviation of the infundibular septum, creating subpulmonary stenosis and a malalignment ventricular septal defect with a large overriding aortic root (Fig. 33-21). Additional ventricular or atrial septal defects, central pulmonary artery hypoplasia, and coronary artery anatomy can usually be delineated by echocardiography but may sometimes require cardiac catheterization for clarification.

Angiography (Fig. 33-22), and often magnetic resonance imaging, may be used to determine presence and anatomy of distal pulmonary artery stenoses and systemic-arterial-to-pulmonary-arterial collaterals.

Differential Diagnosis

The features of cyanosis, a harsh systolic ejection murmur, chest radiographic findings of diminished pulmonary

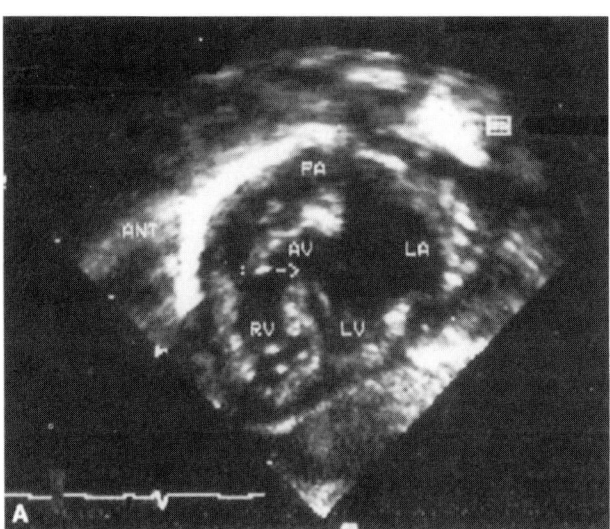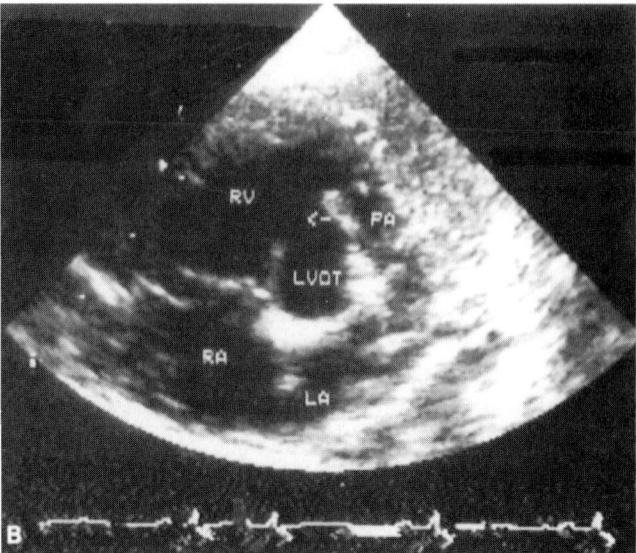

Figure 33-21   Echocardiographic subxiphoid **(A)** and parasternal short-axis **(B)** views of an infant with tetralogy of Fallot. Anterior deviation of the conal septum (above the arrow) is associated with malalignment ventricular septal defect and obstruction of the right ventricular outflow above the pulmonary artery; arrow, ventricular septal defect and narrowed right ventricular outflow; ANT, anterior; AV, aortic valve; LA, left atrium; LV, left ventricle; LVOT, left ventricular outflow tract; PA, pulmonary artery; RA, right atrium; RV, right venticle.

vasculature with a normal-sized heart, and ECG evidence of right ventricular hypertrophy are characteristic of tetralogy of Fallot (see Table 33-12). The same findings with a continuous murmur suggest tetralogy of Fallot with pulmonary atresia. A few infants with tetralogy of Fallot and an underdeveloped pulmonary valve present with a characteristic to-and-fro murmur (i.e., steam engine sound) and severe respiratory distress caused by bronchial or tracheal compression by aneurysmally dilated pulmonary arteries.

Treatment

Initial treatment and timing of surgery depend on the severity of the pulmonary stenosis. If severe cyanosis develops in the newborn, prostaglandin E1 should be employed to reopen the ductus arteriosus, improve pulmonary perfusion and stabilize the infant, and surgery should be done. Cyanotic "tet" spells are much more likely to occur in the infant with a moderate or greater degree of preexisting cyanosis, and echocardiographic findings of severe sub-valvar infundibular stenosis and hypoplasia. Later onset cyanotic "tet" spells should be treated with oxygen, intramuscular or subcutaneous morphine sulfate (0.1 mg/kg), intravenous administration of saline boluses and sodium bicarbonate (approximately 1 mmol/kg), and, if needed, phenylephrine (0.1 mg/kg subcutaneously; 5 to 20 mg/kg by intravenous bolus; 0.1 to 0.5 mg/kg/min by intravenous infusion) titrated to elevate systemic vascular resistance and pressure. Propranolol may be of some value in treating the infant with a reactive infundibulum. The hemoglobin concentration should be maintained high enough to permit adequate

oxygen transport. The occurrence of a single "tet" spell is an indication for surgery, possibly as an emergency procedure.

The newborn with tetralogy of Fallot and little or mild cyanosis can be carefully observed with repeated measurement of transcutaneous systemic oxygen saturation until a stable level is apparent after ductal closure. Many remain asymptomatic through the first 4 to 6 months of life, and can then undergo surgery with greater likelihood of preserving adequate pulmonary valve function. However, because the right ventricular outflow obstruction is often progressive, careful serial follow-up is prudent.

In the past, critically ill infants who required surgery underwent palliative procedures, usually a shunt between the subclavian artery and branch pulmonary artery (Blalock–Taussig). The shunt was ligated during a reparative operation when the child was older. Infants with uncomplicated tetralogy of Fallot requiring surgery now undergo one-stage reparative procedures with excellent results (60). Using sternotomy and cardiopulmonary bypass, the right ventricular outflow tract is enlarged with a pericardial patch, and the ventricular septal defect is closed with a Dacron patch. There are several potential late sequlae, including late dysrhythmias and problematic pulmonary regurgitation, but most patients with uncomplicated tetralogy of Fallot have an asymptomatic course into young-mid adulthood (61). Those with very low birth weight, anomalous origin of the left anterior descending coronary from the right coronary artery and those with pulmonary atresia and hypoplastic-distorted pulmonary arteries may require a palliative shunt with a more definitive repair, entailing a conduit from the right ventricle to the pulmonary artery, when the child is older.

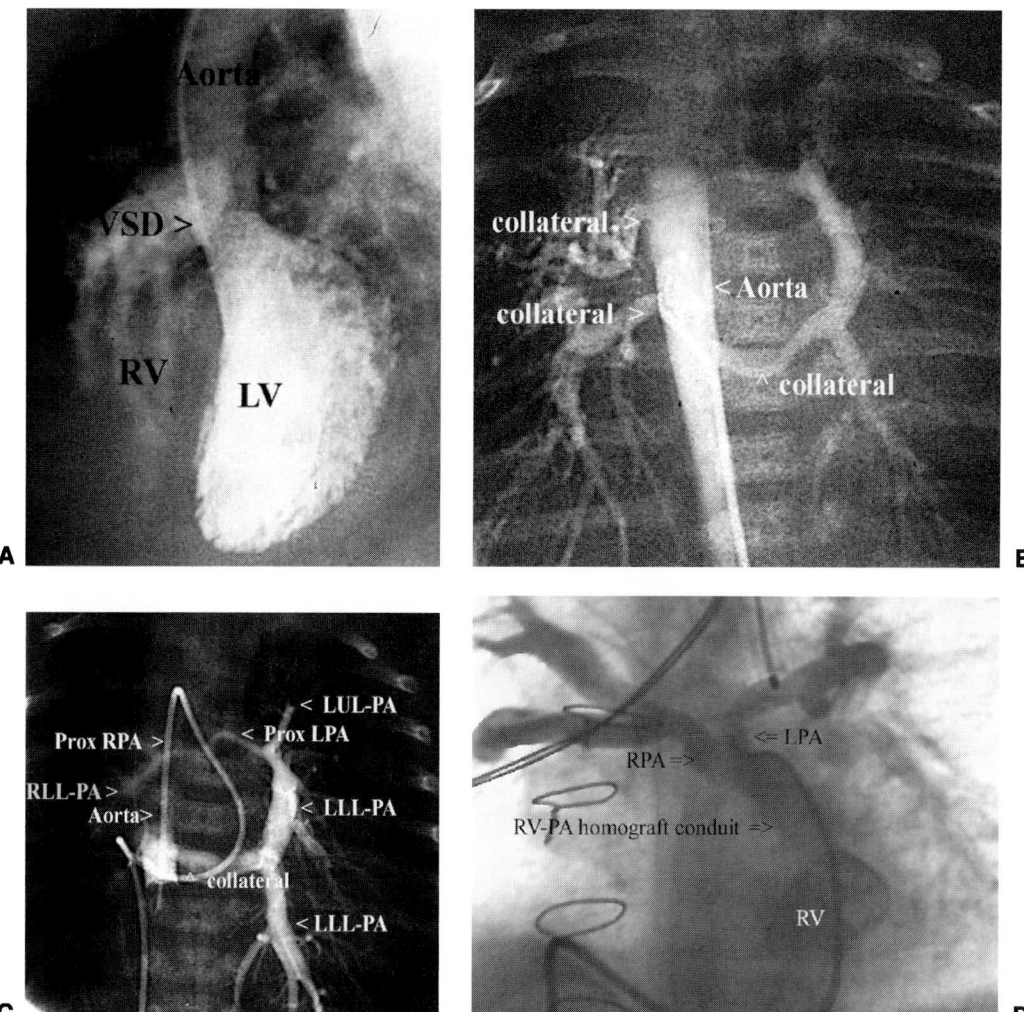

Figure 33-22 Angiograms from a cyanotic infant with complex tetralogy of Fallot with atresia of the right ventricular outflow, pulmonary valve and proximal main pulmonary artery demonstrate the anatomy of the hypoplastic mediastinal pulmonary arteries and collateral vessels that perfuse them. **A.** Left ventricular angiogram demonstrates tetralogy of Fallot with sub-aortic ventricular septal defect and pulmonary outflow atresia. **B.** Balloon occlusion angiography in the descending thoracic aorta demonstrates collateral vessels from the aorta to the right and left lung. **C.** Additional balloon occlusion aortography demonstates the collateral vessel to the left lower pulmonary artery is in continuity with hypoplastic central mediastinal and right pulmonary arteries. Left sublavian arteriography, not shown, demonstrated an additional collateral soley supplying much of the left upper lung lobe. **D.** Right ventricular angiography after surgical implantation of a homograft conduit from right ventricle to the central pulmonary artery, and catheter balloon angioplasties of the left and right pulmonary arteries demonstrates substantial increases in sizes of the pulmonary arteries. LV, left ventricle; LLL-PA, left lower lobe pulmonary artery; LPA, left pulmonary artery; LUL-PA, left upper lobe pulmonary artery; PA, central pulmonary artery; prox, proximal; RLL-PA, right lower lobe pulmonary artery; RPA, right pulmonary artery; RV, right ventricle; VSD, ventricular septal defect.

In general, the earlier severe hypoxemia develops, the more severe is the tetralogy of Fallot, and the poorer the prognosis without surgery. The overall mortality rate without surgery was approximately 35% by 1 year of age.

Pulmonary Stenosis

Pulmonary Valve and Subvalvar Stenosis

Pulmonary valve stenosis is one of the more common intracardiac anomalies detected in the first month of life (Table 33-1). It is usually mild and not progressive. Even mild obstruction (<10 mm Hg systolic pressure gradient across the obstruction) produces a readily audible murmur. Moderate and severe pulmonary valve stenosis detected in the first week of life often progresses for a limited time over the following weeks or months. It generally presents with an isolated murmur radiating to the suprasternal notch, often but not always with an early systolic click resembling a split S1, little or no cyanosis, and no signs of congestive heart failure. A parasternal thrill, high-pitched systolic ejection murmur, and single second heart sound indicate severe pulmonary valve stenosis. Severe valvar obstruction may produce cyanosis (Fig. 33-23)

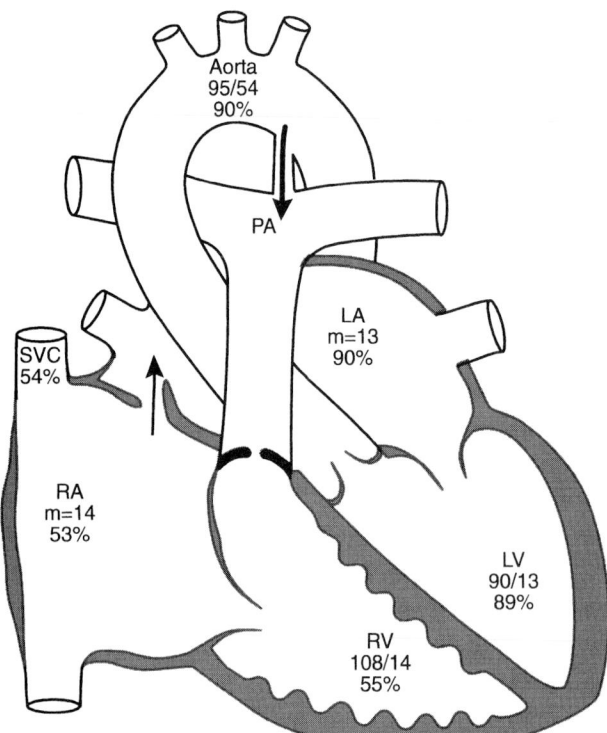

Figure 33-23 Diagram of the cardiac anatomy and physiology in a 3-day-old baby with cyanosis from birth. There was no murmur. The pulmonary valve was nearly atretic with only a tiny orifice. A valvotomy was done, and the cyanosis resolved in 3 weeks. The numbers below the chamber name are pressure measurements (mm Hg) determined at cardiac catheterization; the percentages indicate oxygen saturation. LA, left atrium; LV, left ventricle; PA, pulmonary artery; PV, pulmonary vein; RA, right atrium; RV, right ventricle; SVC, superior vena cava. (Adapted from Mullins CE, Mayer DC. *Congenital heart disease: a diagramatic atlas.* New York: Alan R Liss, 1988, with permission.)

because of right-to-left shunting through a foramen ovale or rarely may present with the findings of right-sided congestive heart failure. In its most severe form, a very immobile, critically stenotic pulmonary valve requires ductal patency for adequate pulmonary blood flow and systemic arterial oxygenation. The right ventricular chamber may be small and noncompliant, resulting in some degree of right-to-left shunting although the foramen ovale, even after removal of the stenosis. Infundibular (i.e., sub-valvar) obstruction as an isolated lesion is rare; its presence usually indicates an associated ventricular defect.

Chest radiography demonstrates normal heart size with fairly normal contour except for occasional upturning of the apex and normal or decreased pulmonary vascular markings. The electrocardiogram is usually normal at birth, although with severe and critical stenosis there may be relative mild left axis deviation for age (R axis 60 to 90 degrees) and increased or decreased right ventricular forces (see Table 33-12).

Echocardiography can determine the valve leaflet mobility, systolic pressure gradient, presence of right ventricular or infundibular hypoplasia, ductal patency, and possible associated anomalies such as atrial septal defect.

Only reassurance and observation are required for the mild stenoses because progressive obstruction is rare. Because moderate obstructions in early infancy often become progressively worse with growth, the patients should be periodically examined with this in mind. The severe and critical obstructions are relieved by catheter balloon dilation (Fig. 33-24) (47,49). Recurrence is unusual. Bacterial endocarditis is rare, but the administration of antibiotics

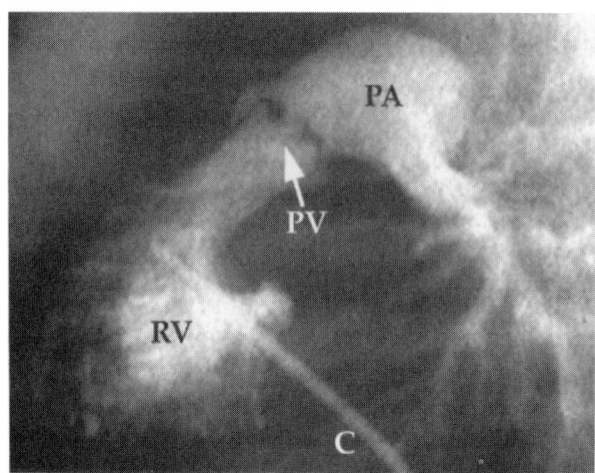

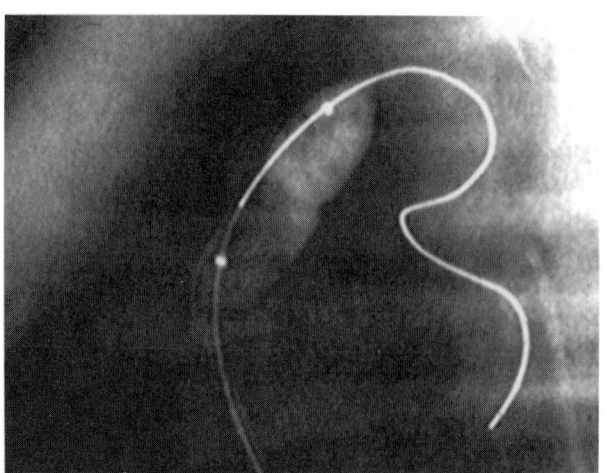

Figure 33-24 **A:** Lateral view of the right ventriculogram of a neonate with mild cyanosis, loud murmur, and severe pulmonary valve stenosis. Cineangiography during injection of contrast through a catheter (C) into the right ventricle (RV) demonstrates a jet of contrast through the small orifice (arrow) of a thickened doming stenotic pulmonary valve (PV). There is poststenotic dilation of the main pulmonary artery. **B:** Immediately following the angiogram seen above, the pulmonary valve was crossed with a catheter, and balloon pulmonary valvuloplasty performed over a guide wire, reducing the peak-to-peak systolic pressure gradient from 82 mm Hg to 2 mm Hg.

for prophylaxis before procedures that may be accompanied by bacteremia is recommended.

Pulmonary Artery Stenosis

Proximal pulmonary artery stenosis is probably the most common form of congenital heart disease discovered by hearing a murmur. The abnormality most often appears to be acute angulation, sometimes with mild narrowing of the proximal pulmonary artery branches. Minimal obstruction produces a readily audible murmur in the left upper sternal border, radiating to the clavicular regions, axillae, and back. Echocardiography can detect proximal pulmonary artery narrowing and pressure gradient and, when bilateral and severe, the presence of right ventricular hypertension. Severe peripheral pulmonary stenosis is rare and is usually associated with other problems such as tetralogy of Fallot, Williams syndrome, Alagille arteriohepatic dysplasia, and infants born of mothers with rubella. Angiography or magnetic resonance imaging is required to visualize the more distal pulmonary arteries. Pulmonary artery stenoses are usually amenable to catheter angioplasty and/or stenting.

Pulmonary Atresia with Intact Ventricular Septum

When the pulmonary valve is atretic and there is no ventricular septal defect, blood cannot pass through the right ventricle in the fetus. Without normal flow, the right ventricle cavity cannot grow normally and changes little in nature and size. If a severely stenotic valve becomes atretic late in gestation, the right ventricle can be near normal and quite adequate in size. However, when atresia occurs earlier in gestation the right ventricle at term is frequently coarsely trabeculated and pea sized. There is membranous pulmonary valvar atresia and, in approximately one-third of the cases, associated infundibular hypoplasia or atresia. The tricuspid valve annulus remains proportionately small and may be stenotic or incompetent. When the atresia occurs early in gestation and the right ventricle is hypoplastic, fistulous tracts connecting the hypertensive right ventricular sinus and the distal coronary arteries often persist, sometimes with proximal coronary artery stenosis. The right ventricle without outflow usually generates supra-systemic pressures. The high pressure probably contributes to the enlargement of fistulas that connect the right ventricle to the coronary arteries. The resultant severe coronary hypertension in utero may cause the coronary arteriopathy, proximal coronary artery stenoses, and myocardial fibrosis frequently seen. The pulmonary arteries are of adequate size and are perfused through a patent ductus arteriosus or, rarely, through aortic-pulmonary collaterals. An unrestrictive interatrial communication is essential to intrauterine survival and is present at birth. Pulmonary atresia with an intact ventricular septum is rarely associated with other cardiovascular or somatic malformations.

Pathophysiology

The major hemodynamic consequence of pulmonary atresia with intact septum is the obligatory right-to-left passage of the total systemic venous return through the foramen ovale to the left atrium. A patent ductus arteriosus provides the only entrance to the pulmonary circulation. As it closes, pulmonary perfusion declines, which results in progressively severe hypoxemia, metabolic acidosis, and death. In those infants with fistulas from the right ventricle to the left anterior descending and/or right coronary arteries and proximal coronary artery stenosis, perfusion of the coronary arteries distal to the stenoses occurs from the high pressure right ventricle through the fistulas. Surgical establishment of continuity between the right ventricle and the pulmonary artery may result in sufficient decrease in the right ventricle pressure to cause hypoperfusion of coronary beds supplied solely by fistulas and produce myocardial infarction. The size of the infarct and its impact directly correlate with the area of distribution of the coronary vessel involved (62).

Clinical Findings

Most infants with pulmonary atresia develop progressively severe cyanosis within the first week of life. As the ductal arteriosus constricts, severe cyanosis, hypotension, bradycardia, hypotonia, and marked acidosis occur. Signs of right-sided failure may develop but are usually absent. The precordium is quiet, and there is no thrill. S2 is single, and there is often a pan-systolic murmur of tricuspid incompetence.

Chest radiography, generally shows normal or mildly enlarged heart size, reduced lung vascular markings, and a left aortic arch (Fig. 33-25). ECG usually reveals a QRS axis in the frontal plane between zero and 80 degrees, absent or diminished right ventricular forces, and a pattern of left ventricular dominance reflecting right ventricular hypoplasia.

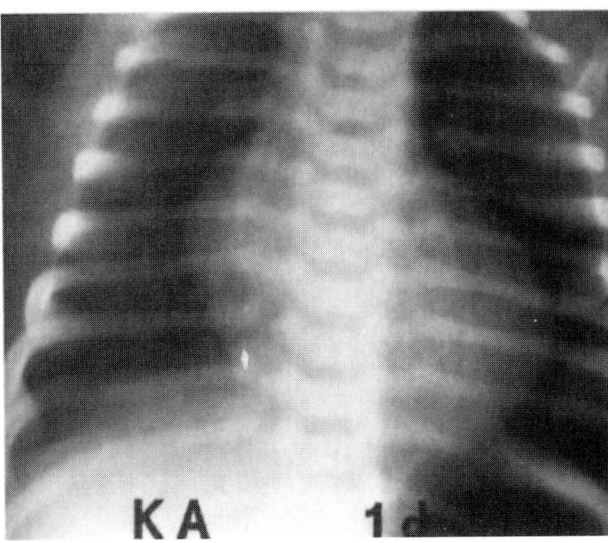

Figure 33-25 A chest radiograph shows decreased pulmonary vascularity and mild cardiomegaly in a 1-day-old infant with pulmonary atresia and an intact ventricular septum.

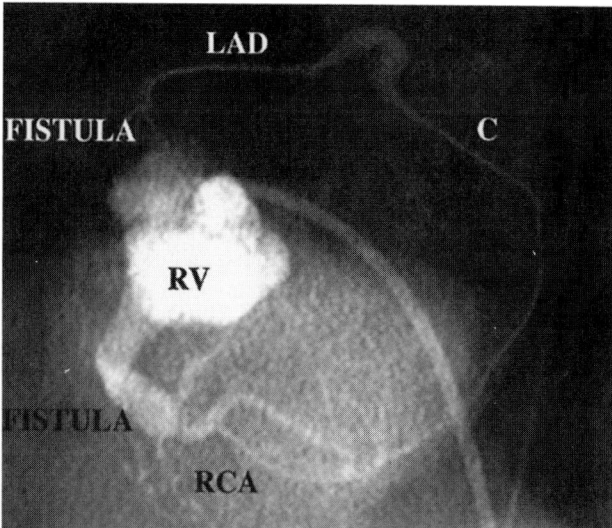

Figure 33-26 Cineangiogram of the right ventricle (RV) in an infant who presented with severe cyanosis, no murmur, single S2, and oligemic pulmonary vascular markings on chest radiograph. Echocardiogram confirmed pulmonary valve atresia, intact interventricular septum, and a closing ductus arteriosus. The aortic origin of the right coronary artery could not be visualized, and there was evidence for coronary fistula. Prostaglandin infusion was started. Selective coronary arteriography and right ventriculography demonstrated atresia of the proximal right coronary artery. A large fistula (FISTULA, black print) from the small right ventricle perfuses the distal right coronary artery and, through collaterals, the circumflex (C). There was also fistula (FISTULA, white print) from the right ventricle to the left anterior descending (LAD). The baby successfully underwent implantation of a modified Blalock-Taussig shunt, with no attempt to connect the right ventricle to the pulmonary artery.

Echocardiographic examination shows normal or somewhat enlarged left-sided structures, a small tricuspid valve and right ventricle, and atresia of the pulmonary valve. If there is membranous atresia of the pulmonary valve, the membrane can move like a critically stenotic valve, and the diagnosis cannot be made with certainty without a careful Doppler flow examination. Limitations in the size of the tricuspid valve and right ventricle and the presence of tricuspid stenosis can be quantified. High-resolution two-dimensional imaging and color Doppler can detect fistulas between the right ventricle and the coronary arteries. After the presumptive clinical diagnosis is made, prostaglandin should be given to dilate and maintain patency of the ductus arteriosus and increase pulmonary blood flow. In those babies diagnosed after ductal constriction, there should be rapid improvement in oxygenation and relief of acidosis.

Cardiac catheterization with selective right ventriculography and ascending aortography is done to determine the presence of fistulas and stenosis in the coronary arteries, essential for planning surgery (Fig. 33-26).

Differential Diagnosis

Pulmonary atresia with an intact septum needs to be differentiated from other cardiac causes of severe cyanosis in the first week of life (see Table 33-12). The combination of peaceful cyanosis, little murmur, single S2, chest radiograph with normal heart size and diminished pulmonary markings, and ECG with R axis of 0 to 80 degrees and diminished V1 R wave amplitude is characteristic. Critical valvar pulmonary stenosis alone, or with tetralogy of Fallot, are accompanied by a systolic ejection murmur, and right ventricular hypertrophy. Tetralogy of Fallot with pulmonary atresia has a continuous murmur and ECG with normal axis for age and prominent right ventricular forces. Transposition of the great arteries with an intact ventricular septum causes peaceful cyanosis and little murmur but is associated with a spilt S2, chest radiograph with cardiomegaly and increased vascular markings, and ECG with normal axis for age and evidence of prominent right ventricular forces. Infants with tricuspid atresia often have a prominent murmur and have a superior frontal plane axis on the ECG. In Ebstein anomaly of the tricuspid valve, the ECG has tall wide P waves and an rsR8S8 pattern, and chest radiograph demonstrates severe cardiac enlargement (Fig. 33-29). Echocardiographic examination differentiates all of these.

Treatment

After stabilization with prostaglandins, the treatment of choice is surgery, which is indicated as soon as feasible after the anatomy is established by catheterization. For infants with an adequately sized right ventricle, pulmonary valvotomy or valvectomy is performed. Some infants may require placement of a patch across the right ventricular outflow tract and valve annulus for adequate relief of obstruction. Often, even when of adequate size, the right ventricle is noncompliant, resulting in persistence of marked right to left atrial shunting. In infants with severe right ventricular noncompliance or hypoplasia a systemic-to-pulmonary shunt also may be necessary for relief of hypoxemia. After a period during which the right ventricular capacity and compliance improve and the pulmonary vascular resistance decreases, these infants may no longer require shunts for maintenance of adequate pulmonary blood flow. Even infants with initially diminutive right ventricular chambers may sometimes demonstrate adequate growth of the chamber if flow through the ventricle is provided by establishing continuity between the right ventricle and pulmonary artery, and the tricuspid valve is adequate. The right ventricle cannot be decompressed in infants who have fistulas between the right ventricle and coronary arteries and stenoses involving at least two separate proximal coronary vessels, without risk of fatal infarction (62). Infants with two or more major coronary stenoses, and those with persistent severe right ventricular hypoplasia, require a staged approach with an initial neonatal shunt and a later Fontan-type cavo-pulmonary anastomosis or transplantation. Without therapy, the malformation is usually fatal, and with surgical treatment, more than 80% to 95% of these newborns survive to 1 year of age.

Tricuspid Atresia

Tricuspid atresia is a relatively uncommon disease that is characterized by absence of the tricuspid valve. Except in rare cases, no valve exists, and tricuspid agenesis is therefore a more precise description of this anomaly.

Pathophysiology

The entire systemic venous return (i.e., cardiac output) enters the right atrium and exits through the foramen ovale to the left heart. The systemic and pulmonary venous streams mix in the left atrium. After passage to the left ventricle, the cardiac output passes to the aorta, and a variable amount gains access to the pulmonary artery through a ventricular septal defect, diminutive right ventricle, and a variable degree of pulmonary stenosis. Flow to the pulmonary artery is limited by the size of the ventricular defect and the amount of infundibular and valvar pulmonary stenosis. The level of cyanosis is determined by the amount of pulmonary blood flow. If no ventricular septal defect is present there is also pulmonary valve atresia and like infants with isolated pulmonary atresia, all pulmonary flow is dependent on the ductus arteriosus. If the ventricular septal defect and right ventricular outflow are small and the infant is very cyanotic in early infancy, the pulmonary blood flow can be increased by maintaining a patent ductus arteriosus and subsequently surgically implanting of a Blalock–Taussig shunt. Some infants have naturally balanced circulations with sufficient flow to the pulmonary arteries to allow an adequate arterial oxygen saturation of 75% to 88%, although not so much regarding cause pulmonary hypertension or congestive heart failure. Infants with a large ventricular septal defect and unobstructed right ventricular outflow are minimally cyanotic and develop congestive heart failure and pulmonary artery hypertension. Occasionally, the great vessels are transposed, with the aorta arising from the right ventricle, and the systemic output may be limited by the size of the ventricular defect. A left superior vena cava is a common associated anomaly of importance to later surgery.

Clinical Findings

Babies are usually discovered to have tricuspid atresia during the first days or weeks of life because of cyanosis. Some have a harsh mixed frequency systolic murmur of left to right flow through the ventricular septal defect or ductus arteriosus, and/or a harsh high-pitched systolic ejection murmur from pulmonary stenosis. The S2 is most often single.

ECG characteristically has features distinguishing it from most other cyanotic lesions. There is a leftward superior axis similar to endocardial cushion defects, but usually with diminished right precordial forces (see Figs. 33-27 and 33-10).

On chest radiograph, the heart is normal size or minimally enlarged and the pulmonary vasculature is diminished when the ventricular septal defect is restrictive, although heart size and pulmonary vascularity are increased when the ventricular septal defect is large and unrestrictive.

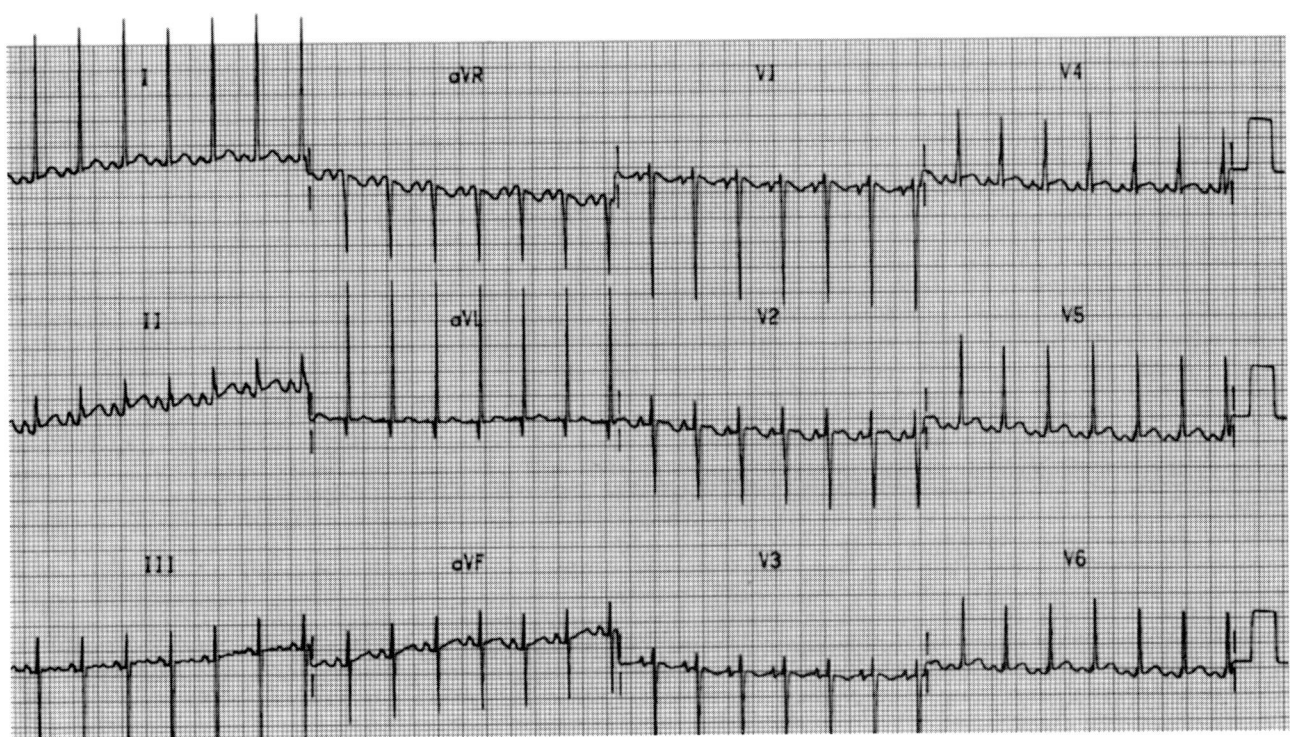

Figure 33-27 Electrocardiogram of a cyanotic newborn with tricuspid atresia shows the characteristic left axis deviation and low right precordial forces.

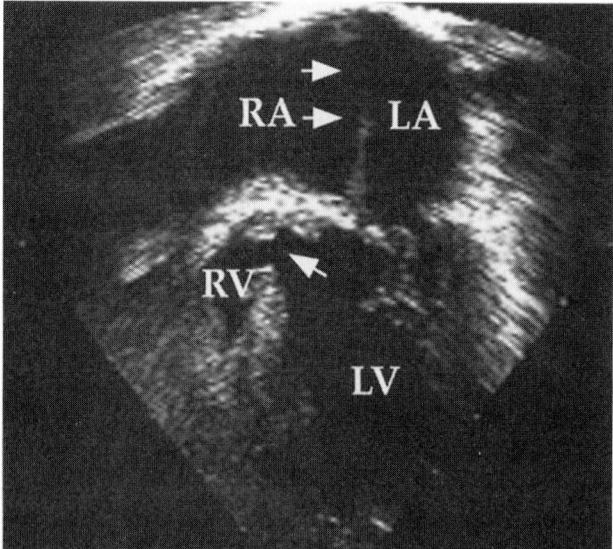

Figure 33-28 Echocardiographic apical four-chamber view in a baby with tricuspid atresia. Systemic venous blood flows from the right atrium (RA) across a widely patent foramen ovale (double arrows) to the left atrium (LA) and into the left ventricle (LV). Some of the outflow of the left ventricle passes through a ventricular septal defect (single arrow) and hypoplastic right ventricle (RV) to the pulmonary arteries (not shown).

The diagnosis is readily confirmed by echocardiographic identification of a diminutive right ventricle, absent tricuspid valve, and right-to-left flow through the foramen ovale (Fig. 33-28). The size of the ventricular septal defect and the degree of sub-valvar and valvar pulmonary stenosis can be accurately determined.

Treatment

Infants with small or no ventricular septal defect and severe obstruction of blood flow through the right ventricle may require infusion of prostaglandin E1 before palliative surgery. Surgical implantation of a modified or classic Blalock–Taussig type shunt from a subclavian or innominate artery to a pulmonary artery provides the means for adequate arterial oxygenation, survival, and growth in those infants with severe intracardiac obstruction to pulmonary blood flow. After several months of age the pulmonary vascular resistance usually decreases sufficiently to permit success of bidirectional Glenn surgery, connecting the upper superior vena cava carrying systemic venous blood return from the upper half of the body directly into the pulmonary artery. Variations on the Fontan operation, in which the systemic venous return from the remainder of the body is directed into the pulmonary arteries, are undertaken at or beyond the age of 1 year (63). More than 75% of infants with tricuspid atresia survive with Fontan physiology (64).

Rarely, in an infant with a large ventricular defect and no pulmonary stenosis, the pulmonary blood flow may be excessive enough to cause congestive heart failure. Anticongestive medications are usually sufficient to allow growth, although a pulmonary artery banding or other procedure may be necessary to diminish pulmonary vascular pressure and resistance.

Ebstein's Anomaly of the Tricuspid Valve

Ebstein's anomaly of the tricuspid valve is encountered rarely in the newborn period. The septal leaflet of the tricuspid valve is displaced downward and adheres to the ventricular septum to various degrees. The result is a dysfunction of the tricuspid valve with regurgitation, and sometimes stenosis, to varying degrees. The dysfunction is compounded by the fact that the right atrium and right ventricle contract at different times, and there is an area of atrialized ventricle or ventricularized atrium, depending on the point of view. This discordant pumping of parts of each chamber contributes to the dysfunction. Those with severe prenatal tricuspid regurgitation often have massive cardiomegaly and may have pulmonary hypoplasia that is rapidly fatal after birth (Fig. 33-4). The effective right ventricular volume is reduced, and there is limited passage of blood through the right ventricle. Some right atrial blood courses through the patent foramen ovale, causing cyanosis. The severity of the defect can be described by the degree of cyanosis that, in the newborn period, can be severe because of the concomitant unresolved elevation of the pulmonary vascular resistance left over from fetal life. As the newborn's pulmonary vascular resistance regresses, the cyanosis often improves, sometimes markedly, although babies with severe regurgitation and pulmonary hypoplasia have a high mortality rate. After surviving the newborn period, the infant has a course determined by the degree of abnormality; some patients survive into late adulthood without important limitation, but others remain cyanotic and prone to supraventricular tachycardia.

Ebstein's disease is recognized because of minimal or prominent systolic low-pitched murmur of tricuspid regurgitation, multiple clicks, and minimal to severe cyanosis.

Chest radiography demonstrates cardiomegaly that may vary from minimal to some of the largest hearts encountered in the newborn period (see Fig. 33-29).

ECG has tall wide P waves and an rsR'S' pattern (see Table 33-12).

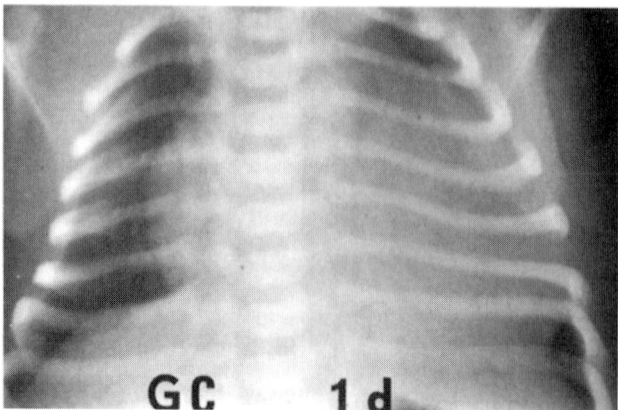

Figure 33-29 A chest radiograph of a 1-day-old cyanotic infant with Ebstein anomaly of the tricuspid valve shows marked cardiomegaly.

Echocardiographic examination confirms the diagnosis and delineates the extent and precise nature of the tricuspid anomaly, the amount of tricuspid regurgitation, the effective right ventricular volume, the atrial septal defect and associated abnormalities. Treatment is usually supportive. A surgical Blalock–Taussig shunt may be required in infants who remain severely cyanotic. Treatment for episodic supraventricular tachycardia may be needed.

Anomalies with Cyanosis as a Result of Complete Mixing of Systemic and Pulmonary Circulations

Hypoplastic Left Heart Syndrome

The hypoplastic left heart syndrome encompasses a variety of specific cardiovascular malformations producing similar hemodynamic and clinical manifestations, including aortic atresia, mitral atresia, premature closure of the foramen ovale, hypoplastic left ventricle with critical mitral stenosis, and aortic stenosis. Some cases of severe complex coarctation, critical aortic valve stenosis, and malaligned atrioventricular canal defects are also included in this category. The left heart chamber is usually very small, and endocardial fibroelastosis in it is common. Hypoplastic left heart syndrome occurs in 10.2% of infants with serious heart disease and is one of the most common lesions presenting in the first week of life (see Tables 33-1, 33-2, and 33-7). It is less common in very premature infants (<1.85 kg). It is usually an isolated lesion, although it has been described in association with trisomy syndromes and in infants of diabetic mothers. Familial cases occur.

Pathophysiology

Obstruction or atresia of the mitral or aortic valves limits or prevents flow through the left heart. The systemic venous return enters the right heart and is ejected into the pulmonary artery. The systemic circulation is largely or totally supplied by right-to-left flow through the ductus arteriosus. Blood traversing the lung enters the left atrium, flows through an atrial septal defect or dilated foramen ovale, and returns to the right atrium to join the incoming systemic venous return. Complete mixing takes place in the right atrium, with similar oxygen saturation measured in the right ventricle, pulmonary artery, and aorta. With little or no egress through the left heart, pulmonary flow must pass left to right through an interatrial communication. Any limitation of flow through the atrial septum produces pulmonary venous hypertension.

The maintenance of adequate systemic circulation requires patency of the ductus arteriosus. In aortic atresia, the ascending aorta, brachiocephalic vessels, and coronary arteries are perfused in a retrograde fashion with blood originating from the patent ductus arteriosus. Spontaneous constriction of the ductus results in flooding of the pulmonary circulation simultaneous with low systemic blood flow, poor coronary perfusion, congestive failure, and shock with metabolic acidosis, electrolyte imbalance, and coagulation abnormalities. Closure of the ductus stops blood flow to the body and causes immediate death.

Clinical Findings

These infants usually become symptomatic within the first week of life. Congestive failure and a shock-like picture may develop precipitously. The baby becomes ashen gray with poor peripheral perfusion, and all pulses are weak. Ductal constriction or flow may appear intermittent, with femoral pulses intermittently palpable. Symptoms and signs of congestive failure are associated with hypotension and, terminally, with bradycardia. S2 is single, and a gallop may be heard.

Chest radiograph shows cardiac enlargement and pulmonary plethora.

ECG can be near-normal, but usually has abnormalities including markedly diminished or absent left ventricular forces, left precordial T wave flattening or inversion, right atrial enlargement, right ventricular hypertrophy, and sometimes right axis deviation (see Fig. 33-30).

Echocardiographic examination demonstrates a small or tiny left ventricle. The ascending aorta is small with retrograde flow in cases of aortic atresia, and there is frequently aortic arch hypoplasia and juxta-ductal coarctation (Fig. 33-31).

Differential Diagnosis

The clinical picture of the hypoplastic left heart syndrome may be simulated by respiratory distress syndrome, interrupted aortic arch, severe complex coarctation, early neonatal myocarditis, isolated critical valvar aortic stenosis, sepsis or some inherited metabolic disorders (see Table 33-12).

Treatment

Without surgery, the mortality rate is 98% by 1 year of age. Surgical therapy consists of converting the circulation to single-ventricle Fontan-type physiology and/or to transplant a new heart. Previously the survival with the first stage of surgical palliation or with attempt to neonatal transplantation was only 1 in 2, or less, and comfort care was often presented as an option. Outcomes have significantly improved; currently survival with stage 1 surgery is 80% to 90% at specialized surgical centers.

Preoperatively the infant must be stabilized with prostaglandin E1, inotropic agents, volume infusion, and bicarbonate. Hyperventilation (i.e., arterial partial pressure of carbon dioxide, $PaCO_2$ < 40 mm Hg) and unnecessary supplemental oxygen administration are avoided. These measures decrease pulmonary vascular resistance and increase preferential flow of the right ventricular output into the pulmonary vascular bed instead of across the ductus to the systemic vasculature, worsening the shock. Often for preoperative stabilization, mechanical hypoventilation with muscle relaxation to maintain the $PaCO_2$ 45 to

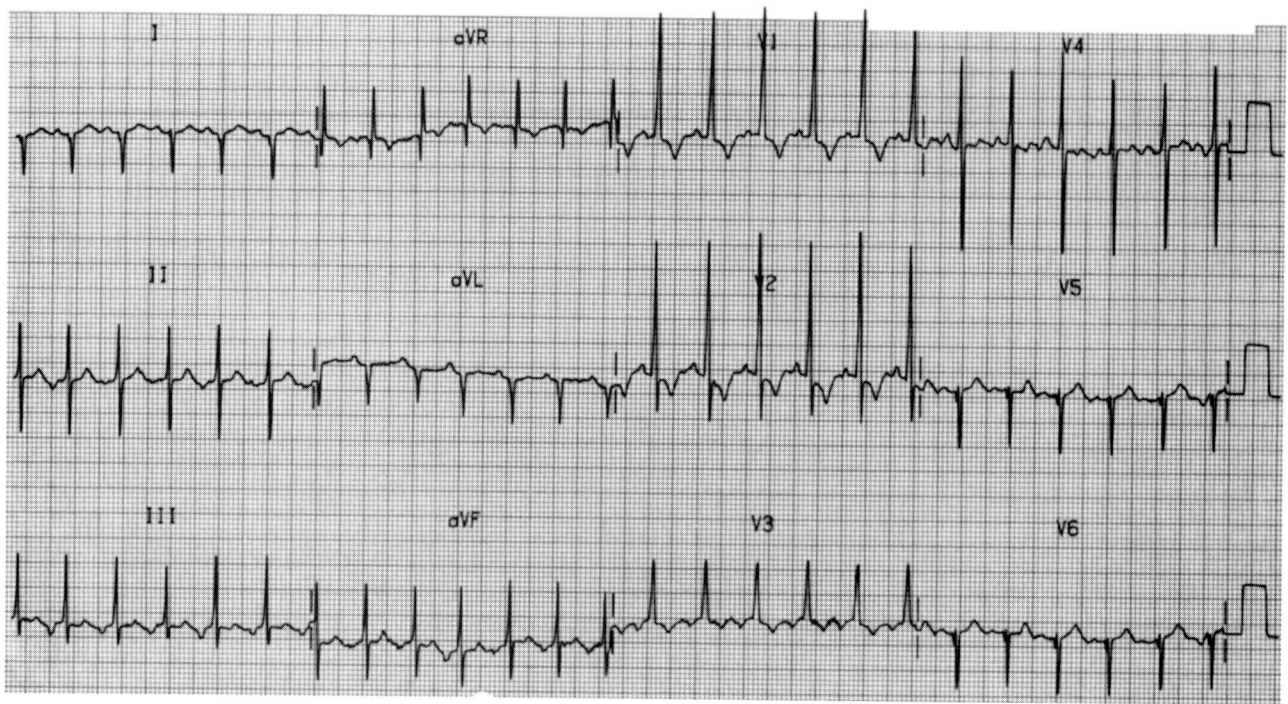

Figure 33-30   Electrocardiogram shows low left precordial forces in a cyanotic newborn with hypoplastic left heart syndrome.

55 mm Hg, and sometimes FiO_2 less than 0.21 to maintain arterial O_2 saturation 70% to 75%, are required to elicit sufficient pulmonary vasoconstriction to induce adequate systemic blood flow.

Palliative surgical therapy consists of staged surgical procedures that convert the circulation to a systemic-right-ventricle perfusing the aorta, with pulmonary arterial Fontan-type physiology. The first-stage, modified Norwood procedure connects the right ventricle to the aorta, recon-

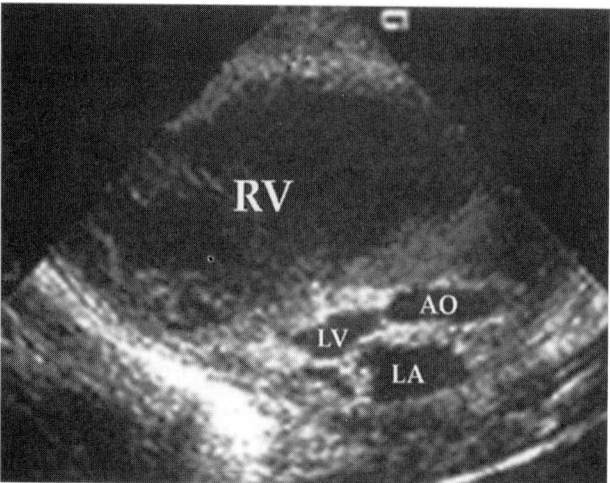

Figure 33-31   Echocardiographic parasternal long-axis view in an infant with hypoplastic left heart syndrome. The right ventricle (RV) is near normal in size. The left atrium (LA), left ventricle (LV) and ascending aorta (AO) are tiny. Both the mitral and aortic valves are atretic.

structs the hypoplastic aortic arch, and provides an interim source of pulmonary blood flow with arterial pressure sufficient to overcome physiologically relatively elevated neonatal pulmonary vascular resistance. Cardiopulmonary bypass is used during cooling of the infant's body temperature to 15 to 18 degrees centigrade and usually temporarily discontinued (i.e., complete deep hypothermic circulatory arrest), the ductus arteriosus is ligated, the obliquely transected main pulmonary artery is anastomosed to the underside of the aortic arch and further augmented with homograft patch, and an atrial septectomy done to allow unimpeded pulmonary venous return to the right atrium. Following re-establishment of cardiopulmonary bypass, blood flow to the pulmonary artery is provided by insertion of a modified Blalock–Taussig, or direct central systemic-to-pulmonary artery shunt, or anastomosis of a small conduit from a superior right ventriculotomy (65).

Several months later, when the pulmonary resistance has dropped from relatively high neonatal values, pulmonary circulation can be supplied relatively directly with systemic venous return. A second-stage bidirectional Glenn procedure is done. The systemic venous return from the upper body is placed directly into the lung through a anastomosis of the upper superior vena cava to the right pulmonary artery, and the systemic-arterial-to-pulmonary-arterial shunt (with its obligate ventricular volume overload) is taken down. Finally, at a third Fontan-type procedure, systemic venous return from the lower body is also diverted directly into the pulmonary artery through a lateral tunnel within or adjacent to the right atrium, directing flow to a second, lower anastomosis of the lower superior vena cava to the pulmonary artery (65). The perinatal and first-stage surgical survival is 85–90%, and with the second and third stage procedures are greater than 98% and 95% to 99%, respectively (66,67). Adult survival is not yet determined.

Cardiac transplantation has been used as an alternative approach with good survival and childhood functional capacity, but there are critical limitations in the timely availability of neonatal donors and long-term morbidities and risks (68–70).

Neither reconstructive surgery leading to a Fontan procedure nor cardiac transplantation can be viewed as curative. Both methods of treatment have high fiscal and emotional costs. However, many survivors eventually do remarkably well in childhood.

Total Anomalous Pulmonary Veins

In the event of failure to connect the common pulmonary vein to the left atrium in the embryo, communications are established with available systemic venous channels that then drain the pulmonary veins. Anatomically abnormal drainage may be supra-cardiac (i.e., into the right or left superior vena cava), intracardiac (i.e., into the coronary sinus, right atrium), or sub-diaphragmatic (i.e., through the inferior vena cava or porta hepatis). Mixed sites of drainage occur in approximately 10% of these patients. A patent foramen ovale or atrial septal defect is invariably present, permitting venous return to the left heart. Anomalous pulmonary venous return is often associated with heterotaxy.

Although isolated total anomalous venous return accounts for only 2% of newborns with serious cardiac disease (see Table 33-2), it is an important lesion because it is potentially curable and often misdiagnosed as pulmonary disease.

Pathophysiology

Infants with anomalous pulmonary venous drainage can be divided into two major categories on the basis of the hemodynamic changes produced: those with unobstructed veins and those with obstructed veins. Unobstructed pulmonary veins entering the systemic venous circulation or directly into the right heart result in a large left-to-right shunt, congestive heart failure, and pulmonary artery hypertension. Systemic output is maintained through right-to-left flow across an interatrial communication. Despite the obligatory right-to-left shunt through the atrium, the large pulmonary blood flow mixing with the systemic venous return at the right atrium allows a reasonable peripheral oxygen tension and produces only mild or moderate cyanosis.

If pulmonary venous return is obstructed, the circulatory effects are drastically different. The obstruction may take the form of increased resistance to flow produced by a long, common, pulmonary venous channel or localized intrinsic or extrinsic obstruction. Sub-diaphragmatic anomalous pulmonary venous return is almost always obstructed by constriction of the ductus venosus, obstructing flow into the inferior vena cava (Fig. 33-32). Obstruction to supra-cardiac pulmonary venous return may occur because of compression of the common pulmonary venous channel between the left primary bronchus and left pulmonary artery or because of narrowing at the entry of the common pulmonary vein into the right superior vena cava. Obstruction at the foramen ovale is uncommon. After birth, significant resistance to flow through the pulmonary veins becomes evident, causing pulmonary venous hypertension, pulmonary edema, marked pulmonary artery hypertension and diminished flow, and severe cyanosis. The arterial

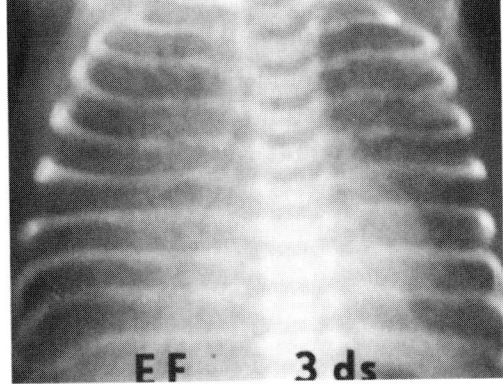 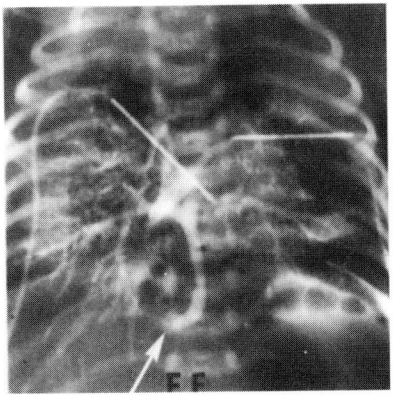

Figure 33-32   A: A chest radiograph of a 3-day-old term infant with obstructed total anomalous pulmonary venous drainage shows a ground-glass appearance of the lungs with normal heart size, similar to the radiographic appearance of respiratory distress syndrome in preterm neonates. **B:** Postmortem angiography shows obstruction of the common pulmonary venous channel below the diaphragm (arrow). **C:** Echocardiographic supra-sternal notch view of another neonate with similar anatomy demonstrated the left lobar pulmonary veins (<) and right lobar pulmonary veins (>) connecting to retro-cardiac posterior confluence, that drained via a vertical vein inferiorly across the diaphragm. Additional images not shown demonstrated intrahepatic connection of the vertical vein through a constricted ductus venosus to the inferior vena cava. The baby did well after emergent surgical anastomosis of the pulmonary venous confluence to the posterior left atrium, ligation of the vertical vein inferiorly, and closure of the formaen ovale.

oxygen tension is low because pulmonary blood flow is markedly reduced, and the relative contribution of fully oxygenated blood to the venous return to the heart mixing in the right atrium is less than in the unobstructed form of this disorder.

Clinical Findings

Infants with total anomalous pulmonary venous return without significant obstruction usually become symptomatic after the neonatal period, when the pulmonary vascular resistance decreases and a large left-to-right shunt and congestive heart failure develop. They are mildly cyanotic with increased respiratory rate and work, often have frank congestive heart failure, and have a large heart revealed on chest radiographs.

Infants with obstructed pulmonary venous return are usually critically ill, severely cyanotic, and tachypneic within the first week of life. There are congestive heart failure and poor peripheral perfusion. In the absence of associated anomalies such as malposition with pulmonary valve or sub-valvar stenosis, there is generally only a relatively soft murmur of a patent ductus arteriosus and/or tricuspid valve regurgitation.

As seen on the chest radiograph, heart size is often normal, and there is evidence of pulmonary edema (Fig. 33-32). The clinical and the radiographic pictures may resemble hyaline membrane disease or diffuse pneumonia complicated by persistent pulmonary hypertension.

ECG at birth may be normal or may show right axis deviation, right atrial hypertrophy, and right ventricular hypertrophy.

Echocardiographic findings include absence of pulmonary venous connections to the left atrium, right-to-left bulging of the atrial septum, right-to-left atrial shunt, and pulmonary venous confluence posterior to the left atrium connecting to a systemic venous channel.

The findings of severe cyanosis, little murmur, and a roentgenographic picture of a normal heart size associated with pulmonary edema are characteristic (see Fig. 33-28A and Table 33-11).

Differential Diagnosis

Respiratory distress syndrome and interstitial pneumonia can be clinically indistinguishable from obstructed total anomalous pulmonary venous connection. Any suggestion of an atypical course mandates echocardiography, particularly in term neonates with equally diffuse involvement of both lungs, a failed or inconclusive hyperoxia test, or a murmur. Two-dimensional echocardiography shows the anomalous common venous connections and obstructions and the presence or absence of other cardiac anomaly.

Treatment

The treatment of total anomalous pulmonary veins is surgical, and success is related to the anatomy (e.g., results are poorer in the mixed variety) and to the age of onset of symptoms, as in patients with the infra-diaphragmatic type. The success rate is better for infants with intracardiac drainage. Using cardiopulmonary bypass and deep hypothermic circulatory arrest, continuity or redirection of the pulmonary venous drainage into the left atrium is established, usually by anastomosis of the retro-atrial common pulmonary venous confluence to a parallel posterior left atriotomy. Although inotropic agents, diuretics, and supportive medical treatment may help temporarily and partially with stabilization, infants with severely obstructed anomalous venous return require immediate surgical intervention. Prostaglandin E1 therapy is not beneficial and can lead to dramatic worsening of the pulmonary edema. In most patients, surgery can be done on the basis of information from echocardiography without the delays involved with cardiac catheterization or magnetic resonance imaging. If there are associated complex congenital anomalies (e.g., heterotaxy syndrome) or intrinsic pulmonary vein stenosis is suspected, preoperative catheterization may sometimes help determine the best management. Those with unobstructed pulmonary veins and congestive heart failure with relatively normal pulmonary artery pressure may be improved with medical treatment, and corrective surgery may be delayed for a few weeks. Among those without additional lesions, the postoperative survivors have an excellent prognosis for a relatively normal life. A few infants develop atrial dysrhythmias postoperatively. Because life threatening, progressive and recurring pulmonary vein obstruction develops in approximately 5% to 10% of infants 1 to 12 months postoperatively, particularly in those with associated heterotaxy syndrome and preoperative pulmonary vein stenosis, initial close follow-up is mandatory.

Truncus Arteriosus

Failure of the cono-truncus to septate into the aorta and main pulmonary artery results in the clinical problem described as truncus arteriosus. It is often associated with microdeletions in a critical region of chromosome 22q11 containing genes responsible for conotruncal development, and with related extra-cardiac anomalies (e.g., DiGeorge syndrome). Other factors can be responsible (28,29). The only artery arising from the heart is the common truncus arteriosus. There is one semilunar valve that may have extra valve leaflets (e.g., four or five) and is often incompetent and rarely stenotic. The pulmonary arteries arise from the left anterior aspect of the truncal root as a single main pulmonary artery, at their bifurcation, or with separate right and left branches. Classifications in vogue are based on the level at which the pulmonary vessels take off, but they are not especially pertinent to the physiology and the clinical picture. Almost universally, there is a ventricular septal defect, usually in the sub-aortic septum, similar to that seen in tetralogy of Fallot. Interrupted aortic arch is an infrequent associated anomaly that should be borne in mind for timely recognition and management.

Pathophysiology

Because of the large ventricular defect and the common arterial trunk, the systemic and pulmonary venous returns are mixed, and the patient is cyanotic. The degree of cyanosis is determined by the pulmonary flow, which is a function of obstruction in the proximal pulmonary arteries. These obstructions are common, rarely severe, and located at the junction of the pulmonary artery and the trunk. If there is no obstruction, which is likely, pulmonary flow exceeds systemic output several-fold, obligating a high-output state and resulting in congestive heart failure and poor survival without surgery. Without surgery, irreversible pulmonary vascular disease is likely to develop as early as the patient's first birthday. Congestive heart failure is less of a problem if there is branch pulmonary artery stenosis, although the degree of cyanosis is greater. Proximal pulmonary artery obstructions frequently develop after surgery. When there is also interrupted aortic arch, a ductus is present, and its untreated closure results in lower body hypotension and hypo-perfusion, followed by death.

Clinical Findings

Infants with truncus arteriosus resemble those with ventricular defect more than the other cyanotic defects. Except cyanosis, which may be mild, development of symptoms is delayed until the pulmonary vascular resistance has resolved enough to allow a large pulmonary flow and the features of a left-to-right shunt. Tachypnea and the other signs of congestion predominate, although cyanosis may be recognized and documented in the first days of life. There is usually a murmur that sounds like a ventricular defect, the peripheral pulses are bounding, and other signs of an aortic runoff are present. The S2 is loud and single, and systolic clicks may be heard. If interrupted aortic arch is also present, diminished pulses, pulse pressure in the lower body, azotemia, and metabolic acidosis develop as the ductus constricts

On chest radiographs, the heart is enlarged, the pulmonary vasculature is engorged, and the aortic arch may be rightward (33%).

ECG inexplicably varies, showing right, left, or combined ventricular hypertrophy (see Table 33-11).

Echocardiographic examination demonstrates the anatomy (Fig. 33-33).

Treatment

Anticongestive measures to control congestion and promote growth have limited effect. Surgical correction is usually undertaken within the first 1 to 6 weeks of life. The later the surgery the more likely that the early postoperative course and survival will be threatened by severe elevation in pulmonary vascular resistance. Although banding of the pulmonary arteries on both sides is possible and is sometimes the only choice, it is easy to understand the difficulty of applying bands on each side equally. For this reason, and because of empirically poor results, most centers perform

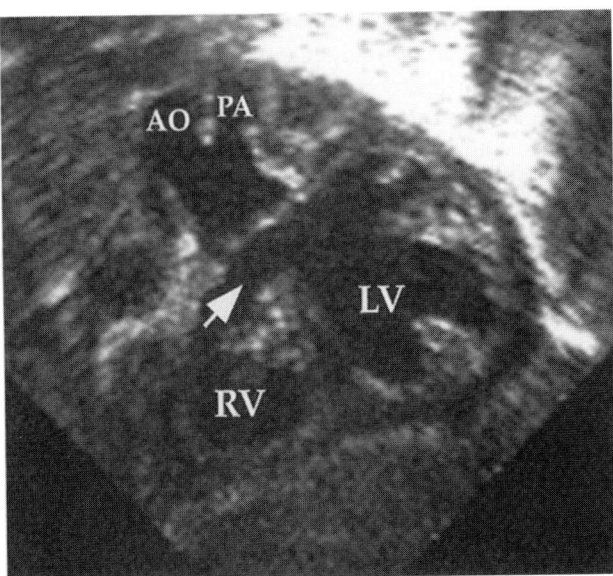

Figure 33-33   Echocardiographic subxiphoid view in a neonate with truncus arteriosus. The right ventricle (RV) and left ventricle (LV) both pump blood through a subaortic ventricular septal defect (arrow) and common truncal valve into the ascending aorta (AO). The main pulmonary artery (PA) arises from the side of the ascending aorta.

one-stage repair in infancy (71). This surgery consists of separating the pulmonary arteries from the trunk, establishing a conduit from the right ventricle to the pulmonary arteries, and closing the ventricular defect. Postoperative management and outcome are aided by the early use of potent pulmonary vasodilators such as nitric oxide. The long-range outcome of this type of repair involves two or three surgical revisions with larger pulmonary artery conduits to accommodate growth during childhood. Severe compression of the conduits and natural or surgery-related proximal pulmonary artery stenoses can develop and require catheter-based interventions in early childhood. The truncal semilunar valve may rarely be sufficiently incompetent to influence the outcome. However, with staged surgical intervention, the long-term survival and outcome are good (72).

Anomalies with Cyanosis with Variable and Mixed Anatomy and Physiology

Single Ventricle

There are few patients who have only one ventricle, with either two atrioventricular valves or a common atrioventricular valve. Most patients characterized as having a single ventricle have one dominant ventricle and a second diminutive structure that is often characterized as an outflow chamber. Because of the similarity of this syndrome to tricuspid atresia, some physicians have preferred the term univentricular heart to describe all patients with a functionally single ventricle, whether they have two atrioventricular valves, tricuspid atresia, or mitral atresia.

Seventy percent of these patients have a single left ventricle with a rudimentary anatomic right ventricular outflow chamber that is left sided (l-transposed position). The ventricular outflow chamber leads to an anterior and leftward aorta, similar to that seen in corrected transposition. Most of the remainder of patients have a single left ventricle with a rudimentary right ventricular outflow chamber that is right-sided (d-transposed position). Pulmonary stenosis coexists in 50% of these patients. In those without pulmonary stenosis, sub-aortic stenosis and coarctation can occur. Almost any other cardiac anomaly may be associated with single ventricle. Single right ventricles also occur, particularly with heterotaxy syndrome.

Pathophysiology

Depending on the presence or absence of pulmonary stenosis, the clinical picture may be dominated by diminished pulmonary flow and cyanosis or by excessive pulmonary flow and high-output congestive heart failure, respectively. Occasionally the pulmonary and systemic flow are balanced, and the patient is only mildly cyanotic and otherwise asymptomatic. The problems peculiar to corrected transposition, such as the tendency to develop complete heart block or develop an incompetent atrioventricular valve (usually the left), are risks. The connection between the single ventricle and the outflow chamber (i.e., ventricular defect) tends to get smaller with time in approximately 50% of patients. This has the physiologic effect of sub-aortic stenosis and must be considered in any management program.

Clinical Findings

The patient usually is visibly cyanotic during the neonatal period. Sometimes those with excessive pulmonary blood flow, minimal cyanosis, and congestive heart failure present later because of growth failure or tachypnea. Most have systolic murmurs from pulmonary stenosis, atrioventricular valve regurgitation, or from other associated defects. The detailed diagnosis is obtained by echocardiographic examination. Catheterization or magnetic resonance imaging are sometimes used preoperatively to delineate anatomic or physiologic details that may influence surgical management.

Treatment

The ultimate goal of management is to separate the pulmonary and systemic circulations by directing all systemic venous return through a cava-pulmonary or atrial-pulmonary anastomosis (e.g., Fontan procedure) and utilizing the single ventricle solely for pumping oxygenated blood to the aorta. Rare patients who have perfectly balanced pulmonary and systemic circulations, and are only mildly cyanotic and virtually asymptomatic, fare well with no surgery for years. Most require a pulmonary artery band to limit pulmonary flow or a shunt procedure to increase pulmonary flow and arterial oxygenation until a modified Fontan procedure (i.e., connection of systemic venous return to the pulmonary arteries) can be performed.

Double-Outlet Right Ventricle

Double-outlet right ventricle is a rare, anatomically and physiologically heterogeneous group of anomalies. The diagnosis is applied when imaging studies demonstrate that both great arteries arise principally from the morphologic right ventricle, invariably in the presence of a ventricular septal defect. A muscular conus commonly underlies both of the great artery outflows. Although various types of double-outlet right ventricle share a common ventricular–arterial relationship, the anatomy of the ventricles, ventricular conotruncal outflows, the relationship of the great arteries, and the presence of additional anomalies are variable. Of primary importance is the relationship of the great arteries to each other and, as a consequence, to the ventricular septal defect. This determines the basic physiology and the surgical management options (73).

Pathophysiology and Clinical Findings

The most common great artery arrangement is a normal relationship, with the aortic valve posterior and rightward and the pulmonary valve leftward and anterior. The ventricular septal defect usually relates to the sub-aortic outflow. Many will have sub-valvar and valvar pulmonary stenosis. Depending on the presence or absence of pulmonary stenosis, the physiology, clinical findings, clinical course, and therapeutic approach are, respectively, like those with tetralogy of Fallot with diminished pulmonary flow or like those with an isolated large sub-aortic ventricular septal defect and pulmonary hyperemia and hypertension.

The second most frequent great artery relationship in double-outlet right ventricle is with the aortic valve to the right, and anterior to or alongside the pulmonary valve, and the great arteries side-by-side. The ventricular septal defect is below the pulmonary outflow. The hemodynamics, clinical findings, and course are as in transposition.

Less common types of double-outlet right ventricle include those with the aorta anterior and leftward, those with a remote uncommitted ventricular septal defect that does relate to either great artery outflow (e.g., atrioventricular inlet type defect), and those with a doubly committed ventricular septal defect that relates to both great artery outflows. Important associated anomalies in those without pulmonary stenosis, with either normally related or side-by-side great arteries, include mitral stenosis or atresia, sub-aortic outflow obstruction, and aortic arch hypoplasia and coarctation. Other less common associated anomalies include heterotaxy with its many related defects (see below and Table 33-13), pulmonary or aortic atresia, multiple ventricular septal defects, and superior–inferior ventricles. These associated anomalies can profoundly influence the hemodynamics, clinical course, and management.

Echocardiographic examination determines the diagnosis by showing the right ventricular–great arteries relationship and can usually determine the great artery and ventricular septal defect relationships and delineate the various associated defects. The need and timing of

TABLE 33-13
COMMON ABNORMALITIES IN ASPLENIA AND POLYSPLENIA SYNDROMES

Asplenia	Polysplenia
Isolated levocardia or dextrocardia	Dextrocardia or levocardia
Visceral isomerism (midline liver and stomach)	Absent inferior vena cava (renal to hepatic segment)
Transposition of the great arteries	Endocardial cushion defect
Double-outlet right ventricle	Total anomalous pulmonary venous return
Total anomalous pulmonary venous return	Coronary sinus rhythm
Endocardial cushion defect	Bilateral epiarterial bronchi
Pulmonary atresia or pulmonary stenosis	
Single ventricle	
Bilateral superior vena cava	
Absent coronary sinus	
Ipsilateral inferior vena cava and abdominal aorta	
P-wave axis of atrial inversion	
Bilateral eparterial bronchi	
Bilateral trilobed lung	

catheterization depend on the anatomy demonstrated by echocardiography and the therapeutic management.

Treatment

Management depends on the specific anatomic abnormalities. Medical and surgical treatment in those with normally related great arteries and no pulmonary stenosis is as with a large ventricular septal defect and in those with pulmonary stenosis as with tetralogy of Fallot. Those infants with side-by-side great arteries and transposition-like physiology may be managed by intracardiac repair or arterial switch procedure. Associated anomalies may require other approaches including systemic-to-pulmonary arterial shunts, Norwood-like procedure, aortic arch repair, and later Fontan-like approach.

l-Transposition of the Great Arteries

In l-transposition of the great arteries with situs solitus, also called corrected transposition, the circulation is often physiologically corrected. The terminology refers to the position of the aorta, which is abnormally positioned, anterior and usually to the left of the pulmonary artery, and to the position of the ventricles. l-Transposition of the great arteries is most commonly associated with ventricular inversion as well, i.e., the ventricles undergo l-looping instead of the usual d-looping. The systemic venous blood enters the right atrium and flows into a right-sided, morphologically left, ventricle and out to the pulmonary artery. Pulmonary venous blood returns to the left atrium and by way of the tricuspid valve into the left-sided, morphologically right, ventricle to the aorta. The aorta is abnormally positioned, anterior and usually to the left of the pulmonary artery. The hemodynamic changes in patients with l-transposition of the great arteries are caused by the commonly associated

cardiac abnormalities that include ventricular septal defect (50%), single ventricle (42%), and pulmonary stenosis or atresia (45%). The latter three result in cyanosis. Left atrioventricular valve regurgitation (23%), conduction disturbances, and arrhythmias, particularly supraventricular tachycardia and complete heart block, are common. This diagnosis should be considered for newborns with complete heart block or supraventricular tachycardia. Medical management and surgery are directed toward correction or palliation of the associated cardiovascular malformations, such as closure of the ventricular septal defect, pulmonary valvotomy, and a cardiac pacemaker if needed.

Malpositions

The term cardiac malposition describes abnormal position of the heart within the thorax or relative to the abdominal viscera. Cardiac position, or malposition, is relatively independent of the intracardiac segmental anatomy or interrelationships. For instance, dextrocardia, positioning of the heart in the right chest, and mesocardia, midline cardiac positioning, may occur with normal positioning of the abdominal viscera and atrial situs as a result of displacement from pulmonary disease or diaphragmatic hernia. Dextrocardia may also occur from genetically orchestrated complete inversion of thoracic and abdominal sidedness (i.e., situs inversus totalis), and with heterotaxic, "ambiguous" malpositioning of the viscera resulting from loss of control of sidedness during embryonic development, (e.g., asplenia and polysplenia syndromes). Cardiac malposition is also present when the heart is in the left thorax (levocardia) when there is heterotaxy or discordant sidedness of the viscera. The term malposition also describes misplacement of the heart as in ectopia cordis.

Fixed cardiac malposition most commonly occurs with heterotaxic malposition of the viscera, as occurs with the asplenia and polysplenia syndromes (Fig. 33-34), and is characterized by discordant sidedness (e.g.., dextrocardia with rightward or midline liver, or levocardia with leftward or midline liver). If the heart is displaced into the right chest or if there is total situs inversus, there is no heterotaxy. Situs inversus totalis is rare, and the heart may be anatomically normal, unlike the more common forms of malposition.

Pragmatically, finding cardiac or abdominal malposition is important as evidence that the patient has a high likelihood of complex combinations of congenital cardiac anomalies. Heterotaxy may be discovered by physical examination or chest radiographs because of abnormal sidedness of the abdominal contents or because the heart is located in the right chest. The cardiac anomalies are remarkably variable, often multiple and complex, and often life-threatening. Table 33-13 shows the anatomic abnormalities encountered in asplenic and polysplenic patients. Incredibly, often all of these occur in combination. For example, a baby with asplenia may have the combination of inferior vena cava crossing from one side of the midline to the other, single left or bilateral superior vena cava, dextrocardia, total and sometimes mixed pulmonary venous connections, single atrium, common atrioventricular valve, single right ventricle with double outlet, and pulmonary stenosis or atresia. Clinically, the initial objective is to determine the details of anatomy and anomaly in each central systemic and pulmonary vein, cardiac chamber, valve, and great artery on a segment-by-segment basis, delineate the interconnections of the various segments of the heart and plan the procedure or sequence of procedures required to repair or optimally palliate the baby's

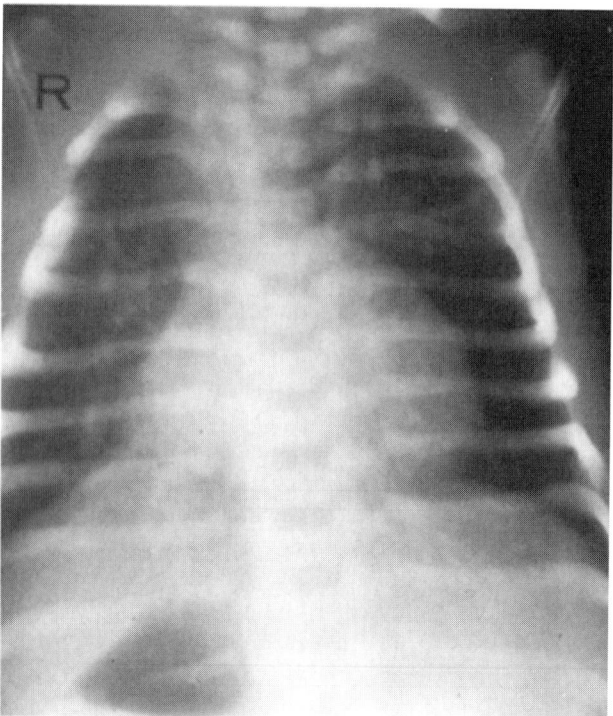

Figure 33-34 A chest radiograph of a neonate with asplenia syndrome, tricuspid atresia, transposition of the great arteries, and a right aortic arch. The liver and stomach are on the right side.

heart. When evidence of cardiac or abdominal malposition are detected, and regardless of the clinical appearance of the baby, it is safest to promptly proceed with a detailed diagnostic evaluation by a cardiac team that has the facilities and experience to accurately determine the anomalies and management. Most patients can be palliated. The overall mortality rate tends to be higher because of the combination of lesions, particularly in those with obstruction of anomalous pulmonary veins (see Table 33-2). Those with asplenia should receive lifetime prophylactic antibiotics because of their propensity for sepsis.

ACYANOTIC LESIONS

Acyanotic diseases associated with normal pulmonary flow include those with systemic outflow obstruction such as coarctation of the aorta and aortic stenosis, mild and moderate pulmonary outflow stenosis, myocardial diseases, and arrhythmias. Acyanotic lesions usually associated with increased pulmonary blood flow include ventricular septal defect, atrial septal defect, endocardial cushion defects, patent ductus arteriosus, aortopulmonary window, and arteriovenous malformations (see Tables 33-14 and 33-15).

Acyanotic Anomalies with Systemic Outflow Obstruction

Coarctation and Interruption of the Aorta

For clinical, prognostic, and probably etiologic reasons, coarctation of the aorta is best considered in two separate categories: simple and complex. Simple coarctation is usually a discrete constriction of the aortic isthmus area, occasionally associated with a patent ductus arteriosus inserting just at or below it. Complex coarctation involves tubular hypoplasia of the aortic arch, with or without discrete aortic narrowing and one or more of the following lesions: patent ductus arteriosus, ventricular septal defect, endocardial cushion defect, aortic stenosis, sub-aortic stenosis, mitral stenosis or regurgitation, hypoplasia of the left ventricle and ascending aorta, other cyanotic anomalies, and endocardial fibroelastosis. In its most severe form the aortic arch may be atretic and completely interrupted as in DiGeorge syndrome. In complex coarctation and interruption of the aorta, the amalgam of left-sided involvement may be secondary to reduced intrauterine flow through the left heart, with consequent underdevelopment and hypoplasia extending from the left atrium to the aortic isthmus. In simple and complex coarctation, there are great variations possible in the extent and location of the coarctation.

Coarctation occurs in 6% to 7% of newborns with heart disease (see Tables 33-1 and 33-2). It is one of the common causes of congestive failure in the neonate (see Tables 33-7). Among symptomatic infants, 82% have complex coarctation, and 18% have simple coarctation. It is more common in male and premature infants. Girls sometimes have Turner

TABLE 33-14

FINDINGS IN ACYANOTIC 0- TO 2-WEEK-OLD NEONATES WITH CONGESTIVE HEART FAILURE[a]

Diagnosis	Physical Examination	Radiographic Findings	Electrocardiographic Findings
Coarctation	↓ Leg pulses and leg BP, soft SEM in back, +/− SRM, +/− click, S₃, +/− differential cyanosis, shocklike sepsis picture	↑ Heart size, pulmonary edema	+/− RVH, develops LVH, BVH
Critical aortic stenosis	Shock, ↓ pulses and perfusion, SEM, click, S₃, single S₂	↑ Heart size, pulmonary edema	LVH, T-wave abnormalities
Patent ductus arteriosus in premature infant	Heave, ↑ pulses, ↑ pulse pressure, continuous or SRM	↑ Heart size (LV, LA), ↑ pulmonary arterial markings	Develops RVH, LVH, BVH
Cardiomyopathy	↓ Pulses, ↓ perfusion, ↓ pulse pressure, ↑ HR, SRM	Large globular heart, pulmonary edema	↓ or ↑ voltage, T-wave changes, Q waves in ALCA
Critical pulmonary stenosis	SEM, click, single S₂, most have cyanosis	Normal or ↓ pulmonary arterial markings, RAE	QRS axis 0°–90°, +/− LVH, develops RVH
Systemic arteriovenous fistula	Heave, ↑ pulses, wide pulse pressure, soft SEM or SRM, bruit, shock, +/− cyanosis	↑ Heart size, ↑ pulmonary arterial markings	Develops RVH, LVH, BVH

[a] Congestive heart failure with cyanosis may be caused by hypoplastic left heart syndrome, transposition of the great arteries, truncus arteriosus, total anomalous pulmonary venous connection, pulmonary atresia with tetralogy, tricuspid atresia, Ebstein malformation, or persistent pulmonary hypertension.
+/−, may or may not be present; ↓, decreased; ↑, increased; ALCA, anamolous left coronary artery; BVH, biventricular hypertrophy; HR, heart rate; LA, left atrium; LV, left ventricle; LVH, left ventricular hypertrophy; RAE, right atrial enlargement; RVH, right ventricular hypertrophy; S₂, second heart sound; S₃, third heart sound; SEM, systolic ejection murmur; SRM, systolic regurgitant murmur.

syndrome. Severe extra-cardiac anomalies, usually renal or gastrointestinal, occur in 6% to 9% of these patients (see Table 33-4).

Pathophysiology

Simple Coarctation. The isthmus is normally smaller than the ascending or descending aorta in newborn infants because only 10% of the combined ventricular output during fetal life passes through the isthmus into the descending aorta, whereas approximately 60% passes through the ductus arteriosus to the descending aorta. After birth, the isthmus gradually grows, but in simple coarctation, there is a constricting band just above the point of connection to the ductus arteriosus. Aortic coarctation may acutely further constrict in the neonatal period, as constriction of the adjacent ductal tissue occurs. During infancy, there may be relative progression of the coarctation from inadequate,

TABLE 33-15

FINDINGS IN ACYANOTIC 2- TO 8-WEEK-OLD NEONATES WITH CONGESTIVE HEART FAILURE[a]

Diagnosis	Physical Examination	Radiographic Findings	Electrocardiographic Findings
Ventricular septal defect	Heave, harsh SRM, +/− S₃, +/− diastolic rumble, normal pulses	↑ Heart size (RV, LV, LA), ↑ pulmonary arterial markings	Develops RAE, RVH, LVH, BVH
Endocardial cushion defect	Same as ventricular septal defect, fixed split S₂	Same as ventricular septal defect	Left axis deviation, develops RAE, RVH, LVH, BVH
Atrial septal defect	Hyperdynamic precordium, soft SEM, fixed split S₂, +/− diastolic rumble	↑ Heart size (RV, normal LA and LV), ↑ pulmonary arterial markings	Develops RAD, RVH
Patent ductus arteriosus in full-term infants	Same as presentation at 0–2 weeks of age		
Cardiomyopathy	Same as presentation at 0–2 weeks of age		

[a] Murmur may be present earlier than 2 weeks of age, and congestive heart failure may occur earlier in premature infants.
+/−, may or may not be present; ↓, decreased; ↑, increased; BVH, biventricular hypertrophy; LA, left atrium; LV, left ventricle; LVH, left ventricular hypertrophy; RAD, right axis deviation; RAE, right atrial enlargement; RV, right ventricle; RVH, right ventricular hypertrophy; S₂, second heart sound; S₃, third heart sound; SRM, systolic regurgitant murmur.

disproportionately small aortic isthmus growth, and perhaps aortic wall hypertrophy and endothelial thickening at the coarctation site. Collateral circulation may be present at birth. In simple coarctation, the increased resistance to flow results in a pressure overload on the left ventricle. If the coarctation is not severe and there is a patent ductus arteriosus, with fall in pulmonary vascular resistance after birth, there is a reversal of flow through the ductus arteriosus from the aorta to the pulmonary artery, and a considerable left-to-right shunt may develop. If the increased pressure and volume load exceed the ability of the heart to compensate by hypertrophy or dilation, congestive failure with diminution of systemic output ensues. Left ventricular end-diastolic pressure is elevated, resulting in increased pulmonary venous pressure and development of pulmonary edema. The increased pulmonary venous pressure also produces pulmonary artery hypertension and right heart failure.

Complex Coarctation and Aortic Interruption. Complex coarctation and aortic interruption are characterized by pulmonary artery hypertension with a ductus arteriosus supplying the descending aorta, usually a large intracardiac left-to-right shunt, and increased pulmonary flow. The right-sided structures are dilated and hypertrophied. There is a pressure and volume overload on both ventricles and congestive heart failure. In those with a large ventricular septal defect and patent ductus arteriosus, the systolic pressures in the pulmonary artery, descending aorta, ascending aorta, and right ventricle are identical. Peripheral pulse pressure is normal, and the pulses are equal throughout. With ductal constriction, the femoral arterial pulsations diminish. If the aortic arch obstruction is severe or complete, perfusion to the lower one-half of the body, previously supplied by the open ductus, is reduced. Manifestations of shock, renal and mesenteric hypoperfusion, and metabolic acidosis develop. Ductus closure causes death.

Clinical Findings

Simple Coarctation. Infants with isolated discrete coarctation may be asymptomatic, although some develop congestive heart failure, often after the age of 1 month. The femoral and pedal pulses are absent or diminished compared with brachial or carotid pulses. Radial and brachial pulses may be decreased if the subclavian artery on that side arises at or below the coarctation. Systolic blood pressure in the upper extremities is higher than in the lower extremities, but marked hypertension is uncommon. Pulse pressure in the lower extremities is narrowed, often 10 to 15 mm Hg. S3 is often present, and there may be an apical systolic ejection click (~ half have a bicuspid aortic valve). A systolic ejection murmur from the coarctation may be heard at the left interscapular area over the back, and at the left upper sternal border. In the neonate a continuous murmur, when present, is usually from a left-to-right shunt across the ductus arteriosus, as collateral vessel flow is generally not audible until older age. Manifestations of congestive heart failure are those of combined left and right heart failure.

Chest radiograph can be nearly normal, but usually shows cardiac enlargement and pulmonary venous congestion.

ECG can be normal, but usually reveals right ventricular hypertrophy in the early months and left ventricular hypertrophy later.

Echocardiographic visualization of the aortic arch usually shows the site, length, and severity of coarctation and the aortic arch branching pattern. There is characteristically a constriction from the outer posterior curvature of the aortic wall, and an anterior peri-ductal shelf may be identified. An instantaneous systolic gradient may be derived from the velocities across the coarctation but may underestimate the severity of the lesion if cardiac output is depressed. The descending aortic flow has a characteristically diminished systolic upstroke velocity and prolonged antegrade flow.

Magnetic resonance and CT imaging can be used to delineate anatomic features not evident with echocardiography (Fig. 33-35).

Complex Coarctation and Aortic Interruption

Infants with severe isolated and complex coarctation usually present with congestive heart failure in the early neonatal period. Generally, the younger the infant, the more severe and complex are the combined malformations. Complete interruption of the aortic arch is usually associated with a ventricular septal defect and a systemic patent ductus arteriosus and is clinically indistinguishable from complicated coarctation. It is frequently seen as part of DiGeorge syndrome, which may have additional manifestations of hypocalcemia, absent thymic shadow on the initial chest radiograph, and possible impaired immune response to transfused viable nonirradiated leukocytes. Besides the findings described for simple coarctation, there is evidence of a large left-to-right shunt and pulmonary artery hypertension. Femoral pulsations may wax and wane, depending on ductal

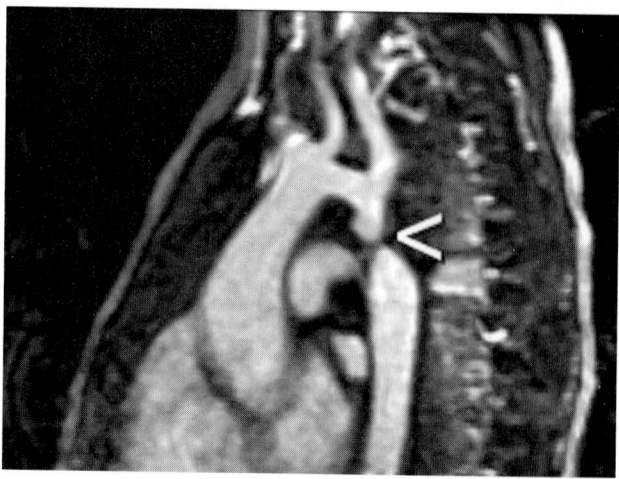

Figure 33-35 Magnetic resonance image of aortic coarctation in a 1 day old. Arrow indicates focal coarctation in the distal end of a hypoplastic aortic arch.

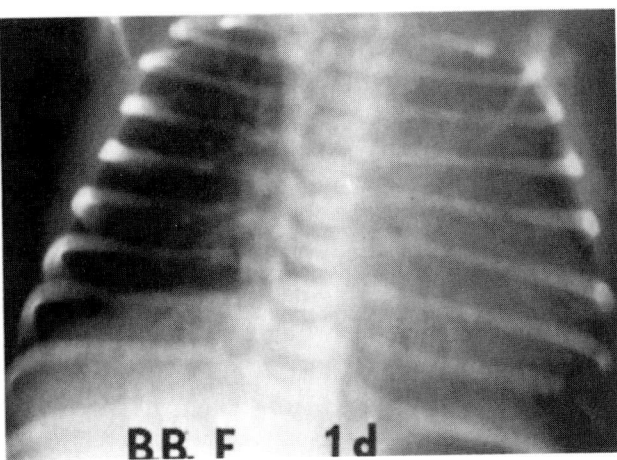

Figure 33-36 A chest radiograph of a 1-day-old infant with complex coarctation of the aorta shows marked cardiac enlargement and pulmonary vascular engorgement.

caliber. A pan-systolic murmur of a septal defect or mitral regurgitation may be found. Ductal closure may result in a critically ill baby with poor perfusion, metabolic acidosis, and possibly disseminated intravascular coagulation, necrotizing enterocolitis, and renal and hepatic dysfunction.

Chest radiographs show considerable cardiac enlargement, pulmonary plethora, and edema (Fig. 33-36).

ECG can be normal, but often has right axis deviation, right atrial hypertrophy, right ventricular hypertrophy, and sometimes diminished left ventricular forces.

Echocardiographic examination delineates the aortic arch anatomy, and reveals associated lesions, including mitral and aortic stenosis, ventricular septal defect, sub-aortic obstruction, and conotruncal abnormalities.

Differential Diagnosis

Aortic arch obstruction should be suspected in any critically ill term baby with a septic-like shock. It should also be suspected as an associated anomaly in young babies with intracardiac anomalies such as ventricular septal defect, single ventricle, truncus arteriosus, and aortic or mitral valve disease who develop signs of poor systemic output. A thorough examination, with careful pulse palpation and blood pressure measurement in all 4 extremities, should lead to the correct diagnosis (see Tables 33-14 and 33-15). Infants presenting before 1 month of age usually have severe or complex coarctation. The presence of a ductus arteriosus supplying the descending aorta may be demonstrated by the finding of a lower arterial PO2 in the legs than in the arms. The hypoplastic left heart syndrome produces a similar shock-like picture or congestive failure in the first week as the ductus arteriosus closes. In these patients, there is cyanosis (See Color Plate), the peripheral pulses are diminished throughout, and the ECG shows marked diminution in left ventricular forces.

Treatment

All neonates with congestive heart failure thought to have coarctation of the aorta should be promptly hospitalized,

treated, and examined by echocardiography. Infants with complex coarctation and aortic interruption become symptomatic because of constriction of the ductus arteriosus. Prostaglandin E1 infusion can dilate the ductus, restore systemic perfusion, improve metabolic abnormalities, and support life during the time needed to study the anatomy and arrange for surgery. Inotropic support with intravenous dopamine or adrenergic agents is often needed. In critically ill babies, there may be adverse ischemic consequences for the gastrointestinal, renal, hepatic, and coagulation systems. Echocardiographic examination usually provides the anatomic detail needed for surgery. If needed, cardiac catheterization, digital subtraction angiography, or magnetic resonance imaging may be useful for additional delineation of the aortic arch and intracardiac anatomy.

If after initial clinical management to effect stabilization, improvement or deterioration occurs, surgery should not be unduly delayed. The surgical procedures employed depend on the severity of the lesion and include resection of the coarctation with primary anastomosis, subclavian or prosthetic patch aortoplasty, or construction of a conduit from ascending to descending aorta; division of the patent ductus arteriosus; and, if needed, intracardiac repair of additional defects such as a large ventricular septal defect. The mortality rate for infants with complicated coarctation is 85% without surgery. Surgery increases the survival rate to 85%. Regardless of the type of coarctation, the mortality is related to age of presentation and is higher for those with duct-dependent descending aortic flow. In some infants with simple and milder coarctation who respond well to medical therapy, surgery may be delayed. Those who undergo surgical coarctation repair early in infancy may develop re-stenosis later, which may require re-operation or catheter balloon dilation. The survivors need close medical supervision throughout childhood and may require other operations for various associated abnormalities later. Catheter balloon dilation of un-operated primary discrete coarctation can offer palliation in the complex critically ill infant, but only in selected infants with an otherwise good size aortic arch does it appear to it provide long-lasting relief (50).

Aortic Stenosis

Fusion of the right-left or right-non commissures of the aortic valve, resulting in a bicommissural, functional "bicuspid" aortic valve, is one of the most common congenital anomalies, occurring in 1.5% of the population. The resulting valve orifice may be diminished, but the effective stenosis is usually mild in neonates. Only very severe aortic valve narrowing produces symptoms or requires intervention in early infancy (Fig. 33-37). Critical isolated aortic valve stenosis is rare, and usually the result of fusion of both the right-non and right-left commissures, with the valve orifice too small to allow adequate cardiac output at physiologically obtainable left ventricular pressures. In this situation, adequate systemic blood flow (before relief of the aortic stenosis) is dependent on a patent ductus arteriosus that

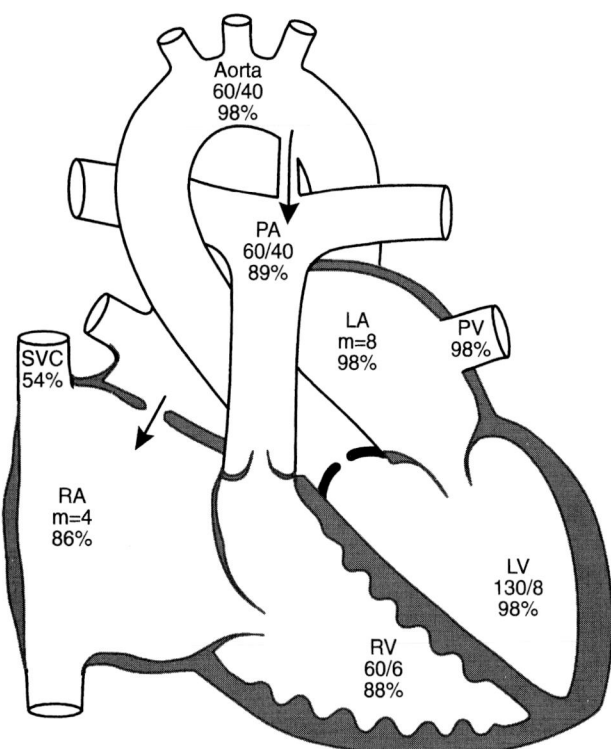

Figure 33-37 Diagram of the cardiac anatomy and physiology in a 1-month-old infant with valvar aortic stenosis had a systolic pressure gradient of 70 mmHg across the aortic valve. The blood passing from left to right through the ductus must return again through the aortic valve, with the excess flow compounding the obstruction. The large atrial shunt, whether a true anomaly or a sprung foramen ovale, elevates left atrial pressure. The numbers below the chamber name are pressure measurements in mmHg determined at cardiac catheterization; the percentages indicate oxygen saturation data. LA, left atrium; LV, left ventricle; PA, pulmonary artery; PV, pulmonary vein; RA, right atrium; RV, right ventricle; SVC, superior vena cava. Adapted from Mullins CE, Mayer DC. *Congenital heart disease: a diagramatic atlas.* New York: Alan R Liss, 1988, with permission.

allows right-to-left blood flow from the pulmonary artery into the aorta.

The symptoms are those of congestive heart failure, pulmonary edema, and sometimes peripheral vascular collapse. The baby may appear ashen and cyanotic if the pulmonary edema is severe. The cardinal features are tachypnea, a blowing systolic murmur at the upper right or middle left sternal border and an apical early systolic click resembling a split S1. If the valve orifice is very small, forward valve flow is small, and the murmur may be soft.

Chest radiographs show cardiac enlargement and pulmonary venous congestion.

ECG usually has biventricular hypertrophy with T-wave changes (see Table 33-14).

Echocardiographic examination demonstrates a deformed immobile aortic valve with commissural fusion. In severe aortic obstruction, trans-valvar flow is diminished, and the systolic murmur and the Doppler-derived pressure gradient are of low amplitude and do not reflect the severity of the lesion. The left ventricle appears hypertrophied and may have decreased or dilated internal dimensions and poor or hyperdynamic systolic function. Some pa-

tients may have coarctation and mitral valve abnormalities. Echocardiography can also identify those neonates with associated hypoplasia of the left ventricular chamber, mitral and aortic annuli and aortic root that do not benefit adequately from valvuloplasty and require a staged hypoplastic left-heart-type surgical approach for survival (51).

Treatment of critical stenosis consists of stabilization with administration of inotropic support, oxygen, and frequently prostaglandin E1 to allow right ventricular support to the systemic circulation; to be followed as soon as feasible by balloon valvuloplasty or surgical valvotomy (52). This provides effective palliation in infancy. Although many require repeat valvuloplasty during childhood, this is usually accomplished with success. Ultimately, and hopefully after childhood growth, many of the worse valves will require surgical replacement with a prosthetic valve or pulmonary autograft (Ross procedure). The asymptomatic infant with auscultatory findings of aortic stenosis and those after valvuloplasty require serial evaluation because, over the long term, valvar aortic stenosis very frequently progresses and recurs to some degree.

Acyanotic Anomalies with Left-to-Right Shunt

Ventricular Septal Defect

Ventricular septal defects may be small or large, single or multiple, and isolated or associated with other cardiovascular malformations. They are an integral part of complex congenital heart disease lesions, such as tetralogy of Fallot, truncus arteriosus, double-outlet right ventricle, and atrioventricular canal, and they have been associated with virtually every other known congenital cardiac malformation. Small, isolated self-closing muscular ventricular septal defects, frequently detectable only by echocardiography, are the most common congenital cardiac anomaly, occurring in 2% to 3% of term newborns (2) and more frequently in infants born prematurely (see Tables 33-1 and 33-2). Large defects occur most commonly singly in the membranous septum, less often in the low portion of the muscular septum, infrequently beneath the pulmonary valve, or posterior next to the tricuspid valve. Even though only 10% of ventricular septal defects cause symptoms, they remain the most common cause of congestive heart failure after the second week of life (see Tables 33-7). Although small defects are usually isolated anomalies, extra-cardiac malformations occur in up to 24% of the patients with large defects. Recognition of a large ventricular septal defect remains paramount because without closure a large defect with pulmonary hypertension can lead to irreversible Eisenmenger-type pulmonary vascular disease by as early as the first birthday.

Pathophysiology

The common small ventricular septal defect has minimal hemodynamic functional effect and does not produce symptoms, but a moderate or large defect in a neonate may cause significant hemodynamic alterations. If the defect is large, right and left ventricular pressures equilibrate, and pulmonary hypertension results (Fig. 33-38). The decreasing pulmonary resistance after birth allows an increasing left-to-right shunt through the defect. The normal regression of pulmonary resistance in the first week of life is usually delayed in these babies. Nonetheless, sufficient reduction in pulmonary resistance occurs by the second week of life to cause symptoms in many patients. Others, with smaller defects or further delay in the reduction of pulmonary vascular resistance, develop symptoms as late as 3 to 4 months of age.

Symptoms are the result of congestive heart failure, sometimes presenting with superimposed pulmonary problems such as bronchiolitis, pneumonia and atelectasis. Congestive heart failure is caused by the obligate high resting cardiac output associated with recirculation of large amounts of blood through the heart and lungs although simultaneously attempting to meet the demand for systemic flow. Cardiac pump reserve for exertions such as feeding is therefore diminished. Excessive pulmonary vascular flow and pressure decrease lung compliance, result-

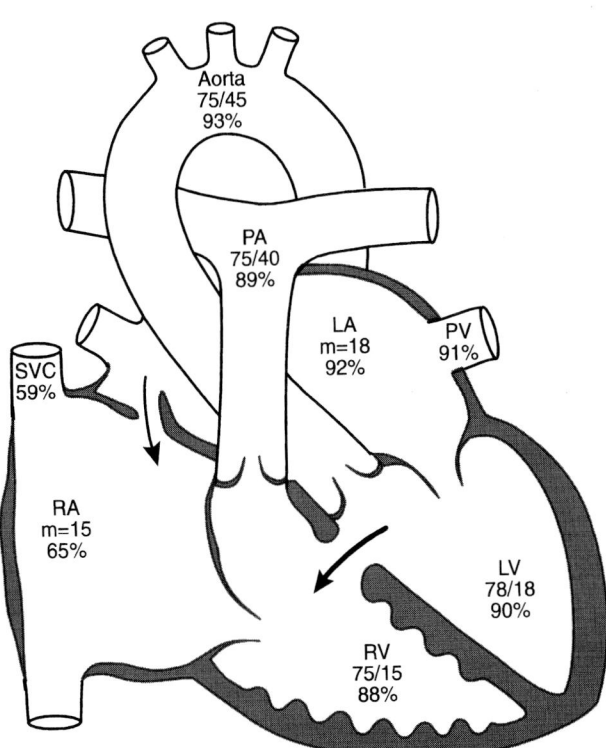

Figure 33-38 Diagram of the anatomy and physiology with a large ventricular septal defect in a 1-month-old baby. The defect allows equilibration of pressure between the two ventricles. With pulmonary resistance much less than systemic resistance, there is a very large left-to-right shunt that caused congestive heart failure, as evidenced by the elevated atrial pressures and the reduced pulmonary venous oxygen saturation because of pulmonary edema. The numbers below the chamber name are pressure measurements in mmHg determined at cardiac catheterization; the percentages indicate oxygen saturation data. LA, left atrium; LV, left ventricle; PA, pulmonary artery; PV, pulmonary vein; RA, right atrium; RV, right ventricle; SVC, superior vena cava. Adapted from Mullins CE, Mayer DC. *Congenital heart disease: a diagramatic atlas.* New York: Alan R Liss, 1988, with permission.

ing in more rapid and labored, but shallower, breaths. The fixed tachypnea impairs feeding and increases caloric expenditure, resulting in diminished growth. Pulmonary congestion may not only decrease the tolerance for but increase susceptibility to recurrent respiratory infections. Enlarged left pulmonary artery and atrium may compress bronchi and result in pulmonary atelectasis. Because pulmonary vascular resistance is lower in premature infants at birth, the development of symptoms from a ventricular septal defect occurs earlier.

Gradual improvement and diminution in pulmonary blood flow in an infant with a moderate or large ventricular defect may occur if there is an anatomic decrease in the size of the defect. Many defects spontaneously close, and most—particularly muscular and membranous defects—become smaller with time. During childhood, but rarely in infancy, there may be progressive and irreversible development of anatomic obstructive changes in the pulmonary arterioles.

Clinical Findings

A small ventricular septal defect is characterized by an isolated mid-higher pitched blowing systolic murmur, which is fairly localized along the left sternal border or at the apex. Infants with large septal defects develop congestive failure in the first few months of life with symptoms of tachypnea (i.e., rate consistently > 60/min), fatigue with feeding, decreased oral intake. Increased respiratory work and retractions, excessive diaphoresis, and recurrent respiratory infections are later manifestations. Weight gain lags considerably behind height maturation. The infant often presents with a respiratory infection that may precipitate or mask underlying congestive failure.

On examination, the infant is scrawny and tachypneic. The cardiac impulse is hyperdynamic. If pulmonary artery hypertension exists, the second heart sound may appear single and loud from early accentuated pulmonary closure. A gallop sound may be heard and is often associated with a mid-diastolic rumble. A mixed frequency holo-systolic murmur, heard best at the lower left sternal border, is soft at birth and usually becomes loud, rough and well transmitted throughout the precordium below the suprasternal notch. There is hepatomegaly and infrequently pulmonary wheezing and rales. Peripheral pulses can be rapid and peripheral edema is rare.

Chest radiograph shows considerable cardiac enlargement, increased pulmonary blood flow, and sometimes pulmonary edema. The main pulmonary artery segment and left atrium are often enlarged. Atelectasis and parenchymal infiltrates are common. ECG usually reveals left ventricular hypertrophy, and if the lesion is associated with pulmonary artery hypertension, right ventricular hypertrophy is detected.

Echocardiographic exam can demonstrate the size, location, and number of ventricular septal defects (Fig. 33-39). Associated lesions not appreciated on physical examination, including atrial septal defect, patent ductus arteriosus,

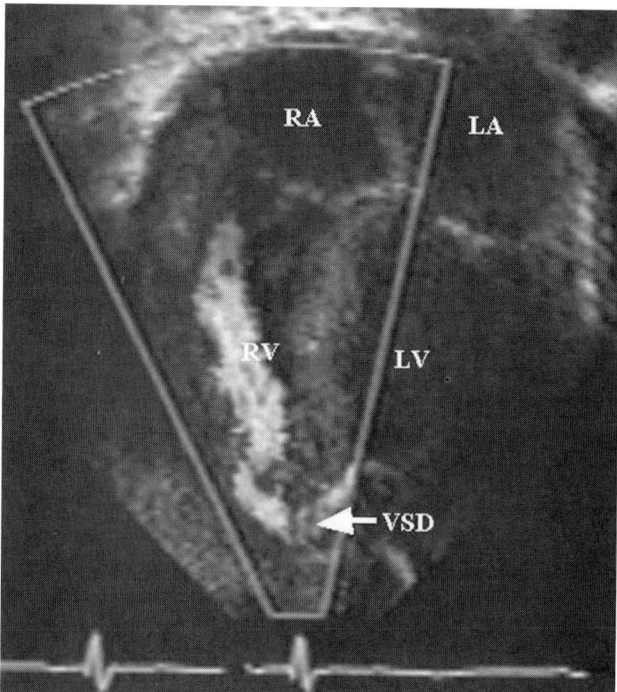

Figure 33-39 Echocardiogram 4 chamber view with color Doppler analysis demonstrates an apical musular ventricular septal defect. (LA, left atrium; LV, left ventricle; RA, right atrium; RV, right ventricle; VSD, ventricular septal defect.)

coarctation of the aorta, and left and right ventricular outflow obstructions, are revealed by echocardiography. Right ventricular and pulmonary hypertension can be assessed both from the curvature of the ventricular septum and by comparison of Doppler measurement of the instantaneous systolic pressure gradient across the defect with simultaneous blood pressure. Often there is at least a trivial degree of tricuspid regurgitation providing means to also estimate right ventricular pressure from the pressure gradient between the right ventricle and right atrium. Defects with a large amount of shunt across them also show evidence of left ventricular volume overload, with large left atrial and left ventricular dimensions and hyperdynamic left ventricular function. Occasionally, an infant with moderate congestive symptoms or findings, or evidence of borderline pulmonary hypertension, or of elevated pulmonary vascular resistance may require cardiac catheterization to delineate the hemodynamics.

Differential Diagnosis

In the neonate, the murmur of a small ventricular septal defect is generally characteristic, but sometimes can be difficult to differentiate from that caused by a small patent ductus arteriosus or tricuspid regurgitation (see Table 33-15). Some infants with large sub-aortic defects have or develop progressive pulmonary stenosis that prohibits left-to-right shunting, cardiomegaly, and congestive heart failure. These babies may develop the features of the tetralogy of Fallot. Later increasing right ventricular hypertrophy on the ECG suggests the development of pulmonary stenosis or increas-

ing pulmonary vascular resistance and the need for careful reevaluation. The coexistence with a large ventricular septal defect of additional malformations resulting in a large left-to-right shunt (e.g., truncus arteriosus) can be difficult to differentiate clinically from isolated large ventricular septal defects; ascertaining their presence often requires echocardiographic examination.

Treatment

An infant with a small ventricular septal defect requires no specific treatment but should be followed. In infants with congestive heart failure, administration of digitalis and diuretics may produce considerable improvement in respiratory symptoms and growth. Systemic afterload reduction with ACE inhibitors (e.g., captopril) moderately decreases the pulmonary/systemic flow ratio and often has additional moderate symptomatic benefit in refractory patients (see Table 33-10). The use of high-caloric formulas, made by supplementation of standard formulas with additional carbohydrate (e.g., corn syrup or polycose) and oil (e.g., corn oil or MCT oil) up to a total of 30 kcal per ounce, is often needed for growth in babies with large defects. The total ad libitum oral intake should not be restricted, because growth failure and small size are a common issue in these infants.

Timely surgical closure of the defect is indicated if the infant does not begin to grow with timely escalation of optimal medical therapy, or has persistent significant pulmonary artery hypertension after 6 months of age. Primary repair in infants entails cardiopulmonary bypass, and, in most patients, atriotomy with patch closure through the tricuspid valve. Some patients require closure through the pulmonary valve or right ventriculotomy. Very low birth weight premature infants and those with multiple large muscular defects may require an initial pulmonary artery banding procedure with corrective surgery done at a later age. Of infants born with isolated large defects requiring closure in the first year of life, mortality is now 1% to 2% or less. Mortality is greater if there are associated severe extra-cardiac congenital anomalies, pulmonary complications, or prematurity. The long-term prognosis after transatrial surgical closure of an isolated ventricular septal defect in the first year of life is excellent, with essentially normal hemodynamics and a small risk for symptomatic dysrhythmias for most patients.

Secundum and Sinus Venosus Atrial Septal Defects

Virtually all babies have a patent foramen ovale at birth. Many foramen ovale functionally close within hours of birth, but many others remain at least partly open for several months and in about 20% the foramen has some blood flow across it throughout life. This is important to the neonatologist, because umbilical vein catheters tend to follow the course of the circulation for the preceding 9 months and may pass through the foramen ovale into the left heart, providing erroneous measures of oxygen levels and allowing passage of intravenously injected air or thrombus to the brain, occasionally with disastrous results.

Pathophysiology and Clinical Features

Secundum atrial septal defects are a common anomaly resulting from an opening in the primum atrial septum around the region of the foramen ovale that rarely causes symptoms or a murmur loud enough to attract attention in infants, and often close spontaneously (2). Much more rare sinus venosus atrial septal defects occur in the atrial septum in which the cavae enter, usually the superior vena cava, often with partial anomalous connection of one or more right pulmonary veins, and are clinically indistinguishable from secundum atrial septal defects. As systolic blood pressure, arterial stiffness, and left ventricular stiffness increase with age, left to right shunting develops across the defect, resulting in increased flow across right heart valves, systolic pulmonary flow murmur at the left upper sternal border and suprasternal notch, diastolic tricuspid flow rumble at the left lower sternal border, persistent delayed closure of the pulmonary valve (and relatively wide fixed splitting of the second heart sound), increased right ventricular workload and increased pulmonary blood flow. Most are found because a murmur of mild pulmonary stenosis is heard and an echocardiographic examination is performed (Fig. 33-40). Others are discovered during evaluation of coexisting cardiac anomaly, or evaluation initiated by extra-cardiac anomalies or failure to thrive. Most small secundum defects (<5 mm diameter), many moderate-size ones (5–8 mm diameter), and some large defects spontaneously close, or nearly close in the first several years of life (2,74). Sinus venosus defects rarely if ever close spontaneously. Because there is rarely significant congestive heart failure, initial management consists of observation and, if the defect persists, it may be closed by surgical or catheter techniques. If a large defect remains open, approximately 10% of those develop Eisenmenger-type pulmonary vascular disease later in life.

Differential Diagnosis

Rarely, a large atrial septal defect is associated with an early decrease in the pulmonary resistance and a large left-to-right shunt in the first months of life. Growth failure and congestive heart failure may raise the question of early cardiac surgery. This is a potentially more complicated and treacherous situation because occult left-sided heart disease (e.g., myocardial disease, aortic stenosis, coarctation) is often responsible for the unusually large imbalance of ventricular compliances, causing a large left-to-right atrial shunt in infancy. Surgical closure of the defect without dealing with the additional problem may have a poor outcome. The simple rule of thumb is to search diligently for associated anomalies and proceed to surgery for isolated atrial septal in early infancy with caution.

Endocardial Cushion Defects

Defects of endocardial cushion development may be partial, resulting in an ostium primum atrial septal defect; complete, resulting in additional total deficiency of the posterior inlet ventricular septum and a common atrioventricular valve (i.e., complete atrioventricular canal); or transitional with a combination of a smaller restrictive defect of the inlet ventricular septum and primum atrial septal defect, (i.e., transitional atrioventricular canal defect). The atrioventricular valves, particularly the anterior mitral valve leaflet, are usually malformed, deficient, or abnormally attached to the ventricular septum. With ostium primum defect, there is usually a cleft in the mitral valve and frequently mitral regurgitation. In complete atrioventricular canal, the primitive atrioventricular valve floats like a sail over both ventricles. This malformation results in a large communication between the right and left atria and the right and left ventricles. Significant atrioventricular valve regurgitation is less common than in those with only an ostium primum defect. Occasionally, but more often in those without trisomy 21, the mitral valve has abnormal chordal attachments and is stenotic. Rarely the large atrioventricular valve is laterally shifted and primarily centered over one ventricle, and the contralateral ventricle is much smaller than normal. Endocardial cushion defects as primary lesions account for 4% of all newborns with serious heart disease (see Tables 33-1 and 33-2).

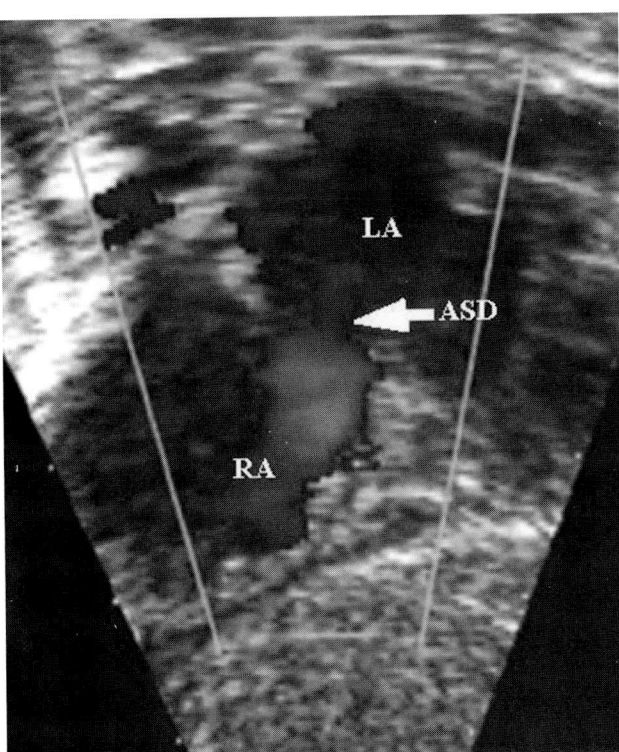

Figure 33-40 Echocardiogram 4 subcostal view with color Doppler analysis demonstrates an secundum atrial septal defect. (ASD, ventricular septal defect; LA, left atrium; RA, right atrium.)

Pathophysiology

The hemodynamic consequence of an ostium primum atrial septal defect is right ventricular volume overload, which is caused by a left-to-right shunt across the atrial septal defect, and variable biventricular volume overload from regurgitation from the left ventricle through the cleft mitral valve to the atria. The volume load, if aggravated by significant mitral regurgitation, can be large and result in congestive heart failure. Streaming of inferior vena cava blood across the large, low-lying defect and cleft common valve leads to mild systemic arterial oxygen desaturation. In complete atrioventricular canal, there is an additional left-to-right shunt through a ventricular septal defect and right ventricular and pulmonary artery hypertension at a systemic level. Infants with pulmonary artery hypertension are particularly susceptible to the development of pulmonary vascular obstructive disease and its complications in later childhood.

Clinical Findings

Isolated primum atrial septal defects without mitral regurgitation results in physical findings similar to secundum and sinus venosus defects with pulmonary flow murmur, fixed second heart sound splitting and sometimes tricuspid diastolic rumble, and is distinguished by ECG left axis deviation. Infants with ostium primum atrial septal defects who are symptomatic in the neonatal period usually have severe mitral regurgitation. Growth retardation may be marked, and weight lags considerably behind height maturation. Recurrent pulmonary infections are common.

With complete atrioventricular canal, there is frequently mild cyanosis. The cardiac impulse is hyperdynamic, and S1 is obscured by a loud pan-systolic murmur audible at the apex or left sternal border. There is usually pulmonary hypertension, and the S2 is accentuated. A S3 and an apical mid-diastolic rumble are often heard. Occasionally, particularly among neonates with Down syndrome, there may be no perceptible auscultatory abnormality. When the murmur is subdued, cardinal features of cardiac anomaly are a hyperdynamic precordium, abnormal second heart sound, and ECG leftward superior axis.

Approximately half of those with isolated complete atrioventricular canal defects have trisomy 21 (75). Forty percent of infants with Down syndrome have congenital heart disease, complete atrioventricular canals being most common. Because babies who have Down syndrome have a tendency to under-ventilate, causing pulmonary venous oxygen desaturation, they may have pulmonary hypertension that, associated with a common atrioventricular canal, may limit left-to-right shunting to amounts that do not produce a murmur (Fig. 33-41). All infants with Down

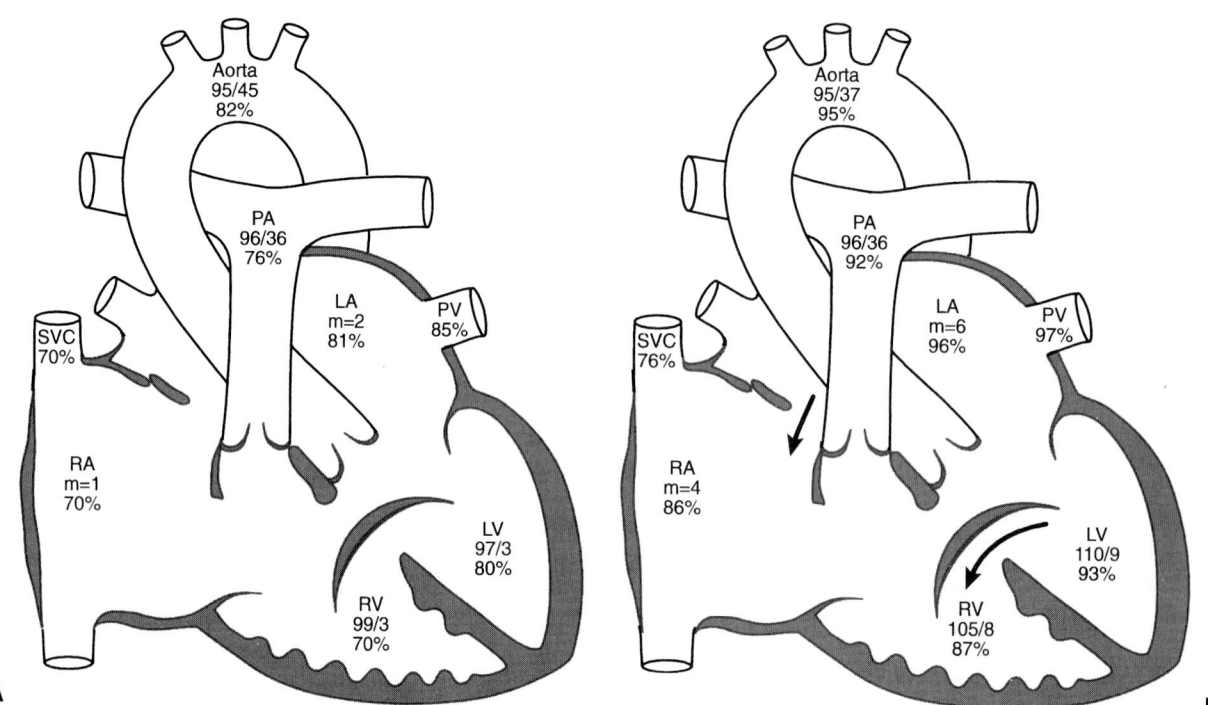

Figure 33-41   Diagram of the anatomy and physiology of an atrioventricular canal in an asymptomatic girl with Down syndrome. There was no murmur. **A:** Although she was breathing room air, the pulmonary resistance was high; there was no left-to-right shunt, and she had arterial oxygen unsaturation. **B:** When breathing oxygen, a large left-to-right shunt developed and the estimated pulmonary resistance fell sharply. The percentages indicate oxygen saturation; the numbers in italics are pressure measurements. The numbers below the chamber name are pressure measurements (mm Hg) determined at cardiac catheterization; the percentages indicate oxygen saturation data. LA, left atrium; LV, left ventricle; PA, pulmonary artery; PV, pulmonary vein; RA, right atrium; RV, right ventricle; SVC, superior vena cava. Adapted from Mullins CE, Mayer DC. *Congenital heart disease: a diagramatic atlas.* New York: Alan R Liss, 1988, with permission.

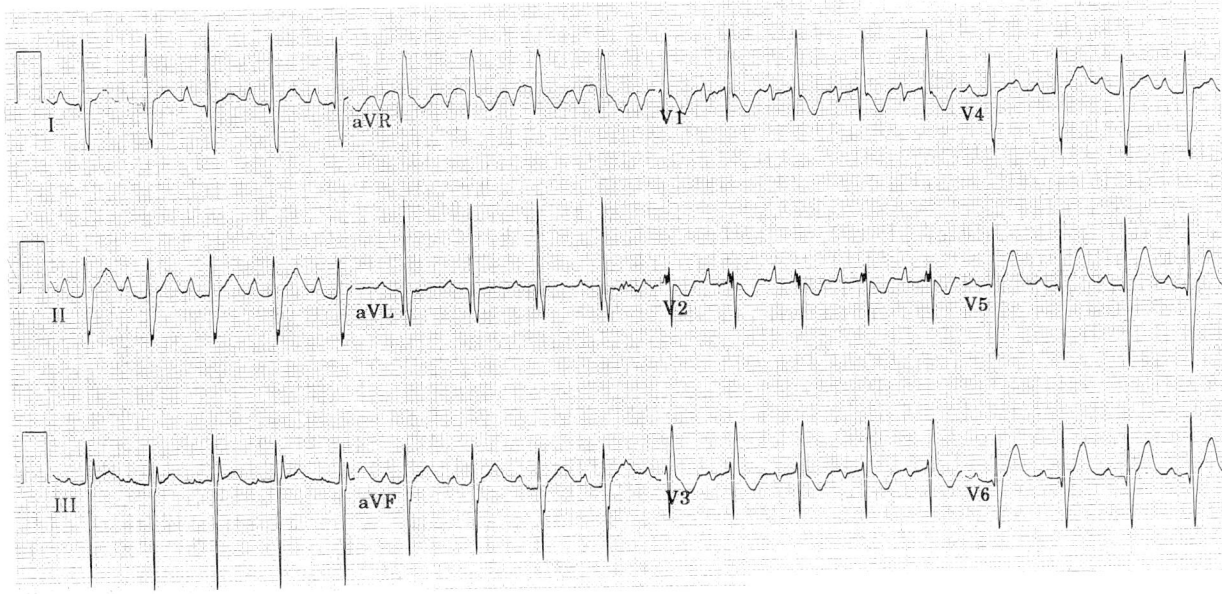

Figure 33-42 Electrocardiogram of infant with atrio-ventricular cushion septal defect shows the characteristic left axis deviation.

syndrome should be evaluated for congenital heart disease by a cardiologist.

Chest radiograph shows cardiac enlargement, sometimes out of proportion to the increased pulmonary vasculature, attributable to the large atria. The main pulmonary artery segment is prominent, and there is pulmonary vascular engorgement.

ECG characteristically shows a left superior QRS axis in the frontal plane, commonly 0° to −60° in primum defects and −60° to −100° in complete canal with a small Q wave in lead aVL (see Fig. 33-42). Significant right ventricular hypertrophy usually indicates right ventricular hypertension (Fig. 33-41).

Echocardiographic examination demonstrates the anatomic features relevant to surgical repair, including the anatomy of the atrioventricular valve with its chordal attachments, papillary muscles, ventricular relationships, possible regurgitation or stenosis of the atrioventricular valves (Fig. 33-43), and possible associated anomalies including systemic and pulmonary venous anomalies, secundum atrial septal defect, muscular ventricular septal defects, ventricular hypoplasia, left or right ventricular outflow stenosis. Preoperative cardiac catheterization is generally not required except to evaluate pulmonary vascular resistance if there is evidence of pulmonary vascular disease.

Treatment

In many patients, palliative or corrective surgery has to be performed in infancy because of refractory congestive heart failure or pulmonary hypertension. Timely treatment with digitalis, diuretics, afterload reduction and caloric supplementation of feedings may result in sufficient improvement in respiratory work and growth to allow substantial

increase in the baby's size and well being for several months before operative repair (see Table 33-10). Infants with refractory symptoms of congestive heart failure should proceed to surgery. In infants with complete atrioventricular canals, there is pulmonary artery hypertension, and surgery is mandatory within the first year to prevent irreversible pulmonary vascular changes.

Primary complete repair is the preferred treatment. This entails cardiopulmonary bypass, atriotomy, patch closure of the atrial and ventricular septal defects, and attachment of the common valve leaflet to the patch or patches. In infants with refractory congestive heart failure weighing less than approximately 2 kg or those with serious

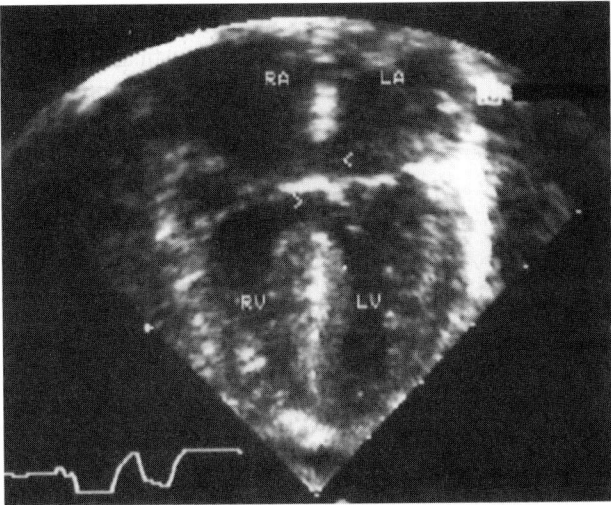

Figure 33-43 Echocardiographic apical four-chamber view of an infant with trisomy 21 and complete atrioventricular canal defect. <, primum atrial septal defect; >, posterior inlet ventricular septal defect; LA, left atrium; LV, left ventricle; RA, right atrium; RV, right ventricle.

confounding noncardiac illness (e.g., duodenal atresia), pulmonary artery banding may be helpful, with complete repair accomplished later. Children with isolated uncomplicated ostium primum atrial septal defects and few symptoms can undergo complete repair at several years of age. The long-term prognosis after surgery in infancy is excellent (76). Late dysrhythmias occasionally occur. There is often some postoperative regurgitation of the atrioventricular valve, but in most infants this is not a significant problem. Systemic vasodilators can reduce the volume of regurgitation and may help preserve ventricular function in patients with significant postoperative mitral regurgitation. When there is severe mitral regurgitation, closure of the septal defect with valvuloplasty may result in clinical improvement, but residual mitral regurgitation may later require valve palliation or replacement. Without surgery, the prognosis is poor. Only 50% of patients with endocardial cushion defects who become symptomatic in the first month of life survive beyond 1 year of age without surgical treatment, and many of these have significant growth failure.

Patent Ductus Arteriosus

The ductus arteriosus, arising from the distal dorsal sixth aortic arch, is well developed by the sixth week of gestation and forms a bridge between the pulmonary artery and the dorsal aorta, inserting at the aortic isthmus. At term, it is a muscular contractile structure. In the full-term infant, functional closure occurs during the first day of life. Persistence of patency of the ductus arteriosus alone or in association with other cardiovascular lesions may produce no symptoms or severe hemodynamic changes, depending on its size.

Isolated patent ductus arteriosus, without hyaline membrane disease, is common, accounting for 4% of all newborns symptomatic with heart disease (4). It is more prevalent in female than male infants. Patent ductus arteriosus is a frequent complication of hyaline membrane disease in the premature infant, in surviving premature infants, and in infants born at high altitudes; in these patients, there is no sex difference. It is common in combination with other congenital heart lesions (e.g., coarctation of the aorta, ventricular septal defect, vascular ring). It occurs in 60% to 70% of infants born with congenital rubella.

Pathophysiology

Ductal closure occurs by constriction and then remodeling with apoptosis (77). At birth, ductal constriction is caused by multiple factors, the most important of which appear to be increased oxygen tension, the levels of prostaglandins, and ductus muscle mass. Prostaglandin E1 is used to dilate a closing ductus in several forms of congenital heart disease in which patency of the ductus arteriosus is necessary to support pulmonary or systemic blood flow (53,54). Delayed closure frequently occurs in premature infants with respiratory distress syndrome. An inhibitor of prostaglandin synthesis (e.g., indomethacin) is used to promote

closure of the ductus in this situation (78,79). The ductus arteriosus that remains patent in the term infant is abnormal and is rarely susceptible to pharmacologic closure.

Within the first hours after birth a small right-to-left or bidirectional shunt may occur. With fall in pulmonary vascular resistance and a rise in systemic resistance, a left-to-right shunt develops through the ductus arteriosus. If spontaneous closure does not occur and the ductus is small, the left-to-right shunt remains small. However, a moderate-sized patent ductus arteriosus is usually associated with a significant left-to-right shunt, increased pulmonary blood flow, left ventricular volume overload, increased left ventricular end-diastolic volume and pressure, elevation of left atrial pressure, and the development of congestive heart failure. The run off of flow from the aorta into the ductus produces wide pulse pressure, and generates bounding peripheral pulsations. A large patent ductus arteriosus produces pulmonary artery hypertension because the pressure is transmitted directly from the aorta to the pulmonary artery through the large defect. Those with moderate and large ducts are prone to the development of pulmonary vascular obstructive disease by 1 year of age or beyond.

The premature infant may develop congestive heart failure earlier because of incomplete development of the medial musculature in the small pulmonary arterioles. The contractile function of the heart, required to handle the increased volume load, may be incompletely developed. Among those with respiratory distress syndrome, there may be an initial period of improvement as the pulmonary status improves, followed by clinical deterioration as left-to-right shunting through the ductus arteriosus increases.

Clinical Findings

Term Infants

In the neonate with a patent ductus arteriosus, as in all left-to-right shunts, the elevated but decreasing pulmonary vascular resistance determines the clinical manifestations. There is usually a crescendo systolic murmur, often with clicks, sometimes detectably spilling into diastole. Often, S2 is not clearly audible. A continuous murmur develops later. The infant with a large patent ductus arteriosus has bounding peripheral pulses, wide pulse pressure (defined as the difference between systolic and diastolic pressure exceeding half of the systolic blood pressure), and hyperactive cardiac impulse at the apex (see Table 33-15). There may be an apical diastolic rumble and symptoms and signs of congestive heart failure, poor weight gain, and recurrent pulmonary infections. In a full-term infant with a large patent ductus arteriosus, overt failure usually does not develop until 3 to 6 weeks of age. If the pulmonary resistance remains high, there may be little murmur.

Chest radiograph shows cardiac enlargement, pulmonary plethora, a prominent main pulmonary artery, and left atrial enlargement. ECG develops left ventricular hypertrophy, occasionally left atrial hypertrophy, and in severe failure, ST-T wave changes.

Echocardiography demonstrates the ductus arteriosus, its size, and the direction of the flow across the defect. Disturbed flow in the pulmonary artery, seen best with color Doppler techniques, is particularly helpful in identifying a patent ductus arteriosus. Continuous-wave Doppler allows measurement of the pressure gradient across the defect and, thereby, estimation of pulmonary pressure (Fig. 33-14). Right ventricular hypertension is also indicated by flattening of the ventricular septum curvature. A large left-to-right shunt is indicated by left heart volume overload and a large left atrium and left ventricle. If there is associated pulmonary disease, the pulmonary resistance may be high, allowing only right-to-left shunting. Right-to-left ductal shunting also occurs with left heart obstructive lesions and coarctation of the aorta.

Preterm Infants

Preterm infants with a patent ductus arteriosus often have the same clinical findings as term babies. Many have a systolic murmur and some have a classic continuous murmur. However, many premature neonates with a large ductus arteriosus have no murmur. Most will have an increase in pulse pressure, at least intermittently. Because arterial pressure varies with age, gestational age, and illness, a rule of thumb for elevation of pulse pressure is when it exceeds half the systolic arterial pressure. Although preterm infants with a large patent ductus arteriosus may develop circulatory overload within the first week of life, some have no specific clinical or radiographic signs discernible from respiratory illness. Unlike term infants, there is no substantial increased incidence of additional cardiac anomalies. However, if examination raises the likelihood of other cardiac or aortic arch anomalies, echocardiographic examination should be done before pharmacologic treatment. Echocardiographic examination of ductal diameter and length, ductal pressure gradient to estimate pulmonary artery pressure, aortic arch anatomy, and possible associated cardiovascular anomalies is indicated prior to surgical closure (Fig. 33-14).

Differential Diagnosis

The infant with congestive failure and a large left-to-right shunt caused by a ventricular septal defect may be clinically indistinguishable from the one with a large patent ductus arteriosus. Other lesions that may result in a large aortic runoff and mimic a patent ductus arteriosus include truncus arteriosus, hemitruncus (i.e., right pulmonary artery from the ascending aorta), aortopulmonary window, aneurysm of the sinus of Valsalva, and large arteriovenous malformations (see Table 33-15). In the sick neonate, clinical differentiation from other lesions is possible using echocardiography.

Treatment

Term Infants. The full-term baby with a persistent patent ductus arteriosus and no evidence of cardiovascular embar-

rassment should be followed, and catheter closure or thoracoscopic or surgical division of the ductus performed later. The choice of method and timing of closure depend on a number of factors, including ductal size. Before therapeutic closure, term infants with congestive heart failure often have symptomatic improvement from treatment with digoxin and diuretics (Table 33-10).

Preterm Infants. Among preterm infants with significant patent ductus arteriosus, indomethacin treatment produces closure in approximately 85% of patients. In symptomatic babies there is a corresponding resolution of findings of congestive heart failure, reduction in required respiratory support and improvement in survival (80). Its use in premature infants with a patent ductus arteriosus who do not yet manifest obvious symptoms from circulatory overload appears to improve many outcome variables including development of congestive failure symptoms, duration of ventilatory and oxygen treatment, and growth (80). Prophylactic administration of indomethacin early after birth in very premature infants decreases the incidence of patent ductus arteriosus, congestive symptoms, cerebral intraventricular hemorrhage, and possibly mortality (81–84). However, until there are data demonstrating an acceptable effect on neurologic function long term, there is uncertainty about the routine prophylactic early use of indomethacin because of the demonstrated negative effects of the drug on neonatal vasoregulation and cerebral blood flow and a theoretical increased risk for cerebral leukomalacia (83). Indomethacin can also cause deterioration of renal and platelet function, and its prophylactic use increases the incidence of oliguria and necrotizing enterocolitis (80,82). It should be avoided if there is significant renal dysfunction, thrombocytopenia, or bleeding. When available, newer prostaglandin synthesis inhibitors such as ibuprofen may have fewer side effects (85). The ductus arteriosus occasionally reopens after initially successful indomethacin treatment and may respond to a second course of treatment. Failure of indomethacin does not adversely affect subsequent surgery (86,87). Avoiding or correcting anemia diminishes the left ventricular volume overload and increases the arterial oxygen content. Surgical interruption of the ductus arteriosus is indicated, regardless of age or weight, in any infant with a persistent hemodynamically significant left-to-right shunt, particularly if there is pulmonary artery hypertension. Surgical mortality is low, and dramatic improvement often occurs. The procedure is performed using a left thoracotomy, or thoracoscope, in the intensive care nursery or the operating room under intravenous or inhalation general anesthesia. Catheter closure is not yet readily technically achievable in small preterm neonates.

Aortopulmonary Window

Defects in the aortopulmonary septum are a rare anomaly resulting in a communication, usually large, between the ascending aorta and main pulmonary artery. Unlike truncus arteriosus, there are usually two normal semilunar valves, and most do not have a ventricular septal defect.

In the approximately half without other cardiovascular anomalies, the physiology and clinical course are similar to truncus arteriosus with large left-to-right shunt, congestive symptoms, and pulmonary hypertension. The half with other cardiovascular anomalies most often have interrupted aortic arch and present with signs of aortic arch obstruction. Anomalous origin of the right pulmonary artery from the aortic trunk (right hemitruncus), anomalous origin of the coronary arteries from the pulmonary trunk, and other anomalies also occur with it. The diagnosis is established by echocardiography. Angiography is sometimes needed to delineate details of the anatomy needed for management. Treatment is surgical (88).

Arteriovenous Malformations

Malformation of the developing peripheral vascular system can result in abnormal connections of arteries, arterioles, and capillaries to the venous system (i.e., arteriovenous fistulae) that create a large shunt. These fistulas can involve vessels of any size and location. Large malformations presenting soon after birth with congestive heart failure occur more often in the liver and head. Capillary hemangiomas involve ongoing abnormal neovascularization. Rarely, infants with prolonged respiratory disease complicated by pneumothorax requiring multiple chest tubes may develop collateral vessels from systemic arteries in the chest wall to the pulmonary arteries. Although most infants with arteriovenous malformations have no other cardiovascular anomaly, abnormal congenital systemic-to-pulmonary vascular corrections can occur with tetralogy of Fallot with pulmonary atresia, partial anomalous pulmonary venous connection (i.e., scimitar syndrome), and bronchopulmonary sequestration.

Pathophysiology

Although most infants do not develop cardiovascular symptoms, a large systemic arteriovenous malformation can result in significant left-to-right shunt and congestive heart failure. Symptomatic babies usually have connections of relatively large arteries and veins in the cerebral or hepatic vasculature. Pulmonary arteriovenous malformations result in an intrapulmonary right-to-left shunt and cyanosis, but they do not produce congestive heart failure.

Clinical Findings

Arteriovenous fistula is one of the few cardiovascular defects that may produce severe congestive heart failure in the first day of life. Cardiovascular shock may be the predominant clinical picture. There may be a hyperdynamic precordium and pulses, flow murmur, severe congestive heart failure, and cyanosis. Bruits over the fontanelle, posterior neck, or abdomen may be audible, and there may be an enlarged head or liver. Echocardiography can demonstrate biventricular dilation and sometimes an enlarged cava with increased flow. Arterial contrast injection demonstrates systemic arteriovenous fistulas. Systemic venous or

pulmonary artery injection of contrast demonstrates pulmonary arteriovenous malformations. Ultrasonography, computed tomography, MRI, and angiography may be useful in finding and delineating the lesion.

Treatment

Malformations causing congestive heart failure usually do not spontaneously improve, except for capillary malformations that may respond to steroid or antiangiogenic drugs such as interferon. Large vessel malformations require mechanical occlusion. Surgery carries a considerable risk, and transcatheter occlusion with a variety of devices, including coils and detachable balloons, has been successful in many, usually older, patients.

Vascular Rings and Slings

A variety of intrathoracic vascular anomalies may encircle the trachea and esophagus and result in symptoms in the neonatal period. Depending on the degree of compression of the trachea or esophagus, several may present in infants with stridor, wheezing, cough, recurrent infections, or feeding difficulties. All of these symptoms are more commonly caused by other abnormalities, such as choanal atresia, tracheomalacia, laryngeal web, hemangioma, or gastroesophageal reflux.

Although uncommon, vascular anomalies may result in serious or life-threatening symptoms and therefore should be considered in any infant with persistent unexplained respiratory symptoms.

Right Aortic Arch with Anomalous Left Subclavian Artery

The spectrum of aortic arch anomalies is most commonly explained by the double arch model first proposed by Edwards and subsequently modified by others (89). This hypothesis explains all observed arch variants by abnormal persistence or regression of portions of a double arch present in embryologic development. The most common of the arch anomalies that has been associated with symptoms in the neonate is the right aortic arch with anomalous left subclavian artery. In this malformation, the aortic arch passes to the right of the trachea over the right mainstem bronchus, then giving rise to the left subclavian artery as the last brachiocephalic branch. A left-sided remnant of the ductus arteriosus connects the pulmonary artery with the descending aorta, resulting in a vascular ring encircling the trachea and esophagus.

Symptoms, when present, are usually not severe and commonly occur beyond the newborn period. The diagnosis may be suspected on plain anterior-posterior chest x-ray by leftward shifting of the trachea from the right-sided arch.

Barium swallow may demonstrate a posterior, oblique indentation of the esophagus from the left subclavian artery.

Echocardiography can demonstrate the position of the arch relative to the trachea and the branching pattern.

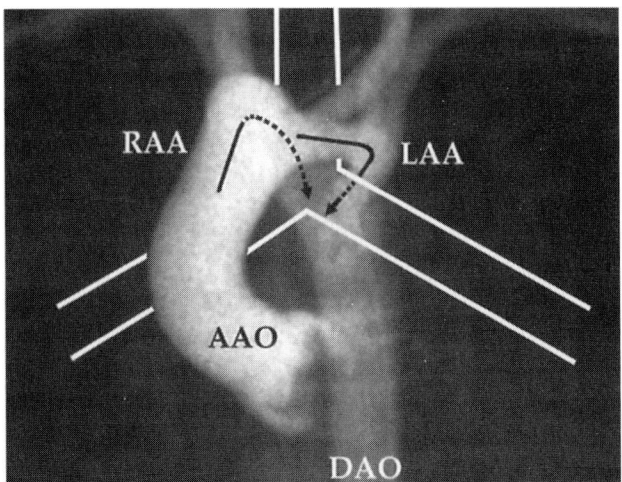

Figure 33-44 Aortogram in the anteroposterior projection in a 2-month-old infant with a history of sudden apnea requiring resuscitation. The anatomy of a typical double aortic arch is displayed. The ascending aorta (AAO) connects to bilateral aortic arches that encircle the airways. The larger and more cephalad right aortic arch (RAA) passes over the right mainstem bronchus. The smaller, lower left aortic arch (LAA) encircles the trachea and passes over the left mainstem bronchus before rejoining the right arch to form the descending aorta (DAO). Solid white lines outline the trachea and mainstem bronchi. Black arrows show the course of the aortic arches.

Associated cardiac malformations, if present, can also be determined at the time of echocardiographic evaluation.

Magnetic resonance imaging has proven to be a useful tool for determining vascular anatomy, and may display evidence of tracheal compression.

Double Aortic Arch

Failure of the normal regression of the embryologic right arch between the right subclavian artery and the descending aorta results in a double aortic arch. The right-sided arch is the larger and more cephalad in approximately 75% of patients. The resulting vascular structure completely encircles the trachea and esophagus.

Symptoms may be dramatic, even life-threatening, and usually occur within the first few months of life.

The plain chest radiograph is generally nondiagnostic. The anatomy can be imaged by echocardiographic examination, magnetic resonance imaging, or angiography (Fig. 33-44).

Barium swallow demonstrates bilateral indentation of the esophagus. If done, bronchoscopy will show the pulsatile compression of the trachea by the vascular ring.

Surgery is indicated in symptomatic infants and consists of division of the smaller arch, usually the left. The postoperative relief of symptoms and prognosis are usually good.

Anomalous Origin of the Left Pulmonary Artery (Pulmonary Sling)

Anomalous origin of the left pulmonary artery is a rare but serious vascular defect, in which the left pulmonary artery arises from the proximal right pulmonary artery and passes between the trachea and the esophagus before supplying the left lung.

Respiratory symptoms are often severe, and there may be associated hypoplasia or stenosis of the trachea or right mainstem bronchus. Swallowing difficulties are uncommon.

Barium esophagram demonstrates anterior compression from the aberrant vessel. Hyperinflation of the right lung as a result of selective compression of the right bronchus may be noted on plain chest radiograph.

Echocardiography will generally demonstrate the key features of the anatomy, although MRI, angiography, and bronchoscopy have been recommended by some to delineate additional details (90,91).

Surgery is indicated and consists of division of the left pulmonary artery with reanastomosis to the main pulmonary artery in a more normal location. Outcome after surgical correction of the pulmonary artery origin has been fair, limited in part by associated lesions and by persistent pulmonary complications related to residual airway abnormalities. Residual left pulmonary artery stenosis is common after surgery.

Anomalous Origin of the Innominate Artery

Compression of the trachea by the innominate artery is a controversial source of respiratory distress in neonates and infants. It has been contended that airway compromise may result if the origin of an otherwise normal innominate artery is more distal than usual, resulting in indentation of the trachea as the vessel courses anteriorly and rightward before splitting into the right subclavian artery and right carotid artery.

Bronchoscopy may reveal a pulsatile mass compressing the distal trachea.

Surgical intervention to suspend the innominate from the anterior chest wall has been advocated, with reported relief of respiratory symptoms in some patients. In some series, this situation has represented a significant portion of infants undergoing surgery for airway compression (92). However, others have disputed this mechanism as a common cause of respiratory distress and suggest conservative management (93).

ACYANOTIC ANOMALIES WITH ABNORMAL CARDIAC FUNCTION OR STRUCTURE

Cardiomyopathy

Sick neonates without cardiac anatomic anomaly often develop symptoms of cardiac and myocardial dysfunction. Systolic and/or diastolic dysfunction most often occur secondary to another abnormality such as sepsis or hypothermia, but occasionally from disorders fundamentally involving myocyte biochemistry. Cardiomyopathy is abnormal myocardial cellular function or structure that occurs with

TABLE 33-16
DILATED CARDIOMYOPATHIES

Infectious causes
  Viral (coxsackie, adenovirus, echo, CMV)
  Bacterial sepsis (endotoxemia, exotoxemia)
Myocardial ischemia
  Asphyxia
  Anomalous origin of left coronary artery
Reversible electrolyte and metabolic causes of myocardial
    dysfunction
  Hypoglycemia
  Hypocalcemia
  Hypophosphatemia
  Hypothermia
  Polycythemia
Work-overload cardiomyopathies
  Tachycardia induced (incessant SVT or VT)
  Severe pulmonary hypertension (H&D)
  Critical aortic valve stenosis (H&D)
Genetic isolated cardiomyopathy
  Dilated cardiomyopathy
    Familial dilated cardiomyopathy (1p, AD)
    Familial dilated cardiomyopathy (AD, AR)
    Familial dilated cardiomyopathy (dystrophin promoter,
      X-linked)
    Arrhythmogenic right ventricular dysplasia (AD)
    Noncompaction of the left ventricle (AD)
    Mitochondrial transfer RNA (tRNA) mutations
      T9997C tRNA Gly
      C3303T tRNA leu
  Restrictive cardiomyopathy
    Familial restrictive cardiomyopathy (AD) (R)
Neuromuscular diseases
  Duchenne muscular dystrophy (X-linked)
  Becker-type muscular dystrophy (X-linked)
  Myotubular myopathy (X-linked, also AR, AD)
  Nemaline rod myopathy (AD, AR) (H&D)
  Multicore myopathy (AR, also possible AD) (D, H, R)
  Friedreich ataxia (AD) (H&D)
  Phytanic acid oxidation disorder (Refsum disease, AR) (H&D)
Metabolic disorders
  Decreased Energy Production
    Disorders of mitochondrial fat oxidation
      Primary carnitine transport protein deficiency (AR) (H&D)
      Primary carnitine palmitoyltransferase II deficiency
        (AR) (H&D)
      Secondary carnitine deficiencies
        (many causes, e.g. methylmalonic and isovaleric
          acidemias, multiple ORT & fat acyl Co-A dehydrogenase
          deficiencies, Kearns-Sayre syndrome, etc.) (H&D)

Disorders of pyruvate metabolism
  Pyruvate dehydrogenase deficiency
    (Leigh necrotizing encephalopathy syndrome, AR) (H&D)
  Pyruvate carboxylase deficiency (Leigh syndrome,
    AR) (H&D)
Disorders of oxidative phosphorylation
  Complex I (NADH-coQ reductase) (AR, mtDNA)
  Complex III (reduced coQ-cytochrome c reductase,
    cytochrome b)
    (AR, mtDNA) (H&D)
  Complex IV (cytochrome c oxidase)
    (Leigh syndrome variants, AR, mtDNA) (H&D)
  Complex V (ATP synthetase)
    (Leigh syndrome variants, AR, mtDNA) (H&D)
  Combined respiratory chain deficiencies (H&D)
    Lethal infantile histiocytoid cardiomyopathy (AR,
      mtDNA) (WPW)
    Lethal infantile mitochondrial disease (mtDNA)
    Mitochondrial transfer RNA (tRNA) mutations
      (H&D) cardiomyopathy and myopathy syndromes
      (multiple mutations in tRNAs for leu, iso, gly, glu, pro)
      (WPW)
    MELAS syndrome (multiple tRNA leu mutations)
      (D, H, WPW)
    MERRF syndrome (multiple tRNA lys mutations) (D, H)
    Kearns-Sayre syndrome (multiple tRNAs leu, asp, cys)
      (HB)
  Mitochondrial DNA (mtDNA) mutations and deletions
    Kearns-Sayre syndrome (multiple mtDNA
      mutations, AD) (HB) others (e.g., 5 kb
      deletion, 7.4 kb deletion)
  Barth syndrome (3-methylglutaconic aciduria type II,
    X-linked) (H&D)
Infiltrative storage disorders
  Glycogen storage disease
    Type IV (Andersen disease, branching enzyme
      deficiency) (D)
  Mucopolysaccharidosis
    Type I (Hurler syndrome) (AR) (H&D)
    Type VI (Maroteaux-Lamy syndrome) (AR)
  Ganglioside degradation disorders
    G_{M2} gangliosidosis (Sandhoff disease, AR) (H&D)
Amino acid and organic acid disorders with toxic metabolites
  Propionic acidemia (AR)
  Ketothiolase deficiency (AR)

D, dilated cardiomyopathy; H, hypertrophic cardiomyopathy; SVT, supraventricular tachycardia; VT, ventricular tachycardia; WPW, Wolf–Parkinson–White syndrome; HB, heart block; AD, autosomal dominant; AR, autosomal recessive.
From refs. 33, 34.

many abnormalities and disorders (see Tables 33-16 and 33-17). Myocardial dysfunction may be grouped by clinical and echocardiographic determination of the cardiovascular pathophysiology, without regard to etiology, as dilated, hypertrophic, and restrictive cardiomyopathy. The nature of appropriate supportive cardiac treatment depends on this cardiovascular physiologic classification. However, the outcome of supportive therapies alone is limited. Additional improvement in outcome may result from determining causation and directed treatment based on etiology.

Dilated Cardiomyopathies

Dilated cardiomyopathies are characterized by diminished cardiac contractility, with ventricular enlargement, abnormal diastolic function, and congestive heart failure. Neonates with dilated cardiomyopathy more frequently have an identifiable cause than is currently achievable in older children and adults (see Table 33-16). These include identifiable infection (e.g., bacterial or viral sepsis, Coxsackie or adenovirus myocarditis, toxoplasmosis), ischemia (e.g.,

TABLE 33-17

HYPERTROPHIC CARDIOMYOPATHY

Hormonal causes
    Maternal diabetes mellitus
    In utero sympathomimetic exposure
    Pheochromocytoma
    Hyperthyroidism
Work overload
    Severe pulmonary hypertension
    Critical aortic valve stenosis
Genetic isolated cardiomyopathy
    Contractile protein mutation
        HCM-1 (myosin heavy chain, AD)
        HCM-2 (troponin T_2, AD)
        HCM-3 (alpha-tropomyosin, AD)
        HCM-4 (myosin binding protein C, AD)
        HCM-5 (AD)
        HCM-6 (AD) (WPW)
        HCM (AR)
    Cardiac phosphorylase kinase deficiency (AR)
    Restrictive cardiomyopathy
        Familial restrictive cardiomyopathy (AD) (R)
Genetic syndromes
    Noonan syndrome (AD)
    Cardio-facio-cutaneous syndrome (AD)
    LEOPARD syndrome (AD)
    Neurofibromatosis (AD)
    Beckwith–Wiedmann syndrome (AD)
    Cutis laxa (X-linked)
Neuromuscular diseases
    Nemaline rod myopathy (AD, AR) (D&H)
    Multicore myopathy (AR, also possible AD) (D, H, R)
    Friedreich ataxia (AD) (D&H)
    Refsum disease (D&H)
Metabolic disorders
    Decreased energy production
        Disorders of mitochondrial fat oxidation
            Primary carnitine transport protein deficiency (AR) (H&D)
            Primary carnitine/acylcarnitine translocase deficiency (AR)
            Primary carnitine palmitoyl-transferase II (AR) (D&H)
            Secondary carnitine deficiencies (H&D)
                many causes, e.g., organic acidemias, multiple ORT & fat acyl Co-A dehydrogenase deficiencies, etc.
            Very-long-chain acyl-CoA dehydrogenase (VLCAD) deficiency
            Long-chain-acyl-CoA dehydrogenase (LCAD) deficiency
            Long-chain 3-hydoxyacyl-CoA dehydrogenase (LCHAD) deficiency
        Disorders of pyruvate metabolism
            Pyruvate dehydrogenase deficiency (Leigh necrotizing encephalopathy syndrome, AR) (H&D)
            Pyruvate carboxylase deficiency (Leigh syndrome, AR) (H&D)

Disorders of oxidative phosphorylation
    Complex II (succinate-coQ reductase) (AR) (WPW)
    Complex III (reduced coQ-cytochrome c reductase, cytochrome b) (AR, mtDNA) (H&D)
    Complex IV (cytochrome c oxidase) (Leigh syndrome variants, AR, mtDNA) (H&D)
    Complex V (ATP synthetase) (Leigh syndrome variants, AR, mtDNA) (H&D)
    Combined respiratory chain deficiencies (D&H&WPW)
    Lethal infantile histiocytoid cardiomyopathy (AR, mtDNA)
    Lethal infantile mitochondrial disease (mtDNA)
    Mitochondrial transfer RNA (tRNA) mutations cardiomyopathy and myopathy syndromes (multiple mutations in tRNAs for leu, iso, gly, glu, pro) (H&D&WPW)
        MELAS syndrome (muliple tRNA leu mutations) (D&H&WPW)
        MERRF syndrome (multiple tRNA lys mutations) (D&H)
        Kearns-Sayre syndrome (multiple tRNAs leu, asp, cys) (HB)
    Mitochondrial DNA (mtDNA) mutations and deletions
        Kearns–Sayre syndrome (multiple mtDNA mutations, AD) (HB)
    Barth syndrome (3-methylglutaconic aciduria type II, X-linked) (H&D)
    Sengers cardiomyopathy with cataracts syndrome (AR)
Infiltrative storage disorders
    Glycogen storage disease
        Type II (Pompe disease, acid maltase deficiency, AR)
        Type III (Cori disease, debranching enzyme deficiency)
        Type IX (Cardiac phosphorylase kinase deficiency)
    Mucopolysaccharidosis
        Type I (Hurler syndrome, AR) (H&D)
        Type II (Hunter syndrome, X-linked)
        Type III (Sanfilippo syndrome, AR)
        Type IV (Morquio syndrome, AR)
        Type VII (Sly syndrome, AR)
    Ganglioside degradation disorders
        G_{M1} gangliosidosis (AR)
        G_{M2} gangliosidosis (Sandhoff disease, AR)
    Glycoprotein metabolic disorder
        Carbohydrate-deficient glycoprotein syndrome (AR)
    Others
        Glycosphingolipid degradation disorder (Fabry, X-linked)
        Globoside degradation disorder (Gaucher disease, AR)
        Phytanic acid oxidation disorder (Refsum disease, AR) (D&H)
        Tyrosinemia (AR)

D, dilated cardiomyopathy; H, hypertrophic cardiomyopathy; SVT, supraventricular tachycardia; VT, ventricular tachycardia; WPW, Wolf–Parkinson–White syndrome; HB, heart block; AD, autosomal dominant; AR, autosomal recessive.
From refs. 33, 34.

birth asphyxia, anomalous left coronary artery origin), hemodynamic work overload (e.g., incessant tachyarrhythmia) and electrolyte or metabolic imbalance (e.g., hypothermia, polycythemia, hypoglycemia, hypocalcemia). Increasingly infants are being recognized with primary biochemical disorders of energy production and metabolism that result in isolated cardiomyopathy or generalized myopathy and encephalopathy (33–35). These infants often have significant deterioration with stress, including that with birth. Caution should be used in attributing permanent or temporary cardiac dysfunction and encephalopathy entirely to "birth asphyxia" in a baby with low Apgar scores without identifiable perinatal cause for asphyxia. Additionally, myocardial diseases that more commonly present in older children, such as those associated with neuromuscular disorders; sometimes have unusually early presentations in infancy.

Pathophysiology

Although the etiologies are diverse, in most dilated cardiomyopathies the clinical course, pathophysiology, and some molecular mechanisms are similar. Myocyte damage, from infection, cytokines, toxic metabolite, or energy deprivation from metabolic block or ischemia, results in myocardial injury. This results in a sequence of molecular and cellular changes with myocardial dysfunction, stunning, apoptosis, necrosis, and interstitial fibrosis, leading to impaired systolic contractility and diastolic compliance. Ventricular enlargement, because of Frank–Starling phenomenon, and tachycardia partially compensate for diminished systolic shortening fraction and support resting cardiac output, but use up reserve in pump function. The impairment in diastolic compliance results in generalized edema and in pulmonary venous engorgement with tachypnea. If cardiac function worsens, resting cardiac output diminishes, and multi-system dysfunction results.

Clinical Findings

The primary manifestations are those of combined right and left heart congestive failure, including diminished activity and feeding, hepatomegaly, tachypnea, retractions, S3, variable systolic regurgitant murmur, and variable signs of low cardiac stroke volume, including tachycardia, narrowed pulse pressure, diminished brachial radial and pedal pulses, systolic hypotension, diminished perfusion, and oliguria.

Chest radiograph shows cardiomegaly and pulmonary edema.

ECG has resting tachycardia, often diffusely diminished voltage amplitude, sometimes diffusely increased voltage amplitude, and often diffuse repolarization changes.

Echocardiographic examination demonstrates ventricular enlargement, generally affecting the left ventricle more than right, and often very severe. Mitral and tricuspid regurgitation, atrial enlargement, and pulmonary hypertension occur frequently. Coronary anomalies, or other cardiac structural anomalies with similar presentation, should be detected.

Because the best hope for successful treatment depends on treating the primary cause, diagnostic evaluation should seek causation. Detailed family history can provide information not elicited by cursory generalized questions. Obstetrical history may provide information about possible infectious causes and events with asphyxia. Physical examination may demonstrate malformations consistent with genetic syndromes, dysmorphic features and organomegaly consistent with peroxisomal or infiltrative storage disorders, encephalopathy and hypotonia consistent with various metabolic disorders and less often with neuromuscular disorders. The absence of noncardiac findings also

provides diagnostic information. Although the history and exam may help point the direction, the diagnosis depends on laboratory studies. Initial evaluation should usually include blood electrolytes with measurement of total CO_2 or bicarbonate, glucose, blood urea nitrogen, creatinine, and complete blood count. If infection is suspected, appropriate bacterial cultures (blood, endotracheal tube aspirate, urine, cerebrospinal fluid), viral cultures (nasopharyngeal, perirectal, cerebrospinal fluid) and serology should be obtained.

Specific Dilated Cardiomyopathies

Although rare, anomalous origin of the left coronary artery from the pulmonary artery should be considered in all children with dilated cardiomyopathy, particularly if there is an ECG pattern of anterolateral myocardial infarction. The anomalous origin of the left coronary artery from the pulmonary artery and retrograde flow in the left anterior descending and left main coronary arteries can usually be seen on echocardiographic examination, although angiography may be needed in some cases. Recognition is key; treatment is surgical, and is usually successful if done promptly after ventricular dysfunction and symptoms appear.

Metabolic disorders can present with either dilated or hypertrophic cardiomyopathy, and often clinically deteriorate with intercurrent infection. If metabolic disease is suspected, additional tests should be done; including measurement of blood ammonia, arterial blood gases, total and free carnitine, lactate, pyruvate, liver function tests, creatine kinase and urine quantitative amino acids, organic acids and, if appropriate, mucopolysaccharide and oligosaccharide levels. Expert consultation from a metabolic disease specialist should be obtained. Chromosomal analysis and skeletal x-ray analysis may be helpful if dysmorphic features are present. Fundoscopic examination for retinal disease and cataracts may help in evaluation for disorders accompanied by these findings. Biopsy of skeletal muscle and/or cardiac muscle for light and electron microscopic examination, mitochondrial genomic studies and biochemical studies are often needed in the evaluation of metabolic disease (33).

Neonatal viral myocarditis is an often fulminant disease, frequently associated with hepatitis and encephalitis. The most commonly identified causes are echovirus, Coxsackie virus, particularly type B, and in some locations rubella virus. In individual cases, the cause may not determined with culturing of nasopharyngeal, tracheal, and stool swabs and serologic tests and PCR analysis may be required for diagnosis. The infection may be acquired perinatally or postnatally. Treatments including immunoglobulin, interferon, steroids, and ribavirin have been under investigation in biopsy-proven myocarditis, but supportive measures are the mainstay of treatment. Several other viruses, bacteria, mycoplasma, rickettsiae, spirochetes, and fungi rarely cause myocarditis. Myocarditis, because of an autoimmune reaction, may occur with maternal lupus erythematosus.

Maternal IgG Ro antibodies cross the placenta, bind to the fetal myocardium, and may block conduction or cause cardiomyopathy. Steroids may be beneficial in this disease.

Chronic supraventricular and ventricular tachycardia can lead to persistent myocardial dysfunction with the picture of cardiomyopathy. Some incessant supraventricular arrhythmias, such as ectopic atrial tachycardia and permanent junctional reciprocating tachycardia can be relatively occult with heart rates of 180–210 per minute, but distinguished from the sinus tachycardia of other dilated cardiomyopathies by abnormal P waves. Again, recognition is key; effective treatment of the cardiomyopathy depends on treatment of the arrhythmia.

Treatment

General acute supportive treatment consists of correction of coexistent electrolyte, calcium, and acid–base abnormalities, providing abundant dextrose intravenously to support potentially jeopardized energy production, judiciously providing fluids to maintain cardiac output although minimizing edema, supporting the myocardial function with intravenous inotropic agents (e.g., dopamine, dobutamine, epinephrine, amrinone) (Table 33-11), and using antiarrhythmic medications as needed. (see Tables 33-18 and 33-19). Additionally, antibiotics, hyperventilation, paralysis, sedation, and vasodilators may be employed. In cases with severe, but presumably self-limited, cardiopulmonary failure refractory to conventional therapy, venoarterial extracorporeal membrane oxygenation (ECMO) has been used with success. Although serious complications continue to exist, ECMO has become a standard treatment for critically ill neonates with self-limited cardiopulmonary failure.

Chronic supportive therapy is aimed at general measures to maximize the strength and longevity of cardiovascular performance, control symptoms of congestive heart failure and control arrhythmias (see Tables 33-10 and 33-19). Optimizing outcome of those more severely effected is often best when done with experience and close monitoring and adjustment. Spironolactone, carefully adjusted doses of angiotensin-converting enzyme (ACE) inhibitors, and judicious use of beta adrenergic receptor blockers (e.g., Carvedilol) can produce significant benefit in hemodynamic function and significantly improve survival. Renal function and potassium levels should be monitored carefully with use of spironolactone and ACE inhibitors, and their dose adjusted for gestational age, postnatal age, and concomitant use. Beta-adrenergic receptor blockers, such as Carvedilol, should be started at very low dose and increased slowly as tolerated using standard regimens. ACE inhibitors and Carvedilol are orally administered, and currently require pharmacy compounding from pills. Digitalization should be carried out with caution and orally if possible in infants with myocarditis, because they may be unduly susceptible to drug-induced arrhythmias. Diuretics can help with symptoms related to pulmonary and systemic edema, but do not appear to influence survival. Cardiac transplantation should be considered if the course appears likely to be fatal despite optimal use of stabilizing measures and treatment of the primary disorder, if there is no irreversible severe dysfunction of other organs, and the underlying primary disease is not likely to recur in the transplanted heart or other organs.

TABLE 33-18
TACHYARRHYTHMIA DIAGNOSIS AND TREATMENT

Type of Arrhythmia	AV Reciprocating Tachycardia	Ectopic Atrial Tachycardia	Atrial Flutter	Atrial Fibrillation	Ventricular Tachycardia
Usual QRS in arrhythmia	Unchanged	Unchanged	Unchanged	Unchanged	Abnormal
Onset and termination	Sudden	Gradual	Sudden	Sudden	Sudden or gradual
Fixed-rate tachycardia	Yes	No	V varies, A fixed	No	yes or no
A:V relationship	1:1	A > V or 1:1	A > V or 1:1	A > V	V > A or 1:1
Mechanism	Reentry	Automaticity	Reentry	Reentry	Reentry or automaticity
May respond to vagal maneuvers	Yes	Rarely	Rarely	No	Rarely
May respond to adenosine	Yes	Rarely	No	No	Rarely
May respond to esophageal pacing	Yes	No	Yes	No	No
May respond to DC countershock	Yes	No	Yes	Yes	Yes, if reentry
Antiarrhythmic agents for acute therapy	Dig, Es, Pro, Proc, Aden	Es, Flec	Dig, Pro, Flec, Sota, Aden	Dig, Pro, Flec, Sota, Aden	Lido, Proc, Es, Bret, Phen
Antiarrhythmic agents for chronic therapy	Dig, Pro, Sota, Flec, Proc, Q, oV, Amio	Pro, Flec, Sota, Amio	Dig, Proc, Q, Flec, Sota, Amio	Dig, Pro, Q, Flec, Sota, Amio	Pro, Proc, Q, Mex, Sota, Amio

A, atrial; V, ventricular; Dig, digoxin; Es, esmolol; Pro, propranolol; Proc, procainamide; Aden, adenosine; Flec, flecainide; Sota, sotalol; Lido, lidocaine; Bret, bretylium; Phen, phenytoin; Q, quinidine; oV, oral verapamil; Mex, mexiletine; Amio, amiodarone.

TABLE 33-19
NEONATAL ANTIARRHYTHMIC DRUGS

Drug (Class)	Currently Commonly Used	Route of Metabolism/ Excretion	Oral Dose	IV Dose	Therapeutic Level	Indications	Contraindications	Toxicity
Adenosine	Yes	Red blood cells and vascular endothelium		0.075–0.10 mg/kg rapid IV push, ↑ to 0.15–0.25 mg/kg after 1 min if not effective		Rx-reentry SVT, DX atrial flutter		Transient AV block, ↓ HR, ↓ BP, and flushing, rare atrial fibrillation
Digoxin	Yes	Renal	Load: 20–30 μg/kg divided in 3 doses, Maintenance: 3–5 μg/kg/12 hours; ↓ w/renal hepatic dysfunction	80% of oral dose	0.8–2.2 ng/mL	SVT, atrial flutter	AV block, VT, many WPW	AV block, ↓ HR, tachyarrhythmias, vomiting, use w/caution w/renal failure, toxicity with hypocalcemia
Quinidine (IA)	Yes	Hepatic	3–15 mg/kg/6 hours; ↓ w/renal or hepatic dysfunction		2–5 μg/mL	SVT, WPW w/ propranolol, PVC, VT	Long QT, known sensitivity, IV use, conduction block, myasthenia gravis	↓ Contractility, ↑ QT, VT, conduction block, vomiting, diarrhea, rash, blood dyscrasias, ↑ HR w/atrial flutter w/o digoxin ↑ digoxin level, need to ↓ digoxin dose by ½
Procainamide (IA)	Yes	Renal, hepatic	2.5–8 mg/kg/4 hours	7 mg/kg over 1 hour Infusion: 20–60 μg/kg/min	Procainamide[a] 4–10 μg/mL	SVT, WPW, PVC, VT	Conduction block, myasthenia gravis	Similar to quinidine, ↓ BP, lupus-like reaction, no effect on digoxin level
Disopyramide (IA)	No	Hepatic, renal	3.5–7.5 mg/kg/6 hours		2–5 μg/mL	SVT, WPW, PVC, VT	Conduction block myasthenia gravis	Similar to quinidine, ↓ contractility, anticholinergic, hypoglycemia, no effect on digoxin level
Lidocaine (IB)	Yes	Hepatic		Bolus: 1 mg/kg/ 5–10 min Infusion: 20–50 μg/kg/min; ↓ w/ cyanosis, hepatic dysfunction	2–5 μg/mL	PVC, VT	Conduction block ↓ junctional and ventricular escape rate	CNS reactions, seizure, ↓ BP, ↓ respiratory drive
Phenytoin (IB)	No	Renal, hepatic	2–3 mg/kg/12 hours; ↓ w/hepatic dysfunction	Load: 10 mg/kg over 30–60 min Maintenance: same as oral	10–20 μg/mL	PVC, VT, digitalis intoxication	Not FDA approved for VT	CNS reactions, ↓ BP, blood dyscrasias, hepatic dysfunction, hypertrichosis, gingival hyperplasia, coarse facies, rash
Flecainide (IC)	No	Renal, hepatic	0.3–2 mg/kg/8 hours; ↓ w/renal, hepatic dysfunction		0.2–1.0 μg/mL	Refractory life-threatening SVT, PJRT, PVC, VT	Conduction block, hepatic dysfunction, myocardial dysfunction	Occasional ↑ SVT frequency w/WPW, ↑ pacing threshold and conduction block, VT, nausea, ↓ contractility
Esmolol (II)	Yes	RBC esterases	IV only	Load: 0.5 mg/kg over 1 min Infusion: 50–100 μg/kg/min		Recurrent, sustained SVT, WPW, VT	As per propranolol	As per propranolol
Propranolol (II)	Yes	Hepatic	0.3–1.0 mg/kg/6 hours; ↓ w/chronic cyanosis, renal, hepatic dysfunction	0.02–0.10 mg/kg over 20 min.		SVT, WPW, PVC, VT, hypertrophic cardiomyopathy, long QT	Use w/verapamil, bronchospasm, conduction block, CHF	↓ HR, conduction block, bronchospasm, ↓ BP, hypoglycemia, depression, ↓ cardiac reflexes w/anesthesia

Drug	Elimination	Dialyzable	Dose	IV Load/Infusion	Therapeutic Level	Indications	Contraindications/Cautions	Side Effects/Comments
Sotalol (II/III)	Renal	No	25–70 mg/m² BSA/8 hours			SVT, WPW & VT with structurally normal heart	Use with verapamil, bronchospasm, conduction block, ? structural heart disease	As per propranolol plus ventricular arrhythmias
Amiodarone (III)	Hepatic	No	5 mg/kg/12 hours for 1 week; then 5 mg/kg/day; ↓ w/hepatic dysfunction	Load: 5 mg/kg over 15–30 min; Infusion: 10–20 µg/kg/min	1–2 mg/L	Refractory, life-threatening, SVT, VT, recurrent VF	Conduction block	Extremely long half-life, corneal deposits, thyroid and hepatic dysfunction, pulmonary fibrosis, may ↑ conduction block and digoxin and quinidine levels, need to ↓ digoxin by ½, hypotension w/IV
Bretylium (III)	Renal	No		Load: 5 mg/kg over 15 min; Infusion: 20–50 µg/kg/min.		Refractory VT, VF		Transient ↑ BP, arrhythmia, then ↓ BP
Verapamil (IV)	Hepatic	No	2–4 mg/kg/8 hours; ↓ w/hepatic, renal dysfunction, neuromuscular disease			Refractory SVT, hypertrophic cardiomyopathy some PVC, VT	IV use, conduction dysfunction, CHF, many WPW, propranolol muscular dystrophy, use w/quinidine, generally avoid in infants	↓ BP, ↓ HR, conduction block, myocardial depression, constipation, may ↑ digoxin level, need to ↓ digoxin dose ⅓ to ½

[a]To differentiate from metabolite measure by some laboratories.
Note: Continuous ECG monitoring should be done during initiation of antiarrhythmic therapy and with IV administration because of potential proarrhythmia and conduction block.
AV arteriovenous; BP, blood pressure; BSA, body surface area; CHF congestive heart failure; CNS, central nervous system; DX, diagnose; FDA, Federal Drug Administration; HR, heart rate; PJRT, permanent junctional reciprocating tachycardia; PVC, premature ventricular contractions; RX, treatment; SVT, supraventricular tachycardia; VF, ventricular fibrillation; VT, ventricular tachycardia; w/, with; WPW, Wolff–Parkinson–White syndrome.

Hypertrophic Cardiomyopathies

Hypertrophic cardiomyopathy is a disorder characterized by inappropriate thickening of the ventricular walls, with normal, hyperdynamic or diminished systolic performance and normal or diminished ventricular chamber size. There are many causes (see Table 33-17). Most commonly, transient cardiomyopathy occurs as secondary disorder in infants of diabetic mother, or with in utero sympathomimetic exposure. Permanent myocardial diseases that more commonly present in older children and adults, such as isolated hypertrophic cardiomyopathy associated with contractile gene mutations, also present in infancy. Hypertrophic cardiomyopathy may occur in infants in association with genetic syndromes (e.g., Noonan syndrome) and infiltrative storage diseases (e.g., Pompe and other glycogen storage diseases, mucopolysaccharidosis). Primary metabolic disorders of energy production (disorders of fatty acid oxidation, nuclear and mitochondrial genome abnormalities in oxidative phosphorylation) cause isolated hypertrophic or dilated cardiomyopathy, or multi-system dysfunction with cardiac and skeletal myopathy and encephalopathy (33,34).

Pathophysiology

Although resulting from diverse etiologies, most hypertrophic cardiomyopathies share certain clinical features and pathophysiology. Specific endocrine, genetic, mitochondrial or metabolite abnormalities elicit a sequence of molecular and cellular changes with myocardial sarcomeric production and often dysfunction, resulting in myocyte thickening, often with interstitial fibrosis, leading to ventricular wall thickening and impaired diastolic compliance. The ventricle walls often become so thick regarding severely narrow ventricular outflow, particularly dynamic with systolic ventricular wall thickening and result in the physiology of aortic stenosis. Sometimes severe thickening of the ventricular walls significantly encroaches and limits ventricular chamber size. Impaired diastolic compliance results in generalized edema and in pulmonary venous engorgement. Metabolic "storage" disorders, such as glycogen storage disease, have ventricular wall thickening from infiltration of the myocardium with accumulated metabolic products, not from deranged myocyte hypertrophy, but present with clinical features of metabolic disease with hypertrophic cardiomyopathy.

Clinical Findings

There may be a history of maternal diabetes, exposure to sympathomimetic or steroid medications, or family history of hypertrophic cardiomyopathy or metabolic disease. A prominent systolic murmur from ventricular outflow stenosis and/or mitral regurgitation are usually present. Signs of right and left heart congestive failure, including diminished activity, hepatomegaly, tachypnea, retractions, and S3, are often present. Signs of low cardiac stroke volume, including tachycardia, narrowed pulse pressure, diffusely diminished pulses, and hypotension may be present. Associated primary conditions may cause dysmorphic features, hypoto-

nia, encephalopathy, and organomegaly seemingly out of proportion to the hemodynamic derangement.

Chest radiograph, in contrast to that seen at older age, often shows cardiomegaly and pulmonary edema.

ECG usually has diffusely increased QRS voltage amplitude and repolarization changes. Additionally, ECG in Pompe's disease characteristically shows a short PR interval.

Echocardiographic examination demonstrates ventricular wall thickening, often extraordinarily severe, variable left and sometimes right ventricular sub-valvar outflow stenosis, and mitral and tricuspid regurgitation. Fixed anatomic sub-aortic stenosis and other structural anomalies that can result in secondary ventricular hypertrophy should be detected.

If there is no family history of known hypertrophic cardiomyopathy and initial laboratory studies screening for metabolic disease are unremarkable, first-degree relatives should be screened with electrocardiography and echocardiography for asymptomatic hypertrophic cardiomyopathy. If physical examination or laboratory studies suggest metabolic disorder, or if echocardiographic evaluation of first degree relatives is negative or unobtainable, then additional laboratory evaluation for metabolic disorder may be helpful (33).

Specific Hypertrophic Cardiomyopathies

Infants of diabetic mothers develop a hypertrophic cardiomyopathy that is generally self-limited, although sometimes is a severe disorder. It results from the myocardial trophic response to fetal hyperinsulinemia provoked by trans-placental passage of high maternal glucose loads. Clinical findings include a systolic ejection murmur, sometimes mild increase in respiratory rate and work and, rarely, evidence of frank congestive heart failure. There is an increased risk of structural heart disease in infants of diabetic mothers.

Echocardiographic examination reveals left ventricular hypertrophy that is sometimes severe, usually with involvement of the septum, and occasionally with outflow obstruction (Fig. 33-45). Treatment is supportive. Inotropes may worsen outflow obstruction and are contraindicated if the obstruction is severe.

The most common permanent hypertrophic cardiomyopathies are genetic disorders in one of the cardiac contractile proteins, most often myosin heavy chain. In 50% of cases it is inherited as an autosomal condition with variable penetrance, and in the others it occurs as a new mutation. This isolated cardiac disorder is characterized by myocyte hypertrophy and disarray, propensity for development of left ventricular outflow or intracavitary systolic pressure gradients, symptoms of congestive heart failure caused by poor diastolic chamber compliance, ventricular arrhythmias, and sudden death. There can be significant progression with time, and a normal echocardiogram at birth does not exclude the possibility for phenotypic expression later in life. Because it can be sub-clinical and cause sudden death in older children and adults, echocar-

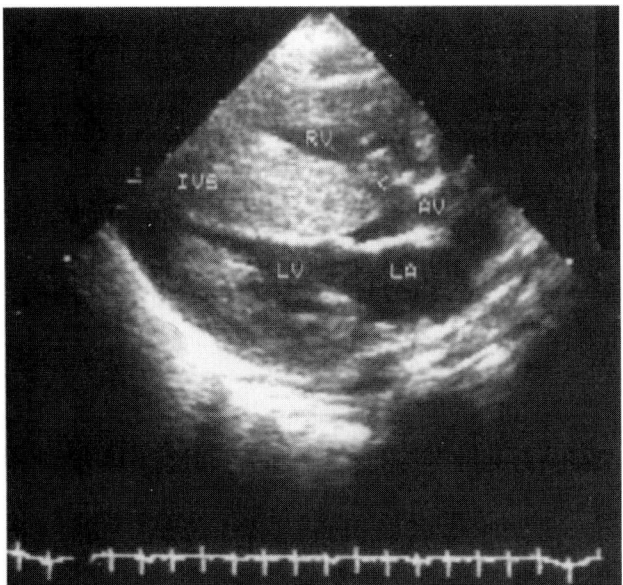

Figure 33-45 Echocardiographic parasternal long-axis view of a diabetic mother's infant with severe hypertrophic cardiomyopathy and subaortic ventricular septal defect. <, ventricular septal defect; AV, aortic valve, IVS, interventricular septum; LA, left atrium; LV, left ventricle; RV, right ventricle.

diograms and electrocardiograms should be obtained in all first-degree relatives and symptomatic relatives. Those presenting at birth appear to have the poorest prognosis. Inotropic agents and diuretics are potentially harmful and generally not used. Calcium channel blockers decrease the systolic pressure gradient, improve diastolic compliance, and may improve survival in adults. Because of hazards associated with calcium channel blockers in infants, their use in infants less than 1 year of age remains investigational. β adrenergic receptor blockers can improve symptoms, but do not appear to affect the progression of hypertrophy or survival. Ventricular septal myomectomy may improve symptoms in those refractory to medical treatment. Holter monitoring for ventricular arrhythmias should be routinely performed, and amiodarone considered in those with ventricular tachycardia. Cardiac transplantation may be required for survival in severely affected, refractory patients.

Metabolic disorders of cellular energy production involving pyruvate metabolism, fatty acid oxidation, and oxidative phosphorylation, and metabolic "storage" disorders, such as glycogen storage disease, may present in early infancy with clinical findings of isolated hypertrophic cardiomyopathy. However, these disorders are particularly likely to be present when there is one or more associated findings such as hypotonia, encephalopathy, cataracts, liver enlargement or dysfunction disproportionate to the hemodynamics, hypoglycemia, metabolic acidosis, elevated ketones, lactate or pyruvate. Treatment options depend on the enzyme affected.

Neonatal Tricuspid Valve Regurgitation

Regurgitation of an anatomically normal tricuspid valve is a common finding in neonates. The regurgitation may be an isolated finding and mild, and cause only a temporary soft regurgitant murmur at the left lower sternal border. Greater degrees of regurgitation of an anatomically normal tricuspid valve often develop with right ventricular myocardial disease, such as cardiomyopathy from asphyxia, and with right ventricular systolic hypertension, as with persistent pulmonary hypertension or pulmonary parenchymal disease. If there is right ventricular diastolic dysfunction, there may be right-to-left shunting through a patent foramen ovale. The explanation for a lower sternal murmur can be documented by echocardiography and managed with observation, because tricuspid regurgitation of this type tends to regress as the underlying right ventricular hypertension or dysfunction resolves (see Fig. 33-15).

Chronic Pulmonary Hypertension and Cor Pulmonale

Cor pulmonale is pulmonary hypertension secondary to ventilatory or pulmonary disease, with right ventricular hypertrophy; it frequently presents as symptoms of congestive heart failure with pulmonary disease. Patients with cor pulmonale have a structurally normal heart, and must be differentiated from those with pulmonary hypertension from intracardiac shunts or pulmonary venous obstruction. The most frequent cause of cor pulmonale in infants has been bronchopulmonary dysplasia, although its incidence has drastically declined in recent years and there are a large number of other causes, including airway obstruction, central hypoventilation, pulmonary hypoplasia, and diaphragmatic abnormalities.

Pathophysiology

Pulmonary artery pressure is controlled by vascular resistance, which is a function of the number of small pulmonary arteries and the average luminal size. The number of vessels may be diminished by congenital pulmonary hypoplasia or acquired parenchymal damage. Additionally, abundant pulmonary artery musculature sufficient to prevent more than minimal pulmonary flow before birth, is present at birth, and can persist and re-constrict in response to certain circumstances, further aggravating pulmonary hypertension. Factors resulting in persisting postnatal pulmonary hypertension include alveolar hypoxia, acidemia, increased pulmonary venous pressure, polycythemia and bacteremia. When pulmonary resistance is fixed, increases in cardiac output with infection or anemia also elevate pulmonary artery pressure. Pulmonary hypertension induces right ventricular hypertrophy and, if severe, causes right ventricular diastolic dysfunction and dilation. In addition to pulmonary hypertension, bronchopulmonary dysplasia also is frequently associated with systemic hypertension and left ventricular hypertrophy. Shifting of the ventricular septal position, elevated ventricular pressure and biventricular hypertrophy, impair biventricular diastolic compliance and increase sensitivity to intravascular volume.

The pulmonary hypertension and cardiac sequelae seen with chronic lung disease generally resolve when the pulmonary parenchymal disease resolves. In contrast, permanent pulmonary vascular change (i.e., Eisenmenger syndrome) occurs in patients with congenital heart disease after 1 year or more of exposure to a large left-to-right shunt with pulmonary artery hypertension.

Clinical Findings

Variable hepatomegaly and systemic venous congestion secondary to right atrial hypertension are predominant findings. Elevated left atrial pressure, especially in the presence of pulmonary parenchymal disease, may predispose to pulmonary symptoms and rales. The right ventricular impulse may be increased and the second heart sound loud and appear single. There may be a relatively soft murmur from tricuspid regurgitation, but a prominent murmur is not common and suggests possible congenital heart disease. Cyanosis (See Color Plate) may result from alveolar dysfunction with intrapulmonary shunting and from right-to-left shunting across a patent foramen ovale. Infants with bronchopulmonary dysplasia appear to be at increased risk for sudden death (10), similar to older patients with primary pulmonary hypertension. The degree of pulmonary artery hypertension and cardiac symptomatology may vary with labile ventilatory or pulmonary conditions. Several echocardiographic methods, some fairly accurate, some not so accurate, and most applicable to particular circumstances, can be used to assess the right ventricular pressure (see Fig. 33-14). Sedation, sometimes necessary for technically acceptable studies in older, active babies, may depress ventilation and should be used with caution.

Differential Diagnosis

In patients with pulmonary hypertension, even those with lung disease, the presence of congenital heart disease should be sought. The absence of a loud murmur does not exclude a septal defect or patent ductus arteriosus in the presence of elevated pulmonary vascular resistance. Because many of the symptoms of cor pulmonale overlap those of congenital heart disease, echocardiographic examination has been useful for excluding occult cardiovascular lesions that could lead to irreversible Eisenmenger syndrome. However, with lung disease ultrasound windows are often poor. These limitations should be realized, and the results correlated with other findings.

Treatment

The treatment of pulmonary hypertension secondary to pulmonary or ventilatory disease is directed primarily at the underlying disorder. Bronchodilators and diuretics may lessen exacerbating abnormalities in alveolar gas exchange and symptoms. Oxygen may be useful not only to prevent cyanosis and exacerbations of pulmonary hypertension, but also as a pulmonary vasodilator. Digitalis has not been found to be beneficial in most infants with congestive symptoms. With resolution of the underlying ventilatory disease, the pulmonary hypertension also resolves.

Cardiac Tumors

Intracardiac tumors in neonates are rare. Rhabdomyoma accounts for most. Fibromas occur much less frequently, and other types occur rarely. Most babies with cardiac rhabdomyoma have tuberous sclerosis (see Table 33-3), and vice versa (94). The presence of one should prompt an investigation for the other. Cardiac rhabdomyoma may be the only manifestation of tuberous sclerosis in neonates. Neonatal cardiac rhabdomyoma are generally multiple and usually regress, often completely. Cardiac tumors 2 mm or more in diameter are readily demonstrated by echocardiography, even in the fetus. Many babies are asymptomatic, even when the tumors are large and multiple, although peri-valvar masses can obstruct valve flow and development. Serious arrhythmias also sometimes occur.

ARRHYTHMIAS

All forms of cardiac arrhythmias can occur in the fetus or newborn. Those most commonly encountered include sinus tachycardia and bradycardia, premature atrial depolarizations, supraventricular tachycardia; and less commonly, atrial flutter, ventricular arrhythmias, and complete heart block. Many arrhythmias are benign, occurring in otherwise normal hearts, and are of no hemodynamic consequence. Others may result in significant acute cardiovascular compromise, particularly if they are very rapid or there is coexistent structural or functional heart disease. Sustained tacharrhythmia can lead to reversible dilated cardiomyopathy (95). Thus, in evaluating patients with arrhythmias it is important to assess the hemodynamic status and cardiac structure and function. Rarely, arrhythmias are the presenting sign of underlying cardiac abnormality such as cardiomyopathy, Ebstein anomaly, or l-transposition of the great arteries. Arrhythmias may also result from noncardiac disease; in neonates, ventricular tachycardia, ventricular fibrillation, sinus arrest, and extreme bradycardia usually occur in association with preceding severe hypoxemia, hypotension, acidosis, electrolyte disturbance, or drug toxicity (e.g., digitalis).

Benign Arrhythmias

Sinus Bradycardia

Many infants have transient bradycardia associated with specific activities such as crying, straining or micturition. Some healthy infants persistently have a heart rate near 80 beats per minute. Sustained bradycardia at less than 70 beats per minute in neonates is abnormal. Noncardiac causes, such as gastroesophageal reflux leading to vagal stimulation, are common. Bradycardia can also be produced by stimulation of the vagus nerve during procedures such as endotracheal, nasogastric and orogastric intubation. Less commonly electrolyte abnormalities, hypothyroidism and exposure to medications (e.g., prenatal beta-adrenergic blockers) are the cause. Isolated persistent sinus bradycardia should prompt careful inspection of an ECG for nonconducted P waves as can occur with nonconducted atrial premature depolarizations, second-degree atrioventricular conduction block, and congenital long QT syndrome (96).

SINUS ARRHYTHMIA

Sinus arrhythmia is the most common cause of an irregular heart rate and rhythm, that is more prominent at slower heart rates, such as in older infants. It represents normal physiologic variability in the sinus rate, in phase with respiration and other variables. The P wave morphology and axis do not change. Once recognized, no further evaluation or treatment is necessary.

Sinus Tachycardia

Sinus tachycardia occurs with serious illness, fever, hypovolemia, anemia, anxiety or pain and sympathomimetic medications (e.g., dopamine, dobutamine, isoproterenol, epinephrine, caffeine, theophylline, and aminophylline), at heart rates up to 230 beats per minute in infants. With a sinus tachycardia, there is more rate variability than seen in many tachyarrhythmias and normal P waves precede the QRS complex, often "merged" into the preceding T wave at heart rates greater than 180 beats per minute (P waves positive in leads I, II, and aVF; negative in lead aVR). Pathologic supraventricular tachyarrhythmias can be differentiated from sinus tachycardia by usually faster rates, abnormal P wave axis or PR interval, and (when present) by an abrupt onset and termination or wide QRS complexes.

Atrial Premature Depolarizations

Premature depolarizations can originate from any conducting tissue. Atrial premature depolarizations occur in up to 30% of newborns (97). The diagnosis is reliably assigned when there is an identifiable, early, nonsinus P wave. However, the P wave may be hidden within the preceding T wave. Atrial premature depolarizations may be conducted to the ventricles normally, or with a bundle branch block pattern resulting in a wide QRS complex (if a bundle branch is refractory from the preceding beat), or may be "blocked" and not conducted to the ventricles (when very early and occurring when the AV node or proximal His bundle is refractory). When frequent, blocked atrial premature depolarizations result in ventricular bradycardia as a result of resetting of the sinus node with each premature atrial depolarization. In neonates with central venous catheters, frequent atrial premature depolarizations may be as a result of contact of the catheter with an atrial wall, and constitute an indication to withdraw the catheter from the atrium. Atrial premature depolarizations might also be secondary to electrolyte abnormalities or drugs (e.g., dopamine, dobutamine, isoproterenol, epinephrine, caffeine, theophylline, and aminophylline). Very rarely are atrial pre-

mature depolarizations secondary to myocarditis or cardiac tumors.

In hemodynamically stable otherwise healthy infants, premature atrial depolarizations generally do not warrant further evaluation. Isolated ectopic atrial depolarizations and atrial bigeminy are only rarely associated with tachycardia, and usually are of no serious consequence. In most infants, these arrhythmias resolve over a few months.

Ventricular Premature Depolarizations

Premature ventricular depolarizations are early QRS complexes with a morphology different from sinus beats and without an identifiable preceding P wave. In newborns, ventricular premature depolarizations may not be much wider than normal QRS complexes. Premature ventricular complexes occur in less than 1% of healthy newborns (98). Although premature ventricular depolarizations are usually benign, their identification should prompt evaluation for possible structural or functional heart disease, electrolyte abnormalities (e.g., hypokalemia, hyperkalemia, and hypocalcemia), hypoglycemia, hypoxia, or the congenital long-QT syndrome. Premature ventricular complexes may also be related to administration of drugs (e.g., dopamine, dobutamine, epinephrine, caffeine, aminophylline, theophylline, digoxin, or other antiarrhythmic medications). In the absence of these problems, they often resolve over a number of months. There are no data to suggest that the daily number or morphology of these complexes influences the prognosis.

ACCELERATED VENTRICULAR RHYTHM

An accelerated ventricular rhythm is a less common arrhythmia. There is a wide QRS rhythm, generally at a rate not more than 10% greater than the underlying sinus rate. This probably represents enhanced automaticity of a ventricular focus. There may be mild accelerations and decelerations of the rate. Atrioventricular dissociation is usually seen. The duration of episodes is variable. Although this arrhythmia generally occurs in otherwise healthy infants, it has been associated with structural heart disease, electrolyte abnormalities, cardiac tumors, intracardiac catheters, maternal heroine and cocaine use, and respiratory distress. Patients are usually asymptomatic and do not need treatment. This arrhythmia generally resolves within months (99).

Tachyarrhythmias

Heart rate alone is not always enough to establish the diagnosis of a pathologic tachycardia. Infants can have a sinus tachycardia with rates up to at least 230 beats/min in response to serious illnesses, fever, hypovolemia, anemia, pain or infusion of inotropic/chronotropic agents. Additionally, some unusual pathologic supraventricular tachycardias can have rates less than 180 beats/min. In assessing a child with a fast heart rate, one should determine if the

QRS complex is narrow or wide during tachycardia, if the rate is fixed or variable, if there is a visible P wave and if so, the P wave axis. Supraventricular tachycardias typically have a narrow (normal) QRS complex. In general, if the QRS complex in tachycardia remains wide, the rhythm should be considered ventricular tachycardia. However, it is not uncommon for the first few beats of SVT to be wide because of aberrant conduction (right or left bundle branch block) before changing to a narrow QRS complex.

A patient with an apparently fixed high heart rate should be carefully assessed. The fixed heart rate could represent a sinus tachycardia secondary to a high-catecholamine state in an otherwise sick infant. An electrocardiogram should be obtained, and the P wave morphology clearly established. If there is no clear P wave, or the P wave does not have a sinus morphology (positive in leads I, II, and aVF; negative in lead aVR) one should strongly consider a pathologic tachycardia or structural heart disease with heterotaxy (see Table 33-17).

All neonates with documented tachyarrhythmias should have a complete cardiac evaluation, including 12-lead ECG (during the tachycardia if hemodynamically stable, and later in sinus rhythm), and echocardiography, to assess cardiac structure and function. It is estimated that between 8% and 25% of infants with SVT have structural heart disease, most often Ebstein malformation of the tricuspid valve, corrected transposition of the great arteries, or hypertrophic cardiomyopathy (100). Cardiac tumors and myocarditis rarely are predisposing causes for ventricular arrhythmias.

The clinical status of infants with tachyarrhythmias depends on the ventricular rate, duration of tachycardia, presence of underlying structural or functional heart disease, and other clinical problems. Patients may be completely asymptomatic, with the arrhythmia noted during an otherwise routine evaluation or although monitored for other reasons. The infant may not have been appearing well, with irritability, poor feeding, restlessness, or respiratory difficulty with tachypnea, retractions and wheezing. With persistent tachyarrhythmia, the child may develop signs and symptoms of congestive heart failure or acidosis, becoming pale and listless. If the tachycardia persists for long enough, heart failure and a secondary dilated car-diomyopathy may develop. In the fetus with persistent or recurrent tachycardia, this is manifest as nonimmune hydrops. Whether a tachycardia related cardiomyopathy develops depends on the ventricular rate, whether the tachyarrhythmia is intermittent or incessant, the frequency of recurrences if intermittent, and the presence of structural heart disease.

Supraventricular Tachycardias

Atrioventricular Reciprocating Tachycardia and Wolff–Parkinson–White Syndrome

The most common type of fetal and neonatal supraventricular tachycardia is atrioventricular reciprocating tachycardia with a reentry circuit via an accessory atrioventricular conduction pathway (101). Most often these accessory conduction pathways persist as isolated anomalies, but they can occur in association with cardiac structural anomalies such as Ebstein anomaly. Accessory atrioventricular conduction pathways resulting in WPW syndrome are rarely inherited as an autosomal dominant trait, sometimes associated with hypertrophic cardiomyopathy (102).

During supraventricular tachycardia there is antegrade conduction from the atria to the ventricles over the AV node and His–Purkinje system, with retrograde conduction over the accessory pathway from the ventricles to the atria. Because antegrade conduction is normal over the AV node and His–Purkinje system, there usually is a normal (narrow) QRS complex during tachycardia. Commonly the accessory atrioventricular conduction pathway conducts only retrograde. Therefore, during sinus rhythm all antegrade conduction is through only the AV node, and the electrocardiogram appears normal.

Atrioventricular reciprocating tachycardia is characterized by the abrupt onset and termination of a fairly fixed heart rate of 230 to 300 beats/min, abnormal or unidentifiable P waves that may be superimposed on the T waves, and usually a normal QRS morphology (see Fig. 33-46 and Table 33-18). The infant may be asymptomatic initially, but then becomes irritable and fussy and refuses feeding, congestive heart failure develops in approximately 20% after 36 hours and in 50% after 48 hours.

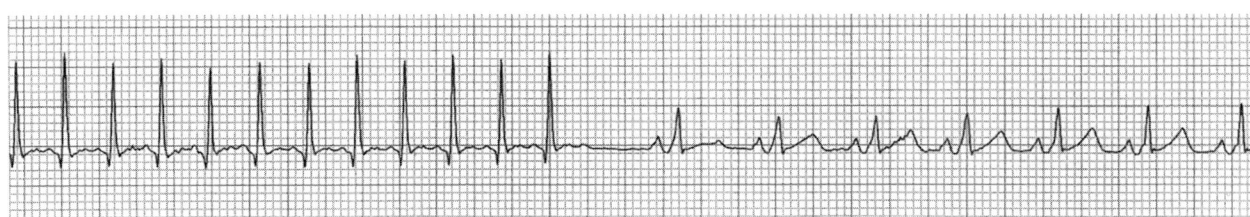

Figure 33-46 Electrocardiogram during conversion of supraventricular tachycardia to sinus rhythm with administration of adenosine. During tachycardia at a rate of 230 beats/min, there is a normal-appearing QRS complex without a delta wave (no ventricular preexcitation), and there is no distinct P wave. After conversion to sinus rhythm, there is a short PR interval (80 milliseconds) and wide up-sloping QRS complex (90 milliseconds) representing ventricular preexcitation, indicative of the Wolff–Parkinson–White syndrome.

Some accessory pathways can conduct impulses in both directions, resulting in the Wolff-Parkinson-White (WPW) syndrome. During sinus rhythm, antegrade atrial-to-ventricular conduction over the accessory pathway results in a short PR interval and wide QRS complex with characteristic delta wave, resulting from rapid "ectopic" depolarization of the ventricles, without the delay in conduction that occurs in the A-V node. Depending on the location of the accessory pathway, and the ECG lead examined, a delta wave may be of variable size and direction. Because antegrade conduction during supraventricular tachycardia is usually through the AV node and His–Purkinje system, the diagnosis of WPW syndrome cannot usually be made during tachycardia. Rarely, an atrioventricular reciprocating tachycardia occurs in patients with WPW syndrome with antegrade conduction over the accessory pathway, and retrograde conduction through the A-V node, resulting in a wide QRS tachycardia, which may be electrocardiographically indistinguishable from ventricular tachycardia. Some patients with WPW syndrome have the potential for very rapid antegrade conduction over their accessory pathway; if those individuals develop a primary atrial tachycardia such as atrial fibrillation, it can lead to ventricular fibrillation (103). Fortunately, atrial fibrillation is rare in children. Patients with WPW syndrome should generally not be treated with digoxin or verapamil, as these medications sometimes enhance antegrade accessory pathway conduction.

Persistent Junctional Reciprocating Tachycardia

One important, but unusual form of accessory pathway has slow retrograde conduction, resulting in a supraventricular tachycardia referred to as persistent junctional reciprocating tachycardia. These tachycardias are usually slower than other supraventricular tachycardias, often less than 200 beats/min in newborns. This often causes an incessant or frequently recurring tachycardia that can result in a reversible dilated cardiomyopathy. Initially this arrhythmia is often well tolerated because of the slower heart rate. It can be recognized by having a fixed rapid heart rate in which there is an abnormal (nonsinus) P-wave axis (usually negative in leads II and aVF, and positive in aVR and aVL). There may be a normal appearing PR interval as a result of slow retrograde conduction, but the abnormal P-wave axis differentiates it from sinus tachycardia. This type of supraventricular tachycardia might terminate with vagal maneuvers, adenosine, atrial pacing or cardioversion, but frequently the arrhythmia rapidly recurs.

Ectopic Atrial Tachycardia

Another potential cause of a dilated cardiomyopathy is an ectopic atrial tachycardia (104). This type of supraventricular tachycardia results from enhanced automaticity of a single cell or small cluster of cells in either atrium. Generally, the P-wave morphology is not normal in at least one lead.

The arrhythmia mechanism does not involve the ventricles. Depending on the atrial rate and possible AV block, there may be a variable A:V relationship (with more atrial than ventricular complexes). This type of SVT is characterized by a variable rate and gradual onset and termination (see Table 33-17). Transiently blocking A-V conduction, with vagal maneuvers or adenosine administration, will not terminate the atrial tachycardia but will demonstrate the diagnosis by the presence of unabated rapid P waves. Ectopic atrial tachycardia also does not terminate with pacing maneuvers or cardioversion, but often improves with beta-adrenergic receptor blockers.

JUNCTIONAL ECTOPIC TACHYCARDIA

Junctional ectopic tachycardia is a rare, often incessant, tachyarrhythmia due do to enhanced automaticity in the A-V node or bundle of His. There is generally a normal (narrow) QRS morphology with variable ventricular rates. If there are visible P-waves, the ventricular rate is greater than the atrial rate and it does not respond to pacing maneuvers or cardioversion, and is often difficult to control with milder antiarrhythmic medications.

Isolated junctional ectopic tachycardia is often familial. Some patients eventually develop complete heart block (105).

Most often junctional ectopic tachycardia is seen early, and temporarily following cardiac surgery in infants, and can result in significant hemodynamic compromise until it is controlled and abates. Intravenous amiodarone may be the best treatment; but cooling the patient down to 33 to 35 C with administration of intravenous procainamide is often helpful.

Atrial Flutter and Fibrillation

Atrial flutter is less common than other types of paroxysmal supraventricular tachycardia in fetuses and neonates. It may be idiopathic, or associated with the same congenital heart lesions as those producing other supraventricular tachycardias. The atrial rate may be 200 to 500 beats/min. The AV node is generally not part of the tachycardia circuit, so that there need not be a 1:1 atrial:ventricular rate relationship. There is often some degree of AV node block resulting in variable conduction, frequently with a 2:1 or 3:1 atrial:ventricular relationship. With a 2:1 block, the ventricular rate at the highest atrial rate would be 250 beats/min, a rate sufficient to produce congestive failure in infancy. The RR interval is constant except when the atrioventricular block changes. The rare infant without AV nodal conduction block may have a very rapid rate and shock. With higher degrees of AV nodal conduction block, a sawtoothed atrial pattern is characteristically seen, often best in leads II or V1. In some patients the diagnosis can not be ascertained from the surface electrocardiogram, especially if there is a 1:1 atrial:ventricular rate relationship. Esophageal recordings may demonstrate the atrial

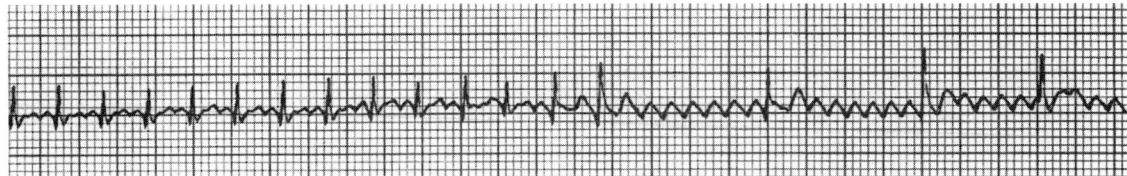

Figure 33-47   Electrocardiogram showing the effect of adenosine on atrial flutter. Before adenosine, there is atrial flutter with 2:1 A–V conduction. The flutter waves are difficult to discern. After adenosine, there is transient slowing of AV node conduction without termination of the atrial flutter. This allows the flutter waves to be readily identified, confirming the diagnosis. The atrial rate during atrial flutter is 500 beats/minute.

activity more clearly, or adenosine might be used to cause transient AV block and demonstrate the flutter waves. Adenosine, although diagnostically helpful, does not convert atrial flutter (Fig. 33-47). Digoxin can be used to slow the ventricular rate, but is unlikely to convert the atrial flutter. Overdrive atrial pacing from the esophagus and, if necessary, cardioversion by DC countershock (initial dose 0.5 to 1 Joule/Kg) can be used to convert the rhythm to sinus. In the absence of structural heart disease, there is generally a benign course once the arrhythmia is converted to sinus rhythm, and subsequent chronic antiarrhythmic therapy is often not necessary (106).

Atrial fibrillation is recognized by an irregularly irregular ventricular rhythm. It is rare in newborns and usually seen in patients with structural heart disease. Digoxin can be used to slow the ventricular rate. Cardioversion by DC countershock (initial dose 0.5 to 1 J/Kg) is usually necessary to convert a sustained episode.

Treatments for Supraventricular Tachycardias

Treatment depends in part on the mechanism of tachycardia (see Tables 33-18 and 33-19) (100). In arrhythmias involving the AV node, such as atrioventricular reciprocating tachycardias without or with the WPW syndrome, transiently slowing or blocking AV node conduction can terminate the tachycardia. Vagal maneuvers are often effective in terminating these types of supraventricular tachycardia. These include the application of ice or very cold damp cloth to the face and rectal stimulation. Ocular compression should not be used as a result of risks to the child's vision.

Rapid bolus of intravenous adenosine (0.1 mg/kg, increased to 0.2 mg/kg if needed) is the treatment of choice for most infants with supraventricular arrhythmias involving the AV node that are refractory to vagal maneuvers. Adenosine is an endogenous nucleoside with a very short half-life that can transiently block AV node conduction, interrupting these arrhythmias, resulting in abrupt conversion to sinus rhythm. It is helpful to record the patient's electrocardiogram during attempts at conversion so that one can see if there was an effect of the intervention on the arrhythmia. There also might be transient evidence of WPW syndrome as the AV node conduction is briefly blocked, in the form of a delta wave from antegrade conduction down an accessory conduction pathway. If there

was transient termination with rapid resumption of the arrhythmia, a longer-acting agent might be necessary to control the arrhythmia. Significant side effects appear to be rare, but include initiation of atrial fibrillation. Rarely, in patients with WPW syndrome, this can cause a ventricular tachycardia or fibrillation. It is therefore recommended that a defibrillator be readily available when administering adenosine. Methylxanthines (e.g., theophylline and caffeine) are competitive antagonists to adenosine, and might make dosing more difficult.

Other antiarrhythmic agents can be used to terminate and control supraventricular tachycardias in infants, in which vagal maneuvers or adenosine have resulted in only a transient termination of the arrhythmia, or for supraventricular tachycardias that do not involve the AV node (i.e., ectopic atrial tachycardia). These might include β blockers (i.e., esmolol or propranolol), class I antiarrhythmic agents (i.e., procainamide or flecainide), digoxin, or class III antiarrhythmic agents (i.e., sotalol or amiodarone). For ectopic atrial tachycardias, a β-blocker is often effective, and intravenous infusion of esmolol is a good first-line therapy until the arrhythmia is controlled. However, class I or class III antiarrhythmic medications may be necessary to adequately suppress ectopic atrial or junctional tachycardias. Intravenous verapamil has been associated with cardiovascular collapse and death in neonates and infants and should not be used in patients under 1 year of age (107).

If available, atrial pacing using an esophageal pacing catheter can be effective in terminating AV reciprocating tachycardias and atrial flutter. Atrial pacing will not terminate ectopic atrial tachycardias or junctional ectopic tachycardias, but the atrial catheter can be helpful in confirming the mechanism of the tachycardia.

If the patient is hemodynamically unstable, DC countershock (starting with 0.5–1.0 Joules/kg) should be attempted for known or suspected reentry-type supraventricular tachycardias, including AV reciprocating tachycardia, atrial flutter, and atrial fibrillation.

Prophylactic antiarrhythmic therapy is prescribed for most infants with supraventricular tachycardia, as there is approximately a 20% recurrence risk of atrioventricular reciprocating tachycardias. Often the recurrence risk diminishes after the first 6 to 12 months, and the medication may be discontinued (108).

Digoxin may be used in patients with atrioventricular reciprocating tachycardia without evident WPW syndrome. The use of digoxin in patients with manifest WPW syndrome is controversial. There is evidence that digoxin can sometimes enhance antegrade accessory pathway conduction, potentially allowing very rapid conduction over the accessory pathway if the patient develops atrial fibrillation, possibly causing a hemodynamically unstable ventricular tachycardia or ventricular fibrillation.

β adrenergic blockers such as propranolol or atenolol are often used in patients with atrioventricular reciprocating tachycardias, especially with WPW syndrome and for ectopic atrial tachycardias. Care may be necessary in using β adrenergic blockers for infants with significant lung disease. For more refractory patients, combination therapy with propranolol and digoxin may be effective (101).

If breakthrough of supraventricular tachycardia occurs, switching to other agents with a greater potency (and toxicity), under the direction of a pediatric cardiologist, may suppress recurrences. These other agents may include drugs with a combination of actions such as sotalol, or others used alone or in combination such as type IA agents (e.g., quinidine, procainamide, disopyramide), type IC agents (e.g., flecainide or propafenone), or amiodarone, and possibly oral verapamil in older infants. The recommended management schemes vary between institutions and will change as more data about existing medications and new medications become available.

Esophageal or intracardiac electrophysiology studies with programmed atrial stimuli can be used to determine probability of recurrence on medications or after medications have been discontinued, for those with reentry supraventricular tachycardia. Rarely, radiofrequency ablation is used in infants with particularly refractory supraventricular tachycardia, often with associated ventricular dysfunction (109). Radiofrequency ablation is more safely and routinely applied in later childhood in those with persistent problematic arrhythmias.

Fetuses with supraventricular tachycardia may be recognized in utero by an unusually rapid heart rate. The mechanism of the arrhythmia can usually be elucidated with echocardiography, and usually involves a reentry mechanism (Fig. 33-6). If the arrhythmia has been present for some time, these fetuses may develop hydrops. Treatment in utero by the administration of digoxin, flecainide, quinidine, procainamide, or sotalol to the mother, or procainamide or amiodarone directly into the umbilical vein, may be effective in terminating or suppressing the arrhythmia.

Ventricular Tachycardias

Wide complex tachyarrhythmias may represent ventricular tachycardia, SVT with aberrant conduction, atrioventricular reciprocating tachycardia in WPW syndrome with antegrade conduction over the accessory pathway and retrograde conduction over the His–Purkinje system and AV node, or any tachycardia in the presence of bundle branch or intraventricular conduction block (e.g., after cardiac surgery, hyperkalemia). In infants, the QRS complex in ventricular tachycardia may be as narrow as 0.06 to 0.11 seconds, but it is always different than in sinus rhythm (Fig. 33-48).

Although dissociation of the ventricles from the atria, with more ventricular beats, is a hallmark of ventricular tachycardia (ventricular:atrial ratio > 1), there may be a 1:1 ventricular:atrial relationship if there is retrograde conduction over the A-V node. For the purposes of initial management, a wide QRS complex tachycardia should be considered ventricular tachycardia unless one has an ECG in sinus rhythm showing the same, wide QRS complex (generally as a result of a fixed bundle branch block). Chronic recurrent ventricular tachycardias are rare in neonates, and are usually associated with structural or functional heart disease. When there is a polymorphic ventricular arrhythmia in the absence of apparent structural or functional heart disease, one should consider torsades de pointes associated with the long-QT syndrome. Very rarely an incessant, monomorphic ventricular tachycardia is found in infants with cardiac tumors (110).

Long-QT syndrome is a generally congenital abnormality of ventricular repolarization that can cause ventricular tachycardia. The congenital long QT syndrome has recently been subdivided into 7 genotypes, caused by mutations in 1 of 6 proteins involved with transmembrane ion currents or in an associated structural anchoring protein (111). It can be inherited in an autosomal dominant fashion (Romano–Ward syndrome, without sensorineural hearing loss), or less often as an autosomal recessive condition (Jervell and Lange-Nielsen syndrome, with sensorineural hearing loss). Patients with this syndrome, including infants, generally have a prolonged

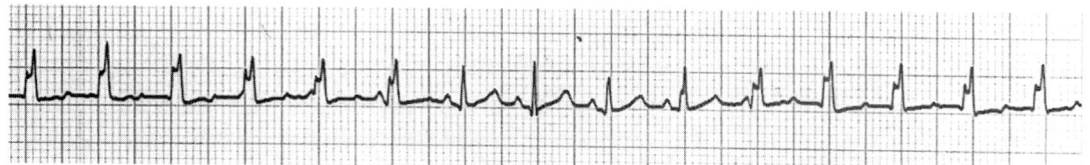

Figure 33-48 Electrocardiogram showing ventricular tachycardia in an infant at a rate of 158 beats/min. Because of retrograde conduction block, occasional sinus beats can be conducted to the ventricles through the AV node and His–Purkinje system, resulting in a normal QRS complex. Note that the QRS complex duration of the ventricular tachycardia measures 0.08 seconds, compared a QRS duration of 0.06 seconds for the conducted sinus beats.

corrected QT interval $(QT \div (RR)^{1/2} > 0.46 \text{ msec})$. Rarely, infants with the long QT syndrome have 2:1 A-V conduction block because the ventricles are refractory when the next atrial impulse conducts through the A-V node and His-Purkinje system (96). Patients with the long QT syndrome are at risk for torsades de pointes (a polymorphic ventricular tachycardia characterized by changing QRS morphology/axis that appears to turn around the baseline point) and sudden death.

To help aid in the diagnosis of the long QT syndrome, a scoring system has been developed based on ECG findings, the patient's arrhytmia (ventricular tachycardia) and symptoms (syncope, aborted sudden death) and family history (112). Care must be made in diagnosing the long QT syndrome in the first few days of life, especially without a family history of long QT syndrome or documented torsades de pointes, because many neonates have a QTc greater than 440 msec in the first few days of life.

Patients identified with the long-QT syndrome should be started on β-blockers, although other antiarrhythmic medications might eventually be preferable for some genotypes. Patients with malignant ventricular tachycardia despite β-blockers occasionally require cervicothoracic sympathectomy, pacemakers, or automatic implantable cardiac defibrillators (113).

Acquired long QT syndrome with risk of torsades de pointes can occur secondary to medications, electrolyte abnormalities (e.g., hypokalemia, hypocalcemia, or hypomagnesemia), endocrine abnormalities (e.g., hyperparathyroidism, hypothyroidism, or pheochromocytoma), or CNS disorders (e.g., encephalitis, head trauma, subarachnoid hemorrhage).

Treatments for ventricular Tachycardias

Because ventricular tachycardia can be life threatening, with the potential for degeneration into ventricular fibrillation, it is safest to treat all wide complex tachycardias as ventricular tachycardia.

If the patient is hemodynamically stable with a monomorphic ventricular tachycardia, antiarrhythmic therapy using lidocaine, procainamide, or amiodarone may suppress the arrhythmia (see Table 33-19). Phenytoin can be especially useful if the arrhythmia is related to digoxin toxicity. For torsades de pointes, treatment should include magnesium sulfate, lidocaine, and possibly isoproterenol or cardiac pacing.

If the patient is, or becomes, hemodynamically unstable, DC cardioversion should be initiated with 1 to 2 Joules/kg initially.

Chronic prophylactic antiarrhythmic therapy should be guided by the type of ventricular tachycardia, any underlying heart disease, and hemodynamic alterations associated with the arrhythmia (see Table 33-19). Radiofrequency ablation is rarely necessary for infants with monomorphic ventricular tachycardia not adequately suppressed by antiarrhythmic medications. Rarely, automatic implantable cardiac defibrillators are necessary for infants with recurrent

life-threatening ventricular arrhythmias despite antiarrhythmic medications.

ATRIOVENTRICULAR BLOCK

First Degree Atrioventricular Block

First degree A-V block is characterized by an abnormally prolonged P-R interval for age and heart rate. Most commonly, this is as a result of enhanced vagal tone and seen during sleep. Rarely this can be secondary to antiarrhythmic medications (e.g., digoxin), hypothermia, increased parasympathetic tone, hypothyroidism, or electrolyte disorders (hypo- or hyperkalemia, hypo- or hypercalcemia, hypoglycemia, and hypomagnesemia). First-degree AV block is generally well tolerated and requires no specific therapy. However, an infant with a muscular dystrophy, Kearns-Sayre syndrome, neonatal lupus, a family history of complete heart block or maternal connective tissue disease should be followed for possible progression of the conduction abnormality.

SECOND-DEGREE ATRIOVENTRICULAR BLOCK

Second-degree AV block is defined as intermittent failure of conduction of some atrial depolarizations to the ventricles. Second-degree AV block is subdivided into Mobitz type I (Wenckebach) and Mobitz type II AV block. In Mobitz type I (Wenckebach) AV block there is progressive delay in A-V conduction before a single atrial beat fails to conduct. Mobitz type I AV block is generally caused by factors similar to those causing first degree A-V block; it is usually well tolerated, and rarely causes symptomatic bradycardia. Mobitz Type II AV block is recognized by the intermittent failure of atrioventricular conduction, without an associated prolongation of the P-R interval. There is often a fixed ratio of atrial to ventricular depolarizations, although this ratio may vary over time. Asymptomatic patients with isolated Mobitz Type II AV block do not require a permanent pacemaker, but should receive close follow-up.

Third-degree (Complete) Atrioventricular Block

Third-degree (complete) atrioventricular (AV) block is defined by the absence of conduction of atrial impulses to the ventricles. The ventricular rhythm may arise from the AV node or His bundle (junctional escape rhythm), in which case there is usually a narrow QRS complex. Alternatively, the ventricular rhythm may arise from the ventricles, resulting in a wide QRS complex. The ventricular rate is related to the origin of the escape rhythm, with AV junctional escape rhythms generally being faster than idioventricular rhythms.

Congenital complete heart block is frequently recognized in utero. It is estimated to occur in 1 of 20,000 live births. In approximately 50% of infants with congenital heart block, there is an associated cardiovascular malformation (e.g., l-transposition of the great arteries, heterotaxy syndrome, endocardial cushion defect). In the absence of structural heart disease, the heart block is usually related to maternal autoantibodies (anti-Ro and/or anti-La) that cross the placenta and interact with the developing conduction system (114). These antibodies are associated with maternal connective tissue disease, particularly lupus erythematosis and Sjögren syndrome. In newborns with heart block and no structural cardiac abnormalities, testing of their mothers for these antibodies is indicated because they may have no signs or symptoms of connective tissue disease.

Occasionally newborns present with second-degree AV block and later progress to complete heart block. Therefore, those infants with persistent second-degree heart block (especially Mobitz type II) should undergo echocardiography to look for structural heart disease, and their mothers should be tested for these antibodies. Rarely myocarditis and fibrosis of the atrioventricular node or His bundle has been implicated as the cause of neonatal heart block. Complete heart block may occur as a complication of cardiac surgery, particularly in the correction of l-transposition, endocardial cushion defects, tetralogy of Fallot, and ventricular septal defects.

Infants with congenital complete heart block generally have a narrow, junctional, escape rhythm between 30 and 110 beats/min. The ventricular rate tends to decrease with increasing age. The stroke volume increases to compensate for the low ventricular rate, to maintain an adequate cardiac output. Examination usually reveals cardiac enlargement from an increased left ventricular end-diastolic volume, and a systolic ejection murmur and apical mid-diastolic rumble from increased stroke flow.

Most infants with isolated congenital complete heart bock without hemodynamically significant cardiac malformation often tolerate the bradycardia well, without symptoms, with normal growth and development, and do not require immediate intervention. Symptoms are usually related to the severity of the associated cardiovascular malformation and the degree of bradycardia. Less often, an infant or fetus with isolated complete heart block develops congestive heart failure or hydrops and some do not survive (115).

Patients with syncope or near syncope (Stokes–Adams attacks), congestive heart failure, or postsurgical block require early initiation of permanent ventricular pacing. Medical therapy with isoproterenol or with transcutaneous or transvenous cardiac pacing is helpful in the acute situation, prior to surgery. The timing of pacemaker implantation in other patients is more controversial. Criteria used to select patients for permanent pacing in infants have included: awake, resting ventricular rates less than 50 beats/min; awake, resting atrial rates greater than 140 beats/min; wide QRS escape rhythms; prolonged QT intervals; frequent, complex ventricular ectopy; or ventricular tachycardia (116).

REFERENCES

1. Mitchell SC, Korones SB, Berendes HW. Congenital heart disease in 56,109 births. *Circulation* 1971;43:323.
2. Hoffman JIE, Kaplan S. The incidence of congenital heart disease. *J Am Coll Cardiol* 2002;39:1890.
3. Fyler DC. Report of the New England Regional Infant Cardiac Program. *Pediatrics* 1980;65(Suppl):375.
4. Hoyert DL, Freedman MA, Strobino DM, Guyer B. Annual summary of vital statistics: 2000. *Pediatrics* 2001;108:1241.
5. Tweddell JS, Hoffman GM, Mussatto KA, at al. Improved survival of patients undergoing palliation of hypoplastic left heart syndrome: lessons learned from 115 consecutive patients. *Circulation* 2002;106:I-82.
6. Newburger JW, Silbert AR, Buckley LP, Fyler DC. Cognitive function and age at repair of transposition of the great arteries in children. *N Engl J Med* 1984;310:1495.
7. Bellinger DC, Jonas RA, Rappaport LA, et al. Developmental and neurologic status of children after heart surgery with hypothermic circulatory arrest or low-flow cardiopulmonary bypass. *N Engl J Med* 1995;332(9):549.
8. Wernovsky G, Newburger J. Neurologic and developmental morbidity in children with complex congenital heart disease. *J Pediatr* 2003;142:6.
9. Pyeritz, RE: Genetics and Cardiovascular Disease. In Braunwald E. *Heart disease: a textbook of cardiovascular medicine*, 6th ed., W. B. Saunders Company, 2001:1977.
10. Clark EB: Mechanisms in the pathogenesis of congenital cardiac malformations. In: Pierpont MEM, Moller JH, eds. *Genetics of cardiovascular disease*. Boston, Martinus Nihjoff, 1986:3.
11. Clark EB. Pathogenetic mechanisms of congenital cardiovascular malformations revisited [review]. *Semin Perinatol* 1996;20(6):465.
12. Lacro RV. *Dysmorphology. Nadas' pediatric cardiology.* Philadelphia: Hanley & Belfus, 1992:37.
13. Ferencz C, Correa-Villasenor A. Epidemiology of cardiovascular malformations: the state-of-the-art. *Cardiol Young* 1991;1:264.
14. Olson EN, Srivastava D. Molecular pathways controlling heart development. *Science* 1996;272:671.
15. Srivastava D, Olson EN. A genetic blueprint for cardiac development. *Nature* 2000;407:221.
16. *Online Mendelian inheritance in man, OMIM (TM).* Baltimore: Center for Medical Genetics, Johns Hopkins University; Bethesda: National Center for Biotechnology Information, National Library of Medicine. World Wide Web URL: http://www.ncbi.nlm.nih.gov/omim/.
17. Gorlin RJ, Cohen MM, Levin LS. *Syndromes of the head and neck,* 3rd ed. Oxford: Oxford University Press, 1990.
18. Jones KL. *Smith's recognizable patterns of human malformation.* 5th ed. Philadelphia: WB Saunders, 1996.
19. Greenwood RD. Cardiovascular malformations associated with extracardiac anomalies and malformation syndromes: patterns for diagnosis. *Clin Pediatr* 1984;23(3):145.
20. Milerad J, Larson O, Hagberg C, Ideberg M. Associated malformations in infants with cleft lip and palate: a prospective, population-based study. *Pediatrics* 1997;100:180.
21. Moore KL, ed. *The developing human: clinically oriented embryology,* 2nd ed. Philadelphia: WB Saunders, 1997.
22. Kurnit DM, Layton WM, Matthysse S. Genetics, chance and morphogenesis. *Am J Human Genet* 1987;41:979.
23. Shaw GM, O'Malley CD, Wasserman CR, Tolarova MM, Lammer EJ. Maternal periconceptional use of multivitamins and reduced risk for conotruncal heart defects and limb deficiencies among offspring. *Am J Med Genet* 1995;59:536.
24. Botto LD, Khoury MJ, Mulinare J, Erickson JD. Periconceptional multivitamin use and the occurrence of conotruncal heart defects: results from a population-based, case-control study. *Pediatrics* 1996;98:911.
25. Hernandez-Diaz S, Werler MM, Walker AM, Mitchell AA. Folic acid antagonists during pregnancy and the risk of birth defects. *N Eng J Med* 2000;343:1608.
26. Junker R, Kotthoff S, Vielhaber H, et al. Infant methylenetetrahydrofolate reductase 677TT genotype is a risk factor for congenital heart disease. *Cardiovasc Res* 2001;51:251.
27. Rosenquist TH, Ratashak SA, Selhub J. Homocysteine induces congenital defects of the heart and neural tube: effect of folic acid. *Proc Natl Acad Sci USA* 1996;93:15227.

28. Kapusta L, Haagmans MLM, Steegers EAP, et al. Congenital heart defects and maternal derangement of homocysteine metabolism. *J Pediatr* 1999;135:773.

29. Dawson BV, Johnson PD, Goldberg SJ, Ulreich JB. Cardiac teratogenesis of trichloroethylene and dichloroethylene in a mammalian model. *J Am Coll Cardiol* 1990;16:1304.

30. Goldberg SJ, Lebwitz MD, Graver EJ, Hicks S. An association of human congenital cardiac malformations and drinking water contaminants. *J Am Coll Cardiol* 1990;16:155.

31. Croen LA, Shaw GM, Sanbonmatsu L, Selvin S, Buffler PA. Maternal residential proximity to hazardous waste sites and risk for selected congenital malformations. *Epidemiology* 1997; 8:347.

32. Richard P, Charron P, Carrier L, et al. EUROGENE Heart Failure Project. Hypertrophic cardiomyopathy: distribution of disease genes, spectrum of mutations, and implications for a molecular diagnosis strategy. *Circulation* 2003;107:2227.

33. Seidman JG, Seidman C. The Genetic Basis for Cardiomyopathy: from Mutation Identification to Mechanistic Paradigms. *Cell* 2001; 104,557.

34. Schwartz ML, Cox GF, Lin AE, et al. Clinical approach to genetic cardiomyopathy in children. *Circulation* 1996;94:2021.

35. Splawski I, Timothy KW, Vincent GM, Atkinson DL, Keating MT. Molecular basis of the long-QT syndrome associated with deafness. *N Engl J Med* 1997;336:1562.

37. Barcroft J. *Researchers of pre-natal life.* Oxford: Blackwell & Mott, 1944.

38. Dawes GS. *Foetal and neonatal physiology: a comparative study of the changes at birth.* Chicago: Year Book, 1969.

39. Lind J, Stern L, Wegelius C. *Human and foetal neonatal circulation.* Springfield, IL: Charles C Thomas, 1964.

40. Rudolph AM. *Congenital diseases of the heart.* Chicago: Year Book, 1974.

41. Friedman D, Buyon J, Kim M, Glickstein JS. Fetal cardiac function assessed by Doppler myocardial performance index (Tei index) *Ultrasound in Obstetrics and Gynecology* 2003;21:33.

42. Budorick NE, Millman SL. New modalities for imaging the fetal heart. *Semin Perinatol* 2000;24:352.

43. Davignon A, Rautaharju P, Boisselle E, et al. Normal ECG standards for infants and children. *Pediatr Cardiol* 1979;1:123.

44. Fowler RS, Finlay CD. The electrocardiogram of the neonate. In Freedom RM, Benson LN, Smallhorn JF, eds. *Neonatal heart disease.* London: Springer-Verlag, 1992.

45. Schwartz PJ, Garson A Jr, Paul T, et al. Guidelines for the interpetation of the newborn electrocardiogram. A task force of the European society of cardiology. *Eur Heart J* 2002;23:1329.

46. Quinones MA, Douglas PS, Foster E, et al. American College of Cardiology. American Heart Association. American College of Physicians-American Society of Internal Medicine. American Society of Echocardiography. Society of Cardiovascular Anesthesiologists. Society of Pediatric Echocardiography.ACC/AHA clinical competence statement on echocardiography: a report of the American College of Cardiology/American Heart Association/American College of Physicians-American Society of Internal Medicine Task Force on Clinical Competence. *J Am College Cardiol* 2003;41:687.

47. Lock JE, Keane JF, Mandell VS, Perry SB. Cardiac catheterization. In Fyler DC, ed. *Nadas' pediatric cardiology.* Philadelphia: Hanley & Belfus, 1992.

48. LaFarge CG, Miettinen OS. The estimation of oxygen consumption. *Cardiovasc Res* 1970;4:23.

49. Kovalchin JP, Forbes TJ, Nihill MR, Geva T. Echocardiographic determinants of clinical course in infants with critical and severe pulmonary valve stenosis. *J Am Coll Cardiol* 1997;29(5):1095.

50. Kaine SF, Smith EO, Mott AR, Mullins, Geva T. Quantitative echocardiographic analysis of the aortic arch predicts outcome of balloon angioplasty of native coarctation of the aorta. *Circulation* 1996;94:1056.

51. Rhodes LA, Colan SD, Perry SB, et al. Predictors of survival in neonates with critical aortic stenosis. *Circulation* 1991;84:2325.

52. Egito ES, Moore P, O'Sullivan J, et al. Transvascular balloon dilation for neonatal critical aortic stenosis: early and midterm results. *J Am Coll Cardiol* 1997;29(2):442.

53. Olley PM, Coceani F, Bodach E. E-type prostaglandins: a new emergency therapy for certain cyanotic congenital heart malformations. *Circulation* 1976;53:728.

54. Lang P, Freed MD, Rosenthal A, et al. The use of prostaglandin E1 in an infant with interruption of the aortic arch. *J Pediatr* 1977; 91:805.

55. Borow K, Green LH, Castaneda AR, et al. Left ventricular function after repair of tetralogy of Fallot and its relationship to age at repair. *Circulation* 1980;61:1150.

56. Jatene AD, Fontes VF, Paulista PP, et al. Anatomic correction of transposition of the great vessels. *J Thorac Cardiovasc Surg* 1976; 72:364.

57. Castaneda AR, Norwood WI, Jonas RA, et al. Transposition of the great arteries and intact ventricular septum: anatomical repair in the neonate. *Ann Thorac Surg* 1984;38:438.

58. Wernovsky G, Mayer JE Jr, Jonas RA, et al. Factors influencing early and late outcome of the arterial switch operation for transposition of the great arteries. *J Thorac Cardiovasc Surg* 1995; 109(2):289.

59. Geva T, Ayres NA, Pac FA, Pignatelli R. Quantitative morphometric analysis of progressive infundibular obstruction in tetralogy of Fallot. A prospective longitudinal echocardiographic study. *Circulation* 1995;92(4):886.

60. Walsh EP, Rockenmacher S, Keane JF, et al. Late results in patients with tetralogy of Fallot repaired during infancy. *Circulation* 1988; 77:1062.

61. Lillehei CW, Varco RL, Cohen M, et al. The first open heart corrections of tetralogy of Fallot. A 26–31 year follow-up of 106 patients. *Ann Surg* 1986;204(4):490.

62. Giglia TM, Mandell VS, Connor AR, Mayer JE Jr, Lock JE. Diagnosis and management of right ventricle-dependent coronary circulation in pulmonary atresia with intact ventricular septum. *Circulation* 1992;86:1516.

63. Franklin RC, Spiegelhalter DJ, Sullivan ID, et al. Tricuspid atresia presenting in infancy. Survival and suitability for the Fontan operation. *Circulation* 1993;87:427.

64. Gentles TL, Mayer JE Jr, Gauvreau K, et al. Fontan operation in five hundred consecutive patients: factors influencing early and late outcome. *J Thorac Cardiovasc Surg* 1997;114:376.

65. Norwood WI, Lang P, Hansen DD. Physiologic repair of aortic atresia—hypoplastic left heart syndrome. *N Engl J Med* 1984; 308:23.

66. Forbess JM, Cook N, Roth SJ, et al. Ten-year institutional experience with palliative surgery for hypoplastic left heart syndrome. Risk factors related to stage I mortality. *Circulation* 1995;92(9 Suppl):II-262.

67. Iannettoni MD, Bove EL, Mosca RS, et al. Improving results with first-stage palliation for hypoplastic left heart syndrome. *J Thorac Cardiovasc Surg* 1994;107:934.

68. Razzouk AJ, Chinnock RE, Gundry SR, et al. Transplantation as a primary treatment for hypoplastic left heart syndrome: intermediate-term results. *Ann Thorac Surg* 1996;62:1.

69. Gutgesell HP, Massaro TA. Management of hypoplastic left heart syndrome in a consortium of university hospitals. *Am J Cardiol* 1995;76:809.

70. Canter C, Naftel D, Caldwell R, et al. Survival and risk factors for death after cardiac transplantation in infants. A multiinstitutional study. The Pediatric Heart Transplant Study. *Circulation* 1997;96:227.

71. Hanley FL, Heinemann MK, Jonas RA, et al. Repair of truncus arteriosus in the neonate. *J Thorac Cardiovasc Surg* 1993;105:1047.

72. Rajasinghe HA, McElhinney DB, Reddy VM, Mora BN, Hanley FL. Long-term follow-up of truncus arteriosus repaired in infancy: a twenty-year experience. *J Thorac Cardiovasc Surg* 1997; 113(5):869–878.

73. Piccoli G, Pacifico AD, Kirklin JW, Blackstone EH, Kirklin JK, Bargeron LM. Changing results and concepts in the surgical treatment of double-outlet right ventricle: analysis of 137 operations in 126 patients. *Am J Cardiol* 1983;52:549.

74. Radzik D, Davignon A, van Doesburg N, et al. Predictive factors for spontaneous closure of atrial septal defects diagnosed in the first 3 months of life [Comment]. *J Am Coll Cardiol* 1994;23:828.

75. Bharati S, Lev M. The spectrum of common atrioventricular orifice (canal). *Am Heart J* 1973;86:553.

76. Hanley FL, Fenton KN, Jonas RA, et al. Surgical repair of complete atrioventricular canal defects in infancy. Twenty-year trends. *J Thorac Cardiovasc Surg* 1993;106:387.

77. Slomp J, Gittenberger-de Groot AC, Glukhova MA, et al. Differentiation, dedifferentiation, and apoptosis of smooth muscle

cells during the development of the human ductus arteriosus. *Arterioscler Thromb Vasc Biol* 1997;17:1003.

78. Friedman WF, Hirschklau MJ, Previtz MP, et al. Pharmacologic closure of patent ductus arteriosus in the premature infant. *N Engl J Med* 1976;295:526.

79. Heymann MA, Rudolph AM, Silverman NH. Closure of the ductus arteriosus in premature infants by inhibition of prostaglandin synthesis. *N Engl J Med* 1976;295:530.

80. Nehgme RA, O'Connor TZ, Lister G, Bracken MB. Patent ductus arteriosus. In Sinclair JC, Bracken MB, eds. *Effective care of the newborn infant.* New York: Oxford University Press, 1992;281.

81. Ment LR, Oh W, Ehrenkranz RA, et al. Low-dose indomethacin and prevention of intraventricular hemorrhage: a multicenter randomized trial. *Pediatrics* 1994;93(4):543.

82. Fowlie PW. Prophylactic indomethacin: systematic review and meta-analysis. *Arch Dis Child* 1996;74:F81.

83. Volpe JJ. Brain injury caused by intraventricular hemorrhage: is indomethacin the silver bullet for prevention? *Pediatrics* 1994;11:673.

84. Reynolds EOR. Prevention of periventricular hemorrhage. *Pediatrics* 1994;11:677.

85. Varvarigou A, Bardin CL, Beharry K, Chemtob S, Papageorgiou A, Aranda JV. Early ibuprofen administration to prevent patent ductus arteriosus in premature newborn infants. *JAMA* 1996;275:539.

86. Wagner HR, Ellison RC, Zierler S, et al. Surgical closure of patent ductus ateriosus in 268 preterm infants. *J Thorac Cardiovasc Surg* 1984;87:870.

87. Gersony WM, Peckham GJ, Ellison RC, et al. Effects of indomethacin in preterm infants with patent ductus arteriosus. Results of a national collaborative study. *J Pediatr* 1983;102:895.

88. Doty DB, Richardson JV, Falkovsky GE, Gordonova MI, Burakovsky VI. Aortopulmonary septal defect: hemodynamics, angiography, and operation. *Ann Thorac Surg* 1981;32:244.

89. Edwards JE. Malformations of the aortic arch system manifested as "vascular rings." *Lab Invest* 1953;2:56.

90. Yeager SB, Chin AJ, Sanders SP. Two-dimensional echocardiographic diagnosis of pulmonary artery sling in infancy. *J Am Coll Cardiol* 1986;7:625.

91. Tonkin IL, Elliot LP, Bargeron LM. Concomitant axial cineangiography and barium esophagography in the evaluation of vascular rings. *Radiology* 1980;135:69.

92. Backer CL, Ilbawi MN, Idriss FS, DeLeon SY. Vascular anomalies causing tracheoesophageal compression. *J Thorac Cardiovasc Surg* 1989;97:725.

93. Swischuk LE. Anterior tracheal indentation in infancy and early childhood: normal or abnormal? *Am J Roentgenol Rad Ther Nucl Med* 1971;112:12.

94. Nir A, Tajik AJ, Freeman WK, et al. Tuberous sclerosis and cardiac rhabdomyoma. *Am J Cardiol* 1995;76:419.

95. De Giovanni JV, Dindar A, Griffith MJ, et al. Recovery pattern of left ventricular dysfunction following radiofrequency ablation of incessant supraventricular tachycardia in infants and children. *Heart* 1998;79:588.

96. Gorgels AP, Al Fadley F, Zaman L, et al. The long QT syndrome with impaired atrioventricular conduction: a malignant variant in infants. *J Cardio Electrophys* 1998;9:1225.

97. Nagashima M, Matsushima M, Ogawa A, et al. Cardiac arrhythmias in healthy children revealed by 24-hour ambulatory ECG monitoring. *Pediatr Cardiol* 1987;8:103.

98. Southall DP, Richards J, Mitchell P, et al. Study of cardiac rhythm in healthy newborn infants. *Brit Heart J* 1980;43:14.

99. Van Hare GF, Stanger P. Ventricular tachycardia and accelerated ventricular rhythm presenting in the first month of life. *Am J Cardiol* 1991;67:42.

100. Snyder CS, Fenrich AL, Friedman RA, et al. Usefulness of echocardiography in infants with supraventricular tachycardia. *Am J Cardiol* 2003;91:1277.

101. Weindling SN, Walsh EP, Saul JP. Efficacy and risks of medical therapy for supraventricular tachycardia in neonates and infants. *Am Heart J* 1996;131:66.

102. Bromberg BI, Lindsay BD, Cain ME, et al. Impact of clinical history and electrophysiologic characterization of accessory pathways on management strategies to reduce sudden death among children with Wolff-Parkinson-White syndrome. *J Am Coll Cardiol* 1996;27:690.

103. Gollob MH, Green MS, Tang AS, et al. Identification of a gene responsible for familial Wolff-Parkinson-White syndrome. *N Eng J Med* 2001;344:1823.

104. Bauersfeld U, Gow RM, Hamilton RM, et al. Treatment of atrial ectopic tachycardia in infants <6 months old. *Am Heart J* 1995;129:1145.

105. Villain E, Vetter V, Garcia JM, et al. Evolving concepts in the management of congenital junctional ectopic tachycardia. *Circulation* 1990;81:1544.

106. Casey FA, McCrindle BW, Hamilton RM, et al. Neonatal atrial flutter: significant early morbidity and excellent long-term prognosis. *Am Heart J* 1997;133:302.

107. Epstein ML, Kiel EA, Victorica BE. Cardiac decompensation following verapamil therapy in infants with supraventricular tachycardia. *Pediatrics* 1985;75:737.

108. Perry JC, Garson A, Jr. Supraventricular tachycardia due to Wolff-Parkinson-White syndrome in children: early disappearance and late recurrence. *J Am Coll Cardiol* 1990;16:1215.

109. Friedman RA, Walsh EP, Silka MJ, et al. NASPE Expert Consensus Conference: Radiofrequency catheter ablation in children with and without congenital heart disease. *Pacing Clin Electrophysiol* 2002;25:1000.

110. Perry JC. Ventricular tachycardia in neonates. *Pacing Clin Electrophysiol* 1997;20:2061.

111. Antzelevitch A. Molecular Genetics of Arrhythmias and Cardiovascular Conditions Associated with Arrhythmias. *Pacing Clin Electrophysiol* 2003;26:2194.

112. Schwartz PJ, Moss AJ, Vincent GM, et al. Diagnostic criteria for the long QT syndrome. An update. *Circulation* 1993;88:782.

113. Hoorntje T, Sreeram N, de Vroet R. Device therapy for malignant neonatal long QT syndrome. *Internat J Cardiol* 1999;71:289.

114. Reed BR, Lee LA, Harmon C, et al. Autoantibodies to SS-A/Ro in infants with congenital heart block. *J Pediatr* 1983;103:889.

115. Buyon JP, Hiebert R, Copel J, et al. Autoimmune-associated congenital heart block: demographics, mortality, morbidity and recurrence rates obtained from a national neonatal lupus registry. *J Am Coll Cardiol* 1998;31:1658.

116. Gregoratos G, Abrams J, Epstein AE, et al. ACC/AHA/NASPE 2002 Guideline Update for Implantation of Cardiac Pacemakers and Antiarrhythmia Devices—summary article: a report of the American College of Cardiology/American Heart Association Task Force on Practice Guidelines. *J Am Coll Cardiol* 2002.

117. Mullins CE, Mayer DC. *Congenital heart disease: a diagramatic atlas.* New York: Alan R Liss, 1988.

Preoperative and Postoperative Care of the Infant with Critical Congenital Heart Disease

34

John M. Costello   *Wayne H. Franklin*

INTRODUCTION

The contemporary strategy of early, complete repair for congenital heart defects originated in the 1970s, as evidenced by the first report in 1976 of complete anatomic correction of d-transposition of the great arteries (d-TGA) with ventricular septal defect (VSD) in early infancy (1). Aided by advances in surgical technique and equipment, myocardial protection, cardiac anesthesia and perioperative care, the strategy of early primary repair is now applied to many other complex congenital heart lesions, such as tetralogy of Fallot and truncus arteriosus (2,3). Furthermore, infants with certain lesions that were considered before the 1980s to be inoperable, such as hypoplastic left heart syndrome (HLHS), currently undergo staged surgical palliation with constantly improving outcomes (4). The first stage of surgical palliation for infants with single ventricle physiology usually must be performed in the neonatal period to minimize early morbidity and mortality, and to optimize the cardiovascular physiology for the subsequent Fontan operation. Early repair or palliation (for single ventricle lesions) benefits infants because prolonged preoperative periods of cyanosis (See Color Plate) and heart failure, and the many associated complications are minimized (5–7). These potential associated complications include impairment of cognitive function as a result of chronic hypoxemia, central nervous system embolic events, and the development of pulmonary vascular obstructive disease. Postoperative complications including pulmonary hypertensive crises are also reduced using a

strategy of early surgical intervention (8). The incidence of vascular complications and infection related to central lines in infants requiring prolonged hospitalization prior to cardiac repair or palliation will also be minimized.

As a result of this early intervention strategy, approximately one-third of all patients with congenital heart defects undergo primary repair or palliation in early infancy. Due to the immaturity of many organ systems, these neonates possess limited physiologic reserve. They have limited ability to increase stroke volume, limited functional residual capacity in the lung, limited fat and carbohydrate reserves, and a limited ability to regulate temperature. Drug metabolism is altered by hepatic and renal immaturity, and total body water content. All of these factors complicate the care of infants in the perioperative period, and some have prolonged intensive care unit (ICU) stays, presenting a challenge for physicians involved with their management.

A variety of pediatric personnel with expertise in pediatric cardiology are involved in the day-to-day management of these patients. These personnel include neonatologists, intensivists, cardiologists, cardiac surgeons, anesthesiologists, nurses, and respiratory therapists. Because of the complexity inherent to this field, and to ensure an optimal outcome for each patient, seamless communication of pertinent anatomic, pathophysiologic, and operational/interventional details is required across all specialties.

This chapter will complement Chapter 33 by providing an overview of the key issues, concepts, and strategies pertaining to the care of infants with critical congenital heart disease. We have allowed some overlap of information between chapters in the interest of clarity. The expected presentation and clinical course of specific congenital heart lesions will be discussed, and the general principles that are widely applied to patient management will be reviewed. This chapter will not provide a comprehensive description of every congenital heart defect and associated variants that may present in infancy. The reader must appropriately apply the concepts and principles discussed in the following pages to each unique patient. The first section will cover general preoperative issues, and the presentation, physiology and management of common types of critical congenital heart disease. The second section will provide an overview of cardiopulmonary bypass (CPB) and its sequelae, followed by a lesion specific discussion of operative intervention, postoperative physiology and common complications.

PREOPERATIVE CARE

Fetal Diagnosis

Fetal echocardiography plays an important role in the management of critical congenital heart disease for a variety of reasons (9). The identification of severe congenital heart disease during the second trimester allows time for family counseling. Fetuses that are likely to require surgical or transcatheter intervention in the neonatal period should ideally be delivered at an institution with a level II or III nursery that is located at or in close proximity to a tertiary care pediatric cardiology center. In the absence of nonimmune hydrops fetalis, fetuses with known critical congenital heart disease should be delivered at term to minimize the potential complications of prematurity, such as respiratory distress syndrome, intraventricular hemorrhage and necrotizing enterocolitis (NEC). As discussed below, infants with unrecognized critical congenital heart disease may develop severe cyanosis (See Color Plate), shock, myocardial dysfunction and end organ damage. Information from the fetal echocardiogram thus guides planning for

initial stabilization upon delivery, such as the need for a prostaglandin E_1 (PGE1) infusion. Prenatal diagnosis is associated with reduced preoperative morbidity and mortality in large series of neonates with HLHS and TGA (10–13). Management strategies may be developed in advance for the uncommon patient with congenital heart disease who may become critically ill in the first few minutes of life, such as some neonates with absent pulmonary valve syndrome, or HLHS with an intact atrial septum. The impact of in utero diagnosis of critical congenital heart disease on postoperative mortality is controversial. Some centers have reported lower postoperative mortality in patients with a fetal diagnosis of HLHS or d-TGA, whereas others found no such impact (12–16).

Known risk factors for congenital heart disease that warrant referral to a pediatric cardiologist for fetal echocardiography are listed in Table 34-1 (17). Even if these screening guidelines are followed, the majority of patients with congenital heart disease will not be detected until after birth. Fetal echocardiography has several known limitations, most notably sub-optimal windows in mothers with large body habitus, and difficulty with precise imaging of extracardiac vessels. Two serious congenital heart lesions that may not be always appreciated with fetal echocardiography deserve comment. Isolated coarctation of the aorta may be difficult to definitively diagnose or exclude in utero as a result of the obligatory presence of the ductus arteriosus (18). Total anomalous pulmonary venous return may also be unrecognized. Thus, any diagnosis of fetal congenital heart disease must be confirmed, and the anatomic details clarified, as soon as possible after birth with a transthoracic echocardiogram.

Routine screening fetal ultrasound studies, which are interpreted by obstetricians, are usually limited to the demonstration of a heart with four chambers. Doppler assessment of blood flow patterns and valvar function is not usually performed, and data regarding longitudinal growth of the ventricular chamber sizes are not available when a single study is performed in the second trimester. Thus, a history of a normal fetal ultrasound does not exclude the possibility of critical congenital heart disease.

TABLE 34-1

RISK FACTORS FOR CONGENITAL HEART DISEASE THAT WARRANT FETAL ECHOCARDIOGRAPHY (SEE ALSO TABLE 33–6)

Maternal Risk Factors	Fetal Risk Factors
1. Family history of congenital heart disease 2. Maternal disease (lupus, diabetes mellitus) 3. Environmental (alcohol, certain viruses, medications)	1. Extracardiac anomalies 2. Chromosomal anomalies 3. Arrhythmia 4. Abnormal fetal growth 5. Fetal distress 6. Obstetrician's suspicion of CHD from screening US

CHD, congenital heart disease; US, ultrasound.

Transitional Circulation

An appreciation of the fetal-placental circulation, and the normal transition from fetal to newborn circulation, is required to understand the timing and presentation of symptoms in the neonate with critical heart disease (19). In the placenta, gas, nutrient, and waste exchange occur between the fetal and maternal circulations. Oxygenated blood then returns from the placenta to the fetus through the umbilical vein and partially bypasses the liver, via the ductus venosus, into the inferior vena cava. The oxygenated blood is preferentially shunted through the foramen ovale to the left atrium (20). The oxygen-rich blood then enters the left ventricle, from where it is pumped out the aorta to supply the coronary circulation and the brain. Deoxygenated blood from the superior vena cava and distal inferior vena cava preferentially enters the right ventricle, and is then pumped to the pulmonary artery. This preferential blood flow phenomenon is known as streaming. Due to the high pulmonary vascular resistance *in utero*, the majority of the deoxygenated pulmonary artery blood bypasses the lungs, and flows through the ductus arteriosus into the descending aorta, supplying the lower body and placenta.

An elegant series of events occur when the umbilical cord is clamped immediately after birth. The ductus venosus functionally closes in large part as a result of decreased flow from the placenta (21). The low resistance placental circulation is gone and thus systemic vascular resistance rises, although pulmonary vascular resistance falls as a result of mechanical expansion of the lungs with respiration and higher oxygen tension (22,23). Blood ejected from the right ventricle now perfuses the lungs rather than entering the ductus arteriosus, and the increased blood returning to the left atrium leads to functional closure of the foramen ovale. The increased oxygen tension also contributes to functional closure of the ductus arteriosus.

When the aforementioned events, in particular the fall in pulmonary vascular resistance and closure of the ductus arteriosus, occur in the setting of critical congenital heart disease, a physiologic state of either inadequate systemic or pulmonary blood flow exists which, if unrecognized, may progress to multi-organ system failure and death.

Presentation of Critical Congenital Heart Disease

Despite the broad spectrum of congenital heart lesions, neonates with critical congenital heart disease undetected in utero present in a limited number of ways: with cyanosis (inadequate pulmonary blood flow), shock (inadequate systemic blood flow) or some combination of these physiologic states. Older neonates and infants with significant left to right shunting at the ventricular or great artery level may present with congestive heart failure. Critical congenital heart disease may be detected prior to the onset of symptoms as a result of abnormal findings on cardiovascular examination or during echocardiographic screening performed in neonates with known chromosomal abnormalities or noncardiac congenital malformations.

Critical coarctation of the aorta, critical aortic valve stenosis, and HLHS are frequently encountered lesions that present in the neonatal period with symptomatic obstruction of the left ventricular outflow tract. In each case, constriction or closure of the ductus arteriosus leads to inadequate systemic blood flow. These patients will typically present within the first week or two of life with feeding difficulties, tachypnea, poor perfusion and metabolic acidosis, a constellation of findings that may be mistaken for septic shock. Due to low systemic cardiac output, findings such as pathologic heart murmurs may not be present and accurate four-extremity blood pressure measurements may be difficult to obtain. Diminished or absent pulses in the lower extremities and an increased right ventricular impulse are more reliable findings on physical examination, and a high index of suspicion is required to make a timely diagnosis.

Critical pulmonary valve stenosis, severe tetralogy of Fallot, and pulmonary atresia are examples of lesions with right ventricular outflow tract obstruction that manifest with progressive cyanosis in the newborn period as constriction of the ductus arteriosus limits pulmonary blood flow.

Lesions with complete intracardiac mixing of the systemic venous and pulmonary venous circulations, such as tricuspid atresia, truncus arteriosus, or complex single ventricles usually have variable degrees of obstruction to either the systemic or pulmonary circulations, depending upon the anatomic details of the individual lesion. Less commonly, they have no obstruction to either systemic or pulmonary blood flow, leading to mild hypoxemia (less commonly clinical cyanosis) but substantial heart failure that presents later in the neonatal period or during early infancy.

d-TGA is a common cyanotic lesion with the unique physiology of systemic and pulmonary circulations that run in parallel. Infants with d-TGA, an intact ventricular septum, and no significant outflow tract obstruction usually present with cyanosis soon after birth. Those with a significant VSD have less desaturation and can present later with congestive heart failure.

The neonate with nonimmune hydrops fetalis may have an underlying cardiac problem. The differential diagnosis includes serious congenital heart disease (particularly with significant atrioventricular valve regurgitation), obstructive cardiac tumors, congenital myocarditis, tachyarrhythmias and bradycardia.

Initial Evaluation and Stabilization of the Neonate with Suspected Congenital Heart Disease

A careful history and cardiovascular examination will often reveal abnormal findings in the infant with critical congenital heart disease, even before the onset of symptoms. Review of maternal records may identify a known risk factor for congenital heart disease (Table 34-1) (17). The course of labor should be reviewed, and factors that suggest acute infection, respiratory distress syndrome, or meconium aspiration should be noted, as they may indicate a primary respiratory cause for hypoxemia. The physical examination focuses on the detection of dysmorphic features, cyanosis, an abnormal precordium, abnormal femoral and peripheral pulses, and/or a pathologic heart murmur. Measurement of blood pressure in all four extremities is useful if an arm-leg gradient of greater than 10 mm Hg is detected, but in the setting of a large patent ductus arteriosus, the pressures may be equal despite the presence of a critical aortic coarctation or interrupted aortic arch. Although respiratory distress may be present in neonates with critical congenital heart disease or pulmonary problems, those with heart disease typically have a shallow rapid respiratory pattern ("quiet tachypnea"), as opposed to the more labored breathing pattern of neonates with a primary pulmonary process.

The term differential cyanosis refers to a condition in which the lower body is visibly more cyanotic than the upper body as a result of right to left shunting at the ductal level. The presence of differential cyanosis, occasionally seen with severe pulmonary hypertension, may also be indicative of aortic arch obstruction or coarctation of the aorta. In neonates with d-TGA, reverse differential cyanosis may be present if aortic arch obstruction or severe pulmonary hypertension also exists. In such patients, oxygenated blood is ejected from the left ventricle to the pulmonary artery, and then passes through the patent ductus arteriosus to the descending aorta.

In newborns that present with cyanosis, a right radial arterial blood gas analysis on room air and 100% inspired oxygen (the "hyperoxia test") is useful for discriminating those with cyanotic heart disease from those with pulmonary disease. The partial pressure of carbon dioxide (pCO_2) is typically mildly decreased in newborns with cardiac disease and mildly elevated in those with pulmonary disease. The arterial oxygen pressure (PaO_2) is often between 25 to 40 mm Hg on room air in both patient groups. In 100% FiO_2, the PaO_2 will usually rise to more than 100 mm Hg in patients with pulmonary disease, provided that significant pulmonary artery hypertension is not present. The PaO_2 will remain unchanged or only increase slightly in most neonates with cyanotic heart disease. There are limitations to the hyperoxia test. Patients with left sided obstructive lesions (e.g., HLHS, critical coarctation of the aorta, critical aortic valve stenosis, interrupted aortic arch) may have a high PaO_2 (>60 mm Hg) in any extremity or a very high PaO_2 (>150 mm Hg) in the right arm with certain anatomic variants. Pulse oximetry should not be used as a substitute for arterial blood gas analysis when performing the hyperoxia test. For example, a neonate receiving 100% fraction of inspired oxygen (FiO_2) may have a pulse oximetry reading of 100%, with a PaO_2 of 80 mm Hg (suggestive of cyanotic heart disease), or a PaO_2 more than 100 mm Hg (suggestive of pulmonary disease). Potential complications exist when performing the hyperoxia test. For example, if the test is continued for a prolonged period of time in neonates with left sided obstructive lesions, pulmonary vascular resistance

may drop further, and the ductus arteriosus may begin to close, leading to clinical deterioration.

Interpretation of a chest radiograph (CXR) and 12-lead electrocardiogram (ECG) may provide insight to the underlying cardiac diagnosis in cyanotic newborns. For example, cyanotic newborns with normal heart size, normal to increased pulmonary arterial markings on CXR, and a normal ECG may have TGA. Cyanotic newborns with normal heart size and decreased pulmonary blood flow on CXR are stratified by the ECG findings: those with right axis deviation (90°–180°) on ECG may have tetralogy of Fallot; those with a normal adult axis (10°–90°) on ECG may have pulmonary atresia with an intact ventricular septum; and those with an ECG with left axis deviation (0° to −90°) and left ventricular hypertrophy may have tricuspid atresia. Infants with a normal to small heart size and increased pulmonary vascular markings on CXR may have total anomalous pulmonary venous return, and those with a large heart with increased pulmonary vascular markings may have truncus arteriosus, or a complex single ventricle lesion with unobstructed pulmonary blood flow. Neonates with a very large heart and decreased pulmonary arterial markings may have Ebstein's anomaly of the tricuspid valve.

If the aforementioned evaluation is consistent with the presence of critical congenital heart disease, it is reasonable to stabilize the infant, including the initiation of a PGE_1 infusion in some cases, and then arrange transport to a pediatric cardiology center in which the initial echocardiogram can be performed. A PGE_1 infusion should be initiated in neonates who present with shock, cyanosis with a minimal increase in PaO_2 during the hyperoxia test, or a fetal diagnosis of ductal dependent congenital heart disease. An echocardiogram may be performed at the presenting institution if the presence of critical congenital heart disease is in doubt, or to guide initial stabilization if the transport time will be prolonged. The echocardiographer and the sonographer must have experience with congenital heart lesions, otherwise false negative and false positive evaluations may occur (24).

The introduction of prostaglandin infusions to maintain ductal patency in the late 1970s represented a major advance for infants with critical congenital heart disease (25,26). While receiving PGE_1, infants can be safely transported over long distances to congenital heart centers. Cardiac surgery can be postponed while infections are treated and other major congenital anomalies identified. Patients who present in shock can be medically managed for several days, allowing time for recovery of end-organ function prior to surgery. Detailed cardiac diagnostic information can be obtained using echocardiography, cardiac catheterization, spiral computed tomography (CT), magnetic resonance imaging (MRI), or electron beam tomography (EBT) to allow optimal planning for intervention.

PGE_1 can be administered through a peripheral intravenous line, although many practitioners prefer to use central venous access to ensure uninterrupted medication delivery. A wide range of dosing of PGE_1 is used depending on the clinical state of the patient. Generally a PGE_1 infusion of 0.1 mcg/kg/min is used when the ductus arteriosus is severely constricted or functionally closed and a state of shock or severe cyanosis exists. Lower doses (0.01–0.05 mcg/kg/min) will maintain ductal patency in neonates with presumed ductal dependent systemic or pulmonary circulation who are otherwise stable (27).

The most troublesome side effect of PGE_1 infusion is apnea, which occurs in approximately one-third of neonates (27,28). Tracheal intubation and mechanical ventilation are usually indicated when PGE_1 is started for neonates who present with severe cyanosis or shock and/or require transfer to another institution. Lower doses of PGE_1 are associated with fewer side effects, particularly apnea (27,29). Patients who are stable upon presentation and are started on a low dose of PGE_1 may be less likely to develop apnea, and their respiratory status may be observed without mechanical ventilation. This strategy may be used in patients who require transfer to another institution, provided that members of the transport team are experienced and prepared to intubate the patient's trachea should the need arise. Preliminary data suggest that aminophylline may be prescribed to minimize the occurrence of apnea in neonates requiring PGE_1 infusion (30). PGE_1 is a potent vasodilator, and hypotension may occur following the initiation of the drug, particularly if narcotics are also administered to facilitate procedures. This problem should be anticipated, and the hypotension usually resolves with a dose reduction of PGE_1 and volume administration. Other common side effects are listed in Table 34-2 (27,28). Although unusual, clinical deterioration may occur following the initiation of a PGE_1 infusion, and in these instances, obstruction to pulmonary venous return (e.g., obstructed total anomalous pulmonary venous return) or left atrial egress (e.g., TGA with intact ventricular septum and a restrictive atrial communication) may be present. These infants require emergent surgical or catheter intervention. Some neonates have congenital absence of the ductus arteriosus (such as those with tetralogy of Fallot with absent pulmonary valve syndrome) or some infants with pulmonary atresia, ventricular septal defect, and major aortopulmonary collateral arteries. A PGE_1 infusion in these patients may worsen cyanosis by lowering systemic vascular resistance and thereby decreasing pulmonary blood flow.

When endotracheal intubation is indicated for a neonate with critical congenital heart disease, the use of medications should be considered to blunt the stress and vagal responses to laryngoscopy, decrease oxygen consumption and thus improve oxygen delivery, and provide pharmacologic paralysis to facilitate the procedure. The choice of specific medications depends on the clinical scenario and the airway skills of the clinician. As mechanical ventilation is initiated, care must be taken in many instances to avoid excessive use of supplemental oxygen and hyperventilation. These maneuvers may lower pulmonary vascular resistance, thereby increasing the ratio of pulmonary to systemic blood flow (Qp/Qs), and "stealing" blood flow from the systemic circulation. This is discussed in greater detail in the HLHS section below.

Stable intravenous access is required for all infants with critical congenital heart disease. The need for arterial and central venous access should be determined on a case-by-case basis, based upon the heart defect, clinical presentation and anticipated preoperative course. Central access may be needed to allow for medication delivery, frequent blood sampling, and the administration of parenteral nutrition. The most accessible vessels in the newborn are the umbilical arteries and veins. The use of umbilical vessels for preoperative stabilization leaves other vessels available for future cardiac catheterizations and surgical procedures. If umbilical lines cannot be placed, the radial or femoral arteries and the femoral veins may be accessed. Some clinicians prefer to avoid placing central venous catheters in the internal jugular or subclavian veins in patients with single ventricle physiology to prevent scarring and clot formation, which may impede venous return following the bidirectional Glenn/hemi-Fontan and Fontan operations.

Adequate cardiac output and oxygen delivery usually exist in infants with critical congenital heart disease following initial stabilization and infusion of PGE_1. Infants who demonstrate signs of inadequate cardiac output may benefit from inotropic infusions, but should be critically reassessed to ensure that the PGE_1 is being delivered correctly, that appropriate oxygenation and ventilation strategies are being employed to prevent pulmonary over-circulation, and that noncardiac etiologies for shock are not present, such as pneumothorax or sepsis. Fetal-maternal hemorrhage, twin-twin transfusion, and blood loss at delivery from delayed cord clamping are examples of perinatal causes of anemia that may necessitate transfusion of packed red blood cells soon after delivery. Most patients with ductal dependent congenital heart disease require a hemoglobin level of 13 to

---

TABLE 34-2

SIDE EFFECTS OF PROSTAGLANDIN E₁ INFUSION

Respiratory	respiratory depression, apnea
Cardiovascular	hypotension, tachycardia
Central nervous system	fever, seizures
Endocrine/metabolic	hypocalcemia, hypoglycemia, cortical hyperostosis*
Gastrointestinal	diarrhea, gastric outlet obstruction*
Hematologic	inhibition of platelet aggregation
Dermatologic	flushing, harlequin rash

* Seen with long-term use.

15 gm/dL. Attention also needs to be given to acid–base status, and blood glucose and calcium levels.

Bacterial pneumonia and sepsis are often considered when an infant presents with cyanosis and shock, and empiric antibiotics may be prescribed before a diagnosis of critical congenital heart disease is confirmed. If no source of bacterial infection is identified, the antibiotics may be discontinued after a 48-hour period. Although it has been suggested that the use of PGE_1 increases the risk of bacterial infection, there is no published evidence to support this concept.

Neonates with critical congenital heart disease require transport to congenital heart centers for further evaluation and intervention. Experienced pediatric transport teams are used when available, and close communication is required with the intensivist and pediatric cardiologist at the congenital heart center throughout the transport process. During transport, care must be taken to maintain a normal patient temperature as hypothermia will increase systemic vascular resistance and may be poorly tolerated. The transport team members must understand that normal ventilation and the avoidance of excessive supplemental oxygen are important to maintain a balanced circulation in many infants with ductal dependent systemic or pulmonary blood flow.

Evaluation at the Congenital Heart Center

Upon arrival to the tertiary care center, the intensivist and nursing staff should obtain a detailed report from the transport team. Historical features that are useful to direct the diagnostic evaluation and initial management include the results of fetal echocardiogram(s), complications of the pregnancy, family history, estimated gestational age of the fetus, severity of cyanosis or shock prior to initial resuscitation, presence of risk factors for infection, and suspected noncardiac congenital anomalies.

A detailed physical examination includes a review of recent and current vital signs. Heart rates are usually within the normal range for age. Four-extremity blood measurements should be obtained. Pulse oximetry results are interpreted in the context of the patient's physiology. The presence of dysmorphic facial features may suggest a specific genetic syndrome. The cardiac examination begins with inspection and palpation of the precordium. An increased right ventricular impulse is often present with significant left ventricular outflow tract obstruction and/or pulmonary hypertension. Auscultation is performed with attention to splitting and quality of the second heart sound, systolic ejection clicks, and the presence of pathologic systolic or diastolic murmurs. The span of the liver is determined, and the quality of the peripheral pulses and perfusion are noted.

The ECG and CXR are reviewed with attention to features that may suggest an underlying cardiac diagnosis as described above. The CXR should also be reviewed to ensure that any tubes or lines placed prior to transport have not migrated. Cardiopulmonary instability in the infant with critical congenital heart disease is often as a

result of noncardiac issues, such as respiratory distress syndrome, tension pneumothorax, or endotracheal tube plugging or malposition.

Even if an echocardiogram has been performed at the referring institution, a complete echocardiogram is obtained upon arrival to the congenital heart center to confirm the diagnosis and clarify anatomic and physiologic details. Complete diagnostic information is obtained in the vast majority of patients with critical congenital heart disease using transthoracic echocardiogram, eliminating the need for diagnostic cardiac catheterization (31,32). Occasionally a critically ill infant with congenital heart disease will not tolerate a prolonged echocardiogram, as a result of temperature instability related to exposure, or hypotension related to abdominal compression during subcostal imaging.

Limited indications exist for diagnostic cardiac catheterization in the current era. For example, infants with pulmonary atresia, VSD and major aortopulmonary collateral arteries (MAPCAs) usually require catheterization to define all sources of pulmonary arterial blood flow. Coronary anatomy can usually be clarified by echocardiography, but occasionally angiography is required, as is the case in some infants with tetralogy of Fallot, pulmonary atresia with intact ventricular septum, or TGA (33). Hemodynamic data, such as pulmonary vascular resistance, may need to be obtained by cardiac catheterization in selected older infants prior to a definitive procedure. Cardiac catheterization is more commonly indicated to perform interventional procedures. For example, neonates with TGA and intact ventricular septum may require enlargement of the atrial communication, and those with HLHS and intact atrial septum require emergent creation of an adequate atrial septal defect (ASD) to allow egress of pulmonary venous blood from the left atrium into the right atrium (34,35). Balloon valvuloplasty of critical aortic or pulmonary valve stenosis is commonly performed in many centers. Cardiac MRI, spiral CT, and electron beam tomography are evolving tools that are currently available in selected centers and are most useful for clarifying anatomy of extracardiac vessels (36,37).

Evaluation of other organ systems is indicated in infants with critical congenital heart disease prior to intervention. Basic laboratory studies are obtained to evaluate acid–base status, oxygenation and ventilation, and the hepatic, renal and hematologic systems. Recovery of end-organ function in infants who present in shock is to be expected in nearly all cases following appropriate resuscitation and stabilization. Infants who are premature or who present with severe cyanosis or shock should have a head ultrasound performed to evaluate for intracranial hemorrhage. If not clear by echocardiography, an abdominal ultrasound is indicated in patients with heart disease associated with heterotaxy syndrome to determine the sidedness of the liver and spleen. An upper gastrointestinal series may be needed in such infants to evaluate for malrotation. Any suspected hematologic issues, such as thrombocytopenia or a bleeding diathesis, should be thoroughly evaluated prior to intervention. Other major birth defects may be seen in up to 25% of patients with significant congenital heart disease. For example, infants with conotruncal heart defects, such as tetralogy of Fallot, pulmonary atresia with VSD, interrupted aortic arch, and truncus arteriosus have an increased risk compared with the general population of having an associated oral cleft, omphalocele, tracho-esophageal fistula, or imperforate anus (38). There is an increased incidence of renal anomalies in infants with congenital heart disease who have other major congenital anomalies, and a screening renal ultrasound may be indicated in this subset of patients (39).

A chromosomal abnormality or easily definable genetic syndrome may be identified in approximately 20% of infants with congenital heart disease. Table 34-3 lists selected common chromosomal abnormalities and genetic syndromes, and the congenital heart lesions with which they are associated (40–42).

Preoperative Supportive Care: General Principles

Cardiopulmonary Management

Infants with ductal dependent congenital heart disease require a "balanced" circulation to achieve adequate systemic and pulmonary blood flow. Those who present with severe cyanosis or shock, or require prolonged interhospital transport are tracheally intubated and mechanical ventilation is provided. Great care must be taken throughout the preoperative period to ensure that appropriate ventilation and oxygenation strategies are used to prevent an iatrogenic imbalance between systemic and pulmonary blood flow. In particular, in patients with ductal dependent systemic blood flow (e.g., HLHS or interrupted aortic arch), hyperventilation and provision of supplemental oxygen will decrease pulmonary vascular resistance, thereby promoting increased pulmonary to systemic flow ratio (Qp/Qs), and "steal" from the systemic and coronary circulations. Such patients will have inappropriately high systemic oxygen saturations (greater than 90%), poor systemic perfusion and are at risk of developing myocardial dysfunction as a result of volume overload and coronary ischemia, renal insufficiency, and/or NEC. Interventions that may be employed to increase pulmonary vascular resistance and improve the balance between systemic and pulmonary circulations, including subambient FiO_2 and hypoventilation, are discussed below in the section on preoperative management of HLHS. Neonates with left ventricular outflow tract obstruction who are stable at presentation may be allowed to spontaneously breathe while awaiting surgical intervention, with close monitoring of their cardiopulmonary status. These neonates will typically have relatively high systemic oxygen saturations (greater than 90%) and "quiet tachypnea," but will maintain adequate peripheral pulses, urine output, and low

TABLE 34-3

SELECTED COMMON CHROMOSOMAL ABNORMALITIES AND GENETIC SYNDROMES ASSOCIATED WITH CONGENITAL HEART DISEASE (SEE ALSO TABLE 33–5)

Patient Group	Incidence of CHD	Most Common Lesions		
		1	2	3
Trisomy 21 (Down S.)	40–50%	AVSD	VSD	ASD
Trisomy 18 (Edwards S.)	90%	VSD	PDA	ASD
Trisomy 13	80%	VSD	PDA	ASD
4p- (Wolf-Hirschhorn S.)	50%	VSD	PDA	ASD
5p- (Cri-du-Chat S.)	30%	variable		
Monosomy X (Turner S.)	20%	CoA	BAV	AS
Noonan S.	66%	PS	HCM	
Holt-Oram S.	90%	ASD	VSD	MVP
Williams S.	75%	supravalvar AS	PPS	PS
22q11 deletion (DiGeorge)	80%	IAA	truncus	TOF
Goldenhar S.	25%	VSD	PDA	TOF
VATER/VACTERL	variable			
CHARGE association	75%	conotruncal		
Beckwith-Wiedmann S.	common	HCM		
Marfan's S.	100% (neonatal)	dilated AAo	MVP/MR	AR

AR, aortic regurgitation; AS, aortic valve stenosis; AAo, ascending aorta; ASD, atrial septal defect; AVSD, atrioventricular septal defect; BAV, bicuspid aortic valve; CHARGE, acronym for coloboma, heart defects, atresia of the posterior choanae, retarded growth/development, genital hypoplasia, ear anomalies/deafness; CoA, coarctation of aorta; HCM, hypertrophic cardiomyopathy; IAA, interrupted aortic arch; MVP, mitral valve prolapse; MR, mitral regurgitation; PDA, patent ductus arteriosus; PPS, peripheral pulmonary stenosis; PS, pulmonary valve stenosis; S, syndrome; TOF, tetralogy of Fallot; VATER/VACTERL, acronyms for vertebral anomalies, anal atresia, cardiac defects, tracheoesophageal fistula, esophageal atresia, renal defects, limb defects; VSD, ventricular septal defect.

lactate levels. Diuretics and low dose inotropic support are occasionally needed to alleviate pulmonary edema and to support the volume-loaded ventricular myocardium. In neonates with right ventricular outflow tract obstruction, the ductus arteriosus is often somewhat stenotic and takes a tortuous course from the aorta to the pulmonary artery, related to the in utero blood flow pattern, which typically will prevent torrential pulmonary blood flow. Thus marked pulmonary overcirculation is less of a clinical concern in ductal-dependent neonates with right ventricular outflow tract obstruction.

Inotropic support is occasionally necessary for neonates with congenital heart disease, particularly those with volume loaded single ventricles, but escalating inotropic or vasopressor requirements often signify a noncardiac problem or inadequate systemic cardiac output as a result of Qp/Qs imbalance. Inotropic agents are discussed in the postoperative section on low cardiac output.

Prematurity

The premature infant with critical congenital heart disease presents a significant challenge. Problems inherent to prematurity, including temperature instability, decreased nutritional reserve, intraventricular hemorrhage, respiratory distress syndrome, infection, and NEC, may develop during the pre- and postoperative course. In preterm infants with critical congenital heart disease, a management strategy of prolonged medical therapy to achieve weight gain prior to surgery is fraught with complications related to infection, heart failure and feeding intolerance (43,44). Advances in cardiopulmonary bypass techniques and miniaturization of surgical equipment allow for the safe conduct of open-heart surgery in these patients. Several reports depict the recent experience with palliative or definitive surgical intervention in premature infants with critical congenital heart disease. Reddy and associates reported the University of California at San Francisco experience with complete (two-ventricle) repair in 102 infants with significant congenital heart disease weighing less than 2,500 grams. These investigators found higher preoperative morbidity in the group of patients having delayed repair. The early and late mortalities were 10 and 8%, respectively, and no patient had postbypass intracranial hemorrhage (44). Investigators from the same center reported a series of 20 very low birth weight (LBW) (< 1,500 gm) infants with symptomatic congenital heart disease who underwent complete repair with only two deaths (10%) (45). Rossi and associates reported a series of infants weighing less than 2 kg, 73% of which were born prematurely. Hospital survival was 83%, and 24% of the patients had neurologic complications (46). Bacha and associates, in a study of 18 infants weighing less than 2 kg with coarctation of the aorta, found that repair can be accomplished with low operative mortality, but the residual or recurrent coarctation rate was 44% (47). Results for single ventricle palliation are less encouraging. The reported mortality for infants weighing less than 2.5 kg at the time of Norwood operation for HLHS or other single ventricle variants is 45% to 51% (48,49). Thus, although prematurity and LBW complicate the care of infants with significant heart disease, early intervention, including corrective surgery, can be performed with acceptable morbidity and mortality.

Nutrition

Although the enteral route is the preferred method for providing nutrition to infants in the intensive care unit, those with critical congenital heart disease awaiting intervention often have several pathophysiologic features that must be considered prior to initiation of enteral feedings. The combination of myocardial dysfunction, cyanosis and falling pulmonary vascular resistance, the later allowing increased diastolic runoff through the ductus arteriosus, may result in inadequate mesenteric oxygen delivery. In one large, retrospective study, approximately 3% of neonates admitted to a busy cardiac intensive care unit developed NEC (50). Independent risk factors for developing NEC were prematurity, a history of resuscitation from severe cyanosis or shock, HLHS, or the presence of diastolic runoff through the ductus arteriosus or other aorto-pulmonary connections (50). In part as a result of the absence of randomized studies, the use of enteral nutrition in infants with ductal-dependent congenital heart disease remains controversial and clinical practice varies widely. The risk-benefit ratio for providing enteral nutrition must be individually determined for each patient. One approach is to avoid enteral feeding in those infants who have one or more of the aforementioned risk factors. It is also reasonable to consider enteral feedings in those infants with an acceptable diastolic blood pressure despite the presence of a patent ductus arteriosus, provided that additional risk factors are not present.

Congenital Complete Heart Block

Congenital complete heart block may be associated with structural heart disease including atrioventricular canal defects and complex lesions with ventricular inversion. In neonates with normal intracardiac anatomy, there is a high incidence of maternal autoimmune disease, particularly systemic lupus erythematosus (51). Congenital complete heart block is diagnosed electrocardiographically when atrioventricular dissociation is present with an atrial rate that is appropriate for age and a slow ventricular rate. The diagnosis may be made in utero by fetal echocardiography and may be associated with hydrops fetalis. Dual chamber epicardial pacemaker placement is indicated when third degree congenital atrioventricular heart block is associated with a wide QRS escape rhythm, complex ventricular ectopy, or ventricular dysfunction. A pacemaker is also indicated in an infant with a ventricular rate less than 50 to 55 beats per minute, or with congenital heart disease and a ventricular rate less than 70 beats per minute (52).

PREOPERATIVE PHYSIOLOGY AND MANAGEMENT: SPECIFIC LESIONS

Right Ventricular Outflow Tract Obstruction

Critical Pulmonary Valve Stenosis

In neonates with critical pulmonary valve stenosis, the pulmonary valve leaflets are thickened and fused to a variable extent, and their mobility is decreased (Fig. 34-1, see also color plate). The pulmonary valve annulus is hypoplastic in severe cases. The pulmonary arteries are usually of normal size, but may be stenotic or dilated. The right ventricle is often hypertrophied and mildly hypoplastic. Significant tricuspid regurgitation, and a right to left atrial shunt are present (53). Infants with isolated critical pulmonary valve stenosis will develop significant cyanosis (See Color Plate) upon closure of the ductus arteriosus. Such infants are dependent on a PGE$_1$ infusion to maintain ductal patency for adequate pulmonary blood flow. Although open surgical valvotomy was routinely performed in the past to relieve right ventricular outflow tract obstruction, most of these infants are candidates for a balloon valvuloplasty in the cardiac catheterization laboratory. Balloon valvuloplasty is successful in approximately 60% to 80% of cases (53–58). Neonates who fail an attempted balloon valvuloplasty may have smaller right heart structures, and are referred for a surgical valvotomy +/− a systemic to pulmonary artery shunt (59,60).

Tetralogy of Fallot

Tetralogy of Fallot, the most common cyanotic congenital heart lesion, is comprised of an anterior malalignment VSD in a heart with two ventricles and aortic to mitral fibrous continuity. Anatomic details that need to be clarified at the time of diagnosis include the severity and location of right ventricular outflow tract obstruction, the pulmonary artery anatomy, the presence of additional VSDs, the sidedness of the aortic arch (rightward in 25%), and the coronary artery anatomy. The left coronary artery may arise from the right coronary artery and cross the right ventricular outflow tract in 5% of cases. Complete anatomic information is usually obtainable by transthoracic echocardiogram (33). If uncertainty exists about the coronary artery anatomy, some surgeons may request a cardiac catheterization, as great care must be taken not to injure the coronary vessels during right ventricular outflow tract reconstruction. Chromosome 22q11 deletion is present in 15% of patients with tetralogy of Fallot, and those with a right aortic arch are at higher risk (41).

In neonates with tetralogy of Fallot, a wide spectrum of presentation exists, depending in large part upon the degree of malalignment of the conal septum into the right ventricular outflow tract. Infants with a minimal degree of obstruction to pulmonary blood flow, commonly referred to as "pink tets," are usually asymptomatic and fairly well oxygenated (systemic saturations > 85%) soon after birth. They are commonly observed in the hospital until the ductus arteriosus closes and then sent home to await surgical repair within the first 6 months of life. Occasionally a "pink tet" will mimic the pathophysiology of an infant with a large VSD and develop congestive heart failure within the first few months of life as pulmonary vascular resistance falls. More commonly these patients develop progressive right ventricular outflow tract obstruction and cyanosis. The exact timing of repair varies depending

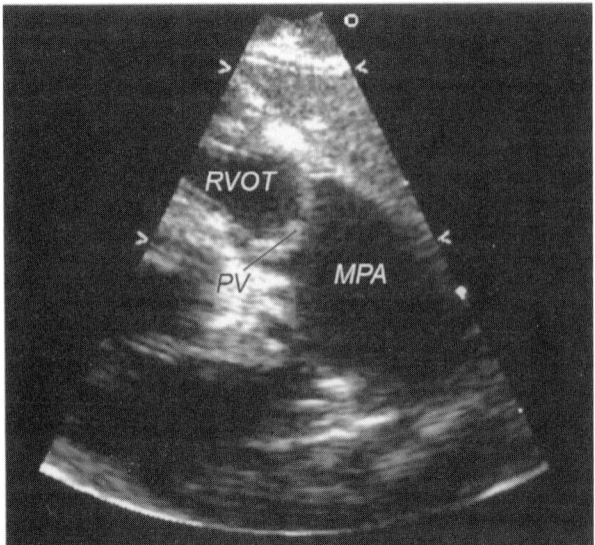

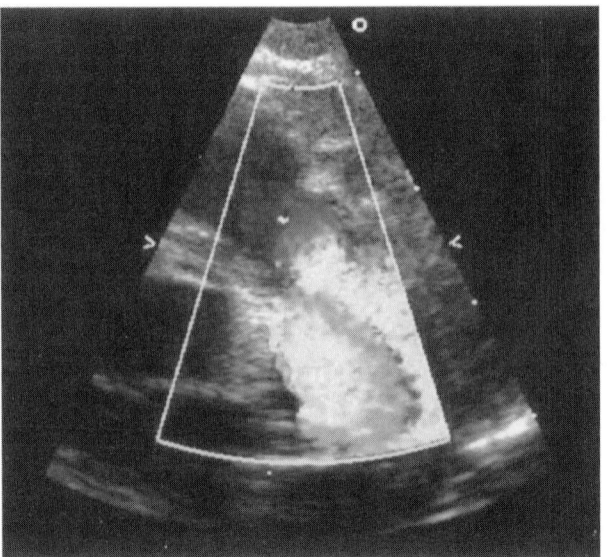

Figure 34-1   Critical pulmonary valve stenosis. **A.** Two-dimensional echocardiogram from the parasternal long axis view demonstrating thickened and doming pulmonary valve leaflets. Note the poststenotic dilation of the main pulmonary artery. **B.** Application of color Doppler during ventricular systole demonstrates a turbulent flow jet originating at the pulmonary valve leaflets and extending into the main pulmonary artery. MPA, main pulmonary artery; PV, pulmonary valve; RVOT, right ventricular outflow tract. (See color plate)

upon several variables including the development of increasing cyanosis, hypercyanotic spells ("TET spells"), and institutional preference (2,61). Infants with tetralogy of Fallot and more severe right ventricular outflow tract obstruction or pulmonary atresia will develop excessive cyanosis (oxygen saturation < 75%–80%) upon closure of the ductus arteriosus. Such patients will require surgical intervention during the initial hospitalization. Either a complete repair or a systemic to pulmonary shunt is performed, depending on the details of the anatomy and surgeon preference (62).

Hypercyanotic episodes, or "TET spells," are potentially life-threatening events notable for significant desaturation and irritability as a result of an acute decrease in pulmonary blood flow. The precise etiology of these spells is unclear but has been attributed to spasm of the infundibular conus, an imbalance between the systemic and pulmonary vascular resistances, increased systemic venous return, and/or tachycardia, all of which may lead to a progressive cycle of decreased pulmonary blood flow, increased cyanosis, and eventually metabolic acidosis. Although TOF spells can occur at any age, the incidence seems to increase after 4 to 6 months of age, which is one of the reasons that early complete repair before this age is commonly recommended. TET spells can be triggered by medical procedures including placement of intravenous catheters and cardiac catheterization. Infants with tetralogy of Fallot have a fixed component of obstruction to pulmonary blood flow, and thus will normally develop transient desaturation with agitation and feeding as a result of increased oxygen consumption and cardiac output. Clinical judgment is required to differentiate a true TET spell from these common and benign desaturation episodes. The absence of a murmur during a true TET spell, signifying a substantial reduction of blood flow across the right ventricular outflow tract, may be useful in this regard. Treatment strategies are implemented with the goal of decreasing patient agitation and heart rate, increasing systemic vascular resistance and pulmonary blood flow, and correcting metabolic acidosis (Table 34-4). Prompt surgical intervention is indicated once an infant has had a TET spell.

Absent pulmonary valve syndrome, identified by the presence of rudimentary pulmonary valve leaflets and free pulmonary insufficiency, is a relatively rare lesion, present in approximately 3% of all patients with tetralogy of Fallot. This lesion is most notable for *in utero* development of aneurysmal dilation of the pulmonary arteries, which may occur as a result of the lack of a ductus arteriosus or as a result of the pulsatile blood flow pattern across the right ventricular outflow tract. When compared with infants with typical tetralogy of Fallot, there may be a higher incidence of chromosome 22q11 deletion in those with absent pulmonary valve (63). A nearly pathognomonic to-and-fro ("sawing wood") murmur is heard as a result of pulmonary annulus stenosis and free pulmonary insufficiency (Fig. 34-2, see also color plate). Such patients may have minimal if any respiratory symptoms and behave much like a "pink tet," or present with severe problems with oxygenation and ventilation soon after birth as a result of compression of the bronchi by the dilated pulmonary arteries (64). Intubation, mechanical ventilation (with judicious use of positive end-expiratory pressure), and deep sedation may be life saving in neonates with symptomatic airway obstruction. Prone positioning may be advantageous as gravity will allow the pulmonary arteries to fall off the mainstem bronchi, thus permitting adequate gas exchange (65). Prompt surgical repair is indicated in symptomatic neonates.

Pulmonary Atresia, Ventricular Septal Defect, Major Aortopulmonary Collateral Arteries

Infants with pulmonary atresia, VSD and MAPCAs represent a challenging subset of infants with pulmonary atresia. This lesion is also referred to as tetralogy of Fallot, pulmonary atresia and MAPCAs. In addition to the anatomic features of tetralogy of Fallot as described above, the true pulmonary arteries are often diminutive or absent, and a variable number of aortopulmonary collaterals arise from the aorta or bracheocephalic vessels to supply pulmonary blood flow. Infants with this lesion will present with either cyanosis or congestive heart failure, depending upon the cardiac anatomy (66). The physical examination may be notable for the presence of a widely radiating continuous murmur produced by the aortopulmonary collateral blood flow. These infants are generally not dependent upon prostaglandin infusion unless a major aortopulmonary

TABLE 34-4

TREATMENT FOR HYPERCYANOTIC EPISODES ("TOF SPELLS")

Intervention	Effect on Pathophysiology
Knee-chest position	↑ systemic vascular resistance
Oxygen	↓ pulmonary vascular resistance
Morphine	↓ agitation
Ketamine	↓ agitation, ↑ systemic vascular resistance
Propranolol	↓ infundibular spasm, ↓ heart rate
Sodium bicarbonate	↓ metabolic acidosis
Phenylephrine	↑ systemic vascular resistance
Cardiopulmonary bypass	rescue therapy when above measures fail

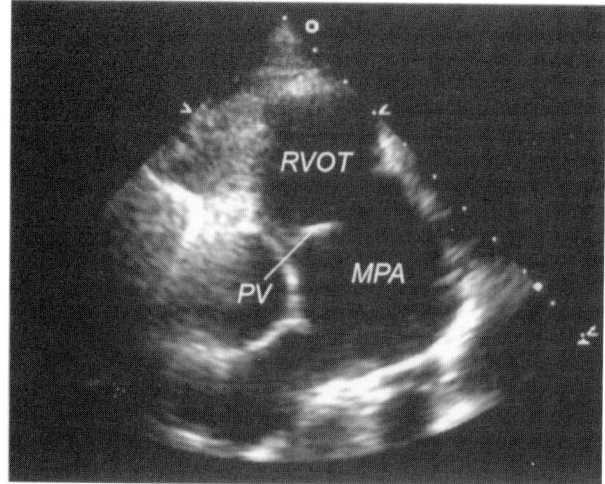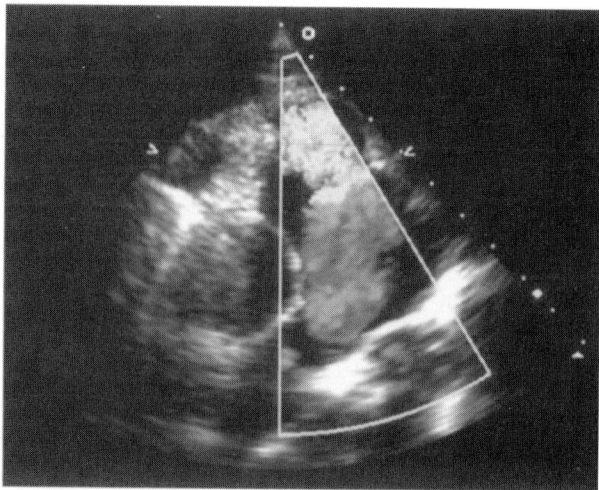

Figure 34-2 Tetralogy of Fallot with absent pulmonary valve. **A.** Two-dimensional echocardiogram from the parasternal long axis view demonstrating rudimentary pulmonary valve leaflets and aneurysmal dilation of the main pulmonary artery. **B.** Application of color Doppler during ventricular diastole revealing free regurgitation from the main pulmonary artery into the right ventricular outflow tract. MPA, main pulmonary artery; PV, pulmonary valve; RVOT, right ventricular outflow tract. (See color plate)

collateral vessel arises from the ductus arteriosus. Cardiac catheterization is required to identify all sources of pulmonary blood flow. Surgical strategy must then be individualized depending upon the pulmonary artery and collateral vessel anatomy. True pulmonary arteries, MAPCAs, or both may supply blood to individual segments of the lungs. The ultimate goal is to encourage true pulmonary artery growth and incorporate as many arterial blood vessels and lung segments into the repair as possible to maximize the effective pulmonary arterial vascular bed, and thus minimize right ventricular hypertension following VSD closure. In situations in which dual blood supply to a lung segment exists, the MAPCAs are coil occluded in the cardiac catheterization laboratory or ligated at the time of surgery to eliminate left to right shunting. As with other conotruncal defects, these infants should undergo genetic testing for chromosome 22q11 deletion.

Pulmonary Atresia with Intact Ventricular Septum

Pulmonary atresia is characterized by a membranous or plate-like obstruction of the right ventricular outflow tract at the level of the pulmonary valve, with variable degrees of hypoplasia of the tricuspid valve and right ventricle, and occasional coronary artery fistulous connections to the right ventricle. Systemic venous return to the right atrium flows through an obligatory atrial communication to the left atrium. Infants with pulmonary atresia and intact ventricular septum will manifest with significant cyanosis upon closure of the ductus arteriosus, and are thus dependent on prostaglandin infusion. Intervention in these patients depends on two key issues: the adequacy of the right ventricular size to support a two-ventricular circulation, and on the presence of "right ventricle dependent coronary circulation."

The right ventricle must have adequate size to support the entire right heart circulation if these patients are to be considered for a two-ventricle repair. The size of the tricuspid valve annulus plays an important role in the decision making process (67). Infants with pulmonary atresia and intact ventricular septum, particularly those with small tricuspid valve annulus size, may have significant fistula communications between the right ventricle and the coronary circulation, known as coronary-cameral fistulae, which may be identified by echocardiogram and further characterized by cardiac catheterization (68,69). If coronary stenoses exist such that a significant amount of coronary blood flow to the myocardium is derived from and dependent upon the coronary cameral fistulae, then "right ventricular dependent coronary circulation" is present. If the right ventricular outflow tract obstruction is relieved in an infant with "right ventricular dependent coronary circulation," coronary perfusion pressure falls and the patient may develop a myocardial infarction. Thus, if the right ventricle is not of adequate size, or if "right ventricle dependent coronary circulation" exists, these patients are referred for a systemic to pulmonary artery shunt in anticipation of an eventual Fontan operation. If a complete two-ventricle repair is deemed appropriate, this may be performed as a primary operation in the neonatal period, although more commonly a systemic to pulmonary artery shunt and right ventricular outflow tract decompression is initially performed to encourage right ventricular growth, with complete repair in later infancy (70). Some infants with membranous pulmonary atresia and intact ventricular septum who meet criteria for a two ventricular repair may undergo perforation of the pulmonary valve using a stiff wire, a radiofrequency ablation catheter, or a laser catheter, followed by balloon valvuloplasty (54,58,71). In well-selected patients, the use of transcatheter intervention may eliminate the need for surgical intervention. The decision to attempt transcatheter intervention is made considering patient size, co-morbidities, anatomic details, and institutional experience.

Ebstein's Anomaly of the Tricuspid Valve

Ebstein's anomaly of the tricuspid valve is a malformation in which the septal and posterior leaflets of the tricuspid valve are displaced to a variable extent into the anatomic right ventricle, and the anterior leaflet, although not inferiorly displaced, is redundant. Tricuspid regurgitation of variable severity occurs (Fig. 34-3, see also Color Plate). One or more accessory connections may be present at the tricuspid valve annulus, creating the necessary substrate for atrio-ventricular reentrant tachycardia. The clinical presentation is usually one of right-sided congestive heart failure and arrhythmias in adolescence or early adulthood. A small subset of infants with Ebstein's anomaly, those with severe tricuspid regurgitation, a large "atrialized" portion of the right ventricle, severe cardiomegaly, and pulmonary hypoplasia are critically ill soon after birth and have a high mortality (72). These neonates will present with severe cyanosis as a result of functional right ventricular outflow tract obstruction, and right to left shunting at the atrial level. Infants with significant cyanosis should be started on PGE_1, and judicious use of positive end-expiratory pressure is required to re-expand the lungs, which are compressed by the generous heart size (73). Additionally, standard measures including inhaled nitric oxide should be employed to decrease pulmonary vascular resistance and cyanosis. In many of these patients, as pulmonary vascular resistance falls over time, forward flow increases across the right ventricular outflow tract, cyanosis decreases, and surgery can be deferred. For those neonates with refractory cyanosis, referral is made

for either a primary complete repair, consisting of a reduction atrioplasty, fenestrated closure of the atrial septum and tricuspid valvuloplasty, or palliation toward the Fontan pathway starting with a systemic to pulmonary artery shunt (73–75).

Left Ventricular Outflow Tract Obstruction

Critical Aortic Valve Stenosis

Isolated congenital aortic valve disease may present in a variety of ways, depending primarily upon the severity of stenosis. A bicuspid aortic valve without stenosis or insufficiency may be an incidental finding in an otherwise healthy patient. At the other extreme, newborns with critical aortic valve stenosis develop shock upon closure of the ductus arteriosus. The murmur is typically softer than expected as a result of the low cardiac output state, and the gradient estimated by echocardiography may not correlate with the severity of the stenosis. Initiation of PGE_1 infusion allows blood from the right ventricle to provide systemic perfusion until an intervention can be performed (76). Once the infant is stabilized, echocardiographic information must be carefully reviewed to predict whether the left ventricle is of adequate size to sustain the systemic circulation following a two-ventricle repair (77). Infants thought to be suitable for a two-ventricle repair usually will be referred for a balloon aortic valvuloplasty; although a surgical aortic valvotomy is an acceptable option (78–80). If hypoplasia of multiple left sided structures suggests that the left ventricle will not be able to support the circulation, then a Norwood operation or heart transplantation may be considered.

Critical Coarctation of the Aorta

A coarctation of the aorta is present when a significant narrowing exists in the thoracic aorta just distal to the left

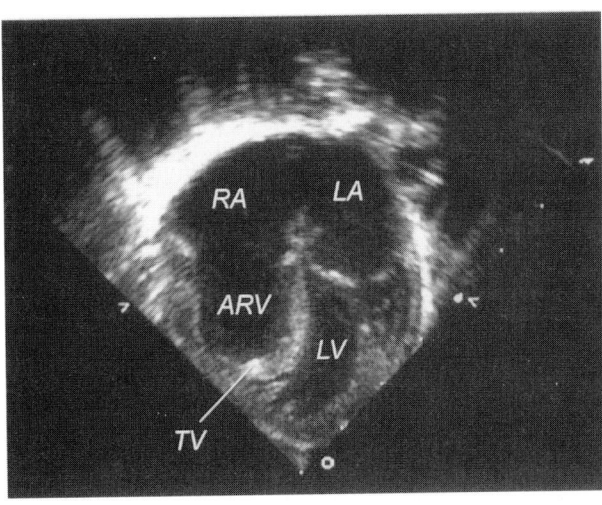

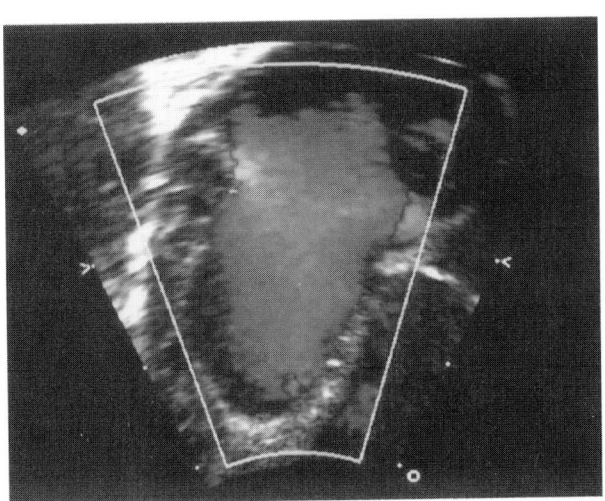

A   **B**

Figure 34-3 Ebstein's anomaly of the tricuspid valve. **A.** Two-dimensional echocardiogram from the apical four-chamber view demonstrating significant displacement of the tricuspid valve leaflets into the right ventricle. **B.** During ventricular diastole, color Doppler demonstrating free retrograde flow across the tricuspid valve annulus. ARV, atrialized right ventricle; LA, left atrium; LV, left ventricle; RA, right atrium; TV, tricuspid valve. (See color plate)

subclavian artery. A "posterior shelf" is present opposite the insertion site of the patent ductus arteriosus. Coarctation of the aorta may exist in isolation or can be associated with aortic arch hypoplasia, a VSD, or other complex intracardiac lesions. When present in isolation, coarctation of the aorta is "critical" when ductal dependent systemic blood flow exists, which represents only about 10% of cases. Neonates with isolated critical coarctation of the aorta also will present with shock if the diagnosis is not made before significant constriction of the ductus arteriosus occurs (Fig. 34-4). Prior to the development of shock, the diagnosis should be suspected by the detection of a brachial-femoral pulse discrepancy, which can be confirmed by measuring an arm-leg blood systolic pressure gradient. A systolic blood pressure gradient between the upper and lower extremities of greater than 10 mm Hg is clinically significant. In approximately 5% of infants with isolated coarctation of the aorta, the right subclavian artery will arise aberrantly from the descending thoracic aorta, distal to the coarctation. Thus it is important to palpate pulses and measure blood pressure in both upper extremities in all infants with suspected coarctation. Occasionally differential cyanosis will be present as the lower body is being perfused by deoxygenated blood from the ductus arteriosus. PGE_1 infusion will almost always reopen the ductus arteriosus and allow recovery of end-organ function prior to surgical repair

(76). In the absence of data from randomized clinical trials, the method of nutritional support for these patients should be individualized and deserves comment. Those neonates with critical coarctation who present in shock with metabolic acidosis and laboratory evidence of end-organ dysfunction should be maintained on bowel rest prior to surgery, and nutritional support is provided with total parenteral nutrition. However, enteral feeds may be considered in the subset of infants who are diagnosed prior to the development of shock, started on PGE_1, and subsequently have reasonable femoral pulses and diastolic blood pressure distal to the coarctation.

Hypoplastic Left Heart Syndrome

HLHS exists when there is severe mitral and aortic valve stenosis or atresia, a diminutive left ventricle, ascending aorta, and aortic arch, and often a juxtaductal coarctation of the aorta. Following birth there are two key communications that need to remain open to permit cardiopulmonary stability. A patent ductus arteriosus (PDA) is necessary to allow blood flow from the pulmonary artery to reach the systemic circulation, and shock will develop once the ductus arteriosus constricts. An adequate ASD is also necessary to allow egress of the pulmonary venous

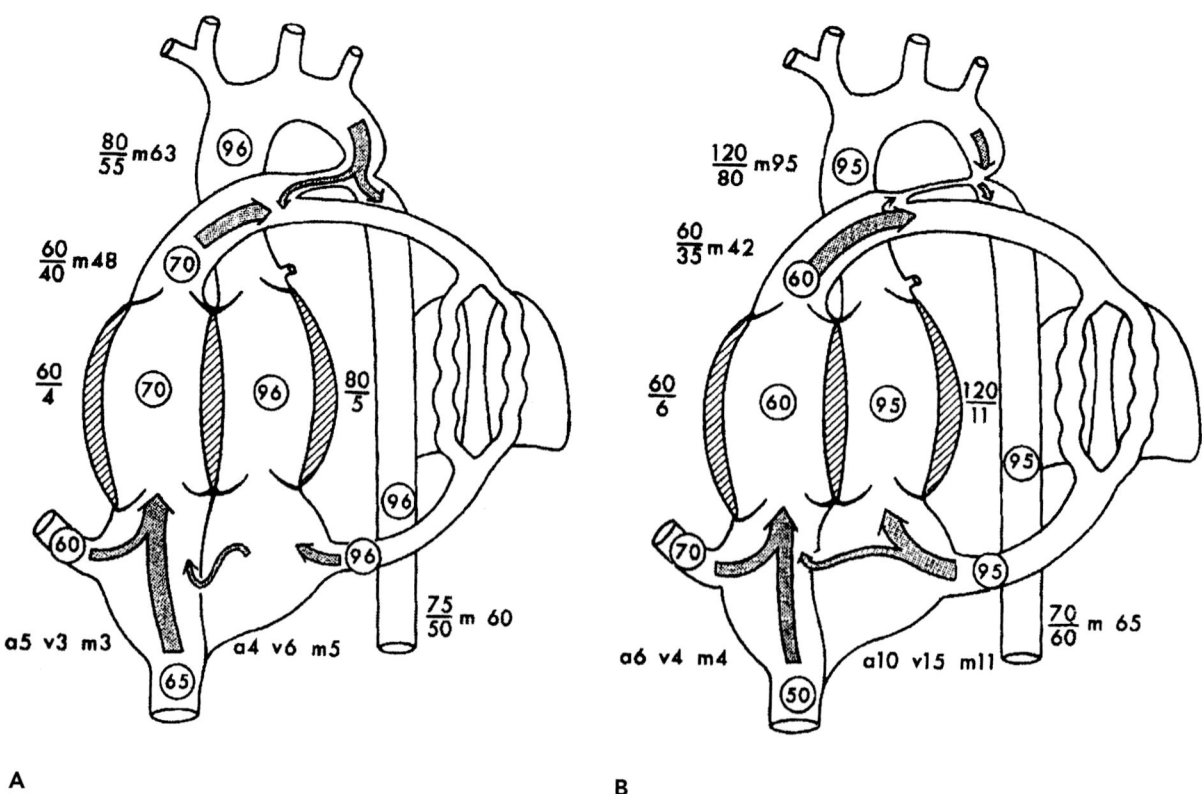

Figure 34-4 Schematic diagram of hemodynamic data and oxygen saturation levels in a neonate with critical coarctation of the aorta. **A:** Hemodynamic data and oxygen saturation levels prior to ductal closure. **B:** Hemodynamic data and oxygen saturation levels following ductal closure. Note the development of systemic hypertension and left atrial hypertension, the persistence of pulmonary hypertension, and the decrease in cardiac output as demonstrated by the lower oxygen saturation level in the inferior vena cava (a, atrial; v, ventricle; m, mean). Reprinted from Rudolph AM. Aortic arch obstruction. In: *Congenital diseases of the heart: clinical-physiological considerations,* 2nd ed. Armonk, NY: Futura, 2001:382–383, with permission.

blood flow from the left atrium to the right atrium. The 5% of infants with HLHS who have a severely restrictive or intact atrial septum will develop profound cyanosis, pulmonary edema, and shock almost immediately following delivery.

Initially, most patients with HLHS (assuming an unrestrictive or mildly restrictive atrial communication) will be hemodynamically stable following the initiation of a PGE_1 infusion. Over several days, however, as pulmonary vascular resistance falls, the ratio of pulmonary to systemic blood flow (Qp/Qs) will increase, leading to an increase in arterial oxygen saturation. Poor systemic circulation may manifest, and the neonate may develop right ventricular volume overload, and coronary and end-organ ischemia. The Qp/Qs may be calculated by the following equation which is derived from the Fick principle: $Qp/Qs = (SaO_2–SvO_2)/(PvO_2–PaO_2)$, in which SaO_2 = aortic saturation; SvO_2 = mixed venous saturation (estimated by the superior vena cava oxygen saturation); PvO_2 = pulmonary venous oxygen saturation (assumed to be > 95% if not directly measured); and PaO_2 = pulmonary artery oxygen saturation (assumed equal to the aortic saturation). Most preoperative neonates will not have a catheter positioned in the superior vena cava to measure SvO_2, and thus the Qp/Qs cannot be precisely calculated. Determination of an absolute value for Qp/Qs is of less importance than having an appreciation for the physiologic disturbance that develops as these neonates become progressively over circulated. Theoretical computer models of newborns with

HLHS demonstrate that, beyond a certain point, slight increases in arterial oxygen saturation are associated with significant decreases in oxygen delivery, and that maximal oxygen delivery occurs at a Qp/Qs less than 1 (Fig. 34-5 and 34.6) (81,82). This model also demonstrates that a SvO_2 less than 40%, or a SaO_2-SvO_2 difference of more than 40%, is likely associated with a severe derangement in systemic oxygen delivery, related to either a high Qp/Qs or low cardiac output (82).

In the typical neonate with HLHS, interventions that lower the pulmonary vascular resistance, such as supplemental oxygen and hyperventilation, may increase Qp/Qs and should be avoided. Patients with pulmonary over-circulation (high Qp/Qs) and evidence of poor end-organ perfusion (e.g., poor urine output, rising lactate levels, diminished peripheral pulses) may be treated with sub-ambient FiO_2, obtained using supplemental inhaled nitrogen to increase pulmonary vascular resistance and thus restore the balance between systemic and pulmonary blood flow (83,84). The supplemental nitrogen may be delivered through the endotracheal tube or through a nasal cannula in neonates who are spontaneously breathing. Pulmonary vascular resistance may also be increased in such patients using supplemental inspired carbon dioxide (CO_2) (85). In a prospective, randomized, crossover study, the impact of hypoxia (17% FiO_2) vs. hypercarbia (2.7% $FiCO_2$) on systemic oxygen delivery in preoperative neonates with HLHS was evaluated (86). All patients were receiving mechanical ventilation, deep sedation or anesthesia, and

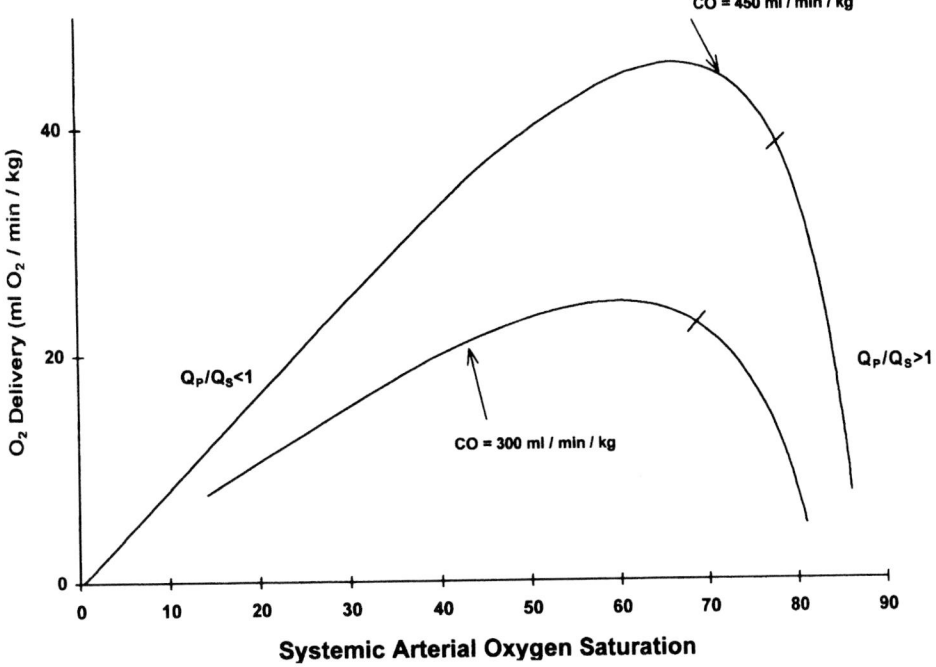

Figure 34-5 Systemic arterial oxygen saturation vs. systemic oxygen (O_2) delivery in the theoretical newborn with hypoplastic left heart syndrome. A computer model was used to generate the curves by setting the cardiac output (CO) at 300 or 450 mL/kg/min and varying Qp/Qs from 0.2 to 10. The short line on each curve represents the point at which Qp/Qs = 1. As SaO_2 increases, oxygen delivery increases and reaches a peak, and then decreases rapidly. Peak oxygen delivery occurs at a Qp/Qs < 1. Reprinted from Barnea O, Santamore WP, Rossi A, et al. Estimation of oxygen delivery in newborns with a univentricular circulation. Circulation 1998;98:1407–13, with permission.

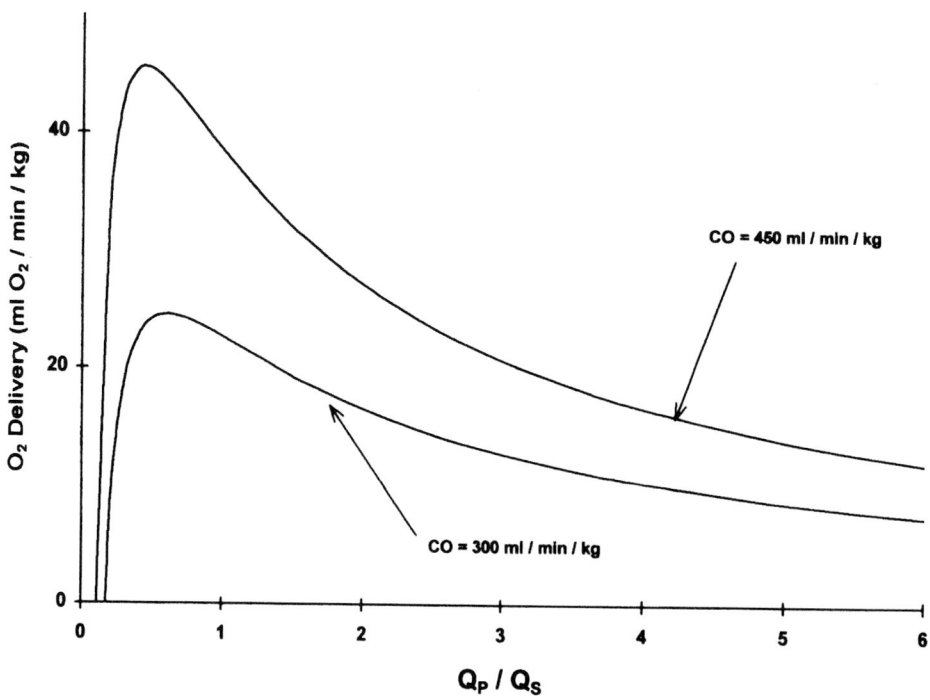

Figure 34-6   Systemic oxygen (O_2) delivery vs. Qp/Qs in the theoretical newborn with hypoplastic left heart syndrome. A computer model was used to generate the curves by setting the cardiac output (CO) at 300 or 450 mL/kg/min. Note that increasing cardiac output can increase oxygen delivery, and that oxygen delivery decreases significantly once Qp/Qs exceeds 1. Reprinted from Barnea O, Santamore WP, Rossi A, et al. Estimation of oxygen delivery in newborns with a univentricular circulation. *Circulation* 1998;98:1407–1413, with permission.

neuromuscular blockade. The study found that both hypoxia and hypercarbia were effective in reducing Qp/Qs ratio (Fig. 34-7). Hypercarbia increased cerebral oxygen saturation, mean arterial blood pressure, oxygen delivery and, although not directly measured, cardiac output, whereas hypoxia did not change these variables, suggesting that hypercarbia may be the preferred therapy (Fig. 34-8) (86,87). However, administration of supplemental CO_2 requires the concurrent use of sedation and paralysis, thus limiting its applicability for most neonates with HLHS prior to surgery.

Neonates with HLHS and myocardial dysfunction should receive inotropic support to improve cardiac output and systemic oxygen delivery. However, care should be taken to avoid inotropic agents that increase systemic vascular resistance because this will favor pulmonary blood flow over systemic blood flow. Low-dose dopamine or milrinone are good inotropic agents for neonates with HLHS and myocardial dysfunction.

The neonate with HLHS and a severely restrictive or intact atrial septum will present with profound cyanosis and shock immediately after birth as a result of obstruction of blood egress from the left atrium. The short- and long-term outlook for such infants has historically been poor, regardless of whether they undergo the Norwood operation or are listed for heart transplantation, due in large part to the in utero development of pulmonary venous hypertension and lymphatic abnormalities that persist following birth (88–90). The immediate management of these criti-

cally ill neonates involves prompt intervention to decompress the left atrium. Emergent surgical intervention, involving either open atrial septectomy or a Norwood procedure, has usually resulted in early death. A Brockenbrough atrial septoplasty (transcatheter, trans-septal needle puncture followed by serial balloon dilation of the new ASD and possibly stent placement) will serve to decompress the left atrium, increase pulmonary venous return and pulmonary blood flow, and alleviate cyanosis (35). Following this procedure, the patient may be medically managed for a few days with a PGE_1 infusion and diuretics to allow pulmonary vascular resistance to fall and pulmonary edema to improve prior to the Norwood operation. This multidisciplinary approach to the neonate with HLHS and severely restrictive or intact atrial septum has resulted in a contemporary 53% survival rate following the Norwood operation, which is better than results obtained with other management strategies for this lesion, but remains poor when compared with the outcome of neonates without atrial obstruction who undergo the Norwood operation (91). Theoretically, alleviation of the left atrial hypertension *in utero* may improve outcome in patients with HLHS and a severely restrictive or intact atrial septum. Fetal intervention to dilate the atrial septum using percutaneous, transcatheter needle puncture of the atrial septum followed by balloon dilation appears to be feasible and is associated with minimal maternal risk, but technical improvements and additional experience will be required before this procedure is widely adopted (92).

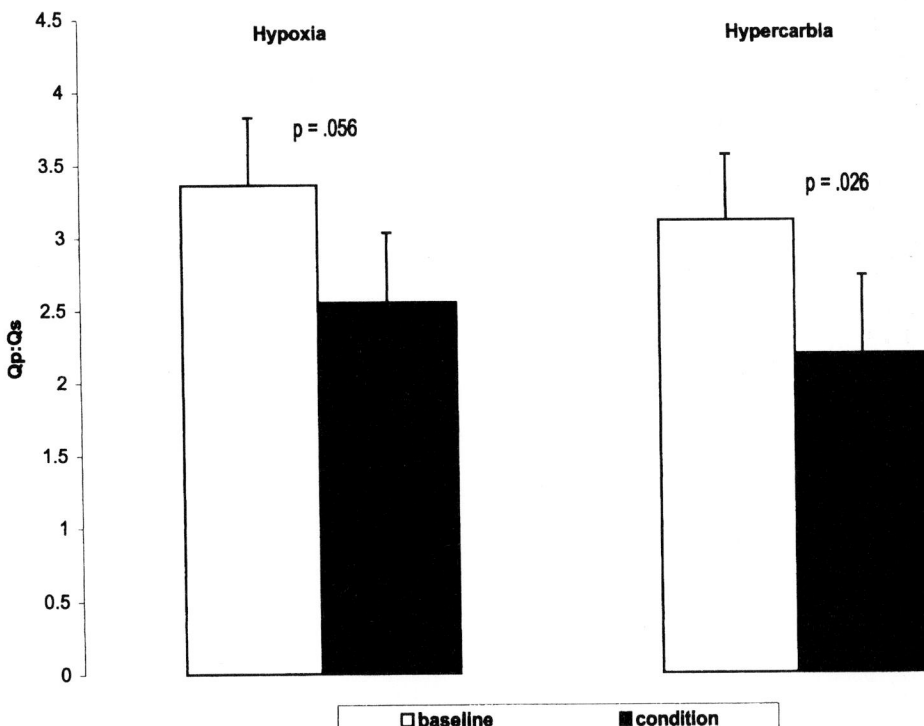

Figure 34-7 Difference in Qp/Qs between condition (either hypoxia or hypercarbia) and baseline (mean ± SEM) in preoperative neonates with hypoplastic left heart syndrome. Reprinted from Tabbutt S, Ramamoorthy C, Montenegro LM, et al. Impact of inspired gas mixtures on preoperative infants with hypoplastic left heart syndrome during controlled ventilation. *Circulation* 2001; 104:I159–I164, with permission.

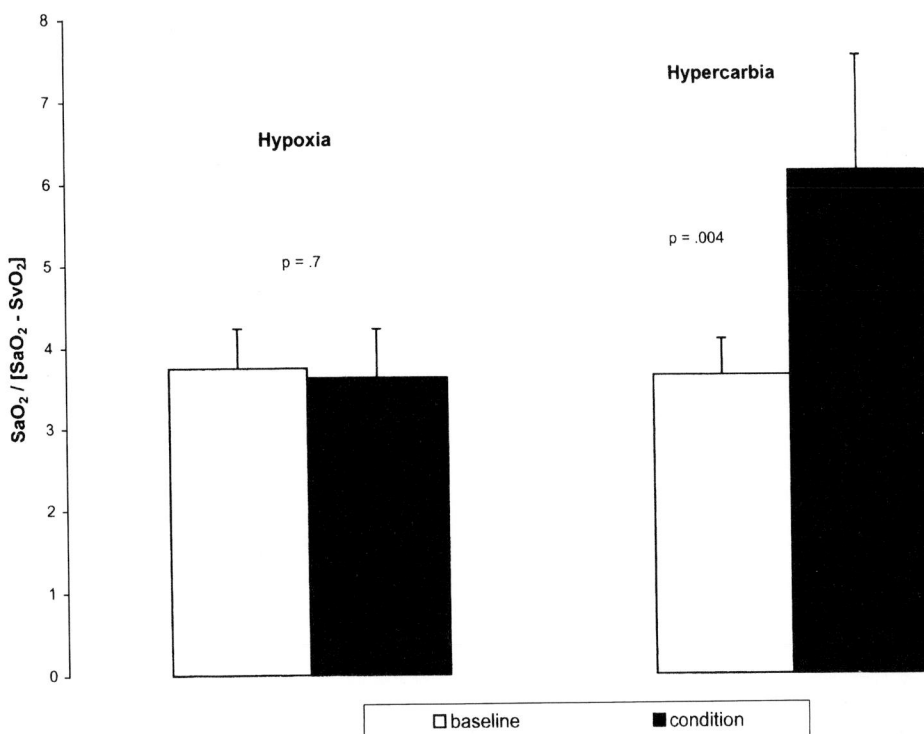

Figure 34-8 Difference in oxygen delivery between condition (either hypoxia or hypercarbia) and baseline (mean ± SEM) in preoperative neonates with hypoplastic left heart syndrome. Oxygen delivery was calculated as $SaO_2 \div (SaO_2\text{-}SvO_2)$, in which SaO_2 and SvO_2 were directly measured. Reprinted from Tabbutt S, Ramamoorthy C, Montenegro LM, et al. Impact of inspired gas mixtures on preoperative infants with hypoplastic left heart syndrome during controlled ventilation. *Circulation* 2001;104:I159–I164, with permission.

Early Survival after S1P by Year of Operation

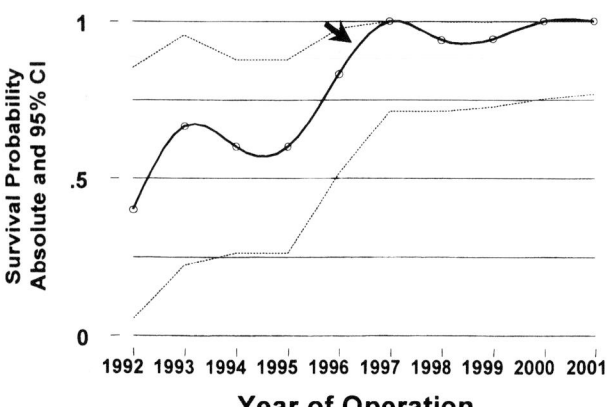

Figure 34-9   Hospital survival following stage 1 palliation in patients with hypoplastic left heart syndrome by year at a single center. Hospital survival improved coincident with the application of new treatment strategies beginning in July of 1996 (arrow). S1P, stage 1 palliation (Norwood operation). Reprinted from Tweddell JS, Hoffman GM, Mussatto KA, et al. Improved survival of patients undergoing palliation of hypoplastic left heart syndrome: lessons learned from 115 consecutive patients. *Circulation* 2002;106: 182–189, with permission.

Initial reports suggested that severe tricuspid regurgitation was a significant risk factor for infants with HLHS (93,94). However, in the preoperative infant with HLHS, the severity of tricuspid regurgitation may be in part related to a high Qp/Qs, with right ventricular volume overload and stretching of the tricuspid valve annulus. Following the Norwood operation, the Qp/Qs may decrease as a result of the fixed resistance to pulmonary blood flow provided by the shunt, and subsequently the degree of tricuspid regurgitation may diminish. Thus, clinical judgment and an appreciation of tricuspid valve morphology are required in such cases.

Several centers have recently reported overall survival rates of more than or equal to 90% following initial surgical palliation for HLHS (Fig. 34-9) (4,95). Contemporary risk factors contributing to higher mortality following the Norwood operation include prematurity, the presence of multiple congenital anomalies, and an intact atrial septum (48,88). Although palliative care is still offered at some centers for neonates with HLHS, fewer clinicians and parents are opting for no intervention given the improving surgical results (96). Some centers offer heart transplantation as a primary option for HLHS (97). Problems with this strategy include the high morbidity and mortality incurred while waiting for a heart to become available from a very limited donor pool, suboptimal neurologic outcome in many patients, and complications inherent to heart transplant (98–100). For these reasons, many pediatric cardiology centers recommend the Norwood operation as the initial surgical intervention in neonates with HLHS, and heart transplantation is typically reserved for the small subset that develop subsequent irreversible myocardial failure.

Interrupted Aortic Arch

An interrupted aortic arch (IAA) is most commonly associated with a VSD, but also is seen with a variety of other congenital cardiac malformations, including truncus arteriosus and TGA (101). If a VSD is not present in a patient with an IAA, an aorto-pulmonary window is likely to be found. IAA is classified by the location of the arch interruption in relation to the bracheocephalic vessels (Fig. 34-10) (102). IAA type B is the most common subtype (>50% of cases), and type C is rare. Chromosome 22q11 deletion is present in approximately 60% of neonates with IAA type B (41). The infant with an unrecognized IAA will present with shock, similar to a critical coarctation, upon closure of the ductus arteriosus. Infants with IAA are dependent upon ductal patency to maintain blood flow to the lower body, and

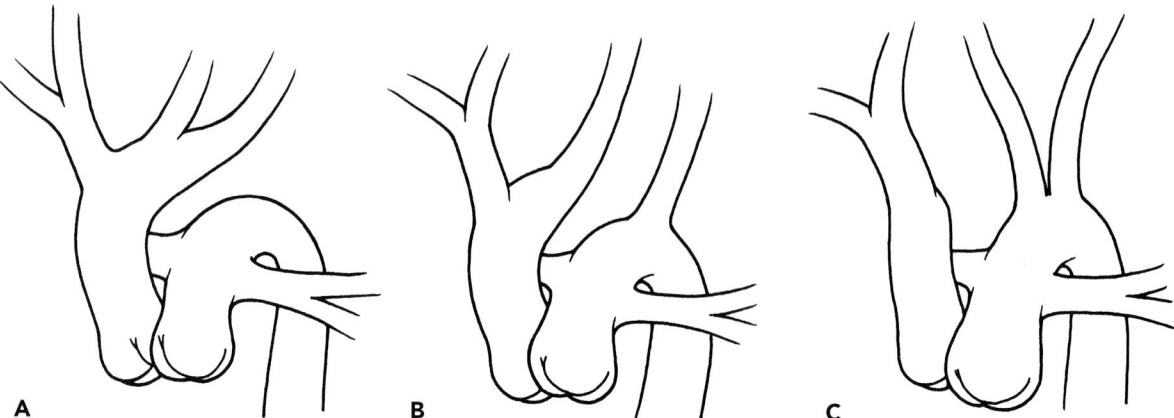

Figure 34-10   The three types of interrupted aortic arch. In type A, the interruption is at the aortic isthmus between the left subclavian artery and the ductus. In type B, the interruption is at the distal aortic arch between the left carotid and left subclavian arteries. In type C, the interruption is at the proximal aortic arch between the innominate and left carotid arteries. Type B is the most common form of this lesion. Type C is rare. Reprinted from Chang AC, Starnes VA. Interrupted aortic arch. In: Chang AC, Hanley FL, Wernovsky G, et al., eds. *Pediatric cardiac intensive care.* Baltimore: Williams and Wilkins, 1998:243–247, with permission.

preoperative management strategies to balance the systemic and pulmonary circulations mimic those used in infants with HLHS. Early surgical intervention is warranted.

Mixing Lesions

Transposition of the Great Arteries

In d-TGA, the aorta arises from the anatomic right ventricle and the pulmonary artery arises from the anatomic left ventricle. Approximately 40% of neonates with TGA have an associated VSD, which occasionally is a malalignment type defect. If anterior malalignment exists, there may be associated right ventricular outflow tract obstruction, aortic valvar stenosis, coarctation of the aorta or rarely an IAA. A posterior malalignment VSD is associated with left ventricular outflow tract obstruction, pulmonary stenosis or atresia. Coronary artery branching abnormalities are present in approximately 30% of cases.

In this unique parallel circulation, deoxygenated systemic venous blood returns to the right heart and is pumped back to the systemic arterial circulation, and oxygenated pulmonary venous blood passes through the left heart and is pumped back to the lungs. Unless there is adequate mixing between these parallel circulations, severe cyanosis, metabolic acidosis and death will occur. Such intercirculatory mixing represents effective pulmonary and systemic blood flows, and may take place at the atrial, ventricular, or great artery level (Fig. 34-11). Infants with TGA and an intact ventricular septum typically have a patent foramen ovale (PFO) or ASD that allows some mixing at the atrial level. However, a PGE_1 infusion is usually necessary to open or maintain patency of the ductus arteriosus, which will increase effective pulmonary blood flow, provided that the pulmonary vascular resistance is lower than the systemic vascular resistance and that there is an adequate atrial communication.

Occasionally infants with TGA may develop severe cyanosis and shock following the initiation of PGE_1 infusion, as a result of increasing blood volume returning to the left atrium and functional closure of the foramen ovale. If this occurs, or if the PFO is restrictive, as assessed by echocardiography, and excessive cyanosis is present, an emergent balloon atrial septostomy should be performed to enlarge the atrial communication (Fig. 34-12, see also Color Plate) (34). The balloon atrial septostomy may be performed at the bedside using echocardiographic guidance, or in the cardiac catheterization laboratory (103). Excessive cyanosis may persist despite a technically successful balloon atrial septostomy. High pulmonary vascular resistance may limit effective pulmonary blood flow, and measures should be taken to lower pulmonary vascular resistance. Because the majority of systemic blood flow comes from the systemic venous circulation in TGA, neonates who remain excessively cyanotic following a balloon atrial septostomy will also improve following maneuvers that will increase the mixed venous oxygen saturation. These include interventions to decrease oxygen consumption, such as sedation and paraly-

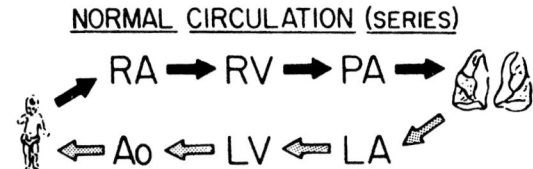

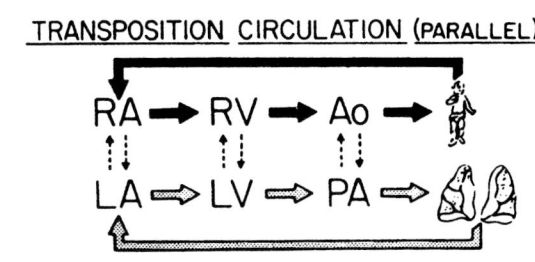

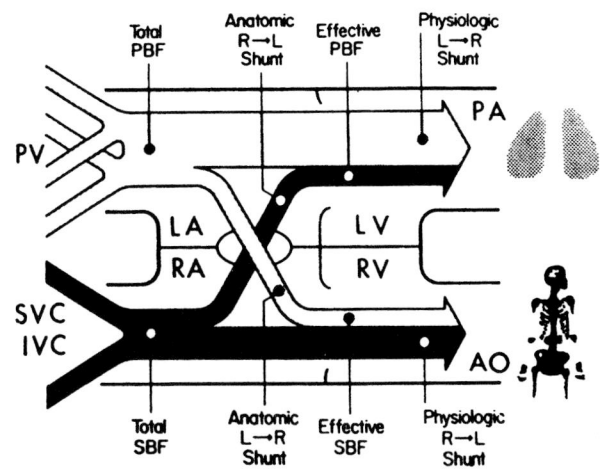

Figure 34-11 The circulation in transposition of the great arteries. **A:** The systemic and pulmonary circulations are in series in the normal circulation, whereas they are in parallel in TGA. Solid arrows, relatively unoxygenated blood; stippled arrows, oxygenated blood; dashed arrows, intercirculatory shunts. **B:** Circulation schema demonstrating flows and shunts in infants with TGA/intact ventricular septum. Note that the anatomic left to right shunt constitutes the effective SBF, and the anatomic right-to-left shunt constitutes the effective PBF. Ao, aorta; IVC, inferior vena cava; LA, left atrium; LV, left ventricle; L → R, left to right; RA, right atrium; RV, right ventricle; R → L, right to left; PA, pulmonary artery; PBF, pulmonary blood flow; PV, pulmonary veins; SBF, systemic blood flow; SVC, superior vena cava. Reprinted from Paul MH, Wernovsky G. Transposition of the great arteries. In: Emmanouilides GC, Riemenschneider TA, Allen HD, et al, eds. *Moss and Adams' heart disease in infants, children and Adolescents, including the fetus and young adult.* Baltimore: Williams & Wilkins, 1995:1154–1225, with permission.

sis, and improve oxygen delivery, such as correcting anemia and administering inotropic agents. To summarize, infants with TGA and intact ventricular septum who remain excessively cyanotic despite the initiation of PGE_1 require a balloon atrial septostomy, and if necessary, interventions to lower pulmonary vascular resistance and increase systemic venous oxygen saturation.

Many clinicians recommend that a semi-elective balloon atrial septostomy be performed in nearly all patients with TGA and intact ventricular septum, even those without

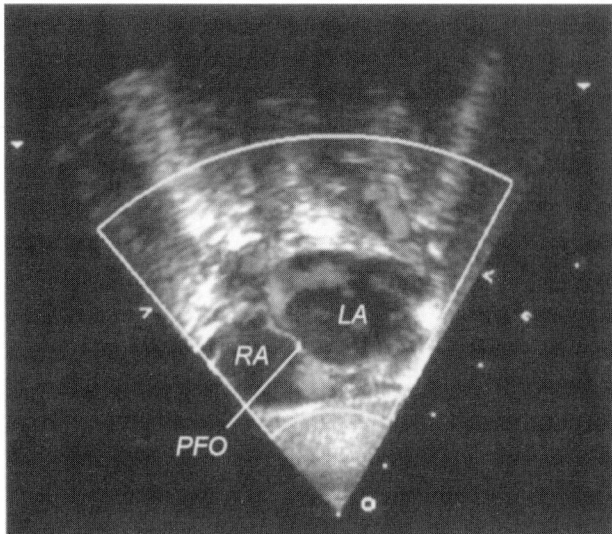
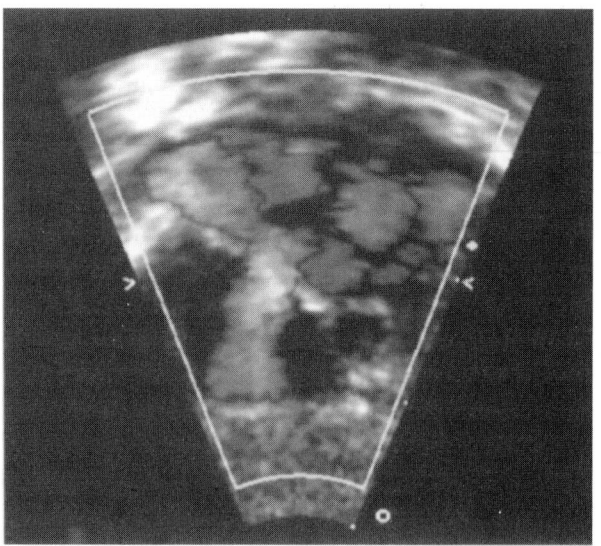

A   B

Figure 34-12   Restrictive atrial septum in a newborn with transposition of the great arteries. **A.** Two-dimensional echocardiogram with color Doppler from the subcostal window demonstrating a tiny patent foramen ovale with left to right flow across the atrial septum. **B.** Following successful balloon atrial septostomy, a wide communication now exists between the left and right atria. LA, left atrium; PFO, patent foramen ovale; RA, right atrium. (See color plate)

excessive cyanosis. Once the atrial septum is enlarged, the PGE_1 can usually be safely discontinued, thus avoiding complications related to that medication and a large ductus arteriosus, such as apnea and NEC. Furthermore, the left atrium is decompressed following a balloon atrial septostomy, which may allow the pulmonary vascular resistance to fall prior to surgery. Finally, the infant may be transferred from the ICU to the general ward to initiate feedings and await surgery. The major risks associated with the performance of a balloon atrial septostomy include myocardial perforation or avulsion of the inferior vena cava from the right atrium during pullback of the balloon, both of which rarely occur. Following initial stabilization of the neonate with TGA and intact ventricular septum, an early arterial switch operation is required before the left ventricle becomes deconditioned.

Infants with TGA and moderate to large VSD generally are well oxygenated and do not require a PGE_1 infusion provided that the ventricular outflow tracts are unobstructed. Early congestive heart failure typically develops, and surgical repair is indicated within the first few weeks of life. A malalignment-type VSD may be associated with clinically significant left or right ventricular outflow tract obstruction. Patients with sub-aortic obstruction may have an associated coarctation of the aorta or an IAA. Such an infant may present with the very unique finding of reverse differential cyanosis, with low oxygen saturation in the right arm and high oxygen saturation in the leg. A PGE_1 infusion is needed, followed by early surgical intervention. Infants with d-TGA and VSD who are referred for surgery after the first few months of life (typically from underdeveloped nations) are at risk for having developed pulmonary vascular obstructive disease. These patients may require a cardiac catheterization to evaluate their pulmonary vascular resistance prior to surgery.

Tricuspid Atresia

Tricuspid atresia is present when there is agenesis of the tricuspid valve and an absent communication between the right atrium and right ventricle. The presentation of infants with this lesion is variable and depends primarily upon the presence and size of a VSD, whether the great arteries are normally related or transposed, and the degree of ventricular outflow tract obstruction (Table 34-5) (104,105). These factors determine which of these neonates will be dependent on a PGE_1 infusion. All of the systemic venous blood must pass through an obligate atrial communication to the left atrium, in which it mixes with the pulmonary venous blood. In the presence of normally looped ventricles and normally related great arteries, the left ventricle then ejects blood to the aorta, and through the VSD, if present, to the pulmonary artery. If the great arteries are transposed, the left ventricle pumps blood to the pulmonary artery (unless pulmonary atresia is present), and through the VSD to the aorta. Although all infants with tricuspid atresia eventually require a Fontan palliation, the type of initial operation depends upon the extent of cyanosis or systemic outflow obstruction. For example, infants with tricuspid atresia, normally looped ventricles and normally related great vessels, a large VSD and no or minimal right ventricular outflow tract obstruction (type I-C) will be well oxygenated and develop early heart failure. In the neonatal period, they require placement of a pulmonary artery band or transection of the pulmonary artery and placement of a systemic to pulmonary artery shunt. Those with a moderate size VSD and a moderate degree of right ventricular outflow tract obstruction (type I-B) will have a balanced circulation with an acceptable amount of cyanosis. Such infants may be discharged home with the expectation of a bi-directional

TABLE 34-5
CLASSIFICATION SYSTEM FOR TRICUSPID ATRESIA

Type and Description	Frequency
Type I: Normally related great arteries A. Intact ventricular septum with pulmonary atresia B. Small ventricular septal defect with pulmonary stenosis C. Large ventricular septal defect without pulmonary stenosis	70%–80%
Type II: d-Transposition of the great arteries A. Ventricular septal defect with pulmonary atresia B. Ventricular septal defect with pulmonary stenosis C. Ventricular septal defect without pulmonary stenosis	12%–25%
Type III: l-Transposition of the great arteries	3%–6%

Glenn or hemi-Fontan operation within the first six months of life. Infants with tricuspid atresia and a small or absent VSD (type I-A or I-B) will have significant cyanosis and thus be dependent on a PGE_1 infusion until a systemic to pulmonary artery shunt is performed. Infants with tricuspid atresia and transposed great arteries, a small or absent VSD (type II-A or II-B) will develop shock unless ductal patency is maintained. These infants require a Damus-Kaye-Stansel operation (aortopulmonary anastomosis) or a modified Norwood operation with a systemic to pulmonary artery shunt.

Total Anomalous Pulmonary Venous Return

Total anomalous pulmonary venous return (TAPVR) is a congenital heart defect in which all four pulmonary veins drain to a systemic vein or the right atrium. TAPVR results from a failure of the common pulmonary vein to fuse with the posterior surface of the left atrium early in fetal life. The pulmonary veins then decompress via the coronary sinus or primitive venous structures, which eventually lead to the right atrium, in which mixing occurs with the systemic venous blood. An anatomic classification system divides TAPVR into supracardiac, cardiac, infracardiac, and mixed, depending upon which primitive venous pathways are employed. Supracardiac TAPVR exists when all of the pulmonary veins come to a confluence behind the left atrium and drain via a vertical vein to the innominate vein or superior vena cava. Occasionally the vertical vein is obstructed as it passes between the left mainstem bronchus and left pulmonary artery. Cardiac TAPVR exists when the pulmonary veins drain to the coronary sinus or right atrium. Obstruction is uncommon in cardiac TAPVR. In infracardiac TAPVR, the pulmonary venous confluence drains inferiorly through the diaphragm and into the portal or hepatic veins, in which obstruction is common. Patients with mixed TAPVR have drainage to more than one site. For example, the left sided pulmonary veins may drain through a vertical vein to the innominate vein, although the right pulmonary veins drain to the right atrium. An obligatory intracardiac (usually atrial) communication exists in neonates with TAPVR to allow some oxygenated blood to reach the left heart and systemic arterial circulation. TAPVR may be associated with significant intracardiac disease as is seen in patients with heterotaxy syndrome, or may exist as an isolated lesion.

The presentation of isolated TAPVR is primarily based upon the presence and degree of obstruction between the pulmonary veins and the right heart. Most patients with infracardiac TAPVR and some with supracardiac TAPVR will have obstructed pulmonary venous pathways that result in pulmonary edema, pulmonary hypertension, cyanosis, and significant respiratory distress soon after birth. The clinical presentation and CXR may mimic those seen with neonatal pneumonia or respiratory distress syndrome, leading to delays in diagnosis. If a venous blood gas is drawn from an umbilical venous catheter positioned just above the liver in a cyanotic newborn, and the oxygen saturation level is in the high 90s, the diagnosis of infracardiac TAPVR should be suspected, as the sample is reflective of pulmonary venous return. The umbilical venous catheter should be removed so that it does not further obstruct pulmonary venous flow and cause clinical decompensation. Stabilization for the neonate with obstructed TAPVR involves mechanical ventilation, sedation and urgent surgical intervention (106). Hypoxemia may be abated somewhat by interventions that increase mixed venous oxygen saturation, including pharmacologic paralysis, correction of anemia, and inotropic support. Although neonates with obstructed TAPVR may be quite cyanotic, measures to lower pulmonary vascular resistance, including the use of hyperventilation and nitric oxide (NO), are usually not beneficial. The use of PGE_1 infusion in such patients is controversial, but generally is discouraged. Some physicians feel that PGE_1 may maintain patency of the ductus venosus in infants with infracardiac obstructed TAPVR, thus allowing for better drainage back to the right heart. Other clinicians believe that maintaining patency of the ductus arteriosus may allow left to right shunting at the arterial level (if the pulmonary vascular resistance is less than the systemic vascular resistance) and thus exacerbate pulmonary edema.

Infants with unobstructed isolated TAPVR and an adequate atrial communication will be mildly hypoxemic without overt clinical cyanosis at birth but develop congestive heart failure (CHF) within a few weeks to months. Surgical repair is performed within the first few days to weeks of life.

Truncus Arteriosus

Truncus arteriosus is present when a single (common) arterial trunk gives rise to the aorta, at least one coronary artery, and at least one pulmonary artery. A single semilunar ("truncal") valve is always present, and an unrestrictive VSD is almost always present. About one-third of patients with truncus arteriosus have a 22q11.2 microdeletion (DiGeorge syndrome) that can be diagnosed with florescent in-situ hybridization (FISH) (107). Several classification systems exist that may be used to describe the origins of the pulmonary arteries from the arterial trunk and the presence or absence of an IAA (108). Newborns with truncus arteriosus who present with mild cyanosis do not require a PGE$_1$ infusion unless an IAA (about 10% of cases) or ductal origin of one of the pulmonary arteries is present.

Infants with truncus arteriosus usually develop too much pulmonary blood flow and congestive heart failure within a few weeks after birth as pulmonary vascular resistance falls and systemic vascular resistance increases, unless stenosis is present at the origin of the pulmonary arteries from the aorta. Supplemental oxygen should be avoided to minimize the risk of decreasing pulmonary vascular resistance. Congestive heart failure is exacerbated in the presence of significant truncal valve insufficiency, which occurs in 50% of cases, or significant truncal valve stenosis (less common). For this reason, and to prevent the development of pulmonary vascular obstructive disease before surgery and minimize the incidence of pulmonary hypertension crises postoperatively, complete surgical repair is generally performed prior to discharge from the nursery (8,109,110).

Left to Right Shunts

Atrial Septal Defect

ASDs may be present in isolation or with nearly any other type of congenital heart defect. ASDs are categorized by location and include secundum, ostium primum and sinus venosus types. The most common type is the secundum ASD, which exists when there is a deficiency in the septum primum in the central portion of the atrial septum. Although secundum ASDs may become smaller and close spontaneously, particularly those that are less than 5 mm in diameter, the ostium primum and sinus venosus defects will always require surgical intervention. The ostium primum defects are located in the inferior region of the atrial septum, and are almost always associated with an additional endocardial cushion abnormality. The sinus venosus defects usually occur at the junction between the superior vena cava and the right atrium, and are almost always associated with partial anomalous pulmonary venous return.

Isolated ASDs only rarely cause symptoms in infants, as significant left to right shunting does not occur until right ventricular compliance falls below left ventricular compliance, and this often takes years to occur. Likewise it is uncommon for patients with large ASDs to require oral medications (digoxin or diuretics). However, clinical judgment regarding the medical management and timing of surgical intervention is required in the neonate with a large ASD and additional medical problems (e.g., chronic lung disease) that complicate the clinical picture. The primary indication for surgery in infancy is the presence of symptoms secondary to left to right shunting. Toddlers require intervention if they have an ostium primum or sinus venosus ASD, or a secundum ASD with evidence for volume overload of the right ventricle. Intervention is indicated in early childhood in asymptomatic patients with significant left to right atrial shunts to prevent late complications including pulmonary vascular obstructive disease, thromboembolic events, arrhythmias, and right heart failure. A variety of devices exist that are used to close secundum ASDs in the catheterization laboratory, but the majority of clinical experience thus far exists with older children (111).

Ventricular Septal Defect

VSDs may be found in a variety of complex congenital heart lesions, or may exist in isolation. VSDs are categorized by location and size. VSDs may be located in the perimembranous, muscular, inlet or conal (outlet, subarterial, supracristal) regions of the ventricular septum, and there may be more than one VSD present. Malalignment of the conal septum may exist, resulting in variable degrees of right or left ventricular outflow tract obstruction. Conal VSDs often develop involvement of the aortic valve over many years (112). The size may be determined by an estimation of the diameter of the VSD in relation to the aortic annulus, and by degree of restriction to blood flow as estimated by Doppler echocardiogram. Perimembranous and muscular VSDs may become smaller or close with time, particularly if the initial diameter of the VSD is less than 5 mm (113). In patients with isolated moderate to large VSDs, congestive heart failure develops over time once an imbalance exists between systemic and pulmonary vascular resistance and a significant left to right shunt develops. Neonates with large VSDs will typically develop pulmonary overcirculation, left ventricular volume overload, and symptoms of congestive heart failure within the first several weeks to months of life as pulmonary vascular resistance falls. Any associated left ventricular outflow tract obstruction, such as coarctation of the aorta, will exacerbate this problem. Premature infants with left to right shunting at the ventricular or great artery level may develop congestive heart failure sooner as a result of decreased musculature in the pulmonary arterioles that allows for a precipitous drop in pulmonary vascular resistance.

A trial of medical management is usually indicated in infants with moderate to large VSDs. Provision of adequate nutrition and administration of medications including loop diuretics and sometimes digoxin and/or angiotensin converting enzyme inhibitors (ACE inhibitors) can often allow surgery to be deferred for a few months (114). Supplemental oxygen and hyperventilation should be avoided, as they will cause pulmonary vascular resistance to fall, and Qp/Qs to rise. Infants who continue to have failure to thrive despite these measures are referred for surgical repair, or in selected cases, transcatheter intervention (115).

Atrioventricular Canal Defect

The presence or absence of a common atrioventricular valve orifice and the relative size of the physiologic VSD characterizes the different types of atrioventricular septal defects, also known as endocardial cushion defects. In patients with an incomplete atrioventricular canal, an ostium primum ASD exists along with a cleft in the mitral valve. There is no physiologic VSD present. A transitional atrioventricular canal defect has an ostium primum ASD, dense attachments of the atrioventricular valve leaflets to the crest of the ventricular septum such that two functionally separate atrioventricular valves exist, and a small physiologic VSD. A complete atrioventricular canal defect has a primum ASD, a common atrioventricular valve and a large inlet VSD. Associate anomalies include a left superior vena cava to the coronary sinus, additional VSDs, and aortic arch obstruction. Uncommonly, right ventricular outflow tract obstruction is seen, and such patients have features of tetralogy of Fallot and an atrioventricular canal (116). In most cases the ventricles are balanced, such that both are of adequate size to support the full cardiac output following surgery. Occasionally one of the ventricles is hypoplastic ("unbalanced"), precluding a two ventricular repair. Such patients may be considered for a one and a half ventricular repair, the single ventricle pathway, or heart transplantation.

Infants with complete atrioventricular canal defects typically develop congestive heart failure within the first few weeks to months of life. The congestive heart failure will be exacerbated if significant atrioventricular valve regurgitation or aortic arch hypoplasia is present. There is an increased incidence of Down syndrome (trisomy 21) in patients with endocardial cushion defects, and such patients are predisposed to the early development of pulmonary vascular obstructive disease. A trial of medical management is indicated in symptomatic infants, as discussed above for patients with large VSDs. Surgical repair is required within the first three to six months of life to eliminate the symptoms of congestive heart failure, prevent the development of pulmonary vascular obstructive disease and minimize the incidence of postoperative pulmonary hypertensive crises. Surgical repair is not commonly performed in the newborn period as a result of the difficulty with suturing the paper-thin atrioventricular valve leaflets.

Infants with incomplete or transitional atrioventricular canal defects often follow the clinical course of patients with isolated ASDs, and these lesions are typically repaired sometime between 6 months and 4 years of age.

Patent Ductus Arteriosus

The ductus arteriosus normally is functionally closed within the first hours to days of life. PDAs may exist in isolation or with many other types of congenital heart disease. An isolated, large PDA will cause symptoms of congestive heart failure once the pulmonary vascular resistance falls, allowing a left to right shunt from the aorta to the pulmonary artery. Left atrial and left ventricular volume overload are present and pulmonary edema may occur. Diastolic runoff exists leading to a "steal" from systemic blood flow, which may contribute to mesenteric ischemia and the development of NEC. PDAs are more common and cause more symptoms in premature infants. Small PDAs typically do not cause symptoms but are a long-term risk for bacterial endocarditis. Symptoms of congestive heart failure may be treated with diuretics, digoxin and the provision of adequate nutrition. Approximately two-thirds of PDAs in premature infants will close following a course of indomethacin or ibuprofen (117). Surgical ligation is indicated for PDAs that do not respond to medical therapy in premature infants, and for PDAs in any symptomatic term infant. Older children with a continuous murmur but no symptoms should have the PDA closed surgically or in the cardiac catheterization laboratory to minimize the risk of endocarditis.

Aortopulmonary Window

An aortopulmonary window is an uncommon, usually large communication between the ascending aorta and pulmonary artery in the presence of two semilunar valves. This lesion usually exists in isolation, but may be associated with IAA, VSD, or other congenital heart defects (118,119). Infants with large aortopulmonary windows will usually develop congestive heart failure at several weeks of life. Prompt surgical repair is indicated in most cases to eliminate the symptoms of congestive heart failure, prevent the development of pulmonary vascular obstructive disease and minimize the incidence of postoperative pulmonary hypertension.

Cardiomyopathy and Heart Transplantation

Cardiomyopathy

A multidisciplinary team, lead by the intensivist, a cardiologist with expertise in heart failure and transplantation, and a congenital heart surgeon, is required to answer several key questions for each infant who presents with a severe cardiomyopathy: What is the primary cause for the cardiomyopathy? Is it treatable or reversible? What level of medical or mechanical support is required? Is the infant a candidate for heart transplantation?

Infants may develop a severe cardiomyopathy from a wide variety of causes, including infection, structural heart disease, chronic arrhythmia, metabolic disorders, and primary myopathies. The broad differential diagnosis for infantile cardiomyopathies is covered in detail in Chapter 33 and will not be repeated here. However, several conditions that may present with severe cardiomyopathy, are difficult to diagnose and are sometimes erroneously referred for heart transplantation, yet are readily treatable deserve comment. Infants born with anomalous left coronary artery from the pulmonary artery (ALCAPA) develop coronary ischemia when the pulmonary artery pressures fall after birth. These patients typically present in the first few weeks to months of life with severe left ventricular dysfunction, mitral regurgitation (as a result of papillary muscle ischemia), and pulmonary edema. The diagnosis may be suspected by the presence of characteristic findings on the electrocardiogram, and confirmed by echocardiography with careful examination of the coronary anatomy and blood flow pattern (120,121). Following reimplantation of the left coronary artery in the aorta, the vast majority of infants with ALCAPA recover left ventricular and mitral valve function (122). Infants with incessant arrhythmias, such as automatic atrial tachycardia, may present with severe cardiomyopathy. The initial rhythm may be thought to be sinus tachycardia secondary to the cardiomyopathy, but the correct diagnosis may be made by careful examination of the P wave morphology on the electrocardiogram. Myocardial function will recover once the arrhythmia is controlled with medications or ablation. Severe viral myocarditis is another condition that may be difficult to differentiate from a primary cardiomyopathy. Myocardial biopsy may provide clarity but is not without risk in sick infants. Many infants with viral myocarditis will recover ventricular function over time with supportive care (123).

Infants with cardiomyopathy may present with congestive heart failure or shock. Many of the principles for supporting cardiac output and monitoring of patients with severe cardiomyopathy are discussed below in the "postoperative care" section, and thus will not be reiterated. Mechanical support, typically with venoarterial extracorporeal membrane oxygenation (ECMO) in infants, may be used as a bridge to recovery or transplantation and is discussed further below. Indications for mechanical support in an infant with severe cardiomyopathy include worsening end-organ function and metabolic acidosis despite maximal medical support.

Heart Transplantation

Heart transplantation is a widely accepted option for many infants with severe congenital heart disease and irreversible cardiomyopathies. Approximately 100 infant heart transplants are reported annually to the registry of the International Society for Heart and Lung Transplantation. Seventy-five percent of these transplants are for congenital heart disease, and the majority of the remainder are for cardiomyopathies (124). Heart transplantation is considered a primary option in some institutions for infants with complex congenital heart disease if surgical intervention is believed to result in an unacceptably high mortality rate (Table 34-6). Transplantation is also an option if uncorrectable anatomical issues and/or irreversible myocardial dysfunction are present following initial surgical intervention. The donor pool is very limited, and as a result as many as 25% of infants will die while waiting for a heart to become available. If more institutions adopted a policy of primary transplantation for the lesions listed in Table 34-6, particularly HLHS, the mortality while waiting for a donor heart to become available would certainly increase. Recent experience with ABO incompatible transplantation has shortened the wait times at a few centers (125). Relative contraindications to heart transplantation include high, fixed pulmonary vascular resistance (>6–8 Woods units per m^2), recent or recurrent malignancy, serious infection, significant systemic disease, other organ system disease (e.g., hepatic, renal, or neurological), and chromosomal, metabolic or genetic abnormalities with a poor long-term prognosis.

Although the 1-year survival following heart transplantation in infancy is lower than that reported for older children, the long-term survival appears to be better, perhaps related to immune tolerance or better compliance with medications (124). The 10-year survival following infant heart transplantation is approximately 60%. Infants who have a successful heart transplant face potential long-term complications related to immunosuppression (i.e., renal insufficiency, infection, diabetes mellitus, and malignancy), transplant coronary artery disease, and rejection (124). In depth conversations about these issues

---

TABLE 34-6

CONGENITAL HEART DEFECTS THAT MAY WARRANT PRIMARY HEART TRANSPLANTATION

Hypoplastic left heart syndrome
Severe Shone's syndrome
Severe Ebstein's anomaly of the tricuspid valve
Atrioventricular septal defects with unbalanced ventricles
Pulmonary atresia/intact ventricular septum with coronary-cameral fistula and myocardial dysfunction
Multiple cardiac tumors with myocardial dysfunction

Adopted from Wong PC, Starnes VA. Pediatric heart and lung transplantation. In Chang AC, Hanley FL, Wernovsky G et al, eds. *Pediatric cardiac intensive care.* Lippincott Williams and Wilkins, Baltimore, 1998, with permission.

with parents are always required before an infant is listed for transplantation.

Comprehensive supportive care is required to maintain patients who are awaiting transplantation in the ICU. An appropriate level of cardiopulmonary support is required to maintain end-organ function. This often entails the use of inotropic agents, vasodilators, and diuretics. Mechanical support, usually ECMO in infants, is occasionally required (126).

Mechanical ventilation may be beneficial to minimize oxygen consumption, and positive end-expiratory pressure will reduce wall stress and thus provide afterload reduction for a failing systemic ventricle. Close attention must also be given to the prevention of infection and the provision of adequate nutrition. Anticoagulation may be indicated for infants with severe myocardial dysfunction to minimize the chance of luminal clot formation.

Management of the infant with HLHS awaiting transplantation deserves comment. Ductal patency is maintained with a low dose PGE_1 infusion, and occasionally these infants can be discharged to home while awaiting transplantation (127). Infants with HLHS awaiting heart transplantation tend to develop pulmonary overcirculation as pulmonary vascular resistance falls over time, which further volume overloads the right ventricle and may exacerbate tricuspid regurgitation. The extended use of subambiant FiO_2, achieved using supplemental inspired nitrogen, to increase pulmonary vascular resistance and limit pulmonary blood flow has been reported in this patient population (84,127). Limitation of pulmonary blood flow by banding of the pulmonary artery, either surgically or using innovative transcatheter techniques, has also been reported (128).

POSTOPERATIVE CARE

Intraoperative and Immediate Postoperative Management

Cardiopulmonary Bypass (CPB)

Selected pediatric cardiac surgical procedures may be performed without the use of CPB such as modified Blalock-Taussig shunt or repair of coarctation of the aorta. However, the majority of cardiac operations performed require CPB. Thus, physicians caring for these patients must be familiar with the equipment and techniques used to perform CPB, its sequelae on end-organ function, and several intraoperative strategies used to minimize the associated morbidities. The primary function of CPB is to temporarily replace the major functions of the heart and lungs while surgical interventions are performed on these organs. A typical CPB circuit used to perform these functions includes venous cannula(s) that drain systemic venous blood from the vena cavae or systemic venous atrium, a reservoir, a heat exchanger, a membrane oxygenator, a roller pump, a filter, and an arterial cannula to return blood to the aorta. Before initiation of CPB, the circu-

lated blood must be modified to provide an appropriate composition of oxygen, carbon dioxide, pH, temperature, hematocrit, oncotic pressure, electrolytes, and glucose (129). The circuit is "primed" with standardized quantities of crystalloid solution, albumin, mannitol, sodium bicarbonate, heparin, calcium, and packed red blood cells. The patient is anticoagulated with heparin for the duration of CPB time, and cooled to a variable extent to minimize metabolic needs and oxygen consumption. Because hypothermia causes increased viscosity and red cell rigidity, hemodilution is used during hypothermic cardiopulmonary bypass.

To obtain a motionless heart for intracardiac repairs, the aorta is cross-clamped and a potassium-rich cardioplegia solution is injected into the proximal ascending aorta. Asystole develops once the cardioplegia solution perfuses the coronary circulation. The combination of cardioplegia and hypothermia provides myocardial protection for several hours. Following placement of the aortic cross clamp, blood from aortopulmonary collaterals will continue to return to the left atrium. To eliminate the left atrial blood return and facilitate certain complex left heart operations, deep hypothermic circulatory arrest (DHCA) may be used. Deep hypothermia refers to cooling of the core temperature to 18°C to 20°C. During circulatory arrest the CPB pump is shut off. In addition to the absence of blood returning to the left atrium, the perfusion cannula may be removed from the surgical field, creating optimal conditions for an accurate repair. Due to concerns about neurologic outcome following DHCA, regional perfusion techniques have recently been designed to minimize or avoid the use of circulatory arrest (130). The neurologic sequelae of CPB and DHCA are discussed in the section on neurologic complications later in this chapter. Following rewarming, weaning and separation from CPB, protamine is administered to reverse the effect of heparin (129). Additional blood components may be required to control bleeding immediately following CPB.

A number of adverse effects from CPB will impact on the postoperative course. During CPB, formed elements of the blood are exposed to artificial surfaces and sheer stress. Ischemia reperfusion injury occurs, as does microembolization of gas bubbles and particulate matter. Hemodilution may cause problems with oxygen delivery and dilution of clotting factors. These events trigger a complex neurohumoral and inflammatory response. CPB is associated with the release of endogenous catecholamines, vasopressin, endothelin, and activation of the renin-angiotensin-aldosterone axis, all of which contribute to elevation of systemic and pulmonary vascular resistances and fluid retention (131–142). A generalized inflammatory response occurs following CPB, and the complement, coagulation and fibrinolytic systems are activated (143–146). Capillary leak also occurs, related to fluid retention, the inflammatory response, and dilution of plasma proteins. White blood cells and platelets are also activated, leading to additional release of inflammatory mediators and proteolytic enzymes (147–149). Pulmonary leukosequestration occurs, as does oxygen free radical generation (150,151). Platelet counts fall following CPB, and clotting factors are diluted (140, 152). Myocardial systolic dysfunction also occurs following CPB in infants and children (153). The end result of these processes is a clinical picture of end-organ dysfunction of variable severity. The cardiovascular, pulmonary, hematologic and renal systems tend to be the most severely affected. Myocardial dysfunction, elevated systemic and pulmonary vascular resistance, abnormal gas exchange and decreased pulmonary compliance, bleeding and fluid retention all may be present in the early postoperative period.

Several pharmacologic agents and management strategies may be employed in the operating room to minimize these adverse effects of CPB. Mannitol is administered to the priming solution to induce an osmotic diuresis and act as an antioxidant (154). Dexamethasone, when administered prior to CPB, has been shown to reduce the inflammatory response to CPB, and is associated with several favorable clinical effects including a reduced need for supplemental fluids, a lower alveolar-arterial oxygen gradient, and decreased duration of mechanical ventilation (155,156). Further studies are needed to determine the optimal timing and dosing of dexamethasone prior to CPB. Aprotinin is a serine protease inhibitor that is used at many centers to attenuate the inflammatory and hemostatic activation related to CPB (157). In a series of pediatric studies, this medication, when used in a high dose regimen, has been demonstrated to safely decrease postoperative bleeding and operative closure time, and improve respiratory function, primarily in infants and in those patients undergoing a repeat sternotomy (158–165). Beneficial effects on the systemic inflammatory response were seen when methylprednisolone was used in addition to aprotinin in adults, but this combination of drugs has not been specifically studied in infants (166). New pharmacologic strategies to further blunt the inflammatory response to CPB are being investigated (167,168).

To aid in the removal of edema and hemoconcentrate the infant's blood, ultrafiltration is typically used during rewarming on CPB. Some surgeons use a technique called modified ultrafiltration (MUF) immediately following CPB, which may be a more efficient method to filter and hemoconcentrate the patient's blood. Following pediatric CPB, MUF has been shown to have favorable effects on hemodynamics, blood product requirements, and total body water balance (169–171). In a study of pediatric patients at risk for postoperative pulmonary hypertension, those receiving MUF had a lower pulmonary to systemic pressure ratio following CPB when compared to the group that had conventional ultrafiltration (171). Modified ultrafiltration has also been demonstrated to improve intrinsic left ventricular systolic function, improve diastolic compliance, increase blood pressure, and decrease inotropic medication use in the early postoperative period in children (172,173). Some investigators have found that the use of MUF is associated with a decrease in mechanical ventilation time following pediatric CPB (174).

Stabilization in the Intensive Care Unit Following Surgery

Ideally, the physicians caring for infants following cardiac surgery will attend preoperative multidisciplinary conferences in which data are presented and discussed to gain familiarity with each patient's anatomic and pathophysiologic issues and the surgical plan. When an infant is returned from the operating room following cardiac surgery, the intensivist must obtain a detailed report from the anesthesiologist and the surgeon. A description must be obtained of the anesthetic regimen, the operative findings and surgical procedure performed, and CPB, aortic cross-clamp and circulatory arrest times. Prolonged CPB times are a risk factor for significant postoperative morbidity and mortality in infants and children (15,175). Circulatory arrest times more than 45 to 50 minutes may be associated with increased postoperative neurologic complications (176). A transesophageal echocardiogram may be performed before and following CPB for complex open heart cases in infants weighing >3 kg, and postoperative findings pertaining to myocardial function and residual lesions should be conveyed to the intensive care unit staff (177,178).

Invasive hemodynamic monitoring is required in nearly all infants following cardiac surgery. Some centers rely heavily on data obtained from invasive hemodynamic monitoring to evaluate myocardial function and detect residual lesions. Other institutions use a combination of minimal invasive monitoring and liberal use of transesophageal echocardiogram to achieve similar information. In any case, it is essential that the clinicians caring for infants following cardiac surgery are familiar with the interpretation and limitations of data obtained from invasive monitoring, and the complications associated with these catheters and pacing wires. A variety of factors may contribute to erroneous data obtained from invasive monitoring, including inappropriate transducer height, and bubbles or clots in the catheters. Information obtained from invasive monitoring cannot be used in isolation, but when placed in the context of the overall clinical picture, can be very useful to guide management in the early postoperative period.

Central venous access is required following CPB in infants, and the anesthesiologist or surgeon will chose a site depending upon the patient's anatomy, anticipated postoperative course and personal preference. For example, physicians may chose to minimize the placement of central venous lines in the subclavian and jugular veins in patients with single ventricle physiology as a result of concerns about thrombosis. Intracardiac lines may be inserted by the surgeon prior to chest closure through the right atrial appendage to the right atrium ("RA line"), or through the right upper pulmonary vein or left atrial appendage to the left atrium ("LA line"). An "OA" line refers to an intracardiac line placed in the common atrium in patients with single ventricle physiology. A pulmonary artery catheter may be placed through the right ventricular outflow tract in patients at high risk for postoperative pulmonary hypertension, residual VSDs, or residual right ventricular outflow tract obstruction. Continuous monitoring of pulmonary artery pressure provides precise knowledge of the severity of pulmonary hypertension, and immediate feedback regarding the effectiveness of interventions to lower pulmonary artery pressure. Significant lability in pulmonary artery pressures during suctioning of the endotracheal tube or awakening from sedation may be a sign that the patient is not ready to be weaned. Measurement of a step-up in oxygen saturation from a superior vena cava or right atrial catheter to a pulmonary artery catheter may be helpful for the detection of significant residual left to right shunting (179). A pullback pressure tracing from the pulmonary artery to the right ventricle may be obtained at the time of removal of the pulmonary artery catheter, which quantifies any residual gradient across the right ventricular outflow tract (179). Some pulmonary artery catheters also have a thermistor tip, thus allowing cardiac output to be calculated by the thermodilution technique.

The report to the intensivist should include information about right and left heart filling pressures, and pulmonary artery pressures (if available) measured before the patient left the operating room. Proper interpretation of these loading conditions is beneficial for the detection of residual lesions, titration of volume administration, and the implementation of interventions that modify vascular tone. Appropriate interpretation of the atrial waveforms may provide insight into the presence of significant atrioventricular valve regurgitation or rhythm disturbances.

Complications associated with intracardiac lines are uncommon but include air embolus, thrombus, infection, bleeding, and catheter retention. Care must be taken when using LA lines in patients with two ventricular repairs, and with any intravenous or intracardiac line in those patients with single ventricle physiology, not to inject air into the systemic circulation. Thus LA lines are only used for monitoring whenever possible, and medication infusions and parenteral nutrition are typically administered through lines that are in the right heart. Although the reported risk of thrombosis or infection is very low with intracardiac catheters, LA and pulmonary artery catheters are removed as soon as possible following surgery, often on the first postoperative day or at the time of chest closure (180,181). Complications at the time of catheter removal include retention and bleeding; the latter has been shown to occur more commonly with pulmonary artery catheters (180,181). Institutional protocols designed to minimize the chance of bleeding at the time of removal of intracardiac lines include guidelines for acceptable coagulation times and platelet counts. Packed red blood cells should be readily available, particularly during the removal of pulmonary artery lines.

Arterial access, necessary for continuous blood pressure monitoring and frequent arterial blood gas sampling, is obtained prior to CPB in the radial, umbilical, femoral, dorsalis pedis or posterior tibial arteries (182–184). Care should be taken to ensure that blood pressure measurements are accurate. If a radial or pedal artery is used for continuous blood pressure monitoring, one must take into account the effect of pulse amplification (higher systolic and lower diastolic blood pressure measured peripherally when compared with central recordings) when interpreting blood pressure values. Dampened waveforms or pressures measured distal to stenotic arteries may give the false impression of hypotension. For example, arm blood pressure measurements in a patient who has, or had in the past, an ipsilateral Blalock-Taussig shunt may be diminished as a result of arterial stenosis. Proper interpretation of the waveform and pulse pressure is important during postoperative management. For example, significant diastolic runoff may produce a wide pulse pressure if an oversized systemic to pulmonary shunt is used, or if severe aortic regurgitation is present. A narrow pulse pressure, along with tachycardia and hypotension, suggests cardiac tamponade. Patients who have had a repair of coarctation or aortic arch reconstruction should have four extremity blood pressure measurements taken to document the absence of a residual gradient.

Accurate assessment of the patient's heart rhythm is an important part of the initial evaluation following surgery. The heart rate and rhythm should be continuously monitored. An electrocardiogram should be obtained in the immediate postoperative period to serve as a new baseline should the infant subsequently develop a tachy-arrhythmia or myocardial ischemia. Atrioventricular synchrony is important for optimizing cardiac output. Temporary pacing wires are commonly placed on the surface of the atrial and/or ventricular myocardium before chest closure, and are tunneled from the mediastinum through the upper abdominal wall where they are secured with tape. These pacing wires may be interrogated when the underlying rhythm is not apparent using the bedside monitor or a 12-lead electrocardiogram (see section on arrhythmias). These wires are quite safe and are usually removed prior to patient discharge (185).

Temperature should be monitored and regulated closely, as high temperature will place increased metabolic demands on the circulatory system, and low temperature will increase systemic vascular resistance (186). Some centers measure central and peripheral temperatures as an indirect estimate of systemic cardiac output. However, a recent investigation found a poor correlation between the core-peripheral temperature gap and lactate levels or hemodynamic parameters, such as cardiac index derived from a pulmonary artery catheter (187).

A directed physical examination should be performed to assess the cardiopulmonary status and adequacy of the surgical repair. Palpation of the precordium should be performed to assess the location and quality of the ventricular impulses. Any murmurs, rubs or gallops should be noted, although dressings and chest tubes may limit the auscultatory findings. It is common to hear a friction rub in the first few days following cardiac surgery, usually as a result of a small accumulation of fluid in the pericardium. The liver span should be noted. Adequate chest rise should be found upon inspiration, and breath sounds should be noted bilaterally. The quality and symmetry of peripheral pulses and warmth of the extremities are useful means of assessing the adequacy of the systemic circulation. Caution must be used when attempting to estimate the adequacy of cardiac output by assessing capillary refill in the postoperative period, as capillary refill time has a poor correlation with cardiac index, systemic vascular resistance index and lactate levels in this setting (187).

Chest tubes should be assessed for location and proper function. Some surgeons will place only a mediastinal chest tube, whereas others will also place pleural tubes. Generally the tubes in infants are removed when drainage falls to less than 20 to 30 cc/day and when there is no evidence for chylothorax or air leak. The stomach should be routinely decompressed postoperatively with a nasogastric tube in all tracheally intubated patients. A CXR should be obtained upon admission to the ICU and daily thereafter, as this practice in infants results in a high percentage of films with an abnormality requiring intervention (188). Particular attention should be given to the location of all tubes and lines, and the heart size and lung fields.

The surgeon will occasionally leave the chest "open" for a few days, with the skin closed either primarily or using a silastic patch, until hemodynamic stability can be achieved, bleeding controlled, and myocardial edema can decrease (189). The sternum is routinely left open in many centers following the Norwood operation (4,190,191). The risk for mediastinitis may be increased when the chest is left open (190). When the chest is eventually closed respiratory compliance may decrease necessitating an increase in ventilatory support (190,192).

Cardiopulmonary interactions play an important role in the physiology of an infant following cardiac surgery (193). Ventilatory manipulations in the early postoperative period of $PaCO_2$, PaO_2, pH and mean airway pressure may be used in the context of the patient's physiology to improve hemodynamics. Mechanical ventilation is also useful to minimize oxygen consumption in infants with limited cardiac reserve. Arterial oxygen saturation is monitored continuously by pulse oximetry. An arterial blood gas analysis is obtained frequently and attention should be given to ensure adequate oxygenation and ventilation for the individual patient's physiology. Ventilator settings used in the operating room are often quite different to those needed in the ICU, primarily as a result of the different ventilators and respiratory tubing used in these settings. Respiratory acidosis has been demonstrated to increase pulmonary vascular resistance in infants following CPB and in most cases should be avoided (193,194). Pulmonary overdistension increases pulmonary vascular resistance and decreases cardiac output (195). A low functional residual capacity following the discontinuation of mechanical ventilation has been associated with increased pulmonary vascular resistance following congenital heart surgery (193). Thus ventilator settings are ordered to maintain relatively normal lung volumes in the early postoperative period. Although early extubation policies have been

reported for older infants and children, most neonates and young infants require at least 12 to 24 hours of mechanical ventilation following congenital heart surgery (196). Criteria for extubation following cardiac surgery in infants include the presence of adequate cardiac output, appropriate mental status to maintain the airway, muscular strength to support respiratory pump function, acceptable gas exchange, and the absence of significant arrhythmias, bleeding or fever.

Standard laboratory values need to be assessed in the early postoperative period. Electrolytes, including magnesium and ionized calcium levels, are monitored and normalized. The complete blood count is obtained daily, and hemoglobin levels are monitored more frequently. In general, a minimum hemoglobin level of 10 to 12 gm/dL is appropriate for infants following a two ventricular repair, and a hemoglobin level of 13 to 15 gm/dL is appropriate for infants following a palliative operation with ongoing cyanosis (See Color Plate). Anemia may place unnecessary workload on the myocardium in the postoperative period. Transfusion of erythrocytes will improve oxygen delivery following pediatric cardiac surgery (197). An excessively high hemoglobin level may increase ventricular afterload or predispose to shunt thrombosis by increasing viscosity (198). Measurement of prothrombin and partial thromboplastin times are obtained initially, and repeated as clinically indicated.

In addition to the physical examination, several clinical parameters may be used to assess the adequacy of cardiac output and oxygen delivery in the immediate postoperative period. The presence of a metabolic acidosis, as quantified by a base deficit or lactate level, suggests inadequate systemic cardiac output and requires investigation. Lactic acidosis develops when inadequate tissue oxygen delivery leads to anaerobic metabolism. Following congenital heart surgery, elevated lactate levels in infants and children upon admission to the ICU are associated with increased morbidity and mortality (175,199–201). Some centers routinely obtain venous blood gases from the superior vena cava to estimate cardiac output. An oxygen extraction ratio (SaO_2–SvO_2/SaO_2) of more than 0.5 at 6 hours after infant cardiac surgery suggests a severe derangement in oxygen transport that may be predictive of mortality (Fig. 34-13) (202). Urine output provides a good estimate of the systemic cardiac output and ideally should be at least 1 cc/kg/hour. Rising blood urea nitrogen (BUN) and creatinine levels (Cr) may be secondary to low cardiac output. Infants often require some inotropic support following CPB, and low dose dopamine is the initial drug of choice at many centers. Additional inotropic support is discussed further in the section below on low cardiac output.

Infants may develop significant fluid retention following CPB, which may impair myocardial, respiratory, and gastrointestinal function. Strategies used to minimize this problem in the operating room, including the use of steroids and ultrafiltration, are discussed earlier. Despite the presence of total body fluid overload,

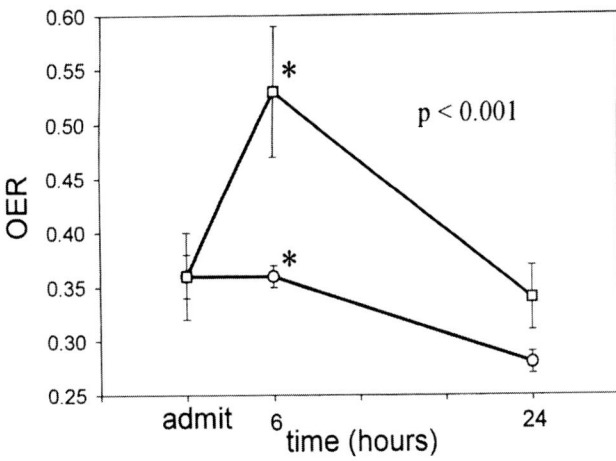

Figure 34-13 Changes in mean oxygen extraction ratio (OER) for survivors and nonsurvivors after infant congenital heart surgery over time (circles = survivors, squares = nonsurvivors). Reprinted from Rossi AF, Seiden HS, Gross RP, et al. Oxygen transport in critically ill infants after congenital heart operations. *Ann Thorac Surg* 1999;67:739–744, with permission from the Society of Thoracic Surgeons.

intravascular volume depletion is common in the first few hours following surgery and several fluid boluses may be required. Furosemide is typically initiated 12 to 24 hours after surgery, either as bolus doses or continuous infusion (203). Additional diuretics with alternative mechanisms of action are used as clinically indicated. Low dose ("renal dose") dopamine is commonly used to augment urine output despite a lack of convincing data supporting its effectiveness in infants. Electrolyte disturbances, particularly hypokalemia, hyponatremia, and a hypochloremic metabolic alkalosis, are commonly encountered as diuresis occurs in the first few days following CPB.

Analgesia is required for all infants following cardiopulmonary bypass. High dose fentanyl is well tolerated and blunts the stress response in neonates following CPB (204–206). Morphine is another narcotic commonly used in the early postoperative period. Benzodiazepines may be given for amnesia and sedation. Either intermittent boluses or continuous infusions of these agents may be used in infants depending on the hemodynamics and perceived risk for pulmonary hypertension. The indications for the use of neuromuscular blocking agents vary at different centers, but these medications may be used to eliminate coughing and minimize oxygen consumption in patients with labile hemodynamics.

Gastrointestinal tract motility is decreased following cardiac surgery in infants as a result of the inflammatory effects of CPB, anesthesia, fluid retention, postoperative use of narcotics and possibly low cardiac output. Furthermore, some neonates may have been exposed to a preoperative period of mesenteric hypoperfusion. If these considerations preclude the initiation of enteral nutrition following surgery, the parenteral nutrition is prescribed. Histamine-2 receptor antagonists are typically administered to minimize

the risk of upper gastrointestinal bleeding until enteral nutrition is established.

Common Postoperative Complications

Low Cardiac Output

The product of heart rate and stroke volume determines cardiac output. Stroke volume is determined by preload, afterload and contractility. Low cardiac output may thus be caused by abnormalities in one or more of these variables. An alteration in the heart rate or rhythm may impact cardiac output, and this is discussed further in the subsequent section on arrhythmias. Decreased preload may occur from hemorrhage, excessive diuresis, insufficient fluid replacement, or cardiac tamponade. Increased afterload may result from pulmonary hypertension, peripheral vasoconstriction or ventricular outflow obstruction. A decrease in myocardial contractility may result from a combination of factors including acidosis, electrolyte imbalance, hypothermia, or myocardial injury secondary to inflammation, a ventriculotomy, inadequate myocardial protection or ischemia reperfusion. Low cardiac output, when defined as a cardiac index less than 2.0 $L/min/m^2$, occurs following approximately 25% of complex two ventricle repairs in infancy (Fig. 34-14) (140). Other signs of low cardiac output include tachycardia, hypotension, poor peripheral perfusion, poor urine output and metabolic acidosis. A detailed assessment must be undertaken to identify the cause of low cardiac output so that proper treatment may be initiated and end-organ failure avoided (207).

A suboptimal surgical repair with significant residual intracardiac shunts, ventricular outflow or aortic obstruction,

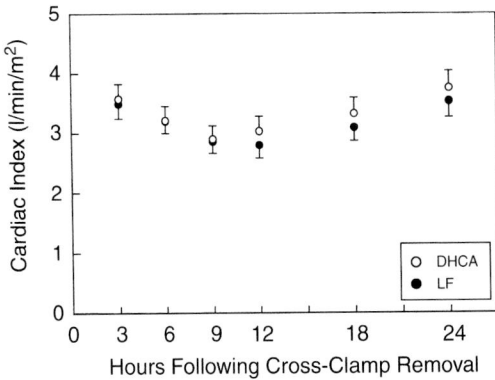

Figure 34-14 Scatterplots showing serial measurements of cardiac index as determined by thermodilution techniques in 122 patients after the arterial switch operation for TGA. Cardiac index fell during the first postoperative night, returning to baseline values by 24 hours after surgery. There was no significant difference between patients randomized to deep hypothermic circulatory arrest (DHCA) and those randomized to low-flow cardiopulmonary bypass (LF). Values are depicted as the mean and one side of each 95% CI. Reprinted from Wernovsky G, Wypij D, Jonas RA, et al. Postoperative course and hemodynamic profile after the arterial switch operation in neonates and infants. A comparison of low-flow cardiopulmonary bypass and circulatory arrest. *Circulation* 1995;92:2226–2235, with permission.

systemic or pulmonary venous stenosis, and/or valvular lesions may be the primary etiology for low cardiac output. The incidence of hemodynamically significant residual lesions following congenital heart surgery has likely decreased in recent years as a result of improving surgical technique and the liberal use of transesophageal echocardiogram immediately following CPB (178). That being said, when an infant develops low cardiac output or follows an atypical clinical course following CPB, a primary responsibility of the intensivist and/or cardiologist is the early detection of residual lesions that require reintervention. Failure to do so will expose the patient to prolonged ICU stays with the associated morbidity and mortality. A combination of factors will lead to the early identification of significant residual lesions, including an appreciation of the anticipated "normal" postoperative course, close attention to data obtained by intracardiac monitoring and physical examination, open communication with the cardiovascular surgeon, and a high index of suspicion (208). Early, focused echocardiography or cardiac catheterization is then required to define the extent of the problem (209,210).

Treatment of low cardiac output in neonates differs from that in older children and adults as a result of differences in cardiovascular physiology. Because neonates have a greater ratio of noncontractile to contractile myocardial mass, ventricular diastolic compliance is diminished, and they have a limited ability to increase their stroke volume, which is fixed at approximately 1.5 cc/kg (211–213). Thus the cardiac output is rate-dependent in this patient population. Heart rate may be optimized by pacing, or by using intravenous infusions of chronotropic agents including dopamine, dobutamine or rarely isoproterenol. For infants with complete heart block, atrioventricular sequential pacing at an appropriate rate is indicated to increase the cardiac output. Other postoperative arrhythmias are discussed in detail below.

Optimization of cardiac loading conditions is a key component to the management of the infant with low cardiac output (214). As described by the Frank-Starling mechanism, augmentation of the end-diastolic volume increases the number of interactions between actin and myosin molecules, resulting in a larger stroke volume and thus higher cardiac output. Conversely, hypovolemia may result in decreased ventricular filling and low cardiac output. Certain cardiac operations in infants, such as repair of tetralogy of Fallot or truncus arteriosus, result in particularly poor right ventricular compliance, which will require additional preload in the early postoperative period to maintain cardiac output. Volume replacement therapy should also be guided by close attention to filling pressures, arterial pressures, and physical examination signs including gallops, liver distention and peripheral pulses. The type and amount of fluid replacement is based upon the hematocrit, albumin level, and percentage of volume loss. Boluses of fluid are given in increments of 5 to 10 ml/kg over several minutes. A left atrial pressure above 14 to 16 mm Hg rarely produces an additional increase in cardiac output, and a left atrial pressure above 20 mm Hg

can cause pulmonary edema (215). Furthermore, as a result of the large venous capacitance of infants, the right atrial pressures may not necessarily reflect the volume administered and should not be used in isolation to estimate preload.

Afterload, defined as the sum of forces that oppose systolic performance, is best quantified by systolic wall stress and vascular impedance, both of which are difficult to measure at the bedside. Afterload may be clinically estimated by using a pulmonary artery catheter to aid in the calculation of the resistance of the systemic and pulmonary vascular beds. An increase in vascular resistance can significantly reduce both stroke volume and the extent and velocity of wall shortening, resulting in decreased cardiac output and ventricular function. Increased vascular resistance is commonly seen following cardiopulmonary bypass in neonates (140). Physiologic factors such as hypoxia, acidosis, hypothermia, and pain may further increase systemic and pulmonary vascular resistance. Increased afterload may also be secondary to residual right or left ventricular outflow tract obstruction. In the setting of decreased cardiac contractility, increased afterload may be a compensatory response necessary to maintain systemic blood pressure.

Vascular resistance, and thus afterload, can be pharmacologically decreased by vasodilatation of the vascular bed(s). Systemic afterload reduction is beneficial for infants with significant aortic or mitral valve regurgitation, left ventricular dysfunction or hypertension. Afterload reduction in the pulmonary circulation is beneficial for infants with tricuspid valve regurgitation, right ventricular dysfunction and pulmonary hypertension. In addition to its inotropic properties, milrinone is a direct vasodilator of the systemic and pulmonary vascular beds (216). The systemic and pulmonary vascular resistances are also effectively lowered by intravenous infusion of sodium nitroprusside or nitroglycerine, which are both NO donors that cause smooth muscle relaxation. With the use of any of these vasodilators, volume augmentation may be necessary to fill the expanded vascular space and maintain adequate preload. Inhaled NO selectively vasodilates the pulmonary vascular bed, thereby decreasing right ventricular afterload and allowing for recovery of right ventricular systolic function (217). Positive pressure ventilation may reduce wall stress and left ventricular afterload in two ventricle hearts provided that preload is maintained (218,219). Occasionally an infant may have vasodilatory shock with inappropriately low systemic vascular resistance following CPB that is refractory to catecholamines. Favorable hemodynamic responses to vasopressin infusions have been described in this setting (220).

Cardiac contractility is the load-independent ability of the myocardium to generate force. Contractility may be chronically impaired preoperatively by pressure and/or volume overload related to the specific cardiac lesion. Contractility may be depressed intraoperatively by medications, anesthesia, myocardial ischemia, an extensive ventriculotomy, or by myocardial resection. Postoperatively, hypoxia, acidosis, and pharmacologic agents may affect contractility. In infants and children the cardiac index tends to reach its nadir approximately 4 hours after CPB, and begins to rise to normal values after 9 to 12 hours (221). The fall in cardiac index and rise in systemic and pulmonary vascular resistance occurring between 6 to 18 hours following the arterial switch operation in neonates with TGA has been well described (140). If the infant still shows evidence of low cardiac output after optimizing the heart rate, the preload, and afterload, myocardial contractility should be enhanced with pharmacologic agents. Several inotropic drugs are currently available, and each has its own characteristic effects that may be more suitable for use in various clinical situations.

Dopamine activates dopaminergic, α, and β-receptors, depending on the dosage used. When prescribed at 1 to 5 mcg/kg/min, dopamine preferentially dilates mesenteric and renal vessels, and increases renal blood flow. Dosing at 5 to 10 mcg/kg/min tends to increase cardiac output with a mild increase in heart rate (222). Higher doses of dopamine (10–20 mcg/kg/min) are usually avoided because of an increase in pulmonary vascular resistance related to alpha-receptor stimulation. Low-dose dopamine is the initial drug of choice to increase inotrope at many centers.

Dobutamine, a synthetic catecholamine, acts primarily on myocardial beta-receptors. Contractility increases with infusion of dobutamine, but there is less effect on heart rate or vascular tone than with dopamine (223–225).

Milrinone is a phosphodiesterase inhibitor that exerts a positive inotropic effect by increasing intracellular levels of cyclic adenosine monophosphate (cAMP), leading to improving cardiac contractility. It also has lusitropic properties, and acts as a direct vasodilator of the systemic and pulmonary vascular beds (216). Milrinone has been shown to decrease the incidence of low cardiac output syndrome in a prospective, randomized clinical trial of pediatric patients less than 6 years of age undergoing biventricular repair, and to improve hemodynamics in neonates with existing low cardiac output (226,227).

Patients who have marked myocardial dysfunction that does not improve with one or a combination of the first line agents listed above may respond to intravenous epinephrine at 0.01 to 0.05 mcg/kg/min. When administered in this dosage range, epinephrine primarily activates β-1 cardiac receptors causing increased inotrope, and β-2 peripheral receptors causing reduced afterload. High-dose epinephrine (>0.1 mcg/kg/min) is not frequently used because of marked α-adrenergic action and adverse effect on renal perfusion. High-dose epinephrine has also been shown to cause myocardial necrosis in neonatal pigs (228).

Infants with refractory low cardiac output, myocardial dysfunction and impending cardiovascular collapse may benefit from having their sternotomy incision reopened in the ICU. The combination of edema of the myocardium and other mediastinal structures, and any fluid or blood collections around the heart may contribute to poor ventricular filling and compliance. Reopening the chest will expand the mediastinal space until edema improves, and any fluid collections or blood clots can be easily removed. Should low cardiac output persist, an open chest allows easy access for cannulation for mechanical support.

In patients with excessive or prolonged inotropic or vasopressor needs following CPB, a state of relative adrenocortical insufficiency may exist. Myocardial β-receptor down regulation has been demonstrated to occur in infants and small children with congenital heart disease in the perioperative period (229). Corticosteroids, probably acting by improving vascular tone and up regulating adrenergic receptors, may allow weaning of high dose catecholamine infusions in infants (230).

Thyroid hormone plays a critical role in the regulation of the cardiovascular system, and decreased levels of tri-iodothyronine (T_3) and thyroxine levels occur in some infants following CPB (231–233). Preliminary data suggest that exogenous supplementation with T_3 is well tolerated and may improve mixed venous oxygen saturation and decrease inotropic requirements following neonatal CPB (234). Favorable changes in hemodynamics have also been reported in older infants and children who were given T_3 following CPB (235,236). Patient enrollment has been completed for a prospective, randomized, double-blind, placebo-controlled clinical trail designed to evaluate the effects of a 72-hour infusion of T_3 on early postoperative outcomes in neonates undergoing the Norwood procedure or repair of IAA at Children's Hospital Boston, and the results will be available in early 2005.

Arrhythmias

The development of a postoperative arrhythmia may severely compromise cardiac output in the infant following CPB. Prolonged CPB and aortic cross clamp times, and higher postoperative serum troponin levels, are associated with the development of arrhythmias in infants and children (237). An accurate diagnosis of the arrhythmia may be obtained with a 12-lead electrocardiogram. However, it is often the case in infants with fast heart rates that the relationship of the P waves to the QRS complex is uncertain on the standard 12-lead ECG, and in these instances, interrogation of temporary atrial pacing wires is very helpful (185,238). Several techniques may be used to interrogate the temporary atrial pacing wires. One such method is to connect the two leg leads of the ECG machine to the temporary atrial pacing wires, and the two arm leads are placed on the patient's arms in the usual fashion. A rhythm strip of leads I, II and III is then recorded from the ECG machine. Lead I will be a surface electrogram, and a sharp atrial electrogram (indicating atrial depolarization) is produced in leads II and III, which may be compared to the surface QRS complex in lead I to determine the relationship of P waves to the QRS complexes. The presence of cannon a-waves may give insight into the presence of an arrhythmia and its mechanism. Cannon a-waves, depicted on the bedside monitor as an increase in amplitude of the atrial pressure waveform obtained by intraatrial lines, occur when the atria contract against a closed atrioventricular valve during various arrhythmias. Nearly any type of arrhythmia may occur following infant CPB. Commonly encountered arrhythmias are discussed in the following paragraphs, and further information may be found in an excellent book on pediatric arrhythmias (239).

Premature atrial complexes (PACs) are occasionally seen and may be related to central lines, electrolyte disturbances or surgical incisions; they are usually benign. Reentrant forms of supraventricular tachycardia (SVT), such as atrial flutter and atrioventricular reentrant tachycardia, are relatively uncommon following infant cardiac surgery. Although rate-related aberrancy and antegrade conduction over accessory connections may occur, in most cases of SVT the QRS complex in tachycardia is similar in morphology and axis to that seen on the baseline postoperative ECG. The baseline QRS complex may be wide if a bundle branch block developed during surgery, as is common following repair of tetralogy of Fallot, VSDs, and complete atrioventricular canal defects. Atrial flutter is more likely to be seen following complex atrial baffling procedures. Atrial flutter is characterized by a rapid, regular atrial rate with variable atrioventricular conduction. Adenosine is helpful diagnostically as the flutter waves will persist in the presence of atrioventricular block. Atrial flutter may be terminated using rapid atrial pacing, via the temporary pacing wires or a transesophageal electrode, or synchronized cardioversion starting at 0.5 to 1 J/kg. Atrioventricular reentrant tachycardia may be seen in infants with accessory connections, such as some patients with Ebstein's anomaly, L-looped ventricular inversion. Pre-excitation (Wolfe-Parkinson-White Syndrome) may be present on the electrocardiogram in sinus rhythm. Atrioventricular reciprocating tachycardia is characterized by retrograde P waves following the QRS complex in a one-to-one relationship, and is terminated with adenosine, rapid atrial pacing, or synchronized cardioversion. Atrioventricular node reentrant tachycardia and atrial fibrillation are rare in infants and will not be discussed further.

Ectopic atrial tachycardia is an uncommon form of SVT following congenital heart surgery. It is characterized by an automatic atrial rhythm with "warm up" and "cool down" behavior at its onset and termination. Infants having disruption of the atrial septum (e.g., tricuspid atresia or TGA following balloon atrial septostomy), longer CPB times, higher inotropic needs, and potassium depletion may be at increased risk for developing this arrhythmia (240). Treatment strategies include normalization of electrolytes and temperature, minimizing inotropic infusions, and administration of a variety of antiarrhythmic agents including beta-blockers and amiodarone.

Junctional ectopic tachycardia (JET) is a common type of SVT seen in the postoperative period in infants, particularly following repair of tetralogy of Fallot or VSDs (241,242). JET is an automatic rhythm originating from the bundle of His, and although thought to be caused by some form of trauma to the atrioventricular (AV) node during surgery, may occasionally be seen following cardiac

surgical interventions distant from the AV node. The occurrence of postoperative JET has been reported to prolong postoperative mechanical ventilation and ICU times (243). Electrophysiological characteristics of JET are as follows: a QRS morphology similar to that seen in sinus rhythm; atrio-ventricular dissociation with the ventricular rate faster than the atrial rate, or 1:1 retrograde conduction; "warm up" behavior as seen with automatic arrhythmias; and failure to respond to adenosine, overdrive pacing or cardioversion (244). Cannon a-waves will have variable amplitude in patients with JET if ventricular-atrial (V-A) dissociation is present, but constant increased amplitude will be seen with JET if the junctional rhythm is conduced to the atria in a 1:1 retrograde pattern. A 12-lead ECG or interrogation of temporary atrial pacing wires will confirm the diagnosis. Although JET usually resolves spontaneously in the first few days following surgery, this arrhythmia will often cause hemodynamic compromise when the ventricular rate exceeds 170 to 180 beats per minute. Treatment strategies must be individualized to the individual patient's heart rate and hemodynamic status and include fever control, provision of adequate analgesia to minimize endogenous catecholamine release, minimizing the use of exogenous catecholamines, normalization of electrolytes and acid-base status, atrial pacing at a rate faster than the junctional rate, and mild hypothermia (245,246). Medications used to treat JET when the above measures fail include amiodarone, esmolol and procainamide (244, 246,247). As these drugs have negative inotropic and chronotropic properties, close monitoring of hemodynamics and back-up pacing capabilities are necessary.

Premature ventricular contractions (PVCs) may reflect myocardial irritability, electrolyte disturbances or hypoxia. Lidocaine is often administered for frequent PVCs or nonsustained ventricular tachycardia (VT). VT is characterized by a fast, wide QRS complex that differs in morphology and axis compared to the postoperative baseline, and has either 1:1 retrograde V-A conduction, or V-A dissociation. The presence of complex ventricular ectopy or VT is suggestive of myocardial ischemia, and those infants who had coronary manipulation as a component of their operation should have a prompt evaluation of coronary blood flow. Sustained VT with hemodynamic compromise may be terminated by synchronized cardioversion starting at 1 J/kg. Pharmacologic therapy, starting with either lidocaine or procainamide, may be considered for patients with hemodynamically stable VT. Ventricular fibrillation (VF) is characterized by a wide complex, irregular rhythm that requires immediate defibrillation, starting at 2 J/kg. Cardiopulmonary resuscitation is required during VF until a perfusing rhythm is reestablished.

Complete heart block typically is apparent when the patient is rewarmed following CPB, but much less commonly may develop in the first few days following surgery. Atrioventricular sequential temporary pacing is used for treatment (248). The capture threshold of the temporary ventricular pacing wire should be determined frequently in patients who have developed or are at high risk for complete heart block. An alternative method of pacing may be required for patients with very high or rapidly rising capture thresholds. If atrioventricular conduction does not return within 7 to 14 days, a permanent pacemaker is placed to prevent low cardiac output and sudden death (52).

Pulmonary Hypertension

Although the movement toward early complete neonatal repair has lead to a decreased incidence of pulmonary hypertensive crises for patients with many congenital heart defects, this complication continues to impede the recovery of infants following complete surgical repair or palliation in the contemporary era (3,8,142,249,250). Severe pulmonary hypertension, defined as a ratio of pulmonary to systemic arterial pressure greater than or equal to 1.0, was present postoperatively in 2% of infants and children having congenital heart surgery at a single center (median age 4.2 months) (251). In this series, severe pulmonary hypertension was associated with an increase in mortality.

Pulmonary hypertension following infant CPB may be caused by a combination of preoperative, intraoperative, and postoperative factors, the sum effect of which may be additive (Table 34-7). The presence of several preoperative clinical features allows for the identification of infants at increased postoperative risk for pulmonary hypertension. Specific lesions, all characterized by having preoperative large left to right shunts or obstructed pulmonary venous return, are associated with postoperative pulmonary hypertension (8,252). Infants with large communications at the ventricular or arterial level by definition have pulmonary hypertension prior to going to the operating room. Infants with obstructed pulmonary venous return, mitral stenosis or left ventricular outflow obstruction (critical aortic valve stenosis or coarctation of the aorta) may have severe preoperative pulmonary hypertension and increased pul-

monary vascular resistance. Down syndrome is also a risk factor for severe postoperative pulmonary hypertension (251).

CPB is associated with increased pulmonary vascular resistance in infants and children (140,141). CPB causes partial ischemia of the pulmonary vasculature, leading to endothelial cell dysfunction and decreased endogenous production of NO (141,253–256). CPB leads to increased plasma levels of catecholamines, endothelin-1 and other pulmonary vasoconstrictors in infants and children (252,257–259). In infants, prolonged CPB time has been associated with increased pulmonary vascular resistance in the postoperative period (142). The presence of significant pulmonary hypertension soon after weaning from CPB is predictive of subsequent pulmonary hypertension in the ICU and the need for prolonged ventilatory support (142,260).

Postoperatively, large residual left to right shunts or obstruction to pulmonary venous or distal pulmonary arterial blood flow, or left ventricular outflow tract obstruction all may cause pulmonary hypertension. Noxious stimuli, particularly suctioning of the endotracheal tube, may trigger a pulmonary hypertensive crisis (261).

Pulmonary hypertension may manifest as low cardiac output following a two-ventricular repair when both septa are completely intact. In infants with a significant risk for pulmonary hypertensive spells, such as those undergoing complete repair of truncus arteriosus, an atrial communication is often intentionally left open so that right to left shunting may occur to preserve cardiac output in the event that pulmonary artery pressures become significantly elevated. In such infants, and those with palliated single ventricle physiology, excessive cyanosis will be present if postoperative pulmonary hypertension occurs. Pulmonary artery catheters, although not commonly used in infants at many congenital heart centers, provide direct and continuous measurement of pulmonary artery pressure following two

TABLE 34-7

FACTORS CONTRIBUTING TO PERIOPERATIVE PULMONARY HYPERTENSION IN INFANTS

Preoperative
left to right shunts
obstructed pulmonary venous return

Intraoperative
microemboli
pulmonary leukosequestration
excess thromboxane production
duration of CPB
endothelial injury

Postoperative
mechanical obstruction to pulmonary blood flow
residual left to right shunt
atelectasis
hypoxic pulmonary vasoconstriction
catecholamines (endogenous and exogenous)

TABLE 34-8

CRITICAL CARE STRATEGIES FOR TREATMENT OF PULMONARY HYPERTENSION

Encourage	Avoid
1. Anatomic investigation	1. Residual anatomic disease
2. Right to left atrial pop off	2. Intact atrial septum
3. Sedation/analgesia	3. Agitation/pain
4. Moderate hyperventilation	4. Respiratory acidosis
5. Moderate alkalosis	5. Metabolic acidosis
6. Adequate inspired oxygen	6. Alveolar hypoxia
7. Normal lung volumes	7. Atelectasis or overdistension
8. Optimal hematocrit	8. Excessive hematocrit
9. Inotropic support	9. Low output and coronary perfusion
10. Pulmonary vasodilators	10. Pulmonary vasoconstrictors

Modified from Wessel DL. Managing low cardiac output syndrome after congenital heart surgery. *Crit Care Med* 2001;29:S220–30, with permission.

ventricular repairs. The severity of pulmonary hypertension may also be estimated echocardiographically by Doppler interrogation of a tricuspid regurgitation jet in the absence of right ventricular outflow tract obstruction.

A combination of relatively simple postoperative strategies should be sufficient to prevent the development of pulmonary hypertensive crises in many at-risk patients (Table 34-8) (262). Adequate oxygenation and ventilation are important in the early postoperative period to maintain low pulmonary vascular resistance, as is the maintenance of relatively normal lung volumes (193–195,263). Deep sedation and analgesia in the immediate postoperative period are also used to minimize the incidence of pulmonary hypertension crises. High dose fentanyl infusions have been shown to reduce the stress response and postoperative morbidity in infants following CPB (257). In particular, fentanyl has been shown to blunt the elevation in pulmonary artery pressure and pulmonary vascular resistance related to endotracheal suctioning following the repair of congenital heart defects in infants (205). Benzodiazepines are commonly used for additional sedation. Prophylactic alpha-receptor blockade and early definitive repair can reduce the incidence of postoperative pulmonary hypertension (8). Although nitric oxide is well tolerated and decreases the incidence of pulmonary hypertensive crises in high-risk infants, this drug is not commonly used for primary prevention of pulmonary hypertension crises in part related to its high cost (250).

Before assuming that increased pulmonary vascular resistance causes pulmonary hypertension, the intensivist must ensure that an anatomic etiology for elevated pulmonary artery pressures is not present. For example, significant residual pulmonary arterial obstruction distal to the point of pulmonary artery pressure measurement will cause pulmonary hypertension, but the pulmonary artery pressure will not fall with medical management including inhaled NO (208).

All of the management strategies mentioned above regarding the prevention of pulmonary hypertension are used in the event of a pulmonary hypertensive crisis. Hyperventilation has been shown to reduce pulmonary artery pressure and pulmonary vascular resistance in infants and children with pulmonary hypertension in the early postoperative period. Although hyperventilation is a first-line intervention for pulmonary hypertensive crises, the following associated effects must be considered. Systemic vascular resistance increases with hyperventilation, as a result of alkalosis, leading to decreased cardiac output (264,265). Depending on the ventilator strategy used to achieve hyperventilation, the mean airway pressure may increase, which may increase pulmonary vascular resistance. Other concerning side effects of hyperventilation include reduced cerebral and coronary blood flow, and a leftward shift of the oxy-hemoglobin dissociation curve.

In an infant with a two-ventricular repair and intact atrial septum who experiences a pulmonary hypertension crisis and develops refractory hypotension, careful infusion of volume through the left atrial line will bypass the pulmonary vascular bed and may temporarily stabilize the blood pressure until the pulmonary vascular resistance is reduced.

Nonselective vasodilators were used in the past to treat severe pulmonary hypertension, however, current standard therapy centers on the use of NO. NO, when produced by the vascular endothelium, diffuses to adjacent smooth muscle cells, in which relaxation occurs by activation of guanylate cyclase, which increases intracellular guanosine 3', 5'-monophosphate (cyclic GMP) (266). Because NO is rapidly inactivated by hemoglobin, it acts as a selective pulmonary vasodilator when delivered by inhalation (267,268). Side effects associated with NO include a rebound effect upon withdrawal of the drug, and methemoglobinemia (269–271). Preliminary observations suggest that sildenafil may be useful to facilitate the weaning of NO in infants who previously demonstrated significant rebound pulmonary hypertension (272).

One randomized study of high-risk infants and young children found that NO did not lower pulmonary artery pressure or prevent pulmonary hypertensive crises. Most patients in the study were receiving nitroprusside, a NO donor, and about one-half were receiving milrinone. Furthermore, this study was not controlled for the use of neuromuscular blockade, and several patients in the study had underlying lung disease (273). However, the vast majority of studies found a beneficial effect of NO in alleviating pulmonary hypertension following CPB in infants and children. In a randomized, double-blind, placebo-controlled clinical trial of infants and children (mostly infants with VSDs or atrioventricular canal defects) who emerged from CPB with a mean pulmonary artery pressure more than 50% of the mean systemic artery pressure, NO was shown to reduce the mean pulmonary artery pressure in the immediate postoperative period (260). Several other nonrandomized reports demonstrate the efficacy and safety of NO for selectively lowering pulmonary artery pressure in infants and young children following CPB (141,274–278). Transient right ventricular dysfunction following repair of congenital heart defects may be exacerbated by pulmonary hypertension. NO improves right ventricular ejection fraction and cardiac output while decreasing pulmonary artery pressure and vascular resistance in infants and young children following a biventricular repair (217). NO also decreases pulmonary artery pressure in infants with single ventricle physiology following the bi-directional Glenn operation (278,279). NO may reduce the need for extracorporeal life support in infants with critical pulmonary hypertension after CPB (280).

The benefits of intravenous prostacycline on pulmonary vascular resistance in children with congenital heart disease are offset by tachycardia and systemic hypotension (281–283). However, more recent studies have found that inhaled prostacycline, which causes vasodilation by increasing intracellular concentrations of cAMP, is as effective as NO for lowering pulmonary vascular resistance following repair of congenital heart disease (284,285). Further clinical investigation and clinical experience are required before inhaled prostacycline can be recommended for widespread clinical use following CPB in infants.

Cyanosis

Excessive cyanosis following surgical repair or palliation may be attributed to a variety of anatomic problems depending upon the individual patient's physiology. In the infant with palliated single ventricle physiology, excessive cyanosis may be attributable to inadequate pulmonary blood low, pulmonary venous desaturation and/or systemic venous desaturation. Decreased pulmonary blood flow may be as a result of stenosis or thrombosis in the systemic to pulmonary artery shunt, or stenosis in the superior vena cava or pulmonary arteries following the bi-directional Glenn or hemi-Fontan operation. If an anatomic problem is suspected with the systemic to pulmonary artery shunt or a bi-directional Glenn, a cardiac catheterization is usually required. Pulmonary hypertension may also cause decreased pulmonary blood flow, which can be attributed to CPB, or impairment of blood egress from the pulmonary

veins (e.g., pulmonary venous obstruction or left atrial outlet obstruction). In palliated single ventricle patients with excessive cyanosis, treatment of pulmonary hypertension includes the use of NO if standard measures to lower pulmonary vascular resistance are ineffective (278,279). Pulmonary venous desaturation may be caused by parenchymal lung disease, pleural effusions, or systemic to pulmonary venous collateral vessels. Systemic venous desaturation, secondary to anemia, low cardiac output or increased oxygen consumption, may also contribute to cyanosis following single ventricle palliation. Similar causes for excessive cyanosis may exist following a two-ventricle repair, particularly if an atrial communication exists allowing right to left shunting. For example, following complete repair of truncus arteriosus, excessive cyanosis related to decreased pulmonary blood flow may be present in the postoperative period as a result of poor right ventricular compliance, right ventricular outflow tract obstruction, or pulmonary hypertension with subsequent right to left shunting at the atrial level. Note that excessive systemic venous desaturation will not contribute to cyanosis following a two-ventricle repair unless a residual intracardiac communication or veno-venous collaterals exist that allow right to left shunting.

Ventilatory management of the infant with excessive cyanosis following the bi-directional Glenn/hemi-Fontan operation deserves special consideration. As pulmonary blood flow is passive and heavily influenced by intrathoracic pressure, ventilator settings that minimize mean airway pressure and maximize exhalation time will enhance pulmonary blood flow. As these operations place the cerebral and pulmonary vascular beds in series, pulmonary blood flow is derived in large part from venous return from the brain to the superior vena cava. Working on the principle that increased partial pressure of CO_2 ($PaCO_2$) results in cerebral arterial vasodilation and increased cerebral blood flow, investigators have demonstrated that hyperventilation decreases SaO_2 following the bi-directional Glenn/hemi-Fontan operation, and the hypoventilation improves SaO_2 (286,287). In addition to CO_2 induced increased cerebral blood flow, however, other uncontrolled factors that may have resulted in improved SaO_2 in these patients included a decrease in mean airway pressure during hypoventilation, and CO_2 stimulated increase in cardiac output leading to increased oxygen saturation in the inferior vena cava (287).

Bleeding

Excessive bleeding may occur from suture lines and/or abnormalities in the coagulation system following CPB (152). Generally accepted risk factors for postoperative bleeding include repeat sternotomy, cyanosis, and operations involving extensive suture lines in the aorta. Excessive bleeding may be defined as greater than 5cc/kg of blood from the chest tube in any given hour or greater than 3 cc/kg/hour × 3 hours. Intraoperative administration of aprotinin may minimize postoperative bleeding, as discussed earlier (164). Aminocaproic acid and tranex-amic acid, both antifibrinolytic agents, may be administered intraoperatively to infants at risk for bleeding (288–291). The platelet count is maintained more than 50,000 to 100,000/mL in the early postoperative period. Fresh frozen plasma is administered for a prothrombin time (PT) more than 25 seconds or for excessive bleeding. Hypertension might exacerbate bleeding and should be controlled. Inadequate neutralization of heparin will be manifested by a prolonged partial thromboplastin time (PTT), and additional protamine is indicated if this diagnosis is suspected.

Bleeding may occur when intracardiac lines are removed. Bleeding is more common following the removal of pulmonary artery catheters and left atrial lines, when compared to right atrial lines (180,181). The pulmonary artery and left atrial lines are generally removed on the first day following surgery if no longer needed clinically, or at the time of chest closure. Coagulation times and platelet counts should be at acceptable levels, and cross-matched blood should be available when these catheters are removed.

Cardiac tamponade may occur when significant bleeding is not evacuated by the chest tube(s). External compression of the heart by blood or blood clots leads to impaired ventricular filling, increased central venous pressure, tachycardia, a narrow pulse pressure and eventually systemic hypotension. The diagnosis can be confirmed by echocardiography, and surgical exploration of the chest is required, either emergently at the bedside, or urgently in the operating room.

Cardiac Arrest

Infants having a cardiac arrest following congenital heart surgery have better survival rate (41% in one series) when compared with other general pediatric intensive care unit patient populations (292). The better survival rate may be attributed to a variety of issues unique to the cardiac population, including the increased incidence of an acute ventricular arrhythmia, the absence of multi-organ system failure in the majority of the cardiac patients, and the common presence of central venous access, arterial access and epicardial pacing wires. Survival to hospital discharge was achieved in 5/22 infants despite resuscitation times >30 minutes in one series of patients, making the use of predetermined resuscitation end points somewhat irrelevant (292). However, the long-term neurologic outcome of these 5 infants was not reported in this study. Algorithms exist for the management of infants experiencing a cardiopulmonary arrest and will not be repeated here (293). If spontaneous circulation has not returned despite a few minutes of resuscitation, the chest may be reopened in infants who have had a recent sternotomy, and open cardiac massage performed. Rapid-deployment extracorporeal membranous oxygenation (ECMO; also see Chapter 32) has been used to salvage some infants receiving ongoing cardiopulmonary resuscitation and is discussed further below (294).

Mechanical Cardiac Support

A recently published textbook includes a detailed discussion of pediatric mechanical cardiac support (295). At most congenital heart centers, postoperative ECMO is used in approximately 3% of infants and children following CPB (296). ECMO is used to provide mechanical cardiopulmonary support in most infants, as aortic balloon pumps and ventricular assist devices currently are not widely available for this patient population as a result of size limitations and other technical issues. Some experience does exist, however, with a centrifugal pump ventricular assist device in infants, including those with isolated left ventricular failure following repair of anomalous origin of the left coronary artery from the pulmonary artery, a lesion that is characterized by having severe but reversible left ventricular systolic dysfunction (297,298).

Following surgical repair or palliation, infants who cannot be weaned from CPB may be converted to an ECMO circuit before leaving the operating room. Once in the ICU, those infants who develop refractory low cardiac output, severe cyanosis, arrhythmias, or pulmonary hypertension despite maximal medical therapy, or have an unexpected cardiac arrest may be candidates for mechanical cardiopulmonary support. Mechanical support may be used as a bridge to myocardial recovery or cardiac transplantation (126,299,300). Venoarterial ECMO is required in nearly all of infants requiring mechanical support for primary cardiac failure, in contrast to neonates with primary respiratory failure who may be supported with venous-venous ECMO. Relative contraindications to ECMO include multiorgan system failure, an irreversible or inoperable disease process, significant neurologic impairment, uncontrolled bleeding, extremes of size and weight, and inaccessible vessels during cardiopulmonary resuscitation (262). The decision to employ ECMO following infant CPB should be made prior to the development of irreversible end-organ failure, as patients who have been placed on ECMO after extended efforts at medical management have been shown to do poorly (301,302).

Although some investigators have found single ventricle physiology to be a risk factor for mortality with cardiac ECMO, relatively good outcomes (50% survival to hospital discharge) were reported in a recent series of patients requiring ECMO after a Norwood palliation (301,302). Management of the systemic to pulmonary artery shunt in infants with single ventricle physiology who require ECMO deserves special consideration. As is the case prior to initiation of mechanical support, the physiology if these patients is such that high flow through the shunt may lead to coronary ischemia, volume overload of the single ventricle and systemic hypoperfusion, all of which will impede efforts to wean from ECMO. If the shunt is left patent when ECMO is initiated, the flow on the ECMO circuit must be increased to compensate. Pulmonary overcirculation may also occur. Partial or complete ligation of the shunt will eliminate the large left to right shunt, but may lead to pulmonary infarction and shunt thrombosis (301,303).

The intensive care management of infants on ECMO has been reviewed elsewhere in great detail and is beyond the scope if this chapter (304). However, two critical issues deserve comment. In infants with biventricular physiology on ECMO, it essential that the left atrium and left ventricle are decompressed to reduce myocardial wall stress and pulmonary edema, thus optimizing the chances for myocardial recovery. Left ventricular distension may be assessed by echocardiogram, and decompression may be accomplished by increasing the ECMO flow rate, using low-dose inotropic agents and afterload reduction to improve myocardial ejection, and/or by decompressing the left atrium by surgically placing a vent. The ventilator strategy used in infants on ECMO for cardiac failure is also important to optimize the probability of myocardial recovery. Even on full venoarterial ECMO flow, the coronary circulation is typically perfused by blood ejected from the left ventricle. Thus a primary goal of ventilator management is to ensure that minimal ventilation-perfusion mismatch occurs in the lungs, so that pulmonary venous blood, which eventually perfuses the myocardium, is adequately oxygenated (304). This is in direct contrast with the typical ventilator strategy used in neonates with primary respiratory failure on ECMO, which focuses on lung rest and avoidance of further lung injury.

Inability to wean from ECMO within 3 to 5 days and the development of renal failure are ominous signs for pediatric cardiac patients (296,302,303,305–307). A high index of suspicion for residual lesions is necessary for infants who fail to wean from ECMO in a timely fashion (306). If transthoracic echocardiographic windows are poor, transesophageal echocardiography may be safely used in infants on ECMO to obtain diagnostic information (308). Cardiac catheterization may also be performed safely with infants on ECMO to evaluate for the presence of residual lesions that may be amenable to transcatheter or surgical intervention, or to decompress the left heart (309).

Rapid-deployment ECMO using a modified circuit and an organized response team may be used to facilitate the resuscitation of infants in full cardiopulmonary arrest following congenital heart surgery. One single center report described a series of 11 infants and children following a mean cardiopulmonary resuscitation time of 55 minutes, with 7 patients (64%) surviving to hospital discharge (294). Other centers have reported similar outcomes for emergent ECMO initiated during a postoperative cardiac arrest (299,303).

Survival to hospital discharge following pediatric cardiac ECMO has been shown to be approximately 40% to 60% in several series (296,299,301,303,307,310,311). Children with viral myocarditis requiring mechanical circulatory support have a higher survival rate (80%) (312). Although the intermediate-term cardiac follow-up is favorable for infants who survive postpericardiotomy ECMO, this patient population may have an increased incidence of significant neurologic deficits when compared with older children who required mechanical support (313,314). The etiology for these neuro-

logical deficits is unclear, but may be related to intraoperative variables such as the use of circulatory arrest, or the complex ECMO circuit that may cause thromboembolic events and requires higher levels of anticoagulation when compared to ventricular assist devices used in older patients.

Pulmonary Complications

Pulmonary dysfunction occurs following CPB as a result of a variety of factors, including the diffuse inflammatory response, increased capillary permeability, fluid overload and microemboli. In an infant animal model of CPB, post-pump pulmonary dysfunction includes an increased pulmonary vascular resistance, alveolar-arterial oxygen gradient, and decreased pulmonary compliance (256). Following CPB, infants have decreased lung compliance and increased total lung resistance (315). A variety of strategies designed to counteract these adverse effects of CPB have been discussed earlier, including the use of MUF, steroids, and strategies to prevent and treat pulmonary hypertension.

The infant who cannot be weaned from mechanical ventilation or extubated in a timely fashion may have a residual cardiac lesion and/or a noncardiac etiology as an explanation for the lack of progress. Non-cardiac reasons for difficult weaning are numerous and include abnormalities in respiratory drive (e.g., central nervous system injury, sedation), respiratory pump (e.g., critical illness polyneuropathy, phrenic nerve injury), gas exchange (e.g., parenchymal lung injury) or increased ventilatory load (e.g., overfeeding, increased dead space).

External compression of the central airways occasionally may complicate the pre- or postoperative course in infants with congenital heart disease. For example, aortic enlargement causing central airway compression may occur in lesions with increased fetal aortic blood flow such as pulmonary atresia (316). Some neonates with tetralogy of Fallot and absent pulmonary valve syndrome have significant pulmonary artery dilation that leads to tracheal and mainstem bronchial compression in the preoperative period, and tracheobronchial malacia may persist following surgery (317). Tracheal stenosis or malacia may develop postoperatively as a result of airway mucosal injury related to the endotracheal tube. Upper airway obstruction will make intrathoracic pressure significantly more negative in the spontaneously breathing patient, and the resultant increased ventricular afterload may be poorly tolerated in the infant with limited cardiac reserve.

The phrenic nerves are at risk for paresis or transection during many infant cardiac surgeries, and paralysis of a hemidiaphragm may make it difficult to wean infants from mechanical ventilation (318). The diagnosis may be confirmed by echocardiogram or fluoroscopy while the infant is spontaneously breathing. Diaphragmatic plication may be required to facilitate weaning from the ventilator (319,320). The recurrent laryngeal nerve may be injured during aortic arch surgery or PDA ligation, resulting in unilateral vocal cord paralysis. Postoperatively, such infants may have problems with maintenance of functional residual capacity and aspiration.

Tracheobronchial ischemia, leading to obstruction of the lower airways, has been reported to occur following unifocalization procedures in infants with pulmonary atresia, ventricular septal defect, and MAPCAs. The tracheobronchial ischemia is probably related to interruption of peribronchial arterial blood supply during mobilization of MAPCAs (321).

The development of a postoperative chylothorax is a relatively infrequent complication (approximately 1%) following congenital heart surgery, but when it occurs it adds morbidity and prolongs hospitalization (322). A chylothorax may develop following thoracic duct injury, and elevated systemic venous pressures or thrombosis of the subclavian veins may exacerbate the condition (323,324). The diagnosis is confirmed by finding elevated triglyceride levels and lymphocyte counts in fluid drained from the pleural cavity (325). Treatment strategies initiate with chest tube drainage and dietary modification with a medium chain triglyceride (MCT) based formula, although many weeks may be required for drainage to stop (325). Prolonged drainage may lead to depletion of plasma proteins (albumin, coagulation factors, immunoglobulins) and lymphocytes, and consideration should be given to replacement with albumin, fresh frozen plasma, and/or intravenous immunoglobulins (IVIG) (323,326). A trial of total parenteral nutrition is warranted for infants not responding to a MCT formula (323). A small randomized animal model and several human case reports and series suggest that chylous drainage may be decreased using medications that decrease splanchnic blood and lymph flow, including somatostatin or octreotide (a synthetic somatostatin analogue) (324,327–331). Surgical options for patients with refractory chylothoraces include thoracic duct ligation, pleuroperitoneal shunt or pleurodesis (325,332,333).

Gastrointestinal Complications

Feeding problems are common in neonates following congenital heart surgery. Many of these patients never had the opportunity to learn to suck and swallow before surgery, and had prolonged periods of oral-tracheal intubation. Nasogastric feedings may be initially required, and input from a speech therapist may be useful.

NEC may occur either before or after congenital heart surgery, particularly in neonates with lesions that produce diastolic runoff, such as single ventricle patients with a systemic to pulmonary artery shunt (50). Because of bowel dysfunction related to anesthesia and narcotics, and the concern for NEC, total parenteral nutrition is commonly started on the first postoperative day in young infants until the intestinal motility returns.

Although significant gastrointestinal bleeding as a result of peptic ulcers or gastritis is rather uncommon following CPB in infants, histamine-2 antagonists are routinely administered until enteral feeding has been established.

Infectious Complications

A variety of factors predispose infants to infection following cardiac surgery. CPB generates a complex pro- and anti-inflammatory response; the latter contributes to a generalized state of immunosuppression (334,335). Neonates in particular may have prolonged pre and postoperative ICU stays following cardiac surgery, during which they are exposed to a variety of indwelling catheters and tubes that predispose to infection. The risk of catheter-related blood stream infection in children increases with the number of central lines used, the duration of catheter use, and the use of ECMO (336). Guidelines for the prevention and management of catheter related infections in children have recently been published (337,338). Prophylactic antibiotics that provide coverage for gram-positive organisms (e.g., a first generation cephalosporin) are administered in the early postoperative period, generally until all of the chest tubes are removed from the patient (339).

The use of delayed sternal closure may be a risk factor for bacterial infections. In a series of children who had delayed sternal closure, the vast majority of whom were infants, the reported incidences are 1% to 7% for surgical site infection, and 0% to 4% for mediastinitis (189,190). Treatment of mediastinitis includes surgical debridement and prolonged parenteral antibiotics.

Renal Insufficiency

CPB is associated with significant fluid retention in infants, and the problem is usually exacerbated by a decline in urine output in the first 12 to 24 hours following surgery. Loop diuretics are used to improve urine output in the early postoperative period. A continuous infusion of furosemide may provide a gentler diuresis in those patients with labile hemodynamics. Spironolactone may be useful for its potassium sparing effect if the enteral route of administration is available.

Significant renal insufficiency may occur in infants with prolonged CPB times or as a result of low cardiac output in the early postoperative period (207). The development of overt renal failure requiring dialysis is associated with 40% to 60% risk of mortality (340,341). Renal perfusion pressure may be calculated by the following equation: renal perfusion pressure = mean arterial pressure − central venous pressure. In general, a renal perfusion pressure of 40 to 50 mmHg in infants is required to maintain urine output. Some surgeons electively place temporary peritoneal dialysis catheters at the time of complex cardiac surgery in infants to allow drainage of postoperative ascites and minimize external compression on the renal veins. Peritoneal dialysis may be performed if needed. Renal function usually recovers following the improvement in cardiac output (340).

Neurologic Complications

Several preoperative, intraoperative, and postoperative factors may contribute to suboptimal neurologic outcomes following cardiac surgery in infancy. Recent reports demonstrate that preoperative neurological abnormalities may be detected on physical examination and brain MRI in some term neonates with congenital heart disease who otherwise had no known risk factors for neurologic injury (342,343).

The use of CPB may result in the embolization of gas bubbles or thrombus, which may contribute to the development of seizures, infarcts, periventricular leukomalacia, and intracranial hemorrhage (343,344). The use of deep hypothermic circulatory arrest (DHCA) for complex neonatal arch reconstruction has been practiced since the 1960s. Data from the 1990s suggests that the use of longer periods of circulatory arrest, when compared to low flow CPB, is associated with an increased incidence of early postoperative seizures (176,345). Both early postoperative seizures and longer circulatory arrest times are associated with neurological deficits following the arterial switch and Norwood operations (346–351). In order to minimize neurologic injury related to the use of circulatory arrest, several centers have recently reported the use of regional low-flow perfusion for complex aortic arch reconstructions (4,130,352,353). Concurrently, however, there have been many advances in the pH and hematocrit strategies used in circulatory arrest that appear to minimize adverse neurologic sequelae (354–356). For example, the incidence of early postoperative clinical seizures following DHCA has decreased dramatically in patients from the current era (2%) as compared to the cohort reported in the 1988–1992 Boston Circulatory Arrest Study (8%) (176,344). Thus it is unclear whether neurological outcomes will be improved using regional perfusion techniques rather than DHCA.

Infants may have additional hypotensive or hypoxic episodes in the intensive care unit following surgery. These postoperative events may exacerbate neurologic insults that occurred prior to or during surgery. Infants with a longer postoperative length of stay appear to have a worse cognitive outcome when assessed at 8 years of age (357).

Early Postoperative Physiology and Management: Specific Lesions

Palliation of the Neonate with a Single Ventricle

Neonates who have cardiac anatomy unsuitable for a two ventricular repair typically have atresia or significant hypoplasia of either of the atrioventricular valves, and/or significant hypoplasia of either ventricle (358). The majority of neonates with single ventricle physiology will eventually undergo Fontan completion as toddlers. Because the Fontan circulation is characterized by passive pulmonary blood flow, this physiology is dependent on low pulmonary artery pressure, and the absence of pulmonary artery distortion, pulmonary venous obstruction, atrioventricular valve regurgitation and ventricular hypertrophy. These requirements dictate the surgical strategy in the newborn period (358). To limit ventricular hypertrophy, unobstructed systemic blood

flow must exist, and if not present at birth, may be achieved using either a Norwood operation or Damus-Kaye-Stansel procedure. Pulmonary blood flow must be tightly regulated to prevent ventricular volume overload, atrioventricular valve regurgitation and pulmonary artery hypertension. This usually requires the placement of a Blalock-Taussig shunt or pulmonary artery band. Care must be taken with both of these procedures to minimize pulmonary artery distortion. Finally, pulmonary venous return must not be obstructed, as this may cause pulmonary artery hypertension. An atrial septectomy is required in some neonates, as is done during the Norwood operation.

Systemic to Pulmonary Artery Shunt

The most common type of systemic to pulmonary artery shunt operation refers to a procedure in which a Gore-Tex™ tube graft is surgically placed between the subclavian or innominate artery and the pulmonary artery, typically without the use of CPB. This operation, also known as the modified Blalock-Taussig shunt, is widely used as the operation of choice to palliate infants with single ventricle physiology and decreased pulmonary blood flow (Fig. 34-15). The operation is also used in selected infants with two-ventricular physiology and obstructed pulmonary blood flow whose complete repair will be deferred. A systemic to pulmonary artery shunt may be performed in isolation or as a part of a larger procedure, such as the Norwood operation for HLHS. In a retrospective, nonrandomized study, Odim and associates reported that performance of the modified Blalock-Taussig operation via a midline sternotomy was technically easier, and was associated with a lower rate of shunt failure when compared with a classic thoracotomy approach (359).

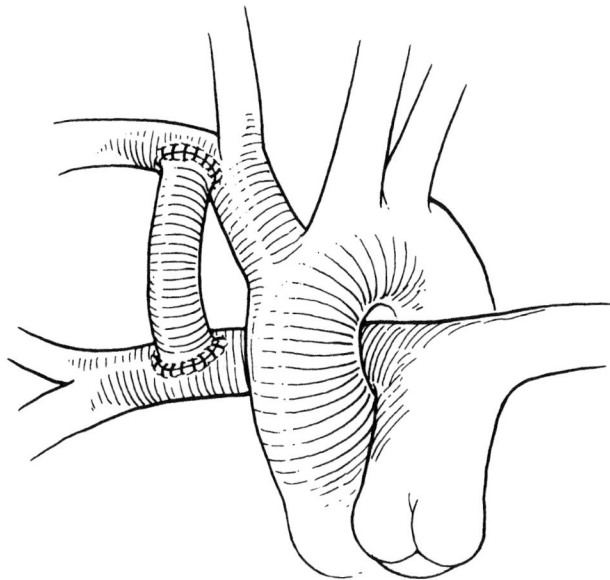

Figure 34-15 The modified Blalock-Taussig shunt operation. Reprinted from Wernovsky G, Bove EL. Single ventricle lesions. In: Chang A, Hanley FL, Wernovsky G, et al., editors. *Pediatric cardiac intensive care.* Baltimore: Williams and Wilkins, 1998:271–287, with permission.

Another type of systemic to pulmonary artery shunt is a central shunt, which involves the placement of a Gore-Tex™ tube between the ascending aorta and pulmonary artery. A central shunt is typically placed only when anatomical issues preclude a modified Blalock-Taussig shunt. Several postoperative complications may occur following the placement of a systemic to pulmonary artery shunt. If the shunt is too large, the systemic ventricle will be subjected to volume overload and congestive heart failure may develop. In patients with single ventricle physiology, elevated pulmonary vascular resistance may exist with the large shunt that may complicate future staging operations. A small shunt will result in excessive postoperative cyanosis. The average shunt diameter is 3.5 mm for a term infant. Distortion or scarring of the pulmonary arteries may also develop at the shunt insertion site. Thrombosis of the shunt is a dreaded postoperative complication that results in the rapid development of severe cyanosis. Most infants are started on aspirin once their chest tubes and lines have been removed. Reported neurologic complications with this shunt include Horner's syndrome, recurrent laryngeal nerve injury, and phrenic nerve injury (359).

Pulmonary Artery Band

In selected infants with single ventricular physiology and unobstructed pulmonary and systemic blood flow, or occasionally in infants with two-ventricular physiology and pulmonary overcirculation, a restrictive band is placed on the main pulmonary artery to decrease Qp/Qs and thus limit symptoms of congestive heart failure, the adverse effects of volume loading on the ventricle(s), and the development of pulmonary vascular obstructive disease (Fig. 34-16). CPB is not required for this procedure. It would be inappropriate to place a pulmonary artery band in an infant who has, or is likely to develop, systemic outflow tract obstruction, as the resultant "doubly obstructed" physiology will lead to the rapid development of ventricular hypertrophy. Placement of a pulmonary artery band, although conceptually simple, requires a great deal of surgical judgment. If the band is placed in an infant with high pulmonary vascular resistance, the patient's systemic oxygen saturation in the operating room may indicate a well-balanced circulation (saturation approximately 80%). However, as the pulmonary vascular resistance falls over the coming weeks, pulmonary blood flow may increase, systemic oxygen saturation will rise, and signs of congestive heart failure will develop. If the pulmonary artery band migrates distally on the main pulmonary artery, distortion of the branch pulmonary arteries may develop, which would have to be corrected before or during the bi-directional Glen/hemi-Fontan operation. The band is removed at the time of complete surgical repair or subsequent palliation.

Damus-Kaye-Stansel Procedure

In children with single ventricular physiology and subaortic stenosis with or without distal aortic arch obstruction, a

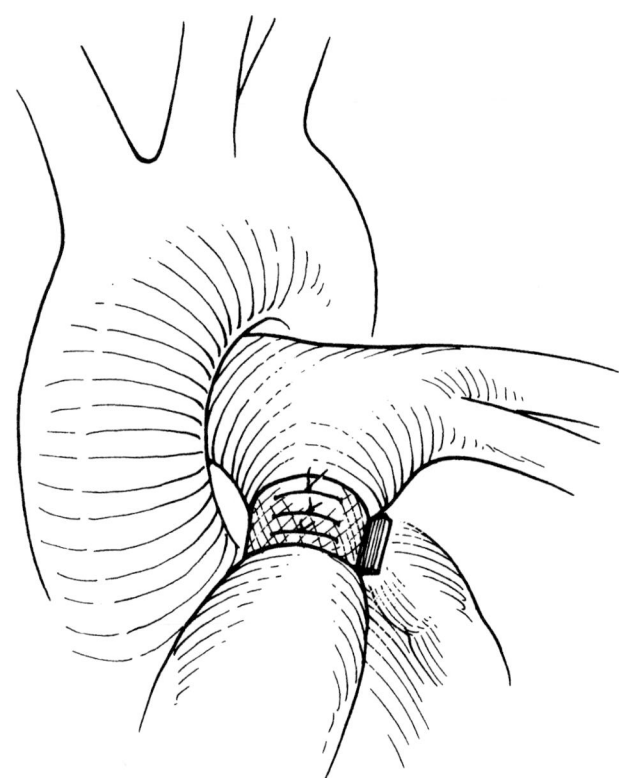

Figure 34-16 Pulmonary artery band. Reprinted from Wernovsky G, Bove EL. Single ventricle lesions. In: Chang A, Hanley FL, Wernovsky G, et al., editors. *Pediatric cardiac intensive care.* Baltimore: Williams and Wilkins, 1998:271–287, with permission.

Damus-Kaye-Stansel palliation may be performed to provide unobstructed systemic blood flow. This procedure involves anastomosis of the proximal main pulmonary artery and ascending aorta, and aortic arch reconstruction if needed. The distal main pulmonary artery is over sewn and a modified Blalock-Taussig shunt is placed to provide pulmonary blood flow. The postoperative physiology and complications are similar to those seen following the Norwood operation, which are discussed in detail below.

Bi-directional Glenn or Hemi-Fontan Operation

The bi-directional Glenn or hemi-Fontan operation involves redirection of the superior vena cava blood flow to both pulmonary arteries (Fig. 34-17). One of these two operations is commonly performed in infants with single ventricle physiology before or at approximately six months of age, in anticipation of a Fontan completion, which is typically done at 2 to 3 years of age (360). Because passive pulmonary blood flow is present following these operations, they cannot be performed when pulmonary vascular resistance is high as in the newborn period (361). The benefits of performing a bidirectional Glenn/hemi-Fontan operation as an intermediate staging procedure before Fontan completion include volume-unloading of the single ventricle, decreased atrioventricular valve regurgitation, and improved systemic oxygen saturation, and decreased

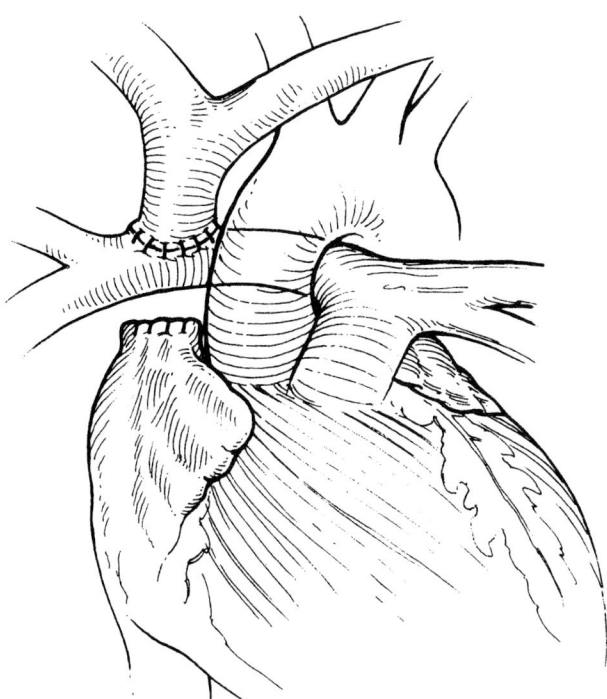

Figure 34-17 Bi-directional Glenn operation. Reprinted from Wernovsky G, Bove EL. Single ventricle lesions. In: Chang A, Hanley FL, Wernovsky G, et al., editors. *Pediatric cardiac intensive care.* Baltimore: Williams and Wilkins, 1998:271–287, with permission.

pleural effusions and mortality following the Fontan completion (360,362–364).

The bi-directional Glenn operation, also known as the bi-directional cavopulmonary shunt operation, involves an end-to-side anastomosis between the superior vena cava and the pulmonary artery. The term "bi-directional" refers to the fact that blood from the superior vena cava perfuses both the left and right pulmonary arteries. The hemi-Fontan operation involves the end-to-side anastomosis between the superior vena cava and the pulmonary artery as described above, but in addition, the proximal superior vena cava is anastomosed to the inferior surface of the pulmonary artery, and a patch is placed at the junction of the superior vena cava and the right atrium. The functional result of this operation is the same as the bi-directional Glenn operation, but it makes the completion Fontan operation simpler if the surgeon ultimately uses a lateral tunnel type of Fontan. There may be an increase risk of sinus node dysfunction following the hemi-Fontan operation related to surgical manipulation. Surgeons that complete the Fontan using an extracardiac conduit perform the bi-directional Glenn shunt as a staging procedure. Any central pulmonary artery stenosis is addressed during the bi-directional Glenn operation.

The bi-directional Glenn operation is associated with minimal morbidity or mortality, and most infants have an unremarkable postoperative course (361,362). Superior vena cava syndrome, identified by the presence of cerebral and upper extremity venous congestion, may develop related to increased pulmonary vascular resistance, and therapies to

reduce pulmonary vascular resistance should then be applied. Infants who are 2 to 3 months of age may have significant cyanosis immediately following the bi-directional Glenn/hemi-Fontan, which usually improves in 24 to 48 hours (360). The evaluation and management of the postoperative bi-directional Glenn/hemi-Fontan patient with excessive hypoxemia is discussed in detail in the previous section on cyanosis.

Fontan completion is generally performed at approximately two years of age. During this operation, the inferior vena cava blood is channeled directly to the pulmonary arteries using several different techniques, functionally bypassing the heart, and thus separating the systemic and pulmonary circulations and essentially eliminating cyanosis. Factors that have been associated with a good outcome following the Fontan operation include low pulmonary vascular resistance, undistorted pulmonary arteries and unobstructed pulmonary veins, and the absence of significant atrioventricular valve regurgitation or ventricular hypertrophy. These factors are greatly influenced be decision making in the neonatal period, as discussed earlier. As this chapter pertains to infancy, the Fontan operation will not be discussed further.

Right Ventricular Outflow Tract Obstruction

Critical Pulmonary Valve Stenosis

The initial intervention in neonates with isolated critical pulmonary valve stenosis is usually a balloon valvuloplasty, performed in the cardiac catheterization laboratory. Infants with critical pulmonary valve stenosis may have very poor right ventricular compliance following balloon valvuloplasty, perhaps related to myocardial ischemia and endocardial fibroelastosis (54). Rather than fill the right ventricle, some systemic venous blood will cross the foramen ovale to the left atrium, resulting in significant cyanosis. To ensure adequate pulmonary blood flow following the procedure, these infants may require several days of a PGE1 infusion (56,57). Occasionally a systemic to pulmonary artery shunt will be required until right ventricular compliance improves (54,59). Placement of a stent in the ductus arteriosus during cardiac catheterization is an alternative. The systemic to pulmonary artery shunt or the stented ductus arteriosus can then be coil embolized or surgically removed at a later date, once the right ventricular compliance has improved. These infants are also at risk for developing infundibular spasm ("suicide right ventricle") following balloon valvuloplasty that manifests as cyanosis and low cardiac output (365). Volume expansion and beta-blockers are the initial treatments should infundibular spasm occur.

Tetralogy of Fallot

Surgical repair of tetralogy of Fallot includes closure of the VSD(s), and reduction or elimination of obstruction to blood flow across the right ventricular outflow tract and pulmonary arteries. Accomplishing this often involves resection of muscle bundles in the right ventricular outflow tract, a pulmonary valvotomy or leaflet resection, and patch augmentation of the proximal pulmonary arteries. In those infants with favorable anatomy, the operation may be accomplished using a transatrial-transpulmonary approach. However, right ventriculotomy with transannular patch is required in some cases to enlarge the right ventricular outflow tract. In infants with tetralogy of Fallot and pulmonary atresia, a ventriculotomy is required if a complete repair is performed using a right ventricle to pulmonary artery conduit.

Right ventricular function and compliance are abnormal following complete repair of tetralogy of Fallot. This is attributable in part to right ventricular hypertrophy that was present prior to surgery, and also to right ventricular myocardial injury related to the subpulmonic resection and VSD closure. Pulmonary regurgitation, if present, will exacerbate the right heart failure. Some surgeons leave the foramen ovale patent so that the right heart may decompress into the left atrium, thus maintaining systemic cardiac output at the expense of mild cyanosis. If the surgeon closed the atrial septum in the operating room, and significant right heart failure exists in the early postoperative period, an atrial communication may be created in the cardiac catheterization laboratory. Inotropic support of the right ventricle is commonly required immediately following surgery, and low dose dopamine and milrinone are commonly used in this regard. Strategies to maintain low pulmonary vascular resistance should be employed. JET is a common rhythm disturbance seen following tetralogy of Fallot repair (242). Following complete repair of tetralogy of Fallot, residual lesions that may complicate the postoperative course include a VSD, right ventricular outflow tract obstruction, and pulmonary artery stenosis.

Neonates with tetralogy of Fallot and significant preoperative cyanosis who have a palliative systemic to pulmonary artery shunt placed may be well saturated but develop congestive heart failure in the postoperative period. The pulmonary blood flow from the shunt plus the native flow across the right ventricular outflow tract may be excessive.

Surgical repair for tetralogy of Fallot with absent pulmonary valve syndrome includes a reduction pulmonary arterioplasty, VSD closure and placement of a valved homograft in the right ventricular outflow tract (317). Replacement of the dilated central pulmonary arteries with bifurcated valved pulmonary homograft is a surgical modification that has been associated in one report with improved survival in neonates who present with respiratory distress (366). A more recently described surgical approach includes translocation of the pulmonary artery anterior to the aorta (Lecompte maneuver) and away from the tracheobronchial tree (367). In addition to the aforementioned issues following tetralogy of Fallot repair, the postoperative course for infants with absent pulmonary valve syndrome may be significantly complicated by airway obstruction as a result of tracheobronchomalacia that

persists even after plication and reduction of the aneurysmal pulmonary arteries (317,368). Case reports suggest that those with refractory tracheobronchomalacia may improve with metallic stenting of the central airways (317). Some of these infants will require a tracheostomy and long-term positive-pressure ventilation until they "outgrow" the malacia.

Pulmonary Atresia, Ventricular Septal Defect, Major Aortopulmonary Collateral Arteries

The goal of surgical intervention in infants with pulmonary atresia, a VSD and MAPCAs is to incorporate blood vessels that supply as many lung segments as possible into the repair, while eliminating any MAPCAs that represent dual blood supply to these segments. The interventional management must be individualized depending on the pulmonary artery anatomy and often involves a series of surgical procedures and transcatheter interventions with balloon dilation of the stenotic branch pulmonary arteries. Surgical options include a staged approach involving bilateral unifocalizations followed by repair using a right ventricular to pulmonary artery conduit (369). A single stage, complete repair is advocated for many of these infants in early infancy at some centers (370). In selected infants with diminutive but confluent pulmonary arteries, a transannular patch to open the right ventricular outflow tract, placement of an right ventricle to pulmonary artery conduit, or an aortopulmonary window may be used to encourage pulmonary artery growth (371). Complete repair including VSD closure is then performed at a later date provided that the pulmonary vascular bed is adequate to accept the entire right ventricular output without the development of severe pulmonary hypertension. The VSD patch may be fenestrated in selected cases to prevent the development of postoperative suprasystemic pulmonary hypertension and right ventricular failure (372).

The postoperative course for infants with pulmonary atresia, ventricular septal defect and MAPCAs is dependent on the operative strategy. Those infants undergoing complete repair including closure of the VSD and placement of a conduit from the right ventricle to the pulmonary artery are at risk for right ventricular failure, secondary to the VSD closure, right ventricular outflow tract muscle bundle resection, ventriculotomy required for conduit placement, and branch pulmonary stenosis. Often the VSD patch is fenestrated, or a foramen ovale is left patient in these patients, which leads to mild postoperative cyanosis, but serves to decompress the right heart and preserve systemic cardiac output (372). Congestive heart failure may persist in the postoperative period if all of the MAPCAs were not incorporated into the repair. Following unifocalization procedures, severe airflow limitation may occur secondary to tracheobronchial ischemia, which may originate from interruption of peribronchial arterial blood supply during mobilization of MAPCAs (321). The intermediate term prognosis is guarded for infants with pulmonary atresia, VSD and MAPCAs secondary to pulmonary hypertension and right ventricular failure (66). Serial cardiac catheterizations with balloon angioplasty of the pulmonary arteries are required for many patients.

Pulmonary Atresia with Intact Ventricular Septum

The postoperative course for infants with pulmonary atresia and intact ventricular septum is highly dependent upon the operation or transcatheter procedure performed. Neonates undergoing a two-ventricular repair may have poor right ventricular compliance, right to left shunting at the foramen and subsequent cyanosis, similar to that seen following repair of tetralogy of Fallot. Those with "right ventricular dependent coronary circulation" may have problems with myocardial ischemia following a systemic to pulmonary artery shunt, even though the right ventricle was not decompressed.

Ebstein's Anomaly of the Tricuspid Valve

Neonates with Ebstein's anomaly who require early surgical intervention are at high risk for mortality as a result of pulmonary hypoplasia, pulmonary hypertension and right heart failure. Surgical options for neonates with refractory symptoms include a primary complete repair, consisting of a reduction atrioplasty, fenestrated closure of the atrial septum and tricuspid valvuloplasty (73). Another approach is to stage the patient toward Fontan palliation with a systemic to pulmonary artery shunt, over sewing of the tricuspid valve annulus and atrial septectomy (74,75). Regardless of the surgical procedure, infants recovering from surgery for Ebstein's anomaly are likely to have problems with pulmonary hypertension related in part to pulmonary hypoplasia. In addition to the usual strategies used to treat pulmonary hypertension, care should be taken to ensure that excessive positive airway pressure is not used to attempt to expand lungs, which may appear small on chest radiograph. Overdistension of the hypoplastic lungs will only lead to further increases in pulmonary vascular resistance. Residual tricuspid regurgitation and right heart failure may also complicate the postoperative course. Atrioventricular reentry tachycardia may occur at any time before or after surgery.

Left Ventricular Outflow Tract Obstruction

Critical Aortic Valve Stenosis

Following the alleviation of critical aortic valve stenosis, either by surgical valvotomy or balloon valvuloplasty, most infants will have a marked improvement in clinical status with recovery of left ventricular function. Note that the gradient across the aortic valve may be minimal immediately following intervention, but will often increase as myocardial function and cardiac output improve. Inotropic support is often required for a few days following the procedure. The PGE_1 infusion may be discontinued once left to right flow is seen at the ductal level by echocardiography.

A small number of infants will do poorly in the postoperative period, as a result of inadequate size of left heart structures or extensive endocardial fibroelastosis. Such patients may require a Norwood palliation, but historically, infants who had a failed attempt at a two-ventricular repair and subsequent attempted Norwood operation have a high mortality (373).

Critical Coarctation of the Aorta

Several operative techniques are available for coarctation repair, including resection with end-to-end anastomoses, patch aortoplasty, subclavian flap aortoplasty. Resection and extended end-to-end anastomosis is a technique that also addresses aortic arch hypoplasia and appears to be associated with a low recoarctation rate (374,375). Due to a significant recoarctation rate and the potential for aneurysm formation, primary balloon angioplasty is generally not recommended in infancy at most congenital heart centers (376,377).

Following repair of an isolated critical coarctation of the aorta, accurate four extremity blood pressure measurements must be obtained to evaluate for the presence of residual aortic arch obstruction. A residual arm-leg blood pressure gradient may be secondary to an inadequate repair, hypoplasia of the aortic arch, or constriction of residual ductal tissue. If a residual coarctation exists, the timing of intervention depends upon the clinical course. Infants who have adequate left ventricular function and who are easily weaned from support may return in 2 to 3 months, after the suture lines have healed, for cardiac catheterization and possible balloon dilation of the obstruction. Those who are unable to be weaned from the ventilator require another procedure during the same hospitalization. Infants who presented in shock may be at risk for mesenteric ischemia and enteral feedings are withheld in the early postoperative period. Infants appear to be at much lower risk for spinal cord ischemia or significant postoperative hypertension following coarctation repair when compared with older children and adults. As with any surgical intervention on the aortic arch, the phrenic and recurrent laryngeal nerves are at risk for injury during coarctation repair.

Hypoplastic Left Heart Syndrome

During the Norwood operation for HLHS, the distal pulmonary artery is over sewn, the proximal pulmonary artery and the aorta are anastomosed, and the aortic arch is reconstructed with pulmonary artery homograft material to allow for unobstructed systemic blood flow (378). An atrial septectomy is performed to allow pulmonary venous return to pass easily to the right atrium, and a modified Blalock-Taussig shunt is placed to provide pulmonary blood flow (Fig. 34-18). Thus following the Norwood operation, the single right ventricle pumps blood to the systemic circulation and coronary arteries, via the reconstructed aorta ("neoaorta"), and to the pulmonary circulation, via the systemic to pulmonary artery shunt.

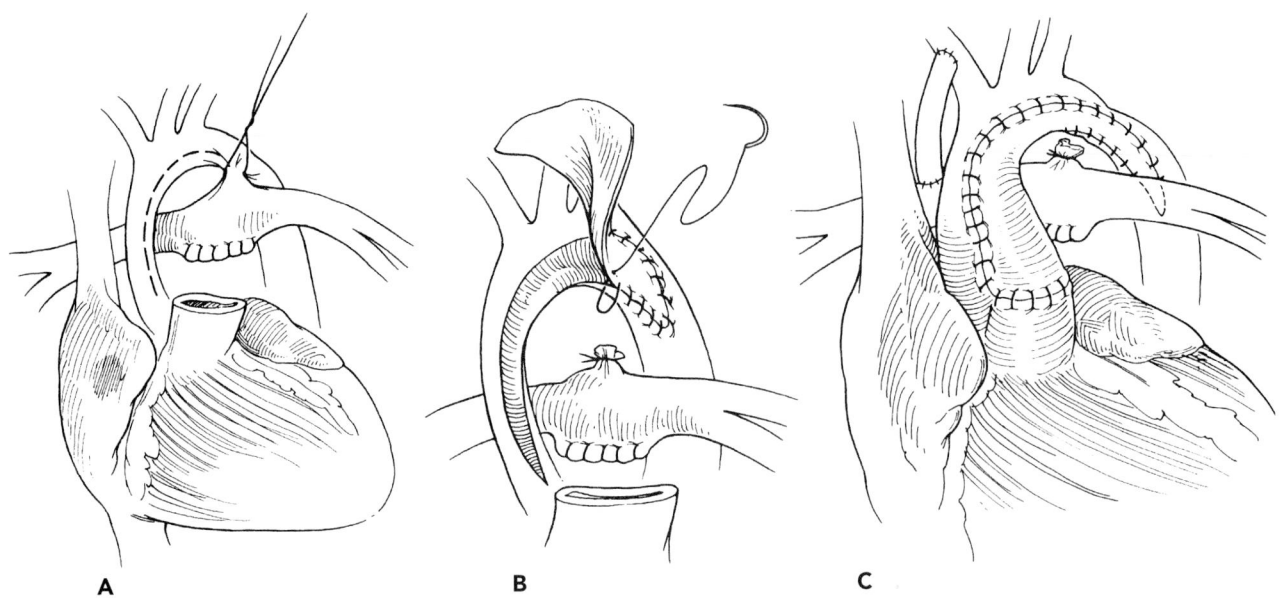

Figure 34-18 Norwood operation for hypoplastic left heart syndrome. The purpose of the Norwood operation for hypoplastic left heart syndrome is to establish reliable, unobstructed outflow to the systemic circulation and to balance the systemic and pulmonary circulations. This is achieved by ligating and dividing the ductus arteriosus and detaching the central and branch pulmonary arteries from the main pulmonary artery as shown in **A**. The hypoplastic aorta is then opened from the descending aorta retrograde to the level of the aortic valve and augmented with a patch of homograft arterial wall. The augmented aorta is then connected to the cardiac end of the main pulmonary artery stump as shown in **B** and **C**. This achieves unobstructed outflow from the single right ventricle through the pulmonary valve to the aorta and systemic vascular bed. Additionally, an atrial septectomy is performed to ensure unobstructed pulmonary venous outflow, and the pulmonary circulation is supplied through the use of a right-sided modified Blalock-Taussig shunt. Reprinted from Wernovsky G, Bove EL. Single ventricle lesions. In: Chang A, Hanley FL, Wernovsky G, et al., editors. *Pediatric cardiac intensive care.* Baltimore: Williams and Wilkins, 1998:271–287, with permission.

A variety of problems may arise following the Norwood operation that often are poorly tolerated as a result of the limited physiologic reserve possessed by these infants. Excessive pulmonary blood flow with inadequate systemic perfusion, similar to that seen in a typical preoperative neonate with HLHS, may be seen but is less common than in prior years due the smaller diameter Blalock-Taussig shunts that are currently used. Others may have problems with myocardial dysfunction, pulmonary hypertension, or the systemic to pulmonary artery shunt.

Ideally, the circulations will be balanced following the Norwood operation such that the Qp/Qs ratio will be approximately 1:1. Pulmonary blood flow will be determined by the pulmonary vascular resistance and the resistance provided by the systemic to pulmonary artery shunt, assuming an unrestrictive, surgically created ASD and unobstructed pulmonary venous blood flow. Systemic blood flow will be determined by the systemic vascular resistance and if present, any residual aortic arch obstruction. The ratio of systemic and pulmonary blood flow may be calculated by the following modified Fick equation: $Qp/Qs = (SaO_2 - SvO_2)/(PvO_2 - PaO_2)$, in which SaO_2 = aortic saturation; SvO_2 = mixed venous saturation (estimated by the superior vena cava oxygen saturation); PvO_2 = pulmonary venous oxygen saturation (assumed to be >95% if not directly measured); and PaO_2 > pulmonary artery oxygen saturation (assumed to equal the aortic saturation). Estimating Qp/Qs using only the arterial PaO_2 or SaO_2 may be misleading without knowledge of SvO_2, estimated by the superior vena cava oxygen saturation, and PvO_2 (Fig. 34-19) (191,379–383). One study documented pulmonary venous desaturation in 11/12 infants following the Norwood operation at some point in the early postoperative period, despite the absence of radiographic abnormalities on chest radiograph (191). Many centers monitor SvO_2 following the Norwood operation, but few monitor PvO_2. Caution must be used when using saturation data for clinical decision-making following the Norwood operation. The CXR must be carefully examined to ensure that the tips of the catheters from which blood gas samples are drawn are in the proper location. The oximetry data cannot be used in isolation and the entire clinical picture must be considered.

Signs of low cardiac output following the Norwood palliation may be attributed to pulmonary overcirculation, myocardial dysfunction, or a combination of the two. An imbalance between the systemic and pulmonary blood flows, particularly a high Qp/Qs, has been implicated as a major factor in the high early postoperative mortality following the Norwood operation. Such infants will have high SaO_2, low SvO_2, and other clinical and laboratory evidence for low cardiac output. Investigators have thus spent

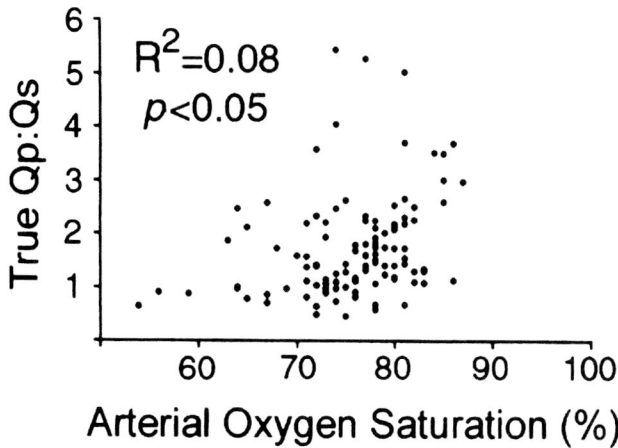

Figure 34-19 Regression analysis of SaO_2 against true Qp/Qs following the Norwood operation. SaO_2 is a poor predictor of Qp/Qs (R2 = 0.08, $p < 0.05$). Variability in Qp/Qs is most pronounced at SaO_2 values in range of 65% to 85%, usual target range for patients after Norwood palliation. Reprinted from Taeed R, Schwartz SM, Pearl JM, et al. Unrecognized pulmonary venous desaturation early after Norwood palliation confounds Qp/Qs assessment and compromises oxygen delivery. *Circulation* 2001; 103:2699–2704, with permission.

considerable effort to study the cardiovascular physiology following the Norwood operation, and several interventions are available that may serve to better "balance" the pulmonary and systemic circulations. In an experimental animal model of postoperative single ventricle physiology with a systemic to pulmonary shunt, addition of carbon dioxide ($PiCO_2$) to the inspired gas resulted in increase pulmonary vascular resistance, even when systemic pH was controlled by administration of tromethamine buffer (Tham) (85). Other investigators have reported the ability to manipulate pulmonary vascular resistance, Qp/Qs, and oxygen delivery in single ventricle animal models by varying the inspired concentrations of oxygen or providing inhaled carbon dioxide or NO (380,384).

The findings from preoperative studies in neonates and postoperative animal models that have evaluated the use of sub-ambient oxygen or inspired carbon dioxide to alter pulmonary vascular resistance should not be extrapolated to neonates recovering from the Norwood operation. Doing so would not account for several important variables, including the fixed resistance provided by the relatively small (3.5 to 4 mm) systemic to pulmonary shunts used in most Norwood operations in the current era as compared to the 6 mm shunts used in some animal models (4,380,385). Although early reports suggest that an imbalance of systemic to pulmonary blood flow may be life threatening to infants following the Norwood operation, several recent postoperative studies suggest that supplemental oxygen or alkalosis do not have deleterious effects on the hemodynamics of most patients with Norwood physiology, presumably as a result of the fixed resistance provided by the systemic to pulmonary shunt (94,191,382,383,386,387). With the above considerations in mind, an infant recovering from the Norwood operation

with signs of isolated pulmonary overcirculation (i.e., high calculated Qp/Qs, pulmonary edema on chest radiograph) should have measures taken to lower systemic vascular resistance and increase pulmonary vascular resistance. Residual aortic arch obstruction must also be excluded in this situation, as such an obstruction will limit systemic blood flow and direct more blood through the shunt.

Several recent reports suggest that myocardial dysfunction may be the dominant hemodynamic disturbance in those infants with low cardiac output following the Norwood operation (201,383,388). Tricuspid valve regurgitation may also contribute to low cardiac output. Isolated myocardial dysfunction is present when the Qp/Qs is calculated to be approximately 1:1, and the SvO_2 is low. An anaerobic threshold is reached when the SvO_2 falls below 30% following the Norwood operation, and efforts to maintain SvO_2 above this value have been associated with very low early mortality (389). Inotropic support and afterload reduction will be beneficial for such patients. A study examining the effect of various inotropic agents in an animal model of single ventricle physiology found that low-dose dopamine and epinephrine had favorable effects on Qp/Qs, and epinephrine improved oxygen delivery, whereas dobutamine increased Qp/Qs and decreased oxygen delivery (390).

The use of phenoxybenzamine, an alpha-adrenergic blocker, may address both the problems of pulmonary overcirculation and myocardial dysfunction following the Norwood operation. In a prospective, nonrandomized study, Tweddell and associates report favorable hemodynamic effects of administering phenoxybenzamine to neonates undergoing the Norwood palliation. Phenoxybenzamine produced lower systemic vascular resistance, resulting in a Qp/Qs that approached unity, and a higher SvO_2 (Fig. 34-20

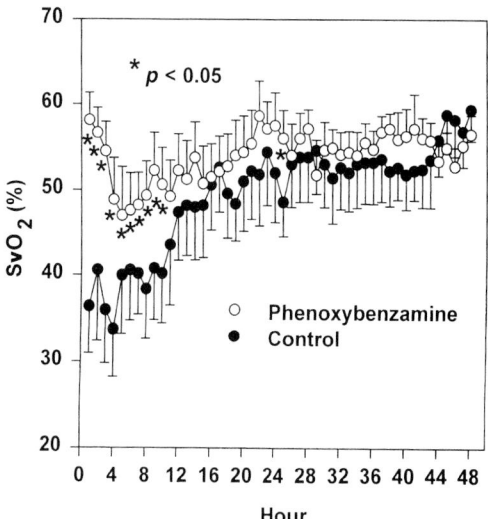

Figure 34-20 Superior vena cava saturation (SvO_2) during the first 48 hours after the Norwood procedure. The SvO_2 was significantly higher in the phenoxybenzamine group than in the control group during hours 1 to 10 and hour 25 ($p < 0.05$, RM ANOVA). Reprinted from Tweddell JS, Hoffman GM, Fedderly RT, et al. Phenoxybenzamine improves systemic oxygen delivery after the Norwood procedure. *Ann Thorac Surg* 1999;67:161–167, with permission from The Society of Thoracic Surgeons.

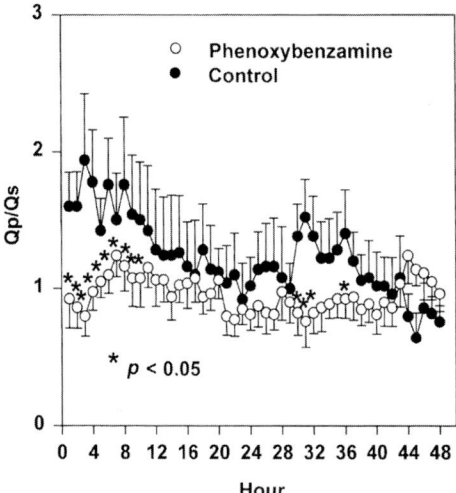

Figure 34-21 Pulmonary to systemic flow ratio (Qp/Qs) during the first 48 hours after the Norwood procedure. The Qp/Qs was significantly higher in the control group than in the phenoxybenzamine group during hours 1 to 10, 30 to 32, and 36 ($p < 0.05$, RM ANOVA). Reprinted from Tweddell JS, Hoffman GM, Fedderly RT, et al. Phenoxybenzamine improves systemic oxygen delivery after the Norwood procedure. *Ann Thorac Surg* 1999;67:161–167, with permission from The Society of Thoracic Surgeons.

and 34.21) (382). In a retrospective study, Tweddell et al found several variables in addition to the use of phenoxybenzamine that may be associated with improved survival following the Norwood operation, including the use of a modified operative technique designed to avoid kinking of the ascending aorta, use of modified ultrafiltration and aprotinin, and postoperative continuous monitoring of SvO$_2$ (4). Phenoxybenzamine has a long half-life, which makes some clinicians reluctant to use the drug.

Excessive desaturation may occur following the Norwood operation, and the differential diagnosis and management strategies are discussed previously in the postoperative cyanosis section. One particular cause for cyanosis following the Norwood operation is inadequate surgical resection of the atrial septum. The septum primum is often displaced posteriorly and to the left. If it is not completely resected, pulmonary venous obstruction may occur.

Recent interest has developed in a surgical variant of the Norwood operation, commonly known as the "Sano modification" (391). In this operation, a right ventricular to pulmonary artery conduit instead of a systemic to pulmonary artery shunt is used to provide pulmonary blood flow, which may improve myocardial function by increasing diastolic blood pressure and thus coronary perfusion pressure (352,392). The postoperative physiology following the Sano modification is somewhat different from the standard Norwood operation and deserves comment. Due to the absence of diastolic runoff through a Blalock-Taussig shunt, infants with "Sano physiology" do not have pulmonary overcirculation (or a large Qp/Qs) and thus, in contrast to patients with typical "Norwood physiology," usually will not benefit from aggressive afterload reduction. In fact, excessive systemic vasodilation may be harmful by creating

inadequate pulmonary blood flow and severe cyanosis, similar to the physiology of a patient with unrepaired tetralogy of Fallot. Early, nonrandomized reports suggest that the Sano modification may improve early survival following stage I palliation of HLHS (391,393). Risks related to this modification center upon the effects of performing a ventriculotomy in an infant with a single right ventricle, and include myocardial dysfunction, arrhythmias, and false aneurysm formation. A multicenter, randomized, clinical trail is planned to compare outcomes following the Sano modification with the standard Norwood operation.

Interrupted Aortic Arch

Complete repair, including VSD closure and reconstruction of the aortic arch, is the preferred operation for newborns with IAA (101). If significant subaortic stenosis is present, a Norwood-type operation may be used to stage the patient for a later biventricular repair (394). Following IAA repair, one must ensure that a residual VSD, sub-aortic obstruction, or aortic arch obstruction does not exist (101,395). Patients with respiratory compromise may have compression of the left mainstem bronchus by the reconstructed aortic arch. Complications related to DiGeorge syndrome, such as hypocalcemia and infection, may also occur.

Mixing Lesions

Transposition of the Great Arteries

In neonates with TGA and no significant outflow tract obstruction, the arterial switch operation is performed and the VSD, if present, is closed (1). The arterial switch operation involves transecting the aorta and pulmonary arteries above the semilunar valves, and anastomosing the aorta to the neoaortic root, such that the left ventricle ejects into the systemic circulation (1). The pulmonary artery is brought anterior to the aorta such that its branches drape over the aorta (Lecompte maneuver), and the pulmonary artery is anastomosed such that it receives blood from the right ventricular outflow tract. The coronary arteries are mobilized with a button of tissue around the ostia and reimplanted into the neoaorta. The VSD (if present) is closed (Fig. 34-22). If significant right ventricular outflow tract obstruction is present in TGA, a Damus-Kaye-Stansel procedure may be performed as an initial palliation, or as a part of the complete repair including closure of the VSD and placement of a right ventricle to pulmonary artery conduit. If significant left ventricular outflow tract obstruction exists, the classic surgical repair is the Rastelli procedure, which involves using a baffle to close the VSD to the aorta and placement a right ventricle to pulmonary artery conduit (396). Other options that do not require a conduit include the Nikaidoh operation (aortic root translocation into the surgically enlarged left ventricular outflow tract, VSD closure, and right ventricular outflow tract reconstruction) or the Réparation à l'Etage ventriculaire ("REV procedure;" involving infundibular resection to enlarge the VSD,

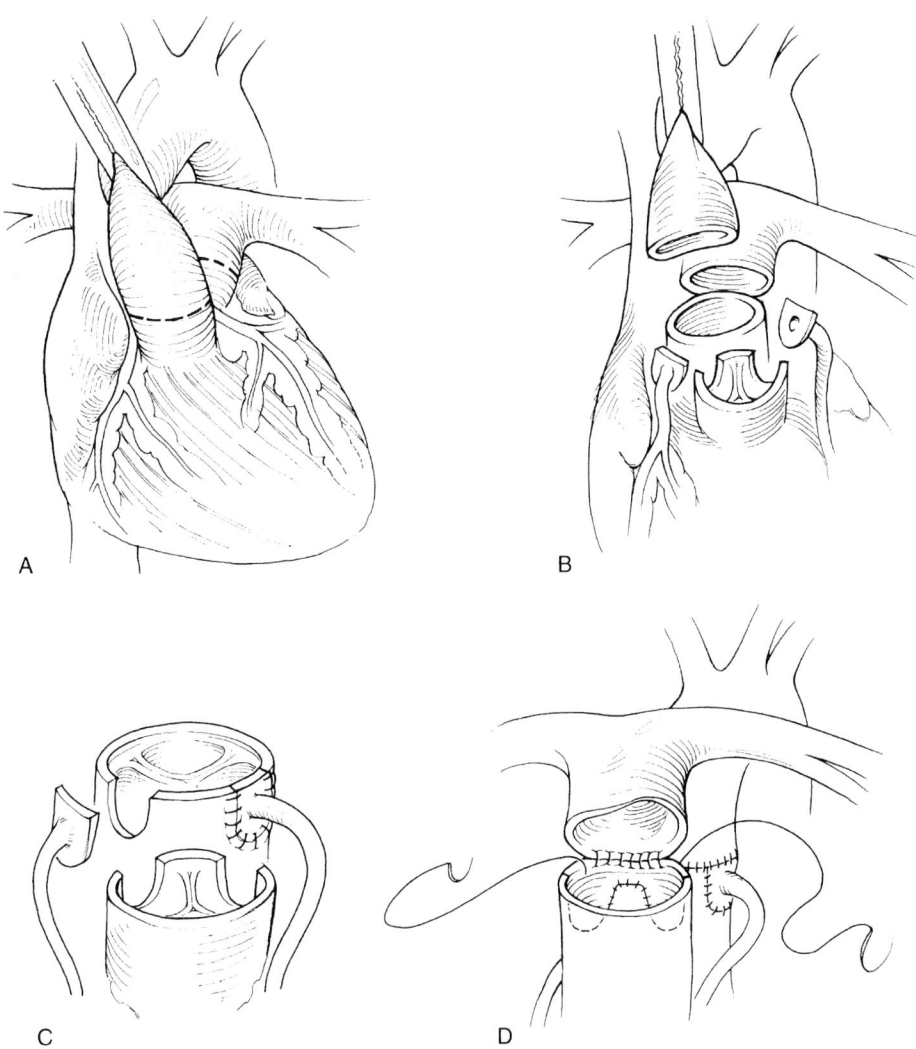

Figure 34-22 Arterial switch operation for transposition of the great arteries (TGA). **A.** The external anatomy is shown. The procedure is performed using cardiopulmonary bypass and either moderate or deep hypothermia with or without circulatory arrest. The broken lines show the sites of transection of the two great vessels. **B.** The aorta and main pulmonary arteries have been surgically transected and the coronary ostia have been removed from the native aortic root. **C.** The coronary buttons are in the process of being transferred to the native aortic root. **D.** The coronary transfer has been completed and the neoaortic root has been anastomosed to the ascending aorta. The coronary explantation sites on the neopulmonary root have been repaired with a patch and the neopulmonary artery is in the process of anastomosis to the distal pulmonary artery. Note, the distal pulmonary artery has been moved anterior to the ascending aorta as described by Lecompte. The procedure also involves closing the atrial septal defect and dividing the patent ductus arteriosus. Reprinted from Wernovsky G, Jonas RA. Other conotruncal lesions. In: Chang A, Hanley FL, Wernovsky G, et al., editors. *Pediatric cardiac intensive care.* Baltimore: Williams and Wilkins, 1998:289–301, with permission.

baffle closure of the VSD directing left ventricular flow to the aorta, the Lecompte maneuver, and right ventricular to pulmonary artery connection using a patch) (397,398).

The expected mortality for the arterial switch operation is very low (399), and many infants will have an unremarkable postoperative course. A period of early low cardiac output has been documented in approximately 25% of these patients (140). Problems with coronary ischemia may occur if there is kinking or stenosis of a coronary artery following reimplantation into the neoaorta. Volume overload in the immediate postoperative period can cause cardiac distension that stretches the newly implanted coronary arteries, resulting in myocardial ischemia and/or infarction. Coronary insufficiency may manifest as low cardiac output with ischemic electrocardiographic changes or ventricular arrhythmias. Significant obstruction of the aortic or pulmonary anastomosis is unusual in the early postoperative period. Residual VSDs and ventricular outflow obstruction can be problematic in complex cases.

Infants with TGA and intact ventricular septum who are referred after 1 to 2 months of age for the arterial switch operation often require placement of a pulmonary artery band to "prepare" the left ventricle before the arterial switch operation (400). A systemic to pulmonary artery shunt is also placed at the time of the pulmonary artery band to ensure adequate pulmonary blood flow. These patients are often critically ill following this operation with biventricular failure (right ventricular failure as a result of the acute volume overload created by the shunt and left ventricular failure related to the acute increase in afterload from the pulmonary artery band) and low cardiac output (400,401). Inotropic support and measures to decrease pulmonary overcirculation are often required for several days until the hemodynamics stabilize. Once the left ventricle is prepared, the patient is returned to the operating room, in which the systemic to pulmonary artery shunt and pulmonary band are removed and the arterial switch operation is performed.

Tricuspid Atresia

The postoperative course following palliation for tricuspid atresia depends upon the operation performed. Infants who require surgery in early infancy will have either a systemic to pulmonary artery shunt or a pulmonary artery band, and the complications associated with these procedures were described earlier. Infants with tricuspid atresia and TGA often require a Damus-Kaye-Stansel procedure, and the postoperative problems are similar to those seen following the Norwood operation as described above. A bi-directional Glenn or hemi-Fontan operation is then performed at around six months of life, and the postoperative course for these operations is also discussed earlier in the chapter.

Total Anomalous Pulmonary Venous Return

In infants with supracardiac and infracardiac total anomalous pulmonary venous return, the pulmonary venous confluence is anastomosed to the back of the left atrium using circulatory arrest, the primitive vertical vein is ligated, and the ASD is closed. If the pulmonary veins drain to the coronary sinus, surgical intervention involves unroofing of the coronary sinus, and closure of the ASD.

Following repair of TAPVR, infants may be predisposed to pulmonary hypertensive crises or persistent pulmonary vein obstruction, in part related to abnormal muscularity of the pulmonary arteries and veins which develops in utero (106,402,403). Pulmonary edema and poor lung compliance may be seen in infants whose pulmonary veins were obstructed preoperatively. The left atrium may be small and poorly compliant, and rapid volume infusions may exacerbate pulmonary edema and pulmonary hypertension in this setting. Deep sedation and the judicious use of positive end-expiratory pressure (PEEP) are indicated in the early postoperative period to facilitate gas exchange. The pulmonary hypertension seen in some infants following repair of TAPVR is very responsive to INO (270).

Truncus Arteriosus

Surgical repair of truncus arteriosus involves VSD closure, removal of the pulmonary arteries from the arterial trunk,

and placement of a conduit from the right ventricle to the pulmonary arteries. If present, surgical attention is also given to the IAA and/or truncal valve insufficiency (404). Care must be taken to identify the origin and course of the coronary arteries so that they are not injured during the operation.

Following repair of truncus arteriosus, infants are at risk for developing right ventricular failure related to pulmonary hypertension, the VSD closure, and the ventriculotomy required for the right ventricle to pulmonary artery conduit. Pulmonary hypertension may be problematic, particularly in patients referred for surgery beyond the neonatal period. Surgeons may leave an atrial communication to decompress the right heart, at the expense of mild postoperative cyanosis. The truncal valve functions as the aortic valve following surgical repair. The severity of preoperative truncal valve stenosis usually is decreased in the postoperative period as the volume overload has been eliminated. Severe truncal valve insufficiency will be poorly tolerated in the postoperative period and may require a surgical valvuloplasty or replacement (109,404). The left ventricle is exposed to increased afterload following surgery as a result of the elimination of the low vascular resistance pulmonary circulation, and the effects of CPB, which may create temporary left ventricular failure. A residual VSD will add a volume load to the left ventricle and contribute to pulmonary hypertension. A state of low cardiac output may exist related to one or more of the above problems. If an IAA was repaired, care must be taken to ensure that residual arch obstruction does not exist and exacerbate myocardial dysfunction and truncal valve insufficiency.

Left to Right Shunts

Atrial Septal Defect

Secundum ASDs may be surgically closed primarily or with a pericardial or Gore-Tex™ patch. Primum ASDs typically require patch closure, and the commonly associated cleft in the mitral valve is usually sutured closed. Sinus venosus ASDs are typically associated with anomalous pulmonary venous drainage of the right pulmonary veins, which must be redirected to the left atrium.

Most patients may be extubated in the operating room or soon after returning to the intensive care unit following ASD closure (405). Atrial arrhythmias may occur following any ASD closure. There is an increase incidence of sinus node dysfunction following sinus venosus ASD repair that is usually transient, however, temporary atrial pacing may be required (406).

Ventricular Septal Defect

The surgical approach to a VSD depends on its location. Perimembranous and inlet VSDs are approached through the right atrium. Tricuspid valve detachment may be required for adequate exposure of the defect (407). Conal VSDs are approached through the pulmonary artery

(408). Muscular VSDs may be approached through the atrium, although apical defects often require a small ventriculotomy (409). Selected infants with large VSDs who are not thought to be candidates from primary repair because of patient size, the presence of multiple VSDs with anticipated difficult surgical exposure, or noncardiac co-morbidities may be palliated with a pulmonary artery band.

The postoperative course following repair of large, isolated VSDs may be complicated by pulmonary hypertension, although this is quite uncommon in the current era as a result of earlier repair. The incidence of a significant residual VSD, which also will cause pulmonary hypertension, is minimized with the routine use of transesophageal echocardiography. Patch dehiscence is a rare complication of VSD closure that may occur once the infant leaves the operating room and thus will be not detected by the transesophageal echocardiogram. Data that would suggest a significant residual VSD include elevated left atrial and pulmonary artery pressures, a step-up of greater than 10% in oxygen saturation from the superior vena cava or right atrium to the pulmonary artery, the presence of low cardiac out syndrome, persistent cardiomegaly and increased pulmonary vascular markings on chest radiograph, and difficulty weaning from the ventilator. JET or surgical heart block may occur following repair of a VSD. Right bundle branch block commonly occurs but does not appear to be of long-term significance.

Atrioventricular Canal Defect

Incomplete and transitional atrioventricular canal defects typically are repaired with a patch closure of the ASD and, commonly, suture closure of the cleft in the mitral valve. The postoperative course is similar to that seen following ASD closure as described above.

Complete atrioventricular septal defect repair may be accomplished using a one or two patch technique to close the primum atrial and inlet ventricular septal defects, dependent on patient anatomy and surgical preference (410). The common atrioventricular valve is divided to create separate tricuspid and mitral valves. All of the postoperative concerns following VSD closure as discussed above also apply to the infant following atrioventricular canal repair. These include pulmonary hypertension, residual VSDs, and arrhythmias (specifically, JET and complete heart block). Additionally, mitral valve regurgitation may occur, causing ventricular volume overload, congestive heart failure, and pulmonary hypertension (411). Mitral regurgitation may be suspected by auscultation and the identification of large ventricular waves on the left atrial line tracing, and further quantified by echocardiography. Afterload reduction should be initiated when significant mitral regurgitation is identified, and volume overload should be avoided. Mitral stenosis is less common, but will cause elevated left atrial pressures and large atrial waves on the left atrial pressure tracing.

Patent Ductus Arteriosus

PDAs may be ligated surgically via a thoracotomy or using a video-assisted thoracoscopic technique (VATS). Specific complications that are uncommonly encountered are related to the injury of nearby structures, including the recurrent laryngeal and phrenic nerves. Coils and occluding devices may be used to close PDAs in the cardiac catheterization laboratory. Hemolysis or obstructions by the coil of the aorta or the proximal left pulmonary artery are rare complications following transcatheter occlusion of a PDA.

Aortopulmonary Window

Although several surgical techniques have been used in the past for aortopulmonary windows, currently the transaortic patch repair is favored by many centers (119). Any associated cardiac lesions are repaired at the same operation. Postoperative problems that may be encountered include pulmonary hypertension and residual left to right shunting. A related and somewhat rare lesion in which one pulmonary artery arises from the ascending aorta and the other from the right ventricle deserves special consideration. Preoperatively, the pulmonary artery that arises from the ascending aorta is exposed to systemic pressures, and the other pulmonary artery receives the entire cardiac output from the right ventricle. This unique combination of high pressure to one pulmonary vascular bed and high flow to the other predisposes these infants to having significant problems with pulmonary hypertension in the immediate postoperative period.

Heart Transplantation

The classical surgical technique used in heart transplantation involves a bi-atrial anastomosis, and connection of the great vessels at the level of the ascending aorta and main pulmonary artery. Many surgeons are now performing a bicaval anastomosis, which eliminates suture lines in the right atrium, includes the donor sinus node in the transplantation, and may reduce the incidence of atrial arrhythmias (412).

Several unique issues must be considered during the early postoperative period following heart transplantation. The characteristics of the donor heart may impact on the postoperative course. The circumstances leading to brain death of the donor, the amount of inotropic support required prior to the organ harvest, and the duration of total ischemic time all impact on myocardial function following transplantation. The size of the donor heart in relation the recipient is also important. For example, a larger donor heart may be useful to overcome pulmonary hypertension in the recipient but may make sternal closure difficult. The condition of the recipient going into the transplant will certainly impact the postoperative course. For example, inadequate nutrition, pulmonary hypertension or renal insufficiency may have been present before surgery and will influence postoperative management.

Immunosuppression is required to prevent rejection and is based on a triple drug regimen including corticosteroids, a calcineurin inhibitor (cyclosporine or tacrolimus) and an antiproliferative agent (azathioprine or mycophenolate mofetil) (413). This strategy suppresses the immune system at multiple different levels while minimizing the toxicity of individual drugs. The use of induction immunotherapy, which refers to the administration of anti-T cell antibodies, may be considered immediately following transplant in patients at high risk for rejection or renal insufficiency (414,415). Induction immunotherapy may allow for dose reduction or delayed introduction of calcineurin inhibitors, allowing time for recovery of renal function. The risk of rejection is highest immediately following transplantation, and thus intense immunosuppression is initiated and then tapered over time. Serial echocardiograms and myocardial biopsies are needed for close surveillance. Signs and symptoms of severe rejection include tachycardia, hypotension, tachypnea, poor perfusion and arrhythmias. Treatment of rejection centers on the augmentation of immune suppression and supportive care until recovery of myocardial function occurs.

Severe pulmonary hypertension may lead to right ventricular failure, and aggressive measures may be required to lower the pulmonary vascular resistance and support the right ventricular systolic function. In patients who are known to be at risk for postoperative hypertension, it may be advantageous to transplant a slightly oversized donor heart. If the donor heart is too large, however, the sternum may need to be left open for several days.

Systemic hypertension is common following heart transplantation related in part to fluid retention, and the side effects of corticosteroids and cyclosporine. Treatment is based on the severity of hypertension and the availability of the enteral route of delivering medications. Intravenous vasodilators and oral antihypertensive agents, such as calcium channel blockers and angiotensin-converting enzyme inhibitors, are commonly used. Seizures may also occur, sometimes related to severe hypertension or cyclosporine toxicity.

The risk of infection following heart transplantation is increased due to a variety of factors. Many infants have prolonged preoperative ICU stays, prolonged exposure to central venous catheters, and malnutrition. Immunosuppression is intense in the early postoperative period. Thus vigilance for infection is high immediately following surgery. In addition to standard surgical antibiotic prophylaxis against gram-positive organisms, additional prophylactic drugs are commonly prescribed to minimize the incidence of infection against cytomegalovirus, herpes viruses and Pneumocystis carinii pneumonia.

CONCLUSION

Neonates and infants with critical congenital heart disease present a tremendous challenge to all medical personnel who are involved in their care. The general pathophysiology, presentations, and management strategies describe

above serve as a starting point to guide physicians toward providing state of the art care. Subtle variations in cardiac anatomy and physiology exist within each type of heart defect, and the importance of developing individualized medical management and interventional plans for each patient cannot be overstated. Optimal outcomes are achieved when problems are anticipated and addressed in a timely fashion (proactive, not reactive management). Frequent reevaluation of response to treatment is essential. Detailed communication across all subspecialties is equally important to achieve optimal outcomes. Perioperative care for infants with congenital heart disease continues to evolve, as new medications, treatment strategies, and surgical and interventional techniques are reported on a routine basis. Fetal heart surgery and transcatheter interventional procedures are still in the developmental stages but are likely to play an expanding role in this patient population, and this trend will certainly present a new set of challenges in the years to come (92,416–418).

REFERENCES

1. Jatene AD, Fontes VF, Paulista PP, et al. Anatomic correction of transposition of the great vessels. *J Thorac Cardiovasc Surg* 1976;72:364.
2. Parry AJ, McElhinney DB, Kung GC, et al. Elective primary repair of acyanotic tetralogy of Fallot in early infancy: overall outcome and impact on the pulmonary valve. *J Am Coll Cardiol* 2000;36:2279.
3. Hanley FL, Heinemann MK, Jonas RA, et al. Repair of truncus arteriosus in the neonate. *J Thorac Cardiovasc Surg* 1993;105:1047.
4. Tweddell JS, Hoffman GM, Mussatto KA, et al. Improved survival of patients undergoing palliation of hypoplastic left heart syndrome: lessons learned from 115 consecutive patients. *Circulation* 2002;106:182.
5. Newburger JW, Silbert AR, Buckley LP, et al. Cognitive function and age at repair of transposition of the great arteries in children. *N Engl J Med* 1984;310:1495.
6. Clapp S, Perry BL, Farooki ZQ, et al. Down's syndrome, complete atrioventricular canal, and pulmonary vascular obstructive disease. *J Thorac Cardiovasc Surg* 1990;100:115.
7. Castaneda AR, Mayer JE Jr, Jonas RA, et al. The neonate with critical congenital heart disease: repair—a surgical challenge. *J Thorac Cardiovasc Surg* 1989;98:869.
8. Bando K, Turrentine MW, Sharp TG, et al. Pulmonary hypertension after operations for congenital heart disease: analysis of risk factors and management. *J Thorac Cardiovasc Surg* 1996;112:1600.
9. Friedman AH, Copel JA, Kleinman CS. Fetal echocardiography and fetal cardiology: indications, diagnosis and management. *Semin Perinatol* 1993;17:76.
10. Verheijen PM, Lisowski LA, Stoutenbeek P, et al. Prenatal diagnosis of congenital heart disease affects preoperative acidosis in the newborn patient. *J Thorac Cardiovasc Surg* 2001;121:798.
11. Eapen RS, Rowland DG, Franklin WH. Effect of prenatal diagnosis of critical left heart obstruction on perinatal morbidity and mortality. *Am J Perinatol* 1998;15:237.
12. Bonnet D, Coltri A, Butera G, et al. Detection of transposition of the great arteries in fetuses reduces neonatal morbidity and mortality. *Circulation* 1999;99:916.
13. Kumar RK, Newburger JW, Gauvreau K, et al. Comparison of outcome when hypoplastic left heart syndrome and transposition of the great arteries are diagnosed prenatally versus when diagnosis of these two conditions is made only postnatally. *Am J Cardiol* 1999;83:1649.
14. Tworetzky W, McElhinney DB, Reddy VM, et al. Improved surgical outcome after fetal diagnosis of hypoplastic left heart syndrome. *Circulation* 2001;103:1269.

15. Kern JH, Hayes CJ, Michler RE, et al. Survival and risk factor analysis for the Norwood procedure for hypoplastic left heart syndrome. *Am J Cardiol* 1997;80:170.

16. Mahle WT, Clancy RR, McGaurn SP, et al. Impact of prenatal diagnosis on survival and early neurologic morbidity in neonates with the hypoplastic left heart syndrome. *Pediatrics* 2001;107:1277.

17. Snider A, Serwer G, Ritter S. Specialized echocardiographic techniques. In: Snider A, Serwer G, Ritter S, eds. *Echocardiography in pediatric heart disease*, 2nd ed. St. Louis: Mosby-Year Book, 1997:76.

18. Sharland GK, Chan KY, Allan LD. Coarctation of the aorta: difficulties in prenatal diagnosis. *Br Heart J* 1994;71:70.

19. Rudolph A. The fetal circulation and postnatal adaptation. In: Rudolph A, ed. *Congenital diseases of the heart: clinical-pathophysiological considerations*, 2nd ed. Armonk, NY: Futura, 2001:3.

20. Edelstone DI, Rudolph AM. Preferential streaming of ductus venosus blood to the brain and heart in fetal lambs. *Am J Physiol* 1979;237:H724.

21. Edelstone DI. Regulation of blood flow through the ductus venosus. *J Dev Physiol* 1980;2:219.

22. Rudolph AM. Fetal and neonatal pulmonary circulation. *Am Rev Respir Dis* 1977;115:11.

23. Teitel DF, Iwamoto HS, Rudolph AM. Changes in the pulmonary circulation during birth-related events. *Pediatr Res* 1990;27:372.

24. Stanger P, Silverman NH, Foster E. Diagnostic accuracy of pediatric echocardiograms performed in adult laboratories. *Am J Cardiol* 1999;83:908.

25. Heymann MA, Berman W Jr, Rudolph AM, et al. Dilatation of the ductus arteriosus by prostaglandin E1 in aortic arch abnormalities. *Circulation* 1979;59:169.

26. Neutze JM, Starling MB, Elliott RB, et al. Palliation of cyanotic congenital heart disease in infancy with E-type prostaglandins. *Circulation* 1977;55:238.

27. Kramer HH, Sommer M, Rammos S, et al. Evaluation of low dose prostaglandin E1 treatment for ductus dependent congenital heart disease. *Eur J Pediatr* 1995;154:700.

28. Lewis AB, Freed MD, Heymann MA, et al. Side effects of therapy with prostaglandin E1 in infants with critical congenital heart disease. *Circulation* 1981;64:893.

29. Hallidie-Smith KA. Prostaglandin E1 in suspected ductus dependent cardiac malformation. *Arch Dis Child* 1984;59:1020.

30. Lim DS, Kulik TJ, Kim DW, et al. Aminophylline for the prevention of apnea during prostaglandin E1 infusion. *Pediatrics* 2003;112:e27.

31. Tworetzky W, McElhinney DB, Brook MM, et al. Echocardiographic diagnosis alone for the complete repair of major congenital heart defects. *J Am Coll Cardiol* 1999;33:228.

32. Kaulitz R, Jonas RA, van der Velde ME. Echocardiographic assessment of interrupted aortic arch. *Cardiol Young* 1999;9:562.

33. Need LR, Powell AJ, del Nido P, et al. Coronary echocardiography in tetralogy of Fallot: diagnostic accuracy, resource utilization and surgical implications over 13 years. *J Am Coll Cardiol* 2000;36:1371.

34. Rashkind WJ, Miller WW. Creation of an atrial septal defect without thoracotomy. A palliative approach to complete transposition of the great arteries. *JAMA* 1966;196:991.

35. Atz AM, Feinstein JA, Jonas RA, et al. Preoperative management of pulmonary venous hypertension in hypoplastic left heart syndrome with restrictive atrial septal defect. *Am J Cardiol* 1999;83:1224.

36. Chung T. Assessment of cardiovascular anatomy in patients with congenital heart disease by magnetic resonance imaging. *Pediatr Cardiol* 2000;21:18.

37. Lardo AC. Real-time magnetic resonance imaging: diagnostic and interventional applications. *Pediatr Cardiol* 2000;21:80.

38. Khoury MJ, Cordero JF, Mulinare J, et al. Selected midline defect associations: a population study. *Pediatrics* 1989;84:266.

39. Murugasu B, Yip WC, Tay JS, et al. Sonographic screening for renal tract anomalies associated with congenital heart disease. *J Clin Ultrasound* 1990;18:79.

40. Towbin J, Greenberg F. Genetic syndromes and clinical molecular genetics. In: Garson A, Bricker J, Fisher D, et al, eds. *The science and practice of pediatric cardiology*. Baltimore, MD: Williams & Wilkins, 1998:2627.

41. Goldmuntz E, Clark BJ, Mitchell LE, et al. Frequency of 22q11 deletions in patients with conotruncal defects. *J Am Coll Cardiol* 1998;32:492.

42. Frohn-Mulder IM, Wesby Swaay E, Bouwhuis C, et al. Chromosome 22q11 deletions in patients with selected outflow tract malformations. *Genet Couns* 1999;10:35.

43. Chang AC, Hanley FL, Lock JE, et al. Management and outcome of low birth weight neonates with congenital heart disease. *J Pediatr* 1994;124:461.

44. Reddy VM, McElhinney DB, Sagrado T, et al. Results of 102 cases of complete repair of congenital heart defects in patients weighing 700 to 2500 grams. *J Thorac Cardiovasc Surg* 1999;117:324.

45. Reddy VM, Hanley FL. Cardiac surgery in infants with very low birth weight. *Semin Pediatr Surg* 2000;9:91.

46. Rossi AF, Seiden HS, Sadeghi AM, et al. The outcome of cardiac operations in infants weighing two kilograms or less. *J Thorac Cardiovasc Surg* 1998;116:28.

47. Bacha EA, Almodovar M, Wessel DL, et al. Surgery for coarctation of the aorta in infants weighing less than 2 kg. *Ann Thorac Surg* 2001;71:1260.

48. Weinstein S, Gaynor JW, Bridges ND, et al. Early survival of infants weighing 2.5 kilograms or less undergoing first-stage reconstruction for hypoplastic left heart syndrome. *Circulation* 1999;100:II167.

49. Pizarro C, Davis DA, Galantowicz ME, et al. Stage I palliation for hypoplastic left heart syndrome in low birth weight neonates: can we justify it? *Eur J Cardiothorac Surg* 2002;21:716.

50. McElhinney DB, Hedrick HL, Bush DM, et al. Necrotizing enterocolitis in neonates with congenital heart disease: risk factors and outcomes. *Pediatrics* 2000;106:1080.

51. Eronen M, Siren MK, Ekblad H, et al. Short- and long-term outcome of children with congenital complete heart block diagnosed in utero or as a newborn. *Pediatrics* 2000;106:86.

52. Gregoratos G, Abrams J, Epstein AE, et al. ACC/AHA/NASPE 2002 Guideline Update for Implantation of Cardiac Pacemakers and Antiarrhythmia Devices—summary article: a report of the American College of Cardiology/American Heart Association Task Force on Practice Guidelines. *J Am Coll Cardiol* 2002;40:1703.

53. Kovalchin JP, Forbes TJ, Nihill MR, et al. Echocardiographic determinants of clinical course in infants with critical and severe pulmonary valve stenosis. *J Am Coll Cardiol* 1997;29:1095.

54. Gournay V, Piechaud JF, Delogu A, et al. Balloon valvotomy for critical stenosis or atresia of pulmonary valve in newborns. *J Am Coll Cardiol* 1995;26:1725.

55. Colli AM, Perry SB, Lock JE, et al. Balloon dilation of critical valvar pulmonary stenosis in the first month of life. *Cathet Cardiovasc Diagn* 1995;34:23.

56. Gildein HP, Kleinert S, Goh TH, et al. Treatment of critical pulmonary valve stenosis by balloon dilatation in the neonate. *Am Heart J* 1996;131:1007.

57. Tabatabaei H, Boutin C, Nykanen DG, et al. Morphologic and hemodynamic consequences after percutaneous balloon valvotomy for neonatal pulmonary stenosis: medium-term follow-up. *J Am Coll Cardiol* 1996;27:473.

58. Weber HS. Initial and late results after catheter intervention for neonatal critical pulmonary valve stenosis and atresia with intact ventricular septum: a technique in continual evolution. *Catheter Cardiovasc Interv* 2002;56:394.

59. Hanley FL, Sade RM, Freedom RM, et al. Outcomes in critically ill neonates with pulmonary stenosis and intact ventricular septum: a multiinstitutional study. Congenital Heart Surgeons Society. *J Am Coll Cardiol* 1993;22:183.

60. Fedderly RT, Lloyd TR, Mendelsohn AM, et al. Determinants of successful balloon valvotomy in infants with critical pulmonary stenosis or membranous pulmonary atresia with intact ventricular septum. *J Am Coll Cardiol* 1995;25:460.

61. Fraser CD Jr, McKenzie ED, Cooley DA. Tetralogy of Fallot: surgical management individualized to the patient. *Ann Thorac Surg* 2001;71:1556.

62. Pigula FA, Khalil PN, Mayer JE, et al. Repair of tetralogy of Fallot in neonates and young infants. *Circulation* 1999;100:II157.

63. Johnson MC, Strauss AW, Dowton SB, et al. Deletion within chromosome 22 is common in patients with absent pulmonary valve syndrome. *Am J Cardiol* 1995;76:66.

64. Lakier JB, Stanger P, Heymann MA, et al. Tetralogy of Fallot with absent pulmonary valve. Natural history and hemodynamic considerations. *Circulation* 1974;50:167.

65. Heinemann MK, Hanley FL. Preoperative management of neonatal tetralogy of Fallot with absent pulmonary valve syndrome. *Ann Thorac Surg* 1993;55:172.

66. Bull K, Somerville J, Ty E, et al. Presentation and attrition in complex pulmonary atresia. *J Am Coll Cardiol* 1995;25:491.
67. Minich LL, Tani LY, Ritter S, et al. Usefulness of the preoperative tricuspid/mitral valve ratio for predicting outcome in pulmonary atresia with intact ventricular septum. *Am J Cardiol* 2000; 85:1325.
68. Satou GM, Perry SB, Gauvreau K, et al. Echocardiographic predictors of coronary artery pathology in pulmonary atresia with intact ventricular septum. *Am J Cardiol* 2000;85:1319.
69. Daubeney PE, Delany DJ, Anderson RH, et al. Pulmonary atresia with intact ventricular septum: range of morphology in a population-based study. *J Am Coll Cardiol* 2002;39:1670.
70. Jahangiri M, Zurakowski D, Bichell D, et al. Improved results with selective management in pulmonary atresia with intact ventricular septum. *J Thorac Cardiovasc Surg* 1999;118:1046.
71. Alwi M, Geetha K, Bilkis AA, et al. Pulmonary atresia with intact ventricular septum percutaneous radiofrequency-assisted valvotomy and balloon dilation versus surgical valvotomy and Blalock Taussig shunt. *J Am Coll Cardiol* 2000;35:468.
72. Celermajer DS, Cullen S, Sullivan ID, et al. Outcome in neonates with Ebstein's anomaly. *J Am Coll Cardiol* 1992;19:1041.
73. Knott-Craig CJ, Overholt ED, Ward KE, et al. Repair of Ebstein's anomaly in the symptomatic neonate: an evolution of technique with 7-year follow-up. *Ann Thorac Surg* 2002;73:1786.
74. Starnes VA, Pitlick PT, Bernstein D, et al. Ebstein's anomaly appearing in the neonate. A new surgical approach. *J Thorac Cardiovasc Surg* 1991;101:1082.
75. Stellin G, Santini F, Thiene G, et al. Pulmonary atresia, intact ventricular septum, and Ebstein anomaly of the tricuspid valve. Anatomic and surgical considerations. *J Thorac Cardiovasc Surg* 1993;106:255.
76. Leoni F, Huhta JC, Douglas J, et al. Effect of prostaglandin on early surgical mortality in obstructive lesions of the systemic circulation. *Br Heart J* 1984;52:654.
77. Lofland GK, McCrindle BW, Williams WG, et al. Critical aortic stenosis in the neonate: a multi-institutional study of management, outcomes, and risk factors. Congenital Heart Surgeons Society. *J Thorac Cardiovasc Surg* 2001;121:10.
78. Cowley CG, Dietrich M, Mosca RS, et al. Balloon valvuloplasty versus transventricular dilation for neonatal critical aortic stenosis. *Am J Cardiol* 2001;87:1125.
79. Gildein HP, Kleinert S, Weintraub RG, et al. Surgical commissurotomy of the aortic valve: outcome of open valvotomy in neonates with critical aortic stenosis. *Am Heart J* 1996;131:754.
80. McCrindle BW, Blackstone EH, Williams WG, et al. Are outcomes of surgical versus transcatheter balloon valvotomy equivalent in neonatal critical aortic stenosis? *Circulation* 2001;104:I152.
81. Barnea O, Austin EH, Richman B, et al. Balancing the circulation: theoretic optimization of pulmonary/systemic flow ratio in hypoplastic left heart syndrome. *J Am Coll Cardiol* 1994;24:1376.
82. Barnea O, Santamore WP, Rossi A, et al. Estimation of oxygen delivery in newborns with a univentricular circulation. *Circulation* 1998;98:1407.
83. Day RW, Tani LY, Minich LL, et al. Congenital heart disease with ductal-dependent systemic perfusion: Doppler ultrasonography flow velocities are altered by changes in the fraction of inspired oxygen. *J Heart Lung Transplant* 1995;14:718.
84. Day RW, Barton AJ, Pysher TJ, et al. Pulmonary vascular resistance of children treated with nitrogen during early infancy. *Ann Thorac Surg* 1998;65:1400.
85. Mora GA, Pizarro C, Jacobs ML, et al. Experimental model of single ventricle. Influence of carbon dioxide on pulmonary vascular dynamics. *Circulation* 1994;90:II43.
86. Tabbutt S, Ramamoorthy C, Montenegro LM, et al. Impact of inspired gas mixtures on preoperative infants with hypoplastic left heart syndrome during controlled ventilation. *Circulation* 2001;104:I159.
87. Ramamoorthy C, Tabbutt S, Kurth CD, et al. Effects of inspired hypoxic and hypercapnic gas mixtures on cerebral oxygen saturation in neonates with univentricular heart defects. *Anesthesiology* 2002;96:283.
88. Rychik J, Rome JJ, Collins MH, et al. The hypoplastic left heart syndrome with intact atrial septum: atrial morphology, pulmonary vascular histopathology and outcome. *J Am Coll Cardiol* 1999;34:554.
89. Graziano JN, Heidelberger KP, Ensing GJ, et al. The influence of a restrictive atrial septal defect on pulmonary vascular morphology in patients with hypoplastic left heart syndrome. *Pediatr Cardiol* 2002;23:146.
90. Canter CE, Moorehead S, Huddleston CB, et al. Restrictive atrial septal communication as a determinant of outcome of cardiac transplantation for hypoplastic left heart syndrome. *Circulation* 1993;88:II456.
91. Vlahos AP, Lock JE, McElhinney DB, et al. Hypoplastic left heart syndrome with intact or highly restrictive atrial septum: outcome after neonatal transcatheter atrial septostomy. *Circulation* 2004; 109:2326.
92. Marshall AC, van der Velde ME, Tworetzky W, et al. Creation of an atrial septal defect in utero for fetuses with hypoplastic left heart syndrome and intact or highly restrictive atrial septum. *Circulation* 2004;110:253.
93. Barber G, Helton JG, Aglira BA, et al. The significance of tricuspid regurgitation in hypoplastic left-heart syndrome. *Am Heart J* 1988;116:1563.
94. Pigott JD, Murphy JD, Barber G, et al. Palliative reconstructive surgery for hypoplastic left heart syndrome. *Ann Thorac Surg* 1988;45:122.
95. Breymann T, Kirchner G, Blanz U, et al. Results after Norwood procedure and subsequent cavopulmonary anastomoses for typical hypoplastic left heart syndrome and similar complex cardiovascular malformations. *Eur J Cardiothorac Surg* 1999; 16:117.
96. Gutgesell HP, Gibson J. Management of hypoplastic left heart syndrome in the 1990s. *Am J Cardiol* 2002;89:842.
97. Razzouk AJ, Chinnock RE, Gundry SR, et al. Transplantation as a primary treatment for hypoplastic left heart syndrome: intermediate-term results. *Ann Thorac Surg* 1996;62:1.
98. Morrow WR, Naftel D, Chinnock R, et al. Outcome of listing for heart transplantation in infants younger than six months: predictors of death and interval to transplantation. *J Heart Lung Transplant* 1997;16:1255.
99. Ikle L, Hale K, Fashaw L, et al. Developmental outcome of patients with hypoplastic left heart syndrome treated with heart transplantation. *J Pediatr* 2003;142:20.
100. Bauer J, Thul J, Kramer U, et al. Heart transplantation in children and infants: short-term outcome and long-term follow-up. *Pediatr Transplant* 2001;5:457.
101. Sell JE, Jonas RA, Mayer JE, et al. The results of a surgical program for interrupted aortic arch. *J Thorac Cardiovasc Surg* 1988;96:864.
102. Backer CL, Mavroudis C. Congenital Heart Surgery Nomenclature and Database Project: patent ductus arteriosus, coarctation of the aorta, interrupted aortic arch. *Ann Thorac Surg* 2000;69:S298.
103. Ashfaq M, Houston AB, Gnanapragasam JP, et al. Balloon atrial septostomy under echocardiographic control: six years' experience and evaluation of the practicability of cannulation via the umbilical vein. *Br Heart J* 1991;65:148.
104. Tandon R, Edwards JE. Tricuspid atresia. A re-evaluation and classification. *J Thorac Cardiovasc Surg* 1974;67:530.
105. Epstein M. Tricuspid atresia. In: Allen H, Gutgesell H, Clark E, et al, eds. *Moss and Adam's heart disease in infants, children, and adolescents.* Philadelphia: Lippincott, Williams & Wilkins, 2001:799.
106. Lupinetti FM, Kulik TJ, Beekman RH 3rd, et al. Correction of total anomalous pulmonary venous connection in infancy. *J Thorac Cardiovasc Surg* 1993;106:880.
107. McElhinney DB, Driscoll DA, Emanuel BS, et al. Chromosome 22q11 deletion in patients with truncus arteriosus. *Pediatr Cardiol* 2003;24:569.
108. Jacobs ML. Congenital heart surgery nomenclature and database project: truncus arteriosus. *Ann Thorac Surg* 2000;69:S50.
109. Bove EL, Lupinetti FM, Pridjian AK, et al. Results of a policy of primary repair of truncus arteriosus in the neonate. *J Thorac Cardiovasc Surg* 1993;105:1057.
110. Thompson LD, McElhinney DB, Reddy M, et al. Neonatal repair of truncus arteriosus: continuing improvement in outcomes. *Ann Thorac Surg* 2001;72:391.
111. Du ZD, Hijazi ZM, Kleinman CS, et al. Comparison between transcatheter and surgical closure of secundum atrial septal defect in children and adults: results of a multicenter nonrandomized trial. *J Am Coll Cardiol* 2002;39:1836.
112. Lun K, Li H, Leung MP, et al. Analysis of indications for surgical closure of subarterial ventricular septal defect without associated aortic cusp prolapse and aortic regurgitation. *Am J Cardiol* 2001;87:1266.

113. Puchalski MD, Brook MM, Silverman NH. Simplified echocardiographic criteria for decision making in perimembranous ventricular septal defect in childhood. *Am J Cardiol* 2002; 90:569.

114. Ross R. Medical management of chronic heart failure in children. *Am J Cardiovasc Drugs* 2001;1:37.

115. Kumar K, Lock JE, Geva T. Apical muscular ventricular septal defects between the left ventricle and the right ventricular infundibulum. Diagnostic and interventional considerations. *Circulation* 1997;95:1207.

116. McElhinney DB, Reddy VM, Silverman NH, et al. Atrioventricular septal defect with common valvar orifice and tetralogy of Fallot revisited: making a case for primary repair in infancy. *Cardiol Young* 1998;8:455.

117. Van Overmeire B, Smets K, Lecoutere D, et al. A comparison of ibuprofen and indomethacin for closure of patent ductus arteriosus. *N Engl J Med* 2000;343:674.

118. McElhinney DB, Reddy VM, Tworetzky W, et al. Early and late results after repair of aortopulmonary septal defect and associated anomalies in infants <6 months of age. *Am J Cardiol* 1998; 81:195.

119. Backer CL, Mavroudis C. Surgical management of aortopulmonary window: a 40-year experience. *Eur J Cardiothorac Surg* 2002;21:773.

120. Johnsrude CL, Perry JC, Cecchin F, et al. Differentiating anomalous left main coronary artery originating from the pulmonary artery in infants from myocarditis and dilated cardiomyopathy by electrocardiogram. *Am J Cardiol* 1995;75:71.

121. Chang RR, Allada V. Electrocardiographic and echocardiographic features that distinguish anomalous origin of the left coronary artery from pulmonary artery from idiopathic dilated cardiomyopathy. *Pediatr Cardiol* 2001;22:3.

122. Schwartz ML, Jonas RA, Colan SD. Anomalous origin of left coronary artery from pulmonary artery: recovery of left ventricular function after dual coronary repair. *J Am Coll Cardiol* 1997; 30:547.

123. Lee KJ, McCrindle BW, Bohn DJ, et al. Clinical outcomes of acute myocarditis in childhood. *Heart* 1999;82:226.

124. Boucek MM, Edwards LB, Keck BM, et al. The Registry of the International Society for Heart and Lung Transplantation: fifth Official Pediatric Report-2001 to 2002. *J Heart Lung Transplant* 2002;21:827.

125. West LJ, Pollock-Barziv SM, Dipchand AI, et al. ABO-incompatible heart transplantation in infants. *N Engl J Med* 2001;344:793.

126. Gajarski R, Mosca R, Ohye R, et al. Use of extracorporeal life support as a bridge to pediatric cardiac transplantation. *J Heart Lung Transplant* 2003;22:28.

127. Bourke KD, Sondheimer HM, Ivy DD, et al. Improved pretransplant management of infants with hypoplastic left heart syndrome enables discharge to home while waiting for transplantation. *Pediatr Cardiol* 2003;24:538.

128. Mitchell MB, Campbell DN, Boucek MM, et al. Mechanical limitation of pulmonary blood flow facilitates heart transplantation in older infants with hypoplastic left heart syndrome. *Eur J Cardiothorac Surg* 2003;23:735.

129. Mayer J. Cardiopulmonary bypass. In: Chang A, Hanley F, Wernovsky G, et al, eds. *Pediatric cardiac intensive care.* Baltimore, MD: Williams & Wilkins, 1998.

130. Pigula FA, Nemoto EM, Griffith BP, et al. Regional low-flow perfusion provides cerebral circulatory support during neonatal aortic arch reconstruction. *J Thorac Cardiovasc Surg* 2000;119:331.

131. Lehot JJ, Villard J, Piriz H, et al. Hemodynamic and hormonal responses to hypothermic and normothermic cardiopulmonary bypass. *J Cardiothorac Vasc Anes* 1992;6:132.

132. Ationu A, Singer DR, Smith A, et al. Studies of cardiopulmonary bypass in children: implications for the regulation of brain natriuretic peptide. *Cardiovasc Res* 1993;27:1538.

133. Stewart JM, Gewitz MH, Clark BJ, et al. The role of vasopressin and atrial natriuretic factor in postoperative fluid retention after the Fontan procedure. *J Thorac Cardiovasc Surg* 1991;102:821.

134. Burch M, Lum L, Elliott M, et al. Influence of cardiopulmonary bypass on water balance hormones in children. *Br Heart J* 1992; 68:309.

135. Philbin DM, Levine FH, Emerson CW, et al. Plasma vasopressin levels and urinary flow during cardiopulmonary bypass in patients with valvular heart disease: effect of pulsatile flow. *J Thorac Cardiovasc Surg* 1979;78:779.

136. Kross J, Dries DJ, Kumar P, et al. Atrial natriuretic peptide may not play a role in diuresis and natriuresis after cardiac operations. *J Thorac Cardiovasc Surg* 1992;103:1168.

137. Kirshbom PM, Tsui SS, DiBernardo LR, et al. Blockade of endothelin-converting enzyme reduces pulmonary hypertension after cardiopulmonary bypass and circulatory arrest. *Surgery* 1995;118:440.

138. Townsend GE, Wynands JE, Whalley DG, et al. Role of renin-angiotensin system in cardiopulmonary bypass hypertension. *Can Anaesth Soc J* 1984;31:160.

139. Bailey DR, Miller ED Jr, Kaplan JA, et al. The renin—angiotensin—aldosterone system during cardiac surgery with morphine—nitrous oxide anesthesia. *Anesthesiology* 1975;42:538.

140. Wernovsky G, Wypij D, Jonas RA, et al. Postoperative course and hemodynamic profile after the arterial switch operation in neonates and infants. A comparison of low-flow cardiopulmonary bypass and circulatory arrest. *Circulation* 1995;92:2226.

141. Wessel DL, Adatia I, Giglia TM, et al. Use of inhaled nitric oxide and acetylcholine in the evaluation of pulmonary hypertension and endothelial function after cardiopulmonary bypass. *Circulation* 1993;88:2128.

142. Schulze-Neick I, Li J, Penny DJ, et al. Pulmonary vascular resistance after cardiopulmonary bypass in infants: effect on postoperative recovery. *J Thorac Cardiovasc Surg* 2001;121:1033.

143. Butler J, Rocker GM, Westaby S. Inflammatory response to cardiopulmonary bypass. *Ann Thorac Surg* 1993;55:552.

144. Mainwaring RD, Lamberti JJ, Hugli TE. Complement activation and cytokine generation after modified Fontan procedure. *Ann Thorac Surg* 1998;65:1715.

145. Kirklin JK, Westaby S, Blackstone EH, et al. Complement and the damaging effects of cardiopulmonary bypass. *J Thorac Cardiovasc Surg* 1983;86:845.

146. Tanaka K, Takao M, Yada I, et al. Alterations in coagulation and fibrinolysis associated with cardiopulmonary bypass during open heart surgery. *J Cardiothorac Anesth* 1989;3:181.

147. Riegel W, Spillner G, Schlosser V, et al. Plasma levels of main granulocyte components during cardiopulmonary bypass. *J Thorac Cardiovasc Surg* 1988;95:1014.

148. Kondo C, Tanaka K, Takagi K, et al. Platelet dysfunction during cardiopulmonary bypass surgery. With special reference to platelet membrane glycoproteins. *ASAIO J* 1993;39:M550.

149. Butler J, Parker D, Pillai R, et al. Effect of cardiopulmonary bypass on systemic release of neutrophil elastase and tumor necrosis factor. *J Thorac Cardiovasc Surg* 1993;105:25.

150. Cavarocchi NC, England MD, Schaff HV, et al. Oxygen free radical generation during cardiopulmonary bypass: correlation with complement activation. *Circulation* 1986;74:III130.

151. Cavarocchi NC, Pluth JR, Schaff HV, et al. Complement activation during cardiopulmonary bypass. Comparison of bubble and membrane oxygenators. *J Thorac Cardiovasc Surg* 1986; 91:252.

152. Kern FH, Morana NJ, Sears JJ, et al. Coagulation defects in neonates during cardiopulmonary bypass. *Ann Thorac Surg* 1992; 54:541.

153. Chaturvedi RR, Lincoln C, Gothard JW, et al. Left ventricular dysfunction after open repair of simple congenital heart defects in infants and children: quantitation with the use of a conductance catheter immediately after bypass. *J Thorac Cardiovasc Surg* 1998;115:77.

154. England MD, Cavarocchi NC, O'Brien JF, et al. Influence of antioxidants (mannitol and allopurinol) on oxygen free radical generation during and after cardiopulmonary bypass. *Circulation* 1986;74:III134.

155. Bronicki RA, Backer CL, Baden HP, et al. Dexamethasone reduces the inflammatory response to cardiopulmonary bypass in children. *Ann Thorac Surg* 2000;69:1490.

156. Schroeder VA, Pearl JM, Schwartz SM, et al. Combined steroid treatment for congenital heart surgery improves oxygen delivery and reduces postbypass inflammatory mediator expression. *Circulation* 2003;107:2823.

157. Mojcik CF, Levy JH. Aprotinin and the systemic inflammatory response after cardiopulmonary bypass. *Ann Thorac Surg* 2001; 71:745.

158. Dietrich W, Mossinger H, Spannagl M, et al. Hemostatic activation during cardiopulmonary bypass with different aprotinin dosages in pediatric patients having cardiac operations. *J Thorac Cardiovasc Surg* 1993;105:712.

159. Carrel TP, Schwanda M, Vogt PR, et al. Aprotinin in pediatric cardiac operations: a benefit in complex malformations and with high-dose regimen only. *Ann Thorac Surg* 1998;66:153.

160. D'Errico CC, Shayevitz JR, Martindale SJ, et al. The efficacy and cost of aprotinin in children undergoing reoperative open heart surgery. *Anesth Analg* 1996;83:1193.

161. Penkoske PA, Entwistle LM, Marchak BE, et al. Aprotinin in children undergoing repair of congenital heart defects. *Ann Thorac Surg* 1995;60:S529.

162. Miller BE, Tosone SR, Tam VK, et al. Hematologic and economic impact of aprotinin in reoperative pediatric cardiac operations. *Ann Thorac Surg* 1998;66:535.

163. Jaquiss RD, Ghanayem NS, Zacharisen MC, et al. Safety of aprotinin use and re-use in pediatric cardiothoracic surgery. *Circulation* 2002;106:I90.

164. Costello JM, Backer CL, de Hoyos A, et al. Aprotinin reduces operative closure time and blood product use after pediatric bypass. *Ann Thorac Surg* 2003;75:1261.

165. Mossinger H, Dietrich W, Braun SL, et al. High-dose aprotinin reduces activation of hemostasis, allogeneic blood requirement, and duration of postoperative ventilation in pediatric cardiac surgery. *Ann Thorac Surg* 2003;75:430.

166. Tassani P, Richter JA, Barankay A, et al. Does high-dose methylprednisolone in aprotinin-treated patients attenuate the systemic inflammatory response during coronary artery bypass grafting procedures? *J Cardiothorac Vasc Anes* 1999;13:165.

167. Clancy RR, McGaurn SA, Goin JE, et al. Allopurinol neurocardiac protection trial in infants undergoing heart surgery using deep hypothermic circulatory arrest. *Pediatrics* 2001;108:61.

168. Schermerhorn ML, Tofukuji M, Khoury PR, et al. Sialyl lewis oligosaccharide preserves cardiopulmonary and endothelial function after hypothermic circulatory arrest in lambs. *J Thorac Cardiovasc Surg* 2000;120:230.

169. Naik SK, Knight A, Elliott M. A prospective randomized study of a modified technique of ultrafiltration during pediatric open-heart surgery. *Circulation* 1991;84:III422.

170. Draaisma AM, Hazekamp MG, Frank M, et al. Modified ultrafiltration after cardiopulmonary bypass in pediatric cardiac surgery. *Ann Thorac Surg* 1997;64:521.

171. Bando K, Turrentine MW, Vijay P, et al. Effect of modified ultrafiltration in high-risk patients undergoing operations for congenital heart disease. *Ann Thorac Surg* 1998;66:821.

172. Davies MJ, Nguyen K, Gaynor JW, et al. Modified ultrafiltration improves left ventricular systolic function in infants after cardiopulmonary bypass. *J Thorac Cardiovasc Surg* 1998;115:361.

173. Chaturvedi RR, Shore DF, White PA, et al. Modified ultrafiltration improves global left ventricular systolic function after open-heart surgery in infants and children. *Eur J Cardiothorac Surg* 1999;15:742.

174. Bando K, Vijay P, Turrentine MW, et al. Dilutional and modified ultrafiltration reduces pulmonary hypertension after operations for congenital heart disease: a prospective randomized study. *J Thorac Cardiovasc Surg* 1998;115:517.

175. Duke T, Butt W, South M, et al. Early markers of major adverse events in children after cardiac operations. *J Thorac Cardiovasc Surg* 1997;114:1042.

176. Newburger JW, Jonas RA, Wernovsky G, et al. A comparison of the perioperative neurologic effects of hypothermic circulatory arrest versus low-flow cardiopulmonary bypass in infant heart surgery. *N Engl J Med* 1993;329:1057.

177. Stevenson JG, Sorensen GK, Gartman DM, et al. Transesophageal echocardiography during repair of congenital cardiac defects: identification of residual problems necessitating reoperation. *J Am Soc Echocardiogr* 1993;6:356.

178. Rosenfeld HM, Gentles TL, Wernovsky G, et al. Utility of intraoperative transesophageal echocardiography in the assessment of residual cardiac defects. *Pediatr Cardiol* 1998;19:346.

179. Lang P, Chipman CW, Siden H, et al. Early assessment of hemodynamic status after repair of tetralogy of Fallot: a comparison of 24 hour (intensive care unit) and 1 year postoperative data in 98 patients. *Am J Cardiol* 1982;50:795.

180. Flori HR, Johnson LD, Hanley FL, et al. Transthoracic intracardiac catheters in pediatric patients recovering from congenital heart defect surgery: associated complications and outcomes. *Crit Care Med* 2000;28:2997.

181. Gold JP, Jonas RA, Lang P, et al. Transthoracic intracardiac monitoring lines in pediatric surgical patients: a ten-year experience. *Ann Thorac Surg* 1986;42:185.

182. Sellden H, Nilsson K, Larsson LE, et al. Radial arterial catheters in children and neonates: a prospective study. *Crit Care Med* 1987;15:1106.

183. Graves PW, Davis AL, Maggi JC, et al. Femoral artery cannulation for monitoring in critically ill children: prospective study. *Crit Care Med* 1990;18:1363.

184. Kocis KC, Vermilion RP, Callow LB, et al. Complications of femoral artery cannulation for perioperative monitoring in children. *J Thorac Cardiovasc Surg* 1996;112:1399.

185. Yabek SM, Akl BF, Berman W Jr, et al. Use of atrial epicardial electrodes to diagnose and treat postoperative arrhythmias in children. *Am J Cardiol* 1980;46:285.

186. Li J, Schulze-Neick I, Lincoln C, et al. Oxygen consumption after cardiopulmonary bypass surgery in children: determinants and implications. *J Thorac Cardiovasc Surg* 2000;119:525.

187. Tibby SM, Hatherill M, Murdoch IA. Capillary refill and core-peripheral temperature gap as indicators of haemodynamic status in paediatric intensive care patients. *Arch Dis Child* 1999;80:163.

188. Quasney MW, Goodman DM, Billow M, et al. Routine chest radiographs in pediatric intensive care units. *Pediatrics* 2001;107:241.

189. McElhinney DB, Reddy VM, Parry AJ, et al. Management and outcomes of delayed sternal closure after cardiac surgery in neonates and infants. *Crit Care Med* 2000;28:1180.

190. Tabbutt S, Duncan BW, McLaughlin D, et al. Delayed sternal closure after cardiac operations in a pediatric population. *J Thorac Cardiovasc Surg* 1997;113:886.

191. Taeed R, Schwartz SM, Pearl JM, et al. Unrecognized pulmonary venous desaturation early after Norwood palliation confounds Qp:Qs assessment and compromises oxygen delivery. *Circulation* 2001;103:2699.

192. Main E, Elliott MJ, Schindler M, et al. Effect of delayed sternal closure after cardiac surgery on respiratory function in ventilated infants. *Crit Care Med* 2001;29:1798.

193. Jenkins J, Lynn A, Edmonds J, et al. Effects of mechanical ventilation on cardiopulmonary function in children after open-heart surgery. *Crit Care Med* 1985;13:77.

194. Chang AC, Zucker HA, Hickey PR, et al. Pulmonary vascular resistance in infants after cardiac surgery: role of carbon dioxide and hydrogen ion. *Crit Care Med* 1995;23:568.

195. Cheifetz IM, Craig DM, Quick G, et al. Increasing tidal volumes and pulmonary overdistention adversely affect pulmonary vascular mechanics and cardiac output in a pediatric swine model. *Crit Care Med* 1998;26:710.

196. Kloth RL, Baum VC. Very early extubation in children after cardiac surgery. *Crit Care Med* 2002;30:787.

197. Seear M, Wensley D, MacNab A. Oxygen consumption-oxygen delivery relationship in children. *J Pediatr* 1993;123:208.

198. Lister G, Hellenbrand WE, Kleinman CS, et al. Physiologic effects of increasing hemoglobin concentration in left-to-right shunting in infants with ventricular septal defects. *N Engl J Med* 1982;306:502.

199. Siegel LB, Dalton HJ, Hertzog JH, et al. Initial postoperative serum lactate levels predict survival in children after open heart surgery. *Intensive Care Med* 1996;22:1418.

200. Cheifetz IM, Kern FH, Schulman SR, et al. Serum lactates correlate with mortality after operations for complex congenital heart disease. *Ann Thorac Surg* 1997;64:735.

201. Charpie JR, Dekeon MK, Goldberg CS, et al. Postoperative hemodynamics after Norwood palliation for hypoplastic left heart syndrome. *Am J Cardiol* 2001;87:198.

202. Rossi AF, Seiden HS, Gross RP, et al. Oxygen transport in critically ill infants after congenital heart operations. *Ann Thorac Surg* 1999;67:739.

203. Singh NC, Kissoon N, al Mofada S, et al. Comparison of continuous versus intermittent furosemide administration in postoperative pediatric cardiac patients. *Crit Care Med* 1992;20:17.

204. Hickey PR, Hansen DD, Wessel DL, et al. Pulmonary and systemic hemodynamic responses to fentanyl in infants. *Anesth Analg* 1985;64:483.

205. Hickey PR, Hansen DD, Wessel DL, et al. Blunting of stress responses in the pulmonary circulation of infants by fentanyl. *Anesth Analg* 1985;64:1137.

206. Anand KJ, Sippell WG, Aynsley-Green A. Randomised trial of fentanyl anaesthesia in preterm babies undergoing surgery: effects on the stress response. *Lancet* 1987;1:62.

207. Rigden SP, Barratt TM, Dillon MJ, et al. Acute renal failure complicating cardiopulmonary bypass surgery. *Arch Dis Child* 1982;57:425.

208. Adatia I, Atz AM, Jonas RA, et al. Diagnostic use of inhaled nitric oxide after neonatal cardiac operations. *J Thorac Cardiovasc Surg* 1996;112:1403.

209. Chang AC, Vetter JM, Gill SE, et al. Accuracy of prospective two-dimensional/Doppler echocardiography in the assessment of reparative surgery. *J Am Coll Cardiol* 1990;16:903.

210. Wolfe LT, Rossi A, Ritter SB. Transesophageal echocardiography in infants and children: use and importance in the cardiac intensive care unit. *J Am Soc Echocardiogr* 1993;6:286.

211. Friedman WF. The intrinsic physiologic properties of the developing heart. *Prog Cardiovasc Dis* 1972;15:87.

212. Romero T, Covell J, Friedman WF. A comparison of pressure-volume relations of the fetal, newborn, and adult heart. *Am J Physiol* 1972;222:1285.

213. Zaritsky A, Chernow B. Use of catecholamines in pediatrics. *J Pediatr* 1984;105:341.

214. Friedman WF, George BL. Treatment of congestive heart failure by altering loading conditions of the heart. *J Pediatr* 1985;106:697.

215. Kouchoukos NT, Kirklin JW, Sheppard LC, et al. Effect of left atrial pressure by blood infusion on stroke volume early after cardiac operations. *Surg Forum* 1971;22:126.

216. Feneck RO. Intravenous milrinone following cardiac surgery. II. Influence of baseline hemodynamics and patient factors on therapeutic response. The European Milrinone Multicentre Trial Group. *J Cardiothorac Vasc Anes* 1992;6:563.

217. Schulze-Neick I, Bultmann M, Werner H, et al. Right ventricular function in patients treated with inhaled nitric oxide after cardiac surgery for congenital heart disease in newborns and children. *Am J Cardiol* 1997;80:360.

218. Grace MP, Greenbaum DM. Cardiac performance in response to PEEP in patients with cardiac dysfunction. *Crit Care Med* 1982;10:358.

219. Pinsky MR, Summer WR, Wise RA, et al. Augmentation of cardiac function by elevation of intrathoracic pressure. *J Appl Physiol* 1983;54:950.

220. Rosenzweig EB, Starc TJ, Chen JM, et al. Intravenous arginine-vasopressin in children with vasodilatory shock after cardiac surgery. *Circulation* 1999;100:II182.

221. Burrows FA, Williams WG, Teoh KH, et al. Myocardial performance after repair of congenital cardiac defects in infants and children. Response to volume loading. *J Thorac Cardiovasc Surg* 1988;96:548.

222. Driscoll DJ, Gillette PC, Duff DF, et al. The hemodynamic effect of dopamine in children. *J Thorac Cardiovasc Surg* 1979;78:765.

223. Driscoll DJ, Gillette PC, Duff DF, et al. Hemodynamic effects of dobutamine in children. *Am J Cardiol* 1979;43:581.

224. Bohn DJ, Poirier CS, Edmonds JF, et al. Hemodynamic effects of dobutamine after cardiopulmonary bypass in children. *Crit Care Med* 1980;8:367.

225. Berg RA, Donnerstein RL, Padbury JF. Dobutamine infusions in stable, critically ill children: pharmacokinetics and hemodynamic actions. *Crit Care Med* 1993;21:678.

226. Hoffman TM, Wernovsky G, Atz AM, et al. Efficacy and safety of milrinone in preventing low cardiac output syndrome in infants and children after corrective surgery for congenital heart disease. *Circulation* 2003;107:996.

227. Chang AC, Atz AM, Wernovsky G, et al. Milrinone: systemic and pulmonary hemodynamic effects in neonates after cardiac surgery. *Crit Care Med* 1995;23:1907.

228. Caspi J, Coles JG, Benson LN, et al. Age-related response to epinephrine-induced myocardial stress. A functional and ultrastructural study. *Circulation* 1991;84:III394.

229. Buchhorn R, Hulpke-Wette M, Ruschewski W, et al. Beta-receptor downregulation in congenital heart disease: a risk factor for complications after surgical repair? *Ann Thorac Surg* 2002;73:610.

230. Shore S, Nelson DP, Pearl JM, et al. Usefulness of corticosteroid therapy in decreasing epinephrine requirements in critically ill infants with congenital heart disease. *Am J Cardiol* 2001;88:591.

231. Klein I, Ojamaa K. Thyroid hormone and the cardiovascular system. *N Engl J Med* 2001;344:501.

232. Mitchell IM, Pollock JC, Jamieson MP, et al. The effects of cardiopulmonary bypass on thyroid function in infants weighing less than five kilograms. *J Thorac Cardiovasc Surg* 1992;103:800.

233. Mainwaring RD, Healy RM, Meier FA, et al. Reduction in levels of triiodothyronine following the first stage of the Norwood reconstruction for hypoplastic left heart syndrome. *Cardiol Young* 2001;11:295.

234. Chowdhury D, Ojamaa K, Parnell VA, et al. A prospective randomized clinical study of thyroid hormone treatment after operations for complex congenital heart disease. *J Thorac Cardiovasc Surg* 2001;122:1023.

235. Bettendorf M, Schmidt KG, Grulich-Henn J, et al. Tri-iodothyronine treatment in children after cardiac surgery: a double-blind, randomised, placebo-controlled study. *Lancet* 2000;356:529.

236. Portman MA, Fearneyhough C, Ning XH, et al. Triiodothyronine repletion in infants during cardiopulmonary bypass for congenital heart disease. *J Thorac Cardiovasc Surg* 2000;120:604.

237. Pfammatter JP, Wagner B, Berdat P, et al. Procedural factors associated with early postoperative arrhythmias after repair of congenital heart defects. *J Thorac Cardiovasc Surg* 2002;123:258.

238. Humes RA, Porter CJ, Puga FJ, et al. Utility of temporary atrial epicardial electrodes in postoperative pediatric cardiac patients. *Mayo Clin Proc* 1989;64:516.

239. Deal BJ, Wolff GS, Gelband H, eds. *Current concepts in diagnosis and management of arrhythmias in infants and children.* Armonk, NY: Futura Publishing, 1998.

240. Rosales AM, Walsh EP, Wessel DL, et al. Postoperative ectopic atrial tachycardia in children with congenital heart disease. *Am J Cardiol* 2001;88:1169.

241. Hoffman TM, Bush DM, Wernovsky G, et al. Postoperative junctional ectopic tachycardia in children: incidence, risk factors, and treatment. *Ann Thorac Surg* 2002;74:1607.

242. Dodge-Khatami A, Miller OI, Anderson RH, et al. Surgical substrates of postoperative junctional ectopic tachycardia in congenital heart defects. *J Thorac Cardiovasc Surg* 2002;123:624.

243. Dodge-Khatami A, Miller OI, Anderson RH, et al. Impact of junctional ectopic tachycardia on postoperative morbidity following repair of congenital heart defects. *Eur J Cardiothorac Surg* 2002;21:255.

244. Laird WP, Snyder CS, Kertesz NJ, et al. Use of intravenous amiodarone for postoperative junctional ectopic tachycardia in children. *Pediatr Cardiol* 2003;24:133.

245. Pfammatter JP, Paul T, Ziemer G, et al. Successful management of junctional tachycardia by hypothermia after cardiac operations in infants. *Ann Thorac Surg* 1995;60:556.

246. Walsh EP, Saul JP, Sholler GF, et al. Evaluation of a staged treatment protocol for rapid automatic junctional tachycardia after operation for congenital heart disease. *J Am Coll Cardiol* 1997;29:1046.

247. Perry JC, Fenrich AL, Hulse JE, et al. Pediatric use of intravenous amiodarone: efficacy and safety in critically ill patients from a multicenter protocol. *J Am Coll Cardiol* 1996;27:1246.

248. Leinbach RC, Chamberlain DA, Kastor JA, et al. A comparison of the hemodynamic effects of ventricular and sequential A-V pacing in patients with heart block. *Am Heart J* 1969;78:502.

249. Hopkins RA, Bull C, Haworth SG, et al. Pulmonary hypertensive crises following surgery for congenital heart defects in young children. *Eur J Cardiothorac Surg* 1991;5:628.

250. Miller OI, Tang SF, Keech A, et al. Inhaled nitric oxide and prevention of pulmonary hypertension after congenital heart surgery: a randomised double-blind study. *Lancet* 2000;356:1464.

251. Lindberg L, Olsson AK, Jogi P, et al. How common is severe pulmonary hypertension after pediatric cardiac surgery? *J Thorac Cardiovasc Surg* 2002;123:1155.

252. Reddy VM, Hendricks-Munoz KD, Rajasinghe HA, et al. Post-cardiopulmonary bypass pulmonary hypertension in lambs with increased pulmonary blood flow. A role for endothelin 1. *Circulation* 1997;95:1054.

253. Koul B, Willen H, Sjoberg T, et al. Pulmonary sequelae of prolonged total venoarterial bypass: evaluation with a new experimental model. *Ann Thorac Surg* 1991;51:794.

254. Beghetti M, Silkoff PE, Caramori M, et al. Decreased exhaled nitric oxide may be a marker of cardiopulmonary bypass-induced injury. *Ann Thorac Surg* 1998;66:532.

255. Schulze-Neick I, Penny DJ, Rigby ML, et al. L-arginine and substance P reverse the pulmonary endothelial dysfunction caused by congenital heart surgery. *Circulation* 1999;100:749.

256. Chai PJ, Williamson JA, Lodge AJ, et al. Effects of ischemia on pulmonary dysfunction after cardiopulmonary bypass. *Ann Thorac Surg* 1999;67:731.

257. Anand KJ, Hickey PR. Halothane-morphine compared with high-dose sufentanil for anesthesia and postoperative analgesia in neonatal cardiac surgery. *N Engl J Med* 1992;326:1.

258. Hiramatsu T, Imai Y, Kurosawa H, et al. Effects of dilutional and modified ultrafiltration in plasma endothelin-1 and pulmonary

vascular resistance after the Fontan procedure. *Ann Thorac Surg* 2002;73:861.

259. Schulze-Neick I, Li J, Reader JA, et al. The endothelin antagonist BQ123 reduces pulmonary vascular resistance after surgical intervention for congenital heart disease. *J Thorac Cardiovasc Surg* 2002;124:435.

260. Russell IA, Zwass MS, Fineman JR, et al. The effects of inhaled nitric oxide on postoperative pulmonary hypertension in infants and children undergoing surgical repair of congenital heart disease. *Anesth Analg* 1998;87:46.

261. Segar JL, Merrill DC, Chapleau MW, et al. Hemodynamic changes during endotracheal suctioning are mediated by increased autonomic activity. *Pediatr Res* 1993;33:649.

262. Wessel DL. Managing low cardiac output syndrome after congenital heart surgery. *Crit Care Med* 2001;29:S220.

263. Atz AM, Adatia I, Lock JE, et al. Combined effects of nitric oxide and oxygen during acute pulmonary vasodilator testing. *J Am Coll Cardiol* 1999;33:813.

264. Morray JP, Lynn AM, Mansfield PB. Effect of pH and PCO_2 on pulmonary and systemic hemodynamics after surgery in children with congenital heart disease and pulmonary hypertension. *J Pediatr* 1988;113:474.

265. Morris K, Beghetti M, Petros A, et al. Comparison of hyperventilation and inhaled nitric oxide for pulmonary hypertension after repair of congenital heart disease. *Crit Care Med* 2000;28:2974.

266. Ignarro LJ, Buga GM, Wood KS, et al. Endothelium-derived relaxing factor produced and released from artery and vein is nitric oxide. *Proc Natl Acad Sci U S A* 1987;84:9265.

267. Frostell C, Fratacci MD, Wain JC, et al. Inhaled nitric oxide. A selective pulmonary vasodilator reversing hypoxic pulmonary vasoconstriction. *Circulation* 1991;83:2038.

268. Rimar S, Gillis CN. Selective pulmonary vasodilation by inhaled nitric oxide is due to hemoglobin inactivation. *Circulation* 1993;88:2884.

269. Miller OI, Tang SF, Keech A, et al. Rebound pulmonary hypertension on withdrawal from inhaled nitric oxide. *Lancet* 1995;346:51.

270. Atz AM, Adatia I, Wessel DL. Rebound pulmonary hypertension after inhalation of nitric oxide. *Ann Thorac Surg* 1996;62:1759.

271. Young JD, Sear JW, Valvini EM. Kinetics of methaemoglobin and serum nitrogen oxide production during inhalation of nitric oxide in volunteers. *Br J Anaesth* 1996;76:652.

272. Atz AM, Wessel DL. Sildenafil ameliorates effects of inhaled nitric oxide withdrawal. *Anesthesiology* 1999;91:307.

273. Day RW, Hawkins JA, McGough EC, et al. Randomized controlled study of inhaled nitric oxide after operation for congenital heart disease. *Ann Thorac Surg* 2000;69:1907.

274. Journois D, Pouard P, Mauriat P, et al. Inhaled nitric oxide as a therapy for pulmonary hypertension after operations for congenital heart defects. *J Thorac Cardiovasc Surg* 1994;107:1129.

275. Miller OI, Celermajer DS, Deanfield JE, et al. Very-low-dose inhaled nitric oxide: a selective pulmonary vasodilator after operations for congenital heart disease. *J Thorac Cardiovasc Surg* 1994;108:487.

276. Curran RD, Mavroudis C, Backer CL, et al. Inhaled nitric oxide for children with congenital heart disease and pulmonary hypertension. *Ann Thorac Surg* 1995;60:1765.

277. Atz AM, Adatia I, Jonas RA, et al. Inhaled nitric oxide in children with pulmonary hypertension and congenital mitral stenosis. *Am J Cardiol* 1996;77:316.

278. Zobel G, Gamillscheg A, Schwinger W, et al. Inhaled nitric oxide in infants and children after open heart surgery. *J Cardiovasc Surg* 1998;39:79.

279. Gamillscheg A, Zobel G, Urlesberger B, et al. Inhaled nitric oxide in patients with critical pulmonary perfusion after Fontan-type procedures and bidirectional Glenn anastomosis. *J Thorac Cardiovasc Surg* 1997;113:435.

280. Goldman AP, Delius RE, Deanfield JE, et al. Nitric oxide might reduce the need for extracorporeal support in children with critical postoperative pulmonary hypertension. *Ann Thorac Surg* 1996;62:750.

281. Bush A, Busst C, Booth K, et al. Does prostacyclin enhance the selective pulmonary vasodilator effect of oxygen in children with congenital heart disease? *Circulation* 1986;74:135.

282. Bush A, Busst C, Knight WB, et al. Modification of pulmonary hypertension secondary to congenital heart disease by prostacyclin therapy. *Am Rev Respir Dis* 1987;136:767.

283. Goldman AP, Delius RE, Deanfield JE, et al. Nitric oxide is superior to prostacyclin for pulmonary hypertension after cardiac operations. *Ann Thorac Surg* 1995;60:300.

284. Rimensberger PC, Spahr-Schopfer I, Berner M, et al. Inhaled nitric oxide versus aerosolized iloprost in secondary pulmonary hypertension in children with congenital heart disease: vasodilator capacity and cellular mechanisms. *Circulation* 2001;103:544.

285. Doctor A, Walsh B, Doorley P, et al. Inhaled prostacycline for acute pulmonary hypertension complicating congenital heart disease. *Pediatr Crit Care Med* 2003;4:A148.

286. Bradley SM, Simsic JM, Mulvihill DM. Hyperventilation impairs oxygenation after bidirectional superior cavopulmonary connection. *Circulation* 1998;98:II372.

287. Bradley SM, Simsic JM, Mulvihill DM. Hypoventilation improves oxygenation after bidirectional superior cavopulmonary connection. *J Thorac Cardiovasc Surg* 2003;126:1033.

288. Zonis Z, Seear M, Reichert C, et al. The effect of preoperative tranexamic acid on blood loss after cardiac operations in children. *J Thorac Cardiovasc Surg* 1996;111:982.

289. Reid RW, Zimmerman AA, Laussen PC, et al. The efficacy of tranexamic acid versus placebo in decreasing blood loss in pediatric patients undergoing repeat cardiac surgery. *Anesth Analg* 1997;84:990.

290. Chauhan S, Kumar BA, Rao BH, et al. Efficacy of aprotinin, epsilon aminocaproic acid, or combination in cyanotic heart disease. *Ann Thorac Surg* 2000;70:1308.

291. Williams GD, Bratton SL, Riley EC, et al. Efficacy of epsilon-aminocaproic acid in children undergoing cardiac surgery. *J Cardiothorac Vasc Anesth* 1999;13:304.

292. Rhodes JF, Blaufox AD, Seiden HS, et al. Cardiac arrest in infants after congenital heart surgery. *Circulation* 1999;100:II194.

293. Anonymous. Guidelines 2000 for Cardiopulmonary Resuscitation and Emergency Cardiovascular Care. Part 10: pediatric advanced life support. *Circulation* 2000;102:I291.

294. Duncan BW, Ibrahim AE, Hraska V, et al. Use of rapid-deployment extracorporeal membrane oxygenation for the resuscitation of pediatric patients with heart disease after cardiac arrest. *J Thorac Cardiovasc Surg* 1998;116:305.

295. Duncan B, ed. *Mechanical support for cardiac and respiratory failure in pediatric patients.* New York: Marcel Dekker, 2001.

296. Walters HL 3rd, Hakimi M, Rice MD, et al. Pediatric cardiac surgical ECMO: multivariate analysis of risk factors for hospital death. *Ann Thorac Surg* 1995;60:329.

297. Thuys CA, Mullaly RJ, Horton SB, et al. Centrifugal ventricular assist in children under 6 kg. *Eur J Cardiothorac Surg* 1998;13:130.

298. del Nido PJ, Duncan BW, Mayer JE Jr, et al. Left ventricular assist device improves survival in children with left ventricular dysfunction after repair of anomalous origin of the left coronary artery from the pulmonary artery. *Ann Thorac Surg* 1999;67:169.

299. Dalton HJ, Siewers RD, Fuhrman BP, et al. Extracorporeal membrane oxygenation for cardiac rescue in children with severe myocardial dysfunction. *Crit Care Med* 1993;21:1020.

300. Kirshbom PM, Bridges ND, Myung RJ, et al. Use of extracorporeal membrane oxygenation in pediatric thoracic organ transplantation. *J Thorac Cardiovasc Surg* 2002;123:130.

301. Kulik TJ, Moler FW, Palmisano JM, et al. Outcome-associated factors in pediatric patients treated with extracorporeal membrane oxygenator after cardiac surgery. *Circulation* 1996;94:II63.

302. Pizarro C, Davis DA, Healy RM, et al. Is there a role for extracorporeal life support after stage I Norwood? *Eur J Cardiothorac Surg* 2001;19:294.

303. Jaggers JJ, Forbess JM, Shah AS, et al. Extracorporeal membrane oxygenation for infant postcardiotomy support: significance of shunt management. *Ann Thorac Surg* 2000;69:1476.

304. Wessel DL, Almodovar MC, Laussen PC. Intensive care management of cardiac patients on extracorporeal membrane oxygenation. In: Duncan BW, ed. *Mechanical support for cardiac and respiratory failure in pediatric patients.* New York: Marcel Dekker, 2001:75.

305. Raithel SC, Pennington DG, Boegner E, et al. Extracorporeal membrane oxygenation in children after cardiac surgery. *Circulation* 1992;86:II305.

306. Black MD, Coles JG, Williams WG, et al. Determinants of success in pediatric cardiac patients undergoing extracorporeal membrane oxygenation. *Ann Thorac Surg* 1995;60:133.

307. Duncan BW, Hraska V, Jonas RA, et al. Mechanical circulatory support in children with cardiac disease. *J Thorac Cardiovasc Surg* 1999;117:529.

308. Marcus B, Atkinson JB, Wong PC, et al. Successful use of transesophageal echocardiography during extracorporeal membrane oxygenation in infants after cardiac operations. *J Thorac Cardiovasc Surg* 1995;109:846.

309. Booth KL, Roth SJ, Perry SB, et al. Cardiac catheterization of patients supported by extracorporeal membrane oxygenation. *J Am Coll Cardiol* 2002;40:1681.

310. Delius RE, Bove EL, Meliones JN, et al. Use of extracorporeal life support in patients with congenital heart disease. *Crit Care Med* 1992;20:1216.

311. Ziomek S, Harrell JE Jr, Fasules JW, et al. Extracorporeal membrane oxygenation for cardiac failure after congenital heart operation. *Ann Thorac Surg* 1992;54:861.

312. Duncan BW, Bohn DJ, Atz AM, et al. Mechanical circulatory support for the treatment of children with acute fulminant myocarditis. *J Thorac Cardiovasc Surg* 2001;122:440.

313. Ibrahim AE, Duncan BW, Blume ED, et al. Long-term follow-up of pediatric cardiac patients requiring mechanical circulatory support. *Ann Thorac Surg* 2000;69:186.

314. Hamrick SEG, Gremmels DB, Keet CA, et al. Neurodevelopmental outcome of infants supported with extracorporeal membrane oxygenation after cardiac surgery. *Pediatrics* 2003;111:e671.

315. DiCarlo JV, Raphaely RC, Steven JM, et al. Pulmonary mechanics in infants after cardiac surgery. *Crit Care Med* 1992;20:22.

316. McElhinney DB, Reddy VM, Pian MS, et al. Compression of the central airways by a dilated aorta in infants and children with congenital heart disease. *Ann Thorac Surg* 1999;67:1130.

317. Dodge-Khatami A, Backer CL, Holinger LD, et al. Complete repair of Tetralogy of Fallot with absent pulmonary valve including the role of airway stenting. *J Card Surg* 1999;14:82.

318. Mok Q, Ross-Russell R, Mulvey D, et al. Phrenic nerve injury in infants and children undergoing cardiac surgery. *Br Heart J* 1991;65:287.

319. Schwartz MZ, Filler RM. Plication of the diaphragm for symptomatic phrenic nerve paralysis. *J Pediatr Surg* 1978;13:259.

320. de Leeuw M, Williams JM, Freedom RM, et al. Impact of diaphragmatic paralysis after cardiothoracic surgery in children. *J Thorac Cardiovasc Surg* 1999;118:510.

321. Schulze-Neick I, Ho SY, Bush A, et al. Severe airflow limitation after the unifocalization procedure: clinical and morphological correlates. *Circulation* 2000;102:III142.

322. Allen EM, van Heeckeren DW, Spector ML, et al. Management of nutritional and infectious complications of postoperative chylothorax in children. *J Pediatr Surg* 1991;26:1169.

323. Bond SJ, Guzzetta PC, Snyder ML, et al. Management of pediatric postoperative chylothorax. *Ann Thorac Surg* 1993;56:469.

324. Pratap U, Slavik Z, Ofoe VD, et al. Octreotide to treat postoperative chylothorax after cardiac operations in children. *Ann Thorac Surg* 2001;72:1740.

325. Buttiker V, Fanconi S, Burger R. Chylothorax in children: guidelines for diagnosis and management. *Chest* 1999; 116:682.

326. McWilliams BC, Fan LL, Murphy SA. Transient T-cell depression in postoperative chylothorax. *J Pediatr* 1981;99:595.

327. Markham KM, Glover JL, Welsh RJ, et al. Octreotide in the treatment of thoracic duct injuries. *Am Surg* 2000;66:1165.

328. Rimensberger PC, Muller-Schenker B, Kalangos A, et al. Treatment of a persistent postoperative chylothorax with somatostatin. *Ann Thorac Surg* 1998;66:253.

329. Cheung Y, Leung MP, Yip M. Octreotide for treatment of postoperative chylothorax. *J Pediatr* 2001;139:157.

330. Ottinger JG. Octreotide for persistent chylothorax in a pediatric patient. *Ann Pharmacother* 2002;36:1106.

331. Rosti L, Bini RM, Chessa M, et al. The effectiveness of octreotide in the treatment of post-operative chylothorax. *Eur J Pediatr* 2002;161:149.

332. Azizkhan RG, Canfield J, Alford BA, et al. Pleuroperitoneal shunts in the management of neonatal chylothorax. *J Pediatr Surg* 1983;18:842.

333. Murphy MC, Newman BM, Rodgers BM. Pleuroperitoneal shunts in the management of persistent chylothorax. *Ann Thorac Surg* 1989;48:195.

334. Tarnok A, Schneider P. Pediatric cardiac surgery with cardiopulmonary bypass: pathways contributing to transient systemic immune suppression. *Shock* 2001;16:24.

335. Allen ML, Peters MJ, Goldman A, et al. Early postoperative monocyte deactivation predicts systemic inflammation and prolonged stay in pediatric cardiac intensive care. *Crit Care Med* 2002;30:1140.

336. Odetola FO, Moler FW, Dechert RE, et al. Nosocomial catheter-related bloodstream infections in a pediatric intensive care unit: risk and rates associated with various intravascular technologies. *Pediatr Crit Care Med* 2003;4:432.

337. O'Grady NP, Alexander M, Dellinger EP, et al. Guidelines for the prevention of intravascular catheter-related infections. *Pediatrics* 2002;110:e51.

338. Mermel LA, Farr BM, Sherertz RJ, et al. Guidelines for the management of intravascular catheter-related infections. *Clin Infect Dis* 2001;32:1249.

339. Maher KO, VanDerElzen K, Bove EL, et al. A retrospective review of three antibiotic prophylaxis regimens for pediatric cardiac surgical patients. *Ann Thorac Surg* 2002;74:1195.

340. Giuffre RM, Tam KH, Williams WW, et al. Acute renal failure complicating pediatric cardiac surgery: a comparison of survivors and nonsurvivors following acute peritoneal dialysis. *Pediatr Cardiol* 1992;13:208.

341. Boigner H, Brannath W, Hermon M, et al. Predictors of mortality at initiation of peritoneal dialysis in children after cardiac surgery. *Ann Thorac Surg* 2004;77:61.

342. Limperopoulos C, Majnemer A, Shevell MI, et al. Neurologic status of newborns with congenital heart defects before open heart surgery. *Pediatrics* 1999;103:402.

343. Mahle WT, Tavani F, Zimmerman RA, et al. An MRI study of neurological injury before and after congenital heart surgery. *Circulation* 2002;106:I109.

344. Menache CC, du Plessis AJ, Wessel DL, et al. Current incidence of acute neurologic complications after open-heart operations in children. *Ann Thorac Surg* 2002;73:1752.

345. Clancy RR, McGaurn SA, Wernovsky G, et al. Risk of seizures in survivors of newborn heart surgery using deep hypothermic circulatory arrest. *Pediatrics* 2003;111:592.

346. Bellinger DC, Jonas RA, Rappaport LA, et al. Developmental and neurologic status of children after heart surgery with hypothermic circulatory arrest or low-flow cardiopulmonary bypass. *N Engl J Med* 1995;332:549.

347. Bellinger DC, Rappaport LA, Wypij D, et al. Patterns of developmental dysfunction after surgery during infancy to correct transposition of the great arteries. *J Dev Behav Pediatr* 1997; 18:75.

348. Rappaport LA, Wypij D, Bellinger DC, et al. Relation of seizures after cardiac surgery in early infancy to neurodevelopmental outcome. *Circulation* 1998;97:773.

349. Bellinger DC, Wypij D, Kuban KC, et al. Developmental and neurological status of children at 4 years of age after heart surgery with hypothermic circulatory arrest or low-flow cardiopulmonary bypass. *Circulation* 1999;100:526.

350. Kern JH, Hinton VJ, Nereo NE, et al. Early developmental outcome after the Norwood procedure for hypoplastic left heart syndrome. *Pediatrics* 1998;102:1148.

351. Mahle WT, Clancy RR, Moss EM, et al. Neurodevelopmental outcome and lifestyle assessment in school-aged and adolescent children with hypoplastic left heart syndrome. *Pediatrics* 2000; 105:1082.

352. Imoto Y, Kado H, Shiokawa Y, et al. Experience with the Norwood procedure without circulatory arrest. *J Thorac Cardiovasc Surg* 2001;122:879.

353. Reddy VM, Hanley FL. Techniques to avoid circulatory arrest in neonates undergoing repair of complex heart defects. *Semin Thorac Cardiovasc Surg* 2001;4:277.

354. Shin'oka T, Shum-Tim D, Jonas RA, et al. Higher hematocrit improves cerebral outcome after deep hypothermic circulatory arrest. *J Thorac Cardiovasc Surg* 1996;112:1610.

355. du Plessis AJ, Jonas RA, Wypij D, et al. Perioperative effects of alpha-stat versus pH-stat strategies for deep hypothermic cardiopulmonary bypass in infants. *J Thorac Cardiovasc Surg* 1997;114:991.

356. Jonas RA. Deep hypothermic circulatory arrest: current status and indications. *Semin Thorac Cardiovasc Surg* 2002;5:3.

357. Newburger JW, Wypij D, Bellinger DC, et al. Length of stay after infant heart surgery is related to cognitive outcome at age 8 years. *J Pediatr* 2003;143:67.

358. Tweddell JS, Litwin SB, Thomas JP Jr, et al. Recent advances in the surgical management of the single ventricle pediatric patient. *Pediatr Clin North Am* 1999;46:465.

359. Odim J, Portzky M, Zurakowski D, et al. Sternotomy approach for the modified Blalock-Taussig shunt. *Circulation* 1995;92:II256.

360. Bradley SM, Mosca RS, Hennein HA, et al. Bidirectional superior cavopulmonary connection in young infants. *Circulation* 1996;94:II5.

361. Reddy VM, McElhinney DB, Moore P, et al. Outcomes after bidirectional cavopulmonary shunt in infants less than 6 months old. *J Am Coll Cardiol* 1997;29:1365.

362. Chang AC, Hanley FL, Wernovsky G, et al. Early bidirectional cavopulmonary shunt in young infants. Postoperative course and early results. *Circulation* 1993;88:II149.

363. Santamore WP, Barnea O, Riordan CJ, et al. Theoretical optimization of pulmonary-to-systemic flow ratio after a bidirectional cavopulmonary anastomosis. *Am J Physiol* 1998;274:H694.

364. Zellers TM, Driscoll DJ, Humes RA, et al. Glenn shunt: effect on pleural drainage after modified Fontan operation. *J Thorac Cardiovasc Surg* 1989;98:725.

365. Galal O, Kalloghlian A, Pittappilly BM, et al. Phentolamine improves clinical outcome after balloon valvoplasty in neonates with severe pulmonary stenosis. *Cardiol Young* 1999;9:127.

366. Hew CC, Daebritz SH, Zurakowski D, et al. Valved homograft replacement of aneurysmal pulmonary arteries for severely symptomatic absent pulmonary valve syndrome. *Ann Thorac Surg* 2002;73:1778.

367. Hraska V, Kantorova A, Kunovsky P, et al. Intermediate results with correction of tetralogy of Fallot with absent pulmonary valve using a new approach. *Eur J Cardiothorac Surg* 2002;21:711.

368. Watterson KG, Malm TK, Karl TR, et al. Absent pulmonary valve syndrome: operation in infants with airway obstruction. *Ann Thorac Surg* 1992;54:1116.

369. Puga FJ, Leoni FE, Julsrud PR, et al. Complete repair of pulmonary atresia, ventricular septal defect, and severe peripheral arborization abnormalities of the central pulmonary arteries. Experience with preliminary unifocalization procedures in 38 patients. *J Thorac Cardiovasc Surg* 1989;98:1018.

370. Reddy VM, McElhinney DB, Amin Z, et al. Early and intermediate outcomes after repair of pulmonary atresia with ventricular septal defect and major aortopulmonary collateral arteries: experience with 85 patients. *Circulation* 2000;101:1826.

371. Rodefeld MD, Reddy VM, Thompson LD, et al. Surgical creation of aortopulmonary window in selected patients with pulmonary atresia with poorly developed aortopulmonary collaterals and hypoplastic pulmonary arteries. *J Thorac Cardiovasc Surg* 2002;123:1147.

372. Marshall AC, Love BA, Lang P, et al. Staged repair of tetralogy of Fallot and diminutive pulmonary arteries with a fenestrated ventricular septal defect patch. *J Thorac Cardiovasc Surg* 2003;126:1427.

373. Rhodes LA, Colan SD, Perry SB, et al. Predictors of survival in neonates with critical aortic stenosis. *Circulation* 1991;84:2325.

374. Dodge-Khatami A, Backer CL, Mavroudis C. Risk factors for recoarctation and results of reoperation: a 40-year review. *J Card Surg* 2000;15:369.

375. Backer CL, Mavroudis C, Zias EA, et al. Repair of coarctation with resection and extended end-to-end anastomosis. *Ann Thorac Surg* 1998;66:1365.

376. Rao PS, Galal O, Smith PA, et al. Five- to nine-year follow-up results of balloon angioplasty of native aortic coarctation in infants and children. *J Am Coll Cardiol* 1996;27:462.

377. Johnson MC, Canter CE, Strauss AW, et al. Repair of coarctation of the aorta in infancy: comparison of surgical and balloon angioplasty. *Am Heart J* 1993;125:464.

378. Norwood WI, Lang P, Hansen DD. Physiologic repair of aortic atresia-hypoplastic left heart syndrome. *N Engl J Med* 1983; 308:23.

379. Rossi AF, Sommer RJ, Lotvin A, et al. Usefulness of intermittent monitoring of mixed venous oxygen saturation after stage I palliation for hypoplastic left heart syndrome. *Am J Cardiol* 1994; 73:1118.

380. Riordan CJ, Randsbeck F, Storey JH, et al. Effects of oxygen, positive end-expiratory pressure, and carbon dioxide on oxygen delivery in an animal model of the univentricular heart. *J Thorac Cardiovasc Surg* 1996;112:644.

381. Riordan CJ, Locher JP Jr, Santamore WP, et al. Monitoring systemic venous oxygen saturations in the hypoplastic left heart syndrome. *Ann Thorac Surg* 1997;63:835.

382. Tweddell JS, Hoffman GM, Fedderly RT, et al. Phenoxybenzamine improves systemic oxygen delivery after the Norwood procedure. *Ann Thorac Surg* 1999;67:161.

383. Rychik J, Bush DM, Spray TL, et al. Assessment of pulmonary/systemic blood flow ratio after first-stage palliation for hypoplastic left heart syndrome: development of a new index with the use of Doppler echocardiography. *J Thorac Cardiovasc Surg* 2000; 120:81.

384. Reddy VM, Liddicoat JR, Fineman JR, et al. Fetal model of single ventricle physiology: hemodynamic effects of oxygen, nitric oxide, carbon dioxide, and hypoxia in the early postnatal period. *J Thorac Cardiovasc Surg* 1996;112:437.

385. Wessel DL. Commentary: simple gases and complex single ventricles. *J Thorac Cardiovasc Surg* 1996;112:655.

386. Mosca RS, Bove EL, Crowley DC, et al. Hemodynamic characteristics of neonates following first stage palliation for hypoplastic left heart syndrome. *Circulation* 1995;92:II267.

387. Bradley SM, Atz AM, Simsic JM. Redefining the impact of oxygen and hyperventilation after the Norwood procedure. *J Thorac Cardiovasc Surg* 2004;127:473.

388. Strauss KM, Dongas A, Hein U, et al. Stage 1 palliation of hypoplastic left heart syndrome: implications of blood gases. *J Cardiothorac Vasc Anes* 2001;15:731.

389. Hoffman GM, Ghanayem NS, Kampine JM, et al. Venous saturation and the anaerobic threshold in neonates after the Norwood procedure for hypoplastic left heart syndrome. *Ann Thorac Surg* 2000;70:1515.

390. Riordan CJ, Randsbaek F, Storey JH, et al. Inotropes in the hypoplastic left heart syndrome: effects in an animal model. *Ann Thorac Surg* 1996;62:83.

391. Sano S, Ishino K, Kawada M, et al. Right ventricle-pulmonary artery shunt in first-stage palliation of hypoplastic left heart syndrome. *J Thorac Cardiovasc Surg* 2003;126:504.

392. Maher K, Pizarro C, Gidding S, et al. Improved hemodynamic profile following the Norwood procedure with right ventricle to pulmonary artery conduit. *Circulation* 2002;106:II.

393. Pizarro C, Malec E, Maher K, et al. Right ventricle to pulmonary artery conduit improves outcome after Norwood procedure for hypoplastic left heart syndrome. *Circulation* 2002; 106:II.

394. Ohye RG, Kagisaki K, Lee LA, et al. Biventricular repair for aortic atresia or hypoplasia and ventricular septal defect. *J Thorac Cardiovasc Surg* 1999;118:648.

395. Apfel HD, Levenbraun J, Quaegebeur JM, et al. Usefulness of preoperative echocardiography in predicting left ventricular outflow obstruction after primary repair of interrupted aortic arch with ventricular septal defect. *Am J Cardiol* 1998;82:470.

396. Moulton AL, de Leval MR, Macartney FJ, et al. Rastelli procedure for transposition of the great arteries, ventricular septal defect, and left ventricular outflow tract obstruction. *Br Heart J* 1981; 45:20.

397. Nikaidoh H. Aortic translocation and biventricular outflow tract reconstruction. A new surgical repair for transposition of the great arteries associated with ventricular septal defect and pulmonary stenosis. *J Thorac Cardiovasc Surg* 1984;88:365.

398. Borromee L, Lecompte Y, Batisse A, et al. Anatomic repair of anomalies of ventriculoarterial connection associated with ventricular septal defect. Clinical results in 50 patients with pulmonary outflow tract obstruction. *J Thorac Cardiovasc Surg* 1988;95:96.

399. Blume ED, Altmann K, Mayer JE, et al. Evolution of risk factors influencing early mortality of the arterial switch operation. *J Am Coll Cardiol* 1999;33:1702.

400. Boutin C, Jonas RA, Sanders SP, et al. Rapid two-stage arterial switch operation. Acquisition of left ventricular mass after pulmonary artery banding in infants with transposition of the great arteries. *Circulation* 1994;90:1304.

401. Wernovsky G, Giglia TM, Jonas RA, et al. Course in the intensive care unit after 'preparatory' pulmonary artery banding and aortopulmonary shunt placement for transposition of the great arteries with low left ventricular pressure. *Circulation* 1992; 86:II133.

402. Haworth SG. Total anomalous pulmonary venous return. Prenatal damage to pulmonary vascular bed and extrapulmonary veins. *Br Heart J* 1982;48:513.

403. Lincoln CR, Rigby ML, Mercanti C, et al. Surgical risk factors in total anomalous pulmonary venous connection. *Am J Cardiol* 1988;61:608.

404. Jahangiri M, Zurakowski D, Mayer JE, et al. Repair of the truncal valve and associated interrupted arch in neonates with truncus arteriosus. *J Thorac Cardiovasc Surg* 2000;119:508.

405. Laussen PC, Reid RW, Stene RA, et al. Tracheal extubation of children in the operating room after atrial septal defect repair as part of a clinical practice guideline. *Anesth Analg* 1996;82:988.
406. Walker RE, Mayer JE, Alexander ME, et al. Paucity of sinus node dysfunction following repair of sinus venosus defects in children. *Am J Cardiol* 2001;87:1223.
407. Aebe R, Katogi T, Hashizume K, et al. Liberal use of tricuspid valve detachment for transatrial ventricular septal defect closure. *Ann Thorac Surg* 2003;76:1073.
408. Backer CL, Idriss FS, Zales VR, et al. Surgical management of the conal (supracristal) ventricular septal defect. *J Thorac Cardiovasc Surg* 1991;102:288.
409. Van Praagh S, Mayer JE Jr, Berman NB, et al. Apical ventricular septal defects: follow-up concerning anatomic and surgical considerations. *Ann Thorac Surg* 2002;73:48.
410. Backer CL, Mavroudis C, Alboliras ET, et al. Repair of complete atrioventricular canal defects: results with the two-patch technique. *Ann Thorac Surg* 1995;60:530.
411. Hanley FL, Fenton KN, Jonas RA, et al. Surgical repair of complete atrioventricular canal defects in infancy. Twenty-year trends. *J Thorac Cardiovasc Surg* 1993;106:387.
412. Dreyfus G, Jebara V, Mihaileanu S, et al. Total orthotopic heart transplantation: an alternative to the standard technique. *Ann Thorac Surg* 1991;52:1181.
413. Costello JM, Pahl E. Prevention and treatment of severe hemodynamic compromise in pediatric heart transplant patients. *Paediatric Drugs* 2002;4:705.
414. Kobashigawa JA, Stevenson LW, Brownfield E, et al. Does short-course induction with OKT3 improve outcome after heart transplantation? A randomized trial. *J Heart Lung Transplant* 1993;12:205.
415. Boucek RJ Jr, Naftel D, Boucek MM, et al. Induction immunotherapy in pediatric heart transplant recipients: a multicenter study. *J Heart Lung Transplant* 1999;18:460.
416. Reddy VM, McElhinney DB. Update on prospects for fetal cardiovascular surgery. *Curr Opin Pediatr* 1997;9:530.
417. Tulzer G, Arzt W, Franklin RC, et al. Fetal pulmonary valvuloplasty for critical pulmonary stenosis or atresia with intact septum. *Lancet* 2002;360:1567.
418. Tworetzky W, Jennings RW, Wilkins-Haug LE, et al. Balloon dilation of severe aortic stenosis in the fetus: technical advances. *J Am Coll Cardiol* 2003;41:496A.

Jaundice

35

M. Jeffrey Maisels

Jaundice is the most common and one of the most vexing problems that can occur in the newborn. As Hansen points out in an elegant historical review (1), "neonatal jaundice must have been noticed by caregivers throughout the centuries . . . ," but the first documented scientific description of neonatal jaundice occurred in the latter part of the eighteenth century when Baumes was awarded a prize from the University of Paris for his description of the clinical course of jaundice in 10 infants (1). Although most jaundiced infants are otherwise perfectly healthy, they make us anxious because bilirubin is potentially toxic to the central nervous system.

Jaundice occurs when the liver cannot clear a sufficient amount of bilirubin from the plasma. When the problem is excessive bilirubin formation or limited uptake and conjugation, unconjugated (i.e., indirect-reacting) bilirubin appears in the blood. When bilirubin glucuronide excretion is impaired (i.e., cholestasis), conjugated monoglucuronide and diglucuronide (i.e., direct-reacting) bilirubin accumulate in plasma and, because of their solubility, also appear in the urine. There is also a fourth bilirubin fraction (unconjugated, monoglucuronide, and diglucuronide are the first three) known as δ-bilirubin, which is formed nonenzymatically from conjugated bilirubin and reacts directly with the diazo reagent (2).

In most jaundiced neonates, only unconjugated bilirubin is found in the blood, and the accumulated bilirubin is distributed by the circulation throughout the body and produces clinical jaundice. It generally is assumed that to cross intact cell membrane barriers the bilirubin must be free, or dissociated, from its albumin binding.

FORMATION, STRUCTURE, AND PROPERTIES OF BILIRUBIN

Detailed reviews of the chemistry and metabolism of bilirubin are found elsewhere (3–7).

Bilirubin is the end product of the catabolism of iron protoporphyrin or heme, of which the major source is circulating hemoglobin (8). The formation of bilirubin from hemoglobin involves removal of the iron and protein moieties, followed by an oxidative process catalyzed by the enzyme microsomal heme oxygenase, an enzyme found in the reticuloendothelial system as well as many other tissues (9). The α-methane bridge of the heme porphyrin ring is opened and carbon monoxide (CO) and biliverdin are formed (Fig. 35-1). One molecule of CO and biliverdin (and, subsequently, bilirubin) is formed for each molecule of heme degraded (4).

Figure 35-2 shows a linear representation of bilirubin. Although conventionally illustrated as in Figs. 35-1 and 35-2, it is likely that the prevalent structure of bilirubin in plasma has the ridge-tile conformation shown in Fig. 35-3, because it is consistent with the biologic properties of bilirubin. In this conformation, the bilirubin polar groups of the molecule are involved in intramolecular hydrogen bonding that restricts solvation and renders the pigment nearly insoluble in water at pH 7.4 but soluble in nonpolar solvents such as chloroform (10). Under these circumstances, bilirubin behaves like other lipophilic substances (e.g., dioxin, polychlorinated biphenyls)—it is difficult to excrete but crosses biologic membranes, such as the placenta, blood–brain barrier, and hepatocyte plasma membrane, easily (10,11). The addition of methanol or ethanol interferes with hydrogen bonding and results in an immediate diazo reaction, the basis for measurement of indirect-reacting bilirubin by the van den Bergh test.

FETAL BILIRUBIN METABOLISM

Bilirubin can be detected in normal amniotic fluid after about 12 weeks of gestation, but it disappears by 36 to 37 weeks' gestation. The ability of human fetal liver to remove bilirubin from the circulation and to conjugate it is severely limited. Between 17 and 30 weeks of gestation, uridine diphosphoglucuronosyl transferase (UDPGT) activity in fetal liver is only 0.1% of adult values, but it increases tenfold to 1% of adult values between 30 and 40 weeks' gestation. After birth, activity increases exponentially, reaching adult levels by 6 to 14 weeks' gestation (Fig. 35-4). This increase is independent of gestation (Table 35-1) (12,13).

The major route of fetal bilirubin excretion is across the placenta. Because virtually all the fetal plasma bilirubin is

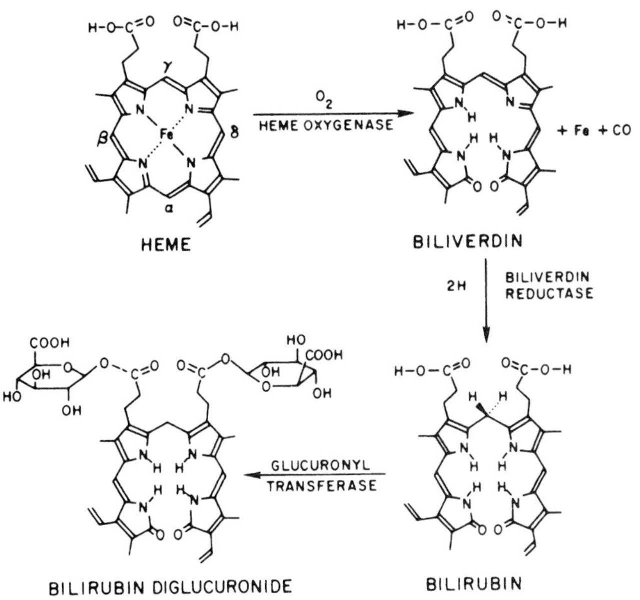

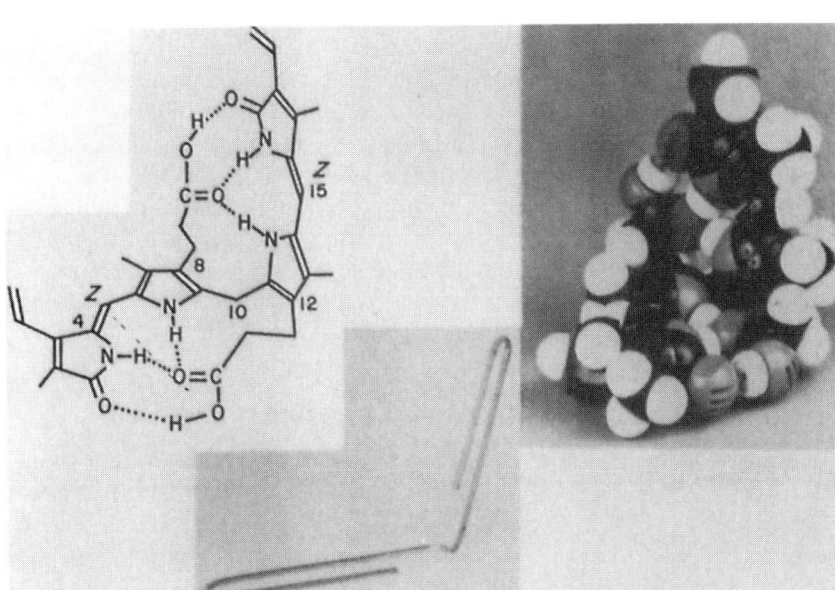

Figure 35-1 Biosynthesis of bilirubin. (From Lightner DA, McDonagh AF. Molecular mechanisms of phototherapy for neonatal jaundice. *Acc Chem Res* 1984;17:417–424, with permission.)

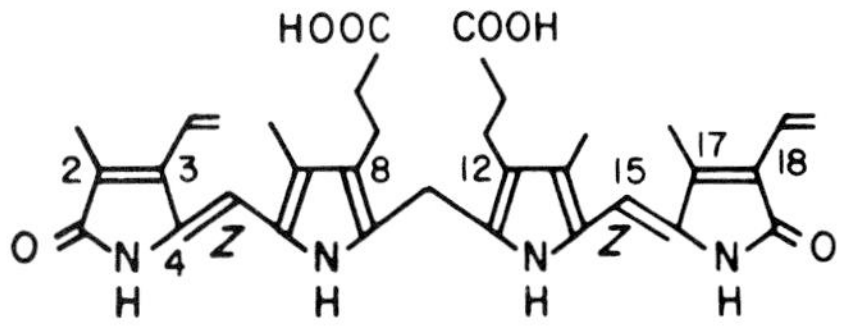

Figure 35-2 The chemical structure of bilirubin. (From McDonagh AF, Lightner DA. "Like a shrivelled blood orange"—bilirubin, jaundice and phototherapy. *Pediatrics* 1985;75:443–455, with permission.)

unconjugated, it is readily transferred across the placenta to the maternal circulation, where it is excreted by the maternal liver. Thus, the newborn rarely is born jaundiced, except in the presence of severe hemolytic disease, when there may be accumulation of unconjugated bilirubin in the fetus. Conjugated bilirubin is not transferred across the placenta, and it also may accumulate in the fetal plasma and other tissues.

Maternal Hyperbilirubinemia and Its Effect on the Fetus

Obstetricians and pediatricians occasionally are confronted with a pregnant mother who has hyperbilirubin-emia as a result of hemolytic anemia or liver disease. Reported cases in the literature provide evidence for transfer of unconjugated bilirubin from the mother to her fetus, but no clear guidelines for management (14–16).

It is possible that prolonged exposure of the fetus to a modest degree of unconjugated hyperbilirubinemia *in utero* could lead to neurologic damage (16).

NEONATAL BILIRUBIN METABOLISM

Bilirubin Production

The normal destruction of circulating erythrocytes accounts for about 75% of the daily bilirubin production in the newborn. Senescent erythrocytes are removed and destroyed in the reticuloendothelial system, where the heme is catabolized and converted to bilirubin (Fig. 35-5). The catabolism of 1 g of hemoglobin yields 35 mg of bilirubin.

A significant contribution (25% or more) to the daily production of bilirubin in the neonate comes from sources other than effete erythrocytes (see Fig. 35-5). This bilirubin consists of two major components:

1. A nonerythropoietic component resulting from the turnover of nonhemoglobin heme protein and free heme, primarily in the liver.

Figure 35-3 Preferred conformation of bilirubin. Chemical structure (**left**); bent paper clip analogy (**middle**); space-filling molecular model (**right**). Each representation is asymmetric and has a nonsuperimposable mirror image, like a D- or L-amino acid. Only one of the two possible mirror-image forms is shown in each representation. (From McDonagh AF, Lightner DA. "Like a shrivelled blood orange" —bilirubin, jaundice and phototherapy. *Pediatrics* 1985;75:443–455 with permission.)

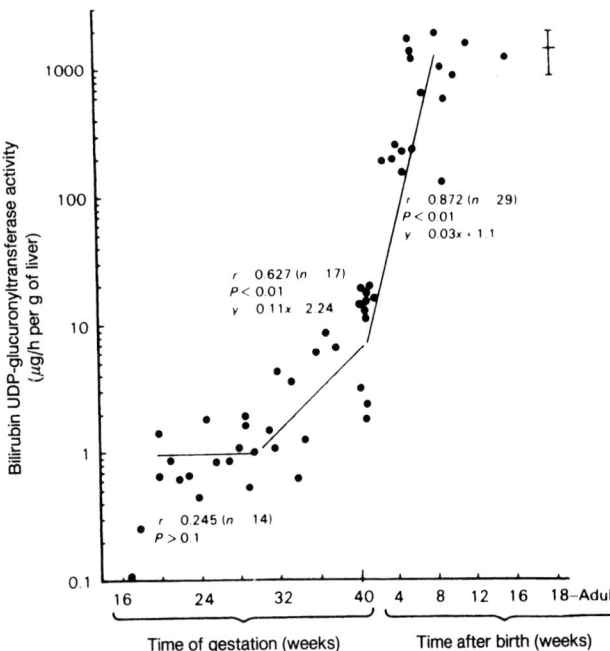

Figure 35-4 Developmental pattern of human hepatic uridine diphosphoglucuronosyl transferase (UDPGT) activity. Samples were obtained from the livers of fetuses after elective abortions, at autopsy from premature and full-term newborns who survived fewer than 7 days, and from liver biopsies of infants, children, and adults undergoing laparotomy. Each point represents the activity of the liver homogenate of a single patient, but results for patients older than 18 weeks of age are shown as a mean ± SD. (From Kawade N, Onishi S. The prenatal and postnatal development of UDP-glucuronyl transferase activity toward bilirubin and the effect of premature birth on this activity in the human liver. *Biochem J* 1981;196:257–260, with permission.)

2. An erythropoietic component arising primarily from ineffective erythropoiesis and the destruction of immature erythrocyte precursors, either in the bone marrow or soon after release into the circulation.

Transport and Hepatic Uptake of Bilirubin

Once bilirubin leaves the reticuloendothelial system, it is transported in the plasma and bound reversibly to albumin. Unconjugated bilirubin is bound tightly to albumin at a primary (high-affinity) binding site as well as a secondary (low-affinity) site. Because binding affinity at the primary binding site is 10^7 to 10^8 L/mol (17), the concentrations of free or unbound bilirubin in plasma are very low, even in the presence of significant hyperbilirubinemia. (The magnitude of the affinity constant was recently

TABLE 35-1
FETAL BILIRUBIN METABOLISM
Bilirubin detected in amniotic fluid at 12 weeks of gestation
Unconjugated bilirubin excreted across placenta
UDPGT activity at term ~1% of adult
UDPGT activity reaches adult levels by 6–14 weeks

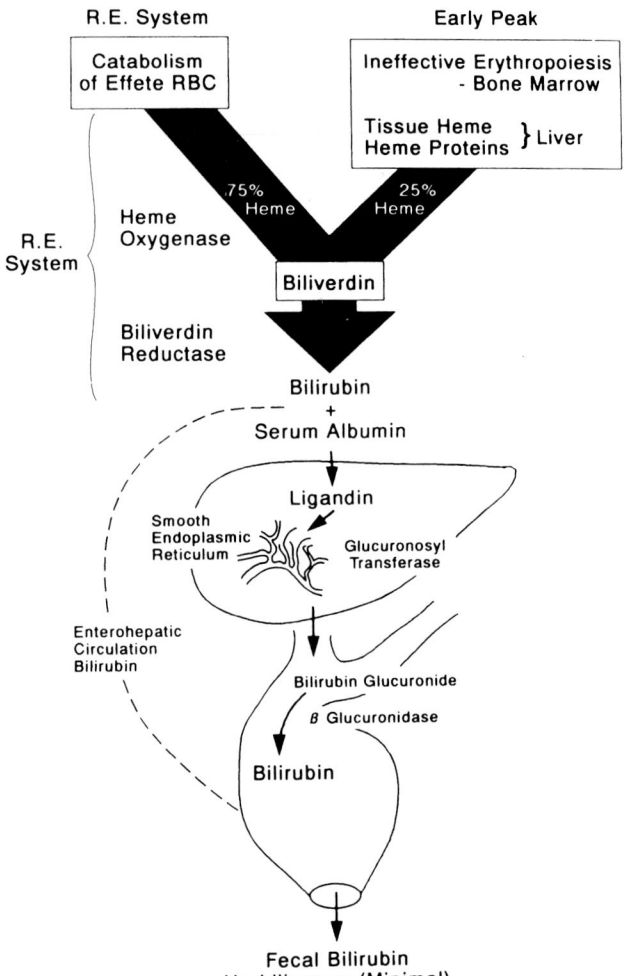

Figure 35-5 Neonatal bile pigment metabolism. RBC, erythrocytes; R.E., reticuloendothelial.

questioned (18).) At pH 7.4, the solubility of bilirubin is very low (about 4 nmol/L [0.24 mg/dL]).

The parenchymal cells of the liver have a selective and highly efficient capacity for removing unconjugated bilirubin from the plasma. When the bilirubin-albumin complex reaches the plasma membrane of the hepatocyte, a proportion of the bilirubin, but not the albumin, is transferred across the cell membrane into the hepatocyte, a process that potentially involves four different transport proteins (3). In the hepatocyte, bilirubin is bound principally to ligandin and possibly other cytosolic-binding proteins (Fig. 35-6) (3). A network of intracellular microsomal membranes may also play an important role in the transfer of bilirubin within the cell and to the endoplasmic reticulum (3,5).

Conjugation and Excretion of Bilirubin

Because of its hydrogen-bonded conformation (see Formation, Structure, and Properties of Bilirubin above), unconjugated (i.e., indirect-reacting) bilirubin is nonpolar and insoluble in aqueous solutions at pH 7.4 and must be converted to its water-soluble conjugate (i.e., direct-

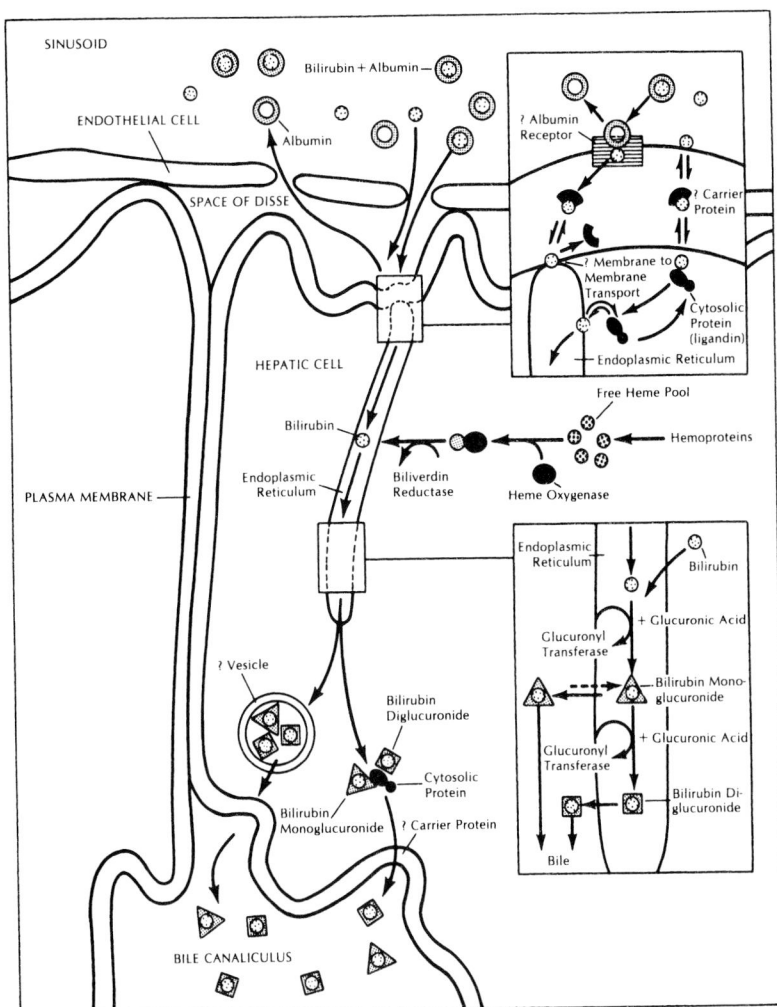

Figure 35-6 Bilirubin transport and conjugation in the hepatocyte. Two mechanisms have been proposed for uptake of bilirubin from the extracellular environment: by means of an albumin receptor or directly. In either case, carrier protein may be involved in transmembrane passage (**upper box**). Transport into the endoplasmic reticulum is facilitated by complexing to ligandin, but direct membrane-to-membrane transfer also may occur. Cytosolic bilirubin is in equilibrium with endoplasmic reticulum bilirubin. The hypothesis of conjugation of insoluble bilirubin to polar glucuronides (**lower box**). Conjugated bilirubin may enter the bile canaliculi by either vesicular transport or carrier-mediated transport. (From Gollan JL, Knapp AB. Bilirubin metabolism and congenital jaundice. *Hosp Pract (Off Ed)* 1985;Feb 15:83–106, with permission.)

reacting bilirubin) before it can be excreted (see Fig. 35-6). This is achieved when bilirubin is combined enzymatically with a sugar, glucuronic acid, producing bilirubin monoglucuronide and diglucuronide pigments that are more water soluble and sufficiently polar to be excreted into the bile or filtered through the kidney.

The presence of elevated bilirubin concentrations *in utero* prematurely induces bilirubin uridine diphosphoglucuronate glucuronosyltransferase (UGT) activity, which suggests that bilirubin plays an important role in the initiation of its own conjugation after birth (19).

Structure and Function of the Uridine Diphosphoglucuronate Glucuronosyltransferase 1A1 Gene

The process of conjugation is catalyzed by a specific hepatic enzyme isoform (1A1) belonging to the UGT family of enzymes. These enzymes metabolize endogenous compounds and various food chemicals in most tissues. Although the UGT1 family contains several isoforms, only the A1 isoform (UGT1A1) participates in the conjugation of bilirubin (20). The glucuronosyltransferase enzyme is synthesized in the hepatocyte and its structure is determined by the UGT1A1 gene (Fig. 35-7 and Table 35-2).

The gene encoding the UGT1 enzyme is located on chromosome 2 at 2q37 (21) and consists of 4 common exons and 13 variable exons (see Fig. 35-7) (22,23). The gene also has a noncoding promoter area (see Fig. 35-7B), which is an upstream regulatory region controlling gene expression. The UGT promoter contains a TATAA box, which is a DNA deoxyribonucleic acid (DNA) sequence of thymine (T) and adenine (A). Mutations in the 1A1 exon or its promoter will affect bilirubin conjugation. Examples of this effect are seen in Gilbert syndrome and the Crigler-Najjar syndromes (see *Pathologic Causes of Jaundice: Decreased Bilirubin Clearance* below). Variations in the promoter sequence can also cause indirect-reacting hyperbilirubinemia.

TABLE 35-2

THE UGT 1A1 GENE

Encodes the UGT1 enzyme
Located on chromosome 2
Consists of 4 common exons (2–5) and 13 variable exons (A1–A13)
Noncoding promoter area controls gene expression
UGT promoter contains TATAA box
Mutations in 1A1 exon or promoter affect bilirubin conjugation
    (e.g., Gilbert and Crigler-Najjar syndromes)

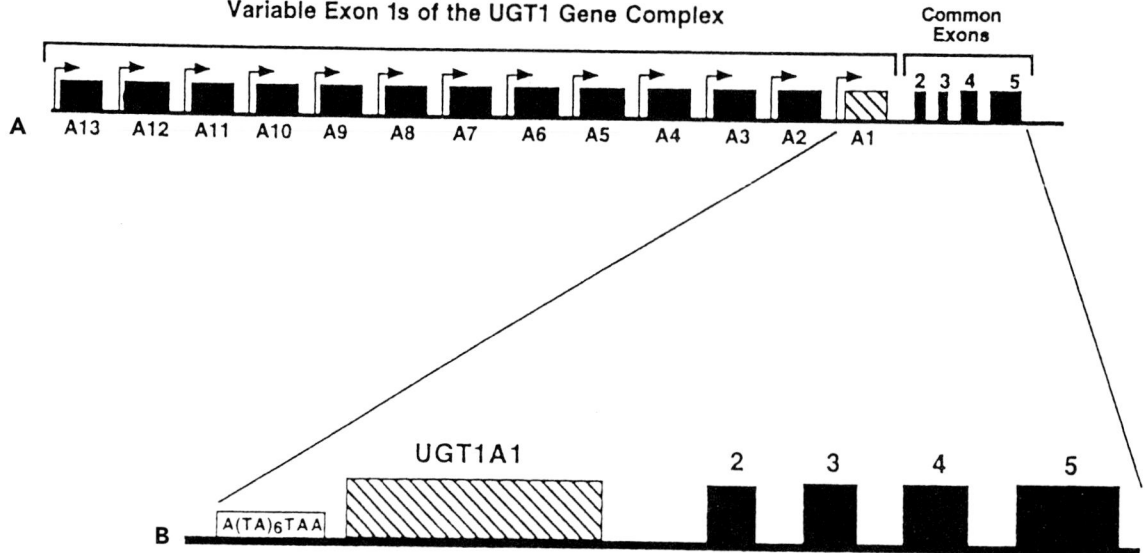

Figure 35-7 The human UGT1 gene locus. **A:** Schematic of the genomic structure of the UGT1 gene complex. **B:** Exploded view of exon 1A1 and common exons 2 to 5 of the gene complex that have been identified as sites for genetic mutations associated with absent or decreased UGT activity that cause deficiencies of bilirubin conjugation. (From Clarke DJ, Moghrabi N, Monaghan G, et al. Genetic defects of the UDP-glucoronosyltransferase-1 (UGT1) gene that cause familial non-haemolytic unconjugated hyperbilirubinemias. *Clinica Chim Acta* 1997;266:63–74, with permission.)

Transfer of Bilirubin into Bile and Intestinal Transport

After conjugation, bilirubin is excreted rapidly into the bile canaliculi by the liver cell, a process that requires metabolic work for the active transport of bilirubin across a large concentration gradient (see Fig. 35-6) (5). Interference with this process is probably responsible for the hyperbilirubinemia associated with hepatocellular disorders such as hepatitis.

Once in the small intestine, conjugated bilirubin is not reabsorbed. In the healthy adult, it is largely reduced by the action of colonic bacteria to a series of colorless tetrapyrroles, collectively known as urobilinogen, and an insignificant amount is hydrolyzed to unconjugated bilirubin and reabsorbed by way of the enterohepatic circulation. In the newborn, however, this enterohepatic circulation of bilirubin is significant and important (see Jaundice in the Healthy Newborn: Physiologic Jaundice below). In addition, in conditions involving high plasma bilirubin levels and poor hepatic excretion, there is a gradient for unconjugated bilirubin from the plasma to the intestinal lumen, and significant amounts of unconjugated bilirubin may be cleared by diffusion across the intestinal wall (24). Figure 35-5 summarizes bile pigment metabolism in the newborn.

PHYSIOLOGIC MECHANISMS OF NEONATAL JAUNDICE

At any time in the infant's first few days after birth, the serum bilirubin level reflects a combination of the effects of bilirubin production, conjugation, and enterohepatic

circulation. Using measurements of blood carboxyhemoglobin (COHb) corrected for ambient CO (COHbc) as an index of bilirubin production and high-performance liquid chromatography (HPLC) measurements of conjugated bilirubin, Kaplan and associates (25) demonstrated that an imbalance between bilirubin production and conjugation is fundamental in the pathogenesis of neonatal bilirubinemia. Several processes account for the bilirubinemia that occurs in virtually all newborns (Table 35-3).

Increased Bilirubin Load on the Liver Cell

Bilirubin Production

CO is produced in equimolar quantities with bilirubin and measurements of CO production show that the normal

---

TABLE 35-3

PHYSIOLOGIC MECHANISMS OF NEONATAL JAUNDICE

Increased bilirubin load on liver cell
  Increased erythrocyte volume
  Decreased erythrocyte survival
  Increased early labeled bilirubin
  Increased enterohepatic circulation of bilirubin
Decreased hepatic uptake of bilirubin from plasma
  Decreased ligandin
Decreased bilirubin conjugation
  Decreased uridine diphosphoglucuronosyl transferase activity
Defective bilirubin excretion
  Excretion impaired but not rate limiting

newborn produces an average of 8 to 10 mg/kg (13.7 to 17.1 μmol/ kg) of bilirubin per day (26,27). This is more than twice the rate of normal daily bilirubin production in the adult and is explained by the fact that the neonate has a higher circulating erythrocyte volume, a shorter mean erythrocyte lifespan, and a larger early labeled bilirubin peak (see Table 35-3). Bilirubin production decreases with increasing postnatal age but is still about twice the adult rate by age 2 weeks (26).

Enterohepatic Circulation

The newborn reabsorbs much larger quantities of unconjugated bilirubin by way of the enterohepatic circulation, than does the adult. Infants have fewer bacteria in the small and large bowel and greater activity of the deconjugating enzyme β-glucuronidase.(28) As a result, conjugated bilirubin, which is not reabsorbed, is not converted to urobilinogen but is hydrolyzed to unconjugated bilirubin, which is reabsorbed, thus increasing the bilirubin load on an already stressed liver (see Fig. 35-5). Studies in newborn humans (29), monkeys (30), and Gunn rats (31) suggest that the enterohepatic circulation of bilirubin is a significant contributor to physiologic jaundice. In the first few days after birth, caloric intake is low, which contributes to an increase in the enterohepatic circulation (32,33).

Decreased Clearance of Bilirubin from the Plasma

Uptake

Ligandin, the predominant bilirubin-binding protein in the human liver cell, is deficient in the liver of newborn monkeys. It reaches adult levels in the monkey by 5 days of age, coinciding with a fall in bilirubin levels, and administration of phenobarbital increases the concentration of ligandin (34). Although this suggests that impaired uptake may contribute to the pathogenesis of physiologic jaundice, uptake does not appear to be rate limiting.

Conjugation

Deficient UGT1A1 activity, with resultant impairment of bilirubin conjugation, has long been considered a major cause of physiologic jaundice. In human infants, the early postnatal increase in serum bilirubin appears to play an important role in the initiation of bilirubin conjugation. (19) In the first 10 days after birth, UGT1A1 activity in full-term and premature neonates usually is less than 1% of adult values (see Fig. 35-4) (12,13). Thereafter, the activity increases at an exponential rate, reaching adult values by 6 to 14 weeks of age (13). The postnatal increase in UGT1A1 activity is independent of the infant's gestation.

Excretion

The absence of an elevated serum level of conjugated bilirubin in physiologic jaundice suggests that, under normal circumstances, the neonatal liver cell is capable of excreting the bilirubin that it has just conjugated.

Nevertheless, the ability of the newborn liver to excrete conjugated bilirubin and other anions (e.g., drugs, hormones) is more limited than that of the older child or adult and may become rate limiting when the bilirubin load is significantly increased. Thus, when intrauterine hyperbilirubinemia occurs, usually as a result of isoimmunization, it is not uncommon to find an elevated serum level of conjugated bilirubin (19).

PHYSIOLOGIC JAUNDICE

Because at some point during the first week of life almost every newborn has a total serum bilirubin (TSB) level that exceeds 1 mg/dL (17 μmol/L, the upper limit of normal for an adult), and two-thirds or more of newborns will appear clinically jaundiced, this type of transient hyperbilirubinemia has been called *physiologic jaundice*. This jaundice results from the interaction of a number of factors (see Table 35-3). The term *physiologic jaundice* generally is applied to newborns whose TSB level falls within the normal range, but because of the significant differences in TSB levels in different populations, it can be difficult to define what is normal or abnormal, physiologic or nonphysiologic. Additionally, defining the term "normal" is, in itself, a difficult task, and depends on whether one chooses a gaussian, percentile, diagnostic, risk factor, or therapeutic definition of the term (35).

In premature newborns, the term *physiologic jaundice* is of little value. If untreated, low-birth-weight infants have exaggerated and prolonged hyperbilirubinemia. Although this may be considered "physiologic" because it occurs in all preterm infants, in very-low-birth-weight infants, TSB levels well within the "physiologic range" are considered potentially hazardous and are treated with phototherapy. Thus, the natural history of hyperbilirubinemia in the very-low-birth-weight infant is never observed, and defining certain bilirubin levels as "physiologic" in this population is misleading and potentially dangerous. Using a diagnostic definition of normal (35), a TSB level of 10 mg/dL (171 μmol/ L) on day 4 in a 750-g neonate would be considered completely "physiologic," and no investigation need be done to identify a cause for this jaundice. Nevertheless, almost all neonatologists would *treat* this infant with phototherapy, implying that this value exceeds the therapeutic definition of normal (i.e., treatment is much more likely to do good than harm). Thus, in today's neonatal intensive care population, the term *physiologic jaundice* has no meaning and no utility and should be abandoned.

BILIRUBIN TOXICITY

Kernicterus

Pathology

The first description of kernicterus (or brain jaundice) in newborns was provided by Hervieux in 1847 (1) and in

TABLE 35-4
COMPARATIVE NEUROPATHOLOGY OF KERNICTERUS

Topography of Lesions	Full-term Infants, Hyperbilirubinemia	Homozygous Gunn Rats	Premature Infants, Low Bilirubin Levels
Globus pallidus	+	+	+
Subthalamus	+	+	+
Hypothalamus	+	−	−
Horn of Ammon	+	+	+
Reticular zone of the substantia nigra	+	+	+
Cranial nerve nuclei	+	+	+
Reticular formation	+		+
Central pontine nuclei			
Interstitial nucleus			
Locus ceruleus	−	+	+
Lateral cuneate nucleus of the medulla	+	+	+
Cerebellum			
Dentate nuclei	+	−	+
Nuclei of roof of fourth ventricle	+	+	+
Purkinje cells	−	+	+
Spinal cord	+	+	+

+, Yellow pigment present; −, yellow pigment absent.
From Ahdab-Barmada M, Moossy J. The neuropathology of kernicterus in the premature neonate: diagnostic problems. *J Neuropathol Exp Neurol* 1984;43:45–56, with permission.

1875, Orth (36) observed bilirubin pigment at autopsy in the brains of infants who were severely jaundiced. Schmorl (37) subsequently described two forms of "brain icterus," the first "characterized by a diffuse yellow coloration of the entire brain substance," and a second form in which "the jaundiced coloration appears to be completely circumscribed and . . . limited to the so-called 'kern' or nuclear region of the brain."

Topography

Full-term infants who die of kernicterus demonstrate bilirubin staining in a characteristic distribution (Table 35-4), although a variety of patterns have been described, grossly and microscopically (38). Kernicteric premature infants and Gunn rats with inherited UGT deficiency display a similar topography of neuronal damage (see Table 35-4) (39). Those regions most commonly affected are the basal ganglia, particularly the subthalamic nucleus and the globus pallidus; the hippocampus; the geniculate bodies; various brainstem nuclei, including the inferior colliculus, oculomotor, vestibular, cochlear, and inferior olivary nuclei; and the cerebellum, especially the dentate nucleus and the vermis (39,40). Ahdab-Barmada has provided a detailed review of the neuropathology of kernicterus, and its anatomic, cytologic, and histologic characteristics (41).

Gross Anatomy

Yellow staining of the brain occurs when it is exposed to elevated levels of bilirubin. Table 35-5 lists the three patterns of bilirubin staining of the brain seen in the newborn (41).

Histology and Cytology

Table 35-6 summarizes the neuropathologic findings of kernicterus. There can be some confusion regarding the diagnosis of kernicterus in the presence of yellow discoloration of the central nervous system. Ahdab-Barmada emphasizes that the diagnosis of kernicterus should only be applied to the incorporation of bilirubin pigment into gangliosides or phospholipids of mature neurons with subsequent damage to the neuron, depending on the amount of pigment trapped within the cell (41). The unique topographic pattern of nuclear involvement is described above (see Topography) and the combination of the bright yellow-orange staining of these brain nuclei, together with evidence of neuronal damage and degeneration within the nuclei, is necessary before a diagnosis of kernicterus can be made (41).

TABLE 35-5
PATTERNS OF BILIRUBIN STAINING OF THE BRAIN IN HYPERBILIRUBINEMIA

Diffuse yellow staining of areas that normally lack a blood–brain barrier, e.g., leptomeninges, ependyma, choroid plexus, cerebrospinal fluid.
Diffuse yellow staining of brain tissues in areas where blood–brain barrier integrity has been compromised (as can occur following hypoxic ischemic encephalopathy, periventricular leukomalacia, ischemic cerebral infarct).
Yellow staining of specific neuronal groups (kernicterus).

From Ahdab-Barmada M. The neuropathology of kernicterus: definitions and debate. In: Maisels MJ, Watchko JF, eds. Neonatal Jaundice. London: Harwood Academic, 2000:75–88.

TABLE 35-6
NEUROPATHOLOGIC FINDINGS OF KERNICTERUS

Early (2–5 Days)	Subacute (6–10 Days)	Late (>10 Days)
Yellow pigment in neuronal cytoplasm	Spongy neuropil within involved nuclei	Neuronal loss with astrocytosis
Moth-eaten appearance of neuronal and nuclear membranes	Hypertrophic, bare astrocytic nuclei	Granular mineralization of residual neuronal membranes in affected nuclei
Pyknotic nucleus	Basophilic neurons with increased nuclear density	Demyelinization of optic tracts and fornix
Loss of Nissl substance	Cellular dissolution of some neurons	Dysmyelination and degeneration of globus pallidus and subthalamic nucleus
Basophilic cytoplasm	Granular mineralization of neuronal cytoplasmic membranes	
Periodic acid-Schiff–positive membrane-bound aggregates within neurons		

From Ahdab-Barmada M, Moossy J. The neuropathology of kernicterus in the premature neonate: diagnostic problems. *J Neuropathol Exp Neurol* 1984;43:45–56, with permission.

Autopsies on jaundiced infants reveal bilirubin staining of the aorta, pleural fluid, and ascitic fluid, or a generalized yellow cast throughout the viscera. The staining usually is not considered a sign of tissue damage unless other cytologic changes are found (38). Bilirubin staining also can be found in necrotic tissue anywhere in the body and has been described in the gastrointestinal tract, lungs (hyaline membranes) (42), kidney, adrenals, and gonads. In infants with hemolytic disease, bile plugs commonly are found in the canaliculi between the hepatocytes, especially in the periportal areas. The kidneys may show bilirubin-stained tubular casts, bilirubin crystals in the small vessels or in edematous interstitium, and renal tubular necrosis. The bilirubin infarcts (i.e., patches of yellow staining in the renal medulla) are probably the result of focal areas of acute tubular necrosis that have been stained by bilirubin (38).

Neuronal necrosis is the dominant histopathologic feature after 7 to 10 days of postnatal life (see Table 35-6). For the most part, its distribution corresponds with the distribution of bilirubin staining, although there are some exceptions to this rule. For example, intense staining develops in the olivary and dentate nuclei, but there is little neuronal necrosis in these regions. The important areas of neuronal injury (as opposed to staining) include the basal ganglia, brainstem oculomotor nuclei, and brainstem auditory (cochlear) nuclei (40). The involvement of these regions explains some of the clinical sequelae of bilirubin encephalopathy (see Clinical Features of Bilirubin Encephalopathy below).

Clinical and Pathologic Correlations

Originally a pathologic diagnosis and later a well-defined acute and chronic neurologic syndrome, kernicterus or

bilirubin encephalopathy appears to be a less-well-circumscribed entity that includes nuclear bilirubin staining of very-low-birth-weight infants who died of other causes and, possibly, a subtle chronic encephalopathy in which extrapyramidal motor disturbances and sensorineural hearing deficit are not the predominant features.

Most, but not all, full-term infants seen today with the pathologic changes described manifest the clinical symptomatology of this disorder, including very high serum bilirubin levels (commonly higher than 30 mg/dL [513 μmol/L]). Exceptions have been described. Perlman and associates (43) recently reported kernicterus at autopsy in two very sick near-term infants with maximum TSB levels of 5.2 and 14.4 mg/dL (89 to 246 μmol/L).

Yellow staining of the brain also has been observed in premature infants who manifested none of the clinical signs of kernicterus during life and in whom TSB levels remained low (44,45). Turkel and colleagues (46) identified 32 infants with kernicterus at autopsy and compared them with 32 control infants of similar gestational ages without kernicterus. In the kernicteric infants, although the gross pattern of staining followed that of classic kernicterus, the typical histologic changes characteristic of kernicterus were found in only three patients. These authors suggest that the bilirubin staining they observed probably was not the same clinicopathologic entity as the kernicterus of posticteric encephalopathy. Instead of the neuronal degeneration typically seen, they found spongy change and gliosis, which both imply nonspecific damage to the brain. This suggests that prior diffuse injury may predispose the brain to bilirubin deposition at relatively low levels of serum bilirubin.

Ahdab-Barmada and Moossy (39) found kernicterus in 97 autopsies of neonates (95 younger than 36 weeks of

TABLE 35-7

COMPARATIVE NEUROPATHOLOGY OF KERNICTERUS AND ANOXIC–ISCHEMIC ENCEPHALOPATHY IN THE PREMATURE NEONATE

Topography of Lesions[a]	Kernicterus	Anoxic–Ischemic Encephalopathy
Cerebral cortex	Absent	Present
Periventricular white matter	Absent	Present
Corpus striatum	Globus pallidus	Putamen and caudate nuclei
Thalamus	Subthalamus	Anterior and lateral nuclei
Horn of Ammon	Resistant sector (H_{2-3})	Sommer sector (H_1)
Midbrain	Interstitial nucleus	Inferior colliculi
	Nuclei of nerve III[b]	Nuclei of nerve III[b]
	Reticular portion of substantia nigra	Compact portion of substantia nigra
Pons	Locus ceruleus	Basal pontine nuclei
	Nuclei of nerves VI, VII	Superior olivary complex
	Reticular formation[b]	Reticular formation[b]
Medulla	Vestibular and cochlear nuclei	Inferior olivary nuclei
		Superior olivary nuclei
Cerebellum	Purkinje cells[b]	Purkinje cells[b]
	Nuclei of roof of fourth ventricle	Granular cells

[a] Only topographic areas considered helpful for differential diagnosis are listed in this table.
[b] Whenever neuronal damage was involved in the same structure in kernicterus and anoxic–ischemic encephalopathy, the cytopathology was different.
From Ahdab-Barmada M. The neuropathology of kernicterus: definitions and debate. In: Maisels MJ, Watchko JF, eds. *Neonatal jaundice*. London: Harwood Academic, 2000:75–88, with permission.

gestation). The neuropathology in these infants was strikingly similar to that of classic kernicterus in the full-term neonate and in the Gunn rat (see Table 35-4). In the National Institute of Child Health and Human Development (NICHHD) cooperative phototherapy study, four low-birth-weight infants had autopsy-proven kernicterus (47). The neuropathologic findings in these infants were those of classic kernicterus. As Table 35-7 shows, the neuropathology of kernicterus is different from that of hypoxic ischemic encephalopathy. Even though hypoxic ischemic insults may predispose the brain to bilirubin deposition in some low-birth-weight infants, in others the typical histologic features of kernicterus will be found.

Pathophysiology of Bilirubin Toxicity

The pathogenesis of kernicterus is highly complex and the risk of developing kernicterus is related to a multiplicity of factors (48), which are discussed below. The cellular and molecular mechanisms of bilirubin toxicity were reviewed by Hansen (49,50) and Volpe (Fig. 35-8) (51).

Bilirubin Chemistry and Neurotoxicity

As discussed in Formation, Structure, and Properties of Bilirubin above, the polar groups of the bilirubin molecule, in its most stable conformation, are involved in intramolecular hydrogen bonding that restricts solvation and renders the pigment nearly insoluble in water at pH 7.4. When doubly ionized in alkaline medium, the molecule is much more soluble. The low water solubility of bilirubin and its tendency to aggregate and precipitate at physiologic pH, particularly acid pH, have long been thought to be key factors in its toxicity. Thus, when the concentration of bilirubin acid exceeds its solubility, bilirubin may gradually aggregate and precipitate from solution (17). Bilirubin crystals have been found in the brain cells of infants who died from kernicterus, and bilirubin concentrations of 2 mg/dL (34 μmol/L) have been observed in kernicteric brains (52). It is likely that even higher local concentrations of pigment exist in the brain in kernicterus and may occur when aggregates precipitate within brain cells (53,54). Wennberg (55) suggested that formation of reversible complexes between bilirubin monoanion and membranes is also important in the development of bilirubin encephalopathy.

Although it is known that bilirubin uncouples oxidative phosphorylation and inhibits cellular respiration and protein phosphorylation, there is no agreement that these are the key mechanisms of bilirubin toxicity *in vivo* (see Fig. 35-8). Bilirubin also inhibits mitochondrial enzymes, interferes with DNA and protein synthesis (56), and alters cerebral glucose metabolism (49,57). Unconjugated bilirubin will initiate a mitochondrial pathway of apoptosis in developing brain neurons (58) and it inhibits the function of N-methyl-D-aspartate-receptor ion channels (59). Bilirubin also binds to lysine sites on albumin and ligandin, proteins that are essential for bilirubin transport and metabolism (49). Consequently, lysine binding may have a role in the pathogenesis of bilirubin toxicity.

It is not known why bilirubin is deposited preferentially in the basal ganglia, but it is possible that regional differences in uptake, tissue binding, metabolism, or cellular

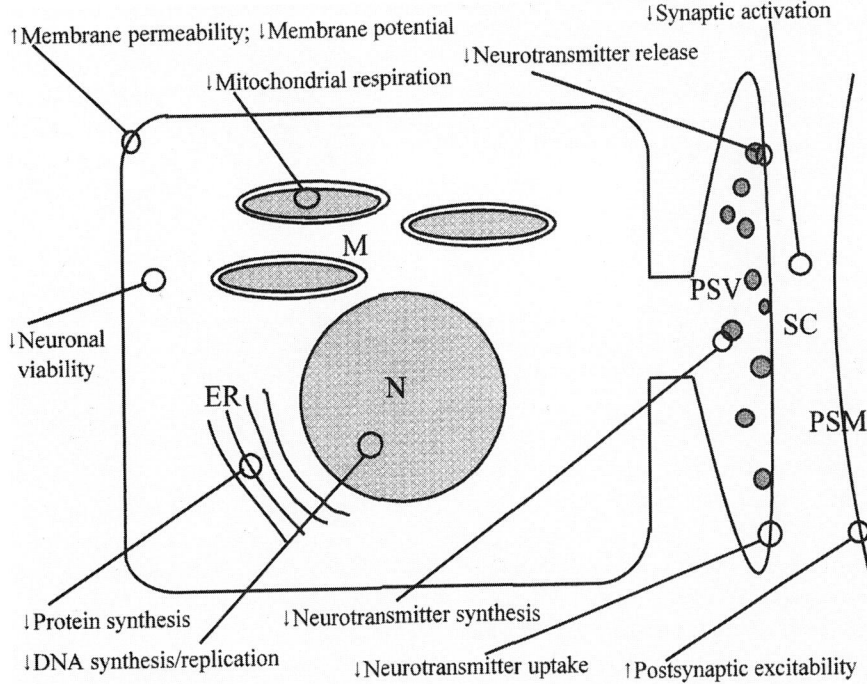

↑Membrane permeability; ↓Membrane potential

↓Mitochondrial respiration

↓Synaptic activation

↓Neurotransmitter release

↓Neuronal viability

M

PSV

SC

ER

N

PSM

↓Protein synthesis

↓DNA synthesis/replication

↓Neurotransmitter synthesis

↓Neurotransmitter uptake

↑Postsynaptic excitability

Figure 35-8 Effects of bilirubin on neurons and neuronal metabolic processes. Bilirubin affects a large number of cellular functions and processes, both *in vivo* and *in vitro*, It decreases neuronal viability; increases membrane permeability and decreases membrane potential; uncouples oxidative phosphorylation; inhibits neurotransmitter release, synthesis, and uptake; inhibits synaptic activation; increases postsynaptic excitability; decreases protein synthesis; and decreases synthesis and replication of DNA. Other bilirubin-affected functions not indicated in the illustration are inhibition of enzyme function and protein phosphorylation. ER, endoplasmic reticulum; M, mitochondrial; N, nucleus; PSM, postsynaptic membrane; PSV, presynaptic vesicles; SC, synaptic cleft. (From Hansen TWR. The pathophysiology of bilirubin toxicity. In: Maisels MJ, Watchko JF, eds. *Neonatal jaundice*. London: Harwood Academic, 2000:89–104, with permission.)

clearance play a role (49). It is also possible that there are regional differences in blood flow or blood brain barrier permeability.

Albumin Binding and the Concept of Free Bilirubin

Bilirubin is transported in the plasma as a dianion bound tightly, but reversibly, to serum albumin and the portion that is unbound or loosely bound (sometimes termed *free bilirubin*) can more readily leave the intravascular space and cross the intact blood brain barrier (60). Albumin has a primary, high-affinity binding site at which the association constant, derived from the equilibrium concentrations of bound and free bilirubin, is about 10^7 to 10^8 moles^{-1} (17). Because of this high binding affinity, equilibrium concentrations of unbound or free bilirubin in plasma are very low. It has been widely accepted that bilirubin toxicity occurs when free bilirubin enters the brain and binds to cell membranes (61) and that the presence of albumin mitigates the *in vivo* and *in vitro* toxic effects of bilirubin (61,62).

The relationship between free bilirubin levels, kernicterus, and developmental outcome is discussed below in the section on the clinical sequelae of hyperbilirubinemia (see Clinical Sequelae of Hyperbilirubinemia : Bilirubin Binding Capacity, Kernicterus, and Developmental Outcome) Drugs

that decrease albumin binding of bilirubin, such as sulfisoxazole, increase the risk of kernicterus (63, 64). These observations are consistent with the hypothesis that bilirubin is able to move freely across the blood-brain barrier, bind to tissues, and damage the cells of the central nervous system.

Ostrow and colleagues have questioned the significance of some published data from *in vitro* models of bilirubin cellular toxicity because of the high concentrations of unconjugated bilirubin that were used (18,65–67). They suggest that bilirubin toxicity might occur at free bilirubin levels that are significantly lower than those previously documented and that precipitation of unconjugated bilirubin in, or on, cells may not be required to produce neurotoxicity (67). These issues cannot be resolved until clinical studies are performed on infants who have had appropriate measurements of free bilirubin as newborns (68) and are then followed into childhood.

Measurement of Free Bilirubin

Although several techniques exist for measuring or estimating free or loosely bound bilirubin and the binding capacity and affinity of bilirubin for albumin (17), changes in free bilirubin concentrations can be transient because there is rapid equilibration and redistribution of bilirubin between the plasma (i.e., albumin) and the tissues. Even under experimental conditions that lead to a significant increase in brain bilirubin content, the differences in free bilirubin concentrations in the serum between control and study animals is small (69) and Brodersen has expressed doubt that the accurate measurement of free bilirubin is possible or clinically useful (17). Nevertheless, there is some evidence to suggest that estimates of unbound bilirubin can provide clinically relevant information regarding changes in auditory brainstem responses (ABRs) (70,71) and in frank kernicterus (72).

There is an extensive literature dealing with bilirubin-binding tests, but no test is currently in general use in the United States in clinical decision making, although a relatively simple semiautomated application of the peroxidase oxidation test is in use in Japan (73) and has been approved in the United States by the Food and Drug Administration (FDA) (74). However, the peroxidase method employs a 40-fold dilution of the sample that can alter intrinsic bilirubin binding (68). Ahlfors developed a test that combines the peroxidase technique with a diazo method for measuring conjugated and unconjugated bilirubin (68). This method uses minimal dilution and should provide more reliable data on free bilirubin levels (68).

Because one molecule of albumin is capable of binding one molecule of bilirubin tightly at the primary binding site, a bilirubin–albumin molar ratio of 1 represents about 8.5 mg of bilirubin per gram of albumin. Thus, a well, full-term infant with a serum albumin concentration of 3 to 3.5 g/dL should be able to bind about 25 to 28 mg/dL of bilirubin (428 to 479 μmol/L) if no other endogenous or exogenous ligands compete for the same site. The albumin-binding capacity of sick low-birth-weight infants is much less than that of full-term infants, and their serum albumin levels often are lower so they are able to bind effectively much less bilirubin. Ahlfors has suggested a range of bilirubin-to-albumin ratios (in mg/g) that can be used as a guide in the process of deciding whether or not to perform an exchange transfusion in term and preterm infants at different levels of risk (75), an approach that has been endorsed by the American Academy of Pediatrics (AAP) (76) (see *Treatment* below). It should be noted, however, that there is significant variability in bilirubin–albumin binding among infants (77), which can affect the validity of the bilirubin-to-albumin ratio. Because binding improves with increasing birth weight, Ahlfors suggests a level of 1.3 μg/dL per kg as a level of free bilirubin at which exchange transfusion should be considered (72), although we have no data relating such free bilirubin levels to long-term outcome. These data are urgently needed.

Factors Affecting the Binding of Bilirubin to Serum Albumin

This subject has been reviewed in detail (17); however, a few of the factors are discussed here.

Fatty Acids

Free fatty acids in plasma may compete with bilirubin for its binding to albumin, but significant interference with bilirubin binding probably does not occur until molar ratios of free fatty acids-to-albumin (F:A) exceed 4:1 (17).

The infusion of 1 g/kg of intralipid over a 15-hour period in infants of less than 30 weeks of gestation produced an F:A ratio of less than 3 and minimal increases in unbound bilirubin concentrations (78). With doses of 2 to 3 g/kg, however, higher ratios were found. Intravenous fat, given as a continuous infusion of 2 g/kg per day for 7 days to infants of 32 weeks or less of gestation (mean birth weight 1,200 g) produced F:A ratios of only 0.1 to 1.8. (79)

pH

The binding of bilirubin to albumin is thought to be unaffected by changes in the serum pH (80,81). Nevertheless, the correction of neonatal acidosis in 11 sick newborns appeared to decrease the serum free bilirubin concentration as measured by a peroxidase technique (82). The role of pH, on the other hand, may be pivotal in determining the binding of bilirubin to cells and partitioning to extravascular tissue and, therefore, its deposition in the central nervous system (55,60).

Drugs

The effect of numerous drugs on bilirubin–albumin binding has been tested *in vitro* using different methods. The measured effect varies with the method used; some systems require much greater concentrations of the drug than others to demonstrate an increase in unbound bilirubin. *In vivo*, of course, the effect of drugs and their potential for inducing kernicterus depends, not simply on their ability to displace bilirubin from albumin, but also on their route and mode of administration. Thus, a displacing drug is likely to be more dangerous when administered intravenously as a bolus than as an infusion. Robertson and colleagues (83) reviewed the bilirubin-displacing effect of drugs used in neonatology (Table 35-8). They arbitrarily chose to consider an increase in the free bilirubin concentration of 5% as potentially dangerous, and they consider a drug to be a potential displacer if it occupies 5% or more of the available albumin. Knowledge of the usual peak serum bilirubin concentrations and the percentage of albumin-bound drug also can be used to calculate the concentration of bound drug. If the bound drug concentration is less than 15 μmol/L, it is unlikely that this drug will cause significant displacement of bilirubin (83).

Robertson and colleagues (83) calculated a maximal displacement factor, δ, from the K_D value, using the following equation:

$$\delta = K_D d + 1$$

where d is the concentration of free drug in the patient's plasma, and K_D is the displacement constant, which represents the competitive effect of the drug with bilirubin for albumin binding. If K_D is 0, then δ = 1, and the drug does not displace bilirubin. If δ = 1.2, there has been a 20% increase of free bilirubin concentration after drug administration. Although an arbitrary value of 1.2 has been suggested as the upper permissible limit for bilirubin displacement,

TABLE 35-8
EFFECT OF DRUGS USED IN NEONATOLOGY ON BILIRUBIN–ALBUMIN BINDING

Agent	δ	Agent	δ
Anticonvulsants		Nafcillin	1.05
Diazepam	1.00	Oxacillin	1.07
Phenobarbital	1.04	Penicillin G	1.06
Phenytoin	1.02	Piperacillin	1.03
Valproate	1.09	Polymyxin B	1.00
Testing not required: lorazepam		Quinine	?
Antihypertensive agents		Spiramycin	1.00
Diazoxide	?	Streptomycin	1.00
Testing not required: hydralazine,		Sulfadiazine	1.18
methyldopa, nitroprusside, reserpine		Sulfamethoxazole	1.69
Cardiac drugs		Sulfisoxazole	2.43
Lidocaine	1.00	Tazobactam	1.00
Procainamide	1.00	Ticarcillin	1.27
Testing not required: bretylium		Trimethoprim	1.01
tosylate, digoxin, disopyramide,		Vancomycin	1.01
quinidine, verapamil		Vidarabine	1.00
Diuretics		Testing not required: amphotericin	
Acetazolamide	1.10	B, ciprofloxacin, erythromycin,	
Bumetanide	1.00	isoniazid, miconazole, netilmicin,	
Chlorothiazide	1.03	pyrimethamine, tobramycin	
Ethacrynic acid	1.27	**Miscellaneous**	
Furosemide	1.07	Calcium chloride	1.00
Hydrochlorothiazide	1.04	Calcium gluconate	1.00
Testing not required: spironolactone		Calcium lactate	1.00
Infectious disease agents		Carnitine	1.00
Acyclovir	1.00	Clofibrate	1.00
Amdinocillin	1.00	Diatrizoate	1.24
Ampicillin	1.08	Indomethacin	1.00
Azlocillin	1.33	Magnesium sulfate	1.00
Aztreonam	1.12	Mannitol	1.00
Carbenicillin	1.35	Tin protoporphyrin	?
Cefamandole	1.07	Tolazoline	1.00
Cefazolin	1.17	Tromethamine	1.00
Cefmenoxime	1.10	Testing not required: bicarbonate,	
Cefmetazole	2.01	cimetidine, dextran, enalapril,	
Cefonicid	1.71	flumecinol, heparin, ketamine,	
Cefoperazone	1.18	metoclopramide, naloxone,	
Ceforanide	1.04	nicardipine, prostaglandin E₁	
Cefotaxime	1.05	**Neuromuscular junction agents**	
Cefotetan	1.74	Pancuronium	1.01
Cefoxitin	?	Testing not required: atracurium	
Ceftazidime	1.02	besylate, neostigmine,	
Ceftizoxime	1.03	tubocurarine, vecuronium	
Ceftriaxone	3.00	**Sedative and analgesic agents**	
Cefuroxime	1.02	Chloral hydrate	1.00
Cephalothin	1.03	Paraldehyde	1.00
Cephapirin	1.03	Pentobarbital	1.03
Cephradine	1.02	Thiopental	1.04
Chloramphenicol	1.02	Testing not required: alfentanil,	
Chloroquine	1.00	chlorpromazine, fentanyl,	
Cilastatin	1.00	meperidine, midazolam, morphine	
Clindamycin	1.00	**Stimulants**	
Fusidate	1.00	Aminophylline	1.24
Imipenem	1.00	Doxapram	1.00
Lincomycin	1.17	**Sympathetic and parasympathetic agents**	
Methicillin	1.00	Edrophonium chloride	1.00
Metronidazole	1.11	Testing not required: atropine	
Mezlocillin		dobutamine, dopamine, epinephrine,	
Moxalactam	1.63	isoproterenol, propranolol	

Drugs are listed according to the category of their use. The symbol δ represents the maximal displacement factor. If δ = 1.2, there is a 20% increase in free bilirubin concentration following drug administration. Drugs listed as not requiring testing have low protein binding or low mean peak serum concentrations. A question mark indicates that the drug requires testing but that the peroxidase technique is not applicable.
From Robertson A, Carp W, Broderson R. Bilirubin displacing effect of drugs used in neonatology. *Acta Paediatr Scand* 1991;80:1119–1127, with permission.

it is recommended that, as much as possible, drugs with the lowest δ values be selected. Table 35-8 lists the effects of drugs used in neonatology on bilirubin–albumin binding. The free drug concentration is calculated from the serum concentration and the percentage of bound drug as taken from existing data in the literature.

Other drugs used (or with potential for use) in the neonatal intensive care unit (NICU) have also been tested. Aminoglycosides have minimal binding to albumin and should have no displacing effect. This has been confirmed for gentamicin (84). The use of ibuprofen has been suggested as an alternative to indomethacin to close the ductus arteriosus in premature newborns. Although indomethacin has some effect on bilirubin–albumin binding, it does so only at plasma levels far greater than those that occur clinically (85). Using the peroxidase–diazo method (68), Ahlfors found a significant increase in the unbound bilirubin concentration at serum ibuprofen levels of 100 µg/mL or greater. This effect was similar to that found with sulfisoxazole. On the first day of life, serum bilirubin levels are very low, but ibuprofen has a long half-life and, over the next few days, could displace bilirubin from its albumin binding and distribute it to the extravascular spaces and cause "low bilirubin" kernicterus. Using a different technique, others have also found significant displacement of bilirubin by ibuprofen (86). Following a dose of 10 mg/kg, plasma ibuprofen levels range from 181 µg/mL on day 1 to 33 µg/mL on day 3 (87,88). These data argue against the use of ibuprofen in the sick, low-birth-weight infant who is already at a greater risk for developing kernicterus.

Benzyl alcohol has been used as a bacteriostatic agent in multidose bottles. A significant association was found between the use of benzyl alcohol and the development of kernicterus and intraventricular hemorrhage (89). Benzyl alcohol is a membrane fluidizer (55) and might act by increasing the permeability of the blood–brain barrier (90). On the other hand, benzoate, a metabolite of benzyl alcohol, is a powerful displacer of bilirubin and leads to an increase in unbound bilirubin levels (91).

Robertson and associates (92) also evaluated the effect of drug combinations on bilirubin–albumin binding. This is important because drug combinations are commonly administered to sick neonates, and the data show that the bilirubin-displacing effect of these combinations cannot be predicted from each drug's effect. For example, the administration of aminophylline with vancomycin increased the displacing effect when compared with either drug alone, but the overall effect was still minimal. In the absence of published data, drugs should be selected that have a low affinity for albumin and that have therapeutic concentrations much lower than the usual concentration of albumin (about 2.8 g/dL in a very-low-birth-weight newborn). Simultaneous treatment with several drugs should be limited as much as possible (92). Finally, as discussed in Blood–Brain and Blood–Cerebrospinal Fluid Barriers below, drugs that do not affect albumin binding of bilirubin may nevertheless affect brain uptake of bilirubin by inhibiting P-glycoprotein (P-gp) function (93).

Other Competing Anions

It is possible that certain unidentified anions interfere with the albumin binding of bilirubin. Evidence for this is suggested by the failure of exchange transfusion to alter significantly the albumin binding of infants' serum, even though the exchange transfusion removes bilirubin, replaces much of the infant's serum albumin with bilirubin-free albumin, and lowers the free bilirubin level (94). Anions that interfere with albumin binding might be present in the extravascular compartment and might not be removed by exchange transfusion.

Clinical Status of the Infant

A relation may exist between bilirubin-binding capacity and the clinical condition and gestational age of the infant. In some studies, very premature and sick infants were able to bind less bilirubin per mole of albumin than were more mature infants (95,96). However, no relation was found between bilirubin-binding ability and gestational age in other studies (97,98).

Finally, while a great deal of attention has focused on the effects of drugs on bilirubin binding and metabolism, relatively little attention has been given to the effects of bilirubin on the pharmacokinetics, efficacy, and toxicities of commonly used drugs.

Bilirubin and the Brain

Under normal circumstances, there is thought to be a constant movement of bilirubin in and out of the brain. Experimentally, however, it is difficult to induce kernicterus or electrical central nervous system changes in healthy animals by infusion of bilirubin, regardless of how much is infused. This may be related to the practical difficulty of preparing homogenous infusates with high bilirubin concentrations, as well as the efficient mechanisms for clearance of bilirubin in experimental animals (99,100). Gross staining of the brain and electrophysiologic changes, however, occur readily in asphyxiated animals and in those subjected to perturbations of the blood–brain barrier or of bilirubin–albumin binding (99,101–106).

Genetic factors may be involved in determining the susceptibility of patients to bilirubin-induced neurotoxicity. For example, in different strains of Gunn rats exposed to similar bilirubin and albumin concentrations, there were significant differences in susceptibility to kernicterus and mortality, suggesting that genetic or other factors may be important in determining individual susceptibility to bilirubin toxicity (107).

Blood–Brain and Blood–Cerebrospinal Fluid Barriers

The blood–brain barrier (BBB) is the barrier that exists between the brain capillary endothelium and the brain parenchyma; it limits the entry of certain substances into the central nervous system (CNS) (Fig. 35-9). The choroid plexus is the barrier between the blood and the cere-

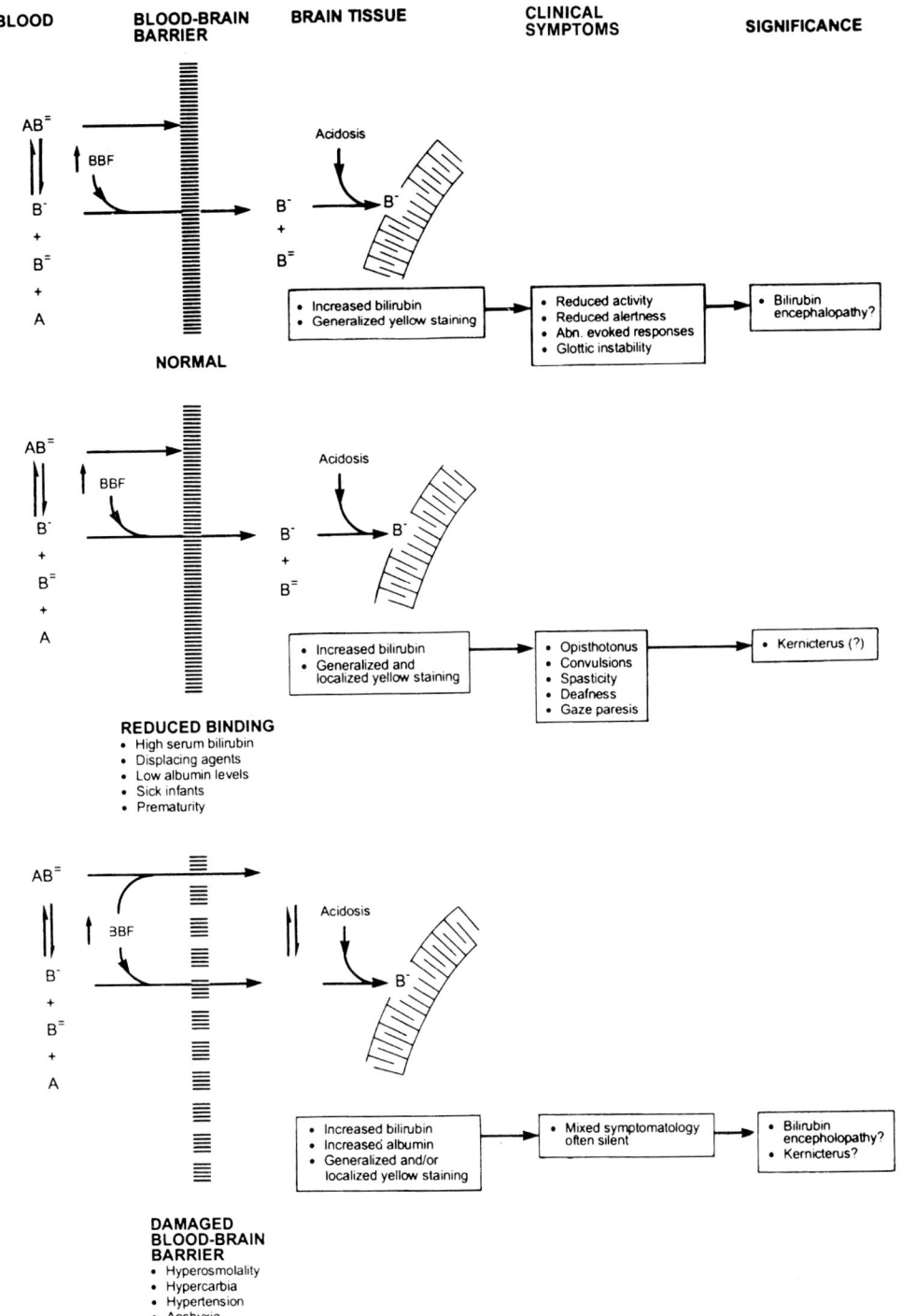

Figure 35-9 Possible mechanisms for bilirubin entry into the brain and for binding to neuronal cell membranes. The different factors affecting this process are indicated. *A*, albumin; *AB*, albumin–bilirubin complex; B^-, bilirubin monoanion; $B^=$, bilirubin dianion; BBF, brain–blood flow. (From Bratlid D. How bilirubin gets into the brain. *Clin Perinatol* 1990;17:449–465, with permission.)

brospinal fluid (CSF) (67). The BBB consists of a continuous lining of endothelial cells connected by tight junctions that restrict intercellular diffusion. The BBB normally excludes most water-soluble substances, proteins, and macromolecules, but is permeable to low-molecular-weight lipid-soluble substances that are not highly protein bound. Large molecules, such as albumin, are excluded from the brain but may enter when the BBB is made permeable by the infusion of a hypertonic solution (62,

101,106). The endothelial cells of the choroid plexus lack tight junctions and are fenestrated, allowing some proteins and their bound ligands to enter the CSF (67). Although the total protein concentration of CSF in the newborn is only approximately 2% of the plasma protein concentration, the ratios of TSB to protein are similar in CSF and plasma, suggesting that the steep concentration gradient from plasma to CSF is the result of the much lower concentration of bilirubin binding protein in the CSF (67).

Opening of the BBB allows albumin-bound bilirubin to bathe the neurons. The partitioning of sufficient bilirubin from albumin to neuronal membranes will produce changes in the electroencephalogram.(62). Disruption of the BBB and increased delivery of bilirubin to the brain may be important in the pathogenesis of bilirubin toxicity.

Protection of Cells from Neurotoxicity and Limiting Bilirubin Access to the Brain. Certain factors—including intracellular binding of unconjugated bilirubin to cytosolic proteins (67,108), neuronal apoptosis inhibitor proteins (NAIPs), and bilirubin oxidation in brain cells (50)—may protect cells of the central nervous system during exposure to elevated concentrations of unconjugated bilirubin. Other factors play a role in limiting bilirubin access to the brain. adenosine triphosphate binding cassette (ABC) transporters are proteins that use adenosine triphosphate (ATP) to translocate substrates across biologic membranes (109) and they play a role in limiting the accumulation of organic anions and other small molecules in the CNS and CSF (67). These are multidrug resistance-associated proteins (MRPs) and multidrug resistance P-glycoproteins (MDR/P-gps). P-gp is a member of the ABC family of membrane transporters and is encoded for by a family of genes known as the multidrug resistance (MDR) genes (MDR1 and MDR2 in humans; mdr1a, mdr1b, and mdr2 in rodents) (67,109,110). P-gp is an ATP-dependent plasma membrane efflux pump expressed in brain capillary endothelial cells and astrocytes of the blood–brain barrier. It limits the passage of lipophilic substrates and, possibly, bilirubin, into the brain (110). Following a high-load bilirubin infusion, P-gp–deficient mice have higher brain bilirubin content than do controls (110). Drugs that inhibit P-gp function increase brain uptake of bilirubin under the same experimental conditions (93). P-gp and other transporters could have an important influence on the deposition of bilirubin in the cells of the CNS (109), but their specific role has yet to be defined.

Lipid Solubility

Lipid-soluble substances that are not protein bound and gases, such as carbon dioxide and oxygen, cross the BBB easily, by simple diffusion, whereas water-soluble substances, proteins, and polar compounds (i.e., ions) do not.

Factors Affecting Blood–Brain Barrier Permeability

Anoxia, hypercarbia, and hyperosmolality open the BBB and increase the deposition of bilirubin and albumin in the brain, producing neurophysiologic and biochemical changes as well as changes in brain physiology and energy metabolism (see Fig. 35-9) (49,60,111). Thus, opening of the BBB is likely to be one important mechanism in the pathogenesis of kernicterus, although other mechanisms undoubtedly exist. For example, during hypercarbia, the increased bilirubin that is deposited in the brain is predominantly in the unbound form, although some is also albumin bound (69,104). The regional deposition of bilirubin in the brain of piglets occurs in areas where hypercarbia produces the greatest increase in regional blood flow (104).

Respiratory acidosis increases bilirubin deposition in the brain but metabolic acidosis does not (103,104).

Effect of Maturity on Blood–Brain Barrier Permeability

Is the BBB of the neonate more permeable to bilirubin and albumin than in older children or adults? The immature brain demonstrates greater passive permeability between the blood and central nervous system for lipid-insoluble molecules (112). Studies in newborn piglets show that the BBB is more permeable to bilirubin in 2-day-old than in 2-week-old piglets, whereas the permeability to albumin does not change (113). Other studies have found that albumin transfer into the brain of newborn Gunn rats decreases with age (114).

Mechanisms by Which Bilirubin Enters the Brain

Bratlid (60) has provided a simplified scheme, not involving membrane transporters for bilirubin entry into the brain, its binding to neuronal cell membranes, and the potential clinical signs that may follow (see Fig. 35-9). Under normal circumstances, bilirubin can enter the brain unaccompanied by albumin. Clinical confirmation of this fact is provided by the observation that even modest elevations of serum bilirubin can sometimes produce clinical and electrophysiologic alterations in healthy full-term infants as demonstrated by changes in behavior (115), characteristics of the cry (116), and changes in the brainstem auditory evoked response (BAER) (117). These symptoms disappear as the bilirubin level decreases (117,118).

The probability of toxic levels of bilirubin entering the brain increases when the serum level of unbound pigment increases, as depicted in the center panel of Fig. 35-9. Finally, if the BBB is disrupted, both albumin and bilirubin can enter the brain; but even in the presence of a damaged BBB, more bilirubin than albumin, on a molar basis, seems to be deposited (69,101–103). In all of these situations, acidosis would increase deposition of bilirubin in brain cells.

Oxidation of Bilirubin in the Brain

There is some evidence that mitochondria in the brain and other tissues contain a bilirubin oxidase that converts bilirubin to biliverdin and other nontoxic products (119, 120). The specificity and clinical relevance of this putative enzyme remains to be established.

CLINICAL FEATURES OF BILIRUBIN ENCEPHALOPATHY

Terminology

Although originally a pathologic diagnosis characterized by bilirubin staining of the brainstem nuclei and cerebellum, the term *kernicterus* has come to be used interchangeably with both the acute and chronic findings of bilirubin encephalopathy. Bilirubin encephalopathy describes the clinical central nervous system findings caused by bilirubin toxicity to the basal ganglia and various brainstem nuclei. To avoid confusion and encourage greater consistency in the literature, the AAP recommends (76) that the term *acute bilirubin encephalopathy* be used to describe the acute manifestations of bilirubin toxicity seen in the first weeks after birth and that the term *kernicterus* be reserved for the chronic and permanent clinical sequelae of bilirubin toxicity. This is the terminology that is used in this chapter. Recently, Johnson and associates suggested the use of the term *bilirubin-induced neurologic dysfunction* (BIND) (121) to describe the changes associated with acute bilirubin encephalopathy; they also proposed a scoring system to quantify the severity of the clinical manifestations.

Acute Bilirubin Encephalopathy

In classic acute bilirubin encephalopathy, markedly jaundiced infants progress through three fairly distinct clinical phases (Table 35-9) (51,122–124). In the early phase, the infant becomes lethargic and hypotonic, and sucks poorly. The intermediate phase is characterized by moderate stupor, irritability, and hypertonia. The infant may develop a fever and a high-pitched cry (51), which might alternate with drowsiness and hypertonia. The hypertonia involves the extensor muscle groups, and most infants exhibit backward arching of the neck (retrocollis) and trunk (opisthotonos) (Fig. 35-10). The fever may be caused by diencephalic involvement. The advanced phase is characterized by pronounced retrocollis-opisthotonos, shrill cry, refusal to feed, apnea, fever, deep stupor to coma, and sometimes seizures and death (51,123,124).

TABLE 35-9
MAJOR CLINICAL FEATURES OF ACUTE BILIRUBIN ENCEPHALOPATHY

Initial phase
  Slight stupor ("lethargic," "sleepy")
  Slight hypotonia, paucity of movement
  Poor sucking; slightly high-pitched cry
Intermediate phase
  Moderate stupor—irritable
  Tone variable—usually increased; some with
    retrocollis-opisthotonos
  Minimal feeding; high-pitched cry
Advanced phase
  Deep stupor to coma
  Tone usually increased; some with retrocollis-opisthotonos
  No feeding; shrill cry

From Volpe JJ. Neurology of the newborn. 4th ed. Philadelphia: WB Saunders, 2001, with permission.

Subsequently, usually after 1 week, hypertonia subsides and is replaced by hypotonia. Infants who manifest hypertonia during the second phase almost always develop the clinical features of chronic bilirubin encephalopathy (122,123) although an emergent exchange transfusion might, in some cases, reverse the CNS changes (125). Van Praagh (123) found that those who were consistently neurologically normal during the first week of life never developed the features of chronic encephalopathy, but other investigators found later evidence of brain damage in some infants in whom no, or equivocal, manifestations of kernicterus were apparent in the newborn (Table 35-10) (122,126,127).

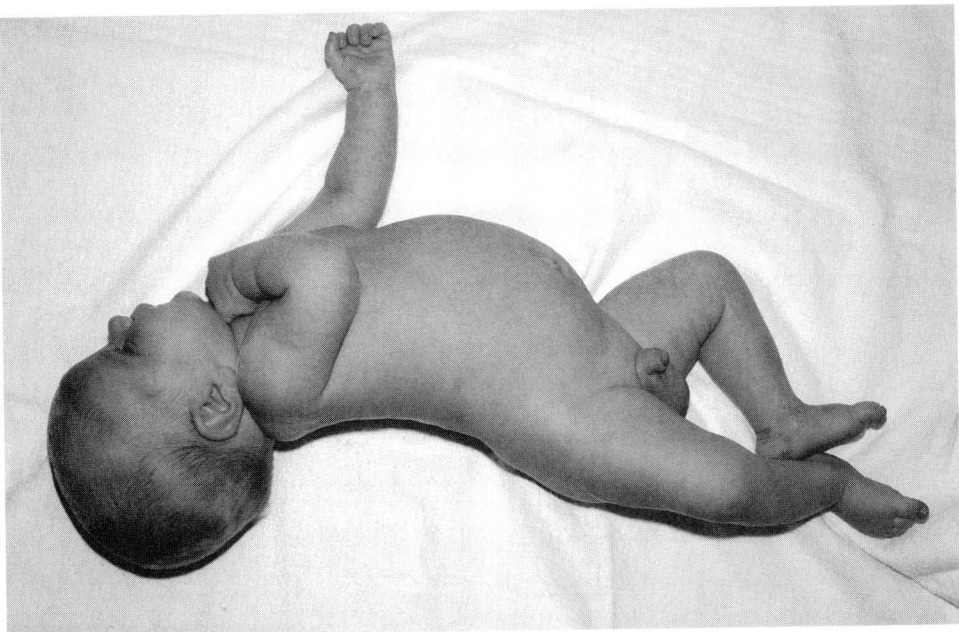

Figure 35-10 This infant presented at age 30 days with a serum bilirubin level of 30 mg/dL (513 μmol/L) secondary to the Crigler-Najjar syndrome type I. He demonstrates retrocollis and opisthotonos, signs of the intermediate to advanced stage of acute bilirubin encephalopathy.

TABLE 35-10

OCCURRENCE OF CLINICAL FEATURES IN ACUTE BILIRUBIN ENCEPHALOPATHY

Clinical Features	Percent (%) of Cases
No definite neurologic signs	15
Equivocal neurologic signs	20–30
Definite neurologic signs	55–65

Adapted from Volpe JJ. Neurology of the newborn. 4th ed. Philadelphia: WB Saunders, 2001; Van Praagh R. Diagnosis of kernicterus in the neonatal period. *Pediatrics* 1961;28:870–876; and Byers RK, Paine RS, Crothers V. Extrapyramidal cerebral palsy with hearing loss following erythroblastosis. *Pediatrics* 1955;15:248.

Kernicterus (Chronic Bilirubin Encephalopathy)

Temporal Evolution

There is a typical temporal evolution of chronic bilirubin encephalopathy after neonatal erythroblastosis fetalis (128). In the first year, infants typically feed poorly, develop a high-pitched cry, and are hypotonic, but have increased deep tendon reflexes, a persistent tonic neck reflex, and motor delay. There is a delay in acquisition of motor skills, although most infants walk alone by 5 years of age. The other typical features of chronic bilirubin encephalopathy usually are not apparent before 1 year of age and often not for several years (51). These children generally are hypotonic at rest for the first 6 or 7 years. By the time they reach their teens, hypertonia has replaced hypotonia (129).

Clinical Features

The classic sequelae of posticteric encephalopathy constitute a tetrad consisting of extrapyramidal disturbances, auditory abnormalities, gaze palsies, and dental dysplasia (Table 35-11) (129).

Extrapyramidal Disturbances

Athetosis (i.e., involuntary, sinuous, writhing movements) may develop as early as 18 months of age, but may be delayed until as late as 8 or 9 years of age (128). If sufficiently severe, athetosis may prevent useful limb function. These movements are described as "uncontrollable, purposeless,

TABLE 35-11

MAJOR CLINICAL FEATURES OF CHRONIC POSTKERNICTERIC BILIRUBIN ENCEPHALOPATHY

Extrapyramidal abnormalities, especially athetosis
Gaze abnormalities, especially of upward gaze
Auditory disturbance, especially sensorineural hearing loss
Intellectual deficits, but minority in mentally retarded range

From Volpe JJ. Neurology of the newborn. 4th ed. Philadelphia: WB Saunders, 2001, with permission.

involuntary, and incoordinate. They may be rapid and jerky (choreiform), slow and worm-like (orthodox athetosis), or so slowed by hypertonicity that the patient may assume momentarily fixed attitudes with stiffness of the extremities (dystonia)" (129). Occasionally, extrapyramidal rigidity may predominate, rather than involuntary motion. In the opinion of Perlstein (129), "the absence of athetosis or of other forms of extrapyramidal dyskinesia, makes the diagnosis of post-icteric encephalopathy dubious, if not untenable." Severely affected children also may have dysarthria, facial grimacing, drooling, and difficulty chewing and swallowing.

Auditory Abnormalities

Some degree of hearing loss is often found in children with kernicterus. Pathologic studies and studies of BAERs indicate that injury to the brainstem, specifically to the cochlear nuclei, is the principal cause of hearing loss, although occasional studies suggest possible involvement of the peripheral auditory system as well (39,73,117,130). It is noteworthy that in some frequently quoted studies, virtually all of the infants who developed severe hearing loss had received prophylactic streptomycin (an ototoxic antibiotic) prior to exchange transfusion (126,131).

Hearing loss is generally most severe in the high frequencies, and an association between moderate hyperbilirubinemia and subsequent sensorineural hearing loss has been described in low-birth-weight infants (see Clinical Sequelae of Hyperbilirubinemia below).

Auditory neuropathy, or auditory dyssynchrony is a recently described entity that is functionally defined as abnormal or absent BAER with normal inner ear function as tested by cochlear microphonic responses or otoacoustic emissions (132). The inner ear or cochlea is normal but the ascending auditory pathway in the nerve or brainstem is abnormal (132). Shapiro has diagnosed auditory neuropathy in ten children with classical kernicterus (132).

Gaze Abnormalities

There may be limitation of upward gaze and other gaze abnormalities although full vertical eye movements during the doll's-eye maneuver are attained in most affected children. This suggests that the lesion is above the level of the oculomotor nuclei (51). Some patients have paralytic gaze palsies. Supranuclear palsies can be explained by bilirubin deposition and neuronal injury in the rostral midbrain, and nuclear palsies can be explained by damage to the oculomotor nuclei (39).

Dental Dysplasia

Approximately 75% of kernicterus children with posticteric encephalopathy have some degree of dental enamel hypoplasia. A smaller percentage have green discoloration of the teeth (129).

Magnetic Resonance Imaging

The diagnosis of acute bilirubin encephalopathy and kernicterus can now be confirmed by magnetic resonance

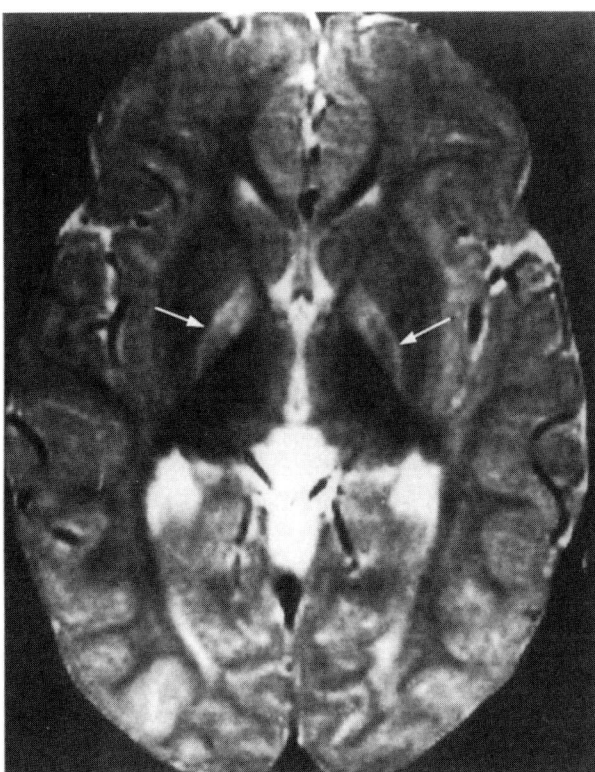

Figure 35-11 Magnetic resonance imaging scan of a 21-month-old male infant who had erythroblastosis fetalis and presented with extreme hyperbilirubinemia and clinical signs of kernicterus at age 54 hours. Note the symmetric, abnormally high-intensity signal from the area of the globus pallidus on both sides (*arrows*). (From Grobler JM, Mercer MJ. Kernicterus associated with elevated predominantly direct-reacting bilirubin. *S Afr Med J* 1997;87:146, with permission.)

imaging (MRI) (133–137). The most characteristic image is a bilateral, symmetric, high-intensity signal in the globus pallidus seen on both T_1- and T_2-weighted images (Fig. 35-11), although it should be noted that similar findings in the globus pallidi have been described in mitochondrial disorders and in pyruvate dehydrogenase deficiency (138). High signal intensity also has been seen in the hippocampus and the thalamus (133). We do not yet know the natural history or time course of the MRI changes of kernicterus, how early these changes will occur, and whether or not they are seen in every case. They have been seen in an 8-day-old infant as well as in a 12-year-old child with a history of severe neonatal jaundice (133,134).

CLINICAL SEQUELAE OF HYPERBILIRUBINEMIA

Although there is no doubt about the relationship between elevated TSB levels and brain damage, the ability of a single peak bilirubin level to predict long-term neurodevelopmental outcomes is poor (139,140). In addition, our conclusions regarding hyperbilirubinemia and neurodevelopmental outcomes are limited by the quality of the published data. In many case reports of kernicterus, analyzed in detail by Ip and associates (139,140), it is impossible to know if the putative

peak TSB levels (measured in some cases more than 7 days after birth) were true peak levels, and many cohort studies have significant problems with blinding of the examiners and dropouts (139–141). For a detailed analysis of the published literature from 1966 to 2001 dealing with these issues, see the evidence reports of Ip and associates (139,140).

Hsia and colleagues (142) and Mollison and Cutbush (143) first established the link between bilirubin levels and brain damage in the early 1950s, when they demonstrated that the risk of kernicterus in infants with Rh hemolytic disease increased dramatically with rising bilirubin levels and that exchange transfusion could markedly reduce the risk. Subsequent studies suggested that, in untreated infants with hemolytic disease, the incidence of kernicterus was much higher than the incidence in markedly jaundiced infants without hemolytic disease (144,145). For many years, there has been considerable disagreement about how jaundice in infants without hemolytic disease should be treated (144–149). Some investigators have described clinical and pathologic kernicterus in premature infants who did not have hemolytic disease and whose TSB levels were well below 20 mg/dL (342 μmol/L) (150,151). In some small, sick infants, yellow staining of the brain was seen at autopsy, with TSB levels less than 10 mg/dL (171 μmol/L) (151). In addition, the finding that gross bilirubin staining of the brain can occur in the absence of the typical microscopic neuronal damage described with kernicterus called into question the meaning of yellow staining of the brain in some very-low-birth-weight infants (46). Unlike the classic form of fatal kernicterus, these very-low-birth-weight infants, although they may have had kernicterus, died of other causes.

Starting in 1967 and continuing into the late 1970s, reports from the Collaborative Perinatal Project (CPP), a study of 53,000 pregnant women and their offspring, linked moderate elevations of neonatal serum bilirubin to lower developmental scores, lower IQ scores, and increased risk of neurologic abnormalities (152). These findings occurred at TSB levels previously presumed to be safe and suggested that acute bilirubin encephalopathy or classic kernicterus was only the most obvious and extreme manifestation of a spectrum of bilirubin toxicity. At the other end of the spectrum might lie more subtle forms of neurotoxicity that occur at much lower bilirubin levels and in the absence of any obvious abnormal clinical findings in the neonatal period; there are some data to support this view (140).

The following section deals with the clinical sequelae of hyperbilirubinemia in different groups of infants.

Rh Hemolytic Disease of the Newborn

In the only controlled clinical trial conducted on the treatment of hemolytic disease of the newborn, Mollison and Walker (153) demonstrated beyond reasonable doubt that exchange transfusion in these infants improved their chance of survival and decreased the risk of fatal kernicterus. The results of these studies, combined with subsequent uncontrolled observations, established exchange transfusion as the standard treatment for preventing kernicterus in infants with erythroblastosis fetalis and showed that kernicterus was unlikely to occur if TSB levels were kept below 20 mg/dL (342 µmol/L), an observation that has been amply confirmed by subsequent experience with the treatment of hemolytic disease (142,143). It is interesting to recall, however, that these studies were performed on infants born in the late 1940s and early 1950s. These infants were commonly asphyxiated and seriously ill, and many were delivered prematurely to prevent stillbirth. Streptomycin, an ototoxic drug was frequently administered to those who received exchange transfusions.

Hsia and associates (142) reported that the incidence of kernicterus in their infants was 8% for those with TSB levels of 19 to 24 mg/dL (325 to 410 µmol/L), 33% for TSB levels of 25 to 29 mg/dL (428 to 496 µmol/L), and 73% for those with bilirubin levels higher than 30 mg/dL (513 µmol/L). Later experience with Rh hemolytic disease was far more encouraging. Johnston and associates (126) studied 129 infants born between 1957 and 1958, all of whom had *indirect-reacting* serum bilirubin levels higher than 20 mg/dL (342 µmol/L). Ninety-two infants with Rh hemolytic disease were followed to age 5 to 6 years and evaluated with detailed psychometric, neurologic, and audiologic evaluations. One of 92 infants had a minimal sensorineural hearing loss (and a normal IQ) and 1 infant had mild athetosis, moderate sensorineural hearing loss, and a normal IQ. Thus, the risk of bilirubin encephalopathy in infants with Rh disease born from 1957 to 1958 with indirect-reacting bilirubin levels higher than 20 mg/dL (342 µmol/L) was 2 of 92 or approximately 2% (126).

In a study of full-term Turkish infants (154), those who had Coombs-positive ABO incompatibility or Rh immunization had a greater risk (vs. infants without hemolytic disease) of neurologic abnormalities and lower IQ scores when their indirect-reacting bilirubin levels exceeded 20 mg/dL (342 µmol/L). These data reinforce the belief that hemolysis is an important risk factor in bilirubin-dependent brain damage. The risk of neurologic abnormalities also was associated with the duration of indirect-reacting hyperbilirubinemia higher than 20 mg/dL (342 µmol/L). In those exposed to these bilirubin levels for less than 6 hours, the incidence of neurologic abnormalities was 2.3%. This increased to 18.7% if the exposure lasted 6 to 11 hours and to 26% with 12 or more hours of exposure (154). These data support earlier observations suggesting that the duration of hyperbilirubinemia is related to the risk of long-term neurodevelopmental outcome (155). It is difficult to define the risk of abnormal outcomes in infants with hemolysis from causes such as red cell membrane defects and glucose-6-phosphate dehydrogenase (G6PD) deficiency, although the risk of bilirubin encephalopathy in G6PD deficiency appears to be similar to that of Rh hemolytic disease (156).

Full-Term and Near-Term Infants Without Hemolysis

Two issues in neonatal medicine that consistently generate controversy are the relationship between hyperbilirubin-

emia and adverse developmental outcome in nonhemolyzing newborns and the indications for treating these infants. These issues are addressed in multiple studies and the reader is referred to extensive reviews for details of the individual studies (124,139,140,144,152). When carefully analyzed, the data tend to demonstrate that, in otherwise healthy neonates without hemolytic disease, TSB levels that do not exceed approximately 25 mg/dL (428 µmol/L) are very unlikely to place these infants at risk of adverse neurodevelopmental consequences. Specifically, in many large studies there has been no convincing demonstration of any adverse effect of such serum bilirubin levels on IQs, definite neurologic abnormalities, or sensorineural hearing loss (124,139,140,144,152).

No studies have looked specifically at infants who are 35 to 37 weeks of gestation, although the data analyzed by Ip and associates (139,140) includes infants of of 34 weeks and older (139,140). In the very large CPP, the study population included all infants with birth weights ≥2,500 g (145,152, 157). Presumably some of these infants were in the 34- to 37-weeks' gestational age category. There are insufficient followup data on infants who had TSB levels of 25 to 30 mg/dL (292 to 513 µmol/L) to draw firm conclusions about this group. Nevertheless, a 21-month followup of 26 Coombs-negative, healthy, term infants with TSB levels of 26.2 to 46.3 mg/dL (446 to 788 µmol/L) revealed no neurodevelopmental abnormalities and no hearing loss (158). Newman identified 11 infants out of 111,009 infants born between 1995 and 1998 with TSB levels ≥30 mg/dL (513 µmol/L); 5 were 35 to 37 weeks' gestation and 5 were 38 to 39 weeks' gestation. They were followed for 1.5 to 5 years and none had neurologic or developmental problems (159).

When they combined both abnormal and suspicious neurologic examination results, Newman and Klebanoff (160), in their analysis of the CPP, did demonstrate a significant increase in abnormalities associated with increasing bilirubin levels. The "suspicious" abnormalities included nonspecific gait abnormalities, awkwardness, an equivocal Babinski reflex, abnormal cremasteric reflex, abnormal abdominal reflex, failure of stereognosis, questionable hypotonia, and gaze abnormalities. The most frequent abnormal findings were awkwardness and abnormal cremasteric reflexes. When the abnormal and suspiciously abnormal children were combined, the risk of abnormalities increased from 14.9% for those whose TSB levels were less than 10.0 mg/dL (171 µmol/L) to 22.4% for those whose TSB levels exceeded 20 mg/dL (340 µmol/L). Because 41,324 infants were enrolled in this study, these differences were statistically highly significant, but this finding should be kept in perspective. Even if the relationship between these findings is causal, we have no evidence that the use of a bilirubin-lowering intervention, such as phototherapy, at these low bilirubin levels would affect the outcome. Finally, as Newman and Klebanoff (160) point out, even if bilirubin levels had been prevented from exceeding 10 mg/dL (171 µmol/L) in every infant, the expected rate of abnormal or suspicious neurologic examination results would only decline from 15.13% to 14.85%.

Less-reassuring information is provided by a study of a group of Israeli army draftees (n = 1,948) in which their preinduction psychological and physical examinations at age 17 years were matched with their newborn bilirubin levels. Seidman and associates (161) found an association between the risk of an IQ below 85 and a TSB level higher than 20 mg/dL (342 μmol/L) in full-term boys (but not with girls) with a negative Coombs test ($p = 0.01$). On the other hand, no association was found between bilirubin levels and mean IQ score, the risk of physical or neurologic abnormality, or hearing loss. In a subsequent analysis of a similar population, Seidman and colleagues (162) found no increase in the risk of an IQ less than 85 with TSB levels higher than 20 mg/dL (342 μmol/L).

Two studies raised concerns regarding "soft signs" of neurologic dysfunction in infants exposed to moderate levels of bilirubin (163,164). In a study performed in the Netherlands, the investigators prospectively evaluated 20 jaundiced infants whose TSB levels ranged from 13.6 to 26 mg/dL (233 to 444 μmol/L) and compared them with a control group of 20, healthy, nonjaundiced infants matched for sex and gestational age (164). At age 1 year, 5 of 8 (63%) infants with TSB levels between 19.6 and 26 mg/dL (335 and 444 μmol/L) demonstrated minor abnormalities in muscle tone and posture compared with 0 of 20 control infants (p < 0.001). In a German study, children at 7 years of age whose neonatal TSB levels had exceeded 20 mg/dL (342 μmol/L) scored significantly worse on a scale designed to measure choreiform and athetoid movements. In that study 8 of 16 (50%) children in the hyperbilirubinemia group versus 3 of 18 (17%) in the control group had abnormal scores (data not found in the original paper but kindly provided by the authors) (141,163). The sample sizes in both the Dutch and German studies were small, but the effect sizes were large. Nevertheless, the outcome measurements are subjective and the blinding was not rigorous.

In a much earlier study, Johnson and Boggs followed 83 infants for 4 years and found abnormal neurologic examinations in 14 of 68 (21%) children whose indirect-reacting bilirubin levels were ≥15 mg/dL (257 μmol/L) versus 0 of 15 in those with TSB levels less than 15 mg/dL (155) (1 tail p = 0.047). Of the 14 children, 11 had "minimal cerebral dysfunction" and 3 had other abnormal signs, including fine and gross motor delay, athetoid movements, and mild mental retardation (it is not stated how many of the 3 infants had some or all of these findings). In that study, however, 53% of the infants had hemolytic disease and 33% were premature, and there is no mention of whether or not the followup evaluations were performed in a blinded fashion (155).

Comorbid Factors and Outcome

In term and near-term infants, there appears to be an increase in the likelihood of neurologic damage if hyperbilirubinemia is accompanied by other risk factors (43,139,140). The risk factors commonly listed include isoimmune hemolytic disease, prematurity, G6PD deficiency, asphyxia, sepsis, acidosis, and hypoalbuminemia (Table 35-12) (139,140).

In the CPP population, Naeye found that infants who were exposed to chorioamnionitis prior to delivery had a higher incidence of low IQ scores and neurologic abnormalities at age 7 years in relationship to increasing bilirubin levels than did those infants who were not exposed to chorioamnionitis (165).

It is long been believed that infants with hemolytic disease are at a greater risk for bilirubin-related brain damage than are those infants who do not have hemolysis. This applies to Rh and ABO hemolytic disease, as well as to G6PD deficiency. Notwithstanding the general agreement on this subject, the data supporting this conclusion are not very strong, nor is there any documented mechanism that explains why a serum bilirubin level of 20 mg/dL in an infant with hemolytic disease should be more dangerous than the same level in an infant without hemolysis. For example, there is no evidence of any difference in the binding of bilirubin to albumin in infants with hemolytic disease as compared with those who are not hemolyzing. Nevertheless, the consensus among experts is that infants who have hemolytic disease should be treated more aggressively than those who do not.

Bilirubin Binding Capacity, Kernicterus, and Developmental Outcome

Because bilirubin that is "free" or loosely bound to albumin is more likely to cross the blood–brain barrier (see Bilirubin Chemistry and Neurotoxicity and Blood–Brain and Blood–Cerebrospinal Fluid Barriers above), our ability to predict the risk of bilirubin encephalopathy might be improved by measurement of unbound bilirubin or the reserve albumin binding capacity. A reduced albumin-binding capacity has been associated with abnormal developmental outcome in some studies (155,166) but not in others (167), although such associations have been found between free bilirubin levels and abnormalities in the BAER (70,71,73,168). Elevated free bilirubin concentrations have also been found in preterm infants with kernicterus (44,72,77,169). Currently there are no bilirubin-binding tests in routine clinical use in the United States, although a semiautomated peroxidase method has been used in Japan (71,73) and a modification of this technique developed in the United States (68). Nevertheless, there are no long-term studies of the developmental outcome of infants in whom binding measurements have been obtained with this technique.

Duration of Hyperbilirubinemia

A relationship has been described between neurologic and psychometric abnormalities and the duration of exposure to TSB levels higher than 15 mg/dL (154,155,166). Many

TABLE 35-12

SUMMARY OF 88 CASE REPORTS OF TERM AND NEAR-TERM (GESTATIONAL AGE ≥34 WEEKS) INFANTS WITH COMORBID FACTORS WHO HAD CLINICAL SIGNS OF ACUTE OR CHRONIC BILIRUBIN ENCEPHALPATHY OR KERNICTERUS DIAGNOSED AT AUTOPSY

	Diagnosis of Kernicterus							
	Clinical							
Comorbidity	Acute Phase Without Followup	Acute Phase but Normal Followup	Chronic Sequelae	Autopsy	Total (N)	Mean Peak TSB ± SD (Range), mg/dL	Mean BW ± SD[a] (Range), g	Gender
ABO incompatibility	6	0	12	1[b]	19	31.6 ± 8.2 (19.0–51.0)	3,118 ± 680 (2,270–4,313)	6 females, 11 males, 2 unknown
Rh incompatibility	3	2	27	1	33	32.1 ± 7.1 (17.7–46.0)	3,063 ± 387 (2,300–3,969)	5 females, 4 males, 24 unknown
G6PD deficiency	10	0	1	2	13	31.8 ± 8.5 (23.0–50.0)	3,353 ± 437 (2,700–4,100)	2 males, 11 unknown
Sepsis or infections	3	1	4	5	13	31.8 ± 9.9 (14.5–47.8)	3,368 ± 586 (2,580–4,360)	7 females, 4 males, 2 unknown
Multiple conditions	3	0	4	3	10	29.1 ± 16.1 (4.0–49.2)	2,913 ± 750 (1,780–3,686)	3 females, 4 males, 3 unknown
Total	25	3	48	12	88	31.6 ± 9.0 (4.0–51.0)	3,155 ± 534 (1,780–4,360)	20 females, 25 males, 42 unknown

BW, birth weight; G6PD, glucose-6-phosphate dehydrogenase; TSB, total serum bilirubin.
[a] Contain some missing data.
[b] This infant had acute phase of kernicterus and chronic kernicterus sequelae and then died at the age of 19 months.
From Ip S, Chung M, Kulig J, et al. An evidence-based review of important issues concerning neonatal hyperbilirubinemia. *Pediatrics* 2004;114:e130–e153, with permission.

of the infants in these studies were either premature or had hemolytic disease. In a Turkish study, exposure to TSB levels greater than 20 mg/dL (342 μmol/L) for less than 6 hours was associated with a 2.3% incidence of neurologic abnormalities. This increased to 18.7% if exposure lasted 6 to 11 hours, and to 26% with 12 or more hours of exposure (154). In the large NICHHD collaborative phototherapy trial, a 6-year followup of 224 control infants who did not receive phototherapy and who had birth weights of less than 2,000 g showed no association between IQ and duration of exposure to bilirubin (170).

An 18-year followup of 55 boys with a history of neonatal hyperbilirubinemia (greater than 15 mg/dL [257 μmol/ L]) was performed in Norway at the time of military draft physical examinations (171). Compared with the total cohort of Norwegian conscripts, there were no significant differences revealed on physical examination or tests of vision, hearing, or IQ. However, seven boys who had a history of positive Coombs tests and bilirubin in excess of 15 mg/ dL (257 μmol/L) for more than 5 days had significantly lower IQ scores than the national average.

Hearing Loss and Audiometric Evoked Responses

The BAER test is an accurate and noninvasive means of assessing the functional status of the auditory nerve and the brainstem auditory pathway. Figure 35-12 shows the BAER tracing of a normal full-term infant. The three positive waveforms labeled in the figure are those most easily identified in the neonate (118). The latency for wave I represents the peripheral conduction time. Latency of waves III and V and the interpeak latency of waves I to III, III to V, and I to V all represent measurements of central conduction time. The interpeak latency I to V is referred to as the brainstem conduction time. Reports also include ampli-

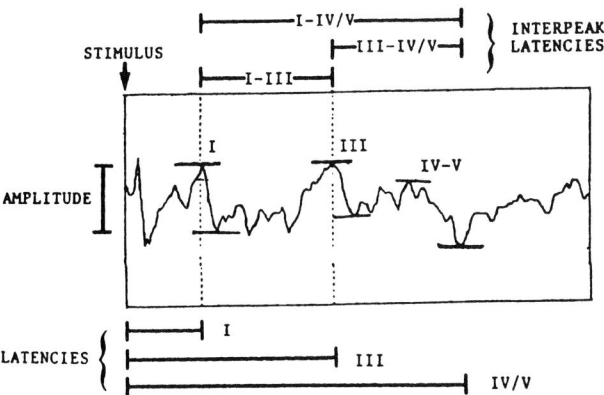

Figure 35-12 A typical tracing of brainstem auditory evoked response has various components. Wave I reflects the response of the peripheral auditory nerve; wave III reflects the superior olive; waves IV to V reflect the inferior colliculus with peak and trough shown. Wave I peak to waves IV to V trough (i.e., interpeak latency) reflects brainstem conduction time. (From Vohr BR. New approaches to assessing the risks of hyperbilirubinemia. *Clin Perinatol* 1990;17:293–306, with permission.)

tudes of the waveforms. These may decrease or be lost in response to various insults.

Several studies have documented a relationship between TSB levels and the BAER (118,132,172), and the acute changes seen in the BAER can be reversed by lowering the TSB level with phototherapy or exchange transfusion (118). Abnormalities of the BAER are more closely related to unbound bilirubin levels than to TSB level (70,71,73,168), but there are no studies relating abnormalities in the BAER to long-term outcome.

Despite evidence for bilirubin damage to the auditory pathway in full-term and preterm infants with classical kernicterus, there is virtually no evidence for a risk of hearing loss related to hyperbilirubinemia in full-term infants who do not have hemolytic disease (152,161,170,173). In a study of almost 17,000 children who received complete hearing and speech evaluations at 8 years of age, the incidence of sensorineural hearing loss in those who had TSB levels 20 mg/dL (342 μmol/L) or higher was 2.2%, and it was also 2.2% in those whose TSB levels were less than 20 mg/dL (342 μmol/L) (152). In the NICHHD phototherapy study, the incidence of sensorineural hearing loss in children followed to age 6 years was identical in the phototherapy and control groups (1.8% vs. 1.9%) (167). Remarkably, in a followup of 36 children with the Crigler-Najjar syndrome, none had evidence of sensorineural hearing loss (173).

Nevertheless, deficits in central hearing, speech, and language can occur in the absence of pure-tone hearing loss (174) and these may be manifestations of *auditory neuropathy* or *dyssynchrony* (132). This recently described entity is defined as abnormal or absent BAER with normal inner ear function as tested by cochlear microphonic responses or otoacoustic emissions (132) and has been diagnosed in children with kernicterus (132).

Cry Analysis

An abnormal cry is a sign of neurologic distress and is associated with acute bilirubin encephalopathy (40). Modest degrees of hyperbilirubinemia also affect the infant's cry (116,118).

Infant Behavior

Investigators have used the Brazelton Neonatal Behavioral Assessment Scale to evaluate the effect of hyperbilirubinemia on infant behavior. Most studies show some effect, although several are confounded by the use of phototherapy (118,140). Jaundiced infants score lower than controls in habituation, orientation, motor performance, regulation of state, and autonomic stability (118).

Premature Infants and Low-Bilirubin Kernicterus

Kernicterus and Developmental Outcome

It is generally believed that premature infants are at greater risk of developing kernicterus or bilirubin encephalopathy than are full-term newborns exposed to similar bilirubin levels.

Watchko and Oski (150) provided a detailed historical review of kernicterus in preterm infants from the 1950s, which has been updated (151). Reports during the years 1950 to 1965 suggested that kernicterus or the clinical sequelae of hyperbilirubinemia were unlikely to develop if exchange transfusions were used to maintain TSB levels below 18 to 22 mg/dL (308 to 376 μmol/L) (150). However, most of the infants in these studies were larger (1,250 to 2,500 g) and more mature (28 to 36 weeks of gestation) than the extremely low-birth-weight infants currently seen in NICUs.

Between 1958 and 1972, a group of studies reported the occurrence of kernicterus at TSB levels well below 20 mg/dL (342 μmol/L) (150). In general, these infants were significantly more premature and of much lower birth weight than those previously observed with kernicterus. Some were exposed to sulfisoxazole, which previously was shown in a controlled trial to be a powerful displacer of bilirubin from its binding to albumin (63,175). As a result of these findings, exchange transfusion in preterm infants was recommended at TSB levels of less than 20 mg/dL (342 μmol/L). Publication of data from the CPP that suggested an association between impaired psychomotor performance and TSB levels higher than 10 to 14 mg/dL (171 to 239 μmol/L) in low-birth-weight infants provided additional support for these recommendations (165,176).

In the NICHHD cooperative phototherapy study (1974 to 1976), infants were randomly assigned to a control group that received no phototherapy or to a group that received phototherapy at predetermined TSB levels. The criteria for exchange transfusion for all infants mandated exchange transfusions at low levels of serum bilirubin (10 mg/dL [171 μmol/L] in high-risk newborns with birth weights less than 1,250 g) (177). Kernicterus was found in 4 of 76 autopsied infants whose birth weights ranged from 760 to 1,270 g (47). Their peak TSB levels ranged from 6.5 to 14.2 mg/dL (111 to 243 μmol/L). All were asphyxiated or had hyaline membrane disease, and all had some degree of periventricular-intraventricular hemorrhage (PIVH). Two had periventricular leukomalacia (PVL) (47).

Surviving infants in the study were followed and evaluated at 6 years of age with the Wechsler Verbal and Performance IQ test. No differences were found between the control and phototherapy groups in the incidence of definite and suspect cerebral palsy, clumsy or abnormal movements, hypotonia, or an IQ lower than 70. There were no differences between the two groups in growth, speech, hearing loss, or evidence of hyperactivity (170).

Scheidt and colleagues (167) also published a 6-year followup of 224 control children from the NICHHD study whose birth weights were lower than 2,000 g. None of these infants received phototherapy, but bilirubin levels were maintained below specified levels by the use of exchange transfusion. No relation was found between serum bilirubin levels and the incidence of cerebral palsy, nor was there any association between maximal bilirubin level and IQ. IQ was not associated with mean bilirubin

level, time and duration of exposure to bilirubin, or measures of bilirubin–albumin binding (167).

Two studies reviewed the risk factors previously suggested to predict the development of kernicterus. They were unable to identify any risk factor or group of factors that was associated with the development of kernicterus in the premature neonate, including birth weight less than 1,500 g, hypothermia, asphyxia, acidosis, hypoalbuminemia, sepsis, meningitis, drug therapy, and TSB levels (178,179).

It is likely that there are some risk factors for the development of kernicterus that are unknown. An excellent example of this possibility was the report from one NICU of an abrupt decrease in kernicterus at autopsy in premature infants. The incidence of kernicterus fell from 31% to 0% when the practice of flushing intravenous catheters with bacteriostatic saline that contained benzyl alcohol was stopped (89). In an earlier study from the same NICU, the incidence of kernicterus diagnosed postmortem among neonates of 25 to 32 weeks of gestation was a remarkably high 25% (39). Benzyl alcohol is an agent that increases membrane fluidity and may facilitate the passage of bilirubin into the brain (55). At the same institution, Watchko and Claasen (160) found only three cases of kernicterus in 72 autopsies performed from 1984 through 1991 on newborns of less than 34 weeks of gestation who lived at least 48 hours. In the 69 newborns who did not have kernicterus, the peak TSB level ranged from 6.3 to 20.6 mg/dL (108 to 352 μmol/L), and 56% had peak TSB values higher than those suggested for exchange transfusion by the NICHHD phototherapy study guidelines (160). This sustained decrease in the incidence of kernicterus confirms the experience in most nurseries that kernicterus in premature newborns is now rare, although it has not disappeared completely.

Sugama and associates documented the surprising observation of the presence of hypotonia and (in one infant) choreoathetosis together with the classical MRI findings of kernicterus in two preterm infants at 31 and 34 weeks gestation (136). Neither of these infants was acutely ill and their TSB levels were 13.1 mg/dL (224 μmol/L) and 14.7 mg/dL (251 μmol/L), respectively (136). Govaert and associates reported MRI findings in five preterm and three term infants with kernicterus. The TSB levels in the term infants ranged from 37.0 to 44.6 mg/dL (632 to 763 μmol/ L), but in the preterm infants (25 to 29 weeks' gestation) peak TSB levels ranged from 8.7 to 11.9 mg/dL (148 to 204 μmol/L). Serum albumin levels in these preterm infants were strikingly low (1.4 to 2.1 g/dL).

Several recent studies have failed to document an association between maximal TSB levels and developmental outcomes in very-low-birth-weight infants (180–183). van de Bor and colleagues (184) found a relation between maximal TSB concentrations in the neonatal period and cerebral palsy (not of the type characteristically found with kernicterus) at a corrected age of 2 years. No relation was found between maximal TSB concentrations and hearing defects. However, in a followup of the same population at 5 years, no significant difference was found in mean maximal TSB concentrations between children with and without handicaps (180) although there was an association between TSB levels and handicap in children who had suffered a grade I intracranial hemorrhage. This effect was not seen in the more severe hemorrhages, but the number of infants with severe hemorrhages was small.

Although these data are reassuring, few of the infants in the reported studies had markedly elevated bilirubin levels (180–183). Most recently, however, peak TSB levels were associated with an increased risk of death, hearing loss and neurodevelopmental impairment in extremely low-birth-weight (ELBW) infants born between 1994 and 1997 (185). Although these associations were statistically significant, the effect sizes were very small. The data in all of these observational studies must be treated with caution because of the multifactorial nature of the causes of adverse neurologic sequelae, the possibility of compounding effects of variables on outcomes, and the difficulty inherent in fully controlling for these variables in such studies.

Some studies suggest an association between hyperbilirubinemia and cystic PVL in low-birth-weight infants (186–188), but others have not found this association (183). Despite the associations described (all from multiple significance testing with the resultant possibility of spurious conclusions), it is unlikely that hyperbilirubinemia is causally related to cystic PVL. PVL is primarily an ischemic lesion, most likely caused by hypoperfusion of the periventricular white matter. Bilirubin normally is not deposited in the periventricular region and primarily is toxic to neurons and not the glial elements that predominate in the periventricular white matter.

Significant associations between peak TSB levels and hearing loss have been documented in low-birth-weight (LBW) infants (189–191) and confirmed recently in a population of ELBW infants (185).

Because of the known role of bilirubin as a powerful antioxidant and the fact that more than 90% of ELBW infants receive phototherapy, the NICHHD neonatal research network has initiated a prospective randomized trial to compare aggressive with conservative phototherapy in a population of ELBW infants (192) (see section on Treatment). The results of this study should provide important information about the association between low TSB levels and developmental outcomes in ELBW infants, as well as the risks and benefits of phototherapy in this highly vulnerable population.

Thus, although kernicterus is currently a very rare event in premature infants hospitalized in NICUs, it is still occurring. Data from the NICHHD trial that is in progress at the time of this writing should be of immense help in guiding our management of the jaundiced ELBW infant (192).

Until further information is available, there seems good reason to believe that the very-low-birth-weight (VLBW) infant's brain is more susceptible to damage from a number of sources and, given that preterm infants have lower serum albumin levels and less-effective albumin binding and are much more likely to be sick than are full-term infants, it makes sense to take a more aggressive approach to maintaining low bilirubin levels in this population (137,185).

Hyperbilirubinemia and Pulmonary Hemorrhage

Studies from the late 1940s and early 1950s suggested an association between pulmonary hemorrhage and kernicterus (90,193,194). All of the infants described died of severe erythroblastosis fetalis. We know that these infants were profoundly anemic, had marked hypoalbuminemia, thrombocytopenia, and disturbances of coagulation, and occasionally were hydropic. It is not surprising that some of these infants developed hemorrhagic pulmonary edema. In an autopsy series of low-birth-weight infants with kernicterus, pulmonary hemorrhage was not found more frequently in the kernicteric infants when compared with those who did not have kernicterus (63). In animal studies, the infusion of bilirubin led to circulatory collapse and anoxia and an increased incidence of hemorrhage, including pulmonary hemorrhages (100). On the other hand, kernicteric Gunn rats showed a significantly lower prevalence of pulmonary hemorrhage when compared with nonkernicteric animals, although the kernicteric group had significantly higher bilirubin levels (195).

THE CLINICAL APPROACH TO THE JAUNDICED NEWBORN

Epidemiology of Neonatal Hyperbilirubinemia

An important first step in the diagnosis and management of any jaundiced newborn is an understanding of the factors that normally affect neonatal bilirubin levels (Table 35-13). Some of these factors have been identified only in large epidemiologic studies and their clinical relevance is questionable, but there are some (designated by asterisks in Table 35-13) that repeatedly have an important influence on TSB levels.

Genetic, Ethnic, and Familial Influences

East Asian and Native American infants have mean maximal TSB concentrations that are significantly higher than those of white infants (196–201). Increased bilirubin production appears to be one factor contributing to the hyperbilirubinemia in these infants (200). In a Hispanic (primarily Mexican) population, 31% of infants had TSB levels greater than 15 mg/dL (202) compared with 3% to 10% of infants in other populations (203,204). Black infants in the United States and Great Britain have lower TSB levels than white infants (197,198,205,206). Neonatal jaundice runs in families (207,208). In a study of 3,301 infants, Khoury and associates (207) found that if a previous sibling had a TSB level higher than 12 mg/dL (205 μmol/L) or higher than 15 mg/dL (257 μmol/L), the risk of similar TSB levels in subsequent siblings was 3.1 and 12.5 times greater, respectively, than in siblings of infants who did not have that degree of jaundice.

TABLE 35-13
EPIDEMIOLOGY OF NEONATAL JAUNDICE

Associated Factors	Effect on Neonatal Serum Bilirubin Levels		
	Increase	Decrease	No Effect
Race	East Asian* Native American Greek Hispanic (Mexican)*	African American*	
Genetic or familial Maternal	Previous sibling with jaundice* Primipara (?) Maternal age ≥25 years Diabetes (if infant macrosomic) Hypertension Oral contraceptive use at time of conception First-trimester bleeding Decreased plasma zinc level	Smoking	
Drugs administered to mother	Oxytocin Diazepam Epidural anesthesia Promethazine	Phenobarbital Meperidine Reserpine Aspirin Chloral hydrate Heroin Phenytoin Antipyrine Alcohol	β-Adrenergic agents
Labor and delivery	Premature rupture of membranes		Fetal distress Low Apgar scores
Infant	Forceps delivery Vacuum extraction* Breech delivery Decreasing gestation* Male gender* Delayed cord clamping Elevated cord blood bilirubin level Jaundice observed before discharge Predischarge TSB level in higher risk zones (Fig. 35.20) Cephalhematoma or bruising* Delayed meconium passage Breast-feeding* Caloric deprivation* Larger weight loss after birth* Low serum zinc and magnesium	Gestation ≥41 weeks* Formula feeding*	
Drugs administered to infant	Chloral hydrate		
Other	Pancuronium Altitude Short hospital stay after birth*		

* Most relevant clinical factors.

Maternal Factors

Smoking

Some studies suggest that infants of mothers who smoke during pregnancy have lower serum bilirubin levels than infants of nonsmokers (197,209), but others have not found this (210,211). These data are confounded by the fact that women who smoke are much less likely to breast-feed, and the likelihood of breast-feeding is inversely related to the number of cigarettes smoked per day (212).

Diabetes

Macrosomic infants of insulin-dependent diabetic mothers are more likely to become jaundiced than are control infants (213). This most likely is the result of an increase in bilirubin production, which is directly related to the degree of macrosomia in these infants (214). These infants have high erythropoietin levels and evidence of increased erythropoiesis, so that ineffective erythropoiesis and polycythemia probably are responsible for the increased bilirubin production (215,216). In addition, diabetic mothers have three times more β-glucuronidase in their breast milk than nondiabetic mothers (216). This enzyme enhances the enterohepatic reabsorption of bilirubin (see Breast-Feeding and Jaundice below).

Events During Labor and Delivery

Induction and Augmentation of Labor by Oxytocin. Multiple studies and several controlled trials have shown an association between the use of oxytocin to induce or augment labor and an increased incidence of neonatal hyperbilirubinemia, although the mechanism for this is unclear (217,218).

Anesthesia and Analgesia. Several studies associate epidural anesthesia, specifically, bupivacaine, with neonatal jaundice (211,219,220). These agents readily cross the placenta and produce measurable levels in the new born (221).

Other Drugs. Tocolytics did not affect neonatal carboxyhemoglobin levels or the need for phototherapy (222,223).

The administration of narcotic agents, barbiturates, aspirin, chloral hydrate, reserpine, and phenytoin sodium to mothers was associated with lower TSB concentrations in their infants, whereas the use of diazepam increased TSB levels by less than 1 mg/dL (224). Antipyrine administered to the mother before delivery decreased TSB levels, and infants of heroin-addicted mothers have lower TSB levels (225). Phenobarbital, if given in sufficient doses to the mother, significantly lowers TSB levels during the first week (217,226).

Delivery Mode. Vaginally delivered term newborns have higher TSB levels than those delivered by cesarean section (227), although this was not found in a controlled trial involving low-birth-weight infants (228). When compared with forceps delivery, the use of vacuum extraction does not increase the number of babies who require phototherapy, although more clinical jaundice is seen with vacuum extraction (229,230).

Placental Transfusion and Hyperviscosity. Although a high hematocrit often is considered a risk factor for neonatal jaundice, controlled trials of an intervention for infants with symptomatic hyperviscosity using partial exchange transfusions showed no differences in the incidence of hyperbilirubinemia in the treated and control groups (231–233). In one study, infants were held 30 cm below the introitus after delivery. If cord clamping was delayed, the mean TSB level at age 72 hours was 7.7 mg/dL (132 μmol/ L) compared with 3.2 mg/dL (55 μmol/L) in the early clamped group (234).

Cord Blood Bilirubin Levels. More than 50 years ago, Davidson and associates (235) found an association between bilirubin levels in cord blood and later neonatal bilirubin concentrations. This observation has been confirmed in infants with and without hemolytic disease (236–238).

Neonatal Factors

Birth Weight and Gestation
Low birth weight and decreasing gestational age are strongly correlated with an increased risk of hyperbilirubinemia (197,206,211,239–241). So-called "near-term" infants of 35 to 38 weeks' gestation are at significantly greater risk of hyperbilirubinemia than are full-term infants (206,211,239,241). Compared with infants at 40 weeks' gestation, infants of 36 to 38 weeks of gestation are 7 to 8 times, and those who are less than 36 weeks are 13 times, more likely to be readmitted to the hospital with severe hyperbilirubinemia (241).

Gender
As a group, male infants consistently have higher bilirubin levels than females (206,211,240–242).

Caloric Intake and Weight Loss
Decreased caloric intake is associated with an increase in serum bilirubin in animals and humans (32). The primary mechanism responsible for this appears to be an increase in the enterohepatic circulation of bilirubin (32,33). A significant association also exists between hyperbilirubinemia and weight loss in the first few days after birth (211, 240–242).

Type of Diet
Infants fed a casein-hydrolysate formula had significantly lower TSB levels from days 10 through 18 than did those infants fed standard casein or whey-predominant formulas (243). The cumulative stool output of the infants fed the casein-hydrolysate was lower than that of the infants fed the other formulas, suggesting that factors other than stool output and its effect on the enterohepatic circulation must explain these observations.

Breast-Feeding and Jaundice
Multiple studies over the last 25 years have found a strong association between breast-feeding and an increased incidence of neonatal hyperbilirubinemia (Figs. 35-13 and 35-14) (244). Although occasional studies have not found this (245,246), a pooled analysis of 12 studies of more than 8,000 newborns showed that breast-fed infants were three times more likely to develop TSB levels of 12 mg/dL (205 μmol) or higher and six times more likely to develop levels of 15 mg/dL (257 μmol) or higher than formula-fed infants (Fig. 35-14) (247). Ninety percent or more of

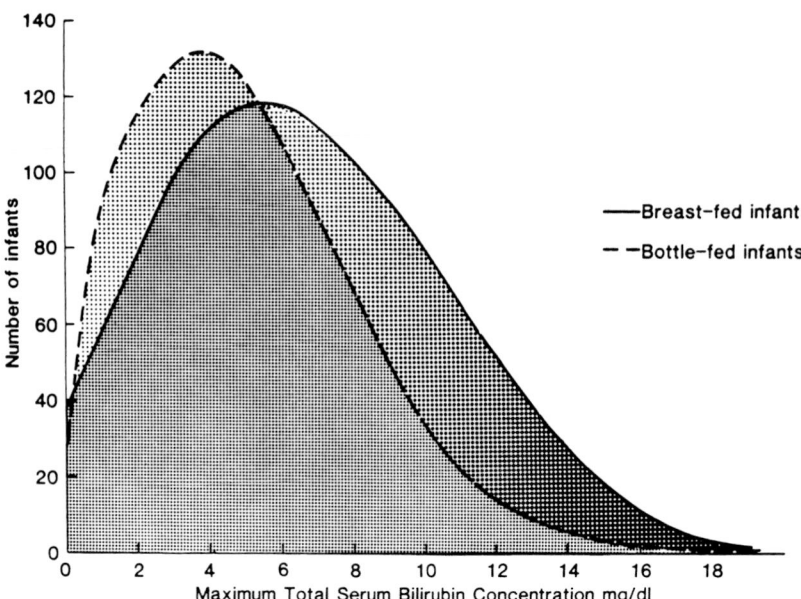

Figure 35-13 Distribution of maximum serum bilirubin concentrations in 1,260 breast-fed and 1,026 formula-fed white newborns with birth weights >2,500 g. TSB levels were measured in every infant on the second or third hospital day and repeated if the concentration exceeded 12.9 mg/dL (221 μmol/L). (From Maisels MJ, Gifford K. Normal serum bilirubin levels in the newborn and the effect of breast feeding. *Pediatrics* 1986;78: 837–843, with permission.)

infants readmitted to hospital in the first 2 weeks of life because of severe hyperbilirubinemia are fully or partially breast-fed (239,241,248,249). In a northern California population, exclusively breast-fed infants were six times more likely than formula-fed infants to develop a TSB greater than 25 mg/dL (428 μmol/L) (206). Of 61 term and near-term infants with kernicterus, 59 were breast-fed (124) (the 2 formula-fed infants were G6PD deficient).

There is some debate about the studies listed above and the data illustrated in Fig. 35-13 (250). Some studies show no differences in TSB levels between formula-fed and breast-fed infants in the first few days after birth. Bertini and associates (246) studied infants in their well baby nursery. Formula supplementation was given to breast-fed infants if a weight loss was considered to be excessive (≥4% after 24 hours, ≥8% after 48 hours, or ≥10% after 72 hours). The investigators found a positive correlation between TSB levels greater than 12.9 mg/dL (221 μmol/L), weight loss after birth, and breast-feeding requiring supplementation with formula. Breast-feeding, *per se* was not associated with hyperbilirubinemia. They concluded that infants who are successfully breast-fed and therefore lose little weight, are not more likely to be jaundiced than formula-fed infants, whereas those who required formula supplementation because of excess weight loss were more likely to be jaundiced. This supports an important role for caloric intake in the development of jaundice and has led some experts to categorize jaundice associated with breast-feeding in the first days after birth as "starvation jaundice" or "breast-nonfeeding jaundice" (250). The implication is that if breast-fed infants were nursed effectively from birth, they would not be more jaundiced than formula-fed infants and there is evidence to support this view (246,251,252).

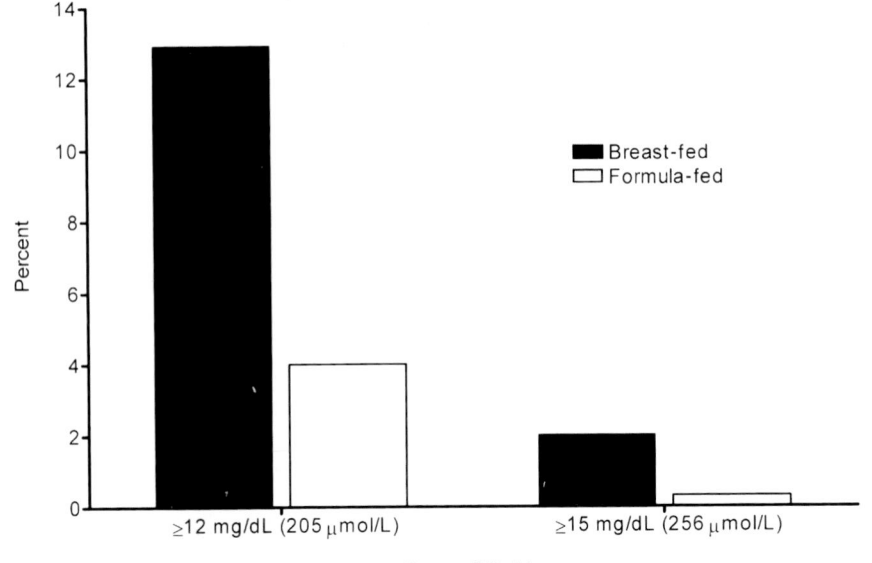

Figure 35-14 Pooled analysis of 12 studies showing the percent of newborns with serum bilirubin levels ≥12mg/dL (205 μmol/L) in breast-fed and formula-fed newborns and, in 6 of the 12 studies, the percent of newborns with serum bilirubin levels ≥15 mg/dL (256 μmol/L) (From Schneider AP. Breast milk jaundice in the newborn. A real entity. *JAMA* 1986;255:3270–3274, with permission.)

Jaundice associated with breast-feeding in the first 2 to 4 days of age has been called "the breast-feeding jaundice syndrome" or "breast-feeding-associated jaundice," and that which appears later (onset at 4 to 7 days of age and prolonged jaundice) has been called the "breast milk jaundice syndrome" (253). There is considerable overlap between these two entities, and evidence to support two distinct syndromes is meager, although calorie deprivation appears to play a major role in the early type of jaundice. In addition to having higher TSB levels in the first 3 to 5 days (see Fig. 35-13) (254), as a group, breast-fed infants have TSB levels that are higher than formula-fed infants for at least 3 to 6 weeks (243,255,256). These are the same infants who have high bilirubin levels in the first week of life, and it is hard to believe that those who are still jaundiced at age 2 to 3 weeks represent a distinct group.

Prolonged indirect-reacting hyperbilirubinemia (beyond 2 to 3 weeks) occurs in 20% to 30% of all breast-feeding infants and, in some infants, may persist for up to 3 months (257). TSB levels were measured at age 28 to 33 days in 282 healthy, breast-fed Turkish infants that were 37 weeks' gestation or older. The TSB was greater than 5 mg/dL (85 µmol/L) in 20.2% and greater than 10 mg/dL (171 µmol/L) in 6% of the infants. (258) Recent evidence suggests that in some infants mutations of the UGT1A1 gene (Gilbert syndrome) play a role in the pathogenesis of this hyperbilirubinemia (259,260).

Pathogenesis of Jaundice Associated with Breast-Feeding. Factors that play a role in the pathophysiology of jaundice associated with breast-feeding are reviewed in detail elsewhere (28,244,253) and are listed in Table 35-14. The primary mechanism for jaundice in the breast-fed infant appears to be an increase in the enterohepatic circulation of bilirubin. Some authors suggest an additional role for inhibitory substances in breast milk, but the data regarding their contribution are conflicting (244).

Intestinal Reabsorption of Bilirubin. Intestinal reabsorption of bilirubin (the enterohepatic circulation) appears to be the most important mechanism responsible for the jaundice associated with breast-feeding (244). Breast-fed infants take in fewer calories than formula-fed

TABLE 35-14
PATHOGENESIS OF JAUNDICE ASSOCIATED WITH BREAST-FEEDING

Increased enterohepatic circulation of bilirubin
  Decreased caloric intake
  Less cumulative stool output and stools contain less bilirubin (compared with formula-fed infants)
  Increased intestinal fat absorption
  Less formation of urobilin in gastrointestinal tract
  Increased activity of β-glucuronidase in breast milk
Mutations of the UGT1A1 gene (Gilbert syndrome)—prolonged breast milk jaundice

infants in the first days after birth and a relationship between decreased caloric intake and an increase in the enterohepatic circulation of bilirubin has been shown (32,33). Breast-fed infants produce lower-weight individual stools, their cumulative stool output (by weight) is lower (243), and their stools contain less bilirubin than those of formula-fed infants (28,261). An increase in stool excretion in the first 21 days is associated with lower TSB levels and in the first 3 weeks, infants fed human milk pass significantly less stool than do infants who are fed casein-predominant formulas (243). Infants fed casein-hydrolysate formulas pass less stool, cumulatively, than those given whey- or casein-predominant formulas (243).

The relationship between fecal bilirubin excretion and TSB levels may be related to the fecal excretion of unabsorbed fat (262). Unconjugated bilirubin apparently associates with unabsorbed fat in the intestinal lumen. When Gunn rats were fed orlistat, a substance that inhibits lipase, they excreted more fat in their stools and their TSB levels were significantly lower (31). This suggests that a substance that increases fecal excretion of fat will decrease the enterohepatic absorption of unconjugated bilirubin and facilitate bilirubin excretion in the gut. Breast-fed infants have higher fat absorption than formula-fed infants (possibly related to the presence of bile salt-stimulated lipase in human milk [263]). It is possible that hyperbilirubinemia could be prevented or mitigated by the administration of orlistat to newborns (31,262). All of these findings support a major role for the enterohepatic circulation in the jaundice associated with breast-feeding.

Urobilinogen Formation. In adults, bilirubin in the gut is reduced rapidly by the action of colonic bacteria to urobilinogen. At birth, the fetal gut is sterile, and although there is an increase in the bacterial content of the gut after delivery, the neonatal intestinal flora do not convert conjugated bilirubin to urobilin. This leaves bilirubin in the bowel and allows it to be deconjugated and thus available for reabsorption. Formula-fed infants excrete urobilin in their stools earlier than breast-fed infants do, perhaps as a consequence of the effect of formula feeding on the intestinal flora (264). Thus, the effect of breast milk on intestinal flora, by slowing the formation of urobilin, further enhances the possibility of intestinal reabsorption of bilirubin.

β-Glucuronidase. β-Glucuronidase is an enzyme that cleaves the ester linkage of bilirubin glucuronide, producing unconjugated bilirubin, which can then be reabsorbed through the gut. Significant concentrations of β-glucuronidase are found in the neonatal intestine, and its activity is higher in human milk than in infant formulas (244).

Gourley and Arend (265) found a positive relation between TSB levels and breast milk β-glucuronidase activity in the first 3 to 4 days after birth, but other researchers have not been able to confirm these findings (257,266).

Meconium Passage

Because the enterohepatic circulation of bilirubin is an important contributor to neonatal hyperbilirubinemia, increasing the rate of bilirubin evacuation from the bowel should decrease the incidence of neonatal jaundice. Two randomized studies showed that the early passage of meconium (stimulated by a rectal thermometer or a suppository) reduced peak TSB levels by about 1 mg/dL (17 μmol) when compared with control groups (267,268).

Phenolic Detergents

The use of phenolic detergents to disinfect incubators and other nursery surfaces was associated with an epidemic of neonatal hyperbilirubinemia in two hospitals (269,270). These detergents should not be used in the nursery.

Altitude

Infants born 3,100 m above sea level are four times more likely to have a bilirubin level above 12 mg/dL (205 μmol/L) than are those born at sea level (271). Both short- and long-term exposure to high altitudes increases TSB levels in adults. The possible mechanisms for these observations include an increase in bilirubin load because of high hematocrits and impaired conjugation and excretion of bilirubin (272–274).

Drugs Administered to the Infant

The use of pancuronium and chloral hydrate in the neonate are associated with an increased risk of hyperbilirubinemia (275–277). Chloral hydrate is metabolized to trichloroa- cetic acrid and the toxic trichloroethanol, both of which accumulate in the tissues of compromised infants. The administration of chloral hydrate is associated with both indirect-reacting and direct-reacting hyperbilirubinemia (276).

Free-Radical Production

Bilirubin appears to have an important physiologic function as an antioxidant and may play a role in the prevention of oxidative membrane damage *in vivo* (see *Physiologic Role of Bilirubin* below) (278). Infants with circulatory failure, sepsis, aspiration syndromes, and asphyxia—conditions believed to enhance free-radical production—had a significantly lower daily rise in mean TSB levels than control infants (279). These finding are consistent with the hypothesis that bilirubin is a free-radical scavenger and is consumed as an antioxidant.

JAUNDICE IN THE HEALTHY NEWBORN

Cord Bilirubin Levels

Mean bilirubin levels in cord blood range from 1.4 to 1.9 mg/dL (24 to 32 μmol/L) (235,280,281), and elevated cord bilirubin levels are associated with an increased risk of hyperbilirubinemia (235,237,280,281).

Normal Serum Bilirubin Levels and the Natural History of Neonatal Jaundice

It is difficult to agree on what represents a "normal bilirubin level" in the term and near-term infant. TSB levels vary considerably, depending on the racial composition of the population, the incidence of breast-feeding, and other genetic and epidemiologic factors (see Table 35-13 and Fig. 35-15). An additional important factor is the large variation found in the laboratory measurements of serum bilirubin, a problem that has been recognized for four decades and currently is unresolved (282–284) (see Laboratory Measurements of Bilirubin below).

Reference to Fig. 35-15 gives some idea of the range of mean bilirubin values found in different populations and the natural history of neonatal jaundice. Since the advent of exchange transfusion and, more recently, phototherapy, it has been impossible to obtain a true picture of the natural history of neonatal bilirubinemia because we treat some infants with rising TSB levels in the first 72 to 96 hours so that what we see is, ultimately, a "damped" picture. Recognizing these limitations, however, some recent studies have helped to clarify the picture (285,286).

An important change in the United States population has been the dramatic increase in breast-feeding at hospital discharge, from 30% in the 1960s to 65% in 2001 (287). In some hospitals, 85% or more of mothers are nursing their

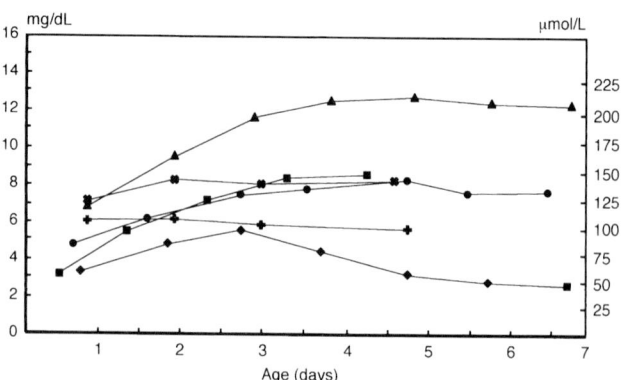

Figure 35-15 Mean total daily bilirubin concentrations in normal full-term and near-term infants. ▲, Fifty healthy Japanese newborn infants, 37 to 42 weeks of gestation, all breast-fed. Excludes Rh and ABO incompatibility (292). ✕, One hundred seventy-six term breast-fed Canadian infants. Excludes Rh hemolytic disease, but includes nine ABO incompatible infants with positive Coombs tests. Seventeen infants received phototherapy. +, One hundred sixty-four Canadian term formula-fed infants, seven ABO incompatible with positive Coombs tests, and three who received phototherapy (280). ■, One thousand eighty-seven term Israeli infants, 78% fully or partially breast-fed (Siedman D, personal communication, 1998) ●, Fifty-six Nigerian term appropriate for gestational age infants. Excludes ABO or Rh incompatibility and G6PD deficiency. Infants were "largely breast-fed" (291). (◆), Twenty-nine full-term American infants, all formula-fed, approximately 50% African American and 50% white (30).

infants on discharge from the hospital. Data from the CPP conducted from 1955 to 1961 (when 30% or fewer mothers breast-fed their infants) and more recent studies (254) found that approximately 95% of all infants had a TSB concentration that did not exceed 12.9 mg/dL (215 μmol/L), and this (95th percentile) became the accepted upper limit of "physiologic jaundice" (205).

More recent data suggest that these values no longer define normal TSB levels in the newborn population (203,288,289). We now see more jaundiced babies, and the TSB levels found in the normal population are significantly higher than previously reported. Three recent studies provide consistent information regarding the upper limits of TSB levels found in the normal population. In a study of 2,840 infants, all of whom had at least one TSB level measured after discharge from hospital, the 95th percentile was a level of 17.5 mg/dL (300 μmol/L) (289). This population was 43% white, 41% black, and 4% Asian; 59% of infants were fully or partially breast-fed. In 11 Kaiser Permanente Northern California Hospitals, the 95th percentile was a TSB level of 17.5 mg/dL (298 μmol/L) (203). In a multicenter study of infants 36 weeks or older in nurseries in the United States, Hong Kong, Japan, and Israel, 2 SD above the mean for the peak TSB levels at 96 ± 6.5 hours was 17 mg/dL (291 μmol/L), and the 95th percentile was 15.5 mg/dL (265 μmol/L) (290). The consistency of these data suggests that we can now accept that the upper limit of "normal" in diverse populations is a TSB level of about 17 to 18 mg/dL (291 to 308 μmol/L). This implies that a 4- to 5-day-old breast-fed infant whose TSB level is 15 to 16 mg/dL (291 μmol/L) does not require any laboratory investigation to find out *why* the infant is jaundiced, although followup is necessary to ensure that the bilirubin levels do not become excessive (289). Data from studies of predominantly breast-fed infants suggest that the normal mean peak TSB level is approximately 8 to 9 mg/dL (137 to 154 μmol/L) (240,280,290,291). In the international, multicenter study, the mean TSB level at 96 ± 6.5 hours was 9.3 mg/dL (290).

In the Japanese population (292) and in other populations of predominantly breast-fed infants, it is clear that the TSB levels are substantially higher, reach their peak later, and remain elevated for much longer than in formula-fed infants. No significant decline in TSB is seen in any of these populations until after the fifth day (see Fig. 35-15).

Figure 35-16 shows "idealized" smoothed curves based on the data from a number of studies that provide a guide to the expected course of bilirubin levels in a primarily breast-fed (60% to 70%) western population (203,235,240, 242,280,289,290). Recognizing all of the limitations to these data already discussed, Fig. 35-16 should be useful for plotting the course of jaundice in an infant and using the velocity of the increase in TSB to make decisions about evaluation, follow-up, and potential intervention.

Bhutani and associates developed a nomogram that defines predischarge risk zones for the subsequent development of hyperbilirubinemia (289) (see Preventing

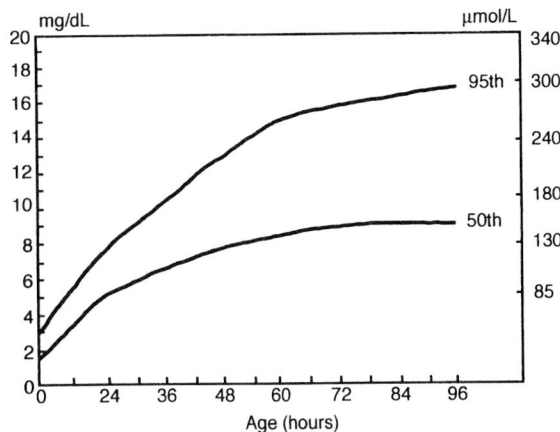

Figure 35-16 Smoothed curves from studies in diverse populations illustrating the expected velocity of total serum bilirubin (TSB) levels and approximate values for the 50th and 95th percentiles. Data for cord blood values come from the studies of Davidson and associates (235) and Saigal and associates (280), values in the first 12 hours are from Frishberg and associates (242), and subsequent values are from Bhutani (289), Seidman (personal communication, 1998), Maisels and associates (290), and Wood and associates (240). Data for the 95th percentile are primarily obtained from the data of Bhutani and associates (289), but also from the studies of Newman and associates (203), and Maisels and associates (290). These data represent values that might be expected in a western, predominantly breast-fed (60% to 70%) population. In view of the significant variations in different populations (see Fig. 35-15), as well as the variations found in laboratory measurement (282,283), the values provided should be used only as rough guidelines. Nevertheless, this graph can be useful in plotting the course of neonatal jaundice, because it will demonstrate when the velocity of the TSB increase deviates significantly from the curves shown. *Note that the values must be plotted according to the infant's age in hours, not days.* Infants who have values that exceed the 95th percentile deserve an evaluation to determine a potential cause for the jaundice, and they require careful surveillance and followup to prevent the development of extreme hyperbilirubinemia. Infants who have none of the epidemiologic risk factors for hyperbilirubinemia (see Table 35-13) but who have TSB values that approach the upper percentiles, also should receive closer scrutiny. Conversely, those whose values fall well below the 50th percentile probably require minimal surveillance and followup for jaundice (289).

Extreme Hyperbilirubinemia and Kernicterus below). Because of sampling bias, however, this nomogram probably does not describe the natural history of bilirubinemia in the newborn (293), although it is a very useful tool for predicting the risk of subsequent hyperbilirubinemia (289) and is recommended by the AAP for this purpose.

PATHOLOGIC CAUSES OF JAUNDICE

Indirect-reacting Hyperbilirubinemia

Table 35-15 lists the causes of pathologic indirect-reacting hyperbilirubinemia in the neonate and Table 35-16 lists the causes of direct-reacting hyperbilirubinemia (cholestatic jaundice). For further discussion of neonatal cholestasis, please see Chapter 40.

TABLE 35-15
CAUSES OF INDIRECT HYPERBILIRUBINEMIA IN NEWBORNS

Increased production or bilirubin load on the liver
  Hemolytic Disease
    Immune mediated
      Rh alloimmunization, ABO and other blood group
        incompatibilities
    Heritable
      Red cell membrane defects
        Hereditary spherocytosis, elliptocytosis,
          pyropoikilocytosis, stomatocytosis
      Red cell enzyme deficiencies
        Glucose-6-phosphate dehydrogenase deficiency,[a]
          pyruvate kinase deficiency, and other erythrocyte
          enzyme deficiencies
      Hemoglobinopathies
        α-Thalassemia, β-thalassemia
      Unstable hemoglobins
        Congenital Heinz body hemolytic anemia
  Other causes of increased production
    Sepsis[a,b]
    Disseminated intravascular coagulation
    Extravasation of blood, hematomas, and pulmonary,
      abdominal, cerebral, or other occult hemorrhage
    Polycythemia
    Macrosomic infants of diabetic mothers
  Increased enterohepatic circulation of bilirubin
    Breast-milk jaundice
    Pyloric stenosis[a]
    Small- or large bowel obstruction or ileus
Decreased Clearance
    Prematurity
    Glucose-6-phosphate dehydrogenase deficiency
  Inborn errors of metabolism
    Crigler-Najjar syndrome, types I and II
    Gilbert syndrome
    Galactosemia[b]
    Tyrosinemia[b]
    Hypermethioninemia[b]
  Metabolic
    Hypothyroidism
    Hypopituitarism[b]

[a] Decreased clearance also part of pathogenesis.
[b] Elevation of direct-reading bilirubin also occurs.

TABLE 35-16
CAUSES OF NEONATAL CHOLESTASIS

Bile duct abnormalities
  Biliary atresia
  Choledochal cyst
  Caroli disease
  Inspissated secretion
  Gallstones
  Spontaneous perforation of bile ducts
  Neonatal sclerosing cholangitis
Infections
  Systemic
    Septicemia
    Urinary tract infection
  Hepatitic
    TORCH (toxoplasmosis, other infections, robella,
      cytomegalovirus, and herpes simplex)
    Echovirus, adenovirus, coxsackievirus
    Human herpes virus-6, varicella-zoster
    HIV, hepatitis B
Inherited and metabolic disorders
  α_1-Antitrypsin deficiency
  Alagille syndrome
  Galactosemia
  Cystic fibrosis
  Niemann-Pick type C
  Progressive familial intrahepatic cholestasis
  Gaucher disease
  Wolman disease
  Tyrosinemia
  Zellweger syndrome
  Carbohydrate-deficient glycoprotein syndrome
  Dubin-Johnson syndrome—deficiency in MRP2 (CMOAT
    [Canalicular multispecific organic anion transporter])
  Rotor syndrome
  Bile acid synthetic disorders
  Aagenaes syndrome
Endocrine disorders
  Hypopituitarism
  Hypothyroidism
  Hypoadrenalism
Chromosomal disorder
  Trisomy 21, 13, 18
  Turner syndrome
Toxic
  Parenteral nutrition
  Chloral hydrate
  Fetal alcohol syndrome
Vascular disorders
  Budd-Chiari syndrome
  Perinatal asphyxia
  Multiple hemangiomata
  Congestive heart failure
Miscellaneous
  Familial hemophagocytic lymphohistiocytosis
  ARC syndrome (arthrogryposis, renal tubular dysfunction, and
    cholestasis)

From McKiernan P. Neonatal cholestasis. *Semin Neonatol* 2002;7:53–165, with permission.

Increased Bilirubin Load: Hemolytic Disease

Immune-Mediated Hemolytic Disease

Rh Erythroblastosis Fetalis. *Pathogenesis.* Hemolytic causes of hyperbilirubinemia are discussed fully in Chapter 46. Most cases of Rh immunization are a result of the Rh (D) antigen although alloimmunization can occur to other fetal red cell surface antigens including the other antigens of the Rh blood-group system (c, C, e, E, cc, and Ce) and those belonging to the Kell, Duffy, Kidd, and MNS systems (294–296). Rh alloimmunization occurs when fetal red blood cells from an Rh (D)-positive fetus cross the placenta into the circulation of an Rh-negative mother and less than 0.1 mL of fetal red cells is sufficient to result in

sensitization. Although Kleihauer-Betke measurements indicate that fetal–maternal hemorrhage occurs in 75% of women, more sensitive molecular detection techniques show that fetal red cells enter the maternal circulation in all pregnancies (296). If the Rh-positive fetus is ABO compatible with its mother, the likelihood of Rh immunization is 16%, but it is only 1.5% to 2% if they are ABO incompatible. This is because the fetal ABO-incompatible red blood cells are rapidly destroyed in the maternal circulation, diminishing the opportunity of the Rh antigen to induce an immune response (294). Once a primary immune response to Rh antigen has been mounted, however, ABO incompatibility between the mother and fetus conveys no protection against a secondary immune response (294). The risk of alloimmunization following induced abortion is 4% to 5%, and it is 2% following spontaneous abortion. Other invasive procedures, such as amniocentesis, chorionic villus sampling, and fetal blood sampling, all increase the risk of fetal maternal hemorrhage and, therefore, alloimmunization (296).

The initial response to the foreign antigen in the maternal circulation is for the maternal immune system to produce immunoglobulin (Ig) M antibodies that do not cross the placenta. This response is followed by production of IgG antibodies, which then cross the placental barrier. The secondary immune response to repeat exposure to the Rh antigen produces anti-D IgG antibodies. This response can be induced with as little as 0.03 ml of D-positive red blood cells (297). The degree of Rh sensitization is related to the dose of antigen exposure and, therefore, to the volume of transplacental hemorrhage (294).

Clinical Course. Approximately 50% of affected infants do not require treatment; they are mildly anemic at birth and never develop severe hyperbilirubinemia. Approximately 25% to 30% will require intervention with phototherapy and/or exchange transfusion and approximately 20% to 25% are so severely affected that they develop hydrops *in utero* (296). About half of this last group become hydropic before 34 weeks' gestation and require direct intravascular fetal transfusion (294). A fetal hematocrit of less than 30% is generally considered an indication for intrauterine transfusion, which is performed, as required, until 34 to 35 weeks' gestation with delivery planned close to term (296).

Prevention of Rh Sensitization. Rh sensitization can almost always be prevented by the administration of Rh immunoglobulin to Rh-negative women at 28 weeks of gestation and again within 72 hours of delivery of an Rh-positive infant (295). In the United States, the dose is 300 µg, but in many other countries it is 100 to 125 µg. If the Kleihauer-Betke test or the fetal red cell assay indicates that there is a transplacental hemorrhage of more than 30 mL of fetal blood (which occurs in 1 in 400 pregnancies) then the dose of Rh (D) immunoglobulin must be at least 10 µg/mL of fetal blood in the maternal circulation (296). Rh immunoglobulin must also be given after abortion or threatened abortion and after amniocentesis or chorionic villus sampling or any other invasive intrauterine procedure. These interventions have dramatically reduced the incidence of erythroblastosis fetalis caused by Rh (D) sensitization, which now has an estimated incidence of about 1 per 1,000 live births (298).

Some laboratories have replaced the Kleihauer-Betke assay with a fetal red blood cell assay (Fetalscreen, Ortho-Clinical Diagnostics, Raritan, NJ) (299). In this assay, an antihemoglobin F antibody is added to the mother's blood to tag hemoglobin F molecules in fetal red cells. Flow cytometry quantifies the number of fetal red cells (of a total of 50,000 maternal cells) so tagged. If less than 0.1% of the maternal cells are tagged it is considered a negative result. Positive results can be quantified to provide the volume of fetal blood in the mother's circulation and the appropriate dose of Rh (D) immunoglobulin to be given.

In mothers who are already sensitized, the administration of intravenous immunoglobulin (IVIg) in early pregnancy has had some benefit in cases of severe fetal alloimmunization (300). The mechanism of action of IVIg appears to involve blockage of Fc receptors on macrophages in the fetal reticuloendothelial system. In one study, fetal survival was 36% higher when high-dose IVIg treatment preceded intrauterine transfusion than it was with transfusion alone (300).

Hydrops Fetalis. The pathogenesis of hydrops fetalis, with its attendant edema and serous effusions, is not clear. It commonly occurs when the fetal hemoglobin drops below 6 to 7 g/dL. The rapid production of severe anemia in fetal sheep produced hydrops associated with an increased central venous pressure and placental edema, whereas the same degree of anemia produced over a longer period did not result in hydrops, placental edema, or an increased central venous pressure (301). In Rh isoimmunization, fetal edema may result from the extensive erythropoiesis that takes place in the fetal liver. This can disrupt the portal circulation and impair albumin synthesis (302,303). Fetuses with severe hydrops also have elevated concentrations of atrial natriuretic factor (304). Hypoxia produces myocardial dysfunction with increased umbilical venous pressure that leads to the release of atrial natriuretic factor (305). Severely affected infants die of progressive cardiorespiratory failure, in which asphyxia and hyaline membrane disease play a major role.

In one hydropic fetus with erythroblastosis fetalis, pulse-Doppler studies of left and right ventricular outputs were obtained over time. Despite severe anemia, cardiac outputs were normal and remained normal after *in utero* percutaneous intravascular transfusions, which reversed the hydrops. These measurements of normal cardiac output *in utero* suggest that high-output failure caused by anemia is not the mechanism for hydrops in these infants and supports the hypothesis that portal hypertension and disruption of normal liver function from extramedullary hematopoiesis is the primary mechanism for the development of hydrops in isoimmune hemolytic disease of the fetus (306).

Treatment of Infants with Rh Hemolytic Disease and Hydrops Fetalis. See sections on Treatment, Phototherapy, and Exchange Transfusion, below.

Late Anemia. A well-known late complication of intrauterine transfusion is the development of anemia in the first months of life. This is commonly seen after about age 2 weeks and is characterized by a persistently low reticulocyte count. Although originally considered to be a hyporegenerative anemia (294,307), there is now some evidence that a decrease in erythropoietin production may not be the primary cause of this late anemia. Recent studies suggest that the anemia is most likely caused by persistence of anti-D antibodies and destruction of red blood cell precursors in the marrow or of reticulocytes in the peripheral circulation (308). In a study of 30 neonates with erythroblastosis, 18 of whom had received intrauterine transfusions and 12 who had not (308), blood samples were analyzed for hemoglobin, erythropoietin, and reticulocytes. As the hemoglobin declined between 10 and 80 postnatal days, there was a matching rise in erythropoietin, which occurred both in infants who had received intrauterine transfusions and those who had not. Thus, intrauterine transfusions, themselves, may not play such an important role in suppressing erythropoiesis. Furthermore, reticulocyte counts remained persistently low despite rising erythropoietin and falling hemoglobin levels. One possible explanation for this is the effect of circulating anti-D antibodies on the erythrocyte precursors in the bone marrow and on the reticulocytes in the peripheral circulation (308).

ABO Hemolytic Disease

Approximately 45% of Americans of western European descent have type O blood, and a similar percentage are type A. Types B and AB make up the balance. African Americans are 50% type O, 29% type A, 17% type B, and 4% AB (309). Hemolytic disease related to ABO incompatibility is generally limited to group A or B infants born to group O mothers, and it tends to run in families. One study found an 88% risk of recurrence of ABO hemolytic disease in ABO incompatible newborns born to parents whose first-born child was similarly affected (310).

In a prospective study of 4,996 consecutive live born infants (311) (Table 35-17), cord blood was analyzed for blood type, hematocrit, and results of the direct antiglobulin test (DAT or Coombs test) and the indirect Coombs test (311). The DAT detects antibodies attached to the red cell, whereas the indirect Coombs test detects IgG antibody in the serum. Only 0.29% of type A, B, or

AB infants who were incompatible with their type A or B mothers had a positive DAT result, whereas 32% of type A or B infants born to type O mothers had positive DATs. A positive DAT was the best predictor of an elevated bilirubin level, but only 20% of infants with a positive DAT developed TSB levels of ≥12.8 mg/dL (224 μmol/L) (311). This large prospective study confirms what was found in other smaller studies: although about one-third of group A or B infants born to group O mothers have anti-A or anti-B antibodies attached to their red cells, only 1 in 5 of those with a positive DAT have a *modest* degree of hyperbilirubinemia.

Consequently, although ABO-incompatible DAT-positive infants are about twice as likely as their compatible peers to have moderate hyperbilirubinemia, severe jaundice in these infants is uncommon (311–315) and ABO hemolytic disease is a relatively rare cause of severe hyperbilirubinemia (Table 35-18).

Diagnosing ABO Hemolytic Disease. There is a wide spectrum of severity in ABO hemolytic disease. Nevertheless, this diagnosis generally should not be made unless there is a positive DAT *and* clinical jaundice within the first 12 to 24 hours. Reticulocytosis and the presence of microspherocytes on the smear help to confirm the diagnosis (Table 35-19).

ABO Incompatibility, Hyperbilirubinemia, and a Negative Direct Antiglobulin Test. Although the epidemiologic data suggest otherwise, most clinicians have seen the occasional ABO-incompatible infant in whom there is an early rising TSB level, yet the DAT is negative. In the past, we have often considered these to be cases of ABO hemolytic disease and have attributed the negative DAT to the technical vicissitudes of Coombs testing in the laboratory. Recent data, however, raise questions about alternative mechanisms.

One obvious possibility is that there is another cause for the hemolysis. Using measurements of end-tidal carbon

---

TABLE 35-17

BILIRUBIN LEVELS IN ABO-INCOMPATIBLE INFANTS ACCORDING TO THE COOMBS TEST

Coombs Test Results	Peak Serum Bilirubin ≥12.8 mg/dL (224 μmol/L)
Direct antiglobulin (Coombs) test positive	46/225 (20.4%)
Indirect Coombs test positive	29/309 (9.4%)
Both tests negative	38/488 (7.8%)

From Ozolek J, Watchko J, Mimouni F. Prevalence and lack of clinical significance of blood group incompatibility in mothers with blood type A or B. *J Pediatr* 1994;125:87–91, with permission.

TABLE 35-18

DISCHARGE DIAGNOSIS IN 306 INFANTS ADMITTED WITH SEVERE HYPERBILIRUBINEMIA[a]

Diagnosis	Number	Percentage
Hyperbilirubinemia of unknown cause or breast-milk jaundice	290	94.8
Cephalhematoma or bruising	3	1.0
ABO hemolytic disease[b]	11	3.6
Anti-E hemolytic disease	1	0.3
Galactosemia	1	0.3
Sepsis	0	0

[a] Infants were readmitted after discharge as newborns. Mean age at admission was 5 days (range, 2 to 17 days), and mean bilirubin level was 18.5 ± 2.8 mg/dL (range, 12.7 to 29.1 mg/dL).
[b] Mother was type O, infant was type A or B, direct Coombs test was positive.
From Maisels MJ, Kring E. Risk of sepsis in newborns with severe hyperbilirubinemia. *Pediatrics* 1992;90:741–743, with permission.

TABLE 35-19

CRITERIA FOR DIAGNOSING ABO HEMOLYTIC DISEASE AS THE CAUSE OF NEONATAL HYPERBILIRUBINEMIA

Mother group O, infant group A or B
  and
Positive DAT
Jaundice appearing within 12–24 hours
Microspherocytes on blood smear
Negative DAT but homozygous for Gilbert's syndrome (317)

monoxide concentration (ETCOc), a direct measurement of heme catabolism, Herschel and associates (316) identified four DAT-negative ABO-incompatible neonates who had elevated ETCOc levels. Further investigation revealed that two of these infants had G6PD deficiency and one had elliptocytosis. Can ABO incompatibility with a negative DAT nevertheless contribute to hyperbilirubinemia? Kaplan and associates (317) found that 43% of DAT-negative, ABO-incompatible infants who were homozygous for the variant UGT promoter associated with Gilbert syndrome, had a TSB level ≥15 mg/dL (256 μmol/L) versus none of the ABO-incompatible DAT-negative infants who were homozygous normal (for the variant promoter) (Fig. 35-17). There was no difference between ABO-incompatible and ABO-compatible DAT-negative newborns, as long as the ABO-incompatible neonates did not have Gilbert syndrome (see Inherited Unconjugated Hyperbilirubinemia). These observations confirm, for the first time, that if another icterogenic factor is present, then ABO-incompatible newborns are at risk for hyperbilirubinemia even if they are DAT negative (317).

Should a blood type and DAT be performed on the cord blood of all infants of group O mothers?

In these days of cost containment, this is a commonly asked question. A recent survey found that 58% of hospital blood banks in the United States were routinely performing Coombs tests and blood typing on newborn cord bloods (318). Approximately 36% of hospitals tested all cord bloods routinely, and 35% tested those of type O or Rh-negative mothers, even though the data suggest that such routine screening is not warranted (311,318). Furthermore, even when such testing is done, there is evidence that it is often ignored by the responsible pediatrician (318,319). The AAP notes that routine cord blood screening for infants of group O, Rh-positive mothers, is an option, but is not required "provided there is appropriate surveillance, and risk assessment before discharge and follow up" (76) so that significantly jaundiced infants are not missed.

Heritable Causes of Hemolysis

Red Cell Membrane Defects

The red cell membrane defects that may produce hemolysis and hyperbilirubinemia in the newborn include *hereditary spherocytosis, elliptocytosis, pyropoikilocytosis, pyknocytosis and stomatocytosis syndromes* (320,321). Detailed descriptions of their clinical presentation and management can be found elsewhere (320–322). The diagnosis of these disorders can be difficult, because newborns commonly exhibit a marked variation in red cell membrane size and shape (322).

In 75% of hereditary spherocytosis patients, inheritance is autosomal dominant so that a positive family history that includes anemia, jaundice, gallstones, and splenectomy can often be elicited. As in G6PD deficiency (see Glucose-6-Phosphate Dehydrogenase Deficiency below), the presence of jaundice severe enough to require phototherapy in newborns with hereditary spherocytosis is strongly related to an interaction with the Gilbert syndrome allele (323). Severe anemia and hydrops fetalis has occurred in

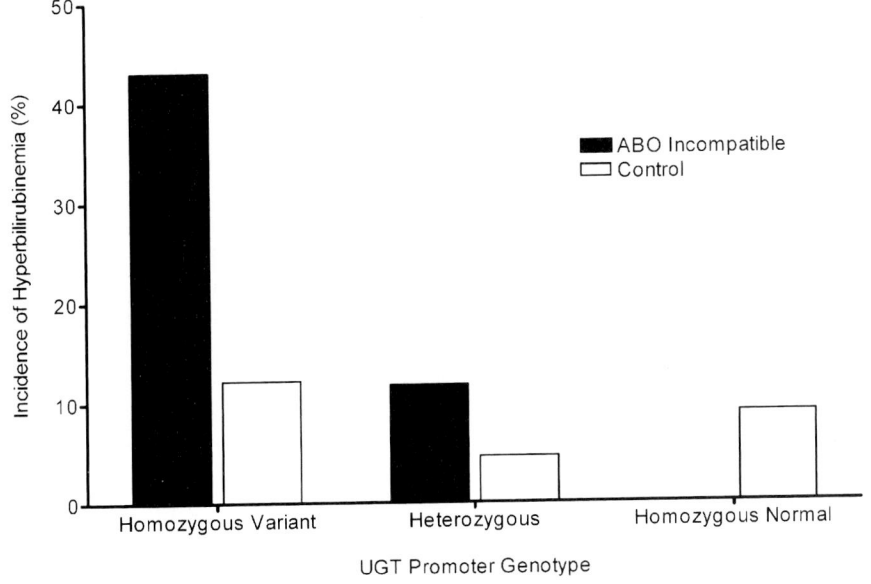

Figure 35-17 Incidence of hyperbilirubinemia defined as TSB ≥15 mg/dL (≥256 μmol/L) in ABO-incompatible and ABO-compatible (control) infants according to the UGT promoter genotype. ABO-incompatible DAT-negative infants who were also homozygous for the variant UGT promoter (Gilbert syndrome) had a significantly higher incidence of hyperbilirubinemia than did ABO-incompatible DAT-negative infants who were homozygous normal for the UGT promoter. The former subgroup also had a significantly greater incidence of hyperbilirubinemia than any of the three UGT promoter genotype subgroups in the control (ABO-compatible) infants. (From Kaplan M, Hammerman C, Renbaum P, et al. Gilbert's syndrome and hyperbilirubinaemia in ABO-incompatible neonates. *Lancet* 2000;356: 652–653, with permission.)

infants with hereditary spherocytosis associated with defective genes for band 3 or spectrin protein (321). The diagnosis can be made using the incubated osmotic fragility test which is a reliable diagnostic tool in newborns when coupled with fetal red cell controls (321,322).

Red Cell Enzyme Deficiencies

Glucose-6-Phosphate Dehydrogenase Deficiency

Epidemiology. G6PD deficiency is the most common, clinically significant, red cell enzyme defect and affects as many as 4,500,000 newborns each year (324). Although known for its prevalence in the populations of the Mediterranean, the Middle East, the Arabian Peninsula, South East Asia, and Africa, immigration and intermarriage have transformed G6PD deficiency into a global problem (156). Nevertheless, most pediatricians in the United States do not think of G6PD deficiency when confronted with a jaundiced infant (325). They should, particularly in black infants. Although African American newborns, as a group, have lower TSB levels than white newborns (197,198, 205,206), G6PD deficiency is found in 11% to 13% of African American newborns. This means that some 32,000 to 39,000 black male G6PD-deficient hemizygote newborns will be born annually in the United States (326), and kernicterus has occurred in some of these infants (124,327– 329). In a recent report, G6PD deficiency was considered to be the cause of hyperbilirubinemia in 19 of 61 (31.5%) infants who developed kernicterus (124).

Clinical Course. Because G6PD deficiency in African American infants is a result of the less-severe Gd A− mutation (326), most of these infants do not develop severe hyperbilirubinemia (326). If subjected to some oxidative stress, however, they can develop acute hemolysis with a sudden increase in the TSB (324). Although previous studies suggested otherwise (326), recent data show that, as a group, black G6PD-deficient infants are significantly more likely than controls to develop hyperbilirubinemia and three times more likely than control infants to require phototherapy (330).

Hemolysis and hyperbilirubinemia in G6PD-deficient neonates can be triggered by exposure to a number of agents (156,324,327). These include naphthalene (found in moth balls), agents for umbilical cord antisepsis, breast milk of a mother who has eaten fava beans (331), and perhaps exposure to a variety of household chemicals (324). Neonatal infection is also a well recognized trigger (156, 332). In most cases, however, no specific triggering agent or condition can be identified and an acute hemolytic event is the exception, rather than the rule (156,333). Most G6PD-deficient neonates have a more gradual onset of hyperbilirubinemia and there is evidence that this hyperbilirubinemia has its origins *in utero* (334).

Pathogenesis of Hyperbilirubinemia in G6PD Deficiency. The G6PD gene (Gd) is located on the X chromosome and hemizygous Gd− males have the full enzyme deficiency and

can be identified by screening tests (324). But female heterozygotes have a wide range of enzyme activity and will frequently be missed by screening tests (335) even though they are also at risk for hyperbilirubinemia (335,336).

In most cases of hyperbilirubinemia in G6PD-deficient neonates, there is no overt evidence of hemolysis such as anemia and reticulocytosis (337,338), although in some populations the usual indices of hemolysis are found (339). Conversely, blood COHb and ETCOc concentrations are consistently elevated in G6PD-deficient infants (339–341). Nevertheless, Kaplan and associates found no difference in COHb levels between hyperbilirubinemic (TSB greater than 15mg/dL [256 μmol/L]) and nonhyperbilirubinemic G6PD-deficient infants (341). These investigators also found that although COHb values were higher in G6PD-deficient neonates than in normal neonates, there was no correlation between TSB levels and COHb values in the G6PD-deficient group (342). All of these observations suggest that while an increase in heme turnover is clearly present in G6PD-deficient neonates, with the exception of those who suffer an acute hemolytic event, hemolysis alone cannot be implicated as the primary mechanism responsible for hyperbilirubinemia.

HPLC measurements of conjugated bilirubin fractions provide an index of the hepatic conjugating capacity. Lower serum conjugated bilirubin fractions relative to serum total bilirubin concentrations indicate diminished conjugating capacity (343). In G6PD-deficient neonates who developed TSB levels greater than 15 mg/dL (256 μmol/L), serum total, mono- and di-conjugated bilirubin fractions were significantly lower than in nonhyperbilirubinemic G6PD-deficient infants (344), suggesting that impaired conjugation plays a role in the pathogenesis of hyperbilirubinemia.

Finally, a remarkable interaction between G6PD deficiency and Gilbert syndrome was demonstrated by Kaplan and associates (345). In this study of Israeli infants, neither the presence of the variant UGT promoter (for Gilbert syndrome) by itself, nor G6PD deficiency alone had a significant effect on the incidence of hyperbilirubinemia (TSB greater than 15 mg/dL [256 μmol/L]), but there was a significant increase in hyperbilirubinemia in G6PD-deficient infants who also had the variant UGT promoter (Fig. 35-18). The incidence of hyperbilirubinemia in G6PD-deficient neonates increased from 9.7% in normal homozygotes to 31.6% in the variant UGT promoter heterozygotes to 50% in homozygotes for the variant promoter. No significant effect of the variant UGT promoter was seen in the G6PD-normal infants (Fig. 35-18). Thus neither G6PD deficiency alone, nor the abnormal UGT promoter alone (Gilbert syndrome), caused an increased incidence of hyperbilirubinemia; both factors were needed to produce a significant increase in TSB levels. It is interesting, however, that in Italian G6PD-deficient neonates, homozygosity for the variant 7/7 promoter did not increase the risk of hyperbilirubinemia (346). Routine screening for G6PD deficiency is currently not performed in the United States, although such screening would be appropriate in the black

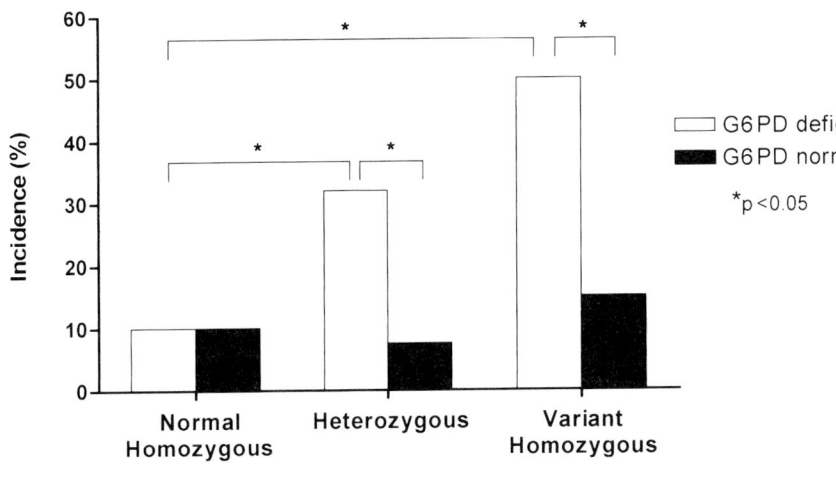

Figure 35-18 Incidence of hyperbilirubinemia, defined as TSB $\geq$ 15.0 mg/dL (256 µmol/L), for G6PD-deficient and control neonates, stratified for the three promoter genotypes of the gene encoding the bilirubin conjugating enzyme UGT1A1. (From Kaplan M, Renbaum P, Levi-Lahad E, et al. Gilbert syndrome and glucose-6-phosphate dehydrogenase deficiency: A dose-dependent genetic interaction crucial to neonatal hyperbilirubinemia. Proc Natl Acad Sci U S A 1997;94:12128–12132, with permission.)

population (326). Table 35-20 summarizes the relationships and mechanisms involved in G6PD deficiency and hyperbilirubinemia.

Treatment. The risk of kernicterus in G6PD-deficient infants with TSB levels above 20 mg/dL (342) µmol/L) appears to be comparable to that associated with Rh disease. Thus, in the presence of G6PD deficiency, more aggressive treatment of these infants is needed (339,347,348).

Pyruvate Kinase Deficiency

This autosomal recessive disorder is less prevalent than G6PD deficiency and, in contrast to G6PD deficiency, typically presents with jaundice, anemia, and reticulocytosis (322). Neonatal hyperbilirubinemia is common and kernicterus has been reported (321). This disorder should be considered in a hyperbilirubinemic neonate with a picture of nonspherocytic, DAT-negative hemolytic anemia (322).

Other Disorders of the Embden-Meyerhof Pathway

Conditions such as *hexokinase deficiency, glucose phosphate isomerase deficiency,* and *phosphofructokinase deficiency* occasionally are associated with hemolysis and neonatal hyperbilirubinemia (321). Jaundice and anemia have also been

---

TABLE 35-20

RESULTS OF STUDIES ON THE PATHOGENESIS OF HYPERBILIRUBINEMIA IN G6PD-DEFICIENT INFANTS

Increased red cell turnover (hemolysis) (339–341) although infants with TSB >15 mg/dL (256 µmol/L) did not have higher COHb levels than those with TSB <15 mg/dL (341)

Decreased conjugating capacity in infants with TSB >15 mg/dL (344)

No increase in TSB >15 mg/dL (vs. G6PD-normal infants) unless deficient infants are also heterozygotes or homozygotes for variant UGT promoter for Gilbert syndrome (345) (found in Israeli but not Italian neonates) (346)

---

described in isolated cases of *2,3-bisphosphoglycerate mutase deficiency* and *phosphoglycerate kinase deficiency* (321).

Hemoglobinopathies

These conditions generally do not present in the newborn period. Fetal hemoglobin (hemoglobin [Hb] F) is composed of alpha (α_2) and gamma (γ_2) chains. *Homozygous α-thalassemia* (complete absence of α chain synthesis) results in profound hemolysis, anemia, hydrops fetalis, and almost always stillbirth or death in the immediate neonatal period (322). As there are no β chains in hemoglobin F, *β-thalassemia* does not manifest itself in neonates. *Sickle cell disease* is asymptomatic in the neonate (349) because of the inhibitory effect of Hb F on Hb S polymerization and cellular sickling (350). The expression of sickle cell disease is thus masked until Hb S levels increase to more than 75% at about 6 months (350).

Extravascular Blood

Cephalhematomas, bruising, intracranial or pulmonary hemorrhage, or any occult bleeding may lead to an elevated TSB level from breakdown of the extravascular erythrocytes (206,351–353). (The catabolism of 1 g of hemoglobin yields 35 mg of bilirubin.) In two reports, severe hyperbilirubinemia followed delayed absorption of intraperitoneal blood in infants who had received intraperitoneal fetal transfusions before birth (351,353). In both reported cases, despite multiple exchange transfusions, hyperbilirubinemia was not controlled until peritoneal lavage was performed. Massive adrenal hemorrhage has also caused severe hyperbilirubinemia (352).

In the VLBW infant, the presence of PIVH is associated with an increase in serum bilirubin levels in some studies (354,355) but not in others (356). Amato and colleagues (356) studied 88 infants with birth weights less than 1,500 g. Phototherapy was initiated only when serum bilirubin levels exceeded 12 mg/dL (205 µmol/L). The incidence of serum bilirubin levels greater than 12 mg/dL was

39% in the PIVH group and 46.8% in the infants without PIVH. There was no difference in the duration of phototherapy in the two groups.

Polycythemia

The catabolism of 1 g of hemoglobin produces 35 mg of bilirubin and it is often assumed that a high hematocrit is a risk factor for neonatal jaundice, because an increase in the erythrocyte mass should increase the bilirubin load presented to the liver. Nevertheless, mean bilirubin levels and the incidence of hyperbilirubinemia were similar in polycythemic infants randomly assigned to receive either partial exchange transfusions or symptomatic treatment (see *Epidemiology of Neonatal Jaundice*) (231–233). In one study, however, infants were held 30 cm below the introitus after delivery. If cord clamping was delayed, the mean TSB level at 72 hours was 7.7 mg/dL (132 µmol/L) compared with 3.2 mg/dL (55 µmol/L) in the early clamped group (234).

Increased Enterohepatic Circulation

(See Physiologic Mechanisms of Neonatal Jaundice, Epidemiology of Neonatal Hyperbilirubinemia, and Breast-feeding and Jaundice for the contribution of the enterohepatic circulation to neonatal jaundice.) Intestinal obstruction or a delay in bowel transit time increases the enterohepatic circulation by decreasing caloric intake and allowing more time for bilirubin deconjugation and reabsorption. Jaundice is common in infants with small-bowel obstruction and occurs in infants with pyloric stenosis (357–359). Correction of the obstruction produces a prompt decline in bilirubin levels.

The pathogenesis of jaundice associated with pyloric stenosis has been debated for many years (358) and it was suggested that caloric deprivation, as well as a decrease in UGT activity, might play an important role (358). In Gilbert syndrome, caloric deprivation produces an increase in TSB levels and a low activity of UGT has been seen in jaundiced infants with pyloric stenosis (358,360). In a report of three formula-fed infants with hypertrophic pyloric stenosis and jaundice (359), two were homozygous for the UGT variant promoter for Gilbert syndrome and one infant was heterozygous for the promoter. These observations confirm a critical role for Gilbert syndrome in the pathogenesis of jaundice associated with pyloric stenosis (see *Gilbert Syndrome* below).

Infants of Diabetic Mothers

Only macrosomic infants of mothers with insulin-dependent diabetes are at increased risk of hyperbilirubinemia (213). This is probably the result of increased bilirubin production (214–216) (see Epidemiology of Neonatal Hyperbilirubinemia: Maternal Factors).

Decreased Bilirubin Clearance

Inherited Unconjugated Hyperbilirubinemia—Inborn Errors of Bilirubin Uridine Diphosphoglucuronate Glucuronosyltransferase Activity

The structure and function of the UGT1A1 gene and the genomics of hyperbilirubinemia have been reviewed in detail (22,23). (See Fig. 35-7 and Structure and Function of the Uridine Diphosphoglucuronate Glucuronosyltransferase 1A1 Gene above) Because a single form of bilirubin UGT accounts for almost all of the bilirubin glucuronidation activity in the human liver, inherited defects of a single enzyme will cause jaundice. Three types of inherited UGT deficiency are recognized.

Crigler Najjar Syndromes. Crigler-Najjar syndromes types I and II (CN-1, CN-2) are caused by one or more mutations in any of the five exons of the UGT1A1 gene (22,23), as well as mutations in the noncoding, intronic region of the gene (see Fig. 35-7 and Table 35-21) (22). More than 30 different genetic mutations have been identified in CN-1 syndrome and the gene frequency for CN-1 is estimated to be 1:1000 (23). Infants with CN-1 have almost

TABLE 35-21
INBORN ERRORS OF HEPATIC BILIRUBIN UGT EXPRESSION

Characteristic	Crigler-Najjar Type 1	Crigler-Najjar Type II (Arias syndrome)	Gilbert Syndrome
Inheritance	Autosomal recessive	Autosomal recessive or dominant	Autosomal dominant or recessive
UGT1 activity	Absent	<10%	50%
Genetics	Nonsense or stop mutation	Missense mutation	Variant promoter
Hyperbilirubinemia	>20 mg/dL	5–15 mg/dL[a]	3–5 mg/dL
Kernicterus	High risk	Low risk[a]	No apparent risk

[a] Marked hyperbilirubinemia can occur in some cases of Arias syndrome, which may place the infant at high risk for kernicterus.
From Watchko JF. Indirect hyperbilirubinemia in the neonate. In: Maisels MJ, Watchko JF, eds. *Neonatal jaundice.* London, UK: Harwood Academic Publishers, 2000:51–66, with permission.

complete absence of bilirubin UGT activity. They develop severe hyperbilirubinemia in the first 2 to 3 days of life and often require exchange transfusion in the first week. Subsequently, intensive home phototherapy controls bilirubin levels to some extent, but as these children get older, increasing skin thickness and pigmentation and a decrease in the surface-area-to-body-mass ratio render phototherapy less effective. A "tanning bed" phototherapy configuration is necessary to obtain adequate irradiance and surface area exposure (see *Phototherapy* below) (361). Brain damage can occur at any time, including adulthood, and plasmapheresis has been used to reduce bilirubin concentrations during acute exacerbations of hyperbilirubinemia (362,363). One 16-year-old boy with CN-1 had 72 plasma exchanges over a period of 28 months before undergoing orthotopic liver transplantation (364). Liver transplantation is currently the only available definitive therapy, and serum bilirubin concentrations decline dramatically within hours of the procedure (365).

Another option is the use of human hepatocyte transplantation (366,367). Because hepatic architecture and function, except for bilirubin UGT activity, are normal in CN-1, transplantation of isolated liver cells is an attractive option. The infusion of hepatocytes (obtained from a donor liver) into the portal vein of a 10-year-old girl with CN-1 decreased TSB levels by 50% (366). Hepatic bilirubin UGT activity increased from 0.4% to 5.5% of mean normal enzyme activity, and more than 30% of the patient's bile pigments were now bilirubin glucuronides. The ultimate treatment of the Crigler-Najjar syndrome, however, lies in the development of effective gene therapy (368), although this has yet to be attempted in a human.

The administration of tin-protoporphyrin and tin-mesoporphyrin to children with CN-1 syndrome (369, 370) reduced TSB levels and the need for phototherapy. Administration of oral calcium phosphate significantly reduced TSB levels in patients with CN-1 who were receiving phototherapy (371).

The diagnosis of Crigler-Najjar syndrome is made by HPLC analysis of serum and duodenal bile, liver biopsy tissue enzyme assay, evaluating the response to phenobarbital (372,373), and by molecular analysis of the UGT1A1 gene (374). In CN-1 disease, phenobarbital has little or no effect on TSB concentrations, whereas in children with CN-2 disease, TSB levels can decrease by 30% to 80% during phenobarbital treatment (375). Phenobarbital acts via a phenobarbital-responsive enhancer module that stimulates the UGT1A1 gene to induce production of glucuronosyltransferase (376). There is now a world registry for the CN-1 syndrome that is a unique source of information about this rare disease (377).

Suresh and Lucey (173) conducted a questionnaire survey of 42 patients ranging in age from 2 months to 21 years who had CN-1. Home phototherapy for 10 to 16 hours, principally at night, was the mainstay of postneonatal therapy. Additional therapies included oral agar, antioxidants, bilirubin oxidase, clofibrate, and cholestyramine, and liver transplantation was performed in 15 of the children. All patients grew normally; in 77% the neurodevelopmental status was normal. Those in school were doing well despite having had TSB levels of 15 to 29 mg/dL (257 to 496 μmol/L) for many years. Although it often is stated that sensorineural hearing loss is the most common form of bilirubin toxicity to the central nervous system, not one of 36 children evaluated had a sensorineural hearing loss, suggesting that bilirubin may not be as ototoxic as commonly believed. In these children it is important to avoid exacerbations of hyperbilirubinemia and to manage intercurrent infections promptly. Albumin infusions and plasmapheresis are effective in dealing with acute exacerbations of jaundice (173,372).

Infants with CN-2 disease (also known as Arias syndrome) generally have less-severe hyperbilirubinemia, although it can occur, and kernicterus has been reported in some infants. There is considerable overlap between CN-1 and CN-2 syndromes. Both infants and adults with CN-2 syndrome respond readily to phenobarbital therapy, with a sharp decline in serum bilirubin levels within 7 to 10 days. This response can be used to differentiate between the two syndromes (372).

Gilbert Syndrome. People with Gilbert syndrome have a mild, benign, chronic or recurrent unconjugated hyperbilirubinemia with no evidence of liver disease or overt hemolysis. There is now evidence, however, that these individuals also have an increase in heme turnover (378) (see below). Gilbert syndrome is common, affecting approximately 6% to 9% of the general population, and both autosomal dominant and recessive patterns of inheritance have been suggested. Typically, the indirect-reacting hyperbilirubinemia is not recognized until after puberty and manifests itself during fasting or intercurrent illness.

The genetic basis for this disorder has been clarified (22,23,379,380) and involves mutations of the UGT1A1 gene promoter (see Fig. 35-7). In whites with Gilbert syndrome there is commonly a variant promoter for the gene encoding UGT1A1. (This is not the case in East Asian populations.) This promoter contains a two base-pair addition (TA) in the TATAA element that gives rise to seven $(TA)_7$ TAA(7/7) rather than the more usual six $(TA)_6$ TAA(6/6) repeats in affected subjects (379). There is an inverse relationship between the number of repeats and the activity of the promoter: as the number of TA repeats increases, UGT activity decreases (379,381). Subjects with Gilbert syndrome are homozygous for the variant promoter, providing a unique genetic marker for this disorder. Heterozygotes have one allele each of the wild-type and variant promoters (6/7) (379). The gene frequency for the 7/7 motif is 0.3 so that 9% of the general population are homozygous and 42% are heterozygous (382). Thus about half of the white population carries a Gilbert promoter on at least one allele.

Although most commonly diagnosed in young adulthood, it is now clear that Gilbert syndrome plays a role in the pathogenesis of neonatal jaundice (22,23). Several investigators have shown that neonates who are homozygous for the

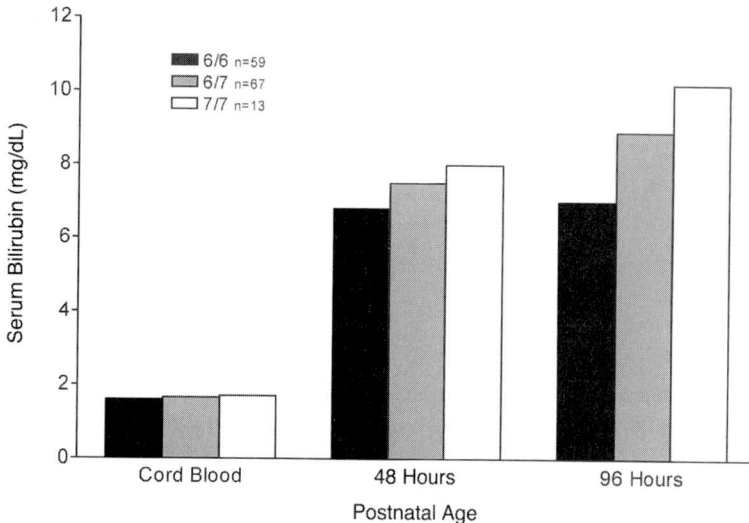

Figure 35-19 Newborn mean serum bilirubin levels as a function of postnatal age and presence of Gilbert promoter abnormality. Homozygous normal UGT genotype (6/6); heterozygous variant UGT genotype (6/7); homozygous variant UGT genotype (7/7). (Redrawn from Watchko JF. Indirect hyperbilirubinemia in the neonate. In: Maisels MJ, Watchko JF, eds. *Neonatal jaundice.* London, UK: Harwood Academic Publishers, 2000:51–66, with permission, from data of Roy-Chowdhury N, Deocharan B, Bejjanki HR, et al. Presence of the genetic marker for Gilbert syndrome is associated with increased level and duration of neonatal jaundice. *Acta Paediatr* 2002;91:100–101.)

variant 7/7 UGT gene promoter have a more rapid rise in their TSB levels (383) and higher TSB levels at age 96 hours (Fig. 35-19) (384). Of neonates with TSB concentrations greater than 13 mg/dL (222 μmol/L) 26.8% were homozygous for the variant 7/7 promoter versus 12.2% of those whose TSB levels were ≤13 mg/dL (385). In a population of Scottish, primarily breast-fed newborns with TSB levels of greater than 5.8 mg/dL (100 μmol/L) after 14 days of life, 31% were homozygous for the 7/7 Gilbert syndrome promoter genotype compared with only 6% of a control group with acute jaundice (259). Of 17 breast-fed Japanese infants with prolonged jaundice, 16 had at least 1 mutation of the UGT1A1 gene, primarily of the G7IR type (260).

Thus, Gilbert syndrome plays an ubiquitous role in the pathogenesis of neonatal hyperbilirubinemia. The combination of the Gilbert genotype with other icterogenic factors such as breast-feeding (259,260), G6PD deficiency (345), ABO incompatibility (317), and pyloric stenosis (359) dramatically increases a newborn's risk of hyperbilirubinemia.

Mutations of the Uridine Diphosphoglucuronate Glucuronosyltransferase 1A1 Gene Coding Area Associated with Gilbert Syndrome. Unlike white populations with Gilbert syndrome, the TATAA promoter variations are rare in East Asian populations (22). In these populations, Gilbert syndrome appears to result from missense mutations in the coding area of the UGT1A1 gene. The most common of these is a G → A transition at nucleotide 211, which causes arginine to replace glycine at position 71 of the corresponding protein product (386,387). This G71R variant is prevalent in Japanese, Korean, and Chinese populations (387) and other mutations have also been reported in association with Gilbert syndrome in these populations (388,389). The presence of these mutations could account for the higher TSB levels found in Japanese and other East Asian newborns.

Heterozygosity for Uridine Diphosphoglucuronate Glucuronosyltransferase 1A1 Noncoding and Coding Area Mutations. Because approximately 50% of the population carry a

Gilbert type promoter on at least one allele, it is not surprising that some individuals may be heterozygous for the variant promoter gene and also heterozygous for a coding region mutation of the gene (22,23). Coinheritance of the Gilbert promoter and a coding region mutation of the gene can also lead to jaundice (23). This is true not only for patients who are homozygous for the Gilbert genotype, but also for compound heterozygotes of a Gilbert type promoter and a structural region mutation of the UGT1A1 (382). A striking example of this situation was recently described in twin girls who developed marked hyperbilirubinemia and kernicterus and were found to be compound heterozygotes for the Gilbert-type UGT promoter and a coding region mutation of the UGT1A1 gene (382).

Based on the gene frequencies for the Gilbert promoter and structural mutations of the UGT1A1 gene, at least 1 in 3,300 infants will be compound heterozygotes for Gilbert and UGT1A1 coding region mutations and at risk for significant hyperbilirubinemia (23,380). Watchko notes that the 1 in 3,300 likelihood of this compound heterozygosity is similar to the frequency of TSB levels greater than 30 mg/dL (greater than 513 μmol/L) (203,288).

We do not know if Gilbert syndrome plays an important role in the pathogenesis of extreme hyperbilirubinemia (TSB levels greater than 30 mg/dL [513 μmol/L]), but the fact that poor feeding and weight loss (a state resembling fasting) (124,390), as well as very low direct-reacting bilirubin fractions, are seen in some of these infants suggests that this is a possibility worthy of investigation.

Other Inborn Errors of Metabolism

Galactosemia. Galactosemia is a rare disease (incidence, 1 in 35,000 to 60,000 live births), and jaundice may be one of the presenting features (391); but infants with significant hyperbilirubinemia caused by galactosemia almost all have some other manifestations of the disease, most often poor feeding, vomiting, excessive weight loss, irritability, and lethargy. Hyperbilirubinemia during the first week of life is almost exclusively unconjugated, and the conjugated fraction tends to rise during the second week, probably reflecting liver damage. The presence of a positive family history, lethargy, poor feeding, or other signs of illness merit additional diagnostic evaluation, including testing the urine for reducing substances using Clinitest (Miles Inc., Diagnostic Division, Elkhart, IN). *Escherichia coli* sepsis is the most devastating complication in the newborn (391).

Tyrosinemia and Hypermethioninemia. The relation between these inborn errors of metabolism and jaundice is primarily a result of the presence of neonatal liver disease, which initially may manifest as indirect-reacting hyperbilirubinemia but which generally is accompanied by some evidence of cholestasis (i.e., direct-reacting hyperbilirubinemia).

Hypothyroidism. Prolonged indirect-reacting hyperbilirubinemia is one of the clinical features of congenital hypothyroidism (392–395), a condition that must be ruled out in any infant who has indirect-reacting hyperbilirubinemia beyond 2 to 3 weeks of age. Although widespread availability of screening programs for congenital hypothyroidism should allow early identification of this problem as a possible cause of jaundice, screening programs do not detect every infant, and errors are more likely to occur with early discharge of infants in whom the thyroxine (T_4) level may still be spuriously elevated.

The pathogenesis of hyperbilirubinemia associated with hypothyroidism is not clear, and administration of triiodothyronine to full-term and preterm infants does not lower peak serum bilirubin levels (396,397). In one infant with prolonged jaundice, UGT activity in a liver biopsy sample was unmeasurable (393), but the jaundice resolved following thyroxine administration. Conversely, when rats underwent thyroidectomy UGT activity *increased* and they also developed cholestasis (398).

Drugs

The use of pancuronium and chloral hydrate is associated with higher bilirubin levels in sick preterm infants (275–277), and chloral hydrate is associated with an increased risk of direct-reacting hyperbilirubinuria (276).

Breast-Milk Jaundice

See Epidemiology of Neonatal Hyperbilirubinemia, Breast-Feeding and Jaundice, above.

Prolonged Indirect-reacting Hyperbilirubinemia

Prolonged indirect-reacting hyperbilirubinemia is defined as indirect-reacting bilirubinemia persisting beyond 2 weeks of age in the full-term infant; Table 35-22 lists its causes. The association of prolonged indirect-reacting hyperbilirubinemia with pyloric stenosis is well described but the pathogenesis of this association has never been clear, although delayed gastric emptying and enterohepatic circulation were thought to play a role. In a report of three infants with pyloric stenosis and hyperbilirubinemia, two were homozygous, and one

TABLE 35-22
CAUSES OF PROLONGED INDIRECT HYPERBILIRUBINEMIA

Breast-milk jaundice	Pyloric stenosis
Hemolytic disease	Crigler-Najjar syndrome
	Gilbert syndrome
Hypothyroidism	Extravascular blood

heterozygous for the variant promoter for Gilbert syndrome (359), implying a key role for Gilbert syndrome in the pathogenesis of the prolonged hyperbilirubinemia that sometimes occurs in pyloric stenosis.

Mixed Forms of Jaundice

Sepsis and Urinary Tract Infection

Jaundice is one sign of bacterial sepsis and some reports suggest that unexplained hyperbilirubinemia may be the only manifestation of sepsis in otherwise healthy-appearing newborns (399–401). Should newborns with unexplained hyperbilirubinemia be subjected to lumbar puncture and blood and urine cultures even if they appear otherwise well? I evaluated 306 newborns admitted within 21 days of birth with indirect-reacting hyperbilirubinemia (peak TSB level 18.5 ± 2.8 mg/dL; range: 12.7 to 29.1 [316 ± 48 μmol/L; range: 217 to 498]) (see Table 35-18). No case of sepsis was diagnosed (249).

In a study of 160 asymptomatic jaundiced infants presenting to an emergency department in Los Angeles, urine cultures (catheter specimens) were positive (greater than 10,000 colony-forming units [cfu]/mL in 12 (7.5%) of the infants (402) (0 of 44 circumcised boys, 9 of 94 uncircumcised boys, and 3 of 62 girls). A positive urine culture was more likely when jaundice was first noted after 8 days of age and if there was an elevated direct-reacting bilirubin concentration (402). The authors recommended that all asymptomatic, jaundiced infants presenting to an emergency department (402) should have a urine culture, but this view has been questioned (403).

Given the prevalence of jaundice in the newborn, the presence of indirect-reacting hyperbilirubinemia as the *only* manifestation of bacteremia or incipient sepsis, must be a very rare occurrence. Furthermore, the finding of a positive blood or urine culture in a newborn with indirect-reacting hyperbilirubinemia does not prove that the infection is the cause of the jaundice. However, infants who appear sick or have late-onset jaundice after the initial icterus has resolved, or infants with direct-reacting hyperbilirubinemia or something else in the history, physical examination, or laboratory investigations that is out of the ordinary, should be evaluated carefully for possible sepsis or urinary tract infection.

Hypopituitarism

Prolonged jaundice that is predominantly cholestatic (elevated direct-reacting bilirubin) has been described in infants with congenital hypopituitarism (404,405), although in some the hyperbilirubinemia is indirect. The pathogenesis of hyperbilirubinemia in this condition remains to be elucidated.

Other Causes

Congenital syphilis, the TORCH (toxoplasmosis, other agents, rubella, cytomegalovirus, and herpes simplex) group of chronic intrauterine infections, and coxsackievirus B infection are the other important causes of mixed jaundice. The clinical features and diagnoses of these conditions are described in Chapter 48.

NEWER DEVELOPMENTS THAT AFFECT OUR APPROACH TO THE JAUNDICED NEWBORN

In the last several years, three factors have emerged that have colored our approach to the evaluation and management of neonatal jaundice. The first is a series of case reports indicating that kernicterus, thought to be almost extinct, is still occurring (124,133,328,329,390,406). The second is the decreasing hospital stay for newborn infants, and the third is an increase in the incidence of neonatal jaundice.

Kernicterus Still Occurs

Neonatologists still see occurrences of kernicterus and reports in the literature (124,133,328,329,390,406) suggest a "resurgence" of this devastating condition. Neverthe-less, there are no appropriate data to support this perception, because there is no uniform surveillance for the reporting of kernicterus over the last 3 to 4 decades, no agreed on case definition for kernicterus, and, most important, no denominators (i.e., population base) for the case reports listed. Nevertheless, the fact that kernicterus, although rare, still occurs, demands our attention because it is nearly always preventable by relatively simple interventions (76).

A preliminary analysis of the reported cases of kernicterus suggests the possible root causes (124,407) listed in Table 35-23.

Early Discharge and the Risk of Jaundice

In addition to the global trend toward a shorter hospital stay for newborns, several studies (239,241,288) but not all (206,408), have found that early discharge itself is associated with an increased risk of significant hyperbilirubinemia and even kernicterus (124,328). Recognizing both the risk of unrecognized jaundice in infants discharged early, as well as the fact that, in infants discharged before 72 hours, the TSB level is almost always still rising, the AAP guidelines for followup of infants discharged before 72 hours are stringent (76) (see section on Preventing Extreme Hyperbilirubinemia and Kernicterus).

It is not clear why infants who are discharged early are at greater risk of developing significant hyperbilirubine-

TABLE 35-23
ROOT CAUSES OF REPORTED CASES OF KERNICTERUS

Early discharge with failure to ensure appropriate followup.
Failure to evaluate the measured TSB level based on the infant's age in hours.
Failure to recognize risk factors for severe hyperbilirubinemia.
Underestimating the severity of jaundice by clinical (i.e., visual) assessment.
Lack of concern regarding the neurotoxic potential of bilirubin.

mia. The vast majority of these hyperbilirubinemic infants are breast-fed, and it is possible that mothers who have longer postpartum stays are more rested, have more time to receive advice and counsel regarding breast-feeding, and are therefore able to nurse their babies more effectively. More frequent and effective lactation, as well as improved caloric intake, decreases the likelihood of hyperbilirubinemia (251,252,409). Early discharge also may have a negative effect on the ability of mothers to assimilate and process the information that they receive regarding lactation and infant care (410). As a result, they may nurse the infants less effectively.

Shorter hospital stays also have necessitated a readjustment in our thinking with regard to the meaning of specific bilirubin levels. To date, this has proved to be a difficult adjustment for pediatricians who are accustomed to using a specific TSB level (irrespective of the infant's age) as an indication for reassurance or concern. The data of Bhutani and associates (289) graphically illustrate this point (Fig. 35-20). Clinicians commonly refer to jaundice occurring on "day 2 or day 3," but reference to the data of Bhutani and associates (see Predischarge Measurement of the Bilirubin Level below) and Fig. 35-20 indicates just how misleading this thought process can be. A TSB level of 8 mg/dL at 24.1 hours is above the 95th percentile and calls for evaluation and close followup, whereas the same level at 47.9 hours is in the low-risk zone and probably requires no further concern—yet both of these values occur on "day 2" (289). One point is worth emphasizing: *If newborns are discharged at less than age 36 hours, their bilirubin levels (with very rare exceptions) can only be going in one direction—up.* The recognition that jaundice is now primarily an outpatient problem requires us to develop a consistent approach to the monitoring and surveillance of these infants if we are to prevent the development of extreme hyperbilirubinemia and kernicterus (76).

More Jaundiced Newborns

There is evidence that the incidence of neonatal jaundice is increasing. In the days of the major CPP (1959 to 1966), only 5% of infants had bilirubin levels ≥13 mg/dL (222 μmol/L) and less than 1% had a peak TSB level of ≥20 mg/dL (342 μmol/L) (205). However, in three more recent studies, the 95th percentile for a population of term and

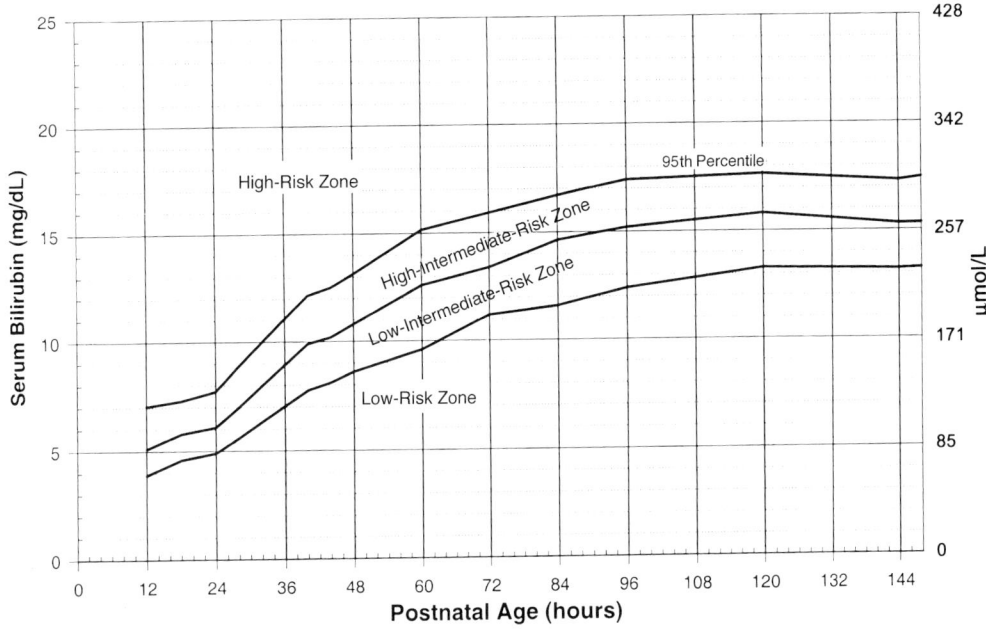

Figure 35-20 Nomogram for designation of risk in 2,840 well newborns ≥36 week's gestational age with birth weight ≥2,000 g or ≥35 weeks' gestational age and a birth weight ≥2,500 g or more based on the hour-specific serum bilirubin values. The serum bilirubin level was obtained before discharge, and the zone in which the value fell predicted the likelihood of a subsequent bilirubin level exceeding the 95th percentile (high-risk zone) as shown in Table 35-27. Note that because of sampling bias (293) this nomogram should not be used to represent the natural history of neonatal hyperbilirubinemia. (From Bhutani VK, Johnson L, Sivieri EM. Predictive ability of a predischarge hour-specific serum bilirubin for subsequent significant hyperbilirubinemia in healthy-term and near-term newborns. *Pediatrics* 1999;103:6–14, with permission.)

near-term infants ranged from 15.5 to 18 mg/dL (289,290, 411). In a study of 11 Kaiser Permanente northern California hospitals, 2% of infants had peak TSB levels ≥20 mg/dL (203). Factors that may be responsible for this increase in jaundice include an increase in the number of infants breast-fed on discharge from the hospital (30% in the 1960s, 65% to 70% in 2001) (412,413) and shorter hospital stays (239,241,288).

PREVENTION, IDENTIFICATION, AND MANAGEMENT OF NEONATAL HYPERBILIRUBINEMIA

The Approach to a Jaundiced Infant

The Institute of Medicine (IOM) issued a report in 2001 that describes a "chasm in health care quality" which needs to be crossed for patients to receive better care (414). The report calls for a "systems approach" drawing on the rapid evolution of knowledge about complex adaptive systems. The IOM report offers 10 "simple rules" to "redesign and improve care" (414) Palmer and associates (415) studied the care of newborns with hyperbilirubinemia in two large managed care organizations and describe how this care might be improved by using practical applications of the ideas about complex adaptive systems.

The recently published guideline of the AAP provides an approach to the evaluation and treatment of hyperbiliru-

binemia in the term and near-term newborn ≥35 weeks of gestation (76). Although bilirubin encephalopathy or kernicterus should almost always be preventable, it is still occurring in this group of infants. Table 35-24 lists the key elements of the recommendations provided in the AAP guideline. The discussion that follows deals primarily with infants ≥35 weeks of gestation, although the basic principles apply to the evaluation and management of hyperbilirubinemia in all infants.

Primary Prevention

Prenatal Testing

Screening for Isoimmunization

All pregnant women should be tested for ABO and Rh (D) typing and undergo a serum screen for unusual isoimmune antibodies (76). If such prenatal testing has not been performed, then a direct Coombs test, a blood type, and an Rh (D) type on the infant's cord blood should be done; this should always be done if the mother is Rh-negative. In addition to identification of potentially Rh-sensitized infants, this testing is obligatory because it identifies Rh-negative mothers who require anti-D gammaglobulin to prevent Rh (D) sensitization.

In infants of group O, Rh-positive mothers, the AAP recommends that routine testing for blood type and Coombs test is optional "provided there is appropriate surveillance

TABLE 35-24

KEY ELEMENTS OF THE AMERICAN ACADEMY OF PEDIATRICS GUIDELINE ON MANAGEMENT OF HYPERBILIRUBINEMIA IN THE NEWBORN INFANT ≥35 WEEKS OF GESTATION

1. Promote and support successful breast-feeding.
2. Establish nursery protocols for the identification and evaluation of hyperbilirubinemia.
3. Measure the TSB or TcB level on infants jaundiced in the first 24 hours.
4. Recognize that visual estimation of the degree of jaundice can lead to errors, particularly in darkly pigmented infants.
5. Interpret all bilirubin levels according to the infant's age in hours.
6. Recognize that infants <38 weeks' gestation, particularly those who are breast-fed, are at higher risk of developing hyperbilirubinemia and require closer surveillance and monitoring.
7. Perform a systematic assessment on all infants prior to discharge for the risk of severe hyperbilirubinemia.
8. Provide appropriate followup based on the time of discharge and the risk assessment.
9. Treat newborns, when indicated, with phototherapy or exchange transfusion.

TcB, transcutaneous bilirubin.
From Maisels MJ, Baltz RD, Bhutani V, et al. Management of hyperbilirubinemia in the newborn infant 35 or more weeks of gestation. *Pediatrics* 2004;114:297–316, with permission.

and risk assessment before discharge and followup (76) so that significantly jaundiced infants are not missed." (See *ABO Hemolytic Disease* above.)

Preventing Hyperbilirubinemia

To prevent severe hyperbilirubinemia, we need to (a) identify infants who are at risk for developing hyperbilirubinemia, (b) follow them closely, and (c) treat them with phototherapy when indicated.

Ensuring Successful Breast-feeding. Because exclusively breast-feeding an infant is strongly associated with an increased risk of hyperbilirubinemia (see Breast-Feeding and Jaundice above), the only *primary* preventive intervention available to us is to ensure the adequacy and success of breast-feeding. In many, but not all, cases of severe hyperbilirubinemia in breast-fed infants, poor caloric intake associated with inadequate breast-feeding (and manifested by increased weight loss) appears to play an important role (218,246,254,390). Exclusively breast-feeding an infant is also a well documented risk factor for dehydration (416), considered by some to be a cause of hyperbilirubinemia, although there is no plausible mechanism for this. It is much more likely that in breast-fed, dehydrated infants, it is the caloric deprivation and its effect on the enterohepatic circulation of bilirubin (see Table 35-14) that is primarily responsible for the severe hyperbilirubinemia (244).

Thus, the clinician's primary role in preventing hyperbilirubinemia is to help ensure that breast-feeding will be successful. The first step is to ask mothers to nurse their infants at least 8 to 12 times per day for the first several days (417), because increasing the frequency of nursing significantly decreases the likelihood of subsequent hyperbilirubinemia (251,252,409). Evidence of adequate intake in breast-fed infants also includes 4 to 6 thoroughly wet diapers within 24 hours and the passage of 3 to 4 stools per day by the fourth day. By the third to fourth day, the stools in adequately breast-fed infants should have changed from meconium to a mustard yellow, mushy stool (418). Weight

loss must also be monitored. Unsupplemented breast-fed infants experience their maximum weight loss by day 3 and, on average, lose 6.1 ± 2.5% (SD) of their birth weight (243,246,251,261,419–422). Thus, approximately 5% to 10% of exclusively breast-fed infants lose 10% or more of their birth weight by day 3, suggesting that adequacy of intake should be evaluated and the infant monitored if weight loss is greater than 10% (423). These assessments will also help to identify breast-fed infants who, because of inadequate intake, are at risk for dehydration.

In many hospitals it is a common practice to provide supplemental feedings of water or dextrose water to breast-fed infants in the mistaken belief that this will lower their TSB levels. As illustrated in Fig. 35-21, this practice does not decrease TSB levels (419,420) but it does interfere with the establishment of effective lactation (424).

Identifying the Jaundiced Newborn

Clinical Assessment

All infants should be monitored routinely for the development of jaundice and nurseries should have established protocols for the assessment of jaundice. In newborns, jaundice is detected by blanching the skin with digital pressure, thus revealing the underlying color of the skin and subcutaneous tissue. It is important for this assessment to be done in a well-lit room or, preferably, in daylight at a window.

The Cephalocaudal Progression of Jaundice

Dermal icterus is seen first in the face and then progresses in a caudal manner to the trunk and extremities so that, for a given bilirubin level, the skin of the face will appear more yellow than that of the foot. First observed more than 100 years ago and confirmed by several investigators using visual observation as well as transcutaneous bilirubinometry, the cephalocaudal progression of dermal icterus is a useful clinical tool but less reliable once the TSB level exceeds 12 mg/dL (205 μmol/L) (425–432).

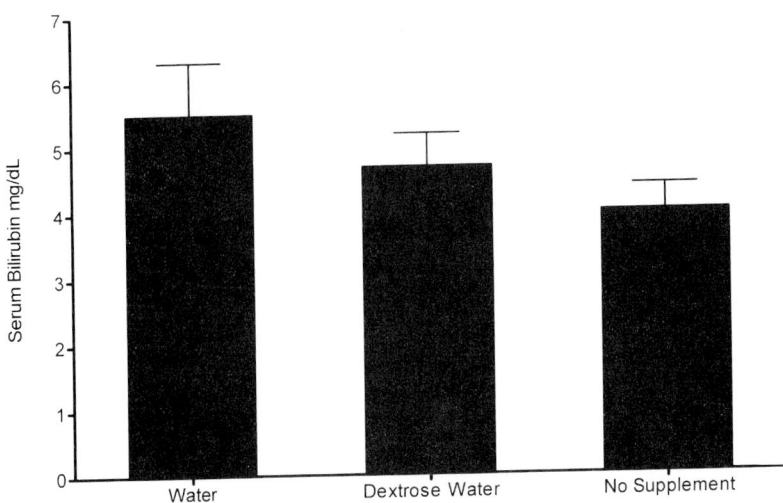

Figure 35-21 Effect of supplementary feeding on serum bilirubin levels on day 6 in breast-fed newborns. Nursing infants were randomly assigned to receive supplemental water (n = 15), dextrose water (n = 17), or no supplement (n = 17). Bilirubin levels on day 6 (mean ± standard error of mean [SEM]) are shown. There were no significant differences between any of the groups. Drawn from the data in Nicoll A, Ginsburg R, Tripp JH. Supplementary feeding and jaundice in newborns. *Acta Pediatr Scand* 1982;71:759–761.

Mechanism of the Cephalocaudal Progression

Knudsen suggests that the cephalocaudal color difference in newborns is best explained by conformational change in the bilirubin–albumin complex (431). Following its formation, bilirubin is bound tightly to albumin, and the initial binding process is extremely rapid (within 10 milliseconds). This is followed by a train of slow, relaxing changes in the conformation of the bilirubin–albumin complex commencing within 1 to 30 seconds, final conformation being reached 8 minutes after the initial binding (433). This time course suggests that initially there is a lower bilirubin-binding affinity to albumin (until the final stage of conformation has occurred) and thus less-effective bilirubin–albumin binding in the blood immediately after it has left the reticuloendothelial system. The affinity increases after the blood reaches the distal portions of the body and the conformational changes in the bilirubin– albumin complex are completed. Knudsen suggests that some of the yellow color of the skin is the result of precipitated bilirubin acid and in the presence of reduced bilirubin-binding affinity to albumin, there is an increased precipitation of bilirubin acid and thus an increase in the yellow color of the skin (431). This is more likely to occur in the proximal parts of the body because of the conformational changes in the young bilirubin–albumin complexes. Consistent with this hypothesis, Knudsen (431) found that there was a significant and linear correlation among the cephalocaudal color difference, the plasma bilirubin concentration, and the square of the hydrogen ion concentration. The cephalocaudal color difference was inversely related to the reserve albumin concentration, thus suggesting that the conformational change in the young bilirubin–albumin complex enhances the precipitation of bilirubin acid in the skin of the proximal parts of the body. If this is the mechanism, then objective measurement of the yellow color of the skin using transcutaneous bilirubinometry could be a better predictor of potential bilirubin encephalopathy than a serum bilirubin measurement.

How Good Is the Visual Assessment of Jaundice?

The ability of clinicians to diagnose jaundice varies widely (235,425,426,434,435), although studies suggest that home health nurses (436) and some neonatologists (435) can effectively evaluate newborns for the presence and severity of jaundice, and that newborns whose TSB levels exceed 12 mg/dL (205 μmol/L) will almost always be identified as "jaundiced" (235,425). Nevertheless, visual estimation of actual bilirubin levels from the degree of jaundice can be unreliable and can certainly lead to errors (235,426,434). Errors are also more likely to occur in darkly pigmented infants. Consequently, a low threshold should be used for measuring the TSB. There is also a problem with relying on visual diagnosis in the first 24 to 36 hours. The difference between a TSB level of 5 mg/dL (85 μmol/L) and 8 mg/dL (137 μmol/L) cannot be perceived by eye, yet this is the difference between a TSB level at the 50th percentile and one that is at the 95th percentile (see Figs. 35-16 and 35-20). The potential errors associated with visual diagnosis have led some experts to recommend that all newborns should have a laboratory measurement of TSB prior to discharge (124) (see Predischarge Measurement of the Bilirubin Level). An alternative is the use of the newer noninvasive (transcutaneous) devices that can provide a valid estimate of TSB levels less than 15 mg/dL (257 μmol/L) (140,204,437,438).

Noninvasive Measurements of Bilirubin

The Ingram Icterometer (Cascade Health Care Products, Salem, OR) is a piece of transparent plastic on which is painted 5 transverse strips of graded yellow hue. The instrument is pressed against the nose, the yellow color of the blanched skin is matched with the appropriate yellow stripe, and a jaundice score is assessed. This device is simple and inexpensive and, remarkably, as a screening tool, it performs as effectively as much more sophisticated instruments (439). It has also been used effectively by nurses and even parents in the home (425,440).

The Minolta Air Shields jaundice meter (Air-Shields, Hatboro, PA) was the first electronic device marketed for transcutaneous bilirubin measurement. With this instrument and its successors (models JM-102 and -103), pressure is applied to a photoprobe and a strobe light is generated by a xenon tube. The light passes through a fiberoptic element, penetrating the blanched skin and entering the subcutaneous tissue. The reflected light returns through a second fiberoptic bundle to the spectrophotometric module where the intensity of the yellow color, corrected for hemoglobin, is measured and displayed. In the original jaundice meter this number was displayed as an arbitrary unit—the transcutaneous bilirubin (TcB) index. The newer model, JM-103, displays a bilirubin value that corresponds closely to the measured TSB level. The JM-103 jaundice meter uses two wavelengths and a dual optical path system (204,438). The principle of operation includes the formation of two beams, one of which reaches only the shallow areas of the subcutaneous tissue, while the other penetrates the deeper layers. The differences between optical densities are detected by blue and green photocells. The measurement of bilirubin accumulated primarily in the deeper subcutaneous tissues should decrease the influence of other skin pigments such as melanin and hemoglobin (438).

Another transcutaneous device, the BiliChek (Respironics, Marietta, GA) employs multiple wavelengths and measures TcB by using the entire spectrum of visible light (380 to 760 nm) reflected by the skin. The absorption of hemoglobin, melanin, and the effect of dermal thickness are isolated mathematically, and absorption of light by bilirubin in the capillary bed and subcutaneous tissues is isolated by spectral subtraction.

To date, studies with the JM-103 and the BiliChek have shown a close correlation between TcB and TSB measurements in mixed racial populations (204,437,441,442). When compared with HPLC measurements of TSB, the BiliChek was as good or better than the TSB measured in the clinical laboratory (441) although the accuracy of the BiliChek in a Hispanic (Mexican) population has been questioned (202). In this population, the BiliChek tended to under estimate the TSB, particularly when the TSB was greater than 10 mg/dL (171 μmol/L) (202). The JM-103 is less precise in black infants than in white infants, although the predominant tendency in black infants is for the TcB value to overestimate TSB levels (204) so that dangerous errors are unlikely to occur.

TcB measurements become less precise with decreasing gestation and are of questionable utility below 30 weeks' gestation (443). Because phototherapy bleaches the skin, both visual assessments of jaundice and TcB measurements in infants undergoing phototherapy are not reliable (444). It might be possible, however, to use existing TcB instruments in infants who are undergoing phototherapy if an area of skin used for TcB measurements is protected from light (444). Data are limited regarding the use of TcB measurements following phototherapy. In one study, TcB measurements 18 to 24 hours after discontinuation of pho-

totherapy correlated well with the TSB and the correlation improved further after an additional 24 hours (444).

Because TcB measurements are so easy to perform, repeated measurements can be obtained over the course of an infant's stay in the nursery. Plotting serial measurements will provide a good indication of whether TcB levels are rising and crossing percentiles and must therefore be followed more closely (see Fig. 35-20) Although the TcB measurement provides a good estimate of the TSB level, as with any laboratory measurement, TcB levels should not be considered in isolation, nor should critical decisions be based on a single measurement.

Both the BiliChek and JM-103 have an acceptable level of diagnostic accuracy, particularly when used as a screening device to place infants in a risk category for followup, or as an indication for obtaining a TSB (445). In some populations, TcB measurements may not be able to identify the precise bilirubin level with an acceptable degree of accuracy ("the wrong job for the tool") (445). Currently, it is probably inadvisable to rely entirely on TcB measurements as a substitute for TSB measurements but they can certainly be helpful in many ways. When used as a screening tool TcB measurements can help us to answer the questions "Should I worry about this infant?" and "Should I obtain a TSB on this infant?" (445). For both of these purposes, the physician can set a value for a TcB measurement (based on the infant's age in hours and other risk factors) above which a TSB level will always be obtained. In our nursery, the nurses currently measure the TcB on all infants and automatically obtain a TSB if the TcB is above the 75th percentile (289). In our study with the JM-103, the chance of a TcB measurement underestimating the TSB level by 3 mg/dL (51.3 μmol/L) or more was only 0.6%, so an alternative approach is to ask, "If the real TSB value is TcB plus 3 mg/dL (51 μmol/L), is there a reasonable chance that this will change my management?" If the answer is yes, a TSB should be measured. This allows the clinician to take into account other risk factors, including the gestation. In this manner, no infant with significant hyperbilirubinemia should be missed and many infants and their families will be spared the trauma, cost, and inconvenience of having a laboratory measurement of serum bilirubin. The ability to measure the TcB in the office or other outpatient settings, including the home, noninvasively and instantaneously, should prove of inestimable value in the monitoring and management of the jaundiced newborn infant and should largely avoid the potential errors associated with clinical estimation of bilirubin levels.

LABORATORY MEASUREMENTS OF BILIRUBIN

Total Serum Bilirubin

This subject has been reviewed in detail (284,446,447) and addressed, most recently by Lo and associates (282). Although this is one of the most commonly performed laboratory measurements in the newborn, the measurement of TSB concentration remains remarkably inaccurate. Repeated surveys over the last 3 decades have disclosed a high level of interlaboratory variation in the measurements of both total and direct-reacting serum bilirubin concentrations in neonatal sera. In a recent study, a sample with a known TSB concentration of 14.8 mg/dL (243 μmol/L) was analyzed in 14 different university hospital laboratories. The mean (± SD) measured TSB was 15.2 ± 2.5 mg/dL (coefficient of variation 16.4%) and the range was 12.1 to 18.5 mg/dL (207 to 316 μmol/L) (283). This remarkably wide range of values in skilled hands suggests that considerable caution is necessary before generalizing bilirubin levels from one institution to the wider universe of newborns. Within-laboratory variation generally is considered to be lower, but in the study of Vreman and associates (283), over time, the coefficient of variation for repeated measurements of the same sample was as high as 17.2% in one laboratory (283).

The most recent analysis of laboratory neonatal TSB measurements was conducted by Lo and associates (282) who examined data submitted by laboratories that participate in the College of American Pathologists (CAP) neonatal bilirubin and chemistry surveys. They compared the data from laboratories throughout the United States with the reference method for measuring TSB (448). They found an acceptable coefficient of variation ranging from 1.9% to 4.5%, in the four most commonly used laboratory instruments. When compared with the reference method, the mean values from these instruments differed from the reference method by −21.6% to 10.9%. The authors attributed these discrepancies to the use of different methods used (primarily with the Vitros instrument, Ortho-Clinical Diagnostics, Raritan, NJ) in the neonatal bilirubin versus the chemistry surveys of the CAP, as well as the presence of a nonhuman protein base and ditaurobilirubin in the survey specimens (115). Lo and associates concluded that it is impossible to evaluate the accuracy of TSB measurements from the CAP surveys because the standard specimens consist of bovine serum containing a mixture of unconjugated bilirubin and ditaurobilirubin. They recommend that survey specimens should consist of human serum enriched with unconjugated bilirubin. The CAP has adopted this recommendation and is now using human-serum-based specimens in their neonatal bilirubin and chemistry surveys (BT Doumas, personal communication, October, 2003).

These variations between laboratories might explain the frequent occurrence in clinical practice of an infant being admitted for treatment of hyperbilirubinemia because an outside laboratory found a high TSB level, but when the test is repeated in the hospital laboratory, the TSB level is 5 or 6 mg/dL (85 to 103 μmol/L) lower. Of course, there is no way of knowing which value is correct. A 16.4% coefficient of variation between laboratories means that if the true serum bilirubin value is 20 mg/dL (342 μmol/L), the 95% confidence limits of a repeat measurement at another laboratory could fall anywhere between 14.4 and 26.6 mg/dL (246 to 455 μmol/L). Because our followup, surveillance, and intervention in jaundiced infants are based on TSB values, spurious underestimation of the TSB concentration might lead to withholding of necessary therapy, and overestimation will produce unnecessary clinical intervention.

Direct-Reacting and Conjugated Bilirubin

Similar concerns exist with regard to measurements of direct-reacting or conjugated bilirubin where laboratory measurements are considered, at best, "only an approximation to the true value" (449). In one study, measurements of direct-reacting bilirubin using the Dupont ACA (automatic clinical analyzer) or Coulter Dacos analyzer produced direct-reacting bilirubin levels in a population of full-term newborns at one hospital that were twice as high as those measured in a similar population at another institution, where a Kodak Ektachem 700 (now known as the Vitros) method was used (450). The Vitros method measures *conjugated bilirubin*, whereas the other methods measure *direct-reacting bilirubin*. Although often used synonymously, direct-reacting bilirubin is not the same as conjugated bilirubin. Direct-reacting bilirubin refers to the bilirubin that reacts directly with diazotized sulfanilic acid (i.e., without the addition of an accelerating agent), whereas conjugated bilirubin refers to bilirubin that has been made water soluble by binding with glucuronic acid in the liver.

Site of Blood Sampling—Capillary Versus Venous Blood Samples

Data regarding the differences in TSB levels when measured in capillary or venous samples are conflicting (451,452). It is useful to recall, however, that virtually all of the published data regarding the relationship of TSB levels to kernicterus or developmental outcome are based on capillary TSB levels. Thus, for the purposes of clinical decision making, capillary blood samples are the gold standard and there is no reason to delay initiation of treatment to obtain a venous blood sample to "confirm" an elevated capillary TSB level.

Sampling Technique

Because of the well-known effects of light on bilirubin, laboratory manuals recommend that blood samples be protected from light until the serum is analyzed. Using serum samples with bilirubin levels of 16.0, 11.8, and 7.9 mg/dL (273, 202, and 135 μmol/L), Sykes and colleagues (453) found that, under the usual clinical conditions, there was no measurable effect of ambient light on serum bilirubin levels for at least 8 hours.

When Is Laboratory Measurement of Bilirubin Indicated?

A TcB and/or TSB level should be done on every infant who is jaundiced in the first 24 hours after birth (407). In a

TABLE 35-25

LABORATORY EVALUATION OF THE JAUNDICED INFANT

Indications	Assessments
Jaundice in first 24 hours	Measure TSB
Jaundice appears excessive for infant's age	Measure TSB
Infant receiving phototherapy or TSB rising rapidly (i.e., crossing percentiles [see Fig. 35-20]) and unexplained by history and physical examination	Blood type and Coomb test, if not obtained with cord blood
	Complete blood count and smear
	Measure direct-reacting or conjugated bilirubin
	It is an option to do reticulocyte count, G6PD, ETCOc, if available
	Repeat TSB in 4–24 hours, depending on infant's age and TSB level
TSB approaching exchange levels or not responding to phototherapy	Do reticulocyte count, G6PD, albumin, and ETCOc, if available
Elevated direct (or conjugated) bilirubin level	Do urinalysis and urine culture; evaluate for sepsis if indicated by history and physical examination
Jaundice present at or beyond age 3 weeks, or sick infant	Total and direct-reacting (or conjugated) bilirubin level; if direct-reacting bilirubin elevated, evaluate for causes of cholestasis
	Check results of newborn thyroid and galactosemia screen; evaluate infant for signs or symptoms of hypothyroidism

ETCOc, end-tidal carbon monoxide corrected for ambient carbon monoxide; G6PD, glucose-6-phosphate dehydrogenase; TSB, total serum bilirubin concentration.
From Maisels MJ, Baltz RD, Bhutani V, et al. Management of hyperbilirubinemia in the newborn infant 35 or more weeks of gestation. *Pediatrics* 2004;114:297–316, with permission.

cohort of 105,384 newborns of ≥2,000 g birth weight and at least 36 weeks' gestational age, jaundice was noted in the medical record in only 2.8% of infants within 18 hours and in 6.7% within 24 hours (454). Compared with those who were not jaundiced on the first day, those jaundiced within 24 hours were much more likely to receive phototherapy (18.9% vs. 1.7%) and were three times more likely to develop a bilirubin level of 25 mg/dL (428 μmol/ L) or higher (454). Thus, the presence of jaundice in the first 24 hours represents a significant risk factor for the subsequent development of severe hyperbilirubinemia and, as recommended by the AAP (76), a TSB should be measured in any infant who is jaundiced in the first 24 hours.

The need for and timing of a repeat TSB or TcB depends on the zone in which the TSB falls (see Fig. 35-20), the age of the infant, other clinical risk factors, and the subsequent evolution of the bilirubin level (Table 35-25). A TcB and/or TSB level should also be done if, at any time, the jaundice appears excessive for the infant's age. Recognizing the risk of error in the visual estimation of bilirubin levels (235,425,426,434), particularly in darkly pigmented infants, and depending on the clinical circumstances, a TSB or TcB should be measured if there is any doubt about the degree of jaundice (76).

Seeking a Cause for the Jaundice

Table 35-25 lists the indications for laboratory evaluation of jaundiced newborns. In some infants, the cause of hyperbilirubinemia is apparent from the history and physical examination. For example, jaundice in a severely bruised infant generally needs no further explanation. In addition, the usual laboratory tests (hematocrit, complete blood count, reticulocyte count, and smear) are neither specific nor sensitive and rarely identify a specific cause for the hyperbilirubinemia (198,254) even in infants who are readmitted to hospital with TSB levels of 18 to 20 mg/dL (308 to 340 μmol/L) or higher (see Table 35-18) (241, 249). One study, however, did find a good correlation between measurements of ETCOc and reticulocyte counts (corrected for the hematocrit) in infants with positive DATs (455). The cause of jaundice should be sought in an infant receiving phototherapy or whose TSB level is rising rapidly, that is, crossing percentiles (see Fig. 35-20), and is not explained by the history and physical examination. Table 35-25 lists the appropriate laboratory tests.

Interpreting the Bilirubin Level

All TSB levels must be interpreted in terms of the infant's age in hours (see Figs. 35-16 and 35-20). An infant with a TSB that exceeds the 95th percentile, or in whom the rate of rise of the TSB crosses percentiles (see Fig. 35-20), or exceeds 0.2 mg/dL per hour deserves further evaluation and followup.

Elevated Direct-Reacting or Conjugated Bilirubin Levels

If the TSB is ≤5 mg/dL (85 μmol/L) or lower a direct-reacting or conjugated bilirubin of greater than 1.0 mg/dL (17.1 μmol/L) is considered elevated. For TSB values greater than 5 mg/dL (85 μmol/L) a direct-reacting or conjugated bilirubin of more than 20% of the TSB is considered abnormal. If the laboratory measures conjugated bilirubin using the Vitros system, any value greater than 1 mg/dL

(17.1 μmol/L) is considered abnormal. An infant who has an elevation of direct-reacting or conjugated bilirubin should have a urinalysis and a urine culture performed because this could be an early sign of urinary tract infection (see Table 35-25). A sepsis evaluation should also be considered. Late onset of jaundice (after the fourth or fifth day) has also been associated with urinary tract infection (402) (see also Pathologic Causes of Jaundice: Sepsis above).

Sick Infants and Infants Jaundiced Beyond Age 3 Weeks

These infants should have a measurement of total and direct-reacting or conjugated bilirubin to identify cholestasis (see Table 35-25). If the direct-reacting or conjugated bilirubin level is elevated then additional evaluation is needed for the causes of cholestasis (see Table 35-16 and Chapter 40). This approach is essential for the early identification of infants with biliary atresia. If these infants are to benefit from the operation of portoenterostomy, surgery should be performed as soon as possible and, ideally, before age 60 days (456). Infants who are jaundiced beyond age 3 weeks should also have the results of the newborn thyroid and galactosemia screen checked. Table 35-22 lists the causes of prolonged indirect-reacting hyperbilirubinemia.

PREVENTING EXTREME HYPERBILIRUBINEMIA AND KERNICTERUS

Most of the cases of kernicterus reported in the last decade did not occur in infants who had ABO or Rh hemolytic disease, but in apparently healthy term and near-term newborns with extremely high bilirubin levels (usually well above 30 mg/dL [513 μmol/L]) (124,390,406), in infants with G6PD deficiency (124,133,328,329), and in very sick newborns with low bilirubin levels (43). If we can prevent extreme hyperbilirubinemia we should be able to prevent almost all cases of kernicterus, but jaundice is very common and extreme hyperbilirubinemia (30 mg/dL [513 μmol/L] or higher) is rare, occurring in only about 1 in 10,000 infants (203). To ensure that we do not miss these rare infants, however, we need to follow and measure serum bilirubin levels in many infants, and treat some infants with phototherapy who will never develop severe hyperbilirubinemia (139,140). Ip and associates have calculated that 5 to 10 infants with TSB levels between 15 and 20 mg/dL (257 to 342 μmol/L) receive phototherapy to prevent 1 infant from reaching a TSB of 20 mg/dL (342 μmol/L) (139,140).

Hospital Policies and Jaundiced Newborns

According to recommendation 2.2 of the AAP Clinical Practice Guideline (76), "clinicians should ensure that all infants are routinely monitored for the development of jaundice, and nurseries should have established protocols for the assessment of jaundice. Jaundice should be assessed whenever the infant's vital signs are measured, but no less than every 8 to 12 hours." Recommendation 2.2.1 states that "protocols for the assessment of jaundice should include the circumstances in which nursing staff can obtain a TcB or order a TSB measurement." Nursing staff have always assumed the responsibility for monitoring infants for jaundice but, for the first time, hospitals are now asked to develop protocols under which nurses can obtain a TcB or TSB without a physician order. Thus a nurse who notices jaundice in an infant who is younger than 24 hours old, will obtain a TcB or TSB and notify the physician of the result. If a TcB measurement is used as a screening tool, TSB measurements can be obtained by nurses whenever the TcB measurement is above a certain bilirubin percentile (see Fig. 35-20 and *Noninvasive Measurements of Bilirubin* above).

Assessing the Risk of Severe Hyperbilirubinemia

Recommendation 5.1 of the AAP Clinical Practice Guideline (76) states: "Before discharge, every newborn should be assessed for the risk of developing severe hyperbilirubinemia, and all nurseries should establish protocols for assessing this risk. Such assessment is particularly important in infants who are discharged before age 72 hours." The guideline continues, "The AAP recommends 2 clinical options used individually or in combination for the systematic assessment of risk: predischarge measurement of the bilirubin level using TSB or TcB and/or assessment of clinical risk factors" (76). This must be followed by appropriate evaluation, monitoring, surveillance, and followup to ensure that severe hyperbilirubinemia is identified early and treated appropriately.

Clinical Risk Factors

Table 35-26 lists the risk factors for the development of hyperbilirubinemia. Almost all of these factors can be identified readily without recourse to the laboratory but, because these risk factors are common and the risk of severe hyperbilirubinemia is small, individually, these factors are of limited use as predictors of severe hyperbilirubinemia. Nevertheless, if no risk factors are present, the risk of severe hyperbilirubinemia is extremely low, and the more risk factors that are present, the greater the risk of severe hyperbilirubinemia (206). Some factors, such as breast-feeding, gestation age below 38 weeks, and significant jaundice (need for phototherapy) in a previous sibling, seem to be particularly important. It is remarkable that almost every recently described case of kernicterus occurred in a breast-fed infant, even when the infant had underlying G6PD deficiency (124,133,328,390).

Decreasing Gestation: The "Near-term" Newborn

Decreasing gestation has been repeatedly identified as a very important contributor to hyperbilirubinemia (197,206,211, 239–241). We found that infants of 36 weeks or less gesta-

TABLE 35-26

RISK FACTORS FOR DEVELOPMENT OF SEVERE HYPERBILIRUBINEMIA IN INFANTS ≥35 WEEKS' GESTATION (IN APPROXIMATE ORDER OF IMPORTANCE)

Major risk factors
    Predischarge TSB or TcB level in the high risk zone (see Fig. 35-20) (289,437)
    Jaundice observed in the first 24 hours (454)
    Blood group incompatibility with positive direct antiglobulin test, other known hemolytic disease (e.g., G6PD deficiency), elevated ETCOc
    Gestational age 35 to 36 weeks (206,241)
    Previous sibling received phototherapy (211,241)
    Cephalhematoma or significant bruising (206)
    Exclusive breast-feeding, particularly if nursing is not going well and weight loss is excessive (206,241)
    East Asian race[a]
Minor risk factors
    Predischarge TSB or TcB in the high-intermediate risk zone (see Fig. 35.20) (289,437)
    Gestational age 37 to 38 weeks (206,241)
    Jaundice observed before discharge (241)
    Previous sibling with jaundice (211,241)
    Macrosomic infant of a diabetic mother (216,582)
    Maternal age ≥25 years (206)
    Male gender (206,241)
Decreased risk (these factors are associated with decreased risk of significant jaundice; listed in order of decreasing importance)
    TSB or TcB in the low risk zone (see Fig. 35-20) (289,437)
    Gestational age ≥41 weeks (206)
    Exclusive bottle feeding (206,241)
    Black race[a] (206)

[a] Race as defined by mother's description.
From Maisels MJ, Baltz RD, Bhutani V, et al. Management of hyperbilirubinemia in the newborn infant 35 or more weeks of gestation. *Pediatrics* 2004;114:297–316, with permission.

tion are 13 times more likely than infants at 40 weeks' gestation to be readmitted for severe jaundice (241). Infants at 38 weeks of gestation are considered term babies yet they are 4 times more likely to develop a TSB. ≥25 mg/dL (428 μmol/L) than those at 40 weeks (206). Although these near-term infants, at 35 to 38 weeks of gestation, are cared for in well-baby nurseries, they are much more likely to nurse ineffectively, receive fewer calories, and have a greater weight loss than their truly term counterparts. When combined with less effective hepatic clearance because of prematurity, it is not surprising that they often become more jaundiced.

Predischarge Measurement of the Bilirubin Level

We know that infants who are clinically jaundiced in the first few days are much more likely to later develop significant hyperbilirubinemia (239,241). Bhutani and associates (289) measured TSB concentrations in 13,003 infants prior to their discharge from the hospital. In 2,840 infants additional TSB levels were measured at least once in the 5 to 6 days following discharge. Infants with ABO incompatibility and positive Coombs tests were excluded, as were Rh-sensitized infants. The investigators plotted the TSB levels against the infant's age in hours and created a nomogram with percentiles that defined a high risk (above 95th percentile), a low risk (values less than 40th percentile), and

an intermediate risk (40th to 95th percentile) zone (289) (see Fig. 35-20) Using this nomogram, these investigators found that of infants whose TSB levels fell in the high-risk zone, 39.5% subsequently had values above the 95th percentile. If the TSB level fell in the low-risk zone no baby subsequently developed a TSB above the 95th percentile. Table 35-27 shows these results. Note, however, that Fig. 35-20 does not describe the natural history of bilirubinemia in the newborn. Because only 2,840 (21.9%) of the 13,003 infants had subsequent TSB levels measured, there is a sampling bias (toward more jaundiced babies) particularly after 48 to 72 hours, so that the lower zones are spuriously elevated (293).

These data do show that obtaining a TSB level prior to discharge is a very useful way of predicting the risk (or absence of risk) of subsequent significant hyperbilirubinemia. The predictive value of a predischarge TSB has been confirmed in several other studies (285,457–459), and it defines a group of infants who, at least as far as hyperbilirubinemia is concerned, may not require an early followup. This information is very useful in situations where early followup is difficult or impossible. Predischarge TSB levels also will alert pediatricians to those infants who, because their TSB levels fall in the high-risk zone, require much more careful surveillance and followup until there is clinical or laboratory evidence supporting a declining bilirubin level.

TABLE 35-27

RISK ZONE AS A PREDICTOR OF HYPERBILIRUBINEMIA

TSB Before Discharge	Newborns (Total = 2,840), n (%)	Newborns Who Subsequently Developed a TSB Level >95th Percentile, n (%)
High-risk zone (>95th percentile)	172 (6.0)	68 (39.5)
High-intermediate-risk zone	356 (12.5)	46 (12.9)
Low-intermediate-risk zone	556 (19.6)	12 (2.26)
Low-risk zone	1756 (61.8)	0

From Bhutani VK, Johnson L, Sivieri EM. Predictive ability of a predischarge hour-specific serum bilirubin for subsequent significant hyperbilirubinemia in healthy-term and near-term newborns. *Pediatrics* 1999;103:6–14, with permission.

Measuring Bilirubin Production

When heme is catabolized, CO is produced in equimolar quantities with bilirubin, and measurement of blood COHb concentration, CO production, or CO excretion provides a measurement of bilirubin production (27,460). The development of a simple noninvasive method for measuring ETCOc, provides a technique for quantifying hemolysis (460) and can identify those infants with high or low rates of bilirubin production. Although the measurement of ETCOc can identify the presence of hemolysis and is useful as a diagnostic test (316,330,461), it has not proved useful as a routine method of screening infants to predict the likelihood of subsequent hyperbilirubinemia (285).

Followup

Identifying the risk of subsequent severe hyperbilirubinemia before the newborn leaves the nursery is of little value unless appropriate follow-up is provided. Recommendation 6.1.1 in the AAP Guideline (76) states that: "All infants should be examined by a qualified health care professional in the first few days following discharge to assess infant well-being and the presence or absence of jaundice. The timing and location of this assessment will be determined by the length of stay in the nursery, presence or absence of risk factors for hyperbilirubinemia (see Table 35-26 and Fig. 35-20) and the risk of other neonatal problems." This examination can take place in an office, clinic or home and can be done by a physician, physician assistant, or nurse. Although written and oral information should be provided to all parents about newborn jaundice, it is unfair and unreasonable to rely only on parents to identify a significantly jaundiced infant.

Table 35-28 provides the AAP recommendations for the timing of followup. If, for geographic, climatic, socioeconomic, or other reasons, appropriate followup cannot be ensured and the predischarge assessment suggests the presence of a significant risk for severe hyperbilirubinemia, it may be necessary to delay discharge either until appropriate followup can be planned, or the period of greatest risk has passed (72 to 96 hours) (76).

At the time of the followup visit, the infant should be assessed for weight gain, adequacy of intake, the pattern of voiding and stooling, and the presence or absence of jaundice. Unless a transcutaneous instrument is available or, at the time of discharge, a followup TSB has already been scheduled, clinical judgment is used to determine the need for a bilirubin measurement. Because of the potential for error in the visual estimation of bilirubin levels, however, a TSB or TcB should be measured if there is any doubt about the degree of jaundice. This is particularly important in darkly pigmented infants where the visual estimation of bilirubin levels can lead to significant error.

Information for Parents

An essential component of insuring the safety of a newborn is to make sure that parents are informed (among other things) about newborn jaundice. The AAP (76) recommends

TABLE 35-28

AAP RECOMMENDATIONS FOR TIMING OF FOLLOWUP VISITS AFTER NEWBORN DISCHARGE

Followup should be provided as follows:

Infant Discharged	Should Be Seen by Age
Before age 24 hours	72 hours
Between 24 and 47.9 hours	96 hours
Between 48 and 72 hours	120 hours

For some newborns discharged before 48 hours, two followup visits may be required; the first between 24 and 72 hours, and the second between 72 and 120 hours. Newborns discharged at 48 to 72 hours should be seen for a followup visit at 72 to 120 hours. Clinical judgment should be used in determining followup. Earlier or more frequent followup should be provided for those who have risk factors for hyperbilirubinemia (see Table 35-26), while those discharged with few or no risk factors can be seen after longer intervals.

From Maisels MJ, Baltz RD, Bhutani V, et al. Management of hyperbilirubinemia in the newborn infant 35 or more weeks of gestation. *Pediatrics* 2004;114:297–316, with permission.

TABLE 35-29

GUIDELINES FOR THE USE OF PHOTOTHERAPY AND EXCHANGE TRANSFUSION IN LOW-BIRTH-WEIGHT INFANTS BASED ON BIRTH WEIGHT

	Total bilirubin level (mg/dL [μmol/L][a])	
Birth Weights (g)	Phototherapy[b]	Exchange Transfusion[c]
≤1,500	5–8 (85–140)	13–16 (220–275)
1,500–1,999	8–12 (140–200)	16–18 (275–300)
2,000–2,499	11–14 (190–240)	18–20 (300–340)

Note that these guidelines reflect ranges used in neonatal intensive care units. They cannot take into account all possible situations. Lower bilirubin concentrations should be used for infants who are sick (e.g., sepsis, acidosis, hypoalbuminemia) or who have hemolytic disease.
[a] Consider initiating therapy at these levels. Range allows discretion based on clinical conditions or other circumstances. Note that bilirubin levels refer to total serum bilirubin concentrations. Direct-reacting or conjugated bilirubin levels should not be subtracted from the total.
[b] Used at these levels and in therapeutic doses, phototherapy should, with few exceptions, eliminate the need for exchange transfusions.
[c] Levels for exchange transfusion assume that bilirubin continues to rise or remains at these levels despite intensive phototherapy.

that "all hospitals should provide written and oral information for parents at the time of discharge. This should include an explanation of jaundice, the need to monitor infants for jaundice and advice on how this should be done." The AAP has produced a parent information document entitled "Jaundice FAQs" (Appendix F) which is available at www.aap.org/family/ jaundicefaw.htm.

TREATMENT

Hyperbilirubinemia can be treated in three ways: (a) exchange transfusion removes bilirubin mechanically; (b) phototherapy converts bilirubin to products that can bypass the liver's conjugating system and be excreted in the bile or in the urine without further metabolism; and (c) pharmacologic agents that interfere with heme degradation and bilirubin production, accelerate the normal metabolic pathways for bilirubin clearance, or inhibit the

enterohepatic circulation of bilirubin. Phototherapy is the most common treatment in use for hyperbilirubinemia; exchange transfusions generally are reserved for phototherapy failures. The bilirubin level at which intervention is necessary is still a contentious issue.

Principles Underlying the Recommendations

Recommendations and guidelines for the use of phototherapy and exchange transfusion in term, near-term and preterm infants are provided in Tables 35-29 to 35-32 and Figs. 35-22 and 35-23. It would be ideal if the guidelines for the implementation of phototherapy and exchange transfusion relied on evidence-based estimates of when the benefit of these interventions exceeded their risks and costs (76). Ideally, these estimates should come from randomized trials or high quality, systematic observational studies but such studies are rare (139,140). Thus, treatment guidelines must rely on relatively uncertain estimates of risks and benefits

TABLE 35-30

GUIDELINES FOR USE OF PHOTOTHERAPY AND EXCHANGE TRANSFUSION IN PRETERM INFANTS BASED ON GESTATIONAL AGE

	Total bilirubin level (mg/dL [μmol/L])		
		Exchange Transfusion	
Gestational Age (Weeks)	Phototherapy	Sick[a]	Well
36	14.6 (250)	17.5 (300)	20.5 (350)
32	8.8 (150)	14.6 (250)	17.5 (300)
28	5.8 (100)	11.7 (200)	14.6 (250)
24	4.7 (80)	8.8 (150)	11.7 (200)

[a] Rhesus disease, perinatal asphyxia, hypoxia, acidosis, hypercapnia.
From Ives NK. Neonatal jaundice. In: Rennie JM, Roberton NRC, eds. *Textbook of neonatology.* New York: Churchill Livingston, 1999:715–732, with permission.

TABLE 35-31

GUIDELINES ACCORDING TO BIRTH WEIGHT FOR EXCHANGE TRANSFUSION IN LOW-BIRTH-WEIGHT INFANTS BASED ON TOTAL BILIRUBIN (mg/dL) AND BILIRUBIN-TO-ALBUMIN RATIO (mg/g) (WHICHEVER COMES FIRST)

	<1,250 g	1,250–1,499 g	1,500–1,999 g	2,000–2,499 g
Standard risk				
Total bilirubin	13	15	17	18
B:A ratio	5.2	6.0	6.8	7.2
High risk[a]				
Total bilirubin	10	13	15	17
B:A ratio	4.0	5.2	6.0	6.8

[a] Risk factors: Apgar <3 at 5 minutes; PaO_2 <40 mm Hg ≥2 h; pH ≤7.15 ≥1 h; birth weight <1,000 g, hemolysis; clinical or central nervous system deterioration; total protein ≤4 g/dL or albumin ≤2.5 g/dL.
B:A ratio, bilirubin-to-albumin ratio.
From Ahlfors CE. Criteria for exchange transfusion in jaundiced newborns. *Pediatrics* 1994;93:488–494, with permission.

and the recognition that using a single TSB level to predict long-term behavioral and developmental outcomes is not reliable and will lead to conflicting results (139,140).

The background to treatment decisions for hyperbilirubinemia has been provided (see section on Bilirubin Toxicity.) The basic principles underlying the recommendations given in Tables 35-29 to 35-32 and Figs. 35-22 and 35-23 are as follows:

- Phototherapy is a highly effective method for preventing and treating hyperbilirubinemia (see Phototherapy below). The main demonstrated value of phototherapy is that it reduces the need for exchange transfusion (177,217, 462,463). Ip and associates have calculated that about 5 to 10 term and near-term infants with TSB levels between 15 and 20 mg/dL (257 to 342 μmol/L) will need to receive phototherapy in order to prevent the TSB in 1 infant from reaching 20 mg/dL (the number needed to treat) (139,140). This means that about 8 to 9 of every 10 infants with these TSB levels will not reach 20 mg/dL (342 μmol/L), even if they are not treated. As phototherapy has proven to be a

generally safe procedure, however, the (unnecessary) treatment of many infants is considered appropriate in order to prevent some infants from reaching TSB levels that are considered potentially dangerous (see Phototherapy below for a discussion of its safety and complications).

- The recommended TSB levels for exchange transfusion are intended to keep TSB levels below those at which kernicterus has been reported (124,139,140), although it is recognized that rare cases of kernicterus have occurred in apparently healthy infants and in sick infants at unexpectedly low TSB levels (43,124,139, 140). With rare exceptions, exchange transfusion is recommended only after intensive phototherapy has failed to keep the TSB level below the exchange transfusion level (76).
- As discussed above (see section on Bilirubin Toxicity) infants (particularly those with the risk factors listed in Tables 35-29 to 35-31 and Figs. 35,22 and 35,23) (43,45,154) and preterm infants (45,150,152,464) are at a greater risk for developing kernicterus at lower bilirubin levels than are well term infants, although

TABLE 35-32

GUIDELINES FOR INITIATING PHOTOTHERAPY AND EXCHANGE TRANSFUSIONS IN NICHHD NEONATAL RESEARCH NETWORK TRIAL (B. MORRIS, PERSONAL COMMUNICATION, 2002)

Birth Weight (g)	Aggressive Management		Conservative Management	
	Phototherapy Begins	Exchange Transfusion	Phototherapy Begins	Exchange Transfusion
501–750	ASAP after enrollment	≥13.0 mg/dL	≥8.0 mg/dL	≥13.0 mg/dL
751–1000	ASAP after enrollment	≥15.0 mg/dL	≥10.0 mg/dL	≥15.0 mg/dL

Enrollment is expected within 12–36 hours after birth, preferably between 12 and 24 hours.
ASAP, as soon as possible.
From Maisels MJ, Watchko JF. Treatment of jaundice in low birthweight infants. *Arch Dis Child Fetal Neonatol Ed* 2003;88:F459–F463, with permission.

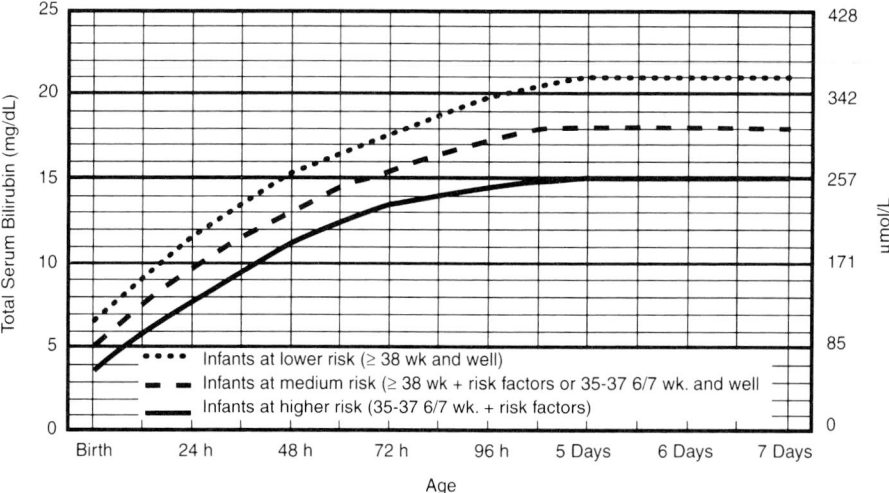

Guidelines for Phototherapy in Hospitalized Infants ≥ 35 Weeks

Note: These guidelines are based on limited evidence and the levels shown are approximations. The guidelines refer to the use of intensive phototherapy which should be used when the TSB exceeds the line indicated for each category.

- Infants at lower risk (≥ 38 wk and well)
- Infants at medium risk (≥ 38 wk + risk factors or 35-37 6/7 wk. and well
- Infants at higher risk (35-37 6/7 wk. + risk factors)

- Use total bilirubin. Do not subtract direct reacting or conjugated bilirubin.
- Risk factors = isoimmune hemolytic disease, G6PD deficiency, asphyxia, significant lethargy, temperature instability, sepsis, acidosis, or albumin < 3.0g/dL (if measured)
- For well infants 35-37 6/7 wk can adjust TSB levels for intervention around the medium risk line. It is an option to intervene at lower TSB levels for infants closer to 35 wks and at higher TSB levels for those closer to 37 6/7 wk.
- It is an option to provide conventional phototherapy in hospital or at home at TSB levels 2-3 mg/dL (35-50mmol/L) below those shown but home phototherapy should not be used in any infant with risk factors.

Figure 35-22   AAP guidelines for phototherapy in hospitalized infants of 35 or more weeks' gestation (76). *Note:* These guidelines are based on limited evidence and the levels shown are approximations. The guidelines refer to the use of intensive phototherapy which should be used when the TSB exceeds the line indicated for each category. Infants are designated as "higher risk" because of the potential negative effects of the conditions listed on albumin binding of bilirubin (77,96), the blood–brain barrier (60), and the susceptibility of the brain cells to damage by bilirubin (55).

"Intensive phototherapy" implies irradiance in the blue-green spectrum (wavelengths of approximately 430 to 490 nm) of at least 30 μW/cm^2 per nm (measured at the infant's skin directly below the center of the phototherapy unit) and delivered to as much of the infant's surface area as possible. Note that irradiance measured below the center of the light source is much greater than that measured at the periphery. Measurements should be made with a radiometer specified by the manufacturer of the phototherapy system.

If total serum bilirubin levels approach or exceed the exchange transfusion line (Fig. 35-23) the sides of the bassinet, incubator, or warmer should be lined with aluminum foil or white material (575). This will increase the surface area of the infant exposed and increase the efficacy of phototherapy (472).

If the total serum bilirubin does not decrease or continues to rise in an infant who is receiving intensive phototherapy, this strongly suggests the presence of hemolysis.

Infants who receive phototherapy and have an elevated direct-reacting or conjugated bilirubin level (cholestatic jaundice) may develop the bronze baby syndrome. See section on phototherapy for the use of phototherapy in these infants. (From Maisels MJ, Baltz RD, Bhutani V, et al. Management of hyperbilirubinemia in the newborn infant 35 or more weeks of gestation. *Pediatrics* 2004;114:297–316, with permission.)

some studies have not confirmed all of these associations (152,178,179). On the other hand, there is no doubt that infants of lower gestation are at a greater risk of developing high TSB levels (203,206).

- Because one of the primary goals of treatment is to prevent further increases in the TSB levels, treatment is recommended at lower TSB levels at younger ages.

It is recognized that it is quite often difficult, and sometimes impossible, to rule out an underlying hemolytic process. There is evidence, for example, that the majority of infants with elevated serum bilirubin levels in the first 2 to 4 days of life have an increase in heme turnover, if not frank hemolysis (465). Although measurements of ETCOc can identify the hemolyzing infant (316,336,455,461,

465), standard diagnostic tests for hemolysis, such as the reticulocyte count, hematocrit, or examination of the peripheral smear, are neither sensitive nor specific (218, 466). Nevertheless, a recent study did find a good correlation between measurements of ETCOc and reticulocyte counts (corrected for the hematocrit) in infants with positive Coombs tests (455).

Most term and near-term infants readmitted with hyperbilirubinemia do not have documented hemolytic disease (241,248,249,467). Of 61 cases of kernicterus, 10 (15%) were considered to have hemolysis and 19 of 61 (32%) were G6PD deficient (124). It is important to note that infants with G6PD deficiency are frequently not anemic and often have none of the classical manifestations of hemolytic disease (326,327).

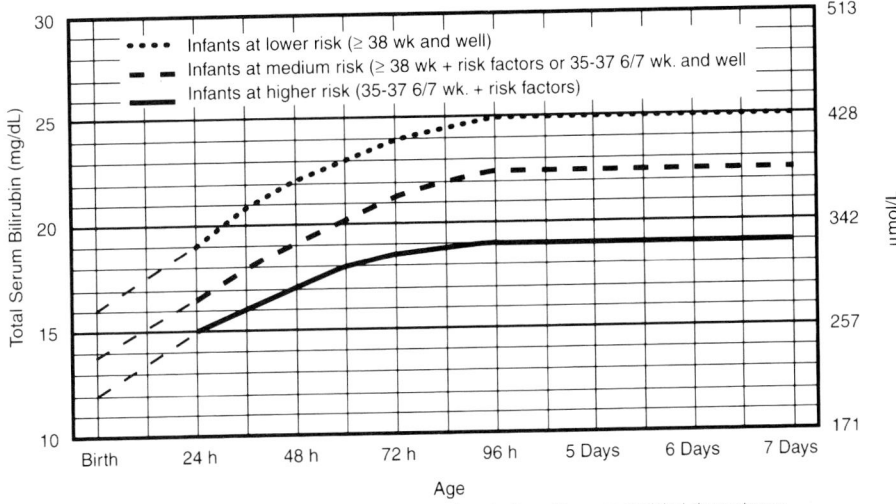

Guidelines for Exchange Transfusion in Infants ≥ 35 Weeks

Note: These guidelines are based on limited evidence and the levels shown are approximations. During birth hospitalization exchange transfusion is recommended if TSB rises to these levels despite intensive phototherapy. For readmitted infants, if TSB is above exchange level, repeat TSB every 2-3hrs and consider exchange if TSB remains above levels indicated after intensive phototherapy for 6 hours.

- The dashed lines for the first 24 hours indicate uncertainty due to a wide range of clinical circumstances and a range of responses to phototherapy.
- Immediate exchange transfusion is recommended if infant shows signs of acute bilirubin encephalopathy (hypertonia, arching, retrocollis, opisthotonos, fever, high pitched cry) or if TSB is ≥5mg/dL (85µmol/L) above these lines.
- Risk factors - isoimmune hemolytic disease, G6PD deficiency, asphyxia, significant lethargy, temperature instability, sepsis, acidosis.
- Measure serum albumin and calculate B/A ratio (See legend)
- Use total bilirubin. Do not subtract direct reacting or conjugated bilirubin
- If infant is well and 35-37 6/7 wk (median risk) can individualize TSB levels for exchange based on actual gestational age.

Risk Category

	B:A Ratio at Which Exchange Transfusion Should be Considered	
	TSB mg/dL/Alb, g/dL	TSB µmol/L/Alb, µmol/L
Infants ≥38 0/7 wk	8.0	0.94
Infants 35 0/7–36 6/7 wk and well or ≥38 0/7 wk if higher risk or isoimmune hemolytic disease or G6PD deficiency	7.2	0.84
Infants 35 0/7 to 37 6/7 wk if higher risk or isoimmune hemolytic disease or G6PD deficiency	6.8	0.80

If the TSB is at or approaching the exchange level, send blood for immediate type and crossmatch. Blood for exchange transfusion is modified whole blood (red cells and plasma) crossmatched against the mother and compatible with the infant (576).

(From Maisels MJ, Baltz RD, Bhutani V, et al. Management of hyperbilirubinemia in the newborn infant 35 or more weeks of gestation. *Pediatrics* 2004;114:297–316, with permission.)

Figure 35-23 AAP guidelines for exchange transfusion in infants who are 35 or more weeks' gestation (76). Note that these suggested levels are based on limited evidence, and the levels shown are approximations. See section on exchange transfusion for risks and complications of exchange transfusion. During birth hospitalization, exchange transfusion is recommended if the TSB rises to these levels despite intensive phototherapy. For readmitted infants, if the TSB level is above the exchange level, repeat TSB measurement every 2 to 3 hours and consider exchange if the TSB remains above the levels indicated after intensive phototherapy for 6 hours. The above bilirubin-to-albumin (B:A) ratios can be used together with, but in not in lieu of the TSB level, as an additional factor in determining the need for exchange transfusion (75).

Risks

When used properly, phototherapy is a very effective and safe method of lowering the serum bilirubin concentration. Its use has drastically decreased the need for exchange transfusion (Figs. 35-24 and 35-25) and it has probably contributed to the virtual disappearance of kernicterus in the low-birth-weight infant.

Conversely, in full-term and near-term newborns, phototherapy can lead to separation of the mother and infant, increase parental concern, decrease the likelihood of successful breast-feeding, and adversely affect the

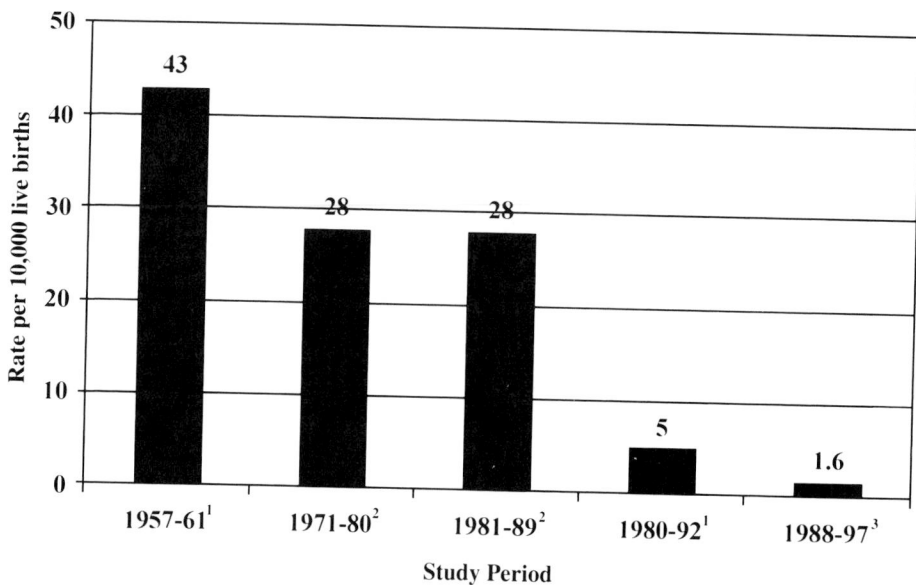

Figure 35-24 Number of infants in different populations who received exchange transfusions between 1957 and 1997. (1) In Athens, Greece, exchange transfusions were performed on 134 infants of 30,830 live births (birth weight ≥2,500 g) between 1957 and 1961 and on 91 infants of 180,594 live births between 1980 and 1992 (577). (2) At the University of Melbourne, Melbourne, Australia, between 1971 and 1980, exchange transfusions were performed in 114 infants of 41,057 live births and between 1981 and 1989, in 134 infants of 47,080 live births (all birth weights) (578). (3) Between 1988 and 1997 exchange transfusions were performed in 8 infants of 55,128 live births at William Beaumont Hospital, Royal Oak, MI (all birth weights) (579).

motherinfant relationship (356). At a time when pediatricians are trying to promote breast-feeding in the face of considerable odds (e.g., early discharge from hospital, the rapid return of mothers to the workforce, commercial marketing of formulas), attention should be given to an intervention that has a negative impact on the nursing mother.

The risks of exchange transfusion include risks from the transfused blood and from the procedure (see section on Exchange Transfusion). Experience with exchange transfusion is decreasing (see Figs. 35-24 and 35-25) and with new types of phototherapy (463) and other interventions in immune hemolytic disease, it is likely to decrease even further (370,468,469). It is now common for a resident to complete a 3-year pediatric training program without ever having performed an exchange transfusion. Under the circumstances, the mortality and morbidity for this procedure is likely to increase in the years ahead.

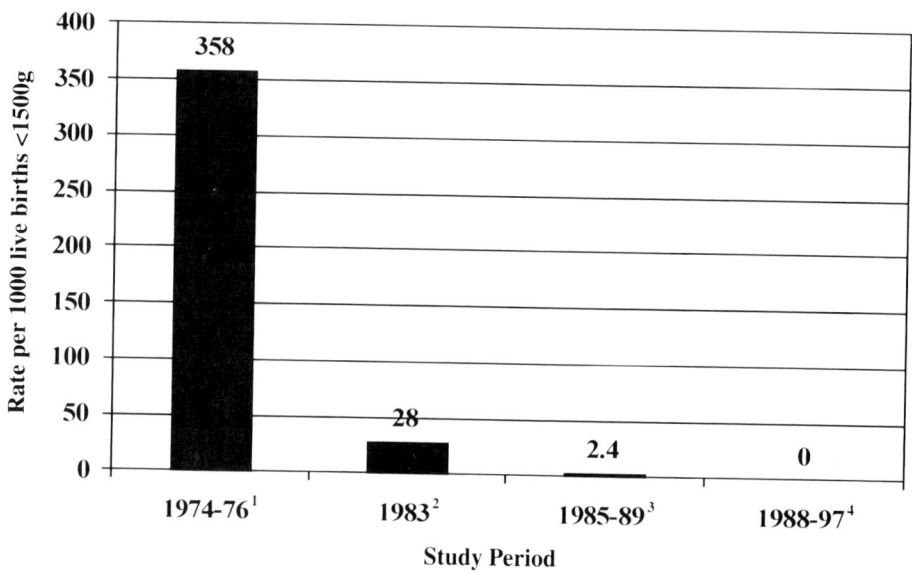

Figure 35-25 Number of infants in different populations with birth weight <1,500 g who received exchange transfusions between 1974 and 1997. (1) A total of 215 newborns weighing <1,500 g in the NICHD Cooperative Phototherapy Trial were assigned to the control group (did not receive phototherapy) (540). Seventy-seven of 215 infants (35.8%) received a total of 161 exchange transfusions. In the phototherapy group, 17 of 196 (8.7%) infants received exchange transfusions. These data are included to illustrate the frequency of exchange transfusion before the introduction of phototherapy. (2) Of a total of 1,338 live births weighing <1,500 g in the Netherlands in 1983, 37 infants (2.8%) required at least 1 exchange transfusion (580). (3) Of 833 live births (weighing 500 to 1,500 g) in a 17-county region in North Carolina, 2 infants required an exchange transfusion (0.24%) (182). (4) No exchange transfusions were performed in 1,213 live births weighing <1,500 g at the William Beaumont Hospital, Royal Oak, MI between 1988 and 1997 (579).

Treating Full-Term and Near-Term Newborns

Most infants who are treated for neonatal jaundice have no identifiable pathology and no evidence of hemolytic disease (see Table 35-18) (218,241,248,249). Approximately 90% are fully or partially breast-fed (249). Guidelines for the treatment of full-term and near-term infants are given in Figs. 35-22 and 35-23. Table 35-33 is an example of a clinical pathway for the management of a newborn readmitted for phototherapy or exchange transfusion.

Breast-Fed Infants

Of infants who develop bilirubin levels high enough to require phototherapy and who do not have evidence of isoimmunization or other obvious hemolytic disease, 80% to 90% are fully or partially breast-fed (218,249). Table 35-34 provides an approach to the prevention and treatment of jaundice associated with breast-feeding. Observational studies show that increasing the frequency of breast-feeding during the first few days after birth decreases TSB levels (251,252,409). We performed a controlled trial in which mothers were randomly assigned to a frequent or demand breast-feeding schedule. We found no significant difference

between the TSB levels measured in the two groups at an average age of 55 hours (470). Given the natural history of jaundice in breast-fed infants, however, it is certain that maximum TSB had not yet been achieved in these infants. However, the observational data of Yamauchi and Yamanouchi (252) show a very strong inverse and linear relationship between the frequency of nursing in the first 24 hours and the probability of hyperbilirubinemia on day 6.

In many hospitals it is a common practice to provide supplemental feedings of water or dextrose water to breast-fed infants in the mistaken belief that this will lower their TSB levels. On the contrary, this practice does not lower TSB levels and should be abandoned (see Fig. 35-21) (419,420). Furthermore, Kuhr and Paneth (424) found that an increase in dextrose water intake in the first 3 days of life was significantly related to a decrease in breast-milk intake on the fourth day.

When the TSB in a breast-fed infant reaches a level at which intervention is being considered, a number of options exist (see Table 35-34). Two randomized controlled trials evaluated some of these interventions. When TSB levels reached 15 mg/dL (257 μmol/L), Amato and associates (471) compared the effect of interrupting breast-feeding ver-

---

TABLE 35-33

EXAMPLE OF A CLINICAL PATHWAY FOR MANAGEMENT OF THE NEWBORN INFANT READMITTED FOR PHOTOTHERAPY OR EXCHANGE TRANSFUSION

Treatment
Use intensive phototherapy and/or exchange transfusion as indicated in Figures 35-22 and 35-23.

Laboratory tests
TSB and direct bilirubin level
Blood type (ABO, Rh)
Direct antibody (Coombs) test
Serum albumin
Complete blood cell count with differential and smear for red cell morphology
Reticulocyte count
ETCOc (if available)
Glucose-6-phosphate dehydrogenase if suggested by ethnic or geographic origin, or if poor response to phototherapy
Urine for reducing substances
If history and/or presentation suggest sepsis, perform blood culture, urine culture, cerebral spinal fluid for protein, glucose, cell count, and culture

Interventions
If TSB ≥25 mg/dL (428 μmol/L) or ≥20 mg/dL (342 μmol/L) in a sick infant or infant <38 weeks' gestation, obtain a type and crossmatch, and request blood in case an exchange transfusion is necessary
In infants with isoimmune hemolytic disease and TSB rising in spite of intensive phototherapy or within 2–3 mg/dL (34–51 μmol/L) of exchange level (see Fig. 35-24), administer intravenous immunoglobulin 0.5–1 g/kg over 2 hours and repeat in 12 hours if necessary
If infant's weight loss from birth is >12%, or if there is clinical or biochemical evidence of dehydration, recommend formula or expressed breast milk; if oral intake is in question, give intravenous fluids

For infants receiving intensive phototherapy
Breast-feed or bottle-feed (formula or expressed breast milk) every 2–3 hours
If TSB ≥25 mg/dL (428 μmol/L) repeat TSB within 2–3 hours
If TSB 20–25 mg/dL (342–428 μmol/L), repeat within 3–4 hours; if TSB <20 mg/dL (342 μmol/L) repeat in 4–6 hours; if TSB continues to fall, repeat in 8–12 hours
If TSB is not decreasing, or is moving closer to level for exchange transfusion, or TSB: albumin ratio exceeds levels shown in Fig. 35-23 consider exchange transfusion; see Fig. 35-23 for exchange transfusion recommendations
When TSB is below 13–14 mg/dL (239 μmol/L) discontinue phototherapy
Depending on the cause of the hyperbilirubinemia, it is an option to measure TSB 24 hours after discharge to check for rebound

From Maisels MJ, Baltz RD, Bhutani V, et al. Management of hyperbilirubinemia in the newborn infant 35 or more weeks of gestation. *Pediatrics* 2004;114:297–316, with permission.

TABLE 35-34

APPROACHES TO THE PREVENTION AND TREATMENT OF JAUNDICE ASSOCIATED WITH BREAST-FEEDING

Prevention
1. Encourage frequent nursing (i.e., at least eight times per day)
2. Do not supplement with water or dextrose water

Treatment options
1. Increase frequency of nursing
2. Continue nursing, administer phototherapy
3. Temporarily interrupt nursing for 48 hours, substitute formula
4. If treating with phototherapy, supplement with expressed breast milk or formula if infant's intake is inadequate, weight loss is excessive, or the infant is dehydrated

sus phototherapy. There was no difference between the groups in the amount of time needed to reduce the bilirubin to less than 12 mg/dL (205 μmol/L). When the TSB level reached 17 mg/dL (291 μmol/L), Martinez and colleagues assigned 125 full-term breast-fed infants to one of four interventions (462); Table 35-35 shows the results. Although discontinuing breast-feeding and using phototherapy was the most effective strategy, in neither of these studies was intensive phototherapy used (472). Notwithstanding the options listed in Table 35-34, any interruption of nursing is undesirable and it is my practice to recommend that breast-feeding be continued while the infant is treated with intensive phototherapy unless very severe hyperbilirubinemia is present (TSB levels in excess of 25 mg/dL [428 μmol/L]) (see Phototherapy below).

Low-Birth-Weight Infants

The management of hyperbilirubinemia in low-birth-weight infants has been reviewed (473) and Tables 35-29 to 35-31 provide suggested guidelines from three different sources. Over the last 2 decades, there has been a remark-able decrease in the incidence of kernicterus found at autopsy in infants who died in NICUs. Some of this may be a result of the liberal use of phototherapy. Certainly, phototherapy has dramatically decreased the necessity for exchange transfusion, which, in low-birth-weight infants, is now almost exclusively carried out in the occasional infant with severe Rh hemolytic disease or extensive bruising (463).

As shown in Tables 35-29 to 35-31, phototherapy generally is used according to a sliding scale: the lower the birth weight, the lower the TSB level at which phototherapy is instituted. In view of the known antioxidant properties of bilirubin, it is possible that maintaining very low TSB levels by the aggressive use of phototherapy might have other, less desirable, consequences (181) (see section on Bilirubin Toxicity–Premature Infants and Low Bilirubin Kernicterus and Physiologic Role of Bilirubin below). To address this and other issues the, NICHHD Neonatal Research Network initiated a trial, the design of which is shown in Table 35-32 (192). The results of this important study should provide guidance with regard to the risks and benefits of phototherapy in the ELBW population.

TABLE 35-35

EFFECT OF INTERVENTIONS FOR JAUNDICE IN BREAST-FED INFANTS

	Group			
	1	**2**	**3**	**4**
	Continue Breast-feeding	**Discontinue Breast-feeding, Substitute Formula**	**Discontinue Breast-feeding, Substitute Formula, Use Phototherapy**	**Continue Breast-feeding, Use Phototherapy**
No.	25	26	38	36
Serum bilirubin ≥20 mg/dL (342 μmol/L)	6 (24%)	5 (19%)	1 (3%)[a]	5 (14%)

When the serum bilirubin reached 17 mg/dL (291 μmol/L), infants were randomly assigned to one of the four interventions above. The number (%) of infants whose bilirubin level subsequently reached or exceeded 20 mg/dL (342 μmol/L) is shown. Conventional (not intensive) phototherapy was used.
[a] Significantly different versus group 1 (p = 0.013) and group 2 (p = 0.036).
From Martinez JC, Maisels MJ, Otheguy L, et al. Hyperbilirubinemia in the breast-fed newborn: a controlled trial of four interventions. *Pediatrics* 1993;91:470–473, with permission.

Elevated Direct-Reacting or Conjugated Bilirubin Levels

There are no helpful data and, as a result, little guidance on how we should deal with the occasional infant who has a high TSB as well as a significant elevation of direct-reacting bilirubin. Because direct-reacting bilirubin is not toxic to the central nervous system, some practitioners have based their decisions for exchange transfusion on the level of indirect-reacting serum bilirubin level (rather than the TSB) as the sole criterion for exchange transfusion (76). The AAP makes a firm recommendation against this practice and notes that the direct-reacting (or conjugated) bilirubin should not be subtracted from the total.

Kernicterus has been described in infants who have elevated TSB levels but in whom the indirect-reacting bilirubin was well below 20 mg/dL (342 µmol/L) (135, 474). One infant had the bronze baby syndrome and another was a 54-hour-old male infant with erythroblastosis fetalis whose TSB level was 45.2 mg/dL (773 µmol/L), of which 31.6 mg/dL (540 µmol/L) was direct reacting. Thus, the total indirect-reacting bilirubin in this infant was only 13.6 mg/dL (135). I have seen the records of other, similar cases. Kernicterus in these infants may be the result of competitive displacement (by direct-reacting bilirubin) of unconjugated bilirubin from its binding site to albumin.

Ebbesen (475) found that infants with elevated direct-reacting bilirubin levels of 6.4 to 9.9 mg/dL (109 to 169 µmol/L) and the bronze baby syndrome had a decrease in reserve albumin-binding capacity. Conversely, some infants with extremely high, but predominantly direct-reacting, serum bilirubin levels have come to no harm.

Hemolytic Disease

As discussed previously, infants with hemolytic disease appear to be at a greater risk of developing bilirubin encephalopathy than are nonhemolyzing infants with similar TSB levels. The reasons for this are not clear. In the early studies of Rh disease, almost all infants were delivered prematurely (to prevent stillbirth); many were asphyxiated and severely ill. It is unlikely that the risk of kernicterus in infants with Rh disease, treated in today's intensive care environment and with similar TSB levels, would be nearly as great. Although it has been suggested that infants with hemolytic disease may have a decrease in their bilirubin-binding capacity, when measured, this has not been found to be the case (476). Similarly, we have no obvious explanation for the increased risk of bilirubin encephalopathy in infants with G6PD deficiency.

Hydrops Fetalis

Hydropic infants generally suffer significant hypoxia *in utero*. Women who are to deliver such infants should be managed exclusively in perinatal centers capable of the full range of obstetric and neonatal intensive care. Hydropic infants, as well as infants who are severely anemic (hematocrit less than 35%) and asphyxiated, require immediate treatment. Exchange transfusion of about 50 mL/kg of packed cells soon after birth raises the hematocrit to approximately 40%. Phlebotomy should not be routinely performed on these infants because they usually are normovolemic and may be hypovolemic (306, 477,478). No manipulations of blood volume should be performed without appropriate measurements of central venous and arterial blood pressures. For accurate monitoring of central venous pressure, however, the umbilical venous catheter must enter the inferior vena cava by way of the ductus venosus. If the catheter is in a portal vein or the umbilical vein, the pressures so measured are meaningless and preclude interpretation of the infant's circulatory status. In addition, before making therapeutic decisions based on measurements of central venous pressure, the physician must also correct acidosis, hypercarbia, hypoxia, and anemia. Serum glucose levels should be monitored carefully, because hypoglycemia is common.

PHOTOTHERAPY

For comprehensive reviews of this subject, the reader is referred to the monograph by Jahrig and associates (479), and to a recent chapter by the author (480).

It helps to understand how phototherapy works if we consider that light is an infusion of discrete photons of energy that correspond to the individual molecules of a drug in a conventional medication. Absorption of these photons by bilirubin molecules in the skin leads to the therapeutic effect in much the same way as binding of drug molecules to a receptor has a desired effect. Tables 35-36 to 35-38 list the factors that influence the dose and efficacy of phototherapy and define the radiometric quantities used in assessing the dose.

Terminology
Light Spectrum

The spectrum of light delivered by the phototherapy unit is determined by the type of light source and any filters used. Because of the optical properties of bilirubin and skin, the most effective lights are those with wavelengths that are predominantly in the blue-green spectrum (481).

TABLE 35-36

FACTORS THAT DETERMINE THE DOSE OF PHOTOTHERAPY

Spectrum of light emitted
Irradiance of light source
Design of phototherapy unit
Surface area of infant exposed to the light
Distance of infant from light source

TABLE 35-37

FACTORS THAT AFFECT THE DOSE AND EFFICACY OF PHOTOTHERAPY

Factor	Mechanism/Clinical Relevance	Implementation and Rationale	Clinical Application
Spectrum of light emitted	Blue-green spectrum most effective; at these wavelengths, light penetrates skin well and is absorbed maximally by bilirubin	Special blue fluorescent tubes or other light sources that have most output in the blue-green spectrum and are most effective in lowering TSB	Use special blue tubes or LED light source with output in blue-green spectrum for intensive PT
Spectral irradiance (irradiance in certain wavelength band) delivered to surface of infant	↑ irradiance → ↑ rate of decline in TSB	Irradiance measured with a radiometer as μW/cm²/nm; standard PT units deliver 8–10 μW/cm²/nm; intensive PT requires ≥30 μW/cm²/nm	If special blue fluorescent tubes used, bring tubes as close to infant as possible to increase irradiance; **Note: cannot do this with halogen lamps because danger of burn;** special blue tubes 10–15 cm above infant will produce an irradiance of at least 35 μW/cm²/nm
Spectral power (average spectral irradiance across surface area)	↑ surface area exposed → ↑ rate of decline in TSB	For intensive PT expose maximum surface area of infant to PT	Place lights above and fiberoptic pad or special blue fluorescent tubesᵃ below infant; for maximum exposure line sides of bassinet, warmer bed, or incubator with aluminum foil
Cause of jaundice	PT likely to be less effective if jaundice caused by hemolysis or if cholestasis present (↑ direct-reacting bilirubin)		When hemolysis present start PT at lower TSB levels. Use intensive PT. Failure of PT suggests hemolysis is cause of jaundice; if ↑ direct-reacting bilirubin, watch for bronze baby syndrome or blistering
TSB level at start of PT	The higher the TSB, the more rapid the decline in TSB with PT		Use intensive PT for higher TSB levels; anticipate more rapid decrease in TSB when TSB >20 mg/dL (342 μmol/L)

LED, light-emitting diode; PT, phototherapy; TSB, total serum bilirubin.
ᵃ Available in Olympic BiliBassinet (Olympic Medical, Seattle, WA).
From Maisels MJ, Baltz RD, Bhutani V, et al. Management of hyperbilirubinemia in the newborn infant 35 or more weeks of gestation. *Pediatrics* 2004;114:297–316, with permission.

There is a common misconception that ultraviolet (UV) light is used for phototherapy. None of the light systems described emit any significant amount of UV radiation, and the small amount of UV light that is emitted by fluorescent tubes is in longer wavelengths (>320 nm) than those that cause erythema (479). In any case, almost all UV light produced is absorbed by the glass wall of the fluorescent tube and by the Plexiglas cover of the phototherapy unit.

Irradiance

Irradiance is the radiant power incident on a surface per unit area of the surface.

The irradiance in a specific wavelength band is called the *spectral irradiance* and is expressed as μW/cm²/nm (see Table 35-38). There is a direct relationship between the efficacy of phototherapy and the irradiance used (Fig. 35-26) (482) and the irradiance is directly related to the distance between the light and the infant (Fig. 35-27) (472).

The Dose–Response Relationship of Irradiance

Figure 35-26 shows that there is a direct relationship between the irradiance used and the rate at which the serum bilirubin declines under phototherapy (482). The data in Fig. 35-26 suggest that there is a saturation point

TABLE 35-38

RADIOMETRIC QUANTITIES USED

Quantity	Dimensions	Usual Units of Measure
Irradiance (radiant power incident on a surface per unit area of the surface)	W/m²	W/cm²
Spectral irradiance (irradiance in a certain wavelength band)	W/m² per nm (or W/m²)	μW/cm² per nm
Spectral power (average spectral irradiance across a surface area)	W/m	mW/nm

From Maisels MJ. Why use homeopathic doses of phototherapy? *Pediatrics* 1996;98:283–287, with permission.

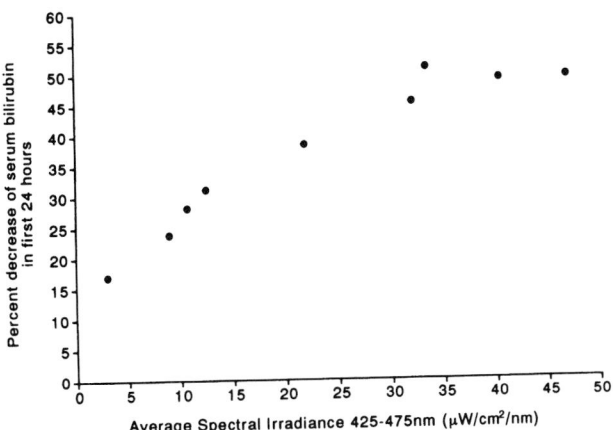

Figure 35-26 Relationship between average spectral irradiance and decrease in serum bilirubin concentration. Full-term infants with nonhemolytic hyperbilirubinemia were exposed to special blue light (Phillips TL 52/20W) of different intensities. Spectral irradiance was measured as the average of readings at the head, trunk, and knees. Drawn from the data of Tan (482). (From Maisels MJ. Why use homeopathic doses of phototherapy? *Pediatrics* 1996;98:283–287, with permission.)

beyond which an increase in the irradiance produces no added efficacy. We do not know, however, that a saturation point exists. As the conversion of bilirubin to excretable photoproducts is partly irreversible and follows first-order kinetics, there may not be a saturation point so we do not know the maximum effective dose of phototherapy.

Effect on Irradiance of the Light Spectrum and the Distance between the Infant and the Light Source.

Figure 35-27 shows that the light intensity (measured as spectral irradiance) is inversely related to the distance from

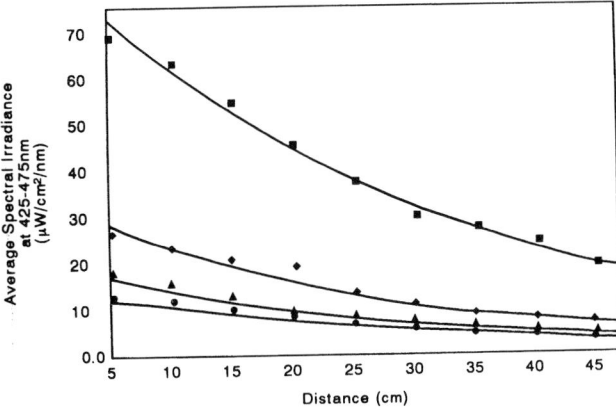

Figure 35-27 Effect of light source and distance from the light source to the infant on average spectral irradiance. Measurements were made across the 425- to 475-nm band using a commercial radiometer (Olympic Bilimeter Mark II). The phototherapy unit was fitted with eight 24-inch fluorescent tubes. (■) Special blue, General Electric 20-W F20T12/BB tube; (◆) blue, General Electric 20-w F20T12/B blue tube; (▲) daylight blue, four General Electric 20-W F20T12/B blue tubes and four Sylvania 20-W F20T1 2/D day light tubes; (●) daylight, Sylvania 20-W F20T12/D daylight tubes. Curves were plotted using linear curve fitting (True Epistat; Epistat Services, Richardson, TX). The best fit is described by the equation $y = Ae^{BX}$. (From Maisels MJ. Why use homeopathic doses of phototherapy? *Pediatrics* 1996;98:283–287, with permission.)

the source. The relationship between intensity and distance is almost (but not quite) linear, indicating that these data do not obey the law of inverse squares, which states that the light intensity will decrease with the square of the distance (472). This law applies only to a point source of light and the light source in phototherapy units has features of a cylindrical and planar source, not a point source. Figure 35-27 also demonstrates the dramatic difference in irradiance produced within the 425- to 475-nm band by different types of fluorescent tubes.

Spectral Power

This is the product of the skin surface irradiance and the spectral irradiance across this surface area. Because irradiance and the surface area of the infant exposed to phototherapy are key elements in determining the efficacy of phototherapy, the use of spectral power is the only meaningful way to compare the dose of phototherapy received by infants under the different phototherapy systems (472). Calculations of spectral power show why a much more effective dose of phototherapy is delivered to the infant by using the appropriate fluorescent tubes than can be delivered using a fiberoptic phototherapy system (472).

Mechanism of Action

Phototherapy detoxifies bilirubin by converting it to photoproducts that are less lipophilic than bilirubin and can bypass the liver's conjugating system and be excreted without further metabolism (10). It is not known exactly where the process of phototherapy takes place, but it probably does not take place in the skin cells. It is more likely that it works on bilirubin bound to albumin in the superficial capillaries or in the interstitial space (483).

Bilirubin Photochemistry

When bilirubin absorbs light, photochemical reactions occur. Although many such reactions have been observed *in vitro*, only three have been shown to occur *in vivo* during phototherapy.

Configurational (Z → E) Isomerization

Isomers are substances that have the same molecular formula but different physicochemical properties. There are four possible configurational isomers of bilirubin (Fig. 35-28). In infants receiving phototherapy, the stable 4Z,15Z isomer is converted predominately to the 4Z,15E isomer (Figs. 35-28 and 35-29).(10) The formation of 4Z,15E bilirubin is spontaneously reversible in the dark and occurs rapidly in bile. Thus the 4Z,15E bilirubin formed in the skin and excreted by the liver is readily converted back to ordinary unconjugated bilirubin. The conversion of the 4Z,15Z isomer to the 4Z,15E isomer is also reversible by light (10).

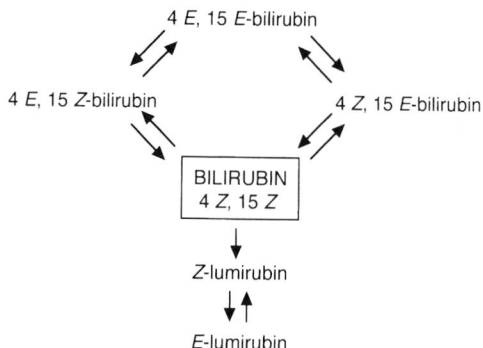

Figure 35-28 Configurational and structural isomers of 4Z, 15Z bilirubin in infants undergoing phototherapy.

When infants are exposed to phototherapy, photoisomerization occurs almost instantaneously, but the clearance of the light-generated 4Z,15E isomer is very slow ($T_{1/2}$ ~15 hours). Thus, although configurational isomerization is extremely rapid and accounts for the bulk of the photochemical outcomes, it probably plays only a minor role in lowering the serum bilirubin concentration because "although it is formed fastest, it has nowhere to go" (484).

Structural Isomerization

In this reaction (Fig. 35-30), intramolecular cyclization of bilirubin (an irreversible process) occurs in the presence of light to form a substance known as lumirubin that can be excreted in bile (without the need for conjugation) and in urine (but at a much lower rate than in bile) (484). During phototherapy, the serum concentration of lumirubin is about 2% to 6% of the TSB, which is much lower than the concentration of the configurational isomers that form about 20% of the total bilirubin. But, because lumirubin is cleared from the serum much more rapidly than the 4Z,15E isomer, it is likely that lumirubin formation is mainly responsible for the phototherapy-induced decline in serum bilirubin in the human infant (484). It is quite possible, however, that the contribution of the other isomers, 4E,15Z and 4E,15E bilirubin, also is important (485).

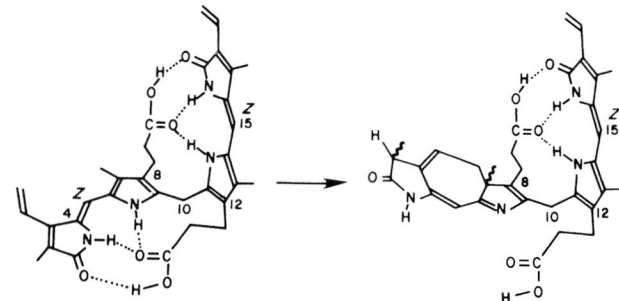

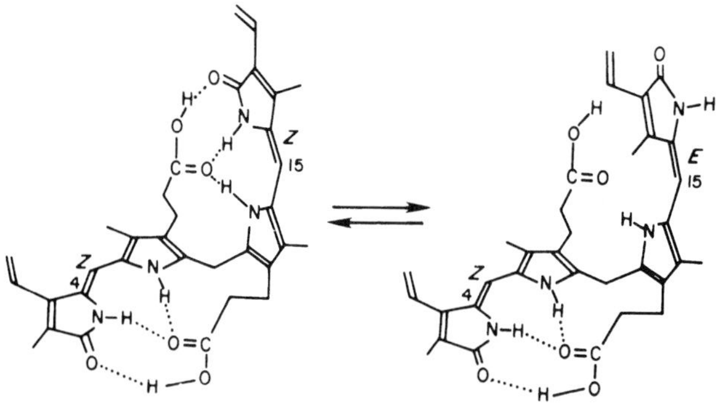

Figure 35-30 Intramolecular cyclization of bilirubin in the presence of light to form lumirubin. (From McDonagh AF, Lightner DA. "Like a shrivelled blood orange"—bilirubin, jaundice and phototherapy. *Pediatrics* 1985;75:443–455, with permission.)

Photooxidation

Bilirubin can be photooxidized to water-soluble, colorless products that can be excreted in the urine. This is a slow process and is probably only a minor contributor to the elimination of bilirubin during phototherapy.

Figure 35-31 summarizes the general mechanisms of phototherapy in neonatal jaundice.

Clinical Use and Efficacy of Phototherapy

There are more than 50 published controlled trials of the clinical use of phototherapy (see Maisels (217) for a description and analysis of these studies), confirming that phototherapy is effective in preventing and treating hyperbilirubinemia and dramatically reduces the need for exchange transfusion (217).

As described previously, there is a clear relationship between the dose of phototherapy and the measured decrement in the serum bilirubin level (see Fig. 35-26) (482). Tables 35-36 and 35-37 list the factors that affect the dose and efficacy of phototherapy. The other important

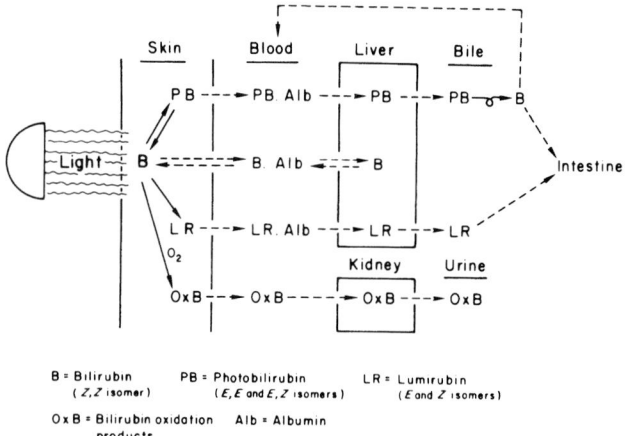

Figure 35-31 General mechanisms of phototherapy for neonatal jaundice. Chemical reactions (*solid arrows*) and transport processes (*broken arrows*) are indicated. Pigments may be bound to proteins in compartments other than blood. Some excretion of photoisomers, particularly lumirubin, in urine also occurs. (From McDonagh AF, Lightner DA. "Like a shrivelled blood orange"—bilirubin, jaundice and phototherapy. *Pediatrics* 1985;75:443–455, with permission.)

Figure 35-29 Z-E carbon–carbon double-bond configurational isomerization of bilirubin in humans. (From McDonagh AF, Lightner DA. "Like a shrivelled blood orange"—bilirubin, jaundice and phototherapy. *Pediatrics* 1985;75:443–455, with permission.)

factors that determine the efficacy of phototherapy are the cause of the hyperbilirubinemia (hemolytic conditions respond less well) and the initial bilirubin level, the rate of decline being proportional to the initial bilirubin concentration (159,486,487).

Light Sources

Fluorescent Tubes

Daylight or cool-white fluorescent tubes provide adequate phototherapy where the objective is to control a slowly rising serum bilirubin level in a preterm or term infant, but they are less effective than "special blue" tubes (see Fig. 35-27). Special blue fluorescent tubes are most effective because they provide light predominantly in the blue-green spectrum. At these wavelengths light penetrates skin well and is absorbed maximally by bilirubin (472,484). The imprint F20-T12/BB (General Electric, Westinghouse, Sylvania) or TL52/20W (Phillips, Eindhoven, The Netherlands) is found on special blue tubes. Note that these are different from regular blue tubes (labeled F20-T12/B) (484). Special blue tubes do impart a bluish tinge to the infant and this may obscure cyanosis. In the term nursery this is of little concern, and if used in the NICU, monitoring by pulse oximetry is all that is necessary. Turquoise fluorescent light (Osram, Denmark) has recently been compared with special blue light in the treatment of preterm infants (488). The emission peak of the turquoise lamps is at 490 nm with a bandwidth of 65 nm. Ebbesen and associates found that these lamps were as effective as special blue lamps but required 23% less irradiance than special blue lamps to produce the same effect on the bilirubin levels (488). They suggest that the use of less irradiance could be associated with fewer side effects.

Light-Emitting Diodes

A new method of delivering high-intensity, narrow-band light has been described (468,489). The use of high-intensity gallium nitride light-emitting diodes (LEDs) permits high irradiance in the spectrum of choice (blue, blue-green, etc.) with minimal heat generation. The device is low weight, low voltage, low power, and portable, and could be an effective means of providing intensive phototherapy in the hospital or at home. Although only limited clinical trials have been performed to date (489), an LED phototherapy unit is commercially available (Natus Inc., San Carlos, CA).

Halogen Lamps

These lamps have the advantage of being more compact than fluorescent systems but, unlike fluorescent lamps, *they cannot be brought close to the infant (to increase the irradiance) without incurring the risk of a burn.* In addition, the surface area covered by most halogen lamps is relatively small, and the spectral power will be less than that produced by a bank of fluorescent lights.

Fiberoptic Systems

These systems consist of a light that is delivered from a tungsten-halogen bulb through a fiberoptic cable and emitted from the sides and ends of the fibers inside a plastic pad (472,490). These systems have the advantage of not requiring eye patches. They are less bulky than conventional phototherapy equipment and provide a convenient way to deliver double phototherapy when it is necessary to expose more of the infant's surface area (see following). They also are useful for home phototherapy. Their major disadvantage is that they have very low spectral power because of their small surface area. This is the result of the inverse relationship between surface area and irradiance. For a given light source, enlarging the pad means that the light must be distributed over a greater area, thus reducing the irradiance (when compared to a small pad and the same light source). To achieve high levels of spectral irradiance, manufacturers must compromise by reducing the size of the pad, which exposes a relatively small surface area of the infant to the light (490). Conversely, because VLBW infants are so small, fiberoptic pads can be used quite effectively in these infants (491–493) and fiberoptic phototherapy does not attenuate the normal post prandial increase in intestinal blood flow (493) (see *Blood Flow* below).

Full-Term and Near-Term Infants—Using Phototherapy Effectively

Phototherapy initially was used in low-birth-weight and full-term infants primarily to prevent slowly rising serum bilirubin levels from reaching levels that might require an exchange transfusion. Today, phototherapy is often used in full-term and near-term infants who have left the hospital and are readmitted on days 4 to 7 for treatment of TSB levels of 20 mg/dL (342 μmol/L) or more. These infants need a full therapeutic dose of phototherapy (now termed *intensive phototherapy*) to get the bilirubin level down as soon as possible (472,487). Intensive phototherapy implies the use of high levels of irradiance in the 425- to 490-nm band (usually ≥30 μW/cm^2 per nm) delivered to as much of the infant's surface area as possible. How this can be achieved is described below. The light spectrum, the irradiance, and the infant's exposed surface area are the key elements in determining the bilirubin response to phototherapy (see Tables 35-36 and 35-37). Thus, to provide the most effective phototherapy for these full-term and near-term infants, we use special blue fluorescent tubes and bring them as close to the infant as possible. To do this, a full-term infant should be in a bassinet, not an incubator, because the top of the incubator prevents the light from being brought sufficiently close to the infant. In a bassinet it is possible to bring the fluorescent lights within about 10 cm of the infant and to produce a spectral irradiance of more than 50 μW/cm^2 per nm (see Fig. 35-27). This does not overheat naked full-term infants. Note, however, that *halogen phototherapy lamps cannot be positioned closer to the infant than recommended by the manufacturers without incurring the risk of a burn.*

To increase the exposed surface area fiberoptic pads should be placed below the infant. This type of "double phototherapy" is approximately twice as effective as single phototherapy in low-birth-weight infants and almost 50% better in full-term infants (494,495). Another way of increasing the surface area of the infant exposed to light is to place a reflecting material (a white sheet or aluminum foil) within or around the bassinet or incubator so that light is reflected onto the infant's skin. Different systems of surrounding the infant with fluorescent lights have been described (487,496,497). Using such a system, Hansen (487) reported declines in serum bilirubins of 10 to 11 mg/dL (170 to 185 µmol/L) within 2 hours. On occasion, I have used two or even three fiberoptic pads to cover almost the entire lower surface of the infant. Although data from Tan (482) suggest that there is a saturation point beyond which an increase in the irradiance produces no added efficacy, we do not know that a saturation point exists. Given that the conversion of bilirubin to excretable photoproducts is partly irreversible and follows first-order kinetics, there may not be a saturation point. Certainly with existing equipment there is probably no such thing as an overdose of phototherapy.

Because phototherapy acts on bilirubin that is present in the extravascular space as well as in the superficial capillaries, it has become a common practice to turn the infant at intervals from supine to prone and back. Two randomized studies suggest that this is not a good idea. Yamauchi and associates (498) found that turning term infants every 6 hours did not improve the efficacy of phototherapy compared with those who are not turned. Shinwell and associates (499) turned infants from prone to supine every 2.5 hours. They found that infants who were not turned had a significantly more rapid decrease in their TSB levels in the first 24 hours of phototherapy than did those who were turned (499).

Measuring the Dose of Phototherapy

Table 35-38 shows the radiometric quantities used in measuring the phototherapy dose. The quantity most commonly reported in the literature is the spectral irradiance. In the nursery, spectral irradiance can be measured using commercially available radiometers. These instruments take a single measurement across a band of wavelengths, typically 425 to 475 nm or 400 to 480 nm. Unfortunately, there is no standardized method for reporting phototherapy dosages in the clinical literature so it is difficult to compare published studies on the efficacy of phototherapy and manufacturer's data for the irradiance produced by different systems. Measurements of irradiance from the same system, using different radiometers, can also produce significantly different results. The width of the phototherapy lamp's emissions spectrum (narrow vs. broad) will affect the measured irradiance. Measurements under lights with a very focused emission spectrum (e.g., blue-light-emitting diode) will vary significantly from one radiometer to another as the response spectra of the radiometers vary from manufac-

turer to manufacturer. Broader-spectrum lights (fluorescent and halogen) have fewer variations among radiometers. Manufacturers of phototherapy systems generally recommend the specific radiometer to be used in measuring the dose of phototherapy when their system is used.

It is also important to recognize that the measured irradiance will vary widely depending on where the measurement is taken. Irradiance measured below the center of the light source can be more than double that measured at the periphery, and this drop off at the periphery will vary with different phototherapy units. Ideally, irradiance should be measured at multiple sites under the area illuminated by the unit and the measurements averaged. The International Electrotechnical Commission (500) defines the *effective surface area* as the intended treatment surface that is illuminated by the phototherapy light. The commission uses 60 × 30 cm as the standard-sized surface.

Is it Necessary to Measure Phototherapy Doses Routinely?

Although it is not necessary to measure spectral irradiance before each use of phototherapy, it is important to perform periodic checks of phototherapy units to make sure that an adequate irradiance is being delivered.

Preterm Infants

Conventional phototherapy with daylight or cool-white fluorescent lights, halogen lamps, or fiberoptic pads have all been effective in decreasing TSB levels and the number of exchange transfusions performed in low-birth-weight infants (see Fig. 35-25) (217). For those with severe bruising or hemolytic disease, however, intensive phototherapy (as described previously) should be used.

Prophylactic Phototherapy in Extremely Low-Birth-Weight Infants

Earlier data suggested that phototherapy, initiated prophylactically from birth in infants weighing less than 1,250 g, was no more effective than phototherapy initiated when the TSB reached 5 mg/dL (85 µmol/L) (501). In a recent study of infants weighing less than 1,000 g, those who received prophylactic phototherapy from birth had significantly lower peak TSB levels than did those who received phototherapy when their TSB levels reached 150 µmol/L (8.8 mg/dL). There was no difference between the groups in the duration of phototherapy (502).

Intermittent Versus Continuous Phototherapy

Clinical studies comparing intermittent with continuous phototherapy have produced conflicting results (479). In practice, on–off cycles complicate nursing care and probably are more trouble than they are worth. There is no doubt, however, that in the majority of circumstances phototherapy does not *need* to be continuous. It can and certainly should be interrupted during feeding or brief parental visits. On the other hand, when bilirubin levels are very high, intensive phototherapy should be administered continuously until a satisfactory decline in the TSB has occurred.

Hydration and Feeding

Breast-fed infants who are readmitted to the hospital with TSB levels commonly have excess weight loss as a result of a combination of mild dehydration and poor caloric intake. In these infants, it makes sense to provide supplemental calories and fluids using a milk-based formula, because formulas inhibit the enterohepatic circulation of bilirubin and help to lower the bilirubin level. Because lumirubin is excreted in the urine, maintaining adequate hydration and good urine output also helps to improve the efficacy of phototherapy. Routine supplementation (with dextrose water) of all infants receiving phototherapy is not indicated.

Biologic Effects and Complications

Even though phototherapy has been used in millions of infants for more than 30 years, reports of significant toxicity are exceptionally rare. Human, animal, and *in vitro* studies suggest that the products of photodecomposition have no neurotoxic effects (503,504).

Skin

Bilirubin is a photosensitizer and, in some circumstances, could act as a photodynamic agent in the presence of light and produce damage. Severe blistering and photosensitivity during phototherapy for jaundice have been described in infants with congenital erythropoietic porphyria (505). The presence of congenital porphyria or a family history of porphyria are absolute contraindications to the use of phototherapy. Rarely, bullous eruptions have occurred in infants with hemolytic disease and transient porphyrinemia who received phototherapy (506,507). All of these infants had significant cholestasis (elevated direct-reacting bilirubin levels), and plasma proto- and coproporphyrin levels were elevated in the two infants in whom they were measured. Other photosensitizers may also be hazardous in infants receiving phototherapy. A 32-weeks' gestation neonate who received intravenous fluorescein for angiography was subsequently exposed to phototherapy (508). This infant developed a partial-thickness burn, which was probably related to the phototoxicity from the fluorescein that produces photosensitization by generation of a superoxide anion when exposed to light at a wavelength of 418 nm in the visible light range (508).

A partial-thickness burn occurred on the back of a 25-weeks' gestation 800-g infant receiving phototherapy with a fiberoptic system (509). This infant required assisted ventilation and inotropic support and died at age 85 hours. There was an extensive, erythematous, denuded area of skin on the back, similar to a partial thickness burn and

from which serous fluid oozed. The Ohmeda Company issued a medical device safety alert on January 26, 1996, in which it reported that four extremely premature infants (≤25 weeks' gestation) had developed purplish-red necrotizing lesions during the use of the BiliBlanket phototherapy system. In all of these infants, conditions were present that might reduce skin integrity such as birth trauma, hypotension, poor perfusion of the skin or bacterial contamination of the incubator or bed. It is unlikely that these were thermal burns although it is important to note that skin of these extremely premature infants is remarkably fragile. Two neonates have been described who developed erythema (one was blistering) following exposure to daylight fluorescent lamps without Plexiglas shielding (510).

Children with the Crigler-Najjar syndrome receiving phototherapy for 2 to 3 years often develop pigmented lesions and tanning as well as skin atrophy.

The Bronze-Baby Syndrome

When infants with cholestatic jaundice are exposed to phototherapy they may develop a grayish-brown discoloration of the skin, serum, and urine known as the bronze baby syndrome (511). The pathogenesis of this syndrome is unknown, but it may be related to an accumulation of porphyrins and other metabolites in the plasma of infants who develop cholestasis (511,512). Although it occurs exclusively in infants with cholestasis, not all infants with cholestatic jaundice develop the syndrome. An animal model of the bronze baby syndrome has been produced by ligating the common bile duct in adult Wistar rats and subjecting them to phototherapy (513).

This syndrome generally has had few deleterious consequences, although a full-term infant with the bronze baby syndrome who died was shown to have kernicterus at autopsy (474). The maximal TSB level in this infant was 18 mg/dL (308 μmol/L) and the direct-reacting bilirubin was 4.1 mg/dL (70 μmol/L). If there is a need for phototherapy, the presence of direct-reacting hyperbilirubinemia should not be considered a contraindication to its use. Because the products of phototherapy are excreted in the bile, the presence of cholestasis will decrease the efficacy of phototherapy. Nevertheless, infants with direct-reacting hyperbilirubinemia often show some response to phototherapy. In infants receiving phototherapy who develop the bronze baby syndrome, exchange transfusion should be considered if the TSB is in the intensive phototherapy range and phototherapy does not promptly lower the TSB. Because of the paucity of data, firm recommendations cannot be made. Note, however, *that the direct-reacting serum bilirubin should not be subtracted from the TSB concentration in making decisions about exchange transfusions* (76) (see Fig. 35-23).

Eye Damage

Because light can be toxic to the retina, the eyes of infants receiving phototherapy should be protected with appropriate eye patches (514). Note that displaced eye patches may obstruct the nares and produce apnea and that shielding infant's eyes and depriving them of visual stimuli could be harmful. The pattern of visual evoked potentials in preterm infants whose eyes had been shielded until they reach 32-weeks postconceptional age where compared with those in infants with unshielded eyes (515). At 41 and 50 weeks post-conception, and at age 3 years, no differences between the groups where found in the visual evoked responses (515). Commercially available eye shields, if properly applied, prevent more than 98% of light transmission (516). Note, however, that in addition to the potential risk of irritation or even corneal abrasion from eye patches, investigators have found an increase in bacterial pathogen isolation and purulent conjunctivitis in infants whose eyes are patched (517).

Insensible Water Loss and Thermal Regulation

Acute changes in the thermal environment occur directly after the initiation of phototherapy (518), and infants receiving phototherapy have an increase in peripheral blood flow that may increase the insensible water loss. Term and preterm infants receiving phototherapy from fluorescent tubes and studied naked in an incubator with an ambient relative humidly of 50% and a servocontrolled environment, showed no increase in water loss from the skin (519). However, a group of Israeli investigators studied 31 preterm infants (gestations 25 to 36 weeks) and measured transepidermal water loss in 7 body areas before and during phototherapy (under fluorescent tubes). They found a mean increase of 26.4% in transepidermal water loss during phototherapy (520). Grünhagen and associates (521) also found an increase in transepidermal water loss of approximately 20% during halogen spotlight phototherapy despite constant skin temperature and relative humidity. These authors suggest that it is appropriate to increase maintenance fluids for preterm infants by 0.35 mL/kg per hour while they are receiving halogen light phototherapy. On the other hand, this may not be necessary if the infant's fluid status is monitored regularly by means of urine output, urine specific gravity, serum electrolytes and change in weight, and fluids adjusted accordingly.

Blood Flow

Under normal circumstances, enteral feedings induce a significant increase in blood flow velocity in the superior mesenteric artery and conventional phototherapy will blunt this postprandial mesenteric blood flow in term and preterm infants (493,522). In preterm infants, Pezzati and associates (493) showed that fiberoptic phototherapy, unlike conventional phototherapy, did not attenuate the post prandial increase in intestinal blood flow. They also found nonstatistically significant increases in the passage of loose, watery, stools and abdominal distention in infants receiving conventional versus fiberoptic phototherapy. They concluded that fiberoptic phototherapy is preferable to conventional phototherapy for treating hyperbilirubinemia in preterm infants.

Cell Damage

Phototherapy can produce DNA strand breaks in cell cultures and DNA strand breakage increases when cells are irradiated in the presence of bilirubin (523). Because light penetrates the thin scrotal skin and perhaps even reaches the ovaries, it has been suggested that shielding the gonads with diapers maybe indicated during phototherapy (524). There is no human or animal evidence, however, to support this practice, and the limited depth of penetration of light makes the possibility of DNA damage to gonads quite unlikely.

Other Complications

The products of photodecomposition have no direct neurotoxic effects. Although phototherapy can produce DNA strand breaks in cell cultures, there is no evidence that this occurs in humans. A relationship has been described between the use of phototherapy and the risk of patent ductus arteriosus in very-low-birth-weight infants (525, 526). The possible mechanisms for this effect are not clear, but may be related to a mechanism similar to nitric oxide-induced vasorelaxation (526).

Intravenous Alimentation

Intravenous alimentation solutions should be protected from phototherapy lights. The exposure of amino acid solutions to light in the blue spectrum produced a significant reduction in tryptophan (527). In addition, when a multivitamin solution was added to the amino acids, a 40% reduction in methionine and 22% reduction in histidine occurred (527).

Diarrhea

Infants receiving phototherapy have an increased incidence of diarrhea (528) and stools become darker and have a greenish tinge (479). These changes are most likely related to the increased excretion of unconjugated bilirubin into the gut.

Home Phototherapy

The economic and social pressures for early discharge of infants from hospital after delivery have led to the widespread use of home phototherapy. Because most of the devices commonly used for home phototherapy do not provide the same degree of irradiance or surface area exposure as those available in the hospital, home phototherapy, of necessity, is used in the prophylactic rather than in the therapeutic mode. Nevertheless, when used appropriately, home phototherapy poses no obvious hazards to the infant and is certainly much cheaper than hospital treatment (529–533). The use of fiberoptic systems and other compact devices has made it easier to administer phototherapy at home.

Figure 35-22 lists the AAP recommendations regarding TSB levels at which home phototherapy is appropriate. Home phototherapy avoids parent–child separation and there is evidence that mothers of infants who receive phototherapy at home are less likely to stop breast-feeding during the period of phototherapy and, if stopped, are more likely to resume breast-feeding than are mothers whose infants are treated in the hospital (534). When compared with other interventions used in the home such as apnea monitors, nasal oxygen, and ventilators, phototherapy must certainly rank among the more benign.

Sunlight Exposure

In their original description of phototherapy, Cremer and associates (535) demonstrated that exposure of newborns to sunlight would lower the serum bilirubin level. Although sunlight provides sufficient irradiance in the 425- to 475-nm band to provide phototherapy, the practical difficulties involved in safely exposing a naked newborn to the sun either inside or outside (and avoiding sunburn) preclude the use of sunlight as a reliable therapeutic tool and it is therefore not recommended.

Crigler-Najjar Syndrome

Other than liver transplantation, the only therapy available to children with the Crigler-Najjar syndrome is phototherapy. This is achieved in most of these children by means of specially designed (noncommercial) home phototherapy devices that provide adequate phototherapy to the growing child and even the adolescent. As the child gets older, phototherapy becomes less effective presumably as a consequence of thickening of the skin, an increase in skin pigmentation, a decrease in surface area relative to body mass, and the need to provide phototherapy only during sleep to allow the normal activities of childhood during the day. The most satisfactory systems provide a "tanning bed" configuration. The child lies on a transparent surface directly above special blue fluorescent tubes. Bubble wrap and plastic "lilos" have been used for this purpose but, because of their low porosity, produce patient discomfort (361,536,537). Job and associates have used a standard mesh or high transmission fabric stretched over an adjustable tension frame (361). This is similar to a traditional hammock and permits adequate transmission of blue light as well as patient comfort.

EXCHANGE TRANSFUSION

Watchko has comprehensively reviewed this subject (538) and Edwards and associates (539) have reviewed the basic indications for, and contraindications to, performing exchange transfusions. A few issues are discussed here. The prevention of Rh hemolytic disease with Rh immunoglobulin and the more effective use of phototherapy has led to a dramatic decline in the number of exchange transfusions

performed (463) (see Figs. 35-24 and 35-25). It is now quite possible for a pediatric resident to complete a 3-year training program without ever having performed an exchange transfusion or even witnessed one. As fewer and fewer of these procedures are done, it is quite likely that the risks of complications will increase.

Exchange Transfusion Risks

Table 35-39 lists potential complications of exchange transfusion and the overall risks of exchange transfusion were reviewed by Ip and associates (139). Reporting the morbidity and mortality associated with exchange transfusion is difficult because both are significantly dependent on the clinical state of the infant before the exchange transfusion. Morbidity and mortality are much lower in term infants with idiopathic hyperbilirubinemia than in sick preterm infants who might be critically ill at the time of the exchange transfusion. In addition, definitions of exchange transfusion-related mortality are not consistent between studies and it is difficult to determine from the literature whether the exchange transfusion procedure itself, or other morbidities were responsible for the deaths of these infants. In addition, many of the published studies refer to infants born before 1970 and there are few U.S. studies of infants born after 1990. Contemporary informa-

TABLE 35-39

POTENTIAL COMPLICATIONS OF EXCHANGE TRANSFUSION

Cardiovascular	Arrhythmias
	Cardiac arrest
	Volume overload
	Embolization with air or clots
	Thrombosis
	Vasospasm
Hematologic	Sickling (donor blood)
	Thrombocytopenia
	Bleeding (overheparinization of donor blood)
	Graft-versus-host disease
	Mechanical of thermal injury to donor cells
Gastrointestinal	Necrotizing enterocolitis
	Bowel perforation
Biochemical	Hyperkalemia
	Hypernatremia
	Hypocalcemia
	Hypomagnesemia
	Acidosis
	Hypoglycemia
Infectious	Bacteremia
	Virus infection (hepatitis, cytomegalovirus)
	Malaria
Miscellaneous	Hypothermia
	Perforation of umbilical vein
	Drug loss
	Apnea

From Watchko JF. Exchange transfusion in the management of neonatal hyperbilirubinemia. In: Maisels MJ, Watchko JF, eds. *Neonatal jaundice*. London, UK: Harwood Academic, 2000:169–176, with permission.

tion on the mortality of exchange transfusions is difficult to obtain, given the infrequency of the procedure. In full-term and near-term infants who are relatively well, the risk of death is low (540–542). The overall mortality is approximately 3 in 1,000 procedures (540,541,543). In the NICHD cooperative phototherapy study (540), morbidity (apnea, bradycardia, cyanosis, vasospasm, thrombosis) was observed in 22 of 328 (6.7%) of exchange transfusions performed. Of the 22 adverse events, however, 6 were mild episodes of bradycardia associated with calcium infusion. Excluding those infants, as well as two who experienced transient arterial spasms, the incidence of significant morbidity associated with the procedure was 5%.

Jackson (541) reported a 15-year experience (1980 to 1995) of exchange transfusion in 106 infants at the Children's Hospital and University of Washington Medical Center in Seattle. Eighty-one were healthy, and there were no deaths in these infants, although one child developed severe necrotizing enterocolitis requiring surgery. There were 25 sick infants, 3 (12%) of whom had serious complications from the exchange transfusion and 2 (8%) died; three additional deaths were considered "possibly due" to the exchange transfusion. Thus, the total number of deaths in sick infants that were possibly caused by the exchange was 5 of 25 (20%). Most recently, adverse events associated with exchange transfusions were reviewed at two perinatal centers in Cleveland, Ohio, between 1992 and 2002 (542). Over a 10.5-year period in two large perinatal centers, only 67 infants were identified who had exchange transfusions for hyperbilirubinemia—an average of about 3 exchange transfusions per year in each institution. The gestational ages ranged from less than 32 weeks (n = 15) to term infants (n = 22). Adverse events occurred in 74% of the exchanges, with thrombocytopenia (44%), hypocalcemia (29%), and metabolic acidosis (24%) being the most common. There were only two serious adverse events, both in infants who had other preexisting, serious neonatal morbidities. The one infant who died was a critically ill 25-weeks' gestation infant with a birth weight of 731 g. The investigators also found that exchange transfusions performed using both umbilical venous and arterial catheters were significantly more likely to be associated with adverse events than when done through the umbilical vein alone or via other routes (542).

Although the risk is very low, exchange transfusion nevertheless carries the usual risk of any blood product. The risk estimates (risk per tested unit) for transfusion transmitted viruses in the United States for the period from 1991 to 1993 were as follows: human immunodeficiency virus, 1:493,000; human T-cell lymphotropic virus, 1:641,000; hepatitis C virus, 1:103,000; and hepatitis B virus, 1:63,000 (544).

Bilirubin Dynamics During and After Exchange Transfusion

During exchange transfusion, bilirubin from the extravascular space is drawn into the plasma, and partial equilibration between extravascular and plasma bilirubin occurs

almost instantaneously (545). Thus, by the end of a double-volume exchange, in which only about 15% of the circulating erythrocytes remain, the serum bilirubin is still 45% to 60% of the preexchange level (545–547). Immediately after the exchange, further equilibration takes plac, which is completed within 30 minutes and produces the early rebound of plasma bilirubin to 60% to 80% of the preexchange level (545).

Repeat Exchange Transfusions

In general, the criteria for repeat exchange transfusions are similar to those used for the initial exchange.

PHARMACOLOGIC TREATMENT

Pharmacologic agents used in the management of hyperbilirubinemia can accelerate the normal metabolic pathways for bilirubin clearance, inhibit the enterohepatic circulation of bilirubin, and interfere with bilirubin formation by either blocking the degradation of heme or inhibiting hemolysis.

Acceleration of Normal Metabolic Pathways for Bilirubin Clearance

Phenobarbital

Phenobarbital is a potent inducer of microsomal enzymes that increases bilirubin conjugation and excretion and increases bile flow. When given in sufficient doses to the mother, the infant, or both, phenobarbital is effective in lowering serum bilirubin levels in the first week of life (226,548). However, concerns about long-term toxicity when given to pregnant women militate against its use for this purpose (549,550).

Decreasing Bilirubin Production by Inhibiting Heme Oxygenase

Tin Mesoporphyrin

As illustrated in Fig. 35-1, the enzyme microsomal heme oxygenase is necessary for the conversion of heme to biliverdin, one of the first steps in the formation of bilirubin from hemoglobin. Certain synthetic metalloporphyrins are powerful competitive inhibitors of heme oxygenase and suppress the formation of bilirubin. The inhibition of heme degradation to bilirubin does not result in the accumulation of heme; the heme is excreted unchanged in the bile in quantities that compensate for the decreased excretion of bilirubin (226).

In a series of controlled clinical trials in Greece and Argentina, Kappas and colleagues demonstrated that tin mesoporphyrin (SnMP) is a potent inhibitor of heme oxygenase and is highly effective in reducing TSB levels and the requirements for phototherapy in term and preterm neonates (370,551,552). They also showed that SnMP in a single dose of 6 μmol/kg was more effective than special blue-light phototherapy in the treatment of term and near-term neonates with established hyperbilirubinemia (551,552). SnMP was equally effective in controlling hyperbilirubinemia in infants with G6PD deficiency (553); a U.S. trial of term and near-term infants showed similar results (554). The only side effect seen so far has been a transient, non–dose-dependent erythema that disappeared without sequelae in infants who received (white light) phototherapy after SnMP administration (555). SnMP has been used in the treatment of the Crigler-Najjar syndrome and has achieved a temporary reduction in TSB levels (369,556), and SnMP has prevented the need for exchange transfusion in Jehovah's Witness newborns with Rh hemolytic disease (557). Kappas reviewed the published controlled clinical trials performed with SnMP (370). Of 279 infants in the control groups, 129 (46%) received phototherapy versus 13 of 443 (3%) of the infants who received SnMP.

The idea of using an inhibitor of bilirubin production is very attractive. It requires no apparatus, infants do not need to be blindfolded, no hospitalization is required, and there is no separation of mother from infant. Phototherapy is a relatively cumbersome and slow method of lowering serum bilirubin levels, whereas SnMP prevents the production of bilirubin and is more efficient than phototherapy. To date, more than 500 newborns have received SnMP in controlled trials, but the drug is still awaiting FDA approval, although it can be obtained for compassionate use (Wellspring Pharmaceu-tical Corp, Neptune, NJ). If approved, SnMP could find immediate application in preventing the need for exchange transfusion in infants who are not responding to phototherapy (557).

Inhibiting the Enterohepatic Circulation of Bilirubin

A number of agents have been administered to infants in an attempt to interrupt the process of the enterohepatic absorption of bilirubin. These include charcoal, agar, and cholestyramine, but they have failed to produce clinically significant reductions in TSB (226). There is evidence that bilirubin in the neonatal gut may be bound to unabsorbed fat (262), and that impairing fat absorption could enhance fecal excretion of unconjugated bilirubin. The administration of orlistat, a substance that binds fat in the intestine, significantly reduced bilirubin levels in Gunn rats (31). To date, there have been no clinical trials of this intriguing concept in the human newborn.

Decreasing Bilirubin Production by Inhibiting Hemolysis

Intravenous Immunoglobulin

Controlled trials have confirmed that the administration of IVIg to infants with Rh hemolytic disease will significantly reduce the need for exchange transfusion (469,558,559). It also is likely that IVIg will help to mitigate the course of severe ABO hemolytic disease (560) and other isoimmune causes of hemolysis. The doses used have ranged from 500 mg/kg given over 2 hours soon after birth to 800 mg/kg given daily for 3 days. In Rh hemolytic disease, anti-D-coated erythrocytes are removed from the circulation through antibody-dependent lysis by cells of the reticuloendothelial system. The mechanism of action of IVIg is unknown, but it is possible that it might alter the course of Rh hemolytic disease by blocking Fc receptors, thereby inhibiting hemolysis. The risks of IVIg therapy are certainly lower than those of exchange transfusion.

PHYSIOLOGIC ROLE OF BILIRUBIN

Despite its potential toxicity, bilirubin may have an important and positive physiologic role (278,561). Bilirubin is a powerful antioxidant *in vitro* (278) and there is a positive relationship between serum bilirubin levels and antioxidant activity in term and preterm infants (562–564). Bilirubin may have a physiologic role as an antioxidant in the human neonate (279,564,565). In sick neonates who have circulatory failure, asphyxia or sepsis, the rate of rise of TSB is less than in control infants (279,565) suggesting that bilirubin is consumed to cope with oxidative stress (561). Because of the possibility that oxidative injury might play a role in the development of retinopathy of prematurity, investigators have evaluated the relationship between bilirubin levels and retinopathy of prematurity (181,181,566–570). Of eight published studies, however, six show no protective effect of an elevated TSB level (567–572). In adults there is clear evidence that decreased TSB levels are associated with an increased risk of coronary artery disease and peripheral vascular disease (561), but we have yet to identify newborns who have suffered a bad outcome because they have too little bilirubin in their serum.

ACKNOWLEDGMENT

I thank Anthony McDonagh, PhD, for his critical review of portions of this chapter.

REFERENCES

1. Hansen TW. Pioneers in the scientific study of neonatal jaundice and kernicterus. *Pediatrics* 2000;106:E15.
2. Weiss JS, Gautam A, Lauff JJ, et al. The clinical importance of protein-bound fraction of serum bilirubin in patients with hyperbilirubinemia. *N Engl J Med* 1983;309:147–150.
3. Tiribelli C, Ostrow JD. New concepts in bilirubin and jaundice: report of the third international bilirubin workshop, April 6–8, 1995. Trieste, Italy. *Hepatology* 1996;24:1296–1311.
4. Berk PD, Noyer C. Structure, formation, and sources of bilirubin and its transport in plasma. *Semin Liver Dis* 1994;14:325–330.
5. Berk PD, Noyer C. Hepatic uptake, binding, conjugation, and excretion of bilirubin. *Semin Liver Dis* 1994;14:331–343.
6. Berk PD, Noyer C. Clinical chemistry and physiology of bilirubin. *Semin Liver Dis* 1994;14:346–351.

7. Hansen TWR. Fetal and neonatal bilirubin metabolism. In: Maisels MJ, Watchko JF, eds. *Neonatal jaundice*. London: Harwood Academic, 2000:3–22.

8. Lightner DA, McDonagh AF. Molecular mechanisms of phototherapy for neonatal jaundice. *Acc Chem Res* 1984;17:417–424.

9. Dennery PA, Rodgers P. Ontogeny and developmental regulation of heme oxygenase. *J Perinatol* 1996;16:S79–S83.

10. McDonagh AF, Lightner DA. "Like a shrivelled blood orange"— bilirubin, jaundice and phototherapy. *Pediatrics* 1985;75: 443–455.

11. Ives NK, Gardner RM. Blood-brain barrier permeability to bilirubin in the rat: studies using intracarotid bolus injection and *in situ* brain perfusion techniques. *Pediatr Res* 1990;27:436.

12. Onishi S, Kawade N, Itoh S, et al. Postnatal development of uridine diphosphate glucuronyl transferase activity towards bilirubin and *o*-aminophenol in human liver. *Biochem J* 1979;194: 705–707.

13. Kawade N, Onishi S. The prenatal and postnatal development of UDP-glucuronyl transferase activity toward bilirubin and the effect of premature birth on this activity in the human liver. *Biochem J* 1981;196:257–260.

14. Dubey AP, Garg A, Bhatia BD. Fetal exposure to maternal hyperbilirubinemia. *Indian Pediatr* 1983;20:527–528.

15. Smith JF, Baker JM. Crigler-Najjar disease in pregnancy. *Obstet Gynecol* 1994;84:670–672.

16. Taylor WG, Walkinshaw SA, Farquharson RG, et al. Pregnancy in Crigler-Najjar syndrome. Case report. *Br J Obstet Gynaecol* 1991; 98:1290–1291.

17. Brodersen R. Binding of bilirubin to albumin. *Crit Rev Clin Lab Sci* 1980;11:305–399.

18. Ostrow JD, Pascolo L, Tiribelli C. Mechanisms of bilirubin neurotoxicity. *Hepatology* 2002;35:1277–1280.

19. Rosenthal P, Blanckaert N, Cabra PM, et al. Formation of bilirubin conjugates in human newborns. *Pediatr Res* 1986;20:947–950.

20. Bosma PJ, Seppen J, Goldhoorn B, et al. Bilirubin UDP-glucuronosyltransferase 1 is the only relevant bilirubin glucuronodating isoform in man. *J Biol Chem* 1994;269:17960–17964.

21. van Es HH, Bout A, Liu J, et al. Assignment of the human UDP-glucuronosyltransferase gene (UGT1A1) to chromosome region 2q37. *Cytogenet Genome Res* 1993;63:114–116.

22. Kaplan M, Hammerman C, Maisels MJ. Bilirubin genetics for the nongeneticist: hereditary defects of neonatal bilirubin conjugation. *Pediatrics* 2003;111:886–893.

23. Watchko JF, Daood MJ, Biniwale M. Understanding neonatal hyperbilirubinaemia in the era of genomics. *Semin Neonatol* 2002;7:143–152.

24. Kotal P, Van der Veere CN, Sinaasappel M, et al. Intestinal excretion of unconjugated bilirubin in man and rats with inherited unconjugated hyperbilirubinemia. *Pediatr Res* 1997;42:195–200.

25. Kaplan M, Muraca M, Hammerman C, et al. Imbalance between production and conjugation of bilirubin: a fundamental concept in the mechanism of neonatal jaundice. *Pediatrics* 2002;4:110.

26. Bartoletti AL, Stevenson DK, Ostrander CR, et al. Pulmonary excretion of carbon monoxide in the human infant as an index of bilirubin production. I. Effects of gestational age and postnatal age and some common neonatal abnormalities. *J Pediatr* 1979;94:952–955.

27. Maisels MJ, Pathak A, Nelson NM, et al. Endogenous production of carbon monoxide in normal and erythroblastotic newborn infants. *J Clin Invest* 1971;50:1–9.

28. Gourley GR. Pathophysiology of breast-milk jaundice. In: Polin RA, Fox WW, eds. *Fetal and neonatal physiology*. Philadelphia: WB Saunders, 1998:1499.

29. Poland RL, Odell GB. Physiologic jaundice: the enterohepatic circulation of bilirubin. *N Eng J Med* 1971;284:1–6.

30. Gartner LM, Lee K-S, Vaisman S, et al. Development of bilirubin transport and metabolism in the newborn rhesus monkey. *J Pediatr* 1977;90:513.

31. Nishioka T, Hafkamp AM, Havinga R, et al. Orlistat treatment increases fecal bilirubin excretion and decreases plasma bilirubin concentrations in hyperbilirubinemic gunn rats. *J Pediatr* 2003;143:327–334.

32. Fevery J. Fasting hyperbilirubinemia: unraveling the mechanism involved. *Gastroenterology* 1997;113:1798–1800.

33. Gärtner U, Goeser T, Wolkoff AW. Effect of fasting on the uptake of bilirubin and sulfobromophthalein by the isolated perfused rat liver. *Gastroenterology* 1997;113:1707–1713.

34. Wolkoff AW, Goresky CA, Sellin J, et al. Role of ligandin in transfer of bilirubin from plasma into liver. *Am J Physiol* 1979; 236:E638.

35. Sackett DL, Haynes RB, Guyatt GH, et al. *Clinical epidemiology: a basic science for clinical medicine*. 2nd ed. Boston: Little Brown, 1991.

36. Orth J. Ueber das vorkommen von bilirubinkrystallen bei neugebornen kindern. *Virchows Arch* 1875;63:447–462.

37. Schmorl G. Zur kenntnis des ikterus neonatorum, insbesondere der dabei auftretenden gehirnveranderungen. *Verh Dtsch Ges Pathol* 1904;15:109–115.

38. Turkel SB. Autopsy findings associated with neonatal hyperbilirubinemia. *Clin Perinatol* 1990;17:381.

39. Ahdab-Barmada M, Moossy J. The neuropathology of kernicterus in the premature neonate: diagnostic problems. *J Neuropathol Exp Neurol* 1984;43:45–56.

40. Volpe JJ. *Neurology of the newborn*. 4th ed. Philadelphia: WB Saunders, 2001.

41. Ahdab-Barmada M. The neuropathology of kernicterus: definitions and debate. In: Maisels MJ, Watchko JF, eds. *Neonatal jaundice*. London: Harwood Academic, 2000:75–88.

42. Valdes-Dapena MA, Nissim JE, Arey JB, et al. Yellow pulmonary hyaline membranes. *J Pediatr* 1976;89:128.

43. Perlman JM, Rogers B, Burns D. Kernicterus findings at autopsy in 2 sick near-term infants. *Pediatrics* 1997;99:612–615.

44. Cashore WJ, Oh W. Unbound bilirubin and kernicterus in low birthweight infants. *Pediatrics* 1982;69:481–485.

45. Gartner LM, Snyder RN, Chabon RS, et al. Kernicterus: high incidence in premature infants with low serum bilirubin concentration. *Pediatrics* 1970;45:906–917.

46. Turkel SB, Miller CA, Guttenberg ME, et al. A clinical pathologic reappraisal of kernicterus. *Pediatrics* 1982;69:267–272.

47. Lipsitz PJ, Gartner LM, Bryla DA. Neonatal and infant mortality in relation to phototherapy. *Pediatrics* 1985;75[Suppl]: 422–426.

48. Ahlfors CE. Bilirubin-albumin binding and free bilirubin. *J Perinatol* 2001;21:S40–S42.

49. Hansen TWR. The pathophysiology of bilirubin toxicity. In: Maisels MJ, Watchko JF, eds. *Neonatal jaundice*. London: Harwood Academic, 2000:89–104.

50. Hansen TWR. Bilirubin brain toxicity. *J Perinatol* 2001;21: S48–S51.

51. Volpe JJ. Bilirubin and brain injury. In: Volpe JJ, ed. *Neurology of the newborn*. Philadelphia: WB Saunders, 2001:521–546.

52. Claireaux A. Icterus of the brain in the newborn. *Lancet* 1953;2:1226.

53. Brodersen R, Robertson A. Chemistry of bilirubin and its interaction with albumin. In: Levine RL, Maisels MJ, eds. *Hyperbilirubinemia in the newborn: report of the 85th Ross Conference on Pediatric Research*. Columbus, OH: Ross Laboratories, 1983: 91–101.

54. Brodersen R, Stern L. Deposition of bilirubin acid in the central nervous system: a hypothesis for the development of kernicterus. *Acta Paediatr Scand* 1990;79:12.

55. Wennberg RP. Cellular basis of bilirubin toxicity. *N Y State J Med* 1991;91:493–496.

56. Chuniaud L, Dessante M, Chantoux F, et al. Cytotoxicity of bilirubin for human fibroblasts and rat astrocytes in culture: effect of the ratio of bilirubin to serum albumin. *Clin Chim Acta* 1996;256:103–114.

57. Roger C, Koziel V, Vert P, et al. Regional cerebral metabolic consequences of bilirubin in rat depend upon post-gestational age at the time of hyperbilirubinemia. *Brain Res Dev Brain Res* 1995;87: 194–202.

58. Rodrigues C, Sola S, Brites D. Bilirubin induces apoptosis via the mitochondrial pathway in developing rat brain neurons. *Hepatology* 2002;35:1186–1195.

59. Hoffman DJ, Zanelli SA, Kubin J, et al. The in vivo effect of bilirubin on the *N*-methyl-D-aspartate-receptor/ion channel complex in the brains of newborn piglets. *Pediatr Res* 1996;40: 804–808.

60. Bratlid D. How bilirubin gets into the brain. *Clin Perinatol* 1990;17:449–465.

61. Wennberg RP, Ahlfors CE, Rasmussen LF. The pathochemistry of kernicterus. *Early Hum Dev* 1979;31:353.

62. Wennberg RP, Hance AJ. Experimental encephalopathy: importance of total bilirubin, protein binding and blood brain barrier. *Pediatr Res* 1986;20:789.

63. Silverman WA. A difference in mortality rate and incidence of kernicterus among premature infants allotted to two prophylactic antibacterial regimens. *Pediatr* 1998;102[Suppl]:225–227.
64. Harris RC, Lucey JF, MacLean JR. Kernicterus in premature infants associated with low concentrations of bilirubin in the plasma. *Pediatrics* 1958;21:875–883.
65. Ostrow JD, Pascolo L, Tiribelli C. Reassessment of the unbound concentrations of unconjugated bilirubin in relation to neurotoxicity in vitro. *Pediatr Res* 2003;54:98–104.
66. Ostrow JD, Tiribelli C. New concepts in bilirubin neurotoxicity and the need for studies at clinically relevant bilirubin concentrations. *J Hepatology* 2001;34:467–470.
67. Ostrow J, Pascolo L, Shapiro S, et al. New concepts in bilirubin encephalopathy. *Eur J Clin Invest* 2003;33:988–997.
68. Ahlfors CE. Measurement of plasma unbound unconjugated bilirubin. *Anal Biochem* 2000;279:130–135.
69. Hansen TWR, Oyasaeter S, Stiris T, et al. Effects of sulfisoxazole, hypercarbia, and hyperosmolality on entry of bilirubin and albumin into brain regions in young rats. *Biol Neonate* 1989;56:22.
70. Amin SB, Ahlfors CE, Orlando MS, et al. Bilirubin and serial auditory brainstem responses in premature infants. *Pediatrics* 2001;107:664–670.
71. Funato M, Tamai H, Shimada S, et al. Vigintiphobia, unbound bilirubin, and auditory brainstem responses. *Pediatrics* 1994;93:50–53.
72. Ahlfors CE, Herbsman O. Unbound bilirubin in a term newborn with kernicterus. *Pediatrics* 2003;111:1110–1112.
73. Nakamura H, Takada S, Shimabuku R, et al. Auditory and brainstem responses in newborn infants with hyperbilirubinemia. *Pediatrics* 1985;75:703–708.
74. Shimabuku R, Nakamura H. Total and unbound bilirubin determination using a automated peroxidase micromethod. *Kobe J Med Sci* 1982;28:91–104.
75. Ahlfors CE. Criteria for exchange transfusion in jaundiced newborns. *Pediatrics* 1994;93:488–494.
76. Maisels MJ, Baltz RD, Bhutani V, et al. Management of hyperbilirubinemia in the newborn infant 35 or more weeks of gestation. *Pediatrics* 2004;114:297–316.
77. Cashore WJ. Free bilirubin concentrations and bilirubin-binding affinity in term and preterm infants. *J Pediatr* 1980;96:521–527.
78. Spear ML, Stahl GE, Paul MH, et al. The effect of 15-hour fat infusions of varying dosage on bilirubin binding to albumin. *JPEN J Parenter Enteral Nutr* 1985;9:144–147.
79. Nizar L, Vyhmeister N, Ross R, et al. A jaundiced look at intravenous fat administration and the risk factor for kernicterus. *Clin Res* 1990;38:197A.
80. Levine RL. Fluorescence quenching studies of the binding of bilirubin to albumin. *Clin Chem* 1972;23:2292.
81. Nelson P, Jacobsen J, Wennberg RP. Effect of pH on the interaction of bilirubin with albumin and tissue culture cells. *Pediatr Res* 1974;8:963.
82. Kozuki K, Oh W, Widness J, et al. Increase in bilirubin binding to albumin with correction of neonatal acidosis. *Acta Paediatr Scand* 1979;68:213.
83. Robertson A, Carp W, Broderson R. Bilirubin displacing effect of drugs used in neonatology. *Acta Paediatr Scand* 1991;80:1119–1127.
84. Brodersen R, Ebbesen F. Bilirubin-displacing effect of ampicillin, indomethacin, chlorpromazine, gentamicin, and parabens *in vitro* and in newborn infants. *J Pharm Sci* 1983;72:248–253.
85. Rasmussen LF, Ahlfors CE, Wennberg RP. Displacement of bilirubin from albumin by indomethacin. *J Clin Pharmacol* 1978;18:477–481.
86. Cooper-Peel C, Brodersen R, Robertson A. Does ibuprofen affect bilirubin-albumin binding in newborn infant serum? *Pharmacol Technol* 1996;79:297–299.
87. Aranda JV, Varvarigou A, Beharry K, et al. Pharmacokinetics and protein binding of intravenous ibuprofen in the premature newborn infant. *Acta Paediatr* 1997;86:289–298.
88. Overmeire BV, Touw D, Schepens PJC, et al. Ibuprofen pharmacokinetics in preterm infants with patent ductus arteriosus. *Clin Pharmacol Ther* 2001;70:336–343.
89. Jardine DS, Rogers K. Relationship of benzyl alcohol to kernicterus, intraventricular hemorrhage, and mortality in preterm infants. *Pediatrics* 1989;83:153–160.
90. Watchko JF. The clinical sequelae of hyperbilirubinemia. In: Maisels MJ, Watchko JF, eds. *Neonatal jaundice*. London: Harwood Academic, 2000:115–138.
91. Ahlfors CE. Benzyl alcohol, kernicterus, and unbound bilirubin. *J Pediatr* 2001;139:317–319.
92. Robertson A, Carp W, Broderson R. Effect of drug combinations on bilirubin–albumin binding. *Dev Pharmacol Ther* 1991;17:95.
93. Hanko E, Tommarello S, Watchko JF, et al. Administration of drugs known to inhibit p-glycoprotein increases brain bilirubin and alters the regional distribution of bilirubin in rat brain. *Pediatr Res* 2003;54:441–445.
94. Valaes T, Hyte M. Effect of exchange transfusion on bilirubin binding. *Pediatrics* 1977;59:881.
95. Cifuentes RF, Nelson AJ, Levine J, et al. Cutaneous bilirubinometry during phototherapy. *Pediatr Res* 1982;16:282A(abst).
96. Cashore WJ, Oh W, Brodersen R. Reserve albumin and bilirubin toxicity index in infant serum. *Acta Paediatr Scand* 1983;72:415–419.
97. Ritter DA, Kenny JD, Norton HJ, et al. A prospective study of free bilirubin and other high-risk factors in the development of kernicterus in premature infants. *Pediatrics* 1982;69:260–266.
98. Robertson A, Sharp C, Karp W. The relationship of gestational age to reserve albumin concentration for binding of bilirubin. *J Perinatol* 1988;8:17.
99. Jirka JH, Duckrow B, Kendig JW, et al. Effect of bilirubin on brainstem auditory evoked potentials in the asphyxiated rat. *Pediatr Res* 1985;19:556–560.
100. Rozdilsky B, Olszewski J. Experimental study of the toxicity of bilirubin in newborn animals. *J Neuropathol Exp Neurol* 1961;20:193–205.
101. Bratlid D, Cashore WJ, Oh W. Effect of serum hyperosmolality on opening of blood brain barrier for bilirubin in rat brain. *Pediatrics* 1983;71:909–912.
102. Bratlid D, Jori G. Mechanism of bilirubin entry into the brain in an animal model. In: Rubaltelli FF, ed. *Neonatal jaundice: new trends in phototherapy*. New York: Plenum Press, 1984:23–24.
103. Bratlid D, Cashore WJ, Oh W. Effects of acidosis on bilirubin deposition in rat brain. *Pediatrics* 1984;73:431–434.
104. Burgess GH, Oh W, Bratlid D, et al. The effects of brain blood flow on brain bilirubin deposition in newborn piglets. *Pediatr Res* 1985;19:691–696.
105. Drummond GS, Kappas A. Chemoprevention of neonatal jaundice: potency of tin- protoporphyrin in an animal model. *Science* 1982;217:1250–1252.
106. Levine RL, Fredericks WR, Rapoport SI. Entry of bilirubin into the brain due to opening of the blood brain barrier. *Pediatrics* 1982;69:255.
107. Stobie PE, Hansen CT, Hailey JR, et al. A difference in mortality between two strains of jaundiced rats. *Pediatrics* 1991;87:5918.
108. Wennberg RP. The blood-brain barrier and bilirubin encephalopathy. *Cell Mol Neurobiol* 2000;20(1):97–109.
109. Watchko JF, Daood MJ, Mahmood B, et al. P-glycoprotein and bilirubin disposition. *J Perinatol* 2001;21:S43-S47.
110. Watchko JF, Daood MJ, Hansen TWR. Brain bilirubin content is increased in P-Glycoprotein-Deficient transgenic null mutant mice. *Ped Res* 1998;44:763–766.
111. Cashore WJ. Bilirubin metabolism and toxicity in the newborn. In: Polin RA, Fox WW, eds. *Fetal and neonatal physiology*. Philadelphia: WB Saunders, 1998:1493–1498.
112. Saunders NR, Mollgard K. Development of the blood-brain barrier. *J Dev Physiol* 1984;6:45.
113. Lee C, Oh W. Permeability of the blood-brain barrier for ^{125}I-albumin-bound bilirubin in newborn piglets. *Pediatr Res* 1989;25:452.
114. Ohsugi M, Sato H, Yamamura H. Transfer of bilirubin covalently bound to ^{125}I-albumin from blood to brain in the Gunn rate newborn. *Biol Neonate* 1992;62:47–54.
115. Escher-Graub DC, Ricker HS. Jaundice and behavioral organization in the full-term neonate. *Helv Paediatr Acta* 1986;41:425–435.
116. Rapisardi G, Vohr B, Cashore W, et al. Assessment of infant cry variability in high-risk infants. *Int J Ped Otorhinolaryngology* 1989;17:19–29.
117. Perlman M, Fainmesser P, Sohmer H, et al. Auditory nerve-brainstem evoked responses in hyperbilirubinemic neonates. *Pediatrics* 1983;72:658–664.
118. Vohr BR. New approaches to assessing the risks of hyperbilirubinemia. *Clin Perinatol* 1990;17:293–306.

119. Hansen TWR, Allen JW. Bilirubin-oxidizing activity in rat brain. *Biol Neonate* 1996;70:289–295.
120. Hansen TWR, Allen JW. Oxidation of bilirubin by brain mitochondrial membranes-dependence on cell type and postnatal age. *Biochem Mol Med* 1997;60:155–160.
121. Johnson L, Brown AK, Bhutani VK. Bind—a clinical score for bilirubin induced neurologic dysfunction in newborns. *Pediatrics* 1999;104:746–747.
122. Gerrard J. Kernicterus. *Brain* 1952;75:526–570.
123. Van Praagh R. Diagnosis of kernicterus in the neonatal period. *Pediatrics* 1961;28:870–876.
124. Johnson LH, Bhutani VK, Brown AK. System-based approach to management of neonatal jaundice and prevention of kernicterus. *J Pediatr* 2002;140:396–403.
125. Harris M, Bernbaum J, Polin J, et al. Developmental follow-up of breastfed term and near-term infants with marked hyperbilirubinemia. *Pediatrics* 2001;107:1075–1080.
126. Johnston WH, Angara V, Baumal R, et al. Erythroblastosis fetalis and hyperbilirubinemia. A five-year follow-up with neurological, physiological and audiological evaluation. *Pediatrics* 1967;39:88–92.
127. Jones MH, Sands R, Hyman CB, et al. Longitudinal study of incidence of central nervous system damage following erythroblastosis fetalis. *Pediatrics* 1954;14:346.
128. Byers RK, Paine RS, Crothers V. Extrapyramidal cerebral palsy with hearing loss following erythroblastosis. *Pediatrics* 1955;15:248.
129. Perlstein MA. The late clinical syndrome of post-icteric encephalopathy. *Pediatr Clin North Am* 1960;7:665.
130. Chin KC, Taylor MJ, Perlman M. Improvement in auditory and visually evoked potentials in jaundiced preterm infants after exchange transfusion. *Arch Dis Child* 1985;60:714–717.
131. Hyman CB, Keaster J, Hanson V, et al. CNS abnormalities after neonatal hemolytic disease or hyperbilirubinemia. A prospective study of 405 patients. *Am J Dis Child* 1969;117:395–405.
132. Shapiro SM, Nakamura H. Bilirubin and the auditory system. *J Perinatol* 2001;21:S52-S55.
133. Penn AA, Enzman DR, Hahn JS, et al. Kernicterus in a full-term infant. *Pediatrics* 1994;93:1003–1006.
134. Martich-Kriss V, Kollias SS, Ball WS. MR findings in kernicterus. *AJNR Am J Neuroradiol* 1995;16:819–821.
135. Grobler JM, Mercer MJ. Kernicterus associated with elevated predominantly direct-reacting bilirubin. *S Afr Med J* 1997;87:146.
136. Sugama S, Soeda A, Eto Y. Magnetic resonance imaging in three children with kernicterus. *Pediatr Neurol* 2001;25:328–331.
137. Govaert P, Lequin M, Swarte R, et al. Changes in globus pallidus with (pre) term kernicterus. *Pediatrics* 2003;112:1256–1263.
138. Hoon AH, Reinhardt EM, Kelley RI, et al. Brain magnetic resonance imaging in suspected extrapyramidal cerebral palsy: observations in distinguishing genetic-metabolic from acquired causes. *J Pediatr* 1997;131:240–245.
139. Ip S, Chung M, Kulig J, et al. An evidence-based review of important issues concerning neonatal hyperbilirubinemia. *Pediatrics* 2004;114:e130–e153.
140. Ip S, Glicken S, Kulig J, et al. *Management of neonatal hyperbilirubinemia.* Rockville, MD: US Department of Health and Human Services, Agency for Healthcare Research and Quality, 2003.
141. Maisels MJ, Newman TB. Bilirubin and neurological dysfunction—do we need to change what we are doing? *Pediatr Res* 2001;50(6):677–678.
142. Hsia DYY, Allen FH, Gellis SS, et al. Erythroblastosis fetalis. VIII. Studies of serum bilirubin in relation to kernicterus. *N Engl J Med* 1952;247:668–671.
143. Mollison PL, Cutbush M. Haemolytic disease of the newborn. In: Gairdner D, ed. *Recent Advances in Pediatrics.* New York: P Blakiston, 1954:110.
144. Newman TB, Maisels MJ. Does hyperbilirubinemia damage the brain of healthy full-term infants? *Clin Perinatol* 1990;17:331–358.
145. Newman TB, Maisels MJ. Evaluation of jaundice in the term newborn: a kinder, gentler approach. *Pediatrics* 1992;89:809–818.
146. American Academy of Pediatrics. Provisional Committee for Quality Improvement and Subcommittee on Hyperbilirubinemia. Practice parameter: management of hyperbilirubinemia in the healthy term newborn. *Pediatrics* 1994;94:558–562.
147. Gartner LM. Management of jaundice in the well baby. *Pediatrics* 1992;89:826–827.
148. Merenstein GB. "New" bilirubin recommendations questioned. *Pediatrics* 1992;89:822–823.
149. Watchko JF, Oski FA. Bilirubin 20 mg/dL = vigintiphobia. *Pediatrics* 1983;71:660–663.
150. Watchko J, Claassen D. Kernicterus in premature infants: current prevalence and relationship to NICHD phototherapy study exchange criteria. *Pediatrics* 1994;93:996–999.
151. Watchko JF, Maisels MJ. Jaundice in low birth weight infants—pathobiology and outcome. *Arch Dis Child Fetal Neonatol Ed* 2003;88;456–459.
152. Watchko JF, Oski FA. Kernicterus in preterm newborns: past, present and future. *Pediatrics* 1992;90:707–715.
153. Mollison PL, Walker W. Controlled trials of the treatment of haemolytic disease of the newborn. *Lancet* 1952;1:429–433.
154. Ozmert E, Erdem G, Topcu M. Long-term follow-up of indirect hyperbilirubinemia in full-term Turkish infants. *Acta Paediatr* 1996;85:1440–1444.
155. Johnson L, Boggs TR. Bilirubin-dependent brain damage: incidence and indications for treatment. In: Odell GB, Schaffer R, Simopoulos AP, eds. *Phototherapy in the newborn: an overview.* Washington, DC: National Academy of Sciences, 1974:122–149.
156. Valaes T. Severe neonatal jaundice associated with glucose-6-phosphate dehydrogenase deficiency: pathogenesis and global epidemiology. *Acta Paediatr* 1994;394[Suppl]:58–76.
157. Martin DH, Thompson W, Pinkerton JHM, et al. A randomized controlled trial of selective planned delivery. *Br J Obstet Gynecol* 1978;85:109–113.
158. Raghubir KV, Fox GF, Inwood S, et al. Follow up of term neonates with extremely high unconjugated bilirubin. *Pediatr Res* 1996;39:276A.
159. Newman TB, Liljestrand P, Gabriel J, et al. Infants with bilirubin levels of 30 mg/dL or more in a large managed care organization. *Pediatrics* 2003;6:1303–1310.
160. Newman TB, Klebanoff MA. Neonatal hyperbilirubinemia and long-term outcome: another look at the collaborative perinatal project. *Pediatrics* 1993;92:651–657.
161. Seidman DS, Paz I, Stevenson DK, et al. Neonatal hyperbilirubinemia and physical and cognitive performance at 17 years of age. *Pediatrics* 1991;88:828–833.
162. Seidman DS, Laor A, Paz I, et al. Neonatal hyperbilirubinemia in healthy term infants and cognitive outcome in late adolescence. *Pediatr Res* 1998;43:194A.
163. Grimmer I, Berger-Jones K, Buhrer C, et al. Late neurological sequelae of non-hemolytic hyperbilirubinemia of healthy term neonates. *Acta Paediatr* 1999;88:661–663.
164. Soorani-Lunsing I, Woltil H, Hadders-Algra M. Are moderate degrees of hyperbilirubinemia in healthy term neonates really safe for the brain? *Pediatr Res* 2001;50:701–705.
165. Naeye RL. Amniotic fluid infections, neonatal hyperbilirubinemia, and psychomotor impairment. *Pediatrics* 1978;62:497–503.
166. Odell GB, Storey GNB, Rosenberg LA. Studies in kernicterus: III. The saturation of serum proteins with bilirubin during neonatal life and its relationship to brain damage at five years. *J Pediatr* 1970;76:12–21.
167. Scheidt PC, Graubard BI, Nelson KB, et al. Intelligence at six years in relation to neonatal bilirubin level: follow-up of the National Institute of Child Health and Human Development Clinical Trial of Phototherapy. *Pediatrics* 1991;87:797–805.
168. Nwaesei CG, Van Aerde J, Boyden M, et al. Changes in auditory brainstem responses in hyperbilirubinemic infants before and after exchange transfusion. *Pediatrics* 1984;74:800–803.
169. Nakamura H, Yonetani M, Uetani Y, et al. Determination of serum unbound bilirubin for prediction of kernicterus in low birth weight infants. *Acta Paediatr Jpn* 1992;54:642–647.
170. Scheidt PC, Bryla DA, Nelson KB, et al. Phototherapy for neonatal hyperbilirubinemia: six year follow-up of the NICHD clinical trial. *Pediatrics* 1990;85:455–463.
171. Nilsen ST, Finne PH, Bergsjo P, et al. Males with neonatal hyperbilirubinemia examined at 18 years of age. *Acta Paediatr Scand* 1984;73:176–180.
172. Shapiro SM. Evoked potentials and bilirubin. In: Maisels MJ, Watchko JF, eds. *Neonatal jaundice.* London: Harwood Academic, 2000:105–114.
173. Suresh G, Lucey J. Lack of deafness in Crigler-Najjar syndrome type 1: a patient survey. *Pediatrics* 2000;100:E9.
174. Johnson L. Hyperbilirubinemia in the term infant: when to worry, when to treat. *N Y State J Med* 1991;91:483–489.

175. Department of Clinical Epidemiology and Biostatistics MUHSC. How to read journals. IV. To determine etiology or causation. *Can Med Assoc J* 1981;124:985.

176. Scheidt PC, Mellits ED, Hardy JB, et al. Toxicity to bilirubin in neonates: infant development during first year in relation to maximum neonatal serum bilirubin concentration. *J Pediatr* 1977;91:292–297.

177. Brown AK, Kim MH, Wu PYK, et al. Efficacy of phototherapy in prevention and management of neonatal hyperbilirubinemia. *Pediatrics* 1985;75:393–400.

178. Kim MH, Yoon JJ, Sher J, et al. Lack of predictive indices in kernicterus. A comparison of clinical and pathologic factors in infants with or without kernicterus. *Pediatrics* 1980;66:852–858.

179. Turkel SB, Guttenberg ME, Moynes DR, et al. Lack of identifiable risk factors for kernicterus. *Pediatrics* 1980;66:502–506.

180. van de Bor M, Ens-Dokkum M, Schreuder AM, et al. Hyperbilirubinemia in low birthweight infants and outcome at 5 years of age. *Pediatrics* 1992;89:359–364.

181. Yeo KL, Perlman M, Hao Y, et al. Outcomes of extremely premature infants related to their peak serum bilirubin concentrations and exposure to phototherapy. *Pediatr* 1998;102(6):1426–1431.

182. O'Shea TM, Dillard RG, Klinepeter KD, et al. Serum bilirubin levels, intracranial hemorrhage, and the risk of developmental problems in very low birth weight infants. *Pediatrics* 1992;90:888–892.

183. Graziani LJ, Mitchell DG, Kornhauser M, et al. Neurodevelopment of preterm infants: neonatal neurosonographic and serum bilirubin studies. *Pediatrics* 1992;89:229.

184. van de Bor M, van Zeben-van der Aa TM, Verloove-Vanhorick SP, et al. Hyperbilirubinemia in very preterm infants and neurodevelopmental outcome at two years of age: results of a national collaborative survey. *Pediatrics* 1989;83:915–920.

185. Oh W, Tyson JE, Fanaroff AA, et al. Association between peak serum bilirubin and neurodevelopmental outcomes in extremely low birth weight infants. *Pediatrics* 2003;112:773–779.

186. Ikonen RS, Kuusinen EJ, Janas MO, et al. Possible etiologic factors in extensive periventricular leucomalacia of preterm infants. *Acta Paeditr Scand* 1988;77:489–495.

187. Trounce J, Shaw DE, Levine MI, et al. Clinical risk factors and periventricular leucomalacia. *Arch Dis Child* 1988;63:17–22.

188. Ikonen RS, Koivkko MJ, Laippala, et al. Hyperbilirubinemia, hypocarbia and periventricular leukomalacia in preterm infants: relationship to cerebral palsy. *Acta Paediatr* 1992;81:802–807.

189. Hack M, Wilson-Costello D, Friedman H, et al. Neurodevelopment and predictors of outcomes of children with birth weights of less than 1000 g 1992–1995. *Arch Pediatr Adolesc Med* 2000;154:725–731.

190. DeVries KL, Lary S, Dubowitz LMS. Relationship of serum bilirubin levels to ototoxicity and deafness in high-risk low-birth-weight infants. *Pediatrics* 1985;76:351–354.

191. DeVries L, Lary S, Whitelaw A. Relationship of serum bilirubin levels and hearing impairment in newborn infants. *Early Hum Dev* 1987;15:269–277.

192. Morris B. A randomized trial of aggressive or conservative phototherapy for extremely low birth weight infants. National Institute of Child Health and Development Neonatal Research Network. Personal communication, 2002.

193. Ahvenainen EK, Call JD. Pulmonary hemorrhage in infants. A descriptive study. *Am J Pathol* 1952;28:1–18.

194. Zuelzer WW, Mudgett RT. Kernicterus: etiologic study based on an analysis of 55 cases. *Pediatrics* 1950;6:452–474.

195. Johnson L, Sarmiento F, Blanc WA, et al. Kernicterus in rats with an inherited deficiency of glucouronyl transferase. *Am J Dis Child* 1960;97:591–608.

196. Horiguchi T, Bauer C. Ethnic differences in neonatal jaundice: comparison of Japanese and Caucasian newborn infants. *Am J Obstet Gynecol* 1975;121:71–74.

197. Linn S, Schoenbaum SC, Monson RR, et. al. Epidemiology of neonatal hyperbilirubinemia. *Pediatrics* 1985;75:770–774.

198. Newman TB, Easterling MJ, Goldman ES, et al. Laboratory evaluation of jaundiced newborns: frequency, cost and yield. *Am J Dis Child* 1990;144:364–368.

199. Munroe M, Shah CP, Badgley R, et al. Birthweight, length, head circumference and bilirubin level in Indian newborns in the Sioux Lookout Zone, Northwestern Ontario. *Can Med Assoc J* 1984;131:453–456.

200. Johnson JD, Angelus P, Aldrich M, et al. Exaggerated jaundice in Navajo neonates: the role of bilirubin production. *Am J Dis Child* 1986;140:889–890.

201. Otterbein L, Mantell L, Choi A. Carbon monoxide provides protection against hyperoxic lung injury. *Am J Physiol Lung Cell Mol Physiol* 1999;20:L688–L694.

202. Engle WD, Jackson GL, Sendelbach D, et al. Assessment of a transcutaneous device in the evaluation of neonatal hyperbilirubinemia in a primarily Hispanic population. *Pediatrics* 2002;110:61–67.

203. Newman TB, Escobar GJ, Gonzales VM, et al. Frequency of neonatal bilirubin testing and hyperbilirubinemia in a large health maintenance organization. *Pediatrics* 1999;104:1198–1203.

204. Maisels MJ, Ostrea EJ Jr, Touch S, et al. Evaluation of a new transcutaneous bilirubinometer. *Pediatrics* 2004;113:1628–1635.

205. Hardy JB, Drage JS, Jackson EC. *The first year of life: the Collaborative Perinatal Project of the National Institutes of Neurological and Communicative Disorders and Stroke.* Baltimore, MD: Johns Hopkins University, 1979.

206. Newman TB, Xiong B, Gonzales VM, et al. Prediction and prevention of extreme neonatal hyperbilirubinemia in a mature health maintenance organization. *Arch Pediatr Adolesc Med* 2000;154:1140–1147.

207. Khoury MJ, Calle EE, Joesoef RM. Recurrence risk of neonatal hyperbilirubinemia in siblings. *Am J Dis Child* 1988;142:1065–1069.

208. Nielsen HE, Haase P, Blaabjerg J, et al. Risk factors and sib correlation in physiological neonatal jaundice. *Acta Paediatr Scand* 1987;76:504–511.

209. Diwan VK, Vaughan TL, Yang CY. Maternal smoking in relation to the incidence of early neonatal jaundice. *Gynecol Obstet Invest* 1989;27:22–25.

210. Knudsen A. Maternal smoking and the bilirubin concentration in the first three days of life. *Eur J Obstet Gynecol Reprod Biol* 1991;25:37–41.

211. Gale R, Seidman DS, Dollberg S, et al. Epidemiology of neonatal jaundice in the Jerusalem population. *J Pediatr Gastroenterol Nutr* 1990;10:82–86.

212. Jones JB. The smoking disease. *Br Med J* 1971;1:228.

213. Jährig D, Jährig K, Striet S, et al. Neonatal jaundice in infants of diabetic mothers. *Acta Paediatr Scand* 1989;360:101–107.

214. Stevenson DK, Ostrander CR, Cohen RS, et al. Pulmonary excretion of carbon monoxide in he human infant as an index of bilirubin production. II. Evidence for the possible effect of maternal prenatal glucose metabolism on postnatal bilirubin production in a mixed population of infants. *Eur J Pediatr* 1981;137:255–259.

215. Widness JA, Susa JB, Garcia JF, et al. Increased erythropoiesis and elevated erythropoietin in infants born to diabetic mothers and in hyperinsulinemic rhesus fetuses. *J Clin Invest* 1981;67:637–642.

216. Berk MA, Mimouni F, Miodovnik M, et al. Macrosomia in infants of insulin-dependent diabetic mothers. *Pediatrics* 1989;83:1029–1034.

217. Maisels MJ. Neonatal Jaundice. In: Sinclair JC, Bracken MB, eds. *Effective care of the newborn infant.* Oxford: Oxford University, 1992:507–561.

218. Maisels MJ, Gifford K, Antle CE, et al. Jaundice in the healthy newborn infant: a new approach to an old problem. *Pediatrics* 1988;81:505–511.

219. Friedman L, Lewis PJ, Clifton P, et al. Factors influencing the incidence of neonatal jaundice. *Br Med J* 1978;1:1235–1237.

220. Brodersen R, Friis-Hansen B, Stern L. Drug-induced displacement of bilirubin from albumin in the newborn. *Dev Pharmacol Ther* 1983;6:217–229.

221. Pedersen H, Morishima HO, Finster M. Uptake and effects of local anesthetics in mother and fetus. *Int Anesthesiol Clin* 1978;16:73–89.

222. Ferguson JE, II, Schutz TE, Stevenson DK. Neonatal bilirubin production after preterm labor tocolysis with nifedipine. *Dev Pharmacol Ther* 1989;12:113–117.

223. Caritis SN, Toig G, Heddinger LA, et al. A double-blind study comparing ritodrine and terbutaline in the treatment of preterm labor. *Am J Obstet Gynecol* 1984;150:7–14.

224. Drew JH, Kitchen WH. The effect of maternally administered drugs on bilirubin concentrations in the newborn infant. *J Pediatr* 1976;89:657–661.

225. Nathenson G, Cohen MI, Litt IF, et al. The effect of maternal heroin addition on neonatal jaundice. *J Pediatr* 1972;81:899–903.

226. Valaes T, Harvey-Wilkes K. Pharmacologic approaches to the prevention and treatment of neonatal hyperbilirubinemia. *Clin Perinatol* 1990;17:245–274.

227. Yamauchi Y, Yamanouchi I. Difference in TcB readings between full term newborn infants born vaginally and by cesarean section. *Acta Paediatr Scand* 1989;79:824–828.

228. Wallace RL, Schifrin BS, Paul RH. The delivery route for very-low-birth-weight infants. A preliminary report of a randomized, prospective study. *J Reprod Med* 1984;29:736–740.

229. Dell DL, Sightler SE, Plauche WC. Soft cup vacuum extraction: a comparison of outlet delivery. *Obstet Gynecol* 1985;66:624–628.

230. Vacca A, Grant A, Wyatt G, et al. Portsmouth operative delivery trial: a comparison of vacuum extraction and forceps delivery. *Br J Obstet Gynaecol* 1983;90:1107–1112.

231. Black VD, Lubchenco LO, Luckey DW, et al. Developmental and neurologic sequelae in the neonatal hyperviscosity syndrome. *Pediatrics* 1982;69:426–431.

232. Black VD, Lubchenco LO, Koops BL, et al. Neonatal hyperviscosity: Randomized study of effect of partial plasma exchange transfusion on long-term outcome. *Pediatrics* 1985;75:1048–1053.

233. Goldberg K, Wirth FH, Hathaway WE, et al. Neonatal hyperviscosity II. Effect of partial plasma exchange transfusion. *Pediatrics* 1982;69:419–425.

234. Saigal S, O'Neill A, Surainder Y, et al. Placental transfusion and hyperbilirubinemia in the premature. *Pediatrics* 1972;49:406–419.

235. Davidson LT, Merritt KK, Weech AA. Hyperbilirubinemia in the newborn. *Am J Dis Child* 1941;61:958–980.

236. Knudsen A, Lebech M. Maternal bilirubin, cord bilirubin and placental function at delivery in the development of jaundice in mature newborns. *Acta Obstet Gynecol Scand* 1989;68:719–724.

237. Rosenfeld J. Umbilical cord bilirubin levels as a predictor of subsequent hyperbilirubinemia. *J Fam Pract* 1986;23:556–558.

238. Risemberg HM, Mazzi E, MacDonald MG, et al. Correlation of cord bilirubin levels with hyperbilirubinemia in ABO incompatibility. *Arch Dis Child* 1977;52:219–222.

239. Soskolne El, Schumacher R, Fyock C, et al. The effect of early discharge and other factors on readmission rates of newborns. *Arch Pediatr Adolesc Med* 1996;150:373–379.

240. Wood B, Culley P, Roginski C, et al. Factors affecting neonatal jaundice. *Arch Dis Child* 1979;54:111–115.

241. Maisels MJ, Kring EA. Length of stay, jaundice and hospital readmission. *Pediatrics* 1998;101:995–998.

242. Frishberg Y, Zelicovic I, Merlob P, et al. Hyperbilirubinemia and influencing factors in term infants. *Isr J Med Sci* 1989;25:28–31.

243. Gourley GR, Kreamer B, Arend R. The effect of diet on feces and jaundice during the first three weeks of life. *Gastroenterology* 1992;103:660.

244. Gourley GR. Breastfeeding, neonatal jaundice and kernicterus. *Semin Neonatol* 2002;7:135–141.

245. Rubaltelli FF. Unconjugated and conjugated bilirubin pigments during perinatal development. IV. The influence of breast-feeding on neonatal hyperbilirubinemia. *Biol Neonate* 1993;64:104–109.

246. Bertini G, Dani C, Trochin M, et al. Is breast feeding really favoring early neonatal jaundice? *Pediatrics* 2001;107.

247. Schneider AP. Breast milk jaundice in the newborn. A real entity. *JAMA* 1986;255:3270–3274.

248. Seidman DS, Stevenson DK, Ergaz Z, et al. Hospital readmission due to neonatal hyperbilirubinemia. *Pediatrics* 1995;96:727–729.

249. Maisels MJ, Kring E. Risk of sepsis in newborns with severe hyperbilirubinemia. *Pediatrics* 1992;90:741–743.

250. Gartner L. Breastfeeding and jaundice. *J Perinatol* 2001;21:S25-S29.

251. De Carvalho M, Klaus MH, Merkatz RB. Frequency of breast-feeding and serum bilirubin concentration. *Am J Dis Child* 1982;136:737–738.

252. Yamauchi Y, Yamanouchi I. Breast-feeding frequency during the first 24 hours after birth in full-term neonates. *Pediatrics* 1990;86:171–175.

253. Auerbach KG, Gartner LM. Breast feeding and human milk: Their association with jaundice in the neonate. *Clin Perinatol* 1987;14:89–107.

254. Maisels MJ, Gifford K. Normal serum bilirubin levels in the newborn and the effect of breast feeding. *Pediatrics* 1986;78:837–843.

255. Kivlahan C, James EJP. The natural history of neonatal jaundice. *Pediatrics* 1984;74:364–370.

256. Maisels MJ, D'Archangelo MR. Breast feeding and jaundice in the first six weeks of life. *Pediatr Res* 1983;17:324A(abst).

257. Alonso EM, Whitington PF, Whitington SH, Rivard WA, Given G. Enterohepatic circulation of non-conjugated bilirubin in rats fed with human milk. *J Pediatr* 1991;118:425–430.

258. Gathwala G, Sharma S. Phototherapy induces oxidative stress in premature neonates. *Indian J Gastroenterol* 2002;21:153–154.

259. Monaghan G, McLellan A, McGeehan A, et al. Gilbert's syndrome is a contributory factor in prolonged unconjugated hyperbilirubinemia of the newborn. *J Pediatr* 1999;134:441–446.

260. Maruo Y, Nishizawa K, Sato H, et al. Prolonged unconjugated hyperbilirubinemia associated with breast milk and mutations of the bilirubin uridine diphosphate glucuronosyltransferase gene. *Pediatrics* 2000;106:e59.

261. De Carvalho M, Robertson S, Klaus M. Fecal bilirubin excretion and serum bilirubin concentration in breast-fed and bottle-fed infants. *J Pediatr* 1985;107:786–790.

262. Verkade HJ. A novel hypothesis on the pathophysiology of neonatal jaundice. *J Pediatr* 2002;141:594–595.

263. Hamosh M. Digestion in the newborn. *Clin Perinatol* 1996;23:191–209.

264. Yoshioka H. Development and differences of intestinal flora in the neonatal period in breast-fed and bottle-fed infants. *Pediatrics* 1983;72:317–321.

265. Gourley GR, Arend RA. Beta-glucuronidase and hyperbilirubinemia in breast-fed and formula-fed babies. *Lancet* 1986;1:644–646.

266. Wilson DC, Afrasiabi M, Reid MM. Breast-milk beta-glucuronidase and exaggerated jaundice in the early neonatal period. *Biol Neonate* 1992;61:232–234.

267. Cottrell BH, Anderson GC. Rectal or axillary temperature measurement: Effect on plasma bilirubin and intestinal transit of meconium. *J Pediatr Gastroenterol Nutr* 1984;3:734–739.

268. Weisman LE, Merenstein GB, Digirol M, et al. The effect of early meconium evacuation on early-onset hyperbilirubinemia. *Am J Dis Child* 1983;137:666–668.

269. Daum F, Cohen MI, McNamara H. Experimental toxicologic studies on a phenol detergent associated with neonatal hyperbilirubinemia. *J Pediatr* 1976;89:853.

270. Wysowski DK, Flynt JW, Goldfield M, et al. Epidemic neonatal hyperbilirubinemia and use of a phenolic disinfectant detergent. *Pediatrics* 1978;61:165.

271. Moore LG, Newberry MA, Freeby GM, Crnic LS. Increased incidence of neonatal hyperbilirubinemia at 3,100 m in Colorado. *Am J Dis Child* 1984;138:157–161.

272. Atland PD, Parker MG. Bilirubinemia and intravascular hemolysis during acclimatization to high altitude. *Int J Biometeorol* 1977;21:165–170.

273. Berendsohn S. Hepatic function at high altitudes. *Arch Intern Med* 1962;109:256–264.

274. Barron ESG. Bilirubinemia. *Medicine (Baltimore)* 1931;10:114–115.

275. Freeman J, Lesko S, Mitchell AA, et al. Hyperbilirubinemia following exposure to pancuronium bromide in newborns. *Dev Pharmacol Ther* 1990;14:209–215.

276. Lambert GH, Muraskas J, Anderson CL, et al. Direct hyperbilirubinemia associated with chloral hydrate administration in the newborn. *Pediatrics* 1990;86:277–281.

277. Reimche LD, Sankaran K, Hindmarsh KW, et al. Chloral hydrate sedation in neonates and infants—clinical and pharmacologic considerations. *Dev Pharmacol Ther* 1989;12:57–64.

278. McDonagh AF. Is bilirubin good for you? *Clin Perinatol* 1990;17:359–369.

279. Benaron DA, Bowen FW. Variation of initial serum bilirubin rise in newborn infants with type of illness. *Lancet* 1991;338:78–81.

280. Saigal S, Lunyk O, Bennett KJ, et al. Serum bilirubin levels in breast- and formula-fed infants in the first 5 days of life. *Can Med Assoc J* 1982;127:985–989.

281. Knudsen A. Prediction of the development of neonatal jaundice by increased umbilical cord blood bilirubin. *Acta Pediatr Scand* 1989;78:217–221.

282. Lo S, Doumas BT, Ashwood E. Performance of bilirubin determinations in US laboratories—revisited. *Clin Chem* 2004;50:190–194.

283. Vreman HJ, Verter J, Oh W, et. al. Interlaboratory variability of bilirubin measurements. *Clin Chem* 1996;42:869–873.

284. Doumas BT, Eckfeldt JH. Errors in measurement of total bilirubin: A perennial problem. *Clin Chem* 1996;42:845–848.

285. Stevenson DK, Fanaroff AA, Maisels MJ, et al. Prediction of hyperbilirubinemia in near-term and term infants. *Pediatrics* 2001;108:31–39.

286. Maisels MJ, Kring EA. The natural history of neonatal bilirubinemia. *Pediatr Res* 2004;55:458A.

287. Li R, Zhao Z, Mokdad A, et al. Prevalence of breastfeeding in the United States: The 2001 national immunization survey. Pediatrics 2003;111:1198–1201.

288. Lee K-S, Perlman M, Ballantyne M. Association between duration of neonatal hospital stay and readmission rate. *J Pediatr* 1995;127:758–766.

289. Bhutani VK, Johnson L, Sivieri EM. Predictive ability of a predischarge hour-specific serum bilirubin for subsequent significant hyperbilirubinemia in healthy-term and near-term newborns. *Pediatrics* 1999;103:6–14.

290. Maisels MJ, Fanaroff AA, Stevenson DK, et al. Serum bilirubin levels in an international, multiracial newborn population. *Pediatr Res* 1999;45:167A.

291. Okolo AA, Omene JA, Scott-Emaukpor AB. Physiologic jaundice in the Nigerian neonate. *Biol Neonate* 1988;53:132–137.

292. Yamauchi Y, Yamanouchi I. Transcutaneous bilirubinometry in normal Japanese infants. *Acta Paediatr Jpn* 1989;31:65–72.

293. Maisels MJ, Newman TB. Predicting hyperbilirubinemia in newborns: the importance of timing. *Pediatrics* 1999;103:493–495.

294. Koenig JM. Evaluation and treatment of erythroblastosis fetalis in the neonate. In: Christensen RD, ed. *Hematologic problems of the neonate*. Philadelphia: WB Saunders, 2000:185–207.

295. Bowman JM. RhD hemolytic disease of the newborn. *N Engl J Med* 1998;339:1775–1777.

296. Bowman JM. The management of alloimmune fetal hemolytic disease. In: Maisels MJ, Watchko JF, eds. *Neonatal jaundice*. London, UK: Harwood Academic Publishers, 2000:23–36.

297. Bowman JM. Immune hemolytic disease. In: Nathan DG, Orkin SH, eds. *Hematology of infancy and childhood*. Philadelphia: WB Saunders, 1998:54–78.

298. Chavez GF, Mulinare J, Edmonds LD. Epidemiology of Rh hemolytic disease of the newborn in the United States. *JAMA* 1991;265:3270–3274.

299. Sebring ES, Polesky HF. Detection of fetal hemorrhage in Rh immune globulin candidates. A rosetting technique using enzyme-treated Rh2Rh2 indicator erythrocytes. *Transfusion* 1982;22:468–471.

300. Voto LS, Mathet ER, Zapaterio JL, et al. High-dose gammaglobulin (IVIG) followed by intrauterine transfusions (IUTs): a new alternative for the treatment of severe fetal hemolytic disease. *J Perinat Med* 1997;25:85–88.

301. Blair DK, Vander Straten MC, Gest AL. Hydrops fetalis in sheep from rapid induction of anemia. *Pediatr Res* 1994;35:560–564.

302. Nicolaides KH, Warenski JC, Rodeck CH. The relationship of fetal plasma protein concentration and hemoglobin level to the development of hydrops in rhesus isoimmunization. *Am J Obstet Gynecol* 1985;152:341–344.

303. Grannum PA, Copel JA, Moya FR, et al. The reversal of hydrops fetalis by intravascular intrauterine transfusion in severe isoimmune fetal anemia. *Am J Obstet Gynecol* 1988;158:914–919.

304. Moya FR, Grannum PA, Riddick L, et al. Atrial natriuretic factor in hydrops fetalis caused by Rh isoimmunization. *Arch Dis Child* 1990;65:683–686.

305. Weiner C. Nonhematologic effects of intravascular transfusion on the human fetus. *Semin Perinatol* 1989;13:338–341.

306. Barss VA, Doubilet PM, St. John-Sutton M, et al. Cardiac output in a fetus with erythroblastosis fetalis: assessment using pulsed Doppler. et al 1987;70:442–444.

307. Ohls RK, Wirkus PEN, Christensen RD. Recombinant erythropoieitin as treatment of late hypo-regenerative anemia of Rh hemolytic disease. *Pediatrics* 1992;90:678–680.

308. Dallacasa P, Ancora G, Miniero R, et al. Erythropoietin course in newborns with Rh hemolytic disease transfused and not transfused in utero. *Pediatr Res* 1996;40:357–360.

309. Giblet ER. Blood groups and blood transfusion. In: Braunwald E, Isselbacher KJ, Petersdorf RG, et al, eds. New York: *Harrison's principles of internal medicine*, 1987:1483–1489.

310. Katz MA, Kanto WP, Korotkin JH. Recurrence rate of ABO hemolytic disease of the newborn. *Obstet Gynecol* 1982;59:611–614.

311. Ozolek J, Watchko J, Mimouni F. Prevalence and lack of clinical significance of blood group incompatibility in mothers with blood type A or B. *J Pediatr* 1994;125:87–91.

312. Kanto WP, Marino B, Godwin AS, et al. ABO hemolytic disease: a comparative study of clinical severity and delayed anemia. *Am J Dis Child* 1978;62:365–369.

313. Osborn LM, Lenarsky C, Oakes RC, et al. Phototherapy in full-term infants with hemolytic disease secondary to ABO incompatibility. *Pediatrics* 1984;74:371–374.

314. Quinn MW, Weindling AM, Davidson DC. Does ABO incompatibility matter? *Arch Dis Child* 1988;63:1258–1260.

315. Serrao PA, Modanlou HD. Significance of anti-A and anti-B isohemagglutinins in cord blood of ABO incompatible newborn infants: correlation with hyperbilirubinemia. *J Perinatol* 1989; 9:154–158.

316. Herschel M, Karrison T, Wen M, et al. Isoimmunization is unlikely to be the cause of hemolysis in ABO-Incompatible but direct antiglobulin test-negative neonates. *Pediatrics* 2002;110: 127–130.

317. Kaplan M, Hammerman C, Renbaum P, et al. Gilbert's syndrome and hyperbilirubinaemia in ABO-incompatible neonates. *Lancet* 2000;356:652–653.

318. Leistikow EA, Collin MF, Savastano GD, et al. Wasted health care dollars. Routine cord blood type and Coombs' testing. *Arch Pediatr Adolesc Med* 1995;149:1147–1151.

319. Maisels MJ, Kring EA. Early discharge from the newborn nursery: effect on scheduling of follow-up visits by pediatricians. *Pediatrics* 1997;100:72–74.

320. Gallagher PG, Forget BG, Lux SE. Disorders of the erythrocyte membrane. In: Nathan DG, Orkin SH, eds. *Hematology of infancy and childhood*. Philadelphia: WB Saunders, 1998:544–664.

321. Gallagher PG. Disorders of erythrocyte metabolism and shape. In: Christensen RD, ed. *Hematologic problems of the neonate*. Philadelphia: WB Saunders, 2000:209–237.

322. Watchko JF. Indirect hyperbilirubinemia in the neonate. In: Maisels MJ, Watchko JF, eds. *Neonatal jaundice*. London, UK: Harwood Academic Publishers, 2000:51–66.

323. Iolascon A, Faienza MF, Moretti A, et al. UGT1 promoter polymorphism accounts for increased neonatal appearance of hereditary spherocytosis. *Blood* 1998;91:1093.

324. Valaes T. Neonatal jaundice in glucose-6-phosphate dehydrogenase deficiency. In: Maisels MJ, Watchko JF, eds. *Neonatal jaundice*. London, UK: Harwood Academic Publishers, 2000:67–74.

325. Brown AK, Damus K, Kim MH, et al. Factors relating to readmission of term and near-term neonates in the first two weeks of life. Early discharge survey group of the Health Professional Advisory Board of the Greater New York Chapter of the March of Dimes. *J Perinat Med* 1999;27:263–275.

326. Kaplan M, Hammerman C. Glucose-6-phosphate dehydrogenase-deficient neonates: A potential cause for concern in North America. *Pediatrics* 2000;106:1478–1480.

327. Kaplan M, Hammerman C. Severe neonatal hyperbilirubinemia: a potential complication of glucose-6-phosphate dehydrogenase deficiency. *Clin Perinatol* 1998;25:575–590.

328. MacDonald M. Hidden risks: early discharge and bilirubin toxicity due to glucose-6-phosphate dehydrogenase deficiency. *Pediatrics* 1995;96:734–738.

329. Washington EC, Ector W, Abboud M, Ohning B, Holden K. Hemolytic jaundice due to G6PD deficiency causing kernicterus in a female newborn. *South Med J* 1995;88:776–779.

330. Herschel M, Kaplan M, Hammerman C, et al. Increased hemolysis in G6PD deficient African American Neonates. *Pediatr Res* 2003;53:399A.

331. Kaplan M, Vreman H, Hammerman C, et al. Favism by proxy in nursing glucose-6-phosphate dehydrogenase-deficient neonates. *J Perinatol* 1998;18(6):477–479.

332. Beutler E. Glucose-6-phosphate dehydrogenase deficiency. *Blood* 1994;84:3613–3636.

333. Kaplan M., Hammerman C. Glucose-6-phosphate dehydrogenase deficiency: a potential source of severe neonatal hyperbilirubinaemia and kernicterus. *Semin Neonatol* 2002;7:121–128.

334. Kaplan M, Algur N, Hammerman C. Onset of jaundice in glucose-6-phosphate dehydrogenase-deficient neonates. *Pediatrics* 2001;108:956–959.

335. Kaplan M., Beutler E, Vreman HJ, et al. Neonatal hyperbilirubinemia in glucose-6-phosphate dehydrogenase deficient heterozygotes. *Pediatrics* 1999;104:68–74.

336. Herschel M, Ryan M, Gelbart T, Kaplan M. Hemolysis and hyperbilirubinemia in an African American neonate heterozygous for glucose-6-phosphate dehydrogenase deficiency. *J Perinatol* 2002;22:577–579.

337. Kaplan M, Abramov A. Neonatal hyperbilirubinemia associated with glucose-6-phosphate dehydrogenase deficiency in Sephardic-Jewish infants: incidence, severity and the effect of phototherapy. *Pediatrics* 1992;90:401–405.

338. Meloni T, Cutillo S, Testa U, Luzatto L. Neonatal jaundice and severity of glucose-6-phosphate dehydrogenase deficiency in Sardinian babies. *Early Hum Dev* 1987;15:317–322.

339. Slusher TM, Vreman HJ, McLaren D, et al. Glucose-6-phosphate dehydrogenase deficiency and carboxy hemoglobin concentrations associated with bilirubin related morbidity and death in Nigerian infants. *J Pediatr* 1995;126:102–108.

340. Necheles TF, Rai US, Valaes T. The role of haemolysis in neonatal hyperbilirubinemia as reflected by carboxyhemoglobin levels. *Acta Paediatr Scand* 1976;65:361–367.

341. Kaplan M, Vreman HJ, Hammerman C, et al. Contribution of haemolysis to jaundice in Sephardic Jewish glucose-6-phosphate dehydrogenase deficient neonates. *Br J Haematol* 1996;93:822–827.

342. Kaplan M, Hammerman C, Renbaum P, et al. Differing pathogenesis of perinatal bilirubinemia in glucose-6-phosphate dehydrogenase-deficient versus normal neonates. *Pediatr Res* 2001; 50:532–537.

343. Muraca M, Rubaltelli FF, Blanckaert N, et al. Unconjugated and conjugated bilirubin pigments during perinatal development. II. Studies on serum of healthy newborns and of neonates with erythroblastosis fetalis. *Biol Neonate* 1990;57:1–9.

344. Kaplan M, Muraca M, Hammerman C, et al. Bilirubin conjugation, reflected by conjugated bilirubin fractions, in glucose-6-phosphate dehydrogenase-deficient neonates: a determining factor in the pathogenesis of hyperbilirubinemia. *Pediatrics* 1998;102(3):e37.

345. Kaplan M, Renbaum P, Levi-Lahad E, et al. Gilbert syndrome and glucose-6-phosphate dehydrogenase deficiency: a dose-dependent genetic interaction crucial to neonatal hyperbilirubinemia. *Proc Natl Acad Sci U S A* 1997;94:12128–12132.

346. Iolascon A, Faienza MF, Perrotta S, et al. Gilbert's syndrome and jaundice in glucose-6-phosphate dehydrogenase deficient neonates. *Haematologica* 1999;84:99–102.

347. Brown WR, Boon WH. Hyperbilirubinemia and kernicterus in glucose-6-phosphate dehydrogenase deficient infants in Singapore. *Pediatrics* 1968;41:1055–1062.

348. Gibbs WN, Gray R, Lowry M. G6PD deficiency and neonatal jaundice in Jamaica. *Br J Hematol* 1979;43:263–274.

349. Bainbridge R, Khoury J, Mimounie F. Jaundice in neonatal sickle cell disease: a case controlled study. *Am J Dis Child* 1988;148: 569.

350. Bard H. Hemoglobin synthesis and metabolism during the neonatal period. In: Christensen RD, ed. *Hematologic problems of the neonate*. Philadelphia: WB Saunders, 2000:365–388.

351. Rajagopalan I, Katz BZ. Hyperbilirubinemia secondary to hemolysis of intrauterine intraperitoneal blood transfusion. *Clin Pediatr* 1984;23:511–512.

352. Rose J, Berdon WE, Sullivan T, et al. Prolonged jaundice as presenting sign of massive adrenal hemorrhage in newborn. *Radiology* 1971;98:263–272.

353. Wright K, Tarr PI, Hickman RO, et al. Hyperbilirubinemia secondary to delayed absorption of intraperitoneal blood following intrauterine transfusion. *J Pediatr* 1982;100:302–304.

354. Epstein MF, Leviton A, Kuban KC, et al. Bilirubin intraventricular hemorrhage and phenobarbital in very low birth weight babies. *Pediatrics* 1988;82:350.

355. Pasnick M, Lucey JF. Serum bilirubin in preterm infants following intracranial hemorrhage. *Pediatr Res* 1983;17:329A.

356. Kemper K, Forsyth B, McCarthy P. Jaundice, terminating breast-feeding, and the vulnerable child. *Pediatrics* 1989;84:773–779.

357. Bleicher MA, Reiner MA, Rapaport SA, et al. Extraordinary hyperbilirubinemia in a neonate with idiopathic hypertrophic pyloric stenosis. *J Pediatr Surg* 1979;14:527.

358. Wooley MM, Felsher BF, Asch MJ, et al. Jaundice, hypertrophic pyloric stenosis, and glucuronyl transferase. *J Pediatr Surg* 1974;9:359.

359. Trioche P, Chalas J, Francoual J, et al. Jaundice with hypertrophic pyloric stenosis as an early manifestation of Gilbert syndrome. *Arch Dis Child* 1999;81:301–303.

360. Labrune P, Myara A, Huguet P, et al. Jaundice with hypertrophic pyloric stenosis: a possible early manifestation of Gilbert syndrome. *J Pediatr* 1989;115:93–95.

361. Job H, Hart G, Lealman G. Improvements in long term phototherapy for patients with Crigler-Najjar syndrome type I. *Phys Med Biol* 1996;41(11):2549–2556.

362. Blumenschein SD, Kallen RJ, Storey P, et al. Familial nonhemolytic jaundice with late onset of neurological damage. *Pediatrics* 1968;42:786.

363. Chalasani N, Roy-Chowdhury N, Roy-Chowdury J, et al. Kernicterus in an adult who is heterozygous for Crigler-Najjar syndrome and homozygous for Gilbert-type genetic defect. *Gastroenterology* 1997;112:2099–2103.

364. Ahmad P, Pratt A, Land VJ, et al. Multiple plasma exchanges successfully maintained a young adult patient with Crigler-Najjar syndrome type I. *J Clin Apheresis* 1989;5:17.

365. Shevell MI, Bernard B, Adelson JW, et al. Crigler-Najjar syndrome type I: Treatment by home phototherapy followed by orthotopic hepatic transplantation. *J Pediatr* 1987;110:429.

366. Fox IJ, Roy-Chowdhury J, Kaufman SS, et al. Treatment of the Crigler-Najjar syndrome type I with hepatocyte transplantation. *N Engl J Med* 1998;338:1422–1426.

367. Roy Chowdhury J, Strom SC, Kaufman SS, et al. Human hepatocyte transplantation: gene therapy and more? *Pediatrics* 1998; 647–648.

368. Kim BH, Takahashi M, Tada K, et al. Cell and gene therapy for inherited deficiency of bilirubin glucuronidation. *J Perinatol* 1996;16:S67–S72.

369. Rubaltelli FF, Guerrini P, Reddi E, et al. Tin-protoporphyrin in the management of children with Crigler-Najjar disease. *Pediatrics* 1989;84:728–731.

370. Kappas A. A method for interdicting the development of severe jaundice in newborns by inhibiting the production of bilirubin. *Pediatrics* 2004;113:119–123.

371. Van der Veere CN, Jansen PLM, Sinaasappel M, et al. Oral calcium phosphate: a new therapy for Crigler-Najjar disease? *Gastroenterology* 1997;112:455–462.

372. Rubaltelli FF, Novello A, Zancan L, et al. Serum and bile bilirubin pigments in the differential diagnosis of Crigler-Najjar disease. *Pediatrics* 1994;94:553–556.

373. Lee W, McKiernan P, Beath S, et al. Bile bilirubin pigment analysis in disorders of bilirubin metabolism in early infancy. *Arch Dis Child* 2001;85:38–42.

374. Sampietro M, Iolascon A. Molecular pathology of Crigler-Najjar type I and II and Gilbert's syndromes. *Haematologica* 1999;84:150–157.

375. Clarke DJ, Moghrabi N, Monaghan G, et al. Genetic defects of the UDP-glucoronosyltransferase-1 (UGT1) gene that cause familial nonhaemolytic unconjugated hyperbilirubinemias. *Clin Chim Acta* 1997;266:63–74.

376. Sugatani J, Kojima H, Ueda A, et al. The phenobarbital response enhancer module in the human bilirubin UDP-glucuronosyltransferase UGT1A1 gene and regulation by the nuclear receptor CAR. *Hepatology* 2001;33:1232–1238.

377. Van der Veere CN, Sinaasappel M, McDonagh AF, et al. Current therapy for Crigler-Najjar syndrome type I: report of a world registry. *Hepatology* 1996;24:311–315.

378. Kaplan M, Hammerman C, Rubaltelli F, et al. Hemolysis and bilirubin conjugation in association with UDP-glucuronosyltransferase 1A1 promoter polymorphism. *Hepatology* 2002;35:905–911.

379. Bosma PJ, Roy-Chowdhury J, Bakker C, et al. The genetic basis of the reduced expression of bilirubin UDP-glucuronosyl transferase 1 in Gilbert's syndrome. *N Engl J Med* 1995;333:1171–1175.

380. Kadakol A, Ghosh SS, Sappal BS, et al. Genetic lesions of bilirubin uridine-diphospho-glucuronate glucuronosyltransferase (UGT1A1) causing Crigler-Najjar and Gilbert syndromes: Correlation of genotype to phenotype. *Hum Mutat* 2000;16:297–306.

381. Monaghan G, Ryan M, Seddon R, et al. Genetic variation in bilirubin UDP-glucuronosyltransferase gene promoter and Gilbert's syndrome. *Lancet* 1996;347:578–581.

382. Kadakol A, Sappal BS, Ghosh SS, et al. Interaction of coding area mutations and the Gilbert-type promoter abnormality of the UGT1A1 gene causes moderate degrees of unconjugated hyperbilirubinemia and may lead to neonatal kernicterus. *J Med Genet* 2001;38:244–249.

383. Bancroft JD, Kreamer B, Gourley GR. Gilbert's syndrome accelerates development of neonatal jaundice. *J Pediatr* 1998;132(4):656–660.
384. Roy-Chowdhury N, Deocharan B, Bejjanki HR, et al. The present of a Gilbert-type promotor abnormality increases the level of neonatal hyperbilirubinemia. *Hepatology* 1997;26:370A.
385. Laforgia N, Faienza MF, Rinaldi A, et al. Neonatal hyperbilirubinemia and Gilbert's syndrome. *J Perinat Med* 2002;30:166–169.
386. Maruo Y, Nishizawa K, Sato H, et al. Association of neonatal hyperbilirubinemia with bilirubin UDP-glucuronosyltransferase polymorphism. *Pediatrics* 1999;103(6):1224–1227.
387. Akaba K, Kimura T, Sasaki A, et al. Neonatal hyperbilirubinemia and mutation of the bilirubin uridine diphosphate-glucuronosyltransferase gene: A common missense mutation among Japanese, Koreans and Chinese. *Biochem Mol Biol Int* 1998;46:21–26.
388. Hsieh S-Y, Wu Y-H, Lin D-Y, et al. Correlation of mutational analysis to clinical features in Taiwanese patients with Gilbert's syndrome. *Am J Gastroenterol* 2001;96:1188–1192.
389. Maruo Y, Sato H, Yamano T, et al. Gilbert syndrome caused by a homozygous missnse mutation (Tyr486Asp) of bilirubin UDP-glucuronosyltransferase gene. *J Pediatr* 1998;132:1045–1047.
390. Maisels MJ, Newman TB. Kernicterus in otherwise healthy, breast-fed term newborns. *Pediatrics* 1995;96:730–733.
391. Berry GT. Inborn errors of carbohydrate, ammonia, aminoacid, and organic acid metabolism. In: Taeusch HW, Ballard RA, eds. *Avery's diseases of the newborn*. Philadelphia: WB Saunders, 1998:245–274.
392. Akerren Y. Prolonged jaundice in the newborn associated with congenital myxedema. A syndrome of practical importance. *Acta Paediatr* 1954;43:411–425.
393. Labrune P, Myara A, Huguet P, et al. Bilirubin uridine diphosphate glucuronosyltransferase hepatic activity in jaundice associated with congenital hypothyroidism. *J Pediatr Gastroenterol Nutr* 1992;14:79–82.
394. Smith DW, Klein AM, Henderson JR, et al. Congenital hypothyroidism - signs and symptoms in the newborn period. *J Pediatr* 1975;87:958–962.
395. Weldon AP, Danks DM. Congenital hypothyroidism and neonatal jaundice. *Arch Dis Child* 1972;(47):469–471.
396. Lees MH, Ruthven CRJ. The effects of triiodothyronine on neonatal hyperbilirubinemia. *Lancet* 1959;2:371–373.
397. Shrand H, Ruthven CRJ. Effect of triiodothyronine on serum bilirubin level in neonatal development of the premature infant. *Lancet* 1960;2:1274–1275.
398. Van Steenbergen W, Fevery J, DeVos R, et al. Thyroid hormones and the hepatic handling of bilirubin. I. Effects of hypothyroidism and hyperthyroidism on the hepatic transport of bilirubin mono- and diconjugates in the Wistar rat. *Hepatology* 1989;9:314–321.
399. Chavalitdhamrong P-O, Escobedo MB, Barton LL, et al. Hyperbilirubinemia and bacterial infection in the newborn. *Arch Dis Child* 1975;50:652–654.
400. Linder N, Yatsiv I, Tsur M, et al. Unexplained neonatal jaundice as an early diagnostic sign of septicemia in the newborn. *J Perinatol* 1988;8:325–327.
401. Rooney JC, Hill DJ, Danks DM. Jaundice associated with bacterial infection in the newborn. *Am J Dis Child* 1971;122:39–41.
402. Garcia FJ, Nager AL. Jaundice as an early diagnostic sign of urinary tract infection in infancy. *Pediatrics* 2002;109:846–851.
403. Maisels MJ, Newman TB. Neonatal jaundice and urinary tract infections. *Pediatrics* 2003;112:1213–1214.
404. Copeland KC, Franks RC, Ramamurthy R. Neonatal hyperbilirubinemia and hypoglycemia and congenital hypopituitarism. *Clin Pediatr* 1981;20:523.
405. Crabtree N, Gerrard J. Perceptive deafness associated with severe neonatal jaundice. *J Laryngol Otol* 1950;64:482–506.
406. Ebbesen F. Recurrence of kernicterus in term and near-term infants in Denmark. *Acta Paediatr* 2000;89:1213–1217.
407. Maisels MJ, Baltz RD, Bhutani VK, et al. Neonatal jaundice and kernicterus. *Pediatrics* 2001;108:763–765.
408. Madden JM, Soumerai SB, Lieu TA, et al. Length-of-stay policies and ascertainment of postdischarge problems in newborns. *Pediatrics* 2004;113:42–49.
409. Varimo P, Similä S, Wendt L, et al. Frequency of breast feeding and hyperbilirubinemia. *Clin Pediatr* 1986;25:112.
410. Eidelman AL, Hoffman MW, Kaitz M. Cognitive deficits in women after childbirth. *Obstet Gynecol* 1993;81:764–767.
411. Newman TB, Escobar GJ, Branch PT, et al. Incidence of extreme hyperbilirubinemia in a large HMO. *Amb Child Health* 1997;3:203(abst).
412. Li R, Zhao Z, Mokdad A, et al. Prevalence of breastfeeding in the United States: the 2001 national immunization survey. *Pediatrcs* 2003;111:1198–1201.
413. Ryan AS, Wenjun MS, Acosta A. Breastfeeding continues to increase into the new millennium. *Pediatrics* 2002;110:1103–1109.
414. Institue of Medicine. *Crossing the quality chasm: a new health system for the 21st century*. Washington, DC: National Academy Press, 2001.
415. Palmer H, Clanton M, Ezhuthachan S, et al. Applying the "10 simple rules" of the Institute of Medicine to management of hyperbilirubinemia in newborns. *Pediatrics* 2003;112:1388–1393.
416. Escobar GJ, Gonzales VM, Armstrong MA, et al. Rehospitalization for neonatal dehydration: a nested case-control study. *Arch Pediatr Adolesc Med* 2002;156:155–161.
417. American Academy of Pediatrics and the American College of Obstetricians and Gynecologists. *Guidelines for perinatal care*. 5th ed. Elk Grove Village, IL: American Academy of Pediatrics, 2002:220–224.
418. Lawrence, RA. Management of the Mother-Infant Nursing Couple. In Lawrence RA. Breast. A guide for the medical profession. ST. Louis: Mosby 1994:215–277.
419. De Carvalho M, Hall M, Harvey D. Effects of water supplementation on physiological jaundice in breast fed babies. *Arch Dis Child* 1981;56:568–569.
420. Nicoll A, Ginsburg R, Tripp JH. Supplementary feeding and jaundice in newborns. *Acta Pediatr Scand* 1982;71:759–761.
421. Butler DA, MacMillan JP. Relationship of breast feeding and weight loss to jaundice in the newborn period: review of the literature and results of a study. *Cleve Clin Q* 1983;50:263–268.
422. Maisels MJ, Gifford K. Breast feeding, weight loss and jaundice. *J Pediatr* 1983;102:117–118.
423. Laing IA, Wong CM. Hypernatraemia in the first few days: is the incidence rising? *Arch Dis Child Neonatal Ed* 2002;87:F158–F162.
424. Kuhr M, Paneth N. Feeding practices and early neonatal jaundice. *J Pediatr Gastroenterol Nutr* 1982;1:485–488.
425. Madlon-Kay DJ. Recognition of the presence and severity of newborn jaundice by parents, nurses, physicians, and icterometer. *Pediatrics* 1997;100:e3.
426. Tayaba R, Gribetz D, Gribetz I, et al. Noninvasive estimation of serum bilirubin. *Pediatrics* 1998;102:e28.
427. Ebbesen F. The relationship between the cephalo-pedal progress of clinical icterus and the serum bilirubin concentration in newborn infants without blood type sensitization. *Acta Obstet Gynaecol Scand* 1975;54:329–332.
428. Kramer LI. Advancement of dermal icterus in the jaundiced newborn. *Am J Dis Child* 1969;118:454–458.
429. Hegyi T, Hiatt M, Gertner I, et al. Transcutaneous bilirubinometry: the cephalocaudal progression of dermal icterus. *Am J Dis Child* 1981;135:547.
430. Knudsen A. The cephalocaudal progression of jaundice in newborns in relation to the transfer of bilirubin from plasma to skin. *Early Hum Dev* 1990;22:23–28.
431. Knudsen A. The influence of the reserve albumin concentration and pH on the cephalocaudal progression of jaundice in newborns. *Early Hum Dev* 1991;25(37).
432. Knudsen A, Broderson R. Skin colour and bilirubin in neonates. *Arch Dis Child* 1989;64:605.
433. Jacobsen J, Brodersen R. Albumin-bilirubin binding mechanism: kinetic and spectroscopic studies of binding of albumin and xanthobilirubic acid to human serum albumin. *J Biol Chem* 1983;10:6319.
434. Moyer VA, Ahn C, Sneed S. Accuracy of clinical judgment in neonatal jaundice. *Arch Pediatr Adolesc Med* 2000;154:391–394.
435. Riskin A, Kuglman A, Abend-Weinger M, et al. In the eye of the beholder: how accurate is clinical estimation of jaundice in newborns? *Acta Paediatr* 2003;92:574–576.
436. Madlon-Kay DJ. Home health nurse clinical assessment of neonatal jaundice. *Arch Pediatr Adolesc Med* 2001;155:583–586.
437. Bhutani V, Gourley GR, Adler S, et al. Noninvasive measurement of total serum bilirubin in a multiracial predischarge newborn population to assess the risk of severe hyperbilirubinemia. *Pediatrics* 2000;106:e17.
438. Yasuda S, Itoh S, Isobe K, et al. New transcutaneous jaundice device with two optical paths. *J Perinat Med* 2003;31:81–88.

439. Schumacher RE, Thornbery J, Gutcher GR. Transcutaneous bilirubinometry: A comparison of old and new methods. *Pediatrics* 1985;76:10–14.
440. Madlon-Kay DJ. Maternal assessment of neonatal jaundice after hospital discharge. *J Fam Prac* 2002;51:445–448.
441. Rubaltelli FF, Gourley G. R., Loskamp N, et al. Transcutaneous bilirubin measurement: a multicenter evaluation of a new device. *Pediatrics* 2001;107:1264–1271.
442. Ebbesen F, Rasmussen LM, Wimberley PD. A new transcutaneous bilirubinometer, bilicheck, used in the neonatal intensive care unit and the maternity ward. *Acta Paediatr* 2002;91:203–211.
443. Knupfer M, Pulzer F, Braun L, et al. Transcutaneous bilirubinometry in preterm infants. *Acta Paediatr* 2001;90:899–903.
444. Tan KL, Dong F. Transcutaneous bilirubinometry during and after phototherapy. *Acta Paediatr* 2003;92:327–331.
445. Schumacher R. Transcutaneous bilirubinometry and diagnostic tests: "the right job for the tool." *Pediatrics* 2002;110:407–408.
446. Sykes E, Epstein E. Laboratory measurement of bilirubin. *Clin Perinatol* 1990;17:397.
447. Doumas BT, Wuu TW. The measurement of bilirubin fractions in serum. *Crit Rev Lab Sci* 1991;29:415–445.
448. Doumas BT, Kwok-Cheung PP, Perry BW, et al. Candidate reference method for determination of total bilirubin in serum: development and validation. *Clin Chem* 1985;31:1779–1789.
449. Watkinson LR, St John A, Penberthy LA. Investigation into paediatric bilirubin analyses in Australia and New Zealand. *J Clin Pathol* 1982;35:52–58.
450. Newman TB, Hope S, Stevenson D. Direct bilirubin measurements in jaundiced term newborns: a re-evaluation. *Am J Dis Child* 1991;145:1305–1309.
451. Eidelman AI, Schimmel, Algur N, et al. Capillary and venous bilirubin values: they are different—and how! *Am J Dis Child* 1989;143:642.
452. Leslie GI, Philips JB, Cassady G. Capillary and venous bilirubin values: are they really different? *Am J Dis Child* 1987;141:1199–1200.
453. Sykes E, Maisels MJ, Kusack S. the effect of ambient light on serum bilirubin levels. *Pediatr Res* 1971;29:326A.
454. Newman TB, Liljestrand P, Escobar GJ. Jaundice noted in the first 24 hours after birth in a managed care organization. *Arch Pediatr Adolesc Med* 2002;156:1244–1250.
455. Javier MC, Krauss A, Nesin M. Corrected end-tidal carbon monoxide closely correlates with the corrected reticulocyte count in coombs' test-positive term neonates. *Pediatrics* 2003;112:1333–1337.
456. Davenport M, Kerkar N., Mieli-Vergani G, et al. Biliary atresia: the King's College Hospital experience (1974–1995). *J Pediatr Surg* 1997;32:479–485.
457. Alpay F, Sarici S, Tosuncuk HD, et al. The value of first-day bilirubin measurement in predicting the development of significant hyperbilirubinemia in healthy term newborns. *Pediatrics* 2000;106:E16.
458. Carbonell X, Botet F, Figueras J, et al. Prediction of hyperbilirubinaemia in the healthy term newborn. *Acta Paediatr* 2001;90:166–170.
459. Kaplan M, Hammerman C, Feldman R, et al. Predischarge bilirubin screening in glucose-6-phosphate dehydrogenase-deficient neonates. *Pediatrics* 2000;105:533–537.
460. Stevenson DK, Vreman HJ. Carbon monoxide production in neonates. *Pediatrics* 1997;100:252–254.
461. Herschel M, Karrison T, Wen M, et al. Evaluation of the direct antiglobulin (Coombs') test for identifying newborns at risk for hemolysis as determined by end-tidal carbon monoxide concentration (ETCOc); and comparison of the Coombs' test with ETCOc for detecting significant jaundice. *J Perinatol* 2002;22:341–347.
462. Martinez JC, Maisels MJ, Otheguy L, et al. Hyperbilirubinemia in the breast-fed newborn: a controlled trial of four interventions. *Pediatrics* 1993;91:470–473.
463. Maisels M. J. Phototherapy—traditional and nontraditional. *J Perinatol* 2001;21:S93–S97.
464. Stern L, Denton RL. Kernicterus in small, premature infants. *Pediatrics* 1965;35:486–485.
465. Maisels M. J., Kring EA, Shumer D. What is the contribution of hemolysis to jaundice in the normal newborn? *Pediatr Res* 2002;51:329A.
466. Newman TB, Easterling MJ. Yield of reticulocyte counts and blood smears in term infants. *Clin Pediatr* 1994;33:71–76.
467. Maisels MJ, Gifford K. Neonatal jaundice in full-term infants: Role of breastfeeding and other causes. *Am J Dis Child* 1983;137:561–562.
468. Vreman HJ, Wong RJ, Stevenson DK. Light-emitting diodes: A novel light source for phototherapy. *Pediatr Res* 1998;44:804–809.
469. Rubo J, Albrecht K, Lasch P, et al. High-dose intravenous immune globulin therapy for hyperbilirubinemia caused by Rh hemolytic disease. *J Pediatr* 1992;121:93–97.
470. Maisels MJ, Vain N, Acquavita AM, et al. The effect of breast-feeding frequency on serum bilirubin levels—a randomized controlled trial. *Am J Obstet Gynecol* 1994;170:880–883.
471. Amato M, Howald H, von Muralt G. Interruption of breast-feeding vs. phototherapy as treatment of hyperbilirubinemia in full term infants. *Helv Paediatr Acta* 1985;40:127–131.
472. Maisels MJ. Why use homeopathic doses of phototherapy? *Pediatrics* 1996;98:283–287.
473. Maisels MJ, Watchko JF. Treatment of jaundice in low birthweight infants. *Arch Dis Child Fetal Neonatol Ed* 2003;88:F459–F463.
474. Clark CF, Torii S, Hamamoto Y, et al. The "bronze baby" syndrome: postmortem data. *J Pediatr* 1976;88:461–464.
475. Ebbesen F. Low reserve albumin for binding of bilirubin in neonates with deficiency of bilirubin excretion and bronze baby syndrome. *Acta Paediatr Scand* 1982;71:415–410.
476. Catterton Z, Carp W, Bunyaten C, et al. Bilirubin binding capacity in ABO hemolytic disease of the newborn. *Clin Res* 1979;27:817A.
477. Phibbs RH, Johnson P, Tooley WH. Cardiorespiratory status of erythroblastotic newborn infants. II. Blood volume, hematocrit, and serum albumin concentration in relation to hydrops fetalis. *Pediatrics* 1974;53:13–23.
478. Nicolaides KH, Clewell WH, Rodeck CH. Measurement of human fetoplacental blood volume in erythroblastosis fetalis. *Am J Obstet Gynecol* 1987;157:50–53.
479. Jährig K, Jährig D, Meisel P, eds. *Phototherapy: treating neonatal jaundice with visible light.* München: Quintessenz Verlags-GmbH, 1998.
480. Maisels MJ. Phototherapy. In: Maisels MJ, Watchko JF, eds. *Neonatal jaundice.* London, UK: Harwood Academic Publishers, 2000:177–204.
481. Agati G, Fusi F, Donzelli GP, et al. Quantum yield and skin filtering effects on the formation rate of lumirubin. *J Photochem Photobiol B* 1993;18(2–3):197–203.
482. Tan KL. The pattern of bilirubin response to phototherapy for neonatal hyperbilirubinemia. *Pediatr Res* 1982;16:670–674.
483. Christensen T, Kinn G. Bilirubin bound to cells does not form photoisomers. *Acta Paediatr* 1993;82(1):22–25.
484. Ennever JF. Blue light, green light, white light, more light: treatment of neonatal jaundice. *Clin Perinatol* 1990;17:467–481.
485. McDonagh AF, Maisels MJ. Photoisomerization of bilirubin in Crigler-Najjar patients. In: Kappas A, Lucey J, eds. *Treatment of Crigler-Najjar syndrome, conference proceedings.* New York City: Rockefeller University, 1996.
486. Jährig K, Jährig D, Meisel P. Dependence of the efficiency of phototherapy on plasma bilirubin concentration. *Acta Paediatr Scand* 1982;71(2):293–299.
487. Hansen TWR. Acute management of extreme neonatal jaundice—the potential benefits of intensified phototherapy and interruption of enterohepatic bilirubin circulation. *Acta Paediatr* 1997;86:843–846.
488. Ebbesen F, Agati G, Pratesi R. Phototherapy with turquoise versus blue light. *Arch Dis Child Fetal Neonatal Ed* 2003;88:F430–F431.
489. Seidman DS, Moise J, Ergaz Z. A new blue light-emitting phototherapy device: a prospective randomized controlled study. *J Pediatr* 2000;136:771–774.
490. ECRI. Fiberoptic phototherapy systems. *Health Devices* 1995;24:134–150.
491. Costello SA, Nyikal J, Yu VY, et al. BiliBlanket phototherapy system versus conventional phototherapy: a randomized controlled trial in preterm infants [see comments]. *J Paediatr Child Health* 1995;31:11–13.
492. Donzelli GP, Moroni M, Pratesi S, et al. Fibreoptic phototherapy in the management of jaundice in low birthweight neonates. *Acta Paediatr* 1996;85:366–370.
493. Pezzati M, Biagiotti R, Vangi V, et al. Changes in mesenteric blood flow response to feeding: conventional versus fiberoptic phototherapy. *Pediatrics* 2000;105:350–353.

494. Holtrop PC, Ruedisueli K, Maisels MJ. Double versus single phototherapy in low birth weight newborns. *Pediatrics* 1992;90:674–677.
495. Tan KL. Efficacy of bidirectional fiberoptic phototherapy for neonatal hyperbilirbinemia. *Pediatrics* 1997;99:e13:5.
496. Tan KL, Lim GC, Boey KW. Efficacy of "high-intensity" blue-light and "standard" daylight phototherapy for non-haemolytic hyperbilirubinemia. *Acta Paediatr* 1992;81(11):870–874.
497. Garg AK, Prasad RS, Hifzi IA. A controlled trial of high-intensity double-surface phototherapy on a fluid bed versus conventional phototherapy in neonatal jaundice. *Pediatrics* 1995;95:914–916.
498. Yamauchi Y, Casa N, Yamanouchi I. Is it necessary to change the babies' position during phototherapy? *Early Hum Dev* 1989;20:221–227.
499. Shinwell ES, Sciaky Y, Karplus M. Effect of position changing on bilirubin levels during phototherapy. *J Perinatol* 2002;22:226–229.
500. International Electrotechnical Commission. Medical electrical equipment, part 2-50: particular requirements for the safety of infant phototherapy equipment. IEC 60601-2-50 available at http://www.iec.ch.2000. Accessed 9/5/2004.
501. Curtis-Cohen M, Stahl GE, Costarino AT, et al. Randomized trial of prophylactic phototherapy in the infant with very low birth weight. *J Pediatr* 1987;107:121–124.
502. Jangaard KA, Vincer MJ, Allen AC. A randomized trial of prescribed phototherapy for established hyperbilirubinemia in infants weighing <1500 grams: a regimen as effective as prophylactic phototherapy? *Pediatr Res* 2003;53:366A.
503. Haddock JH, Nadler HL. Bilirubin toxicity in human cultivated fibroblasts and its modification by light treatment. *Proc Soc Exp Biol Med* 1970;134(1):45–48.
504. Silberberg DH, Johnson L, Schutta H, et al. Effects of photodegradation products of bilirubin on myelinating cerebellum cultures. *J Pediatr* 1970;77:613.
505. Tonz O, Vogt J, Filippini L, et al. Severe light dermatosis following phototherapy in a newborn infant with congenital erythropoietic urophyria. *Helv Paediat Acta* 1975;30:47–56.
506. Mallon E, Wojnarowska F, Hope P, Elder G. Neonatal bullous eruption as a result of transient porphyrinemia in a premature infant with hemolytic disease of the newborn. *J Am Acad Dermatol* 1995;33:333–336.
507. Paller AS, Eramo LR, Farrell EE, et al. Purpuric phototherapy-induced eruption in transfused neonates: relation to transient porphyrinemia. *Pediatrics* 1997;100:360–364.
508. Kearns GL, Williams BJ, Timmons OD. Fluorescein phototoxicity in a premature infant. *J Pediatr* 1985;107:796–798.
509. Hussain K, Sharief N. Dermal injury following the use of fiberoptic phototherapy in an extremely premature infant [see comments]. *Clin Pediatr (Phila)* 1996;35(8):421–422.
510. Siegfried EC, Stone MS, Madison KC. Ultraviolet light burn: a cutaneous complication of visible light phototherapy of neonatal jaundice. *Pediatr Dermatol* 1992;9:278–282.
511. Rubaltelli FF, Jori G, Reddi E. Bronze baby syndrome: a new porphyrin-related disorder. *Pediatr Res* 1983;17:327–330.
512. Meisel P, Jahrig D, Theel L, et al. The bronze baby syndrome: consequence of impaired excretion of photobilirubin? *Photochem Photobiol* 1982;3:345–352.
513. Jori G, Reddi E, Rubaltelli FF. Bronze baby syndrome: an animal model. *Pediatr Res* 1990;27:22–25.
514. Messner KH, Maisels MJ, Leure-DuPree AE. Phototoxicity to the newborn primate retina. *Invest Ophthalmol Vis Sci* 1978;17(2):178–182.
515. Roy M-S, Caramelli C, Orquin J, et al. Effects of early reduced light exposure on central visual development in preterm infants. *Acta Paediatr* 1999;88:459–461.
516. Robinson J, Moseley MJ, Fielder A, et al. Light transmission measurements in phototherapy eye patches. *Arch Dis Child* 1991;66:59–61.
517. Fok TF, Wong W, Cheung KL. Eye protection for newborns under phototherapy: Comparison between a modified headbox and the conventional eyepatches. *Ann Trop Paediatrics* 1997;17:349–354.
518. Dollberg S, Atherton HD, Hoath SB. Effect of different phototherapy lights on incubator characteristics and dynamics under three modes of servocontrol. *Am J Perinatol* 1995;12(1):55–60.
519. Kjartansson S, Hammarlund K, Sedin G. Insensible water loss from the skin during phototherapy in term and preterm infants. *Acta Paediatr* 1992;81:764–768.
520. Maayan-Metzger A, Yosipovitch G, Hadad E, et al. Transepidermal water loss and skin hydration in preterm infants during phototherapy. *Am J Perinatol* 2001;18:393–396.
521. Grunhagen DJ, De Boer MGJ, De Beaufort AJ, et al. Transepidermal water loss during halogen spotlight phototherapy in preterm infants. *Pediatr Res* 2002;51:402–405.
522. Yao AC, Martinussen M, Johansen OJ, et al. Phototherapy-associated changes in mesenteric blood flow response to feeding in term neonates. *J Pediatr* 1994;124(2):309–312.
523. Rosenstein BS, Ducore JM. Enhancement by bilirubin of DNA damage induced in human cells exposed to phototherapy light. *Pediatr Res* 1984;18(1):3–6.
524. Speck WT. Effect of phototherapy on fertilization and embryonic development. *Pediatr Res* 1979;13:506.
525. Rosenfeld W, Sadhev S, Brunot V, et al. Phototherapy effect on the incidence of patent ductus arteriosus in premature infants: prevention with chest shielding. *Pediatrics* 1986;78:10–14.
526. Barefield ES, Dwyer MD, Cassady G. Association of patent ductus arteriosus and phototherapy in infants weighing less than 1000 grams. *J Perinatol* 1993;13(5):376–380.
527. Bhatia J, Mims LC, Roesel RA. The effect of phototherapy on amino acid solutions containing multivitamins. *J Pediatr* 1980;96:284.
528. Drew JH, Marriage KJ, Bayle VV, et al. Phototherapy—short and long-term complications. *Arch Dis Child* 1976;54:454.
529. Schuman AJ, Karush G. Fiberoptic vs conventional home phototherapy for neonatal hyperbilirubinemia. *Clin Pediatr (Phila)* 1992;31(6):345–352.
530. Slater L, Brewer MF. Home versus hospital phototherapy for term infants with hyperbilirubinemia: a comparative study. *Pediatrics* 1984;73:515–519.
531. Rogerson AG, Grossman ER, Gruber HS, et al. Fourteen years of experience with home phototherapy. *Clin Pediatr (Phila)* 1986;25(6):296–299.
532. Meropol SB, Luberti AA, De Jong AR, et al. Home phototherapy: use and attitudes among community pediatricians. *Pediatrics* 1993;91(1):97–100.
533. Plastino R, Buchner DM, Wagner EH. Impact of eligibility criteria on phototherapy program size and cost. *Pediatrics* 1990;85(5):796–800.
534. James J, Williams SD, Osborn LM. Home phototherapy for treatment of exaggerated neonatal jaundice enhances breast-feeding. *Am J Dis Child* 1990;144:431–432(abst).
535. Cremer RJ, Perryman PW, Richards DH. Influence of light on the hyperbilirubinemia of infants. *Lancet* 1958;1:1094–1097.
536. Hughes-Benzie R, Uttley DA, Heick HM. Crigler-Najjar syndrome type I: management with phototherapy crib mattress [Letter]. *Arch Dis Child* 1993;69(4):470.
537. Yohannan MD, Terry HJ, Littlewood JM. Long-term phototherapy in Crigler-Najjar syndrome. *Arch Dis Child* 1983;58(6):460–462.
538. Watchko JF. Exchange transfusion in the management of neonatal hyperbilirubinemia. In: Maisels MJ, Watchko JF, eds. *Neonatal jaundice*. London, UK: Harwood Academic, 2000:169–176.
539. Edwards MC, Fletcher MA. Exchange transfusions. In: Fletcher MA, MacDonald MG, eds. *Atlas of procedures in neonatology*. Philadelphia: JB Lippincott, 1993:363–372.
540. Keenan WJ, Novak KK, Sutherland JM, et al. Morbidity and mortality associated with exchange transfusion. *Pediatrics* 1985;75[Suppl]:417–421.
541. Jackson JC. Adverse events associated with exchange transfusion in healthy and ill newborns. *Pediatrics* 1997;99:e7.
542. Patra K, Storfer-Isser A, Siner B, et al. Adverse events associated with neonatal exchange transfusion in the 1990s. *J Pediatr* 2004;144:626–631.
543. Ellis MI, Hey EN, Walker W. Neonatal death in babies with rhesus isoimmunization. *Q J Med* 1979;48:211–225.
544. Schreiber GB, Busch MP, Kleinman SH, et al. The risk of transfusion-transmitted viral infections. *N Engl J Med* 1996;334:1685–1690.
545. Valaes T. Bilirubin distribution and dynamics of bilirubin removal by exchange transfusion. *Acta Paediatr Scand (Suppl)* 1963;52:149.
546. Veall N, Mollison PL. The rate of red cell exchange in replacement transfusion. *Lancet* 1951;2:792–797.
547. Brown AK, Zuelzer WW, Robinson AR. Studies in hyperbilirubinemia. II. Clearance of bilirubin from plasma and extra vascular space in newborn infants during exchange transfusion. *Am J Dis Child* 1957;93:274–286.

548. Valaes T. Pharmacological approaches to the prevention and treatment of neonatal hyperbilirubinemia. In: Maisels MJ, Watchko J. F., eds. *Neonatal jaundice*. London, UK: Harwood Academic Publishers, 2000:205–214.

549. Yaffe SJ, Dorn LD. Effects of prenatal treatment with phenobarbital. *Dev Pharmacol Ther* 1990;15:215.

550. Reinisch JM, Sanders SA, Mortensen EL, et al. *In utero* exposure to phenobarbital and intelligence deficits in adult men. *JAMA* 1995;15:18–25.

551. Kappas A, Drummond G, Henschke C, et al. Direct comparison of Sn-mesoporphyrin, an inhibitor of bilirubin production, and phototherapy in controlling hyperbilirubinemia in term and near-term newborns. *Pediatrics* 1995;95:468–474.

552. Martinez JC, Garcia HO, Otheguy L, et al. Control of severe hyperbilirubinemia in full-term newborns with the inhibitor of bilirubin production Sn-mesoporphyrin. *Pediatrics* 1999;103:1–5.

553. Valaes T, Drummond GS, Kappas A. Control of hyperbilirubinemia in glucose-6-phosphate dehydrogenase-deficient newborns using an inhibitor of bilirubin production, Sn-mesoporphyrin. *Pediatrcs* 1998;101(5).

554. Bhutani VK, Meloy LD, Poland RL, et al. Randomized placebo-controlled clinical trial of stannsoporfin (Sn-MP) to prevent severe hyperbilirubinemia in term and near-term infants. *Pediatr Res* 2004;55:448A.

555. Valaes T, Petmezaki S, Henschke C, et al. Control of jaundice in preterm newborns by an inhibitor of bilirubin production: studies with tin-mesoporphyrin. *Pediatrics* 1994;93:1–11.

556. Galbraith RA, Drummond GS, Kappas A. Suppression of bilirubin production in the Crigler-Najjar type I syndrome: studies with the heme oxygenase inhibitor tin-mesoporphyrin. *Pediatrics* 1992;89:175.

557. Kappas A, Drummond GS, Munson DP, et al. Sn-mesoporphyrin interdiction of severe hyperbilirubinemia in Jehovah's Witness newborns as an alternative to exchange transfusion. *Pediatrics* 2001;108:1374–1377.

558. Dagoglu T, Ovali F, Samanci N, et al. High-dose intravenous immunoglobulin therapy for haemolytic disease. *J Int Med Res* 1995;23:264–271.

559. Voto LS, Sexer H, Ferreiro G, et al. Neonatal adminstration of high-dose intravenous immunoglobulin and rhesus hemolytic disease. *J Perinat Med* 1995;23:443–451.

560. Hammerman C, Kaplan M, Vreman HJ, Stevenson DK. Intravenous immune globulin in neonatal ABO isoimmunization: factors associated with clinical efficacy. *Biol Neonate* 1996;70:69–74.

561. Sedlak TW, Snyder SH. Bilirubin benefits: cellular protection by a biliverdin reductase antioxidant cycle. *Pediatrics* 2004;113:1776–1782.

562. Hammerman C, Goldstein R, Eiran M, et al. Antioxidant potential of bilirubin in the premature infant. *Pediatr Res* 1997;41:152A.

563. Belanger S, Lavoie JC, Chessex P. Influence of bilirubin on the antioxidant capacity of plasma in newborn infants. *Biol Neonate* 1997;71:233–238.

564. Gopinathan V, Miller NJ, Milner AD, et al. Bilirubin and ascorbate antioxidant activity in neonatal plasma. *FEBS Lett* 1994;349:197–200.

565. Hegyi T, Goldie E, Hiatt M. The protective role of bilirubin in oxygen radical disease of the preterm infant. *J Perinatol* 1994;14:296–300.

566. Heyman E, Ohisson A, Girschek P. Retinopathy of prematurity and bilirubin (letter). *N Engl J Med* 1989;320:256.

567. DeJonge MH, Khuntia A, Maisels MJ, et al. Bilirubin levels and severe retinopathy of prematurity in 23–26 week estimated gestational age infants. *J Pediatr* 1999;135:102–104.

568. Gaton DD, Gold J, Axer-Siegel R, et al. Evaluation of bilirubin as possible protective factor in the prevention of retinopathy of prematurity. *Br J Ophthalmol* 1991;75:532–534.

569. Hosono S, Ohno T, Kimoto H, et al. No clinical correlation between bilirubin levels and severity of retinopathy of prematurity. *J Pediatr Ophthalmol Strabismus* 2002;39:151–156.

570. Milner JD, Aly HZ, Ward LB, et al. Does elevated peak bilirubin protect from retinopathy of prematurity in very low birthweight infants. *J Perinatol* 2003;23:208–211.

571. Fauchére JC, Meier-Gibbons FE, Koerner F, et al. Retinopathy of prematurity and bilirubin - no clinical evidence for a beneficial role of bilirubin as a physiological antioxidant. *Eur J Pediatr* 1994;153:358–362.

572. Boynton BR, Boynton CA. Retinopathy of prematurity and bilirubin [Letter]. *N Engl J Med* 1989;321:193–194.

573. Gollan JL, Knapp AB. Bilirubin metabolism and congenital jaundice. *Hosp Pract (Off Ed)* 1985;Feb 15:83–106.

574. Roy-Chowdhury N, Deocharan B, Bejjanki HR, et al. Presence of the genetic marker for Gilbert syndrome is associated with increased level and duration of neonatal jaundice. *Acta Paediatr* 2002;91:100–101.

575. Eggert P, Stick C, Schroder H. On the distribution of irradiation intensity in phototherapy. Measurements of effective irradiance in an incubator. *Eur J Pediatr* 1984;142:58–61.

576. American Association of Blood Banks Technical Manual Committee. Perinatal issues in transfusion practice. In: Brecher M, ed. *Technical manual*. Bethesda, MD: American Association of Blood Banks, 2002:497–515.

577. Valaes, Koliopoulos C, Koltsidopoulos A. The impact of phototherapy in the management of neonatal hyperbilirubinemia: comparison of historical cohorts. *Acta Paediatr* 1996;85:273–276.

578. Guaran R, Drew JH, Watkins A. Jaundice: clinical practice in 88,000 liveborn infants. *Aust NZ J Obstet Gynaecol* 1992;32:186–192.

579. Maisels MJ. Is exchange transfusion for hyperbilirubinemia in danger of becoming extinct? *Pediatr Res* 1999;45:210A.

580. van de Bor, van Zeben-van der Aa TM, Verloove-Vanhorick SP, et al. Hyperbilirubinemia in preterm infants and neurodevelopmental outcome at 2 years of age: results of a national collaborative survey. *Pediatrics* 1989;83:915–920.

581. McKiernan P. Neonatal cholestasis. *Semin Neonatol* 2002;7:153–165.

582. Peevy KJ, Landaw SA, Gross SJ. Hyperbilirubinemia in infants of diabetic mothers. *Pediatrics* 1980;66:417–419.

583. Ives NK. Neonatal jaundice. In: Rennie JM, Roberton NRC, eds. *Textbook of neonatology*. New York: Churchill Livingston, 1999:715–732.

36

Calcium and Magnesium Homeostasis

Winston W. K. Koo   *Reginald C. Tsang*

Calcium (Ca) is the most abundant mineral in the body and, together with phosphorus (P), forms the major inorganic constituent of bone. Magnesium (Mg) is the fourth most abundant cation and is the second most common intracellular electrolyte in the body. The maintenance of Ca and Mg homeostasis requires a complex interaction of hormonal and nonhormonal factors; adequate functioning of various body systems, particularly the renal, gastrointestinal, and skeletal systems; and adequate dietary intake. From a clinical perspective, mineral homeostasis is reflected in the maintenance of circulating concentrations of Ca and Mg in the normal range and integrity of the skeleton.

In the circulation, the amount of Ca and Mg is less than 1% of their respective total body content; however, disturbances in serum concentrations of these minerals are associated with disturbances of physiologic function manifested by numerous clinical symptoms and signs. Chronic and severely lowered serum concentrations of these minerals also may reflect the presence of a deficiency state.

At all ages, the total body content of Ca and Mg in the skeleton are about 99% and 60%, respectively. Thus, the skeleton is a reservoir for mineral homeostasis in addition to its role providing structural and mechanical support; disturbances in mineral homeostasis can result in osteopenia and rickets in infants and children, and osteomalacia and osteoporosis in adults.

The mechanisms to maintain mineral homeostasis in neonates are the same as for children and adults. However, the newborn infant has a number of unique challenges to maintain mineral homeostasis during adaptation to extrauterine life and to continue a rapid rate of growth. These include an abrupt discontinuation of the high rate of intrauterine accretion of Ca (approximately 120 mg/kg/day) and Mg (approximately 4 mg/kg/day) during the third trimester; a smaller skeletal reservoir available for mineral homeostasis; a delay in establishment of adequate nutrient intake for at least a few days or longer, particularly in sick and preterm infants; and a high requirement for Ca and Mg for the most rapid period of postnatal skeletal growth, with an average gain in length of more than 25 cm during the first year. There also may be diminished end-organ responsiveness to hormonal regulation of mineral homeostasis, although the functional capacity of the gut and kidney improves rapidly within days after birth. The effects of these issues are exaggerated in infants with heritable disorders of mineral metabolism, such as extracellular calcium-sensing receptor (CaR) mutations, and in infants who have experienced adverse antenatal events such as maternal diabetes, intrapartum problems such as perinatal asphyxia or maternal Mg therapy, or postnatal problems such as immature functioning of multiple organs from premature birth.

Increased understanding of the physiology and molecular basis of mineral metabolism allows a better understanding of the pathophysiology of the resultant clinical disorder. This in turn allows a more rational management to minimize the adverse impact from disturbed mineral homeostasis and to prevent iatrogenic causes precipitating or prolonging these problems.

TISSUE DISTRIBUTION

In the fetus, about 80% of minerals are accrued between 25 weeks of gestation and term. During this period, the estimated daily accretion per kilogram of fetal body weight is 2.3 to 2.98 mmol (92 to 119 mg) Ca and 0.1 to 0.14 mmol (2.51 to 3.44 mg) Mg. The peak accretion rates occur at 36 to 38 weeks of gestation. In newborn term infants, the total body Ca and Mg contents average approximately 28 grams and 0.7 grams, respectively (1,2).

After birth, 99% of total body Ca is in bone. The tissue distribution of Mg varies according to the extent of bone mineralization and rate of soft tissue growth. Near the end of the third trimester, however, about 60% of the body's Mg is in bone, 20% in muscle, and most of the remainder is found in the intracellular space of other tissues.

CIRCULATING CONCENTRATION

Calcium

Serum Ca (1 mmol/L = 4 mg/dL) occurs in three forms: approximately 40% is bound, predominantly to albumin; approximately 10% is chelated and complexed to small molecules such as bicarbonate, phosphate, or citrate; and approximately 50% is ionized. Complexed and ionized Ca are ultrafiltrable.

Total Ca concentrations (tCa) in cord sera increase with increasing gestational age. Serum tCa may be as high as 3 mmol/L in cord blood of infants born at term, and the concentrations are significantly higher than paired maternal values at delivery (3–6). Serum tCa reaches a nadir during the first 2 days after birth (7–13); thereafter, concentrations increase and stabilize at a level generally above 2 mmol/L (14). In infants exclusively fed human milk, the mean serum tCa increases from 2.3 to 2.7 mmol/L over the first 6 months postnatally. Normally serum tCa in children and adults remains stable, with a diurnal range of less than 0.13 mmol/L. During the third trimester of pregnancy, a modest reduction in maternal serum tCa concentration (average 0.1 mmol/L) is associated with a decrease in serum albumin concentration.

Serum ionized Ca (iCa) concentration is the best indicator of physiologic blood Ca activity. Measurement of serum iCa is firmly established in clinical medicine, and simple, rapid, and direct determination of iCa from whole blood, plasma, and serum by ion-selective electrodes is freely available. Whole-blood iCa analyzers are gaining popularity because they are adaptable for "point of care" testing. However, some differences exist in values from different iCa analyzers, particularly for whole-blood iCa values (15), as a result of differences in the design of the reference electrode, formulation of calibrating solutions, and lack of a reference system for iCa. Thus, normative data should be generated according to the subject's age, the instrument, and the type of sample used for iCa measurement.

Serum iCa decreases in the presence of high serum albumin, P, bicarbonate, and heparin. Serum iCa increases with increased Mg and is inversely related to blood pH. The effect of the latter may be minimized by the immediate analysis of serum samples for iCa. Freezing serum samples in 5% carbon dioxide-containing tubes may minimize the impact of pH variations if measurement of iCa is delayed for 1 week.

One report showed a wide range of cord whole-blood iCa of 0.4 to 1.85 mmol/L from apparently normal pregnancies (16). This is a much wider range compared with multiple reports based on cord sera, although the range for whole-blood iCa becomes much narrower within hours after birth and similar to serum iCa values. Cord-serum iCa increases with increasing gestational age and is higher than values in paired maternal sera. In healthy term neonates, serum iCa averages 1.25 mmol/L with 95% confidence limits of 1.1 to 1.4 mmol/L (4.4 to 5.6 mg/dL), and there is

a decline in serum iCa in the first 48 hours of life with a nadir at 24 hours (17). Serum iCa generally changes in parallel with tCa in healthy humans. However, serum iCa is stable and normal during pregnancy in contrast to a slight reduction in tCa. Serum tCa and iCa are correlated in infants and adults, but the correlation is inadequate to predict one from the other with sufficient accuracy.

The concentration of iCa is critical to many important biologic functions with the extracellular Ca concentration normally maintained within a narrow range. The Ca ion is well established as an intracellular second messenger, but identification of the extracellular CaR has established that iCa also functions as a messenger outside cells. Ca homeostasis also involves the maintenance of an extremely large Ca concentration gradient across the cellular plasma membrane. In the cell, distribution of Ca is not uniform. The cytosolic compartment contains 50 to 150 nmol of Ca per liter of water; a larger intramitochondrial Ca pool contains 500 to 10,000 nmol of Ca per liter of cell water. In contrast, the concentration of iCa in extracellular fluid is 1 million nmol/L (1 mmol/L). There are at least two adenosine triphosphate-dependent mechanisms involved in the maintenance of the Ca concentration gradient across the plasma membrane. The measurement of intracellular Ca continues to improve with better instrumentation and probes, but it is not yet freely available.

Magnesium

Approximately 30% of serum Mg (1 mmol/L = 2.4 mg/dL) is in the protein-bound form, with the remainder in the ultrafiltrable portion. Seventy percent to 80% of ultrafiltrable Mg is in ionic form, and the remainder is complexed to anions, particularly phosphate, citrate, and oxalate. Cord-serum total Mg (tMg) is higher than paired maternal values. Serum tMg of 0.92 ± 0.13 mmol/L (mean $\pm$ 2 SD) in children is slightly higher than the adult values of 0.88 ± 0.13 mmol/L (18). Ion-selective electrodes are used in the measurement of ionized Mg (iMg) in whole blood and sera. iMg concentrations average 62% to 70% of the tMg concentration in cord and postnatal sera. Cord-serum iMg is also higher than that in maternal serum (19–21). The clinical role of iMg (versus tMg) in a number of disease states appears limited (22).

Cellular Mg content of most tissues is 6 to 9 mmol/kg wet weight, and most of this Mg is localized in membrane structures (e.g., microsome, mitochondria, plasma membrane). The much smaller pool of free Mg in the cell is maintained at about 1 mmol/L and is in an exchanging equilibrium with membrane-bound Mg. Unbound intracellular Mg has a critical role in cellular physiology and catalyzes enzymatic processes concerned with the transfer, storage, and use of energy. Intracellular Mg usually remains stable despite wide fluctuations in serum Mg. In Mg-deficient states, however, the intracellular content of Mg can be low despite normal serum concentrations. The measurement of intracellular Mg continues to improve with better instrumentation and probes but is not freely available.

PHYSIOLOGIC CONTROL

Calciotropic hormones, including parathyroid hormone (PTH), 1,25 dihydroxyvitamin D [1,25(OH)$_2$D], and possibly calcitonin (CT), appear to maintain Ca homeostasis by intermodulation of their physiologic effects on each other and on the classic target organs: kidney, intestine, and bone. Dietary intake of Ca, Mg, P, and other nutrients including sodium, glucose, and protein also may significantly contribute to the regulation of mineral homeostasis. PTH serves as the major component of the rapid response to hypocalcemia, whereas 1,25(OH)$_2$D, with its major effect on elevating intestinal absorption of Ca, is responsible for a slower but more sustained contribution to the maintenance of normocalcemia. CT, on the other hand, appears to function in the opposite role to PTH but with the capacity to stimulate the production of 1,25(OH)$_2$D, which in theory may serve an additional regulatory role in the maintenance of Ca homeostasis.

In contrast, the control of Mg homeostasis by calciotropic hormones under physiologic conditions appears to be limited. However, Mg is critical to the maintenance of Ca homeostasis since Mg regulates the production and secretion of PTH, acts as a cofactor for the 25-hydroxyvitamin D 1α hydroxylase enzyme in the production of 1,25(OH)$_2$D, and maintains adequate sensitivity of target tissues to PTH. Furthermore, Mg is considered a mimic/antagonist of Ca as it often functions synergistically with Ca, yet competes with it in the gut and kidney for transport and other metabolic pathways.

Parathyroid Hormone

In humans, parathyroid glands are derived from the third and fourth pharyngeal pouch. The PTH gene, along with the genes for insulin, β-globulin, and CT, is located on chromosome 11p15 (23), and restriction site polymorphisms near the PTH gene have been detected. The initial translational product of the mRNA is a 115-amino-acid prepro-PTH. Prepro-PTH then undergoes proteolytic cleavage in the endoplasmic reticulum to remove a 25-residue amino-terminal signal sequence to form pro-PTH. The prohormone-specific region is cleaved further during subsequent intracellular processing to generate the 84-amino-acid secreted form of the intact hormone with a relative molecular mass (M$_r$) of 9,500. PTH is synthesized by the chief cells and stored in secretory granules. It is colocated and secreted with chromogranin A, a protein that may act in autocrine- or paracrine-regulated release of PTH.

About 50% of the newly generated PTH is proteolytically degraded intracellularly, and some of the inactive fragments are also secreted. After release into the circulation, the intact PTH molecule has a serum half-life of 5 to 8 minutes and undergoes a series of cleavages by endopeptidases in the liver and kidney. The amino-terminal fragments contain the biologically active fractions, with the 1–34 fragment having the most calcemic activity; modifications at the amino terminal, particularly at the first two

residues, can abolish its biologic activity. The midregion and carboxyl-terminal fragments are biologically inert, although the latter may have some *in vitro* biological activity.

Circulating immunoreactive PTH is a complex mixture of intact 1–84 PTH, multiple peptide fragments from the amino- and carboxyl-terminals, and mid-molecular regions. Normally there are greater amounts of middle and carboxyl fragments than intact hormone in the circulation because of metabolic breakdown of the short-lived, intact hormone, coupled with glandular secretion of inactive fragments. The fragments are cleared from the blood virtually exclusively by glomerular filtration. Intact PTH and amino-terminal fragments constitute less than 20% of PTH immunoreactivity in the peripheral circulation. PTH molecules reactive in the widely used commercial immunoradiometric assays (IRMA), designed to detect both amino- and carboxyl-terminal epitopes of the peptide, have been considered as "intact" PTH (IPTH). However, there have been reports that the large 7–84 fragment of PTH is also detected by these assays. This large fragment is biologically inactive and present in greater concentrations in uremic states or hyperparathyroidism. The conventional IPTH technique increases the PTH concentration by 30% to 50%, compared to the latest chemiluminescence or IRMA techniques that measure the "whole" or "bio-intact" PTH. Therefore, the treatment of secondary hyperparathyroidism based on data from conventional IPTH assays theoretically may lead to overtreatment and oversuppression of biologically active PTH, although the clinical significance of this possibility remains to be defined. In any case, consistency of the PTH assay methodology and serial measurements are critical to the interpretation and management of pathologic states.

PTH concentrations in cord blood frequently are low and do not correlate with PTH concentrations in maternal sera (4,24). Earlier studies of higher levels of bioactive PTH in cord sera from cytochemical assays may be related to elevated concentrations of parathyroid hormone-related protein (PTHrP), since PTH-like bioactivity was tightly correlated with levels of PTHrP in sheep and pig. Small amounts (approximately 5%) of perfused fragments (35–84, 44–68, and 65–84 amino acids) but probably not the whole PTH molecule are reported to cross the human placenta. Serum PTH concentrations increase postnatally coincidentally with the fall in serum Ca in both term and preterm infants (4,24–27). The rise in serum IPTH is greater for preterm infants with hypocalcemia compared to term infants reflecting appropriate PTH response. Serum PTH concentrations are similar for children and adults but are increased in the elderly. Serum concentrations of intact PTH as measured by IRMA showed no change during normal pregnancy. In adults, serum intact PTH is present in picomolar concentrations. It has a significant circadian periodicity, spontaneous episodic pulsatility with distinct peak property and a significant temporal coupling with serum iCa and P concentrations and prolactin secretion.

PTH effects on end-organ systems appear to be mediated through its binding to specific receptors. The type 1 PTH/PTHrP receptor has been identified in bone, cartilage, kidney, intestine, aorta, urinary bladder, adrenal gland, brain, and skeletal muscle. It binds equally to PTH and PTHrP and belongs to a superfamily of guanine-nucleotide-binding (G) protein-coupled cell membrane receptors (GPCR) including those for CT, secretin, growth hormone-releasing hormone, corticotrophin-releasing hormone, glucagon, vasoactive intestinal polypeptide, and others. Another PTH receptor (type 2) responds only to PTH, although its main endogenous ligand appears to be a 39-amino-acid peptide, hypothalamic tubular infundibular peptide. It has been found in the brain, pancreas, and intestines, but the physiologic significance of this receptor remains ill defined.

The gene for the PTH/PTHrP receptor is located on chromosome 3p21.1-p24.2. It contains 17 exons and encodes a mature glycoprotein of 593 amino acids (28). The type 1 PTH receptor consists of extended extracellular, ligand-binding amino-terminal and intracellular G-protein–associated carboxyl-terminal domains and seven transmembrane domains. Signal transduction mediated by G proteins results in multiple second messenger pathways to affect both stimulatory and inhibitory end-organ responses. The strongest and best-characterized second messenger signaling pathway is the PTH-stimulated coupling of the type 1 PTH receptor to the stimulating G protein (G_s; composed of 3 subunits: α, β, and γ, and encoded by the GNAS1 gene localized to 20q13.3), which activates adenyl cyclase, an enzyme that generates cyclic AMP (cAMP). However, coupling of the type 1 PTH receptor to the G_q class protein activates phospholipase C, which generates inositol phosphate (IP_3) and diacylglycerol (DAG). These second messengers in turn lead to stimulation of protein kinases A and C and Ca transport channels and result in a variety of hormone-specific tissue responses.

In physiologic terms, PTH acts synergistically with $1,25(OH)_2D$ and is the most important regulator of extracellular Ca concentration. PTH acts directly on bone and kidney, and indirectly on intestine. Immediate control of blood Ca is probably due to PTH-induced mobilization of Ca from bone and increased renal distal tubular reabsorption of Ca. PTH also decreases proximal tubular and thick ascending limb reabsorption of sodium, Ca, phosphate, and bicarbonate. PTH effects on kidney are mediated primarily through stimulation of sodium/calcium exchange, calcium transport proteins and renal 25 OHD-1α-hydroxylase, but a decrease in sodium-dependent phosphate cotransporter, NPT-2. Maintenance of steady-state Ca balance is probably from increased intestinal Ca absorption secondary to increased $1,25(OH)_2D$ production. PTH increases acutely within minutes the rate of Ca release from bone into blood. Chronic effects of PTH are to increase the numbers of osteoblasts and osteoclasts and to increase the remodeling of bone. Continuous exposure to elevated concentrations of PTH leads to increased osteoclastic resorption of bone. In contrast to its classic action on Ca mo-

bilization from bone, the amino-terminal fragments of PTH and PTHrP, and small pulses of PTH have an anabolic effect on bone, independent of its resorptive action. Other PTH effects on bone include enhanced collagen synthesis, activities of alkaline phosphatase, ornithine and citrate decarboxylases, and glucose-6-phosphate dehydrogenase; DNA, protein and phospholipid synthesis.

Extracellular Ca is the most potent regulator of PTH secretion and is mediated by the cell-surface CaR, which detects minute perturbations in the extracellular iCa concentration and responds with alterations in cellular function that normalize iCa. Thus, iCa functions as extracellular as well as intracellular messenger. The human CaR gene is located on chromosome 3q13.3-q21 and encodes a cell-surface protein of 1,078 amino acids. The CaR gene is developmentally upregulated, and CaR transcripts are present in numerous tissues including chief cells of the parathyroid glands, kidneys (in particular the thick ascending limb), brain and nerve terminals, breast, lung, intestine, adrenal and skin, and also the precursor and mature osteoblasts and osteoclasts. CaR is a member of the GPCR superfamily with a seven-member membrane-spanning domain. It contains at least seven exons, of which six encode the large (approximately 600-amino-acid) amino-terminal extracellular domain and/or its upstream untranslated regions, while a single exon codes for the remainder of the receptor including a cytoplasmic carboxyl-terminal intracellular domain. Signal transduction mediated by G proteins results in activation of phospholipase C that generates IP_3 and DAG, and subsequent stimulation of protein kinase C (PKC) and Ca transport channels.

Low or falling serum Ca concentrations result in active secretion of preformed PTH within seconds. There is a sigmoidal type of PTH secretion in response to decreased serum Ca, which is most pronounced when serum Ca is in the mildly hypocalcemic range. PTH secretion is 50% of maximal at a serum iCa of about 1 mmol/L (4 mg/dL); this is considered the calcium set point for PTH secretion (29). Sustained hypocalcemia increases PTH mRNA within hours. Protracted hypocalcemia leads within days to cellular replication and increased gland mass. High serum Ca suppresses PTH secretion via activation of CaR. It in turn activates phospholipase C and generation of IP_3 and DAG and probably increases the proteolytic destruction of preformed PTH. Hyperphosphatemia stimulates PTH secretion, probably by lowering the serum Ca concentration.

In the kidney, CaR decreases the basal and PTH-stimulated paracellular reabsorption of Ca, Mg, and sodium via multiple mechanisms including inhibition of cAMP accumulation; stimulation of phospholipase A2 activity. The release of free arachidonic acid is promoted which is metabolized via the lipooxygenase pathway to P450 metabolites that inhibit the activities of the sodium-potassium-chloride cotransporter and potassium channel; and possibly affect renal water regulation by inhibition of vasopressin-abated water flow. In chronic renal failure, downregulation in the expression of renal CaR may account for the development of secondary hyperparathyroidism (30), and downregulation of PTH receptors may account for the skeletal resistance to the calcemic effect of PTH (31). Extracellular Ca exerts numerous other actions on parathyroid function, including modulation of the intracellular degradation of PTH, cellular respiration, membrane voltage, and the hexose monophosphate shunt.

Maintenance of Ca homeostasis through other organs also may be possible, for example, through the presence of CaR in intestinal cells (32), and probable modulation of CT secretion from changes in intracellular Ca (33). Furthermore, expression of CaR in gastrin-secreting G cells and acid-secreting parietal cells, together with data indicating that CaR exhibits selectivity for L-aromatic amino acids, appears to provide a molecular explanation for amino acid sensing in the gastrointestinal tract, regulation of PTH secretion and urinary Ca excretion, and the physiologic interaction between Ca and protein metabolism.

Decrease in serum Mg concentration stimulates PTH secretion (34,35), although chronic hypomagnesemia inhibits secretion of PTH (34,36). Hypomagnesemia is also associated with an increased target tissue resistance to PTH probably from inactivity of adenylate cyclase, a Mg-requiring enzyme. Hypermagnesemia rapidly decreases the secretion of PTH *in vivo* in human subjects, and PTH concentration remains depressed despite concomitant hypocalcemia, presumably in part due to stimulation of CaR by other divalent cations such as Mg. Vitamin D and its metabolites, 25-hydroxyvitamin D (25-OHD) and $1,25(OH)_2D$, acting through vitamin D receptors, decrease the level of PTH mRNA. Additional systemic factors (growth hormone, insulin-like growth factor 1, estrogen, progesterone, CT, cortisol, catecholamines, prostaglandins, and somatostatin) and local factors (interleukin-l [IL-1]) modulate PTH secretion and function, although their role in the regulation of Ca and Mg metabolism under physiologic conditions is not clear.

Calcitonin

CT is secreted primarily from thyroid C cells and also from many extrathyroidal tissues including placenta, brain, pituitary, mammary gland, and other tissues. Developmentally, CT-containing cells and parathyroid gland cells are thought to derive from the same tissue source as the neural crest. In the rat, the number of thyroid C cells and secretion of CT increase from fetal life to suckling, a period of rapid growth (37). There is probably no placental crossover of CT; the human placental tissue is able to produce CT in response to the presence of Ca in the culture medium. In human neonates, the CT content in crude tissue preparations of thyroid is larger than that of the adult thyroid (38).

There are two calcitonin genes, α and β, located on chromosome 11p15.2 near the genes for β-globulin and PTH. Two different RNA molecules are transcribed from the α gene. It is comprised of six exons with the fourth exon translated into the precursor for CT and the fifth

translated into the precursor for CT gene-related peptide-I (CGRP-I). The initial translational product of the mRNA is prepro-CT, a 141-amino-acid peptide. It is cleaved by endopeptidase at the endoplasmic reticulum to form pro-CT, a 13-kDa 116-amino-acid peptide. CT (between the sixtieth and ninety-first positions of the pro-CT peptide) and equimolar amounts of non-CT secretory peptides, corresponding to the flanking peptides linked to the amino and carboxyl terminals of the prohormone, are generated during precursor processing. Further structural modifications to the CT molecule occur intracellularly prior to release into the circulation. These modifications include formation of a disulfide bridge between two cysteine remnants in position 1 and 7, and hydroxylation of the C-terminal proline residue; both are essential for binding of CT to its receptor. The CT monomer is a 32-amino-acid peptide (M_r 3,400). CGRP-I is synthesized wherever the CT mRNA is expressed, e.g., in medullary carcinoma of thyroid, although there is no translational product from the CGRP-I sequence.

The β or CGRP-II gene is transcribed into the mRNA for CGRP predominantly in nerve fibers in the central and peripheral nervous systems, blood vessels, thyroid and parathyroid glands, liver, spleen, heart, lung, and possibly bone marrow. CGRP, a 37-amino-acid peptide (M_r 4,000), is also generated from the larger precursor molecule pro-CGRP, a 103-amino-acid peptide. Seventy-five amino-terminal residues of the preprohormones for CT and CGRP are predicted to be identical.

Classic bioactivity of human CT (hCT) is present in the full 32-amino-acid structure or its smaller fragments, such as hCT 8–32 and hCT 9–32; the ring structure of CT enhances, but is not essential for, hormone action. Basic amino acid substitutions confer a helical structure in this region as found in salmon and other nonmammalian CT, resulting in greater potency in lowering serum Ca and probably a longer circulating half life. The kidney appears to be the dominant organ in the metabolism of human CT. A small percentage of the metabolic clearance rate of CT in humans may be accounted for by enzymatic degradation in blood. Injected hCT monomer disappears from the blood *in vivo* with a half-life of approximately 10 minutes; in contrast, the half-life of hCT in plasma incubated *in vitro* at 37°C may be longer than 20 hours (39). Depending on the animal species, other sites such as the liver, intestine, and bone may be involved in the metabolism of CT.

Circulating immunoreactive CT and CGRP are a heterogeneous mixture of different molecular forms and are recognized as long as the antigenic epitopes recognized by the antiserum are expressed. Immunoreactive CT or CGRP concentration is expressed in gravimetric or molar equivalents of synthetic CT or CGRP. Sample preparation with initial extraction, gel chromatography, and high-performance liquid chromatography separation, and the use of two-site immunoassay can improve the sensitivity and specificity of CT measurements. Serum CT concentrations during pregnancy are variable. They are high at birth compared to paired maternal CT concentrations (40).

Serum CT further increases during the first few days after birth and may reach levels five- to ten-fold higher than adult CT concentrations. Serum CT concentrations decrease progressively during infancy; however, in preterm infants up to 3 months after birth, the mean serum CT concentrations may remain twice the adult value. There is also a small peak of serum CT concentration during late childhood. In human adults, the basal serum CT concentration may be lower in women than in men, but the concentration is not affected by increasing age. The CT secretory response to Ca infusion is lower in women and with increasing age. In human adults, serum CT and CGRP concentrations are found in the picomolar range. Diurnal variability has been reported for serum CGRP but not for serum CT. In normal individuals, larger precursor molecules of CT such as procalcitonin are not detected.

CT function is mediated by binding to receptors linked to G proteins, members of the GPCR superfamily, and by activation of adenylate cyclase and phospholipase C (41). CT receptors (CTR) have been identified in the central nervous system, testes, skeletal muscle, lymphocytes, and placenta. The function of CTR can be influenced by accessory proteins, receptor isoforms, genetic polymorphisms, developmental and/or transcriptional regulation, feedback inhibition, and the specific cellular or tissue background. The CTR gene is located on chromosome 7q2l.2-q21.3 and encodes a 490-amino-acid G-protein–linked receptor with seven transmembrane domains. Two isoforms of human CTR arise by alternative splicing of an exon of 48 nucleotides that encodes a l6-amino-acid insertion within the first intracellular loop. The isoform with the insertion (hCTR-l) activates only adenylate cyclase, whereas the other isoform (hCTR-2) activates both adenylate cyclase and phospholipase C. CGRP functions are also mediated by receptors (42).

The presence of receptor-activity-modifying proteins (RAMPs) can posttranslationally modify the initially orphan calcitonin receptor-like (CL) receptor and CTR to exhibit different receptor functions, i.e., functional modification of G-protein–coupled receptors is possible. RAMP1, 2, and 3 thus far identified are single transmembrane domain proteins with intracellular C-terminals of up to 10 amino acids and extracellular N-terminals of about 120 amino acids. Noncovalent association of a RAMP with the CL receptor or CTR results in heterodimeric RAMP/receptor complexes at the cell surface. The CL receptor functions as a CGRP receptor when coexpressed with RAMP1, whereas CL receptor/RAMP2 and CL receptor/RAMP3 are adrenomedullin 1 and 2 receptor subtypes, respectively. CTR, with 60% homology to the CL receptor, predominantly recognizes CT in the absence of RAMP. When CTR is coexpressed with RAMP1, it transforms into an amylin/ CGRP receptor. When CTR is coexpressed with RAMP3, it interacts only with amylin. Thus, two class II G-protein– coupled receptors, the CL receptor and CTR, are associated with three RAMPs to form high-affinity receptors for CGRP, adrenomedullin, or amylin.

Secretion of CT is stimulated by an increase in serum Ca and Mg concentrations and by gastrin, glucagon, and cholecystokinin (along with several other structural analogues of these hormones, e.g., pentagastrin, prostaglandin E2), glucocorticoid, norepinephrine, and CGRP; secretion is suppressed by hypocalcemia, propranolol and other adrenergic antagonists, somatostatin, chromogranin A and vitamin D. CT gene transcription is positively regulated by glucocorticoids and negatively regulated by PKC, Ca, and vitamin D. Calcitonin may activate the l-hydroxylase system independent of PTH (43), whereas $1,25(OH)_2D$ decreases CT gene expression in adult rats but is ineffective in 13-day-old suckling rats (44). The latter observation may be related to fewer $1,25(OH)_2D$ receptors in C cells of immature rats. Calcitonin induces refractoriness to its own actions by downregulation, and functional reduction of receptor mRNA is a well-known phenomenon. Clinically, it is manifested as the "escape" phenomenon during therapy with calcitonin.

In humans, changes in Ca (and P) metabolism are not seen despite extreme variations in CT production. In the neonate, there is neither an identifiable hypocalcemic response to the postnatal surge in serum CT nor a blunting of CT secretion in the presence of hypocalcemia. In adults, there are no definite effects attributable to CT deficiency (e.g., totally thyroidectomized patients receiving only replacement thyroxin) or CT excess (e.g., patients with medullary carcinoma of thyroid), except for the chronic suppression of bone remodeling. The clinical significance of CT is related to its use as a tumor marker in the management of medullary carcinoma of the thyroid and its pharmacologic effect to inhibit osteoclast-mediated bone resorption and increase renal Ca clearance. The pharmacologic activities of CT are useful for the suppression of bone resorption in Paget disease, for limited use in the treatment of osteoporosis, and for early phase treatment of severe hypercalcemia. In addition, CT also increases renal clearance of Mg, P, and sodium and free water clearance. The net effect of CT is a lowering of serum Ca and P concentrations. Thus, the bioactivity of CT on calcium metabolism frequently is opposite that of PTH; CT probably modulates the effect of PTH on target organs.

Noncalcium-related actions of CT and associated molecules are increasingly being discovered. For example, CT and CTR may play important roles in a variety of processes as wide ranging as embryonic development and sperm function/physiology. In addition, pro-CT detectable in the plasma is not produced in the C cells of the thyroid and is being explored as a marker of bacterial-induced inflammation/sepsis. Production of pro-CT after exposure to bacterial endotoxin and inflammatory cytokines tumor necrosis factor (TNF) and IL-6 appears to be primarily from neuroendocrine cells in the lung and intestine. Cells of neuroendocrine origin express all proteins related to CT (CGRP-I and -II and amylin) derived from the same family of genes, and it is speculated that "inflammatory" pro-CT may be coded by the same gene family. There are no enzymes in the plasma that can break down pro-CT, and when it is secreted into the circulation, it has a half-life of 25 to 30 hours, thus increasing serum pro-CT. After administration of endotoxin, the peak circulating concentrations of TNF, IL-6, pro-CT, and C-reactive protein occur at approximately 90 minutes, 180 minutes, 6 to 8 hours, and 24 hours, respectively.

CGRP primarily affects catecholamine release, vascular tone and blood pressure, and cardiac contractility. Its clinical role probably also lies in its potential pharmacologic effect. The influence of CGRP on Ca and P homeostasis is minor compared to that of CT. However, amylin, a pancreatic islet-derived or synthetic 37-amino-acid peptide, is a member of the CGRP family with a potent hypocalcemic effect despite sharing only 15% of its amino acid sequence with human CT. The hypocalcemic effect of amylin is probably mediated by the CTR on osteoclasts, and it is 100-fold more potent than CGRP (45). Both CT and CGRP inhibit gastric acid secretion and food intake.

Vitamin D

Vitamin D (M_r 384) can be obtained from diet or synthesized endogenously. It must undergo several metabolic transformations primarily in the liver and kidney to form the physiologically most important metabolite, $1,25(OH)_2D$, which functions as a hormone in the maintenance of mineral homeostasis. Under *in vivo* conditions, there are more than 30 other vitamin D metabolites, with and without putative functions.

Dietary vitamin D (1 μg = 40 IU) is derived from plants as ergocalciferol (vitamin D_2) and from animals as cholecalciferol (vitamin D_3). Dietary vitamin D is absorbed from the duodenum and jejunum into lymphatics, and about 50% of the vitamin D in chylomicron is transferred to vitamin D-binding protein (DBP) in blood before uptake by the liver.

In animals, vitamin D_3 can be synthesized endogenously in the skin (46). During exposure to sunlight, the high-energy UV photons (290 to 315 nm) penetrate the epidermis and photochemically cleave the bond between carbons 9 and 10 of the sterol B-ring of 7-dehydrocholesterol (7-DHC or provitamin D_3) to produce previtamin D_3. It then undergoes a thermally induced isomerization to vitamin D_3 that takes 2 to 3 days to reach completion. Thus, cutaneous synthesis of vitamin D_3 continues for many hours after a single sun exposure. Previtamin D_3 is photolabile; continued exposure to sunlight causes the isomerization of previtamin D_3 to biologically inert products, principally lumisterol. No more than 10% to 20% of the initial provitamin D_3 concentrations ultimately end up as previtamin D_3, thus preventing excessive production of previtamin D_3 and vitamin D_3.

Vitamin D_3 synthesis in the skin is directly dependent on the amount of sunlight exposure and is affected by time of day, season, and latitude. Peak sunlight at midday, in summer, and at lower latitudes are optimal conditions; the amount of skin area exposed and duration of sunlight exposure directly affect vitamin D_3 synthesis. Melanin in the skin competes with 7-DHC for ultraviolet photons, but the production of vitamin D_3 can be adjusted by increasing

the duration of sunlight exposure. Use of topical sunscreen blocks ultraviolet photons, and aging decreases the capacity for cutaneous synthesis of vitamin D_3.

The term "vitamin D" is frequently used generically to describe vitamins D_2 and D_3 and their metabolites. In mammals, vitamins D_2 and D_3 appear to metabolize along the same pathway, and there is little functional difference between their metabolites. However, differences in affinity to DBP and receptors between D_2 and D_3 and their metabolites support the contention that vitamin D_3 is more bioavailable than D_2.

In the circulation, vitamin D and its metabolites are bound to proteins, mainly DBP (approximately 85%) and albumin (approximately 15%). The DBP gene is located on chromosome 4q11-13. It is a member of the albumin multigene family of proteins that includes albumin and α-fetoprotein. DBP is an approximately 53-kDa globulin in humans, and its x-ray crystallographic structure has been determined (47). Plasma DBP concentration (4 to 8 μM) is approximately 20-fold higher than that of the total circulating vitamin D metabolites (approximately 100 nM), i.e., it is normally less than 5% saturated with vitamin D metabolite. The amount of unbound or free 25-OHD and $1,25(OH)_2D$, important in determining bioactivity, is less than 1% of the total concentration.

In the liver, vitamin D is hydroxylated at carbon 25 to 25-OHD. Quantitatively, 25-OHD (1 nmol/L = 0.4 ng/mL) is the most abundant vitamin D metabolite in the circulation and is a useful index of vitamin D reserve. Regulation of 25-hydroxylase activity is limited, and there are few limitations to the production of 25-OHD. However, *in vivo* administration of $1,25(OH)_2D$ (48) inhibits hepatic production of 25-OHD, and Ca deficiency (49) increase the metabolic clearance of 25-OHD with subsequently decrease circulating 25-OHD.

In the kidney, 25-OHD is hydroxylated further to $1,25(OH)_2D$ by 25-OHD-1α-hydroxylase (CYP1α), and to 24,25-dihydroxyvitamin D ($24,25(OH)_2D$) by 25-OHD-24-hydroxylase (CYP24). The hydroxylation occurs primarily in the mitochondria of renal proximal tubules. The genes for these enzymes have been localized to chromosome 12q13-14 and 20q13.3, respectively. The human gene encoding CYP1α is 5 kb in length and is comprised of nine exons and eight introns; its exon/intron organization is similar to other cloned mitochondrial P450 enzymes.

The activity of CYP1α and therefore production of $1,25(OH)_2D$ are tightly regulated. It is the rate-limiting hormonally regulated step in the bioactivation of vitamin D. PTH increases transcriptional activity of the CYP1α gene promoter and therefore increases mRNA for $1,25(OH)_2D$. Decreases in serum or dietary Ca or P increase mRNA for and serum concentration of $1,25(OH)_2D$ independent of PTH (49–51). However, hypophosphatemia in renal wasting disorders does not elicit appropriate phosphate conservation or an increase in $1,25(OH)_2D$ production. These disorders include X-linked hypophosphatemic rickets (XLH), autosomal-dominant hypophosphatemic rickets (ADHR), and tumor-induced osteomalacia. They have similar phenotypic manifestations characterized by hypophosphatemia, decreased renal phosphate reabsorption, normal (and thus inappropriately low) or low serum calcitriol concentrations, normal serum Ca and PTH, and defective skeletal mineralization.

XLH results from mutations in the PHEX (phosphate-regulating gene with homologies to endopeptidases on the X chromosome, Xp22.1) gene, which encodes a membrane-bound endopeptidase (52), whereas ADHR is associated with mutations of the gene encoding fibroblast growth factor 23 (FGF23) and is linked to chromosome 12p13.3 (53). The latter is a small heat-sensitive molecule less than 25 kDa that inhibits sodium-dependent phosphate wasting and probably inhibits CYP1α. The endopeptidase, PHEX, degrades native FGF23 which provides the biochemical link among these clinical syndromes. XLH rickets also has been associated with mutations in CLCN5, a voltage-gated chloride channel gene located on Xp11.22.

Other factors that enhance 1,25(OH)$_2$D production include estrogen, prolactin, growth hormone, insulin-like growth factor I, and PTHrP. 1,25(OH)$_2$D production is feedback regulated and is inhibited by chronic deficiency of or low circulating Mg (36). Mg deficiency also lowers serum 1,25(OH)$_2$D response to a low-Ca diet but does not appear to limit 1,25(OH)$_2$D production in animals (54). The effect of Mg on 1,25(OH)$_2$D metabolism is presumably related in part to its role as a cofactor of the CYP1α enzyme. In contrast to the rapid increase within minutes in the secretion and serum concentration of PTH, measurable alterations in serum 1,25(OH)$_2$D concentrations usually occur hours after exposure to an appropriate stimulus. Extrarenal production of 1,25(OH)$_2$D in macrophages, particularly in granulomatous disease states, may not be tightly regulated; is stimulated by γ-interferon (55), but is not responsive to changes in dietary Ca intake.

The degradation of 1,25(OH)$_2$D is also tightly regulated. 1,25(OH)$_2$D strongly induces the enzyme 25-hydroxyvitamin D-24 hydroxylase (CYP24) in all target cells for vitamin D. CYP24 catalyzes several steps of 1,25(OH)$_2$D degradation, collectively known as the C24 oxidation pathway, which starts with 24-hydroxylation and culminates in the formation of the biliary excretory form, calcitroic acid. CYP24 expression is inhibited by PTH and by dietary phosphate restriction. In the kidney and intestine in particular, upregulation of the CYP24 enzyme in response to 1,25(OH)$_2$D treatment is rapid and occurs within 4 hours (56). Physiologic production of 24,25(OH)$_2$D is therefore an important means to regulate the circulating concentration of 1,25(OH)$_2$D and catabolism of vitamin D, although it may also have a role in bone integrity and fracture healing in the chick model. Most of the other vitamin D metabolites are derived primarily from further metabolic alterations to 25-OHD and 1,25(OH)$_2$D through oxidation or side chain cleavage and have poorly defined physiologic functions. However, many analogues of vitamin D metabolites are being studied for the numerous potential pharmacologic actions that involve less calcemic-inducing and more maturation and differentiation effects.

Like other steroid hormones, 1,25(OH)$_2$D function is mediated primarily through modulation of the cellular genome by binding to a specific nuclear receptors, vitamin D receptor, VDR, a 424-amino-acid phosphoprotein for which the x-ray crystallographic structure has been determined (47). The VDR gene contains nine exons and is located on chromosome 12q13-14 near the site of the gene for CYP1α (57). VDR is a member of the subfamily of nuclear receptors with ligand-binding domains that bind classic hormones including thyroid hormone, androgens, estrogens, progesterone, glucocorticoids, aldosterone, hormonal forms of vitamin A, and 1,25(OH)$_2$D. It has several functional domains including a 110-residue N-terminal DNA-binding domain with two zinc fingers, C-terminal hormone-binding domain, and hinge region important for nuclear localization. The VDR interacts with the 9-*cis* retinoic acid nuclear receptor retinoid X receptor (RXR) to form a heterodimeric RXR-VDR complex that binds to specific DNA sequences, termed vitamin D-responsive elements (VDREs). After 1,25(OH)$_2$D binds to the receptor, it induces conformational changes (58) that result in the recruitment of a multitude of transcriptional coactivators that stimulate the transcription of target genes. VDR also can adopt a dual role as a repressor in the absence of ligand and then subsequently as a coactivator when a ligand binds. VDR is upregulated by 1,25(OH)$_2$D at both the mRNA and protein levels and is increased during growth, gestation, and lactation; however, it shows an age-dependent decrease in mature animals and humans, supporting the notion that VDR may be up- or downregulated, depending on Ca needs.

Although 1,25(OH)$_2$D regulates more than 60 genes whose actions include those associated with Ca homeostasis and immune responses, as well as cellular growth, differentiation, and apoptosis, two basic clinical functions define the major classic actions of vitamin D. The first is that vitamin D is required to prevent rickets in children and osteomalacia in adults. The second is the prevention of hypocalcemic tetany. These functions are maintained by 1,25(OH)$_2$D through its effect on a number of target tissues, primarily intestine, kidney, and bone, with modulating effects from other hormones including PTH and CT.

The genomic action of 1,25(OH)$_2$D can be preceded by more rapid nongenomic actions that occur in minutes and involve membrane-associated events such as increased Ca transport, and PKC and mitogen-activated protein kinase activation. This nongenomic rapid increase in cytosolic Ca within seconds to minutes is reported to occur in various cell types from the intestine and parathyroid, osteoblasts, myocytes, and leukemic cells (59).

Quantification of vitamin D and its metabolites has been achieved by several different methods, including high-performance liquid chromatography, with detection by ultraviolet absorbance or binding assays, and immunoassays based on antibodies raised to vitamin D metabolite conjugates. Values from different laboratories cannot be compared without making direct comparison of their assay procedures. Interlaboratory coefficients of variation for the measurement of 25-OHD, 24,25(OH)$_2$D, and l,25(OH)$_2$D may range between 35% and 52%. Furthermore, differences between the affinities of vitamins D$_2$ and D$_3$ to DBP and VDR, and different chromatographic behavior on various preparative chromatographic systems demand that great care be taken with assay techniques when dealing with patients who have significant vitamin D$_2$ intake. To ensure reliable results, appropriate vitamin D standards must be used for standard curve generation in performing competitive protein binding assays of these compounds.

Maternofetal transfer of vitamin D and its metabolites varies, depending on the species. In humans, the cord-serum vitamin D concentration is very low and may be undetectable; the 25-OHD concentration is directly correlated with, but is lower than, maternal values, consistent with placental crossover of this metabolite; and 1,25(OH)$_2$D concentrations also are lower than maternal values, but there is no agreement on the maternofetal relationship of this and other dihydroxylated vitamin D metabolites (3,60–62). However, the placenta, like the kidney, produces 1,25(OH)$_2$D, making it difficult to ascertain just how much fetal 1,25(OH)$_2$D results from placental crossover versus placental synthesis. 24,25(OH)$_2$D also crosses the placenta, and its concentration in the sera of mothers and newborns varies with the seasons, being highest in autumn. It appears that the human fetus receives the bulk of its vitamin D already metabolized to 25-OHD.

Seasonal and racial variations in serum 25-OHD concentrations occur, presumably from variations in endogenous production. The concentration of serum 25-OHD, as with 24,25(OH)$_2$D, is lower in winter. These changes may be reflected in cord-serum values. In normal adults, serum 1,25(OH)$_2$D concentrations are relatively constant and maintained within approximately 20% of the overall 24-hour mean, and show no seasonal variation, which is consistent with the tightly regulated CYPlα activity. African American mothers, infants, and young children tend to have lower 25-OHD and higher 1,25(OH)$_2$D concentrations than their white counterparts. Serum 1,25(OH)$_2$D in the newborn becomes elevated within 24 hours after delivery and appears to vary with to Ca and P intake.

The circulating half-life of vitamin D is about 24 hours and for 25-OHD is 2 to 3 weeks, although the latter half-life is decreased in vitamin D-deficient individuals. 1,25(OH)$_2$D has a much shorter half-life of 3 to 6 hours. Metabolites of 25-OHD and 1,25(OH)$_2$D may undergo enterohepatic circulation after exposure to intestinal β-glucuronidase. The physiologic role of enterohepatic circulation of vitamin D metabolites has not been precisely quantitated.

NONCLASSIC CONTROL OF CALCIUM AND MAGNESIUM HOMEOSTASIS

Factors other than the classic calciotropic hormones, PTH, CT, and 1,25(OH)$_2$D, whether acting systemically or locally on multiple effector organs, are increasingly being recognized as important to the maintenance of mineral homeostasis in certain circumstances. The ultimate effect on mineral homeostasis often involves bone formation and/or resorption and flux of Ca and Mg between extracellular fluid and bone, with or without direct involvement by calciotropic hormones. Skeletal health, particularly in the growing skeleton, requires the integrated actions of classic calciotropic hormones, endocrine modulators of growth, numerous cytokines and growth factors and their receptors and endogenous modulators.

Many factors, such as growth hormone, insulin-like growth factor I, estrogen, progesterone, cortisol, and TNF, can affect the secretion or function of one or more of the calciotropic hormones. In turn, many factors such as insulin-like growth factor I; transforming growth factor-β$_1$; IL-1, -2, -4, and -6; TNF-α, and interferon-γ (IFN-γ) can be modulated by calciotropic hormones.

Local factors such as transforming growth factor-β$_1$, lymphotoxin, TNF-α, IFN-γ, IL-1, and IL-6 acting in a paracrine (i.e., cell-to-cell) or autocrine (i.e., cell-to-self) fashion may influence Ca flux of bone cells. The effects on Ca flux based on these interactions are probably more important under pathologic situations. IFN-γ from activated macrophages (55,63) stimulates CYP1α mRNA and enzyme production, with little or no feedback inhibition by 1,25(OH)$_2$D, which potentially may compromise Ca homeostasis.

Interaction between systemic and local factors can occur, and some factors such as PTHrP may act both systemically and locally (64). PTHrP is also known as PTH-like peptide, PTH-like protein, or human humoral hypercalcemic factor. PTHrP and PTH genes appear to be members of the same gene family. PTHrP mRNA encodes a 177-amino-acid protein consisting of a 36-amino-acid precursor segment and 141-amino-acid mature peptide. The mature PTHrP contains several structural or functional domains. The N-terminal 1–13 region has eight of 13 residues in common with PTH. The amino acids 34–111 segment is highly conserved among species while amino acid 118 to the C-terminus is poorly conserved. PTHrP gene expression is found in an extensive variety of endocrine and nonendocrine tissues. PTHrP biologic activity and immunoreactivity for PTHrP mRNA have been found in many tissues, by as early as 7 weeks of gestation, including the fetus, placenta, lactating breasts, and milk in human and in various tissues in the sheep (65) and pig (66). Both PTH and PTHrP appear to bind to the same G-protein–linked receptor. Synthetic and recombinant PTHrPs can mimic the effects of PTH on the classic PTH target organs, involving activation of adenylate cyclase and other second messenger systems.

Several PTHrP assays with varying sensitivities and specificities have been developed which account for the variability reported between assays (67). The stability of PTHrP in plasma samples may be enhanced if sample collection is done in the presence of protease inhibitors. Circulating immunoreactive PTHrP concentrations are low or undetectable in normal subjects. Serum PTHrP is increased during pregnancy (5,6) and is similar to or lower than umbilic cord PTHrP concentrations. In cord sera, PTHrP concentration is 10- to 15-fold higher than that of PTH. Amniotic fluid PTHrP concentrations at midgestation and at term are 13- to 16-fold higher than the cord or maternal levels (68), and the concentration of PTHrP in milk is 100-fold higher. PTHrP concentrations correlate positively with total milk calcium (69).

PTHrP concentrations in the circulation of individuals with humoral hypercalcemia of malignancy (HHM) are elevated (67). The amino-terminal fragment PTHrP 1–74 appears to be specific for HHM, whereas the carboxyl-terminal fragment PTHrP 109–138 is elevated in the serum of patients with HHM or renal failure. The levels of PTHrP in these patients are similar to the concentration of PTH (10^{-12} to 10^{-11} mol/L).

Clinically, PTHrP is the humoral mediator secreted by tumors that results in the syndrome of HHM, and the measurement of PTHrP is of clinical utility primarily as a tumor marker in HHM. Physiologically, PTHrP is an important paracrine regulator of several tissue-specific functions that may directly or indirectly affect fetal and neonatal mineral homeostasis, probably through its effect on smooth muscle relaxation, placental Ca transport, lactation, fetal bone development, and control of cellular growth and differentiation.

DISTURBANCES IN SERUM MINERAL CONCENTRATIONS

Hypocalcemia

Neonatal hypocalcemia may be defined as a serum tCa concentration of less than 2 mmol/L (8 mg/dL) in term infants and 1.75 mmol/L (7 mg/dL) in preterm infants with iCa below 1.0 to 1.1 mmol/L (4.0 to 4.4 mg/dL), depending on the particular ion-selective electrode used. Whole-blood iCa shows similar values to serum iCa and is often used to determine hypocalcemia. However, the appropriate range used is also subject to the type of instrument used (15).

The definition of hypocalcemia is based on the clinical perspective because serum Ca concentrations are maintained within narrow ranges under normal circumstances, and the potential risk for disturbances of physiologic function increases as the serum Ca concentration decreases below the normal range. Furthermore, improvements in physiologic function, e.g., changes in cardiac contractility, blood pressure, and heart rate, are reported in hypocalcemic infants undergoing Ca therapy (70–72), and a higher mortality rate has been reported for children with hypocalcemia in pediatric intensive care settings (73).

Clinically, there are two peaks in the occurrence of neonatal hypocalcemia. An early form typically occurs during the first few days after birth, with the lowest concentrations of serum Ca being reached at 24 to 48 hours of age; late neonatal hypocalcemia occurs toward the end of the

first week. These findings reflect in part the traditional clinical practice of screening for biochemical abnormalities in small or sick hospitalized infants during the first few days, and in symptomatic infants during hospitalization and after hospital discharge. However, the nadir of serum Ca concentration may occur at less than 12 hours (9 to 12) or not until some weeks after birth (74,75), and many neonates, particularly those with genetic defects in Ca metabolism, may be hypocalcemic but remain asymptomatic and undetected during the early neonatal period. This also may contribute to the less frequent diagnosis of late neonatal hypocalcemia compared to early neonatal hypocalcemia. Additionally, increased understanding of the mechanisms of disturbed Ca metabolism would support the approach to neonatal hypocalcemia based on risk factors and pathophysiologic basis rather than the traditional "early" or "late" onset.

Pathophysiology

Multiple risk factors for neonatal hypocalcemia (Table 36-1) support the existence of varied and frequently interrelated pathophysiologic mechanisms (Table 36-2). However, the pathophysiologic mechanisms are not fully defined for all cases of hypocalcemia. In most cases of neonatal hypocalcemia, there is a decrease in both tCa and iCa, although iCa may be decreased without lowering tCa.

There are common bases for the occurrence of hypocalcemia, particularly for "early" onset hypocalcemia. These include the abrupt discontinuation of placental Ca supply at birth, limited or no dietary Ca, transient limited increase

TABLE 36-1
RISK FACTORS FOR NEONATAL HYPOCALCEMIA

Maternal
    Insulin-dependent diabetes
    Hyperparathyroidism
    Vitamin D or magnesium deficiency
    Medications: calcium antacid and anticonvulsant (?)
    Narcotic use (?)

Peripartum
    Birth asphyxia

Infant
    Intrinsic
    • Prematurity
    • Malabsorption
    • Malignant infantile osteopetrosis
    • Parathyroid hormone: impaired synthesis, secretion, regulation, or responsiveness
    • Mitochondrial fatty acid disorder (?)
    Extrinsic
    • Diet
        ■ Inadequate calcium
        ■ Excess phosphorus
    • Enema: phosphate
    • Exchange transfusion with citrated blood
    • Infectious diarrhea (?)
    • Clinical therapy (?): phototherapy, alkali, high rate of intravenous lipid

TABLE 36-2
PATHOPHYSIOLOGY OF NEONATAL HYPOCALCEMIA

Physiologic Basis	Mechanism	Clinical Association
Calcium (Ca)	Decreased reserves	Prematurity
	Decreased intake or absorption	Prematurity, malabsorption syndrome
	Increased Ca complex	Chelating agent (e.g., citrated blood for exchange transfusion, long-chain free fatty acid)
Magnesium (Mg)	Decreased tissue store	IDM, maternal hypomagnesemia
	Decreased intake or absorption	Prematurity, malabsorption syndrome, specific Mg malabsorption (rare)
	Increased loss	Intestinal fistula, enterostomy, or renal (primary or secondary)
Phosphorus (P)	Increased load	Exogenous (e.g., dietary, enema) phosphate loading
pH	Increased	Respiratory or metabolic alkalosis (e.g., shifts Ca from ionized to protein-bound fraction)
Parathyroid hormone (PTH)	Inadequate or defective synthesis or secretion	Maternal hypercalcemia, DiGeorge association, hypoparathyroidism, hypomagnesemia, PTH gene mutations
	Impaired regulation	CaR activating mutations, autosomal-dominant or sporadic hypocalcemia with hypercalciuria
	Impaired responsiveness	Chronic hypomagnesemia, type 1 PTH receptor inactivating mutation (?), pseudohypoparathyroidism
Calcitonin	Increased	IDM, birth asphyxia, prematurity
Vitamin D	Deficiency	Severe maternal deficiency
	Decreased response to $1,25(OH)_2D$	Prematurity
Osteoclast activity	Absent	Malignant infantile osteopetrosis
Miscellaneous	Increased anabolism	Hungry bone/refeeding syndrome
	Others ?	Mitochondrial fatty acid disorder, rotavirus diarrhea, phototherapy, narcotic withdrawal

$1,25(OH)_2D$, 1,25-dihydroxyvitamin D; IDM, infant of insulin-dependent diabetic mother; CaR, calcium-sensing receptor

in the serum PTH concentration, possibly end-organ resistance to PTH and $1,25(OH)_2D$, and elevated serum CT concentration. Many illnesses may preclude early enteral feeding but many clinicians do not use parenteral nutrition that contains Ca for 1 or more days after birth, thus increasing the risk for hypocalcemia. Even in healthy term infants, the amount of Ca retention from milk feeds probably is less than 20 mg/kg body weight on the first day, rising to at least 45 to 60 mg/kg on the third day; these amounts are significantly lower than the daily *in utero* Ca accretion of more than 100 mg/kg during the third trimester (2).

Hypocalcemia (in varying degrees of severity) may occur in association with "transient" congenital hypoparathy- roidism (TCHP), i.e., suppression of fetal and neonatal parathyroid function from maternal hyperparathyroidism (74,75) and maternal use of high doses of calcium carbonate (76) as antacid, and thus, impaired PTH response to the interruption of placental supply of Ca at birth. Neonatal hypocalcemia is often the first manifestation that leads to the diagnosis of maternal hyperparathyroidism.

In the neonate, hypocalcemia frequently occurs in the presence of rising concentrations of PTH in the circulation. It is possible that this represents either a relative inade-

quate response of the parathyroid gland or end-organ resistance to PTH. Resistance to pharmacologic doses of $1,25(OH)_2D$, demonstrated *in vitro* (77) and *in vivo* in infants (11,12), may also contribute to hypocalcemia.

Despite the hypocalcemic effects of CT, the role of CT in the development of neonatal hypocalcemia remains uncertain. Serum CT concentrations continue to increase after birth in neonates of normal and diabetic pregnancies (9,26) irrespective of the variation in serum Ca; in neonates with birth asphyxia (9); and in preterm infants (25). The stimulus for the postnatal rise in serum CT, despite falling serum Ca, is unknown. There are conflicting reports on the effect of Ca supplementation to suppress the postnatal surge in CT secretion. However, serum CT is increased after an intravenous bolus of Ca during exchange blood transfusion (78).

The above problems are exaggerated in the preterm infant and account for the inverse relationship between the frequency of hypocalcemia versus birth weight and gestational age; more than 50% of preterm very-low-birth-weight neonates may have hypocalcemia (10–12). Infants with intrauterine growth retardation may have hypocalcemia if they are also preterm or have birth asphyxia; otherwise, there is apparently no increased incidence of hypocalcemia related to growth retardation (13).

Hypomagnesemia may be contributory to hypocalcemia in infants of mothers with insulin-dependent diabetes (79) , although gestational diabetics may (80) or may not (81) have disturbed mineral metabolism. Both hypocal- cemia and hypomagnesemia may be the result of a common insult from the diabetic pregnancy, and rigid control of maternal glucose levels during pregnancy may significantly diminish these complications (82). Severe and persistent hypomagnesemia from any cause can result in hypocalcemia (see hypomagnesemia section). Deficiency of various minerals, including Ca, Mg, and trace minerals such as zinc, can result from chronic intestinal malabsorption and fistula or enterostomy loss. During infancy, congenital or acquired short-bowel syndrome and any chronic diarrheal condition, especially if associated with steatorrhea, are leading causes of malabsorption and possibly impaired enterohepatic circulation of vitamin D and vitamin D metabolites.

Excessive P load can result in hypocalcemia. Cow milk and even "humanized" cow-milk–derived formulae (83,84) with "lower" P content compared with cow milk but higher compared with human milk, and cereals which usually have high P content are typical sources of dietary P load. Accidental overdose of oral phosphate supplement (85) or phosphate-containing enema (86) are less frequent causes of excessive P load.

Neonatal hypocalcemia from impaired synthesis or secretion of PTH in the newborn may be secondary to maternal hypercalcemia or to developmental defects of the parathyroid gland. A variety of mutations of PTH or CaR genes, some with Mendelian modes of inheritance, can affect the synthesis, metabolism, and function of PTH and result in hypocalcemia.

Relative inadequacy or the transient nature of the PTH response to the abrupt withdrawal of the placental transfer of Ca contributes to the fall in serum Ca after birth. This also may be responsible for the hypocalcemia induced by exchange transfusion using citrated blood (78,87) or feeding of the relatively high P content of cow-milk formula (83,84). The ability of the neonatal parathyroid glands to respond to hypocalcemic stress increases with postnatal age. Neonates with TCHP may have prolonged hypocalcemia that requires treatment until late infancy or early childhood, and hypoparathyroidism may recur in later childhood (88–90).

Hypoparathyroidism in the infant is a heterogeneous group of disorders and may occur sporadically or with differing Mendelian modes of inheritance (91–93). Synthesis of defective PTH can occur in the autosomal-dominant form with a point mutation in the signal peptide-encoding region for prepro-PTH. The autosomal-recessive form is associated with a mutation in the donor splice site leading to transcriptional loss of the second exon and prevention of translation. The X-linked recessive form is associated with embryonic dysgenesis of parathyroid glands. Hypoparathyroidism from fetal parathyroid hypoplasia or dysgenesis usually requires lifelong treatment to prevent hypocalcemia.

Deletion of chromosome 22q11.2 is associated with varied phenotypic manifestations including DiGeorge and velocardiofacial/Shprintzen syndromes. Both syndromes may represent different degrees of the same disorder with partial or complete absence of derivatives of the third, fourth, and possibly fifth pharyngeal pouches, and are often associated with defective development of the third, fourth, and sixth aortic arches. It is estimated that up to 30% of these patients may have hypoparathyroidism, although far fewer patients develop hypocalcemia (94). Delayed motor development, cognition and neurodevelopment, and behavior and temperament problems are frequently reported in more than 50% of affected patients (95,96). Early screening and intervention for these problems are advised. Multiple other organ systems (94,97) may be involved and include some combination of congenital heart disease, primarily involving the aortic arch, decreased T-cell number or function, and possibly thyroid C-cell deficiency. DiGeorge association may be inherited in an autosomal-dominant fashion (98).

Dysregulation of PTH can result from activating mutations of CaR with a reduction in EC_{50} (concentration of extracellular Ca required to elicit half of the maximal increase in intracellular inositol phosphate) to suppress PTH synthesis. It is manifested as autosomal dominant or as sporadic cases of hypocalcemia with hypercalciuria (99,100). The latter is an effect of the mutated CaR in the kidneys. Hypocalcemia is usually mild and asymptomatic, and diagnosis is often delayed beyond the neonatal period, although hypocalcemia was likely present during the immediate newborn period.

Relative defective response to PTH can result in neonatal hypocalcemia. The inactivating mutation of the type 1 PTH receptor gene, as documented in Blomstrand chondrodystrophy, is present in the prenatally lethal form of short-limb dwarfism (101). Theoretically this defective response to PTH may result in hypocalcemia but the regulation of serum Ca has not been evaluated *in vivo*.

Impaired end-organ response to PTH occurs with chronic hypomagnesemia and may involve simultaneous impairment in both PTH and $1,25(OH)_2D$ pathways (36). End-organ unresponsiveness to PTH associated with genetic defect is classically manifested as pseudohypoparathyroidism type 1a (PHP-1a) or Albright hereditary osteodystrophy. The biochemical basis of the defect is proximal to cAMP production (102). It is inherited in an autosomal-dominant fashion with heterozygous inactivating mutations in the maternal GNAS1 exons that encode the α subunit of G_s ($G_s\alpha$). The gene GNASl is located on chromosome 20q13.3 and encodes 13 exons that are alternatively spliced to yield four $G_s\alpha$ proteins. Multiple mutations have been reported and include abnormalities in splice junctions associated with deficient mRNA production and point mutations that result in diminished amounts and activities of the G proteins. The inactivating mutation of the gene impairs the production of the adenylate cyclase second messenger system, leading to resistance to multiple hormones (including PTH, vasopressin, and thyrotropin) that activate $G_s\alpha$. Clinical manifestations include short stature, round face, brachymetacarpals and brachymetatarsals, dental dysplasia, subcutaneous calcifications, abnormalities in taste, smell, hearing, and vision, and developmental delay. Biochemical abnormalities include hypocalcemia, hyperphosphatemia, increased circulating PTH, and insensitivity to the administration of exogenous PTH (unaltered urinary Ca, P, and cAMP) in the absence of compromised renal function. The extent of resistance to other hormones is variable, and the complete biochemical picture is usually not evident until 2 to 3 years after birth.

Parent-specific methylation with parental imprinting of the GNAS1 gene, involving selective inactivation of either the maternal or paternal allele, is possible and leads to different phenotypic expression. In the case of the $G_s\alpha$ gene, it is paternally imprinted (silenced) so that the disease PHP-1a is not inherited from the father carrying the defective allele but only from the mother (103). However, the defective allele is not imprinted or silenced in all tissues and reflects haplotype insufficiency. For example, PHP-1b is characterized by isolated resistance to PTH without the accompanying skeletal manifestations. Paternal isodisomy of chromosome 20q in patients that lack the maternal-specific methylation pattern within GNAS1 results in normal $G_s\alpha$ protein and activity in the fibroblast but not in the renal proximal tubules (104). There is a third type, PHP-1c, reported in a few patients that differs from PHP-1a only in having normal erythrocyte levels of $G_s\alpha$; presumably there is a post-$G_s\alpha$ defect in adenyl cyclase stimulation. All type 1 PHP individuals show a deficient urinary cAMP response to the administration of exogenous PTH. Individuals with pseudopseudohypoparathyroidism have typical clinical manifestation of PHP-1a but have normal serum Ca and normal response of urinary cAMP to exogenous PTH. The mutated GNAS1 gene is inherited from the father, i.e., paternal imprinting, with suppression of the mutant copy in selected tissues, and there is a 50% reduction in the amount of $G_s\alpha$.

Infants with neonatal hypocalcemia seizures and "transient" biochemical features of pseudohypoparathyroidism have been reported (105). These infants have elevated serum PTH and P with hypocalcemia at diagnosis. Administration of exogenous human PTH 1–34 showed little phosphaturic effect although there was brisk response in plasma and urine cAMP and alkaline phosphatase. After initial treatment for hypocalcemia, the serum Ca and PTH spontaneously normalized before 6 months of age.

Maternal anticonvulsant therapy with phenytoin and phenobarbital also may result in neonatal hypocalcemia, presumably from increased clearance of vitamin D secondary to the induction of the hepatic cytochrome P450 enzyme system. However, other maternal factors including seasonal variation in sunlight exposure, increased maternal age and parity, and poor socioeconomic status, may contribute to development of neonatal hypocalcemia, presumably in part from varied and probably deficient maternal vitamin D. Furthermore, there is no seasonal variation in the rate of early neonatal hypocalcemia (106) despite seasonal variation in maternal and fetal vitamin D status, as indicated by maternal and cord 25-OHD concentrations. Thus, maternal vitamin D or Mg deficiency probably predisposes to but is not the primary cause of hypocalcemia in the neonate.

Malignant infantile osteopetrosis may present with neonatal hypocalcemia, presumably reflecting continued Ca uptake from unopposed bone formation (107). Rapid replenishment of nutrients in severe deficiency, including prolonged starvation, often leads to disturbed blood biochemistries including hypokalemia, -phosphatemia, -magnesemia and -calcemia. This is known as the "refeeding syndrome" or "hungry bone syndrome" with excessively rapid shift of electrolytes and minerals intracellularly in various tissues, particularly muscle and bone (108,109).

The pathophysiology in some situations with hypocalcemia remains ill defined. Approximately 40% of infants with severe diarrhea from rotavirus have hypocalcemia, and it resolves with symptomatic support and improvement in diarrhea (110). Mitochondrial fatty acid disorders have been associated with severe metabolic anomalies including hypoglycemia, hypocalcemia, hyperkalemia and metabolic acidosis, and organ dysfunction including hepatic and cardiac failure (111).

Decreases in serum iCa can occur without decreases in serum tCa. Agents that complex Ca in the blood would be expected to decrease iCa. Such agents include citrate, which is used as an anticoagulant for blood storage. During "exchange blood transfusion," iCa can decrease to 0.5 mmol/L in spite of administration of conventional amounts of Ca (i.e., 0.5 to 1 mL of 10% Ca gluconate for each 100 mL of blood exchanged) during the transfusion. Increased levels of long-chain free fatty acids from intravenous lipid emulsion can complex Ca and reduce iCa *in vitro*; thus, hypocalcemia potentially can occur with excessive rates of intravenous lipid infusion. Alkalosis can result in shifts of Ca from the ionized state to the protein-bound fraction. Because alkalosis increases neuromuscular hyperirritability, the combination of decreased serum iCa and alkalosis may precipitate clinical tetany in an infant with borderline serum Ca status. In clinical practice, administration of sodium bicarbonate in the therapy of metabolic acidosis often occurs in situations with high risk of hypocalcemia such as prematurity or perinatal asphyxia, but it is not known if it has an independent role in the development of hypocalcemia. The mechanisms for hypocalcemia in some situations are not known. For example, neonates with severe hyperbilirubinemia tend to have lower iCa (112), the use of phototherapy may be associated with hypocalcemia (113), and infants born to narcotic-using mothers are reported to have a lower serum iCa if they manifest withdrawal symptoms (114).

Diagnosis

Suspicion of hypocalcemia must be confirmed by measurement of serum tCa and iCa since clinical manifestations are

TABLE 36-3
DIAGNOSTIC WORKUP FOR NEONATAL HYPOCALCEMIA

History
  Screen for risk factors (Table 36-1)

Physical examination
  General examination with focus on peripheral and central nervous and cardiovascular systems
  Associated features, e.g., infant of a diabetic mother, prematurity, birth asphyxia, congenital heart disease, pseudohypoparathyroidism, etc.

Investigations[a,b,c]
  Serum total and ionized calcium (tCa and iCa), magnesium (Mg), phosphorus (P), total protein and albumin, and simultaneous "intact" or "whole" parathyroid hormone (PTH)
  Acid–base status
  Complete blood count (lymphocyte count)
  Electrocardiogram (Q-Tc >0.4 sec or Q$_o$-Tc >0.2 sec)
  Chest x-ray (thymic shadow, aortic arch)
  Urine Ca, P, Mg, and creatinine
  Meconium and urine screen for narcotics
  Maternal serum +Ca and iCa, Mg and P, urine Ca and P, if suspect maternal or heritable calcium disorder is suspected, particularly in persistent neonatal hypocalcemia
  Additional workup as indicated: vitamin D metabolites, T-cell number and function, malabsorption studies, response to exogenous PTH, molecular genetic studies (deletion of 22q11.2, PTH receptor and end-organ responsiveness abnormalities, and calcium-sensing receptor defects, etc.) and family screening.

[a] If serum tCa and iCa are normal, diagnostic workup should focus on non-calcium related causes of clinical symptomatology, e.g., serum glucose, sepsis workup, screen for excretion of illicit drugs, neuroimaging studies, etc.
[b] Resolution of clinical symptomatology when serum tCa or iCa has been normalized confirms the role of hypocalcemia.
[c] Maternal and family screening for calcium disorders is indicated in the absence of specific diagnosis for the neonatal hypocalcemia.

many and varied and may be indistinguishable from other common neonatal diseases (Table 36-3). Confirmation of hypocalcemia as the cause of clinical manifestations is its reversibility when serum tCa or iCa has been normalized.

The less mature the infant, the more subtle and varied are the clinical manifestations; in addition, the infant is frequently asymptomatic. Clinical manifestations may include irritability, jitteriness or lethargy, poor feeding with and without feeding intolerance, abdominal distention, apnea, cyanosis, and seizures, which may be confused with manifestations of hypoglycemia, sepsis, meningitis, anoxia, intracranial bleeding, and narcotic withdrawal. The degree of irritability of the infants does not appear to correlate with serum Ca values. Frank convulsions are seen more commonly with "late" neonatal hypocalcemia. In newborn infants, the classic signs of tetany from peripheral hyperexcitability of motor nerves, including carpopedal spasm (spasm of the wrists and ankles, Trousseau sign), facial spasm (Chvostek sign), and laryngospasm (spasm of the vocal cords), are uncommon.

The level of iCa that determines which feature of tetany will be manifested varies among individuals and is affected by other components of the extracellular fluid, e.g., hypomagnesemia and alkalosis lower, whereas hypokalemia and acidosis raise, the threshold for tetany. At physiologic concentrations of hydrogen and potassium ions, tetany may develop in older infants at an iCa less than 0.8 mmol/L (3.2 mg/dL), and will almost always be manifested (with the possible exception of preterm infants) at an iCa less than 0.6 mmol/L (2.4 mg/dL). If serum albumin concentrations are normal, the corresponding serum tCa concentrations usually are less than 1.8 mmol/L (7.2 mg/dL). In the preterm infant, serum iCa may not decrease to the same extent as tCa, presumably in part because of the sparing effect of lower serum albumin and acidosis found frequently in these infants. This also may partially explain the frequent lack of clinical signs of hypocalcemia in preterm infants. The measurement of electrocardiographic QT intervals, corrected for heart rate, and standard nomograms relating serum tCa and total protein to iCa, have little value for the prediction of neonatal serum iCa. Serum tCa is correlated with iCa but is also inadequate for the prediction of one from the other.

Management

Symptomatic hypocalcemia, manifested as seizures for example, should be treated promptly with parenteral Ca. It is possible that neonatal hypocalcemia may resolve spontaneously. However, asymptomatic hypocalcemia probably also should be corrected, as Ca potentially can alter important cellular functions in which Ca serves either as a first or second messenger in cellular activity.

Any neonate with seizures should have blood drawn for diagnostic tests before therapy. Intravenous administration of Ca salts is the most effective and most rapid means of elevating serum Ca concentrations. Gradual or abrupt decreases in heart rate during the infusion is an indication to slow or stop the infusion. In neonates, 10% Ca gluconate (0.45 mmol [18 mg] elemental Ca/kg) can effectively increase serum iCa, heart rate, cardiac contractility, and blood pressure (70–72) (Table 36-4). In children, small equimolar doses (0.07 mmol [2.8 mg] elemental Ca/kg) of 10% Ca chloride compared to 10% Ca gluconate may result in higher mean arterial blood pressure with a slightly greater mean increase (0.06 mmol/L [0.2 mg/dL]) in the measured serum iCa (115). Prolonged use of Ca chloride in high doses may be associated with acidosis and probably should be avoided. With intravenous Ca therapy, bolus infusion may be associated with a transient slight decrease in blood pH and serum P and with hypercalcemia. Continuous infusion probably is more efficacious than intermittent therapy because renal loss of Ca may be greater with the latter method; a dose of 1.25 to 2.0 mmol (50 to 80 mg) elemental Ca/kg/day has been used successfully in the treatment and prevention of neonatal hypocalcemia. Intravenous Ca supplements should be rapidly weaned or replaced with Ca-containing parenteral nutrition if the infant is not expected to tolerate enteral feeding.

Arterial infusion of Ca in high concentrations is potentially fraught with many dangers and should be avoided.

TABLE 36-4

MANAGEMENT OF NEONATAL HYPOCALCEMIA

Acute phase therapy

- Correction of hypomagnesemia, acid–base problem, etc, if possible
- Intravenous 10 to 20 mg elemental Ca/kg as 10% Ca gluconate or 10% Ca chloride (provides 9 mg elemental Ca/mL or 27.2 mg/mL, respectively) with dextrose water or normal saline infused over 5 to 10 minutes under constant ECG monitoring; repeat as necessary until resolution of severe symptomatology, such as seizures.
- In infants who are not fed enterally, this is followed by intravenous continuous infusion at 50 to 75 mg elemental Ca/kg/d. Alternately, parenteral nutrition containing 50 mg elemental Ca/100 mL is preferred and continued until feeding
- In asymptomatic infants, oral 50 to 75 mg elemental Ca/kg/d in 4 to 6 divided doses. One mL of calcium carbonate, glubionate, gluceptate, gluconate, lactate, or chloride contains 40, 23, 18, 9, 13, and 27 mg elemental Ca, respectively.
- Once serum tCa is normalized, cut the dose of the Ca supplement in half daily for 2 days, then discontinue
- Serial serum tCa (+/−iCa) every 12–24 hours until clinically stable, every 24 hours until normalized, and at 24 hours after Ca supplement discontinued

Maintenance therapy: treat underlying disorder, if possible

- Low phosphorus (P) formula if serum P is high (>2.6 mmol/L or 8 mg/dL) until serum Ca and P normalized
- Prolonged and higher Ca doses, and 1,25(OH)$_2$D may be needed, e.g., hypoparathyroidism
- 1,25 (OH)$_2$D, 1,25-dihydroxyvitamin D; ECG, electrocardiogram.

Massive sloughing of soft tissue may occur in the distribution of the arterial supply; for example, inadvertent administration into a mesenteric artery theoretically can lead to necrosis of intestinal tissues. If an umbilic venous catheter is used, the tip should be in the inferior vena cava and not intracardiac, as administration of Ca directly into the heart may result in arrhythmia. Parenteral nutrition solutions containing standard mineral (including Ca) content can be safely infused through appropriately positioned umbilic venous or arterial catheters. Direct admixture of Ca preparations with bicarbonate or phosphate solutions will result in precipitation and must be avoided.

Oral Ca supplements at a similar dosage to parenteral Ca (1.87 mmol [75 mg] elemental Ca/kg per day in four to six divided doses) should be started if the infant is expected to tolerate it, and the serum Ca is normalizing after the initial intravenous Ca therapy. All oral Ca preparations are hypertonic, and there is a theoretical potential for precipitating necrotizing enterocolitis in infants at risk for this condition. Oral Ca preparations generally contain higher Ca concentration than intravenous preparations, for example, Ca glubionate, gluceptate, and carbonate have respectively 2.88, 2.25 and 2.5 mmol (115, 90, and 200 mg) elemental Ca per 5 mL, and are useful for infants, particularly those requiring fluid restriction. Syrup-based oral Ca preparations have high sucrose content that may constitute a significant car-

bohydrate and osmolar load for small preterm infants, and may be associated with an increase in frequency of bowel movements. Alternately, an intravenous preparation can be used orally if the fluid volume is tolerated. Treatment of asymptomatic hypocalcemia can be instituted with oral Ca supplement in the same dosage.

The duration of supplemental Ca therapy depends on the underlying cause of hypocalcemia and usually lasts several days for most cases of neonatal hypocalcemia, or may be prolonged as in the case of hypocalcemia caused by malabsorption or hypoparathyroidism. The serum Ca concentrations should be measured daily during the first few days of treatment and for 1 or 2 days after discontinuation, until serum tCa and iCa concentrations are stabilized. Persistently low serum Ca concentrations should prompt further investigations even in the absence of suspicious history or physical features associated with pathologic causes of hypocalcemia.

Vitamin D metabolites, 1,25(OH)$_2$D at 0.05 to 0.2 μg/kg/day intravenously or orally and 1α-hydroxyvitamin D at 0.33 μg bid orally, and exogenous PTH have been used in the treatment of neonatal hypocalcemia. However, there is no practical advantage to the use of these agents in place of Ca for the treatment of acute hypocalcemia.

For severe persistent hypocalcemia, vitamin D or one of its analogues is often used in addition to Ca supplementation. The use of 1,25(OH)$_2$D is preferred because it can raise serum Ca within 1 to 2 days after initiation of therapy and leaves no residual effects within several days of its discontinuation. Vitamin D has a slower onset of action of 2 to 4 weeks and the residual effect also lasts several weeks after its discontinuation, thus making dosage adjustment more difficult.

Successful management of neonatal hypocalcemia also depends on the resolution, if possible, of the primary cause of hypocalcemia. For example, a poor response to Ca therapy may often result from concurrent Mg deficiency. Hypomagnesemia, if present, must be treated to obtain maximal response to Ca therapy. In phosphate-induced hypocalcemia, high-phosphate formulae and solids should be discontinued, and human milk or low-phosphate formula should be substituted. Use of aluminum hydroxide gel to bind intestinal phosphate should be avoided because of potential risk for aluminum toxicity (116).

Early milk feeding and the use of Ca-containing parenteral nutrition within hours after birth are the best means to minimize the development and recurrence of hypocalcemia, and they may negate the need for Ca supplementation. Delaying premature delivery and minimizing perinatal asphyxia, judicious use of bicarbonate therapy and mechanical ventilation, for example, during intentional induction of alkalosis in the treatment of persistent pulmonary hypertension, are also useful measures to minimize neonatal hypocalcemia. Maintenance of normal maternal vitamin D status with exogenous vitamin D supplement, if needed, in theory may be helpful in maintaining normal fetal vitamin D status and may secondarily prevent hypocalcemia in some neonates. Early feeding and provision of Ca to the gut in the neonate may be important to enhancing the ability of vitamin D metabolites to prevent hypocalcemia.

Pharmacologic prevention of neonatal hypocalcemia has focused primarily on the prophylactic use of Ca salts or vitamin D metabolites. In newborn infants, Ca supplementation results in sustained lowering of serum IPTH concentrations compared to unsupplemented controls (27). Theoretically, Ca supplementation may decrease the metabolic stress from hypocalcemia and minimize the potential for depletion of tissue Ca stores. Early studies used up to 1.8 to 2.0 mmol (72 to 80 mg)/kg/day of oral Ca supplement and about half this amount intravenously to prevent hypocalcemia. However, it should be noted that a similar amount of Ca can be provided from an intake of 150 to 200 mL/kg/day of standard term infant formula or human milk. Standard preterm infant formula can provide almost 5 mmol (200 mg) of Ca/kg/day, and parenteral nutrition with 1.25 to 1.5 mmol (50 to 60 mg) Ca/100 mL can easily provide 1.5 mmol (60 mg) of Ca/kg/day. These amounts of Ca are well tolerated as they have been the standard practice in most neonatal nurseries for more than a decade. Early feeding or parenteral nutrition must be considered as the best means to prevent neonatal hypocalcemia, particularly for the preterm infant. Vitamin D_3 and its metabolites have been used in attempts to prevent neonatal hypocalcemia with variable degrees of success. In small preterm infants, serum Ca was normalized only at pharmacologic doses of $1,25(OH)_2D$.

Complications of hypocalcemia vary with the clinical manifestations and may be related to the therapy and underlying pathophysiology. Acute complications are associated with clinical manifestations, including seizure, apnea, cyanosis and hypoxia, bradycardia, and hypotension. Therapy-related complications, such as cardiac arrhythmia, arterial spasm, tissue necrosis, and extravasation of Ca solution, can be avoided by continuous electrocardiogram monitoring during Ca infusion, avoiding infusion of Ca into the arterial line, and checking for venous patency before Ca infusion. There is also a risk for metastatic calcification from aggressive Ca treatment in the presence of hyperphosphatemia. In situations in which PTH is absent or nonfunctional, its protective hypocalciuric action cannot occur; therefore, markedly raising the serum Ca concentration may cause hypercalciuria, renal stones, nephrocalcinosis, and possible renal damage. These complications were reported during therapy in patients with an activating CaR mutation, even while the patients were normocalcemic (100). Isolated transient hypocalcemia even in symptomatic cases has not been associated with long-term sequelae. Long-term outcomes depend on the underlying causes, for example, patients with 22q11.2 deletion syndromes frequently have defects of multiple organ systems and neurodevelopmental delay unrelated to hypocalcemia (94–97).

Regular clinical follow-up and laboratory monitoring such as for serum Ca and IPTH are necessary in infants with "transient" hypoparathyroidism since some of these infants are at risk for "recurrence" of hypoparathyroidism and hypocalcemia as late as adolescence (88–90).

Hypercalcemia

Hypercalcemia in infants occurs much less frequently than hypocalcemia. However, it is increasingly being diagnosed because serum Ca is usually part of a panel of chemistry tests and because of increasing knowledge of its pathogenesis. Hypercalcemia is present when serum tCa is greater than 2.75 mmol/L (11 mg/dL) or when iCa is greater than 1.4 mmol/L (5.6 mg/dL), depending on the particular ion-selective electrode used. In pathologic hypercalcemia, elevation of serum iCa usually occurs simultaneously with elevation of tCa; however, elevated tCa may occur without elevation of iCa. Elevation of protein available to bind Ca (e.g., prolonged application of tourniquet before venipuncture, with resultant transudation of plasma water into tissues, shown in adult patients with multiple myeloma and possibly adrenal insufficiency) may result in elevation of serum tCa. A change in serum albumin of 1 g/dL generally results in a parallel change in tCa of about 0.2 mmol/L. Conversely, reduced albumin binding of Ca may result in normal serum tCa in the presence of elevated iCa.

Pathophysiology

Hypercalcemia may occur within hours after birth or be delayed for weeks or months. It may result from increased intestinal or renal Ca absorption, increased bone turnover, or iatrogenic causes.

In the neonatal intensive care setting, hypercalcemia is often iatrogenic from inadequate provision of dietary phosphate during and after hospitalization, as with the use of low- or no-phosphate parenteral nutrition or human milk without fortifier in very-low-birth-weight infants (117–121) (Table 36-5). Phosphate deficiency or hypophosphatemia stimulates CYP1α and synthesis of $1,25(OH)_2D$, which enhances intestinal absorption and renal reabsorption of Ca and P. Increased Ca absorbed in the presence of increased $1,25(OH)_2D$ cannot be deposited in bone in the absence of phosphate and contributes to hypercalcemia. Hypercalcemia is more likely if there is concomitant use of Ca supplements, a common practice for the prevention or treatment of hypocalcemia in preterm infants. Decreased renal Ca excretion in the neonate or from underlying illness also may exaggerate the extent of hypercalcemia.

Neonatal hyperparathyroidism frequently results in marked hypercalcemia. It may be a sporadic congenital occurrence, show Mendelian inheritance, or be secondary to maternal hypocalcemia.

Hereditary primary hyperparathyroidism manifested in neonates is associated with inactivating mutations of CaR. The severity of hypercalcemia is related to the extent of CaR mutation. Mild hypercalcemia (serum tCa less than 3.0 mmol/L [12 mg/dL]) associated with heterozygous mutated CaR is manifested clinically in most patients with familial hypocalciuric hypercalcemia (FHH). The normal urinary Ca excretion despite hypercalcemia is an effect of the mutated CaR in the kidneys. Serum PTH is usually

TABLE 36-5

PATHOPHYSIOLOGY OF NEONATAL HYPERCALCEMIA

Phosphate deficiency
  Low or no phosphate, but calcium-containing parenteral nutrition
  Very-low-birth-weight infants fed human milk or, less commonly, standard formula
Parathyroid related
  Hereditary primary hyperparathyroidism
  • Calcium-sensing receptor inactivating mutations: familial hypocalciuric hypercalcemia, neonatal severe hyperparathyroidism
  • Parathyroid hormone receptor activating mutation
  Secondary hyperparathyroidism
  • Maternal: hypocalcemia, renal tubular acidosis
  • Neonatal: renal tubular acidosis
Parathyroid hormone-related protein-secreting tumors
Vitamin D
  Excessive intake
  • Mother: high-dose vitamin D
  • Neonate: high-dose vitamin D prophylaxis, overfortification of milk
  Increased 1,25-dihydroxyvitamin D
  • Subcutaneous fat necrosis
  • Histiocytic disorders, disseminated tuberculosis with septic shock and hemophagocytic syndrome (?)
Calcitonin response impairment (?) in congenital hypothyroidism
Vitamin A excess
Uncertain pathophysiologic mechanism
  Chromosomal/gene abnormalities
  • Idiopathic infantile hypercalcemia/Williams syndrome
  • Severe infantile hypophosphatasia
  • Microdeletion of 4q
  Heritable metabolic defect
  • Blue diaper syndrome
  • Glycogen storage disease type 1a, congenital lactase or sucrase-isomaltase deficiency, disaccharidase deficiency
  Extracorporeal membrane oxygenation therapy

within the normal range but is higher than expected for the degree of hypercalcemia. FHH has been reported in patients from 2 hours to 82 years of age and is usually diagnosed in infants as part of a screening procedure after diagnosis of a family member with hypercalcemia or familial multiple endocrine neoplasia. It is inherited as an autosomal-dominant trait with a high degree of penetrance (122). There usually is significant hypophosphatemia and a modest increase in serum Mg concentration, and functional parathyroid glands are needed for full expression. Neonatal hyperparathyroidism associated with FHH that resolves spontaneously over several months has been reported (123). More severe hypercalcemia with serum tCa of 3 to 3.3 mmol/L (12 to 13 mg/dL) has been attributed to coexpression of the normal and mutated CaR, with the latter having a functional equivalent of a "dominant-negative" effect. The most marked hypercalcemia (serum Ca greater than 4 mmol/L [16 mg/dL]) occurs in neonatal severe hyperparathyroidism with homozygous inactivating

germline mutations of the CaR gene. This severe disorder can be lethal within the first few weeks after birth (124, 125).

Activating mutations of the PTH/PTHrP receptor gene in Jansen metaphyseal dysplasia presumably have the receptor defects in the kidney, bone, and chondrocytes at the growth plate. The clinical manifestations include postnatal-onset short-limb dwarfism with radiographic rachitic changes, and mild hypercalcemia occurs in about 50% of the affected patients (126).

Neonatal hyperparathyroidism may be secondary to various causes of maternal hypocalcemia including maternal hypoparathyroidism (127) and maternal (128) or neonatal (129) renal tubular acidosis. Presence of metabolic acidosis independently increases bone resorption and enhances the renal effects of hyperparathyroidism; the hypercalcemic effects are augmented by decreased renal excretory capacity of the neonate.

Elevated serum PTHrP and hypercalcemia are found in increasing numbers of infants with a variety of tumors (130–133), including malignant hepatic sarcoma, infantile fibrosarcoma, renal adenoma, and rhabdoid tumors. There is also associated mortality in some cases, although the relative contribution to death from hypercalcemia versus the underlying disease is not clear.

Hypercalcemia was reported in 34% of neonates and infants from intermittent high-dose vitamin D (600,000 IU every 3 to 5 months) prophylaxis (134). Hypercalcemia also has been reported in infants given human milk with very high vitamin D content (7,000 IU/L), from high-dose vitamin D therapy for maternal hypoparathyroidism, from milk with excessive vitamin D fortification from errors during processing, and in preterm infants given chronic vitamin D supplementation in addition to high-Ca and high-P milk formulae. Neonates with extensive subcutaneous fat necrosis often have a history of perinatal asphyxia and may develop hypercalcemia after a period of low or normal serum Ca concentrations (135). There is an anecdotal report that body cooling for the treatment of birth asphyxia may augment the development of subcutaneous fat necrosis. Hypercalcemia is reported to occur between 2 and 16 weeks, most commonly at 6 to 7 weeks after the development of subcutaneous fat necrosis. Increased prostaglandin E activity, increased release of Ca from fat and other tissues, and unregulated production of $1,25(OH)_2D$ from macrophages infiltrating fat necrotic lesions, have been postulated to be responsible for the hypercalcemia in this condition. Histiocytic disorders and disseminated tuberculosis with septic shock and hemophagocytic syndrome may be complicated with hypercalcemia in infants; it is not known if this is also related to nonrenal production of $1,25(OH)_2D$. Vitamin A toxicity is associated with hypercalcemia, presumably secondary to the retinoic acid stimulation of osteoclastic activity and bone resorption. Vitamin A toxicity in infants may occur at intakes as low as 2,100 IU/100 kcal and can be fatal (136).

Hypercalcemia may develop before and during thyroxine therapy of infants with congenital agoitrous hypothyroidism

(137). In theory, deficient CT response to Ca loading or an increased degradation of CT may be responsible for the hypercalcemia.

Neonatal hypercalcemia is reported in other situations in which the pathophysiology remains uncertain. Idiopathic infantile hypercalcemia, often considered as part of Williams syndrome, is associated with varying manifestations including hypercalcemia, mental retardation, elfin facies, and supravalvular aortic stenosis. There also may be prenatal and postnatal growth failure. The presence of hypercalcemia in infants with Williams syndrome is variable, and serum Ca may be normal, but the presence of nephrocalcinosis and soft-tissue calcifications in some of these infants suggests that hypercalcemia may have occurred previously. An exaggerated response to pharmacologic doses of vitamin D_2 and a blunted CT response to Ca loading and PTH infusion may contribute to the pathogenesis of hypercalcemia in idiopathic infantile hypercalcemia. Several genetic defects in idiopathic infantile hypercalcemia, including hemizygosity at the elastin gene on the long arm of chromosome 7, have been reported (138,139). No mutations of the CT/CGRP gene has been detected. However, the cellular mechanism that leads to the phenotypic expression remains unknown.

Severe infantile hypophosphatasia is associated with hypercalcemia. It is a rare autosomal-recessive disorder associated with decreased synthesis of tissue-nonspecific alkaline phosphatase from a deletion or point mutation in its gene located on chromosome 1. These patients have severe bone demineralization, low serum alkaline phosphatase, and elevated urinary pyrophosphate and phosphoethanolamine. The condition may be lethal *in utero* or shortly after birth because of inadequate bony support of the thorax and skull, although milder phenotypes are compatible with survival to adulthood (140).

Microdeletion of the long arm of chromosome 4 has been associated with hypercalcemia and cardiac failure (141).

Blue diaper syndrome is a rare familial disorder with impaired intestinal transport of tryptophan. The blue discoloration of the urine results from the hydrolysis and oxidation of urinary indican, an end product of intestinal degradation of unabsorbed tryptophan and hepatic metabolism of its intermediate metabolites. Blue discoloration of the urine has been reported within weeks after birth, although hypercalcemia and nephrocalcinosis are not reported until some months after birth. Glycogen storage disease type 1a, congenital lactase deficiency, and congenital sucrase-isomaltase deficiency with chronic diarrhea have been associated with hypercalcemia and nephrocalcinosis. Hypercalcemia apparently resolves without specific treatment following treatment for disaccharidase deficiency.

Transient hypercalcemia occurs in infants during extracorporeal membrane oxygenation (ECMO) therapy varying in frequency from less than 5% to about 30%, depending on whether the cut-off point used is greater than 2.5 or 2.25 mmol (12 mg/dL or 11 mg/dL), respectively (142, 143).

Diagnosis

Neonates with hypercalcemia may be asymptomatic despite the onset of hypercalcemia at birth. In these cases, there are often delays of weeks or months before diagnosis is made, coincidental to a chemistry panel screening during the course of other illness or because of hypercalcemia in another family member.

The presence of a family history of Ca disorders or anatomic anomalies (e.g., elfin facies, evidence of congenital heart disease, subcutaneous fat necrosis) on physical examination of the infant may be helpful in arriving at the diagnosis (Table 36-6).

Symptoms and signs are frequently nonspecific and include lethargy, irritability, poor feeding with or without feeding intolerance, constipation, polyuria, dehydration, and failure to thrive. Hypertension associated with hypercalcemia may occur in infants, although it may be in part linked to treatment-related relative fluid overload, as in many infants who require ECMO therapy.

Management

Therapy depends on the extent of elevation of serum Ca and whether the infant is symptomatic. For mildly elevated

---

TABLE 36-6

DIAGNOSTIC WORKUP FOR NEONATAL HYPERCALCEMIA

History
- Familial or maternal disturbances in calcium (Ca) or phosphorus (P) metabolism
- Gestational age, difficult labor, extracorporeal membrane oxygenation (ECMO) therapy and pre-ECMO therapy
- Mother's and infant's intake of Ca, P, vitamins D and A

Physical examination
- General examination with focus on growth parameters, hydration status, heart rate, blood pressure, cornea for band keratopathy (rare)
- Associated features (e.g., subcutaneous fat necrosis, elfin facies, congenital heart disease, developmental delay)

Investigations
- Serum total and ionized Ca, magnesium, P, creatinine (Cr), total protein and albumin, alkaline phosphatase (total and bone specific), simultaneous "intact" or "whole" parathyroid hormone (PTH), 25-hydroxyvitamin D and 1,25 dihydroxyvitamin D
- Acid–base status
- Urine Ca, P, Cr, amino acids
- X-ray of chest, hands, and long bones
- Ultrasound of kidneys and abdomen, ophthalmologic examination, electrocardiogram (shortened QT interval, bradycardia) for complications
- If the above do not yield diagnosis, other tests depend on associated history and symptomatology
  - Parental (both parents) serum and urine Ca, P, and Cr
  - Molecular studies
  - Family screening depends on the primary diagnosis
  - Serum PTH-related protein and screen for occult tumors
  - Screen for metabolic defects and unusual dietary supplements

serum tCa (less than 12 mg/dL) in the presence of an iatrogenic cause, e.g., phosphate-free parenteral nutrition or the use of Ca supplements without any dietary phosphate intake, resolution of the underlying cause should also clear up the Ca problem. Hypercalcemia induced by dietary P deficiency is becoming less common with the increasing use of commercial fortifier for human milk fed to preterm infants and the use of high Ca- and high P-containing infant formulae and parenteral nutrition for the preterm infant. In patients with low serum P concentrations, large amounts of phosphate supplement may cause hypocalcemia and the possibility of metastatic calcification. Phosphate supplements given orally may result in diarrhea.

With moderate to severe hypercalcemia, the initial treatment is nonspecific with expansion of the extracellular fluid compartment (10 to 20 mL/kg of 0.9% sodium chloride intravenously) and furosemide (2 mg/kg)-induced diuresis (Table 36-7). Care should be taken to avoid fluid and electrolyte imbalance with careful monitoring of fluid balance and serum Ca, Mg, sodium, potassium, and osmolality at 6- to 12-hour intervals. Furosemide therapy may be repeated at 4- to 6-hour intervals. Prolonged diuresis also requires replacement of Mg losses.

Minimal information is available on the use of hormonal and other drug therapy for neonatal hypercalcemia. Nonmammalian sources of CT, e.g., salmon CT (4 to 8 IU/kg every 12 hours subcutaneously or intramuscularly), have greater hypocalcemic effects and longer durations of action, compared with recombinant hCT. However, salmon CT has greater potential for allergic reaction and induction of antibody formation. The hypocalcemic effect decreases after a few days of any CT treatment. Steroid (prednisone 0.5 to 1 mg/kg per day) therapy may result in significant problems including hypertension, hyperglycemia, and gastrointestinal hemorrhage, and thus is not recommended for long-term therapy. Bisphosphonates, oral etidronate (25 mg bid), and intravenous pamidronate (0.5 mg/kg) have been used for hypercalcemia in the mother and neonate. Long-term use of pamidronate in infants and children with osteogenesis imperfecta decreases serum iCa with a compensatory increase in PTH (144). The effects on growth plate, bone production, and mineralization remains unknown, and its use should be restricted to acute short-term therapy. Dialysis in the neonate is not without technical or metabolic complications. Rarely, parathyroidectomy may be necessary, although it is not always effective. Development of calcimimetic agents able to amplify the sensitivity of the CaR to iCa and suppress PTH levels, with a resulting decrease in blood iCa, offer potential for noninvasive therapy of hypercalcemia.

Treatment for chronic conditions also includes restriction of dietary intake of vitamin D and Ca and minimizing exposure to sunlight to decrease endogenous vitamin D production. A low-Ca, low-vitamin D_3, low-iron infant formula is available for the management of hypercalcemia in infants. This formula contains only trace amounts of Ca (less than 10 mg/100 kcal) and no vitamin D. Long-term

TABLE 36-7
MANAGEMENT OF NEONATAL HYPERCALCEMIA

Acute
- Remove etiologic factor, if possible, e.g., discontinue vitamin D and calcium (Ca) supplements
- Intravenous normal saline (20 mL/kg) and loop diuretic (furosemide 2 mg/kg). Reassess and repeat every 4 to 6 hours as necessary. Monitor fluid balance and serum Ca, magnesium (Mg), sodium, potassium, phosphorus (P), and osmolality every 6 to12 hours. Prolonged diuresis may require Mg and potassium replacement
- Use lower Ca content milk or parenteral nutrition, if possible, to maintain nutrition
- In neonates with low serum P (<1.3 mmol/L; 4 mg/dL), oral phosphate supplement at 0.5 to 1 mmol (15 to 30 mg) elemental P/kg/day in 4 divided doses given judiciously may normalize serum P and Ca. In infants not being fed, use parenteral nutrition containing usual amount of phosphate (1 to 1.5 mmol [31 to 46 mg]/100 mL) but no Ca until serum Ca returned to normal
- Minimal data on the use of hormones, e.g., subcutaneous or intramuscular recombinant human calcitonin (4 to 8 IU/kg every 6 hours), +/− oral glucocorticoid (prednisone 0.5 to 1 mg/kg/day). Other drugs, e.g., bisphosphonates (oral etidronate 25 mg bid, intravenous pamidronate 0.5 mg/kg) are experimental
- Peritoneal or hemodialysis with a low-Ca dialysate may be considered in severely symptomatic patients refractory to medical therapy
- Parathyroidectomy may be needed when patient is clinically stablized

Maintenance
- Depends on underlying cause
- Additional general therapy may be needed: low Ca, no vitamin D infant formula (Calcilo XD, Abbott Laboratories Columbus, OH); keep in minimize sunlight exposure to lower endogenous synthesis of vitamin D

use of this formula alone will lead to calcium depletion; iatrogenic vitamin D deficiency is also a concern in this situation, and both can result in deleterious consequences.

Complications of hypercalcemia vary with the clinical manifestations at presentation. Persistent hypercalcemia may result in ectopic calcification, which involves the ectopic deposition of a solid phase of calcium and phosphate in walls of blood vessels and in connective tissue about the joints, gastric mucosa, renal parenchyma, and cornea, especially when accompanied by normal or elevated levels of serum P. Prolonged therapy, such as severe limitation of Ca and vitamin D intake, may be associated with hypocalcemia and bone demineralization (145). Severe hypercalcemia can be fatal, although some of the infants have other potentially lethal underlying conditions. Long-term complications usually depend on the underlying cause of hypercalcemia, including failure to thrive and nephrocalcinosis.

Neonatal hypercalcemia may not develop until some weeks after the onset of the insult and may resolve spontaneously, as in subcutaneous fat necrosis. Therefore, serum Ca should be monitored at regular intervals in certain situations to determine the onset of hypercalcemia and to determine the continued need for treatment. Family screening for hypercalcemia should be done unless a specific nonfamilial cause for hypercalcemia is established in the index case.

Hypomagnesemia

Hypomagnesemia is present when serum tMg is less than 0.6 mmol/L (1.5 mg/dL). There are no data on the level of iMg during hypomagnesemia. Tissue Mg deficiency, however, may be present despite normal serum Mg concentrations.

Pathophysiology

Decreased tissue accretion of Mg is a major cause of hypomagnesemia (Table 36-8). The compensatory response at birth of abrupt termination of placental transfer of Mg will be impaired if there is reduced tissue Mg. The severity and prevalence of hypomagnesemia in infants of insulin-dependent diabetic mothers is directly related to the severity of maternal diabetes, which is thought to reflect the severity of maternal Mg deficiency (146). Mg infusion in infants results in greater increases in serum Ca and PTH in those with initially low serum Mg concentrations and in children with insulin-dependent diabetes, compared to normal control subjects.

Maternal hyperparathyroidism has been associated with neonatal hypomagnesemia (147). Negative Mg balances may occur with hyperparathyroidism, which may account for neonatal hypomagnesemia. Alternately, neonatal hypoparathyroidism in this situation may lead to hypomagnesemia from reduced PTH mobilization of bone Mg to extracellular fluid.

In theory, chronic maternal Mg deficiency from any cause may result in decreased tissue Mg accretion for the

TABLE 36-8
NEONATAL HYPOMAGNESEMIA

Decreased tissue accretion
  Infants of mothers with insulin-dependent diabetes or
    hyperparathyroidism
  Small-for-gestational-age infants
  Chronic maternal magnesium deficiency
Decreased absorption
  Extensive small-intestine resection
  Specific intestinal magnesium malabsorption
Increased loss
  Intestinal fistula or diarrhea
  Hepatobiliary disorders
  Decreased renal tubular reabsorption
  • Primary: transient receptor potential channel protein
    mutation, renal tubulopathies with hypo- or hypercalciuria
  • Secondary: extracellular fluid compartment expansion,
    osmotic diuresis, drugs (e.g., loop diuretic,
    aminoglycoside, ibuprofen overdose)
Others
  Increased phosphate intake
  Exchange transfusion with citrated blood

fetus. Hypomagnesemia occurs more frequently in infants with intrauterine growth retardation compared to infants with appropriate weight for gestational age.

Intestinal resection, particularly of the jejunum and ileum, the major sites of Mg absorption; malabsorption; and rapid intestinal transit time may lead to Mg deficiency and hypomagnesemia. Mg content in bile, gastric fluid, and pancreatic secretion varies from 0.2 to 5.0 mmol/L (0.5 to 12 mg/dL). Diarrheal Mg content may be as high as 7.1 mmol/L (17 mg/dL). Thus, chronic losses from diarrhea, intestinal fistula, or enterostomy may be associated with significant Mg loss.

Infants with congenital biliary atresia and neonatal hepatitis may have low serum Mg concentrations. This is thought to be partly related to increased aldosterone-related renal Mg losses.

Hypomagnesemia can occur as a primary defect in Mg transport in the intestine or kidney or in conjunction with a variety of inherited hypokalemic salt-losing tubulopathies.

Mutation in a member of the long transient receptor potential channel protein TRPM6, which encodes for a bifunctional protein that combines Ca- and Mg-permeable cation channel properties with protein kinase activity and is expressed in intestinal epithelia and kidney tubules, can result in hypomagnesemia (148). Genetic mapping and analysis of a balanced translocation breakpoint have localized some cases of recessively inherited familial hypomagnesemia to chromosome 9q (149).

Renal tubulopathies may be subclassified further into a hypercalciuric group consistent with classic Bartter syndrome, which usually presents in infancy with failure to thrive and episodes of dehydration. Mutations in PCLN-1, which encodes the renal tight junction protein paracellin-1 (claudin-16), resulting in impaired tubular reabsorption of Mg and Ca in the thick ascending limb of Henle's loop have been reported (150). These patients typically present with urinary tract infection, polyuria, hematuria, hypomagnesemia, hypercalciuria, nephrocalcinosis, and progressive renal failure. A variant syndrome with hypocalciuria is thought to present later with short stature, substantially lower serum Mg, and more episodes of tetany.

Secondary defects in renal tubular reabsorption of Mg may result from extracellular fluid expansion caused by excessive glucose, sodium, or fluid intake, or from osmotic diuresis, diuretics such as furosemide, high doses of aminoglycosides such as gentamicin, and ibuprofen overdose.

Increased phosphate intake may lead to decreased Mg absorption, and infants on high-phosphate milk preparations have lowered serum Mg concentrations. Elevation of serum phosphate concentrations decreases serum Mg. It is not known if these changes are related to decreased Mg absorption or to the shift of Mg from extracellular to intracellular compartments. In infants with uremia, serum Mg concentrations may be decreased, possibly in relation to higher blood phosphate concentrations (151). Patients with renal failure, however, become hypermagnesemic at Mg loads that do not affect people with normal renal function.

Exchange blood transfusions using citrate as an anticoagulant result in complexing of citrate with Mg, which leads to hypomagnesemia, especially after multiple exchanges (87,152).

Diagnosis

Suspicion of hypomagnesemia must be confirmed by measurement of serum tMg and iMg, if available, since clinical manifestations are many and varied and may be indistinguishable from those of other common neonatal diseases. The less mature the infant, the more subtle and varied are the clinical manifestations, and the infants frequently are asymptomatic.

The typical deficit required to produce symptomatic hypomagnesemia is approximately 0.5 to 1.0 mmol (12 to 24 mg)/kg of body weight. However, critical assessment of Mg deficiency is difficult because more than 99% of total body Mg is found in intracellular fluids or is complexed in the skeleton. It has been proposed that high Mg retention after a Mg load may be a test to reflect Mg deficiency. Infants generally retain large amounts of infused Mg, however, and there are large variations in response; the clinical utility of this test thus appears limited in infancy. Confirmation of hypomagnesemia as the cause of clinical manifestations is its reversibility when serum tMg or iMg has been normalized.

Infants with hypomagnesemia associated with malabsorption, or increased losses from the gut or kidney, also are at risk for concurrent hypocalcemia, hypokalemia, and possible disturbance of the acid–base status. The loss of other nutrients such as zinc also may be considerable. Symptoms and signs of hypomagnesemia, which often coexists with hypocalcemia, may be indistinguishable. Thus, simultaneous measurement of serum Ca (total and ionized, if available), P, potassium, sodium, chloride and bicarbonate, urea nitrogen and creatinine, and zinc status may be indicated. Measurement of urine and intestinal fluid content of Mg also may be helpful in diagnosis and management. Additional investigations depend on the underlying etiology, and the status of other nutrients also may need to be considered.

Typically, hypomagnesemia is associated with decreased circulating PTH concentrations, decreased production of active vitamin D metabolites, in particular $1,25(OH)_2D$, and resistance to PTH and $1,25(OH)_2D$. When hypomagnesemia coexists with hypocalcemia, a trial infusion of 6 mg of elemental Mg/kg over 1 hour with pre- and postinfusion measurements of total and ionized Ca and PTH may be helpful in the diagnosis of the primary defect. An increase in serum PTH after Mg infusion is indicative of hypoparathyroidism and hypocalcemia secondary to Mg deficiency, whereas no change or a decrease in serum PTH supports the diagnosis of hypocalcemia unrelated to Mg deficiency.

Management

Clinical manifestations of symptomatic hypomagnesemia such as seizures should be treated promptly with parenteral Mg. Asymptomatic hypomagnesemia probably also should be corrected, as Mg potentially can alter important cellular functions and may lead secondarily to hypocalcemia with its attendant complications. Hypocalcemia occurring under this circumstance is corrected only when the Mg disturbance is corrected.

Any neonate with seizures should have blood drawn for diagnostic tests before therapy. The treatment of choice for acute hypomagnesemic seizures is 50% Mg sulfate, 0.05 to 0.1 mL/kg (0.1 to 0.2 mmol/kg or 2.5 to 5.0 mg of elemental Mg/kg) given by slow intravenous infusion over 15 to 20 minutes, or by intramuscular route. The frequency of Mg administration depends on the clinical response and rate of increase in serum Mg. Repeat doses may be given at 2- to 12-hour intervals. Infants receiving parenteral Mg therapy should receive continuous cardiorespiratory monitoring. Serum Mg concentrations should be measured daily or more frequently as clinically indicated to evaluate efficacy and safety until values are stable.

Concomitantly, oral Mg supplements can be started if oral fluids are tolerated. Fifty percent Mg sulfate can be given at a dose of 0.2 mL/kg per day. In specific Mg malabsorption, daily oral doses of 1 mL/kg per day may be required. Oral Mg salts are not well absorbed, and large doses may cause diarrhea. The maintenance Mg supplement should be diluted five- to six-fold to allow for more frequent administration, maximizing gut absorption and minimizing side effects. Some oral preparations of Mg (e.g., Mg L-lactate dihydrate), especially those in a sustained-release form, may have greater bioavailability than other sources of Mg (e.g., Mg oxide, hydroxide, citrate). However, practical experience with the use of Mg salts other than Mg sulfate in infancy is limited.

Potassium and zinc deficiency frequently coexists with Mg-deficient states, especially when there are abnormal gastrointestinal losses or malabsorption. Appropriate replacement therapy is needed. Treatment of underlying disorders (e.g., closure of gastrointestinal fistula) should be pursued actively. Chronic Mg therapy is needed if the underlying cause persists, such as a genetic defect in Mg transport.

Complications of hypomagnesemia vary with clinical manifestations and may be related to therapy and underlying pathophysiology. Prolonged dietary Mg deprivation in human adults leads to personality change, tremor, muscle fasciculations, spontaneous carpopedal spasm, and generalized spasticity, as well as hypomagnesemia, hypocalcemia, and hypokalemia. Mg depletion in pregnant rats results in fetal mortality, malformations, hypomagnesemia, decreased skeletal Mg content, hemolytic anemia, hypoproteinemia, and edema.

In infants, acute complications are associated with clinical manifestations including seizure, apnea, cyanosis, hypoxia, bradycardia, and hypotension. Possible complications of intravenous infusion include systemic hypotension and prolongation or even blockade of sinoauricular or atrioventricular conduction. Isolated transient hypomagnesemia even in symptomatic cases has not been associated with long-term sequelae. Long-term outcome of neonatal hypomagnesemia depends on the underlying cause and adequacy of therapy, and severe neurodevelopmental deficit has been reported, presumably from suboptimal therapy and recurrent seizures.

Hypermagnesemia

Hypermagnesemia is present when serum Mg is more than 1.04 mmol/L (greater than 2.5 mg/dL). There are insufficient data to define hypermagnesemia based on the measurement of serum iMg alone.

Pathophysiology

Hypermagnesemia may result from a combination of excessive Mg load and a relatively low capacity for renal excretion of Mg (Table 36-9). Neonatal hypermagnesemia most commonly occurs after maternal Mg sulfate administration for preeclampsia. In mothers given Mg sulfate, serum Mg concentrations have been reported from 1.1 to 5.8 mmol/L (2.6 to 14.0 mg/dL), with umbilic cord-serum Mg concentrations from 0.8 to 4.8 mmol/L (2.0 to 11.5 mg/dL) (153,154); concomitant maternal hypocalcemia also may occur secondarily to decreased serum PTH concentrations. Variations in parenteral Mg intake (118,119, 155) resulting from high Mg content or high rate of infusion of parenteral nutrition fluids may result in hypermagnesemia, particularly in critically ill neonates. The use of Mg-containing antacids or enemas can cause hypermagnesemia. Prematurity and perinatal asphyxia may aggravate hypermagnesemia, presumably because of decreased renal Mg excretion.

Diagnosis

Most neonates with hypermagnesemia, particularly preterm infants, are asymptomatic, even at serum Mg concentrations of more than 1.25 mmol/L (3 mg/dL) (118,119,153–155). Clinical signs may not correlate with serum Mg concentrations, although there does appear to

be a correlation with the duration of maternal Mg sulfate therapy, possibly representing tissue Mg content. With judicious use of Mg sulfate in the mother, however, signs of Mg intoxication should be uncommon in the infant. In adults with hypermagnesemia, hypotension and urinary retention occur at serum Mg concentrations of 1.67 to 2.5 mmol/L (4.0 to 6.0 mg/dL); central nervous system depression, hyporeflexia, and electrocardiographic abnormalities (i.e., increased atrioventricular and ventricular conduction time) at 2.5 to 5.0 mmol/L (6.0 to 12.0 mg/dL); and respiratory depression, coma, and cardiac arrest above 5.0 mmol/L (12.0 mg/dL). Clinical signs of neuromuscular depression with floppiness, lethargy, and respiratory depression are frequent manifestations of severe neonatal hypermagnesemia. Acute hypotonia, apnea, hypotension, and refractory bradycardia mimicking septic shock syndrome have been reported in premature infants accidentally overdosed with Mg in parenteral nutrition (156).

Serum Ca concentrations may be normal, increased, or decreased and should be measured in all infants with suspected hypermagnesemia. Hypermagnesemia might in theory displace bound Ca in the circulation and lead to elevation of serum iCa concentration. Hypermagnesemia may suppress PTH and 1,25(OH)$_2$D production and may result in lower serum Ca concentrations (157,158). Rickets has been reported when maternal Mg therapy is prolonged (e.g., in tocolysis to prevent preterm delivery). It is speculated that excess Mg interferes with normal mineralization of fetal bone.

In newborn infants, a delay in passage of meconium (i.e., meconium plug syndrome) has been thought to be related to neonatal hypermagnesemia. In pregnant and newborn rats and dogs, however, hypermagnesemia does not have an effect on intestinal motility or the consistency of meconium.

Management

In asymptomatic infants with normal renal function, serum Mg generally returns to normal within several days after adequate hydration and nutritional support and elimination of further Mg intake. These infants should be cared for in a facility that can provide cardiorespiratory support in case additional complications develop.

For symptomatic infants, intravenous Ca given in the same dosage as for treatment of hypocalcemia may be useful for acute therapy, since Ca is a direct antagonist of Mg. Loop diuretics (e.g., furosemide) with adequate fluid intake may hasten Mg excretion. Exchange blood transfusion with citrated blood is an effective treatment for severely depressed hypermagnesemic infants. Citrated donor blood is particularly useful because the complexing action of citrate will expedite removal of Mg from the infant. Peritoneal and hemodialysis may be considered in refractory patients.

In infants, acute complications are associated with clinical manifestations including respiratory depression and hypoxia, bradycardia, and hypotension; and potential

TABLE 36-9
NEONATAL HYPERMAGNESEMIA

Increased load
  Maternal magnesium sulfate administration
  Neonatal magnesium therapy
    • Parenteral nutrition
    • Antacid
    • Enema

Decreased excretion
  Prematurity and asphyxia

complications associated with therapy such as exchange transfusion. Isolated transient hypermagnesemia even in symptomatic cases has not been associated with long-term sequelae.

SKELETAL MANIFESTATIONS OF DISTURBED MINERAL HOMEOSTASIS

Pathophysiology

Skeletal manifestations of disturbed mineral metabolism in infants usually present as osteopenia or rachitic changes on standard radiographs. True fetal or congenital rickets is rare. It may result from severe maternal nutritional osteomalacia associated with Ca and vitamin D deficiency, maternal hypo- or hyperparathyroidism, or prolonged maternal treatment with Mg sulfate or phosphate-containing enemas (74,75,159–163) (Table 36-10).

The most frequent cause of skeletal abnormalities in infancy is nutritional deficiency, although it may occur secondarily to disorders of metabolism of multiple organs including gut, pancreas, liver, and kidney. In the Western world, rickets and osteopenia presenting during infancy occur most frequently in small preterm infants and may occur in more than 30% of extremely low-birth-weight (less than 1 kg) infants. The rate of occurrence depends on the nutrient intake and is associated most frequently with prolonged low-Ca and/or low-P parenteral nutrition and

prolonged intake of soy formula or unfortified human milk (2). The primary underlying cause in preterm infants appears to be mineral deficiency, particularly Ca and P, which was demonstrated more than 2 decades ago (164) and confirmed by many investigators (2); vitamin D deficiency is of secondary importance. Unfortified human milk fed to preterm infants or standard milk formula for term infants often have low serum concentrations of 25-OHD. The major reason for the low serum 25-OHD in these situations is the increased metabolism of 25-OHD with mineral deficiency. Unfortunately, vitamin D deficiency secondary to mineral deficiency is still frequently misdiagnosed as the primary cause of osteopenia, fracture, and rickets in preterm infants, and is treated with more vitamin D supplement without improving the mineral and general nutritional support.

Chronic diuretic therapy, commonly used in infants with bronchopulmonary dysplasia may aggravate the Ca deficiency. Contamination of nutrients with toxins such as aluminum is an added risk factor (116). The extent, however, to which each specific risk factor is responsible for the development of osteopenia, fractures, and rickets is difficult to define in critically ill infants receiving multiple therapies and suboptimal nutritional support (2). Isolated nutritional deficiency of copper and ascorbic acid has been reported in preterm infants with clinical and radiographic manifestations similar to rickets.

In infants born at term, insufficient endogenous production or exogenous supply of vitamin D is important in the cause of rickets and osteopenia. In one report, almost all children with vitamin D deficiency had ethnocultural risk factors, and 80% of the mothers were also vitamin D deficient (165). However, Ca deficiency also is important in older infants and young children (166). Clinical risk factors thus include prolonged exclusive human milk feeding, limited sunshine exposure, macrobiotic diet, and prolonged total parenteral nutrition.

Acquired and heritable forms of rickets that develop despite adequate availability of vitamin D usually are associated with renal tubular disorders and metabolic defects in vitamin D and PTH metabolism. Both hypo- and hyperphosphatasia are autosomal-recessive disorders associated with disturbed bone resorption and formation. These causes of rickets are rare, but their skeletal manifestations may present during infancy.

TABLE 36-10

RISK FACTORS FOR DEVELOPMENT OF OSTEOPENIA AND RICKETS IN INFANTS

in utero
- Severe maternal nutritional osteomalacia (i.e., vitamin D +/−calcium deficiency)
- Maternal hypoparathyroidism and hyperparathyroidism
- Prolonged maternal magnesium or phosphate treatment
- Birth weight <1 kg

Postnatal
- Prolonged organ dysfunction: intestine, kidney, liver, pancreas
- Nutritional
  - Preterm infants
    - Prolonged low calcium and/or low phosphate total parenteral nutrition
    - Soy formula or unfortified human milk for small preterm infants
    - Chronic loop diuretic therapy given to preterm infants
  - Term infants
    - Vitamin D deficiency
    - Calcium deficiency
    - Macrobiotic diet
  - Toxin contamination: aluminum (?)
- Inherited Defects
  - Renal tubular disorder
  - Disorders of vitamin D or parathyroid hormone metabolism
  - Hypo- or hyperphosphatasia

Diagnosis

A history of significant nutritional defects in the mother, either from self-selected dietary restriction or cultural habits, e.g., extensive covering of the body with lack of sunlight exposure or a family history of metabolic disorders and disturbed bone mineral metabolism, should raise the awareness of the potential for nutritional and skeletal problems in both the mother and infant.

Infants with congenital rickets may be asymptomatic at birth, leading to a delay in diagnosis unless investigations are performed as part of the workup for disturbances in maternal mineral metabolism. Most postnatal cases of rickets and osteopenia are diagnosed incidentally during the radiographic investigation of skeletal complications such as fractures, or nonskeletal problems such as respiratory illness. Radiographic features such as generalized bone demineralization and widening, cupping, and fraying of the distal metaphyses confirm the presence of osteopenia and rickets. Some investigators have derived a scoring system for the assessment of osteopenia and rickets based on the extent of radiographic changes (167–169). The use of dual-energy x-ray absorptiometry (DXA) allows a more accurate quantification of the degree of bone mineralization (170,171), although its role in the diagnosis of bone disorders remains to be defined.

Classic clinical features of rickets such as severe skeletal deformities, including kyphoscoliosis and bowing of the legs, may not be present if the diagnosis is made early in infancy, before significant growth and weight-bearing have occurred. This is particularly true for the preterm infant whose skeletal problems typically are diagnosed between 2 and 6 months postnatally (172). With the current practice of early discharge of preterm infants from neonatal units, it is possible that some nutritional rickets could be diagnosed after hospital discharge; if there are associated fractures, it may be misdiagnosed as child abuse, as is the case with fractures from other medical illnesses. Clinical hypotonia is probably due to a decrease in the intracellular phosphate pool of the skeletal muscle.

Serial biochemical changes (117,173,174) commonly include persistently low serum inorganic phosphate, elevated serum alkaline phosphatase activity more than five times the normal adult upper limit, and elevation of other bone turnover markers in serum and urine. Serum Ca is usually normal except in late severe nutritional vitamin D deficiency rickets. Vitamin D deficiency as indicated by low or undetectable serum 25-OHD is possible; however, it is more likely in preterm infants to be secondary to mineral deficiency. There may be elevated serum 1,25(OH)$_2$D and IPTH. The elevated IPTH and 1,25(OH)$_2$D still may be relatively insufficient to maintain Ca and P homeostasis if the Ca and P intake remain low. Urine changes may reflect increased serum IPTH with increased urine P excretion and Ca conservation. However, in chronic P deficiency, urine findings may reflect changes of P-deficiency–related PTH resistance, in which case urine P would be minimal while there is calciuria. Measurement of specific trace mineral status may be useful if deficiency is suspected (175,176). Additional investigations are needed if inherited renal tubular disorders or disorders of vitamin D and PTH metabolism are suspected.

Treatment and Prevention

Rickets and fractures from nutritional deficiencies respond well to adequate nutrient intake. The best treatment for nutritional osteopenia, fractures, and rickets is prevention. For preterm infants, the use of high Ca and high P parenteral nutrition, until establishment of enteral feeding

with human milk containing commercial fortifiers, or formulae designed specifically for preterm infants is appropriate (2,177,178). Human milk alone is likely to be inadequate in a number of nutrients including protein, sodium, Ca, P, and possibly other nutrients for the needs of the very small preterm infant. All human-milk–fed small preterm infants, particularly those with birth weights less than 1,500 grams, should receive commercial fortifier containing multiple nutrients in human milk during their hospital stay and probably posthospital discharge.

The use of Ca and P supplementation alone is inappropriate for the treatment or prevention of osteopenia with or without fractures or rickets, since bone growth requires protein and multiple other nutrients for matrix formation and mineralization. In addition, further large increases in Ca and P intake beyond the current recommended intake is probably not advisable because of the risks of bezoar and even intestinal obstruction with excessive oral intake, and hyperphosphatemia with intravenous intake. In preterm infants, most fractures have significant callus formation at diagnosis and only require splinting support; short-term analgesia is needed if the fracture is recent and without callus formation.

Human milk or standard infant formulae should provide adequate amounts of Ca and P for healthy term infants. Other appropriate nutrients also should be introduced during the latter half of infancy to maintain adequate nutritional status for all infants.

In preterm infants receiving infant formulae with lower Ca and P content (compared to the preterm infant formulae currently available in the United States), normal vitamin D status as indicated by serum 25-OHD concentrations has been reported in infants who received daily supplements of 400 to 2,000 IU vitamin D. However, for enterally fed preterm infants given adequate volumes of high Ca-, high P-, and vitamin D-fortified preterm infant formula, or human milk fortified with commercial human milk fortifiers, a daily total intake of 400 IU vitamin D should be adequate; additional vitamin D supplementation may be excessive.

Prophylactic vitamin D supplementation has been recommended for all breastfed term infants (179) since adequate endogenous production of vitamin D cannot be assured with infants living in varied geographic regions and in families with varied ethnocultural practices.

For infants who require parenteral nutrition as the major source of nutritional support, 25 to 40 IU vitamin D/dL of parenteral nutrition solution with a maximum total daily intake of 400 IU is sufficient to maintain vitamin D status regardless of the gestational age of the infant (180).

For infants with established nutritional vitamin D deficiency, a daily supplementation of 400 IU vitamin D (181) in addition to adequate overall nutritional support is also adequate. Provision of pharmacologic doses of vitamin D to the infants is associated with hypercalcemia, nephrocalcinosis, and hypertension.

Specific therapies are required for inherited renal tubular disorders and disorders of vitamin D and PTH metabolism, and usually include one or more of the following: Ca, phosphate, and 1,25(OH)$_2$D.

Monitoring and Followup

The goal is for the affected infants to grow normally without residual defect. Regular clinical assessment and growth measurements are essential. On followup during infancy (172,173,181), there were no major residual physical deformities with the use of 400 IU vitamin D for the treatment of rickets for infants born at term or preterm. Skeletal maturation as assessed by ossification centers of the wrists for preterm infants is similar to term infants at 1 year of age (172). However, long-term linear growth in the extremely low-birth-weight infants may remain delayed, suggesting that bone mineral status in the smallest preterm infants still may be suboptimal (182) despite the relatively uncommon occurrence of radiographic rickets and fractures on followup. Current data on DXA-measured total body bone mineral content in the small preterm infant are difficult to interpret because of inconsistencies in the techniques used among different studies (183,184).

Biochemical monitoring of nutritional rickets includes measurement of serum Ca, P, and alkaline phosphatase and avoiding hypercalciuria (less than 0.15 mmol [6 mg/kg/day], especially in human-milk–fed preterm infants) at 1- to 2-week intervals until stable and then at 1- to 2-month intervals. Bone turnover markers, IPTH, vitamin D metabolites, and any other abnormal biochemical parameters should be monitored at 1- to 2-month intervals. All biochemical monitoring should be continued until standard radiographs show completion of healing and remodeling of skeletal defects. Radiographs of the wrists and fracture site(s) should be taken at 2- to 4-month intervals. Standardization of the DXA measurement in infants with serial measurements at 2- to 3-month intervals should provide an added means to better understand bone mineral status in the developing skeleton (185,186). Screening for other affected family members and molecular studies may be warranted in heritable conditions. Other specific monitoring depends on the underlying cause of the skeletal defect.

REFERENCES

1. Ziegler EE, O'Donnell AM, Nelson SE, et al. Body composition of the reference fetus. *Growth* 1976;40:329–341.
2. Koo WWK, Steichen JJ. Osteopenia and rickets of prematurity. In: Polin R, Fox W, eds. *Fetal and neonatal physiology*, 2nd ed. Philadelphia: WB Saunders, 1998:2335–2349.
3. Steichen JJ, Tsang RC, Gratton TL, et al. Vitamin D homeostasis in the perinatal period: 1,25-dihydroxyvitamin D in maternal, cord and neonatal blood. *N Engl J Med* 1980;302:315–319.
4. Saggese G, Baroncelli GI, Bertelloni S, et al. Intact parathyroid hormone levels during pregnancy, in healthy term neonates and in hypocalcemic preterm infants. *Acta Paediatr Scand* 1991;80:36–41.
5. Thiebaud D, Janisch S, Koelbl H, et al. Direct evidence of a parathyroid related protein gradient between the mother and the newborn in humans. *Bone Miner* 1993;23:213–221.
6. Seki K, Wada S, Nagata N, et al. Parathyroid hormone-related protein during pregnancy and the perinatal period. *Gynecol Obstet Invest* 1994;37:83–86.
7. Tsang RC, Oh W. Neonatal hypocalcemia in low birth weight infants. *Pediatrics* 1970;45:773–781.
8. Snodgrass GJ, Stemmler L, Went J, et al. Interrelations of plasma calcium, inorganic phosphate, magnesium and protein over the first week of life. *Arch Dis Child* 1973;48:279–285.
9. Venkataraman PS, Tsang RC, Chen IW, et al. Pathogenesis of early neonatal hypocalcemia: studies of serum calcitonin, gastrin, and plasma glucagon. *J Pediatr* 1987;110:599–603.
10. David L, Salle BL, Putet G, et al. Serum immunoreactive calcitonin in low birth weight infants. Description of early changes; effect of intravenous calcium infusion; relationships with early changes in serum calcium, phosphorus, magnesium, parathyroid hormone and gastrin levels. *Pediatr Res* 1981;15:803–814.
11. Venkataraman PS, Tsang RC, Steichen JJ, et al. Early neonatal hypocalcemia in extremely preterm infants: high incidence, early onset, and refractoriness to supraphysiologic dose of calcitriol. *Am J Dis Child* 1986;140:1004–1008.
12. Koo WWK, Tsang RC, Poser JW, et al. Elevated serum calcium and osteocalcin levels from calcitriol in preterm infants. A prospective randomized study. *Am J Dis Child* 1986;140:1152–1158.
13. Nelson N, Finnstrom O, Larsson L. Plasma ionized calcium, phosphate and magnesium in preterm and small for gestational age infants. *Acta Paediatr Scand* 1989;78:351–357.
14. Soldin SJ, Hicks JM. Calcium and ionized calcium. In: Soldin SJ, Hicks JM, eds. *Pediatric reference ranges*. Washington, DC: American Association for Clinical Chemistry Press, 1995:38–39.
15. Murthy JN, Hicks JM, Soldin SJ. Evaluation of i-STAT portable clinical analyzer in a neonatal and pediatric intensive care unit. *Clin Biochem* 1997;30:385–389.
16. Dollberg S, Bauer R, Lubetzky R, et al. A reappraisal of neonatal blood chemistry reference ranges using the Nova M electrodes. *Am J Perinatol* 2001;18:433–440.
17. Loughead JL, Mimouni F, Tsang RC. Serum ionized calcium concentrations in normal neonates. *Am J Dis Child* 1988;142:516–518.
18. Lowenstein FW, Stanton MF. Serum magnesium levels by age, sex and two racial groups in the United States, First National Health and Nutrition Examination Survey (NHANES I), 1971–1974. *J Am Coll Nutr* 1986;5:399–414.
19. Handwerker SM, Altura BT, Jones KY, et al. Maternal-fetal transfer of ionized serum magnesium during the stress of labor and delivery: a human study. *J Am Coll Nutr* 1995;14:376–381.
20. Koo B, Sauser K, Hammami M, et al. Neonatal magnesium homeostasis with and without maternal magnesium treatment. *Clin Chem* 1996;42:S309.
21. Marcus JC, Valencia GB, Altura BT, et al. Serum ionized magnesium in premature and term infants. *Pediatr Neurol* 1998;18:311–314.
22. Sanders GT, Huijgen HJ, Sanders R. Magnesium in disease: a review with special emphasis on the serum ionized magnesium. *Clin Chem Lab Med* 1999;37:1011–1033.
23. Kronenberg HM, Igarashi T, Freeman MW, et al. Structure and expression of the human parathyroid hormone gene. *Recent Prog Horm Res* 1986;42:641–663.
24. Rubin LP, Posillico JT, Anast CS, et al. Circulating levels of biologically active and immunoreactive intact parathyroid hormone in human newborns. *Pediatr Res* 1991;29:201–207.
25. Venkataraman PS, Blick KE, Fry HD, et al. Postnatal changes in calcium-regulating hormones in very-low-birth-weight infants. Effect of early neonatal hypocalcemia and intravenous calcium infusion on serum parathyroid hormone and calcitonin homeostasis. *Am J Dis Child* 1985;139:913–916.
26. Mimouni F, Loughead J, Tsang R, et al. Postnatal surge in serum calcitonin concentrations: no contribution to neonatal hypocalcemia in infants of diabetic mothers. *Pediatr Res* 1990;28:493–495.
27. Dilena BA, White GH. The responses of plasma ionised calcium and intact parathyrin to calcium supplementation in preterm infants. *Acta Paediatr Scand* 1991;80:1098–1100.
28. Gelbert L, Schipani EA, Juppner H, et al. Chromosomal localization of the parathyroid hormone/parathyroid hormone-related protein receptor gene to human chromosome 3p21.1-p24.2. *J Clin Endocrinol Metab* 1994;79:1046–1048.

29. Brown EM. Four-parameter model of the sigmoidal relationship between parathyroid hormone release and extracellular calcium concentration in normal and abnormal parathyroid tissue. *J Clin Endocrinol Metab* 1983;56:572–581.

30. Mathias RS, Nguyen HT, Zhang MY, et al. Reduced expression of the renal calcium-sensing receptor in rats with experimental chronic renal insufficiency. *J Am Soc Nephrol* 1998;9:2067–2074.

31. Drueke TB. Abnormal skeletal response to parathyroid hormone and the expression of its receptor in chronic uremia. *Pediatr Nephrol* 1996;10:348–350.

32. Chattopadhyay N, Cheng I, Rogers K, et al. Identification and localization of extracellular Ca^{2+}-sensing receptor in rat intestine. *Am J Physiol* 1998;274:G122–G130.

33. Eckert RW, Scherubl H, Petzelt C, et al. Rhythmic oscillations of cytosolic calcium in rat C-cells. *Mol Cell Endocrinol* 1989;64:267–270.

34. Zofkova I, Kancheva RL. The relationship between magnesium and calciotropic hormones. *Magnes Res* 1995;8:77–84.

35. Toffaletti J, Cooper DL, Lobaugh B. The response of parathyroid hormone to specific changes in either ionized calcium, ionized magnesium, or protein-bound calcium in humans. *Metabolism* 1991;40:814–818.

36. Fatemi S, Ryzen E, Flores J, et al. Effect of experimental human magnesium depletion on parathyroid hormone secretion and 1,25-dihydroxyvitamin D metabolism. *J Clin Endocrinol Metab* 1991;73:1067–1072.

37. Garel JM, Besnard P, Rebut-Bonneton C. C cell activity during the prenatal and postnatal periods in the rat. *Endocrinology* 1981;109:1573–1577.

38. Wolfe HJ, DeLellis RA, Volkel EF, et al. Distribution of calcitonin-containing cells in the normal neonatal human thyroid gland: a correlation of morphology with peptide content. *J Clin Endocrinol Metab* 1975;41:1076–1081.

39. Huwyler R, Born W, Ohnhaus EE, et al. Plasma kinetics and urinary excretion of exogenous human and salmon calcitonin in man. *Am J Physiol* 1979;236:E15–E19.

40. Samaan NA, Anderson GD, Adam-Mayne ME. Immunoreactive calcitonin in the mother, neonate, child and adult. *Am J Obstet Gynecol* 1975;121:622–625.

41. Purdue BW, Tilakaratne N, Sexton PM. Molecular pharmacology of the calcitonin receptor. *Receptors Channels* 2002;8:243–255.

42. Juaneda C, Dumont Y, Quirion R. The molecular pharmacology of CGRP and related peptide receptor subtypes. *Trends Pharmacol Sci* 2000;21:432–438.

43. Shinki T, Ueno Y, DeLuca HF, et al. Calcitonin is a major regulator for the expression of renal 25-hydroxyvitamin D_3-1α-hydroxylase gene in normocalcemic rats. *Proc Natl Acad Sci USA* 1999;96:8253–8258.

44. Besnard P, el M'Selmi A, Jousset U, et al. Effects of 1,25-dihydroxycholecalciferol and calcium on calcitonin mRNA levels in suckling rats. *Mol Cell Endocrinol* 1991;79:45–52.

45. Wimalawansa SJ, Gunasekera RD, Datta HK. Hypocalcemic actions of amylin amide in humans. *J Bone Miner Res* 1992;7:1113–1116.

46. Holick MF. Photosynthesis of vitamin D in the skin: effect of environmental and life-style variables. *Fed Proc* 1987;46:1876–1882.

47. Mizwicki MT, Norman AW. Two key proteins of the vitamin D endocrine system come into crystal clear focus: comparison of the x-ray structures of the nuclear receptor for $1_α$, 24(OH)$_2$ vitamin D_3, the plasma vitamin D binding protein, and their ligands. *J Bone Miner Res* 2003;18:795–806.

48. Bell NH, Shaw S, Turner RT. Evidence that 1,25-dihydroxyvitamin D_3 inhibits the hepatic production of 25-hydroxyvitamin D in man. *J Clin Invest* 1984;74:1540–1544.

49. Clements MR, Johnson L, Fraser DR. A new mechanism for induced vitamin D deficiency in calcium deprivation. *Nature* 1987;325:62–65.

50. Yoshida T, Yoshida N, Monkawa T, et al. Dietary phosphorus deprivation induces 25-hydroxyvitamin D_3 1α-hydroxylase gene expression. *Endocrinology* 2001;142:1720–1726.

51. Portale AA, Halloran BP, Morris RC Jr. Physiologic regulation of the serum concentration of 1,25-dihydroxyvitamin D by phosphorus in normal man. *J Clin Invest* 1989;83:1494–1499.

52. The HYP Consortium. A gene (PEX) with homologies to endopeptidases is mutated in patients with X-linked hypophosphatemic rickets. *Nat Genet* 1995;11:130–136.

53. Shimada T, Kakitani M, Yamazaki Y, et al. Targeted ablation of Fgf23 demonstrates an essential physiological role of FGF23 in phosphate and vitamin D metabolism. *J Clin Invest* 2004;113:561–568.

54. Weaver VM, Welsh J. 1,25-Dihydroxycholecalciferol and the genesis of hypocalcaemia in magnesium-deficient chicks. *Magnes Res* 1990;3:171–177.

55. Adams JS, Sharma OP, Gacad MA, et al. Metabolism of 25-hydroxyvitamin D_3 by cultured pulmonary alveolar macrophages in sarcoidosis. *J Clin Invest* 1983;72:1856–1860.

56. Shinki T, Jin CH, Nishimura A, et al. Parathyroid hormone inhibits 25 hydroxyvitamin D_3-24-hydroxylase mRNA expression stimulated by 1α,25-dihydroxyvitamin D_3 in rat kidney but not in intestine. *J Biol Chem* 1992;267:13757–13762.

57. Miyamoto K, Kesterson RA, Yamamoto H, et al. Structural organization of the human vitamin D receptor chromosomal gene and its promoter. *Mol Endocrinol* 1997;11:1165–1179.

58. Yamada S, Yamamoto K, Masuno H, et al. Three-dimensional structure-function relationship of vitamin D and vitamin D receptor model. *Steroids* 2001;66:177–187.

59. Norman AW, Bishop JE, Bula CM, et al. Molecular tools for study of genomic and rapid signal transduction responses initiated by 1α,25(OH)$_2$-vitamin D_3. *Steroids* 2002;67:457–466.

60. Verity CM, Burman D, Beadle PC, et al. Seasonal changes in perinatal vitamin D metabolism: maternal and cord blood biochemistry in normal pregnancies. *Arch Dis Child* 1981;56:943–948.

61. Hollis BW, Pittard WB III. Evaluation of the total fetomaternal vitamin D relationship at term: evidence for racial differences. *J Clin Endocrinol Metab* 1984;59:652–657.

62. Nehama H, Weintroub S, Eisenberg Z, et al. Seasonal variation in paired maternal newborn serum 25 hydroxyvitamin D and 24,25 dihydroxyvitamin D concentrations in Israel. *Isr J Med Sci* 1987;23:274–277.

63. Overbergh L, Decallonne B, Valckx D, et al. Identification and immune regulation of 25-hydroxyvitamin D-1-α-hydroxylase in murine macrophages. *Clin Exp Immunol* 2000;120:139–146.

64. Martin TJ, Moseley JM, Williams ED. Parathyroid hormone-related protein: hormone and cytokine. *J Endocrinol* 1997;154:S23–S37.

65. MacIsaac RJ, Caple JW, Danks JA, et al. Ontogeny of parathyroid hormone-related protein in the ovine parathyroid gland. *Endocrinology* 1991;129:757–764.

66. Abbas SK, Ratcliff WA, Moniz C, et al. The role of parathyroid hormone-related protein in calcium homeostasis in the fetal pig. *Exp Physiol* 1994;79:527–536.

67. Bilezikian JP. Clinical utility of assays for parathyroid hormone-related protein. *Clin Chem* 1992;38:179–181.

68. Dvir R, Golander A, Jaccard N, et al. Amniotic fluid and plasma levels of parathyroid hormone-related protein and hormonal modulation of its secretion by amniotic fluid cells. *Eur J Endocrinol* 1995;133:277–282.

69. Law F, Moate PJ, Leaver DD, et al. Parathyroid hormone-related protein in milk and its correlation with bovine milk calcium. *J Endocrinol* 1991;128:21–26.

70. Salsburey DJ, Brown DR. Effect of parenteral calcium treatment on blood pressure and heart rate in neonatal hypocalcemia. *Pediatrics* 1982;69:605–609.

71. Mirro R, Brown DR. Parenteral calcium treatment shortens the left ventricular systolic time intervals of hypocalcemic neonates. *Pediatr Res* 1984;18:71–73.

72. Venkataraman PS, Wilson DA, Sheldon RE, et al. Effect of hypocalcemia on cardiac function in very-low-birth-weight preterm neonates: studies of blood ionized calcium, echocardiography and cardiac effect of intravenous calcium therapy. *Pediatrics* 1985;76:543–550.

73. Broner CW, Stidham GL, Westenkirchner DF, et al. Hypermagnesemia and hypocalcemia as predictors of high mortality in critically ill pediatric patients. *Crit Care Med* 1990;18:921–928.

74. Hanukoglu A, Chalen S, Kowardski AA. Late onset hypocalcemia, rickets and hypoparathyroidism in an infant of a mother with hyperparathyroidism. *J Pediatr* 1988;112:751–754.

75. Thomas AK, McVie R, Levine SN. Disorders of maternal calcium metabolism implicated by abnormal calcium metabolism in the neonate. *Am J Perinatol* 1999;16:515–520.

76. Robertson WC Jr. Calcium carbonate consumption during pregnancy: an unusual cause of neonatal hypocalcemia. *J Child Neurol* 2002;17:853–855.

77. Ravid A, Koren R, Rotem C, et al. Mononuclear cells from human neonates are partially resistant to the action of 1,25 dihydroxyvitamin D. *J Clin Endocrinol Metab* 1988;67:755–759.

78. Dincsoy MY, Tsang RC, Laskarzewski P, et al. Serum calcitonin response to administration of calcium in newborn infants during exchange blood transfusion. *J Pediatr* 1982;100:782–786.

79. Mimouni F, Tsang, RC, Hertzberg VS, et al. Polycythemia, hypomagnesemia and hypocalcemia in infants of diabetic mothers. *Am J Dis Child* 1986;140:798–800.

80. Banerjee S, Mimouni FB, Mehta R, et al. Lower whole blood ionized magnesium concentrations in hypocalcemic infants of gestational diabetic mothers. *Magnes Res* 2003;16:127–130.

81. Sarkar S, Watman J, Seigel WM, et al. A prospective controlled study of neonatal morbidities in infants born at 36 weeks or more gestation to women with diet-controlled gestational diabetes (GDM-class Al). *J Perinatol* 2003;23:223–228.

82. Schwartz R, Teramo KA. Effects of diabetic pregnancy on the fetus and newborn. *Semin Perinatol* 2000;24:120–135.

83. Specker B, Tsang R, Ho M, et al. Low serum calcium and high parathyroid hormone levels in neonates fed humanized cow's milk-based formula. *Am J Dis Child* 1991;145:941–945.

84. Venkataraman PS, Tsang RC, Greer FR, et al. Late infantile tetany and secondary hyperparathyroidism in infants fed humanized cow milk formula. Longitudinal follow-up. *Am J Dis Child* 1985;139:664–668.

85. Perlman JM. Fatal hyperphosphatemia after oral phosphate overdose in a premature infant. *Am J Health Syst Pharm* 1997;54: 2488–2490.

86. Davis RF, Eichner JM, Bleyuer WA, et al. Hypocalcemia, hyperphosphatemia and dehydration following a single hypertonic phosphate enema. *J Pediatr* 1977;90:484–485.

87. Dincsoy MY, Tsang RC, Laskarzewski P, et al. The role of postnatal age and magnesium on parathyroid hormone responses during "exchange" blood transfusion in the newborn period. *J Pediatr* 1982;100:277–283.

88. Bainbridge R, Mughal Z, Mimouni F, et al. Transient congenital hypoparathyroidism: how transient is it? *J Pediatr* 1988;111: 866–868.

89. Kooh SW, Binet A. Partial hypoparathyroidism: a variant of transient congenital hypoparathyroidism. *Am J Dis Child* 1991;145: 877–880.

90. Greig F, Paul E, DiMartino-Nardi J, et al. Transient congenital hypoparathyroidism: resolution and recurrence in chromosome 22q11 deletion. *J Pediatr* 1996;128:563–567.

91. Arnold A, Horst SA, Gardella TJ, et al. Mutation of the signal peptide-encoding region of the preproparathyroid hormone gene in familial isolated hypoparathyroidism. *J Clin Invest* 1990;86: 1084–1087.

92. Bilous RW, Murty G, Parkinson DB, et al. Autosomal dominant familial hypoparathyroidism, sensorineural deafness, and renal dysplasia. *N Engl J Med* 1992;327:1069–1074.

93. Sunthornthepvarakul T, Churesigaew S, Ngowngarmratana S. A novel mutation of the signal peptide of the preproparathyroid hormone gene associated with autosomal recessive familial isolated hypoparathyroidism. *J Clin Endocrinol Metab* 1999;84: 3792–3796.

94. Taylor SC, Morris G, Wilson D, et al. Hypoparathyroidism and 22q11 deletion syndrome. *Arch Dis Child* 2003;88:520–522.

95. Swillen A, Devriendt K, Legius E, et al. The behavioural phenotype in velo-cardio-facial syndrome (VCFS): from infancy to adolescence. *Genet Couns* 1999;10:79–88.

96. Gerdes M, Solot C, Wang PP, et al. Taking advantage of early diagnosis: preschool children with the 22q11. 2 deletion. *Genet Med* 2001;3:40–44.

97. Greenhalgh KL, Aligianis IA, Bromilow G, et al. 22q11 deletion: a multisystem disorder requiring multidisciplinary input. *Arch Dis Child* 2003;88:523–524.

98. Keppen LD, Fasules JW, Burks AW, et al. Confirmation of autosomal dominant transmission of the DiGeorge malformation complex. *J Pediatr* 1988;113:506–508.

99. Baron J, Winer KK, Yanovski JA, et al. Mutations in the Ca^{2+}-sensing receptor gene cause autosomal dominant and sporadic hypoparathyroidism. *Hum Mol Genet* 1996;5:601–606.

100. Pearce SH, Williamson C, Kifor O, et al. A familial syndrome of hypocalcemia with hypercalciuria due to mutations in the calcium sensing receptor. *N Engl J Med* 1996;335:1115–1122.

101. Zhang P, Jobert AS, Couvineau A, et al. A homozygous inactivating mutation in the parathyroid hormone/parathyroid hormone-related peptide receptor causing Blomstrand chondrodysplasia. *J Clin Endocrinol Metab* 1998;83:3365–3368.

102. Ringel MD, Schwindinger WF, Levine MA. Clinical implications of genetic defects in G proteins: The molecular basis of McCune Albright syndrome and Albright hereditary osteodystrophy. *Medicine* 1996;75:171–184.

103. Linglart A, Carel JC, Garabedian M, et al. GNAS1 lesions in pseudohypoparathyroidism Ia and Ic: genotype phenotype relationship and evidence of the maternal transmission of the hormonal resistance. *J Clin Endocrinol Metab* 2002;87:189–197.

104. Bastepe M, Lane AH, Juppner H. Paternal uniparental isodisomy of chromosome 20q and the resulting changes in GNAS1 methylation as a plausible cause of pseudohypoparathyroidism. *Am J Hum Genet* 2001;68:1283–1289.

105. Minagawa M, Yasuda T, Kobayashi Y, et al. Transient pseudohypoparathyroidism of the neonate. *Eur J Endocrinol* 1995;133: 151–155.

106. Mimouni F, Mimouni CP, Loughead JL, et al. A case control study of hypocalcemia in high risk neonates: racial, but no seasonal differences. *J Am Coll Nutr* 1991;10:196–199.

107. Srinivasan M, Abinun M, Cant AJ, et al. Malignant infantile osteopetrosis presenting with neonatal hypocalcemia. *Arch Dis Child Fetal Neonatal Ed* 2000;83:F21–F23.

108. Crook MA, Hally V, Panteli JV. The importance of the refeeding syndrome. *Nutrition* 2001;17:632–637.

109. Weinsier RL, Krumdieck CL. Death resulting from overzealous total parenteral nutrition: the refeeding syndrome. *Am J Clin Nutr* 1980;34:393–399.

110. Foldenauer A, Vossbeck S, Pohlandt F. Neonatal hypocalcaemia associated with rotavirus diarrhoea. *Eur J Pediatr* 1998;157: 838–842.

111. Wasant P, Matsumoto I, Naylor E, et al. Mitochondrial fatty acid oxidation disorders in Thai infants: a report of 3 cases. *J Med Assoc Thai* 2002;85(Suppl 2):S710–S719.

112. Sarici SU, Serdar MA, Erdem G, et al. Evaluation of plasma ionized magnesium levels in neonatal hyperbilirubinemia. *Pediatr Res* 2004;55:243–247.

113. Romagnoli C, Polidori G, Cataldi L, et al. Phototherapy induced hypocalcemia. *J Pediatr* 1979;94:815–816.

114. Oleske JM. Experience with 118 infants born to narcotic-using mothers: does a lower serum ionized calcium level contribute to the symptoms of withdrawal? *Clin Pediatr* 1977;16:418–423.

115. Broner CW, Stidham GL, Westenkirchner DF, et al. A prospective, randomized, double-blind comparison of calcium chloride and calcium gluconate therapies for hypocalcemia in critically ill children. *J Pediatr* 1990;117:986–989.

116. Koo WWK, Kaplan LA. Aluminum and bone disorders: with specific reference to aluminum contamination of infant nutrients. *J Am Coll Nutr* 1988;7:199–214.

117. Koo WWK, Antony G, Stevens LH. Continuous nasogastric phosphorus infusion in hypophosphatemic rickets of prematurity. *Am J Dis Child* 1984;138:172–175.

118. Koo WWK, Tsang RC, Steichen JJ, et al. Parenteral nutrition for infants: effect of high versus low calcium and phosphorus content. *J Pediatr Gastroenterol Nutr* 1987;6:96–104.

119. Koo WWK, Tsang RC, Succop P, et al. Minimal vitamin D and high calcium and phosphorus needs of preterm infants receiving parenteral nutrition. *J Pediatr Gastroenterol Nutr* 1989;8:225–233.

120. Lyon AJ, McIntosh N, Wheeler K, et al. Hypercalcemia in extremely low birthweight infants. *Arch Dis Child* 1984;59: 1141–1144.

121. Kimura S, Nose O, Seino Y, et al. Effects of alternate and simultaneous administrations of calcium and phosphorus on calcium metabolism in children receiving total parenteral nutrition. *J Parenter Enteral Nutr* 1986;10:513–516.

122. Pearce SH, Trump D, Wooding C, et al. Calcium-sensing receptor mutations in familial benign hypercalcaemia and neonatal hyperparathyroidism. *J Clin Invest* 1995;96:2683–2692.

123. Wilkinson H, James J. Self limiting neonatal primary hyperparathyroidism associated with familial hypocalciuric hypercalcemia. *Arch Dis Child* 1993;69:319–321.

124. Ross AJ, Cooper A, Attie MF, et al. Primary hyperparathyroidism in infancy. *J Pediatr Surg* 1986;21:493–499.

125. Pollak M, Chou Y, Marx S, et al. Familial hypocalciuric hypercalcemia and neonatal severe hyperparathyroidism. Effects of mutant gene dosage on phenotype. *J Clin Invest* 1994;93: 1108–1112.

126. Schipani E, Langman C, Parfitt AM, et al. Constitutively activated receptors for parathyroid hormone and parathyroid hormone–related peptides in Jansen's metaphyseal chondrodysplasia. *N Engl J Med* 1996;335:708–714.

127. Loughead J, Mughal F, Mimouni F, et al. Spectrum and natural history of congenital hyperparathyroidism secondary to maternal hypocalcemia. *Am J Perinatol* 1990;7:350–355.

128. Savani R, Mimouni F, Tsang R. Maternal and neonatal hyperparathyroidism as a consequence of maternal renal tubular acidosis. *Pediatrics* 1993;91:661–663.

129. Rodriguez-Soriano J, Garcia-Fuentes M, Vallo A, et al. Hypercalcemia in neonatal distal renal tubular acidosis. *Pediatr Nephrol* 2000;14:354–355.

130. Lakhdir F, Lawson D, Schatz D. Fatal parathyroid hormone–related protein–induced humoral hypercalcemia of malignancy in a 3-month old infant. *Eur J Pediatr* 1994;153:718–720.

131. Michigami T, Yamato H, Mushiake S, et al. Hypercalcemia associated with infantile fibrosarcoma producing parathyroid hormone-related protein. *J Clin Endocrinol Metab* 1996;81:1090–1095.

132. Mahoney C, Cassady C, Weinberger E, et al. Humoral hypercalcemia due to an occult renal adenoma. *Pediatr Nephrol* 1997;11:339–342.

133. Amar AM, Tomlinson G, Green DM, et al. Clinical presentation of rhabdoid tumors of the kidney. *J Pediatr Hematol Oncol* 2001;23:105–108.

134. Markestad T, Hesse V, Siebenhuner M, et al. Intermittent high-dose vitamin D prophylaxis during infancy: effect on vitamin D metabolites, calcium, and phosphorus. *Am J Clin Nutr* 1987;46:652–658.

135. Hicks MJ, Levy ML, Alexander J, et al. Subcutaneous fat necrosis of the newborn and hypercalcemia: case report and review of the literature. *Pediatr Dermatol* 1993;10:271–276.

136. Bush ME, Dahms BB. Fatal hypervitaminosis A in a neonate. *Arch Pathol Lab Med* 1984;108:838–842.

137. Tau C, Garabedian M, Farriaux JP, et al. Hypercalcemia in infants with congenital hypothyroidism and its relation to vitamin D and thyroid hormones. *J Pediatr* 1986;109:808–814.

138. Telvi L, Pinard J, Ion R, et al. De novo t(X; 21) (q28; q11) in a girl with phenotypic features of Williams-Beuren syndrome. *J Med Genet* 1992;29:747–749.

139. Nickerson E, Greenberg F, Keating MT, et al. Deletions of the elastin gene at 7q11.23 occur in 90% of patients with Williams syndrome. *Am J Hum Genet* 1995;56:1156–1161.

140. Whyte MP. Hypophosphatasia and the role of alkaline phosphatase in skeletal mineralization. *Endocr Rev* 1994;15:439–461.

141. Strehle EM, Ahmed OA, Hameed M, et al. The 4q– syndrome. *Genet Couns* 2001;12:327–339.

142. Zwischenberger JB, Nguyen TT, Upp JR Jr, et al. Complications of neonatal extracorporeal membrane oxygenation. Collective experience from the Extracorporeal Life Support Organizations. *J Thorac Cardiovas Surg* 1994;107:838–848.

143. Fridriksson JH, Helmrath MA, Wessel JJ, et al. Hypercalcemia associated with extracorporeal life support in neonates. *J Pediatr Surg* 2001;36:493–497.

144. Rauch F, Plotkin H, Travers R, et al. Osteogenesis imperfecta types I, III, and IV: effect of pamidronate therapy on bone and mineral metabolism. *J Clin Endocrinol Metab* 2003;88:986–992.

145. Mathias RS. Rickets in an infant with Williams syndrome. *Pediatr Nephrol* 2000;14:489–492.

146. Mimouni F, Tsang RC. Perinatal magnesium metabolism: personal data and challenges for the 1990s. *Magnes Res* 1991;4:109–117.

147. Monteleone JA, Lee JB, Tashjian AH Jr, et al. Transient neonatal hypocalcemia, hypomagnesemia and high serum parathyroid hormone with maternal hyperparathyroidism. *Ann Intern Med* 1975;82:670–672.

148. Schlingmann KP, Weber S, Peters M, et al. Hypomagnesemia with secondary hypocalcemia is caused by mutations in *TRPM6*, a new member of the *TRPM* gene family. *Nat Genet* 2002;31:166–170.

149. Walder RY, Shalev H, Brennan TM, et al. Familial hypomagnesemia maps to chromosome 9q, not to the X chromosome: genetic linkage mapping and analysis of a balanced translocation breakpoint. *Hum Mol Genet* 1997;6:1491–1497.

150. Weber S, Schneider L, Peters M, et al. Novel paracellin-1 mutations in 25 families with familial hypomagnesemia with hypercalciuria and nephrocalcinosis. *J Am Soc Nephrol* 2001;12:1872–1881.

151. Ghazali S, Hallett RJ, Barratt TM. Hypomagnesemia in uremic infants. *J Pediatr* 1972;81:747–750.

152. Bajpai PC, Sugden D, Stern L, et al. Serum ionic magnesium in exchange transfusion. *J Pediatr* 1967;70:193–199.

153. Stone SR, Pritchard JA. Effect of maternally administered magnesium sulfate on the neonate. *Obstet Gynecol* 1970;35:574–577.

154. Lipsitz PJ. The clinical and biochemical effects of excess magnesium in the newborn. *Pediatrics* 1971;47:501–509.

155. Koo WWK, Fong T, Gupta JM. Parenteral nutrition in infants. *Aust Paediatr J* 1980;16:169–174.

156. Ali A, Walentik C, Mantych GJ, et al. Iatrogenic acute hypermagnesemia after total parenteral nutrition infusion mimicking septic shock syndrome: two case reports. *Pediatrics* 2003;112:e70–e72.

157. Cholst IN, Steinberg SF, Tropper PJ, et al. The influence of hypermagnesemia on serum calcium and parathyroid hormone levels in human subjects. *N Engl J Med* 1984;310:1221–1225.

158. Donovan EF, Tsang RC, Steichen JJ, et al. Neonatal hypermagnesemia: effect on parathyroid hormone and calcium homeostasis. *J Pediatr* 1980;96:305–310.

159. Lamm CI, Norton KI, Murphy RJ, et al. Congenital rickets associated with magnesium sulfate infusion for tocolysis. *J Pediatr* 1988;113:1078–1082.

160. Russell JGB, Hill LF. True fetal rickets. *Br J Radiol* 1974;47:732–734.

161. Park W, Paust H, Kaufmann HJ, et al. Osteomalacia of the mother—rickets of the newborn. *Eur J Pediatr* 1987;146:292–293.

162. Anatoliotaki M, Tsilimigaki A, Tsekoura T, et al. Congenital rickets due to maternal vitamin D deficiency in a sunny island of Greece. *Acta Paediatr* 2003;92:389–391.

163. Rimensberger P, Schubiger G, Willi U. Congenital rickets following repeated administration of phosphate enemas in pregnancy: a case report. *Eur J Pediatr* 1992;151:54–56.

164. Steichen JJ, Gratton T, Tsang RC. Osteopenia of prematurity: the cause and possible treatment. *J Pediatr* 1980;96:528–534.

165. Nozza JM, Rodda CP. Vitamin D deficiency in mothers of infants with rickets. *Med J Aust* 2001;175:253–255.

166. Thacher TD, Fischer PR, Pettifor JM, et al. A comparison of calcium, vitamin D, or both for nutritional rickets in Nigerian children. *N Engl J Med* 1999;341:563–568.

167. Koo WWK, Gupta JM, Nayanar VV, et al. Skeletal changes in premature infants. *Arch Dis Child* 1982;57:447–452.

168. James JR, Congdon PJ, Truscott J, et al. Osteopenia of prematurity. *Arch Dis Child* 1986;61:871–876.

169. Lyon AJ, McIntosh N, Wheeler K, et al. Radiological rickets in extremely low birthweight infants. *Pediatr Radiol* 1987;17:56–58.

170. Koo WWK, Hammami M, Hockman EM. Use of fan beam dual energy x-ray absorptiometry to measure body composition of piglets. *J Nutr* 2002;132:1380–1383.

171. Chauhan S, Koo WWK, Hammami M, et al. Fan beam dual energy x-ray absorptiometry body composition measurements in piglets. *J Am Coll Nutr* 2003;22:408–414.

172. Koo WWK, Sherman R, Succop P, et al. Fractures and rickets in very low birth weight infants: conservative management and outcome. *J Pediatr Orthop* 1989;9:326–330.

173. Koo WWK, Sherman R, Succop P, et al. Serum vitamin D metabolites in very low birth weight infants with and without rickets and fractures. *J Pediatr* 1989;114:1017–1022.

174. Koo WWK. Laboratory assessment of nutritional metabolic bone disease in infants. *Clin Biochem* 1996;29:429–438.

175. Koo WWK, Succop P, Hambidge KM. Serum alkaline phosphatase and serum zinc concentrations in preterm infants with rickets and fractures. *Am J Dis Child* 1989;143:1342–1345.

176. Koo WWK, Succop P, Hambidge KM. Sequential concentrations of copper and ceruloplasmin in serum from preterm infants with rickets and fractures. *Clin Chem* 1991;37:556–559.

177. Koo WWK, Warren L. Calcium and bone health in infants. *Neonatal Netw* 2003;22:23–37.

178. Koo WWK, McLaughlin K, Saba M. Nutrition support for the neonatal intensive care patients. In: *The ASPEN nutrition support practice manual*. Washington DC: American Society for Parenteral and Enteral Nutrition (*in press*).

179. Gartner LM, Greer FR, for the Section on Breastfeeding and Committee on Nutrition, American Academy of Pediatrics: prevention of rickets and vitamin D deficiency: new guidelines for vitamin D intake. *Pediatrics* 2003;111:908–910.

180. Koo WWK, Tsang RC, Steichen JJ, et al. Vitamin D requirement in infants receiving parenteral nutrition. *J Parenter Enteral Nutr* 1987;11:172–176.
181. Venkataraman PS, Tsang RC, Buckley DD, et al. Elevation of serum 1,25-dihydroxyvitamin D in response to physiologic doses of vitamin D in vitamin D deficient infants. *J Pediatr* 1983;103:416–419.
182. Hack M, Taylor HG, Klein N, et al. School-age outcomes in children with birth weights under 750 g. *N Engl J Med* 1994;331: 753–759.
183. Koo WWK, Hockman EM, Hammami M. Dual energy X ray absorptiometry measurements in small subjects: conditions affecting clinical measurements. *J Amer Coll Nutr* 2004;23: 212–219.
184. Koo WWK, Hammami M, Shypailo RJ, et al. Bone and body composition measurements of small subjects: discrepancies from software for fan-beam dual energy X-ray absorptiometry. *J Amer Coll Nutr* (*in press*).
185. Koo WWK, Walters J, Bush AJ, et al. Dual energy x-ray absorptiometry studies of bone mineral status in newborn infants. *J Bone Miner Res* 1996;11:997–1002.
186. Koo WWK, Bush AJ, Walters J, et al. Postnatal development of bone mineral status during infancy. *J Amer Coll Nutr* 1998;17: 65–70.

Carbohydrate Homeostasis

Edward S. Ogata

Glucose homeostasis results from the net balance between systemic organ requirements and the production and regulation of glucose. The neonate's ability to maintain glucose homeostasis is less well developed than the older child or adult because it is in a metabolic transition period. The abrupt switch from intrauterine life, in which glucose and metabolic fuels are provided in a well-regulated manner, to a situation in which meals are intermittent and which necessitates regulation of exogenous glucose and production of endogenous glucose. As the capability to perform these functions continues to develop in the neonate, clinical disorders that can afflict the neonate may perturb this balance, resulting in hypoglycemia or hyperglycemia. In addition, antecedent intrauterine events can alter the development of glucoregulatory capabilities in the fetus, resulting in altered neonatal glucose homeostasis.

To understand the processes responsible for glucose homeostasis in the normal neonate, an appreciation of the development of glucoregulatory capabilities in the fetus is necessary. This chapter reviews this information and its relation to the clinical disorders associated with altered neonatal glucose homeostasis. Information on the perinatal aspects of diabetes in pregnancy also is presented.

MATERNAL METABOLISM DURING PREGNANCY

Although the metabolic alterations that develop in the pregnant woman throughout gestation favor the growth and development of the fetus, the first half of gestation is also a critical period for maternal anabolism. The increased calories ingested by the woman during early gestation sustain fetal growth and facilitate maternal fat deposition. This is important preparation for the second half of gestation, a period of exponential fetal growth during which these maternal stores are mobilized to meet fetal needs. The storage of maternal energy stores is facilitated by the increased secretion of insulin that occurs in women with normal carbohydrate metabolism (1–5).

Changes in maternal insulin secretion and action are dramatic during the second half of pregnancy. During the first half, basal insulin secretion is normal, and insulin secretion mediates the laying down of metabolic fuels (6). In the second half of gestation, insulin secretion is greatly exaggerated (7,8). Intravenous glucose tolerance testing indicates that by the third trimester, normal pregnant women secrete three times the insulin than they do in the nonpregnant state (1).

The development of insulin resistance during the second half of pregnancy is responsible for this exaggerated insulin secretion. Responsiveness to insulin develops 40% to 60% during the second half of gestation (7,8). The conceptus causes this insulin resistance in part by the generation of human placental lactogen, progesterone, and estrogen which become available in ever increasing amounts as gestation progresses (9–11). These directly antagonize the effect of maternal insulin. Insulin resistance increases in liver, adipose tissue, and skeletal muscle (12). Insulin binding appears to be normal during late gestation, indicating that insulin resistance is mediated by events distal to receptor/insulin binding. It is possible that tyrosine kinase inhibition may also contribute to insulin resistance (12,13).

Preexisting maternal diabetes potentiates the effects of the antiinsulin factors, causing an excessive provision of glucose and other metabolic fuels to the fetus. This is the basic perturbation responsible for the problems of the infant of the diabetic mother (Fig. 37-1) (1,14).

Metabolic fuel availability is guaranteed to the fetus even during brief maternal fasting. After an overnight fast, pregnant women have significantly lower plasma glucose concentrations than fasted nongravid women (8,15); however, glucose production in the mother is significantly increased (16,17). This increased production ensures the provision of glucose to the fetus.

Prolonged maternal fasting does alter fuel provision to the fetus. As the fast progresses, maternal ketogenesis progressively increases (15,18). The human fetal brain at early gestation can use ketones (Fig. 37-2) (19). However, this ability to use an alternative fuel may be harmful rather than beneficial to the fetus. Offspring of mothers who were ketotic during pregnancy appear to have an increased incidence of cognitive and psychomotor delay at 3 and

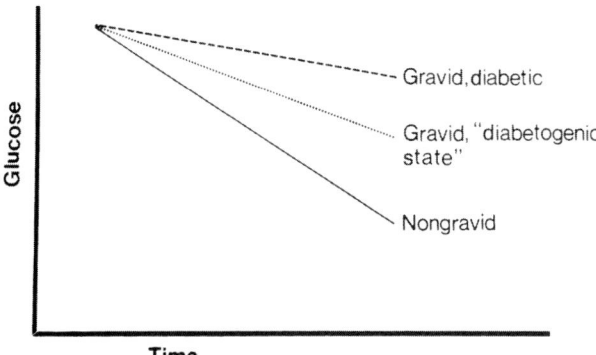

Figure 37-1 Plasma glucose changes after glucose challenge in nongravid, gravid, and gravid diabetic women. Compared to the nongravid woman, the pregnant woman with normal carbohydrate metabolism demonstrates delayed glucose clearance from midgestation onward as a result of antiinsulin factors that develop during pregnancy. The delay in glucose clearance from the maternal circulation assures glucose provision to the fetus, particularly during the postprandial period. The blunting of maternal glucose clearance is exaggerated by the counterinsulin factors in the woman with diabetes mellitus. The decreased clearance of glucose and other metabolic fuels stimulates fetal insulin production and is responsible for many of the problems of the infant of the diabetic mother.

5 years of age (20). The mechanisms responsible for this potential association between ketone body oxidation and impaired brain function are unknown. Because of this uncertainty, maternal fasting, even foregoing breakfast, should be avoided during pregnancy.

DEVELOPMENT OF GLUCOSE-PRODUCING AND GLUCOREGULATORY CAPABILITIES IN THE FETUS

To understand the problems of neonatal glucose homeostasis, the development of glucose production and regulatory capabilities in the fetus must be understood.

Glycogen

The third trimester of the human pregnancy is the first period in gestation during which some of the energy and substrate available to the fetus can be channeled from meeting needs for ongoing growth and development to energy storage. As the third trimester progresses, fat deposition and hepatic glycogen storage increase (21). The human fetus can synthesize and mobilize glycogen and respond to the signals that regulate these processes as early as the ninth week of gestation (22). However, only minute quantities of hepatic glycogen are present in early gestation as the great bulk of hepatic glycogen accumulates during the third trimester (22,23).

Several types of infants are at risk for neonatal hypoglycemia as a result of limited hepatic glycogen stores. Infants delivered prematurely have an abbreviated or no third trimester and thus have limited glycogen stores. Fetuses who

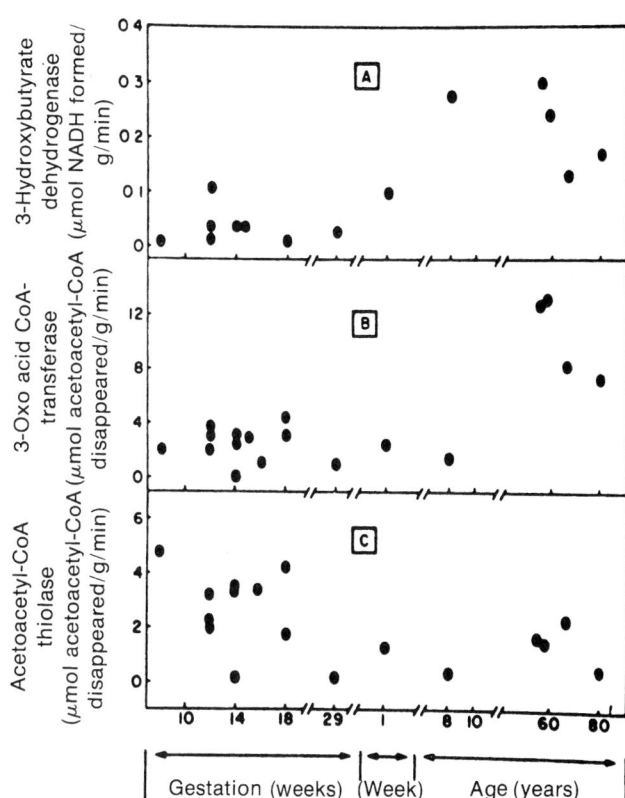

Figure 37-2 Enzymatic activity of the three key enzymes necessary for the oxidation of ketones (i.e., [A5]β-hydroxybutyrate and acetoacetate). The activities of these enzymes are present in substantial quantities in the human fetal brain during early gestation. (From Felig P, Lynch V. [Starvation in human pregnancy: hypoglycemia, hypoinsulinemia, and hyperketonemia.] *Science* 1970; 170:990–992, with permission.)

are growth-retarded (i.e., small-for-gestational-age [SGA]) on the basis of limited metabolic fuel availability and diminished gaseous exchange (i.e., uteroplacental insufficiency) will use these fuels for growth and not for glycogen synthesis. Perinatal stress causes neonatal hypoglycemia in part because of catecholamine-stimulated mobilization of hepatic glycogen stores. This can occur at birth or during the antepartum period. In the latter situation, fetuses might recover from stress and be delivered without difficulty. As newborns, such infants have depleted glycogen stores and are at risk for hypoglycemia.

Gluconeogenesis

For many years, it was believed that maternally derived glucose was the sole metabolic fuel for the fetus and that the fetus could not produce glucose. As indicated, the fetus can use other fuels such as the ketones and can, under special circumstances, mobilize hepatic glycogen. The fetus also can carry out gluconeogenesis to a limited degree, although it is likely that under normal circumstances it does not need to call on this function. Data from human abortuses have demonstrated that the four key gluconeogenic enzymes are present in fetal liver by 2 to 3 months of gestation (24,25). The activities of these enzymes are believed to increase throughout gestation and the neonatal period. Thus, all appropriately grown newborns, including the very premature, probably have some degree of gluconeogenic capability. However, the growth-retarded neonate may have impaired gluconeogenic capability.

Endocrine Regulation

Insulin and glucagon, important hormones for regulating glucose, can be measured in fetal plasma as early as 12 weeks of gestation (26). Although plasma concentrations of these hormones are low, the relative content of these hormones in the fetal pancreas is quite high (27,28). These high concentrations may result from the limited ability of the fetal islets to secrete these hormones. Both premature and term infants have limited capacity to secrete these hormones in response to a glucose challenge in the newborn period. This indicates that the fetus also has limited secretory capability (Fig. 37-3) (28-30). Of note, amino acids have a greater effect in stimulating insulin and limiting glucagon secretion than glucose in the fetus (31,32).

Insulin may be more important for enhancing growth than for regulating metabolic fuels during fetal life. Insulin stimulates the growth of specific tissues (e.g., adipose, hepatic, connective, skeletal, cardiac muscle) (33,34).

Excessive insulin secretion during fetal life resulting from such conditions as maternal diabetes causes the disproportionate growth of insulin-sensitive tissues, resulting in macrosomia (1,14,35,36). A lack of insulin, as in infants with transient neonatal diabetes mellitus, always is accompanied by fetal growth retardation.

Glucagon or a critical glucagon/insulin ratio is important for inducing gluconeogenic enzymes. Glucagon stimulates the induction of gluconeogenic enzymes *in vitro* and *in vivo* (37,38). Fetal plasma glucagon concentrations increase progressively during fetal life, and this is associated with a concomitant increase in gluconeogenic enzyme activity. At birth, plasma glucagon concentrations surge, coinciding with the rapid postnatal increase in gluconeogenic activity (39). Insulin may modulate glucagon's effect because it can inhibit gluconeogenic enzyme induction (37). Thus, a balance between these two hormones controls gluconeogenic enzyme induction during perinatal life.

Adrenergic mechanisms can stimulate hepatic glycogenolysis during fetal life, much as in the adult. As labor progresses, fetal sympathoadrenal activity increases, resulting in a considerable increase in circulating catecholamine levels (40,41). Cord clamping triggers an increase in glucagon secretion (42). As plasma glucose concentrations plummet with cord clamping, insulin secretion slowly decreases. These adjustments, particularly the remarkable increase in catecholamine secretion, stimulate glycogenolysis and gluconeogenesis in the neonate (Fig. 37-4).

Islet cell function remains unresponsive for several weeks of neonatal life in term infants. Newborn infants increase insulin and limit glucagon secretion sluggishly in response to glucose challenge. Limited data indicate that these responses become adult-like between the first and second weeks of life (43). This adaptation is critically important because the neonate, unlike the fetus, must

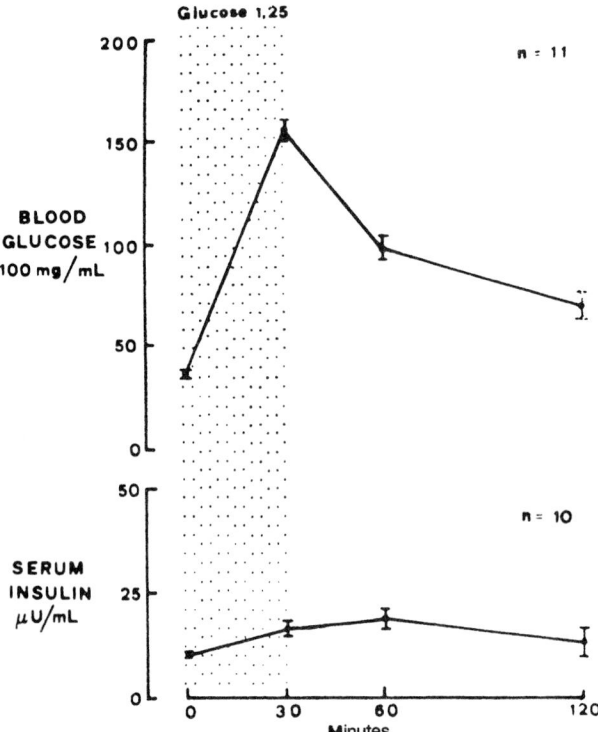

Figure 37-3 Insulin secretion after glucose challenge in premature infants. Whereas normal adults secrete insulin briskly in response to glucagon, premature infants in the neonatal period secrete insulin only sluggishly. (From Assan R, Buillet J. Pancreatic glucagon and glucagon-like material in tissues and plasma from human fetuses 6 to 26 weeks old. In: Jonxis JHP, Visser HKA, Troelstra JA, eds. *Metabolic processes in the fetus and newborn infant, nutrition symposium.* Baltimore: Williams & Wilkins, 1971: 210–212, with permission.)

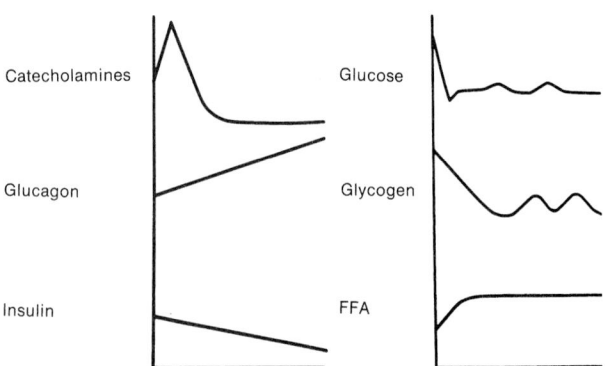

Figure 37-4 Levels of hormones and metabolic fuels change after birth. At birth, the counterregulatory hormones (i.e., catecholamines and glucagon) increase greatly, whereas insulin secretion decreases. Neonatal plasma glucose concentrations plummet as a result of cord clamping. The changes in counter regulatory hormones and insulin favor mobilization of glucose and fat and stimulate gluconeogenesis. These changes assure adequate neonatal glucose production. FAA, free fatty acids. (From Kalhan SC, Bier DM, Savin SM, et al. Estimation of glucose turnover and 13C recycling in the human newborn by simultaneous [1-13C]glucose and [6,6-1H2]glucose tracers. *J Clin Endocrinol Metab* 1980;50:456–460, with permission.)

regulate glucose production and storage through feeding and fasting cycles. Little is known about the premature infant's ability to regulate glucose in the neonatal period. The ability to modulate insulin and glucagon secretion probably develops as the neonatal period progresses.

Glucose Transporters

Glucose transporters (Glut) are a family of structurally similar proteins encoded by a family of genes and expressed in a tissue-specific manner in most mammalian tissues (44). Several isoforms have been described in the human fetus and placenta. Because Gluts facilitate transfer of glucose from the maternal to fetal circulation and also uptake of glucose by most fetal and neonatal tissues, they are critically important for growth and development.

Glut$_1$ is the dominant isoform in most fetal tissues and the placenta (45,46). Insulin, insulin-like growth factors, and other hormones and peptides regulate its activity and expression. The Gluts are developmentally regulated. The appearance of Glut isoforms varies in time of appearance and type (Glut$_2$ in liver, Glut$_4$ in muscle) during intrauterine and neonatal life (47). Glut$_1$ and Glut$_3$ are expressed in various tissues, including the placenta. Ambient glucose can affect both glucose transport activity and expression of Glut genes. Glut$_1$ expression appears to increase with gestation. In placentas of women with diabetes, Glut$_3$ decreases with gestation, suggesting an attempt by the placenta to limit glucose transport in the face of maternal hyperglycemia (48).

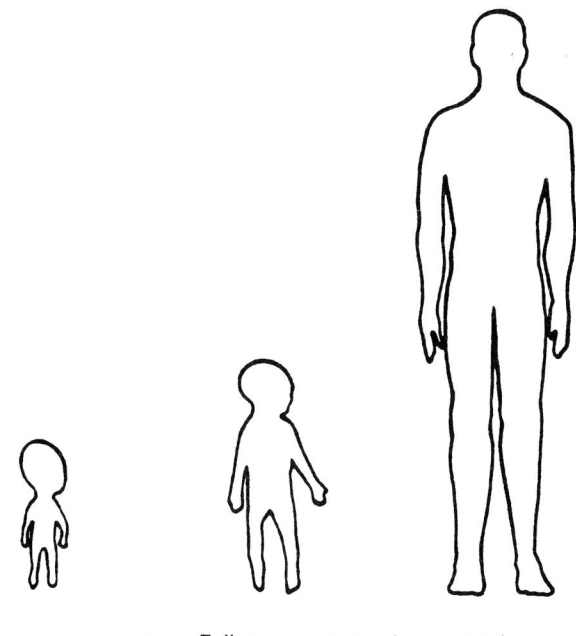

Premature neonate
5 to 6 mg/kg/min

Full-term neonate
3 to 5 mg/kg/min

Adult
2 to 3 mg/kg/min

Figure 37-5 Glucose turnover in premature and term neonates and the adult. When related to body weight, glucose turnover is greatest in the premature infant and least in the adult. The increased turnover in neonates results in part from their relatively increased brain-to-body mass ratio. (From Kalhan SC, Bier DM, Savin SM, et al. Estimation of glucose turnover and 13C recycling in the human newborn by simultaneous [1-13C]glucose and [6,6-1H2]glucose tracers. *J Clin Endocrinol Metab* 1980;50:456–460, with permission.).

NEONATAL GLUCOSE REQUIREMENTS

The clinician makes a leap of faith in using the chemical or paper strip determination of plasma or blood glucose concentration to judge the adequacy of tissue glucose provision in the neonate. A normal plasma concentration is interpreted to mean that glucose supply to the brain and other organs is adequate for ongoing metabolic needs. To appreciate glucose requirements, glucose kinetics must be understood.

Glucose turnover represents the rate of production of glucose by the liver and other organs and the simultaneous use or uptake of glucose by the brain and other organs. Turnover is usually expressed as milligrams of glucose per kilogram of body weight per minute. Although stable isotope technology has allowed quantification of glucose turnover in neonates, this methodology cannot be directly applied for clinical purposes. Thus, the clinician must rely on the measurements of glucose concentrations, which are static, as representative of the dynamic rate of glucose production and use in a neonate. In general, plasma glucose concentrations roughly correlate with glucose turnover. Diminished plasma glucose concentrations suggest that glucose production is limited or that glucose use is increased (i.e., need is outstripping production). Elevated plasma glucose concentrations suggest that either produc-

tion is excessive or, more likely, organ uptake and use are diminished. These are the dynamic physiologic conditions that define hypoglycemia and hyperglycemia.

In the neonate, glucose production correlates directly with brain and body mass, confirming the critical role of glucose as a metabolic fuel (49–52). This holds even in the most immature of premature infants (53). Glucose turnover for newborn infants, when related to body mass, significantly exceeds that of adults (Fig. 37-5). Premature infants have even greater turnover values than term neonates. This in part reflects the ratio of brain to body mass, which is greatest in premature infants and least in adults. These relations emphasize the importance of glucose as the primary fuel for the brain (Fig. 37-6).

Neonatal Hypoglycemia

A variety of blood and plasma glucose concentration values based on screening of neonates or clinical experience have been recommended as values defining hypoglycemia (54,55). All of these are somewhat arbitrary because they cannot be correlated directly with glucose use rate or severity of symptoms. Because plasma or blood glucose concentrations only roughly reflect glucose turnover, a plasma glucose concentration less than 40 mg/dL should be used to define hypoglycemia. When glucose turnover is sufficient to meet the needs of the organism, concentrations usually

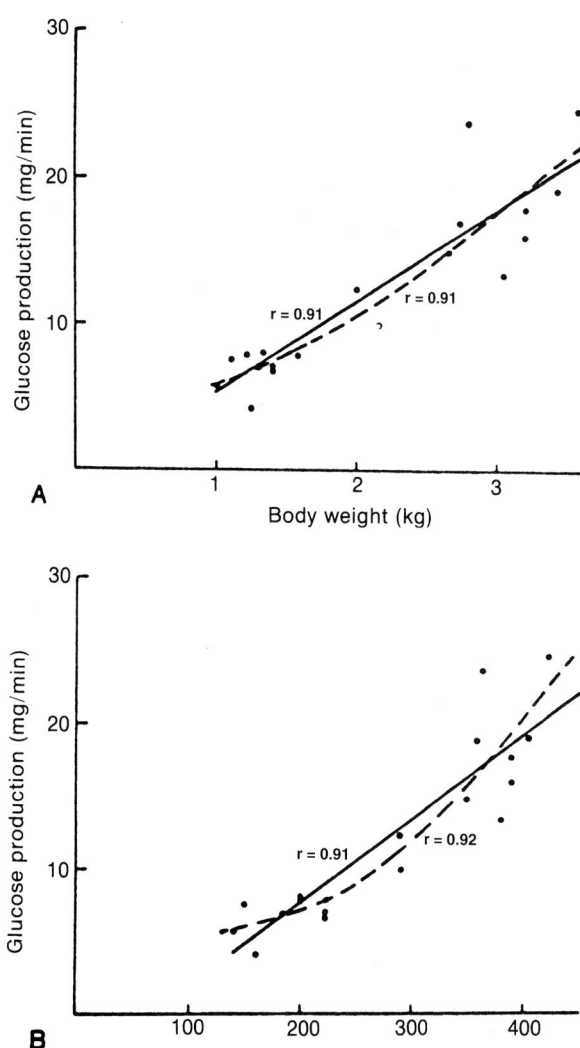

A Body weight (kg)

B Estimated brain weight (grams)

Figure 37-6 Linear and curvilinear regression analyses indicate strong relations between glucose turnover and body mass (A), and between glucose turnover and brain mass (B), in newborn human infants. (From Devaskar SU, Mueckler MM. The mammalian glucose transporters. *Pediatr Res* 1992;31:1–13, with permission.)

exceed this value. It also is important to note that values somewhat less than 40 mg/dL still can be associated with adequate glucose provision.

The chemical definition of hypoglycemia must take into account the methodology of glucose determination. Glucose concentration in whole blood is approximately 10% to 15% lower than that in plasma. Delay in determination after blood sampling may result in glucose oxidation by erythrocytes, causing falsely low values. Although the use of paper strip methods to estimate glucose concentrations quickly is acceptable, their results should be corroborated by true chemical determinations.

The clinical manifestations of inadequate glucose provision to the neonatal brain range from no symptoms to lethargy or mild tremors to frank convulsions (Table 37-1). The degree of glucose limitation necessary to cause brain damage is unknown. The lack of clearly defined data on this problem and the prevailing opinion concerning the

TABLE 37-1
SYMPTOMS OF HYPOGLYCEMIA
Jitteriness
Tremors
Apnea
Cyanosis
Limpness/lethargy
Seizures

potentially damaging effects of hypoglycemia mandate that infants at risk be monitored and that asymptomatic and symptomatic infants be appropriately treated.

All conditions associated with the development of hypoglycemia in the neonate result from one or a combination of two basic mechanisms: inadequate production or excessive tissue use. Inadequate glucose production results from a lack of glycogen stores, an inability to synthesize glucose, or both (Fig. 37-7). Excessive tissue use results from increased insulin secretion. Table 37-2 categorizes infants at risk for hypoglycemia in relation to these basic mechanisms.

Inadequate Glucose Production as a Result of Limited Glycogen Stores

Premature Infants

As indicated, the third trimester of pregnancy is an important period for hepatic glycogen deposition. An infant delivered prematurely without the benefit of part of or the entire third trimester will have limited hepatic glycogen stores. The greater the degree of prematurity, the less glycogen will be present. SGA premature infants are at extremely

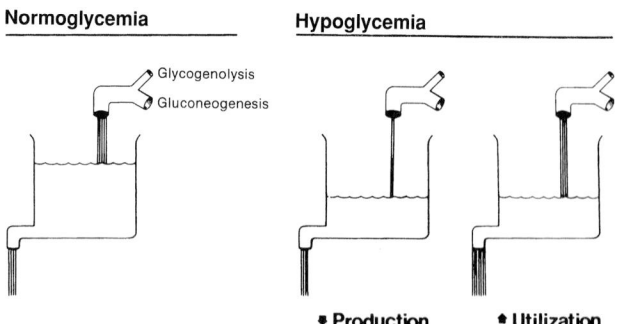

Figure 37-7 The rates of glucose production and utilization are represented by the faucet and drain of the sink. The level in the sink is equivalent to plasma or blood glucose concentrations. If production from glycogenolysis and gluconeogenesis is adequate, and use is not excessive, normoglycemia exists and the plasma or blood glucose concentration (i.e., the level in the sink) is normal. Hypoglycemia develops if production is inadequate to meet body needs or if use outstrips production. This results in decreased glucose concentrations (i.e., diminished level in sink). (From Kalhan SC, Bier DM, Savin SM, et al. Estimation of glucose turnover and 13C recycling in the human newborn by simultaneous [1-13C]glucose and [6,6-1H2]glucose tracers. *J Clin Endocrinol Metab* 1980; 50:456–460, with permission.)

TABLE 37-2
INFANTS AT RISK FOR HYPOGLYCEMIA[a]

Diminished production
  Limited glycogen
    SGA
    Prematurity
    Birth stress
    Glycogen storage disorders
  Limited gluconeogenesis
    SGA
    Inborn errors
Increased utilization
  Hyperinsulinism
    IDM
    Beckwith-Wiedemann syndrome
    Nesidioblastosis or pancreatic adenoma
    Erythroblastosis fetalis
    Exchange transfusion, chlorpropamide, benzothiazides,
      β-sympathomimetics, malpositioned UA catheter
Unknown
  LGA infants who are not IDM
  Sepsis
  Polycythemia or hyperviscosity syndrome
  Congenital hypopituitarism

[a] IDM, infant of diabetic mother; LGA, large for gestational age; SGA, small for gestational age; UA, umbilical artery.

high risk for development of hypoglycemia because available nutrients during intrauterine life are channeled toward growth, with little set aside for glycogen storage. For this reason, SGA premature infants have extremely limited glycogen stores (55–57).

Infants Who Have Suffered Perinatal Disease

Infants who are stressed *in utero* are at increased risk for development of hypoglycemia as neonates. Hypoxia, acidosis, and alterations in fetal blood pressure and flow can stimulate catecholamine secretion *in utero*, which in turn will mobilize hepatic glycogen stores. In addition, hypoxia increases the rate of anaerobic glycolysis, thereby accelerating glucose use. These events deplete fetal glycogen stores and place the infant at risk for hypoglycemia after delivery.

Glycogen Storage Disease

Intrinsic defects in glycogen synthesis, storage, or breakdown result in complex metabolic problems (see Chapter 41). Several types of glycogen storage disease (e.g., Ia, I, VI, 0) include hypoglycemia as one of many associated complications (54,58).

Inadequate Glucose Production as a Result of Limited Gluconeogenesis

Small-for-Gestational-Age Infants

Full-term and premature SGA neonates are at great risk for development of hypoglycemia as a result of inadequate

hepatic glycogen stores. With treatment, the hypoglycemia is usually short lived. Approximately 1% of SGA infants in whom hypoglycemia develops have a prolonged course requiring intravenous therapy for days. A delay in the induction of gluconeogenic capability probably is responsible for this prolonged hypoglycemia. These SGA neonates have elevated plasma concentrations of gluconeogenic precursors, suggesting an inability to convert exogenous gluconeogenic precursors, such as alanine, to glucose (59,60).

In animal models of intrauterine growth retardation, the induction of one gluconeogenic enzyme, phosphoenolpyruvate carboxykinase, is delayed (61,62). This occurs despite appropriate increases in glucagon and decreases in insulin; these relations should favor enzyme induction. Why some SGA infants fail to induce gluconeogenic capability is unclear. Corticosteroid therapy can be used to treat prolonged hypoglycemia. The success of this practice probably results in part from the ability of corticosteroids to induce hepatic gluconeogenic enzymes.

Many SGA infants have heightened metabolic requirements during the neonatal period. The mechanisms for this are not understood, but they may represent an attempt to compensate for the preceding intrauterine deprivation (63). This may explain the increased glucose requirements demonstrated by some hypoglycemic SGA infants.

Congenital Absence of Gluconeogenic Capability

Unlike SGA infants in whom gluconeogenic capability eventually develops, a few infants have been reported to have permanent congenital lack of gluconeogenic enzymes (64). A single infant who was unable to secrete glucagon also has been reported (65).

Excessive Tissue Use or Hyperinsulinism

A variety of disorders are associated with fetal and neonatal hyperinsulinism. In some disorders, the mechanisms for heightened beta-cell function are well understood, whereas in others, the pathogenesis is unclear. In the former category are infants of diabetic mothers (IDM) and infants with altered pancreatic islets caused by conditions such as nesidioblastosis and pancreatic adenoma. Those for whom an etiology is not clear include infants with erythroblastosis and Beckwith-Wiedemann syndrome. The finding of a hypoglycemic infant who is macrosomic and requires high rates of glucose infusion (10 to 20 mg/kg body weight per minute) suggests a hyperinsulinemic state.

Infants of Diabetic Mothers

IDM are at great risk for development of hypoglycemia as a result of the carryover of the fetal hyperinsulinemic state into neonatal life. They have elevated plasma insulin concentrations and release insulin briskly in response to glucose challenge. The problems of the IDM are presented in the following sections.

Nesidioblastosis—Persistent Hyperinsulinemic Hypoglycemia of Infancy

This condition is characterized by macrosomia and profound prolonged neonatal hypoglycemia due to hyperinsulinism. Several different accidents of development at the cell morphologic and molecular level cause persistent fetal and neonatal hyperinsulinism. Classically, in nesidioblastosis, pancreatic ductular cells are found in acinar tissue. In persistent hyperinsulinemic hypoglycemia, there can be focal hyperplasia of pancreatic islet cells or diffuse lesions of the entire pancreas (66–68). Focal lesions correspond to somatic defects and are, in some cases, related to mutations of sulfonylurea receptor 1 (69–71). Other forms of persistent hyperinsulinemic hypoglycemia of infancy include mutations of the potassium-linked ATP channel in beta cells (72).

Nesidioblastosis or persistent hyperinsulinemic hypoglycemia of infancy should be considered whenever a macrosomic infant has hypoglycemia with elevated plasma insulin concentrations over several days. Rebound hypoglycemia in response to excessive glucose administration is another characteristic. Increased insulin/glucose ratios and glucose requirements exceeding 10 mg/kg/min support the possibility of nesidioblastosis.

Surgical excision of a portion of the pancreas can provide definitive diagnosis and therapy. However, over the long term this may result in the development of diabetes mellitus in the patient. Both somatostatin and diazoxide have been used successfully to limit insulin secretion for as long as several months and may produce remission (73,74)

Unexplained Neonatal Hyperinsulinemia and Hypoglycemia

Infants with Beckwith-Wiedemann syndrome, erythroblastosis fetalis, and those whose mothers took chlorpropamide or benzothiazides are at risk for development of hypoglycemia as a result of hyperinsulinism. In 1964 Beckwith and colleagues (75) and Lazarus and associates (76) independently reported exophthalmos-macroglossia-gigantism syndrome. Such infants frequently have omphalocele, muscular macroglossia, macrosomia, and neonatal hypoglycemia. The hypoglycemia and macrosomia are caused by hyperinsulinism resulting from beta-cell hypertrophy. Some of the morbidity and mortality originally associated with this syndrome was related to unrecognized hypoglycemia. Thus, early recognition and prevention of hypoglycemia is mandatory. The gene responsible for many of the features of this syndrome is found on chromosome 11p15.5 (77). Because the insulin and insulin-like growth factor genes are closely located, combined gene dosage imbalance probably also contributes to the development of hyperinsulinism and hypoglycemia (78).

Infants with erythroblastosis fetalis caused by Rh incompatibility were reported in the past to be at risk for hypoglycemia from hyperinsulinism secondary to beta-cell hyperplasia (79). The mechanisms responsible for islet cell hyperplasia are unknown, although it was proposed that elevated plasma glutathione concentrations may stimulate the fetal beta cell to increase insulin secretion (80). The advent of direct intravascular transfusion of Rh-affected fetuses may reduce the risk of hypoglycemia. With this therapy, severely affected Rh fetuses that receive serial intravascular transfusions by the percutaneous umbilic technique are normoinsulinemic despite originally having elevated glutathione concentrations. Hypoglycemia does not develop in these fetuses after birth (81).

It is important to note that infants undergoing exchange transfusion are at risk for development of hypoglycemia because of stimulation of insulin secretion by glucose in stored erythrocytes (74). Checking for hypoglycemia during and after an exchange transfusion is therefore important.

Maternal use of chlorpropamide and benzothiazide can directly increase insulin secretion in the neonate (82,83). β-sympathomimetic agents used to stop premature labor have been reported to cause neonatal hypoglycemia (84). These drugs stimulate glycogen breakdown and gluconeogenesis in the mother and fetus (85). Both the increased availability of maternal glucose and the β-sympathomimetic agent that crosses the placenta stimulate fetal insulin secretion, resulting in neonatal hyperinsulinism and hypoglycemia. For these reasons, infants whose mothers received tocolytic therapy shortly before delivery should be monitored for hypoglycemia.

Some debate exists as to whether glucose administered to the mother during labor and delivery stimulates fetal beta-cell secretion and causes neonatal hyperinsulinism and hypoglycemia. Acute maternal glucose loading may stimulate fetal insulin secretion and increase the risk of neonatal hypoglycemia (86). If glucose infusion is well controlled, the likelihood of this is minimized. Control of maternal glucose administration is particularly important in situations in which the fetus is suspected of having heightened beta-cell sensitivity (e.g., maternal diabetes, Rh incompatibility) because under these circumstances even moderate excursions of glucose may stimulate fetal insulin secretion.

Malposition of the tip of an umbilic artery catheter at a level between the tenth thoracic and second lumbar vertebrae may result in glucose-stimulated hyperinsulinism. Several infants have been reported in whom hypoglycemia was relieved only when the tip of the umbilic artery catheter was repositioned. It has been proposed that glucose from the malpositioned catheter flows into the celiac axis, thereby stimulating insulin secretion (87). Animal studies have confirmed this possibility (88), which should be considered in unexplained cases of hypoglycemia.

Large-for-gestational-age (LGA) infants whose mothers do not have diabetes mellitus are at risk for transient hypoglycemia. This is particularly true of LGA infants of obese women (89). The mechanisms responsible for hypoglycemia are unknown, although limited data suggest that hyperinsulinism is not a major factor.

Sepsis in a neonate is often heralded by hypoglycemia or hyperglycemia. The mechanisms for this are not understood. Several studies have indicated rapid glucose disposal rates after intravenous challenge in septic term neonates. Although this suggests a hyperinsulinemic state, insulin secretion in these neonates was normal (90,91). The hyperglycemia and hypoglycemia that often precede the other signs of sepsis in premature infants may be catecholamine mediated.

Hypoglycemia is a well-acknowledged complication of neonatal polycythemia-hyperviscosity syndrome (92). Although polycythemia is more likely to occur in SGA and LGA infants who are at risk for hypoglycemia for other reasons, hypoglycemia also occurs at an increased rate in polycythemic appropriately grown infants. Animal studies have documented diminished cerebral glucose uptake with polycythemia; however, the mechanisms responsible for decreasing glucose provision are unknown (93). The increased erythrocyte mass is not sufficient to reduce glucose availability. The diminished plasma volume resulting from polycythemia may limit glucose provision. These possibilities remain to be confirmed.

Congenital hypopituitarism is a rare disorder in the neonate resulting from a spectrum of developmental accidents (94,95). Congenital absence of the anterior pituitary is the common cause of this disorder, although holoprosencephaly and optic disk dysplasia also have been associated. Affected male neonates have microphallus, whereas girls have normal external genitalia (96). Neonatal hypoglycemia often develops and can be severe. The endocrine alterations resulting from congenital hypopituitarism are complex, and the mechanisms by which they cause hypoglycemia are not understood. Congenital syphilis has been reported to cause hypopituitarism and this syndrome (97). Growth hormone is important in this regard because it can reverse hypoglycemia. Because hypoglycemia can develop later in the postnatal period, infants should have growth hormone therapy initiated for the long term.

Infants who have suffered hypothermia are at increased risk for development of hypoglycemia (98). This may result from increased availability of catecholamines (99), which would deplete glycogen reserves. Tissue use of glucose might also be increased under these conditions.

Other unusual clinical conditions reported in association with hypoglycemia include salicylate administration (100), congenital adrenal hyperplasia (101), and trisomy 13 mosaicism (102). The mechanisms for these phenomena are not known.

Hypoglycemia has been noted to sometimes occur in infants who suffer poor calorie intake for prolonged periods as a consequence of inadequate maternal breast milk production. The mechanisms for this are not known but probably involve glycogen depletion and diminished release of gluconeogenic precursors by striated muscle. Severe hepatic damage, most likely a result of impaired substrate transport and gluconeogenic capability, can also cause hypoglycemia. Disruption of intravenous glucose administration or rapid reduction in the rate of a glucose infusion can be associated with rebound hypoglycemia as a result of sluggish beta-cell responsiveness; insulin secretion may not decrease with appropriate rapidity and in response to cessation of exogenous glucose.

Neonatal Hyperglycemia

Hyperglycemia occurs primarily in three major groups of infants: those who are very premature, those who have neonatal diabetes mellitus, and those who are septic. Altered glucoregulation in response to sepsis was discussed in the preceding section (see Unexplained Neonatal Hyperinsulinemia and Hypoglycemia) (103,104).

The Very Premature Infant

Advances in perinatal care have improved the survival rate of the very premature infant. With this, the problem of glucose intolerance has greatly increased because the risk of hyperglycemia is at least 18 times greater in infants weighing under 1,000 grams than in those weighing more than 2,000 grams. Depending on the definition, age at screening, and type of intravenous solution administered, the incidence of hyperglycemia in very premature infants has been reported to range from 20% to 86% (103,104). In general, the smaller and more premature an infant, the greater the likelihood that he or she will not tolerate exogenous glucose at maintenance rates (4 to 6 mg/kg/minute). It is not uncommon to administer glucose at 1 to 2 mg/kg/minute or less and still observe plasma glucose concentrations exceeding 200 mg/dL.

Several basic mechanisms are probably responsible for glucose intolerance in very premature infants. Many probably do not secrete glucoregulatory hormones appropriately. In addition, end-organ response to these hormones may be blunted. Thus, endogenous glucose production may continue while tissue glucose uptake is limited despite intravenous glucose therapy. Limited data indicate that the premature infant will only slowly increase insulin secretion in response to glucose challenge (105–109). The amount secreted may not be sufficient to regulate glucose. Such infants may (108) or may not (110) decrease glucagon in response to glucose. In addition, very premature infants can be resistant to insulin (111). This resistance is accentuated by catecholamines, which are often quite elevated. These factors contribute to the limited ability of the premature infant to reduce glucose production in the same manner as the adult when exogenous glucose is provided (Fig. 37-8).

Neonatal Diabetes Mellitus

This is a rare disorder characterized by hypoinsulinism, progressive wasting, polyuria, and glycosuria during the neonatal period. Such infants usually are not ketotic. Of note, they are always SGA (112,113). The intrauterine growth

(mg·kg⁻¹min⁻¹)

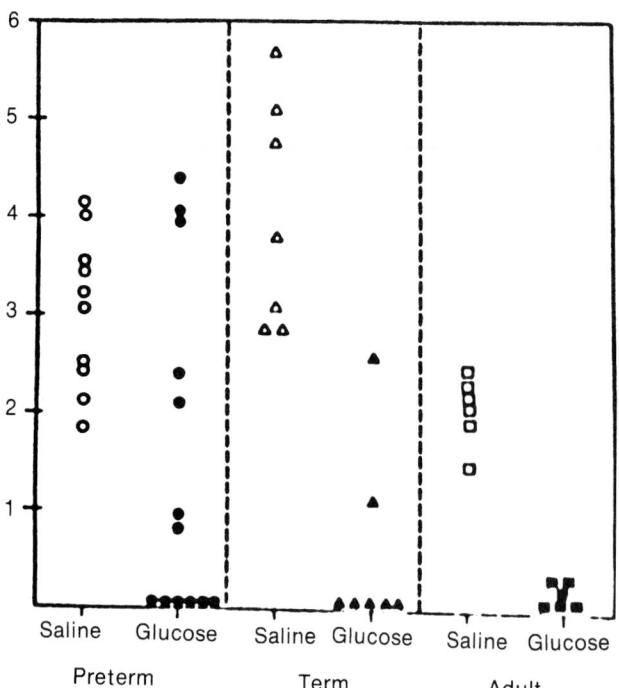

Figure 37-8 Hepatic glucose production rates in human premature neonates, full-term neonates, and adults during either saline (open symbols) or glucose (closed symbols) infusion. With glucose infusion, adults and full-term infants but not preterm infants reduce endogenous glucose production. Many preterm infants are apparently unable to regulate glucose production; this contributes to the development of hyperglycemia in these infants. (From Bower BD, Jones LF, Weeks MM. Cold injury in the newborn. A study of 70 cases. *Br Med J* 1960;5169:303–309, with permission.)

retardation results from limited fetal insulin secretion and exemplifies the importance of insulin as a fetal growth-stimulating hormone. This disorder may be heterogeneous with respect to etiology. Synthesis of an abnormal, poorly functioning insulin molecule or receptor deficiencies are other possible causes. Neonatal diabetes mellitus usually is transient; the early acute period calls for standard diabetic therapy (i.e., monitoring caloric intake and administering exogenous insulin).

DIAGNOSIS AND TREATMENT

Hypoglycemia

All infants at risk for development of hypoglycemia should undergo frequent plasma glucose determinations. The commercially available paper strip indicators are widely used. Because their accuracy is fair, it is desirable to confirm values close to hypoglycemia or hyperglycemia with laboratory chemical determinations. Infants at risk for hypoglycemia should be checked frequently during the first 4 hours of life and then at 4-hour intervals until the risk period has passed. If an infant is feeding, blood

sampling should be done before feeding. For IDM and SGA infants, the screening should continue for at least 24 hours.

Infants who have borderline asymptomatic hypoglycemia, who do not have respiratory distress syndrome (RDS) or other serious disorders, and who are capable of enteral feedings may receive either 5% dextrose solution or formula as their initial treatment. In general, this approach can be used for infants at term who are LGA or SGA. However, because this mode of therapy is not always successful, plasma or blood glucose concentrations must be checked shortly after feeding.

Intravenous administration of glucose in a quantity sufficient to meet tissue requirements is the treatment of choice for hypoglycemia. The administration of 10% or 15% dextrose solution at 5 to 10 mL/kg body weight, followed by a continuous infusion at 5 to 6 mg/kg body weight/minute, will increase plasma glucose concentrations to 40 mg/dL or greater and acutely meet tissue requirements. The maintenance rates may require adjustment depending on the etiology of hypoglycemia.

Glucagon and epinephrine increase glucose production. Because both mobilize hepatic glycogen stores, their efficacy in treating hypoglycemia is variable, particularly in infants with limited hepatic stores. The numerous cardiovascular effects of epinephrine also limit its usefulness in infants.

Infants who are hypoglycemic for prolonged periods as a result of an inability to produce glucose can be treated with corticosteroids (hydrocortisone 5 mg/kg/day every 12 hours; prednisone 2 mg/kg/day orally). Steroids exert some of their effects by inducing gluconeogenic enzyme activity.

Hyperglycemia

Hyperglycemia in low-birth-weight infants traditionally has been treated by reducing the rate of administration of exogenous glucose. This is something of a clinical paradox because such a reduction can theoretically limit glucose availability to the brain. Attempts in the past to provide exogenous insulin as a means to regulate glucose met with variable success, primarily because of technical difficulties in providing insulin (111,114,115). New insulin delivery systems designed for children and adults provide the means to deliver minute amounts of insulin under controlled conditions. These systems have finely tuned programmable pumps and tubing that does not bind insulin (116). Application of this technology has met with preliminary success (117). Individualized continuous insulin infusion to infants at 26 weeks of gestation weighing 700 to 800 grams enhanced glucose infusion and parenteral energy intake. Weight gain was significantly greater over 7 to 21 days compared with infants managed conventionally (Fig. 37-9). If further studies confirm these observations and clarify the potential metabolic consequences of this therapy, this method may prove beneficial in treating hyperglycemia in low-birth-weight infants.

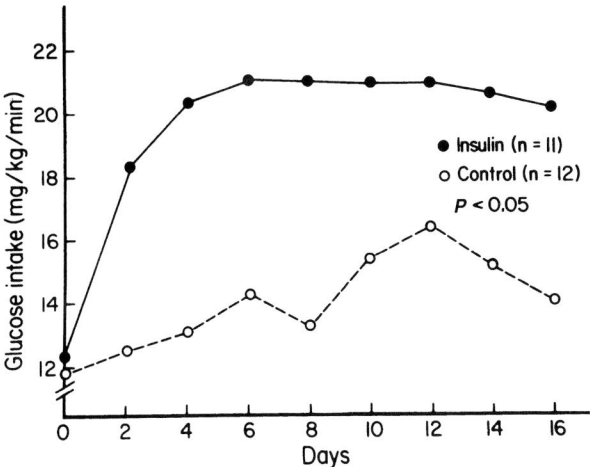

Figure 37-9 Mean glucose infusion rates per day in insulin-treated (solid line) and control (dashed line) very-low-birth-weight infants. The controlled administration of insulin significantly increased glucose infusion from day 2 to 16. (From Johansson EDB. Plasma levels of progesterone in pregnancy measured by a rapid competitive binding technique. *Acta Endocrinol (Copenh)* 1969;61: 607–617, with permission.)

CONSEQUENCES

Hypoglycemia

The clinical manifestations of inadequate glucose provision to the brain range from no symptoms to mild tremors to seizures. The issue of potential long-term sequelae of hypoglycemia remains unclear. This issue is complicated by the fact that hypoglycemia often occurs in infants who have coexisting conditions that also can cause brain damage. The observations suggesting that asymptomatic hypoglycemia poses less of a risk compared to symptomatic hypoglycemia are limited, as are the observations that associate prolonged hypoglycemia with a greater risk of brain damage than brief hypoglycemia. Limited data suggest that seizures associated with hypoglycemia worsen prognosis (118–127). Because of the uncertainty in this area, all hypoglycemic infants, symptomatic or not, should be appropriately treated.

Hyperglycemia

Hyperglycemia has been associated with an increased incidence of mortality, intracranial hemorrhage, and developmental delay in very premature infants. Whether hyperglycemia causes these problems or is merely associated with their development is unclear. Increased serum osmolarity resulting from hyperglycemia might disrupt cell-serum balance and cause cell injury (103). In addition, hyperglycemia can alter cell glucose transport, which may perturb cell metabolic functions.

Infants of Diabetic Mothers

Table 37-3 lists the frequently occurring problems of IDM categorized according to proposed mechanisms. The fetal

TABLE 37-3
PROBLEMS OF THE INFANT OF A DIABETIC MOTHER

Macrosomia or birth stress
Hypoglycemia
Respiratory distress syndrome
Intrauterine growth retardation
Hypocalcemia
Hyperbilirubinemia
Polycythemia or hyperviscosity
Cardiomyopathy
Congenital anomalies
Hyperinsulinism
Altered metabolic fuels, uteroplacental insufficiency
Decreased parathormone
Increased erythrocyte destruction, bruising

and neonatal hyperinsulinism central to many of these problems results from exaggerated provision of maternal metabolic fuels to the fetus, resulting in pancreatic beta-cell hypertrophy, hyperplasia, and hyperfunction (1,14). The alterations in maternal metabolism resulting from diabetes mellitus that are responsible for these and other effects on the fetus have been reviewed.

Altered Fetal Growth

Macrosomia, a clinical term suggesting excessive weight for gestational age, is a well-known characteristic of IDM (Fig. 37-10). Macrosomia in IDM results primarily from increased adiposity because IDM have both adipocyte hyperplasia and adipocyte hypertrophy (128). IDM also have excess nonfatty tissue. The liver and heart often are enlarged, and skeletal muscle increased. Much of this excess tissue is located in the shoulders and intrascapular area. Because IDM have normal brain growth, this results in a disproportionality between head and shoulder size and greatly increases the risk of shoulder dystocia (Fig. 37-11). This

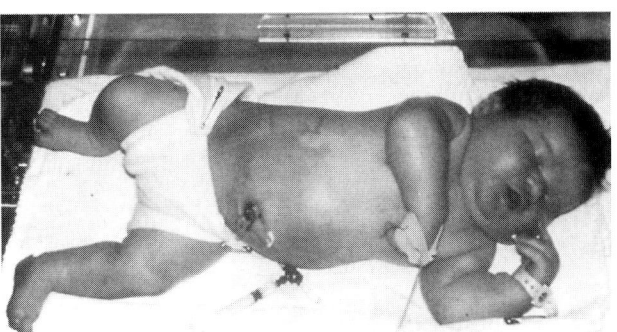

Figure 37-10 A macrosomic infant of a diabetic mother (IDM) has head circumference and length that are at the 90th percentile; the IDM's body weight greatly exceeds the 90th percentile. The IDM has considerable fat deposition in the shoulder and intrascapular area.

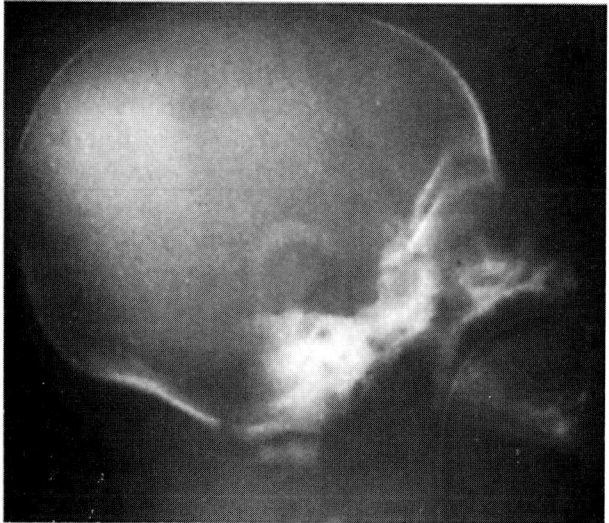

Figure 37-11 Lateral skull and neck radiograph of an infant of a diabetic mother after a difficult vaginal delivery. Infants of diabetic mothers are at extreme risk for shoulder dystocia, which can result in severe complications, such as separation of the C1-C2 cervical spine.

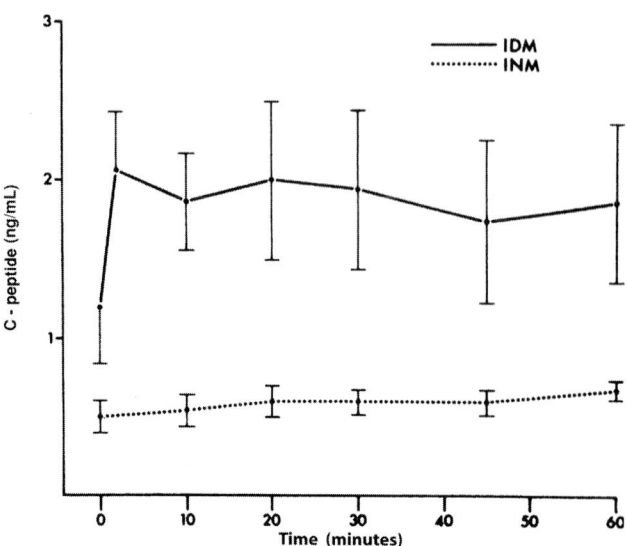

Figure 37-12 Beta-cell response to intravenous glucose challenge in infants of diabetic mothers (IDM) and infants of mothers with normal carbohydrate metabolism (INM). C-peptide is cleared from the proinsulin molecule when the beta cell is stimulated to secrete insulin. The measurement of C-peptide represents insulin on an equimolar basis and is a more accurate measure of beta-cell secretion than insulin in IDM. IDM exuberantly secrete insulin in response to glucose challenge. This adult-like response differs greatly from the normally expected sluggish insulin response of the INM. The significantly increased insulin concentration in IDM before glucose challenge (i.e., 0 minutes) indicates that basal insulin secretion also is elevated. The increased beta-cell function in IDM is responsible for their high incidence of hypoglycemia.

birth complication occurs far more frequently in macrosomic IDM than in large infants of mothers who do not have diabetes. Macrosomia is responsible for the great risk of birth trauma, meconium aspiration syndrome, persistent pulmonary hypertension, and high incidence of cesarean section delivery of IDM.

Because insulin has both mitogenic and anabolic effects in the fetus, the fetal hyperinsulinemic state is central to the development of macrosomia. The augmented production of insulin by the fetus stimulates the growth of insulin-sensitive tissues (e.g., adipose, muscle, connective) to cause macrosomia. Hepatic glycogen storage is exaggerated. The effect of insulin probably is mediated to some extent through stimulation of insulin-like growth factors (129). It is not surprising that head growth is normal in IDM during intrauterine life because insulin does not stimulate brain growth to any great extent.

The excess fat in IDM develops during the third trimester; IDM delivered before 30 weeks of gestation rarely are LGA. Serial fetal ultrasound measurements confirm that the fetal IDM does not exceed normal growth limits until 28 to 30 weeks of gestation (30). Despite improved maternal therapy, 20% to 30% of insulin-dependent diabetic women continue to bear macrosomic infants (130). Women with gestational diabetes, the mildest form of carbohydrate intolerance, have as great an incidence of macrosomia as women with preexisting diabetes.

Intrauterine growth retardation is another well-known complication of diabetes in pregnancy. The development of growth retardation has been attributed to maternal vascular disease, causing uteroplacental insufficiency. More recent data suggest that growth retardation may result from alterations in maternal metabolic fuel availability during early gestation (131).

Hypoglycemia

Approximately 25% to 50% of all IDM who manifest hypoglycemia will do so within the first 24 hours of life. Hypoglycemia is particularly likely to occur in macrosomic IDM because hyperinsulinism is responsible for both fetal overgrowth and hypoglycemia (Fig. 37-12) (132). Several studies also suggest that these IDM may fail to release glucagon or catecholamines in response to hypoglycemia (133). These hormonal alterations result in both increased glucose clearance and diminished glucose production.

Hypocalcemia and Hypomagnesemia

Hypocalcemia develops in 10% to 20% of IDM during the neonatal period. This usually occurs in association with hyperphosphatemia and occasionally with hypomagnesemia. Parathormone concentrations are significantly lower in IDM than in infants of nondiabetic mothers during the first 4 days of life (Fig. 37-13). This may be a result of hypomagnesemia, which limits parathormone secretion even in the presence of hypocalcemia. Maternal hypomagnesemia, which may occur from increased renal loss secondary to diabetes, is believed responsible for fetal and neonatal hypomagnesemia (134,135). Birth asphyxia, which frequently occurs in IDM, also causes hypocalcemia.

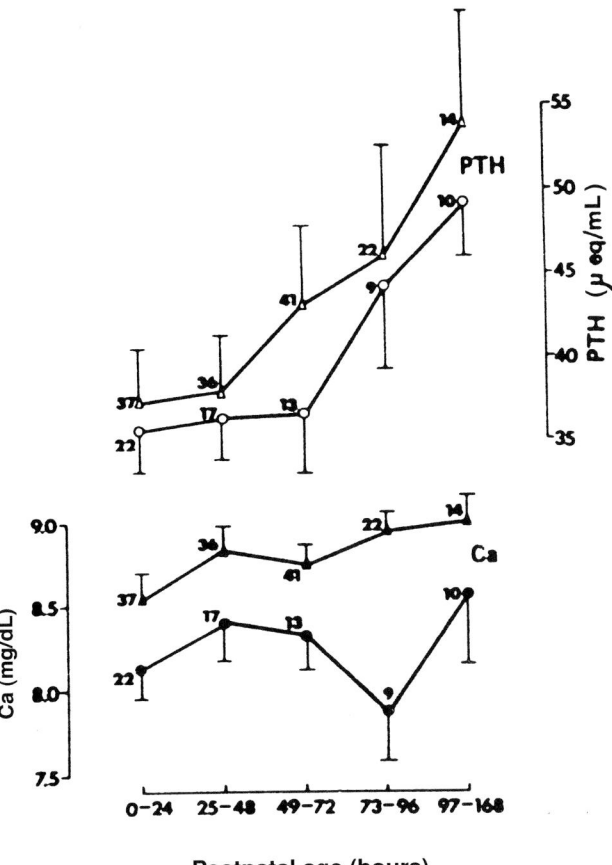

Figure 37-13   Parathormone (PTH) and calcium concentration in infants of diabetic mothers (circles) and full-term control (triangles) infants. Infants of diabetic mothers have lower plasma calcium and PTH concentrations during the first 6 days of life. (From Lucas A, Morley R, Cole TJ. Adverse neurodevelopmental outcome of moderate neonatal hypoglycaemia. *BMJ* 1988;297:1304–1308, with permission.)

Hyperbilirubinemia

Indirect hyperbilirubinemia develops in 20% to 25% of IDM. Their carbon monoxide production is increased as a result of increased hemoglobin breakdown and bilirubin production (136). The increased rate of erythrocyte breakdown in IDM is probably linked to altered erythrocyte membrane composition resulting from changes in maternal fuel availability. Polycythemia frequently occurs in IDM, and the normal breakdown of this increased erythrocyte mass also causes hyperbilirubinemia. Macrosomic IDM are often bruised at birth; the resultant resorption of blood also contributes to hyperbilirubinemia.

Hyperviscosity

IDM have a 10% to 20% risk of being polycythemic and developing neonatal hyperviscosity syndrome. Several factors are responsible for this. The hematocrit of umbilic-cord blood at birth tends to be elevated, probably as a result of increased erythropoiesis (137).

The increased incidence of renal vein thrombosis reported in IDM may be related to hyperviscosity, although this disorder does occur in IDM with normal hematocrits.

Unexpected Fetal Death

In the past, a high incidence of unexpected fetal death occurred in late gestation. Improvement in metabolic control of maternal diabetes throughout pregnancy and new methods to assess fetal status have decreased the incidence of this tragic complication. The mechanisms of unexpected fetal death are not completely understood. In the fetal sheep, sustained hyperglycemia is associated with increased insulin secretion, elevated fetal oxygen consumption, acidosis, and death (138). This could explain the association between poor maternal metabolic control and the increased risk of fetal death.

Respiratory Distress Syndrome

IDM are at increased risk of developing RDS. In the past, IDM were at a four- to six-fold greater risk for RDS than infants of nondiabetic mothers (139). This incidence has been reduced substantially by the recent emphasis on tight control of maternal metabolism. The increased risk of RDS in poorly regulated diabetic women is due in great part to fetal hyperinsulinism. Insulin adversely affects fetal lung maturation by inhibiting the development of enzymes necessary for the synthesis of the phospholipid components of surfactant (140). Standard methods to assess fetal lung maturity antenatally may not be applicable to a diabetic pregnancy. The measurement of phosphotidylglycerol has greatly improved this capability.

Cardiomyopathy

IDM are at increased risk for various cardiomyopathies (141). Many have thickening of the interventricular septum and left or right ventricular wall. The increased cardiac muscle mass results from the fetal hyperinsulinemic state. Most of these infants are asymptomatic, and the thickening is detected by electrocardiogram or echocardiogram. In a small fraction of infants, outflow obstruction severe enough to cause left ventricular failure may occur. These abnormalities generally regress over 3 to 6 months, and the condition appears to have no permanent effect on the myocardium. Those infants with congestive heart failure who survive the initial period with medical management also improve spontaneously.

Occasionally, IDM have severe congestive heart failure at birth. Frequently, these infants have suffered intrapartum asphyxia and are hypoglycemic and hypocalcemic. Such infants generally respond to assisted ventilation and correction of their metabolic abnormalities and usually recover completely. It is unclear whether heart failure results from the combined effects of hypoglycemia, hypocalcemia, and asphyxia on an inherently normal myocardium, or whether the myocardium is abnormal and therefore more susceptible to failure.

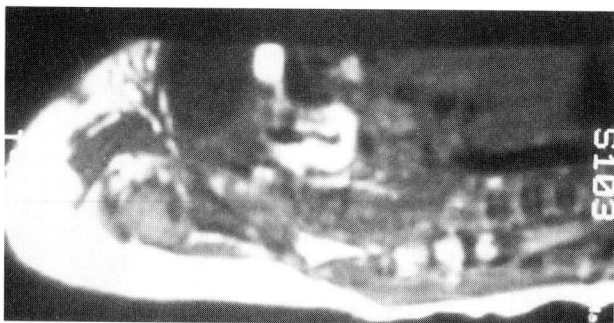

Figure 37-14 Magnetic resonance image of an infant of a diabetic mother. The infant has spinal agenesis-caudal regression syndrome. The spinal cord is interrupted, and hip-femur relationships are malformed.

Congenital Abnormalities

Major congenital malformations occur two to four times more frequently in IDM than in infants born to nondiabetic women. Although many abnormalities occur in IDM, ventricular septal defects, transposition of the great arteries, and spinal agenesis-caudal regression syndrome occur with particular frequency (Fig. 37-14). Neural tube defects, gastrointestinal atresia, and urinary tract malformations also are relatively common. A transient anomaly unique to IDM is known as the neonatal small left colon, microcolon, or lazy colon syndrome. This condition presents as gastrointestinal obstruction, and barium contrast studies suggest congenital aganglionic megacolon. Unlike infants with Hirschsprung disease, these infants have normal innervation of the bowel and ultimately have normal bowel function.

Poor control of maternal diabetes during the first trimester, a critical period of organogenesis, has been proposed as the mechanism for the increased incidence of malformations (142,143). IDM with congenital abnormalities generally have normal karyotypes (144). *In vitro* studies using embryos of laboratory animals have demonstrated that altering metabolic fuels can produce profound malformations (145). Clinical studies, however, have not confirmed a relation between birth defects and alterations in maternal metabolic variables (146).

Postnatal Problems

The postnatal problems of IDM are consistent in the Barker hypothesis which links intrauterine disorders with adverse adult outcomes (147). IDM are at increased risk for development of obesity in later life, compared to infants of mothers with normal carbohydrate metabolism (148). Studies suggest that *in utero* hyperinsulinism may be responsible for this postnatal phenomenon. IDM who become obese during childhood have the severest hyperinsulinism *in utero* (149).

Whether maternal diabetes adversely affects the long-term cognitive development of the offspring remains unanswered. In the past, the increased incidence of birth trauma and neonatal disorders probably contributed to an increased risk of poor outcome. Studies suggest that altered maternal metabolic fuel availability also may have an effect. An inverse correlation has been reported between childhood IQ and degree of abnormality of second- and third-trimester maternal lipid metabolism (150). This is consistent with the potential detrimental effect of ketones on fetal brain development.

A yet unanswered question is whether IDM develop diabetes mellitus during postnatal life. Children and adults who were IDM have an increased incidence of diabetes mellitus. Limited data suggest that offspring of fathers with insulin-dependent diabetes have a five-fold greater risk for development of diabetes mellitus than offspring of insulin-dependent diabetic mothers. Although diabetes is in part a genetic disorder, it has not been possible to delineate precisely the mode of inheritance in IDM. It is possible that the altered metabolic state of the diabetic pregnancy may modulate this genetic predisposition. Noninsulin-dependent diabetes mellitus occurs by age 20 years in 45.5% of infants of insulin-dependent diabetic mothers but in only 8.6% and 1.4% of prediabetic and nondiabetic mothers, respectively. The mechanisms by which alterations in maternal glucose and other metabolic fuels alter fetal beta-cell function are unknown.

REFERENCES

1. Freinkel N. Banting lecture 1980. Of pregnancy and progeny. *Diabetes* 1980;29:1023–1035.
2. Hytten ET, Leitch I. *The physiology of human pregnancy*, 2nd ed. Oxford: Blackwell Scientific, 1971.
3. Kalkhoff R, Schalch DS, Walker JL, et al. Diabetogenic factors associated with pregnancy. *Trans Assoc Am Physicians* 1964;77:270–280.
4. Lind T, Billewicz WZ, Brown G. A serial study of changes occurring in the oral glucose tolerance test during pregnancy. *J Obstet Gynaecol Br Commonw* 1973;80:1033–1039.
5. Spellacy WN, Goetz FC. Plasma insulin in normal late pregnancy. *N Engl J Med* 1963;268:988–991.
6. Catalano PM, Tyzbir ED, Roman NM, et al. Longitudinal changes in insulin release and insulin resistance in nonobese pregnant women. *Am J Obstet Gynecol* 1991;165:1667–1672.
7. Spellacy WN, Goetz FC, Greenberg BZ, et al. Plasma insulin in normal "early" pregnancy. *Obstet Gynecol* 1965;25:862–865.
8. Bleicher SJ, O'Sullivan JB, Freinkel N. Carbohydrate metabolism in pregnancy. V. The interrelations of glucose, insulin and free fatty acids in late pregnancy and post-partum. *N Engl J Med* 1964;271:866–872.
9. Grumbach M, Kaplan SL, Sciarra JJ, et al. Chronic growth hormone- prolactin (CGP) secretion; disposition, biologic activity in man, and postulated function as the "growth hormone" of the second half of pregnancy. *Ann N Y Acad Sci* 1968;148:501–531.
10. Johansson EDB. Plasma levels of progesterone in pregnancy measured by a rapid competitive binding technique. *Acta Endocrinol (Copenh)* 1969;61:607–617.
11. Buchanan TA, Catalano PM. The pathogenesis of GDM: implications for diabetes after pregnancy. *Diabetes Rev* 1995;3:584–601.
12. Tsibris JCM, Raynor LO, Buhi WC, et al. Insulin receptors in circulating erythrocytes and monocytes from women on oral contraceptives or pregnant women near term. *J Clin Endocrinol Metab* 1980;51:711–717.
13. Moore P, Kolterman O, Weyant J, et al. Insulin binding in human pregnancy: comparisons to the postpartum, luteal, and follicular states. *J Clin Endocrinol Metab* 1981;52:937–941.

14. Pedersen J. *The pregnant diabetic and her newborn*, 2nd ed. Baltimore: Williams & Wilkins, 1977.

15. Felig P, Lynch V. [Starvation in human pregnancy: hypoglycemia, hypoinsulinemia, and hyperketonemia.] *Science* 1970; 170:990–992.

16. Kalhan SC, D'Angelo LJ, Savin SM, et al. Glucose production in pregnant women at term gestation. Sources of glucose for human fetus. *J Clin Invest* 1979;63:388–394.

17. Ogata ES, Metzger BE, Freinkel N. Carbohydrate metabolism in pregnancy. XVI. Longitudinal estimates of the effects of pregnancy on D-(6-3H) glucose and D-(6-14C) glucose turnovers during fasting in the rat. *Metabolism* 1981;30:487–492.

18. Scow RO, Chernick SS, Brinley MS. Hyperlipemia and ketosis in the pregnant rat. *Am J Physiol* 1964;206:796–804.

19. Patel MS, Johnson CA, Rajan R, et al. The metabolism of ketone bodies in developing human brain: development of ketone-body-utilizing enzymes and ketone bodies as precursors for lipid synthesis. *J Neurochem* 1975;25:905–908.

20. Churchill JA, Berendes HW, Nemore J. Neuropsychological deficits in children of diabetic mothers. *Am J Obstet Gynecol* 1969;105:257–268.

21. Shelley HJ. Glycogen reserves and their changes at birth and in anoxia. *Br Med Bull* 1961;17:137–143.

22. Schwartz AL, Rall TW. Hormonal regulation of incorporation of alanine-U-14C into glucose in human fetal liver explants. Effect of dibutyryl cyclic AMP, glucagon, insulin, and triamcinolone. *Diabetes* 1975;24:650–657.

23. Schwartz AL, Rall TW. Hormonal regulation of glycogen metabolism in human fetal liver. II. Regulation of glycogen synthase activity. *Diabetes* 1975;24:1113–1122.

24. Greengard O. Enzymatic differentiation of human liver: comparison with the rat model. *Pediatr Res* 1977;11:669–676.

25. Raiha NC, Lindros KO. Development of some enzymes involved in gluconeogenesis in human liver. *Ann Med Exp Biol Fenn* 1969;47:146–150.

26. Kaplan SL, Grumbach MM, Shepard TH. The ontogenesis of human fetal hormones. I. Growth hormone and insulin. *J Clin Invest* 1972;51:3080–3093.

27. Assan R, Buillet J. Pancreatic glucagon and glucagon-like material in tissues and plasma from human fetuses 6 to 26 weeks old. In: Jonxis JHP, Visser HKA, Troelstra JA, eds. *Metabolic processes in the fetus and newborn infant, nutrition symposium*. Baltimore: Williams & Wilkins, 1971:210–.

28. Schaeffer LD, Wilder ML, Williams RH. Secretion and content of insulin and glucagon in human fetal pancreas slices in vitro. *Proc Soc Exp Biol Med* 1973;143:314–319.

29. Grasso S, Distefano G, Messina A, et al. Effect of glucose priming on insulin response in the premature infant. *Diabetes* 1975;24:291–294.

30. Milner RDG. The development of insulin secretion in man. In: Jonxis JHP, Visser HKA, Troelstra JA, eds. *Metabolic processes in the fetus and newborn infant, nutrition symposium*. Baltimore: Williams & Wilkins, 1971:310.

31. Grasso S, Messina A, Distefano G, et al. Insulin secretion in the premature infant. Response to glucose and amino acids. *Diabetes* 1973;22:349–353.

32. Wise JK, Lyall SS, Hendler R, et al. Evidence of stimulation of glucagon secretion by alanine in the human fetus at term. *J Clin Endocrinol Metab* 1973;37:341–344.

33. Hill DE. Effect of insulin on fetal growth. *Semin Perinatol* 1978;2:319–328.

34. Susa JB, McCormick KL, Widness JA, et al. Chronic hyperinsulinemia in the fetal rhesus monkey: effects on fetal growth and composition. *Diabetes* 1979;28:1058–1063.

35. Ogata ES, Sabbagha R, Metzger BE, et al. Serial ultrasonography to assess evolving fetal macrosomia. Studies in 23 pregnant diabetic women. *JAMA* 1980;243:2405–2408.

36. Pedersen J. Weight and length at birth of infants of diabetic mothers. *Acta Endocrinol (Copenh)* 1954;16:330–342.

37. Girard JR, Caquet D, Bal D. Control of rat liver phosphorylase, glucose-6-phosphatase and phosphoenolpyruvate carboxykinase activities by insulin and glucagon during the perinatal period. *Enzyme* 1973;15:272–285.

38. Girard JR, Ferré A, Kervran A, et al. Role of the insulin/glucagon ratio in the changes of hepatic metabolism during development of the rat. In: Foa PP, Bajaj JS, Foa NL, eds. *Glucagon: its role in physiology and clinical medicine*. New York: Springer-Verlag, 1977:563–581.

39. Sperling MA, DeLamater PV, Phelps D, et al. Spontaneous and amino acid-stimulated glucagon secretion in the immediate postnatal period. Relation to glucose and insulin. *J Clin Invest* 1974;53:1159–1166.

40. Padbury J, Agata Y, Ludlow J, et al. Effect of fetal adrenalectomy on catecholamine release and physiologic adaptation at birth in sheep. *J Clin Invest* 1987;80:1096–1103.

41. Agata Y, Padbury JF, Ludlow JK, et al. The effect of chemical sympathectomy on catecholamine release at birth. *Pediatr Res* 1986; 20:1338–1344.

42. Grajwer LA, Sperling MA, Sack J, et al. Possible mechanisms and significance of the neonatal surge in glucagon secretion: studies in newborn lambs. *Pediatr Res* 1977;11:833–836.

43. Molsted-Pedersen L. Aspects of carbohydrate metabolism in newborn infants of diabetic mothers. II. Neonatal changes in K values. *Acta Endocrinol (Copenh)* 1972;69:189–194.

44. Bell GI, Kayano T, Buse JB, et al. Molecular biology of mammalian glucose transporters. *Diabetes Care* 1990;13:198–208.

45. Devaskar SU, Mueckler MM. The mammalian glucose transporters. *Pediatr Res* 1992;31:1–13.

46. Takata K, Kasahara T, Kasahara M, et al. Localization of erythrocyte/Hep G2 type glucose transport (GLUT1) in human placental villi. *Cell Tissue Res* 1992;267:407–412.

47. Simmons RA, Flozak A, Ogata ES. The effect of insulin and insulin-like growth factor-I on glucose transport in normal and small for gestational age fetal rats. *Endocrinology* 1993;133:1361–1368.

48. Sciullo E, Cardellini G, Baroni MG, et al. Glucose transporter (Glut1, Glut3) mRNA in human placenta of diabetic and non-diabetic pregnancies. *Early Pregnancy* 1997;3:172–182.

49. Bier DM, Arnold KJ, Sherman WR, et al. In-vivo measurement of glucose and alanine metabolism with stable isotopic tracers. *Diabetes* 1977;26:1005–1015.

50. Bier DM, Leake RD, Haymond MW, et al. Measurement of "true" glucose production rates in infancy and childhood with 6,6-dideuteroglucose. *Diabetes* 1977;26:1016–1023.

51. Kalhan SC, Bier DM, Savin SM, et al. Estimation of glucose turnover and 13C recycling in the human newborn by simultaneous [1-13C]glucose and [6,6-1H2]glucose tracers. *J Clin Endocrinol Metab* 1980;50:456–460.

52. Kalhan SC, Savin SM, Adam PAJ. Measurement of glucose turnover in the human newborn with glucose-1-13C. *J Clin Endocrinol Metab* 1976;43:704–707.

53. Sunebag A, Ewald U, Larsson A, et al. Glucose production rate in extremely immature neonate (<28 weeks) studied by use of deuterated glucose. *Pediatr Res* 1993;33:97–100.

54. Cornblath M, Schwartz R. *Disorders of carbohydrate metabolism in infancy*, 3rd ed. Boston: Blackwell Scientific, 1991.

55. Pagliara AS, Karl IE, Haymond M, et al. Hypoglycemia in infancy and childhood: parts I and II. *J Pediatr* 1973;82:365–379,558–577.

56. Ogata ES. Carbohydrate metabolism in the fetus and neonate and altered neonatal glucoregulation. *Pediatr Clin North Am* 1986;33:25–45.

57. Lubchenco LO, Bard H. Incidence of hypoglycemia in newborn infants classified by birth weight and gestational age. *Pediatrics* 1971;47:831–838.

58. Greene HL. Glycogen storage disease. *Semin Liver Dis* 1982;2: 291–301.

59. Haymond MW, Karl IE, Pagliara AS. Increased gluconeogenic substrates in the small-for-gestational-age infant. *N Engl J Med* 1974;291:322–328.

60. Mestyan J, Soltesz G, Schultz K, et al. Hyperaminoacidemia due to the accumulation of gluconeogenic amino acid precursors in hypoglycemic small-for-gestational age infants. *J Pediatr* 1975; 87:409–414.

61. Bussey ME, Finley S, LaBarbera A, et al. Hypoglycemia in the newborn growth-retarded rat: delayed phosphoenolpyruvate carboxykinase induction despite increased glucagon availability. *Pediatr Res* 1985;19:363–367.

62. Pollak A, Susa JB, Stonestreet BS, et al. Phosphoenolpyruvate carboxykinase in experimental intrauterine growth retardation in rats. *Pediatr Res* 1979;13:175–177.

63. Sinclair JC, Silverman WA. Intrauterine growth in active tissue mass of the human fetus, with particular reference to the undergrown baby. *Pediatrics* 1966;38:48–62.

64. Vidnes J, Sovik O. Gluconeogenesis in infancy and childhood. II. Studies on the glucose production from alanine in three cases

of persistent neonatal hypoglycaemia. *Acta Paediatr Scand* 1976; 65:297–305.

65. Vidnes J, Oyasaeter S. Glucagon deficiency causing severe neonatal hypoglycemia in a patient with normal insulin secretion. *Pediatr Res* 1977;11:943–949.

66. Garces LY, Drash A, Kenny FM. Islet cell tumor in the neonate. Studies in carbohydrate metabolism and therapeutic response. *Pediatrics* 1968;41:789–796.

67. Heitz PU, Kloppel G, Hacki WH, et al. Nesidioblastosis: the pathologic basis of persistent hyperinsulinemic hypoglycemia in infants. Morphologic and quantitative analysis of seven cases based on specific immunostaining and electron microscopy. *Diabetes* 1977;26:632–642.

68. Salinas ED Jr, Mangurten HH, Roberts SS, et al. Functioning islet cell adenoma in the newborn. Report of a case with failure of diazoxide. *Pediatrics* 1968;41:646–653.

69. Otonkoski T, Ammala C, Huopio H, et al. A point mutation inactivating the sulfonylurea receptor causes the severe form of persistent hyperinsulinemic hypoglycemia of infants in Finland. *Diabetes* 1999;48:408–415.

70. Fournet JC, Verkarre V, De Longlay P, et al. Loss of imprinted genes and paternal SUR1 mutations lead to hyperinsulinism in focal adenomatous hyperplasia. *Ann Endocrinol (Paris)* 1998;59: 485–491.

71. de Lonlay-Debeney P, Fournet JC, Martin D, et al. [Persistent hyperinsulinemic hypoglycemia in the newborn and infants.] *Arch Pediatr* 1998;5:1347–1352.

72. Aguilar-Bryan L, Bryan J. Molecular biology of adenosine triphosphate-sensitive potassium channels. *Endocr Rev* 1999;20: 101–135.

73. Otonkoski T, Andersson S, Simell O. Somatostatin regulation of beta-cell function in the normal human fetuses and in neonates with persistent hyperinsulinemic hypoglycemia. *J Clin Endocrinol Metab* 1993;76:184–188.

74. Leibowitz G, Glaser B, Higazi AA, et al. Hyperinsulinemic hypoglycemia of infancy (nesidioblastosis) in clinical remission: high incidence of diabetes mellitus and persistent beta-cell dysfunction at long-term follow-up. *J Clin Endocrinol Metab* 1995;80:386–392.

75. Beckwith JB. Macroglossia, omphalocele, adrenal cytomegaly, gigantism, and hyperplastic visceromegaly. *Birth Defects* 1969;5:188–196.

76. Lazarus L, Young JD, Friend JC. EMG syndrome and carbohydrate metabolism. *Lancet* 1968;2:1347–1348.

77. Normal AM, Read AP, Clayton-Smith J, et al. Recurrent Wiedemann-Beckwith syndrome with inversion of chromosome (11) (p11.2p15.5). *Am J Med Genet* 1992;42:638–641.

78. Weksburg R, Shen DR, Fei YL, et al. Disruption of insulin-like growth factor 2 imprinting in Beckwith-Wiedemann syndrome. *Nat Genet* 1993;5:143–150.

79. Barrett CT, Oliver TK Jr. Hypoglycemia and hyperinsulinism in infants with erythroblastosis fetalis. *N Engl J Med* 1968;278: 1260–1262.

80. Steinke J, Gries FA, Driscoll SG. In vitro studies of insulin inactivation with reference to erythroblastosis fetalis. *Blood* 1967;30: 359–363.

81. Socol ML, Dooley SL, Ney JA, et al. Absence of hyperinsulinemia in isoimmunized fetuses treated with intravascular transfusion. *Am J Obstet Gynecol* 1991;165:1737–1740.

82. Senior B, Slone D, Shapiro S, et al. Benzothiadiazines and neonatal hypoglycaemia. *Lancet* 1976;2:377.

83. Zucker P, Simon G. Prolonged symptomatic neonatal hypoglycemia associated with maternal chlorpropamide therapy. *Pediatrics* 1968;42:824–825.

84. Brazy JE, Pupkin MJ. Effects of maternal isoxsuprine administration on preterm infants. *J Pediatr* 1979;94:444–448.

85. Ogata ES. Isoxsuprine infusion in the rat: alterations in maternal, fetal and neonatal glucose homeostasis. *J Perinat Med* 1981;9:293–301.

86. Kenepp NB, Kumar S, Shelley WC, et al. Fetal and neonatal hazards of maternal hydration with 5% dextrose before caesarean section. *Lancet* 1982;1:1150–1152.

87. Nagel JW, Sims S, Aplin CE 2nd, et al. Refractory hypoglycemia associated with a malpositioned umbilical artery catheter. *Pediatrics* 1979;64:315–317.

88. Cowett RM, Tenenbaum DG, Fatoba O, et al. The effects of arterial glucose infusion above the celiac axis in the neonatal lamb. *Biol Neonate* 1985;47:179–185.

89. Kliegman R, Gross T, Morton S, et al. Intrauterine growth and postnatal fasting metabolism in infants of obese mothers. *J Pediatr* 1984;104:601–607.

90. Leake RD, Fiser RH Jr, Oh W. Rapid glucose disappearance in infants with infection. *Clin Pediatr (Phila)* 1981;20:397–401.

91. Yeung CY, Lee VWY, Yeung CM. Glucose disappearance rate in neonatal infection. *J Pediatr* 1973;82:486–489.

92. Wiswell TE, Cornish JD, Northam RS. Neonatal polycythemia: frequency of clinical manifestations and other associated findings. *Pediatrics* 1986;78:26–30.

93. Rosenkrantz TS, Philipps AF, Skrzypczak PS, et al. Cerebral metabolism in the newborn lamb with polycythemia. *Pediatr Res* 1988;23:329–333.

94. Lovinger RD, Kaplan SL, Grumbach MM. Congenital hypopituitarism associated with neonatal hypoglycemia and microphallus: four cases secondary to hypothalamic hormone deficiencies. *J Pediatr* 1975;87:1171–1181.

95. Johnson JD, Hansen RC, Albritton WL, et al. Hypoplasia of the anterior pituitary and neonatal hypoglycemia. *J Pediatr* 1973; 82:634–641.

96. Kauschansky A, Genel M, Smith GJ. Congenital hypopituitarism in female infants. Its association with hypoglycemia and hypothyroidism. *Am J Dis Child* 1979;133:165–169.

97. Daaboul JJ, Kartchner W, Jones KL. Neonatal hypoglycemia caused by hypopituitarism in infants with congenital syphilis. *J Pediatr* 1993;123:983–985.

98. Bower BD, Jones LF, Weeks MM. Cold injury in the newborn. A study of 70 cases. *Br Med J* 1960;5169:303–309.

99. Schiff D, Stern L, Leduc J. Chemical thermogenesis in newborn infants: catecholamine excretion and the plasma non-esterified fatty acid response to cold exposure. *Pediatrics* 1966;37:577–582.

100. Pickering D, Ellis H. Neonatal hypoglycaemia due to salicylate poisoning. *Proc R Soc Med* 1968;61:1256.

101. Gemelli M, De Luca F, Barberio G. Hypoglycaemia and congenital adrenal hyperplasia. *Acta Paediatr Scand* 1979;68:285–286.

102. Smith VS, Giacoia GP. Hyperinsulinaemic hypoglycaemia in an infant with mosaic trisomy 13. *J Med Genet* 1985;22:228–230.

103. Pildes RS. Neonatal hyperglycemia. *J Pediatr* 1986;109:905–907.

104. Dweck HS, Cassady G. Glucose intolerance in infants of very low birth weight. I. Incidence of hyperglycemia in infants of birth weights 1,100 grams or less. *Pediatrics* 1974;53:189–195.

105. Cowett RM, Oh W, Schwartz R. Persistent glucose production during glucose infusion in the neonate. *J Clin Invest* 1983;71: 467–475.

106. Hertz DG, Karn CA, Liu YM, et al. Intravenous glucose suppresses glucose production but not proteolysis in extremely premature newborns. *J Clin Invest* 1993;92:1752–1758.

107. Lilien LD, Rosenfield RL, Baccaro MM, et al. Hyperglycemia in stressed small premature neonates. *J Pediatr* 1979;94:454–459.

108. Massi-Benedetti F, Falorni A, Luyckx A, et al. Inhibition of glucagon secretion in the human newborn by simultaneous administration of glucose and insulin. *Horm Metab Res* 1974;6: 392–396.

109. Zarif M, Pildes RS, Vidyasagar D. Insulin and growth-hormone responses in neonatal hyperglycemia. *Diabetes* 1976;25:428–433.

110. Grasso S, Fallucca F, Mazzone D, et al. Inhibition of glucagon secretion in the human newborn by glucose infusion. *Diabetes* 1983;32:489–492.

111. Goldman SL, Hirata T. Attenuated response to insulin in very low birthweight infants. *Pediatr Res* 1980;14:50–53.

112. Gentz JCH, Cornblath M. Transient diabetes of the newborn. *Adv Pediatr* 1969;16:345–363.

113. Hutchison JH, Keay AJ, Kerr MM. Congenital temporary diabetes mellitus. *Br Med J* 1962;5302:436–440.

114. Vaucher YE, Walson PD, Morrow G 3rd. Continuous insulin infusion in hyperglycemic, very low birth weight infants. *J Pediatr Gastroenterol Nutr* 1982;1:211–217.

115. Binder ND, Raschko PK, Benda GI, et al. Insulin infusion with parenteral nutrition in extremely low birth weight infants with hyperglycemia. *J Pediatr* 1989;114:273–280.

116. Ostertag SG, Jovanovic L, Lewis B, et al. Insulin pump therapy in the very low birth weight infant. *Pediatrics* 1986;78:625–630.

117. Collins JW Jr, Hoppe M, Brown K, et al. A controlled trial of insulin infusion and parenteral nutrition in extremely low birth weight infants with glucose intolerance. *J Pediatr* 1991;118: 921–927.

118. Creery RDG. Hypoglycaemia in the newborn: diagnosis, treatment and prognosis. *Dev Med Child Neurol* 1966;8:746–754.
119. Haworth JC. Neonatal hypoglycemia: how much does it damage the brain? *Pediatrics* 1974;54:3–4.
120. Haworth JC, McRae KN. Neonatal hypoglycemia: a six-year experience. *J Lancet* 1967;87:41–45.
121. Haworth JC, Vidyasagar D. Hypoglycemia in the newborn. *Clin Obstet Gynecol* 1971;14:821–839.
122. Koivisto M, Blanco-Sequeiros M, Krause U. Neonatal symptomatic and asymptomatic hypoglycaemia: a follow-up study of 151 children. *Dev Med Child Neurol* 1972;14:603–614.
123. Pildes RS, Cornblath M, Warren I, et al. A prospective controlled study of neonatal hypoglycemia. *Pediatrics* 1974;54:5–14.
124. Pildes R, Forbes AE, O'Connor SM, et al. The incidence of neonatal hypoglycemia—a completed survey. *J Pediatr* 1967;70:76–80.
125. Raivio KO. Neonatal hypoglycemia. II. A clinical study of 44 idiopathic cases with special reference to corticosteroid treatment. *Acta Paediatr Scand* 1968;57:540–546.
126. Griffiths AD, Bryant GM. Assessment of effects of neonatal hypoglycaemia. A study of 41 cases with matched controls. *Arch Dis Child* 1971;46:819–827.
127. Lucas A, Morley R, Cole TJ. Adverse neurodevelopmental outcome of moderate neonatal hypoglycaemia. *BMJ* 1988;297:1304–1308.
128. Fee BA, Weil WB Jr. Body composition of infants of diabetic mothers by direct analysis. *Ann N Y Acad Sci* 1963;110:869–897.
129. Roth S, Abernathy MP, Lee WH, et al. Insulin-like growth factors I and II peptide and messenger RNA levels in macrosomic infants of diabetic pregnancies. *J Soc Gynecol Investig* 1996;3:78–84.
130. Ogata ES, Freinkel N, Metzger BE, et al. Perinatal islet function in gestational diabetes: assessment by cord plasma C-peptide and amniotic fluid insulin. *Diabetes Care* 1980;3:425–429.
131. Eriksson UJ, Lewis NJ, Freinkel N. Growth retardation during early organogenesis in embryos of experimentally diabetic rats. *Diabetes* 1984;33:281–284.
132. Sosenko IR, Kitzmiller JL, Loo SW, et al. The infant of the diabetic mother: correlation of increased cord C-peptide levels with macrosomia and hypoglycemia. *N Engl J Med* 1979;301:859–862.
133. Stern L, Ramos A, Leduc J. Urinary catecholamine excretion in infants of diabetic mothers. *Pediatrics* 1968;42:598–605.
134. Schedewie HK, Odell WD, Fisher DA, et al. Parathormone and perinatal calcium homeostasis. *Pediatr Res* 1979;13:1–6.
135. Noguchi A, Eren M, Tsang RC. Parathyroid hormone in hypocalcemic and normocalcemic infants of diabetic mothers. *J Pediatr* 1980;97:112–114.
136. Stevenson DK, Bartoletti AL, Ostrander CR, et al. Pulmonary excretion of carbon monoxide in the human infant as an index of bilirubin production. II. Infants of diabetic mothers. *J Pediatr* 1979;94:956–958.
137. Widness JA, Susa JB, Garcia JF, et al. Increased erythropoiesis and elevated erythropoietin in infants born to diabetic mothers and in hyperinsulinemic rhesus fetuses. *J Clin Invest* 1981;67:637–642.
138. Philips AF, Dubin JW, Matty PJ, et al. Arterial hypoxemia and hyperinsulinemia in the chronically hyperglycemic fetal lamb. *Pediatr Res* 1982;16:653–658.
139. Robert MF, Neff RK, Hubbell JP, et al. Association between maternal diabetes and the respiratory-distress syndrome in the newborn. *N Engl J Med* 1976;294:357–360.
140. Bourbon JR, Farrell PM. Fetal lung development in the diabetic pregnancy. *Pediatr Res* 1985;19:253–267.
141. Gutgesell HP, Speer ME, Rosenberg HS. Characterization of the cardiomyopathy in infants of diabetic mothers. *Circulation* 1980;61:441–450.
142. Miller E, Hare JW, Cloherty JP, et al. Elevated maternal hemoglobin A1c in early pregnancy and major congenital anomalies in infants of diabetic mothers. *N Engl J Med* 1981;304:1331–1334.
143. Fuhrmann K, Reiher H, Semmler K, et al. Prevention of congenital malformations in infants of insulin-dependent diabetic mothers. *Diabetes Care* 1983;6:219–223.
144. Simpson JL, Elias S, Martin AO, et al. Diabetes in pregnancy, Northwestern University series (1977–1981). I. Prospective study of anomalies in offspring of mothers with diabetes mellitus. *Am J Obstet Gynecol* 1983;146:263–270.
145. Freinkel N, Lewis NJ, Akazawa S, et al. The honeybee syndrome—implications of the teratogenicity of mannose in rat-embryo culture. *N Engl J Med* 1984;310:223–230.
146. Mills JL, Knopp RH, Simpson JL, et al. Lack of relation of increased malformation rates in infants of diabetic mothers to glycemic control during organogenesis. *N Engl J Med* 1988;318:671–676.
147. Barker DJ, Eriksson JG, Forsen T, et al. Fetal origins of adult disease: strength of effects and biological basis. *Int J Epidemiol* 2002;31:1235–1239.
148. Vohr BR, Lipsitt LP, Oh W. Somatic growth of children of diabetic mothers with reference to birth size. *J Pediatr* 1980;97:196–199.
149. Metzger BE, Silverman BL, Freinkel N, et al. Amniotic fluid insulin concentration as a predictor of obesity. *Arch Dis Child* 1990;65:1050–1052.
150. Rizzo T, Metzger BE, Burns WJ, et al. Correlations between antepartum maternal metabolism and child intelligence. *N Engl J Med* 1991;325:911–916

Congenital Anomalies

38

Scott Douglas McLean

Much of our practice of pediatrics and neonatology is geared toward the provision of acute care, such as resuscitation, antibiotics, and intravenous fluids. When we encounter a newborn with one or more birth defects, this acute-care paradigm remains—and appropriately so—in the forefront of our clinical perspective. However, the child with a congenital anomaly must also be simultaneously considered from a different perspective, one that looks far back and far forward in time. When did this structural abnormality have its origin? Was there a teratogenic exposure during a critical period of organogenesis? Has a new mutation occurred in one of the parents' germ cells? Are some of the DNA alterations in this newborn ancient relics that only now reveal themselves in the living world? Is this congenital anomaly a clue to the presence of other pathology? Will our best efforts have a reasonable chance of ensuring long-term health? Will siblings or offspring be similarly affected?

Over the past several decades, research has dramatically improved our insights into the genetic and environmental causes of many isolated birth defects, multiple congenital anomaly syndromes, and other genetic conditions. In some instances, the molecular pathology has been dissected in impressive detail, such as for cystic fibrosis (CF) and the CF transmembrane regulator gene on chromosome 7q31. For other conditions, such as the VACTERL association, we have yet to understand the genomic origins but have accumulated much clinical and epidemiologic data that allow us to formulate helpful diagnostic criteria, predict prognosis, and estimate recurrence risks. For any individual newborn with a congenital anomaly, establishing an accurate diagnosis is the key to intelligent clinical management in both the short and long term.

In a busy nursery, caring for a newborn with a congenital malformation is nearly a daily activity. Although the consultative services of a clinical geneticist or dysmorphologist often are quite helpful, this resource may not be available, and the attending pediatrician or neonatologist must assume that role, at least temporarily. Naturally, such a task brings many challenges—cognitive, managerial, and emotional—for which the practitioner often feels underprepared. Useful tools include a careful prenatal history, three-generation pedigree, meticulous physical examination, and sensitivity for the emotional and social impact of the birth of a malformed child. A dramatically visible departure from the norm multiplies a parent's fear, concern, worry, and guilt and might also become very stressful for nurses and physicians. Consequently, to optimize care for the infant and to instill confidence and control in an intrinsically unsettling situation, the clinical leaders of the health care team should prepare themselves by becoming familiar with a general strategy for diagnosis and management of an infant with congenital malformations.

In aggregate, birth defects are ubiquitously common and have likely been so throughout human history. Epidemiologic studies consistently place the incidence of major malformations in newborns at 2% to 3% (1,2). Many other neonates harbor occult anomalies that are eventually detected later in childhood, giving a cumulative rate of major birth defects of approximately 4%, or one of every 25 newborn children. In the United States, 150,000 children with birth defects are born each year. Congenital anomalies are the leading cause of infant mortality and the second leading cause of death in children between the ages of 1 and 4 years (3). Excluding the intangible costs of pain and suffering, the lifetime economic cost per child in 1992 ranged from $75,000 to $503,000 (4). The Centers for Disease Control and the National Birth Defects Prevention Network conduct and facilitate a number of research and surveillance activities, central to which is the commitment of individual practitioners to diagnose and report all congenital defects accurately and reliably.

DEFINITIONS AND CLASSIFICATIONS

A congenital anomaly is any alteration, present at birth, of normal anatomic structure. It may be major or minor, isolated or part of a larger constellation of defects, of clear or uncertain cause. Several genetic and environmental etiologies are well delineated (Table 38-1), but the fundamental etiology of nearly half of all birth defects is unknown (5).

The nomenclature for various birth defects and malformation syndromes can be a source of confusion for both the novice and veteran clinician alike. Categories of anomalies

TABLE 38-1
CAUSES OF MALFORMATIONS IN NEWBORNS[a]

	Percent
Chromosome abnormalities	10.1
Single mutant genes	3.1
Familial	14.5
Multifactorial inheritance	23.0
Teratogens	3.2
Uterine factors	2.5
Twinning	0.4
Unknown cause	43.2

[a] Modified from Nelson K, Holmes LB. Malformations due to presumed spontaneous mutations in newborn infants. N Engl J Med 1989; 320:19, with permission.

may seem arbitrary and capricious, but a developmental or embryologic perspective often will cast light on the rationale behind a particular designation. The term "birth defect," enjoys wide usage and conveys immediate meaning for parents. "Congenital anomaly" is fundamentally equivalent, indicating an abnormality of anatomic structure present at birth and may be further refined in terms of severity ("major" and "minor"), pathogenesis ("malformation," "deformation," "disruption," "dysplasia"), or pattern ("isolated," "syndromic"). These terms are defined in Table 38-2.

The great majority of congenital anomalies occur in isolation, as a single phenomenon, and are postulated to arise because of a primary, intrinsic malformation of a fetal structure that occurs at 10 weeks of gestation or earlier. On occasion, other family members are similarly affected, implying the presence of a single gene mutation that behaves as an autosomal dominant, autosomal recessive, or X-linked trait. More commonly, however, the family history is entirely bereft of other affected individuals. Classic mendelian genetics does not adequately explain this situation, but another model—multifactorial inheritance—has proven quite useful.

In the multifactoral model, a constellation of influences, including multiple genes inherited from each parent, and poorly defined environmental influences, seems to allow a developing fetal structure to cross a threshold of "liability," beyond which morphogenesis proceeds abnormally (6). These birth defects tend to recur at a low rate, approximately 3% to 5% for each subsequent pregnancy for the parents of one affected child, 10% to 15% if two siblings have previously been similarly affected.

Multiple congenital malformations, on the other hand, are caused by a very different spectrum of fundamental problems. For a child with several major anomalies, the underlying cause is more likely to be a malformation sequence, developmental field defect, association, or syndrome, each of which may in turn may be caused by a chromosomal anomaly, a single-gene mutation, a teratogen, or unknown factors. Minor anomalies deserve special attention because, in terms of diagnostic significance, they are frequently the equals of the major malformations (7), often providing the linchpin of clinical recognition of a rare

TABLE 38-2
TERMINOLOGY

Major anomaly	An anatomic abnormality severe enough to reduce normal life expectancy or compromise normal function; e.g., neural tube defect, cleft lip.
Minor anomaly	A structural alteration that either requires no treatment or can be corrected in a straightforward manner, with no permanent consequences, and present in less than 4% of the normal population; e.g., preauricular skin tag, small ventricular septal defect.
Minor variant	A physical feature, often familial, that is present in only a small proportion (1%–5%) of normal individuals, e.g., simian crease of the palm, epicanthal folds.
Malformation	A morphologic defect of an organ, part of an organ, or region due to an *intrinsically abnormal developmental process*; e.g., microphthalmia, ectrodactyly.
Deformation	An abnormal form, shape, or position of a part of the body caused by *unusual mechanical forces on normal tissue*; e.g., club foot, plagiocephaly.
Disruption	A morphologic defect due to extrinsic interference with a normal developmental process resulting in *breakdown of normal tissue*; e.g., amniotic band sequence, fetal alcohol syndrome.
Sequence	Several anomalies that occur due to a cascade of events, caused by a single initiating event or anomaly; e.g., Potter sequence, Pierre Robin sequence.
Developmental field defect	A set of morphologic defects that share a common or contiguous region during embryogenesis; e.g., hemifacial microsomia.
Association	A nonrandom set of anomalies in which the specific components occur together more frequently than would be expected by chance and for which cause is not established; e.g., VACTERL association, CHARGE association.
Syndrome	A recognizable pattern of anomalies that "run together;" e.g., Down syndrome, Smith–Lemli–Opitz syndrome.

VACTERL: Vertebral defects, imperforate Anus, congenital Cardiac anomalies, TracheoEsophageal fistula, Radial defects, Renal dysplasia, and other Limb malformations.
CHARGE: Coloboma, Heart disease, Atresia choanae, Retarded growth and development and/or CNS anomalies, Genital hypoplasia, and Ear anomalies or deafness.

syndrome. A single minor anomaly is present in 13% of neonates, but more than one is decidedly less common—two minor anomalies occur in only 1%, and three minor anomalies in just 0.05% (8). As the numbers of minor anomalies increase, the search for occult major anomalies and the consideration that a syndromic diagnosis is possible should increase proportionately.

MANAGEMENT STRATEGY

Since the last edition of this textbook, the American College of Medical Genetics (ACMG), under the sponsorship of the New York State Department of Health, has published clinical guidelines for health care practitioners who care for newborn infants with one or more birth defects (9). This document incorporates expert opinion from a broad array of disciplines and describes practical, detailed components of the history, physical examination, differential diagnosis, diagnostic stratagem, genetic counseling, and record keeping. As such, the ACMG guidelines represent a significant step forward in promoting a national standard of care with which neonatologists, pediatricians, and family practitioners should become familiar.

The fundamental approach to managing an infant with one or more congenital anomalies is much the same as the management of any other clinical scenario. Effective clinical intervention is organized around an understanding of the natural history of the condition at hand. History taking begins with conception and includes a detailed three-generation pedigree. Physical features must be scrutinized, measured, and documented with precision, and confirmatory studies must be carefully chosen and accurately interpreted. Common pitfalls include incomplete ascertainment of all relevant information, impetuous diagnosis and prognostication, and failure to communicate with parents in a straightforward and compassionate manner.

Neonates with congenital malformations present with extremely variable clinical needs, so a "one size fits all" strategy for management has limited practical value. However, a number of algorithmic approaches have proven useful. In the ACMG clinical management algorithm (Fig. 38-1), an early determination of whether the malformation is isolated or multiple helps organize subsequent clinical activity. Beyond this, the major thrust of activity is devoted to pursuing and establishing a precise diagnosis, the essential starting point for understanding natural history, designing effective intervention, and educating the family about recurrence risks and prenatal management options for subsequent pregnancies. Another, more integrated approach suggested by Dr. Judith Hall (10) delineates three parallel and simultaneous lines of activity, as outlined in Fig. 38-2. Urgent interventions for the infant are undertaken immediately. Also, from the outset, the family is provided with support in the form of information, preliminary interpretation, and acknowledgment of their distress and concern. The third concurrent activity is data collection—history, physical, laboratory studies and imaging, and preliminary definition of

the nature of the problem. All efforts should be made to verify information and to amass a complete database.

History

Prenatal information, beginning with conception, must be specifically sought from both the mother and her obstetric records. The nature and timing of maternal illnesses, such as rubella or cytomegalovirus infections, including febrile episodes, can suggest a direct infectious disruption. Maternal use of alcohol, drugs, medications, or tobacco—degree, gestational timing, and duration—should be documented. Quickening, the date at which there is maternal sensation of fetal movement, and the subsequent vigor and frequency of fetal activity, reflects central nervous system integrity and peripheral muscular function. Prenatal ultrasonography, especially if performed serially and in detail, may yield critical information regarding the amount of amniotic fluid and malformations of the kidneys, brain, heart, skeleton, and gastrointestinal system. Recent reports have suggested an association between in vitro fertilization and several genetic conditions, such as Angelman syndrome (11), retinoblastoma (12) and Beckwith-Wiedemann syndrome (13). Chorionic villus sampling has previously been suspected to cause limb-reduction deformities, but recent studies by the World Health Organization affirm its safety for first-trimester prenatal diagnosis (14). A review of the ultrasound studies and the obstetric record, and a discussion with the attending obstetrician or perinatologist, can save valuable time and effort. Maternal serum and amniotic fluid α-fetoprotein levels and prenatal chromosome studies should be verified and documented in the infant's medical record. Late trimester problems with fetal position, such as transverse or breech lie, potentially indicate neuromuscular or structural abnormalities of the fetus. Fetuses with significant neuromuscular problems often encounter perinatal distress and have a poor transition to extrauterine life. Finally, it often is useful to inquire about any prenatal event or factors that the parents suspect, even remotely, may have caused their infant's problems. Concerns about witnessing a solar or lunar eclipse, for example, are best made explicit, if only for the purpose of assuaging guilt.

Family History

A systematic and detailed inquiry into the age, health, development, and congenital anomalies of all members of the immediate family comprises the core of an adequate family history. All second-degree relatives, such as grandparents, aunts, uncles, nieces, and nephews, should be considered, and more distant relatives may contribute valuable data. A three-generation pedigree provides a concise picture of patterns of inheritance. One must specifically clarify the biologic parentage for each individual. Spontaneous abortions, miscarriages, stillbirths, and infant deaths clearly are germane, but parents typically omit this information unless the interviewer specifically inquires. Consanguinity also should be directly but tactfully questioned. A "quick pedigree" is an

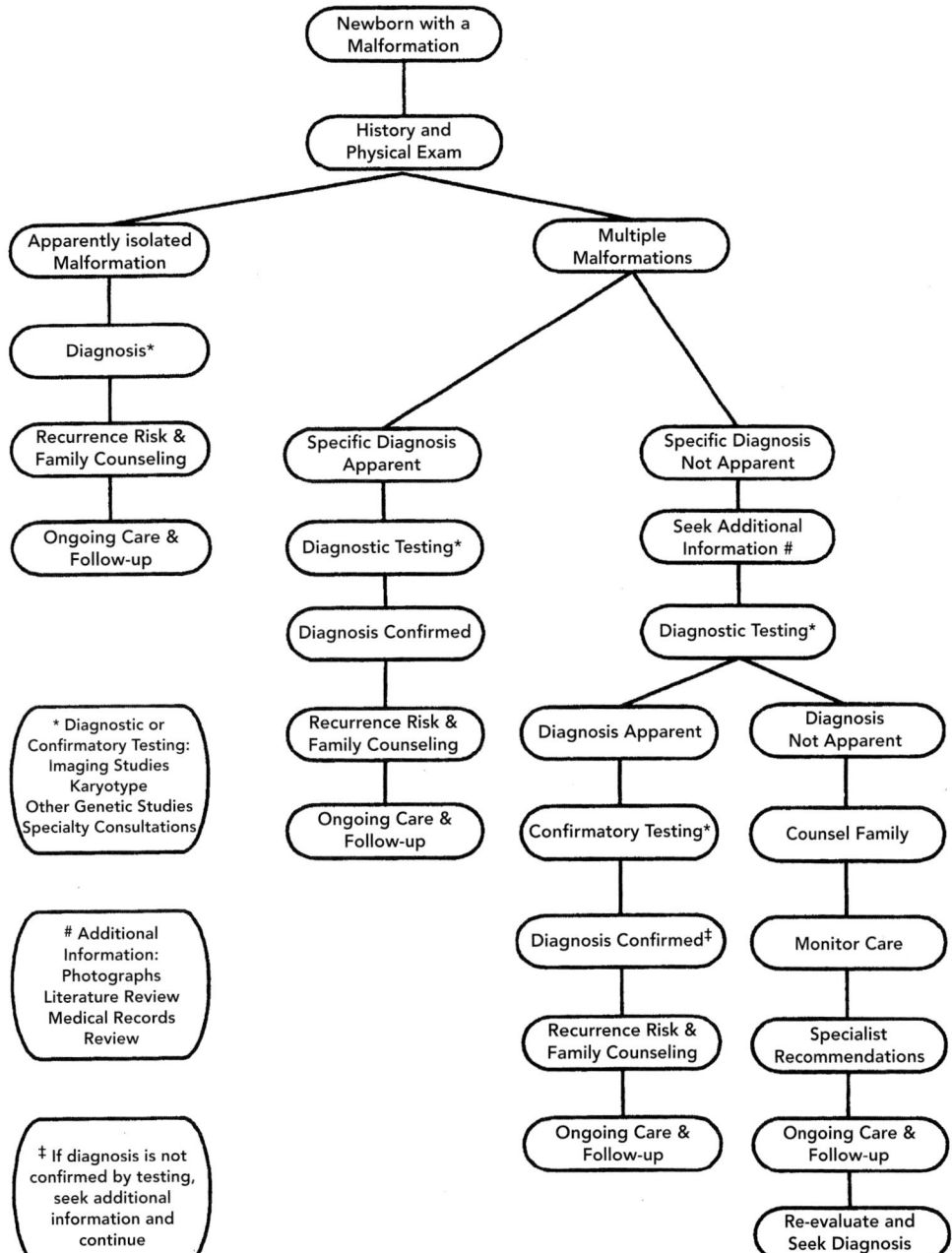

Figure 38-1 Management algorithm for the infant with multiple congenital anomalies. Reprinted from American College of Medical Genetics Foundation, sponsored by the New York State Department of Health. Evaluation of the newborn with single or multiple congenital anomalies: a clinical guideline. May 1999. Available at http://www.health.state.ny.us/nysdoh/dpprd/main.htm. Accessed 1/1/05, with permission.

oxymoron; routinely the entire process requires patience and time. With this in mind, the interviewer will be sympathetic, on the day of delivery, to parents who are understandably terrified, exhausted, and disoriented. After rest, time, and a chance to speak with relatives, they may be more prepared to help refine and expand on their complete family history.

Physical Examination

It is axiomatic that a proper newborn physical examination is detailed and complete. The careful observer, especially

one who repeats the examination several times, will recognize departures from the norm. Several points are worth keeping in mind when examining infants with a malformation or a generalized dysmorphic appearance.

- Be alert. There is a heightened chance that additional, initially unsuspected anomalies are present. Although a malformation may be minor in severity, it might represent the most important, critical clue to the diagnosis.
- Collect "clues" systematically, by closely examining each topographical segment of the body and by scrutinizing progressively more detailed regions. For example, on

Gather Data	Therapeutic Intervention	Psychosocial Support
History	**Resuscitation**	family
prenatal		staff
perinatal	**Urgent procedures**	**Within 24 hours**
family		meet with family
Physical examination	**Formulate overall plan**	define anomalies
detailed		discuss
multisystem	**Define long-term issues**	investigation
measurements		intervention
family members	**Preventive measures**	**At regular intervals**
Ancillary studies	Genetic counseling	review diagnosis
photographs		reformulate plans
radiographs	**Reevaluate** plans and	continue support
cytogenetics	therapies regularly	
DNA analysis		
Define problem(s)		
categorize process		
<u>diagnosis</u>		

Figure 38-2 Integrated approach to management. Modified from reference 48.

initial observation it may be noted that the fingers are disproportionately short; a closer examination may reveal that the fourth and fifth fingers are stiff and rigidly extended, with faint flexion creases, especially at the distal interphalangeal joints, that the nails are short and narrow, almost absent on the fifth finger. The placenta may be examined with the obstetrician or pathologist to seek evidence of cryptic twinning, umbilical cord anomalies, or amniotic bands.

■ Document the examination with great care, using appropriate morphologic terms and sufficient detail, and strongly consider supplementing written findings with clinical photographs. Parental consent for photographs should be documented.

■ Measure those features that are obviously or potentially abnormal in size, shape, position, or symmetry. Normal standards are available for virtually any anatomic structure, encompassing all ages from preterm infant to adulthood (15,16). Hall (7) admonishes, "Never make a clinical judgment on a measurable parameter without measuring it."

■ Examine both parents, if possible, seeking any signs of similar anomalies. Dominant conditions frequently manifest a subtle but distinctive phenotype in adults.

Adjunctive Investigations

The emerging clinical picture will dictate imaging studies and consultations with pediatric subspecialists. For exam-

ple, a newborn with Down syndrome, even when a cardiac murmur is absent, merits the attention of a pediatric cardiologist, because significant structural defects of the heart are present in 50% but may be missed on clinical examination. A newborn girl with puffy hands and feet, a webbed neck, and coarctation of the aorta also should receive a renal ultrasound, because kidney malformations commonly are associated with Turner syndrome. When the diagnosis is unclear and several malformations are present, occult anomalies of the central nervous system, heart, kidneys, vertebrae, and eyes are reasonable to pursue, especially when the known birth defects are multiple and severe. Renal ultrasounds are often ordered when the neonate has a single umbilical artery or an ear malformation, such as a preauricular pit. In the absence of supporting findings, such as other malformations, a family history of deafness or renal anomalies, or maternal diabetes, this investigation is unlikely to be useful (17). Skeletal films, to include hands, feet, long bones, pelvis, vertebrae, chest, and cranium, are helpful when length is less then the 5th percentile for gestational age or when the limbs are disproportionately short. These studies often require interpretation by a pediatric radiologist skilled in this area.

Chromosomal Analysis

Forty-six chromosomes are present in most normal human cells. Formation of ova and sperm, however, is a surprisingly error-prone process: nearly two-thirds of all fertilizations result in aneuploidy or abnormal chromosomal number or structure, with subsequent reproductive loss. Some of this prenatal loss occurs late enough to be recognized as a miscarriage or spontaneous abortion, but most wastage is occult. Ninety-eight percent of these chromosomal defects are lethal (13).

An abnormal karyotype occurs in one of 170 liveborn infants. Among chromosomally abnormal neonates, one-third have an extra sex chromosome with mild or no phenotypic manifestations in the newborn period, one-fourth have trisomy of an autosome, such as trisomy 21 or trisomy 18, and 40% have a variation of chromosomal structure, such as a deleted or duplicated segment or a translocation. Of the latter, most (79%) are balanced and generally do not cause birth defects. Approximately 10% of infants who die in the perinatal period secondary to multiple congenital malformations have abnormal cytogenetic studies (13).

Which infants deserve chromosomal studies? Truly isolated malformations are very infrequently caused by a cytogenetic defect. On the other hand, neonates with multiple major malformations or a generalized dysmorphic appearance, and stillborn infants, with or without malformations, should have cytogenetic testing. Between these extremes lies a sizable gray area. Factors in favor of chromosomal testing include intrauterine growth retardation, an abnormal neurologic exam, a major malformation accompanied by several minor malformations, and a history of multiple pregnancy losses for the mother or in close relatives.

Peripheral blood lymphocytes are the tissue of choice for most cytogenetic analysis, but many other tissues can be used, including skin fibroblasts, bone marrow, placenta, and pericardium, usually harvested postmortem. Two to three milliliters of venous or arterial blood, collected in a sodium heparin (green top) tube, are generally sufficient and should be kept at room temperature or refrigerated, never frozen, in transit. The cells usually will remain viable for 1 or 2 days, but the shortest possible transit time increases the chances for useful results. If the sample is shipped, an overnight courier is recommended. The lymphocytes are separated, incubated in the presence of a mitogen to stimulate cell division, which is then abruptly halted with colchicine, and the cell membranes are disrupted gently while being placed on a glass slide. After enzymatic preparation and staining, the "spread" of chromosomes is analyzed in approximately 20 cells. Generally, 550 or more bands are visible with Giemsa staining of 46 chromosomes at metaphase. Several cells are photographed and arranged in standard groupings, a karyotype. Turnaround time for cytogenetic analysis is typically three to four days, although some laboratories are able to provide results in slightly less time. Because of the high percentage of dividing cells in bone marrow, karyotypes from this tissue may be obtained in a matter of hours, although the quality of the banding frequently is inadequate for high-resolution analysis of small or subtle abnormalities. To achieve the latter, a special request for prometaphase analysis should accompany a peripheral blood sample.

In the past several years, an increasing number of syndromic conditions have been found to be caused by very small chromosomal deletions that are not visible by routine karyotyping, even at pro-metaphase levels of detail. Molecular probes that will hybridize at these loci with great specificity have been developed. These DNA probes are complexed with a fluorescent marker and become powerful tools for detecting submicroscopic chromosomal deletions. This technique, termed fluorescent in situ hybridization (FISH), has also been adapted for whole, entire chromosomes and can identify the nature of many chromosomal anomalies, such as translocations. A metaphase spread can, in essence, be painted with several single-locus or whole-chromosome FISH probes simultaneously, providing a highly specific, and colorful, picture of genomic structure.

Among children with mental retardation of unknown etiology, in whom extensive investigations, including standard cytogenetic studies, are normal, approximately 5% harbor very small, occult chromosomal deletions or unbalanced translocations. A recently developed technique—subtelomeric probe analysis—uses FISH and/or other molecular tools to ascertain whether the regions just proximal to the tips of each of the 46 chromosomes are present in their normal locations. Although initially designed to investigate subnormal intelligence in older children, subtelomeric analysis appears to also be useful for some infants with congenital anomalies in whom standard investigations have not been fruitful. This technology seems to have better diagnostic success for individuals with intrauterine growth retardation, microcephaly, and a positive family history (19).

Metabolic Studies

Inborn errors of metabolism are often assumed to have a purely biochemical or neurologic phenotype, but metabolic disease is well recognized as an occasional cause of dysmorphic facial features and congenital malformations (20). For instance, ambiguous genitalia are seen in some cases of 21-hydroxylase deficiency and other types of congenital adrenal hyperplasia, and infants with pyruvate dehydrogenase deficiency may have agenesis of the corpus callosum and facial features that resemble fetal alcohol syndrome. A number of the congenital disorders of glycosylation feature congenital malformations of the heart, limbs, and central nervous system (21). Many peroxisomal conditions result in distinctive phenotypes: Zellweger syndrome, also known as cerebro-hepato-renal syndrome, and rhizomelic chondrodysplasia punctata (RCDP) exemplify this class of disease. For the Zellweger spectrum of peroxisomal abnormalities, serum levels of very long chain fatty acids will be elevated; in RCDP the very long chain fatty acids are normal but phytanic acid is elevated.

Synthesis and Analysis of Data

Every clinician develops a unique, individual strategy of diagnosis. Acquiring a deep and broad fund of knowledge is arguably fundamental and, oftentimes, sufficient in itself. Unfortunately, the sheer numbers of conditions and syndromes impose some limits on the "brute force" approach; the London Dysmorphology Database, for instance, contains over 3,000 multiple congenital anomaly syndromes (22).

Precise diagnosis is neither possible nor necessary in the immediate newborn period for many neonates with a multiple congenital anomaly syndrome. More than half of all individuals with congenital anomalies never receive a firm diagnosis, even after the most definitive of workups, and remain an "unknown." Categorization of an anomaly as a malformation, disruption, or deformation, however, is a feasible and useful first step. These terms have been defined and discussed previously. An isolated major anomaly in the absence of any similarly affected relative would suggest a multifactoral etiology. If there are multiple malformations, one of the following strategies may be useful:

- Instant recognition, or gestalt diagnosis, which depends on the clinician's previous experience and strength of visual memory. Certain caveats apply, however: many disorders have a considerable range of phenotypic variation, and other conditions, or phenocopies, may mimic the one that has instantly come to mind.

- Perusal of an atlas or illustrated text, such as Smith's Recognizable Patterns of Human Malformation, to match a photograph with the patient. This simple strategy often yields excellent results.

- Pattern analysis, in which all phenotypic and clinical "problems" are enumerated, grouped, combined, recombined, and weighed to discern developmental relationships, sequences, and influences. Major organ systems or classes of disease (e.g., skeletal dysplasias) then become entry points for further comparison, matching the patient's pattern against published descriptions while attempting to take into account phenotypic variability.
- Focusing the initial investigation on the anomaly that is most distinctive, rare, or unusual. Clinodactyly of the fifth finger is very common, but a coloboma of the iris is fairly unusual. A variety of texts or electronic databases then can be consulted and a relatively short list of diagnostic possibilities generated.

Once a preliminary analysis has generated a differential diagnosis, all reasonable efforts are made to test each competing hypothesis. Often, a clinical finding can corroborate a possibility. For instance, a lateral radiograph of the knee may allow confirmation of chondrodysplasia punctata by demonstrating the typical stippled, punctate mineralization of the epiphyses. Although many diagnoses are purely clinical, molecular tools are becoming extremely helpful. An electronic literature search or querying an internet resource, such as Online Mendelian Inheritance in Man, can help determine whether a novel approach using direct deoxyribonucleic acid (DNA) sequence analysis, FISH, or linkage analysis has been developed for the disease in question.

More often than not, the diagnostician will not be able to establish an etiology. When this is the case, there is a temptation to "force" a diagnosis, analogous to hammering a somewhat square peg into a slightly round hole. This may not be in the best interests of the patient so that, in these situations, there is honor in admitting ignorance. Certain characteristics of many syndromic conditions, such as the so-called "elfin" facies of Williams syndrome, are not apparent in the newborn period. The most useful diagnostic decision may be to wait and start afresh at a later time, recollecting data, recombining features into new patterns, and researching the literature. The assistance of a clinical geneticist or dysmorphologist during all phases of evaluation frequently optimizes the diagnostic process. If such services are not immediately available via direct consultation, telephonic or telemedicine consultation may be highly effective.

Other Management Issues

Communication with the parents of a child with congenital anomalies requires a compassionate, timely, and honest presentation of the facts. One's choice of terminology is important but often challenging. Many parents find it quite helpful for the principal caregiver to examine the infant in their presence, pointing out the features that seem to be unusual, and delineating those that are normal. Parents naturally feel responsible for the birth defect, which they might interpret as a reflection of their own shortcomings, real or imagined. Guilt is as common for the parents of a malformed child as pride is for the parents of a normal newborn. Although it is not always possible to convince parents to set aside unreasonable guilt, they can at least be reassured that they had no control over the events causing the abnormality and that they have permission to not feel guilty.

Expect the full spectrum of grief from both parents. They have experienced the loss of a much-anticipated "normal" child. Shock, denial, bargaining, and acceptance will all occur, even when their child does not have a lethal condition. The physicians and nursing personnel involved in the care of the malformed infant work as a team to keep track of this process and be alert for dysfunctional grief. Social work services, clergy, and support groups are important adjuncts. The National Organization for Rare Disorders, the Alliance of Genetic Support Groups, and specific support groups can provide up-to-date information and lay contacts for interested parents.

Not uncommonly, parents and relatives seek and find extensive information about birth defects, syndromes, chromosomal anomalies, and teratogenic conditions on the internet. In some cases, this information is more detailed and current than that available to a busy clinician who relies on brief textbook entries. Based on this information, parents may become firm, even strident and argumentative, demanding specific tests and management. This situation requires judgment, tact, and an open mind on the part of the attending physician, because this information may be quite useful, and parents who remain your allies will positively influence the entire spectrum of medical management. As correct and cutting edge as this information may be, parents will appreciate your pointing out that the clinical acumen and experience of the neonatal team is essential to assess the extent to which generic recommendations may be helpful for any particular patient. An imperative component of this process will be to verify the reliability of the information and ascertain whether it is based on credible scientific data.

If the malformed infant dies and there is any question regarding the precise diagnosis, a full, unrestricted autopsy can prove extremely useful. Visceral, central nervous system, and skeletal anomalies frequently come to light at postmortem examination. Clinical photography and cytogenetic analysis of fibroblasts obtained from sterile skin biopsy, fascia, or pericardium also may yield important insights. Tissue, cells in culture, and extracted DNA can be stored in a long-term repository and later reanalyzed in light of new research or collaboration.

Families often are reluctant to grant permission for an autopsy. In many instances, however, this procedure has profound implications for the parents' reproductive options and even those of distant relatives. Cultural and social beliefs and practices must, of course, be carefully respected regarding the care of the child's body after death. Nevertheless, an autopsy can be recast in the light of a final gift of the child to his family, perhaps even to the world, if in fact a diagnosis is thereby established or medical science advanced.

SELECTED EXAMPLES

Teratogenic Conditions

A teratogen, from the Greek root teras, meaning monster or marvel, is any environmental factor that causes a structural or functional abnormality in the developing fetus or embryo. These environmental agents include infections, medications, drugs, chemicals, and maternal metabolites, such as phenylalanine (Table 38-3). By their very nature, teratogens induce a disruption or sequence of disruptions of inherently normal tissue. Extensive compendia of these agents have been studied in humans and laboratory animals, and several excellent resources are available for the clinician. Additionally, both professionals and patients can access regional teratogen hot lines.

Ethanol, the most common human teratogen, is estimated to affect as many as 1 in 300 newborns, primarily as a neurotoxin, with consequences ranging from cerebral palsy to learning disability. Up to one-fifth of mental retardation (usually mild) is attributable to fetal alcohol syndrome (FAS), but numerous structural anomalies have also been reported (Table 38-4). Although the syndrome has been recognized for over 30 years, the dysmorphisms and other clinical signs of FAS are still often overlooked in the newborn nursery (23).

Multifactoral Disorders

The multifactorial model of inheritance, as previously discussed, provides a conceptual basis for understanding the pathogenesis and recurrence risks of isolated, nonsyndromic congenital malformations. The central concept of this model is that multiple genes and environmental factors influence whether a particular anatomic structure may develop abnormally. The susceptibility, or genetic liability, of a malformation in a population is described in terms of

TABLE 38-3
SELECTED TERATOGENS AND THEIR EFFECTS

Teratogen	Anomalies	Comments
Phenytoin (Dilantin)	Growth deficiency Wide anterior fontanelle Hypertelorism Cleft lip and palate Hypoplastic distal phalanges Small nails	Similar facial features seen with exposure to carbamazepine, valproate, mysoline, phenobarbital. Full spectrum in 10%, milder effects in one-third.
Warfarin (Coumadin)	Nasal hypoplasia Stippled epiphyses Short fingers Seizures	Critical period between 6 and 9 week's gestation. One-third of exposed fetuses are affected.
Retinoic acid (Accutane)	Microtia or anotia Hypertelorism Micrognathia Conotruncal cardiac defects Hydrocephalus Microcephaly Cortical, cerebellar dysplasia	If exposed more than 15 days after conception, one-third have embryopathy.
Rubella	Growth deficiency Microcephaly Deafness Cataracts Microphthalmia Chorioretinitis Cardiac septal defects Patent ductus arteriosus Peripheral pulmonic stenosis	Fifty-percent chance of effects if exposed in first trimester, but risk extends into second trimester. May have late, persistent infectious sequelae, e.g., diabetes mellitus.
Varicella	Mental deficiency Seizures Cortical atrophy/microcephaly Growth deficiency Limb hypoplasia/club foot Cutaneous scars	One to two percent with effects when exposed between 8 and 20 week's gestation; wide spectrum of severity.
Maternal phenyketonuria	Mental retardation (73% to 92%) Hypertonia Low birth weight (52%) Microcephaly (73%) Cardiac defects (15%) Spontaneous abortion (30%)	Even when "on diet," phenylalanine levels may rise above 4 to 10 mg/dL, the apparent threshold for fetal effects. Percentages cited here are for levels >16 mg/dL. Normal is <2.

TABLE 38-4
STRUCTURAL ANOMALIES IN FETAL ALCOHOL SYNDROME

Growth deficiency of prenatal onset
Mental retardation
Microcephaly
Short palpebral fissures
Maxillary hypoplasia
Cervical vertebral malformations (10%–20%)
Short nose
Smooth philtrum
Thin upper lip
Ventricular septal defect, atrial septal defect
Small distal phalanges
Small fifth fingernails

a continuous distribution of susceptibility factors in which there is a point, or threshold, beyond which, in an all-or-none fashion, a structural defect will occur. Table 38-5 lists some common multifactoral disorders and their recurrence risks. This type of multifactoral heritability is postulated to account for most isolated malformations.

The neural tube defects (NTDs) result from failed neural tube folding before 28 days' gestational age and comprise a spectrum of malformations ranging from anencephaly at one extreme to simple meningocele at the other. A number of genetic and environmental (e.g., ethanol, valproic acid) causes are well delineated. Seventy percent to 80% of NTDs have traditionally been considered to be isolated phenomena with recurrence risks of the usual order of magnitude for multifactoral disorders: 3% to 5%. Over the past decade, although, epidemiologic studies have demonstrated that seventy percent of isolated NTDs can be avoided by adequate maternal intake of folic acid in the periconceptual period (24). Numerous public health and professional organizations recommend that all women of childbearing age take 0.4 mg of folic acid per day. Women who have previously borne an affected child should take folic acid at an increased dosage, 4.0 mg/d, beginning 1 month prior to conception and continuing through at least the third month of gestation (25).

TABLE 38-5
MULTIFACTORAL DISORDERS

Disorder	Empiric Recurrence Risk
Cleft lip with or without cleft palate	4%–5%
Cleft palate	2%–6%
Ventricular septal defect	3%–4%
Pyloric stenosis	3%
Hirschsprung anomaly	3%–5%
Clubfoot	2%–8%
Congenital hip dysplasia	3%–4%
Neural tube defects	3%–5%
Atrial septal defect (secundum)	2%–3%

Chromosomal Abnormalities

Since 1956, when Tjio and Levan demonstrated that the normal diploid number of human chromosomes (46), seemingly innumerable permutations of abnormal chromosome number and structure have been described. Many of these are unique, but others are recurrent and produce readily recognized phenotypes. Most trisomies, such as trisomy 16, the most common trisomy in humans, are uniformly lethal in the prenatal period. Other rearrangements, such as most balanced translocations, have no phenotypic consequences unless a breakpoint disrupts a gene. Aneuploidy that adds or deletes enough genetic material to be cytogenetically visible commonly causes multiple congenital anomalies in several developmental fields.

Trisomy 21

Down Syndrome is the most common chromosomal aberration recognized at birth, with an incidence of about 1 per 700 live births. Only one of four conceptions that result in trisomy 21 is viable (27). The phenotype is quite variable, but distinctive facies (Fig. 38-3) and some degree of mental retardation are always present. Gestalt recognition of Down syndrome usually is uncomplicated, but diagnosis may be difficult if the infant is seriously ill or has atypical findings. Conversely, between 13 and 18 percent of children referred to a clinical geneticist because of suspected Down syndrome actually have another diagnosis (28).

An individual infant with Down syndrome will almost certainly lack one or several "classic" findings, such as a wide gap between the first and second toes. Keep in mind that a single feature, such as the simian crease, falls well short of being pathognomonic, but the overall constellation of major and minor anomalies suggests the diagnosis. Tables 38-6 and 38-7 list the major and minor anomalies, respectively, that have been observed in children with Down syndrome. Although major heart defects are present in about half of Down syndrome infants, a heart murmur and other signs of cardiovascular pathology may be quite subtle in the immediate newborn period. Atrioventricular canal can be particularly tricky to diagnose by auscultation. An echocardiogram is recommended for all newborns with suspected or confirmed Down syndrome, ideally prior to discharge, certainly by 1 month of age. If for any reason the cardiac ultrasound is delayed or unavailable before hospital discharge, an electrocardiogram should be obtained. Leftward deviation of the QRS axis to between zero and −90 degrees is characteristic of an endocardial cushion defect.

For 90% of newborns with Down syndrome, nondisjunction during maternal meiosis results in the formation of a gamete with two copies of chromosome 21 (27). The well-recognized relationship between trisomy 21 and maternal age (Table 38-8) has yet to be well-explained. Although risk increases with age, most Down syndrome infants are born to younger mothers because their birth rate is much greater than that of older mothers. Translocation of

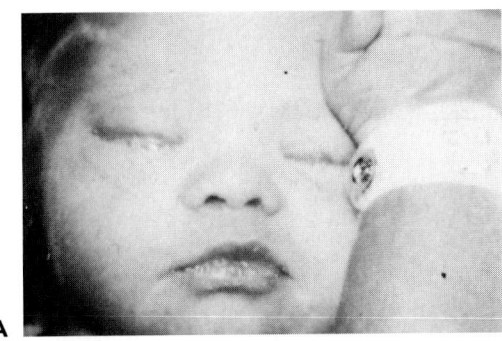

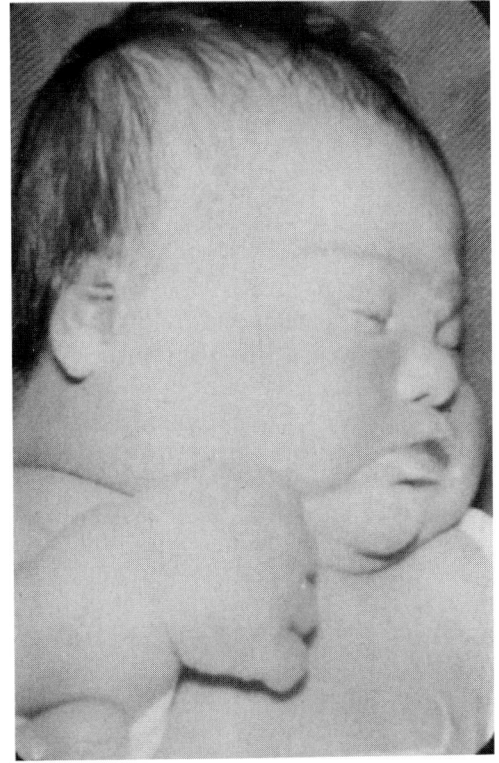

Figure 38-3 A Trisomy 21. B Down syndrome.

TABLE 38-6		
MAJOR ANOMALIES AT BIRTH IN DOWN SYNDROME		
Cardiac: all types		40%
Atrioventricular canal	16%–20%	
Ventricular septal defect	16%	
Patent ductus arteriosus	3%–5%	
Atrial septal defect	4%–10%	
Gastrointestinal: all types		10%–18%
Duodenal stenosis/atresia	3%–5%	
Imperforate anus	2%	
Other	6%	
Hematologic: leukemoid reaction		Common
Hypothyroidism (congenital)		1%

From refs. 17a–17c.

guidelines that address the needs of Down syndrome children and their parents from birth to adulthood (30).

Trisomy 18

Described by Edwards and associates (31) in 1960, trisomy 18 affects 1 of 5,000 newborns. Girls outnumber boys at a 4:1 ratio, and a maternal age effect is well established: de novo nondisjunction during meiosis accounts for 90%. One-tenth represent mosaicism, and various translocations and isochromosomal anomalies occasionally are seen. Life expectancy is markedly reduced, with nearly 90% mortality in the first year and frequent demise in the neonatal period (32). The congenital anomalies in trisomy 18 neonates usually are multiple, severe, and associated with consider-

chromosome 21 to another acrocentric chromosome occurs in 1 of 30 Down syndrome neonates, and other mechanisms of abnormal gametogenesis can also give rise to an extra copy of this chromosome. Accordingly, these possibilities must be evaluated via karyotyping, to provide accurate genetic counseling. Any chromosomal pattern other than trisomy 21 mandates analysis of parental karyotypes. For example, if an isochromosome 21 is present in the infant, parental chromosomal analysis may disclose that a parent carries the same isochromosome. Recurrence risk for that parent is then 100%. Straightforward trisomy 21 in the infant is not associated with chromosomal abnormalities of either parent and their testing is unnecessary. Recurrence risks are then 1% plus the age-related maternal risk.

Improvement in routine health care and advances in cardiac surgery have improved both the quality and longevity of life for individuals with Down syndrome. Median life expectancy is now 58.6 years (29). The American Academy of Pediatrics has published helpful health supervision

TABLE 38-7	
MINOR ANOMALIES IN DOWN SYNDROME	
Microbrachycephaly	75%
Upslanting palpebral fissures[a]	80%
Epicanthal folds	59%
Speckling of iris (Brushfield spots)[b]	56%
Flat facial profile[a]	90%
Low nasal bridge	68%
Small ears[b]	100%
Mildly dysplastic ears[a]	50%
Short neck	61%
Excess skin at nape of neck[a,b]	80%
Protruding tongue	47%
Narrow palate	76%
Open mouth	58%
Short hands and fingers	
Clinodactyly (curving) of the fifth finger[a]	60%
Simian crease[a]	45%
Wide gap between the first and second toes[b]	68%
Poor Moro reflex[a]	85%
Hyperflexibility of joints[a]	80%
Hypotonia[a]	80%

[a] Among the ten cardinal features cited by Bryan Hall from ref. 7.
[b] From ref. 28 as having superior discriminative efficacy and power.

TABLE 38-8

INCIDENCE OF DOWN SYNDROME AS A FUNCTION OF MATERNAL AGE

Maternal Age (yr)	Incidence
20	1:1667
25	1:1250
30	1:952
35	1:385
36	1:295
37	1:227
38	1:175
39	1:137
40	1:106
41	1:82
42	1:64
43	1:50
44	1:38
45	1:30
46	1:23
47	1:18
48	1:14
49	1:11

From ref. 27.

able morbidity. Severe psychomotor retardation always is present. Fig. 38-4 demonstrates typical facial features.

Considerable overlap with trisomy 13 syndrome may result in frequent diagnostic uncertainty in the newborn period, pending cytogenetic analysis. Table 38-9 lists some features that are common to both conditions, and Table 38-10 includes those findings that are more common to trisomy 18. Careful communication with the cytogenetic laboratory will ensure that chromosomal data are available as soon as possible, a helpful adjunct for decision-making when the clinical management options include expectant care and minimal intervention. In selected instances, there may be considerable benefit from rapid analysis via FISH probes for chromosome 13 and 18 markers. Bear in mind, however, that, on occasion, these modalities may not detect trisomic states that involve translocations or partial duplication and that full chromosomal analysis is superior and definitive. These results usually are available 48 to 72 hours after the laboratory receives the specimen.

Trisomy 13

This is the third most common autosomal trisomy recognized at birth, affecting 1 of 12,000 newborns, and initially was delineated in 1960 by Patau and associates (33). Three-fourths are straightforward trisomy 13; a maternal age effect is apparent. Twenty percent are caused by translocations, mostly Robertsonian, in which the long arm of the acrocentric chromosome 13 becomes attached via the centromere to another acrocentric chromosome, commonly chromosome 14. A small percentage of these translocations are familial, so parental karyotyping is

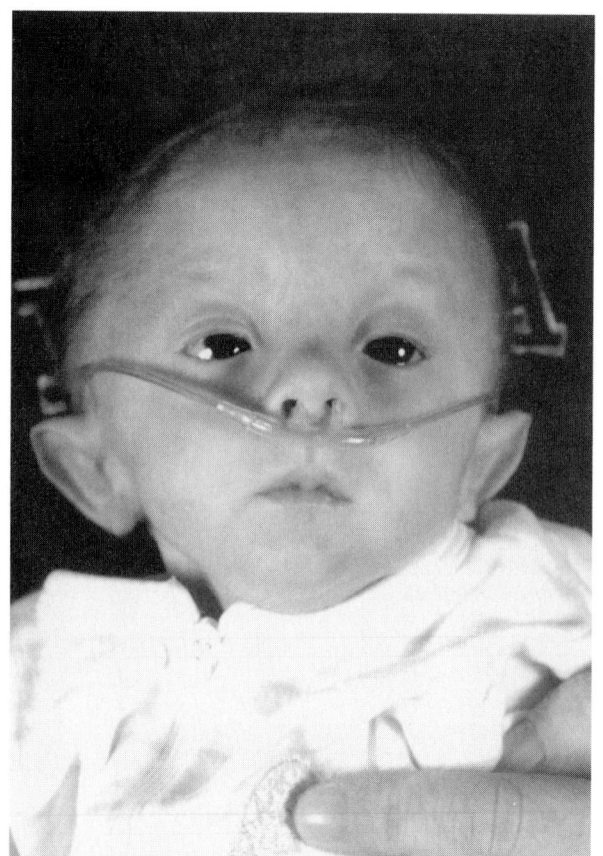
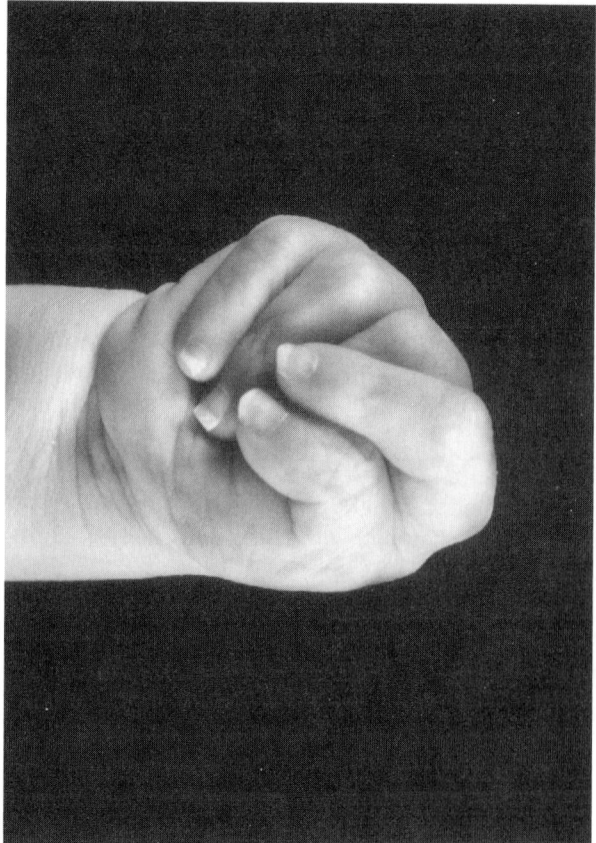

Figure 38-4   A,B: Trisomy 18.

TABLE 38-9
ANOMALIES COMMON TO BOTH TRISOMY 13 AND TRISOMY 18

Growth deficiency
Severe developmental retardation
Microcephaly
Ear anomalies
Microphthalmia
Highly arched palate
Micrognathia
Excessive neck skin
Congenital heart defects, various
    Ventricular septal defect, patent ductus arteriosus
Umbilical hernia
Renal anomalies
    Cystic kidneys
Cryptorchidism
Overlapping, flexed fingers
Prominent heels

TABLE 38-11
FINDINGS MORE COMMON TO TRISOMY 13

Scalp defects
Holoprosencephaly
Sloping forehead
Capillary hemangiomas
Ocular hypotelorism
Iris coloboma
Prominent nasal bridge
Cleft lip
Cleft palate
Short neck
Hypoplastic nipples
Cardiac: dextrocardia
Polydactyly (postaxial)
Apnea

essential for adequate recurrence risk counseling. Mosaicism is seen in 5%. For both trisomy 13 and trisomy 18, the median age of death is 10 days and 91% die within the first year. As with trisomy 18, cognitive and motor development is profoundly affected. Table 38-11 lists some of the anomalies that tend to be encountered more commonly in trisomy 13. Figure 38-5 shows typical facies.

The Support Organization for Trisomy 18, 13, and Related Disorders (34) is a consumer-oriented, lay group that serves as an excellent resource for parents, professionals, and other interested parties regarding trisomies 13 and 18 in particular.

Abnormalities of the Sex Chromosomes

With the exception of Turner syndrome, sex chromosome aneuploidies tend to be phenotypically bland in newborn children. Klinefelter syndrome, 47,XXY, is associated with a few, occasional congenital anomalies, such as cryptorchidism and hypospadias. Variants with more than one Y or more than two X chromosomes tend to have greater mental deficiency and more malformations, both minor and major.

Turner syndrome is caused by complete or partial absence of one X chromosome and occurs in 1 of 2,500 newborn girls. One half have a 45,X karyotype; a large

TABLE 38-10
FINDINGS MORE COMMON TO TRISOMY 18

Prominent occiput
Narrow palpebral fissures
Small mouth
Short sternum
Widely spaced nipples
Cardiac: polyvalvular disease
Prominent clitoris
Hypoplastic labia
Hip dislocation
Clubfoot
Hypoplastic nails
Syndactyly between toes 2 and 3
Hammertoes
Seizures

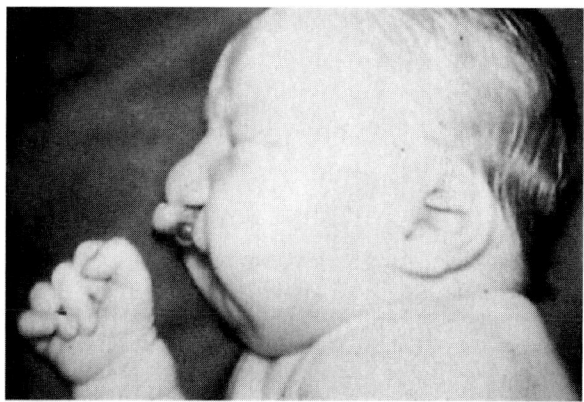

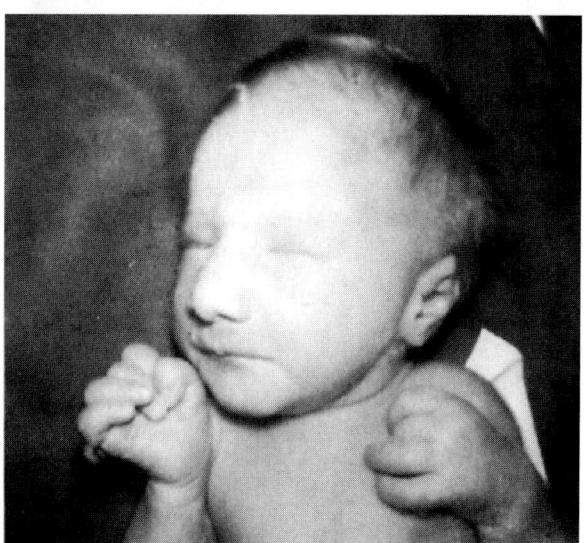

Figure 38-5   A,B: Trisomy 13.

number of other X chromosome anomalies, ranging from various isochromosome X patterns to simple deletions, ring chromosomes, and mosaics, account for the remainder. Almost all conceptuses with Turner syndrome are spontaneously aborted but, of those that are live born, only one-third are recognized in the newborn period. Clinical findings may include prominent ears, low posterior hairline, webbed neck, broad chest with widely spaced nipples, and puffiness of the dorsa of the hands and feet (Fig. 38-6). Although short stature is common in older girls, mean birth length is 47 cm, just within two standard deviations of the population mean. Ovarian dysgenesis (greater than 90%), renal anomalies (40% to 60%, horseshoe kidney in particular), and cardiac malformations (10%–20%, especially coarctation of the aorta) will require directed investigations once this diagnosis is suspected (35). An AAP health supervision guideline (36) summarizes the age-specific evaluations for girls with Turner syndrome. For neonates, recommendations include careful examination for hip dysplasia, hearing screening, pediatric cardiology consultation, comparison of systolic blood pressures in the arms and legs, renal ultrasonography, and consultation with pediatric endocrinology.

Partial Aneusomies

Deletions, duplications, and translocations of any segment, small or large, of any chromosome are possible. The resulting partial monosomy, partial trisomy, or combination of the two often causes multiple major and minor anomalies, intrauterine growth retardation, and a dysmorphic facial appearance. The deleted or duplicated segment may be interstitial, involving the midsection of one of the arms of a chromosome, or terminal. As a general rule, the larger the deletion or duplication, the more severe the somatic and functional effects. For example, deletion of the short arm of chromosome 5 (sometimes designated 5p- or 5p minus) is one of the most common autosomal deletion syndromes, with an incidence of 1 in 20,000 births. Also called cri-du-chat syndrome because of the high-pitched cry of affected infants, 5p- results in a distinctive phenotype: microcephaly; round facies; hypertelorism; broad nasal bridge, epicanthal folds; posteriorly rotated, malformed ears; preauricular skin tags, and small chin (Fig. 38-7). Various other malformations may be present, including cleft lip with or without cleft palate, heart defects, and megacolon. Hypotonia and mental retardation are typical. The severity of cri-du-chat syndrome can be correlated roughly with the location and extent of the deletion: absence of band 5p15.2 is associated with severe mental retardation; deletion of band 5p15.3 causes the typical cat cry (37). Other common partial aneusomies are summarized in Table 38-12.

Many chromosomal rearrangements occur de novo as spontaneous events in a single egg or sperm. These are unlikely to recur. Some, however, are the consequence of a balanced translocation or other rearrangement, such as pericentric inversion, in one parent. Generally, balanced translocations do not cause problems because most of the human genome consists of long stretches of DNA between genes. Breaks and rejoinings in these noncoding regions will have neutral consequences. If the break falls within a

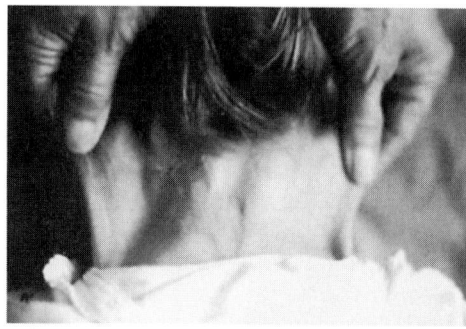
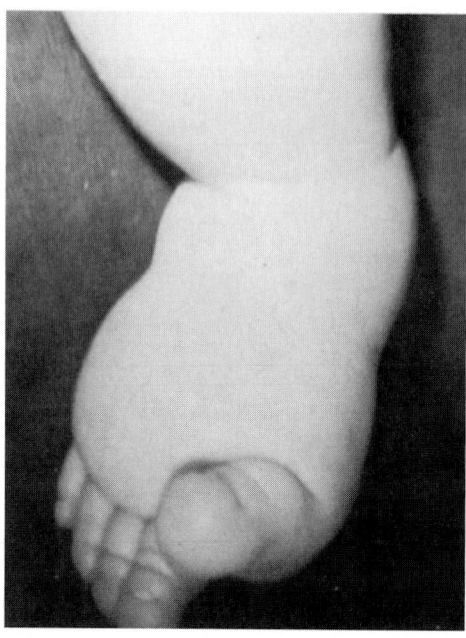

Figure 38-6   A,B: Turner syndrome.

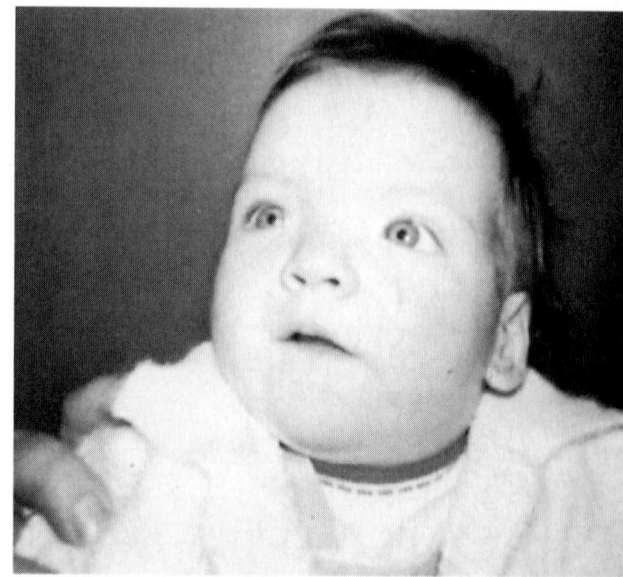

Figure 38-7   Cri-du-chat syndrome (5p-).

TABLE 38-12
SELECTED CHROMOSOMAL ANOMALY SYNDROMES

Karyotype	Features
4p-	Poor growth, microcephaly, prominent glabella, hypertelorism, downturned corners of mouth, micrognathia, cleft lip/palate, cryptorchidism, heart defects, profound developmental retardation. May involve only a small region, to include 4p16, requiring high-resolution banding or FISH for confirmation. Also known as the Wolf–Hirschhorn syndrome.
Dup 9p	Poor growth, macrocephaly, hypertelorism, downslanting palpebral fissures, prominent nose, downturned corners of mouth, cupped ears, short fingers and toes, developmental retardation.
Del 11p13	Mental deficiency, poor growth and microcephaly, aniridia, cataracts, blindness, cryptorchidism, hypospadias, Wilms tumor (50%). The interstitial deletion encompasses a tumor-suppressor gene and provides the *de facto* "first hit" in tumorigenesis.
13q-	Growth deficiency, mental deficiency, microcephaly, prominent nasal bridge, hypertelorism, microphthalmia, colobomata, bilateral retinoblastoma, micrognathia, anomalous auricles, hypoplastic thumbs, congenital heart disease, genitourinary anomalies. Band q14 is the locus of the RB gene, a tumor-suppressor gene implicated in retinoblastoma.
18p-	Mild growth deficiency and microcephaly, psychomotor retardation, ptosis, epicanthal folds, hypertelorism, wide mouth, protruding ears, small hands and feet, pectus excavatum.
18q-	Short-stature hypotonia, variable mental deficiency, conductive deafness, auricular anomalies, long hands, tapering digits, cardiac defects.
Dup 22q	Highly variable, also known as cat-eye syndrome, after the bilateral inferotemporal colobomata of the irides, which also may involve the choroid and retina. Mild developmental delays, normal growth, slight hypertelorism, downslanting palpebral fissures, preauricular tags or pits, cardiac defects, anal atresia, renal agenesis. Forty-seven chromosomes are present: the "extra" chromosome is composed of one or two chromosome 22 fragments, joined by their acrocentric short arms, creating trisomy or tetrasomy 22 q. FISH provides confirmation of the nature of the small "marker" chromosome. Parental karyotypes are necessary because a mildly affected parent also may have the marker.

gene, some phenotypic effects may ensue. Careful analysis of balanced translocations has, in fact, provided the critical link for mapping and cloning several important genes.

Not uncommonly, an unbalanced translocation in a newborn with multiple congenital anomalies is the consequence of a balanced translocation in a parent. During formation of eggs or sperm at meiosis, balanced rearrangements often yield gametes that have significant deletions, duplications, or more complex anomalies, with serious consequences for the offspring. Unbalanced translocations, in which there is both a duplicated chromosomal segment and a deletion, produce phenotypes that are unique, because they are a blending of a partial monosomy and a partial trisomy. Chromosomal studies on both mother and father then are critical for providing adequate recurrence risk counseling.

Microdeletion Syndromes

An increasing number of dysmorphologic syndromes are proving to be caused by fairly subtle interstitial or terminal chromosomal deletions. These are sometimes detectable via chromosome studies, especially if high-resolution or prometaphase analysis is employed, but more often the deleted region is submicroscopic and must be specifically investigated via specialized cytogenetic and molecular techniques, most commonly FISH. Although these microdeletions seem almost trivially small, they amount to a loss of several thousand of base pairs of DNA, usually resulting in haploinsufficiency of several contiguous genes. In some instances, microdeletions may be transmitted from parent

to child as an autosomal dominant trait, but most occur de novo, with unaffected parents, as a consequence of imprecise alignment of homologous chromosomes and unequal crossing over during meiosis. Another technique, comparative genomic hybridization (38), can also delineate small deletions. Table 38-13 lists several common microdeletion syndromes, their loci, and general features.

22q11.2 Deletion Syndrome has emerged over the last several years as the most commonly diagnosed microdeletion syndrome. Also known as Shprintzen syndrome, velo-cardio-facial syndrome (VCFS), DiGeorge syndrome (DGS), or conotruncal anomaly face syndrome, this condition may be manifest by congenital heart defects, especially those affecting the conotruncal structures (tetralogy of Fallot, conal ventricular septal defect, persistent truncus arteriosus, or interrupted aortic arch), and palate abnormalities, ranging from complete cleft palate as a result of the Pierre Robin sequence to submucous clefting or velopharyngeal insufficiency. Hypocalcemia as a result of parathyroid dysplasia, thymic hypoplasia with diminished T-cell production, developmental delays and mental retardation, renal malformations, subnormal growth, and a characteristic craniofacial appearance may be apparent in many affected individuals. Minor ear malformations, a bulbous nasal tip, malar hypoplasia, and long facies are frequently encountered in children and adults; however, these typical facial features may not be present in newborns, especially African-American infants (39). Consequently, the concurrence of cardiovascular and palatal anomalies should prompt FISH studies for the 22q11 submicroscopic deletion. Because other chromosomal defects can resemble

TABLE 38-13
MICRODELETION SYNDROMES

Chromosome Locus	Syndrome	Clinical Features
1p36		Hypotonia, growth retardation, developmental delays, deep-set eyes, pointed chin, seizures, cardiomyopathy, deafness
4p16	Wolf–Hirschhom	Hypotonia, microcephaly, hypertelorism, prominent glabella, severe mental deficiency
5p16	Cri du chat	Low birth weight, cat-like cry, microcephaly, downslanting palpebral fissures
7p13	Grieg cephalopolysyndactyly	Polydactyly, syndactyly, frontal bossing.
7q11.23	Williams	Supravalvular aortic stenosis, hyperacussis, stellate irides, prominent lips, mild mental retardation
8q24	Langer–Giedion	Multiple exostoses, bulbous nose, protruding ears, loose skin in infancy
11q13	WAGR	Wilms tumor, Aniridia, Genital anomalies, growth Retardation
13q14.11	Retinoblastoma	Retinoblastoma, growth deficiency, microcephaly, prominent nasal bridge, hypoplastic thumbs, cardiac defects
15q12	Prader–Willi	Paternal deletion in 70%, maternal 15q disomy in 30%, hypotonia, hypogonadism, poor growth in infancy, hyperphagia and obesity in childhood, behavioral difficulties
15q12	Angelman	Maternal deletion in 60%, paternal disomy in 5%, severe mental retardation, seizures, ataxic gait, microcephaly, paroxysmal laughter
16p13.3	ATR-16	Alpha thalassemia, mild mental retardation
16p13.3	Rubinstein–Taybi	CBP gene deletion in 25%, growth deficiency, mental retardation, small mouth, beaked nose, broad thumbs and toes
17p13	Miller–Dieker	Lissencephaly, high forehead with vertical furrowing while crying
17p11.2	Smith–Magenis	Brachycephaly, broad nasal bridge, short philtrum, prominent jaw, broad hands
20p11.23	Alagile	Deep-set eyes, broad forehead, chronic cholestasis, vertebral defects, peripheral pulmonary artery stenosis
22q11.2	DiGeorge, Shprintzen, Velo-cardio-facial	Aortic arch anomalies, parathyroid and thymic deficiency leading to hypocalcemia and diminished cellular immunity, cleft palate, prominent nose with narrow alar base, conotruncal cardiac defects, tapering fingers

22q11 deletion syndrome, cytogenetic testing should routinely be submitted simultaneously. In about 15% of individuals with the VCFS/ DGS phenotype, 22q11.2 FISH is normal; in some, atypical or other cytogenetic deletions can be identified. Should testing be considered for infants with apparently isolated palatal clefting or conotruncal anomalies? Many authorities advocate a low threshold for testing. Our appreciation of the incidence of 22q11.2 deletion syndrome continues to grow, FISH analysis is sensitive and specific, and our considerable insights into the natural history of this condition allow for practical and beneficial management (40).

Single Gene Disorders

Achondroplasia

The most common skeletal dysplasia recognized at birth, achondroplasia is an autosomal dominant condition characterized by short limbs, frontal bossing, a large head, mid-

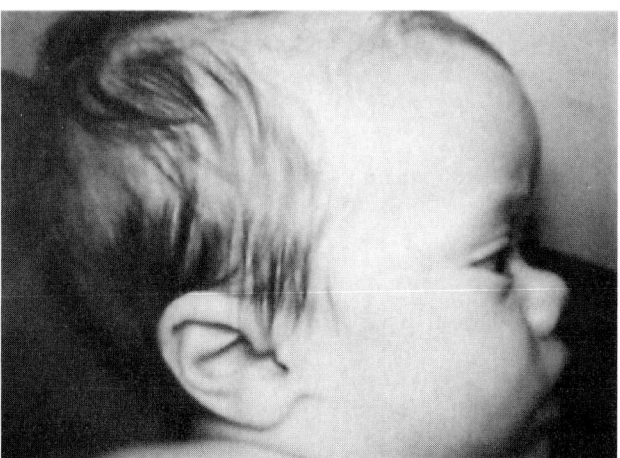

Figure 38-8 Achondroplasia.

face hypoplasia, and distinctive radiographic findings. In
the newborn period, a thoracolumbar gibbus, or sharp
kyphotic angulation of the vertebrae, may be present, followed in early childhood by lumbar lordosis. Midface
hypoplasia, a low nasal root, and relative prognathism
(Fig. 38-8) are apparent at birth and become more pronounced in childhood. The limb shortening is of the rhizomelic type, involving the humeri and femurs more than
the distal extremities. There may be limitation of elbow
extension, yet other joints may be relatively hyperextensible.
The fingers often display a trident pattern, with a splay or
gap between the third and fourth digits. Mild hypotonia is
common. The enlarged head circumference is associated
with mild ventriculomegaly in some cases, and in older
children and adults a narrow foramen magnum has, on
occasion, caused symptomatic cervicomedullary compression. Cognitive development is normal.

Achondroplasia is caused by specific mutations of the
fibroblast growth factor receptor-3 gene (FGFR3) on chromosome 4p16.3. Heterozygosity for a point mutation at
nucleotide 1138, converting a glycine residue to either a
arginine or cysteine, is responsible for 99% of cases (41).

Smith–Lemli–Opitz Syndrome

For this inborn error of metabolism, a deficiency of
7-dehydrocholesterol reductase results in a distinctive pattern of multiple congenital anomalies (42). Like most
other enzyme deficiencies, this SLOS is inherited in an
autosomal recessive fashion. The reductase, which maps to
chromosome 7q32.1, is responsible for the last step in
cholesterol synthesis. Consequently, serum cholesterol
tends to be low, although in 10% it falls within normal
limits, and the immediate precursor, 7-dehydrocholesterol,
is markedly elevated. A variable spectrum of anomalies
may be seen, including microcephaly, various central nervous system structural defects, hypotonia, growth deficiency, and distinctive facies with a high, square forehead,
ptosis, a short nose, anteverted nares, and micrognathia
(Fig. 38-9). Peripheral and central neural myelinization is

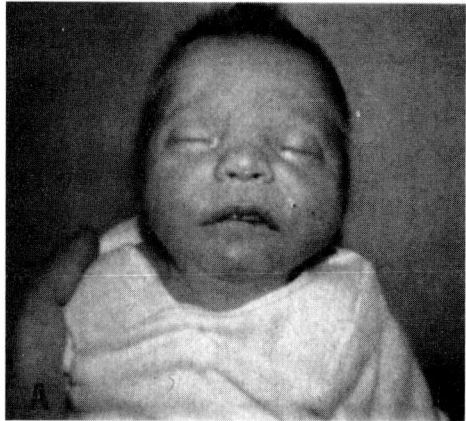 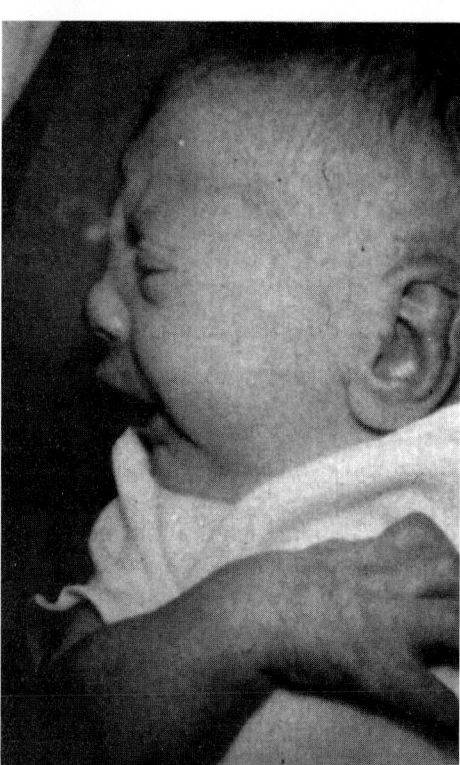

Figure 38-9 A,B: Smith–Lemli–Opitz syndrome.

reduced. About three-fourths of genotypic XY males have
genital anomalies—cryptorchidism, ambiguous genitalia,
even complete sex reversal. Polydactyly and syndactyly
between the second and third toes is very common. More
severely affected individuals may have visceral defects,
such as renal cysts or agenesis, cardiac anomalies, pancreatic hyperplasia, hepatic dysfunction, cataracts, severe
growth retardation, postaxial polydactyly, and may be stillborn or die in the neonatal period.

Chondrodysplasia Punctata, Rhizomelic Type

Rhizomelic chondrodysplasia punctata, an autosomal
recessive inborn error of peroxisome metabolism as a
result of mutations of the peroxin 7 (PEX7) gene on chromosome 6q22-24, is manifest as a distinctive skeletal dysplasia with mental retardation and poor long-term survival

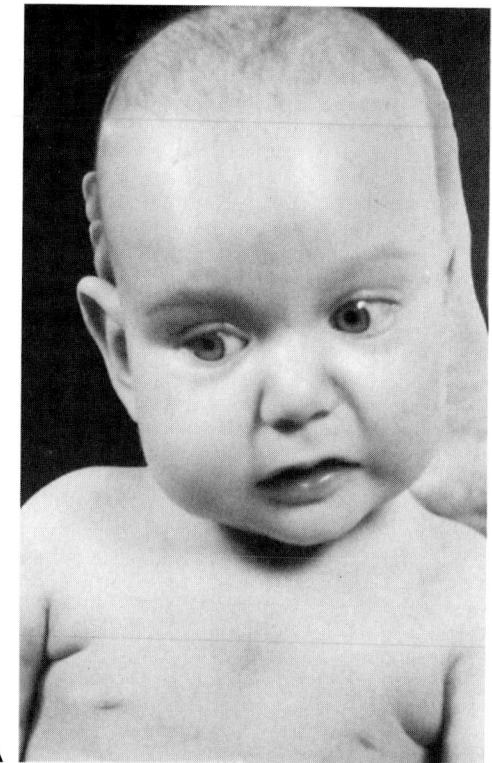
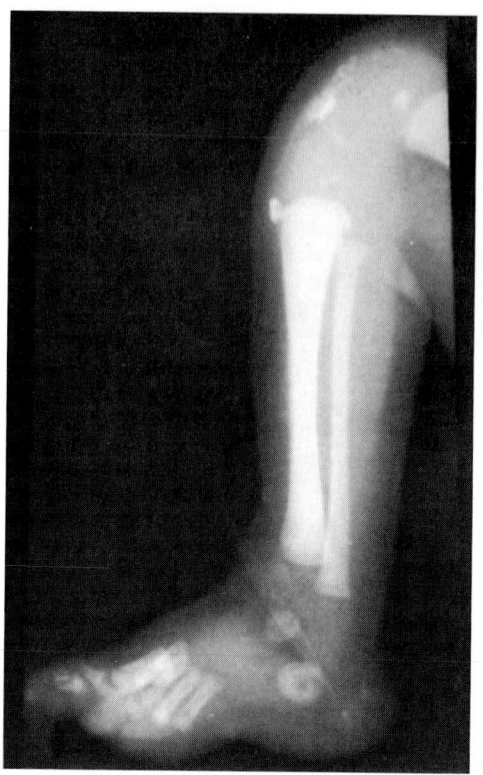

Figure 38-10   A,B: Rhizomelic chondrodysplasia punctata.

(43). Birth length is reduced and the proximal limbs are shortened. Additionally, there is microcephaly, full cheeks, a depressed nasal bridge, cataracts, ichthyosis, coronal clefts of the vertebral bodies, and congenital heart disease (Fig. 38-10). In the neonatal period, punctate calcific stippling of the epiphyses is readily apparent on lateral radiographs of the knee. Severe psychomotor retardation is the rule, and death usually occurs in the first year of life. Serum phytanic acid is increased and plasmalogen biosynthesis is deficient. Ultrastructural studies of hepatocytes demonstrate that peroxisomes are absent or markedly abnormal.

Treacher Collins Syndrome

Also known as mandibulofacial dysostosis, this autosomal dominant condition was first described in the mid-1800s. Clinical features vary within and between families but typically include a narrow face with downslanting palpebral fissures, zygomatic underdevelopment, a small chin, and an extension of scalp hair onto the cheek (Fig. 38-11). The lower eyelids are notched at the outer third; medially the eyelashes are sparse or absent. The ears often are crumpled and small. One-third lack the external auditory canal and/or have ossicular anomalies of the middle ear that cause conductive hearing loss. Ear tags and preauricular fistulae are common. The mouth is wide, and overt or occult palatal clefts are common. Intelligence is usually normal. In the early 1990s, several investigators localized the gene to chromosome 5q32-33.2 using linkage analysis and FISH. In 1996, the gene, designated TCOF1, was positionally cloned (44). The gene product, named "treacle" (British

for "molasses"), is truncated in most TCOF1 patients as a result of the introduction of a premature termination codon via various deletions, insertions, and splicing alterations.

Apert Syndrome

This autosomal dominant craniosynostosis syndrome is readily recognized by the combination of an unusual head shape and characteristic limb anomalies. Premature fusion of coronal sutures bilaterally leads to acro-brachycephaly—a short yet tall cranial shape—with a full forehead, flat occiput, flat midface, shallow orbits, and downslanting palpebral fissures. There is a mitten-like syndactyly of the fingers and toes, both cutaneous and osseous, and broad thumbs (Fig. 38-12). Other anomalies may involve the cardiac, gastrointestinal, central nervous, and genitourinary systems. Most infants with Apert syndrome are born to unaffected parents: in a single germ cell, a new mutation occurs in the fibroblast growth factor receptor-2 (FGFR2) gene on chromosome 10q25-26. Other FGFR2 mutations cause several other dominant craniosynostosis syndromes, such as Crouzon syndrome and Pfeiffer syndrome (45).

Malformation Sequences

A malformation sequence represents the ultimate consequence of a precise cascade of fetal events. Initiated by one primary event, which is often a mechanical or vascular disruption of a specific developmental field, a sequence may stand alone as a recognizable entity or may be a component

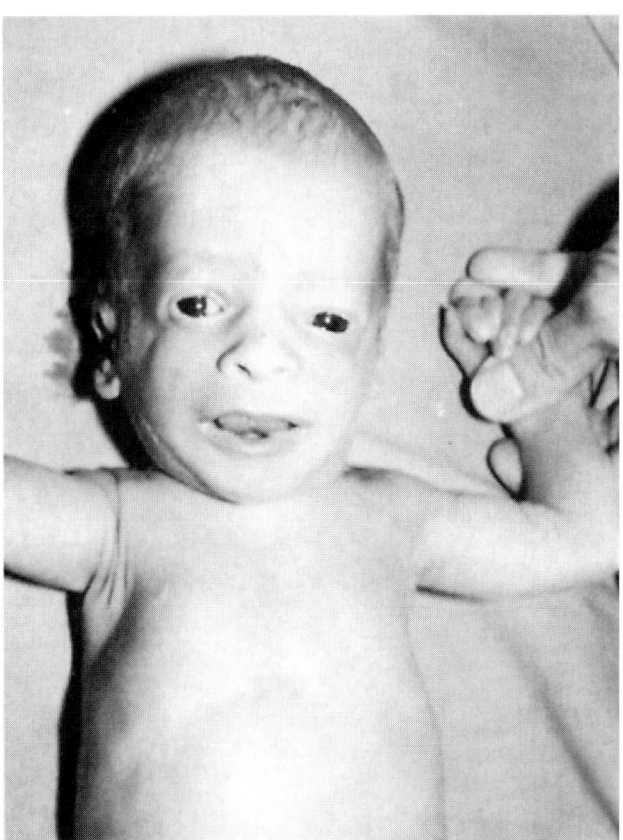

Figure 38-11 Treacher Collins–Franceschetti syndrome.

of a larger picture, associated with a chromosomal defect, microdeletion, or single-gene disorder. The Pierre Robin sequence, for example, is recognized as a cleft of the posterior palate, often in the shape of a "U," in a child with a markedly retruded, small mandible. At 5 to 9 weeks' gestation, the malpositioned jaw allows the tongue to interfere

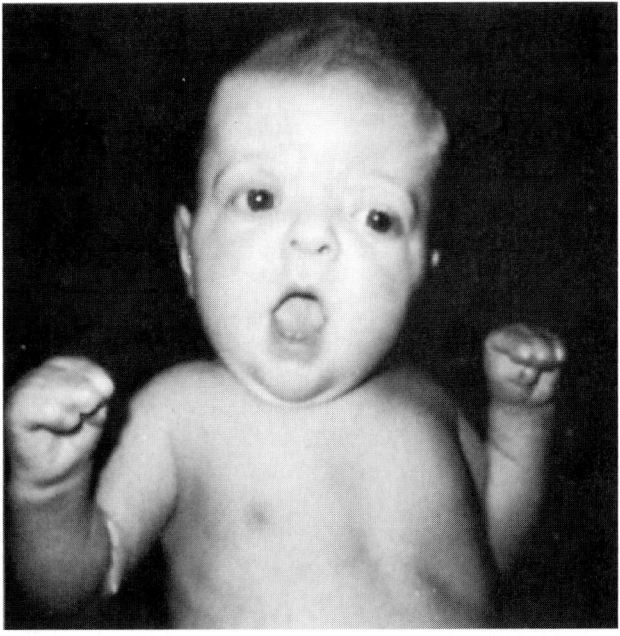

Figure 38-12 Apert syndrome.

with the medial apposition of the posterior palatal shelves as they migrate toward the midline, thereby mechanically prohibiting their fusion. The newborn can quickly develop significant airway obstruction and will require very close observation and occasional surgical intervention. The Robin sequence may be isolated but, compared to other orofacial clefts, has a relatively high association with chromosomal anomalies and syndromic diagnoses, such as trisomy 18, 22q11 deletion Beckwith–Wiedemann syndrome, Miller–Dieker syndrome, fetal alcohol syndrome, and many others.

Other Mechanisms

Uniparental disomy involves the inheritance of both copies of a particular chromosome or chromosome segment from only one parent and has been observed in cystic fibrosis, Russell–Silver syndrome, Prader–Willi syndrome, and Angelman syndrome, among others. Imprinting refers to how a gene may function differently, depending on whether it is inherited from the mother or the father, and is often mediated via methylation of DNA sequences that regulate gene expression.

Beckwith–Wiedemann syndrome (BWS) is a complex condition that may be caused by several mechanisms affecting a multigenic region on the short arm of chromosome 11, including mutations of the CDKN1C gene, abnormal methylation, paternal uniparental disomy, and chromosome 11p15 duplications. Diagnosis of BWS, however, remains clinical: frequent features include somatic overgrowth, macroglossia, omphalocele, visceromegaly, and dysplasia of the renal medulla. Transitory, symptomatic hypoglycemia is present in 30%, and a number of neoplasms, including Wilms tumor, adrenal cortical carcinoma, and hepatoblastoma, are common, especially in individuals with hemihypertrophy, which affects about 13% of patients. Glabellar nevus flammeus, linear grooves of the ear lobes, and posterior helical ear pits are valuable diagnostic signs (Fig. 38-13). About 85% of cases are sporadic, 15% familial. About 1% to 2% have either a small, interstitial duplication of chromosome 11 involving band p15.5 or an inversion or translocation in this region; invariably the duplicated region is paternal in origin. Other individuals derive both 11p15.5 regions from their father. They have the normal number of chromosomes— that is, they are disomic for this region—but have inherited both segments from only one parent, i.e., uniparental disomy. These data also suggest that BWS is caused by a dosage effect related to a gene or genes that are differentially expressed in maternally and paternally derived alleles, i.e., imprinting. Recently, two genes, KCNQ1OT1 and H19, have been found to have abnormal methylation in 2/3 cases of BWS, and direct DNA analysis of the CDKN1C gene, which is available on a research basis, can uncover mutations many individuals. The recurrence risk depends on the nature of the genetic mutation. For instance, if an 11p15 inversion is inherited from the mother, the recurrence risk is 50%, but paternal uniparental disomy has a

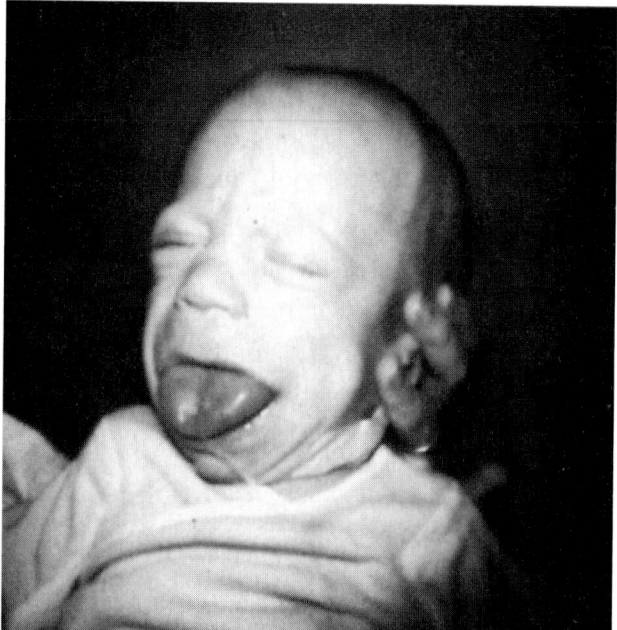

Figure 38-13 Beckwith–Wiedemann syndrome.

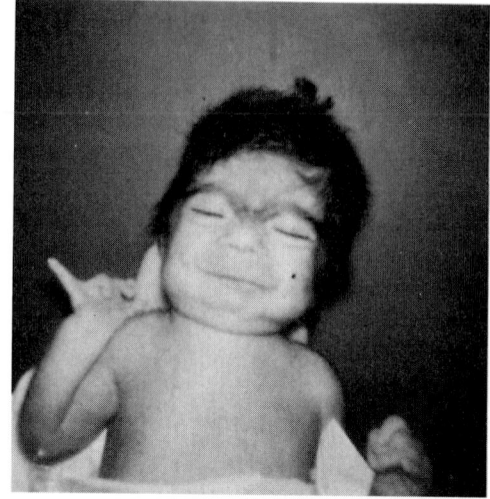

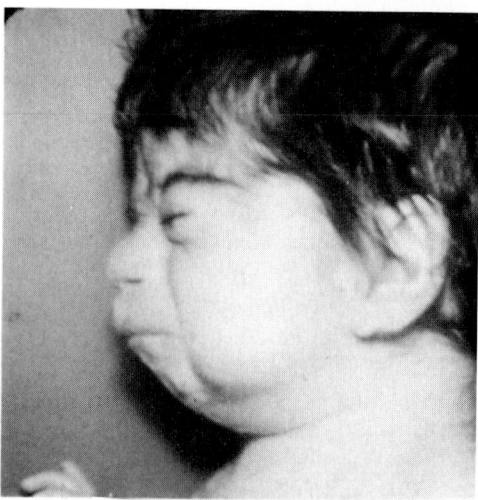

Figure 38-14 A,B: Cornelia de Lange syndrome.

very low chance of recurrence. Some genotype-phenotype associations have been delineated. Individuals with cytogenetic abnormalities may have some degree of mental retardation; uniparental disomy and H19 hypermethylation are associated with an increased risk for Wilms tumor (46).

Disorders of Unknown Etiology

Cornelia de Lange syndrome is a sporadic condition of unknown etiology that can be recognized by the facial gestalt. The eyebrows are crescent shaped, neatly defined, and often meet in the midline (synophrys); the anterior hairline is low; the nose is short and the nostrils upturned; and the lips are thin with down turned corners, like that of a carp (Fig. 38-14). Microcephaly and mental retardation are common but not invariable. Growth is deficient prenatally and postnatally. About one-fourth have upper limb anomalies, which can range from proximally placed thumbs to severe reduction defects. Empiric recurrence risk is estimated to be 2% to 5%. Duplication of the long arm of chromosome 3 causes a very similar malformation pattern (phenocopy) and must be excluded.

GENETIC COUNSELING

Throughout human history, various astrologers, wise men, shamans, village elders, high priestesses, court jesters, and mothers in law have paid close attention to birth defects. Curiosity has naturally inspired us to theorize, to attempt to find meaning and significance, and then to communicate the "truth" about a congenital anomaly to parents, relatives, communities, and rulers. As an omen or prophecy, the malformation of a newborn has been inferred to be the visitation of a god, of celestial forces, of bad seed or bad

morals, sure to portend either a bright future or ruin to the bearer of bad fruit. From these basic impulses to understand and to predict has grown the modern discipline of genetic counseling.

The term "counseling" has the unfortunate connotation of giving authoritative advice, a fairly formal process in which information and directive statements flow in one direction, from counselor to consultand. Genetic counseling seeks to eschew these misconceptions. It is a process of communication between a genetic counselor or counseling team and an individual, couple, or family about what exactly has caused a genetic problem, how they might understand it, and what options they have for the future—in which they can find additional educational resources, support groups, research studies, what modifications to the usual health maintenance activities might be able to prevent potential problems, whether a similar problem could affect other family members, how one could detect this prenatally or after birth, the risks and benefits of doing so, and the options for prenatal management. Informally, many clinicians perform these activities as an integral component of routine care giving. Formally, however, genetic counseling is a complex and comprehensive activity that has blossomed as a discipline in its own right. It is learned didactically and practically via postgraduate programs in medical genetics and genetic counseling, with board certification (and recertification) incumbent on thoroughly documented case workups, close supervision by experienced preceptors, and successful performance on rigorous, standardized examinations. There are 27 American Board of Genetic Counseling (ABGC) accredited programs in the United States and Canada; nearly 2500 individuals have received ABCG certification since 1993. Additionally, physicians who have completed formal postgraduate training in clinical genetics, via fellowship or, in the past decade, through residency training, and who obtain board certification through the ABMG are also qualified to provide genetic counseling.

The goals of genetic counseling have evolved over the past several decades. The provision of advice regarding reproductive choice and behavior, with an eye toward reducing the amount of genetic disease in future generations, has been superseded by other aims. The genetic counselor fundamentally seeks to provide information with clarity, sensitivity, and support to enable the person seeking information, the consultand, to understand well and decide capably. Emphasis is placed on the psychological and cultural aspects of this interactive process, and support and follow-up are key elements. Genetic counseling requires that the diagnosis be established with as much precision as possible, that an accurate and full pedigree be obtained, and that up-to-date information regarding the diagnosis be researched. Recurrence risk calculations may be simple and straightforward, or they may require more sophisticated tools, such as Bayesian analysis. Bayes' theorem, created more than 200 years ago, allows the laws of probability to be applied to a specific clinical scenario and quantifies the risk of recurrence by incorporating multiple observations into a complex formula (47). These data, the natural history of the disorder in question, management options, and the full spectrum of reproductive options are discussed in detail with the consultand, often with explicit attention to the significance these have for that individual, the psychological and practical burden perceived in the context of the social structure, finances, and personal experience. Principles of genetic counseling also include a commitment to strive for a nondirective approach, truth telling, avoidance of paternalism, respect for autonomy and dignity, and anticipation of ongoing psychological needs and issues. A concerted effort is made to identify and facilitate outside sources of information and support, such as from clergy, genetic support groups, and social services.

Difficult Decisions

Some infants are born with anomalies that are irreparable and incompatible with life. For these newborns, the decision to limit intervention, although deeply saddening, is clear. Bilateral renal agenesis and anencephaly are salient examples—no amount of intervention will help; solace and support are the only options. Other newborns, whose malformations are profound, but who may respond to heroic therapy, demand greater courage on the part of parents and clinicians—courage to analyze carefully in the face of chaos, in the context of a health care system whose bias is to act, simply because action is possible, and without much time in which to reach a decision. A clinical genetics consultation that incorporates rapid dysmorphologic analysis and directed, confirmatory testing will usually clarify the key issues of this decision making process.

The central importance of an accurate diagnosis is difficult to overstate. For a neonate with multiple major anomalies, the neurologic prognosis cannot always be predicted solely on the basis of the severity of the obvious malformations. For instance, in the case of VACTERL association, the tracheo-esophageal fistula and anal atresia will require urgent, life-saving surgery, the vertebral abnormalities can seem grimly bizarre, and the overall picture may appear dismal. However, these children typically have normal cognitive development, our surgical and rehabilitation medicine colleagues have much to offer, and prognosis may be quite good. On the other hand, some infants with trisomy 13 or trisomy 18 have remarkable few major anomalies—parents may even have strong doubts about the diagnosis—but the neuro-developmental progress will be minimal.

The dignity of the child compels the caregiver to have as clear a vision of the future as possible, to deal with decisions such as whether or not to intubate, transplant an organ, etc. The infant with thanatophoric dysplasia may well live, with extraordinary care, to several years of age, as has been reported in a few children, and one in ten infants with trisomy 18 lives to the first birthday, albeit with significant psychomotor retardation. However, these facts are a starting point for an individualized analysis, shared between family and physician, and not the foundation of policy to either routinely offer maximal intervention or insist that care be denied.

The parents of some profoundly disabled children perceive them as interactive and capable of both receiving and giving affection. For these families, the rationale to limit medical support, because the long-term prognosis is not good, is specious. They counter that they find richness and reward in their child, which they feel is reciprocated, and that any judgment regarding "quality of life" is theirs, and theirs alone, to make. Of course, the parents of a newborn with, for instance, trisomy 13 have had only the limited experience of the pregnancy to develop an appreciation for their baby's human worth. If they have had prenatal genetic testing and counseling, they may have been aware of this diagnosis for more than 5 months, have made a conscious decision to not terminate the pregnancy, and have become well-read and quite sophisticated regarding options for intervention and support. These parents will be seeking a neonatal and pediatric team with whom they can be partners, not adversaries. If there is disagreement regarding prognosis or intervention, medical or surgical, the clinician may do worse than fall back on basic principles—complete ascertainment of facts, diagnostic precision, and solid understanding of the natural history. One cannot underestimate the power of careful and frequent communication with the family, with the dual aims of appreciating the family's points of view and of presenting, with clarity, the medical point of view.

Recommended Resources

Suggested Internet Bookmarks

- http://www.health.state.ny.us/nysdoh/dpprd/main.htm
  Evaluation of the newborn with single or multiple congenital anomalies: a clinical guideline, American College of Medical Genetics Foundation and the New York State Department of Health. See reference 9 below and text. Thorough familiarity with this resource is highly recommended.
- http://www.kumc.edu/gec/geneinfo.html.
  Information for Genetic Professionals, University of Kansas Medical Center. This is one of the original online clearinghouses of practical genetic information. Thousands of internet links to other genetic web sites are available via this starting point. Particularly useful is the section on support groups.
- http://www.ncbi.nlm.nih.gov/entrez/query.fcgi?db=OMIM
  Online Mendelian Inheritance in Man (OMIM), National Center for Biotechnology Information-Johns Hopkins University. Originally published in print by Dr. Victor McKusick, this catalogue reigns as one of the most definitive and current sources of information for over 14,000 mendelian disorders, with search capabilities and links to MEDLINE, graphics, and clinical photographs, and access to DNA sequence data.
- http://www.geneclinics.org/
  GeneTests, funded by the National Institutes of Health, the Health Resources and Services Administration, and the Department of Energy. Originally a database of laboratories offering esoteric DNA tests, GeneTests still specializes in connecting clinicians and over 500 molecular testing laboratories. Additionally, this site incorporates GeneReviews, a compendium of definitive treatises, written and updated by leading authorities, of about 300 genetic diseases for which diagnostic DNA testing is available. Also at this site, GeneClinics can locate genetics professionals and services in the United States.
- http://www.geneticalliance.org/
  Genetic Alliance, The Alliance of Genetic Support Groups. For current information on support groups and information that can be understood by patients and their families, this site is the definitive resource. Additionally, the Alliance can provide expert information about the ethical, social, and legal issues for genetic medicine in general and specific conditions. Families, researchers, policymakers, health care professionals and industry are invited to participate as partners "to make the promise of genetics real."
- http://www.aap.org/visit/gencomp.htm
  Genetics Compendium, The American Academy of Pediatrics, has numerous links to information from the AAP, especially the Committee on Genetics, including policy statements and health supervision guidelines for many conditions and scenarios.

For Your Library

- Smith's Recognizable Patterns of Human Malformation, 5th Edition.
  First published in 1970, the 1997 edition, written by Kenneth Lyon Jones, continues to provide a classic tool for diagnosis, education, and reference, with hundreds of clinical descriptions, detailed photographs, and definitive chapters on clinical strategy and dysmorphology. W.B. Saunders Company.
- Syndromes of the Head and Neck, 4th Edition.
  Despite the title, this text goes far beyond the head and neck. Robert J. Gorlin, D.D.S, M.S. D.Sc., M. Michael Cohen, Jr., D.M.D., Ph.D., and Raoul C.M. Hennekam, M.D., Ph.D. Oxford University Press, 2001.
- Teratogenic Effects of Drugs, 2nd Edition.
  J. M. Friedman, M.D., Ph.D. and Janine E. Polifka, Ph.D. Johns Hopkins University Press, 2000.

REFERENCES

1. Chung CS, Myrianthopoulos NC. Congenital anomalies: mortality and morbidity, burden and classification. *Am J Med Genet* 1987; 27:505.
2. Van Regemorter N, Dodion J, Druart C. Congenital malformations in 10,000 consecutive births in a university hospital: need for genetic counseling and prenatal diagnosis. *J Pediatr* 1984;104:386.
3. MacDorman MF, Minino AM, Strobino DM, et al. Annual summary of vital statistics–2001. *Pediatrics* 2002;110:1037.
4. Economic costs of birth defects and cerebral palsy—United States, 1992. *MMWR Morb Mortal Wkly Rep* 1995;44:694–699.
5. Nelson K, Holmes LB. Malformations due to presumed spontaneous mutations in newborn infants. *N Engl J Med* 1989;320:19.
6. Risch NJ. Genetic Epidemiology. In: Rimoin DL, Connor JM, Pyeritz RE, et al, eds. *Principles and Practice of Medical Genetics* London: Churchill Livingstone, 2002: 457–458.
7. Hall BD. The state of the art of dysmorphology. *Am J Dis Child* 1993;147:1184.
8. Stevenson RE, Hall JG. Terminology. In: Stevenson RE, Hall JG, Goodman RM, eds. *Human malformations and related anomalies*, vol 1. New York: Oxford University Press, 1993:21.
9. American College of Medical Genetics Foundation, sponsored by the New York State Department of Health. Evaluation of the newborn with single or multiple congenital anomalies: a clinical guideline. May 1999. Available at http://www.health.state.ny.us/nysdoh/dpprd/main.htm. Accessed 1/1/05.
10. Hall JG. An approach to malformation syndromes. In: Berg K, ed. *Medical genetics: past, present, future.* New York: Alan R. Liss, 1985:275.
11. Cox GF, Burger J, Lip V, et al. Intracytoplasmic sperm injection may increase the risk of imprinting defects. *Am J Hum Genet* 2002;71:162.
12. Moll AC, Imhof SM, Schouten-van Meeteren AY, et al. Retinoblastoma is associated with in-vitro fertilization. *Lancet* 2003;361:309.
13. DeBaun MR, Niemitz EL, Feinberg AP. Assisted Reproductive Technology may increase the risk of Beckwith Wiedemann syndrome. *Am J Hum Genet* 2003;72:156.
14. Elias S, Simpson JL, Shulman LP. Techniques for prenatal diagnosis. In: Rimoin DL, Connor JM, Pyeritz RE, et al, eds. *Principles and Practice practice of Medical medical genetics.* London: Churchill Livingstone, 2002:810.
15. Hall JG, Froster-Iskenius UG, Allanson JE. *Handbook of normal physical measurements.* Oxford: Oxford University Press, 1989.

16. Saul RA, Seaver LH, Sweet KM, et al. *Growth references: third trimester to adulthood.* Greenwood, SC: Keys Printing, 1998.
17. Wang RY, Earl DL, Ruder RO, et al. Syndromic ear anomalies and renal ultrasounds. *Pediatrics* 2001;108:E32.
18. Opitz JM. Study of the malformed fetus and infant. *Pediatr Rev* 1981;3:57.
19. De Vries BBA, Winter R, Schinzel A, et al. Telomeres: a diagnosis at the end of the chromosomes. *J Med Genet* 2003;40:385.
20. Burton BK. Inborn errors of metabolism in infancy: a guide to diagnosis. *Pediatrics* 1998;102. Available at http://www.pediatrics.org/cgi/content/full/102/6/e69. Accessed 1/1/05.
21. Westphal V, Srikrishna G, Freeze HH. Congenital disorders of glycosylation: have you encountered them? *Genet Med* 2000;2:329.
22. Winter RM, Baraitser M. *London dysmorphology database, vol 3.0.* Oxford: Oxford University Press, 2001.
23. Thackray HM, Tifft C. Fetal alcohol syndrome. *Pediatr Rev* 2001;22:47.
24. Hall JG, Solehdin F. Genetics of neural tube defects. *Ment Retard Dev Disabil Res Rev* 1998;4:269.
25. American Academy of Pediatrics, Committee on Genetics. Folic acid for the prevention of neural tube defects. *Pediatrics* 1999;104:325.
26. Tjio JH, Levan A. The chromosome number of man. *Hereditas* 1956;42:1.
27. Hook EB. Chromosome abnormalities: prevalence, risks, and recurrence. In: Brock DH, Rodeck CH, Ferguson-Smith MA, eds. *Prenatal diagnosis and screening.* Edinburgh: Churchill Livingstone, 1992:351.
28. Rex AP, Preus M. A diagnostic index for Down syndrome. *J Pediatr* 1982;100:903.
29. Glasson EJ, Sullivan SG, Hussain R, et al. The changing survival profile of people with Down's syndrome: implications for genetic counselling. *Clin Genet* 2002;62:390.
30. American Academy of Pediatrics, Committee on Genetics. Health supervision for children with Down syndrome. *Pediatrics* 2001:107:442.
31. Edwards JH, Harnden DG, Cameron AH. A new trisomic syndrome. *Lancet* 1960;1:787.
32. Rasmussen SA, Wong L-Y C, Yang Q, et al. Population-based analyses of mortality in trisomy 13 and trisomy 18. *Pediatrics* 2003;111:777.
33. Patau K, Smith DW, Therman E, et al. Multiple congenital anomalies caused by an extra autosome. *Lancet* 1960;1:790.
34. S.O.F.T., 2982S Union St., Rochester, NY 14624; (716) 594-4621. Available at http://www.trisomy.org. Accessed 1/1/05.
35. Robinson A, de la Chapelle A. Sex chromosome abnormalities. In: Emery AEH, Rimoin DL, eds. *Principles and practice of medical genetics*, 2nd ed, vol 1. Edinburgh: Churchill Livingstone, 1990:973.
36. Frias JL, Davenport ML, AAP Committee on Genetics, AAP Section on Endocrinology. Health supervision for children with Turner syndrome. *Pediatrics* 2003;111:692.
37. Cerruti Mainardi P, Perfumo C, Cali A, et al. Clinical and molecular characterization of 80 patients with 5p deletion: genotype-phenotype correlation. *J Med Genet* 2001;38:151.
38. Levy B, Dunn TM, Kaffe S, et al. Clinical applications of comparative genomic hybridization. *Genet Med* 1998;1:4.
39. McDonald-McGinn DM, Driscoll DA, Emanuel BS, et al. The 22q11 deletion in African American patients: an underdiagnosed population. *Am J Hum Genet* 1996;59:90(A).
40. McDonald-McGinn DM, Emanuel BS, Zackai EH. 22q11 deletion syndrome. *GeneReviews* 1999;(Sept 23). Available at http://www.geneclinics.org. Accessed 1/1/05.
41. Francomano CA. Achondroplasia. Gene Reviews 2001;(Mar 8). Available at http://www.geneclinics.org. Accessed 1/1/05.
42. Kelly RI, Hennekam RCM. The Smith-Lemli-Opitz syndrome. *J Med Genet* 2000;37:321.
43. White AL, Modaff P, Holland-Morris F, et al. Natural history of rhizomelic chondrodysplasia punctata. *Am J Med Genet* 2003;118A: 332.
44. The Treacher Collins Syndrome Collaborative Group. Positional cloning of a gene involved in the pathogenesis of Treacher Collins syndrome. *Nat Genet* 1996;12:130.
45. Robin NH, Falk MJ. Craniosynostosis syndromes (FGFR-related). *GeneReviews* 2003;(Feb 13). Available at http://www.geneclinics.org. Accessed 1/1/05.
46. Shuman C, Weksberg R. Beckwith-Wiedemann syndrome. *GeneReviews* 2003;(Apr 10). Available at http://www.geneclinics.org. Accessed 1/1/05.
47. Young ID. Risk estimation in genetic counseling. In: Rimoin DL, Connor JM, Pyeritz RE, eds. *Principles and practice of medical genetics*, 3rd ed, vol 1. Edinburgh: Churchill Livingstone, 1996:521.
48. Hall JG. When a child is born with congenital abnormalities. *Contemp Pediatr* 1988; August:78.

39

Endocrine Disorders of the Newborn

Mary M. Lee   *Thomas Moshang, Jr.*

From the moment of conception, physiologic endocrine processes are actively involved in growth and development of the human fetus. Disturbances in the interplay of these complex hormonal processes during intrauterine life can cause somatic or biochemical alterations in the fetus and newborn infant. Clinical disorders of endocrine function in the neonate therefore, can reflect an altered physiologic state in the fetus, the mother, or the fetal-maternal unit. Moreover, the occurrence of these perturbations of endocrine function at varying stages of fetal development results in diverse clinical manifestations. Knowledge of the ontogeny of the endocrine glands and their physiologic function during fetal development facilitates understanding disorders of endocrine function in the newborn.

DISORDERS OF SEXUAL DIFFERENTIATION

Normal Sexual Differentiation

The normal regulation of sexual differentiation is broadly illustrated in Fig. 39-1. All embryos are initially undifferentiated with a bipotential gonad and the anlagen for both male and female reproductive tracts and genitalia (1). Differentiation of the gonads as testes or ovaries dictates the subsequent development of the internal and external genitalia. The gonad forms when germ cells migrate from the dorsal endoderm of the yolk sac to populate the genital ridges. At the fifth to sixth week of gestation, these primitive bipotential gonads consist of both cortical (ovarian) and medullary (testicular) components. The genital ridge is composed of three cell types: (a) germ cells destined to become prespermatogonia in the male or oogonia in the female, (b) supporting epithelial cells destined to become Sertoli cells (male) or granulosa cells (female) and (c) mesenchymal cells destined to become the steroid-producing Leydig cells (male) or theca cells

(female). Development of the supporting cells as Sertoli or follicular are a critical determinant in whether the germ cells differentiate as spermatogonia or oogonia.

Of the genes that are critical for gonadal development, mutations in two have been clearly associated with gonadal dysgenesis. Mutations of the Wilms tumor gene (2) (WT1), are associated with three related syndromes (the WAGR contiguous gene syndrome, and Denys-Drash and Frasier) that affect renal function and gonadal development and mutations in the transcription factor, steroidogenic factor 1 (3) (SF-1), cause agenesis of the adrenals and gonads.

Sexually dimorphic differentiation of the gonads and reproductive system commences when the testis-determining gene is first expressed. In 1959, Ford and colleagues determined that the Y chromosome was necessary for male development (4); in 1966, the critical region for testis determination was localized to the short arm of the Y chromosome (5); and in 1990, the primary testis-determining gene was definitively identified at Yp11.3 by positional cloning in patients with sex reversal (6). This gene, termed SRY (sex-determining region of the Y chromosome), is a member of the Sox family of transcription factors that all contain a high mobility group (HMG) DNA-binding motif (6). Activation of SRY initiates differentiation of the bipotential gonad as a testis. Loss of function mutations in SRY or a delay in its onset of expression can cause XY sex reversal with gonadal dysgenesis, although a gain of function mutation in SRY causes XX sex reversal associated with incomplete testicular development.

SOX9, a presumptive target for SRY, is a related HMG box gene that induces the supporting cells of the gonadal ridge to differentiate as Sertoli cells (7). Inactivating mutations of SOX9 cause the skeletal anomalies of camptomelic dysplasia that is associated with variable penetrance of 46,XY sex reversal and testicular dysgenesis (8). A role for additional downstream genes in testicular determination is supported by the absence of identifiable SRY or SOX9 mutations in

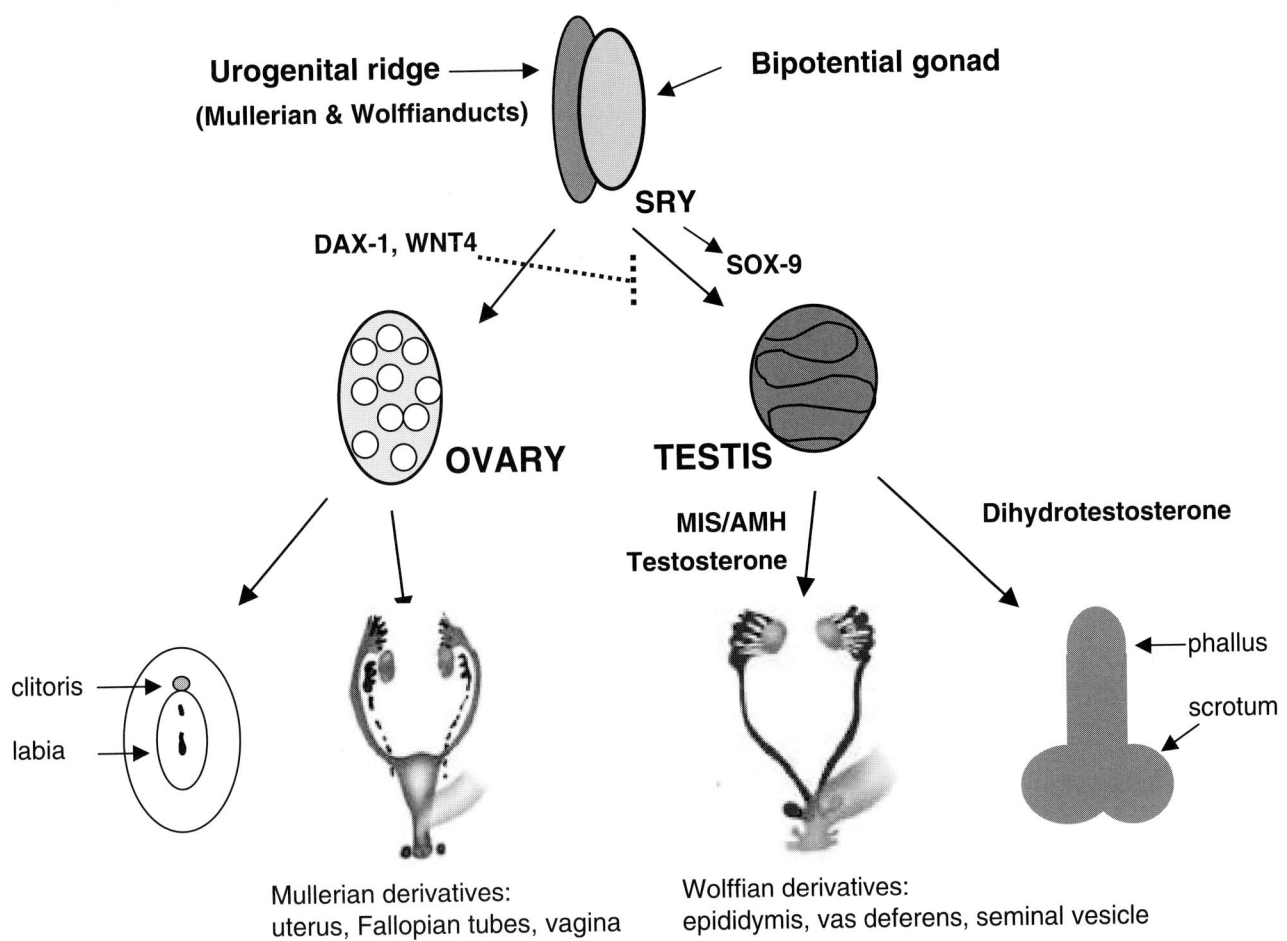

Figure 39-1   Schematic of the sex differentiation pathway. The urogenital ridge and gonad are initially undifferentiated. In male embryos, the induction of SRY expression initiates testis determination. The testicular hormones, MIS/AMH and androgens stimulate male phenotypic development of the internal and external genitalia. In female embryos, the absence of SRY in concert with the expression of genes that inhibit testicular determination enables the gonad to develop as an ovary. In the absence of androgens and MIS/AMH, the internal and external genitalia differentiate as female.

some cases of sex reversal and the association of sex reversal and dysgenetic gonads with other autosomal deletions.

At least two genes, Wnt-4, a locally secreted signaling glycoprotein, and Dax-1, a nuclear hormone receptor in the DSS region of the X-chromosome, are critical for ovarian development, perhaps by suppressing testicular genes. A duplication of either of these genes interferes with normal testicular development to cause a dosage sensitive form of 46,XY sex reversal (3,9).

Sexually dimorphic differentiation of the wolffian (male anlagen) and mullerian (female anlagen) internal genital tracts depends on the hormonal milieu established by the somatic cells. If SRY is expressed, the primary sex cords develop into testes and the somatic cells differentiate as Sertoli and Leydig cells. The Sertoli cells secrete Mullerian inhibiting substance (MIS), a 140-kd glycoprotein in the TGF-β family of proteins. MIS causes degeneration of the mullerian ducts by inducing apoptotic cell death of the ductal epithelial cells.

The Leydig cells secrete testosterone, which stimulates the wolffian ducts to differentiate into the vas deferens, seminal vesicle, and epididymis and virilizes the external genitalia.

Differentiation of the external genitalia requires the activation of testosterone by 5α-reductase-2 to its more active metabolite, dihydrotestosterone (DHT). DHT stimulates fusion of the urethral folds and the labioscrotal swellings to form the corpus spongiosa and scrotum. DHT also stimulates growth of the genital tubercle and prostate. Sexually dimorphic differentiation of the internal ducts and the external genitalia is complete by 12 weeks of gestation. Subsequently, during the latter part of gestation, the testes descend into the scrotum and the phallus enlarges as testosterone production increases under the stimulus of pituitary gonadotropins.

In 46,XX embryos, the primary sex cords become follicles by 10 weeks gestation and the germ cells differentiate to oogonia. Both X chromosomes are needed for maintenance of the ovary. In the absence of one X chromosome, as in Turner syndrome, the ovaries form initially, but regress before birth. In females, fetal ovaries do not secrete MIS, thus the mullerian ducts differentiate to form the uterus, fallopian tubes and upper vagina. The absence of testosterone and DHT production by the fetal ovary cause the wolffian ducts to degenerate and enables the external genitalia to differentiate as female.

DISORDERS OF CHROMOSOMAL SEX

A number of sex chromosome aberrations have been reported (see Chapter 38): some are embryonic lethal (e.g., 45,YO), others cause minimal somatic or hormonal manifestations in the newborn (e.g., 47,XXY), and a few perturb gonadal and genital development (45,X/46,XY,45,X0). In contrast to the autosomes, extra genetic material from the X chromosome can be tolerated with minor untoward effects as a result of inactivation of the second and additional X chromosomes. Although ovarian formation and function are intact in patients with X polyploidy, early menopause may occur (10). In contrast, a Y chromosome is generally necessary for testicular development, although rare cases of sex-reversed 46,XX males with normal testicular function and male genitalia are reported (11).

The classic sex chromosomal anomalies occur relatively frequently as determined by newborn screening. In the New Haven Study, 47,XXY occurred once in 545 males, 47,XYY occurred once in 728 males, 47,XXX occurred once in 727 females, and 45,XO occurred once in 2181 female newborns (12). The incidence of 45,XO if higher than this, but leads to increased fetal demise and is found in 1 in 15 spontaneous abortions (13). The diagnosis of Turner syndrome, however, is made with greater frequency than the other sex chromosomal aberrations because of the associated somatic abnormalities.

Turner Syndrome

The classic and most common chromosomal abnormality is total loss of one X chromosome. Over 50% of girls with Turner syndrome have a 45,XO karyotype, 17% have mosaicism with an isochromosome 46,X,i(Xq), 8% are chimeras with 45,X0/46,XX, and the remainder have other forms of mosaicism with loss of X material (14). The presence of a mosaic 46,XX cell line has little bearing on stature or somatic abnormalities, but does influence gonadal development. Goldberg and associates reported spontaneous female sexual development in 3 of 25 patients with mosaic karyotypes, but in none in those with 45,X0 (15).

The Turner phenotype in the newborn is secondary to lymphangiectasia and lymphedema. The webbed neck is most often seen as redundant folds about the posterior neck. The lymphedema involves the dorsa of the hands and feet. A host of associated somatic defects have been described in this syndrome (14,16), most of which become more evident with increasing age. The most common are triangular facies with low-set ears, high-arched palate, low hairline, shield-like chest with widespread and hypoplastic areolae, and cubitus valgus. Coarctation of the aorta is the typical cardiovascular abnormality; however the more benign condition of bicuspid aortic valves occurs more frequently. Miscellaneous renal malformations are observed. Skin manifestations include hemangiomas, cutis laxa, pigmented nevi, dysplastic nails, and tendency to keloid formation. Skeletal abnormalities include "beaking" of the medial tibial condyle, drumstick-shaped distal phalanges, vertebral anomalies, and short metacarpals (17). Dermatoglyphic abnormalities include palmar simian creases, distal axial triradius, and an increased number of digital ulnar whorls. Declining growth can manifest in young children and is the most consistent characteristic in the older child.

After diagnosis, screening for associated disorders such as cardiac and renal defects is needed (16). Therapy is focused on the specific developmental anomaly, such as coarctation of the aorta, and on providing education about potential associated problems, such as recurrent otitis media, chronic lymphocytic thyroiditis, and idiopathic hypertension. The incidence of mental retardation is slightly increased with specific X chromosome rearrangements. In most children with Turner syndrome however, cognition is normal with good verbal skills and selected spatial deficits.

A major concern for girls with Turner syndrome is extreme short stature with a mean adult height of 148 cm. Recombinant growth hormone increases final height and is approved for treatment of short stature in Turner syndrome. The combination of early use of growth hormone (before 5 years of age) and low dose estrogen replacement at an appropriate age is thought to give the best outcome in terms of height and pyschosexual development (18). Estrogen/progesterone therapy at the appropriate age is indicated for the treatment of sexual infantilism.

Questions regarding fertility may arise even in the newborn period because primary gonadal failure occurs in more than 90% of individuals with Turner syndrome. Women with Turner syndrome, however, have successfully carried offspring to term using donor oocytes, at a rate similar to couples with other causes of infertility (19).

The presence of Y material in the karyotype raises concerns about testicular elements that are at risk for malignant transformation. In patients with mosaicism that includes Y material, gonadectomy is therefore recommended, both to eliminate the risk for gonadoblastoma and to avoid the virilizing effects of hormonally active residual testicular elements (20).

DISORDERS OF GONADAL DETERMINATION

Disorders of gonadal determination can occur in association with autosomal or sex chromosomal anomalies and/or loss of function mutations or deletions of SRY and

SOX-97. Mutations have also been identified in other genes essential for gonadal formation such as WT-1 and SF-1. The clinical phenotype of these single gene mutations varies from complete gonadal dysgenesis to lesser degrees of testicular damage. Teratogens such as radiation, viruses, and drugs have also been implicated in *in utero* gonadal damage. Differentiation and development of the internal ducts and external genitalia in these infants depend on the timing and extent of insult to the developing gonad.

Complete Gonadal Dysgenesis

Complete dysgenesis of the genital ridges results in normal female genitalia with no associated somatic findings, thus the diagnosis is often not suspected during infancy. Infants with 46,XY complete gonadal dysgenesis may be identified as a result of genitalia that are discordant with the prenatal karyotype. Affected girls tend to be tall with eunuchoid proportions and often present with primary amenorrhea and sexual infantilism. An autosomal recessive form of 46,XX gonadal dysgenesis is associated with sensory neural deafness (21). The majority of 46,XY gonadal dysgenesis is sporadic but familial forms can be sex-limited autosomal recessive, X-linked, or autosomal dominant in inheritance (22).

Partial Gonadal Dysgenesis

Incomplete loss of function of genes essential for testicular differentiation, or exposure to teratogens that damage the developing testis cause partial gonadal dysgenesis. Testicular loss after 9-10 weeks of gestation will not interfere with involution of the mullerian structures because the critical time for exposure to MIS is at 7 to 10 weeks, but will perturb mid-line fusion and development of the external genitalia, which is dependent on on-going testosterone production by the testes. Thus the external genitalia are female or severely undervirilized, but the gonads, uterus and fallopian tubes are absent and the wolffian structures are incompletely developed.

True Hermaphroditism

In true hermaphroditism, both ovarian and testicular elements are present. Findings may consist of an ovary on one side and a testis on the contralateral side, an ovary or a testis and a contralateral ovotestis, or two ovotestes (23). Most patients with true hermaphroditism have ambiguous external genitalia, although differentiation of the internal duct structures and external genitalia depend on the amount of functioning testicular tissue. In those reared as female, the testicular component of the gonad may secrete androgens at puberty to cause unwanted virilization, thus gonadectomy should be performed early. Although some patients have sex chromosome abnormalities, 46,XX is the most common karyotype, followed by 46,XY. The pathogenesis of true hermaphroditism is not well understood, but is not consistently linked to alterations in SRY expression.

DISORDERS OF PHENOTYPIC SEX

Disorders of phenotypic sex result when the anatomic development of the external genitalia does not correspond to the chromosomal and gonadal sex. The external genitalia may be truly ambiguous—that is, the sex of the infant cannot be ascertained by physical examination. Alternatively, the phenotype may be normal male or female, but inappropriate for the genotype. These conditions may be secondary to genetic defects affecting hormonal synthesis or action, problems in timing or regulation or hormonal secretion, defects in receptor binding or signaling defects, or teratogens or maternal hormones that perturb reproductive tract development. A genotypic (46,XY) male with testes and inadequate virilization falls in the category of male pseudohermaphroditism. A virilized genotypic (46,XX) female with ovaries is considered to have female pseudohermaphroditism.

Female Pseudohermaphroditism

The female fetus can be virilized by fetal adrenal androgens or maternal androgens transferred across the placenta. Exposure to androgens prior to week 12 of gestation results in fusion of the urogenital sinus and genital folds. Exposure to androgens after week 12 of gestation or after birth causes milder manifestations of clitoral enlargement, labial hyperpigmentation, and posterior labial fusion.

Congenital Adrenal Hyperplasia

The major cause of virilization in a female is congenital adrenal hyperplasia (CAH) as a result of steroidogenic enzyme defects in cortisol biosynthesis. The more common inherited enzymatic deficiencies of adrenal biosynthesis (21-hydroxylase, 11-hydroxylase, and 3β-hydroxysteroid dehydrogenase defects) all virilize the female. The gonads are ovaries, thus internal genital duct development is female—the wolffian ducts regress and the mullerian structures are normally formed. The excess adrenal androgens, however, promote fusion of the labia and the urogenital sinus, and phallic enlargement. Rarely, the virilization is severe enough to cause complete external masculinization. The 21-hydroxylase and 3β-hydroxysteroid dehydrogenase forms of CAH are complicated by associated mineralocorticoid deficiency that may present as a salt-losing adrenal crisis. The enzymatic defects causing CAH are more fully discussed in the section on adrenal disorders.

Drug-Induced Female Pseudohermaphroditism

A number of female newborns have been virilized by progestational agents used to prevent spontaneous abortion or other medications with androgenic potency (24). When these drugs are used during the first trimester, the labioscrotal folds are fused with formation of a urogenital sinus and clitoromegaly. When fetuses are exposed after the first trimester, they develop only clitoral enlargement, without labioscrotal fusion. In contrast to untreated infants with CAH, there is neither progressive virilization nor continued acceleration of growth and skeletal maturation after birth. No medical intervention is needed as androgens are not elevated but surgical correction might be warranted. These children will feminize normally at puberty and achieve normal fertility.

Virilizing Disorders in the Mother

Virilization of a female fetus by an androgen-producing maternal tumor is rare. These tumors almost always are caused by an ovarian lesion-arrhenoblastomas, Krukenberg tumors, luteomas, lipoid or stromal cell tumors, although adrenal adenomas are also reported (25). The tumors cause clitoromegaly, acne, deepening of the voice, decreased lactation and hirsutism in the mothers and are associated with elevated serum androgens and elevated excretion of urinary 17-ketosteroids (26).

Aromatase Deficiency

Rare genetic defects in the fetal or placental aromatase gene impair aromatization of maternal and placental androgens to estrogens and cause in utero elevations of androgens (27). Both fetal and maternal virilization can occur.

Idiopathic Female Pseudohermaphroditism

Idiopathic virilization may be caused by nonhormonal factors as exposure to androgens cannot be documented. This can occur in isolation or in conjunction with congenital anomalies of the gastrointestinal (GI) and urinary tracts that include imperforate anus, renal agenesis, urinary tract obstructions, urethrovaginal fistulas, and/or defective mullerian duct formation.

Male Pseudohermaphroditism

Incomplete masculinization of the male fetus can be as a result of a myriad of causes that disrupt either androgen action or the response of target tissues to androgens during sexual differentiation. The differential diagnosis of male pseudohermaphroditism is extensive, including enzymatic defects of testosterone synthesis, unresponsiveness to testosterone action (androgen-resistance syndromes), hypothalamic or pituitary dysfunction, and vascular or teratogenic insult to the testis.

Defects in Testosterone Biosynthesis

Male fetuses are undervirilized when in utero testosterone production is reduced as a result of a genetic mutation in one of the testosterone synthetic enzymes (28). The phenotype varies according to the specific gene affected. Defects in 17α-hydroxylase/lyase and 17β-hydroxysteroid

dehydrogenase primarily affect testosterone production although defects in enzymes needed for both testosterone and cortisol synthesis cause a form of CAH associated with incomplete masculinization. Steroidogenic acute regulatory protein (StAR) and 3β-hydroxysteroid dehydrogenase mediate early steps in cortisol and aldosterone synthesis. Mutations in either of these genes can result in a severe salt-losing syndrome and insufficient masculinization of the genitalia. The full details of these disorders, including diagnosis and treatment, are outlined in the section on adrenal hyperplasia.

Syndromes of Androgen Resistance

This is a group of disorders characterized by undervirilized genitalia with normal mullerian duct regression and normal testosterone synthesis (29). The term androgen resistance encompasses androgen receptor or postreceptor defects (androgen insensitivity syndrome [AIS]) and 5α-reductase deficiency in which the conversion of testosterone to its more active metabolite, DHT is affected. In both conditions, MIS is produced normally by the fetal testis and causes involution of the mullerian structures. In AIS, although testosterone is produced, the defect resides in the receptor or its signaling, thus target tissue response is compromised. Consequently, all aspects of male development mediated by androgens, including development of the wolffian structures and external genitalia are affected.

In contrast, in 5α-reductase deficiency, sufficient testosterone is produced for differentiation of the wolffian structures, but not for complete virilization of the external genitalia, which requires DHT (30). DHT is needed for mid-line fusion and phallic growth, thus patients with 5α-reductase deficiency typically have a blind vaginal pouch, a small phallic structure with chordee, a hooded prepuce, and perineoscrotal hypospadias. At puberty, the increase in secretion of testosterone and induction in expression of 5α-reductase and the androgen receptor in genital tissues stimulate growth of pubic hair, penile enlargement, and descent of the testes. 5α-reductase deficiency is suspected in 46,XY patients with perineoscrotal hypospadias and an elevated testosterone to DHT ratio of more than 35 under basal conditions and more than 74 after human chorionic gonadotropin (hCG) stimulation. The diagnosis is confirmed by finding reduced 5α-reductase activity in fibroblasts from genital skin.

Complete AIS (CAIS), an X-linked condition, was previously referred to as the testicular feminization syndrome (31). Affected patients have a 46,XY karyotype, normal female external genitalia with a blind vaginal pouch, absent wolffian and mullerian structures, and abdominal or inguinal testes. Unlike patients with 5α-reductase deficiency, virilization does not occur at puberty but peripheral conversion of the high testosterone concentrations to estradiol stimulates good breast development and estrogenization of the vaginal mucosa. Most patients have little pubic hair and some have total absence of sexual hair. In all other respects, including height, habitus, voice, breast development, and gender identity, these individuals are feminine. The diagnosis is made in infancy or childhood as a result of female genitals that are discrepant with an 46,XY karyotype, or to the discovery of testicular tissue during hernia repair. Adolescent patients frequently present with primary amenorrhea. Genetic mutations of the androgen receptor are identified in only two thirds of individuals with suspected AIS. The gonads in CAIS have a 9% risk for malignant transformation to neoplasia, thus should be removed surgically.

A wide spectrum of phenotypes is observed in individuals with incomplete forms of androgen insensitivity. Partial or mild AIS (PAIS) can range from a female phenotype with clitoromegaly and posterior labial fusion to a male phenotype with infertility and sparse pubic hair. Sex assignment may be difficult in patients with PAIS. In some cases, assessment of responsiveness of the phallus to androgens is helpful.

OTHER CONDITIONS INVOLVING GENITOURINARY DEVELOPMENT

Male or Female Genital Phenotype Inconsistent with Genotype

A problem ensues at birth when the phenotype is inconsistent with the chromosomal sex determined by prenatal cytogenetic analysis. A repeat karyotype after birth may reveal an error in the prenatal cytogenetic analysis. A number of intersex conditions, however, can present at birth with external genitalia that are normal in appearance but discordant with chromosomal sex (Table 39-1). In general, these children should be raised according to the phenotypic sex.

Hypospadias and Cryptorchidism

Isolated hypospadias occurs in 0.8% of newborn infants and isolated cryptorchidism is present in approximately 5% of full-term and up to 15% of premature infants. Generally, neither condition by itself is associated with an endocrine abnormality. The incidence of intersex conditions however,

is greater if the hypospadias is severe (on the shaft or perineum), or if the testes are nonpalpable. If cryptorchidism and hypospadias are both present, 25% of infants have a disorder of intersex.

Micropenis

Isolated micropenis with otherwise normally formed genitalia generally is not considered as ambiguous genitalia. This condition is associated with insufficient testosterone secretion during the third trimester. The evaluation of micropenis is discussed under hypopituitarism, the most common treatable cause of this condition.

EVALUATION

The evaluation of a newborn with ambiguous genitalia should be managed expediently by a team of experienced providers. Parents should be reassured that incomplete or excessive differentiation of the genitals occurred as part of a continuum in the developmental process and that the appropriate sex will be determined within several days. It is our general philosophy not to discuss pending studies in detail because there are occasions for gender assignment that are inconsistent with either chromosomal or gonadal sex and presentation of all data available enables a more cohesive explanation. As in any diagnostic problem, the approach to the child with ambiguous genitalia should begin with a thorough history, a careful physical examination, and appropriate laboratory and radiologic testing. Table 39-2 outlines the different causes of sexual ambiguity.

A history of drug ingestion, particularly in the first trimester, or recent androgenic changes in the mother might suggest the cause of female pseudohermaphroditism. First trimester infections or exposure to teratogens might suggest gonadal dysgenesis. A family history of an unexplained neonatal death or siblings with virilization or precocious puberty, might suggest the diagnosis of CAH although a history of female relatives with sexual infantilism suggests X-linked causes such as AIS.

A thorough physical examination is important, but on no account should a diagnosis be based on the physical

TABLE 39-1
ETIOLOGY OF MALE OR FEMALE GENITAL PHENOTYPE INCONSISTENT WITH THE GENOTYPE

Disorder	Genotype	Phenotype	Etiology
Pure gonadal dysgenesis	XY	Female	mutations in SRY, SOX9 WT1, SF-1
46,XX Males	XX	Male	SRY translocation
46,XY Females	XY	Female	SRY deletion
Congenital lipoid hyperplasia	XY	Female	CAH (StAR)
17,20-Lyase deficiency	XY	Female	CAH (17-βHSD)
17-Hydroxylase deficiency	XY	Female	CAH (p450c17)
Androgen resistance syndrome	XY	Female	mutation in AR

TABLE 39-2
ETIOLOGY OF AMBIGUOUS GENITALIA

Disorders of gonadal determination
  Complete or partial gonadal dysgenesis
  Sex reversal
  True hermaphroditism
Virilization of females
  Congenital adrenal hyperplasia
    21-Hydroxylase deficiency
    11-Hydroxylase defiency
    3β-Hydroxysteroid dehydrogenase deficiency
  Chromosomal aberrations
    XO/XY
    XX/XY
    Variants
  Maternal virilization
    Drug-induced
    Excess androgen production by mother
  Aromatase deficiency
  Idiopathic
    Isolated
    Associated with midline congenital anomalies
Inadequate masculinization of males
  Defects in testosterone biosynthesis
    17-hydroxylase deficiency
    17-β-hydroxysteroid dehydrogenase
  Congenital adrenal hyperplasia
    StAR
    3β-hydroxysteroid dehydrogenase deficiency
  Androgen resistance syndromes
    5α-Reductase deficiency
    Androgen receptor defects
  Congenital anorchia/vanishing testis
  Teratogenic insult
  Idiopathic
    Isolated
    Associated with midline congenital anomalies

findings. The presence or absence of palpable gonads helps to differentiate the major categories of intersex conditions. In general, gonads lacking testicular elements will not descend below the inguinal region. Thus, a palpable gonad excludes the diagnosis of female pseudohermaphroditism in which the gonads are ovaries by definition. Measurement of the length and diameter of the penis is valuable both for prognostic information and also as a baseline if treatment is given to enlarge the penis. The urethral opening should be identified and the existence or absence of a vagina should be determined. The degree of fusion of the labial-scrotal folds and the presence of associated urinary or GI tract anomalies should be assessed.

The physical examination can help direct the laboratory and radiologic investigation. Certain tests are obtained as soon as it is apparent that there is sexual ambiguity, although others may be required at a later stage to make an accurate diagnosis (Table 39-3). For example, serum 17-hydroxy-progesterone and electrolytes are useful initial screening tests for congenital adrenal hyperplasia but other steroid precursors and genetic studies may help establish the specific diagnosis. In the newborn period, testosterone,

follicle-stimulating hormone (FSH), and luteinizing hormone (LH) should be drawn to assess the hypothalamic-pituitary-gonadal axis. Serum testosterone can be elevated from either gonadal or adrenal production and should be interpreted in the context of the examination and other laboratory studies. Measurement of MIS may help determine the presence of testicular tissue (32). It should be stressed that sex assignment does not require that all studies leading to a final diagnosis be completed (e.g., the exact type of congenital adrenal hyperplasia may be important for genetic counseling and future prenatal diagnosis, but not for sex assignment). The karyotype can help determine whether the infant is a virilized female or an inadequately virilized male. This, however, should not be used as the primary criteria for sex assignment as other factors such as gonadal function, sensitivity to androgens, future sexual function and potential for fertility or pregnancy (even if by *in vitro* fertilization) are also critical.

Pelvic ultrasound to evaluate the internal genital structures and gonads should be performed by an experienced radiologist. Ultrasonography may identify nonpalpable gonads, and may be able to define the echogenic pattern as either ovarian or testicular tissue (33). The presence of a uterus indicates a lack of MIS action and probable absence of functioning testicular tissue in early gestation, and usually indicates that the child should be raised as a female. Conversely, the absence of mullerian structures implies the presence of functioning testicular tissue that secreted MIS at 7 to 9 weeks of gestation. This is consistent with sex-determining region Y (SRY) expression and suggestive of an XY karyotype, but is not a major determinant for male sex assignment. The karyotype, phallic size and degree of hypospadias, internal genital structures, gonadal pathology, and etiology of the intersex condition are all part of the equation in gender determination.

TABLE 39-3
STUDIES TO EVALUATE AMBIGUOUS GENITALIA

Immediate studies
  Karyotype
  Pelvic ultrasonography
  Serum
    Electrolytes
    17-Hydroxyprogesterone
    17-OH pregnenolone
    Testosterone
    11-Deoxycortisol
    Dihydrotestosterone
    Mullerian inhibiting substance
    FSH/LH
Follow-up studies
  hCG stimulation testing
  Cortrosyn stimulation testing
  Genito-urethrogram and other radiologic studies
  Exploratory laparotomy and gonadal biopsy
  Skin biopsy to evaluate androgen action
  Genetic/molecular studies for specific mutations

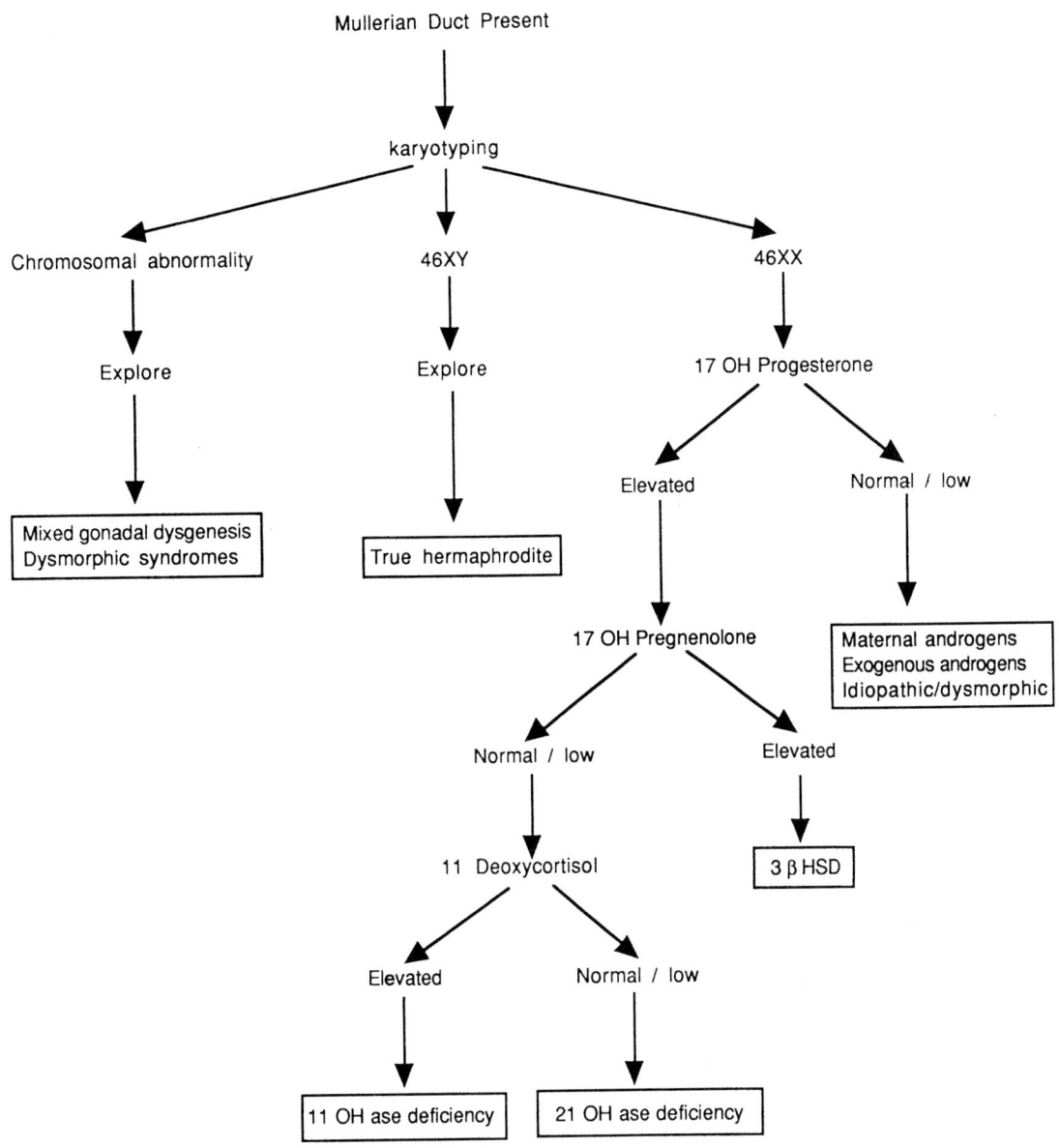

Figure 39-2 An algorithm for evaluating sexual ambiguity in infants with mullerian structures.

To evaluate further the specific etiology of the sexual ambiguity, secondary studies may be necessary. The algorithms in Figs. 39-2 and 39-3, which are based on the initial ultrasound findings, delineate the steps that may be necessary to make a definitive diagnosis. These algorithms do not include patients with normal male or female phenotypes that are discordant with the genotype. Surgical exploration frequently will be required in cases of true hermaphroditism or partial gonadal dysgenesis but may be done at a later time. It should be stressed that the final histopathologic diagnosis is not necessary for sex assignment.

After the evaluation is complete, including consultations from an endocrinologist and an urologist, the appropriate sex assignment is determined by a consensus of opinion from the team that might also include a geneticist, a psychiatrist or psychologist, the pediatrician, and clergy or other support personnel. Parental input is also considered in the decision, especially in cases in which the appropriate sex assignment is uncertain. Gender identity, and future sexual function and fertility are major determining factors. The attending physician should discuss the condition fully with the parents, including expectations for future sexual function and fertility and whether any hormonal medications or surgery are recommended.

Gender assignment for most infants with ambiguous genitalia is straightforward when chromosomal sex and gonadal sex correlate with the internal structures. The external genitalia may require reconstructive surgery to improve function and cosmetic appearance. The timing of surgery has become controversial and highly politicized as a result of heightened concerns about ethical issues of informed consent by the child, the possibility of gender dysphoria and sex reassignment, and the risk for postsurgical loss of genital sensation. With little long-term data to support early vs. late reconstructive surgery, it may be prudent to postpone surgery until gender identity is clear and

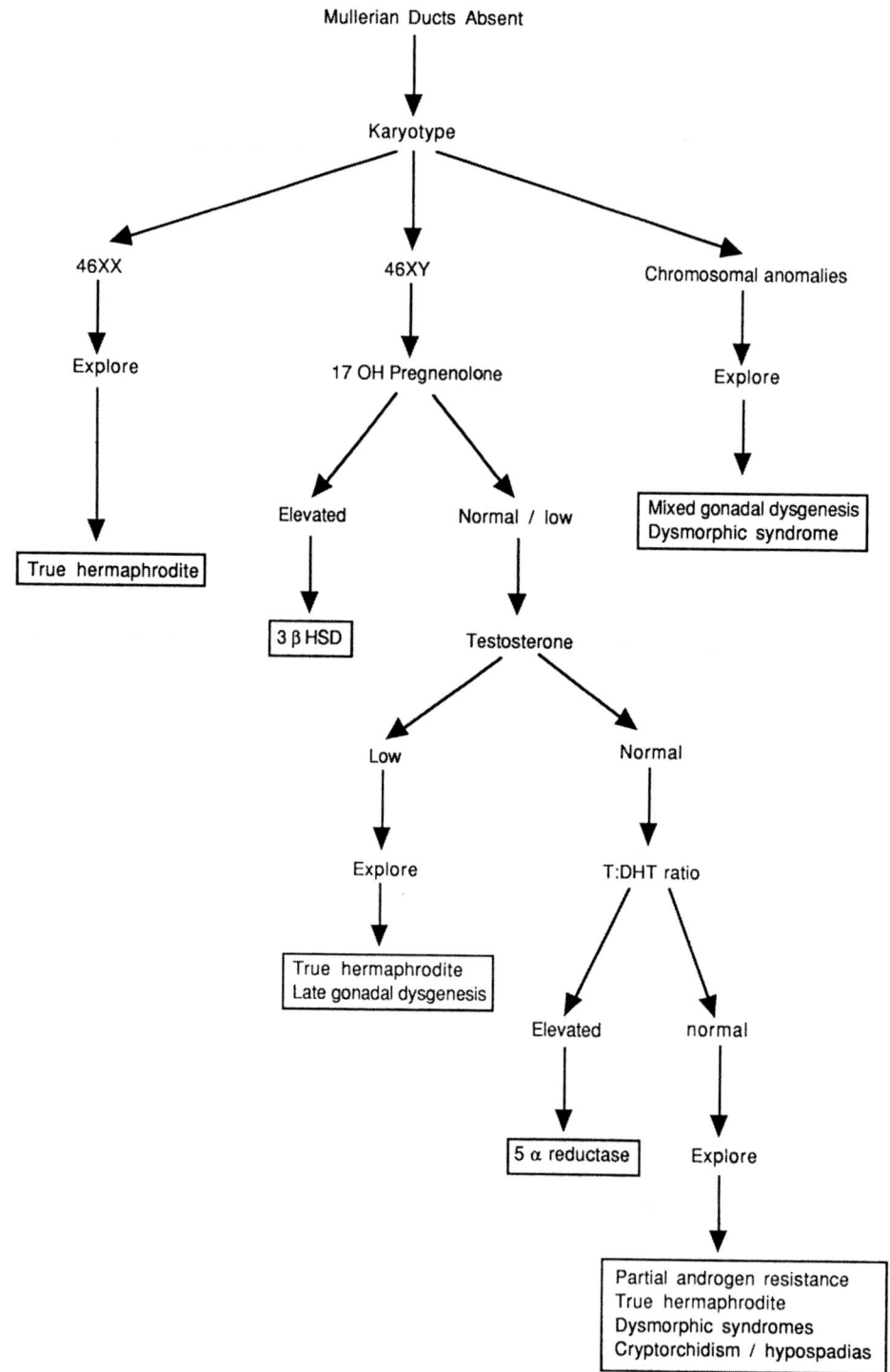

Figure 39-3 An algorithm for evaluating sexual ambiguity in infants without mullerian structures.

to have the full participation of the family (and child) in the decision. Hormonal therapy may be required to induce secondary sexual maturation, but is usually not needed during the neonatal period. Rarely, as in cases of partial androgen resistance syndromes, true hermaphroditism, or mixed gonadal dysgenesis, gender assignment contrary to chromosomal or gonadal sex must be considered. In these cases, careful consideration must be given to the likelihood of gender role and sexual function as an adult (34).

Severe micropenis or agenesis previously warranted a female sex assignment despite the presence of testes or a normal 46,XY karyotype, but this approach is now under reappraisal. Recent reports of dissatisfaction with a female sex assignment in some 46,XY individuals with cloacal exstrophy or other nonhormonally mediated causes of aphallia reinforce the need to explore new paradigms for sex assignment. These paradigms will need to include other factors that affect adult gender identity such as the role of prenatal hormones on central nervous system (CNS) sex differentiation.

DISORDERS OF THE HYPOTHALAMUS AND PITUITARY

Development of the Hypothalamic-Pituitary Axis

The hypothalamus arises by proliferation of neuroblasts in the intermediate zone of the diencephalic wall and formation of the supraoptic and periventricular nuclei. The anterior pituitary, or adenohypophysis, arises embryonically from an invagination of the oral ectodermal cavity called the Rathke pouch. This diverticulum arises at 3 weeks of gestation, and by 5 weeks has migrated upward to its final position and separated completely from the oral cavity. Concordantly, the posterior pituitary, or neurohypophysis, is formed from a downward invagination of the floor of the diencephalon. Neural fibers migrate from the hypothalamus down to the posterior pituitary to form the neurohypophyseal tract. The hypothalamus regulates the pituitary by secreting both stimulatory and inhibitory hormones. The stimulatory hormones include growth hormone-releasing hormone (GHRH), thyrotropin-releasing hormone (TRH), corticotropin-releasing hormone (CRH), and gonadotropin-releasing hormone (GnRH). The main inhibitory hormones are somatostatin, which inhibits growth hormone release and prolactin inhibitory factor, which inhibits prolactin release. In response to these hypothalamic hormones, the anterior pituitary secretes prolactin, growth hormone (GH), thyroid-stimulating hormone (TSH), adrenocorticotropic hormone (ACTH), LH, and FSH. The posterior pituitary secretes vasopressin and oxytocin. The hypothalamic and pituitary glands are functional after week 12 of gestation.

Most disorders of the hypothalamic-pituitary axis in the newborn period, except for the syndrome of inappropriate secretion of antidiuretic hormone (SIADH), are those of insufficiency related to malformations, trauma, infection or genetically inherited disorders, as outlined in Table 39-4. This differs from older children and adults who may have either functionally active tumors that secrete pituitary hormones or infiltrative disease or tumors that interfere with normal pituitary function.

DISORDERS OF THE ANTERIOR PITUITARY

Anterior pituitary dysfunction is difficult to detect in the newborn. The predominant features of anterior pituitary insufficiency are hypoglycemia, micropenis and, occasionally, cholestatic jaundice. The hypoglycemia may be quite severe and comparable to that seen in infants with congenital hyperinsulinism. The infants may even have a brisk glycemic response to glucagon causing further confusion (35). The cholestatic jaundice is initially unconjugated, then becomes predominantly conjugated, and will often only resolve after hormone replacement. There may be combined deficiency of multiple pituitary hormones or isolated deficiency of a single hormone. The molecular basis of multiple hormone deficiency is established for a number of genetic defects and was reviewed recently by Parks and associates (36). Evidence for the importance of the POU family of pituitary transcription factors in establishing pituitary lineages came from identifying the roles of Pit-1 in the Snell dwarf mouse (37), Prop-1 in the Ames dwarf mouse (38) and P-Lim knockout mice (39). In humans P-Lim is associated with deficiencies of all anterior pituitary hormones except ACTH in conjunction with retinal colobomas. Pit-1 mutations cause pituitary gland hypoplasia and deficiencies of GH, TSH, and prolactin. Prop-1 (Prophet of Pit-1) is essential for Pit-1 expression, and therefore has an identical clinical picture. Hypopituitarism in conjunction with optic nerve hypoplasia and absence of the septum pellucidum comprise the syndrome of Septo-optic dysplasia (SOD). Pituitary function can vary from intact to panhypopituitarism including diabetes insipidus. Mutations in a homeodomain protein, HESX-1, have been found in some patients with SOD associated with mild panhypopituitarism or isolated GH deficiency (40). SOD is often suggested by wandering nystagmus in the newborn, reflective of optic nerve hypoplasia and blindness.

Growth Hormone Deficiency

Growth hormone deficiency in the neonate may present as hypoglycemia, micropenis, or both. Micropenis is defined as penile size less than 2.5 cm stretched length in the term

---

TABLE 39-4
ETIOLOGY OF DISORDERS OF THE HYPOTHALAMIC-PITUITARY AXIS

Malformations
    Cleft lip and palate
    Optic nerve atrophy
    Septooptic dysplasia
    Transphenoidal encephalocele
    Holoprosencephaly
    Anencephaly
Trauma associated with breech delivery
Congenital infection
    Rubella
    Toxoplasmosis
Tumor
    Hypothalamic hamartoblastoma (i.e., Pallister Hall syndrome)
    Rathke pouch cyst
    Craniopharyngioma
    Glioblastoma
Isolated or combined familial or idiopathic pituitary hormone deficiency
    Autosomal recessive or X-linked recessive familial panhypopituitarism

infant. Congenital deficiency of growth hormone does not cause intrauterine growth retardation and often does not affect linear growth until 6 to 9 months of age. Intrauterine growth is primarily determined by maternal factors, including nutritional status, placental function, and gestational infection or drugs. During early postnatal life, thyroid hormone, insulin, and nutrition are more important growth determinants than growth hormone. A family history of short stature is pertinent because familial autosomal dominant inheritance of growth hormone deficiency is well recognized.

Gonadotropin Deficiency

Gonadotropin deficiency can occur as either isolated hypogonadotropic hypogonadism or combined multiple pituitary hormone deficiency. Although infants with combined deficiencies present with micropenis, those with isolated gonadotropin deficiency may not be recognized at birth. The genitalia can be normal male in Kallmans syndrome (hypogonadotropic hypogonadism and anosmia), a syndrome caused by mutations in the KAL gene encoding anosmin-1. Female infants are asymptomatic at birth and may not be identified until puberty fails to occur. Other causes of micropenis associated with gonadotropin deficiency include syndromic conditions, such as Noonan syndrome and Prader-Willi syndrome.

Adrenocorticotropic Hormone Deficiency

Adrenocorticotropic hormone deficiency rarely presents as an acute adrenal crisis; the cortisol insufficiency is typically mild and may cause hypoglycemia or hyponatremia without hyperkalemia, and occasionally, prolonged direct hyperbilirubinemia. Isolated ACTH deficiency is extremely rare but has been linked to the CRH gene locus (41). The combination of both growth hormone and ACTH deficiency may cause hypoketotic hypoglycemia of such severity that it is difficult to differentiate from congenital hyperinsulinism (35).

Thyroid-Stimulating Hormone Deficiency

Thyroid-stimulating hormone deficiency is essentially asymptomatic in the newborn. On newborn screening tests, the serum thyroxine (T4) concentration is low or low normal with the TSH in the normal range. This finding may be misinterpreted as the euthyroid sick syndrome (see Disorders of the Thyroid) in a stressed neonate. Furthermore, secondary hypothyroidism may be missed if primary TSH screening is used. TSH deficiency is usually associated with other pituitary deficiencies and rarely occurs in isolation. In an infant with any of the CNS abnormalities outlined in Table 39-4, secondary hypothyroidism should be considered and may be missed with routine newborn screening procedures.

Diagnosis

The diagnosis of hypothalamic and pituitary deficiency may require stimulation testing if random values are non-diagnostic. Growth hormone is tonically elevated in the first few days of life, thus a random growth hormone greater than 10 ng/mL suggests adequate growth hormone secretion. If a random value is low, growth hormone provocative testing is needed to confirm deficiency. In normal newborn infants, growth hormone values increase to greater than 25 ng/mL with stimulation testing. ACTH deficiency causing adrenal insufficiency is unlikely if a random cortisol is greater than 20 mcg/dL, because serum cortisol is low in newborns, without diurnal variation. In general, ACTH or CRH stimulation testing is necessary to test the hypothalamic-pituitary-adrenal axis. Random sex steroids, FSH, and LH may be diagnostic at 1 to 3 months of age when the hypothalamic-pituitary-gonadal axis is active transiently, otherwise gonadotropin-releasing hormone stimulation testing is needed to assess LH and FSH secretion.

In those infants suspected of anterior pituitary deficiency, ultrasonography through the open fontanelle may discern mid-line malformations of the brain, although magnetic resonance imaging or computed tomography scanning is more sensitive. If septo-optic dysplasia is a consideration, ophthalmologic examination should be performed.

Treatment

Anterior pituitary deficiency may not be detected clinically during the neonatal period if the hypoglycemia is mild, the micropenis, obviously not a clinical feature in hypopituitary females, is marginal, and jaundice is not severe. Treatment considerations, therefore, are based on the severity of symptoms. The child who is severely hypoglycemic will require immediate growth hormone and glucocorticoid replacement albeit at relatively modest doses. Recombinant growth hormone is injected subcutaneously, at a dose of 0.04 mg/kg daily. Glucocorticoid replacement with 8 to 10 mg/m² of oral hydrocortisone per day is often sufficient. This dose should be at least tripled for acute illness. If the testes are nonpalpable, MIS determination will ascertain their presence (32). An MIS value in the normal male range for age verifies the presence of testes. In male infants with micropenis, testosterone enanthate at a dose of 25 mg every month can be administered to stimulate penile growth. If the penile response is inadequate after a three month course, this can be repeated.

DISORDERS OF THE POSTERIOR PITUITARY

Vasopressin or antidiuretic hormone (ADH) and oxytocin are the two major posterior pituitary endocrine hormones. Oxytocin has no known function in the neonate although

ADH helps to regulate intravascular volume and osmolality. ADH is synthesized in the supraoptic and periventricular nuclei of the hypothalamus by 12 weeks of gestation. It is bound to neurophysin and is transported along the neurons of the neurohypophyseal tract to the posterior pituitary, where it is stored and released as necessary. ADH increases the permeability of the collecting tubules of the kidney to water and urea. Its secretion is stimulated by hyperosmolar states and volume depletion and inhibited predominantly by volume overload. The two main disorders of ADH secretion are diabetes insipidus and the syndrome of inappropriate SIADH.

Diabetes Insipidus

Diabetes insipidus (DI) in the newborn may be as a result of central ADH insufficiency or renal unresponsiveness to ADH (nephrogenic DI). This section will discuss only central DI.

DI in the neonate may present with failure to thrive, irritability, fever, vomiting, hypernatremia, and a history of polyhydramnios. Polyuria is difficult to appreciate in newborn infants because healthy newborn infants can void up to 20 times a day (42). However, sustained urine outputs greater than 60% of fluid input, and single-void volumes of greater than 6 mL/kg suggest DI. In a child with hyperosmolar serum, the diagnosis is confirmed by finding inappropriately dilute urine that becomes more concentrated after vasopressin administration. Failure to respond to vasopressin is suggestive of renal DI. Water deprivation tests should not be done in newborns as acute dehydration and hypernatremia may cause permanent CNS injury.

A list of causes of central DI is given in Table 39-5. Secondary DI is more common than primary in the neonatal period and should be strongly suspected in infants with certain malformations.

TABLE 39-5
ETIOLOGY OF CENTRAL DIABETES INSIPIDUS

Primary
  Familial
    X-linked recessive
    Autosomal dominant
  Idiopathic
Secondary
  Malformation sequences
    Optic atrophy
    Septooptic dysplasia
    Holoprosencephaly
  Birth trauma
  Periventricular hemorrhage
  Infection
    Meningitis
    Encephalitis
  Infiltrative disease (in older infants)
    Histiocytosis X
    Granulomatous disease
  Germ cell tumors (in older children)

Treatment

Treatment of DI requires strict management of fluid balance. Infants with DI require enormous quantities of free water; it is not unusual to provide several times the usual maintenance quantities of water as 5% glucose intravenously, although providing nutrition and electrolytes by the oral route. Desmopressin is a long-acting analogue of vasopressin. A number of different formulations are available; oral or subcutaneous may be easiest in infants. Sublingual administration can be helpful in patients with cleft lip and palate. Sublingual or subcutaneous dosing starts at 1 to 2 mcg once or twice daily and oral doses are about 10- to 20-fold higher. The dose and dose interval must be carefully titrated in each child by monitoring fluid intake, urine output, serum electrolytes and osmolality, and state of hydration. Management should include a "breakthrough" period of diuresis daily to avoid fluid overload although providing sufficient milk intake to meet caloric needs. Rapid shifts in the serum sodium caused by excessive fluid input or urine output should be avoided. An alternative approach, which minimizes the risk of water overload, is to use a diluted formula without administering any vasopressin. This treatment is based on the principle that hunger rather than thirst is the driving force behind fluid intake in the neonate. Providing the total daily caloric intake as one-third strength formula will usually result in stable fluid balance. This approach requires two to three hourly feeding even during the night, thus sleep may be disrupted. Moreover the volume of fluid needed can compromise growth in some infants. For emergency treatment of severe dehydration, intravenous aqueous pitressin infusion, instead of desmopressin, is recommended as the short half life of pitressin allows precise control of fluid balance.

Syndrome of Inappropriate Antidiuretic Hormone Secretion

The secretion of ADH is normally higher in premature infants (43) but can be further increased in sick premature infants for the reasons outlined in Table 39-6. A common mechanism in many pathologic cases is intravascular volume depletion, which is detected by stretch receptors in the left atrium. Thus, the elevated ADH levels are appropriate for the volume status, but inappropriate for the osmolar status. SIADH, by definition, occurs in a volume replete or overloaded state when there is dilutional hyponatremia associated with inappropriately concentrated urine with continued sodium loss (urine sodium >20–30 mEq/L). This occurs in the absence of volume depletion, renal failure, or adrenal insufficiency. True SIADH is uncommon in neonates (44), and should be differentiated from hyponatremia caused by ADH levels that are appropriately elevated in response to volume depletion. It is vitally important to limit water and sodium intake and prevent hyponatremia in SIADH, but equally important to adequately treat the volume depletion states associated with appropriately increased ADH secretion.

TABLE 39-6

CAUSES OF ELEVATED LEVELS OF ANTIDIURETIC HORMONE IN THE NEWBORN

Birth asphyxia
Acute deterioration of hyaline membrane disease and
    bronchopulmonary dysplasia
Respiratory syncytial virus infection
Pneumothorax
Pulmonary interstitial emphysema
Artificial ventilation
Acute blood loss
Periventricular hemorrhage
Surgery
Pain
Syndrome of inappropriate ADH secretion

ADH, antidiuretic hormone.

Hyponatremia occurs commonly in newborn premature infants who have a higher fractional excretion of sodium than term infants. The most common nonphysiological cause of hyponatremia is renal sodium wasting as a result of diuretics. The differential diagnosis of hyponatremia in the newborn includes prerenal failure, renal failure, adrenal insufficiency and SIADH. The SIADH, if it occurs, is associated more commonly with sepsis and central nervous system infection in older infants, but perhaps in critically ill neonates as well. Unlike volume depletion states, SIADH is treated by fluid restriction. If volume depletion is evident, combined with polyuria, urinary sodium loss, and hyponatremia, salt wasting should be suspected.

DISORDERS OF THE ADRENAL GLAND

Development and Function of the Adrenal Gland

The adrenal gland consists of a cortex and medulla, which each function independently and secrete two different classes of hormones. The fetal adrenal cortex is of mesodermal origin, whereas the chromaffin cells of the adrenal medulla are of neuroectodermal origin. Diseases of the adrenal medulla during the neonatal period are extremely rare, thus this section will focus on disorders of the adrenal cortex.

The anlage of the adrenal cortex arises as two large masses on either side of the aorta, at the level of the first thoracic nerve, immediately adjacent to the medullary cells that have migrated from the neural crest. Fetal adrenal cortical cells can be identified by 4 weeks gestation. By 7 weeks of gestation, the medullary cells begin to migrate to the interior of the adrenal cortex. The coelomic epithelium envelops the original cortical cells and remains as an outer shell. The fetal adrenal gland is steroidogenically active and large during gestation, but involutes during the latter half of pregnancy and especially after birth, suggesting a role in the maintenance of pregnancy. The adult adrenal cortex slowly develops from the outer shell although the fetal zone undergoes involution. DAX-1, a gene on the X chromosome, is essential for development of the definitive zone of the adrenal cortex (3). Mutations in this gene are responsible for congenital adrenal hypoplasia.

The trophic hormonal control of the fetal adrenal is not clear. In anencephalic fetuses, the fetal adrenal appears to develop normally during the first 12 weeks of gestation, then involutes. In patients with enzymatic defects of cortisol biosynthesis however, the hyperplasia and increased activity of the adrenal glands during the first 12 weeks of gestation suggests that ACTH must play some role during that time.

The adrenal cortex secretes three main types of steroid hormones, glucocorticoids, mineralocorticoids, and androgens. The glucocorticoids, of which cortisol (hydrocortisone) is the most important, exert their major physiologic effects on carbohydrate, protein, and fat metabolism. The mineralocorticoids, desoxycorticosterone and aldosterone, maintain salt and water balance by promoting sodium retention in exchange for hydrogen and potassium in the distal convoluted tubules of the kidney. The adrenal androgens, dehydroepiandrosterone (DHEA), δ4-androstenedione, and 11β-hydroxyandrostenedione, are anabolic and responsible for the development of sexual hair in girls at puberty. The slightly higher levels of adrenal androgens during the neonatal period may be secondary to the relative deficiency of 3β-hydroxysteroid dehydrogenase in the fetal zone of the fetal adrenal cortex, which is reflected in the higher concentrations of δ5 steroids (e.g., DHEA, 17-OH pregnenolone) especially in premature infants.

The production of adrenocortical steroids is controlled by a hypothalamic-pituitary-adrenal homeostatic mechanism. Hypothalamic CRH stimulates release of pituitary ACTH, which in turn, stimulates cortisol biosynthesis. Increased levels of cortisol exert down-regulation of the axis, probably at the level of the hypothalamus.

Aldosterone secretion is controlled by the renin-angiotensin system rather than ACTH. Acute changes in pressure receptors control the release of renin from the juxtaglomerular cells of the kidney. Circulating renin, in turn, increases angiotensin II, which acts on the zona glomerulosa of the adrenal cortex to stimulate aldosterone secretion and vascular contractility. The increased blood volume and higher pressures within the arterial receptors exert negative-feedback inhibition of the renin-angiotensin system. Secondary mechanisms such as a low sodium or high potassium intake also increase aldosterone excretion. ACTH will cause a transient, albeit unsustained, increase in aldosterone excretion, and aldosterone secretion will be diminished in the absence of ACTH. Finally, cortisol itself may have a permissive role in aldosterone action at the tissue level.

ADRENAL INSUFFICIENCY

The disorders of the adrenal cortex during the neonatal period consist almost entirely of those conditions that cause adrenal insufficiency. The inborn errors of steroid biosynthesis (CAH) can cause excessive production of various steroids, but Cushing syndrome or cortisol excess is rare during the neonatal period. Cushing syndrome may occur secondary to exogenous steroids such as dexamethasone, but Cushing disease has not been described in the very young infant. Adrenal cortical tumors occur in older infants but have not been reported in the neonate. Adrenal insufficiency can result from hypopituitarism, adrenal hemorrhage and other adrenal injury, ACTH receptor abnormalities, inherited degenerative disorders, or inborn errors of steroid biosynthesis.

Adrenocorticotropic Hormone Insufficiency

In a number of neonatal deaths associated with shock and peripheral vascular collapse in conjunction with severe hyponatremia and hyperkalemia, the adrenal glands were noted to be hypoplastic at autopsy. Because some of these cases were reported in infants with anencephaly or with partial or total pituitary aplasia, the lack of ACTH was thought to be responsible for the failure of development of the definitive zone after birth. The possibility, however, of another critical trophic factor is suggested by the findings in patients with congenital hypopituitarism. These patients have decreased cortisol production, but normal mineralocorticoid function and rarely develop hyperkalemia. They develop hypoglycemia, poor feeding, and failure to thrive, but can, in general, maintain water and electrolyte balance and respond to sodium deprivation with an increase in aldosterone excretion.

Familial isolated glucocorticoid insufficiency. This is an autosomal recessive disorder that can present during the neonatal period or later in childhood with shock, hyperpigmentation, hypoglycemia, and failure to thrive. These patients have cortisol insufficiency and cannot increase serum cortisol or urinary 17-hydroxysteroid excretion in response to ACTH stimulation. They can, however, respond to sodium deprivation with increased aldosterone excretion and decreased sodium excretion. Some pedigrees have a defect in the melanocortin-2 receptor (ACTH receptor) although others may have postreceptor defects (45). In one family with five affected siblings, two had intact glucocorticoid function during early infancy and developed glucocorticoid deficiency at a later age, suggesting an inherited degenerative process of the adrenal glands as the pathogenetic basis in this family (46).

Damage

Adrenal insufficiency can occur during the newborn period as a result of damage to the relatively large and hyperemic adrenal glands. Trauma in association with a difficult delivery, particularly breech delivery; hemorrhagic diseases; or infectious processes can damage the adrenal glands. Minor hemorrhage or unilateral damage may not cause adrenal insufficiency, and may present subsequently as calcification of the adrenal glands detected on an abdominal radiograph obtained for other purposes. All patients with shock in association with hyponatremia should be suspect for adrenal insufficiency. The highly sensitive ACTH determinations, using monoclonal antibodies and immunoradiometric assays, can detect elevated levels of plasma ACTH that are diagnostic of primary adrenal insufficiency.

Congenital Adrenal Hyperplasia

CAH is a genetic disorder involving a deficiency of one of several enzymes required for normal steroid biosynthesis. Deficient cortisol synthesis secondary to an enzymatic deficiency causes increased ACTH production, which in turn, stimulates a compensatory hypertrophy of the adrenal cortex and increase in steroidogenesis. This partially compensates for the block in the biosynthetic pathway, but also leads to the increased production and accumulation of precursor steroids preceding the enzymatic defect. Although ACTH chiefly regulates the glucocorticoid pathway, the synthesis of mineralocorticoids and androgens are variably affected depending on the specific enzyme involved.

The principal biochemical reactions in the conversion of cholesterol into active adrenocortical steroids require a series of hydroxylations (Fig. 39-4) that are mediated by cytochrome P450 oxidases. The initial step requires that the StAR protein form contact sites between the outer and inner membranes of mitochondria to transport cholesterol into the mitochondria and start the steroidogenic process. Five enzymes are necessary for the synthesis of cortisol: P450scc, P450c17, P450c21, P450c11, and 3β-hydroxysteroid dehydrogenase enzymes (47). The genes for all of these enzymes have been cloned and defects in any of them can cause insufficient glucocorticoid production and CAH. The clinical manifestations of this syndrome correspond to the particular enzyme affected and are summarized in Table 39-7.

Virilization

Virilization of the female is secondary to the elevated adrenal androgens caused by those enzymatic defects subsequent to 17-hydroxylation. In most cases, the labioscrotal folds are partially fused with clitoral enlargement, which may be bound down by chordee. Occasionally, virilization may be so severe that a phallic urethra develops. In male infants, virilization is generally is not apparent during the neonatal period, and, the diagnosis in the milder nonsalt-losing forms of this disorder, can be undetected for several years. Boys can present later with secondary sexual changes, increased somatic growth, and well-developed musculature. The classic, and most prevalent virilizing form of CAH is a defect in cytochrome P450c21 (21-hydroxylase deficiency), accounting for almost 90% of recognized cases (48).

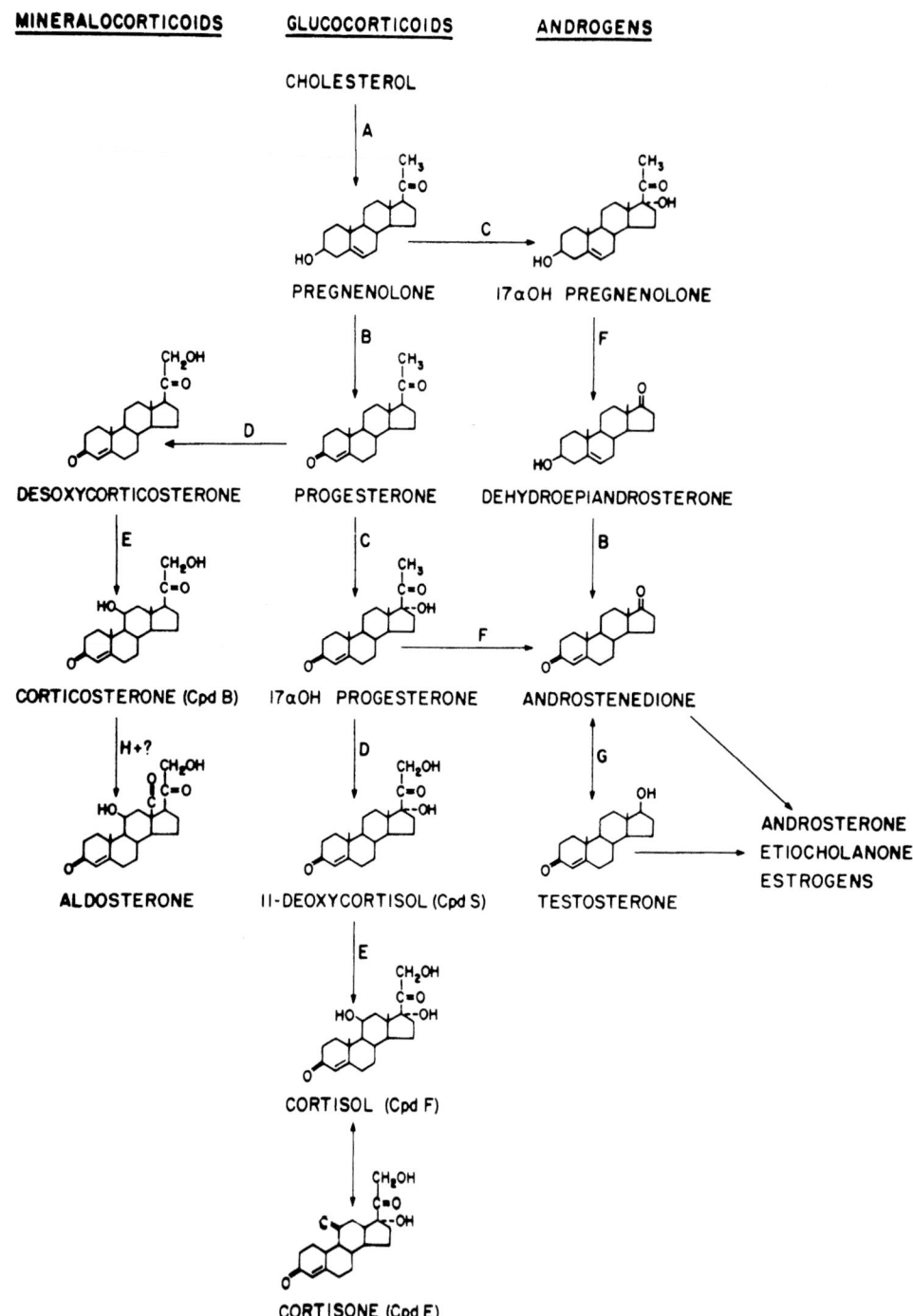

Figure 39-4 The biosynthetic pathway of adrenal steroid. The classic enzyme terminology is represented by the alphabetical letters with the appropriate cytochrome P450 oxidases in parentheses. A, 20,22-desmolase (P450scc); B, 3β-hydroxysteroid dehydrogenase: C, 17α-hydroxylase (P450c17); D, 21-hydroxylase (P450c21); E, 11-hydroxylase (P450c11); F, 17,20-lyase (P450c17); G, 17-keto reductase; H+, 18-hydroxylase + 18-oxidase (P450c11).

Mutations in P450c11 and 3β-hydroxysteroid dehydrogenase also cause female virilization.

Incomplete Masculinization

Failure of complete masculine development occurs in those forms of adrenal hyperplasia in which the androgen pathway is affected. Incomplete masculinization in the male, which requires fetal testosterone production, sug-

gests that the enzymatic defects occur in both the adrenal gland and the testis (28). In the 3β-hydroxysteroid dehydrogenase defect, secreted steroids consist almost entirely of compounds with δ5-3α-hydroxy configuration (49). Fetal testosterone production by the testis is also impaired, causing incomplete masculinization in the male (50). The marked elevation of δ5-3β-hydroxyadrenal androgens, especially DHEA, however, is converted periph- erally to active androgens that virilize the female infant. Elevation

TABLE 39-7

CLINICAL AND BIOCHEMICAL FINDINGS OF THE COMMON VARIANTS OF CONGENITAL ADRENAL HYPERPLASIA

Enzyme Deficiency (Classic)	Phenotype		Other Clinical Manifestations	Predominant Steroids
	46XX	46XY		
Congenital lipoid hyperplasia	Female	Female	Salt-wasting crisis	Low level–all steroids No response to ACTH
3β-Hydroxysteroid dehydrogenase deficiency	Virilized	Hypospadias	Salt-wasting crisis	Dehydroepiandrosterone 17-OH pregnenolone Increased Δ^5-Δ^4 ratio of steroids
21-Hydroxylase deficiency	Virilized	Male	Pseudoprecocious puberty in male Late virilization in female Salt-wasting crisis	17-OH progesterone Androstenedione Testosterone
11α-Hydroxylase deficiency	Virilized	Male	Pseudoprecocious puberty in male Hypertension	11-Deoxycortisol 11-Deoxycorticosterone Androstenedione Low renin
17α-Hydroxylase deficiency	Female	Female	Sexual infantilism Hypertension	Corticosterone 11-Deoxycorticosterone (Low renin)

ACTH, adrenocorticotrophic hormone.

of serum 17-hydroxypregnenolone is diagnostic of 3β-hydroxysteroid dehydrogenase deficiency, although 17-hydroxyprogesterone concentrations also are markedly elevated (50).

Hypertension

Hypertension has been associated with enzymatic blocks resulting in excessive secretion of mineralocorticoids. A defect of cytochrome P450c11 (11-hydroxylase deficiency) causes an accumulation of desoxycorticosterone, a potent mineralocorticoid, and 11-deoxycortisol (47). The P450c17 defect (17α-hydroxylase deficiency) blocks 17-hydroxylation of progesterone, interfering with cortisol and androgen biosynthesis, and shunting steroid production to the mineralocorticoid pathway (51). Genital development in females is unaffected but males are undervirilized. The hypertension resulting from excess mineralocorticoid production, however, is an inconstant feature and it is not known if hypertension is present during the newborn period. Whether the hypertension is related to the duration of excessive secretion of mineralocorticoid, the severity of the defect, or variations in sodium intake is also unclear.

Salt Loss

Mineralocorticoid insufficiency and severe sodium loss are seen in the salt-losing form of 21-hydroxylase deficiency, and 3β-hydroxysteroid dehydrogenase deficiency. The electrolytes initially are normal, but, within the first week of life, serum sodium will slowly decrease with a concomitant rise in serum potassium. These infants may manifest acute adrenal crisis with shock, peripheral collapse, and dehydration, by a week of age.

The underlying metabolic defects for two clinical variants of the 21-hydroxylase enzyme defect are now understood. Bongiovanni and Eberlein postulated that both are the result of the same enzymatic defect (52). In the salt-loser, there is almost complete 21-hydroxylase deficiency, whereas in the simple form, there is sufficient 21-hydroxylase to permit aldosterone synthesis. A single gene mediates the hydroxylation of both progesterone and 17-hydroxyprogesterone. Different mutations of the P450c21 gene account for the heterogeneity of 21-hydroxylase deficiency disorders, including the nonclassic late-onset variant, although there is phenotypic variability with the same genotype (47,48).

A few instances of aldosterone deficiency caused by a specific defect of 18-dehydrogenase, the last enzymatic process in aldosterone synthesis, have been described (53,54). There is salt and water loss, without the other clinical consequences of congenital adrenal hyperplasia. These disorders are secondary to mutations of the P450c11 enzyme.

Congenital Lipoid Hyperplasia

Previously, this disorder was thought to be as a result of a deficiency of the enzyme, 20,22 desmolase (P450scc) that mediates the conversion of cholesterol to pregnenolone. The etiology is now recognized as a genetic defect of the StAR protein, a mitochondrial protein needed for transport of cholesterol across the mitochondrial membrane. StAR is needed for acute steroidogenesis, thus in some individuals, glucocorticoid production is initially preserved, but the accumulation of cholesterol esters causes continuing destruction of the adrenal and onset of adrenal insufficiency at older ages (55). Male and females both have female appearing external genitalia, hyponatremia, hyperkalemia and dehydration. However, the age at presentation varies from the newborn period to several months of age and later. No steroids are produced and the adrenal glands are markedly enlarged, filled with cholesterol esters.

Prenatal Diagnosis and Treatment of Congenital Adrenal Hyperplasia

CAH, 21-hydroxylase deficiency, can be diagnosed prenatally using molecular techniques. Once the diagnosis of 21-hydroxylase deficiency has been established in a propositus, molecular analysis of the P450c21 gene should be done in the propositus and the parents. The parents should have ACTH stimulation testing to confirm biochemically that they are genetic heterozygotes for 21-hydroxylase deficiency. The management of the pregnancy, the techniques used for diagnosis, the treatment of the female fetus with 21-hydroxylase deficiency, and the problems with these techniques have been reviewed (56,57). In brief, the mother is started on dexamethasone early in the first trimester and, subsequently, chorionic villus sampling or amniocentesis is performed to determine the sex and genetic studies. If molecular and genetic techniques confirm the diagnosis and the fetus is female, dexamethasone treatment is continued to term. Long-term consequences of prenatal steroids remain unknown and therapy can be associated with cushingoid symptoms in the mother, thus prenatal management and therapy should be monitored closely and performed at centers with expertise.

Diagnosis of Adrenal Insufficiency

The diagnosis of acute adrenal insufficiency is difficult to make in the newborn. There must be a high index of suspicion in any acutely ill infant with shock, peripheral collapse, and a rapid and weak pulse, and in any infant with poor feeding, failure to thrive, intermittent pyrexia, or even hypoglycemia and convulsions. A subtle sign of congenital adrenal hypoplasia is hyperpigmentation, especially in the extensor creases and genitalia; however, this sign is seldom recognized until the diagnosis has been made. Decreased serum sodium and chloride and increased serum potassium levels are suggestive of mineralocorticoid deficiency. Isolated hyponatremia does not exclude glucocorticoid insufficiency, and should be viewed as a possible sign of adrenal insufficiency. Certainly, ambiguous external genitalia at birth always should suggest the possibility of CAH.

Serum cortisol levels are low in all newborns, especially in premature infants and lack diurnal variation, therefore random cortisol determinations usually are not diagnostic. In clinical situations highly suggestive of adrenal insufficiency, it is recommended that a rapid, 1-hour low dose ACTH stimulation test be performed and that pharmacologic doses of glucocorticoids be administered, along with fluid and electrolyte resuscitation, after testing. Plasma concentrations of ACTH are elevated in those infants with primary adrenal insufficiency, including CAH. A plasma sample for ACTH determination should be obtained before ACTH testing.

Delineation of the specific enzyme defect in CAH can be determined by measuring serum concentrations of the various steroidal precursors (see Table 39-7). Cord blood concentrations of 17-hydroxyprogesterone are normally elevated to the range of 900 to 5,000 ng/dL. Serum values rapidly decrease by the second or third day of life to less than 100 ng/dL in newborns (58), but can increase to greater than 200 ng/dL at 1 to 2 months of age in male infants. Newborn values above 1,000 ng/dl are of concern although 17-hydroxyprogesterone values are higher in stressed newborns, especially preterm sick newborns, in whom they can be greater than 600 ng/dL (59). These values, however remain significantly lower than those in patients with 21-hydroxylase deficiency, which are often markedly above 2,000 ng/dL. Serum 17-hydroxyprogesterone is used for newborn screening for CAH using a filter paper technique (60). It is important to recognize that elevated serum concentrations of 17-hydroxyprogesterone are not diagnostic of the 21-hydroxylase defect. Serum 17-hydroxyprogesterone can be mildly elevated in the 11-hydroxylase defect and can be markedly elevated in the 3β-hydroxysteroid dehydrogenase defect secondary to peripheral conversion of 17-hydroxypregnenolone to 17-hydroxyprogesterone (50). Serum values of 17-hydroxypregnenolone are especially elevated in the premature infant, and values up to 2,000 ng/dL are normal (59).

Treatment of Adrenal Insufficiency

The immediate need of a critically ill infant in adrenal crisis is for cortisol. If possible, cortisol should be withheld until the diagnosis can be established, either by ACTH testing or by obtaining serum for determination of the appropriate steroids and ACTH. However, if a newborn infant is in shock and in extremis, glucocorticoids should be immediately given as a lifesaving measure. In the usual situation, salt and water alone will relieve the clinical crisis. Intravenous isotonic saline in 5% glucose water should be infused at a rate of 100 to 120 mL/kg during the first 24 hours. If the infant is in severe shock, the use of plasma or 5% albumin, 10 to 20 mL/kg to restore intravascular volume, and cortisol, is often necessary. Hydrocortisone hemisuccinate or phosphate, 1.5 to 2 mg/kg, should be given intravenously immediately. Constant infusion of hydrocortisone hemisuccinate or phosphate (50 mg/m² /day) should be continued. Hydrocortisone hemisuccinate, 2 mg/kg, can be given intramuscularly if intravenous access is a problem. The infant with severe shock may require a vasopressor, although vasopressor drugs may not be efficacious until hydrocortisone is administered.

Hydrocortisone or cortisone acetate, 10 to 12 mg/m²/day, is the mainstay for long-term treatment of patients with adrenal insufficiency. For acute illness, stress doses of hydrocortisone should be given parenterally at triple the maintenance dose.

Often a mineralocorticoid is a necessary adjunct for the chronic treatment of adrenal insufficiency. The dose of the oral mineralocorticoid, 9α-fludrocortisone (Florinef) is 0.05 to 0.1 mg/day, which is sufficient for most forms of adrenal insufficiency. In the salt-losing forms of congenital adrenal hyperplasia, occasionally higher doses of fludrocortisone are necessary. Even the compensated (nonsalt-losing) variant may benefit from low dose mineralocorticoid.

Iatrogenic Adrenal Insufficiency

During the neonatal period, pharmacologic doses of glucocorticoids are often needed for adjunctive treatment of a number of diseases, such as bronchopulmonary dysplasia. The dose and duration of glucocorticoid therapy that will cause iatrogenic adrenal insufficiency is not known, particularly in infants. High-dose glucocorticoid therapy for a brief duration ($<$ 1 week) probably will not cause adrenal insufficiency, therefore a slow taper is not needed unless the clinical course of the primary condition deteriorates. Treatment longer than 14 days may result in at least transient adrenal insufficiency. After a prolonged course, the dose of glucocorticoids can be decreased by one-half every several days until a physiologic replacement dose (10 mg of hydrocortisone/m^2/day orally) is achieved. The dose can then be lowered more gradually, by 20% every 4 or 5 days.

Adrenal function may be suppressed for some time after prolonged pharmacologic glucocorticoid therapy. Again, there are no studies correlating dose, duration of pharmacologic treatment, and time needed for recovery of adrenal function after high-dose glucocorticoid therapy in infants. There are anecdotal reports of adrenal crisis occurring during stress more than 6 months after discontinuation of pharmacologic glucocorticoid therapy. Although it is possible to evaluate periodically the adrenal response to exogenous ACTH to determine when iatrogenic adrenal insufficiency has resolved, alternatively, pharmacologic doses of glucocorticoids can be used empirically during situations of stress for at least a year after discontinuation of prolonged high-dose glucocorticoid therapy. A minimal dose of glucocorticoid to be used during stress situations is 30 mg of hydrocortisone/m^2/day, orally.

DISORDERS OF THE THYROID

Development and Function of the Thyroid

The fetal thyroid begins as a thickening of epithelium at the base of the tongue that migrates down the trachea, leaving the thyroglossal duct as an embryonic remnant. During its caudal migration, the thyroid assumes a more bilobate shape. The developing thyroid is able to concentrate iodide by 12 weeks of gestation, and to organify iodide and synthesize thyroxine (T4) and triiodothyronine

(T3) by 14 weeks of gestation. Free T4 and, more so, T3 can cross the placenta in either direction. It is probable that the gradient is from mother to fetus during the first 12 weeks and then the gradient in transfer of thyroid hormones is from fetus to mother except in the hypothyroid fetus (61,62). There is no placental transfer of maternal or fetal TSH, although thyroid-stimulating immunoglobulins (TSI) will cross the placenta. The hypothalamic-pituitary feedback mechanisms are operative by the latter part of gestation. The hypothalamus secretes a tripeptide, TRH, which stimulates pituitary secretion of TSH. TSH, in turn, stimulates thyroid hormone production by regulating every step of thyroid hormone biosynthesis and release, from iodide accumulation to proteolysis of thyroglobulin. The thyroid hormones exercise negative feedback control of TSH response to TRH at the pituitary level but also inhibits at the hypothalamic level.

The biosynthesis of thyroid hormones is illustrated in Fig. 39-5. Circulating plasma iodide is concentrated by the thyroid gland, then oxidized by a thyroid peroxidase and bound to tyrosine to form monoiodotyrosine (MIT) and diiodotyrosine (DIT). The iodotyrosines are held by peptide linkage to thyroglobulin and coupled to form T3 and T4. T3 and T4 are then cleaved from thyroglobulin by thyroid proteases and secreted into the circulatory system. A large percentage of circulating T3 arises by deiodination of T4 by diodinases 1, 2, and 363. Diodinase 1 (D1) and Diodinase 2 (D2) are differentially localized in the pituitary and peripheral tissues. At the pituitary level, D2 partially regulates TSH production by modulating T3 concentrations. Diodinase 3 (D3) converts T4 to reverse T3 and T2, biologically inactive iodothyronines. Within the thyroid, iodotyrosines and iodothyronines are deiodinated by dehalogenase enzymes and remain within the intrathyroidal iodide pool to be reused. The iodide released from peripheral deiodination enters the circulatory system to be reconcentrated by the thyroid gland or excreted by the kidneys. The iodothyronines are transported in the plasma by proteins. Thyroxine-binding globulin (TBG), an α-globulin, is the major carrier of T4, but binds T3 to a lesser extent. Thyroxine also is bound by T4-binding prealbumin and by albumin. At the cellular level, the unbound, free T3 and T4 are biologically active. Genetic disorders, acquired conditions, or drugs that quantitatively change the concentration of TBG will alter circulating total T4 without affecting the physiologic thyroid status.

THYROID FUNCTION TESTS

Thyroid function tests in infants are elevated compared to values in older children. This is secondary to the cold-stimulated surge of TSH and TRH in the immediate postnatal period and the higher TBG concentrations secondary to maternal estrogen effect. Total T4 ranges from 7.3 to 22.9 mcg/dL during the first month of life, with mean values greater than 10 mcg/dL (Tables 39-8 and 39-9). Thyroid function tests normally are lower in premature and sick newborns

EXTRACELLULAR FLUID   THYROID

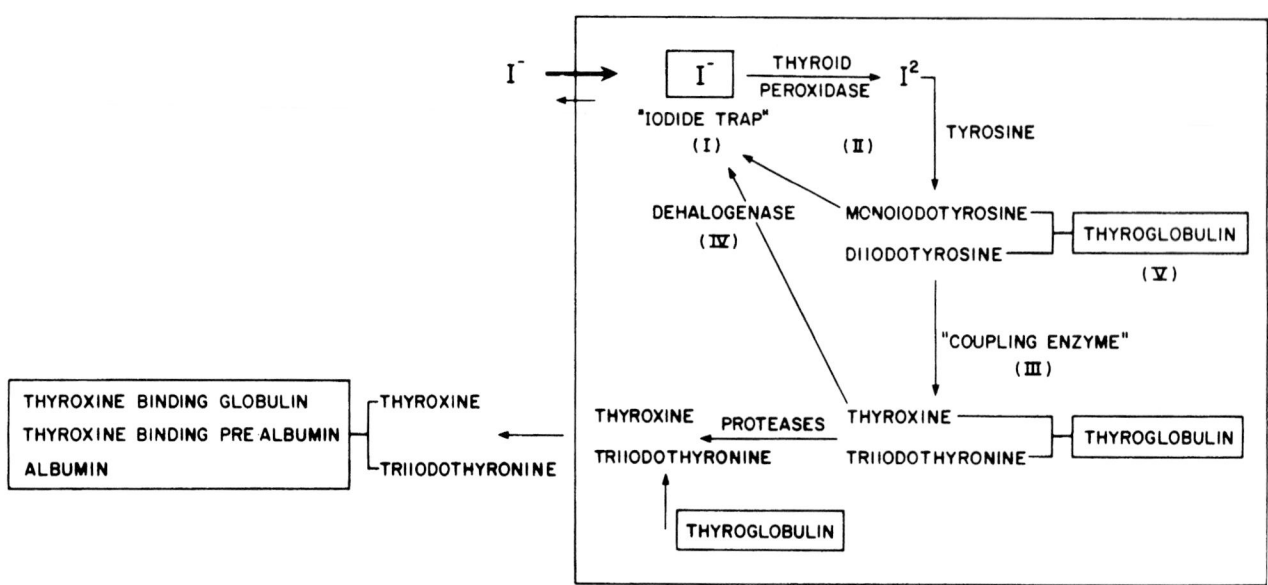

Figure 39-5 Thyroid hormone synthesis. The roman numerals represent described enzymatic defects of thyroxine synthesis.

than in healthy term newborn infants (Table 39-10), as a result of lower concentrations of TBG (64,65).

Congenital Hypothyroidism

The causes of congenital hypothyroidism are many and include genetic and sporadic disorders of embryogenesis, inborn errors of T4 biosynthesis, and environmental factors. Congenital hypothyroidism can be classified into the following subgroups:

- agenesis (athyrotic cretinism) or dysgenesis of the thyroid gland (thyroid hypoplasia, thyroid ectopia)
- endemic goitrous hypothyroidism
- inborn errors of T4 synthesis (familial goitrous cretinism)
- drug-induced hypothyroidism
- thyroid hormone resistance
- thyroid unresponsiveness to TSH
- secondary hypothyroidism (pituitary hypothyroidism)
- tertiary hypothyroidism (hypothalamic hypothyroidism).

Agenesis or Dysgenesis of the Thyroid Gland

Disordered embryogenesis of the thyroid gland is the most frequent cause of congenital hypothyroidism in the United States. Although congenital endemic goitrous hypothyroidism may have been more prevalent throughout the world at one time, the frequency of this disorder has declined with the introduction of iodine into endemic areas.

Genetic mutations in thyroid transcription factors have been identified in familial forms of thyroid agenesis, although athyrosis generally is a sporadic disorder (66). Thyroid antibodies have been detected with increased incidence among mothers of children with hypothyroidism and may cause either transient or persistent congenital hypothyroidism (67). Most mothers with thyroid antibodies have unaffected children, however, and, conversely, most mothers of children with congenital hypothyroidism do not have thyroid antibodies. Thyroid hypoplasia has been reported in children with congenital toxoplasmosis,

TABLE 39-8

RANGE OF MEAN VALUES FOR THYROID AND THYROID-STIMULATING HORMONES DURING THE NEONATAL PERIOD IN FULL-TERM INFANTS

	T_4 (μg/dL)	T_3 (ng/dL)	TBG (mg/dL)	TSH (μU/mL)
Cord blood	10.9 (7–13)	48 (12–90)	5.4 (1.2–9.6)	9.5 (2.4–20)
2 h of age	22.1	217		86
24–72 h of age	17.2 (12.4–21.9)	125 (89–256)	5.4	7.3(<2.5–16.3)
2 wk of age	12.9 (8.2–16.6)	250	5 (1–9)	
6 wk of age	10.3 (7.9–14.4)	163 (114–189)	4.8 (2–7.6)	2.5 (<2.5–6.3)

T_3, triiodothyronine; T_4, thyroxine; TBG, thryoxine-binding globulin; TSH, thyroid-stimulating hormone.

TABLE 39-9

THE UPPER LIMIT OF NORMAL FOR MEASUREMENTS OF THYROID-STIMULATING HORMONE IN THE FIRST 5 DAYS OF LIFE[a]

Age at Collection (d)	Standard TSH Cutoff		Age-adjusted TSH Cutoff	
	No. of Infants	TSH Value (mU/L)	No. of Infants	TSH Value (MU/L)
0–1	19	>20	8	>30
2	54	>20	26	>25
3	136	>20	45	>25
4	30	>20	30	>20
5	34	>20	34	>20
Total	273		143	

Retrospective study of 37,927 infants with definite abnormal results during a 6-month period (1988–1989).
TSH, thyroid-stimulating hormone.
[a] From Allen DB, Sieger JE, Litsheim T, Duck SC. Age-adjusted thyrotropin criteria for neonatal screening of hypothyroidism. *J Pediatr* 1990;117:310, with permission.

but in utero infectious disorders have not been implicated commonly as a cause of thyroid dysgenesis.

Endemic Goitrous Hypothyroidism

Although endemic goiter is one of the widespread nutritional diseases in the world, the introduction of iodine into various foods, including infant formulas, has markedly decreased the incidence of endemic goitrous hypothyroidism. The dietary requirements for iodine vary, but 40 to 100 mcg/day is sufficient for most children. In areas with endemic goiters, factors other than iodine (e.g., enzymatic defects, other genetic factors, and other dietary factors such as goitrogens), probably contribute to goiter formation. Such factors are suggested by the evidence that females are more commonly afflicted than males, that not everyone within the endemic area is afflicted despite similar iodine intake, and the variable incidence of endemic cretinism in different areas. In the Alps, deaf-mutism is a common finding in association with endemic cretinism, suggesting possibly an associated enzymatic defect of organification of iodide. When cretinism occurs in conjunction with an endemic goiter, the signs and symptoms are similar to the dysgenetic form of cretinism except for the presence of a goiter and an elevated radioactive iodine uptake.

TABLE 39-10

MEAN VALUES FOR THYROID AND THYROID-STIMULATING HORMONES IN CORD BLOOD OF FULL-TERM AND PREMATURE INFANTS

	T_4 (μg/dL)	T_3 (ng/dL)	TSH (μU/mL)
Term	10.9	48	9.5
35 wk of gestation	9.5	29	12.7
32 wk of gestation	7.6	15	

T_3, triiodothyronine; T_4, thyroxine; TSH, thyroid-stimulating hormone.

Inborn Errors of Thyroxine Synthesis

The inherited disorders of T4 synthesis involve deficiencies in one or more of the enzymes necessary for hormonogenesis or release of thyroid hormones, resulting in hypothyroidism (69). A compensatory increase in TSH production produces hyperplasia and enlargement of the thyroid gland, creating the clinical picture of familial goitrous cretinism.

Iodide Trap Defect

The thyroid gland has the ability to concentrate iodide, so that the intrathyroidal iodide concentration may be 40-fold greater than in serum. In this rare inherited defect of T4 synthesis, this ability is lost. As would be anticipated, the 24-hour radioactive iodine uptake is negligible. Thyroid scans do not demonstrate the presence of thyroid tissue, although there may be some uptake, but the gland is detected by ultrasonography. Several other organs, including the salivary glands, share the ability to concentrate iodide, and this defect can be distinguished from athyrosis because the salivary iodide concentration also is low and there usually is a goiter that can be detected by ultrasonography. This defect essentially reflects iodine deficiency, and can be compensated using high doses of iodide, although treatment with thyroxine is easier and probably more effective.

Organification or Peroxidase Defect

A defect in the organification of iodide is one of the more frequent disorders of hormonogenesis. In this defect, the thyroid has an increased uptake of iodide but is unable to oxidize it or combine it with tyrosine. This leads to the accumulation of free iodide in the gland that can be discharged or released with administration of anions such as perchlorate or thiocyanate, although iodine bound to tyrosine or thyronines cannot be discharged. These findings have led to a simple test for the organification defect. The patient is given a tracer amount of radioactive iodine, which is rapidly concentrated into the gland in a patient with the organification defect. When the radioactivity over the gland has stabilized, a potassium perchlorate or thiocyanate given orally (0.5–1 g) will displace the unorganified iodine, causing a rapid discharge of the radioactive iodine from the thyroid gland.

A variant of this form of familial goiter secondary to a defect in organification is associated with neurosensory hearing loss (or Pendred syndrome). The clinical picture differs from the full organification defect, in that patients with the Pendred syndrome often have only small goiters and the perchlorate discharge is incomplete.

Coupling Defect

Coupling of MIT and DIT into T4 and T3 is a complex intermediate step involving several processes, and should not be considered a defined single enzymatic deficiency. The inability of the thyroid gland to couple MIT and DIT into T4 and T3 leads to the accumulation of large amounts of MIT and DIT in the gland, with the small amounts of T4 and T3 synthesized being immediately released into the circulation. Radioactive iodine uptake by the thyroid gland is rapid and high. Definitive diagnosis requires thyroid biopsy and chromatographic analysis of the iodotyrosines and iodothyronines. Chromatographic analysis of thyroid gland tissue detects large amounts of MIT and DIT with only trace quantities of T4 and T3.

Dehalogenase Defect

The deiodination of the iodotyrosines and iodothyronines occurs within the thyroid and in the liver, kidneys, and other organs. The inherited inability of the thyroid to deiodinate MIT and DIT causes leakage of these precursors from the gland and depletion of iodide stores. This loss of iodide causes decreased hormone synthesis, resulting in a compensatory rise in TSH, thyroid hyperplasia, and increased synthesis of MIT, DIT, and iodothyronines. The goitrous hypothyroidism in this defect is not caused by a biosynthetic block but by iodine deficiency, which can be treated with large amounts of iodine. However, equally efficacious and easier is to use thyroid hormone replacement therapy. Radioactive iodine is rapidly accumulated and turned over. Because this defect is extrathyroidal and intrathyroidal, radioactive MIT and DIT appears unchanged in the urine.

Abnormal Thyroglobulin

Thyroglobulin is synthesized exclusively within the thyroid. The defects of thyroglobulin formation incorporate a group of disorders, including errors of thyroglobulin synthesis, and decreased synthesis. Deficient protease activity for thyroglobulin degradation also has been postulated to result in deficiency of thyroid hormone release. These disorders are characterized by abnormal circulating and intrathyroidal iodoproteins. These peptides sometimes have been described as albumin-like, and have been identified as the iodoalbumin thyroalbumin, in which the major iodinated compounds appear to be monoiodohistadines and diiodohis-

tadines (70,71). The thyroglobulin abnormality is thought to cause iodination of inappropriate proteins, mainly albumin, with a subsequent low yield of T4. A compensatory increase in TSH secretion causes thyroid hyperplasia and a rapid turnover of T4 or albumin. Proteolysis of the iodohistadinethyroalbumin results in a high secretion of iodohistadine, which can be detected in the urine.

Drug-induced Neonatal Goiter

Many drugs have been demonstrated to be goitrogenic. In the newborn infant, the most commonly implicated drugs are iodides and thiourea derivatives used for treatment of maternal thyrotoxicosis. The use of these drugs not only has caused goiter in the newborn but also has been associated with scattered reports of hypothyroidism (72). Although the correlation between the dose of the drug and the occurrence of goiter is poor, prolonged administration of thiourea drugs to the mother increases the risk of fetal goiter. One recommendation for minimizing this risk is to lower the dose of thiourea drugs during the last trimester and add thyroid hormone concurrently (73). In infants of hyperthyroid mothers, it is necessary to distinguish the drug-induced goiter from the TSI-induced goiter. A low T4 suggests that the goiter is secondary to the drug, whereas a high T4 is more compatible with a TSI-induced goiter and maternal antibody mediated neonatal hyperthyroidism. A mixed picture can also occur with an initially low T4 that increases within a few days as serum concentrations of the drug decline sufficiently. The stimulating effects of TSI antibodies, which have a much longer half-life, can manifest as thyrotoxicosis at a few days to a week of age (discussed under congenital thyrotoxicosis). Treatment usually is not necessary for the infant with a drug-induced goiter unless the goiter is asphyxiating or, more rarely, the infant is hypothyroid. Thyroid hormone will cause the goiter to subside.

Concerns have been raised regarding the appropriate use of antithyroid agents in the lactating mother. Propylthiouracil (PTU) is the preferred drug (74), but if alternatives are needed because of adverse drug reactions, carbimazole and methimazole are only transmitted at low levels in breast milk and also appear to be safe (75,76). Nonetheless, thyroid function should be monitored in the infant.

RESISTANCE TO THYROID HORMONES

Refetoff and associates reported a family with deaf-mutism, stippled epiphyses, delayed bone age and goiter that appeared clinically euthyroid (77). Serum T4 was elevated but thyroid hormone-binding proteins and hormone biosynthesis were normal. This family had the variant of thyroid hormone resistance characterized by generalized tissue unresponsiveness to thyroid hormone. Other patients with primarily central resistance of the hypothalamus and pituitary gland to thyroid hormone are mildly hyperthyroid during infancy and childhood (78). Mutations in the α isoform of the thyroid hormone receptor have been identified in a number of families with both peripheral and central resistance to thyroid hormones (79).

UNRESPONSIVENESS TO THYROID-STIMULATING HORMONE

Stanbury and associates reported a severely retarded 8-year-old boy with a normal thyroid gland, a low PBI, normal radioactive iodine uptake, and high endogenous levels of biologically active TSH (80). Exogenous TSH neither stimulated the thyroid gland in vivo nor increased glucose metabolism by thyroid slices *in vitro*. Thyroid-stimulating hormone unresponsiveness of the thyroid gland was postulated by these investigators as an explanation for this clinical syndrome. Mutations in the TSH receptor have now been identified as the cause of TSH resistance (79). Patients can be either euthyroid or present with congenital hypothyroidism.

SECONDARY AND TERTIARY HYPOTHYROIDISM

Central hypothyroidism is caused by the failure of secretion of TSH and TRH from the pituitary and hypothalamus, respectively. Newborn infants with these disorders may be missed in newborn screening programs, which rely on primary TSH screening or those directed to primary hypothyroidism, by screening for both low T4 and elevated TSH levels. All patients with the midline abnormalities outlined in Table 41-4 should be suspected of possible secondary or tertiary hypothyroidism. Therefore, they should have more complete thyroid studies (including a free T4 determined by dialysis and ultra sensitive TSH level) because of the risk that they might be missed by the newborn screening test. Isolated TSH deficiency is rare and identification of central hypothyroidism should lead to evaluation of other pituitary functions.

SYMPTOMS OF HYPOTHYROIDISM

Symptoms of agenesis of the thyroid gland are readily detectable by 6 weeks of age; however, some infants will have clinical manifestations at birth or during the immediate neonatal period (81). Infants with ectopic or residual thyroid tissue or inborn errors of T4 synthesis often will produce enough thyroid hormone to delay the onset of clinical symptoms and are typically asymptomatic when identified by newborn screening. The signs during the early neonatal period are subtle and include prolonged neonatal jaundice, mottling of the skin, poor suck, poor feeding, lethargy, umbilical hernia, bradycardia, constipation, and intermittent cyanosis. Occasionally infants with congenital hypothyroidism can demonstrate severe respiratory distress. Later, the more classic symptoms of cretinism appear. The

progressive myxedema causes coarsening of the facies, with puffy eyelids, flattened nasal bridge, and enlarged tongue. The cry is hoarse secondary to myxedema of the larynx and epiglottis. Lethargy, hypotonia, constipation, poor feeding, poor weight gain, dry hair, and pallor become more notable with time.

There is considerable evidence for the essential role of the thyroid hormones in the growth and development of the central nervous system (82). The final outcome of mental development in children with congenital hypothyroidism depends on the severity and duration of thyroid insufficiency and the time of initiation of therapy and dose of hormone administered. The prognosis appears to be worse if signs of hypothyroidism are clinically evident at diagnosis. Thus, a delay in treatment until three months of age is associated with a poorer cognitive outcome than those treated earlier (83). Klein and associates found no differences in IQ testing or other psychometric parameters in children with congenital hypothyroidism treated before 1 month of age as compared to matched normal controls (84). Others have found developmental delay even in those infants treated within 1 month of age who had severe hypothyroidism as defined by a thyroxine concentration less than 2 mcg/dL and retarded bone maturation (85). In general although, the prognosis for cognitive outcome is good in those children with congenital hypothyroidism are started on adequate doses of thyroid hormone within the first month of life.

DIAGNOSIS

The incidence of congenital hypothyroidism has been estimated to be 1 in 4,000 births. In view of the desirability of early diagnosis and treatment, newborn screening using filter paper spots is standard in the United States (86). Previously, it was a common approach is to use an initial T4 screen. If the T4 is in the lowest 10% of the samples being tested or below a specific value, a repeat T4 and a TSH are determined on the same sample. If the repeat T4 is still low (<10 mcg/dL) or the TSH is elevated, confirmatory tests are requested. More recently, many of the states are using an approach to detect primary hypothyroidism, screening for elevation of TSH. This latter approach provides better detection of primary hypothyroidism, eliminating the infants who are premature, euthyroid sick or have thyroxine binding protein deficiency. The potential problems with newborn screening for congenital hypothyroidism have been reviewed (87). Following a positive screen, a serum sample should be obtained for more specific thyroid functions. The diagnosis should be confirmed by serum free T4, TSH, and thyroid hormone binding index.

In those states still using T4 as a primary screen, almost 34% of low T4 values detected by newborn screening are not the result of true hypothyroidism, but represent diminished levels of TBG in patients with TBG deficiency or prematurity. In those cases suggestive of deficient thyroid hormone

TABLE 39-11

INCIDENCE OF VARIOUS FORMS OF CONGENITAL HYPOTHYROIDISM

Disorder	Incidence
Congenital thyroid agenesis or dysgenesis	1:4000
Inborn errors of thyroxine synthesis	1:30,000
Hypothalamic-hypopituitary hypothyroidism	1:66,000[a]

[a] Hypothalamic-hypopituitary hypothyroidism incidence is based on newborn screening studies so may be underdetected.

binding, a direct measurement of TBG should be determined and a test such as the T3 resin uptake to evaluate for problems of thyroxine binding other than TBG deficiency. A low T4 and a normal TSH may represent secondary or tertiary hypothyroidism or TBG deficiency. Thyroxine-binding globulin deficiency is an X-linked disorder and occurs in 1 in 2,000 screening studies of boys. Low T4 levels also are found normally in premature infants and severely ill newborn infants, and are not necessarily indicative of hypothyroidism (see Euthyroid Sick Syndrome). A T4 greater than 7 mcg/dL is regarded as normal in premature or sick infants (65,86). Note the need to avoid using specimens obtained in the first 24 to 48 hours after birth because of the normal surge of TSH (see Tables 39-8 and 39-9). Radiographic skeletal age is often useful, because 50% of full-term infants with congenital hypothyroidism will not have the osseous centers normally present at birth. It is important to perform a thyroid scan or ultrasound on all patients with congenital hypothyroidism to identify those patients with inborn errors of T4 synthesis so that appropriate genetic counseling may be given.

The incidence figures for various forms of congenital hypothyroidism, as determined by the newborn screening studies, are listed in Table 39-11. It is probable that the hypothalamic-hypopituitary forms of hypothyroidism have been underestimated by the newborn screening studies, because many of the TSH-deficient patients have normal serum T4 concentrations at birth. Also, the syndromes of T4 resistance and thyroid resistance to TSH can be missed by the newborn screening method. Probably the most common cause of undetected congenital hypothyroidism is omitting the screening study. This is more likely to occur in intensive care situations, because of the magnitude of other ongoing problems.

TREATMENT AND PROGNOSIS

The dose of thyroid hormone prescribed should be sufficient to achieve high euthyroid levels of serum T4 within 2 weeks of starting therapy. During the newborn period, the starting dose of l-thyroxine is 10–12 mcg/kg/day, which usually equals 37.5 mcg/day for most full-term infants. Serum T4 normalizes before the serum TSH, therefore serum T4 should be used to guide therapy during the first 4 weeks to avoid overdosing with L-thyroxine. After 4 to 6 weeks of therapy, however, TSH level is the best measure for monitoring treatment. If the TSH remains elevated, the dose of l-thyroxine should be increased.

Recently controversy has arisen over the issue of transient hypothyroxinemia in preterm infants and neurological outcome. A retrospective analysis of T4 levels in premature infants suggested that severe transient hypothyroxinemia during the immediate neonatal period was associated with problems in neurologic and mental development at two years of age (88). None of the infants were subsequently diagnosed as having permanent hypothyroidism. Despite adjusting for many variables it is still not clear whether those children with the impaired neurologic and mental outcome had lower thyroxine levels causing the worse outcome or because these children were sicker which resulted in the worse outcome and lower thyroxine levels. Perhaps the answer lies in a paper, which showed that thyroid replacement in a randomized double blind, placebo controlled study of 200 infants, less than 30 weeks gestation did not improve developmental outcome (89). No firm recommendations may be made at this time and further studies are awaited.

EUTHYROID SICK SYNDROME

The euthyroid sick syndrome is a reflection of adaptive physiologic processes that occur during acute and chronic illness. Thyroid hormones increase basal metabolism, cardiac output, and oxygen consumption. Reduced production of thyroid hormones, especially T3, which reduces oxygen consumption and basal metabolic rate, is beneficial for certain illnesses (e.g., catabolic or hypoxic conditions). In animal studies, hypophysectomized rats survive longer during oxygen deprivation than intact animals. The euthyroid sick syndrome has been noted in both premature and full-term sick newborn infants.

The euthyroid sick syndrome is characterized by a low normal T4 concentration, an extraordinarily low T3 concentration, and a normal TSH level. The latter two findings distinguish the euthyroid sick syndrome from primary and secondary hypothyroidism. T3 levels generally are in the low normal range in both primary and secondary hypothyroidism, with TSH levels markedly elevated in primary hypothyroidism. Unlike older infants and children, reverse T3 is not useful in the diagnosis of euthyroid sick syndrome, because it is elevated normally in the newborn infant. Euthyroid sick syndrome does not require any treatment other than correction of the primary disease.

CONSUMPTIVE HYPOTHYROIDISM SECONDARY TO GIANT HEMANGIOMA

Infants with large hemangioma may develop hypothyroidism, which is not present at birth, and therefore is not detected by newborn screening studies (90). The location of the hemangioma may be in the liver and ectodermally.

The infants develop hypothyroidism as the hemangioma grows during early infancy (within a few months to a year), which is detrimental to brain development if undetected. The cause of the hypothyroidism is as a result of markedly increased activity of the type D3 iodothyronine deiodinase that rapidly converts T4 to reverse T3 and T3 to T2. Both reverse T3 and T2 are biologically inactive, resulting in insufficient T4 and T3 for metabolic needs and increased TSH. This "consumption" of T4 and T3 ameliorates with involution of the giant hemangioma, which sometimes need to be surgically excised. The hypothyroidism must be treated with significant doses of synthetic thyroxine to overcome the rapid inactivation of T4.

CONGENITAL THYROTOXICOSIS

Thyrotoxicosis in the neonatal period is relatively uncommon. Affected infants almost always are born of mothers who have either active or a previous history of Graves disease. Neonatal thyrotoxicosis may also present in infants born to mothers with Hashimoto thyroiditis. Fewer than 5% of infants born to mothers with Graves disease will have thyrotoxicosis in the newborn period. Neonatal thyrotoxicosis is caused by the placental transfer of maternal thyroid stimulating immunoglobulins, which can be demonstrated in over 90% of studied cases (91).

Neonatal thyrotoxicosis is manifested by poor weight gain or excessive weight loss, goiter, irritability, tachycardia, flushing, and exophthalmos. A number of these infants tend to be small for gestational age. The infant of a thyrotoxic mother with a high normal T4 should be followed closely. A low or suppressed TSH is further evidence of neonatal thyrotoxicosis. The onset of symptoms usually occurs within the first week of life, but may be delayed until the second week, particularly if the mother has been on antithyroid drugs that can also cross the placenta. Arrhythmias, such as paroxysmal atrial tachycardia, cardiac failure, and rarely death have been reported with severe thyrotoxicosis (92). In several reported cases, there has been a rapid advance in skeletal maturation, with advanced bone age and premature closure of the cranial sutures (93,94). Neonatal thyrotoxicosis is a self-limiting condition and abates as the levels of TSI antibodies decrease, thus the prognosis is good. Most infants are asymptomatic by 2 months of age and most cases will have resolved by 9 months.

Major therapeutic concerns in neonatal thyrotoxicosis are tracheal obstruction secondary to goitrous encroachment, and cardiac failure. Subtotal thyroidectomy is rarely required to relieve tracheal obstruction. Iodide (one drop every 8 hours of saturated solution of potassium iodide), along with a β-adrenergic blocking agent such as propranolol hydrochloride, can be used to control the thyrotoxicosis. Iodide has the advantage of interfering not only with T4 synthesis but also with the release of thyroid hormones. In the most severe cases, digitalis, sedation, or glucocorticoids may be necessary to prevent cardiovascular collapse.

REFERENCES

1. Tilmann C, Capel B. Cellular and molecular pathways regulating mammalian sex determination. *Recent Prog Horm Res* 2002;57:1.
2. Little M, Wells C. A clinical overview of WT1 gene mutations. *Hum Mutat* 1997;9:209.
3. Achermann JC, Meeks JJ, Jameson JL. Phenotypic spectrum of mutations in DAX-1 and SF-1. *Mol Cell Endocrinol* 2001;185:17.
4. Ford CE, Jones KW, Polani PE, et al. A sex-chromosome anomaly in a case of gonadal dysgenesis. *Lancet* 1959;1:711.
5. Jacobs PA, Ross A. Structural abnormalities of the Y chromosome in man. *Nature* 1966;210:352.
6. Sinclair AH, Berta P, Palmer MS, et al. A gene from the human sex determining region encodes a protein with homology to a conserved DNS binding motif. *Nature* 1990;346:240.
7. Clarkson MJ, Harley VR. Sex with two SOX on: SRY and SOX9 in testis development. *Trends Endocrinol Metab* 2002;13:106.
8. Kwoc C, Weller PA, Guioli S et al. Mutations in SOX9, the gene responsible for campomelic dysplasia and autosomal sex reversal. *Am J Hum Genet* 1995;57:1028.
9. Jordan BK, Mohammed M, Ching ST, et al. Up-regulation of WNT-4 signaling and dosage-sensitive sex reversal in humans. *Am J Hum Genet* 2001;68:1102.
10. Johnston AW, Ferguson-Smith MA, Handmaker SD Jr, et al. The triple-X syndrome: clinical, pathological and chromosomal studies in three mentally retarded cases. *Br Med J* 1961;2:1047.
11. Zenteno-Ruiz JC, Kofman-Alfaro S, Mendez JP. 46,XX sex reversal. *Arch Med Res* 2001;32:559.
12. Lus HA, Rudd FH. Chromosomal abnormalities in the human population: estimation of rates based on New Haven Newborn Study. *Science* 1970;169:496.
13. Carr DH, Gedeon M. Population cytogenetics in human abortuses. In: Hook EB, Porter IH, eds. *Population cytogenetics.* New York: Academic Press, 1977:1.
14. Palmer CG, Reichmann A. Chromosomal and clinical findings in 110 females with Turner syndrome. *Hum Genet* 1976;35:35.
15. Goldberg MD, Scully AL, Solomon IL, et al. Gonadal dysgenesis in phenotypic female subjects. *Am J Med* 1968;45:529.
16. Saenger P, Albertsson Wikland K, Conway GS, et al. Recommendations for the diagnosis and management of Turner syndrome. *J Clin Endocrinol Metab* 2001;86:3061.
17. Preger L, Steinbach HL, Moskowitz P. Roentgenographic abnormalities in phenotypic females with gonadal dysgenesis. *A J Radiology* 1968;104:899.
18. Quigley CA, Crowe BJ, Anglin G, et al. Growth hormone and low dose estrogen in Turner syndrome: results of a United States multi-center trial to near-final height. *J Clin Endocirnol Metab* 2002;87:393.
19. Serhal PF, Craft IL. Oocyte donation in 61 patients. *Lancet* 1989;1:1185.
20. Moshang T, Vallet HL, Cintron C, et al. Gonadal function in XO/XY or XX/XY Turner's syndrome. *J Pediatr* 1972;80:460.
21. Pallister PD, Opitz JM. The Perrault syndrome: autosomal recessive ovarian dysgenesis with facultative, non-sex-limited sensorineural deafness. *Am J Med Genet* 1979;4:239.
22. Sternberg WH, Barclay DL, Kloepfer HW. Familial XY gonadal dysgenesis. *N Engl J Med* 1968;278:695.
23. Krob G, Braun A, Kuhnle U. True hermaphroditism: geographical distribution, clinical findings, chromosomes and gonadal histology. *Eur J Pediatr* 1994;153:2.
24. Grumbach MM, Ducharme J, Moloshok RE. On the fetal masculinizing action of certain oral progestins. *J Clin Endocrinol Metab* 1959;19:1369.
25. Murset G, Zachman M, Prader A, et al. Male external genitalia of a girl caused by virilizing adrenal tumor in the mother. *Acta Endocrinol* 1970;65:627.
26. Haymond MW, Weldon VV. Female pseudohermaphroditism secondary to a maternal virilizing tumor. *J Pediatr* 1973;82:682.
27. Shozu M, Akasofu K, Harada T, et al. A new cause of female pseudohermaphroditism: placental aromatase deficiency. *J Clin Endocrinol Metab* 1991;72:560.
28. Miller WL. Disorders of androgen biosynthesis. *Semin Reprod Med* 2002;20:205.
29. McPhaul MJ. Androgen receptor mutations and androgen insensitivity. *Mol Cell Endocrinol* 2002;198:61.

30. Imperato-McGinley J. 5alpha-reductase-2 deficiency and complete androgen insensitivity: lessons from nature. *Adv Exp Med Biol* 2002;511:121, discussion 131-134.
31. Quigley CA, De Bellis A, Marschke KB, et al. Androgen receptor defects: historical, clinical, and molecular perspectives. *Endocr Rev* 1995;16:271.
32. Lee MM, Donahoe PK, Silverman BL, et al. Measurements of serum mullerian inhibiting substance in the evaluation of children with nonpalpable gonads. *N Engl J Med* 1997;336:1480.
33. Eberenz W, Rosenberg HK, Moshang T, et al. True hermaphroditism: sonographic determination of ovotestes. *Radiology* 1991;179:429.
34. Diamond M, Sigmundson HK. Sex reassignment at birth. Long term review and clinical implications. *Arch Pediatr Adolesc Med* 1997;151:298.
35. Stanley CA. Hyperinsulinism in infants and children. *Pediatr Clin North Am* 1997;44:363.
36. Parks JS, Brown MR, Hurley DL, et al. Heritable Disorders of the Pituitary. *J Clin Endocrin Metab* 1999;84:4362.
37. Pfaffle R, Kim C, Otten et al. Pit-1: clinical aspects. *Horm Res* 1996;45[Suppl]:25.
38. Sornson MW, Wu W, Dasen JS, et al. Pituitary lineage determination by the Prophet of Pit-1 homeodomain factor defective in Ames mouse. *Nature* 1996;384:327.
39. Bach I, Rhodes SJ, Pearse RV II, et al. P-Lim, a LIM homeodomain factor is expressed during pituitary organ and cell committment andsynergizes with Pit-1. *Proc Natl Acad Sci U S A* 1995;92:2720.
40. Thomas PQ, Dattani MT, Brickman JM, et al. Heterozygous HESX1 mutations associated with isolated congenital pituitary hypoplasia and septo-optic dysplasia. *Hum Mol Genet* 2001;10:39.
41. Kyllo J, Collins MM, Vetter KL, et al. Linkage of congenital isolated adrenocorticotropic hormone deficiency to corticotropin releasing hormone locus using sequence repeat polymorphisms. *Am J Med Genetics* 1996;62:262.
42. Goellner MH, Ziegler EE, Fomon SI. Urination during the first three years of life. *Nephron* 1981;28:174.
43. Rees L, Brook CGD, Shaw JCL, et al. Hyponatremia in the first week of life in preterm infants: parts I and II. *Arch Dis Child* 1984;59:414.
44. Judd BA, Haycock GB, Dalton N, et al. Hyponatremia in premature babies and following surgery in older children. *Acta Paediatr Scand* 1987;76:385.
45. Clark AJL, Weber A. Adrenocorticotropin insensitivity syndromes. *Endocrine Rev* 1998;19:828.
46. Moshang T Jr, Rosenfield RL, Bongiovanni AM, et al. Familial glucocorticoid insufficiency. *J Pediatr* 1973;82:821.
47. Miller WL, Levine LS. Molecular and clinical advances in congenital adrenal hyperplasia. *J Pediatr* 1987;111:1.
48. White PC, Speiser, PW. Congenital adrenal hyperplasia due to 21-hydroxylase deficiency. *Endocr Rev* 2000;21:245.
49. Simard J, Rheaume E, Sanchez R, et al. Molecular basis of congenital adrenal hyperplasia due to 3β-hydroxysteroid dehydrogenase deficiency. *Mol Endocrinol* 1993;7:716.
50. Cara J, Moshang T, Bongiovanni AM. Elevated 17 hydroxyprogesterone and testosterone in a newborn male with 3β-hydroxysteroid dehydrogenase deficiency. *N Engl J Med* 1985;313:618.
51. Auchus RJ. The genetics, pathophysiology, and management of human deficiencies of P450c17. *Endocrinol Metab Clin NA* 2001;30:101.
52. Eberlein WR, Bongiovanni AM. Defective steroidal biogenesis in congenital adrenal hyperplasia. *Pediatrics* 1958;21:661.
53. Ulick S, Gautier E, Vetterik K, et al. An aldosterone biosynthetic defect in a salt-losing disorder. *J Clin Endocrinol Metab* 1964;24:669.
54. Visser HK, Cost WS. A new hereditary defect in the biosynthesis of aldosterone: urinary C 21-corticosteroid pattern in three related patients with a salt-losing syndrome, suggesting an 18-oxidation defect. *Acta Endocrinol* 1964;47:589.
55. Bose HS, Sugawara, Strauss JF III, et al. The pathophysiology and genetics of congenital lipoid hyperplasia. *N Engl J Med* 1996;335:1870.
56. Pang S, Pollack MS, Marshall RN, et al. Prenatal treatment of congenital adrenal hyperplasia due to 21-hydroxylase deficiency. *N Engl J Med* 1990;322:111.
57. Speiser PW, Laforgia N, Kato K, et al. First trimester prenatal treatment and molecular genetic diagnosis of congenital adrenal

hyperplasia (21-hydroxylase deficiency). *J Clin Endocrinol Metab* 1990;70:838.
58. Weiner D, Smith J, Dahlem S, et al. Serum adrenal steroid levels in full term infants. *J Pediatr* 1987;110:122.
59. Lee MM, Rajagopalen L, Berg GJ, et al. Serum adrenal steroid concentrations in premature infants. *J Clin Endocrinol Metab* 1989;69:1133.
60. Pang S, Wallace MA, Hofman L, et al. Worldwide experience in newborn screening for classical congenital adrenal hyperplasia due to 21-hydroxylase deficiency. *Pediatrics* 1988;81:866.
61. Vulsma T, Gons MH, Vijlder JJM. Maternal-fetal transfer of thyroxine in congenital hypothyroidism due to a total organification defect or thyroid agenesis. *N Engl J Med* 1989;321:13.
62. Dussault J, Row VV, Lickrish G, et al. Studies of serum triiodothyronine concentration in maternal and cord blood: transfer of triiodothyronine across the human placenta. *J Clin Endocrinol Metab* 1969;29:595.
63. Pittman CS, Chambers JB Jr, Read VH. The extrathyroidal conversion rate of thyroxine to triiodothyronine in normal man. *J Clin Invest* 1971;50:1187.
64. Fisher DA. Thyroid function in premature infants. *Clin Perinat* 1998;25:999.
65. Adams LM, Emery JR, Clark SJ, et al. Reference ranges for newer thyroid function tests in premature infants. *J Pediatr* 1995;126:122.
66. Macchia PE, De Delice M, Di Lauro R. Molecular genetics of congenital hypothyroidism. *Curr Opin Genet Dev* 1999;9:289.
67. Blizzard RM, Chandler RW, Landing BH, et al. Maternal autoimmunization to thyroid as a probable cause of athyrotic cretinism. *N Engl J Med* 1960;262:327.
68. Zakaria M, McKenzie JM, Eidson MS. Transient neonatal hypothyroidism: characterization of maternal antibodies to the thyrotropin receptor. *J Clin Endocrinol Metab* 1990;70:1239.
69. de Vijlder JJ, Ris-Stalpers C, Vulsma T. Inborn errors of thyroid hormone biosynthesis. *Exp Clin Endocrinol Diabetes* 1997;105:32.
70. Savoie JC, Thompoulos P, Savoie F. Studies on mono and di-iodohistidine: I. The identification of histadines from thyroidal iodoproteins and their peripheral metabolism in the normal man and rat. *J Clin Invest* 1973;52:106.
71. Savoie JC, Massin JP, Savoie F. Studies on mono and di-iodohistidine: II. Congenital goitrous hypothyroidism with thyroglobulin defect and iodohistidine-rich iodoalbumin production. *J Clin Invest* 1973;52:116.
72. Burrow GN. Neonatal goiter after maternal propylthiouracil therapy. *J Clin Endocrinol Metab* 1965;5:403.
73. Herbst AL, Selenkow JA. Hyperthyroidism during pregnancy. *N Engl J Med* 1965;273:627.
74. Kampmann JP, Johansen K, Hansen JM, et al. Propylthiouracil in human milk: revision of a dogma. *Lancet* 1980;1:736
75. Lamberg BA, Ikonen E, Osterlund K, et al. Antithyroid treatment of maternal hyperthyroidism during lactation. *Clin Endocrinol* 1984;21:81.
76. Azizi F. Effect of methimazole treatment of maternal thyrotoxicosis on thyroid function in breastfeeding infants. *J Pediatr* 1996;128:855.
77. Refetoff S, DeWind LT, DeGroot LJ. Familial syndrome combining deaf-mutism, stippled epiphyses, goiter, and abnormally high PBI: possible target organ refractoriness to thyroid hormone. *J Clin Endocrinol Metab* 1967;27:279.
78. Bode HH, Danon M, Weintraub BD, et al. Partial target organ resistance to thyroid hormone. *J Clin Invest* 1973;52:776.
79. Refetoff S, Weiss RE, Usala SJ. The syndromes of resistance to thyroid hormone. *Endocrin Rev* 1993;14:348.
80. Stanbury JB, Rocmans P, Butler UK, et al. Congenital hypothyroidism with impaired thyroid response to thyrotropin. *N Engl J Med* 1968;279:1132.
81. Lowrey GH, Aster RH, Carr EA, et al. Early diagnostic criteria of congenital hypothyroidism. *Am J Dis Child* 1958;96:131.
82. Oppenheimer JH, Schwartz JH. Molecular basis of thyroid hormone-dependent brain development. *Endocrinol Rev* 1997;18:462.
83. Klein AH, Meltzer S, Kenny FM. Improved prognosis in congenital hypothyroidism treated before age 3 months. *J Pediatr* 1972;81:912.
84. New England Congenital Hypothyroidism Collaborative. Characteristics of infantile hypothyroidism discovered on neonatal screening. *J Pediatr* 1984;102:539.

85. Glorieux J, Desjardins M, Letarte J, et al. Useful parameters to predict the eventual mental outcome of hypothyroid children. *Pediatr Res* 1988;24:6.
86. Committee on Genetics, American Academy of Pediatrics. Screening for congenital deficiency of thyroid hormone. *Pediatrics* 1977;60:389.
87. Willi SM, Moshang T Jr. Diagnostic dilemmas: results of screening tests for congenital hypothyroidism. *Pediatr Clin North Am* 1991:38;555
88. Reuss ML, Paneth N, Pinto-Martin JA, et al. The relation of transient hypothyroxinemia in preterm infants to neurologic development at two years of age. *N Engl J Med* 1996;334;821.
89. van Wassenaer AG, Kok JH, de Vijlder JJ, et al. Effects of thyroxine supplementation on neurologic development in infants born at less than 30 weeks' gestation. *N Engl J Med* 1997;336:21.
90. Huang SA, Tu HM, Harney JW, et al. Severe hypothyroidism caused by type 3 iodothyronine deiodinase in infantile hemangiomas. *N Engl J Med* 2000;343:185-189.
91. Foley TP Jr, White C, New A. Juvenile Graves' disease: usefulness and limitations of thyrotropin receptor antibody determinations. *J Pediatr* 1989;110:378.
92. Riopel DA, Mullins CE. Congenital thyrotoxicosis with paroxysmal atrial tachycardia. *Pediatrics* 1972;50:140.
93. Farrehi C. Accelerated maturity in fetal thyrotoxicosis. *Clin Pediatr* 1968;7:134.
94. Hollingsworth DR, Mabry CC, Eckard JM. Hereditary aspects of Grave's disease in infancy and childhood. *J Pediatr* 1972;81:446.

Gastrointestinal Disease

40

Jon A. Vanderhoof   *Terence L. Zach*   *Thomas E. Adrian*

Although most pediatric gastroenterologists are uncomfortable with primary care of the sick premature infant, they often are valuable consultants to the neonatologist. In evaluating a complex gastrointestinal (GI) or hepatobiliary problem, a gastroenterologist often uses an organ system-specific developmental pathophysiologic approach. In looking at a problem from a somewhat different perspective than the neonatologist, the opinion of the consultant may augment the analysis of the primary physician. It remains the responsibility of the neonatologist to put the consultant's view into perspective as it relates to the other complex problems of the sick infant.

The gastroenterologist also may offer his or her skills in invasive procedures to aid in the diagnosis of GI and liver disease. Upper and lower GI endoscopy, liver biopsy, rectal suction biopsy, esophageal, antroduodenal, and anorectal motility studies, and even endoscopic retrograde cholangiopancreatography can be performed in term infants and, depending on the skill and training of the gastroenterologist, in premature infants as well. Small diameter neonatal endoscopes are now available which facilitate obtaining small bowel biopsies from the distal duodenum and jejunum.

In some institutions, gastroenterologists with special expertise in nutrition provide assistance in nutritional support of parenteral nutrition-dependent or malnourished infants. Their role becomes especially important in infants with GI or liver disease who may require long-term follow-up, such as the infant with progressive liver disease, or home on parenteral nutrition, such as the infant with short bowel syndrome.

DEVELOPMENT OF THE GASTROINTESTINAL TRACT

Subsequent to the development of the individual organs of the GI tract, specialized features of the system begin to become apparent, mostly in the second and third trimesters (1). At approximately 14 weeks of gestation, differentiation of the pancreatic endocrine and exocrine tissues begins, and crypts and villi begin to form in the small intestine. A few weeks later, the colon, initially populated with villi similar to those in the small intestine, begins to develop its more characteristic surface, with gradual loss of villi. As these morphologic changes occur, numerous functional processes begin, some of which mature early *in utero*, some only at birth, and some during the first year of life.

Carbohydrate Absorption

The functional maturation of the digestive process is complex (2). There are marked differences in maturation of the digestive and absorptive processes of different nutrients (Table 40-1). In the neonate, most dietary carbohydrate is presented in the form of lactose, the predominant carbohydrate in virtually all mammalian milk. Lactose and other disaccharides are digested by enzymes located on the brush border membrane in mature enterocytes; those located on the distal and midportions of the small intestinal villi. Component monosaccharides are released after hydrolysis by disaccharidases. Lactase hydrolyzes lactose to glucose and galactose, and both subsequently are transported by active carrier-mediated transport. Other disaccharidases include maltase, which hydrolyzes maltose to two glucose units, glucoamylase, which hydrolyzes glucose oligosaccharides to glucose monomers, and sucrase, which hydrolyzes sucrose to fructose and glucose. Sucrase is actually a double enzyme, the other part of the molecule being isomaltase, which hydrolyzes a-1-6 bonds of a-limit dextrins. Disaccharidase activities are highest in the proximal and midjejunum and decrease distally.

Lactase activity develops later in gestation than the other disaccharidases. Lactase activity is low until the final weeks of gestation. Although other disaccharidase levels can be detected somewhat earlier in gestation and reach nearly adult levels between 26 and 34 weeks of gestational age, lactase levels are only 30% of full-term levels by that point in gestation. Because of the delayed maturation of lactase, specialized infant formulas for preterm infants have been designed, with a significant percentage of carbohydrate presented as sucrose or glucose polymers rather than lactose. Alternatively, the addition of lactase to formulas for

TABLE 40-1

DIGESTIVE AND ABSORPTIVE FUNCTION IN INFANTS RELATIVE TO ADULTS

Process	Premature Infant	Full-term Infant	Adult
Salivary enzymes	Normal	Normal	Normal
Gastric acid production	$\varnothing$	$\varnothing$ to normal	Normal
Bile acid secretion	$\varnothing\varnothing$	$\varnothing$	$\varnothing$
Pancreatic enzyme production	$\varnothing\varnothing$	$\varnothing$	Normal
Lactase production	$\varnothing$	Normal	Normal
Sucrase and isomaltase production	Normal	Normal	Normal

preterm infants may enhance weight gain (3). The predominant enzyme for digestion of starches and glucose polymers is pancreatic amylase, which is nearly absent during the first 4 to 6 months of life and gradually matures during the latter half of the first year. An alternative pathway therefore must exist for the digestion of these glucose polymers (4,5).

Salivary glands produce an amylase that may be important in the digestion of complex carbohydrates in the newborn. This enzyme is detectable at 20 weeks of gestation and is present in significant quantities in premature infants. As with pancreatic amylase, however, the ability of the newborn to secrete salivary amylase is substantially reduced and matures throughout the first year of life. Salivary amylase is inactivated by gastric acid, but probably retains some activity in the stomach of premature infants. Glucoamylase is a brush border enzyme capable of digesting glucose units from the nonreducing ends of starch and dextrin. Glucoamylase is present in neonates and infants at 50% to 100% of adult levels.

Finally, it is probable that some malabsorbed carbohydrate is digested in the colon through the colon salvage pathway. Colonic anaerobic bacteria are capable of metabolizing carbohydrates to produce short-chain fatty acids that then are absorbed through the colonic mucosa. Considering the relative pancreatic insufficiency and lactase deficiency in the newborn infant, the colon salvage pathway may be an important mechanism by which infants absorb carbohydrates.

Fat Absorption

Fat absorption is a complex process, primarily because fat is insoluble in the aqueous environment of the small intestinal lumen (6). Solubilization, therefore, is an important part of the fat assimilation process. The first phase of fat absorption is that of enzymatic digestion or lipolysis. Because most dietary fat is present in the form of triglycerides, otherwise known as triacylglycerols, these first must be hydrolyzed by pancreatic lipase.

Phospholipids are hydrolyzed concurrently by pancreatic phospholipase. Colipase, a cofactor secreted by the pan-

creas, also is required, facilitating the action of lipase by binding to bile salt–lipid surfaces and improving the interaction of lipase with triglyceride. The efficiency of this process is augmented by the release of cholecystokinin (CCK) from the duodenal epithelium, which occurs in response to the presence of lipid and protein in the duodenum. Cholecystokinin stimulates pancreatic secretion, gallbladder contraction, and simultaneous relaxation of the sphincter of Oddi, to mix large quantities of bile acids and digestive juices with lipids. Pancreatic lipase levels are reduced in preterm infants and intrauterine growth-retarded infants, significantly impairing lipolysis (7). Lingual lipase, secreted from the salivary glands, may facilitate lipolysis in the premature infant and partially compensate for the infant's relative pancreatic insufficiency (8). Nonetheless, fat absorption is significantly impaired in newborn infants and, to a greater extent, in premature infants, due at least in part to pancreatic insufficiency.

Closely linked with the process of enzymatic digestion of fats is micellar solubilization by bile acids (9). Bile acid molecules are complex structures with both hydrophobic and hydrophilic ends. Bile acids interface with lipids to render them water soluble by positioning the hydrophobic portion in close proximity to the lipid globules although allowing the hydrophilic portion to remain free to interact with the aqueous environment. Lipids then become enclosed in disc-shaped water-soluble micelles that contain fatty acids, monoglycerides, phospholipids, cholesterol, and fat-soluble vitamins.

Solubilization is particularly important because of the presence of the intestine's unstirred water layer. This stagnant layer of water overlies the microvillus membrane of the intestinal epithelial cells and is the primary barrier to lipid transport. The actual thickness of the unstirred water layer is complex and difficult to measure, but the layer is significantly reduced by the constant agitation of the fluid in the GI tract as a result of gut motility and villus contraction. Because of the convolutions in the small intestine caused by the presence of villi and microvilli, the total surface area available to interface between the intestinal surface and the unstirred layer is much greater than the interface between the unstirred water layer and the aqueous intraluminal environment. Penetration through the unstirred layer by the disc-shaped micelles is the rate-limiting step for lipid absorption. Disease processes that increase the unstirred layer thickness will markedly inhibit fat absorption in much the same manner as disease states that render the supply of bile acids inadequate for micellar solubilization. Bile acids commonly are deficient in cholestatic liver diseases, such as neonatal hepatitis or biliary atresia, and in rare cases of congenital bile acid deficiency. Bile acids are deconjugated rapidly and reabsorbed in the presence of small intestinal bacterial overgrowth. Bile acid deficiency therefore may occur in patients with disorders that cause intestinal stasis and bacterial overgrowth, such as short bowel syndrome. In disorders of mucosal injury, the unstirred layer thickness may be increased, making penetration of the fat-containing micelles difficult and further exacerbating fat malabsorption.

Bile acids are extremely important in the fat absorption process. In the absence of bile acids, only about one-third of dietary triglycerides, a very small percentage of fatty acids, and virtually no cholesterol or fat-soluble vitamins are absorbed. Medium-chain triglycerides may be better absorbed because of their enhanced water solubility, which allows penetration of the unstirred water layer without micellar solubilization. In both preterm and term infants, bile acid synthesis is limited and the bile salt pool size is low (10). Moreover, preterm infants may have an ineffective bile salt transport process in the distal ileum, resulting in impaired enterohepatic circulation of bile salts (11). Consequently, the bile acid concentration may be less than adequate for the formation of micelles and solubilization of fat. Thus, penetration of the unstirred layer is less efficient in the term infant and further impaired in the preterm infant compared to adults.

After lipids are enclosed in the bile acid micelle and reach the lipid bilayer membrane of the small intestinal mucosal cell, absorption into the cell occurs by passive diffusion. Because of the convolutions of the GI tract, a large surface area exists for lipid assimilation. In the absence of disease, this process progresses in the term and preterm infant relatively uninhibited. In disorders in which the absorptive surface area is reduced or damaged, however, such as short bowel syndrome or any form of diffuse enterocolitis, fat, carbohydrate, and, to a limited degree, protein are malabsorbed.

Within the enterocyte, monoglycerides and esterified fatty acids are immediately resynthesized to triglycerides. These triglycerides, along with apoproteins, phospholipids, free cholesterol, some diglycerides, and esterified cholesterol, are stabilized within chylomicrons. The outer structure of the chylomicron then fuses with the basolateral membrane and is extruded into the lamina propria, in which it is carried by the lacteals and lymphatic channels and deposited into the blood stream.

Protein Absorption

The assimilation of protein begins in the stomach through the action of hydrochloric acid and pepsin. The maturational aspects of this process have been the subject of substantial study and some controversy. Conflicting data exist regarding the status of acid secretion in the newborn infant. Newborn infants appear to be capable of secreting acid, although the process is somewhat immature (12). In premature infants, it is probable that the process is impaired to a greater extent (13). Pepsinogen, the proenzyme for pepsin, which facilitates protein digestion in the stomach, is secreted in preterm infants, but in much lower concentrations than in term infants (14).

The gastric aspects of protein digestion are relatively inconsequential, compared to the much more complete process in the small intestine. Enterokinase, produced in the duodenal mucosa, activates the pancreatic proteolytic enzyme trypsinogen, converting it to trypsin, which then activates essentially all of the other enzymes involved in protein digestion. Enterokinase levels have been demonstrated in human fetuses as early as 21 weeks of gestation (15). Enterokinase expression is diminished during fetal development, however, and is only 10% of adult levels in the term newborn. Additionally, pancreatic and duodenal proteolytic enzymes are present in preterm and term infants in lower concentrations than in older children and in adults. These enzymes initiate hydrolysis of proteins, and the hydrolysis process is completed by brush border and cytosolic peptidases. Protein is absorbed in the form of amino acids and dipeptides through active transport processes that appear to be well developed by 28 weeks of gestational age. Despite the relative immaturity of multiple phases of the protein assimilation process, both preterm and term infants are quite capable of absorbing adequate quantities of dietary protein. In small infants, the protein malabsorption resulting from mucosal injury is probably far less consequential than the malabsorption of the other major macronutrients.

Micronutrient Absorption

Absorption of micronutrients matures at varying rates in infancy. Water is absorbed passively in response to sodium and other electrolytes, as it is in older children and adults (16). Experimental evidence suggests that the intestinal epithelium may be more secretory during early infancy, and the increased susceptibility of infants to diarrheal disorders probably is at least partially related to this process.

Mineral absorption depends on the form in which the mineral is presented to the infant. Iron, for example, is absorbed extremely well from breast milk. Even the preterm infant is capable of absorbing nearly 50% of the iron in breast milk, whereas only a small percentage of iron is absorbed from cow-milk formulas, necessitating iron supplementation. Calcium and phosphorous also are well absorbed from breast milk (17,18). Magnesium, copper, and, to a lesser extent, zinc are well absorbed by both term and preterm infants (19). In general, minerals are absorbed somewhat better from breast milk than from cow milk. Most vitamins appear to be absorbed adequately in both term and preterm infants, although fat-soluble vitamin deficiency is common in disorders affecting fat absorption, especially disorders causing bile acid deficiency.

Gut Motility

Although nutrient assimilation is heavily dependent on the development of digestive and absorptive function, actual feeding depends greatly on the maturation of gut motility (20–22). Neuroblasts migrate in a cranial-to-caudal direction between weeks 5 and 12 of gestation. There is gradual maturation of gut motility throughout the fetal period and the first several years of postnatal life. In the fetus, normal propulsive motility in the gut probably does not appear until approximately 30 weeks of age. Interdigestive phenomena, known as migrating motor complexes, can be demonstrated by approximately 33 weeks of gestation. Motor activity in the neonatal gut differs significantly from that in adults, in that the propagation rate of the migrating motor complex is substantially slower in neonates, and the complex is not abolished by feeding as in older children.

Sucking and swallowing reflexes begin early during fetal development, but the maturation of the process is not completed until after birth. The fetus is able to swallow amniotic fluid as early as 11 to 12 weeks of gestation. Actual sucking probably does not occur until approximately 18 to 24 weeks. This type of sucking is termed nonnutritive sucking, differentiating it from the more effective nutritive sucking mechanism that develops by 34 to 35 weeks of gestation. The onset of nutritive sucking closely parallels a rapid increase in growth of the fetal stomach (23) and the acquisition of mature patterns of gastric antral and small intestinal motility.

By the time a term infant is born, sucking movements are followed in an orderly progression by swallowing, esophageal peristalsis, relaxation of the lower esophageal sphincter, and relaxation of the gastric fundus. The first stage of swallowing is an involuntary reflex in both the term and preterm infant. Early introduction of oral feeds may accelerate the time from gavage to full nipple feeding (24).

Some data suggest that nonnutritive sucking may play an important role in weight gain in preterm infants. The mechanism of this effect may be related to maturational changes in the infant GI tract, and sucking may facilitate gastric emptying and other GI functions, primarily through stimulation of secretion of GI regulatory peptides.

Maturation of GI motility may have important implications for a number of conditions. Gastroesophageal reflux is common in both term and preterm infants, and probably relates to diminished lower esophageal sphincter function or inappropriate relaxation of the lower esophageal sphincter, often in association with delayed gastric emptying. The maturation of both lower esophageal sphincter function and gastric emptying has been studied extensively, with somewhat equivocal results. Depending on the technique used to measure sphincter function, the lower esophageal sphincter tone has been shown to be either low or normal in both preterm and term infants (25). Hypertonic carbohydrate solutions appear to delay gastric emptying in infants, much as they do in adults.

GASTROINTESTINAL HORMONES AND ENTERIC NEUROPEPTIDES

GI peptide hormones appear to play an important role in the structural and functional development of the gut, and in the control of alimentary functions. The function of a vast endocrine system is integrated with that of the enteric nervous system, which itself uses other regulatory peptides as local messengers.

Endocrine cells producing gastrin, somatostatin, motilin, and glucose-dependent insulinotropic peptide (GIP) are detectable in the fetus at 8 weeks of gestation, with gastrin- and somatostatin-producing cells being most numerous (26). By 14 weeks, all of the endocrine cell types are present in the intestinal mucosa, although the anatomic distribution is more widespread than that seen in the adult (26). By the end of the second trimester, the distribution of gut endocrine cells resembles that of the adult (26). Peptidergic nerves are first demonstrable in the myenteric plexus at about 12 weeks of gestation, correlating with the known developmental pattern of enteric nerve plexuses (26). These enteric nerves then migrate through to the submucous plexus. By the third trimester, all of the regulatory peptide systems are well developed (27). At birth, the molecular forms of the GI regulatory peptides and their distribution in the gut are similar to those of the adult (27).

Surges of gut hormones appear to be responsible for the marked growth and functional change that occur in the alimentary tract in early neonatal life. Substantial changes in GI hormone secretion are seen during this period, triggered by the switch from intravenous to enteral feeding (28).

Gastrin is an important regulator of gastric secretion and is trophic to the gastric mucosa. At birth, cord blood levels of gastrin are already four to five times higher than those in the adult, and prefeed basal levels remain elevated for several weeks (29,30). Furthermore, gastrin levels increase in response to the first milk feed (31). After 3 to 4 weeks of life, basal gastrin levels decline, a change accompanied by development of marked elevation of levels following feeding (29,32). Gastric acid is detectable in the stomach at birth and reaches a peak in the first day or two of life (30,33). Thereafter, acid output decreases for a period of about 1 month despite the hypergastrinemia and rapid growth of the stomach. It has been suggested that the lack of responsiveness to gastrin could be as a result of a lack of receptors in the oxyntic gland mucosa. Perhaps a more likely explanation, however, is that secretion is suppressed by an inhibitor, such as peptide YY (PYY) or neurotensin, thus enabling gastrin to stimulate growth of the gastric mucosa without hyperstimulation of acid secretion (34,35).

Basal levels of the duodenal hormone, secretin, are higher at birth than in adults, and, during the first 3 weeks of life, a more marked postprandial response develops than is seen in the adult (36). Because secretin is considered to be a major factor in triggering the neutralization of acid chyme entering the duodenum, the increase in circulating secretin levels may be of considerable importance in mucosal protection during this period. It is notable that the postnatal surge of secretin, unlike that of the other alimentary hormones, occurs even in the absence of feeding, indicating the importance of this mucosal cytoprotective function (32).

Cholecystokinin, released from the upper small intestine, stimulates pancreatic enzyme secretion and contracts the gallbladder. Additionally, CCK has marked trophic effects on the pancreas and appears to be responsible for regeneration after resection or acute pancreatitis (37). The observed postnatal surge of plasma CCK concentrations, therefore, may be of importance in stimulating growth of this organ (38). Interestingly, CCK levels decrease during kangaroo care in the NICU setting, in contrast to the increase seen with nasogastric tube feeding (39).

Also released from the small intestine, motilin is a hormonal peptide with powerful motor functions. These motor functions include acceleration of gastric emptying and stimulation of the interdigestive myoelectric complexes (MMC) during the interprandial period. The motilin receptor-mediated induction of phase III of the MMC occurs by 32 weeks of gestational age. Motilin concentrations are low in cord blood, but preprandial basal concentrations show a massive postnatal surge that peaks at around 2 weeks of postnatal life (32). This peak is enhanced, but delayed, in preterm neonates. It is likely that this increase in circulating motilin concentrations is responsible for the known increase in motor activity of the gut that occurs during the neonatal period. Interdigestive motor complexes appear normal at birth in the term infant, but interdigestive cycles are incomplete in preterm neonates (40). Premature babies exhibit abnormal motor activity, with periods of motor quiescence and nonpropagating contractions. Thus, motor activity is more immature in preterm infants than in term infants (40). The relationship between maturation of the migrating motor complexes and the late postnatal surge of motilin in preterm neonates is not clear.

The jejunal hormone, GIP, is thought to be largely responsible for the postprandial increase in circulating insulin levels (41). Basal GIP concentrations are low at birth and increase gradually throughout the first month of life, together with the development of a marked postfeeding GIP response similar to that seen in the adult after ingestion of a mixed meal (32,42). The development of the GIP response to feeding in neonates is mirrored by the postprandial insulin response, which increases through the first month of life to maintain glucose homeostasis (42).

Neurotensin is an ileal peptide that has inhibitory effects on gastric secretion and motility. Plasma neurotensin concentrations are higher in the neonate than in the adult, and an enhanced postprandial response develops in the first month of life (43). Both reduction of gastric secretion and slowing of the rate of gastric emptying will decrease the rate at which acid chyme enters the duodenum and, therefore, will result in a more steady absorption of nutrients from the gut. Thus, neurotensin may be important in the adaptation of the neonate to enteral nutrition. PYY is an important hormone from the distal intestine that inhibits gastric emptying and slows small bowel transit (44). PYY also inhibits gastric and small bowel secretion, leading to an increase in net absorption (34). Concentrations of PYY are elevated in cord blood and rise postnatally to a peak within the first 2 weeks postpartum (35). At their peak, plasma PYY concentrations are about 50 times higher than fasting levels in normal adults (35). There is evidence to suggest that gastric emptying and intestinal transit are rapid during the first week of life, both in term and

preterm infants. The triggering mechanism for the changes that then take place is unknown, but it is likely that factors such as PYY play a role (44). Additionally, the very potent inhibitory effect of PYY on gastric secretion may account for the prevention of hypersecretion of acid during the early neonatal period, despite the marked hypergastrinemia (34). A truncated form of PYY (PYY7-36 amide) is produced by proteolytic cleavage of the 36 amino acid peptide. A recent study demonstrated that this truncated form of PYY potently inhibits food intake.

Enteroglucagon is one of three biologically active peptides produced by posttranslational processing of the glucagon gene product in the small and large intestine. Glucagon-like peptides I and II (GLP-I and GLP-II) are the two other peptides secreted in parallel with enteroglucagon, which can serve as a marker for production of all three. GLP-I has incretin effects and physiologically enhances insulin secretion in response to ingested nutrients in the same manner as GIP and is also a satiety hormone. GLP-II, on the other hand, is a trophic peptide that increases growth of the small intestinal mucosa (45,46). Plasma enteroglucagon concentrations show a very marked postnatal surge, which peaks within the first week and is associated with the development of a marked postprandial response (29,32). Because an increased rate of small intestinal growth occurs in the early neonatal period, it is likely that GLP-II is important in neonatal alimentary maturation. The resulting mucosal growth increases the absorptive area for the uptake of nutrients from the gut lumen.

Temporally, the postnatal surges of gut hormones parallel the changes in GI function that accompany the introduction of enteral feeding in the infant. It is therefore of considerable interest that these surges are not seen in infants who have never received enteral feeding nor with nonnutritive suckling (32,47). Concentrations of all gut hormones, with the exception of secretin, remain low in infants receiving only parenteral nutrition (32,47).

Precise mechanisms control the secretion of each gut hormone, and the amount of a particular peptide liberated by a meal is adequate to stimulate the appropriate digestive response (48). For example, a meal rich in long-chain triglycerides will evoke a large CCK response, not seen with medium-chain fats (49). The high circulating levels of CCK in turn stimulate pancreatic enzyme secretion and, by gallbladder contraction, release of the bile salts necessary for digestion of the long-chain fat. Medium-chain triglycerides, on the other hand, are rapidly hydrolyzed by lingual and gastric lipases; they are water soluble, do not require micelle formation, and are absorbed rapidly. Thus, bile salts and pancreatic enzymes are not required for digestion of medium-chain triglycerides, and a large CCK response is not seen when they are ingested (49). The gut endocrine system, with its sparse distribution of overlapping cell types, is designed to produce an integrated digestive response to the discontinuous stimulation of ingested food (48). Because the type of food presented can influence the integrated hormonal response, it is apparent that differences in nutrition in early neonatal life may result in changes in the growth and functional development of the neonatal alimentary tract.

Although the fetus makes little demand on its GI tract, the situation changes dramatically at birth, when demand for nutrients necessitates the rapid maturation of the alimentary tract. This development of the GI tract is characterized by the integrated maturation of its many functions. The observation, however, that premature infants make a satisfactory transition from intravenous nutrition through the placenta to extrauterine enteral feeding suggests that external influences can exert a substantial influence. The massive postnatal surges in circulating levels of hormones, which have trophic and secretory and motor functions, is compelling circumstantial evidence of a profound gut endocrine influence on alimentary development (32). This is supported further by the observation that these hormonal surges are not seen in sick infants who are on parenteral nutrition and have not been fed orally (47). It is likely that failure of secretion of trophic gut hormones is responsible for the hypoplastic gut and pancreas that accompany parenteral nutrition. Appropriate enteral stimuli or hormone replacement eventually may alleviate this problem. Indeed, early minimal enteral feeding, sufficient to stimulate hormonal surges appears to have beneficial effects without any abdominal complications.

ABNORMALITIES OF THE GASTROINTESTINAL TRACT

To avoid repetition, an attempt has been made to confine the abnormalities described in this section to those that might require consultation by a pediatric gastroenterologist. Some overlap with general surgery has been allowed, however, to avoid extensive cross-referencing (see Chapter 44).

Abdominal Wall Defects

Major defects of the abdominal wall, omphalocele and gastroschisis, occur in approximately 1 of 6,000 live births (50–52). In either case, a portion of the infant's GI tract remains outside the abdominal cavity at birth. Omphalocele is a failure of the extraembryonic intestine to reenter the abdominal cavity through the umbilicus, a developmental anomaly that occurs between weeks 10 and 12 of gestational age. The defect includes the umbilicus, and the viscera typically are covered with a peritoneal sac. Occasionally, the sac may rupture, making the disorder difficult to distinguish clinically from gastroschisis.

Omphalocele can be an isolated defect; however, omphalocele is often associated with other congenital anomalies or syndromes. Genetic evaluation of patients with omphalocele may provide information regarding causation or recurrence risk. Periconceptional multivitamin use may reduce the risk of nonsyndromic omphalocele (53).

Gastroschisis is an actual defect in the abdominal wall that occurs lateral to the umbilicus. The infant with gastroschisis has a normal umbilical cord not involved in the defect. The defect usually occurs to the right of the umbilical cord. Both omphalocele and gastroschisis may occur in the presence of other intestinal anomalies. Malrotation is present in association with omphalocele. Although intestinal atresias more commonly are found in gastroschisis, atresias may be associated with either anomaly. Abdominal wall defects frequently are diagnosed prenatally by fetal ultrasound (54). The preferred route of delivery remains controversial and may depend on the size of the defect (55). Vaginal delivery may be acceptable for small defects, and cesarean section may be preferred in cases with large defects (56).

Gastroschisis or omphalocele requires immediate pediatric surgical consultation. Fluid losses and hypothermia are of primary immediate concern, especially in the case of gastroschisis because no membrane covers the bowel. Large fluid and heat losses are common, and intravenous fluid replacement should be initiated immediately. The defect should be wrapped, using warm, sterile, moist saline gauze or a sterile transparent plastic bag. Care must be taken to prevent twisting and infarction of the bowel. A nasogastric tube should be inserted to minimize intestinal distention.

Postoperative management includes sedation and mechanical ventilation for at least 48 to 72 hours because of increased intraabdominal pressure. Careful monitoring of fluids and electrolytes is essential. High fluid intake is required (57). During the postoperative period, gut motility is slow to return, especially in the case of gastroschisis. Patients with gastroschisis may demonstrate sluggish motility for up to 8 months, and a protracted course of parenteral nutrition commonly is required. Delayed onset of necrotizing enterocolitis (NEC) is not uncommon and should be suspected if bloody stools are observed.

Disorders of the Esophagus

Gastroesophageal Reflux

Gastroesophageal reflux is the most common esophageal disorder in the neonatal period (58). Gastric contents normally are retained within the stomach through the action of the lower esophageal sphincter, a zone of high pressure in the distal esophagus that remains tonically contracted except during deglutition (59). The anatomy of the stomach and esophagus, and their relationship to the diaphragm and related structures, may play a secondary role in retaining gastric contents within the stomach. Although considerable controversy exists, there is evidence to suggest that the lower esophageal sphincter may be fully functional in the normal full-term infant. Some evidence suggests that sphincter pressure may be decreased, either continuously or intermittently, in infants with gastroesophageal reflux, facilitating reflux of gastric contents into the esophagus. There is considerable controversy over the incidence of reflux in the premature infant. Reflux appears relatively more common, but some data suggest that the lower esophageal sphincter may be competent. Delayed gastric emptying and other motility problems also may play a role in reflux in premature infants.

In adults and older children, chronic esophagitis as a result of reflux of acid into the distal esophagus is the major concern with gastroesophageal reflux. During the neonatal period, however, esophagitis rarely occurs. Reflux typically presents with continual regurgitation and spitting up or vomiting of small quantities of formula after eating. The association between reflux and apnea of prematurity remains controversial (60,61). Recurrent aspiration during reflux episodes may occasionally result in pneumonitis or exacerbation of preexisting neonatal pulmonary disease. If enough formula is regurgitated, the infant may fail to thrive. In neonates, reflux also may be associated with delayed gastric emptying. Delayed gastric antral distention occurs in some very premature infants in the early postnatal period (62). Such delays in antral distention could contribute to gastroesophageal reflux and feeding intolerance commonly seen in premature infants less than 32 weeks' gestation. As in older children, reflux is encountered more frequently in infants with neurologic abnormalities.

Gastroesophageal reflux may exist as a primary disorder as a result of lower esophageal sphincter incompetence or intermittent relaxation, or it may be a manifestation of another disorder. First of all, it must be realized that gastroesophageal reflux may occur physiologically in all infants, although not with the frequency and severity of pathologic reflux. Any disorder that limits gastric emptying or causes a partial proximal small intestinal obstruction, such as annular pancreas or pyloric stenosis, will result in some gastroesophageal reflux. Small bowel disorders, including milk protein enterocolitis or infectious enteritis, will cause vomiting and regurgitation—in essence, gastroesophageal reflux. Finally, a variety of systemic disorders, including certain inborn errors of metabolism, chronic infection, chronic renal disease, and increased intracranial pressure, may result in chronic emesis similar to gastroesophageal reflux. Drugs, such as xanthines, which may be given because of apnea or lung disease, decrease lower esophageal sphincter pressure and may exacerbate or even cause reflux.

Several diagnostic studies are available to diagnose gastroesophageal reflux in infants; however, these studies as a rule do not separate primary from secondary causes. For example, an infant with milk protein enterocolitis or pyloric stenosis will have a positive test result for gastroesophageal reflux by any of the available studies. The most widely available test for reflux is an upper GI series, which is preferable to a barium swallow, because the latter only examines esophageal motility. The stomach must be filled with barium to assess the patient accurately for reflux. Unfortunately, assessing a child for gastroesophageal reflux radiographically lacks sensitivity because of the short time interval during which the child is observed, and it lacks specificity because of the likelihood of physiologic reflux occurring during performance of an upper GI series. Therefore, the primary role of an upper GI series is to exclude gastric outlet lesions such as pyloric stenosis, or proximal small bowel partial obstructions such as duodenal webs or annular pancreas.

Twenty-four-hour potential of hydrogen (pH) monitoring is the most widely accepted means of assessing gastroesophageal reflux (63). The pH probe is placed approximately 2 cm proximal to the lower esophageal sphincter, and distal esophageal pH is recorded over a 24-hour period. The infant must be bolus-fed during the study, to ensure adequate gastric distention to simulate the physiologic state. Considerable controversy exists over appropriate feeding for children during 24-hour pH monitoring. The inconsistency of acid secretion in small infants makes the procedure much less reliable during the neonatal period, and, consequently, simultaneous measurement of intragastric pH often is helpful in determining the validity of the study.

A 99Tc scintiscan may be used to screen for gastroesophageal reflux, although this technique is not considered as reliable as 24-hour pH monitoring. The technique is useful, however, for measuring gastric emptying delay, which may coexist with gastroesophageal reflux in a number of infants. Endoscopy with biopsy is a useful technique for detecting reflux in older infants; however, endoscopic biopsies are less useful during the neonatal period because pathologic reflux has not had sufficient time to cause esophageal mucosal injury. In older children, the presence of intraepithelial eosinophils suggests reflux, but this sign cannot be relied on in neonates, and biopsy specimens frequently are normal. Contrary to earlier belief, eosinophils are now recognized as being strongly associated with allergic disease of the gut, especially if present in the esophagus in large numbers. Most such cases however appear later in childhood.

Treatment of gastroesophageal reflux is based on the severity of symptoms. If the child is thriving well and the major complaint is frequent regurgitation and spitting, the infant may be placed prone on an incline at approximately 30 degrees with the head higher than the feet. It has been demonstrated that children positioned in this manner will reflux less frequently. Although it may take several weeks for symptoms to resolve, the risk of esophagitis is lessened and reflux tends to resolve more quickly. If the volume of reflux is severe and the infant is chronically irritable, has evidence of esophagitis, or is failing to thrive, then inhibition of gastric acid secretion with agents such as antacids or histamine-2 (H2)-receptor antagonists may be necessary. Cimetidine and ranitidine are available in liquid preparations, and they both work well. Data suggest that aluminum antacids may elevate serum aluminum levels in small infants (64). Proton pump antagonists such as omeprazole are even more potent suppressors of acid secretory activity than H2-receptor antagonists. Suppression of gastric acidity may actually be harmful as it increases gastric colonization which could lead to increased risk of sepsis and pneumonia (65). Bethanechol, a parasympathomimetic agent, has been demonstrated to increase lower esophageal sphincter resting tone and improve weight gain in infants with failure to thrive secondary to gastroesophageal reflux (66). Unfortunately, bethanechol may have associated central nervous system side effects, such as irritability and sleeplessness. Metoclopramide also has been used to treat gastroesophageal reflux in infants. The effectiveness of metoclopramide is controversial, and it probably is most helpful when delayed gastric emptying coexists with reflux. Some clinicians thicken infants' formula with cereal. Although this may reduce spitting, it usually does not reduce reflux or its complications and results in nutrient imbalance in the infant's carefully formulated diet. Infant formulas containing rice starch as part of the carbohydrate component have been shown to have a modest beneficial effect in gastroesophageal reflux in infants. They have a distinct advantage over addition of rice cereal in that they maintain an appropriate macronutrient balance.

Gastroesophageal reflux may be treated successfully at any age with surgical fundoplication in approximately 95% of cases. The most common surgical procedures include the Nissen fundoplication, in which the stomach is wrapped and sutured 360 degrees around the distal esophagus, and the Thal fundoplication, which consists of a 270-degree wrap. Complications, including gaseous distention of the stomach and dumping syndrome, may be less common with the Thal procedure. Many surgeons now perform fundoplications laparoscopically. Indications for an operation for gastroesophageal reflux include recurrent aspiration pneumonia, failure to thrive secondary to severe vomiting unresponsive to in-hospital medical management, or apparent life-threatening apnea events associated with gastroesophageal reflux (67). Such procedures may be performed laparoscopically by competently trained pediatric surgeons.

Differential diagnosis of the typical neonate with chronic recurrent vomiting includes, in addition to gastroesophageal reflux, two major categories of disease. The first is upper GI anomalies, including pyloric stenosis. Virtually all of these can be eliminated by upper GI contrast studies; pyloric stenosis can be excluded adequately by ultrasonography in the hands of an experienced pediatric ultrasonographer. The second major diagnostic category is formula protein intolerance. Infants with formula protein intolerance commonly vomit, especially those with significant small bowel mucosal disease. Such infants often are irritable and usually have loose, Hematest-positive (Ames, Elkhart, IN) stools. Proctoscopic examinations of the rectum usually demonstrate colitis. This disorder is discussed in detail later in this chapter.

Esophageal Anomalies

The other major category of esophageal disease that presents in the neonatal period is tracheoesophageal fistula or esophageal atresia (68). These anomalies occur in approximately 1 in 4,000 live births. In addition to a prenatal history of polyhydramnios, increased salivation with coughing, choking, and cyanosis shortly after birth should raise the suspicion of tracheoesophageal fistula–esophageal atresia. The most common variety is that of atresia with the distal esophageal pouch connected to the trachea through a

fistula. Such infants frequently have a stomach distended with air and respiratory symptoms as a result of tracheal aspiration of refluxed gastric acid. Immediate pediatric surgical consultation is required (see Chapter 44).

After surgery, gastroesophageal reflux is a virtual certainty. Patients with tracheoesophageal fistula or esophageal atresia have incompetent lower esophageal sphincter function and aperistaltic contractions in the midesophagus. Although swallowing usually proceeds without much difficulty, gastroesophageal reflux with chronic esophagitis and occasionally stricture formation are frequent long-term complications. Subsequent esophageal dilatations and fundoplication may be necessary.

Disorders of the Stomach and Duodenum

Congenital Anomalies

Congenital anomalies of the upper GI tract frequently present with vomiting. The most common is pyloric stenosis, which occurs in approximately 1 in every 500 live births (69,70). The disease is most common in Caucasian males. A positive family history often is present. Pyloric stenosis usually presents with nonbilious projectile vomiting during the third to fourth week of life. The disorder often is insidious in onset. After emesis, infants are hungry and will attempt to eat to compensate for malnutrition. It is now clear that pyloric stenosis is caused by the selective inadequate development of inhibitory neurons in the myenteric plexus of the pyloric region that utilize vasoactive intestinal polypeptide and nitric oxide as neurotransmitters to relax the sphincter. Eventually, nutrition deteriorates and infants become dehydrated and alkalotic secondary to chronic vomiting of the acidic gastric contents. Unconjugated hyperbilirubinemia is present in a small percentage. Patients with pyloric stenosis have normal or firm stools, in contrast to infants with formula protein intolerance, who usually have loose stools with evidence of malabsorption, inflammation, or both. Serum electrolytes reveal potassium and chloride deficiency and metabolic alkalosis. Prior to the availability of modern imaging techniques, the failure of a silver salt added to the infant's urine to produce a white precipitate of silver chloride was a means of differentiating pyloric stenosis from salt-losing adrenal hyperplasia. Physical examination demonstrates visible peristalsis in the epigastric region. Careful palpation of the abdomen while feeding may reveal a pyloric olive. The olive can be felt best when the stomach is empty, particularly just after vomiting. Diagnosis usually is confirmed by an upper GI series or ultrasonography, or both in the case of ambiguity, before proceeding with surgical intervention (71).

Before operative correction of the pyloric stenosis, infants should be rehydrated intravenously and the electrolyte imbalance and alkalosis corrected. Surgical correction consists of longitudinal incision of the hypertrophied muscle (i.e., pyloromyotomy). After the operation is completed, the patient usually can be fed within 6 to

12 hours. Rarely, if there has been prolonged gastric distention as a result of delayed diagnosis, time to full refeeding may be prolonged. Pyloric stenosis has been noted to recur in rare cases. Nonoperative medical management of pyloric stenosis, consisting of anticholinergic drugs and small frequent feedings, occasionally may be helpful. This therapy, sometimes used in Europe, is rarely used in North America because of the excellent results of surgical intervention.

Other rare gastric anomalies also may present in the neonatal period. Various forms of gastric atresia or hypoplasia have been described, most of which present with vomiting at or shortly after birth. Congenital microgastria may occur in association with a variety of other anomalies, including limb abnormalities, asplenia, megaesophagus, situs inversus, midgut malrotation, and cardiac anomalies. After major reconstructive surgery of the stomach, prognosis may be quite good.

Acid Peptic Disease

Acid peptic disease may be seen in newborn infants (72–74). Ulcers in children occur most commonly in the neonatal period or during the second decade of life. In newborn infants, ulcers, whether gastric or duodenal, usually present with hematemesis. Occasionally, blood loss may be substantial, manifested by symptoms of hypovolemia and shock. Differential diagnosis of hematemesis in the newborn includes swallowed maternal blood, or blood ingested from a cracked nipple through breastfeeding. Detection of swallowed maternal blood can be determined by assaying for adult hemoglobin in the gastric contents with the Apt test.

Diagnosis of peptic ulcer disease in the neonate requires endoscopy. Radiographic studies rarely are useful because the lesions are quite superficial and difficult to image radiographically. Endoscopy can be performed easily in a newborn infant by a skilled pediatric endoscopist using appropriate equipment. The smallest pediatric upper GI endoscopes can be used safely in term infants under conscious sedation. The minimum size of the infant in whom endoscopy can be performed safely varies with the skill of the endoscopist, but endoscopy often also can be performed safely in larger premature babies. A bronchoscope can be used in smaller infants, although the examination usually is unsatisfactory. Neonatal upper GI endoscopes are now available which facilitate diagnosis significantly. Although ulcerations may be identified anywhere in the stomach and the duodenum, multiple superficial gastric lesions are most common in newborn infants. Ulcers may be primary, or they may be secondary, as in the case of drugs known to irritate the upper GI tract, such as steroids or theophylline. Treatment with antacids, or preferably H1-receptor antagonists such as cimetidine or ranitidine, for a period of 2 to 6 weeks results in complete healing of the lesion. Secondary ulcers may be treated in a similar fashion. In this instance, continuation of the offending agent requires careful assessment of the risk-to-benefit ratio, because lesions will heal more rapidly if the agents are discontinued. Neonatal infection with Helicobacter pylori is a rare phenomenon (75).

Spontaneous gastric perforation is a rare occurrence in the newborn. It occurs most commonly during the first 5 days of life, especially in infants subjected to severe stress or hypoxia (76). The constellation of symptoms typically includes a sudden deterioration in clinical status between the second and fifth day of life, characterized by refusal to eat, vomiting, abdominal distention, and respiratory distress. Free intraperitoneal air (usually a large volume) and fluid are demonstrable on plain radiographs of the abdomen. Immediate surgical consultation should be sought.

Disorders of the Small Intestine

Congenital Anomalies

Of the various small intestinal disorders that present in the neonatal period, congenital anomalies that produce obstruction are likely to present earliest. Patients present with bilious vomiting, abdominal distention, and occasionally obstipation. Bilious vomiting indicates obstruction distal to the ampulla of Vater. Bilious vomiting associated with the passage of blood through the rectum suggests vascular compromise of the small intestine, necessitating immediate surgical intervention.

Malrotation or nonrotation of the gut is an anatomic defect produced by incomplete rotation and fixation of the embryonic intestine after return from its extraabdominal location at about week 10 of gestation (77). During development, the intestine rotates 270 degrees around the axis of the superior mesenteric artery to place the cecum in the right lower quadrant. When the cecum fails to rotate completely, the mesenteric attachment of the small intestine is limited to that supporting the superior mesenteric artery and vein. This permits the bowel to twist on itself and produces a midgut volvulus. In the malrotated colon, adhesive bands, otherwise known as Ladd bands, stretch anteriorly from the right peritoneal gutter over the duodenum, in which they can produce obstruction. Rotational anomalies may be associated with other intestinal anomalies, usually duodenal stenosis or atresia or other small intestinal atresias. Cardiac, esophageal, urinary, and anal anomalies also may be present. Rotational abnormalities should be considered in the differential diagnosis of a high intestinal obstruction identified radiographically. Unfortunately, the diagnosis often is missed by plain abdominal radiographs because air may be present in several loops of bowel distal to the obstruction. Rotational abnormalities are identified more easily with an upper GI series, or barium enema. The radiographic hallmark of malrotation is the identification of the cecum in the upper abdomen or to the left of the midline. Symptomatic rotational abnormalities require urgent surgical exploration, because a volvulus may result in loss of the entire midgut within hours of presentation as a result of vascular occlusion. Intestinal dysmotility is common following operative repair of a malrotation with or without an associated volvulus (78).

Jejunal or ileal atresias range from membranous obstructions to complete atresia. Atresias can be single or multiple (79,80). An apple peel or Christmas tree deformity of the superior mesenteric artery results in an extensive jejunal atresia followed by multiple ileal atresias that are vascularly supplied by a branch of the ileocolic artery. Unlike duodenal atresia, relatively few anomalies are associated with ileal atresia. Cystic fibrosis, however, is present in approximately 20% of infants with jejunoileal atresia.

Small intestinal atresias in the neonatal period present with bilious vomiting. The degree of abdominal distention varies with the site of the atresia. If the atresia is distal, vomiting may be delayed for up to 24 hours after birth. Depending on the location of the atresia, varying numbers of dilated loops of bowel with air–fluid levels may be present on abdominal radiographs. Because it is difficult to differentiate small intestine from colon on plain abdominal radiographs in newborns, a contrast enema should be performed to exclude colonic lesions and obstructions. Contrast enemas also are helpful in excluding disorders such as meconium plug syndrome or associated rotational abnormalities.

Meconium Ileus

Meconium ileus occurs almost exclusively in patients with cystic fibrosis. It is caused by abnormally viscid mucus glycoprotein in meconium (81). Approximately 10% to 20% of patients with cystic fibrosis have meconium ileus as the first sign of their disease. Pathologically, the lumen of the distal small intestine is obstructed by an accumulation of abnormal meconium. Infants present with bilious vomiting and abdominal distention during the first 2 days of life. A palpable sausage-like mass may be present, and rectal examination may identify hard, dry, gray-tan meconium. Abdominal radiographs demonstrate some evidence of complete obstruction, but the radiologic hallmark is the soap-bubble appearance of trapped air within the tenacious meconium in the distal small bowel. A water-soluble contrast enema occasionally is therapeutic in disrupting the meconium obstruction. Care should be taken to avoid dehydration, because contrast substances are hypertonic and can result in massive pooling of fluid within the bowel lumen. Surgical intervention is required if the contrast enema is unsuccessful. When the diagnosis of meconium ileus is made, patients should be thoroughly evaluated for cystic fibrosis.

Other disorders related to meconium may be seen in the neonatal period. Meconium peritonitis may occur when intrauterine bowel perforation, secondary to obstruction, has resulted in leakage of sterile meconium into the peritoneal cavity. Common causes include atresia, volvulus, stenosis, cystic fibrosis, meconium ileus, and Hirschsprung's disease. Small flecks of intraabdominal calcification may be identified radiographically. Ascites occasionally occurs, but may resolve spontaneously unless secondary infection develops. In severe cases, meconium peritonitis can result in adhesions that require surgical intervention.

Necrotizing Enterocolitis

The most serious GI disorder occurring in neonates is NEC (79,80). Because NEC appears predominantly in sick, low-birth-weight infants, the incidence has increased in recent years as the mortality rate for the very-low-birth-weight infant has decreased. It has been estimated that 90% of cases occur in premature infants and that NEC may develop in 1% to 10% of infants hospitalized in neonatal intensive care units (84). Significant intercenter differences in the prevalence of NEC have been reported (79). The mortality rates vary from 10% to 50%. The age of onset of NEC is related to birth weight and gestational age. Smaller, more immature infants (less than 28 weeks of gestation) tend to have NEC at an older age than larger, more mature (greater than 31 weeks of age) infants (85). Thus, the more premature the infant, the longer the duration of risk. A diagnosis of NEC in a premature infant significantly increases the patient's length of stay and imposes added financial burden (86).

The etiology of NEC is not fully known (87). Multiple factors appear to be involved, including hypoxia, acidosis, and hypotension, which may lead to ischemic damage of the mucosal barrier of the small intestine (88). Secondary bacterial invasion of the mucosa may be involved in the pathogenesis of pneumatosis intestinalis. Moreover, NEC has been observed to occur in epidemics in neonatal intensive care units, further supporting the role of microbial agents in pathogenesis. A number of conditions may predispose the larger infant to development of NEC, including cyanotic congenital heart disease, obstructive lesions of the systemic cardiac outflow (e.g., hypoplastic left heart, coarctation of the aorta), polycythemia, umbilical catheters, exchange transfusions, perinatal asphyxia, maternal preeclampsia, and maternal use of cocaine. Infants with patent ductus arteriosus also seem to be at greater risk. In this case, oxygenated blood is shunted from the intestine. All of these factors suggest that mucosal injury and ischemia are important in the development of NEC. The role of inflammatory mediators, such as tumor necrosis factor-α and platelet-activating factor, oxygen free radicals, and local nitric oxide synthesis also have received attention (89–92).

Rapid onset of enteral feeding may be a risk factor for NEC, because of changes in enteric blood flow and oxygen requirements during feeding (93,94). Early introduction of small volumes of enteral feeding appears to significantly reduce the risk of necrotizing enterocolitis when compared to aggressive advancement of enteral feeding in at risk preterm infants. NEC occasionally is reported in infants who have never been enterally fed. Several factors related to enteral feeding have been studied, and a number of theories have been proposed on how enteral feedings might precipitate NEC. Hyperosmolar formulas have been implicated in the production of NEC, but these formulas differed from standard formulas in other ways as well. Additionally, most hyperosmolar formulas have been reformulated to minimize this risk. Formula feedings seem to predispose to NEC more than breast-feeding, suggesting that breast milk factors, including growth factors, antibodies, and cellular immune factors, might be protective. It also is likely that formula within the GI tract may provide a substrate for bacterial proliferation. The role of bacterial invasion in this disease has been well recognized, but is likely to be a secondary event after compromise of the intestinal mucosal barrier. Enterobacter sakazakii, a rare infection in premature infants which is occasionally associated with the feeding of powdered formula has been seen in some infants with necrotizing enterocolitis but a causal relationship has not been established (95).

The shunting of blood away from the intestine in a fashion similar to the diving reflex in aquatic mammals has been postulated as a potential mechanism for producing the initial gut ischemia. This reflex might occur in response to a hypoxic episode and has been studied extensively in animal models.

The association of NEC with prematurity implicates immaturity of the intestinal mucosal barrier. A number of factors that affect the mucosal barrier are immature in premature infants, including acid output, intestinal motility, and enzyme production. Immaturity of the microvillus membrane itself, and differences in the mucus secreted by the small intestine, may play a significant role. The mucosal immune system is immature, and less secretory IgA is produced. Some interest has arisen in the possible role of oral immunoglobulin administration for prophylaxis against NEC (96).

The reported GI hormone abnormalities in NEC patients are difficult to interpret because of the spectrum of ages at which the disease develops, the randomness of blood sample timing, and the variation in quantity of enteral feedings. Concentrations of GIP, neurotensin, and enteroglucagon in infants with NEC are lower than those normally fed infants of comparable age, but gastrin, motilin, and pancreatic polypeptide (PP) levels appear to be normal (97).

Clinical presentations vary widely. Abdominal distention usually is one of the earliest and most consistent clinical signs. Other symptoms include bloody stools, apnea, bradycardia, lethargy, shock, and retention of gastric contents as a result of poor gastric emptying. Thrombocytopenia, neutropenia, and metabolic acidosis may develop during bowel ischemia. Not every patient has every sign, however, and clinical presentation may vary markedly. Diagnosis is confirmed by radiographic demonstration of pneumatosis intestinalis or portal hepatic venous air. Nonspecific radiographic findings include thickening of the bowel wall, dilated loops of bowel, and ascites. The presence of reducing substances in the stool, as a result of carbohydrate malabsorption, may be an early finding in NEC, as may increased α1-antitrypsin levels, which indicate protein-losing enteropathy.

Suspicion of NEC dictates that all enteral feedings should be discontinued. An orogastric tube is placed routinely to relieve distention of the alimentary tract. Intravenous access must be secured to provide fluid, electrolytes, and nutrition, because the patient will not be fed enterally for an extended period of time. Intravenous antibiotics are administered to provide coverage for enteric organisms. Inclusion of specific antianaerobic agents does not appear to be helpful (98). The duration of oral intake restriction depends on the clinical status. Patients who merely have poor feeding with increased residuals, and the presence of minimal radiographic findings, may be fed within 48 to 72 hours. In the presence of pneumatosis intestinalis and marked abdominal distention, 2 weeks of parenteral nutrition may be required before judicious gradual reintroduction of enteral feedings is considered.

Throughout the course of the disease, frequent radiographic evaluation of the abdomen for evidence of intestinal perforation is required. Apnea, bradycardia, abdominal wall discoloration or edema, or a sudden increase in intraabdominal girth should give rise to the suspicion of bowel perforation. Frequent laboratory evaluations include a complete blood count and platelet count to look for thrombocytopenia and neutropenia, both of which suggest deterioration. In infants with severe inflammation of the small intestine, large volumes of fluid and electrolytes or blood products may be required to maintain perfusion and blood pressure. This is especially true in infants in whom severe metabolic acidosis develops secondary to poor perfusion. Ventilatory support usually is necessary. Exploratory laparotomy with resection of dead bowel has been the traditional surgical approach to patients with evidence of perforation or gangrenous bowel. Peritoneal drainage prior to laparotomy may be of benefit in extremely low birth weight infants or hemodynamically unstable patients (99).

Infants who require surgical intervention are at risk for postoperative complications and complications associated with total parenteral nutrition (TPN). The most common complications after surgery for NEC are sepsis, intestinal strictures, short bowel syndrome, and wound infections (100). Intraabdominal abscesses are relatively rare. In a number of infants, the mucosal inflammatory process may progress to transmural necrosis that may, if it does not lead to perforation, result in fibroblast proliferation, granulation tissue, and stricture formation. Some clinicians routinely study the GI tract radiographically after NEC has been treated medically. It is not uncommon to find asymptomatic ileal stenosis or colonic stenosis in such patients. If symptoms of partial obstruction, such as abdominal distention, failure to thrive, or poor feeding develop in infants who have recovered from a bout of NEC, contrast studies are indicated; however, it should be noted that ileal stenosis may not be detected by these studies.

Localized Intestinal Perforation

Localized intestinal perforation has recently been recognized as a clinical entity distinct from NEC (101). Localized intestinal perforations are similar to NEC in that they occur almost exclusively in premature infants. In contrast, patients with localized intestinal perforations are less likely to have symptoms of a severe illness, such as metabolic acidosis or leukopenia, than patients with NEC (101). Patients with localized intestinal perforations are more likely to survive to discharge than patients with NEC.

The etiology of localized intestinal perforation is not known. Interruption of regional blood flow to the bowel has been hypothesized. Patients with localized perforation are more likely to have received higher dosages of indomethacin or had an umbilical artery catheter in place shortly before the perforation than patients with NEC (101,102).

Short Bowel Syndrome

Short bowel syndrome is defined as a malabsorptive state that occurs after bowel resection. Infants with short bowel syndrome fall into two categories: those with congenital anomalies (e.g., gastroschisis, apple peel anomaly of the superior mesenteric artery, intestinal atresia) and anatomically normal patients who undergo bowel resection for NEC. The latter group tends to have fewer complications and a better prognosis, when equal lengths of residual small intestine remain.

After massive resection of the small intestine, the remaining small bowel undergoes an adaptation process characterized by epithelial hyperplasia (103). Within 1 to 2 days after resection, enterocytes begin replicating in the crypts. Gradual morphologic changes occur in the small intestine, including a marked lengthening of villi that results in increased mucosal surface area. This is followed by an increase in absorptive capacity that eventually enables many to survive without parenteral nutrition. The adaptation process is gradual, however, and may require weeks to years.

The major gut hormone changes seen after ileal resection are marked increases in plasma levels of PYY, enteroglucagon, and motilin (103,104). Increases of enteroglucagon (which reflect parallel changes in the enterotropic hormone, GLP-II and of PYY, which inhibits gastric acid secretion and small intestinal secretion, enhances absorption and delays gastric emptying and intestinal transit, are appropriate responses in this condition. Preservation, or even enhancement, of the PYY response would be valuable in diminishing the rapid transit and diarrhea associated with this condition. Studies in experimental animals have revealed that improvements in transit and fluid absorption are temporally related to the increase in PYY response that occurs after bowel resection (105,106).

Hypergastrinemia also accompanies intestinal resection and is responsible for the increased gastric secretion seen postoperatively. The increase of gastrin levels is triggered by the reduction in small intestinal inhibitory factors and usually subsides after a few weeks, when intestinal adaptation has taken place. Mucosal hyperplasia does not occur in the absence of enteral nutrition. In fact, mucosal atrophy may result if the patient is nourished only parenterally

(107). Enteral nutrition stimulates intestinal adaptation by several mechanisms (108). Highly unsaturated long-chain fats stimulate intestinal adaptation to a greater extent than protein or carbohydrate; the mechanism by which this occurs is poorly understood. Nonetheless, careful attention to the provision of adequate enteral nutrition is important.

Management of the short bowel syndrome is a multistage process (109). During the early postoperative period, use of parenteral nutrition and careful attention to fluid and electrolyte abnormalities are essential. High-volume ostomy losses must be replaced with a solution of comparable electrolyte content to obviate the need for frequent changes in electrolyte concentration in parenteral nutrition solutions.

The presence of an ostomy may create additional problems. These vary somewhat, depending on whether the ostomy is in the ileum, from which the volume output is likely to be much greater, or in the colon, in which case stool consistency may vary markedly based on whether the ostomy was placed proximally or distally. If available, the services of an enterostomal therapist, with special training in rehabilitation of infants and children with ostomies, will assist the parents in understanding the implications of the ostomy. In general, as would be expected, caring for an infant with a small intestinal ostomy requires meticulous monitoring of fluid and electrolyte balance which implies equally meticulous planning if home care is considered. The ostomy should be placed away from sites such as the iliac crest, costal margin, or umbilicus, so that ostomy appliances will fit easily.

Most ostomy devices consist of an adhesive, nonallergenic wafer device with a flange that allows the transparent drainage pouch to be secured to it over the stoma. The pouch can be removed easily for draining by snapping it off the wafer, or it can be emptied through a drainage port at the bottom of the bag. When leakage occurs beneath the wafer, the device should be removed, and careful skin care around the ostomy is necessary. The skin should be washed gently with a soft cloth moistened with mild soap and tepid water. The skin should be dried thoroughly after cleansing. Many protective ointments and powders are available to apply around the stoma area to prevent skin breakdown. If skin irritation is present, tincture of benzoin or steroid preparations available in spray form may be used. The pouches often are reusable and may be washed with mild soap and water and soaked in a deodorant solution to control odor problems. Appropriate teaching will prevent many of the other problems encountered by ostomy patients, such as skin excoriation, minor stoma bleeding, stoma prolapse, and odor. Additional ostomy problems include prolapse and stenosis. The latter should be suspected in the presence of abdominal distention and vomiting. In either situation, the surgeon should be notified.

When enteral feeds are started, a slow continuous infusion of an extensively hydrolyzed protein formula generally works best. Formulations such as Alimentum (Ross Laboratories, Columbus, OH) or Pregestimil (Mead Johnson

Laboratories, Evansville, IN), which contain significant quantities of long-chain fats, are ideal. These lactose-free preparations with hydrolyzed protein are absorbed rapidly, yet provide adequate stimulation of intestinal adaptation. Stool losses must be monitored carefully. If there is significant concern about allergic disease, an amino acid based formula such Neocate, (Scientific Hospital Supplies, Liverpool UK) may be advantageous. A marked increase in fluid losses or significant evidence of carbohydrate malabsorption manifested by a low stool pH or positive stool-reducing substances are contraindications for further increasing the enteral infusion. Enteral infusions are increased as tolerated, and parenteral nutrition is decreased in a gradual isocaloric fashion. Patients then can be weaned to intermittent parenteral nutrition and prepared for home parenteral nutrition therapy (110). Intermittent parenteral nutrition allows provision of parenteral nutrients at night, primarily for the convenience of caregivers. Parenteral nutrition initially is discontinued only for short periods of time, usually 4 to 6 hours, each day. In small infants, this usually is delayed until the patient can tolerate approximately 20% of calorie intake enterally to avoid hypoglycemia when he or she is not receiving parenteral nutrition. The duration of parenteral nutrition can be decreased gradually until all parenteral nutrition infuses over 10 to 12 hours at night. It is wise to taper the parenteral nutrition rates up and down when placing a patient on or off of parenteral nutrition, to prevent fluctuation in serum glucose levels.

Home parenteral nutrition has markedly reduced the cost of long-term management of short bowel syndrome patients and has decreased family stresses and nosocomial infections (111). It has become a standard therapy in patients with short bowel syndrome, and prolonged hospitalizations rarely are necessary. To minimize complications, careful training of home nursing personnel is essential, and coordination of activity between physician and nursing staff must be tightly controlled.

Continuous enteral infusions are used in patients with short bowel syndrome for several reasons. The percentage of calories absorbed from the continuous infusion is greater than that possible with bolus feedings, because transport carrier proteins are continually saturated. Continuous infusion provides constant stimulation of mucosal adaptation and reduces the need for parenteral calories, decreasing the risk of parenteral nutrition liver disease. Children should be fed small quantities of formula orally to learn to suck and swallow. Eventually, solids can be fed around the nasogastric tube. These manipulations often will speed the transition from continuous enteral to oral feeding later in the course of therapy.

Numerous chronic complications arise in the treatment of short bowel syndrome, including bacterial overgrowth, nutritional deficiency states, watery diarrhea, parenteral nutrition liver disease, and catheter-related problems. Bacterial overgrowth is defined as increased bacterial content in the small intestine (112). Complications from bacterial overgrowth include increased malabsorption, δ-lactic

acidosis, and colitis-like or ileitis-like syndrome. Normal small bowel bacterial counts vary from 103/mL proximally to much greater numbers in the ileum. Normal antegrade peristalsis and gastric and mucosal immune factors prevent excess bacterial proliferation. In short bowel syndrome, because of disruption of normal anatomy and motility, overgrowth is likely and bacterial counts usually exceed 105/mL. Bacterial overgrowth should be suspected whenever motility is slowed, the bowel is dilated, or the ileocecal valve is absent. Organisms typically include facultative bacteria and anaerobes. Bacteria deconjugate bile salts, causing them to be reabsorbed, depleting the bile salt pool, impairing micelle solubilization, and resulting in steatorrhea and malabsorption of fat-soluble vitamins. More important, bacterial overgrowth causes mucosal inflammation, exacerbating malabsorption of all nutrients. Protein-losing enteropathy and loss of immunoglobulins may occur. Bacteria may compete with the host for nutrients, such as vitamin B12.

Screening for bacterial overgrowth can be done with a fasting breath hydrogen or glucose breath hydrogen test, or by detecting the presence of indican in the urine. Measurement of breath hydrogen is a simple test in infants and children, although collection of samples in the neonate requires special care. A fasting breath hydrogen level greater than 42 ppm is seen only in small bowel bacterial overgrowth (113). A breath hydrogen level greater than 20 ppm after the administration of 2 g/kg of oral glucose, with measurement at 15-minute intervals after ingestion, suggests bacterial overgrowth. Measurement of indican in the urine is a simple screening test for bacterial overgrowth, because bacteria convert dietary tryptophan to indican. Unfortunately, indicanuria may occur in other conditions, and the technique lacks sensitivity (114). Bacterial overgrowth can be diagnosed definitively by culture of aspirates from the small intestine, although this technique is difficult to interpret as contamination and culture techniques may frequently overestimate or underestimate the extent of overgrowth. Small intestinal biopsies demonstrating inflammatory changes suggest bacterial overgrowth.

Accumulation of d-lactate in the blood stream results in neurologic symptoms varying from frank disorientation to coma (115). Bacterial overgrowth may cause colitis-like or ileitis-like syndrome with large ulcerations characteristic of Crohn's disease, but without granulomas (116). Broad-spectrum oral antibiotics (e.g., metronidazole, trimethoprim-sulfamethoxazole (TMP-SMZ), gentamicin) and anti-inflammatory agents often are beneficial. Broad-spectrum antimicrobial coverage should be directed at the organisms present, usually anaerobes. Antimotility agents may improve nutrient contact with the mucosa by lengthening transit time, but tend to exacerbate bacterial overgrowth and should be used with caution. Recently, use of probiotic bacteria has been proposed for the treatment of certain patients with small bowel bacterial overgrowth (117). However, the overall experience with probiotic therapy in bacterial overgrowth has been somewhat disappointing.

Secretory diarrhea may be a problem in some children with short bowel syndrome. This may be related to hypergastrinemia, which often occurs after resection. Because the tight junctions in the ileum are less permeable than the jejunum, the ileum plays a major role in fluid and electrolyte conservation, and ileal resections are more likely to result in major fluid and electrolyte losses than jejunal resections. Because most infants with NEC have ileal disease, this is a major problem in neonates after bowel resection. Ileal resection also results in malabsorption of bile acids, because the ileum is the primary site for bile acid reabsorption. Malabsorption of bile acids into the colon may cause fluid secretion and watery diarrhea, which may respond to a bile acid-binding resin such as cholestyramine. Unfortunately, cholestyramine may further deplete the bile acid pool, exacerbating steatorrhea.

Nutritional deficiency states may occur after parenteral nutrition is discontinued, including deficiencies of fat-soluble vitamins A, D, and E, and the minerals iron, zinc, calcium, and magnesium.

Parenteral nutrition hepatobiliary tract disease is the major complication that may result in death in infants with short bowel syndrome (111). The mechanism by which the liver injury occurs is unknown. In most instances, enteral administration of a significant percentage of calories, usually between 20% and 30% of total requirements, reduces the risk of parenteral nutrition liver disease.

Cholelithiasis develops in approximately 20% of infants receiving parenteral nutrition for short bowel syndrome because of malabsorption of bile acids, altered bilirubin metabolism, and gallbladder stasis. Cholangitis may occur in the presence of partial obstruction. Early cholecystectomy should be considered if patients are symptomatic with elevated direct bilirubin and liver enzymes.

Catheter-related infections and thrombosis are common in infants requiring long-term parenteral nutrition (118). In our experience, catheter-related infections rarely are as a result of intestinal bacterial overgrowth and most commonly are related to catheter care technique. Diligent parental instruction in catheter care and in the signs and symptoms of sepsis is extremely important.

During later stages of therapy, additional surgery may be indicated (119). One of the first questions usually concerns whether to close a stoma that was formed at the time of initial surgery. If the colon remains, and especially if ileum exists as well, reconnecting an ostomy may substantially conserve fluid and electrolytes, but also may result in perianal disease. In infants with dilated segments of proximal bowel, resecting a tight anastomosis or tapering the bowel to improve flow of luminal contents often reduces bacterial overgrowth. A number of procedures have been designed to slow transit time, including reverse segments of bowel, one-way valves, or colon interposition, but none is considered reliably effective, and all may increase bacterial overgrowth.

A procedure to increase the length of the bowel has been devised that involves transecting the bowel longitudinally, preserving the blood supply to both sides of the bowel, and creating a segment about twice the length and one-half of the diameter. This allows reducing the diameter of the bowel without any loss of mucosal surface area. Because it does not actually increase the mucosal surface area, it is indicated primarily to reduce bacterial overgrowth without losing absorptive surface in infants with dilated bowel. Our experience has been quite rewarding with this procedure, with 12 of 14 recent patients demonstrating significant improvement and several becoming independent of parenteral nutrition after surgery (120). More simplified techniques of intestinal lengthening have recently been described. In general, these procedures should not be, performed in neonates, because they are likely to be successful only after significant bowel dilation has occurred.

Intestinal transplantation has now become a reality. Well over 100 patients now have been transplanted at a number of centers in the United States and Europe (121). Patients with short bowel syndrome with evidence of parenteral nutrition-induced liver dysfunction should be referred early for intestinal transplantation. Recent evidence suggests that isolated intestinal transplantation prior to the development of irreversible parenteral nutrition-induced liver disease may be an attractive alternative to the combined liver/bowel transplantation, which has traditionally been utilized for such patients. However, long-term survival 5 years following intestinal transplantation has only been in the range of 50%.

It is possible for infants to survive without transplantation or permanent parenteral nutrition with surprisingly short segments of bowel (122,123). As a general rule, patients with greater than 25 cm of normal bowel at the time of neonatal resection who have an ileocecal valve, or with greater than normal 40 cm of normal bowel at the time of neonatal resection who have no ileocecal valve, have a reasonable chance of eventually becoming independent of parenteral nutrition. The ileocecal valve appears to play a major role in determining the long-term prognosis, primarily because of its ability to exclude colonic bacteria from entering the small bowel and perhaps also because of its ability to delay transit through the small intestine.

Mucosal Injury Disorders

Because of the limited small intestinal reserve in small infants, small intestinal disease perhaps is most catastrophic in infancy. In small intestinal injury, all nutrients are malabsorbed. Most symptoms, however, are related to carbohydrate malabsorption because of the osmotic diarrhea produced when these malabsorbed molecules are broken down further by intestinal bacteria into smaller and smaller osmotically active particles. The osmotic gradient overrides the ability of the ileum and colon to reabsorb fluid effectively, and watery diarrhea ensues.

Measurement of stool pH and reducing substances is an ideal means to screen for small bowel mucosal disease in infancy. When carbohydrates are malabsorbed and broken down into organic acids by colonic bacteria, the stool pH drops below 5.5. Stool pH can be measured easily with litmus paper, simply by inserting the paper into the stool. Measurement of reducing substances in stool can be done by placing five drops of stool and ten drops of water into a test tube and dropping in a Clinitest (Ames) tablet. Positive reducing substances in stool confirms the presence of carbohydrate malabsorption. Patients receiving formulas that are predominantly sucrose are less likely to demonstrate positive reducing substances in their stools because sucrose is a nonreducing carbohydrate.

Infectious Diarrhea

During the neonatal period, infectious diseases of the small intestine are relatively uncommon. A number of viruses may cause diarrhea in small infants, including rotavirus, enteric adenoviruses, and enteroviruses. Viral gastroenteritis usually presents with watery stools, with evidence of carbohydrate malabsorption. The predominant mucosa injury in viral gastroenteritis is in the proximal jejunum, in which carbohydrates are absorbed. In contrast, bacterial pathogens generally produce more distal injury that involves the colon and results in Hematest-positive stools that contain leukocytes (Table 40-2). Bacterial causes of diarrhea include Salmonella sp, Shigella sp, invasive *Escherichia coli*, and *Campylobacter jejuni*. *Clostridium difficile* infection predominantly involves the large intestine and, in severe cases, produces pseudomembranous colitis. Infection with *C. difficile* usually follows a course of broad-spectrum antibiotics. Severe watery or bloody diarrhea and colonic perforation may occur. Diagnosis is difficult in neonates, because a very high percentage of small infants carry *C. difficile* without evidence of disease.

Human Immunodeficiency Virus-Associated Disease

Human immunodeficiency virus (HIV) infection in infants results in a variety of GI problems. Failure to thrive is common. Chronic diarrhea and generalized lymphadenopathy often are present. Other common presentations include asymptomatic hepatosplenomegaly, which may occur in conjunction with severe interstitial pneumonia and hypergammaglobulinemia.

TABLE 40-2
SCREENING STOOL STUDIES IN INFECTIOUS DIARRHEA

	Bacterial	Viral
Clinitest	−	±
pH	≥5.5	£5.5
Hematest	+++	−
Leukocytes	+++	−

−, negative; ±, negative or positive, +++, strongly positive.

Chronic diarrhea in infants with acquired immunodeficiency syndrome (AIDS) presents a very difficult management problem. Diarrhea in older children may result from opportunistic infections, tumors, including Kaposi's sarcoma and lymphoma, and direct HIV infection of the gut. Opportunistic organisms include viral agents (e.g., cytomegalovirus, rotavirus, herpes simplex, coxsackievirus, adenovirus), bacterial pathogens (e.g., Salmonella sp, Campylobacter-like organisms, Listeria sp, Mycobacterium avium-intracellulare, *Plesiomonas shigelloides*), fungal pathogens (e.g., Candida sp, Aspergillus sp), and parasitic pathogens (e.g., cryptosporidium, Strongyloides sp, Giardia sp, amoebas, *Isospora belli*). A broad spectrum of endoscopic and histologic findings is possible because of the diverse nature of the disease. Extensive viral and bacterial cultures and examinations for ova and parasites are warranted in infants and children with AIDS.

Treatment consists of therapy directed at any specific infectious pathogen identified, coupled with use of parenteral and enteral nutrition. As in almost all chronic enteropathies, primary attention should be given to continuous enteral infusion with an elemental diet or protein hydrolysate formula. If malabsorption develops in the patient, as indicated by stools testing positive for reducing substances or manifesting a pH below 5.5, supplemental parenteral nutrition is needed to provide the remainder of caloric and other nutritional needs. The presence of a significant secretory component of the diarrhea may make treatment difficult, complicate the use of continuous enteral infusion, and require careful attention to intake and output of fluid and electrolytes to maintain biochemical homeostasis.

Hormonal Changes in Diarrhea

Infective diarrhea in infants is associated with a massive increase in circulating concentrations of motilin, enteroglucagon, and PYY (124,125). These abnormalities resolve once the patients are better. The gut endocrine system in infants, however, responds in a manner different from that of adults. In infants with diarrhea, plasma motilin concentrations exceed those that are known to accelerate gastric emptying and increase small bowel motility (125). Motilin is therefore likely to be involved in the motor abnormalities associated with this condition. A hormonally triggered increase in transit rate may constitute a defense mechanisms to rid the bowel of pathogens and secreted toxins. The extremely high enteroglucagon levels in neonatal infective diarrhea appear to be related to the extent of mucosal injury and its repair (126). Measurement of selected gut hormones may give information on the extent of mucosal damage or the presence of ongoing pathologic change.

Formula Protein Intolerance

One of the most common causes of chronic diarrhea in small infants is formula protein-induced enterocolitis

(127,128). Small bowel involvement (i.e., enteritis), colon involvement (i.e., colitis), or concomitant small bowel and colon involvement are possible with this disorder. Protein-induced mucosal injury has been reported with cow-milk protein, soy protein, breast milk, and even beef protein. A number of infants who are intolerant of protein hydro-lysate formulas, have responded well to an amino acid–based infant formula, Neocate (129).

Infants typically present before 3 months of age with bright red blood in the stool, which may be normal or loose in consistency depending on the extent of inflammation. Sigmoidoscopic examination may reveal gross friability or may appear normal until the mucosa is wiped with a cotton swab, at which time the mucosa readily bleeds. Rectal biopsy confirms inflammation, with the combination of polymorphonuclear leukocytes and eosinophils in the lamina propria. Stools may test positive for occult blood and may contain leukocytes. If the inflammation extends into the small intestine, carbohydrate malabsorption may occur, infants will have watery diarrhea, and stools will be acidic (pH less than 5.5) and test positive for reducing substances. Small intestinal biopsy will demonstrate varying degrees of mucosal injury, with shortening and blunting of the villi, inflammatory infiltrates, and an increase in mitotic activity in the crypts. Disaccharidase levels in the mucosal biopsies often are reduced.

Other symptoms that may occur as a result of formula protein-induced enterocolitis are vomiting and irritability. Infants with formula protein intolerance commonly vomit, especially those with small intestinal disease. It often is difficult to differentiate this disorder from gastro-esophageal reflux, because both groups may present with irritability; however, babies with formula protein sensitivity commonly have loose stools and abnormal sigmoido-scopic examinations. This is an important distinction because the treatment is vastly different. Irritability, not dissimilar from infantile colic, may occur in infants with formula protein intolerance. In infantile colic, the irritability classically occurs at a specific time of the day and responds symptomatically to repetitive stimuli. Infants with irritability secondary to formula protein intolerance usually are inconsolably irritable, often feed poorly, have loose stools, spit up, and have abnormal sigmoidoscopic examinations or other evidence of small intestinal or colonic inflammation. A careful history and physical examination and appropriate laboratory studies can be quite specific in differentiating the two disorders.

Infants who manifest signs and symptoms of formula protein intolerance should be placed on a protein hydro-lysate formula such as Nutramigen, Pregestimil, or Alimentum, because a high percentage also will be intolerant of soy formula. A small percentage of infants who do not respond to these formulas may improve on an amino acid formulation such as Neocate.

Most infants with formula protein intolerance will out-grow their sensitivity by 1 year of age. Powell (130) has described a specific challenge procedure to confirm the diagnosis of cow-milk protein intolerance. Patients should not have received the suspected antigen for at least 2 weeks before testing and should be asymptomatic. A standard dose (100 mL of cow milk or soy formula) is administered and the child is monitored carefully for reaction. Stool specimens are analyzed for occult blood, leukocytes, and reducing sugars, and a leukocyte count is obtained 6 to 8 hours later. The test result is considered positive if diarrhea develops within 24 hours, leukocytes or blood appear in stools, or the leukocyte count rises by more than 4,000 cells/mL over baseline. Approximately 20% of the infants have a delayed reaction. If the child originally had evidence of severe milk protein sensitivity, it is wise to hospitalize the infant, start with small volumes (5 to 10 mL) of formula, and gradually increase the volume to avoid severe mucosal injury, anaphylaxis, and shock. Skin testing rarely is useful in children with formula protein intolerance who have predominantly GI symptoms.

Intractable Diarrhea of Infancy

A state of persistent diarrhea and malabsorption despite the institution of a protein hydrolysate formula and in the absence of infectious pathogens is referred to as intractable or protracted diarrhea of infancy (131). These patients demonstrate a variety of histologic abnormalities on small intestinal biopsy, including blunting or flattening of the villi, increased mononuclear cells with occasional poly-morphonuclear infiltrates, cuboidalization of the surface epithelium, and a mild-to-moderate increase in mitotic activity in the crypts. Histologic lesions vary substantially, however, and correlate poorly with ultimate prognosis (132). Such infants have chronic weight loss and progressive malnutrition unless appropriate therapy is instituted. Initial therapy involves slow institution of a continuous enteral infusion of a diluted extensively hydrolyzed protein formula such as Pregestimil or Alimentum (133). The rate is rapidly advanced to approximately 150 mL/kg/d or more, provided the child is not on supplemental parenteral nutrition. The concentration of the formula then is advanced sequentially over 3 to 4 days, until the patient is tolerating full caloric requirements and gaining weight. During this time, stool pH and reducing substances are monitored, and evidence of carbohydrate malabsorption suggests failure of enteral feedings. If this occurs, a period of parenteral nutrition is indicated, usually through a central venous catheter, with gradual reintroduction of enteral feedings by continuous infusion. In treating such infants, it is important to avoid using formulas that contain intact milk or soy protein, because the likelihood of protein sensitivity in such infants is high and further mucosal injury may result. Lengthy periods of parenteral or continuous enteral infusion may be necessary, but the ultimate prognosis is good.

In addition to intractable (i.e., protracted) diarrhea associated with formula protein intolerance, other rare syndromes have been reported to result in mucosal injury and chronic diarrhea. One is congenital microvillus atrophy or microvillus inclusion disease, a disorder with hypoplastic atrophy of the villi and shortening or depletion of microvilli (134). This disorder requires electron microscopic diagnosis and has a very poor prognosis. A similar disorder has been recognized electron microscopically and has been associated with "tufting" of the microvilli, hence, the term "tufting enteropathy" (135). A number of patients also have been described with an intractable diarrhea-like syndrome in association with a mild immune defect, stiff unmanageable hair, and peculiar facies (136). All of these conditions are quite rare. Severe protracted diarrhea also may be associated with autoimmune enteropathy; however, this disorder usually presents outside the immediate neonatal period (137). Mucosal lesions are severe and the prognosis is poor. Infants with this disorder often have multiorgan autoantibodies, including gut epithelium, and frequently have pancreatic involvement with hyperglycemia or hypoglycemia.

Disorders of the Colon

Congenital Anomalies

There is substantial overlap in small bowel and colonic disease in neonates. Many of the congenital anomalies involve both the small and large intestines, and certain mucosal injury disorders, including formula protein enterocolitis and NEC, can involve both the small intestine and colon. There are some disorders that primarily affect the colon. Most are congenital and involve anatomic obstructions, such as atresias, or dysmotility, such as Hirschsprung's disease.

Anatomic Lesions

Colonic stenosis or atresia is a rare event, often associated with other skeletal anomalies. Colonic duplication also is a rare entity, which may present with delayed symptoms of obstruction. Duplications usually are cystic, gradually enlarging masses, located posterior to the rectum, which may be confused with tumors (138).

Motility Disorders

More frequent are the disorders that present with delayed passage of meconium secondary to dysmotility. Meconium plug syndrome is one such entity, in which inspissated meconium in the distal colon results in obstruction and dilatation proximally. Delayed passage of meconium is the presenting symptom, and barium enema examination reveals a large plug of meconium that often is evacuated after the barium enema. Normal feeding and stooling usually follows removal of the obstruction, but 20% to 30% of patients with meconium plug syndrome have Hirschsprung's disease. If symptoms recur after removal of the meconium plug, rectal suction biopsy is indicated.

Delayed passage of meconium also may occur with the neonatal small left colon syndrome. Radiographic examination of these infants demonstrates normal-to-dilated proximal colon with constricted or smaller distal colon, with the constricted area usually beginning around the splenic flexure. The line of demarcation is much more abrupt than is seen in neonatal Hirschsprung's disease. The disorder is more common in infants of diabetic mothers (139). It usually resolves spontaneously, although placement of a colostomy may be necessary until normal motility returns. Colonic motility eventually will return, usually within 2 to 12 weeks, and the colostomy may be closed at that time.

Hirschsprung's disease, or congenital aganglionic megacolon, occurs in approximately 1 in 5,000 live births, more commonly in males than in females (140). The risk of recurrence in families is reported to be as high as 10%; higher in infants with total aganglionosis. The frequency is ten times higher in infants with trisomy 21. The disease is caused by a congenital absence of the ganglion cells in both the submucous and myenteric plexuses. Ganglion cells regulate normal colonic peristaltic activity. The absence of ganglion cells results in an inability of the bowel to undergo coordinated relaxation. Impaired migration of neural crest cells into the distal colon is thought to be the mechanism through which Hirschsprung's disease develops, although there is some controversy about this. The disorder almost always involves the distal rectum, but the extent varies substantially. There also is controversy regarding whether or not skip areas can occur. A few such cases have been reported, but they appear to be extremely rare. In most instances, involvement does not extend proximal to the sigmoid colon. In very rare instances, the involvement may extend beyond the colon into the small intestine. The further the lesion extends, the more difficult the medical management becomes.

Most cases of Hirschsprung's disease are not diagnosed in the neonatal period. When they are, the most common clinical presentation is delayed passage of meconium, with passage of the first stool beyond 24 hours of age. This presentation probably is common but often overlooked. Infants also may appear irritable, with poor feeding and failure to thrive, which, unfortunately, is the typical presentation of a wide variety of small bowel and colonic disorders.

Some infants with Hirschsprung's disease may present with a life-threatening complication—acute enterocolitis (141). Toxic megacolon is common. Although enterocolitis may occur in the newborn period, it more commonly presents at 2 to 3 months of age. Mortality remains around 50%. The disorder presents with sudden or gradual onset of diarrhea, followed by bloody stools and eventually the clinical appearance of sepsis. The clinical overlap between infectious enterocolitis or formula protein-induced enterocolitis is such that Hirschsprung's enterocolitis also must be considered in the differential diagnosis of these more common entities. Patients who present with bloody diarrhea in infancy and have negative stool cultures, and who do not respond quickly to protein hydrolysate formula, need to have a rectal biopsy performed. If Hirschsprung's disease is suspected, surgical consultation should be obtained immediately, and attempts should be made to decompress the colon with a rectal tube or rectal irrigation. Controversy continues in the surgical literature regarding what is the best operation for Hirschsprung's disease (142).

Diagnosis of Hirschsprung's disease usually rests with rectal suction biopsy. A small biopsy tube is inserted into the rectum and a small piece of tissue is removed from a point 2 cm proximal to the mucocutaneous junction. If the biopsy is obtained higher, patients with low-segment Hirschsprung's disease may be missed. If the biopsy is taken more distally, it will be obtained in the hypoganglionic zone, an area in which ganglion cells are normally sparse, resulting in a false-positive biopsy for Hirschsprung's disease. The biopsy must be deep enough to contain sufficient submucosa to identify ganglion cells. Superficial biopsies are inadequate to diagnose Hirschsprung's disease. Because ganglion cells are sparse, the biopsy must be serially sectioned, and 60 to 80 sections of tissue examined. Ganglion cells in newborns are somewhat immature and difficult to identify. Thus, a rectal suction biopsy is a reliable diagnostic tool, provided the biopsy is obtained from an appropriate location and depth and an experienced gastroenterologist or pathologist interprets the biopsy. If results are equivocal, a full-thickness biopsy may be performed to establish the diagnosis.

Diagnosis also can be made by inflating a balloon in the distal rectum and measuring relaxation of the internal anal sphincter, a process impaired in Hirschsprung's disease. Although this technique is performed less commonly, those who are skillful in its use believe it is as reliable as rectal biopsy. In contrast, barium enema examination in the newborn is highly unreliable in the diagnosis of Hirschsprung's disease because the transition zone has yet to develop. Therefore, proximal colonic dilation usually is not apparent in the neonate, and the clinician must look for irregular contractions in the rectosigmoid as the primary hallmark of Hirschsprung's disease.

Treatment begins with placement of a decompressing colostomy proximal to the transition zone between ganglionic and aganglionic bowel. Definitive surgery usually is done at 8 to 12 months of age. A number of different operations have been devised in which the aganglionic bowel is removed and the ganglionic bowel attached into the distal rectum. Surgical treatment generally is successful in restoring long-term fecal continence (143).

Patients with total colonic Hirschsprung's disease present major difficulties in postoperative fluid and electrolyte balance. Infants frequently require prolonged courses of parenteral nutrition. Parents should be warned about the protracted nature of the disease, and infants should be observed closely for fluid, electrolyte, and nutritional problems.

Several other intestinal motility disorders present in the neonatal period. Transient hypomotility occurs in some premature infants and is characterized by markedly delayed gastric emptying and absent or diminished small bowel motility. In most instances, these abnormalities gradually resolve with time; support with parenteral nutrition coupled with intermittent attempts at feeding is all that is indicated. Alterations in calcium and magnesium metabolism such as parathyroid dysfunction or hypothyroidism can cause diminished motility, and these disorders should be excluded in infants with apparent motility disorders. Occasionally, infants with chronic idiopathic intestinal pseudoobstruction syndrome can present during infancy. This term applies to a number of neuropathic and myopathic disorders that result in chronic progressive GI hypomotility. A variety of histologic lesions have been described, and the prognosis for improvement is poor. Occasionally, the disorder also may involve the urinary tract, with associated megacystis and megaureter (144).

Pancreatic Disorders

Cystic Fibrosis

Disorders of the pancreas uncommonly present during the neonatal period. The most common is cystic fibrosis, which occurs in approximately 1 in 1,600 Caucasian live births (145). This autosomal recessive disorder usually presents later in childhood with failure to thrive or chronic pulmonary disease, but may present with meconium ileus in the neonatal period. After the obstruction has been relieved, therapy consists of compensating for the pancreatic insufficiency through use of extensively hydrolyzed protein formulas such as Pregestimil or Alimentum, which contain -medium-chain triglycerides as part of their lipid component. Medium-chain triglycerides do not require digestion by pancreatic enzymes for absorption and, consequently, may facilitate nutrient assimilation in infants with pancreatic insufficiency. Despite the use of elemental formulas, replacement pancreatic enzyme therapy from birth is necessary to aid the digestion of endogenously secreted proteins.

In children with pancreatic insufficiency as a result of cystic fibrosis, the release of the pancreatic hormone polypeptide (PP) is almost totally abolished. Fasting PP levels are low and the normal response to milk feeding is absent (146). Plasma insulin and GIP responses are reduced significantly in cystic fibrosis patients compared to control subjects, even though the early glucose rise is greater in the former group (141). Reduced GIP secretion in response to feeding may exacerbate the glucose intolerance that accompanies pancreatic destruction. Although plasma enteroglucagon concentrations are elevated in cystic fibrosis, levels of other hormones such as gastrin, secretin, motilin, and glucagon are quite normal (146).

The second most common cause of pancreatic insufficiency in infancy is Shwachman syndrome, an autosomal recessive disorder characterized by pancreatic insufficiency and bone marrow dysfunction with cyclic neutropenia (145,148). This rare disorder should be considered in infants with steatorrhea and neutropenia. Extremely rare isolated defects in pancreatic enzyme secretion, including trypsinogen and lipase, also have been reported.

Liver Disease

Development

The liver is a complex organ serving multiple metabolic functions. From a digestive standpoint, its primary function is that of an exocrine organ producing bile for the emulsification of fats. Postnatally, the liver receives its blood from two separate sources, approximately 25% from the hepatic artery and 75% from the portal vein. The portal vein drains the splanchnic bed and allows the liver the opportunity to regulate and metabolize substances absorbed by the intestine and hormones produced in the GI tract.

Bile is composed primarily of water. The concentration of solids in the bile are increased threefold by the gallbladder. The fetal liver is capable of synthesizing bile acids from cholesterol slowly, and the rate of synthesis increases progressively throughout gestation. The major bile salt in newborns is taurocholate. Conjugation of bile salts with glycine in preference to taurine gradually increases, and, by adulthood, most bile salts are conjugated with glycine. The bile acid pool is very small in the preterm infant, but gradually increases in the newborn and matures throughout infancy. This relatively small bile acid pool results in reduced bile salt secretion and, in addition to the relative pancreatic insufficiency, plays a role in the less efficient absorption of fat in the newborn infant. Bile acids are reabsorbed in the ileum through an active transport mechanism. There is some passive transport of bile acids in the jejunum and colon as well. In the fetus, taurocholate is absorbed passively and active ileal transport appears after birth.

Cholestatic Liver Disease

Most liver diseases in the neonatal period present with cholestasis, or conjugated hyperbilirubinemia (149,150). Although elevation of the amino transferase (i.e., transaminase) enzymes is considered the hallmark of hepatocellular injury in older children and adults, neonates may have significant hepatocellular injury even in the presence of normal amino transferase levels. There are many causes of prolonged conjugated hyperbilirubinemia in the neonatal period. These can be subdivided into general categories, including the following: infectious disorders; toxic insults such as parenteral nutrition and sepsis; metabolic disorders; anatomic disorders, including congenital hepatic fibrosis and choledochal cyst; and idiopathic infantile cholangiopathies, including primarily biliary atresia and neonatal hepatitis (151).

Neonatal Hepatitis and Biliary Atresia

After extensive evaluation of the infant with cholestasis, a diagnosis of either extrahepatic biliary atresia or idiopathic neonatal hepatitis is made in 70% to 80% of cases (152, 153). Current thinking suggests that neonatal hepatitis and biliary atresia form a continuum of a pathophysiologic process directed at various levels of the hepatobiliary tract. Inflammation in the bile duct epithelium may result in sclerosis and obliteration of the bile ducts and manifest itself as extrahepatic biliary atresia. Primary hepatocellular inflammation is more likely to result in neonatal hepatitis. Reovirus type III has been found in a number of infants with both idiopathic neonatal hepatitis and biliary atresia. This virus has been implicated as a causative agent in both disorders, although there is evidence that raises questions about this hypothesis (154–156).

Idiopathic neonatal hepatitis is slightly more common than biliary atresia. Both sporadic and familial varieties exist. Neonatal hepatitis, unlike biliary atresia, is more common in low-birth-weight infants. Jaundice develops during the first week of life in most cases. A wide variety of clinical presentations may occur, from severe failure to thrive or fulminant hepatic failure to asymptomatic jaundice. Acholic stools are uncommon, but may occur if cholestasis is severe. Physical examination reveals a firm, enlarged liver and occasionally splenomegaly. The presence of other signs of congenital infection may point toward a more specific diagnosis. Liver biopsy may be helpful in making the diagnosis, but the histologic findings are relatively nonspecific. In most cases, neonatal hepatitis can be differentiated successfully from biliary atresia by percutaneous liver biopsy. Clinical management is directed toward nutritional support and medical management of clinical complications such as ascites or pruritus. The prognosis is variable, with one-half of the cases resolving with little or no sequelae. Life-threatening chronic liver disease may necessitate liver transplantation.

Extrahepatic biliary atresia accounts for about one-third of cases of neonatal cholestasis. Familial cases are uncommon, as are cases in premature infants. Patients typically present with jaundice during the first or second week of life. Acholic stools are more common than in neonatal hepatitis. The liver is firm and enlarged, and splenomegaly may be present, as in neonatal hepatitis. Infants often appear clinically well, although progressive liver injury results in nutritional deficiencies, failure to thrive, and ascites.

Differentiation between neonatal hepatitis and biliary atresia has been the subject of controversy over the years. Serum amino transferase (i.e., transaminase) levels are notoriously unreliable indicators of neonatal liver disease and may be normal even in some patients with neonatal hepatitis. Extremely elevated γ-glutamyltransferase levels are suggestive of the marked bile ductular proliferation found in biliary atresia (157). Liver biopsy demonstrates inflammatory obliteration of the extrahepatic biliary tree, with bile stasis and bile ductular proliferation in the liver. Histologic features may overlap with neonatal hepatitis, particularly early in the course of the disease, making it difficult to differentiate. Histologic transition from neonatal hepatitis to biliary atresia has been reported and may be a relatively common phenomenon. The duodenal intubation and aspiration test is a simple, rapid, inexpensive method to check for patency of the extrahepatic biliary tree. Collection of 12 2-hour aliquots of duodenal drainage from a feeding tube placed in the duodenum over a 24-hour period suggests biliary atresia if no yellow fluid is present. Aspiration of bile-stained fluid from the duodenum suggests patency of the extrahepatic biliary tract. This test is sensitive and specific for the evaluation of infantile cholestasis (158). The test has reliability comparable to, or better than, radionuclide imaging with scans, which may give abnormal results in neonatal hepatitis during periods of severe cholestasis. Reliability of the radionuclide studies may be improved by measurement of duodenal fluid counts collected by a simple string test, in which infants swallow a string that absorbs fluid from the small intestine that later can be analyzed (159). The combination of liver biopsy and imaging study or duodenal drainage usually is used to determine whether the patient is more likely to have biliary atresia or neonatal hepatitis. If bile drainage cannot be confirmed or the typical histologic picture of neonatal hepatitis is not apparent on liver biopsy, then surgical exploration and intraoperative cholangiography usually is performed to establish a final diagnosis.

If the patient has biliary atresia, a hepatoportoenterostomy with Roux-en-Y enteroanastomosis (i.e., Kasai procedure) is performed to attempt bile drainage. The Kasai procedure rarely alters the long-term outcome of biliary atresia (160, but may delay the necessity of liver transplantation. Some advocate not performing a Kasai procedure. Most, however, believe that performing the procedure does not worsen the prognosis at transplant and may allow the child to live longer so that a more suitable liver donor may be located before transplantation. For those infants with progressive liver disease after the Kasai procedure, every attempt must be made to optimize their condition before transplantation. Deficient absorption must be corrected by vitamin supplementation (i.e., A, D, E, and K) require supplementation. Salt and protein restriction may become necessary, as liver failure progresses.

Hepatic transplantation is the definitive treatment for biliary atresia and results in long-term survival in 70% to 85% of infants.

Other Causes of Cholestasis

Rare causes of cholestasis must be excluded before confirming the diagnosis of neonatal hepatitis or biliary atresia (Table 40-3) (151). Infectious diseases such as cytomegalovirus, hepatitis B, HIV, rubella, herpes, toxoplasmosis, and syphilis should be excluded by standard serologic or culture techniques. Metabolic disorders to be considered include tyrosinemia, galactosemia, and hereditary fructose intolerance. Obtaining urine for reducing substances to exclude galactosemia and hereditary fructose intolerance, and succinyl acetone to exclude tyrosinemia should be done immediately. Anatomic disorders such as choledochal cysts can be diagnosed by ultrasonography. Other causes such as TPN cholestasis or sepsis should be considered, based on the clinical presentation.

TABLE 40-3
STEPS IN EVALUATING NEONATAL CHOLESTASIS

1. Determine that hyperbilirubinemia is predominantly direct
2. Exclude metabolic and infectious causes of cholestasis
3. Perform ultrasound to exclude anatomic lesions
4. Obtain percutaneous liver biopsy and hepatobiliary scan or duodenal drainage study
5. Explore whether studies suggest biliary atresia and perform Kasai procedure if indicated

Occasionally, liver biopsy will demonstrate a marked reduction in the number of intrahepatic bile ducts, revealing a disorder known as paucity of the intrahepatic bile ducts or intrahepatic biliary hypoplasia. Some of these patients fall into the category of Alagille syndrome, also known as syndromatic paucity or arteriohepatic dysplasia (161). These patients exhibit unusual facial characteristics, ocular abnormalities including posterior embryotoxon (i.e., prominent Schwalbe line), pulmonic stenosis, and vertebral arch defects, including anterior vertebral arch fusion with butterfly vertebrae. Careful cardiac examination, examination of the eyes by an ophthalmologist, and radiographic examination of the lumbosacral spine should be obtained in patients with suspected Alagille syndrome who have a paucity of intralobular bile ducts. Prognosis for long-term survival in syndromatic patients is relatively good.

There are patients with nonsyndromatic paucity who have liver biopsy findings similar to those with Alagille syndrome. In general, these patients have a much poorer prognosis than those with syndromatic paucity. Life-threatening cirrhosis develops in many, and these patients may require hepatic transplantation. As in biliary atresia, liver transplantation has markedly changed the prognosis for these patients.

A number of infectious disorders, both viral and bacterial, may present during the neonatal period, and a specific diagnosis should be sought in such instances. Hepatitis B typically is found in infants whose mothers were infected during the third trimester. As many as 60% to 90% of infants born to hepatitis B surface antigen-positive mothers may be infected. Transmission from mother to infant most commonly occurs at the time of delivery. Mothers who are hepatitis B antigen-positive are at extremely high risk to transmit hepatitis B virus to their infants. Additionally, mothers who are chronic carriers of hepatitis B surface antigen also may infect their infants. Most hepatitis B in infancy is asymptomatic. Abnormal liver tests develop at approximately 6 to 8 weeks of age and may persist for up to 1 year. Nearly 50% of these children remain hepatitis B surface antigen-positive and are at risk for developing hepatocellular carcinoma. Such children should be screened annually with α-fetoprotein levels for evidence of liver cancer, unless their hepatitis B surface antigen determinations revert to negative. Maternal screening for hepatitis B surface antigen is essential to prevent perinatal transmission of hepatitis B. Neonates born to mothers who are hepatitis B antigen-positive should receive hepatitis B hyperimmune globulin, 0.5 mL intramuscularly at the time of birth, and hepatitis B vaccine within 12 hours of birth. Booster immunizations with hepatitis B vaccine are recommended at 1 and 6 months of age (162).

Several other viruses may produce hepatitis during the neonatal period. Hepatitis A may develop in infants of mothers with active icteric hepatitis A at the time of delivery. Hepatitis C commonly is transmitted through blood contact and produces a clinical spectrum similar to hepatitis B. Serologic tests and viral RNA assays are available to detect hepatitis C. infants with hepatitis B or C run substantial risks for chronic liver disease. Recent experience has been gained with the use of α-interferon in the treatment of chronic hepatitis B and C, and with lamivudine in hepatitis B. Preliminary results look promising, but more experience is needed. Other viruses, such as Epstein–Barr virus, cytomegalovirus, HIV, rubella, herpes simplex, coxsackievirus, and adenoviruses may cause a wide spectrum of neonatal liver disease (163). In most instances, infection with these viruses results in spontaneous resolution without chronic injury.

Bacteria also may produce neonatal liver injury, because invasion of the liver may occur. Specific hepatic infection may result from certain bacterial diseases such as syphilis and listeriosis, and the parasitic disorder toxoplasmosis.

A number of metabolic diseases may present with neonatal cholestasis. The most common is α1-antitrypsin deficiency. α1-Antitrypsin is the major protease inhibitor in the hepatocyte. Deficiency of α1-antitrypsin occurs in a number of inheritable phenotypes. These Pi or protease inhibitor phenotypes can be determined. Type ZZ produces the most complete deficiency state and most cases of liver disease. It is estimated that 10% to 20% of type ZZ patients develop liver disease (164). Isolated cases of type MZ and MS also have been reported with liver injury (165). The ZZ phenotype is inherited through an autosomal recessive mechanism and occurs in 1 in 2,000 live births. Patients can be identified by the measurement of a very low α1-antitrypsin level in the blood. Diagnosis is confirmed by the determination of the ZZ phenotype, plus the classic histologic findings of periodic-acid–Schiff-positive, diastase-resistant granules on liver biopsy.

Liver disease may develop in patients with cystic fibrosis, although very few of these present during the neonatal period. Measurement of sweat chloride and specific mutational analysis to exclude cystic fibrosis should be part of the evaluation of neonatal liver disease.

Three metabolic diseases present with rather fulminant neonatal liver disease. (See also Chapter 41.) These include galactosemia, hereditary fructose intolerance, and tyrosinemia. These disorders should be expected when coagulation abnormalities appear inappropriately severe relative to the apparent degree of liver disease. Fructose intolerance does not present in the neonatal period unless the infants is on a sucrose containing formula (sucrose is metabolized to glucose and fructose). Patients with galactosemia have positive urinary reducing substances if they are being fed lactose at the time of screening. Patients with hereditary fructose intolerance also may test positive. Patients with tyrosinemia can be screened by measuring succinyl acetone content in the urine. Plasma and urine amino acids will demonstrate marked elevations of tyrosine, although this may be a nonspecific finding in any infant with neonatal liver disease. Patients with galactosemia respond to a galactose-free diet, and liver injury usually resolves spontaneously. Neonatal sepsis, particularly gram negative sepsis, is a frequent occurrence in these infants, and precautions should be taken. Patients with tyrosinemia commonly undergo progressive liver and renal dysfunction and are candidates for emergent liver transplantation once the diagnosis is made.

Several lipid storage diseases produce neonatal liver disease. Niemann–Pick disease, Wolman disease, cholesterol-ester storage disease, and Gaucher disease are included in this group. Most present with an insidious onset later in life.

A number of disorders exist in which paroxysmal dysfunction occurs. The most common is Zellweger syndrome, the cerebrohepatorenal syndrome. These patients present with cholestasis, hepatomegaly, hypotonia, and dysmorphic features, and may be diagnosed by demonstration of very-long-chain fatty acids in the serum.

Defects in the urea cycle may present with hyperammonemia during the first 2 days of life. A sepsis-like picture with vomiting, lethargy, seizures, and coma suggests this diagnosis. The most common form is ornithine transcarbamylase deficiency. Serum ammonia levels are very high, provided the infant is being fed protein. Diagnosis depends on plasma and urinary amino acid levels, and liver biopsy must be assayed for specific enzymes (see Chapter 41). Protein intake should be restricted and liver transplantation should be considered. Transient hyperammonemia of the newborn also has been reported with spontaneous resolution and no long-term neurologic sequelae. Permanent resolution of the hyperammonemia usually occurs by 2 weeks of age.

Another cause of acute liver failure in the neonate is neonatal hemochromatosis or neonatal iron storage disease (166,167). This rare, apparently inherited disorder of iron storage and metabolism may present with acute and rather fulminant liver failure characterized by severe cholestasis and coagulopathy. A variety of histologic findings have been observed in the livers of these patients, but they consistently have increased iron deposition in the liver and in other organs. Salivary gland biopsy may be used to establish the diagnosis. The disorder is rapidly progressive and often fatal unless transplantation can be performed early. Recently, antioxidant cocktails have been advocated for such patients, and some success has been reported (168).

Cholestasis may occur in any patient on chronic parenteral nutrition, but it is far more common in sick premature infants who receive parenteral nutrition for long periods of time (169,170). The mechanism by which the liver injury occurs is unknown and perhaps multifactorial (171). Several risk factors have been identified, however, including recurrent infections, prematurity, and lack of enteral feeding. Certain components of parenteral solutions have been implicated in causing liver injury. Excessive caloric administration may play a role. Certain amino acids may be more hepatotoxic, although many of these data are derived from animal studies. Higher doses of protein may result in a more rapid rise in bilirubin, but does not appear to alter ultimate risk of development of liver disease. Available intravenous lipid preparations do not appear to cause cholestasis and may, in fact, be beneficial in this regard.

The reason premature infants are more susceptible to liver disease while on parenteral nutrition probably is related to developmental immaturity of several hepatobiliary processes. These infants have reduced and altered bile acid synthesis, decreased bile acid pool size, and, therefore, decreased intraluminal bile acids. Gallbladder function also is impaired. Bile acid reabsorption from the small bowel is underdeveloped. The premature liver also is less capable of detoxifying potentially toxic secondary bile acids.

Lack of enteral feeding definitely predisposes to parenteral nutrition cholestasis. GI hormones that stimulate bile flow depend on enteral feeding for their release. Reduced gut motility in the unused bowel may contribute to bacterial proliferation and the resultant production of toxic secondary bile acids. Infection, especially GI, and GI surgery may potentiate the liver injury through related mechanisms. Limited amounts of enteral feeding, as tolerated, may be very beneficial in preventing liver injury in the parenteral nutrition-dependent infant.

Diagnosis of parenteral nutrition liver disease depends on exclusion of other causes of cholestasis in the parenteral nutrition-dependent patient. Separation of this disorder from other causes of cholestasis is difficult using standard laboratory tests. Histologic study is nonspecific, but may be helpful in making the diagnosis (172). The disease often is reversible once parenteral nutrition is discontinued. It occasionally may progress to cirrhosis, and hepatocellular carcinoma has been reported.

Treatment is accomplished best by discontinuing parenteral nutrition. If this cannot be accomplished, the following steps should be taken:

1. Reevaluate solutions to ensure they are appropriately formulated and balanced.
2. Use low-dose enteral feedings as tolerated to stimulate bile flow and gut motility.
3. Cycle the parenteral nutrition so that it is given over only part of the day.
4. Use amino acid solutions specially formulated for infants.

Other potential therapies, yet unproven, include choleretics such as Phenobarbital or ursodeoxycholic acid, hormone stimulation of bile flow, and bowel prokinetic agents.

Success with combined intestinal-liver transplants suggests that this procedure may play an important role in infants with end-stage parenteral nutrition liver disease (173).

REFERENCES

1. Lebenthal E, Keung YK. Alternative pathways of digestion and absorption in the newborn. In: Lebenthal E, ed. *Textbook of gastroenterology and nutrition in infancy*, 2nd ed. New York: Raven Press, 1989:3.
2. Lebenthal E, Tucker N. Carbohydrate digestion: development in early infancy. *Clin Perinatol* 1986;13:37.
3. Erasmus HD, Ludwig-Auser HM, Paterson PG, et al. Enhanced weight gain in preterm infants receiving lactase-treated feeds: a randomized, double-blind, controlled trial. *J Pediatr* 2002;141:532.
4. Cicco R, Holzman I, Brown D, et al. Glucose polymer intolerance in premature infants. *Pediatrics* 1981;67:498.
5. Lebenthal E, Lee PC. Alternate pathways of digestion and absorption in early infancy. *J Pediatr Gastroenterol Nutr* 1984;3:1.
6. Watkins JB. Lipid digestion and absorption. *Pediatrics* 1985;75: [Suppl]:151.
7. Boehm G, Bierbach U, Seuger H, et al. Activities of lipase and trypsin in duodenal juice of infants small for gestational age. *J Pediatr Gastroenterol Nutr* 1991;12:324.
8. Jensen RG, Clark RM, de Jong FA, et al. The lipolytic triad: human lingual, breast milk and pancreatic lipases: physiological implications of their characteristics in digestion of dietary fats. *J Pediatr Gastroenterol Nutr* 1982;1:243.
9. Watkins JB, Ingall D, Szczepanik P, et al. Bile salt metabolism in the newborn. *N Engl J Med* 1973;288:431.
10. Balistreri WF, Heubi JE, Suchy FJ. Immaturity of the enterohepatic circulation in early life: factors predisposing to "physiologic" malabsorption and cholestasis. *J Pediatr Gastroenterol Nutr* 1983;2:346.
11. Acra SA, Ghishan FK. Active bile salt transport in the ileum: characteristics and ontogeny. *J Pediatr Gastroenterol Nutr* 1990;10:421.
12. Euler AR, Byrne WJ, Meis PJ, et al. Basal and pentagastrin stimulated acid secretion in human newborn infants. *Pediatr Res* 1979;13:36.
13. Hyman PE, Clarke DD, Everett SL, et al. Gastric acid secretory function in preterm infants. *J Pediatr* 1985;106:467.
14. Agunod M, Yamaguchi N, Lopez R, et al. Correlative study of hydrochloric acid, pepsin and intrinsic factor secretion in newborns and infants. *Am J Digest Dis* 1969;14:400.
15. Antonowicz I, Lebenthal E. Developmental pattern of small intestinal enterokinase and disaccharidase activities in the human fetus. *Gastroenterology* 1977;723:1299.
16. Younoszai MK, Sapario RS, Laughlin M, et al. Maturation of jejunum and ileum in rats: water and electrolyte transport during in vivo perfusion of hypertonic solutions. *J Clin Invest* 1978;62:271.
17. Southgate DAT, Widdowson EM, Smits BJ, et al. Absorption and excretion of calcium and fat by young infants. *Lancet* 1969;1:487.
18. Senterre J, Putet G, Salle B, et al. Effects of vitamin D and phosphorus supplementation on calcium retention in preterm infants fed banked human milk. *J Pediatr* 1983;103:305.
19. Voyer M, Davakis M, Antener I, et al. Zinc balances in preterm infants. *Biol Neonate* 1982;42:87.
20. Tomomasa R, Hyman PE, Itoh K, et al. Gastroduodenal motility in neonates: response to human milk compared with cow's milk formula. *Pediatrics* 1987;80:434.
21. Berseth CL. Gestational evolution of small intestine motility in preterm infants. *J Pediatr* 1989;115:646.
22. Worniak ER, Fenton TR, Milla PJ. The development of fasting small intestine motility in human neonates. In: Roman C, ed. *Gastrointestinal motility*. London: Lancaster Press, 1983:265.
23. Nagata S, Koyanagi T, Horimoto N, et al. Chronological development of the fetal stomach assessed using real-time ultrasound. *Early Hum Dev* 1990;22:15.
24. Simpson C, Schanler RJ, Lau C. Early introduction of oral feeding in preterm infants. *Pediatrics* 2002;110(3):517.

25. Vanderhoof JA, Rappoport PJ, Paxson CL Jr. Manometric diagnosis of lower esophageal sphincter incompetence in infants: use of a small, single-lumen perfused catheter. *Pediatrics* 1978;62:805.

26. Buchan AMJ, Bryant MG, Polak JM, et al. Development of regulatory peptides in the human fetal intestine. In: Bloom SR, Polak JM, eds. *Gut hormones*. New York: Churchill-Livingston, 1981:119.

27. Bryant MG, Buchan AMJ, Gregor M, et al. Development of intestinal regulatory peptides in the human fetus. *Gastroenterology* 1982;83:47.

28. Lucas A, Bloom SR, Aynsley-Green A. Development of gut hormone responses to feeding in neonates. *Arch Dis Child* 1980; 55:678.

29. Lucas A, Adrian TE, Christofides ND, et al. Plasma motilin, gastrin and enteroglucagon and feeding in the human newborn. *Arch Dis Child* 1980;55:673.

30. Euler AP, Byrne WJ, Cousins LM, et al. Increased serum gastrin concentrations and gastric hyposecretion in the immediate newborn period. 1977;72:1271.

31. Aynsley-Green A, Lucas A, Bloom SR. The effects of feeds of differing composition on entero-insular hormone secretion in the first hours of life in human neonates. *Acta Paediatr Scand* 1979;68: 265.

32. Lucas A, Bloom SR, Aynsley-Green A. Postnatal surges in plasma gut hormones in term and preterm infants. *Biol Neonate* 1982; 41:63.

33. Miller BA. Observations on the gastric acidity during the first month of life. *Arch Dis Child* 1941;16:22.

34. Adrian TE, Savage AJ, Sagor GR, et al. Effect of peptide YY on gastric, pancreatic and biliary function in humans. *Gastroenterology* 1985;89:494.

35. Adrian TE, Smith HA, Calvert SA, et al. Elevated plasma peptide YY in human neonates and infants. *Pediatr Res* 1986;20:1225.

36. Lucas A, Adrian TE, Bloom SR, et al. Plasma secretin in neonates. *Acta Paediatr Scand* 1980;69:205.

37. Johnson LR. Regulation of gastrointestinal growth. In: Johnson LR, ed. *Physiology of the gastrointestinal tract*, 2nd ed. New York: Raven Press, 1987:301.

38. Calvert SA, Soltesz G, Jenkins PA, et al. Feeding premature infants with human milk or preterm milk formula: effects on postnatal growth, intermediary metabolism and regulatory peptides. *Biol Neonate* 1985;47:189.

39. Tornhage CJ, Serenius F, Uvnas-Moberg K, et al. Plasma somatostatin and cholecystokinin levels in preterm infants during kangaroo care with and without nasogastric tube feeding. *J Pediatr Endocrinol Metab* 1998;11(5):645.

40. Berseth CL. Gestational evolution of small intestine motility in preterm and term infants. *J Pediatr* 1989;115:646.

41. Sarson DL, Wood SM, Holder D, et al. The effect of glucose-dependent insulinotropic polypeptide infused at physiological concentrations on the release of insulin in man. *Diabetologia* 1982;22:33.

42. Lucas A, Sarson DL, Bloom SR, et al. Developmental aspects of gastric inhibitory polypeptide (GIP) and its possible role in the enteroinsular axis in neonates. *Acta Paediatr Scand* 1980;69:321.

43. Lucas A, Aynsley-Green A, Blackburn AN, et al. Plasma neurotensin in term and preterm neonates. *Acta Paediatr Scand* 1981;17:201.

44. Savage AP, Adrian TE, Carolan G, et al. Effects of peptide YY (PYY) on mouth to cecum transit time and on the rate of gastric emptying in healthy volunteers. *Gut* 1987;70:166.

45. Drucker DJ, Ehrlich P, Asa SL, et al. Induction of epithelial proliferation by glucagon-like peptide 2. *Proc Natl Acad Sci U S A* 1996;92:7911.

46. Chance WT, Foley-Nelson T, Thomas I, et al. Prevention of parenteral nutrition-induced hypoplasia by coinfusion of glucagon-like peptide-2. *Am J Physiol* 1997;273:G559.

47. Lucas A, Bloom SR, Aynsley-Green A. Metabolic and endocrine consequences of depriving preterm infants of enteral nutrition. *Acta Paediatr Scand* 1983;72:245.

48. Adrian TE, Bloom SR. Effect of food on the hormones of the gastrointestinal tract. In: Hunter JO, Jones V, eds. *Food and the gut*. Philadelphia: Bailliére Tindall, 1985:13.

49. Isaacs PET, Ladas S, Forgacs IC, et al. A comparison of the effects of ingested medium- and long-chain triglyceride on gallbladder volume and the release of cholecystokinin and other gut peptides. *Dig Dis Sci* 1987;32:481.

50. Martin LW, Torres AM. Omphalocele and gastroschisis. *Surg Clin North Am* 1985;65:1235.

51. Meller JL, Reyes HM, Loeff DS. Gastroschisis and omphalocele. *Clin Perinatol* 1989;16:113.

52. Yazbeck S, Ndoye M, Khan AH. Omphalocele: a 25 year experience. *J Pediatr Surg* 1986;21:761.

53. Botto LD, Mulinare J, Erickson JD. Occurrence of omphalocele in relation to maternal multivitamin use: a population-based study. *Pediatrics* 2002;109(5):904.

54. Dykes EH. Prenatal diagnosis and management of abdominal wall defects. *Semin Pediatr Surg* 1996;5:90.

55. Quirk JG, Forney J, Collins HB, et al. Outcomes of newborns with gastroschisis: the effects of mode of delivery, site of delivery, and interval from birth to surgery. *Am J Obstet Gynecol* 1996; 174:1134.

56. Lenke RR, Hatch EI Jr. Fetal gastroschisis: a preliminary report advocating the use of cesarean section. *Obstet Gynecol* 1986; 67:395.

57. Langer JC. Gastroschisis and omphalocele. *Semin Pediatr Surg* 1996;5:124.

58. Herbst JJ. Gastroesophageal reflux in infants. *J Pediatr Gastroenterol Nutr* 1985;4:163.

59. Werlin SL, Dodds WJ, Hogan WJ, et al. Mechanisms of gastroesophageal reflux in children. *J Pediatr* 1980;97:244

60. Peter CS, Sprodowski N, Bohnhorst B, Silny J, Poets CF. Gastroesophageal reflux and apnea of prematurity: no temporal relationship. *Pediatrics* 2001;109(1):8.

61. Barrington KJ, Tan K, Rich W. Apnea at discharge and gastroesophageal reflux in the preterm infant. *J Perinatol* 2002;22:8.

62. Carlos MA, Babyn PS, Marcon MA, et al. Changes in gastric emptying in early postnatal life. *J Pediatr* 1997;130:931.

63. Sondheimer JM. Continuous monitoring of distal esophageal pH: a diagnostic test for gastroesophageal reflux in infants. *J Pediatr* 1980;93:804.

64. Tsou VM, Young RM, Hart MH, et al. Elevated plasma aluminum levels in normal infants using antacids containing aluminum. *Pediatrics* 1991;87:148.

65. Mehall JR, Nothrop R, Saltzman DA, et al. Acidification of formula reduces bacterial translocation and gut colonization in a neonatal rabbit model. *J Pediatr Surg* 2001;36:56.

66. Strickland AD, Chang JHT. Results of treatment of gastroesophageal reflux with bethanechol. *J Pediatr* 1983;103:311.

67. Jolley SG, Halpern LM, Tunell WP, et al. The risk of sudden infant death from gastroesophageal reflux. *J Pediatr Surg* 1991; 26:691.

68. Raffensperger JG. Esophageal atresia and tracheoesophageal stenosis. In: Raffensperger JG, ed. *Swenson's pediatric surgery*, 5th ed. Norwalk, CT: Appleton and Lange, 1990:697.

69. Benson CD, Lloyd JR. Infantile pyloric stenosis: a review of 1120 cases. *Am J Surg* 1964;107:429.

70. Dodge JA. Genetics of hypertrophic pyloric stenosis. *Clin Gastroenterol* 1973;2:523.

71. Hernanz-Schulman M, Sells LL, Ambrosino MM, et al. Hypertrophic pyloric stenosis in the infant without a palpable olive: accuracy of sonographic diagnosis. *Radiology* 1994;193: 771.

72. Nord KS. Peptic ulcer disease in the pediatric population. *Pediatr Clin North Am* 1988;35:117.

73. Drumm B, Rhoads JM, Stringer DA, et al. Peptic ulcer disease in children: clinical findings, and clinical course. *Pediatrics* 1988;82: 410.

74. Murphy MS, Eastham EJ. Peptic ulcer disease in childhood: long-term prognosis. *J Pediatr Gastroenterol Nutr* 1987;6:721.

75. Guelrud M, Mujica C, Jaen D, et al. Prevalence of Helicobacter pylori in neonates and young infants undergoing ERCP for diagnosis of neonatal cholestasis. *J Pediatr Gastroenterol Nutr* 1994; 18(4):461.

76. Bell JJ. Perforation of the gastrointestinal tract and peritonitis in the neonate. *Surg Gynecol Obstet* 1985;160:20.

77. Smith EI. Malrotation of the intestine. In: Welch KJ, Randolph JG, Ravitch MM, et al, eds. *Pediatric surgery*, 4th ed. Chicago: Year Book, 1986:882.

78. Feitz R, Vos A. Malrotation: the postoperative period. *J Pediatr Surg* 1997;32:1322.

79. Grosfeld JL. Jejunoileal atresia and stenosis. In: Welch KJ, Randolph JG, Ravitch MM, et al, eds. *Pediatric surgery*, 4th ed. Chicago: Year Book, 1986:838.

80. Martin LW, Zerella JT. Jejunoileal atresia: a proposed classification. *J Pediatr Surg* 1967;11:399.
81. Holgersen LO, Stanly-Brown EG. Idiopathic post-operative intussusception in infants and childhood. *Am Surg* 1978;44:305.
82. Brown EG, Sweet AY. Neonatal necrotizing enterocolitis. *Pediatr Clin North Am* 1982;29:1149.
83. Kliegman RM, Fanaroff AA. Necrotizing enterocolitis. *N Engl J Med* 1984;310:1093.
84. Hack M, Horbar JK, Malloy MH, et al. Very low birth weight outcomes of the National Institute of Child Health and Human Development Neonatal Network. *Pediatrics* 1991;87:587.
85. Uauy RD, Fanaroff AA, Korones SB, et al. Necrotizing enterocolitis in very low birth weight infants: biodemographic and clinical correlates. *J Pediatr* 1991;119:630.
86. Bisquera JA, Cooper TR, Berseth CL. Impact of necrotizing enterocolitis on length of stay and hospital charges in very low birth weight infants. *Pediatrics* 2002;109(3):423.
87. Kliegman RM, Walsh M. Neonatal necrotizing enterocolitis: pathogenesis, classification and spectrum of illness. *Curr Probl Pediatr* 1987;17:213.
88. Ballance WA, Dahms BB, Shenker N, et al. Pathology of neonatal necrotizing enterocolitis: a ten-year experience. *J Pediatr* 1990; 117[Suppl 1, Pt 2]:S6.
89. Kliegman RM. Neonatal necrotizing enterocolitis: bridging the basic science with clinical disease. *J Pediatr* 1990;117:833.
90. Caplan MS, Sun X-M, Hsueh W, et al. Role of platelet activating factor and tumor necrosis factor-alpha in neonatal necrotizing enterocolitis. *J Pediatr* 1990;116:960.
91. Amin HJ, Zamora SA, McMillan DD, et al. Arginine supplementation prevents necrotizing enterocolitis in the premature infant. *J Pediatr* 2002;140:425.
92. Neu J. Arginine supplementation and the prevention of necrotizing enterocolitis in very low birth weight infants. *J Pediatr* 2002; 140:389.
93. Anderson DM, Kliegman RM. The relationship of neonatal alimentation practices to the occurrence of endemic necrotizing enterocolitis. *Am J Perinatol* 1991;8:62.
94. Covert RF, Neu J, Elliott MJ, et al. Factors associated with age of onset of necrotizing enterocolitis. *Am J Perinatol* 1989;6:455.
95. van Acker J, de Smet F, Muyldermans G, et al. Outbreak of necrotizing enterocolitis associated with Enterobactr sakazakii in powdered milk formula. *J Clin Microbiol* 2001;39(1):293.
96. Eibl MM, Wolf HM, Furnkranz H, et al. Prophylaxis of necrotizing enterocolitis by oral IgA-IgG: review of a clinical study in low birth weight infants and discussion of the pathogenic role of infection. *J Clin Immunol* 1990;10[Suppl 6]:72S.
97. Aynsley-Green A, Lucas A, Lawson GR, et al. Gut hormones and regulatory peptides in relation to enteral feeding, gastroenteritis, and necrotizing enterocolitis in infancy. *Arch Dis Child* 1990; 117[Suppl]:24.
98. Faix RG, Polley TZ, Grasela TH. A randomized controlled trial of parenteral clindamycin in neonatal necrotizing enterocolitis. *Pediatrics* 1988;112:271.
99. Morga LJ, Shochat SJ, Hartman GE. Peritoneal drainage as primary management of perforated NEC in the very low birth weight infant. *J Pediatr Surg* 1994;29:310.
100. Horwitz JR, Lally KP, Chen HW, et al. Complications after surgical intervention for necrotizing enterocolitis: a multicenter review. *J Pediatr Surg* 1995;30:994.
101. Buchheit JP, Stewart DL. Clinical comparison of localized intestinal perforation and necrotizing enterocolitis in neonates. *Pediatrics* 1994;93:32.
102. Fujii AM, Brown E, Mirochnick M, et al. Neonatal necrotizing enterocolitis with intestinal perforation in extremely premature infants receiving early indomethacin treatment for patnet ductus arteriosus. *J Perinatol* 2002;22:535.
103. Dowling RH, Booth CC. Structural and functional changes following small intestinal resection in the rat. *Clin Sci* 1967;32:139.
104. Adrian TE, Savage AP, Fuessl HS, et al. Release of peptide YY (PYY) after resection of small bowel, colon or pancreas in man. *Surgery* 1987;101:715.
105. Besterman HS, Adrian TE, Mallinson CN, et al. Gut hormone release after intestinal resection. *Gut* 1982;23:854.
106. Armstrong DN, Ballantyne GH, Adrian TE, et al. Adaptive increase in peptide YY and enteroglucagon after proctocolectomy and pelvic ileal reservoir reconstruction. *Dis Colon Rectum* 1991;34:119.
107. Wilmore DW, Dudrick SJ, Daly JM, et al. The role of nutrition in the adaptation of the small intestine after massive resection. *Surg Gynecol Obstet* 1971;132:673.
108. Vanderhoof JA. Short bowel syndrome. In: Lebenthal EB, ed. *Gastroenterology and nutrition in early infancy*, 2nd ed. New York: Raven Press, 1990:793.
109. Vanderhoof JA. Short bowel syndrome. In: Kassirer JP, ed. *Current therapy in internal medicine*, 3rd ed. Philadelphia: BC Decker, 1991:550.
110. Vanderhoof JA. Clinical management of the short bowel syndrome. In: Balistreri WF, Vanderhoof JA, eds. *Pediatric gastroenterology and nutrition*. London: Chapman and Hall, 1990:24.
111. Goulet OJ, Revillon Y, Jan D, et al. Neonatal short bowel syndrome. *J Pediatr* 1991;119[Suppl 1, Pt 1]:18.
112. Gracey M. The contaminated small bowel syndrome: pathogenesis, diagnosis and treatment. *Am J Clin Nutr* 1979;32:234.
113. Perman JA, Modler S, Barr RG, et al. Fasting breath hydrogen concentration: normal values and clinical adaptation. *Gastroenterology* 1984;87:1358.
114. Aarbakke J, Schjonsby H. Value of urinary simple phenol and indican determinations of the stagnant loop syndrome. *Scand J Gastroenterol* 1976;2:409.
115. Hudson M, Packnee R, Mowat NA. D-lactic acidosis in short bowel syndrome: an examination of possible mechanisms. *Q J Med* 1990;74:157.
116. Taylor SF, Sondheimer JM, Sokol RJ, et al. Noninfectious colitis associated with short gut syndrome in infants. *J Pediatr* 1991; 119:24.
117. Young RJ, Vanderhoof JA. Probiotic therapy in children with short bowel syndrome and bacterial overgrowth. *Gastroenerology* 1997;112:A916.
118. Caniano DA, Starr J, Ginn-Pease ME. Extensive short-bowel syndrome in neonates: outcome in the 1980s. *Surgery* 1989;105: 119.
119. Thompson JS. Recent advances in the surgical treatment of the short-bowel syndrome. *Surg Ann* 1990;22:107.
120. Thompson J, Pinch L, Murray N, et al. Experience with intestinal lengthening procedures. *J Pediatr Surg* 1991;26:721.
121. Vanderhoof JA. Short bowel syndrome in children and small intestinal transplantation. *Pediatr Clin North Am* 1996;43:533.
122. Cooper A, Floyd TS, Ross AJ, et al. Morbidity and mortality of short bowel syndrome acquired in infancy: an update. *J Pediatr Surg* 1984;19:711.
123. Dorney SFA, Ament ME, Berquist WE, et al. Improved survival in very short small bowel of infancy with use of long-term parenteral nutrition. *J Pediatr* 1985;106:521.
124. Adrian TE, Savage AP, Bacarese-Hamilton AJ, et al. Peptide YY abnormalities in gastrointestinal disease. *Gastroenterology* 1986; 90:379.
125. Besterman HS, Christofides ND, Welsby PD, et al. Gut hormones in acute diarrhea. *Gut* 1983;24:665.
126. Lawson GR, Nelson R, Laker MF, et al. Gut regulatory peptides and intestinal permeability in acute infantile gastroenteritis. *Arch Dis Child* 1992;67:272.
127. Walker-Smith J, Harrison M, Kilby A, et al. Cow's milk-sensitive enteropathy. *Arch Dis Child* 1978;53:375.
128. Walker-Smith J. Cow's milk protein intolerance: transient food intolerance of infancy. *Arch Dis Child* 1975;50:347.
129. Vanderhoof JA, Murray ND, Kaufman SS, et al. Intolerance to protein hydrolysate infant formulas, an under-recognized cause of gastrointestinal symptoms in infants. *J Pediatr* 1997;131:741.
130. Powell GK. Milk- and soy-induced enterocolitis of infancy. *J Pediatr* 1978;93:553.
131. Avery GB, Villavicencio O, Lilly JR, et al. Intractable diarrhea in early infancy. *Pediatrics* 1968;41:712.
132. Goldgar CM, Vanderhoof JA. Lack of correlation of small bowel biopsy and clinical course of patients with intractable diarrhea of infancy. *Gastroenterology* 1986;90:527.
133. Orenstein SR. Enteral versus parenteral therapy for intractable diarrhea of infancy: a prospective, randomized trial. *J Pediatr* 1986;109:277.
134. Schmitz J, Ginies JL, Arnaud-Battandier F, et al. Congenital microvillous atrophy, a rare cause of neonatal intractable diarrhoea. *Pediatr Res* 1982;16:1014.
135. Patey N, Scoazec JY, Cuenod-Jabri B, et al. Distribution of cell adhesion molecules in infants with intestinal epithelial dysplasia (tufting enteropathy). *Gastroenterology* 1997;113:833.

136. Girault D, Goulet O, L-Ldeist F, et al. Intractable infant diarrhea associated with phenotypic abnormalities and immunodeficiency. *J Pediatr* 1994;125:36.

137. Unsworth J, Hutchins P, Mitchell J, et al. Flat small intestinal mucosa and autoantibodies against the gut epithelium. *J Pediatr Gastroenterol Nutr* 1982;1:503.

138. Holcomb GW III, Gheissari A, O'Neill JA Jr, et al. Surgical management of alimentary tract duplications. *Ann Surg* 1989;209:167.

139. Davis WS, Campbell JB. Neonatal small left colon syndrome. Occurrence in asymptomatic infants of diabetic mothers. *Am J Dis Child* 1975;129(9):1024.

140. Martin LW, Torres Am. Hirschsprung's disease. *Surg Clin North Am* 1985;65:1171.

141. Bill AJ, Chapman ND. The enterocolitis of Hirschsprung's disease: its natural history and treatment. *Am J Surg* 1962;103:70.

142. Swenson O. Hirschsprung's disease: A review. *Pediatrics* 2002;109(5):914.

143. Heikkinen M, Rintala R, Luukkonen P. Long-term anal sphincter performance after surgery for Hirschsprung's disease. *J Pediatr Surg* 1997;32:1443.

144. Granata C, Puri P. Megacystis-microcolon-intestinal hypoperistalsis syndrome. *J Pediatr Gastroenterol Nutr* 1997;25:12.

145. Durie PR, Forstner GG. Pathophysiology of the exocrine pancreas in cystic fibrosis. *J R Soc Med* 1989;18[Suppl 16]:2.

146. Adrian TE, McKiernan J, Johnstone DI, et al. Hormonal abnormalities of the pancreas and gut in cystic fibrosis. *Gastroenterology* 1980;79:460.

147. Aggett PJ, Cavanagh NPC, Matthew DJ, et al. Schwachman's syndrome. *Arch Dis Child* 1980;55:331.

148. Ip WE, Dupuis A, Ellis L, et al. Serum pancreatic enzymes define the pancreatic phenotype in patients with Shwachman-diamod syndrome. *J Pediatr* 2002;141:259.

149. Alagille D. Management of chronic cholestasis in childhood. *Semin Liver Dis* 1985;5:254.

150. Balistreri WF. Neonatal cholestasis. In: Lebenthal E, ed. *Textbook of gastroenterology and nutrition in infancy.* New York: Raven Press, 1981:1081.

151. Sokol RJ. Medical management of neonatal cholestasis. In: Balistreri WF, Stocker JT, eds. *Pediatric hepatology.* New York: Hemisphere Publishing, 1990:41.

152. Balistreri WF. Neonatal cholestasis: medical progress. *J Pediatr* 1985;106:171.

153. Balistreri WF. Neonatal cholestasis: lessons from the past, issues for the future. *Semin Liver Dis* 1987;7:61.

154. Morecki R, Glaser JH, Cho S, et al. Biliary atresia and reovirus type 3 infection. *N Engl J Med* 1982;307:481.

155. Morecki R, Glaser J. Reovirus 3 and neonatal biliary disease: discussion of divergent results. *Hepatology* 1989;10:515.

156. Fischler B, Haglund B, Hjern A. A population-based study on the incidence and possible pre- and perinatal etiologic risk factors of biliary atresia. *J Pediatr* 2002;141:217.

157. Maggiore G, Bernard O, Hadchouel M, et al. Diagnostic value of serum gamma-glutamyl transpeptidase activity in liver diseases in children. *J Pediatr Gastroenterol Nutr* 1991;12:21.

158. Faweya AG, Akinyinka OO, Sodeinde O. Duodenal intubation and aspiration test: utility in the differential diagnosis of infantile cholestasis. *J Pediatr Gastroenterol Nutr* 1991;13:290.

159. Rosenthal P, Miller JH, Sinatra FR. Hepatobiliary scintigraphy and the string test in the evaluation of neonatal cholestasis. *J Pediatr Gastroenterol Nutr* 1989;8:296.

160. Raffensperger JG. A long-term follow-up of three patients with biliary atresia. *J Pediatr Surg* 1991;26:176.

161. Alagille D, Odievre M, Gautier M, et al. Syndromic paucity of interlobular bile ducts (Alagille syndrome or arteriohepatic dysplasia): review of 80 cases. *J Pediatr* 1987;110:195.

162. Tajiri H, Nose O, Shimizu K, et al. Prevention of neonatal HBV infection with the combination of HBIG and HBV vaccine and its long-term efficacy in infants born to HBeAg positive HBV carrier mothers. *Acta Paediatr Jpn* 1989;31:663.

163. Hart MH, Kaufman SS, Vanderhoof JA, et al. Neonatal hepatitis and extrahepatic biliary atresia associated with cytomegalovirus infection in twins. *Am J Dis Child* 1991;145:302.

164. Povey S. Genetics of alpha-1-antitrypsin deficiency in relation to neonatal liver disease. *Mol Biol Med* 1990;7:161.

165. Pittschieler K. Liver disease and heterozygous alpha-1-antitrypsin deficiency. *Acta Paediatr Scand* 1991;80:323.

166. Egawa H, Berquist W, Garcia-Kennedy R, et al. Rapid development of hepatocellular siderosis after liver transplantation for neonatal hemochromatosis. *Transplantation* 1996;62:1511.

167. Barnard JA, Manci E. Idiopathic neonatal iron-storage disease. *Gastroenerology* 1991;101:1420.

168. Witzleben CL, Uri A. Perinatal hemochromatosis: entity or end result? *Hum Pathol* 1989;20:335.

169. Bell RL, Ferry GD, Smith EO, et al. Total parenteral nutrition-related cholestasis in infants. *J Parenter Enteral Nutr* 1986;10:356.

170. Merritt RJ. Cholestasis associated with total parenteral nutrition. *J Pediatr Gastroenterol Nutr* 1986;5:9.

171. Balistreri WF, Novak DA, Farrell MK. Bile acid metabolism, total parenteral nutrition, and cholestasis. In: Lebenthal E, ed. *Total parenteral nutrition: indications, utilization, complications and pathophysiological considerations.* New York: Raven Press, 1986:319.

172. Cohen C, Olsen MM. Pediatric total parenteral nutrition, liver histopathology. *Arch Pathol Lab Med* 1981;105:152.

173. Vanderhoof JA, Langnas AN, Pinch LW, et al. Short bowel syndrome: a review. *J Pediatr Gastroenterol Nutr* 1992;14:359.

Inherited Metabolic Disorders

Barbara K. Burton

Major advances in the recognition and treatment of inborn errors of metabolism have made it more essential than ever that the neonatologist be familiar with the clinical presentation of these disorders. Many of the diseases in this group are associated with symptoms in the neonatal period, and many affected infants find their way into neonatal intensive care units. The likelihood of establishing a diagnosis often is directly related to the level of awareness of the neonatologist responsible for the infant's care. Although many of the individual inborn errors of metabolism occur infrequently, collectively, they are not rare. There is no doubt that a significant number of children with these disorders are undiagnosed. Every geneticist has had the experience of diagnosing an inborn error of metabolism in a child and discovering that the parents have had one or more other children who died in early infancy of vague or undetermined causes. In such cases, it is reasonable to assume that the other children were similarly affected but undiagnosed. Autopsy findings in such cases are often nonspecific and unrevealing unless special biochemical studies are done. Infection often is suspected as the cause of death, and sepsis is a common accompaniment of inherited metabolic disorders.

The significance of the precise diagnosis of metabolic disease cannot be overemphasized. Increasingly, these disorders are lending themselves to successful medical management. If treatment means the prevention of significant mental retardation or death, even when the numbers are small, the diagnosis is clearly worth pursuing. However, the success of most treatment regimens depends on the earliest possible institution of therapy, stressing the importance of early clinical diagnosis. Even when no effective therapy exists or an infant cannot be salvaged, diagnosis is critical for purposes of genetic counseling.

Inborn errors of metabolism are all genetically transmitted, typically in an autosomal recessive or X-linked recessive fashion, and there is usually a substantial risk of recurrence. Prenatal diagnosis is available for many conditions in this group. Awareness of the diagnosis before birth of an at-risk infant can lead to earlier therapy and an improved prognosis.

This chapter defines the constellation of findings in the newborn that should alert the clinician to the possibility of inherited metabolic disease. The discussion is confined to the disorders for which manifestations are observed in the first few months of life and does not include the many disorders (e.g., most lysosomal storage diseases) that typically present in later infancy or childhood. The laboratory tools used to evaluate infants suspected of having inherited metabolic disease are discussed. Treatment of important groups of metabolic disorders are addressed, focusing on the stabilization and acute management of patients with these conditions.

A list of the major inborn errors of metabolism that have been described clinically in early infancy is shown in Table 41-1. This table cannot be considered complete because it includes only the disorders for which manifestations in the first few months of life have been documented in the literature. It is likely that disorders typically occurring later in childhood occasionally may present as early as the first month of life. New disorders causing neonatal disease undoubtedly will continue to be described. A single literature reference is listed for each disorder in the table, and detailed information about most of the disorders listed can be found in recent editions of reference textbooks (1,2).

CLINICAL MANIFESTATIONS OF INBORN ERRORS OF METABOLISM

Acute Metabolic Encephalopathy

Several groups of inherited metabolic disorders, most notably the organic acidemias, urea cycle defects, and certain disorders of amino acid metabolism, typically present with acute life-threatening symptoms in the neonatal period. Because they are associated with protein intolerance, symptoms usually begin after feedings have been instituted.

TABLE 41-1	
INBORN ERRORS OF METABOLISM THAT PRESENT IN EARLY INFANCY	

Disorder	Reference
Disorders of Carbohydrate Metabolism	
Galactosemia (i.e., galactose-1-phosphate uridyl transferase deficiency)	39
Hereditary fructose intolerance (i.e., fructose-1-phosphate aldolase deficiency)	40
Fructose-1,6-bisphosphatase deficiency	41
Glycogen storage disease type I (i.e., von Gierke disease, glucose-6-phosphate deficiency)	42
Glycogen storage disease type II (i.e., Pompe disease, alpha-glucosidase deficiency)	43
Glycogen storage disease type III (i.e., limit dextrinosis, debrancher deficiency)	42
Glycogen storage disease type IV (i.e., amylopectinosis, brancher deficiency)	44
Disorders of Amino Acid Metabolism	
Maple syrup urine disease	45
Homocystinuria	46
Nonketotic hyperglycinemia	47
Phenylketonuria	48
Hereditary tyrosinemia	49
Hyperornithinemia–hyperammonemia–homocitrullinuria syndrome	50
Lysinuric protein intolerance	51
Methylene tetrahydrofolate reductase deficiency	52
Pyridoxine dependency with seizures (i.e., presumed glutamic acid decarboxylase deficiency)	53
Organic Acidemias	
Methylmalonic acidemia	54
Methylmalonic acidemia with homocystinuria	55
Propionic acidemia	56
Isovaleric acidemia	57
3-Methyl crotonyl CoA carboxylase deficiency	58
Holocarboxylase synthetase deficiency (i.e., early-onset multiple carboxylase deficiency)	59
Biotinidase deficiency (i.e., late-onset multiple carboxylase deficiency)	60
Glutaric acidemia type I	61
Glutaric acidemia type II (i.e., multiple acyl CoA dehydrogenase deficiency, severe)	62
Ethylmalonic-adipic aciduria (i.e., later-onset glutaric acidemia type II, multiple acyl CoA dehydrogenase deficiences, mild)	63
3-Hydroxy-3-methylglutaric acidemia	64
2-Methylacetoacetyl-CoA thiolase deficiency	65
Mevalonic aciduria	66
Pyroglutamic aciduria	67
3-Hydroxyisobutyric aciduria	68
3-Methylglutaconic aciduria	69
2-Methylbutyryl CoA dehydrogenase deficiency	70
Urea Cycle Disorders	
Carbamyl phosphate synthetase deficiency	71
Ornithine transcarbamylase deficiency	71
Citrullinemia	71
Argininosuccinic aciduria	71
Arginase deficiency	72
N-Acetylglutamate synthetase deficiency	73
Fatty Acid Oxidation Defects	
Short-chain acyl CoA dehydrogenase deficiency	74
Medium-chain acyl CoA dehydrogenase deficiency	75
Very-long-chain acyl CoA dehydrogenase deficiency	76
Long-chain 3-hydroxyacyl-CoA dehydrogenase deficiency	77
Carnitine-acylcarnitine translocase deficiency	78
Carnitine transporter deficiency (i.e., primary systemic carnitine deficiency)	79
Carnitine palmitoyl transferase II deficiency	80
Isobutyryl-CoA dehydrogenase deficiency	81
Lactic Acidemias	
Pyruvate dehydrogenase deficiency	32
Pyruvate carboxylase deficiency	82

(continued)

TABLE 41-1
(continued)

Disorder	Reference
Phosphoenolpyruvate carboxykinase deficiency	83
Mitochondrial encephalomyopathies	84
Transport Disorders	
Cystic fibrosis	85
Infantile free sialic acid storage disease	86
Hartnup disease	87
Lysosomal Storage Disorders	
GM$_1$ gangliosidosis type I (i.e., generalized gangliosidosis, beta-galactosidase deficiency)	88
Gaucher disease type II (i.e., glucocerebrosidase deficiency)	89
Niemann–Pick disease types A and B (i.e., sphingomyelinase deficiency)	90
Niemann–Pick disease type C	91
Mannosidosis (i.e., a-mannosidase deficiency)	92
Fucosidosis (i.e., a-fucosidase deficiency)	93
Farber disease (i.e., acid ceramidase deficiency)	94
Wolman disease (i.e., acid lipase deficiency)	95
Krabbe disease (i.e., galactocerebrosidase deficiency)	96
Mucopolysaccharidosis type VI (i.e., Maroteaux-Lamy syndrome, arylsufatase B deficiency)	97
Mucopolysaccharidosis type VII (i.e., beta-glucuronidase deficiency)	98
Mucolipidosis type II (i.e., I-cell disease)	99
Mucolipidosis type IV	100
Multiple sulfatase deficiency	101
Sialidosis type II (i.e., neuraminidase deficiency)	102
Peroxisomal Disorders	
Zellweger syndrome	103
Neonatal adrenoleukodystrophy	103
Rhizomelic chondrodysplasia punctata	103
Disorders of Metal Metabolism	
Menke kinky hair disease	104
Molybdenum cofactor deficiency	105
Sulfite oxidase deficiency	106
Neonatal hemochromatosis	107
Other Disorder	
Congenital adrenal hyperplasia	108
Carbohydrate deficient glycoprotein syndrome	109
Hereditary orotic aciduria	110
Hypophosphatasia	111
Crigler–Najjar syndrome	112
A$_1$–antitrypsin deficiency	113
Canavan disease (i.e., aspartoacylase deficiency)	114
Steroid sulfatase deficiency	115
Senger syndrome	116
Smith–Lemli–Opitz syndrome	32
Lowe syndrome	117

Affected infants are typically full term and usually appear normal at birth. The interval between birth and clinical symptoms ranges from hours to weeks. The initial findings are usually those of lethargy and poor feeding, as seen in almost any sick infant. Although sepsis is often the first consideration in infants who present in this way, these symptoms in a full-term infant with no specific risk factors strongly suggest a metabolic disorder. Infants with inborn errors of metabolism may rather quickly become debilitated and septic; therefore, it is important that the presence of sepsis not preclude consideration of other possibilities. The lethargy associated with these conditions is an early symptom of a metabolic encephalopathy that may progress to coma. Other signs of central nervous system (CNS) dysfunction, such as seizures and abnormal muscle tone, may also exist. Evidence of cerebral edema may be observed, and intracranial hemorrhage occasionally occurs (3).

An infant with an inborn error of metabolism who presents more abruptly or in whom the lethargy and poor feeding go unnoticed may first come to attention because of

TABLE 41-2

LABORATORY STUDIES FOR AN INFANT SUSPECTED OF HAVING AN INBORN ERROR OF METABOLISM

Complete blood count with differential
Urinalysis
Blood gases
Electrolytes
Blood glucose
Plasma ammonia
Urine reducing substances
Urine ketones if acidosis or hypoglycemia is present
Plasma and urine amino acids, quantitative
Urine organic acids
Plasma lactate

apnea or respiratory distress. The apnea is typically central in origin and a symptom of the metabolic encephalopathy, but tachypnea may be a symptom of an underlying metabolic acidosis, as occurs in the organic acidemias. Infants with urea cycle defects and evolving hyperammonemic coma initially exhibit central hyperventilation, which leads to respiratory alkalosis. Indeed, the finding of respiratory alkalosis in an infant with lethargy is virtually pathognomonic of hyperammonemic encephalopathy.

Vomiting is a striking feature of many of the inborn errors of metabolism associated with protein intolerance, although it is less common in the newborn than in the older infant. If persistent vomiting occurs in the neonatal period, it usually signals significant underlying disease. Inborn errors of metabolism should always be considered in the differential diagnosis. It is common for an infant to be diagnosed as having a metabolic disorder after having undergone surgery for suspected pyloric stenosis (4). Formula intolerance frequently is suspected, and many affected infants have numerous formula changes before a diagnosis finally is established.

The basic laboratory studies that should be obtained for an infant who has acute life-threatening symptoms consistent with an inborn error of metabolism are listed in Table 41-2.

HYPERAMMONEMIA

Among the most important laboratory findings associated with inborn errors of metabolism presenting with an acute encephalopathy is hyperammonemia. A plasma ammonia level should be obtained for any infant with unexplained vomiting, lethargy, or other evidence of an encephalopathy. Significant hyperammonemia is observed in a limited number of conditions. Inborn errors of metabolism, including urea cycle defects and many of the organic acidemias, are at the top of the list. Also in the differential diagnosis is a condition referred to as transient hyperammonemia of the newborn (THAN) (5). Ammonia levels in these conditions frequently exceed 1,000 μmol/L. The finding of marked hyperammonemia provides an important clue to diagnosis and indicates the need for urgent treatment to reduce the

ammonia level. The degree of neurologic impairment and developmental delay subsequently observed in infants with urea cycle defects depends on the duration of the neonatal hyperammonemic coma (6).

A flow chart for the differentiation of conditions producing significant hyperammonemia in the newborn is shown in Fig. 41-1. The timing of the onset of symptoms may provide an important clue. Infants with urea cycle defects typically do not become symptomatic until after 24 hours of age. Patients with some of the organic acidemias, such as glutaric acidemia type II, or with pyruvate carboxylase deficiency may exhibit symptomatic hyperammonemia during the first 24 hours. Symptoms in the first 24 hours are characteristic of THAN, a condition that is poorly understood but apparently not genetically determined. The typical patient with this disorder is a large premature infant (mean gestational age of 36 weeks) who has symptomatic pulmonary disease, often from birth, and severe hyperammonemia. Survivors do not have recurrent episodes of hyperammonemia and may or may not exhibit neurologic sequelae, depending on the extent of the neonatal insult. There are some affected infants who survive with normal intelligence despite extraordinarily high ammonia levels (5). The disorder has become extremely rare in recent years for unknown reasons.

Infants who develop severe hyperammonemia after 24 hours of age usually have a urea cycle defect or an organic acidemia; infants with organic acidemias typically exhibit a metabolic acidosis and ketonuria as well. Urine organic acids should always be obtained, regardless of whether or not acidosis is present. Metabolic acidosis is not a feature of the urea cycle defects. Plasma amino acid analysis is helpful in the differentiation of the specific defects in this group. Characteristic amino acid abnormalities provide a definitive diagnosis of citrullinemia and argininosuccinic aciduria. Although no diagnostic amino acid elevations are observed in carbamyl phosphate synthetase deficiency or ornithine transcarbamylase deficiency, a low or undetectable level of plasma citrulline is observed in both of these conditions. This finding is helpful in differentiating these two conditions from THAN, in which the plasma citrulline level is normal. However, plasma citrulline is not accurately measured in all laboratories performing amino acid analysis, probably because it is important in few other clinical settings. In clinical situations in which this is a critical diagnostic test, samples should be sent to laboratories with expertise in the differentiation of urea cycle defects. Carbamyl phosphate synthetase deficiency and ornithine transcarbamylase deficiency may be differentiated by measuring urine orotic acid, which is low in the former and elevated in the latter. The pattern of inheritance of the two may also help to differentiate them; ornithine transcarbamylase deficiency, an X-linked disorder, rarely produces severe hyperammonemia in a female infant, whereas carbamyl phosphate synthetase deficiency, an autosomal recessive disorder, occurs with equal frequency in the two genders.

Although the clinical and laboratory evaluation outlined should lead to a specific tentative diagnosis for virtually

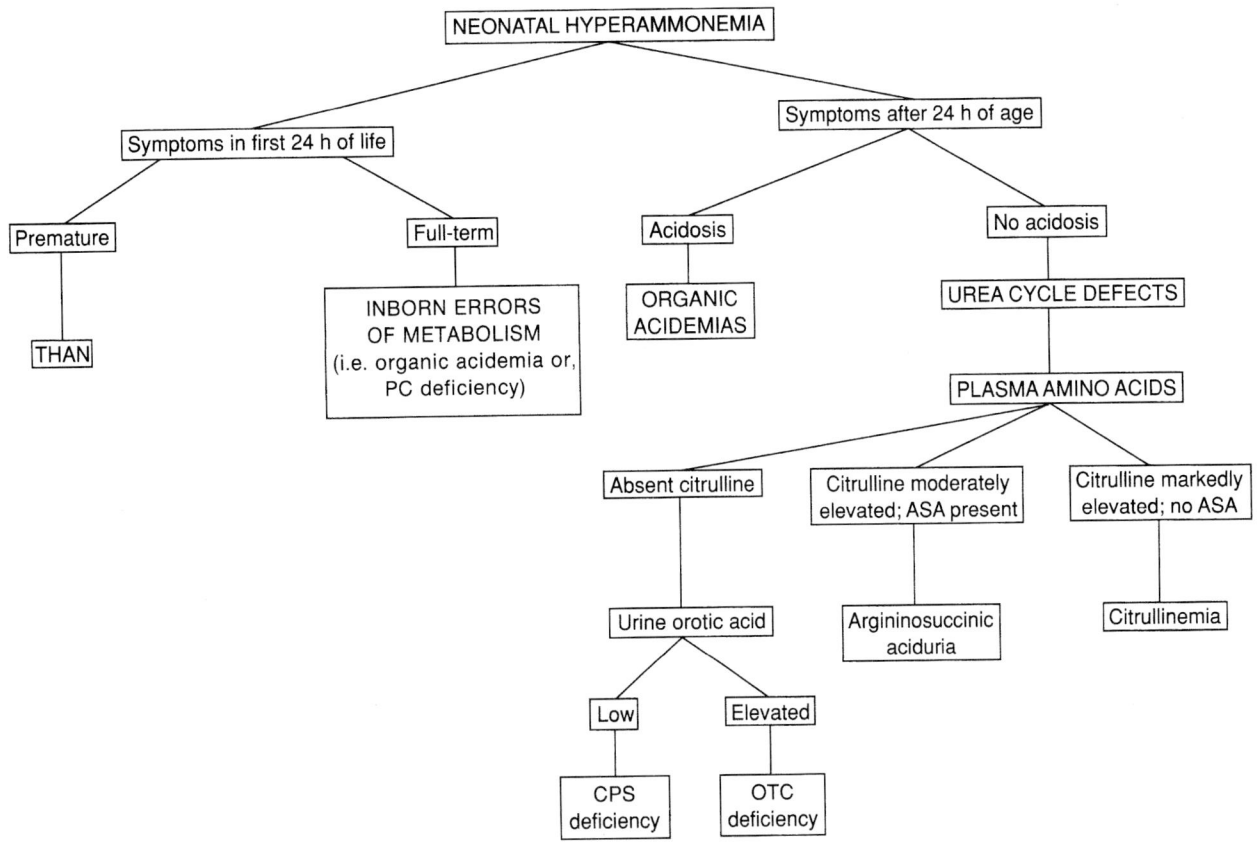

Figure 41-1   Differentiating between conditions that produce severe neonatal hyperammonemia. ASA, argininosuccinic acid; CPS, carbamyl phosphate synthetase; OTC, ornithine transcarbamylase; PC, pyruvate carboxylase; THAN, transient hyperammonemia of the newborn.

all patients, liver biopsy may be indicated for enzymatic confirmation of the diagnoses of carbamyl phosphate synthetase and ornithine transcarbamylase deficiencies, because these diagnoses dictate rigid lifelong therapy or consideration of hepatic transplantation. Acute treatment should be based on the presumptive diagnosis, with biopsy considered only after the infant is stabilized.

Less significant elevations of plasma ammonia than those associated with inborn errors of metabolism and THAN can be observed in a variety of other conditions associated with liver dysfunction, including sepsis, generalized herpes simplex infection, and perinatal asphyxia. Liver function studies should be obtained in evaluating the significance of moderate elevations of plasma ammonia. However, even in cases of severe hepatic necrosis, it is rare for ammonia levels to exceed 500 µmol/L (7). Mild transient hyperammonemia with ammonia levels as high as twice normal is relatively common in the newborn, especially in the premature infant, and is usually asymptomatic. It appears to be of no clinical significance, and there are no long-term neurologic sequelae (8).

METABOLIC ACIDOSIS

The second important laboratory feature of many of the inborn errors of metabolism during acute episodes of illness

is metabolic acidosis with an increased anion gap, readily demonstrable by measurement of arterial blood gases or serum electrolytes and bicarbonate. A flow chart for the evaluation of infants with this finding is shown in Fig. 41-2. An increased anion gap (greater than 16) is observed in many inborn errors of metabolism and in most other conditions producing metabolic acidosis in the neonate. The differential diagnosis of metabolic acidosis with a normal anion gap essentially is limited to two conditions, diarrhea and renal tubular acidosis. Among the inborn errors, the largest group typically associated with overwhelming metabolic acidosis in infancy is the group of organic acidemias, including methylmalonic acidemia, propionic acidemia, and isovaleric acidemia. The list of disorders in this group has expanded dramatically as new disorders have been defined through the use of organic acid analysis.

In addition to specific organic acid intermediates, plasma lactate often is elevated in organic acidemias as a result of secondary interference with coenzyme A (CoA) metabolism. Neutropenia and thrombocytopenia commonly are observed and further underscore the clinical similarity of these disorders to neonatal sepsis. Hyperammonemia, sometimes as dramatic as that associated with urea cycle defects, is seen commonly but not uniformly in critically ill neonates with organic acidemias.

The metabolic acidosis associated with organic acidemias and certain other inborn errors of metabolism may have

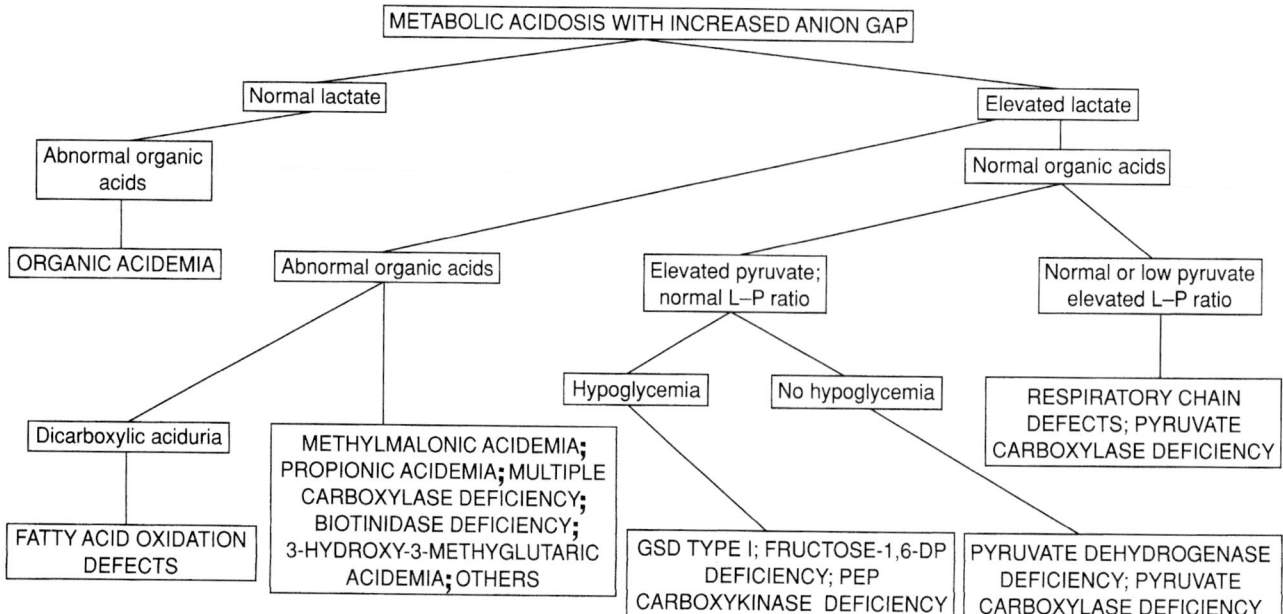

Figure 41-2 Evaluating metabolic acidosis in the young infant. fructose-1,6-DP, fructose-1,6-bisphosphatase; GSD, glycogen storage disease; L/P, lactate/pyruvate.

significant adverse impact on many different organ systems, which may lead to the erroneous diagnosis of a wide variety of seemingly unrelated disorders. I had the experience of caring for an infant with isovaleric acidemia who presented at 10 days of age with respiratory distress, severe metabolic acidosis, a dilated heart, and poor cardiac output. The infant was suspected of having the hypoplastic left heart syndrome or other severe congenital heart disease. Cardiac catheterization was performed, even though members of the nursing staff had observed that the infant had a strong unpleasant odor, reminiscent of sweaty feet. Personnel in the catheterization laboratory also noticed that the blood had a strong peculiar odor, but it was not until 18 hours later, long after significant heart disease had been ruled out, that the diagnosis of metabolic disease was first considered. Despite attempts at therapy with dialysis and other measures, the child succumbed to the disease. In this case, the metabolic acidosis led to poor function of the myocardium and not the reverse.

Another child subsequently found to have methylmalonic acidemia was admitted through the emergency room with severe metabolic acidosis and a tight, distended abdomen with evidence of multiple air–fluid levels on X-ray films. The history revealed that the child had fed poorly since birth and had repeated episodes of vomiting despite several formula changes. Intestinal obstruction was suspected, and the child was taken to the operating room, in which most of the small intestine was found to be infarcted, presumably secondary to the acidosis and poor tissue perfusion. No anatomic abnormalities were found. Postoperatively, metabolic disease was considered, and the diagnosis of a vitamin B12-responsive form of methylmalonic acidemia was made. The infant died of complications of the disease even though the early diagnosis and

treatment of this disorder, before the terminal episode, should have been associated with a good prognosis.

Defects in pyruvate metabolism or in the respiratory chain may lead to primary lactic acidosis presenting as severe metabolic acidosis in infancy (9,10). Unlike most of the other conditions presenting acutely in the newborn, the clinical features of these disorders are unrelated to protein intake. Disorders in this group should be considered in patients with lactic acidosis who have normal or nondiagnostic urine organic acids. Differentiation of the various disorders in this group can be facilitated by measuring plasma pyruvate and calculating the lactate/pyruvate ratio. A normal ratio (less than 25) suggests a defect in pyruvate dehydrogenase (PDH) or in gluconeogenesis, and an elevated ratio (greater than 25) suggests pyruvate carboxylase deficiency or a mitochondrial respiratory chain defect.

Not all infants with life-threatening metabolic disease have metabolic acidosis or hyperammonemia. For example, patients with nonketotic hyperglycinemia typically present in the neonatal period with evidence of severe and progressive CNS dysfunction, but do not exhibit metabolic acidosis or hyperammonemia (11). Even patients with galactosemia rarely may present with symptoms of acute CNS toxicity, which may progress to cerebral edema, when galactose-1-phosphate levels rise precipitously. Therefore, a series of laboratory studies designed to screen for inborn errors of metabolism should be obtained for any infant with clinical findings suggesting an inborn error of metabolism, even if metabolic acidosis and hyperammonemia are not present. These studies are listed in Table 41-2. Most are self-explanatory. Although not available in many hospital laboratories, amino acid and organic acid analysis can be obtained in any part of the country through reference

TABLE 41-3

DISORDERS ASSOCIATED WITH NONGLUCOSE REDUCING SUBSTANCES IN URINE

Disorder	Compound
Galactosemia	Galactose
Hereditary fructose intolerance	Fructose
Hereditary tyrosinemia	p-Hydroxy-phenylpyruvic acid
Galactokinase deficiency	Galactose
Essential fructosuria	Fructose
Pentosuria	Xylulose
Severe liver disease with secondary galactose intolerance	Galactose

laboratories or through referral of samples to medical center genetics units. It is important to insist that any reference laboratory used for this purpose provide prompt test results and reference ranges and provide interpretation of abnormal results.

Urine testing for reducing substances should be performed using Benedict reagent (Clinitest tablets, Miles, Elkhart, IN). If the result is positive, the urine should be tested for glucose by dipstick. A nonglucose reducing substance in the urine is probably galactose, but there are other possibilities (Table 41-3).

Several disorders associated with an acute metabolic encephalopathy in the neonate deserve special mention because they typically are not associated with hyperammonemia or metabolic acidosis. One of these is nonketotic hyperglycinemia, a condition that typically results in severe and progressive CNS dysfunction, including obtundation, seizures, and altered muscle tone. Routine laboratory studies all yield normal findings. The first diagnostic clue is usually the finding of elevated glycine on plasma amino acid analysis. The diagnosis is confirmed by measurement of cerebrospinal fluid (CSF) glycine and demonstration of an elevated CSF to plasma glycine ratio. Although therapy of infants with nonketotic hyperglycinemia has been attempted with dietary protein restriction, sodium benzoate, and a variety of other drugs, the results have been disappointing. Most infants with this disorder die or exhibit significant neurologic impairment.

A second disorder that produces a progressive encephalopathy with no clues on routine laboratory studies is molybdenum cofactor deficiency. The neurologic findings in the affected infant are virtually indistinguishable from those associated with hypoxic-ischemic encephalopathy. Surviving infants exhibit similar neurologic sequelae including cerebral palsy, mental retardation, and seizures. The diagnosis may be suggested by the finding of hypouricemia or, beyond the neonatal period, by ectopia lentis noted on ophthalmologic examination. If it is suspected, urine should be screened for the presence of sulfites, a finding attributable to a deficiency of the enzyme sulfite oxidase, which accompanies the disorder.

The inborn errors of metabolism most likely to be associated with an acute encephalopathy in the newborn are summarized in Table 41-4. The typical laboratory findings in each condition or group of conditions also are listed.

EMERGENCY TREATMENT OF THE INFANT WITH AN ACUTE METABOLIC ENCEPHALOPATHY

When an inborn error of metabolism, such as an organic acidemia or urea cycle defect, is suspected in a critically ill infant, immediate treatment should be initiated even if a definitive diagnosis may not yet be established. Within 48 to 72 hours, the results of amino acid and organic acid analyses should be available, allowing diagnostic confirmation in

TABLE 41-4

MAJOR INBORN ERRORS OF METABOLISM PRESENTING IN THE NEONATE AS AN ACUTE ENCEPHALOPATHY

Disorders	Characteristic Laboratory Findings
Organic acidemias (includes MMA, PA, IVA, MCD and many less common conditions)	Metabolic acidosis with increased anion gap; elevated plasma and urine ketones; variably elevated plasma ammonia and lactate; abnormal urine organic acids
Urea cycle defects	Respiratory alkalosis, no metaboalic acidosis; markedly elevated plasma ammonia; elevated urine orotic acid in OTCD; abnormal plasma amino acids
Maple syrup urine disease	Metabolic acidosis with increased anion gap; elevated plasma and urine ketones; abnormal plasma amino acids
Non-ketotic hyperglycinemia	No acid–base or electrolyte abnormalities; normal ammonia; abnormal plasma amino acids
Molybdenum cofactor deficiency	No acid–base or electrolyte abnormalities; normal ammonia; normal amino and organic acids; low serum uric acid; elevated sulfites in urine

IVA, isovaleric acidemia; MCD, multiple carboxylase deficiency; MMA, methylmalonic acidemia; OTCD, ornithine transcarbamylase deficiency; PA, propionic acidemia.

most cases. Appropriate and aggressive treatment before the confirmation of a diagnosis may be life saving and may avert or reduce the neurologic sequelae of some of these disorders. The immediate treatment of infants with disorders in this group has two primary goals. The first is the removal of accumulated metabolites, such as organic acid intermediates or ammonia. At the first suspicion of a disorder associated with protein intolerance, protein intake in the form of breast milk, infant formula, or hyperalimentation should be discontinued immediately. In critically ill infants with hyperammonemia, arrangements should be made for hemodialysis. Although peritoneal dialysis, continuous arteriovenous hemoperfusion, and exchange transfusion all have been used in the past to lower plasma ammonia levels, all are substantially less effective than hemodialysis (12). In infants who are comatose, ventilator dependent, or exhibit evidence of cerebral edema, dialysis should be instituted immediately without waiting to see if there is a response to dietary manipulation, medication, or other less aggressive therapy. Maximal supportive care should be provided simultaneously. In patients suspected of having a urea cycle defect because of significant hyperammonemia without acidosis, an infusion of 6 cc/kg of 10% arginine hydrochloride (HC1) (0.6 g/kg) can be given intravenously over 90 minutes. In patients with citrullinemia and argininosuccinic aciduria, this often results in a precipitous drop in the plasma ammonia level. An intravenous arginine preparation is commercially available and should be readily accessible from any hospital pharmacy.

If an organic acidemia is suspected, vitamin B12 (1 mg) should be given intramuscularly in case the patient has a vitamin B12-responsive form of methylmalonic acidemia. Biotin (10 mg) should be given orally or by nasogastric tube, because some patients with multiple carboxylase deficiency are biotin responsive. If acidosis exists, intravenous bicarbonate should be administered liberally. Calculations of bicarbonate requirements appropriate for the treatment of other conditions rarely are adequate in these disorders because of ongoing production of organic acids or lactate. The acid–base status should be monitored frequently, with therapy adjusted accordingly.

After removing toxic metabolites, the second major goal of therapy in infants with inborn errors of metabolism should be to prevent catabolism. Ten percent glucose should be liberally administered intravenously, because it is important to provide as many calories as possible. Intravenous lipids can be given to infants with urea cycle defects and other disorders in which dietary fat plays no role. Protein should not be withheld indefinitely. If clinical improvement is observed and a final diagnosis has not been established, some amino acid intake should be provided after 2 to 3 days of complete protein restriction. Essential amino acids or total protein can be provided orally or intravenously at an initial dose of 0.5 g protein/kg body weight/24 hours. This should be increased incrementally to 1.0 g/kg/24 hours and held at that level until the diagnostic evaluation is complete and plans can be made for definitive long-term therapy. Therapy should be planned in conjunction with a geneticist or specialist in metabolic disease. Until then, supplemental calories and nutrients can be provided orally using protein-free diet powder (Product 80056, Mead Johnson, or Prophree, Ross Laboratories).

The chronic therapy of urea cycle defects and most of the organic acidemias involves restriction of dietary protein. Depending on the specific diagnosis, this may be accomplished by simple restriction of total protein intake in breast milk or standard infant formula or by use of special formulas designed for individual inborn errors of metabolism. Formulas have been developed for many of the more common metabolic disorders and are commercially available. These specialized formulas typically are deficient in one or several specific amino acids. Dietary treatment alone may be effective in management of some patients with organic acidemias and in several disorders of amino acid metabolism, such as maple syrup urine disease.

In several of the vitamin-responsive disorders, such as methylmalonic acidemia, multiple carboxylase deficiency, and homocystinuria, dietary protein restriction may be combined with specific cofactor therapy. In the organic acidemias and certain other disorders, l-carnitine, usually beginning with a dose of 100 mg/kg/d, may be given. Acyl-CoAs accumulating in these disorders combine with carnitine to produce acylcarnitine that are water soluble and excreted in the urine. Without treatment, many patients with these disorders develop a secondary carnitine deficiency. Treatment with exogenous carnitine prevents the development of symptoms of carnitine deficiency and provides a measure of protection against recurrent episodes of metabolic decompensation by providing an augmented mechanism for excretion of accumulated metabolites.

Patients with urea cycle defects require supplementation with oral arginine or, in some cases, citrulline, which is converted to arginine in the body. In normal persons, adequate amounts of arginine are synthesized via the urea cycle. Patients with a defect in urea synthesis have deficient arginine production and must depend on dietary supplementation. In the case of carbamyl phosphate synthetase and ornithine transcarbamylase deficiencies, the most severe of the urea cycle defects, drug therapy also is required. These disorders were formerly almost uniformly lethal in the neonatal period. The development of novel drugs that provide an alternate pathway for waste nitrogen excretion has allowed survival of many affected infants (13). Sodium benzoate and sodium phenylacetate were the agents originally used, but these have been replaced largely for oral use by sodium phenylbutyrate.

Despite rigorous therapy and intensive surveillance, patients with urea cycle defects remain at risk for intercurrent episodes of hyperammonemia, which may result in death or neurologic sequelae. The risk appears to be greatest for patients with carbamyl phosphate synthetase and ornithine transcarbamylase deficiency. Liver transplantation should be considered seriously for patients with these disorders, if they can be stabilized.

HYPOGLYCEMIA

Hypoglycemia and its associated symptoms occasionally may be seen in infants with disorders of protein intolerance, but it more commonly is seen in disorders of carbohydrate metabolism or of fatty acid oxidation. Among the best known inborn errors of metabolism associated with hypoglycemia are the glycogen storage diseases, of which types I and III are the most likely to be associated with manifestations in the neonatal period. The hypoglycemia in these disorders is related to the inability of the liver to release glucose from glycogen, and it is most profound during periods of fasting. Hypoglycemia, hepatomegaly, and lactic acidosis are prominent features of these disorders. Hypoglycemia is not a feature of glycogen storage disease type II (Pompe disease) because cytoplasmic glycogen metabolism and release are normal in this disorder, in which glycogen accumulates within lysosomes as a result of the deficiency of the lysosomal enzyme a-1,4-glucosidase. The clinical manifestations of this disorder include macro-glossia, hypotonia, cardiomegaly with congestive heart failure, and hepatomegaly. Cardiomegaly is the most striking and may be apparent in the neonatal period. Congestive heart failure is the cause of death in most cases.

A disorder that presents clinically with findings virtually indistinguishable from the hepatic glycogen storage diseases types I and III is fructose-1,6-bisphosphatase deficiency, a disorder of gluconeogenesis. Several other disorders of gluconeogenesis have been described. The basic immediate treatment of all of these disorders is frequent feedings and glucose administration. The definitive diagnosis is made by liver biopsy and assay of appropriate hepatic enzymes. In some cases, enzymatic assays can be performed using lymphocytes or cultured skin fibroblasts.

A number of inherited defects in fatty acid oxidation have been identified in infants presenting with hypoglycemia. Although many of the disorders in this group typically present after 2 months of age, neonatal manifestations may be observed. These disorders are important because of their apparent frequency and because of the variability of the initial presentation. Affected infants have an impaired capacity to use stored fat for fuel during periods of fasting and readily deplete their glycogen stores. Despite the development of hypoglycemia, acetyl CoA production is diminished, and ketone production is impaired. The hypoglycemia occurring in these conditions typically is characterized as nonketotic, although small amounts of ketones may be produced. Hypoglycemia may occur as an isolated finding or may be accompanied by many of the other biochemical derangements typically associated with Reye's syndrome, such as hyperammonemia, metabolic acidosis, and elevated transaminases. Hepatomegaly may or may not be present. Any infant presenting with findings suggesting Reye's syndrome should be evaluated for fatty acid oxidation defects. As the incidence of true Reye's syndrome has decreased, most children presenting at any age with this constellation of findings have an inherited metabolic disorder.

The most common of the fatty acid oxidation defects is medium-chain acyl-CoA dehydrogenase deficiency, which is estimated to occur in 1 of 15,000 births, an incidence similar to that observed for phenylketonuria (PKU) (14, 15). It is among the most common inborn errors of metabolism. In addition to presenting as nonketotic hypoglycemia or a Reye's-like syndrome, it may present as sudden death or an acute life-threatening event. Many infants diagnosed as having medium-chain acyl-CoA dehydrogenase deficiency have a history of a sibling who died of sudden infant death syndrome (16). Fat accumulation in the liver or muscle of any infant who dies unexpectedly should strongly suggest the possibility of this or a related disorder of fatty acid oxidation. Very-long-chain fatty acyl-CoA dehydrogenase deficiency is associated with similar clinical findings, although there may be evidence of a significant cardiomyopathy. Infants with this defect may present with cardiac arrhythmias or unexplained cardiac arrest. Defects in the carnitine cycle or in carnitine uptake also may lead to a profound defect in fatty acid oxidation and result in sudden neonatal death.

The accumulation of fatty acyl-CoAs in patients with fatty acid oxidation defects leads to a secondary carnitine deficiency, probably as a result of excretion of excess acylcarnitine in the urine (17,18). Urine organic acid analysis and measurement of serum carnitine and analysis of the plasma acylcarnitine profile are the most helpful laboratory studies in the initial screening for defects in fatty acid oxidation. These studies are sufficient to establish the diagnosis of medium-chain acyl-CoA dehydrogenase deficiency, which is associated with the presence of a characteristic metabolite, octanoylcarnitine, on the acylcarnitine profile. Enzymatic assays may be necessary for the definitive diagnosis of some of the fatty acid oxidation defects. As is true for the defects in carbohydrate metabolism leading to hypoglycemia, treatment of the fatty acid oxidation defects involves avoidance of fasting and provision of adequate glucose. Restriction of dietary fat intake and supplemental l-carnitine therapy at a dose of 50 to 100 mg/kg/d is recommended. With appropriate therapy, patients with medium-chain acyl-CoA dehydrogenase deficiency appear to have an excellent prognosis. The prognosis for the other fatty acid oxidation defects is more variable.

JAUNDICE AND LIVER DYSFUNCTION

Jaundice or other evidence of liver dysfunction may be the presenting finding in a number of inherited metabolic disorders in the neonatal period. These are listed in Table 41-5, along with the laboratory studies useful in diagnosis. For most of the inborn errors of metabolism associated with jaundice, the elevated serum bilirubin is of the direct-reacting type. This generalization does not include those inborn errors of erythrocyte metabolism, such as

TABLE 41-5
INBORN ERRORS OF METABOLISM ASSOCIATED WITH NEONATAL LIVER DISEASE AND LABORATORY STUDIES USEFUL IN DIAGNOSIS

Disorder	Laboratory Studies
Galactosemia	Urine reducing substances; red blood cell galactose-1-phosphate uridyl transferase
Hereditary tyrosinemia	Plasma quantitative amino acids; urine succinylacetone
a_1-antitrypsin deficiency	Quantitative serum alpha$_1$-antitrypsin; protease inhibitor (Pi) typing
Neonatal hemochromatosis	Serum ferritin; liver biopsy; buccal biopsy
Zellweger syndrome	Plasma very long chain fatty acids
Niemann-Pick disease type C	Skin biopsy for fibroblast culture; studies of cholesterol esterification and accumulation
Glycogen storage disease type IV (brancher deficiency)	Liver biopsy for histology and biochemical analysis or skin biopsy with assay of branching enzyme in cultured fibroblasts

glucose-6-phosphate dehydrogenase deficiency or pyruvate kinase deficiency, which occasionally are responsible for hemo-lytic disease in the newborn. The best-known metabolic disease associated with jaundice is galactosemia, in which the deficiency of the enzyme galactose-1-phosphate uridylyl transferase results in an accumulation of galactose-1-phosphate and other metabolites, such as galactitol, which are thought to have a direct toxic effect on the liver and on other organs. Jaundice and liver dysfunction in this disorder are progressive and usually appear at the end of the first or during the second week of life, with vomiting, diarrhea, poor weight gain, and eventual cataract formation if the infant is receiving breast milk or a galactose-containing formula. Hypoglycemia may be observed. The disease may present initially with indirect hyperbilirubinemia resulting from hemolysis secondary to high levels of galactose-1-phosphate in erythrocytes. Alternatively, the effects of acute galactose toxicity on the brain rarely may cause the CNS symptoms to predominate and, in some cases, *Escherichia coli* sepsis is the presenting problem.

If galactosemia is suspected, the urine should be tested simultaneously with Benedict reagent and with a glucose oxidase method. The glucose oxidase method is specific for glucose, and Benedict reagent can detect any reducing substance. A negative dipstick for glucose with a positive Benedict reaction means that a nonglucose reducing substance is present. With appropriate clinical findings, this is most likely to be galactose. Paper or thin-layer chromatography can be used to identify positively the reducing substance. If a child with galactosemia has been on intravenous fluids and recently has not been receiving galactose in the diet, galactose may not be present in the urine.

If the diagnosis of galactosemia is suspected, whether or not reducing substances are found in the urine, galactose-containing feedings should be discontinued immediately and replaced by soy formula or other lactose-free formula, pending the results of appropriate enzyme assays on erythrocytes to confirm the diagnosis. Untreated galactosemics, if they survive the neonatal period, have persis-

tent liver disease, cataracts, and severe mental retardation. Many affected infants die of *E. coli* sepsis in the neonatal period, and the early onset of sepsis may alter the presentation of the disorder (19).

Treatment of the disorder by maintenance of strict dietary restriction of galactose, if started early, results in complete reversal of liver disease and enables many affected individuals to develop normal or near-normal intelligence. Unfortunately, there continues to be an increased incidence of mental retardation even among treated patients. Additionally, there are some late sequelae of the disorder that appear to be unaffected by current therapy. These include premature ovarian failure in females and a late-onset neurologic syndrome involving ataxia and tremors in both genders (20,21). Many states have newborn screening programs for galactosemia, but clinical manifestations of the disorder often appear before the results of screening studies are available; therefore, it is critical that physicians remain alert to this possibility.

Another inborn error of metabolism that occasionally presents in the newborn period with jaundice, hepatomegaly, and the presence of reducing substances in the urine is hereditary fructose intolerance, which is characterized by episodes of profound hypoglycemia, vomiting, and metabolic acidosis. This disorder is seen uncommonly in the neonate, because most newborns are not exposed immediately to a fructose-containing diet unless they have been given a soy formula with sucrose as the carbohydrate source. In the uncommon event that an infant who has been receiving fructose should present with these findings, this diagnosis should be considered. Analysis of the urine reveals the presence of a nonglucose reducing substance that can be demonstrated by chromatography to be fructose. Treatment involves elimination of fructose from the diet and results in complete resolution of all clinical signs and symptoms. Confirmation of the diagnosis is by assay of the deficient enzyme fructose-1-phosphate aldolase in liver tissue, but this rarely is necessary.

a1-Antitrypsin deficiency, a puzzling disorder that is among the most common of all inherited metabolic diseases, also may present with neonatal jaundice (22). The clinical manifestations of this disorder may be identical to those of traditional neonatal or giant cell hepatitis, and a determination of serum a1-antitrypsin should be a part of the initial evaluation of all children presenting with this syndrome. Infants with deficient levels of a1-antitrypsin on quantitative analysis should have protease inhibitor typing performed to confirm the diagnosis. There is no specific treatment for the liver disease associated with a1-antitrypsin deficiency, but approximately one-half of all affected infants eventually exhibit complete resolution of the liver dysfunction. Others may progress to end-stage disease and require liver transplantation. A history of chronic pulmonary disease in adult family members may be obtained.

Hereditary tyrosinemia is another disorder that presents with liver disease in early infancy. The biochemical hallmarks of this disorder include marked elevations of plasma tyrosine and methionine and generalized amino-aciduria with a disproportionate increase in the excretion of tyrosine. However, these findings are relatively nonspecific and may be observed as a secondary phenomenon in other forms of liver disease. Hereditary tyrosinemia once was among the most difficult of inborn errors of metabolism to diagnose clinically. The finding of succinylacetone in the urine of patients with this disease has led to a helpful diagnostic test for the disorder (23). It also has become possible to establish the diagnosis definitively by demonstrating a deficiency of the enzyme fumarylacetoacetate fumarylhydrolase in lymphocytes and cultured skin fibroblasts of affected individuals (24).

Neonatal hemochromatosis, a recently described and poorly understood disorder, may be the most common cause of congenital cirrhosis. Its fulminating course distinguishes it from many of the other metabolic disorders associated with neonatal liver disease. In addition to being associated with severe liver failure from birth, the disorder is characterized by distinctive hepatic morphology and hepatic and extrahepatic parenchymal iron deposition. Serum ferritin and iron typically are elevated, whereas total transferrin is low, but these findings are not diagnostic. The definitive diagnosis is established by liver biopsy or autopsy. If liver biopsy is contraindicated because of a secondary coagulopathy, biopsy of the salivary glands or buccal mucosa is a useful alternative. Most affected infants succumb to the disorder during the early weeks of life. The only clearly effective mode of therapy is liver transplantation; intensive chelation therapy may be attempted but largely has been unsuccessful. At present, it is not clear whether iron storage is the primary defect or is secondary to fetal liver disease that may be causally heterogeneous. There are familial recurrences, so at least some cases appear to have a genetic basis, although the mode of inheritance is not well established.

Less common metabolic causes of neonatal liver dysfunction include Niemann–Pick disease type C and glycogen storage disease type IV. Infants with Niemann–Pick disease type C exhibit cholestatic jaundice, which typically resolves by several months of age. They then are clinically normal for a period of months to years before developing findings of a degenerative neurologic disorder. Infants with glycogen storage disease type IV accumulate an abnormal form of glycogen in the liver as a result of a deficiency of the glycogen branching enzyme. This leads to progressive cirrhosis and generalized hepatic dysfunction. Hypoglycemia is not a prominent feature, as it is in some other forms of glycogen storage disease.

Zellweger syndrome, formerly referred to as the cerebrohepatorenal syndrome, is another cause of neonatal jaundice and hepatic dysfunction, but it usually is recognizable clinically because of the associated hypotonia and dysmorphic features. It is the prototype of the peroxisome assembly disorders and is associated with generalized peroxisomal dysfunction.

In contrast to disorders in which there is an elevation of the direct-reacting bilirubin, a persistent elevation of indirect bilirubin beyond the limits of physiologic jaundice, without evidence of hemolysis, suggests the diagnosis of the Crigler–Najjar syndrome. The hyperbilirubinemia in this disorder is related to a partial or complete deficiency of glucuronyl transferase, the liver enzyme responsible for the normal conjugation of bilirubin to bilirubin diglucuronide. There is no effective long-term therapy for all patients with this disorder, but the standard modalities of phototherapy and exchange transfusion may prevent the development of kernicterus in the neonatal period (25,26). Hepatic transplantation has been performed successfully in patients with this disorder. Patients with a partial deficiency of the enzyme may respond to phenobarbital therapy (26).

FINDINGS SUGGESTIVE OF A STORAGE DISEASE

Many of the well-known lipid storage diseases typically do not present in the neonatal period. Among those that occasionally may be associated with hepatosplenomegaly in the neonatal period are GM1-gangliosidosis type I, Gaucher disease, Niemann–Pick disease, and Wolman disease. The glycogen storage diseases that are associated with hepatomegaly in the newborn have previously been discussed in reference to hypoglycemia. Infants with the most common mucopolysaccharidoses, such as the Hurler and Hunter syndromes, uncommonly exhibit clinical abnormalities in the first month of life. Newborns with the typical features of these syndromes, such as coarse facial features, hepatosplenomegaly, skeletal abnormalities, and hernias, are more likely to have GM1-gangliosidosis or a mucolipidosis, such as I-cell disease. Beta-glucuronidase deficiency, also classified as mucopolysaccharidosis type VII, may present in the neonatal period with features virtually indistinguishable clinically from those seen later in the Hurler and Hunter syndromes. An infantile form of sialidosis (i.e., neuraminidase deficiency) typically is associated with findings at birth. The clinical manifestations of several of these conditions may be so severe in utero that fetal hydrops develops.

If one of these disorders is suspected, urine screening tests for mucopolysaccharides and oligosaccharides should be performed. These can be helpful diagnostically, but negative results do not rule out the possibility of a storage disorder. False-positive mucopolysaccharide spot tests are commonly observed in neonates. The definitive diagnosis of most disorders of lipid or mucopolysaccharide metabolism is made by appropriate biochemical studies on leukocytes or cultured skin fibroblasts.

ABNORMAL ODOR

Abnormal body or urinary odor, more commonly observed by nurses or mothers rather than physicians, is an important but often overlooked clue to the diagnosis of several of the inborn errors of metabolism and may be the most specific clinical finding in these patients. It is best described for PKU, for which the urine was found to have a peculiar musty odor years before the biochemical basis of the disease was understood. In the acutely ill neonate with an abnormal odor, isovaleric acidemia, glutaric acidemia type II, and maple syrup urine disease are the most likely entities to be encountered. In maple syrup urine disease, the urine has a distinctive sweet odor, said to be reminiscent of maple syrup or burnt sugar. The odor associated with isovaleric acidemia and glutaric acidemia type II is pungent and unpleasant and similar to that of sweaty feet.

DYSMORPHIC FEATURES

There formerly appeared to be a clear distinction between inborn errors of metabolism and dysmorphic syndromes, both of which may be inherited in a similar fashion. Infants with inherited metabolic disease were thought to be phenotypically normal at birth, with no evidence of major or minor structural anomalies. It is becoming increasingly apparent that inherited metabolic disorders may be associated with consistent patterns of birth defects, suggesting that metabolic derangements in utero may disrupt the normal process of fetal development.

This phenomenon is illustrated clearly by the group of disorders associated with multiple defects in peroxisomal enzymes, including those involved in fatty acid oxidation and plasmalogen synthesis (27,28). These include Zellweger syndrome, neonatal adrenoleukodystrophy, and several variant conditions, all of which are associated with congenital hypotonia and dysmorphic features, such as epicanthal folds, Brushfield spots, large fontanels, simian creases, and renal cysts. Patients with glutaric acidemia type II, one of the organic acidemias, have a characteristic phenotype, including a high forehead,

hypertelorism, low-set ears, abdominal wall defects, palpably enlarged kidneys, hypospadias, and rocker bottom feet (29,30). An energy-deficient mechanism, referred to as fuel-mediated teratogenesis, similar to that postulated for maternal diabetes mellitus, has been suggested to explain these findings. Several of the other organic acidemias, such as mevalonic aciduria, and 3-hydroxy-isobutyric aciduria, have been associated with multiple dysmorphic features.

Some infants with pyruvate dehydrogenase (PDH) deficiency have dysmorphic facial features resembling those observed in the fetal alcohol syndrome (FAS) (31). The specific findings observed include a narrow forehead with frontal bossing, a broad nasal bridge, short nose with anteverted nostrils, and a long philtrum. The resemblance to FAS has been explained by suggesting that there is a common mechanism in the two disorders, involving a deficiency of PDH activity. It has been postulated that, in FAS, acetaldehyde from the maternal circulation inhibits fetal PDH, which leads to malformations.

The Smith–Lemli–Opitz syndrome is an autosomal recessive disorder associated with a wide range of malformations, including dysmorphic facies, cleft palate, congenital heart disease, hypospadias, polydactyly, and 2–3 syndactyly of the feet. Recent observations have revealed that this disorder is an inborn error of cholesterol biosynthesis. Affected infants have decreased levels of plasma cholesterol accompanied by markedly elevated levels of the cholesterol precursor 7-dehydrocholesterol (32).

Isolated malformations may be even more commonly associated with inherited metabolic disorders than are specific malformation patterns. Patients with nonketotic hyperglycinemia frequently have agenesis of the corpus callosum and may have gyral malformations related to defects in neuronal migration as well (33). Patients with PDH deficiency also may exhibit agenesis of the corpus callosum (34). It is not uncommon for patients with almost any of the inborn errors of metabolism to exhibit one or more dysmorphic features or anomalies that are nonspecific. The observation of dysmorphic features in an infant in no way should preclude consideration of an inherited metabolic disorder. In selected circumstances, it may heighten the clinical suspicion.

ABNORMAL EYE FINDINGS

Abnormal eye findings typically are associated with many of the inborn errors of metabolism, although they are not always found at the time of initial presentation. Cataracts classically are associated with galactosemia and other disorders of galactose metabolism, but also are observed in disorders such as Zellweger syndrome and Lowe syndrome. Dislocated lenses, seen in homocystinuria, molybdenum cofactor deficiency, and sulfite oxidase deficiency, may be found as early as the first month of life and are an important clue to diagnosis. Retinal degenerative changes are typical of the peroxisomal disorders, including Zellweger syndrome

TABLE 41-6

EYE ABNORMALITIES ASSOCIATED WITH INBORN ERRORS OF METABOLISM

Eye Finding	Associated Disorders
Cataracts	Galactosemia
	Homocystinuria
	Lowe syndrome
	Zellweger syndrome
	Rhizomelic chondrodysplasia punctata
	Senger syndrome
	Hypophosphatasia
Ectopia lentis	Homocystinuria
	Molybdenum cofactor deficiency
	Sulfite oxidase deficiency
Cherry red spot	Niemann–Pick disease types A and B
	Gaucher disease type II
	GM_2 gangliosidosis (Tay–Sachs; Sandhoff)
	Sialidosis type II
	Farber disease
Corneal clouding	Mucopolysaccharidoses
	Mucolipidoses
	Lowe syndrome
	Homocystinuria
Pigmentary retinopathy	Zellweger syndrome
	Neonatal adrenoleukodystrophy
	Long-chain 3-hydroxyacyl-CoA dehydrogenase deficiency

and neonatal adrenoleukodystrophy, and are observed in several other conditions. Other abnormalities that may be associated with inborn errors of metabolism include corneal clouding and congenital glaucoma. A careful eye examination, preferably by an ophthalmologist, should be performed whenever an inherited metabolic disorder is suspected. A summary of some of the inherited metabolic disorders associated with specific ocular abnormalities is shown in Table 41-6.

SAMPLES TO OBTAIN FROM A DYING CHILD WITH A SUSPECTED INBORN ERROR OF METABOLISM

If death appears imminent in a child suspected of having an inborn error of metabolism, it is important to obtain the appropriate samples for postmortem analysis. This is critical for resolution of the cause of death and is essential for subsequent genetic counseling and prenatal diagnosis. The following samples should be collected and stored: urine, frozen; plasma, separated from whole blood and frozen; and a small snip of skin obtained using sterile technique and stored at room temperature or 37°C in tissue culture medium, if available, or sterile saline. The latter sample can be obtained by slipping a 25-gauge needle under the skin, lifting the skin, and snipping a 2- to 3-mm ellipse with a sterile scissors, which can be found in a suture removal tray. The skin should be cleansed with alcohol. If an autopsy is performed, a sample of unfixed liver

tissue should be obtained as soon as possible after death and frozen at −20°C for subsequent biochemical studies. Additional tissue should be preserved for electron microscopy. If consent for autopsy is denied, consent for a postmortem needle biopsy of the liver should be requested. The liver tissue should be frozen in total or in part if histologic studies appear to be indicated. As soon as possible after death, the case should be reviewed with a metabolic specialist and plans made for the transport of samples to the appropriate laboratory.

NEWBORN SCREENING FOR INHERITED METABOLIC DISORDERS

All 50 states and the District of Columbia in the United States and many other countries have newborn screening programs in place for genetic disorders. However, there are significant state-to-state differences in the disorders that are included, the methods of screening, and follow-up. Therefore, physicians must become familiar with the newborn screening protocol in the state or country in which they are practicing. The recent development of the technology of tandem mass spectroscopy has led many states to reexamine their newborn screening practices and many are now moving toward implementation of expanded newborn screening using this technology. Tandem mass spectroscopy (MS/MS) allows for the performance of a complete acylcarnitine profile and amino acid profile on the filter paper blood specimen and is being used in an increasing number of states and countries to screen for organic acid and fatty acid oxidation disorders and an increased number of amino acid disorders, including maple syrup urine disease, homocystinuria, and hereditary tyrosinemia. Phenylketonuria is also detected through MS/MS, replacing testing methods previously used for this disorder which was routinely screened for in all states and the District of Columbia.

The only other disorder that is a routine component of newborn screening in all 50 states and the District of Columbia is congenital hypothyroidism. Hemoglobinopathies and galactosemia are included in the newborn screening panel of most states. Testing methods vary from state to state for each of these individual disorders. In the case of many metabolic disorders such as PKU, the levels of the abnormal metabolite do not begin to rise in the infant's circulation until the umbilical cord is cut and therefore testing is not recommended until the infant is at least 24 hours of age. In the case of infants discharged before 24 hours of age, most states recommend that a sample be obtained at discharge and subsequently repeated. In the case of sick infants who are not being fed, the initial newborn screening sample should not be withheld indefinitely but should be submitted at the recommended time, often 7 days, because screening for some other disorders, such as hypothyroidism, is not affected by the feeding history. For PKU screening and screening for some other disorders, however, another specimen should be submitted after feedings are instituted. Confirmation of positive new-born screening test results is always necessary to establish a definitive diagnosis regardless of the type of screening method utilized. Even with tandem mass spectroscopy, false positive test results occur. Each state or country has developed a system for the evaluation of infants with positive results which may or may not include submission of repeat specimens to a central laboratory.

As newborn screening for metabolic disorders is expanded, an increasing number of inborn errors of metabolism will be diagnosed presymptomatically. This should not in any way discourage the neonatologist from considering the diagnosis of an inborn error of metabolism in an infant presenting with appropriate signs and symptoms. Many infants with conditions such as galactosemia, maple syrup urine disease and many of the organic acidemias will become symptomatic before the results of newborn screening tests are available. Additionally, there are many important inherited metabolic disorders, such as ornithine transcarbamylase deficiency that will not be detected by newborn screening, even with tandem mass spectroscopy. Therefore, it will be important to continue to have a high index of suspicion for metabolic disease in any infant who presents with findings suggestive of such a disorder.

MATERNAL METABOLIC DISORDERS

With advances in therapy for inborn errors of metabolism, it is now common for patients with many of these disorders to reach adult life with normal or near-normal intelligence and the desire to have families of their own. This has led to serious concerns about the potential adverse effects of maternal metabolic derangements on fetal growth and development. The real potential for adverse consequences is illustrated by the experience that has accumulated with maternal PKU. In the past, patients with PKU were severely retarded and did not reproduce. This changed completely with the initiation of newborn screening programs and early dietary management. Dietary therapy was once maintained until 5 to 6 years of age and then discontinued. Treatment now is continued indefinitely in most cases, because it has been demonstrated that some patients exhibit neurologic deterioration and loss of intelligence quotient (IQ) points after discontinuation of the diet. Nonetheless, many patients with PKU who are now adults have been off the diet for years and have high phenylalanine levels. After women with PKU began reproducing, it became clear that the maternal metabolic environment in this condition had extremely harmful effects on fetal development. A spectrum of findings referred to as "maternal PKU syndrome" is observed in a large percentage of exposed infants, most of whom do not themselves have PKU (35,36). More than 90% of exposed infants exhibit mental retardation, and microcephaly occurs in 72%, growth retardation in 40%, and congenital heart disease in 12%. Altered facial features, similar to those observed in FAS, may be observed. Mothers with hyperphenylala-

ninemia, a condition that is associated with lower phenylalanine levels than classical PKU and does not always require treatment, may also be at increased risk for fetal abnormalities.

There is evidence that dietary treatment of pregnant women before conception and throughout pregnancy, with careful control of phenylalanine levels, reduces the risk to the fetus (38). This is a difficult goal to achieve, however, because the phenylalanine-restricted diet is an onerous one to patients who have ever been on a normal diet, and some adult patients, despite early therapy, may have borderline intellectual functioning. There has been no evidence for an increased risk of birth defects or any other problems in infants born to fathers with PKU.

Pregnancies have been reported in mothers with a variety of other inherited metabolic disorders, including several forms of glycogen storage disease, propionic acidemia, isovaleric acidemia, homocystinuria, hereditary orotic aciduria, and several others, with no adverse outcomes clearly attributable to the maternal disorder. The collaborative experience with many disorders, however, is limited to single cases or small numbers of patients. It is probable that other maternal metabolic disorders will be identified that adversely affect fetal development.

REFERENCES

1. Scriver CR, Beaudet AL, Valle D, et al, eds. *The metabolic and molecular basis of inherited disease,* 8th ed. New York: McGraw-Hill, 2001.
2. Rimoin DL, Conner JM, Pyeritz RE, et al, eds. *Emery and Rimoin's principles and practice of medical genetics,* 4th ed. New York: Churchill Livingston, 2002.
3. Fischer AQ, Challa VR, Burton BK, et al. Cerebellar hemorrhage complicating isovaleric acidemia: a case report. *Neurology* 1981; 31:746.
4. Nyhan WL. Patterns of clinical expression and genetic variation in the inborn errors of metabolism. In: Nyhan WL, ed. *Heritable disorders of amino acid metabolism.* New York: John Wiley and Sons, 1974.
5. Ballard RA, Vinocur B, Reynolds JW, et al. Transient hyperammonemia of the preterm infant. *N Engl J Med* 1978;299:920.
6. Msall M, Batshaw ML, Suss R, et al. Neurologic outcome in children with inborn errors of urea synthesis. *N Engl J Med* 1984; 310:1500.
7. Goldberg RN, Cabal LA, Sinatra FR, et al. Hyperammonemia associated with perinatal asphyxia. *Pediatrics* 1979;64:336.
8. Batshaw ML, Wachtel RC, Cohen L, et al. Neurologic outcome in premature infants with transient asymptomatic hyperammonemia. *J Pediatr* 1986;108:271.
9. Robinson BH, Taylor J, Sherwood WG. The genetic heterogeneity of lactic acidosis: occurrence of recognizable inborn errors of metabolism in a pediatric population with lactic acidosis. *Pediatr Res* 1980;14:956.
10. Robinson BH, Glerum DM, Chow W, et al. The use of skin fibroblast cultures in the detection of respiratory chain defects in patients with lactic acidemia. *Pediatr Res* 1990;28:549.
11. Dalla Bernardina B, Aicardi J, Goutieres F, et al. Glycine encephalopathy. *Neuropadiatrie* 1979;10:209.
12. Wiegand C, Thompson T, Bock GH, et al. The management of life-threatening hyperammonemia: a comparison of several therapeutic modalities. *J Pediatr* 1980;96:142.
13. Batshaw ML, Brusilow SW, Waber L, et al. Treatment of inborn errors of urea synthesis: activation of alternative pathways of waste nitrogen synthesis and excretion. *N Engl J Med* 1982; 306:1387.

14. Matsubara Y, Narisawa K, Tada K, et al. Prevalence of K329E mutation in medium-chain acyl-CoA dehydrogenase gene determined from Guthrie cards. *Lancet* 1991;1:552.

15. Ziadeh R. Medium chain acyl-CoA dehydrogenase deficiency in Pennsylvania: neonatal screening shows high incidence and unexpected mutation frequencies. *Pediatr Res* 1995;37:675.

16. Duran M, Hofkamp M, Rhead WJ, et al. Sudden child death and "healthy" affected family members with medium-chain acyl coenzyme A dehydrogenase deficiency. *Pediatrics* 1986;78:1052.

17. Stanley CA, Hale DE, Coates PM, et al. Medium chain acyl-CoA dehydrogenase deficiency in children with non-ketotic hypoglycemia and low carnitine levels. *Pediatr Res* 1983;17:877.

18. Engel AG, Rebouche CJ. Carnitine metabolism and inborn errors. *J Inherit Metab Dis* 1984;1[Suppl 7]:38.

19. Levy HL, Sepe SJ, Shih VE, et al. Sepsis due to Escherichia coli in neonates with galactosemia. *N Engl J Med* 1977;297:823.

20. Kaufman FR, Kogut MD, Donnell GN, et al. Hypergonadotropic hypogonadism in female patients with galactosemia. *N Engl J Med* 1981;304:994.

21. Friedman JH, Levy HL, Boustany RM. Late onset of distinct neurologic syndromes in galactosemic siblings. *Neurology* 1989;39:741.

22. Cutz E, Cox DW. Alpha1-antitrypsin deficiency: the spectrum of pathology and pathophysiology. *Perspect Pediatr Pathol* 1979;5:1.

23. Lindbland B, Lindstedt S, Stein G. On the enzymic defects in hereditary tyrosinemia. *Proc Natl Acad Sci U S A* 1977;74:4641.

24. Kvittingen EA, Halvorsen S, Jellum E. Deficient fumarylacetoacetate fumarylhydrolase activity in lymphocytes and fibroblasts from patients with hereditary tyrosinemia. *Pediatr Res* 1983;14:541.

25. Karon M, Imach D, Schwartz A. Effective phototherapy in congenital non-obstructive non-hemolytic jaundice. *N Engl J Med* 1970;282:377.

26. Gorodischer R, Levy G, Krasner J, et al. Congenital non-obstructive non-hemolytic jaundice: effect of phototherapy. *N Engl J Med* 1970;282:375.

27. Schutgens RB, Heymans HS, Wanders RJ, et al. Peroxisomal disorders: a newly recognized group of genetic diseases. *Eur J Pediatr* 1986;144:430.

28. Wilson GN, Holmes RD, Hajra AK. Peroxisomal disorders: clinical commentary and future prospects. *Am J Med Genet* 1988;30:771.

29. Sweetman L, Nyhan WL, Trauner DA, et al. Glutaric aciduria type II. *J Pediatr* 1980;96:1020.

30. Chalmers RA, Tracy BM, King GS, et al. The prenatal diagnosis of glutaric acidemia type II using quantitative gas chromatography–mass spectroscopy. *J Inherit Metab Dis* 1985;2:145.

31. Robinson BH, McMillan H, Petrova-Benedict R, et al. Variable clinical presentation in patients with deficiency of pyruvate dehydrogenase complex. A review of 30 cases with a defect in the E component of the complex. *J Pediatr* 1987;111:525.

32. Opitz JM, de la Cruz F. Cholesterol metabolism in the RSH/Smith–Lemli–Opitz syndrome: summary of an NICHD conference. *Am J Med Genet* 1994;50:326.

33. Dobyns WB. Agenesis of the corpus callosum and gyral malformations are frequent manifestations of nonketotic hyperglycinemia. *Neurology* 1989;39:817.

34. Wick H, Schweizer KK, Baumgartner R. Thiamine dependency in a patient with congenital lactic acidemia due to pyruvate dehydrogenase deficiency. *Agents Actions* 1977;7:405.

35. Wilcken B, Wiley V, Hammond J, et al. Screening newborns for inborn errors of metabolism by tandem mass spectrometry. *N Engl J Med* 2003;348:2304.

36. Lenke RR, Levy HL. Maternal phenylketonuria and hyperphenylalaninemia. An international survey of untreated and treated pregnancies. *N Engl J Med* 1980;303:1202.

37. Levy HL, Waisbren SE. Effects of untreated maternal phenylketonuria and hyperphenylalaninemia on the fetus. *N Engl J Med* 1983;309:1269.

38. Koch R, Friedman E, Azen C, et al. The International Collaborative Study of Maternal Phenylketonuria: status report 1998. *Eur J Pediatr* 2000;[Suppl 2]:S156.

39. Fishler K, Koch R, Donnell GN, et al. Developmental aspects of galactosemia from infancy to childhood. *Clin Pediatr* 1980;19:38.

40. Baerlocher K, Gitzelmann R, Steinmann B, et al. Hereditary fructose intolerance in early childhood: a major diagnostic challenge. Survey of 20 symptomatic cases. *Helv Paediatr Acta* 1978;33:465.

41. Pagliara AS, Karl IE, Keating JP, et al. Hepatic fructose-1,6-diphosphatase deficiency. A cause of lactic acidosis and hypoglycemia in infancy. *J Clin Invest* 1972;51:2115.

42. Chen Y-T. Glycogen storage diseases. In: *Harrison's principles of internal medicine*, 14th ed. New York, McGraw Hill, 1998:2176.

43. Huijing F, van Creveld S, Losekoot G. Diagnosis of generalized glycogen storage disease (Pompe's disease). *J Pediatr* 1963;63:984.

44. Levin B, Burgess EA, Mortimer PE. Glycogen storage disease type IV: amylopectinosis. *Arch Dis Child* 1968;43:548.

45. Clow CL, Reade TM, Scriver CR. Outcome of early and long-term management of classical maple syrup urine disease. *Pediatrics* 1981;68:856.

46. Mudd SH, Skovby F, Levy HL, et al. The natural history of homocystinuria due to cystathionine beta-synthase deficiency. *Am J Hum Genet* 1985;37:1.

47. Baumgartner R, Ando T, Nyhan WL. Nonketotic hyperglycinemia. *J Pediatr* 1969;75:1022.

48. Smith I, Wolff OH. Natural history of phenylketonuria and influence of early treatment. *Lancet* 1974;2:540.

49. Kvittingen EA. Hereditary tyrosinemia type I—an overview. *Scand J Clin Lab Invest* 1986;46:27.

50. Fell V, Pollitt RJ, Sampson GA, et al. Ornithinemia, hyperammonemia and homocitrullinuria. A disease associated with mental retardation and possibly caused by defective mitochondrial transport. *Am J Dis Child* 1974;127:752.

51. Simell O, Perheentupa J, Rapola J, et al. Lysinuric protein intolerance. *Am J Med* 1975;59:229.

52. Fowler B. Genetic defects of folate and cobalamin metabolism. *Eur J Pediatr* 1998;157:S60.

53. Scriver CR, Whelan DT. Glutamic acid decarboxylase (GAD) in mammalian tissue outside the central nervous system, and its possible relevance to hereditary B6 dependency with seizures. *Ann N Y Acad Sci* 1969;166:83.

54. Matsui SM, Mahoney MJ, Rosenberg LE. The natural history of the inherited methylmalonic acidemias. *N Engl J Med* 1983;308:857.

55. Mitchell GA, Watkins D, Melancon SB, et al. Clinical heterogeneity in cobalamin C variant of combined homocystinuria and methylmalonic aciduria. *J Pediatr* 1986;108:410.

56. Wolf B, Hsia YE, Sweetman L, et al. Propionic acidemia: a clinical update. *J Pediatr* 1981;99:835.

57. Newman CGH, Wilson BDR, Callaghan P, et al. Neonatal death associated with isovaleric acidemia. *Lancet* 1967;2:439.

58. Finnie MDA, Cottrall K, Seakins JWT, et al. Massive excretion of 2-oxoglutaric acid and 3-hydroxyisovaleric acid in a patient with a deficiency of 3-methylcrotonyl-CoA carboxylase. *Clin Chim Acta* 1976;73:513.

59. Burri BJ, Sweetman L, Nyhan WL. Heterogeneity of holocarboxylase synthetase in patients with biotin-responsive multiple carboxylase deficiency. *Am J Hum Genet* 1985;37:326.

60. Wolf B, Heard GS, Weissbecker KA, et al. Biotinidase deficiency: initial clinical features and rapid diagnosis. *Ann Neurol* 1985;18:614.

61. Leibel RL, Shih VE, Goodman SI, et al. Glutaric acidemia: a metabolic disorder causing progressive choreoathetosis. *Neurology* 1980;30:1163.

62. Goodman SI, Stene DO, McCabe ERB, et al. Glutaric acidemia type II: clinical, biochemical and morphologic considerations. *J Pediatr* 1982;100:946.

63. Mantagos S, Genel M, Tanaka K. Ethylmalonic-adipic aciduria: in vivo and in vitro studies indicating deficiency of activities of multiple acyl-CoA dehydrogenases. *J Clin Invest* 1979;64:1580.

64. Wysocki SJ, Hahnel R. 3-Hydroxy-3-methylglutaryl-CoA lyase deficiency: a review. *J Inherit Metab Dis* 1986;9:225.

65. Robinson BH, Sherwood WG, Taylor J, et al. Acetoacetyl CoA thiolase deficiency: a cause of severe ketoacidosis in infancy simulating salicylism. *J Pediatr* 1979;95:228.

66. Hoffmann G, Gibson KM, Brandt IK, et al. Mevalonic aciduria—an inborn error of cholesterol and nonsterol isoprene biosynthesis. *N Engl J Med* 1986;314:1610.

67. Hagenfeldt L, Larsson A, Zetterstrom R. Pyroglutamic aciduria. Studies of an infant with chronic metabolic acidosis. *Acta Paediatr Scand* 1974;63:1.

68. Ko FJ, Nyhan WL, Wolff J, et al. 3-Hydroxyisobutyric aciduria: an inborn error of valine metabolism. *Pediatr Res* 1991;30:322.

69. Kelley RI, Cheatham JP, Clark BJ, et al. X-linked dilated cardiomyopathy with neutropenia, growth retardation, and 3-methylglutaconic aciduria. *J Pediatr* 1991;119:738.

70. Gibson KM, Burlingame TG, Hogema B, et al. 2-methylbutyryl-Coenzyme A dehydrogenase deficiency: a new inborn error of L-isoleucine metabolism. *Pediatr Res* 2000;47:830.

71. Hudak ML, Jones MD Jr, Brusilow SW. Differentiation of transient hyperammonemia of the newborn and urea cycle enzyme defects by clinical presentation. *J Pediatr* 1985;107:712.

72. Cederbaum SD, Shaw KNF, Valente M. Hyperargininemia. *J Pediatr* 1977;90:569.

73. Bachmann C, Krahenbühl S, Colombo JP, et al. N-acetylglutamate synthetase deficiency: a disorder of ammonia detoxification. *N Engl J Med* 1981;304:543.

74. Amendt BA, Greene C, Sweetman L, et al. Short chain acyl-CoA dehydrogenase deficiency: clinical and biochemical studies in two patients. *J Clin Invest* 1987;79:1303.

75. Stanley CA. New genetic defects in mitochondrial fatty acid oxidation and carnitine deficiency. *Adv Pediatr* 1987;34:59.

76. Strauss AW. Molecular basis of human mitochondrial very-long-chain acyl-CoA dehydrogenase deficiency causing cardiomyopathy and sudden death in childhood. *Proc Natl Acad Sci U S A* 1995;92:10496.

77. Sewell AC. Long chain 3-hydroxyacyl-CoA dehydrogenase deficiency: a severe fatty acid oxidation disorder. *Eur J Pediatr* 1994;153:745.

78. Chalmers RA, Stanley CA, English N, et al. Mitrochondrial carnitine-acylcarnitine translocase deficiency presenting as sudden neonatal death. *J Pediatr* 1997;131:220.

79. Rinaldo P, Stanley CA, Hsu BYL, et al. Sudden neonatal death in carnitine transporter deficiency. *J Pediatr* 1997;131:304.

80. Hug G, Bove KE, Soukup S. Lethal neonatal multiorgan deficiency of carnitine palmitoyl-transferase II. *N Engl J Med* 1991; 325:1862.

81. Nguyen TV, Andresen BS, Corydon TJ, et al. Identification of isobutyryl-CoA dehydrogenase and its deficiency in humans. *Mol Genet Metab* 2002;77:68.

82. Robinson BH, Oei J, Sherwood WG, et al. The molecular basis for the two different clinical presentations of classical pyruvate carboxylase deficiency. *Am J Hum Genet* 1984;36:283.

83. Clayton PT, Hyland K, Brand M, et al. Mitochondrial phosphoenolpyruvate carboxikinase deficiency. *Eur J Pediatr* 1986; 145:46.

84. Munnich A, Rustin P. Clinical spectrum and diagnosis of mitochondrial disorders. *Amer J Med Genet* 2001;106:4.

85. The Cystic Fibrosis Genotype-Phenotype Consortium. Correlation between genotype and phenotype in patients with cystic fibrosis. *N Engl J Med* 1993;329:1308.

86. Stevenson RE, Lubinsky M, Taylor HA, et al. Sialic acid storage disease with sialuria: clinical and biochemical features in the severe infantile type. *Pediatrics* 1983;72:441.

87. Scriver CR, Mahon B, Levy HL, et al. The Hartnup phenotype: mendelian transport disorder, multifactorial disease. *Am J Hum Genet* 1987;40:401.

88. O'Brien JS. Generalized gangliosidosis. *J Pediatr* 1969;75:167.

89. Barranger JA, Murray GJ, Ginns EI. Genetic heterogeneity of Gaucher's disease. In: Barranger JA, Brady RO, eds. *Molecular basis of lysosomal storage disorders*. New York: Academic Press, 1984:311.

90. Besley GT, Elleder M. Enzyme activities and phospholipid storage patterns in brain and spleen samples from Niemann–Pick disease variants: a comparison of neuropathic and non-neuropathic forms. *J Inherit Metab Dis* 1986;9:59.

91. Funk JK, Filling-Katz MR, Sokol J, et al. Clinical spectrum of Niemann-Pick disease type C. *Neurology* 1989;39:1040.

92. Autio S, Louhimo T, Helenius M. The clinical course of mannosidosis. *Ann Clin Res* 1982;14:93.

93. Dawson G, Spranger JW. Fucosidosis: a glycosphingolipidosis. *N Engl J Med* 1971;285:122.

94. Antonarakis SE, Valle D, Moser HW, et al. Phenotypic variability in siblings with Farber disease. *J Pediatr* 1984;104:406.

95. Young LW, Sty JR, Babbitt JP. Wolman's disease. *Am J Dis Child* 1979;133:959.

96. Clarke JTR, Ozere RL, Krause VW. Early infantile variant of Krabbe globoid cell leukodystrophy with lung involvement. *Arch Dis Child* 1981;8:640.

97. Spranger JW, Koch F, Mekusick VA, et al. Mucopolysaccharidosis VI (Maroteaux–Lamy's disease). *Helv Paediatr Acta* 1970;25: 337.

98. Nelson A, Peterson L, Frampton B, et al. Mucopolysaccharidosis VII (beta-glucuronidase deficiency) presenting as nonimmune hydrops fetalis. *J Pediatr* 1982;101:574.

99. Leroy JG, Spranger JW, Feingold M, et al. I-cell disease: a clinical picture. *J Pediatr* 1971;79:360.

100. Amir N, Zlotogora J, Bach G. Mucolipidosis type IV: clinical spectrum and natural history. *Pediatrics* 1987;79:953.

101. Burk RD, Valle D, Thomas GH, et al. Early manifestations of multiple sulfatase deficiency. *J Pediatr* 1984;104:574.

102. Aylsworth AS, Thomas GH, Hood JL, et al. A severe infantile sialidosis: clinical, biochemical and microscopic features. *J Pediatr* 1980;96:662.

103. Wilson GN, Holmes RD, Hajra AK. Peroxisomal disorders: clinical commentary and future prospects. *Am J Med Genet* 1988; 30:771.

104. Danks DM, Stevens BJ, Campbell PE, et al. Menkes kinky hair syndrome: an inherited defect in copper absorption with widespread effects. *Pediatrics* 1972;50:188.

105. Arnold GL, Greene CL, Stout JP, et al. Molybdenum cofactor deficiency. *J Pediatr* 1993;4:595.

106. Mudd SH, Irreverre F, Laster L. Sulfite oxidase deficiency in man: demonstration of the enzymatic defect. *Science* 1967;156:1599.

107. Verlos A, Temple IK, Hubert A-F, et al. Recurrence of neonatal haemochromatosis in half sibs born of unaffected mothers. *J Med Genet* 1996;33:444.

108. White PC, New MI, Dupont B. Congenital adrenal hyperplasia. *N Engl J Med* 1987;316:1580.

109. Jaeken J, Stibler H, Hagberg B. The carbohydrate-deficient glycoprotein syndrome: a new inherited multisystemic disease with severe central nervous system involvement. *Acta Paediatr Scand Suppl* 1991;375:1.

110. McClard RW, Black MJ, Jones ME, et al. Neonatal diagnosis of orotic aciduria: an experience with one family. *J Pediatr* 1983; 102:85.

111. Kozlowski K, Sutcliffe J, Barylak A, et al. Hypophosphatasia: review of 24 cases. *Pediatr Radiol* 1976;5:103.

112. Berk PD, Jones EA, Howe RB, et al. Disorders of bilirubin metabolism. In: Bondy, PK, Rosenberg LE, eds. *Metabolic control and disease*, 8th ed. Philadelphia: WB Saunders, 1980:1009.

113. Sveger T. Liver disease in alpha1-antitrypsin deficiency detected by screening of 200,000 infants. *N Engl J Med* 1976;294:1316.

114. Matalon R, Michals K, Sebesta D, et al. Aspartoacylase deficiency and N-acetylaspartic aciduria in patients with Canavan disease. *Am J Med Genet* 1988;29:463.

115. Shapiro LJ, Weiss R, Buxman MM, et al. Enzymatic basis of typical X-linked ichthyosis. *Lancet* 1978;2:756.

116. Cruysberg JRM, Sengers RCA, Pinckers A, et al. Features of a syndrome with congenital cataracts and hypertrophic cardiomyopathy. *Am J Ophthalmol* 1986;102:740.

117. Charmas LR, Bernardini I, Rader D, et al. Clinical and laboratory findings in the oculocerebrorenal syndrome of Lowe, with special reference to growth and renal function. *N Engl J Med* 1991;324:1318.

Renal Disease

42

Suhas M. Nafday   **Luc P. Brion**   **Corinne Benchimol**
Lisa M. Satlin   **Joseph T. Flynn**   **Chester M. Edelmann, Jr.**

DEVELOPMENTAL PHYSIOLOGY

The kidneys play a central role in the physiologic transition from fetal to postnatal life. Whereas homeostasis *in utero* is maintained largely by the placenta, adaptation to the extra uterine environment requires that the kidneys assume the responsibility of regulating water and solute balance. Although the neonatal kidney traditionally has been characterized as dysfunctional, closer analysis indicates that this organ functions at a level that is appropriate to the physiologic needs of the growing infant, except in the very-low-birth-weight (VLBW) infant.

Embryology

The metanephros, the definitive mammalian kidney, first appears at 5 weeks postconceptional age and begins to produce urine by 10 weeks postconceptional age (1–3). The ureteric bud, an offshoot of the mesonephric duct, induces formation of nephrons within the metanephric blastema. The nephroblastic cells of the blastema, on contact with the ureteric bud, differentiate into the glomerulus, proximal convoluted tubule, loop of Henle, and distal convoluted tubule. The ureteric bud ultimately forms the ureter, pelvis, calyces, and collecting ducts of the metanephros.

The processes of induction, morphogenesis and differentiation of the metanephros occurs in a centrifugal pattern, proceeding from the center to the periphery (4–6). Thus, the first nephrons to develop are those residing in the juxtamedullary region, whereas the youngest are located in the nephrogenic zone just under the renal capsule.

The full complement of approximately 1 million nephrons per kidney in the human is achieved by about 35 weeks' gestational age (GA), or a body weight of about 2,300 g (6). When birth occurs before this age, the formation of new nephrons (nephronogenesis) continues until a full complement is achieved. Once complete, nephronogenesis is never resumed, even after extensive loss of renal tissue. Thus, the full-term infant is born with as many nephrons as he or she will ever have.

Physiologic, biochemical, and enzymatic maturation of newly formed nephrons may lag behind anatomic maturation by weeks or months. Thus, the immature kidney is characterized by structural and functional heterogeneity arising from the concurrent presence of nephrons in varied stages of differentiation.

Renal Physiology

Urine produced by the fetal metanephric kidneys contributes to the formation of amniotic fluid (3,6). Although renal function is not necessary for long-term regulation of fetal water and electrolyte homeostasis, it is important for normal growth (7), lung development (8), and protection from acute changes in fetal vascular volume (9). The hourly rate of urine production in normal fetuses is about 5 mL at 20 weeks, 10 mL at 30 weeks, increasing to up to 50 mL at 40 weeks (3,10).

Renal Blood Flow

Low rates of fetal and neonatal renal blood flow (RBF) exist in a variety of animal species, whether normalized to body weight, surface area or kidney weight. RBF in the human fetus, estimated by Doppler ultrasonography, increases from 20 mL/min at 25 weeks GA to more than 60 mL/min at 40 weeks and reaches adult levels by 2 years of age (11,12). The effective renal plasma flow (RPF) has traditionally been calculated from the renal clearance of the organic acid para-aminohippurate (PAH), corrected for the fraction of PAH extracted by the kidney (12); the value for effective RPF divided by (100 − hematocrit [%])/100 provides an estimate of RBF. The effective RPF increases rapidly between 30 and 40 weeks GA, reaching adult values by 24 months of postnatal life (12) (Fig. 42-1).

Because the renal extraction ratio for PAH varies with age, calculated values of effective RPF must be interpreted with caution in the fetus and neonate. The rate of extraction of PAH in the 1-week-old full-term newborn is only about 60%, reaching the adult value of 90% by 5 months (13). PAH clearance averages 148 mL/min/1.73 M^2 body surface

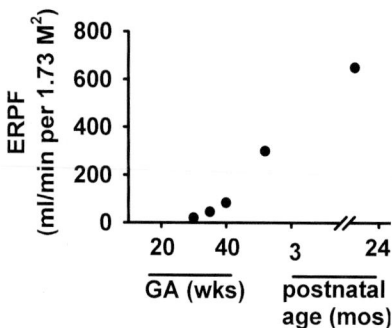

Figure 42-1 Developmental changes in effective renal plasma flow (ERPF), calculated from the renal clearance of para-aminohippurate (PAH) and corrected for the fraction of PAH extracted by the kidney. The ERPF, used to estimate RBF, increases rapidly between 30 and 40 weeks GA, reaching adult values by 24 months of postnatal life (From ref. 12, with permission).

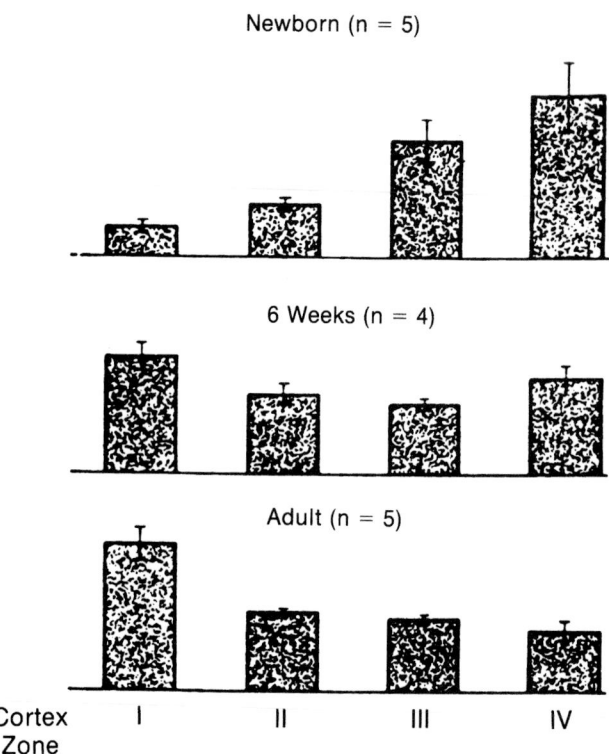

Figure 42-2 Postnatal changes in the intrarenal distribution of blood flow. Relative rates of blood flow per glomerulus in the four cortical zones of the canine kidney. Zone I represents the most superficial region, and zone IV represents the deepest. The total height of the bars in each age group is equal. At birth, the blood flow to the superficial cortex was lowest, with most blood flow perfusing the deep cortex. By 6 weeks of age, this pattern was reversed. Maturation is accompanied by an increase in blood flow to the outer cortex, due primarily to a decrease in renal vascular resistance (From ref. 17, with permission).

area (BSA) in full-term infants at 2 weeks of life, increasing to 200 mL/min/1.73 M^2 by 3 months (14). PAH clearance, corrected for BSA, reaches adult levels sometime between 1 and 2 years of age (12). The incomplete PAH extraction early in life appears to be as a result of relatively greater blood flow to juxtamedullary nephrons and efferent arteriovenous shunting in cortical nephrons, thereby allowing blood to bypass PAH-transporting segments of the nephron. Additionally, the organic acid secretory pathways in the proximal tubule are immature early in development (15). Thus, RBF and RPF will be underestimated by PAH clearance alone in neonates, particularly in premature infants, in the absence of determination of the PAH extraction ratio.

RBF is determined by cardiac output and the ratio of renal to systemic vascular resistance. Developmental changes in both hemodynamic variables contribute to the postnatal increase in RBF. Adult kidneys (which comprise 0.5% of total body mass) receive approximately 20% to 25% of the total cardiac output, corresponding to a RBF of 4 mL/min/g kidney weight. In contrast, the previable fetus receives only about 5% of the cardiac output, and the 1-week-old term infant receives about 9% (16).

The perinatal increase in RBF is gradual (13,17,18), consistent with the premise that clamping of the umbilical cord and the immediate imposition of functional demands at birth do not in themselves account for the postnatal increase in RBF. The maturational increase in RBF cannot be completely explained by increases in renal mass (19) or by nephronogenesis, which is complete well before maximal levels of RBF are achieved.

The intrarenal distribution of RBF in the newborn differs from that in the adult, reflecting the relative size, number, and maturity of glomeruli present in the different regions of the kidney at that stage of development. RBF in the newborn is distributed primarily to the inner cortex and medulla. Maturation is accompanied by a redistribution of blood flow toward the superficial cortex, so that the ratio of inner cortical to outer cortical blood flow becomes progressively smaller than in the fetus (18,20–22) (Fig. 42-2). At

maturity, about 93% of RBF goes to the cortex, which constitutes about 75% of the renal mass, whereas only 7% is distributed to the renal medulla and perirenal fat.

The primary factor responsible for the maturational increase and change in intrarenal distribution in RBF is a decrease in renal vascular resistance (RVR) (23), with the rise in cardiac output and mean arterial blood pressure (MAP) only partially accounting for these postnatal changes in renal hemodynamics (23–25,27). The balance of afferent and efferent arteriolar resistances ultimately determines the RVR, RBF, glomerular capillary pressure and glomerular filtration rate (GFR). The intrarenal vascular resistance, localized both at the afferent and efferent arterioles (26), is much higher in the newborn than in the adult (19,23). The postnatal fall in RVR occurs at a time when the systemic vascular resistance increases about 6-fold (23).

Anatomic factors also contribute to the developmental increase and redistribution of RBF. The intrarenal vascular system distal to the afferent arteriole in the neonate differs from that in the adult. Variability in the complexity of the glomerular capillary network exists early in postnatal life (28). Inner cortical glomeruli at this age generally have a smaller number of capillaries than the in adult, although they appear similar in overall structure. Few efferent arterioles descend into the medulla; most connect directly to the venous system (arteriovenous shunting) (29), bypassing the proximal tubules (26).

A variety of vasoactive substances have been implicated in the developmental regulation of RBF and GFR. The most important factors are discussed below. Changes in the balance of the vasoconstrictor renin-angiotensin system (RAS) and renal sympathetic nervous systems, both of which are highly active in early development, and vasodilatory humoral factors, including nitric oxide (NO), are believed to mediate, at least in part, the developmental reduction in RVR and increase in RBF.

Renin-Angiotensin System

All components of the RAS are present in the fetal metanephric kidney (30–34) (Fig. 42-3). Renin, angiotensinogen and angiotensin-converting enzyme (ACE) are first detected in fetal metanephros by ~6 weeks gestation. The site of localization of renin within the kidney is developmental-stage specific. Whereas the majority of renin-containing cells are located in the juxtamedullary apparatus in both the newborn and adult, renin message and protein in the fetus are also present in the arcuate and interlobular arteries and glomeruli (35).

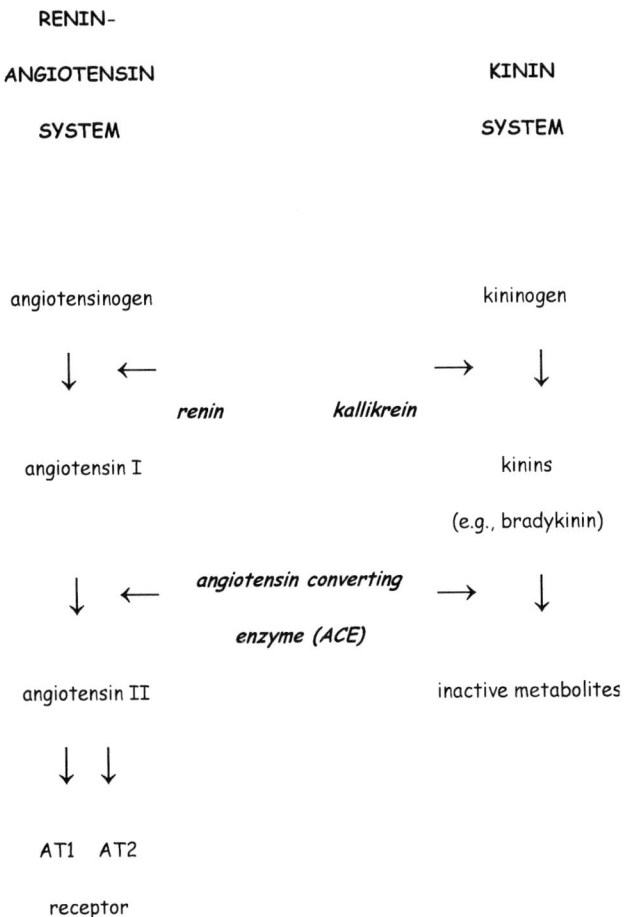

Figure 42-3 Relationship between the renin-angiotensin and kinin systems. See text for details.

The RAS is very active in the fetus and newborn. The fetus produces renin as early as 17 weeks GA (36). Plasma renin activity (PRA) is inversely related to GA in the fetus and newborn, decreasing from 60 ng/mL/h at 30 weeks to about 10 to 20 ng/mL/h at term (37). PRA is 3-to-5 times higher in human infants (38–44) than in adults. Changes in PRA in the fetus in response to several stimuli (increase after volume depletion or hypoxia, and decrease after volume expansion or after administration of a β-adrenergic antagonist or of a prostaglandin synthetase inhibitor [PGSI]) are similar to those observed in adults.

The high levels of PRA in neonates are generally associated with circulating levels of angiotensin II (ANG II) and aldosterone that exceed those measured in the adult (45–50). These high levels may reflect high rates of secretion or low metabolic clearance rates relative to body size. The reason for these high levels may be a relative end-organ unresponsiveness to aldosterone (51,52). Circulating levels of plasma ANG II decrease during postnatal life in parallel with PRA (53).

The observation that administration of ACE inhibitors during late gestation can result in anuria and oligohydramnios, renal tubular abnormalities, pulmonary hypoplasia, growth retardation, and increased fetal loss (54–56) underscores the pivotal role of the RAS in normal fetal growth and development. Genetic disruption of the genes encoding angiotensinogen (57), ACE (58), or ANG II type 1 receptor is also associated with profound abnormalities in kidney morphology.

The significance of the RAS in the maintenance of renal hemodynamics in the perinatal period remains uncertain. However, as identified above, a number of observations suggest that this axis may be important under conditions of stress in the near-term fetus. An acute reduction in blood volume or onset of hypoxia in the fetus or neonate significantly increases renin and ANG II levels (10,59,60). ACE inhibition blocks the increase in RVR and reduction in RBF experienced by near-term fetuses in response to hemorrhage (61,62).

Kinins

Bradykinins are potent vasodilator peptides generated from the protein precursor kininogen by the proteolytic enzyme kallikrein (Fig. 42-3). The kinins are inactivated by kininase I, which is a carboxypeptidase, and the peptidyl dipeptide hydrolase kininase II, which is ACE. Thus, ACE inhibitors not only decrease ANG II production but also prevent the breakdown of kinins.

Premature infants have undetectable levels of urinary kinins (63); urinary excretion of kallikreins and kinins is lower in newborns than older children (64). The role of these substances in modulating the function of the immature kidney remains unclear.

Prostaglandins

Prostaglandins (PGs) contribute to the maintenance of RBF and GFR, especially during conditions of enhanced vasoconstrictor activity. Complex interactions between PGs and the RAS and kinin systems exist, making it difficult to identify the specific effects of PGs on regulation of blood pressure, RBF, and electrolyte and water homeostasis. PG synthesis from arachidonic acid requires cyclooxygenase (COX), the inhibitory target of aspirin and various non-steroidal antiinflammatory drugs (65). Two isoforms of COX have been identified, each representing a different gene product and subject to differential regulation. COX-1 has been proposed to participate in glomerulogenesis (66), whereas COX-2 regulates renal perfusion and glomerular hemodynamics (67). Differences in intrarenal COX-1 and -2 localization between the adult and fetal human kidney may account for the variable renal responses to PG inhibition observed between the two groups (66).

Urinary excretion of PGs is high in the fetus (68,69), presumably reflecting a high rate of renal synthesis. Urinary excretion of PGE2 and prostacyclin metabolites in the premature infant is five times that noted at term and 20 times that measured in older children (70). Although rates of excretion decrease after birth, urinary PG excretion remains significantly higher in neonates than in children or adults (71,72).

PGs produced by the fetal and neonatal kidney may contribute to the regulation of renal perfusion and glomerular hemodynamics. Maternal administration of indomethacin, a nonselective COX inhibitor, reduces RBF in the fetus, and is associated with an increase in RVR and MAP (73). Intrauterine exposure of the human fetus to COX inhibitors can lead to a decrease in GFR with consequent reduction in fetal urine output and oligohydramnios (74–77). Postnatal administration of a PGSI to preterm infants (78,79) to close a patent ductus arteriosus (PDA) may also compromise renal function, leading to a reduction in RBF, GFR and urine volume.

Renal Nerves and the Adrenergic System

The renal vascular bed of the fetus is less reactive to renal nerve stimulation than that of the newborn and adult (80,81). In contrast to observations made in adult animals, several studies have demonstrated that renal nerve stimulation in the fetal and newborn kidney activates noradrenergic pathways, norepinephrine stimulates β2-adrenoceptors to produce renal vasodilation, and maturation of the renal adrenergic system is associated with downregulation of the renal β-adrenoceptor response (80–82).

Circulating catecholamine levels, particularly norepinephrine, are very high just before and immediately after birth (83), falling to adult values within a few days of life. The high plasma levels of catecholamines act directly to increase afferent arteriolar tone and indirectly, via stimulation of renin and ANG II release, to increase efferent resistance, possibly contributing to the maintenance of the high RVR characteristic of the neonatal kidney (84). The fetal and neonatal kidney demonstrates enhanced sensitivity to catecholamines compared to the adult, related in part to developmental differences in adrenergic receptor density (85,86).

Nitric Oxide

Endogenous NO is a major vasodilator in the developing kidney, contributing to the maintenance of intrarenal vascular tone and serving to buffer the highly activated endogenous vasoconstrictor state (87,88). The sensitivity of renal hemodynamics in the fetal and neonatal kidney to inhibition of NO synthesis is significantly greater than that of the adult kidney.

Dopamine and Dopamine Receptors

The fetal and neonatal kidneys are less sensitive than their adult counterparts to the renal vasodilatory and the natriuretic effects of dopamine (89,90). Exogenous administration of dopamine, which results in an increase in RBF in the adult, has no effect in the young animal unless there also is an increase in systemic blood pressure and cardiac output (81,91,92). This blunted response is considered to reflect the limited generation of the vasodilatory second messenger cyclic adenosine monophosphate (cAMP) (89,91) and a low density of renal dopamine-1-like receptors in the neonatal kidney (93).

The pharmacological effects of dopamine are dose-dependent. Whereas the renal response to low concentrations of dopamine generally reflects dopaminergic receptor-mediated effects, high concentrations stimulate α-adrenergic receptors. Thus, the renal vasoconstriction observed following intrarenal dopamine infusion in fetal and neonatal animals (94,95) likely reflects dopamine binding to α-adrenoceptors, which are abundant by term (96,97).

Arginine Vasopressin

The plasma concentration of arginine vasopressin (AVP) in neonates increases abruptly after birth and is highest in infants whose mothers labored before vaginal delivery (98). Although AVP has the potential to contribute to the high RVR characteristic of the neonate through its action on vascular and glomerular V1 receptors, its role in regulating basal renal hemodynamics remains poorly defined. Infusion of synthetic AVP does not alter RBF and RVR in fetal sheep (99). However, AVP may play a role in certain stress-induced responses. For example, during hemorrhage, but not during hypoxemia, the marked decrease in RBF and increase in RVR correlate closely with the rise in plasma AVP (10,59,100).

Atrial Natriuretic Factor

ANF acts on the mature kidney to increase sodium excretion and GFR, antagonize renal vasoconstriction, and inhibit renin secretion (101). ANF release from atrial cardiocytes is stimulated in the fetus by an increase in intracardiac pressure and atrial distention (102–105), and levels fall in response to a decrease in central venous pressure, as during hemorrhage (106). The natriuretic and diuretic response to systemically infused ANF in newborns is attenuated compared to adults (107–111). Whereas specific ANF receptors have been identified on near-term fetal glomerular membranes, the ANF binding capacity is age-dependent, increasing 7-fold between fetal and adult life (112). The blunted response of the immature subject to ANF has been attributed to ineffective production of the second messenger cyclic GMP (108,113), a rapid systemic clearance of ANF (107,108), and a greater ANF-induced reduction in RBF in fetuses and newborns than in adults (107).

Glomerular Filtration

Initiation of glomerular filtration in the human fetus occurs between 9 and 12 weeks of GA (114,115). It has been suggested that the functional demand placed on the neonatal kidney by cessation of placental function at birth stimulates GFR to increase. However, estimates of GFR correlate well with GA, a relationship that persists whether the fetus remains in utero or is born prematurely (116–119). Specifically, GFR averages approximately 8 to 10 mL/min/ 1.73 M^2 at 28 weeks of GA and increases only slightly before 34 weeks postmenstrual age, although body size and kidney weight increase appreciably during this time. After about 34 weeks postmenstrual age, at which time GFR averages 25 mL/min/1.73 M^2 regardless of postnatal age, GFR increases rapidly, often by threefold to fivefold within 1 week (116,118,120), coincident with completion of nephronogenesis (Fig. 42-4). Thus, an infant born prematurely at 28 weeks of GA shows little increase in GFR until the infant is about 6 weeks old, i.e., until a postmenstrual age of 34 weeks is attained and nephrogenesis has been completed (121). The GFR of neonates who are small

for GA is similar to that of infants whose body weight is appropriate for the same GA.

During the first 4 months of life, GFR increases rapidly relative to body size, kidney weight, and BSA (11). Thereafter, a slower rise is noted until adult values, determined on the basis of BSA, are reached by 2 years of age (11,122,123). The postnatal increase in GFR in premature infants may lag behind that observed in full-term newborns; at 9 months of age, the GFR of VLBW infants is approximately 70% of that measured in full-term infants of identical postnatal age (121).

Glomeruli are formed in the nephrogenic zone of the kidney. With maturation, these glomeruli migrate to deeper zones of the renal cortex. At birth, the more mature glomeruli in the juxtamedullary cortex, which are nearly as large as glomeruli in the adult kidney, have higher filtration rates than the most recently formed glomeruli in the superficial cortex, some of which may not begin filtration for some time. Thus, GFR, similar to RBF, matures centrifugally. As nephrons enlarge and forces that regulate filtration permit, GFR increases, with most of the surge as a result of enhanced perfusion of superficial nephrons (18,24,124) (Fig. 42-2), related temporally to the increase in total RBF and its centrifugal redistribution within the renal cortex.

The addition of newly functioning nephrons is insufficient, however, to account for the large increases in GFR observed during maturation. A substantial rise in single nephron GFR occurs (125). The process of urine formation starts with ultrafiltration of plasma through the glomerular capillary membrane. The rate of filtration depends on filtration characteristics of the membrane and on the net ultrafiltration pressure, represented by the difference between the mean glomerular transcapillary hydraulic, i.e., glomerular capillary minus the Bowman's space hydraulic pressures and mean colloid osmotic pressures over the length of the glomerular capillary, and the glomerular plasma flow. The capillary hydrostatic pressure promotes filtration, whereas both the colloid osmotic pressure within the capillary and the hydrostatic pressure in the Bowman's space oppose it. The postnatal increase in GFR may result from changes in all of these variables, in addition to the surface area available for filtration, and the permeability of the filtering membrane.

Autoregulation of Renal Blood Flow and Glomerular Filtration Rate

Autoregulation in the mature kidney allows for constancy of RBF and GFR as the MAP and renal perfusion pressure vary over a wide range, from about 80 to 150 mmHg. Autoregulation is accomplished primarily by changes in the RVR at the level of the afferent and efferent arterioles. Although systemic blood pressure in the fetus (i.e., 40–60 mmHg) and neonate is less than the lower limit of autoregulatory range defined for adults, experimental evidence suggests that the fetus and newborn are able to autoregulate RBF efficiently at their prevailing low arterial pressure,

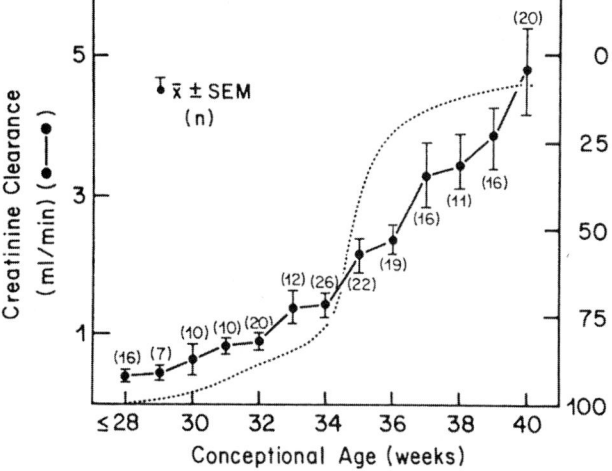

Figure 42-4 Changes in glomerular filtration rate (mL/min), estimated by creatinine clearance, and nephrogenic activity in the kidney cortex (%) are plotted as a function of postconceptional age in the human infant. There is a temporal relationship between the accelerated rate of increase in glomerular filtration rate and completion of nephrogenesis after 34 weeks of gestation (From Arant BS. Neonatal adjustments to extrauterine life. In: Edelmann CM Jr, ed. *Pediatric kidney disease.* Boston: Little, Brown and Company, 1992:1021).

albeit at a lower perfusion set point than in the adult (126–128). In support of this notion is the observation that a 16% increase in fetal arterial blood pressure elicited by AVP infusion does not alter RBF (129). The autoregulatory response is considered to be mediated in part by a myogenic response of the renal afferent arteriole (130,131), which constricts to limit any rise in glomerular hydrostatic pressure, and the tubuloglomerular feedback control mechanism (132,133) (see below). As MAP falls, the renal afferent arteriole dilates and the efferent arteriole constricts, the latter effect due, at least in part, to stimulation of renin release and ANG II generation (134,135). The balance of theses two responses maintains glomerular capillary hydrostatic pressure and preserves RBF and GFR.

Tubuloglomerular Feedback

Tubuloglomerular feedback serves to maintain a constant rate of water and salt delivery to distal segments of the nephron in which reabsorption is regulated to maintain fluid balance. A stimulus (e.g., tubular flow rate, ion concentration) at the macula densa is transmitted to vascular structures of the nephron that control GFR to elicit a change of single nephron GFR. Tubuloglomerular feedback is maximally sensitive in a range that corresponds to normal values of single nephron GFR and tubular flow rate. As GFR increases with maturation, the maximal response and flow range of maximum sensitivity also increase, so that the relative sensitivity of the tubuloglomerular feedback mechanism is unaltered during growth (136,137). An intact RAS appears to be critical for this signaling pathway (157) and NO may play a modulatory role (138,139).

Tubular Function

The axial and polarized (apical vs. basolateral) distribution of transport proteins along sequential segments of the nephron allows the kidney to reabsorb the bulk of glomerular filtrate proximally and then, in more distal segments, adjust the solute and water content of the urine to maintain homeostasis. The fully differentiated kidney is generally a reabsorptive organ. However, transport of some ions and solutes by individual nephron segments is bidirectional. Thus, sodium, bicarbonate, phosphate, amino acids, and glucose are reabsorbed, hydrogen ions are secreted, and potassium and organic acids are both reabsorbed and secreted. In general, the kidney of the full term, but not necessarily preterm, neonate is uniquely suited to meet the developmental stage-specific metabolic demands.

Sodium

Term infants are in a state of positive sodium balance, a requisite for somatic growth, particularly of bone. Although the sodium intake per unit of BSA is generally smaller in the newborn than in the adult, the magnitude of this positive balance remains relatively constant within a wide range of sodium intakes (140,141). The tendency of the neonatal

kidney to retain sodium may become problematic under conditions of salt loading. Exogenous administration of a sodium load to an adult is followed by immediate expansion of the extracellular fluid (ECF) space. This signals the kidney to decrease tubular sodium reabsorption, resulting in increased excretion of sodium and a relatively rapid return of the ECF space to the baseline condition. Full-term newborn infants given a sodium load in excess of 12 mEq/kg/d experience a rise in serum sodium levels, abnormal increase in weight, and generalized edema (142). The limited capacity of the neonatal kidney to excrete a sodium load compared to its mature counterpart appears to be due more to factors related to tubular sodium reabsorption than to the low GFR (143).

The fractional excretion of sodium (FENa) is the ratio of the sodium clearance to the creatinine clearance, expressed as a percent. It is obtained from the following formula:

$$\text{FENa (\%)} = 100 \times U_{na}/U_{cr} \times P_{cr}/P_{Na}$$

in which U_{Na} is the urinary concentration of sodium (mEq/L), U_{cr} is the urinary concentration of creatinine (mg/dL), P_{Na} is the plasma sodium concentration (mEq/L), and P_{cr} is the plasma creatinine concentration (mg/dL). FENa, which may be as high as 20% during early fetal life, decreases progressively during gestation (144–146), so that the FENa in the full-term newborn generally averages about 0.2% (146,147). After the first few hours of postnatal life, the FENa and urinary sodium excretion decline rapidly, possibly secondary to contraction of the ECF volume (144). Premature infants of less than 30 weeks of GA continue to show elevated values of FENa, similar to those observed in the fetus, which may exceed 5% during the first few days of life (146,148,149). In these infants, excessive urinary sodium losses exceeding dietary sodium intake (e.g., breast milk, low-salt formula) often create a state of negative sodium balance and loss of body weight during the first 2 weeks of life (i.e., hyponatremia of prematurity). These infants may require at least 2 mEq/kg/d of supplemental sodium to maintain a normal sodium concentration and remain in positive balance (150,151).

Sodium is freely filtered at the glomerulus. The initial two-thirds of the proximal tubule of the suckling rat absorbs ~50% of the filtered load of sodium and water (143,152–154), values only slightly less that those reported in the adult (152,153,155). Studies in several mammalian species ingesting a normal salt intake demonstrate parallel and proportionate increases in GFR and the reabsorptive capacity of the proximal tubule after birth, consistent with maintenance of glomerulotubular balance during postnatal development (125,156,157). Functional glomerulotubular imbalance may exist in the premature infant in whom the reabsorptive capacity of the proximal tubule lags behind the capacity for glomerular filtration (158,159).

The fractional reabsorption of sodium along the loop of Henle, expressed as a percentage of load, increases by about 20% during postnatal development (153), consistent with functional maturation of this nephron segment. Sodium is absorbed in this segment through the furosemide- and bumetanide-sensitive Na-K-2Cl cotransporter located in the urinary membrane and is extruded from the cell at the basolateral membrane by the Na-K-ATPase transporter. In contrast, the fractional reabsorption of sodium along the distal tubule is greater in younger than in older animals, thereby explaining the sodium retention and blunted response to sodium loading characteristic of the young animal (143,160).

Clearance studies in human infants (151–155,158, 159,161–166) suggest that the percent of filtered sodium reabsorbed by the proximal tubule increases by about 5% between 28 and 34 wks GA, whereas the percent of distal sodium reabsorption increases by more than 15% during this same period. However, because the proximal tubule reabsorbs more than 70% of the filtered load of sodium, the small percentage increase in fractional reabsorption in this segment contributes to the postnatal increase in renal sodium retention as much as the larger percentage increase in the distal tubule.

Distal sodium reabsorption occurs in the cortical collecting duct (CCD) by apical sodium entry into principal cells through the amiloride-sensitive sodium channel ENaC and its extrusion at the basolateral membrane by the Na-K-ATPase. The avidity of the distal nephron for sodium reabsorption, may be related to the high levels of aldosterone that prevail in early postnatal life (44). Cellular effects of aldosterone within the fully differentiated distal nephron (specifically the CCD) include increases in the density of ENaC channels and stimulation of Na-K-ATPase activity (167–169). The net effect of these actions is the stimulation of sodium absorption.

Plasma aldosterone concentrations in the premature infant and newborn are high compared to those in the adult (50,170). However, clearance studies in premature infants (50,171) and investigations in neonatal laboratory animals (172,173) reveal a blunted responsiveness of the immature kidney to aldosterone. The density of aldosterone binding sites, receptor affinity, and degree of nuclear binding of hormone-receptor appear to be similar in mature and immature rats (18), suggesting that the early hyposensitivity to aldosterone represents a postreceptor phenomenon. Premature infants can augment their renin secretion in response to negative sodium balance, but aldosterone production initially fails to respond adequately to this stimulation (174). The resulting relative hypoaldosteronism results in an inability to conserve sodium, manifested clinically by weight loss and hyponatremia.

Paradoxically, preterm infants of about 34 to 36 weeks GA excrete a sodium load more efficiently than do term newborns, but not as efficiently as adults (118,148,171). The sodium wasting characteristic of the preterm infant may be as a result of paucity of ENaC channels in the urinary membrane of the distal nephron (175).

Urinary sodium excretion during maturation is regulated not only by the RAS, but also by circulating catecholamines, renal sympathetic innervation, atrial natri-

uretic factor (ANF), PGs, dopamine, and glucocorticoids. Direct renal nerve stimulation in fetal and newborn sheep leads to sodium retention (176), a response qualitatively similar to that observed in adult animals and attributed to norepinephrine acting on α-adrenergic receptors (177). Studies in newborns indicate a relatively poor natriuretic response to ANF compared to their adult counterparts (108,178,179). Renal PGE2, PGD2, and PGI2 reduce sodium and water absorption in the adult, promoting a natriuresis and diuresis, responses that are blocked by administration of indomethacin. In contrast, administration of this inhibitor to fetal sheep causes a natriuresis, despite a decrease in fetal RBF (73). Dopamine inhibits sodium reabsorption in the nephron by activation of D1-like dopamine receptors. The natriuretic effect of dopamine is less pronounced in the fetal and neonatal kidney of many species, including man, compared to the adult as a result of blunted renal hemodynamic and tubular effects (171,173,180–182).

Circulating levels of glucocorticoids, including cortisol and corticosterone, surge in many species during or just before the period of weaning (183–186). Both endogenous gluco- and mineralocorticoids bind to the mineralocorticoid receptor with equal affinity (187). Although blood glucocorticoid concentrations are ~100-fold higher than aldosterone concentrations, the metabolism of cortisol into inactive derivatives by 11β-hydroxysteroid dehydrogenase type 2 (11-β-HSD2) protects the mineralocorticoid receptor from glucocorticoids (187). The presence of ENaC, mineralocorticoid receptor and low levels of 11-β-HSD2 in the CCD suggest that glucocorticoids may act as sodium retaining steroids during early postnatal life (188,189).

Potassium

Potassium is transported actively across the placenta from mother to fetus (190). Indeed, fetal potassium is maintained at levels exceeding 5 mEq/L even in the face of maternal potassium deficiency (190,191).

Unlike adults, who are in zero balance, growing infants maintain a state of positive potassium balance (50,192). The relative conservation of potassium early in life generally is associated with higher plasma potassium values than in the adult (153,159,192,193). These levels average 5.2 mEq/L from birth to age 4 months, decreasing to 4.2 mEq/L by 3 years of age (193). The renal clearance of potassium in the infant is less than in the older child, even when corrected for GFR (193). Children and adults ingesting a regular diet containing sodium in excess of potassium excrete urine with a sodium-to-potassium ratio greater than 1, as expected. Although the sodium-to-potassium ratio of breast milk and commercial infant formulas averages 0.5, the urinary sodium-to-potassium ratio of the newborn also is greater than 1, consistent with significant potassium retention.

Infants, like adults, can excrete potassium at a rate that exceeds its glomerular filtration when given a potassium load, indicating the capacity for net tubular secretion (194); however, the rate of potassium excretion per unit body weight in response to exogenous potassium loading is less in newborn than older animals (195). Clearance studies in saline-expanded dogs also provide indirect evidence for a diminished secretory and enhanced reabsorptive capacity of the immature distal nephron to potassium (196). In general, the limited potassium secretory capacity of the immature kidney becomes clinically relevant only under conditions of potassium excess. Under normal circumstances, potassium retention by the newborn kidney is appropriate and a requirement for growth.

Potassium is freely filtered at the glomerulus. Approximately 50% of the filtered load is reabsorbed along the proximal tubule in both newborns and adults (153). Up to 40% of the filtered load of potassium reaches the superficial distal tubule of the newborn, in contrast to about 10% in mature animals, providing evidence for functional immaturity of the loop of Henle (153,197).

Urinary potassium excretion is derived almost entirely from secretion in distal segments of the nephron, including the CCD. The low rates of potassium excretion characteristic of the newborn kidney are due, at least in part, to a low potassium secretory capacity of this segment (198). In contrast to the high rates of potassium secretion observed in adult CCDs, neonatal segments show no significant baseline potassium transport (199). An increase in tubular fluid flow rate does not stimulate potassium secretion in the neonatal CCD of the rabbit, as it does in the fully differentiated segment, until after weaning (199,200). Baseline and flow-stimulated potassium secretion appear to be limited early in life by a paucity of small-conductance (SK) (201) and calcium-activated maxi-K channels (200), respectively, in the urinary membrane of the CCD. The developmental expression of immunodetectable ROMK, the molecular correlate of the SK channel (202,203), and shortly thereafter, the maxi-K channel, immediately precedes the appearance of baseline and flow-stimulated potassium secretion in the CCD.

As stated above, fetal and neonatal kidneys are relatively insensitive to aldosterone. Chronic administration of exogenous aldosterone to fetal sheep increases sodium absorption and decreases PRA, yet fails to increase urinary potassium excretion (204). However, administration of the aldosterone antagonist spironolactone or sodium channel blocker amiloride, both without consistent effect on sodium excretion, inhibit renal potassium excretion in fetal sheep, suggesting that endogenous mineralocorticoids influence renal potassium excretion in utero (205).

Acid–Base

The acid–base status of the fetus is maintained by placental function and maternal mechanisms. The fetal kidney in the second one-half of pregnancy, however, is able to acidify the urine (206,207). Immediately after birth, the acid–base state of the full-term newborn is characterized by a metabolic acidosis (208); respiratory compensation generally occurs within 24 hours in the full-term infant (209).

The normal range for serum bicarbonate is lower for preterm infants (16 to 20 mmol/L) and full-term infants (19 to 21 mEq/L) than for children and adults (24 to 28 mmol/L). The lower levels of buffer base concentration in the blood of infants can be accounted for in part by the inability to completely excrete the byproducts of growth and metabolism (210,211). The load of endogenous acid generated by the metabolism of protein and deposition of calcium into the skeleton is larger in the infant than in the adult (212–215).

The concentration of bicarbonate in plasma is determined predominantly by the renal bicarbonate threshold, which is lower in preterm and term infants than adults (194,216–219). The low bicarbonate threshold characteristic of the newborn is considered to reflect nephron heterogeneity and/or a low fractional reabsorption of bicarbonate in the immature kidney (50,220), the latter attributed in part to the relatively large proportion of total body water in the infant.

Postnatal maturation of the proximal tubular capacity for bicarbonate absorption has been proposed to be as a result of increases in activity of the sodium-hydrogen (Na/H) exchanger (NHE) and H+-ATPase localized to the urinary membrane of this segment (221,222). Experimental evidence further suggests that neonatal bicarbonate reabsorption is limited by low activity of carbonic anhydrase. Carbonic anhydrase facilitates renal acidification by catalyzing the interconversion of carbon dioxide and water to carbonic acid. The two major renal isoforms are cytosolic carbonic anhydrase II (95%) and membrane-bound carbonic anhydrase IV (5%). Carbonic anhydrase activity is present in the early human fetal kidney (223–225). The newborn kidneys of several experimental animals (226–228) exhibit less carbonic anhydrase activity than do mature kidneys. Postnatal increases in carbonic anhydrases II and IV likely contribute to the developmental increase in bicarbonate absorption observed in the maturing proximal tubule (226,229).

The renal response to acid loading increases with advancing gestational and postnatal ages. When compared to adult subjects given a comparable acid load, the infant exhibits a larger fall in blood potential of hydrogen (pH) and bicarbonate concentration, a smaller and slower fall in urine pH, and much smaller increase in urinary titratable acid and ammonium excretion per M2 (230–233). Premature infants born at 34 to 36 weeks of GA and studied 1 to 3 weeks after birth exhibit rates of excretion of net acid, titratable acid, and ammonium that are about 50% lower than term babies of similar postnatal age; net acid excretion increases to levels observed in term newborns only after 3 weeks of age (219,233). In response to acid loading with ammonium chloride, urinary pH values of less than 6 are rarely observed in premature infants until the second month of life (234). In contrast, by the end of the second postnatal week, urinary pH values of 5.0 or lower, comparable to those in the adult, are consistently observed in term infants (235,236).

The capacity of the neonatal kidney for the excretion of net acid is blunted, due in part to a limited excretion of urinary buffers, including phosphate and ammonium ions.

The rates of ammonia synthesis and excretion are low in the neonate (237) and, in response to acid loading, do not increase to mature values until 2 months of age (218, 235,238). Phosphate loading, administration of cow milk that is rich in protein and phosphate instead of breast milk, or high-protein feeding enhances the ability of the newborn to excrete titratable acids and ammonia (236,239).

The final site of urinary acidification is the renal collecting duct. Functional immaturity of this segment and the acid–base transporting intercalated cells therein may further limit the ability of the neonate to eliminate an acid load (240,241). Postnatal differentiation of intercalated cells has been shown to include changes in the morphology and function of these specialized cells with an increase in density.

Up to 10% of preterm infants develop a partially compensated hyperchloremic metabolic acidosis during weeks 1 to 3 of life, i.e., late metabolic acidosis (218), despite an otherwise healthy appearance. Typically, spontaneous remission occurs in the subsequent 2 weeks. These infants are characterized further by an apparent delay in postnatal weight gain despite ample dietary intake, suggesting a high rate of endogenous acid formation in infants whose dietary intake exceeds their anabolic capacity (212). Although infants provided supplemental sodium bicarbonate to maintain acid–base homeostasis showed greater increases in length than controls, there were no differences in weight gain between the two groups (217,242).

Calcium

The state of positive calcium balance characteristic of growing individuals is sustained by the coordinated interaction of bone, intestine and kidney. Urinary excretion of calcium varies inversely with GA in the first week of life and varies directly with urine flow and sodium excretion (243). High rates of calcium excretion may contribute in part to early neonatal hypocalcemia, which occurs in the first 24 to 48 hours of life (244). The urinary calcium-to-creatinine ratio in full-term infants ranges from 0.05 to 1.2 mg/mg during the first week of life, but may exceed 2 in premature neonates (243,245). In children more than 1 year of age, the ratio is approximately 0.2, and in adults, the ratio is less than 0.11 (246). The high fractional excretion of calcium in preterm infants may be related to maturational changes in the tubular handling of calcium. Approximately 50% of filtered calcium is reabsorbed along the superficial proximal tubule in mature rats, yet only 1% of filtered calcium is excreted (153), suggesting that, in the adult, almost one-half of the filtered calcium is reabsorbed at a site beyond the proximal tubule or in deep nephrons (153). The fractional reabsorption of calcium in the loop of Henle, like that for sodium, potassium, and chloride, is low in newborn rats, increasing significantly with advancing postnatal age (153,247). Absorption in both proximal tubule and thick ascending limb of the loop of Henle (TALH) is predominantly coupled to sodium absorption and is a passive process through the paracellular pathway.

Calcium reabsorption within the distal nephron is active, transcellular and is regulated independently of sodium (248). Furosemide, methylxanthines, and dexamethasone increase urinary calcium excretion, thus increasing the risk for nephrocalcinosis and nephrolithiasis (249,250).

The principal hormones that regulate renal calcium excretion in the adult are parathyroid hormone (PTH), 1,25-dihydroxyvitamin D3 and calcitonin (251). A reduction in the serum calcium concentration results in the secretion of PTH from the parathyroid glands, a response leading to the conservation of calcium by the kidney and the enhanced uptake of calcium by the intestine, which occurs indirectly through the PTH-induced synthesis of the active vitamin D metabolite 1,25-dihydroxyvitamin D. The net effect is to return the serum calcium back toward its normal baseline level. In mature animals and in adults, PTH decreases urinary calcium excretion by stimulating calcium reabsorption across the cortical TALH and collecting duct (252–258). PTH-responsive adenylate cyclase has been found in renal cortical homogenates from preterm rabbits (259) and in the TALH in 2-day-old puppies (260). It has been suggested that neonatal hypocalcemia may be as a result of end-organ unresponsiveness to PTH. In premature and full-term newborns, however, the administration of exogenous PTH increases urinary excretion of cAMP (261,262), results in a calcemic response, but affects calciuria and phosphaturia only minimally (263). Vitamin D stimulates calcium reabsorption in the distal tubule via binding to vitamin D receptors (VDRs). Renal production of 1,25-dihydroxyvitamin D increases rapidly after birth, provided that the concentration of the substrate, 25-hydroxyvitamin D, is adequate (264). VDR are present in cells of branching ureteral buds by 15 days GA and at later developmental stages in glomerular and tubular cells (265).

Systemic calcium homeostasis is controlled in large part by the extracellular G protein-coupled calcium-sensing receptor (CaSR), located on parathyroid and kidney cells in which it senses the extracellular calcium concentration and in turn alters the rate of secretion of PTH and renal calcium (and sodium and chloride) reabsorption in the TALH and early distal nephron (266–269). There is little expression of CaSR in the fetal kidney (270). Steady state abundance of CaSR messenger ribonucleic acid (mRNA) and protein increase significantly during the first week of life, related principally to an increase in expression of the receptor in the TALH and, to a lesser extent, in the collecting duct (270).

Phosphate

In contrast to most other transport processes, the capacity of the kidney of the neonate to reabsorb phosphate is far greater than in the adult and progressively declines with advancing age (271,272). The fractional reabsorption of phosphate increases from 85% of the filtered load at 28 weeks GA to 99% at term, decreasing thereafter to approximately 85% between 3 and 20 months of age (273). The high renal reabsorptive capacity for phosphate early in life allows the infant to retain a large portion of phosphate absorbed from the gut and sustain a state of positive balance (273), as is required for growth and development. Note that phosphate is a major constituent of bone, muscle, and membrane phospholipids and is critical for cellular processes involving ATP. Human neonates and older infants have a higher serum phosphate concentration than adults.

Studies in experimental animals also demonstrate enhanced renal tubular reabsorption of phosphate early in life (168,169). Younger subjects have a higher maximal net reabsorption of phosphate per unit glomerular filtrate than adults (274,275). The fractional reabsorption of phosphate in the newborn proximal tubule and distal nephron is higher than that in the adult (276,277). The high intrinsic rate of sodium phosphate transport measured in neonatal proximal tubules has been attributed to an abundance of a growth-related sodium-phosphate cotransporter protein in the luminal membrane (278), a high membrane fluidity of the immature nephron (279), a low intracellular phosphate concentration (174), and the hormonal milieu prevailing in the perinatal period (279,280). Nephron heterogeneity may also explain, in part, the limited urinary phosphate excretion observed in the rapidly growing animal. Because deep nephrons reabsorb more phosphate than cortical nephrons (281,282), and nephronogenesis begins in the juxtamedullary region, the kidney of the immature animal may contain a relatively greater number of functioning nephrons with a high capacity for phosphate reabsorption.

Renal phosphate transport is regulated by a number of factors, including dietary intake, PTH, growth hormone, insulin-like growth factor 1, and glucocorticoids (283,284). The sensitivity of the renal response to these factors is developmental-stage specific. Growth hormone stimulates proximal tubular phosphate transport (283). The high reabsorptive capacity of the juvenile kidney for phosphate persists after parathyroidectomy (275,285). Serum levels of PTH are low immediately after birth, increasing substantially thereafter to levels in infancy exceeding those observed in later childhood (286,287). Although exogenous PTH administered to humans or experimental animals results in a blunted response in the immediate postnatal period (259,274), 1-wk-old full term infants exhibit a prompt phosphaturic response and an increase in urinary cAMP excretion after PTH administration (261–263).

Magnesium

Ninety-seven percent of the filtered magnesium is reabsorbed by the mature nephron, largely (~60%) in the TALH (288). Micropuncture analysis of magnesium transport in developing rats shows efficient renal tubular reabsorption of magnesium in this segment early in life (153). The proximal tubule of the adult animal reabsorbs only about 10% of the filtered magnesium, whereas that of the young rat reabsorbs about 60% of the filtered load (153).

Postnatal maturation is associated with a decrease in the fractional reabsorption of magnesium in the proximal tubule (153). The avid retention of magnesium by the immature kidney likely contributes to the inverse relationship noted between plasma magnesium and somatic maturity in early postnatal life (289).

Magnesium reabsorption is regulated by a number of hormones, including PTH, calcitonin, glucagon, and AVP (290–295). Additionally, dietary magnesium restriction or loading stimulates or inhibits magnesium reabsorption, as appropriate, a response mediated by the CaSR in the cortical TALH and distal tubule (296,297). Loop diuretics such as furosemide inhibit magnesium absorption and increase magnesium excretion as a result of their inhibition of sodium chloride transport and modification of the transepithelial voltage in the TALH (298).

Glucose

Premature infants of less than 34 weeks of GA have a higher urinary glucose concentration, higher fractional excretion of glucose, and lower maximal reabsorption of glucose than full-term infants and older children (116). However, the maximal reabsorption of glucose factored by GFR, the fractional reabsorption of glucose, is similar in neonates and in adults (116,299,300). These results provide additional evidence for preservation of glomerulotubular balance, at least in term infants. The lower renal threshold for glucose in newborns compared to their adult counterparts is believed to reflect a greater degree of nephron heterogeneity early rather than later in life (299).

The neonatal proximal tubule possesses both high- and low-affinity sodium-coupled glucose transporters that mediate reabsorption of filtered glucose; interestingly, only the low-affinity high-capacity system is present in adults (301–303). It is not clear when during maturation the high-affinity system disappears, but its presence early in life may enable the anatomically immature kidney to efficiently reabsorb sugar from the glomerular filtrate.

Organic Acids

Organic acids, including PAH (see RBF) and endogenously produced uric acid, are eliminated by filtration and proximal tubular secretion. Organic acids are transported from the peritubular circulation across the basolateral surface of the proximal tubule to the tubular fluid. The renal clearance of organic acids is low in the neonate, even when corrected for body size, and increases gradually with age (17,304,305). As discussed previously, the limitation in tubular excretion of weak acids may be due in part to the preponderance of blood flow to the juxtamedullary region, bypassing tubular secretory sites. Additional variables that may account for the limited clearance of organic acids include the low GFR, limited energy for transport, and restricted expression of organic anion transporter proteins (306).

Amino Acids

The renal reabsorption of many amino acids, including threonine, serine, proline, glycine, and alanine, is lower in newborn animals and humans than in adults, often resulting in aminoaciduria (307,308). This does not appear to be a generalized defect in amino acid reabsorption, because other filtered amino acids (e.g., methionine, isoleucine, leucine, tyrosine) are reabsorbed more completely. Specific transporters for acidic, basic, and neutral amino acids have been identified in the urinary membrane of proximal tubules in newborn kidneys (309–312). The transient limitation in net transtubular reabsorption of amino acids characteristic of the neonate may arise from intrinsic differences in activity and transport capacity of these discrete transport systems, and/or a lower rate of amino acid efflux out of the cell into the peritubular circulation in the neonate compared to the adult, a mechanism that also would account for the high intracellular concentrations of amino acids observed early in life (309).

Urinary Concentration and Dilution

The fetal metanephric kidney of a variety of species, including man, produces large volumes of hypotonic urine that contribute significantly to the volume and composition of amniotic fluid (144,158,313–315). Yet, the fetal nephron is able to concentrate urine under conditions of stress, such as that induced by maternal water deprivation (316), hemorrhage (61), or infusion of AVP (317,318). However, the maximum urine osmolality that can be achieved is only about 20% of that in the adult (129,319).

Urinary Concentration

Urine voided at or shortly after birth generally is hypotonic with respect to plasma (313,320). The maximal urinary concentrating ability ($\sim$1,000–1,200 mOsm/kg) of children and adults is generally not attained by the neonate before 6 to 12 months of age (321,322). After fluid deprivation for 12 to 24 hours, the maximal urine osmolality achieved in premature and full-term newborns is 600 to 800 mOsm/kg, respectively (321,322). A few 1- to 2-month-old infants may be able to generate a urine osmolality as high as 1,000 mOsm/kg (323,324).

Urinary concentration requires a corticomedullary osmotic gradient, the pituitary release of AVP and the ability of the collecting duct to increase its water permeability in response to AVP. The limited urinary concentrating ability of the infant appears to be due primarily to an inability to generate a corticomedullary osmotic gradient and diminished responsiveness of the distal nephron to AVP (323,324).

Corticomedullary Gradient

The capacity to concentrate the urine has been directly related to elongation of the loops of Henle and their penetration into the medulla (325). The inner medulla and renal papillae are poorly developed in the immature kidney. In the rat, the 1.6-fold increase in length of the renal medulla correlates well with the 1.5-fold increase in urine osmolality observed between 10 and 20 days of age (325). In addition to anatomic maturation of the loops of Henle, urinary concentration requires the generation of a high interstitial solute concentration gradient in the medulla, which is underdeveloped early in life (321,326,327). Generation of the corticomedullary osmotic gradient necessitates the postnatal maturation of several processes involved in urinary concentration: sodium reabsorption and urea sequestration by the TALH and functional activation of aldose reductase, an enzyme necessary for generation of intracellular osmolytes, important for maintenance of cell function in the concentrated milieu (326,328,329). These structural and functional limitations of the countercurrent multiplication and exchange systems prevent build-up and maintenance of a medullary gradient in the immature kidney.

Antidiuretic Hormone

The limited ability of the immature kidney to concentrate urine is not as a result of an inability to synthesize and secrete AVP. Circulating levels of antidiuretic hormone (ADH) are elevated in preterm and term infants and decrease rapidly in term infants within 24 hours of birth (98,330,331). Studies in fetal and newborn animals (59,332,333), and in human infants (331,334), indicate a qualitatively appropriate response to osmolar or volume stimuli known to affect AVP release. Furthermore, exogenous administration of AVP or 1-des-amino-8-d-AVP (DDAVP) to healthy 1- to 3-week-old newborns leads to a response, albeit of shorter duration and reduced magnitude than that observed at 4 to 6 weeks (335). Cumulative evidence suggests that the blunted sensitivity of the fetal and neonatal kidney to AVP and limited concentrating ability of the neonatal animal is not as a result of a paucity of V2 receptors (receptor to which ADH binds in the collecting duct) (336,337), aquaporin channels involved in water transport across renal tubule epithelia (338), or efficiency of coupling to second messengers (adenylate cyclase and protein kinase A activity) (339–341) after the first week of postnatal life, but is limited primarily by the poorly developed corticomedullary osmotic gradient.

Urinary Dilution

Premature infants (less than 35 weeks of GA) studied under conditions of maximal water diuresis decrease urine osmolality to 70 mOsm/kg, whereas infants more than 35 weeks of GA are able to reduce urine osmolality to 50 mOsm/kg (159). Although there is greater proximal sodium rejection in preterm than term infants, the high avidity of the distal nephron for sodium reabsorption allows the neonate, especially the preterm infant, to generate a free water clearance greater than that in adults (143,196,342). Despite the greater capacity for free water clearance, the ability of the neonate to excrete a hypotonic load is limited, presumably as a result of the low GFR.

CLINICAL EVALUATION OF RENAL FUNCTION AND DISEASE

Early diagnosis of a renal anomaly may help to prevent complications, including those related to the kidney itself (e.g., progressive loss of renal function as a result of systemic hypertension, obstructive or reflux uropathy, or infection) and those related to other organs (e.g., cerebral hemorrhage, seizures or congestive heart failure [CHF] secondary to hypertension, ventricular arrhythmia secondary to hyperkalemia, urosepsis). In this section, clinical and laboratory features that should raise suspicion of a renal problem are reviewed and an approach to establish the correct diagnosis is presented.

Incidence of Renal and Urinary Tract Malformations

The incidence of renal and urinary tract malformations varies in different studies depending on the methodology used for detection: 0.2% to 0.6% by abdominal palpation (343–345), 7% to 9% in autopsy series (Table 42-1)

(346,347), 0.1% to 1.4% by prenatal ultrasonography (US) (348–352), and 1% to 2% in prospective studies using US screening (353–357). A similar incidence (1.3%) was found using a perinatal approach that combined family history, prenatal US, physical examination, and case-oriented neonatal imaging (356). In one large series, the male-to-female ratio for hydronephrosis was 2.4:1, compared to 1.4:1 for parenchymal anomalies (358).

History

Family History

Positive family history should be sought for hereditary disease, including renal cystic disease, tubular disorders, and nephrotic syndrome. There is a 9% incidence of asymptomatic renal malformations—most often unilateral renal agenesis—in the first-degree relatives of infants with agenesis or dysgenesis of both kidneys or agenesis of one kidney and dysgenesis of the other (359). A study using US has confirmed that, in some families, bilateral agenesis or dysplasia is inherited as an autosomal dominant trait

TABLE 42-1

INCIDENCE OF RENAL AND URINARY TRACT MALFORMATIONS IN INFANCY

Author	No. of Subjects	Selection Criteria	Method of Screening	Most Common Anomalies (Final Diagnosis)	No. of Subjects with Anomalies (% of Total)
Sherwood 1956	12,160	Consecutive NN	Palpation confirmation by IVU	Ectopia (7), horseshoe/fused kidneys (5), obstruction (6), Wilms (1)	22(0.2%)
Museles 1971	12,150	Consecutive NN	Palpation confirmation by IVU	Ectopia (7), horseshoe (4), agenesis (3)	22(0.2%)
Brion 1984	1,200	Consecutive NN	Prenatal US (2/3), physical examination, US screening for various indications	Hypoplasiaiagenesis (4), obstructive uropathy (8), reflux (1)	15(1.3%)
Helm 1986	11,986	Consecutive pregnancies	Prenatal US	Hydronephrosis (9), VUR (3), mild dilatation (10), cystic disease (3)	33(0.3%)
Steinhart 1988	437	Healthy infants	US	VUR (3), obstructive uropathy (3)	6(1.4%)
Gillerot 1988	900	NN autopsies	Autopsy	Dysplasia/agenesis (30), polycystic kidneys (18), obstructive uropathy (11), cloacal exstrophy (4)	63(7%)
Scott 1991	1,061	NN in well-baby nursery	Postnatal US, followed by appropriate workup	Duplex kidney (1), solitary kidney (2), hydronephrosis	11(1.0%)
Scott 1993	242,628	Northern Region Fetal Abnormality Survey	Population survey including both prenatal US and postnatal US	Hydronephrosis (97), VUR (16), renal agenesis (33), MKD (15), dysplasia (6), PKD (11), duplex kidney (15), megaureter (10), urethral valves	451(2%)
Jelen 1993	1,021	Consecutive neonates	Postnatal US	Hydronephrosis (6), MKD (2), duplication (4), agenesis (2)	20(2%)
Fugelseth 1994	22,310	Consecutive pregnancies	Prenatal US at 17 and 32 wk	Hydronephrosis (24), MKD (10)	47(0.2%)
Gunn 1995	3,856	Consecutive pregnancies	Prenatal US after 28 wk, confirmed by postnatal US at 6 d to 6 wk	Transient pylectasis (216), obstructive uropathy (23), VUR (14), MKD (8), urethral valves (3)	54(1.4%)
Kim 1996	5,442	Consecutive pregnancies	Prenatal US confirmed by US	Hydronephrosis (37), MKD (5), PKD (2), renal agenesis (2), ectopic kidney (1), hypoplastic kidney (1)	48(0.9%)

IVU, intravenous urography; MKD, multicystic kidney dysplasia; NN, newborn infants; PKD, polycystic kidney disease; US, ultrasonography; VUR, vesicoureteral reflux.

(renal adysplasia) (360). The clinician should keep in mind that some autosomal dominant diseases have variable penetrance or time of presentation (e.g., adult-type polycystic disease) and that a new mutation may occur. Additionally, the history for prior fetal loss should be carefully reviewed, preferably with an autopsy review.

The risk of renal or urinary tract malformation or renal failure is increased by maternal diabetes and by certain medications or drugs, including trimethadione, thalidomide, cocaine, PGSIs and ACE inhibitors (see Appendix G–2). Maternal diabetes, especially in poorly controlled cases, is associated with a higher incidence of urogenital malformations (2.6% vs. 1.2% in controls) (361) and neonatal renal vein thrombosis. The risk for renal or urinary tract malformations is higher in an infant of a diabetic mother with a caudal regression syndrome or a femoral hypoplasia– unusual facies syndrome (see Appendix G–2). Fetal alcohol syndrome is associated with unilateral renal agenesis, renal hypoplasia, ureteral duplication, and hydronephrosis (362). A meta-analysis showed that maternal cocaine abuse is associated with an odds ratio of genitourinary malformations of 5.0 (95% confidence interval 1.1 to 23.6); the odds ratio was 6.1 (95% confidence interval 1.2 to 31.3) in studies comparing cocaine–polydrug users to polydrug users without cocaine (363).

Pregnancy

The diagnosis of a urologic problem may be obtained by US performed as a routine examination or as a part of the workup for another anomaly. A high maternal serum or amniotic alpha-fetoprotein (AFP) concentration is associated with several anomalies, including bladder exstrophy or myelodysplasia (which are associated with urinary tract malformations, see Appendix G–2), and with congenital nephrotic syndrome of the Finnish type (CNF). Increased maternal serum AFP concentration is associated with pyelectasis and thick-walled bladder (364). Oligohydramnios may result from amniotic sac rupture, prolonged leaking or from fetal oligoanuria. The latter can result from bilateral congenital renal disease, bilateral urinary tract obstruction, acquired fetal renal disease secondary to maternal administration of indomethacin or ACE inhibitors (365–367), or severe pregnancy-induced hypertension. Among many causes, polyhydramnios may be the first clue to the diagnosis of a nephrogenic defect of urinary concentration, whereas fetal hydrops may be the first sign of congenital nephrotic syndrome.

PHYSICAL EXAMINATION

Dysmorphism

Renal and Urinary Tract Anomalies Associated with Multiple Congenital Anomalies

Any dysmorphic feature (e.g., abnormal ears) should lead the clinician to look for other anomalies and structural defects. Appendix I–1 lists the major signs of multiple congenital anomalies associated with renal and urinary tract anomalies (see Chapters 38 and 43). The most typical sequence related to kidney disease is the oligohydramnios sequence, i.e., Potter syndrome, which may result from prolonged leakage of amniotic fluid or from intrauterine oligoanuria. Fetal deformation caused by severe oligohydramnios includes Potter facies, which is characterized by a redundant, wrinkled skin, flat nose, low-set ears, bilateral skin folds arising at the inner canthus, receding chin, and malposition of the hands and feet (368). Lung hypoplasia results from fetal compression as a result of the oligohydramnios (369) and, in some cases, massive abdominal distention. Even a short duration (1 week) of oligohydramnios can induce hypoplasia of the lung during the pseudoglandular period (12 to 16 weeks of GA) and the canalicular period (17 to 28 weeks of GA) (368–371).

Associations of Renal and Urinary Tract Anomalies with Single Signs

Upper urinary tract anomalies may be associated with several isolated anomalies (e.g., abnormal vertebrae, anorectal malformations) (see Appendix G–3); however, some of these associations are controversial (372–374). Ultrasonographic screening of infants with isolated single umbilical artery (UA) showed urinary tract malformations in 8/112 (7%) (373). A meta-analysis of studies using a more extensive urologic workup found a higher incidence (33/204, or 16.2 %); however, additional anomalies detected by this more extensive investigation were only minor (375). The presence of specific index signs should raise the suspicion of a known multiple congenital anomaly; the presence of vertebral or anorectal anomalies can suggest a possible VATER syndrome. Urinary tract abnormalities were detected in 6 infants with isolated preauricular tags (6/70; 8.6%) (376). Some signs may be an indication for performance of US only in some families (e.g., preauricular pits) (374). The risk of finding renal or urinary tract anomalies increases with the number of additional system anomalies and, in the case of hypospadias, with its severity (372).

Thus, it appears justified to obtain a US in newborn infants with specific types of single anomalies and in those with recognized multiple congenital anomalies.

Vital Signs and General Examination

Shock and asphyxia can lead to prerenal or intrinsic renal failure. Tachycardia, peripheral vasoconstriction, hypotension, or narrowing of the pulse pressure suggests hypovolemia or low-output cardiac failure, which places the infant at risk for prerenal failure. Tachyarrhythmia, premature ventricular contractions, or abnormal QRS complexes on cardiac monitoring may be the first sign of hyperkalemia, which may be as a result of, or related to, renal immaturity or renal failure. Seizures or coma may be as a result of hypertension or complications of renal failure.

Measurement and Evolution of Blood Pressure in the Neonatal Period

Accurate blood pressure measurement is obviously crucial not only to the evaluation of hypertension (see below), but also to the ongoing assessment of any neonate. Many neonates will have their blood pressure measured directly through an indwelling umbilical or radial artery catheter; this technique provides the most accurate method of measuring blood pressure, minor artifacts (such as from air bubbles or blood clots in the tubing) notwithstanding (377). Indwelling catheters also are helpful in the management of infants with hypertension as they make it possible to obtain frequent blood pressure determinations. This is discussed in more detail below.

The most commonly used indirect method of blood pressure measurement is the oscillometric technique, which directly measures mean arterial pressure (MAP) based on the oscillations of the arterial wall; systolic and diastolic blood pressure are then back-calculated from the MAP using manufacturer-specific algorithms. These devices are usually sufficiently accurate for routine clinical use, although it is important to note that the readings obtained by oscillometric devices may differ between 1 to 5 mm Hg compared to directly measured blood pressure (378). Shock may also lead to inaccurate oscillometric measurements (379). Despite these issues oscillometric devices clearly are useful for measuring blood pressure in infants without indwelling arterial catheters, and in infants that have been discharged from the nursery.

Selection of a proper sized cuff is also crucial for correct indirect blood pressure measurement. As discussed in the Fourth Report of the National High Blood Pressure Education Program (380), the length of the cuff bladder should be 80% to 100% of the arm circumference and the length of the cuff bladder should be 80% to 100% of the arm circumference. Leg blood pressures tend to be higher than those obtained in the arm (381–384); therefore it is important to have the nursing staff document in which extremity an infant's blood pressure is being measured so that trends can be accurately followed over time.

Many studies have examined the pattern of normal blood pressure in normal and premature infants (384–386). Most recently, Zubrow and colleagues examined blood pressures obtained in over 600 infants of varying birth weights (BWs) and GAs admitted to 14 neonatal intensive care units (NICUs) (387). They found that blood pressure at birth is closely correlated with GA and BW (Appendix G1a&b). There is then a predictable increase in blood pressure over the first 5 days of life that is independent of these factors. Thereafter, blood pressure continues to rise gradually, with the most important determining factor being post conceptual age (Appendix G1c). These data provide a clinically useful method of determining whether an infant's blood pressure is normal or elevated (388) (see Hypertension).

Blood pressure increases with the awake state, in the knee–chest position, with crying, pain, and during physical examination and procedures, or even during feeding (382,389–391). In some infants, blood pressure follows a circadian pattern (392). Tracking of blood pressure begins during the first months of life (393).

Chest

A small chest suggests hypoplastic lungs, which can be associated with renal and urinary tract malformations. Previous data suggesting an association of kidney and urinary tract malformations with polythelia, i.e., supernumerary nipples were not confirmed by a large study on 200 asymptomatic infants (394). Prerenal failure may result from CHF, PDA, and severe respiratory distress.

Abdomen

The physical examination of a newborn infant should include bimanual palpation of the abdomen for the presence of a normal kidney in each flank (212,213,225). The examination is easiest in the delivery room, before the bowel is filled with gas; later on, it is facilitated by relaxation of the abdominal wall musculature obtained, for instance, by eliciting the sucking reflex. Several characteristics of the kidneys should be evaluated, including location (normally in the flank; an ectopic kidney may be located in the pelvis), size (the normal size for a 3.3 ± 0.5 [mean ± SD] kg infant is 4.2 to 4.3 ± 0.5 cm) (395), and long axis (normally cephalocaudal). A horseshoe kidney may be suspected if the lower pole is closer to the midline than the upper pole. The consistency of a normal kidney is firm, in contrast to a cystic or a hydronephrotic kidney, which may be depressible. The surface normally is smooth, but large cysts can be palpated in multicystic or autosomal dominant polycystic kidneys.

Two thirds of abdominal masses are genito-urinary in origin and may be as a result of a polycystic/multicystic kidney, renal vein thrombosis, congenital or acquired hydronephrosis (e.g., as a result of a fungus ball or papillary necrosis), or a renal tumor (396,397). A suprapubic mass suggests bladder distention, which may result from lower urinary tract obstruction or an occult spinal cord lesion. In some patients, one or both kidneys cannot be palpated. This may be as a result of a less than optimal examination (e.g., absence of patient relaxation, bowel distention), unilateral renal agenesis, renal malposition (in which case the kidney may be felt at another place in the abdomen), or renal hypoplasia or aplasia. Some abnormalities of the abdominal wall, such as bladder exstrophy, cloacal exstrophy, and prune-belly syndrome, are associated with renal anomalies. Sphincter dysfunction may suggest an occult spinal dysraphism.

The umbilical cord should be checked for the presence of a single umbilical artery. Ano-rectal anomalies or ambiguous genitalia, including severe hypospadias (372), should raise the suspicion of associated renal or urologic malformations. Percussion of the abdomen may disclose ascites or a large bladder. In the absence of hydrops fetalis, neonatal ascites commonly is as a result of the rupture of an obstructed urinary tract (398).

Limbs

Motor and sensory dysfunction of the lower limbs suggests an occult spinal dysraphism. Several limb anomalies are part of syndromes or sequences associated with renal or urinary tract malformations, such as skeletal dysplasia, caudal regression syndrome, radial aplasia, femoral hypoplasia, rocker bottom feet, compression deformation, polydactyly, syndactyly, and hemihypertrophy.

Hydration

Serial measurements of net body weight should be compared to the normal evolution of postnatal weight (399). Signs of dehydration include weight loss, dry skin and mucosae, sunken fontanelle, and signs of hypovolemia. In newborn infants, generalized edema usually starts around the eyes, at the perineum, and on the lateral sides of the trunk. Edema may be a sign of renal failure or nephrotic syndrome, among other causes.

Clinical Observations

Time of the First Postnatal Voiding

With early feeding, 97% of all infants void within 24 hours after birth (including in the delivery room) (400). Urine produced in utero normally is dilute, with an average osmolality less than 200 mOsm/kg. Higher osmolality in utero may result from obstructive urinary tract disease, poor tubular reabsorption of sodium, administration of oxytocin or indomethacin to the mother, or intrauterine asphyxia. In contrast, urine produced after birth usually is isotonic or hypertonic, probably as a result of increased release of oxytocin and ADH.

Urine Output

In full-term infants, urine output after the first day of life increases progressively, in parallel with daily intake. In low BW (LBW) and VLBW infants, three phases occur in the early postnatal period: an oliguric phase, during which the urine output is always lower than the intake; a polyuric phase starting between 24 and 72 hours of age, during which the output exceeds the intake; and an adaptive phase, during which the kidney adjusts to the rate of fluid intake (401,402). A diuretic phase is observed in most infants, regardless of respiratory status or environment. The diuretic phase is associated with a high excretion of sodium and chloride, and, in much smaller amounts, potassium and bicarbonate (403).

Characteristics of Urination

The baby should be observed for dribbling or persistence of a large bladder after urination, suggesting either posterior urethral valves or neurogenic bladder. Urination through an abnormal location suggests hypospadias, epispadias, ambiguous genitalia, or both. Additional discussion can be found in Chapter 43.

Urinalysis

Urinalysis at the bedside includes the dipstick, which can help diagnose proteinuria, excretion of hemoprotein (hematuria, hemoglobinuria or myoglobinuria), glucosuria, and leukocyturia, and the measurement of urine specific gravity (SG) by refractometry. Urine SG is inversely proportional to the urine output. In neonates, the relationship between SG and osmolarity differs from that in older subjects (404), and dipsticks do not provide a reliable assessment of urine osmolarity (405). The rate of physiologic proteinuria in the neonate changes with GA and postnatal age (Table 42-2). The differential diagnosis of pink urine and of hemoprotein is discussed later in this chapter (see Differential Diagnosis of Hematuria). Massive glucosuria may occur when glycemia is greater than 150 mg/dL, whereas mild glucosuria is common in VLBW infants even when glycemia is normal.

Laboratory Evaluation

Measurement of Glomerular Filtration Rate

GFR may be expressed in mL/min; mL/min/1.73 m^2 of BSA; mL/min/kg of body weight; or mL/min/kg of lean body mass; which of these units is most appropriate for infants is controversial (406).

To be an adequate marker for GFR, a substance must not be metabolized, must be completely filtered through the glomerulus, must not be secreted by the tubule, and must be eliminated from the body only by the kidney, unless GFR is determined by a classic clearance method (407). Adequate markers include inulin, polyfructosan, radionuclides such as 99mTechnetium-diethylenetriaminepentacetic acid (DTPA) and Cystatin C (408).

In the clinical setting, GFR often is estimated by creatinine clearance or by comparing Pcr to normal values for

TABLE 42-2
PROTEINURIA DURING THE FIRST DAYS OF LIFE

Gestational Age (wk)	No. of Infants	Mean and Range (mg/m²/h)
≤28	5	0.86 (0.2–1.33)
30	12	2.08 (0–9.4)
32	15	2.32 (0–5.22)
34	15	2.48 (0–13.07)
36	17	1.27 (0–4.60)
40	26	1.29 (0–6.14)

From Jose PA, Slotkoff LM, Lilienfield LS, et al. Sensitivity of neonatal renal vasculature to epinephrine. *Am J Physiol* 1974;226:796–799, with permission.

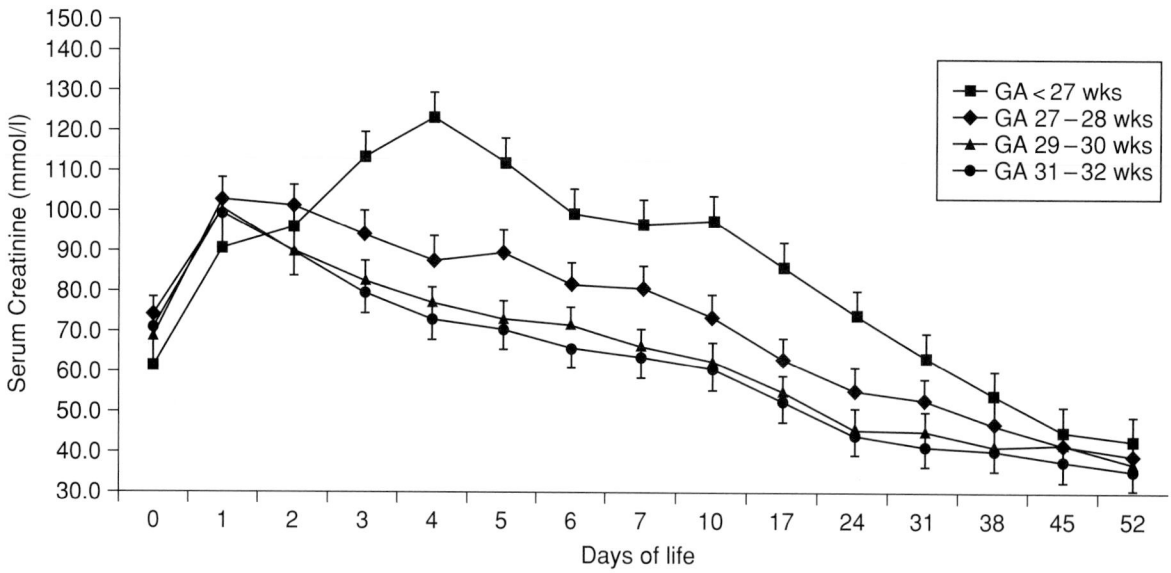

Figure 42-5   Postnatal evolution of serum creatinine concentration (umol/L) in preterm infants. Values are given as mean and standard error (From ref. 411, with permission).

GA and postnatal age (Figs. 42-5 and 42-6). Limitations of creatinine clearance as an assessment of GFR have been attributed to inaccurate determination of Pcr, effect of maternal creatinine load on creatinine concentration, tubular secretion of creatinine, passive back-diffusion of creatinine across leaky tubules in extremely preterm infants, and difficulty in obtaining complete urine collections in newborn infants, especially in girls. Cord blood creatinine concentration is almost equivalent to the maternal level. In full-term infants, Pcr decreases exponentially after birth (409), whereas in VLBW infants, it increases in the first 36 to 96 hours of life and then gradually decreases.

In the most immature infants, the increase in Pcr is higher and the decrease is more gradual, probably as a result of a slower progression of glomerular function and a greater backflow across the immature tubular and vascular structures (410,411) (Figures 42-5 and 42-6).

If measured reliably, Pcr is correlated with the half-life of medications eliminated by glomerular filtration (412–414). Nevertheless, the relationship between GFR and Pcr is hyperbolic, so that a fall in GFR of 50% may not be detectable by a change in Pcr. Thus, the clinician usually can use Pcr for routine estimation of GFR in most newborn infants, except immediately after birth or during sudden

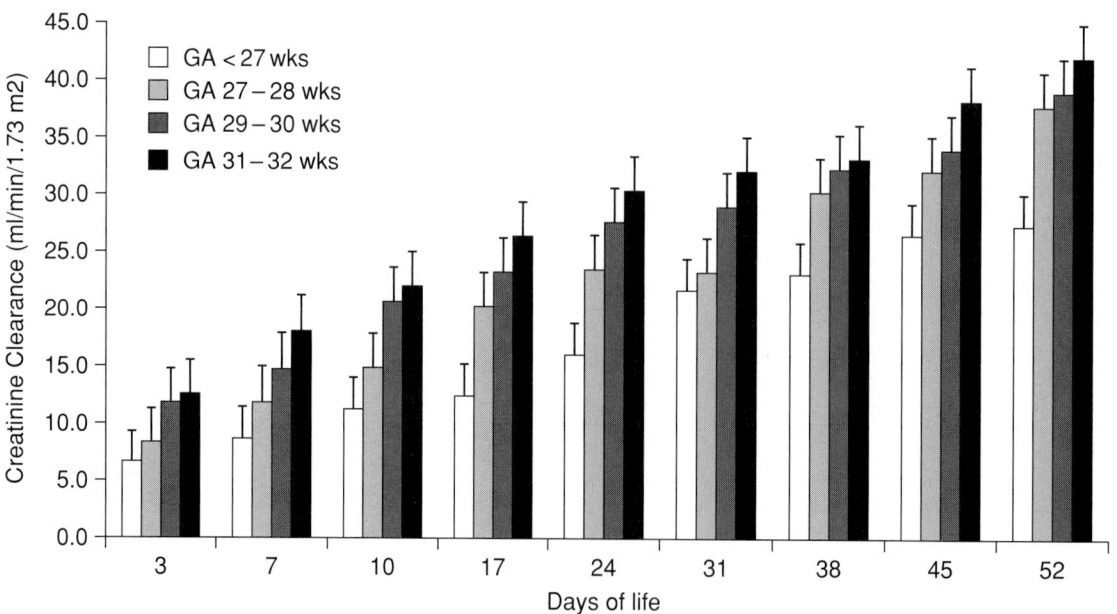

Figure 42-6   Postnatal evolution of creatinine clearance (mL/min/1.73 m^2) in preterm infants. Values are given as mean and standard error (From ref. 411, with permission).

changes in GFR. Formal measurements of creatinine clearance or GFR are recommended for patients with renal impairment.

A reasonably accurate estimation of GFR can be made by using an empirically derived formula (409), which has been applied to normal preterm and term infants (409,415)

a. Preterm infants: Estimated GFR (ml/min per 1.73 m^2) = 0.33 × length (cm)/Pcr (mg/dl)
b. Term infants: Estimated GFR (ml/min per 1.73 m^2) = 0.45 × length (cm)/Pcr (mg/dl)

Blood Urea Nitrogen

A high value of blood urea nitrogen (BUN) can result from catabolism, dehydration, high protein load (e.g., oral, intravenous, gastrointestinal bleeding), or renal failure. A low value of BUN can result from ECF expansion or decreased production of urea. The latter may be observed in association with anabolism, low protein intake, urea cycle disorder, liver failure, or liver immaturity (416).

Uric Acid

Serum concentration of uric acid is higher in cord blood than in maternal blood. Urinary uric acid concentration in full-term infants drops to its lowest value by the 7th day; its concentration in preterm infants remains significantly higher than in full-term babies during the first month of life (417). A high urinary uric acid to creatinine ratio is a marker of perinatal asphyxia (418).

Plasma Renin Activity

The most common indication for the measurement of PRA is the evaluation of hypertension. Normal levels of PRA are higher in the newborn infant than in older children or adults. This is discussed further in the section on Hypertension.

Genetic, Biochemical, and Molecular Diagnosis

The number of tests available for the diagnosis of congenital disorders is rapidly increasing (see Chapters 10, 12, 38, and 41). Classic chromosome analysis can be enhanced by high-resolution methods. Biochemical diagnosis is possible either by measuring enzyme activity or a chemical in a biologic fluid (e.g., high AFP concentration in maternal serum or amniotic fluid suggesting a diagnosis of congenital nephrotic syndrome in a high-risk family) or in cultured cells obtained from chorionic villi, amniotic cells, or fibroblasts (e.g., for diagnosing cystinosis).

There are a number of methods used in genetic analysis (see Chapter 38). In many disorders, the gene has been mapped to a specific chromosomal locus and is genetically linked to DNA markers. Genetic diagnosis is then possible on amniotic fluid, chorionic villous, or blood samples, if

one or more specific alleles are informative, i.e., characteristic for the disease in a given family or in a given population (e.g., in CNF, see later in this chapter). If the gene responsible for a particular disease has been cloned and sequenced, the specific mutation in an affected individual or family can be determined by polymerase chain reaction (PCR), followed by sequence analysis or another method. Molecular diagnosis may be complicated by the fact that a similar phenotype may result from mutations of one of two or more genes, e.g., autosomal dominant polycystic kidney disease (ADPKD) (chromosomes 16, 4, and 2) (419–423) and for nephrogenic diabetes insipidus (NDI).

Urinary Acidification

Immaturity of renal tubular acidification results in a significantly lower value of serum bicarbonate concentration in VLBW infants than in full-term infants. In parallel, the serum base excess is often between −5 and −10 mEq/L in VLBW infants, compared with 0 to −5 mEq/L in full-term infants, and the anion gap, is normally 15 to 22 mEq/L in premature infants, compared to 12 ± 2 mEq/L (less than 15 mEq/L) in full-term infants. In newborn infants, metabolic acidosis often is secondary to asphyxia, hypoxia, shock, or sepsis. If metabolic acidosis is persistent, an inborn error in metabolism or a defect in tubular acidification, among other diagnoses, should be suspected. Measurement of urine pH, and of urine-to-blood carbon dioxide tension gradient is indicated to rule out distal renal tubular acidosis (RTA) (424) (see Tubular Function).

Microscopic Examination of Urine

The shape of erythrocytes in freshly voided urine should be observed under the microscope. The presence of deformed cells suggests hematuria of glomerular origin, whereas undeformed cells predominate in either massive hematuria or lower urinary tract disease. Leukocyturia is common in normal infants during the first few days of life (425); yet, leukocyturia may be lacking in a newborn infant with a positive urine culture, in contrast to older children. The presence of bacteria on a Gram stain is a better predictor of urinary tract infection (UTI). The presence of erythrocyte casts in the urine suggests the diagnosis of glomerulopathy, and leukocyte casts can be observed during UTI.

Urine Electrolytes and Osmolality

The measurement of urinary and blood osmolality, urea, creatinine, and electrolytes is indicated for the differential diagnosis of polyuria, hyponatremia and for the early diagnosis of oligoanuria.

Proteinuria

Maturation is associated with a decrease in the daily rate of proteinuria (see Table 42-2) and with qualitative changes, which can be analyzed by two-dimensional gel electrophoresis (426). The first voided urine in 22- to 28-week-old infants contains many proteins and peptides, whereas urine in full-term infants contains much less polypeptides. Urinary excretion of lysosomal and brush border enzymuria and that of low molecular weight (LMW) proteins follow specific developmental patterns (427). LMW proteins i.e., beta2-microglobulin, myoglobin, and retinol-binding globulin, are filtered through the glomerulus, reabsorbed, and catabolized by the tubule. As the tubular reabsorption of β2-microglobulin increases with maturation, its fractional excretion decreases until 2 years of age (428). The urinary concentration of LMW proteins is a sensitive indicator of renal tubular damage as a result of asphyxia or medications (see Acute Renal Failure).

Imaging of the Kidney and the Urinary Tract

Ultrasonography and Doppler Flow Analysis

Ultrasonography is performed to screen for renal and urologic malformations or as one of the first steps in the workup of renal failure, oligoanuria, hypertension, UTI, or hematuria (429). Indications for the performance of neonatal US are shown in Table 42-3. Ultrasonography (US) has been found to be a sensitive and reliable method for the detection of nephrocalcinosis (NC). The bright foci are almost always located in the medulla, rarely in the pyelocalyceal system, and hardly ever in the cortex (430,431). NC can present as white dots or white flecks and diminishes gradually over a period of months to years. NC does not influence kidney length in the first 2 years of life (432, 433).

Recently, high-resolution images obtained with high frequency linear array transducers have allowed excellent characterization of renal parenchymal architecture and pathological conditions. In neonates, the US appearances are distinctive, because the renal cortex has echogenicity equal to or greater than that of liver and spleen, whereas in older children the cortex is hypoechoic relative to other organs (434). The differential diagnosis of US anomalies is presented in Table 42-4 (435–438).

Blood flow through renal vessels can be assessed by Doppler US, which is indicated for the evaluation of hematuria, hypertension, and acute renal failure (ARF), especially in a patient with UA catheterization. Pulsed-Doppler flow analysis i.e., duplex scanning, allows the measurement of blood flow velocity, which gives an assessment of RBF, and calculation of the ratio of end-diastolic minimum velocity to systolic peak velocity (i.e., diastolic-to-systolic ratio), thereby helping in the assessment of RVR (439–441).

Voiding Cystourethrogram

Vesicoureteral reflux (VUR) and bladder obstruction should be ruled out in patients with hydronephrosis, renal

TABLE 42-3
INDICATIONS FOR ULTRASONOGRAPHY TO RULE OUT RENAL-URINARY TRACT MALFORMATIONS AND/OR ACQUIRED RENAL DISEASE IN NEWBORN INFANTS

History[a]
  Family history
    First-degree relative with potter's syndrome (bilateral renal agenesis/dysgenesis), autosomal dominant polycystic kidney disease
    Sibling with autosomal recessive polycystic kidney disease
  Abnormal prenatal ultrasonography (kidney, bladder, ascites)
  Oligohydramnios, unless normal postnatal renal function and oligohydramnios attributed to
    Prolonged rupture of the membranes
    Postdate delivery, subacute fetal distress
Physical examination or evidence for other congenital anomaly[a,b]
  Syndrome, sequence or field defect described in Appendix I-1[b]
  Any part of a possible VATER syndrome (vertebral anomalies, anorectal anomalies, tracheoesophageal fistula)
  Preauricular pits, if family history
  Supernumerary nipples
  Congenital diaphragmatic hernia with additional anomalies
  Lung hypoplasia, symptomatic spontaneous pneumothorax
  Abnormal abdominal examination
    Abnormal kidney palpation
    Abdominal mass Bruit[c]
  Ascites
  Single umbilical artery
  Second- or third-degree hypospadias
  Ambiguous genitalia
Evidence for renal disease
  Renal failure, oligoanuria[c]
  Systemic hypertension[c]
  Urinary tract infection
  Hematuria[c]
  Significant proteinuria
  Nephrotic syndrome
  Nephrocalcinosis and nephrolithiasis in preterm infants on prolonged diuretic therapy

[a] The best timing of ultrasonography remains to be determined. A negative test immediately after birth does not rule out hydronephrosis and/or vesicoureteral reflux. A repeat test should be obtained within a few weeks (or earlier if clinically indicated).
[b] The frequency of urinary tract anomalies in many of these entities has not been determined. Because a cost-benefit analysis has not been performed, the indication for neonatal ultrasonographic screening should be decided on an individual basis. The frequency of fetal urinary tract anomalies in association with maternal diabetes or cocaine use is probably too low to justify neonatal ultrasonography in asymptomatic infants.
[c] These patients also should have Doppler ultrasonography.

dysplasia or anomaly, trabeculated bladder, bladder distention, or myelomeningocele (442). Lateral views of the male urethra are mandatory for the diagnosis of posterior urethral valves (443). In a neonate with symptomatic UTI, US should be done initially to assess the presence of obstructive uropathy and signs of renal involvement. If no dilatation is seen and there is a good response to treatment, voiding cystourethrogram (VCUG) can be delayed. If US demonstrates an abnormal bladder, VCUG should be undertaken as soon as possible.

TABLE 42-4

RENAL ULTRASONOGRAPHIC PATTERNS IN NEWBORN INFANTS

Normal appearance
  Prerenal failure
  Renal artery thrombosis
  Congenital renal disease, e.g., renal tubular acidosis
  Renal cystic disease (in which cysts develop late)
  Developing hydronephrosis or vesicoureteral reflux
Increased cortical echogenicity
  With increased corticomedullary differentiation in large kidneys
    Beckwith-Wiedemann syndrome
  With normal corticomedullary differentiation
    Prerenal failure
    Renal ischemia
    Mild renal dysplasia
    Congenital nephrotic syndrome, Finnish type
  With loss of corticomedullary differentiation in normal to small kidneys[a]
    Severe renal dysplasia
    Pyelonephritis, including renal candidiasis
      (often heterogeneous)
    Renal tubular dysgenesis/glomerular dysgenesis[b]
  With loss of corticomedullary differentiation in large kidneys[a]
    Renal vein thrombosis
      Edema results in decreased echoes
      Hemorrhage results in increased echoes
    Corticomedullary necrosis[c]
    Autosomal recessive polycystic kidney disease
    Renal glomerular dysgenesis/tubular dysgenesis
    Transient nephromegaly (benign)
    Contrast nephropathy
    Lymphangioma
    Mesoblastic nephroma[d]
Cysts(s)[e]
  See Appendix 1–3
Increased medullary echogenicity
  Nephrocalcinosis
  Medullary cystic disease
  Tamm-Horsfall proteinuria, acute tubular necrosis
  Medullary sponge kidney
Intrapyelic echogenicity
  Renal candidiasis ("fungus ball")
  Lithiasis
Hydronephrosis

This list does not include findings shown by Doppler ultrasonography.
[a] Diffuse or heterogenous hyperechogenicity of cortex or whole kidney.
[b] Renal size may be enlarged.
[c] Renal size may be normal or enlarged.
[d] Solid mass causing distortion of intrarenal collecting system, with occasional cystic areas corresponding to necrosis or hemorrhage.
[e] Absence of cysts visualized by ultrasonography does not rule out a renal cystic disease in a newborn infant. Some entities result in development of cysts later in life, whereas others (e.g., autosomal recessive polycystic kidney disease) result in hyperechogenicity.
Modified from DeVane GW, Porter JC. An apparent stress-induced release of arginine vasopressin by human neonates. *J Clin Endocrinol Metab* 1980;51:1412–1416, with permission.

Renal Radionuclide Scan

Mercaptoacetyl triglycine (MAG 3) has become the isotope of choice in neonates and infants. It has a high protein binding and thus remains in the blood pool rather than being distributed in the extra vascular space, as does 99mTc-DTPA. The renal extraction of MAG 3 is virtually double that of DTPA (443,444). In contrast, 99mTc-dimercaptosuccinic acid (DMSA) binds to the proximal convoluted tubules and is only minimally excreted into the urine; it is preferred for the analysis of renal morphology and differential function. Typical indications for radionuclide studies include renovascular hypertension, lack of visualization of a kidney by US, preoperative evaluation of the severity of urinary tract obstruction, and evaluation of differential renal function. In normal newborn infants, routinely measuring GFR using radionuclides is not ethically justifiable, even though the amount of radioactivity is minimal. Therefore, normal values for age are not available.

Computed Tomography and Magnetic Resonance Imaging

Computed tomography (CT) and magnetic resonance imaging (MRI) are indicated in the diagnosis of renal tumors, renal abscess, and nephrolithiasis. MRI T2-weighted images (which emphasize the difference in transverse relaxation times between different tissues) are independent of renal function, and provide images in which water is bright, and with excellent contrast between normal and abnormal tissues (444). MRI offers many advantages: the contrast medium, gadolinium chelate, is not nephrotoxic, no ionizing radiation is used, and high resolution three dimensional images can be obtained (445). Lack of nephrotoxicity makes MRI the ideal modality to follow renal transplants (446). Additionally, MRI appears to be more sensitive than US in detecting a tethered cord in a patient with bladder distention and lack of VUR or urethral stenosis on VCUG. Gadolinium-enhanced magnetic resonance (MR) angiography using a fast three-dimensional gradient echo sequence allows a good depiction of the major vessels. However need for sedation, relatively high cost, and good results from US and scintigraphy have limited the use of MRI.

Other Investigations

Intravenous urography is no longer indicated in the neonatal period. Percutaneous antegrade pyelography may be diagnostic in some cases of cystic disease or urinary tract obstruction (447). Contrast angiography used formerly for the diagnosis of renovascular hypertension, aortic thrombus, or an abdominal tumor has been replaced by the less invasive modality of MR angiography.

Renal Pathology

Renal biopsy is indicated in nephrotic syndrome and may be indicated in polycystic kidney disease, hematuria, or persistent severe renal failure of unclear origin. Major contraindications to renal biopsy include bleeding diathesis, anticoagulant therapy, moderate or severe hypertension, solitary kidney, and intrarenal tumor (448). The technique involves visualization of the kidney using US, radioisotope, or radiopaque contrast. The most common complication is macroscopic hematuria, which occurs in 5% to 7% of biopsies.

ACUTE RENAL FAILURE AND OLIGOANURIA

ARF, usually defined as an acute deterioration in the ability of the kidneys to maintain the homeostasis of body fluids (449), is associated with an acute decrease in the rate of glomerular filtration, as opposed to isolated acute tubular dysfunction. Because the placenta fulfills that role in utero, congenital malformations associated with limitation of renal function will not lead to renal failure until birth. ARF in newborn infants is suggested by a progressive increase in the infant's serum creatinine above normal values for age in the context of normal maternal renal function (Fig. 42-5) (450,451).

Incidence

The incidence of intrinsic oliguric ARF in newborn infants admitted to the NICU ranges between 1% and 6% in retrospective studies, and between 6% and 8% in prospective studies (450–452).

Diagnosis

Intrauterine oligoanuria can be suspected when oligohydramnios develops in the absence of amniotic fluid leakage or rupture of the amniotic membranes; it can be as a result of a congenital urinary tract anomaly (e.g., urinary tract obstruction, renal agenesis, dysgenesis), to toxins (e.g., ACE inhibitors, indomethacin) (235,453,454), or to intrauterine asphyxia. If urine output alone is used to assess renal function, ARF often will be either overlooked or over diagnosed. Indeed, normal urine output is found in approximately one-third of neonates with ARF (450, 455), although low urine output may occur in the absence of ARF. Infants who have been subjected to perinatal asphyxia, shock, hypoxemia, or various nephrotoxins are at risk of development of ARF. Clinical signs of ARF include syndromes or signs suggestive of renal or urogenital malformations, oligoanuria, polyuria, hematuria, proteinuria, fluid overload, dehydration, cardiac arrhythmia, and systemic hypertension. Other signs include decreased activity, seizures, anemia, vomiting, and anorexia. Sometimes ARF is suspected on the basis of electrolyte abnormalities or elevated plasma levels of medications (e.g., aminoglycosides).

ARF is characterized by decreased GFR and renal tubular function compared to normal values for either postconceptional age or GA and postnatal age. Although the diagnosis of ARF is strongly suggested by a Pcr that is above the upper limit of normal, during the first days of life such an elevation also may result from abnormal maternal renal function. Thus, measuring GFR or following Pcr over time is required to diagnose ARF in a newborn infant during the first few days of life. Because renal tubular function

changes with maturation, it is important to use criteria appropriate for age; indices developed for more mature subjects are not indicative of intrinsic renal failure in VLBW infants.

Etiology

A wide variety of malformations and prenatal, perinatal, and postnatal events may cause neonatal renal failure (Table 42-5) (451–462). The most common type of acute intrinsic renal failure is ATN, which is discussed in the next section.

Pathophysiology of Acute Tubular Necrosis

The evolution of acute tubular necrosis (ATN) is characterized by three successive phases: initiation, maintenance, and recovery. Although ATN may be precipitated by a single event, its development is multifactorial and involves vascular, i.e., hemodynamic, nephronal, and cellular, i.e., metabolic factors (449).

Vasoconstriction of the afferent arterioles plays a major role in the initiation phase of ATN (463–465). Increased renal vascular resistance results from changes in the relative concentrations of vasoconstrictive agents such as PRA, adenosine, thromboxane, endothelin, and platelet activating factor, and vasodilator agents such as natriuretic peptides, NO, PGs, and prostacyclin. The increase in PRA, which results from the stimulation of the juxtaglomerular apparatus by the high solute content of damaged tubules, helps maintain glomerular filtration by vasoconstricting the efferent arteriole. During the maintenance phase of ATN, the main factors are nephronal and cellular. The main cellular injury comes in the form of programmed cell death (apoptosis). Renal cellular injury is accompanied by release of free oxygen radicals, changes in intracellular calcium metabolism, phospholipid breakdown, altered cell polarity, and secondarily, loss of tight cell junctions between cells, loss of the cell brush border, and disruption of the cytoskeleton, leading to disruption of major cellular functions, e.g., Na+/K+-ATPase, and cell swelling. All these processes, except damage caused by free oxygen radicals, are accompanied by cellular ATP depletion, thereby limiting cellular restoration with reperfusion, an energy consuming process. When cellular ATP decreases, the concentration of intracellular heat shock transcription factor rises. Proximal tubular cells loaded with heat shock protein and then exposed to ischemic damage had significantly less ATP release after ischemia than nonheat shock protein-loaded cells and a marked reduction in apoptosis. Generation of heat shock protein and lactic dehydrogenase after anoxic injury in neonatal kidneys provides a better defense mechanism against ischemic renal injury compared to adult kidneys.

The production of local growth factors decreases during the early phase of ATN; the tubular epithelium only regenerates during the recovery phase. GFR initially increases in parallel with a decrease in intratubular pressure and casts; GFR then increases in parallel with RPF and urine output

TABLE 42-5
ETIOLOGIC CLASSIFICATION OF ACUTE NEONATAL RENAL FAILURE

Parenchymal malformation[a]
  Renal agenesis
  Renal hypoplasia
    Simple hypoplasia
    Oligonephronic hypoplasia
  Renal dysplasia
    Multicystic
    Hypoplastic
    Aplastic
    Associated with urinary tract obstruction or
      vesicoureteral reflux
  Nephron dysgenesis
    Tubular dysgenesis: congenital hypernephronic
      nephromegaly with tubular dysgenesis =
      congenital tubular dysgenesis = isolated
      congenital renal tubular immaturity
    Glomerular dysgenesis:
      Idiopathic
      Secondary to maternal administration of
        indomethacin or angiotensin-converting enzyme
        inhibitors
  Polycystic kidney disease
    Adult type (autosomal dominant)
    Infant type (autosomal recessive)
    Other
Acquired renal dysfunction or lesion[b]
  Asphyxia/hypoxia/ischemia
    Functional (may lead to prenal or intrinsic renal failure)
      Systemic hypotension, shock, hypovolemia, severe
        dehydration
      Renal artery vasoconstriction, e.g., nephrotoxins,
        endotoxin, endothelin
      Reverse diastolic blood flow (preeclampsia, patent
        ductus arteriosus)

  Prenatal/perinatal/postnatal asphyxia
    Respiratory distress, hypoxemia
    Sepsis
    Heart failure, extracorporeal membrane oxygenation,
      cardiopulmonary bypass surgery
    Hyperviscosity, polycythemia
    Severe anemia
  Vascular
    Arterial/arteriolar thrombosis/embolism/stenosis
    Cortical/medullary necrosis, renal infarction
    Venous thrombosis
  Urinary tract obstruction (see Table 42-7)
  Urinary tract infection
  Disseminated intravascular coagulation
  Drugs
    Antibiotics (aminoglycosides, amphotericin, acyclovir)
    Non steroid anti-inflammatory agents
    Tolazoline
    Alpha-Adrenergic agents
    Angiotensin-converting enzyme inhibitors
    Radiocontrast agents
    Cyclosporine
  Toxins
    Hemoglobinuria
    Myoglobinuria
    Hyperoxaluria
    Benzyl alcohol
    Polysorbate
    Ethylene glycol
    Uric acid nephropathy
  Glomerular disease
    Membranous glomerulonephritis (IgG-mediated)
    Congenital syphilis
    Diffuse mesangial sclerosis

[a] May not cause acute renal failure until after the neonatal period.
[b] May occur *in utero*.

(452). Unless enough fluid is provided to compensate for the large amounts of urine lost during the polyuric phase, hypovolemia may develop and slow the recovery or even cause a secondary deterioration of renal function. Randomized trials are needed to determine strategies to reduce the severity of ARF with the least side effects (466). Although many candidate drugs have been studied, none have proven effective in clinical trials.

Renal Blood Flow

Decreased RBF may result from multiple mechanisms such as reverse diastolic flow, hypotension, heart failure, and vasoconstriction (Table 42-5). In mothers with preeclampsia, absent or retrograde diastolic blood flow in the fetal aorta and UA predicts several perinatal complications, including renal failure (467).

RBF velocity remains low for at least 1 week in VLBW infants with intrauterine growth retardation (468). Prevention of prenal failure includes correction of any abnormality in and maintenance of adequate oxygenation,

ventilation, blood pressure, cardiac output, hydration (see Chapter 21), blood glucose, and hematocrit, and prevention and early treatment of sepsis. Preliminary data suggest that indomethacin-mediated renal vasoconstriction and ARF may be reduced by using prior volume expansion and by using a low dose and a slow infusion of indomethacin (469). Although furosemide increases urine output in patients receiving indomethacin for treating a PDA, the routine use of furosemide in these patients cannot be recommended (470,471).

Urine Output

In asymptomatic low-risk full-term infants receiving routine care, low or even absent urine output (detected by checking the number of wet diapers) during the first 24 hours of life is a normal event, assuming adequate fluid intake. If spontaneous urination is not observed within an additional 12 hours, i.e., at 36 hours of life, the baby should be reexamined for possible urinary retention, and the bladder should be catheterized.

In contrast, in premature infants and in patients with suggestive history, symptoms, or abnormal physical examination, urine output should be measured from birth. If there is no urine by 24 hours of life or if subsequent output is less than 1 mL/kg/h, the bladder should be catheterized; suprapubic pressure (i.e., the Credé maneuver) should be avoided, because of the risk of VUR, and rarely for bladder or renal rupture (472). Patients at high risk for renal failure (e.g., shock, extracorporeal membrane oxygenation [ECMO], or major surgery) should have their bladder catheterized to measure the hourly urine output.

If polyuria develops, possible diagnoses include hypervolemia, tubular dysfunction, diabetes insipidus, glucose overload, the polyuric phase of ATN, and the polyuric phase of postrenal failure (e.g., after decompression of the bladder by catheterization).

Perinatal Asphyxia

The risk for and severity of ARF increases with the severity of asphyxia (473–475). ARF associated with asphyxia is predominantly nonoliguric (474). Thus, unless Pcr is monitored daily in the severely asphyxiated neonate, renal failure will be easily missed. Early diagnosis of ARF secondary to perinatal asphyxia is suggested by the finding of increased tubular LMW proteinuria immediately after birth (476–478). Asphyxiated infants with a urine output less than 1 mL/kg/h for 36 hours usually have a high urinary concentration of beta2-microglobulin and clinical signs of hypoxic–ischemic encephalopathy. A dipstick may help detect hematuria, myoglobinuria, and proteinuria. Oligoanuria in these infants may result from prerenal, i.e., functional–mediated failure mediated in part by endothelin (479), intrinsic renal failure (e.g., ATN), or syndrome of inappropriate secretion of ADH (SIADH).

Prevention and Early Diagnosis of Acute Renal Failure

The first step is to identify infants at high risk for renal failure or oligoanuria immediately after birth or after predisposing events (Figs. 42-5 and 42-6). In these infants, urine collection should be initiated right away, and vital signs, electrolytes, and renal function should be followed serially. If urinary tract anomalies are suspected, a complete urologic workup should be considered (see Chapter 43). Decompression of the urinary tract by bladder catheterization or surgical intervention, or both, may be indicated. Oliguric renal failure develops in 22% of patients on venoarterial ECMO and may develop in patients on venovenous ECMO in the absence of changes in cardiac output, blood pressure, or hypoalbuminemia; the exact pathophysiology of the renal dysfunction in such infants remains to be elucidated (480,481).

General Approach in Oligoanuria

The diagnosis of oligoanuria, i.e., urinary output less than 0.5 to 1.0 mL/kg/h should be confirmed by demonstrating the absence of urine by bladder catheterization. Delayed micturition has been described in association with transient bladder distention attributed to severe perinatal asphyxia (482). Bladder puncture should be avoided because of the high likelihood of causing trauma.

Once oligoanuria is confirmed, the history should be reviewed for severe asphyxia, respiratory failure, hypotension, shock, and renal toxins. Intake and output over the last few days should be reviewed. The physical examination should seek evidence of weight change, dehydration, malformations, respiratory failure, CHF, shock, hypotension, and central nervous system disease. General care should be optimized, including measures to support ventilation, oxygenation, cardiac output, functional circulatory volume, and ECF volume.

Urine and Blood Analysis

The differential diagnosis of oligoanuria includes not only renal failure but also SIADH and decreased urine production secondary to the administration of ADH or its analogs (Table 42-6). The differentiation between prerenal and true renal ARF is presented in Table 42-7.

Urine should be examined promptly for protein, cellular elements and crystals, electrolytes, creatinine, and SG or osmolality. A blood sample should be obtained for

TABLE 42-6
DIFFERENTIAL DIAGNOSIS OF OLIGOANURIA

Renal failure
  Prerenal (see Table 42-7)
  Intrinsic (see Table 42-7)
  Postrenal
    Bladder retention
      Urethral valves
      Meningomyelocele, tethered cord
      Massive vesicoureteral reflux
    Bilateral ureteral obstruction
      Ureteropelvic junction obstruction
      Ureterovesical junction obstruction, ureterocele
      Lithiasis
      Fungus ball
    Extrinsic compression
    Uroascites (i.e., ruptured urinary tract)
      Secondary to urinary tract obstruction
      Bladder perforation (umbilical artery catheterization or direct bladder trauma)
Syndrome of inappropriate secretion of antidiuretic hormone
Exogenous administration (to the mother or the newborn infant) of
  Antidiuretic hormone, desmopressin
  Oxytocin
  Non steroidal anti-inflammatory agents
Acute bladder distension without renal failure
  Curarization
  Neurogenic bladder
  Hematoma of the anterior wall of the bladder (traumatic suprapubic aspiration)

TABLE 42.7

DIFFERENTIAL DIAGNOSIS: PRERENAL VS. INTRINSIC OLIGURIC RENAL FAILURE[a]

	Prerenal	Intrinsic
FENa(%)	≤1	>3
UNa (mmol/L)	≤20	>50
U_{SG}	>1,025	<1,014
U Osm (mOsm/kg)	≥500	≤300
U/P osm[b]	≥1.2	0.8–1.2
U/Pcr	High (>40)	Low (9.7 ± 3.6)
BUN/Pcr (mg/mg)	>30	<20
Renal failure index[c]	Low (<1)	High (>4)
Ultrasonography[d]	Normal	May be abnormal[d]
Response to challenge[e]	UO >2 mL/kg/h	No↑UO

[a] FENa is obtained by dividing sodium clearance by glomerular filtration rate and multiplying by 100. FENa and UNa are high (falsely suggesting an intrinsic renal failure) after diuretic administration, volume expansion, urinary excretion of nonabsorbable solutes (glycosuria, mannitol, glycerol, bicarbonate [in metabolic alkalosis]), adrenal insufficiency, or gestational age <28 wk. FENa increases transiently in normal full-term infants immediately after birth and in premature infants during the diuretic phase. FENa is also high in case of prolonged urinary tract obstruction and in chronic renal failure. Conversely, FENa and UNa are low (falsely suggesting prerenal failure) in acute renal failure due to severe vasoconstriction (e.g., indomethacin, radiocontrast nephropathy, sepsis, early phase of myoglobinuria), in acute urinary tract obstruction, and in some cases of nonoliguric ATN.
[b] Although plasma osmolality can be estimated using the formula:
Posm: 2 × PNa (mEq/L) + gl (mg/dL)/18 + BUN (mg/dL)/2.8
Where PNa is plasma sodium concentration, gl is glycemia and BUN is blood urea nitrogen, the measured value of Posm is preferable, especially in critically ill patients, because of large differences in the case of sick cell syndrome (leaking cellular membranes), and in infants with a birth weight <1,000 g (Giacoia 1992).
[c] Renal failure index = U Na × Pcr/Ucr
[d] The ultrasonography in "intrinsic" renal failure may show increased echogenicity of the pyramids, which probably corresponds to precipitation of Tamm-Horsfall protein, signs of renal vein thrombosis, renal artery thrombosis, adrenal hemorrhage, hydronephrosis, cystic kidney disease, renal dysplasia , hypoplasia, or other pathology (see Table 42-5).
[e] The challenge corresponds to the administration of 20 mL/kg of crystalloid (more should be given if there is evidence of hypovolemia) and/or 1 mg/kg of furosemide. Normalization of the urine output after such a challenge may correspond to a prerenal failure or to the polyuric phase following an oliguric renal failure. See text for additional comments.
FENa, fractional excretion of sodium; UNa, urinary sodium concentration; U_{SG}, urine specific gravity; Uosm, urine osmolality; U/P osm, ratio of urine to plasma osmolality; U/Pcr, Urine to plasma creatinine ratio; BUN/Pcr, ratio of blood urea nitrogen to plasma creatinine concentration; UO, urine output

hematocrit, electrolytes, creatinine, BUN, and glucose; other tests (e.g., serum concentration of xanthine or uric acid, oxaluria) may be indicated based on history or initial results. Plasma osmolality can be either measured or calculated from the following formula:

$$Posm (mOsm/kg) = 2 \times Na (mEq/L) + glucose (mg/dL)/18 + BUN (mg/dL)/2.8.$$

Use of this formula is not recommended for infants with a BW less than 1,000 g, in whom it may substantially underestimate true osmolality (483).

While waiting for the results of these tests and ordering a renal US, and in some instances a renal scan, an initial therapeutic decision often can be made. This is especially important in patients in whom no urine can be obtained for analysis. Prerenal failure is a reasonable presumptive diagnosis in the presence of respiratory failure, CHF, dehydration, or shock, if osmolality or SG is high in the absence of casts in the urine. Rapid correction of the problem may be the only therapeutic intervention needed. The SIADH can be suspected in cases of severe neurologic dysfunction,

pneumothorax, or pleural effusion, with weight gain, oligoanuria, high urinary SG and hyponatremia.

The urine obtained initially, i.e., before any diuretic or fluid challenge should be sent for urinalysis and urine chemistry for the assessment of tubular function. Various indices and tests have been proposed to differentiate ATN from prerenal or functional failure, by the presence of tubular dysfunction in ATN (484,485). FENa is the preferred index. A FENa greater than 3% (>6 % in preterm <32 weeks) (485) suggests a diagnosis of intrinsic failure and a value less than 2.5% a prerenal failure; however, several exceptions exist (Table 42-7). Renal failure index (RFI) is sometimes used as an alternative to FENa:

$$RFI = UNa \times Pcr/Ucr.$$

Cutoff points for diagnosis of ATN are RFI more than 4 in term and more than 8 in preterm infants less than 32 weeks.

Asphyxiated newborn infants may manifest transient tubular dysfunction associated with a normal or mildly decreased GFR and a normal or decreased urine output. Their tubular dysfunction is characterized by a positive dipstick test for blood, moderate tubular proteinuria, i.e., LMW proteins and N-acetyl-β-D-glucosaminidase [NAG], and a FENa that is either normal or mildly increased (476,477,486–488). In contrast, ATN is associated with marked proteinuria, markedly decreased GFR, and often oligoanuria. Urinary concentration of myoglobin and retinol-binding protein, but not NAG, can be used to differentiate between normal transient tubular dysfunction and ATN (476,477). Renal and bladder US may establish a diagnosis of urinary tract obstruction, uro-ascites, or renal cystic disease (see Appendix G–4), suggest renal vein or artery thrombosis, adrenal hemorrhage, or show abnormal cortical, medullary, or pyelocalicial echogenicity (see Table 42-4) (435–438,489–491). One common finding is increased echogenicity of the pyramids (494,495), which may correspond to the precipitation of Tamm–Horsfall protein in patients with ATN.

The diagnosis of SIADH is suggested by a plasma osmolality less than 280 mOsm/kg, a ratio of urinary to plasma osmolality that is greater than 1, high urine SG, and an inappropriate increase in weight. The strict criteria used for the diagnosis of SIADH in adults rarely are met in newborn infants. In most instances, inappropriate levels of ADH are found in patients with abnormal renal function, because asphyxia is a common cause of both problems. The treatment of SIADH usually includes fluid restriction with a normal sodium intake; hypertonic glucose may be necessary to treat severe hypoglycemia secondary to drastic fluid restriction, and furosemide (with careful replacement of the sodium lost in the urine) may be needed in patients with severe CHF secondary to fluid overload. Hypertonic saline is indicated to raise natremia to 125 mEq/L in patients developing central nervous system signs (e.g., seizures, coma) associated with severe hyponatremia.

Challenge Test

A challenge test is indicated only if the etiology of the renal failure is not evident from the assessment of risk factors, clinical signs, US, and urine indices (see Table 42-7). This can be a fluid challenge (20 mL/kg of crystalloid solution, e.g., isotonic saline) followed by a diuretic challenge (usually furosemide 1 mg/kg intravenously) in a nondehydrated infant. Although patients who fail to respond to furosemide may respond to bumetanide (5 mg/kg/dose intravenously), a more potent loop diuretic, this medication has not been evaluated prospectively in acute neonatal oliguria.

A diuretic challenge test should be done first in patients thought to be hypervolemic or in heart failure, whereas a fluid challenge should be done first in those thought to be hypovolemic. If the first challenge test does not yield a satisfactory response, defined by a normal urine output, the other test should be considered. Although normalization of the urine output is most commonly observed in prerenal failure, it also may be coincidental with the beginning of the polyuric phase of an intrinsic renal failure, or with the transformation of an oliguric into a nonoliguric renal

failure (492). The correct diagnosis may be suggested by renal US and by the rapidity of GFR recovery, rather than by the FENa, which is increased by the challenge itself. In any of these situations, the prognosis usually is good. In contrast, if anuria persists despite optimization of general care and double-challenge test, the diagnosis of intrinsic renal failure is likely, severe fluid restriction is indicated, and the prognosis is guarded.

Nonoliguric Renal Failure

Nonoliguric renal failure is characterized by a sudden decrease in GFR and tubular function in the absence of oligoanuria. Thirty to fifty percent of neonates with ARF are nonoliguric (450,493). The ARF observed in one third of patients who receive cardiopulmonary bypass surgery typically is nonoliguric (456). Renal failure without oliguria may be overlooked in the absence of routine measurement of blood chemistries and urinalysis (450,451). It may be confused initially with the polyuric phase of an intrinsic or postrenal renal failure, especially after an undiagnosed oligoanuria episode, or with prerenal failure that has been treated by the administration of fluids for hypovolemia (492). Although the prognosis of nonoliguric renal failure usually is better than oliguric renal failure (455), it can be complicated by symptomatic hyperkalemia (484).

Treatment of Acute Renal Failure

Supportive Treatment and Prevention of Complications

In our experience, prompt treatment of ARF and its complications avoids the need for renal replacement therapy (e.g., dialysis, continuous arteriovenous hemofiltration [CAVH]) in most patients. Some researchers, however, argue that early institution of replacement therapy may result in improved mortality and morbidity.

Supportive treatment of infants with ARF should be aimed at maintaining homeostasis of all vital systems. Some patients may need major respiratory and cardiovascular support (495), and all such patients require adequate fluid and electrolyte balance and adjustment of the dosage of medications that are eliminated by the kidney (450,496,497). Early diagnosis and treatment may help prevent many complications of ARF, such as water or medication intoxication and hyperkalemia. The prognosis of ARF depends not only on the severity and the duration of the renal injury, but also, and perhaps mainly, on the overall status of the patient.

Use of low dose dopamine for improving renal function remains controversial. In hypotensive premature infants (29–34 weeks of GA) with respiratory distress syndrome, non randomized trials suggest that the infusion of dopamine at a rate of 5 to 20 μg/kg/min results in a transient elevation in blood pressure compared to controls, followed by increases in urine output, creatinine clearance, and natriuresis (498,499). A systematic review failed to provide enough evidence to recommend routine use of low dose dopamine for improving renal function and urine volume in critically ill neonates (500). Two small randomized trials have assessed the effect of low-dose dopamine in preterm infants (501,502). Cuevas and associates (502) found that in preterm infants with respiratory distress syndrome and a GA greater than or equal to 30 weeks, dopamine at 1 or 2.5 µg/kg/min increased blood pressure and natriuresis but did not significantly increase GFR and urine output compared with controls. Lynch and associates (501) found that in oliguric preterm infants with BW greater than 1250 grams, dopamine infusion at a dose of 2.5 µg/kg/min did not affect blood pressure but increased GFR and urine output and that a dose of 7.5 µg/kg did not affect blood pressure min or GFR but increased urine output compared with controls receiving a dose of 0.5 µg/kg/min.

In severely asphyxiated newborn infants, one prospective randomized study showed that infusion of dopamine at low dose (2 to 5 µg/kg/min) increased systolic blood pressure and urine output and decreased the incidence of abnormal Pcr (503). Another randomized clinical trial showed that theophylline (antiadenosine effect) improved renal function in asphyxiated full term neonates; additional data are needed before recommending routine use of theophylline in asphyxiated term neonates for improving renal function (504,505).

Fluid and Electrolytes

Water and sodium metabolism: In the presence of oligo-anuria refractory to the initial fluid and diuretic challenge, fluid restriction is indicated. Fluid intake is limited to ongoing sensible losses, i.e., gastrointestinal losses, urinary output, third-space losses, drainage, plus 25 mL/kg/24 hours in a full-term infant, and 50 to 100 mL/kg/24 hours in a LBW or VLBW infant to replace insensible water loss. Neither sodium nor potassium should be administered routinely during this phase. However, babies with nonoliguric renal failure may have very large sodium losses, up to 10 mEq/kg/day, and these must be replaced on the basis of serial sodium measurements and clinical assessment. If fluid restriction is not initiated early in the course of ARF, fluid overload will result, with potential CHF, pulmonary edema, and pulmonary hemorrhage. If massive fluid overload leads to severe CHF, hemo (dia) filtration may be indicated.

Hyperkalemia: Patients with ARF often develop hyperkalemia, i.e., a potassium concentration greater than 6.5 mEq/L (506,507). Factitious hyperkalemia can result from hemolysis or clot formation during sampling, i.e., release of potassium from erythrocytes or platelets or from interference with the measurement of potassium concentration by benzalkonium released from a heparin-coated umbilical catheter (508). If hyperkalemia is associated with hyponatremia, hypoglycemia, and hypotension, a diagnosis of adrenal insufficiency should be considered (see Chapter 39). This most often results either from congenital adrenal hyperplasia or from bilateral adrenal hemorrhage;

the latter may be suspected on the basis of anemia with thrombocytopenia, jaundice, and bilateral abdominal masses, and confirmed by US.

The treatment of hyperkalemia includes discontinuing any potassium intake; discontinuing any medication that could cause hyperkalemia (e.g., indomethacin, ACE inhibitors, potassium-sparing diuretics); and correcting hypovolemia using isotonic saline to promote tubular secretion of potassium. Simultaneous administration of several forms of therapy (Table 42-8) often is required for treating life-threatening hyperkalemia (501,506,509–516). The use of glucose-insulin, albuterol and cation-exchange resins for treating hyperkalemia has been assessed by randomized trials in neonates.

If electrocardiographic changes are associated with hyperkalemia, administration of calcium chloride or calcium gluconate is indicated; this will rapidly, but only transiently, decrease myocardial cell excitability, but will not decrease potassium concentration (see Table 42-8) (510). Thus, the administration of calcium should be followed immediately by at least one method to decrease the potassium concentration.

Several methods (Table 42-8) have been proposed to induce cellular uptake of potassium, including the combination of glucose and insulin, albuterol, bicarbonate, and exchange transfusion with washed packed cells. Glucose-insulin infusion is more efficient in correcting hyperkalemia than bicarbonate or cation exchange resins, and equally efficient as albuterol. If glucose and insulin are infused, the initial ratio for VLBW infants (500 to 1,000 g) should be approximately 2.2 g/U (511); the ratio should be adjusted (range 1–3 g/U) according to the evolution of the glycemia.

Albuterol increases cellular uptake of potassium by inducing Na+/K+-ATPase activity through cAMP, independently of the action of insulin or aldosterone, and by inducing an increase in serum insulin level (517). A randomized trial in preterm neonates showed that nebulized albuterol (400 µg) decreases potassium level by 0.7 mEq/L within 4 hours and 1.1 mEq/L within 8 hours vs. no significant change in the saline group (517). Intravenous albuterol infusion (4 µg/kg over 5 minutes) reduces serum potassium by 1.48 ± 0.5 mEq/L and 1.64 ± 0.5 mEq/L at 40 and 120 minutes, respectively, in hyperkalemic children (512,518). However, a serious word of caution is required because albuterol administration increases serum potassium during the first 3 minutes, presumably through alpha-receptor stimulation (517,519). Nebulized albuterol transiently increases serum potassium by more than 0.1 mEq/L (up to 0.4 mEq/L) in half the adult patients with renal failure and intravenous albuterol transiently increases potassium by 0.65 mEq/L in baboons (519,520). Therefore albuterol should not be used as the first line of treatment, and calcium should be available in case an acute arrhythmia develops.

Although sodium bicarbonate (1 mEq/kg) has been recommended for treating hyperkalemia; its efficacy in patients with renal failure is controversial: one study showed

TABLE 42-8

TREATMENT OF HYPERKALEMIA IN RENAL FAILURE

Medication	Dose (iv Unless Otherwise Specified)	Mechanism	Onset of Action	Duration
Calcium chloride	0.25–0.5 mEq/kg over 5–10 min	Modifies myocardial excitability	1–3 min	30–60 mm
Calcium gluconate	0.5–1 mEq/kg over 5–10 mm			
Sodium bicarbonate	1 mEq/kg over 10–30 mm	Intracellular uptake of K	5–10 min	2 h
Glucose	0.5 g/kg/h	Intracellular uptake of K	30 min	4–6 h
+Insulin	1 U/2.2 g glucose (1–3)[a]			
Albuterol	4–5 µg/kg over 15–20 min[c]	Intracellular uptake of K	30–40 mm	>120 min
Cation exchange resin (Na/Ca polystyrene sulfonate)	1 g/kg intrarectally q 6 h[b]	Exchange of K for Na or Ca	1–2 h	6 h
Exchange transfusion[d]	2/3 washed RBCs reconstituted with 5% albumin	Uptake of K by RBCs	Minutes[e]	>12 h
Peritoneal dialysis	Use a dialysate with low K concentration	Dialysis	Minutes[e]	No limit
Hemo(dia)filtration		Filtration (and dialysis)	Minutes[e]	Days

[a] The preparation of an insulin drip requires saturating the plastic tubing with the insulin solution before infusing to the patient. The average ratio of glucose to insulin associated with maintenance of normal glycemia in very-low-birth-weight infants is 2.2 ± 0.6 g/U (mean ± SD) (Lui).
[b] Oral administration of polystyrene resin should be avoided in very-low-birth-weight infants and those with poor peristalsis (risk for concretions) (Ohlson). Substantial load of calcium or sodium may result from the respective resin. The effect on potassium concentration is slower than glucose insulin combination.
[c] Since administration of albuterol may cause a transient increase in serum potassium concentration, it should not be used as the first medication to treat hyperkalemia (see text for details). The iv preparation is not available in the United States. Albuterol is also efficient by aerosol.
[d] Many blood banks do not wash red blood cells anymore
[e] These techniques are both rapid and extremely effective in correcting potassium levels. The time to set them up may be the limiting factor: other techniques may be used to stabilize the infant initially.
Modified from ref 510.

lower efficacy than either glucose-insulin or albuterol (521) and another study showed no efficacy (522). Repeated doses of bicarbonate may result in hypernatremia. Furthermore, addition of bicarbonate to other therapies (insulin-glucose or albuterol) does not increase their efficacy. Until randomized trials are available, bicarbonate administration is indicated to treat acidosis related to renal failure, but its potential benefits on hyperkalemia (reduction of serum potassium by H/K exchange in mineral acidosis) should be weighed against the potential risk for intraventricular hemorrhage (IVH).

Exchange transfusion with washed, packed erythrocytes reconstituted with plasma or albumin may reduce potassium concentration efficiently and for as long as 12 hours (516); however, many blood banks no longer perform this procedure. Hyperkalemic infants requiring red blood cell transfusions should receive either fresh blood or blood passed through a sodium polystyrene sulfonate filter, which removes most of the potassium (523).

Although cation-exchange resins offer the potential advantage of removing potassium permanently from the body rather than increasing cellular uptake, their use in neonates is not recommended because of low efficacy and safety. Hyperkalemic neonates treated with cation-exchange resins have a slow onset of potassium response (514), more prolonged hyperkalemia and more frequent IVH than those treated with glucose-insulin (524). Side effects of these resins include sodium overload (if using sodium polystyrene sulfonate but not if using a resin with calcium

instead of sodium), bowel obstruction, perforation and bleeding (515).

Renal replacement therapy, especially CAVH, is the procedure of choice for hyperkalemic infants with severe oliguric ARF and for those on ECMO (525).

Acid–Base and Mineral Disturbances

Metabolic acidosis develops rapidly in most infants with ARF. It may require the administration of large doses of sodium bicarbonate, which may aggravate fluid overload.

Hypocalcemia develops rapidly in almost all patients with ARF. It may result from hyperphosphatemia and increased deposition of calcium in injured tissues, especially in rhabdomyolysis; skeletal resistance to PTH, which results from decreased hydroxylation of vitamin D (526); and, in aminoglycoside-induced ARF, parathyroid dysfunction secondary to hypomagnesemia, which is as a result of increased tubular loss (527). Hypercalcemia may occur as a late complication of rhabdomyolysis, as a result of reabsorption of calcium deposited in necrotic tissues. Hyperphosphatemia is as a result of tissue damage (e.g., severe asphyxia, shock, and rhabdomyolysis) and decreased urine excretion (526). Additionally, ARF usually causes hypermagnesemia, which may result from decreased excretion and from shift from the intracellular space (528).

During the oliguric phase, no intake of magnesium (e.g., antacids) or phosphate should be provided, to limit both hypermagnesemia and hyperphosphatemia. The polyuric phase of ATN is associated with increased urinary excretion of phosphate and magnesium. Intravenous calcium may be required to treat severe hypocalcemia (low ionized calcium with either symptoms or electrographic changes) or hyperkalemia with electrocardiographic changes; however, additional intravenous calcium should not be given routinely until the plasma phosphate level has been reduced to normal, to limit the risk of ectopic calcification. The hyperphosphatemia is managed by the addition of calcium carbonate to feeds. This binds phosphate, rendering it insoluble and thereby reducing its absorption. Aluminum hydroxide is not used anymore as a phosphate binder because of the risk of neurotoxicity.

Polyuric Phase

The oliguric phase of ARF is followed by a polyuric phase. During this phase, serial measurements of urine electrolytes and hourly monitoring of the urine output are imperative to adequately replace urinary losses and prevent dehydration, hyponatremia, and hypokalemia. In some cases, bicarbonate, phosphate, and magnesium need to be given to replace urinary losses. When GFR approaches normal levels, fluid intake should be decreased gradually and carefully, although following weight, serum chemistries, and urine output. Replacing the urine output volume for volume for an indefinite duration would cause an adaptive persistence of the polyuria. However, some patients may not recover a normal urinary concentrating ability despite normalization of GFR; these patients still need high fluid intake (529).

Nutrition

If fluid restriction is required, glucose intake often is minimal, and severe hypoglycemia may develop unless a hypertonic solution of glucose is infused through a central venous catheter. If refractory hypoglycemia occurs because of low glucose intake, steroids or a continuous infusion of glucagon can be given. If this is unsuccessful, hemofiltration should be initiated. This technique will allow increased fluid and glucose intake while rapidly correcting the hypervolemia.

Adequate nutrition should be provided to assure anabolism, thereby reducing renal load (530). Breast milk or low-protein formula should be initiated as soon as possible; if the infant cannot be fed, total parenteral nutrition (TPN) should be initiated. If the ARF is severe, the usual amino acid solution should be replaced by essential *L*-amino acids supplemented with *L*-histidine (Levamin Essential; Leiras, Turku, Finland), initially given at a dose of 0.5 to 1 g/kg/d.

Hematologic Disturbances

Anemia associated with ARF may result from several factors, including decreased erythropoietin production, abnormal or ineffective erythropoiesis, impaired iron use, and short-

ened erythrocyte survival. Transfusion of packed erythrocytes may be necessary. Bleeding tendency may result from abnormal platelet function and, in some patients (e.g., those with renal venous thrombosis), from thrombocytopenia.

Adjustment of Medication Dosage

The interval of administration of medications with renal elimination (e.g., antibiotics, paralyzing agents, theophylline, antiepileptic drugs, and digoxin) should be adjusted to actual renal function (spontaneous or renal replacement therapy) to avoid toxic levels. The latter might, in turn, increase the severity of the renal failure (see Nephrotoxicity). Although there are insufficient data to calculate adjustment of dosage in newborn infants, predictions can be made from the relationship between Pcr and the half-life of serum concentration of a particular drug (412–414). Monitoring drug levels will allow additional adjustments. When possible, medications with minimal or no renal toxicity should be chosen.

Renal Replacement Therapy

Renal replacement therapy is indicated for failure of conservative management to improve severe fluid overload, hyperkalemia, metabolic acidosis, hyperphosphatemia, hypocalcemia, or hypertension, or for allowing provision of adequate nutrition and drug administration (518,531). Modalities include peritoneal dialysis, hemodialysis, hemofiltration, and hemodiafiltration (532–538).

Peritoneal dialysis is contraindicated in patients with respiratory failure and should be used with caution in those with peritonitis (533). In patients with liver failure, the dialysis solution should contain bicarbonate (instead of lactate) (534). The other techniques require either heparinization, which is contraindicated in premature infants because of the risk of intraventricular hemorrhage, or prostacyclin (536). CAVH, first used in neonates in 1985, is the technique of choice for the treatment of massive fluid overload. Availability of large-bore intravascular catheters in a patient on ECMO makes this technique particularly easy to initiate. Pump-assisted venovenous hemofiltration is now preferred in most pediatric centers over arteriovenous hemofiltration. If renal failure persists beyond the neonatal period, chronic dialysis and renal transplantation may be necessary (see Chronic Renal Failure).

Before renal replacement therapy is initiated, serious consideration should be given to the possibility that the patient may have either a dysmorphic syndrome with a very poor prognosis regarding the future quality of life, or severe irreversible multiorgan failure. Immediate survival depends mostly on nonrenal problems, whereas ultimate prognosis also depends on the severity of bilateral renal parenchymal disease (537,538).

Prognosis

The short-term prognosis for neonatal ARF depends on the general condition of the infant and the status of all major organs and systems. A team approach to management is crucial and should include a neonatologist, nephrologist, urologist, geneticist, and radiologist.

Acquired Renal Failure

In one series, the mortality rate in patients with oliguric ARF as a result of acquired conditions, i.e., asphyxia and sepsis was 60% and even higher in those with congenital heart disease (451). A similar mortality rate (61%) was observed in a series of infants requiring peritoneal dialysis in the first 60 days of life (532). For newborn infants in whom ARF develops although on ECMO, the prognosis is grim. In contrast, the prognosis for nonoliguric renal failure or for prerenal failure is excellent, unless major arrhythmia secondary to hyperkalemia develops or multiorgan failure develops. Long-term abnormalities in GFR and in tubular function are common in acquired and congenital causes of ARF. In one series, limited urinary concentrating ability tested using DDAVP was observed at 1 to 36 months of age in 11% of patients who had a neonatal Pcr more than or equal to 1.5 mg/dL (529). Fanconi syndrome has been reported as a sequela of renovascular accident in the neonatal period (539).

Congenital Urinary Tract Malformations

Congenital malformations of the kidney and the urinary tract are important not only in the immediate neonatal period, but also they constitute a major cause of chronic renal failure. The reader is referred to Chapter 13 for the description of specific malformations.

Immediate mortality of infants with congenital urinary tract malformations depends primarily on the severity of respiratory failure associated with lung hypoplasia and pulmonary hypertension (540). Infants with severe pulmonary hypoplasia, often associated with typical Potter syndrome, die within the first postnatal hours or days. The presence of bilateral renal parenchymal disease is the major factor predicting poor renal function in cases with congenital renal or urinary tract malformations. Patients with prenatal diagnosis of bilateral urinary tract obstruction should have a comprehensive assessment, including family history, ultrasonography, karyotype, AFP, specific biochemical or genetic tests as indicated, and serial urine biochemical analyses (Table 42-9) (541–543a). Malformations of the kidney and the urinary tract have been linked to mutations of paired homeobox-2 gene (PAX-2) and the angiotensin type 2-receptor gene located on the X chromosome (544). If prenatal assessment demonstrates severe urinary tract obstruction with oligohydramnios in a fetus without a lethal disease and without evidence for renal dysfunction suggestive of bilateral renal dysplasia (541), intervention may be indicated to alleviate oligohydramnios and thus limit or prevent lung hypoplasia. Depending on GA, one may then consider either intrauterine decompression of the urinary tract or elective premature delivery after steroid administration to the mother. Serial determinations of urine indicators

appear more reliable in predicting long-term renal function than single measurements (541–543). Chronic renal failure (CRF) may develop despite early surgical intervention for urinary tract obstruction or reflux (545).

Special Considerations

Structural anomalies of the kidneys and urinary tract are discussed in Chapter 43.

Tubular Dysgenesis

Several cases of perinatal ARF have been described in association with immature nephrons, predominantly with either glomerular lesions or tubular lesions. Oligohydramnios developed in most patients during the second trimester. These infants died in utero or soon after birth.

The administration of ACE inhibitors during pregnancy can result in oligohydramnios, lung hypoplasia, and neonatal renal failure with oligoanuria for 3 to 9 days, hypotension, hypoplasia of the calvaria, and, in many cases, perinatal death (453,454). Pathologic examination may show tubular dysgenesis with abundant presence of renin in glomeruli and preglomerular arterioles, suggesting up-regulation of the renin-angiotensin system (RAS) (546). Similar lesions may occur in one kidney, with renal artery stenosis secondary to arteritis or medial arterial calcinosis (547).

Oberg and associates found signs of renal tubular dysgenesis in 11 of 21 donor twins with twin-to-twin transfusion but in none of the 17 recipient twins (548). Pathophysiology in the donor twin presumably involves reduction in renal perfusion and glomerular filtration with secondary up regulation of renin synthesis. The histological features of tubular dysgenesis are similar to that seen in fetuses exposed to ACE inhibitors during pregnancy. In contrast, the recipient kidney shows downregulation of RAS and histology shows kidneys with multiple hemorrhagic infarcts and hypertrophy of mesangial cells as seen in hypertensive nephropathy.

Intrauterine growth restriction is associated with congenital oligonephropathy and with an increased incidence of hypertension, type II diabetes, hyperlipidemia, CRF, and coronary heart disease in adulthood (549). Congenital oligonephropathy is characterized by a significantly reduced number of glomeruli, which may adversely affect renal development. Animal studies support a role of abnormal maturation of RAS (550).

Prenatal administration of both cyclo-oxygenase type 1 and 2 (COX-1 & 2) inhibitors (e.g., indomethacin, nimesulide) has been associated with perinatal death, bleeding diathesis, ileal perforation, premature ductal closure, fetal oligoanuria, oligohydramnios, and transient or prolonged neonatal renal failure (requiring chronic dialysis) with hematuria and casts (551,552). Pathology may show immature tubules and glomeruli, massive cortical necrosis, or ischemic changes in the cortex associated with cystic dilation of the superficial nephrons and increased intrarenal renin (367).

TABLE 42-9
ASSESSMENT OF THE FETUS WITH BILATERAL RENAL MASS

Procedure	Significance and Interpretation
Family history	Autosomal dominant polycystic kidney disease, autosomal recessive polycystic kidney disease, hereditary renal dysplasia
Comprehensive ultrasonography	Dysmorphic syndrome (e.g., skeletal dysplasia)
	Lung hypoplasia (secondary to abdominal mass, oligohydramnios, or both)
	Abnormality of central nervous system, spinal cord, heart, gastrointestinal tract, limbs
	Tumor (obstructing urinary flow)
	Hydrops, ascites
	Oligohydramnios, polyhydramnios
	Cortical cysts or abnormal echogenicity suggest renal dysplasia; however, hydronephrosis may be difficult to differentiate from cystic dysplasia
	Large trabeculated bladder in a male suggests a diagnosis of posterior urethral valves
DNA analysis	Fetal karyotype to rule out trisomy 13, 18, 9
	Molecular genetics (for specific diagnoses)
Alpha-fetoprotein	If abnormal for gestational age:
	Low: consider diagnosis of trisomy
	High: consider myelomeningocele
Assessment of renal function[a]	Abnormal fetal urine composition (especially progressive worsening on serial analysis) predicts poor long-term renal function and thus is a contraindication to fetal intervention
	Sodium >95th percentile for gestational age (100 mEq/L at 20 wk)[b]
	Chloride >90 mEq/L
	Osmolality >210 mOsm/kg
	Calcium >2 mmol/L (8 mg/dL)
	Phosphate >2 mmol/L
	Beta 2-microglobulin >4 mg/L
	Protein >20 mg/dL
	Urine output <2 mL/h
	Abnormal amino acid concentration for gestational age
	High fetal serum level of beta$_2$-microglobulin: >4.9 mg/L (95% confidence interval at 18–39 wk) or >5.6 mg/L

[a] Serial measurements of urine biochemistry are more predictive of long-term outcome than a single measurement, because serial results show more pronounced deviation from the normal with increasing gestation in fetuses with renal dysplasia.[543]
[b] The 95th percentile is approximately 120, 90,70 and 60 mEq/L at 18, 21, 24 and 27 weeks, respectively.[543]

Renal Artery Thrombosis

The clinical presentation of renal artery thrombosis is a variable combination of hyperreninemic systemic hypertension, hematuria, thrombocytopenia, severe oligoanuric ARF (if the lesion is bilateral), and loss of femoral pulses and of blood flow to the lower extremities. Renal artery thrombosis is often but not always (553) associated with a history of UA catheterization (554–557). Although mechanical injury and alteration of blood flow in the relatively small arteries of neonates is the major stimulus, other contributing factors may include an immature fibrinolytic system, partly as a result of physiologic deficiency in protein C, or plasminogen, hemodynamic factors, and inherited deficiencies of the naturally occurring circulating anticoagulants (hereditary antithrombin III deficiency) (558). The incidence of thrombi in infants with a UA catheter in place ranges between 24% and 95% (559,560). These thrombi may become symptomatic when massive or when embolism occurs.

Real-time US may be normal or show increased cortical echogenicity or nephromegaly. The diagnosis of renal artery thrombosis is confirmed by MR angiography or color Doppler sonography. MR angiography is superior to color Doppler sonography in the evaluation of renal vasculature (561).

ARF associated with bilateral renal artery thrombosis may require prolonged replacement therapy (e.g., peritoneal dialysis) (555). The indications for surgical treatment are not clear (562,563). Systemic anticoagulation, thrombolysis and, if it fails, thrombectomy should be considered for patients with refractory hypertension and those with massive aortic thrombus resulting in major complications (e.g., compromised limb perfusion, renovascular hypertension or anuria) (555,562,563). The other patients usually can be treated with antihypertensive agents and symptomatic management of the complications of ARF; heparinization may help limit further extension of the thrombus. Although renal artery thrombosis often results in localized or diffuse renal hypotrophy, renal function often improves to a level that is close to normal, and hypertension resolves in most patients within a few months (564,565). Fanconi syndrome may occur in rare patients (565).

Renal Venous Thrombosis

Neonatal renal venous thrombosis is an uncommon condition. It may be associated with polycythemia; severe perinatal asphyxia; severe dehydration, sometimes with shock; maternal diabetes; angiography for congenital cyanotic heart disease; and adrenal hemorrhage (566,567). Suboptimal fibrinolysis in stressed newborn infants may be an important factor (568). Renal venous thrombosis presents clinically as the association of a unilateral or bilateral palpable flank mass with hematuria, proteinuria, and, in some cases, oligoanuria.

Ultrasonography of the kidney shows a typical image, characterized by enlargement of the kidney, loss of definition of the corticomedullary junction, abnormal focal or generalized increase in echo amplitude of the renal parenchyma, and decrease in the size and echo amplitude of the central echo complex (567). The diagnosis of renal venous thrombosis is confirmed by MR angiography or color Doppler sonography. In cases in which patency of the IVC is unclear on MR angiography, color Doppler sonography should also be performed (561).

Ultrasonography and Doppler studies show whether the thrombosis extends to the inferior vena cava. The acute complications of renal venous thrombosis include ARF, systemic hypertension, and disseminated intravascular coagulation. The lesion ultimately may result in renal atrophy (569,570). Thrombophilia should be ruled out with appropriate investigations.

Conservative and supportive therapies are indicated. The indications for surgery are not clear. Although unproven, in the presence of consumption coagulopathy, administration of heparin may be considered. The therapeutic decision should take into account the risk of disseminated bleeding and intraventricular hemorrhage, especially in premature infants (571).

In cases associated with bilateral renal venous thrombosis or inferior vena cava thrombosis, similar results have been reported using either thrombectomy or thrombolysis (572,573).

Cortical Necrosis and Medullary Necrosis

Renal cortical or medullary necrosis is the most severe type of ARF. The most common causes of renal necrosis include severe asphyxia and shock (574,575). Idiopathic arterial calcification is a rare cause of renal infarction (576). The symptomatology is not specific and includes oligoanuric ARF, proteinuria, and hematuria that is often grossly apparent. The kidneys often are enlarged; renal US shows homogeneously hyperechoic kidneys, with loss of sharp corticomedullary definition (437). The renal scan shows either very poor renal function or nonvisualization of the kidneys. Calcifications may become visible both on the US and the abdominal radiography. The treatment is similar to that described previously for ATN. The prognosis of bilateral global cortical necrosis is dismal; the diagnosis has been made most often at autopsy. Patients with focal or unilateral necrosis may recover, but often have chronic hypertension and CRF. Infants with medullary necrosis typically have persistent limitations in urinary concentrating ability.

Postrenal Failure

Postrenal failure may result from urinary tract anomalies, extrinsic compression of the urinary tract, fungal infection (fungus ball) or, rarely, urolithiasis (577) (see Hypercalciuria, Nephrocalcinosis, and Nephrolithiasis, and Chapter 43). The medical treatment of postrenal failure is similar to that of intrinsic renal failure. Decompression of the urinary tract (see Chapter 43) often results in an increase in GFR and a polyuric phase, which usually is transient. During the polyuric phase, severe dehydration, hyponatremia, and hyperkalemia may develop despite adequate increase of serum aldosterone levels (578). Sequential adjustment of fluid and electrolyte intake to these losses may help prevent or limit such complications. When GFR comes to baseline within 1 week after corrective surgery, fluid intake should be reduced slowly and carefully, taking into account the fact that limited urine-concentrating ability is expected in association with dysplastic kidneys. The evolution of renal function depends on the degree of renal dysplasia, which is very common in congenital urinary tract obstruction, and the frequency of UTI, which is related to VUR, urinary stasis, and the presence of an indwelling catheter.

NEPHROTOXICITY

Several agents that cross the placenta (see Chapter 15) can damage the fetal kidney, including aminoglycosides, ACE inhibitors, heavy metals, and organic solvents (Table 42-10) (579). Chapters 15 and 56 provide a discussion of the relevant pharmacokinetics. Nephrotoxicity may result from renal ischemia or direct cytotoxicity, or both. Direct cytotoxicity is related to the concentration of drug or metabolite in renal tubular cells, which depends on the concentration of free drug in the plasma, GFR, and tubular transport.

Nephrotoxicity may present as oligoanuria, ARF, drug toxicity caused by decreased clearance of a medication with renal excretion, hypotension, hematuria, proteinuria, RTA, nephrocalcinosis or nephrolithiasis, polyuria, abnormal plasma electrolyte concentrations, or cardiac arrhythmia (see Table 42-10). Because most NICU patients are exposed to multiple drugs as well to episodes of hypoxemia and ischemia, it often is very difficult to determine whether a particular drug is the major renal offender.

TABLE 42-10
NEPHROTOXIC EFFECTS OF VARIOUS AGENTS

Substance	Renal Side Effects
Drugs	
Aminoglycosides	Proteinuria, increased urinary excretion of Na, K, Mg, and glucose, Fanconi syndrome, myelin figures, decreased concentrating ability, decreased RBF, polyuric ARF, ATN, interstitial nephritis
Methicillin	Interstitial nephritis
Amphotericin B	Hyperkaliuria, hyposthenuria, NDI, hypernatriuria, ATN, oliguria, RTA, nephrocalcinosis
Acyclovir	Crystalluria, obstructive nephropathy
Indomethacin	Decreased RBF, ATN, oligoanuria, hyponatremia, hyperkalemia, nephron dysgenesis, and oligohydramnios (*in utero*)
Tolazoline	Hypotension and hypoxemia resulting in decreased GFR, ATN, oliguria, hematuria
Adrenergic agents	Decreased RBF, ATN
ACE inhibitors	Hypotension, decreased RBF, ATN, nephron dysgenesis (*in utero*)
Radiocontrast agents	Decreased RBF, oliguric ATN, Tamm-Horsfall proteinuria, nephromegaly with US similar to ARPKD, increased urinary excretion of uric acid
Cyclosporine	Renal vasoconstriction, decreased RBF and GFR, interstitial nephritis
Loop diuretics	Nephrocalcinosis, nephrolithiasis
Ifosfamide	Fanconi syndrome
Toxins	
Hemoglobin	ATN
Myoglobin	ATN
Oxalate	Nephrocalcinosis, nephrolithiasis, oxalosis with ARF
Benzyl alcohol	Cardiovascular collapse, ATN
Polysorbate (in iv tocopherol)	ATN
Uric acid	Crystalluria, ATN
Organic solvents (toluene)	Fanconi syndrome, aminoaciduria, hyperchloremic acidosis
Alcohol (fetal alcohol syndrome)	Distal RTA
Ethylene glycol (in paracetamol)	ARF, metabolic acidosis

ACE, angiotensin-converting enzyme; ARF, acute renal failure; ARPKD, autosomal recessive polycystic kidney disease; ATN, acute tubular necrosis; GFR, glomerular filtration rate; NDI, nephrogenic diabetes insipidus; RBF, renal blood flow; RTA, renal tubular acidosis.

Prevention of nephrotoxicity includes avoiding teratogens during pregnancy, adjusting the daily dose of medications excreted by the kidney according to measured or predicted GFR and to serum drug levels, avoiding known toxins (458,580,581), and avoiding, if possible, nephrotoxic drugs, especially synergistic combinations.

Specific Considerations

Aminoglycosides

Aminoglycosides cause renal vasoconstriction mediated by thromboxane B2 (582) and direct cellular toxicity, especially in the proximal tubule, which absorbs the drug and stores it in lysosomes. Eventually, tubular necrosis, tubular atrophy, intratubular myeloid bodies, and interstitial nephritis may develop (583,584).

Aminoglycoside nephrotoxicity often presents as isolated proteinuria, reversible polyuric ARF with a high FENa, or transient tubular dysfunction (585,586). Laboratory findings may include proteinuria, decreased GFR, decreased urine-concentrating ability, glucosuria, increased urinary excretion of sodium, potassium, calcium, and magnesium, alterations in tubular transport of organic acids, and, rarely, a Fanconi syndrome (528,585–589). The most

sensitive indicator of nephrotoxicity is the detection of proteinuria (initially brush border enzymes, e.g., trehalase, and LMW proteins; after 1 week of therapy, cytoplasmic and lysosomal enzymes, e.g., NAG) (590,591) or phospholipiduria (592).

Gentamicin, kanamycin, and tobramycin are more nephrotoxic than amikacin or netilmicin (584,590). Studies in infants and children, in contrast with those in adults, have failed to show an additive toxicity of vancomycin and aminoglycosides (593–595). The daily dose of aminoglycosides should be adjusted according to Pcr and to serum drug levels. Pcr, serum electrolytes, urinalysis, and urine output should be followed serially in high-risk patients; sodium and potassium intake should be adjusted to urine losses. In patients with severe nephrotoxicity and in those with renal failure, a less toxic antibiotic should be used. A number of studies have compared the safety of the traditional multiple daily dosing of gentamicin (2.5 mg/kg) to the higher dose (4–5 mg/kg) extended dose interval in neonates. The trials did not report any nephrotoxic events for either regimen (596,597). An association was reported between single dose gentamicin regimen (4 mg/kg every 24 hours) and clinically significant hypocalcemia in full-term neonates (598).

NONSTEROIDAL ANTIINFLAMMATORY AGENTS

Vasoactive forms of nonsteroidal antiinflammatory agents such as indomethacin, aspirin and ibuprofen can induce renal hypoperfusion in neonates, especially preterm neonates, resulting in usually reversible, oliguric ARF (79). These drugs abolish the vasodilatory effects of prostaglandins, which maintain an effective GFR. Nonsteroidal antiinflammatory agents, when used during pregnancy for preventing toxemia and preterm birth or for treating polyhydramnios, easily pass the placenta. Postnatally these agents may be infused for closing a PDA or given orally for specific tubular disorders (see section on tubular dysfunction). Indomethacin has traditionally been the choice, but recently, ibuprofen has been advocated for its less severe renal toxicity (596). A systematic review (600) has shown that administration of ibuprofen reduced the risk of oliguria (urine output <1 ml/kg/hour) (relative risk 0.22, 95% confidence interval 0.09, 0.51) but increased the risk for oxygen requirement at 28 days, as compared to indomethacin.

Indomethacin is excreted into the urine through the organic secretory pathway of the proximal tubule, which explains higher levels in more immature patients (601). Indomethacin administration was found to transiently decrease RBF in premature infants with symptomatic PDA (440). Some patients develop transient renal dysfunction, associated with a fall of PRA from the high levels that are attributed to renal hypoperfusion before closure of the PDA, and a transient rise in the plasma level of AVP (602). During prolonged administration of indomethacin, i.e., up to 1 week, hormonal levels normalize, and renal function tends to improve (602,603). Indomethacin causes NAG enzymuria and increases the proximal tubular reabsorption of solutes (e.g., Na+), the corticomedullary gradient, and the hydroosmotic effect of ADH. The latter two changes result in an increased ratio of urine to plasma osmolality and decreased free water clearance, leading to water retention and dilutional hyponatremia (604–606). Indomethacin administration may also cause oliguric ARF and decreased renal K+ excretion, resulting in hyperkalemia. The latter may result from hyporeninemic hypoaldosteronism, decreased Na+ delivery to the distal tubule, or ARF. Maternal administration of indomethacin may induce nephron dysgenesis (see Acute Renal Failure) (551,552), oligohydramnios, and neonatal renal failure (604). However, perinatal indomethacin does not seem to affect long-term renal growth, structure or function in children born at less than 33 weeks of gestation (607).

Indomethacin is contraindicated if Pcr is elevated, i.e., Pcr greater than 1.8 mg/dL and in the presence of oligoanuria or hyperkalemia. The incidence of nephrotoxicity is increased by the combination of indomethacin with other nephrotoxins. One randomized trial showed that decrease in renal blood flow velocity and in urine output is observed with bolus indomethacin administration but not with continuous infusion (608). Two systematic reviews of randomized clinical trials found no evidence to support the use of

dopamine (609) or furosemide (610) to prevent renal dysfunction in indomethacin treated preterm neonates.

During a course of indomethacin, Pcr, serum electrolyte concentrations, and urine output should be monitored. The interval of drug administration should be adjusted according to Pcr or GFR, and fluid intake should be adjusted according to urine output. If oligoanuria develops, a challenge dose of furosemide should be given; fluid restriction should be initiated if oligoanuria persists.

Amphotericin B

Amphotericin B causes nephrotoxicity by renal vasoconstriction (611) and by its affinity to sterols, which are important components of membranes. Functional tubular alterations include an increase in urinary pH, in fractional excretion of Na+, K+, and phosphate, and in NAG enzymuria (612). Prolonged administration results in glomerular lesions, interstitial edema, focal tubular atrophy, and nephrocalcinosis (613). In newborn infants, amphotericin administration often increases Pcr and BUN, and transiently reduces serum potassium level (614); increasing potassium intake can prevent hypokalemia. Acute signs of nephrotoxicity may include decreased RBF and GFR, azotemia, oligoanuria, increased urinary excretion of Na+, K+, phosphate and bicarbonate, and hyposthenuria. Later complications may include NDI, distal RTA, and nephrocalcinosis (613,615). The incidence and prognosis of renal damage depend on the total dose of amphotericin administered (613). Nephrotoxicity may be limited by using a slow infusion (616), adjusting the daily dose to GFR and to minimum inhibitory and fungicidal concentrations (617), and avoiding hypercholesterolemia (618). If oligoanuric ARF develops, amphotericin should be withheld temporarily and restarted later, either at a lower dose or preferentially using a liposomal formulation at a similar or higher dose (619). Liposomal amphotericin has limited toxicity and is well tolerated in neonates including VLBW babies (620–622).

Acyclovir

Acyclovir administration may result in an increase in urine beta2-microglobulin and an obstructive nephropathy mediated by crystalluria that may lead to ARF (623). The risk of nephropathy can be minimized by adjusting the interval of administration for GA and renal function, by using a slow infusion, and by providing sufficient fluid intake to maintain adequate urinary output (623,624). If acyclovir is considered in a patient who also needs fluid restriction, the urine should be checked regularly for crystalluria and increased Pcr. If renal dysfunction is observed, the dose of acyclovir should be withheld or decreased, and fluid intake increased temporarily.

Radiocontrast Agents

Radiocontrast agents may cause ischemia, direct toxicity, and tubular obstruction by Tamm–Horsfall protein (625) or by uric acid crystals resulting from increased uricosuria (626). The signs of radiocontrast nephrotoxicity may include poor visualization or a prolonged nephrogram, proteinuria with casts, and oliguric ARF (625). In newborn infants who need angiography or CT with contrast, a low-osmolality agent is preferred. Adequate hydration should be provided before the procedure.

Angiotensin-converting Enzyme Inhibitors

Administration of ACE inhibitors during pregnancy has been associated with tubular dysgenesis, oliguric ARF, hypotension, hypoplasia of the calvaria, and perinatal death, and is therefore contraindicated (see Acute Renal Failure) (365,366,454). Neonates born in ARF after maternal ACE inhibition have a high mortality rate using conservative management; peritoneal dialysis may be considered to treat the ARF and to remove the ACE inhibitor (454). Postnatal ACE inhibition may cause profound hypotension, decreased RBF, and oliguric ARF (627,628), especially in association with hypovolemia. These hypotensive events respond to massive volume expansion but not to inotropes. ACE inhibition also enhances the renal toxicity of aminoglycosides (582).

Myoglobinuria–Hemoglobinuria

Rhabdomyolysis causes major shifts between intra- and extracellular electrolytes, shock, severe renal vasoconstriction, hyperuricemia, thrombi in the glomerular capillary tufts as a result of disseminated intravascular coagulation, intratubular hemoprotein casts, formation of free radicals, and peroxidation of lipids (629,630). The low incidence of neonatal rhabdomyolysis (631,632) may result from the low myoglobin content of immature muscle, especially in premature infants (633). Myoglobinuria should be suspected in severely asphyxiated full-term infants with a strongly positive reaction for heme in the absence of microscopic hematuria.

Chronic Renal Failure

The definition of chronic kidney disease (CKD) in infants and children, levels of severity of CKD, and recommended practice guidelines for management of pediatric CKD have recently been refined through the National Kidney Foundation's Kidney Disease Outcomes Quality Initiative (K/DOQI) process (634). A patient can be considered to have CKD if either of the following criteria is present:

- a) Kidney damage for ≥3 months, as defined by structural or functional abnormalities of the kidney, with or without decreased glomerular filtration rate (GFR); or
- b) GFR ≤60 mL/min/1.73 m² for ≥3 months, with or without other signs of kidney damage.

The levels of severity of pediatric CKD are outlined in Table 42-11.

TABLE 42-11
STAGES OF CHRONIC KIDNEY DISEASE[1]

Stage	GFR (ml/min/1.73 m²)	Description
1	≥90	Kidney damage with normal or increased GFR
2	60–89	Kidney damage with mild reduction of GFR
3	30–59	Moderate reduction of GFR
4	15–29	Severe reduction of GFR
5	<15 (or dialysis)	Kidney failure

[1] Adapted from reference 634
Abbreviations used in table: GFR, glomerular filtration rate.

Incidence

The incidence of pediatric end-stage renal disease (ESRD) is three to eight cases per one million children (age range 0 to 16 years) (635–637). Only 6% of children with ESRD are under 3 years of age (637). Renal transplantation is the preferred treatment modality for infants and children with ESRD, and is performed more commonly in children than in adults (638). As of 2003, of the 8399 renal transplants in children between 0 and 18 years of age registered in the North American Pediatric Renal Transplant Cooperative Study (NAPRTCS), only 5% were performed in children under 1 year of age (639). For those infants and children not receiving renal transplants, peritoneal dialysis is more common overall than hemodialysis, especially in the youngest age groups (638).

Etiology

As might be expected, inherited/congenital etiologies of renal failure are common in infants and children with CKD. A recent review of 10 years of data collected from pediatric nephrology centers in Britain and Ireland demonstrated that most children reaching ESRD under the age of 2 had such underlying diagnoses as renal dysplasia, structural problems, and other inherited conditions, with relatively few having acquired conditions such as glomerulonephritis or cortical necrosis (Table 42-12) (640). Structural disease also compromised the majority of children less than 1 year of age entered into the NAPRTCS chronic renal insufficiency database (639). These forms of renal disease are usually characterized by slow rates of progression, meaning that preemptive renal transplantation can usually be planned.

MANAGEMENT OF CKD IN INFANCY

Infant CKD is a complex condition requiring intensive, specialized management to avoid the many complications of renal insufficiency and promote normal growth and development. Management can be generally divided into two categories—conservative management, which encompasses

TABLE 42-12

DIAGNOSES OF CHILDREN WHO REACHED END STAGE RENAL FAILURE BEFORE THE AGE OF 2 YEARS DURING THE 10 YEARS 1988–97 INCLUSIVE[1]

Diagnosis	Treated	Not Treated	Antenatal Diagnosis (%)
Renal dysplasia	57	7	40
Posterior urethral valves	44	0	84
Finnish congenital nephrotic syndrome	26	2	8
Cortical necrosis	12	1	
Diffuse mesangial sclerosis and nephrotic syndrome	8	1	
Recessively inherited polycystic kidney disease	6	2	25
Prune belly syndrome	4	0	50
Renal vein thrombosis	4	0	
Nephronophthisis	3	0	
Hemolytic uremic syndrome	3	0	
Hyperoxaluria type I	2	2	
Interstitial nephritis	2	0	
Wilms tumor	2	1	
Cloaca, aortic thrombosis, glomerular fibrosis, glomerulonephritis	1 each	0	
Total	177	15	

[1] Reprinted with permission from Reference 640.

all of the medical therapies short of dialysis and transplantation, and renal replacement therapy, which include both dialysis and transplantation. Table 42-13 summarizes the many problems encountered in infants with CKD and the usual approaches to management of each problem.

The most crucial aspect of managing an infant with CKD is ensuring adequate nutrition. As mentioned previously, most infants with CKD have underlying structural renal disease as the etiology of their CKD. These conditions are characterized by tubular dysfunction leading to salt and water wasting, which in turn produces unique requirements not only for adequate caloric intake, but also for adequate intake of sodium and water to achieve normal growth rates (see the earlier discussion on sodium balance). A recent report demonstrated that infants and young children with CKD who were fed with dilute, sodium-supplemented feedings had superior growth compared to similar patients who were fed with high caloric density formulas (640).

TABLE 42-13

CONSERVATIVE MANAGEMENT OF INFANTS WITH CKD

Problem	Usual Therapy	Comment
Acidosis	Alkali (Na citrate, NaHCO$_3$)	Correction of acidosis necessary to maintain anabolism and promote normal growth
Anemia	Recombinant erythropoietin	Iron supplementation always necessary during erythropoietin treatment
Anorexia	Nasogastric or gastrostomy feeds	Nearly all infants with CKD require supplemental feedings
Hyperphosphatemia	Low-phosphate formula; phosphate binders	CaCO$_3$ most commonly used phosphate binder in infancy; avoid aluminum containing binders
Secondary hyperparathyroidism	Vitamin D analogues (DHT, calcitriol)	Maintain serum intact PTH in normal range in pre-dialysis CKD patients; avoid calcium*phosphorous product >70
Uremia	Low-protein diet	Do not restrict protein intake below RDA for age; infants with CNS require increased protein intake
Growth failure	Supplemental feedings; rHGH	Correction of all above problems must be achieved prior to instituting rHGH treatment
Neurodevelopmental delay	"Early intervention" services	Most infants require some combination of physical, occupational and speech/feeding therapies

Abbreviations used in table:
CaCO$_3$, calcium carbonate; CKD, chronic kidney disease; CNS, congenital nephrotic syndrome; DHT, dihydrotachysterol; Na, sodium; NaHCO$_3$, sodium bicarbonate; RDA, recommended daily allowance; rHGH, recombinant human growth hormone.

Most infants with CKD will require placement of a feeding gastrostomy to maintain adequate intake of fluid, formula, and medications.

Other aspects of the management of CKD in infants and children have been reviewed elsewhere (641–645). It should be noted that common complications of acute renal failure, such as hyperkalemia and hypertension as a result of fluid overload, are uncommon in infants with CKD because of the polyuria that accompanies the structural forms of renal disease that occur in infancy (645). No matter what the underlying etiology, infants with CKD require the services of a multidisciplinary team consisting of pediatric nephrologists, pediatric renal dietitians, pediatric surgeons and other medical personnel geared toward meeting their unique needs.

Infant Dialysis

As with acute renal failure, once conservative measures prove insufficient to control the manifestations of CKD, then renal replacement therapy becomes necessary. The most common indication for the elective institution of dialysis in infancy is growth failure; the most common nonelective indication is probably persistent renal insufficiency following neonatal acute renal failure.

Peritoneal dialysis is by far and away the most common dialysis modality employed in infants requiring chronic renal replacement therapy (638–640,645). The reasons for this are multiple, but include the relative ease of achieving access compared to hemodialysis, avoidance of exposure to blood products, and the ability to provide care in the home setting. Even with meticulously provided care, complications of peritoneal dialysis in infants are common and include infection (especially peritonitis) and catheter malfunction (640,645–647). Chronic hemodialysis is technologically feasible in infancy, but in most pediatric nephrology centers it is reserved for infants who have failed peritoneal dialysis, or for the rare infant in whom peritoneal dialysis is impossible for surgical or social reasons.

It should be emphasized that in infants, chronic dialysis is almost universally considered a temporary measure until renal transplantation can be performed. One of the major reasons for this is the poor survival rates of infants on dialysis compared to older children: According to the NAPRTCS dialysis registry, survival of children less than or equal to 1 years of age at the initiation of dialysis was 86.6% after 1 year, 76% after 2 years and 70.5% after 3 years, compared to survival rates of 97.9%, 94.9% and 92% at the same time intervals for children more than or equal to 12 years of age at the initiation of dialysis (639). This comparatively poor survival is for the most part a consequence of other co-morbid conditions in many infants who require chronic dialysis (647,648).

Withholding care is still sometimes considered when an infant is found to have severe CKD requiring renal replacement therapy (649,650). The usual reasons cited in such cases are the enormous demands on the infant's family and

the historically uncertain long-term outcome of such infants. However, as documented in numerous series over the past decade, infants receiving chronic dialysis can be reasonably expected to maintain normal growth rates and achieve near-normal neurodevelopmental progress (640,646,647,651). Advances in the success of renal transplantation in infants (643,649,652) add further weight in favor of providing dialysis when an infant is found to have irreversible CKD. Although it is true that this requires an enormous commitment on the part of the infant's family and medical team, it can be said that provision of chronic dialysis is now the standard of care for infants with severe CKD, and that withholding or withdrawing dialysis should be considered only in unusual circumstances (645,650,653).

Renal Transplantation

The advantages of renal transplantation in infants and children with CKD are numerous. Chief among them are improved growth and development compared to long-term dialysis, and a more normal quality of life (640,643, 654–656). These benefits explain why renal transplantation is considered the preferred renal replacement modality for infants and children with ESRD, and why it is performed more commonly in children than in adults. Transplantation in infancy remains a somewhat rare event, however; only 5% of the pediatric renal transplants reported to the NAPRTCS registry were performed in children under 1 year of age (639). The success of renal transplantation in infancy has increased markedly compared to one or two decades ago (643,649,652). This improvement has occurred in parallel with numerous improvements in all aspects of transplant medicine, especially advancements in pretransplant management and in immunosuppressive regimens.

It should be noted that undertaking renal transplantation before the age of 1 year remains somewhat controversial, primarily because of historically poor rates of graft and patient survival. The most recent NAPRTCS data show that recipient age continues to have a significant impact on graft survival for cadaveric transplants, with recipients less than or equal to 1 year of age having a 5-year graft survival of just 54% compared to 70% for older children (639). However, no similar difference in graft survival was seen for recipients of transplants from living donors. Long-term allograft renal function appears to be unaffected by recipient age for both cadaveric and living-donor transplants (639). However, posttransplant patient survival is markedly lower for infants (<24 months old at transplant), particularly for recipients of cadaver donor grafts. Fortunately, this has been improving over time: the 3-year patient survival for recipients of cadaver grafts has increased from 78% between 1987 and 1994 to 94% in 1995 and later. For infants receiving living donor grafts, 3-year survival also improved from 88% in 1987 to 1994 to 95% in 1995 and beyond (639). This improvement in patient survival adds further impetus to pursuing a goal of transplantation for infants with irreversible CKD, and should, over time, make this goal less controversial and more accepted as standard of care.

SUMMARY

As can be deduced from the preceding sections, the overall prognosis for infants with CKD has improved considerably over the last 2 to 3 decades. This may have resulted not only from changes in treatment but also from a change in the patient population associated with an earlier diagnosis. As indicated in Table 42-12, many infants with structural forms of CKD are now routinely diagnosed antenatally (640), thus enabling planning for the future. When such infants are identified, multidisciplinary teams consisting of an obstetrician, neonatologist, pediatric nephrologist and pediatric surgeon or urologist can meet with the family to discuss the infant's short- and long-term prognoses, thereby helping the family to make informed decisions about the infant's postnatal care.

HYPERTENSION

Definition

In newborn and premature infants, systemic hypertension is best defined as systolic and/or diastolic blood pressure that persistently exceeds the mean + 2 standard deviations for infants of similar postconceptual age (388). The graphs published by Zubrow et al. (Appendix G1c) are probably most useful in this regard (387). After one month of age, hypertension is defined as systolic and/or diastolic blood pressure >95th percentile for that infant's age and gender (380). These normative values can be found in the curves published in the Second Task Force report (657) (Appendix G1d).

As with older children, the diagnosis of hypertension should not be made based on a single reading. If the infant is critically ill and continuous blood pressure monitoring reveals sustained blood pressure elevation over several hours, then hypertension should be diagnosed and appropriate investigation and intervention initiated. For less critically ill infants still in the NICU, a pattern of elevated readings over 1 to 2 days should be sufficient to make the diagnosis of hypertension. For older infants who are being followed as outpatients, then at least three elevated readings should be documented over 1 to 2 weeks before a diagnosis of hypertension is made (380).

Incidence

Although one recent series found that 28% of infants with BWs less than 1,500 grams had at least one elevated blood pressure documented during their NICU stay (658), the actual incidence of hypertension in neonates is very low, ranging from 0.2% in healthy newborns to between 0.7% and 2.5% in high-risk newborns (659–663). Certain categories of infants are at significantly higher risk, however. For example, hypertension is relatively common in patients with a history of UA catheterization (3%) (664) and those with bronchopulmonary dysplasia (BPD) (as high as 43%)

(660). In one series, it also was associated with PDA and intraventricular hemorrhage (663). On the other hand, hypertension is so uncommon in otherwise healthy term infants that routine blood pressure determination is not even recommended (665).

Etiology and Pathophysiology

Although numerous conditions are known to cause hypertension in the neonate or older infant (Appendix G1e), a clear etiology can be determined in only approximately one-third of hypertensive newborn infants (661,666). The most important categories of causes of neonatal hypertension include renovascular hypertension, renal disease, and bronchopulmonary dysplasia (388,661).

Renovascular Hypertension

The most common cause of neonatal renovascular hypertension is aortic or renal thromboembolism related to UA catheterization (664). This was first demonstrated in the 1970's by Ford and associates (667) and Bauer and associates (668). Hypertension may develop either while the catheter is in place or long after its removal (669) and may be associated with a history of renal failure or hematuria. Associated signs may include ARF in patients with bilateral involvement, hematuria, and loss of femoral pulses and blood flow to the lower extremities in patients with extensive aortic thrombosis.

Although there have been several studies that have examined duration of line placement and line position ("low" vs. "high") as factors involved in thrombus formation, these data have not been conclusive (670–672). Thus, the assumption has been made that the cause of hypertension in such cases is related to thrombus formation at the time of line placement, probably related to disruption of the vascular endothelium of the umbilical artery. Such thrombi may then embolize to the kidneys, causing areas of infarction and increased renin release. A similar phenomenon has been reported in infants with dilatation of the ductus arteriosus (673).

The Cochrane Group has recently attempted to resolve the controversy regarding UA catheter placement (674). They analyzed 11 randomized clinical trials and one study using alternate assignments to compare the incidence of morbidity and mortality for high vs. low catheter tip placement. The placement of a catheter tip was defined as high when located in the descending aorta above the diaphragm and low when placed in the descending aorta above the bifurcation but below the renal arteries. The reviewers concluded that high catheter position causes fewer clinically obvious ischemic complications and possibly decreases the frequency of aortic thrombosis. As far as hypertension was concerned, however, it was concluded that it seems to appear with equal frequency among infants with high or low placement.

Congenital vascular anomalies responsible for neonatal renovascular hypertension include stenosis or hypoplasia of the renal artery (675,676) and segmental intimal hyperplasia (677). All these conditions may involve the aorta and the renal arteries. Unilateral renovascular stenosis may cause a reversible syndrome characterized by hypokalemic alkalosis, salt-losing syndrome, and hyperechogenicity of the contralateral kidney (678).

Hypertension may rarely result from two types of infiltration of the arterial wall. Idiopathic arterial calcification of infancy is characterized by calcium deposits in all layers of the arteries, including the aorta and the coronary arteries, and in the heart valves (679–682). Some of these deposits may be visible on a plain radiogram. Most cases have been diagnosed at autopsy. Hypertension typically fails to respond to standard antihypertensive medication and to nephrectomy; biphosphonate, calcium antagonists, or PGE1 may be successful (681,683). Galactosialidosis may result in intimal infiltration by sialyloligosaccharides and hyperreninemic hypertension (684).

Other causes of renovascular hypertension include neonatal renal arterial embolism in the absence of UA catheterization (673), intramural hematoma of the renal artery (685), renal venous thrombosis (686), external compression of the renal artery by a hydronephrotic kidney (687), adrenal hemorrhage (688), and urinoma (689). Finally, a neonate with hypertension as a result of an aneurysm of the abdominal aorta was recently reported (690); this fortunately rare condition may present with intractable congestive heart failure.

Bronchopulmonary Dysplasia

Many infants with BPD develop hypertension (653,691). This phenomenon was first described in the mid-1980s by Abman and colleagues (653). In a study of 65 infants discharged from a neonatal intensive care unit, the instance of hypertension in infants with BPD was 43%, vs. an incidence of 4.5% in infants without BPD. Investigators were unable to identify a clear cause of hypertension, but postulated that hypoxemia might be involved. Over half of the infants with BPD who developed hypertension did not display it until after discharge from the NICU, highlighting the need for measurement of blood pressure in NICU "graduates," whether or not they have lung disease (666).

Abman's findings have been reproduced by other investigators, most recently in 1998 by Alagappan (692), who found that hypertension was twice as common in VLBW infants with BPD compared to the incidence in all VLBW infants. Because all of the hypertensive infants required supplemental oxygen and aminophylline, development of hypertension appeared to be correlated with the severity of pulmonary disease. Anderson and colleagues have demonstrated that the more severe the bronchopulmonary dysplasia (defined as a greater need for diuretics and bronchodilators), the higher the likelihood of the development of increased blood pressure (693).

These observations reinforce the impression that infants with severe BPD are clearly at increased risk and need close monitoring for the development of hypertension. This is especially true in infants who require ongoing treatment with theophylline preparations and/or corticosteroids; as many as 30% of infants receiving dexamethasone for BPD manifest hypertension (694). If severe hypertension develops, the risk of intraventricular hemorrhage, CHF, and renal failure may outweigh the possible beneficial effects of steroids on the lung disease.

Renal Causes of Hypertension

Hypertension is a common complication of renal anomalies and diseases such as polycystic kidney disease (PKD) (695), renal hypodysplasia (696), hydronephrosis (697), and interstitial nephritis (661). It is well known that both autosomal dominant and autosomal recessive polycystic kidney disease (PKD) may present in the newborn period with severe nephromegaly and hypertension (695,698,699). With recessive PKD, the median age of onset of hypertension was recently reported to be 16 days (700); the majority of affected infants will be discovered to be hypertensive during the first year of life (698). The most severely affected infants with recessive PKD are at risk for development of congestive heart failure as a result of severe, malignant hypertension. Bilateral nephrectomy may be life saving in such infants.

Although much less common than in PKD, hypertension has also been reported in infants with multicystic dysplastic kidneys (661,701,702). This is somewhat paradoxical, as such kidneys are usually thought to be nonfunctioning. In fact, the case has been made that hypertension in such patients is the result of another coexisting urologic abnormality such as parenchymal scarring (703). Another possible explanation is increased renin production by macrophages within the dysplastic kidney (704).

Renal obstruction may be accompanied by hypertension, even when there is no compression of the renal artery. This has been seen for example in infants with congenital ureteropelvic-junction obstruction (661,663), and sometimes may persist following surgical correction of the obstruction (705). Hypertension has also been described in infants with congenital primary megaureter (706). Ureteral obstruction by other intraabdominal masses may also be accompanied by hypertension. The mechanism of hypertension in such instances is unclear, although the RAS has been implicated (707,708). Finally, unilateral renal hypoplasia may also present with hypertension (696), although this is uncommon.

Hypertension as a result of acquired renal parenchymal disease is less common than that as a result of congenital renal abnormalities. However, severe ATN, interstitial nephritis, or cortical necrosis may be accompanied by significant hypertension (661,663), usually as a result of fluid and sodium overload or hyperreninemia. Hemolytic-uremic syndrome, which has been described in both term and preterm infants (709), is usually also accompanied by hypertension. Such hypertension may be extremely difficult to control, requiring treatment with multiple agents (709).

Genetic Causes of Hypertension

Genetic forms of hypertension that may present in the neonatal period fall into two broad categories, namely hypertension resulting from a single-gene disorder, and hypertension occurring as one feature of a malformation syndrome. Single-gene disorders causing hypertension with reported cases in infancy include Liddle's Syndrome (710,711), glucocorticoid-remediable aldosteronism (GRA) (712,713), and Gordon's Syndrome (pseudohypoaldosteronism type II) (663).

Liddle's syndrome is an autosomal dominant, low-renin form of hypertension characterized by elevated renal sodium reabsorption that results from activating mutations in the β or γ subunit of ENaC. These mutations result in an increased number and prolonged half-life of channels at the cell surface (714,715). The genetic defect has been localized to a single segment of chromosome 16 that encodes the ENaC subunits; several different mutations have been described, all of which either cause a frameshift mutation or introduce premature stop codons (716). This condition must be differentiated from 11-β-HSD2 deficiency (see Chapter 41). The treatment, i.e., the administration of KCl and an aldosterone-independent K-sparing diuretic, such as triamterene or amiloride, results in normalization of the electrolyte and acid–base balance and the blood pressure.

GRA is an autosomal dominant disease characterized by early onset of hypertension with normal or elevated aldosterone levels despite suppressed plasma renin activity (717). GRA is caused by a chimeric gene that results from unequal crossing-over the aldosterone synthase and 11β-hydroxylase genes on chromosome 8. The resulting chimeric gene is expressed in the adrenal fasiculata and encodes a protein product with aldosterone synthase enzymatic activity whose expression is regulated by ACTH. Consequently, aldosterone synthase activity is thus ectopically expressed in the adrenal fasciculata under control of ACTH rather than ANG II. Aldosterone secretion becomes inexorably linked to cortisol secretion, and maintenance of normal cortisol levels results in constitutive aldosterone secretion, which leads to expanded plasma volume and hypertension (718).

Gordon's syndrome (pseudohypoaldosteronism type II) is an autosomal dominant disorder characterized by hypertension, hyperkalemia and metabolic acidosis. It may rarely be diagnosed during the neonatal period in patients with a family history (719). It has been linked to mutations of genes on chromosomes 1, 17 and 12 that encode the WNK kinases, a family of serine-threonine kinases (720,721). These mutations lead to increased expression of WNK1 and WNK 4 in the distal nephron. Although the exact mechanism by which these mutations produce hypertension is unclear, hyperactivity of the Na–K–Cl cotransporter of the loop of Henle has been postulated.

Malformation syndromes that may cause hypertension include Williams Syndrome (renal artery stenosis), Turner's Syndrome (aortic coarctation), neurofibromatosus and Cockayne Syndrome (722). Usually the hypertension in these syndromes presents beyond the neonatal period, but infantile presentations with hypertension have been described.

Other Causes of Hypertension

Coarctation of the thoracic aorta (see Chapters 33 and 34) is easily detected in the newborn period based on decreased pulses and lower blood pressures in the lower extremities compared to the upper extremities (723). It has been reported in numerous case series of neonatal hypertension (659,661,663,666,724). Hypertension may persist in these patients even after surgical repair of the coarctation (725). Repair early in infancy seems to lead to an improved long-term outcome compared to delayed repair (723).

Endocrine disorders, particularly congenital adrenal hyperplasia, hyperaldosteronism and hyperthyroidism constitute easily recognizable clinical entities that have been reported to cause hypertension in neonates (726–729). Several adrenal disturbances can induce hypertension directly; they should be differentiated from Liddle's syndrome. Hyperthyroidism is associated with systolic hypertension and sustained tachycardia and, sometimes, with episodes of supraventricular tachycardia (729).

Tumors, including neuroblastoma, Wilms tumor, and mesoblastic nephroma may all present in the neonatal period and may produce hypertension, either because of compression of the renal vessels or ureters, or because of production of vasoactive substances such as renin or catecholamines (730–734).

Neurologic causes of hypertension include intracranial hypertension, drug withdrawal, seizures, and familial dysautonomia. Seizures are common complications of severe hypertension; in turn, blood pressure may increase transiently during seizure episodes (735). Narcotic withdrawal should be treated as described in Chapter 56. Appropriate pain relief should be given before and after surgical procedures (see Chapter 57). A discussion of treatment of intracranial hypertension is presented elsewhere (see Chapter 51).

Iatrogenic causes of neonatal hypertension are usually obvious but important to consider. If the infant is hypervolemic secondary to excessive administration of sodium or fluids, intake should be restricted and a diuretic administered. It is imperative to eliminate hidden sources of sodium, such as isotonic saline used to flush an arterial line and sodium-containing medications (e.g., antibiotics). If fluid restriction is not possible and severe hypertension with CHF is present, hemofiltration should be strongly considered.

If hypertension is induced by a medication, one may consider withholding it, decreasing the dose, or using an infusion instead of repeated injections. As noted earlier, dexamethasone may cause blood pressure elevation relatively commonly (694,736,737); if this occurs, a decision must be made regarding the possible benefits of continued steroid treatment vs. the risks of hypertension. Hypertension induced by pancuronium probably is mediated by release of catecholamines (738–740); blood pressure may normalize after replacing pancuronium with vecuronium.

Hypertension develops in 11% to 92% of neonates receiving ECMO (741–743), and may result in serious complications, including intracranial hemorrhage (741) and increased mortality (744). Despite extensive investigation, the exact pathogenesis of this form of hypertension remains poorly understood. Fluid overload, altered handling of sodium and water, and derangements in atrial baroceptor function have all been proposed as causative factors (741,742). Nicardipine infusions are commonly used to treat this form of hypertension (745–747).

Hypertension may develop after surgery. Of four patients who developed hypertension after surgical repair of an abdominal wall defect, three had edema of the lower extremities and normal PRA, and one had evidence for ureteropelvic obstruction and high PRA (748). The duration of hypertension in these patients ranged from 12 days to 6 months. Hypertension appearing after primary closure for bladder exstrophy may be related to traction for skeletal immobilization (749).

Clinical Features and Investigation

Mild-to-moderate hypertension may be asymptomatic (750,751). Symptomatic presentations, such as congestive heart failure, seizures, poor feeding and lethargy, are nonspecific and may be as a result of the underlying disease, the hypertension itself, or its complications (e.g., neurologic, cardiovascular).

The first step in the evaluation is to determine whether the infant is indeed hypertensive, or if the blood pressure rises only during periods of agitation, pain, crying, feeding, or performance of procedures. As discussed earlier, only infants with persistent blood pressure elevation should have the "diagnosis" of hypertension made and diagnostic work-ups initiated.

A relatively focused history should be obtained, paying attention to determining whether there were any pertinent prenatal exposures, and to the particulars of the infant's nursery course and any concurrent conditions. The procedures that the infant has undergone (e.g., umbilical catheter placement) should be reviewed, and the current medication list should be scrutinized. Easily identifiable causes of hypertension such as fluid overload or medication-induced hypertension should be able to be identified at this stage, and appropriate measures taken to correct the problem.

The physical examination should similarly focus on identifying obvious problems that may be causing the blood pressure elevation. Blood pressure readings should be obtained in all four extremities to rule out coarctation of the thoracic aorta. The general appearance of the infant should be assessed, with particular attention paid to the

TABLE 42-14
PHYSICAL EXAM FINDINGS IN HYPERTENSIVE INFANTS

Finding	Probable Cause of Hypertension
Abdominal bruit	Renal artery stenosis
Ambiguous genitalia	Congenital adrenal hyperplasia
Bilateral flank masses	PKD; UPJ obstruction (bilateral); tumor
Bulging anterior fontanelle	Intracranial hemorrhage
Diminished LE pulses	Aortic coarctation
Edema	Fluid overload; Congenital Nephrotic Syndrome
Elfin facies	Williams Syndrome (renovascular)
Unilateral flank mass	UPJ obstruction; tumor
Widely spaced nipples; neck folds	Turner's Syndrome (coarctation)

Abbreviations used in Table 42-14: LE, lower extremity; PKD, polycystic kidney disease; UPJ, Ureteropelvic junction.

presence of dysmorphic features. Careful cardiac and abdominal examinations should be performed. Table 42-14 lists physical exam findings associated with specific causes of hypertension.

All hypertensive neonates should have a urinalysis and routine blood chemistry tests (see Appendix G1f). If hypertension appears to be iatrogenic or secondary to drug withdrawal, specific therapy can be tried before additional investigations are performed. If no cause is evident, or if a renal or renovascular etiology is suspected, the workup usually will include US of the kidneys, adrenals, aorta, and bladder, with a flow study, i.e., Doppler US, of the aorta and the renal arteries. Renal scans, angiography, MRI, or CT may be indicated in specific patients. If there is any suspicion of hydronephrosis or reflux, urine obtained by suprapubic aspiration or bladder catheterization should be sent for bacterial and fungal culture. Of 17 patients with fungal uropathy, hypertension was one of the presenting signs in seven (752).

PRA should be obtained as part of the work-up in most hypertensive infants. If PRA is elevated compared to age-appropriate normal values for the same laboratory, consideration should be given to obtaining a renal scan in addition to the renal US and Doppler. Renal microemboli from a UA catheter, however, can elude detection by any of these means. High PRA may be secondary to the administration of diuretics or adrenergic medications or to severe respiratory disease; mild elevations of PRA may be seen in normal infants. Conversely, one normal value of PRA does not exclude hyperreninemic hypertension.

Treatment

Treatment of neonatal hypertension should be tailored to the severity of the hypertension and the infant's overall clinical status. For example, critically ill infants with acute onset of severe hypertension should be treated with an intravenous agent administered by continuous infusion, as this will allow the greatest control over the magnitude and rapidity of the blood pressure reduction. These infants should have their blood pressure lowered by no more than 25% over the first eight hours to prevent cerebral ischemia (753,754). On the other hand, relatively well infants with mild hypertension may be treated with oral antihypertensive agents. Recommended doses for intravenous and oral antihypertensive drugs can be found in Tables 42.15 and 42-16.

Of the many intravenous antihypertensive agents available, nicardipine has emerged as the most useful for management of severe neonatal hypertension (746,747,755, 756). It can be precisely titrated to the desired antihypertensive effect, and may be continued for prolonged periods of time without loss of antihypertensive efficacy (746). Alternative agents that may be given by continuous infusion include esmolol, hydralazine, labetalol and sodium nitroprusside. Esmolol and labetalol may be contra-indicated in infants with lung disease, and nitroprusside can only be used for limited periods of time (usually <72 hours) because of the accumulation of thiocyanate (757). Intravenous agents that can be administered by intermittent bolus injection include hydralazine and labetalol. The intravenous ACE inhibitor enalaprilat has been reported to be effective in cases of severe neonatal hypertension (758);

however, our anecdotal experience suggests that this agent may cause sudden, oliguric acute renal failure similar to that reported for oral enalapril (759,760)—given this, we do not recommend use of enalaprilat in neonates.

The choice of oral antihypertensive medications is more controversial. Whereas ACE inhibitors are considered the drugs of choice for adults and children with renovascular hypertension and some centers have had good success in neonates as well (388), many neonatologists have serious concerns about the potential major side effects (761). Other medications, such as a β-blocker or, in the case of a hypertensive crisis, a potent vasodilator, should be tried first. The advantage of a β-blocker such as propranolol is that it reduces the secretion of renin and the release of norepinephrine; however, it may also cause bronchoconstriction or hypoglycemia, making its use problematic in some infants.

Of the available vasodilators, the calcium channel blockers isradipine and amlodipine have found widespread use (762–764). Both may be compounded into stable extemporaneous suspensions (765,766). Older vasodilating agents such as hydralazine and minoxidil may also be useful in selected infants, or when the newer agents are not available.

Surgery is indicated for treatment of neonatal hypertension in a limited set of circumstances (767). In particular, hypertension caused by ureteral obstruction or aortic coarctation is best approached surgically. For infants with

TABLE 42-15

INTRAVENOUS ANTIHYPERTENSIVE AGENTS

Drug	Class	Dose	Route	Comments
Diazoxide	Vasodilator (arteriolar)	2–5 mg/kg/dose	RAPID bolus injection	NOT RECOMMENDED. Slow injection ineffective; duration unpredictable.
Enalaprilat	ACE Inhibitor	15 ± 5 mcg/kg/dose Q 8–24 hr	Bolus injection	NOT RECOMMENDED. May cause prolonged hypotension and acute renal insufficiency.
Esmolol	β blocker	Drip: 100–300 mcg/kg/min	Continuous infusion	Very short-acting; continuous infusion necessary.
Hydralazine	Vasodilator (arteriolar)	Bolus: 0.15–0.6 mg/kg/dose Q4 hr Drip: 0.75–5.0 mcg/kg/min	Bolus or continuous infusion	Tachycardia frequent side-effect; Must administer Q4hr when given IV bolus
Labetalol	α & β blocker	Bolus: 0.20–1.0 mg/kg/dose Drip: 0.25–3.0 mg/kg/hr	Bolus or continuous infusion	Heart failure, lung disease relative contra-indications
Nicardipine	Ca^{++} channel blocker	Drip: 0.5–4 mcg/kg/min	Continuous infusion	May cause reflex tachycardia
Sodium Nitroprusside	Vasodilator (arteriolar & venous)	Drip: 0.5–10 mcg/kg/min	Continuous Infusion	Thiocyanate toxicity can occur with prolonged (>72 hr) use or in renal failure.

Abbreviations and symbols used in Table 42-15:
a, alpha; ACE, angiotensin converting enzyme; β, beta; Ca^{++}, calcium; hr, hour; IV, intravenous; kg, kiligram; mcg, micrograms; mg, milligrams; Q, every.

TABLE 42-16
ORAL ANTIHYPERTENSIVE AGENTS

Drug	Class	Initial Dose	Interval	Maximum Dose	Comments
Amlodipine	Ca^{++} channel blocker	0.06 mg/kg	QD-BID	0.6 mg/kg/day	May have slow/gradual onset of effect
Captopril	ACE Inhibitor	0.01 mg/kg/dose	TID	2 mg/kg/day	1st dose may cause rapid drop in BP; monitor serum creatinine and K$^+$
Chlorothiazide	Thiazide diuretic	5 mg/kg/dose	BID	30 mg/kg/day	Monitor electrolytes
Clonidine	Central α agonist	0.05–0.1 mg/kg/dose	BID-TID	Not established	May produce dry mouth & sedation; rebound HTN with abrupt discontinuation
Enalapril	ACE inhibitor	0.08 mg/kg/dose	QD-BID	0.58 mg/kg/day	Monitor serum creatinine and K$^+$
Hydralazine	Vasodilator (arteriolar)	0.25–1.0 mg/kg/dose	TID-QID	7.5 mg/kg/day	Tachycardia & fluid retention common side-effects
Hydrochloro-thiazide	Thiazide diuretic	1 mg/kg/dose	QD	3 mg/kg/day	Monitor electrolytes
Isradipine	Ca^{++} channel blocker	0.05 mg/kg/dose	TID-QID	0.8 mg/kg/day	Suspension may be compounded; useful for both acute & chronic HTN
Labetalol	α and β blocker	2 mg/kg/dose	BID	20 mg/kg/day	Monitor heart rate; avoid in infants with BPD
Minoxidil	Vasodilator (arteriolar)	0.1–0.2 mg/kg/dose	BID-TID	1 mg/kg/day	Most potent oral vaso-dilator; excellent for refractory HTN
Propranolol	β-blocker	0.5–1.0 mg/kg/dose	TID	8–10 mg/kg/day	Monitor heart rate; avoid in infants with BPD
Spironolactone	Aldosterone antagonist	0.5 mg/kg/dose	BID	3.3 mg/kg/day	Potassium "sparing;" monitor electrolytes.

Abbreviations and symbols used in Table 42–16:
α, alpha; ACE, angiotensin converting enzyme; β, beta; BID, twice daily; BPD; bronchopulmonary dysplasia; Ca^{++}, calcium; HTN, hypertension; K$^+$, potassium; kg, kilogram; mg, milligrams; QD, once daily; QID, four times daily; TID, three times daily.

renal arterial stenosis, it may be necessary to manage the infant medically until it has grown sufficiently to undergo definitive repair of the vascular abnormalities (768). Infants with hypertension secondary to Wilms tumor or neuroblastoma will require surgical tumor removal, possibly following chemotherapy. A case has also been made by some authors for prophylactic removal of multicystic-dysplastic kidneys because of the risk of development of hypertension (769), although this is controversial (770).

Prognosis

The prognosis of neonatal hypertension depends on etiology, timing of the diagnosis, presence of complications, and response to therapy. Patients in whom hypertension is diagnosed on the basis of neurologic, cardiovascular, or renal decompensation have a high mortality rate. The mortality rate of patients with idiopathic calcification of the arteries or with massive aortic thrombosis remains high despite aggressive therapy. The long-term prognosis for newborn infants with thromboembolism of the renal artery or the aorta is good, often with progressive resolution of the

hypertension within a year and only mild-to-moderate decrease in renal function (770–772). Hypertension in patients with BPD tends to resolve after 6 months of age (773). On the other hand, patients with polycystic kidney disease are likely to have persistent hypertension throughout childhood (700,774). And as noted earlier, infants who undergo repair of aortic coarctation are at risk for persistent or recurrent hypertension (725).

Diuretics

The effects of diuretics on water and solute excretion are summarized in Table 42-17. The pharmacology of diuretics is described in detail in Chapter 56. This section reviews the strategy in using diuretics in neonates.

The choice of diuretic depends on the acuity of hypertension or fluid overload, the adequacy of renal function, and the expected side effects. For emergencies (e.g., cardiovascular or respiratory failure as a result of fluid overload), loop diuretics are the best choice because of their rapidity of action and their potency. In most patients, fluid restriction should be initiated along with diuretic therapy.

TABLE 42-17

EFFECTS OF VARIOUS TYPES OF DIURETICS ON URINE AND SOLUTE EXCRETION

Type of Diuretic	Site of Major Action	Elimination	FeNa (%)	Urine Characteristics							
				Volume	CH_2O	K^+	Ca^{2+}	Mg^{2+}	$H_2PO_4^-$	Cl	HCO_3^-
CA inhibitors	PCT	Secretion	3–6	+	+	+++	0,+	0,+	++	0	+++
Osmotic	Loop	Filtration	>10	++	+	+	+	+	++	+	+++
Loop	TAl > PCT[a]	Secretion	15–30	+++	+, –[b]	++	+++	++	++	+++	+[c]
Thiazides	DCT > PCT	Secretion	5–10	++	0	++	–, +[d]	++	++	+++	+, –[c]
Metolazone	DCT > PCT	Secretion	4–7	+++	0,–	0	–	+	++	+++	0
Spironolactone	CD	Metabolization	2–3	+	0	–	++	+	+	+	0
Other K-Sparing	CD > DCT[e]	Variable[f]	2–3	+	0	–	–	–	+	+	+

Most of these studies were performed in adults,

+, increase; 0, no change; –, decrease.

CA, carbonic anhydrase; CD, connecting tubule and collecting duct; CH_2O, free water clearance; DCT, distal convoluted tubule; FeNa, fractional excretion of sodium; loop, thin Henle's loop; PCT, proximal convoluted tubule; TAL, thick ascending loop of Henle.

[a] Ethacrynic acid at usual doses does not have any significant effect on proximal tubule reabsorption. Note that ethacrynic acid is not recommended because of its ototoxicity.

[b] Decreased CH_2O during water loading and increased CH_2O during dehydration.

[c] Despite decreased reabsorption of bicarbonate related to the inhibition of carbonic anhydrase, the acute result is a "contraction" alkalosis. Chronic administration results in increased urine acidification in the distal part of the nephron (see text).

[d] Thiazides may be associated with hypercalciuria after salt loading.

[e] Amiloride causes mild metabolic acidosis by decreasing Na/H exchange, especially in the DCT.

[f] Amiloride is not metabolized and acts on the luminal side. Triamterene is hydroxylated in the liver.

Modified from ref. 67.

Hyponatremia is a common complication when thiazides are initiated without fluid restriction, because they do not impair urinary concentrating ability. Mild hyponatremia (130–135 mEq/L) does not justify additional sodium intake; the latter would initiate the vicious cycle of diuretic–low serum sodium concentration–increased sodium intake–more hypertension or lung edema–more diuretic. However, potassium and chloride depletion should be prevented.

Both hypokalemia and hypochloremic metabolic alkalosis may occur during thiazide or loop diuretic administration, unless the patient has renal failure or appropriate preventive therapy is initiated (775). Acute thiazide or loop diuretic administration results in a "contraction" alkalosis because of a reduction of the ECF volume and a relatively low bicarbonate concentration in the urine (776,777). During chronic diuretic administration, metabolic alkalosis results from increased distal urine acidification, which may be as a result of hypokalemia, mineralocorticoid excess, and increased delivery of Na+ to the distal convoluted tubule, in which protons are secreted in exchange for Na+. There is serious concern about the effects of metabolic alkalosis associated with diuretic therapy in patients with chronic lung disease (776). Thus, KCl should be added as soon as diuretic therapy is initiated, except in the presence of renal failure, to prevent potassium depletion and metabolic alkalosis.

Resolution of peripheral edema is neither an emergency nor a priority. An effective circulatory volume and a normal blood pressure should be maintained at all times; this is especially critical during vasodilation (e.g., antihypertensive medications, general anesthesia). In a patient with low circulatory volume and abnormally low serum protein concentration (e.g., postoperative phase, third-space losses, nephrotic syndrome, hydrops fetalis) with visceral (e.g., pleural, peritoneal, pericardiac) fluid accumulation, the circulatory volume should be expanded with colloids before administration of diuretics.

Thiazides (or metolazone if CRF) have been used as first choice for chronic diuretic therapy, to minimize bone calcium loss and prevent nephrocalcinosis and nephrolithiasis.

However, this calcium-sparing effect disappears after sodium load during sodium replacement and with the addition of spironolactone. During chronic therapy, the efficacy of a single diuretic decreases progressively, because of compensatory mechanisms that increase sodium reabsorption at other sites of the nephron (778,779). Thus, the combination of two diuretics with different sites of action may be required. The addition of spironolactone to a thiazide has not been conclusively proven to be beneficial (780,781).

Intermittent doses of furosemide can be added to this regimen when necessary. In refractory patients, the association of metolazone and furosemide should be considered (778). Patients on chronic diuretic therapy should have regular US screening (see Nephrocalcinosis and Nephrolithiasis).

BACTERIURIA AND URINARY TRACT INFECTIONS

In infants, bacteriuria can be diagnosed with certainty only by culturing samples obtained by invasive techniques (bladder catheterization or suprapubic aspiration). There is no consensus, however, about the magnitude of bacteriuria required to reach significance (Table 42-18). Bacteriuria in newborn infants can be either asymptomatic or an indication of pyelonephritis, which is characterized by local and systemic inflammatory response. Similarly, candiduria can be asymptomatic, cause hydronephrosis, or be part of a disseminated infection. Lower UTI, i.e., cystitis usually cannot be diagnosed on clinical grounds in newborn infants, except when associated with hematuria.

Frequency in Newborn Infants

The frequency of bacteriuria ranges between 0% and 2.0% in an unselected neonatal population and between 0.6% and 10% in an NICU population (782–788). Risk factors include prematurity (frequency of bacteriuria is 0.1%–10%) (783,785,787,788), male gender (male-to-female ratio

TABLE 42-18

METHODS OF DIAGNOSING BACTERIURIA/URINARY TRACT INFECTION IN NEWBORN INFANTS

Method	Bacteria/ml	Organism Species	Interpretation
Suprapubic Aspiration	Any	One	Positive
Catheterization	1,000–10,000	One	Positive only if pt symptomatic or if dilute urine sample
	1,000–10,000	Two or more	Contaminated
	>10,000	One	Positive
Clean-catch	10,000–100,000	One	Positive only if pt symptomatic or if dilute urine sample
	10,000–100,000	Two or more	Contaminated
	>100,000	One	Positive

ranges from 1:1 to 9:1 in newborn infants) and urinary tract anomalies (785–788). The higher incidence of UTI in boys than in girls in infancy results from the higher frequency of structural abnormalities (785,786) in males and from the higher bacterial counts and higher prevalence of *Escherichia coli* in uncircumcised infants (789). Circumcision reduces the risk for UTI in infancy (790) to a rate that is similar to that in females (786). However, the risk for UTI rises for 2 weeks after ritual Jewish circumcision (791). VUR is less frequent in extremely LBW infants who developed UTI than in infants weighing 1001–1500g (792). UTI often occurs in association with neonatal sepsis (785). In one series, Candida spp were responsible for 25 of 60 (42%) hospital-acquired UTI in a NICU (793).

Pathophysiology

The risk of UTI depends on bacteriologic factors (see Chapter 48) and host characteristics. Periurethral cultures obtained in uncircumcised infants show higher total bacterial counts, and a higher prevalence of *E. coli* than cultures obtained in circumcised infants (789). The normal defense against UTI includes maintenance of an adequate flow of urine; complete emptying of the bladder, and presence of an anatomic barrier, i.e., the bladder outlet. These defense mechanisms may be compromised by urinary tract obstruction, VUR (see Chapter 43), bladder dysfunction (e.g., neurogenic bladder), or manipulation (e.g., prolonged or repeated bladder catheterization) (794,795). Immune defenses in general are described in Chapter 45. In the case of pyelonephritis, endocytosis of bacteria is performed by inflammatory cells and by proximal tubular cells.

Pathology

Acute pyelonephritis is characterized by the presence of polymorphonuclear leukocytes in the glomeruli, tubules, and interstitium (796). Some glomeruli are completely destroyed, whereas others are infiltrated with leukocytes and surrounded by fibrin. The tubules are necrotic, dilated, and their lumens are filled with leukocytes and bacteria. Suppuration may develop in the kidney, often with multiple abscesses, and in other parts of the genitourinary tract. Chronic or recurrent pyelonephritis is characterized by infiltration of inflammatory cells, loss or hyalinization of glomeruli, and atrophy of tubules, with obstruction of the lumen with colloid casts. The development of renal scars may not occur until after 1 year of life.

Clinical Presentation

The clinical presentation of UTI in newborn infants may include one or more of the following signs:

- Growth failure and gastrointestinal symptoms. Failure to thrive, excessive weight loss, poor feeding, diarrhea, and vomiting are the most common clinical features of neonatal UTI.

- Jaundice. The hyperbilirubinemia observed in newborn infants with UTI may be either direct or indirect and sometimes is associated with hemolytic anemia. It is commonly the main clinical feature at presentation and may be the only sign of UTI in some infants (797).
- Temperature instability or fever (temperature ≥38°C). UTI has been reported in 7.5% to 11% of febrile infants presenting to the emergency room during the first 8 to 12 weeks of life (798,799).
- Irritability, lethargy.
- Abnormal urination. This includes poor urinary stream, malodorous urine, and polyuria, which may lead to severe dehydration.
- Signs associated with bacteremia (e.g., respiratory distress) or with focal infection (e.g., mucocutaneous candidiasis, omphalitis).
- Hypertension. This may develop as a result of hydronephrosis associated with the UTI (see Complications) (800).

Laboratory Features

Urinalysis

Based on specimens obtained by bladder catheterization or suprapubic aspiration, only one-half of febrile outpatients with documented UTI during the first 3 months of life had an abnormal urinalysis, defined either by the presence of more than five leukocytes per high power field or by the presence of any bacteria (798). The positive predictive value of pyuria on samples obtained by suprapubic aspiration ranges between 71% (pyuria greater than 10 leukocytes/mm^3) (782) and 96% (pyuria ≥20 leukocytes/mm^3) (787). Thus, the presence of pyuria, at least on a sample obtained by suprapubic aspiration, is suggestive of UTI, whereas the absence of pyuria is insufficient to rule it out (788,801,802). Microscopic demonstration of yeast cells in urine obtained by suprapubic aspiration or bladder catheterization is very suggestive of candiduria.

Urine Culture

The incidence of UTI during the first 3 days of life is very low, making urine culture superfluous during an evaluation for sepsis at that age (802,803). If antibiotic therapy is to be started immediately because of suspicion of sepsis in an infant who is more than 3 days of age, urine should be obtained by suprapubic aspiration or by bladder catheterization (See Table 42-18) (805). Agents most commonly responsible for neonatal UTI include *E. coli* and other gram-negative rods such as Klebsiella, Enterobacter, Citrobacter, and Serratia. Common gram-positive organisms causing UTI include *Staphylococcus aureus* and *Enterococcus*. The incidence of early onset group B Streptococcus infections has decreased as a result of the use of intrapartum antibiotic prophylaxis (806). Candida species are a frequent cause of UTI acquired in the NICU (807).

Complications

Acute complications of UTI in newborn infants include bacteremia, suppuration, VUR, urolithiasis, urinary tract obstruction, sometimes associated with hypertension or ARF, severe hydromineral imbalance (808), methemoglobinemia (809) and ARF, which may result from urinary tract obstruction or massive VUR. Bacteremia develops in 29% of infants with UTI under 1 month of age and in 31% to 43% of neonates with UTI (810–812). Occasionally, UTI is also associated with meningitis. Among NICU patients with hospital-acquired UTI (VLBW infants), bacteremia was present in only 3 of 35 cases (8%), whereas candidemia was present in 13 of 25 (52%) infants with candidal UTI (807). Suppurative complications of UTI, extremely rare in newborn infants, may occur in the kidney, the perirenal area, the prostate, and other genitourinary organs (813,814).

Vesicoureteral reflux is observed commonly during the acute stage of UTI (815); it often decreases or disappears after treatment and may reappear at the time of recurrent infections (816). Intraparenchymal reflux is associated with a high risk of renal scarring (see Chapter 43). Bacterial UTI can be associated with urolithiasis or with hypertension in hydronephrotic infants (817). As many as one third infants with mycotic UTIs develop fungus balls (807), which may obstruct the renal pelvis or the bladder outlet (800,817–819). This obstruction may lead to the development of an abdominal mass, systemic hypertension, or anuria.

Investigation

Pyelonephritis vs. Bacteriuria

Pyelonephritis, which presents a high risk for renal scarring, should be differentiated from asymptomatic bacteriuria, which presents a low risk. Clinical and laboratory features suggesting the diagnosis of pyelonephritis include fever, an increase in blood leukocyte count with a left shift, an elevated sedimentation rate, an increase in the serum concentration of C-reactive protein, and renal tubular dysfunction (820–822). Unfortunately, none of these tests, alone or in combination, can reliably establish the diagnosis or predict the development of renal scars (820). Neonates with UTI should be evaluated for sepsis.

Imaging

Imaging for UTI includes US, followed by VCUG or DMSA scan, or both (823). Ultrasonography of the entire urinary tract may detect urinary tract malformations, hyperechogenic areas suggestive of pyelonephritis (437,819), and renal pyelectasis or ballooning during voiding, both suggestive of VUR (823,824). The American Academy of Pediatrics routinely recommends postnatal US in 2-month to 2-year old children with febrile UTI (825), although this examination may be avoided in those with normal, late-pregnancy US, normal voiding pattern, no abdominal mass, and good response to treatment of the UTI and a normal basic metabolic panel when rehydrated (826) Routine early postnatal US in young children with a postnatal age at least equal to one month and with febrile UTI has a low yield (826) and has minimal impact in patient care (827). Color Doppler cystogram may show signals from the bladder to the ureter during the course of bladder filling (828). Whereas US and color Doppler are sensitive to detect VUR, the sensitivity of US to detect pyelonephritis has not been evaluated.

The VCUG may be done immediately after documenting sterilization of the urine. Alternatively, if the US is negative, the VCUG may be delayed for approximately 1 month, i.e., after resolution of transient, low-grade, UTI-related VUR (816). Significant VUR is very unlikely, and VCUG may be avoided, if US (especially with color Doppler cystography) and DMSA scan are all normal (823–825,828,829).

Cortical defects observed on DMSA scans performed 1 month after a UTI are associated with pyelonephritis, VUR, and the development of renal scars (830–832). Because 99mTc-DMSA binds to the proximal tubules and is excreted only minimally into the urine, it yields excellent visualization of the parenchyma and detection of cortical defects (833). The presence of areas of decreased cortical uptake of DMSA is a reliable indicator of pathologic inflammatory changes of acute pyelonephritis (830). The role of VCUG and DMSA scan in extremely LBW infants with UTI has not been established (834).

Renal Function

Renal glomerular and tubular function should be assessed at the time of the diagnosis and during treatment and follow-up. Especially in patients with obstructive urinary tract disease, UTI can result in transient or permanent decrease in GFR or in tubular dysfunction, characterized by RTA, pseudohypoaldosteronism, decreased urine concentrating ability, or increased NAG enzymuria (835).

Treatment

The treatment of UTI is discussed in Chapter 47. The interval of administration of the antibiotics may have to be adjusted according to their levels and to GFR (412). Third-generation cephalosporins, piperacillin, and aztreonam (836) are alternatives to the ampicillin–gentamicin combination and are chosen according to local epidemiology. A repeat urine culture should be obtained during treatment and after completion of the antibiotic therapy. In the case of failure to respond to treatment, US should be repeated, antibiotic therapy may have to be adjusted, and a systemic infection or other foci should be ruled out. Low-dose antibiotic therapy may be indicated after the initial 10-day course until the VCUG or the DMSA scan is performed, at least in those patients with abnormal US (837). Long-term prophylaxis may be used in patients with high risk of recurrence (e.g., severe VUR).

Therapy for asymptomatic bacteriuria in the absence of bacteremia can be given orally after the first few days. It is possible that shorter courses for the treatment of asymptomatic bacteriuria may be adequate (837), but this has not been evaluated in newborn infants. Although most neonatologists recommend treating bacteriuria regardless of the presence or absence of symptoms (838,839), growing evidence supports simple observation of infants and children with asymptomatic bacteriuria (837,840). However, additional experience in newborn infants must be obtained before withholding therapy for asymptomatic bacteriuria can be recommended.

Surgical intervention may be required for patients with severe VUR and those with urinary tract obstruction (see Chapter 43) (841–843). If a fungus ball is associated with urinary tract obstruction or does not disappear during systemic treatment, daily washings with amphotericin B through a bladder catheter or a nephrostomy tube may be necessary (842,843).

Long-term Complications and Follow-Up

In patients with pyelonephritis or urinary tract anomalies, GFR, urinary concentrating ability, and tubular acidification should be assessed serially. Additionally, US may demonstrate the formation of urolithiasis (844–846). The development of renal failure, once a common complication of UTI in small children, is observed only rarely, except in patients with major urinary tract malformations and renal dysplasia.

Although the association between segmental hypoplasia of the kidney, i.e., Ask–Upmark kidney, VUR and UTI has been known for years (847,848), the development of renal scars remains a serious potential complication (849). In patients in whom UTI develops before 1 year of age, approximately one-half of the kidneys with VUR will develop renal scars, and 70% of the kidneys that eventually develop scars have VUR (829). Several risk factors for formation of renal scars can be identified early, including UTI associated with specific strains of E. coli (824), grades III to IV VUR, especially if complicated by recurrent infections (849,850), and abnormal DMSA scan at the time of the UTI (831). In the piglet model, the DMSA scan was shown to have a sensitivity of 85% and a specificity of 97% for detection of scars caused by VUR and UTI (851). Infants at risk for chronic renal scarring need long-term follow-up by a nephrologist and a urologist, including repeat urine cultures and sequential isotopic scans, and they should be considered for prophylactic antibiotic therapy (816).

Prevention

Although circumcised male infants have a decreased incidence of UTI (786–788), routine circumcision has not been recommended by the American Academy of Pediatrics (852). Infants with neurogenic bladder associated with myelodysplasia often receive intermittent bladder catheterizations and anticholinergic medication. This method has

been shown to result in a lower frequency of long-term deterioration of the radiologic appearance of the kidney, despite a relatively high incidence (19% to 42%) of bacteriuria–UTI (853,854).

A recent meta-analysis of subjects with VUR comparing trials with antibiotics alone or a combined approach with reimplantation surgery/chemoprophylaxis demonstrated a reduction of UTI in the combined approach only up to 2 years of age. Subsequently, the frequency of all forms of UTI was similar in these 2 groups (855). Prophylactic antibiotics include low dose Amoxicillin or Cephalexin as a daily or twice daily dose up to 6 weeks to 2 months of age and subsequently replaced by Co-trimoxazole (1–2 mg/kg of trimethoprim component) or nitrofurantoin (1–2 mg/kg) given as a single evening dose. Data from another study indicate that children without VUR of grade 3 or greater are not at a higher risk of UTI in the absence of prophylactic antibiotics (856). Neonatal VUR resolves or improves in a large majority of patients by 4 years without somatic growth restriction or hypertension (76% in low grade and 59% in high grade reflux)(857).

TUBULAR DYSFUNCTION

This section deals with tubular disorders that present commonly in the neonatal period, including those for which early onset of treatment during the neonatal period may modify or delay the evolution toward renal failure. The reader is referred to other sources for discussion of uncommon disorders not included here (858).

Hypercalciuria, Nephrocalcinosis, and Nephrolithiasis

Normal values of the urinary calcium-to-creatinine ratio in full-term infants are less than 0.86 mg/mg (2.42 mMol/mMol) between 5 days and 7 months (859). Nephrocalcinosis and nephrolithiasis are increasingly recognized in infants with hypercalciuria, most often in premature infants (see next section) (Table 42-19). Prenatal development of nephrocalcinosis has been detected in neonatal familial hyperparathyroidism (860). Hypercalciuria may result from increased calcium intake or ingestion, decreased tubular reabsorption (861) (see sections on Renal Tubular Acidosis and Hypokalemic Salt Losing Nephropathies), or increased bone calcium reabsorption or uptake. Nephrocalcinosis and nephrolithiasis also may result from the precipitation of calcium phosphate or oxalate in the absence of hypercalciuria (see Primary Oxaluria type I and Oxalosis). Finally, nephrolithiasis may result from high urinary concentrations of cystine (see Cystinuria), uric acid (see Uric Acid), xanthine (see Xanthinuria), 2,8-dihydroxyadenine (see Adenine Phosphoribosyltransferase Deficiency), or acyclovir (see Nephrotoxicity), and may occur in association with UTI (see Urinary Tract Infection) and with obstructive urinary tract malformations (844–846). Nephrocalcinosis may decrease renal tubular function, whereas

TABLE 42-19
MECHANISMS OF NEPHROCALCINOSIS AND NEPHROLITHIASIS IN INFANCY

Hypercalciuria
  Increased calcium intake or absorption with/without hypercalcemia
    Excessive calcium intake (P0 or IV)
    Rapid calcium infusion
    Hypervitaminosis D
    Fanconi syndrome if excessive vitamin D administration
    Phosphate depletion, low phosphate intake
    X-linked hypophosphatemia (during phosphate and vitamin D administration)
  Decreased renal tubular reabsorption
    Diuretics (loop diuretics, spironolactone, thiazides if sodium intake or extracellular volume is increased)
    Osmotic diuresis
    Distal renal tubular acidosis (RTA type I)
    Arthrogryposis multiplex congenita with renal and hepatic anomalies
    Bartter's syndrome and related syndromes
    Autosomal dominant hypocalcemia
    Dent's disease (hypercalciuric nephrolithiasis)[a]
  Increased bone reabsorption or decreased bone uptake
    Primary hyperparathyroidism (including neonatal familial hyperparathyroidism)
    Secondary hyperparathyroidism
    Acidosis
    Chronic corticosteroid therapy
    Hypophosphatasia
    Hyperthyroidism
  Idiopathic hypercalcemia
Other mechanisms
  Factors facilitating precipitation of calcium phosphate/oxalate
    Low urine output
    Alkaline urine
    Absence of inhibitors: citrate, inorganic phosphate, magnesium
    Oxaluria (primary or secondary)
  Other causes of nephrolithiasis
  Cystinosis
  Cystinuria
  Oxaluria (primary or secondary)
  Hyperuricemia
  Classical hereditary xanthinuria
  Adenine phosphoribosyltransferase deficiency (2,8-dihydroxyadenine lithiasis)
  Acyclovir
  Urinary tract infection
  Obstructive urinary tract malformations

[a] Youngest patient described is 1 yr old.

nephrolithiasis may cause hematuria, colic, dysuria, UTI, hydronephrosis, ARF, and CRF. The treatment of asymptomatic urolithiasis is high fluid intake and specific therapy when available; lithotripsy and surgical treatment are discussed in Chapter 43.

Nephrocalcinosis and Nephrolithiasis in Premature Infants

Nephrocalcinosis or nephrolithiasis, detected by ultrasonography in 20% to 60% of premature infants with a GA less than 32 weeks, is predominantly as a result of hypercalciuria (862–867). Hypercalciuria may result from increased calcium intake or gastrointestinal absorption, decreased renal tubular calcium reabsorption, and abnormal regulation of bone mineral content (Table 42-19) (868). Chronic use of discontinuous daily calcium infusions is associated with recurrent periods of hypercalcemia and hypercalciuria. High enteral calcium intake may be associated with hypercalciuria in the absence of hypercalcemia (869). Insufficient phosphate intake may result in hypophosphatemia, hypercalcemia, hypercalciuria, and osteopenia of prematurity (870). Increasing the phosphate intake in these patients reduces calcemia and calciuria (871). Several authors have found a significant association between administration of furosemide and hypercalciuria in LBW infants (863,865,872). Hypercalciuria also may be induced by spironolactone (873,874) or by thiazides in patients with increased sodium intake or extracellular volume (868,875,876). Addition of acetate to the TPN reduces calciuria without affecting serum levels of calcium, PTH, or vitamin D (877). Acute and chronic acidosis induce bone calcium reabsorption and hypercalciuria.

Other factors may contribute to the development of nephrocalcinosis. One study using multivariate analysis showed that risk factors for nephrocalcinosis included duration of ventilation, toxic gentamicin or vancomycin levels, low fluid intake during week 3, and male gender (878). The risk for lithiasis and nephrocalcinosis increases with high saturation levels, which result from low urine output or high urinary oxalate or urate (879,880). To prevent hypercalciuria, VLBW infants should receive enough phosphate and should receive neither discontinuous calcium infusions nor excessive doses of vitamin D. If chronic diuretic therapy is indicated, the drug of choice is a thiazide (or metolazone if CRF), without sodium supplementation, and renal US should be done to assess for possible nephrocalcinosis or nephrolithiasis. Nephrocalcinosis appears to resolve spontaneously in 40% to 50% of cases on follow up, but can be associated with recurrent UTI, renal colic, and hematuria. Patients with persistent calcifications at 1 to 2 years of age show signs of tubular dysfunction, including a decrease in tubular reabsorption of phosphate, increase in FENa, and limitation of distal renal tubular acidification (881). Thus, hypercalciuric patients with nephrolithiasis or nephrocalcinosis should receive a thiazide without sodium supplementation; if an additional diuretic is required, amiloride or triamterene may be considered (882).

Primary Hyperoxaluria TYPE I and Oxalosis

Primary hyperoxaluria type I, i.e., glycolic aciduria is an autosomal recessive disorder as a result of a functional deficiency of the hepatic peroxisomal enzyme alanine: glyoxylate aminotransferase (AGT) (883), which leads to oxalosis, i.e., progressive accumulation of calcium oxalate in various tissues. The AGT gene has been cloned and mapped to chromosome 2q36-37 (884–886). The diagnosis is strongly suggested by a high oxalate-to-creatinine ratio in the urine (887–890) in the absence of secondary causes for oxaluria (e.g., TPN or vitamin B6 deficiency), and is further supported by measuring glycolic aciduria and L-glyceric aciduria (889,891). Definitive diagnosis is possible by measuring AGT in a liver biopsy or by DNA analysis. Approximately 12% of patients present in infancy, with anorexia, failure to thrive, vomiting, dehydration, and fever; presentation in the neonatal period is rare (892–894). Renal damage includes nephrocalcinosis, urolithiasis, and renal failure. In pyridoxine-responsive patients, therapy includes pyridoxine, inhibitors of calcium oxalate precipitation, large fluid intake (2 L/m^2/d), and later dialysis and renal transplantation (895–897). In pyridoxine-resistant patients, the treatment of choice is either early liver transplantation or combined hepatorenal transplantation for end stage renal disease (898).

Disorders of Purine Metabolism

Two disorders of purine metabolism may lead to nephrolithiasis in infancy: classic xanthinuria and adenine phosphoribosyltransferase deficiency.

Classic Xanthinuria

Classic xanthinuria is an autosomal recessive disorder with two genotypes. Type I is an isolated defect of the xanthine dehydrogenase (XDH) gene, which has been mapped to chromosome 2p22–23 (899,900). Classic xanthinuria type II is a combined defect of XDH and aldehyde oxidase (900a), which results from a functional defect of the human molybdenum cofactor sulfurase gene (HMCS) gene (901). Both disorders cause severe neonatal encephalopathy, lens dislocation, and microcephaly. Additionally, xanthinuria may result from the administration of allopurinol (inhibitor of xanthine oxidase) to a patient with high uric acid production, i.e., Lesch–Nyhan syndrome or treatment of malignancy. Classic xanthinuria may present with complications of xanthine urolithiasis or with ARF; some patients eventually develop CRF, duodenal ulcers, myopathy, or arthropathy, whereas others remain asymptomatic. The association of ARF with a history of hematuria or red-brown deposits on the diaper or in the urine sediment should raise the suspicion of classic xanthinuria (902). US may show the lithiasis. Classic xanthinuria is diagnosed by demonstrating high levels of xanthine and hypoxanthine and low-to-undetectable levels of uric acid in plasma and urine. Early treatment of xanthinuria with high fluid intake, a diet low in purines and adequate therapy of nephrolithiasis and its complications yields an excellent prognosis.

Adenine Phosphoribosyltransferase Deficiency

Adenine phosphoribosyltransferase deficiency is an autosomal recessive disorder as a result of mutations of the adenine phosphoribosyltransferase deficiency gene, which has

been cloned and mapped to chromosome 16q24 (903). Two types have been characterized: patients with type I (mainly Caucasians) have no enzyme activity in their erythrocyte lysates, whereas those with type II (Japanese) have some residual activity. DNA analysis shows that these two types correspond to different mutations (904). The defect causes an increase in urinary excretion of 2,8-dihydroxy-adenine, which is very poorly soluble. The disease presents with the complications of lithiasis, which can develop even in the neonatal period. The diagnosis can be suspected by visualizing round brown crystals in the urine sediment and confirmed by measuring erythrocyte adenine phosphoribosyltransferase deficiency activity and by DNA analysis. The treatment of this disorder includes a high fluid intake, allopurinol, alkali, and a diet low in purines. The prognosis depends on renal function at the time of the diagnosis; patients with ESRD require renal transplantation in addition to disease-specific therapy.

Familial Hypocalciuric Hypercalcemia

Familial hypocalciuric hypercalcemia (FHH) may correspond to three different genotypes. Type I, the most common, is an autosomal dominant disorder resulting from a defect in the human calcium sensor receptor (CaSR) gene, which has been cloned and mapped to chromosome 3q21-q24 (905–907). Type II has been mapped to chromosome 19p13.3, and type III to chromosome 19q13 (908–910). Inactivating mutations of the CaSR gene increase both the parathyroid calcium set point, i.e., serum calcium concentration that results in a 50% reduction in maximum PTH release and the set point for renal tubular reabsorption of calcium. Analysis of several families has shown that FHH is the heterozygous, benign form, whereas neonatal severe hyperparathyroidism is the life-threatening homozygous form (911,912). In contrast, activating mutations of the CaSR gene result in autosomal dominant hypocalcemia, which is associated with urolithiasis (see Table 42.19) (861).

The diagnosis of FHH is based on family history of hypercalcemia, a low urine calcium-to-creatinine ratio (less than 0.03 mg/mg), a low fractional excretion of calcium (less than 0.016, or 1.6%), and high magnesium and low phosphate concentrations in the serum (913–915). Hypercalcemia and hypermagnesemia result from an increase in their tubular reabsorption and in their release from bone, whereas hypophosphatemia results from a decrease in renal tubular reabsorption. In most patients with FHH, PTH levels are within normal limits for normocalcemic controls but inappropriately high for the serum Ca2+ concentration. The differential diagnosis includes other causes of neonatal hypercalcemia (see section on Nephrocalcinosis and Nephrolithiasis and Chap. 36), and multiple endocrine neoplasia syndromes (see Chapter 39). FHH is usually a benign disorder that fails to respond to parathyroidectomy (916). However, some patients with FHH have recurrent pancreatitis. Some neonates with FHH have transient self-limited hyperparathyroidism (917). In contrast, those with neonatal severe hyperparathyroidism have severe hypercalcemia, high serum alkaline phosphatase activity, and typical radiographic bone changes; these patients may require total parathyroidectomy followed by administration of 1,25(OH)2D3 (918,919).

Fanconi Syndrome

Fanconi syndrome is characterized by generalized dysfunction of the proximal tubule. The cardinal signs are renal glucosuria, renal phosphaturia, and generalized aminoaciduria; other features, present inconsistently, include proximal RTA (pRTA), tubular proteinuria, increased urinary excretion of urate, sodium, potassium, and calcium, and decreased ability to concentrate the urine and to secrete PAH (919a). In some cases, distal tubular dysfunction is present, and the disease evolves toward renal failure, with less evidence of tubular dysfunction.

Because several transport systems are deficient in this syndrome, the pathophysiologic process presumably involves a global disturbance, such as an alteration of the integrity of the tubular membranes or of sulfhydryl-requiring enzymes (919a).

Idiopathic cases of Fanconi syndrome most often are sporadic, although autosomal recessive, autosomal dominant, and X-linked recessive transmission have been described (920). Fanconi syndrome occurs in association with a variety of disorders (Table 42-20), the most common of which is cystinosis (921). Disorders associated with late-onset renal dysfunction will not be reviewed here. General discussion of inborn errors of the metabolism can be found in Chapter 41.

The clinical presentation of Fanconi syndrome includes polyuria, polydipsia, dehydration, and failure to thrive. Signs include acidosis, hypophosphatemia, and rickets. The diagnosis is confirmed by the demonstration of glucosuria in the presence of a normal glycemia (less than 120 to 150 mg/dL), decreased tubular reabsorption of phosphate, and generalized hyperaminoaciduria. The prognosis of Fanconi syndrome depends on the underlying disorder.

The treatment includes administration of sodium citrate or bicarbonate, and as required, water, potassium, phosphate, and carnitine (922). Once rickets has developed, careful administration of vitamin D is required; excess vitamin D may result in hypercalciuria and nephrocalcinosis. Indomethacin, a PGSI, has been given successfully to some patients (923,924). Specific dietary therapy for fructose intolerance, galactosemia, or tyrosinemia results in disappearance of the Fanconi syndrome. In many other diseases, treatment serves only to slow the deterioration of renal function.

Special Considerations

Cystinosis

The reported incidence of cystinosis ranges between 1:20,000 and 1:326,000 (858). It is an autosomal recessive lysosomal transport disorder, characterized by accumulation of cystine, as a result of a defect in the carrier-mediated transport of cystine from the lysosomes to the cytosol (925). Cystinosis results from inactivating mutation of the CTNS gene, mapped to the short arm of chromosome 17p13 (926), which encodes cystinosin, a lysosomal cystine transporter. The infantile, i.e., nephropathic type of cystinosis is the most severe form (858,927) and is characterized by fluid and electrolyte loss, aminoaciduria, glycosuria, phosphaturia, RTA, rickets, and growth restriction, with onset of symptoms generally between 6 and 12 months of age. At birth, patients with cystinosis appear normal except for lighter skin and hair pigmentation than siblings. In some patients, the initial presentation may suggest a diagnosis of Bartter syndrome or of nephrogenic diabetes

TABLE 42-20
CAUSES OF FANCONI SYNDROME IN INFANCY

Idiopathic		Secondary	
	Inherited Disease of the Metabolism (AR unless specified)		Acquired
Isolated	GRACILE syndrome		Renovascular accident in neonatal period
ARC syndrome (AR)	Cystinosis		Interstitial nephritis
	Fructose-1-phosphate aldolase deficiency		Medications: valproate, aminoglycosides, ifosfamide[a]
	Hepatorenal tyrosinemia type 1		Renal transplantation
	Galactosemia		Toluene, heavy metal poisoning
	Glycogenosis with Fanconi S (Fanconi-Bickel S)		Vitamin D deficiency rickets
	Oculocerebrorenal (Lowe) syndrome (X-linked)		Dysproteinemia
	Vitamin D-dependent rickets		Nephrotic syndrome
	Disorders of the energy metabolism		
	Pearson's syndrome (maternofetal transmission)		
	Cytochrome-c oxidase deficiency		
	Pyruvate carboxylase deficiency		
	Carnitine palmitoyl transferase I deficiency		

[a] Fanconi syndrome also has been reported after administration of other medications in older patients. S, syndrome.
Abbreviations: AR, autosomal recessive; ARC, arthrogryposis, renal tubular dysfunction and cholestasis

insipidus (NDI) (927). Retinopathy may be detected within the first weeks of life (928), whereas characteristic corneal opacities appear only after 1 year. Laboratory findings include urinary excretion of typical cystine crystals, besides features of Fanconi syndrome. Progressive deterioration of the GFR leads to ESRD at a median age of 9.2 years (929).

PCR detection assays have been established, providing basis for rapid molecular diagnosis of cystinosis (930). Prenatal diagnosis is made by direct measurement of cystine in cultured amniocytes or chorionic villi cells. The mutational spectrum varies with different populations (931). Genetic counseling could be offered to families of specific ethnic backgrounds by screening of the most common mutation, e.g., G339R in Jewish-Moroccan and Amish-Mennonite populations (931).

The treatment of cystinosis in infancy includes alkalinization and supplementation of water, potassium, carnitine (922), phosphate, and vitamin D. Indomethacin, a PGSI, may reduce urinary losses and improve growth; however, it also may transiently decrease GFR (923,924). The treatment of choice is the administration of cysteamine, i.e., β-mercaptoethylamine hydrochloride (which is poorly tolerated and has persistent nauseating odor) or phosphocysteamine (which lacks the foul taste and odor of cysteamine). These agents help deplete cells of cystine (932). Treatment improves growth and delays the progression toward renal failure (933,934), especially if initiated soon after birth (935).

Arthrogryposis, Renal Tubular Dysfunction, and Cholestasis Syndrome

This is an autosomal recessive syndrome seen predominantly in Pakistanis. Renal tubular dysfunction ranges from isolated RTA to complete Fanconi syndrome, and hepatic histology shows various combinations of cholestasis, intrahepatic biliary hypoplasia, giant cell hepatitis, lipofuscin deposition, and fibrosis. Additional features observed in some patients include failure to thrive, NDI, neurogenic muscular atrophy (resulting in arthrogryposis), cerebral malformations, ichthyosis, dysmorphism, nerve deafness, and abnormality in platelet morphology (936). At least 2 candidate genes (FIC1 and HNF1) have been identified (937).

Glycogen Storage Disease with Fanconi Syndrome (Fanconi–Bickel Syndrome)

More than 112 patients have been described with Fanconi–Bickel syndrome, i.e., glycogen storage disease [GSD] with Fanconi syndrome. This syndrome is caused by homozygous or compound heterozygous mutations within GLUT2, the gene encoding the most important facilitative glucose transporter in hepatocytes, pancreatic β cells, enterocytes, and renal tubular cells. It is characterized by the association of hepatomegaly secondary to glycogen accumulation, glucose and galactose intolerance, fasting hypoglycemia, Fanconi syndrome, and severely stunted growth (938). In the kidney, glycogen accumulation is limited to the proximal tubule, with maximal levels in the straight part. This syndrome should be differentiated from phosphorylase b kinase deficiency (939) or from GSD type I (often as a result of glucose-6-phosphatase deficiency), which is associated with late onset of proximal tubular dysfunction in approximately 15% of the cases (940).

Fever, vomiting, growth failure, and rickets develop in the patients within 6 weeks to 10 months of birth, followed by hepatomegaly, protuberant abdomen, moon-shaped face, and fat deposition around the shoulders and the abdomen (920,941). Kidneys of most patients are relatively large. Laboratory findings include glucosuria on the first day of life, galactosemia on the fourth day, and hypophosphatemia by the eighth week. The Fanconi syndrome, initially severe, tends to improve. Hepatic glycogenosis causes a tendency toward hypoglycemia, ketonuria, hypercholesterolemia, and hypertriglyceridemia, but no lactic acidosis. Particular attention should be given to treating possible acute decompensations at the time of surgery or infections. Hypoglycemia can be prevented by frequent protein-enriched feedings, by uncooked cornstarch (942), and restriction of galactose intake. The treatment of the nephropathy is nonspecific.

Growth Retardation, Aminoaciduria, Cholestasis, Iron Overload, Lactic Acidosis, and Early Death Syndrome

Growth retardation, aminoaciduria, cholestasis, iron overload, lactic acidosis, and early death (GRACILE) syndrome is an autosomal recessive metabolic disorder of Finnish disease heritage, characterized by fetal growth retardation, lactic acidosis, Fanconi type aminoaciduria, cholestasis, and iron overload. It is caused by a missense mutation in the BCS1L gene, which is located on chromosome 2q33–37 and encodes a mitochondrial protein needed for the assembly of the mitochondrial chain complex III. Prenatal diagnosis can be performed on linkage analysis in families with at least one affected child. Typical histological changes may be present in early fetal life (943–945).

Galactose-1-Phosphate Uridyl Transferase Deficiency

Galactosemia (see Chapter 39) is an autosomal recessive disorder that results in intracellular accumulation of galactose-1-phosphate in various tissues, including the kidney. The galactose 1-phosphate uridyltransferase gene has been cloned and mapped to chromosome 9p13 (946–948). Most neonatal screening programs routinely measure the activity of the red blood cell enzyme. Symptoms of the severe form often develop in the neonatal period, soon after initiating lactose intake, i.e., milk, and include hypoglycemia, anorexia, vomiting, diarrhea, hepatomegaly, jaundice, and hypoprothrombinemia (949). Renal dysfunction develops within 2 weeks after initiation of galactose intake; it is characterized by severe proteinuria, generalized aminoaciduria, and a significant defect in transport of phosphate, bicarbonate, and PAH (949–951). Lactose intake leads to galactosuria, which produces a positive test for reducing substances but no glucosuria. Removing lactose and galactose from the diet results in rapid resolution (949).

Hereditary Fructose Intolerance

Hereditary fructose intolerance (HFI) is an autosomal recessive disorder as a result of deficiency in fructose-1-phosphate aldolase (liver aldolase B), which normally is present in the liver, small intestine, and renal cortex (see Chap. 41). Mutations lie within exon 5 of the aldolase B gene. This gene has been cloned and mapped to chromosome 9q21.3-q22.2 (952,953). In patients with HFI, ingestion of fructose results in the accumulation of fructose-1-phosphate in these tissues. Although fructose is not part of the normal diet in the neonatal period, the routine use of sucrose has been recommended for sedation during neonatal procedures (954,955). In patients with HFI, a single dose of fructose will induce serious hypoglycemia, hypophosphatemia, generalized hyperaminoaciduria, RTA, proteinuria, and phosphaturia, and transient fructosuria or glucosuria, or both (956,957). The diagnosis of HFI is suggested by the history of fructose or sucrose intake, the presence of reducing substances in the urine, hyperaminoaciduria, and high plasma concentrations of methionine and tyrosine, and by the clinical response to removal of fructose and sucrose from the diet. HFI can be diagnosed by measuring aldolase activity in liver biopsy specimens or by screening for mutations using reverse dot-blot procedure (958). Removal of fructose and sucrose from the diet results in normalization of tubular function within 2 weeks.

Hepatorenal Tyrosinemia

Hereditary tyrosinemia type I, i.e., hepatorenal tyrosinemia, tyrosinosis (see Chap. 41) is an autosomal recessive disorder as a result of a deficiency in fumarylacetoacetate hydrolase (FAH or fumarylacetoacetase) (959). The disorder is most common in the Saguenay-Lac St.-Jean region of the province of Quebec and in Scandinavia (960). The gene coding for this enzyme has been cloned and mapped to chromosome 15q23-q25 (961–963). Approximately 35 mutations have been described so far (964). Renal tubular dysfunction results from the accumulation of succinyl-acetoacetate and succinylacetone. Prenatal diagnosis is possible by measurement of succinylacetone in amniotic fluid and of FAH activity in amniocytes or chorionic villi and by restricted fragment length polymorphism in informative families (961–963). Hepatorenal tyrosinemia can be differentiated from transient neonatal tyrosinemia by a high blood concentration of succinylacetone in the former.

Clinical presentation includes failure to thrive, a cabbage-like odor, vomiting, diarrhea, severe metabolic acidosis, hepatomegaly, jaundice, melena, ascites, edema, fever, and tubular dysfunction (965,966). Renal dysfunction includes hyperaminoaciduria, severe phosphaturia, and variable degrees of RTA, glucosuria, and proteinuria (965,966). Early presentation (less than 2 months) of tyrosinemia type I is associated with liver failure and death by the age of 1 year in most untreated patients. Removal of phenylalanine, tyrosine, and methionine from the diet normalizes tubular function but does not prevent death from liver failure, recurrent bleeding, hepatocellular carcinoma, or porphyria-like syndrome with respiratory failure (967,968). Liver transplantation has considerably changed the survival rate; these patients have normal GFR but tubular dysfunction (968). Promising results suggest that administration of 2-(2-nitro-4-trifluoromethylbenzoyl)-1,3-cyclohexanedione (NTBC) may decrease the production of succinylacetone, the incidence of crises, and the need for liver transplantation (969,970).

Oculocerebrorenal Syndrome of Lowe

Oculocerebrorenal (OCRL) syndrome of Lowe is a rare X-linked disorder caused by mutations of the OCRL1 gene, which has been cloned and mapped to chromosome Xq25-q26 (971–973). Deficiency in the OCRL1 gene product, a phosphatidylinositol 4, 5-bisphosphate (PIP2)-5-phosphatase, raises intracellular concentration of PIP2, leading in turn to decreased actin stress fibers and abnormal distribution of actin binding proteins, and disruption of tight junctions and adherens junctions (974).

The phenotype includes major abnormalities in the eyes (including cataracts), nervous system (mental retardation), and kidneys (Fanconi syndrome) (see Appendix G–2) (975). Glomerular involvement develops progressively in childhood and eventually leads to renal failure in the second to fourth decade (976,977). Lowe syndrome can be diagnosed prenatally by identification of defective mRNA expression of the OCRL1 gene in cultured amniocytes (978). Urinary trehalase protein concentration and trehalase catalytic activity by ELISA has recently been used to help in the diagnosis of renal tubular damage in Lowe syndrome, Dent's disease, and congenital nephrotic syndrome (979). Treatment of the Fanconi syndrome includes alkalinization therapy (Polycitra) with carnitine supplements, supplementation of phosphate once serum alkaline phosphatase increases (suggesting bone resorption) and, in some patients, supplementation with potassium or calcium.

Disorders of Energy Metabolism

These disorders have a wide range of presentation, including multiorgan dysfunction, lactic acidosis, hematologic disturbances (e.g., pancytopenia), growth failure, liver failure, pancreatic insufficiency, myopathy, cardiopathy, nervous system and sensorial disturbances, and nephropathy (see Chapter 41). Some of the genes involved are coded by nuclear deoxyribonucleic acid (DNA), whereas other genes are coded by mitochondrial DNA, resulting in maternal inheritance (980). Renal involvement most often consists of Fanconi syndrome, although some patients develop RTA, Bartter syndrome, chronic tubulointerstitial nephritis, nephrotic syndrome, or renal failure (981). Pathology may show cytoplasmic vacuolization of tubular cells and giant mitochondria. Neonatal or infantile involvement of the kidney may occur in several disorders, including Pearson's marrow-pancreas syndrome (maternal inheritance), fatal infantile mitochondrial myopathy, cytochrome c oxidase deficiency, pyruvate carboxylase deficiency, carnitine palmitoyl transferase I deficiency, and phosphoenolpyruvate carboxykinase deficiency (980–989).

Nephrogenic Diabetes Insipidus

NDI is a rare inherited disease characterized by the failure of kidney to respond to AVP because of a receptor or postreceptor defect, despite raised serum concentrations of AVP (990). Congenital NDI is most often transmitted as an X-linked trait, as a result of mutations of the vasopressin receptor (AVPR2) gene (991), coding for the basolateral vasopressin V2 receptor in the collecting duct (992). The gene has been cloned and mapped to chromosome Xq28 by linkage analysis (993). In some families, NDI is an autosomal recessive trait, which results from mutations of the apical aquaporin-2 water channels (994).

Symptoms of congenital NDI include polyuria, dehydration, fever, constipation, and failure to thrive. Pertinent laboratory findings include a persistently low urine osmolality despite hypernatremic dehydration, without other tubular dysfunction. In the past, severe episodes of dehydration with hypertonic encephalopathy resulted in a 16% prevalence of long-term neurologic problems (995). Although a more recent series showed a 14% risk for cognitive delay and a 47% risk for attention deficit hyperactivity disorder, there was no association between test performances and hypernatremia (996).

The differential diagnosis of NDI includes several entities causing polyuria (Table 42-21). The diagnosis of NDI is confirmed by the failure to concentrate the urine and to increase urinary cAMP in response to intranasal administration of DDAVP, in contrast to patients with central diabetes insipidus, i.e., ADH deficiency (997). Patients with defective V2 receptors, but not those with defective aquaporin 2, have abnormal extra renal response of the V2 receptors to administration of DDAVP or desmopressin (994). Aquaporin 2 cannot be detected in the urine from patients with mutations in the aquaporin-2 gene and is found at lower concentration than normal in those with mutations of the V2 receptor (998). Diagnosis in utero can be made by linkage analysis if other family members have the disease (993). Female carriers of the X-linked trait are asymptomatic, but may have mild impairment of urine-concentrating ability.

Treatment of acute hypernatremic dehydration includes correction of the free-water deficit, i.e.:

$$\text{Water deficit} = 0.6 \times \text{body weight} \times [(Na/140) - 1],$$

Where water deficit is in liters, body weight is in kg, and Na is plasma sodium concentration in mM/L.

Chronic therapy to reduce urine output most often includes the combination of chlorothiazide, indomethacin, and potassium supplements (999,1000). Preliminary data suggest that an alternative treatment may be the use of amiloride (0.3 mg/kg/day po three times a day) and hydrochlorothiazide, without potassium supplements (993,1001). Gene therapy holds promise in the treatment of NDI (1002).

Hypokalemic Alkalosis

The differential diagnosis of hypokalemic alkalosis in infancy is given in Table 42-22. The discussion in this section is limited to the renal causes.

Hypokalemic Salt Losing Tubulopathies (Bartter-like Syndromes)

This group of closely related hereditary tubulopathies share hypokalemic metabolic alkalosis, hyperreninemic

---

TABLE 42-21
ETIOLOGY OF NEPHROGENIC DEFECT IN URINARY CONCENTRATION

	Decreased Effect of Antidiuretic Hormone on Tubular Permeability to Water	Decreased Corticomedullary Concentration Gradient

Congenital	Nephrogenic diabetes insipidus
	Hypokalemia
	   Bartter syndrome and related syndromes
	   Pseudohypoaldosteronism
	   Proximal renal tubular acidosis
	   Duplication of the mitochondrial genome
		Medullary cystic disease, polycystic kidney disease
		Bilateral dysplastic kidneys
		Urinary tract obstruction

Acquired	Drug: PGE_2, PGE_1, amphotericin, lithium Hypokalemia Hypercalcemia	Polyuria: water/osmotic diuresis Obstructive disease (before and after treatment) Chronic/acute renal failure Pyelonephritis Nephrocalcinosis Medullary necrosis Malnutrition

PG, prostaglandin.

TABLE 42-22
DIFFERENTIAL DIAGNOSIS OF HYPOKALEMIC ALKALOSIS

Inadequate intake
    Cl^--deficient diet
    Insufficient K and Cl in iv
Gastrointestinal losses
    Vomiting, pyloric stenosis
    Gastric suction
    Cl^- diarrhea
Kidney
    Diuretics: loop diuretics, thiazides
    Hypovolemia + other cause for hypokalemia (e.g., proximal
        RTA, cystinosis)
    Bartter syndrome and related syndromes
    Liddle syndrome (pseudohyperaldosteronism)
    Unilateral renovascular disease (rarely)
Endocrine
    Primary hyperaldosteronism
    Cushing syndrome
    Congenital adrenal hyperplasia (with hypertension):
        11 β-hydroxylase deficiency
        17 β-hydroxylase deficiency
        11 β-hydroxysteroid dehydrogenase deficiency
Cystic fibrosis

hyperaldosteronism with normal blood pressure, hyperplasia of the juxtaglomerular apparatus, and impaired urinary-concentrating ability (1003). These tubulopathies, all transmitted as autosomal recessive traits, have been classified into three types of phenotypic entities: the antenatal variant, the classical variant, and the Gitelman syndrome.

Neonatal or antenatal Bartter syndrome (hyperprostaglandin E syndrome), the most severe form, is characterized by polyhydramnios, premature birth, life threatening episodes of salt and water loss in the neonatal period, hypokalemic alkalosis, and failure to thrive, and hypercalciuria and early onset nephrocalcinosis (1004). Some patients have a distinctive appearance: thin with small muscles and a triangular facies characterized by prominent forehead, large eyes, protruding ears, and drooping mouth. Strabismus is frequently present. Increased urinary PGE2 excretion has been considered a characteristic feature (1005). This condition is genetically heterogeneous. Type I results from loss-of-function mutations of the SLC12A1 gene, which has been mapped to chromosome 15q 15–21 and encodes the renal bumetanide-sensitive Na-K-2Cl co transporter (also termed NKCC2, BSC1, and ENCC2) of the TALH. Type II results from loss-of-function mutations of the KCNJ1 gene, which is located on chromosome 11q24–25 and encodes ROMK, a potassium channel expressed in the TALH and in the CCD (1006). A third type of antenatal Bartter syndrome, with sensorineural deafness, has been described in nine consanguineous families, and mapped to chromosome 1p31; the gene responsible for this syndrome has not yet been determined (1007,1008). Patients with type I present during early

neonatal period with massive NaCl wasting, hypokalemia, and metabolic alkalosis (1009). In contrast, neonates with type II, especially those prematurely (1010), may present with mild NaCl wasting and a biochemical picture mimicking pseudohypoaldosteronism type I, i.e. hyponatremia, hyperkalemia, and metabolic acidosis. In these patients, the typical features of Bartter syndrome may manifest within 3 to 6 weeks; however renal potassium loss is less pronounced than in NKCC2-deficient patients. The association of pseudohypoaldosteronism-1 (PHA-I) with polyhydramnios has been controversial, thus postnatal transient hyperkalemia in the context of polyhydramnios and prematurity should raise the diagnosis of ROMK mutations (1011). Prenatal diagnosis has been made in the past by high Cl content of the amniotic fluid. Amniotic fluid Na, K, Ca, and PGE2 are normal. Trophoblastic DNA analysis will soon allow early and accurate diagnosis.

Classical Bartter syndrome (Type III) occurs in infancy or early childhood. It is characterized by marked salt wasting and hypokalemia, leading to polyuria, polydipsia, volume contraction, muscle weakness, and failure to thrive. Hypercalciuria and nephrocalcinosis may occur (1012). This syndrome results from mutations of the CLCNKB gene, mapped to chromosome 1p36, which encodes the renal chloride channel C1C-Kb (1010,1013).

Gitelman syndrome (Type IV) is a Bartter-like condition with hypomagnesemia and hypocalciuria, and mild presentation usually in older children and adults (1010).

In the immediate neonatal period, dehydration and electrolyte imbalance often require continuous saline infusion. Administration of indomethacin in the early postnatal period is not only unnecessary but also dangerous in patients with type II, and has potential side effects, e.g., NEC and renal failure. Prenatal treatment with indomethacin is also useless and dangerous for the fetus. However, at 4–6 weeks of age, the patient will benefit greatly from this therapy and eventually, of KCl supplementation. Long-term prognosis is guarded and lack of therapeutic control may lead to slow progression to chronic renal failure (1006).

Renal Tubular Acidosis

Plasma bicarbonate (HCO_3^-) concentrations normally are lower than subsequent values in the term newborn and even lower in premature or VLBW infants (1014). Metabolic acidosis in newborn infants usually is normochloremic, with an increased serum anion gap. The most common cause is lactic acidosis resulting from asphyxia, ischemia, hypoxemia, or local tissue damage. Less commonly, it is as a result of a congenital metabolic disorder (see Chapter 41) or to renal failure.

The diagnosis and classification of RTA has traditionally been made on the basis of functional studies. Four types of RTA have been described: classic distal, i.e., type I, pRTA, i.e., type II, hyperkalemic distal, i.e., type IV, which is the most common type of RTA, and mixed proximal and distal, i.e., type III (Table 42-23) (1015). Application of molecular

TABLE 42-23
ETIOLOGY OF RENAL TUBULAR ACIDOSIS IN INFANCY

Proximal RTA (Type 2)	Hyperkalemic RTA (Type 4)	Distal RTA (Type 1)	Mixed (Type 3)

Primary
AR, AD
  Sporadic transient
	Early childhood hyperkalemic
	  RTA
		With bicarbonate wasting in
		  infancy and early childhood)
		Sporadic
		With cystic fibrosis
			Familial hyperparathyroidism with
			  hypercalciuria and RTA (Nishiyama)
			  VLBW infant

Secondary
  Fanconi syndrome
  Metachromatic
    leukodystrophy[a]
  Mitochondrial diseases
  Hereditary nephritis
  Tetralogy of Fallot[a]
  Vitamin D deficiency
  Vascular accident in
    NN period
  Hereditary nephritis
  Carbonic anhydrase
    inhibition
  Carbonic anhydrase II
    deficiency with
    osteopetrosis (AR)
  Drugs and toxins:
    valproic acids,
    heavy metals
  Deficiency in NBC-1
    (pRTA with glaucoma)
	1: Primary hypoaldosteronism,
	  adrenal insufficiency
	2–3: Hyporeninemic
	  hypoaldosteronism[b] with
	  chronic renal disease
	4: Pseudohypoaldosteronism-1
	  with or without salt wasting
	5: Partial unresponsiveness
	  to aldosterone
	Tubulointerstitial disease
	Urinary tract obstruction, UTI
	Unilateral dysplastic
	  kidney or RVT
	Drugs (e.g., KCl, K-sparing
	  diuretics, heparin, ACE
	  inhibitors, PGSI, cyclosporine)
	Toxins
		Hypergammaglobulinemia (i.e.,
		  maternal Sjögren syndrome)
		Fetal alcohol syndrome
		Toluene, amphotericin B, lithium
		Hypercalcemic hyperthyroidism
		Vitamin D intoxication
		Nephrocalcinosis
		Medullary sponge kidney
		Urinary tract obstruction
		Carnitine palm itoyltransferase
		  type I deficiency (1)
		Carbonic anhydrase II deficiency
		  with osteopetrosis (AR)
		AR with sensorineural deafness:
		  deficiency in B1 subunit of
		  H^+-ATPase
		AR without sensorineural deafness:
		  deficiency in A-4 subunit of
		  H^+-ATPase
		AD: mutation of SLC4A1 gene:
		  deficiency in Cl^-/HCO_3^-
		  exchanger AE1
			Carbonic anyhdrase II deficiency
			  (with osteopetrosis) (AR)
			Hype rparathyroidism
			Nephrocalcinosis and Fanconi
			  syndrome
			Renal transplantation

Renal tubular acidification also may be deficient in the case of renal failure (i.e., normochloremic metabolic acidosis) or of acute diarrhea (hypochloremic metabolic acidosis) (see text).
[a] The only patients with this type of RTA were diagnosed after 12 mo of age.
[b] Types 2 and 3, associated with hyporeninemic hypoaldosteronism, are seen mostly in adults.
ACE, angiotensin-converting enzyme; AD, autosomal dominant; AR, autosomal recessive; H^+-ATPase, proton pump (ATPase); NBC-1, Na-HCO_3 co-transporter, NN, neonatal; PGSI, prostaglandin synthetase inhibitor, pRTA, proximal renal tubular acidosis; RTA, renal tabular acidosis; RVT, renal venous thrombosis; UTI, urinary tract infection; VLBW, very low birth weight.

biology techniques has opened a new perspective to understanding the pathophysiology of inherited cases of RTA (1016).

Clinical presentation of RTA includes polyhydramnios, polyuria with episodes of dehydration, failure to thrive, vomiting, and serum biochemical disturbances. Failure to thrive appears to be a direct consequence of acidosis; correction of acidosis often results in catch-up growth, unless other complications (e.g., rickets, renal failure) have developed.

Differential Diagnosis

The differential diagnosis of metabolic acidosis depends on the findings of hypertension, hyponatremia and salt wasting, hyperkalemia, generalized proximal tubular dysfunction, decreased ability to acidify the urine, UTI, nephrocalcinosis, or urinary tract malformation. Further workup (e.g., measurement of urinary ammonium, titratable acid, or PCO_2; ammonium chloride, sodium sulfate, or bicarbonate loading) may be required in specific cases, in consultation with a nephrologist (1015,1017,1018).

Proximal Renal Tubular Acidosis

pRTA or RTA type II is characterized by hyperchloremic metabolic acidosis as a result of impaired capacity of proximal tubule to reabsorb HCO_3^- (1014). pRTA could potentially result from loss-of-function mutations of one of three Na+/HCO_3^- co-transporters (NBC 1–3), apical membrane-bound and cytosolic carbonic anhydrase isozymes, or apical NHE3 (1004,1014). pRTA may occur as a manifestation of a generalized proximal tubular dysfunction (Fanconi syndrome), as part of mixed acidosis (type III), or as an isolated disease. Primary isolated pRTA is usually transient, whereas persistent pRTA may be associated with ocular abnormalities. A mutation in the SLC4A4 gene mapped to chromosome 4q21 and encoding the Na+-HCO_3^- co transporter (NBC-1), has been described in pRTA with bilateral glaucoma (1019).

The diagnosis of pRTA is suspected when the serum bicarbonate concentration is low for age and urinary pH is inadequately low (except if RTA is mixed) in the presence of mild-to-moderate acidosis. The diagnosis is confirmed either by the presence of a Fanconi syndrome or by measuring the urinary concentration of bicarbonate at various serum levels during a bicarbonate infusion. Alternatively, the serum bicarbonate can be raised to normal by administration of bicarbonate or citrate supplement, with subsequent observation of the serum bicarbonate level at which the urine becomes acid.

Treatment consists of the administration of sodium bicarbonate or citrate (initially 5 to 10 mEq/kg/d) and potassium citrate. In some patients, acidosis will persist despite administration of high doses of alkali; hydrochlorothiazide or PGSI may be beneficial. Patients with Fanconi syndrome require additional therapy (see Fanconi Syndrome).

Distal Renal Tubular Acidosis

Several criteria have been proposed for the diagnosis of defects in distal RTA (dRTA) (1020–1022), including the inability to decrease urinary pH below 5.5 during metabolic acidosis, limited urinary ammonium concentration, limited urinary PCO_2, and decreased difference between urinary and arterial blood PCO_2. dRTA is almost always observed in children as a primary entity, which may be inherited either as a recessive or dominant form. Autosomal dominant dRTA has been associated with mutations in the SLC4A1 gene encoding the Cl^-/HCO_3^- exchanger AEI (1023). Most patients with autosomal recessive dRTA and nerve deafness have mutations in the ATP6B1 gene encoding the B-1 subunit of H+-ATPase (1023). Autosomal recessive dRTA without deafness may result from mutations of the ATP6VOA4 gene encoding the A-4 subunit of the H+-ATPase (1024).

In classic or type I RTA, there is no defect of potassium secretion; nephrocalcinosis and nephrolithiasis are common (1025). The development of nephrocalcinosis is attributed to the association of hypercalciuria, high urine pH, and hypocitraturia (1026). Idiopathic RTA type I in infants can be associated with bicarbonate wastage. It can be hereditary and may be associated with several other conditions (see Table 42-23). The treatment includes the administration of sodium bicarbonate or citrate and potassium citrate. Administration of citrate is important for the prevention of nephrolithiasis.

Hyperkalemic dRTA or type IV is the most common type of dRTA. It results from the association of defects in K+ and H+ secretion at the level of the collecting duct. Primary type IV RTA or early childhood hyperkalemic RTA has been described in some infants and children who presented with failure to thrive and frequent vomiting (1027). These patients had isolated signs of dRTA with hyperkalemia, without nephrocalcinosis, and responded well to alkali therapy. Secondary cases of type IV RTA can be divided into five groups, which include hypoaldosteronism and impaired or absent renal response to aldosterone (see Table 42-23) (1017,1025). Type IV RTA is also common in patients with obstructive uropathy. The treatment of type IV RTA includes correction of the metabolic acidosis, limitation of potassium intake, and specific therapy for each specific disorder, e.g., surgical correction of obstructive uropathy (1017).

Mixed Renal Tubular Acidosis

In some disorders, both proximal and distal RTA is present; this is known as mixed RTA or type III (see Table 42-23). VLBW infants during the first days or weeks of life have a mild degree of mixed tubular acidosis, with lower normal values of serum bicarbonate concentration and higher urine pH despite metabolic acidosis (see Renal Physiology). Patients with the carbonic anhydrase II deficiency syndrome may have proximal, distal, or mixed RTA. This autosomal recessive disorder results from one of several mutations of the CA2 gene, which has been cloned and mapped to chromosome 8q22 (1028,1029). Patients with this disorder develop metabolic acidosis, osteopetrosis, growth retardation, mental retardation, and cerebral calcifications (1030). The majority of patients come from the Mediterranean area and the Middle East.

Pseudohypoaldosteronism

PHA consists of unresponsiveness of the collecting duct to mineralocorticoids. PHA type I (PHA-11) is an autosomal recessive or dominant disorder characterized by severe neonatal salt wasting, hyperkalemia, and metabolic acidosis. The clinical presentation may include polyuria, anorexia, failure to thrive, and vomiting (1031). Patients often develop hypercalciuria and nephrocalcinosis (1032). Although polyhydramnios has been attributed to PHA1, it is likely that most cases may have been as a result of undiagnosed antenatal Bartter syndrome as a result of ROMK mutation.

Autosomal recessive PHA-1 results from a mutation of either one of the three subunits (α, β, γ) of ENaC (1033, 1034). The disease locus maps to chromosome 16p12.2–13.11 in some families and to 12p13.1-pter in other families. This type of PHA1 also causes respiratory symptoms, which may include cough, rhinorrhea, and recurrent respiratory infections, and in one case report, RDS unresponsive to surfactant (1035–1037).

Autosomal dominant PHA-1, caused by loss-of-function mutations in the mineralocorticoid receptor gene (MLR), (1038) is a milder form, wherein symptoms are limited to the kidney.

The differential diagnosis of hyponatremia with hyperkalemia and metabolic acidosis with normal anion gap includes adrenal insufficiency and hypoaldosteronism (see Chapter 41), acquired partial PHA (or unresponsiveness to aldosterone), and antenatal Bartter syndrome as a result of a mutation of ROMK (See Table 42-23). Laboratory findings in PHA include hyperreninemia, hyperaldosteronism, and increased urinary excretion of aldosterone and tetrahydroaldosterone; in contrast, urinary excretion of 17-hydroxy- and 17-ketosteroids should be interpreted cautiously (1031,1039). Prenatal diagnosis of PHA may be suggested by polyhydramnios with high concentrations of sodium and aldosterone in the amniotic fluid (1031). The treatment of PHA consists of administering large amounts of sodium chloride although limiting potassium intake. Indomethacin administration may help reduce urine output, natriuresis, calciuria, and nephrocalcinosis; however, it also may decrease GFR (1039).

Hyperphosphaturic Syndromes

Hyperphosphaturia results from decreased proximal tubular reabsorption. Whereas severe hyperphosphaturia may result from hyperparathyroidism or Fanconi syndrome, mild hyperphosphaturia occurs after administration of diuretics (e.g., loop diuretics, carbonic anhydrase inhibitors, thiazides) or from drugs or toxins that are toxic to the proximal tubule. Other causes of hypophosphatemia (e.g., rickets and phosphate depletion) are discussed in Chapter 36. We will review briefly the hereditary forms of hyperphosphaturia that are pertinent to infancy.

X-linked Hypophosphatemia

X-linked hypophosphatemia (XLH), also called familial hypophosphatemic rickets or vitamin-D–resistant rickets, is the most common disease associated with hyperphosphaturia in infancy. It is as a result of a mutation of the PHEX gene, a phosphate-regulating gene that is flanked by RFLPs. It is mapped to chromosome Xp22.1 and has been cloned (1040–1042). Clinical signs, including bone deformations, usually appear after the first year of life. In neonates from affected families, hypophosphatemia and low tubular reabsorption of phosphate can already be detected during the first month of life (1043). The treatment includes oral phosphate supplementation and 1(OH)D3 or 1,25(OH)2D3. This therapy improves but does not cure the bone disease, causes nephrocalcinosis in 60% of the patients (1044,1045), and may cause renal failure or hyperparathyroidism. Preliminary results suggest beneficial effects of using 24,25(OH)2D3 instead of 1,25(OH)2D3 (1046). Thiazide diuretics decrease urinary calcium excretion and prevent progression of nephrocalcinosis in children with XLH (1047).

Hypophosphatemic Rickets with Hypercalciuria

Hypophosphatemic rickets with hypercalciuria (HHRH; OMIM 241530) is an autosomal recessive disorder with rickets, bone pain, muscle weakness, failure to thrive, hypophosphatemia with hyperphosphaturia, normocalcemia with hypercalciuria, high plasma 1,25(OH)2-D3 concentration, low PTH concentration, and elevated plasma alkaline phosphatase activity. The treatment consists of the administration of supplemental phosphate (1048,1049). Possible candidate genes for HHRH include those encoding renal phosphate transporters or their regulators, except NPT2 (1050).

Autosomal Dominant Hypophosphatemic Rickets

Autosomal dominant hypophosphatemic rickets (ADHR, OMIM 193100) is a rare, less severe disorder, with autosomal dominant inheritance with variable penetrance (1051).

Patients with early presentation show phosphate wasting. Low serum phosphorus concentrations, rickets, osteomalacia, and lower extremity deformities characterize this condition as early as 1 year. Other features include short stature, bone pain, and dental abscesses. ADHR results from missense mutations in a gene encoding a new member of the fibroblast growth factor (FGF) family, FGF23 (1052). Treatment consists of administration of vitamin D, with phosphate supplementation in some patients.

Vitamin-D–Dependent Rickets Type I

Vitamin-D–dependent rickets type I (VDDR I) is an autosomal recessive disorder, also called pseudo vitamin D deficiency type I (PDDR) or hereditary selective deficiency of 1,25-alpha-(OH)2D3. VDDR I results from mutations in the 25-hydroxyvitamin D 1-alpha hydroxylase gene, mapped to 12q4 by linkage analysis (1052). Increased phosphaturia results from hyperparathyroidism, in turn as a result of a defect of 1-alpha-hydroxylation of vitamin D in the proximal tubule (1053).

Infants with this disorder present with the typical signs of rickets, including hypotonia, tetany, irritability, motor retardation, deformations, and growth failure. Serum levels of 1,25(OH)2D3 are very low or undetectable, resulting in decreased gastrointestinal absorption of calcium. This disorder should be differentiated from other causes for deficiency in 1-alpha-hydroxylase (e.g., Fanconi syndrome, RTA, or X-linked hypophosphatemia). Patients with VDDR I respond to the administration of physiologic doses of 1-alpha-OHD3 or 1,25-alpha-(OH)2D3 (1053).

Hereditary Generalized Resistance to 1,25(OH)2D3

Hereditary generalized resistance to 1,25(OH)2D3 is an autosomal recessive disorder, also called vitamin-D–dependent rickets type II (VDDR II), hypocalcemic vitamin D-resistant rickets (HVDRR), or vitamin D dependency type II or pseudo vitamin D deficiency type II. In patients with this disorder, lack of sensitivity of target organs to 1,25(OH)2D3 (1054) results from heterogeneous mutations of the vitamin D receptor (VDR) gene (1055,1056). This gene has been cloned and mapped to chromosome 12q13–14, i.e., close to the gene for VDDR I (1055,1057). Patients present with rickets and some with alopecia by 2 to 12 months of life (1058). Serum levels of 1,25(OH)2D3 are very high. Rickets in these patients responds with limited success to high doses of oral calcium and supraphysiologic doses of 1,25(OH)2D3 (1058). In some patients, vitamin D analogs may partially or completely restore the responsiveness of the mutated VDR (1059).

Glucosuria

Several disorders are associated with renal glucosuria: an isolated defect, or primary glucosuria, which is a benign condition, congenital glucose-galactose malabsorption,

Fanconi syndrome, and other rare entities. They all are associated with mild-to-moderate glucosuria, which does not require specific therapy (1060,1061).

Neonates with glucose-galactose malabsorption develop severe, watery, acidic diarrhea and dehydration. This disorder is as a result of one of several mutations of the intestinal Na–D-glucose co transporter (SGLT1). The corresponding gene, mapped to chromosome 22q13.1, has been cloned; mutations can be detected prenatally (1062–1064).

In VLBW infants, the incidence of glucosuria is increased because of two factors: decreased tubular reabsorption of glucose (see Renal Physiology) and instability of glycemia (1065). At a mean GA of 29 weeks, glucosuria appears when glycemia exceeds 152 ± 8 mg/dL (1065). Massive glucosuria is uncommon in VLBW infants; however, it may lead to osmotic diuresis and, thus, dehydration and loss of electrolytes (1065,1066).

Uric Acid

Hyperuricemia

Hyperuricemia may result from a decrease in urinary excretion of uric acid, from an increase in its production, or from both. Uric acid excretion decreases after administration of several drugs (e.g., diazoxide, diuretics, dopamine, ethambutol), during lactic acidosis, and in association with maternal toxemia, ECF contraction, renal failure, hypertension, and lead intoxication. Decrease in urinary excretion of uric acid may result in higher serum levels but not in renal toxicity.

Increased production of uric acid is observed after perinatal asphyxia, after fructose administration (especially in patients with fructose intolerance), in Down syndrome, neoplasia, hypoxanthine-guanine phosphoribosyltransferase deficiency (Lesch–Nyhan syndrome), superactivity of 5-phosphoribosyl-a-1-pyrophosphate synthetase, and type I glycogenosis. In the latter condition, hyperuricemia results both from an increased production and from decreased excretion as a result of lactic acidosis. Because the risk of uric acid precipitation is favored by a high urinary concentration and a low urine pH, the newborn infant is at relatively low risk for tubular obstruction by uric acid crystalluria, despite low ability of the immature renal tubule to reabsorb uric acid. The prevention of uric acid nephropathy in patients at high risk includes maintaining a high tubular flow rate by the administration of high volumes of alkaline fluids (1067). Uric acid crystalluria with tubular obstruction has been described rarely in newborn infants with ARF secondary to perinatal asphyxia (1068). ARF may be observed also in Lesch–Nyhan syndrome (577). Allopurinol is indicated for infants with hyperuricemia secondary to neoplasia and should be given before chemotherapy in specific patients (1069).

Defects of Tubular Handling of Uric Acid

Increased urinary excretion of uric acid may result from various medications (e.g., ascorbic acid, glycine, citrate, and iodinated radiocontrast agents) and from rare defects in tubular handling of uric acid. These disorders may be suspected on the basis of family history, low serum concentration of uric acid, or crystalluria. Early diagnosis may allow specific therapy and prevention of urolithiasis, which may develop later in childhood.

Amino Acidurias

Several systems of tubular transport of amino acids are known. For many of the defects of these transporters, a firm diagnosis can be made only after a few months of age, i.e., when the normally high excretion of amino acids in infants starts to decrease. We discuss here only those disorders of amino acid transport that may cause symptoms in infancy, i.e., Fanconi syndrome (see corresponding section in this chapter), cystinuria, and lysinuric protein intolerance (LPI).

Cystinuria

Cystinuria is an autosomal recessive disorder as a result of a defect of the D2H or human rBAT protein, which is responsible for renal and gastrointestinal transport of the dibasic amino acids cystine, lysine, arginine, and ornithine (858,1070). Cystinuria has been classified into three phenotypes, based on the degree of intestinal uptake of cystine by homozygotes and the level of urinary dibasic amino acids in heterozygotes (1071): type I (silent carriers), type II (marked elevation) and type III (mild elevation). Mutations in the SLC3A1 gene, which has been mapped to chromosome 2p21 and encodes rBAT, cause type I cystinuria (1070,1072–1075). Mutations of the SLC7A9 gene, which have been mapped to chromosome 19q13.1 and encodes b0.+AT (a putative subunit of rBAT that normally heterodimerizes with rBAT), cause nontype I cystinuria (i.e., types II and III) (1076). Urolithiasis usually develops within the first 2 decades, but rarely may occur by the end of the first year of life. Urinary cystine calculi may produce considerable morbidity including urinary obstruction, colic, and infection and, in severe cases, loss of kidney function (1004).

Neonatal urinary screening programs have shown an average prevalence of approximately 1 in 7,000, with a range of 1:2,000 in England to 1:15,000 in the United States (1077). Neonatal screening offers the possibility of monitoring children before formation of cystine stones; this is particularly important for patients at highest risk for lithiasis (type I/I homozygous cystinuria) (1078). Prevention of stone formation includes hydration and alkalinization of the urine; D-penicillamine and a-mercaptopropionylglycine are effective in decreasing the rate of stone formation in patients with lithiasis (1079).

Lysinuric Protein Intolerance

Lysinuric protein intolerance (LPI, hyperdibasic aminoaciduria type 2, or familial protein intolerance) is an autosomal recessive disorder as a result of a defect of the basolateral transport of the cationic amino acids lysine, arginine, and ornithine in the renal tubule and the gastrointestinal tract (858). LPI results from loss-of-function mutations of the SLC7A gene on chromosome 14q12 which encodes the $\gamma+L$ amino acid transporter-1 ($\gamma+LAT-1$) (1080–1082). Half of the patients with LPI have been described in Finland, where the prevalence is 1:60,000. Most breast-fed infants are asymptomatic, although some may develop symptoms of hyperammonemia during the neonatal period. Within 1 week of weaning or increase in the protein intake, most infants affected with this disorder develop nausea, vomiting, and mild diarrhea. Later on, patients present with poor feeding, failure to thrive, severe hypotonia, hepatosplenomegaly, osteoporosis, seizures, coma and developmental delay. Some may develop interstitial pulmonary infiltration, alveolar proteinosis, or severe renal involvement, including glomerular and tubular damage, which progresses rapidly to CRF (1083,1084).

Demonstrating markedly increased lysinuria in contrast to only moderate increase in ornithine and arginine establishes the diagnosis. Other findings include abnormal plasma amino acid concentrations, anemia, leukopenia, thrombocytopenia, and postprandial increases in urinary orotic acid and plasma ammonia. The treatment consists of administering a low-protein diet supplemented with citrulline. Hyperammonemic episodes are treated with ornithine, arginine, or citrulline, sodium benzoate, and sodium phenylacetate.

Storage Disorders

Storage disorders that may affect the neonatal kidney include ARC syndrome and Fanconi–Bickel syndrome (see Fanconi Syndrome), and two lysosomal storage disorders, i.e., sialidosis and galactosialidosis.

Sialidosis Type II

Sialidosis is an autosomal recessive disorder as a result of mutations of the lysosomal sialidase gene, mapped to chromosome 6p21.3 (1085), and encoding sialidase (alpha-N-acetyl-neuraminidase), an enzyme that catalyzes the catabolism of sialoglycoconjugates (858). The deficiency of sialidase results in lysosomal accumulation of sialylglycoproteins and oligosaccharides. Patients with sialidosis type II develop Hurler-like phenotype, dysostosis multiplex, mental retardation, and hepatosplenomegaly, and may later develop cherry red spot macula and myoclonus. Patients with the congenital form develop ascites and/or hydrops fetalis and die either in the neonatal period or during infancy. Some patients develop nephrosialidosis, which is characterized by severe proteinuria and progressive nephrotic syndrome. Pathology consists of foamy enlargement of glomerular and tubular epithelial cells (1086). Prenatal diagnosis is possible by demonstrating absence of neuraminidase activity in amniotic or chorionic villi cells (1087).

Neuraminidase Deficiency with β-Galactosidase Deficiency (Galactosialidosis)

Galactosialidosis is an autosomal recessive disorder as a result of a defect of a lysosomal protein, called protective protein/cathepsin A (PPCA), which normally forms a complex with β-galactosidase and neuraminidase, thereby protecting these two enzymes from proteolysis (858). The gene coding for PPCA has been mapped to chromosome 20q13.1 and cloned (1088,1089). Deficiency in PPCA results in the accumulation of sialyloligosaccharides. Patients with the early infantile form of this disease develop fetal hydrops, visceromegaly, ascites, and skeletal dysplasia and die early. The renal lesion usually consists of membrane-bound vacuoles in the glomerulus and in tubular cells; additionally, endothelial vacuolization may occur, leading to hyperreninemic hypertension (684). Prenatal diagnosis may be suggested by a high concentration of sialyloligosaccharides in the amniotic fluid (a nonspecific finding) (1090) and confirmed by measuring b-galactosidase and neuraminidase in cultured amniotic cells (1091). Additionally, cultured fibroblasts (and one patient's amniotic and chorionic villi cells) from 12 patients with the early infantile form had almost no cathepsin A activity of the protective protein, whereas those from eight patients with later presentation of the disease had 2% to 5% residual activity (1092).

CONGENITAL NEPHROTIC SYNDROME

Nephrotic syndrome is defined by the association of marked proteinuria (more than 1 g/m2/d) with hypoalbuminemia (less than 2.5 g/dL), hyperlipidemia and edema. A nephrotic syndrome is called congenital if it presents within the first 3 months of life. This definition is based on the natural history of the Finnish type, the most common type of nephrotic syndrome in newborn infants.

Finnish Type (CNF or NPHS 1, OMIM 256300)

The incidence of CNF is estimated to be 1.2 per 10,000 births in Finland (1093), but is considerably less frequent in other countries (e.g. 1:50,000 in North Americans) (1094a). CNF should be suspected if there is a history of CNF in a sibling, hydrops fetalis or edema of the placenta, i.e., placental weight greater than 25% of BW, or an elevated AFP or total protein concentration in the amniotic fluid. Because the disease begins *in utero* in all patients, an increased AFP (more than 10 SD above the mean amniotic fluid concentration during the second trimester) is a reliable indicator of the disease (1093).

CNF is an autosomal recessive disorder caused mainly by mutations in the nephrin gene (NPHS1), mapped to chromosome 19q13.1, which encodes nephrin, a putative transmembrane protein belonging to the immunoglobulin superfamily of adhesion molecules (1095). In Finnish families, four main CNF haplotype categories have been observed (1096). Analysis of nonFinnish families suggests that most patients with CNF share the same disease locus (1097).

The natural history of the disease is based on experience before the availability of renal transplantation in young patients (1093,1096–1101). The mean GA was 36.6 ± 1.8 weeks (mean ± SD), and 42% of the infants were premature (less than 37 weeks of GA). Many infants were small for GA, especially those with a GA at or above 37 weeks. In some patients, the typical signs of nephrotic syndrome (i.e., edema, proteinuria, hypoalbuminemia) did not develop until the third month of life. The disease was resistant to steroids or cytotoxic medications (1098). Complications included severe failure to thrive and ascites in all patients, severe bacterial infections in 85%, hypothyroidism, pyloric stenosis in 12%, and thrombotic events in 10% (1098). An increase in Pcr or BUN was observed in 20% of the patients, but none had frank uremia. One-half of the patients died by 6 months of life, and all of them by 4 years.

The proteinuria, initially very selective, i.e., almost entirely albumin as a result of increased permeability of the glomerulus only for small proteins, increases progressively and becomes nonselective, corresponding to increased sieving coefficient and to tubular damage (1101). Blood chemistry is significant for low serum albumin concentration and total thyroxine concentration (as a result of urine loss of thyroxine-binding globulin) (1102), a normal or mildly elevated Pcr, and hyperlipidemia. Ultrasonography shows enlarged kidneys, increased echogenicity of the renal cortex, decreased differentiation between cortex and medulla and poor visualization of the pyramids (1103). Tubular dilations may be misinterpreted as other causes of cystic disease, including autosomal recessive PKD (1104).

The diagnosis of CNF can be confirmed by linkage analysis or by renal biopsy. The latter shows irregularities of the glomerular basement membrane and thinning of the lamina densa (1105), followed by fusion of the epithelial cell foot processes, all of which are similar to the findings in minimal-change, steroid-sensitive nephrotic syndrome. On light microscopy, changes include obliteration of capillary loops and glomerular hyalinization, and dilated tubules from both proximal and distal origin (microcystic disease).

Infants with CNF require intensive management, which includes repetitive administration of albumin and diuretics for ascites, thyroxin, anticoagulation, oral and parenteral hyperalimentation, and the treatment of multiple complications (1098). Chronic renal insufficiency develops between 6 and 23 months of age. As a consequence, most patients eventually receive dialysis while waiting for transplantation. Aggressive therapy, including bilateral nephrectomy (performed in one series at a mean age of 1.2 years) and peritoneal dialysis until transplantation when the infant reaches about 10 kg, allows normal growth and development, a patient survival rate of 97%, and a graft survival rate of 94%, 81% and 81% at 1, 3, and 5 years after transplant (1106). Recently, conservative management of CNF with captopril and indomethacin, sometimes in combination with unilateral nephrectomy, has been described to significantly improve plasma albumin concentration, reduce the need for albumin infusion and duration of hos-

pitalization, maintain normal growth and allow delay of dialysis, and transplantation for at least three years (1107).

Other Causes

Differential Diagnosis

The entities associated with congenital nephrotic syndrome may be differentiated by the natural history of the disease; by the presence of associated anomalies (e.g., in Denys-Drash syndrome),; by maternal and neonatal serology (TORCH syndrome and lupus); by measuring AFP concentration in the amniotic fluid, which is consistently elevated only in CNF; by DNA analysis in specific families; and by renal biopsy. Nevertheless, classification of a patient into one of the major entities may not be possible (1100). Specific therapy may be available for some patients (e.g., those with congenital infection).

Diffuse Mesangial Sclerosis

The second most common cause of congenital nephrotic syndrome is diffuse mesangial sclerosis (DMS), which appears to represent a heterogenous group of disorders (1100). The onset varies between the second trimester of gestation and 33 months of age. In contrast to CNF, CRF develops rapidly in these patients and is the major cause of death in the absence of dialysis and renal transplantation. Renal venous thrombosis is a frequent complication. In most families, DMS is transmitted as an autosomal recessive trait. Histologic examination of the glomeruli shows mesangial cells embedded in a periodic acid-Schiff–positive and silver-positive fibrillar network occluding the capillaries. Tubular changes are similar to those seen in CNF, and interstitial fibrosis is more pronounced than in CNF. Patients with DMS present with proteinuria (with or without nephrotic syndrome), sometimes hematuria, often arterial hypertension, and progressive CRF leading to ESRD within a few months to 2 years from the onset.

In some infants, DMS is part of Denys-Drash syndrome, which also includes ambiguous genitalia—most often male pseudohermaphroditism, i.e., 46XY karyotype—and Wilms tumor (1108). Denys-Drash syndrome is associated with mutations of the Wilms tumor suppressor gene (WT1) (1109). In these patients, the WT1 expression is abnormal and is associated with increased expression of PAX2 gene, which encodes a transcription factor normally expressed early during development. Increased expression of PAX2 is associated with podocyte hyperplasia (1110). Several patients have presented with incomplete forms of Denys-Drash syndrome (i.e., only two of the three signs of the triad) (1108). DMS is also common in Galloway–Mowat syndrome, an autosomal recessive disorder that includes microcephaly, abnormal gyral pattern, developmental delay, and nephrotic syndrome. Renal pathology in this syndrome may show diffuse mesangial sclerosis, focal segmental sclerosis, mesangial proliferation, or basement membrane and tubular anomalies (1111,1112). In a consanguineous family with previously affected siblings, prenatal diagnosis may be suggested by demonstration of enlarged hyperechogenic kidneys with amniotic fluid at the upper limit of normal and normal amniotic fluid concentration of AFP (1113).

Congenital Infection

Nephrotic syndrome as a result of congenital infection is seen most commonly in congenital syphilis (1114,1115), in which case the lesion is characterized by epimembranous or proliferative glomerulopathy, with diffuse deposits of immunoglobulin and treponemal antigen along the glomerular capillaries and sub epithelial electron-dense deposits (1114). The condition responds very well to the administration of penicillin. The nephrotic syndrome associated with congenital toxoplasmosis is less common (1116,1117). The lesion is characterized by the deposition in the glomeruli of immunoglobulin, complement, and Toxoplasma antigen and antibody. It may respond to administration of pyrimethamine, sulfadiazine, and steroid. Congenital nephrotic syndrome has also been reported in a few patients with congenital cytomegalovirus infection (1118,1119).

Other Causes

Some cases of congenital nephrotic syndrome are associated with dysmorphic features, such as pachygyria, microcephaly, buphthalmos, or disturbances of neuronal migration. Nephrotic syndrome may result from sialidosis type II (see Sialidosis) or from type I carbohydrate-deficient glycoprotein syndrome (1120–1123). Transient cases of congenital nephrotic syndrome have been described as a result of maternal transmission (1124), intoxication with mercury, or nail patella syndrome (1125). Of three infants reported to have infantile systemic lupus erythematosus and congenital nephrotic syndrome, one had steroid-responsive membranous glomerulopathy (1126,1127).

Hematuria and Proteinuria

Differential Diagnosis of Hematuria

Pink or red urine or coloration of the diaper may result from hematuria, hemoglobinuria, myoglobinuria, uric acid, porphyria, or bile pigments. Red-brown deposits on the diaper may result from xanthinuria. The presence of blood on the diaper also may result from rectal bleeding or vaginal mucoid sanguinous discharge caused by maternal hormone withdrawal. On a dipstick test, the reagent strip based on the orthotolidine peroxidase reaction will give a positive reaction with hemoglobinuria, myoglobinuria, hematuria, or other oxidants, such as hydrogen peroxide and ascorbic acid. A dipstick can detect 5 to 20 intact erythrocytes per microliter of urine, and 0.05 to 0.3 mg of free hemoglobin per 100 mL of urine, which corresponds to 2 to 10 lysed erythrocytes per microliter. The diagnosis of hematuria requires visualization of an excessive number of erythrocytes in an uncontaminated specimen of urine (usually >5 RBC's/hpf).

Incidence

Gross hematuria during the first month of life occurred in 35 of 132,050 admissions (0.21 of 1000) to a major tertiary center between 1950 and 1967 (1128). In a more recent series, the incidence of hematuria during the first 48 hours of life was much lower in normal full-term infants (0 of 63) than in patients admitted to the NICU (48 of 78); none of these patients, however, had abnormalities on physical examination or had proteinuria, hypertension, or abnormal values of Pcr or BUN (1129). Transient hematuria was found in 76% of asphyxiated newborns (1130). In another series, hematuria was estimated to occur in 62% of newborn infants with UA catheter in place and US evidence of an arterial clot, and in 25% in those without evidence for a clot (1131). Hematuria was present in one-half of infants with ARF secondary to cardiac surgery and in two-thirds of newborn infants with irreversible ARF (1132,1133).

Etiology

Hematuria may occur in a wide variety of diseases, including bleeding diatheses and renal and postrenal disorders. PGSI-mediated hematuria may be as a result of platelet dysfunction, ATN, or tubular dysfunction. Congenital infections (e.g., syphilis, toxoplasmosis, cytomegalovirus) may cause thrombocytopenia or, rarely, glomerulonephritis. Common congenital causes of hematuria include hydronephrosis, PKD, tumors, and sponge kidneys. Acquired causes include asphyxia, coagulation abnormalities, infectious and vascular disorders, and nephrotoxicity.

Evaluation

The first step is to confirm the diagnosis of hematuria by the demonstration of erythrocytes in fresh urine voided spontaneously or after gentle suprapubic pressure (Fig. 42-7). Suprapubic aspiration is contraindicated, because it can cause microscopic or macroscopic hematuria. If the patient is anuric, despite treating possible conditions that might be causing prerenal failure and despite a diuretic challenge and a fluid challenge (see Acute Renal Failure), the bladder should be catheterized using a lubricated 3.5Fr to 5Fr catheter; however, one should take into account that this procedure could in itself cause hematuria.

The history may disclose familial nephritis. Maternal history may be positive for diabetes (suggesting renal venous thrombosis, infection, thrombocytopenia, glomerulonephritis), autoimmune disease, or recent use of PGSI. The patient's history should be reviewed, especially for asphyxia, sepsis, shock, hypertension, renal failure, medications, and placement of a UA line. Pertinent points in the physical examination include hypertension, bruising, edema (suggesting ARF or glomerulonephritis), an abdominal mass that may indicate hydronephrosis, cystic disease, adrenal hemorrhage, and, rarely, renal trauma and bruit (suggesting renovascular disease). In some patients, the presumptive etiology is obvious (e.g., bleeding disorder, blad-

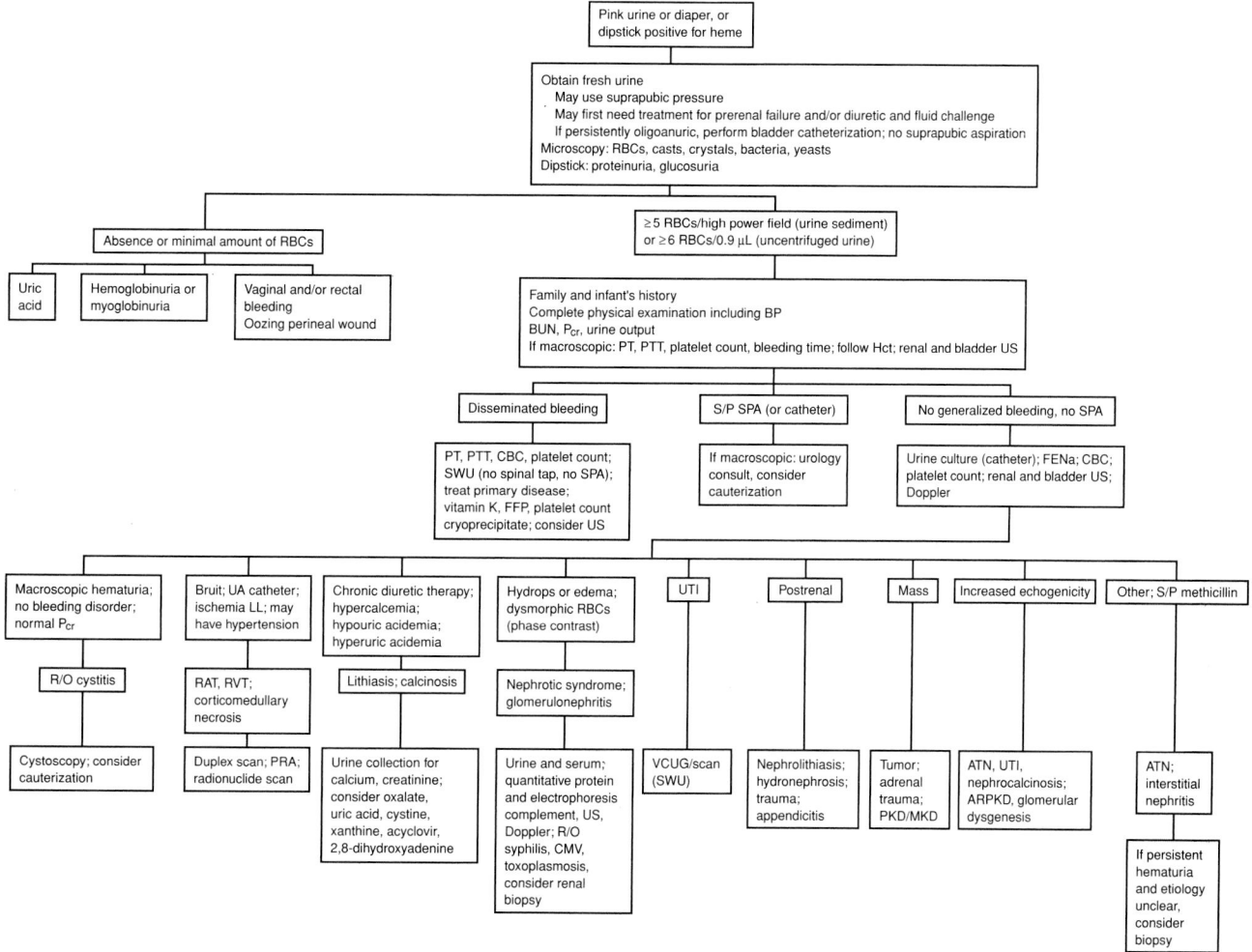

Figure 42-7   Differential diagnosis of hematuria. ARF, acute renal failure; ARPKD, autosomal recessive polycystic kidney disease; ATN, acute tubular necrosis; BP, blood pressure; BUN, blood urea nitrogen; CBC, complete blood count; CMV, Cytomegalovirus; FeNa, fractional excretion of sodium; Hct, hematocrit; LL, lower limbs; MKDIPKD, multicystic/polycystic kidney disease; P_{cr}, plasma creatine concentration; PRA, plasma renin activity; PT, prothrombin time; PTT, partial thromboplastin time; RAT, renal artery thrombosis; RBC, erythrocyte; R/O, rule out; RVT, renal venous thrombosis; S/P, status post; SPA, suprapubic aspiration; SWU, sepsis workup; UA, umbilical artery; UO, urine output; US, ultrasonography; UTI, urinary tract infection; VCUG, voiding cystourethrogram.

der trauma, severe asphyxia, ATN, renovascular disease, glomerulonephritis, nephrotic syndrome).

The initial workup should include a microscopic examination of the urine, dipstick test, and measurement of urine output, BUN, and Pcr (see Fig. 42-7). Most patients should have a bladder and renal US and a urine culture. Microscopic examination of the urine may show dysmorphic erythrocytes or erythrocyte casts indicating glomerulonephritis, bacteriuria, yeast forms, or crystalluria. The latter may be the first clue to a diagnosis of urolithiasis. The dipstick may show glucosuria or proteinuria. If either of these is present, additional specific investigations should be obtained. If a glomerular disease is suspected, fresh urine should be examined using phase contrast microscopy, which is the method of choice for identifying the presence of dysmorphic erythrocytes; however, this method is unreliable in determining the origin of massive hematuria.

Transient microscopic hematuria during the first 48 hours of life may be insignificant (1129), as long as the infant is asymptomatic, i.e., has no bleeding diathesis and does not exhibit other evidence of a renal lesion (e.g., no familial renal disease; normal physical examination, blood pressure, urine output, Pcr, BUN and US; no erythrocyte casts in the urine).

In patients with macroscopic hematuria, the first diagnoses to exclude are bleeding disorder, trauma, and cystitis. In those patients, coagulation tests, platelet count, and bleeding time should be assessed, and a renal and bladder US should be obtained. Purpura, excessive bleeding after venipuncture, or thrombocytopenia suggests that hematuria is as a result of a bleeding disorder. Specific treatment for sepsis or endocarditis and the bleeding disorder should be initiated. If renal function and urine output are normal, and hematuria disappears after resolution of the bleeding diathesis, no additional renal workup is required. It should be remembered, however, that thrombocytopenia with hematuria may occur in association with renal diseases, such as renal venous thrombosis and UTI with sepsis. Macroscopic hematuria also may occur after suprapubic aspiration or catheterization of the bladder; if hematuria disappears rapidly, US is normal, and urine output, BUN, and Pcr remain normal, no additional investigations are required. In patients with massive hematuria in whom a bleeding disorder has been excluded, cystoscopy should be performed, unless the presumptive etiology is renal.

All other patients should have a urine culture, and a renal and bladder US, which may disclose an intravascular thrombus, renal venous or arterial thrombosis, cystic kidney disease, lithiasis or nephrocalcinosis, hydronephrosis, adrenal hemorrhage, or other anomalies. The association of hematuria with UA catheterization, an abdominal bruit, or blanching of the lower extremities, especially with hypertension, strongly suggests the diagnosis of a renovascular etiology (1131,1134). Hematuria is an unusual complication of nephrolithiasis or nephrocalcinosis during the neonatal period; it has been reported in one 10-week-old patient with familial hypercalciuria (1135).

Glomerulonephritis is a rare occurrence in newborn infants. It should be suspected if the patient has either hydrops or generalized edema with massive proteinuria or erythrocyte casts or dysmorphic erythrocytes. These patients should be assessed for possible congenital syphilis, toxoplasmosis, cytomegalovirus infection, various causes of nephrotic syndrome, familial nephritis, and immune-mediated glomerulonephritis. Consultation with a pediatric nephrologist should be obtained, and a renal biopsy should be considered.

For the other patients, the differential diagnosis includes a wide range of diseases; US is the most important initial investigation. Further workup depends on the clinical presentation (e.g., hypertension, ARF) or presumed etiology (e.g., ATN, cystic disease, tumor). If hematuria persists without obvious etiology, a renal biopsy should be considered.

Differential Diagnosis of Proteinuria

Proteinuria may be suggested by a positive (1+) dipstick test. The degree of proteinuria can be quantified by a timed collection or spot urine protein:creatinine ratio. Abnormal proteinuria is defined according to normal values for age (see Table 42-2).

Incidence

Increased proteinuria occurs frequently in newborn infants admitted to the NICU; it is associated with various types of renal injury. The detection of increased tubular proteinuria is a sensitive screening test for renal damage after perinatal asphyxia (1136), and for tubular damage as a result of nephrotoxicity (see Acute Renal Failure; Nephrotoxicity).

Etiology

Proteinuria of tubular origin, the most common type, never is massive. It includes LMW proteins, i.e., <60,000 kD, which are freely filtered through the glomerulus. Additionally, in some patients, lysosomal proteins such as NAG can be found in the urine. Although tubular proteinuria can be isolated, it is associated most often with perinatal asphyxia or renal ischemia, UTI, ARF, Fanconi syndrome, or nephrotoxicity (see Acute Renal Failure; Tubular Dysfunction).

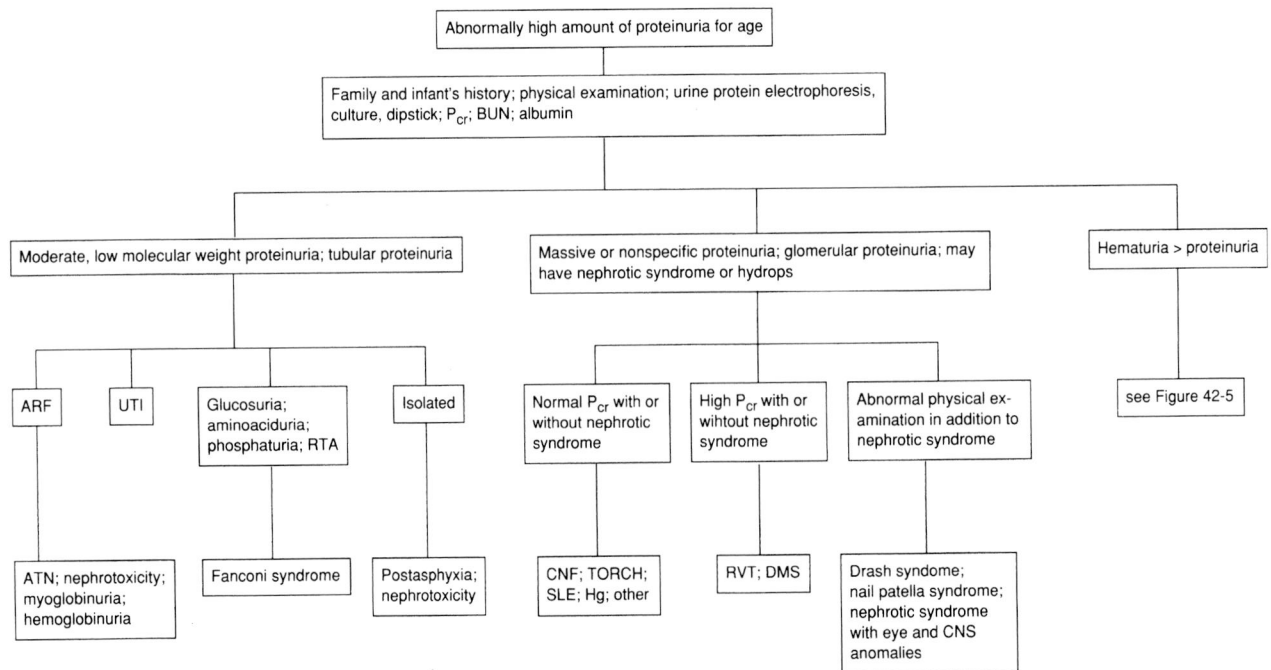

Figure 42-8 Differential diagnosis of proteinuria. AFR, acute renal failure; ATN, acute tubular necrosis; BUN, blood urea nitrogen; CNF, congenital nephrotic syndrome (Finnish type); DMS, diffuse mesangial sclerosis; Hg, mercury intoxication; P_{cr}, plasma creatine concentration; RTA, renal tubular acidosis; RVT, renal venous thrombosis; SLE, systemic lupus erythematosus; UTI, urinary tract infection.

In contrast, proteinuria of glomerular origin includes proteins with higher molecular weight such as albumin. It may become massive and lead to nephrotic syndrome (see Congenital Nephrotic Syndrome, above).

Evaluation

Because proteinuria occurs frequently, an extensive workup is not indicated unless there is evidence for renal disease. Apart from the history and physical examination, a major step in the differential diagnosis is the differentiation between tubular and glomerular proteinuria. This can be obtained by electrophoresis of urinary proteins or by quantitative measurement of specific LMW proteins and albumin (Fig. 42-8). Additionally, there may be evidence of tubular damage (e.g., glucosuria, RTA). Discussions of specific disorders are provided elsewhere in this chapter.

REFERENCES

1. Saxén L. *Organogenesis of the kidney.* Cambridge, MA: Harvard University Press, 1987.
2. De Martino C, Zamboni L. A morphologic study of the mesonephros of the human embryo. *J Ultrastruct Res* 1966;16:399–427.
3. Rabinowitz R, Peters MT, Vyas S, et al. Measurement of fetal urine production in normal pregnancy by real-time ultrasonography. *Am J Obstet Gynecol* 1989;161:1264–1266.
4. Evan AP, Gattone VHD, Schwartz GJ. Development of solute transport in rabbit proximal tubule. II. Morphologic segmentation. *Am J Physiol* 1983;245:F391–F407.
5. Evan AP, Satlin LM, Gattone VHD, et al. Postnatal maturation of rabbit renal collecting duct. II. Morphologic observations. *Am J Physiol* 1991;261:F91–F107.
6. Potter EL, Thierstein ST. Glomerular development in the kidney as an index of foetal maturity. *J Pediatr* 1943;22:695–706.
7. Thorburn GD. The role of the thyroid gland and kidneys in fetal growth. In: Elliott K, Knight J, eds. *Ciba Found Symp 27. Symposium on Size at Birth.* Amsterdam: Elsevier, Excerpta Medica, 1974;27:185–214.
8. Perlman M, Levin M. Fetal pulmonary hypoplasia, anuria, and oligohydramnios: clinicopathologic observations and review of the literature. *Am J Obstet Gynecol* 1974;118:1119–1123.
9. Gomez RA, Meernick JG, Kuehl WD, et al. Developmental aspects of the renal response to hemorrhage during fetal life. *Pediatr Res* 1984;18:40–46.
10. Wladimiroff JW, Campbell S. Fetal urine production rates in normal and complicated pregnancy. *Lancet* 1974;1:151–154.
11. Veille JC, Hanson RA, Tatum K, et al. Quantitative assessment of human fetal renal blood flow. *Am J Obstet Gynecol* 1993;169:1399–1402.
12. Rubin MI, Bruck E, Rapoport MJ. Maturation of renal function in childhood: clearance studies. *J Clin Invest* 1949;28:1144.
13. Calcagno PL, Rubin MI. Renal extraction of para-aminohippurate in infants and children. *J Clin Invest* 1963;42:1632–1639.
14. Barnett HL, Hare WK, McNamara H, et al. Influence of postnatal age on kidney function of premature infants. *Proc Soc Exp Biol Med* 1948;69:55–57.
15. Schwartz GJ, Goldsmith DI, Fine LG. p-Aminohippurate transport in the proximal straight tubule: development and substrate stimulation. *Pediatr Res* 1978;12:793–796.
16. Rudolph AM, Heymann MA, Teramo KAW, et al. Studies on the circulation of the previable human fetus. *Pediatr Res* 1971;5:452.
17. Aperia A, Broberger O, Herin P, et al. Renal hemodynamics in the perinatal period: a study in lambs. *Acta Physiol Scand* 1977;99:261–269.
18. Robillard JE, Weismann DN, Herin P. Ontogeny of single glomerular perfusion rate in fetal and newborn lambs. *Pediatr Res* 1981;15:1248–1255.
19. Ichikawa I, Maddox DA, Brenner BM. Maturational development of glomerular ultrafiltration in the rat. *Am J Physiol* 1979;236:F465–F471.
20. Kleinman LI, Reuter JH. Maturation of glomerular blood flow distribution in the newborn dog. *J Physiol (Lond)* 1973;228:91–103.
21. Olbing H, Blaufox MD, Aschinberg LC, et al. Postnatal changes in renal glomerular blood flow distribution in puppies. *J Clin Invest* 1973;52:2885–2895.
22. Aschinburg LC, Goldsmith DI, Olbing H, et al. Neonatal changes in renal blood flow distribution in puppies. *Am J Physiol* 1975;228:1453–1461.
23. Gruskin AB, Edelmann CM Jr, Yuan S. Maturational changes in renal blood flow in piglets. *Pediatr Res* 1970;4:7–13.
24. Aperia A, Broberger O, Herin P. Maturational changes in glomerular perfusion rate and glomerular filtration rate in lambs. *Pediatr Res* 1974;8:758–765.
25. Spitzer A, Edelmann CM Jr. Maturational changes in pressure gradients for glomerular filtration. *Am J Physiol* 1971;221:1431–1435.
26. Spitzer A, Schwartz GJ. The kidney during development. In: Windhager E, ed. *The handbook of physiology. Section 8. Renal physiology.* Oxford and New York: Oxford Unviersity and American Physiology Society. 1992;475–544.
27. Jose PA, Logan AG, Slotkoff LM, et al. Intrarenal blood flow distribution in canine puppies. *Pediatr Res* 1971;5:335–344.
28. Vernier RL, Birch-Andersen A. Studies of the human fetal kidney. I. Development of the glomerulus. *J Pediatr* 1962;60:754–768.
29. Evan AP, Stoeckel JA, Loemker V, et al. Development of the intrarenal vascular system of the puppy. *Anat Rec* 1979;194:187–199.
30. Butkus A, Albiston A, Alcorn D, et al. Ontogeny of angiotensin II receptors, type 1 and 2, in ovine mesonephros and metanephros. *Kidney Int* 1997;52:628–636.
31. Gomez RA, Chevalier RL, Carey RM, et al. Molecular biology of the renal renin-angiotensin system. *Kidney Int Suppl* 1990;30:S18–S23.
32. Lumbers ER. Functions of the renin-angiotensin system during development. *Clin Exp Pharmacol Physiol* 1995;22:499–505.
33. Schutz S, Le Moullec JM, Corvol P, et al. Early expression of all the components of the renin-angiotensin-system in human development. *Am J Pathol* 1996;149:2067–2079.
34. Wintour EM, Alcorn D, Butkus A, et al. Ontogeny of hormonal and excretory function of the meso- and metanephros in the ovine fetus. *Kidney Int* 1996;50:1624–1633.
35. Graham PC, Kingdom JCP, Raweily EA, et al. Distribution of renin-containing cells in the developing human kidney: an immunohistochemical study. *Br J Obstet Gynaecol* 1992;99:765–769.
36. Ljungqvist A, Wagermark J. Renal juxtaglomerular granulation in the human foetus and infant. *Acta Pathol Microbiol Scand* 1966;67:257–266.
37. Richer C, Hornych H, Amiel-Tison C, et al. Plasma renin activity and its postnatal development in preterm infants. *Biol Neonate* 1977;31:301–304.
38. Kotchen TA, Strickland AL, Rice TW, et al. A study of the renin–angiotensin system in newborn infants. *J Pediatr* 1972;80:938–946.
39. Broughton Pipkin F, Smales OR, O'Callaghan M. Renin and angiotensin levels in children. *Arch Dis Child* 1981;56:298–302.
40. Dillon MJ. Renin-angiotensin-aldosterone system. *Eur J Clin Pharmacol* 1980;18:105–108.
41. Godard C, Geering JM, Geering K, et al. Plasma renin activity related to sodium balance, renal function and urinary vasopressin in the newborn infant. *Pediatr Res* 1979;13:742–745.
42. Richer C, Hornych H, Amiel-Tison C, et al. Plasma renin activity and its postnatal development in preterm infants. Preliminary report. *Biol Neonate* 1977;31:301–304.
43. Sulyok E, Nemeth M, Tenyi I, et al. Postnatal development of renin-angiotensin-aldosterone system, RAAS, in relation to electrolyte balance in premature infants. *Pediatr Res* 1979;13:817–820.
44. Van Acker KJ, Scharpe SL, Deprettere AJR, et al. Renin-angiotensin–aldosterone system in the healthy infant and child. *Kidney Int* 1979;16:196–203.
45. Catt KJ, Cain MD, Coghlan JP, et al. Metabolism and blood levels of angiotensin II in normal subjects, renal disease, and essential hypertension. *Circ Res* 1970;27[Suppl 2]:177–193.

46. Pipkin FB, Kirkpatrick SM, Mott JC. Angiotensin II-like activity in arterial blood in new-born lambs. *J Physiol (Lond)* 1971;218:61P–62P.

47. Pipkin FB, Mott JC, Roberton NR. Resting concentration of angiotensin II-like activity in the arterial blood of rabbits of different ages. *J Physiol (Lond)* 1971;214:21P–22P.

48. Pipkin FB, Kirkpatrick SM, Lumbers ER, et al. Renin and angiotensin-like levels in Foetal, new-born and adult sheep. *J Physiol (Lond)* 1974;241:575–588.

49. Siegel SR, Fisher DA, Oh W. Serum aldosterone concentrations related to sodium balance in the newborn infant. *Pediatrics* 1974;53:410–413.

50. Sulyok E, Nemeth M, Tenyi I, et al. Relationship between maturity, electrolyte balance and the function of the renin–angiotensin–aldosterone system in newborn infants. *Biol Neonate* 1979;35:60–65.

51. Beitins IZ, Bayard F, Levitsky L, et al. Plasma aldosterone concentration at delivery and during the newborn period. *J Clin Invest* 1972;51:386–394.

52. Kowarski A, Katz H, Migeon CJ. Plasma aldosterone concentration in normal subjects from infancy to adulthood. *J Clin Endocrinol Metab* 1974;38:489–491.

53. Arant BS Jr, Stephenson WH. Developmental change in systemic vascular resistance compared with prostaglandins and angiotensin II concentration in arterial plasma of conscious dogs. *Pediatr Res* 1982;16:120A.

54. Broughton Pipkin F, Symonds EM, Turner SR. The effect of captopril (SQ14,225) upon mother and fetus in the chronically cannulated ewe and in the pregnant rabbit. *J Physiol (Lond)* 1982;323:415–422.

55. Guron G, Adams MA, Sundelin B, et al. Neonatal angiotensin-converting enzyme inhibition in the rat induces persistent abnormalities in renal function and histology. *Hypertension* 1997;29:91–97.

56. Pryde PG, Sedman AB, Nugent CE, et al. Angiotensin-converting enzyme inhibitor fetopathy. *J Am Soc Nephrol* 1993;3:1575–1582.

57. Niimura F, Labosky PA, Kakuchi J, et al. Gene targeting in mice reveals a requirement for angiotensin in the development and maintenance of kidney morphology and growth factor regulation. *J Clin Invest* 1995;96:2947–2954.

58. Hilgers KF, Reddi V, Krege JH, et al. Aberrant renal vascular morphology and renin expression in mutant mice lacking angiotensin-converting enzyme. *Hypertension* 1997;29: 216–221.

59. Robillard JE, Weitzman RE, Fisher DA, et al. The dynamics of vasopressin release: blood volume regulation during fetal hemorrhage in the lamb fetus. *Pediatr Res* 1979;13:606–610.

60. Nakamura KT, Ayres NA, Gomez RA, et al. Renal responses to hypoxemia during renin–angiotensin system inhibition in fetal lambs. *Am J Physiol* 1985;249:R116–R124.

61. Gomez RA, Meernik JG, Kuehl WD, et al. Developmental aspects of the renal response to hemorrhage during fetal life. *Pediatr Res* 1984;18:40–46.

62. Gomez RA, Robillard JE. Developmental aspects of the renal response to hemorrhage during converting-enzyme inhibition in fetal lambs. *Circ Res* 1984;54:301–312.

63. Tortorolo G, Porcelli G, Cuatalo P. Urinary kallikreins in premature, small at term and normal newborns and in children. In: Pisano JJ, Austen KF, eds. *Chemistry and biology of kallikrein: kinin system in health and disease*. Washington: PHEW (National Institutes of Health), 1974:76.

64. Godard C, Vallotton MB, Favre L. Urinary prostaglandins, vasopressin, and kallikrein excretion in healthy children from birth to adolescence. *J Pediatr* 1982;100:898–902.

65. Vane JR, Bakhle YS, Botting RM. Cyclooxygenases 1 and 2. *Annu Rev Pharmacol Toxicol* 1998;38:97–120.

66. Komhoff M, Grone HJ, Klein T, et al. Localization of cyclooxygenase-1 and -2 in adult and fetal human kidney: implication for renal function. *Am J Physiol* 1997;272:F460–F468.

67. Zang MZ, Wang JL, Cheng HF, et al. Cyclooxygenase-2 in rat nephron development. *Am J Physiol* 1997;273:F994–F1002.

68. Walker DW, Mitchell MD. Prostaglandins in urine of foetal lambs. *Nature* 1978;271:161–162.

69. Walker DW, Mitchell MD. Presence of thromboxane B2 and 6-keto-prostaglandin F1-a in the urine of fetal sheep. *Prostaglandins Med* 1979;3:249–250.

70. Arant BS Jr. Renal disorders of the newborn infant. *Pediatr Nephrol* 1984;12:111.

71. Robillard JE, Weismann DN, Gomez RA, et al. Renal and adrenal responses to converting-enzyme inhibition in fetal and newborn life. *Am J Physiol* 1983;244:R249–R256.

72. Benzoni D, Vincent M, Betend B, et al. Urinary excretion of prostaglandins and electrolytes in developing children. *Kidney Int* 1981;20:386–388.

73. Matson JR, Stokes JB, Robillard JE. Effects of inhibition of prostaglandin synthesis on fetal renal function. *Kidney Int* 1981;20:621–627.

74. Hendricks SK, Smith JR, Moore DE, et al. Oligohydramnios associated with prostaglandin synthetase inhibitors in preterm labour. *Br J Obstet Gynaecol* 1990;97:312–316.

75. Kaplan BS, Restaino I, Raval DS, et al. Renal failure in the neonate associated with in utero exposure to non-steroidal anti-infalmmatory agents. *Pediatr Nephrol* 1994;8:700–704.

76. Kirshon B, Moise KJ Jr, Wasserstrum N, et al. Influence of short-term indomethacin therapy on fetal urine output. *Obstet Gynecol* 1988;72:51–53.

77. van den Anker JN, Hop WC, de Groot R, et al. Effects of prenatal exposure to betamethasone and indomethacin on the glomerular filtration rate in the preterm infant. *Pediatr Res* 1994;36:578–581.

78. Seyberth HW, Rascher W, Hackenthal R, et al. Effect of prolonged indomethacin therapy on renal function and selected vasoactive hormones in very-low-birth-weight infants with symptomatic patent ductus arteriosus. *J Pediatr* 1983;103: 979–984.

79. Chamaa NS, Mosig D, Drukker A, et al. The renal hemodynamic effects of ibuprofen in the newborn rabbit. *Pediatr Res* 2000;48:600–605.

80. Robillard JE, Nakamura KT, Wilkin MK, et al. Ontogeny of renal hemodynamic response to renal nerve stimulation in sheep. *Am J Physiol* 1987;252:F605–F612.

81. Nakamura KT, Matherne GP, Jose PA, et al. Ontogeny of renal b-adrenoceptor mediated vasodilation in sheep: comparison between endogenous catecholamines. *Pediatr Res* 1987;22: 465–470.

82. Robillard JE, Nakamura KT, DiBonna GF. Effects of renal denervation on renal responses to hypoxemia in fetal lambs. *Am J Physiol* 1986;250:F294–F301.

83. Lagercrantz H, Bistoletti P. Catecholamine release in the newborn infant at birth. *Pediatr Res* 1973;11:889–893.

84. Jose PA, Slotkoff LM, Lilienfield LS, et al. Sensitivity of neonatal renal vasculature to epinephrine. *Am J Physiol* 1974;226: 796–799.

85. McKenna OC, Angelakos ET. Development of adrenergic innervation in the puppy kidney. *Anat Rec* 1970;167:115–125.

86. McKenna OC, Angelakos ET. Adrenergic innervation of the canine kidney. *Circ Res* 1968;22:345–354.

87. Solhaug MJ, Ballevre LD, Guignard JP, et al. Nitric oxide in the developing kidney. *Pediatr Nephrol* 1996;10:529–539.

88. Simeoni U, Zhu B, Muller C, et al. Postnatal development of vascular resistnace of the rabbit isolated perfused kidney: modulation by nitric oxide and angiotensin II. *Pediatr Res* 1997;42:550–555.

89. Felder RA, Felder CC, Eisner GM, et al. The dopamine receptor in adult and maturing kidney. *Am J Physiol* 1989;257: F315–F327.

90. Pelayo JC, Fildes RD, Jose PA. Age-dependent renal effects of intrarenal dopamine infusion. *Am J Physiol* 1984;247:R212–R216.

91. Feltes TF, Hansen TN, Martin CG, et al. The effects of dopamine infusion on regional blood flow in newborn lambs. *Pediatr Res* 1987;21:131–136.

92. Driscoll DJ, Gillette PC, Lewis RM, et al. Comparative hemodynamic effects of isoproterenol, dopamine, and dobutamine in the newborn dog. *Pediatr Res* 1979;13:1006–1009.

93. Tenore G, Barili P, Sabbatini M, et al. Postnatal development of dopamine D1-like and D2-like receptors in the rat kidney: a radioligand binding study. *Mech Ageing Dev* 1997;95:1–11.

94. Breyer MD, Harris RC. Cyclooxygenase 2 and the kidney. *Curr Opin Nephrol Hypertens* 2001;10:89–98.

95. Buckley NM, Brazeau P, Fraiser ID. Cardiovascular effects of dopamine in developing swine. *Biol Neonate* 1983;43:50–60.

96. Fildes RD, Eisner GM, Calcagno PL, et al. Renal a-adrenoceptors and sodium excretion in the dog. *Am J Physiol* 1985;248:F128–F133.

97. Felder RA, Pelayo JC, Calcagno PL, et al. Alpha adrenoceptors in the developing kidney. *Pediatr Res* 1983;17:177–180.
98. Pohjavuori M, Fyhrquist F. Hemodynamic significance of vasopressin in the newborn infant. *J Pediatr* 1980;97:462–465.
99. Robillard JE, Weitzman RE. Developmental aspects of the fetal response to exogenous arginine vasopressin. *Am J Physiol* 1980;238:F407–F414.
100. Weismann DN, Robillard JE. Renal hemodynamic responses to hypoxemia during development: relationship to circulatory vasoactive substances. *Pediatr Res* 1988;23:155–162.
101. Maack T. Role of atrial natriuretic factor in volume control. *Kidney Int* 1996;49:1732–1737.
102. Robillard JE, Weiner C. Atrial natriuretic factor in the human fetus: effect of volume expansion. *J Pediatr* 1988;113:552–555.
103. Panos MZ, Nicolaides KH, Anderson JV, et al. Plasma atrial natriuretic peptide in human fetus: response to intravascular blood transfusion. *Am J Obstet Gynecol* 1989;161:357–361.
104. Ross MG, Ervin MG, Lam RW, et al. Plasma atrial natriuretic peptide response to volume expansion in the ovine fetus. *Am J Obstet Gynecol* 1987;157:1292–1297.
105. Ross MG, Ervin MG, Lam RW, et al. Fetal atrial natriuretic factor and arginine vasopressin responses to hyperosmolality and hypovolemia. *Pediatr Res* 1988;24:318–321.
106. Cheung CY, Brace RA. Hemorrhage-induced reductions in plasma atrial natriuretic factor in the ovine fetus. *Obstet Gynecol* 1991;165:474–481.
107. Robillard JE, Nakamura KT, Varille VA, et al. Ontogeny of the renal response to natriuretic peptide in sheep. *Am J Physiol* 1988;254:F634–F641.
108. Chevalier RL, Gomez RA, Carey RM, et al. Renal effects of atrial natriuretic peptide infusion in young and adult rats. *Pediatr Res* 1988;24:333–337.
109. Hargrave BY, Iwamoto HS, Rudolph AM. Renal and cardiovascular effects of atrial natriuretic peptide in fetal sheep. *Pediatr Res* 1989;26:1–5.
110. Semmekrot BA, Wiesel PH, Monnens LA, et al. Age differences in renal response to atrial natriuretic peptide in rabbits. *Life Sci* 1990;46:849–856.
111. Tulassay T, Rascher W, Seyberth HW, et al. Role of atrial natriuretic peptide in sodium homeostasis in premature infants. *J Pediatr* 1986;109:1023–1027.
112. Castro R, Leake RD, Ervin MG, et al. Ontogeny of atrial natriuretic factor receptors and cyclic GMP response in rabbit renal glomeruli. *Pediatr Res* 1991;30:45–49.
113. Muchant DG, Thornhill BA, Belmonte DC, et al. Chronic sodium loading augments natriuretic response to acute volume expansion in the preweaned rat. *Am J Physiol* 1995;269:R15–R22.
114. Altschule MD. The changes in the mesonephric tubules of human embryos seven to twelve weeks old. *Anat Rec* 1930;46:81.
115. Gersh I. The correlation of structure and function in the developing mesonephros and metanephros. *Contrib Embryol* 1937;153:35.
116. Arant BS Jr. Developmental patterns of renal functional maturation compared in the human neonate. *J Pediatr* 1978;92:705–712.
117. Coulthard MG. Maturation of glomerular filtration in preterm and mature babies. *Early Hum Dev* 1985;11:281–292.
118. Aperia A, Broberger O, Elinder G, et al. Postnatal development of renal function in pre-term and full-term infants. *Acta Paediatr Scand* 1981;70:183–187.
119. Leake RD, Trygstad CW, Oh W. Inulin clearance in the newborn infant. Relationship to gestational and postnatal age. *Pediatr Res* 1976;10:759–762.
120. Oh W, Arcilla RA, Oh MA, et al. Renal and cardiovascular effects of body tilting in the newborn infant: a comparative study of infants born with early and late cord clamping. *Biol Neonate* 1966;10:76–92.
121. Vanpee M, Blennow M, Linne T, et al. Renal function in very low birth weight infants: normal maturity reach during early childhood. *J Pediatr* 1992;121:784–788.
122. Barnett HL. Renal physiology in infants and children. I. Method for estimation of glomerular filtration rate. *Proc Soc Exp Biol Med* 1940;44:654–658.
123. Arant BS Jr. Postnatal development of renal function during the first year of life. *Pediatr Nephrol* 1987;1:308–313.
124. Aperia A, Herin P. Development of glomerular perfusion rate and nephron filtration rate in rats 17–60 days old. *Am J Physiol* 1975;228:1319–1325.
125. Spitzer A, Brandis M. Functional and morphologic maturation of the superficial nephrons: relationship to total kidney function. *J Clin Invest* 1974;53:279–287.
126. Jose PA, Slotkoff LM, Montgomery S, et al. Autoregulation of renal blood flow in the puppy. *Am J Physiol* 1975;229:983–988.
127. Buckley NM, Brazeau P, Frasier ID. Renal blood flow autoregulation in developing swine. *Am J Physiol* 1983;245:H1–H6.
128. Aperia A, Herin P. Effect of arterial blood pressure reduction on renal hemodynamics in the developing lamb. *Acta Physiol Scand* 1976;98:387–394.
129. Robillard JE, Weitzman RE. Developmental aspects of the fetal renal response to exogenous arginine vasopressin. *Am J Physiol* 1980;238:F407–F414.
130. Semple SJG, deWardener HE. Effect of increased venous pressure on circulatory "autoregulation" of isolated dog kidneys. *Circ Res* 1959;7:643–648.
131. Gilmore JP, Cornish KG, Rogers SD, et al. Direct evidence for myogenic autoregulation of the renal microcirculation in the hamster. *Circ Res* 1980;47:226–230.
132. Moore LC. Interaction of tubuloglomerular feedback and proximal nephron reabsorption in autoregulation. *Kidney Int Suppl* 1982;12:S173–S178.
133. Schnermann J, Traynor T, Yang T, et al. Tubuloglomerular feedback: new concepts and developments. *Kidney Int Suppl* 1998;67:S40–S50.
134. Arendshorst WJ, Brannstrom K, Ruan X. Actions of angiotensin II on the renal microvasculature. *J Am Soc Nephrol* 1999;10[Suppl 11]:S49–S61.
135. Badr KF, Ichikawa I. Prerenal failure: a deleterious shift from renal compensation to decompensation. *N Engl J Med* 1988;319:623–629.
136. Briggs JP, Schubert G, Schnermann J. Quantitative characterization of the tubuloglomerular feedback response: effect of growth. *Am J Physiol* 1984;247:F808–F815.
137. Muller-Suur R, Ulfendahl HR, Persson AEG. Evidence for tubuloglomerular feedback in juxtamedullary nephrons of young rats. *Am J Physiol* 1983;244:F425–F431.
138. Welch WJ, Wilcox CS, Thomson SC. Nitric oxide and tubuloglomerular feedback. *Semin Nephrol* 1999;19:251–262.
139. Wilcox CS, Welch WJ, Murad F, et al. Nitric oxide synthase in macula densa regulates glomerular capillary pressure. *Proc Natl Acad Sci U S A* 1992;89:11993–11997.
140. Gordon HH, Levine SZ, Marples E, et al. Water exchange of premature infants: comparison of metabolic (organic) and electrolyte (inorganic) methods of measurement. *J Clin Invest* 1939;18:187–194.
141. McCance RA, Widdowson EM. The response of the newborn puppy to water, salt and food. *J Physiol (Lond)* 1958;141:81–87.
142. Aperia A, Broberger O, Thodenius K, et al. Renal response to an oral sodium load in newborn full-term infants. *Acta Paediatr Scand* 1972;61:670–676.
143. Aperia A, Elinder G. Distal tubular sodium reabsorption in the developing rat kidney. *Am J Physiol* 1981;240:F487–F491.
144. Nakamura KT, Matherne GP, McWeeny OJ, et al. Renal hemodynamics and functional changes during the transition from fetal to newborn life in sheep. *Pediatr Res* 1987;21:229–234.
145. Robillard JE, Sessions C, Kennedey RL, et al. Interrelationship between glomerular filtration rate and renal transport of sodium and chloride during fetal life. *Am J Obstet Gynecol* 1977;128:727–734.
146. Siegel SR, Oh W. Renal function as a marker of human fetal maturation. *Acta Paediatr Scand* 1976;65:481–485.
147. Engelke SC, Shah BL, Vasan U, et al. Sodium balance in very low birth-weight infants. *J Pediatr* 1978;93:837–841.
148. Aperia A, Broberger O, Thodenius K, et al. Developmental study of the renal response to an oral salt load in preterm infants. *Acta Paediatr Scand* 1974;63:517–524.
149. Delgado MM, Rohatgi R, Khan S, et al. Sodium and potassium clearances by the maturing kidney: clinical-molecular correlates. *Pediatr Nephrol* 2003;18:759–767.
150. Lorenz JM, Kleinman LI, Kotagal UR, et al. Water balance in very low-birth-weight infants: relationship to water and sodium intake and effect on outcome. *J Pediatr* 1982;101:423–432.

151. Al-Dahhan J, Haycock GB, Nichol B, et al. Sodium homeostasis in term and preterm neonates. III. The effect of salt supplementation. *Arch Dis Child* 1984;59:945–950.

152. Celsi G, Larsson L, Aperia A. Proximal tubular reabsorption and Na-K-ATPase activity in remnant kidney of young rats. *Am J Physiol* 1986;251:F588–F593.

153. Lelievre-Pegorier M, Merlet-Benichou C, Roinel N, et al. Developmental pattern of water and electrolyte transport in rat superficial nephrons. *Am J Physiol* 1983;245:F15–F21.

154. Solomon S. Absolute rates of sodium and potassium reabsorption by proximal tubule of immature rats. *Biol Neonate* 1974;25:340–351.

155. Corman B, Roinel N. Single-nephron filtration rate and proximal tubule reabsorption in aging rats. *Am J Physiol* 1991;260: F75–F80.

156. Elinder G. Effect of isotonic volume expansion on proximal tubular reabsorption of Na and fluid in the developing rat kidney. *Acta Physiol Scand* 1981;112:83–88.

157. Horster M, Valtin H. Postnatal development of renal function: micropuncture and clearance studies in the dog. *J Clin Invest* 1971;50:779–795.

158. Merlet-Benichou C, de Rouffignac C. Renal clearance studies in fetal and young guinea pigs: effect of salt loading. *Am J Physiol* 1977;232:F178–F185.

159. Rodriguez-Soriano J, Vallo A, Oliveros R, et al. Renal handling of sodium in premature and full-term neonates: a study using clearance methods during water diuresis. *Pediatr Res* 1983;17: 1013–1016.

160. Schoeneman MJ, Spitzer A. The effect of intravascular volume expansion of proximal tubular reabsorption during development. *Proc Soc Exp Biol Med* 1980;165:319–322.

161. Sulyok E, Varga F, Gyory E, et al. Postnatal changes in proximal and distal tubular sodium reabsorption in healthy very-low-birth-weight infants. *J Pediatr* 1979;95:787–792.

162. Broberger U, Aperia A, Thodenius K, et al. Renal function in infants with hyperbilirubinemia. *Acta Paediatr Scand* 1979;68: 75–79.

163. Aperia A, Bergqvist G, Brogerger O, et al. Renal function in newborn infants with high hematocrit values before and after isovolemic haemodilution. *Acta Paediatr Scand* 1974;63: 878–884.

164. Harkavy KL, Scanlon JW, Jose P. The effects of theophylline on renal function in the premature newborn. *Biol Neonate* 1979;35:126–130.

165. Rodriguez-Soriano J, Vallo A, Castillo G, et al. Renal handling of water and sodium in infancy and childhood: a study using clearance methods during hypotonic saline diuresis. *Kidney Int* 1981;20:700–704.

166. Leslie GI, Arnold JD, Gyory AZ. Postnatal changes in proximal and distal tubular sodium reabsorption in healthy very-low-birth-weight infants. *Biol Neonate* 1991;60:108–113.

167. Pacha J, Frindt G, Antonian L, et al. Regulation of Na channels of the rat cortical collecting tubule by aldosterone. *J Gen Physiol* 1993;102:25–42.

168. Masilamani S, Kim GH, Mitchell C, et al. Aldosterone-mediated regulation of ENaC alpha, beta, and gamma subunit proteins in rat kidney. *J Clin Invest* 1999;104:R19–R23.

169. Ikeda U, Hyman R, Smith TW, et al. Aldosterone-mediated regulation of Na+, K+-ATPase gene exprexion in adult and neonatal rat cardiocytes. *J Biol Chem* 1991;266:12058–12066.

170. Van Acker KJ, Scharpe SL, Deprettere AJ, et al. HM. Renin-angiotensin-aldosterone system in the healthy infant and child. *Kidney Int* 1979;16:196–203.

171. Aperia A, Broberger O, Herin P, et al. Sodium excretion in relation to sodium intake and aldosterone excretion in newborn preterm and full term infants. *Acta Paediatr Scand* 1979;68: 813–817.

172. Vehaskari VM. Ontogeny of cortical collecting duct sodium transport. *Am J Physiol* 1994;267:F49–F54.

173. Stephenson G, Hammet M, Hadaway G, et al. Ontogeny of renal mineralocorticoid receptors and urinary electrolyte responses in the rat. *Am J Physiol* 1984;247:F665–F671.

174. Siegel SR, Oaks G, Palmer S. Effects of angiotensin II on blood pressure, plasma renin activity, and aldosterone in the fetal lamb. *Dev Pharmacol Ther* 1981;3:144–149.

175. Satlin LM, Palmer LG. Apical Na+ conductance in maturing rabbit principal cell. *Am J Physiol* 1996;270:F391–F397.

176. Robillard JE, Nakamura KT. Neurohormonal regulation of renal function during development. *Am J Physiol* 1988;254:F771–F779.

177. Hayashi Y, Chiba K, Matsuoka T, et al. Renal nerve stimulation induces alpha2-adrenoceptor-mediated antinatriuresis under inhibition of prostaglandin synthesis in anesthetized dogs. *Tohoku J Exp Med* 1999;188:335–346.

178. Brace RA, Bayer LA, Cheung CY. Fetal cardiovascular, endocrine, and fluid responses to atrial natriuretic factor infusion. *Am J Physiol* 1989;257:R580–R587.

179. Semmekrot BA, Wiesel PH, Monnens LAH, et al. Age differences in renal response to atrial natriuretic peptide in rabbits. *Life Sci* 1990;46:849–856.

180. Segar JL, Smith FG, Guillery EN, et al. Ontogeny of renal response to specific dopamine DA1–receptor stimulation in sheep. *Am J Physiol* 1992;263:R868–R873.

181. Jaton T, Thonney M, Gouyon JB, et al. Renal effects of dopamine and dopexamine in the newborn anesthetized rabbit. *Life Sci* 1992;50:195–202.

182. Kaneko S, Albrecht F, Asico LD, et al. Ontogeny of DA1 receptor-mediated natriuresis in the rat: in vivo and in vitro correlations. *Am J Physiol* 1992;263:R631–R638.

183. Henning SJ. Plasma concentration of total and free corticosterone during development in the rat. *Am J Physiol* 1978;235: E451–E456.

184. Henning SJ. Postnatal development: coordination of feeding, digestion, and metabolism. *Am J Physiol* 1981;241:G199–G214.

185. Malinowska KW, Hardy RN, Nathanielsz PW. Plasma adrenocorticosteroid concentrations immediately after birth in the rat, rabbit and guinea-pig. *Experientia* 1972;28:1366–1367.

186. Malinowska KW, Natanielsz PW. Plasma aldosterone, cortisol and corticosterone concentrations in the new-born guinea-pig. *J Physiol* 1974;236:83–93.

187. Farman N. Molecular and cellular determinants of mineralocorticoid selectivity. *Curr Opin Nephrol Hypertens* 1999;8:45–51.

188. Bostanjoglo M, Reeves WB, Reilly RF, et al. 11Beta–hydroxysteroid dehydrogenase, mineralocorticoid receptor, and thiazide-sensitive Na-Cl cotransporter expression by distal tubules. *J Am Soc Nephrol* 1998;9:1347–1358.

189. Farman N. Steroid receptors: distribution along the nephron. *Semin Nephrol* 1992;12:12–17.

190. Serrano CV, Talbert LM, Welt LG. Potassium deficiency in the pregnant dog. *J Clin Invest* 1964;43:27–31.

191. Dancis J, Springer D. Fetal homeostasis in maternal malnutrition: potassium and sodium deficiency in rats. *Pediatr Res* 1970;4:345–351.

192. Sulyok E. The relationship between electrolyte and acid–base balance in the premature infant during early postnatal life. *Biol Neonate* 1971;17:227–237.

193. Satlin LM. Maturation of renal potassium transport. *Pediatr Nephrol* 1991;5:260–269.

194. Tuvdad F, McNamara H, Barnett HL. Renal response of premature infants to administration of bicarbonate and potassium. *Pediatrics* 1954;13:4–11.

195. McCance RA, Widdowson EM. The response of the new-born piglet to an excess of potassium. *J Physiol* 1958;141:88–96.

196. Kleinman LI, Banks RO. Segmental nephron sodium and potassium reabsorption in newborn and adult dogs during saline expansion. *Proc Soc Exp Biol Med* 1983;173:231–237.

197. Zink H, Horster M. Maturation of diluting capacity in loop of Henle of rat superficial nephrons. *Am J Physiol* 1977;233: F519–F524.

198. Giebisch G. Renal potassium transport: mechanisms and regulation. *Am J Physiol* 1998;274:F817–F833.

199. Satlin LM. Postnatal maturation of potassium transport in rabbit cortical collecting duct. *Am J Physiol* 1994;266:F57–F65.

200. Woda CB, Miyawaki N, Ramalakshmi S, et al. Ontogeny of flow-stimulated potassium secretion in rabbit cortical collecting duct: functional molecular aspects. *Am J Physiol Renal Physiol* 2003;285:F629–F639.

201. Satlin LM, Palmer LG. Apical K+ conductance in maturing rabbit principal cell. *Am J Physiol* 1997;272:F397–F404.

202. Ho K, Nichols CG, Lederer WJ, et al. Cloning and expression of an inwardly rectifying ATP-regulated potassium channel. *Nature* 1993;363:31–38.

203. Zhou H, Tate SS, Palmer LG. Primary structure and functional properties of an epithelial K channel. *Am J Physiol* 1994;266: C809–C824.

204. Robillard JE, Nakamura KT, Lawton WJ. Effects of aldosterone on urinary kallikrein and sodium excretion during fetal life. *Pediatr Res* 1985;19:1048–1052.
205. Kairaitis K, Lumbers ER. The influence of endogenous mineral-corticoids on the composition of fetal urine. *J Dev Physiol* 1990;13:347–351.
206. Vaughn D, Kirschbaum TH, Bersentes T, et al. Fetal and neonatal response to acid loading in the sheep. *J Appl Physiol* 1968;24:135–141.
207. Smith FG Jr, Schwartz A. Response of the intact lamb fetus to acidosis. *Am J Obstet Gynecol* 1970;106:52–58.
208. Weisbrot IM, James LS, Prince CE, et al. Acid–base homeostasis of the new-born infant during the first 24 hrs of life. *J Pediatr* 1958;52:395–403.
209. Smith CA. *The physiology of the newborn infant.* Springfield, IL: CC Thomas, 1959:320.
210. Schwartz G. Acid-base homeostasis. In: Edelman CM, ed. *Pediatric kidney disease.* Boston: Little, Brown, 1969:201–230.
211. Edelman CM Jr, Spitzer A. The maturing kidney. A modern view of well-balanced infants with imbalanced nephrons. *J Pediatr* 1969;75:509–519.
212. Kildeberg P, Engel K, Winters RW. Balance of net acid in growing infants: endogenous and transintestinal aspects. *Acta Paediatr Scand* 1969;58:321–329.
213. Svenningsen NW, Lindquist B. Incidence of metabolic acidosis in term, preterm and small-for-gestational age infants in relation to dietary protein intake. *Acta Paediatr Scand* 1973;62:1–10.
214. Kildeberg P, Winters RW. Balance of net acid: concept, measurement and applications. *Adv Pediatr* 1978;25:349–381.
215. Wamberg S, Kildeberg P, Engel K. Balance of net base in the rat. II. Reference values in relation to growth rate. *Biol Neonate* 1976;28:171–190.
216. Pitts R, Ayer J, Schiess W. The renal regulation of acid-base balance in man III. The reabsorption and excretion of bicarbonate. *J Clin Invest* 1949;28:35–44.
217. Schwartz GJ, Haycock GB, Edelmann CM Jr, et al. Late metabolic acidosis: a reassessment of the definition. *J Pediatr* 1979;95:102–107.
218. Edelmann CM Jr, Rodriguez-Soriano J, Boichis H, et al. Renal bicarbonate reabsorption and hydrogen ion excretion in normal infants. *J Clin Invest* 1967;46:1309–1317.
219. Svenningsen NW. Renal acid–base titration studies in infants with and without metabolic acidosis in the postneonatal period. *Pediatr Res* 1974;8:659–672.
220. Friis-Hansen B. Body water compartment in children: changes during growth and related changes in body composition. *Pediatrics* 1961;28:169–181.
221. Shah M, Gupta N, Dwarakanath V, et al. Ontogeny of Na+/H+ antiporter activity in rat proximal convoluted tubules. *Pediatr Res* 2000;48:206–210.
222. Baum M, Quigley R. Maturation of proximal tubular acidification. *Pediatr Nephrol* 1993;7:785–791.
223. Day R, Franklin J. Renal carbonic anhydrase in premature and mature infants. *Pediatrics* 1951;7:182–185.
224. Larsson L, Lonnerholm G. Carbonic anhydrase in the metanephrogenic zone of the human fetal kidney. *Biol Neonate* 1985;48:168–171.
225. Lonnerholm G, Wistrand PJ. Carbonic anhydrase in the human fetal kidney. *Pediatr Res* 1983;17:390–397.
226. Brion LP, Zavilowitz BJ, Rosen O, et al. Changes in soluble carbonic anhydrase activity in response to maturation and NH4Cl loading in the rabbit. *Am J Physiol* 1991;261:R1204–R1213.
227. Fisher DA. Carbonic anhydrase activity in fetal and young rhesus monkeys. *Proc Soc Exp Biol Med* 1961;107:359–363.
228. Maren TH. Carbonic anhydrase: chemistry, physiology, and inhibition. *Physiol Rev* 1967;47:595–781.
229. Schwartz GJ, Olson J, Kittelberger AM, et al. Postnatal development of carbonic anhydrase IV expression in rabbit kidney. *Am J Physiol* 1999;276:F510–F520.
230. Fomon S, Harris D, Jensen R. Acidification of the urine in infants fed human milk and whole cow's milk. *Pediatrics* 1959;23:113–120.
231. Gordon H, McNamara H, Benjamin H. The response of young infants to ingestion of ammonium chloride. *Pediatrics* 1948;2:290–302.
232. Hatemi N, McCance R. Renal aspects of acid-base control in the newly born. III. Response to acidifying drugs. *Acta Paediatr Scand* 1961;50:603–616.
233. Kerpel-Fronius E, Heim T, Sulyok E. The development of the renal acidifying processes and their relation to acidosis in low-birth-weight infants. *Biol Neonate* 1970;15:156–168.
234. Sulyok E, Heim T. Assessment of maximal urinary acidification in premature infants. *Biol Neonate* 1971;19:200–210.
235. Ranlov P, Siggaard-Andersen O. Late metabolic acidosis in premature infants. Prevalence and significance. *Acta Paediatr Scand* 1965;54:531–540.
236. Svenningsen NW, Lindquist B. Postnatal development of renal hydrogen ion excretion capacity in relation to age and protein intake. *Acta Paediatr Scand* 1974;63:721–731.
237. Goldstein L. Ammonia metabolism in kidneys of suckling rats. *Am J Physiol* 1971;220:213–217.
238. Peonides A, Levin B, Young WF. The renal excretion of hydrogen ions in infants and children. *Arch Dis Child* 1965;40:33–39.
239. McCance RA, Widdowson EM. Renal aspects of acid–base control in the newly born. I. Natural development. *Acta Paediatr Scand* 1960;49:409–414.
240. Satlin LM, Schwartz GJ. Postnatal maturation of rabbit renal collecting duct: intercalated cell function. *Am J Physiol* 1987;253:F622–F635.
241. Mehrgut FM, Satlin LM, Schwartz GJ. Maturation of HCO3 transport in rabbit collecting duct. *Am J Physiol* 1990;259:F801–F808.
242. Radde IC, Chance GW, Bailey K. Growth and mineral metabolism in very low birth-weight infants. I. Comparison of the effects of two modes of NaHCO3 treatment of late metabolic acidosis. *Pediatr Res* 1975;9:564–568.
243. Arant BS Jr. Renal handling of calcium and phosphorus in normal human neonates. *Semin Nephrol* 1983;2:94–99.
244. Brown DR, Steranka BH. Renal cation excretion in the hypocalcemic premature human neonate. *Pediatr Res* 1981;15:1100–1104.
245. Karlen J, Aperia A, Zetterstrom R. Renal excretion of calcium and phosphate in preterm and term infants. *J Pediatr* 1985;106:814–819.
246. Ghazali S, Barratt TM. Urinary excretion of calcium and magnesium in children. *Arch Dis Child* 1974;49:97–101.
247. Wittner M, Desfleurs E, Pajaud S, et al. Calcium and magnesium transport in the cortical ascending limb of henle's loop: influence of age and gender. *Pflügers Arch* 1997;434:451–456.
248. Friedman PA. Codependence of renal calcium and sodium transport. *Annu Rev Physiol* 1998;60:179–197.
249. Zanardo V, Dani C, Trevisanuto D, et al. Methylxanthines increase renal calcium excretion in preterm infants. *Biol Neonate* 1995;68:169–174.
250. Kamitsuka MD, Williams MA, Nyberg DA, et al. Renal calcification: a complication of dexamethasone therapy in preterm infants with bronchopulmonary dysplasia. *J Perinatol* 1995;15:359–363.
251. Friedman PA. Mechanisms of renal calcium transport. *Exp Nephrol* 2000;8:343–350.
252. Jahan I, Pitts RF. Effect of parathyroid on renal tubular reabsorption of phosphate and calcium. *Am J Physiol* 1948;155:42–49.
253. Gesek FA, Friedman PA. On the mechanism of parathyroid hormone stimulation of calcium uptake by mouse distal convoluted tubule cells. *J Clin Invest* 1992;90:749–758.
254. Bourdeau JE, Burg MB. Effect of PTH on calcium transport across the cortical thick ascending limb of Henle's loop. *Am J Physiol* 1980;239:F121–F126.
255. Greger R, Lang F, Oberleithner H. Distal site of calcium reabsorption in the rat nephron. *Pflügers Arch* 1978;374:153–157.
256. Shareghi GR, Stoner LC. Calcium transport across segments of the rabbit distal nephron in vitro. *Am J Physiol* 1978;235:F367–F375.
257. Shimizu T, Yoshitomi K, Nakamura M, et al. Effects of PTH, calcitonin, and cAMP on calcium transport in rabbit distal nephron segments. *Am J Physiol* 1990;259:F408–F414.
258. Suki WN, Rouse D. Hormonal regulation of calcium transport in thick ascending limb renal tubules. *Am J Physiol* 1981;241:F171–F174.

259. Linarelli LG, Bobick J, Bobick C. The effect of parathyroid hormone on rabbit renal cortex adenyl cyclase during development. *Pediatr Res* 1973;7:878–882.

260. Imbert-Teboul M, Chabardes D, Clique A, et al. Ontogenesis of hormone-dependent adenylate cyclase in isolated rat nephron segments. *Am J Physiol* 1984;247:F316–F325.

261. Mallet E, Basuyau J-P, Brunelle P, et al. Neonatal parathyroid secretion and renal receptor maturation in premature infants. *Biol Neonate* 1978;33:304–308.

262. Linarelli LG. Nephron urinary cyclic AMP and developmental renal responsiveness to parathyroid hormone. *Pediatrics* 1972; 50:14–23.

263. Tsang RC, Light IJ, Sutherland JM, et al. Possible pathogenetic factors in neonatal hypocalcemia of prematurity. *J Pediatr* 1973;82:423–429.

264. Senterre J, Salle B. Renal aspects of calcium and phosphorus metabolism in preterm infants. *Biol Neonate* 1988;53: 220–229.

265. Johnson JA, Grande JP, Roche PC, et al. 1 alpha, 25-dihydroxyvitamin D3 receptor ontogenesis in fetal renal development. *Am J Physiol* 1995;269:F419–F428.

266. Brown EM, MacLeod RJ. Extracellular calcium sensing and extracellular calcium signaling. *Physiol Rev* 2001;81:239–297.

267. Brown EM, Gamba G, Riccardi D, et al. Cloning and characterization of an extracellular Ca(2+)-sensing receptor from bovine parathyroid. *Nature* 1993;366:575–580.

268. Brown EM, Pollak M, Hebert SC. The extracellular calcium-sensing receptor; its role in health and disease. *Annu Rev Med* 1998;49:15–29.

269. Riccardi D, Hall AE, Chattopadhyay N, et al. Localization of the extracellular Ca2+/polyvalent cation-sensing protein in rat kidney. *Am J Physiol* 1998;274:F611–F622.

270. Chattopadhyay N, Baum M, Bai M, et al. Ontogeny of the extracellular calcium-sensing receptor in rat kidney. *Am J Physiol* 1996;271:F736–F743.

271. Smith FG Jr, Adams FH, Borden N, et al. Studies of renal function in the intact fetal lamb. *Am J Obstet Gynecol* 1966;96: 240–246.

272. Brodehl J, Gellisen K, Weber HP. Postnatal development of tubular phosphate reabsorption. *Clin Nephrol* 1982;17: 163–171.

273. Hohenauer I, Rosenberg TF, Oh W. Calcium and phosphorus homeostasis on the first day of life. *Biol Neonate* 1970;15: 49–56.

274. Johnson V, Spitzer A. Renal reabsorption of phosphate during development: whole kidney events. *Am J Physiol* 1986;251: F251–F256

275. Caverzasio J, Bonjour JP. Fleisch H. Tubular handling of Pi in young growing and adult rats. *Am J Physiol* 1982;242:F705–F710.

276. Kaskel FJ, Kumar AM, Feld LG, et al. Renal reabsorption of phosphate during development: tubular events. *Pediatr Nephrol* 1988;2:129–134.

277. Spitzer A, Barac-Nieto M. Ontogeny of renal phosphate transport and the process of growth. *Pediatr Nephrol* 2001;16: 763–771.

278. Neiberger RE, Barac-Nieto M, Spitzer A. Renal reabsorption of phosphate during development: transport kinetics in BBMV. *Am J Physiol* 1989;257:F268–F274.

279. Segawa H, Kaneko I, Takahashi A, et al. Growth-related renal type II Na/Pi cotransporter. *J Biol Chem* 2002;277: 19665–19672.

280. Prabhu S, Levi M, Dwarakanath V, et al. Effect of glucocorticoids on neonatal rabbit renal cortical sodium-inorganic phosphate messenger RNA and protein abundance. *Pediatr Res* 1997;41:20–24.

281. Haas JA, Berndt T, Knox FG. Nephron heterogeneity of phosphate reabsorption. *Am J Physiol* 1978;234:F287–F290.

282. Haramati A, Haas JA, Knox FG. Nephron heterogeneity of phosphate reabsorption: effect of parathyroid hormone. *Am J Physiol* 1984;246:F155–F158.

283. Hammerman MR, Karl IE, Hruska KA. Regulation of canine renal vesicle Pi transport by growth hormone and parathyroid hormone. *Biochim Biophys Acta* 1980;603:322–335.

284. Arar M, Levi M, Baum M. Maturational effects of glucocorticoids on neonatal brush-border membrane phosphate transport. *Pediatr Res* 1994;35:474–478.

285. Haramati A, Mulroney SE, Webster SK. Developmental changes in the tubular capacity for phosphate reabsorption in the rat. *Am J Physiol* 1988;255:F287–F291.

286. Arnaud SB, Goldsmith RS, Stickler GB, et al. Serum parathyroid hormone and blood minerals: interrelationships in normal children. *Pediatr Res* 1973;7:485–493.

287. David L, Anast CS. Calcium metabolism in newborn infant: the interrelationship of parathyroid function and calcium, magnesium, and phosphorus metabolism in normal sick and hypocalcemic newborns. *J Clin Invest* 1974;54:287–296.

288. Quamme GA, Dirks JH. Intraluminal and contraluminal magnesium on magnesium and calcium transfer in the rat nephron. *Am J Physiol* 1980;238:F187–F198.

289. Ariceta G, Rodriguez-Soriano, Vallo A. Magnesium homeostasis in premature and full-term neonates. *Pediatr Nephrol* 1995; 9:423–427.

290. Wittner M, di Stefano A, Wangemann P, et al. Differential effects of ADH on sodium, chloride, potassium, calcium and magnesium transport in cortical and medullary thick ascending limbs of mouse nephron. *Pflügers Arch* 1988;412: 516–523.

291. Dai LJ, Ritchie G, Kerstan D, et al. Magnesium Transport in the Renal Distal Convoluted Tubule. *Physiol Rev* 2001;81:51–84.

292. Bailly C, Roinel N, Amiel C. Stimulation by glucagon and PTH of Ca and Mg reabsorption in the superficial distal tubule of the rat kidney. *Pflügers Arch* 1985;403:28–34.

293. Bailly C, Imbert-Teboul M, Roinel N, et al. Isoproterenol increases Ca, Mg, and NaCl reabsorption in mouse thick ascending limb. *Am J Physiol* 1990;258:F1224–F1231.

294. Di Stefano A, Wittner M, Nitschke R, et al. Effects of parathyroid hormone and calcitonin on Na+, Cl−, K+, Mg2+ and Ca2+ transport in cortical and medullary thick ascending limbs of mouse kidney. *Pflügers Arch* 1990;417:161–167.

295. Kang HS, Kerstan D, Dai LJ, et al. Beta-adrenergic agonists stimulate Mg(2+) uptake in mouse distal convoluted tubule cells. *Am J Physiol Renal Physiol* 2000;279:F1116–F1123.

296. Shafik IM, Quamme GA. Early adaptation of renal magnesium reabsorption in response to magnesium restriction. *Am J Physiol* 1989;257:F974–F977.

297. Hebert SC, Brown EM, Harris HW. Role of the Ca(2+)-sensing receptor in divalent mineral ion homeostasis. *J Exp Biol* 1997;200:295–302.

298. Di Stefano A, Roinel N, de Rouffignac C, et al. Transepithelial Ca2+ and Mg2+ transport in the cortical thick ascending limb of Henle's loop of the mouse is a voltage-dependent process. *Ren Physiol Biochem* 1993;16:157–166.

299. Arant BS Jr, Edelmann CM Jr, Nash MA. The renal reabsorption of glucose in the developing canine kidney: a study of glomerulo-tubular balance. *Pediatr Res* 1974;8:638–646.

300. Robillard JE, Sessions C, Kennedy RL, et al. Maturation of the glucose transport process by the fetal kidney. *Pediatr Res* 1978;12:680–684.

301. Roth KS, Hwang SM, Yudkoff M, et al. The ontogeny of sugar transport in kidney. *Pediatr Res* 1978;12:1127–1131.

302. Beck JC, Lipkowitz MS, Abramson RG. Characterization of the fetal glucose transporter in rabbit kidney: comparison with the adult brush border electrogenic Na+-glucose symporter. *J Clin Invest* 1988;82:379–387.

303. You G, Lee WS, Barros EJ, et al. Molecular characteristics of Na(+)-coupled glucose transporters in adult and embryonic rat kidney. *J Biol Chem* 1995;270:29365–29371.

304. Horster M, Lewy JE. Filtration fraction and extraction of PAH during neonatal period in the rat. *Am J Physiol* 1970;219: 1061–1065.

305. Friis C. Postnatal development of renal function in piglets: glomerular filtration rate, clearance of PAH and PAH extraction. *Biol Neonate* 1979;35:180–187.

306. Lopez-Nieto CE, You G, Bush KT, et al. Molecular cloning and characterization of NKT, a gene product related to the organic cation transporter family that is almost exclusively expressed in the kidney. *J Biol Chem* 1997;272:6471–6478.

307. Brodehl J, Gellissen K. Endogenous renal transport of free amino acid in infancy and childhood. *Pediatrics* 1968;42: 395–404.

308. Webber WA, Cairns JA. A comparison of the amino acid concentrating ability of the kidney cortex of newborn and mature rats. *Can J Physiol Pharmacol* 1968;46:165–169.

309. Chesney RW, Jones D, Zelikovic I. Renal amino acid transport: cellular and molecular events from clearance studies to frog eggs. *Pediatr Nephrol* 1993;7:574–584.

310. Roth KS, Hwang SM, London JW, et al. Ontogeny of glycine transport in isolated rat renal tubules. *Am J Physiol* 1977;233: F241–F246.

311. Hwang SM, Serabian MA, Roth KS, et al. l-proline transport by isolated renal tubules from newborn and adult rats. *Pediatr Res* 1983;17:42–46.

312. Segal S, Smith I. Delineation of separate transport systems in rat kidney cortex for l-lysine and l-cystine by developmental patterns. *Biochem Biophys Res Commun* 1969;35:771–777.

313. McCance RA, Widdowson EM. Renal function before birth. *Proc R Soc Lond B Biol Sci* 1953;141:489–497.

314. McCance RA, Stainer MW. The function of the metanephros of foetal rabbits and pigs. *J Physiol* 1960;11:1937–1947.

315. Robillard JE, Matson JR, Sessions C, et al. Developmental aspects of renal tubular reabsorption of water in the lamb fetus. *Pediatr Res* 1979;13:1172–1176.

316. Ross MG, Sherman DJ, Ervin MG, et al. Maternal dehydration-rehydration: fetal plasma and urinary responses. *Am J Physiol* 1988;255:E674–E679.

317. Horne RS, MacIssac RJ, Moritz KM, et al. Effect of arginine vasopressin and parathyroid hormone-related protein on renal function in the ovine foetus. *Clin Exp Pharmacol Physiol* 1993; 20:569–577.

318. Woods LL, Cheung CY, Power GG, et al. Role of arginine vasopressin in fetal renal response to hypertonicity. *Am J Physiol* 1986;251:F156–F163.

319. Lingwood B, Hardy KJ, Horacek I, et al. The effects of antidiuretic hormone on urine flow and composition in the chronically-cannulated ovine fetus. *Q J Exp Physiol Cogn Med Sci* 1978;63:315–330.

320. Strauss J, Daniel SS, James LS. Postnatal adjustment in renal function. *Pediatrics* 1981;68:802–808.

321. Edelmann CM Jr, Barnett HL, Troupkou V. Renal concentrating mechanisms in newborn infants: effect of dietary protein, and water content, role of urea and responsiveness to antidiuretic hormone. *J Clin Invest* 1960;39:1062–1069.

322. Polacek E, Vocel J, Neugebauerova L, et al. The osmotic concentrating ability in healthy infants and children. *Arch Dis Child* 1965;40:291–295.

323. Siga E, Horster MF. Regulation of osmotic water permeability during differentiation of inner medullary collecting duct. *Am J Physiol* 1991;260:F710–F716.

324. Horster MF, Zink H. Functional differentiation of the medullary collecting tubule: influence of vasopressin. *Kidney Int* 1982;22:360–365.

325. Trimble ME. Renal response to solute loading in infant rats: relation to anatomical development. *Am J Physiol* 1970;219: 1089–1097.

326. Edelmann CM Jr, Barnett HL, Stark H. Effect of urea on concentration of urinary nonurea solute in premature infants. *J Appl Physiol* 1966;21:1021–1025.

327. Rane S, Aperia A, Eneroth P, et al. Development of urinary concentrating capacity in weaning rats. *Pediatr Res* 1985;19: 472–475.

328. Horster MF, Gilg A, Lory P. Determinants of axial osmotic gradients in the differentiating counter-current system. *Am J Physiol* 1984;246:F124–F132.

329. Schwartz GJ, Zavilowitz BJ, Radice AD et al. Maturation of aldose reductase expression in the neonatal rat inner medulla. *J Clin Invest* 1992;90:1275–1283.

330. Hadeed AJ, Leake RD, Weitzman RE, et al. Possible mechanisms of high blood levels of vasopressin during the neonatal period. *J Pediatr* 1979;94:805–808.

331. Rees L, Forsling ML, Brook CGD. Vasopressin concentrations in the neonatal period. *Clin Endocrinol* 1980;12:357–362.

332. Leake RD, Weitzman RE, Weinberg JA, et al. Control of vasopressin secretion in the new-born lamb. *Pediatr Res* 1979;13: 257–260.

333. Weitzman RE, Fisher DA, Robillard JE, et al. Arginine vasopressin response to an osmotic stimulus in the fetal sheep. *Pediatr Res* 1978;12:35–38.

334. DeVane GW, Porter JC. An apparent stress-induced release of arginine vasopressin by human neonates. *J Clin Endocrinol Metab* 1980;51:1412–1416.

335. Svenningsen NW, Aronson AS. Postnatal development of renal concentration capacity as estimated by DDAVP-test in normal and asphyxiated neonates. *Biol Neonate* 1974;25:230–241.

336. Rajerison RM, Butlen D, Jard S. Ontogenic development of antidiuretic hormone receptors in rat kidney: comparison of hormonal binding and adenylate cyclase activation. *Mol Cell Endocrinol* 1976;4:271–285.

337. Ostrowski NL, Young WS, Knepper MA, et al. Expression of vasopressin V1a and V2 receptor messenger ribonucleic acid in the liver and kidney of embryonic, developing, and adult rats. *Endocrinology* 1993;133:1849–1859.

338. Bonilla-Felix M, Jiang W. Aquaporin-2 in the immature rat: expression, regulation, and trafficking. *J Am Soc Nephrol* 1997; 8:1502–1509.

339. Schlondorff D, Weber H, Trizna W, et al. Vasopressin responsiveness of renal adenylate cyclase in newborn rats and rabbits. *Am J Physiol* 1978;234:F16–F21.

340. Imbert-Teboul M, Chabardes D, Clique A, et al. Ontogenesis of hormone-dependent adenylate cyclase in isolated rat nephron segments. *Am J Physiol* 1984;247:F316–F325.

341. Gengler WR, Forte LR. Neonatal development of rat kidney adenyl cyclase and phosphodiesterase. *Biochim Biophys Acta* 1972;279:367–372.

342. Kleinman LI. Renal sodium reabsorption during saline loading and distal blockade in newborn dogs. *Am J Physiol* 1975;228: 1403–1408.

343. Museles M, Gaudry CC Jr, Bason WM. Renal anomalies in the newborn found by deep palpation. *Pediatrics* 1971;47:97–100.

344. Sherwood DW, Smith RC, Lemmon RH, et al. Abnormalities of the genitourinary tract discovered by palpation of the abdomen of the newborn. *Pediatrics* 1956;18:782–789.

345. Perlman M, Williams J. Detection of renal anomalies by abdominal palpation in newborn infants. *Br Med J* 1976;2: 347–349.

346. Gillerot Y, Koulischer L. Major malformations of the urinary tract: anatomic and genetic aspects. *Biol Neonate* 1988;53: 186–196.

347. Rubenstein M, Meyer R, Bernstein J. Congenital abnormalities of the urinary system. I. A postmortem survey of developmental anomalies and acquired congenital lesions in a children's hospital. *J Pediatr* 1961;58:356–366.

348. Helin I, Persson PH. Prenatal diagnosis of urinary tract abnormalities by ultrasound. *Pediatrics* 1986;78:879–883.

349. Livera LN, Brookfield DSK, Egginton JA, et al. Antenatal ultrasonography to detect fetal renal abnormalities: a prospective screening programme. *Br Med J* 1989;298:1421–1423.

350. Gunn TR, Mora JD, Pease P. Antenatal diagnosis of urinary tract abnormalities by ultrasonography after 28 weeks' gestation: incidence and outcome. *Am J Obstet Gynecol* 1995;172: 479–486.

351. Kim EK, Song TB. A study on fetal urinary tract anomaly: antenatal ultrasonographic diagnosis and postnatal follow-up. *J Obstet Gynaecol Res* 1996;22:569–573.

352. Fugelseth D, Lindemann R, Sande HA, et al. Prenatal diagnosis of urinary tract anomalies. The value of two ultrasound examinations. *Acta Obstet Gynaecol Scand* 1994;73:290–293.

353. Scott JES, Lee REJ, Hunter EW, et al. Ultrasound screening of newborn urinary tract. *Lancet* 1991;2:338:1571–1573.

354. Rubecz I, Kodela I, Gasztonyi V, et al. Postnatal screening examination of renal developmental anomalies: classical diagnosis, screening of risk group and routine screening. *Orv Hetil* 1991;132:585–589.

355. Steinhart JM, Kuhn JP, Eisenberg B, et al. Ultrasound screening of healthy infants for urinary tract abnormalities. *Pediatrics* 1988;82:609–614.

356. Brion L, Rondia G, Avni FE, et al. Importance of deep abdominal palpation in the perinatal diagnosis of urologic malformations. *Biol Neonate* 1984;46:215–219.

357. Jelen Z. The value of ultrasonography as a screening procedure of the neonatal urinary tract: a survey of 1021 infants. *Int Urol Nephrol* 1993;25:3–10.

358. Scott JE, Renwick M. Urological anomalies in the Northern Region Fetal Abnormality Survey. *Arch Dis Child* 1993;68: 22–26.

359. Roodhooft AM, Birnholz JC, Holmes LB. Familial nature of congenital absence and severe dysgenesis of both kidneys. *N Engl J Med* 1984;310:1341–1345.

360. McPherson E, Carey J, Kramer A, et al. Dominantly inherited renal adysplasia. *Am J Med Genet* 1987;26:863–872.

361. Neave C. Congenital malformation in offspring of diabetics. *Perspect Pediatr Pathol* 1984;8:213–222.

362. Havers W, Majewski F, Olbing H, et al. Anomalies of the kidneys and genitourinary tract in alcohol embryopathy. *J Urol* 1980;124:108–110.

363. Lutiger B, Graham K, Einarson TR, et al. Relationship between gestational cocaine use and pregnancy outcome: a meta-analysis. *Teratology* 1991;44:405–414.

364. Petrikovsky BM, Nardi DA, Rodis JF, et al. Elevated maternal serum alpha-fetoprotein and mild fetal uropathy. *Obstet Gynecol* 1991;78:262–264.

365. Barr M Jr, Cohen MM Jr. ACE inhibitor fetopathy and hypocalvaria: the kidney–skull connection. *Teratology* 1991;44:485–495.

366. Cunniff C, Jones KL, Phillipson J, et al. Oligohydramnios sequence and renal tubular malformation associated with maternal enalapril use. *Am J Obstet Gynecol* 1990;162:187–189.

367. van der Heijden BJ, Carlus C, Narcy F, et al. Persistent anuria, neonatal death, and renal microcystic lesions after prenatal exposure to indomethacin. *Am J Obstet Gynecol* 1994;171:617–623.

368. Thomas IT, Smith DW. Oligohydramnios, cause of the nonrenal features of Potter's syndrome, including pulmonary hypoplasia. *J Pediatr* 1974;84:811–815.

369. Nimrod C, Varela-Gittings F, Machin G, et al. The effect of very prolonged membrane rupture on fetal development. *Am J Obstet Gynecol* 1984;148:540–543.

370. Moessinger AC, Collins MH, Blanc WA, et al. Oligohydramnios-induced lung hypoplasia: the influence of timing and duration in gestation. *Pediatr Res* 1986;20:951–954.

371. Thibeault DW, Beatty EC Jr, Hall RT, et al. Neonatal pulmonary hypoplasia with premature rupture of fetal membranes and oligohydramnios. *J Pediatr* 1985;107:273–277.

372. Khuri FJ, Hardy BE, Churchill BM. Urologic anomalies associated with hypospadias. *Urol Clin North Am* 1981;8:565–571.

373. Bourke WG, Clarke TA, Mathews TG, et al. Isolated single umbilical artery—the case for routine renal screening. *Arch Dis Child* 1993;68:600–601.

374. Lachiewicz AM, Sibley R, Michael AF. Hereditary renal disease and preauricular pits: report of a kindred. *J Pediatr* 1985;106:948–950.

375. Thummala MR, Raju TN, Langenberg P. Isolated single umbilical artery anomaly and the risk for congenital malformations: a meta-analysis. *J Pediatr Surg* 1998;33:580–585.

376. Kohelet D, Arbel E. A prospective search for urinary tract abnormalities in infants with isolated preauricular tags. *Pediatr* 2000;105:e61.

377. Rothe CF, Kim KC. Measuring systolic arterial blood pressure: possible errors from extension tubes or disposable transducer domes. *Crit Care Med* 1980;8:683–689.

378. Low JA, Panagiotopoulos C, Smith JT, et al. Validity of newborn oscillometric blood pressure. *Clin Invest Med* 1995;18:163–167.

379. Kimble KJ, Darnall RA Jr, Yelderman M, et al. An automated oscillometric technique for estimating mean arterial pressure in critically ill newborns. *Anesthesiology* 1981;54:423–425.

380. National High Blood Pressure Education Program Working Group on High Blood Pressure in Children and Adolescents. The Fourth report on the diagnosis, evaluation and treatment of high blood pressure in children and adolescents. National Heart, Lung, and Blood Institute, Bethesda, Maryland.

381. de Swiet M, Peto J, Shinebourne EA. Difference between upper and lower limb blood pressure in neonates using Doppler technique. *Arch Dis Child* 1974;49:734–735.

382. Park MK, Lee D. Normative arm and calf blood pressure values in the newborn. *Pediatrics* 1989;83:240–243.

383. Crapanzano MS, Strong WB, Newman IR, et al. Calf blood pressure: clinical implications and correlations with arm blood pressure in infants and young children. *Pediatrics* 1996;97:220–224.

384. Versmold HT, Kitterman JA, Phibbs RH, et al. Aortic blood pressure during the first 12 hours of life in infants with birth weight 610 to 4,220 grams. *Pediatrics* 1981;67:607–613.

385. Tan KL. Blood pressure in very low birth weight infants in the first 70 days of life. *J Pediatr* 1988;112:266–270.

386. Hegyi T, Carbone MT, Anwar M, et al. Blood pressure ranges in premature infants. I. The first hours of life. *J Pediatr* 1994;124:627–633.

387. Zubrow AB, Hulman S, Kushner H, et al. Determinants of blood pressure in infants admitted to neonatal intensive care units: a prospective multicenter study. *J Perinatol* 1995;15:470–479.

388. Flynn JT. Neonatal hypertension: diagnosis and management. *Pediatr Nephrol* 2000;14:332–341.

389. de Swiet M, Fayers P, Shinebourne EA. Systolic blood pressure in a population of infants in the first year of life: the Brompton study. *Pediatrics* 1980;65:1028–1035.

390. Spahr RC, MacDonald HM, Mueller-Heubach E. Knee–chest position and neonatal oxygenation and blood pressure. *Am J Dis Child* 1981;135:79–80.

391. Sinkin RA, Phillips BL, Adelman RD. Elevation in systemic blood pressure in the neonate during abdominal examination. *Pediatrics* 1985;76:970–972.

392. Gemelli M, Manganaro R, Mami C, et al. Circadian blood pressure pattern in full-term newborn infants. *Biol Neonate* 1989;56:315–323.

393. Zinner SH, Lee YH, Rosner B, et al. Factors affecting blood pressures in newborn infants. *Hypertension* 1980;2(4 Pt 2):99–101.

394. Grotto I, Browner-Elhanan K, Mimouni D, et al. Occurrence of supernumerary nipples in children with kidney and urinary tract malformations. *Pediatr Dermatol* 2001;18:291–294.

395. Scott JES, Hunter EW, Lee REJ, et al. Ultrasound measurement of renal size in newborn infants. *Arch Dis Child* 1990;65:361–364.

396. Longino LA, Martin LW. Abdominal masses in the newborn infant. *Pediatrics* 1958;596–604.

397. Pinto E, Guignard JP. Renal masses in the neonate. *Biol Neonate* 1995;68(3):175–184.

398. Griscom NT, Colodny AH, Rosenberg HK, et al. Diagnostic aspects of neonatal ascites: report of 27 cases. *AJR Am J Roentgenol* 1977;128:961–969.

399. Shaffer SG, Quimiro CL, Anderson JV, et al. Postnatal weight changes in low birth weight infants. *Pediatrics* 1987;79:702–705.

400. Brion LP, Satlin LM, EdelmannCM Jr. In: Avery GB, Fletcher MA, McDonald MG, eds. *Renal disease in neonatology-pathophysiology & management of the newborn*, 5th ed. Lippincott, Williams & Wilkins, 1999:902–973.

401. Bidiwala KS, Lorenz JM, Kleinman LI. Renal function correlates of postnatal diuresis in preterm infants. *Pediatrics* 1988;82:50–58.

402. Lorenz JM, Kleinman LI, Ahmed G, et al. Phases of fluid and electrolyte homeostasis in the extremely low birth weight infant. *Pediatrics* 1995;96:484–489.

403. Ramiro-Tolentino SB, Markarian K, Kleinman L. I. Renal bircarbonate excretion in extremely low birth weight infants. *Pediatrics* 1996;98:256–261.

404. Benitez OA, Benitez M, Stijnen T, et al. Inaccuracy in neonatal measurement of urine concentration with a refractometer. *J Pediatr* 1986;108:613–616.

405. Gouyon JB, Houchan N. Assessment of urine specific gravity by reagent strip in newborn infants. *Pediatr Nephrol* 1993;7:77–78.

406. Coulthard MG, Hey EN. Weight as the best standard for glomerular filtration in the newborn. *Arch Dis Child* 1984;59:373–375.

407. Coulthard MG, Ruddock V. Validation of inulin as a marker for glomerular filtration in preterm babies. *Kidney Int* 1983;23:407–409.

408. Stickle D, Cole B, Hock K, et al. Correlation of plasma concentrations of cystatin C and creatinine to inulin clearance in a pediatric population. *Clin Chem* 1998;44:1334–1338.

409. Schwartz GJ, Feld LG, Langford DJ. A simple estimate of glomerular filtration rate in full term infants during the first year of life. *J Pediatr* 1984;104:849–854.

410. Guignard JP, Drukker A. Why do newborn infants have a high plasma creatinine? *Pediatrics* 1999;103:e49.

411. Gallini F, Maggio L, Romagnoli C, et al. Progression of renal function in preterm neonates with gestational age < or = 32 weeks. *Pediatr Nephrol* 2000;15:119–124.

412. Brion LP, Fleischman AR, Schwartz GJ. Gentamicin interval in newborn infants determined by renal function and postconceptional age. *Pediatr Nephrol* 1991;5:675–679.

413. Koren G, James A, Perlman M. A simple method for the estimation of glomerular filtration rate by gentamicin pharmacokinetics during routine monitoring in the newborn. *Clin Pharmacol Ther* 1985;38:680–685.

414. Kildoo CW, Lin LM, Gabriel MH, et al. Vancomycin pharmacokinetics in infants: relationship to postconceptional age and serum creatinine. *Dev Pharmacol Ther* 1990;14:77–83.

415. Brion L, Fleischman AR, McCarton C, et al. A simple estimate of glomerular filtration rate in low birth weight infants during the first year of life: non invasive assessment of body composition and growth. *J Pediatr* 1986;109:698–707.

416. Oyanagi K, Nakamura K, Sogawa H, et al. A study of urea-synthesizing enzymes in prenatal and postnatal human liver. *Pediatr Res* 1980;14:236–241.

417. Tsukahara H, Hiraoka M, Hori C, et al. Urinary uric acid excretion in term and premature infants. *J Paediatr Child Health* 1996;32:330–332.

418. Bader D, Gozal D, Weinger-Abend M. Neonatal urinary uric acid/creatinine ratio as an additional marker of perinatal asphyxia. *Eur J Pediatr* 1995;154:747–749.

419. Germino GG, Barton NJ, Lamb J, et al. Identification of a locus which shows no genetic recombination with the autosomal dominant polycystic kidney disease gene on chromosome 16. *Am J Hum Genet* 1990;46:925–933.

420. Saris JJ, Breuning MH, Dauwerse HG, et al. Rapid detection of polymorphism near gene for adult polycystic kidney disease. *Lancet* 1990;335:1102–1103.

421. International Polycystic Kidney Disease Consortium. Polycystic kidney disease: the complete structure of the PKD1 gene and its protein. *Cell* 1995;81:289–298.

422. Fossdal R, Bothvarsson M, Asmundsson P, et al. Icelandic families with autosomal dominant polycystic kidney disease: families unlinked to chromosome 16p13.3 revealed by linkage analysis. *Hum Genet* 1993;91:609–613.

423. Kimberling WJ, Kumar S, Gabow PA, et al. Autosomal dominant polycystic kidney disease: localization of the second gene to chromosome 4q13-q23. *Genomics* 1993;18:467–472.

424. Lin JY, Lin JS, Tsai CH. Use of the urine-to-blood carbon dioxide tension gradient as a measurement of impaired distal tubular hydrogen ion secretion among neonates. *J Pediatr* 1995;126:114–117.

425. Aas K. The cellular excretion in the urine of normal newborn infants. *Acta Paediatr* 1961;50:361–370.

426. Kronquist KE, Crandall BF, Tabsh KM. Characterization of fetal urinary proteins at midgestation and term. *Biol Neonate* 1984;46:267–275.

427. Simeoni U. Specific developmental profiles of lysosomal and brush border enzymuria in the human. *Biol Neonate* 1994;65:1–6.

428. Van Oort A, Monnens L, van Munster P. Beta-2-microglobulin clearance, an indicator of renal tubular maturation. *Acta Clin Belg* 1980;35[Suppl 10]:30.

429. Gordon I, Barratt TM. Imaging the kidneys and urinary tract in the neonate with acute renal failure. *Pediatr Nephrol* 1987;1:321–329.

430. Alon U, Brewer WH, Chan JC. Nephrocalcinosis: detection by ultrasonography. *Pediatrics* 1983;71:970–973.

431. Cramer B, Husa L, Pushpanathan C. Nephrocalcinosis in rabbits—correlation of ultrasound, computed tomography, pathology and renal function. *Pediatr Radiol* 1998;28:9–13.

432. Dick P, Shuckett B, Tang B, et al. Observer reliability in grading nephrocalcinosis on ultrasound examinations in children. *Pediatr Radiol* 1999;29:68–72.

433. Schell-Feith EA, Holscher SC, Zonderland HM, et al. Ultrasonographic features of nephrocalcinosis in preterm neonates. *Br J Radiol* 2000;73:1185–1191.

434. Mercado-Deane MG, Beeson JE, John SD. US of renal insufficiency in neonates. *Radiographics* 2002;22:1429–1438.

435. Slovis TL. Pediatric renal anomalies and infections. *Clin Diagn Ultrasound* 1989;24:157–185.

436. Lusiri A, Salinas-Madrigal L, Noguchi A, et al. Renal tubular dysgenesis. *AJR Am J Roentgenol* 1991;157:383–384.

437. Shackelford GD, Kees-Folts D, Cole BR. Imaging the urinary tract. *Clin Perinatol* 1992;19:85–119.

438. Shultz PK, Strife JL, Strife CF, et al. Hyperechoic renal medullary pyramids in infants and children. *Radiology* 1991;181:163–167.

439. Glickstein J, Friedman D, Schacht R, et al. Renal artery Doppler waveforms in neonates with umbilical artery catheters. *Clin Res* 1991;39:669A.

440. Cleary GM, Higgins ST, Merton DA, et al. Developmental changes in renal artery blood flow velocity during the first three weeks of life in preterm neonates. *J Pediatr* 1996;129:251–257.

441. Van Bel F, Guit GL, Schipper J, et al. Indomethacin-induced changes in renal blood flow velocity waveform in premature infants investigated with color Doppler imaging. *J Pediatr* 1991;118:621–626.

442. Gaum LD, Wese FX, Alton DJ, et al. Radiologic investigation of the urinary tract in the neonate with myelomeningocele. *J Urol* 1982;127:510–512.

443. Gordon I, Riccabona M. Investigating the new born kidney-update on imaging techniques. *Semin Neonatol* 2003;8:269–278.

444. Bruyn RD, Gordon I. Postnatal investigation of fetal renal disease. *Prenat Diagn* 2001;21:984–991.

445. Norton KI. New imaging applications in the evaluation of pediatric renal disease. *Curr Opin Pediatr* 2003;15:186–190.

446. Huber A, Heuck A, Scheidler J, et al. Contrast–enhanced MR angiography in patients after renal transplantation. *Eur Radiol* 2001;11:2488–2495.

447. Kullendorff CM, Salmonson EC, Laurin S. Diagnostic cyst puncture of multicystic kidney in neonates. *Acta Radiol* 1990;31:287–289.

448. Edelmann CM Jr, Churg J, Gerber MA, et al. Renal biopsy: indications, technique, and interpretation. In: Edelmann CM Jr, ed. *Pediatric kidney disease*, 2nd ed. Boston: Little, Brown, 1992:499–527.

449. Simon EE. Review: new aspects of acute renal failure. *Am J Med Sci* 1995;310:217–221.

450. Chevalier RL, Campbell F, Brenbridge AG. Prognostic factors in neonatal acute renal failure. *Pediatrics* 1984;74:265–272.

451. Stapleton FB, Jones DP, Green RS. Acute renal failure in neonates: incidence, etiology and outcome. *Pediatr Nephrol* 1987;1:314–320.

452. Norman ME, Asadi FK. A prospective study of acute renal failure in the newborn infant. *Pediatrics* 1979;63:475–479.

453. Hanssens M, Keirse MJNC, Vankelecom F, et al. Fetal and neonatal effects of treatment with angiotensin-converting enzyme inhibitors in pregnancy. *Obstet Gynecol* 1991;78:128–135.

454. Bhatt-Mehta V, Deluga KS. Fetal exposure to lisinopril: neonatal manifestations and management. *Pharmacotherapy* 1993;13:515–518.

455. Grylack L, Medani C, Hultzen C, et al. Non oliguric acute renal failure in the newborn: a prospective evaluation of diagnostic indexes. *Am J Dis Child* 1982;136:518–520.

456. Asfour B, Bruker B, Kehl HG, et al. Renal insufficiency in neonates after cardiac surgery. *Clin Nephrol* 1996;46:59–63.

457. McCrory WW. Congenital malformations causing renal failure in the neonatal period. *Contrib Nephrol* 1979;15:55–66.

458. Arrowsmith JB, Faich GA, Tomita DK, et al. Morbidity and mortality among low birth weight infants exposed to an intravenous vitamin E product, E-Ferol. *Pediatrics* 1989;83:244–249.

459. Tack ED, Perlman JM. Renal failure in sick hypertensive premature infants receiving captopril therapy. *J Pediatr* 1988;112:805–810.

460. Parchoux B, Bourgeois J, Gilly J, et al. Hypertrophic kidneys in utero and neonatal renal failure by diffuse mesangial sclerosis. *Pédiatrie* 1988;43:219–222.

461. Nauta J, de Heer E, Baldwin WM III, et al. Transplacental induction of membranous nephropathy in a neonate. *Pediatr Nephrol* 1990;4:111–116.

462. Ridgen SP, Barratt TM, Dillon MJ, et al. Acute renal failure complicating cardiopulmonary bypass surgery. *Arch Dis Child* 1982;57:425–430.

463. Isenberg G, Racelis D, Oh J, et al. Prevention of ischemic renal damage with prostacyclin. *Mt Sinai J Med* 1982;49:415–417.

464. Schramm L, Heidbreder E, Lukes M, et al. Endotoxin-induced acute renal failure in the rat: effects of urodilatin and diltiazem on renal function. *Clin Nephrol* 1996;46:117–124.

465. Schramm L, Heidbreder E, Lopau K, et al. Influence of nitric oxide on renal function in toxic acute renal failure in the rat. *Miner Electrolyte Metab* 1996;22:168–177.

466. Hammerman MR. New treatments for acute renal failure: growth factors and beyond. *Curr Opin Nephrol Hypertens* 1997;6:7–9.

467. Yoon BH, Lee CM, Kim SW. An abnormal umbilical artery waveform: a strong and independent predictor of adverse perinatal outcome in patients with preeclampsia. *Am J Obstet Gynecol* 1994;171:713–721.

468. Kempley ST, Gamsu HR, Nicolaides KH. Renal artery blood flow velocity in very low birth infants with intrauterine growth retardation. *Arch Dis Child* 1993;68:588–590.

469. Leititis JU, Burghard R, Gordjani N, et al. Effect of a modified fluid therapy on renal function during indomethacin therapy for persistent ductus arteriosus. *Acta Paediatr Scand* 1987;76:789–794.

470. Yeh TF, Wilks A, Singh J, et al. Furosemide prevents the renal side effects of indomethacin in premature infants with patent ductus arteriosus. *J Pediatr* 1982;101:433–437.

471. Romagnoli C, Zecca E, Papacci P, et al. Furosemide does not prevent indomethacin-induced renal side effects in preterm infants. *Clin Pharmacol Ther* 1997;62:181–186.

472. Reinberg Y, Fleming T, Gonzalez R. Renal rupture after the Credé maneuver. *J Pediatr* 1994;124:279–281.

473. Martín-Ancel A, García-Alix A, Cabañas FGF, et al. Multiple organ involvement in perinatal asphyxia. *J Pediatr* 1995;127:786–793.

474. Karlowicz MG, Adelman RD. Nonoliguric and oliguric acute renal failure in asphyxiated term neonates. *Pediatr Nephrol* 1995;9:718–722.

475. Elçioglu Sirin A, Can G, et al. Renal function disorders in newborns with perinatal asphyxia. *Geburtshilfe Frauenheilkd* 1995;55:160–163.

476. Perlman JM, Tack ED. Renal injury in the asphyxiated newborn infant: relationship to neurologic outcome. *J Pediatr* 1988;113:875–879.

477. Roberts DS, Haycock GB, Dalton RN, et al. Prediction of acute renal failure after birth asphyxia. *Arch Dis Child* 1990;65:1021–1028.

478. Kojima T, Kobayashi T, Matsuzaki S, et al. Effects of perinatal asphyxia and myoglobinuria on development of acute, neonatal renal failure. *Arch Dis Child* 1985;60:908–912.

479. Proverbio MR, Di Pietro A, Coletta M. Studio delle modificazioni dell'emodinamica renale in corso di insufficienza renale acuta nel neonato anossico. *Pediatr Med Chir* 1996;18:33–35.

480. Kelly RE, Phillips JD, Foglia RP. Pulmonary edema and fluid mobilization as determinants of the duration of ECMO support. *J Pediatr Surg* 1991;26:1016–1022.

481. Roy BJ, Cornish JD, Clark RH. Venovenous extracorporeal membrane oxygenation affects renal function. *Pediatrics* 1995;95:573–578.

482. Ivey HH. The asphyxiated bladder as a cause of delayed micturition in the newborn. *J Urol* 1978;120:498–499.

483. Giacoia GP, Miranda R, West KI. Measured vs calculated plasma osmolality in infants with very low birth weights. *Am J Dis Child* 1992;146:712–717.

484. Ellis EN, Arnold WC. Use of urinary indexes in renal failure in the newborn. *Am J Dis Child* 1982;136:615–617.

485. Mathew OP, Jones AS, James E, et al. Neonatal renal failure: usefulness of diagnostic indices. *Pediatrics* 1980;65:57–60.

486. Tack ED, Perlman JM, Robson AM. Renal injury in sick newborn infants: a prospective evaluation using urinary b2-microglobulin concentrations. *Pediatrics* 1988;81:432–440.

487. Cole JW, Portman RJ, Lim Y, et al. Urinary β2-microglobulin in full-term newborns: evidence for proximal tubular dysfunction in infants with meconium-stained amniotic fluid. *Pediatrics* 1985;76:958–964.

488. Tsukahara H, Yoshimoto M, Saito M, et al. Assessment of tubular function in neonates using urinary β2-microglobulin. *Pediatr Nephrol* 1990;4:512–514.

489. Chiara A, Chirico G, Comelli L, et al. Increased renal echogenicity in the neonate. *Early Hum Dev* 1990;22:29–37.

490. Avni EF, Spehl-Robberecht M, Lebrun D, et al. Transient acute tubular disease in the newborn: characteristic ultrasound pattern. *Ann Radiol (Paris)* 1983;26:175–182.

491. Dmochowski RR, Crandell SS, Corriere JN Jr. Bladder injury and uroascites from umbilical artery catheterization. *Pediatrics* 1986;77:421–422.

492. Myers BD, Moran SM. Hemodynamically mediated acute renal failure. *N Engl J Med* 1986;314:97–105.

493. Medani CR, Davitt MK, Huntington DF, et al. Acute renal failure in the newborn. *Contrib Nephrol* 1979;15:47–54.

494. Brion LP, Schwartz GJ, Campbell D, et al. Early hyperkalemia in very low birthweight infants in the absence of oliguria. *Arch Dis Child* 1989;64:270–272.

495. Gibbons MD, Horan JJ, Dejter SW. Extracorporeal membrane oxygenation: an adjunct in the management of the neonate with severe respiratory distress and congenital urinary tract anomalies. *J Urol* 1993;150:434–437.

496. Finn WF. Diagnosis and management of acute tubular necrosis. *Med Clin North Am* 1990;74:873–891.

497. Karlowicz MG, Adelman RD. Acute renal failure in the neonate. *Clin Perinatol* 1992;19:139–158.

498. Seri I, Tulassay T, Kiszel J, et al. Cardiovascular response to dopamine in hypotensive preterm neonates with severe hyaline membrane disease. *Eur J Pediatr* 1984;142:3–9.

499. Tulassay T, Seri I, Machay T, et al. Effects of dopamine on renal functions in premature neonates with respiratory distress syndrome. *Int J Pediatr Nephrol* 1983;4:19–23.

500. Prins I, Plotz FB, Uiterwaal C, et al. Low dose dopamine in neonatal and pediatric intensive care: a systematic review. *Intensive Care Med* 2001;27:206–210.

501. Lynch S, Lemley K, Polak M. The effect of dopamine on glomerular filtration rate in normotensive, oliguric premature neonates. *Pediatr Nephrol* 2003;18:649–652.

502. Cuevas L, Yeh TF, et al. The effect of low-dose dopamine infusion on cardiopulmonary and renal status in premature newborns with respiratory distress syndrome. *Am J Dis Child* 1991;145:799–803.

503. DiSessa TG, Leitner M, Ti CC, et al. The cardiovascular effects of dopamine in the severely asphyxiated neonate. *J Pediatr* 1981;99:772–776.

504. Toth-Heyn P, Drukker A, Guignard JP. The stressed neonatal kidney: from pathophysiology to clinical management of neonatal vasomotor nephropathy. *Pediatr Nephrol* 2000;14:227–239.

505. Jenik AG, Ceriani Cernadas JM, Gorenstein A, et al. A randomized, double-blind, placebo-controlled trial of the effects of prophylactic theophylline on renal function in term neonates with perinatal asphyxia. *Pediatrics* 2000;105:E45.

506. Lackmann GM, Mader R, Tollner U. Serumkaliumspiegel bei asphyktischen und gesunden Neugeborenen in den ersten 144 Lebensstunden. *Klin Padiatr* 1991;203:399–402.

507. Shaffer SG, Kilbride HW, Hayen LK, et al. Hyperkalemia in very low birth weight infants. *J Pediatr* 1992;121:275–279.

508. Gaylord MS, Pittman PA, Bartness J, et al. Release of benzalkonium chloride from a heparin-bonded umbilical catheter with resultant factitious hypernatremia and hyperkalemia. *Pediatrics* 1991;87:631–635.

509. Gruskay J, Costarino AT, Polin RA, et al. Nonoliguric hyperkalemia in the premature infant weighing less than 1000 grams. *J Pediatr* 1988;113:381–386.

510. Smith JD, Bia MJ, DeFronzo RA. Clinical disorders of potassium metabolism. In: Arieff AI, DeFronzo RA, eds. *Fluid, electrolyte, and acid–base disorders*, vol 1. New York: Churchill-Livingstone, 1985:413–509.

511. Lui K, Thungappa U, Nair A, et al. Treatment with hypertonic dextrose and insulin in severe hyperkalaemia of immature infants. *Acta Paediatr* 1992;81:213–216.

512. Murdoch IA, Dos Anjos R, Haycock GB. Treatment of hyperkalemia with intravenous salbutamol. *Arch Dis Child* 1991;66:527–528.

513. Kemper MJ, Harps E, Müller-Wiefel DE. Hyperkalemia: therapeutic options in acute and chronic renal failure. *Clin Nephrol* 1996;46:67–69.

514. Malone TA. Glucose and insulin versus cation-exchange resin for the treatment of hyperkalemia in very low birth weight infants. *J Pediatr* 1991;118:121–123.

515. Ohlsson A, Hosking M. Complications following oral administration of exchange resins in extremely low-birth-weight infants. *Eur J Pediatr* 1987;146:571–574.

516. Setzer ES, Ahmed F, Goldberg RN, et al. Exchange transfusion using washed red blood cells reconstituted with fresh-frozen plasma for treatment of severe hyperkalemia in the neonate. *J Pediatr* 1984;104:443–446.

517. Allon M, Shanklin N. Effect of bicarbonate administration on plasma potassium in dialysis patients: interactions with insulin and albuterol. *Am J Kid Dis* 1996;28:508–514.

518. Haycock GB. Management of acute and chronic renal failure. *Semin Neonatol* 2003;8:325–334.

519. Du Plooy WJ, Hay L, Kahler CP, et al. The dose-related hyper- and-hypokalaemic effects of salbutamol and its arrhythmogenic potential. *Br J Pharmacol* 1994;111:73–76.

520. Mandelberg A, Krupnik Z, Houri S, et al. Salbutamol metered-dose inhaler with spacer for hyperkalemia: how fast? How safe? *Chest* 1999;115:617–622.

521. Singh BS, Sadiq HF, Noguchi A, et al. Efficacy of albuterol inhalation in treatment of hyperkalemia in premature neonates. *J Pediatr* 2002;141:16–20.

522. Ngugi NN, McLigeyo SO, Kayima JK. Treatment of hyperkalaemia by altering the transcellular gradient in patients with renal failure: effect of various therapeutic approaches. *East Afr Med J* 1997;74:503–509.

523. Inaba S, Nibu K, Takano H, et al. Potassium-adsorption filter for RBC transfusion: a phase III clinical trial. *Transfusion* 2000;40:1469–1474.

524. Hu P-S, Su B-H, Peng C-T, et al. Glucose and insulin infusion versus Kayexalate for the early treatment of no-oliguric hyperkalemia in very–low birth-weight infants. *Acta Paediatr Tw* 1999;40:314–318.

525. Sell LL, Cullen ML, Whittlesey GC, et al. Experience with renal failure during extracorporeal membrane oxygenation: treatment with continuous hemofiltration. *J Pediatr Surg* 1987;22:600–602.

526. Llach F, Felsenfeld AJ, Haussler MR. The pathophysiology of altered calcium metabolism in rhabdomyolysis-induced acute renal failure: interactions of parathyroid hormone, 25-hydroxy-cholecalciferol and 1,25-dihydroxycholecalciferol. *N Engl J Med* 1981;305:117–123.

527. Patel R, Savage A. Symptomatic hypomagnesemia associated with gentamicin therapy. *Nephron* 1979;23:50–52.

528. Arieff AI, Massry SG. Calcium metabolism of brain in acute renal failure. Effects of uremia, hemodialysis, and parathyroid hormone. *J Clin Invest* 1974;53:387–392.

529. Zaramella P, Zorzi C, Pavanello L, et al. The prognostic significance of acute neonatal renal failure. *Child Nephrol Urol* 1991;11:15–19.

530. Kekömaki M. Uremic catabolism in a neonate: reversal by parenteral nutrition. *J Pediatr Surg* 1981;16:35–41.

531. Coulthard MG, Vernon B. Managing acute renal failure in very low birthweight infants. *Arch Dis Child* 1995;73:F187–F192

532. Matthews DE, West KW, Rescorla FJ, et al. Peritoneal dialysis in the first 60 days of life. *J Pediatr Surg* 1990;25:110–115.

533. Mattoo TK, Ahmad GS. Peritoneal dialysis in neonates after major abdominal surgery. *Am J Nephrol* 1994;14:6–8

534. Nash MA, Russo JC. Neonatal lactic acidosis and renal failure: the role of peritoneal dialysis. *J Pediatr* 1977;91:101–105.

535. Bishof NA, Welch TR, Strife CF, et al. Continuous hemodiafiltration in children. *Pediatrics* 1990;85:819–823.

536. Zobel G, Ring E, Müller W. Continuous arteriovenous hemofiltration in premature infants. *Crit Care Med* 1989;17:534–536.

537. Coulthard MG, Sharp J. Haemodialysis and ultrafiltration in babies weighing under 1000 g. *Arch Dis Child* 1995;73:F162–F165.

538. Blowey DL, McFarland K, Alon U, et al. Peritoneal dialysis in the neonatal period: outcome data. *J Perinatol* 1993;13:59–64.

539. Stark H, Geiger R. Renal tubular dysfunction following vascular accidents of the kidney in the newborn period. *J Pediatr* 1973;83:933–940.

540. Callan NA, Blakemore K, Park J, et al. Fetal genitourinary tract anomalies: evaluation, operative correction, and follow-up. *Obstet Gynecol* 1990;75:67–74.

541. Glick PL, Harrison MR, Golbus MS, et al. Management of the fetus with congenital hydronephrosis. II. Prognostic criteria and selection for treatment. *J Pediatr Surg* 1985;20:376–387.

542. Elder JS, O'Grady JP, Ashmead G, et al. Evaluation of fetal renal function: unreliability of fetal urinary electrolytes. *J Urol* 1990;144:574–578.

543. Nicolini U, Fisk NM, Rodeck CH, et al. Fetal urine biochemistry: an index of renal maturation and dysfunction. *Br J Obstet Gynaecol* 1992;99:46–50.

543a. Muller F, Parvy P, Dommergues M, et al. Acides aminés libres de l'urine foetale et pronostic de la fonction rénale dans les uropathies obstructives bilatérales. *Ann Biol Clin* 1994;52:651–655.

544. Pohl M, Bhatnagar V, Mendoza SA, et al. Toward an etiological classification of developmental disorders of the kidney and upper urinary tract. *Kidney Int* 2002;61:10–19.

545. Bensman A, Baudon JJ, Jablonski JP, et al. Uropathies diagnosed in the neonatal period: symptomatology and course. *Acta Paediatr Scand* 1980;69:499–503.

546. Bernstein J, Barajas L. Renal tubular dysgenesis: evidence of abnormality in the renin-angiotensin system. *J Am Soc Nephrol* 1994;5:224–227.

547. Landing BH, Ang SM, Herta N, et al. Labeled lectin studies of renal tubular dysgenesis and renal tubular atrophy of postnatal renal ischemia and end-stage kidney disease. *Pediatr Pathol* 1994;14:87–99.

548. Oberg KC, Pestaner JP, Bielamowicz L, et al. Renal tubular dysgenesis in twin-twin transfusion syndrome. *Pediatr Dev Pathol* 1999;2:25–32.

549. Robinson R. The fetal origins of adult disease. *BMJ* 2001;322:375–376.

550. Battista MC, Oligny LL, St-Louis J, et al. Intrauterine growth restriction in rats is associated with hypertension and renal dysfunction in adulthood. *Am J Physiol Endocrinol* Metab 2002;283:E124–E131.

551. Kaplan BS, Restaino I, Raval DS, et al. Renal failure in the neonate associated with in utero exposure to non-steroidal anti-inflammatory agents. *Pediatr Nephrol* 1994;8:700–704.

552. Sawdy R, Lye S, Fisk N, et al. A double blind randomised study of fetal side effects during and after the short-term maternal administration of indomethacin, sulindac and nimesulide for treatment of preterm labor. *Am J Obstet Gynecol* 2003;188:1046–1051.

553. Durante D, Jones D, Spitzer R. Neonatal renal arterial embolism syndrome. *J Pediatr* 1976;89:978–981.

554. Malin SW, Baumgart S, Rosenberg HK, et al. Nonsurgical management of obstructive aortic thrombosis complicated by renovascular hypertension in the neonate. *J Pediatr* 1985;106:630–634.

555. Payne RM, Martin TC, Bower RJ, et al. Management and follow-up of arterial thrombosis in the neonatal period. *J Pediatr* 1989;114:853–858.

556. Kennedy LA, Drummond WH, Knight ME, et al. Successful treatment of neonatal aortic thrombosis with tissue plasminogen activator. *J Pediatr* 1990;116:798–801.

557. Seibert JJ, Northington FJ, Miers JF, et al. Aortic thrombosis after umbilical artery catheterization in neonates: prevalence of complications on long-term follow-up. *AJR Am J Roentgenol* 1991;156:567–569.

558. Ellis D, Kaye RD, Bontempo FA. Aortic and renal artery thrombosis in a neonate: recovery with thrombolytic therapy. *Pediatr Nephrol* 1997;11:641–644.

559. Umbilical Artery Catheter Trial Study Group. Relationship of intraventricular hemorrhage or death with the level of umbilical artery catheter placement: a multicenter randomized clinical trial. *Pediatrics* 1992;90:881–887.

560. Schmidt B, Andrew M. Neonatal thrombotic disease: prevention, diagnosis, and management. *J Pediatr* 1988;113:407–410.

561. Pfluger T, Czekalla R, Hundt C, et al. MR angiography versus color Doppler sonography in the evaluation of renal vessels and the inferior vena cava in abdominal masses of pediatric patients *AJR Am J Roentgenol* 1999;173:103–108.

562. Caplan MS, Cohn RA, Langman CB, et al. Favorable outcome of neonatal aortic thrombosis and renovascular hypertension. *J Pediatr* 1989;115:291–295.

563. Vailas GN, Brouillette RT, Scott JP, et al. Neonatal aortic thrombosis: recent experience. *J Pediatr* 1986;109:101–108.

564. Seibert JJ, Northington FJ, Miers JF, et al. Aortic thrombosis after umbilical artery catheterization in neonates: prevalence of complications on long-term follow-up. *AJR Am J Roentgenol* 1991;156:567–569.

565. Adelman RD. Long-term follow-up of neonatal renovascular hypertension. *Pediatr Nephrol* 1987;1:35–41.

566. Rasoulpour M, McLean RH. Renal venous thrombosis in neonates. Initial and follow-up abnormalities. *Am J Dis Child* 1980;134:276–279.

567. Lam AH, Warren PS. Ultrasonographic diagnosis of neonatal renal venous thrombosis. *Ann Radiol* 1981;24:7–12.

568. Corrigan JJ Jr, Jeter MA. Tissue-type plasminogen activator, plasminogen activator inhibitor, and histidine-rich glycoproteins in stressed human newborns. *Pediatrics* 1992;89:43–46.

569. Evans DJ, Silverman M, Bowley NB. Congenital hypertension due to unilateral renal vein thrombosis. *Arch Dis Child* 1981;56:306–308.

570. Mocan H, Beattie TJ, Murphy AV. Renal venous thrombosis in infancy: long-term follow-up. *Pediatr Nephrol* 1991;5:45–49.

571. Weinschenk N, Pelidis M, Fiascone J. Combination thrombolytic and anticoagulant therapy for bilateral renal vein thrombosis in a premature infant. *Am J Perinatol* 2001;18:293–297.

572. Clark AGB, Saunders A, Bewick M, et al. Neonatal inferior vena cava and renal venous thrombosis treated by thrombectomy and nephrectomy. *Arch Dis Child* 1985;60:1076–1077.

573. Bromberg WD, Firlit CF. Fibrinolytic therapy for renal vein thrombosis in the child. *J Urol* 1990;143:86–88.

574. Kurnetz R, Bernstein J. Neonatal blood loss and hematuria. *J Pediatr* 1974;84:452–455.

575. Anand SK, Northway JD, Smith JA. Neonatal renal papillary and cortical necrosis. *Am J Dis Child* 1977;131:773–777.

576. Van Reempts PJ, Boven KJ, Spitaels SE, et al. Idiopathic arterial calcification of infancy. *Calcif Tissue Int* 1991;48:1–6.

577. Jenkins EA, Hallett RJ, Hull RG. Lesch-Nyhan syndrome presenting with renal insufficiency in infancy and transient neonatal hypothyroidism. *Br J Rheumatol* 1994;33:392–396.

578. Terzi F, Assael BM, Claris-Appiani A, et al. Increased sodium requirement following early postnatal surgical correction of congenital uropathies in infants. *Pediatr Nephrol* 1990;4:581–584.

579. Lindemann R. Congenital renal tubular dysfunction associated with maternal sniffing of organic solvents. *Acta Paediatr Scand* 1991;80:882–884.

580. Brown WJ, Buist NR, Gipson HT, et al. Fatal benzyl alcohol poisoning in a neonatal intensive care unit. *Lancet* 1982;1:1250.

581. Gershanik J, Boeckler B, Enlsey H, et al. The gasping syndrome and benzyl alcohol poisoning. *N Engl J Med* 1982;307:1384–1388.

582. Klotman PE, Boatman JE, Volpp BD, et al. Captopril enhances aminoglycoside nephrotoxicity in potassium-depleted rats. *Kidney Int* 1985;28:118–127.

583. Cronin RE, Bulger RE, Southern P, et al. Natural history of aminoglycoside nephrotoxicity in the dog. *J Lab Clin Med* 1980;95:463–474.

584. Cojocel C, Dociu N, Ceacmacudis E, et al. Nephrotoxic effects of aminoglycoside treatment on renal protein reabsorption and accumulation. *Nephron* 1984;37:113–119.

585. Cojocel C, Hook JB. Aminoglycoside nephrotoxicity. *Trends Pharmacol Sci* 1983;4:174–179.

586. Giapros VI, Andronikou S, Cholevas VI, et al. Renal function in premature infants during aminoglycoside therapy. *Pediatr Nephrol* 1995;9:163–166.

587. Heimann G. Renal toxicity of aminoglycosides in the neonatal period. *Pediatr Pharmacol* 1983;3:251–257.

588. Russo JC, Adelman RD. Gentamicin-induced Fanconi syndrome. *J Pediatr* 1980;96:151–153.

589. Casteels-Van Daele M, Corbeel L, Van de Casseye W, et al. Gentamicin-induced Fanconi syndrome. *J Pediatr* 1980;97:507–508.

590. Rajchgot P, Prober CG, Soldin S, et al. Aminoglycoside-related nephrotoxicity in the premature newborn. *Clin Pharmacol Ther* 1984;35:394–401.

591. Ylitalo P, Mörsky P, Parviainen MT, et al. Nephrotoxicity of tobramycin: value of examining various protein and enzyme markers. *Methods Find Exp Clin Pharmacol* 1991;13:281–287.

592. Ibrahim S, Langhendries JP, Bernard A. Urinary phospholipids excretion in neonates treated with amikacin. *Int J Clin Pharm Res* 1994;14:149–156.

593. Nahata MC. Lack of nephrotoxicity in pediatric patients receiving concurrent vancomycin and aminoglycoside therapy. *Chemotherapy* 1987;33:302–304.

594. Swinney VR, Rudd CC. Nephrotoxicity of vancomycin-gentamicin therapy in pediatric patients. *J Pediatr* 1987;110:497–498.

595. Goren MP, Baker DK Jr, Shenep JL. Vancomycin does not enhance amikacin-induced tubular nephrotoxicity in children. *Pediatr Infect Dis J* 1989;8:278–282.

596. Glover ML, Shaffer CL, Rubino CM, et al. A Multicenter evaluation of Gentamicin therapy in neonatal intensive care unit. *Pharmacotherapy* 2001;21:7–10.

597. Avent ML, Kinney JS, Istre GR, et al. Gentamicin and Tobramicin in neonates: comparison of a new extended dosing Interval regimen with a traditional multiple daily dosing regimens. *Am J Perinatol* 2002;19:413–420.

598. Jackson GL, Sendelbach DM, Stehel EK, et al. Association of hypocalcemia with a change in gentamicin administration in neonates. *Pediatr Nephrol* 2003;18:653–656.

599. Van Overmeire B, Smets K, Lecoutere D, et al. A comparison of ibuprofen and indomethacin for closure of patent ductus arteriosus. *N Engl J Med* 2000;343:674–681.

600. Ohlsson A, Walia R, Shah S. *Ibuprofen for the treatment of patent ductus arteriosus in preterm and/or low birth weight infants (Cochrane Review).* In: The Cochrane Library, Issue 3, 2003. Oxford: Update Software.

601. Bhat R, Vidyasagar D, Vadapalli M, et al. Disposition of indomethacin in preterm infants. *J Pediatr* 1979;95:313–316.

602. Seyberth HW, Rascher W, Hackenthal R, et al. Effect of prolonged indomethacin therapy on renal function and selected vasoactive hormones in very-low-birth-weight infants with symptomatic patent ductus arteriosus. *J Pediatr* 1983;103:979–984.

603. Hammerman C, Aramburo MJ. Prolonged indomethacin therapy for the prevention of recurrences of patent ductus arteriosus. *J Pediatr* 1990;117:771–776.

604. vd Heijden AJ, Provoost AP, Grose W, et al. Renal functional impairment in preterm neonates related to intrauterine indomethacin exposure. *Pediatr Res* 1988;24:644–648.

605. John EG, Vasan U, Hastreiter AR, et al. Intravenous indomethacin and changes of renal function in premature infants with patent ductus arteriosus. *Pediatr Pharmacol* 1984;4:11–19.

606. Hammerman C, Zaia W, Wu HH. Severe hyponatremia with indomethacin: a more serious toxicity than previously realized? *Dev Pharmacol Ther* 1985;8:260–267.

607. Ojala R, Houhala A, Harmoinen A, et al. Renal follow up of premature infants with and without indomethacin exposure. *Arch Dis Child Fetal Neonatal Ed* 2001;84:F28–F33.

608. Christmann V, Liem KD, Semmekrot BA, et al. Changes in cerebral, renal and mesenteric blood flow velocity during continuous and bolus infusion of indomethacin. *Acta Paediatr* 2002;91:369–370.

609. Barrington K, Brion LP. *Dopamine versus no treatment to prevent renal dysfunction in indomethacin-treated preterm newborn infants (Cochrane Review).* In: The Cochrane Library, Issue 3, 2003. Oxford: Update Software.

610. Brion LP, Campbell DE. *Furosemide for prevention of morbidity in indomethacin-treated infants with patent ductus arteriosus (Cochrane Review).* In: The Cochrane Library, Issue 3, 2003. Oxford: Update Software.

611. Heyman SN, Clark BA, Kaiser N, et al. In-vivo and in-vitro studies on the effect of amphotericin B on endothelin release. *J Antimicrob Chemother* 1992;29:69–77.

612. Joly V, Dromer F, Barge J, et al. Incorporation of amphotericin B (AMB) into liposomes alters AMB-induced acute nephrotoxicity in rabbits. *J Pharmacol Exp Ther* 1989;251:311–316.

613. Reynolds ES, Tomkiewicz ZM, Dammin GJ. The renal lesion related to amphotericin B treatment for coccidioidomycosis. *Med Clin North Am* 1963;47:1149–1154.

614. Baley JE, Meyers C, Kliegman RM, et al. Pharmacokinetics, outcome of treatment, and toxic effects of amphotericin B and 5-fluorocytosine in neonates. *J Pediatr* 1990;116:791–797.

615. Leenders AC, de Marie S. The use of lipid formulations of amphotericin B for systemic fungal infections. *Leukemia* 1996;10:1570–1575.

616. Rubin SI, Krawiec DR, Gelberg H, et al. Nephrotoxicity of amphotericin B in dogs: a comparison of two methods of administration. *Can J Vet Res* 1989;53:23–28.

617. Baley JE, Kliegman RM, Fanaroff AA. Disseminated fungal infections in very-low-birth-weight infants: therapeutic toxicity. *Pediatrics* 1984;73:153–157.

618. Vadiei K, Lopez-Berestein G, Luke DR. Disposition and toxicity of amphotericin-B in the hyperlipidemic Zucker rat model. *Int J Obes* 1990;14:465–472.

619. Lopez-Berestein G, Bodey GP, Frankel LS, et al. Treatment of hepatosplenic candidiasis with liposomal-amphotericin B. *J Clin Oncol* 1987;5:310–317.

620. Friedlich PS, Steinberg I, Fujitani A. Renal tolerance with the use of intralipid-amphotericin B in low-birth-weight neonates. *Am J Perinatol* 1997;14:377–383.

621. Juster-Reicher A, Leibovitz E, Linder N, et al. Liposomal amphotericin B (AmBisome) in the treatment of neonatal candidiasis in very low birth weight infants. *Infection* 2000;28: 223–226.

622. Weitkamp JH, Poets CF, Sievers R, et al. Candida infection in very low birth-weight infants: outcome and nephrotoxicity of treatment with liposomal amphotericin B (AmBisome). *Infection* 1998;26:11–15.

623. Bianchetti MG, Roduit C, Oetliker OH. Acyclovir-induced renal failure: course and risk factors. *Pediatr Nephrol* 1991;5: 238–239.

624. Englund JA, Fletcher CV, Balfour HH. Acyclovir therapy in neonates. *J Pediatr* 1991;119:129–135.

625. Berdon WE, Schwartz RH, Becker J, et al. Tamm-Horsfall proteinuria: its relationship to prolonged nephrogram in infants and children and to renal failure following intravenous urography in adults with multiple myeloma. *Radiology* 1969;92: 714–722.

626. Sleasman JE, Stapleton FB, Tonkin II. Marked uricosuric effect of contrast media during cardiac catheterization in children. *Pediatr Res* 1986;17:219A(abst).

627. Wood EG, Bunchman TE, Lynch RE. Captopril-induced reversible acute renal failure in an infant with coarctation of the aorta. *Pediatrics* 1991;88:816–818.

628. Perlman JM, Volpe JJ. Neurologic complications of Captopril treatment of neonatal hypertension. *Pediatrics* 1989;83:47–52.

629. Ward MM. Factors predictive of acute renal failure in rhabdomyolysis. *Arch Intern Med* 1988;148:1553–1557.

630. Martin W, Villani GM, Jothianandan D, et al. Selective blockade of endothelium-dependent and glyceryl trinitrate-induced relaxation by hemoglobin and by methylene blue in the rabbit aorta. *J Pharmacol Exp Ther* 1985;232:708–716.

631. Haftel AJ, Eichner J, Haling J, et al. Myoglobinuric renal failure in a newborn infant. *J Pediatr* 1978;93:1015–1016.

632. Turner MC, Naumburg EG. Acute renal failure in the neonate: two fatal cases due to group B streptococci with rhabdomyolysis. *Clin Pediatr* 1987;26:189–190.

633. Kagen LJ, Christian CL. Immunologic measurements of myoglobin in human adult and fetal skeletal muscle. *Am J Physiol* 1966;211:656–660.

634. Hogg RJ, Furth S, Lemley KV, et al. National Kidney Foundation's Kidney Disease Outcomes Quality Initiative. National Kidney Foundation's Kidney Disease Outcomes Quality Initiative clinical practice guidelines for chronic kidney disease in children and adolescents: evaluation, classification, and stratification. *Pediatrics* 2003;111:1416–1421.

635. Potter DE, Holliday MA, Piel CF, et al. Treatment of end stage renal disease in children: a 15-year experience. *Kidney Int* 1980;18:103–109.

636. Pistor K, Olbing H, Schärer K. Children with chronic renal failure in the Federal Republic of Germany. I. Epidemiology, modes of treatment, survival. *Clin Nephrol* 1985;23:272–277.

637. Foreman JW, Chan JCM. Chronic renal failure in infants and children. *J Pediatr* 1988;113:793–800.

638. Pediatric ESRD. In: *U.S. Renal Data System, USRDS 2002 Annual Data Report: Atlas of End-Stage Renal Disease in the United States*. National Institutes of Health, National Institute of Diabetes and Digestive and Kidney Diseases: Bethesda, MD, 2002: 121–134.

639. *North American Pediatric Transplant Cooperative Study.* 2003 Annual Report. Rockville, MD: The EMMES Corporation, 2003.

640. Coulthard MG, Crosier J. Outcome of reaching end stage renal failure in children under 2 years of age. *Arch Dis Child* 2002;87:511–517.

641. Hanna JD, Foreman JW, Chan JCM. Chronic renal insufficiency in infants and children. *Clin Pediatr* 1991;30:365–384.

642. Tapper D, Watkins S, Burns M, et al. Comprehensive management of renal failure in infants. *Arch Surg* 1990;125:1276–1281.

643. Harmon WE. Nephrology forum. Treatment of children with chronic renal failure. *Kidney Int* 1995;47:951–961.

644. Chan JCM, Williams DM, Roth KS. Kidney failure in infants and children. *Pediatr Rev* 2002;23:47–60.

645. Rees L. Management of the infant with end-stage renal failure. *Nephrol Dial Transplant* 2002;17:1564–1567.

646. Verrina E, Zacchello G, Perfumo F, et al. Clinical experience in the treatment of infants with chronic peritoneal dialysis. *Adv Perit Dial* 1995;11:281–284.

647. Ledermann SE, Scanes ME, Fernando ON, et al. Long-term outcome of peritoneal dialysis in infants. *J Pediatr* 2000;136: 24–29.

648. Ellis EN, Pearson D, Champion B, et al. Outcome of infants on chronic peritoneal dialysis. *Adv Perit Dial* 1995;11:266–269.

649. Neu AM, Warady BA. Dialysis and renal transplantation in infants with irreversible renal failure. *Adv Ren Replace Ther* 1996;3:48–59.

650. Shooter M, Watson A. The ethics of withholding and withdrawing dialysis therapy in infants. *Pediatr Nephrol* 2000;14: 347–351.

651. Warady BA, Belden B, Kohaut E. Neurodevelopmental outcome of children initiating peritoneal dialysis in early infancy. *Pediatr Nephrol* 1999;13:759–765.

652. Humar A, Nevins TE, Remucal M, et al. Kidney transplantation in children younger than 1 year using cyclosporine immunosuppression. *Ann Surg* 1998;228:421–428.

653. Bunchman TE. Infant dialysis: the future is now. *J Pediatr* 2000;136:1–2.

654. So SK, Chang PN, Najarian JS, et al. Growth and development in infants after renal transplantation. *J Pediatr* 1986;110: 343–350.

655. Davis ID, Chang PN, Nevins TE. Successful renal transplantation accelerates development in young uremic infants. *Pediatrics* 1990;86:594–600.

656. Najarian JS, Almond PS, Mauer M, et al. Renal transplantation in the first year of life: the treatment of choice for infants with end-stage renal disease. *J Am Soc Nephrol* 1992;2:S228–S233.

657. National Heart, Lung and Blood Institute Task Force on Blood Pressure Control in Children. *Report of the Second Task Force on blood pressure control in children—1987. National Institutes of Health.* January, 1987.

658. Al-Aweel I, Pursley DM, Rubin LP, et al. Variations in prevalence of hypotension, hypertension and vasopressor use in NICUs. *J Perinatol* 2001;12:272–278.

659. Inglefinger JR. Hypertension in the first year of life. In: Inglefinger JR, ed. *Pediatric hypertension.* Philadelphia, WB Saunders, 1982:229–240.

660. Abman SH, Warady BA, Lum GM, et al. Systemic hypertension in infants with bronchopulmonary dysplasia. *J Pediatr* 1984; 104:929–931.

661. Buchi KF, Siegler RL. Hypertension in the first month of life. *J Hypertens* 1986;4:525–528.

662. Skalina MEL, Kliegman RM, Fanaroff AA. Epidemiology and management of severe symptomatic neonatal hypertension. *Am J Perinatol* 1986;3:235–239.

663. Singh HP, Hurley RM, Myers TF. Neonatal hypertension: incidence and risk factors. *Am J Hypertens* 1992;5:51–55.

664. Adelman RD, Merten D, Vogel J, et al. Nonsurgical management of renovascular hypertension in the neonate. *Pediatrics* 1978;62:71–76.

665. American Academy of Pediatrics Committee on Fetus and Newborn. Routine evaluation of blood pressure, hematocrit and glucose in newborns. *Pediatrics* 1993;92:474–476.

666. Friedman AL, Hustead VA. Hypertension in babies following discharge from a neonatal intensive care unit: a 3-year follow-up. *Pediatr Nephrol* 1987;1:30–34.

667. Ford KT, Teplick SK, Clark RE. Renal artery embolism causing neonatal hypertension. *Radiology* 1974;113:169–170.

668. Bauer SB, Feldman SM, Gellis SS, et al. Neonatal hypertension: a complication of umbilical-artery catheterization. *N Engl J Med* 1975;293:1032–1033.

669. Merten DF, Vogel JM, Adelman RD, et al. Renovascular hypertension as a complication of umbilical arterial catheterization. *Radiology* 1978;126:751–757.

670. Goetzman BW, Stadalnik RC, Bogren HG, et al. Thrombotic complications of umbilical artery catheters: a clinical and radiographic study. *Pediatrics* 1975;56:374–379.

671. Wesström G, Finnström O, Stenport G. Umbilical artery catheterization in newborns. I. Thrombosis in relation to catheter type and position. *Acta Paediatr Scand* 1979;68:575–581.

672. Stork EK, Carlo WA, Kliegman RM, et al. Neonatal hypertension appears unrelated to aortic catheter position. *Pediatr Res* 1984;18:321A(abst).

673. Durante D, Jones D, Spitzer R. Neonatal arterial embolism syndrome. *J Pediatr* 1976; 89:978–981.

674. Barrington KJ. *Umbilical artery catheters in the newborn: effects of position of the catheter tip (Cochrane Review)*. In: The Cochrane Library, Issue 4. Oxford: Update Software, 2001.

675. Angella JJ, Sommer LS, Poole C, et al. Neonatal hypertension associated with renal artery hypoplasia. *Pediatrics* 1968;41: 524–526.

676. Wilson DI, Appleton RE, Coulthard MG, et al. Fetal and infantile hypertension caused by unilateral renal arterial disease. *Arch Dis Child* 1990;65:881–884.

677. Schmidt DM, Rambo ON Jr. Segmental intimal hyperplasia of the abdominal aorta and renal arteries producing hypertension in an infant. *Am J Clin Pathol* 1965;44:546–555.

678. Castello Girona F, Yeste Fernandez D, Porta Ribera R, et al. Renovascular hypertension due to unilateral renal artery stenosis with hypokalemic alkalosis, the hyponatraemic syndrome and reversible hyperechogenicity of the contralateral kidney. A study of two infants. *An Esp Pediatr* 1996;45:49–52.

679. Milner LS, Heitner R, Thomson PD, et al. Hypertension as the major problem of idiopathic arterial calcification of infancy. *J Pediatr* 1984;105:934–938.

680. Van Dyck M, Proesmans W, Van Hollebeke E, et al. Idiopathic infantile arterial calcification with cardiac, renal and central nervous system involvement. *Eur J Pediatr* 1989;148:374–377.

681. Meradji M, de Villeneuve VH, Huber J, et al. Idiopathic infantile arterial calcification in siblings: radiologic diagnosis and successful treatment. *J Pediatr* 1978;92:401–405.

682. Van Reempts PJ, Boven KJ, Spitaels SE, et al. Idiopathic arterial calcification of infancy. *Calcif Tissue Int* 1991;48:1–6.

683. Ciana G, Colonna F, Forleo V, et al. Idiopathic arterial calcification of infancy: effectiveness of prostaglandin infusion for treatment of secondary hypertension refractory to conventional therapy: case report. *Pediatr Cardiol* 1997;18:67–71.

684. Nordborg C, Kyllerman M, Conradi N, et al. Early-infantile galactosialidosis with multiple brain infarctions: morphological, neuropathological and neurochemical findings. *Acta Neuropathol* 1997;93:24–33.

685. Takahashi G, Nakano H, Ueda K, et al. Neonatal renovascular hypertension: haematoma within the renal arterial wall: a case report. *Z Kinderchir* 1984;39:341–343.

686. Evans DJ, Silverman M, Bowley NB. Congenital hypertension due to unilateral renal vein thrombosis. *Arch Dis Child* 1981;56:306–308.

687. Davis RS, Manning JA, Branch GL, et al. Renovascular hypertension secondary to hydronephrosis in a solitary kidney. *J Urol* 1973;110:724–727.

688. Bensman A, Neuenschwander S, Lavollay B, et al. Hypertension artérielle et compression du pédicule vasculaire rénal par un hématome de la surrénale chez un nouveau-né. *Ann Pediatr (Paris)* 1982;29:670.

689. Patel MR, Mooppan MM, Kim H. Subcapsular urinoma: unusual form of "page kidney" in newborn. *Urology* 1984;23: 585–587.

690. Kim ES, Caitai JM, Tu J, et al. Congenital abdominal aortic aneurysm causing renovascular hypertension, cardiomyopathy and death in a 19-day-old neonate. *J Pediatr Surg* 2001;36: 1445–1449.

691. Sheftel DN, Hustead V, Friedman A. Hypertension screening in the follow-up of premature infants. *Pediatrics* 1983;71: 763–766.

692. Alagappan A, Malloy MH. Systemic hypertension in very low-birth weight infants with bronchopulmonary dysplasia: incidence and risk factors. *Am J Perinatol* 1998;15:3–8.

693. Anderson AH, Warady BA, Daily DK, et al. Systemic hypertension in infants with severe bronchopulmonary dysplasia: associated clinical factors. *Am J Perinatol* 1993;10:190–193.

694. Ferrara TB, Couser RJ, Hoekstra RE. Side effects and long-term follow-up of corticosteroid therapy in very low birthweight infants with bronchopulmonary dysplasia. *J Perinatol* 1990;10: 137–142.

695. Cole BR, Conley SB, Stapleton FB. Polycystic kidney disease in the first year of life. *J Pediatr* 1987;111:693–699.

696. Tokunaka S, Takamura T, Osanai H, et al. Severe hypertension in an infant with unilateral hypoplastic kidney. *Urology* 1987;29:618–620.

697. Munoz AI, Baralt JF, Melendez MT. Arterial hypertension in infants with hydronephrosis: report of six cases. *Am J Dis Child* 1977;131:38–40.

698. Zerres K, Rudnik-Schöneborn S, Deget F, et al. Autosomal recessive polycystic kidney disease in 115 children: clinical presentation, course and influence of gender. *Acta Paediatr* 1996; 85:437–435.

699. Fick GM, Johnson AM, Strain JD, et al. Characteristics of very early onset autosomal dominant polycystic kidney disease. *J Am Soc Nephrol* 1993;3:1863–1870.

700. Guay-Woodford LM, Desmond RA. Autosomal recessive polycystic kidney disease: the clinical experience in North America. *Pediatrics* 2003;111:1072–1080.

701. Susskind MR, Kim KS, King LR. Hypertension and multicystic kidney. *Urology* 1989;34:362–366.

702. Angermeier KW, Kay R, Levin H. Hypertension as a complication of multicystic dysplastic kidney. *Urology* 1992;39: 55–58.

703. Husmann DA. Renal dysplasia: the risks and consequences of leaving dysplastic tissue in situ. *Urology* 1998;52:533–536.

704. Liapis H, Doshi RH, Watson MA, et al. Reduced renin expression and altered gene transcript profiles in multicytic dysplastic kidneys. *J Urol* 2002;168:1816–1820.

705. Gilboa N, Urizar RE. Severe hypertension in newborn after pyeloplasty of hydronephrotic kidney. *Urology* 1983;22: 179–182.

706. Oliveira EA, Diniz JS, Rabelo EA, et al. Primary megaureter detected by prenatal ultrasonography: conservative management and prolonged follow-up. *Urol Nephrol* 2000;32:13–18.

707. Cadnapaphornchai P, Aisenbrey G, McDonald KM, et al. Prostaglandin-mediated hyperemia and renin-mediated hypertension during acute ureteral obstruction. *Prostaglandins* 1978;16:965–971.

708. Riehle RA Jr, Vaughan ED Jr. Renin participation in hypertension associated with unilateral hydronephrosis. *J Urol* 1981; 126:243–246.

709. Wilson BJ, Flynn JT. Familial, atypical hemolytic uremic syndrome in a premature infant. *Pediatr Nephrol* 1998;12:782–784.

710. Vania A, Tucciarone L, Mazzeo D, et al. Liddle's syndrome: a 14-year follow-up of the youngest diagnosed case. *Pediatr Nephrol* 1997;11:7–11.

711. Assadi FK, Kimura RE, Subramanian U, et al. Liddle syndrome in a newborn infant. *Pediatr Nephrol* 2002;17:609–611.

712. Field ML, Roy S 3rd, Stapleton FB. Low-renin hypertension in young infants. *Am J Dis Child* 1985;139:823–825.

713. Dluhy RG, Anderson B, Harlin B, et al. Glucocorticoid-remediable aldosteronism is associated with severe hypertension in early childhood. *J Pediatr* 2001;138:715–720.

714. Snyder PM, Price MP, McDonald FJ, et al. Mechanism by which Liddle's syndrome mutations increase activity of a human epithelial Na+ channel. *Cell* 1995;83:969–978.

715. Shimkets RA, Lifton RP, Canessa CM. The activity of the epithelial sodium channel is regulated by clathrin-mediated endocytosis. *J Biol Chem* 1997;272:25537–25541.

716. Hansson JH, Nelson-Williams C, Suzuki H, et al. Hypertension caused by a truncated epithelial sodium channel gamma subunit: genetic heterogeneity of Liddle syndrome. *Nat Genet* 1995;11:76–82.

717. Lifton RP. Genetic determinants of human hypertension. *Proc Natl Acad Sci USA* 1995;92:8545–8551.

718. Lifton RP, Dluhy RG, Powers M, et al. Hereditary hypertension caused by chimeric gene duplications and ectopic expression of aldosterone synthase. *Nat Genet* 1992;2:66–74.

719. Gereda JE, Bonilla-Felix M, Kalil B, et al. Neonatal presentation of Gordon syndrome. *J Pediatr* 1996;129:615–617.

720. Wilson FH, Disse-Nicodeme S, Choate KA, et al. Human hypertension caused by mutations in WNK kinases. *Science* 2001;293:1107–1112.

721. Disse-Nicodeme S, Achard JM, Desitter I, et al. A new locus on chromosome 12p13.3 for pseudohypoaldosteronism type II, an autosomal dominant form of hypertension. *Am J Hum Genet* 2000;67:302–310.

722. Higginbottom MC, Griswold WR, Jones KL, et al: The Cockayne syndrome: an evaluation of hypertension and studies of renal pathology. *Pediatrics* 1979;64:929–934.

723. Beekman RH. Coarctation of the aorta. In: Emmanouilides GC, Riemenschneider TA, Allen HD, et al, eds. *Moss and Adams' heart disease in infants, children and adolescents: including the fetus and young adult*, 5th ed. Baltimore, MD: Williams & Wilkins, 1995:1111–1133.

724. Arar MY, Hogg RJ, Arant BS, et al. Etiology of sustained hypertension in children in the southwestern United States. *Pediatr Nephrol* 1994;8:186–189.

725. O'Sullivan JJ, Derrick G, Darnell R. Prevalence of hypertension in children after early repair of coarctation of the aorta: a cohort study using casual and 24 hour blood pressure measurement. *Heart* 2002;88:163–166.

726. Mimouni M, Kaufman H, Roitman A, et al. Hypertension in a neonate with 11 beta-hydroxylase deficiency. *Eur J Pediatr* 1985;143:231–233.

727. White PC. Inherited forms of mineralocorticoid hypertension. *Hypertens* 1996;28:927–936.

728. Pozzan GB, Armanini D, Cecchetto G, et al. Hypertensive cardiomegaly caused by an aldosterone-secreting adenoma in a newborn. *J Endocrinol Invest* 1997;20:86–89.

729. Schonwetter BS, Libber SM, Jones D Jr, et al. Hypertension in neonatal hyperthyroidism. *Am J Dis Child* 1983;137:954–955.

730. Chan HS, Cheng MY, Mancer K, et al. Congenital mesoblastic nephroma: a clinicoradiologic study of 17 cases representing the pathologic spectrum of the disease. *J Pediatr* 1987;111:64–70.

731. Malone PS, Duffy PG, Ransley PG, et al. Congenital mesoblastic nephroma, renin production and hypertension. *J Pediatr Surg* 1989;24:599–600.

732. Weinblatt ME, Heisel MA, Siegel SE. Hypertension in children with neurogenic tumors. *Pediatrics* 1983;71:947–951.

733. Steinmetz JC. Neonatal hypertension and cardiomegaly associated with a congenital neuroblastoma. *Pediatr Pathol* 1989;9:577–582.

734. Haberkern CM, Coles PG, Morray JP, et al. Intraoperative hypertension during surgical excision of neuroblastoma: case report and review of 20 years' experience. *Anesth Analg* 1992;75:854–858.

735. Perlman JM, Volpe JJ. Seizures in the premature infant: effects on cerebral blood flow velocity, intracranial pressure and arterial blood pressure. *J Pediatr* 1983;102:288–293.

736. Smets K, Vanhaesebrouck P. Dexamethasone associated systemic hypertension in low birth weight babies with chronic lung disease. *Eur J Pediatr* 1996;155:573–575.

737. Stark AR, Carlo WA, Tyson JE, et al. Adverse effects of early dexamethasone treatment in extremely-low-birth-weight infants. *N Engl J Med* 2001;344:95–101.

738. Bancalari E, Gerhardt T, Feller R, et al. Muscle relaxation during IPPV in prematures with RDS. *Pediatr Res* 1980;14:590.

739. Greenough A, Gamsu HR, Greenall F. Investigation of the effects of paralysis by pancuronium on heart rate variability, blood pressure and fluid balance. *Acta Paediatr Scand* 1989;78:829–834.

740. Cabal LA, Siassi B, Artal R, et al. Cardiovascular and catecholamine changes after administration of pancuronium in distressed neonates. *Pediatrics* 1985;75:284–287.

741. Sell LL, Cullen ML, Lerner GR, et al. Hypertension during extracorporeal membrane oxygenation: cause, effect, and management. *Surgery* 1987;102:724–730.

742. Boedy RF, Goldberg AK, Howell CG Jr, et al. Incidence of hypertension in infants on extracorporeal membrane oxygenation. *J Pediatr Surg* 1990;25:258–261.

743. Roy BJ, Cornish JD, Clark RH. Venovenous extracorporeal membrane oxygenation affects renal function. *Pediatrics* 1995;95:573–578.

744. Becker JA, Short BL, Martin GR. Cardiovascular complications adversely affect survival during extracorporeal membrane oxygenation. *Crit Care Med* 1998;26:1582–1586.

745. Tobias JD, Pietsch JB, Lynch A. Nicardipine to control mean arterial pressure during extracorporeal membrane oxygenation. *Paediatr Anaesth* 1996;6:57–60.

746. Flynn JT, Mottes TA, Brophy PB, et al. Intravenous nicardipine for treatment of severe hypertension in children. *J Pediatr* 2001;139:38–43.

747. McBride BF, White CM, Campbell M, et al. Nicardipine to control neonatal hypertension during extracorporeal membrane oxygen support. *Annals Pharmacother* 2003;37:667–670.

748. Adelman RD, Sherman MP. Hypertension in the neonate following closure of abdominal wall defects. *J Pediatr* 1980;97:642–644.

749. Husmann DA, McLorie GA, Churchill BM. Hypertension following primary bladder closure for vesical exstrophy. *J Pediatr Surg* 1993;28:239–241.

750. Guignard JP, Gouyon JB, Adelman RD. Arterial hypertension in the newborn infant. *Biol Neonate* 1989;55:77–83.

751. Rasoulpour M, Marinelli KA. Systemic hypertension. *Clin Perinatol* 1992;19:121–137.

752. Baetz-Greenwalt B, Debaz B, Kumar ML. Bladder fungus ball: a reversible cause of neonatal obstructive uropathy. *Pediatrics* 1988;81:826–829.

753. Deal JE, Barratt TM, Dillon MJ. Management of hypertensive emergencies. *Arch Dis Child* 1992;67:1089–1092.

754. Adelman RD, Coppo R, Dillon MJ. The emergency management of severe hypertension. *Pediatr Nephrol* 2000;14:422–427.

755. Gouyon JB, Geneste B, Semama DS, et al. Intravenous nicardipine in hypertensive preterm infants. *Arch Dis Child* 1997;76:F126–F127.

756. Milou C, Debuche-Benouachkou V, Semama DS, et al. Intravenous nicardipine as a first-line antihypertensive drug in neonates. *Intensive Care Med* 2000;26:956–958.

757. Linakis JG, Lacouture PG, Woolf A. Monitoring cyanide and thiocyanate concentrations during infusion of sodium nitroprusside in children. *Pediatr Cardiol* 1991;12:214–218.

758. Wells TG, Bunchman TE, Kearns GL. Treatment of neonatal hypertension with enalaprilat. *J Pediatr* 1990;117:664–667.

759. Schilder JL, Van den Anker JN. Use of enalapril in neonatal hypertension. *Acta Paediatr* 1995;84:1426–1428.

760. Dutta S, Narang A. Enalapril-induced acute renal failure in a newborn infant. *Pediatr Nephrol* 2003;18:570–572.

761. Perlman JM, Volpe JJ. Neurologic complications of captopril treatment of neonatal hypertension. *Pediatrics* 1989;83:47–52.

762. Johnson CE, Jacobson PA, Song MH. Isradipine therapy in hypertensive pediatric patients. *Ann Pharmacother* 1997;31:704–707.

763. Flynn JT, Warnick SJ. Isradipine treatment of hypertension in children: a single-center experience. *Pediatr Nephrol* 2002;17:748–753.

764. Flynn JT, Smoyer WE, Bunchman TE. Treatment of hypertensive children with amlodipine. *Am J Hypertens* 2000;13:1061–1066.

765. MacDonald JL, Johnson CE, Jacobson P. Stability of isradipine in an extemporaneously compounded oral liquid. *Am J Hosp Pharm* 1994;51:2409–2411.

766. Nahata MC, Morosco RS, Hipple TF. Stability of amlodipine besylate in two liquid dosage forms. *J Am Pharm Assoc* 1999;39:375–377.

767. Hendren WH, Kim SH, Herrin JT, et al. Surgically correctable hypertension of renal origin in childhood. *Am J Surg* 1982;143:432–442.

768. Bendel-Stenzel M, Najarian JS, Sinaiko AR. Renal artery stenosis: long-term medical management before surgery. *Pediatr Nephrol* 1995;10:147–151.

769. Webb NJA, Lewis MA, Bruce J, et al. Unilateral multicystic dysplastic kidney: the case for nephrectomy. *Arch Dis Child* 1997;76:31–34.

770. Seibert JJ, Northington FJ, Miers JF, et al. Aortic thrombosis after umbilical artery catheterization in neonates: prevalence of complications on long-term follow-up. *AJR Am J Roentgenol* 1991;156:567–569.

771. Adelman RD. Long-term follow-up of neonatal renovascular hypertension. *Pediatr Nephrol* 1987;1:35–41.

772. Caplan MS, Cohn RA, Langman CB, et al. Favorable outcome of neonatal aortic thrombosis and renovascular hypertension. *J Pediatr* 1989;115:291–295.

773. Emery EF, Greenough A. Blood pressure levels at follow-up of infants with and without chronic lung disease. *J Perinat Med* 1993;21:377–383.

774. Roy S, Dillon MJ, Trompeter RS, et al. Autosomal recessive polycystic kidney disease: long-term outcome of neonatal survivors. *Pediatr Nephrol* 1997;11:302–306.

775. Perlman JM, Moore V, Siegel MJ, et al. Is chloride depletion an important contributing cause of death in infants with bronchopulmonary dysplasia? *Pediatrics* 1986;77:212–216.

776. Cannon PJ, Heinemann HO, Albert MS, et al. "Contraction" alkalosis after diuresis of edematous patients with ethacrynic acid. *Ann Intern Med* 1965;62:979–990.

777. Loon NR, Wilcox CS, Kanthanatana S, et al. Metabolic alkalosis during furosemide infusion in man: roles of volume contraction and acid excretion. *Kidney Int* 1987;31:208(abst).

778. Segar JL, Robillard JE, Johnson KJ, et al. Addition of metolazone to overcome tolerance to furosemide in infants with bronchopulmonary dysplasia. *J Pediatr* 1992;120:966–973.

779. Mirochnick MH, Miceli JJ, Kramer PA, et al. Renal response to furosemide in very low birth weight infants during chronic administration. *Dev Pharmacol Ther* 1990;15:1–7.

780. Brion LP, Primhak RA, Ambrosio-Perez I. Diuretics acting on the distal renal tubule for preterm infants with (or developing) chronic lung disease. *Cochrane Database Syst Rev* 2002;(1): CD001817.

781. Hoffman DJ, Gerdes JS, Abbasi S. Pulmonary function and electrolyte balance following spironolactone treatment in preterm infants with chronic lung disease: a double-blind, placebo-controlled, randomized trial. *J Perinatol* 2000;20:41–45.

782. Gower PE, Husband P, Coleman JC, et al. Urinary infection in two selected neonatal populations. *Arch Dis Child* 1970;45: 259–263.

783. Edelmann CM Jr, Ogwo JE, Fine BP, et al. The prevalence of bacteriuria in full-term and premature newborn infants. *J Pediatr* 1973;82:125–132.

784. Drew JH, Acton CM. Radiological findings in newborn infants with urinary infection. *Arch Dis Child* 1976;51:628–630.

785. Maherzi M, Guignard JP, Torrado A. Urinary tract infection in high-risk newborn infants. *Pediatrics* 1978;62:521–523.

786. Wiswell TE, Hachey WE. Urinary tract infections and the uncircumcised state: an update. *Clin Pediatr* 1993;32:130–134.

787. Olusanya O, Owa JA, Olusanya OI. The prevalence of bacteriuria among high risk neonates in Nigeria. *Acta Paediatr Scand* 1989;78:94–99.

788. Vilanova Juanola JM, Canos Molinos J, Rosell Arnold E, et al. Urinary tract infection in the newborn infant. *An Esp Pediatr* 1989;31:105–109.

789. Wiswell TE, Miller GM, Gelston HM, et al. Effect of circumcision status on periurethral bacterial flora during the first year of life. *J Pediatr* 1988;113:442–446.

790. Lerman SE, Liao JC. Neonatal circumcision. *Pediatr Clin North Am* 2001;48:1539–1557.

791. Cohen HA, Drucker MM, Vainer S, et al. Postcircumcision urinary tract infection. *Clin Pediatr* 1992;31:322–324.

792. Bauer S, Eliakim A, Pomeranz A, et al. Urinary tract infection in very low birth weight preterm infants. *Pediatr Infect Dis J* 2003;22:426–429.

793. Phillips JR, Karlowicz MG. Prevalence of Candida species in hospital-acquired urinary tract infections in a neonatal intensive care unit. *Pediatr Infect Dis J* 1997;16:190–194.

794. Fernandez Escribano A, Garcia Meseguer C, Pastor Abascal I, et al. Neonatal pelvic ectasia. *An Esp Pediatr* 1989;31:570–574.

795. Ehrlich O, Brem AS. A prospective comparison of urinary tract infections in patients treated with either clean intermittent catheterization or urinary diversion. *Pediatrics* 1982;70: 665–669.

796. Neumann CG, Pryles CV. Pyelonephritis in infants and children. *Am J Dis Child* 1962;104:215–219.

797. Moraga Llop FA, del Alcázar Muñoz R, Casado Toda M, et al. Jaundice associated with urinary infection in the first three months of life: study of 66 cases. *An Esp Pediatr* 1980;13:5–16.

798. Crain EF, Gershel JC. Urinary tract infections in febrile infants younger than 8 weeks of age. *Pediatrics* 1990;86:363–367.

799. Krober MS, Bass JW, Powell JM, et al. Bacterial and viral pathogens causing fever in infants less than 3 months old. *Am J Dis Child* 1985;139:889–892.

800. Pappu LD, Purohit DM, Bradford BF, et al. Primary renal candidiasis in two preterm neonates: report of cases and review of the literature on renal candidiasis in infancy. *Am J Dis Child* 1984;138:923–926.

801. Newman CGH, O'Neill P, Parker A. Pyuria in infancy, and the role of suprapubic aspiration of urine in diagnosis of infection of urinary tract. *Br Med J* 1967;2:277–279.

802. Bonadio WA. Urine culturing technique in febrile infants. *Pediatr Emerg Care* 1987;3:75–78.

803. Visser VE, Hall RT. Urine culture in the evaluation of suspected neonatal sepsis. *J Pediatr* 1979;94:635–638.

804. DiGeronimo RJ. Lack of efficacy of the urine culture as part of the initial sepsis workup of suspected neonatal sepsis. *Pediatr Infect Dis J* 1992;11:764–766.

805. Nelson JD, Peters PC. Suprapubic aspiration of urine in premature and term infants. *Pediatrics* 1965;36:132–134.

806. Schrag SJ, Zywicki S, Farley MM, et al. Group B streptococcal disease in the era of intrapartum antibiotic prophylaxis. *N Engl J Med* 2000;342:15–20.

807. Phillips JR, Karlowicz MG. Prevalence of Candida species in hospital-acquired urinary tract infections in a neonatal intensive care unit. *Pediatr Infect Dis J* 1997;16:190–194.

808. Vaid YN, Lebowitz RL. Urosepsis in infants with vesicoureteral reflux masquerading as the salt-losing type of congenital adrenal hyperplasia. *Pediatr Radiol* 1989;19:548–550.

809. Luk G, Riggs D, Luque M. Severe methemoglobinemia in a 3-week-old infant with a urinary tract infection. *Crit Care Med* 1991;19:1325–1327.

810. Wiswell TE, Geschke DW. Risks from circumcision during the first month of life compared with those for uncircumcised boys. *Pediatrics* 1989;83:1011–1015.

811. Ginsburg CM, McCracken GH Jr. Urinary tract infections in young infants. *Pediatrics* 1982;69:409–412.

812. Goldman M, Barr J, Bistritzer T. Urinary tract infection following ritual Jewish circumcision. *Isr J Med Sci* 1996;32:1098–1102.

813. Crawford DB, Rasoulpour M, Dhawan VM, et al. Renal carbuncle in a neonate with congenital nephrotic syndrome. *J Pediatr* 1978;93:78–80.

814. Walker KM, Coyer WF. Suprarenal abscess due to group B streptococcus. *J Pediatr* 1979;94:970–971.

815. Wang SF, Huang FY, Chiu NC, et al. Urinary tract infection in infants less than 2 months of age. *Acta Paediatr Sin* 1994;35: 294–300.

816. Edwards D, Normand ICS, Prescod N, et al. Disappearance of vesicoureteral reflux during long-term prophylaxis of urinary tract infection in children. *Br Med J* 1977;2:285–288.

817. Munoz AI, Baralt JF, Melendez MT. Arterial hypertension in infants with hydronephrosis: report of six cases. *Am J Dis Child* 1977;131:38–40.

818. Yadin O, Gradus Ben-Ezer D, Golan A, et al. Survival of a premature neonate with obstructive anuria due to Candida: the role of early sonographic diagnosis and antimycotic treatment. *Eur J Pediatr* 1988;147:653–655.

819. Tung KT, MacDonald LM, Smith JC. Neonatal systemic candidiasis diagnosed by ultrasound. *Acta Radiol* 1990;31:293–295.

820. Hellerstein S, Duggan E, Welchert E, et al. Serum C-reactive protein and the site of urinary tract infections. *J Pediatr* 1982;100:21–25.

821. Johnson CE, Shurin PA, Marchant CD, et al. Identification of children requiring radiologic evaluation for urinary tract infection. *Pediatr Infect Dis* 1985;4:656–663.

822. Pylkkänen J, Vilska J, Koskimies O. The value of level diagnosis of childhood urinary tract infection in predicting renal injury. *Acta Paediatr Scand* 1981;70:879–883.

823. Rickwood AM, Carthy HM, McKendrick T, et al. Current imaging of childhood urinary tract infections: prospective survey. *Br Med J* 1992;304:663–665.

824. Dremsek PA, Gindl K, Voitl P, et al. Renal pyelectasis in fetuses and neonates: diagnostic value of renal pelvis diameter in pre- and postnatal sonographic screening. *AJR Am J Roentgenol* 1997;168:1017–1019.

825. Haberlik A. Detection of low-grade vesicoureteral reflux in children by color Doppler imaging mode. *Pediatr Surg Int* 1997;12:38–43.

826. Hoberman A, Charron M, Hickey R, et al. Imaging studies after a first febrile urinary tract infection in young children. *N Engl J Med* 2003;348:195–202.

827. Stapleton FB. Imaging studies for childhood urinary infections. *N Engl J Med* 2003;16:348:251–252.

828. Hiraoka M, Kasuga K, Hori C, et al. Ultrasonic indicators of ureteric reflux in the newborn. *Lancet* 1994;343:519–520.

829. Gleeson FV, Gordon I. Imaging in urinary tract infection. *Arch Dis Child* 1991;66:1282–1283.

830. Rushton HG, Majd M, Chandra R, et al. Evaluation of 99-technetium-dimercapto-succinic acid renal scans in experimental acute pyelonephritis in piglets. *J Urol* 1988;140: 1169–1174.

831. Verber IG, Meller ST. Serial 99mTc dimercaptosuccinic acid (DMSA) scans after urinary infections presenting before the age of 5 years. *Arch Dis Child* 1989;64:1533–1537.

832. Rossleigh MA, Wilson MJ, Rosenberg AR, et al. DMSA studies in infants under one year of age. *Contrib Nephrol* 1990;79: 166–169.

833. Ash JM, Antico VF, Gilday DL, et al. Special considerations in the pediatric use of radionuclides for kidney studies. *Semin Nucl Med* 1982;12:345–369.

834. Eliakim A, Dolfin T, Korsetz A, et al. Urinary tract infection in premature infants: the role of imaging studies and prophylactic therapy. *J Perinatol* 1997;17:305–308.

835. Rodríguez-Soriano J, Vallo A, Oliveros R. Transient pseudohypoaldosteronism secondary to obstructive uropathy in infancy. *J Pediatr* 1983;103:375–380.

836. Constantopoulos A, Thomaidou L, Loupa H, et al. Successful response of severe neonatal gram-negative infection to treatment with aztreonam. *Chemotherapy* 1989;35[Suppl 1]:101–105.

837. Feld LG. Urinary tract infections in childhood: definition, pathogenesis, diagnosis, and management. *Pharmacotherapy* 1991;11:326–335.

838. Zhanel GG, Harding GK, Guay DR. Asymptomatic bacteriuria: which patients should be treated? *Arch Intern Med* 1990;150:1389–1396.

839. Leung AK, Robson WL. Urinary tract infection in infancy and childhood. *Adv Pediatr* 1991;38:257–285.

840. Wettergreen B, Hellstrom M, Stokland E, et al. Six year follow up of infants with bacteriuria on screening. *Br Med J* 1990;13:845–848.

841. Dore B, Irani J, Istin A, et al. Vesicorenal reflux in children under age 2: indications and results of surgery. *J Urol (Paris)* 1990;96:365–371.

842. Rehan VK, Davidson DC. Neonatal renal candidal bezoar. *Arch Dis Child* 1992;67:63–64.

843. Matsumoto AH, Dejter SW Jr, Barth KH, et al. Percutaneous nephrostomy drainage in the management of neonatal anuria secondary to renal candidiasis. *J Pediatr Surg* 1990;25:1295–1297.

844. Rickwood AMK, Reiner I. Urinary stone formation in children with prenatally diagnosed uropathies. *Br J Urol* 1991;68:541–542.

845. Naoumis A, Dumas R, Belon C, et al. La lithiase urinaire de l'enfant. Enquête étiologique. *Arch Fr Pédiatr* 1989;46:347–349.

846. Royer P, Lévy M. La lithiase urinaire du nourrisson. *Acq Méd Récent* 1969:51–59.

847. Arant BS Jr, Sotelo-Avila C, Bernstein J. Segmental "hypoplasia" of the kidney (Ask-Upmark). *J Pediatr* 1979;95:931–939.

848. Welch TR, Nogrady MB, Outerbridge EW. Roentgenologic sequelae of neonatal septicemia and urinary tract infection. *Am J Roentgenol Radium Ther Nucl Med* 1973;118:28–38.

849. Holland NH, Jackson EC, Kazee M, et al. Relation of urinary tract infection and vesicoureteral reflux to scars: follow-up of thirty-eight patients. *J Pediatr* 1990;116:S65–S71.

850. Majd M, Rushton HG, Jantausch BG, et al. Relationship among vesicoureteral reflux, P-fimbriated Escherichia coli, and acute pyelonephritis in children with febrile urinary tract infection. *J Pediatr* 1991;119:578–585.

851. Arnold AJ, Brownless SM, Carty HM, et al. Detection of renal scarring by DMSA scanning—an experimental study. *J Pediatr Surg* 1990;25:391–393.

852. American Academy of Pediatrics–Circumcision policy statement. *Pediatr* 1999;103:686–693.

853. Joseph DB, Bauer SB, Colodney AH, et al. Clean, intermittent catheterization of infants with neurogenic bladder. *Pediatrics* 1989;84:78–82.

854. Kasabian NG, Bauer SB, Dyro FM, et al. The prophylactic value of clean intermittent catheterization and anticholinergic medication in newborns and infants with myelodysplasia at risk of developing urinary tract deterioration. *Am J Dis Child* 1992;146:840–843.

855. Wheeler D, Vimalachandra D, Hodson EM. Antibiotics and surgery for vesicoureteric reflux: a meta-analysis of randomised controlled trials. *Arch Dis Child* 2003;88:688–694.

856. Hellerstein S, Nickell E. Prophylactic antibiotics in children at risk for urinary tract infection. *Pediatr Nephrol* 2002;17:506–510.

857. Upadhyay J, McLorie GA, Bolduc S, et al. Natural history of neonatal reflux associated with prenatal hydronephrosis: long-term results of a prospective study. *J Urol* 2003;169:1837–1841.

858. Scriver CR, Beaudet AL, Sly WS, et al, eds. *The metabolic and molecular basis of inherited disease*. New York: McGraw-Hill, 1995.

859. Sargent JD, Stukel TA, Kresel J, et al. Normal values for random urinary calcium to creatinine ratios in infancy. *J Pediatr* 1993;123:393–397.

860. Nishiyama S, Tomoeda S, Inoue F, et al. Self-limited neonatal familial hyperparathyroidism associated with hypercalciuria and renal tubular acidosis in three siblings. *J Pediatr* 1990;86:421–427.

861. Pearce SH, Williamson C, Kifor O, et al. A familial syndrome of hypocalcemia with hypercalciuria due to mutations in the calcium-sensing receptor. *N Engl J Med* 1996;335:1115–1122.

862. Hufnagle KG, Khan SN, Penn D, et al. Renal calcifications: a complication of long-term furosemide therapy in preterm infants. *Pediatrics* 1982;70:360–363.

863. Jacinto JS, Modanlou HD, Crade M, et al. Renal calcification incidence in very low birth weight infants. *Pediatrics* 1988;88:31–35.

864. Noe HN, Bryant JF, Roy S 3rd, et al. Urolithiasis in pre-term neonates associated with furosemide therapy. *J Urol* 1984;132:93–94.

865. Short A, Cooke RWI. The incidence of renal calcification in preterm infants. *Arch Dis Child* 1991;66:412–417.

866. Woolfield N, Haslam R, Le Quesne G, et al. Ultrasound diagnosis of nephrocalcinosis in preterm infants. *Arch Dis Child* 1988;63:86–88.

867. Saarela T, Vaarala A, Lanning P, et al. Incidence, ultrasonic patterns and resolution of nephrocalcinosis in very low birth weight infants. *Acta Paediatr* 1999;88:655–670.

868. Coe FL, Bushinsky DA. Pathophysiology of hypercalciuria. *Am J Physiol* 1984;16:F1–F13.

869. Rowe JC, Goetz CA, Carey DE, et al. Achievement of in utero retention of calcium and phosphorus accompanied by high calcium excretion in very low birth weight infants fed a fortified formula. *J Pediatr* 1987;110:581–585.

870. Senterre J, Salle B. Renal aspects of calcium and phosphorus metabolism in preterm infants. *Biol Neonate* 1988;53:220–229.

871. Chessex P, Pineault M, Zebiche H, et al. Calciuria in parenterally fed preterm infants: role of phosphorus intake. *J Pediatr* 1985;107:794–796.

872. Ezzedeen F, Adelman RD, Ahlfors CE. Renal calcification in preterm infants: pathophysiology and long-term sequelae. *J Pediatr* 1988;113:532–539.

873. Atkinson SA, Shah JK, McGee C, et al. Mineral excretion in premature infants receiving various diuretic therapies. *J Pediatr* 1988;113:540–545.

874. Fischer AF, Parker BR, Stevenson DK. Nephrolithiasis following in utero diuretic exposure: an unusual case. *Pediatrics* 1988;81:712–714.

875. Brickman AS, Massry SG, Coburn JW. Changes in serum and urinary calcium during treatment with hydrochlorothiazide: studies on mechanisms. *J Clin Invest* 1972;51:945–954.

876. Costanzo LS, Windhager EE. Calcium and sodium transport by the distal convoluted tubule of the rat. *Am J Physiol* 1978;235:F492–F506.

877. Berkelhammer CH, Wood RJ, Sitrin MD. Acetate and hypercalciuria during total parenteral nutrition. *Am J Clin Nutr* 1988;48:1482–1489.

878. Narendra A, White MP, Rolton HA, et al. Nephrocalcinosis in preterm babies. *Arch Dis Child Fetal Neonatal Ed* 2001;85:F207–F213.

879. Campfield T, Braden G, Flynn-Valone P, et al. Urinary oxalate excretion in premature infants: effect of human milk versus formula feeding. *Pediatrics* 1994;94:674–678.

880. Hoppe B, Hesse A, Neuhaus T, et al. Urinary saturation and nephrocalcinosis in preterm infants: effect of parenteral nutrition. *Arch Dis Child* 1993;69:299–303.

881. Downing GJ, Egelhoff JC, Daily DK, et al. Kidney function in very low birth weight infants with furosemide-related renal calcifications at ages 1 to 2 years. *J Pediatr* 1992;120:599–604.

882. Leppla D, Browne R, Hill K, et al. Effect of amiloride with or without hydrochlorothiazide on urinary calcium and saturation of calcium salts. *J Clin Endocrinol Metab* 1983;57:920–924.

883. Watts RWE. Alanine glyoxylate aminotransferase deficiency: biochemical and molecular genetic lessons from the study of a human disease. *Adv Enzyme Regul* 1992;32:309–327.

884. Danpure CJ, Purdue PE, Fryer P, et al. Enzymological and mutational analysis of a complex primary hyperoxaluria type 1 phenotype involving alanine:glyoxylate aminotransferase peroxisome-to-mitochondrion mistargeting and intraperoxisomal aggregation. *Am J Hum Genet* 1993;53:417–432.

885. Takada Y, Kaneko N, Esumi H, et al. Human peroxisomal L-alanine:glyoxylate aminotransferase. Evolutionary loss of a mitochondrial targeting signal by point mutation of the initiation codon. *Biochem J* 1990;268:517–520.

886. Danpure CJ. Molecular and clinical heterogeneity in primary hyperoxaluria type 1. *Am J Kidney Dis* 1991;17:366–369.

887. von Schnakenburg C, Byrd DJ, Latta K, et al. Determination of oxalate excretion in spot urines of healthy children by ion chromatography. *Eur J Clin Chem Clin Biochem* 1994;32:27–29.

888. Sonntag J, Schaub J. The identification of hyperoxaluria in very low-birthweight infants—which urine sampling method? *Pediatr Nephrol* 1997;11:205–207.

889. Morgenstern BZ, Milliner DS, Murphy ME, et al. Urinary oxalate and glycolate excretion patterns in the first year of life: a longitudinal study. *J Pediatr* 1993;123:248–251.

890. Reusz GS, Dobos M, Byrd D, et al. Urinary calcium and oxalate excretion in children. *Pediatr Nephrol* 1995;9:39–44.

891. Johnson SA, Rumsby G, Cregeen D, et al. Primary hyperoxaluria type 2 in children. *Pediatr Nephrol* 2002;17:597–601.

892. De Zegher FE, Wolff ED, vd Heijden AJ, et al. Oxalosis in infancy. *Clin Nephrol* 1984;22:114–120.

893. Morris MC, Chambers TL, Evans PW, et al. Oxalosis in infancy. *Arch Dis Child* 1982;57:224–228.

894. Furuta M, Torii S. Congenital oxalosis: first report of two neonatal cases. *Ann Paediatr Jpn* 1967;13:42.

895. Rose GA, Arthur LJH, Chambers TL, et al. Successful treatment of primary hyperoxaluria in a neonate. *Lancet* 1982;1:1298–1299.

896. Leumann EP, Wegmann W, Largiader F. Prolonged survival after renal transplantation in primary hyperoxaluria of childhood. *Clin Nephrol* 1978;9:29–34.

897. Allen AR, Thompson EM, Williams G, et al. Selective renal transplantation in primary hyperoxaluria type 1. *Am J Kidney Dis* 1996;27:891–895.

898. Jamieson NV, the European PH1 Transplantation Study Group. The European Primary Hyperoxaluria Type 1 Transplant Registry report on the results of combined liver/kidney transplantation for primary hyperoxaluria 1984–1994. *Nephrol Dial Transplant* 1995;10[Suppl 8]:33–37.

899. Rytkönen EM, Halila R, Laan M, et al. The human gene for xanthine dehydrogenase (XDH) is localized on chromosome band 2p22. *Cytogenet Cell Genet* 1995;68:61–63.

900. Levartovsky D, Lagziel A, Sperling O. XDH gene mutation is the underlying cause of classical xanthinuria: a second report. *Kidney Int* 2000;57:2215–2220.

900a. Reiter S, Simmonds HA, Zöllner N, et al. Demonstration of a combined deficiency of xanthine oxidase and aldehyde oxidase in xanthinuric patients not forming oxipurinol. *Clin Chim Acta* 1990;187:221–234.

901. Ichida K, Matsumura T, Sakuma R. Mutation of human molybdenum cofactor sulfurase gene is responsible for classical xanthinuria type II. *Biochem Biophys Res Commun* 2001;282:1194–1200.

902. Badertscher E, Robson WL, Leung AK, et al. Xanthine calculi presenting at 1 month of age. *Eur J Pediatr* 1993;152:252–254.

903. Broderick TP, Schaff DA, Bertino AM, et al. Comparative anatomy of the human APRT gene and enzyme: nucleotide sequence divergence and conservation of a non-random CpG dinucleotide arrangement. *Proc Natl Acad Sci U S A* 1987;84:3349–3353.

904. Kambayashi T, Nakanishi T, Suzuki K, et al. Two siblings with 2,8-dihydroxyadenine urolithiasis. *Hinyokikka Kiyo* 1994;40:1097–1101.

905. Garrett JE, Capuano IV, Hammerland LG. Molecular cloning and functional expression of human parathyroid calcium receptor cDNAs. *J Biol Chem* 1995;270:12919–12925.

906. Janicic N, Soliman E, Pausova Z, et al. Mapping of the calcium-sensing receptor gene (CASR) to human chromosome 3q13.3–21 by fluorescence in situ hybridization, and localization to rat chromosome 11 and mouse chromosome 16. *Mamm Genome* 1995;6:798–801.

907. Pollak MR, Brown EM, Chou YH, et al. Mutations in the human Ca2+-sensing receptor gene cause familial hypocalciuric hypercalcemia and neonatal severe hyperparathyroidism. *Cell* 1993;75:1297–1303.

908. Heath H 3rd, Jackson CE, Otterud B, et al. Genetic linkage analysis in familial benign (hypocalciuric) hypercalcemia: evidence for locus heterogeneity. *Am J Hum Genet* 1993;53:193–200.

909. Trump D, Whyte MP, Wooding C, et al. Linkage studies in a kindred from Oklahoma, with familial benign (hypocalciuric) hypercalcaemia (FBH) and developmental elevations in serum parathyroid hormone levels, indicate a third locus for FBH. *Human Genet* 1995;96:183–187.

910. Lloyd SE, Pannett AA, Dixon PH, et al. Localization of familial benign hypercalcemia, Oklahoma variant (FBHOk), to chromosome 19q13. *Am J Hum Genet* 1999;64:189–195.

911. Pollak MR, Chou YH, Marx SJ, et al. Familial hypocalciuric hypercalcemia and neonatal severe hyperparathyroidism. Effects of mutant gene dosage on phenotype. *J Clin Invest* 1994;93:1108–1112.

912. Marx SJ, Fraser D, Rapoport A. Familial hypocalciuric hypercalcemia. Mild expression of the gene in heterozygotes and severe expression in homozygotes. *Am J Med* 1985;78:15–22.

913. Law WM, Heath H. Familial benign hypercalcemia (hypocalciuric hypercalcemia). Clinical and pathogenetic studies in 21 families. *Ann Intern Med* 1985;102:511–519.

914. Kristiansen JH, Brochner-Mortensen J, Pedersen KO. Renal tubular function in familial hypocalciuric hypercalcemia. *Contrib Nephrol* 1987;56:210–214.

915. Watanabe H, Sutton RAL. Renal calcium handling in familial hypocalciuric hypercalcemia. *Kidney Int* 1983;24:353–357.

916. Marx SJ, Stock JL, Attie MF, et al. Familial hypocalciuric hypercalcemia: recognition among patients referred after unsuccessful parathyroid exploration. *Ann Intern Med* 1980;92:351–356.

917. Page LA, Haddow J. Self-limited neonatal hyperparathyroidism in familial hypocalciuric hypercalcemia. *J Pediatr* 1987;111:261–264.

918. Dezateux CA, Hyde JC, Hoey HM, et al. Neonatal hyperparathyroidism. *Eur J Pediatr* 1984;142:135–136.

919. Hauache OM. Extracellular calcium-sensing receptor: structural and functional features and association with diseases. *Braz J Med Biol Res* 2001;34:577–584.

919a. Roth KS, Foreman JW, Segal S. The Fanconi syndrome and mechanisms of tubular transport dysfunction. *Kidney Int* 1981;20:705–716.

920. Manz F, Bickel H, Brodehl J, et al. Fanconi-Bickel syndrome. *Pediatr Nephrol* 1987;1:509–518.

921. Wrong OM, Norden AG, Feest TG. Dent's disease: a familial proximal renal tubular syndrome with low-molecular-weight proteinuria, hypercalciuria, nephrocalcinosis, metabolic bone disease, progressive renal failure and a marked male predominance. *Q J Med* 1994;87:473–493.

922. Gahl WA, Bernardini IM, Dalakas MC, et al. Muscle carnitine repletion by long-term carnitine supplementation in nephropathic cystinosis. *Pediatr Res* 1993;34:115–119.

923. Usberti M, Pecoraro C, Federico S, et al. Mechanism of action of indomethacin in tubular defects. *Pediatrics* 1985;75:501–507.

924. Haycock GB, Al-Dahhan J, Mak RHK, et al. Effect of indomethacin on clinical progress and renal function in cystinosis. *Arch Dis Child* 1982;57:934–939.

925. Gahl WA, Tietze F, Bashan N, et al. Defective cystine exodus from isolated lysosome-rich fractions of cystinotic leucocytes. *J Biol Chem* 1982;257:9570–9575.

926. The cystinosis collaborative research group. Linkage of the gene for cystinosis to markers on the short arm of chromosome 17. *Nat Genet* 1995;10:246–248.

927. Lemire J, Kaplan BS. The various renal manifestations of the nephropathic form of cystinosis. *Am J Nephrol* 1984;4:81–85.

928. Wong VG, Lietman PS, Seegmiller JE. Alterations of pigment epithelium in cystinosis. *Arch Ophthalmol* 1967;77:361–369.

929. Gretz N, Manz F, Augustin R, et al. Survival time in cystinosis: a collaborative study. *Proc Eur Dialys Transplant Assoc* 1982;19:582–589.

930. Kalatzis V, Antignac C. New aspects of the pathogenesis of cystinosis. *Pediatr Nephrol* 2003;18:207–215.

931. Mason S, Pepe G, Dall'Amico R, et al. Mutational spectrum of the CTNS gene in Italy. *Eur J Hum Genet* 2003;11:503–508.

932. Gahl WA, Thoene J, Schneider J. Cystinosis: a disorder of lysosomal membrane transport. In: Scriver CJ, Beaudet AL, Sly WS, et al, eds. *The metabolic and molecular bases of inherited disease*. New York: McGraw–Hill, 2001:5085–5108.

933. Gahl WA, Reed GF, Thoene JG, et al. Cysteamine therapy for children with nephropathic cystinosis. *N Engl J Med* 1987;316:971–977.

934. Clark KF, Franklin PS, Reisch JS, et al. Effect of cysteamine-HCl and phosphocysteamine dosage on renal function and growth in children with nephropathic cystinosis. *Clin Res* 1992;40:113A.

935. Reznik VM, Adamson M, Adelman RD, et al. Treatment of cystinosis with cysteamine from early infancy. *J Pediatr* 1991;119:491–493.

936. Coleman RA, Van Hove JL, Morris CR. Cerebral defects and nephrogenic diabetes insipidus with the ARC syndrome: additional findings or a new syndrome (ARCC-NDI)? *Am J Med Genet* 1997;72:335–338.

937. Eastham KM, McKiernan PJ, Milford DV, et al. ARC syndrome: an expanding range of phenotypes. *Arch Dis Child* 2001;85:415–420.

938. Santer R, Steinmann B, Schaub J. Fanconi-Bickel syndrome-a congenital defect of facilitative glucose transport. *Curr Mol Med* 2002;2:213–227.

939. Sanjad SA, Kaddoura RE, Nazer HM, et al. Fanconi's syndrome with hepatorenal glycogenosis associated with phosphorylase b kinase deficiency. *Am J Dis Child* 1993;147:957–959.

940. Chen YT, Scheinman JI, Park HK, et al. Amelioration of proximal renal tubular dysfunction in type I glycogen storage disease with dietary therapy. *N Engl J Med* 1990;323:590–593.

941. Garty R, Cooper M, Tabachnik E. The Fanconi syndrome associated with hepatic glycogenosis and abnormal metabolism of galactose. *J Pediatr* 1974;85:821–823.

942. Lee PJ, Van't Hoff WG, Leonard JV. Catch-up growth in Fanconi-Bickel syndrome with uncooked cornstarch. *J Inherit Metab Dis* 1995;18:153–156.

943. Fellman V. The GRACILE Syndrome, a neonatal lethal metabolic disorder with iron overload. *Blood Cells Mol Dis* 2002;29:444–450.

944. Visapaa I, Fellman V, Vesa J, et al. GRACILE syndrome, a lethal metabolic disorder with iron overload, is caused by a point mutation in BCS1L. *Am J Hum Genet* 2002;71:863–876.

945. Fellman V, Visapaa I, Vujic M, et al. Antenatal diagnosis of hereditary fetal growth retardation with aminoaciduria, cholestasis, iron overload, and lactic acidosis in the newborn infant. *Acta Obstet Gynecol Scand* 2002;81:398–402.

946. Sparkes RS, Sparkes MC, Funderburk SJ, et al. Expression of GALT in 9p chromosome alterations: assignment of GALT locus to 9cenÆ9p22. *Ann Hum Genet* 1980;43:343–347.

947. Reichardt JK, Berg P. Cloning and characterization of a cDNA encoding human galactose-1-phosphate uridyl transferase. *Mol Biol Med* 1988;5:107–122.

948. Flach JE, Reichardt JK, Elsas LJ II. Sequence of a cDNA encoding human galactose-1-phosphate uridyl transferase. *Mol Biol Med* 1990;7:365–369.

949. Komrower GM, Schwarz V, Holzel A, et al. A clinical and biochemical study of galactosemia: a possible explanation of the nature of the biochemical lesion. *Arch Dis Child* 1956;31:254–264.

950. Yi-Yung Hsia, Hsia H-H, Green S, et al. Amino-aciduria in galactosemia. *Am J Dis Child* 1954;88:458–465.

951. Darling S, Mortensen O. Aminoaciduria in galactosaemia. *Acta Paediatr* 1954;43:337–341.

952. Dreyfus JC, Schapira F, Besmond C, et al. Study of hereditary fructose intolerance by methods of molecular biology. *Ann Méd Int* 1985;136:456–458.

953. Lebo RV, Tolan DR, Bruce BD, et al. Spot-blot analysis of sorted chromosomes assigns a fructose intolerance disease locus to chromosome 9. *Cytometry* 1985;6:478–483.

954. Pacifiers, passive behaviour, and pain [Editorial]. *Lancet* 1992;1:275–276.

955. Blass EM, Hoffmeyer LB. Sucrose as an analgesic for newborn infants. *Pediatrics* 1991;87:215–218.

956. Levin B, Snodgrass GJ, Oberholzer VG, et al. Fructosaemia. *Arch Dis Child* 1968;45:826–838.

957. Mass RE, Smith WR, Walsh JR. The association of hereditary fructose intolerance and renal tubular acidosis. *Am J Med Sci* 1966;251:516–523.

958. Lau J, Tolan DR. Screening for hereditary fructose intolerance mutations by reverse dot-blot. *Mol Cell Probes* 1999;13:35–40.

959. La Du BN. The enzymatic deficiency in tyrosinemia. *Am J Dis Child* 1967;113:54–57.

960. Bergeron P, Laberge C, Grenier A. Hereditary tyrosinemia in the province of Québec: prevalence at birth and geographic distribution. *Clin Genet* 1974;5:157–162.

961. Grompe M, St.-Louis M, Demers SI, et al. A single mutation of the fumarylaceto-acetate hydrolase gene in French Canadians with hereditary tyrosinemia type I. *N Engl J Med* 1994;331:353–357.

962. Labelle Y, Phaneuf D, Leclerc B, et al. Characterization of the human fumarylacetoacetate hydrolase gene and identification of a missense mutation abolishing enzymatic activity. *Hum Mol Genet* 1993;2:941–946.

963. Demers SI, Phaneuf D, Tanguay RM. Hereditary tyrosinemia type I: strong association with haplotype 6 in French Canadians permits simple carrier detection and prenatal diagnosis. *Am J Hum Genet* 1994;55:327–333.

964. Russo PA, Mitchell GA, Tanguay RM. Tyrosinemia: a review. *Pediatr Dev Pathol* 2001;4:212–221.

965. Halvorsen S, Pande H, Loken AC, et al. Tyrosinosis: a study of 6 cases. *Arch Dis Child* 1966;41:238–249.

966. Gentz J, Jagenburg R, Zetterström R. Tyrosinemia: an inborn error of tyrosine metabolism with cirrhosis of the liver and multiple renal tubular defects (de Toni-Debré-Fanconi syndrome). *J Pediatr* 1965;66:670–696.

967. van Spronsen FJ, Thomasse Y, Smit GPA, et al. Hereditary tyrosinemia type I: a new clinical classification with difference in prognosis on dietary treatment. *Hepatology* 1994;20:1187–1191.

968. Laine J, Salo MK, Krogerus L, et al. The nephropathy of type I tyrosinemia after liver transplantation. *Pediatr Res* 1995;37:640–645.

969. Lindstedt S, Holme E, Lock EA, et al. Treatment of hereditary tyrosinaemia type I by inhibition of 4-hydroxyphenylpyruvate dioxygenase. *Lancet* 1992;340:813–817.

970. Kvittingen EA. Tyrosinaemia—treatment and outcome. *J Inherit Metab Dis* 1995;18:375–379.

971. Silver DN, Lewis RA, Nussbaum RL. Mapping the Lowe oculocerebrorenal syndrome to Xq24-q26 by use of restriction fragment length polymorphisms. *J Clin Invest* 1987;79:282–285.

972. Attree O, Olivos IM, Okabe I, et al. The Lowe's oculocerebrorenal syndrome gene encodes a novel protein highly homologous to inositol polyphosphate-5-phosphatase. *Nature* 1992;358:239–242.

973. Nussbaum RL, Orrison BM, Jänne PA, et al. Physical mapping and genomic structure of the Lowe syndrome gene OCRL1. *Hum Genet* 1997;99:145–150.

974. Suchy SF, Nussbaum RL. The deficiency of PIP2 5-Phosphatase in Lowe syndrome affects Actin polymerization. *Am J Hum Genet* 2002;71:1420–1427.

975. Charnas LR, Bernardini I, Rader D, et al. Clinical and laboratory findings in the oculocerebrorenal syndrome of Lowe, with special reference to growth and renal function. *N Engl J Med* 1991;324:1318–1325.

976. Van Acker KJ, Roels H, Beelaerts W, et al. The histologic lesions of the kidney in the oculo-cerebro-renal syndrome of Lowe. *Nephron* 1967;4:193–214.

977. Witzleben CL, Schoen EJ, Tu WH, et al. Progressive morphologic renal changes in the oculo-cerebro-renal syndrome of Lowe. *Am J Med* 1968;44:319–324.

978. Tsuru T, Yamagata T, Momoi MY, et al. Prenatal diagnosis of Lowe syndrome by OCRL I messenger RNA analysis. *Prenat Diagn* 1999;19:269–270.

979. Ishihara R, Taketani S, Sasai-Takedatsu M, et al. ELISA for urinary trehalase with monoclonal antibodies: a technique for assessment of renal tubular damage. *Clin Chem* 2000;46:636–643.

980. Rötig A, Cormier V, Blanche S, et al. Pearson's marrow-pancreas syndrome. A multisystem mitochondrial disorder in infancy. *J Clin Invest* 1990;86:1601–1608.

981. Niaudet P, Rötig A. Renal involvement in mitochondrial cytopathies. *Pediatr Nephrol* 1996;10:368–373.

982. DiMauro S, Mendell JR, Sahenk Z, et al. Fatal infantile mitochondrial myopathy and renal dysfunction due to cytochrome-c-oxidase deficiency. *Neurology* 1980;30:795–804.

983. Ogier H, Lombes A, Scholte HR, et al. De Toni-Fanconi-Debré syndrome with Leigh syndrome revealing severe muscle cytochrome c oxidase deficiency. *J Pediatr* 1988;112:734–739.

984. Gruskin AB, Patel MS, Linshaw M, et al. Renal function studies and kidney pyruvate carboxylase in subacute necrotizing

encephalomyopathy (Leigh's syndrome). *Pediatr Res* 1973;7: 832–841.

985. Buist NR. Is pyruvate carboxylase involved in the renal tubular reabsorption of bicarbonate? *J Inherit Metab Dis* 1980;3: 113–116.

986. Falik-Borenstein ZC, Jordan SC, Saudubray JM, et al. Brief report: renal tubular acidosis in carnitine palmitoyl transferase I deficiency. *N Engl J Med* 1992;327:24–27.

987. Clayton PT, Hyland K, Brand M, et al. Mitochondrial phospho-enolpyruvate carboxykinase deficiency. *Eur J Pediatr* 1986;145: 46–50.

988. Rötig A, Bessis JL, Romero N, et al. Maternally inherited duplication of the mitochondrial genome in a syndrome of proximal tubulopathy, diabetes mellitus, and cerebellar ataxia. *Am J Hum Genet* 1992;50:364–370.

989. Rotig A. Renal disease and mitochondrial genetics. *J Nephrol* 2003;16:286–292.

990. Bichet DG, Oksche A, Rosenthal W. Congenital nephrogenic diabetes insipidus. *J Am Soc Nephrol* 1997;8:1951–1958.

991. Wildin RS, Antush MJ, Bennett RL, et al. Heterogenous AVPR2 gene mutations in congenital nephrogenic diabetes insipidus. *Am J Hum Genet* 1994;55:266–277.

992. Anderson JG, Notmann DD, Springer J. Studies in nephrogenic diabetes insipidus. *Clin Res* 1969;27:477A.

993. Knoers NV, van der Heyden H, van Oost BA, et al. Linkage of X-linked nephrogenic diabetes insipidus with DXS52, a polymorphic DNA marker. *Nephron* 1988;50:187–190.

994. van Lieburg AF, Knoers VVAM, Mallmann R, et al. Normal fibrinolytic responses to 1-desamino-8-D-arginine vasopressin in patients with nephrogenic diabetes insipidus caused by mutations in the aquaporin 2 gene. *Nephron* 1996;72: 544–546.

995. Macaulay D, Watson M. Hypernatraemia in infants as a cause of brain damage. *Arch Dis Child* 1967;42:485–491.

996. Hoekstra JA, van Lieburg AF, Monnens LAH, et al. Cognitive and psychosocial functioning of patients with congenital nephrogenic diabetes insipidus. *Am J Med Genet* 1996;61: 81–88.

997. Ohzeki T. Urinary adenosine 3858-monophosphate (cAMP): response to antidiuretic hormone in diabetes insipidus (DI): comparison between congenital nephrogenic DI type 1 and 2, and vasopressin sensitive DI. *Acta Endocrinol* 1985;108: 485–490.

998. Deen PM, van Aubel RA, van Lieburg AF, et al. Urinary content of aquaporin 1 and 2 in nephrogenic diabetes insipidus. *J Am Soc Nephrol* 1996;7:836–841.

999. Libber S, Harrison H, Spector D. Treatment of nephrogenic diabetes insipidus with prostaglandin synthesis inhibitors. *J Pediatr* 1986;108:305–311.

1000. Rascher W, Rosendahl W, Henrichs IA, et al. Congenital nephrogenic diabetes insipidus-vasopressin and prostaglandins in response to treatment with hydrochlorothiazide and indomethacin. *Pediatr Nephrol* 1987;1:485–490.

1001. Kirchlechner V, Koller DY, Seidl R, et al. Treatment of nephrogenic diabetes insipidus with hydrochlorothiazide and amiloride. *Arch Dis Child* 1999;80:548–552.

1002. Schöneberg T, Sandig V, Wess J, et al. Reconstitution of Mutant V2 Vasopressin Receptors by Adenovirus-mediated Gene Transfer—Molecular Basis and Clinical Implication. *J Clin Invest* 1997;100:1547–1056.

1003. Bartter FC, Pronove P, Gill JR Jr, et al. Hyperplasia of the juxtaglomerular complex with hyperaldosteronism and hypokalemic alkalosis: a new syndrome. *Am J Med* 1962;33: 811–828.

1004. Zelikovic I. Molecular pathophysiology of tubular transport disorders. *Pediatr Nephrol* 2001;16:919–935.

1005. Seyberth HW, Rascher W, Schweer H, et al. Congenital hypokalemia with hypercalciuria in preterm infants: a hyperprostaglandinuric tubular syndrome different from Bartter syndrome. *J Pediatr* 1985;107:694–701.

1006. Rodriguez-Soriano J. Bartter and related syndromes: the puzzle is almost solved. *Pediatr Nephrol* 1998;12:315–327.

1007. Vollmer M, Jeck N, Lemmink HH, et al. Antenatal Bartter syndrome with sensorineural deafness: refinement of the locus on chromosome 1p31. *Nephrol Dial Transplant* 2000;15: 970–974.

1008. Brennan TM, Landau D, Shalev H, et al. Linkage of infantile Bartter syndrome with sensorineural deafness to chromosome 1p. *Am J Hum Genet* 1998;62:355–361.

1009. Simon DB, Karet FE, Hamdan JM, et al. Bartter's syndrome, hypokalaemic alkalosis with hypercalciuria, is caused by mutations in the Na-K-2Cl cotransporter NKCC2. *Nat Genet* 1996; 13:183–188.

1010. Peters M, Jeck N, Reinalter S, et al. Clinical presentation of genetically defined patients with hypokalemic salt-losing tubulopathies. *Am J Med* 2002;112:183–190.

1011. Finer G, Shalev H, Birk O, et al. Transient neonatal hyperkalemia in the antenatal (ROMK defective) Bartter syndrome. *J Pediatr* 2003;142:318–323.

1012. Guay-Woodford LM. Bartter syndrome: unraveling the pathophysiologic enigma. *Am J Med* 1998;105:151–161.

1013. Shaer AJ. Inherited primary renal tubular hypokalemic alkalosis: a review of Gitelman and Bartter syndromes. *Am J Med Sci* 2001;322:316–332.

1014. Drukker A, Guignard JP. Renal aspects of the term and preterm infant: a selective update. *Curr Opin Pediatr* 2002;14: 175–182.

1015. Carlisle EJF, Donnelly SM, Halperin ML. Renal tubular acidosis (RTA): recognize the ammonium defect and pHorget the urine pH. *Pediatr Nephrol* 1991;5:242–248.

1016. Rodriguez-Soriano J. New insights into the pathogenesis of renal tubular acidosis—from functional to molecular studies. *Pediatr Nephrol* 2000;14:1121–1136.

1017. Rodríguez-Soriano J, Vallo A, Oliveros R, et al. Transient pseudohypoaldosteronism secondary to obstructive uropathy in infancy. *J Pediatr* 1983:103:375–380.

1018. Svenningsen NW. Renal acid-base titration studies in infants with and without metabolic acidosis in the postneonatal period. *Pediatr Res* 1974;8:659–672.

1019. Igarashi T, Inatomi J, Sekine T, et al. Novel nonsense mutation in the $Na+/HCO_3^-$ cotransporter gene (SLC4A4) in a patient with permanent isolated proximal renal tubular acidosis and bilateral glaucoma. *J Am Soc Nephrol.* 2001;12:713–718.

1020. Dubose TD Jr. Hydrogen ion secretion by the collecting duct as a determinant of the urine to PCO_2 gradient in alkaline urine. *J Clin Invest* 1982;69:145–156.

1021. Wrong O. Distal tubular acidosis: the value of urinary pH, pCO_2 and NH4+ measurements. *Pediatr Nephrol* 1991;5:249–255.

1022. Alon U, Hellerstein S, Warady BA. Oral acetazolamide in the assessment of (urine-blood) PCO_2. *Pediatr Nephrol* 1991;5: 307–311.

1023. Karet FE, Finberg KE, Nelson RD, et al. Mutations in the gene encoding B1 subunit of H+-ATPase cause renal tubular acidosis with sensorineural deafness. *Nat Genet* 1999;21:84–90.

1024. Stover EH, Borthwick KJ, Bavalia C, et al. Novel ATP6V1B1 and ATP6V0A4 mutations in autosomal recessive distal renal tubular acidosis with new evidence for hearing loss. *J Med Genet* 2002;39:796–803.

1025. Mcsherry E. Renal tubular acidosis in childhood. *Kidney Int* 1981;20:799–809.

1026. Brenner RJ, Spring DB, Sebastian A, et al. Incidence of radiographically evident bone disease, nephrocalcinosis, and nephrolithiasis in various types of renal tubular acidosis. *N Engl J Med* 1982;307:217–221.

1027. Norman ME, Feldman NI, Cohn RM, et al. Urinary citrate excretion in the diagnosis of distal renal tubular acidosis. *J Pediatr* 1978;92:394–400.

1028. Nakai H, Byers MG, Venta PJ, et al. The gene for human carbonic anhydrase II (CA 2) is located at chromosome 8q22. *Cytogenet Cell Genet* 1987;44:234–235.

1029. Hu PY, Lim EJ, Ciccolella J, et al. Seven novel mutations in carbonic anhydrase II deficiency syndrome identified by SSCP and direct sequencing analysis. *Hum Mutat* 1997;9:383–387, corrections 576.

1030. Sly WS, Hewett-Emmett D, Whyte MP, et al. Carbonic anhydrase II deficiency identified as the primary defect in the autosomal recessive syndrome of osteopetrosis with renal tubular acidosis and cerebral calcification. *Proc Natl Acad Sci U S A* 1983;80:2752–2756.

1031. Abramson O, Zmora E, Mazor M, et al. Pseudohypoaldosteronism in a preterm infant: intrauterine presentation as hydramnios. *J Pediatr* 1992;120:129–132.

1032. Shalev H, Ohali M, Abramson O. Nephrocalcinosis in pseudo-hypoaldosteronism and the effect of indomethacin therapy. *J Pediatr* 1994;125:246–248.

1033. Chang SS, Grunder S, Hanukoglu A, et al. Mutations in subunits of the epithelial sodium channel cause salt wasting with hyperkalaemic acidosis, pseudohypoaldosteronism type 1. *Nat Genet* 1996;12:248–253.

1034. Strautnieks SS, Thompson RJ, Gardiner RM, et al. A novel splice-site mutation in the subunit of the epithelial sodium channel gene in three pseudohypoaldosteronism type 1 families. *Nat Genet* 1996;13:248–250.

1035. Kerem E, Bistritzer T, Hanukoglu A, et al. Pulmonary epithelial sodium-channel dysfunction and excess airway liquid in pseudohypoaldosteronism. *N Engl J Med* 1999;41:156–162.

1036. Thomas CP, Zhou J, Liu KZ, et al. Systemic pseudohypoaldosteronism from deletion of the promoter region of the human Beta epithelial Na+ channel subunit. *Am J Respir Cell Mol Biol* 2002;27:314–319.

1037. Akcay A, Yavuz T, Semiz S, et al. Pseudohypoaldosteronism type 1 and respiratory distress syndrome. *J Pediatr Endocrinol Metab* 2002;15:1557–1561.

1038. Geller DS, Rodriguez-Soriano J, Vallo Boado A, et al. Mutations in the mineralocorticoid receptor gene cause autosomal dominant pseudohypoaldosteronism type I. *Nat Genet* 1998;19:279–281.

1039. Wolthers BG, Kraan GP, van der Molen JC, et al. Urinary steroid profile of a newborn suffering from pseudohypoaldosteronism. *Clin Chim Acta* 1995;236:33–43.

1040. Tenenhouse HS, Scriver CR. X-linked hypophosphatemia: a phenotype in search of a cause. *Int J Biochem* 1992;24:685–691.

1041. The HYP Consortium. A gene (PEX) with homologies to endopeptidases is mutated in patients with X-linked hypophosphatemic rickets. *Nat Genet* 1995;11:130–136.

1042. Rowe PSN, Goulding J, Read A, et al. Refining the genetic map for the region flanking the X-linked hypophosphatemic rickets locus (Xp22. 1-22.2). *Hum Genet* 1994;93:291–294.

1043. Chan JCM, Alon U, Hirschman GM. Renal hypophosphatemic rickets. *J Pediatr* 1985;106:533–544.

1044. Reusz GS, Latta K, Hoyer PF, et al. Evidence suggesting hyperoxaluria as a cause of nephrocalcinosis in phosphate-treated hypophosphataemic rickets. *Lancet* 1990;335:1240–1243.

1045. Alon U, Donaldson DL, Hellerstein S, et al. Metabolic and histologic investigation of the nature of nephrocalcinosis in children with hypophosphatemic rickets and in the Hyp mouse. *J Pediatr* 1992;120:899–905.

1046. Carpenter TO, Keller M, Schwartz D, et al. Dihydroxyvitamin D supplementation corrects hyperparathyroidism and improves skeletal abnormalities in X-linked hypophosphatemic rickets—a clinical research center study. *J Clin Endocrinol Metab* 1996;81:2381–2388.

1047. Seikaly MG, Baum M. Thiazide diuretics arrest the progression of nephrocalcinosis in children with X-linked hypophosphatemia. *Pediatrics* 2001;108:E6.

1048. Tieder M, Modai D, Samuel R, et al. Hereditary hypophosphatemic rickets with hypercalciuria. *N Engl J Med* 1985;312:611–617.

1049. Tieder M, Modai D, Shaked U, et al. "Idiopathic" hypercalciuria and hereditary hypophosphatemic rickets. Two phenotypical expressions of a common genetic defects. *N Engl J Med* 1987;316:125–129.

1050. Jones A, Tzenova J, Frappier D, et al. Hereditary hypophosphatemic rickets with hypercalciuria is not caused by mutations in the Na/Pi cotransporter NPT2 gene. *J Am Soc Nephrol* 2001;12:507–514.

1051. Econs MJ, McEnery PT. Autosomal dominant hypophosphatemic rickets/osteomalacia: clinical characterization of a novel renal phosphate-wasting disorder. *J Clin Endocrinol Metab* 1997;82:674–681.

1052. The ADHR Consortium: autosomal dominant hypophosphataemic rickets is associated with mutations in FGF23. *Nat Genet* 2000;26:345–348.

1053. Delvin EE, Glorieux FH, Marie PJ, et al. Vitamin D dependency: replacement therapy with calcitriol. *J Pediatr* 1981;99:26–34.

1054. Brooks MH, Bell NH, Love L, et al. Vitamin-D-dependent rickets type II: resistance of target organs to 1,25-dihydroxyvitamin D. *N Engl J Med* 1978;298:996–999.

1055. Hughes MR, Malloy PJ, Kieback DG, et al. Point mutations in the human vitamin D receptor gene associated with hypocalcemic rickets. *Science* 1988;242:1702–1705.

1056. Takeda E, Yamamoto H, Taketani Y, et al. Vitamin D-dependent rickets type I and type II. *Acta Paediatr Jpn* 1997;39:508–513.

1057. Labuda M, Fujiwara M, Ross MV, et al. Two hereditary defects related to vitamin D metabolism map to the same region of human chromosome 12q13-14. *J Bone Miner Res* 1992;7:1447–1453.

1058. Balsan S, Garabedian M, Liberman UA, et al. Rickets and alopecia with resistance to 1,25-dihydroxyvitamin D: two different clinical courses with two different cellular defects. *J Clin Endocrinol Metab* 1983;57:803–811.

1059. Gardezi SA, Nguyen C, Malloy PJ, et al. A rationale for treatment of hereditary vitamin D-resistant rickets with analogs of 1 alpha,25-dihydroxyvitamin D(3). *J Biol Chem* 2001;276:29148–29156.

1060. Elsas LJ, Hillman RE, Patterson JH, et al. Renal and intestinal hexose transport in familial glucose–galactose malabsorption. *J Clin Invest* 1970;49:576–585.

1061. Horowitz L, Schwarzer S. Renal glycosuria: occurrence in two siblings and a review of the literature. *J Pediatr* 1955;47:634–639.

1062. Turk E, Martín MG, Wright EM. Structure of the human Na+/glucose cotransporter gene SGLTI. *J Biol Chem* 1994;269:15204–15209.

1063. Martín MG, Turk E, Lostao MP, et al. Defects in Na+/glucose cotransporter (SGLT1) trafficking and function cause glucose-galactose malabsorption. *Nat Genet* 1996;12:216–220.

1064. Martín MG, Turk E, Kerner C, et al. Prenatal identification of a heterozygous status in two fetuses at risk for glucose-galactose malabsorption. *Prenat Diagn* 1996;16:458–462.

1065. Stonestreet BS, Rubin L, Pollak A, et al. Renal functions of low birth weight infants with hyperglycemia and glucosuria produced by glucose infusions. *Pediatrics* 1980;66:561–567.

1066. Wilkins BH. Renal function in sick very low birthweight infants. 4. Glucose excretion. *Arch Dis Child* 1992;67:1162–1165.

1067. Conger JD, Falk SA. Intrarenal dynamics in the pathogenesis and prevention of acute urate nephropathy. *J Clin Invest* 1977;59:786–793.

1068. Ahmadian Y, Lewy PR. Possible urate nephropathy of the newborn infant as a cause of transient renal insufficiency. *J Pediatr* 1977;91:96–100.

1069. Krakoff IH, Murphy ML. Hyperuricemia in neoplastic disease in children: prevention with allopurinol, a xanthine oxidase inhibitor. *Pediatrics* 1968;41:52–56.

1070. Pras E, Raben N, Golomb E, et al. Mutations in the SLC3A1 transporter gene in cystinuria. *Am J Hum Genet* 1995;56:1297–1303.

1071. Zelikovic I. Aminoaciduria and glycosuria. In: Barratt TM, Avner ED, Harmon D, eds. *Pediatric nephrology*, 4th ed. Baltimore, MD: Lippincott, Williams & Wilkins, 1999:507–527.

1072. Gasparini P, Calonge MJ, Bisceglia L, et al. Molecular genetics of cystinuria: identification of four new mutations and seven polymorphisms, and evidence for genetic heterogeneity. *Am J Hum Genet* 1995;57:781–788.

1073. Pras E, Sood R, Raben N, et al. Genomic organization of SLC3A1, a transporter gene mutated in cystinuria. *Genomics* 1996;36:163–167.

1074. Purroy J, Bisceglia L, Calonge MJ, et al. Genomic structure and organization of the human rBAT gene (SLC3A1). *Genomics* 1996;37:249–252.

1075. Zhang XX, Rozen R, Hediger MA, et al. Assignment of the gene for cystinuria (SLC3A1) to human chromosome 2p21 by fluorescence in situ hybridization. *Genomics* 1994;24:413–414.

1076. The consortium for Cystinuria Non-type I Cystinuria caused by mutations in SCL7A9, coding for a subunit(+AT) of rBAT. *Nat Genet* 1999;23:52–57.

1077. Levy HL. Genetic screening. In: Harris H, Hirschhorn K, eds. *Advances in human genetics*. New York: Plenum Press, 1973;4:1–104.

1078. Goodyer PR, Clow C, Reade T, et al. Prospective analysis and classification of patients with cystinuria identified in a newborn screening program. *J Pediatr* 1993;122:568–572.

1079. Chow GK, Streem SB. Medical treatment of cystinuria: results of contemporary clinical practice. *J Urol* 1996;156:1576–1578.

1080. Sperandeo MP, Bassi MT, Riboni M, et al. Structure of the SLC7A7 gene and mutational analysis of patients affected by lysinuric protein intolerance. *Am J Hum Genet* 2000;66:92–99.

1081. Palacin M, Bertran J, Zorzano A. Heteromeric amino acid transporters explain aminoacidurias. *Curr Opin Nephrol Hypertens* 2000;9:547–553.

1082. Mykkanen J, Toivonen M, Kleemola M, et al. Promoter analysis of the human SLC7A7 gene encoding y+L amino acid transporter-1 (y+LAT-1). *Biochem Biophys Res Commun* 2003; 301:855–861.

1083. DiRocco M, Garibotto G, Rossi GA, et al. Role of haematological, pulmonary and renal complications in the long-term prognosis of patients with lysinuric protein intolerance. *Eur J Pediatr* 1993;152:437–440.

1084. Parenti G, Sebastio G, Strisciuglio P, et al. Lysinuric protein intolerance characterized by bone marrow abnormalities and severe clinical course. *J Pediatr* 1995;126:246–251.

1085. Pshezhetsky AV, Richard C, Michaud L, et al. Cloning, expression and chromosomal mapping of human lysosomal sialidase and characterization of mutations in sialidosis. *Nat Genet* 1997;15:316–320.

1086. Maroteaux P, Humbel R, Strecker G, et al. Un nouveau type de sialidose avec atteinte rénale: La néphrosialidose, 1. Etude clinique, radiologique et nosologique. *Arch Fr Pédiatr* 1978;35: 819–829.

1087. Johnson WG, Thomas GH, Miranda AF, et al. Congenital sialidosis: biochemical studies: clinical spectrum in four sibs; two successful prenatal diagnoses. *Am J Hum Genet* 1980;32:43A.

1088. Fukuhara Y, Takano T, Shimmoto M, et al. A new point protection of protective protein gene in two Japanese siblings with juvenile galactosialidosis. *Brain Dysfunct* 1992;5:319.

1089. Galjart NJ, Gillemans N, Harris A, et al. Expression of cDNA encoding the human "protective protein" associated with lysosomal b-galactosidase and neuraminidase: homology to yeast proteases. *Cell* 1988;54:755–764.

1090. Kleijer WJ, Hoogeveen A, Verheijen FW, et al. Prenatal diagnosis of sialidosis with combined neuraminidase and beta-galactosidase deficiency. *Clin Genet* 1979;16:60–61.

1091. Sewell AC, Pontz BF. Prenatal diagnosis of galactosialidosis. *Prenat Diagn* 1988;8:151–155.

1092. Kleijer WJ, Geilen GC, Janse HC, et al. Cathepsin A deficiency in galactosialidosis: studies of patients and carriers in 16 families. *Pediatr Res* 1996;39:1067–1071.

1093. Huttunen NP. Congenital nephrotic syndrome of Finnish type: study of 75 patients. *Arch Dis Child* 1976;51:344–348.

1094. Albright SG, Warner AA, Seeds JW, et al. Congenital nephrosis as a cause of elevated alpha protein. *Obstet Gynecol* 1990;76: 969–971.

1095. Kestilä M, Lenkkeri U, Männikkö M. Positionally cloned gene for a novel glomerular protein nephrin is mutated in congenital nephrotic syndrome. *Mol Cell* 1998;1:575–582.

1096. Männikkö M, Kestilä M, Holmberg C. Fine mapping and haplotype analysis of the locus for congenital nephrotic syndrome on chromosome 19q13.1. *Am J Hum Genet* 1995;57:1377–1383.

1097. Männikkö M, Lenkkeri U, Kashtan CE, et al. Haplotype analysis of congenital nephrotic syndrome of the Finnish type in non-Finnish families. *J Am Soc Nephrol* 1996;7:2700–2703.

1098. Mahan JD, Mauer SM, Sibley RK, et al. Congenital nephrotic syndrome: evolution of medical management and results of renal transplantation. *J Pediatr* 1984;105:549–557.

1099. Kestilä M, Männikkö M, Holmberg C, et al. Congenital nephrotic syndrome of the Finnish type maps to the long arm of chromosome 19. *Am J Hum Genet* 1994;54:757–764.

1100. Norio R, Rapola J. Congenital and infantile nephrotic syndromes. In: Bartsocas CS, ed. *Genetics of kidney disorders.* New York: Alan R. Liss, 1989:179.

1101. Huttunen NP, Vehaskari M, Viikari M, et al. Proteinuria in congenital nephrotic syndrome of the Finnish type. *Clin Nephrol* 1980;13:12–19.

1102. Mattoo TK. Hypothyroidism in infants with nephrotic syndrome. *Pediatr Nephrol* 1994;8:657–659.

1103. Lanning P, Uhari M, Koulavainen K, et al. Ultrasonic features of the congenital nephrotic syndrome of the Finnish type. *Acta Paediatr Scand* 1989;78:717–720.

1104. Bratton VS, Ellis EN, Seibert JT. Ultrasonographic findings in congenital nephrotic syndrome. *Pediatr Nephrol* 1990;4: 515–516.

1105. Autio-Harmainen H, Rapola J. The thickness of the glomerular basement membrane in congenital nephrotic syndrome of the Finnish type. *Nephron* 1983;34:48–50.

1106. Holmberg C, Laine J, Ronnholm K, et al. Congenital nephrotic syndrome. *Kidney Int* 1996;49[Suppl 53]:S51–S56.

1107. Kovacevic L, Reid CJD, Rigden SPA. Management of congenital nephrotic syndrome. *Pediatr Nephrol* 2003;18:426–430.

1108. Habib R, Loirat C, Gubler MC, et al. The nephropathy associated with male pseudohermaphroditism and Wilms' tumor (Drash syndrome): a distinctive glomerular lesion—report of 10 cases. *Clin Nephrol* 1985;24:269–278.

1109. Schumacher V, Scharer K, Wuhl E, et al. Spectrum of early onset nephrotic syndrome associated with WT1 missense mutations. *Kidney Int* 1998;53:1594–1600.

1110. Barisoni L, Mundel P. Podocyte biology and the emerging understanding of podocyte diseases. *Am J Nephrol* 2003;23: 353–360.

1111. Garty BZ, Eisenstein B, Sandbank J, et al. Microcephaly and congenital nephrotic syndrome owing to diffuse mesangial sclerosis: an autosomal recessive syndrome. *J Med Genet* 1994; 31:121–125.

1112. Cooperstone BG, Friedman A, Kaplan BS. Galloway-Mowat syndrome of abnormal gyral patterns and glomerulopathy. *Am J Med Genet* 1993;47:250–254.

1113. Hofstaetter C, Neumann I, Lennert T, et al. Prenatal diagnosis of diffuse mesangial glomerulosclerosis by ultrasonography: a longitudinal study of a case in an affected family. *Fetal Diagn Ther* 1996;11:126–131.

1114. Wiggelinkhuizen J, Kaschula RO, Uys CJ, et al. Congenital syphilis and glomerulonephritis with evidence for immune pathogenesis. *Arch Dis Child* 1973;48:375–381.

1115. Papaioannou AC, Asrow GG, Schuckmell NH. Nephrotic syndrome in early infancy as a manifestation of congenital syphilis. *Pediatrics* 1961;27:636–641.

1116. Shahin B, Papadopoulou ZL, Jenis EH. Congenital nephrotic syndrome associated with congenital toxoplasmosis. *J Pediatr* 1974;85:366–370.

1117. Couvreur J, Alison F, Boccon-Gibod L, et al. Rein et toxoplasmose. *Ann Pediatr (Paris)* 1984;31:847–852.

1118. Amir G, Hurvitz H, Neeman Z, et al. Neonatal cytomegalovirus infection with pancreatic cystadenoma and nephrotic syndrome. *Pediatr Pathol* 1986;6:393–401.

1119. Batisky D, Roy S 3rd, Gaber LW. Congenital nephrosis and neonatal cytomegalovirus infection: a clinical association. *Pediatr Nephrol* 1993;7:741–743.

1120. Shapiro LR, Duncan PA, Farnsworth PB, et al. Congenital microcephaly, hiatus hernia and nephrotic syndrome: an autosomal recessive syndrome. *Birth Defects* 1976;12: 275–278.

1121. Robain O, Deonna T. Pachygyria and congenital nephrosis disorder of migration and neuronal orientation. *Acta Neuropathol* 1983;60:137–141.

1122. Palm L, Hägerstrand I, Kristofferssen U, et al. Nephrosis and disturbances of neuronal migration in male siblings: a new hereditary disorder? *Arch Dis Child* 1986;61:545–548.

1123. van der Knaap MS, Wevers RA, Monnens L, et al. Congenital nephrotic syndrome: a novel phenotype of type I carbohydrate-deficient glycoprotein syndrome. *J Inherit Metab Dis* 1996;19:787–791.

1124. Lagrue G, Branellec A, Niaudet P, et al. Transmission of nephrotic syndrome to two neonates: spontaneous regression. *Presse Med* 1991;20:255–257.

1125. Similä S, Vesa L, Wasz-Höckert O. Hereditary onycho-osteodysplasis (the nail-patella syndrome) with nephrosis-like renal disease in a newborn boy. *Pediatrics* 1970;46:61–65.

1126. Ty A, Fine B. Membranous nephritis in infantile systemic lupus erythematosus associated with chromosomal abnormalities. *Clin Nephrol* 1979;12:137–141.

1127. Massengill SF, Richard GA, Donnelly WH. Infantile systemic lupus erythematosus with onset simulating congenital nephrotic syndrome. *J Pediatr* 1994;124:27–31.

1128. Emmanuel B, Aronson N. Neonatal hematuria. *Am J Dis Child* 1974;208:204–206.

1129. Cramer A, Steele A, Wishne P, et al. Transient hematuria in premature and sick neonates. *Pediatr Res* 1981;15:692.

1130. Thullen JD, Fanaroff AA, Makker SP. Renal manifestations of perinatal asphyxia. *Pediatr Res* 1979;13:380.

1131. Seibert JJ, Taylor BJ, Williamson SL, et al. Sonographic detection of neonatal umbilical-artery thrombosis: clinical correlation. *AJR Am J Roentgenol* 1987;148:965–968.

1132. Chesney RW, Kaplan BS, Freedom RM, et al. Acute renal failure: an important complication of cardiac surgery in infants. *J Pediatr* 1975;87:381–388.

1133. Pillion G, Sonsino E, Beaufils F. Insuffisance rénale aiguë du nouveau-né. *J Annu Pédiatr (Paris)* 1982;29.

1134. Willis J, Duncan C, Gottschalk S. Paraplegia due to peripheral venous air embolus in a neonate: a case report. *Pediatrics* 1981;67:472–473.

1135. Kalia A, Travis LB, Brouhard BH. The association of idiopathic hypercalciuria and asymptomatic gross hematuria in children. *J Pediatr* 1981;99:716–719.

1136. Miltényi M, Pohlandt F, Boka G, et al. Tubular proteinuria after perinatal hypoxia. *Acta Paediatr Scand* 1981;70:399–403.

Structural Abnormalities of the Genitourinary Tract

George W. Kaplan   Irene M. McAleer

A discussion of neonatal pediatric urology in essence encompasses most of pediatric urology. Although, there are age-specific problems that do not present in early infancy, problems present primarily or specifically in the neonatal period. It is these latter lesions on which this discussion will focus. The almost universal use of antenatal ultrasonography, especially with Doppler and 3-dimensional (3D) imaging, has had a profound effect on detection, management, and understanding of many lesions of the urinary tract. Genitourinary anomalies account for approximately 50% of all antenatally sonographically detected lesions; hydronephrosis represents about two-thirds of these genitourinary abnormalities (1). Information from ultrasonography has been further complemented with magnetic resonance imaging (MRI) imaging, fetal bladder urine specimen measurements of electrolytes, osmolality, and β2-microglobulin. *In utero* surgical therapy is also possible with improved fetal surgical techniques, although the benefits derived from fetal surgery are not clear (2,3,4,5).

To properly understand and interpret the symptoms and findings seen in most congenital urologic problems, understanding the significant events of embryogenesis of the lesions seen is essential. Abnormalities of embryogenesis will be addressed as the resulting anomalies are covered.

The ureteral bud arises from the mesonephric duct at 4 to 5 weeks of gestation, the kidney begins to form at 6 weeks, and the bladder develops during the sixth to seventh week. The Wolffian duct is then incorporated into the bladder (Fig. 43-1). It is not until week 10 of gestation that urine production begins, and it is usually not until 14 to 16 weeks of gestation that the urinary tract is evident on antenatal ultrasonography (6). A number of anomalies may result from disordered embryogenesis of the ureter or kidney. Most genitourinary anomalies seem to occur sporadically, although some of the abnormalities are familial and others are related to chromosomal abnormalities.

IMAGING

The overall incidence of detection of fetal anomalies is currently about 1%. Urologic diagnostic imaging in the fetus, the newborn, and, to some extent, in the infant, is limited by the renal function (see Fig. 43-1). Neonatal renal functional parameters may be sufficient to maintain homeostasis: they may not suffice to produce the accuracy of diagnosis as expected from some imaging examinations used in older children and adults.

Ultrasonography and voiding cystourethrography are not dependent on renal function and, hence, assume even greater diagnostic import than in other age groups. Improved ultrasonographic equipment, resolution, and techniques are identifying fetal anomalies with greater accuracy resembling similar studies obtained in children and adults. Doppler imaging of the renal vessels in utero can suggest the presence of 1 or 2 functioning kidneys and Doppler imaging of the hypogastric vessels can delineate the presence or absence of the bladder if there is difficulty in reliably locating the bladder. Intravenous urography and, to a lesser extent, renal scintigraphy depend on renal function to produce images and consequently may be less reliable than in the adult; newer scintigraphic agents and techniques have made evaluation of the neonatal kidneys more reproducible and reliable (Fig. 43-2).

ANOMALIES OF THE KIDNEY

With normal embryogenesis as background, the anomalies and problems that may be encountered can be anticipated, because most have an embryologic basis. Some are incompatible with life, which may lead to an early demise; some are of no clinical significance, but most are potential sources of morbidity that can be minimized if the children are treated at an early age.

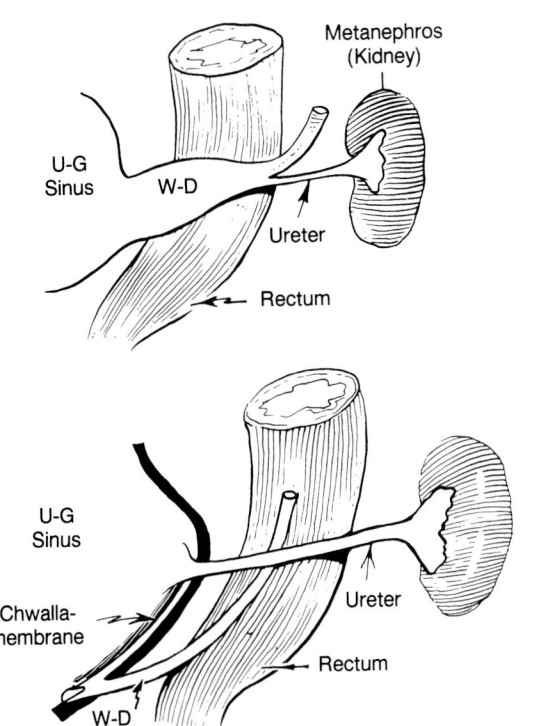

Figure 43-1 Incorporation of the wolffian (i.e., mesonephric) duct (W-D) into the urogenital sinus (U-G). From Kelalis PP, King LR, Belman AB, eds. *Clinical pediatric urology*, vol. 1. Philadelphia: WB Saunders, 1976:504, with permission.

Renal anomalies include the cystic diseases and abnormalities of number, position, and rotation. If the pronephros fails to develop, the mesonephros will not develop, resulting in renal and ureteral agenesis and absence of the ipsilateral genital ducts in the male. If the mesonephric duct develops but the mesonephros does not, there will be renal agenesis but the genital ducts will be present and there might be a blind-ending ureter.

Nephrogenesis is induced by the ureter; therefore, normal nephrogenesis depends on the ureteral bud meeting normal metanephrogenic blastema (7). If the ureter fails to meet the metanephric blastema, a blind-ending ureter might result. When the ureter meets a degenerating portion of the metanephrogenic blastema (i.e., the cephalic or caudal end of the blastema), renal dysplasia may result (7).

Renal Agenesis

Renal agenesis can be unilateral or bilateral. Bilateral renal agenesis obviously is incompatible with extrauterine life. In cases of bilateral renal agenesis, there is no in utero urine production; thus, there is marked oligohydramnios and the affected fetus may exhibit the deformational changes of Potter syndrome (8). Adequate amniotic fluid is required for normal lung development so the lungs may be hypoplastic. The incidence of bilateral renal agenesis is roughly 1 in

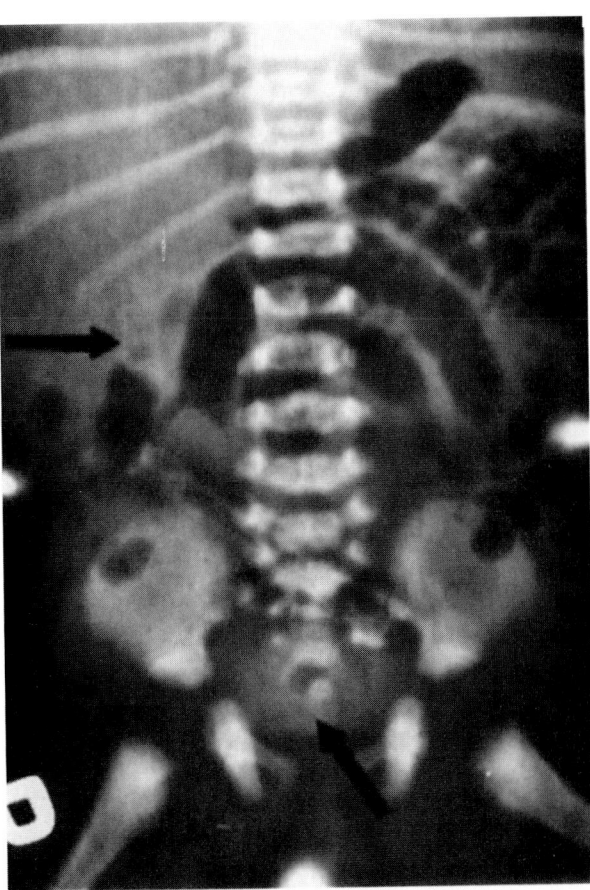

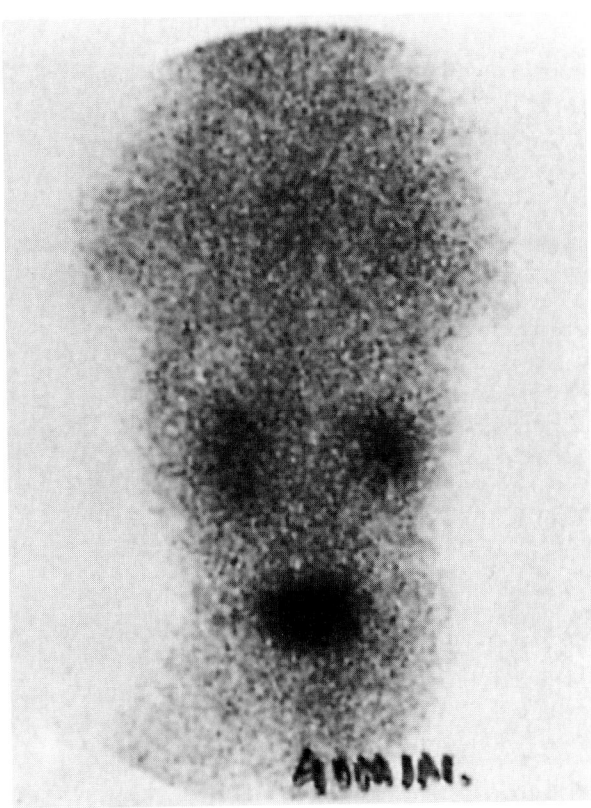

Figure 43-2 **A:** An excretory urogram in a newborn infant. The right kidney barely concentrates contrast (arrow); there is no evidence of the left kidney. Contrast is apparent in the bladder (arrow). **B:** An isotope renal scan the next day demonstrates the presence and function of two kidneys. The child was normal.

4,000 to 5,000 births (8). Renal agenesis sometimes may be associated with sirenomelia (8). Bilateral renal agenesis can be diagnosed antenatally by a combination of sonographic findings that include lack of identifiable renal masses, no demonstrable renal vessels on Doppler imaging, absent bladder, and severe oligohydramnios (6). For reasons that are unclear, some infants with this diagnosis have normal or near-normal levels of amniotic fluid. Renal agenesis must be considered postnatally when Potter facies are noted, when there is no urinary output within 24 to 48 hours, or when there is evidence of ventilatory failure with small lungs on chest radiograph. The postnatal diagnosis can be inferred ultrasonographically by the absence of identifiable kidneys or renal vessels with Doppler and the absence of urine in the bladder. Renal scintigraphy is used to prove that there is no identifiable functioning renal tissue. When the postnatal diagnosis of bilateral renal agenesis is made and confirmed, attempts at life support, which may have been initiated because of respiratory distress, should, in our opinion, be abandoned. There may be a familial inheritance of bilateral renal agenesis, with one review reporting up to 3% of siblings of probands having bilateral renal agenesis (9).

The incidence of unilateral renal agenesis is roughly 1 in 500 to 1,500 (8,10). There is a higher incidence of contralateral renal abnormality in patients with unilateral renal agenesis when compared to the general population, being generally obstructive or refluxing in nature. One-third of the patients with a solitary kidney in one series required some form of surgical procedure on the solitary unit (11). Unilateral renal agenesis may be associated with congenital scoliosis and with vaginal and uterine agenesis (12,13). It is the most common nonskeletal anomaly seen with imperforate anus (14). Unilateral renal agenesis previously was not thought to affect longevity or health as long as the contralateral kidney was normal. Recent experimental studies have suggested that renal injury may be produced in the solitary kidney by hyperfiltration and that a reduced protein diet may be somewhat protective. Clinical studies of patients with a solitary kidney (e.g., transplant donors, trauma victims) have, at this point, failed to confirm this (15).

Brenner and associates have noted that most people with unilateral renal agenesis do not develop progressive renal disease but longstanding hyperfiltration in most people with a solitary kidney from any etiology may cause glomerular hypertension which may be the culprit for developing progressive glomerular damage with subsequent proteinuria and renal insufficiency (16). Goldfarb and associates reviewed renal function in donor nephrectomy patients and found that renal function was well preserved in most donors over a prolonged follow-up averaging 25 years with some increase in proteinuria found in some patients but with only marginal significance in the group as a whole (17).

Renal Ectopia and Fusion

Failure of renal ascent will result in a pelvic kidney and may be associated with vaginal or vertebral anomalies (12). If the two metanephrogenic masses come into contact with each other in the pelvis, they may fuse and form a pancake or a horseshoe kidney (13). The embryogenesis of crossed ectopia, with or without fusion, is harder to explain but might result from lateral bending and rotation of the tail bud of the embryo, thereby altering the course of ascent (13).

Renal malrotation, or incomplete rotation, occurs when the ascending kidney, maintains its early fetal orientation and its renal pelvis is directed anteriorly. Malrotation is routinely present in fusion anomalies and in pelvic and crossed ectopias, and is also occasionally seen in kidneys located in the renal fossa. Incomplete rotation is of no clinical significance, but may cause difficulties in some imaging study interpretation: it may also be important in planning reconstructive procedures.

Abnormalities of renal position (i.e., ectopia) are interesting anomalies that generally, are of no clinical import but may become apparent because of trauma (i.e., hematuria), a palpable mass, or associated urologic abnormality. The ectopic kidney may be located in the chest or the pelvis. Thoracic kidneys usually are associated with eventration of the diaphragm and are of no clinical significance except as a finding on a chest radiograph (18). Pelvic ectopia is the most common of the abnormalities of position and often is associated with vesicoureteral reflux or ureteropelvic junction obstruction (19). Additionally, girls with müllerian anomalies have an increased incidence of pelvic kidney compared to the general population; hence, the finding of a pelvic kidney in a girl warrants further investigation of the genital tract to uncover associated anomalies (20).

Fusion anomalies, such as horseshoe or pancake kidneys, may present in the same way that anomalies of position present. Horseshoe kidneys are found with increased frequency in girls with Turner syndrome (21). There is an increased incidence of ureteropelvic junction obstruction in horseshoe kidneys (19). Some patients with horseshoe kidneys may have increased stone formation, as a result of relative urinary stasis with drainage from the nondependent renal pelvis. Crossed ectopia with or without fusion (i.e., one kidney is found on the opposite side of the side of ureteral bud development) is uncommon. When crossed ectopia occurs, the left kidney more commonly crosses to the right side than vice versa (22). By definition, the ipsilateral ureteral orifice is located on the anatomically appropriate side of the body (i.e., the left ureter is on the left side of the trigone and the right ureter is on the right side of the trigone). There is an increased incidence of vesicoureteral reflux and of ureteropelvic junction obstruction in crossed ectopic kidneys (19). Patients with crossed ectopia have an increased incidence of skeletal and cardiac abnormalities (14).

Supernumerary Kidney

The presence of a supernumerary (i.e., third) renal mass is a very rare anomaly; the clinical significance of this is determined by associated pathologic conditions (23). The supernumerary kidney usually is small, and more often caudal than cranial to the normally placed kidney. Many patients and some physicians confuse a supernumerary kidney with duplication of the collecting system and incorrectly, refer to ureteral duplication as a third kidney.

Cystic Disease

Renal cystic diseases are a group of disorders seen in pediatric urologic practice that frequently will present in the neonatal period. Because there is no uniform system of classification, there can be difficulty in communication between disciplines. An accurate diagnosis is needed for prognosis and for genetic counseling. It is for this reason that communication must be clear. Table 43-1 is a classification scheme that has been clinical useful in our practice.

Autosomal recessive polycystic kidney disease (ARPCKD), as the name implies, is an inherited disorder whose mode of transmission follows a mendelian recessive pattern. Its reported incidence is between 1 in 6,000 to 1 in 14,000 pregnancies. In this disorder, formerly known as infantile polycystic disease, the kidneys are very large and often occupy the entire retroperitoneum (Fig. 43-3). The cysts are small and are actually enlargements of the collecting ducts (24). The liver almost always is abnormal. At times there will be periportal hepatic fibrosis as a significant part of this complex. Death in the neonatal period is secondary to either renal or pulmonary failure. Those who survive the neonatal period usually will exhibit decreased renal function and hypertension, but at times liver failure as a result of hepatic fibrosis may be the most prominent part of the clinical picture (25). Imaging studies such as antenatal or postnatal ultrasonography, computed tomography (CT) or intravenous urography usually are diagnostic with very large kidneys demonstrating a sunburst streaking pattern.

ADPCKD is inherited in a mendelian dominant fashion and is more common than the recessive form. It usually

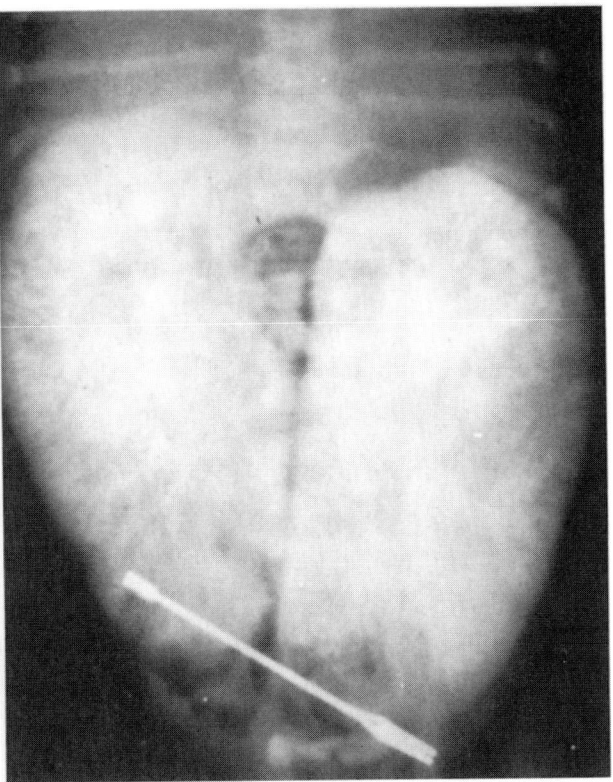

Figure 43-3 An excretory urogram in a 2-day-old girl with autosomal recessive polycystic kidney disease shows the sunray appearance of the contrast material and the enormous renal size. From Kelalis PP, King LR, Belman AB, eds. *Clinical pediatric urology*, vol. 2. Philadelphia: WB Saunders, 1976:686, with permission.

TABLE 43-1
CLASSIFICATION OF RENAL CYSTIC DISEASE

Polycystic disease
    Autosomal recessive
    Autosomal dominant
Renal cortical cysts in hereditary syndromes
    Tuberous sclerosis
    von Hippel–Lindau disease
    Meckel syndrome
    Zellweger cerebrohepatorenal syndrome
    Jeune asphyxiating thoracic dysplasia
    Syndromes of multiple malformations that include cortical cysts
Renal medullary cysts
    Familial juvenile nephronophthisis
    Medullary cystic disease
    Renal retinal dysplasia
    Medullary sponge disease
Renal dysplasia
    Multicystic kidney disease
    Other cystic dysplasias
    Multilocular mesoblastic nephroma
Other cystic diseases
    Simple cysts, single or multiple
    Unilateral segmental cystic disease

does not present until adult life, hence its former name, adult polycystic disease. These patients usually present with hypertension, hematuria, urinary tract infection, or renal failure. When this problem presents in childhood, it may do so as an abdominal mass or may be found with ultrasound as either antenatal evaluation, screening for polycystic disease, or coincidentally when an ultrasound is being obtained for some other evaluation. Imaging studies will prove diagnostic, because multiple large cysts that splay and distort the collecting system will be present. Although there often are associated hepatic cysts, liver failure is not usually a clinical feature of this disorder. Microdissection studies have shown that the cysts are as a result of abnormal branching of the collecting tubules and cystic dilations of portions of the nephron (26). Generally, detectable cysts may not develop until middle to late adult life; hence, the disease is undetectable clinically until they appear.

Tuberous sclerosis can mimic both autosomal recessive and autosomal dominant polycystic disease in that lesions grossly similar to either form of polycystic disease can be found in the tuberous sclerosis complex (27). Microscopically, lesions characteristic of tuberous sclerosis will be seen on biopsy of the affected kidneys. Angiomyolipomas (i.e., renal hamartomas), are the more commonly seen renal lesions in patients with tuberous sclerosis.

Multicystic kidney disease, with a frequency of 1 in 3,000 pregnancies (11), is the most common form of cystic disease seen in neonates. Originally defined by Spence and associates (28), this is a unilateral (or bilateral) lesion in which the entire kidney is replaced by cysts of varying sizes. Grossly, there is no recognizable renal tissue present, but microscopically there may be dysplastic renal elements in the septa between the cysts (Fig. 43-4). Bilateral multicystic

kidney disease is incompatible with life. Multicystic kidney disease is sporadic and is not inherited. Some multicystic kidneys involute, probably by absorption of the cyst fluid. This can occur antenatally or in the first few months of life. It is likely that many cases of presumed renal agenesis are multicystic kidneys that have undergone involution.

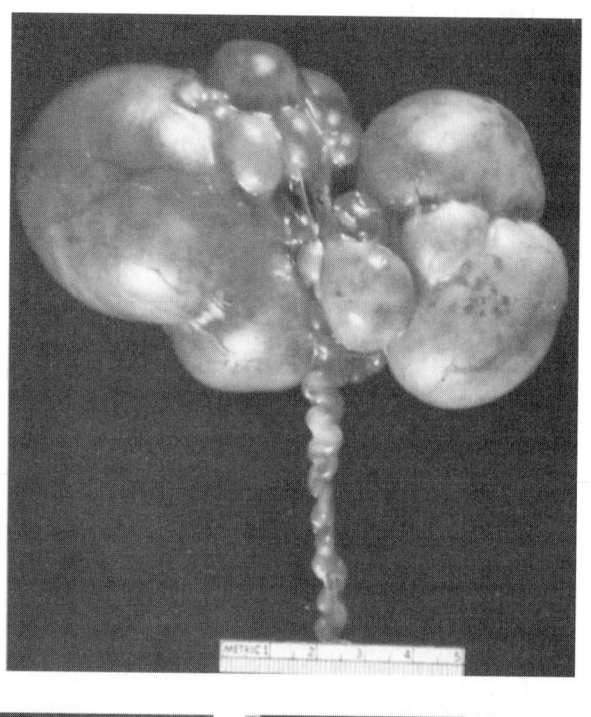

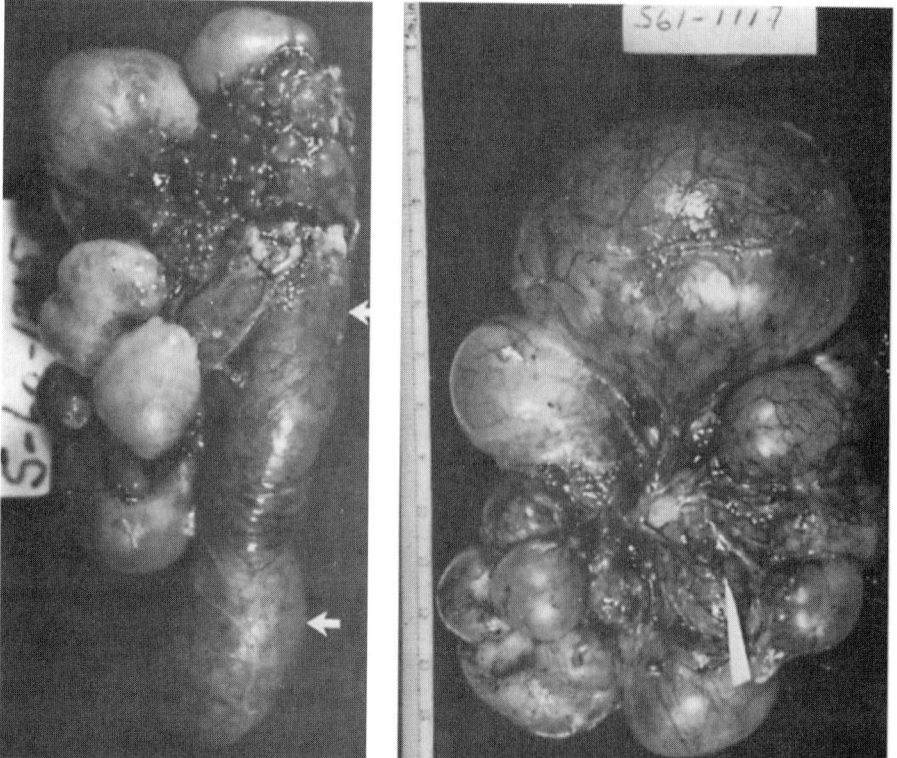

Figure 43-4 Three examples of the variety of multicystic diseases. **A:** Multicystic kidney with a torturous atretic ureter. The cysts vary in size and appear to be held together by fibrous tissue. **B:** Multicystic kidney in a 1-month-old girl. The dilated pelvis and proximal ureter are indicated (arrows). **C:** Multicystic kidney in a 4-day-old girl. No ureter was found during the nephrectomy. From Kelalis PP, King LR, Belman AB, eds. *Clinical pediatric urology*, vol. 2. Philadelphia: WB Saunders, 1976:210, with permission.

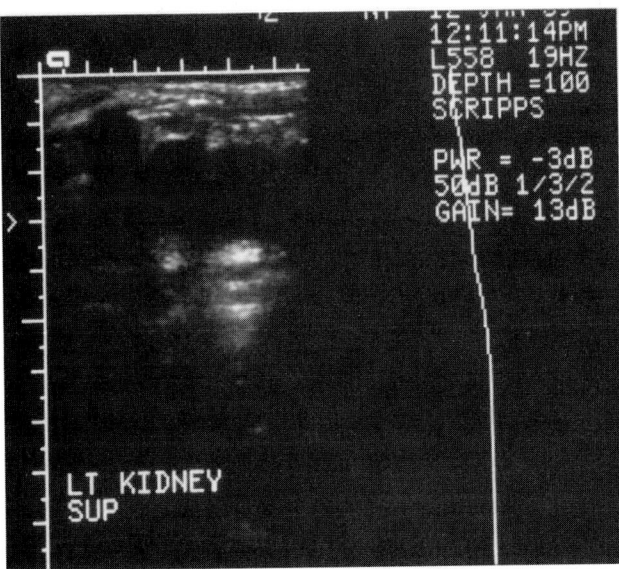

Figure 43-5 An abdominal ultrasonographic study carried out in an infant with multicystic (i.e., cystic dysplastic) kidney.

Multicystic kidneys usually are detectable with antenatal ultrasonography, but occasionally can present during infancy as palpable masses. Ultrasonography will demonstrate multiple, variably sized cysts in a random pattern (Fig. 43-5), and the affected kidney is generally without function on renal scan or intravenous urography.

There is a great deal of controversy surrounding the management of these lesions; traditional therapy had been nephrectomy, but many pediatric urologists advocate observation because the incidence of sequelae such as infection, pain, hypertension, or malignancy is very low. Nephrectomy seems a reasonable alternative to lifelong follow-up, however, and is our current recommendation if the kidney does not completely involute within 6 to 12 months. At the present time, a Multicystic Kidney Registry is collecting data on cases that are followed with observation. Roughly 25% of the patients with multicystic kidney disease have an obstructive lesion such as ureteropelvic junction obstruction on the contralateral side, and it is this fact that will determine the patient's ultimate prognosis. Since the inception of the Multicystic Kidney Registry, vesicoureteral reflux has been found to be more common than obstruction. Involution, if it occurs, may take many years to occur; up to 50% of those followed for 3 to 5 years had no change in the multicystic kidney appearance on ultrasound (29).

ANOMALIES OF THE URETERS AND BLADDER

Duplication and Triplication of the Ureters

Multiple ureteral buds or premature division of the ureteral bud could produce ureteral duplication or triplication (30). If there are multiple ureteral buds, one bud is likely to meet

degenerating rather than normal nephrogenic tissue. This could account for the increased incidence of renal dysplasia in the upper pole of a duplicated system (4). Duplication of the urinary collecting system is one of the more common abnormalities seen in the urinary tract; its occurrence is about 0.8% (30). Approximately 12% of sibs and parents were affected with ureteral duplication when reviewing family inheritance probands. (9) Duplication can be either complete or incomplete. Incomplete duplication is usually of no clinical significance, there can be ureteroureteral reflux between the two limbs of the partial duplication resulting in dilation of one of the ureters, usually the lower one. Complete duplication occurs once in every 500 cases (30). Complete duplication, generally of no clinical significance, is associated with a higher incidence of other abnormalities in the urinary system. These abnormalities include both vesicoureteral reflux and obstruction.

Vesicoureteral reflux probably is the more common of the anomalies associated with ureteral duplication, and usually occurs into the lower moiety of a duplicated system (Fig. 43-6). Duplication is seen in approximately one in five people with vesicoureteral reflux, which is much higher than its incidence in the general population (31). The grade of reflux associated with a complete duplication usually is greater than that seen with a single system. Obstruction is common when the upper moiety of a complete duplication is abnormal, Both obstruction and vesicoureteral reflux associated with duplications may present as either mass lesions or urosepsis; many of these duplications are diagnosed in utero, with hydronephrosis seen in the upper or lower segments of the duplicated systems.

If the ureteral bud arises from a locus that is more cranial or caudal than normal, ureteral ectopia, vesicoureteral reflux, or paraureteral diverticula might be produced (32). Ectopic ureteroceles probably result from abnormalities of the ureteral bud and ureteral ectopia (33). Simple ureteroceles are thought to be produced by persistence of the Chwalla membrane (i.e., the membrane covering the distal end of the ureter during development) (34).

Ureteral obstruction occurs primarily at the ureteropelvic and ureterovesical junctions. These obstructions usually are intrinsic in nature, and the ureter may be of normal or reduced caliber externally (35,36). Multicystic kidney disease has been said to result from ureteral obstruction early in gestation or may be secondary to disordered induction of the metanephrogenic mass by a faulty ureteral bud (37). Kitagawa and associates demonstrated an animal model for development of a multicystic kidney by obstructing the fetal lamb urethra (male) or ureter (female) at 60 days gestation, and proposed that the cysts developed only when the obstruction occurs after the glomeruli start to produce urine. (38)

Bladder Anomalies

Agenesis of the bladder could result if the allantoic stalk failed to develop (39); it also could occur if there was bilateral failure of ureteral migration with bilateral ureteral

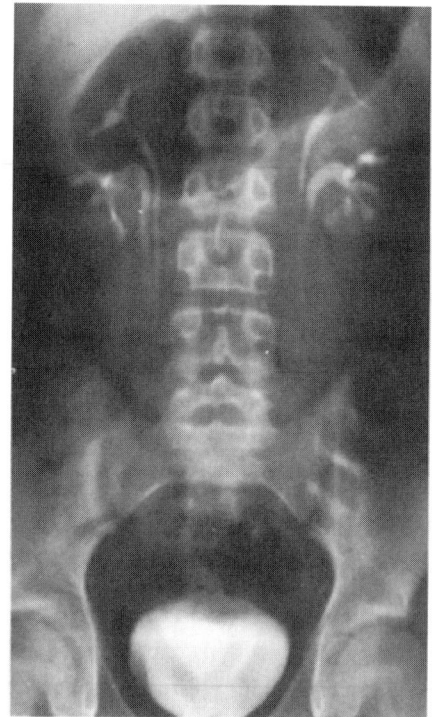
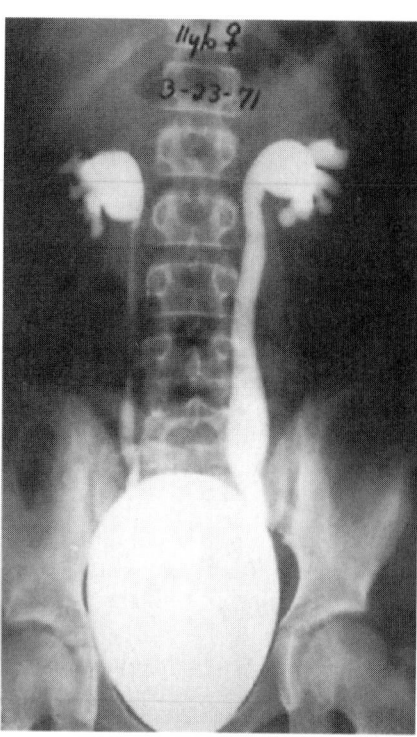

Figure 43-6 **A:** An intravenous urogram in a girl with complete, bilateral duplication of the collecting system. Note the blunting of the lower calyces. **B:** A cystogram in the same child demonstrates reflux into both lower collecting systems only. From Belman AB. The clinical significance of vesicoureteral reflux. *Pediatr Clin North Am* 1976;23:707, with permission.

ectopia, because migration of the ureters is necessary for formation of the trigone, which may be necessary for enlargement of the allantoic stalk (40). Urachal anomalies occur because of a general mesodermal failure, as in the prune-belly syndrome, or because of delayed closure of the urachus (41). Duplications of the bladder and urethra often are associated with duplications of the hindgut and lower spinal cord. Hence, it would seem that splitting of the hind end of the embryo might be responsible for this type of anomaly (42).

Posterior urethral valves probably result from abnormal insertion and persistence of the mesonephric ducts distal to the Müllerian tubercle (type I), or from persistence of the cloacal membrane (type III) (43). Type II valves probably do not exist as an obstructing lesion (see Fig. 43-17).

Ureteral Ectopia

Ureteral ectopia exists when the ureter opens in a position other than its normal location at the corner of the trigone. Ectopia may occur in ureters of single or duplex kidneys (Fig. 43-7). The most common form of ureteral ectopia is lateral ureteral ectopia, in which the ureteral orifice lies within the bladder lateral to its normal position. This is the etiologic mechanism for primary vesicoureteral reflux (see Vesicoureteral Reflux). Significant medial or distal ureteral ectopia, less common than lateral ureteral ectopia, will cause clinical pathologic conditions that vary depending on the location of the ureteral orifice and the gender of the patient. An abnormal proximal budding locus on the mesonephric duct allows the ureteral bud to remain in prolonged contact with the Wolffian duct, so that the medially ectopic ureteral orifice may open anywhere along

the course of the Wolffian duct (Fig. 43-8). In males, this includes the posterior urethra, seminal vesicles, vas deferens, or epididymis (44). In females, the ectopic ureter may open into the urethra, the uterus, or proximal vagina, or along the course of Gartner's duct in the anterolateral wall of the vagina. If a medially ectopic ureter opens within the confines of the bladder, no clinical abnormality occurs. If, however, the ureter opens within the confines of the bladder neck mechanism, obstruction of the involved renal unit or vesicoureteral reflux may occur.

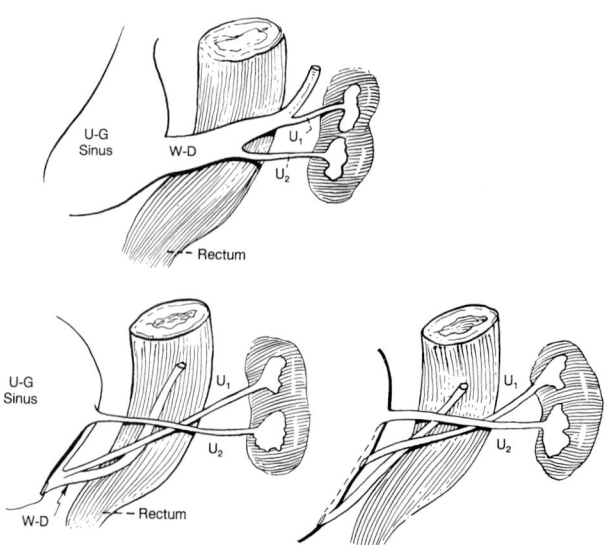

Figure 43-7 Development of ectopic ureter. U, ureter; U-G, urogenital; W-D, Wolffian duct. From Kelalis PP, King LR, Belman AB, eds. *Clinical pediatric urology*, vol. 1. Philadelphia: WB Saunders, 1976:510, with permission.

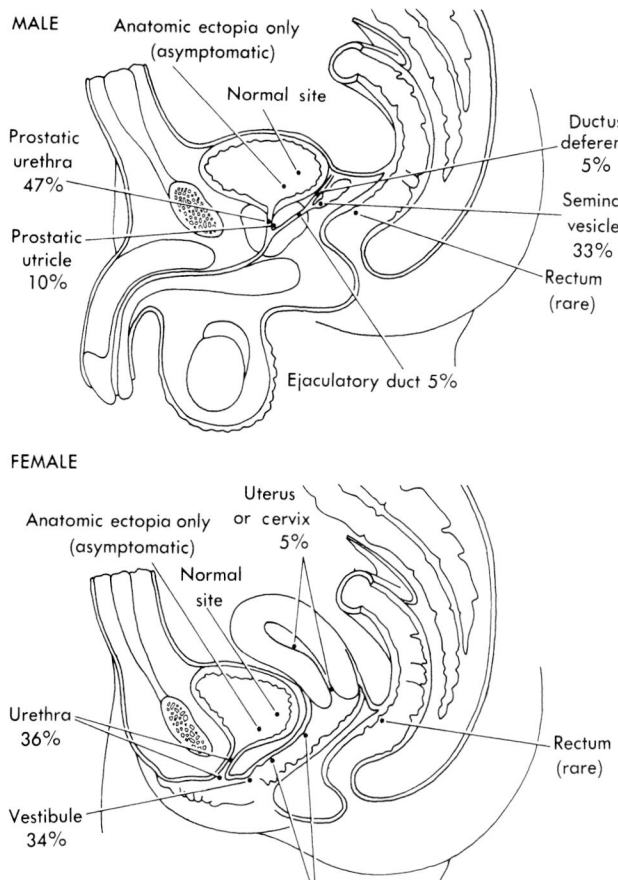

Figure 43-8 Sites of ectopic ureteral orifices and their relative frequencies of occurrence in men and women. From Gray SW, Skandalakis JE. *Embryology for surgeons*. Philadelphia: WB Saunders, 1972:536, with permission.

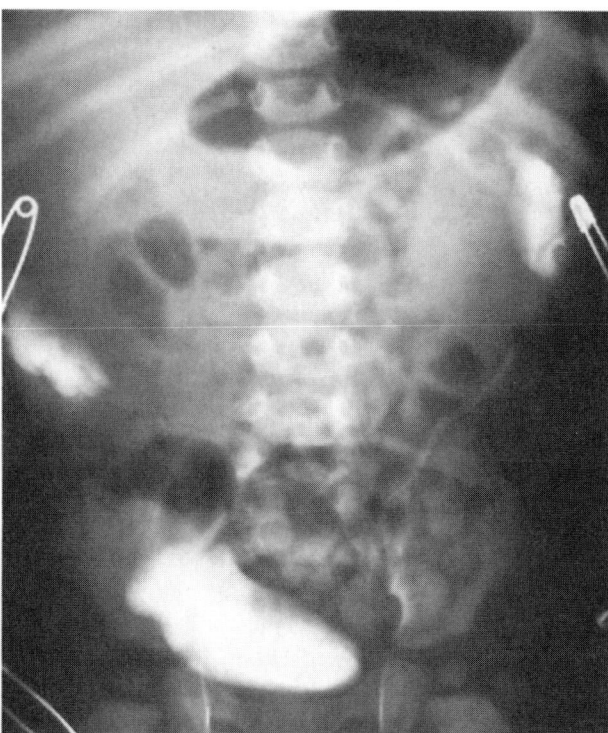

Figure 43-9 Excretory urogram in an infant with ureteral duplication. Ectopic ureters from upper segments produced massive displacement of lower segments, leading to a misdiagnosis of abdominal mass and neuroblastoma. From Kelalis PP, King LR, Belman AB, eds. *Clinical pediatric urology*, vol. 1. Philadelphia: WB Saunders, 1976:518, with permission.

In females, ectopic ureteral orifices that lie distal to the internal sphincter mechanism of the bladder neck can cause incontinence (45). Older girls usually present with constant dampness that is associated with an otherwise symptom-free, normal voiding pattern. Infant girls may be constantly wet or have a purulent discharge if the system is infected. Physical examination suggests the diagnosis if urine can be seen welling up in the vagina or if a spurt of urine is seen coming from the perineal ectopic ureteral orifice. Many are not diagnosed by physical findings alone. Eighty percent of these ectopic ureters arise from the upper pole segment of a total ureteral duplication, and CT, MRI, or diuretic renography with radionuclide agents will better delineate the anatomy. Occasionally, intravenous urography may suggest the diagnosis (45). However, the ectopic segment frequently functions poorly and it may not be visible on excretory urography even with delayed radiographs. A high index of suspicion and an awareness of the radiographic clues to a nonvisible duplication (i.e., the drooping lily sign) often will lead to the diagnosis (Fig. 43-9). Because an ectopic vaginal ureter may drain a poorly functioning and thus non-visualizable single renal unit, congenital absence of one kidney in a girl with incontinence must not be accepted as a

diagnosis without a thorough investigation. This investigation should include abdominal sonography, nuclear renal scan; occasionally computed tomography or MRI may be the only way to define the anatomy (46).

Treatment of the ectopic ureter depends on the presence or absence of significant function in the involved renal unit. If the ureter drains an otherwise healthy system, ureteral reimplantation into the bladder will correct the problem and preserve maximal renal function. If the ureteral anomaly is associated with a duplex kidney and there is good function in both segments of the kidney, ipsilateral ureteroureterostomy is indicated. Generally, the involved renal unit functions poorly, so excision of the involved segment is indicated. The distal ureteral stump is left undisturbed to avoid compromise of the normal sphincter mechanisms. The male infant with an ectopic ureter frequently presents with an antenatal ultrasound finding suggestive of ureteral dilatation, a mass, urinary tract infection, or epididymitis (44). In boys, an ectopic ureter will arise more frequently from a nonduplicated kidney, and can drain into the male genital tract anywhere from the prostatic urethra to the epididymis. Treatment is similar to that for females.

Ureterocele

A ureterocele is a cystic dilation of the distal submucosal or intravesical portion of a ureter. Ureteroceles account for a broad spectrum of associated or secondary pathologic conditions, and constitute one of the more complex and confusing groups of anomalies of the lower urinary tract (47).

Ureteroceles in children most commonly involve the end of the upper pole ureter of a duplex kidney (i.e., ectopic ureterocele), but may less commonly involve a single-system ureter (i.e., simple ureterocele) (48). The etiology of ureteroceles is uncertain. Failure of reabsorption of the Chwalla membrane from over the ureteral orifice has been proposed as an obstructive etiology (34). It seems more likely that ureteroceles result from an intrinsic defect in the ureteral bud itself, and from faulty or delayed incorporation of the ureteral bud into the urethra and bladder base (45).

Ureteroceles associated with a single-system ureter (i.e., simple ureteroceles) tend to be intravesical and in the normal position. Intravesical ureteroceles in children often are also associated with hydronephrosis of varying degrees (49).

Ureteroceles may be associated with significant derangement of the upper and lower urinary tract. The ureterocele most commonly originating from the upper pole ureter of a duplex kidney is associated with secondary pathology; the most frequently noted associated condition is hydronephrosis, with impaired function or dysplasia of the upper pole system and obstruction or reflux in the ipsilateral lower pole system (Fig. 43-10). Contralateral reflux or obstruction also may occur. The pathophysiology of the associated findings is easily understood by recognizing that a ureterocele may dissect under the trigonal epithelium and deform the ipsilateral or contralateral ureterovesical junction, causing various combinations of vesicoureteral

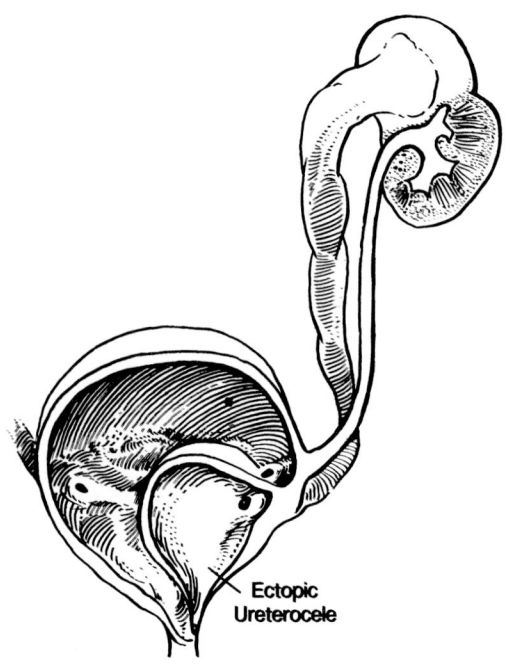

Figure 43-10   Ectopic ureterocele. From Malek RS, Kelalis PP, Burke EC, et al. Simple and ectopic ureterocele in infancy and childhood. *Surg Gynecol Obstet* 1972;134:611, with permission.

reflux or obstruction in any or all of the ureters (50). Ten percent of ureteroceles occur bilaterally (47). If the ureterocele prolapses into, or otherwise occludes, the bladder outlet, bilateral hydronephrosis and relative bladder outlet obstruction may occur.

Ureteroceles occur more commonly in females and usually manifest in early childhood; the ratio of occurrence in males and females is 1:6 cases (47). Most of our patients have presented during the first year of life. Most are now diagnosed antenatally with ultrasound but, historically, the most common presentation was that of a febrile infant found to have a urinary tract infection. If the ureterocele prolapses into the urethra, difficult voiding or azotemia may prompt evaluation. Ureterocele is the most common cause of urinary retention in the female infant. Rarely, a ureterocele will prolapse through the external urethral meatus in a female and present as an introital mass.

Classically, the diagnosis of a ureterocele is fairly straightforward. Renal and bladder ultrasonography will reveal the upper tract dilation and the wall of the ureterocele in the bladder (51). This can be seen antenatally. The intravenous urogram, if obtained, commonly shows complete ureteral duplication with upper pole hydronephrosis and the characteristic lucency of the ureterocele in the bladder. Cystography is necessary to establish the presence or absence of associated vesicoureteral reflux and to assess the integrity of the detrusor muscle backing the ureterocele. A diuretic renal scan can outline the function of the involved upper pole segment and any measurable obstruction of any of the segments, and is helpful in determining the best surgical approach.

The choice of treatment of a ureterocele depends on several factors. The age and clinical condition of the patient, the presence or absence of significant function in the involved renoureteral unit, and the presence of reflux or obstruction in the ipsilateral or contralateral uninvolved ureters all influence the choice of therapy. In the critically ill, septic infant, transurethral or transvesical unroofing or puncture of the ureterocele may provide decompression and allow stabilization of the child until his or her clinical condition allows definitive treatment. Alternatively, placement of a temporary percutaneous nephrostomy into the involved renal unit often can be done without the need for general anesthesia. The best form of definitive treatment has been debated over the years. If an intravesical ureterocele is associated with a single kidney and minimal hydronephrosis, simple excision of the ureterocele and reimplantation of the involved ureter should suffice. However, cystoscopic puncture of the ureterocele may also correct the problem without need for further surgical intervention (52). Even if the system is duplex, an en bloc ureteral reimplantation can be performed if the ureters are not too dilated (47).

Generally, definitive management of the hydronephrotic upper tract associated with a ureterocele depends on the function of the obstructed segment. If sufficient function exists in the involved unit, pyeloureterostomy or ureteroureterostomy to the ipsilateral uninvolved unit is appropriate (47). In the most common situation, however, function usually is so poor that removal of the involved upper pole unit may be necessary (47). Some patients have had. distal ureterocele reconstruction without hemi-nephrectomy with good initial results. The upper pole should be followed for resolution of the hydronephrosis. Some centers have described definitive endoscopic treatment of the ureterocele by puncturing the ureterocele with an electrocautery probe (53). Initially promising success rates have not proven to be as good as predicted (52). Woodard found that 80% of his patients required further surgery when transurethral puncturing of ureteroceles was used as primary therapy (178). Puncture of the ureterocele is appropriate initial management for unstable or septic patients and in select patients with intravesical ureteroceles as potentially definitive treatment. Debate centers over the management of the distal ureter and ureterocele itself. If upper pole nephrectomy has been performed, the distal ureter and ureterocele may collapse, alleviating any associated pathologic condition caused by the mass effect of the ureterocele. If there is significant reflux into the ureter associated with the ureterocele (which is uncommon), or if the ureterocele tends to evert into the dilated ureter prior to initial surgical intervention, excision of the involved ureter and marsupialization of the ureterocele is preferred. Depending on the function of the upper pole moiety, either heminephrectomy or upper to lower pole uretero-ureterostomy generally is also necessary. This obviates the need for a secondary, delayed surgical excision of the ureterocele because of recurrent urinary tract infections or persistent reflux (50). At times, preliminary cutaneous diversion of the involved ureter with delayed reconstruction is warranted, to allow maximal recovery of function before deciding on the need for nephrectomy vs. reconstruction (47).

Ureteropelvic Junction Obstruction

Obstruction at the ureteropelvic junction probably is the most common cause of a palpable abdominal mass in the newborn, and is the most common cause of antenatal

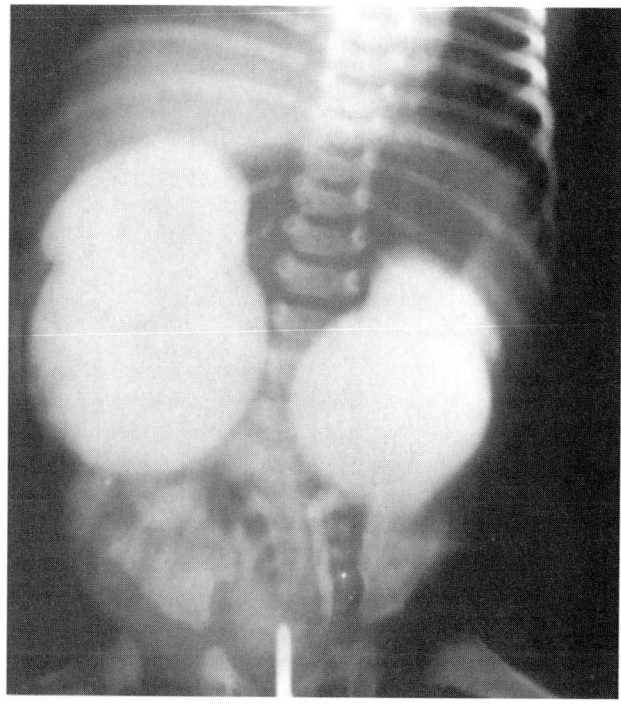

Figure 43-11 Severe bilateral hydronephrosis secondary to ureteropelvic junction obstructions.

hydronephrosis. This lesion usually is the result of narrowing of the ureter at the junction of the renal pelvis with the ureter. Because the renal pelvis is compliant, there can be a great deal of renal preservation despite massive dilation of the kidney behind the obstruction (Fig. 43-11) (54).

The diagnosis of ureteropelvic junction obstruction can be made sonographically because there is a sonolucent central mass within the renal area surrounded by thin renal parenchyma (Fig. 43,12A). A grading system has been suggested by the Society for Fetal Urology to better standardize terminology and interpretation of renal ultrasound findings (55). The system is based on the severity of renal pelvis and calyceal dilatation and the renal parenchymal thickness (Fig. 43-13). Vesicoureteral

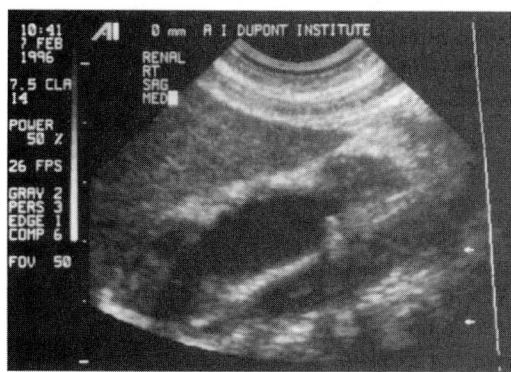

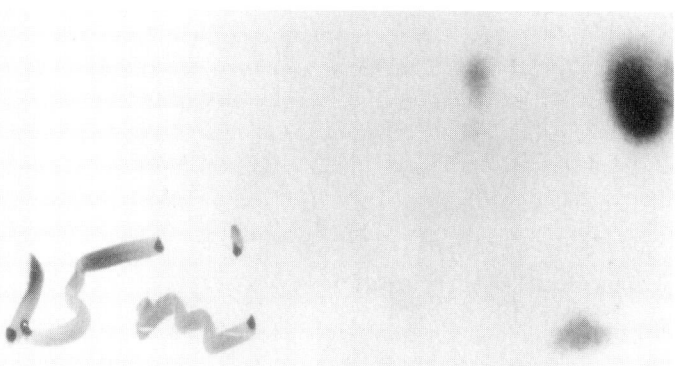

A   **B**

Figure 43-12 **A:** An abdominal ultrasonogram in a newborn infant demonstrates a single, large echo-free region consistent with hydronephrosis. **B:** A delayed renal scan in a newborn infant with right hydronephrosis secondary to ureteropelvic junction obstruction.

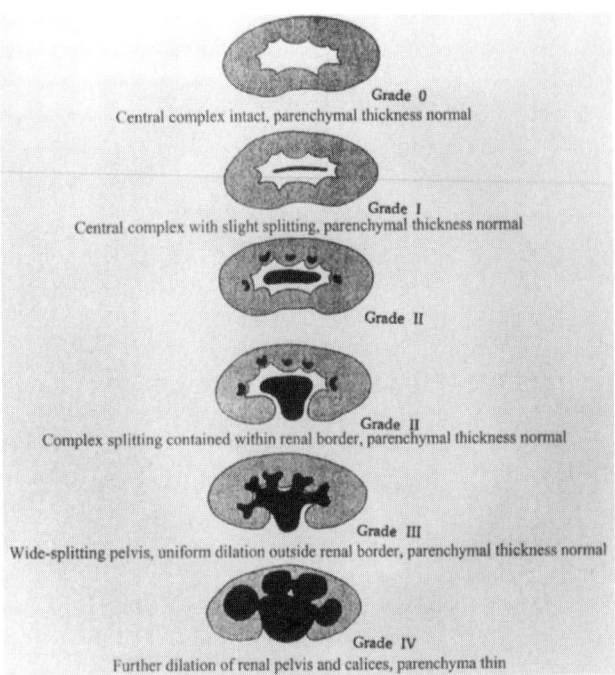

Grade 0
Central complex intact, parenchymal thickness normal

Grade I
Central complex with slight splitting, parenchymal thickness normal

Grade II

Grade II
Complex splitting contained within renal border, parenchymal thickness normal

Grade III
Wide-splitting pelvis, uniform dilation outside renal border, parenchymal thickness normal

Grade IV
Further dilation of renal pelvis and calices, parenchyma thin

Figure 43-13 Society for Fetal Urology grading system for ultrasonographically detected hydronephrosis. From Baskin LS. Prenatal hydronephrosis. In: Baskin LS, Kogan BA, Duckett JW, eds. *Handbook of pediatric urology.* Philadelphia: Lippincott–Raven, 1997:11, with permission. Modified by Curt Powell, M.D.

reflux must be excluded from the differential diagnosis using voiding cystography. The function of the obstructed kidney can be determined by radionuclide scanning (Fig. 43-12B). One of the advantages of radionuclide scintigraphy is that the physiologic significance of dilatation can be determined by administering furosemide (56). If the dilatation is of significance, there will be retention of the radionuclide behind the obstruction, whereas if there is no physiologic significance to the hydronephrosis, the administered diuretic will cause the radionuclide to wash out rapidly from the dilated system. To obtain valid results, the patient must be adequately hydrated and have adequate bladder drainage to prevent false interpretation of obstruction on the scan as a result of dehydration or bladder distention (57). It is becoming apparent, in some instances, that presumed significant hydronephrosis in the newborn is physiologically insignificant and may with time, stabilize or improve and require no treatment. Those instances that are physiologically significant, may require repair, generally dismembered pyeloplasty, resulting in improved drainage and renal function in some instances (54).

Ureterovesical Obstruction

Obstruction at the ureterovesical junction is not nearly so common as obstruction at the ureteropelvic junction, but it is far from rare (36). Lower ureteral obstruction may present as marked hydroureteronephrosis (i.e., a mass), but may sometimes present as urinary infection (Fig. 43-14).

As with ureteropelvic obstruction, it has become apparent that not all ureterovesical obstructions are physiologically significant and some require no treatment. Radionuclide scanning with diuretics is helpful in making the diagnosis of a physiologic obstruction (56). At times, however, an antegrade pyelogram with a pressure perfusion study is necessary to determine the significance or lack of significance of an apparent narrowing at the ureterovesical junction (58). These lesions, if identified as obstructive, are treated by excision of the obstructing segment, tailoring or tapering of the dilated ureter, and reimplantation of the ureter into the bladder (59).

Vesicoureteral Reflux

Vesicoureteral reflux is the most common abnormality of the urinary system seen in children; it may occur in 1 of 100 births (12). The actual incidence is unknown, but it is at least as common as cryptorchidism or hypospadias. Genome mapping, performed on families with primary vesicoureteral reflux who also have associated reflux nephropathy, has found an association with a locus on chromosome 1 which is also seen in some families with vesicoureteral reflux (60). Vesicoureteral reflux is known to

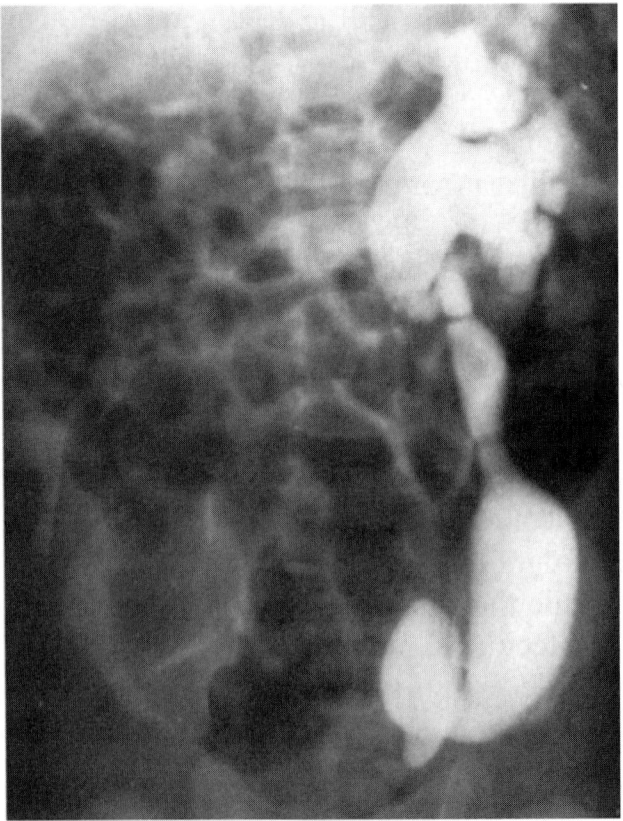

Figure 43-14 Left ureterovesical obstruction in a 3-month-old boy who presented with unresponsive diarrhea. Urine culture was positive, and radiographic evaluation demonstrated significant pathology, as is evident in this illustration. The diarrhea resolved with treatment of the urinary infection. The ureterovesical obstruction was treated surgically. From Kelalis PP, King LR, Belman AB, eds. *Clinical pediatric urology,* vol. 1. Philadelphia: WB Saunders, 1976:276, with permission.

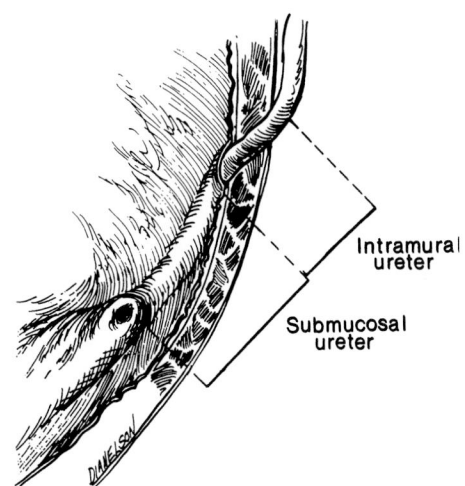

Figure 43-15 Normal ureterovesical junction. From Harrison JH, et al, eds. *Campbell's urology*, 4th ed. Philadelphia: WB Saunders, 1979:1597, with permission.

be a familial problem. When one child in a family is identified as having reflux, as many as 30% to 50% of the siblings of that child may have vesicoureteral reflux (61). For that reason, it is thought that all younger siblings of any proband identified to have reflux should be screened (62). It also has been found that transmission of reflux from a previously refluxing parent to his or her children is approximately 66% (61). The normal ureterovesical junction is a relatively efficient mechanism that allows egress of urine into the lumen of the bladder, but, because of its oblique course through the ureteral wall, prevents the bladder urine from reentering the ureter (Fig. 43-15) (63). It is obvious that there is maturation of the ureterovesical junction with both time and growth, because infants have a much higher incidence of vesicoureteral reflux than do older children (64).

Reflux is graded on an international grading scale of 1 to 5 (65). The major significance of this grading system is that the higher the grade of reflux, the more likely it is that reflux will persist despite somatic growth, and the more likely that there is associated or eventual reflux nephropathy. Conversely, the lower the grade of reflux, the more likely there will be spontaneous resolution of the vesicoureteral reflux without reflux nephropathy (66).

Although the presence of hydronephrosis suggests an abnormality in the urinary tract, many patients with significant vesicoureteral reflux will have a normal ultrasound study. The radiologic confirmation of vesicoureteral reflux is accomplished by voiding cystourethrography. Generally, this should not be performed while the child is actively infected; if an infection has been the presenting sign, voiding cystography may be performed once the urine is sterile and the patient afebrile and under treatment,. Because renal scarring is produced easily in the neonate, it is especially important to establish the presence or absence of vesicoureteral reflux before discontinuing antibiotics in patients who have presented with urinary infection.

Once reflux is demonstrated, especially in the infant, the patient should be maintained on low-dose antibacterial therapy until resolution of the reflux, hopefully preventing urinary tract infections. The choices of agents are limited in the newborn, but amoxicillin is a reasonable alternative until hepatobiliary maturation is sufficient to allow the use of sulfa or nitrofurantoin. A reasonable initial daily suppression dose would be 10 to 25 mg/kg of amoxicillin. With growing concerns of bacterial resistance to amoxicillin, low dose sulfamethoxasole-trimethoprim or nitrofurantoin may be used if carefully monitored. Breakthrough infection, while the patient is on antibacterial suppression or if there is poor parental compliance, suggests the need for surgical repair, either with open surgical techniques or endoscopic techniques.

Exstrophy

Exstrophy of the bladder is a rare, but extremely significant, abnormality (Fig. 43-16). It affects roughly 1 child in every 25,000 live births. Exstrophy is not commonly associated with abnormalities in other organ systems, and the remainder of the urinary tract usually is normal in these children. Functional reconstruction of the exstrophic bladder can be a formidable surgical undertaking, but in experienced hands can result in a continent child with a relatively normal upper urinary tract (67). The major factor affecting the success of closure in terms

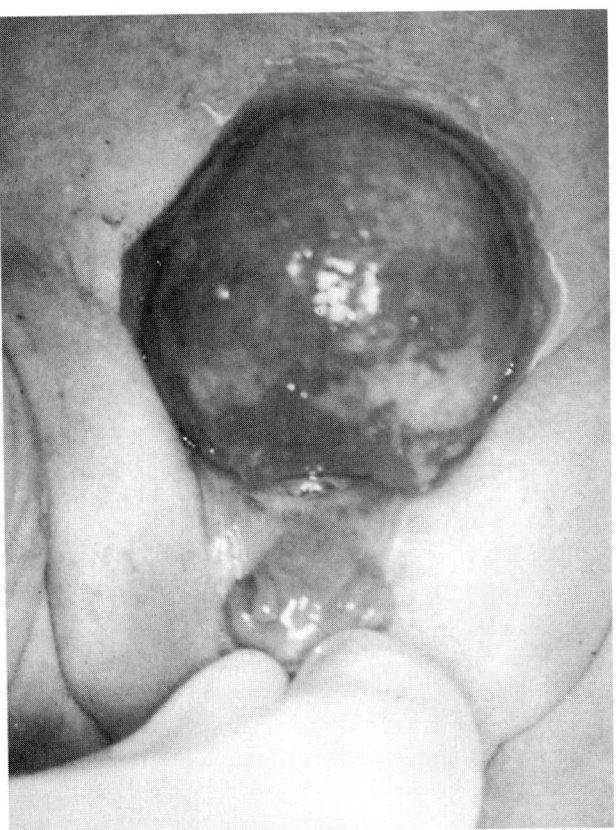

Figure 43-16 Complete bladder exstrophy in a male child. Note that the penis is epispadiac, short, and stubby.

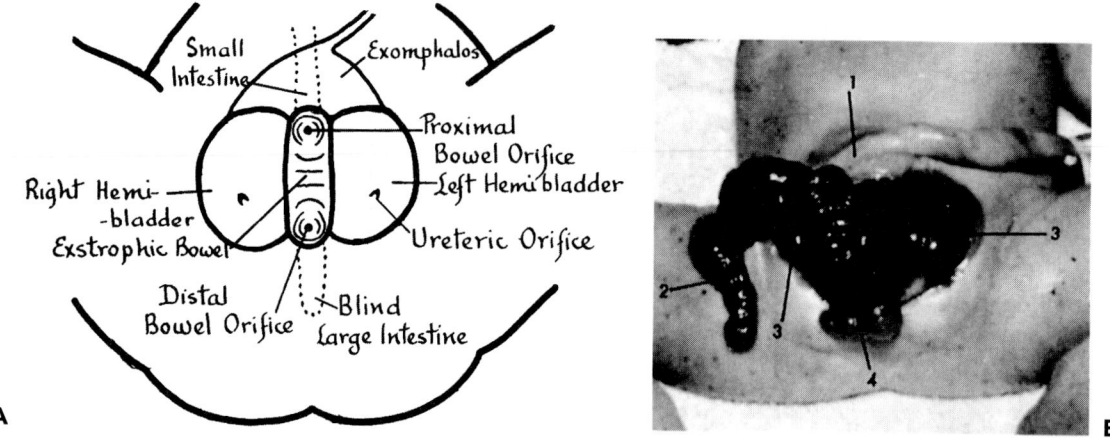

Figure 43-17 Exstrophy of the cloaca. **A:** Diagram of the external anatomy. **B:** In a patient with exstrophy of the cloaca, the anatomic features as numbered include exomphalos (1), ileum that has prolapsed through the proximal bowel orifice (2), and the hemibladders lying on either side of the exstrophic bowel (3). Note the absence of an anus (4) and of definable external genitalia. From Paquin AJ. Ureterovesical anastomosis: the description and evaluation of a technique. *J Urol* 1954;82:573, with permission.

of continence seems to be the size of the exstrophic bladder at presentation.

The epithelium of the exstrophic bladder is grossly normal at birth, but becomes hyperplastic very shortly thereafter if the bladder is not closed. It is preferable, if possible, that the exstrophic bladder be left uncovered and kept moist using plastic wrap pending closure, assuming that closure can be accomplished in the newborn period. Gauze or petroleum gauze should not be used, as these can dry the bladder surface and denude the urothelium.

Functional closure of exstrophy is traditionally a staged procedure. In the first stage, iliac osteotomies are performed to facilitate closure. Even though osteotomy can be omitted, especially in newborns, success rates are higher when osteotomy is used (68). The exstrophic bladder is dissected free from the anterior abdominal wall, closed into a sphere, and dropped back into the pelvis. The abdominal wall then is closed over the bladder. There is no attempt at the first stage to produce urinary continence. After 2 to 3 years, a second-stage procedure is performed in an attempt to produce urinary control. Mitchell has recently advocated bladder closure and epispadias repair as a one-stage procedure, with good initial results that include continence after the single procedure in a significant number of the patients so treated (69).

In the past, ureterosigmoidostomy was used as an alternative to functional closure. In this operation, the ureters were anastomosed to the colon and the patient voided a mixture of urine and stool. There are metabolic abnormalities (e.g., hyperchloremic acidosis) associated with this form of diversion, and it has become apparent that patients who have been treated by ureterosigmoidostomy have an increased risk for development of adenocarcinoma of the colon at some time after their diversion (70). These patients should have routine surveillance colonoscopy. Similarly, the unclosed exstrophic bladder is at high risk

for development of adenocarcinoma of the bladder in the second or third decade of life (71). Functional closure seems to obviate this latter risk.

Exstrophy of the cloaca is a severe anomaly, once thought incompatible with long-term survival. In this anomaly, two halves of an exstrophic bladder are separated by a midline strip of exteriorized cecum (Fig. 43-17) (72). The ileum may prolapse through the bowel plate. Additionally, the child has an imperforate anus with almost no colon present distal to the exstrophic bowel plate. The small intestine is often short, and there may be a malrotation anomaly. The genital tubercle is split and widely separated. Hence, it is very difficult to produce a functional penis in boys with this anomaly (73). Genetic males with cloacal exstrophy were previously raised as females, but this practice is now questioned as some gender reassigned patients have expressed the view that they are uncomfortable with their assigned role (74). Some of these individuals are now being reassigned based on their genotypic karyotype. Each patient's ultimate gender of rearing should be carefully discussed and determined with the parents, with great thought and open discussion about these complexities. These children often have spinal dysraphism and a neurogenic bladder and bowel. For this reason, and the very short colon, a functional anus is almost impossible to produce, and permanent colostomy, incorporating the exstrophic bowel, is the bowel diversion of choice. Because the colon is short, it is best to preserve as much as possible to improve water reabsorption. Permanent ileostomy, although used in the past, may lead to problems with dehydration and short gut syndrome. Because of the problems with a short gut, a staged reconstruction is generally recommended by addressing the bowel problems with initial colostomy and considering further reconstruction once patient survival and bowel function is better determined. Ultimate bladder closure uniting the two halves of the exstrophic bladder, utilizes iliac osteotomy before anterior closure. Although normal urinary control usually is not possible, dryness provided by clean intermittent catheterization is a reasonable goal.

Patent Urachus

The urachus is a tube that connects the urogenital sinus and the allantois between months 3 and 5 of intrauterine life. The urachus normally regresses first to a small-caliber, epithelialized tube and then into a sealed, obliterated cord by term or during the neonatal period. It may remain patent up to the infraumbilical area in the premature infant (75). Thirty-two percent of all bladders have tubular remnants of the urachus noted at necropsy (76). Significant urachal anomalies are rare; they occur twice as often in males as in females (76).

Complete failure of obliteration of the urachus results in a persistent communication between the bladder and the umbilicus that leaks urine intermittently or continuously. It is the most common urachal anomaly encountered. The etiology of this condition is unknown. It has been suggested that bladder outlet obstruction may be a contributing factor, although the chronology of embryologic events suggests that the urachal lumen obliterates before urethral tubularization. Ultrasonography can frequently diagnose a persistent tract up to the umbilicus. The diagnosis may ultimately be confirmed by retrograde fistulography, instillation of methylene blue into the tract or intravesically, or injection of indigo carmine intravenously. A voiding cystourethrogram occasionally will demonstrate the communication, but is more useful to look for other associated lower urinary tract anomalies such as obstruction or vesicoureteral reflux. A persistent omphalomesenteric duct must be considered in the differential diagnosis. In infants with minimal umbilical drainage that causes a small stain on the diaper, an umbilical granuloma or a patch of gastric mucosa may be at fault (77). Iatrogenic creation of a vesicoumbilical fistula, during an umbilical artery cutdown, has been reported (75). Treatment of a patent urachus consists of complete extraperitoneal excision of the urachus with an attached cuff of bladder to completely remove any urachal remnant in the bladder and prevent possible cancer development in residual tissue. Attempts should be made to preserve the umbilicus.

Megacystis Microcolon Intestinal Hypoperistalsis Syndrome

Megacystis microcolon intestinal hypoperistalsis syndrome (MMIHS) was first described in 1976 and is considered rare (78). The disorder, thought to be an autosomal recessive trait, affects females more than males (4:1 preponderance) and generally is fatal within the first year of life. In a large review of 72 patients only 10 survived, with 9 on parenteral nutrition. Most patients die from sepsis, liver failure and postoperative complications (79). Presentation includes abdominal distention, an abdominal mass (i.e., a distended bladder), and functional intestinal obstruction

characterized by bilious vomiting and absent or decreased bowel sounds. The small bowel is short, dilated, and hypoactive, and may have associated malrotation and an accompanying microcolon but no anatomic obstruction. The abdominal musculature generally is lax. Many of these patients are now presumptively diagnosed prenatally with ultrasonography demonstrating a large bladder, generally with a thin wall, bilateral hydroureteronephrosis, with normal or increased amniotic fluid (thought to be as a result of the microcolon) (80).

The etiology is unknown. Treatment consists of parenteral alimentation and urinary diversion by means of a cutaneous vesicostomy. Patients with Ochoa urofacial syndrome also may present with megacystis in infancy (81).

Posterior Urethral Valves

The most common lesion obstructing the lower urinary tract in a boy is the lesion termed posterior urethral valves, occurring in 1:8000 to 1:25000 live births (82) (Fig. 43-18). The name is a misnomer, because the valves are really a diaphragm or membrane that traverses the urethra from a point just distal to the verumontanum in which it connects with urothelial folds (71,84). Dewan and colleagues have extensively studied the anatomy of this membrane with videocystourethrography, and prefer to classify this anomaly as a congenital posterior urethral membrane (COPUM) as a result of its variable morphological expression (84). Embryologically, these membranes occur because there is an abnormal anterior insertion and persistence of the distal extent of the Wolffian duct (43). To understand the clinical picture of urethral valves, one must consider the dynamics and pathophysiologic consequences of the obstruction itself. The valves are best considered as a rigid membrane, despite their frequently flimsy nature. The vesical neck also is a relatively rigid area. With antegrade flow of fluid, this membrane obstructs. When obstruction is present, the urethra dilates proximally and elongates. The detrusor hypertrophies, with resultant trabeculation and sacculation in response to the extra work involved in voiding. Detrusor hypertrophy also produces relative hypertrophy of the vesical neck.

The prostatic urethra becomes dilated in a fusiform manner between the two relatively rigid points, creating a subvesical chamber. If there is a primary abnormality of the ureterovesical junction, or if a paraureteral saccule develops, vesicoureteral reflux may result. The presence of bilateral vesicoureteral reflux increases the possibility that renal failure will eventually occur. Hydroureteronephrosis may develop, with or without reflux. Renal parenchymal damage in the form of renal dysplasia or interstitial nephritis, with or without superimposed pyelonephritis, often is concomitant or a result of the urethral obstruction. Renal dysplasia is frequently present at birth in infants with posterior urethral valves, and has been found at as early as 15 weeks of gestational age in the fetus (85).

Osathanondh and Potter (86) state that dysplasia is a consequence of intrauterine urinary obstruction. In

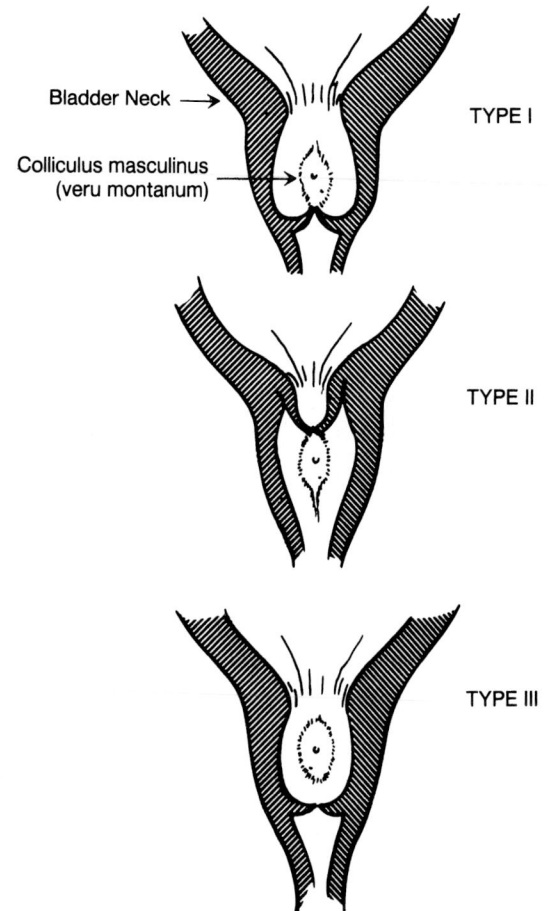

Bladder Neck →

Colliculus masculinus
(veru montanum) →

TYPE I

TYPE II

TYPE III

Figure 43-18 Young classified valves into three types. The type II valve probably does not exist. From Kelalis PP, King LR, Belman AB, eds. *Clinical pediatric urology*, vol. 1. Philadelphia: WB Saunders, 1976:306, with permission.

experimental animals, intrauterine urethral obstruction early in gestation usually has led to a patent urachus, without hydronephrosis or dysplasia—a situation that does not correspond to the clinical sequence in humans (87). Later in gestation, experimental intrauterine urethral obstruction results in hydronephrosis without dysplasia (88). Recent experimentation creating urethral obstruction or ureteral obstruction at different stages in gestation in the lamb may produce a kidney similar to a MCDK (if earlier in gestation) or an obstructed hydronephrotic kidney similar to those seen with posterior urethral valves (if later in gestation) (38).

Clinically, dysplasia is found more often in association with severe vesicoureteral reflux (89). Additionally, dysplasia often is unilateral and not bilateral, as one would expect if it resulted from intrauterine urethral obstruction. Maizels and Simpson (90), using chick embryos, showed that dysplasia results from problems associated with the renal blastema and not from obstruction of the ureter. Dysplasia, when present, may represent a primary abnormality of the ureterorenal unit and may have no direct causal relationship to the presence of intrauterine urethral obstruction.

The clinical presentation of the infant with posterior urethral valves often is related to the severity of the obstruction. Virtually all of the signs and symptoms seen in the boy with posterior urethral valves are secondary to the obstructive nature of the valves, the effect of intrauterine oligohydramnios, or the presence of superimposed urinary infection or azotemia (10,91). Routine use of ultrasonography has increased the detection of a thick walled bladder with a keyhole configuration, with or without hydroureteronephrosis, and oligohydramnios suggestive of posterior urethral valves however postnatal confirmation of valves is only about 39% to 40% (4).

If not detected antenatally, 25% to 50% of boys with posterior urethral valves present during the neonatal period (92). The nonrenal features of Potter syndrome may be seen in newborns with posterior urethral valves, including intrauterine growth deficiency, pulmonary hypoplasia, limb positioning defects (e.g., talipes equinovarus), and the characteristic Potter facies. All are thought to be as a result of a deficiency of amniotic fluid and subsequent fetal compression. The incidence of other organ system anomalies not directly attributable to urethral obstruction is low (93). A palpably enlarged bladder, urinary tract infection, ascites, pulmonary difficulties, such as isolated pneumothorax, failure to thrive, or gastrointestinal disturbances may lead to investigation. A strong urinary stream does not preclude the diagnosis of posterior urethral obstruction (94). Pulmonary hypoplasia will present with respiratory distress, especially with spontaneous pneumothorax or pneumomediastinum, which is an unusual but important symptom of valves in newborns. Any full-term boy with respiratory distress should be suspect for a renal problem. Hydronephrosis is present in 90% of infants with valves (94).

Boys who present with posterior urethral valves in infancy have a poorer prognosis than children who present symptomatically at an older age, especially if serum creatinine levels are higher than 0.8 mg% or 1.0 mg% at 1 month after treatment of the valves. Presumably, this is because there is a high incidence of renal dysplasia associated with this type of presentation.

Urinary ascites is a less common presentation for children with posterior urethral valves (95). The presence of ascitic fluid in a newborn infant should prompt investigation of the urinary tract, because urinary ascites is responsible for one-third of all cases of neonatal ascites (96). Ascites is rarely as a result of frank perforation of the urinary tract (97); most often it is as a result of leakage of urine through the renal fornices and transudation of fluid across the peritoneal membrane into the peritoneal cavity (98). The ascitic fluid usually has a chemical content equivalent to that of serum, because the peritoneal membrane has passively dialyzed the high urea and creatinine content of urine into the vascular system. These children may not have marked hydronephrosis because the urinary tract has been decompressed by leakage of urine (98). These boys often present as extremely ill infants, but occasionally appear to be initially healthy except for abdominal distention. Their prognosis regarding renal preservation often is better than that of a child who does not present with urinary ascites, presumably because the leakage of urine from the distended system protects the upper urinary tract from the ravages of high intraluminal pressure (98). Occasionally, a localized retroperitoneal urinoma will form. The diagnosis of urinary ascites usually is made clinically, and confirmed by ultrasound examination or a plain radiograph of the abdomen demonstrating bowel displaced to the central abdomen and a ground-glass appearance of the remainder of the abdomen.

Twenty-five to 50% of patients with posterior urethral valves have vesicoureteral reflux at presentation (10,99). In one-half of cases, the reflux is bilateral. When there is massive unilateral vesicoureteral reflux associated with posterior urethral valves, the kidney on the refluxing side often is dysplastic and does not function at presentation or subsequently. This is the so-called VURD syndrome (valves, unilateral reflux, and dysplasia). VURD syndrome was initially thought to have a protective effect on the nonrefluxing kidney, but recent long term follow up of some patients with VURD have found that only 25% of the boys between ages 5 and 8 years had normal renal function (100). Marked hydronephrosis without vesicoureteral reflux usually carries a better prognosis for long-term renal function than does the presence of bilateral vesicoureteral reflux. In patients with posterior urethral valves, if reflux is present, it will resolve with relief of obstruction in one-third to one-half of cases (99).

Obstructive uropathy will be suggested on ultrasonography by findings such as bilateral hydronephrosis or by a distended, thick-walled bladder. Patients with posterior urethral valves often have a dilated and elongated posterior urethra that can be imaged sonographically and has been termed the keyhole bladder. Perirenal urinoma or ascites also can be detected.

The single most important study in the diagnosis of infravesical obstruction is the voiding cystourethrogram. An adequate study requires complete visualization of the urethra from the bladder neck to the meatus and oblique and lateral projections of the urethra during voiding without a catheter in the urethra, because an indwelling catheter may obscure the lesion.

Posterior urethral valves appear as a sharply defined transverse or oblique lucency, with proximal urethral elongation and distention and diminution of flow distal to the valve. The bladder neck may be secondarily thickened and collar-like. The bladder usually is trabeculated with saccules or diverticula, especially paraurethral diverticula (Fig. 43-19). Vesicoureteral reflux is often present at diagnosis, and the refluxing ureters frequently are grossly dilated and tortuous.

Functional imaging studies of the upper urinary tracts will determine the degree of upper tract damage produced by lower tract obstruction. Historically, intravenous urography has been used routinely in upper tract imaging but may be inconclusive, especially if renal function is poor. If

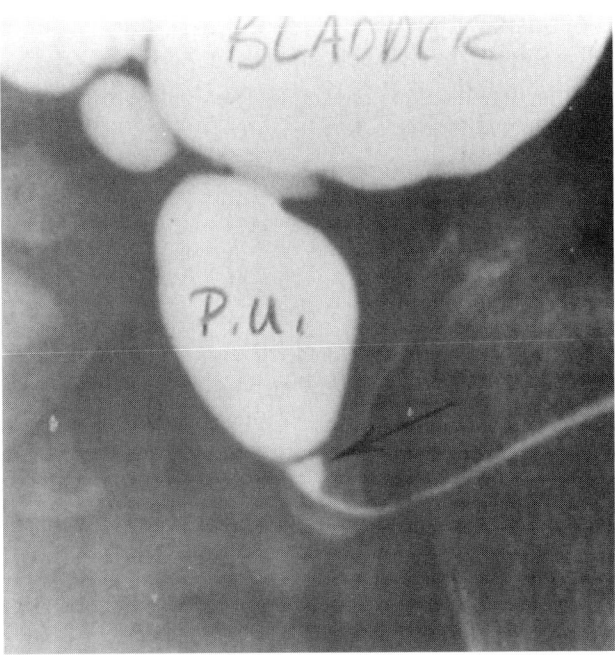

Figure 43-19 Voiding cystourethrogram in a newborn boy with posterior urethral value (arrow). The prostatic urethra (PU) is dilated, and the bladder is trabeculated with multiple diverticula (upper left).

function is sufficient for radiographic visualization and if delayed radiographs are obtained, marked hydroureteronephrosis should be evident. Delayed filling, visualizing a poorly functioning renal unit, may be secondary to vesicoureteral reflux rather than evidence of renal function. In the newborn or azotemic infant in whom obstruction is suspected, a radionuclide renal scan usually provides more information than excretory urography. A scan allows estimation of differential renal function. Scintigraphy also is safer than excretory urography because it eliminates the need for iodinated contrast agents, which have a risk for associated morbidity.

When these infants first present, resuscitative measures may be necessary to treat associated urinary infection, replace fluid and electrolytes, and, most important, drain the urinary tract. A small intraurethral catheter (e.g., a feeding tube) often will suffice to drain the urinary tract for a few days. Once the child is stable, the valves must be either transurethrally resected primarily or the urinary tract should be drained for a prolonged period using a cutaneous vesicostomy. Many of these infants are anticipated in advance because of suggestive antenatal imaging; they can be followed closely immediately after birth and may not require resuscitative measures, because the child generally is evaluated almost immediately after birth.

The long-term outlook for infants who present with posterior urethral valves is only fair, because approximately 50% of boys who present with posterior urethral valves eventually will progress to renal failure and transplantation despite treatment (101). This does not mean that a fatalistic attitude must be adopted, but, nonetheless, expectations must be realistic. If the serum creatinine is normal at 2 years of age, the prognosis for long-term normal renal function is good but not perfect (102). In a long-term follow-up of 11 to 22 years of children with urethral valves, one-third had poor renal function: 10% who survived childhood had died of renal failure; 21% had end-stage renal disease or chronic renal failure; and 46% had diurnal enuresis. Diurnal enuresis increased the likelihood that there would be progression to renal failure (103).

In utero intervention, with vesicoamniotic shunts or primary fetal endoscopic ablation of valves, has not improved survival or renal function in this group of patients; many expire before delivery as a result of premature rupture of membranes or sepsis, and many of those who survive go on to develop chronic renal failure and renal transplantation (3,4,5,104).

Renal Tumors

Fortunately, tumors of the urinary tract are rare in infancy and those that do occur tend to exhibit a benign behavior. Variants of Wilms' tumor can be seen in the neonatal period and include mesoblastic nephroma (105), nephroblastomatosis (106), and benign cystic nephroma (107). With the advent of frequent in utero ultrasonographic screening, many of these lesions are found as abnormally large kidneys or kidneys with a recognizable mass on ultrasound. Otherwise, they usually will present in infancy as a palpable flank mass and occasionally can produce hypertension (108).

Mesoblastic nephroma is the most frequent of these tumors. This recognized variant of Wilms' tumor behaves in an almost uniformly benign manner (105). Histologically, mesoblastic nephroma is composed largely of mesenchymal stroma with spindle-shaped fibrous or leiomyomatous cells. Ultrasonography will demonstrate a solid intrarenal mass. Computerized tomography will better delineate the mass characteristics, and may demonstrate tumor extension outside the renal bed. Although rarely obtained, radionuclide scans will show the mass as nonfunctioning tissue, and intravenous urography will reveal distortion of the calyceal architecture by the tumor. Ultrasound and computerized tomography will demonstrate the tissue characteristics more clearly than scintigraphy or pyelography. MRI with gadolinium may be necessary to better delineate subtle lesions. Nephrectomy is curative, but there have been a few reports of local recurrence and rare reports of distant metastasis (105). Chemotherapy and radiation therapy are not necessary adjuncts to therapy.

Nephroblastomatosis can be diffuse or nodular (106). Diffuse nephroblastomatosis usually presents as marked enlargement of both kidneys. The kidneys are grossly enlarged and have a whitish hue. Biopsy reveals primitive metanephric epithelium resembling that seen in Wilms' tumor. This lesion usually responds to chemotherapy (i.e., actinomycin D). Nodular renal blastoma consists of microscopic foci of primitive metanephric epithelium and often

is an incidental autopsy finding in infants. It is thought that Wilms' tumor may, in some instances, arise from foci of nodular renal blastema.

Benign cystic nephroma occasionally is classified with the cystic diseases, but more properly belongs with the renal tumors because elements of Wilms' tumor may be found in the septa between the cysts (109). As with the other tumors, patients with cystic nephroma present with a palpable mass. Ultrasonography will identify the mass as multiple cysts or as complex (i.e., mixed cystic and solid). Although enucleation of the mass is a theoretical therapeutic option, nephrectomy usually is the treatment of choice. Despite the presence of Wilms' tumor elements in the septa, chemotherapy is not necessary for cure.

Renal Vein Thrombosis

Another renal lesion that has a definite predilection for the neonatal period is renal vein thrombosis (110). This problem usually results from hemoconcentration secondary to dehydration, and is often seen in infants of diabetic mothers. It also may be seen in infants with cyanotic congenital heart disease, sickle-cell disease, or perinatal stress or sepsis. Sludging in the intrarenal venules occurs, with subsequent thrombosis. The thrombus then tends to propagate centrally. The infants present with a palpable mass, hematuria, albuminuria, and thrombocytopenia. If both kidneys are involved, the infant will become uremic. Treatment is supportive and involves correction of the underlying problems. Surgery (i.e., nephrectomy) was once thought essential to survival; however, it is recognized that nephrectomy is unnecessary and that, if collateral circulation is present, there may be renal recovery. Thrombectomy is of no help because the problem is in the peripheral rather than the central veins. Thrombolytic agents developed for clot lysis may be considered for treatment of bilateral renal vein thrombosis.

Adrenal Hemorrhage

At times, either spontaneously or in association with renal vein thrombosis, there may be hemorrhage into the adrenal gland (111). Hemorrhage also can occur following a traumatic delivery, sepsis, or asphyxia. The infant may present with icterus (from absorption of hemoglobin) and an abdominal mass. Ultrasonography will demonstrate a sonolucent or solid mass above the kidney. This may also be detected with antenatal ultrasonography as an adrenal mass. It must be followed postnatally to differentiate it from a congenital neuroblastoma or neural crest tumor (CT may be required to differentiate an adrenal tumor from an adrenal hemorrhage). Over the course of a few weeks, the mass, if as a result of adrenal hemorrhage, will be reabsorbed or, rarely, will form an adrenal pseudocyst (112). If the latter occurs, percutaneous drainage is the preferred mode of therapy. Otherwise, no therapy is necessary. Adrenal calcification often is seen several weeks after an adrenal hemorrhage. Adrenal hemorrhage can occur bilaterally in 10% of patients, and it occurs more commonly on the right side.

Prenatal Ultrasonography

The advent of high-resolution, real-time ultrasonography has allowed the antenatal diagnosis of many anomalies of the urinary tract. It has become apparent with time, however, that diagnostic accuracy in utero is not complete and that the natural history of some lesions is not as clear-cut as once thought (113). The hope that antenatal intervention might result in improvement in outcome has proven ill-founded (114). The maternal risk of morbidity with intervention has been reported to be as high as 4% to 5% (115), and there are no clear-cut examples of improvement in fetal outcome as a result of such interventions (10,116). Studies of the results of postnatal treatment after antenatal identification of lesions have, however, clearly demonstrated improved outcome (115). There seems to be no advantage to early delivery; thus, the timing of delivery in fetuses with hydronephrosis generally is determined best by obstetric factors rather than fetal concerns (117).

As stated earlier, the fetal kidneys can be identified in the early part of the second trimester of pregnancy. Dilation of the renal pelvis and calices in a nonduplex system, without identification of a dilated ureter, suggests the presence of ureteropelvic obstruction. It has become apparent that some instances of hydronephrosis resolve spontaneously and completely in utero, whereas most that are present at birth will stabilize or improve with time. Conversely, some seem to dilate progressively with time. Hence, not all dilations of the upper urinary tract are obstructive in nature (113). Most of those that are of significance prove to be secondary to narrowing at the ureteropelvic junction. In the hope of standardizing the descriptive terminology for the ultrasound findings with hydronephrosis, the Society for Fetal Urology has graded the severity of the hydronephrosis based on the extent of renal pelvis and calyceal dilatation and parenchymal thinning or atrophy (58).

In a duplicated system, there can be dilation of either the lower pole system or the upper pole system. Dilations of the lower pole system usually are as a result of ureteropelvic junction obstruction or to vesicoureteral reflux. Obstructions of the upper pole system usually are associated with hydroureter and often are accompanied by a ureterocele or an obstructed ectopic ureter. Solid intrarenal lesions most commonly are mesoblastic nephromas, with neuroblastoma occurring infrequently.

Ureteral dilation can, at times, be massive and may be confused with bowel on sonography; however, following the ureter from a dilated upper system down to the bladder usually will distinguish the dilated ureter from bowel because dilated ureters often do not demonstrate peristalsis. Although bilateral hydroureter may be associated with bilateral ureterovesical obstruction, it is more likely as a result of either high-grade vesicoureteral reflux, posterior urethral valves, or the prune-belly syndrome.

In a male fetus, a thick-walled, enlarged bladder often is secondary to posterior urethral valves or the prune-belly syndrome, especially if a keyhole posterior urethra is identified. In females, an enlarged bladder is more likely as a result of the megalocystis microcolon hypoperistalsis syndrome. Ureteroceles also can be identified by sonography in the bladder. No identifiable bladder on serial ultrasonography or on MRI imaging, suggests bilateral renal agenesis, bilateral single ureteral ectopy, or exstrophy of the bladder.

Lesions associated with hydronephrosis and normal amounts of amniotic fluid generally carry a good prognosis, whereas those associated with increased renal echogenicity and decreased amounts of amniotic fluid generally carry a poor prognosis for pulmonary maturation and renal function (118).

Abdominal Masses

The finding of an abdominal mass is not infrequent in the newborn nursery. An unselected series of infants in the newborn nursery revealed abdominal masses arising from the genitourinary tract in approximately 1 in every 500 admissions (119). It is quite clear from multiple reports that the urinary tract often is the source of a palpable abdominal mass in infants (120,121). In most reported series, approximately two-thirds of the infants presenting with an abdominal mass are found to have lesions in the urinary tract. In infancy, hydronephrosis and cystic kidneys are the most common lesions producing abdominal masses, whereas in older children tumors are more common (122). The obvious inference from these data is that ultrasonography, because the urinary tract is easily visualized, is the study most likely to identify the source of a palpable abdominal mass; frequently CT is required to better delineate solid abdominal masses. The physical and radiographic characteristics of the common abdominal masses of renal origin are listed in Table 43-2.

Hematuria

Hematuria in the infant can be a sign of renal vein thrombosis, acute tubular necrosis, renal calculi, urinary infection, or urinary tract obstruction (123). The presence of hematuria must be confirmed by examination of the urine, both chemically and microscopically. A positive chemical test may reflect hemoglobinuria, rather than hematuria, which implies the presence of cellular elements in the urine. Even more common than the presence of hematuria or hemoglobinuria, however, is concern about a red diaper in an infant. Two relatively common causes for red diapers are the presence of urates in the urine, giving a pink hue to the urine, especially in the diaper, and the growth of Serratia sp. on urine-soaked cloth diapers left standing. Obviously, these latter two situations are of no clinical consequence, but must be separated from true hematuria or hemoglobinuria in diagnostic considerations.

TABLE 43-2

ABDOMINAL MASSES OF RENAL ORIGIN

Mass	Texture	Renal Scan or Excretory Urogram	Ultrasonogram
Hydronephrosis	Smooth	Delayed drainage	Sonolucent
Multicystic kidney	Irregular	Nonfunction	Multiple large and small cysts (i.e., cystic dysplasia)
Polycystic kidney	Smooth (recessive); irregular or smooth (dominant)	Delayed function; distortion of collecting system Multiple large and small cysts (dominant)	Diffuse small cysts (recessive)
Tumor	Smooth	Distortion of collecting system	Solid
Renal vein thrombosis	Smooth	Poor function to nonfunction	Relatively normal renal architecture; enlarged kidney

GENITAL ABNORMALITIES

Cryptorchidism

Undescended testes are a very common finding in the newborn period, affecting perhaps as many as 1 in every 50 newborn males (124). Most testes that are undescended at birth, however, will descend during the first 6 to 9 months of life, so that the incidence of cryptorchidism at 1 year of age is approximately 0.7% to 0.8%, which is exactly the same incidence that has been found in postpubertal males (124). The newborn examination is important in determining testicular position, because the cremasteric reflex at that time is weak to absent (125). If the testis is well descended in a newborn, it is unlikely that there will be problems with true cryptorchidism later in life. Optimal results from treatment of cryptorchidism are thought to be produced by interventions after the possibility of testicular descent has passed (i.e., beyond 6 months of age) and before adverse effects of testicular nondescent are seen histologically (i.e., approximately 1.5 to 2 years of age), hence before 18 months of age (126). Many children are now undergoing surgical treatment of cryptorchidism between 6 to 9 months old with good surgical and anesthetic results. There appears to be increased mobility of the cord structures at this age, even with very high inguinal or abdominal testes, which facilitates the relocation of the testis to the scrotum.

Penile Agenesis

Although many of the penile anomalies are common, some, such as agenesis of the penis, are rare, occurring in 1 in 10 to 30 million live births (Fig. 43-20). Penile agenesis suggests an early embryologic failure in the development of the genital tubercle. The urethra usually exits on the perineum or near the anal verge. Previously these children were raised as females, with castration and reconstruction of the external genitalia performed at an early age (127). Management of this and other previously sex reassigned conditions continues to be controversial, as some reports on long-term follow-up of these patients have called the practice of gender reassignment into question (74).

Penile Duplication

Penile duplication (i.e., true diphallia) is a rare anomaly that also may involve duplications of the urethra and bladder (Fig. 43-21) (128). Reconstruction of these anomalies involves complex decisions about functional capability of the urinary, genital, and gastrointestinal tracts, and appearance.

Microphallus

The boy born with an abnormally small phallus presents a true therapeutic dilemma. Most cases of microphallus are as a result of hypogonadism (128) and will respond to testosterone, but an occasional patient with microphallus has end-organ failure and will not respond to exogenous testosterone. It is notable that, despite the relatively common finding of microphallus in the newborn nursery, it is an extremely rare event to find an adult with a phallus so small that it is incapable of sexual function.

The normal full-term newborn phallus measures approximately 3 to 3.5 cm in stretched length; the definition of microphallus requires a phallus that is less than 2.5 cm in stretched length, excluding ambiguous genitalia or the penis with hypospadias or chordee (129). To determine whether or not microphallus will respond to hormonal stimulation, 25 mg of testosterone enanthate is administered intramuscularly every 4 weeks for a total of 75 mg (see Chapter 39) (130). Some element of response usually is evident after the first dose. In most instances, after the course is completed, the child has a relatively normal phallus. If there is no response to testosterone, gender reassignment can be considered, but male gender assignment may still be preferable in most infants with micropenis (131).

In a recent long term review of patients with micropenis raised as either male or female, then reassessed as adults, half of the men were dissatisfied with their genitalia but generally satisfied with their gender of rearing, whereas most who were raised as women (80%) were

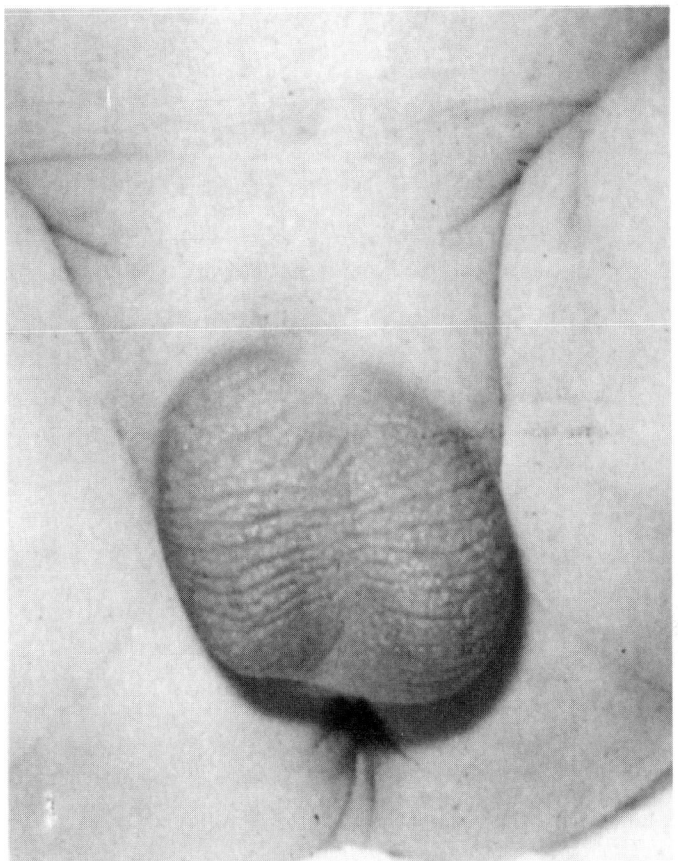

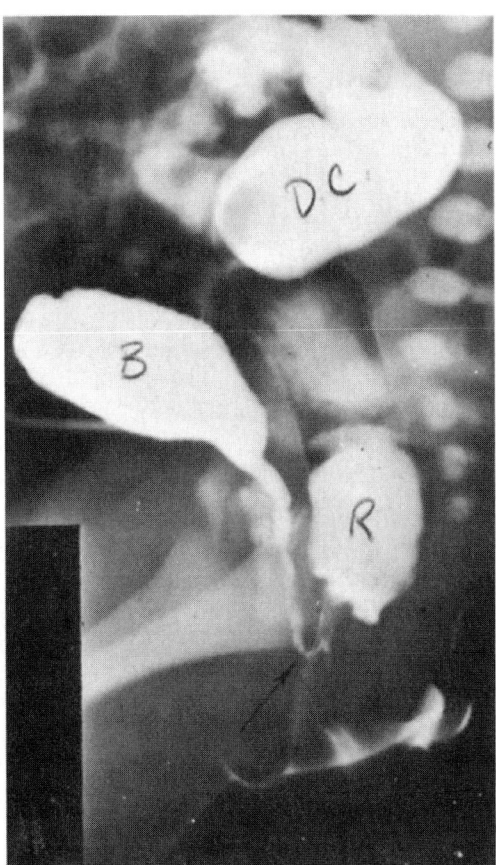

Figure 43-20 **A:** Genetic boy born with complete penile agenesis. **B:** An antegrade cystourethrogram in a genetic boy with penile agenesis. The bladder is full (B), and there is communication between the urethra and rectum (arrow). The rectum (R) and descending colon (DC) are filled with voided contrast material.

dissatisfied with their genitalia and required several surgeries to gender convert to female appearance. Interestingly, those raised as female were also satisfied with their sex of rearing. (131)

Hypospadias

The term hypospadias, by definition, refers to the abnormal location of the urethral meatus somewhere ventral to the normal glanular tip (Fig. 43-22); however, the term actually encompasses a complex that includes chordee (i.e., a ventral curvature of the penis on erection) and an abnormality of the prepuce or torsion of the penis. Although it is traditional in some circles to categorize hypospadias by degrees (i.e., first, second, and third), it is more helpful to describe hypospadias by the location of the meatus and the presence or absence of chordee (Fig. 43-23). At times, the hypospadiac meatus is quite stenotic and can be very difficult to see, especially in the newborn.

It has become obvious that the sibling of a child with hypospadias has an increased (14%) chance of having hypospadias (132). It is thought that hypospadias is inherited as a multifactorial problem. The historic incidence of hypospadias is 1 in 300 live births. The apparent incidence of hypospadias, particularly more proximally located hypospadias, appears to be increasing over the past few

decades in the United States and some Scandinavian countries but it does not appear to have an increased occurrence in all countries (133,134). There has also been a reported 5-fold increased incidence of hypospadias in males conceived by in vitro fertilization; this may be as a result of maternal progesterone use but a definite etiology has not been determined (135). It once was thought that there might be associated abnormalities of the upper urinary tract in children with hypospadias, but critical analysis of series of children with hypospadias who have been uniformly investigated reveals that there is no increased incidence of upper tract abnormalities when children with hypospadias are compared to those of the general population (136). Routine karyotype evaluation of patients with hypospadias and cryptorchidism does not seem warranted, except in more severe cases of perineal hypospadias or ambiguous genitalia (137).

Most forms of hypospadias can be surgically corrected and, if the patient's health warrants, it is preferable to perform this surgery in the first year of life, typically after 6 months of age. Circumcision should be delayed in children with hypospadias as the foreskin is commonly used for the repair of these problems.. Physical findings suggesting hypospadias are an abnormality of the foreskin, an incomplete foreskin, and penile torsion or chordee. Whenever these abnormalities are noted, circumcision should be

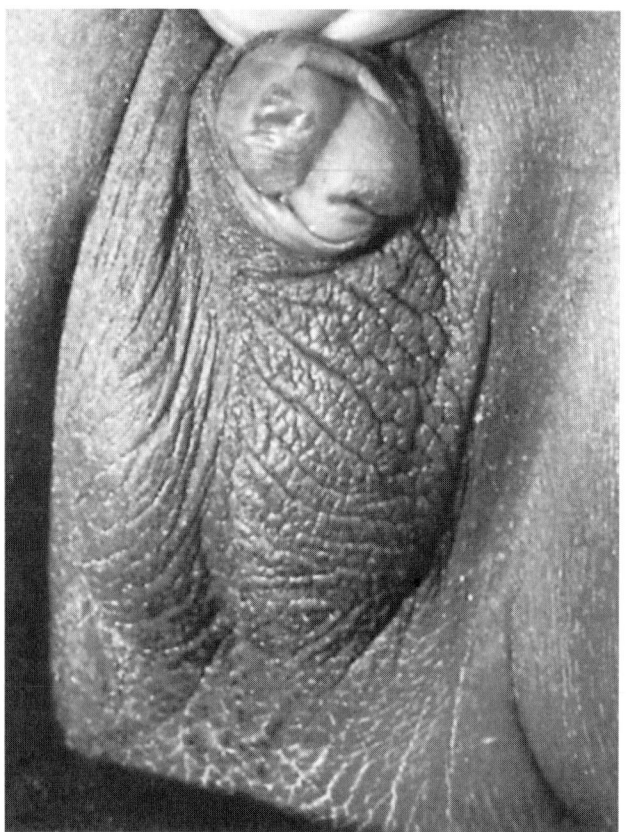

Figure 43-21 Duplication of the glans in a 2-year-old boy. From Kossow JH, Morales PA. Duplication of bladder and urethra and associated anomalies. *Urology* 1973;1:71, with permission.

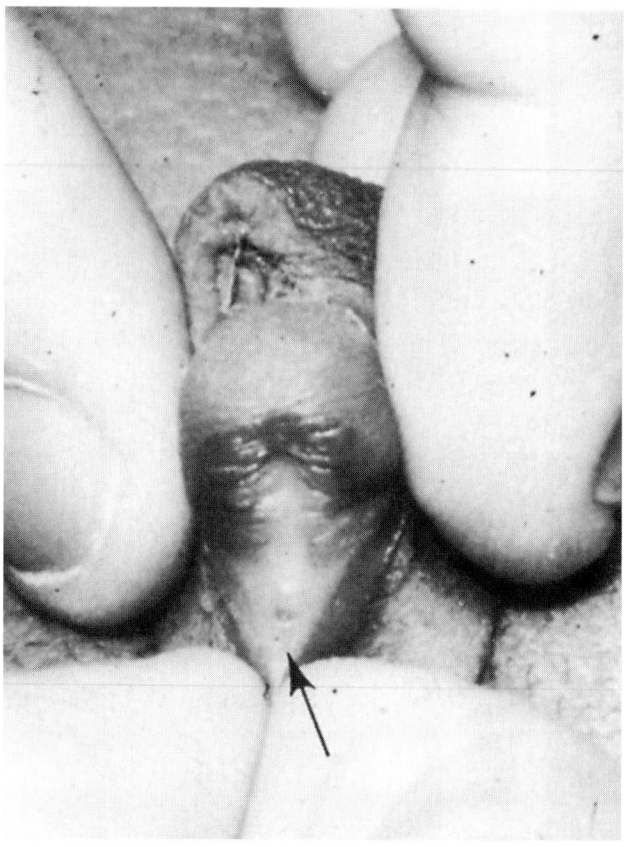

Figure 43-22 The hypospadiac meatal position (arrow) is demonstrated by pulling the ventral shaft of skin away from the penis.

delayed until the child can be assessed by a hypospadiologist who can determine whether the foreskin will be necessary for the repair or if a repair is even necessary.

Epispadias

Epispadias usually is associated with exstrophy, but occasionally appears as an isolated defect (Fig. 43-24). The inci-

dence of isolated epispadias previously reported as 1 in 100,000 live births has now been estimated as occurring in 1 in 40,000 live births (138). The repair of this lesion is moderately difficult. The more severe degrees of epispadias usually are associated with urinary incontinence and are more common than those associated with continence. In incontinent cases, the bladder neck must be reconstructed. Children with epispadias tend to have a relatively short

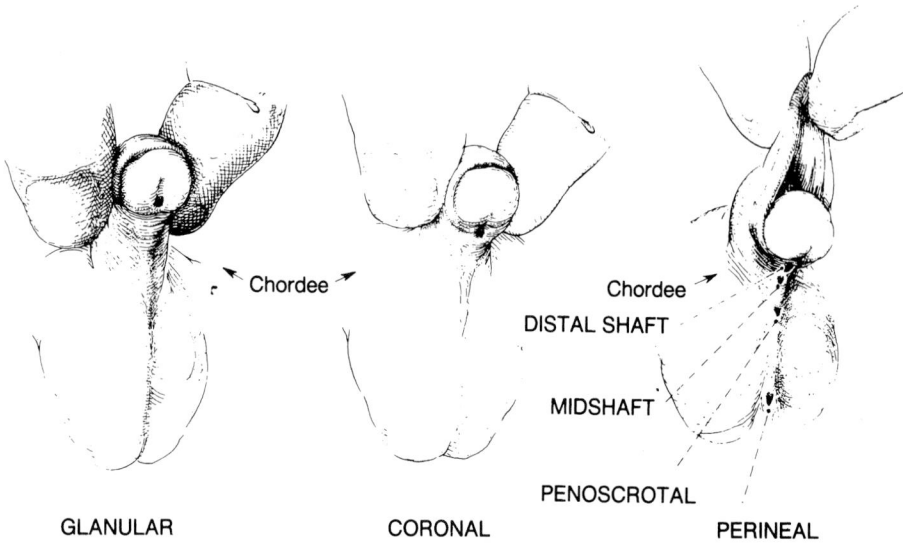

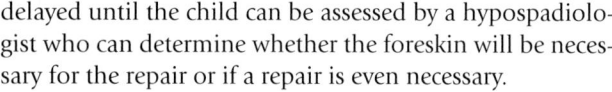

Figure 43-23 Classification of hypospadias based on anatomic location of the urethral meatus. The associated chordee is best described in terms of its severity (mild, moderate, or severe). From Kelalis PP, King LR, Belman AB, eds. *Clinical pediatric urology*, vol. 1. Philadelphia: WB Saunders, 1976:577, with permission.

GLANULAR   CORONAL   PERINEAL

Chordee

Chordee
DISTAL SHAFT

MIDSHAFT

PENOSCROTAL

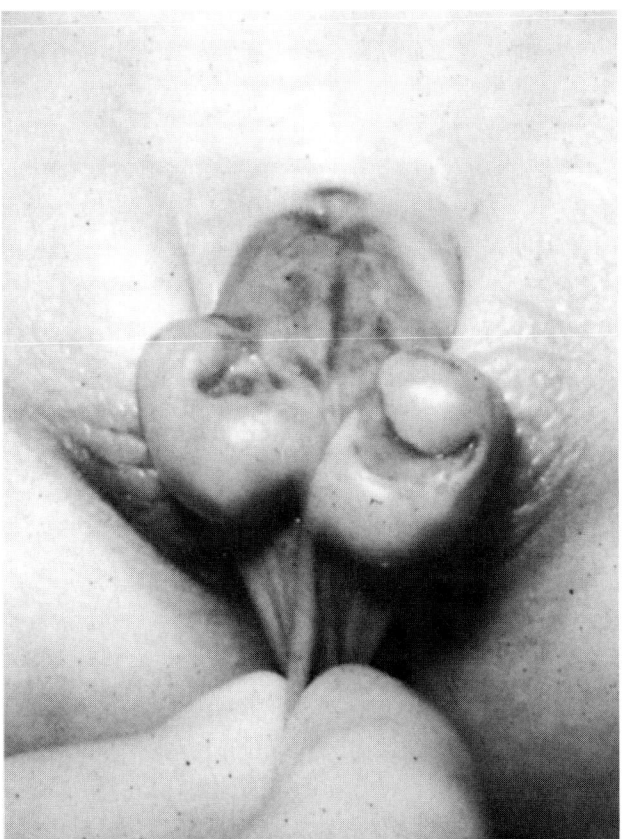

Figure 43-24 Isolated epispadias without exstrophy. The bladder neck is intact in this child, who has good but not excellent urinary continence. Note also the incomplete duplication of glans.

phallus and, although attempts at lengthening the phallus are somewhat helpful, this aspect of the problem sometimes defies correction.

Urethral Duplication

Urethral duplication is an uncommon anomaly, more commonly noted in boys, which can present either as a partial or complete duplication. When there is a duplication it is more common that the urethras are oriented in an anteroposterior plane, rather than lying side by side. The more ventral urethra usually is the functional urethra, and the dorsal urethra often is stenotic and unusable (139). Repair of these anomalies must be tailored to the individual situation. Generally, duplication of the urethra in the female is seen with bladder duplication and is oriented side by side. Urethral duplication in a female with a dorsal urethra and a secondary vaginal urethra is very rare, generally presenting with urinary tract infections; the functioning female urethra is the more ventral urethral structure just as in the male (140).

Another variant of a duplicated urethra, or possibly an exstrophy variant, is the congenital prepubic sinus, which can occur in males or females as a small orifice located just above the pubis. The tract generally is removed surgically and can be traced down to the bladder or urethra in those cases described (141).

Ambiguous Genitalia

Ambiguity of the external genitalia is a quandary encountered with some regularity in the newborn nursery (see Chapter 39). These patients often pose difficult diagnostic and therapeutic challenges. It is important to establish a diagnosis rapidly. On physical examination, the presence or absence of palpable gonads is very helpful. If a gonad is palpably present, it almost certainly is a testis. Hence, bilaterally palpable gonads suggest very strongly that the patient is a genetic male. If a gonad is palpable only unilaterally, there probably is a testis on that side. There could conceivably be a normal testis, a streak gonad, or an ovary on the other side. If no testes are palpable, the patient could be an XX female, an XY male with abdominal testes or mixed gonadal dysgenesis, or a true hermaphrodite.

Chromosomal gender is established by karyotype. An XY male who is undervirilized could have Klinefelter syndrome, true hermaphroditism, 5a-reductase deficiency, hypopituitarism, 17-hydroxylase deficiency, or 3b-hydroxy steroid deficiency.

If the patient is an XX female, ambiguity could be produced by excessive maternal androgens or the adrenogenital syndrome, which is most commonly caused by a 21-hydroxylase deficiency. This latter must be considered in any phenotypically male patient with nonpalpable gonads, even if the genitalia appear completely masculinized, to avoid an Addisonian crisis in a patient with a salt-losing adrenogenital syndrome (Fig. 43-25).

Gender assignment (i.e., gender of rearing) should be accomplished as soon as possible after appropriate endocrinologic, karyotypic and anatomic evaluation, to assure that life threatening conditions do not occur and to avoid excessive parental anxiety. A team approach with neonatology, endocrinology, psychology, genetics and pediatric urology or surgery input will help the parents make as informed selection of the sex of rearing as possible with the information available at the time of review. Anxiety produced by indecision over gender assignment is exponentially increased by changes in gender assignment. The elements that should be considered are potential fertility, capacity for future psychosexual function, and the possibility for satisfactory reconstruction. This last factor mandates that an experienced surgeon participate in the decision regarding gender of rearing so that the parents will understand the surgical options, potential complications or multiplicity of procedures and lifelong medical treatments that might be required for either sex for chosen gender assignment. Psychological implications of reports of patient dissatisfaction with gender reassignment are that these feelings are typically expressed most strongly in adolescence and adulthood. Long-term surveys of 46 XY adults with ambiguous genitalia or micropenis at presentation have found that most individuals are rather satisfied with their sex of rearing either as male or female but each group has different psychosexual or surgical experiences that has affected their overall satisfaction with the appearance of their external genitalia. In a recent review, 46 XY individuals with newborn ambiguous genitalia who were raised as females generally

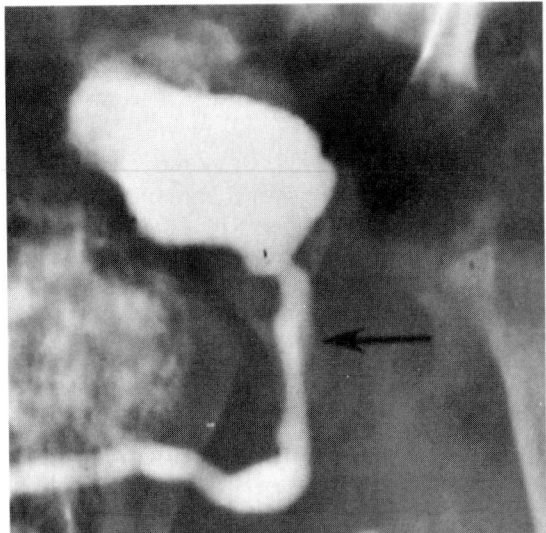
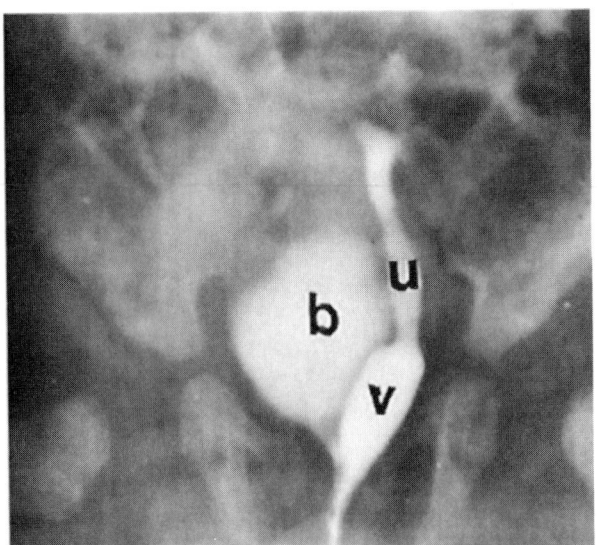

Figure 43-25 Voiding cystourethrogram in a genetic girl who was totally masculinized by adrenal hyperplasia. **A:** Utriculus masculinus (arrow), as would normally be expected in a male. **B:** Retrograde vaginohistogram reveals a normal vagina (v) and uterus (u), and an overflow of contrast into the urinary bladder (b).

had more acceptable appearing female genitalia and required fewer surgical procedures to achieve that appearance than those 46 XY individuals raised as males. The opposite case was found when surveying 46 XY micropenis patients and their external genitalia appearance and surgical experience (131,142,143). Unfortunately, the choice of appropriate gender of rearing is made more difficult as more information is available with research in this area. Ongoing human and animal study may shed some light and facilitate decision making for gender assignment (144).

Development of the Prepuce and Circumcision

The prepuce forms as a roll of epithelium that fuses ventrally at the frenulum. If there is failure of urethral development, this will interfere with development of the prepuce, so that abnormalities of the prepuce are very suggestive of other penile abnormalities (e.g., hypospadias, chordee, epispadias). Once the prepuce has covered the glans, its inner epithelial surface fuses with the epithelium of the glans and does not separate from it until some time in childhood (145). It is unusual for a male to have a completely retractable foreskin at birth. In the process of separation of the inner epithelial layer from the glans, cystic spaces form between the two layers and sometimes are filled with desquamated epithelial cells that form white, pearl-like beads or infantile smegma that can be seen through the overlying skin. Occasionally areas of infantile smegma may become inflamed or infected, although most drain spontaneously.

Because circumcision is so common in the United States, the natural history of preputial development has been lost, and one must depend on observations made in countries in which circumcision usually is not practiced.

The foreskin in the newborn normally is not retractable. In a large series from Denmark, the foreskin was not completely retractable in most boys until puberty (146). Phimosis is defined as the inability to retract the foreskin. In early childhood, this is the normal physiologic state. Although by definition this may be phimosis, most children will develop normally and will not have problems as a result of the temporary inability to retract the foreskin. Forcible retraction of the prepuce tends to produce tears in the preputial orifice, resulting in scarring that may lead to pathologic phimosis.

Circumcision is performed for a multitude of reasons. Medically, carcinoma of the penis, pathologic phimosis, paraphimosis, some sexually transmitted diseases, and some urinary infections in infancy may be prevented by circumcision (147). If the overall population is considered on a public health or economic basis, the advantages to the individual patient perhaps may be mitigated by the cost of circumcising the entire male population to prevent problems in a minority. The cost of circumcision is further increased by the routine use of local anesthesia (see Chapter 57).

The benefits of circumcision are occasionally offset by complications that may arise from the procedure, just as they may arise after any other surgical procedure (148). The most common complications seen are hemorrhage and wound infection. Both are generally easily treated, minor annoyances. Serious complications including sepsis, amputation of part of the glans, loss of the entire penis, urethrocutaneous fistulas, bands of scar between the shaft and the glans (Fig. 43-26), denudation of the skin of the entire shaft of the penis, recurrent phimosis (Fig. 43-27), and urethral fistulas (Fig. 43-28) occur rarely (149). At times, parents are very unhappy with the cosmetic appearance of the penis even though the functional result is good.

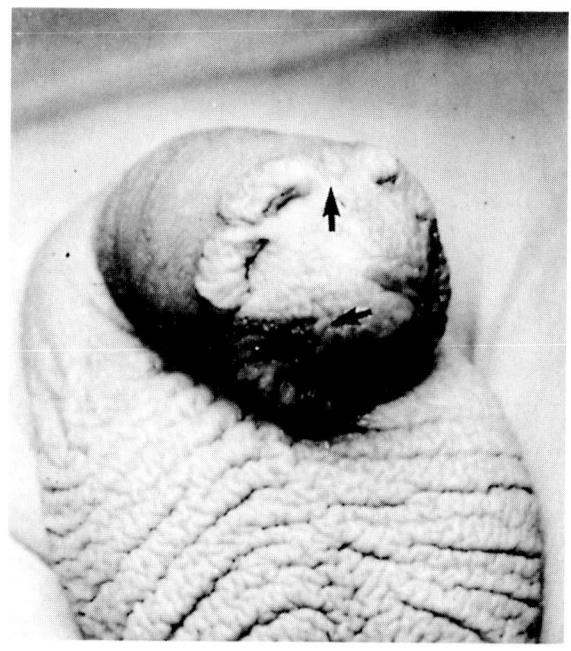
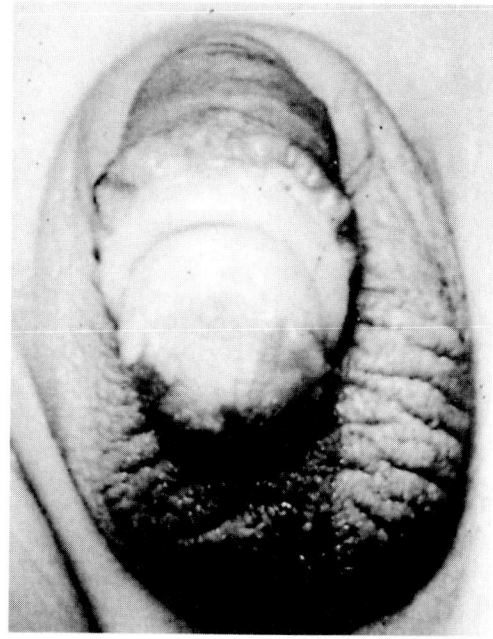

Figure 43-26   Adhesions (arrows) between the distal foreskin and glans penis before (**A**) and after (**B**) surgical transection.

Testicular Torsion

Torsion of the testis in the newborn usually presents as a firm, slightly enlarged testis. There rarely is much abnormality of the overlying skin. Neonatal torsion seems to be painless, and actually may be an antenatal event in as many as 72% of the cases (150,151). Twenty-eight percent

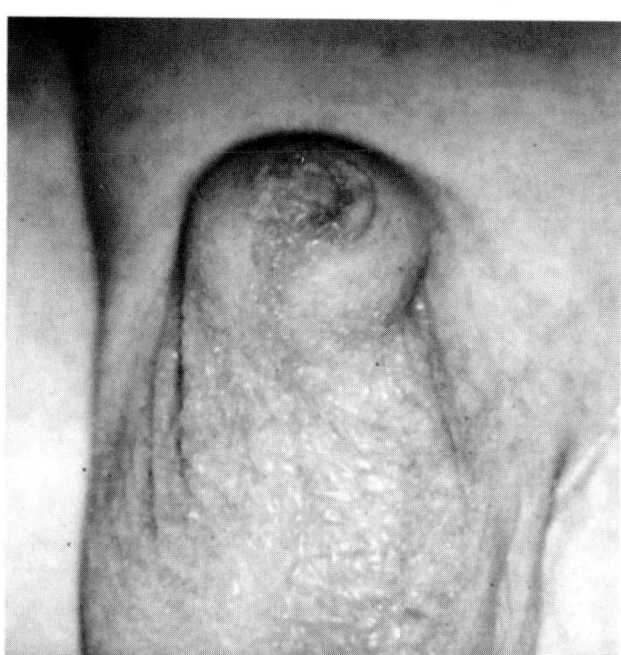

Figure 43-27   In this patient with circumcision injury, excessive removal of skin from the shaft resulted in skin regeneration over the retracted glans, obscuring the glans. The appearance is that of amputation of the glans. From Belman AB. The penis. *Urol Clin North Am* 1978;5:17, with permission.

of the neonatal cases develop in the postnatal period. Exploration of the testis that has undergone torsion in the newborn period probably is of limited value, because it generally is too late for testicular salvage (152). Ten percent of neonatal torsions are bilateral; some are asynchronous, and some are of the intravaginal rather than the extravaginal type. Exploration for neonatal torsion is warranted if the changes are found shortly after birth and performed expeditiously (less than 6 hours from the time of change in testicular examination). In one series, using an inguinal approach, up to 20% of testes torsed acutely in the neonatal period were salvaged (153); this may overrepresent actual salvage rates in the newborn time period. In the case of an obviously infarcted testis, contralateral exploration and testicular fixation when the infant is stable may prevent contralateral torsion (154).

Testicular Tumors

Tumors of the testis occasionally present at birth or in early infancy (155). Teratomas of the testis, occurring in 19.7% of cases registered in the Prepubertal Testicular Tumor Registry, are benign and are treated by excision (156). On some occasions, this can be excision of the tumor only, leaving the remainder of the testis in situ; orchiectomy is necessary if the entire testis has been replaced by teratoma. A common tumor presenting in the newborn testis is one of the gonadal stromal tumors, with Sertoli cell tumors being the most common (156,157). Although these tumors histologically may appear malignant, in infancy they invariably exhibit a benign behavior, and orchiectomy is curative. This is not the case when gonadal stromal tumors appear in later childhood because malignant behavior has been documented.

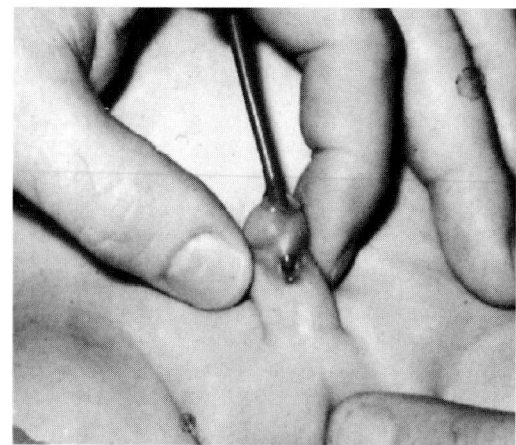
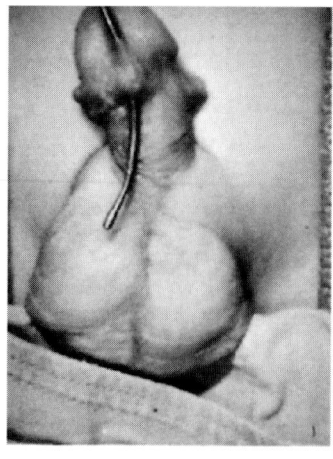

A

B

Figure 43-28 A, B: Two examples of circumcision injuries with secondary coronal fistulas. From Belman AB. The penis. *Urol Clin North Am* 1978; 5:17, with permission.

Yolk sac tumors occur in infancy; approximately 30% of reported yolk sac tumors of the testis are identified in infancy. These malignant tumors are best treated by radical orchiectomy. As long as there is no evidence of metastatic disease, adjunctive chemotherapy, node dissection, or radiation therapy is thought to be unwarranted (158). A-fetoprotein (AFP) levels are elevated in patients with yolk sac tumors, AFP levels are normally elevated in infancy but should not be elevated in adults. Age-adjusted AFP levels will improve the usefulness of AFP measurements as a tumor marker in infants (159).

URINARY TRACT INFECTION

Infancy is one period of life during which there is reversal in the gender incidence of bacteriuria. The overall incidence of neonatal urinary tract infections is somewhere between 1.5 to 5 cases per 1,000 live births. The male-to-female ratio is somewhere between 3:1 and 5:1 (160), whereas later in childhood and until later adult life, there is a female preponderance of patients with urinary infections. It has been documented that uncircumcised males are more likely to have urinary infections than are circumcised males (161). The incidence of urinary infection in uncircumcised males approximates 1 per 100. At times, the source of the urinary infection is hematogenous rather than ascending (162).

It is imperative that there be radiographic evaluation of any newborn with culture documented bacteriuria. Vesicoureteral reflux is present in approximately one-half of those evaluated, and obstructive uropathy is not an unusual finding (163). Therefore, at a minimum, urinary tract evaluation with voiding cystourethrography and ultrasonography is indicated.

UROLOGIC ASPECTS OF MYELODYSPLASIA

Almost any child with myelodysplasia will have involvement of the urinary tract. This may be of little consequence in the newborn period, but it is essential that the patient be appropriately evaluated shortly after birth and that a surveillance program be instituted. It was thought that hydronephrosis was found at birth, in roughly 10% of children with myelodysplasia, but studies have suggested that some of the hydronephrosis formerly detected actually was a result of spinal shock after closure of the neurologic lesion and in many children resolved spontaneously (164). Although manual expression of the bladder (Credé maneuver) has been used to empty the bladders of children with myelodysplasia, it is not recommended because the intravesical pressures that are produced can be quite high, which can lead to upper tract deterioration, especially in patients with associated vesicoureteral reflux (165). Intermittent catheterization can be used successfully in both male and female infants if needed, and, in which these procedures are not successful or acceptable and bladder emptying is thought to be necessary, temporary cutaneous vesicostomy is a proven management modality (166). Children with myelodysplasia, if at all possible, should be managed by a multidisciplinary team that includes neurologists, neurosurgeons, urologists, and orthopedic surgeons. With this approach, these children have an excellent chance of survival and development as productive citizens in modern society. In utero closure of the meningomyelocele defect has been done in several U.S. medical centers with mixed results (167).

PRUNE-BELLY SYNDROME

This lesion is a spectrum of abnormalities characterized by the triad of abdominal wall deficiency, hydronephrosis, and, in males, cryptorchidism. It is the abdominal wall defect that gives the characteristic appearance leading to its name. The incidence of this lesion has been estimated to be 1 per 35,000 to 50,000 live births (10,168). Males are affected ten times more frequently than females (169). There is no clear-cut evidence that this is an inherited disorder. Theories of embryogenesis include obstructive uropathy and mesenchymal dysplasia (170).

There can be massive hydroureteronephrosis and the bladder often is very dilated. Because there is prostatic hypoplasia with dilation of the prostatic urethra, antenatal studies may not differentiate these patients from boys with posterior urethral valves. The kidneys often are dysplastic, and this dysplasia will determine prognosis (171). Although some affected children die in infancy, many today will survive. Reconstruction of the urinary tract, orchiopexy, and repair of the abdominal wall defect often are helpful in altering the outlook for these children (172).

UROLOGIC IMPLICATIONS OF IMPERFORATE ANUS

Because of the intimate relationships of the lower urinary and gastrointestinal tract development, the urinary tract will commonly be affected in a high proportion of children with imperforate anus; the higher the lesion, the greater the chance of urinary involvement (173). It is for this reason that all newborns with imperforate anus should be screened for urinary tract abnormalities with ultrasonography and a voiding cystourethrogram. Often there is a constellation of other associated anomalies which has come to be known as the VACTERRL association (vertebral, anorectal, cardiac, tracheoesophageal, renal, radial, and limb abnormalities). Because three elements qualify as the association, when two elements are present, a third should be sought. This is a nongenetic, sporadically occurring lesion.

FEMALE GENITAL ABNORMALITIES

The female reproductive system is formed by the Müllerian or paramesonephric ducts. The Müllerian system differentiates into a female organ system when Müllerian inhibitory substance is absent. During the sixth to eighth week of gestation, the Müllerian ducts will form lateral to the wolffian ducts, cross medially, and fuse in the midline incorporating the urogenital (UG) sinus to form the uterovaginal canal by the tenth week of gestation. The fallopian tubes develop from the lateral ends of the Müllerian ducts. The vagina develops from the fused Müllerian ducts and the UG sinus. It is believed that the upper four-fifths of the vagina is Müllerian derived and the lower fifth is from the UG sinus. Vaginal formation is completed by the fifth month of gestation.

The external genitalia differentiates *in utero* during the 12th to 16th weeks. Passive development of the genital tubercle into the clitoris, the urethral folds into the labia minora, and the genital swellings into the labia majora occurs in the absence of fetal androgens.

Vaginal Agenesis

Vaginal agenesis (Meyer–Rokitansky–Kuster–Hauser Syndrome) occurs when the vaginal plate does not canalize. The incidence is reported as 1 in 4,000 to 5,000 live female

births (174). The patients generally are 46XX females presenting with primary amenorrhea but having normal secondary female sex features. The ovaries and the external genitalia generally are normal, but the vaginal plate is not canalized and the uterus may be rudimentary. It is common to have associated genitourinary anomalies; renal anomalies are seen in 34% of the patients (175). Renal agenesis and ectopia are the most common findings. Patients also may have skeletal anomalies, particularly in the spine and ribs. Combinations of these anomalies has been termed as the MURCS association (Müllerian duct aplasia, renal aplasia, and cervicothoracic somite malformations). Surgical correction is individualized based on the location and development of the uterine and vaginal remnants (175).

Hydrocolpos and Hydrometrocolpos

If the vaginal canalization is incomplete, the hymen may be imperforate or a high transverse vaginal septum may be present. The infant may then present with distention of the vagina with glandular secretions stimulated by maternal estrogens, known as hydrocolpos, or distention of the vagina and the uterus with the same secretions, known as hydrometrocolpos. With current antenatal ultrasonography, this can be found prior to delivery, but many infants still present with an abdominal mass, possible urinary obstruction, and a bulging introital mass. Ultrasound imaging may demonstrate a fluid-filled or mixed density fluid-filled pelvis mass, and possibly a distended bladder with or without hydroureteronephrosis, if there is secondary urinary obstruction (Fig. 43-29).

Definitive treatment depends on the extent of vaginal canalization; this can be a simple hymenotomy or vaginoplasty or vaginal pull-through if there is a high septal defect. CT or MRI imaging with T2 weighted imaging may better delineate the remaining vaginal plate but occasionally, needle aspiration of the fluid with radiographic contrast injection and imaging is necessary to delineate the length of the vaginal plate.

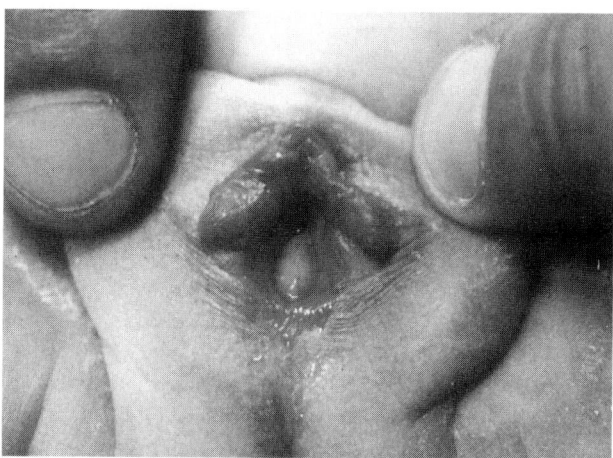

Figure 43-29 Newborn female with imperforate hymen.

Duplication or Fusion Anomalies

Duplication of the uterus and vagina occur if fusion of the Müllerian ducts is incomplete. The child may have two uteri, one or two cervices with either a single vagina or two separate vaginas, or one or both vaginas may be open to the perineum. These malformations can be identified early in life by ultrasonography, but frequently will not present until adolescence. The typical presentation is a menstruating female having cyclic pelvic pain associated with menses and an enlarging pelvic mass. Treating vaginal duplication usually only requires incising the longitudinal vaginal septum. Successful pregnancies have been reported in some women with duplicated uteri.

Urogenital Sinus and Cloacal Abnormalities

Having a common urogenital sinus is a normal part of development in both sexes. If Müllerian ductal development arrests during the first trimester, a persistent urovaginal confluence or common UG sinus will be found at birth. Varying locations for the junction of the vagina and urethra occur, depending on the degree of vaginal differentiation. The earlier the arrest occurs, the higher the connection will be located. The anus may be located in its normal location or may be more anteriorly placed. These infants are found to have a common introital opening for urethra and vagina and a second opening for the anus. A flush genitogram will delineate the length of the common urogenital channel and the connections of the urethra and vagina. This is performed by placing a feeding tube or urethral catheter just inside the common opening and injecting contrast material in a retrograde fashion. The type of surgical reconstruction required is determined by the length of the common channel and the location of the urethral vaginal junction. This corrective surgery can be performed during the first year of life in most lesions (175). Total urogenital mobilization can be used to bring a high junction lesion to the perineum, generally without incontinence (176,177).

A combined urogenital sinus and anorectal malformation is termed a cloacal anomaly. By 4 to 6 weeks of gestation, the urorectal septum should divide the common allantoic–hindgut confluence. If this does not occur, a common cloaca will be present at birth. Because of the imperforate anus, these infants have abdominal distention and a single perineal opening. Delineating the anatomy is important for appropriate surgical management. This generally requires a combined approach with pediatric general surgery and urology input. These infants typically will require diverting colostomy as initial treatment. A flush genitogram can define the urethral, vaginal, and bowel junctions to better plan ultimate reconstruction with bowel pull-through, formal vaginoplasty, and urethroplasty or a simple cutback vaginoplasty. Complete reconstruction can be contemplated during infancy and may be easier near 1 year of age. Delaying reconstruction until late childhood or puberty generally is more difficult, as a result of previous scarring from anal pull-through and the deeper, less mobile pelvis present in older girls (Fig. 43-30).

Ovarian Cysts

Ovarian cysts develop in the presence of hormonal stimulation and more commonly are seen after puberty. The fetal ovary is stimulated by fetal gonadotrophins, maternal estrogens, and placental chorionic gonadotrophin and may develop cysts during fetal development and infancy. Ovarian cysts are being found more frequently with the advent of prenatal ultrasonographic imaging. More than 250 cysts have been reported since 1975 (178). Many of these infants underwent surgical therapy with oophorectomy, cystectomy, or cyst aspiration because of the risk of ovarian torsion as a result of the cyst increasing the ovarian size and concerns about the occasional ovarian tumor. If discovered in utero by ultrasonography, the cysts can be followed until delivery. Vaginal delivery is possible in most cases, with cesarean section being reserved for very large cysts. Postnatally, small ovarian cysts (< 4 cm) can be

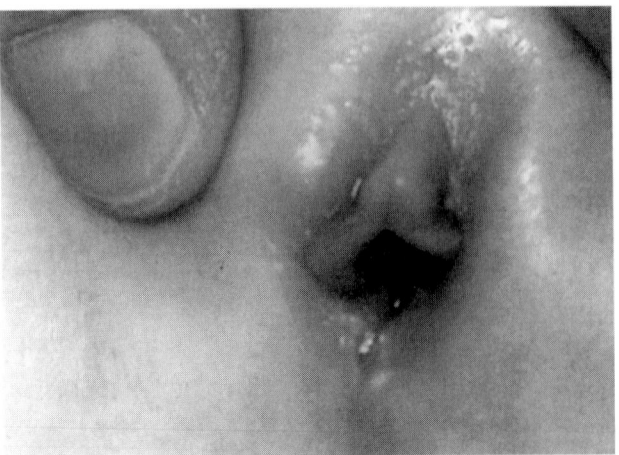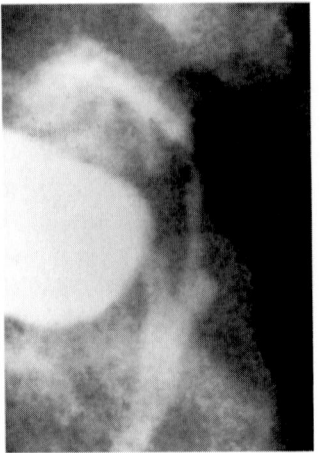

Figure 43-30   **A:** Newborn female with cloacal anomaly. Note single perineal orifice. **B:** Flush genitogram demonstrating a high confluence of the bladder, vagina, and bowel into a common cloaca.

followed with serial ultrasonography, because most cysts will regress in the first 3 to 4 months of life. Larger cysts can be followed for involution or can be aspirated to provide conservation of the ovary. Laparoscopic or open surgery should be contemplated if there are complex ovarian cysts, symptomatic cysts, or cysts recur after aspiration. Conserving ovarian tissue by removing or unroofing the cyst is generally how most of these lesions are handled.

Introital Masses

Introital masses generally are determined at the first examination of the infant. The differential diagnosis for introital masses in female infants include imperforate hymen, prolapsing ureterocele, and Skene's or Gartner's cysts. Prolapsing ureteroceles may extrude through the urethral meatus. Paraurethral cysts (Skene's or Gartner's) also are present in newborn girls, and present with lateral displacement of the urethral meatus. These cysts involute or rupture spontaneously fairly quickly, so treatment usually is unnecessary.

ACKNOWLEDGMENT

The authors would like to thank A. Barry Belman for his generosity in allowing the republication of illustrations from his chapter in the third edition of this book.

REFERENCES

1. Mandell J, Peters CA, Retik AB. Current concepts in the perinatal diagnosis and management of hydronephrosis. *Urol Clin North Am* 1990;17:247.
2. Baskin LS. Prenatal hydronephrosis. In: Baskin LS, Kogan BA, Duckett JW, eds. *Handbook of pediatric urology*. Philadelphia: Lippincott–Raven, 1997:11.
3. Fowler SF, Sydorak RM, Albanese CT, et al. Fetal endoscopic surgery: lessons learned and trends reviewed. *J Pediatr Surg* 2002 Dec;37(12):1700.
4. Holmes N, Harrison MR, Baskin LS. Fetal surgery for posterior urethral valves: long-term postnatal outcomes. *Pediatrics* 2001 Jul;108(1):e7.
5. Freedman AL, Johnson MP, Smith CA, et al. Long-term outcome in children after antenatal intervention for obstructive uropathies. *Lancet* 1999;Jul31;354(9176):374.
6. Townsend RR, Manlo-Johnson M. Prenatal diagnosis of urinary tract abnormalities with ultrasound: a review. *Scand J Urol Nephrol* 1991;138[Suppl]:13.
7. Mackie GG, Stephens FD. Duplex kidneys: a correlation of renal dysplasia with position of the ureteral orifice. *J Urol* 1979; 114:274.
8. Potter EL. *Normal and abnormal development of the kidney*. Chicago: Year Book, 1972:86.
9. Carter CO. The genetics of urinary tract malformations. *J Genet Hum* 1984;31(1):23.
10. Cendron M, Elder JS, Duckett JW. Perinatal urology. In: Gillenwater JY, Grayhack JT, Howards SS, et al, eds. *Adult and pediatric urology*, 3rd ed. St. Louis: Mosby-Year Book, 1996:2075–2170.
11. Emanuel B, Nachman R, Aronson N, et al. Congenital solitary kidney: a review of 74 cases. *Am J Dis Child* 1974;127:17.
12. McGee MD, Lucey DT, Fried FA. A new embryologic classification for urogynecological malformations: the syndrome of mesonephric duct induced Müllerian deformities. *J Urol* 1979; 121:265.
13. Cook WA, Stephens FD. Fused kidneys: morphologic study and theory of embryogenesis. In: Bergsma D, Duckett JW, eds. Urinary system malformations in children. *Birth defects: original article series*. New York: March of Dimes, 1977:327.
14. Belman AB, King LR. Urinary tract abnormalities associated with imperforate anus. *J Urol* 1972;108:823.
15. Brenner B, Meyer TW, Hostetter TH. Dietary protein intake and the progressive nature of kidney disease: role of hemodynamically mediated glomerular injury in the pathogenesis of progressive glomerular sclerosis in aging, renal ablation and intrinsic renal disease. *N Engl J Med* 1983;307:652.
16. Brenner BM, Lawler EV, Mackenzie HS. The hyperfiltration theory: a paradigm shift in nephrology. *Kidney Int* 1996;49:1974.
17. Goldfarb DA, Matin SF, Braun WE, et al. Renal outcome 25 years after donor nephrectomy. *J Urol* 2001;166(6):2043.
18. Burke EC, Wenzel JE, Utz DC. The intrathoracic kidney: report of a case. *Am J Dis Child* 1967;113:487.
19. Kelalis PP, Malek RS, Segura JW. Observations on renal ectopia and fusion in children. *J Urol* 1973;110:588.
20. Leduc B, Van Campenhout J, Simaro R. Congenital absence of the vagina: observations on 25 cases. *Am J Obstet Gynecol* 1968; 100:512.
21. Elli F, Stalder G. Malformations of kidney and urinary tract in common chromosomal aberrations. *Hum Genet* 1973;18:1.
22. McDonald JH, McClellan DS. Crossed renal ectopia. *Am J Urol* 1957;93:995.
23. N'Guessan G, Stephens FD. Supernumerary kidney. *J Urol* 1983; 130:649.
24. Osathanondh V, Potter EL. Pathogenesis of polycystic kidneys: type I due to hyperplasia of interstitial portions of collecting tubules. *Arch Pathol* 1964;77:466.
25. Blythe H, Ockenden BG. Polycystic disease of kidneys and liver presenting in childhood. *J Med Genet* 1971;8:257.
26. Osathanondh V, Potter EL. Pathogenesis of polycystic kidneys: type 3 due to multiple abnormalities of development. *Arch Pathol* 1964;77:485.
27. Stapleton FB, Johnson DL, Kaplan GW, et al. The cystic renal lesion in tuberous sclerosis. *J Pediatr* 1980;97:574.
28. Spence HM, Baird SS, Ware EW Jr. Cystic disorders of the kidney: classification, diagnosis, treatment. *JAMA* 1957;163:1466.
29. Wacksman J, Phipps L. Report of multicystic kidney registry: preliminary findings. *J Urol* 1993;150:1870.
30. Campbell MF. Embryology and anomalies of the urogenital tract. In: Campbell MF, ed. *Clinical pediatric urology*. Philadelphia: WB Saunders, 1951:198.
31. Ambrose SS, Nicholson WP. Ureteral reflux into duplicated ureters. *J Urol* 1964;92:439.
32. Stephens FD, Lenaghan D. The anatomical basis and dynamics of vesicoureteral reflux. *J Urol* 1962;87:669.
33. Stephens FD. Caecoureterocele and concepts of the embryology and aetiology of ureteroceles. *Aust N Z J Surg* 1971;40:239.
34. Chwalla R. The process of formation of cystic dictations of the vesical end of the ureter and of diverticula at the ureteral ostium. *Urol Cutan Rev* 1927;31:499.
35. Johnston JH. The pathogenesis of hydronephrosis in children. *Br J Urol* 1969;41:724.
36. McLaughlin AP III, Pfister RC, Leadbetter WF, et al. Pathophysiology of primary megaureter. *J Urol* 1973;109:805.
37. Osathanondh V, Potter EL. Pathogenesis of polycystic kidneys: type 2 due to inhibition of ampullary activity. *Arch Pathol* 1964; 77:459.
38. Kitagawa H, Pringle KC, Koike J, et al. Different phenotypes of dysplastic kidney in obstructive uropathy in fetal lambs. *J Pediatr Surg* 2001;36(11):1698.
39. Glenn JF. Agenesis of the bladder. *JAMA* 1959;169:2016.
40. Williams DI. The development of the trigone of the bladder. *Br J Urol* 1951;23:123.
41. Bauer SB, Retik AB. Urachal and related umbilical disorders. *Urol Clin North Am* 1978;5:195.
42. Satler EJ, Mossman HW. A case of double bladder and double urethra in the female child. *J Urol* 1968;79:274.
43. Stephens FD. *Congenital malformations of the urinary tract*. New York: Praeger, 1983.
44. Das S, Amar AD. Extravesical ureteral ectopia in male patients. *J Urol* 1981;125:842.
45. Brock WA, Kaplan GW. Voiding dysfunction in children. *Curr Probl Pediatr* 1980;2:10.

46. Weiss JP, Duckett JW, Snyder HM. Single unilateral vaginal ectopic ureter: is it really a rarity? *J Urol* 1984;132:1177.
47. Brock WA, Kaplan GW. Ectopic ureteroceles in children. *J Urol* 1978;119:800.
48. Mandel J, Colodny AH, Lebowitz R, et al. Ureteroceles in infants and children. *J Urol* 1980;123:921.
49. Snyder HM, Johnston JH. Orthotopic ureteroceles in children. *J Urol* 1978;119:543.
50. Scherz HC, Kaplan GW, Packer MG, et al. Ectopic ureteroceles: surgical management with preservation of continence: review of 60 cases. *J Urol* 1989;142:538.
51. Somner TE, Crowe JE, Resnick MI. Diagnosis of ectopic ureterocele using ultrasound. *Urology* 1980;15:82.
52. Cooper CS, Passerini-Glazel G, Hutcheson JC, et al. Long-term followup of endoscopic incision of ureteroceles: Intravesical versus extravesical. *J Urol* 2000;(Sep):164:1097.
53. Blyth B, Passerini-Glazel G, Camuffo C, et al. Endoscopic incision of ureteroceles: intravesicle versus ectopic. *J Urol* 1993; 149:556.
54. White JM, Kaplan GW, Brock WA. Ureteropelvic junction obstruction in children. *Am Fam Physician* 1984;29:211.
55. Maizels M, Reisman ME, Flum ES, et al. Grading nephroureteral dilatation detected in the first year of life: correlation with obstruction. *J Urol* 1992;148:609.
56. Koff SA, Thrall JH, Keyes JW Jr. Assessment of hydroureteronephrosis in children using diuretic radionuclide urographs. *J Urol* 1980;132:531.
57. Conway JJ, Maizels M. The "well tempered" diuretic renogram: a standard method to examine the asymptomatic neonate with hydronephrosis or hydroureteronephrosis. A report from combined meeting of The Society for Fetal Urology and members of The Pediatric Nuclear Medicine Council-The Society of Nuclear Medicine. *J Nucl Med* 1992;33(11):2047.
58. Whitaker RH. Methods of assessing obstruction in the dilated ureter. *Br J Urol* 1973;45:15.
59. Johnston JH. Reconstructive surgery of megaureter in childhood. *Br J Urol* 1967;39:17.
60. Feather SA, Malcolm S, Woolf AS, et al. Primary, nonsyndromic vesicoureteric reflux and its nephropathy is genetically heterogeneous, with a locus on chromosome 1. *Am J Hum Genet* 2000; (Apr):66(4):1420.
61. Noe HN, Wyatt RJ, Peeden JN, et al. The transmission of vesicoureteral reflux from parent to child. *J Urol* 1992;148:1869.
62. Dwoskin JY. Sibling uropathology. *J Urol* 1976;115:726.
63. Paquin AJ. Ureterovesical anastomosis: the description and evaluation of a technique. *J Urol* 1954;82:573.
64. Baker R, Maxted W, Maylith J, et al. Relation of age, sex, and infection to reflux: data indicating high spontaneous cure rate in pediatric patients. *J Urol* 1966;95:27.
65. Levitt SA, Duckett J, Spitzer A, et al. Medical versus surgical treatment of primary vesicoureteral reflux: report of the International Reflux Study Committee. *Pediatrics* 1981;67:392.
66. Dwoskin JY, Perlmutter AD. Vesicoureteral reflux in children: a computerized review. *J Urol* 1973;109:888.
67. Jeffs RD. Exstrophy and cloacal exstrophy. *Urol Clin North Am* 1978;5:127.
68. Scherz HC, Kaplan GW, Sutherland DH, et al. Fascia late and early apica casting as adjuncts in closure of bladder exstrophy. *J Urol* 1990;144:550.
69. Grady RW, Mitchell ME. Complete primary repair of exstrophy: surgical technique. *Urol Clin North Am* 2000;(Aug):27(3):569.
70. Eraklis A, Folkman J. Adenocarcinoma at the site of ureterosigmoidostomies for exstrophy of the bladder. *J Pediatr Surg* 1978; 13:730.
71. McIntosh JF, Worley G Jr. Adenocarcinoma arising in exstrophy of the bladder: report of two cases and review of the literature. *J Urol* 1955;73:820.
72. Johnston JH, Penn IA. Exstrophy of the cloaca. *Br J Urol* 1966; 38:302.
73. Tank ES, Lindenauer SM. Principles of management of exstrophy of the cloaca. *Am J Surg* 1970;119:95.
74. Diamond M, Sigmundson HK. Sex Reassignment at birth: long term review and clinical implications. *Arch Pediatr Adolesc Med* 1997;151:298.
75. Waffarn F, Devasker UP, Hodgman JE. Vesico-umbilical fistula: a complication of umbilical artery cutdown. *J Pediatr Surg* 1980; 15:211.
76. Walden TB, Karafin L, Kendall AR. Urachal diverticulum in a 3 year old boy. *J Urol* 1979;122:554.
77. Bambirra EA, Miranda D. Gastric polyp of the umbilicus in an 8 year old boy. *Clin Pediatr* 1980;19:430.
78. Berdon WE, Baker DH, Becker JA, et al. Megacystis—microcolon intestinal hypoperistalsis syndrome: a new cause of intestinal obstruction: report of radiologic findings in five newborn girls. *AJR Am J Roentgenol* 1976;126:957.
79. Granata C, Puri P. Megacystis-microcolon-intestinal hypoperistalsis syndrome. *J Pediatr Gastroenterol Nutr* 1997;25:12.
80. Lashley DB, Masliah E, Kaplan GW, et al. Megacystis microcolon hypoperistalsis syndrome: bladder distention and pyelectasis in the fetus without anatomic outflow obstruction. *Urology* 2000; 55(5):774.
81. Ochoa B, Curlin RJ. Urofacial (Ochoa) syndrome. *Am J Med Genet* 1987;27:661.
82. Dinneen MD, Duffy PG. Posterior urethral valves. *Br J Urol* 1996; 78:275.
83. Robertston WB, Hayes JA. Congenital diaphragmatic obstruction of the male posterior urethra. *Br J Urol* 1969;41:592.
84. Dewan PA, Keenan RJ, Morris LL, et al. Congenital urethral obstruction: Cobb's collar or prolapsed congenital obstructive posterior urethral membrane (COPUM). *Br J Urol* 1994; 73(1):91.
85. Rattner WH, Meyer R, Bernstein J. Congenital abnormalities of the urinary system: IV. Valvular obstruction of the posterior urethra. *J Pediatr* 1963;63:94.
86. Osathanondh V, Potter EG. Pathogenesis of polycystic kidneys: type 4 due to urethral obstruction. *Arch Pathol* 1964;77:502.
87. Javadpour N, Graziano MF, Terrill R. Experimental induction of patent allantoic duct by intrauterine bladder outlet obstruction. *J Surg Res* 1974;17:341.
88. Tanagho EA. Surgically induced partial urinary obstruction in the fetal lamb: II. Urethral obstruction. *Invest Urol* 1972;10:25.
89. Johnston JH. Vesicoureteral reflux with urethral valves. *Br J Urol* 1979;51:100.
90. Maizels M, Simpson SB Jr. Primitive ducts of renal dysplasia induced by cultured ureteral buds and condensed renal mesenchyme. *Science* 1983;219:509.
91. Churchill BM, McLorie MD, Khoury AE, et al. Emergency treatment and long-term follow up of posterior urethral valves. *Urol Clin North Am* 1990;17:343.
92. Cass AS, Stephens FD. Posterior urethral valves: diagnosis and management. *J Urol* 1974;112:519.
93. Sheldon CH, Gonzales R, Bauer MS, et al. Obstructive uropathy, renal failure, and sepsis in the neonate: a surgical emergency. *Urology* 1980;16:457.
94. Egami K, Smith ED. A study of the sequelae of posterior urethral valves. *J Urol* 1982;127;84.
95. Scott TW. Urinary ascites secondary to posterior urethral valves. *J Urol* 1976;116:87.
96. Tank ES, Carey TC, Seifert NL. Management of neonatal urinary ascites. *Urology* 1980;16:270.
97. Weller MH, Miller KE. Unusual aspects of urine ascites. *Radiology* 1973;129:665.
98. Parker RM. Neonatal urinary ascites: a potentially favorable sign in bladder outlet obstruction. *Urology* 1974;3:589.
99. Johnston JH. Vesicoureteral reflux with urethral valves. *Br J Urol* 1979;51:100.
100. Cuckow PM, Dinneen MD, Risdon RA, et al. Long-term renal function in the posterior urethral valves, unilateral reflux and renal dysplasia syndrome. *J Urol* 1997;158(3 Pt 2):1004.
101. Johnston JH, Kulatilake AE. The sequelae of posterior urethral valves. *Br J Urol* 1971;43:743.
102. Mayor G, Genton N, Tobrado A, et al. Renal function in obstructive uropathy: long-term effect of reconstructive surgery. *Pediatrics* 1975;56:740.
103. Parkhouse HF, Barratt TM, Dillon MJ, et al. Long term outcome of boys with posterior urethral valves. *Br J Urol* 1988;62:59.
104. McLorie G, Farhat W, Khoury A, et al. Outcome analysis of vesicoamniotic shunting in a comprehensive population. *J Urol* 2001;166(3):1036.
105. Howell CG, Othersen HB Jr, Kiviat NE, et al. Therapy and outcome in 51 children with mesoblastic nephroma: a report of the National Wilms' Tumor Study. *J Pediatr Surg* 1982;6:826.
106. Machin GA. Persistent renal blastema (nephroblastomatosis) as a frequent precursor of Wilms' tumor: a pathological and clinical

review: 2. Significance of nephroblastomatosis in the genesis of Wilms' tumor. *Am J Pediatr Hematol Oncol* 1980;2:253.

107. Gonzalez-Cirraso F, Kidd JM, Hernandez RJ. Cystic nephroma: morphologic spectrum and implications. *Urology* 1982;20:88.

108. Ganguly A, Gribble J, Tune B, et al. Renin-secreting Wilms' tumor with severe hypertension: report of a case and brief review of renin-secreting tumors. *Ann Intern Med* 1973;79:835.

109. Joshi VV, Banarsee AK, Yadak K, et al. Cystic partially differentiated nephroblastoma: a clinicopathologic entity in the spectrum of infantile renal neoplasia. *Cancer* 1977;40:789.

110. Belman AB, King LR. The pathology and treatment of renal vein thrombosis in the newborn. *J Urol* 1972;107:852.

111. Khuri FJ, Alton DJ, Hardy BE, et al. Adrenal hemorrhage in neonates: report of 5 cases and review of the literature. *J Urol* 1980;124:684.

112. Levin S, Collins D, Kaplan GW, et al. Neonatal adrenal pseudo-cyst mimicking metastatic disease. *Ann Surg* 1974;174:186.

113. Blane CE, Koff SA, Bowerman RA, et al. Non-obstructive fetal hydronephrosis: sonographic recognition and therapeutic implications. *Radiology* 1983;147:95.

114. Elder JS, Duckett JW Jr, Snyder HM. Intervention for fetal obstructive uropathy: has it been effective? *Lancet* 1987;2:1007.

115. Murphy JL, Kaplan GW, Packer MG, et al. Prenatal diagnosis of severe urinary tract anomalies improves renal function and growth. *Child Nephrol Urol* 1988;89:290.

116. Manning FA, Harrison MR, Rodeck C, et al. Catheter shunts for fetal hydronephrosis: report of the International Fetal Surgery Registry. *N Engl J Med* 1985;315:336.

117. Montana MA, Cyr DR, Lenke RR, et al. Sonographic detection of fetal ureteral obstruction. *AJR Am J Roentgenol* 1985;145:595.

118. Glick PL, Harrison MR, Golbus MS, et al. Management of the fetus with congenital hydronephrosis: II. Prognostic criteria and selection for treatment. *J Pediatr Surg* 1985;20:376.

119. Sherwood DW, Smith RC, Lemmon RH, et al. Abnormalities of the genitourinary tract discovered by palpation of the abdomen of the newborn. *Pediatrics* 1956;18:782.

120. Wedge JJ, Grosfeld JL, Smith JP. Abdominal masses in the newborn: 63 cases. *J Urol* 1971;106:770.

121. Raffensberger J, Abdusleiman A. Abdominal masses in children under one year of age. *Surgery* 1968;63:514.

122. Melicow MM, Uson AC. Palpable abdominal masses in infants and children: a report based on a review of 653 cases. *J Urol* 1959;81:705.

123. Emanuel B, Nachman R, Aronson N, et al. Congenital solitary kidney. *Am J Dis Child* 1974;127:17.

124. Scorer CG. The descent of the testicle. *Arch Dis Child* 1964; 39:605.

125. Scorer CG, Farrington GH. *Congenital deformities of the testis and epididymis.* London: Butterworths, 1971;4:45.

126. Kogan JJ, Tennenbaum SY, Gill B, et al. Efficacy of orchiopexy by patient age 1 year for cryptorchidism. *J Urol* 1990;144:508.

127. Kessler WO, McLaughlin AP. Agenesis of the penis: embryology and management. *Urology* 1973;1:226.

128. Rodriguez C. Report of a case of diphallus. *J Urol* 1965;94: 436.

129. Lee PA, Mazur T, Danish R, et al. Micropenis: criteria, etiologies, and classification. *Johns Hopkins Med J* 1980;146:156.

130. Burstein S, Grumbach MM, Kaplan SL. Early determination of androgen responsiveness is important in the management of microphallus. *Lancet* 1979;2:983.

131. Wisniewski AB, Migeon CJ, Gearhart JP, et al. Congenital micropenis: long-term medical, surgical and psychosexual follow up of individuals raised male or female. *Horm Res* 2001;56:3.

132. Bauer SB, Retik AB, Colodny AH. Genetic aspects of hypospadias. *Urol Clin North Am* 1981;8:559.

133. Paulozzi LJ, Erickson JD, Jackson RJ. Hypospadias trends in two US surveillance systems. *Pediatrics* 1997;100(5):831.

134. Anderson B, Mitchell M. Recent advances in hypospadias: current surgical technique and research in incidence and etiology. *Curr Urol Rep* 2001;2(2):122.

135. Silver RI, Rodriguez R, Chang TSK, et al. In vitro fertilization is associated with an increased risk of hypospadias. *J Urol* 1999; 161:1954.

136. Cerasaro TS, Brock WA, Kaplan GW. Upper urinary tract anomalies associated with congenital hypospadias: is screening necessary? *J Urol* 1986;135:537.

137. McAleer IM, Kaplan GW. Is routine karyotyping necessary in the evaluation of hypospadias and cryptorchidism? *J Urol* 2001; 165:2029.

138. Canning DA, Koo HP, Duckett JW. Anomalies of the bladder and cloaca. In: Gillenwater JY, Grayhack JT, Howards SS, et al, eds. *Adult and pediatric urology*, 3rd ed. St. Louis: Mosby-Year Book, 1996:2445–2488.

139. Williams DI, Kenawi MM. Urethral duplications in the male. *Eur Urol* 1975;1:209.

140. Bonney WW, Young HH II, Levin D, et al. Complete duplication of the urethra with vaginal stenosis. *J Urol* 1975;113(1):132.

141. Soares-Oliveira M, Juliá V, Garcia Aparicio L, et al. Congenital Prepubic Sinus. *J Pediatr Surg* 2002;37(8):1225.

142. Migeon CJ, Wisniewski AB, Brown TR, et al. 46, XY intersex individuals: phenotypic and etiologic classification, knowledge of condition, and satisfaction with knowledge in adulthood. *Pediatrics* 2002;110(3):e32.

143. Migeon CJ, Wisniewski AB, Gearhart JP, et al. Ambiguous genitalia with penoscrotal hypospadias in 46, XY individuals: long-term medical, surgical and psychosexual outcome. *Pediatrics* 2002;110(3):e31.

144. Hrabovsky Z, Hutson, JM. Androgen imprinting of the brain in animal models and humans with intersex disorders: Review and recommendations. *J Urol* 2002;168:2142.

145. Gairdner D. The fate of the foreskin: a study of circumcision. *Br Med J* 1949;2:1433.

146. Oster J. Further fate of the foreskin. *Arch Dis Child* 1968;43:200.

147. Wiswell TE. Routine neonatal circumcision: a reappraisal. *Am Fam Physician* 1990;41:859.

148. MacDonald MG. Circumcision. In: Fletcher MA, MacDonald MG, eds. *Atlas of procedures in neonatology*, 3rd ed. Philadelphia: Lippincott, Williams and Wilkins, 2002:361.

149. Kaplan GW. Complications of circumcision. *Urol Clin North Am* 1983;10:543.

150. Burge DM. Neonatal testicular torsion and infarction: etiology and management. *Br J Urol* 1987;59:70.

151. Das S, Singer A. Controversies in perinatal torsion of the spermatic cord: a review, survey and recommendations. *J Urol* 1990; 143:231.

152. Jerkins GR, Noe HN, Hollabauch RS, et al. Spermatic cord torsion in the neonate. *J Urol* 1983;129:121.

153. Pinto KJ, Noe HN, Jerkins GR. Management of neonatal torsion. *J Urol* 1997;158:1196.

154. Kaplan GW, Silber I. Neonatal torsion: to pex or not? In: King LR, ed. *Neonatal problems in urology*. Philadelphia: JB Lippincott, 1988:386.

155. Kaplan GW. Prepubertal testicular tumors. *World J Urol* 1984; 2:238.

156. Kay R. Prepubertal testicular tumor registry. *Urol Clin North Am* 1993;20:1.

157. Kaplan GW, Chromie WJ, Kelalis PP, et al. Gonadal stromal tumors: a report of the Prepubertal Testicular Tumor Registry. *J Urol* 1986;136:300.

158. Kaplan GW, Chromie WJ, Kelalis PP, et al. Prepubertal yolk sac testicular tumors: report of the Testicular Tumor Registry. *J Urol* 1988;140:1109.

159. Wu JT, Book L, Sudar K. Serum alpha-fetoprotein (AFP) levels in normal infants. *Pediatr Res* 1981;15:50.

160. Drew JH, Acton CK. Radiologic findings in newborn infants with urinary infection. *Arch Dis Child* 1976;51:628.

161. Wiswell TE, Smith FR, Bass JW. Decreased incidence of urinary tract infections in circumcised male infants. *Pediatrics* 1985; 75:401.

162. Stamey TA. *Urinary infections.* Baltimore: Williams & Wilkins, 1972.

163. Bergstrom T, Larson H, Lincoln K, et al. Studies of urinary tract infections in infancy and childhood: XII. Eighty consecutive patients with neonatal infection. *J Pediatr* 1972;80:858.

164. Chiaramonte RM, Horowitz EM, Kaplan GW, et al. Implications of hydronephrosis in the newborn with myelodysplasia. *J Urol* 1986;136:147.

165. Barbalias GA, Klauber GT, Blaivas JG. Critical evaluation of the Credé maneuver: a urodynamic study of 207 patients. *J Urol* 1983;130:720.

166. Cohen JS, Harbach LS, Kaplan GW. Cutaneous vesicostomy for temporary diversion in infants with neurogenic bladder dysfunction. *J Urol* 1978;119:120.

167. Harrison MR. Fetal surgery: trials, tribulation and turf. *J Pediatr Surg* 2003;38(3):275.
168. Garlinger P, Ott J. Prune belly syndrome: possible genetic implications. *Birth Defects Res Part A Clin Mol Teratol* 1974;10:173.
169. Rabinowitz R, Schillinger JF. Prune belly syndrome in the female subject. *J Urol* 1977;118:454.
170. Silverman FM, Huang N. Congenital absence of the abdominal muscle associated with malformation of the genitourinary and alimentary tracts: report of cases and review of literature. *Am J Dis Child* 1950;80:9.
171. Williams DI, Parker RM. The role of surgery in the prune belly syndrome. In: Johnston JH, Goodwin WF, eds. *Review of pediatric urology*. Amsterdam: Excerpta Medica, 1974:315.
172. Woodard JR, Parrott TS. Reconstruction of the urinary tract in prune belly syndrome. *J Urol* 1978;119:824.
173. Fleisher MH, McLorie GA, Churchill BM, et al. The yield of investigation of the urinary tract in imperforate anus. *J Urol* 1985; 133:142.
174. Hensle TW. Genital anomalies. In: Gillenwater JY, Grayhack JT, Howards SS, et al, eds. *Adult and pediatric urology*, 3rd ed. St. Louis: Mosby-Year Book, 1996:2529.
175. Brandt ML, Luks FI, Filiatrault D, et al. Surgical indications in antenatally diagnosed ovarian cysts. *J Pediatr Surg* 1991;26:276.
176. Pena A. Total Urogenital mobilization- an easier way to repair cloacas. *J Pediatr Surg* 1997;(Feb):32(2):263.
177. Rink RC, Pope JC, Kropp BP, et al. Reconstruction of the high urogenital sinus: early perineal approach without division of the rectum. *J Urol* 1997;158:1293.
178. Smith C, Gosalbez R, Parrott TS, et al. Transurethral puncture of ectopic ureteroceles in neonates and infants. *J Urol* 1994;152:2110.

Surgical Care of Conditions Presenting in the Newborn

Gary E. Hartman   **Michael J. Boyajian**   **Sukgi S. Choi**
Martin R. Eichelberger   **Kurt D. Newman**   **David M. Powell**

Successful management of newborns with surgical conditions requires close cooperation among neonatologist, surgeon, anesthesiologist, and radiologist. The fragile nature and limited reserve of these infants are superimposed on the stress of the surgical condition and its operative correction. In addition to the physiologic concerns related to the surgical condition, special attention must be directed toward (a) temperature regulation, (b) fluid, blood, and glucose administration, and (c) monitoring of respiratory and cardiovascular performance.

Venous and arterial access for fluid administration and monitoring may be challenging. Peripheral venous access with a 22- or 24-gauge catheter provides adequate access for the most vigorous fluid resuscitation. Central venous access may be necessary in the unstable newborn or if peripheral access is unsuccessful. Umbilical artery catheterization provides vascular access and arterial monitoring and is a well-established procedure in even the smallest prematures. The umbilical catheter may be maintained in most operative procedures. Peripheral arterial access may be obtained using radial, ulnar, or posterior tibial puncture or cutdown.

Fluid requirements are usually significantly greater than maintenance, especially in situations with intestinal obstruction, peritonitis, or gastroschisis. Before the operation there may be extraordinary losses from the gastrointestinal (GI) tract or inflamed peritoneum. These losses continue in the postoperative period and are superimposed on the sodium and water retention associated with the stress response. The endocrine, metabolic, and cytokine response to operative stress, which has been well documented in adults, has been confirmed in neonates (1–3). Postoperatively, decreased urine volume may result from the surge in antidiuretic hormone, intravascular volume depletion, or both, limiting the utility of urine volume alone as a monitor of adequacy of fluid replacement. Additional assessments including skin temperature, quality of peripheral pulses, serial measurements of weight, he-matocrit, and serum electrolytes and osmolality supplement urine volume as indicators of adequate volume replacement (4).

Temperature maintenance is a critical concern for all newborns, but in particular for those undergoing diagnostic studies and operative procedures in radiology and operating suites. A variety of means of temperature support may be utilized, including warming the environment, heat lamps, heating blankets, scalp and extremity wrapping, heated intravenous fluids and blood products, and heated inhaled anesthetic agents and surgical irrigating fluids. Temperature must be constantly monitored, and every effort made to minimize exposure to cold stress. Hypothermia is a potentially lethal condition, and the importance of temperature support cannot be overemphasized (5).

Anesthetic and postoperative pain management can minimize the magnitude of the stress response and accelerate the neonate's return to normal homeostasis in terms of cortisol, catecholamine, and insulin modulation (6). The expertise of all the specialists involved may be the advantage necessary to achieve survival and mandates close collaboration.

LESIONS OF THE HEAD AND NECK

Congenital abnormalities of the head and neck occur commonly in the newborn. Because of the short, fat neck of the baby, some of these lesions are not immediately apparent, and the examiner must be alert to their possibility to detect them.

Cleft Lip

Clefts of the lip or palate occur in approximately one of every 600 to 700 Caucasian newborns. The frequency is doubled in Asians and halved in African Americans. Cleft lip occurs somewhat more often in male patients and on the left side. The defect probably results from lack of the mesodermal reinforcement of the junction of the naso-medial and lateral facial processes that normally takes place in the sixth to seventh week of gestation. Multiple genetic influences seem to be more important than environmental factors. The cleft deformity ranges from minor notching to complete separation of the entire lip and nasal floor (Fig. 44-1). The defect may involve the lip, the lip and palate, or only the palate, and it may be unilateral or bilateral. Median cleft lip is rare and is usually associated with hypotelorism, microcephaly, and early death.

Airway obstruction is not typically a consequence of isolated cleft lip or palate. Initial care focuses on feeding the infant and counseling the parents. Swallowing and airway protection should be normal, but the negative pressure of the normal suck is vented through the cleft, resulting in inadequate inflow. Fatigue during feeding is common and may mimic satiation. Although suckling is not altogether discouraged, a baby with a complete cleft lip or any degree of cleft palate should be expected to suffer mechanical feeding difficulty. The solution may be to rely on an enlarged nipple aperture, a compressible bottle, or a syringe

feeder. With the use of a positive-pressure delivery system, the feeding schedule should be normal.

Lip closure is usually carried out at around 3 months of age. The major goals are muscle continuity, balanced lip height, the normal Cupid's-bow lip shape, a smooth and pout-free lip margin, a good nasal sill, adequate sulcus lining, and a minimal, well-placed scar. The wide, complete unilateral and the complete bilateral clefts present greater challenges. Preliminary lip adhesion for the unilateral case or presurgical orthodontics can improve anatomic associations and facilitate the definitive surgery. Residual nasal deformity is often a stubborn problem and may require secondary surgery.

Cleft Palate

The embryologic palatal shelves initially hang vertically and then rise to meet and fuse from front to back between weeks 7 and 12 of gestation. Interference with this process may result in complete, incomplete, or submucous cleft of the palate. Initial care is discussed in the section on cleft lip.

The major significance of this defect is the effect on speech. Normal modulation of speech requires reliable, dynamic palatal separation of the mouth from the nose. This requires a palate of adequate length, suppleness, and muscle power. Velopharyngeal incompetence or incomplete nasal closure results in hypernasal speech and significant communication disability.

Chronic or recurrent effusion and infection in an otherwise normal ear is common in the child with a cleft palate because eustachian tube function is compromised. This child usually needs myringotomies and ventilation tubes.

Early surgery seems to have a negative effect on facial growth, but the trend is toward closure during infancy because of the improved speech results. Most American surgeons choose 9 to 12 months of age as optimal timing for a single-stage closure.

Palatal closure is accomplished with local soft tissue. Mucoperiosteal flaps are mobilized and closed in the midline, with oral and nasal lining, effecting muscle apposition and retroposition. No bone reconstruction is involved. The goal is normal speech, and this is achieved in approximately 85% of patients. A second operation produces good results for almost all the remaining infants.

An essential concept in the treatment of these children is a multidisciplinary approach. The patient should be followed through adolescence by a team consisting of a plastic surgeon, otolaryngologist, audiologist, pedodontist, orthodontist, speech pathologist, geneticist, pediatrician, and social worker.

Pierre–Robin Sequence

The Pierre–Robin sequence is characterized by retrognathia or microgenia (i.e., small or recessed jaw or chin), glossoptosis, airway obstruction, and cleft palate. The lack of forward support of the tongue allows it to fall back and

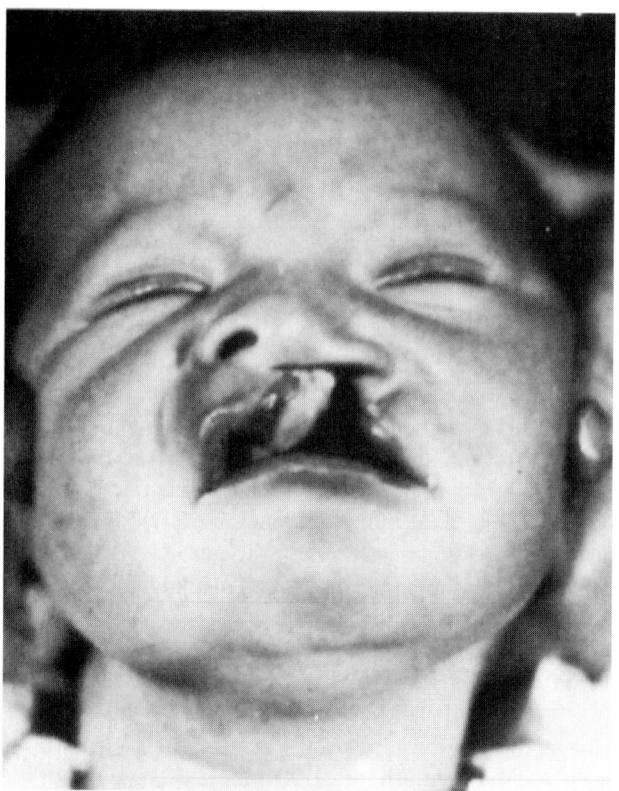

Figure 44-1 Complete congenital cleft of the lip with associated cleft of the palate that extends forward through the alveolar ridge.

compromise the airway. The basic defect may result from intrauterine restriction of mandibular growth.

Intensive monitoring, including a home apnea monitor, is necessary for many patients. The airway can usually be maintained by conservative measures. Prone positioning allows the tongue to fall forward. An appropriately apertured board may facilitate this positioning, and a nasal airway may be useful. Early gavage feedings may obviate hazardous oral feedings. A lip–tongue adhesion may be performed in more difficult cases, but its effectiveness varies. Tracheostomy should be avoided, if possible, but it is sometimes the only safe choice. Management should be as conservative as the clinical situation permits. The airway problem is typically self-limited, resolving as the child grows.

MASSES IN THE NECK

Masses in the neck are common in children and may be congenital, infectious, or neoplastic. Thyroglossal duct remnants, branchial apparatus anomalies, and lymphangiomas (i.e., cystic hygromas) are the most common congenital pediatric lesions in the neck.

Thyroglossal Duct Remnants

Thyroid tissue left behind in an abnormal location during normal developmental descent can result in a thyroglossal duct cyst, which presents in the midline of the neck. Infection may lead to a cutaneous salivary fistula. After appropriate therapy for infection, treatment consists of resection of the cyst, the central portion of the hyoid bone, and dissection of the tract up to its origin at the foramen cecum (Sistrunk operation) (7–9).

Branchial Cleft Anomalies

Branchial clefts with their corresponding arches and pouches are embryologic structures that give rise to many of the components of the lower face and neck. Abnormal persistence of any portion of the branchial apparatus leads to specific anomalies about the face and neck (10,11).

Preauricular Tabs and Sinuses

These lesions are not true branchial cleft remnants because they originate from an abnormal formation of the ear rather than a branchial cleft component. The preauricular sinus almost always ends blindly, and excision is indicated to prevent recurrent infection in later years.

Cervical Fistulas

Fistulas that originate from the first branchial arch present in the neck just below the ear and communicate with the external auditory canal. A fistula originating from the second branchial arch is the most common branchial cleft

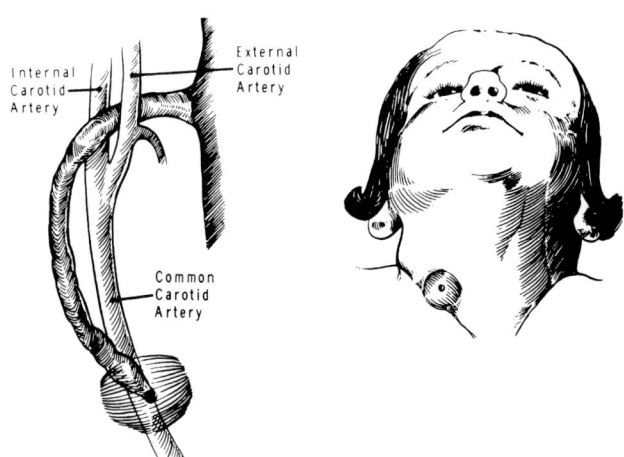

Figure 44-2 Brachial cleft cyst, which presents low in the neck as a mass or an opening in the skin, extends upward and laterally in the neck, and passes between the branches of the carotid artery to connect with the pharynx below the tonsillar facia. From Nardi GL, Zuidema GD. *Surgery*, 3rd ed. Boston: Little, Brown, 1972, with permission.

remnant. The fistula usually extends from the skin of the lower neck upward along the sternocleidomastoid muscle and then passes inward between the internal and external carotid arteries to attach to the posterolateral pharynx just below the tonsillar fossa (Fig. 44-2). The presenting complaint is usually related to persistent or intermittent drainage onto the neck. Complete surgical extirpation is necessary for cure. A large incision in the neck can be avoided by the use of two or three small, neat, transverse stair-step incisions.

Branchial Cyst

Approximately 10% of persistent branchial deformities are cystic. These invariably arise low in the anterior triangle of the neck and present as smooth cysts anterior to the sternocleidomastoid muscle. Dissection with excision is curative.

Cervical Cutaneous Tabs

Occasionally, a baby presents with a cutaneous tab in the skin of the anterior aspect of the neck. A small, irregular mass of cartilage may be contained in the skin tab. The cartilage is never associated with a fistula, and removal of this small appendage is not urgent.

Cystic Hygroma

Cystic hygroma (i.e., lymphangioma) is a congenital deformity arising from abnormal development of lymphatic channels (Fig. 44-3) (12). About 80% of these watery cysts occur in the neck, and most are located posterior to the sternocleidomastoid muscle. Other sites of occurrence are the groin, the axilla, and the mediastinum. The term "hygroma" suggests the watery fluid contained in the

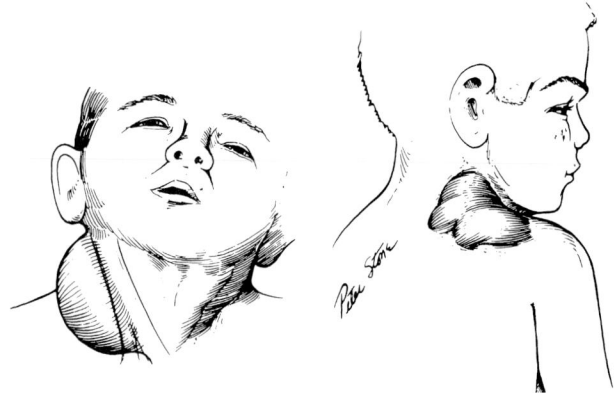

Figure 44-3 The typical cystic hygroma occurs in the lateral neck. The mass may extend into the scapular, axillary, or thoracic compartments, or the hygroma may present separately in any of these locations. Although depicted here as a single cyst, the hygroma is often a multiloculated, ill-defined mass. From Nardi GL, Zuidema GD. *Surgery*, 3rd ed. Boston: Little, Brown, 1972, with permission.

endothelium-lined spaces. The cyst may be unilocular, but more often there are numerous cysts of various sizes that permeate the surrounding structures and distort the local anatomy. Supporting connective tissue often shows extensive lymphocytic infiltration. Except in the case of a single large cyst, no definite cleavage plane is found between hygroma and normal tissue.

The lesion is usually evident at birth. Occasionally, the mass occupies the entire submandibular region, distorting the subglottic area and compromising the airway. A supra-clavicular mass may become prominent with the Valsalva maneuver. This form of cystic hygroma is usually associated with a mediastinal component. Some cystic hygromas contain nests of poorly supported vascular channels that are prone to bleeding and may produce sudden enlargement and discoloration of the lesion.

Symptoms are related entirely to the location and size of the mass. Disfigurement is often severe. Infection in the mass may lead to dangerous regional cellulitis, but after the infection subsides, the resultant intracystic fibrosis and scar may significantly reduce the size of the tumor mass. Prenatal ultrasonography has been used to diagnose cystic hygroma (13). This modality has demonstrated a hidden mortality with a high incidence of associated anomalies, including abnormal karyotypes and hydrops fetalis, when lymphangiomas are detected before 30 weeks of gestation.

Repeated aspiration of the cyst with injection of sclerosing agents is not recommended because any surgical excision that is subsequently required is rendered significantly more difficult by the sclerosing procedure. Elective surgical excision between 4 and 12 months of age is indicated for asymptomatic patients. Airway compression or recurrent infections may necessitate removal at an earlier age (14). Total excision is often impractical because of the extent of the hygroma and its proximity to vital structures. Important nerves and vascular structures must not be sacrificed in an attempt to achieve total excision of this benign lesion;

multiple excisions of the residual hygroma are preferable. Postoperative wound drainage using closed-suction drains may reduce recurrence.

UPPER AIRWAY OBSTRUCTION CAUSING RESPIRATORY DISTRESS

A neonate is essentially an obligate nasal breather for the first several months of life. (Recently this belief has been challenged, and some investigators have proposed that a neonate is a preferential nasal breather [15].) Therefore, during the first few months of an infant's life, any nasal condition causing obstruction can cause respiratory difficulties. Typically a neonate with nasal obstruction presents with cyclic cyanosis (See Color Plate).

A newborn's epiglottis is softer and bulkier than that of older children and adults and is often tubular in shape. Excessive and redundant mucosa over the epiglottis and arytenoids can contribute to inspiratory stridor. The larynx in a newborn is a well-developed organ; however, it is one-third the size of an adult larynx. The subglottis of a neonate measures approximately 4.5 mm in diameter. Because of the smaller dimension, 1 mm of circumferential edema in the subglottis can reduce the cross-sectional area of a neonate's airway by more than 60% (16). The trachea and bronchi are also smaller in dimensions and are shorter than those in an adult. In addition to these anatomic differences, the airway structures in a neonate are more pliable, and its mucosa more reactive. Therefore, conditions that affect the airway such as epiglottitis and croup can have proportionately greater effect on a small infant's airway.

Evaluation of airway obstruction begins with a careful history regarding the characteristics of the stridor or other upper airway noises, voice quality, severity of airway symptoms, feeding difficulties, previous intubation history or other manipulation of the airway, other associated anomalies, and symptoms of gastroesophageal reflux or aspiration. The great majority of airway abnormalities causing obstructive symptoms can be identified from the history alone (17). History is supplemented by physical examination and other evaluation modalities. High-kilovolt anterior–posterior and lateral soft tissue film of the neck can help in evaluation of the areas from nasal cavity to subglottis. Posterior–anterior and lateral chest x-rays can help to delineate tracheal and bronchial pathology. Other studies such as computed tomography (CT) scans and magnetic resonance imaging (MRI) may be needed to evaluate airway obstruction involving the nasal cavity, nasopharynx, and trachea.

Flexible nasopharyngoscopy and laryngoscopy can be performed at the bedside with monitoring. Areas from nasal vestibule to the vocal cords can be evaluated for functional and anatomic abnormalities. Flexible bronchoscopy with sedation is often suboptimal for evaluation of the subglottic, tracheal, and bronchial airways and is inferior to rigid endoscopy. Rigid endoscopy is usually performed in the operating room under general anesthesia but with spontaneous ventilation (no paralysis). This type of anesthesia enables the surgeon to evaluate the dynamics of the airway and any anatomic abnormalities.

Nasal Obstruction

Nasal Pyriform Aperture Stenosis

Congenital nasal pyriform aperture stenosis (anterior nasal stenosis) is secondary to the overgrowth of the nasal process of the maxilla (18). In this condition, the entrance into the nasal cavity known as the pyriform aperture is reduced to a slit-like opening. Because the pyriform aperture is the narrowest part of the nasal airway, even small changes in the cross-sectional area at this level can result in significant increase in nasal airway resistance and airway obstruction. Clinically, nasal obstruction causes apneic episodes and cyclic cyanosis, which is relieved by crying. Physical examination shows a bony, shelf-like projection of the posterior portion of the vestibule that almost completely obstructs the nasal cavity. The CT scan is the study of choice and helps to confirm the diagnosis and to define the anatomy of the nasal cavity and posterior choanae. Association of anterior nasal stenosis with midfacial dysostosis and endocrine and central nervous system abnormalities has been reported (19). Therefore, a genetic consult should be considered.

The infant is initially managed with a McGovern nipple or an oral airway with close monitoring. Gavage feeding may be necessary. If the infant is doing well, then discharge to home with an apnea monitor and a plan for close follow-up evaluations can be considered. If the infant does not tolerate an oral airway or continues to have significant nasal obstruction despite conservative management, then surgical intervention is necessary before discharge from the hospital. Sublabial approach with the use of microinstruments to remove portions of the nasal process of the maxilla is recommended (18). When the obstruction is mucosal rather than bony in nature, the diagnosis is likely to be stuffy nose syndrome, and it requires symptomatic medical treatment only.

Deviated Nasal Septum

Careful intranasal examination shows some septal deformities in as many as 70% of newborns, which may be secondary to intrauterine or birth trauma (20,21). Significant deviation of nasal septum secondary to traumatic delivery or the use of forceps is seen in approximately 1% of neonates. Physical examination shows tilted columella, deviation of the nasal septum and asymmetry of the nasal alae. Radiographic studies are not helpful. Closed reduction of the nasal septum by the use of gentle traction should be carried out during the first week of life. Careful examination of the nasal cavities to detect septal hematoma is essential. If this is present, a septal hematoma must be evacuated emergently because hematoma can lead to abscess formation and saddle nose deformity. Parents should be counseled that nasal growth disturbances can

occur following trauma and that further nasal surgery may be necessary when the child is older.

Choanal Atresia

The simplest and the most widely held theory regarding pathogenesis of choanal atresia is that it results from the persistence of bucconasal membranes that normally involute during the seventh week of gestation. The incidence of choanal atresia is approximately one in 5,000 to 8,000 live births. Unilateral choanal atresia is twice as frequent as bilateral choanal atresia. Ninety percent of the atresia is bony; 10% is membranous. The female-to-male ratio is reported to be 2:1. In approximately 50% of the patients with choanal atresia, other associated anomalies are seen. The most common anomaly associated with choanal atresia is the CHARGE association (coloboma, heart disease, atresia of the choana, retarded growth and development, genitourinary anomalies, ear anomalies and/or deafness) (22). For these reasons, a genetic consultation may be indicated for patients diagnosed with choanal atresia.

In cases of unilateral atresia, unilateral mucoid nasal rhinorrhea may be seen; however, significant respiratory distress is usually absent. In bilateral choanal atresia, characteristic cyclic respiratory obstruction is seen. Nasal obstruction leads to increasing respiratory effort and distress until the child cries and the nasal obstruction is bypassed temporarily. Diagnosis is established by the inability to pass a 6-Fr suction catheter through the nostril beyond 3 to 4 cm into the nasopharynx. The atretic plate can also be visualized using a fiberoptic nasopharyngoscope. The best method of delineating the atresia is by CT scan.

A neonate with bilateral choanal atresia is initially managed with oral airway or McGovern nipple and gavage feedings. Tracheotomy is rarely needed. Choanal atresia can be addressed by transnasal, transpalatal or endoscopic approaches (23,24). Emergent surgical correction for bilateral choanal atresia is seldom required and is reserved for those infants that can not be managed conservatively. Under these circumstances, a transnasal repair can be performed with a staged definitive transpalatal repair when the child is older. In a neonate who is easily managed by conservative means alone, surgical correction can be deferred for 1 to 2 years. Restenosis requiring revision surgery is not uncommon.

Congenital Midline Nasal Masses

Encephaloceles and gliomas arise from faulty closure of the foramen caecum at the third week of fetal development (25). Gliomas are locally aggressive lesions that can cause symptoms by enlargement and pressure effects on the surrounding structures. Approximately 30% of gliomas are intranasal and thus can cause nasal obstruction and septal deviation. Fifteen percent of gliomas have a fibrous connection to the dura. Basal encephaloceles herniate through a defect in the cribriform plate and usually present as intranasal masses and cause nasal obstruction.

Congenital midline nasal masses are best evaluated by a combination of CT scan and MRI. Depending on whether there is a connection to the dura, gliomas may require a combined approach by the neurosurgery and otolaryngology services. Encephaloceles always have an intracranial connection and thus require an intracranial exploration. Early surgical intervention is advised to decrease the risk of meningitis and further enlargement of the mass with resulting cosmetic deformity.

Oropharyngeal Obstruction

Glossoptosis

Pierre–Robin sequence (PRS) consists of micrognathia, glossoptosis, and U-shaped cleft palate; it represents the best-known cause of glossoptosis. Pierre–Robin sequence results secondary to arrest in development of mandible at the seventh to the 11th week of gestation, which then leads to high position of tongue in the oral cavity and prevention of fusion of palatal shelves (26). It may present as an isolated anomaly or as a part of a syndrome such as Stickler's syndrome (see Chapter 38). Genetic consultation is advised.

Airway obstruction in neonates with PRS occurs because of the micrognathia, which causes posterior displacement of the tongue base. Obstruction is more severe in supine position and worsens during sleep or induction of anesthesia. Airway obstruction can be managed by positioning, placement of a nasopharyngeal airway, intubation, and tracheotomy (27). Most patients without other significant airway or neurologic deficits can be managed conservatively (28). For neonates with severe airway symptoms who do not respond to positioning or nasopharyngeal airway, a tracheotomy is required. Once it is performed, the tracheotomy tube remains in place until the cleft palate repair is completed.

Macroglossia

Macroglossia is seen in neonates with Beckwith–Wiedemann syndrome (BWS). Additionally, patients with BWS may have omphalocele, adrenal cytomegaly, and visceromegaly (29). BWS occurs secondary to sporadic mutation and has a mortality rate of over 20%. The airway obstruction seen in these patients is secondary to macroglossia. Initial management consists of tracheotomy, followed by a tongue reduction procedure at a later date.

True macroglossia and relative macroglossia (a small oral cavity) can also be seen in neonates with Down syndrome; however, the size of the tongue rarely necessitates surgical intervention.

Laryngeal Obstruction

Laryngomalacia

Laryngomalacia is the most common cause of stridor in infants (30). Laryngomalacia describes the collapse of supraglottic structures on inspiration. The pathophysiology of laryngomalacia is unknown. Usually, it is a self-limited condition with mild symptoms that resolve by age 18 to 24 months.

Infants with laryngomalacia present with variable inspiratory stridor that worsens with crying, feeding, and upper respiratory infections and improves with prone position. A small number of infants have more severe symptoms of airway obstruction consisting of retraction, feeding difficulties, failure to thrive, and cyanosis. Diagnosis is confirmed by flexible laryngoscopy, which shows inward collapse of the epiglottis, aryepiglottic folds, and the mucosa over the arytenoids during inspiration. In fewer than 5% of the infants, surgery is indicated to relieve severe obstruction and prevent pulmonary and cardiac complications (31). Surgery consists of trimming the supraglottic tissue with carbon dioxide laser or by sharp dissection (32). A tracheotomy is an alternative to supraglottoplasty (epiglottoplasty).

Vocal Cord Paralysis

Vocal cord paralysis accounts for approximately 10% of all congenital laryngeal anomalies (30). Unilateral paralysis does not cause significant airway symptoms; however, the infant may have a hoarse and breathy cry. Surgical intervention is usually not required. An infant with bilateral vocal cord paralysis (BVCP) presents with normal voice and cry, but with an inspiratory stridor. Central nervous system anomalies, in particular Arnold–Chiari malformation, are often associated with BVCP (30,33). The diagnosis of BVCP is made by flexible laryngoscopy. Radiographs of the airway and chest and, if indicated, CT scan of the brain should be obtained.

In BVCP associated with Arnold–Chiari malformation, neurosurgical decompression will result in resolution of BVCP. In most infants with idiopathic BVCP, tracheotomy is required to establish an airway. During tracheotomy, the entire airway should be inspected to exclude any additional airway anomalies. Definitive vocal cord lateralizing procedures can be done at a later date, if spontaneous resolution of the paralysis does not occur (34).

Laryngeal Atresia/Web

During embryogenesis, epithelium temporarily obliterates the laryngeal lumen. This epithelial plug is then resorbed during the seventh to eighth week of gestation (35). Failure of this resorption process can result in laryngeal web, subglottic stenosis (SGS), and laryngeal atresia. Laryngeal atresia is a rare and life-threatening condition that must be recognized in the delivery room and must be followed by an emergent placement of tracheotomy tube if the infant is to survive.

The most common laryngeal web is seen at the glottic level and affects the vocal cords (36). The web may be thick, causing severe obstruction, or thin and membranous. Infants with laryngeal web present with abnormal cry, stridor, and respiratory distress. Laryngeal web can cause cyanosis or unexplained airway obstruction at birth, which requires intubation or a tracheotomy. Laryngeal web is often associated with SGS. Diagnosis is made by airway films and rigid endoscopy. Definitive treatment options to allow decannulation include dilation, endoscopic microsurgical or laser division of the web, and an open repair (36).

Posterior Laryngeal Cleft

Posterior laryngeal cleft is often associated with other congenital anomalies such as esophageal atresia, tracheoesophageal fistula, and tracheal and bronchial stenosis. Posterior laryngeal cleft is difficult to diagnose, particularly if the cleft is limited to the interarytenoid region. Posterior laryngeal cleft has been classified into four types, with type 1 being a mild interarytenoid cleft above the level of the vocal cords and type 4 representing a complete laryngotracheoesophageal cleft (37).

Presenting symptoms depend on the extent of the cleft. Airway obstruction is not a prominent feature. Rather, aspiration, choking, cyanosis, and feeding difficulties are seen commonly. Stridor and voice abnormalities can be seen but are not common. Diagnosis is made by careful inspection of the posterior glottis during endoscopy. Laryngeal cleft can be repaired endoscopically or by an external approach using laryngofissure or lateral pharyngotomy.

Subglottic Stenosis

SGS is defined as narrowing of the airway at the level of the cricoid to less than 4 mm in a full-term infant and 3 mm in a premature infant. It is considered to be congenital if there has not been any previous airway manipulation. The stenosis may be cartilaginous or membranous. Many of the infants with congenital SGS may have only mild symptoms and go undiagnosed, whereas others may get intubated and thus diagnosed as having acquired SGS. Thus, the true incidence of congenital SGS is unknown. Acquired SGS is most commonly secondary to prolonged endotracheal intubation. One percent to 8% of infants who require prolonged intubation may acquire SGS (38). The injury to the subglottis is related to the duration of intubation, the size of the endotracheal tube (ETT), the degree of ETT motion, and the number of reintubations.

Infants with SGS can present with stridor, respiratory distress, and croupy barking cough. Others present with recurrent or prolonged croup and inability to be extubated after intubation, or obstructive apnea. Airway radiographs can show narrowing of the subglottic airway; however, the definitive diagnosis is made on rigid endoscopy. For infants who have severe airway obstruction and fail repeated attempts at extubation, a tracheotomy or anterior cricoid split (ACS) can be considered. An ACS can be performed only in infants without other underlying airway abnormalities that contribute to the airway obstruction and who have good pulmonary reserve (39). Any need for ventilatory support, oxygen requirement over 30%, congestive

heart failure, and respiratory infection are contraindications to ACS.

Anterior cricoid split involves opening of the upper two tracheal rings, cricoid cartilage, and lower half of the thyroid cartilage in the anterior midline and presumably works by decompressing the airway. Postoperative intubation for 7 to 10 days and meticulous care to avoid ETT plugging and accidental extubation are imperative. Systemic corticosteroid is administered beginning 24 hours preextubation and continues for 72 hours postextubation. If ACS is successful, a tracheotomy can be avoided. Patients who fail ACS can undergo revision ACS or a tracheotomy followed by a formal laryngotracheal reconstruction at a later date.

Subglottic Hemangioma

Hemangiomas represent malformation of vasoformative tissue. Hemangioma in the airway usually occurs in the submucosa of the subglottic region; it increases in size over 6 to 18 months, followed by involution (40). Hemangioma may extend beyond the airway into the mediastinum. Approximately 50% of infants with airway hemangioma have cutaneous hemangioma in the head and neck region.

Infants with subglottic hemangioma present with inspiratory stridor, hoarseness, barky cough, and airway obstruction. Airway film shows soft tissue swelling in the subglottis, which is often asymmetric. Endoscopy shows a lesion that is localized to the posterior subglottis and is soft and compressible. Biopsy is usually not necessary unless diagnosis is in question, and the endoscopist should be prepared to manage possible hemorrhage into the airway. Treatment of subglottic hemangioma depends on the degree of airway obstruction and the extent of airway involved by the hemangioma. Treatment options include tracheotomy followed by expectant waiting for involution of the hemangioma, corticosteroids, and laser excision. More recently, interferon-a2a administration has been introduced as a treatment for airway hemangiomas (41).

Tracheal Obstruction

Tracheal Stenosis

Tracheal stenosis may be secondary to mucosal webs of variable thickness without any gross deformity of the underlying cartilage. Stenosis of the trachea can also be caused by complete tracheal rings of variable length. The segment with complete tracheal rings lacks the posterior membranous portion of the trachea.

Symptoms of airway obstruction from tracheal stenosis depends on the diameter of the narrowed airway lumen. Neonates with tracheal stenosis can present with persistent cough, respiratory distress, expiratory stridor, and wheezing. Symptoms tend to worsen following an upper respiratory infection, and sudden and complete obstruction can occur from mucus plugging of the narrowed segment. Many patients also tend to have feeding difficulties. The diagnosis is suggested by history, airway films, and fluoroscopy; however, a definitive diagnosis is made by endoscopic evaluation. Mucosal web may respond to dilation alone. Short segments of tracheal stenosis are resected with end-to-end anastomosis (42). Long segments of stenosis require tracheoplasty using pericardial and/or cartilage grafts (43). These surgical procedures are associated with high morbidity and mortality rates.

Tracheomalacia

In tracheomalacia there is increased flaccidity of the tracheal walls, which leads to anterior–posterior collapse of the airway and obstruction (44). Primary tracheomalacia is an isolated finding that usually resolves by age 2 years. Secondary tracheomalacia is seen in neonates with tracheoesophageal fistula (TEF) or external vascular compression. In primary tracheomalacia and in secondary tracheomalacia associated with TEF, deficiency in the tracheal cartilage may cause the abnormal collapse of the trachea (44,45).

Clinical symptoms of tracheomalacia range from mild to severe. Common features of severe cases include inspiratory and/or expiratory stridor, wheezing, persistent coughing, recurrent respiratory infections, reflex apnea, and difficulty with clearing airway secretions. Reflex apnea describes a respiratory arrest that can progress to a cardiac arrest and is seen in patients with tracheobronchial compression (46). Diagnosis of tracheomalacia can be suggested by fluoroscopy, but a definitive diagnosis can only be made by endoscopic examination of the airway under spontaneous ventilation. Widened semicircular cartilages, ballooning of the posterior membranous wall, and collapse of tracheal lumen are seen. In severe cases tracheotomy is required until the condition resolves. The use of positive airway pressure through the tracheotomy tube may be necessary to maintain patency of the airway below the tracheotomy tube (47).

Vascular Compression

Innominate artery compression of the trachea can occur when there is an anomalous distal origin of the innominate artery from the aortic arch. The innominate artery crosses the trachea in a left-inferior-to-right-superior direction and causes compression of the trachea. Infants with this condition present with stridor, recurrent respiratory infections, feeding difficulties, and reflex apnea. Diagnosis is best made by endoscopy and MRI. Surgery is necessary only in infants with severe stridor or reflex apnea. Suspension of the innominate artery through thoracotomy or median sternotomy and reimplantation of the innominate artery are available surgical options (48).

Other less common vascular anomalies causing airway obstruction include double aortic arch, right aortic arch with left ligamentum arteriosum, and pulmonary artery sling. Evaluation of these conditions includes chest radiographs, MRI, and endoscopy. In symptomatic infants, the appropriate surgical procedure should be undertaken by a cardiothoracic surgeon.

THORACIC LESIONS CAUSING RESPIRATORY DISTRESS

Congenital Lobar Emphysema

Congenital lobar emphysema can be severe or life-threatening as a result of hyperexpansion of a single lobe of the lung. Air is permitted into the involved lobe but denied egress. The lobe becomes emphysematous, resulting in compression of adjacent pulmonary parenchyma and mediastinal displacement. Symptoms may appear shortly after birth and invariably develop before 4 months of age (49). The cause is unknown. An inherent, cartilaginous defect in the bronchus has been postulated, but the bronchial abnormality is not always recognizable in the resected specimen.

A chest radiograph is characteristic, showing hyperaeration of the involved lobe with mediastinal shift away from the affected side. The lobar distribution of the hyperaeration can be appreciated, and adjacent pulmonary parenchyma is compressed. The upper lobes are most frequently involved, but the condition may be seen in the middle lobe. Rarely, the lesion is bilateral (50).

Treatment is surgical, and prompt thoracotomy and lobectomy are undertaken after the diagnosis is made. An infant may remain compensated for some weeks and then deteriorate rapidly from acute hyperinflation of the involved lobe. There is no place for expectant management of congenital lobar emphysema.

An identical clinical picture may be seen in the neonate who has been ventilated for a prolonged time and develops a large pneumatocele as a result of respiratory tract barotrauma. It is often difficult for the physician to determine whether respiratory distress is caused by the pneumatocele or by generalized pulmonary parenchymal disease. Surgical excision of the pneumatocele is indicated if the lesion is enlarging and the respiratory status is worsening without another apparent cause.

Cystic Adenomatoid Malformation

Cystic adenomatoid malformation (CAM) is a pulmonary maldevelopment that presents with cystic replacement of pulmonary parenchyma. If the cysts are small (i.e., microcystic CAM) and constitute a small portion of one lung, the child may be asymptomatic. If the lesion is microcystic and replaces a large portion of the lung, the fetus may develop hydrops, and the prognosis is poor (51). If the cysts are macroscopic and the child is in respiratory distress at birth, the problem may be misdiagnosed as congenital diaphragmatic hernia. Appropriate therapy for the symptomatic neonate with CAM is thoracotomy and resection of the involved lung. Postoperative support with extracorporeal membrane oxygenation (ECMO) has been necessary for infants developing severe persistent pulmonary hypertension after CAM excision (52).

Bronchogenic Cyst

Bronchogenic cyst is another lung bud anomaly in which the normal bronchiole-to-bronchiole communication is absent or atretic, resulting in a mucus-producing cyst that may obstruct the trachea, bronchus, or esophagus. This seldom causes severe problems in the neonate, but it must be considered if a space-occupying lesion is detected on a chest x-ray film obtained for investigation of respiratory distress. Excision of the bronchogenic cyst is the preferred treatment.

Iatrogenic Airway Injury

As aggressive management of the pulmonary disease of newborns has developed, there has been a concurrent increase in injury to the airway or pulmonary parenchyma. Long-term intubation and high peak inspiratory pressure settings on the ventilator place these children at an increased risk of airway injury. It has been known since 1976 that perforation of bronchi, particularly the bronchus of the right lower lobe, can be prevented by careful measurement of suction catheters so that they do not extend more than 1 cm beyond the carina (53). The development of a bronchopulmonary fistula after chest tube evacuation of a pneumothorax can be life-threatening and may require surgical closure of the fistula, although some children have been successfully treated nonoperatively (54).

Complications of high-pressure ventilation include development of interstitial emphysema and bronchopulmonary dysplasia. The interstitial emphysema is usually self-limited, although some infants may benefit from a surgical approach to the problem (55). Surgery can be curative for granulomas within the airway of chronically intubated neonates, particularly if the lesions contribute to air trapping or stenosis. The best management for iatrogenic airway injury is prevention, and although not totally avoidable, careful attention to ventilator management and suction techniques should reduce the incidence and severity of these problems.

Diaphragmatic Hernia

Development of the diaphragm is generally complete the 12th week of gestation, by which time the bowel has returned to the abdominal cavity. Failure of the development of the posterolateral portion of the diaphragm results in persistence of the pleuroperitoneal canal or foramen of Bochdalek, which allows the viscera to occupy the chest cavity, and the abdomen is underdeveloped and scaphoid. Both lungs are hypoplastic, more so on the side of the hernia. Bronchial branching, lung weight, and lung volume are decreased. The pulmonary arteries are hypoplastic (56,57). The lesion occurs in one of every 3,000 live births, with equal frequency in male and female infants. Sporadic

occurrence is the rule, but a familial pattern has been reported (58,59).

The prenatal diagnosis of congenital diaphragmatic hernia (CDH) can be made using fetal sonography as early as 15 weeks of gestation (60). Sonographic findings include herniated abdominal viscera, abnormal anatomy of the upper abdomen, and mediastinal shift away from the herniated viscera (61). The high-risk fetus is identified by a diagnosis early in gestation, a dilated stomach in the chest, low lung-to-thorax ratio, low lung-to-head ratio, and polyhydramnios. Amniocentesis with a fetal karyotype identifies chromosomal defects; trisomy 18 and 21 are most common. More than 40% of newborns with CDH have associated anomalies of the heart, brain, limbs, genitourinary system, or craniofacial region (62).

Typically, babies with congenital Bochdalek hernia present dramatically with cyanosis (See Color Plate) and severe respiratory distress immediately after birth. Because the abdominal viscera are dislocated through the defect into the chest, the abdominal contour is scaphoid. Breath sounds are diminished or absent, and because the mediastinal structures have been displaced, the heart sounds are heard in the right chest. As the bowel fills with gas, respiration and cardiac action are further compromised, hypoxia and respiratory acidosis are increased, and death is inevitable unless appropriate intervention is undertaken. Congenital diaphragmatic hernia is no longer considered a surgical emergency unless the viability of the herniated bowel is in question. In some instances, the infants remain relatively asymptomatic in the early hours and days of life, and rarely, a diaphragmatic hernia is an incidental finding in an older child. The respiratory symptoms demand an immediate x-ray film, which is diagnostic. The hernia is on the left side in 90% of these infants, and the air-filled bowel is seen occupying the left hemithorax, with resultant displacement of the mediastinum to the right (Fig. 44-4). The abdomen is gasless. Additional x-ray films are unnecessary, and contrast studies for additional confirmation are contraindicated.

Many newborns with CDH have respiratory failure within minutes of birth, and urgent stabilization is mandatory to reverse hypoxia, hypercarbia, and metabolic acidosis. Prompt and aggressive preoperative care is essential (63,64). This generally includes mechanical ventilation with 100% oxygen, sedation with narcotics, muscle paralysis, controlled alkalosis with hyperventilation and intravenous sodium bicarbonate, and vasopressors. Permissive hypercarbia and gentle ventilation have proven effective in a number of centers. Regardless of the mode of therapy, the goal is to reverse the baby's persistent pulmonary hypertension with right-to-left shunting of oxygen-poor blood across the open foramen ovale and the ductus arteriosus.

Some infants do not improve despite aggressive therapy, and many centers use ECMO before hernia repair to stabilize these desperately ill infants (65,66). Venovenous or venoarterial bypass is used, depending on the infant's hemodynamic stability. Bypass is continued until the pulmonary hypertension is reversed and lung function is

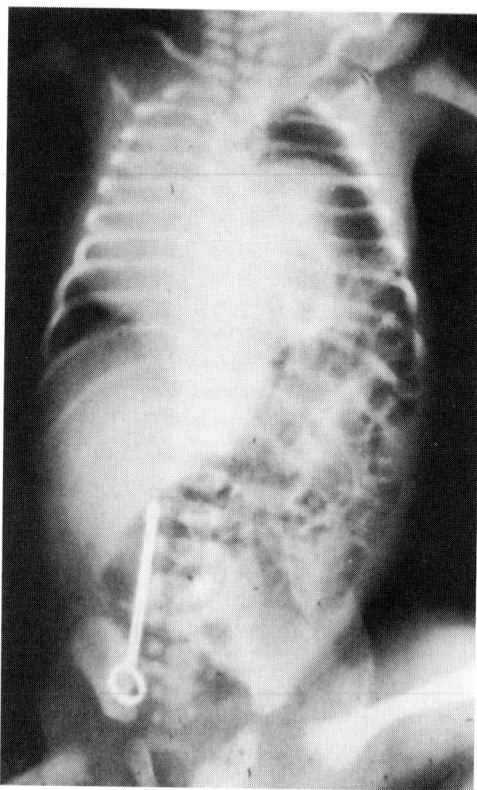

Figure 44-4   X-ray film of left diaphragmatic hernia with loops of bowel well up into the chest. Although most diaphragmatic hernias do not have a sac, the smooth curve of the sac in this instance is visible. Notice that the heart is displaced to the border of the right chest.

improved. Most infants respond within 7 to 10 days, but some require up to 3 weeks of support. Newborns who have not improved after this time probably have such severe pulmonary hypoplasia that further extracorporeal life support is futile.

There are no absolute respiratory criteria that exclude newborns with CDH from consideration for ECMO support (67,68). Approximately 60% of infants with CDH who are supported by ECMO are expected to survive (see Chap. 32).

The surgical findings are usually those of a posterolateral defect in the left diaphragm, with most or all of the abdominal viscera in the chest. The surgeon reduces the hernia gently by withdrawing the viscera from the chest. If a sac is present, it is delivered and excised. There may be adequate diaphragmatic tissue to accomplish direct suture repair. If a significant portion of the diaphragm is lacking, prosthetic material is used to close the defect. Before completion of the repair, a small chest tube may be placed in the left hemithorax and brought out through an intercostal space.

The temptation to expand the compressed lung at the time of initial surgery must be resisted. Aggressive attempts at expansion can result in pneumothorax on the contralateral side, which, if unrecognized, is a disastrous complication.

The abdominal viscera have been located in the thorax throughout most of the developmental period of the fetus; thus, there is insufficient room within the abdomen to accommodate the intestine without dangerously increasing the intraabdominal pressure, compressing the vena cava, and compromising respirations by elevating the diaphragm. To avoid these potential problems, the surgeon may omit anatomic closure of the abdominal wall. Skin flaps are quickly mobilized, and only the skin is closed, or the abdomen is closed by creating a silastic silo as for gastroschisis or a large omphalocele. The ventral pouch created accommodates the intraabdominal organs; diaphragmatic action and venous return are unimpeded. The ventral hernia is repaired after the infant has been weaned off the ventilator and is in stable clinical condition.

Ten percent of infants with Bochdalek hernias present with the defect on the right side. The difference in incidence on the two sides may be explained by the presence of the liver, which partially blocks the pleuroperitoneal canal and limits the amount of bowel that can herniate into the chest. Symptoms in babies with right-sided hernias may be less severe, but when a right diaphragmatic hernia of Bochdalek presents as an emergency, it is managed as described.

After CDH repair and removal from ECMO, ventilation is continued with ventilation rates and oxygen concentrations necessary to maintain adequate oxygenation. Continuous transcutaneous oxygen monitoring of upper and lower body areas is useful. To avoid relapse into pulmonary hypertension, weaning from the ventilator should be achieved by making small incremental changes in the inspired oxygen and ventilator rate.

New modalities being investigated may offer an increased chance of survival for infants with CDH. These include surfactant replacement therapy, liquid ventilation, intratracheal pulmonary ventilation, and pulmonary lobar transplantation (69,70). Prenatal repair of the diaphragmatic hernia has been abandoned, as there was no improvement in survival or morbidity in a randomized trial. Current prenatal therapy of CDH is directed at occluding the trachea, which results in enlargement of the lungs with retained fluid. The baby is then delivered by planned cesarean section, at which time the trachea is repaired or intubated, with the baby remaining on placental support. Initial discouraging results with this technique have been improved with recent modifications; however, fetal tracheal plugging remains an experimental procedure that is being evaluated in a limited number of centers (71,72).

Babies who present after the first day of life with signs and symptoms prompting a diagnosis of diaphragmatic hernia are almost always hardier patients and have greater pulmonary reserve, and they can be expected to make a satisfactory recovery.

The anterior retrosternal hernia of Morgagni is rarely encountered in the newborn. The diagnosis is confirmed by chest radiograph in the lateral projection. The standard treatment is surgical reconstruction, beginning with an abdominal approach through a thoracoabdominal incision. The prognosis is usually favorable, and these lesions are not associated with the severe cardiopulmonary complications seen with Bochdalek hernias in the neonatal period.

Eventration of the Diaphragm

Eventration of the diaphragm may be congenital or acquired. The congenital presentation may mimic that of a congenital diaphragmatic hernia with a sac. The acquired lesion results from paralysis of the diaphragm, most commonly caused by operative trauma or birth injury (73).

Large eventrations and diaphragmatic paralysis are poorly tolerated by infants (74). Paradoxic cephalad motion of the diaphragm on inspiration produces a shift of the mobile, neonatal mediastinum that limits the function of the contralateral lung. Moderate or severe respiratory distress is evident; many newborns with eventration require ventilatory support.

Diagnosis is suggested by a marked elevation of a hemidiaphragm on a chest radiograph. Fluoroscopic examination identifies paradoxic movement of the diaphragm. Treatment is plication of the diaphragm with nonabsorbable sutures that reef up or overlap the diaphragm. The taut diaphragm results in less abnormal motion and improved ventilation.

LESIONS OF THE ESOPHAGUS

Esophageal Atresia and Associated Anomalies

The success story of the management of infants born with esophageal atresia and tracheoesophageal fistula is one of the most dramatic and satisfying that the pediatric surgeon, the neonatologist, and the pediatrician can point to. In the early 1900s, virtually all babies born with esophageal atresia and tracheoesophageal fistula died. In 1941, Haight and Towsley were the first to bring an infant with esophageal atresia and tracheoesophageal fistula successfully through the rigors of primary transthoracic reconstruction (75). This landmark accomplishment occurred before antibiotics, respiratory support, or sophisticated intravenous nutrition were available. This surgical approach formed the basis of modern operative and postoperative care of infants born with this anomaly. Fifty years after the first survivor was announced, every baby born with atresia of the esophagus who is spared coexisting fatal abnormalities and is offered appropriate care has an excellent chance of leading a normal life.

Embryologic and Genetic Considerations

The cause of esophageal atresia is unknown, but it is related to the common origin of the esophagus and trachea (76). The embryonic trachea and esophagus are first recognized as a ventral diverticulum of the foregut approximately 22 or 23 days after fertilization (77). As the diverticulum elongates, a proliferation of endodermal cells appears on the lateral walls. These cell masses become ridges of tissue that ultimately divide the foregut into tracheal and esophageal channels. The division into separate tubes is completed between 34 and 36 days after fertilization. Many embryologic studies indicate that interruption of development in the fourth fetal week allows persistence of fistulas and clefts between the esophagus and trachea and permits incomplete development of the esophagus.

There are reports of familial occurrences of esophageal atresia, which raises the possibility of a heritable genetic factor. Numerous accounts of twins and siblings with esophageal atresia have been reported (78). Conversely, certain commonly coexistent anomalies, such as the VACTERL (i.e., vertebral, anal, cardiac, tracheal, esophageal, renal, and limb anomalies) association (see Chapter 38) and other malformations, strongly suggest that the developing fetus is affected by a teratogen or defect of embryogenesis (79).

In many babies with esophageal atresia, it is the associated anomalies that alter treatment and affect survival. Congenital heart defects and chromosomal abnormalities are the most worrisome. Major anomalies that may seriously affect the infant but that are not usually fatal include imperforate anus and other congenital obstructions of the gut. Grosfeld and Ballantine found that 31 (37%) of 84 infants had cardiac anomalies; 18 (21.4%) had GI malformations, of whom 11 (13%) had imperforate anus; and six (7%) had the VACTERL association (80). A ventricular septal defect is the most common cardiac lesion, followed in frequency by patent ductus arteriosus and tetralogy of Fallot. Piekarski and Stephens suggest that the high incidence of coexisting anomalies is a reflection of generalized damage to the mesenchymal tissue in the fourth week of gestation (81).

Esophageal Atresia with Tracheoesophageal Fistula

Esophageal atresia occurs in approximately one of 3,000 to 4,500 births. In the most common form of esophageal anomaly (86% of patients), the blind-ending upper esophageal segment usually extends into the upper portion of the thorax, and the lower portion of the esophagus is connected to the trachea at or just above the tracheal carina (Fig. 44-5) (82). This connection is 3 to 5 mm in diameter and easily admits inspired air or, in a retrograde fashion, acidic gastric secretions. The earliest clinical sign of esophageal atresia is excessive oral secretions or regurgitation of saliva. The saliva pools in the blind-ending esophagus and then accumulates until it is apparent around the lips as excessive mucus. The first feeding is followed by choking, coughing, and regurgitation. Abdominal distension is a prominent feature, occurring as inspired air is transmitted through the fistula and distal esophagus into the stomach. Gastric juice may pass upward in the distal esophagus, traversing the tracheoesophageal fistula and spilling into the trachea and lungs, leading to chemical

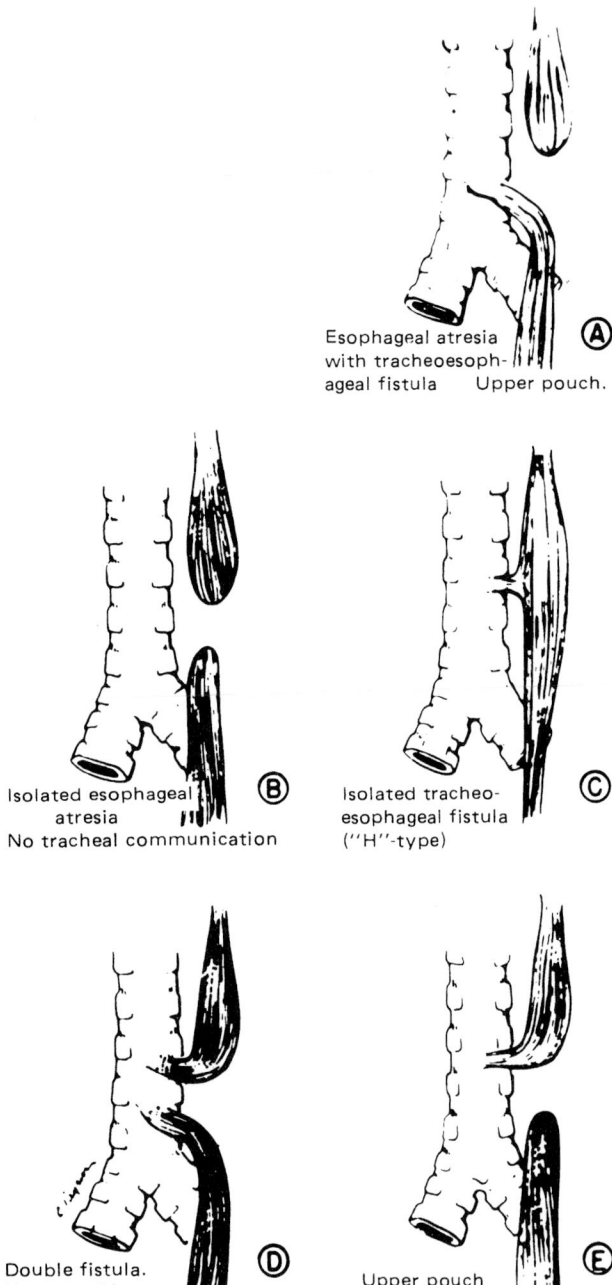

Esophageal atresia with tracheoesophageal fistula   Upper pouch. (A)

Isolated esophageal atresia   No tracheal communication (B)

Isolated tracheoesophageal fistula ("H"-type) (C)

Double fistula. Upper and lower esophagus. (D)

Upper pouch fistula (E)

Figure 44-5 The various forms of esophageal malformations are shown in the order of the frequency in which they occur. From Nardi GL, Zuidema GD. *Surgery*, 3rd ed. Boston: Little, Brown, 1972, with permission.

pneumonia. Pulmonary difficulties are compounded by atelectasis and diaphragmatic elevation secondary to gastric distension.

Diagnosis

The diagnosis of many infants with esophageal atresia is made prenatally. Polyhydramnios is the most frequent finding, particularly in infants with pure esophageal atresia. Those with a tracheoesophageal fistula may not de-

velop polyhydramnios if the communication is large enough to permit swallowing of the amniotic fluid through the fistula. An additional finding on a prenatal ultrasound is failure to identify the fetal stomach, which should raise the suspicion for esophageal atresia. The prenatal diagnosis of esophageal atresia permits the search for other anatomic anomalies and possible chromosomal defects. Appropriate prenatal counseling and preparation of the family can be initiated, specifically with arrangement for postnatal correction, unless contraindicated by coexistent abnormalities.

Once the infant is born, attentive members of the nursing staff who are feeding the baby are often the first to suspect the esophageal blockage. Esophageal atresia may not be obvious on the initial newborn examination unless an attempt is made to pass a tube into the stomach. Thin, flexible feeding catheters should be avoided because they may coil up in the esophagus and give the misleading impression that they have passed into the stomach. A larger, stiffer catheter carefully advanced will meet the obstruction. Occasionally, a tube dissects into the wall of a normal esophagus, leading to a misdiagnosis of esophageal atresia, particularly in a premature infant. A contrast x-ray film rules this out and confirms the diagnosis of atresia; a lateral projection with 1 mL of dilute barium or an isoosmolar contrast agent (e.g., metrizamide) shows the length of the upper pouch, defines its precise extension into the chest, and demonstrates the rare upper pouch fistula (Fig. 44-6A,B). Air seen in the bowel confirms the presence of a tracheoesophageal fistula. The existence of pneumonia or atelectasis also can be demonstrated on the initial radiographs.

Evaluation of the heart and great vessels with echocardiography is important to identify potential cardiac anomalies and verify the aortic arch position. A right-sided arch may alter the surgical approach and exposure. Bronchoscopy is useful to identify the level of the fistula and to exclude upper pouch fistulas and laryngotracheoesophageal clefts.

Management

After the diagnosis is secure, the following measures should be instituted promptly:

- Basic supportive measures, such as an infant warmer.
- Place the infant in a 30- to 40-degree head-up position.
- Give nothing orally.
- Provide intravenous antibiotics for possible aspiration.
- Place a sump suction catheter in the upper pouch to remove the excess secretions (Fig. 44-7).
- Consult with the appropriate pediatric surgical service.

The traditional approach to the timing of surgical repair was based on the increased risk of operating on infants with low birth weight and pneumonia. However neonatal care has evolved to the point that neither low birth weight nor the presence of pneumonia is a risk factor for poor survival (83). Severe anomalies and their consequences are now the crucial determinants of survival. Therefore, at Children's National Medical Center (CNMC), each baby admitted with esophageal atresia is managed according to

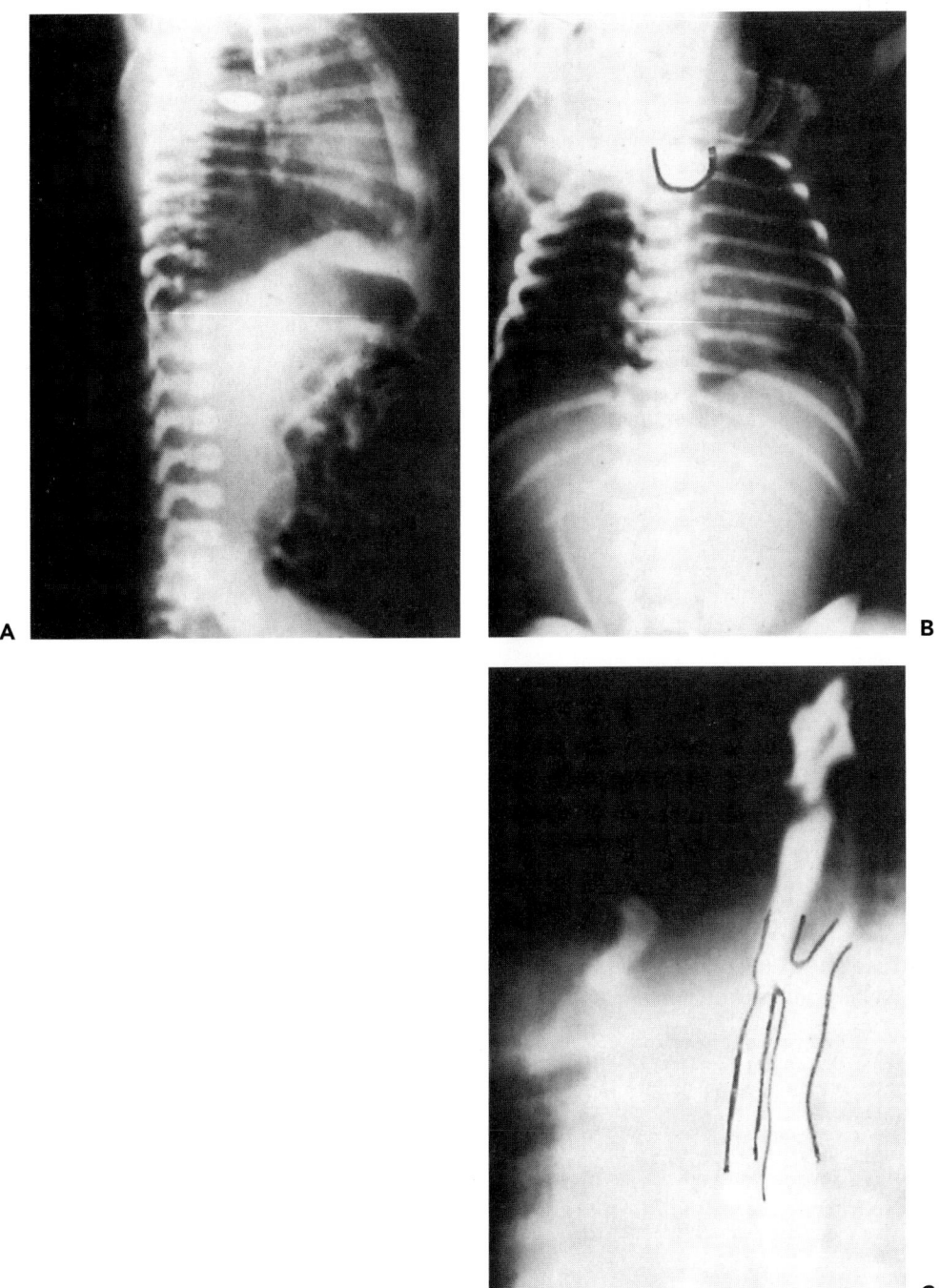

Figure 44-6 **A:** Lateral radiograph of a baby with esophageal atresia and tracheoesophageal fistula reveals a small meniscus of barium in the upper pouch. Gas is present in the stomach and intestinal tract because of the fistulous connection to the trachea. In this radiograph, some air in the lower esophageal segment can be seen in the posterior mediastinum. **B:** In a radiograph of a patient with isolated esophageal atresia, the upper pouch is outlined by barium. There is no air below the diaphragm. **C:** In a barium swallow in a patient with H-type isolated tracheoesophageal fistula, a normal-sized lumen of the esophagus is seen. Dye has spilled into the trachea, outlining the upper trachea and larynx. The fistula is at the level of the clavicle.

his or her physiologic status alone (84). If the infant is stable, immediate primary repair is undertaken. If unstable, surgery is delayed until the clinical status is stabilized, the impact of associated anomalies is determined, and the infant can be anesthetized and operated on safely.

Of historic interest, a classification developed by Waterston and colleagues in 1962 was useful in the stratification of patients for different management plans and the comparison of outcomes (85). The infants were classified as follows:

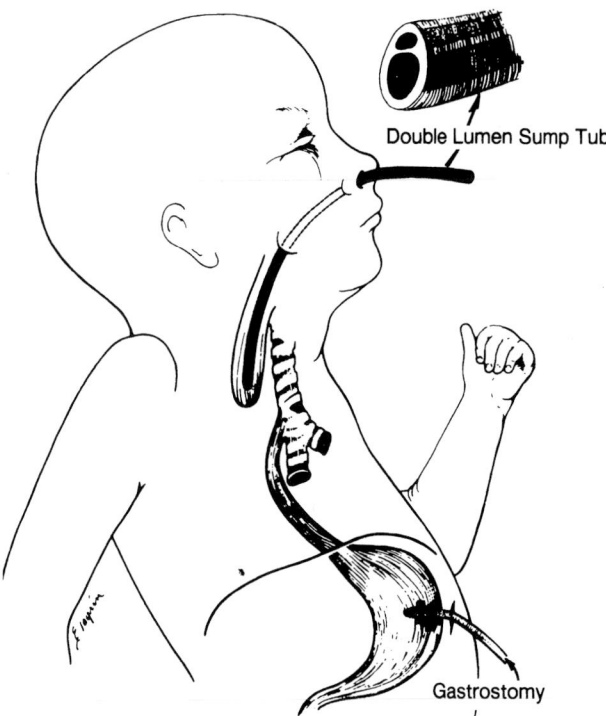

Figure 44-7 Temporary care of a patient with esophageal atresia and tracheoesophageal fistula is performed with the patient in the upright position. A gastrostomy is in the stomach, and a double-lumen sump tube is in the upper pouch to clear secretions and saliva.

- Category A: Birth weight over 2.5 kg (5.5 lb) and otherwise well
- Category B: Birth weight of 1.8 to 2.5 kg and well, or higher birth weight but moderate pneumonia and other congenital anomalies
- Category C: Birth weight under 1.8 kg, or higher birth weight but severe pneumonia and severe congenital anomaly.

Immediate Operative Repair

A thoracic incision provides exposure of the upper pouch and tracheoesophageal fistula. A right thoracotomy is standard unless the aortic arch is on the right, which would interfere with the dissection. A retropleural approach affords protection of the lung by maintaining its pleural envelope. If an anastomotic leak occurs, it will not communicate with the pleural cavity but can be drained posteriorly from the mediastinum with less morbidity.

The fistula is identified and carefully divided from the trachea. The tracheal opening is closed with several sutures, with care to avoid narrowing the tracheal lumen. Although some centers have advocated simple ligation of the fistula, this procedure is rarely performed because it is associated with an unacceptably high rate of recurrence (86).

The circumference of the lower esophageal fistula is usually small and is enlarged by trimming and spatulating its open end. The tip of the upper pouch is mobilized extensively and cut across to expose the lumen. Most surgeons employ a single-layer circumferential anastomosis to approximate the two ends instead of the classic two-layer Haight anastomosis (87).

Avoiding undue tension on the repair and averting compromise of the blood supply to the two ends are key factors in obtaining good results. The upper pouch is more amenable to mobilization than the distal fistula because the blood supply comes submucosally from the neck. The blood supply to the distal fistula is more easily compromised because it derives from tiny branches off the aorta. If the ends do not come together easily, there are surgical techniques available for extending the length of the upper pouch (88).

Although once routine, gastrostomy is now rarely used in stable infants. Postoperatively, infants are maintained on intravenous nutrition. Some surgeons employ a transanastomotic feeding tube so that early enteral feedings can be initiated. A chest tube is placed to drain the mediastinum and pleural space if necessary. The chest tube is connected to suction and monitored for evidence of air leak, blood loss, or saliva, which indicate an anastomotic leak. Postoperative management requires meticulous care to avoid potential disruption of the tracheal suture line, particularly if suctioning or reintubation is required. A contrast swallow is usually obtained on the fifth or sixth postoperative day. If all looks well, and there is no leak, feedings are begun and quickly advanced. Some surgeons routinely dilate the esophagus of all infants before discharge to prevent potential stricture formation.

Delayed Primary Repair and Staged Repair

If the infant is unstable, an intermediate plan allows correction of minor difficulties before repair. This plan involves delay of the surgical repair for several days. Management of these babies includes upper pouch suction with a Replogle tube, head-up position, antibiotics, and parenteral nutrition. These maneuvers provide for stabilization, improvement of pulmonary status, and diagnosis and management of certain higher-priority malformations, particularly cardiac lesions. Primary retropleural repair, as described previously, is undertaken when the infant's condition is stable and the risk of surgery has been reduced.

Unstable infants with serious coexisting anomalies or severe prematurity have diminished chances for survival. For these infants, a gastrostomy is placed, and repair is postponed. This approach uses early retropleural fistula division without anastomosis, gastrostomy feedings, and continuous sump suction of the upper pouch. Division of the fistula is important to prevent reflux of gastric contents. In some premature infants with noncompliant lungs, division of the fistula is required to allow adequate ventilation, in essence closing off the lower-resistance pathway through the fistula and stomach. Immediate closure of the fistula may be lifesaving in these instances.

Gastrostomy and fistula division without anastomosis requires constant, intensive nursing care, but it can be safely maintained for many weeks. Coupled with the holding pattern provided by suction of the upper pouch and gastrostomy drainage, infants with esophageal atresia and tracheoesophageal fistula can be maintained indefinitely by intravenous nutrition although weight and pulmonary status are improved and other congenital anomalies are studied and corrected. Later, the definitive transthoracic operation is performed, and the esophageal anastomosis is accomplished electively.

Results

At the CNMC in Washington, D.C., over 150 patients with a blind upper esophageal pouch and a fistula arising from the bifurcation of the trachea were treated between 1966 and 1997. Approximately 90% of these patients survived. Since 1982, the physiologic status of the infant has been the sole guide to therapy. The survival for infants who were classified as stable and had primary repair is 100%. Survival in the unstable group who had staged repair is 60%. The deaths were from associated anomalies, including congenital diaphragmatic hernia and hypoplastic left heart. As a result of this experience with high-risk infants, we concluded that a staged procedure, even one that abandons the esophagus, is preferable to primary repair for selected infants in the highest-risk group. This decision is controversial. Most pediatric surgeons eschew the staged approach, preferring primary repair in most infants with esophageal atresia and tracheoesophageal fistula.

Complications

Complications are not uncommon and require scrupulous diagnostic evaluation. Strictures, gastroesophageal reflux, poor motility, recurrent fistula, and tracheomalacia produce similar respiratory symptoms and may be difficult to differentiate.

Gastroesophageal reflux after repair of esophageal atresia has become increasingly recognized as a clinical problem because of more sensitive diagnostic tools, such as 24-hour potential of hydrogen (pH) monitoring. Werlin and coworkers showed that all of the 14 postoperative esophageal atresia patients they studied exhibited severe esophageal motor dysfunction. Only five of the 14 had a swallowing problem (89). In 1980, Jolley and others studied 25 young patients between 3 and 83 months after repair of esophageal atresia and tracheoesophageal fistula. Seventeen of 25 had significant gastroesophageal reflux demonstrated by prolonged pH monitoring, and 12 of these patients had significant symptoms in the form of vomiting, respiratory difficulty, or esophagitis (90). Wheatley and Coran concluded that esophageal dysmotility and gastroesophageal reflux were serious problems in combination and recommended fundoplication in selected patients (91).

Esophageal stricture is a common complication (31% in our series) after the anastomosis of the esophagus. Stricture may present early with an inability to swallow, choking, or failure to thrive, but symptoms may develop later, particularly at the time of transition to solid foods. In most infants esophageal dilation is successful, but some require repetitive dilations as often as every 2 weeks

for 1 year. Occasionally, a recalcitrant stricture requires operative resection.

Anastomotic disruption with leakage of saliva, gastric juice, and swallowed liquid into the mediastinum or thoracic space was once a dreaded complication after surgery. It is no longer universally fatal because of improvements in nutrition and antibiotics. The leak may be identified on a contrast study obtained before feeding or by an increase in the output from the chest tube or the drainage of saliva through the chest tube. If the operative repair has been accomplished with a retropleural approach and the pleura remains intact, external drainage posteriorly from the mediastinum is a relatively simple matter. If transthoracic repair is followed by esophageal disruption, the leak is best treated by extensive drainage, parenteral nutrition, and delayed surgical intervention. If the baby is deteriorating, it may be wise to abandon the esophagus and create a diverting cervical esophagostomy.

Recurrent fistulas may develop in a few infants (92). Usually, there is a history of a perioperative leak. The symptoms are often those of recurrent respiratory problems, such as bronchitis or pneumonia, related to silent aspiration. Reoperation is required to divide the fistula.

Tracheomalacia is an uncommon complication, but it is difficult to manage. It may be related to a congenital weakness of the trachea or operative injury. The spectrum of presentation ranges from complete collapse of the airway, with an inability to ventilate without positive pressure, to mild tracheal compromise. Bronchoscopy reveals the level and degree of collapse. In severe cases, operative suspension of the aorta and trachea is curative.

Esophageal Atresia without Fistula

Esophageal atresia may occur without a fistulous connection to the respiratory tract. This variant accounts for approximately 8% of esophageal malformations. As with other forms of esophageal atresia, these babies cannot swallow food or saliva. Because there is no tracheoesophageal fistula, air is absent from the GI tract, and the abdomen is noticeably scaphoid. The radiologic findings of a blind upper pouch coupled with the absence of air below the diaphragm are pathognomonic of isolated esophageal atresia.

For many years, the standard treatment of isolated esophageal atresia included cervical esophagostomy and gastrostomy. At a later time, a feeding pathway would be created with a segment of small bowel or colon or with construction of a reversed gastric tube. This time-proven practice still has a place in the treatment of pure esophageal atresia. Since the mid-1970s, new methods for bridging the gap between the disparate esophageal segments have evolved. Howard and Myers reported a technique for elongating the blind upper pouch using daily stretching by bougie dilators, allowing the two esophageal ends to be successfully united after several months (93). Mechanical stretching of the pouches may not be necessary. Natural growth in the first months of life produces impressive elongation of the esophageal pouches. During the interval, meticulous nursing care is required to prevent aspiration of saliva and ensure adequate nutrition. In many infants, the wisest course may still be cervical esophagostomy and gastrostomy, with later esophageal replacement (94). This course is even more appropriate for the premature infant, especially if respiratory distress proves troublesome.

The decision to preserve or abandon the esophagus rests on the patient's weight, pulmonary status, presence of other serious anomalies, and general hardiness during the early diagnostic and sustaining maneuvers. Our experience has led us to treat the last 20 consecutive infants who presented with isolated atresia of the esophagus by cervical esophagostomy and gastrostomy, reconstructing the esophagus at 1 year of age using a reversed gastric tube. The latter is a tube created from the greater curve of the stomach, brought up through the chest, and anastomosed to the upper esophageal segment. Nineteen of the 20 infants survived and are growing well.

Isolated Tracheoesophageal Fistula

Isolated (i.e., H-type) tracheoesophageal fistula is a rare lesion, representing approximately 4% of esophageal anomalies. Although congenital tracheoesophageal communication without atresia may be found at any level, most of these fistulas occur in the upper portion of the trachea and the esophagus, at or above the level of the second thoracic vertebra (95). Larger fistulas and communications extending throughout the length of the trachea have been seen, defects appropriately called laryngotracheoesophageal clefts.

The infant suffering from congenital tracheoesophageal fistula usually chokes and coughs with feeding. Prompt relief may be achieved by gavage feeding. Frequently the diagnosis is not made in infancy because the symptoms can be subtle. Pneumonitis often develops in the early days of life and recurs frequently as patchy bronchopneumonia. With continued aspiration through the fistula, a constant state of bronchopneumonia supervenes, attended by all of the manifestations of chronic infection. For any child with recurrent pneumonia, a wide variety of disease entities must be considered, but the list should include H-type tracheoesophageal fistula.

A contrast esophageal swallow with a dilute or isoosmolar medium may reveal the fistula (see Fig. 44-6C). Tracheobronchoscopy is usually successful in demonstrating this anomaly, but simultaneous esophagoscopy may be required. The fistula can be exposed through a cervical collar incision in most instances. A thoracic approach is necessary in 10% to 15% of patients. Surgery produces complete cures for most patients.

Laryngotracheoesophageal Cleft

Although once uniformly fatal, laryngotracheoesophageal clefts can now be repaired with good results. Early diagno-

sis is essential to prevent repeated aspiration through the communication between the trachea and esophagus below the vocal cords. Bronchoscopy allows identification of the cleft and its severity. Defects range from those involving only the upper trachea to those extending the entire length and beyond the carina. Management involves tracheostomy and an antireflux procedure to prevent aspiration, with later repair of the defect (96).

Gastroesophageal Reflux

In 1947, Berenberg and Neuhauser defined a condition they called "chalasia," or abnormal relaxation of the gastroesophageal junction (97). The affected babies manifest relentless regurgitation that may present as spitting, mild vomiting, or vigorous vomiting after every feeding. The deleterious effects of gastroesophageal reflux in infants have been recognized with increasing frequency (98–100). The spectrum of symptoms caused by gastroesophageal reflux in the infant is distinctly different from that seen in the adult. In infants, the main symptoms of gastroesophageal reflux are regurgitation, significant growth retardation, aspiration pneumonia, apneic spells, stridor, and esophagitis (91,92,101,102). The abnormality is the absence of a normal valvular mechanism at the gastroesophageal junction that allows unimpeded reflux of gastric content. Associated medical conditions affect many infants. Congenital or acquired central nervous system disorders are most frequent, including severe asphyxia, cerebral palsy, chromosomal anomalies, and microcephaly.

Infants with repaired esophageal atresia and tracheoesophageal fistula may have reflux that leads to anastomotic strictures, poor weight gain, or aspiration pneumonias.

Most infants with gastroesophageal reflux have some form of vomiting from birth. In some babies, the vomiting suggests the diagnosis of pyloric stenosis. Retardation of growth and development is the second most common presenting symptom, occurring in approximately 50% of our patients. These babies rank below the tenth percentile on their growth chart or show a marked falling off of growth progression. Recurrent aspiration with pneumonia occurs in approximately one-third of infants with pernicious gastroesophageal reflux. Reflux may also be the underlying cause of severe apnea in some infants (100).

A barium swallow demonstrates reflux in about 75% of symptomatic patients. However, reflux can also be shown in many otherwise normal, healthy infants, and radiologists have understandable difficulty in defining gastroesophageal reflux that is pathologic. Gastroesophageal reflux can be documented and quantified with radionuclide material. This examination permits an accurate appraisal of the pathophysiologic effects of reflux in most patients. It has proved adaptable to infants, and when serial observations are extended over several hours, normal reflux can usually be differentiated from pathologic reflux. Gastric emptying is also measured by this scan.

Monitoring of pH at different levels of the esophagus can demonstrate gastric acid reflux. With timed studies, physicians can now chart reflux in relation to sleeping, various body positions, and during eating, documenting episodes that lead to characteristic symptoms or life-threatening incidents (103). Esophagoscopy helps physicians to document the presence of esophagitis in selected infants.

Every effort should be made to reverse the consequences of pernicious gastroesophageal reflux by conservative therapy. Medical therapy of symptomatic infants with gastroesophageal reflux consists of maintaining a semiupright posture and small frequent feedings of thickened material. Bethanechol has yielded little or no benefit, but metaclopramide, which increases the tone and amplitude of gastric contraction, relaxes the pyloric sphincter, and accelerates gastric emptying, has proved more helpful.

In rare instances, the extent of a baby's nutritional depletion or chronic pneumonitis may demand hospitalization. In infants sick enough to be hospitalized, 3 weeks is an ample period to determine whether their symptoms can be controlled by intensive medical measures. Infants less severely affected should be evaluated in an outpatient setting over 2 to 4 months. If symptoms are controlled by medical means, reflux usually disappears by 15 months, coincident with the development of upright posture. In our experience, medical therapy fails for approximately 15% of patients.

With worsening or protraction of symptoms despite adherence to conservative treatment, surgical correction is recommended if the infant fails to gain weight and grow adequately, has recurrent pneumonitis, has life-threatening apnea spells, or has esophagitis. Prompt operative correction is thought appropriate without medical trial for those patients with thoracic translocation of a significant portion of the stomach and esophageal stricture.

Surgical intervention is undertaken to place the gastroesophageal junction well below the diaphragm (i.e., lengthen the intraabdominal esophagus), recreate an acute angle of His, and create a valve-like mechanism to force the fundus of the stomach against the esophagus. The Nissen fundoplication involves wrapping the fundus of the stomach completely around the esophagogastric junction (Fig. 44-8). In the Thal procedure, the wrap is partial (i.e., 210 to 270 degrees). Postoperative problems such as dysphagia and inability to burp and vomit (i.e., gas-bloat syndrome) appear less likely with the Thal procedure (102). Gastroesophageal reflux is discussed in more detail in Chapter 37.

ABDOMINAL SURGERY

The indications for abdominal surgery are distension and bilious vomiting. To these should be added the scaphoid contour seen if there is high intestinal obstruction or the abdominal viscera are in an ectopic location, as in infants with congenital diaphragmatic hernia. Extreme degrees of abdominal distension are associated with intestinal and gastric perforation. Tenderness signifying peritoneal irritation can be elicited by careful examination. A tender erythematous abdominal wall is a reliable sign of an intraab-

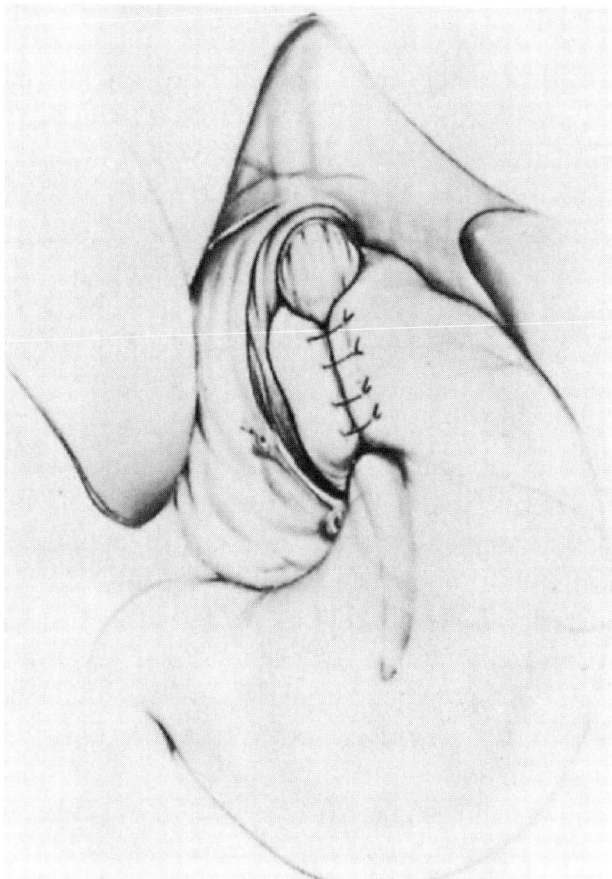

Figure 44-8 A successful method for the surgical correction of gastroesophageal reflux employs gastric fundoplication as described by Nissen.

dominal catastrophe with resultant peritonitis and ischemic intestine. Reliance on bowel sounds can be misleading. Peristalsis can exist despite peritonitis or be absent when intestinal distension is caused by mechanical obstruction.

Pertinent radiologic studies to be obtained in all cases of suspected intraabdominal surgical lesions are the flat and upright views of the abdomen. The left lateral decubitus radiograph may be substituted for the upright radiograph if pneumoperitoneum is suspected. Intestinal obstruction can be diagnosed and the level of obstruction determined by the configuration of the air–fluid levels. Pneumoperitoneum is usually readily appreciated on abdominal x-ray films. Supine radiographs may show the football sign produced by superimposition of the falciform ligament on a large bubble of free air (Fig. 44-9). The bowel wall may be outlined by air outside and inside the bowel lumen. The left lateral decubitus radiograph may show air around the liver. Not infrequently, the findings on radiographs may be subtle and require an alert physician to make the diagnosis. Distended bowel and the absence of air–fluid levels in intestinal loops of various sizes suggest obstruction secondary to meconium ileus. Calcifications scattered within the abdomen indicate intrauterine perforation with meconium peritonitis.

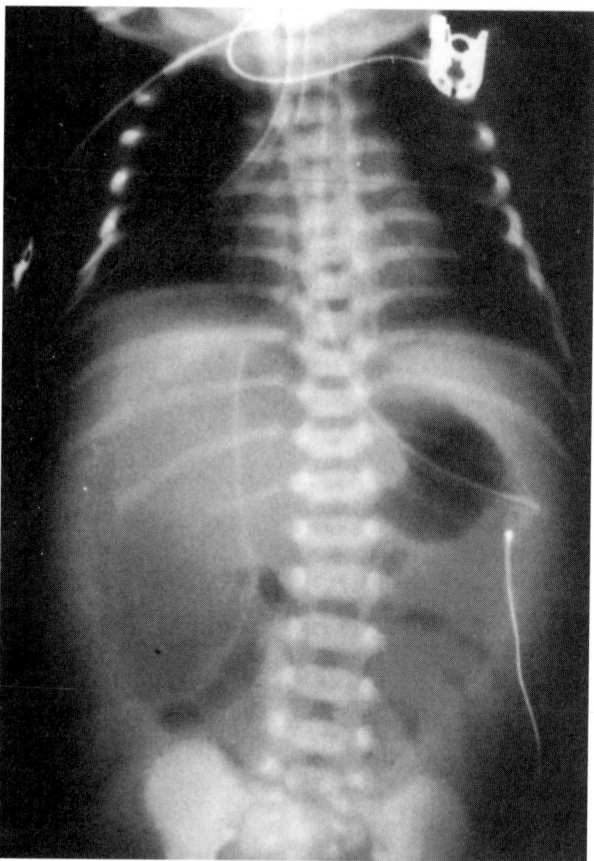

Figure 44-9 Supine abdominal x-ray film demonstrates a massive intraperitoneal air collection. The air is seen as a large central bubble on which is superimposed a dense linear opacity produced by the falciform ligament. The falciform ligament forms the lace for the football sign.

Unless precluded by a deteriorating clinical condition, a contrast enema, usually of isoosmotic Gastrografin initially, requires only a short delay that is usually justified by the information obtained. The enema need not be an elaborate study in these precarious subjects.

The diagnosis of malrotation is most accurately made with a small amount of contrast placed into the stomach to confirm the position of the ligament of Treitz. Incomplete obstructions of the GI tract, such as those caused by congenital stenosis or intraluminal web, are often the most difficult congenital lesions to diagnose and require contrast studies of the upper GI (UGI) tract with careful attention to every centimeter of intestine on fluoroscopy.

Pneumoperitoneum: Gastric Perforation

Spontaneous perforation of a hollow viscus is most frequently seen in distressed neonates who have undergone resuscitation immediately after birth. The presence of free air in the peritoneal cavity may be secondary to perforation anywhere in the GI tract and is a surgical emergency. The surgeon approaching the infant with pneumoperitoneum must be prepared to investigate systematically the entire GI tract and anticipate problems such as Hirschsprung dis-

ease, gastric perforation, necrotizing enterocolitis (NEC), or other ischemic insults to the intestine resulting in perforation (104–106).

After perforation, egress of air into the peritoneal cavity usually leads to impressive abdominal distension. Elevation of the diaphragm occurs with potential embarrassment of the infant's respiratory dynamics. A temporary but lifesaving maneuver is needle aspiration of the peritoneal cavity, which diminishes air under pressure, allowing the diaphragm to return to a more normal position. There is usually dramatic relief of abdominal distension and respiratory distress. It is not hazardous to insert a needle adapted to a 50-mL syringe through the anterior abdominal wall. The bowel is usually compressed against the posterior parietes and is not likely to be injured by this maneuver.

Surgical intervention must be prompt. When massive distension of the abdomen occurs, a gastric perforation can be anticipated. Typically, the rent occurs high on the greater curvature of the stomach. Because the perforation may be located on the posterior wall, thorough exploration of relatively inaccessible areas of the stomach must be carried out. Although it has been suggested that perforation of the stomach results from congenital deficiency of musculature in the gastric wall, this explanation is questionable. The apparent absence of musculature at the margin of the perforation probably represents retraction of the muscles of an overdistended stomach, with a ballooning of mucosa between the muscle fibers.

Repair is accomplished by primary closure in two layers after debridement of the margins of the perforation. A gastrostomy tube, inserted through a noninvolved area of the stomach, is advisable to ensure postoperative decompression. The subsequent course of the infant is usually uncomplicated if the underlying problem for which resuscitation was required is controlled. Cautious feedings can be started within a few days of surgical repair. For diagnosis and management of perforations occurring elsewhere in the GI tract, see Meconium Peritonitis and Necrotizing Enterocolitis.

Temporary Diversion of the Intestinal Tract

Newborn intestinal emergencies often demand a temporary vent or enterostomy. Although not as desirable as an end-to-end union of the bowel, these measures may be lifesaving in fragile infants who are critically ill as the result of intestinal obstruction or peritonitis or who are threatened by serious congenital defects. An abdominal stoma in the infant does not carry the same implications as in the adult; the physician must stress this fact to allay the fears and doubts of a worried parent. Most enterostomies are temporary, and the outlook for restoration of complete intestinal continuity is good.

Gastrostomy

The stomach requires venting for two reasons. First, decompression of the GI tract is necessary in the face of any abdominal catastrophe. Placement of the gastrostomy obviates the need for a nasogastric tube. It is more efficient and eliminates the danger of pressure necrosis of the alar cartilage of the infant's nose and the respiratory hazards that attend nasogastric tubes. Second, the gastrostomy tube provides access for feeding a depleted neonate.

Gastrostomy can be performed under local anesthesia, although it is usually done under general anesthesia. Frequently, the procedure complements a primary abdominal operation. A simple Stamm gastrostomy is preferred, and it is not difficult to remove or replace the tube as an office procedure. If the gastrostomy tube is to be maintained for a long time, it may be replaced after 1 month with a gastrostomy button, which is easier for the parents to care for at home (107).

Ileostomy

Temporary ileostomy is less desirable than primary union of the bowel, but there are clinical circumstances in which its creation as a temporary diverting procedure is prudent, including inflammatory necrosis of the distal small bowel with intraperitoneal soiling and peritonitis, ischemic insult with marginal viability of the bowel, and marked disparity in lumen size, as in intestinal atresia or meconium ileus.

A properly performed ileostomy is usually well tolerated and rarely causes skin breakdown. With appropriate supportive care, weight gain and healing proceed, and intestinal reconstruction can be carried out electively with greater safety for the infant. We recommend closure of the ileostomy when the infants weigh 2.5 to 3.0 kg to minimize fluid and electrolyte imbalances that these babies may develop (108).

In very sick infants or in babies with other underlying conditions such as meconium ileus, the double-barrel enterostomy of Mikulicz has proved valuable. The common wall that has been created is gradually crushed with a special clamp, partly reestablishing intestinal continuity. Complete closure of the bowel can be achieved without reentering the peritoneal cavity. Another effective technique of intestinal venting that permits access to the distal GI tract is the end-to-side enteroenterostomy described by Bishop and Koop (109). This technique has particular application for lesions in the proximal GI tract, such as jejunal and high ileal atresia.

Colostomy

The four usual indications for colostomy in the neonate are impending or actual perforation of the colon, colonic atresia with huge disparity of the bowel lumen, Hirschsprung's disease, and high imperforate anus. The loop colostomy has the advantage of simplicity and speed in critically ill babies. An end-colostomy is mechanically sound, easily managed, and avoids spillage into the distal loop, which is an advantage in treating Hirschsprung disease and imperforate anus. A diaper neatly covers the colostomy during the early months of life, until definitive surgical correction of the primary problem is accomplished and the colostomy can be closed (see Chapter 37).

Rotational Abnormalities

Malrotation

In the developing embryo, the elongating intestine must undergo rotation as it returns to the celomic cavity so that it can be accommodated within the confines of the abdominal cavity. The proximal small intestine assumes the characteristic C-shaped contour, and the duodenum is fixed to the left of the midline at the ligament of Treitz. The cecum takes a counterclockwise rotation, reaching its final location in the right lower abdomen (110). Incomplete intestinal rotation with consequent inadequate fixation of the intestinal mesentery may be an asymptomatic occurrence, may give rise to subtle symptoms difficult to diagnose, or may present as a life-threatening intraabdominal catastrophe. An understanding of the mechanism by which the lesion becomes symptomatic is necessary if the physician is to recognize and prevent the devastating complications that can accompany midgut volvulus.

If rotation is abnormal, bands are formed between the ectopic cecum, located in the right upper quadrant, and the right lateral abdominal wall. As these bands course from the cecum to the abdominal wall, they traverse the duodenum and can cause intermittent, incomplete duodenal obstruction. Symptoms of partial duodenal obstruction are often baffling. The infant may experience intervals of normal feeding pattern that are interspersed with exasperating episodes of vomiting. Because the obstruction is high in the GI tract, abdominal distension does not occur. The telltale sign of an underlying mechanical problem is bile in the vomitus. This lesion, more than any other, supports the contention that bile-stained vomitus in an infant necessitates a thorough diagnostic workup to detect a malrotation and subsequent midgut volvulus. More than 50% of babies present with symptoms before 1 week of age, but 10% remain asymptomatic until after 1 year of age (111).

The most reliable diagnostic study is a UGI series for localization of the ligament of Treitz. Surgical correction of malrotation of the colon prevents a future volvulus of the midgut and relieves the partial duodenal obstruction. The bands binding the cecum to the right abdominal wall are lysed, and the large bowel is freed and transposed to the left side of the abdomen. The duodenum is mobilized on its medial aspect, in which the narrow mesentery is intimately associated with the superior mesenteric artery. As the mesentery of the small bowel is freed medially, it assumes a broad position over the posterior abdominal wall. With the mesentery splayed, the potential for torsion is eliminated. It is unnecessary to fix the intestine in its new position with sutures (112). The appendix, because it now lies on the left side of the abdomen, is usually removed or inverted. Operative correction of malrotation in this manner is known as the Ladd procedure.

Malrotation with Midgut Volvulus

If fixation of the mesentery of the small bowel has not occurred normally, the intestine is subject to torsion on the axis of the superior mesenteric artery. This mechanism of obstruction must be considered for an infant with bile-stained vomiting, especially if there is no abdominal distension. Abdominal tenderness is an ominous finding.

Roentgenographic abnormalities are often characteristic, with evidence of duodenal obstruction and scanty gas distributed through the remainder of the bowel. The air–fluid levels typical of intestinal obstruction elsewhere in the GI tract are not usually associated with this malrotation. An airless abdomen is an ominous sign and usually indicates that infarction of the intestine has already taken place. Bloody stools imply that significant compromise to the intestinal vasculature has occurred. A UGI series shows a corkscrew-like constriction of the third portion of the duodenum.

If midgut volvulus is diagnosed or suspected as the underlying mechanism for the infant's illness, emergency surgical exploration is undertaken. If the findings are favorable and the bowel is viable, the torsion is reduced by counterclockwise rotation, and a Ladd procedure is carried out as described for the treatment of malrotation without volvulus. The prognosis is favorable as long as the viability of the intestine is not in question. However, if the diagnosis has been delayed or the volvulus has been an intrauterine event, intestinal ischemia, infarction, or both may be encountered in the distribution of the superior mesenteric artery. Initial judgments regarding the viability of the intestine are not easy; intestinal resection at the time of initial exploration is contraindicated. The ischemic intestine must be given every opportunity to recover after the torsion has been reduced. The first operation consists of untwisting the small bowel and establishing a gastrostomy.

Reexploration is undertaken 24 to 36 hours later, and areas of obvious infarction are identified. These are resected, and appropriate enterostomies are brought out to the abdominal wall; anastomosis is contraindicated. Any intestine of marginal viability is retained in hope that it will recover. Reexploration to determine recovery or further loss of small bowel is repeated after another interval of 36 to 48 hours. After the full extent of intestinal loss has been established and the margins of viable bowel exteriorized, the surgeon is faced with the management of a desperately ill infant at risk from sepsis, disseminated intravascular coagulation, and the inevitable nutritional crisis attending a short-bowel syndrome.

A central venous catheter for total parenteral alimentation is established, and nourishment is provided by this technique throughout the early postoperative weeks. After the infant has achieved positive nitrogen balance and the reestablishment of intestinal continuity is complete, there is then a difficult period of weaning from parenteral onto oral feedings. About 40 cm of residual small intestine seems to be required for successful adaptation of the intestine in full-term infants, although adaptation has been reported for children with considerably less than 40 cm of intestine (113). If the distal ileum and ileocecal valve are intact, slightly less bowel may be tolerated. Infant formulas that are fat-free and contain monosaccharides and hydrolyzed protein should be used to feed these babies because these formulas require only a minimal absorptive surface and little enzyme activity for assimilation. Gradually, the volume and concentration of these substances may be increased until all calories are taken orally. The process of weaning the infant from total intravenous to total oral alimentation may take months. This underscores the devastating complications of a midgut volvulus and indicates the need for vigilance by pediatrician and surgeon in the pursuit of the diagnosis of malrotation.

Hypertrophic Pyloric Stenosis

Pyloric stenosis occurs in approximately one of 300 to 1,000 live births. Its cause is obscure. Boys are affected about four times as frequently as girls, and the disease seems to have a predilection for the first-born child. There is a familial tendency, with a 2.5% to 20% incidence of pyloric stenosis in children of affected parents; the variation in incidence depends on the genders of the affected parent and child (114). It has been speculated that hypertrophy of the circular muscles of the pylorus results from propulsion of milk curds against the spastic pyloric canal, producing edema, additional spasm, and subsequent hypertrophy of the musculature, leading to complete obstruction. Some researchers have postulated that the muscle hypertrophy is a response to vagal stimulation. This is somewhat substantiated by the observation that infants undergoing surgery for esophageal atresia and tracheoesophageal fistula seem to have a higher incidence of pyloric stenosis, a result perhaps of vagal nerve irritation in the operative field. No infectious agent has been isolated despite the apparent seasonal incidence of the disease. The clinical onset of bile-free projectile vomiting at 2 to 8 weeks of age in a first-born boy strongly suggests the diagnosis of congenital hypertrophic pyloric stenosis. Occasionally, the onset is insidious, and these babies can present to the pediatrician as perplexing feeding problems. A typical history reveals intermittent vomiting that gradually increases in frequency and intensity over a week, until the baby vomits most ingested feedings with impressive force.

Abdominal examination is carried out with the stomach empty. If the infant has not just vomited, the physician may need to use a nasogastric tube to ensure an adequate examination. The baby can be given a pacifier for relaxation. Visible peristalsis may be observed moving across the upper abdomen. The examiner stands to the left, elevating the baby's feet with his left hand to relax the abdominal muscles and then palpates gently in the right upper quadrant. The pyloric olive is palpable to the experienced examiner in 90% of patients, and radiographic studies are usually not needed. If pyloric stenosis is suspected but the olive cannot be palpated, the diagnostic procedure of choice is abdominal ultrasonography, which is more than

90% accurate in centers experienced with this technique (115). A UGI series is usually reserved for those patients with vomiting but a normal ultrasonographic examination, in whom another cause of obstruction is suspected. Hyperbilirubinemia is seen in 8% of babies with pyloric stenosis. Almost all the bilirubin is of an indirect type and may be related to a decreased level of hepatic glycuronyl transferase (116). Jaundice clears after pyloromyotomy.

Infants with pyloric stenosis are conveniently grouped according to their clinical condition at the time they are seen by the surgeon. About one-half are well hydrated and in a satisfactory nutritional state. Serum electrolytes are normal, and the urine, although concentrated, is of adequate volume. These babies can undergo surgical correction without preoperative preparation. For the remaining infants, preparation before surgery is necessary. The typical pattern of electrolyte disturbance is that of mild or moderate metabolic alkalosis. The hypokalemia may not be reflected in the serum electrolytes, but potassium supplements must be provided before the alkalosis can be corrected. Salt-losing adrenogenital syndrome can present with symptoms identical to pyloric stenosis. However, this condition is characterized by an elevated serum potassium and metabolic acidosis.

These moderately dehydrated infants usually can be corrected within 12 hours with 5% dextrose–half-normal saline solution at a rate half to twice that of maintenance. After urine production is certain, potassium should be replaced at 2 mEq/kg for the 12-hour period of therapy.

A few infants present with severe dehydration and malnutrition and are often well below their birth weight. In this group, extensive rehydration is mandatory before surgery. The infants are profoundly alkalotic and potassium deficient. Their protein stores are depleted, urine is scanty, and they may be anemic. Intensive therapy for 2 to 3 days is required to bring these infants into metabolic balance. Fluids, electrolytes, colloid, and even blood may be necessary. Fortunately, it is rare to see such children today.

A Ramstedt–Fredet pyloromyotomy is usually performed through a transverse skin incision placed in the right upper quadrant of the abdomen. However, a circumbilical incision or laparoscopic approach have gained popularity. This short, safe, surgical procedure accomplishes division of the hypertrophic circular muscles of the gastric outlet and reestablishes patency of the pyloric channel (Fig. 44-10). In most cases, glucose water feedings can be reinstituted 6 to 8 hours postoperatively. If the child tolerates the first feeding, slow advancement of the volume of his regular formula is encouraged. The infant commonly vomits a few times postoperatively, but this should not alter his feeding advancement. Explanation to the parents that this vomiting is common can allay their anxiety. The child is generally ready for discharge on the second or third postoperative day, when he attains adequate oral intake. Typically, the babies enjoy a growth spurt in the immediate postoperative weeks, much to the satisfaction of the parents.

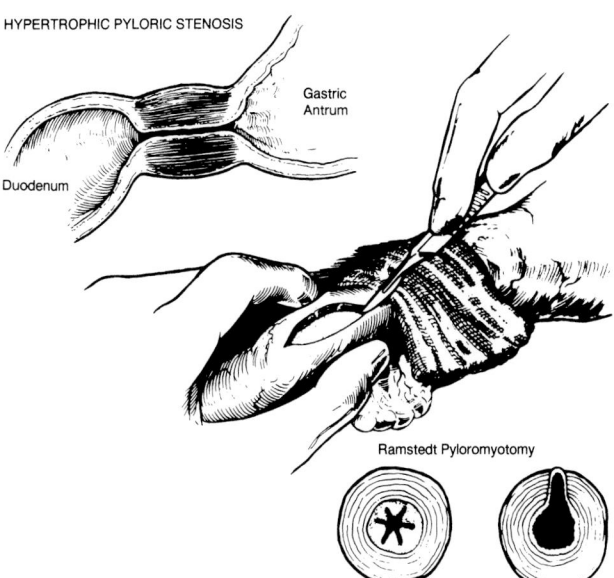

Figure 44-10 A Ramstedt pyloromyotomy is made through all layers of the pylorus except the mucosa. The cross section demonstrates how the mucosa of the pylorus expands into the defect created, enlarging the cross-sectional diameter of the pyloric channel.

Duodenal Atresia, Stenosis, and Annular Pancreas

Duodenal obstruction may be complete or partial and results from intrinsic causes or external compression (117). An intraluminal diaphragm can cause partial, intermittent obstruction that is difficult to recognize. Only a carefully performed UGI series outlines an intraluminal web and determines the site of obstruction. Annular pancreas, duodenal stenosis, and congenital bands are other causes of partial duodenal obstruction in which the need for early surgical intervention is more apparent.

Duodenal atresia results in complete obstruction. In instances of complete duodenal obstruction, swallowed air is prevented from passing beyond the duodenum, and the middle and lower abdomen are scaphoid. The characteristic x-ray finding is that of a double bubble of ingested air filling the stomach and blind-ending duodenum (Fig. 44-11). Duodenal atresia is often associated with trisomy 21.

Unless the underlying cause of obstruction is related to malrotation, an initial period of nasogastric drainage and resuscitation with intravenous fluids and electrolytes is appropriate before duodenal obstruction is surgically corrected. Surgical therapy is tailored to the particular lesion encountered. The intraluminal web can be resected through a transduodenal approach. It may be necessary for the surgeon to perform a gastrotomy or duodenotomy, through which a Foley catheter with the balloon minimally inflated is passed, to identify the site at which the web is attached.

Some stenotic lesions can be managed by local duodenoplasty, but obstruction from duodenal atresia requires bypass for relief. Obstruction secondary to duodenal atresia or annular pancreas is best treated by creating a

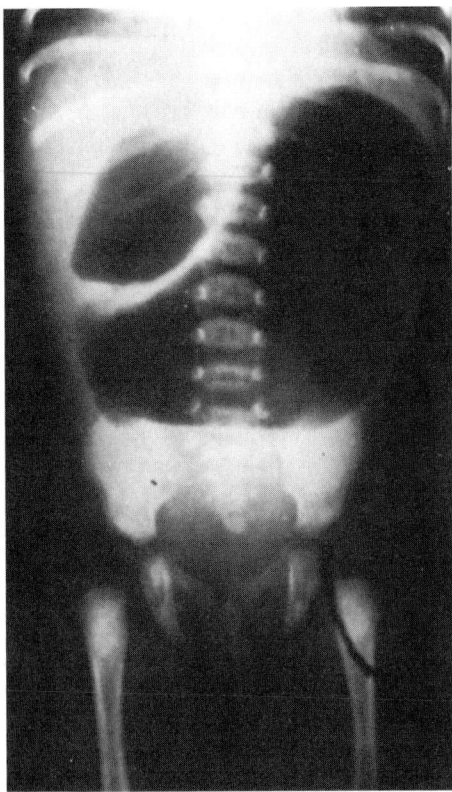

Figure 44-11   Characteristic double bubble of congenital duodenal obstruction.

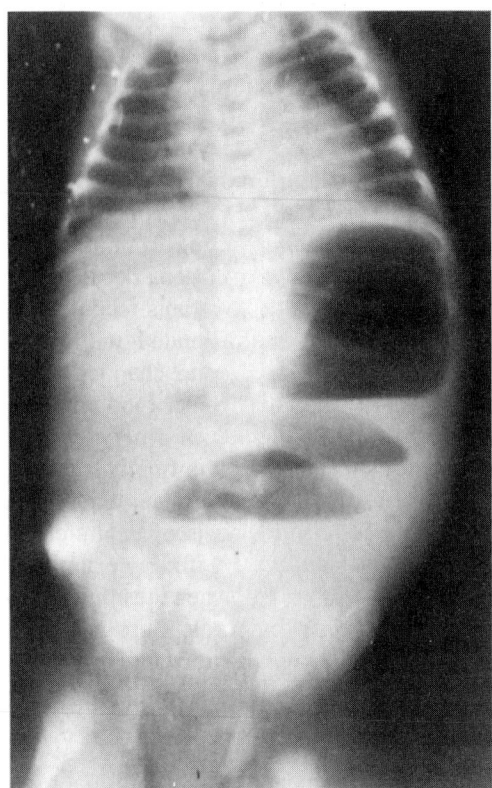

Figure 44-13   An upright abdominal x-ray film of a patient with jejunal atresia shows gastric distension and approximately three loops of bowel with no gas beyond the obstruction.

duodenoduodenostomy (118). A duodenojejunostomy is an alternative method to establish intestinal continuity.

Jejunoileal Atresia

Atresia of the bowel probably results from an ischemic insult to the intestine during its development (119). The atresia may be discrete, involving only a short segment of jejunum or ileum (Fig. 44-12), or it may involve the intestine over many centimeters (120). Atretic areas are some-

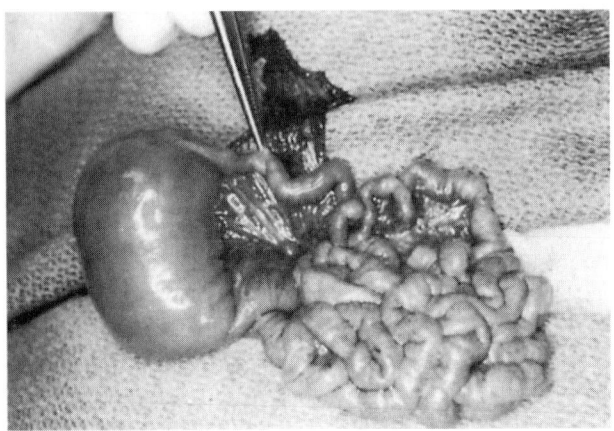

Figure 44-12   In this patient with jejunal atresia, a dilated proximal segment and a narrow distal jejunum are evident.

times multiple, and although the intervening bowel is normal, considerable length may be missing. Abdominal distension and bile-stained vomitus are the usual presenting symptoms. Radiographs show air–fluid levels distributed throughout the abdomen (Fig. 44-13). In cases of distal ileal obstruction, the contrast enema adds confirmation, showing the typical microcolon.

A short period of restoration with fluids, electrolytes, and colloid may be necessary, but this should never exceed a few hours. The method of surgical correction depends on the intraoperative findings. If the intestinal length is normal, the dilated proximal end is excised back to near-normal-caliber bowel, and an end-to-back anastomosis is performed. In the infant with a large-gap atresia, the proximal end is tapered, and anastomosis is then accomplished (121,122). The end-to-side reconstruction, described by Bishop and Koop, has proved safe and effective and has the added advantage of providing access to the GI tract for irrigations postoperatively (109). This type of repair is particularly helpful if there is a major disparity in the size of the ends of the intestine. A Mikulicz enterostomy or simple end-enterostomy may be lifesaving in critically ill, depleted newborns with distal bowel obstruction.

Incomplete obstruction resulting from stenosis of the bowel can be puzzling and hazardous because there is a confusing clinical picture. The infants feed poorly, occasionally vomit, or become distended without pattern. These symptoms continue despite changes in the formula.

The pediatrician may consider food allergies, nonspecific failure to thrive, and even a nervous mother as underlying causes. The obstruction finally becomes complete, or the bowel perforates. Surgical exploration may be needed to confirm a diagnosis of ileal stenosis, and this approach is considered even if x-ray examinations of the intestine have been normal when the clinical course of the infant suggests this diagnosis. Cure is achieved by appropriate intestinal tailoring procedures such as a Y–V plasty or longitudinal incision and transverse closure (i.e., Heineke–Mikulicz principle).

Meconium Plug Syndrome

The meconium plug syndrome is a benign form of colon obstruction in the neonate caused by a firm white plug of mucus. These babies usually present with abdominal distension. Abdominal x-ray films reveal distended loops of bowel. A barium enema shows a long radiolucency within the descending colon. The plug is passed after the barium enema or a saline rectal irrigation. Although meconium plug syndrome is found in otherwise completely normal infants, it can be difficult to differentiate from Hirschsprung disease and to rule out cystic fibrosis, so many surgeons routinely perform a rectal biopsy and obtain a sweat chloride test in infants with meconium plug syndrome.

Meconium Peritonitis

Meconium peritonitis usually follows antenatal intestinal obstruction and perforation of the bowel above the obstruction in conditions such as bowel atresia, volvulus, meconium ileus, and neonatal Hirschsprung's disease. If it occurs early in gestation, the perforation may have sealed off, but the chemical peritonitis gives rise to tiny scattered foreign-body reactions that may become calcified and be visible radiographically. If the perforation occurs closer to birth, calcifications are usually not seen on radiographs, and chemical peritonitis may be followed by bacterial peritonitis. More frequently, the presenting signs are those of intestinal obstruction.

Meconium Ileus

Intestinal obstruction resulting from viscid meconium impacted in the terminal ileum is seen as the earliest manifestation of cystic fibrosis. This problem affects about 10% of the cystic fibrosis population. Infants with meconium ileus subsequently develop other complications of their underlying disease, but the later respiratory sequelae are not necessarily more severe (123).

The clinical presentation of meconium ileus is not unlike that seen with other forms of distal intestinal obstruction. Abdominal distension and bile-stained vomitus are characteristic. The upright radiograph of the abdomen is especially helpful in this form of intestinal obstruction in the newborn. The characteristic soap bubble mass in the right lower abdomen and a paucity of air–fluid levels despite the pres-

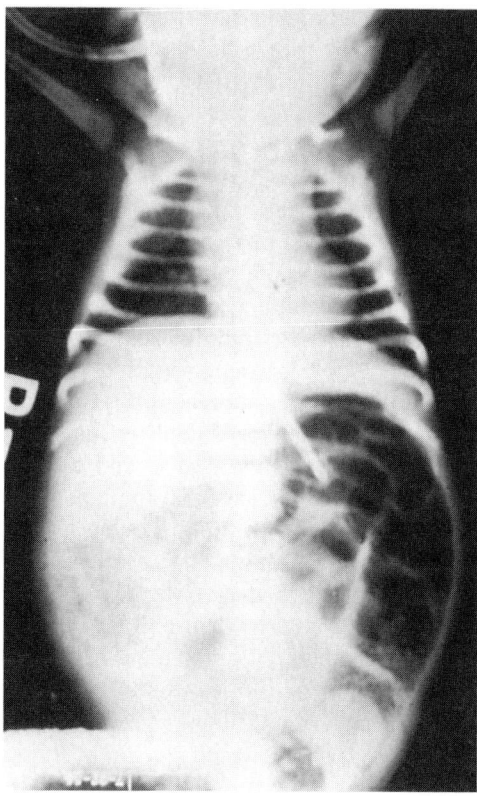

Figure 44-14 An x-ray film of a newborn infant with meconium ileus reveals many gas-filled loops, but little fluid is seen. The right lower quadrant is filled with a large loop of intestine distended by meconium. Gas trapped in the meconium gives the typical ground-glass appearance.

ence of many gas-filled loops of intestine is pathognomonic (Fig. 44-14). The air–fluid levels characteristic of obstruction do not develop because air is trapped by the tenacious meconium, and a clear interface is not produced. The contrast enema shows a microcolon, unused because of the distal ileal obstruction. Concretions of meconium in the terminal ileum immediately proximal to the ileocecal valve are often seen.

Surgical intervention may be required for relief of obstruction, but enemas of Gastrografin often eliminate the obstructing mass of meconium (124). At our institution, the Gastrografin is diluted 1:4 with saline so that the complications of a hyperosmolar fluid enema are avoided. This radiopaque contrast material contains a wetting agent (Tween 80) in which the thick meconium is soluble. If the Gastrografin can be successfully advanced through the microcolon and into the obstructed distal ileum, there is reasonable expectation that meconium will be passed spontaneously with relief of obstruction (125). When the first attempt moves some meconium out, but the infant's obstruction is not completely relieved, a second enema is justified several hours later. Complete removal of the meconium may take several Gastrografin enemas over a few days. If these maneuvers fail to relieve the obstruction, or if meconium peritonitis is present, surgical exploration is the only acceptable treatment.

If surgical correction is necessary, technical problems associated with evacuating the tar-like meconium from the distended ileum and establishing intestinal continuity between the dilated proximal intestine and the distal microcolon have been solved in various ways. Irrigation through an ileostomy with dilute acetylcysteine has proved effective in some infants. A rapid and safe anastomosis involving the Bishop–Koop technique is well suited for this problem (109). A Mikulicz enterostomy has the virtue of speed although providing decompression and establishment of continuity. These techniques allow access to the distal intestine for postoperative irrigations with acetylcysteine. With use, the colon has the potential to function normally, and the vent established by the Mikulicz or Bishop–Koop procedure is closed surgically. In selected infants, resection and primary anastomosis can be performed at the first operation. In the postoperative period, the infant is subject to respiratory difficulty secondary to impacted secretions. These may require tracheal suctioning or bronchoscopy for relief. When oral feedings are instituted, exogenous pancreatic supplements are provided so that digestion and use of calories are ensured.

Duplications

An uncommon cause of intestinal obstruction in the newborn is that arising secondary to duplications of the bowel. These can exist at any level of the intestine and may cause obstruction when the lumen is compromised by the gradually expanding duplication or by the duplication acting as a focus for segmental intestinal volvulus. Because they occur on the mesenteric aspect of the bowel, duplications are intimately involved with the blood supply to the normal intestine. Small, cystic duplications are easily resected with a segment of the adjacent bowel (126). However, extensive fusiform or intramural duplications may tax the surgeon's ingenuity. In these instances, resection of the common wall, with creation of a single conduit, may enable the surgeon to preserve an extensive segment of normal intestine (127). Gastric mucosa can exist within a duplication and result in GI hemorrhage (128). This cause of GI bleeding is considered in the evaluation of a baby with melena.

Hirschsprung's Disease

The clinical presentation of Hirschsprung's disease (i.e., aganglionic megacolon) may be subtle and go unrecognized for months or years until the classic symptoms of constipation and abdominal distension are unmistakable. However, the history of constipation goes back to the early days of life in most patients with Hirschsprung's disease. The consequences of aganglionosis can be life-threatening in the newborn period (129). The absence of ganglion cells modifies neuromuscular conduction and prevents proper evacuation of the bowel. Abdominal distension or debilitating enterocolitis brings the infant to the surgeon's attention.

Failure of an infant to pass meconium in the first 36 hours of life should alert the pediatrician to the possibility of Hirschsprung's disease. Retention of a meconium plug requiring mechanical assistance for its evacuation is another presumptive sign that the colon may be aganglionic. A positive barium enema, even in a newborn, can be a reliable indication of Hirschsprung's disease (130). The characteristic terminal narrow segment, with transition to dilated bowel in the area of the rectosigmoid, is a classic finding in older children but may not be present in neonates. Anal dilation produced by a rectal examination may confuse the findings. A normal barium enema in the neonate does not exclude the diagnosis of aganglionosis, and confirmatory evidence must be obtained by rectal biopsy.

Several techniques of biopsy have been described, but any one that provides an adequate specimen of the rectal wall can establish the diagnosis. The absence of ganglion cells in the submucosal or muscular plexus confirms the diagnosis. Experienced pathologists can interpret the more superficial biopsies, which include only the submucosal tissue. The advantage of partial-thickness biopsy is that there is less intramural scarring to complicate the definitive surgical procedure for correction of Hirschsprung disease. A suction biopsy technique is available that is readily adapted for use in infants (131). This bedside procedure provides adequate submucosal tissue for interpretation by an experienced pediatric pathologist. A histochemical technique estimating acetylcholinesterase activity has been helpful in establishing the diagnosis in some centers and has the added advantage of requiring only tiny fragments of bowel tissue (132).

The clinical presentation of Hirschsprung disease varies. Intestinal obstruction is not always typical. Enterocolitis is often the presenting complaint in a newborn, and this may be confused with NEC, seen primarily in premature infants with respiratory distress. The effects of enterocolitis associated with Hirschsprung disease can be devastating unless recognized and treated appropriately (133). Enterocolitis often presents with diarrhea and signs of collapse. Sepsis may be fatal if not promptly recognized and treated. The enterocolitis can sometimes be controlled by careful rectal lavage with normal saline. It is vital that the volume of solutions instilled be recovered during the lavage.

Whether the symptoms are those of obstruction or enterocolitis, after the infant has been resuscitated, the safest course of action is the performance of a colostomy in an area of bowel containing ganglion cells. Most babies have a transition somewhere in the rectosigmoid, and a high sigmoid colostomy usually ensures normal innervation (134). The presence of ganglion cells at the site of the colostomy should be verified by biopsy at the time of colostomy formation. In desperately ill infants, the condition may preclude a controlled laparotomy with frozen-section confirmation of the transition area. In these babies, a right transverse colostomy ensures that ganglionic bowel has been exteriorized in 98%. The few remaining infants have total colonic aganglionosis or aganglionic small bowel and present special problems in management. In these infants, barium enema is helpful, showing marked foreshortening of the entire colon. The basic surgical principle is to achieve exteriorization of the most distal normally innervated bowel.

Definitive surgical therapy is deferred until the infants are managed through the initial crisis and have achieved a weight of about 7 to 9 kg. At that time, the ganglionic intestine is transposed to the anus by one of the several pull-through techniques now available. These include the classic operation described by Swenson (135) and the modification popularized by Duhamel (136). Many centers favor the endorectal pull-through procedure of Soave (137). Several centers have advocated surgery in the newborn period with a pull-through operation and no colostomy (138). The early results are promising, but the follow-up period has been too short to allow proper scrutiny.

If the physician suspects Hirschsprung disease, the diagnosis is made early. The outlook for these infants is favorable because currently available operations have now become standardized (139). Minor constipation is the most frequent sequela of surgery. Most babies with congenital megacolon achieve excellent functional results (140).

Necrotizing Enterocolitis

Necrotizing enterocolitis is a condition predominantly seen in premature infants. It is characterized by partial- or full-thickness intestinal ischemia, usually involving the terminal ileum. The cause is unknown, but the common pathway appears to be a combination of factors that leads to intestinal ischemia (141). Studies suggest that the combination of ischemia and reperfusion injury may be a factor in the development of NEC (142). Known risk factors include prematurity, neonatal stress, formula feedings, and surgery in the newborn period. Other factors considered to increase the risk of NEC are umbilical artery catheterization, infection with certain types of bacteria, and hypoalbuminemia (143).

Although the cause is uncertain, the histopathology is well established. Initially, the disease begins as mucosal ischemia, with resultant sloughing of this layer. As the disease progresses, gas develops within the muscular layers (Fig. 44-15) and may be seen on x-ray films as pneumatosis cystoides intestinalis. If full-thickness necrosis occurs, perforation and peritonitis develop. The rapidity of disease progression differs in each patient, but those who perforate usually do so within the first few days of the disease.

The diagnosis of NEC is based on clinical assessment and x-ray studies. The earliest signs are often an intolerance of feedings with vomiting. In about one-half of the patients, the vomitus is bile stained. Abdominal distension is a common early finding. Hematest-positive stools help confirm the diagnosis, but blood may be absent or a late finding. Abdominal wall erythema and a palpable abdominal mass are commonly late findings and signify more extensive disease. The use of paracentesis to choose surgical candidates has been advocated by Kosloske (144) and Ricketts (145).

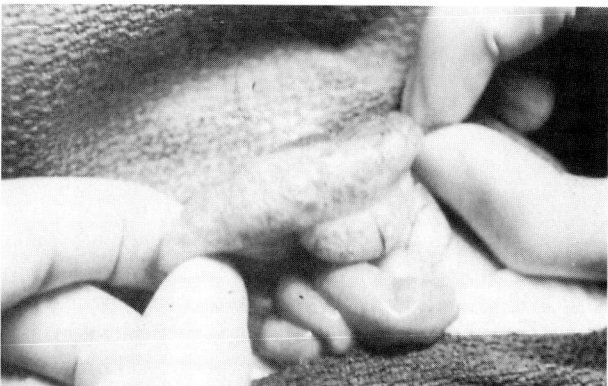

Figure 44-15 Operative photograph of a loop of intestine affected by necrotizing enterocolitis. The gas in the seromuscular layer distorts the segment of intestine. Normal loops of uninvolved intestine also are evident.

Radiographic findings in early NEC may show only separated loops of distended intestine, suggesting bowel wall thickening. Pneumatosis cystoides intestinalis is pathognomonic for NEC and may be present early in the disease process. A persistent large loop of intestine seen on a series of x-ray films has been used by some as an indication for surgery, but in our experience, many children with persistent loops have been successfully treated medically.

Hepatic portal venous gas usually implies a particularly severe or extensive form of the disease, and more than 80% of children with this finding required surgery. Free intraperitoneal air is an absolute indication for surgery, although pneumoperitoneum from air dissecting down from the chest in the ventilator-dependent child must be ruled out so that an unnecessary laparotomy is not performed (dissecting air − PO_2 of air in abdomen = FiO_2 provided to infant by the ventilator; pneumoperitoneum − PO_2 of air in abdomen = 21 torr).

Initial management of the child with NEC without pneumoperitoneum is standardized. The child receives nothing orally, the stomach is decompressed with a gastric sump tube, and intravenous antibiotics are begun. Antibiotics must cover gram-negative and gram-positive aerobic organisms, but anaerobic bacteria coverage is less necessary (146). Fungal infection is common after surgical treatment of NEC, and oral nystatin (Mycostatin) is recommended postoperatively (147). The best method of determining which babies require surgery consists of repeated physical examinations by the same examiner; flat and left lateral decubitus abdominal radiographs every 4 to 6 hours for detection of pneumoperitoneum; careful monitoring of the respiratory status and acid–base balance; and monitoring of the leukocyte and platelet counts for signs of sepsis.

In our experience, indications for surgery include pneumoperitoneum, persistent metabolic acidosis (i.e., pH less than 7.2), rapidly worsening pulmonary status, and unremitting neutropenia or thrombocytopenia (148). Because many of our patients with hepatoportal venous gas come to surgery, we operate on these children if they do not improve promptly on medical therapy. Our experience is similar to that of others in that mortality is higher in patients who have perforated before surgery, and it is therefore better to operate before perforation has occurred.

Surgery in these infants should be expeditious and conservative. The frankly necrotic or perforated intestine should be removed, and ileostomies formed. Although routine primary anastomosis in NEC has been advocated by some, most surgeons prefer ileostomy formation in almost all patients (149). When massive resection is necessary, the chance for the child's survival is limited, but the premature infant's intestine still has potential for growth and adaptation, and rarely is the entire intestine involved in the disease. Drainage of the peritoneum under local anesthesia in the infant weighing under 1,500 g has been advocated for perforated NEC by Ein and colleagues, although many babies managed by this method eventually require formal laparotomy (150).

If ileostomy is performed, the mucous fistula should be exteriorized close to the functioning ileostomy, and closure should be planned when the child is large enough (i.e., approximately 2 kg) and at a sufficient time after the event (i.e., at least 4 to 6 weeks) to minimize the possibility of recurrence (151). Because of a 20% incidence of stricture after medical or surgical treatment of NEC in our patients, barium enema is performed in all our surgical patients before ileostomy closure and in any medical patients with feeding difficulties. Other physicians have advocated a UGI study for all babies with medically treated NEC before feeding (152).

The children are not fed orally for at least 2 to 3 weeks after the onset of NEC, and it frequently takes more than 1 month for those patients successfully treated medically to attain adequate oral caloric intake. Hyperalimentation is mandatory in these children as soon as NEC is diagnosed, and we prefer central intravenous alimentation for most children with NEC.

The long-term success rate for treatment for NEC has been good despite long hospitalization for GI adaptation when massive resection is necessary. The quoted survival rate for children with medically treated NEC is now more than 80%, and the survival rate for those requiring surgery is approximately 50%. At CNMC, the survival rate for NEC has steadily increased since 1980 and is 80% for the surgical and medical groups combined (148). Successful medical treatment may be followed by late-onset intestinal obstruction as a result of scarring, and an interesting long-term complication of ileocolic anastomosis in infancy is the development of anastomotic ulcers. These ulcers present as painless rectal bleeding or melena years after the NEC surgery (153). Necrotizing enterocolitis is discussed in more detail in Chapter 40.

Imperforate Anus

Imperforate anus affects male and female infants with equal frequency and occurs in approximately one of every 20,000 live births. The lesion results from a failure of dif-

ferentiation of the urogenital sinus and cloaca. Associated anomalies include urogenital, cardiac, spinal cord, and esophageal malformations, especially esophageal atresia and tracheoesophageal fistula. The latter lesion occurs in 10% of patients with imperforate anus (154).

Imperforate anus can be broadly classified as high or low, depending on the relationship of the distal rectal pouch to the levator complex. High imperforate anus in either gender implies that the rectal pouch is above the sphincter muscle complex. Low imperforate anus implies that the rectum has descended past this level, with an abnormal location in the perineum. Because the levator musculature is actually funnel shaped, these associations are somewhat approximate and should be considered as guidelines. Infants with low imperforate anus can be expected to have rectal continence after repair. The sphincter muscle complex must be precisely located and preserved in infants with high imperforate anus, and a normal relationship to the rectum established surgically for continence to be achieved.

Eighty percent of girls with imperforate anus have the low type. Usually, the rectum terminates by means of a fistula anterior to the normal location of the anus on the perineum (Fig. 44-16A), on the vaginal fourchette (Fig. 44-16B), or low in the vagina. Because the termination of the colon is accessible and colostomy is not necessary, early therapy can be directed at decompression of the bowel by catheter irrigation and dilation of the fistula.

It is possible to transpose the anus from the posterior vagina or perineum to its normal position in the newborn period. This is not always necessary if the bowel is easily decompressed or the baby can stool spontaneously through the fistula. A judicious interval is appropriate to allow the baby to grow before surgery is carried out. Definitive repair usually can be accomplished by means of perineal operation because the rectum is properly related to the muscles of continence. In instances in which the fistula cannot be identified, it is usually high in the vagina and not accessible to dilation or surgical revision in the newborn period. In this 20% of female infants, a colostomy is necessary. Definitive therapy for high imperforate anus in the female infant is deferred until the baby weighs 7 to 9 kg.

In boys, the incidences of high and low imperforate anus are equal. Approximately one-half of the babies present with a fistula placed ectopically on the perineum, anterior to the normal location of the anus. The fistula can terminate as far forward as the penoscrotal junction. At birth, the opening of the fistula is not always apparent, and an interval of 12 to 24 hours may be required until the bowel fills with air or meconium reaches the most distal point in the GI tract (Fig. 44-17A). When a spot of meconium or beads of mucus can be identified on the perineum, there is assurance that the rectal pouch is low, implying that the rectum has traversed the sphincter muscle complex, and continence is expected after repair. In babies with these findings, a perineal anoplasty in the newborn period accomplishes decompression of the bowel, and no colostomy is needed.

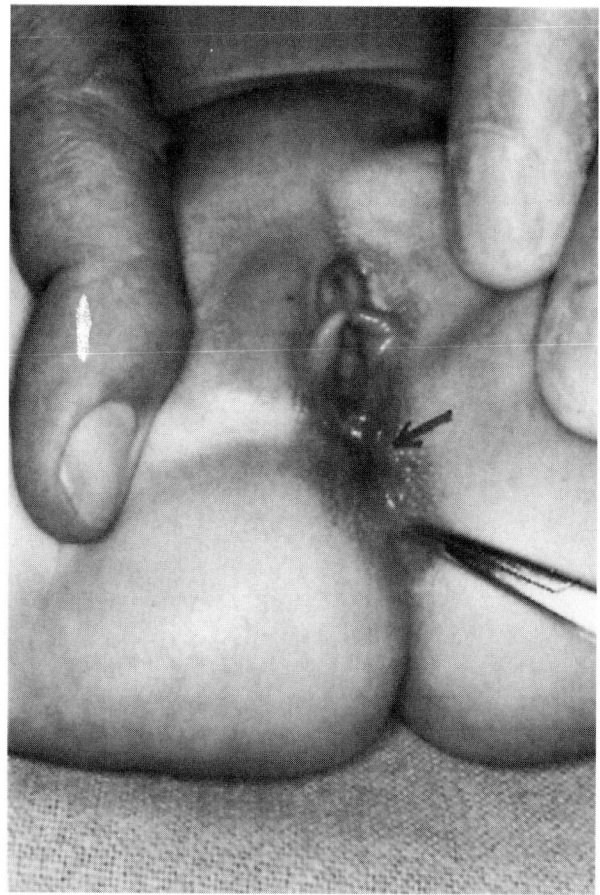
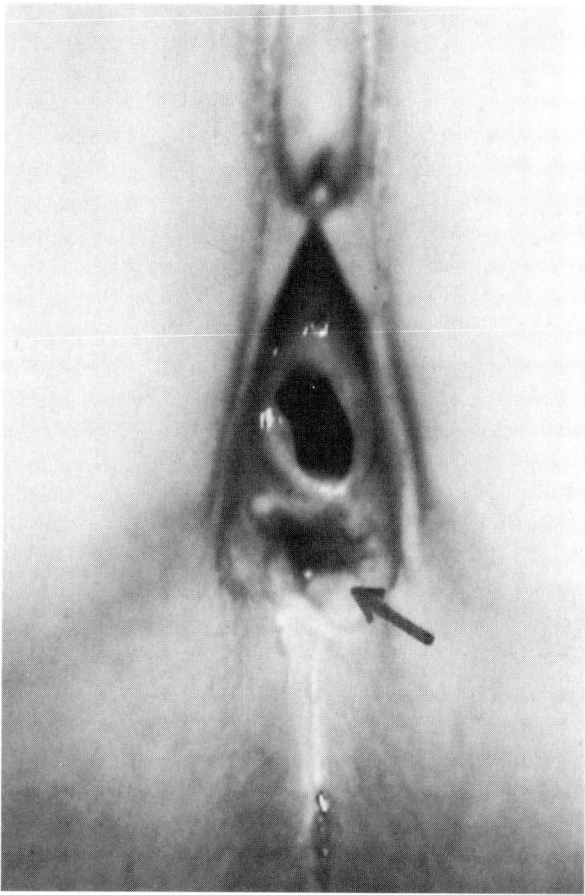

Figure 44-16   **A:** Female infant with an imperforate anus. The arrow demonstrates the opening of the perineal fistula. The clamp is at the point where a normal anus would open. **B:** Close-up photograph of imperforate anus and an introital fistula just inside the labia minora and immediately beneath the hymenal ring. This is the most common form of fistulous opening in a female imperforate anus.

If no fistula is visible on the perineum, the male infant can be presumed to have a high imperforate anus. The fistula usually communicates with the posterior urethra. A colostomy is needed for decompression, and the definitive pull-through operation is generally deferred until the baby is about 1 year of age. Improved results in children with high imperforate anus are being reported with the use of the posterior sagittal anoplasty, described by Pena and DeVries, at approximately 1 year of age (155).

The value of an x-ray film with the infant in the upside-down position (i.e., Wangensteen–Rice position) is limited in the diagnosis of the level of imperforate anus (Fig. 44-17B) and is primarily of historic interest (156). Although it may help when it shows the rectal pouch at or near the perineum, it can also be misleading if the distal rectum is filled with meconium that prevents air from reaching the most distal aspect of this pouch, and complete reliance on this view for the selection of therapy is ill advised. Ultrasonography may be helpful in locating the rectal pouch.

Needle aspiration for detecting meconium in the blind perineum, with or without injection of contrast material,

has been advocated by some physicians but should be performed only by the pediatric surgeon responsible for the child's care (157). If there is no fistula, and a low imperforate anus cannot be diagnosed with certainty, a colostomy is advised. Risk of a colostomy performed for a low imperforate anus is preferable to prejudicing the chances of a successful pull-through procedure by an ill-advised perineal exploration in the newborn period. With realization of the importance of the accurate transposition of the rectal pouch to the perineum, successful functional restoration has become the rule.

DISORDERS OF THE GENITALIA

Vaginal and Uterine Anomalies

Anomalies of the female reproductive tract range from simple imperforate hymen to complex forms of vaginal atresia and uterine malformations (158). These anatomic abnormalities result from errors in müllerian duct or urogenital sinus development. In the newborn, because of obstruction

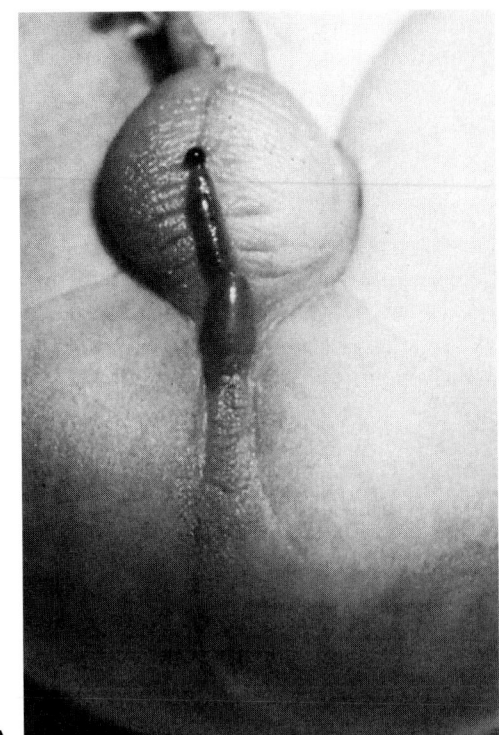
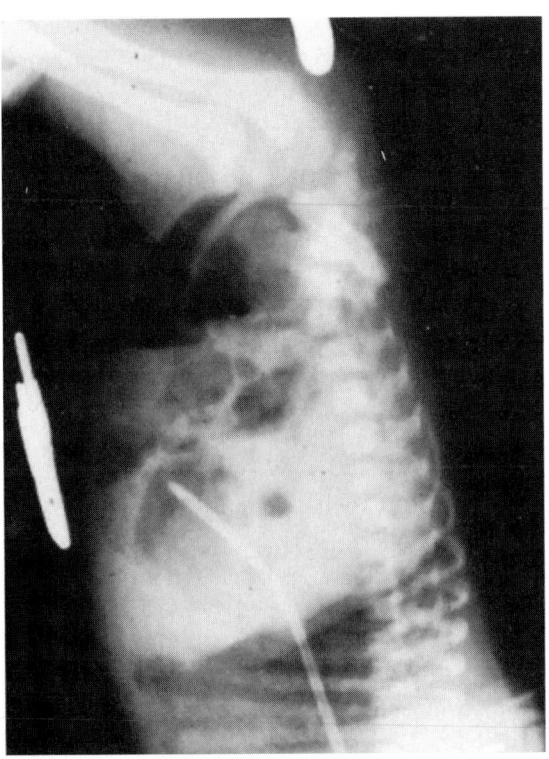

A

B

Figure 44-17 **A:** Imperforate anus and partly covered perineal fistula that opens on the scrotum always occurs with a low pouch. The rectum has traversed the levator sling musculature properly. **B:** Upside-down radiographic technique of Wangensteen–Rice using a metal marker at the anus shows the distance between the rectal pouch and the anal skin. It is clearly above a line drawn between the pubis and lower border of the sacrum. There is a second gas-containing space anterior to the rectum. This indicates the presence of a rectourethral fistula with air trapped in the bladder.

and accumulation of reproductive tract secretions, these conditions usually present during physical exam with either an abnormal perineum or a pelvic mass. In babies with imperforate hymen, the bulging hymen is easily identified, and hymenectomy or hymenotomy via a perineal approach provides relief of the distal vaginal obstruction. More proximal anomalies require additional ultrasonographic, radiographic, or endoscopic investigation to determine the location of the obstruction. The subsequent surgical strategy depends on the severity of the defect and may include a combined abdominal and perineal approach with complex reconstructive techniques. In children with vaginal agenesis, a neovagina is created from a segment of colon.

Ovarian Masses

The use of prenatal ultrasound has led to the increased detection of ovarian cysts in newborns (159). Formed in response to maternal hormones, presumably many of these cysts will resolve spontaneously following birth. For simple cysts, the decision regarding treatment, therefore, lies in the increased risk of ovarian torsion. Small cysts, less than 5 cm in size, should be followed with serial ultrasound examinations. Larger cysts and all complex ovarian masses should be excised, with care taken to preserve ipsilateral ovarian tissue.

Ambiguous Genitalia

Disruption of the orderly molecular and biochemical events in sexual differentiation lead to incomplete anatomic differentiation and clinically manifest as intersex abnormalities. These may be classified as true hermaphroditism (ovarian and testicular tissue present), male pseudohermaphroditism (testicular feminizaton), female pseudohermaphroditism (congenital adrenal hyperplasia), and mixed gonadal dysgenesis (160).

Optimal care of the infant born with ambiguous genitalia requires a team approach with input from parents, neonatologists, endocrinologists, and pediatric surgeons. When a newborn presents with ambiguous genitalia, the diagnostic and therapeutic goals include immediate determination of the type of abnormality based on physical examination of the gonads and cytologic analysis (Table 44-1), prompt gender assignment based on the type of abnormality and external anatomic considerations, and early medical management of congenital adrenal hyperplasia. These goals should be accomplished if possible within the first 24 hours of life. Genetically female infants should be assigned the female gender regardless of the degree of virilization. For genetically male babies, assignment depends largely on the size of the phallus because satisfactory surgical techniques do not exist to reconstruct an adequate phallus.

TABLE 44-1
DIAGNOSIS OF INTERSEX ABNORMALITY BASED ON CHROMOSOME ANALYSIS AND GONAD PHYSICAL EXAMINATION

	Symmetric Gonads	Asymmetric Gonads
XY	Male pseudohermaphroditism (testicular feminization)	Gonadal dysgenesis
XX	Female pseudohermaphroditism (congenital adrenal hyperplasia)	True hermaphroditism

However, follow-up studies have indicated a high incidence of emotional problems among genetic males assigned as females.

The timing or type of surgical intervention is determined by gender assignment and subsequent radiographic or endoscopic investigations. Gonads associated with gonadal dysgenesis or inconsistent with gender assignment are excised to prevent malignant degeneration and contradictory hormone secretion, respectively. Reconstructive procedures such as clitiroplasty and vaginoplasty must take into account preservation of sensation and function and the location and division of a urethrovaginal fistula. Infants assigned the male gender require hypospadias repair.

OBSTRUCTIVE JAUNDICE

A variety of neonatal cholestatic syndromes overlap in presentation with obstructive jaundice from biliary atresia. Many conditions causing direct hyperbilirubinemia have been grouped under the term "neonatal hepatitis." To some extent, this is misleading because hepatitis implies an inflammatory process within the liver. It is preferable to separate the infants into one group with cholestatic syndromes and another group with extrahepatic obstruction, such as biliary atresia. In the former group, specific disease entities are further identified by serologic testing or metabolic screening (see Chapters 35 and 40). A common metabolic condition that causes neonatal jaundice is a1-antitrypsin deficiency. Screening for this inherited disorder is recommended for all infants with conjugated hyperbilirubinemia. Infants with cystic fibrosis may present with obstructive jaundice that mimics biliary atresia, and infants receiving intravenous hyperalimentation for weeks or months may develop cholestatic jaundice.

Advances in hepatobiliary imaging using 99mTc scans have made it possible to differentiate cholestatic from obstructive jaundice with a high degree of accuracy, particularly after administration of phenobarbital for 5 days before the scan (161). Numerous diagnostic blood tests have been recommended, but none is completely reliable, and most represent unnecessary procrastination. The infant who has an obstructive profile on liver function tests and

hepatic scan, with a negative evaluation for cystic fibrosis and a1-antitrypsin deficiency, should be evaluated with an abdominal ultrasound to identify the gallbladder and extrahepatic biliary ducts and with a percutaneous liver biopsy. Absence of the extrahepatic duct on ultrasound and the finding of extrahepatic cholestasis on biopsy mandate surgical exploration.

An initial exploration is made through a limited right subcostal incision. If a normal gallbladder is seen, a transcholecystic cholangiogram is obtained. If the extrahepatic biliary tree appears normal, a liver biopsy is obtained, and the incision is closed.

If the gallbladder is atretic, or the liver is obviously cirrhotic, suggesting an obstructive process, the incision is enlarged so that the extrahepatic biliary system can be formally explored. Any remnant of the gallbladder or extrahepatic biliary duct through which a cholangiogram can be performed is used. In the infant with extrahepatic biliary atresia, only thread-like remnants of the biliary tree are identified. The atretic ducts are transected at their confluence, deep into the porta hepatis, and an anastomosis is created to a segment of the small intestine. This procedure is called a portoenterostomy (Kasai procedure). When the operation is performed in infants younger than 3 months of age, there is reasonable expectation that bile will drain into the intestine (162). Children who fail to drain bile after the portoenterostomy may be rescued by liver transplantation before 1 year of age, although the complication rate in these infants is higher than in older children with liver transplants (163).

Other causes of jaundice that can be relieved surgically are choledochal cysts, common duct stones, and inspissated sludge in the bile ducts. True choledochal cysts are rarely encountered in the newborn period but should be treated by cyst excision and intestinal drainage of the hepatic duct, using a technique similar to the Kasai procedure. Bile peritonitis after spontaneous rupture of the bile duct may resemble a choledochal cyst to the unwary surgeon. These babies require only drainage of the area, with anticipation that the perforation will heal spontaneously although the infant is maintained on antibiotics (164,165).

Biliary hypoplasia is a descriptive term for the radiologic finding of a diminutive extrahepatic ductal system. This may be a secondary condition resulting from intrahepatic cholestasis. Biliary hypoplasia has been associated with intrahepatic disease conditions, such as the cholestasis seen in a1-antitrypsin deficiency (166). A cholangiogram confirms the patency of these structures and their narrow caliber. Liver biopsy invariably shows cholestasis, and there is often a paucity of intrahepatic bile ducts. Speculation that there is an inflammatory component associated with biliary hypoplasia and that it represents a phase of a dynamic process, leading perhaps to total biliary obstruction, has prompted the use of corticosteroids for treatment. In some instances of steroid therapy, the jaundice resolved, and subsequent biopsies reverted to normal.

With the increased use of abdominal ultrasonography, cholelithiasis has been diagnosed in infants with increasing frequency, particularly in infants with ileal resection or long-term intravenous hyperalimentation (167). In the asymptomatic baby, observation often is rewarded with spontaneous disappearance of the gallstones, although symptomatic cholelithiasis should be managed by cholecystectomy (168). Obstructive jaundice is discussed in more detail in Chapters 35 and 40.

HERNIA AND HYDROCELE

Inguinal hernia and hydrocele occur commonly, especially in male infants. They result from the persistence of a patent processus vaginalis, a finger-like projection of the peritoneum accompanying the testicle as it descends into the scrotum. In the female infant, the peritoneal extension accompanies the round ligament and can remain patent, becoming a potential hernia sac. A hydrocele is often associated with an inguinal hernia, or it may be an isolated finding. The fluid may be in communication with the peritoneal cavity, and the hydrocele may therefore wax and wane in size, or it may be separated and completely isolated in the scrotum, in the inguinal canal, or, in female infants, the canal of Nuck. A hydrocele presents a smooth, cylindric contour, with the superior margin generally distinct. It is not tender and is often asymptomatic. The hernia is often large enough that it is easily appreciated as a swelling in the groin or scrotum. The mass can usually be reduced back into the abdominal cavity.

The special anatomic associations of infants puts them at particular risk for incarceration of a hernia. The internal inguinal ring is narrow, and intestine finding its way into the hernia sac in the inguinal canal can become trapped and be reduced only with great difficulty. The incidence of inguinal hernia is dramatically increased in children born earlier than 36 weeks of gestation, with as many as 35% of them developing hernias.

In premature infants in our neonatal unit, we repair the hernias before discharge. If the premature infant has a hernia that freely moves in and out of the inguinal canal, has no history of incarceration, and is first seen as an outpatient, we prefer to delay elective repair until the baby is at least 46 weeks of gestation to minimize postoperative apnea (6), especially in the anemic child (169). If a troublesome hernia in a premature infant must be repaired earlier than the elective 46 weeks of gestational age, we prefer to use spinal anesthesia rather than general anesthesia to minimize the risk of postoperative apnea (6).

If there is diagnostic confusion between an incarcerated hernia and a hydrocele, a rectal examination with bimanual palpation of the internal inguinal ring delineates the structures passing through the ring into the inguinal canal. The vas deferens is a constant reference point, and the intestine adjacent to the vas and between the examining fingers confirms the diagnosis of a hernia. Surgical repair is indicated in all cases of inguinal hernia.

If incarceration of a hernia occurs, moderate bimanual pressure, applied by compressing the sac from below

although providing a gentle downward counterforce with the hand above the inguinal ring, usually achieves reduction. Occasionally, these hernias reduce spontaneously after sedation is given and struggling and crying are terminated. If the hernia fails to reduce, or if there is obvious intestinal obstruction and systemic toxicity, emergency surgical reduction and repair are necessary.

An inguinal hernia in a female infant is often diagnosed by palpation of a nontender ovoid mass in the groin. The mass represents an ovary herniated into the open sac. Although the gonad can usually be reduced back into the abdomen, it often prolapses in and out until surgical repair is carried out. If the inguinal hernia is apparent unilaterally, the opposite side is routinely explored in all children younger than 1 year of age because the incidence of bilateral hernias in these children is approximately 50%.

ABNORMALITIES OF THE UMBILICUS AND ABDOMINAL WALL

Umbilical Hernia

Umbilical hernia is a common condition of the newborn, presenting as a central fascial defect beneath the umbilicus. Incarceration is a rare complication in patients with umbilical hernia, but it occurs more commonly in patients with smaller defects of the fascia, such as those seen in the neonate. Umbilical hernias are more common in African-Americans, in premature infants, and in patients with congenital deficiencies of thyroid hormone.

Most babies with umbilical hernia require no surgical treatment because the hernia disappears spontaneously up to 9 years of age. With persistence of the hernia until 4 years of age, repair is indicated. In a few patients, there is progressive enlargement of the skin of the umbilicus until a prominent proboscis is produced. Surgical repair is indicated early. A simple repair suffices for all these patients and can be accomplished through a small semilunar incision made in the curve of the umbilicus. Complicated fascial flap repairs, such as may be required in adults, are unnecessary and contraindicated in young patients. The umbilicus is never excised.

Adhesive dressings with coins and metallic or plastic objects have no place in the management of umbilical hernia because they are ineffective and merely cover the defect at the expense of irritating the surrounding skin.

Primary Infection of the Umbilicus

With the advent of prenatal care, the incidence of infection around the umbilicus (i.e., omphalitis) has been markedly reduced. Potentially serious complications can result from infections in this area. Cellulitis of the abdominal wall, with direct spread into the peritoneal cavity and resultant peritonitis of the newborn, has been recorded. The most serious consequence is ascending infection along the umbilical vein to the portal system and liver. Before antibiotics, the resultant multiple hepatic abscesses were often fatal. A more common sequela is portal vein thrombosis, which is a major cause of portal hypertension in children. In the past, this was a significant cause of esophageal varices in young patients, and although this condition now occurs less often, it must be avoided by prompt local and systemic antibiotic treatment of suspected infections in and around the umbilicus.

UMBILICAL GRANULOMA

The formation of weeping granulation tissue at the umbilicus is common in the newborn. Failure of the umbilical epithelium to grow over the severed stump of the umbilicus results in a persistent crusting mass of granulomatous tissue. Cauterization with silver nitrate is diagnostic and therapeutic. Applications of silver nitrate twice weekly for 1 month clear most umbilical granulations. With persistence of fluid at the umbilicus, a patent omphalomesenteric duct or patent urachus should be considered.

Patent Omphalomesenteric Duct

During fetal development, the omphalomesenteric duct forms a connection from the intestinal tract to the placenta. If this duct fails to involute, a tubular attachment persists between the ileum and the abdominal wall (Fig. 44-18). Liquid ileal content refluxes out of this duct.

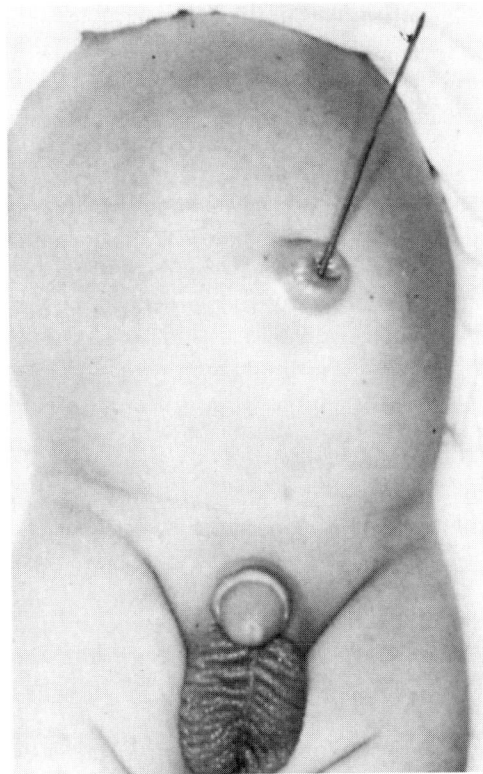

Figure 44-18 A probe indicates that the umbilical opening which connects with the intestinal tract (i.e., patent omphalomesenteric duct).

Diagnosis of a congenital fistula at the umbilicus is made by inspection, sonography, and probing of the tract. The introduction of radiopaque material into the ostium at the umbilicus demonstrates a connection to the intestinal lumen on lateral x-ray films of the abdomen.

Treatment for patent omphalomesenteric duct is elective abdominal exploration with division and closure of the fistula at its origin in the ileum and total excision of the fistula, including its attachment to the undersurface of the umbilicus. This procedure must not be postponed because there is a potential for intestinal volvulus to occur around the postlike attachment between the umbilicus and the ileum.

In rare instances, if the patent omphalomesenteric duct opening is large, the peristaltic activity of the bowel can result in eversion of proximal intestine, as in intussusception, through the opening onto the abdominal wall. Clinically, this appears as a mucosa-covered extrusion, and the resulting mass is easily confused with a small ruptured omphalocele. Careful inspection of the neck of the defect at the border of the abdominal skin discloses the true nature of the lesion. The bowel has in effect turned inside out and prolapsed through the patent omphalomesenteric duct. Immediate operation, with reduction and repair, is indicated.

Patent Urachus

During embryologic development, there is free communication between the urinary bladder and the abdominal wall. Persistence of this tract establishes a communication between the urinary bladder and the umbilicus through which urine may pass. Although this passage is small, the umbilicus is constantly wet. The first sign of a patent urachus may be urinary infection. In some patients, a portion of the urachus has obliterated with only a partially patent remnant or cyst remaining beneath the umbilicus. Urachal cysts may present after the newborn period as an infected infraumbilical mass caused by colonization with skin organisms from the umbilicus; sonography reveals this anatomy.

In the diagnostic workup of a newborn suspected of having a patent urachus, the cystogram in lateral projection demonstrates the abnormal tract. Another diagnostic technique is the introduction of a colored dye into the bladder through the urethral catheter. The appearance of dye on the abdominal wall confirms the connection between the umbilicus and the bladder. Extraperitoneal surgical exploration of the infraumbilical area allows complete excision of the urachal tract and closure of the bladder. Partial urachal remnants, sinus tracts, and cysts are easily excised.

Omphalocele

Developmental arrest of those somites that form the peritoneal, muscular, and ectodermal layers of the abdominal wall results in a central defect called an omphalocele. The

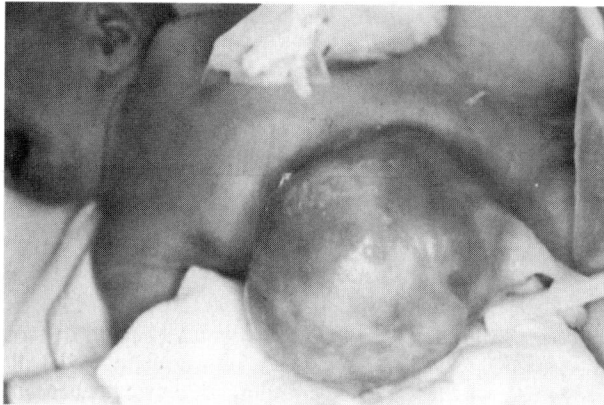

Figure 44-19   Large omphalocele. Notice the covering of the sac and its relation to the umbilicus, which protrudes from the lower portion.

defect is covered by a translucent membrane overlying the bowel and solid viscera and may vary in size from a small hernia of the cord that is 1 or 2 cm in diameter to a huge mass containing essentially all the abdominal viscera (Fig. 44-19). Usually, the sac remains intact, but it is occasionally ruptured during delivery.

The diagnosis of this lesion is made entirely by inspection because it is readily apparent immediately after delivery of the baby. The abdomen is wrapped carefully with well-padded, saline-soaked gauze and an outer dry layer in preparation for transport. Placement of a nasogastric tube to decompress the stomach and attention to maintenance of a normal core temperature are essential initial maneuvers. No pressure is placed on the omphalocele in an attempt to reduce it. This is hazardous to the integrity of the sac, may interfere with venous return, and may impede the infant's respiratory efforts.

Small omphaloceles are usually amenable to complete one-stage surgical repair. For larger omphaloceles (6 cm), a sheet of Silastic with interwoven Marlex can be sewn around the edge of the defect to envelop the omphalocele (170,171). Steady pressure on the prosthesis and a reduction in size over several days bring about gradual reduction of the omphalocele so that surgical closure can be accomplished. Irrigation with povidone–iodine (Betadine) solution or coverage with a layer of silver sulfadiazine (Silvadene) has been effective in reducing surface contamination throughout the time for which the prosthesis is required.

Coexisting anomalies, such as exstrophy of the cloaca or congenital heart disease, may make surgical closure inappropriate. Painting the omphalocele sac with 4% mercurochrome promotes a firm, strong crust to cover the defect. This protection serves until the natural process of epithelialization occurs. Although success with a plastic prosthesis has obviated the need for the painting method, it is still a useful treatment in rare instances; mercury toxicity is possible.

Congenital malrotation of the colon usually occurs in patients born with omphalocele. Although it is in itself not a serious defect, the anomaly can lead to midgut volvulus, and symptoms of intestinal obstruction in a baby who has previously recovered from treatment of omphalocele must be considered a dire emergency.

Gastroschisis

Originally confused as a type of omphalocele, gastroschisis is now recognized as a separate entity. It differs embryologically in that the abdominal wall has completed its development but a defect remains at the base of the umbilical stalk, through which a portion of the intestinal tract has escaped. Gastroschisis always occurs as a defect lateral to the base of the umbilicus, and the defect may represent an isolated congenital defect in the abdominal wall. An alternative theory of the embryogenesis of gastroschisis holds that closure of the celomic cavity has been completed although a portion of the intestinal tract remained trapped outside the abdomen in the base of the umbilical cord. It is postulated that this hernia of the cord then ruptures, allowing the intestine to float freely in the amnion although the umbilical arteries and vein remain attached to the baby.

The escape of the intestine into the amniotic cavity can occur at different times in fetal development. This conclusion follows the observation that in some infants the intestines are glistening and normal looking, as if they had escaped a celomic envelope just before birth. Many infants with gastroschisis, however, are born with edematous and matted intestinal loops that appear to have been exposed to the amniotic fluid for many weeks (Fig. 44-20).

Immediate treatment in the delivery room consists of wrapping the baby and the exteriorized intestine in saline-soaked gauze and dry sterile dressings. Prompt surgical repair is undertaken. In about one-half of the patients, the viscera can be returned to the abdomen and secure closure obtained. In favorable cases, peristalsis returns in a few days, and normal bowel function can be expected. If the

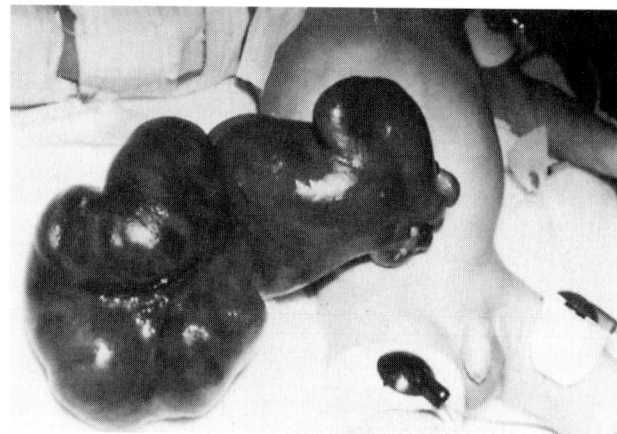

Figure 44-20   Patient with gastroschisis. The edematous, matted bowel is the result of the intestines floating freely in the amniotic fluid. Remarkably, these distorted viscera ultimately fit back into the abdominal cavity and assume normal appearance and function.

bowel is matted and edematous, it may take many weeks before intestinal function recovers. Nutrition can be successfully supported during this interval by intravenous hyperalimentation. Previously, many of these babies died of malnutrition before intestinal function returned.

If the abdominal wall cannot be closed without undue tension, which interferes with respiration and venous return, an extraabdominal prosthetic compartment must be fashioned. As in staged omphalocele repair, Silastic-covered Marlex is well suited for this purpose because its surface is inert and does not adhere to the bowel. After the prosthesis is fastened to the fascial margins, the capacity of the plastic compartment is gradually reduced until complete surgical closure is possible, usually within 7 to 10 days. This staged maneuver, coupled with intravenous alimentation, has resulted in an increased percentage of survivors from a previously lethal anomaly (172). Intestinal atresia occurs in about 10% of patients with gastroschisis. In these babies, the clinical course is one of early complete obstruction, which requires abdominal exploration if the lesion has been inadvertently overlooked at the time of initial repair of the gastroschisis.

Congenital Deficiency of the Abdominal Muscle

The prune-belly syndrome consists of three major anomalies:

1. Deficiency of the abdominal musculature
2. Dilation of the urinary collecting system
3. Bilateral cryptorchidism.

By definition, all patients with this syndrome are male, but a similar condition has been reported in female patients. In severely affected infants, there is marked wrinkling of the skin of the abdomen and no muscular substance beneath (Fig. 44-21). Lower abdominal musculature is most frequently and severely involved.

The bladder is characteristically large, and the ureters are dilated and tortuous. The kidneys may be hypoplastic,

but usually there is enough renal parenchyma for adequate function from at least one side. There is an increased incidence of patent urachus, particularly if the renal function is poor.

The cause of the condition is unknown. It has been proposed that all these infants have some degree of urethral obstruction, with resultant overdistension of the bladder and abnormal pressure on the developing muscular somites (173). Others have suggested that the primary deficiency is in the abdominal musculature, allowing overdistension of the bladder with secondary changes in the urinary collecting system. It is probable that neither of these explanations is completely valid and that some more comprehensive explanation exists for the coexistence of the unusual abdominal deficiency and the distortion of the collecting system.

The treatment of these infants is conservative and nonoperative if their renal function is good (174). If the renal function is poor, urinary diversion may be necessary in the neonatal period to eliminate pressure in the collecting system. Abdominal wall reconstruction and bilateral orchiopexy can be performed between 1 and 2 years of age if the renal function is stable. Reconstruction of the abdominal wall is best performed through a low transverse incision so that the use of normal upper abdominal musculature is maximized (175).

SACROCOCCYGEAL TERATOMA

A sacrococcygeal teratoma is an unusual tumor that is usually detected in the newborn or neonate (176). Most teratomas present as a large mass arising from the coccyx. The mass is made of mature and immature elements of different cell types. The mass may be several centimeters in diameter, or it may rival the size of the newborn infant (177). In the newborn period, the tumor is usually benign; however, when it is discovered later, the incidence of malignancy rises (178).

The diagnosis is frequently made at the time of prenatal ultrasound (179). A large solid or cystic mass is observed in the sacral region. The maternal serum alpha-fetoprotein level may be elevated. Occasionally, the blood flow through the tumor is large enough to produce heart failure and hydrops in the fetus (180). Langer and colleagues proposed using a large mass and heart failure as an indication for fetal surgery to arrest the tumor growth (181). If a sacrococcygeal teratoma is diagnosed prenatally, a multidisciplinary approach to the pregnancy and delivery is indicated (182).

The key to the management of an infant born with a sacrococcygeal teratoma is an expeditious surgical resection. The infant is stabilized, with careful attention to high-output cardiac failure. Hypothermia can be a major problem in the nursery and the operating room because of the large surface area of the mass. After a search for coexisting anomalies, and after appropriate resuscitation, the mass is resected. Complete resection is usually possible without long-term sequelae, although bowel continence can be a

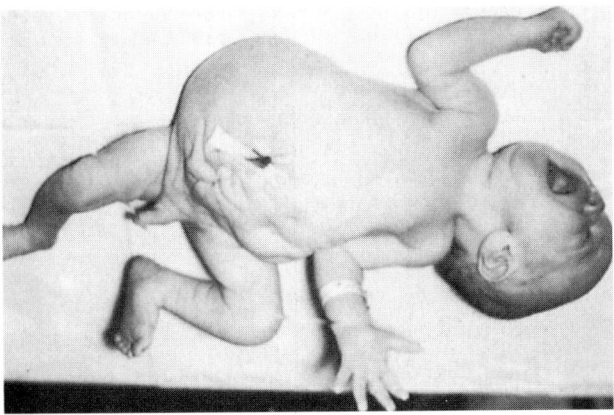

Figure 44-21 An infant with congenital deficiency of the abdominal musculature shows the typical prune-belly appearance.

problem if the sphincter mechanism is disturbed by the tumor or the surgery. It is important to remove the coccyx to prevent recurrence. The tumors are rarely malignant in the newborn period, and complete surgical resection is curative.

VASCULAR ACCESS

An excellent text, Atlas of Procedures in Neonatology, is recommended for an in-depth review of vascular access techniques in the infant (183). The traditional method of maintaining vascular access in the neonate for blood sampling, medications, and parenteral nutrition has been to use an umbilical vessel catheter. When the umbilical vessel catheter must be maintained for an extended period of time, the risk of complications, such as emboli, thrombosis, and infections, becomes prohibitive, and the line must be removed. The use of transcutaneous pulse oximetry has reduced the need for arterial umbilical lines in neonates with pulmonary problems. When arterial access is required, the right radial artery is a useful alternative because its preductal location accurately reflects intracerebral blood oxygenation.

Even in the smallest babies, a radial artery line can be placed by cutdown with optical magnification. Placing an arterial line percutaneously is preferable to the cutdown technique, with the aim of maintaining future arterial patency. However, multiple attempts to access the radial artery percutaneously should be discouraged to avoid damage to the artery, preventing access by cutdown. The posterior tibial artery is an alternate site for arterial lines in neonates. More proximal arterial lines in the brachial artery have been used in selected patients, although the risk of extremity ischemia is substantial with this location. Access via the femoral artery is contraindicated.

Establishing reliable venous access in the preterm infant has become one of the most common procedures done by pediatric surgeons. The placement of a catheter into the central venous circulation allows the use of more concentrated intravenous solutions and eliminates the risk of subcutaneous infiltration of solutions and resultant skin sloughs. In the past, central venous catheters were placed predominantly by a percutaneous approach; this is now restricted to larger neonates, using a Seldinger technique. In preterm infants, a Silastic catheter is placed by cutdown, with a Dacron cuff attached to the catheter placed beneath the skin to prevent catheter infection and accidental removal. A percutaneous ultrathin Silastic catheter that can be threaded from a peripheral vein to the central venous system is used with increasing frequency at the CNMC, but many children continue to require the cutdown technique.

The site of venous catheter placement depends on patient anatomy, disease, location of previous catheters, and surgeon preference. The sites of choice are the external jugular or facial vein to avoid damage to the internal jugular vein. In the infant weighing less than 1,000 g, the internal jugular vein may be the only one of adequate size, and its use unilaterally should not cause serious problems. When the line is placed in the neck, the tip of the catheter should be in the superior vena cava just cephalad to the right atrium. Silastic catheters within the atrium may cause atrial thrombus formation, atrial perforation, or dysrythmias.

If the superior vena caval system cannot be used, the saphenous vein, at its junction with the femoral vein, can usually be cannulated, even in infants weighing less than 1,000 g. If the saphenous vein is used, it is best to keep the catheter tip caudad to the renal veins (i.e., below the level of L1 to L2).

Central venous catheters in neonates are plagued with complications. Infection remains the most common complication, occurring in approximately 10% of infants. Although catheter infection can be successfully treated with intravenous antibiotics, it is better to remove the catheter, give intravenous medications and nutrition temporarily through a peripheral intravenous line, and replace the central line, if still needed, after all cultures are free of infection. Most of the organisms that contaminate central venous lines originate from the infant's skin or from careless decontamination of the connecting tubing before line changes or the administration of medication.

Central vein thrombosis is a serious problem that may lead to superior vena caval syndrome, which includes head and arm swelling and pleural effusions as a result of obstruction of the thoracic duct drainage. Babies weighing less than 1,000 g are at particularly high risk of developing thrombus (184). Management of vena caval thrombosis with thrombolytic agents, such as urokinase, may be beneficial, but the risk of systemic anticoagulation must always be considered. Some reduction in the risk of thrombosis may be achieved by the use of 1 U of heparin per 1 mL of intravenous solution.

REFERENCES

1. Anand KJ, Brown MJ, Causon RC, et al. Can the human neonate mount an endocrine and metabolic response to surgery? *J Pediatr Surg* 1985;20:41.
2. Tsang TM, Tam PK. Cytokine response of neonates to surgery. *J Pediatr Surg* 1994;29:794.
3. Kucukaydin OH, Ustdal KM. The endocrine and metabolic response to surgical stress in the neonate. *J Pediatr Surg* 1995; 30:625.
4. Rowe MI, Lloyd DA, Lee M. Is the refractometer specific gravity a reliable index for pediatric fluid management? *J Pediatr Surg* 1986;21:580.
5. Roe CF, Santulli RV, Blair CS. Heat loss in infants during general anesthesia and operations. *J Pediatr Surg* 1966;1:266.
6. Welborn LG, Rice LJ, Hannallah RS, et al. Postoperative apnea in former preterm infants: prospective comparison of spinal and general anesthesia. *Anesthesiology* 1990;72:838.
7. Gross RE, Connerly JL. Thyroglossal cysts and sinuses. *N Engl J Med* 1940;223:616.
8. Brown PM, Judd ES. Thyroglossal cysts and sinuses: results of radical (Sistrunk) operation. *Am J Surg* 1961;102:494.
9. Athow AC, Fagg NL, Drake DP. Management of thyroglossal cysts in children. *Br J Surg* 1989;76:811.
10. Gray SW, Skandalakis JE. The pharynx and its derivatives. In Gray SW, Skandalakis JE, eds. *Embryology for surgeons: the embryologic*

basis for the treatment of congenital defects. Philadelphia: WB Saunders, 1972.

11. Bill AH Jr, Vadheim JL. Cysts, sinuses, and fistulas of the neck arising from the first and second branchial clefts. *Ann Surg* 1955;142:904.
12. Gray SW, Skandalakis JE. The lymphatic system. In Gray SW, Skandalakis JE, eds. *Embryology for surgeons: the embryologic basis for the treatment of congenital defects.* Philadelphia: WB Saunders, 1972.
13. Langer JC, Fitzgerald PG, Desa D, et al. Cervical cystic hygroma in the fetus: clinical spectrum and outcome. *J Pediatr Surg* 1990; 25:58.
14. Grosfeld JL, Weber TR, Vane DW. One stage resection for massive cervicomediastinal hygroma. *Surgery* 1982;92:693.
15. Rodenstein DO, Perlmutter N, Stanescu DC. Infants are not obligatory nasal breathers. *Am Rev Respir Dis* 1985;131:343–347.
16. Eckenhoff JE. Some anatomic considerations of the infant larynx influencing endotracheal anesthesia. *Anesthesiology* 1951;12: 401–410.
17. Wiseman NE, Sanchez I, Powell RE. Rigid bronchoscopy in the pediatric age group: diagnostic effectiveness. *J Pediatr Surg* 1992; 27:1294–1297.
18. Brown OE, Myer CM, Manning SC. Congenital nasal aperture stenosis. *Laryngoscope* 1989;99:86–91.
19. Arlis H, Ward RF. Congenital nasal pyriform aperture stenosis. *Arch Otolaryngol Head Neck Surg* 1992;118:989–991.
20. Hinderer KH. Nasal problems in children. *Pediatr Ann* 1976;52: 499–509.
21. Kirchner JA. Traumatic nasal deformity in the newborn. *Arch Otolaryngol* 1955;62:139–142.
22. Pagon RA, Graham JM Jr, Zonana J, et al. Coloboma, congenital heart disease, and choanal atresia with multiple anomalies: CHARGE association. *J Pediatr* 1981;99:223–227.
23. Stankiewicz JA. The endoscopic repair of choanal atresia. *Otolaryngol Head Neck Surg* 1990;103:931–937.
24. Theogaraj SD, Hoehn JG, Hagan KF. Practical management of congenital choanal atresia. *Plast Reconstr Surg* 1983;72: 634–642.
25. Hengerer AS, Yanofsky SD. Congenital malformation of the nose and paranasal sinuses. In: Bluestone CD, Stool SE, Kenna MA, eds. *Pediatric otolaryngology.* Philadelphia: WB Saunders, 1996: 831–842.
26. Sadewitz VL. Robin sequence: changes in thinking leading to changes in patient care. *Cleft Palate Craniofac J* 1992;29:246–253.
27. Benjamin B, Walker P. Management of airway obstruction in the Pierre Robin sequence. *Int J Pediatr Otorhinolaryngol* 1991;22:29–37.
28. Tomaski SM, Zalzal GH, Saal HM. Airway obstruction in the Pierre Rob sequence. *Laryngoscope* 1995;105:111–114.
29. Gorlin RJ Cohen MM, Levin LS. Overgrowth syndromes and postnatal onset obesity syndromes. In: Corlin RJ, Pindborg JJ, Cohen MM, eds. *Syndromes of the head and neck,* 3rd ed. New York: Oxford University Press, 1990:323–352.
30. Holinger LD, Holinger PC, Holinger PH. Etiology of bilateral abductor vocal cord paralysis: a review of 389 cases. *Ann Otol Rhinol Laryngol* 1976;85:428–436.
31. Mancuso RF, Choi SS, Zalzal GH, Grundfast KM. Laryngomalacia: the search for the second lesion. *Arch Otolaryngol Head Neck Surg* 1996;122:302–306.
32. Holinger LD, Konior RJ. Surgical management of severe laryngomalacia. *Laryngoscope* 1989;99:136–142.
33. Cohen SR, Geller KA, Birns JW, et al. Laryngeal paralysis in children: a long-term retrospective study. *Ann Otol Rhinol Laryngol* 1982;91:417–424.
34. Bower CM, Choi SS, Cotton RT. Arytenoidectomy in children. *Ann Otol Rhinol Laryngol* 1994;103:271–278.
35. Tucker JA, O'Rahilly R. Observations on the embryology of the human larynx. *Ann Otol Rhinol Laryngol* 1972;81:520–523.
36. Cohen SR. Congenital glottic webs in children: a retrospective review of 51 patients. *Ann Otol Rhinol Laryngol* 1985;14:2–16.
37. Benjamin B, Ingles A. Minor congenital laryngeal clefts: diagnosis and classification. *Ann Otol Rhinol Laryngol* 1989;98:417–420.
38. Ratner I, Whitfield J. Acquired subglottic stenosis in the very-low-birth-weight infant. *Am J Dis Child* 1983;137:40–43.
39. Cotton RT, Seid AB. Management of the extubation problem in the premature child: anterior cricoid split as an alternative to tracheotomy. *Ann Otol Rhinol Laryngol* 1980;89:508–511.
40. Sie KC, McGill T, Healy GB. Subglottic hemangioma: ten years experience with the carbon dioxide laser. *Ann Otol Rhinol Laryngol* 1994;103:167–172.
41. Ohlms LA, Jones DT, McGill TJ, et al. Interferon alpha-2a therapy for airway hemangiomas. *Ann Otol Rhinol Laryngol* 1994;103: 1–8.
42. Grillo HC, Zannini P. Management of obstructive tracheal disease in children. *J Pediatr Surg* 1984;19:414–416.
43. Idriss FS, DeLeon SY, Ilbawi MN, et al. Tracheoplasty with pericardial patch for extensive tracheal stenosis in infants and children. *J Thorac Cardiovasc Surg* 1984;88:527–536.
44. Benjamin B. Tracheomalacia in infants and children. *Ann Otol Rhinol Laryngol* 1984;93:438–442.
45. Wailoo MP, Emery JL. The trachea in children with tracheo-esophageal fistula. *Histopathology* 1979;3:329–338.
46. Fearon B, Shortreed R. Tracheobronchial compression by congenital cardiovascular anomalies in children: syndrome of apnea. *Ann Otol Rhinol Laryngol* 1963;72:949–969.
47. Wiseman NE, Duncan PG, Cameron CB. Management of tracheobronchomalacia with continuous positive airway pressure. *J Pediatr Surg* 1985;20:489–493.
48. Hawkins JA, Bailey WW, Clark SM. Innominate artery compression of the trachea: treatment of reimplantation of innominate artery. *J Thorac Cardiovasc Surg* 1992;103:817–820.
49. Murray GF. Congenital lobar emphysema. *Surg Gynecol Obstet* 1967;124:611.
50. Ekkelkamp S, Vos A. Successful surgical treatment of a newborn with bilateral congenital lobar emphysema. *J Pediatr Surg* 1987; 22:1001.
51. Adzick NS, Harrison MR, Glick PL, et al. Fetal cystic adenomatoid malformation: prenatal diagnosis and natural history. *J Pediatr Surg* 1985;20:483.
52. Atkinson JB, Ford EG, Kitagawa H, et al. Persistent pulmonary hypertension complicating cystic adenomatoid malformation in neonates. *J Pediatr Surg* 1992;27:54.
53. Anderson KD, Chandra R. Pneumothorax secondary to perforation of sequential bronchi by suction catheters. *J Pediatr Surg* 1976;11:687.
54. Gangitano ES, Pomerance JJ, Gans SL. Successful surgical repair of iatrogenic lung perforation in a neonate. *J Pediatr Surg* 1981; 16:70.
55. Zerella JT, Trump DS. Surgical management of neonatal interstitial emphysema. *J Pediatr Surg* 1987;22:34.
56. Geggel RL, Murphy JD, Langleben D. Congenital diaphragmatic hernia: arterial structural changes and persistent pulmonary hypertension after surgical repair. *J Pediatr Surg* 1985;92:805.
57. Levin DL. Morphologic analysis of the pulmonary vascular bed in congenital left-sided diaphragmatic hernia. *J Pediatr Surg* 1978;92:805.
58. Crane JP. Familial congenital diaphragmatic hernia: prenatal diagnostic approach and analysis of twelve families. *Clin Genet* 1979;16:244.
59. Cannon C, Dildy GA, Ward R, et al. A population-based study of congenital diaphragmatic hernia in Utah: 1988–1994. *Obstet Gynecol* 1996;87:959.
60. Adzick NS, Vacanti JP, Lillehei CW. Fetal diaphragmatic hernia: ultrasound diagnosis and clinical outcome in 38 cases. *J Pediatr Surg* 1989;24:654.
61. Adzick NS, Harrison MR, Glick PL. Diaphragmatic hernia in the fetus: prenatal diagnosis and outcome in 94 cases. *J Pediatr Surg* 1985;20:357.
62. Benjamin DR, Juul S, Siebert JR. Congenital posterolateral diaphragmatic hernia: associated malformations. *J Pediatr Surg* 1988;23:899.
63. Nakayama DK, Motoyama EK, Tagge EM. Effect of preoperative stabilization on respiratory system compliance and outcome in newborn infants with congenital diaphragmatic hernia. *J Pediatr Surg* 1991;118:793.
64. Frenckner B, Ehren H, Granholm T, et al. Improved results in patients who have congenital diaphragmatic hernia using preoperative stabilization, extracorporeal membrane oxygenation, and delayed surgery. *J Pediatr Surg* 1997;32:1185.
65. Breaux CW, Rouse TM, Cain WS, et al. Improvement in survival of patients with congenital diaphragmatic hernia utilizing a strategy of delayed repair after medical and/or extracorporeal membrane oxygenation stabilization. *J Pediatr Surg* 1991;26:333.

66. Connors RH, Tracy T, Bailey PV, et al. Congenital diaphragmatic hernia repair on ECMO. *J Pediatr Surg* 1990;25:1043.

67. Van Meurs KP, Newman KD, Anderson KD. Effect of extracorporeal membrane oxygenation on survival of infants with congenital diaphragmatic hernia. *J Pediatr Surg* 1990;117:954.

68. Newman KD, Anderson KD, Van Meurs K, et al. Extracorporeal membrane oxygenation and congenital diaphragmatic hernia: should any infant be excluded? *J Pediatr Surg* 1990;25:1048.

69. Wilson JM, Thompson JR, Schnitzer JJ, et al. Intratracheal pulmonary ventilation and congenital diaphragmatic hernia: a report of two human cases. *J Pediatr Surg* 1993;28:484.

70. Crombleholme TM, Adzick NS, Hardy K, et al. Pulmonary lobar transplantation in neonatal swine: a model for treatment of congenital diaphragmatic hernia. *J Pediatr Surg* 1990;25:11.

71. Harrison MR, Langer JC, Adzick NS. Correction of congenital diaphragmatic hernia in utero: initial clinical experience. *J Pediatr Surg* 1990;25:47.

72. VanderWall KJ, Skarsgard ED, Filly RA, et al. Fetendo-clip: a fetal endoscopic tracheal clip procedure in a human fetus. *J Pediatr Surg* 1997;32:970.

73. Haller JA, Pickard LR, Tepas JJ, et al. Management of diaphragmatic paralysis in infants with special emphasis on selection of patients for operative plication. *J Pediatr Surg* 1979;14:779.

74. Langer JC, Filler RM, Coles J, et al. Plication of the diaphragm for infants and young children with phrenic nerve palsy. *J Pediatr Surg* 1988;23:749.

75. Haight C, Towsley HA. Congenital atresia of the esophagus with tracheo-esophageal fistula. Extrapleural ligation of fistula and end to end anastomosis of esophageal segments. *Surg Gynecol Obstet* 1943;76:672.

76. Tondury G. Embryology of esophageal atresia. *Z Kinderchir* 1975;17:6.

77. Skandalakis, Gray SW, Ricketts R. The esophagus. In Gray SW, Skandalakis JE, eds. *Embryology for surgeons*, 65. Baltimore: Williams and Wilkins, 1994.

78. Pfeiffer RA. Genetic and epidemiologic aspects of esophageal atresia. In: Willital GH, Nihoul-Fekete C, Myers N, eds. *Management of esophageal atresia*, vol 2. Munich: Urban & Schwarzenburg, 1990.

79. Rokitansky A, Kolankayah A, Bichler B, et al: Analysis of 309 cases of esophageal atresia for associated congenital malformations. *Am J Perinatol* 1994;11:123.

80. Engum SA, Grosfeld JL, West KW, et al. Analysis of morbidity and mortality in 227 cases of esophageal atresia and/or tracheoesophageal fistula over 2 decades. *Arch Surg* 1995;130:502.

81. Piekarski DH, Stevens FD. The association and embryogenesis of tracheoesophageal and anorectal anomalies. *Prog Pediatr Surg* 1976;9:63.

82. Holder TM, Cloud DT, Lewis JE Jr, et al. Esophageal atresia and tracheoesophageal fistula. A survey of its members by the Surgical Section of the American Academy of Pediatrics. *Pediatrics* 1961;34:542.

83. Pohlson EC, Schaller R, Tapper D. Improved survival with primary anastomosis in the low birth weight neonate with esophageal atresia and tracheoesophageal fistula. *J Pediatr Surg* 1988;23:418.

84. Randolph JG, Newman K, Anderson KD. Current results and repair of esophageal atresia with tracheoesophageal fistula using physiologic status as a guide to therapy. *Ann Surg* 1989;209:525.

85. Waterston DJ, Bonham-Carter RE, Aberdeen E. Oesophageal atresia: tracheoesophageal fistula—a study of survival in 218 infants. *Lancet* 1962;1:819.

86. Spitz L. Esophageal atresia: past, present and future. *J Pediatr Surg* 1996;31:19.

87. Manning P, Morgan RA, Coran A, et al. 50 years' experience with esophageal atresia in tracheoesophageal fistula. *Ann Surg* 1987;204:446.

88. Livaditas A. Esophageal atresia, a method of overbridging large segmental gaps. *Z Kinderchir* 1973;13:298.

89. Werlin SC, Dodds WJ, Hogan WJ, et al. Esophageal function in esophageal atresia. *Dig Dis Sci* 1981;26:796.

90. Jolley SJ, Johnson DG, Roberts CC, et al. Patterns of gastroesophageal reflux in children following repair of esophageal atresia and distal tracheoesophageal fistula. *J Pediatr* Surg 1980;15: 857.

91. Wheatley MJ, Coran AG, Wesley JR. Efficacy of the Nissen fundoplication in the management of gastroesophageal reflux following esophageal atresia repair. *J Pediatr Surg* 1993;28:53.

92. Ghandour KE, Spitz L, Brereton RJ, et al. Recurrent tracheoesophageal fistula: experience with 24 patients. *J Paediatr Child Health* 1990;26:89.

93. Howard R, Myers NA. Esophageal atresia: a technique for elongating the upper pouch. *Surgery* 1965;58:725.

94. Ein SH, Shandling B. Pure esophageal atresia: a 50 year review. *J Pediatr Surg* 1994;29:1208.

95. Schneider JM, Becker JM. The H-type tracheoesophageal fistula in infants and children. *Surgery* 1962;51:677.

96. Donahoe PK, Gee PE. Complete laryngotracheoesophageal cleft: management and repair. *J Pediatr Surg* 1984;19:143.

97. Neuhauser EBD, Berenberg W. Cardioesophageal relaxation as cause of vomiting in infants. *Radiology* 1947;48:480.

98. Randolph JG, Lilly JR, Anderson KD. Surgical treatment of gastroesophageal reflux in infants. *Ann Surg* 1974;180:479.

99. Foglia RM, Fonkalsrud EW, Ament ME, et al. Gastroesophageal fundoplication for management of chronic pulmonary disease in children. *Am J Surg* 1980;140:72.

100. Leape LL, Holder TM, Franklin JD, et al. Respiratory arrest in infants secondary to gastroesophageal reflux. *Pediatrics* 1977;50:924.

101. Nielson DW, Heldt GP, Tooley WH. Stridor and gastroesophageal reflux in infants. *Pediatrics* 1990;85:1034.

102. Randolph JG. Experience with the Nissen fundoplication for correction of gastroesophageal reflux in infants. *Ann Surg* 1983;198:579.

103. Halpern LM, Jolley SG, Tunell WP, et al. The mean duration of gastroesophageal reflux during sleep as an indicator of respiratory symptoms from gastroesophageal reflux in children. *J Pediatr Surg* 1991;26:686.

104. Holgersen LO. The etiology of spontaneous gastric perforation of the newborn: a reevaluation. *J Pediatr Surg* 1981;16:608.

105. Bell MJ. Perforation of the gastrointestinal tract and peritonitis in the neonate. *Surg Gynecol Obstet* 1985;160:20.

106. Tan CE, Krily EM, Agrawal M, et al. Neonatal gastrointestinal perforation. *J Pediatr Surg* 1989;24:888.

107. Gauderer MWL, Olsen MM, Stellato TA, et al. Feeding gastrostomy "button"—experience and recommendations. *J Pediatr Surg* 1988;23:24.

108. Gertler JP, Seashore JH, Touloukian RJ. Early ileostomy closure in necrotizing enterocolitis. *J Pediatr Surg* 1987;22:140.

109. Bishop HC, Koop CE. Management of meconium ileus: resection, Roux-en-Y anastomosis and ileostomy irrigation with pancreatic enzymes. *Ann Surg* 1957;145:410.

110. Moore K. *The developing human*, 3rd ed. Philadelphia: WB Saunders, 1981.

111. Ford EG, Senac MO, Srikanth MS, et al. Malrotation of the intestine in children. *Ann Surg* 1992;215:172.

112. Stauffer UG, Herrmann P. Comparison of late results in patients with corrected intestinal malrotation with and without fixation of the mesentery. *J Pediatr Surg* 1980;15:9.

113. Cooper A, Floyd TF, Ross AJ, et al. Morbidity and mortality of short-bowel syndrome acquired in infancy: an update. *J Pediatr Surg* 1984;19:711.

114. Carter CO, Evans KA. Inheritance of congenital pyloric stenosis. *J Med Genet* 1969;6:233.

115. Tunell WP, Wilson PA. Pyloric stenosis: diagnosis by real time sonography, the pyloric muscle length method. *J Pediatr Surg* 1984;19:795.

116. Woolley MM, Feesher BF, Asch MJ, et al. Jaundice, hypertrophic pyloric stenosis and hepatic glucuronyl transferase. *J Pediatr Surg* 1974;9:359.

117. Fonkalsrud EW, deLorimier AA, Hays DM. Congenital atresia and stenosis of the duodenum—a review compiled from the members of the surgical section of the American Academy of Surgery. *Pediatrics* 1969;43:79.

118. Merrill JR, Raffensperger JG. Pediatric annular pancreas: twenty year experience. *J Pediatr Surg* 1976;11:921.

119. Louw JH, Barnard CN. Congenital intestinal atresia: observations on its origin. *Lancet* 1955;1:1065.

120. de Lorimier AA, Fonkalsrud EW, Hays DM. Congenital atresia and stenosis of the jejunum and ileum. *Surgery* 1969;65:819.

121. Thomas CG. Jejunoplasty for the correction of jejunal atresia. *Surg Gynecol Obstet* 1969;129:545.

122. Weber TR, Vane DW, Grosfeld JL. Tapering enteroplasty in infants with bowel atresia and short gut. *Arch Surg* 1982;117:684.

123. LoPresti JM, Altman RP, Kulczychi L. Meconium ileus: operative therapy and pulmonary complications in the newborn. *Clin Proc Child Hosp DC* 1972;28:221.

124. Noblett HR. Treatment of uncomplicated meconium ileus by Gastrografin enema: a preliminary report. *J Pediatr Surg* 1969;4:190.

125. Mabogunje OA, Wang CI, Mahour H. Improved survival of neonates with meconium ileus. *Arch Surg* 1982;117:37.

126. Bishop HC, Koop CE. Surgical management of duplication of the alimentary tract. *Am J Surg* 1964;107:434.

127. Wrenn EL. Tubular duplication of the small intestine. *Surgery* 1962;52:494.

128. Leape LL. Case records of the Massachusetts General Hospital: Duplication of the ileum. *N Engl J Med* 1980;302:958.

129. Fraser GC, Berry C. Mortality of neonatal Hirschsprung's disease: with particular reference to enterocolitis. *J Pediatr Surg* 1967;2:205.

130. Taxman TL, Ulish BS, Rothstein FC. How useful is the barium enema in the diagnosis of infantile Hirschsprung's disease? *Am J Dis Child* 1986;140:881.

131. Campbell PE, Noblett HR. Experience with rectal suction biopsy in the diagnosis of Hirschsprung's disease. *J Pediatr Surg* 1969;4:410.

132. Huntley CC, Shaffner LdeS, Challa VR, et al. Histochemical diagnosis of Hirschsprung's disease. *Pediatrics* 1982;69:755.

133. Teich S, Schisgall RM, Anderson KD, et al. Ischemic enterocolitis as a complication of Hirschsprung's disease. *J Pediatr Surg* 1986;21:143.

134. Harrison MW, Dytes DM, Campbell JR, et al. Diagnosis and management of Hirschsprung's disease. *Am J Surg* 1986;152:49.

135. Swenson O, Bill AH Jr. Resection of rectum and rectosigmoid with preservation of the sphincter for benign spastic lesions producing megacolon. An experimental study. *Surgery* 1948;24:212.

136. Duhamel B. Retrorectal and transanal pullthrough procedure for the treatment of Hirschsprung's disease. *Dis Colon Rectum* 1964;7:455.

137. Soave F. Hirschsprung's disease: a new surgical technique. *Arch Dis Child* 1964;39:116.

138. Carcassonne N, Guys J, Morisson-Lacombe G, et al. Management of Hirschsprung's disease: curative surgery before 3 months of age. *J Pediatr Surg* 1989;24:1032.

139. Foster P, Cowan G, Wrenn EL, et al. 25 years' experience with Hirschsprung's disease. *J Pediatr Surg* 1990;25:531.

140. Sherman JO, Snyder ME, Weitzman JJ, et al. A 40-year multinational retrospective study of 880 Swenson procedures. *J Pediatr Surg* 1989;24:833.

141. Touloukian RJ, Posch JN, Spencer R. The pathogenesis of ischemic gastroenterocolitis of the neonate: selective gut mucosal ischemia in asphyxiated neonatal piglets. *J Pediatr Surg* 1972;7:194.

142. Czyrko C, Steigman C, Turley DL, et al. The role of reperfusion injury in occlusive intestinal ischemia of the neonate: malon-aldehyde-derived fluorescent products and correlation of histology. *J Surg Res* 1991;51:1.

143. Atkinson SD, Tuggle DW, Tunell WP. Hypoalbuminemia may predispose infants to necrotizing enterocolitis. *J Pediatr Surg* 1989;24:674.

144. Kosloske AM, Lilly JR. Paracentesis and lavage for diagnosis of intestinal gangrene in neonatal necrotizing enterocolitis. *J Pediatr Surg* 1978;13:315.

145. Ricketts RR. The role of paracentesis in the management of infants with necrotizing enterocolitis. *Am Surg* 1986;52:61.

146. Mollitt DL, Tepas JJ, Talbert JL. The microbiology of neonatal peritonitis. *Arch Surg* 1988;123:176.

147. Smith SD, Tagge EP, Miller J, et al. The hidden mortality in surgically treated necrotizing enterocolitis: fungal sepsis. *J Pediatr Surg* 1990;25:1030.

148. Buras R, Guzzetta P, Avery GB, et al. Acidosis and hepatic portal venous gas: indications for surgery in necrotizing enterocolitis. *Pediatrics* 1986;78:273.

149. Harberg FJ, McGill CW, Saleem MM, et al. Resection with primary anastomosis for necrotizing enterocolitis. *J Pediatr Surg* 1983;18:743.

150. Ein SH, Shandling B, Wesson D, et al. A 13-year experience with peritoneal drainage under local anesthesia for necrotizing enterocolitis perforation. *J Pediatr Surg* 1990;25:1034.

151. Musemeche CA, Kosloske AM, Ricketts RR. Enterostomy in necrotizing enterocolitis: an analysis of techniques and timing of closure. *J Pediatr Surg* 1987;22:479.

152. Radhakrishnan J, Blechman G, Shrader C, et al. Colonic strictures following successful medical management of necrotizing enterocolitis: a prospective study evaluating early gastrointestinal contrast studies. *J Pediatr Surg* 1991;26:1043.

153. Parashar K, Kyawhla S, Booth IW, et al. Ileocolic ulceration: a long term complication following ileocolic anastomosis. *J Pediatr Surg* 1988;23:226.

154. Kiesewetter WB. Rectum and anus. In: Ravitch MM, Welch KJ, Benson CD, et al, eds. *Pediatric surgery*, vol 2. Chicago: Year Book, 1979:1059.

155. Pena A, DeVries PA. Posterior sagittal anoplasty: important technical considerations and new applications. *J Pediatr Surg* 1982;17:796.

156. Wangensteen OH, Rice CO. Imperforate anus: a method of determining the surgical approach. *Ann Surg* 1930;92:77.

157. Danis RK, Graviss ER. Imperforate anus: avoiding a colostomy. *J Pediatr Surg* 1978;13:759.

158. Reynolds, M. Neonatal disorders of the external genitalia and vagina. *Semin Pediatr Surg* 1998;7:2.

159. Brandt ML, Luks FI, Filiatrault D, et al. Surgical indications in antenatally diagnosed ovarian cysts. *J Pediatr Surg* 1991;26:276.

160. Donahoe PK, Powell DM, Lee MM. Clinical management of intersex abnormalities. *Curr Probl Surg* 1991;28:519.

161. Majd M, Reba RC, Altman RP. Effect of phenobarbital on 99mTc-IDA scintigraphy in the evaluation of neonatal jaundice. *Semin Nucl Med* 1981;11:194.

162. Karrer FM, Lilly JR, Stewart BA, et al. Biliary atresia registry, 1976 to 1989. *J Pediatr Surg* 1990;25:1076.

163. Stevens LH, Emond JC, Piper JB, et al. Hepatic artery thrombosis in infants: a comparison of whole livers, reduced-size grafts, and grafts from living-related donors. *Transplantation* 1992;53:396.

164. Lilly JR, Weintraub WW, Altman RP. Spontaneous perforation of the extrahepatic bile ducts and bile peritonitis in infancy. *Surgery* 1974;75:664.

165. Megison SM, Votteler TP. Management of common bile duct obstruction associated with spontaneous perforation of the biliary tree. *Surgery* 1992;111:237.

166. Altman RP, Chandra R. Biliary hypoplasia consequent to alpha-1-antitrypsin deficiency. *Surg Forum* 1976;37:377.

167. King DR, Ginn-Pease ME, Lloyd TV, et al. Parenteral nutrition with associated cholelithiasis: another iatrogenic disease of infants and children. *J Pediatr Surg* 1987;22:593.

168. Jacir NN, Anderson KD, Eichelberger MR, et al. Cholelithiasis in infancy: resolution of gallstones in three of four infants. *J Pediatr Surg* 1986;21:567.

169. Welborn LG, Hannallah RS, Luban NLC, et al. Anemia and postoperative apnea in former preterm infants. *Anesthesiology* 1991;74:1003.

170. Schuster SR. A new method for the staged repair of large omphaloceles. *Surg Gynecol Obstet* 1967;125:837.

171. Yazbeck S, Ndoye M, Khan AH. Omphalocele: a 25-year experience. *J Pediatr Surg* 1986;21:761.

172. Caniano DA, Brokaw B, Ginn-Pease ME. An individualized approach to the management of gastroschisis. *J Pediatr Surg* 1990;25:297.

173. Moerman P, Fryns JP, Goddeeris P, et al. Pathogenesis of the prune-belly syndrome: a functional urethral obstruction caused by prostatic hypoplasia. *Pediatrics* 1984;73:470.

174. Tank ES, McCoy G. Limited surgical intervention in the prune-belly syndrome. *J Pediatr Surg* 1983;18:688.

175. Randolph J, Cavett C, Eng G. Surgical correction and rehabilitation for children with "prune-belly" syndrome. *Ann Surg* 1981;193:757.

176. Tapper D, Lack EE. Teratoma in infancy in childhood: a 54-year experience at the Children's Hospital Medical Center. *Ann Surg* 1983;198:389.

177. Altman RP, Randolph JG, Lilly, JR. Sacrococcygeal teratoma: American Academy of Pediatric Surgical Section Survey. *J Pediatr Surg* 1974;9:389.

178. Billmire DF, Grosfeld JL. Teratomas in childhood: analysis of 142 cases. *J Pediatr Surg* 1986;21:548.

179. Sepulveda WH. Prenatal sonographic diagnosis of congenital sacrococcygeal teratoma and management. *J Perinat Med* 1989;17:93.

180. Smith KG, Silverman NH, Harrison MR, et al. High output cardiac failure in fetuses with large sacrococcygeal teratoma: diagnosis by echocardiography and Doppler ultrasounds. *J Pediatr* 1989;114:1023.

181. Langer JC, Harrison MR, Schmidt KG, et al. Fetal hydrops and deaths from sacrococcygeal teratoma: rational for fetal surgery. *Am J Obstet Gynecol* 1990;163:682.

182. Nakayama DK, Killian A, Hill LM, et al. The newborn with hydrops and sacrococcygeal teratoma. *J Pediatr Surg* 1991;26:1435.

183. MacDonald MG, Ramasethu J, eds. *Atlas of procedures in neonatology*, 3rd edition, Philadelphia, Lippincot Williams & Wilkins, 2002.

184. Mehta S, Connors AF, Danish EH, et al. Incidence of thrombosis during central venous catheterization of newborns: a prospective study. *J Pediatr Surg* 1992;27:18.

Immunology of the Fetus and Newborn

45

Joseph A. Bellanti   *Barbara J. Zeligs*   *Yung-Hao Pung*

Immunology has come a long way since 1905, when the Russian biologist Eli Metchnikoff prophetically wrote, "Within a very short period, immunity has been placed in possession not only of a host of medical ideas of the highest importance, but also of effective means of combating a whole series of maladies of the most formidable nature in man and the domestic animal Science is far from having said its last word, but the advances already made are amply sufficient to dispel pessimism in so far as this has been suggested by the fetal of diseases and the feeling that we are powerless to struggle against them" (1).

Once the branch of medicine that dealt exclusively with the study of protection of the host against microorganisms, immunology now enjoys a much broader biologic scope and is concerned with the host processes that recognize and eliminate foreignness. Immunologic responses serve three functions: defense, i.e., resistance to infection by microorganisms, homeostasis, i.e., removal of worn-out host cells, and surveillance, i.e., perception and destruction of mutant cells (2). Although not fully developed, the cells of the immunologic system of the fetus and neonate manifest a striking capacity for response to the environment. However, the fetus and newborn appear to be particularly vulnerable to injury caused directly by immunologic mechanisms or inflicted by infectious agents that take advantage of the relatively immature and inexperienced immune system. Immaturity refers to the genetically programmed low response or lack of response of the fetal and newborn immune system. Inexperience refers to the fact that the newborn immune system has not yet had its first immunologic encounter. Those who care for newborns must understand these processes because they form the basis for the prevention, diagnosis, and treatment of many diseases that afflict these patients (Table 45-1).

DEVELOPMENT OF THE IMMUNE SYSTEM

Role of the Environment

The development of the immune response may be visualized as a series of adaptive cellular responses to an ever-changing and potentially hostile environment. Development can be considered at several levels: the species, the individual, or the cell (Table 45-2). From an evolutionary standpoint, the effect of a hostile macroenvironment provided the selective pressures leading to the survival of those life forms within the species that were best adapted to that environment (i.e., phylogeny). Within the developing fetus, the microenvironment in which undifferentiated progenitor cells exist (e.g., thymus, bursa of Fabricius) provides yet another type of inductive environment, permitting the full expression of immunity within the developing infant. The immunologically mature person may be considered as the best-selected form resulting from this type of development (i.e., ontogeny). The molecular environment (i.e., antigen) in which immunologically reactive cells exist provides the best-studied inductive stimulus leading to the proliferative and differentiating events commonly associated with cellular immune responses. Memory cells may be considered the best-adapted form for this environment. Fetal and neonatal development of the immunologic system is best understood in terms of the developing host responding to his environment. The cells and functions that constitute the immune system appear early in fetal life, but at least some of them are fully activated only after birth, after interaction of the neonate with his environment. Under certain circumstances (e.g., intrauterine infections), the environment of the developing fetus may be so altered that the immune system begins activation *in utero*. The neonatologist and others entrusted with the care of the newborn must be concerned

TABLE 45-1
APPLICATIONS OF IMMUNOLOGY FOR THE NEONATOLOGIST

Type	Example of Immunologic Procedure	Disease
Prevention	Rhogam	Hemolytic disease of the newborn
Diagnosis	Elevated IgM globulins in cord serum	Intrauterine infections
Therapy	Fresh blood transfusions	Acute sepsis of the newborn

with the deleterious effect of factors introduced to the fetus from the ever-changing and complex external environment. Threatening agents that may gain access to the fetus during prenatal development include maternal drugs, infecting organisms, and antibiotics. The obstetrician and the neonatologist, who have already made significant contributions to the understanding of teratogenic effects of these agents, must be made aware of their effects on the developing immunologic system.

The glucocorticoids, toxic agents which are frequently administered to human fetuses and newborns for prevention of respiratory distress syndrome, also act on their immune system. Glucocorticoid administration results in the inhibition of several cellular and humoral systems including cytokine production and T-cell activation, both of which are already significantly decreased in the newborn. Additionally, neonatal immune cells are more sensitive to glucocorticoids than adult immune cells (3). Further, it has long been noted that sex hormones appear to play a significant role in modulation of immune function (4). It has been repeatedly observed in studies of serious bacterial infections in infants, i.e., sepsis, pneumonia, and meningitis, that a preponderance of male infants exists over females (5,6,7,8). There are variety of humoral and cellular deficiencies compared to the adult levels which may contribute to this susceptibility including the following: lower numbers of white blood cells and polymorphonuclear neutrophil leukocytes (PMN) in males (9); lower numbers of CD3 and CD4 cells and higher numbers of CD8 and natural killer (NK) cells in males (10); higher immunoglobulin M (IgM) levels in females (11); and greater antimicrobial antibody responses which have longer duration persist in females (12).

Development of Components

For ease of discussion, the immunologic system may be considered under two major headings. The innate immune system, which functions primarily during inflammatory responses, includes the phagocytic cell system, i.e., PMNs, mononuclear phagocytes, i.e., monocytes and macrophages, and several amplification systems, including complement, coagulation, and kinin systems. The adaptive immune system consists of cell-mediated, i.e., T-cell and humoral, i.e., B-cell systems. It is important to stress that the innate and adaptive systems are intimately interrelated and interdependent. For example, the activation of the complement system by immunoglobulins, i.e., IgM and immunoglobulin G [IgG] or the production of chemotactic factors and other cytokines plays a significant role in the whole inflammatory response. The monocyte or macrophage may function in inflammatory responses and play a significant role in the processing of antigen, steps that are essential to the induction of the specific immune response. The macrophage forms part of the innate and adaptive immune systems and is important to the afferent and efferent limbs of the immune response. The cytokines are other products secreted by cells that play a role in innate and adaptive immune mechanisms. Several abnormalities of innate immunity may affect the newborn infant, including abnormalities of quantitative and qualitative factors of cellular function (e.g., neutrophils, mononuclear phagocytes) and humoral factors (e.g., specific antibody, complement, fibronectin) (13,14,15). The quantitative cellular abnormalities are related to size and ability to regenerate mature cells for the storage pools of phagocytic cells in the fetal liver, neonatal spleen, bone marrow, and local sites such as

TABLE 45-2
EFFECT OF ENVIRONMENT ON THE DEVELOPMENT OF THE IMMUNE RESPONSE

Target	Inductive Environment	Process	Selected Form
Species	Macroenvironment	Phylogeny	Existing life forms
Individual	Microenvironment	Ontogeny	Immunologically mature
Individual Cell	Molecular environment (antigen)	Induction of immune response	"Memory" cells

TABLE 45-3

DEFICIENCIES IN NEONATAL HOST DEFENSES PREDISPOSING TO INFECTION

Anatomic barriers
Injuries during delivery (e.g. skin abrasions)
Invasive procedures in the nursery (e.g. umbilical artery
    catheters, endotracheal tubes)

Phagocytic cells
Small polymorphonuclear leukocyte storage pool
Decreased polymorphonuclear leukocyte adherence
Decreased polymorphonuclear leukocyte and monocyte
    chemotaxis
Decreased polymorphonuclear leukocyte intracellular killing in
    stressed neonates
Decreased phagocytosis in stressed neonates

Complement
Decreased levels of complement
Decreased expression of complement receptors

Cytokines
Decreased levels of cytokines, particularly IFN-γ, TNF-α and IL-12

Cellular immunity
Maturational deficiencies in T-cell immunoregulation, i.e., Th2
    skewing, and antigen presenting system

Humoral immunity
Decreased IgA, IgM
Decreased IgG in premature neonates
Impaired antibody function
Decreased levels of fibronectin
Decreased levels of cytokine (e.g. IFN-γ, TNF)

lung and skin. The qualitative cellular abnormalities are related to the adherence and directed migration, i.e., chemotaxis of phagocytic cells in response to and toward a chemoattractant that is exogenous, e.g., bacterial proteins or endogenous, e.g., cellular or plasma products, the attachment and internalization, i.e., phagocytosis of the source of the inflammation after its precoating, i.e., opsonization by specific plasma factors such as antibody or complement, and the inactivation, i.e., microbicidal activity and digestion, i.e., antigen processing of the phagocytosed material. The deficiencies in the neonatal phagocytic cell system that may predispose to infection are summarized in Table 45-3.

INFLAMMATORY RESPONSE

After tissue injury or invasion by microorganisms, a cascade of systemic and local events is triggered. This generalized response to injury is referred to as an inflammatory response. The febrile response is believed to reflect enhanced metabolic activity and to be related to the release of endogenous pyrogens (i.e., cytokines interleukin-1 [IL-1] and tumor necrosis factor alpha [TNFα]) from the host's leukocytes, which then trigger a hypothalamic response (16). Because these pathways are not particularly well developed in the neonate, fever is not a valuable sign of

infection in this age group. Similarly, leukocytosis and an increased rate of sedimentation, commonly associated with bacterial infections in the older infant and child, are not particularly useful predictive markers of inflammation in neonates. However, other parameters in the inflammatory response, such as the increase in α- and β-globulins with the elevation of C-reactive protein, occur in the neonatal period and are commonly used in the diagnosis of infectious diseases in the neonate. An elevation in total neutrophil count is an inconsistent and unreliable index of neonatal sepsis; neutropenia during sepsis is more common in the neonate. If neutropenia reflects storage pool exhaustion, it is a poor prognostic sign, even with appropriate antibiotic therapy (17,18,19). An important event accompanying innate immune responses in the newborn is the activation of the coagulation system, with disseminated intravascular coagulation, as seen in bacterial sepsis. The measurement of clotting factors and fibrin split products may provide another marker for infection.

CELLULAR COMPONENTS

The cellular responses are carried out primarily by phagocytic cells, such as PMNs, monocytes, and macrophages, and secondarily by eosinophils and lymphocytes. The storage pool size and the function of PMNs play a critical role in the inflammatory response.

POLYMORPHONUCLEAR

Polymorphonuclear Leukocyte Storage Pools

Leukocytes are first produced in the liver at about 2 months of gestation. By 5 months of gestation, the bone marrow has become the primary hematopoietic center, and liver production has diminished (20). PMN storage pools are considerably smaller per kilogram of body weight in the premature and full-term newborn than in adults (21,22). Neonates are less capable of increasing their PMN numbers because the proliferative rate of their progenitor cells is already near maximum compared with adults (23).

Polymorphonuclear Leukocyte Adherence, Mobility, and Chemotaxis

The skin of the newborn is relatively deficient in expressions of innate immunity. After introduction of a foreign substance into the skin, several inflammatory cells begin to adhere to the wall of vessels near the substance and move in a directed fashion toward it in response to a chemical released from the foreign material or surrounding tissue. This adherence phenomenon is now recognized to occur through the action of cell surface receptors that function as adhesion molecules (i.e. adhesins) which include integrins, immunoglobulin superfamily, selectins and other adhesion molecules which are described below. Normally circulating

PMNs express certain glycoproteins on their surfaces which function as adhesion molecules, i.e., L-selectins. During the initial inflammatory response, soluble mediators including the cytokines, i.e., TNF-alpha (TNF-α) and IL-1, induce the expression of molecules on the surface of endothelial cells i.e., E-selectins, which serve as a counteracting receptor for certain blood group antigens, i.e., sialyl Lewis X and Lewis X found on PMNS. This interaction aided by the L-selectins on PMNs results in "leukocyte rolling," a phenomenon in which loose PMN-endothelial cell adhesions are made and broken permitting loose cell associations resulting in rotation of the PMN along the endothelial surface. As further activation occurs, intercellular adhesion molecule-1 (ICAM-1) is expressed on the endothelial cells together with the $\beta 2$ integrin adhesion receptor on PMNs. This results in a high avidity spreading of the PMNs and the release of their L-selectins, which initiates their transendothelial migration.

An absence of leukocyte adhesins is seen in an autosomal recessive disorder, the leukocyte adhesion deficiency-1 (LAD-1). This is associated with a mutation of the gene on chromosome 21q22.3 encoding CD18, the 95kD $\beta 2$ integrin subunit, which occurs on PMNs, monocytes, macrophages, and certain lymphocytes and is associated with impaired cell adhesion. It is clinically seen in infants with delayed separation of the umbilical cord, and in recurrent bacterial and fungal life-threatening infections. In the adult inflammatory response, a prominent PMN infiltration occurs during the first 4 to 12 hours, followed by a predominant mononuclear response consisting of macrophages and lymphocytes. In the newborn, the shift from a PMN response to a mononuclear cell response is slower and less intense than in the adult, reflecting maturational deficiency. In some studies, a curiously high percentage of eosinophils is observed in the 2- and 4-hour exudate of newborns older than 24 hours but not in those younger than 24 hours. Although the precise mechanisms for this eosinophilic response are unknown, it is of interest that the lesions of erythema toxicum, well known to neonatologists, consist primarily of eosinophilic leukocytes. Mobility or movement encompasses a series of cellular events that are decreased in the neonate and include cell responsiveness to chemoattractants (24,25,26,27,28). The latter reflects expression of cell surface receptors (particularly complement receptor [CR]) (3), adherence, deformability, and aggregation, all of which are necessary for normal chemotaxis (29,30,31,32,33,34,35,36). Chemotaxis does not appear to reach adult levels until 16 years of age (37). Neonatal PMNs exhibit less chemotactic activity than do adult cells because of deficiencies of intrinsic cellular factors and extrinsic humoral factors. The primary deficient humoral factors are complement components C5 (38).

PHAGOCYTOSIS

Once mobilized, the phagocytic cells mount an attack on their target by a process of phagocytosis. In the adult, many foreign substances, such as damaged tissue or nonvirulent organisms, may be ingested by phagocytic cells through unenhanced processes involving cell receptors (e.g., integrins, fibronectin), nonspecific plasma, and tissue factors. More virulent organisms require opsonization by a specific antibody or complement. The newborn may have compromised cellular and humoral factors involved in phagocytosis. Of the immunoglobulins, only IgG globulins are transmitted across the placenta. The complement factors do not cross the placenta (39). Complement and fibronectin levels are deficient in the neonate (40). Several investigations of phagocytosis in the neonate have had conflicting results. In some studies, phagocytosis by neonatal leukocytes is abnormal when they are suspended in neonatal serum. Normal activity is restored when the same cells are resuspended in adult serum. However, under certain in vitro and in vivo conditions, neonatal PMNs are deficient in phagocytic capacity compared with the adult PMN (41). For example, if the concentration of adult serum is varied or if phagocytes are taken from sick full-term infants, phagocytic activity is deficient relative to that in normal full-term neonates. The decreased phagocytic activity may be related to the decreased expression of the complement receptor CR3 in the newborn, which is reported to reach only 60% to 70% of adult levels during stimulation. This receptor is important for complement-dependent adherence, surface adherence with albumin and fibronectin, and penetration of PMN into tissues. Decreased expression of C3 may contribute to the relatively poor adherence and chemotaxis of neonatal cells. Further, the reported deficiency in the newborn of IL-1 and TNF-α (42), critical in the expression of E-selectins on endothelial cells and the $\beta 2$ integrin adhesion receptors on PMNs, could also contribute to the relatively poor adherence and chemotaxis of neonatal cells.

Microbicidal and Metabolic Activity

After particle uptake by phagocytes, there is an increase in oxygen consumption and in glucose use by the hexose monophosphate pathway (HMP), events that are collectively referred to as the "respiratory burst." The formation of hydrogen peroxide, the result of increased HMP activity, is considered to be of major importance in the killing of many bacteria by the oxygen-dependent antimicrobial system. A second antimicrobial system, which is oxygen-independent and granule associated, plays an important role in phagocytic cell function.

Oxygen-Dependent Systems

Phagocytic leukocytes, such as PMNs, respond to a particulate or soluble stimulus with a respiratory burst of increased oxygen consumption and the production of toxic microbicidal oxygen radicals, including superoxide (O_2^-), hydrogen peroxide (H_2O^2), and hydroxyl radicals. When the cell membrane is stimulated, nicotinamide adenine dinucleotide phosphate (NADPH) oxidase, i.e., membrane-associated oxidative enzymatic system, which consists of the oxidase and nonmitochondrial flavoprotein and cytochrome components, is activated and transfers electrons to molecular oxygen, reducing it to the free-radical superoxide anion (43). Chronic granulomatous disease (CGD) is a genetic disorder in which the PMNs and monocytes are incapable of generating the oxidative burst necessary to produce the antimicrobial oxygen metabolites, i.e., hydrogen peroxide and related compounds. This is the result of a deficiency of one of the components of the NADPH oxidase complex. The consequent loss of the important antibacterial mechanisms of the human host defense is the basis for recurrent bacterial and fungal infections in these children. There has been marked clinical improvement in CGD patients treated with interferon-γ (IFN-γ). The production of high-energy oxygen radicals and superoxide by the newborn's PMNs is evaluated differently by various researchers. The O_2^- generation system seems to be efficient in the normal newborn and human fetus (44,45). There is some evidence that the NADPH oxidase system in granulocytes generating O_2^- is completely developed during fetal life, but triggering mechanisms are probably deficient. The release by fetal and newborn bone marrow of many immature phagocytic cells with significantly reduced phagocytic function into the peripheral blood and the relatively rapid exhaustion of this cell reservoir may explain the defect in granulocyte function observed in stressed and infected newborns (46).

Oxygen-Independent Systems

The oxygen-independent microbicidal system is demonstrated by the ability of phagocytic cells to kill organisms in anaerobic conditions and by non-O_2-dependent microbicidal activity of the cells from patients with CGD. The active components of the O_2-independent system reside in the phagocytic cell granules. In the PMN, the primary (i.e., azurophilic) granules contain acid hydrolases, neutral proteases, lysozyme, bactericidal cationic protein, and myeloperoxidase, a critical component in the O_2-dependent system, which catalyses the generation of toxic oxyhalide (HOCl$-$) from H_2O_2. The specific granules contain vitamin B12-binding protein, phospholipase-A2, collagenase, more lysozyme, and lactoferrin, which has an important role in OH generation by the O_2-dependent system. The secondary granules contain stores of cell receptors for complement components (e.g., CR3) and chemoattractant. It is clear from the contents of the granules that degranulation plays a key role in both microbicidal systems and that deficiencies in granule population could result in a poor inflammatory response. This is particularly demonstrated by the role that the first granules to be released play in the amplification of the complement cascade, generation of chemoattractant C5a, release of a monocyte chemoattractant, and promotion of PMN adherence to endothelial cells (47). The granule complement is established early in cell differentiation. Primary granules appear in the promyelocyte stage and secondary granules in the myelocyte

stage. Except under extreme conditions, when very immature cells are released from the bone marrow (e.g., severe neonatal sepsis), the granule content of neonatal phagocytes is similar to that of the adult. The results obtained in studies of bactericidal activity of neonatal PMNs are similar to those found in studies of phagocytosis; results obtained under apparently normal conditions differ from those obtained under stress. A deficient bactericidal activity has been shown in PMNs from neonates with a variety of clinical abnormalities, including sepsis, meconium aspiration, respiratory distress syndrome, hyperbilirubinemia, and premature rupture of the membranes (48). When subjected to the demands of adjustment to extrauterine life, relative deficiencies of the bactericidal activities of PMNs contribute significantly to the compromised host defense mechanisms of the neonate.

MONOCYTES AND MACROPHAGES

The other major phagocyte system involved in immunologic processes is the mononuclear phagocyte system, which consists of circulatory monocytes and tissue macrophages. Tissue macrophages comprise a wide network of phagocytic cells, including alveolar and gastrointestinal tract macrophages important for initial defense at major portals of entry and dendritic cells important in antigen processing and presentation of antigen at local sites (i.e., Langerhans cells in the skin). Liver (i.e., Kupffer cells) and spleen macrophages are vital for the systemic clearance of microorganisms, cellular debris, and immunocomplexes. Monocytes-macrophages perform a variety of functions, from microbicidal activity to secreting over 100 molecules important in inflammatory regulation (49). These secretory products include cytokines, growth factors, eicosanoids, enzymes, enzyme inhibitors, clotting factors, complement components, plasma-binding proteins, and low-molecular-weight reactive oxygen and nitrogen products.

Macrophages play a vital role in angiogenesis and wound healing. Inflammation, which is a vital part of the immune defense, is marked by the rapid movement of monocytes out of the circulation in response to several factors, including bacterial protein, complement components, fibrinopeptides, and several cytokines (e.g., transforming growth factor [TGF], platelet-derived growth factor [PDGF], IL-1, TNF, IL-2). During this inflammatory response, the monocytes may be further primed by cytokines (e.g., IFN-γ), IL-2, granulocyte-macrophage colony-stimulating factor [GM-CSF]). Interferon-γ activated macrophages are more bactericidal, tumoricidal, and express more major histocompatibility complex class II (MHC II) molecules on their surface. They are enabled to present antigens to lymphocytes and are primed to release cytokines (e.g., TNF-α). Monocytes-macrophages can express several plasma membrane receptors, such as those for immunoglobulin (i.e., Fc receptor [FcR]) and complement components (i.e., CR1 and CR3), that enhance their function, and carbohydrate receptors (e.g., MMR on resident macrophages only).

Although studies of Fc and C3b receptors on newborn monocytes reflect a level similar to those in adult cells, cord blood monocytes are less efficient in the phagocytosis of group B streptococci and intracellular killing of Staphylococcus aureus and group B streptococci (50). The reason for this defective intracellular killing is unknown, but the characteristic susceptibility of the newborn to group B streptococcal (GBS) infections may depend, in part, on the immunologic immaturity of the mononuclear phagocyte system. Monocytes, particularly cytokine-activated macrophages, are the first and the most important defense against many intracellular microorganisms (e.g., *Toxoplasma gondii*). Although the antibacterial activity of the newborn's monocytes is comparable to that of the adult, these cells probably have only an initial role in limiting infection. The high incidence (65%) of congenital toxoplasmosis after maternal infection during the third trimester and the significant incidence of serious tissue damage in the fetus may result from a deficient activation of the fetal tissue macrophages. Decreased generation by neonatal lymphocytes of IFN-γ, which is necessary for killing of intracellular pathogens, for the increased expression of MHC II and cytokine production, and for normal inflammatory response and antigen presentation, may facilitate the survival and replication of *T. gondii* in fetal tissues (51,52). Macrophage function is deficient in the neonate (53). This may be related to decreased cytokine production. Investigation has focused on the functional capabilities of monocytes in neonates, including chemotaxis, phagocytosis, microbial killing, and antibody-dependent cellular cytotoxicity (ADCC). Only chemotaxis has been shown to be primarily deficient, although the total number and the function of alveolar macrophages has been reported to be deficient in the neonatal period (54). This observation may partially explain the newborn's susceptibility to GBS pneumonia.

HUMORAL COMPONENT

Complement System

The complement system is a key component in the production of innate or natural resistance to infection in vertebrates. Deficiencies of complement components can contribute to the susceptibility of the neonatal host to infection. Despite its significant biologic role, relatively little is known about the complement system in the neonate, except that it is deficient in this period and the components do not cross the placenta from mother to fetus (39). The third component of complement, C3, can be synthesized in different tissues in the human conceptus, beginning as early as 290 days of gestation (55). The sites of synthesis for C3 appear to be the fibroblast, the lymphoid cell, and the macrophage. There is some evidence that the liver is the major producer of C3 in adults. Serum concentration of C3 in the fetus rises almost exponentially, from 1.9 mg/dL at 5.5 weeks of gestation to between 52 and 167

mg/dL at 28 to 41 weeks. The mean level in cord blood is approximately 90 mg/dL, one-half the maternal levels. Studies of C3 phenotypes indicate that C3 is synthesized in utero. The concentration of complement in the newborn falls slightly after birth and recovers before the infant is 3 weeks of age. By 6 months of age, C3 reaches adult levels. Phagocytosis of bacterial products enhances production of complement components. It can be deduced that antigen stimulation after birth may play a role in the induction of complement synthesis. Complement components C3, C4, and C5 are deficient in premature and full-term infants compared with maternal and adult standards. Propp and colleagues found that C1q, C3, C4, and C5 in cord blood from full-term neonates were approximately 50% of the respective maternal levels (56). Low levels of properdin, factor B(C3PA), C1, C2, C3, and C4 also have been reported in cord blood. Levels of C1q, C2, C3, C4, C5, factor B (C3PA), properdin, and total hemolytic complement are lower in the neonatal period. Most of the biologic effects of complement, including opsonization, immune adherence, complement-dependent viral neutralization, generation of anaphylactic and chemotactic factors, and production of cell membrane lesions, require only the first five complement components. Because the fetus can synthesize each of these components in biologically active form within the first trimester of development, but in smaller quantities than the adult, all these immunologic functions could be affected to some degree by complement levels. There is a decreased expression of CR3, the receptor for the complement component C3bi on neonatal PMNs, which is important in a variety of adhesion reactions, such as cell adherence, mobility, and phagocytosis.

FIBRONECTIN AND ADHESION MOLECULES

Fibronectin is a nonimmune opsonin that exists in an insoluble form on most cells and in a soluble form in plasma and interstitial fluid. Newborn infants have fibronectin levels in the plasma that are one-third to one-half those found in the adult. These levels are further reduced in premature infants and under various pathologic conditions in the newborn (e.g., sepsis, malnutrition, respiratory distress syndrome, asphyxia) (57). Fibronectin is a glycoprotein with a molecular weight of 450,000 that promotes the clearance by phagocytic cells of fibrin, platelets, immune complexes, and collagenous debris. Fibronectin is also an important opsonic factor for numerous pathogenic microorganisms, including *Staphylococcus aureus*, Streptococcus sp., and some gram-negative bacteria. It functions as a chemoattractant for phagocytic cells alone, as for macrophages, or by increasing the response in PMNs. Fibronectin induces the expression of the complement receptors, i.e., CR1 and CR3, amplifying functions of the phagocytic cell system. Low levels of fibronectin may contribute to hypofunction of the neonatal phagocytic cell system, predisposing to the development of sepsis. Adhesion molecules are a group of glycoproteins on cells that mediate cell-to-cell or cell-to-matrix (e.g., fibronectin, basement membrane) attachments. These include four groups of adhesin molecules, i.e., integrins, immunoglobulin superfamily molecules, selectins and other adhesin molecules. The attachment occurs through ligand-receptor interaction, as with ICAM-1, vascular cell adhesion molecule-1 (VCAM-1), and endothelial leukocyte adhesion molecule-1 (ELAM-1) on endothelial cells with the integrins LFA-1 (CD11a/CD18), Mac-1 (CD11b/CD18), p150,95 (CD11c/CD18), VLA-4, and slex integrin-adhesin molecules on phagocytic cell plasma membranes. This binding facilitates recruitment of these cells into inflammatory sites. Activation of phagocytic cells by a variety of events, including adherence, and by cytokines such as TNF-α and IL-1, induces the expression of the adhesion molecules. If the cytokine production is deficient, the adhesion molecule expression may also be reduced. Deficient cytokine production may be responsible for the decreased inflammatory response seen in newborns.

CYTOKINES

There are a group of hormonelike proteins, or glycoproteins, secreted primarily by lymphocytes and macrophages and a variety of other cells, that act as mediators of systemic inflammatory and immune responses by being molecular messengers between participating cells. Some of these were previously referred to as lymphokines or monokines, based on their cellular origin, but they are all generically referred to as cytokines. A summary of the major cytokines appears in Table 45-4, listing their primary cell sources and principal functions. In the neonatal period, there are deficiencies in two very important cytokines that may be key in the age-dependent susceptibility of the infant to viral and bacterial infections. These include IFN-γ and TNF-α, both of which display reduced mRNA expression and protein production (58,59). The primary deficiency appears to result from an immaturity in T-cell function, particularly in the production of IFN-γ in the neonate, which is reported to be 10-fold less than in the adult. Interferon- has antiviral effects and is an important immune cell modulator. It increases MHCII expression and the cellular functions, particularly of NK cells, PMNs, and microbicidal activity of macrophages. It induces T-cell differentiation and IgG and TNF production, which augments antimicrobial activity of phagocytic cells. In the neonate, the T-cell production of TNF is 50% less than in the adult, and IFN-γ-enhanced mononuclear phagocyte production of TNF is 7% less than adult levels. Tumor necrosis factor plays a major role in enhancing phagocytic cell function and inducing a variety of other antimicrobial, inflammatory, and immune functions, such as the expression of adhesion molecules (i.e., integrins ICAM-1, VCAM-1, ELAM-1 on endothelial cells and phagocytic cells) alone or by inducing the production of other

cytokines. A study has reported that both IL-12 mRNA expression by cord blood mononuclear cells and IL-12 production are greatly reduced compared to adult levels. IL-12 is an important cytokine in the regulation of NK and T-cell function. It is hypothesized that the impaired capacity of IL-12 production in the neonate may contribute to the decreased production of IFN-γ and NK cytotoxicity (60). Further, Zola and associates (61) have reported significantly lower expression of some of the cytokine receptors on CD4 and CD8 T lymphocytes and on B lymphocytes. These include the following, decreased IL-2(p55) and TNFR(p75) on CD4, CD8 T cells, and on B cells; decreased IL-2(p75) on CD4 and CD8 T cells; decreased IL-6 and IL-7 on CD4 T cells; decreased IFN-γ on CD8T cells and decreased IL-4 on B cells (62). Collectively, these deficiencies in the neonatal cytokine repertoire may, in part, contribute to the immaturity of the immune response of the newborn and may play a major role in their increased susceptibility to infections.

ANTIBODIES

Antibodies react with antigens, and they appear to play a significant role in events mediating inflammatory responses, such as phagocytosis, chemotaxis, and the release of mediators. The extent to which the antibodies affect these functions in the fetus and newborn depends on the permeability of the placenta to a given antibody and maturation of the antibody-producing system. Silverstein and colleagues studied the maturation of immunologic capability and lymphoid tissues in the normal fetal lamb in utero (Fig. 45-1) (63). They established the sequence of the antibody response to different antigens. Bacteriophage OX174 given on day 37 elicited the earliest antibody response, at 41 days

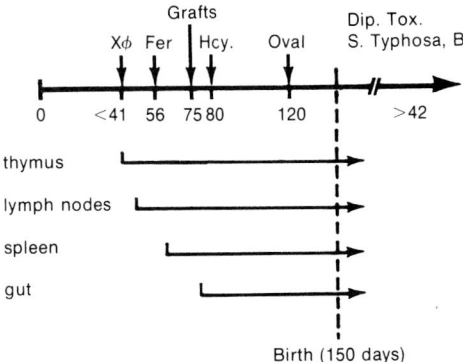

Figure 45-1 Comparison of immunologic and lymphoid development in the fetal lamb. Numbers on the upper horizontal axis show the earliest times at which antibody responses and graft rejection could be detected. The order in which lymphocytes appear in different tissues is as follows: bacteriophage (X ϕ), horse ferritin (Fer); snail hemocyanin (Hcy); hen albumin (Oval); diptheria toxoid (Dip Tox). (Adapted from Silverstein A, Prendergast R. The maturation of lymphoid tissue structure and function in ontogeny. From Lindahl-Kiessling K, Alm G, Hanna MG Jr, eds. *Morphological and functional aspects of immunity*. New York, Plenum Press, 1971, with permission.

TABLE 45-4

CHARACTERISTICS OF MAJOR CYTOKINES

Cytokine	Primary Cell Source	Activity	Principal Effects
IL-1	Macrophages, NK and B cells, Endothelial cells	Immunoaugmentation: activates T cells by enhancing production of IL-2 and expression of IL-2 receptors; augments B cell proliferation and Ig synthesis; activates macrophages	Inflammation, immunostimulatory, fever
IL-2	T lymphocytes and large granular lymphocytes (LGL)	T, B and NK cell growth factor	Activates cytotoxic T cells, B cells, NK cells and macrophages
IL-3	T lymphocytes	Hematopoietic growth factor	Promotes growth of early myeloid progenitor cells
IL-4	T helper lymphocytes, eosinophils, basophils, possibly mast cells	T and B cell growth factor; promotes IgE production	Enhances antigen-presenting capacity of B cells; Promotes immunoglobulin switch from IgM to IgE; influences T lymphocytes growth, differentiation and survival; drives naive T-helper cells towards a Th2 phenotype
IL-5	Th cells	B cells and eosinophil growth factor and stimulator	Promotes IgA switch and eosinophilia
IL-6 Polyclonal	Monocytes, macrophages, T and B cells, Fibroblasts, endothelial cells, hepatocytes	Hybridoma growth factor; augments inflammation	Mediates T cell activation, growth and differentiation; Growth factor for B cells and immunoglobulin production; Induces fever and production of acute-phase proteins; Inhibits IL-1 and TNF synthesis
IL-7	Stromal cells	Lymphopoietin	Growth factor for B and T cell precursors
IL-8	Monocytes, macrophages, endothelial and epithelial cells	Most important chemoattractant for neutrophils, activates PMN, chemoattractant for lymphocytes	Regulates lymphocyte homing and neutrophil infiltration
IL-9	Eosinophils and Th2 lymphocytes	T and B cell growth factor; Mast cell growth factor; stimulation of hematopoiesis	Together with IL-2 increases fetal thymocyte proliferation; stimulates erythroid precursor cell proliferation; synergistic with IL-4 to produce IgE, synergistic with IL-5 to enhance production of eosinophils
IL-10	Monocytes, B and T lymphocytes (Th1 and Th2) and thymocytes	Proliferation of cytotoxic T-cells, B-cells and mast cells; inhibition of cytokine synthesis by Th1 cells; inhibiton of cytokine synthesis by Th2 cells; inhibition of IFN-γ and TNF by NK cells; IL-10 shows homology with EBV proteins	Inhibits cytokines associated with cellular immunity and allergic inflammation and stimulates humoral and cytotoxic immune responses; down-regulates production of pro-inflammatory cytokines
IL-11	Bone marrow stroma cells, stromal fibroblasts	Functions as cofactor in hematopoiesis; B cell regulator of stem cell cycle; has stimulatory function on connective tissue cells; cytoprotective for skin, bowel mucosa and joint inflammation	Synergistic with other growth factors to produce erythrocytes, platelets and mast cells; stimulates Ig synthesis in the presence of T cells; contributes to lymphoid production in bone marrow
IL-12	Monocytes, macrophages, B cells and others	Activates NK cells, induces CD4 T cell differentiation to Th1-like cells; induces proliferation of T helper and cytotoxic lymphocytes	Induces IFN-γ secretion, activates macrophages, enhances cell mediated cytotoxicity
IL-13	T cells	B cell growth and inhibits macrophage inflammatory cytokine production	Homologous to IL-4; Promotes T cell growth and proliferation; stimulates B cell growth and differentiation; promotes IgE production
IL-14	B cell of non Hodgkin's lymphoma	B cell growth factor (BCGF)	Stimulates rapid proliferation of non-Hodgkin's lymphoma B cell; inhibits Ig synthesis
IL-15	Monocytes, macrophages, neutrophils, fibroblasts, epithelium	IL-2 like, stimulates growth of intestinal epithelium and modulates epithelial changes in celiac disease	Stimulates T and B cell growth and proliferation; chemotactic for T cells; differentiation of NK cells
IL-16	CD8+ T cells, mast cells, respiratory epithelial cells, CD4+ T cells, eosinophils	Potent chemoattractant for CD4+ T cells, monocytes and eosinophils	Chemoattractant; modulator of T cell activation; inhibitor of HIV replication, induces IL-2 receptors in CD4+ cells

(continued)

TABLE 45-4
(continued)

Cytokine	Primary Cell Source	Activity	Principal Effects
IL-17	Activated CD4+ T cells, eosinophils	Stimulates macrophages, fibroblasts and stromal cells to produce PGE2, cytokines (IL-6, IL-8, IL-11, G-CFS) and nitric oxide	Stimulates cytokine production and induces expression of ICAM-1
IL-18	Stromal cells, activated macrophages	Growth factor and stimulator of Th1 proliferation	Synergistic with IL-12 to induce IFN-γ and GM-CFS in activated T cells, upregulates cytokine receptors
IL-19	Monocytes	Member of the IL-10 family	Can be induced by LPS and GM-CSF
IL-20	Keratinocytes	Member of the IL-10 family	Overexpressed in psoriasis
IL-21	Activated T lymphocytes	Homologous to IL-2 and IL-15	Activates NK cells; promotes proliferation of B and T lymphocytes
IL-22	T cells, mast cells	Member of the IL-10 family	Induced by IL-9 and LPS; induces acute phase response
IL-23	Activated dendritic cells	Homologous with an IL-12 subunit	Induces of IFN-γ; contributes to Th1-like differentiation
IL-24	Th2 lymphocytes	Member of the IL-10 family	Induced by IL-4
IL-25	Th2-like lymphocytes	Contibutes to IgE secretion	Stimulates release of IL-4 and IL-13
G-CSF	Monocytes, T cells, endothelium and fibroblasts	Myeloid growth factor	Generates neutrophils
M-CSF	Monocytes, fibroblasts, endothelium	Macrophage growth factor	Generates macrophages
GM-CSF	T cells and others (endothelium, fibroblasts, monocytes)	Monomyelocytic growth factor	Myelopoiesis
IFN-α	Monocytes, macrophages, B lymphocytes and NK cells	Antiviral, antiproliferative and immunomodulating, mediation of antitumor activity	Stimulates NK and phagocytic cells, upregulates MHC class I antigens
IFN-β	Fibroblasts	Antiviral, antiproliferative and immunomodulating, mediation of antitumor activity	Stimulates NK and phagocytic cells, upregulates MHC class I antigens
IFN-γ	Th lymphocytes, NK cells and macrophages	Immunomodulating, antiproliferative	Induce cell membrane antigen expression (i.e., MHC class I and II); primary cytokine responsible for cell-mediated immunity; inhibits IL-4 or IL-13 induced IgE production
TNF-α	Mononuclear phagocytes	Inflammatory, immunoenhancing and tumoricidal	Induces anti-tumor immune responses; induces expression of adhesion molecules; potent activator of neutrophils; responsible for severe cachexia; causes vascular thomboses, tumor necrosis and enhances phagocytic cell function, induces apoptosis of many cells; induces secondary production of cytokines by stromal cells
TNF-β = LT	T lymphocytes	Stimulates antitumor immunity	Induces anti-tumor immune responses; induces expression of adhesion molecules
TGF-β	Chondrocytes, osteocytes, fibroblasts, platelets, monocytes and some T cells	Anti-inflammatory; induces formation of extracellular matrix; causes immunosuppression by inhibiting B and T cells	Wound healing, scar formation and bone remodeling; supports IgA isotype class switch; plays major role in immune nonresponsiveness (tolerance) in the gut

B, bursal dependent; EBV, Epstein-Barr virus; G-CSF, granulocyte-colony-stimulating factor; GM-CSF, granulocyte-macrophage-colony-stimulating factor; IL, interleukin; IFN, interferon; LGL, large granular lymphocytes; M-CSF, macrophage-colony-stimulating factor; MHC, major histocompatibility complex; NK, natural killer; T, thymus derived; TGF, transforming growth factor; TH, thymic; TNF, tumor necrosis factor.

of gestation. This is a remarkable observation, because the fetal sheep has little organized lymphoid tissue at this stage. At approximately 66 days of gestation, the fetus becomes able to respond to the protein ferritin, but not until 125 days of gestation can it respond to egg albumin. Antibodies against Salmonella typhi or bacillus Calmette-Guerin appear only after birth. The researchers were unable to induce tolerance until the lamb reached the age at which it was able to recognize the antigen and produce antibody. It is possible to draw an analogy between this phenomenon and the poor response of human newborn infants to the polysaccharide antigens. These phenomena must be understood

TABLE 45-5

DEVELOPMENT OF THE IMMUNE SYSTEM IN THE FETUS

Gestation (Wk)	Findings
4	First blood centers appear in yolk sac
5.5	Synthesis of complement is detected
7	Lymphocytes appear in peripheral blood, about 1000/mm^3
7–9	Lymphocytes appear in thymus
11	CD2 receptors (i.e., E rosette) develop in thymus lymphocytes; B-cell maturation occurs in liver and spleen, with IgG, IgA, IgM, and IgD surface markers; serum IgM levels can be detected
12	Antigen recognition is demonstrable
13	Graft-versus host reactivity is present
14	Phytohemagglutinin responses by thymus lymphocytes occurs
17	Serum IgM levels can be detected
20	Secondary lymphoid complex is present
20–25	Lymphocytes in blood number about 10,000/mm^3
22	Complement levels detectable in serum
30	IgA level detectable in serum

Adapted from Cauchi MN. Immunological aspects of pregnancy and the newborn. In: Cauchi MN, Gilbert GL, Brown JB, eds. *The clinical pathology of pregnancy and the newborn infant*. London: Edward Arnold Publishers, 1984:325, with permission.

in the human if adequate immunization techniques are to be developed and allergic diseases are to be prevented (Table 45-5).

OPSONIC CAPACITY

The opsonic capacity of blood refers to the enhancement of phagocytosis and includes the activities of antibodies, complement, and other proteins that are not well defined. IgM appears to have the greatest opsonic activity. Full-term and premature human newborns appear to be relatively deficient in opsonic activity toward a variety of agents. The degree of deficiency varies with different agents and probably particularly involves antibodies of the IgM type. This deficiency of antibodies may account for the susceptibility of the newborn to gram-negative infections, because IgM antibodies do not traverse the placenta. However, Miller observed that addition of purified IgM to neonatal sera does not enhance opsonization of yeast particles. Complement and other heat-labile factors amplify the opsonic activity of IgM to a much greater extent than they amplify IgG opsonic activity. The deficit in opsonic activity derives from deficiencies of complement, particularly of components C3, C5, and C3PA. In the premature infant, lowered levels of IgG may play a role in the opsonic deficiency (64). Rigorously controlled studies of the opsonic capacity of the fetus and newborn are needed so that the usefulness of potentially harmful treatments, such as fresh plasma transfusion in the septicemic neonate, can be determined. One

of the important clinical sequelae of deficient antimicrobial antibody is seen in GBS infection of the newborn. The increased susceptibility of newborns to GBS infection has been correlated with deficiency of maternal antibody directed against the type-specific polysaccharides of the organism.

ADAPTIVE IMMUNE MECHANISMS

The maturation of adaptive immune responses in the human begins in utero between 8 and 12 weeks of gestation. The differentiation of cells destined to perform these functions appears to arise from a population of progenitor cells, referred to as stem cells, that are located within the yolk sac, fetal liver, and bone marrow of the developing embryo (Fig. 45-2). Depending on the type of microchemical environment surrounding these cells, differentiation occurs along at least two avenues: hematopoietic and lymphopoietic.

HEMATOPOIETIC DIFFERENTIATION

One type of microchemical environment leads to the proliferation and differentiation of stem cells into myeloid, erythroid, and megakaryocyte precursors. The products of these cell lines are the monocytes, granulocytes, erythrocytes, and platelets of the circulation. In the human, granulocytic cells are first observed in the liver of the fetus in the second month of gestation. Leukocyte production by the fetal liver declines at about the fifth month of gestation, when the bone marrow activity increases.

LYMPHOPOIETIC DIFFERENTIATION

Classically, the lymphoid system develops along two independent pathways leading to morphologically and functionally distinct populations of immune lymphocytes: the thymus-derived system of cell-mediated immunity (CMI), whose principal effector cells are the T lymphocytes, and the bursal-dependent system of antibody-mediated immunity, which is effected by the B lymphocytes. The T lymphocyte is commonly identified by the T-cell receptor-CD3 (TCR-CD3) complex or CD2 surface marker (i.e., binding site for sheep erythrocytes). The B lymphocyte is recognized primarily by its surface CD19 or CD20 markers or immunoglobulin.

The immune system of the human derives from gut-associated tissue in the embryo. The first appearance of pluripotential hematopoietic stem cells in the yolk sac is at 2.5 to 3 wk of gestational age and these cells migrate to the fetal liver at 5 wk of gestation; later, they reside in the bone marrow, in which they remain throughout life. The lymphoid stem cells develop from these precursor cells and depending on the organs or tissues to which the stem cells traffic, differentiate into T, B, or NK cells. During the middle

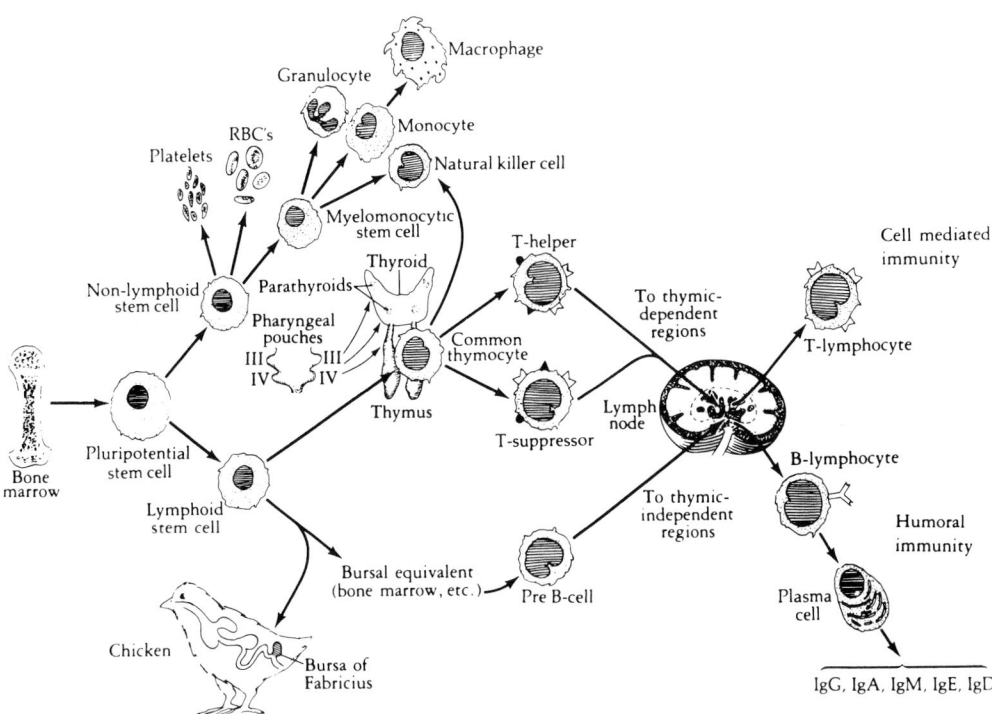

Figure 45-2 Ontogeny of immune response, showing differentiation of progenitor cells into hematopoietic and immunocompetent cells. From Bellanti JA. *Immunology III*. Philadelphia, WB Saunders, 1985:48, with permission.

of the first trimester of gestation, primary lymphoid organ (thymus and bone marrow) development begins and proceeds rapidly, followed by secondary lymphoid organ (spleen, lymph nodes, tonsils, Peyer patches, and lamina propria) development. Throughout life these organs continue to serve as sites of differentiation of T, B, and NK lymphocytes from stem cells. Both the initial organogenesis and the continued cell differentiation occur as a consequence of the interaction of a vast array of lymphocytic and microenvironmental cell surface molecules and proteins secreted by the involved cells. The complexity and number of such cell surface molecules led to the development of an international nomenclature and classification of these differentiation antigens, which are now referred to as clusters of differentiation (CD) (65) (Table 45-6).

T-CELL SYSTEM

The basic cell type differentiates into lymphoid cells when the progenitor cells are influenced by certain microchemical environments. The first is the thymus, which leads to the differentiation of T cells (66,67). The thymus gland is derived from the epithelium of the third and fourth pharyngeal pouches at about the sixth week of fetal life. The parathyroid glands also begin their development at about this time from the same pouches. With further differentiation, a caudal migration of epithelium occurs, and beginning in the eighth week, blood-borne stem cells enter the gland and begin lymphoid differentiation. With further

development, the thymus is infiltrated with lymphocytes and is differentiated into a dense cortex containing many small lymphocytes and a less dense, central medulla with relatively more epithelial elements. Thymocyte precursors are probably derived from multipotential hematopoietic precursors in the fetal liver and later in the bone marrow (68,69,70). Under the influence of thymic epithelium-derived chemoattractants, pro-T cells initially localize to the thymic corticomedullary junction. These CD4-negative, CD8-negative T-cell precursors undergo extensive gene rearrangement, phenotypic alteration, and biochemical modification to yield the population of thymocytes that undergoes intrathymic selection. First, precursor T cells with affinity for self MHC (i.e., usually CD4-positive and CD8-positive) are positively selected in the cortex of the thymus. Subsequently, in the medulla, they undergo negative selection, and those that recognize self-antigens are deleted. More than 95% of the thymocytes, which include cells that have not been positively selected and those that have been negatively selected, proceed to programmed cell death, a process called apoptosis. The selected mature thymocytes, usually bearing mature TCRs with CD8 or CD4 molecules (i.e., single positive), seed the peripheral lymphoid tissue. In the developing thymus, there exists a dynamic interplay of cytokines that act in a coordinated and temporal manner to control the passage of the precursor cell through different stages of development in the thymus (Fig. 45-3). In particular, IL-1, IL-2, IL-4, and IL-7 may play central roles in precursor proliferation and differentiation (71). T-cell differentiation within

TABLE 45-6

CLASSIFICATION OF LYMPHOCYTE SURFACE MOLECULES; CLUSTERS OF DIFFERENTIATION (CD)

CD Number	Other Names	Tissue/Lineage	Function
CD1	T6	Cortical thymocytes; Langerhans cells	Antigen presentation to TCRγδ cells
CD2	SRBC receptor	T and NK cells	Alternative pathway of T cell activation; binds LFA-3 (CD58)
CD3	T3, Leu 4	T cells	Transduces signals from TCR (TCR-associated)
CD4	T4, Leu3a	Helper T cell subset	Receptor for HLA class II antigens; associated with p56 lck tyrosine kinase
CD7	3A1, Leu 9	T and NK cells and their precursors	Co-mitogenic for T lymphocytes
CD8	T8, Leu2a	Cytotoxic T cell subset; also on 30% of NK cells	Receptor for HLA class I antigens; associated with p56 lck tyrosine kinase
CD10	cALLA	B cell progenitors	Peptide cleavage
CD11a	LFA-1a α chain	T, B, and NK cells	Ligand for ICAMS 1, 2, and 3 with CD 18
CD11b,c	MAC-1,CR3; CR4	NK cells	With CD18, receptors for C3bi
CD16	FcRγIII	NK cells	FcR for IgG
CD19	B4	B cells	Regulates B cell activation
CD20	B1	B cells	Mediates B cell activation
CD21	B2	B cells	C3d and the EBV receptor; CR2
CD34	My10	Precursor cells	Unknown
CD40	CD40	B cells and monocytes	Initiates isotype switching when ligated
CD45	Leukocyte common antigen, T200	All leukocytes	Tyrosine phosphatase that regulates lymphocyte activation; CD45R0 isoform on memory T cells, CD45RA isoform on naive T cells
CD56	N-CAM; NKH-1	NK cells	Mediates NK homotypic adhesion
CD154	CD40 ligand, gp39	Activated CD4 T cells	Ligates CD40 on B cells and initiates isotype switching

CD = clusters of differentiation. Adapted from Buckley RH. The T-, B-, and NK-cell system. In: Behrman RE, Kliegman RM, Jenson HB, eds. Nelson Textbook of pediatrics, 17th ed. Philadelphia: Saunders-Elsevier, 2004:683, with permission.

the thymus appears to be regulated by several factors synthesized by the thymic epithelial cells. Several peptides have been described, and they share some properties that may result from their relative impurity (72). One of the best characterized of these thymic hormones is thymopoietin (molecular weight, 5562), which promotes prothymocyte to thymocyte differentiation, as demonstrated in the appearance of typical T-cell surface markers (73). Some synthetic polypeptide molecules that seem to have all the differentiation-inducing properties of the original molecule are being evaluated. Although the characterization of hormones is preliminary, the use of thymosin has intriguing applications in clinical medicine as a replacement therapy for immunoincompetence. The clinical importance of the simultaneous embryogenesis of the parathyroid and thymus is seen in one of the immunologic deficiency disorders of infancy, the DiGeorge anomaly. The DiGeorge anomaly is a developmental defect in which derivatives of pharyngeal pouches III and IV do not arise, usually because of inadequate neural crest contributions resulting in congenital aplasia of the thymus and the parathyroids. The condition presents in the early newborn period with hypocalcemic tetany, characteristic facies and

cardiovascular defects and a propensity to infections which result from T cell deficiency, e.g., canidiasis. Recently, a spectrum of disorders resembling the DiGeorge syndrome has been described all associated with a deletion of the long arm of the 22 chromosome (74). This gamut of disorders has been referred to as the Catch 22 and include a cluster of developmental anomalies including velocardiofacial (VCF) or Shprintzen syndrome, conotruncal atresia and the DiGeorge syndrome. There is no known feature that uniformly occurs, and the diagnosis of DiGeorge anomaly is usually based on two or more of the following: (a) typical facies (e.g., hypoplastic mandible, short philtrum, hypertelorism, ears low set or malformed or both) (b) characteristic heart lesion (e.g., conotruncal malformation, usually interrupted aortic arch [IAA] type B) (c) persistent hypocalcemia with onset in the first month of life (d) documented inability to identify the thymus at surgery or autopsy (e) decrease in T-cell response to mitogens (f) decrease in T-cell number (75,76). Two rare conotruncal anomalies, type B IAA and truncus arteriosus, account for over one-half of the cardiac lesions seen in DiGeorge anomaly. Of all patients with IAA type B, 68% had DiGeorge anomaly; of all patients with truncus arteriosus,

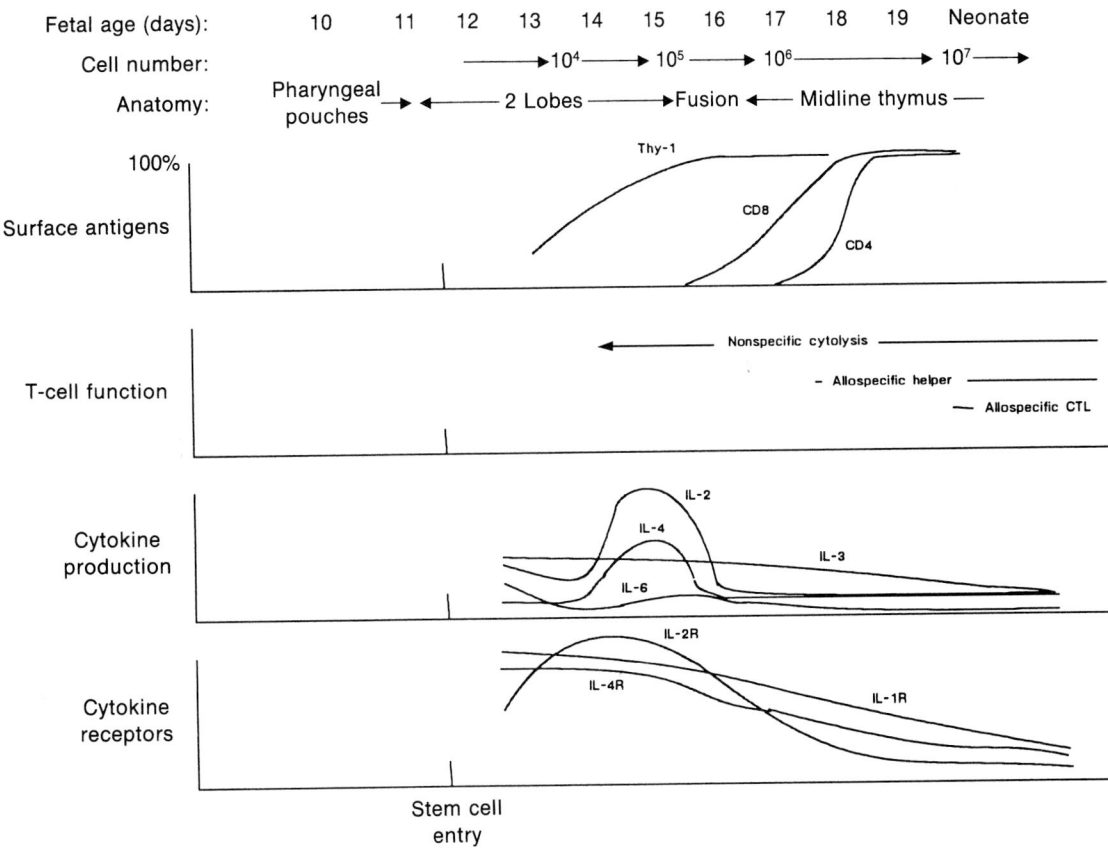

Figure 45-3 Temporal relations among the production of cytokines, expression of cytokine receptors, and the differentiating events occurring in precursor cells in the murine fetal thymus during T-cell ontogeny (CTL, cytotoxic T lymphocytes). Adapted from Carding SR, Haydan AC, Bottomly K, et al. Cytokines in T-cell development. *Immunol Today* 1991;12:240, with permission.

33% had DiGeorge anomaly. Failure of descent of the thymus is extremely common in DiGeorge anomaly, but immunodeficiency that requires correction occurs in only approximately 25% of the patients. The term, complete DiGeorge anomaly, should be reserved for patients with complete absence of the thymus and parathyroids who are in need of reconstitution of the immune system without which life is incompatible. The physician can identify patients requiring treatment of the thymic defect by T-cell enumeration and in vitro proliferation assays. Two alternatives for therapy are thymus transplantation and bone marrow transplantation from a HLA-matched sibling. After emigration of the T cells from the thymus, they circulate through the lymphatic and vascular systems as the long-lived lymphocytes (i.e., the recirculating pool), which then populate certain restricted regions of the lymph nodes, the thymic-dependent subcortical areas, and the periarteriolar regions of the spleen. Removal of the thymus in neonatal mice renders them deficient in the number of circulating T cells and leads to depletion of the thymic-dependent areas in lymphoid tissue. The long-lived nature of these lymphocytes and the degree of competence in the human may explain in part why, after thymectomy, immediate deficits are not usually seen in the newborn period, although they may become apparent later in life. After birth, the thymus

plays a continually changing role in relation to body size. It is largest compared with body size during fetal life, and at birth, it weighs 10 to 15 g. The gland continues to increase in size, reaching a maximum of 30 to 40 g at puberty, after which involution occurs. The increased incidence of autoimmunity and malignancy with aging has been associated with senescence of thymic function.

T CELLS

The stages in the life history of T cells are marked by the gradual appearance of a variety of membrane-bound glycoproteins (Fig. 45-4). Many of them have been identified by employing monoclonal antibodies. Immature thymocytes are characterized by the expression of some surface markers acquired during intrathymic development, such as transferrin receptor (CD71), CD1, CD2, CD4, CD8, and the CD3/TCR complex. After the T cells enter the circulation, they lose the transferrin receptor and CD1 molecule. In the peripheral blood, approximately 70% of T cells express the CD4 marker, and CD8 is found on approximately 30%. T cells that acquire helper activity characteristically express CD4, and suppressor T cells have CD8 but not CD4 on their surface. The CD4 receptor with

THYMUS

LYMPHOID TISSUES

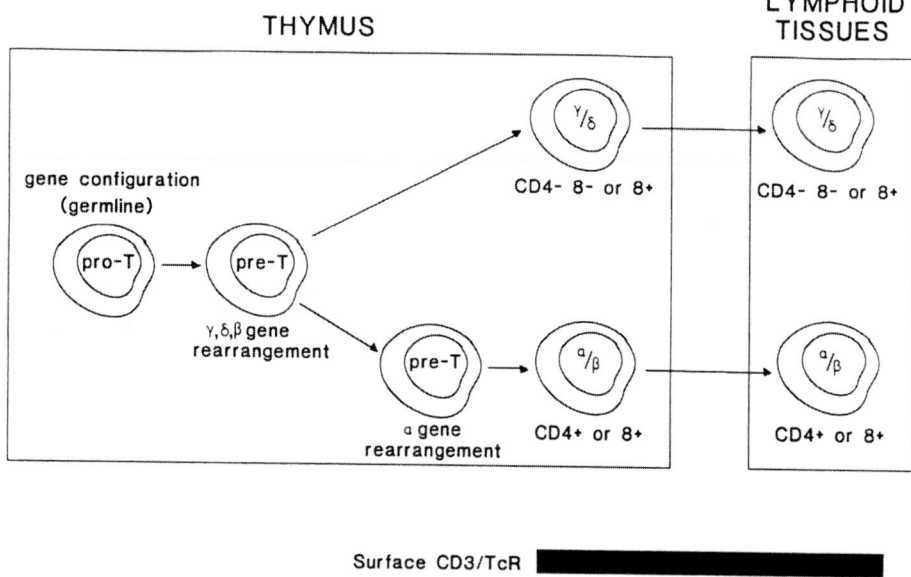

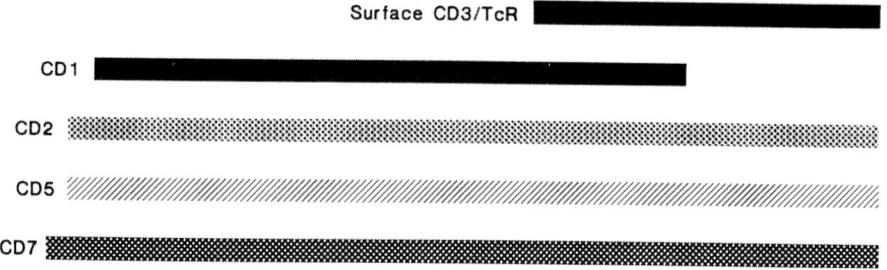

Figure 45-4 Temporal relation among T-cell maturation, differentiation, and cell surface antigen expression.

antigen-specific TCR/CD3 complex allows the helper T cell to recognize antigens combined with antigen-presenting cell surface MHC II molecules. Helper T cells are induced to undergo blast transformation and cell division after interaction with antigen and MHC II molecules on the macrophage and other antigen-presenting cells. T-cell activation leads to the production of a variety of cytokines (e.g., IL-2, IL-3, IL-4, IL-5, IL-6, GM-CSF, IFN-γ, TNF), cell proliferation, and increased cell surface receptor expression (e.g., CD71, IL-2 receptor). Significantly decreased production of IL-4 and IFN-γ by neonatal T cells has been observed after activation (77). T helper cell populations have been further subdivided into Th1 and Th2 subsets. These subsets are identified by their different patterns of cytokine production: Th1 produces IFN-γ, IL-2, TNF-β; Th2 produces IL-4, IL-5, IL-6, IL-9, IL-10, IL-13 (78). The functions of Th1 and Th2 cells appear to correlate with their distinctive cytokine production, i.e., Th1 cells are involved in cell-mediated immune reactions and delayed type hypersensitivity; Th2 cells are involved in antibody production and atopic disease (79).

The T cell population in the cord blood of newborns is skewed largely toward a Th2 phenotype (80). This is the result of the production of Th2 stimulating factors from the placenta that leads to the induction of the cytokines IL-4, Il-5, IL-13, and the reduced production of IFN-γ. The decreased Th1 function during pregnancy is consistent with the survival advantage imparted to the fetus during his/her intrauterine existence. At birth, the lymphocyte system of the neonate is primarily dominated by cells with a Th2 phenotype that results in a suppression of cell-mediated responses. In the early postnatal period, the normal infant continues to show a Th2 skewing, but by the end of the first year (81) there is a shift to Th1 predominance (Fig. 45-5).

Consequently 60% to 70% of normal children exhibit no reactivity to allergens by the age of five years. In contrast, the allergic infant continues to show a prominent Th2 skewing with a delayed acquisition of Th1 function (82) (Fig. 45-5). Studies of cord blood mononuclear cells (CBPM) showed that T cells produce a minimal Th1-like response (83). Further, the diminished capacity of the infant's T cells to produce IFN-γ is not primarily caused by an intrinsic cellular defect. The ability of allergens to induce specific proliferative responses by cord blood mononuclear cells at birth indicates that intrauterine lymphocyte "priming" has occurred. This does not indicate that all newborns who have come into contact with allergens during the prenatal period, and have mounted a specific Th2 immune response, subsequently will become atopic infants. Thus the presence of a specific allergen mediated proliferative response at birth cannot necessarily be considered a predictive marker for the subsequent appearance of allergic illnesses. A study by Prescott and associates (84), showed that future atopics have paradoxically lower values in all types of Th2 cytokines. This suggests that maintenance of a Th2 cytokine pattern would require either the presence of Th2-enhancing stimuli that have a booster effect and/or the lack of down-regulating

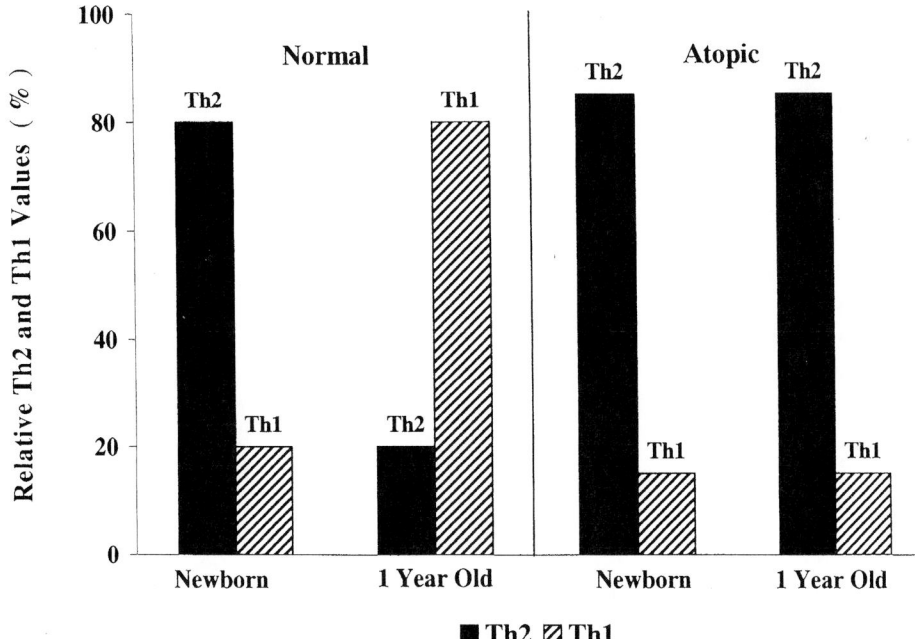

Figure 45-5 Schematic representation of hypothetical changes in Th1 and Th2 values in the normal infant during postnatal development showing the Th2 skewing in early infancy and the acquisition of normal Th1. In contrast, the atopic infant shows the Th2 skewing in early infancy but a delayed acquisition of normal Th1 values. Adapted from Bellanti JA, Malka-Rais J, Castro HJ, Mendez de Inocencio J, Sabra A. Developmental immunology: clinical application to allergy-immunology. *Ann Allergy Asthma Immunol* 2003;90:2, with permission.

stimuli capable of shifting the immune system toward the production of a predominate Th1 type cytokine pattern (85) (Fig. 45-5).

The mechanisms that favor "immune shifting" are not well known. The progressive maturation of the antigen presenting cells, especially dendritic cells, which are immature at birth may play a role. The Th2 skewing in the newborn (86) may in part be the result of the diminished capacity of antigen presenting cells to produce IL-12 at the time of antigen presentation which is necessary to induce T cells to favor their differentiation toward a Th1 phenotype, and NK cells to produce IFN-γ (87). This may result in a production of predominant Th2 cell clones when antigens are presented to the antigen presenting cell system during the immature phase. Subsequent contact with these antigens may predispose to a Th2 response in the first few months of life (Fig. 45-5).

Increase in Atopic Diseases and the Role of Decreased Infection in Industrialized Countries: the Hygiene Hypothesis

In recent years there has been an alarming increase in the prevalence of the atopic diseases, i.e., those which are characterized by a familial predilection and increased IgE production and which include allergic rhinitis, asthma and infantile (atopic) eczema. Although no satisfactory explanation has been found, at least two hypotheses have been offered to explain this increase (88). These include: (a) a change in nutritional patterns or increased exposure to environmental pollutants as a result of our modern technologies and industrialization; and (b) changes in lifestyle in affluent developed countries in which as a result of improved sanitation there has been a reduction in the Th1 inductive influences as a result of minimized exposure

to infectious agents or their byproducts, e.g., endotoxin. One of the earliest observations that supported an antiallergic effect by some infections came from reports suggesting a reduction in allergic disease in children with tuberculosis and following bacillus Calmette-GuC)rin (BCG) immunization. In a study by Shirakawa and associates (89), an inverse correlation between asthma, allergic symptoms, IgE levels and Th2 cytokine production was found with positive tuberculin tests in children at 6 and 12 years of age. Others have been unable to find a beneficial effect of measles or BCG (90,91). It has been reported that exposure to some viral infections very early in life appears to offer some protection against asthma (92), atopic sensitization within the first 12 months of life and children who come from large sibships also are reported to have a decrease in allergies at school (93,94, 95). It has been suggested that in the affluent Western societies, in which infectious disease has decreased, that the Th1-promoting effect of these infections has been lost. This theory is known as the "hygiene hypothesis" and has been proposed to explain the remarkable increases in atopic diseases in these societies (96).

Another important factor that has been identified is bacterial endotoxin, which is a potent stimulator of IL-12 production. In turn, Il-12 elicits IFN-γ production and evokes a Th1 response from naïve helper T cells (97,98). Further evidence for the atopy preventing Th1 favoring effects of endotoxin exposure was shown in a study which reported lower prevalence of atopy in farm-residing children compared with nonfarm-residing children in Germany, Austria and Switzerland (99,100). Additionally, it has been reported that children living in homes, during the first year of life, with 2 or more dogs or cats, known sources of endotoxin, have a decreased risk of atopic sensitization at age 6 to 7 years (101). Thus, in addition to factors which influence the maturation of the antigen presenting cell system in early childhood there are other inductive influences may be responsible for establishing a mature Th1 response and in protecting against early allergic sensitization.

T-cell helper function in newborns is quite low, but it develops almost to adult levels by 6 months of age. T-cell-mediated suppression of immune responsiveness is somewhat higher in the infant than in the adult. The percentage of putative suppressors with the CD8 phenotype is lower in cord blood than in adult blood (102). However, in functional assays, neonatal T cells elicit increased spontaneous suppressor activity compared with adult T cells. Moreover, suppressor T cells exert a strong cytostatic effect on adult B- and T-cell proliferation, probably to prevent graft-vs.-host (GVH) reaction by maternal cells transferred to the fetus. Natural killer CD3-negative CD56-positive cell activity is extremely low in the neonatal period, and it reaches the adult level by between 1 to 5 months of age. Although the percentage of NK cells in the peripheral mononuclear cell population is decreased in neonates, the absolute number of these cytotoxic NK cells is high in infancy and even higher from 1 month to 4 years of age compared with that in adults (103). The increased number of NK cells with adequate cytotoxic abilities present from 1 month to 4 years of age indicates the predominance of NK immunity during infancy to early childhood, in the presence of immaturity in other aspects of immunologic system. In the neonatal period, the decreased NK cell activity predisposes to increased severity of viral infections. As a general rule, T cells acquire immunocompetence (i.e., strong proliferation in mixed lymphocyte culture [MLC] and antigen binding) early during fetal life, even though their functional capacities are not always comparable to those of the adult. Newborns, particularly premature infants, have a significantly lower rate and degree of skin sensitization to dinitrochlorobene (DCNB), and rejection of skin allografts is slower in newborns than in normal adults. Delayed hypersensitivity can be induced in newborns during the first month of life. The newborn's inconsistency in this capacity appears to be caused more by a decreased inflammatory response and macrophage function than by depressed T-cell activity. A depressed T-cell function may be a consequence of neonatal viral infection, hyperbilirubinemia, corticosteroid therapy, or maternal medications taken late during pregnancy. Specific T-cell immunity can result from antigenic exposure in utero to certain antigens such as penicillin, mumps virus, Escherichia coli, diphtheria and tetanus toxoid, and dental plaque in the mother. There are some suggestions that specific CMI can be acquired from the ingestion of T cells contained in colostrum or breast milk or transferred through the placenta. The proliferative capabilities of immature lymphocytes are well developed early in gestation and, at the time of birth, are equal to or may exceed those of adult lymphocytes; the inflammatory response and macrophage functions, however, appear to be impaired in the newborn period.

B-CELL SYSTEM

If the progenitor cells fall under the influence of a second type of microchemical environment, differentiation produces a population of lymphocytes and plasma cells concerned with humoral immunity or antibody synthesis (see Fig. 45-2). This B-cells population comes under the influence of the bursa of Fabricius in birds (104). In humans, bone marrow constitutes one of the equivalents of the bursa, but all available evidence indicates that the human fetal liver is the analog of the bursa of Fabricius in humans. The process of B-cell differentiation from a multipotent stem cell begins in fetal liver between 8 and 9 weeks of gestation, with the appearance of pre-B cells. Pre-B cells have MHC II antigens on their surface and the CD19 receptors (i.e., pan-B cell marker) shown in Fig. 45-6. These cells begin to synthesize the cytoplasmic , the heavy chain of IgM, that later becomes the surface IgM that appears on "baby" or immature B cells. CD21, which is the receptor for complement C3d and Epstein-Barr virus (EBV), also begins to appear on the immature B-cell surface. Although these cells continue to express surface IgM, they begin to express one of the surface immunoglobulins (i.e., IgA, IgG, IgD) shown in Fig. 45-7.

Recently, a new molecular ligand has been described which governs the IgM-IgG isotype class switch referred to as the CD40 receptor (CD40-R) found on the T cells which binds to a CD40 ligand on B cells. A deficiency of the CD40 ligand has been described in hyperimmunoglobulin M syndrome. The CD40 ligand is deficient developmentally in the newborn and accounts for the prominent IgM responses of the fetus and newborn as described below (105,106). After stimulation by antigen, and helper T cells through CD40/CD40 ligand, the immature cells become mature plasma cells or memory cells (107). As in T-cell development, B-cell development involves several cytokines, such as IL-3, IL-4, IL-5, IL-6, and IL-7. These cytokines influence B-cell growth and differentiation but also regulate, with CD40/CD40 ligand interaction, the immunoglobulin class switch and secretion. The cytokines that are responsible for isotype switching from IgM have been partially elucidated; IL-10 induces the switch to IgG1 or IgG3; transforming growth factor induces the switch to IgA1 or IgA2 and IL-4 associated with IL-13 induces the

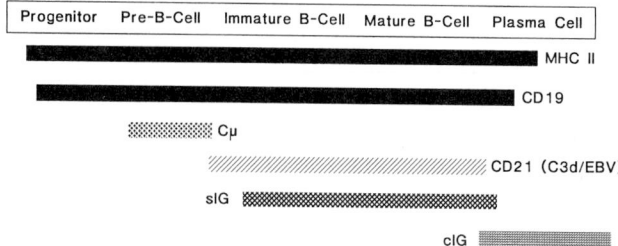

Figure 45-6 Temporal relation among B-cell maturation, differentiation, and cell surface marker or antigen expression, with permission.

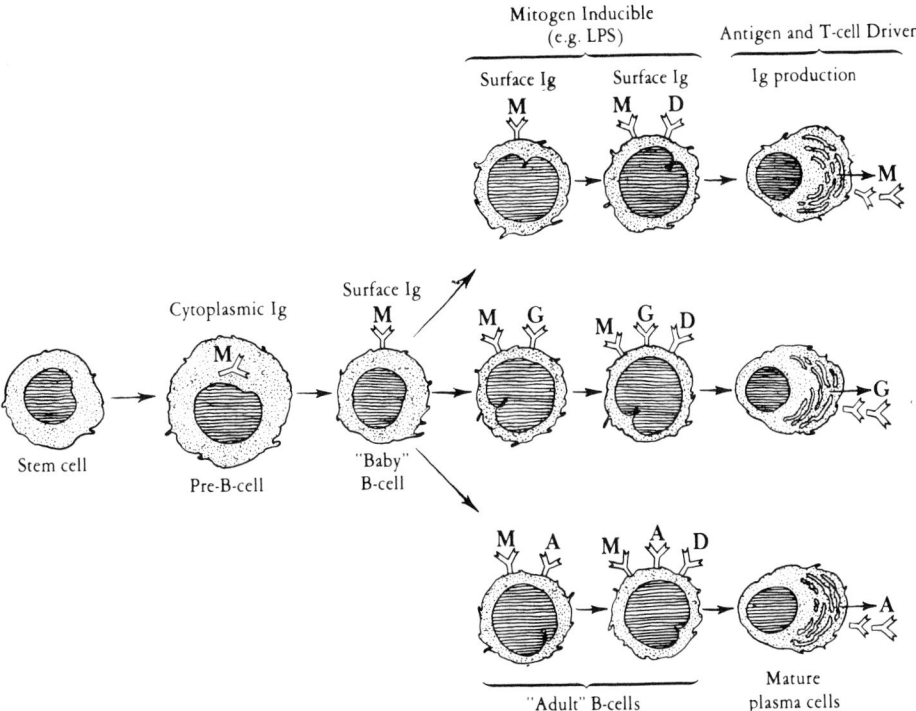

Figure 45-7 Mammalian B-cell differentiation model. B cells differentiate from a stem cell to a rapidly dividing pre-B cell lacking functional antibody receptors. These cells initially synthesize cytoplasmic IgM that later becomes surface IgM (i.e., baby B cells). These baby B cells can easily be made tolerant and are pivotal for further differentiation of immunoglobulin-producing cells. While they continue to express surface IgM, they begin to express one of the surface IgG subclasses or IgA, followed later by the appearance of surface IgD. When these double or triple cells are triggered by antigen, helper T cells, or B-cell mitogens, they become mature plasma cells or memory cells (not illustrated in this figure). The antigen-dependent T-cell-driven stage requires the presence of surface IgD that is lost after antigenic stimulation. (LPS, lipopolysaccharide). Adapted from Cooper MD, Seligmann M. In: Bellanti JA, ed. *Immunology III.* Philadelphia: WB Saunders, 1985, with permission.

switch to IgE and IgG4 (108). IL-6 induces the committed B cells to become a mature immunoglobulin-secreting plasma cell. The first surface immunoglobulin expressed by a B cell is an IgM; at 13 weeks of fetal life, most B cells express IgM and IgD. In the next differentiation step, B-cell clones start to express IgG (i.e., subclasses 1, 2, 3, 4), IgA (i.e., subclasses 1, 2), or IgE. Full-term babies probably have a complete repertoire of B-cell clones, and they can theoretically synthesize each type of immunoglobulin. However, human newborns fail to respond efficiently to all antigens; for example, they are unable to mount an antibody response to polysaccharide antigens. Infants respond to protein antigens (i.e., T-dependent antigens), mainly with IgM production and a slow progression, compared with that of the adult, to IgG response. Children younger than 18 months fail to respond with an IgG2 production to Hemophilus influenzae type b capsular antigen (Hib); this deficient synthesis of IgG2, which is the predominant subclass of antibody against *H. influenzae*, may explain the frequent appearance of H. influenzae infections in young children. The acquisition of adult levels of immunoglobulins is achieved by approximately 1 year of age for IgM, at 5 to 7 years for IgG, and at 10 to 14 years for immunoglobin A (IgA) (109). The reasons for this defective antibody

response are believed to be related in part to diminished expression of CD40 ligand (CD40L) by activated neonatal T cells and decreased production of cytokines. Additionally, the expression of CD40L is a function of age; reduced at birth, increasing during the first few months and reaching a plateau in the second decade. This is reportedly as a result of maturation of the CD4+ subset and has been correlated with expression of CD45RO antigen. Excessive suppressor T-cell activity in newborn blood, defective regulatory cytokine production, and a partial immaturity of the B cell have been suggested as limiting factors in the perinatal response (110,111). The relative deficiency of antibody responses of infants less than 2 years of age to polysaccharide antigens has been overcome by vaccines which utilize carrier proteins with the polysaccharide antigen, e.g., Hib vaccine. The fetal liver occupies the central role in B-cell development, as it probably does in T-cell development. The B cells constitute a much smaller part of the recirculating pool of lymphocytes than the T cells and populate the thymic-independent regions of the lymphoid tissue, including the germinal centers of lymph nodes. Removal of the bursa or its mammalian equivalent leads to a profound deficiency of γ-globulin with little or no effect on CMI (112). Antibody provides a major defense against encapsulated high-grade pyogenic pathogens including *Streptococcus pneumoniae*, *H. influenzae*, and *Neisseria meningitidis*. The development of immunity in the fetus and the newborn must not be considered separate from maternal influences.

The Mucosa-Associated Lymphoid Tissues: Anatomic Organization

It is now generally recognized that there exists in the human, a highly integrated and finely regulated common mucosal immune system referred to as the mucosa-associated lymphoid tissues (MALT), which consists of an extensive network of cells and cell products found on the vast domain of mucosal surfaces which interface with the external environment and which protect us from entry of foreign substances. Although originally conceived of as a "local" immune system only found at body surfaces, separate and distinct from a "peripheral" immune system, it is now clear that the MALT is but one component of a broader unified immune system. The mucosa-associated lymphoid tissues performs immune exclusion by inhibiting colonization of pathogens and penetration of harmful soluble antigens. The neonatal period is particularly criti-

cal because the newborn is immediately exposed to a large number of microorganisms, foreign proteins and chemicals.

Shown in Fig. 45-8 is a schematic representation of the unique features of the MALT and its relationship to the total immunologic system. Immunologically activated T and B lymphocytes derived from the generalized lymphatic drainage are comingled in the lymph with counterpart T and B lymphocytes derived from stimulation at mucosal and skin sites and enter the blood through the thoracic duct. From there, this collection of lymphocytes forms a recirculating pool which can "home" back to their original mucosal sites of sensitization or to other mucosal sites. This recirculating pool of sensitized T and B lymphocytes in the blood can also percolate back into the lymph in primary lymphoid tissues in lymph nodes and other secondary lymphoid tissues at mucosal sites through unique structures called postcapillary venules. Thus, lymphocytes enter the lymph through both the vascular and the lymphatic channels and form a continuously recirculating pool of lymphocytes prepared to function at internal sites and at mucosal surfaces.

Included within MALT are the mucosal surfaces of the gastrointestinal, respiratory and genitourinary systems

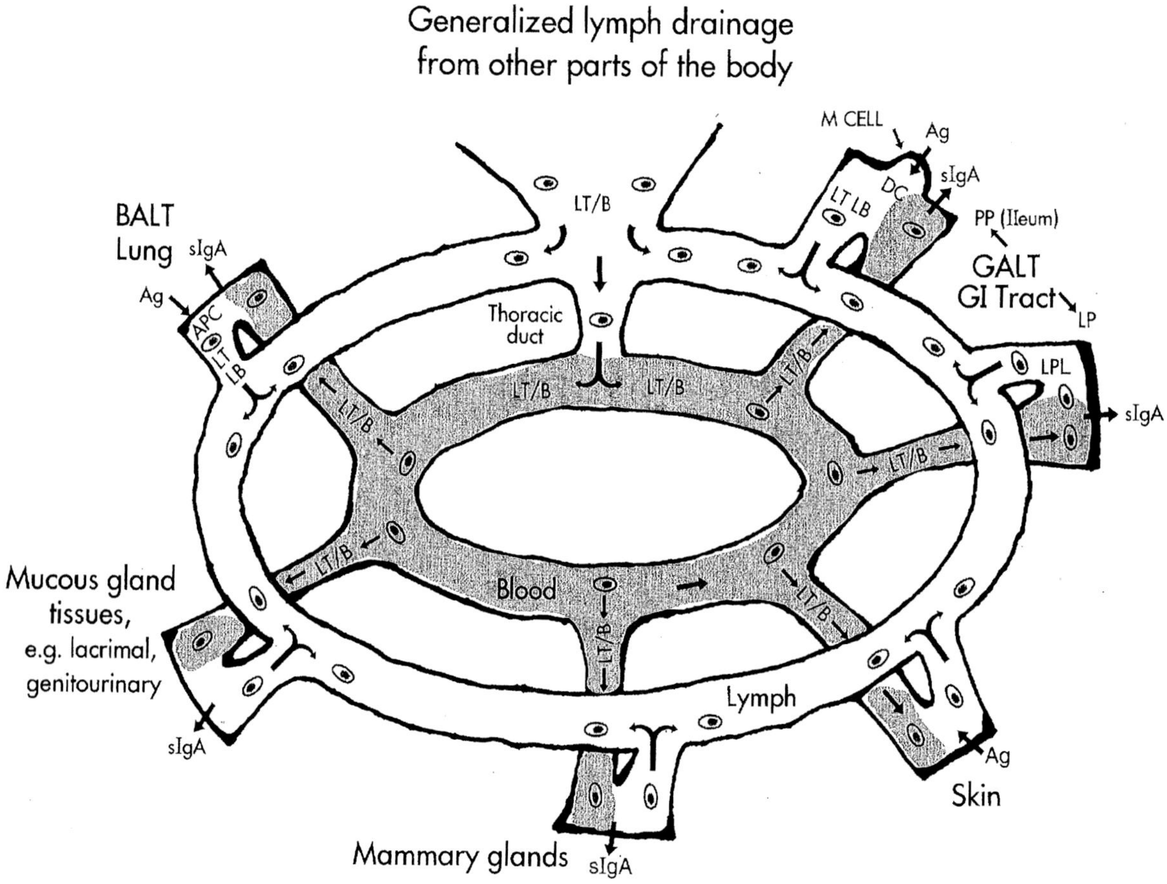

Figure 45-8 Schematic representation of the unique features of the mucosa-associated lymphoid tissues (MALT) and its relationship to the total immunologic system. Reproduced with permission from Bellanti JA, Sabra A, Zeligs BJ, et al. Gastrointestinal Immunopathology. *Ann Allergy Asthma Immunol* 2004; 93:26–32.

and all tissues that interface with the external environment (Fig. 45-8). For ease of discussion, the various components of MALT have been classified into clusters of anatomically organized sites shown in Fig. 45-8 and which include: (a) the gut-associated lymphoid tissues (GALT); (b) the skin-associated lymphoid tissues (SALT); the mammary-associated lymphoid tissues; (c) other mucous gland-secreting tissues, e.g., lacrimal, genitourinary systems; and (d) the bronchus-associated lymphoid tissues (BALT) and the nasopharyngeal-associated lymphoid tissues (NALT).

The Enteromammary Circulation

Lactating mammary glands are another part of the mucosal immune system and in the human participate in a set of remarkable immunologic events which links the inductive sites of the GALT, BALT, and mammary-associated lymphoid tissues of the mother with the effector sites of gut and the upper airways of the breast fed infant (113) (Fig. 45-9).

After initial sensitization to food antigens or microflora found in the GALT and BALT of the mother, primed B and T lymphocytes from Peyer's patches or peribronchial lymphoid tissues leave these sites via lymph and peripheral blood and home to the lactating mammary gland in which local production of secretory antibodies (secretory IgA [sIgA] and secretory IgM [sIgM]) specific for these antigens occurs. Breast milk, therefore, contains a boutique of specialized antibodies resulting from antigenic stimulation in the inductive sites of MALT both in gut and airways of the mother. This has been documented by showing that sIgA from breast milk exhibits antibody specificity for a wide range of common intestinal and respiratory pathogens. The secretory antibodies are thus highly targeted against infectious agents in the mother's environment, which are those likely to be encountered by the infant during its first weeks of life. In addition to its role in infectious disease the benefits of breast feeding in prevention of allergic disease in the infant are well documented. Thus, breast-feeding represents a unique immunological integration of the mucosal immunologic systems of the mother and child, which has biologic significance both in the protection afforded the breast fed infant against infectious disease and in the prevention of allergic disease.

MATERNAL, FETAL, AND NEONATAL INTERACTIONS

In the human, the predominant transfer of antibody occurs by way of the passage of the IgG immunoglobulins from the maternal circulation to that of the fetus. This is accomplished by means of an active transport of this immunoglobulin molecule by virtue of a receptor located on one portion of the molecule referred to as the Fc fragment. In this manner, the fetus receives a library of preformed antibody from his or her mother, reflecting most of her experiences with infectious agents. The sIgA immunoglobulins found in breast milk also

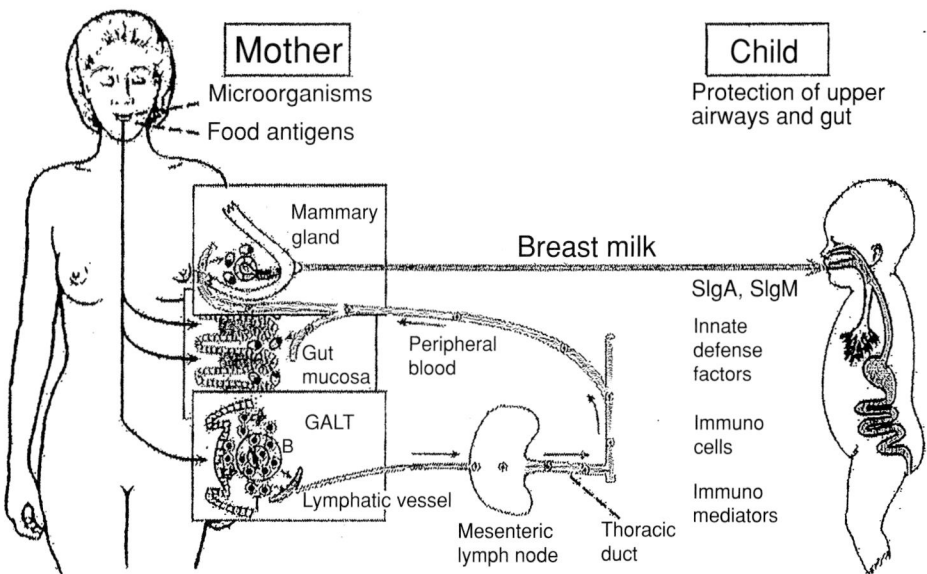

Figure 45-9 Integration of mucosal immunity between mother and the newborn, showing the linkage of the mucosal immunologic systems of the mother and child. After initial sensitization to the food antigens and microflora found in the GI tract of the mother, primed B and T lymphocytes from Peyer's patches leave via lymph and peripheral blood to the lactating mammary gland in which local production of secretory antibodies (SIgA and SIgM) specific for enteric antigens (microorganisms and food proteins) occurs. By this mechanism, the breast-fed infant receives relevant secretory antibodies directed against the antigens found in the maternal GI tract reflecting her intestinal microenvironment and hence the infant is better protected both in the gut and in the upper airways in the same way as the mother's gut mucosa is protected by similar antibodies. Reproduced with permission from Brandtzaeg P. Mucosal immunity: integration between mother and the breast-fed infant. *Vaccine.* 2003;21:3382–3388, with permission.

provide local protection of the mucous membranes of the gastrointestinal tract. Although these antibodies are not absorbed, their unique structure renders them more effective in these sites and may explain the lower incidence of enteric infections seen in breast-fed infants. It has been shown that as much as 11 g of sIgA may be delivered initially to the breast-fed newborn infant in 24 hours, based on total output in the early colostrum. Subsequently, total sIgA output appears to decrease significantly, and between 3 and 50 days postpartum, as much as 3 g of sIgA may be delivered to the breast-fed infant (114). The fate of ingested sIgA has not been clearly defined. A small amount may be absorbed from the intestine and appear in the circulation within the first 24 hours of life (115). Significant numbers of granulocytes, macrophages, and B and T lymphocytes appear in breast milk (116). The B lymphocytes in human milk can produce IgA antibodies. Secretory antibodies in milk are directed against antigens occurring in the gastrointestinal tract: *Escherichia coli*, O. and *K.* antigens, *Shigella O* antigen, *Vibrio cholerae O* antigen, *E. coli* and *V. cholerae* enterotoxins, poliovirus, and rotavirus. There appears to be a direct relation between the extent of intestinal antigenic exposure and the level of specific secretory antibodies in milk. It is possible that, after antigenic stimulation, the lymphoid cells from the Peyer patches of the gastrointestinal tract home by way of the mesenteric lymph nodes and the blood to the mammary gland tissue and appear in the milk. As a result of this homing mechanism, human milk contains secretory IgA antibodies against many microorganisms harbored in the maternal intestine at the time of lactation (i.e., microorganisms that the baby is most likely to be exposed to after birth). Because of the same homing mechanism, human milk contains IgA antibodies to many food protein antigens (e.g., cow-milk

proteins). It is possible, particularly in infants with atopic predisposition, that the frequency and magnitude of food allergy may be decreased by a prolonged period of breast-feeding (117). In the early period of life, when the infant's own secretory IgA system is maturationally deficient, breast-feeding may provide the infant with antibodies that support the local immune defense system. Decreasing the antigenic exposure or influencing the infant immune response by prolonged breast-feeding may prevent or delay the development of atopic disease. Other protective factors are present in human milk, such as lactoferrin, lactoperoxidase, Lacto bacillus bifidus factor, complement components, and leukocytes. Necrotizing enterocolitis, a disease seen primarily in premature infants who have suffered severe perinatal stress, affects predominantly formula-fed infants. Neonatal rats subjected daily to a short period of hypoxia developed a reproducible model of the disease. All animals died as a result of necrotizing enterocolitis if they were formula-fed, but not if breast-fed. The viable macrophages in their breast-feedings appear to have afforded the survivors protection and to have prevented the mortality seen in control animals. However, studies carried out after naturally acquired maternal cytomegalovirus infection or other viral and bacterial infections have demonstrated acquisition of neonatal infections in breast-feeding babies of infected mothers (118). Occasionally, fetal cells or other proteins may gain access to the maternal circulation and actively immunize the mother to the paternal allotypes found on these substances. This process, referred to as isoimmunization, may lead to serious disease in the infant, such as hemolytic disease of the newborn, thrombocytopenia, and leukopenia. The development of serum immunoglobulins during intrauterine life and postnatally is shown in Fig. 45-10. The amount and type

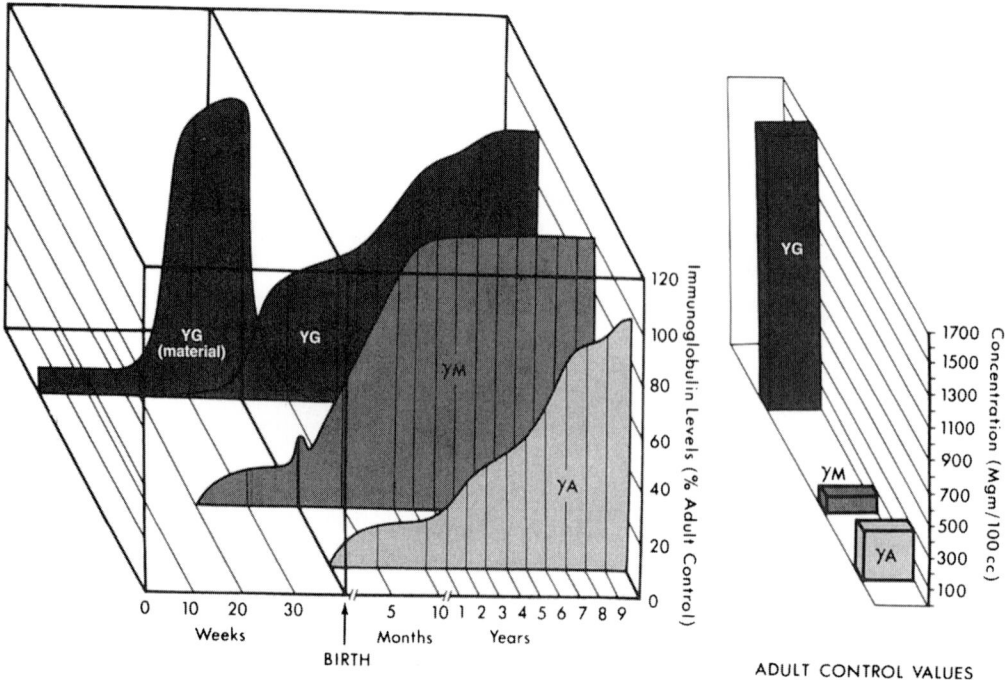

Figure 45-10 Development of serum immunoglobulins in the human during maturation. From Bellanti JA. *Immunology III.* Philadelphia: WB Saunders, 1985:49, with permission.

of -globulin found in the blood of the newborn at birth is higher than those of the mother and are made up almost exclusively of the IgG immunoglobulins. There are few or no IgA and IgM globulins in cord sera because the fetus is usually protected in utero from antigenic stimuli. If challenged *in utero* as a consequence of immunization of the mother with Salmonella vaccine or infection (e.g., congenital rubella, cytomegalic inclusion disease, toxoplasmosis), the fetus responds with antibody production, largely of the IgM variety. The exclusion of other classes of antibody is beneficial to the fetus in many cases. For example, the exclusion of the IgM isohemagglutinins, leukoagglutinins, or the IgE antibodies of allergy prevents disease that may be produced by these antibodies. However, it also prevents the passage of other maternal antibodies that would be beneficial to the newborn, such as the IgM antibodies important in bacterial defense (e.g., opsonins, agglutinins, bactericidal antibodies) against gram-negative bacteria. This may explain the increased susceptibility of the newborn to infection with gram-negative organisms such as *E. coli*. There is great variability in the types of antibodies that are obtained transplacentally by the fetus (Table 45-7). This reflects the quantity of antibodies in the maternal circulation and of their molecular sizes. For example, low-molecular-weight IgG antibodies (e.g., rubeola antibody), present in high concentrations in maternal serum, are readily transferred. IgG antibodies in lower concentrations (e.g., Bordetella pertussis) are poorly transferred, and macroglobulin antibodies (e.g., Wasser mann antibody) are completely excluded. Because the IgG immunoglobulins are passively transferred, they have a finite half-life, between 20 and 30 days, and their concentration in serum falls rapidly within the first few months of life, reaching its lowest level between the second and fourth months. This period is referred to as physiologic hypogammaglobulinemia. During the course of the first few years, the levels of globulin increase because of exposure of the maturing infant to antigens in the environment. There appears to be a sequential development in the -globulins at different rates. The IgM globulins attain adult levels by 1 year of age. Under physiologic conditions, little or no IgA synthesis is observed *in utero*. Plasma cells appear in the intestinal lamina propria of the neonate shortly after birth. IgA is not detectable in the serum or in the secretions during the first 2 to 3 days of life, although IgA is frequently present in the secretions after the fourth day of life. The secretory IgA concentration matures rapidly, reaching adult levels by 4 to 6 weeks of life. Serum IgA levels rise more slowly, and adult levels are observed after 10 to 14 years. This pattern of appearance of immunoglobulins recapitulates that seen in phylogeny and appears to parallel that seen after antigenic exposure during the primary immune response. In addition to providing protection to the newborn, passively acquired IgG antibodies may interfere with active antibody synthesis after immunization procedures. Several studies have confirmed that passively acquired antibody to diphtheria and to pertussis may actually inhibit active antibody formation after active immunization. This occurs in the case of killed vaccines, appears to be dose related, and can be overcome by increasing the inoculum size. In the case of immunization with live virus vaccines, the effect of passively acquired antibody is to neutralize the vaccine virus, inhibiting successful immunization with parenteral live vaccines. Immunization at 2 to 3 months of age with killed vaccines (e.g., diphtheria, pertussis, tetanus) does not appear to be appreciably inhibited by this passive antibody. Live virus immunization procedures are usually delayed until the end of the first year of life because of the inhibitory effect of the passive antibody. Another situation in which passive acquired antibody may interfere with active antibody synthesis is the natural immunity acquired by the newborn infant from breast milk. IgA in breast milk may interfere with successful immunization with live poliovirus vaccines by neutralizing virus in the gastrointestinal tract.

TABLE 45-7

RELATION OF ANTIBODY TYPE AND TRANSPLACENTAL TRANSFER

Good Passive Transfer	Poor Passive Transfer	No Passive Transfer
Diphtheria antitoxin	*Hemophilus influenzae*	Enteric somatic (i.e., O)
Tetanus antitoxin	*Bacillus pertussis*	antibodies (*Salmonella sp.,*
Antierythrogenic toxin	Dysentery	*Shigella sp., Escherichia coli*)
Antistaphylococcal	Streptococcus MG	Skin-sensitizing antibody
antibody		Heterophile antibody
Salmonella flagella (H)		Wasserman antibody
antibody		
Antistreptolysin		
All the antiviral antibodies		
Present in maternal		
circulation (e.g., rubeola,		
rubella, mumps,		
poliovirus)		
VDRL antibodies		

VDRL, venereal disease research laboratory.

TABLE 45-8

MATERNAL ANTIBODIES THAT CAN PRODUCE HARMFUL EFFECTS IN THE INFANT

Maternal Disease	Antibodies	Effect on Infant
Hyperthyroidism	LATS	Transient hyperthyroidism
Idiopathic Thrombocytopenia	Platelet antibodies	Transient thrombocytopenia
Isoimmunization (e.g., platelets, neutrophils, red blood cells)	Platelet, neutrophil, isohemagglutinins, $Rh_O(D)$ antibodies	Transient thrombocytopenia, neutropenia, anemia
Lupus erythematosus	Autoantibodies to blood elements (e.g., LE-cell factor, Coombs test, platelets)	Transient LE-cell phenomenon, neutropenia, thrombocytopenia, congenital heart disease (i.e., AV block)
Myasthenia gravis	Cholinergic receptor antibody	Transient neonatal myasthenia gravis

AV, atrioventricular; LATS, long-acting thyroid stimulator; LE, lupus erythematosus
Adapted from Bellanti JA, ed. *Immunology III.* Philadelphia: WB Saunders, 1985:579, with permission.

Poliovirus immunizations are not usually delayed, even in breast-fed infants, because active immunization follows sequential poliovirus administration according to recommended immunization schedules for infants and children. Maternal antibodies can have harmful effects, as shown in Table 45-8.

Preliminary studies have reported that nucleotides added to human formulas at concentrations similar to that in human milk enhanced the development of the immune system during infancy. (119). Responses to vaccines were evaluated in full term healthy infants receiving milk based control formula with or without nucleotides added and compared with infants fed human milk. The nucleotide group had significantly higher antibody titers to Haemophilus influenzae type b polysaccharide and diphtheria toxoid immunization but responses to tetanus toxoid or oral polio virus immunization were not enhanced.

IMMUNOLOGIC CONSEQUENCES OF INTRAUTERINE INFECTIONS

The possibility of intrauterine infection should be suspected in a newborn infant if there is a known exposure of the mother to an infectious disease during pregnancy or if the infant is small for gestational age or fails to thrive. Manifestations of intrauterine infection include petechiae, hepatosplenomegaly, congenital malformation, inguinal hernia, thrombocytopenia, and unusual skin rash (see Chapter 47). An IgM concentration greater than 20 mg/dL in the cord blood or in the infant serum is considered abnormal. It should be pointed out that an elevated IgM level may be the result of leakage of maternal blood into the fetus; under these circumstances, the infant's IgA level usually exceeds the IgM level, reflecting the IgA-IgM ratio in maternal blood. IgM concentration test repeated after 3 to 4 days disclose a significant fall in the case of maternal transfusion, but the amount of IgM actively synthesized by the newborn will have increased. Congenital infections fre-

quently become chronic and persist for weeks or years with signs and symptoms that are not seen in children or adults with the same infection. The agents that produce persistent infection of the human fetus exhibit a predilection for the reticuloendothelial system. Impaired function of reticuloendothelial cells may be associated with the development of immunodeficiency. In the congenital rubella syndrome, infection results from transmission of the virus from the pregnant mother to the fetus in the first 5 months of gestation. The infection of the child continues after birth for 6 months to 3 years, despite passive antibody acquired from the mother and active antibody synthesis by the infant. After birth, the child may continue to shed virus while making antibody. A variety of abnormal antibody responses have been reported in children with congenital rubella, including increased levels of IgM with low IgG and absent IgA and low levels of IgM with low levels of IgG and absent IgA (120,121). Reports have appeared of poor antibody responses in patients with congenital rubella as determined by delayed appearance of isohemagglutinins, suboptimal vaccine responses, immune paresis with no response to tetanus or Salmonella typhi vaccines, and impaired CMI as demonstrated by impaired lymphoproliferative responses to phytohemagglutinin and decreased lymphocytotoxicity (122,123,124). These abnormal responses have been associated with an increased frequency of infections. Many of the alterations reverted to normal responses later, when the child was no longer excreting virus (125). This could represent a form of immunologic blockade while the child is shedding virus, reversal of which may be linked to the maturity of the immunologic systems. Cytomegalovirus and herpesviruses produce infections that persist for years or throughout life, when infection is acquired in utero. Cell-mediated immunity appears to be particularly important in these infections. In one study, eight infants with congenital cytomegalovirus infection and six of their mothers showed decreased specific CMI (126). The decreased CMI in the mothers may have contributed to the transmission of the infection to the infant. The earlier the infection, the more devastating is the effect on the ontogeny of the immune system. If an insult occurs to the thymus in the first trimester, the normal development of T-cell function is affected; if the insult occurs in the third trimester, no resulting damage should be expected. Viral infection of the fetus may be limited by the degree of cellular immune competence, as exemplified by the infants with proven congenital infection and intact cellular responses who are no longer shedding virus at birth. The cellular competence of the fetus may also modulate the manifestations of intrauterine infection. Intrauterine syphilis, for example, presents in late pregnancy, at which time the body mounts a brisk cellular immune response to the spirochete. Infection occurring early in gestation may go unnoticed because the spirochete has neither a toxic nor a teratogenic effect on the fetus. The spirochete is teratogenic only when the immune response to the organism is activated. In contrast, rubella in very early gestation has primarily teratogenic effects (e.g., congenital defects). In later pregnancy (2–4 months), a primarily inflammatory effect is seen (e.g., hepatitis, iridocyclitis, meningitis). These differences may result from an intact cellular immune response characteristic of the older fetus, but in some cases, the immune response of the child may fail to limit or clear these infections.

IMMUNOLOGIC EVALUATION

The functional significance of the two-compartment system is important in clinical medicine. It provides a useful basis on which understanding of the primary immunodeficiency disorders rests and a framework for a more logical approach to the management of maturational deficiencies in the newborn period. Selective deficiencies of the thymic-independent B system (i.e., agammaglobulinemias) present with recurrent bacterial infections. Selective deficiencies of the thymic-dependent tissues are associated with fungal and viral infections. Patients with combined B- and T-cell defects have the most serious of all the immunodeficiency syndromes, with profound deficiencies in cell-mediated and antibody-mediated functions; they present with a diversity of infections. Evaluation of the immune system during the perinatal period is not an easy task. The evaluator must take into consideration the dynamic, rapidly growing, and adaptive parameters of the immune function in response to a changing internal and external environment. Table 45-9 shows some of the major classes of immunodeficiencies that can be diagnosed in the newborn period, with their time of onset and associated infections. A detailed history, with emphasis on family background and a careful physical examination, should offer a solid foundation for interpretation of clinical and research laboratory data. Table 45-10 presents some suggestions for the clinical evaluation of the newborn. Table 45-11 lists some of the pertinent clinical and historic information that could be useful in the diagnosis of immunodeficiency disorders in the newborn period. Although most

immunologic defects are not clinically apparent until postnatal life, it is not unlikely that in certain instances the result of immunologic deficiency may be intrauterine infection with a resultant damaged baby at birth or an aborted conceptus. Cohen and Zuelzer and others have shown maternal blood-formed elements in fetal circulation (127). Theoretically, early passage of immunologically active mononuclear cells from the mother to the fetus could be responsible for GVH reaction. Although direct proof of GVH reactions in the fetus is lacking, several clinical situations suggest that such processes may occur in the newborn and fetus. Among these can be cited the report of an XX/XY chimerism in a 12-week-old abortus of a mother who had several repeated spontaneous abortions (128). A case was reported by Naiman and colleagues, in which, after three exchange transfusions, the infant developed jaundice, aplastic anemia, and marked histiocytosis (129). This infant also showed chimerism of the mononuclear cells, with one line representing donor cells.

NEONATAL IMMUNE RESPONSE TO HUMAN IMMUNODEFICIENCY VIRUS

The immune response to human immunodeficiency virus (HIV) infection in neonates is described in greater detail in Chapter 47. The complexity of the immune response to HIV infection seen in the adult is equal or greater in the newborn. Human immunodeficiency virus has a tropism for human CD4-positive T cells and bone-marrow-derived dendritic cells, megakaryocytes, cells of monocyte-macrophage lineage, and the macrophage-microglial and endothelial cells of the central nervous system. A characteristic depletion of CD4-positive cell numbers is seen in HIV infections, after which there is a continuous but variable rate of decline of CD4 cells. In adults there is acute loss of CD4-positive T cells around the time of seroconversion and in the late symptomatic phase of disease. There are several proposed mechanisms to explain the depletion of CD4 cells, because infection of the cell is not necessarily cytopathic. One possible mechanism is that discharge of virions may be vigorous enough to disrupt the cell and cause death, depleting cell numbers. Alternatively, expression of viral antigens on the cell surface can result in CMI cytotoxicity. These losses may be compounded by the inability of the bone marrow to respond appropriately to replenish CD4 cells. Because CD4 cells play a pivotal role in many immunoregulatory functions, the loss in these cells is responsible for a reduction in their helper-inducer function and a decrease in other T-cell, B-cell, and monocyte activities, resulting in wide-ranging functional defects in cellular and humoral immunity. Immune dysregulation and innate immune activation are features of HIV disease. Generalized immune activation evidenced by polyclonal hypergammaglobulinemia and elevated activation markers (e.g., $\beta 2$-microglobulin, neopterin) is recognized, and the levels of these activation markers are used to predict disease progression. Human immunodeficiency virus encoding a super-

TABLE 45-9

IMMUNODEFICIENCY DISORDERS THAT CAN BE DIAGNOSED IN THE NEONATAL PERIOD

Disorder	Example	Genetics	Time of Onset	Type of Infection
Phagocytic Cell Disorders				
Quantitative	Neutropenia	Variable	At birth	Virulent bacteria
	Congenital asplenia	Variable	At birth or later	Gram-negative
Qualitative	Chronic granulomatous disease	X-linked, autosomal recessive	At birth	Less virulent bacteria
	Leukocyte adhesion deficiency	Mutation of gene on 21q22.3	At birth, delayed separation of umbilical cord	Virulent bacteria, fungal
Disorders of antibody-forming cells				
	Agammaglobulinemia	Variable	>6 mo of age, earlier if infant is premature or small for dates	Virulent bacteria
Disorders of T-cells and/or B-cells				
T-cell immunodeficiency (i.e., cell-mediated or delayed hypersensitivity)	Catch 22 (Congenital aplasia of thymus), i.e., DiGeorge syndrome, VCFS, conotruncal anomaly	Variable	At birth	Fungal, viral
	Chronic mucocutaneous candidiasis	Sporadic forms, autosomal recessive		Fungal
	Pediatric acquired immunodeficiency syndrome	None	At birth or later	Bacterial, fungal, protozoal, viral, *Pneumocystis Carinii*
Combined B- and T-cell immunodeficiency	Severe combined immunodeficiency	X-linked recessive, autosomal recessive, sporadic forms	6 mo	Bacterial, fungal, viral, *Pneumocystis carinii*
	Cellular immunodeficiency with abnormal immunoglobulins (i.e., Nezelof syndrome)	Variable	Variable	Bacterial, viral, fungal
Complex (i.e., multisystem) immunodeficiencies	Immunodeficiency with ataxia and telangiectasia	Autosomal recessive	>6 mo	Bacterial, viral, fungal
	Immunodeficiency with eczema and thrombocytopenia (i.e., Wiskott-Aldrich syndrome)	X-linked Recessive	>6 mo	Bacterial, fungal, viral, *Pneumocystis carinii*
Disorders of early and late components of complements				
	Deficiency of C1, C2, C4 and later components of complement have been described	Variable	At birth	Gram-negative

antigen has been suggested; this may play a role in the generalized polyclonal activation and subsequent clonal deletion of T cells. One of the most perplexing clinical problems for the pediatrician and neonatologist is the diagnosis of acquired immunodeficiency syndrome in children younger than 15 months of age, because maternal IgG antibody to HIV is passively transferred across the placenta and may persist until 15 to 18 months of age in uninfected infants. Detection of HIV antibody is therefore not reliable for infants younger than 15 months of age. Moreover, viral culture and P24 antigen assays have a low sensitivity (i.e.,

viral culture detects approximately 50% of infected neonates). Although potentially useful, polymerase chain reaction (PCR) assay is limited by the high false positives as a result of contamination or carryover during testing, the complexity of the test and required laboratory facilities, and the cost. With improved quality control, PCR can identify as many as 50% of asymptomatic perinatally infected infants at birth. Viral-specific IgA antibody (i.e., HIV-IgA) immunoblot assay has a high sensitivity (99.4%) and high specificity (99.7%) for children older than 3 months of age but a much lower sensitivity in neonates. As a practical

TABLE 45-10
CLINICAL EVALUATION OF THE IMMUNE SYSTEM IN NEONATES

History
  Previous newborn deaths in the family; history of immune diseases
  Previous isoimmunization in mother (e.g., due to pregnancy or transfusions [Rh, ABO] or to γ-globulin administration)
  Previous diseases in the mother (e.g., autoimmune diseases: SLE, thyroiditis, myasthenia gravis, idiopathic thrombocytopenic purpura)
  History of medications in mother (e.g., quinine, guinidine, Sedormid, chlorpromazine)
  History of infections during pregnancy (e.g., rubella, cytomegalic inclusion diseases, toxoplasmosis, syphilis, herpes simplex, UTI, vaginal infections, TB)
Physical Examination
  General appearance (i.e., assess degree of activity: if there is hyperactivity, consider hyperthyroidism, passive transfer of LATS; if there is hypoactivity or muscle weakness, consider myasthenia gravis with transfer of antibodies to muscle; if there is purpura, consider thrombocytopenia due to the passive transfer of antibodies to platelets)
  Skin (e.g., jaundice in first 24 h of life, petechiae are characteristic of isoimmunization such as erythroblastosis fetalis)
  Eyes (e.g., exopthalmos due to LATS)
  Chest (e.g., pneumonitis seen in many intrauterine infections)
  Cardiovascular (e.g., evaluate for congenital heart disease, congenital heart block in infants of mothers with SLE)
  Abdomen (e.g., hepatosplenomegaly seen in severe erythroblastosis fetalis, in congenital intrauterine infections, in GVH reactions, and in the absence of spleen)
  Extremities (e.g., deformities and other birth defects)
  Neurologic (e.g., convulsions, weakness)

GVH, graft-versus host; LATS, long-acting thyroid stimulator; SLE, systemic lupus erythematous; TB, tuberculosis; UTI, urinary tract infection. From Bellanti JA, ed. *Immunology III.* Philadelphia: WB Saunders, 1985:578, with permission.

TABLE 45-11
DIAGNOSTIC CLUES FOR IMMUNODEFICIENCY DISORDERS IN NEONATES

Findings	Comments
Hypocalcemic tetany Absence of thymic shadow Candidiasis	Catch 22, DiGeorge syndrome-characteristic features are in vitro lymphocyte stimulation with phytohemagglutinin and MLR
History of immunodeficiency in other family members	Most immunologic defects genetically determined; gender-linked most common
Agammaglobulinemia	Quantitative immunoglobulins not useful because of passive transfer of IgG; determination after 2 to 4 mo helpful in establishing diagnosis; allotypes helpful; B-cell (CD19) enumeration
Chronic granulomatous Disease	NBT helpful as screening test only because there may be nonspecific elevation; tests of bactericidal function fail to reach normal values in presence of adult sera
Poor growth, splenomegaly, hepatomegaly, diffuse dermatitis, diarrhea	GVH-laboratory findings include anemia, decrease in serum complement, hysticocytic infiltration of bone marrow, and erythrophagocytosis; skin biopsy shows mummified cells
Howell-Jolly bodies in peripheral smear, absence of spleen, shadow in x-ray film	Congenital absence of spleen and other associated Malformations
Seborrheic dermatitis	C5 deficiency (i.e., Leiner disease)
Chronic diarrhea	Defect in phagocytosis of baker's yeast particles secondary to failure of sera to opsonize yeast

GVH, graft-versus host; MLR, mixed lymphocyte reaction; NBT, nitroblue tetrazine

approach, identification of the infected infant relies on identification of the infected mother, followed by careful clinical and laboratory monitoring of the infant throughout the first year of life. Suggested laboratory tests include serial HIV antibody testing (i.e., ELISA and immunoblot); serial P24 antigen testing; HIV culture; immunoglobulin levels; T-cell numbers and subsets, remembering that neonates have significantly higher T-cell numbers than older children; and one or more other diagnostic techniques (e.g., PCR, HIV-IgA, immunoblot assay). The aim is to diagnose HIV infection before the onset of severe opportunistic infection, especially Pneumocystis carinii pneumonia.

EVALUATION OF THE HUMORAL IMMUNE SYSTEM

Table 45-12 summarizes the evaluation of the humoral immune system. Pure humoral immunodeficiency syndromes are not clinically manifested in the prenatal period because of the protective effect of maternal IgG. However, very premature infants, particularly those born at less than 32 weeks of gestation, may have IgG serum levels below 400 mg/dL. Small-for-gestational-age infants also have decreased IgG, some impairment of specific antibody responses (e.g., to attenuated polio virus), reduction in specific IgG secretory antibody responses, and an increased incidence of antibodies to food (130). Another factor to be considered is hypogammaglobulinemia in the mother, which, although rare, can lead to inadequate levels of IgG in the newborn.

EVALUATION OF THE CELL-MEDIATED IMMUNE SYSTEM

Table 45-13 summarizes the evaluation of the CMI system of the newborn. Evaluation of the CMI system begins with a total and differential leukocyte count. Lymphopenia is seen in most of the CMI deficiencies, but the lymphocyte count may be normal in some patients. The number of T

TABLE 45-12

DIAGNOSTIC TESTS FOR EVALUATION OF THE HUMORAL IMMUNE FUNCTION IN NEONATES

Test	Comment
Practical	
Quantitative measurement of immunoglobulins	May reveal elevated IgM or IgA; does not distinguish maternal from fetally produced IgG
IgG subclass determination	IgG3 increases in prenatal period and reaches adult levels after 3 months; IgG1, IgG2, IgG4 close to adult levels many months (years) later
Determinations of total number B and T cells by CD markers	Does not necessarily correlate with decreased Ig synthesis; helpful to elucidate level of B cell defect
Specialized	
Specific antibody responses de novo sensitization (e.g., Salmonella)	O antigen induces IgM; H antigen induces IgG
Regional lymph node biopsy after immunization	Helpful for humoral as well as CMI

TABLE 45-13

DIAGNOSTIC TESTS FOR EVALUATION OF CELL-MEDIATED IMMUNITY IN NEONATES

Test	Comments
Practical	
WBC and differential	Normal lymphocyte count does not rule out CMI deficiency; low count compatible but not diagnostic
Determination of absolute number of T cell by CD2/CD3 marker; T cell subsets by CD4 and CD8	No functional test but correlates well with CMI status
Mitogen stimulation of lymphocytes, e.g., PHA and/or measurement of cytokine production	Optimal, suboptimal, and overoptimal concentrations of PHA should be used
Specific antigen stimulation of lymphocytes and/or measurement of cytokine production	Previously known exposure required (e.g. Candida)
Specialized	
Skin testing with DNCB	Positive result practically rules out CMI deficiency
Lymph node biopsy after stimulation with de novo organism	To determine whether dependent areas are normal
Biopsy of thymus	To be performed in patients with obvious CMI; helps elucidate different types of CMI deficiencies that could orient new therapeutic measures
MHC I and MHC II antigen expression	Such as bare lymphocyte syndrome (i.e., MHC II deficiency)

cells, B cells, CD4 helper cells, and CD8 suppressor cells can be ascertained by flow cytometry, using specific monoclonal antibody for individual cell markers (e.g., CD3 for T cells, CD19 or CD20 for B cells). In vitro lymphoblastogenic responses of T cells to specific antigens also are informative for host CMI, provided the antigens have been encountered previously (e.g., Candida for a baby with history of thrush). Tests of lymphoproliferative responses should be performed with different concentrations of T-cell mitogens, such as concanavalin A and phytohemagglutinin. Newborn lymphocytes seem to respond better than those of adults at low dosages of mitogens; at higher concentrations, they are less responsive than adult lymphocytes (131). Mixed lymphocyte culture reactions may be helpful in diagnosing CMI deficiencies. A dissociation of low phytohemagglutinin, with normal MLC, can be seen in some patients with CMI deficiency. On the basis of phylogeny and ontogeny, it can be speculated that such a defect originates at a higher level of T-cell differentiation. Lack of MLC responses suggests a defect occurring earlier in ontogenic development. Determinations of enzymes, such as adenine deaminase and nucleoside phosphorylase, may help clarify some of the cases of severe combined immunodeficiency and motivate the clinician to investigate enzyme replacement therapy or possible gene therapy. Skin testing with fungal, bacterial, and viral antigens for delayed hypersensitivity has not proved useful in the newborn. Skin testing with PHA is claimed to be somewhat more sensitive (132). Contact sensitization to DNCB offers advantages over intradermal testing. Dinitrochlorobenzene is positive in 90% of normal persons. Viral infections sometimes depress CMI, and some of the patients who are

referred to us may show anergy because of persistent viral infections. In these cases, sound medical judgment, patience, and repeated studies are necessary. Fetal growth retardation and malnutrition also depress CMI and humoral responses for several months after birth (Error! Bookmark not defined.). Evaluation of the innate immune responses in the newborn is almost limited to testing PMN function with the Rebuck skin-window technique (Table 45-14), which has not yet been standardized for the newborn. The nitroblue tetrazine test may be used as a screening test for CGD; the results should be confirmed by bactericidal assay. Lowered numbers of complement components have been described in the prenatal and cord blood. The extent to which these reflect actual functional abnormalities of complements is uncertain. Phagocytic tests should include evaluation of influences of C3 and C5. Separate evaluation of the complement effects on phagocytosis, chemotaxis, and bactericidal activities must be made. A functional deficiency of C5 activity has been described in Leiner disease. Monocyte function, although important, is not usually clinically evaluated because of a lack of adequate methods. Poplack and colleagues have shown that in humans, ADCC activity

TABLE 45-14

DIAGNOSTIC TESTS FOR POLYMORPHONUCLEAR LEUKOCYTE FUNCTION IN NEONATES

Test	Comment
Peripheral blood count and differential	Often of help, count important (e.g., neutropenia); morphology of cells important (e.g., Chediak-Higashi syndrome)
Rebuck skin window	May give general clue to defect of inflammatory function, particularly ability to marshal leukocytes to site of infection
Phagocytosis	Results vary with assay used; particle being phagocytized critical; assay used must distinguish humoral and cellular components of process
Chemotaxis	Decreased in cellular and humoral activity during neonatal period
Quantitative NBT	Screening test; if normal or high, does not rule out CGD
Flow cytometry for cell surface markers	Can detect absence of CD11 for diagnosis of LAD1 or absence of CD15 for LAD2; can detect CGD by employing rhodamine dye assay
Bactericidal activity	Measured by direct killing assay; CGD can be diagnosed during neonatal period
Measurement of specific leukocyte Enzymes	Not done routinely

against erythrocytes depends only on the monocyte (133). It is hoped that this test will prove significant in the evaluation of the monocyte in the fetus and newborn infant.

IMMUNOLOGIC THERAPY

Because newborn infants are less immunologically competent than adults and premature infants are even more susceptible to serious infections than full-term infants, several replacement therapies have been tried with variable results.

PREVENTION OF INFECTION IN LOW BIRTH WEIGHT INFANTS

There is little transport of maternal IgG to the fetus before 32 weeks of gestation, and endogenous synthesis does not begin until about 24 weeks after birth (134,135,136,137). In low-birth-weight infants, serum IgG levels by 3 months of age are only 60 to 150 mg/dL, compared with 100 to 350 mg/dL for infants born at term (138,139,140). It is reasonable to consider intravenous immunoglobulin (IVIG) prophylaxis in premature infants. Some pilot studies indicated a lower rate of severe infection in IVIG-treated low birth weight infants compared with placebo-treated

patients (141,142,143,144). In a randomized, double-blind, placebo-controlled trial involving 588 infants with birth weights of 500 to 1750 g, mortality was not significantly reduced among IVIG recipients (145). However, the number of infections was significantly reduced among IVIG recipients. There was some evidence that the beneficial effect may vary by birth-weight category, and significantly more placebo patients were small for gestational age. Information about long-term results (less than 56 days) is not available from this trial. Preliminary analysis of other trials indicates no significant differences in infection rates between IVIG recipients and placebo recipients (146,147). Another multicenter, randomized, controlled trial, involving more than 2000 neonates with birth weights between 500 and 1500 g, has been completed (148). Intravenous immunoglobulin was initiated at less than 72 hours of age, and continued every 2 weeks until hospital discharge or a weight of 1.8 kg. No significant difference was seen in the rate of nosocomial infection or in the mortality rate between control and treated groups.

The disparity in these results may be as a result of several variables. For instance, these studies are complicated by the fact that multiple factors contribute to the predisposition to infection in premature neonates and that different predominant pathogens occur in different nurseries. There are differences in the titers of antibodies to various pathogens, especially GBS infection, in different lots of IVIG preparations. Moreover, differences in the study design and IVIG dosage and schedule make direct comparison of the various trials difficult. At this time, IVIG cannot be recommended as standard prophylaxis for low-birth-weight infants.

TREATMENT OF PRESUMED NEONATAL INFECTION

Small trials using primarily historic controls have yielded mixed results. Questions remain concerning dose, schedule, and patient selection. Sidiropoulos and colleagues treated successively admitted infants suspected of neonatal sepsis with antibiotics or antibiotics plus IVIG (0.5–1.0 g/day for 6 days) (149). A reduction of mortality was found. Two of 20 infants treated with antibiotics plus IVIG died, compared with 4 of 15 infants treated with antibiotics alone (10% vs. 26%; $p = 0.16$). Among premature infants weighing less than 2500 g, IVIG made a significant difference. Four (44%) of 9 patients who received antibiotics alone died, compared with 1 (9%) of the 11 who received antibiotics plus IVIG ($p < 0.05$). Haque and associates studied 60 preterm infants of 28–37 weeks of gestation who were suspected of having bacterial sepsis (150). One-half of the group was treated with antibiotics alone and one-half was treated with antibiotics plus IgM-enriched IVIG. The doses were 190 mg/kg/day of IgG and 30 mg/kg/day of IgM for 4 days. Six (20%) of the 30 infants who received antibiotics alone died, compared with 1 (3.3%) of the 30 who received antibiotics plus IVIG, a statistically significant difference.

Christensen and associates used IVIG plus antibiotics in neonates with clinical signs of sepsis. They found IVIG recipients to have a more rapid correction of neutropenia, a more rapid appearance of immature neutrophils in the peripheral circulation suggesting release of neutrophils from marrow storage pools, and an increase in arterial oxygen tension compared with control infants receiving albumin (151). There were no deaths in either group, and no difference in mortality rates were observed. These studies suggest, but do not prove, that IVIG is a valuable form of therapy in septic premature newborns.

GROUP B STREPTOCOCCAL INFECTION

Group B streptococcal infection is one of the serious diseases in the newborn period. The use of IVIG in this condition has been addressed by Fischer (152,153,154) and Santos (155). Some of these preparations are opsonic for multiple strains of group B streptococci in vitro and protect animals against experimental GBS disease. Such passively administered IgG could ensure that premature infants who are at high risk of infection or already ill are protected by antibody to group B streptococci, even if little of it has been obtained transplacentally. However, not all GBS strains are uniformly susceptible to opsonization by antibody to group B streptococci. Lot-to-lot variation in antibody activity to group B streptococci has been observed. To ensure that an appropriate quantity of antibody is administered, screening of immunoglobulin lots for functional activity and pharmacokinetic studies in neonates are necessary. Studies by Hill and colleagues indicated that administration of IVIG in neonatal rats improved the outcome of GBS pneumonia and sepsis by increasing opsonization and by enhancing PMN migration (156). The mechanisms of these actions are unclear, but antibody may prevent neutrophil depletion by localizing bacteria to the lung in which they can be phagocytized by pulmonary leukocytes and may generate inflammatory mediators, causing the release of PMNs from the marrow (157,158). Combined use of other plasma factors may provide even better protection against bacterial pathogens. Neonatal rats with GBS infection had significantly lower mortality rates if given IVIG and fibronectin than if given fibronectin alone. If IVIG is used, it seems reasonable to normalize the IgG level to between 700 and 1000 mg/dL, using frequent infusions and determination of IgG levels. A dose of 100 mg/kg usually raises serum IgG by about 100 mg/dL.

An alternative method of transferring specific GBS antibody to the newborn by maternal immunization in late gestation (30–32 weeks) has been extensively investigated by Baker, Rench, and McInnes (159) who found that a GBS-tetanus-conjugate vaccine elicited good levels of functional antibody in mothers and their infants in whom levels persisted for at least 2 months. Recently, although the commonly used practice of intrapartum antimicrobial prophylaxis has been successful in lowering the incidence of early onset GBS sepsis, there are concerns that this prophylactic use of antibiotics may raise the incidence of non-GBS antimicrobial-resistant infection (160).

SPECIFIC ANTIBODY REPLACEMENT THERAPY

Variability in IVIG preparations and lots creates several difficulties in predicting results of treatment for specific organisms. There is a potential role for directed preparations containing specific antibodies. Intravenous immunoglobulin apparently has minimal short-term side effects or complications. Nevertheless, large, multicenter studies must be completed before possible long-term problems such as hepatitis or inhibition of subsequent antibody synthesis can be identified or ruled out. The fact that IVIG has known immunomodulating properties should be kept in mind when one is considering its use in persons without antibody deficiency (161). Passively administered antibodies are potent antigen-specific immunosuppressive agents, as illustrated by the high degree of efficacy of Rho(D) immune globulin (RhoGAM) in preventing sensitization of Rh-negative women to the Rh-D antigen on the erythrocytes of their Rh-positive fetuses. Recent studies in patients with systemic vasculitis demonstrated a 51% decrease in antineutrophil cytoplasm antibodies after high-dose therapy with IVIG, and this decrease was maintained during follow-up (162). Although there are no controlled clinical studies of the suppression of immune responses to other antigens by passively administered antibody, there is no reason to believe that antibodies to the Rh-D and neutrophil cytoplasm antigens are unique in this regard. There is evidence from animal and in vitro studies that IVIG can suppress antibody formation, T-cell proliferation and the activity of NK cells (163,164,165,166,167). In addition to the masking of antigens, IVIG has many potential mechanisms for suppressing the immune response, including interaction with Fc receptors on the membranes of various cells of the immune system and the combination of antiidiotypic antibodies with antibody-producing cells or secreted antibodies (168). Antiidiotypic antibodies in IVIG could impair the capacity of B cells from even immune hosts to secrete antibody. Blockade of the Fc receptor by high doses of IVIG, as in the treatment of idiopathic thrombocytopenic purpura, or by the formation of immune complexes of IVIG with antigens could also impair the normal clearance of opsonized infectious agents and lead to overwhelming infection. There are many reasons not to administer IVIG unless there is a demonstrated broad antibody-deficiency state or other accepted clinical indications. Furthermore, studies in neonatal animals have shown that, in some situations, survival rates are reduced with high concentrations of IVIG plus antibiotic compared with antibiotic alone. The routine use of IVIG as adjuvant therapy of neonatal infections cannot be recommended at this time (169).

SUMMARY OF RECENT CONSIDERATIONS CONCERNING THE USE OF INTRAVENOUS IMMUNOGLOBULIN IN NEONATAL SEPSIS

A review of studies of IVIG therapy by Weisman and associates (170) reports that although it is safe, the studies do not prove efficacy in treatment or prevention of neonatal bacterial infection. It suggests that pathogen-specific antibody IVIG products are required and larger and more careful trials need to be performed. In support of this, a more recent report of the safety and efficacy of monthly prophylaxis with respiratory syncytial virus immune globulin (RSV-IVIG) showed positive results. This was a randomized study of 510 children with bronchopulmonary dysplasia and/or prematurity. The children received 750 mg/kg of RSV-IVIG or placebo intravenously every 30 days. The results suggest that monthly administration was safe well tolerated and reduced the hospitalization by 41% in children receiving RSV-IVIG treatment (171). Following this study the use of RSV-IVIG was approved by the FDA for prevention of severe RSV infections in infants younger than 24 months with bronchopulmonary dysplasia or history of premature birth (172).

ACTIVE IMMUNIZATION OF PREGNANT WOMEN

Although the results of specific antibody replacement therapies seems promising, the availability and delay of the initiation of therapy (i.e., using it only when the condition is clinically suspected) are of concern. If pregnant women could be safely immunized at the beginning of the third trimester, producing high levels of protective antibody which then cross the placental barrier, this would probably give protection to neonates early enough to significantly decrease the incidence of the infection. Group B streptococcal sepsis develops in approximately 3 neonates per 1000 live births, resulting in approximately 11,000 cases annually in the United States. Mortality and morbidity from these infections continue to be substantial (173,174, 175,176). Because human immunity to group B streptococci correlates with type-specific anticapsular antibodies and low levels of these antibodies predict susceptibility to invasive disease, to actively immunize women with capsular polysaccharide antigens of group B streptococci to stimulate production of type-specific, IgG antibody for transplacental protection of the fetus might be a valuable therapeutic or prophylactic approach (177,178, 179,180). Baker and associates immunized 40 pregnant women, at a mean gestation of 31 weeks, with a single 50 g dose of the type III capsular polysaccharide of group B streptococci (181). Twenty-five women (63%) responded to the vaccine. Of the infants born to these women, 80% continued to have protective levels of antibody (e.g., IgG-specific antibody, 2 g/mL) at 1 month of age, and 64% had protective levels at 3 months. Serum samples from infants with

2 g/mL of antibody to type III group B streptococci uniformly promoted efficient opsonization, phagocytosis, and bacterial killing in vitro of type III strains. This effect may be mediated exclusively by the alternative complement pathway. Although this vaccine, with an overall response rate of 63%, is not optimally immunogenic, this study suggests that maternal immunization is feasible and can provide passive immunity against systemic infection with type III group B streptococci in most newborns. Larger trials with better vaccines are required to evaluate the safety and clinical effectiveness of this strategy.

USE OF RECOMBINANT HUMAN GRANULOCYTE-COLONY STIMULATING FACTOR OR GRANULOCYTE-MACROPHAGE COLONY-STIMULATING FACTOR

Recently several studies have investigated the use of recombinant human granulocyte-colony stimulating factor (rh G-CSF) or recombinant human granulocyte-macrophage colony-stimulating factor (rh GM-CSF) in newborn infants with presumed sepsis. This is based on the reported lower levels of these cytokines in the premature infant and an inability of the mononuclear cells of the neonate to produce significant amounts after stimulation (182,183). The first study consisted of 42 newborn infants 26 to 40 weeks of age with presumed bacterial sepsis within 3 days of life which were randomized to receive either placebo or varying doses of rh G-CSF, i.e., 1, 5, or 10 micrograms/Kg every 24 hours or 5 or 10 micrograms/Kg every 12 hours. The results showed that rh G-CSF was well-tolerated and induced a significant dose dependent increase in peripheral blood and bone marrow absolute neutrophil concentration and in C3bi expression. A 2-year follow-up of neonates treated with rh G-CSF showed that there were no associated long term adverse effects (184). In a second study, 20 very low birth weight (VLBW) neonates 72 hours old were randomized to receive either placebo or rh GM-CSF at varying doses intravenously per day. The results revealed that in infants receiving rh GM-CSF there was a significant increase in the circulating absolute neutrophil count and their C3bi receptor expression and monocyte count. In addition there was a significant increase in bone marrow absolute neutrophil concentration. One important consideration for the use of G-CSF or GM-CSF in the prevention of neonatal infection is that the use of these cytokines alone only stimulates an increase in phagocytic cell numbers. This may not be sufficient, and prevention may require the use of antimicrobial specific antibody and/or complement, e.g. fresh plasma, as a source of opsonins. A recent review of clinical trials employing G-CSF and GM-CSF for treatment or prevention of neonatal infections by Carr, Modi and Dore, although promising, concluded that there is currently insufficient evidence to support the introduction of either modality into neonatal practice (185).

PLASMA COMPONENT TRANSFUSION

Neonates have significant impairment in humoral and cellular immune factors. Augmentation of deficient humoral factors by transfusion of transfer factor, fresh frozen plasma, antibody, or whole blood has been protective in humans or neonatal animals with infection 186,187,188,189,190,191,192,193,194). Because of the extensive interaction between cellular and humoral factors, the positive effect of these therapies is thought to be produced, at least partially, by their improvement of neonatal neutrophil function. One study showed that replacement of humoral factors and PMNs is superior to replacement of humoral factors alone. Transfer factor is a dialyzable extract from human leukocytes with chemoattractant activity. The results of its use in patients with chemotactic defects vary. Some investigators found that transfer factor corrected the PMN chemotactic defect in patients with candidiasis and the hyper-IgE syndrome, but others found that it suppressed PMN function in several patients with the hyper-IgE syndrome. Fresh frozen plasma contains antibody, complement, fibronectin, and other proteins that help protect against infection and have been found to be deficient in the neonate, especially the premature infant (195,196,197). Fresh frozen plasma infusions are commonly given to neonates with hypotension and are well tolerated. A preliminary study suggests that fresh frozen plasma transfusions improve PMN chemotaxis in newborn infants. Whether this improvement results in decreased morbidity or mortality from infection is unknown.

NEUTROPHIL TRANSFUSION THERAPY

Bone marrow reserve for PMN in neonates is limited, and bone marrow pool exhaustion during neonatal infection is common. The most direct way to correct the impairment in neonatal PMN function and reserve is to transfuse adult PMNs into newborn infants. Several studies of the efficacy of the use of transfused adult PMNs in human neonates with sepsis have produced varying results (198,199,200,201,202,203). The first clinical trial of PMN transfusion in human neonates was carried out by Laurenti and associates. In this nonrandomized study, the mortality rate was 10% in the transfused group and 72% in the nontransfused group. No untoward effects of the transfusions were observed. The striking improvement in morbidity and mortality rates in the transfused group suggested that PMN transfusions could benefit septic newborns. Christensen and colleagues carried out a prospective trial of adult PMN transfusion in 26 septic neutropenic neonates. Ten neonates with moderate or no depletion of their marrow PMN reserve did not receive PMN transfusion, and none died. Eight (89%) of 9 neonates with severe depletion of marrow PMN reserve who did not receive PMN transfusion died. These data indicate that septic neutropenic neonates with normal marrow PMN reserve who are given standard antibiotic and supportive care are likely to survive without PMN transfusion. In contrast, septic neutropenic neonates with severe marrow PMN depletion have a high mortality rate despite antibiotics and supportive care and can probably benefit from adult PMN transfusions. Two studies of the use of transfusion of PMNs from whole blood buffy coat layers failed to demonstrate a beneficial effect in septic neonates. Baley and associates conducted a prospective, randomized, controlled trial of PMN transfusions for septic neonates that failed to demonstrate any improvement in survival. Several researchers have recommended bone marrow examination before neonatal PMN transfusion to detect bone marrow exhaustion. Neonates with marrow exhaustion have a poor prognosis and may benefit most from PMN transfusion. Because this procedure is invasive and delays delivery of PMNs to neonates with fulminant infection, a rapid, accurate, and easily performed test to document marrow exhaustion would be useful. There are several potential problems associated with PMN transfusion. Polymorphonuclear leukocyte sequestration in the lung, resulting in pulmonary decompensation (e.g., decreased PaO_2), occurs in adults and children (204,205). Graft vs. host disease has been reported after PMN transfusion in the immunocompromised host (206). Irradiation of leukocytes with minimum of 3000 cGy should be sufficient to impair lymphocyte function and prevent GVH disease without altering PMN number and function. Human immunodeficiency virus transmission from PMN transfusion is another potential concern. Although minimized with current antibody screening programs, an estimated 1 in 100,000 to 1,000,000 units of antibody-negative blood may contain transmissible virus as a result of recent HIV infection in the donor (207). It is unknown if the risk of HIV transmission is greater with PMN transfusion than with whole blood or packed cell transfusions. Cytomegalovirus, EBV, and hepatitis virus are other infectious agents that may be transmitted by PMN transfusion. Use of one of the recipient's parents, preferably the mother, as the PMN donor minimizes the risk of viral transmission. Although the results of studies of PMN transfusion in neonates appear promising, large prospective randomized trials must be carried out before it can be concluded that the potential benefits of PMN transfusion outweigh the risks. Polymorphonuclear leukocyte transfusion cannot be recommended for routine adjunctive therapy of neonatal sepsis at this time (208). Polymorpho-nuclear leukocyte transfusion can be considered for the subgroup of septic neonates with neutrophil storage pool depletion, because this group of high-risk infants appear to be the most likely to benefit. Although the use of granulocyte transfusions has been hampered by limitation in collecting adequate quantities of leucocytes, recently the potential use of G-CSF to stimulate normal donor production of granulocytes has stimulated renewed interest and may address this drawback (209).

REFERENCES

1. Metchnikoff E. *Immunity in infective diseases.* London: Cambridge University Press, 1905.
2. Bellanti JA. *Immunology III.* Philadelphia, WB Saunders, 1985.
3. Kavelaars A, Zijlstra J, Bakker J, et al. Increased dexamethasone sensitivity of neonatal leukocytes: different mechanisms of glucocorticoid inhibition of T cell proliferation in adult and neonatal cells. *Eur J Immunol* 1995;25:1346.
4. Bellanti JA, Zeligs BJ, MacDowell AL. The maternal-neonatal interaction: role of gender and hormonal effects on the maturational deficiency in newborn phagocytic cell function. *Pediatr Res* 1997;41:745.
5. Bakwin, H. The sex factor in infant mortality. *Hum Biol* 1920;1:90.
6. Ciocco, A. Sex differences in morbidity and mortality. *Q Rev Biol* 1940;15:59.
7. Schlegel RJ, Bellanti JA. Increased susceptibility of males to infection. *Lancet* 1969;ii:826.
8. Washburn TC, Medearis DN, Childs B. Sex differences in susceptibility to infection. *Pediatrics* 1965;35:57.
9. Ohlsson A, Wang E, Myhr T, et al. The interaction of maternal smoking in pregnancy and newborn sex on total white blood cell counts (TWBC) and total neutrophil counts (TNC) in the first 24 hours (HRS) of life. *Pediatr Res* 1997;40:218A.
10. Motley D, Meyer MP, King RA, et al. Determination of lymphocyte immunophenotypic values for normal full-term cord blood. *Am J Clin Pathol* 1996;105:38.
11. Afoke AO, Eeg-Olofsson O, Hed J, et al. Seasonal variations and sex differences of circulating macrophages, immunoglobulins and lymphocytes in healthy school children. *Scand J Immunol* 1993;37:209.
12. Terres G, Morrison SL, Habicht GS. A quantitative difference in immune response between male and female mice. *Proc Soc Exp Biol Med* 1968;127:664.
13. Baker CJ. Group B streptococcal infections in newborns. *Pediatr Rev* 1979;64:5.
14. McCracken GH, Mize SG. A controlled study of intrathecal antibiotic therapy in gram-negative enteric meningitis of infancy. *J Pediatr* 1976;89:66.
15. Polin RA. Role of fibronectin in diseases of newborn infants and children. *Rev Infect Dis* 1990;12:428.
16. Vogel SN, Nogan MM. Role of cytokines in endotoxin-mediated host responses. In: Opperheim JJ, Shevach EM, eds. *Immunophysiology. The role of cells and cytokines in immunity and inflammation.* New York: Oxford University Press, 1990:238.
17. Christensen RD, Bradley PP, Rothstein G. The leukocyte left shift in clinical and experimental neonatal sepsis. *J Pediatr* 1981;98:101.
18. Christensen RD, Rothstein G, Anstall HB, et al. Granulocyte transfusions in neonates with bacterial infection, neutropenia, and depletion of mature marrow neutrophils. *Pediatrics* 1982;70:1.
19. Krause PJ, Herson VC, Eisenfeld L, et al. Enhancement of neutrophil function for treatment of neonatal infections. *Pediatr Infect Dis J* 1989;8:362.
20. Playfair JHL, Wolfendale MR, Kay HEM. The leukocytes of peripheral blood in the human foetus. *Br J Hematol* 1963;9:336.
21. Cartwright GE, Athens JW, Wintrobe MM. The kinetics of granulopoiesis in normal man. *Blood* 1964;24:780.
22. Erdman SH, Christensen RD, Bradley PP, et al. The supply and release of storage neutrophils: a developmental study. *Biol Neonate* 1982;41:132.
23. Christensen RD, Hill HR, Rothstein G. Granulocyte stem cell (CFUc) proliferation in experimental group B streptococcal sepsis. *Pediatr Res* 1983;17:278.
24. Abramson JS, Wheeler JG, Quie PG. The polymorphonuclear phagocytic system. In: Stiehm, ER, ed. *Immunologic disorders in infants and children.* Philadelphia: WB Saunders, 1989.
25. Anderson DC, Hughes BJ, Edwards, M, et al. Impaired chemotaxigenesis by type III group B streptococci in neonatal sera: relationship to diminished concentration of specific anticapsular antibody and abnormalities of serum complement. *Pediatr Res* 1983;17:496.
26. Miller ME. Phagocytic function in the neonate: selected aspects. *Pediatrics* 1979;64(Suppl):709.
27. Mohandes AE, Touraine JL, Osman M, et al. Neutrophil chemotaxis in infants of diabetic mothers and in preterms at birth. *J Clin Lab Immunol* 1982;8:117.
28. Sacchi F, Rondini G, Mingrat G, et al. Different maturation of neutrophil chemotaxis in term and preterm newborn infants. *J Pediatr* 1982;101:273.
29. Anderson DC, Becker, Freeman KL, et al. Abnormal stimulated adherence of neonatal granulocytes: impaired induction of surface MAC-1 by chemotactic factors or secretagogue. *Blood* 1987;70:740.
30. Anderson DC, Hughes BJ, Smith CW. Abnormal mobility of neonatal polymorphonuclear leukocytes. *J Clin Invest* 1981; 68:683.
31. Bruce MC, Baley JE, Medvik K, et al. Impaired surface membrane expression of C3bi but not C3b receptors on neonatal neutrophils. *Pediatr Res* 1987;21:306.
32. Krause PJ, Maderazo EG, Scroggs M. Abnormalities of neutrophil adherence in newborns. *Pediatrics* 1982;69:184.
33. Miller MH. Cell elastimetry in the study of normal and abnormal movement of human neutrophils. *Clin Immunol Immunopathol* 1979;14:502.
34. Nunoi H, Endo F, Chikazawa S, et al. Chemotactic receptor of cord blood granulocytes to the synthesized chemotactic peptide N-formyl-methionyl-leucyl-phenylalanine. *Pediatr Res* 1983; 17:57–6.
35. Olson TA, Ruymann FB, Cook BA, et al. Newborn polymorphonuclear leukocyte aggregation: a study of physical properties and ultrastructure using chemotactic peptides. *Pediatr Res* 1983;17:993.
36. Yasui K, Masuda M, Matsuoka T, et al. Abnormal membrane fluidity as a cause of impaired functional dynamics of chemoattractant receptors on neonatal polymorphonuclear leukocytes: lack of modulation of the receptors by a membrane fluidizer. *Pediatr Res* 1988; 24:442.
37. Klein RB, Fischer TJ, Gard SE, et al. Decreased mononuclear and polymorphonuclear chemotaxis in human newborns, infants and young children. *Pediatrics* 1977;60:467.
38. Miller ME. Chemotactic function in the human neonate: humoral and cellular function. *Pediatr Res* 1971;5:487.
39. Berger M. Complement deficiency and neutrophil dysfunction as risk factors for bacterial infection in newborns and the role of granulocyte transfusion in therapy. *Rev Infect Dis* 1990;12[Suppl 4]: S401.
40. Roth P, Polin RA. Adherence of human newborn infants' monocytes to matrix-bound fibronectin. *J Pediatr* 1992;121:285.
41. Miller ME. Phagocytosis in the newborn infant: humoral and cellular factors. *J Pediatr* 1969;74:255.
42. Varis I, Deneys V, De Bruyère M, et al. TNF-α and IL-1β production in cord blood monocytes. *Bone Marrow Transplant* 2000; 25(Suppl 1):S146.
43. Gallin JI. Interferon-γ in the management of chronic granulomatous disease. *Rev Inf Dis* 1991;13:973.
44. Ambruso DR, Altenburger KM, Johnston RB Jr. Defective oxidative metabolism in newborn neutrophils: discrepancy between superoxide anion and hydroxyl radical generation. *Pediatrics* 1979;64:722.
45. Newburger PE. Superoxide generation by human fetal granulocytes. *Pediatr Res* 1982;16:373.
46. Shigeoka AO, Charette RP, Wyman ML, et al. Defective oxidative metabolic responses of neutrophils from stressed neonates. *J Pediatr* 1981;98:392.
47. Falloon J, Gallin JI. Neutrophil granules in health and disease. *J Allergy Clin Immunol* 1986;77:653.
48. Wright WC Jr, Ank BJ, Herbert J, et al. Decreased bactericidal activity of leukocytes of stressed newborn infants. *Pediatrics* 1975; 56:578.
49. Stein M, Keshav S. The versatility of macrophage. *Clin Exp Allergy* 1992;22:19.
50. Marodi L, Leijh PCJ, Van Furth R. Characteristics and functional capacities of human cord blood granulocytes and monocytes. *Pediatr Res* 1984;18:1127.
51. Wilson CB, Haas JE. Cellular defenses against Toxoplasma gondii in newborns. *J Clin Invest* 1984;73:1606.
52. Wilson CB, Lewis DB. Basis and implications of selectively diminished cytokine production in neonatal susceptibility to infection. *Rev Infect Dis* 1990;12(Suppl 4):S410.
53. Blaese RM. Macrophages and the development of immunocompetence. In: Bellanti JA, Dayton DH, eds. *The phagocytic cell in host resistance.* New York: Raven Press, 1975:309.
54. Weston WL, Carson BS, Barkin RM, et al. Monocyte-macrophage function in the newborn. *Am J Dis Child* 1977;131:1291.

55. Gitlin D, Biasucci A. Development of gamma G, gamma M, beta 1c, beta 1a, C1 esterase inhibitor, ceruloplasmin, transferrin, hemopexin, haptoglobin, fibrinogen, plasminogen, alpha-1-antitrypsin, orosomucoid, beta-lipoprotein, α2-macroglobin and pre-albumin in the human conceptus. *J Clin Invest* 1969;48:1433.

56. Propp RP, Alper CA. C3 synthesis in the human fetus and lack of transplacental passage. *Science* 1968;162:672.

57. Zimmerman GA, Prescott SM, McIntyre TM. Endothelial cell interactions with granulocytes: tethering and signaling molecules. *Immunol Today* 192;13:93.

58. English K, Burchett S, English J, et al. Production of lymphotoxin and tumor necrosis factor by human neonatal mononuclear cells. *Pediatr Res* 1988;24:717.

59. Weatherstone K, Rich E. Tumor necrosis factor/cachectin and interleukin-1 secretion by cord blood monocytes from premature and term neonates. *Pediatr Res* 1989;25:342.

60. Lee SM, Suen Y, Chang L, et al. Decreased interleukin-12 (IL-12) from activated cord versus peripheral blood mononuclear cells and upregulation of interferon-γ, natural killer, and lymphokine-activated killer activity by IL-12 in cord blood mononuclear cells. *Blood* 1996;88:945.

61. Zola H, Fusco M, Weedon H, et al. Reduced expression of the interleukin-2-receptor chain on cord blood lymphocytes: relationship to functional immaturity of the neonatal immune response. *Immunology* 1996;87:86.

62. Zola H, Fusco M, Macardle PJ, et al. Expression of cytokine receptors by human cord blood lymphocytes: comparison with adult blood lymphocytes. *Pediatr Res* 1995;38:397.

63. Silverstein A, Uhr J, Kramer K, et al. Fetal response to antigenic stimulus: II. Antibody production by the fetal lamb. *J Exp Med* 1963;117:799.

64. Froman ML, Stiehm ER. Impaired opsonic activity but normal phagocytosis in low birth-weight infants. *N Engl J Med* 1969;281:926.

65. Buckley RH. The T-, B-, and NK-cell system. In: Behrman RE, Kliegman RM, Jenson HB, eds. *Nelson textbook of pediatrics*, 17th ed. Philadelphia: Saunders-Elsevier, 2004:683.

66. August CS, Berkel AJ, Driscoll B, et al. Onset of lymphocyte function in the human fetus. *Pediatr Res* 1971;5:539.

67. Stites DP, Carr MC, Fudenberg HH. Development of cellular immunity in the human fetus: dichotomy of proliferative and cytotoxic responses of lymphoid cells to phytohemagglutinin. *Proc Natl Acad Sci U S A* 1972;69:1440.

68. Boyd RL, Hugo P. Towards an integrated view of thymopoiesis. *Immunol Today* 1991;12:71.

69. Finkel TH, Kubo RT, Cambier JC. T-cell development and transmembrane signaling: changing biological responses through an unchanging receptor. *Immunol Today* 1991;12:79.

70. Nikolic-Zugic J. Phenotypic and functional stages in the intrathymic development of αβT cells. *Immunol Today* 1991;12:65.

71. Carding SR, Hayday AC, Bottomly K. Cytokines in T-cell development. *Immunol Today* 1991;12:239.

72. Low TL, Goldstein AL. Thymic hormones: an overview. *Methods Enzymol* 1985;116:213.

73. Goldstein G, Scheid M, Boyse EA, et al. Thymopoietin and bursopoietin: induction signals regulating early lymphocyte differentiation. *Cold Spring Harbor Symp Quant Biol* 1977;41:5.

74. Leana-Cox J, Pangkanon S, Eanet KR, et al. Familial DiGeorge/velocardiofacial syndrome with deletions of chromosome area22q11.2: report of five families with a review of the literature. *Am J Med Genet* 1996;65:309.

75. Bastian J, Law S, Vogler L, et al. Prediction of persistent immunodeficiency in the DiGeorge anomaly. *J Pediatr* 1989;115:391.

76. Hong R. The DiGeorge anomaly. *Immunodef Rev* 1991;3:1.

77. Lew DB, Yu CC, Meyer J, et al. Cellular and molecular mechanisms for reduced interleukin 4 and interferon- production by neonatal T cells. *J Clin Invest* 1991;87:194.

78. Romagnani S, Parronchi P, D'Elios MM, et al. An update on human Th1 and Th2 cells. *Int Arch Allergy Immunol* 1997;113:153.

79. Mosmann TR, Sad S. The expanding universe of T-cell subsets: Th1, Th2 and more. *Immunol Today* 1996;17:138.

80. Prescott SL, Macaubas C, Holt BJ, et al. Transplacental priming of the immune system to environmental allergens: universal skewing of initial T cell responses toward the Th2 cytokine profile. *J Immunol* 1998;160:4730.

81. Reen DJ. Activation and functional capacity of human neonatal CD4 T-cells. *Vaccine* 1998;16:1401.

82. Bellanti JA, Malka-Rais J, Castro HJ, et al. Developmental immunology: clinical application to allergy-immunology. *Ann Allergy Asthma Immunol* 2003;90S:2.

83. Ridge JP, Fuchs EJ, Matzinger P. Neonatal tolerance revisited: turning on newborn T cells with dendritic cells. *Science* 1996; 271:1723.

84. Prescott SL, Macaubas C, Smalla Combe T, et al. Development of allergen-specific T cell memory in atopic and normal children. *Lancet* 1999;353:196.

85. Jones CA, Holloway JA, Warner JO. Does atopic disease start in foetal life? *Allergy* 2000;55:2.

86. Lee SM, Suen Y, Chang L, et al. Decreased interleukin-12 (IL-12) from activated cord versus adult peripheral blood mononuclear cells and upregulation of interferon-gamma, natural killer, and lymphokine-activated killer activity by IL-12 in cord blood mononuclear cells. *Blood* 1996;88:945.

87. Martinez F. Maturation of immune response at the beginning of asthma. *J Allergy Clin Immunol* 1999;103:355.

88. McGeady SJ Immunocomptetence and allergy. *Pediatrics* 2004; 113:1107.

89. Shirakawa T, Enomoto T, Shimazu S, et al. The inverse association between tuberculin responses and atopic disorder. *Science* 1997;275:77.

90. Paunio M, Heinonen OP, Virtanen M, et al. Measles history and atopic diseases: a population-based cross-sectional study. *JAMA* 2000;283:343.

91. Alm JS, Lilja G, Pershagen G, et al. Early BCG vaccination and development of atopy. *Lancet* 1997;350:400.

92. Illi S, von Mutius E, Lau S, et al. Early childhood infectious diseases and the development of asthma up to school age: a birth cohort study. *BMJ* 2001;322:390.

93. Strachan DP, Harkins LS, Johnston ID, et al. Childhood antecedents of allergic sensitization in young British adults. *J Allergy Clin Immunol* 1997;99:6.

94. von Mutius E, Martinez FD, Fritzsch C, et al. Skin test reactivity and number of siblings. *BMJ* 1994;308:692.

95. Svanes C, Jarvis D, Chinn S, et al. Childhood environment and adult atopy: results from the European Community Respiratory Health Survey. *J Allergy Clin Immunol* 1999;103:415.

96. Strachan DP. Hay fever, hygiene, and household size. *BMJ* 1989; 299:1259.

97. von Mutius E. Environmental factors influencing the development and progression of pediatric asthma. *J Allergy Clin Immuno* 2002;109:S525.

98. Liu AH. Endotoxin exposure in allergy and asthma: reconciling a paradox. *J Allergy Clin Immunol* 2002;109:379.

99. Riedler J, Braun-Fahrlander C, Eder W, et al. Exposure to farming in early life and development of asthma and allergy: a cross-sectional survey. *Lancet* 2001;358:1129.

100. Braun-Fahrlander C, Riedler J, Herz U, et al. Environmental exposure to endotoxin and its relation to asthma in school-age children. *N Engl J Med* 2002;347:869.

101. Ownby DR, Johnson CC, Peterson EL. Exposure to dogs and cats in the first year of life and risk of allergic sensitization at 6 to 7 years of age. *JAMA* 2002;288:963.

102. Haywood AR, Loyword L, Lyslyard PM, et al. Fc receptor heterogeneity of human suppressor T cells. *J Immunol* 1978;121:1.

103. Yabuhara A, Kawai H, Komiyama A. Development of natural killer cytotoxicity during childhood: marked increases in number of natural killer cells with adequate cytotoxic abilities during infancy to early childhood. *Pediatr Res* 1990;28:316.

104. Cooper MD, Lawton AR. The mammalian "bursa equivalent": does lymphoid differential along plasma cell lines begin in the gut-associated lymphoepithelial tissues (GALT) of mammals? In: Hanne MG, ed. *Contemporary topics in immunobiology*. New York: Plenum Press, 1972:49.

105. Brugnoni D, Airo P, Graf D, et al. Ontogeny of CD40L expression by activated peripheral blood lymphocytes in humans. *Immunol Lett* 1996;49:27.

106. Nonoyama S, Penix LA, Edwards CP, et al. Diminished expression of CD40 ligand by activated neonatal T cells. *J Clin Invest* 1995;95:66.

107. Lindhout E, Koopman G, Pals ST, et al. Triple check for antigen specificity of B cells during germinal centre reactions. *Immunol Today* 1997;18:573.

108. Caligaris-Cappio F, Ferranini M. B cells and their fate in health and disease. *Immunol Today* 1996;17:206.

109. Rosen FS, Cooper MD, Wedgewood RJP. The primary immuno-deficiencies. *N Engl J Med* 1984;311:235.
110. Andersson U, Bird G, Britton S. Cellular mechanisms of restricted immunoglobulin formation in the human neonate. *Eur J Immunol* 1980;10:888.
111. Gathings WE, Kubagawa H, Cooper MD. A distinctive pattern of B cell immaturity in perinatal human. *Immunol Rev* 1981;57:107.
112. Cooper MD, Lawton AR, Kincade PW. A two stage model for development of antibody producing cells. *Clin Exp Immunol* 1972;2:143.
113. Brandtzaeg P. Mucosal immunity: integration between mother and the breast-fed infant. *Vaccine* 2003;21:3382.
114. Losonsky GA, Ogra PL. Development of immunocompetence in the products of lactation. In: Ogra PL, ed. *Monograph on neonatal infections: nutritional and immunologic interactions.* New York: Grune & Stratton, 1983:48.
115. Ogra SS, Weintraub D, Ogra PL. Immunologic aspects of human colostrum and milk. III. Fate and absorption of cellular and soluble components in the gastrointestinal tract of newborns. *J Immunol* 1977;119:245.
116. Smith EV, Goldman AS. The cell of human colostrum: I. In vitro studies of morphology and functions. *Pediatr Res* 1968;2:103.
117. Hanson LA, Ahlstedt S, Carlsson B, et al. Secretory IgA antibodies against cow's milk proteins in human milk and their possible effect in mixed feeding. *Int Arch Allergy Appl Immunol* 1977;54:457.
118. Ogra PL, Greene HL. Human milk and breast feeding: an update on the state of the art. *Pediatr Res* 1982;16:266.
119. Pickering LK, Granoff DM, Erickson JR, et al. Modulation of the immune system by human milk and infant formula containing nucleotides. *Pediatrics* 1998;101:242.
120. Alford CA Jr. Studies on antibody in congenital rubella infections. *Am J Dis Child* 1965;110:455.
121. Bellanti JA, Artenstein MS, Olson LC, et al. Congenital rubella: clinicopathologic, virologic, and immunologic studies. *Am J Dis Child* 1965;110:464.
122. Fuccillo DA, Steele RW, Henson SA, et al. Impaired cellular immunity to rubella virus in congenital rubella. *Infect Immun* 1974;9:81.
123. Michaels RH. Suspension of antibody response in congenital rubella. *J Pediatr* 1972;80:583.
124. South MA, Montgomery JR, Rowls WE. Immune deficiency in congenital rubella and other viral infections. *Birth Defects Orig Artic Ser* 1975;9:234.
125. Stern LM, Forbes IJ. Dysgammaglobulinemia and temporary immune paresis in case of congenital rubella. *Aust Paediatr J* 1975;77:38.
126. Rola-Pleszczynski M, Frenkel LD, Fuccillo DA, et al. Specific impairment of cell-mediated immunity in mothers and infants with congenital infection due to cytomegalovirus. *J Infect Dis* 1977;135:386.
127. Cohen F, Zuelzer WW. Mechanism of isoimmunization. II. Transplacental passage and postnatal survival of fetal erythrocytes in heterospecific pregnancy. *Blood* 1967;30:796.
128. Taylor AI, Polani PE. XX/XY mosaicism in man. *Lancet* 1965;1:1226.
129. Naiman TL, Punnet HH, Lischner HW, et al. Possible graft-versus-host-reaction after intrauterine transfusion for Rh erythroblastosis fetalis. *N Engl J Med* 1969;281:697.
130. Chandra RH. Fetal malnutrition and postnatal immunocompetence. *Am J Dis Child* 1975;129:450.
131. Stites DP, Wybran J, Carr MC, et al. Development of cellular immunocompetence in man. In: Porter R, Knight J, eds. *Ontogeny of acquired immunity. Ciba Foundation symposium.* Amsterdam, North Holland: Elsevier, 1972:113.
132. Bonforte RJ, Topilsky M, Siltzbach LE, et al. Phytohemagglutinin skin test: a possible in vivo measure of cell-mediated immunity. *J Pediatr* 1972;81:775.
133. Poplack DG, Bonnard GD, Holiman BJ, et al. Monocyte-mediated antibody-dependent cellular cytotoxicity: a clinical test of monocyte function. *Blood* 1976;48:809.
134. Ballow M, Cates KL, Rowe JC, et al. Development of the immune system in very low birth weight (less than 1500 g) premature infants: concentrations of plasma immunoglobulins and patterns of infections. *Pediatr Res* 1986;20:899.
135. Hobbs JR, Davis JA. Serum-globulin levels and gestational age in premature babies. *Lancet* 1967;1:757.
136. Stiehm ER. Role of immunoglobulin therapy in neonatal infections: where we stand today. *Rev Infect Dis* 1990;12(Suppl):S439.
137. Yoder MC, Polin RA. Immunotherapy of neonatal septicemia. *Pediatr Clin North Am* 1990;33:481.
138. Noya FJD, Rench MA, Courtney JT, et al. Pharmacokinetics of intravenous immunoglobulin in very low birth weight neonates. *Pediatr Infect Dis J* 1989;8:759.
139. Noya FJD, Rench MA, Garcia-Prats JA, et al. Disposition of an immunoglobulin intravenous preparation in very low birth weight neonates. *J Pediatr* 1988;112:278.
140. Sasidharan P. Postnatal IgG levels in very-low-birth weight infants: preliminary observations. *Clin Pediatr (Phila)* 1988;27:271.
141. Buaael JB. Intravenous gammaglobulin in the prophylaxis of late sepsis in very-low-birth weight infants: preliminary results of a randomized, double-blind, placebo-controlled trial. *Rev Infect Dis* 1990;12(Suppl):s2457.
142. Chiricl G, Rondini G, Plebani A, et al. Intravenous gammaglobulin therapy for prophylaxis of infection in high-risk neonates. *J Pediatr* 1987;110:437.
143. Clapp DW, Kliegman RM, Baley JE, et al. Use of intravenously administered immune globulin to prevent nosocomial sepsis in low birth weight infants: report of a pilot study. *J Pediatr* 1989;115:973.
144. Haque KN, Zaidi MH, Haque SK, et al. Intravenous immunoglobulin for prevention of sepsis in preterm and low birth weight infants. *Pediatr Infect Dis* 1986;5:622
145. Baker CJ, Melish ME, Hall RT, et al. Intravenous immune globulin for the prevention of nosocomial infection in low-birth-weight neonates. *N Engl J Med* 1992;327:213.
146. Magny J-F, Bremard-Oury C, Brault D, et al. Intravenous immunoglobulin therapy for prevention of infection in high-risk premature infants: report of a multicenter, double-blind study. *Pediatrics* 1991;88:437.
147. Stabile A, Sopo SM, Romanelli V, et al. Intravenous immunoglobulin for prophylaxis of neonatal sepsis in premature infants. *Arch Dis Child* 1988;63:441.
148. Fanaroff A, Wright E, Korones S, et al. A controlled trial of prophylactic intravenous immunoglobulin (IVIG) to reduce nosocomial infection (N.I.) in VLBW infants. *Pediatr Res* 1992;33: 202A(abst).
149. Sidiropoulos D, Boehme U, Von Muralt G, et al. Immunoglobulin supplementation in prevention or treatment of neonatal sepsis. *Pediatr Infect Dis* 1986;5:s193.
150. Haque KN, Zaidi MH, Bahakim H. IgM-enriched intravenous immunoglobulin therapy in neonatal sepsis. *Am J Dis Child* 1988;142:1293.
151. Christensen RD, Brown MS, Hall DC, et al. Effect on neutrophil kinetics and serum opsonic capacity of intravenous administration of immune globulin to neonates with clinical signs of early-onset sepsis. *J Pediatr* 1991;118:606.
152. Fischer GW, Hemming VG, Hunter KW, et al. Intravenous immunoglobulin in the treatment of neonatal sepsis: therapeutic strategies and laboratory studies. *Pediatr Infect Dis* 1986;5:S171.
153. Fisher GW, Hunter KW, Wilson SR. Modified human immune serum globulin for intravenous administration: in vitro opsonic activity and in vivo protection against group B streptococcal disease in suckling rats. *Acta Paediatr Scand* 1982;71:639.
154. Fisher GW, Hunter KW, Wilson SR, et al. The role of antibody in group B streptococcal disease. In: Alving BM, Finlayson JS, eds. *Immunoglobulins: characteristics and uses of intravenous preparations.* vol 1. Washington DC: US Government Printing Office, 1980:81.
155. Santos JI, Shigeoka AO, Rote NS, et al. Protective efficacy of a modified immune serum globulin in experimental group B streptococcal infections. *J Pediatr* 1981;99:873.
156. Hill HR, Shigeoka AO, Pineus S, et al. Intravenous IgG in combination with other modalities in the treatment of neonatal infection. *Pediatr Infect Dis* 1986;5:S180.
157. Hall RT, Shigeoka AO, Hill HR. Serum opsonic activity and peripheral neutrophil counts before and after exchange transfusion in infants with early onset Group B streptococcal septicemia. *Pediatr Infect Dis* 1983;2:356.
158. Stiehm ER. Intravenous immunoglobulins in neonates and infants: an overview. *Pediatr Infect Dis* 1986;5:S217.
159. Baker CJ, Rench MA, McInnes P. Immunization of pregnant women with Group B streptococcal type III capsular polysaccharide-tetanus conjugate vaccine. *Vaccine* 2003;21:3468.
160. Alarcon A, Pena P, Salas S, et al. Neonatal early onset Escherichia coli sepsis: trends in incidence and antimicrobial resistance in

the era of intrapartum antimicrobial prophylaxis. *Pedatr Infect Dis J* 2004;23:295.

161. Dwyer JM. Intravenous therapy with gamma globulin. *Adv Intern Med* 1987;32:111.

162. Jayne DRW, Davies MJ, Fox CJV, et al. Treatment of systemic vasculitis with pooled intravenous immunoglobulin. *Lancet* 1991; 337:1137.

163. Bussel J, Pahwa S, Porges A, et al. Correlation of in vitro antibody synthesis with the outcome of intravenous γ-globulin treatment of chronic idiopathic thrombocytopenic purpura. *J Clin Immunol* 1986;6:50.

164. Engelhard D, Waner JL, Kapoor N, et al. Effect of intravenous immune globulin on natural killer cell activity: possible association with autoimmune neutropenia and idiopathic thrombocytopenia. *J Pediatr* 1986;108:77.

165. Hashimoto F, Sakiyama Y, Matsumoto S. The suppressive effect of gammaglobulin preparations on in vitro pokeweed mitogen-induced immunoglobulin production. *Clin Exp Immunol* 1986; 65:409.

166. Kawada K, Terasaki PI. Evidence of immunosuppression by high-dose gammaglobulin. *Exp Hematol* 1987;15:133.

167. Stohl W. Cellular mechanisms in the in vitro inhibition of pokeweed mitogen-induced B cell differentiation by immunoglobulin for intravenous use. *J Immunol* 1986;136:4407.

168. Bussel JB. Intravenous immunoglobulin therapy for the treatment of idiopathic thrombocytopenic purpura. *Prog Hemost Thromb* 1986;8:103.

169. NIH Consensus Conference. Intravenous immunoglobulin. *JAMA* 1990;264:3189.

170. Weisman LE, Cruess DF, Fischer GW. Standard versus hyperimmune intravenous immunoglobulin in preventing or treating neonatal bacterial infections. *Clin Perinatol* 1993;20:211.

171. The PREVENT Study Group. Reduction of respiratory syncytial virus hospitalization among premature infants and infants with bronchopulmonary dysplasia using respiratory syncytial virus immune globulin prophylaxis. *Pediatrics* 1997;99:93.

172. American Academy of Pediatrics Committee on Infectious Disease, Committee on Fetus and Newborn. Respiratory syncytial virus immune globulin intravemous: indication for use. *Pediatrics* 1997;99:645.

173. Baker CJ, Edwards MS. Group B streptococcal infections. In: Remington JS, Klein JO, eds. *Infectious diseases of the fetus and newborn infant.* 2nd ed. Philadelphia: WB Saunders 1983: 820.

174. Dillon HC Jr, Khare S, Gray BM. Group B streptococcal carriage and disease: a 6-year prospective study. *J Pediatr* 1987;110:31.

175. Institute of Medicine, National Academy of Sciences. *New vaccine development: establishing priorities. vol 1. Diseases of importance in the United States.* Washington, DC: National Academy Press, 1985:424.

176. Wald ER, Bergman I, Taylor HG, et al. Long-term outcome of group B streptococcal meningitis. *Pediatrics* 1986;77:217.

177. Baker CJ, Kasper DL. Correlation of maternal antibody deficiency with susceptibility to neonatal group B streptococcal infection. *N Engl J Med* 1976;294:753.

178. Baker CJ, Kasper DL, Tager IB, et al. Quantitative determination of antibody to capsular polysaccharide in infection with type III strains of group B streptococcus. *J Clin Invest* 1977;59:810.

179. Boyer KM, Gotoff SP. Prevention of early-onset neonatal group B streptococcal disease with selective intrapartum chemoprophylaxis. *N Engl J Med* 1986;314:1665.

180. Stewardson-Kreiger PB, Albrandt K, Nevin T, et al. Perinatal immunity to group B beta-hemolytic Streptococcus type Ia. *J Infect Dis* 1977;136:619.

181. Baker CJ, Rench MA, Edwards MS, et al. Immunization of pregnant women with a polysaccharide vaccine of Group B streptococcus. *N Engl J Med* 1988;319:1180.

182. Cairo MS, Christensen R, Sender LS, et al. Results of a phase I/II trial of recombinant human granulocyte-macrophage colony-stimulating factor in very low birthweight neonates: significant induction of circulatory neutrophils, monocytes, platelets, and bone marrow neutrophils. *Blood* 1995;86:2509.

183. Gillan ER, Christensen RD, Suen Y, et al. A randomized, placebo-controlled trial of recombinant human granulocyte colony-stimulating factor administration in newborn infants with presumed sepsis: significant induction of peripheral and bone marrow neutrophilia. *Blood* 1994;84:1427.

184. Rosenthal J, Healey T, Ellis R, et al. A two-year follow-up of neonates with presumed sepsis treated with recombinant human granulocyte colony-stimulating factor during the first week of life. *J Pediatr* 1996;128:135.

185. Carr R, Modi N, Dore C. G-CSF and GM-csf for treating or preventing neonatal infections. *Cochrane Database Syst Rev* 2003; 3:CD003066.

186. Bortulussi R, Fischer GW. Opsonic and protective activity of immunoglobulin, modified immunoglobulin and serum against neonatal E. coli K1 infection. *Pediatr Res* 1986;20:175.

187. Eisenfeld L, Krause PJ, Herson VC, et al. *Enhancement of neonatal polymorphonuclear leukocyte (PMN) motility with adult fresh frozen plasma (FFP).* Abstract 1409. Washington, DC: The Society for Pediatric Research Meetings, 1986.

188. Friendenberg WR, Marx JJ Jr, Hensen RL, et al. Hyperimmunoglobulin E syndrome: response to transfer factor and ascorbic acid therapy. *Clin Immunol Immunopathol* 1979;12:132.

189. Givner LB, Edwards MS, Baker CJ. A polyclonal woman Ig preparation hyperimmune for type III Group B Streptococcus: in vitro opsonophagolytic activity and efficacy in experimental models. *J Infect Dis* 1988;158:724.

190. Harper TE, Christensen RD, Rothstein G, et al. Effect of intravenous immunoglobulin G on neutrophil kinetics during experimental Group B streptococcal infection in neonatal rats. *Rev Infect Dis* 1986;8:S401.

191. Santos JI, Shigeoka AO, Hill HR. Functional leukocyte administration protection against experimental neonatal infection. *Pediatr Res* 1980;14:1408.

192. Shigeoka AD, Gobel RJ, Janatova J, et al. Neutrophil mobilization induced by complement fragments during experimental Group B streptococcal (GBS) infection. *Am J Pathol* 1988;133:623.

193. Shigeoka AO, Hall RT, Hill HR. Blood transfusion in Group B streptococcal sepsis. *Lancet* 1978;1:636.

194. Snyderman R, Altman LC, Frankel A. Defective mononuclear leukocyte chemotaxis: a previously unrecognized immune dysfunction. Studies in a patient with chronic mucocutaneous candidiasis. *Ann Intern Med* 1973;78:509.

195. Cates KL, Rowe JC, Ballow M. The premature infant as a compromised host. *Curr Probl Pediatr* 1983;13:63.

196. Gerdes JS, Yoder MC, Douglas SD, et al. Decreased plasma fibronectin in neonatal sepsis. *Pediatrics* 1983;72:877.

197. Miller ME, Stiehm ER. Immunology and resistance to infection. In: Remington JS, Klein JO, eds. *Infectious diseases of the fetus and newborn infant.* Philadelphia: Saunders, 1983:27.

198. Baley JE, Stork EK, Warentin PI, et al. Buffy coat transfusions in neutropenic neonates with presumed sepsis, a prospective randomized trial. *Pediatrics* 1987;80:712.

199. Cairo MS, Rucker R, Bennetts GA, et al. Improved survival of newborns receiving leukocyte tranfusions for sepsis. *Pediatrics* 1984;74:887.

200. Cairo MS, Worcester C, Rucker R, et al. Role of circulating complement and polymorphonuclear leukocyte transfusion in treatment and outcome in critically ill neonates with sepsis. *J Pediatr* 1987;110:935.

201. Laing IA, Boulton FE, Hume R. Polymorphonuclear leukocyte transfusion in neonatal septicaemia. *Arch Dis Child* 1983; 58:1003.

202. Laurenti F, Ferro R, Giancarlo I, et al. Polymorphonuclear leukocyte transfusion for the treatment of sepsis in the newborn infant. *J Pediatr* 1981;98:118.

203. Wheeler JG, Chauvenet AR, Johnson CA, et al. Buffy coat transfusion in neonates with sepsis and neutrophil storage depletion. *Pediatrics* 1987;79:411.

204. Strauss RG, Connett JE, Gale RP, et al. A controlled trial of prophylactic granulocyte transusion during induction chemotherapy for acute myelogenous leukemia. *N Engl J Med* 1981; 305:597.

205. Wright DG, Robichaud KJ, Pizzo PA, et al. Lethal pulmonary reactions associated with the combined use of amphotericin B and leukocyte transfusions. *N Engl J Med* 1981;304:1185.

206. Rosen RC, Huestis DW, Corrigan JJ. Acute leukemia and granulocyte transfusion: fatal graft-versus-host reaction following transfusion cells obtained from normal donors. *J Pediatr* 1978; 93:268.

207. Friedland GH, Klein RS. Transmission of the human immunodeficiency virus. *N Engl J Med* 1987;317:1125.

208. Hill HR. Phagocyte transfusion: ultimate therapy of neonatal disease? *J Pediatr* 1981;98:59.

209. Briones MA, Josephson CD, Hillyer CD. Granulocyte transfusion: revisited. *Curr Hemaol Rep* 2003;2:522.

Hematology

46

Victor Blanchette   Yigal Dror   Anthony Chan

ANEMIAS

Erythroid Development

Early hematopoietic cells originate in the yolk sac. By the eighth week of gestation, more definitive fetal erythropoiesis is taking place in the liver. The liver remains the primary site of erythroid production throughout the early fetal period. By 6 months of gestation, the bone marrow becomes the principal site of erythroid cell development. Later during gestation, a switch occurs in the type of hemoglobin being formed, with adult hemoglobin (HbA) replacing fetal hemoglobin (HbF). The site of production of erythropoietin (EPO) switches from the less sensitive hepatic to the more sensitive renal site (1).

The earliest characterized erythroid precursor is the burst-forming unit (BFU-E), which gives rise to colony-forming units (CFU-E). These are identified by their growth characteristics in culture. Neonatal BFU-E and CFU-E are as sensitive as their adult counterparts to EPO stimulation (2,3). Earlier development is a function of other factors, including interleukin-3 and stem cell factor. The numbers of BFU-E progressively decline along the series of fetal blood, cord blood, adult bone marrow, and adult blood. More than 40 times the number of BFU-E can be cultured from fetal blood as from an equivalent volume of adult blood (1). Measurement of the peripheral blood pool does not indicate the size of the total body pool, so it cannot be inferred that the fetus has a markedly greater erythropoietic potential than an adult does (4). It is probably at least comparable.

The major difference between fetal and adult erythropoiesis is in the response to EPO. Erythropoiesis is controlled by a feedback loop involving EPO. A decrease in erythrocyte mass is reflected by an increase in EPO, which drives erythropoiesis to increase erythrocyte mass and diminish EPO production. The expected correlation between EPO and measures of oxygen delivery (e.g., hemoglobin level, mixed venous oxygen tension, and available oxygen) can be detected in premature neonates, providing evidence that the same feedback loop exists (5–7). The measured levels of EPO are much lower than those of older children and adults with corresponding degrees of anemia. Brown and colleagues (7) presented evidence that the magnitude of the EPO response was lowest in the least mature infant (27 to 31 weeks of gestation). Forestier and associates (8) found low EPO values in cordocentesis samples from infants between 18 and 37 weeks of gestation. Surprisingly, there was no correlation between gestational age and EPO level. This poor EPO response persists through the neonatal period, resulting in a reduced erythropoietic stimulus and lower hemoglobin levels in premature infants.

Normal Hemoglobin Levels

In the newborn period, the hemoglobin concentration is undergoing constant physiologic change. A clear definition of the normal hemoglobin range is therefore important for proper evaluation and management.

Normal hemoglobin values at birth have been determined through measurement of levels in cord blood of newborn infants. In a review of normal blood values in the newborn, Oski and Naiman (9) cited a range of 13.7 to 20.1 g/dL, with a mean of 16.8 g/dL. Blanchette and Zipursky (10) obtained similar results in studies of healthy newborns, yielding cord hemoglobin values (mean ± 1 SD) of 16.9 ± 1.6 g/dL in full-term infants and 15.9 ± 2.4 g/dL in premature infants. Definitive values for premature infants are known as a result of cordocentesis sampling. Data from Forestier and colleagues (8) for 18 to 29 weeks of fetal life and our data for fetuses older than 36 weeks of gestation are given in Table 46-1. Based on these data, cord hemoglobin levels less than 13.0 g/dL should be considered abnormal in term and premature (<36 weeks of gestation) neonates. In the very premature infant (<26 weeks of gestation), values as low as 12.0 g/dL may be acceptable. If anemia is confirmed, a prompt and careful search for the cause should be initiated.

One factor that can significantly influence the hemoglobin level in newborn infants is the amount of placental transfusion. At birth, blood is rapidly transferred from the placenta to the infant, with one-fourth of the placental transfusion occurring within 15 seconds of birth and one-half by the end of the first minute (11). The placental

TABLE 46-1				
NORMAL ERYTHROCYTE VALUES DURING GESTATION[a]				
Weeks of Gestation	**Erythrocytes (×10¹²/L)**	**Hemoglobin (g/dL)**	**Hematocrit (%)**	**Mean Corpuscular Volume (fL)**
18–21	2.85 ± 0.36	11.7 ± 1.3	37.3 ± 4.3	131.11 ± 10.97
22–25	3.09 ± 0.34	12.2 ± 1.6	38.6 ± 3.9	125.1 ± 7.84
26–29	3.46 ± 0.41	12.9 ± 1.4	40.9 ± 4.4	118.5 ± 7.96
>36	4.7 ± 0.4	16.5 ± 1.5	51.0 ± 4.5	108 ± 5

[a] Values are means ±1 standard deviation.

vessels contain 75 to 125 mL of blood at birth.(12) Usher and associates (13) demonstrated that the blood volume of an infant could be increased by as much as 61% by delayed cord clamping. In that study, the average erythrocyte mass in a group of infants with delayed cord clamping was 49 mL/kg at 72 hours of age compared with 31 mL/kg in a group in whom the cord was clamped immediately after birth. Although infants delivered after delayed cord clamping have higher hemoglobin values, it should be recognized that the placental transfusion may be markedly reduced or prevented if the infant is held above the level of the placenta at the time of delivery; in this situation, it is possible for an infant to lose blood into the placenta and be born anemic (14).

Anemia in the Newborn Period

Anemia at birth or appearing during the first few weeks of life can be broadly categorized into three major groups. The anemia may be the result of blood loss, hemolysis, or underproduction of erythrocytes.

Physiological Anemia and the Anemia of Prematurity

The hemoglobin concentration of healthy full-term and premature infants undergoes typical changes during the first weeks of life (15–18). After birth, there is a transient increase in hemoglobin concentration as plasma moves extravascularly to compensate for the placental transfusion and an increase in circulating erythrocyte volume that occurs at the time of delivery (19). Thereafter, the hemoglobin concentration gradually falls, to reach minimal levels of 11.4 ± 0.9 g/dL in term infants by 8 to 12 weeks of age and 7.0 to 10.0 g/dL in premature infants by 6 weeks of age (Fig. 46-1) (18).

There are several reasons for the fall in hemoglobin. The first is the decline in erythrocyte production that occurs in the first few days of life and is evidenced by a fall in reticulocyte counts during that time (Fig. 46-2). Normally, reticulocyte counts may be elevated during the first 1 or 2 days of life (200 to 300 × 10⁹/L) but then fall to low levels (in the order of 50 × 10⁹/L) through the remainder of the neonatal period. This diminution of erythropoiesis is probably related to decreased EPO production. The reduced

EPO response persists until approximately 6 weeks of age, at which time erythrocyte production increases, as evidenced by a sharp rise in reticulocyte numbers in the blood and an increase in total body hemoglobin (Fig. 46-2). Other factors that contribute to the physiologic anemia in newborns, particularly the more profound anemia in premature infants, are the shortened survival of neonatal erythrocytes and rapid body growth (Fig. 46-2) (20,21).

The effect of rapid body growth on hemoglobin levels is unique to neonates and deserves special mention. Healthy premature infants are in a phase of rapid growth when

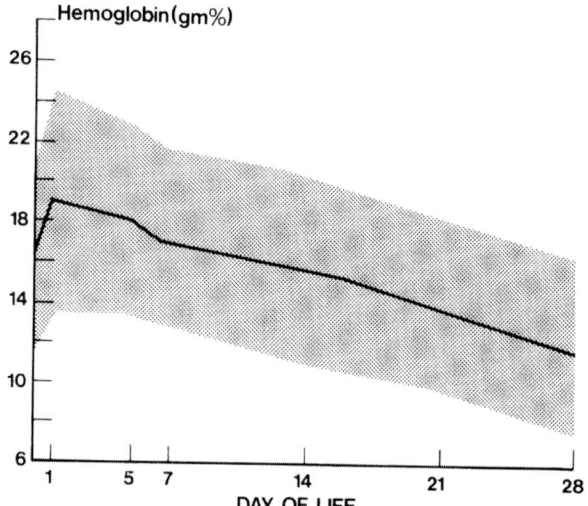

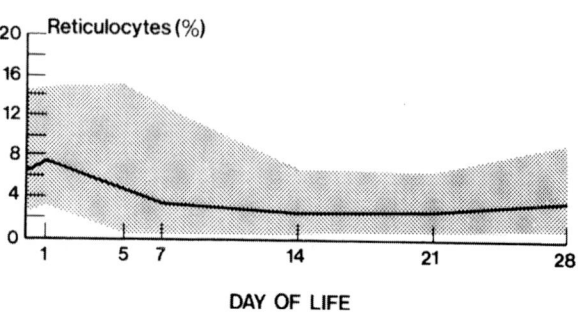

Figure 46-1 Hemoglobin values of 178 normal premature infants ≤36 weeks of gestation. Data at the first point, day 0, are cord blood values. Subsequent points represent data from capillary blood samples on 1, 5, 7, 14, and 28 days of life. The dark line represents the mean value, and the shaded area includes 95% of all values.

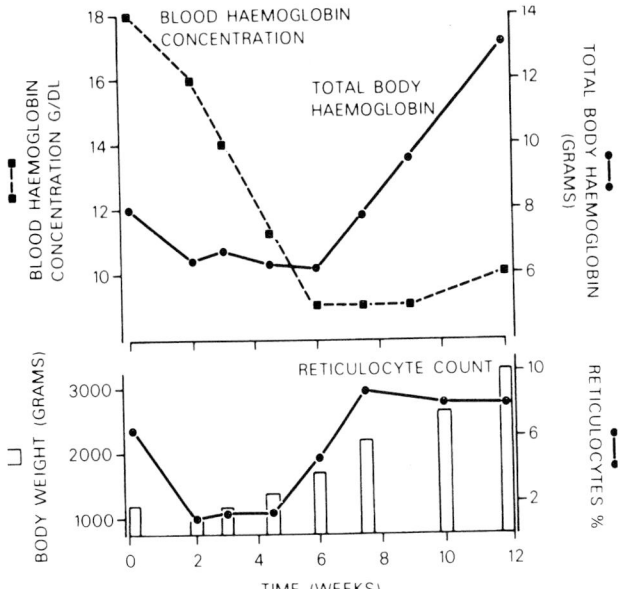

Figure 46-2 Changes in total body hemoglobin, blood hemoglobin concentration, reticulocyte count, and body weight in a representative premature infant. The vertical bars represent the infant's body weight. During the first 6 weeks of life, the blood hemoglobin concentration and total body hemoglobin fall as a result of decreased erythrocyte production, as evidenced by the low reticulocyte count. The more rapid decline in blood hemoglobin concentration from the third to the sixth week is the result of the increasing body size and dilution of the hemoglobin mass. After 6 weeks of age, hemoglobin production increases, as evidenced by the increased reticulocyte count and the rapid increase in total body hemoglobin. The blood hemoglobin concentration during that period may rise slightly, or not at all, because the total body size increases at approximately the same rate as the total hemoglobin mass.

active erythropoiesis, as evidenced by a mild reticulocytosis, resumes at 6 to 8 weeks of age. Associated with this rapid gain in body weight is an obligatory increase in the total circulating blood volume. The resultant hemodilution may cause a peripheral hemoglobin concentration that is static or even falls slightly. The apparent paradox of a stable or falling hemoglobin concentration despite active erythropoiesis (i.e., mild reticulocytosis and an increasing erythrocyte mass) gradually corrects, and the peripheral hemoglobin concentration increases (see Fig. 46-2). Failure to recognize the important effect of rapid body growth on the peripheral hemoglobin concentration may lead to inappropriate investigation and treatment of apparent anemia (16,22).

The signs and symptoms of this early anemia in premature infants are nonspecific and reflect changes in metabolic rate or cardiorespiratory function and perfusion. Controversy exists about whether tachycardia, tachypnea, periodic breathing, and apnea are reliable indicators of anemia (23–29). Stockman and Clark (30) demonstrated an improvement in weight gain after transfusion in premature infants in infants with poor weight gain. Others have not confirmed these observations (27–29). Lactate measurements and cardiac output can be shown to decrease following transfusion, but neither measurement on its own can be considered a surrogate for diagnosing anemia (27,31).

Trials of folate, iron, and vitamin E have not shown any evidence of benefit in preventing the physiological anemia of infancy (32). Optimal protein supplementation is important for maintaining good hematopoiesis (33–38).

Several groups have tested blood transfusion as therapy for the anemia of prematurity. Blank and associates (39) and Meyer and associates (40) were unable to demonstrate clinical benefit in transfused versus nontransfused neonates other than an improved hematocrit. In both studies several children were transfused for tachycardia, apnea, bradycardia, or other clinical signs interpreted as signs and symptoms of anemia. Others have shown benefit in these clinical parameters from transfusion in selected asymptomatic infants (41–43), although hemoglobin values are not necessarily the best indicator of need (41). Surveys of blood product use in neonatal units show that most transfusion practices are based on a preset hemoglobin value or what the clinician interprets as signs and symptoms of anemia (apnea, poor weight gain, etc.) (44). Similar clinical criteria have been incorporated into guidelines for the transfusion of premature infants (45). Trials of transfusion therapy at arbitrary values have not demonstrated clear benefit and may expose infants to infectious agents (e.g., cytomegalovirus [CMV], hepatitis, human immunodeficiency virus [HIV]) (46) and other risks from blood products (e.g., graft-versus-host disease). Future trials of transfusion therapy for anemia in premature infants require better defined end points before they can yield definitive results. Prevention of anemia would be a better strategy.

The desire to avoid the use of blood products coupled with the need to treat symptomatic anemia has led to trials of recombinant EPO in premature newborns. Low plasma EPO levels are a major contributing factor in the pathogenesis of anemia of prematurity. This is caused by reduced responsiveness of the liver compared to the kidney to tissue hypoxia and increased clearance of EPO in premature infants (1). When plated in clonogenic assays, erythroid progenitors from neonates demonstrate good responsiveness to EPO with an increase in BFU-E and CFU-E colonies (2,3). Furthermore, EPO in sufficient doses combined with adequate iron and protein supplements can induce an increase in the hemoglobin concentration in neonates. However, it remains unclear if these findings can be translated into a clinically meaningful reduction in the need for red blood cell (RBC) transfusions in premature neonates. In clinical trials reported to date, EPO has been started either early (within the first week of life) (47–53) or late (about 3 weeks of age) (34,36,54–61). In general, infants receiving larger EPO doses at both time points have shown improvement in reticulocyte counts and hemoglobin levels and a decrease in the number of transfusions per infant. Of importance, however, early initiation of EPO therapy was not associated with a significant reduction in the number of infants transfused, and in groups treated later most red blood cell exposures occurred before the start of EPO therapy.

In a recent meta-analysis Vamuakas and Strauss (62) analyzed 21 prospective controlled trials of EPO in newborn infants published during the period 1990 through 1999. The clinically relevant end points were a reduction in the number and volume of RBC transfusions. The investigators found that treatment with EPO reduced RBC transfusions by an average of 11ml/kg, a value that was statistically significant ($p < 0.001$). However, there was extreme variation among trials. The variability in the studies included birth weight of study subjects, postnatal age at study entry, frequency and dose of EPO, use of iron supplementation, and triggers for RBC transfusion. Unfortunately, even among studies in which these variables were similar there were differences in results.

In another meta-analysis by Garcia and associates (63) the authors analyzed 8 randomized placebo-controlled studies that administered EPO or placebo after the first week of life and focused on erythrocyte transfusion needs after the third week of life ("late" transfusions). In this specific group of patients they found that neonates in the EPO group received significantly fewer transfusions proportional to the dose of EPO administered. Based on these two analyses, it remains unclear whether EPO treatment should be universally recommended for all premature babies as a means to prevent clinically significant anemia that will require RBC transfusion. It is also unclear whether the cost of the RBC transfusions that are avoided by treatment with EPO is higher than the cost of EPO. Furthermore, although no adverse effects of EPO could be demonstrated by 1 year of age (53) the long term side effects of EPO in premature infants is unknown. Recently development of neutralizing antierythropoietin antibodies was demonstrated in patients with chronic renal failure who developed pure red cell aplasia following treatment with EPO. These patients were adults who received EPO treatment for 3 to 67 months. The condition resolved several months after cessation of EPO treatment during which time the patients required multiple RBC transfusions. Whether neonates who are treated with EPO for less than 3 months can develop neutralizing antibodies remains to be determined (64), and this potential complication of EPO therapy should be taken into consideration when assessing the risk:benefit of EPO therapy in newborn infants (65).

In summary, the overall incremental benefit of EPO therapy in neonates in the setting of rigorous transfusion guidelines and effective strategies to minimize iatrogenic (phlebotomy) blood losses, plus appropriate iron and protein supplementation is not clear and requires further study in carefully designed prospective clinical trials. Alternative transfusion strategies, discussed in detail later in this chapter, may be equally effective in preventing multiple donor exposure and may be more cost-effective. Currently, the most prudent approach is for individual neonatal units to assess the impact of newer transfusion strategies in their population before implementing routine EPO therapy (66).

If a decision is made to administer recombinant EPO to decrease RBC transfusions to ill extremely low birth weight infants (birth weight <1,000 g) Calhoun and colleagues have recommended that a dose of 200 U/kg/day of EPO

plus iron supplementation be given for two weeks; if the goal is to decrease or possibly eliminate the need for late transfusions to very low birth weight infants (birth weight <1,500 g) with the anemia of prematurity or the late anemia of Rhesus hemolytic disease the investigators recommend giving 400 U/kg of EPO three times per week subcutaneously for 2 weeks with added iron (67).

Anemia Caused by Blood Loss

Blood loss resulting in anemia may occur prenatally, at the time of delivery, or postnatally. Blood loss may be the result of occult hemorrhage before birth, obstetric accidents, internal hemorrhages, or excessive blood sampling for diagnostic studies (Table 46-2). Faxelius and colleagues (68) associated a low erythrocyte volume with a maternal history of bleeding in the late third trimester, placenta previa, abruptio placentae, nonelective cesarean section, deliveries associated with cord compression, Apgar scores less than 6, an early central venous hematocrit less than 45%, and a mean arterial pressure less than 30 mm Hg.

Occult Hemorrhage Before Birth

Occult hemorrhage before birth may be caused by bleeding of the fetus into the maternal circulation or by the bleeding of one fetus into another in multiple pregnancies. In approximately 50% of all pregnancies, some fetal cells can

TABLE 46-2
TYPES OF HEMORRHAGE IN THE NEONATE

Occult hemorrhage before birth
Fetomaternal
    Traumatic amniocentesis
    Spontaneous
    After external cephalic version
Twin-to-twin
Obstetric accidents, malformations of the placenta and cord
Nuchal cord with placental blood trapping
Rupture of a normal umbilical cord
    Precipitous delivery
    Entanglement
Hematoma of the cord or placenta
Rupture of an abnormal umbilical cord
    Varices
    Aneurysm
Rupture of anomalous vessels
    Aberrant vessel
    Velamentous insertion
    Communicating vessels in multilobed placenta
Incision of placenta during cesarean section
Placenta previa
Abruptio placentae
Internal hemorrhage
Intracranial
Giant cephalhematoma
Subgaleal
Retroperitoneal
Laceration of the liver
Ruptured spleen
Pulmonary

be demonstrated in the maternal circulation (69). In about 8% of pregnancies, from 0.5 to 40.0 mL of blood is transferred from the fetus to the mother at birth, and in 1% of pregnancies, the blood loss exceeds 40 mL. Fetomaternal hemorrhages are more common after traumatic diagnostic amniocentesis or external cephalic version.

Fetomaternal Hemorrhage

The clinical manifestations of a fetomaternal hemorrhage depend on the volume of the hemorrhage and the rapidity with which it has occurred. A sudden and unexpected decrease in fetal movements may be a warning sign of an acute, massive fetomaternal hemorrhage (70). The prognosis for such cases is poor and may be improved by prompt delivery and a neonatal transfusion, or if the fetus is premature by cord sampling and an intrauterine transfusion (71–73). If the hemorrhage has been prolonged or repeated during the course of the pregnancy anemia develops slowly giving the fetus an opportunity to develop hemodynamic compensation. These infants may manifest only pallor at birth. After acute hemorrhage just before delivery, the infant may be pale and sluggish, with gasping respirations and signs of circulatory shock.

The degree of anemia varies. Usually, the hemoglobin is less than 12.0 g/dL before the physician recognizes signs and symptoms of anemia. Hemoglobin values as low as 3.0 to 4.0 g/dL have been recorded in infants who were born alive and survived. If the hemorrhage has been acute, and particularly in hypovolemic shock, the hemoglobin value may not reflect the magnitude of the blood loss. Several hours may elapse before hemodilution occurs and the magnitude of the hemorrhage is appreciated. In general, a loss of 20% of the blood volume acutely is sufficient to produce signs of shock and is reflected in a fall in hemoglobin concentration within 3 hours of the event.

In acute and chronic hemorrhage, the erythrocytes usually appear normochromic and normocytic. Rarely in chronic hemorrhage, the cells appear hypochromic and microcytic, indicating fetal iron deficiency anemia (74).

If anemia is a direct result of a fetomaternal hemorrhage, the Coombs test is negative, and the infant is not jaundiced. Infants with anemia secondary to blood loss generally have lower than average bilirubin values throughout the neonatal period as a consequence of their reduced erythrocyte mass.

The diagnosis of a fetomaternal hemorrhage great enough to result in anemia at birth can be made with certainty only by the demonstration of fetal cells in the maternal circulation. The Kleihauer technique of acid elution is the simplest and most commonly employed method for the detection of fetal cells (75). The test is based on the property of HbF to resist elution from the cell in an acid medium. The acid elution technique can be relied on with certainty for diagnosis only when other conditions capable of producing elevations in maternal HbF levels are absent. These include maternal thalassemia minor, sickle-cell anemia, hereditary persistence of HbF, and in some normal women, a pregnancy-induced rise in HbF production (76).

In these conditions, the appearance of the Kleihauer test, with many cells containing variable amounts of HbF, is easily differentiated from that of a true transplacental hemorrhage, in which the fetal cells containing high concentrations of HbF are readily differentiated from the maternal cells containing no HbF.

The diagnosis of a fetomaternal hemorrhage may be missed in situations in which the mother and infant are incompatible in the ABO blood group system. In such instances, the infant's A or B cells are rapidly cleared from the maternal circulation by the maternal anti-A or anti-B and may not be seen in the Kleihauer preparation.

Twin-to-twin Transfusion

Twin-to-twin transfusion is observed in 13% to 33% of monozygotic multiple births with monochorial placentas (77). In approximately 70% of monozygotic twin pregnancies, a monochorial placenta exists. Blood exchange between twins may produce anemia in the donor and polycythemia in the recipient. If a significant hemorrhage has occurred, the difference in hemoglobin between the twins exceeds 5.0 g/dL. There is a maximal discrepancy of 3.3 g/dL in cord blood hemoglobin concentration in dizygotic twins. The anemic twin may develop congestive heart failure and hydrops, and the plethoric twin may manifest symptoms and signs of the hyperviscosity syndrome, disseminated intravascular coagulation (DIC) and hyperbilirubinemia.

The hemorrhage may be acute or chronic. Tan and associates (77), on the basis of a review of 482 twin pairs in which 35 were found to have the transfusion syndrome, pointed out how the difference in weight of the twins could be used to establish the timing of the hemorrhage. If the weight difference exceeded 20% of the weight of the larger twin, the transfusion was chronic, and the smaller infant was invariably the donor. The anemic, smaller twin displayed reticulocytosis. If the difference in the weight of the twins did not exceed 20% of the weight of the larger twin, the larger twin was the donor in almost 50% of cases. In these presumably acute transfusions around the time of birth, significant reticulocytosis was not observed in the anemic donor.

If twin-to-twin transfusion is suspected, attempts to confirm it by placental examination should be made. The placentas of all multiple pregnancies should be routinely examined for purposes of genetic counseling. If hematologic evidence has not been obtained, and the infants have died, other findings may suggest the diagnosis, including polyhydramnios of the recipient's amniotic sac and oligohydramnios of the donor and marked differences in the size and organ weights of the twins.

With the advent of accurate ultrasound assessment of the fetus, the diagnosis of twin-to-twin transfusion in utero has become possible, and a careful assessment of chorionicity in twins undergoing first trimester ultrasound scanning is recommended (78). The early detection of monochorionic twins identifies a high-risk pregnancy that should be managed in obstetric centers experienced in dealing with such cases. In cases of severe twin to twin transfusion, the donor (anemic) twin is smaller, and there is associated oligohydramnios; the recipient (polycythemic, hypervolemic) twin is larger, and there is associated polyhydramnios. Intrauterine diagnosis is therefore dependent on identification of same sex, size difference, oligohydramnios/polyhydramnios, and a monochorionic placenta. When diagnosed in utero, twin-to-twin transfusion syndrome can be classified into five discreet stages (79). Stage I is defined by the finding of isolated discrepancy in amniotic fluid volumes between fetuses; absence of a urine filled bladder in the donor fetus defines Stage II, absent or reversed end-diastolic flow in the umbilical artery of the donor fetus or abnormal venous Doppler pattern in the recipient, such as reversed flow in the ductus venosus or pulsatile umbilical venous flow Stage III, hydrops fetalis Stage IV and demise of one or both fetuses Stage V. Perinatal outcomes correlate with disease severity as assessed by the stage at presentation and gestational age at delivery; overall the perinatal mortality rate for the twin-to-twin transfusion syndrome is 30% to 50% (80). Therapy has included repeated amniocentesis to reduce polyhydramnios, photocoagulation of placental vascular anastomoses, amniotic septostomy, and selected feticide by cord occlusion (78).

Obstetric Accidents and Complications

Obstetric accidents and malformations of the placenta and cord may be responsible for major blood loss at the time of delivery. These accidents may be unreported to the pediatrician and may result in diagnostic confusion about the cause of shock in the early hours of life or the presence of pallor and unexplained anemia during the second or third day of life.

The obstetric conditions that can produce neonatal hemorrhage are listed in Table 46-2. Severe and often fatal fetal hemorrhage may accompany placenta previa, abruptio placentae, or accidental incision of the placenta or umbilical cord during a cesarean section. A tight nuchal cord may cause venous obstruction leading to excessive blood trapping in the placenta and resulting in severe hypovolemia (81) and anemia (82). A prospective study of red cell mass suggested that babies born with a tight nuchal cord had a significantly lower red cell mass than controls (83).

In women with late-third-trimester bleeding, Clayton and associates (84) were able to anticipate the birth of a possible anemic infant by examining the vaginal blood for the presence of fetal erythrocytes, employing the acid elution technique of Kleihauer (75,84).

It is good pediatric practice to obtain a hemoglobin measurement routinely at the time of delivery of all babies born of women with late third-trimester bleeding. This determination should be repeated in 6 to 12 hours to observe the expected fall in hemoglobin resulting from the hemodilution that follows recent blood loss.

Severe bleeding as a result of an obstetric accident or complication of delivery often results in the birth of a pale, limp infant. Respirations, which usually commence spontaneously, are often irregular and gasping. They are not associated with retraction, as in conditions accompanied by primary pulmonary disease. Cyanosis is minimal, and the infant's pale color is not improved by oxygen administration. The peripheral pulses are weak or absent, and the blood pressure is reduced. The venous pressure measured after the insertion of an umbilical catheter is found to be extremely low.

Internal Hemorrhage

Anemia that appears in the first 24 to 72 hours of life and is not associated with significant jaundice is commonly caused by hemorrhage at the time of birth or by a postnatal internal hemorrhage. Traumatic deliveries may result in subdural or subarachnoid hemorrhages or cephalhematomas of sufficient magnitude to produce anemia. Subaponeurotic or subgaleal hemorrhages are relatively common after vacuum extraction and may lead to significant neonatal anemia.

Breech deliveries may be associated with hemorrhage into the adrenals, kidney, spleen, or retroperitoneal area. Rupture of the liver or subcapsular hemorrhage into the liver may occur more commonly than is clinically recognized (85–87). An infant with a ruptured liver may appear well for the first 24 to 48 hours of life and then suddenly go into shock. The abdomen may appear distended, and a mass contiguous with the liver is often palpable. Shifting dullness on abdominal percussion can often be demonstrated, and an elevation of the right hemidiaphragm may be seen on the radiograph. Splenic rupture may occur after a difficult delivery or as a result of the extreme distension of the spleen that is often seen in babies with severe erythroblastosis fetalis. The physician should always suspect a rupture of the spleen when an anemic, and often hydropic, infant with erythroblastosis is found to have a low initial venous pressure at the time of exchange transfusion. The diagnosis of intraabdominal hemorrhage is readily made with ultrasonography.

In infants with birth weights less than 1,500 g, bleeding into the cerebral ventricles, subarachnoid space, and parenchyma can also produce significant decreases in hemoglobin concentration.

Iatrogenic Anemia due to Blood Sampling

Anemia appearing during the first week of life is often caused by blood removal for diagnostic studies required for the frequent monitoring of critically ill infants. Removal of more than 20% of a subject's blood volume produces anemia. In an infant of 1,500 g, this represents a blood loss of only 25 mL. If frequent blood sampling is necessary, a flow sheet should be used to record the amount removed at any given time. This simple technique often converts a diagnosis of idiopathic anemia to one of iatrogenic anemia.

Despite the use of micromethods using small volumes of blood by most laboratories, cumulative blood losses through sampling for laboratory monitoring are often surprisingly large in small infants. Blanchette and Zipursky

(88) reported an average blood loss of 22.9 mL of packed cells from 59 premature infants studied through the first 6 weeks of life. Forty-six % (26 of 57) of the infants studied had cumulative losses that exceeded their circulating erythrocyte mass at birth (Fig. 46-3); in a few cases, losses were equivalent to two or three times the infants' initial circulating erythrocyte masses. Because these losses must be replaced, at least in part, by erythrocyte transfusions, some infants had the equivalent of a double- or triple-volume exchange transfusion simply as a result of blood sampling for laboratory tests. Approximately 10% of all blood loss during sampling for laboratory monitoring was hidden and represented blood on cotton swabs or in the dead space of syringes or tubing of butterfly sets used to collect blood samples (89).

There is a strong correlation between the volume of blood sampled and that transfused (Fig. 46-4), suggesting that much of the erythrocyte transfusion requirements of ill, premature infants is a direct consequence of blood loss for essential laboratory monitoring (88). In the study by Blanchette and Zipursky (88), significantly more blood was sampled from infants judged to be clinically ill than from healthy premature infants. Iatrogenic blood loss through sampling was significant in both groups (mean ± 1 SD = 26.9 ± 9 and 14.6 ± 5 mL, respectively). These comparative volumes may not appear large, but the actual values must be compared with a total erythrocyte mass that varies between 32.3 and 45.5 mL/kg (90–94). The removal of 1 mL of blood from a 1-kg infant is equivalent to removing 70 mL of blood from an average adult, and it is therefore not surprising that repeated blood sampling, even with capillary samples, can have a profound effect on the hemoglobin concentration of small, premature infants. Ballin and colleagues have demonstrated that, if the erythrocytes that are discarded from samples drawn in which only the plasma was used were instead reinfused, the fall in hemoglobin concentration could be substantially reduced (95).

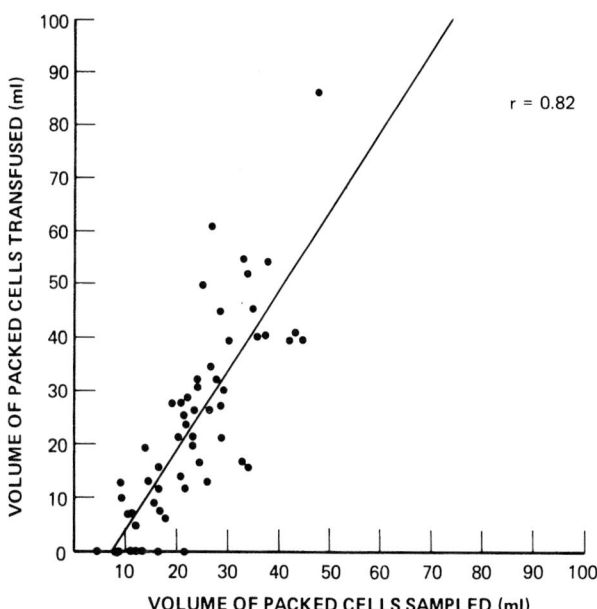

Figure 46-4   Relation during the first 6 weeks of life between the cumulative volumes of blood sampled from and transfused into 57 premature infants who had birth weights less than 1,500 g. Volumes represent milliliters of packed erythrocytes (r, correlation coefficient).

Treatment of Anemia Secondary to Blood Loss

The treatment of anemia secondary to blood loss depends on the degree of anemia and the acuteness of the hemorrhage. For acute hemorrhage, the following measures must be employed:

1. If the infant is pale and limp at birth, clear the airway, administer oxygen, and intubate if necessary.
2. Obtain venous access immediately. In some circumstances, this may best be achieved by the insertion of an umbilical venous line. Blood specimens for hematologic determinations and crossmatching should be drawn. If an umbilical line is placed, it may be possible to measure a central venous pressure.
3. As soon as it is apparent that pallor is a result of hypovolemic shock or profound anemia and not a consequence of asphyxia, administer 15 to 20 mL/kg, in order of preference and depending on ready availability, of O Rh-negative packed RBCs, plasma, 5% albumin, or isotonic saline. Infants with acute external blood loss usually demonstrate dramatic improvement after such a procedure. Infants with massive internal hemorrhages show less evidence of response.
4. A repeat injection of 10 to 20 mL/kg of whole blood or reconstituted whole blood (packed RBCs plus fresh frozen plasma [FFP]) may be appropriate after the first transfusion, particularly if whole blood was not administered initially and the venous pressure and arterial pressure have not returned to normal.

After resuscitating the infant, make efforts to determine the cause of blood loss. Examine the placenta and cord for evidence of abnormalities. Obtain a blood sample from the

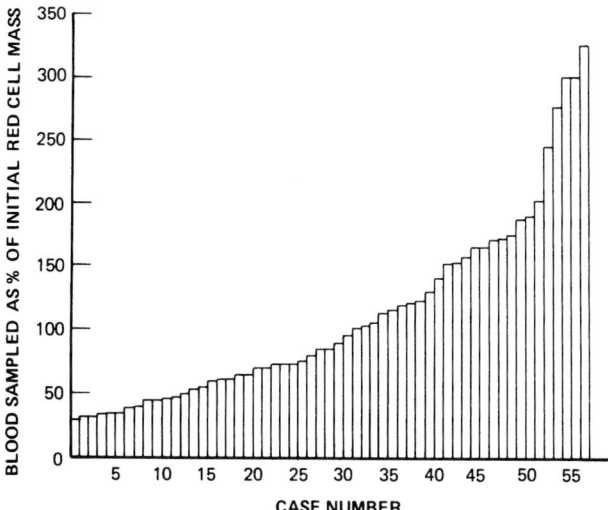

Figure 46-3   Cumulative blood losses through sampling in premature infants, expressed as a percentage of their erythrocyte mass at birth. Infants were studied during the first 6 weeks of life, and each vertical bar represents a single infant.

mother for the detection of a fetomaternal hemorrhage. The infant who is mildly anemic at birth as a consequence of chronic blood loss and who is in no distress may not require transfusion.

For anemic infants still requiring intensive support, especially mechanical ventilation, it is probably appropriate to treat anemia with blood transfusion. The decision to transfuse must be based on the hemoglobin level and on the clinical condition of the baby.

Hemolytic Anemia

Anemia as a consequence of a hemolytic process is common in the newborn period and has multiple causes. Hemolysis is almost always associated with elevation of the serum indirect bilirubin value to 170 µmol/L (10 mg/dL) or greater. In general, a hemolytic process is first detected during the investigation of jaundice occurring during the first week of life.

Difficulties in Diagnosing Hemolytic Disease in Newborn Infants

Detection and diagnosis of hemolytic disease in newborn infants may be difficult because many of the tests used in older children and in adults are of little value during the first days of life. Hemolytic disease in adults is diagnosed if there is evidence of a rapidly falling hemoglobin con-

centration, increased erythrocyte production in the absence of hemorrhage, abnormal erythrocyte morphology, and increased erythrocyte destruction within the bloodstream with the release of free hemoglobin or within the reticuloendothelial system with production of bilirubin. In the newborn infant, these signs of a hemolytic process are of limited value and require additional interpretation.

Evidence of Increased Erythrocyte Production

In adults, an increased reticulocyte count with a stable or falling hemoglobin concentration is evidence of increased erythrocyte production and, in the absence of hemorrhage, is diagnostic of a hemolytic process. The reticulocyte count in normal newborns has a wide range, limiting its value except in severe hemolytic disease.

Erythrocyte Morphology

The shape of erythrocytes in newborns differs from that in adults. Abnormally shaped cells are frequently seen in blood smears of newborn infants, particularly premature infants. The various abnormally shaped cells in full-term and premature infants are shown in Fig. 46-5 and their percentages are detailed in Table 46-3. Accordingly, erythrocytes in newborns can have distorted morphology without any pathological hemolysis.

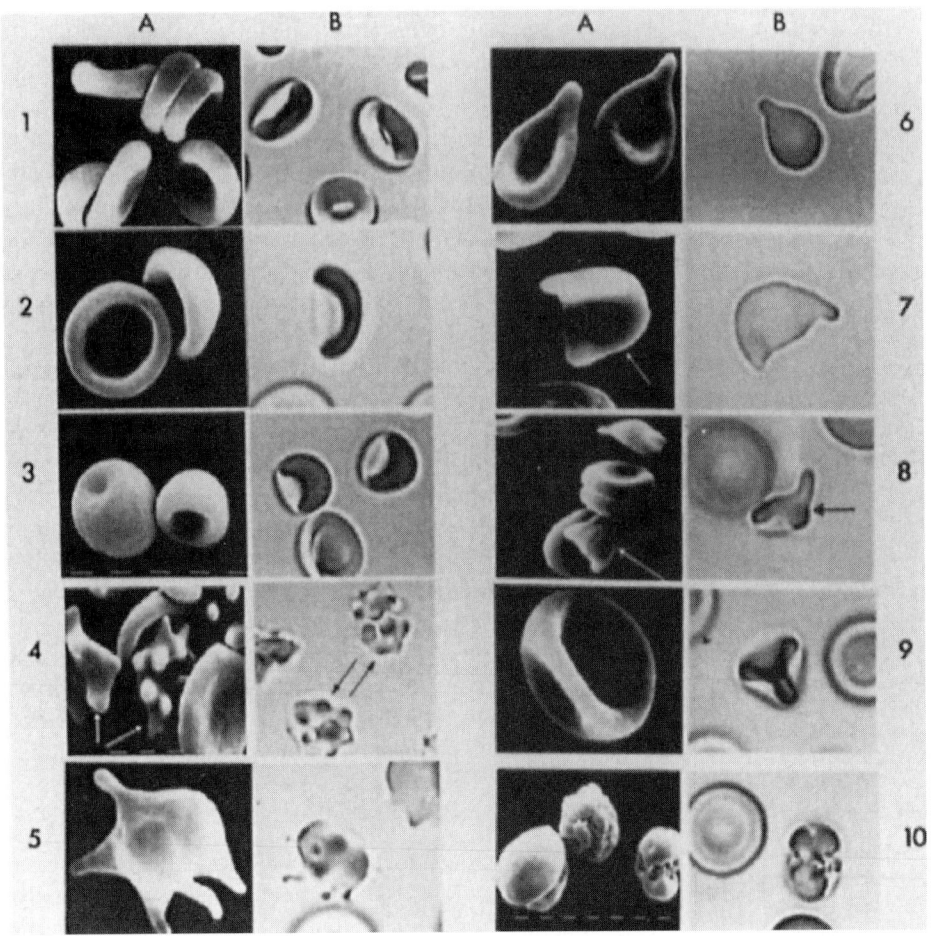

Figure 46-5 The three-dimensional appearance of erythrocytes as seen by scanning electron microscopy **(A)** and by light microscopy **(B)** of glutaraldehyde-fixed cells. (1, discocytes; 2, bowls; 3, spherocytes; 4, echinocytes; 5, acanthocytes; 6, dacrocytes; 7, keratocytes; 8, schizocytes; 9, knizocytes; 10, immature erythrocytes).

TABLE 46-3
ERYTHROCYTE DIFFERENTIAL COUNTS IN ADULTS AND NEONATES

Erythrocytes	Median (5%–95%)[a]		
	Adults	**Full-Term Infants[b]**	**Premature Infants[c]**
Number studied	53	31	52
Disks	78 (42–94)	43 (18–62)	39.5 (18–57)
Bowls	18 (4–50)	40 (14–58)	29 (13–53)
Ratio of disks to bowls	2 (0–4)	2 (0–5)	3 (0–10)
Spherocytes	0 (0–0)	0 (0–1)	0 (0–3)
Echinocytes	0 (0–3)	1 (0–4)	5.5 (1–23)
Acanthocytes	0 (0–1)	1 (0–2)	0 (0–2)
Dacrocytes	0 (0–1)	1 (0–3)	1 (0–5)
Keratocytes	0 (0–1)	2 (0–5)	3 (0–7)
Schizocytes	0 (0–1)	0 (0–2)	2 (0–5)
Knizocytes	1 (0–4)	3 (0–8)	1 (0–6)
Others	1 (0–4)	3 (0–7)	4 (1–11)

[a] All values are expressed as a median plus the 5% to 95% range, because the distribution of most values was nongaussian.
[b] Of the sample, 29 were ABO compatible, 1 was AB with an A mother, and 1 was AB with a B mother.
[c] Includes ABO-compatible and ABO-incompatible infants.

Evidence of Erythrocyte Destruction

The catabolism of erythrocytes results in the equimolar production of bilirubin and carboxyhemoglobin (96,97). A rapid increase in the degree of hyperbilirubinemia is a cardinal sign of erythrocyte destruction. The measurement of blood carboxyhemoglobin or in the rate of carbon monoxide excretion (98) also correlates with hemolysis (99–101).

In adults and children, intravascular hemolysis is evidenced by increased levels of hemoglobin in the plasma (i.e., hemoglobinemia), a fall in serum haptoglobin, and the appearance of hemoglobinuria and methemalbuminemia. In the normal newborn, haptoglobin levels may be zero, and plasma hemoglobin levels are above those found in adults. Gross elevations in plasma hemoglobin and hemoglobinuria are evidence of intravascular hemolysis, but the value of these tests in detecting mild hemolysis in newborn infants is limited.

When erythrocytes are destroyed in the reticuloendothelial system, bilirubin is produced, with elevation of indirect bilirubin in the blood. In the newborn, there are many other causes of hyperbilirubinemia (see Chapter 35). In newborns, unlike adults, indirect hyperbilirubinemia is not a specific sign of hemolytic disease. Unusually rapid appearance of jaundice, particularly in the first 24 hours, suggests hemolytic disease. Because there are many causes of indirect hyperbilirubinemia, all newborns with abnormally high indirect bilirubin levels must be studied for evidence of hemolytic disease.

Alloimmune Hemolytic Disease

Hemolytic disease in the newborn as a consequence of alloimmunization of the mother is caused by the passage of fetal erythrocytes into the maternal circulation, in which they stimulate the production of antibody. Antibodies of the IgG class return to the fetal circulation, attach to antigenic sites on the surface of the erythrocyte, and cause its rapid removal by the fetal reticuloendothelial system. The incidence and clinical manifestations of alloimmunization depend on the type of blood group incompatibility between the mother and fetus. This topic has been the subject of many comprehensive reviews (102–105).

Rh Hemolytic Disease. The incidence of Rh incompatibility in a population depends, in large part, on the prevalence of the Rh-negative antigens. The prevalence of the Rh-negative genotype ranges from approximately zero in Japanese, Chinese, and North American Indian populations to 5.5% among African-Americans and 15% among American Caucasians (106–108). Among Caucasian women, it has been estimated that in approximately 9% of all pregnancies, an Rh-negative woman carries an Rh-positive fetus. In 6% of pregnancies at risk, alloimmunization of the mother occurs if there is no immunoprophylaxis.

The severity of Rh hemolytic disease varies greatly from infant to infant. It is estimated that, without antenatal diagnosis and treatment, the perinatal mortality in this disease would be approximately 17.5%, with stillbirths accounting for about 14% of deaths (105). The degree of hemolytic disease tends to be more severe in subsequent pregnancies than in the initial one in which sensitization has occurred.

Pathogenesis. The entry of fetal cells into the maternal circulation is the cause of Rh isoimmunization. As few as 0.05

to 0.1 mL of cells, particularly if transferred repeatedly, are sufficient to produce immunization. Rh immunization tends to occur more frequently in pregnancies that have been complicated by toxemia, cesarean section, or manual removal of the placenta, because transplacental hemorrhages occur with greater frequency and in greater volume under these circumstances. It is estimated that 1% of Rh-negative women develop antibodies as a consequence of these transplacental hemorrhages before the delivery of their first child. An additional 7.5% manifest evidence of sensitization within 6 months of the delivery of their first child, and another 7.5% show no evidence of immunization 6 months after delivery but develop antibodies during their next pregnancy if their fetus is Rh-positive, presumably as a consequence of a sensitization during the first pregnancy.

Destruction of Fetal Erythrocytes by Anti-D. The transfer of antibody from the mother into the fetal circulation is responsible for the clinical manifestations of the hemolytic process. The erythrocyte, coated with an antibody of the IgG class, is removed primarily in the spleen of the fetus. The rate of destruction is generally proportional to the amount of antibody on the cell. At very high levels of antibody, the cell may be destroyed by intravascular hemolysis and splenic sequestration.

Before birth, the chief danger of excess erythrocyte destruction is profound anemia. After birth, the infant is primarily at risk from the toxic products of erythrocyte breakdown, such as bilirubin. In utero, the infant responds to the increased breakdown of cells by increasing the rate of erythrocyte production. This is reflected by an elevation of reticulocyte count and the presence of nucleated erythrocytes in the peripheral circulation. This accelerated demand for erythrocytes results in active erythropoiesis in non-marrow sites such as the liver, spleen, and lung. A major portion of the hepatosplenomegaly observed in infants with hemolytic disease is a result of this extramedullary erythropoiesis.

In infants with severe Rh incompatibility, the liver and pancreas exhibit pathologic changes. Islet cell hyperplasia can be observed in the pancreas, and focal cellular necrosis with cholestasis may be seen in the liver.

The most severely affected infants manifest hydrops fetalis. This massive edema with pleural effusions and ascites is not strictly related to the hemoglobin level of the infant. Other factors play a role in the development of hydrops, including intrauterine hypoxia, hypoproteinemia, and a lowering of the nonprotein oncotic pressure of the plasma. Hydrops fetalis has been observed in a variety of other conditions (Table 46-4).

Clinical Manifestations. The main signs of hemolytic disease in the newborn are jaundice, pallor, and enlargement of the liver and spleen. Jaundice usually becomes evident during the first 24 hours of life, frequently within the first 4 to 5 hours of life, and becomes maximal by the third or

TABLE 46-4
SOME CAUSES OF HYDROPS FETALIS

Severe chronic anemia *in utero*
  Parvovirus infection
  Erythroblastosis fetalis
  Homozygous alpha-thalassemia
  Chronic fetomaternal transfusion or twin-to-twin transfusion
  Glucose-6-phosphate dehydrogenase deficiency (rarely)
Cardiac failure
  Severe congenital cardiomyopathy or myocarditis
  Premature closure of foramen ovale
  Large arteriovenous malformation (e.g., hemangioma)
  Intrauterine arrhythmias
Hypoproteinemia
Renal disease
  Congenital nephrosis
  Renal vein thrombosis
Congenital hepatitis
Intrauterine infections
  Syphilis
  Toxoplasmosis
  Cytomegalovirus
Miscellaneous
  Maternal diabetes mellitus
  Parabiotic syndrome of multiple pregnancies
  Sublethal umbilical or chorionic vein thrombosis
  Fetal neuroblastoma
  Cystic adenomatoid malformation of the lung
  Pulmonary lymphangiectasia
  Chorioangioma of the placenta
  Transient leukemia of Down syndrome

fourth day. Jaundice and the metabolism of bilirubin are extensively discussed in Chapter 35.

The degree of anemia reflects the severity of the hemolytic process and the infant's capacity to respond to it with increased erythrocyte production. Late anemia may develop in infants with Rh alloimmunization. This is observed in two clinical settings. In one, the infant does not become sufficiently jaundiced in the initial newborn period to require exchange transfusion. This is more common since the advent of phototherapy, which may control the jaundice even though the hemolytic process continues. Continued erythrocyte destruction occurs, and the infant can develop severe or fatal anemia between 7 and 21 days of life. The other, more common situation occurs in infants who have had exchange transfusions. In these infants, a gradual fall in hemoglobin may be observed, with hemoglobin values of 5 to 6 g/dL being reached by 4 to 6 weeks of life. This results from the continued presence of IgG anti-D in the neonatal circulation with destruction of residual and newly formed Rh-positive cells. Spontaneous correction can be expected by 6 to 8 weeks of age.

Petechiae and purpura may be observed in infants with severe anemia as a result of thrombocytopenia and a disturbance in the intrinsic system of coagulation. This disturbance may result from DIC or from hepatic dysfunction with consequent inability to synthesize the vitamin K-dependent factors (109,110).

Laboratory Findings. Decreased hemoglobin concentration, increased reticulocyte count, and increased numbers of nucleated erythrocytes in the peripheral blood reflect the presence of the hemolytic process. Hemoglobin determinations performed on venous samples most accurately reflect the severity of the hemolytic process. Values less than 13 g/dL in the cord blood should be regarded as abnormal. The reticulocyte count is usually greater than 6% and may reach 30% to 40%. In the peripheral blood, nucleated erythrocytes may be observed in addition to some degree of polychromasia and anisocytosis. Spherocytes are not found in patients with Rh hemolytic disease.

The erythrocytes of infants with Rh hemolytic disease test positive on direct Coombs testing, indicating the presence of maternal IgG on the erythrocyte surface. An eluate obtained from cord red blood cells, if available, should confirm presence of anti-D. Of note, affected infants may type as Rh-negative at birth as a result of maternal anti-D blocking the Rh antigen on cord or neonatal red blood cells reacting with the Rh typing reagent.

Prevention. The prevention of Rh hemolytic disease focuses primarily on the administration of anti-D immune globulin to the mother in the antenatal period, usually at the 28th week of gestation and in some countries at the 34th week of gestation, and after delivery, abortion, and invasive procedures. For immunized women the focus is on the prevention of fetal hydrops and death by intrauterine transfusion until safe delivery can be assured, usually at the 36th week of gestation. Some recent reviews are worth noting (111–113).

The early proposals for the use of anti-Rh immunoglobulin were based on the observation that ABO incompatibility offered protection against the development of Rh sensitization, probably by allowing destruction of the fetal erythrocytes in the mother before they could stimulate Rh antibody formation. Because most major transfers of fetal erythrocytes occur at the time of delivery, efforts were undertaken to destroy such cells soon after delivery. The development of a human immunoglobulin concentrate of anti-D (WinRho) greatly facilitated application of this means of prevention. Prevention of Rh sensitization is now about 90% effective with the use of anti-D immune globulin at the time of delivery. Failures may reflect fetomaternal transfusions that occur before term, or massive transfusions that occur at the time of delivery in which the amount of anti-D immunoglobulin administered is inadequate to destroy the large numbers of fetal cells that have entered the circulation, or because of prior sensitization of the mother following transfusion of Rh positive RBCs. Prior sensitization of a Rh negative mother caused by maternal–fetal transfusion from her Rh positive mother has been reported. The physician can detect massive hemorrhages at delivery by examining maternal blood for fetal erythrocytes by the Kleihauer technique. It has been estimated that approximately one in 250 deliveries involves a transplacental hemorrhage of

more than 30 mL (105). In such instances, a larger dose of anti-D immunoglobulin should be given, and is based on the volume of fetal blood detected by the Kleihauer test.

Immunization before delivery occurs in approximately 1% of women at risk (105) and can be prevented by the antenatal administration of anti-D immunoglobulin at week 28 or 34 of gestation (111–114). It has been suggested that this may not be cost-effective therapy; however, it is the recommendation of some experts that all Rh-negative women with Rh-positive partners should be treated antenatally with anti-D immunoglobulin to prevent Rh immunization (115).

Stillbirths are prevented by intrauterine transfusions or by the early termination of pregnancy. The pregnant woman at risk for delivery of an infant with Rh(D) hemolytic disease is one who is Rh (D)-negative, has an Rh (D)-positive partner, and has anti-D antibodies in her serum. All such women must be followed carefully during pregnancy (102,116).

Intrauterine Diagnosis and Treatment. The most accurate assessment of severity of disease in the at-risk fetus is the estimation of amniotic fluid bilirubin levels. Amniotic fluid is normally clear and colorless. It acquires a yellow pigmentation in cases of severe hemolytic disease because of the passage of bilirubin into it. The amount of bile pigment in the amniotic fluid more accurately reflects the degree of fetal involvement than does the maternal antibody titer. The concentration of bilirubin pigments, usually measured by spectrophotometry of amniotic fluid, is approximately 350 to 700 nm. Normal amniotic fluid, when plotted on a logarithmic scale, describes a straight line, but when a pigment is present, a bulge appears at approximately 450 nm. This can be measured, and the change in optical density (OD) as a function of gestational age can be employed to gauge the severity of the hemolytic process (116,117). Women who should be considered for amniocentesis are those with a history of hemolytic disease in previous infants and those whose anti-D titers are greater than 0.125 by the indirect Coombs test, remembering that titers may vary from laboratory to laboratory.

Fetal Rh(D) typing using DNA extracted from amniotic fluid cells can identify the fetus at risk (118) and thus avoid the need for fetal blood sampling to determine the Rh status of the fetus. At-risk pregnant women determined to be carrying an Rh-negative fetus can then be referred back to the care of local physicians/obstetricians for routine antenatal monitoring.

For the Rh positive fetus, analysis of the amniotic fluid indicates whether the fetus is suffering from severe disease, and this is used as a guide to management, which may include continued observation with amniocentesis at 2-week intervals, premature induction after 33 weeks of gestation, or intrauterine blood transfusion. Measurement of medial cerebral artery velocity using Doppler ultrasound may be used as an indicator of anemia (119,120).

In severely affected cases, allogenic blood should be made available (i.e., on hand) at the time of delivery to transfuse immediately if needed. Also, if hydrops is present, platelets should be available for transfusion because splenic platelet sequestration can cause significant thrombocytopenia (platelet count <50,000 μL).

The treatment of severe hemolytic disease in utero has been by intrauterine transfusions into the peritoneum of the fetus. The preferred method now is direct intrauterine transfusion through the umbilical vein. With intrauterine diagnosis (e.g., amniotic fluid, fetal DNA genotyping, or fetal blood analyses), most fetuses with severe Rh disease can be salvaged. Those who reach 36 weeks of gestation can be induced prematurely, and the survival rate is expected to be the same as for a full-term infant with Rh disease. For those with more severe disease who would not survive to 36 weeks of gestation, intrauterine transfusion beginning at 20 to 22 weeks of gestation results in salvage of as many as 87% of patients (121).

Blood for intrauterine transfusion should be O negative, fresh (<7 days old) and CMV safe. Before transfusion a fetal hemoglobin level should be obtained, a direct Coomb's test performed and the fetal red blood cell antigen status confirmed. The amount of blood to be transfused is then calculated and the fetal hemoglobin level rechecked at the midway point of the placental transfusion; additional blood is then transfused as appropriate given the final target hemoglobin level (122,123). For the fetus with hydrops fetalis and severe anemia the transfusion is often split over a few days with the first transfusion calculated to increase the hemoglobin level to 100 g/L.

Management. Newborns with Rh hemolytic disease are at risk of death or neurological damage, primarily from anemia or hyperbilirubinemia. As soon as the infant has been delivered and respirations have been established, the infant should be carefully examined and an assessment of pallor, organomegaly, petechiae, edema, ascites, respiratory rate, pulse, and blood pressure made in an attempt to judge the severity of the hemolytic process. Cord blood samples should be analyzed for hemoglobin concentration, reticulocyte count, nucleated erythrocyte count, blood type, direct Coombs reaction, and serum bilirubin concentration, conjugated and unconjugated.

In the infant with a positive-reacting Coombs test, the major initial decision is whether to perform an immediate exchange transfusion or to observe the infant's clinical status. In many instances, the outcome of previous pregnancies and the result of amniocentesis during the current pregnancy provide valuable information about what to anticipate in the way of severity. Except for the obviously pale or edematous child, the decision to perform an immediate exchange transfusion is based on laboratory findings.

It has been suggested that a cord hemoglobin less than 11.0 g/dL or a cord bilirubin higher than 4.5 mg/dL is an indication for immediate exchange transfusion (121). The value of immediate transfusion is that it is more efficient to remove a "potential bilirubin load" (i.e., antibody-coated erythrocytes) than to allow hemolysis to occur, with distribution of bilirubin throughout the tissues, from which it is removed with greater difficulty by exchange transfusion.

For less severely affected infants, exchange transfusion is indicated if it becomes apparent that the rate of bilirubin rise is such that total indirect bilirubin will exceed 20 mg/dL (330 μmol/L) in otherwise healthy full-term infants (124). The physician needs to use lower maximal bilirubin levels in sick or premature infants (see Chapter 35).

The potential role of high dose intravenous immunoglobin G (IVIG) therapy in infants with Rh(D) hemolytic disease merits discussion. In a multicenter controlled trial of IVIG therapy to reduce the need for exchange transfusions in neonates with Rh hemolytic disease, Rubo and associates (125) randomly assigned 34 patients with Rh incompatibility to receive conventional treatment including phototherapy, with or without IVIG therapy (dose 500 mg/kg). They found that 12.5% of the children in the IVIG group required exchange transfusions compared to 69% of the control group ($p < 0.005$). No side effects of IVIG were observed. Gottstein and Cooke (126) reviewed randomized and quasi-randomized controlled trials comparing IVIG and phototherapy with phototherapy alone in neonates with Rh and/or ABO incompatibility. They found that significantly fewer infants required exchange transfusion in the IVIG treated group. The duration of phototherapy and of hospitalization were also significantly reduced. Therefore, it seems that IVIG therapy reduces serum bilirubin levels and the need for blood exchange transfusions in children with alloimmune hemolytic disease.

ABO Hemolytic Disease. ABO hemolytic disease results from the action of maternal anti-A or anti-B antibodies on fetal erythrocytes of the corresponding blood group. Although approximately 20% of all pregnancies are associated with ABO incompatibility between the mother and fetus, the incidence of severe hemolytic disease is low. Anti-A and anti-B antibodies are found in the IgA, IgM, and IgG fractions of plasma. Only the IgG antibodies cross the placenta and are responsible for the production of disease. These naturally occurring antibodies result from continuous immune stimulation by A and B substances that exist in foods and gram-negative bacteria. Anti-A and anti-B titers are low or absent in most pregnancies and it is not understood why some women develop high anti-A or anti-B titers. They may be the result of repeated, asymptomatic bacterial infections. ABO hemolytic disease tends to occur in the newborns of mothers with high levels of IgG anti-A or anti-B titers.

Fewer A or B antigenic sites are present on the erythrocytes of the newborn, which is responsible for the weakly reactive Coombs test in infants with ABO hemolytic disease. The sparse distribution of A and B sites on the erythrocytes of the newborn also explains why the erythrocyte life span in ABO hemolytic disease is only slightly shortened. Adult group A erythrocytes transfused into a baby with maternally acquired anti-A antibody are rapidly destroyed and may produce severe intravascular hemolysis. For this reason group O RBCs are used for transfusion support of infants with severe ABO hemolytic disease of the newborn. Another factor that explains the low incidence of severe ABO hemolytic disease in neonates is the fact that fetal and newborn blood contains soluble blood group A and B substances that neutralize transplacentally acquired antibodies.

The diagnosis of ABO hemolytic disease is often difficult and may first require the exclusion of other causes of hyperbilirubinemia. Usually, the diagnosis is suspected when hyperbilirubinemia appears in the group A or B baby of a blood group O mother. The disease is more common and more severe in infants of African descent. Jaundice appearing in the first 24 hours (icterus praecox) is particularly characteristic of ABO hemolytic disease. Anemia may be mild or may not be present. Evidence of alloimmunization is difficult to interpret because the Coombs test may be negative or only weakly positive. It has been observed that one-third of all A or B babies of O mothers have a positive direct Coombs test (127); in approximately two-thirds of these babies, an elution test demonstrated anti-A or anti-B on the surfaces of their erythrocytes (127). However, the Coombs and elution tests are not specific for ABO hemolytic disease because these tests are frequently positive in infants who are not affected with disease.

The diagnosis of ABO hemolytic disease is supported by the finding of increased numbers of spherocytes; these are best detected by evaluating the three-dimensional shape of the erythrocyte (Fig. 46-6). Increased erythrocyte production is also demonstrated by an increased reticulocyte count. The diagnosis of ABO hemolytic disease is supported by the following tests and findings:

1. Indirect (unconjugated) hyperbilirubinemia.
2. Jaundice appearing during the first 24 hours of life.
3. A Group A or B baby of a Group O mother.
4. Increased numbers of spherocytes in the blood.
5. Increased erythrocyte production evidenced by reticulocytosis or an elevated carboxyhemoglobin concentration.
6. The presence of IgG, anti-A, or anti-B in cord plasma or serum.

The levels of IgG anti-A, or anti-B in the mothers of babies with ABO hemolytic disease are significantly higher than those in mothers whose infants do not have the disease. These tests are often not available and, unfortunately, are not high in specificity or sensitivity in the diagnosis of ABO hemolytic disease.

Treatment of this disease is directed primarily toward the prevention of hyperbilirubinemia. Phototherapy reduces the need for exchange transfusion (128). Prophylactic phototherapy may be beneficial when the cord bilirubin is at least 4 mg/dl (129).

Hemolytic Disease Resulting From Minor Blood Group Incompatibility. Hemolytic disease related to maternal erythrocyte antibodies other than anti-D, anti-A, or anti-B is relatively uncommon. In one study, minor group antibodies were found in 121 (0.08%) of 142,800 pregnant women (130). The principal antibodies found were anti-E, anti-c, and anti-K (Kell). In a report of 30 cases of hemolytic disease of the newborn, the following antibodies were responsible: 14 anti-c, nine anti-E, two anti-Ce, two anti-K, one anti-Fy^a, one anti-Jk^a, and one anti-U (131). Anti-K antibodies may cause severe hemolytic disease in newborn infants, including hydrops fetalis and neonatal death (132). Of interest, the severity of hemolytic disease of the newborn does not correlate with the anti-K titre (133). These antibodies are known to inhibit fetal erythropoiesis (134,135). Based on the above it is recommended that all pregnant women should have their blood screened for antibodies at least once during pregnancy before week 34 of gestation.

Inherited Defects of the Erythrocyte

Inherited defects of erythrocyte metabolism, membrane function, and hemoglobin synthesis all may manifest themselves in the newborn period. Defects of erythrocyte metabolism include glucose-6-phosphate dehydrogenase (G6PD) deficiency and less common disorders such as pyruvate kinase deficiency.

Glucose-6-Phosphate Dehydrogenase Deficiency. The major function of the erythrocyte is the delivery of oxygen to the tissues. The cell is constantly exposed to oxygen, and the erythrocyte membrane and cytoplasm are subjected to oxidative damage. Oxidation causes the formation of precipitates of denatured hemoglobin (Heinz bodies), which appear to be associated with a shortened erythrocyte life span in vivo (Fig. 46-7). The erythrocyte has a metabolic system that can prevent oxidative damage (Fig. 46-8). Glucose-6-phosphate dehydrogenase is an enzyme in this system; if it is absent, there is a risk of oxidative damage to the erythrocyte, particularly if the

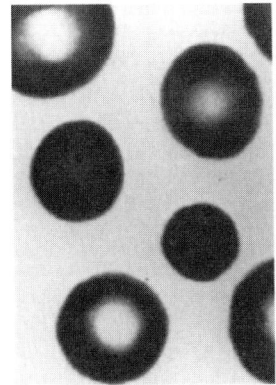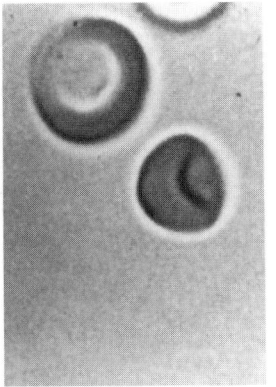

Figure 46-6 The erythrocytes of a patient with hereditary spherocytosis, as seen on a stained blood smear **(A)** and by three-dimensional viewing **(B)** of glutaraldehyde-fixed cells.

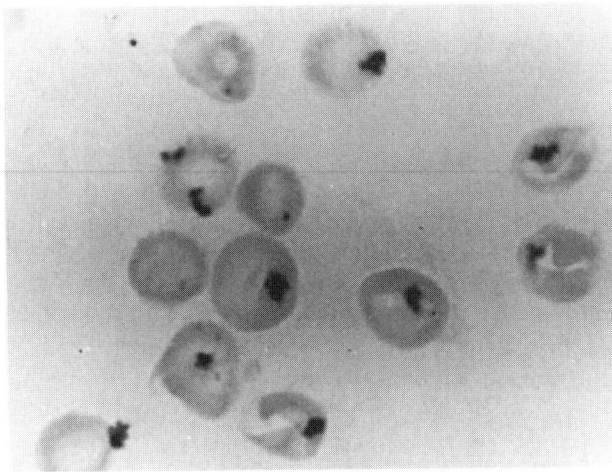

Figure 46-7 Heinz bodies in a newborn who developed hemolytic anemia after exposure to naphthalene in mothballs.

cell is stressed by chemicals or drugs capable of oxidative damage (Table 46-5).

Glucose-6-phosphate dehydrogenase deficiency is a common genetic disorder affecting millions of people in the world (136). There are three major types of deficiency, all of which are inherited as a gender-linked recessive disorder. The most severe deficiency occurs rarely and is associated with a chronic hemolytic anemia. With this type of deficiency, the person has a mild or moderate anemia throughout life and may have severe hemolytic disease as a newborn. The second type affects Asians (e.g., 5.5% of Chinese) and many populations in the Middle East and Mediterranean region (e.g., 0.7% to 3% of Greeks, with the highest incidence of 53% among Kurds). These persons are healthy but are at risk of developing hemolytic anemia when exposed to oxidative drugs or chemicals (e.g., sulfa drugs, fava beans). The anemia may be of sudden onset and may be severe. In the absence of

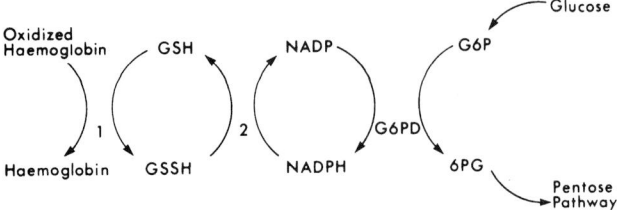

Figure 46-8 Protection against oxidative stress in erythrocytes. The erythrocyte is constantly exposed to oxygen; as a result, there is formation of hydrogen peroxide (H_2O_2), lipid peroxides in the membrane, and oxidized products of hemoglobin such as methemoglobin and Heinz bodies. To prevent the formation of, and to reduce, the levels of these oxidized products, the erythrocyte has a system by which a series of enzyme steps link the metabolism of glucose through the pentose pathway to the reduction of oxidized products (1, glutathione peroxidase; 2, glutathione reductase; G6PD, glucose-6-phosphate dehydrogenase; 6PG, 6-phosphogluconate; G6P, glucose-6-phosphate ; GSH, reduced glutathione; GSSH, oxidized glutathione; NADP, nicotinamide-adenine dinucleotide phosphate; NADPH, nicotinamide-adenine dinucleotide phosphate, reduced)

TABLE 46-5
DRUGS, CHEMICALS, AND OTHER FACTORS THAT CAUSE GLUCOSE-6-PHOSPHATE DEHYDROGENASE DEFICIENCY HEMOLYTIC DISEASE

Antimalarials
  Primaquine
  Pamaquine
  Pentaquine
Antipyretics and analgesics
  Aspirin[a]
  Acetanilid
  Acetophenetidin (phenacetin)[a]
  Acetaminophen[a]
Diabetic acidosis
Vitamin K analogs
Infections
  Respiratory viruses
  Infectious hepatitis
  Infectious mononucleosis
  Bacterial pneumonia
Nitrofurans
  Nitrofurantoin (Furadantin)
  Furazolidone (Furoxone)
  Furaltadone (Altafur)
  Nitrofurazone (Furacin)
Sulfonamides
  Sulfanilamide
  N^2-Acetylsulfanilamide
  Sulfacetamide (Sulamyd)
  Sulfamethoxazole (Gantanol)
  Salicylazosulfapyridine (Azulfidine)
Sulfones
  Thiazolesulfone
Others
  Methylene blue
  Toluidine blue
  Naphthalene
  Phenylhydrazine
  Acetylphenylhydrazine
  Fava beans
  Nalidixic acid (Neggram)
  Niridazole (Ambilhar)
  Chloramphenicol

[a] Of doubtful significance.

fava beans or drug exposure, hemoglobin levels are normal, although there is evidence that the erythrocyte life span is slightly shorter than normal. The third type of deficiency affects individuals of African descent (e.g., 10% to 14% of African Americans), in whom the severity of the defect usually is not as great as in those with the other two types. Anemia appears only with drug exposure, is less severe than that of the Asian–Mediterranean type, and tends to be self-limited.

Glucose-6-Phosphate Dehydrogenase Deficiency and Neonatal Jaundice. Because their erythrocytes have a diminished capacity to deal with oxidative stress as a result of lower levels of glutathione peroxidase and catalase and a relative deficiency of vitamin E, newborn infants with G6PD deficiency are at greater risk of developing hemolytic anemia than are adults. It appears that G6PD deficiency is associated with an increased incidence of neonatal hyperbilirubinemia, especially in the more severe type affecting the Asian and Mediterranean groups. Hyperbilirubinemia in G6PD-deficient boys has been reported in newborns in Greece, Italy, Singapore, and Thailand (137,138). Full-term African American infants with G6PD deficiency do not develop hyperbilirubinemia more frequently than normal infants do, although the incidence in premature infants may be slightly higher (139). It has been reported, however, that male infants of African descent with G6PD deficiency have a significantly higher incidence of hyperbilirubinemia than do controls (140). Although the hyperbilirubinemia is associated with G6PD deficiency, there is a tendency for the jaundice to occur more frequently in particular families and communities, indicating that genetic and environmental factors must influence the incidence of the disease.

In this group of patients, jaundice may be severe and may lead to kernicterus (101,141–143). In most cases, however, hemoglobin and reticulocyte counts are normal, although in some affected infants the cord blood contains increased bilirubin and decreased hemoglobin levels, suggesting the presence of a mild hemolytic process in utero. There is no evidence of intravascular hemolysis in most of these patients. Slusher and associates (144) demonstrated elevated carboxyhemoglobin (a sensitive indicator of hemolysis) values in Nigerian children with G6PD deficiency and hyperbilirubinemia. Studies of Sephardic-Jewish neonates have yielded opposite results, with no elevation of carboxyhemoglobin values over nonjaundiced G6PD-deficient controls (145,146). The latter observation has been coupled with data suggesting deficient hepatic bilirubin conjugation in neonates with G6PD deficiency (147).

Clinical Manifestations. The jaundice that occurs in these infants usually appears to be an accentuation of the physiologic jaundice of newborns with a late peak (around 5–6 days), although jaundice may appear in some during the first 24 hours of life. There is seldom evidence of a hemolytic process. Abnormal erythrocyte morphology has been documented during hemolytic episodes in adults, but this is seldom described in newborns. However, a more severe hemolytic anemia may appear, with evidence of abnormal erythrocyte morphology, Heinz bodies in the peripheral blood, and intravascular hemolysis. This may be the result of infection or exposure to drugs or chemicals (e.g., naphthalene in mothballs) (148). However, it is unusual to elicit the latter from the perinatal history.

Diagnosis. The presence of unexplained hyperbilirubinemia in an infant of a high-risk (racial intermarriage must be taken into account) population may suggest G6PD deficiency. The enzyme defect can be detected by one of many screening tests (149,150), based on changes in either fluorescence or color resulting from the activity of NADPH, thus indirectly measuring the activity of G6PD. Current

screening tests are very effective, yielding good sensitivity and specificity, but an abnormal result should be followed up with a definitive measurement of G6PD activity based on spectrophotometric measurement of the reduction of NADP+ to NADPH (151). A false normal screen result can occur in infants with significant hemolysis, which destroys the older, more G6PD-deficient red blood cells.

The finding of G6PD deficiency in a jaundiced infant does not in itself prove that the jaundice was caused by the enzyme defect. Other causes of jaundice must be excluded. In a study on Sephardic-Jewish neonates, neonates with both ABO incompatibility and G6PD deficiency showed no increased evidence of hemolysis when compared with neonates with only ABO incompatibility (152). Glucose-6-phosphate dehydrogenase deficiency is most severe and frequent in male infants because it is a recessive gender-linked disorder. However, female infants may be affected because they have two populations of erythrocytes, one with normal and one with low levels of G6PD, in keeping with the Lyon hypothesis. Given the high gene frequency, it is also possible for a female infant to be homozygous for the deficiency.

Treatment. Treatment is the same as that for hyperbilirubinemia described in Chapter 35. Drugs and chemicals likely to produce hemolytic anemia (Table 46-5) should be avoided by these patients.

Other Glycolytic Enzyme Defects of the Erythrocyte.
Other abnormalities are far less common than G6PD deficiency and are unusual causes of a hemolytic process during the newborn period. Virtually all of the recognized defects have been associated with jaundice and anemia in neonates. Of this group, erythrocyte pyruvate kinase deficiency appears to be most commonly responsible for a severe hemolytic process during the first week of life. These disorders are usually characterized by the presence of a normal osmotic fragility of unincubated blood, few or no spherocytes in the peripheral blood smear, and failure of splenectomy in later life to correct the hemolytic process. Unless the infant is a member of a high-risk group (the Amish population in the United States), it is practical to defer diagnosis of these infants until approximately 3 months of life, after it has been established that the hemolytic process observed in the neonatal period is chronic and that the more common reasons for it have been excluded.

Abnormalities of the Erythrocyte Membrane

Hereditary Spherocytosis. In approximately 50% of patients with hereditary spherocytosis, a history of neonatal jaundice can be obtained. Hyperbilirubinemia may require exchange transfusions. Untreated hyperbilirubinemia has resulted in kernicterus in infants with hereditary spherocytosis.

Although most patients with hereditary spherocytosis are anemic, the degree of anemia, reticulocytosis, and hyperbilirubinemia is quite variable. The hemoglobin may fall rapidly during the first several weeks of life, reaching values of 5.0 to 7.0 g/dL by 1 month of age. Neither the hematologic values observed during the immediate newborn period nor the values observed during the first several months of life are reliable indicators of the eventual severity of the disease. Hemoglobin levels of 4.0 to 7.0 g/dL during the first several months of life may subsequently stabilize in the range of 7.0 to 10.0 g/dL. Repeated transfusions are then rarely needed except during the course of infections or aplastic crises. Splenectomy, if indicated, should be deferred if possible, until at least 5 or 6 years of age so that the risk of postsplenectomy infections is minimized.

Hereditary spherocytosis can be diagnosed during the newborn period. Examination of the peripheral blood reveals characteristic microspherocytes, and the osmotic fragility of erythrocytes is increased. The osmotic fragility of the erythrocytes of normal newborn infants is lower than that of adults' erythrocytes, and if an infant is suspected of having spherocytosis, the osmotic fragility should be compared with normal newborn standards. The osmotic fragility test should be deferred, if possible, until the child can readily spare the necessary blood volume for the test. Family studies are extremely useful in confirming the diagnosis, although an affected parent is identified in only approximately 70% of cases.

Hereditary Elliptocytosis. Hereditary elliptocytosis may manifest in the newborn period as a hemolytic anemia. Only 12% to 15% of newborns with this morphologic abnormality have a shortened erythrocyte survival in later life, but many more appear to have a hemolytic anemia during the first several weeks or months of life. In the newborn period, hereditary elliptocytosis may manifest as hyperbilirubinemia and anemia associated with the presence of fragmented and deformed erythrocytes in the circulation. This is referred to as neonatal poikilocytosis. The erythrocytes of these infants are unusually susceptible to fragmentation after heating. This defect disappears within the first few months of life, and the erythrocytes assume an elliptic appearance, usually with no or minimal evidence of hemolytic disease. As in hereditary spherocytosis, demonstration of an affected parent or sibling helps to establish the diagnosis.

Most patients do not require treatment, although an exchange transfusion may be required for infants with hyperbilirubinemia. For patients with persistent hemolytic anemia, splenectomy has proved beneficial, but as in hereditary spherocytosis, it should be deferred, if possible, until the patient is at least 5 or 6 years of age.

Disorders of Hemoglobin Synthesis. The predominant hemoglobin in the newborn infant is HbF ($\alpha2\gamma2$); therefore, it is not surprising that abnormalities in β-chain production (e.g., sickle-cell disease, β-thalassemia) do not manifest during the first month of life. Thalassemia has been diagnosed as early as the second month of life (153).

Patients with sickle-cell disease are usually found to be anemic by 3 months of age, but cases of jaundice and systemic signs during the neonatal period have been reported (154).

Early identification of infants with severe sickle cell syndromes e.g. homozygous sickle cell disease, sickle β-thalassemia through universal newborn screening programs are strongly recommended because morbidity and mortality from sepsis in infants in sickle cell disease can be substantially reduced by early identification of affected infants, enrollment in comprehensive care and prophylactic treatment with penicillin (155–157). Red blood cell transfusion before sampling as part of a newborn screening program can impair detection of sickle cell disease and it is therefore recommended that repeat screening be performed in such infants 120 days following the last transfusion (158).

Abnormalities in γ-chain production have been described during the first month of life, although most of these are not clinically significant. Heinz body hemolytic anemia with an unstable γ-chain abnormality has been reported (159). Cases of microcytic anemia in newborns with reduced γ-chain synthesis have been described as part of a γ-β-thalassemia syndrome (160–163).

Alpha-chain disorders occur frequently in the newborn period. Most are clinically insignificant although some forms of α-thalassemia that manifest in the newborn period can be serious. The α-thalassemia group of diseases represents abnormalities in the synthesis of the α-chains of hemoglobin. Synthesis of these chains is determined by two pairs of α-genes. A deletion of one or more of these four α-genes results in one of the α-thalassemia disorders. The severity of the disease in the newborn and in the adult depends on the number of genes deleted. If one gene is lacking, the patient is hematologically normal unless he or she is a newborn, in which case there is a slight elevation of Bart hemoglobin ($\gamma4$). If two genes are absent (i.e., two missing from one chromosome or one missing from each of the two chromosomes), the patient has α-thalassemia trait, which manifests as microcytosis in the newborn (mean corpuscular volume <95 μm^3/cell) and elevation of Bart hemoglobin. If three genes are deleted, the patient has hemoglobin H (HbH; $\beta4$) disease, a lifelong hemolytic anemia that manifests in the newborn as jaundice and anemia. If all four genes are absent, the patient can form no α-chains and cannot form HbA or HbF. As a result, the infant is usually born dead or severely hydropic, with death occurring several hours after birth. There are now several examples of such children being maintained on transfusion therapy (164). The hemoglobin of these infants is predominantly Bart hemoglobin.

In patients with HbH disease, one parent is lacking one α-gene (i.e., a silent carrier), and the other is lacking two α-genes on one chromosome (i.e., α-thalassemia trait). In the patient with homozygous α-thalassemia, each parent is lacking two genes on one chromosome. It is now thought that the α-thalassemia trait that is found in 2% to 10% of individuals of African descent is in the trans form in which one abnormal gene is present on each of the two chromosomes (i.e., $-\alpha,-\alpha$), and that the cis form ($--,\alpha\alpha$) does not occur in such individuals but does occur with various frequencies in populations in Southeast Asia and the Mediterranean region. This is the reason homozygous α-thalassemia and HbH disease are not found in individuals of African descent.

The incidence of α-thalassemia can be determined through measurement of levels of Bart hemoglobin in newborns. Silent carriers (i.e., $-\alpha,\alpha\alpha$) have as much as 2% of Bart hemoglobin. Those with α-thalassemia trait ($--,\alpha\alpha$ or $-\alpha,-\alpha$) have 2% to 9% Bart hemoglobin. Those with HbH disease ($-\alpha,--$) have up to 20% of Bart hemoglobin.

Acquired Defects of the Erythrocyte

Infections. Infections can induce a hemolytic anemia in the newborn infant who has no underlying inherited defect of erythrocyte metabolism. Such cases manifest with hyperbilirubinemia, which initially may be indirect and subsequently include direct hyperbilirubinemia. Severe hemolytic anemia infrequently complicates sepsis. One exception is Clostridium welchii sepsis, in which anemia is associated with microspherocytosis.

Congenital syphilis, toxoplasmosis, cytomegalic inclusion disease, rubella, generalized coxsackie B infections, and *Escherichia coli septicemia* are examples of infections in which anemia and jaundice are common. Some of the nonhematologic manifestations of these diseases (e.g., rash, chorioretinitis, purpura, and hepatosplenomegaly) are useful in differentiating these disorders from alloimmunization or other primary erythrocyte abnormalities.

Drugs. The erythrocytes of the newborn infant are particularly sensitive to the toxic effects of oxidant drugs. Those, particularly of premature babies, demonstrate increased numbers of Heinz bodies, marked glutathione instability, and an increased tendency to develop methemoglobinemia when incubated with acetylphenylhydrazine or menadione. In many respects, the cells of these infants mimic the metabolic abnormalities observed in cells from patients with G6PD deficiency. Severe Heinz body hemolytic anemia (Fig. 46-7), which occurs in infants with severe G6PD deficiency, is also seen in normal newborns who are exposed to oxidant drugs. The best and most frequent example of this is naphthalene-induced hemolytic anemia caused by exposure to mothballs. This disease is associated with a severe hemolytic anemia, hemoglobinuria, and the presence of fragmented erythrocytes and spherocytes in the circulation. If these are detected, a careful search for exposure to naphthalene or other oxidant drugs (Table 46-5) should be carried out. This increased susceptibility to oxidative damage may be related to the low levels of antioxidants, including glutathione peroxidase, catalase, and vitamin E, in the newborn infant. Idiopathic Heinz body hemolytic anemia probably reflects a similar mechanism, resulting in hyperbilirubinemia and anemia with Heinz bodies present, but the infant has normal G6PD levels, a normal hemoglobin electrophoresis, and a negative heat test for the presence of unstable hemoglobins (165). Evaluation of the family yields no evidence of an inherited disorder, and in the affected neonate, the disorder appears to be self-limited, disappearing within the first several months of life. Vitamin C supplementation may be a factor in the etiology of idiopathic Heinz body hemolytic anemia; however, a randomized controlled trial of vitamin C in small premature newborns was unable to demonstrate hemolysis in supplemented infants (166).

Anemia Caused by Impaired Erythrocyte Production

Diamond–Blackfan Syndrome

Inherited impaired erythrocyte production is a rare cause of anemia in the newborn. The most common cause is the Diamond–Blackfan syndrome, also known as congenital hypoplastic anemia or pure red cell aplasia. The incidence is 4 to 7 cases per million live births. In approximately one-third of infants with this abnormality, anemia is detected at birth (167), and most patients are diagnosed in the first year of life. The leukocyte count and platelet count are usually normal. In 15 to 20% of cases there is a positive family history consistent with either recessive (autosomal or possibly X-linked) or autosomal dominant inheritance (168). In 25% of cases the disease is associated with mutations in the *RPS19* gene on chromosome 19q13.2, and in about 40% the disease is associated with an as yet unidentified gene on 8p23 (169).

Low birth weight affects about 10% of these patients. Physical anomalies are found in about one third of patients. Anomalies apparent at birth include microcephaly, cleft palate, eye defects, web neck, and abnormalities of the thumb including absent or triphalangeal thumbs (170).

The diagnosis may be established by demonstrating anemia, reticulocytopenia, and a marked decrease in the bone marrow erythroid–myeloid ratio in an otherwise healthy newborn. Erythroid to myeloid ratios range from 1:6 to more than 1:200. Clonogenic assays show decreased CFU-E and BFU-E progenitors (171). Molecular diagnosis based on the finding of mutations for the *RPS19* gene is available, but will identify only one quarter of all affected patients.

Spontaneous remissions are rare and unpredictable and most patients require treatment for severe anemia. The majority of the patients will respond to prednisone, which is the recommended initial treatment. Response, reflected by a reticulocytosis and a rise in the hemoglobin level, often occurs within 2 weeks. After the hemoglobin has reached its maximum, the medication is reduced to the lowest dose necessary to maintain a hemoglobin level in the acceptable range. Unfortunately, only about 30 to 40% of the patients remain responsive to prednisone and can be maintained on acceptably low doses. Most patients require a lifelong transfusion program. Hematopoietic stem cell transplantation from a matched sibling donor is successful in up to 80% of the patients (172). There is a slightly increased risk of myelodysplasia, leukemia and solid tumors (173,174).

Congenital Sideroblastic Anemia

Sideroblastic anemias are inherited or acquired disorders of mitochondrial iron utilization resulting in accumulation of iron in the mitochondria of red blood cell precursors. This can be diagnosed by Perl's Prussian-blue iron staining showing greater than 10% cells with circular or ringed staining around the nucleus. Among the inherited sideroblastic anemias are X-linked sideroblastic anemia (associated with the *ALAS2* gene) (175,176); X-linked sideroblastic anemia with ataxia (associated with the *ABC7* gene) (177,178); thiamine responsive megaloblastic anemia (associated with the *SLC19A2* gene) (179,180); and Pearson marrow pancreatic syndrome (associated with the heteroplasmic mitochondrial DNA deletions). The associated genes encode for proteins involved in the transport of iron across the mitochondrial membrane and its utilization.

Diagnosis is facilitated by the presence or absence of nonhematological manifestations, and can be confirmed by molecular testing. Treatment depends on the specific syndrome. Patients with X-linked sideroblastic anemia respond to pyridoxine and patients with thiamine responsive megaloblastic anemia respond to pharmacological doses of thiamine. In the other types of congenital sideroblastic anemia RBC transfusions are the mainstay of treatment. Hematopoietic stem cell transplantation is curative (181). In Pearson syndrome the cytopenia improves with age and hematopoietic stem cell transplantation may not be required.

Congenital Dyserythropoietic Anemia

Congenital dyserythropoietic anemias (CDA) are inherited disorders with ineffective erythropoiesis and striking morphological dyserythropoiesis. Three main types of CDA exist: CDA I, II, and III, which differ in marrow morphology, serologic findings and inheritance patterns. CDA I, II, and III disorders were linked to 15q15, 20q11.2, and 15q21-q25 chromosomal sites respectively, but only the gene for CDA I has been identified and cloned (182).

Most patients with CDA are diagnosed in late childhood or adolescence; however, some patients present in the neonatal period with variable splenomegaly, jaundice, and normocytic or macrocytic anemia. Cases of hydrops fetalis have also been described (183–185).

Most patients have mild anemia and do not require chronic therapy. In cases with severe anemia splenectomy, a chronic RBC transfusion program or hematopoietic stem cell transplantation should be considered. Later in life patients can develop iron overload necessitating iron chelation as a result of ineffective erythropoiesis and multiple transfusions.

Parvovirus Infection

Parvovirus B19 is a single stranded DNA virus, which can bind directly to the P antigen on red blood cells. The expression of P antigen on erythroid and placental tissues may mediate transplacental fetal erythroid infection; however, there is accumulating evidence for the existence of a putative cellular coreceptor for efficient entry of parvovirus B19 into human cells (186).

Fetal parvovirus B19 infection may cause anemia, abortion, or stillbirth or be asymptomatic. Hydrops fetalis with lack of congenital malformations is the typical clinical presentation (187). Approximately 18% of cases of nonimmune hydrops fetalis are caused by parvovirus infection (188). Hydrops fetalis usually manifests during the second trimester of pregnancy and reflects a profound reduction of erythrocyte production in the fetal liver and marrow. This may result in severe anemia, high-output cardiac failure, and death. Myocarditis may also occur and contribute to the accumulation of fluids (189).

Bone marrow aspirates show a paucity of red blood cell precursors, with occasional giant pronormoblasts with large eosinophilic nuclear inclusion bodies, cytoplasmic vacuolization and, occasionally, "dog-ear" projections (190). Diagnosis of parvovirus infection in older immunocompetent children can be made by positive IgM serology. However, this test is unreliable in infants, in which the diagnosis should be based on detection of viral DNA in peripheral blood or bone marrow samples by dot blot hybridization or polymerase chain reaction (PCR) (191,192). Viral studies of amniotic fluid or fetal blood may also be helpful in making the diagnosis before birth (193).

Cordocentesis allows fetal blood sampling for hemoglobin measurement and PCR testing for parvovirus. During the procedure the anemia can be corrected by intravenous RBC transfusion, which can lower the mortality rate from approximately 50% to 18% (194). Postnatal monitoring of the hemoglobin level and judicious transfusions result in resolution of the condition in the majority of cases with a good long term outcome. Although rare, failure of red cell production has sometimes continued after birth (195).

Vitamin Deficiencies

Specific vitamin deficiencies may cause anemia in newborn infants because of decreased erythrocyte production, increased erythrocyte destruction, or a combination of these two mechanisms.

Nutritional anemia secondary to iron or folate deficiency is uncommon in neonates (196). Studies by Seip and Halvorsen (197) indicate that stainable iron disappears from bone marrow aspirates by 12 weeks of age in premature infants and by 20 to 24 weeks in term infants, and it is only after this period that iron deficiency manifests in infants who do not receive supplemental iron. To prevent the development of iron deficiency, premature infants should receive supplemental iron from no later than 2 months of age. Although most premature infants have low serum folate levels by 1 to 3 months of age, they rarely manifest evidence of a megaloblastic anemia. Cases of megaloblastic anemia resulting from folate deficiency typically involve infants receiving goat's milk or phenytoin therapy and infants with chronic diarrhea or infection. Folic acid and vitamin B12 deficiencies are rare disorders of later infancy and have been reviewed by Shojania (198).

A syndrome thought to have been vitamin E deficiency anemia in newborn infants was first described by Hassan and associates (199) in 1966 and typically occurred in premature infants (birth weight <1,500 g) at 6 weeks of age. Characteristic features included anemia, reticulocytosis, thrombocytosis, decreased serum vitamin E levels (<0.5 mg/dL), increased fragility of erythrocytes in the presence of dilute solutions of hydrogen peroxide, and shortened erythrocyte survival (200). Damage to the erythrocyte membrane by lipid peroxides, formed naturally during peroxidation of polyunsaturated fatty acids (PUFA) in the erythrocyte membrane, was thought to be the mechanism of the anemia; vitamin E, a biological antioxidant, inactivates lipid peroxides and protects against erythrocyte damage. The anemia may be exaggerated by increasing the PUFA content of the diet, particularly if infants are also given supplemental iron, a catalyst in the autooxidation of PUFA to free radicals and lipid peroxides (201). After the association among the PUFA content of the diet, iron supplementation, and the vitamin E requirement of premature infants was recognized, the PUFA content of infant formulas was reduced. Vitamin E deficiency as described above has become rare in premature infants, and there is no evidence that routine vitamin E supplementation is of benefit in preventing the anemia of prematurity (202).

Evaluation of Anemia in Neonates

Anemia is characterized by an abnormally low erythrocyte mass; in clinical practice, the hemoglobin concentration is assumed to reflect the circulating erythrocyte mass, and an abnormally low hemoglobin concentration defines the anemic state. After diagnosis, causes of anemia are traditionally considered under the pathophysiologic categories of decreased erythrocyte production, increased destruction (i.e., hemolysis), and blood loss. In newborn infants, this classic approach to anemia is complicated by a hemoglobin concentration that undergoes constant physiologic change during the first few weeks of life. The site of blood sampling, quantity of blood sampled for laboratory monitoring, and the effect of rapid growth can significantly influence the hemoglobin values observed in newborn infants. Failure to consider these factors may lead to errors in diagnosis and result in unnecessary investigation and therapy.

Accuracy of Capillary Hemoglobin Levels

Blanchette and Zipursky (88) compared capillary hemoglobin values obtained by duplicate puncture of the right and left heels of 35 healthy full-term infants. The standard deviation of the difference in hemoglobin concentration of the duplicate samples was 0.8 g/dL; in an infant with a hemoglobin concentration of 17.0 g/dL, 95% of hemoglobin values obtained fall between 15.4 and 18.6 g/dL. It is evident that a difference as large as 1.5 g/dL of hemoglobin in consecutive laboratory reports may reflect the error inherent in the technique of capillary blood sampling in the newborn infant.

Effect of the Sampling Site on Hemoglobin Levels

In newborn infants, hemoglobin levels measured in capillary blood samples may be significantly higher than values obtained from simultaneously collected venous blood samples. Oettinger and Mills (203) found an average difference of 3.6 g/dL between simultaneous capillary and venous hemoglobin determinations in 24 infants studied on the first day of life. Other investigators have reported similar differences (Fig. 46-9) (88,204,205). These differences have been found in term and premature infants, and they persist through the first 6 weeks to 3 months of life (88,206). The difference in capillary and venous hemoglobin levels is most marked in the more premature infants (206). Linderkamp and colleagues (205) suggested that warming of the heel reverses the poor circulation and stasis in peripheral vessels that is largely responsible for capillary and venous differences. If the heel is prewarmed before collection of a capillary sample, the difference in capillary and venous hemoglobin values decreases significantly (204).

Correlation of Capillary Hematocrit Levels and Total Erythrocyte Mass

Erythrocyte mass is probably the best measurement of anemia. In adults, it correlates directly with hemoglobin values, which can be used as a valid means of determining anemia. In infants, the correlation between erythrocyte mass and hemoglobin values, although statistically significant, is poor (68,88). Fig. 46-10 and 46-11 show the results of measurements made using a microtechnique using ^{51}Cr to measure erythrocyte mass in premature infants in the first and sixth weeks of life (88). Extremely wide variations in erythrocyte mass occur for any given hematocrit value.

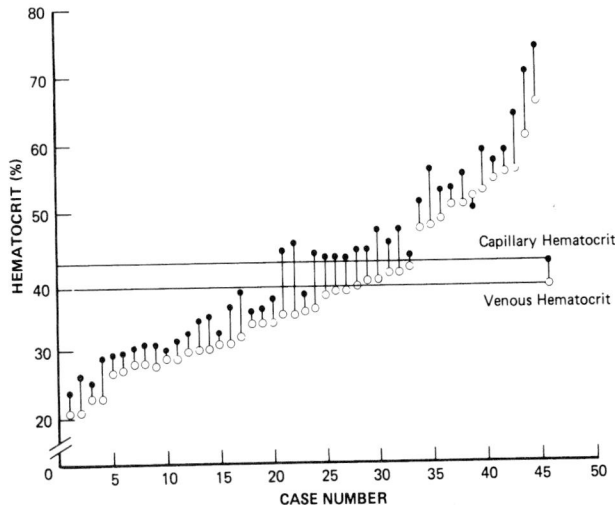

Figure 46-9 Simultaneous capillary (dark circles) and venous (open circles) hematocrit levels in 45 premature infants studied during the first 6 weeks of life. Each vertical line represents values for 1 infant, and the horizontal solid line represents mean capillary and venous hematocrit levels for the whole group. Data are not shown for 5 infants in whom capillary and venous hematocrit levels were identical.

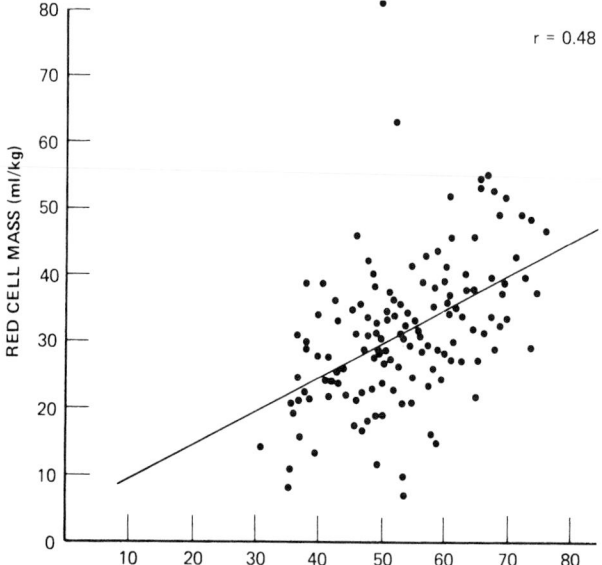

Figure 46-10 Simultaneous capillary hematocrit and circulating erythrocyte mass levels in 135 premature infants who had birth weights less than 1500 g and were studied during the first week of life (r, correlation coefficient)

The capillary hematocrit is often a poor reflection of the circulating erythrocyte mass in newborn infants. This is particularly true for ill infants, in whom a poor peripheral circulation may exaggerate capillary and venous hematocrit differences, and for premature infants during periods of rapid body growth, when increases in the total circulating blood volume may influence hemoglobin levels through hemodilution (205).

Of the many techniques available for measuring erythrocyte mass, the use of chromium-labeled erythrocytes (^{51}Cr) remains the gold standard (207). This technique allows

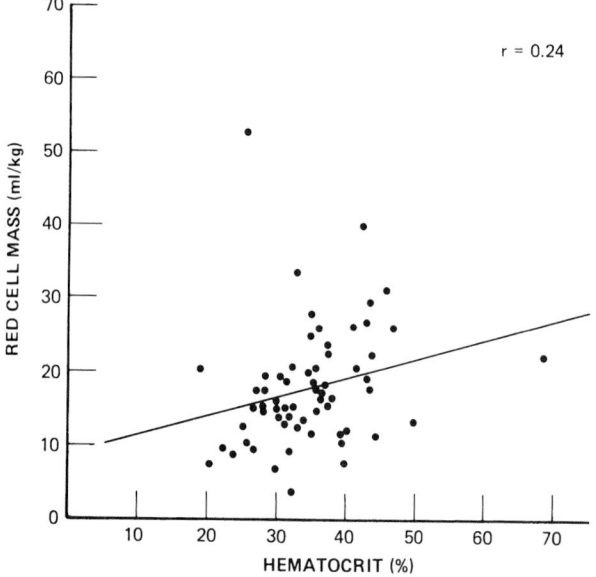

Figure 46-11 Simultaneous capillary hematocrit and circulating erythrocyte mass levels in 63 premature infants who had birth weights less than 1500 g and were studied at 6 weeks of age (r, correlation coefficient)

a direct measurement of erythrocyte mass and does not depend on approximations involving the use of measured plasma volumes, body weights, hematocrit values, or dilution of fetal hemoglobin after transfusion. The values shown in Fig. 46-10 agree with those obtained by other researchers (90–94). A nonradioactive technique involving the use of biotinylated erythrocytes has been applied in neonates and yields values similar to those obtained with ^{51}Cr (208,209).

Work Up of a Newborn Infant with Anemia

At no other time does such a variety of disorders result in anemia as in the first week of life. The need for rapid treatment often adds to the diagnostic confusion. It is because of the multiple causes and the need for prompt therapy that the fundamentals of diagnosis should be appreciated and practiced without delay. Attempts at diagnosis begin with a history if the cause is not immediately apparent. In the family history, attention should be paid to anemia in other members of the family or to unexplained episodes of anemia, jaundice, cholelithiasis, or splenectomy. A positive family history is frequently obtained in cases of infants with hereditary spherocytosis, and a history of affected siblings may be encountered in cases of patients with enzymatic defects of the erythrocyte.

In the maternal history, information should be obtained concerning both her and her husband's ethnic origins and her medication history near term. Information about drugs known to initiate hemolysis in cases of G6PD deficiency should be sought and especially any history of recent exposure to mothballs containing naphthalene.

The obstetric history should provide information about vaginal bleeding during pregnancy, placenta previa, abruptio placentae, vasa previa, and cesarean section. Additional questions should be answered. Was the birth traumatic? Did the cord rupture? Was it a multiple birth?

The age at which anemia is first noticed is also of diagnostic value. Marked anemia at birth is usually the result of hemorrhage or severe alloimmunization. Anemia manifesting itself during the first 2 days of life is frequently caused by external or internal hemorrhages, but anemia appearing after the first 48 hours of life is most commonly hemolytic and is usually associated with jaundice.

One approach to the differential diagnosis of anemia in the newborn period is presented in Fig. 46-12. The physician should first decide whether the low hemoglobin level can be explained by blood loss from sampling. Cumulative losses, particularly in ill premature infants, may be extremely large, and correct interpretation of rapid changes in hemoglobin level can be made only if careful attention is paid to exact volumes of blood sampled and transfused. If the cause of anemia remains unknown, several laboratory tests may aid in diagnosis: reticulocyte count, a direct antiglobulin test (i.e., Coomb's test) of the infant's blood, examination of a peripheral blood smear, and examination of the maternal blood smear for fetal erythrocytes. Ultrasound examination of the head or abdomen is useful to detect occult blood loss. From these studies and the history,

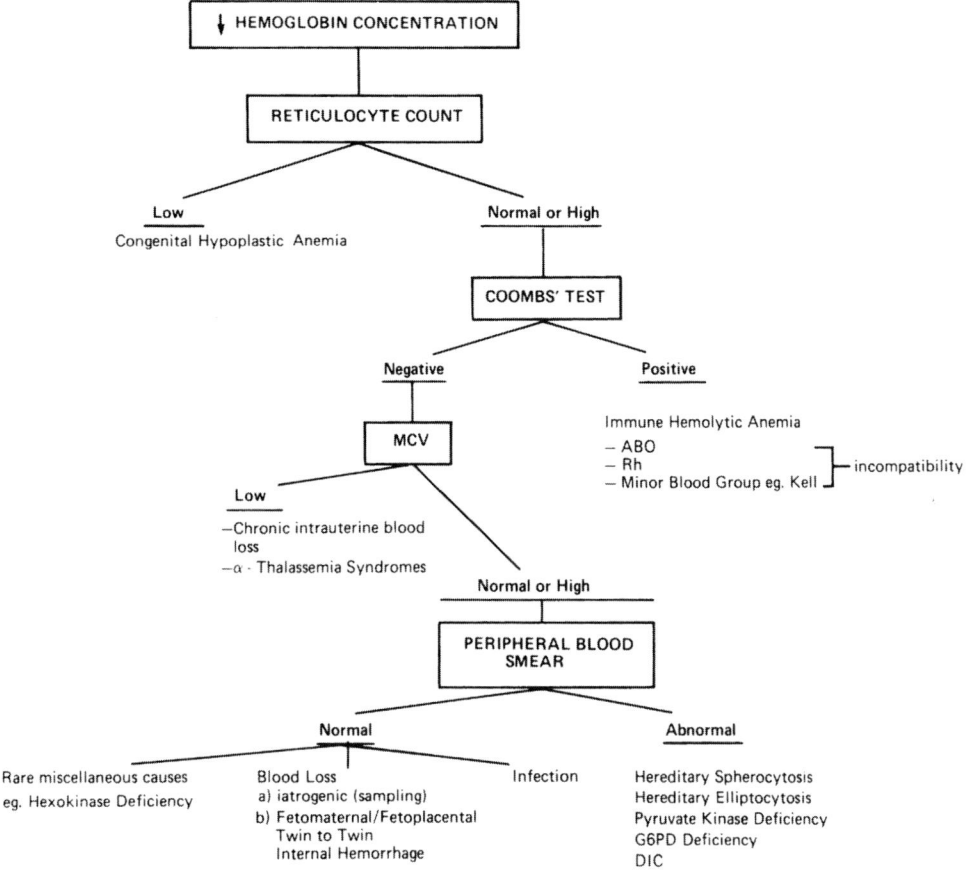

Figure 46-12   Diagnostic approach to anemia in the newborn infant.

a diagnosis often can be made, or at least the list of diagnostic possibilities can be greatly shortened.

Bone marrow aspiration is rarely needed in the neonatal period for the work-up of a baby with anemia. However, if anemia persists without evidence for hemolysis or blood loss a bone marrow should be considered to rule out conditions such as Diamond-Blackfan anemia.

Polycythemia

A venous hemoglobin exceeding 22.0 g/dL or a venous hematocrit more than 65% during the first week of life should be regarded as polycythemia. Although neonatal polycythemia may be the result of fetal disorders such as twin-to-twin transfusion, placental insufficiency, and certain metabolic disorders (Table 46-6), most cases occur in otherwise normal infants. Most of these infants have been full-term, appropriate for gestational age, and without asphyxia at birth. Polycythemia occurs in 1.5% to 4% of newborn infants (210–212).

The symptoms observed in the polycythemic infant appear to be primarily a consequence of hypervolemia and an increase in blood viscosity. After the central venous hematocrit reaches 60% to 65%, the increase in blood viscosity becomes much greater as a result of the exponential relationship between hematocrit and viscosity (213). Plasma and erythrocyte factors also affect the viscosity of neonatal blood (214–216).

Respiratory distress, thrombocytopenia, cyanosis, congestive heart failure, convulsions, priapism, jaundice, renal vein thrombosis, hypoglycemia, and hypocalcemia appear to be more common in infants with polycythemia (212). Many infants with polycythemia are asymptomatic.

TABLE 46-6
NEONATAL POLYCYTHEMIA

Possible causes by placental hypertransfusion
  Twin-to-twin transfusion
  Maternofetal transfusion
  Delayed cord clamping
    Intentional
    Unassisted home delivery
Possible associations
  Placental insufficiency
    Small-for-gestational-age infants
    Postmaturity birth
    Toxemia of pregnancy
  Placental previa
  Endocrine and metabolic disorders
    Congenital adrenal hyperplasia
    Neonatal thyrotoxicosis
    Maternal diabetes
  Miscellaneous
    Trisomies 13, 19, and 21
    Hyperplastic visceromegaly (i.e., Beckwith syndrome)
    Erythroderma icthyosiforme congenita

In addition to supportive care, partial exchange transfusion has been used for the treatment of polycythemia. Reduction of the venous hematocrit to less than 60% may improve symptoms, but it has not been shown to improve long-term neurologic outcome (217–219).

Fetal Hemoglobin, Neonatal Erythrocytes, and 2,3-Diphosphoglycerate

Human tissue metabolism depends critically on an adequate supply of oxygen. The oxygen transport system in humans is the erythrocyte, which contains the iron–protein conjugate hemoglobin. The erythrocyte's primary function is to bring oxygen to the tissues in adequate quantities at a partial pressure sufficient to permit its rapid diffusion from the blood. The ultimate supply of oxygen to the cell is determined by a number of factors, including the content of oxygen in the inspired air, the pulmonary and alveolar ventilation, the diffusion of oxygen from the alveolar air to the capillary bed, the cardiac output, the blood volume, the hemoglobin concentration, and the passive diffusion of oxygen from the capillaries to the cells. The initial passive diffusion of oxygen from the lungs and its final release to the tissues are largely determined by the affinity of hemoglobin for oxygen.

The oxygen–hemoglobin equilibrium curve reflects the affinity of hemoglobin for oxygen (Fig. 46-13). As blood circulates in the normal lung, arterial oxygen tension rises from 40 mm Hg and reaches approximately 110 mm Hg, sufficient to ensure at least 95% saturation of the arterial blood. The shape of the curve is such that a further increase in the oxygen tension in the lung results in only a small increase in the degree of saturation of the blood. As blood travels from the lung, the oxygen tension falls as oxygen is released to the tissues from hemoglobin. In the normal adult, when the oxygen tension has fallen to approximately 27 mm Hg, at a pH of 7.4 and a temperature of 37°C, 50% of the oxygen bound to hemoglobin has been released. The P50, the whole-blood oxygen tension at 50% oxygen saturation, is 27 mm Hg. If the affinity of hemoglobin for oxygen is reduced, more oxygen is released to the tissues at a given oxygen tension. In such situations, the oxygen–hemoglobin equilibrium curve is shifted to the right of normal. It has long been recognized that increases in blood acidity, carbon dioxide content, ionic concentration, and temperature are capable of decreasing the affinity of hemoglobin for oxygen and shifting the curve to the right. If the affinity of hemoglobin for oxygen is increased, as occurs with alkalosis or a decrease in temperature, the equilibrium curve appears shifted to the left, and the tension must drop lower than normal before the hemoglobin releases an equivalent amount of oxygen.

The oxygen dissociation curve of the erythrocytes of newborn infants is shifted to the left, reflecting an increase in the affinity of the hemoglobin for oxygen, compared with the blood of adults (Fig. 46-13). This shift results primarily from the fact that binding of 2,3-diphosphoglycerate to HbF is less than that to HbA (220). As a result, the

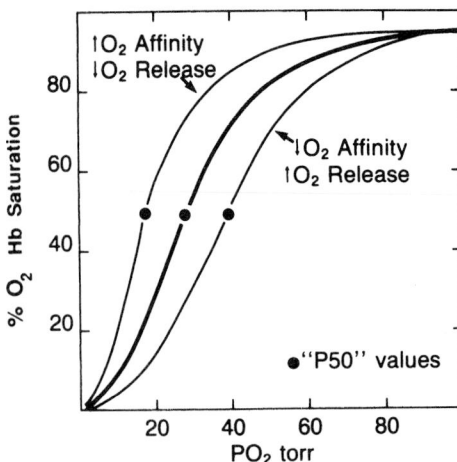

Figure 46-13   The oxygen dissociation curve of normal adult blood. The oxygen tension at 50% oxygen saturation (P50) is approximately 27 torr. As the curve shifts to the right, the oxygen affinity of the hemoglobin decreases, and more oxygen is released at a given oxygen tension. With a shift to the left, the opposite effects are observed. A decrease in pH or an increase in temperature decreases the affinity of hemoglobin for oxygen.

unloading of oxygen in the tissues requires a greater fall of oxygen tension in the newborn than in adults. Conversely, the uptake of oxygen in the lung is enhanced in newborns. It is not clear whether this phenomenon is a benefit or handicap to newborns; presumably, its role in intrauterine life is to permit greater movement of oxygen from the mother to the fetus. There is no evidence that provision of blood containing HbA improves tissue oxygenation in the newborn.

BLEEDING DISORDERS

The hemostatic system is not completely developed at birth, and this affects normal laboratory ranges and interpretation of bleeding disorders in neonates. There is little evidence to suggest that the immature hemostatic system places neonates at increased risk of hemorrhage. However, in the neonatal period, many hemorrhagic problems appear as a result of the diseases and disorders that occur at that time of life. The study of hemorrhagic disorders in the newborn period requires an understanding of the development of the hemostatic system, of congenital and acquired factors that can affect it, and appreciation of the role of disease in producing disturbances in the system.

Because of the incomplete development of the hemostatic system in neonates, interpretation of laboratory tests in any given infant requires knowledge of normal ranges for healthy infants of similar gestational and postnatal age, as detailed in Tables 46-7 and 46-8 (221). Ideally, each institution should develop their own normal ranges to account for variations that may be caused by the use of different reagents and coagulation analyzers (222). To minimize iatrogenic blood losses associated with multiple

TABLE 46-7

REFERENCE VALUES FOR COAGULATION TESTS IN HEALTHY FULL-TERM INFANTS DURING THE FIRST SIX MONTHS OF LIFE

	Day 1		Day 5		Day 30		Day 90		Day 180		Adult	
	M	B	M	B	M	B	M	B	M	B	M	B
PT (s)	13.0	(10.1–15.9)*	12.4	(10.0–15.3)*†	11.8	(10.0–14.3)*†	11.9	(10.0–14.2)*	12.3	(10.7–13.9)*	12.4	(10.8–13.9)
INR	1.00	(0.53–1.62)	0.89	(0.53–1.48)	0.79	(0.53–1.26)	0.81	(0.53–1.26)	0.88	(0.61–1.17)	0.89	(0.64–1.17)
APTT (s)	42.9	(31.3–54.5)	42.6	(25.4–59.8)	40.4	(32.0–55.2)	37.1	(29.0–50.1)*	35.5	(28.1–42.9)*	33.5	(26.6–40.3)
TCT (s)	23.5	(19.0–28.3)*	23.1	(18.0–29.2)†	24.3	(19.4–29.2)*	25.1	(20.5–29.7)*	25.5	(19.8–31.2)*	25.0	(19.7–30.3)
Fibrinogen (g/L)	2.83	(1.67–3.99)*	3.12	(1.62–4.62)*	2.70	(1.62–3.78)*	2.43	(1.50–3.87)*†	2.51	(1.50–3.87)*†	2.78	(1.56–4.00)
FII (U/ml)	0.48	(0.26–0.7)	0.63	(0.33–0.93)	0.68	(0.34–1.02)	0.75	(0.45–1.05)	0.88	(0.60–1.16)	1.08	(0.70–1.46)
FV (U/ml)	0.72	(0.34–1.08)	0.95	(0.45–1.45)	0.98	(0.62–1.34)	0.90	(0.45–1.32)	0.91	(0.55–1.27)	1.06	(0.62–1.50)
FVII (U/ml)	0.66	(0.28–1.04)	0.89	(0.35–1.43)	0.90	(0.42–1.38)	0.91	(0.39–1.43)	0.87	(0.47–1.27)	1.05	(0.67–1.43)
FVIII (U/ml)	1.00	(0.50–1.78)*†	0.88	(0.50–1.54)*†	0.91	(0.50–1.57)*†	0.79	(0.50–1.25)*†	0.73	(0.50–1.09)†	0.99	(0.50–1.49)
vWF (U/ml)	1.53	(0.50–2.87)†	1.40	(0.50–2.54)†	1.28	(0.50–2.46)†	1.18	(0.50–2.06)†	1.07	(0.50–1.97)†	0.92	(0.50–1.58)†
FIX (U/ml)	0.53	(0.15–0.91)	0.53	(0.15–0.91)	0.51	(0.21–0.81)	0.67	(0.21–1.13)	0.86	(0.36–1.36)	1.09	(0.55–1.63)
FX (U/ml)	0.40	(0.12–0.68)	0.49	(0.19–0.79)	0.59	(0.31–0.87)	0.71	(0.35–1.07)	0.78	(0.38–1.18)	1.06	(0.70–1.52)
FXI (U/ml)	0.38	(0.10–0.66)	0.55	(0.23–0.87)	0.53	(0.27–0.79)	0.69	(0.41–0.97)	0.86	(0.49–1.34)	0.97	(0.67–1.27)
FXII (U/ml)	0.53	(0.13–0.93)	0.47	(0.11–0.83)	0.49	(0.17–0.81)	0.67	(0.25–1.09)	0.77	(0.39–1.15)	1.08	(0.52–1.64)
PK (U/ml)	0.37	(0.18–0.69)†	0.48	(0.20–0.76)	0.57	(0.23–0.91)	0.73	(0.41–1.05)	0.86	(0.56–1.16)	1.12	(0.62–1.62)
HMWK (U/ml)	0.54	(0.06–1.02)	0.74	(0.16–1.32)	0.77	(0.33–1.21)*	0.82	(0.30–1.46)*	0.82	(0.36–1.28)*	0.92	(0.50–1.36)
FXIII$_a$ (U/ml)	0.79	(0.27–1.31)	0.94	(0.44–1.44)*	0.93	(0.39–1.47)*	1.04	(0.36–1.72)*	1.04	(0.46–1.62)*	1.05	(0.55–1.55)
FXIII$_b$ (U/ml)	0.76	(0.30–1.22)	1.06	(0.32–1.80)*	1.11	(0.39–1.73)*	1.16	(0.48–1.84)*	1.10	(0.50–1.70)*	0.97	(0.57–1.37)
Plasminogen (CTA U/ml)	1.95	(1.25–2.65)	2.17	(1.41–2.93)	1.98	(1.26–2.70)	2.48	(1.74–3.22)	3.01	(2.21–3.81)	3.36	(2.48–4.24)

Abbreviations: PT = prothrombin time; s = seconds; INR = International Normalized Ratio; APTT = activated partial thromboplastin time; TCT = thrombin clotting time; g/L = grams/litre; F = factor; vWF = von Willebrand factor; PK = prekallikrein; HMWK = high molecular weight kininogen.

All factors except fibrinogen are expressed as units per millilitre (U/ml) where pooled plasma contains 1.0 U/ml. All values are expressed as mean (M) followed by the lower and upper boundary encompassing 95% of the population (B). Between 40 and 77 samples were assayed for each value in each population.

Reproduced with permission from Andrew M. The relevance of developmental hemostasis to hemorrhagic disorders of newborns. *Semin Perinatol* 1997;21:70–85.

TABLE 46-8

REFERENCE VALUES FOR COAGULATION TESTS IN HEALTHY PREMATURE INFANTS (30–36 WEEKS GESTATION) DURING THE FIRST SIX MONTHS OF LIFE

	Day 1		Day 5		Day 30		Day 90		Day 180		Adult	
	M	B	M	B	M	B	M	B	M	B	M	B
PT (sec)	13.0 (10.6–16.2)*		12.5 (10.0–15.3)*†		11.8 (10.0–13.6)*		12.3 (10.0–14.6)*		12.5 (10.0–15.0)*		12.4 (10.8–13.9)	
APTT (sec)	53.6 (27.5–79.4) ‡		50.5 (26.9–74.1)‡		44.7 (26.9–62.5)		39.5 (28.3–50.7)		37.5 (27.2–53.3)*		33.5 (26.6–40.3)	
TCT (sec)	24.8 (19.2–30.4)*		24.1 (18.8–29.4)*		24.4 (18.8–29.9)*		25.1 (19.4–30.8)*		25.2 (18.9–31.5)*		25.0 (19.7–30.3)	
Fibrinogen (g/L)	2.43 (1.50–3.73)*†‡		2.80 (1.60–4.18)*†‡		2.54 (1.50–4.14)*†		2.46 (1.50–3.52)*		2.28 (1.50–3.60)†		2.78 (1.56–4.00)	
FII (U/ml)	0.45 (0.20–0.77)†		0.57 (0.29–0.85)‡		0.57 (0.36–0.95)†‡		0.68 (0.30–1.06)		0.87 (0.51–1.23)		1.08 (0.70–1.46)	
FV (U/ml)	0.88 (0.41–1.44)*†‡		1.00 (0.46–1.54)*		1.02 (0.48–1.56)		0.99 (0.59–1.39)		1.02 (0.58–1.46)		1.06 (0.62–1.50)	
FVII (U/ml)	0.67 (0.21–1.13)		0.84 (0.30–1.38)		0.83 (0.21–1.45)		0.87 (0.31–1.43)		0.99 (0.47–1.51)*		1.05 (0.67–1.43)	
FVIII (U/ml)	1.11 (0.50–2.13)*†		1.15 (0.53–2.05)*†‡		1.11 (0.50–1.99)*†‡		1.06 (0.58–1.88)*†‡		0.99 (0.50–1.87)*†‡		0.99 (0.50–1.49)	
vWF (U/ml)	1.36 (0.78–2.10) †		1.33 (0.72–2.19)†		1.36 (0.66–2.16)†		1.12 (0.75–1.84)*†		0.98 (0.54–1.58)*†		0.92 (0.50–1.58)	
FIX (U/ml)	0.35 (0.19–0.65)*‡		0.42 (0.14–0.74)*†‡		0.44 (0.13–0.80)†		0.59 (0.25–0.93)		0.81 (0.50–1.20)†		1.09 (0.55–1.63)	
FX (U/ml)	0.41 (0.11–0.71)		0.51 (0.19–0.83)		0.56 (0.20–0.92)		0.67 (0.35–0.99)		0.77 (0.35–1.19)		1.06 (0.70–1.52)	
FXI (U/ml)	0.30 (0.08–0.52)†‡		0.41 (0.13–0.69)‡		0.43 (0.15–0.71)‡		0.59 (0.25–0.93)‡		0.78 (0.46–1.10)		0.97 (0.67–1.27)	
FXII (U/ml)	0.38 (0.10–0.66)‡		0.39 (0.09–0.69)‡		0.43 (0.11–0.75)		0.61 (0.15–1.07)		0.82 (0.22–1.42)		1.08 (0.52–1.64)	
PK (U/ml)	0.33 (0.09–0.57)		0.45 (0.26–0.75)†		0.59 (0.31–0.87)		0.79 (0.37–1.21)		0.78 (0.40–1.16)		1.12 (0.62–1.62)	
HK (U/ml)	0.49 (0.09–0.89)		0.62 (0.24–1.00)‡		0.64 (0.16–1.12)‡		0.78 (0.32–1.24)		0.83 (0.41–1.25)*		0.92 (0.50–1.36)	
XIII$_a$ (U/ml)	0.70 (0.32–1.08)		1.01 (0.57–1.45)*		0.99 (0.51–1.47)*		1.13 (0.71–1.55)*		1.13 (0.65–1.61)*		1.05 (0.55–1.55)	
XIII$_b$ (U/ml)	0.81 (0.35–1.27)		1.10 (0.68–1.58)*		1.07 (0.57–1.57)*		1.21 (0.75–1.67)		1.15 (0.67–1.63)		0.97 (0.57–1.37)	
Plasminogen (CTA U/ml)	1.70 (1.12–2.48)‡		1.91 (1.21–2.61)‡		1.81 (1.09–2.53)		2.38 (1.58–3.18)		2.75 (1.91–3.59)‡		3.36 (2.48–4.24)	

Abbreviations: PT = Prothrombin time; s = seconds; INR = international normalized ratio; APTT = activated partial thromboplastin time; TCT = thrombin clotting time; g/L = grams per litre; F = Factor; vWF = von Willebrand factor; PK = prekallikrein; HMWK = high molecular weight kininogen.

All factors except fibrinogen are expressed as units per millilitre (U/ml) where pooled plasma contains 1.0 U/ml. All values are given as means (M) followed by the lower and upper boundary encompassing 95% of the population (B). Between 40 to 96 samples were assayed for each value for the newborn.

* Values that are indistinguishable from those of the adult.

† These measurements are skewed because of a disproportionate number of high values. The lower limit that excludes the lower 2.5% of the population has been given (B). The lower limit for factor VIII was 0.50 U/mL at all points for the infant.

‡ Values are different from the fullterm infant

Reproduced with permission from Andrew M. The relevance of developmental hemostasis to hemorrhagic disorders of newborns. *Semin Perinatol* 1997;21:70–85.

sampling of ill, very low birth weight infants, coagulation laboratories that service neonatal intensive care units (NICUs) should develop microtechniques for the assessment of the hemostatic system (223).

There are several important features of the coagulation system in the newborn (Tables 46-7 and Table 46-8) (221). The prothrombin time (PT) and international normalized ratio (INR) of full-term and premature infants is only slightly outside the adult range (224,225). However, the partial thromboplastin time (PTT), which is frequently used as a screening test in adults, is much longer in newborn infants, particularly premature infants (224,225). Prolongation of the PTT in newborns often results from a reduction in contact factors XI and XII and may not pose a bleeding problem. Factors XI and XII are low in premature infants (a mean of 30% and 38%, respectively), increasing to 38% and 53%, respectively, in full-term infants (224, 225). Substantial prolongation of the PTT (by depression of factors XI and XII) has been observed in children with sepsis without evidence of hemorrhage, leading to the conclusion that the PTT is of limited value in the sick newborn. The two-unit thrombin time is a valuable screening test because it can detect heparin contamination and fibrinogen deficiency. Bleeding disorders in newborn infants are best separated into local bleeding problems and generalized hemorrhagic diatheses.

Local Bleeding Problems in Newborn Infants

Bleeding can occur from the cord, into the scalp, into the gastrointestinal tract, into the abdomen (e.g., liver, adrenal glands), and into the lung. There is little evidence to suggest that the physiologically low levels of coagulation factors in the newborn play any role in the genesis of these disorders.

Intraventricular hemorrhage (IVH) is a major problem of premature infants (see Chapter 50). There is little evidence to suggest that a hemorrhagic diathesis is a major initiating factor in neonates, and therapeutic trials of plasma or coagulation factor concentrates have been equivocal or unsuccessful. It appears likely that IVH occurs as a result of local phenomena related to hypoxia, hemodynamic changes and prematurity. However, it is reasonable to assume that abnormalities in hemostasis could contribute to extension of IVH once such an event has occurred, and that affected infants should receive appropriate supportive care (e.g. FFP, cryoprecipitate, platelets) designed to correct clinically significant abnormalities such as DIC and/or severe thrombocytopenia.

Hemorrhagic Disorders

Acquired Hemorrhagic Diathesis

Major causes of generalized acquired hemorrhagic diatheses as a result of blood coagulation factor deficiency in the newborn period are vitamin K deficiency, hemorrhagic disease of the newborn, DIC, and liver disease.

Vitamin K Deficiency. It was shown many years ago that the administration of vitamin K at birth prevented hemorrhagic disease of the newborn, the classic form of which occurs in the first week of life. It has become an accepted procedure to administer 1 mg of vitamin K1 oxide intramuscularly at birth, and as a result, hemorrhagic disease in the newborn has virtually disappeared. However, there has been controversy about the question of vitamin K deficiency in newborns and the need for prophylactic treatment. Vitamin K is a cofactor necessary for the γ-carboxylation of a prothrombin precursor to active prothrombin. In the absence of vitamin K, this precursor (proteins induced by vitamin K absence [PIVKA]) may be detected in the plasma (226,227). Because PIVKA was found in only one-third of term infants, it has been suggested that not all infants are vitamin K-deficient, and not all need to receive prophylactic vitamin K (228). However, evidence exists that many newborn infants are vitamin K deficient, even though elevated PIVKA levels are not found in all of them (227). Because it is not possible to select babies who are likely to bleed, it is recommended that all babies receive 1 mg of vitamin K1 at birth.

Babies born to mothers who are on anticonvulsant medication are at particularly high risk of having vitamin K deficiency (e.g., early hemorrhagic disease of the newborn), and these mothers should receive vitamin K before delivery (229). Late hemorrhagic disease of newborns (i.e., vitamin K deficiency hemorrhagic disease) manifests at 4 to 6 weeks of age. Infants with this disease characteristically have not received vitamin K prophylaxis at birth; have been maintained on breast milk, which has a low content of vitamin K; and may have suffered from diarrhea or cholestatic liver disease (230). This disorder continues to be reported from areas in which routine prophylaxis is not given (231) or in which oral vitamin K has been used as a single dose during the first days of life (232). Oral vitamin K is effective in preventing early but not late hemorrhagic disease (233–235). These observations provide additional support for the recommendation that vitamin K should be given intramuscularly to all infants at birth to prevent hemorrhagic disease of the newborn (232). There have been concerns that intramuscular administration of vitamin K prophylactic therapy in newborns may increase the risk of malignant disease in childhood. However, recent reports on this topic do not suggest that intramuscular injection of vitamin K is linked to childhood cancer (236).

Disseminated Intravascular Coagulation (DIC). There have been many reports of DIC in newborn infants associated with a variety of diseases. Some reports suggest that most cases of DIC in neonates are caused by cardiovascular collapse (237). This refers to those infants who have had an episode of cardiac arrest, an Apgar score of 0 to 1, or an episode of profound hypotension.

The infant is found to have a generalized hemorrhagic diathesis with bleeding from venipuncture sites, bruising, and widespread internal hemorrhage. Blood studies reveal prolongation of screening tests (e.g., PT or INR, PTT, thrombin time), elevated fibrin split products or D-dimers, depressed factor V levels, and hypofibrinogenemia. Platelet counts may be normal or only slightly depressed. The findings in this syndrome should be differentiated from those observed in sepsis or necrotizing enterocolitis, in which thrombocytopenia is severe, coagulation factors may be normal or slightly reduced, and bleeding is minimal (237).

Management of DIC in the newborn requires aggressive treatment of the underlying cause (e.g., cardiovascular collapse) plus supportive care with hemostatic factors if coagulation factor levels are severely depressed or bleeding is a problem. In such situations replacement therapy with cryoprecipitate (a source of fibrinogen and factor VIII), FFP (a source of all labile coagulation factors) and platelets should be given. The aim should be to maintain a fibrinogen level of 1.0 g/dL or above and a platelet count above 100×10^9/L until the condition resolves and laboratory evidence of severe DIC has disappeared. The recommended initial dose of cryoprecipitate is 0.5 Units/kg (10 ml/kg). During the initial phases affected neonates should be monitored frequently (at approximately 4 hour intervals) with screening coagulation tests (PT/INR and PTT) plus measurement of fibrinogen levels and platelet counts. Presence of a low fibrinogen level and/or significant thrombocytopenia is evidence that DIC is ongoing.

The syndrome of DIC typically complicates a serious illness in an infant. Diagnosis and treatment of the hemorrhagic diathesis is generally relatively straightforward. Unfortunately, the underlying disease and the ischemic damage caused by DIC results in high mortality rates (237).

Localized Intravascular Coagulation (Kasabach-Merritt Syndrome). The clinical and hematologic features of the Kasabach-Merritt syndrome include: an enlarging infantile vascular lesion, most often a hemangioendothelioma or a tufted angioma; thrombocytopenia; a consumptive coagulopathy characterized by a low fibrinogen level; and a microangiopathic hemolytic anemia. Although most affected infants have cutaneous lesions, the syndrome can be caused by visceral hemangioma. This possibility should always be considered in neonates with unexplained thrombocytopenia and coagulopathy (238). Affected infants may manifest high output cardiac failure as a result of increased blood flow through the vascular lesion(s). Management of infants with the Kassabach-Merritt syndrome is often challenging (239,240) and includes supportive care; management of heart failure if present; judicial use of FFP, cryoprecipitate/fibrinogen concentrates and platelet transfusions to maintain hemostatic levels of platelets and fibrinogen in association with more specific therapy targeted at the vascular lesion such as corticosteroids, and/or vincristine (241); second line therapeutic interventions include use of interferon and antifibrinolytic agents; however, because of the risk of therapy associated spastic diplegia interferon should be reserved for life-threatening cases only and used for short periods with close monitoring of neurological status (239). In selected cases embolization may be of help.

Other Causes of Acquired Bleeding Disorders. Profound liver disease can produce a hemorrhagic diathesis as a result of vitamin K deficiency or a primary failure of production of coagulation factors.

Despite the use of heparin to maintain intravenous and intraarterial catheters, a hemorrhagic diathesis from heparin therapy is unusual. The frequency of IVH has not been shown to be affected by heparinization of the infusate through arterial lines, but the confidence intervals are wide and even a major increase in the incidence of grade 3 and 4 IVH would not have been detected (242). However, it is not uncommon in studies of newborn infants for blood samples to be contaminated with heparin. All laboratories studying blood coagulation in newborns should be able to detect heparin contamination. High doses of heparin can be inadvertently administered through peritoneal dialysis.

Congenital Hemorrhagic Disorders in the Neonatal Period

Hemophilia A (factor VIII deficiency) and hemophilia B (factor IX deficiency) may present with bleeding symptoms in the newborn period (243). Because of gender-linked inheritance, male infants and only extremely rarely female infants, are affected. All cases of hemophilia A can be diagnosed at birth because the lower limit of the reference range for factor VIII (<50% or 0.5 U/mL) is similar to the adult value. Although the severe (<1%) and moderate (1%–5%) forms of hemophilia B can be confidently diagnosed in the neonatal period, boys with the mild form may require investigation in later infancy because their levels of factor IX may fall within the lower limit of the reference range for full-term and premature infants at birth (Tables 46-7 and 46-8) (221). The delay in confirming the diagnosis is usually of no consequence because children with mild deficiencies of factor IX are not at risk for spontaneous bleeding.

The bleeding manifestations of neonatal hemophilia include scalp hematomas, prolonged bleeding from venipuncture sites or from surgical procedures such as circumcision, and intracranial hemorrhage (ICH). Management of bleeding involves the infusion of factor VIII (hemophilia A cases) or IX (hemophilia B cases) to restore hemostasis; the replacement product of first choice, if available, is a recombinant factor VIII or IX concentrate (244). If recombinant products are not available a plasma derived factor VIII or IX concentrate treated during preparation to inactivate the HIV and hepatitis viruses should be used (245). In countries where these products are not available FFP (a source of factor VIII and IX), cryoprecipitate (a source of factor VIII), or even fresh whole blood may have to be used. Prothrombin complex concentrates containing factors II, VII, IX, and X should not be used in newborns other than those with known deficiencies of these factors because of the risk of inducing thrombosis.

Severe, isolated deficiencies of factors II, V, VII, X, XI, and fibrinogen are rare and are inherited in an autosomal manner (246). The homozygous forms of the disorders may present with bleeding in the newborn period. Delayed bleeding from the umbilical stump is characteristic of homozygous factor XIII deficiency. The PT/INR, PTT, and thrombin times are normal in patients with factor XIII deficiency, and the diagnosis should be suspected based on the finding of an increased solubility of the patient's recalcified plasma clot in urea or monochloroacetic acid and confirmed by quantitation of the factor XIII level. Treatment of these coagulation factor deficiencies involves infusion of stored plasma (except for factor V), FFP, or specific factor concentrates.

Bleeding is uncommon in newborns with von Willebrand disease (vWD) (247). With the exception of the rare form of severe (type 3) vWD, a diagnosis of vWD cannot be made with confidence in the newborn period because levels of von Willebrand factor are elevated at birth, masking the presence of the most common forms of vWD (248).

PLATELET DISORDERS

A platelet count less than 150×10^9/L is abnormal in term and premature infants (249). The level of platelets in the blood reflects a balance between their production and destruction. Thrombocytopenia may result from decreased production, increased destruction, sequestration, or some combination of these mechanisms. Examination of a well-stained smear of peripheral blood to assess platelet morphology and number, and of bone marrow to assess megakaryocyte morphology and number, has traditionally yielded important information concerning the mechanism of thrombocytopenia in older children. Decreased numbers of platelets and megakaryocytes indicate a production defect, and megakaryocytic hyperplasia and the presence of megathrombocytes (young large platelets) in a peripheral blood smear are characteristic of thrombocytopenic states in which there is increased peripheral destruction of platelets. In newborn infants these indices have not proved as useful as in older children because bone marrow sampling is more challenging and an adequate specimen is often not obtained. Recently, however, Sola and colleagues (250) have published a technique for bone marrow biopsies in neonates that yields small but high-quality specimens thus allowing accurate assessment of cellularity and megakaryocyte numbers.

There are many causes of thrombocytopenia in the newborn. The most common of these disorders are highlighted in Table 46-9 and have been reviewed elsewhere (249,251–254). Some of these disorders, selected because of their frequency or relative importance, are reviewed in detail below.

Neonatal Immune Thrombocytopenia

Immune thrombocytopenia occurs when antibody-sensitized platelets are prematurely destroyed in the reticuloendothelial system, particularly the spleen. Characteristic laboratory features include isolated thrombocytopenia and an increased number of immature megakaryocytes in a bone marrow aspirate.

TABLE 46-9
CAUSES OF NEONATAL THROMBOCYTOPENIA

Decreased production of platelets
  Inherited thrombocytopenias
    Thrombocytopenia–absent radius syndrome
    Wiskott–Aldrich syndrome
    Other X-linked, dominant or recessively transmitted
      thrombocytopenias
  Congenital leukemias and histiocytoses
Increased destruction of platelets
  Immune thrombocytopenias
    Neonatal alloimmune thrombocytopenia
    Neonatal autoimmune thrombocytopenia
    Drug-induced thrombocytopenia
  Giant hemangioma syndrome
  Other states with disseminated intravascular coagulation
Both decreased production and increased destruction of platelets
  Infections
    Congenital, usually viral
    Acquired, usually bacterial
  Osteopetrosis

A variety of conditions are associated with the transplacental passage of maternal antiplatelet antibodies into the fetus, resulting in immunologic destruction of platelets and fetal thrombocytopenia. The antibody may be formed against an antigen on the platelets of the infant (isoimmune or alloimmune thrombocytopenia, in which case the mother's platelet count is normal) or an antigen present on the platelets of the mother (autoimmune thrombocytopenia, in which case both the mother and child may have thrombocytopenia), as occurs in maternal immune thrombocytopenic purpura (ITP) or thrombocytopenia associated with a collagen vascular disorder such as systemic lupus erythematosus.

Neonatal Alloimmune Thrombocytopenia. In neonatal alloimmune thrombocytopenia, the infant possesses a platelet antigen of paternal origin that is lacking in the mother. Typically, the infant's platelets cross the placenta into the maternal circulation during pregnancy or at the time of delivery and cause immunization of the mother, with the formation of antibodies against the foreign platelet antigen. Less frequently, the cause of immunization is exposure of an antigen-negative mother to antigen-positive platelets during transfusion. During pregnancy, transplacental passage of the maternal IgG antibodies leads to sensitization of fetal platelets. Sensitized platelets are rapidly destroyed in the fetal reticuloendothelial system, particularly the spleen, and the result may be thrombocytopenia in utero and in the infant at the time of delivery. This mechanism is analogous to that causing hemolytic disease of the newborn.

The platelet-specific antigen system most often involved in cases of neonatal alloimmune thrombocytopenia is HPA-1a (Pl^{A1}) (Table 46-10) (255). Other platelet-specific antigens are involved less frequently (256–264). In the largest series of cases of suspected neonatal alloimmune

TABLE 46-10

PLATELET-SPECIFIC ALLOANTIGENS

Nomenclature		Glycoprotein	Phenotype Frequency%	
New	Old	(GP) Localization	Caucasian	Japanese
HPA-1a	Pl[A1]	IIIa	97.9	99.9
-1b	Pl[A2]	IIIa	26.5	3.7
HPA-2a	Ko[b]	Ibα	99.3	ND
-2b	Ko[a]	Ibα	14.6	25.4
HPA-3a	Bak[a]	IIb	87.7	78.9
-3b	Bak[a]	IIb	64.1	70.7
HPA-4a	Pen[a]	IIIa	99.9	99.9
-4b	Pen[b]	IIIa	<0.02	1.7
HPA-5a	Br[b]	Ia	99.2	99.8
-5b	Br[a]	Ia	20.6	8.7

Adapted from Blanchette VS, Johnson J, Rand M. The management of alloimmune neonatal thrombocy-topenia. *Baillieres Best Pract Res Clin Haematol* 2000;13:365–390, with permission.
ND = no data

thrombocytopenia, 91% (120 of 132) of serologically proven cases involved HPA-1a (Pl[A1]) alloantibodies (265). Of the remaining 12 cases, the pathologic alloantibodies were anti-HPA 5b (Br[a])-9, anti-HPA-1b (Pl[A2])-1, anti-HPA-3[a] (Baka) with HLA antibody-1, and blood group B isoag-glutinins-1. Although HLA alloantibodies often develop as a result of pregnancy, they rarely are the cause of severe neonatal thrombocytopenia.

The incidence of neonatal alloimmune thrombocytope-nia, based on data collected in prospective studies, is esti-mated to be in the order of 1 in 1800 live-born infants (255). In 85% of cases in which serological information was available, neonatal alloimmune thrombocytopenia reflected fetomaternal incompatibility for the HPA-1a (Pl[A1]) alloantigen. Prospective studies of HPA-1a (Pl[A1]) antigen negative pregnant women provide complementary information reviewed in (255). Fifty-seven of 851 HPA-1a negative women were found to have HPA-1a alloantibod-ies, 48 during pregnancy and 9 in the postpartum period yielding an overall incidence of HPA-1a (Pl[A1]) alloimmu-nization of approximately 1 per 650 pregnancies. Thirty infants manifested thrombocytopenia suggesting an inci-dence of neonatal alloimmune thrombocytopenia as a result of HPA-1a (Pl[A1]) alloantibodies in the order of 1 per 1200 pregnancies in a Caucasian population. Two impor-tant points emerge from these prospective screening stud-ies: first, not all pregnancies involving an HPA-1a (Pl[A1]) alloimmunized mother will result in a thrombocytopenic fetus/neonate; and second, the appearance of HPA-1a (Pl[A1]) alloantibodies, similar to red blood cell alloantibod-ies in cases of hemolytic disease of the newborn, may occur for the first time in the postpartum period.

The typical infant with neonatal alloimmune thrombo-cytopenia is term, and thrombocytopenia is unexpected. Cutaneous manifestations of severe thrombocytopenia (e.g., bruising, a petechial rash) are often the only abnor-malities found on physical examination. A complete blood count shows severe isolated thrombocytopenia with a nor-mal hemoglobin and leukocyte count.

Affected infants are at risk of serious hemorrhage, par-ticularly into the central nervous system (CNS). In a review by Pearson and colleagues (266), the incidence of fatal hemorrhage was 10% to 15%. In some cases, CNS hemor-rhage occurs in utero before delivery (267–271). Bussell and associates (272) estimated that as many as 25% of CNS hemorrhage cases of associated with neonatal alloim-mune thrombocytopenia occur antenatally.

Early diagnosis and effective therapy of infants with neonatal alloimmune thrombocytopenia is important. The disorder should be suspected in all infants with severe, iso-lated thrombocytopenia in whom a specific cause for the thrombocytopenic state cannot be identified (e.g., sepsis, DIC, and skeletal anomalies such as absent radii) and if the maternal platelet count is normal. These infants should receive antigen-negative, compatible platelets harvested from the mother or a phenotyped blood donor. If maternal platelets are used, supernatant plasma with pathologic anti-body should be removed by centrifugation or washing, and the compatible maternal platelets infused after irradiation. In clinical practice, severely thrombocytopenic infants (i.e., platelet counts <30 × 10⁹/L) are often initially transfused with a unit of random donor platelets; in such cases, the platelet response is of diagnostic value (273,274). Because most individuals of European descent type positively for the HPA-1a (Pl[A1]) and HPA-3[a] (Bak[a]) antigens (98% and 88%, respectively), most random donor platelets are in-compatible in cases of neonatal alloimmune thrombocy-topenia involving these alloantigens in a European based population, and their infusion fails to produce a satisfac-tory post transfusion platelet increment, defined as a platelet count of at least 30,000/μL. In other ethnic groups, other platelet-specific alloantigens should be considered.

The rarity of the HPA-1a (Pl[A1] negative) phenotype in individuals of African and Oriental descent explains why neonatal alloimmune thrombocytopenia as a result of HPA-1a (Pl[A1]) fetomaternal incompatibility, the common cause of this disorder in a Caucasian population, is extremely rare in these populations. In Japanese patients the majority of cases of neonatal alloimmune thrombocytopenia are caused by antibodies to HPA-4b (Pen[b]) (275).

In situations in which alloimmune thrombocytopenia is clinically suspected, the lack of response to random donor platelets provide additional evidence for the diagnosis, and it is then most important that severely affected infants receive compatible antigen-negative platelets collected from the mother or blood donors of known antigen type. Regional blood centers serving large NICUs should be encouraged to develop a small bank of blood donors phenotyped for relevant platelet antigens who are readily available for donation. In a Caucasian based population, transfusion with HPA-1a and HPA-5b negative platelets will be effective in over 95% of cases of fetomaternal alloimmune thrombocytopenia and are the initial product of choice for this condition (276). In selected cases, it may be useful to harvest and store in the frozen state the platelets from mothers or antigen-negative donors for immediate use if an affected infant is anticipated (277).

Other therapeutic interventions for neonatal alloimmune thrombocytopenia include exchange transfusion to remove pathologic antibody and intravenous administration of large doses of immunoglobulin G (HDIVIG). This latter strategy is of proven benefit in children with ITP and has been used with variable success in infants with alloimmune thrombocytopenia (278–283). However, if compatible platelets can be quickly obtained, these additional therapeutic interventions are rarely indicated. If compatible platelets cannot be obtained, or if a significant delay can be anticipated before this ideal product will be available, the therapy of choice is a trial of HDIVIG. Current practice is to administer a total dose of 2 g/kg of body weight, given as 1g/kg over 6 to 8 hours on each of two consecutive days. Corticosteroid therapy (e.g., prednisone) is of no proven benefit if used in the traditional dose of 1 to 2 mg/kg/day.

The risk of this disorder recurring in a subsequent pregnancy of a sensitized HPA-1a (Pl[A1]) negative woman is high, and is dependent on the platelet genotype of the pregnant woman's partner. If the partner is homozygous (HPA-1a/1a) the rate of recurrence is essentially 100%, whereas the risk is 50% of the partner in heterozygous (HPA-1a/1b). This has led to the recommendation that in at-risk pregnancies, and especially in cases in which there is a history of a previously affected infant, fetal platelet antigen typing should be performed on fetal DNA obtained from amniocytes obtained following amniocentesis at 15 to 18 weeks gestation (reviewed in 255). If the fetus is determined to be HPA-1a (Pl[A1]) negative no further intervention is needed. If the fetus is HPA-1a (Pl[A1]) positive a cordocentesis should be planned at 20 to 24 weeks gestation to determine the fetal platelet count and to guide antenatal management (284). Options include weekly administration of intravenous immunoglobulin G to the mother with or without the addition of corticosteroids (the preferred approach in North American centers), or repeated intrauterine transfusions of compatible antigen negative platelets (the preferred approach in some European centers) (284,285).

The route of delivery is determined by the fetal platelet count obtained following cordocentesis before delivery. If the fetal platelet count is less than 50×10^9/L, delivery by cesarean section is recommended. At the time of delivery, a cord blood platelet count should be obtained, and thrombocytopenia should be verified in a peripheral blood sample obtained shortly after delivery. If the infant is severely thrombocytopenic, compatible antigen-negative platelets should be infused immediately. These high-risk pregnancies should be managed by a team of perinatologists, neonatologists, and hematologists.

Neonatal Autoimmune Thrombocytopenia. Clinical and laboratory features of neonatal autoimmune thrombocytopenia parallel those of the alloimmune state. In both disorders, the observation of ecchymoses, a petechial rash, or both in an otherwise well infant may be the first clue to the disorder. Measurement of a maternal platelet count and examination of a peripheral blood smear obtained from the mother can help to differentiate autoimmune from alloimmune neonatal thrombocytopenia. In neonatal alloimmune thrombocytopenia, the maternal peripheral blood smear and platelet count are normal, whereas in the autoimmune condition (e.g., mothers with autoimmune ITP), the platelet count is reduced, and the existing platelets are often large (i.e., megathrombocytes). Occasionally, the finding of unexpected thrombocytopenia in an infant may lead to the diagnosis of previously unrecognized ITP in the mother. Autoimmune thrombocytopenia may occur in infants of mothers with ITP who have normal platelet counts after splenectomy. Occasionally in mothers with ITP, increased bone marrow activity can compensate for accelerated destruction of antibody-sensitized platelets. These women may have normal platelet counts, but their infants are at risk of developing acquired thrombocytopenia.

Management of infants with autoimmune neonatal thrombocytopenia differs from that of those with the alloimmune form of the disease. Compatible platelets cannot be found because platelet autoantibodies react with all donor platelets. Therapeutic options include exchange transfusion to remove passively acquired maternal autoantibodies, corticosteroids, and HDIVIG. In infants with significant thrombocytopenia (i.e., platelet counts $<50 \times 10^9$/L) or clinical bleeding, the authors favor administration of immunoglobulin G in a dose of 1 g/kg daily for two consecutive days. A marked increment in platelet count can be anticipated within 24 to 48 hours in 75% of patients (286,287). If this response is not observed, corticosteroid therapy should be started (e.g., prednisone or an equivalent corticosteroid at a dose of 3 to 4 mg/kg/day initially, with rapid tapering once the platelet count increased above 50×10^9/L). Exchange transfusion to remove pathologic antibodies or splenectomy should not be considered in newborn infants unless there is a real clinical emergency with life-threatening bleeding e.g., bleeding into the CNS, and for whom front line therapies such as high-dose IVIG and corticosteroids have proved ineffective.

The same considerations apply to the route of delivery as have been outlined in the discussion of neonatal alloimmune thrombocytopenia. The maternal platelet count and levels of platelet-bound IgG and serum platelet antibody do not predict with certainty which infants will be thrombocytopenic (288–290). The management of the pregnant woman with chronic ITP (or ITP in remission after splenectomy) has been controversial. Studies indicate that the severity of the disease in the fetus is much less than previously reported and that the occurrence of ICH is rare (291,292). Reflecting these observations some experts advise that antenatal determination of the fetal platelet count is not justified in all pregnant women with ITP, and that Cesarean section should be reserved for obstetric indications only (293). If a decision is made to measure the fetal platelet count as a guide to the mode of delivery, cordocentesis is preferred over scalp vein sampling because of the poor reliability of this latter technique (293). The platelet count of affected infants should be monitored carefully in the first few days of life because values may fall to low levels requiring treatment with platelet-enhancing therapies such as IVIG and/or corticosteroids.

Decreased Production of Platelets

Decreased production of platelets in the bone marrow in the neonatal period can be as a result of various causes including perinatal infections (prenatal, natal, or postnatal), maternal drug use (e.g. azathioprine), metabolic defects (e.g. branched amino acid metabolism defects) or inherited marrow failure syndromes.

Inherited Thrombocytopenia. Several inherited marrow failure syndromes are associated with thrombocytopenia. In some of them (e.g. thrombocytopenia absent radii syndrome) only defects in thrombopoiesis are manifest. In others (e.g. congenital amegakaryocytic thrombocytopenia or Fanconi anemia) the first manifestation is usually thrombocytopenia but later on the complete stem cell phenotype is affected with the appearance of multilineage cytopenia.

The genes associated with some of the reported syndromes are known: *WASP* for Wiskott-Aldrich syndrome and X-linked thrombocytopenia (XLT) (294), *CBFA2* for familial thrombocytopenia with a predisposition to acute myeloid leukemia (295), *MYH9* in May-Hegglin/ Sebastian/ Fechtner/Epstein/Alport syndromes (296), *C-MPL* in congenital amegakaryocytic thrombocytopenia (297), *GATA1* in thrombocytopenia with dyserythropoiesis (298), *FLJ14813* in autosomal dominant nonsyndromic familial thrombocytopenia (299), and *HOXA11* in thrombocytopenia associated with radioulnar synostosis (300).

Clues for the specific diagnosis of the inherited marrow failure syndrome can be provided by a family history suggestive of an inherited pattern (e.g., autosomal recessive in

amegakaryocytic thrombocytopenia and autosomal dominant in familial thrombocytopenia with a predisposition to acute myelogenous leukemia); age at diagnosis (e.g., birth in thrombocytopenia absent radii syndrome and adulthood in thrombocytopenia with a predisposition to acute myelogenous leukemia); associated nonhematological manifestations (e.g., limb abnormalities in thrombocytopenia–absent radius and radio-ulnar synostosis syndromes, and renal anomalies in Alport syndrome) (301).

A battery of tests, including bone marrow aspiration and biopsy, is usually required to establish a diagnosis and early referral to a hematologist is advisable. An algorithm to assist clinicians in the diagnosis of the inherited thrombocytopenia has been reported (302). Management varies from supportive care during surgical procedures and avoidance of anti-platelet agents to hematopoietic stem cell transplantation. The efficacy of thrombopoietic growth factors in this group of patients has not yet been determined.

Thrombocytopenia in Premature Newborn Infants

The commonest example of thrombocytopenia in neonates is that seen in premature low birth-weight infants admitted to NICUs. In this patient population the frequency of thrombocytopenia, defined by a platelet count of less than $150 \times 10^9/L$, is of the order of 25% (303–305). In the prospective study of 807 consecutive newborn infants reported by Castle and associates (304) the incidence of thrombocytopenia was 22%; in 38% of thrombocytopenic infants the platelet count was 50 to $100 \times 10^9/L$, and in 20% the platelet count was less than $50 \times 10^9/L$.

A practical classification of thrombocytopenia in neonates has been proposed by Roberts and associates (253) and Murray (254). In this classification a distinction is made between early onset and late-onset thrombocytopenia. Early onset thrombocytopenia is present at birth or occurs within 72 hours of life. Only a minority of these cases will have immunological disorders (e.g., neonatal auto-/alloimmune thrombocytopenia) or coagulopathy (e.g., DIC) as a cause for thrombocytopenia. The vast majority of cases are preterm infants born following pregnancies complicated by placental insufficiency or fetal hypoxia e.g. maternal pregnancy-induced hypertension (PIH), fetal intrauterine growth retardation and maternal diabetes (253). Typically these infants have modest thrombocytopenia (platelet counts $100–150 \times 10^9/L$). Following birth their platelet count falls, reaching a nadir by postnatal day 4 to 5 before recovering to greater than $150 \times 10^9/L$ by 7 to 10 days of age (304). Although earlier studies suggested that, on the one hand, decreased platelet production (303), and on the other hand, increased platelet destruction (304) were the major cause of thrombocytopenia in neonates admitted to NICUs, more recent evidence suggests that early onset thrombocytopenia in low birth weight infants is primarily the result of a transient impairment of megakaryocytopoiesis (306). In contrast, late-onset neonatal thrombocytopenia defined by a platelet count of less than $150 \times 10^9/L$ occurring after the first 72 hours of life almost always results from sepsis or necrotizing enterocolitis (NEC). This late-onset thrombocytopenia has a significant natural history (254). Thrombocytopenia usually progresses rapidly with a platelet nadir that is reached within 24 to 48 hours and is frequently severe with the platelet nadir often falling below 50×10^9/L. Affected infants often require platelet transfusion support. Platelet recovery is slow, occurring over 5 to 7 days as sepsis or NEC is controlled. Neonates with this type of thrombocytopenia initially require careful monitoring of their platelet count (at least every 12 hours) to track their platelet nadir and to time appropriate intervention with platelet transfusions. In neonates with NEC a rapid fall in platelet count to a level well below 100×10^9/L may be a useful marker of intestinal gangrene (307). Finally, in neonates with thrombocytopenia and no apparent cause, thrombosis should be considered.

Evaluation of the Neonate with Thrombocytopenia

An approach to the multiple diagnostic possibilities is outlined in Fig. 46-14. In this schema, it is as important to study the mother as it is to study the infant and to examine the placenta (for multiple hemangiomas). Points requiring specific inquiry include a history of previous bleeding in the form of purpura, bruising, or nose bleeds that might suggest a diagnosis of maternal ITP at some time in the past; ingestion of drugs that may cause thrombocytopenia in the mother and infant (e.g. quinidine, quinine); previous siblings affected with purpura, suggesting one of the immune or inherited thrombocytopenias; and skin rash or

exposure to rubella in the first 8 weeks of pregnancy. Serologic evidence of congenital infections (e.g., syphilis, CMV, herpesvirus, toxoplasmosis) should be sought and recorded. An accurate maternal platelet count should be performed as soon as possible after delivery so that immune neonatal thrombocytopenia caused by maternal ITP can be differentiated from that caused by platelet alloimmunization, in which case the mother's platelet count is normal.

Physical findings of importance in the differential diagnosis of the affected newborn include hepatosplenomegaly and congenital anomalies. Hepatosplenomegaly is often accompanied by jaundice and suggests an infectious process as the most likely cause of thrombocytopenia. In some cases, congenital leukemia may have to be considered. Among the congenital anomalies associated with neonatal thrombocytopenia, the commonest group recognizable at birth is that occurring in the rubella syndrome (congenital heart defects, cataracts, and microcephaly). Deformity and shortening of the forearms should suggest bilateral absence of the radii, with associated amegakaryocytic thrombocytopenia. A single large hemangioma or multiple smaller hemangiomas point to possible platelet trapping and should prompt a search for bruits produced by internal hemangiomas.

A complete blood count on the infant should include a hemoglobin determination, leukocyte count, platelet count, and a blood smear. Associated anemia may result from blood loss, concurrent hemolysis (e.g., infection associated with), or marrow infiltration caused by congenital leukemia. Leukocytosis of a mild degree may accompany infection or blood loss, but if this exceeds 40,000 to

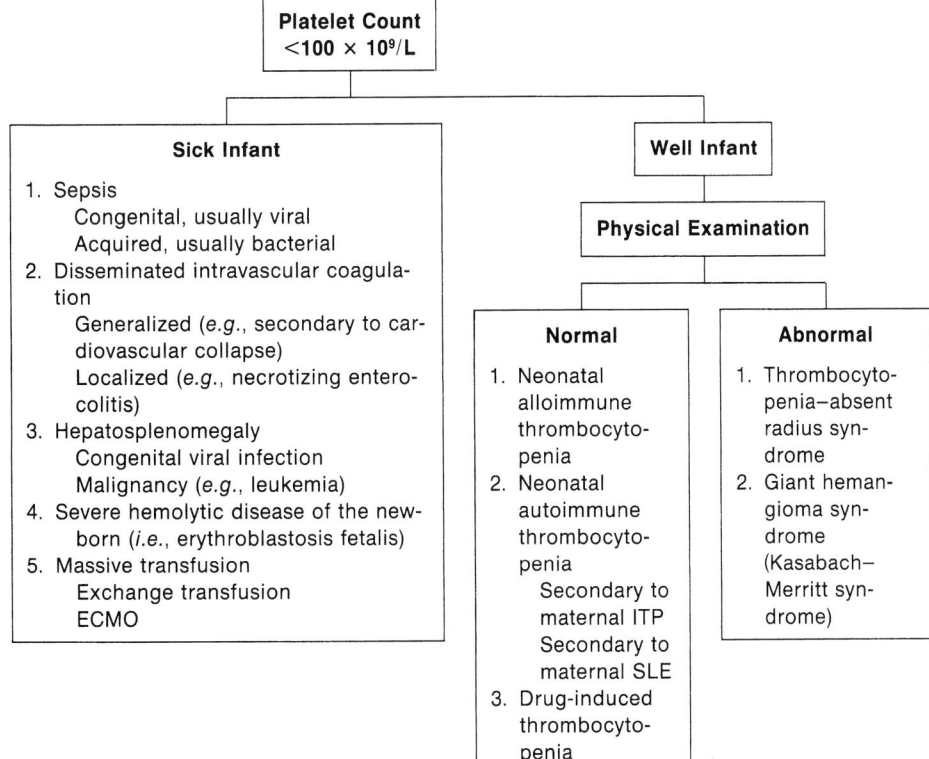

Figure 46-14 Approach to the diagnosis of the thrombocytopenic newborn (ECMO, extracorporeal membrane oxygenation; ITP, immune thrombocytopenic purpura; SLE, systemic lupus erythematosus).

50,000/μL, it may point to congenital leukemia. Bone marrow examination should be considered if thrombocytopenia is persistent and a specific cause cannot be identified. Serologic tests for platelet antibodies and platelet antigen typing are generally only available in reference laboratories. If alloimmune thrombocytopenia is suspected by the finding of an otherwise normal newborn with thrombocytopenia and a healthy mother with a normal platelet count, blood should be drawn from the parents soon after delivery for serologic testing. Characteristically, the maternal serum contains an antibody reactive against paternal platelets. Platelet antigen typing should be performed on both parents, if available; in cases of neonatal alloimmune thrombocytopenia, the mother will type negative and the father positive for the pathologic platelet-specific antigen. In this situation, the infant's platelet type is assumed to be identical to that of the father because it is usually not possible to obtain sufficient blood from severely thrombocytopenic newborn infants for extensive serologic testing. Results of platelet studies may not be available for some time, and therapy should not be delayed pending their results.

LEUKOCYTES

Neutrophil Disorders

A diverse group of leukocyte disorders is encountered in newborn infants. Different blood cells are involved (e.g., neutrophils, lymphocytes, eosinophils), and the disorders may be quantitative or qualitative in nature. This section focuses on abnormalities that are particularly relevant to newborn infants because of the frequency with which they are encountered (e.g., neutrophil changes associated with bacterial infections) or because they are unique to this age group (e.g., congenital leukemia or neonatal alloimmune neutropenia).

Normal Leukocyte Count in the Neonatal Period

The morphologic definition of a mature neutrophil is a cell in which the nucleus is distinctly segmented into two or more lobes connected by a thin filament. Cells with no lobulation and those in which the width of the narrowest segment of the nucleus is greater than one-third the width of the broadest segment are referred to as nonsegmented neutrophils or bands (Fig. 46-15). During the first two weeks of life for full-term and premature infants, a band to segmented neutrophil ratio greater than 0.3 should be considered abnormal (308). Examination of a peripheral blood smear during the first few days of life characteristically reveals an excess of polymorphonuclear neutrophils. Particularly in premature infants, some immature forms (e.g., promyelocytes, myelocytes) may be seen. Sometime between the fourth and seventh days of life, the lymphocyte becomes the predominant cell and remains so until the fourth year of life.

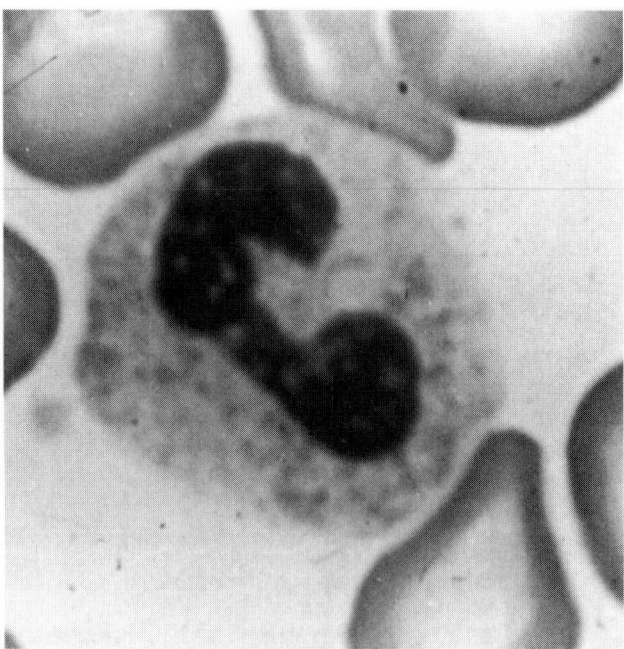

Figure 46-15   A band neutrophil.

Counts of segmented and band (i.e., nonsegmented, young) neutrophils of full-term and very low-birth weight infants have been reported by a number of investigators (308–314). The lower limit of normal for neutrophil counts in very low-birth weight infants are significantly below those for term infants, and the data most widely used for defining neutropenia in NICUs is that generated from the University of Texas Southwestern Medical Center at Dallas by Manroe (312) and Mouzinho (314) (Figs. 46-16, 46-17, and 46-18).

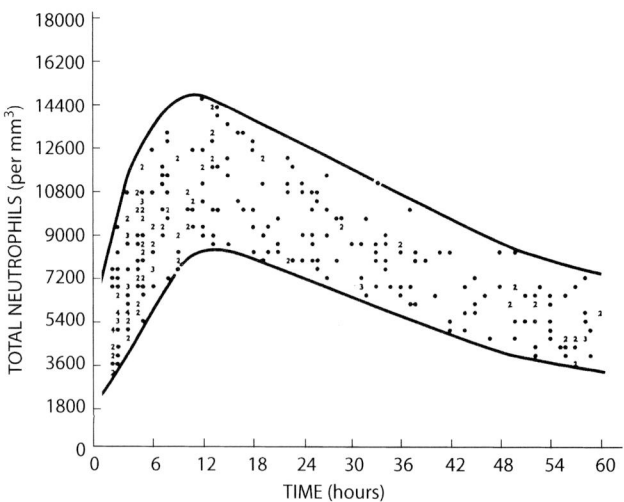

Figure 46-16   The total neutrophil count reference range in the first 60 hours of life. Subjects were 434 newborn infants (birth weight 2685 ± 683g; range 29-44 weeks gestational age) Solid circles represent single values; numbers represent the number of values at the same point. Heavy lines represent the envelope bounding these data. Reproduced with permission from Manroe BL, Weinberg AG, Rosenfeld CR, et al. The neonatal blood count in health and disease. I. Reference values for neutrophilic cells. *J Pediatr* 1979;95:89–98.

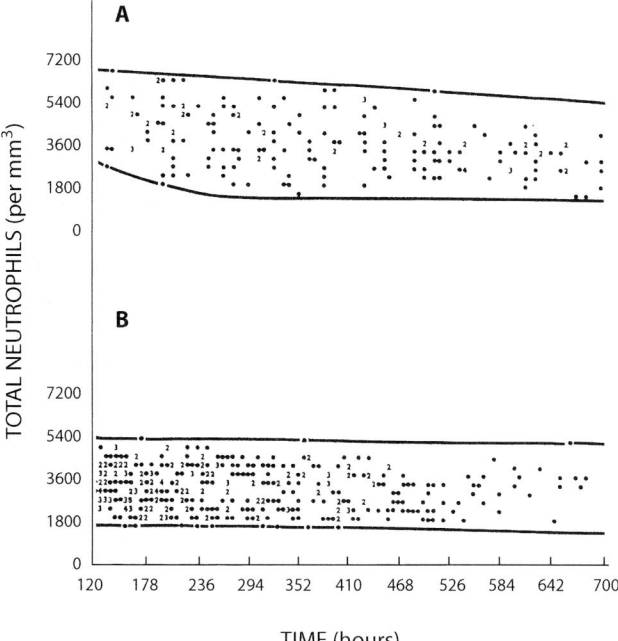

Figure 46-17   The reference range for the total neutrophil count for **(A)** infants 60 to 120 hours of life and **(B)** 120 hours to 28 days. Subjects were 434 newborn infants (birth weight 2685 ± 683g; range 29-44 weeks gestational age) Solid circles represent single values; numbers represent the number of values at the same point. Heavy lines represent the envelope bounding these data. Reproduced with permission from Manroe BL, Weinberg AG, Rosenfeld CR, et al. The neonatal blood count in health and disease. I. Reference values for neutrophilic cells. J Pediatr 1979;95:89–98.

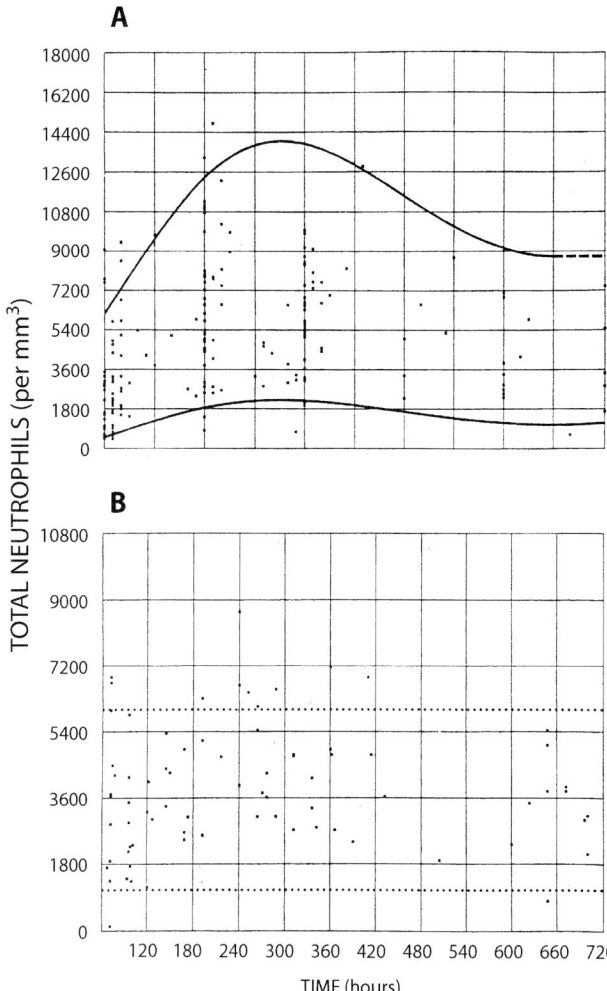

Figure 46-18   Revised reference ranges for total neutrophil values in very low birth weight infants from **(A)** birth to 60 hours of life and **(B)** 61 hours to 28 days of life. Subjects were 193 newborn infants: 50 at 1000g and 143 at 1001–1500g. Bold **(A)** and dotted **(B)** lines represent the envelopes bounding these data, respectively. Reproduced with permission from Mouzinho A, Rosenfeld CR, Sanchez PJ, et al. Revised reference ranges for circulating neutrophils in very-low-birth-weight neonates. Pediatrics 1994;94:76–82.

Although the definition of neutropenia is essentially a statistical consideration based on data obtained from studies of healthy term and premature newborn infants, there is consensus among experts that absolute neutrophil counts above 1,000/μL are not likely to place neonates at risk of acquiring clinically significant infections (315). In our experience it is a helpful rule of thumb to consider an absolute band plus neutrophil count below 1,000/μL to be "clinically significant" in full-term and premature newborn infants.

Physiological neutrophilia is common in neonates in the first week of life. According to Thilaganathan and associates (316) total leukocyte counts in umbilical cord blood ranged between 7.25 to 48 × 10^9/L with a mean of 13.8 × 10^9/L. After birth neutrophil counts increase to levels up to 23,000 at 16 hours post labour and then gradually decrease to less than 9.5 × 10^9/L at 5 days of age.

The mechanism for the physiological neutrophilia seems to be a surge in cytokine secretion. Barak and associates (317) found that serum and urinary colony-stimulating activity levels were significantly increased (3–5 fold) on the first and fourth days of life, but declined to normal values by the 14th and 28th days. Ishii and associates (318) found that G-CSF and M-CSF levels were significantly higher on day 1 after birth and then gradually decreased. Granulocyte-macrophage colony-stimulating factor (GM-

CSF) levels did not change significantly during the neonatal period. Interestingly, these investigators found that granulocyte colony-stimulating (G-CSF) and GM-CSF produced in the placenta (trophoblasts and decidual stromal cells) are the major cause of physiological leukocytosis in newborn infants at birth.

Neutropenia

Causes of neutropenia in newborn infants include decreased production of neutrophils, increased destruction, or a combination of both mechanisms (Table 46-11). Most episodes occur during the first week of life and are related to low gestational age, low birth weight, infections, pregnancy induced hypertension, severe neonatal asphyxia, drug therapy, or other perinatal events (319). Late-onset neutropenia, defined as an absolute neutrophil count of

TABLE 46-11
CAUSES OF NEONATAL NEUTROPENIA

Decreased Production of Neutrophils
Infants of hypertensive women
Donors of twin-twin transfusion
Rhesus hemolytic disease
Kostmann syndrome*
Reticular dysgenesis*
Cyclic neutropenia*
Shwachman-Diamond syndrome*
Cartilage-hair hypoplasia*
Glycogen storage disease type 1b*
Chédiak-Higashi syndrome*
Barth syndrome*
Neutropenia associated with immunodeficiency syndromes
Excessive Neutrophil Margination
Endotoxemia (e.g., necrotizing enterocolitis)
Increased Destruction of Neutrophils
Neonatal alloimmune neutropenia
Neonatal autoimmune neutropenia
Drug induced neutropenia
Decreased Production and Increased Destruction of Neutrophils
Infections
   Congenital, usually viral
   Acquired, usually bacterial
Drug induced neutropenia

* Extremely rare causes of neutropenia in newborn infants.

less than 1,500/μL at a postnatal age of more than 3 weeks has been reported in well, very low birth-weight infants with anemia of prematurity, and reticulocytosis (320). It is speculated that a requirement of progenitor cells for enhanced erythropoiesis associated with the physiological anemia of prematurity limits their availability for granulopoiesis leading to a decrease in neutrophil production. This condition should be considered physiological and is not generally associated with an increased risk of infection.

The various causes of neutropenia in neonates are summarized in Table 46-11. The commonest causes include neutropenia associated with infection, neutropenia in premature infants, neutropenia in infants of hypertensive mothers, and allo-autoimmune neutropenia (321). Other causes for destruction or underproduction of neutrophils are rare, and include inherited marrow failure syndromes.

Changes in Blood Neutrophils During Bacterial Infection

Neutropenia frequently occurs in the setting of neonatal sepsis. It can be the cause of sepsis, but more commonly it is a consequence of infection. It is noteworthy that neutrophil function, particularly chemotaxis and phagocytosis, is reduced in newborn infants and may contribute to susceptibility to infection (322). In neonates, clinical signs of infection may be minimal, and the speed of evolution of disease may be rapid. Changes in neutrophil number and appearance are often helpful in the diagnosis of bacterial infections in this age group (310).

Changes in Neutrophil Numbers

In infants with systemic bacterial infection, the total neutrophil count is usually decreased (i.e., neutropenia), but may also be increased (i.e., neutrophilia), or normal. In a study of 24 newborn infants with proven bacterial sepsis (positive bacterial cultures from the blood, cerebrospinal fluid, bladder-tap urine, or peritoneal fluid), neutropenia was observed in five, neutrophilia in three, and normal neutrophil counts in the remaining 16 (309). Although neutrophilia is a relatively nonspecific finding and may occur in conditions other than sepsis, the finding of neutropenia is highly significant in newborn infants and may be the first clue to bacterial infection. In the study of Manroe and associates (312) neutropenia was observed in 77% of neonates with confirmed or suspected bacterial disease. Neutrophilia was absent almost as often in infected infants (42%) as it was present (58%). In a more recent study the frequency of neutropenia in newborn infants, defined by reference ranges established by Manroe (312) and Mouzinho (314), was 8.1% (135/1662 cases) (319). In 65% (41/63 cases) of neonates neutropenia was present on the day of the clinical onset of sepsis. In 13% (8/63 cases) neutropenia developed within 3 days of the onset of sepsis, and in 22% (14/63 cases) neutropenia was present before the clinical onset of sepsis. Seventy-seven % of the neutropenic episodes occurred during the first week of life; in 75% of affected neonates the duration of neutropenia ranged from 0 to 8 days, with 75% having neutropenia for less than 24 hours. In addition to neutropenia, increased numbers of immature neutrophils (band forms) and an elevated band to segmented neutrophil ratio are seen in neonates with sepsis. Although Baley and colleagues (323) did not find the immature:total neutrophil ratio to be of value in the identification of sepsis in neonates others have found the opposite and have stressed the potential clinical importance of hematologic changes in the assessment of sepsis in neonates (309,310). In a study of premature infants with proven bacterial infection 73% (11 of 15) of infants had elevated band counts and a reversed band to segmented neutrophil ratio (310).

Changes in Neutrophil Morphology

In addition to numerical changes in neutrophils, morphological changes may appear. During infection, the neutrophils of newborn infants have increased numbers of Döhle bodies (i.e., aggregates of rough endoplasmic reticulum), vacuoles, and toxic granules (310). Rodwell and colleagues (324) have proposed a hematologic scoring system for use in the early diagnosis of sepsis in neonates (Table 46-12). In their studies the combination of a neutrophil count less than or equal to 500/mm^3 and scores more than or equal to 3 identified a poor prognostic group (325).

Neutropenia of Prematurity

The most common example of neutropenia seen in NICUs occurs in premature infants, particularly those of VLBW. The mechanisms underlying postnatal neutropenia in such

TABLE 46-12
HEMATOLOGIC SCORING SYSTEM IN NEONATES WITH SUSPECTED SEPSIS

	Abnormality	Score
Immature : total neutrophil ratio[a]	↑	1
Total neutrophil count[a,b]	↑ or ↓	1
I : M ratio	≥0.3	1
Immature PMN count	↑	1
Total WBC count[c]	↑ or ↓	1
Degenerative changes in PMNs[d]	≥3+[e]	1
Platelet count	<150,000/mm^3	1

[a] normal values as defined by Manroe et al (312)
[b] if no mature neutrophils are seen on the blood film, score 2 rather than 1 for total PMN count
[c] ≤5,000/mm^3 or ≥25,000, 30,000 and 21,000/mm^3 at birth, 12–24 hours and day 2 onward, respectively
[d] quantitated on 0 to 4+ scale according to classification by Zipursky et al (310)
[e] for vacuolization, toxic granulation, or Döhle bodies
Abbreviations: 1 = immature; M = mature; PMN = polymorphonuclear leukocytes; WBC = white blood cell

infants appears to be a combination of reduced total body neutrophil mass, together with reduced numbers of committed neutrophil precursors in the bone marrow at birth and an inability to increase granulopoiesis in response to sepsis (326). The role of recombinant hematopoietic growth factors, in particular granulocyte colony-stimulating factor (rhG-CSF) and GM-CSF remains controversial. There is now substantial data indicating that intravenous or subcutaneous administration of these growth factors at daily doses of 5 to 10 μg/kg produces significant increases in the level of circulating neutrophils (G-CSF), or both neutrophils and monocytes (GM-CSF), without significant clinical toxicity. The use of GM-CSF was found by one group to be associated with fewer episodes of postnatal neutropenia and septicemia (327), but not by another (328). Results of prospective, controlled randomized clinical trials are summarized in Table 46-13 (327–332). Although some studies have shown a significant decrease in nosocomial infection rates in treated newborn infants as compared to controls, most studies have failed to demonstrate a significant benefit in overall mortality for treated infants. As a result routine administration of growth factors to extremely low (<1,000 g) or very low (<1,500 g) birth-weight infants at risk for neutropenia and sepsis cannot, as yet, be considered standard of care (333–335). Definitive answers regarding the role of growth factors, administered either prophylactically or as part of treatment of infection in newborn infants, must await the results of future prospective, randomized controlled trials with adequate numbers of subjects to answer clinically important end-points such as morbidity, mortality, and cost.

Less frequent causes of neutropenia in newborn infants as a result of either decreased production or increased destruction are summarized below.

Rare Causes of Neutropenia

Increased Destruction of Neutrophils

Neonatal Alloimmune Neutropenia. Neonatal alloimmune neutropenia is the neutrophil counterpart of the erythrocyte disorder hemolytic disease of the newborn. Estimates of the frequency of alloimmune neutropenia vary widely, with figures ranging from one in 500 to one in 2,000 newborn infants (336–338). Alloimmune neutropenia occurs when a mother becomes sensitized to a foreign antigen present on the neutrophils of her infant and is then stimulated to form specific immunoglobin G (IgG) antibody directed against this fetal antigen of paternal origin. Transplacental passage of IgG antibody into the fetal circulation results in accelerated destruction of neutrophils in the reticuloendothelial system with consequent neutropenia. Because neutropenia is the direct consequence of transplacentally acquired maternal IgG, the condition is self-limiting, and neutropenia persists for only a few weeks or months. The severity of neutropenia is influenced by the titer and subclass of the maternal IgG neutrophil antibody, the phagocytic activity of the infant's reticuloendothelial system, and the capacity of the infant's marrow to compensate for the shortened survival of antibody-sensitized neutrophils.

Investigation of infants with neonatal alloimmune neutropenia has contributed much to the current knowledge of neutrophil-specific antigens (Table 46-14) (339,340), and the antigen systems most often involved are NA1, NA2, and NB1. In approximately one-half of cases the responsible neutrophil-specific antigen system remains unidentified. Although human leukocyte antigen (HLA) antigens are present on granulocytes, and alloimmunization to these antigens is common in pregnancy, HLA antibodies are not thought to be a significant cause of neutropenia in newborn infants. It appears that maternal HLA antibodies are effectively absorbed by HLA antigens in placental tissue; the antibodies that reach the fetus are neutralized by soluble antigens or weakened by having to react with antigens on various cells distributed in the blood and other tissues. In contrast, neutrophil-specific antibodies cross the placenta without any obstacle and concentrate on the target antigen, which occurs only on the relatively small mass of mature neutrophils.

The clinical course of infants with alloimmune neutropenia is of interest. Neutropenia is usually severe and symptomatic infants may present with delayed separation of the umbilical cord, skin infections, otitis media, or pneumonia within the first two weeks of life. In a review of 19 affected infants reported before 1974, Lalezari and associates (341) found that 12 infants had total absence of circulating neutrophils for at least part of their course. The duration of neutropenia ranged from 2 to 17 weeks, with a mean of 7 weeks. Infections were common, and most were caused by *Staphylococcus aureus*. Two infants died, one with staphylococcal septicemia and the other with pneumonia and possible meningitis. Whilst most infections in newborn infants with neonatal alloimmune neutropenia are

TABLE 46-13

RANDOMIZED TRIALS OF RECOMBINANT GROWTH FACTORS (rhG-CSF AND rhGM-CSF) IN NEWBORN INFANTS

Study Aim	Investigator	Number of Study Subjects	Characteristics of Study Group	Study Design	Study Outcome
Treatment	Schibler 1998 (329)	20	• <3 days old • early onset sepsis • neutropenia	rhG-CSF i.v. 10 μg/kg/d IV × 3 days vs placebo	• no difference in circulating neutrophil counts, morbidity or mortality between treatment and control groups
Prophylaxis	Cairo 1999 (328)	264	• birth weight 501–1000 g • age <72 h	rhGM-CSF 8 μg/kg/d i.v. × 7 days then on alternate days × 10 doses vs placebo	• no difference in the incidence of nosocomial infections or morbidity/mortality between treatment and control groups
Prophylaxis	Carr 1999 (327)	75	• birth weight 500–1500 g • postnatal age <72 h • absolute neutrophil counts (×10⁹/L)	rhGM-CSF sq 10 μg/kg/d × 5 days vs no rhGM-CSF	• treated infants did not develop post-natal neutropenia and had fewer episodes of septicemia (11/36 vs 18/39, NS) than did controls
Treatment	Bedford-Russel 2001 (330)	28	• birth weight ≥500–≤1500 g • clinical signs of sepsis • ANC <5 × 10⁹/L • postnatal age ≤28 d	rhG-CSF i.v. 10 μg/kg/d × 14 days or until discontinuation of antibiotics vs placebo	• significantly faster increase in ANC in rhG-CSF group vs controls • significant decrease in mortality at 6 and 12 months in study group • decreased but not significantly different neutrophil counts, duration of mechanical ventilation, duration of stay in NICU, death during first 42 d
Treatment	Miura 2001 (331)	44	• <37 wk GA • birth weight 500–2000 g • postnatal age <5 d • early onset bacterial sepsis	i.v. rhG-CSF 10 μg/kg/d × 3 d vs placebo	• fewer nosocomial infections in treatment vs controls (2/22 vs 9/19) p < 0.02 • higher neutrophiil counts in treatment vs control groups • no difference in mortality between treatment vs control groups
Treatment	Bilgin 2001 (332)	60	• birth weight 1100–3500 g • clinical signs of sepsis • ANC <1.5 × 10⁹/L	rhGM-CSF sq 5 μg/kg/d × 7 d vs no rhGM-CSF	• mortality in rhGM-CSF group significantly lower than controls (10% vs 30%, p < 0.05) • ANC and monocyte counts significantly higher in treated vs control groups

Abbreviations: GA = gestational age; g = grams; μg = micrograms; kg = kilogram; d = days; wk = week; h = hour; IV = intravenous; subcutaneous = sq; rhGM-CSF = recombinant human granulocyte macrophage colony-stimulating factor; rhG-CSF = recombinant human granulocyte colony-stimulating factor; ANC = absolute neutrophil count, NS = not significant.

mild, affected infants with severe neutropenia are at risk for serious bacterial infections, and therapeutic intervention should be considered. In the past, in addition to intravenous antibiotic therapy for infants with suspected or proven infection, therapies included exchange transfusion to remove passively acquired maternal neutrophil antibodies, transfusion with compatible antigen-negative granulocytes harvested from the mother or known antigen-negative blood donors, corticosteroids, and high-dose intravenous immunoglobulin (HDIVIG).

There is little evidence that corticosteroids are of value in this condition. The response to intravenous IgG therapy is variable and of the order of 50% (342). The preferred treatment for neonates with severe alloimmune neutrope-

nia is administration of the growth factor, rhG-CSF. The dose recommended is 10 μg/kg per day given by intravenous or subcutaneous injection for 3 days with titration of additional doses to keep the blood neutrophil count greater than 1000/μL (338). The response to rhG-CSF is usually rapid and evident within 24 to 48 hours; generally 2 to 3 weeks treatment is sufficient. It is important that infants be monitored for recurrence of neutropenia once rhG-CSF therapy is stopped (343). For infants who fail to respond to initial therapy with rhG-CSF, a trial of IVIG (1 g/kg/day for 2 to 5 days) alone or in combination with rhG-CSF should be considered. The use of exchange transfusion or transfusion with compatible antigen-negative neutrophils should be reserved for those rare infants who

TABLE 46-14
HUMAN NEUTROPHIL ANTIGENS (HNA)

Antigen	Location	Polymorphisms	Older Terminology
HNA-1	FcγRIIIb	HNA-1a	NA1
		HNA-1b	NA2
		HNA-1c	SN
HNA-2	GP 50	HNA-2a	NB1
HNA-3	GP 70–95	HNA-3a	5b
HNA-4	CD11b(MAC-1)	HNA-4a	MART
HNA-5	CD11a(LFA-1)	HNA-5a	OND

Modified from Bux J. Molecular genetics of granulocyte polymorphisms. *Vox Sang* 2000;78 [Suppl 2]:125–130, with permission.

have failed an adequate trial of HDIVIG (1 to 2 g/kg/day for 2 to 5 days) and rhG-CSF (10 μg/kg/day or higher doses), who are clinically extremely ill and who are not responding to broad-spectrum intravenous antibiotic therapy. As the condition may recur in subsequent pregnancies we would recommend testing the next baby's neutrophil counts immediately after birth and at 1 week of age. However, asymptomatic babies may not need treatment.

Rare cases of alloimmune neutropenia have been reported in newborn infants following transfusion of blood components or IVIG. In the case reported by Wallis and associates (344) neutropenia occurred in a newborn infant following a RBC transfusion; pathologic antibodies to the neutrophil specific antigen, HNA1b, were subsequently detected in the donor plasma of the transfused unit. A similar mechanism was speculated in the cause of neutropenia in newborn infants following infusion of IVIG for neonatal thrombocytopenia (345).

Neonatal Autoimmune Neutropenia. Transient neutropenia in the neonatal period may reflect transfer of IgG neutrophil antibodies from mother to fetus during pregnancy (346). In these cases, the maternal serum contains the pathologic neutrophil antibodies, and the mother may be neutropenic and may have a history of an autoimmune disorder, such as systemic lupus erythematosus (347,348). Most children are asymptomatic and the neutropenia resolves spontaneously by the 3rd to 4th months of life.

Autoimmune Neutropenia of Infancy. Autoimmune neutropenia of infancy typically occurs in children between the ages of 3 to 30 months (348,349). The mechanism involves production of autoreactive antibodies usually against antigens of the NA1 or NA2 antigens on the Fcγ receptor IIIb (350). Rarely it can be seen in the neonatal period (351). In such cases an underlying immunodeficiency should be ruled out. The disorder is self-limiting, and only 5 to 10% of the children require treatment with G-CSF or IVIG (342).

Decreased Production of Neutrophils.

Infants of Hypertensive Women. Neutropenia can be seen in infants born to mothers with PIH. The mechanism is reduced production as a result of an inhibitor interfering with normal granulopoiesis (352). Neutropenia resolves spontaneously in 3 to 5 days.

Kostmann Syndrome. Congenital neutropenia is severe in patients with Kostmann syndrome; cases are reported in which there was striking neutropenia (usually $<0.2 \times 10^9$/L) from the first day of life (353). Bone marrow smears typically reveal normal cellularity, with a maturation arrest at the promyelocyte-myelocyte level. Inheritance is autosomal dominant, and is associated with activating mutations in one copy of the *ELA2* gene (354), causing abnormally activated neutrophil elastase with exclusive membrane localization (355) and increased apoptosis of myeloid precursors (356). Cases associated with mutation in either the *ELA-2* repressor gene *GFI1* (357) or the *WASP* gene (358) were also described. Severe bacterial infections occur early in life, in 50% of patients within the first month of life, and the disorder is usually fatal. Treatment with G-CSF increases neutrophil counts and prevents infection in 90% of cases (359). In patients non responsive to G-CSF alone addition of low dose prednisone to the G-CSF regimen (360), or hematopoietic stem cell transplantation (361) may be successful.

Cyclic Neutropenia. Cyclic neutropenia is a sporadic or familial disorder characterized by a regular, repetitive decrease in peripheral blood neutrophils at approximately 21-day intervals (362,363). It is caused by *ELA2* gene mutations at the active site of neutrophil elastase causing defective membrane localization of the enzyme (355) and a cycling increase in apoptosis of myeloid precursors (356). Patients may develop severe infection and mouth sores during the neutrophil nadir leading to chronic gingivitis. Diagnosis requires the demonstration of regular neutrophil cycles and thus is usually made after the neonatal period. Treatment with G-CSF improves symptoms in most patients.

Glycogen Storage Disease Type Ib. Patients with this autosomal recessive disorder have classical features of glycogen storage disease type Ia, which includes hepatomegaly and metabolic crisis with hypoglycemia and lactic acidosis. Additionally, they have neutropenia and impaired neutrophil chemotaxis and respiratory burst. Granulocytes are reduced and dysfunctional probably because they are apoptotic with translocation and activation of the Bax proapoptotic protein (364). The genetic defect is different from glycogen storage disease type Ia, and resides in the gene encoded for the glucose 6-phosphate translocase enzyme. Neutropenia may be severe and cause serious infection and inflammatory bowel disease. Most patients require G-CSF, which successfully increases the neutrophil counts, improves function, and prevents infection (365).

Barth Syndrome. Barth syndrome is an X linked-recessive disorder with dilated cardiomyopathy, skeletal myopathy,

3-methylglutaconic aciduria, and neutropenia (366). The disorder is associated with the *TAZ* gene mutation, which encodes 10 different proteins called "taffazins" of still unknown function (367). Neutropenia varies from mild to very severe. The mechanism for the neutropenia is unclear. Marrow specimens are of normal cellularity but with maturation arrest at the myeloid stage. Most patients do not require treatment for their neutropenia. However, in our experience, in cases with severe bacterial infections, G-CSF can be given with a very good response.

Neutropenia Associated with Immunodeficiency Syndromes. Neutropenia may occur in association with immunodeficiency syndromes. Therefore, it is imperative to assess lymphopoiesis in patients with neutropenia, particularly as some of these disorders need urgent change in management. Immune abnormalities, typical features and inheritance patterns that help identify the cause of the neutropenia and the molecular defects are summarized in Table 46-15.

Agammaglobulinemia. Approximately one-third of patients with agammaglobulinemia develop neutropenia in the first year of life during periods of infection. Typically patients with agammaglobulinemia have low or absent

IgG production; however, the passage of IgG from the mother to the fetus may result in detectable IgG in the first months of life. In contrast, detection of IgM, which does not cross the placenta, is a reliable indicator of B cell function even at an early age. In most cases the disorder is caused by a defect in the expression or function of the Bruton tyrosine kinase (*BTK*) gene in B cells. In recent years, mutations in other genes responsible for B cell development have been identified as a cause of a similar phenotype (368). These genes are important for B lymphocyte development, however because B cells normally constitute only 5% to 20% of total lymphocytes, lymphopenia is usually not evident.

Hyper IgM Syndrome. Neutropenia is often observed in patients with the hyper IgM (HIGM) syndrome in which defects in the immunoglobulin class switch recombination and somatic mutation prevent generation of an appropriate antibody repertoire. Typically IgM levels are high with low or near normal IgG and IgA levels. Recently, mutations in several genes have been identified as causing the hyper IgM syndrome. HIGM type 1 is inherited as an X linked recessive trait as a result of abnormal T cell expression of the CD40 ligand. Affected males suffer from recurrent bacterial and

TABLE 46-15
NEUTROPENIA ASSOCIATED WITH IMMUNODEFICIENCIES

Disorder	Typical Immune Abnormalities	Associated Features	Inheritance Pattern	Genetic Defect
Agammaglobulinemia	Low/Absent IgG	None	X-linked; autosomal recessive	*BTK*
Common Variable Immunodeficiency	Low IgG	None	Variable	Unknown
IgA deficiency	Low IgA	None	Autosomal resessive/dominant	Unknown
Hyper IgM syndrome	High IgM. Low/normal IgG	Liver disease, ectodermal dysplasia	X-linked; autosomal recessive	*CD40 ligand, AID, CD40, NEMO-IKK*
Wiskott-Aldrich syndrome	Variable T/B cell counts	Eczema, small platelets thrombocytopenia	X-linked	*WASP*
Cartilage-hair hypoplasia	Variable T/B cell counts	Dwarfism, fine hair	Autosomal recessive	*RMRP*
Shwachman-Diamond syndrome	Variable T/B cell counts	Pancreatic insufficiency	Autosomal recessive	*SBDS*
Griscelli disease	T cell	Albinism; HLH	Autosomal recessive	*RAB27a*
Autoimmune lymphoproliferative syndrome (ALPS)	Variable T/B cell count	Hepatosplenomegaly, lymphadenopathy	Autosomal dominant	*CD95, CD95 ligand, caspase 8, caspase 10*
Chediak-Higashi syndrome	NK cells	Bleeding, albinism, cytoplasmic granules	Autosomal recessive	*LYST*
HLH	T cells	Hepatoslenomegaly, lymphadenopathy, fever	Variable	*Perforin, IL-2R gamma, PNP, RAB27a*
WHIM syndrome	Low IgG	Warts, myelokathexis	Autosomal dominant	*CXCR4*
Dyskeratosis congenita	Variable T/B cell count	Skin pigmentation, nail dystrophy, dental abnormalities, pancytopenia	X-linked; autosomal dominant/recessive	*DKCI, TERC*
Reticular dysgenesis	SCID	None	Autosomal recessive	Unknown

Abbreviations: HLH = hemophagocytic lymphohistocytosis; NK = natural killer cells; SCID = severe combined immunodeficiency

opportunistic infections (e.g., pneumocystis carinii pneumonia and watery diarrhea as a result of cryptosporidium infection) from a young age. Severe liver disease is also a feature of the disorder. Patients with the autosomal recessive HIGM type 2 disorder present with enlarged tonsils and lymph nodes, sinopulmonary infections but without opportunistic infections. HIGM type 2 is caused by mutations in the activation-induced cytosine deaminase gene. Patients with defects in the B cell receptor CD40 have been recently described and are designated HIGM type 3; their clinical condition is similar to type 1 cases. A fourth form of HIGM affects males and is characterized by the association of hypogammaglobulinemia with hypohidrotic ectodermal dysplasia. These conditions are caused by mutations of the gene in *NEMO/IKK (γ)*, which is the same gene responsible for incontinentia pigmenti in heterozygous females (369).

Wiskott-Aldrich Syndrome. Up to one-quarter of males with Wiskott-Aldrich syndrome manifest neutropenia (370). Characteristic features of the disorder include eczema and thrombocytopenia with small (pin-point) platelets on a peripheral blood smear (371). The identification of the gene responsible for the Wiskott-Aldrich Syndrome (*WASP*) facilitates the diagnosis especially in cases without typical features, and has revealed that in some instances neutropenia may be the only symptom (372).

Cartilage Hair Hypoplasia. Severe and persistent neutropenia can occur in cartilage hair-hypoplasia (CHH). The disorder is characterized fine hair, short limbed dwarfism, metaphyseal dysplasia (not often evident in the first year of life) and T cell abnormalities. This autosomal recessive condition is caused by mutations in the *RMRP* gene (373). Although common in the Finish and Amish, the disorder has been reported in other populations (374). In those patients with severe immunodeficiency, hematopoietic stem cell transplantation can correct the immune dysfunction.

Another familial disease involving bone formation, neutropenia and immunodeficiency was recently described (375). In affected subjects severe congenital neutropenia and hypogammaglobulinemia were associated with infantile osteoporosis with multiple bone fractures.

Chediak-Higashi Syndrome. Chediak-Higashi syndrome is an autosomal recessive disorder caused by mutations in the lysosomal trafficking regulator gene. It is characterized by variable degrees of oculocutaneous albinism, easy bruising and bleeding as a result of platelet dysfunction. Patients suffer from recurrent infections as a result of neutropenia, impaired chemotaxis and bactericidal activity and abnormal natural killer (NK) cell function. The hallmark of the disease is the presence of large cytoplasmic granules in circulating granulocytes (376).

Griscelli Disease. Patients with Griscelli disease have some features similar to those with the Chediak-Higashi syndrome including partial albinism, frequent episodes of fever and pyogenic infections, neutropenia and thrombocy-

topenia (377). Their immune abnormalities may lead to uncontrolled T lymphocyte and macrophage activation syndrome. However, affected patients lack abnormal cytoplasmic granules. The disorder is caused by mutations in the *RAB27A* gene (378).

Hemophagocytic Lymphohistiocytosis. Hemophagocytic lymphohistiocytosis (HLH) is characterized by pancytopenia, fever, hepatosplenomegaly, neurologic findings, liver and coagulation abnormalities and elevated triglyceride and ferritin levels. Mutation in several genes important for immune function have been found among patients with familial HLH (379).

Autoimmune Lymphoproliferative Syndrome. Neutropenia is a frequent finding in patients with autoimmune lymphoproliferative syndrome (ALPS). In this disorder, neutropenia is often associated with other autoimmune disorders. In some patients defects in genes associated with lymphocyte apoptosis have been identified (380).

WHIM Syndrome. Patients with autosomal dominant WHIM (Warts, Hypogammaglobulinemia, Infections, and Myelokathexis) syndrome may present in the first months of life. The neutropenia results from a defective release of marrow cells into the peripheral blood. Fever, stress and possibly G-CSF administration may temporarily overcome the confinement of neutrophils to the marrow (381). Recently, mutations in the chemokine receptor gene *CXCR4* were identified as the cause of the WHIM syndrome (382).

Reticular Dysgenesia. Reticular dysgenesia, the cause of which is still unknown, is one of the rarest and most extreme forms of neutropenia associated with severe combined immunodeficiency (SCID). It is characterized by congenital agranulocytosis, lymphopenia and lymphoid and thymic hypoplasia (383). Neutrophil counts usually do not improve with administration of G-CSF and the patients often die within the first weeks of life unless they receive hematopoietic stem cell transplantation (384).

Congenital Leukemia in Infants

Leukemia in infants is a rare disorder (385,386). Infants show a larger proportion of the predominant form of congenital acute myeloid leukemia, commonly either monoblastic or myelomonocytic leukemia; whereas leukemia in older children is typically lymphoblastic. The clinical presentation is defined by a high white blood cell count, hepatosplenomegaly and in many cases central nervous system involvement. Skin involvement is common in myeloid but not in lymphoid leukemia.

In 60% to 70% of cases of infants with acute lymphoblastic leukemia (ALL) the leukemic blasts harbor a chromosomal translocation, internal duplication or deletion involving the mixed lineage leukemia (*MLL*) gene (also called *ALL1* or *HRX*) encoded at chromosome band

11q23 (387). Among the numerous translocations involving MLL, t(4;11) is most frequent in infant ALL (388). Despite the high intensity of multiagent chemotherapy protocols developed for infant ALL, the prognosis remains unfavorable and long-term survival is achieved in only 25% to 50% of cases (386). Particularly poor outcomes are associated with an age of less than 6 months at diagnosis or the presence of MLL gene rearrangement. Hematopoietic stem cell transplantation has not been shown to improve the dismal outcome of infants with ALL and t(4;11) (388). In contrast to ALL, young age and the presence of 11q23/MLL abnormalities have no clear adverse prognostic value in infant AML (386). A megakaryoblastic phenotype of the blasts and the t(1;22) (389–392) are thought to be associated with a less favorable prognosis (393). Treatment outcomes in infants with AML do not appear to be different from older children, in whom event-free survival rates between 40% and 50% can be achieved (211).

The study of newborns has significantly advanced our understanding of leukemia. The prenatal origin of leukemia became evident from studies showing that ALL may arise in monozygotic twins from a prenatally shared population of leukemic blasts after a variable latency period (394). Back tracking experiments demonstrate that specific translocations present in the leukemic blasts of childhood ALL such as the t(12;21), which results in the expression of the TEL-AML1 fusion protein, are in fact already detectable at birth in neonatal blood spots of approximately 75% of cases (395).

Transient leukemia (transient myeloproliferative disorder) in infants with Down syndrome

Children with Down syndrome (constitutional trisomy 21) have a 10- to 20-fold increased overall risk of developing ALL or acute myeloid leukemia (AML) (396). Acute megakaryoblastic leukemia, a form of AML, is estimated to occur with a 500 fold increased frequency (397,398). Contrary to previously held opinions chemotherapy of AML in children with Down syndrome results in superior outcomes with the probability of event-free survival exceeding 70% when compared to the general pediatric population (399,400). This favorable response has at least in part been attributed to the greater sensitivity of leukemic blasts derived from individuals with Down syndrome to chemotherapeutic agents such as cytosine arabinoside (401). Children with Down syndrome and ALL have outcomes comparable to their general pediatric population when they are treated appropriately despite their propensity for complications such as mucositis and pulmonary infections (402).

Unique to individuals with Down syndrome, a transient myeloproliferative syndrome (TMD), also transient leukemia (TL), is observed in at least 10% of newborns (reviewed in 403). Classically these infants are well and show in their peripheral blood circulating blasts that are indistinguishable from those of acute megakaryoblastic leukemia. The number of blasts may exceed 100,000/mm³ or may be barely detectable. Some infants have hepa-

tosplenomegaly or skin infiltrates. Remarkably, the blasts of TL/TMD in Down syndrome disappear spontaneously in the majority of cases in the first 3 to 4 months of life. After this spontaneous resolution of the TMD/TL, however, approximately 20% of these children go on to develop acute megakaryoblastic leukemia later in life (403). Of note, TL/TMD may also develop in phenotypically normal appearing newborn infants with mosaicism for trisomy 21. At present therapeutic intervention is reserved for the approximately 15% to 20% of cases of TMD/TL who develop life-threatening complications such as hyperleukocytosis, pericardial or pleural infusions, and acute liver failure (404). Progressive liver failure as a result of blast infiltration or fibrosis is frequently fatal (405) despite therapeutic reduction of the circulating and infiltrating blasts.

Inactivating mutations within the gene encoding the hematopoietic transcription factor GATA1 were recently shown to be specific for the blasts of acute megakaryoblastic leukemia in Down syndrome (406). These mutations are also present in the blasts of TL/TMD of Down syndrome (407–411) supporting a pathogenic concept in which prenatal mutations of GATA1 give rise to TL/TMD (412,413). Second, as yet undetermined, events eventually result in the transformation of a clone of TMD/TL blasts to acute megakaryoblastic leukemia (408,414).

Management of newborns with Down syndrome should include a complete blood count with a careful review of the blood smear. Immunophenotyping and cytogenetic evaluation of any blast population is recommended. Although observation is sufficient for the majority of newborns with Down syndrome and TL/TMD, neonatologists need to be aware of the potential complications and the availability of chemotherapeutic intervention (415).

Juvenile Myelomonocytic Leukemia

Juvenile myelomonocytic leukemia (JMML), previously referred to as juvenile chronic myelogenous leukemia (JCML) or chronic myelomonocytic leukemia (CMML) is a rare myeloproliferative disorder in the neonatal period and early infancy (416). Suggestive clinical features include hepatosplenomegaly, lymphadenopathy, pallor, fever and skin rash (417,418). The peripheral blood shows leukocytosis with immature myeloid cells and monocytosis. Fetal hemoglobin may be elevated. Clonal chromosomal abnormalities, for example monosomy 7, support the diagnosis. The Philadelphia chromosome and BCR-ABL fusion transcript, which are typical of adult chronic myelogenous leukemia are absent in JMML. In vitro bone marrow cultures show growth factor-independent growth (419) and hypersensitivity to granulocyte macrophage-colony stimulating factor (420). JMML is associated with neurofibromatosis (417) and Noonan syndrome (421) as a result of germ line mutations of the NF1 and PTPN11 genes respectively. Somatic mutations of NF1 (422) and PTPN11 (421) have also been found in nonsyndromic cases of JMML. Clinical responses can be introduced with 13-cis-retinoic acid and novel agents such as farnesyltransferase inhibitors are being evaluated (423). However, at present hematopoietic stem cell transplantation is the only curative therapy for JMML.

Neutrophilia and Neonatal Leukemoid Reactions

The incidence of leukemoid reactions with leukocyte counts more than 50×10^9/L among neonates in the NICU varies between 1.3 to 15% (424–427). It is most commonly seen in the first week of life. The most common causes include administration of betamethasone antenatally, infection, and transient leukemoid reactions of Down syndrome. However, Rastogi and associates (425) did not find concurrent pathology in nine cases with leukemoid reaction in a retrospective study of 60 preterm infants. The mechanism involves accelerated neutrophil production. Serum cytokine measurement did not show a consistent increase in G-CSF or GM-CSF, thus, marrow paracrine secretion or other mechanisms are possible. The leukemoid reaction resolves within several days to weeks, and the main clinical significance is the possibility of an underlying pathology. Rastogi and associates (425) noted that the neonates who had been able to mount a leukemoid response had a better chance of survival than those who did not. Recently, an association has been reported between leukemoid reaction with leukocyte counts more than 50×10^9/L and the development of bronchopulmonary dysplasia and chronic lung disease (427). Congenital infections such as CMV disease, toxoplasmosis, and syphilis may manifest as hepatosplenomegaly with a pronounced leukemoid response in the peripheral blood. Severe bacterial infections also may be associated with a leukemoid blood picture.

Evaluation of the Infant with Neutropenia

The unexpected finding of neutropenia in a newborn infant should prompt consideration of bacterial infection. A peripheral blood smear should be carefully examined for Döhle bodies, vacuolization, and toxic granulation, and the band to segmented neutrophil ratio should be determined. In infants with some combination of neutropenia, an increased band to segmented neutrophil ratio, and morphology suggestive of bacterial infection, empirical broad-spectrum antibiotic therapy should be started until the results of cultures are known. If there is no clinical or laboratory evidence of infection, other causes of neutropenia must be considered; however, it is still prudent to utilize broad-spectrum antibiotic coverage until it is clear from cultures and the infant's clinical course that sepsis is not the etiology of the neutropenia. As noted, preeclampsia and/or hypertension in the mother is a common cause of neutropenia and should be considered in the differential diagnosis. A maternal history, including a drug history, and a maternal neutrophil count should be obtained to exclude maternal illness (e.g., systemic lupus erythemato-

sus) as a cause of neutropenia. The physician should obtain a careful family history asking specifically about family members with documented neutropenia or a history of severe or unusual infections or early neonatal deaths. Early neonatal deaths may be caused by overwhelming infection secondary to neutropenia before any diagnosis is made. This information may provide an important clue to the possibility of an inherited neutropenic syndrome (e.g. Kostmann syndrome). Physical examination of affected infants suggests or excludes hypersplenism and congenital viral infections as the likely cause of neutropenia. In well infants with no apparent cause for the neutropenic state, neonatal alloimmune neutropenia should be considered. In such cases, a search should be made for neutrophil antibodies in a sample of maternal and/or baby's serum and neutrophil-specific antigen typing of the biologic parents of the affected neonate should be requested. These tests are best performed in neutrophil reference laboratories and require inclusion of the granulocyte agglutination test, the granulocyte immunofluorescence test, and the monoclonal antibody immobilization of granulocyte antigens assay for optimal detection of known antibodies (338,341). Ideally samples are obtained from the affected neonate (or biologic father acting as a surrogate) and the mother. It is important to stress that treatment of the infant should not be delayed whilst confirmatory serologic studies are in progress. Finally, a bone marrow aspirate and biopsy should be considered if neutropenia is severe (<500/μL), unresponsive to medical therapy, and persists for longer than one week.

Lymphopenia

Lymphocytes account for approximately 30% of the circulating white blood cells in newborn infants. Lymphopenia should always be considered when the total lymphocyte count is below the lower 5th percentile for age and particularly if the absolute lymphocyte count is less than 1,500/μL (428). Lymphopenia may occur in a number of immunodeficiency diseases, during infections or as part of an autoimmune process. Disorders in which lymphopenia is often diagnosed with neutropenia are detailed in the section neutropenia associated with immunodeficiency although those in which isolated lymphopenia is the hallmark of the disease are reviewed below. Of importance in the investigation of these disorders is the assessment of lymphocyte subsets and function. The values must be compared to age adjusted normal ranges (429). Usually in the newborn, 35% to 64% of lymphocytes express CD4 and are designated as "helper" T lymphocytes and 12% to 18% of lymphocytes express CD8 which is a marker for "suppressor/cytotoxic" T-lymphocytes. CD19 (a B cell marker) is found on 6% to 32% of lymphocytes and CD16/56 which designate natural killer cells is detected on 4% to 18% of cells. Typical laboratory features that may help to clarify the etiology of lymphopenia in newborn infants and the molecular defects are summarized in Table 46-16.

TABLE 46-16
LYMPHOPENIA IN THE NEONATAL PERIOD

Disorder	Typical Immune Abnormalities	Associated Features	Inheritance	Genetic Defect
SCID, gamma, Common chain deficiency type	SCID (T−, NK−, B+)	None	X-linked recessive	IL-2R gamma
SCID, Jak-3 deficiency type	SCID (T−, NK−, B+)	None	Autosomal recessive	JAK-3
SCID, IL-7 R alpha deficiency type	SCID (T−, NK+, B+/−)	None	Autosomal recessive	IL-7R alpha
SCID, CD3 TCR deficiency type	SCID (T−, NK+, B+)	None	Autosomal recessive	CD3 epsilon/gamma/delta
SCID, CD45 deficiency type	SCID (T−, NK+, B+)	None	Autosomal recessive	CD45
SCID, ZAP-70 deficiency type	SCID (CD8−, NK+, B+)	None	Autosomal recessive	ZAP-70
Di-George syndrome	Variable (T+/−, NK+, B+)	Hypocalcemia, cardiac abnormalities	Autosomal dominant, Autosomal recessive	22q11.2 chromosome deletion
SCID, Omenn's type	SCID (T+/−, NK+, B−)	Erythroderma, splenomegaly, lymphadenopathy	Autosomal recessive	RAG1, RAG2, Artemis
SCID, ADA deficiency type	SCID (T−, NK−, B−)	Bone dysplasia	Autosomal recessive	ADA
AT	Variable T/B cells	Ataxia, increased AFP, telangiectasia	Autosomal recessive	ATM
Nijmegen syndrome	Variable T/B cells	Microcephaly	Autosomal recessive	nibrin
Hyper-IgM syndrome	High IgM, low/normal IgG	Liver disease, ectodermal dysplasia	X-linked recessive, Autosomal recessive	CD40 ligand, AID, CD40, NEMO-IKK
Wiskott-Aldrich syndrome	Variable T/B cells	Eczema, thrombocytopenia, small platelets	X-linked recessive	WAS

Abbreviations: SCID = Severe combined immunodeficiency syndrome; AT = Ataxia telangiectasia; ADA = Adenosine deaminase deficiency; AFP = Alpha fetoprotein; NK = natural kille

Severe Combined Immunodeficiency Syndrome

One disorder, severe combined immunodeficiency (SCID) deserves special mention. This rare but serious disorder carries a grave prognosis unless recognized early in life and treated promptly. The most frequently identified cause of SCID is abnormal expression or function of the gamma (also known as common) chain of the interleukin (IL)-2 receptor. Because the gene is located on the X chromosome only males are affected and they often present in the first months of life with life-threatening infections and lymphopenia. T and NK cell numbers and/or function are significantly decreased (430). B cell numbers and immunoglobulin levels can be reduced, normal, or elevated. The thymus is often undetected by chest radiograph or ultrasound, and lymphatic tissue such as lymph nodes or tonsils are absent. The only definitive treatment is bone marrow transplantation. Recently replacing the abnormal protein by viral mediated gene therapy has been achieved. If newborn infants with SCID require blood transfusions they should be given only irradiated blood products so that graft versus host disease does not develop.

Mutations in Jak-3, which is a signaling molecule downstream of the IL-2 receptor, may cause a similar phenotype both in males and females (431). Defects in another lymphocyte receptor, the alpha chain of the IL-7 receptor, can also result in SCID with low T cell numbers, variable B cell numbers, but normal NK activity (432). Mutations in several components of the CD3 complex expressed on T cells result in abnormal T cell development with normal B and NK cell function (433). Similarly, mutations in the transmembrane protein tyrosine phosphase (CD45) result in diminished T cell number and function and normal B cell number; however, patients also have decreased serum immunoglobin levels (434). Mutations in another T cell signaling molecule, ZAP-70 affect primarily CD8 development (435).

Abnormal adenosine deaminase (ADA) enzyme activity has been observed in approximately 15% of patients with SCID. Infants with ADA deficiency have a more profound lymphopenia than do children with other types of SCID, because the accumulation of ADA substrates or their metabolites is toxic to T, B, and NK cells. Patients with ADA deficiency may have chondroosseous dysplasia, which is evidenced by the presence of multiple skeletal abnormalities on radiographic examination, including flaring of the costochondral junctions. Enzyme replacement therapy with polyethylene glycol-modified bovine ADA or bone marrow transplantation has resulted in some clinical and immunologic improvement, and recently, successful correction of the defect by therapy has been reported (436).

Other Disorders

In a few of the immunodeficiency disorders associated with lymphopenia, there are clinical features that may aid in the diagnosis. Di-George syndrome, also referred to as velo-cardio-facial syndrome, is often caused by microdeletion in the 22q11.2 region. It occurs with an estimated frequency of 1 in 4,000 and is accompanied by reduced T cell numbers in more than 50% of affected patients. In the minority of subjects, complete absence of T cells was reported and bone marrow or thymus transplantation were attempted (437). The commonly associated hypocalcemia, cardiac defects and typical facial dysmorphism assist in the diagnosis.

Omenn's syndrome, which is often caused by mutations in the recombinant activating genes (*RAG*), may present with erythroderma, hepatosplenomegaly, lymphadenopathy and eosinophilia. Although some *RAG* mutations result in severely reduced B and T cell numbers, several missense mutations in the gene allow limited T cell development. Recently, abnormal function of another gene involved in recombination, *Artemis*, was identified as leading to an early arrest of both B and T cell maturation (438,439).

Patients with ataxia-telangiectasia (AT) often present in the 3rd to 4th year of life with cerebella ataxia followed by the appearance of cutaneous telangiectasia, and variable, humoral and cellular immunodeficiencies. A minority of patients may present in the first year of life with increased susceptibility to infection and lymphopenia (440). Elevated serum α fetoprotein is characteristic and assists in the diagnosis that should be made as early as possible to minimize any exposure to radiation. Ataxia-telangiectasia is caused by defects in the *ATM* gene. Patients with Nijmegen breakage syndrome caused by defects in the *NBS1* gene also have an increased sensitivity to ionizing radiation. Similar to patients with ataxia-telangiectasia, they too may present very early in life with lymphopenia. However, those with Nijmegen breakage syndrome often have microcephaly and normal serum α fetoprotein levels which allows a distinction between to two diseases (441).

Other immunodeficiencies, such as hyper-IgM syndrome, Wiskott-Aldrich syndrome, cartilage hair hypoplasia, Schwachman-Diamond syndrome, dyskeratosis congenita and reticular dysgenesis which may cause lymphopenia and neutropenia are reviewed elsewhere in this chapter.

Eosinophilia

An elevated eosinophil count is common in premature infants. Normal values for a group of healthy premature infants studied by us are illustrated in Fig. 46-19. The upper limit of normal (95th percentile) for absolute eosinophil counts in a group of 167 full-term infants was 1,016/μL, 1,323/μL, and 1,372/μL at 0, 1, and 5 days, respectively. The corresponding mean values were 475/μL, 496/μL, and 540/μL. In a prospective study of 45 premature infants, Bhat et al (442) found the incidence of eosinophilia to be 75.5%. Similar results have been

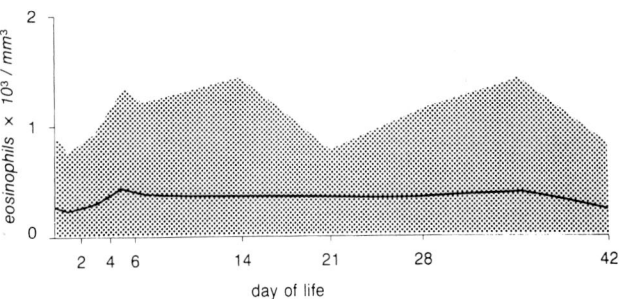

Figure 46-19 Eosinophil counts in 142 healthy, premature infants. Data at the first point, day 0 are cord blood values. Subsequent points represent data from capillary blood samples on 1, 5, 7, 14, 28, 35, and 42 days of life. The heavy line represents the mean of each point. The shaded area includes 95% of the infants studied, excluding the top and bottom 2.5% of the group.

reported by other investigators (443–445). In Bhat's study, an absolute eosinophil count of more than 700/μL was considered to be abnormal. The frequency and severity of eosinophilia were greatest in the subgroup of infants younger than 30 weeks gestational age. There was a significant association between the development of eosinophilia and number of blood transfusions administered, use of parenteral nutrition, and duration of intubation. The causative nature of these associations is uncertain because these features are common in ill, premature infants. Prolonged processing of antigens at the cellular level is required for the development of eosinophilia, and the investigators suggested that eosinophilia in the premature infant may be a physiological process needed to handle foreign antigens. The fact that eosinophilia is more frequent in premature infants than in term infants may reflect immaturity of barrier mechanisms in the gastrointestinal tract, respiratory tract, or both.

Pancytopenia

Shwachman-Diamond Syndrome

Shwachman-Diamond syndrome is a multisystemic autosomal recessive disease characterized by varying degrees of bone marrow failure and cytopenia, most commonly neutropenia (446). Exocrine pancreatic dysfunction, metaphyseal dysplasia, neutropenia and various B, T and natural killer (NK) cell abnormalities characterize Shwachman Diamond Syndrome (447). Patients may present in the neonatal period with failure to thrive, a small chest with thoracic dystrophy or infection as a result of neutropenia. The bone marrow may show hypocellularity with maturation arrest of myeloid elements, but from our experience it may also appear completely normal in the first several years of life. The cytopenia may progress to pancytopenia and severe aplasia as a result of increased apoptosis through the Fas pathway (448) and abnormal marrow stromal function. The syndrome is associated with the *SBDS* gene mutation (449). Patients with SDS are susceptible to recurrent viral, bacterial and fungal infections. Overwhelming sepsis is a well recognized fatal complication of the disorder particularly early in life (447). Transfusions or cytokine therapy may be required to treat the cytopenia in addition to pancreatic replacement enzymes; however, the only curative treatment is allogeneic hematopoietic stem cell transplantation.

Fanconi Anemia

Fanconi's anemia is an inherited marrow failure syndrome with a defect in DNA repair and accelerated apoptosis. At least 11 different genes are associated with the disease (*FANCA,B,C,D1[BRCA2],D2,E,F,G,I,J,L*); nine of them were identified as of June 2004 (450). Some children present with only hematological abnormalities, although others have multiple congenital anomalies including thumbs, kidneys, cardiac and skin defects. Patients may have characteristic facies. Diagnosis is usually made at the age of 4 to 8 years, when children develop cytopenia, macrocytosis, and a high fetal hemoglobin. However, early diagnosis is possible if the characteristic nonhematological manifestations are evident at birth. Further, approximately 4% of the children have cytopenia in the neonatal period (451) and some develop congenital tumors (452). The chromosomal fragility test is positive in almost all patients. Treatment of the cytopenia includes transfusion, cytokines and androgens, but only allogeneic hematopoietic stem cell transplantation is curative.

Dyskeratosis Congenita

Typically patients have cytopenia, macrocytosis, high fetal hemoglobin, mucous membrane leukoplakia, dystrophic nails, reticulated skin pigmentation and increased lacrimation as a result of atresia of the lacrimal ducts which appear in early or late childhood (453). From our experience and others (453) severe cases can present in the neonatal period with thrombocytopenia, immunodeficiency and varying CNS malformations. In some of these patients T cell abnormalities and opportunistic infection have been reported (454,455). At least 3 genes are associated with the diseases: *DKC1* (X-linked recessive), *hTR* (autosomal dominant) (456) and an unknown autosomal recessive gene. The gene products are involved in telomere maintenance (456). Treatment of the hematological complications include transfusions and cytokines, but only allogeneic hematopoietic stem cell transplantation is curative (453,457).

Congenital Amegakaryocytic Thrombocytopenia

Children with this disorder present with thrombocytopenia at birth, which gradually progresses to pancytopenia. Initially the bone marrow shows a paucity of megakaryocytes, but later on varying degrees of decreased cellularity develops. Nonhematological manifestations can occur, but are not frequent. This disorder is associated with mutations in the gene (*C-mpl*) encoding for the thrombopoietin receptor (458,459). The only curative treatment is allogeneic hematopoietic stem cell transplantation from a sibling (460) or an unrelated donor (461).

Cytopenia Related to Metabolic Disorders

Neutropenia can be seen in inherited defects in the metabolism of branched amino acids such as propionic aciduria and methylmalonic aciduria. The neutropenia is probably related to a toxic effect of specific metabolites whose serum levels are increased causing underproduction (462). Deterioration in the cytopenia can occur with episodes of metabolic crisis. Pearson disease is caused by deletional mutations in mitochondrial DNA (463), and is associated with variable degrees of pancreatic dysfunction, pancytopenia, and metabolic acidosis (464). Marrow aspirates show ring sideroblasts and vacuoles in myeloid and erythroid precursors. The cytopenia tends to improve with age (465,466).

TRANSFUSION OF BLOOD AND BLOOD PRODUCTS

Transfusions of blood products to newborn infants are essential in many clinical situations, and guidelines for transfusion practice in this patient population have been published and updated (467,468). However, guidelines simply provide a list of acceptable clinical situations in which transfusions may be given, and they should not serve as absolute indications for transfusion therapy. In all cases, the responsible physician should take into account the general condition of the infant. The decision to transfuse blood products should reflect careful consideration of the risk-benefit ratio for the individual patient. Physicians should clearly document, in writing, the indication for each transfusion administered and perform an assessment of the efficacy of the transfusion (e.g. relief of symptoms of anemia, cessation of bleeding). Informed consent from a parent or guardian (if appropriate), a process that includes discussion of risks, benefits and alternatives to transfusion, should be obtained in accordance with all applicable local, state and national regulatory requirements (468).

Erythrocyte Transfusions

Transfusion of erythrocytes in newborn infants, particularly in premature newborns, is a common practice. The indications are those that hold for any other time of life; hypovolemia and anemia. Transfusion for anemia has created much controversy. Anemia is defined as a hemoglobin concentration lower than that which is normal for the given patient. This concept of normality is difficult to apply to the premature infant, who as part of his/her normal course may require respiratory assistance, may have apneic spells, and may have much blood sampled for laboratory tests. There is significant controversy about whether a low hemoglobin concentration is harmful to infants or whether transfusions to maintain an arbitrary hemoglobin concentration improve their clinical condition. Guidelines for administering a RBC transfusion are presented in Table 46-17 and, although lacking definitive proof, are provided as an aid with the recognition that

TABLE 46-17

GUIDELINES FOR TRANSFUSION OF RED BLOOD CELLS IN PATIENTS LESS THAN FOUR MONTHS OF AGE

1. Hct <20% with *low reticulocyte* count and symptoms of anaemia*

2. Hct <30% with an infant:
   - on <35% hood O_2
   - on O_2 by nasal cannula
   - on continuous positive air way pressure and/or intermittent mandatory ventilation with mechanical ventilation with mean air way pressure <6 cm H_2O
   - with *significant* apnea or bradycardia†
   - with *significant* tachycardia or tachypnea‡
   - with low weight gain ▲

3. Hct <35% with an infant:
   - on >35% hood O_2
   - on continuous positive air way pressure/ intermittent mandatory ventilation with mean airway pressure ≥6–8 cm H_2O

4. Hct <45% with an infant:
   - on ECMO
   - with congenital cyanotic heart disease

---

* Tachycardia, tachypnea, poor feeding.
† More than six episodes in 12 hr or two episodes in 24 hr requiring bag and mask ventilation while receiving therapeutic doses of methylxanthines.
‡ Heart rate >180 beats/min for 24 hr; respiratory rate >80 breaths/min for 24 hr. ▲ Weight gain of <10 g/day observed over 4 days while receiving ≥100 kcal/kg/day

practice is variable and that criteria should be developed and updated as required by an appropriate process at each local institution.

In newborn infants almost all RBC transfusions are packed RBCs as compared to whole blood or reconstituted whole blood which should be considered a special request and indicated only in specific clinical situations (Table 46-18).

Small volume (10–15 ml/kg) transfusions of packed RBCs are frequently required in extremely low birth weight (<1000 g) or very low birth weight (<1500 g) newborn infants. There are two phases of RBC transfusion need following preterm delivery: (a) early, in infants requiring

TABLE 46-18

GUIDELINES FOR TRANSFUSION OF WHOLE BLOOD OR RECONSTITUTED WHOLE BLOOD

1. **Exchange Transfusion for:**
   - hemolytic disease of the newborn
   - hyperbilirubinemia with risk of kernicterus

2. **After cardiopulmonary bypass**

3. **Extracorporeal membrane oxygenation (ECMO)**

4. **Massive transfusion***

---

* Defined as transfusion of >1 blood volume in 24 hr

major surgery or intensive care; and (b) later, during the period of the physiologic anemia of prematurity. Factors that influence the need for RBC transfusion in premature infants include (a) the initial endowment of the infant with blood at birth reflected by the initial red cell mass; (b) the magnitude of iatrogenic blood losses, related to the degree and duration of intensive care; and (c) failure of erythropoiesis (469). As a result of the impact of placental transfusion at birth (a source of autologous blood) (470,471), more restrictive practices for RBC transfusion in LBW infants (472,473), and the elimination of a fixed iatrogenic blood loss as a "trigger" for RBC transfusion, significantly fewer small volume RBC transfusions are given to low birth-weight infants (473–475). As an example in the study reported by Widness and colleagues (475) the percentage of infants with a birth weight of 1.0 to 1.5 kg who were given RBC transfusions was 83% in 1982, 67% in 1989 and 34% in 1993; the average number of RBC transfusions (15 ml/kg) given per patient was 7.0 in 1982, 5.0 in 1987, and 2.3 in 1993. In a more recent study of extremely low birth weight infants (birth weight <1000 g) reported by Maier and colleagues (473) the median number of RBC transfusions decreased from 7 in the period 1989 to 1991 to 2 in the period 1995 to 1997 with a corresponding reduction in the median number of blood donors per infant from 5 to 1; impressively, the percent of extremely low birth weight (ELBW) infants not transfused with packed RBC in the same periods increased from 3% (1989–1991) to 25% (1995–1997). These changes in transfusion practices need to be taken into consideration when evaluating the results of erythropoietin (EPO) trials in newborn infants, and there is general consensus among experts that, based on available data, the more liberal transfusion practices of the 1980s and early 1990s can be replaced by a more restrictive transfusion policy in small preterm infants without any significant adverse short-term affects; future trials of RBC transfusion and EPO administration in low birth weight infant should focus on long-term outcomes such as neurological development (472). Efforts to reduce iatrogenic blood loss by restricting phlebotomy, miniaturized analyses in the laboratory and transcutaneous blood gas monitoring in ill, small preterm infants need to be stressed (473).

The type of RBC product for use in small volume (15 + 5 ml/kg) transfusions has been reviewed in detail by Strauss and colleagues (476). Based on a critical review of available literature, it is apparent that a dedicated single-donor system, in which RBCs are collected into AS-1 or AS-3 anticoagulant from either unrelated donors or biologic parents, and stored for up to 42 days, is able to supply all small volume RBC transfusions needed by individual patients without adverse effects (476). Their protocol at the University of Iowa Hospital and Clinics is of interest in this regard; depending on the anticipated RBC needs of individual preterm infants up to 50% of a fresh RBC unit is reserved for use by each infant throughout the 42 days of RBC storage. With this dedicated single-donor system, 88%

of transfused preterm infants received RBCs from only one donor, with the remaining 12% being exposed to only two donors. The ideal goal of only one donor per infant was almost achieved without compromising safety (476), and with acceptable cost-effectiveness (477). In addition to recommending use of RBCs stored in extended-storage anticoagulant or preservative solutions to limit donor exposures (as compared to relatively fresh RBCs), Strauss and colleagues (476) recommended the use of CMV safe (CMV seronegative or leukocyte-reduced RBCs) to minimize and potentially eliminate transfusion-transmitted CMV, and γ-irradiation to prevent transfusion-associated graft versus host disease (TA GVHD).

One area of interest is the choice of blood products in newborn infants with activation of the Thomsen-Friedenreich neoantigen (T antigen), a condition often reported in association with NEC. The condition may be associated with hemolysis and is thought to reflect exposure of the Thomsen-Friedenreich cryptantigen (T antigen) by removal of *N*-acetylneuraminidase acid (also known as sialidase). Neuraminidase is produced by a large number microbial agents including bacteria, viruses and protozoa. *In vivo* T activation has been reported in association with anaerobic, particularly clostridial sepsis, and other infections. In one recent study 48 of 375 (12.8%) neonates admitted to a tertiary referral center were found to have T or t-variant activated RBCs (478). Thirteen of the 48 infants (27%) developed at least one episode of sepsis and 9 (19%) NEC during their hospital stay; however, T-activation was not always temporally associated with NEC or sepsis. Twenty-three of the 48 (48%) of infants with T-activated RBCs received standard blood products without evidence of transfusion-associated hemolysis. Based on these observations the investigators concluded that, in the neonatal population, routine screening for T-activation of infants with sepsis or NEC is not justified and that the routine provision of low-titer anti-T blood components, washed RBCs or platelet suspended in additive is not warranted and should be considered only in the very small percentage of infants with true T-activation (as compared to T-variant activation) and clinically significant transfusion-associated hemolysis (478). These findings and recommendations are at slight variance to those of Williams and colleagues who reported an incidence of 11% of T-antigen activation in 72 infants with NEC, four of whom experienced hemolysis (one severe) associated with the transfusion of standard blood products (479). The investigators proposed a transfusion protocol that included the use of washed RBCs/platelets or blood components with low anti-T reactivity. Although it is clear that prudence should be exercised in selecting blood components for neonates with RBC T-activation, it is important that such infants, many of whom are small and ill, not be denied the benefits of essential hemostatic components (e.g. plasma, cryoprecipitate, platelets) because of a perceived potential risk of hemolysis from standard donor products that are likely to contain anti-T antibodies (480).

Preparation of Blood for Transfusion and Crossmatching

There are several principles of blood transfusion and crossmatching that should be understood by those caring for neonates. First, omission of the crossmatch for initial and subsequent transfusions of neonates is recommended if the initial antibody screen does not demonstrate unexpected antibodies and the erythrocytes transfused are of an ABO and Rh type that is compatible with the baby and mother. This recommendation reflects the fact that newborn infants appear unable to form alloantibodies to erythrocyte antigens (481,482). Repeated blood sampling for pretransfusion testing only contributes to phlebotomy losses for small newborn infants. Second, the practice of using FFP to adjust erythrocyte preparations to a predetermined hematocrit value for small-volume transfusions (i.e., not exchange transfusion) may lead to exposure of newborn infants to two different donors pre transfusion. This practice should be discouraged (483). If necessary, isotonic saline should be used to adjust hematocrit.

Exchange Transfusions

The authors recommend that blood for exchange transfusion be as fresh as possible and less than 5 days old. Because extracellular potassium increases rapidly during storage of erythrocyte concentrates at 4°C, it is recommended that erythrocyte units for exchange transfusion of ill premature infants be saline washed before reconstitution with FFP. Manual and automated saline wash processes are effective (484). This maneuver effectively eliminates any chance of iatrogenic hyperkalemia, a complication reported in ill premature infants after exchange transfusion (485).

Platelet Transfusions

A platelet count less than 150×10^9/L in a newborn infant is abnormal and requires investigation. In older children and adults, the risk of serious internal hemorrhage, particularly ICH, increases significantly when the platelet count falls below 20,000/μL. Donor platelets are usually infused prophylactically when this degree of thrombocytopenia occurs. The situation in newborn infants is less clear. Particularly in ill premature infants, in whom the risk of hemorrhage into the CNS is high, factors other than the absolute platelet count may play a role. Many of these infants are on medications, such as antibiotics, that may impair platelet function. Immaturity of blood vessels in the periventricular area and changes in cerebral blood flow and pressure associated with fluid and ventilation therapy may play a role. Alternatively, IVH may be the final result of cerebral infarction, perhaps related to asphyxia, with hemorrhage into the infarcted area. The clinical impact of significant neonatal thrombocytopenia (i.e., platelet counts $<100 \times 10^9$/L) in infants weighting less than 1,500 g at birth has been studied prospectively by Andrew and associates (486). The incidence of IVH in 97 thrombocytopenic infants was 78%, compared with 48% in non-thrombocytopenic control infants. The more severe grades

TABLE 46-19
GUIDELINES FOR TRANSFUSION OF PLATELET CONCENTRATES IN NEONATES[a]

Premature infants (gestational age <37 weeks)
  Blood platelets $<30 \times 10^9/L$ in a stable infant
  Blood platelets $<50 \times 10^9/L$ in a sick infant
All other infants
  Blood platelet count $<20 \times 10^9/L$
  Blood platelet count $<50 \times 10^9/L$ with active bleeding or the need for an invasive procedure
  Blood platelet count $<100 \times 10^9/L$ with active bleeding plus DIC or *other coagulation abnormalities*[b]
  Bleeding with *qualitative platelet defect* and *marked prolongation* of bleeding time, regardless of the platelet count
  Cardiovascular bypass surgery with unexplained *excessive bleeding*, regardless of the platelet count

[a] Adapted from Blanchette VS, Hume HA, Levy GJ, et al. Guidelines for auditing pediatric blood transfusion practices. *Am J Dis Child* 1991;145:787–796, with permission.
[b] Statements in *italics* require additional definition by a local transfusion committee.

TABLE 46-20
ESTIMATED RISK OF TRANSFUSION

Risk Factor	Estimated Risk per Unit Transfused
Viral Infection	
Hepatitis B	1/220,000
Hepatitis C	1/800,000–1.6 million
HIV	<1/1.4–2.4 million
Bacterial Contamination	
Red cells	1/500,000
Platelets	1/2,000
Immune	
Acute hemolytic reaction	1/250,000–1 million
Delayed hemolytic reaction	1/1,000
Transfusion-related acute lung injury	1/8,000
Transfusion associated graft-versus-host disease	1/500,000–1 million

Adapted from Goodnough LT. Risks of blood transfusion. *Crit Care Med* 2003;31:S678–S686, with permission.

of IVH (i.e., grades III and IV) were more frequent in the thrombocytopenic infants. Despite this, a trial of platelet transfusion for platelet counts less than $150 \times 10^9/L$ during the first 7 days of life failed to decrease the incidence of developing or extending IVH in sick premature infants (487).

Guidelines for transfusion of platelet concentrates are outlined in Table 46-19. The standard platelet product available from blood banks is harvested from a single whole-blood donation of approximately 450 mL. After centrifugation of this whole-blood unit, platelet-rich plasma (PRP) is separated from the erythrocyte fraction, and the PRP is further centrifuged to yield 1 unit of FFP and 1 unit of random donor platelets. Each platelet concentrate contains approximately 0.7×10^{11} platelets in a volume of 50 mL; this product can be stored for as long as 5 days at 22°C. The objective of most platelet transfusions is to increase the infant's platelet count to more than $100 \times 10^9/L$. This can be achieved by the infusion of 10 mL of a standard platelet concentrate per kilogram of body weight. Generally, this volume is not excessive, providing intake of other fluids is monitored and adjusted as needed. Although methods exist to reduce the volume of platelet concentrates, additional processing should be performed with care because of possible platelet loss, clumping, and dysfunction caused by the additional handling (488). Platelets should be administered through a standard 170-μm blood filter as rapidly as the infant's overall condition permits and certainly within 2 hours. A microaggregate filter should not be used because it will trap a large number of platelets.

Granulocyte Transfusions

Although granulocyte transfusions have been beneficial in some forms of neutropenia (489), they are now rarely used in neonatal units. The reasons for this are the difficulty in obtaining fresh granulocytes and the apparent efficacy of G-CSF in rapidly elevating neutrophil counts in neutropenic infants with sepsis (490), alloimmune neutropenia (338), or other causes of neutropenia (491),

Risks

Potential complications of blood transfusion have been reviewed by Mollison (492). For newborn infants, posttransfusion hepatitis, CMV infection, HIV infection, and graft-versus-host disease are of particular concern. Because of these potential complications (Table 46-20), it is important that physicians order blood or blood product support for newborns only in situations in which the infant will clearly benefit from such therapy.

Hepatitis. Transfusion-associated hepatitis may be caused by the hepatitis A or B viruses or more commonly by the hepatitis C virus (HCV) (493,494). Cases of HCV were previously classified as non-A, non-B hepatitis. Available information indicates that neonates given blood before anti-HCV screening (introduced in the early 1990s) were at substantial risk for posttransfusion hepatitis C and may constitute a sizable proportion of those with chronic HCV infection who were infected during childhood (495). Infection in neonates seems to be clinically silent and biochemical abnormalities may be minimal or absent. However, although it appears that chronic hepatitis C is clinically milder in children than adults, the long-term outcome of individuals infected with hepatitis C in the newborn period is unknown (495). Of note, parents/guardians of children and particularly neonates transfused immediately or shortly after birth and not requiring ongoing transfusion support may be unaware of their child's previous transfusion history and risk status for hepatitis C (496). Some have therefore urged that neonatologists become partners in lookback programs by reviewing their files to identify at-risk patients transfused as neonates so that they (or their parents) can be contacted to offer hepatitis C testing (495). Children identified to have continuing HCV infection through such programs will require ongoing follow-up for their condition and encouragement to maintain a lifestyle that minimizes the risk of progression of their infection. In particular, excessive alcohol use and needle sharing should be avoided. It is very important that they be vaccinated to prevent co-infection with the hepatitis A and B viruses (497), because severe and even life-threatening fulminant hepatitis has been described in individuals with chronic hepatitis C who became superinfected with acute hepatitis A (498),

Cytomegalovirus Infection. Transfusion-acquired CMV infection can occur when at-risk CMV antibody-negative infants are infused with CMV antibody-positive blood products. In the study by Yeager and colleagues (499), 13.5% (10 of 74) of seronegative infants who received CMV antibody-positive erythrocytes developed CMV infection. Infection did not occur in 90 seronegative infants who received only CMV antibody-negative blood. Two of the ten infected infants in this series died, and three others developed serious symptoms including pneumonia, hepatitis, hemolytic anemia, and thrombocytopenia. All of the fatal or other serious infections occurred in infants with a birth weight less than 1,200 g; infection was more common in infants who received 50 mL or more of blood. Similar data have been reported by Adler and colleagues (500), and other reports have stressed the morbidity and mortality that may be associated with transfusion-acquired CMV infection in neonates (501,502).

Based on these studies, it has been recommended that CMV antibody-negative blood products be made available to preterm infants of birth weight 1,250 g or less who are CMV antibody-negative. A study by Preiksaitis and associates (503) challenges this recommendation for all neonates. In this prospective study of 120 seronegative infants, only one case of acquired CMV infection was observed. Because no mortality and little morbidity could be attributed to transfusion-acquired CMV, the investigators did not recommend that all neonatal units provide specialized blood components for the prevention of CMV infection (503). The indications for use of CMV-seronegative blood products in newborn infants currently include: low birth weight neonates (birth weight <1,500 g) born to seronegative mothers in centers that have documented a high incidence of transfusion- acquired CMV infection in neonates; low birth weight neonates born to seronegative or seropositive mothers and who require granulocyte transfusions; and neonates receiving extracorporeal membrane oxygenation (ECMO).

The importance of breast milk as a source of CMV infection in newborn infants has also been stressed (504,505). In future studies of transfusion-acquired CMV infection in newborn infants, it will be important to control for this variable, particularly in nurseries in which pooled breast milk is used. If a decision to transfused CMV low-risk blood products to selected low birth weight infants is made, and CMV-seronegative erythrocytes are not available, products that are associated with a low risk transmitting CMV infection include frozen, deglycerolized erythrocytes; washed erythrocytes; and filtered erythrocytes (506–508).

It is now recommended that to avoid transfusion-induced CMV infection newborns should receive either blood products from CMV-negative donors or filtered blood, which in recent studies appears to be highly effective in preventing CMV infection even in immunosuppressed patients (509). Furthermore, transfusion of prestorage leukocyte-reduced packed RBCs was associated with improvement in several clinical outcomes in premature infants (510).

Acquired Immunodeficiency Syndrome. Since the first report of AIDS in 1981, much has been learned about the disorder (511). The causative agent of the syndrome is now known to be the HIV-1 virus. The virus can be grown in culture, and antibody to the virus can be detected with immunologic techniques, such as an enzyme-linked immunosorbent assay. Blood donations are routinely screened for evidence of antibodies to the HIV-1 virus, and the risk of HIV-1 transmission by blood products is extremely small. However, HIV-1 transmission has occurred in newborn infants, and this potentially fatal complication demands that blood or blood component therapy be restricted to situations in which therapy is clinically indicated and is likely to be of benefit to the newborn infant (512–514). The potential complication of HIV infection is a major reason to limit the number of blood donors to whom a given newborn infant is exposed.

Graft-Versus-Host Disease. Graft-versus-host disease has been reported in congenitally immunodeficient infants, after blood transfusion in premature infants, after ECMO, and in apparently normal infants with Rh isoimmunization who have received intrauterine transfusions followed by exchange transfusion (515–519). Features of transfusion-associated graft-versus-host disease (TAGVHD), usually a fatal disorder, include fever, generalized rash, diarrhea, hepatitis and pancytopenia. Irradiation of blood products to prevent graft-versus-host disease is recommended for the following groups:

- Neonates with known or suspected cellular immune deficiencies
- Neonates requiring intrauterine transfusions
- Neonates who receive intrauterine transfusions and who require transfusion postnatally
- Recipients of cellular blood products from first-degree blood relatives
- Premature infants weighting less than 1,200 g at birth

Data supporting the last recommendation are not available. However, very-low-birth-weight infants (<1,200 g) may have an associated immunodeficiency, and it is reasonable to offer protection to this group of infants (468). White blood cell reduction has not been shown to prevent TAGVHD. The only known method of preventing TAGVHD is irradiation at 2500 cGy using a device approved for blood irradiation of the FDA (468). The shelf life of irradiated RBCs is reduced to 28 days after irradiation as a result of acceleration of the storage lesion (468).

Plasma Derivatives

Albumin

Albumin is available in 5% and 25% solutions. Although albumin infusion has been recommended as a means of drawing more bilirubin into the intravascular space before exchange transfusion, convincing data in support of such a practice is lacking.

Fresh-Frozen Plasma

Centrifugation of a single donor unit of whole blood within 6 hours of collection yields a concentrate of erythrocytes and 1 unit of FFP. If stored at −30°C, the plasma product has a shelf life of 12 months and contains all coagulation factors.

Cryoprecipitate

Cryoprecipitate is prepared from FFP derived from multiple donors by slow thawing at 2°C to 4°C. Each unit of cryoprecipitate contains approximately 80 units of factor VIII and 250 mg of fibrinogen in 5 to 10 mL of plasma. If stored at −30°C, the product has a shelf life of 12 months. Cryoprecipitate also contains various amounts of factor XIII.

Factor VIII and IX Concentrates

Concentrates of factors VIII and IX are commercially manufactured from large pools (2,000–20,000 donors) of plasma. Each concentrate lot is assayed for coagulation factor activity, and this value is stated in units on each vial. Traditionally, concentrates of factors VIII and IX have not been used in newborn infants or young children because of the increased risk of hepatitis associated with infusion of factor VIII and IX concentrates, and of DIC and thrombotic complications associated with infusion of factor IX concentrates because of thrombogenic materials in such concentrates and low antithrombin III levels in newborns. Disseminated intravascular coagulation is particularly likely if liver dysfunction occurs. The introduction of very high-purity, virus-inactivated, plasma derived and recombinant factor concentrates appears to have eliminated the risk of HIV-1 infection and to have significantly reduced the incidence of hepatitis, altering the previous general recommendations. However, factor IX concentrates are not recommended for use in newborns other than those with proven congenital factor IX deficiency (hemophilia B). Most North American hemophilia centers now recommend that infants with newly diagnosed severe hemophilia immediately receive hepatitis B immunization, and that they receive very high purity, virus inactivated plasma derived or recombinant factor concentrates, as clinically indicated for prevention or control of bleeding (245).

Hyperimmune Serum Globulin

Prevention of Hepatitis B Virus Infection. Infants of mothers who are positive for hepatitis B surface antigen (HBsAg) are frequently infected with hepatitis B virus. Infection is most likely to occur if mothers are also positive for hepatitis Be antigen. Approximately 90% of infants whose mothers are positive for both markers will become infected, and most of these infants will be permanent carriers of the hepatitis B virus. It is estimated that one in four infants who are chronic carriers after perinatal infection will later develop cirrhosis or hepatocellular carcinoma (520).

Infants receive greatest protection from a combination of active immunization with three doses of hepatitis B vaccine, together with passive immunization using hepatitis B immune globulin (HBIG). The following schedule is recommended: at birth, 0.5 mL of HBIG and 10 µg of hepatitis B vaccine (520). Both the vaccine and the immunoglobulin are given intramuscularly and can be administered at the same time if separate sites are used. At 1 and 6 months, 10 µg of hepatitis B vaccine is given. Infants should be tested for presence of anti-HBsAg at 9 months. If they are found to be negative (<10% of all cases), a repeat dose of the vaccine should be given.

Prevention of Cytomegalovirus Infection. The administration of CMV hyperimmune globulin to CMV antibody-negative patients who undergo bone marrow transplantation decreases the incidence of transfusion-acquired CMV infection. Whether a similar approach may be beneficial for the CMV antibody-negative premature infant exposed to multiple blood products is unknown.

THROMBOSIS AND EMBOLISM

Thromboembolism (TE) is uncommon in the neonatal period. However, TE can cause significant morbidity and mortality. Neonatal TE represents approximately 50% of the TE in the pediatric population (521). The reported incidence of symptomatic TE in newborn infants is approximately one case per 400 admissions to a NICU (522), or one case per 20,000 births (523).

Risk Factors and Pathogenesis

Three major factors contribute to the formation of thrombi (Virchow's triad): abnormalities of the vessel wall, disturbances of blood flow, and changes in blood coagulation.

Abnormalities of the Vessel Wall

Intravascular Catheters

Although the vessel walls of aorta and inferior vena cava are shown to have antithrombotic properties in the young compared to adults (524,525), these vessels can often be damaged by intravascular catheters in sick newborns. Indeed, intravascular catheters have become the single most important risk factor for neonatal thrombotic disease (522). The placement of such catheters carries a potential risk of thrombosis, regardless of which vessel is used; possibly because of their widespread use, umbilical catheters have received the most attention to date. In a retrospective review of 4,000 infants who underwent umbilical artery catheterization in the 1970s, severe symptomatic vessel obstruction was observed in approximately 1% of patients (526). Clinically silent thromboses have been detected more often at autopsy or during contrast angiography in asymptomatic infants with an umbilical artery catheter in place. Between 3% and 59% of cases have had postmortem evidence of catheter-related thrombosis (527–533). In six prospective angiographic studies, thrombosis was demonstrated in 10% to 95% of patients (534–539). Very recently, thrombi associated with a correctly placed umbilical venous catheter were documented venographically at the time of elective catheter removal in 30% (14/47) of asymptomatic infants (540). In the same study, it was found that real-time and Doppler flow ultrasonography was not sufficiently accurate to diagnose such thrombi. Before this report, neonatal thrombosis, which was associated with central venous catheters, had been estimated to occur in approximately 14% of asymptomatic infants, based on serial echocardiography (541,542).

Abnormal chorionic vessels are present in a range of maternal disorders such as PIH or placental infection. These abnormal blood vessels predispose to the development of chorionic thrombi, which can embolize into the fetal circulation, particularly into the pulmonary arteries and portal veins (543). Paradoxic emboli have also been reported as the cause of neonatal cerebral infarction (544,545).

Abnormal Blood Flow

Blood flow is a critical determinant of thrombus formation. Increased blood viscosity (as a consequence of polycythemia or dehydration) has been implicated in cases of neonatal thrombotic disease (522,523). Hyperviscosity caused by polycythemia is also thought to contribute to the alleged thrombotic tendency in infants with diabetic mothers (546). Shock is another example of a severe disturbance of blood flow, predisposing to thrombosis (547). The presence of a catheter within the lumen of blood vessels attenuates blood flow and is the commonest predisposition of a thrombus in neonate (522).

Abnormal Blood Coagulation

Epidemiologic studies in adults have confirmed several hereditary disorders and coexistent genetic defects as risk factors for thromboembolism (548,549). Much less is known about hereditary thrombophilia in newborn infants. The occurrences of homozygous protein C and S deficiencies have been strongly linked with severe neonatal thrombotic disease (550,551). Heterozygous deficiencies of antithrombin, factor V Leiden (resistance to activated protein C), prothrombin G20210A mutations and, elevated lipoprotein (a), polymorphisms (677C→T)of methylenetetrahydrofolate reductase (MTHFR) have also been associated with neonatal thrombosis and purpura fulminans in isolated case reports and series (552–554). Whether a congenital prothrombotic state contributes to the development of thrombosis in the presence of a strong stimulus such as venous catheters remained controversial (555).

Clinical Features

Neonatal TE can occur in either the venous or arterial system. In the Canadian Registry, thrombosis was venous, arterial, and mixed in 62, 34, and 4 %, respectively (522). The vessels affected are numerous; they include renal, adrenal, portal, hepatic, and cerebral veins; peripheral, cerebral, pulmonary, coronary, renal, and mesenteric arteries; and the aorta, vena cava, and right atrium (546). The clinical presentation of thrombosis is variable. Signs and symptoms may be fairly specific, such as a cool, pale, and pulseless limb in the case of peripheral arterial obstruction. Often, however, the clinical presentation is very nonspecific: examples include respiratory insufficiency and profound hypoxemia caused by pulmonary emboli (556) and seizures caused by arterial stroke or cerebral venous thrombosis (557–561). Occasionally, thrombosis is suspected only retrospectively when sequelae of vessel occlusion become apparent (e.g., portal hypertension as a consequence of portal vein thrombosis). Table 46-21 summarizes the major sites of thrombotic vessel obstruction and their clinical symptoms and signs in the newborn infant.

The most common predisposing factor for thrombosis is the presence of a catheter (522,523). In thrombosis unrelated to a catheter, renal vein thrombosis is the most common (523). Thrombocytopenia often accompanies thrombosis in newborns. Patients should be evaluated for a thromboembolic disorder if thrombocytopenia cannot be explained by other conditions.

Purpura fulminans is characterized by ecchymotic lesions that increase in a radial fashion and become purplish black with bullae, and then necrotic and gangrenous. In the presence of purpura fulminans, protein C or protein S deficiencies should be considered.

Management

The literature on neonatal thrombotic disease consists almost entirely of case reports and case series (562). Such anecdotal observations are poor guides to management, as they are uncontrolled and fraught with bias (562). Extrapolation of findings in adult patients to newborn infants may be inappropriate because the etiology, the localization of thrombi, the coagulation system and its response to antithrombotic and fibrinolytic agents differ markedly between the two age-groups. Current approaches to the management of neonatal thrombosis remain to be validated in future clinical trials. Updated information on the use of antithrombotic agents are published regularly by American College of Chest Physicians (563).

Diagnosis

Whenever thrombotic disease is suspected in the newborn, every effort should be made to confirm or refute the

TABLE 46-21
CLINICAL PRESENTATION OF THROMBOEMBOLIC DISEASE IN NEWBORN INFANTS

Site of Vessel Obstruction	Clinical Signs and Symptoms
Venous	
Vena cava inferior	May be associated with renal venous thrombosis; edema and cyanosis of legs
Vena cava superior	Soft-tissue edema of head, neck, and chest; chylothorax
Cerebral	Seizures
Renal	Enlarged kidney(s); hematuria
Adrenal	Often associated with adrenal hemorrhagic necrosis
Portal and hepatic	Mainly clinically silent during acute phase
Arterial	
Aorta	Congestive heart failure; systolic gradient between upper and lower limbs; decreased femoral pulses; renal failure
Peripheral	Pulselessness; fall in skin temperature; discoloration
Cerebral	Prolonged apnea; seizures
Pulmonary	Respiratory distress; pulmonary hypertension
Coronary	Congestive heart failure; cardiac shock
Renal	Systemic hypertension (usually self-limiting if microemboli in end arterioles); congestive heart failure
Mesenteric	Signs of "necrotizing enterocolitis"

diagnosis. Contrast angiography with the use of non-ionic contrast media is the "gold standard" imaging technique for the confirmation of thrombosis before embarking on thrombolytic or surgical therapy. Other, less invasive tests such as real-time ultrasonography or Doppler flow studies may be helpful adjunctive measures, but their precision and accuracy in neonatal thrombotic disease are still uncertain (564). The advantages of this technique are that it is noninvasive, does not require exposure to ionizing radiation, and can be performed at the bedside.

The accuracy of ultrasound may be reduced by the presence of a catheter because reduced compressibility of the vessel lumen by the ultrasound probe (a sign of thrombosis) is difficult to assess (565). Low pulse pressure in preterm and sick newborns may also limit the interpretation of Doppler flow study. In one series of 47 infants with umbilical venous catheters, the accuracy of Doppler echocardiography was poor compared to contrast venography in detecting asymptomatic thrombus (540). Thrombi were detected by venogram in 14 patients (30%). The sensitivity and specificity of echocardiographic diagnosis for the three cardiologists who interpreted both studies ranged from 21 to 43% and 76 to 94%, respectively. However, the relative accuracy of these techniques to detect symptomatic thrombosis is not known.

For diagnosis of cerebral venous thrombosis, angiogram remains the gold standard. However, magnetic resonance imaging (MRI) with venography or Doppler flow ultrasound through the anterior fontanelle may also be used. For the diagnosis of arterial ischemic stroke, MRI is more sensitive to small or early infarcts that are frequently missed by computed tomography (CT) scan (565,566).

For neonates that are diagnosed to have a thrombus, whether a prothrombotic workup needs to be done is controversial (567). In most circumstances, the diagnosis of a prothrombotic state does not alter the management of the patient, except for protein C, protein S or antithrombin deficiencies. For patients with purpura fulminans, spontaneous thrombotic events or extensive thrombosis, prothrombotic workup including protein C, protein S and antithrombin level should be done. Parents should be counseled before testing is done. The clinical utility of testing for other prothrombotic state such as factor V Leiden, prothrombin G20210A mutations, elevated lipoprotein (a), point mutation (677→T) of MTHFR, and elevated homocysteine need to be assessed on an individual basis and ideally in a study context.

Treatment

Organ or limb dysfunction as a result of thrombosis is the most compelling indication for active intervention. The lack of strong evidence for the benefits and safety of antithrombotic therapy in this population does not usually justify aggressive therapy for asymptomatic thrombosis. In the absence of well-designed studies to address the efficacy and safety of intervention, supportive care alone may be appropriate for asymptomatic thrombosis. Catheters should be removed in catheter related thrombosis. Objective monitoring of the thrombus should be undertaken if supportive care only is chosen.

Intracranial hemorrhage or hemorrhagic infarction should be ruled out by suitable imaging techniques before anticoagulant or fibrinolytic drugs are prescribed. In all infants who receive antithrombotic therapy, the platelet count should be maintained above 50×10^9/L, and the fibrinogen concentration greater than 1 g/L (564).

Anticoagulation Therapy

Anticoagulation therapy in neonate usually involves the use of unfractionated heparin (UFH) or low molecular weight heparin (LMWH).

Unfractionated Heparin

Unfractionated heparin is a glycosaminoglycan (GAG) composed of a heterogeneous mixture of polysaccharide chains of varying lengths (3,000–30,000 Daltons). Un-fractionated heparin catalyzes the inactivation of various clotting factors, such as factor Xa and thrombin, by antithrombin. The binding of antithrombin to heparin is mediated by a unique pentasaccharide sequence that is randomly distributed along the heparin chains (568). The inactivation of thrombin, but not factor Xa, requires the formation of a ternary complex in which heparin binds to both antithrombin and thrombin (569). This ternary complex (containing heparin, antithrombin, and thrombin) forms only on pentasaccharide-containing chains with at least 18 saccharide units. The inactivation of factor Xa by heparin only requires the presence of pentasaccharide with no minimum requirement of the chain length on the heparin molecule.

Unfractionated heparin (UFH) offers the advantages of rapid reversibility and low cost. Unpredictable pharmacokinetic response and resultant requirement for frequent monitoring are the disadvantages of UFH.

The use of a dedicated intravenous catheter for UFH infusion avoids interruption of anticoagulation therapy and minimizes the risk of inadvertent flushing of the catheter that may lead to excessive anticoagulation.

Dose. The dose of heparin therapy in newborns is based on a prospective cohort study of UFH treatment in 65 children with thrombosis, of whom 29 were less than one year of age, including 13 newborns (570). Heparin is administered intravenously with a loading dose of 75 U/kg and an initial maintenance dose of 28 U/kg per hour. Dosing is adjusted to maintain an aPTT of 60 to 85 sec, which corresponds to an antifactor Xa activity of 0.35 to 0.7 U/mL (563). The dose can be adjusted according to a published nomogram (571). The therapeutic range is an extrapolation from adult data. The therapeutic range for UFH in neonates may be different from adults because the plasma concentrations of prothrombin and antithrombin in neonates are decreased compared to adults (572).

The duration of therapy is uncertain. One approach is to monitor the thrombus with ultrasound and continue therapy until the thrombus has resolved for a maximum of three months of therapy. Low molecular weight heparin can be used for prolong therapy.

Adverse Effects

The major side effects of UFH are bleeding, heparin-induced thrombocytopenia (HIT), and osteoporosis (573). The risk of bleeding in newborns is uncertain. In one pediatric prospective study of which 13 were newborns, none

had significant bleeding (95% CI, 0%–25%) (570). As in adults, bleeding likely relates to the concentration of heparin and presence of underlying disorders that predispose to bleeding (574). If bleeding occurs, UFH should be discontinued. For heparin reversal, 1 mg of protamine sulfate can inactivate 100 U heparin. The dose of protamine depends on the amount of heparin being given, and is calculated by assuming the half-life of heparin to be 1 hour.

Heparin-induced thrombocytopenia is a well-recognized complication of heparin therapy in adults (575–578). Two major mechanisms cause this thrombocytopenia. One mechanism appears to be a direct effect of heparin on platelet activation. In most of these cases, the fall in platelet count occurs within the first two days after heparin initiation, often returns to normal with continued heparin administration, and is of no clinical consequence, at least in adults. The incidence of this type is estimated at 10% to 20% of adults receiving UFH. The second type is mediated by antibodies to a heparin-platelet factor 4 complex, which results in platelet activation and aggregation and enhanced generation of thrombin (579,580). This occurs in 3% or less of adults receiving UFH for more than 4 days (576,578,581).

Heparin-induced thrombocytopenia has been described in newborns (582). However, it is difficult to evaluate the incidence because critically ill newborns have many reasons to have thrombocytopenia and/or thrombosis. One report described 34 newborns (mean gestational age 29 weeks) who developed thrombocytopenia (platelet count <70,000/μL, $n = 23$), a precipitous fall of 30 to 50% in the platelet count ($n = 5$) or thromboses ($n = 6$) while receiving heparin (583). Heparin-associated antiplatelet antibodies were found in 14 patients; these patients had clinical characteristics comparable to the 20 infants without antibodies, including the presence of an umbilical artery catheter in all but one patient in each group. Among those who had abdominal ultrasonography, aortic thrombosis occurred in 11 of 13 (84%) infants with and 5 of 20 (25%) without antibodies. Bleeding was not observed. However, the sensitivity of ultrasound to detect an asymptomatic thrombus in newborns is poor (540). Thus, the relationship between antibody formation and thrombosis in this population remains uncertain. In a more recent randomized controlled trial with 138 newborns who received prophylactic doses of UFH, none of the patients developed HIT (97.5% CI, 0%–2.6%) (584). Heparin-induced thrombocytopenia should be considered in a newborn receiving UFH with thrombocytopenia of no apparent cause, although the condition is uncommon and thrombocytopenia from other causes occurs frequently in ill LBW infants.

Osteoporosis has been reported in adult patients receiving UFH for more than 6 months (585). Bone loss is thought to occur because of decreased bone formation, increased bone resorption, or both. However, there is no information on this complication in newborns (565).

Low Molecular Weight Heparin

Low molecular weight heparin is prepared from UFH by chemical or enzymatic degradation. Like UFH, LMWH potentiates the inactivation of factor Xa by AT. However, the effect of LMWH on the AT inhibition of thrombin is decreased compared to UFH because most of the molecules in LMWH do not contain enough saccharide units to form the ternary complex in which thrombin and AT are bound simultaneously (573). As a result, LMWH in the usual therapeutic dose does not prolong the aPTT. The aPTT can be prolonged by higher doses of LMWH, but not to the same extent as UFH.

Limited information is available on the efficacy and safety of LMWH in newborns (586–588). One prospective cohort study included 173 children who were treated with the LMWH preparation enoxaparin because they had or were at high risk for thromboembolic events (587). Patients ranged in age from one day to 18 years; 21 (14.5%) were less than 36 weeks gestational age and 48 (33.5%) were less than 3 months postnatal age when treatment was initiated. Thrombi resolved clinically in 94% of patients who received therapeutic doses. In those receiving prophylaxis, 96% had no symptoms of new or recurrent TEs. Major bleeding occurred in seven (4%) of patients, of whom four were newborns. In a more recent report, the incidence of bleeding in neonates treated with enoxaparin is estimated to be 6% (588).

Over the last few years, LMWH has been used more frequently than UFH in neonates. The advantages of using LMWH are more predictable pharmacokinetics, ease of administration, at least equal efficacy and safety compared to UFH and probably decreased risk of HIT and osteoporosis. Low molecular weight heparin can be administered subcutaneously and requires minimal laboratory monitoring and dose adjustment; these are important for newborns with poor venous access (589).

Dose. There are several LMWH preparations and they should not be used interchangeably (590). In the United States, four preparations (enoxaparin, dalteparin, ardeparin, and tinzaparin) are currently approved by the FDA for different clinical indications. Dosing in pediatric patients has been reported for enoxaparin (586), dalteparin (591), clivarin (592), and tinzaparin (593). For neonates, the most experience lies in the use of enoxaparin.

For treatment of thrombosis, enoxaparin can be initiated in a dose of 1.5 mg/kg per dose subcutaneously twice each day (588,594). Dalteparin is initiated in a dose of 150 IU/kg per dose once each day (590). Doses are adjusted to maintain an antifactor Xa concentration (measured four hours after the dose) of 0.5 to 1 U/mL, the therapeutic range established in adults (595).

For prophylaxis, enoxaparin is initiated at 0.75 mg/kg per dose twice each day. Dalteparin is initiated at 100 IU/kg per dose once each day. The target concentration of antifactor Xa (0.1–0.3 U/mL) is lower for prophylaxis than for treatment (594).

The duration of therapy is uncertain. Our approach is to monitor the thrombus with ultrasound and continue therapy until the thrombus has resolved or, if still present, for up to 3 months.

If bleeding occurs, LMWH should be discontinued. The dose of protamine sulfate for reversal of heparin effect depends on the dose of LMWH and the time since LMWH was last administered. If LMWH was given within four hours, the maximum dose of protamine is 1 mg per 100 U LMWH, given by slow intravenous push. If LMWH was given more than four hours previously, a lower dose of protamine should be used. However, protamine only partially neutralizes the effects of LMWH (596).

Adverse Effects. The major adverse effect of LMWH is bleeding. The largest reported cohort of neonates that had been treated with enoxaparin showed a bleeding risk of 6% (95% CI 1.8%– 15.7%). The premature neonates are probably at increased risk compared to term neonates (588). The incidence of HIT related to the use of LMWH in neonates is unknown but is likely to be less than 1%.

Warfarin

Warfarin is not recommended in the neonatal period because of the potential risk of bleeding (565). The effect of warfarin is mediated through reduction of the functional plasma concentration of the vitamin K-dependent coagulation factors (factors II, VII, IX, and X). However, the concentration of these factors is physiologically reduced in newborns and is often similar to those of adults receiving warfarin therapy. Breast-fed newborns are especially sensitive to the effect of warfarin because human milk has low concentrations of vitamin K. On the other hand, formula-fed babies are relatively warfarin resistant because of vitamin K supplement in infants formula.

Warfarin is only available in tablet form. Splitting or crushing the tablet into powder may cause variability in the dose. Additionally, treatment with warfarin requires frequent monitoring of the INR.

Thrombolytic Agents

There is limited experience in using fibrinolytic agents in newborn infants (597,598). Over the years, a gradual shift seems to have occurred from streptokinase to urokinase and, more recently, to tissue plasminogen activator (tPA) (597). A wide range of doses, both with or without boluses, have been used with variable successes and failures (522, 523,597,598). In the absence of any controlled data in this population on the superiority of one thrombolytic agent over the others, the choice of drug should be determined by familiarity and cost.

Any clinician who is contemplating thrombolytic therapy in sick neonates must weigh the risk of prolonged vessel occlusion and the uncertain drug benefits against the infant's risk of suffering from serious bleeding complications. Contraindications should be seriously considered before the initiation of the thrombolytic therapy (599).

Dose. The dose of tPA in newborns is extrapolated from doses in older children and adults. For systemic therapy, tPA can be given as a continuous infusion at a rate of 0.1 to 0.5 mg/kg per hour for six hours, without a loading dose

(563). The drug can be given through a central or peripheral venous catheter.

Transfusion of FFP before initiation of thrombolytic therapy may decrease the risk of bleeding. Furthermore, FFP provides plasminogen, which may enhance the effect of the tPA. Fresh frozen plasma and/or cryoprecipitate can be given if the fibrinogen concentration is <1 g/L or if there is bleeding (563).

Aside from resolution of the thrombus, there is no easy way to measure the effectiveness of the tPA infusion. The presence of d-dimers or fibrin/fibrinogen degradation products only indicates a fibrinolytic state.

Treatment of bleeding following use of tPA includes use of cryoprecipitate to increase the fibrinogen concentration, stopping the tPA infusion if possible, and administration of platelets if needed.

Adverse Effects. Bleeding is the most concerning side effect of fibrinolytic therapy. However, as a result of the variety of dosing regimens and whether contraindications for the use of fibrinolytic therapy are followed, the bleeding risk associated with the use of fibrinolytic therapy remains unclear but certainly may be major.

Surgery. The main objectives of surgical intervention in neonatal large vessel thrombosis have been, first, to remove the occluding clot and, second, to resect a nonviable product of the vessel obstruction (amputation for limb gangrene; resection of necrotic bowel). Thrombectomy may be used in selected cases, particularly if the thrombus obstructs a major artery.

Because of the devastating functional loss with all ensuing problems, amputation in peripheral arterial occlusion should be postponed as long as possible. The main aim is to prevent superimposed secondary infection. Ideally, surgical intervention should be delayed until the necrotic parts are well demarcated. In some cases, surgery is not necessary at all because autoamputation occurs, which results in the least possible loss of tissue.

Prognosis. The vast majority of infants with thrombotic disease survive; mortality rates are highest among infants with aortic thrombosis or with central venous catheter–associated TEs affecting the right atrium or the superior vena cava (522). In the Canadian Registry, for example, the mortality rates for both aortic and right atrial or superior vena cava thrombosis were 33%. In the Netherlands Registry, the mortality rate was 15% but none of the deaths were directly related to the TEs (523). Data on long-term follow-up of neonatal TEs are very limited. The outcome of the following conditions is relatively better studied.

Renal Vein Thrombosis

A total of 58 neonates with renal venous thrombosis have been followed for 0.1 to 17 years by four different investigator teams (600). Persistent hypertension was found in 28% of all children, and 21% had residual renal tubular

defects (600). In another study, 26 out of 39 affected kidneys were atrophic (601).

Aortic Thrombosis

The available follow-up data on survivors of aortic thrombosis suggests that blood pressure and renal function are likely to normalize during early childhood, but persistent hypertension, leg-growth discrepancies, and abnormalities in renal size and function have been described (602–605).

Cerebral Venous Thrombosis

The best available data on the outcome showed 77% of the newborns surviving sinovenous thrombosis are neurologically normal (606).

Arterial Ischemic Stroke

One third of the neonates with arterial ischemic stroke are normal with the rest having neurological deficits. Lesions that involve the motor cortex, internal capsule, and basal ganglia together are associated with increased disability as compared to lesions limited to the cortex or basal ganglia alone (565). Prothrombotic states such as Factor V Leiden were associated with a worse neurological outcome in perinatal arterial infarction (607).

Prophylaxis

To reduce the risk of TE disease in the newborn, intravascular catheters should be used judiciously, and blood flow should be optimized at all times.

Arterial Catheters

In a systematic review of five clinical trials, heparinization decreased the risk of catheter occlusion (relative risk 0.20, 95% CI, 0.11–0.35) (242). However, the risk of aortic thrombosis, IVH, death, or clinical ischemic events did not appear to be affected. Therefore, fluid infused through an umbilical arterial catheter should contain UFH in a concentration of 0.5 to 1.0 units/mL.

Although data are limited in newborns, use of UFH prolongs the patency of peripheral arterial catheters (608–610). Fluid infused through a peripheral arterial catheter should also be heparinized, using a similar concentration.

Central Venous Catheters

Fluid infused through a central venous catheter should contain heparin in a concentration of 0.5 units/mL to prevent thrombosis and catheter occlusion. However, heparinization of central venous catheters (umbilical or peripherally placed percutaneous) has not been studied in well designed trials (611). At the present time, there is no data to support systemic anticoagulant prophylaxis to prevent catheter related thrombosis and thus this approach cannot be recommended.

ACKNOWLEDGMENTS

The authors are grateful to Dr. Hans Hitzler (Division of Hematology/Oncology, The Hospital for Sick Children,

Toronto, Canada); Dr. Eyal Grunebaum (Division of Immunology, The Hospital for Sick Children, Toronto, Canada); Dr. Greg Denomme (Canadian Blood Services, Toronto, Canada) for their useful contributions to the chapter and to Dr Alvin Zipursky for his critical review and comments during the preparation of this manuscript. This chapter was prepared with the editorial assistance of Lu Ann Brooker.

REFERENCES

1. Brown MS. Fetal and neonatal erythropoiesis. In: Stockman JA, Pochedly C, eds. *Developmental and Neonatal Hematology.* New York: Raven Press, 1988:39–56.
2. Shannon KM, Naylor GS, Torkilson JC, et al. Circulating erythroid progenitors in the anemia of prematurity. *N Engl J Med* 1987;317:728–733.
3. Rhondeau SM, Christensen RD, Ross MP, et al. Responsiveness to recombinant human erythropoietin of marrow erythroid progenitors from infants with the "anemia of prematurity". *J Pediatr* 1988;112:935–940.
4. Christensen RD. Hematopoiesis in the fetus and neonate. *Pediatr Res* 1989;26:531–535.
5. Stockman JA III, Garcia JF, Oski FA. The anemia of prematurity. Factors governing the erythropoietin response. *N Eng J Med* 1977;296:647–650.
6. Stockman JA III, Graeber JE, Clark DA, et al. Anemia of prematurity: determinants of the erythropoietin response. *J Pediatr* 1984;105:786–792.
7. Brown MS, Garcia JF, Phibbs RH, et al. Decreased response of plasma immunoreactive erythropoietin to "available oxygen" in anemia of prematurity. *J Pediatr* 1984;105:793–798.
8. Forestier F, Daffos F, Catherine N, et al. Developmental hematopoiesis in normal human fetal blood. *Blood* 1991;77:2360–2363.
9. Oski FA, Naiman JL. Normal blood values in the newborn period. In: Oski FA, Naiman JL, eds. *Hematologic Problems in the Newborn*, 3rd ed. Philadelphia: WB Saunders, 1982:11.
10. Blanchette VS, Zipursky A. Neonatal hematology. In: Avery GB, ed. Neonatology: *Pathophysiology and management*, 3rd ed. Philadelphia: JB Lippincott, 1987:638–686.
11. Yao AC, Moinian M, Lind J. Distribution of blood between infant and placenta after birth. *Lancet* 1969;2:871–873.
12. Colozzi AE. Clamping of the umbilical cord: its effect on the placental transfusion. *N Engl J Med* 1954;250:629–632.
13. Usher R, Shephard M, Lind J. The blood volume of the newborn infant and placental transfusion. *Acta Paediatr* 1963;52:497–512.
14. Gunther M. The transfer of blood between baby and placenta in the minutes after birth. *Lancet* 1957;1:1277–1280.
15. Schulman I, Smith CH, Stern GS. Studies on the anemia of prematurity. *Am J Dis Child* 1954;88:567–595.
16. O'Brien RT, Pearson HA. Physiologic anemia of the newborn infant. *J Pediatr* 1971;79:132–138.
17. Stockman JA III. Anemia of prematurity. *Clin Perinatol* 1977;4:239–257.
18. Stockman JA III, Oski FA. Physiological anaemia of infancy and the anaemia of prematurity. *Clin Hematol* 1978;7:3–18.
19. Gairdner D, Marks J, Roscoe JD. Blood formation in infancy. Part II. Normal erythropoiesis. *Arch Dis Child* 1952;27:214–221.
20. Pearson HA. Life-span of the fetal red blood cell. *J Pediatr* 1967;70:166–171.
21. Bratteby LE, Garby L, Groth T, et al. Studies on erythrokinetics in infancy. XIII. The mean life span and life span frequency function of red blood cells formed during foetal life. *Acta Paediatr Scand* 1968;57:311–320.
22. Schulman I. The anemia of prematurity. *J Pediatr* 1959;54:663–672.
23. Joshi A, Gerhardt T, Shandloff P, et al. Blood transfusion effect on the respiratory pattern of preterm infants. *Pediatrics* 1987;80:79–84.
24. Keyes WG, Donohue PK, Spivak JL, et al. Assessing the need for transfusion of premature infants and the role of hematocrit, clinical signs, and erythropoietin level. *Pediatrics* 1989;84:412–417.

25. Sasidharan P, Heimler R. Transfusion-induced changes in the breathing pattern of healthy preterm anemic infants. *Pediatr Pulmonol* 1992;12:170–173.
26. Bifano EM, Smith F, Borer J. Relationship between determinants of oxygen delivery and respiratory abnormalities in preterm infants with anemia. *J Pediatr* 1992;120:292–296.
27. Izraeli S, Ben-Sira L, Harell D, et al. Lactic acid as a predictor for erythrocyte transfusion in healthy preterm infants with anemia of prematurity. *J Pediatr* 1993;122:629–631.
28. Lachance C, Chessex P, Fouron J-C, et al. Myocardial, erythropoietic, and metabolic adaptations to anemia of prematurity. *J Pediatr* 1994;125:278–282.
29. Böhler T, Janecke A, Linderkamp O. Blood transfusion in late anemia of prematurity: effect on oxygen consumption, heart rate, and weight gain in otherwise healthy infants. *Infusionsther Transfusionsmed* 1994;21:376–379.
30. Stockman JA III, Clark DA. Weight gain: a response to transfusion in selected preterm infants. *Am J Dis Child* 1984;138:828–830.
31. Möller JC, Schwarz U, Schaible TF, et al. Do cardiac output and serum lactate levels indicate blood transfusion requirements in anemia of prematurity? *Inten Care Med* 1996;22:472–476.
32. Doyle JJ, Zipursky A. Neonatal blood disorders. In: Sinclair JC, Bracken MB, eds. *Effective care of the newborn infant.* Oxford: Oxford University, 1992:425–453.
33. Rönnholm KAR, Siimes MA. Haemoglobin concentration depends on protein intake in small preterm infants fed human milk. *Arch Dis Child* 1985;60:99–104.
34. Bechensteen AG, Hågå P, Halvorsen S, et al. Erythropoietin, protein, and iron supplementation and the prevention of anaemia of prematurity. *Arch Dis Child* 1993;69:19–23.
35. Kivivuori SM, Järvenpää AL, Salmenperä L, et al. Erythropoiesis of very-low-birth-weight infants is dependent on prenatal growth rate and protein status. *Acta Paediatr* 1994;83:13–18.
36. Rønnestad A, Moe PJ, Breivik N. Enhancement of erythropoiesis by erythropoietin, bovine protein and energy fortified mother's milk during anaemia of prematurity. *Acta Paediatr* 1995;83:809–811.
37. Brown MS, Shapiro H. Effect of protein intake on erythropoiesis during erythropoietin treatment of anemia of prematurity. *J Pediatr* 1996;128:512–517.
38. Bechensteen AG, Halvorsen S, Hägä P, et al. Erythropoietin (Epo), protein and iron supplementation and the prevention of anaemia of prematurity: effects on serum immunoreactive Epo, growth and protein and iron metabolism. *Acta Paediatr* 1996;85:490–495.
39. Blank JP, Sheagren TG, Vajaria J, et al. The role of RBC transfusion in the premature infant. *Am J Dis Child* 1984;138:831–833.
40. Meyer J, Sive A, Jacobs P. Empiric red cell transfusion in asymptomatic preterm infants. *Acta Paediatr* 1993;82:30–34.
41. Alverson DC, Isken VH, Cohen RS. Effect of booster blood transfusions on oxygen utilization in infants with bronchopulmonary dysplasia. *J Pediatr* 1988;113:722–726.
42. Ross MP, Christensen RD, Rothstein G, et al. A randomized trial to develop criteria for administering erythrocyte transfusions to anemic preterm infants 1 to 3 months of age. *J Perinatol* 1989;9:246–253.
43. Stute H, Greiner B, Linderkamp O. Effect of blood transfusion on cardiorespiratory abnormalities in preterm infants. *Arch Dis Child Fetal Neonatal Ed* 1995;72:F194–F196.
44. Levy GJ, Strauss RG, Hume H, et al. National survey of neonatal transfusion practices: I. Red cell therapy. *Pediatrics* 1993;91:523–529.
45. Fetus and Newborn Committee Canadian Pediatric Society. Guidelines for transfusion of erythrocytes to neonates and premature infants. *Can Med Assoc J* 1992;147:1781–1792.
46. Goodnough LT. Risks of blood transfusion. *Crit Care Med* 2003;31:S678–S686.
47. Obladen M, Maier R, Segerer H, et al. Efficacy and safety of recombinant human erythropoietin to prevent anaemias of prematurity. European randomized multicenter trial. *Contrib Nephrol* 1991;88:314–326.
48. Carnielli V, Montini G, Da Riol R, et al. Effect of high doses of human recombinant erythropoietin on the need for blood transfusions in preterm infants. *J Pediatr* 1992;121:98–102.
49. Emmerson AJB, Coles HJ, Stern CMM, et al. Double blind trial of recombinant human erythropoietin in preterm infants. *Arch Dis Child* 1993;68:291–296.

50. Soubasi V, Kremenopoulos G, Diamandi E, et al. In which neonates does early recombinant human erythropoietin treatment prevent anemia of prematurity? Results of a randomized controlled study. *Pediatr Res* 1993;34:675–679.

51. Maier RF, Obladen M, Scigalla P, et al. The effect of epoetin beta (recombinant human erythropoietin) on the need for transfusion in very-low-birth-weight infants. European Multicentre Erythropoietin Study Group. *N Engl J Med* 1994;330:1173–1178.

52. Ohls RK, Osborne KA, Christensen RD. Efficacy and cost analysis of treating very low birth weight infants with erythropoietin during their first two weeks of life: a randomized, placebo-controlled trial. *J Pediatr* 1995;126:421–426.

53. Soubasi V, Kremenopoulos G, Diamanti E, et al. Follow-up of very low birth weight infants after erythropoietin treatment to prevent anemia of prematurity. *J Pediatr* 1995;127:291–297.

54. Shannon KM, Mentzer WC, Abels RI, et al. Recombinant human erythropoietin in the anemia of prematurity: results of a placebo-controlled pilot study. *J Pediatr* 1991;118:949–955.

55. Ohls RK, Christensen RD. Recombinant erythropoietin compared with erythrocyte transfusion in the treatment of anemia of prematurity. *J Pediatr* 1991;119:781–788.

56. Shannon KM, Mentzer WC, Abels RI, et al. Enhancement of erythropoiesis by recombinant human erythropoietin in low birth weight infants: a pilot study. *J Pediatr* 1992;120:586–592.

57. Meyer MP, Meyer JH, Commerford A, et al. Recombinant human erythropoietin in the treatment of the anemia of prematurity: results of a double-blind, placebo-controlled study. *Pediatrics* 1994;93:918–923.

58. Shannon KM, Keith JI, Mentzer WC, et al. Recombinant human erythropoietin stimulates erythropoiesis and reduces erythrocyte transfusions in very low birth weight preterm infants. *Pediatrics* 1995;95:1–8.

59. Chen J-Y, Wu T-S, Chanlai S-P. Recombinant human erythropoietin in the treatment of anemia of prematurity. *Am J Perinatol* 1995;12:314–318.

60. Donato H, Rendo P, Vivas N. Recombinant human erythropoietin in the treatment of anemia of prematurity; a randomized double-blind, placebo-controlled trial comparing three different doses. *Int J Pediatr Hematol/Oncol* 1996;3:279–285.

61. Bader D, Blondheim O, Jonas R, et al. Decreased ferritin levels, despite iron supplementation, during erythropoietin therapy in anaemia of prematurity. *Acta Paediatr* 1996;85:496–501.

62. Vamvakas EC, Strauss RG. Meta-analysis of controlled clinical trials studying the efficacy of rHuEPO in reducing blood transfusions in the anemia of prematurity. *Transfusion* 2001;41:406–415.

63. Garcia MG, Hutson AD, Christensen RD. Effect of recombinant erythropoietin on "late" transfusions in the neonatal intensive care unit: a meta-analysis. *J Perinatol* 2002;22:108–111.

64. Casadevall N, Nataf J, Viron B, et al. Pure red-cell aplasia and antierythropoietin antibodies in patients treated with recombinant erythropoietin. *N Engl J Med* 2002;346:469–475.

65. Zipursky A. The risk of hematopoietic growth factor therapy in newborn infants. *Pediatr Res* 2002;51:549.

66. Doyle JJ. The role of erythropoietin in the anemia of prematurity. *Semin Perinatol* 1997;21:20–27.

67. Calhoun DA, Christensen RD, Edstrom CS, et al. Consistent approaches to procedures and practices in neonatal hematology. *Clin Perinatol* 2000;27:733–753.

68. Faxelius G, Raye J, Gutberlet R, et al. Red cell volume measurements and acute blood loss in high-risk newborn infants. *J Pediatr* 1977;90:273–281.

69. Zipursky A, Hull A, White FD, et al. Foetal erythrocytes in the maternal circulation. *Lancet* 1959;1:451–452.

70. Giacoia GP. Severe fetomaternal hemorrhage: a review. *Obstet Gynecol Surv* 1997;52:372–380.

71. Fischer RL, Kuhlman K, Grover J, et al. Chronic, massive fetomaternal hemorrhage treated with repeated fetal intravascular transfusions. *Am J Obstet Gynecol* 1990;162:203–204.

72. Rouse D, Weiner C. Ongoing fetomaternal hemorrhage treated by serial fetal intravascular transfusions. *Obstet Gynecol* 1990;76:974–975.

73. Thomas A, Mathew M, Unciano ME, et al. Acute massive fetomaternal hemorrhage: case reports and review of the literature. *Acta Obstet Gynecol Scand* 2003;82:479–480.

74. Pai MK, Bedritis I, Zipursky A. Massive transplacental hemorrhage: clinical manifestations in the newborn. *Can Med Assoc J* 1975;112:585–589.

75. Kleihauer E, von Braun H, Betke K. Demonstration von fetalem Hamoglobin in den Erythrocyten eines Blutausstrichs. *Klin Wochenschr* 1957;35:637.

76. Pembrey ME, Weatherall DJ, Clegg JB. Maternal synthesis of haemoglobin F in pregnancy. *Lancet* 1973;1:1350–1354.

77. Tan KL, Tan R, Tan SH, et al. The twin transfusion syndrome. Clinical observations on 35 affected pairs. *Clin Pediatr* 1979;18:111–114.

78. Lewi L, Van Schoubroeck D, Gratacos E, et al. Monochorionic diamniotic twins: complications and management options. *Curr Opin Obstet Gynecol* 2003;15:177–194.

79. Quintero RA, Morales WJ, Allen MH, et al. Staging of twin-twin transfusion syndrome. *J Perinatol* 1999;19:550–555.

80. Duncombe GJ, Dickinson JE, Evans SF. Perinatal characteristics and outcomes of pregnancies complicated by twin-twin transfusion syndrome. *Obstet Gynecol* 2003;101:1190–1196.

81. Vanhaesebrouck P, Vanneste K, de Praeter C, et al. Tight nuchal cord and neonatal hypovolaemic shock. *Arch Dis Child* 1987;62:1276–1277.

82. Shepherd AJ, Richardson CJ, Brown JP. Nuchal cord as a cause of neonatal anemia. *Am J Dis Child* 1985;139:71–73.

83. Cashore WJ, Usher RH. Hypovolemia resulting from a tight nuchal cord at birth. *Pediatr Res* 1975;7:399.

84. Clayton EM, Pryor JA, Wierdsma JG, et al. Fetal and maternal components in third-trimester obstetric hemorrhage. *Obstet Gynecol* 1964;24:56–60.

85. Henderson JL. Hepatic hemorrhage in stillborn and newborn infants; A clinical and pathological study of forty-seven cases. *J Obstet Gynaecol Br Commonw* 1941;48:377–388.

86. Holmberg E. Rupture of liver in newborn observed at General Lying in Hospital in Helsingfors from 1924 to 1932. *Finska Lak-Sallsk Handl* 1933;75:1067–1096.

87. Potter EL. Fetal and neonatal deaths: a statistical analysis of 2000 autopsies. *JAMA* 1940;115:996–1001.

88. Blanchette VS, Zipursky A. Assessment of anemia in newborn infants. *Clin Perinatol* 1984;11:489–510.

89. Bell EF, Nahmias C, Sinclair JC. The assessment of anemia in small premature infants. *Pediatr Res* 1977;11:467a.

90. Mollison PL, Veall N, Cutbush M. Red cell and plasma volume in newborn infants. *Arch Dis Child* 1950;25:242–253.

91. Bratteby L-E. Studies on erythro-kinetics in infancy. XI. The change in circulating red cell volume during the first five months of life. *Acta Paediatr Scand* 1968;57:215–224.

92. Bratteby L-E. Studies on erythro-kinetics in infancy. X. Red cell volume of newborn infants in relation to gestational age. *Acta Paediatr Scand* 1968;57:132–136.

93. Dyer NC, Brill AB, Faxelius G. Blood volume and hemorrhage timing in newborn infants with respiratory distress using the stable tracer ^{50}Cr. *Proc Am Nucl Soc* 1971;5:46.

94. Francoual C, Relier J-P, Thérain F. Interet de la mesure du volume globulaire total chez le nouveau-né en detresse respiratoire. *Arch Franc Péd* 1977;34:34–83.

95. Ballin A, Arbel E, Kenet G, et al. Autologous umbilical cord blood transfusion. *Arch Dis Child Fetal Neonatal Ed* 1995;73:F181–F183.

96. Schacter BA. Heme catabolism by heme oxygenase: physiology, regulation, and mechanism of action. *Semin Hematol* 1988;25:349–369.

97. Rodgers PA, Vreman HJ, Dennery PA, et al. Sources of carbon monoxide (CO) in biological systems and applications of CO detection technologies. *Semin Perinatol* 1994;18:2–10.

98. Ostrander CR, Cohen RS, Hopper AO, et al. Paired determinations of blood carboxyhemoglobin concentration and carbon monoxide excretion rate in term and preterm infants. *J Lab Clin Med* 1982;100:745–755.

99. Bjure J, Fallström SP. Endogenous formation of carbon monoxide in newborn infants. I. Non-icteric and icteric infants without blood group incompatibility. *Acta Padiatr Scand* 1963;52:361–366.

100. Alden ER, Lynch SR, Wennberg RP. Carboxyhemoglobin determination in evaluating neonatal jaundice. *Am J Dis Child* 1974;127:214–217.

101. Necheles TF, Rai US, Valaes T. The role of haemolysis in neonatal hyperbilirubinaemia as reflected in carboxyhaemoglobin levels. *Acta Paediatr Scand* 1976;65:361–367.

102. Queenan JT. *Modern management of the Rh problem.* New York: Harper and Row, 1967.

103. Liley AW. Diagnosis and treatment of erythroblastosis in the fetus. *Adv Pediatr* 1968;15:29–63.

104. Naiman JL. Current management of hemolytic disease of the newborn infant. *J Pediatr* 1972;80:1049–1059.

105. Zipursky A. Hemolytic anemia of the newborn In: Nathan DG, Oski FA, eds. *Hematology of infancy and childhood.* Philadelphia: WB Saunders, 1974:46–99.

106. Shao C-P, Maas J-H, Su Y-Q, et al. Molecular background of Rh D-positive, D-negative, D(el) and weak D phenotypes in Chinese. *Vox Sang* 2002;83:156–161.

107. Ekman GC, Billingsly R, Hessner MJ. Rh genotyping: avoiding false-negative and false-positive results among individuals of African ancestry. *Am J Hematol* 2002;69:34–40.

108. Daniels G, Green C, Smart E. Differences between RhD-negative Africans and RhD-negative Europeans. *Lancet* 1997;350:862–863.

109. Hathaway WE. Coagulation problems in the newborn infant. *Pediatr Clin North Am* 1970;17:929–942.

110. Chessells JM, Wigglesworth JS. Haemostatic failure in babies with rhesus isoimmunization. *Arch Dis Child* 1971;46:38–45.

111. Bowman J. Thirty-five years of Rh prophylaxis. *Transfusion* 2003;43:1661–1666.

112. Fung Kee Fung K, Eason E, Crane J, et al. Prevention of Rh alloimmunization. *J Obstet Gynaecol* Can 2003;25:765–773.

113. Fung Kee Fung K. Prevention of Rh alloimmunization: are we there yet? *J Obstet Gynaecol Can* 2003;25:716–719.

114. Lee D, Contreras M, Robson SC, et al. Recommendations for the use of anti-D immunoglobulin for Rh prophylaxis. British Blood Transfusion Society and the Royal College of Obstetricians and Gynaecologists. *Transfus Med* 1999;9:93–97.

115. Torrance GW, Zipursky A. Cost-effectiveness of antepartum prevention of Rh immunization. *Clin Perinatol* 1984;11:267–281.

116. Bowman JM, Friesen RF. Hemolytic disease of the newborn. In: Gellis SS, Kogan BM, eds. *Current pediatric therapy* (vol 4). Philadelphia: WB Saunders, 1970:405–411.

117. Bowman JM, Pollack JM. Amniotic fluid spectrophotometry and early delivery in the management of erythroblastosis fetalis. *Pediatrics* 1965;35:815–835.

118. Bennett PR, Le Van KC, Colin Y, et al. Prenatal determination of fetal RhD type by DNA amplification. *N Engl J Med* 1993; 329:607–610.

119. Stiller RJ, Ashmead GG, Paul D, et al. Fetal blood flow measurements in severe rhesus isoimmunization. A case report. *J Reprod Med* 1987;32:453–455.

120. Whitecar PW, Moise KJ Jr. Sonographic methods to detect fetal anemia in red blood cell alloimmunization. *Obstet Gynecol Surv* 2000;55:240–250.

121. Zipursky A, Bowman JM. Isoimmune hemolytic diseases In: Nathan DG, Oski FA, eds. *Hematology of infancy and childhood.* Philadelphia: WB Saunders, 1993:44–73.

122. Nicolaides KH, Soothill PW, Rodeck CH, et al. Rh disease: intravascular fetal blood transfusion by cordocentesis. *Fetal Ther* 1986;1:185–192.

123. Nicolaides KH, Clewell WH, Rodeck CH. Measurement of human fetoplacental blood volume in erythroblastosis fetalis. *Am J Obstet Gynecol* 1987;157:50–53.

124. American Academy of Pediatrics, Provisional Committee for Quality Inprovement and Subcommittee on Hyperbilirubinemia. Practice parameter: management of hyperbilirubinemia in the healthy term newborn. *Pediatrics* 1994;94:558–565.

125. Rubo J, Albrecht K, Lasch P, et al. High-dose intravenous immune globulin therapy for hyperbilirubinemia caused by Rh hemolytic disease. *J Pediatr* 1992;121:93–97.

126. Gottstein R, Cooke RW. Systematic review of intravenous immunoglobulin in haemolytic disease of the newborn. *Arch Dis Child Fetal Neonatal Ed* 2003;88:F6-F10.

127. Desjardins L, Blajchman MA, Chintu C, et al. The spectrum of ABO hemolytic disease of the newborn infant. *J Pediatr* 1979;95:447–449.

128. Kaplan E, Herz F, Scheye E, et al. Phototherapy in ABO hemolytic disease of the newborn infant. *J Pediatr* 1971;79:911–914.

129. Risemberg HM, Mazzi E, MacDonald MG, et al. Correlation of cord bilirubin levels with hyperbilirubinaemia in ABO incompatibility. *Arch Dis Child* 1977;52:219–222.

130. Kornstad L. New cases of irregular blood group antibodies other than anti-D in pregnancy. Frequency and clinical significance. *Acta Obstet Gynecol Scand* 1983;62:431–436.

131. Giblett ER. Blood group antibodies causing hemolytic disease of the newborn. *Clin Obstet Gynecol* 1964;7:1044–1055.

132. Pepperell RJ, Barrie JU, Fliegner JR. Significance of red-cell irregular antibodies in the obstetric patient. *Med J Aust* 1977;2:453–456.

133. Caine ME, Mueller-Heubach E. Kell sensitization in pregnancy. *Am J Obstet Gynecol* 1986;154:85–90.

134. Vaughan JI, Manning M, Warwick RM, et al. Inhibition of erythroid progenitor cells by anti-Kell antibodies in fetal alloimmune anemia. *N Engl J Med* 1998;338:798–803.

135. Daniels G, Hadley A, Green CA. Causes of fetal anemia in hemolytic disease due to anti-K. *Transfusion* 2003;43:115–116.

136. Beutler E. G6PD deficiency. *Blood* 1994;84:3613–3636.

137. Lu T-C, Wei H, Blackwell RQ. Increased incidence of severe hyperbilirubinemia among newborn Chinese infants with G6PD deficiency. *Pediatrics* 1966;37:994–999.

138. Doxiadis SA, Karaklis A, Valaes T, et al. Risk of severe jaundice in glucose-6-phosphate dehydrogenase deficiency of the newborn. Differences in population groups. *Lancet* 1964;14:1210–1212.

139. Eshaghpour E, Oski FA, Williams M. The relationship of erythrocyte glucose-6-phosphate dehydrogenase deficiency to hyperbilirubinemia in Negro premature infants. *J Pediatr* 1967;70:595–601.

140. Bienzle U, Effiong C, Luzzatto L. Erythrocyte glucose 6-phosphate dehydrogenase deficiency (G6PD type A) and neonatal jaundice. *Acta Paediatr Scand* 1976;65:701–703.

141. Fessas PH, Doxiadis SA, Valaes T. Neonatal jaundice in glucose-6-phosphate dehydrogenase deficient infants. *Br Med J* 1962;2:1359–1362.

142. Olowe SA, Ransome-Kuti O. The risk of jaundice in glucose-6-phosphate dehydrogenase deficient babies exposed to menthol. *Acta Paediatr Scand* 1980;69:341–345.

143. Kaplan M, Renbaum P, Levy-Lahad E, et al. Severe neonatal icterus in some glucose-6-phosphate dehydrogenase (G-6-PD)-deficient infants is explained by the combined effect of G-6-PD deficiency and the UDP-glucoronyltransferase 1 (UDPGT1) promoter polymorphism of Gilbert's syndrome. A new paradigm for multigenic disease. *Blood* 1997;90,8a.

144. Slusher TM, Vreman HJ, McLaren DW, et al. Glucose-6-phosphate dehydrogenase deficiency and carboxyhemoglobin concentrations associated with bilirubin-related morbidity and death in Nigerian infants. *J Pediatr* 1995;126:102–108.

145. Kaplan M, Abramov A. Neonatal hyperbilirubinemia associated with glucose-6-phosphate dehydrogenase deficiency in Sephardic-Jewish neonates: incidence, severity, and the effect of phototherapy. *Pediatrics* 1992;90:401–405.

146. Kaplan M, Vreman HJ, Hammerman C, et al. Contribution of haemolysis to jaundice in Sephardic Jewish glucose-6-phosphate dehydrogenase deficient neonates. *Br J Haematol* 1996;93:822–827.

147. Kaplan M, Rubaltelli FF, Hammerman C, et al. Conjugated bilirubin in neonates with glucose-6-phosphate dehydrogenase deficiency. *J Pediatr* 1996;128:695–697.

148. Valaes T, Doxiadis SA, Fessas P. Acute hemolysis due to naphthalene inhalation. *J Pediatr* 1963;63:904–915.

149. Beutler E, Mitchell M. Special modifications of the fluorescent screening method for glucose-6-phosphate dehydrogenase deficiency. *Blood* 1968;32:816–818.

150. Motulsky AG, Campbell-Kraut JM. Population genetics of glucose-6-phosphate dehydrogenase deficiency of the red cell. In: Blumber BS, ed. *Proceedings of the conference on genetic polymorphism and geographic variations in disease.* New York: Grune and Stratton, 1961:159.

151. Kaplan M, Leiter C, Hammerman C, et al. Comparison of commercial screening tests for glucose-6-phosphate dehydrogenase deficiency in the neonatal period. *Clin Chem* 1997;43:1236–1237.

152. Kaplan M, Vreman HJ, Hammerman C, et al. Combination of ABO blood group incompatibility and glucose-6-phosphate dehydrogenase deficiency: effect on hemolysis and neonatal hyperbilirubinemia. *Acta Paediatr* 1998;87:455–457.

153. Erlandson ME, Hilgartner M. Hemolytic disease in the neonatal period and early infancy. *J Pediatr* 1959;54:566–585.

154. Hegye T, Delphin ES, Bank A, et al. Sickle cell anemia in the newborn. *Pediatrics* 1977;60:213–216.

155. Consensus Development Panel. Newborn screening for sickle cell disease and other hemoglobinopathies. *JAMA* 1987;258:1205–1209.

156. Pass KA, Lane PA, Fernhoff PM, et al. US newborn screening system guidelines II: follow-up of children, diagnosis, management, and evaluation. Statement of the Council of Regional Networks for Genetic Services (CORN). *J Pediatr* 2000;137:S1–S7.

157. Joiner CH. Universal newborn screening for hemoglobinopathies. *J Pediatr* 2000;136:145–146.

158. Reed W, Lane PA, Lorey F, et al. Sickle-cell disease not identified by newborn screening because of prior transfusion. *J Pediatr* 2000;136:248–250.

159. Lee-Potter JP, Deacon-Smith RA, Simpkiss MJ, et al. A new cause of haemolytic anaemia in the newborn. A description of an unstable fetal haemoglobin: F Poole, $\alpha_2{}^G\gamma_2$ 130 tryptophan-glycine. *J Clin Pathol* 1975;28:317–320.

160. Kan YW, Forget BG, Nathan DG. Gamma-beta thalassemia: a cause of hemolytic disease of the newborn. *N Engl J Med* 1972;286:129–134.

161. Oort M, Roos D, Flavell RA, et al. Haemolytic disease of the newborn and chronic anaemia induced by delta-beta-gamma thalassaemia in a Dutch family. *Br J Haematol* 1981;48:251–262.

162. Pirastu M, Kan YW, Lin CC, et al. Hemolytic disease of the newborn caused by a new deletion of the entire beta-globin cluster. *J Clin Invest* 1983;72:602–609.

163. Fearon ER, Kazazian HH Jr, Waber PG, et al. The entire beta-globin gene cluster is deleted in a form of gamma delta beta-thalassemia. *Blood* 1983;61:1273–1274.

164. Olivieri NF. Fetal erythropoiesis and the diagnosis and treatment of hemoglobin disorders in the fetus and child. *Semin Perinatol* 1997;21:63–69.

165. Ballin A, Brown EJ, Zipursky A. Idiopathic Heinz body hemolytic anemia in newborn infants. *Am J Pediatr Hematol Oncol* 1989;11:3–7.

166. Doyle J, Vreman HJ, Stevenson DK, et al. Does vitamin C cause hemolysis in premature newborn infants? Results of a multicenter double-blind, randomized, controlled trial. *J Pediatr* 1997;130:103–109.

167. Diamond LK, Wang WC, Alter BP. Congenital hypoplastic anemia. *Adv Pediatr* 1976;22:349–378.

168. Halperin DS, Freedman MH. Diamond Blackfan anemia: etiology, pathophysiology, and treatment. *Am J Pediatr Hematol Oncol* 1989;11:380–394.

169. Gazda H, Lipton JM, Willig TN, et al. Evidence for linkage of familial Diamond-Blackfan anemia to chromosome 8p23.3-p22 and for non-19q non-8p disease. *Blood* 2001;97:2145–2150.

170. Aase JM, Smith DW. Congenital anemia and triphalangeal thumbs: a new syndrome. *J Pediatr* 1969;74:471–474.

171. Freedman MH, Amato D, Saunders EF. Erythroid colony growth in congenital hypoplastic anemia. *J Clin Invest* 1976;57:673–677.

172. Vlachos A, Federman N, Reyes-Haley C, et al. Hematopoietic stem cell transplantation for Diamond Blackfan anemia: a report from the Diamond Blackfan Anemia Registry. *Bone Marrow Transplant* 2001;27:381–386.

173. Wasser JS, Yolken R, Miller DR, et al. Congenital hypoplastic anemia (Diamond-Blackfan syndrome) terminating in acute myelogenous leukemia. *Blood* 1978;51:991–995.

174. Lipton JM, Federman N, Khabbaze Y, et al. Osteogenic sarcoma associated with Diamond-Blackfan anemia: a report from the Diamond-Blackfan Anemia Registry. *J Pediatr Hematol Oncol* 2001;23:39–44.

175. Rundles RW, Falls HF. Hereditary (? sex-linked) anemia. *Am J Med Sci* 1946;211:641–658.

176. Cotter PD, Baumann M, Bishop DF. Enzymatic defect in "X-linked" sideroblastic anemia: molecular evidence for erythroid delta-aminolevulinate synthase deficiency. *Proc Natl Acad Sci U S A* 1992;89:4028–4032.

177. Pagon RA, Bird TD, Detter JC, et al. Hereditary sideroblastic anaemia and ataxia: an X linked recessive disorder. *J Med Genet* 1985;22:267–273.

178. Allikmets R, Raskind WH, Hutchinson A, et al. Mutation of a putative mitochondrial iron transporter gene (ABC7) in X-linked sideroblastic anemia and ataxia (XLSA/A). *Hum Mol Genet* 1999;8:743–749.

179. Porter FS, Rogers LE, Sidbury JB Jr. Thiamine-responsive megaloblastic anemia. *J Pediatr* 1969;74:494–504.

180. Fleming JC, Tartaglini E, Steinkamp MP, et al. The gene mutated in thiamine-responsive anaemia with diabetes and deafness (TRMA) encodes a functional thiamine transporter. *Nat Genet* 1999;22:305–308.

181. Urban C, Binder B, Hauer C, et al. Congenital sideroblastic anemia successfully treated by allogeneic bone marrow transplantation. *Bone Marrow Transplant* 1992;10:373–375.

182. Dgany O, Avidan N, Delaunay J, et al. Congenital dyserythropoietic anemia type I is caused by mutations in codanin-1. *Am J Hum Genet* 2002;71:1467–1474.

183. Carter C, Darbyshire PJ, Wickramasinghe SN. A congenital dyserythropoietic anaemia variant presenting as hydrops fetalis. *Br J Haematol* 1989;72:289–290.

184. Wickramasinghe SN, Illum N, Wimberley PD. Congenital dyserythropoietic anaemia with novel intra-erythroblastic and intra-erythrocytic inclusions. *Br J Haematol* 1991;79:322–330.

185. Williams G, Lorimer S, Merry CC, et al. A variant congenital dyserythropoietic anaemia presenting as a fatal hydrops foetalis. *Br J Haematol* 1990;76:438–439.

186. Weigel-Kelley KA, Yoder MC, Srivastava A. (alpha)5(beta)1 integrin as a cellular coreceptor for human parvovirus B19: requirement of functional activation of β1 integrin for viral entry. *Blood* 2003;102:3927–3933.

187. Public Health Laboratory Service Working Party on Fifth Disease. Prospective study of human parvovirus (B19) infection in pregnancy. *Br Med J* 1990;300:1166–1170.

188. Jordan JA. Identification of human parvovirus B19 infection in idiopathic nonimmune hydrops fetalis. *Am J Obstet Gynecol* 1996;174:37–42.

189. Wright C, Hinchliffe SA, Taylor C. Fetal pathology in intrauterine death due to parvovirus B19 infection. *Br J Obstet Gynaecol* 1996;103:133–136.

190. Koduri PR. Novel cytomorphology of the giant proerythroblasts of parvovirus B19 infection. *Am J Hematol* 1998;58:95–99.

191. Wattre P, Thirion V, Bellagra N, et al. PCR value in the diagnosis of feto-placental human parvovirus B19 hydrops fetalis: apropos of 10 cases. *Ann Biol Clin (Paris)* 1997;55:327–331.

192. Dieck D, Schild RL, Hansmann M, et al. Prenatal diagnosis of congenital parvovirus B19 infection: value of serological and PCR techniques in maternal and fetal serum. *Prenat Diagn* 1999;19:1119–1123.

193. Zerbini M, Musiani M, Gentilomi G, et al. Comparative evaluation of virological and serological methods in prenatal diagnosis of parvovirus B19 fetal hydrops. *J Clin Microbiol* 1996;34:603–608.

194. Schild RL, Bald R, Plath H, et al. Intrauterine management of fetal parvovirus B19 infection. *Ultrasound Obstet Gynecol* 1999;13:161–166.

195. Brown KE, Green SW, Antunez de Mayolo J, et al. Congenital anaemia after transplacental B19 parvovirus infection. *Lancet* 1994;343:895–896.

196. Dallman PR. Iron, vitamin E, and folate in the preterm infant. *J Pediatr* 1974;85:742–752.

197. Seip M, Halvorsen S. Erythrocyte production and iron stores in premature infants during the first months of life. The anemia of prematurity-aetiology, pathogenesis, iron requirement. *Acta Paediatr* 1956;45:600–617.

198. Shojania AM. Folic acid and vitamin B12 deficiency in pregnancy and in the neonatal period. *Clin Perinatol* 1984;11:433–459.

199. Hassan H, Hashim SA, van Itallie TB, et al. Syndrome in premature infants associated with low plasma vitamin E levels and high polyunsaturated fatty acid diet. *Am J Clin Nutr* 1966;19:147–157.

200. Oski FA, Barness LA. Vitamin E deficiency: a previously unrecognized cause of hemolytic anemia in the premature infant. *J Pediatr* 1967;70:211–220.

201. Williams ML, Shott RJ, O'Neal PL, et al. Role of dietary iron and fat on vitamin E deficiency anemia of infancy. *N Engl J Med* 1975;292:887–890.

202. Zipursky A, Brown EJ, Watts J, et al. Oral vitamin E supplementation for the prevention of anemia in premature infants: a controlled trial. *Pediatrics* 1987;79:61–68.

203. Oettinger L Jr, Mills WB. Simultaneous capillary and venous hemoglobin determinations in the newborn infant. *J Pediatr* 1949;35:362–365.

204. Oh W, Lind J. Venous and capillary hematocrit in newborn infants and placental transfusion. *Acta Paediatr Scand* 1966;55:38–40.

205. Linderkamp O, Versmold HT, Strohhacker I, et al. Capillary-venous hematocrit differences in newborn infants. I. Relationship to blood volume, peripheral blood flow, and acid base parameters. *Eur J Pediatr* 1977;127:9–14.

206. Rivera LM, Rudolph N. Postnatal persistence of capillary-venous differences in hematocrit and hemoglobin values in low-birth-weight and term infants. *Pediatrics* 1982;70:956–957.
207. International Committee for Standardization in Haematology. Recommended methods for measurement of red-cell and plasma volume. *J Nucl Med* 1980;21:793–800.
208. Hudson IRB, Cavill IAJ, Cooke A, et al. Biotin labeling of red cells in the measurement of red cell volume in preterm infants. *Pediatr Res* 1990;28:199–202.
209. Cavill I, Trevett D, Fisher J, et al. The measurement of the total volume of red cells in man: a non-radioactive approach using biotin. *Br J Haematol* 1988;70:491–493.
210. Wirth FH, Goldberg KE, Lubchenco LO. Neonatal hyperviscosity: I. Incidence. *Pediatrics* 1979;63:833–836.
211. Stevens K, Wirth FH. Incidence of neonatal hyperviscosity at sea level. *J Pediatr* 1980;97:118–119.
212. Wiswell TE, Cornish JD, Northam RS. Neonatal polycythemia: frequency of clinical manifestations and other associated findings. *Pediatrics* 1986;78:26–30.
213. Shohat M, Reisner SH, Mimouni F, et al. Neonatal polycythemia: II. Definition related to time of sampling. *Pediatrics* 1984;73:11–13.
214. Linderkamp O, Wu PY, Meiselman HJ. Deformability of density separated red blood cells in normal newborn infants and adults. *Pediatr Res* 1982;16:964–968.
215. Riopel L, Fouron J-C, Bard H. Blood viscosity during the neonatal period: the role of plasma and red blood cell type. *J Pediatr* 1982;100:449–453.
216. Linderkamp O, Versmold HT, Roegel KP, et al. Contributions of red cells and plasma to blood viscosity in preterm and full-term infants and adults. *Pediatrics* 1984;74:45–51.
217. Black VD, Lubchenco LO, Koops BL, et al. Neonatal hyperviscosity: randomized study of effect of partial plasma exchange transfusion on long-term outcome. *Pediatrics* 1985;75:1048–1053.
218. Black V, Camp BW, Roberts L, et al. Neonatal hyperviscosity. Outcome at school age following a randomized trial of partial plasma exchange. *J Dev Behav Pediatr* 1986;7:202.
219. Black VD, Camp BW, Lubchenco LO. Neonatal hyperviscosity is associated with lower achievement and IQ scores at school age. *Pediatr Res* 1988;23,442a.
220. Bauer C, Ludwig M, Ludwig I. Different effects of 2,3-diphosphoglycerate and adenosine triphosphate on the oxygen affinity of adult and foetal human hemoglobin. *Life Sci* 1968;7:1339.
221. Andrew M. The relevance of developmental hemostasis to hemorrhagic disorders of newborns. *Semin Perinatol* 1997;21:70–85.
222. Monagle P, Ignjatovic V, Barnes C, et al. Reference ranges for hemostatic parameters in children. *J Thromb Haemostas* 2003;1(Suppl 1):P0076.
223. Johnston M, Zipursky A. Microtechnology for the study of the blood coagulation system in newborn infants. *Can J Med Technol* 1980;42:159–164.
224. Andrew M, Paes B, Milner R, et al. Development of the human coagulation system in the full-term infant. *Blood* 1987;70:165–172.
225. Andrew M, Paes B, Milner R, et al. Development of the human coagulation system in the healthy premature infant. *Blood* 1988;72:1651–1657.
226. Bloch CA, Rothberg AD, Bradlow BA. Mother-infant prothrombin precursor status at birth. *J Pediatr Gastroenterol Nutr* 1984;3:101–103.
227. Dreyfus M, Lelong-Tissier MC, Lombard C, et al. Vitamin K_1 deficiency in the newborn. *Lancet* 1979;1:1351.
228. Shearer MJ, Rahin S, Barkhan P, et al. Plasma vitamin K in mothers and their newborn babies. *Lancet* 1982;2:460–463.
229. Blayer WA, Skinner AL. Fatal neonatal hemorrhage after maternal anticonvulsant therapy. *JAMA* 1976;235:626–627.
230. Loughnan PM, McDougall PN. Epidemiology of late onset haemorrhagic disease: a pooled data analysis. *J Paediatr Child Health* 1993;29:177–181.
231. Ekelund H. Late haemorrhagic disease in Sweden 1987–89. *Acta Paediatr Scand* 1991;80:966–968.
232. Zipursky A. Vitamin K at birth. *Br Med J* 1996;313:179–180.
233. Sann L, Leclercq M, Guillaumont BS, et al. Serum vitamin K1 concentrations after oral administration of vitamin K1 in low birth weight infants. *J Pediatr* 1985;107:608–611.
234. Hathaway WE, Isarangkura PB, Mahasandana C, et al. Comparison of oral and parenteral vitamin K prophylaxis for prevention of late hemorrhagic disease of the newborn. *J Pediatr* 1991;119:461–464.
235. von Kries R. Neonatal vitamin K. *Br Med J* 1991;303:1083–1084.
236. American Academy of Pediatrics Committee on the Fetus and Newborn. Controversies concerning vitamin K and the newborn. *Pediatrics* 2003;112:191–192.
237. Zipursky A, deSa D, Hsu E, et al. Clinical and laboratory diagnosis of hemostatic disorders in newborn infants. *Am J Pediatr Hematol Oncol* 1979;1:217–226.
238. Byard RW, Burrows PE, Izakawa T, et al. Diffuse infantile haemangiomatosis: clinicopathological features and management problems in five fatal cases. *Eur J Pediatr* 1991;150:224–227.
239. Hall GW. Kasabach-Merritt syndrome: pathogenesis and management. *Br J Haematol* 2001;112:851–862.
240. Mulliken JB, Anupindi S, Ezekowitz AB, et al. Case records of the Massachusetts General Hospital. Weekly clinicopathological exercises. Case 13-2004. A newborn girl with a large cutaneous lesion, thrombocytopenia, and anemia. *N Engl J Med* 2004;350:1764–1775.
241. Haisley-Royster C, Enjolras O, Frieden IJ, et al. Kasabach-Merritt phenomenon: a retrospective study of treatment with vincristine. *J Pediatr Hematol Oncol* 2002;24:459–462.
242. Barrington KJ. Umbilical artery catheters in the newborn: effects of heparin. *Cochrane Database Syst Rev* 2000;CD000507.
243. Baehner RL, Strauss HS. Hemophilia in the first year of life. *N Engl J Med* 1966;275:524–528.
244. Mannucci PM, Tuddenham EG. The hemophilias—from royal genes to gene therapy. *N Engl J Med* 2001;344:1773–1779.
245. Brettler DB, Levine PH. Factor concentrates for treatment of hemophilia: which one to choose? *Blood* 1989;73:2067–2073.
246. Blanchette VS, Dean JS, Lillicrap D. Rare congenital hemorrhagic disorders. In: Lilleyman JS, Hann IM, Blanchette V, eds. *Pediatric Hematology.* London: Churchill Livingstone, 1999:611–628.
247. Croizat P, Revol L, Favre-Gilly J, et al. Les hémorrhagies néonatales dans les dietheses hemorrhagiques congénital. *Nouv Rev Fr Hematol* 1964;4:181–182.
248. Katz JA, Moake JL, McPherson PD, et al. Relationship between human development and disappearance of unusually large von Willebrand factor multimers from plasma. *Blood* 1989;73:1851–1858.
249. Andrew M, Kelton J. Neonatal thrombocytopenia. *Clin Perinatol* 1984;1:359–391.
250. Sola MC, Rimsza LM, Christensen RD. A bone marrow biopsy technique suitable for use in neonates. *Br J Haematol* 1999;107:458–460.
251. Pearson HA, McIntosh S. Neonatal thrombocytopenia. *Clin Haematol* 1978;7:111–122.
252. Sola MC, Del Vecchio A, Rimsza LM. Evaluation and treatment of thrombocytopenia in the neonatal intensive care unit. *Clin Perinatol* 2000;27:655–679.
253. Roberts IAG, Murray NA. Management of thrombocytopenia in neonates. *Br J Haematol* 1999;105:864–870.
254. Murray NA. Evaluation and treatment of thrombocytopenia in the neonatal intensive care unit. *Acta Paediatr Suppl* 2002;91:74–81.
255. Blanchette VS, Johnson J, Rand M. The management of alloimmune neonatal thrombocytopenia. *Baillieres Best Pract Res Clin Haematol* 2000;13:365–390.
256. von dem Borne AE, von Riesz E, Verheugt FW, et al. Bak^a, a new platelet-specific antigen involved in neonatal allo-immune thrombocytopenia. *Vox Sang* 1980;39:113–120.
257. Friedman JM, Aster RH. Neonatal alloimmune thrombocytopenic purpura and congenital porencephaly in two siblings associated with a "new" maternal antiplatelet antibody. *Blood* 1985;65:1412–1415.
258. Mueller-Eckhardt C, Becker T, Weisheit M, et al. Neonatal alloimmune thrombocytopenia due to fetomaternal Zw^b incompatibility. *Vox Sang* 1986;50:94–96.
259. Shibata Y, Miyaji T, Ichikawa Y, et al. A new platelet antigen system, Yuk^a/Yuk^b. *Vox Sang* 1986;51:334–336.
260. Kiefel V, Santoso S, Katzmann B, et al. A new platelet-specific alloantigen Br^a. Report of 4 cases with neonatal alloimmune thrombocytopenia. *Vox Sang* 1988;54:101–106.
261. Kroll H, Kiefel V, Santoso S, et al. Sr^a, a private platelet antigen on glycoprotein IIIa associated with neonatal alloimmune thrombocytopenia. *Blood* 1990;76:2296–2302.
262. Kaplan C, Morel-Kopp MC, Kroll H, et al. HPA-5b [Br(a)] neonatal alloimmune thrombocytopenia: clinical and immunological analysis of 39 cases. *Br J Haematol* 1991;78:425–429.

263. Jallu V, Meunier M, Brement M, et al. A new platelet polymorphism Duv(a+), localized within the RGD binding domain of glycoprotein IIIa, is associated with neonatal thrombocytopenia. *Blood* 2002;99:4449–4456.
264. Santoso S, Kiefel V, Richter IG, et al. A functional platelet fibrinogen receptor with a deletion in the cysteine-rich repeat region of the beta(3) integrin: the Oe(a) alloantigen in neonatal alloimmune thrombocytopenia. *Blood* 2002;99:1205–1214.
265. Mueller-Eckhardt C, Kiefel V, Grubert A, et al. 348 cases of suspected neonatal alloimmune thrombocytopenia. *Lancet* 1989;1:363–366.
266. Pearson HA, Shulman NR, Marder VJ, et al. Isoimmune neonatal thrombocytopenic purpura; clinical and therapeutic considerations. *Blood* 1964;23:154–177.
267. Herman JH, Jumbelic MI, Ancona RJ, et al. In utero cerebral hemorrhage in alloimmune thrombocytopenia. *Am J Pediatr Hematol Oncol* 1986;8:312–317.
268. Lester RB, Sty JR. Prenatal diagnosis of cystic CNS lesions in neonatal isoimmune thrombocytopenia. *J Ultrasound Med* 1987;6:479–481.
269. Burrows RF, Caco CC, Kelton JG. Neonatal alloimmune thrombocytopenia: spontaneous in utero intracranial hemorrhage. *Am J Hematol* 1988;28:98–102.
270. Manson J, Speed I, Abbott K, et al. Congenital blindness, porencephaly, and neonatal thrombocytopenia: a report of four cases. *J Child Neurol* 1988;3:120–124.
271. de Vries LS, Connell J, Bydder GM, et al. Recurrent intracranial haemorrhages in utero in an infant with alloimmune thrombocytopenia. Case report. *Br J Obstet Gynaecol* 1988;95:299–302.
272. Bussel JB, Berkowitz RL, McFarland JG, et al. Antenatal treatment of neonatal alloimmune thrombocytopenia. *N Engl J Med* 1988;319:1374–1378.
273. Gill FM, Schwartz E. Platelet transfusion as a diagnostic and therapeutic aid in the newborn. *Pediatr Res* 1971;5:409–411.
274. McIntosh S, O'Brien RT, Schwartz AD, et al. Neonatal isoimmune purpura: response to platelet infusions. *J Pediatr* 1973;82:1020–1027.
275. Matsui K, Ohsaki E, Goto A, et al. Perinatal intracranial hemorrhage due to severe neonatal alloimmune thrombocytopenic purpura (NAITP) associated with anti-Yuk^b (HPA-4^a) antibodies. *Brain* Dev 1995;17:352–355.
276. Ranasinghe E, Walton JD, Hurd CM, et al. Provision of platelet support for fetuses and neonates affected by severe fetomaternal alloimmune thrombocytopenia. *Br J Haematol* 2001;113:40–42.
277. McGill M, Mayhaus C, Hoff R, et al. Frozen maternal platelets for neonatal thrombocytopenia. *Transfusion* 1987;27:347–349.
278. Massey GV, McWilliams NB, Mueller DG, et al. Intravenous immunoglobulin in treatment of neonatal isoimmune thrombocytopenia. *J Pediatr* 1987;111:133–135.
279. Suarez CR, Anderson C. High-dose intravenous gammaglobulin (IVG) in neonatal immune thrombocytopenia. *Am J Hematol* 1987;26:247–253.
280. Beck R, Reid DM, Lazarte R. Intravenous gammaglobulin therapy for neonatal alloimmune thrombocytopenia. *Am J Perinatol* 1988;5:79–82.
281. Kaplan M, Abramov A, Goren A. Repeated single-dose intravenous immunoglobulin therapy for neonatal passive immune thrombocytopenia. *Isr J Med Sci* 1987;23:844–845.
282. Mueller-Eckhardt C, Kiefel V, Grubert A. High-dose IgG treatment for neonatal alloimmune thrombocytopenia. *Blut* 1989;59:145–146.
283. Pietz J, Kiefel V, Sontheimer D, et al. High-dose intravenous gammaglobulin for neonatal alloimmune thrombocytopenia in twins. *Acta Paediatr Scand* 1991;80:129–132.
284. Skupski DW, Bussel JB. Alloimmune thrombocytopenia. *Clin Obstet Gynecol* 1999;42:335–348.
285. Bussel J, Kaplan C, McFarland J. Recommendations for the evaluation and treatment of neonatal autoimmune and alloimmune thrombocytopenia. The Working Party on Neonatal Immune Thrombocytopenia of the Neonatal Hemostasis Subcommittee of the Scientific and Standardization Committee of the ISTH. *Thromb Haemost* 1991;65:631–634.
286. Ballin A, Andrew M, Ling E, et al. High-dose intravenous gammaglobulin therapy for neonatal autoimmune thrombocytopenia. *J Pediatr* 1988;112:789–792.
287. Hanada T, Saito K, Nagasawa T, et al. Intravenous gammaglobulin therapy for thromboneutropenic neonates of mothers with systemic lupus erythematosus. *Eur J Haematol* 1987;38:400–404.
288. Kelton JG, Inwood MJ, Barr RM, et al. The prenatal prediction of thrombocytopenia in infants of mothers with clinically diagnosed immune thrombocytopenia. *Am J Obstet Gynecol* 1982;144:449–454.
289. Cines DB, Dusak B, Tomaski A, et al. Immune thrombocytopenic purpura and pregnancy. *N Engl J Med* 1982;306:826–831.
290. Kelton JG. Management of the pregnant patient with idiopathic thrombocytopenic purpura. *Ann Intern Med* 1983;99:796–800.
291. Karpatkin M, Porges RF, Karpatkin S. Platelet counts in infants of women with autoimmune thrombocytopenia: effects of steroid administration to the mother. *N Engl J Med* 1981;305:936–939.
292. Christiaens GC, Nieuwenhuis HK, von dem Borne AE, et al. Idiopathic thrombocytopenic purpura in pregnancy: a randomized trial on the effect of antenatal low dose corticosteroids on neonatal platelet count. *Br J Obstet Gynaecol* 1990;97:893–898.
293. Gill KK, Kelton JG. Management of idiopathic thrombocytopenic purpura in pregnancy. *Semin Hematol* 2000;37:275–289.
294. Zhu Q, Watanabe C, Liu T, et al. Wiskott-Aldrich syndrome/X-linked thrombocytopenia: WASP gene mutations, protein expression, and phenotype. *Blood* 1997;90:2680–2689.
295. Song W-J, Sullivan MG, Legare RD, et al. Haploinsufficiency of CBFA2 causes familial thrombocytopenia with propensity to develop acute myelogenous leukaemia. *Nat Genet* 1999;23:166–175.
296. Seri M, Pecci A, Di Bari F, et al. MYH9-related disease: May-Hegglin anomaly, Sebastian syndrome, Fechtner syndrome, and Epstein syndrome are not distinct entities but represent a variable expression of a single illness. *Medicine* 2003;82:203–215.
297. van den Oudenrijn S, Bruin M, Folman CC, et al. Mutations in the thrombopoietin receptor, Mpl, in children with congenital amegakaryocytic thrombocytopenia. *Br J Haematol* 2000;110:441–448.
298. Nichols KE, Crispino JD, Poncz M, et al. Familial dyserythropoietic anaemia and thrombocytopenia due to an inherited mutation in GATA1. *Nat Genet* 2000;24:266–270.
299. Gandhi MJ, Cummings CL, Drachman JG. FLJ14813 missense mutation: a candidate for autosomal dominant thrombocytopenia on human chromosome 10. *Hum Hered* 2003;55:66–70.
300. Thompson AA, Nguyen LT. Amegakaryocytic thrombocytopenia and radio-ulnar synostosis are associated with HOXA11 mutation. *Nat Genet* 2000;26:397–398.
301. Greenhalgh KL, Howell RT, Bottani A, et al. Thrombocytopenia-absent radius syndrome: a clinical genetic study. *J Med Genet* 2002;39:876–881.
302. Balduini CL, Cattaneo M, Fabris F, et al. Inherited thrombocytopenias: a proposed diagnostic algorithm from the Italian Gruppo di Studio delle Piastrine. *Haematologica* 2003;88:582–592.
303. Mehta P, Vasa R, Neumann L, et al. Thrombocytopenia in the high-risk infant. *J Pediatr* 1980;97:791–794.
304. Castle V, Andrew M, Kelton J, et al. Frequency and mechanism of neonatal thrombocytopenia. *J Pediatr* 1986;108:749–755.
305. Beiner ME, Simchen MJ, Sivan E, et al. Risk factors for neonatal thrombocytopenia in preterm infants. *Am J Perinatol* 2003;20:49–54.
306. Watts TL, Murray NA, Roberts IA. Thrombopoietin has a primary role in the regulation of platelet production in preterm babies. *Pediatr Res* 1999;46:28–32.
307. Ververidis M, Kiely EM, Spitz L, et al. The clinical significance of thrombocytopenia in neonates with necrotizing enterocolitis. *J Pediatr Surg* 2001;36:799–803.
308. Xanthou M. Leucocyte blood picture in healthy full-term and premature babies during neonatal period. *Arch Dis Child* 1970;45:242–249.
309. Akenzua GI, Hui YT, Milner R, et al. Neutrophil and band counts in the diagnosis of neonatal infections. *Pediatrics* 1974;54:38–42.
310. Zipursky A, Palko J, Milner R, et al. The hematology of bacterial infections in premature infants. *Pediatrics* 1976;57:839–853.
311. Coulombel L, Dehan M, Tchernia G, et al. The number of polymorphonuclear leukocytes in relation to gestational age in the newborn. *Acta Paediatr Scand* 1979;68:709–711.
312. Manroe BL, Weinberg AG, Rosenfeld CR, et al. The neonatal blood count in health and disease. I. Reference values for neutrophilic cells. *J Pediatr* 1979;95:89–98.
313. Lloyd BW, Oto A. Normal values for mature and immature neutrophils in very preterm babies. *Arch Dis Child* 1982;57:233–235.

314. Mouzinho A, Rosenfeld CR, Sanchez PJ, et al. Revised reference ranges for circulating neutrophils in very-low-birth-weight neonates. *Pediatrics* 1994;94:76–82.

315. Christensen RD, Calhoun DA, Rimsza LM. A practical approach to evaluating and treating neutropenia in the neonatal intensive care unit. *Neonat Hematol* 2000;27:557–601.

316. Thilaganathan B, Athanasiou S, Ozmen S, et al. Umbilical cord blood erythroblast count as an index of intrauterine hypoxia. *Arch Dis Child Fetal Neonatal Ed* 1994;70:F192-F194.

317. Barak Y, Leibovitz E, Mogilner B, et al. The in vivo effect of recombinant human granulocyte-colony stimulating factor in neutropenic neonates with sepsis. *Eur J Pediatr* 1997;156: 643–646.

318. Ishii E, Masuyama T, Yamaguchi H, et al. Production and expression of granulocyte- and macrophage-colony-stimulating factors in newborns: their roles in leukocytosis at birth. *Acta Haematol* 1995;94:23–31.

319. Funke A, Berner R, Traichel B, et al. Frequency, natural course, and outcome of neonatal neutropenia. *Pediatrics* 2000;106: 45–51.

320. Chirico G, Motta M, Villani P, et al. Late-onset neutropenia in very low birthweight infants. *Acta Paediatr Suppl* 2002;91: 104–108.

321. Christensen RD, Calhoun DA, Rimsza LM. A practical approach to evaluating and treating neutropenia in the neonatal intensive care unit. *Clin Perinatol* 2000;27:577–601.

322. Wolach B, Sonnenschein D, Gavrieli R, et al. Neonatal neutrophil inflammatory responses: parallel studies of light scattering, cell polarization, chemotaxis, superoxide release, and bactericidal activity. *Am J Hematol* 1998;58:8–15.

323. Baley JE, Stork EK, Warkentin PI, et al. Neonatal neutropenia. Clinical manifestations, cause, and outcome. *Am J Dis Child* 1988; 142:1161–1166.

324. Rodwell RL, Leslie AL, Tudehope DI. Early diagnosis of neonatal sepsis using a hematologic scoring system. *J Pediatr* 1988;112: 761–767.

325. Rodwell RL, Taylor KM, Tudehope DI, et al. Hematologic scoring system in early diagnosis of sepsis in neutropenic newborns. *Pediatr Infect Dis J* 1993;12:372–376.

326. Christensen RD, Harper TE, Rothstein G. Granulocyte-macrophage progenitor cells in term and preterm neonates. *J Pediatr* 1986;109:1047–1051.

327. Carr R, Modi N, Dore CJ, et al. A randomized, controlled trial of prophylactic granulocyte-macrophage colony-stimulating factor in human newborns less than 32 weeks gestation. *Pediatrics* 1999;103:796–802.

328. Cairo MS, Agosti J, Ellis R, et al. A randomized, double-blind, placebo-controlled trial of prophylactic recombinant human granulocyte-macrophage colony-stimulating factor to reduce nosocomial infections in very low birth weight neonates. *J Pediatr* 1999;134:64–70.

329. Schibler KR, Osborne KA, Leung LY, et al. A randomized, placebo-controlled trial of granulocyte colony-stimulating factor administration to newborn infants with neutropenia and clinical signs of early-onset sepsis. *Pediatrics* 1998;102:6–13.

330. Bedford Russell AR, Emmerson AJ, Wilkinson N, et al. A trial of recombinant human granulocyte colony stimulating factor for the treatment of very low birthweight infants with presumed sepsis and neutropenia. *Arch Dis Child Fetal Neonatal Ed* 2001;84: F172-F176.

331. Miura E, Procianoy RS, Bittar C, et al. A randomized, double-masked, placebo-controlled trial of recombinant granulocyte colony-stimulating factor administration to preterm infants with the clinical diagnosis of early-onset sepsis. *Pediatrics* 2001;107: 30–35.

332. Bilgin K, Yaramis A, Haspolat K, et al. A randomized trial of granulocyte-macrophage colony-stimulating factor in neonates with sepsis and neutropenia. *Pediatrics* 2001;107:36–41.

333. Calhoun DA, Christensen RD. The role of haemopoietic growth factors in neonatal neutropenia and infection. *Semin Neonatol* 1999;4:17–26.

334. Bernstein HM, Pollock BH, Calhoun DA, et al. Administration of recombinant granulocyte colony-stimulating factor to neonates with septicemia: a meta-analysis. *J Pediatr* 2001;138: 917–920.

335. La Gamma EF, De Castro MH. What is the rationale for the use of granulocyte and granulocyte-macrophage colony-stimulating

336. factors in the neonatal intensive care unit? *Acta Paediatr Suppl* 2002;91:109–116.

336. Levine DH, Madyastha PR. Isoimmune neonatal neutropenia. *Am J Perinatol* 1986;3:231–233.

337. Minchinton RM, McGrath KM. Alloimmune neonatal neutropenia—a neglected diagnosis? *Med J Aust* 1987;147:139–141.

338. Maheshwari A, Christensen RD, Calhoun DA. Immune neutropenia in the neonate. *Adv Pediatr* 2002;49:317–339.

339. Bux J. Molecular genetics of granulocyte polymorphisms. *Vox Sang* 2000;78[Suppl 2]:125–130.

340. Bux J, Chapman J. Report on the second international granulocyte serology workshop. *Transfusion* 1997;37:977–983.

341. Lalezari P, Radel E. Neutrophil-specific antigens: immunology and clinical significance. *Semin Hematol* 1974;11:281–290.

342. Bux J, Behrens G, Jaeger G, et al. Diagnosis and clinical course of autoimmune neutropenia in infancy: analysis of 240 cases. *Blood* 1998;91:181–186.

343. Girlando P, Zuppa AA, Romagnoli C, et al. Transient effect of granulocyte colony-stimulating factor in allo-immune neonatal neutropenia. *Biol Neonate* 2000;78:277–280.

344. Wallis JP, Haynes S, Stark G, et al. Transfusion-related alloimmune neutropenia: an undescribed complication of blood transfusion. *Lancet* 2002;360:1073–1074.

345. Lassiter HA, Bibb KW, Bertolone SJ, et al. Neonatal immune neutropenia following the administration of intravenous immune globulin. *Am J Pediatr Hematol Oncol* 1993;15:120–123.

346. Kameoka J, Funato T, Miura T, et al. Autoimmune neutropenia in pregnant women causing neonatal neutropenia. *Br J Haematol* 2001;114:198–200.

347. Neiman AR, Lee LA, Weston WL, et al. Cutaneous manifestations of neonatal lupus without heart block: characteristics of mothers and children enrolled in a national registry. *J Pediatr* 2000;137: 674–680.

348. Lalezari P, Khorshidi M, Petrosova M. Autoimmune neutropenia of infancy. *J Pediatr* 1986;109:764–769.

349. Conway LT, Clay ME, Kline WE, et al. Natural history of primary autoimmune neutropenia in infancy. *Pediatrics* 1987;79:728–733.

350. Bruin MC, von dem Borne AE, Tamminga RY, et al. Neutrophil antibody specificity in different types of childhood autoimmune neutropenia. *Blood* 1999;94:1797–1802.

351. Calhoun DA, Rimsza LM, Burchfield DJ, et al. Congenital autoimmune neutropenia in two premature neonates. *Pediatrics* 2001;108:181–184.

352. Koenig JM, Christensen RD. The mechanism responsible for diminished neutrophil production in neonates delivered of women with pregnancy-induced hypertension. *Am J Obstet Gynecol* 1991;165:467–473.

353. Kostman-R. Infantile genetic agranulocytosis. A review with presentation of ten new cases. *Acta Paediatr Scand* 1975;64:362–368.

354. Dale DC, Person RE, Bolyard AA, et al. Mutations in the gene encoding neutrophil elastase in congenital and cyclic neutropenia. *Blood* 2000;96:2317–2328.

355. Benson KF, Li FQ, Person RE, et al. Mutations associated with neutropenia in dogs and humans disrupt intracellular transport of neutrophil elastase. *Nat Genet* 2003;35:90–96.

356. Aprikyan AA, Kutyavin T, Stein S, et al. Cellular and molecular abnormalities in severe congenital neutropenia predisposing to leukemia. *Exp Hematol* 2003;31:372–381.

357. Person RE, Li FQ, Duan Z, et al. Mutations in proto-oncogene GFI1 cause human neutropenia and target ELA2. *Nat Genet* 2003;34:308–312.

358. Devriendt K, Kim AS, Mathijs G, et al. Constitutively activating mutation in WASP causes X-linked severe congenital neutropenia. *Nat Genet* 2001;27:313–317.

359. Boxer LA, Hutchinson R, Emerson S. Recombinant human granulocyte-colony-stimulating factor in the treatment of patients with neutropenia. *Clin Immunol Immunopathol* 1992;62:S39-S46.

360. Dror Y, Ward AC, Touw IP, et al. Combined corticosteroid/granulocyte colony-stimulating factor (G-CSF) therapy in the treatment of severe congenital neutropenia unresponsive to G-CSF: activated glucocorticoid receptors synergize with G-CSF signals. *Exp Hematol* 2000;28:1381–1389.

361. Zeidler C, Welte K, Barak Y, et al. Stem cell transplantation in patients with severe congenital neutropenia without evidence of leukemic transformation. *Blood* 2000;95:1195–1198.

362. Page AR, Good RA. Studies on cyclic neutropenia. A clinical and experimental investigation. *Am J Dis Child* 1957;94:623.

363. Guerry D, Dale DC, Omine M, et al. Periodic hematopoiesis in human cyclic neutropenia. *J Clin Invest* 1973;52:3220–3230.

364. Kuijpers TW, Maianski NA, Tool AT, et al. Apoptotic neutrophils in the circulation of patients with glycogen storage disease type 1b (GSD1b). *Blood* 2003;101:5021–5024.

365. Calderwood S, Kilpatrick L, Douglas SD, et al. Recombinant human granulocyte colony-stimulating factor therapy for patients with neutropenia and/or neutrophil dysfunction secondary to glycogen storage disease type 1b. *Blood* 2001;97:376–382.

366. Barth PG, Van't Veer-Korthof ETH, Van Delden L, et al. An X-linked mitochondrial disease affecting cardiac muscle, and skeletal muscle and neutrophil leukocytes. In: Busch HFM, Jennekens FGI, Schotte HR, eds. *Mitochondria and muscular diseases.* Beetsterzwaag: Mefar, 2004:161–164.

367. Bione S, D'Adamo P, Maestrini E, et al. A novel X-linked gene, G4.5. is responsible for Barth syndrome. *Nat Genet* 1996;12:385–389.

368. Conley ME. Early defects in B cell development. *Curr Opin Allergy Clin Immunol* 2002;2:517–522.

369. Gulino AV, Notarangelo LD. Hyper IgM syndromes. *Curr Opin Rheumatol* 2003;15:422–429.

370. Dupuis-Girod S, Medioni J, Haddad E, et al. Autoimmunity in Wiskott-Aldrich syndrome: risk factors, clinical features, and outcome in a single-center cohort of 55 patients. *Pediatrics* 2003;111:e622-e627.

371. Ochs HD. The Wiskott-Aldrich syndrome. *Semin Hematol* 1998;35:332–345.

372. Imai K, Nonoyama S, Ochs HD. WASP (Wiskott-Aldrich syndrome protein) gene mutations and phenotype. *Curr Opin Allergy Clin Immunol* 2003;3:427–436.

373. Makitie O, Pukkala E, Kaitila I. Increased mortality in cartilage-hair hypoplasia. *Arch Dis Child* 2001;84:65–67.

374. Nakashima E, Mabuchi A, Kashimada K, et al. RMRP mutations in Japanese patients with cartilage-hair hypoplasia. *Am J Med Genet* 2003;123A:253–256.

375. Elhasid R, Hofbauer LC, Ish-Shalom S, et al. Familial severe congenital neutropenia associated with infantile osteoporosis: a new entity. *Am J Hematol* 2003;72:34–37.

376. Ward DM, Shiflett SL, Kaplan J. Chediak-Higashi syndrome: a clinical and molecular view of a rare lysosomal storage disorder. *Curr Mol Med* 2002;2:469–477.

377. Ménasché G, Fischer A, de Saint Basile G. Griscelli syndrome types 1 and 2. *Am J Hum Genet* 2002;71:1237–1238.

378. Menasche G, Pastural E, Feldmann J, et al. Mutations in RAB27A cause Griscelli syndrome associated with haemophagocytic syndrome. *Nat Genet* 2000;25:173–176.

379. Grunebaum E, Roifman CM. Gene abnormalities in patients with hemophagocytic lymphohistiocytosis. *Isr Med Assoc J* 2002;4:366–369.

380. Rieux-Laucat F, Le Deist F, Fischer A. Autoimmune lymphoproliferative syndromes: genetic defects of apoptosis pathways. *Cell Death Differ* 2003;10:124–133.

381. Gorlin RJ, Gelb B, Diaz GA, et al. WHIM syndrome, an autosomal dominant disorder: clinical, hematological, and molecular studies. *Am J Med Genet* 2000;91:368–376.

382. Hernandez PA, Gorlin RJ, Lukens JN, et al. Mutations in the chemokine receptor gene CXCR4 are associated with WHIM syndrome, a combined immunodeficiency disease. *Nat Genet* 2003;34:70–74.

383. DeVaal OM, Seynhaeve V. Reticular dysgenesia. *Lancet* 1959;2:1123–1125.

384. Bertrand Y, Muller SM, Casanova JL, et al. Reticular dysgenesis: HLA non-identical bone marrow transplants in a series of 10 patients. *Bone Marrow Transplant* 2002;29:759–762.

385. Felix CA, Lange BJ. Leukemia in infants. *Oncologist* 1999;4:225–240.

386. Biondi A, Cimino G, Pieters R, et al. Biological and therapeutic aspects of infant leukemia. *Blood* 2000;96:24–33.

387. Ernst P, Wang J, Korsmeyer SJ. The role of MLL in hematopoiesis and leukemia. *Curr Opin Hematol* 2002;9:282–287.

388. Pui CH, Gaynon PS, Boyett JM, et al. Outcome of treatment in childhood acute lymphoblastic leukaemia with rearrangements of the 11q23 chromosomal region. *Lancet* 2002;359:1909–1915.

389. Mercher T, Coniat MB, Monni R, et al. Involvement of a human gene related to the Drosophila spen gene in the recurrent t(1;22) translocation of acute megakaryocytic leukemia. *Proc Natl Acad Sci U S A* 2001;98:5776–5779.

390. Ma Z, Morris SW, Valentine V, et al. Fusion of two novel genes, RBM15 and MKL1, in the t(1;22)(p13;q13) of acute megakaryoblastic leukemia. *Nat Genet* 2001;28:220–221.

391. Carroll A, Civin C, Schneider N, et al. The t(1;22) (p13;q13) is nonrandom and restricted to infants with acute megakaryoblastic leukemia: a Pediatric Oncology Group Study. *Blood* 1991;78:748–752.

392. Lion T, Haas OA, Harbott J, et al. The translocation t(1;22) (p13;q13) is a nonrandom marker specifically associated with acute megakaryocytic leukemia in young children. *Blood* 1992;79:3325–3330.

393. Bernstein J, Dastugue N, Haas OA, et al. Nineteen cases of the t(1;22)(p13;q13) acute megakaryoblastic leukaemia of infants/children and a review of 39 cases: report from a t(1;22) study group. *Leukemia* 2000;14:216–218.

394. Ford AM, Ridge SA, Cabrera ME, et al. In utero rearrangements in the trithorax-related oncogene in infant leukaemias. *Nature* 1993;363:358–360.

395. Greaves MF, Wiemels J. Origins of chromosome translocations in childhood leukaemia. *Nat Rev Cancer* 2003;3:639–649.

396. Hasle H, Clemmensen IH, Mikkelsen M. Risks of leukaemia and solid tumours in individuals with Down's syndrome. *Lancet* 2000;355:165–169.

397. Zipursky A, Brown EJ, Christensen H, et al. Transient myeloproliferative disorder (transient leukemia) and hematologic manifestations of Down syndrome. *Clin Lab Med* 1999;19:157–167.

398. Zipursky A, Peeters M, Poon A. Megakaryoblastic leukemia and Down's syndrome: a review. *Pediatr Hematol Oncol* 1987;4:211–230.

399. Ravindranath Y, Abella E, Krischer JP, et al. Acute myeloid leukemia (AML) in Down's syndrome is highly responsive to chemotherapy: experience on Pediatric Oncology Group AML Study 8498. *Blood* 1992;80:2210–2214.

400. Gamis AS, Woods WG, Alonzo TA, et al. Increased age at diagnosis has a significantly negative effect on outcome in children with Down syndrome and acute myeloid leukemia: a report from the Children's Cancer Group Study 2891. *J Clin Oncol* 2003;21:3415–3422.

401. Taub JW, Matherly LH, Stout ML, et al. Enhanced metabolism of 1-beta-D-arabinofuranosylcytosine in Down syndrome cells: a contributing factor to the superior event free survival of Down syndrome children with acute myeloid leukemia. *Blood* 1996;87:3395–3403.

402. Dordelmann M, Schrappe M, Reiter A, et al. Down's syndrome in childhood acute lymphoblastic leukemia: clinical characteristics and treatment outcome in four consecutive BFM trials. Berlin-Frankfurt-Munster Group. *Leukemia* 1998;12:645–651.

403. Zipursky A. Transient leukaemia—a benign form of leukaemia in newborn infants with trisomy 21. *Br J Haematol* 2003;120:930–938.

404. Al Kasim F, Doyle JJ, Massey GV, et al. Incidence and treatment of potentially lethal diseases in transient leukemia of Down syndrome: Pediatric Oncology Group Study. *J Pediatr Hematol Oncol* 2002;24:9–13.

405. Schwab M, Niemeyer C, Schwarzer U. Down syndrome, transient myeloproliferative disorder, and infantile liver fibrosis. *Med Pediatr Oncol* 1998;31:159–165.

406. Wechsler J, Greene M, McDevitt MA, et al. Acquired mutations in GATA1 in the megakaryoblastic leukemia of Down syndrome. *Nat Genet* 2002;32:148–152.

407. Groet J, McElwaine S, Spinelli M, et al. Acquired mutations in GATA1 in neonates with Down's syndrome with transient myeloid disorder. *Lancet* 2003;361:1617–1620.

408. Hitzler JK, Cheung J, Li Y, et al. GATA1 mutations in transient leukemia and acute megakaryoblastic leukemia of Down syndrome. *Blood* 2003;101:4301–4304.

409. Mundschau G, Gurbuxani S, Gamis AS, et al. Mutagenesis of GATA1 is an initiating event in Down syndrome leukemogenesis. *Blood* 2003;101:4298–4300.

410. Rainis L, Bercovich D, Strehl S, et al. Mutations in exon 2 of GATA1 are early events in megakaryocytic malignancies associated with trisomy 21. *Blood* 2003;102:981–986.

411. Xu G, Nagano M, Kanezaki R, et al. Frequent mutations in the GATA-1 gene in the transient myeloproliferative disorder of Down syndrome. *Blood* 2003;102:2960–2968.

412. Ahmed M, Sternberg A, Hall G, et al. Natural history of GATA1 mutations in Down Syndrome. *Blood* 2004;103:2480–2489.

413. Shimada A, Xu G, Toki T, et al. Fetal origin of the GATA1 mutation in identical twins with transient myeloproliferative disorder and acute megakaryoblastic leukemia accompanying Down syndrome. *Blood* 2004;103:366.

414. Gurbuxani S, Vyas P, Crispino JD. Recent insights into the mechanisms of myeloid leukemogenesis in Down syndrome. *Blood* 2004;103:399–406.

415. Gamis AS, Hilden JM. Transient myeloproliferative disorder, a disorder with too few data and many unanswered questions: does it contain an important piece of the puzzle to understanding hematopoiesis and acute myelogenous leukemia? *J Pediatr Hematol Oncol* 2002;24:2–5.

416. Arico M, Biondi A, Pui CH. Juvenile myelomonocytic leukemia. Blood 1997;90:479–488.

417. Niemeyer CM, Arico M, Basso G, et al. Chronic myelomonocytic leukemia in childhood: a retrospective analysis of 110 cases. European Working Group on Myelodysplastic Syndromes in Childhood (EWOG-MDS). *Blood* 1997;89:3534–3543.

418. Pinkel D. Differentiating juvenile myelomonocytic leukemia from infectious disease. *Blood* 1998;91:365–367.

419. Freedman MH, Estrov Z, Chan HS. Juvenile chronic myelogenous leukemia. *Am J Pediatr Hematol Oncol* 1988;10:261–267.

420. Emanuel PD, Bates LJ, Castleberry RP, et al. Selective hypersensitivity to granulocyte-macrophage colony-stimulating factor by juvenile chronic myeloid leukemia hematopoietic progenitors. *Blood* 1991;77:925–929.

421. Tartaglia M, Niemeyer CM, Fragale A, et al. Somatic mutations in PTPN11 in juvenile myelomonocytic leukemia, myelodysplastic syndromes and acute myeloid leukemia. *Nat Genet* 2003;34:148–150.

422. Side LE, Emanuel PD, Taylor B, et al. Mutations of the NF1 gene in children with juvenile myelomonocytic leukemia without clinical evidence of neurofibromatosis, type 1. *Blood* 1998;92:267–272.

423. Emanuel PD, Snyder RC, Wiley T, et al. Inhibition of juvenile myelomonocytic leukemia cell growth in vitro by farnesyltransferase inhibitors. *Blood* 2000;95:639–645.

424. Calhoun DA, Kirk JF, Christensen RD. Incidence, significance, and kinetic mechanism responsible for leukemoid reactions in patients in the neonatal intensive care unit: a prospective evaluation. *J Pediatr* 1996;129:403–409.

425. Rastogi S, Rastogi D, Sundaram R, et al. Leukemoid reaction in extremely low-birth-weight infants. *Am J Perinatol* 1999;16:93–97.

426. Zanardo V, Savio V, Giacomin C, et al. Relationship between neonatal leukemoid reaction and bronchopulmonary dysplasia in low-birth-weight infants: a cross-sectional study. *Am J Perinatol* 2002;19:379–386.

427. Nakamura T, Ezaki S, Takasaki J, et al. Leukemoid reaction and chronic lung disease in infants with very low birth weight. *J Matern Fetal Neonatal Med* 2002;11:396–399.

428. Nicholson JF, Pesce MA. Reference ranges for laboratory tests and procedures. In: Behrman RE, Kliegman RM, Jenson HB, eds. *Nelson textbook of pediatrics*, 17th ed. Philadelphia: WB Saunders, 2004:2396–2426.

429. Shearer WT, Rosenblatt HM, Gelman RS, et al. Lymphocyte subsets in healthy children from birth through 18 years of age: the Pediatric AIDS Clinical Trials Group P1009 study. *J Allergy Clin Immunol* 2003;112:973–980.

430. Buckley RH. Primary immunodeficiency diseases due to defects in lymphocytes. *N Engl J Med* 2000;343:1313–1324.

431. Notarangelo LD, Mella P, Jones A, et al. Mutations in severe combined immune deficiency (SCID) due to JAK3 deficiency. *Hum Mutat* 2001;18:255–263.

432. Puel A, Leonard WJ. Mutations in the gene for the IL-7 receptor result in T(−)B(+)NK(+) severe combined immunodeficiency disease. *Curr Opin Immunol* 2000;12:468–473.

433. Dadi HK, Simon AJ, Roifman CM. Effect of CD3delta deficiency on maturation of alpha/beta and gamma/delta T-cell lineages in severe combined immunodeficiency. *N Engl J Med* 2003;349:1821–1828.

434. Kung C, Pingel JT, Heikinheimo M, et al. Mutations in the tyrosine phosphatase CD45 gene in a child with severe combined immunodeficiency disease. *Nat Med* 2000;6:343–345.

435. Arpaia E, Shahar M, Dadi H, et al. Defective T cell receptor signaling and CD8+ thymic selection in humans lacking zap-70 kinase. *Cell* 1994;76:947–958.

436. Aiuti A, Slavin S, Aker M, et al. Correction of ADA-SCID by stem cell gene therapy combined with nonmyeloablative conditioning. *Science* 2002;296:2410–2413.

437. Markert ML, Sarzotti M, Ozaki DA, et al. Thymus transplantation in complete DiGeorge syndrome: immunologic and safety evaluations in 12 patients. *Blood* 2003;102:1121–1130.

438. Chapel H, Geha R, Rosen F. Primary immunodeficiency diseases: an update. IUIS PID (Primary Immunodeficiencies) Classification Committee *Clin Exp Immunol* 2003;132:9–15.

439. Moshous D, Callebaut I, de Chasseval R, et al. Artemis, a novel DNA double-strand break repair/V(D)J recombination protein, is mutated in human severe combined immune deficiency. *Cell* 2001;105:177–186.

440. Meyts I, Weemaes C, Wolf-Peeters C, et al. Unusual and severe disease course in a child with ataxia-telangiectasia. *Pediatr Allergy Immunol* 2003;14:330–333.

441. Maraschio P, Spadoni E, Tanzarella C, et al. Genetic heterogeneity for a Nijmegen breakage-like syndrome. *Clin Genet* 2003;63:283–290.

442. Bhat AM, Scanlon JW. The pattern of eosinophilia in premature infants. A prospective study in premature infants using the absolute eosinophil count. *J Pediatr* 1981;98:612.

443. Gibson EL, Vaucher Y, Corrigan JJ Jr. Eosinophilia in premature infants: relationship to weight gain. *J Pediatr* 1979;95:99–101.

444. Lawrence R, Jr., Church JA, Richards W, et al. Eosinophilia in the hospitalized neonate. *Ann Allergy* 1980;44:349–352.

445. Rothberg AD, Cohn RJ, Argent AC, et al. Eosinophilia in premature neonates. Phase 2 of a biphasic granulopoietic response. *S Afr Med J* 1983;64:539–541.

446. Dror Y, Freedman MH. Shwachman-Diamond syndrome. *Br J Haematol* 2002;118:701–713.

447. Dror Y, Freedman MH. Shwachman-Diamond syndrome: an inherited preleukemic bone marrow failure disorder with aberrant hematopoietic progenitors and faulty marrow microenvironment. *Blood* 1999;94:3048–3054.

448. Dror Y, Freedman MH. Shwachman-Diamond syndrome marrow cells show abnormally increased apoptosis mediated through the Fas pathway. *Blood* 2001;97:3011–3016.

449. Boocock GR, Morrison JA, Popovic M, et al. Mutations in SBDS are associated with Shwachman-Diamond syndrome. *Nat Genet* 2003;33:97–101.

450. D'Andrea AD, Grompe M. The Fanconi anaemia/BRCA pathway. *Nat Rev Cancer* 2003;3:23–34.

451. Alter BP, Young NS. The bone marrow failure syndromes. In: Nathan DG, Oski SH, eds. *Nathan and Oski's Hematology of infancy and childhood*. 5th ed. Philadelphia: WB Saunders, 1998:237–335.

452. Halperin EC. Neonatal neoplasms. *Int J Radiat Oncol Biol Phys* 2000;47:171–178.

453. Dokal I. Dyskeratosis congenita in all its forms. *Br J Haematol* 2000;110:768–779.

454. Lee BW, Yap HK, Quah TC, et al. T cell immunodeficiency in dyskeratosis congenita. *Arch Dis Child* 1992;67:524–526.

455. Marrone A, Mason PJ. Dyskeratosis congenita. *Cell Mol Life Sci* 2003;60:507–517.

456. Vulliamy T, Marrone A, Dokal I, et al. Association between aplastic anaemia and mutations in telomerase RNA. *Lancet* 2002;359:2168–2170.

457. Dror Y, Freedman MH, Leaker M, et al. Low-intensity hematopoietic stem-cell transplantation across human leucocyte antigen barriers in dyskeratosis congenita. *Bone Marrow Transplant* 2003;31:847–850.

458. Ballmaier M, Germeshausen M, Schulze H, et al. c-mpl mutations are the cause of congenital amegakaryocytic thrombocytopenia. *Blood* 2001;97:139–146.

459. Ihara K, Ishii E, Eguchi M, et al. Identification of mutations in the c-mpl gene in congenital amegakaryocytic thrombocytopenia. *Proc Natl Acad Sci U S A* 1999;96:3132–3136.

460. Lackner A, Basu O, Bierings M, et al. Haematopoietic stem cell transplantation for amegakaryocytic thrombocytopenia. *Br J Haematol* 2000;109:773–775.

461. Kudo K, Kato K, Matsuyama T, et al. Successful engraftment of unrelated donor stem cells in two children with congenital amegakaryocytic thrombocytopenia. *J Pediatr Hematol Oncol* 2002;24:79–80.

462. Corazza F, Blum D, Clercx A, et al. Erythroblastopenia associated with methylmalonic aciduria. Case report and in vitro studies. *Biol Neonate* 1996;70:304–310.

463. Rotig A, Cormier V, Blanche S, et al. Pearson's marrow-pancreas syndrome. A multisystem mitochondrial disorder in infancy. *J Clin Invest* 1990;86:1601–1608.

464. Pearson HA, Lobel JS, Kocoshis SA, et al. A new syndrome of refractory sideroblastic anemia with vacuolization of marrow precursors and exocrine pancreatic dysfunction. *J Pediatr* 1979; 95:976–984.

465. De Vivo DC. The expanding clinical spectrum of mitochondrial diseases. *Brain Dev* 1993;15:1–22.

466. Muraki K, Nishimura S, Goto Y, et al. The association between haematological manifestation and mtDNA deletions in Pearson syndrome. *J Inherit Metab Dis* 1997;20:697–703.

467. Blanchette VS, Hume HA, Levy GJ, et al. Guidelines for auditing pediatric blood transfusion practices. *Am J Dis Child* 1991;145: 787–796.

468. Roseff SD, Luban NL, Manno CS. Guidelines for assessing appropriateness of pediatric transfusion. *Transfusion* 2002; 42:1398–1413.

469. Maier RF, Obladen M, Messinger D, et al. Factors related to transfusion in very low birthweight infants treated with erythropoietin. *Arch Dis Child Fetal Neonatal Ed* 1996;74:F182-F186.

470. Ibrahim HM, Krouskop RW, Lewis DF, et al. Placental transfusion: umbilical cord clamping and preterm infants. *J Perinatol* 2000;20:351–354.

471. Rabe H, Wacker A, Hulskamp G, et al. A randomised controlled trial of delayed cord clamping in very low birth weight preterm infants. *Eur J Pediatr* 2000;159:775–777.

472. Franz AR, Pohlandt F. Red blood cell transfusions in very and extremely low birthweight infants under restrictive transfusion guidelines: is exogenous erythropoietin necessary? *Arch Dis Child Fetal Neonatal Ed* 2001;84:F96-F100.

473. Maier RF, Sonntag J, Walka MM, et al. Changing practices of red blood cell transfusions in infants with birth weights less than 1000 g. *J Pediatr* 2000;136:220–224.

474. Boulton JE, Jeffries AL, O'Brien KK, et al. Changing transfusion practices in the NICU. *Pediatr Res* 1996;39,197a.

475. Widness JA, Seward VJ, Kromer IJ, et al. Changing patterns of red blood cell transfusion in very low birth weight infants. *J Pediatr* 1996;129:680–687.

476. Strauss RG. Data-driven blood banking practices for neonatal RBC transfusions. *Transfusion* 2000;40:1528–1540.

477. Hilsenrath P, Nemechek J, Widness JA, et al. Cost-effectiveness of a limited-donor blood program for neonatal red cell transfusions. *Transfusion* 1999;39:938–943.

478. Boralessa H, Modi N, Cockburn H, et al. RBC T activation and hemolysis in a neonatal intensive care population: implications for transfusion practice. *Transfusion* 2002;42:1428–1434.

479. Williams RA, Brown EF, Hurst D, et al. Transfusion of infants with activation of erythrocyte T antigen. *J Pediatr* 1989;115: 949–953.

480. Crookston KP, Reiner AP, Cooper LJ, et al. RBC T activation and hemolysis: implications for pediatric transfusion management. *Transfusion* 2000;40:801–812.

481. Floss AM, Strauss RG, Goeken N, et al. Multiple transfusions fail to provoke antibodies against blood cell antigens in human infants. *Transfusion* 1986;26:419–422.

482. Ludvigsen CW, Jr, Swanson JL, Thompson TR, et al. The failure of neonates to form red blood cell alloantibodies in response to multiple transfusions. *Am J Clin Pathol* 1987;87:250–251.

483. Sacher RA, Strauss RG, Luban NL, et al. Blood component therapy during the neonatal period: a national survey of red cell transfusion practice, 1985. *Transfusion* 1990;30:271–276.

484. Blanchette VS, Gray E, Hardie MJ, et al. Hyperkalemia after neonatal exchange transfusion: risk eliminated by washing red cell concentrates. *J Pediatr* 1984;105:321–324.

485. Scanlon JW, Krakaur R. Hyperkalemia following exchange transfusion. *J Pediatr* 1980;96:108–110.

486. Andrew M, Castle V, Saigal S, et al. Clinical impact of neonatal thrombocytopenia. *J Pediatr* 1987;110:457–464.

487. Andrew M, Vegh P, Caco C, et al. A randomized, controlled trial of platelet transfusions in thrombocytopenic premature infants. *J Pediatr* 1993;123:285–291.

488. Moroff G, Friedman A, Robkin-Kline L, et al. Reduction of the volume of stored platelet concentrates for use in neonatal patients. *Transfusion* 1984;24:144–146.

489. Christensen RD, Rothstein G, Anstall HB, et al. Granulocyte transfusions in neonates with bacterial infection, neutropenia,

and depletion of mature marrow neutrophils. *Pediatrics* 1982;70:1–6.

490. Gillan ER, Christensen RD, Suen Y, et al. A randomized, placebo-controlled trial of recombinant human granulocyte colony-stimulating factor administration in newborn infants with presumed sepsis: significant induction of peripheral and bone marrow neutrophilia. *Blood* 1994;84:1427–1433.

491. Makhlouf RA, Doron MW, Bose CL, et al. Administration of granulocyte colony-stimulating factor to neutropenic low birth weight infants of mothers with preeclampsia. *J Pediatr* 1995; 126:454–456.

492. Mollison PL. *Blood transfusion in clinical medicine.* London: Blackwell Scientific Publications, 1979.

493. Giacoia GP, Kasprisin DO. Transfusion-acquired hepatitis A. *South Med J* 1989;82:1357–1360.

494. Azimi PH, Roberto RR, Guralnik J, et al. Transfusion-acquired hepatitis A in a premature infant with secondary nosocomial spread in an intensive care nursery. *Am J Dis Child* 1986;140: 23–27.

495. Aach RD, Yomtovian RA, Hack M. Neonatal and pediatric posttransfusion hepatitis C: a look back and a look forward. *Pediatrics* 2000;105:836–842.

496. Goldman M, Juodvalkis S, Gill P, et al. Hepatitis C lookback. *Transfus Med Rev* 1998;12:84–93.

497. Committee on Infectious Diseases. Hepatitis C virus infection. American Academy of Pediatrics. *Pediatrics* 1998;101:481–485.

498. Vento S, Garofano T, Renzini C, et al. Fulminant hepatitis associated with hepatitis A virus superinfection in patients with chronic hepatitis C. *N Engl J Med* 1998;338:286–290.

499. Yeager AS, Grumet FC, Hafleigh EB, et al. Prevention of transfusion-acquired cytomegalovirus infections in newborn infants. *J Pediatr* 1981;98:281–287.

500. Adler SP, Chandrika T, Lawrence L, et al. Cytomegalovirus infections in neonates acquired by blood transfusions. *Pediatr Infect Dis* 1983;2:114–118.

501. de Cates CR, Roberton NR, Walker JR. Fatal acquired cytomegalovirus infection in a neonate with maternal antibody. *J Infect* 1988;17:235–239.

502. Weston PJ, Farmer K, Croxson MC, et al. Morbidity from acquired cytomegalovirus infection in a neonatal intensive care unit. *Aust Paediatr J* 1989;25:138–142.

503. Preiksaitis JK, Brown L, McKenzie M. Transfusion-acquired cytomegalovirus infection in neonates. A prospective study. *Transfusion* 1988;28:205–209.

504. Rawls WE, Wong CL, Blajchman M, et al. Neonatal cytomegalovirus infections: the relative role of neonatal blood transfusion and maternal exposure. *Clin Invest Med* 1984;7:13–19.

505. Wu J, Tang ZY, Wu YX, et al. Acquired cytomegalovirus infection of breast milk in infancy. *Chin Med J (Engl)* 1989;102:124–128.

506. Taylor BJ, Jacobs RF, Baker RL, et al. Frozen deglycerolyzed blood prevents transfusion-acquired cytomegalovirus infections in neonates. *Pediatr Infect Dis* 1986;5:188–191.

507. Luban NL, Williams AE, MacDonald MG, et al. Low incidence of acquired cytomegalovirus infection in neonates transfused with washed red blood cells. *Am J Dis Child* 1987;141:416–419.

508. Gilbert GL, Hayes K, Hudson IL, et al. Prevention of transfusion-acquired cytomegalovirus infection in infants by blood filtration to remove leucocytes. Neonatal Cytomegalovirus Infection Study Group. *Lancet* 1989;1:1228–1231.

509. Bowden RA, Slichter SJ, Sayers M, et al. A comparison of filtered leukocyte-reduced and cytomegalovirus (CMV) seronegative blood products for the prevention of transfusion-associated CMV infection after marrow transplant. *Blood* 1995;86:3598–3603.

510. Fergusson D, Hebert PC, Lee SK, et al. Clinical outcomes following institution of universal leukoreduction of blood transfusions for premature infants. *JAMA* 2003;289:1950–1956.

511. Shannon KM, Ammann AJ. Acquired immune deficiency syndrome in childhood. *J Pediatr* 1985;106:332–342.

512. Ammann AJ, Cowan MJ, Wara DW, et al. Acquired immunodeficiency in an infant: possible transmission by means of blood products. *Lancet* 1983;1:956–958.

513. Shannon K, Ball E, Wasserman RL, et al. Transfusion-associated cytomegalovirus infection and acquired immune deficiency syndrome in an infant. *J Pediatr* 1983;103:859–863.

514. McCarthy VP, Charles DL, Unger JL. Transfusion-associated HIV infection in a neonate from a seronegative donor. *Am J Dis Child* 1987;141:1145–1146.

515. Seemayer TA, Bolande RP. Thymic involution mimicking thymic dysplasia: a consequence of transfusion-induced graft versus host disease in a premature infant. *Arch Pathol Lab Med* 1980;104:141–144.

516. Berger RS, Dixon SL. Fulminant transfusion-associated graft-versus-host disease in a premature infant. *J Am Acad Dermatol* 1989;20:945–950.

517. Funkhouser AW, Vogelsang G, Zehnbauer B, et al. Graft versus host disease after blood transfusions in a premature infant. *Pediatrics* 1991;87:247–250.

518. Hatley RM, Reynolds M, Paller AS, et al. Graft-versus-host disease following ECMO. *J Pediatr Surg* 1991;26:317–319.

519. Bastian JF, Williams RA, Ornelas W, et al. Maternal isoimmunisation resulting in combined immunodeficiency and fatal graft-versus-host disease in an infant. *Lancet* 1984;1:1435–1437.

520. Brunell PA, Bass JW, Daum RS, et al. American Academy of Pediatrics Committee on Infectious Diseases: prevention of hepatitis B virus infections. *Pediatrics* 1985;75:362–364.

521. van Ommen CH, Heijboer H, Buller HR, et al. Venous thromboembolism in childhood: a prospective two-year registry in The Netherlands. *J Pediatr* 2001;139:676–681.

522. Schmidt B, Andrew M. Neonatal thrombosis: report of a prospective Canadian and international registry. *Pediatrics* 1995;96:939–943.

523. Nowak-Gottl U, von Kries R, Gobel U. Neonatal symptomatic thromboembolism in Germany: two year survey. *Arch Dis Child Fetal Neonatal Ed* 1997;76:F163-F167.

524. Nitschmann E, Berry L, Bridge S, et al. Morphological and biochemical features affecting the antithrombotic properties of the aorta in adult rabbits and rabbit pups. *Thromb Haemost* 1998;79:1034–1040.

525. Nitschmann E, Berry L, Bridge S, et al. Morphologic and biochemical features affecting the antithrombotic properties of the inferior vena cava of rabbit pups and adult rabbits. *Pediatr Res* 1998;43:62–67.

526. O'Neill JA Jr, Neblett WW III, Born ML. Management of major thromboembolic complications of umbilical artery catheters. *J Pediatr Surg* 1981;16:972–978.

527. Cochran WD, Davis HT, Smith CA. Advantages and complications of umbilical artery catheterization in the newborn. *Pediatrics* 1968;42:769–777.

528. Gupta JM, Roberton NR, Wigglesworth JS. Umbilical artery catheterization in the newborn. *Arch Dis Child* 1968;43:382–387.

529. Wigger HJ, Bransilver BR, Blanc WA. Thromboses due to catheterization in infants and children. *J Pediatr* 1970;76:1–11.

530. Egan EA, Eitzman DV. Umbilical vessel catheterization. *Am J Dis Child* 1971;121:213–218.

531. Symansky MR, Fox HA. Umbilical vessel catheterization: indications, management, and evaluation of the technique. *J Pediatr* 1972;80:820–826.

532. Marsh JL, King W, Barrett C, et al. Serious complications after umbilical artery catheterization for neonatal monitoring. *Arch Surg* 1975;110:1203–1208.

533. Tyson JE, deSa DJ, Moore S. Thromboatheromatous complications of umbilical arterial catheterization in the newborn period. Clinicopathological study. *Arch Dis Child* 1976;51:744–754.

534. Neal WA, Reynolds JW, Jarvis CW, et al. Umbilical artery catheterization: demonstration of arterial thrombosis by aortography. *Pediatrics* 1972;50:6–13.

535. Goetzman BW, Stadalnik RC, Bogren HG, et al. Thrombotic complications of umbilical artery catheters: a clinical and radiographic study. *Pediatrics* 1975;56:374–379.

536. Olinsky A, Aitken FG, Isdale JM. Thrombus formation after umbilical arterial catheterisation. An angiographic study. *S Afr Med J* 1975;49:1467–1470.

537. Saia OS, Rubaltelli FF, D'Elia R et al. Clinical and aortographic assessment of the complications of arterial catheterization. *Eur J Pediatr* 1978;128:169–179.

538. Wesstrom G, Finnstrom O, Stenport G. Umbilical artery catheterization in newborns. I. Thrombosis in relation to catheter type and position. *Acta Paediatr Scand* 1979;68:575–581.

539. Mokrohisky ST, Levine RL, Blumhagen JD, et al. Low positioning of umbilical-artery catheters increases associated complications in newborn infants. *N Engl J Med* 1978;299:561–564.

540. Roy M, Turner-Gomes S, Gill G, et al. Accuracy of Doppler echocardiography for the diagnosis of thrombosis associated with umbilical venous catheters. *J Pediatr* 2002;140:131–134.

541. Mehta S, Connors AF Jr, Danish EH, et al. Incidence of thrombosis during central venous catheterization of newborns: a prospective study. *J Pediatr Surg* 1992;27:18–22.

542. Tanke RB, van Megen R, Daniels O. Thrombus detection on central venous catheters in the neonatal intensive care unit. *Angiology* 1994;45:477–480.

543. Rayne SC, Kraus FT. Placental thrombi and other vascular lesions. Classification, morphology, and clinical correlations. *Pathol Res Pract* 1993;189:2–17.

544. Parker MJ, Joubert GI, Levin SD. Portal vein thrombosis causing neonatal cerebral infarction. *Arch Dis Child Fetal Neonatal Ed* 2002;87:F125-F127.

545. Kraus FT, Acheen VI. Fetal thrombotic vasculopathy in the placenta: cerebral thrombi and infarcts, coagulopathies, and cerebral palsy. *Hum Pathol* 1999;30:759–769.

546. Schmidt B, Zipursky A. Thrombotic disease in newborn infants. *Clin Perinatol* 1984;11:461–488.

547. Shama A, Patole SK, Whitehall JS. Low molecular weight heparin for neonatal thrombosis. *J Paediatr Child Health* 2002;38:615–617.

548. Seligsohn U, Zivelin A. Thrombophilia as a multigenic disorder. *Thromb Haemost* 1997;78:297–301.

549. Crowther MA, Kelton JG. Congenital thrombophilic states associated with venous thrombosis: a qualitative overview and proposed classification system. *Ann Intern Med* 2003;138:128–134.

550. Marlar RA, Montgomery RR, Broekmans AW. Diagnosis and treatment of homozygous protein C deficiency. Report of the Working Party on Homozygous Protein C Deficiency of the Subcommittee on Protein C and Protein S, International Committee on Thrombosis and Haemostasis. *J Pediatr* 1989;114:528–534.

551. Mahasandana C, Suvatte V, Marlar RA, et al. Neonatal purpura fulminans associated with homozygous protein S deficiency. *Lancet* 1990;335:61–62.

552. Jochmans K, Lissens W, Vervoort R, et al. Antithrombin-Gly 424 Arg: a novel point mutation responsible for type 1 antithrombin deficiency and neonatal thrombosis. *Blood* 1994;83:146–151.

553. Pipe SW, Schmaier AH, Nichols WC, et al. Neonatal purpura fulminans in association with factor V R506Q mutation. *J Pediatr* 1996;128:706–709.

554. Heller C, Schobess R, Kurnik K, et al. Abdominal venous thrombosis in neonates and infants: role of prothrombotic risk factors—a multicentre case-control study. For the Childhood Thrombophilia Study Group. *Br J Haematol* 2000;111:534–539.

555. Revel-Vilk S, Chan A, Bauman M, et al. Prothrombotic conditions in an unselected cohort of children with venous thromboembolic disease. *J Thromb Haemost* 2003;1:915–921.

556. Levin DL, Weinberg AG, Perkin RM. Pulmonary microthrombi syndrome in newborn infants with unresponsive persistent pulmonary hypertension. *J Pediatr* 1983;102:299–303.

557. de Vries LS, Groenendaal F, Eken P, et al. Infarcts in the vascular distribution of the middle cerebral artery in preterm and full-term infants. *Neuropediatrics* 1997;28:88–96.

558. Estan J, Hope P. Unilateral neonatal cerebral infarction in full term infants. *Arch Dis Child Fetal Neonatal Ed* 1997;76:F88-F93.

559. Barron TF, Gusnard DA, Zimmerman RA, et al. Cerebral venous thrombosis in neonates and children. *Pediatr Neurol* 1992;8:112–116.

560. Rivkin MJ, Anderson ML, Kaye EM. Neonatal idiopathic cerebral venous thrombosis: an unrecognized cause of transient seizures or lethargy. *Ann Neurol* 1992;32:51–56.

561. deVeber G, Andrew M. Cerebral sinovenous thrombosis in children. *N Engl J Med* 2001;345:417–423.

562. Roy M, Schmidt B. Neonatal thrombosis: are we doing the right studies? *Semin Thromb Hemost* 1995;21:313–341.

563. Monagle P, Chan A, Massicotte P, et al. Anti thrombotic therapy in children. The seventh ACCP conference on anti thrombotic and thrombolytic therapy. *Chest* 2004 126 (3 suppl); 645S–687S.

564. Schmidt B, Andrew M. Report of Scientific and Standardization Subcommittee on Neonatal Hemostasis Diagnosis and Treatment of Neonatal Thrombosis. *Thromb Haemost* 1992;67:381–382.

565. Andrew ME, Monagle P, deVeber G, et al. Thromboembolic disease and antithrombotic therapy in newborns. *Hematology (Am Soc Hematol Educ Program)* 2001;358–374.

566. Michaels LA. A response to laboratory testing for thrombophilia in pediatric patients. *Thromb Haemost* 2003;89:204–205.

567. Manco-Johnson MJ, Grabowski EF, Hellgreen M, et al. Laboratory testing for thrombophilia in pediatric patients. On behalf of the Subcommittee for Perinatal and Pediatric Thrombosis of the Scientific and Standardization Committee of the International Society of Thrombosis and Haemostasis (ISTH). *Thromb Haemost* 2002;88:155–156.

568. Choay J, Petitou M, Lormeau JC, et al. Structure-activity relationship in heparin: a synthetic pentasaccharide with high affinity for antithrombin III and eliciting high anti-factor Xa activity. *Biochem Biophys Res Commun* 1983;116:492–499.

569. Danielsson A, Raub E, Lindahl U, et al. Role of ternary complexes, in which heparin binds both antithrombin and proteinase, in the acceleration of the reactions between antithrombin and thrombin or factor Xa. *J Biol Chem* 1986;261:15467–15473.

570. Andrew M, Marzinotto V, Massicotte P, et al. Heparin therapy in pediatric patients: a prospective cohort study. *Pediatr Res* 1994;35:78–83.

571. Andrew M, deVeber G. *Pediatric thromboembolism and stroke protocols.* Hamilton: BC Decker, 1999.

572. Schmidt B, Buchanan MR, Ofosu F, et al. Antithrombotic properties of heparin in a neonatal piglet model of thrombin-induced thrombosis. *Thromb Haemost* 1988;60:289–292.

573. Weitz JI. Low-molecular-weight heparins. *N Engl J Med* 1997;337:688–698.

574. Juergens CP, Semsarian C, Keech AC, et al. Hemorrhagic complications of intravenous heparin use. *Am J Cardiol* 1997;80:150–154.

575. Warkentin TE, Kelton JG. Heparin-induced thrombocytopenia. *Prog Hemost Thromb* 1991;10:1–34.

576. Warkentin TE, Levine MN, Hirsh J, et al. Heparin-induced thrombocytopenia in patients treated with low-molecular-weight heparin or unfractionated heparin. *N Engl J Med* 1995;332:1330–1335.

577. Demasi R, Bode AP, Knupp C, et al. Heparin-induced thrombocytopenia. *Am Surg* 1994;60:26–29.

578. Schmitt BP, Adelman B. Heparin-associated thrombocytopenia: a critical review and pooled analysis. *Am J Med Sci* 1993;305:208–215.

579. Visentin GP, Ford SE, Scott JP, et al. Antibodies from patients with heparin-induced thrombocytopenia/thrombosis are specific for platelet factor 4 complexed with heparin or bound to endothelial cells. *J Clin Invest* 1994;93:81–88.

580. Ziporen L, Li ZQ, Park KS, et al. Defining an antigenic epitope on platelet factor 4 associated with heparin-induced thrombocytopenia. *Blood* 1998;92:3250–3259.

581. Warkentin TE, Aird WC, Rand JH. Platelet-endothelial interactions: sepsis, HIT, and antiphospholipid syndrome. *Hematology (Am Soc Hematol Educ Program)* 2003;497–519.

582. Ranze O, Ranze P, Magnani HN, et al. Heparin-induced thrombocytopenia in paediatric patients—a review of the literature and a new case treated with danaparoid sodium. *Eur J Pediatr* 1999;158[Suppl 3]:S130–S133.

583. Spadone D, Clark F, James E, et al. Heparin-induced thrombocytopenia in the newborn. *J Vasc Surg* 1992;15:306–311.

584. Klenner AF, Fusch C, Rakow A, et al. Benefit and risk of heparin for maintaining peripheral venous catheters in neonates: a placebo-controlled trial. *J Pediatr* 2003;143:741–745.

585. Hirsh J, Warkentin TE, Raschke R, et al. Heparin and low-molecular-weight heparin: mechanisms of action, pharmacokinetics, dosing considerations, monitoring, efficacy, and safety. *Chest* 1998;114:489S–510S.

586. Massicotte P, Adams M, Marzinotto V, et al. Low-molecular-weight heparin in pediatric patients with thrombotic disease: a dose finding study. *J Pediatr* 1996;128:313–318.

587. Dix D, Andrew M, Marzinotto V, et al. The use of low molecular weight heparin in pediatric patients. *J Pediatr* 2000;136(4):439–445.

588. Streif W, Goebel G, Chan AK, et al. Use of low molecular mass heparin (enoxaparin) in newborn infants: a prospective cohort study of 62 patients. *Arch Dis Child Fetal Neonatal Ed* 2003;88:F365-F370.

589. Albisetti M, Andrew M. Low molecular weight heparin in children. *Eur J Pediatr* 2002;161:71–77.

590. van der Heijden JF, Prins MH, Buller HR. For the initial treatment of venous thromboembolism: are all low-molecular-weight heparin compounds the same? *Thromb Res* 2000;100:V121–V130.

591. Nohe N, Flemmer A, Rumler R, et al. The low molecular weight heparin dalteparin for prophylaxis and therapy of thrombosis in childhood: a report on 48 cases. *Eur J Pediatr* 1999;158[Suppl 3]:S134–S139.

592. Massicotte P, Julian JA, Gent M, et al. An open-label randomized controlled trial of low molecular weight heparin compared to heparin and coumadin for the treatment of venous thromboembolic events in children: the REVIVE trial. *Thromb Res* 2003;109:85–92.

593. Kuhle S, Massicotte MP, Dinyari M, et al. A dose-finding study of Tinzaparin in pediatric patients. *J Thromb Haemostas* 2003;1[Suppl 1]:P1887.

594. Dix D, Andrew M, Marzinotto V, et al. The use of low molecular weight heparin in pediatric patients: a prospective cohort study. *J Pediatr* 2000;136:439–445.

595. Cruickshank MK, Levine MN, Hirsh J, et al. A standard heparin nomogram for the management of heparin therapy. *Arch Intern Med* 1991;151:333–337.

596. Crowther MA, Berry LR, Monagle PT, et al. Mechanisms responsible for the failure of protamine to inactivate low-molecular-weight heparin. *Br J Haematol* 2002;116:178–186.

597. Corrigan JJ Jr. Neonatal thrombosis and the thrombolytic system: pathophysiology and therapy. *Am J Pediatr Hematol Oncol* 1988;10:83–91.

598. Leaker M, Massicotte MP, Brooker LA, et al. Thrombolytic therapy in pediatric patients: a comprehensive review of the literature. *Thromb Haemost* 1996;76:132–134.

599. Manco-Johnson MJ, Grabowski EF, Hellgreen M, et al. Recommendations for tPA thrombolysis in children. On behalf of the Scientific Subcommittee on Perinatal and Pediatric Thrombosis of the Scientific and Standardization Committee of the International Society of Thrombosis and Haemostasis. *Thromb Haemost* 2002;88:157–158.

600. Mocan H, Beattie TJ, Murphy AV. Renal venous thrombosis in infancy: long-term follow-up. *Pediatr Nephrol* 1991;5:45–49.

601. Bokenkamp A, von Kries R, Nowak-Gottl U, et al. Neonatal renal venous thrombosis in Germany between 1992 and 1994: epidemiology, treatment and outcome. *Eur J Pediatr* 2000;159:44–48.

602. Adelman RD. Long-term follow-up of neonatal renovascular hypertension. *Pediatr Nephrol* 1987;1:35–41.

603. Caplan MS, Cohn RA, Langman CB, et al. Favorable outcome of neonatal aortic thrombosis and renovascular hypertension. *J Pediatr* 1989;115:291–295.

604. Payne RM, Martin TC, Bower RJ, et al. Management and follow-up of arterial thrombosis in the neonatal period. *J Pediatr* 1989;114:853–858.

605. Seibert JJ, Northington FJ, Miers JF, et al. Aortic thrombosis after umbilical artery catheterization in neonates: prevalence of complications on long-term follow-up. *AJR Am J Roentgenol* 1991;156:567–569.

606. deVeber GA, MacGregor D, Curtis R, et al. Neurologic outcome in survivors of childhood arterial ischemic stroke and sinovenous thrombosis. *J Child Neurol* 2000;15:316–324.

607. Mercuri E, Cowan F, Gupte G, et al. Prothrombotic disorders and abnormal neurodevelopmental outcome in infants with neonatal cerebral infarction. *Pediatrics* 2001;107:1400–1404.

608. Rais-Bahrami K, Karna P, Dolanski EA. Effect of fluids on life span of peripheral arterial lines. *Am J Perinatol* 1990;7:122–124.

609. Butt W, Shann F, McDonnell G, et al. Effect of heparin concentration and infusion rate on the patency of arterial catheters. *Crit Care Med* 1987;15:230–232.

610. Randolph AG, Cook DJ, Gonzales CA, et al. Benefit of heparin in peripheral venous and arterial catheters: systematic review and meta-analysis of randomised controlled trials. *Br Med J* 1998;316:969–975.

611. Shah P, Shah V. Continuous heparin infusion to prevent thrombosis and catheter occlusion in neonates with peripherally placed percutaneous central venous catheters. *Cochrane Database Syst Rev* 2001;CD002772.

47

Bacterial and Fungal Infections

Robert L. Schelonka   *Bishara J. Freij*   *George H. McCracken, Jr.*

Infections cause significant mortality and long-term morbidity in neonates, especially for premature infants of very low birth weight (1–6). Temporal and geographic differences in the relative frequencies of various neonatal pathogens are well recognized (7–11). In North America in the 1930s and 1940s, gram-positive cocci such as group A β-hemolytic streptococci and *Staphylococcus aureus* were the most common bacterial isolates from neonates with sepsis, with *Escherichia coli* accounting for most of the remaining cases. *S. aureus* and *E. coli* became the major pathogens in the 1950s, but since the late 1960s, group B β-hemolytic streptococci and *E. coli* have predominated. Coagulase-negative staphylococci emerged in the 1980s and have surpassed *S. aureus* and gram-negative enteric bacilli as the bacteria most frequently associated with nosocomial infections in many neonatal intensive care units (NICUs), and several *Candida* species have increased in frequency to become major neonatal pathogens in the 1990s. This has largely been a consequence of the survival of very-low-birth-weight (VLBW) infants who require lengthy hospitalizations and considerable mechanical and nutritional support (12,13). Since the 1990s there has been an emerging problem of multiple-drug-resistant gram-positive and gram-negative enteric bacilli in NICUs (14–17).

The outcome of neonatal infections may be improved if illness is recognized early and appropriate antimicrobial agents are administered promptly. This chapter presents pertinent epidemiologic and pathogenetic concepts of specific infections, clinical manifestations, and diagnostic evaluations of patients with these diseases, with a rational approach to therapy of neonatal infections.

EPIDEMIOLOGY

The two principal sources of newborn infection are the mother and the nursery environment. Infection is acquired from the mother transplacentally, at the time of delivery, or in the postnatal period. The infant may acquire infection postnatally from environmental sources, such as nursery personnel, respiratory equipment, sinks, contaminated total parenteral nutrition solutions or medication vials, and incubators. Infections manifesting within the first week of life are usually the result of exposure to microorganisms of maternal origin, but infections presenting later can have a maternal or environmental source.

Myriad aerobic and anaerobic bacteria, mycoplasmas, chlamydiae, fungi, viruses, and protozoa can be found in the maternal genital tract. Some of these organisms pose little threat to the newborn infant (e.g., *Lactobacillus*, α-hemolytic streptococci, *Veillonella*), and others are infrequent causes of neonatal disease (e.g., *Streptococcus pneumoniae*, *Neisseria meningitidis*) (18–20). More commonly, organisms such as groups A and B β-hemolytic streptococci, *E. coli*, *Listeria monocytogenes*, *Haemophilus influenzae*, *Neisseria gonorrhoeae*, cytomegalovirus, and herpes simplex virus are responsible for serious neonatal infections (3,4).

Within a few days after birth, α-hemolytic streptococci, *S. epidermidis*, and gram-negative enteric bacilli colonize the throat, nose, umbilicus, and stool (21–23). The gastrointestinal (GI) tract of newborns becomes heavily colonized by lactobacilli. Infants in NICUs tend to have delayed colonization, which probably is related to early antimicrobial therapy for possible sepsis, and are more likely to acquire nosocomial strains of gram-negative bacilli such as *Klebsiella*, *Enterobacter*, *Citrobacter*, and *E. coli* (24–26). Colonization of the scalp, axilla, and groin by coagulase-negative staphylococci is universal by 48 hours of age (12). In a prospective study of 18 premature infants admitted to a NICU, *S. epidermidis* as the only coagulase-negative staphylococcal species isolated from the axilla, ear, nasopharynx, and rectum was found in about 11% of infants during their first postnatal day; this increased to 100% by 4 weeks of age. None of these infants had a predominant *S. epidermidis* biotype on the first day compared with 89% by 4 weeks of age. The prevalence of slime production and multi-drug resistance among isolates rose from 68% to 95% and from 32% to 82%, respectively, during the 4-week study period (27).

Postnatal fungal colonization is more likely to occur in low-birth-weight (LBW) infants. An estimated 10% of term infants have GI Candida colonization within the first 5 days of life; infants weighing less than 1,500 g have colonization rates of about 60% (28). Early colonization (less than 2 weeks of age) is more common, involves the GI and respiratory tracts, and is with *Candida albicans* or *C. tropicalis*, unlike late colonization (≥2 weeks of age), which usually involves the skin and is more likely to be with *C. parapsilosis* (29). *C. albicans* colonization of infants is usually of maternal origin, whereas *C. parapsilosis* colonization is acquired from exogenous sources such as the hands of nursery personnel (30). Cutaneous colonization with *Malassezia (Pityrosporum) furfur*, a lipophilic yeast best known as the cause of tinea versicolor, is common and is found in as many as two-thirds of all critically ill newborns; fewer than 3% of healthy newborns and young infants have skin colonization by this fungus (31–33). The use of water-in-oil emollient creams (e.g., Eucerin Creme) as a moisturizer for premature infants does not appear to alter colonization patterns by bacteria or fungi (34), but in a randomized controlled trial of topical emollient cream there was an 5% absolute increased risk (25.8% vs. 20.4%; RR: 1.26; 95% CI: 1.02,1.54) of acquiring nosocomial bacterial sepsis. This increase in infection rates due mostly to an increase in the number of coagulase-negative staphylococci infection (35). The vagina or cervix of asymptomatic, sexually active women is colonized by *Ureaplasma urealyticum* in 40% to 80% and by *Mycoplasma hominis* in 21% to 53%. Vertical transmission rates from 45% to 66% for preterm and term neonates have been reported for *U. urealyticum* (36). By 3 months of age, about 33% to 68% of these infants continue to have detectable pharyngeal, ocular, or vaginal colonization (37). Vertical transmission rates for infants born to women with cervical *Chlamydia trachomatis* infections have been estimated at 40% to 70%; about 35% of untreated infants continue to be infected at one or more sites (e.g., conjunctiva, nasopharynx, oropharynx, rectum, vagina) at 12 months of age (38–40).

In the United States, bacterial sepsis affects up to 32,000 infants annually, and the incidence of neonatal sepsis is from 1 to 8 cases per 1,000 live births (41–43). The average national incidence rate for nursery-acquired infections is about 1.4%, but figures reported for NICUs are considerably higher and range from 5% to 30% (3,44–47). The most important risk factors for acquiring a nosocomial infection are low birth weight and gestational age; others include prolonged hospitalization, invasive procedures, placement of indwelling devices such as central venous catheters or ventriculoperitoneal shunts, bacterial or fungal colonization, and overcrowded nurseries.

PHARMACOLOGIC BASIS OF ANTIMICROBIAL THERAPY

Selection of antimicrobial therapy for neonatal infections must be based on pharmacokinetic properties of antibiotics in newborn infants of different gestational and postnatal ages, antimicrobial susceptibilities of commonly encountered pathogens within each nursery, and the natural history of the infectious disease being treated (48).

Combining two or more antibiotics is the usual clinical practice when initiating therapy for presumed systemic bacterial disease (e.g., ampicillin and an aminoglycoside are combined to treat suspected early onset septicemia or meningitis before identification of the pathogen). After a bacterium has been identified and its susceptibility to various antimicrobial agents is determined, a single appropriate antibiotic usually is satisfactory for treating most infections.

Although antibiotics are used commonly to prevent infection, they are effective prophylactically only if directed against a single pathogen. For example, a single dose of penicillin G given intramuscularly at birth reduces the colonization rate and incidence of early- onset group B streptococcal (GBS) disease, except in infants who acquire the infection *in utero* (49). However, if antibiotics are used as broad-spectrum coverage against many potential pathogens, they rarely are effective. This umbrella method of chemoprophylaxis encourages the emergence of resistant strains among previously susceptible bacteria and alters the normal flora of the GI and respiratory tracts with overgrowth of potentially virulent organisms. Broad-coverage prophylaxis may partially suppress a bacterium, masking the development of clinical disease and causing neglect of important surgical measures or serious delay in administering more effective therapy.

SEPSIS NEONATORUM

The term sepsis neonatorum describes a disease of infants who are younger than 1 month of age, are clinically ill, and have positive blood cultures. The presence of clinical manifestations differentiates this condition from the transient bacteremia observed in some healthy neonates.

The bacteria responsible for neonatal sepsis vary geographically. GBS and *E. coli* predominate in the United States, whereas *S. aureus* and gram-negative bacilli are much more common in developing countries (8). The bacterial etiology of sepsis also varies by the postnatal age of the infant. In a study of a cohort of 6,956 VLBW infants (401 to 1,500 g) admitted to 15 medical centers in the United States during a 32-month period between 1998 and 2000, the incidence of early- onset sepsis (occurring during the first 72 hours of life) was 1.5% and that of late-onset sepsis (occurring after 3 days of age) was 25%. The nature of the pathogens associated with the early-onset and late-onset infections differed markedly, with *E. coli* predominating (44% of cases) in the former and coagulase-negative staphylococci (48% of cases) in the latter (Table 47-1) (3,4).

TABLE 47-1

DISTRIBUTION OF PATHOGENS IN A COHORT OF 5,447 (EARLY-ONSET) AND 6,956 (LATE-ONSET) VERY-LOW-BIRTH-WEIGHT INFANTS (401–1,500 G) IN THE UNITED STATES FROM SEPTEMBER 1,1998 TO AUGUST 1, 2000.

Organism	Early-Onset Sepsis (N = 84)	Late-Onset Sepsis (N = 1,313)
Gram-postive bacteria		
Group B streptococci	9 (11)	30 (2)
Streptococcus viridans	3 (4)	NS
Other streptococci	4 (5)	NS
Enterococcus/group D streptococci	NS	43 (3)
Coagulase-negative staphylococci	9 (11)	629 (48)
Staphylococcus aurerus	1 (1)	103 (8)
Other	3 (4)	117 (9)
Gram-negative bacteria		
Escherichia coli	37 (44)	64 (5)
Haemophilus influenzae	7 (8)	NS
Klebsiella	NS	52 (4)
Pseudomonas	NS	35 (3)
Enterobacter	NS	33 (3)
Other	7 (8)	18 (1)
Fungi		
Candida albicans	2 (2)	76 (6)
Candida parapsilosis	0 (0)	54 (4)
Other	0 (0)	30 (2)

Values are given as number (percent).
NS, not specified

Pathogenesis

Maternal, environmental, and host factors determine which infants exposed to a potentially pathogenic organism will develop sepsis, meningitis, or other serious invasive infections.

Many prepartum and intrapartum obstetric complications have been associated with increased risk of infection in the newborn, the most significant of which are premature onset of labor, prolonged rupture of fetal membranes, chorioamnionitis, and maternal fever. In one study of 963 pregnancies complicated by premature rupture of membranes, the incidence of clinical sepsis increased from 2% among infants born within 23 hours of membrane rupture to 7% and 11% among those delivered 24 to 47 hours and 48 to 71 hours after rupture, respectively. The risk was highest for the premature, LBW infants (50). The incidence of infection has been estimated at 8.7% for infants born to mothers with prolonged rupture of membranes (≥24 hours) and clinical chorioamnionitis (51). Intraamniotic infection is associated with a higher incidence of sepsis among infants weighing less than 2,500 g at birth compared with those weighing 2,500 g or more (16% and 4%, respectively). Death from sepsis is greater in the LBW group (11% and 0%, respectively) (52). Isolation of bacteria from the chorioamnion has been associated with an increased risk of neonatal death among preterm infants (53). Maternal urinary tract infections, low parity, and the use of internal monitoring devices are risk factors for chorioamnionitis (54). Concurrent maternal and neonatal bacteremia has been documented for many microorganisms (55–57).

With improved supportive care of the sick neonate has come increased opportunity for microorganisms of relatively low virulence to cause systemic disease. The use of arterial and venous umbilical catheters, central venous catheters, indwelling urinary catheters, and endotracheal tubes provides access to the debilitated infant for organisms in the respiratory, GI, or genitourinary tract, on the skin, or in respiratory support equipment.

Bacterial colonization of the skin and mucosal surfaces precedes invasive disease in most infants with sepsis. Type III strains of GBS, the ones most commonly associated with early-onset septicemia and with meningitis at any age in early infancy, adhere better to vaginal and neonatal buccal epithelial cells *in vitro* than do other GBS strains (58,59). Bloodstream invasion generally follows local multiplication of the organism at sites of colonization. Aspiration of infected amniotic fluid is another proposed route for fetal infection among infants born to mothers with chorioamnionitis.

Animals have been used to define the host-bacteria interactions that determine pathogenesis of disease. Bloodstream infection in infant rats or mice caused by *E. coli* K1 or any of the GBS serotypes can be prevented by pretreatment with type-specific capsular polysaccharide antibody (60,61). The orogastric route for *E. coli* K1 in the infant rat and the intratracheal installation of GBS in the rhesus monkey or rat produce illnesses that closely parallel the human syndromes (62–64).

Several investigations of the host-parasite association of humans with GBS have focused on measurement of specific antibody in the serum of infected and colonized persons. Protective concentrations of antibody to GBS serotype III were found in 73% of women whose newborn infants were well but in only 17% of women whose neonates developed sepsis or meningitis caused by this organism (65). The amount of antibody to GBS serotype III was considerably lower in ill infants than in healthy neonates born to mothers with vaginal colonization (65). Levels of GBS serotype III antibodies correlate with *in vitro* opsonic activity and in vivo protection of animals experimentally infected with these strains (66,67). The administration of standard intravenous immunoglobulin preparations with activities against GBS, of human GBS monoclonal antibodies, or of GBS hyperimmune polyclonal antibodies provides significant protection to animals experimentally infected with this pathogen (68,69). Asymptomatic colonization also is associated with antibody formation (70,71). Although less extensively studied, similar observations have been made for other GBS serotypes (69,72–75).

Evidence suggests that antibodies to the K1 *E. coli* antigen are protective against infection by this organism, but this is not firmly established (76). Neonatal serum has been shown to be inefficient in killing *E. coli* because of a deficiency of nonimmunoglobulin G serum components, such as complement factor 9 (77,78).

Physiologic deficiencies of the classic and alternative pathways of complement activation in neonates contribute to inefficient bacterial opsonization (79,80). Organisms such as GBS and *E. coli* that have high capsular sialic acid content tend to be poor activators of the alternative complement pathway (81).

Fibronectin is a multifunctional glycoprotein found in the plasma and on the surface of certain epithelial cells, basement membranes, and connective tissues. In plasma, fibronectin acts as a nonspecific opsonin that enhances clearance of invading bacteria (82). Fibronectin is deficient in neonatal plasma, and its concentration varies inversely with gestational age (82,83). Septic infants have been shown to have significantly lower plasma concentrations of this glycoprotein than healthy, age-matched controls (84). The soluble form of fibronectin binds poorly to GBS (85). Fibronectin enhances phagocyte function *in vitro* and *in vivo* (82).

Quantitative and qualitative deficiencies in neonatal neutrophils contribute to the immaturity of the immune system of newborns. The abnormalities become most pronounced at times of stress or during infections and include impaired chemotaxis, decreased deformability, reduced C3bi receptor expression, depressed bacterial killing by phagocytes, and oxidative metabolic abnormalities. The neutrophil storage pool of neonates is markedly depleted compared with that of adults (86). Stem cell proliferative rates are at near maximal capacity and cannot increase appreciably in response to infection (87).

Clinical Manifestations

Most infants with septicemia present with nonspecific signs that are usually observed first by the nurse or mother rather than by the physician. The most common of these vague signs are temperature instability, lethargy, apnea, and poor feeding (88). Although hypothermia is more common, a temperature elevation above 37.8°C is significant in the neonate and frequently associated with bacterial infections, especially with temperatures higher than 39°C (89). The clinical signs in some infants may suggest respiratory or GI disease (e.g., tachypnea and cyanosis or vomiting, diarrhea, and abdominal distention). Septicemia must always be included in the differential diagnosis when evaluating an infant with these findings (88).

Clinical manifestations of sepsis in very-low-birth weight infants (501–1,500 g) include increasing apnea (55%), feeding intolerance, abdominal distension, or heme-positive stools (43%), increased respiratory support (29%), and lethargy and hypotonia (23%). Abnormal white blood cell count, unexplained metabolic acidosis, and hyperglycemia are noted in 46%, 11%, and 10%, respectively (47).

Although it is tempting to recommend an evaluation for septicemia in all infants with nonspecific clinical manifestations, this is impractical and unnecessary in many cases. A complete history and physical examination, coupled with clinical experience, are the best guides to determine the extent of the evaluation. If septicemia cannot be reasonably excluded on clinical grounds, a blood culture should be obtained and empiric antibiotics administered. Hepatosplenomegaly, jaundice, and petechiae are classic signs of neonatal infection but represent late manifestations.

Streptococcal Disease

In the 1970s, Group B β-hemolytic streptococci infections emerged a leading infectious cause of morbidity and mortality in the United States (90,91). By the 1980s, GBS were the most common gram-positive bacteria isolated from blood of infants with septicemia in North America (92). Although control measures such as intrapartum antibiotic therapy which were in widespread practice in the 1990s have reduced the incidence of early onset Group B streptococcal (GBS) disease, GBS remains an important cause of neonatal sepsis. GBS accounts for 10% to 40% of sepsis cases occurring in the first week of life (3,93,94).

In the mid 1980s, clinical trials demonstrated that administering intrapartum intravenous antibiotics could prevent early onset neonatal GBS sepsis (95). In response to these findings, the American Academy of Pediatrics in 1992 provided guidelines recommending intrapartum antibiotic prophylaxis (IAP) of selected GBS carriers (96). In 1996, with additional data and the collaborative efforts of clinicians, researchers, professional organizations and the public health community, the Centers for Disease Control and Prevention (CDC) issued consensus guidelines recommending IAP to prevent GBS maternal-infant transmission

(97,98). The 1996 national guidelines recommended that women colonized with GBS at 35 weeks or more of gestation or women with intrapartum risk factors (delivery <37 weeks gestation, intrapartum temperature ≥100.4°F or rupture of membranes ≥18 h) should be offered intrapartum chemoprophylaxis. Additionally, women having a previous infant with invasive GBS disease or women with GBS bacteriuria during pregnancy should also be offered intrapartum chemoprophylaxis. Because of the routine implementation of IAP, the incidence of early onset neonatal infections decreased by 65 percent, from 1.7 per 1000 live births in 1993 to 0.6 per 1000 in 1998 (99). With the decline in early onset GBS disease, there has been a concomitant rise in *E. coli* and ampicillin-resistant *E. coli* sepsis in very low birth weight and preterm infants (4). The CDC and the American College of Obstetricians and Gynecologists have recommended universal screening at 35 or more weeks of gestation and IAP for GBS-colonized women (100,101).

The epidemiology, pathogenesis, and clinical features of GBS disease have been defined (102). The organism is a common inhabitant of the female genital tract and can be isolated from vaginal and anorectal cultures of as many as 35% of asymptomatic pregnant women (102–105). Risk factors for maternal GBS colonization include lower parity, higher frequency of intercourse, multiple sexual partners, and concurrent colonization with *Candida* spp (104). Peripartum GB S colonization of the lower urogenital tract has been associated with several maternal complications including preterm labor, premature rupture of membranes, endometritis, chorioamnionitis, urinary tract infection, intrapartum or postpartum fever, late abortions, and invasive infections, such as bacteremia or meningitis (57,106). The identical serotype can be isolated frequently from urethral cultures of the sexual partners of these culture-positive women (107). Although most infected pregnant women have normal, healthy infants, 1% to 2% of pregnancies involving maternal infection result in stillbirths or infants with neonatal disease. Vertical transmission of group B Streptococci occurs in approximately 50% to 70% of mother-infant pairs, resulting in neonatal colonization rates of from 8% to 25%. Transmission is most likely to occur among infants born to heavily colonized mothers (108). The early-onset GBS syndrome occurs within the first 72 hours of life (mean age of onset 20 hours), and 65% of reported cases involve premature infants. There is often a history of other maternal obstetric complications (Table 47-2) (106). Onset is sudden and follows a fulminant course, with the primary focus of inflammation in the lungs, although meningitis can develop. Respiratory distress is the most common initial sign among infants with early onset meningitis (109). Apnea, hypotension, and disseminated intravascular coagulation cause rapid deterioration and often lead to the patient's demise within 24 hours. It is difficult to identify the infant with respiratory distress caused by GBS infection, because in 60% of infected patients, the chest radiograph shows a reticulogranular pattern with air bronchograms indistinguishable from that seen with uncomplicated hyaline membrane disease. The mortality

TABLE 47-2

RISK FACTORS FOR EARLY-ONSET GROUP B STREPTOCOCCAL DISEASE

Premature Delivery
Low Birth Weight
Increased interval between membrane rupture and delivery
Rupture of membranes before labor onset
Amnionitis and intrapartum fever
Maternal group B streptococcal rectovaginal colonization (especially heavy colonization)
African American race
Young (<20 yr) maternal age
Group B streptococcal bacteriuria during current pregnancy
Low level of capsular polysaccharide type-specific antibodies
Previous stillbirth or spontaneous abortion
Multiple gestation
Previous delivery of infant with group B streptococcal disease
Prolonged duration of intrauterine monitoring

Adapted from Schuchat A. Epidemiology of group B Streptococcal disease in the United States: Shifting paradigms. Clin Microbial Rev 1998; 11:497.

rate is approximately 6% and is inversely correlated with birth weight (110,111). All five GBS serotypes have been incriminated in early-onset disease in roughly similar proportions. A similar syndrome has been associated with groups D and G streptococci (112,113).

A late-onset syndrome caused by GBS or *L. monocytogenes* occurs most frequently at 2 to 4 weeks of age, but it may be seen as late as 16 weeks. The onset is insidious; poor feeding and fever are the most frequent presenting signs. A fulminant illness with rapid onset and progressive deterioration occasionally is encountered (114). Meningitis is seen in approximately 60% of infants with the late-onset syndrome, and GBS serotype III accounts for about 95% of these cases (102). Rarely, infants with late-onset meningitis caused by GBS present with hydrocephalus. These infants may appear to have uncomplicated hydrocephalus with normal lumbar cerebrospinal fluid (CSF). Examination of ventricular fluid reveals pleocytosis, and the organism is recovered on culture. Spinal fluid cultures of infants with meningitis caused by gram-positive organisms usually are sterile within 24 to 36 hours of therapy, and the mortality rate is 10% to 15%.

Approximately 20% of neonatal infections caused by GBS do not fit into the early- or late-onset syndromes and extend over a broad clinical spectrum involving many different organ systems. Several manifestations have been observed (102,115,116):

- Cellulitis
- Scalp abscess
- Impetigo
- Fasciitis
- Breast abscess
- Adenitis
- Supraglottitis
- Conjunctivitis
- Orbital cellulitis

- Ethmoiditis
- Otitis media
- Pneumonia complicated by empyema
- Myocarditis
- Endocarditis
- Hepatitis
- Septic arthritis
- Osteomyelitis
- Bursitis
- Urinary tract infection
- Omphalitis
- Peritonitis
- Asymptomatic transient bacteremia.

The transient bacteremia is remarkable because these infants appear clinically well and are cultured because of a history of maternal obstetric complications. A repeat blood culture before the institution of antibiotic therapy frequently is sterile.

Both relapses and reinfections can occur after invasive GBS infections (102). Reasons for relapse may include an inadequate penicillin dose, a short duration of therapy of the initial episode, or unrecognized foci of infection (e.g., endocarditis, brain abscess). Reinfection can occur because of maternal GBS mastitis (117). Rifampin (20 mg/kg/d for 4–7 days) has been used to eradicate GBS carriage in infants with recurrent disease and is given after completion of systemic penicillin therapy (117).

Coagulase-Positive Staphylococcal Disease

The phage group I S. aureus, which was common in the late 1950s, still exists in some nurseries and occasionally causes serious systemic neonatal disease. The pathogenicity of this organism is based on its ability to invade the skin and musculoskeletal system, producing furuncles, breast abscesses, adenitis, and osteomyelitis. Septicemia usually is secondary to local invasion. After S. aureus is recovered from blood cultures of neonates, a careful search should be made for a primary focus. Some group I S. aureus strains produce toxic shock syndrome toxin-1, formerly known as enterotoxin F or pyrogenic toxin C, and have caused toxic shock syndrome in older neonates (118,119). Clinical characteristics of this disease include the sudden onset of fever, diarrhea, shock, mucous membrane hyperemia, and a diffuse erythematous macular rash with subsequent desquamation of the hands and feet, commencing on about the fifth or sixth day of illness.

In the early 1970s, phage group II coagulase-positive staphylococci emerged as a common cause of neonatal infection. Although this organism may be invasive, pathogenicity depends principally on production of exotoxins (e.g., exfoliative or epidermolytic toxins A and B). Common areas of primary infection include the umbilical stump, conjunctiva, and throat; infection of a surgical wound has been described (120). The exfoliative toxins act on the zona granulosa of the epidermis and cause epidermal splitting through activity of the toxins on the desmosomes (121). Clinical disease may take one of several forms,

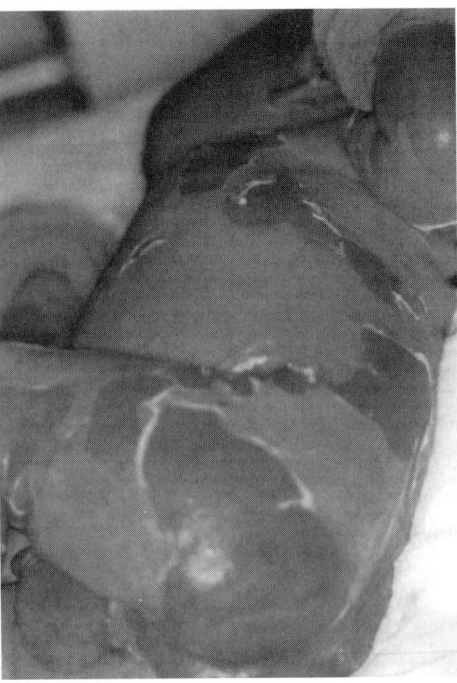

Figure 47-1 A 10-day-old Caucasian boy with staphylococcal scalded skin syndrome. He was treated with fluids, oral dicloxacillin, and wound care. His skin healed completely and without scarring within 2 weeks of this photograph being taken.

including bullous impetigo, toxic epidermal necrolysis (Ritter disease), and nonstreptococcal scarlatina. Collectively, these diseases have been referred to as the expanded scalded skin syndrome (Fig. 47-1) (122).

The initial finding in Ritter disease is generalized erythema associated with edema and tenderness on palpation, usually noticed between days 3 and 16 of life (123). After several days, a distinctive desquamation of large sheets of epidermis occurs, which is different from the fine desquamation observed in the second and third weeks of streptococcal scarlet fever. Large flaccid bullae commonly observed in Ritter disease will, on rupture, leave a tender, weeping erythematous base. Some infants may appear quite toxic with the generalized form of disease. A rare, congenital form of staphylococcal scalded skin syndrome has been described (124). Spread within a nursery can occur, and its recognition warrants the prompt institution of infection control measures to limit the spread of the toxigenic strain of S. aureus (125).

Umbilical venous or arterial catheters and central venous lines are well-recognized risk factors for staphylococcal bacteremia. S. aureus is second only to coagulase-negative staphylococci as a cause of catheter-related infections (126).

The mortality rate for neonates with S. aureus bacteremia is about 20%. LBW infants are at highest risk of death from this infection (127).

Coagulase-Negative Staphylococcal Disease

The isolation of coagulase-negative staphylococci from blood, CSF, or urine of newborns with clinical signs of sepsis can be significant, and these bacteria should not be dismissed as contaminants. Of the at least 30 recognized coagulase-negative staphylococcal species, *S. epidermidis* is clinically the most significant for neonates (128–130). Experience indicates that these bacteria are responsible for about 10% to 27% of all cases of sepsis in NICUs, but can account for as many as 48% of late-onset sepsis cases in VLBW infants (3,92) Coagulase-negative staphylococcal infections are nosocomial in origin and result in substantially longer hospitalizations for affected infants (131,132). Risk of infection with these organisms increases with decreasing gestational age and birth weight (133–136).

Clinical manifestations of coagulase-negative staphylococcal infections are similar to those caused by other pathogens and include apnea, bradycardia, temperature instability (e.g., hypothermia, hyperthermia), respiratory distress (e.g., tachypnea, retractions, cyanosis), GI manifestations (e.g., poor feeding, abdominal distention, bloody stools), lethargy, and metabolic acidosis (12,129). Clinical illnesses include septicemia, meningitis with or without CSF abnormalities, necrotizing enterocolitis, pneumonia, omphalitis, soft tissue abscesses associated with persistent bacteremia, endocarditis, and scalp abscesses and osteomyelitis at insertion sites of fetal monitoring electrodes (133–144).

Risk factors for coagulase-negative staphylococcal infections include the presence of foreign bodies, such as central venous lines, ventriculoperitoneal shunts, or peritoneal dialysis catheters, prior antibiotic therapy, and intravenous infusion of lipid emulsions for nutritional support (129, 145,146). The organisms travel along catheter tracks from colonization sites. They eventually adhere to, and proliferate on, certain biosynthetic materials and later cause local or systemic reactions. The mechanism by which adherence occurs appears initially to involve hydrophobic and electrostatic interactions between the bacteria and the biopolymers (129). Once attached, a viscous exopolysaccharide referred to as slime is formed. Slime covers the bacteria to form a surface biofilm that protects them from such environmental factors as antibiotics and host defenses although allowing continued access to nutrition (129). The density of the biofilm may be increased if the organisms are exposed to subinhibitory concentrations of antibiotics to which they are susceptible (e.g., vancomycin) (147). Slime appears to inhibit neutrophil chemotaxis and phagocytosis and the lymphoproliferative responses of mononuclear cells to mitogens (148,149). Slime-producing strains account for most coagulase-negative staphylococci isolated from infants with invasive infections (135). Ineffective opsonophagocytosis as a result of intrinsic deficiencies in neonatal host defenses contributes to the increased susceptibility of LBW infants to infection with these organisms (150,151).

Coagulase-negative staphylococci produce a variety of toxins that may serve as virulence factors, including hemolysins, proteases, urease, and fibrinolysin (12). Most fecal isolates produce a hemolysin that functionally and immunologically is identical to the delta toxin produced by *S. aureus* (152). This toxin causes severe mucosal necrosis

and hemorrhage when injected into ligated infant rat bowel loops and may play a role in the pathogenesis of neonatal necrotizing enterocolitis (153–154).

Listeria monocytogenes Disease

The incidence of perinatal listeriosis decreased by about 51% between 1989 and 1993, from 17.4 to 8.6 per 100,000 persons younger than 1 year of age (155–156). This reduction was related temporally with industry, regulatory, and educational efforts to aggressively enforce food monitoring policies.

The pathogenesis of clinical diseases caused by *L. monocytogenes* is similar to those caused by GBS. A fulminant, disseminated disease (granulomatosis infantiseptica) may occur during the first several days of life. The pathogen is acquired transplacentally or by aspiration at the time of vaginal delivery, and multiple organ systems (e.g., liver, spleen, kidneys, lungs, brain, and skin) are involved; 35% to 55% of infants die of their infection (157,158). The infant frequently presents with hypothermia, lethargy, and poor feeding. Early passage of meconium in a premature infant suggests *Listeria* infection (159). A characteristic rash consisting of small, salmon-colored papules scattered primarily on the trunk can be observed in some infants. The chest roentgenogram shows parenchymal infiltrates suggestive of aspiration pneumonitis in most infants. A miliary-type of bronchopneumonia can be seen in some cases. *Listeria* serotypes Ia, Ib, and IVb produce the early onset disease, whereas serotype IVb is the predominant type in late-onset meningitic disease (160).

A delayed form of neonatal listeriosis occurs during the second through fifth weeks of life and primarily involves the meninges (160,161). The infected infant usually is the full-term product of an uncomplicated labor and delivery. Onset of symptoms and signs is relatively insidious and indistinguishable from those observed with meningitis caused by other pathogens. The source of the organism in late-onset disease is unclear. Although acquisition of *Listeria* may occur during passage through an infected birth canal, it appears that most cases result from postpartum horizontal spread. In favor of the latter route of infection are several reported clusters of neonatal listeriosis and the demonstration of cross-infections between newborns using enzyme electrophoretic typing and DNA fingerprinting (157,162–164).

The peripheral leukocyte count usually shows a brisk leukocytosis, with a predominance of polymorphonuclear leukocytes in the differential count (165). A significant elevation in the number of monocytes, to 7% to 21% of the total leukocyte count, has been documented on admission laboratory evaluation of infected infants. A monocytosis of this magnitude can be demonstrated in most remaining infants on repetitive testing of the peripheral leukocyte count, but monocytes typically are not found in the spinal fluid of infants infected with *L. monocytogenes*. Polymorphonuclear leukocytes predominate in about 75% of cases, with a relative lymphocytosis in the remaining 25%. In contrast, adults with *Listeria* meningoencephalitis may have CSF monocytosis of 80% to 90% (158). As with other pyogenic meningitides, hypoglycorrhachia and elevated protein concentrations are frequent findings. Examination of the stained smear of spinal fluid has not been rewarding in more than 50% of cases. This is a reflection of the relatively low concentrations of organisms in the fluid. The bacteriology laboratory should be forewarned of the clinical suspicion of *Listeria* meningitis, because these microorganisms occasionally are discarded as contaminants because of their tinctorial and morphologic similarities with diphtheroids. Overnight refrigeration of spinal fluid specimens frequently enhances growth of this organism.

Enterococcal Infection

Group D streptococci were formerly divided into enterococcal and nonenterococcal types. The enterococci are now included in the new genus *Enterococcus*; most neonatal infections are caused by *Enterococcus faecalis* and, to a lesser extent, by *E. faecium* (166–168).

Early onset enterococcal disease (less than 7 days of age) is relatively mild and presents clinically with respiratory distress or diarrhea. No associations with underlying conditions, invasive procedures, or maternal obstetric complications have been observed (169). Late-onset disease (≥7 days of age) most commonly afflicts low-birth weight infants with complicated clinical problems that often require surgical procedures (e.g., bowel resection), central venous catheters, or prior treatment with antimicrobials. Clinical manifestations of late-onset disease include apnea, bradycardia, circulatory failure, meningitis, pneumonia, scalp abscesses, catheter-related bacteremia, and necrotizing enterocolitis-associated septicemia (169). About 20% of enterococcal blood isolates represent skin contamination; clinical correlation is needed to differentiate contamination from true infection (167).

Enterococci can spread rapidly within a nursery (170). Nosocomial outbreaks of enterococcal septicemia in NICUs are well documented (168,171). The mortality rate is estimated at 6% to 11%, but it can be as high as 17% in infants with necrotizing enterocolitis-associated septicemia (167,169).

The importance of identifying *Enterococcus* as the etiologic agent in septicemia primarily relates to selection of proper antimicrobial agents. The enterococci are moderately resistant to penicillin alone, as a result of certain properties of their penicillin-binding proteins (167,172). Some enterococcal strains have acquired new mechanisms of antibiotic resistance that include β-lactamase production and high-level aminoglycoside resistance (minimal inhibitory concentrations [MIC] ≥2,000 μg/mL) (170,173,174). Strains resistant to the glycopeptides vancomycin and teicoplanin (glycopeptide-resistant enterococci) were first described in 1987 and since have emerged as major nosocomial pathogens (175–179). Nonenterococcal group D streptococci continue to be susceptible to penicillin (167).

Gram-Negative Bacterial Infection

In North America, *E. coli* is the most common gram-negative organism causing septicemia during the neonatal period. *Klebsiella* and *Enterobacter* strains are second (3,92). In contradistinction to illness caused by GBS and *L. monocytogenes*, *E. coli* infections do not fit into distinct clinical syndromes of early- and late-onset disease. Approximately 40% of *E. coli* strains causing septicemia possess K1 capsular antigen, and strains identical with those isolated from blood cultures usually can be identified in the patient's nasopharynx or rectal cultures. The clinical features of *E. coli* sepsis generally are similar to those observed in infants with disease caused by other pathogens. Respiratory distress is noted in about 73% with *E. coli* sepsis occurring during the first week of life (180). Localized *E. coli* infections have included breast abscess, cellulitis, pneumonia, lung abscess, empyema, osteomyelitis, septic arthritis, urinary tract infection, ascending cholangitis, and otitis media.

An increase in the proportion of neonatal *E. coli* sepsis cases caused by ampicillin-resistant strains has been noted by several investigators (3,180–181) This shift occurred as maternal intrapartum prophylaxis for the prevention of early onset GBS sepsis was being implemented more widely by obstetricians at these medical centers. Most deaths were seen in neonates infected with ampicillin-resistant *E. coli* strains.

Pseudomonas septicemia may present with a characteristic violaceous papular lesion or lesions that, after several days, develop central necrosis. Although these skin lesions most commonly are seen in *Pseudomonas* infection, they may be associated with other organisms (182). *Pseudomonas* typically is encountered in late-onset sepsis, although occasional newborns with an early-onset form of this infection have been reported.

Neonatal infections caused by *H. influenzae* biotype IV have increased in frequency in the last 20 years and currently account for about 8% of early-onset sepsis in very LBW infants (401–1,500 g) (3,183). These strains are nontypeable, have a distinct multilocus enzyme genotype revealed by clonal analysis, express peritrichous fimbriae and a variant P6 outer membrane protein, and have a characteristic outer membrane electrophoretic profile. Genetic analysis suggests that these strains represent a cryptic genospecies only distantly related to *H. influenzae* or *Haemophilus haemolyticus* (183–184).

Anaerobic Infections

Anaerobes account for up to 25% of all bacteria isolated from blood cultures of neonates with suspected septicemia in various studies (185–188). A recent retrospective review of neonatal bacterial infections suggests that the incidence of anaerobic isolates is about 1% (189). Bacteroides spp, primarily *Bacteroides fragilis*, and clostridia are most commonly recovered (187). *Peptostreptococcus* spp, *Veillonella* spp, *Propionibacterium acnes*, *Eubacterium* spp, and Fusobacterium spp occur relatively infrequently. Anaerobes are found mixed in cultures with aerobic bacteria in about one-third of cases. Clinical illnesses include transient bacteremia, fulminant septicemia, postoperative infections, and intrauterine death associated with septic abortion (185). Localized diseases such as omphalitis, cellulitis, and necrotizing fasciitis are seen commonly with clostridia (190). Conditions predisposing to anaerobic septicemia include prolonged rupture of membranes, chorioamnionitis, prematurity, and GI disease.

Anaerobes isolated from blood within the first 2 days of life are usually gram-positive and penicillin G-susceptible, but those isolated from older newborns tend to be gram-negative and penicillin G-resistant (186). Gram-positive anaerobes are more likely to be recovered from blood of infants with sepsis associated with chorioamnionitis, whereas gram-negative anaerobes predominate in necrotizing enterocolitis-associated bacteremia (186). The mortality rates for reported cases of anaerobic septicemia are about 35% for illnesses caused by *Bacteroides* spp and 12% for other anaerobes (187).

Genital Mycoplasmas

M. hominis and *U. urealyticum* occasionally are isolated from the blood of neonates with sepsis. Cassell and colleagues (36) observed concomitant bacteremia in 40% and 26% of preterm infants with positive endotracheal cultures for *M. hominis* and *U. urealyticum*, respectively. Other investigators were unable to recover genital mycoplasmas from the blood or CSF of neonates with suspected sepsis (191–192). An association between persistent pulmonary hypertension and *U. urealyticum* sepsis and pneumonia has been observed (193).

Fungal Infections

Fungal sepsis occurs in as many as 12% of LBW infants (3). Most cases are as a result of *Candida* spp, particularly *C. albicans* (194–196). *C. tropicalis, C. parapsilosis, C. lusitaniae,* and *C. glabrata* also cause systemic candidiasis (196). Congenital candidiasis is uncommon and results from ascending infection through intact membranes. It usually manifests with early skin lesions (e.g., maculopapular rash, pustules, vesicles, desquamation, skin abscesses), but disseminated and life-threatening infections can occur (197–198).

The incidence of candidemia in NICUs is increasing steadily. In one such unit in Norfolk, Virginia, the rate of candidemia increased over 11-fold in the 15-year period between 1981 and 1995. Additionally, *C. parapsilosis* was responsible for 60% of all candidemias during the last 5 years of the study period (199).

Risk factors for late-onset systemic candidiasis include prematurity, low birth weight, use of broad-spectrum antimicrobial agents, H2 blocker therapy, steroid therapy, central vascular catheters, parenteral hyperalimentation, intralipid infusions, prolonged endotracheal intubation, necrotizing enterocolitis, and immunologic immaturity

(200–202). The most important of these factors appears to be the number of prior antibiotics and the duration of therapy (203–204). LBW infants in whom mucocutaneous candidiasis develops are at considerable risk of subsequent invasive disease (203–205). Infants with invasive candidiasis caused by *C. albicans* are more likely to have antecedent candidal thrush or perineal dermatitis and to die of their infection than neonates with severe *C. parapsilosis* infections (199,206). Clinical manifestations vary and are indistinguishable from those caused by other pathogens. A fungal cause for sepsis should be considered strongly in an infant weighing less than 1,500 g who has been hospitalized for a prolonged period, is receiving parenteral hyperalimentation through a central vascular catheter, and previously has been treated with multiple antibiotics; a history of GI disease or surgery adds to the clinical suspicion. Diseases caused by *Candida* spp include, but are not limited to, pneumonia, endocarditis, endophthalmitis, meningitis, cerebral abscesses, pyelonephritis, renal mycetoma (fungal balls), peritonitis, hepatosplenic abscesses, arthritis, and osteomyelitis (194,207–215).

Malassezia furfur causes invasive neonatal fungal disease. Most infections involve chronically ill premature infants who are receiving lipid emulsions through a central venous catheter (216). The most commonly reported presenting signs include fever (50%) and respiratory distress (50%). Pathologic analysis reveals mycotic thrombi around catheter tips, endocardial vegetations, and lung lesions that include mycotic emboli with occlusion of pulmonary arteries, septic thrombi, pulmonary vasculitis, and alveolitis (216). Involvement of other organs is uncommon. *Malassezia pachydermatis* is a recently recognized human pathogen that has been incriminated in NICU outbreaks of bloodstream, urinary tract, and central nervous system infections. In one reported outbreak, the source of *M. pachydermatis* was the contaminated hands of health care workers who were colonized from their pet dogs at home (217). Systemic infections as a result of other fungi such as *Torulopsis glabrata, Hansen ula anomala, Aspergillus* spp, *Cryptococcus neoformans, Coccidioides immitis, Blastomyces* spp, and *Trichosporon beigelii* are rare (218–221).

Laboratory Tests and Findings

Since the early 1970s, several screening tests and scoring systems have been described that are purported to aid the physician in making the diagnosis of neonatal infection. Although a few are helpful in identifying the infant at high risk of developing infection, the diagnosis of septicemia can be made only by recovery of the organism from blood cultures or other normally sterile body fluids (221,222). It is imperative that these cultures be obtained by strict aseptic technique. Blood should be obtained from a peripheral vein rather than from the umbilical vessels, the outer several millimeters of which are contaminated frequently with bacteria. Femoral vein aspiration may result in cultures contaminated with coliform organisms from the perineum. Heelstick samples have low sensitivities. The skin overlying the vein to be punctured should be cleansed with an antiseptic solution, such as an iodophor, and allowed to dry for maximal antiseptic effect. The amount of blood drawn is critical; 1 to 2 mL of blood is required for optimal results (223). The sensitivity of a single blood culture in identifying septicemia is only 80% (222). Obtaining blood cultures from multiple sites may enhance the yield and aid in identifying false-positive results (224). Quantitative blood cultures, if available, are helpful in differentiating true pathogens from culture contaminants (225,226). Routine blood culture methods are sufficient for the detection of *Candida* septicemia (227); however, if *M. furfur* is a suspected pathogen, the microbiology laboratory should be alerted so that blood can be inoculated onto special media that provide for the organism's absolute nutritional requirement for medium-chain fatty acids (196).

It frequently is helpful to obtain cultures of other sites before initiating antimicrobial therapy. For example, percutaneous bladder aspiration of urine for culture can be helpful in identifying the urinary tract as the focus of infection. This is particularly true for illness occurring after the third postnatal day. Nasopharyngeal, skin, umbilical cord, gastric, and rectal cultures frequently are positive in the early septicemic form of listeriosis and GBS disease. However, these colonization sites are not predictive of the cause of bloodstream infection and should not be used to guide antimicrobial therapy (228). All clinically stable infants with suspected septicemia should have CSF obtained for examination and culture before therapy. This practice has been challenged for infants younger than 7 days of age because of its low yield; the yield from a lumbar puncture is much higher when performed on infants older than 1 week of age (229–235). Practitioners opting to forego performing a lumbar puncture for infants with suspected early onset sepsis should anticipate that, on occasion, the diagnosis of meningitis will be delayed or missed because not all newborns with bacterial meningitis have positive blood culture results (234,236).

The peripheral leukocyte count is the most frequently used indirect indicator of bacterial infection. After correction for the nucleated erythrocyte count, the total absolute neutrophil count and the ratio of immature to total neutrophilic forms are compared with normal standard values for age. In the absence of maternal hypertension, severe asphyxia, periventricular hemorrhage, maternal fever, or hemolytic disease, absolute total neutropenia and an elevated ratio of immature to total neutrophilic forms suggest bacterial infection (237,238). Infants born in high-altitude areas have higher total and immature neutrophil counts (239). Wide interreader differences in band neutrophil identification have been observed, thereby limiting the utility of the immature to total neutrophil ratio in actual clinical practice (240). Repeating complete blood counts within 24 hours of birth may enhance the value of the test as a screen for sepsis high-risk infants (239). In the absence of clinical signs of sepsis, leukocyte values are unlikely to rule out infection. In a prospective, observational study of 856 near-term or term neonates without clinical signs of

sepsis who were exposed to maternal chorioamnionitis, 99% had at least 1 abnormal neutrophil value based on published reference values (237–242). Single or serial neutrophil values did not assist in the diagnosis of early onset infection or determination of duration of antibiotic therapy in the at risk but culture-negative infants (243).

Gastric aspirate stains and culture, erythrocyte sedimentation rate, C-reactive protein (CRP), and the nitroblue tetrazolium test have not proved useful as indicators of bacterial infection, although in combination these tests may offer some guidance (244). CRP values appear not to be influenced by perinatal asphyxia, hyperbilirubinemia, periventricular hemorrhage, or respiratory distress syndrome (245). Serial CRP measurements may be helpful in identifying infants not likely to be infected and in whom antibiotics can be safely stopped (246). The detection of interleukin-6 (IL-6) in serum, especially in conjunction with an elevated CRP or procalcitonin measurement, may be useful in the early diagnosis of neonatal infection (243–252). The levels of granulocyte colony-stimulating factor, neutrophil CD11b expression, circulating intracellular adhesion molecule-1, interleukin-1 receptor antagonist (IL-1ra), serum procalcitonin, and interleukin-8 are all elevated in newborns with sepsis, but how these laboratory findings can best be utilized for the diagnosis of neonatal sepsis is yet to be defined (247,249,250,253,254). In one study, IL-1ra and IL-6 levels were found to be elevated (a 15-fold median maximal increase) 2 days before a diagnosis of sepsis was made (250).

Detection of the soluble antigens of *E. coli* Kl, GBS, *H. influenzae* type b, *N. meningitidis*, and *S. pneumoniae* by latex particle agglutination (LPA) is useful for identifying the infant infected with these pathogens. The absence of antigen does not rule out infection by these organisms. Substantial sensitivity differences have been found among the commercially available LPA assays for GBS antigen (255). False-positive LPA test results for GBS in urine specimens can result from contamination of bag specimens with these bacteria from perineal and rectal colonization, cross-reacting antigens, or absorption of antigen from the GI tract (256,257). Similar false-positive test results may be obtained for the other bacteria. Rapid diagnosis of invasive *Candida* infection by detection of its circulating cell wall (e.g., mannan), cytoplasmic (e.g., enolase), or heat-labile antigens is possible, although the reliability of these tests is yet to be proved (258).

Therapy

After septicemia is suspected, suitable cultures should be obtained and therapy with ampicillin and an aminoglycoside started immediately. If meningitis has been excluded, ampicillin is administered intravenously or intramuscularly in individual doses of 50 mg/kg given every 12 hours, or 8 hours for infants weighing <2,000 g or ≥2,000 g, respectively. The frequency is increased 3 or 4 times daily for infants 1 to 4 weeks of age, depending on their birth weight. The selection of the aminoglycoside antibiotic should be based on antimicrobial susceptibilities of enteric organisms isolated from infants in each nursery. Gentamicin is the drug of choice for treatment of infections caused by susceptible gram-negative organisms and is administered intravenously or intramuscularly in a dosage of 4 to 5 mg/kg at 24 to 48 hour intervals depending on the infant's postmenstrual and postnatal age (259).

Aminoglycoside-resistant E. coli have been encountered in some nurseries in North America. In these nurseries or in an infant from whom an isolate is shown to be resistant to kanamycin or gentamicin, amikacin or cefotaxime should be used. Studies have demonstrated no significant ototoxicity in infants and children who were treated in the neonatal period with kanamycin or gentamicin (48). However, in premature infants and in those receiving these drugs for prolonged periods, brainstem evoked response audiometry should be performed whenever possible. Serum concentrations of the aminoglycosides should be monitored in LBW premature infants because of erratic absorption and elimination of the drugs in these infants. Although cefotaxime should not be used routinely for initial empiric therapy of neonatal sepsis, it is an effective agent when used alone or combined with an aminoglycoside for infections caused by coliform bacilli.

When the type of skin lesions or historic experience suggests the possibility of Pseudomonas infection, ceftazidime, piperacillin or ticarcillin with or without an aminoglycoside is the therapy of choice. Although not approved for use in neonates by the Food and Drug Administration, we have successfully used ticarcillin-clavulanate and piperacillin-tazobactam for treatment of sepsis caused by multiresistant gram-negative enteric bacilli, Pseudomonas, and anaerobic bacteria.

If S. aureus sepsis is suspected but not proved, parenteral methicillin or nafcillin should be substituted for penicillin or ampicillin, because approximately 80% of these staphylococci will be penicillin-resistant. Although gentamicin and kanamycin possess activity against most staphylococci, these agents cannot be recommended because there are no studies of their efficacy in neonatal staphylococcal disease. For disease caused by coagulase negative staphylococci or multiresistant S. aureus strains, vancomycin is the preferred therapy. Peak and trough serum vancomycin concentrations should be monitored because of the drug's narrow therapeutic index.

After the pathogen is identified and its antimicrobial susceptibilities are known, the most appropriate drug or drugs should be selected. As a general rule, gentamicin alone or in combination with ampicillin, or cefotaxime alone or in combination with an aminoglycoside, should be used for susceptible E. coli, Klebsiella spp, and Enterobacter spp; amikacin alone or in combination with cefotaxime for gentamicin-resistant coliform bacteria; ceftazidime, piperacillin, ticarcillin, pipercillin-tazobactam, or ticarcillin-clavulanate, with or without an aminoglycoside, for Pseudomonas; ampicillin alone or in combination with an aminoglycoside for P. mirabilis, enterococci, and L. monocytogenes; and penicillin for other gram-positive organisms, except for penicillin-resistant S. aureus, for which methi-

cillin or nafcillin is the drug of choice. Vancomycin is used for coagulase-negative staphylococci and MRSA. Rarely, coagulase-negative staphylococcal strains that are resistant to vancomycin can emerge during treatment with this agent (260). S. aureus strains with reduced susceptibility to vancomycin (glycopeptide-intermediate S. aureus [GISA]) have been isolated from a few patients with a variety of infections. The first such clinical isolate was described in a 4-month-old Japanese infant with a nosocomial surgical site infection (261–262). No GISA strains have been identified in newborns to date. Treatment of GISA-related infections generally requires the use of drugs such as linezolid. The MIC and minimal bactericidal concentration (MBC) of penicillin and ampicillin should be determined for GBS because a small percentage of these organisms are tolerant (i.e., have an MBC to MIC ratio greater than 32) to these antibiotics (263). These strains are best treated with a penicillin-aminoglycoside combination. Penicillin resistant and vancomycin-tolerant pneumococci have been reported in newborn infants in France but not yet in North America (264). The therapeutic options for vancomycin-resistant enterococcal infections in neonates are seriously limited. Some strains may be susceptible to a combination of penicillin or ampicillin and an aminoglycoside. Chloramphenicol or tetracyclines may be effective against some strains, but these drugs have serious toxicities for neonates. Nitrofurantoin is active against many vancomycin-resistant enterococcal strains and has been used to treat enterococcal urinary tract infections in adults. Dalfopristin-quinupristin is approved for use in adults, but there are no data on its use in infants. Several investigational ketolides, oxazolidinones, glycylcyclines, and even newer semisynthetic glycopeptides with in vitro activities against vancomycin-resistant enterococci are being evaluated (265). U. urealyticum infections are treated with erythromycin (266).

Three classes of antifungals are commonly used in the treatment of systemic fungal infections in neonates: the polyene macrolides (amphotericin B [deoxycholate and lipid preparations]); the azoles (fluconazole); and the fluorinated pyrimidines (flucytosine). The drug of choice for systemic fungal infections is amphotericin B, with or without flucytosine (194,267). The half-life and serum concentrations of amphotericin B are highly variable during the neonatal period (268). The drug appears to be better tolerated by infants than older children and adults, but renal and hepatic functions should be monitored carefully (194,269). The optimal daily dosage of amphotericin B is not universally agreed on. The most commonly used dosage regimen is to begin with 0.5 mg/kg of the drug on the first day and, if tolerated, to increase the daily dosage to 1.0 mg/kg by the second or third day of treatment. The cumulative dosage of amphotericin B needed for the adequate treatment of systemic Candida infection is not well defined, but it is estimated to be 20 to 30 mg/kg (194). Resistance to amphotericin B among Candida species is not a major clinical problem (270). Amphotericin B frequently is combined with flucytosine for the treatment of central nervous system fungal infection because of flucytosine's excellent CSF penetration and the *in vitro* synergy of this drug combination against *Candida*. GI intolerance, myelosuppression, and hepatotoxicity are common side effects of flucytosine (194).

Experience with the use of liposomal amphotericin B preparations in newborns is growing (271–276). Linder and colleagues (275) compared the effectiveness and tolerability of three antifungal preparations, amphotericin B, liposomal amphotericin B (LamB) and amphotericin B colloidal dispersion (ABCD), for the treatment of 52 neonates with Candida bloodstream infection. Sterilization of the blood was achieved with amphotericin B in 68% of patients, LamB in 83% and ABCD in 57%, when used as monotherapy; with the addition of a second antifungal agent, success rates were 100%, 83.3%, and 92.8%, respectively. There were no differences between the groups in the time to resolution of fungemia. No patients had immediate local or systemic adverse events and none showed deterioration in renal function. Juster-Reicher and colleagues (276) evaluated high-dose (5–7 mg/kg/day) liposomal amphotericin B in 37 very low birth weight infants with systemic candidiasis. Candidiasis was as a result of *C. parapsilosis* in 17 cases, and *C. albicans* in 15 cases. Fungal eradication was achieved in (95%) episodes; median duration of therapy until fungal eradication was 8.7 ± 4.5 days. The authors concluded that high-dose liposomal amphotericin B was effective and safe in the treatment of neonatal candidiasis. Additionally, fungal eradication was more rapid in patients treated early with high doses and in patients who received high-dose liposomal amphotericin B as first-line therapy. At present, lipid formulations of amphotericin B do not appear to be more efficacious than conventional amphotericin B deoxycholate, and their use should be limited to patients who are either refractory to, or intolerant of, the regular amphotericin B preparation (277).

The use of fluconazole for the treatment of neonatal candidiasis is increasing slowly, but the cumulative published experience is meager (278–280). Wenzl and colleagues (280) successfully treated three premature infants (gestational ages 24 to 29 weeks) with *C. albicans* sepsis using oral fluconazole at doses of 4.5 to 6 mg/kg once daily for 4 to 6 weeks. Huttova and associates (279) from the Slovak Republic treated 40 newborns with fluconazole, 28 of whom weighed less than 1,500 g at birth. All infants had fungemia with *C. albicans*. Fluconazole was administered as a single daily intravenous dose of 6 mg/kg for a total of 6 to 48 days. A cure rate of 80% was achieved; 10% died as a direct consequence of their infection. Mild elevations of liver enzyme concentrations were noted in 5% of neonates. The same group has subsequently reported their experience in 40 neonates with breakthrough fungemias as a result of *C. albicans* and *C. parapsilosis* appearing although receiving fluconazole therapy even though initial antifungal susceptibility testing demonstrated that the isolates were susceptible to fluconazole (281). At present, there is little evidence to support the use of fluconazole as monotherapy in neonatal fungal sepsis.

Guidelines for determining duration of therapy in the neonatal period often are lacking, because objective evidence of illness may be minimal. Culture of the blood should be repeated 24 to 48 hours after initiation of therapy; if positive, alteration of therapy may be necessary. In the absence of deep tissue involvement or abscess formation, treatment usually is continued 5 to 7 days after clinical improvement. If multiple organs are involved or clinical response is slow, treatment may need to be continued for 2 to 3 weeks.

Suspected central venous catheter-related bacterial sepsis can be managed initially with the intraluminal infusion of vancomycin combined with ceftazidime or an aminoglycoside. After infection is confirmed and the pathogen identified, single-drug therapy usually is sufficient. Reported cure rates with antibiotics alone without catheter removal have ranged from 50% to more than 90% for pediatric patients. Persistently positive blood cultures after 2 to 4 days of appropriate antimicrobial therapy warrants catheter removal. A continuous infusion of a low dose of urokinase for 24 hours may help in clearing catheter-related infections in some infants who fail conventional antibiotic therapy but this product is no longer available (282). Patients responding to antibiotic therapy should be treated for 2 to 3 weeks or at least for 10 days from the time of the first negative blood culture. Catheter-related fungal infections are rarely cured without catheter removal (283).

Immunotherapy of neonatal sepsis is discussed in Chapter 46. Extracorporeal membrane oxygenation for newborns with persistent pulmonary hypertension as a result of overwhelming early onset GBS sepsis may improve their survival (284).

Prevention

The identification of high-risk GBS-carrier mothers and the subsequent interruption of vertical transmission by intrapartum maternal chemotherapy can prevent many cases of early-onset neonatal GBS disease (43,49,99,110). Many approaches have been suggested and some have been tested. They range from giving penicillin prophylaxis to all newborns or ceftriaxone prophylaxis to all women in labor, to screening all pregnant women for GBS carriage at one or more points in pregnancy and treating antepartum or intrapartum with penicillin or ampicillin, to only offering intrapartum antibiotics to women who meet certain criteria that place them at high risk of delivering an infant with early onset GBS disease. Currently, the CDC and the American College of Obstetricians and Gynecologists recommend universal screening to detect maternal GBS colonization and treatment of those gravidas who are positive with intrapartum antibiotics (Table 47-3).

Intrapartum antibiotic prophylaxis-related adverse effects include the small but real risk of death from anaphylaxis for women (estimated risk of 0.001%) and an increase in the proportion of infants with sepsis caused by ampicillin-resistant bacteria (4). A recent study examined the susceptibility profile of 119 colonizing and 8 invasive GBS strains

TABLE 47-3

SUMMARY OF CENTERS FOR DISEASE CONTROL AND PREVENTION RECOMMENDATIONS FOR THE PREVENTION OF NEONATAL EARLY-ONSET GROUP B STREPTOCOCCAL SEPSIS

- All pregnant women should be screened at 35–37 weeks' gestation for vaginal and rectal GBS colonization. At the time of labor or rupture of membranes, intrapartum chemoprophylaxis should be given to all pregnant women identified as GBS carriers.
- Women with GBS isolated from the urine in any concentration during their current pregnancy should receive intrapartum chemoprophylaxis.
- Women who have previously given birth to an infant with invasive GBS disease should receive intrapartum chemoprophylaxis.
- If the result of GBS culture is not known at the onset of labor, intrapartum chemoprophylaxis should be administered to women with any of the following risk factors: gestation <37 weeks, duration of membrane rupture ≥18 hours, or a temperature of ≥100.4°F (≥38.0°C).
- Women with threatened preterm (<37 weeks' gestation) delivery should be assessed for need for intrapartum prophylaxis to prevent perinatal GBS disease.
- GBS-colonized women who have a planned cesarean delivery performed before rupture of membranes should not routinely receive intrapartum chemoprophylaxis for perinatal GBS disease prevention.
- For intrapartum chemoprophylaxis, the following regimen is recommended for women without penicillin allergy: penicillin G, 5 million units intravenously initial dose, then 2.5 million units intravenously every 4 hours until delivery. An alternative regimen is ampicillin, 2 g intravenously initial dose, then 1 g intravenously every 4 hours until delivery.
- Intrapartum chemoprophylaxis for penicillin-allergic women but not at high risk for anaphylaxis should be given cefazolin, 2 g intravenously initial dose, then 1 g intravenously every 8 hours until delivery. Women at high risk for anaphylaxis should be given either clindamycin, 900 mg intravenously every 8 hours until delivery, OR erythromycin, 500 mg intravenously every 6 hours until delivery.
- Routine use of antimicrobial prophylaxis for newborns whose mothers received intrapartum chemoprophylaxis for GBS infection is not recommended.

Adapted from Schrag S, Gorwitz R, Fultz-Butts K, et al. Prevention of perinatal group B streptococcal disease. Revised guidelines from CDC. *MMWR Recomm Rep* 2002;51:1, with permission.

collected from two hospitals in Birmingham, Alabama, between January 1996 and September 1997 from predominantly vaginally delivered term newborns and found that the GBS isolates almost universally were penicillin susceptible, with only a small minority of the strains showing moderate penicillin or ampicillin susceptibility (285). However, between 16% to 21% of GBS isolates are erythromycin resistant and 4% to 15% are clindamycin resistant, which raises concerns about the possible inadequacy of currently recommended alternatives for penicillin-allergic women (285,286).

The rectovaginal swabs for GBS cultures should be placed in a transport medium that will maintain GBS viability, unless direct inoculation into a selective broth medium is possible. One study suggests that rectovaginal swabs placed in standard transport media can be used as long as the specimens subsequently are transferred to selective growth media within 2 hours of collection (287).

The management of infants born to women given intrapartum antimicrobial prophylaxis depends on their clinical status. If signs or symptoms suggestive of sepsis are present, then a full diagnostic evaluation is performed and empiric antibiotic therapy is started. If the neonate has no clinical signs of sepsis at birth but is less than 35 weeks of gestation, or if the infant is more than or equal to 35 weeks of gestation but intrapartum antibiotic prophylaxis was given 4 hours or less before delivery, then a complete blood count and differential and a blood culture should be obtained and the infant should be observed for at least 48 hours. If sepsis subsequently is suspected based on clinical signs, then a full diagnostic workup and empiric therapy are initiated. No evaluation or therapy is needed for

neonates without signs of sepsis born at more than or equal 35 weeks of gestation and whose mothers had received intrapartum antibiotic prophylaxis more than 4 hours before delivery. These infants should be observed for at least 48 hours for signs suggestive of sepsis (99). The timing of intrapartum penicillin or ampicillin administration is important. In one study from Spain, the rate of GBS colonization of neonates born to carrier mothers was 46%, 29%, 2.9%, and 1.2% when ampicillin was given less than 1 hour, 1 to 2 hours, 2 to 4 hours, and more than 4 hours before delivery, respectively (288).

Immunologic approaches to prevention include passive or active immunization of mothers, with transplacental passage of protective antibodies to the fetus. A number of vaccines are currently being development against Group B streptococcal capsular polysaccharide antigens of serotypes Ia, Ib, II, III and V (289–292). Although these tetanus toxoid conjugate vaccines appear to be safe and immunogenic, they have not been evaluated extensively during pregnancy, and are not currently available outside of clinical trials.

SYPHILIS

T. pallidum subsp pallidum, the causative agent of syphilis, is a motile, nonculturable, gram-negative, microaerophilic spirochete that is too slender to be observed by light microscopy. The laboratory differentiation of *T. pallidum* from the other pathogenic treponemes that cause yaws (*T. pallidum* subsp *pertenue*), endemic syphilis (*T. pallidum* subsp *endemicum*), or pinta (*T. carateum*) is difficult.

Ultrastructurally, *T. pallidum* has an outer cell membrane (i.e., envelope), periplasmic flagella that arise at each end of the cell, cell wall, and a multilayer cytoplasmic membrane; a capsulelike amorphous layer coats the organism (293). Several outer membrane-associated proteins have been identified, and these are present in 100-fold lower amounts than typically is found in gram-negative bacteria. This property has been related to the chronicity of syphilitic infection (294).

Person-to-person transmission of *T. pallidum* occurs primarily through contact with infectious lesions during sexual activity. The organism enters the body through sites of minor trauma that disrupt mucosal or epithelial barriers (295). Fibronectin receptors appear to mediate the attachment of *T. pallidum* to epithelial or mucosal cells (296). Parenteral transmission of this spirochete through transfusions is rare because of routine serologic screening of blood or blood products, but intravenous drug users occasionally acquire syphilis by sharing needles contaminated with *T. pallidum*-infected blood (297). Intrauterine transmission from an infected mother to her developing fetus accounts for most congenitally infected infants; rarely, infection is acquired at birth through contact with a genital lesion (298). *In utero* transmission can occur as early as 9 to 10 weeks of gestation. The most important determinant for the risk of fetal infection is the maternal stage of syphilis. Mothers with primary, secondary, early latent, or late latent stages of syphilis have at least a 50%, 50%, 40%, or 10% risk, respectively, of delivering an infant with congenital syphilis (CS) (298). The risk of fetal infection also may be higher in more advanced stages of pregnancy (299). Concomitant maternal infection with *T. pallidum* and HIV-1 may enhance the transplacental spread of either pathogen to the fetus (298).

Natural and experimental *T. pallidum* infections elicit complex cellular and humoral immune responses. Most antitreponemal antibodies produced during the course of a syphilitic infection cross-react with antigens from nonpathogenic treponemes (i.e., culturable treponemes that are part of the normal oral, intestinal, or genital flora) and are not pathogen specific (300–301). Antibodies directed against integral membrane lipoproteins with molecular masses of 47, 44.5, 17, and 15.5 kilodaltons appear to be *T. pallidum* specific; their detection on Western immunoblot assays indicates syphilitic infection (302–304). A variety of other host immunologic defenses are activated after *T. pallidum* infection, including infiltration of inoculation sites with polymorphonuclear leukocytes that contain treponemicidal peptides (defensins), T-lymphocyte activation and proliferation with interferon production, cytokine secretion, macrophage-mediated phagocytosis and intracellular killing of opsonized *T. pallidum*, and complement activation (305–308). Autoantibodies to blood cells, serum components, fibronectin, and collagen also are generated (309). Some treponemes manage to evade these clearance mechanisms during the acute phase of untreated infection, which allows them to disseminate and establish a chronic infection (307,310).

Congenital Syphilis

Epidemiology

The number of cases of CS reported to the CDC increased steadily between 1980 and 1991, reflecting a true increase in the number of primary and secondary maternal syphilis cases and a change since 1989 in the surveillance case definition for CS (311). The new surveillance case definition was implemented to provide guidelines for reporting but not for making a clinical diagnosis of CS (312). In essence, the change involved considering stillbirths and infants born to women with untreated syphilis as presumptively infected, regardless of symptoms or results of subsequent follow-up evaluations. Because vertical transmission of *T. pallidum* does not occur in all instances, the new definition leads to the inclusion of a number of uninfected infants in the "presumptive case" category (312). The older surveillance case definition led to underestimates of the true incidence of CS. Many infants in whom the diagnosis could not be made at birth were treated presumptively but not reported because the diagnosis could not be confirmed; others were reported inconsistently or lost to follow-up. The new case definition improved sensitivity at the expense of specificity (313,314). Compared with traditional criteria for diagnosis, the new definition results in about a five-fold increase in the reported number of CS cases (298,315).

The CDC analyzed national surveillance data for CS. During 2000 to 2002, the rate of CS decreased 21.1%, from 14.2 to 11.2 cases per 100,000 live births with an absolute reduction of CS cases from 578 cases in 2000 to 451 cases in 2002. During 2000 to 2002, the rate of CS declined in all racial/ethnic minority populations in the United States. The rate of CS declined 50.6% among American Indian/Alaska Native infants, 22.4% among Hispanic infants, 21.4% among Asian/Pacific Islander infants, and 19.8% among non-Hispanic black infants; the rate remained unchanged among non-Hispanic white infants. Additionally, rates of CS declined in all regions of the United States except the Northeast. The rate of CS declined 29.5% in the South, 22.9% in the West, and 12.5% in the Midwest; the rate increased 0.9% in the Northeast. Among the 451 cases of CS reported in 2002, a total of 333 (73.8%) occurred because the mother had no documented treatment or received inadequate treatment for syphilis before or during pregnancy. In 63 (14.0%) cases, the mother was treated adequately but did not have an adequate serologic response to therapy, and the infant was evaluated inadequately for CS. In 39 (8.6%) cases, the mother was treated adequately but did not have an adequate serologic response to therapy, and the infant's evaluation revealed laboratory or clinical signs of CS. A total of 16 (3.6%) cases were reported for other reasons (316).

Clinical Manifestations

The pathologic and morphologic alterations of CS are as a result of host immune and inflammatory responses to spirochetal fetal invasion (317–319). The most prominent histopathologic abnormalities are vasculitis with resultant necrosis and fibrosis (320). Syphilitic stillbirths usually are macerated with *T. pallidum*-rich vesiculobullous cutaneous lesions, hepatosplenomegaly, and protuberant abdomen.

Most infants with CS do not show signs of disease at birth. Infants who develop clinical manifestations during the first 2 years of life are considered to have early CS, whereas features that appear later, usually near puberty, comprise late CS (320).

The placenta may be larger and paler than normal. The main histopathologic abnormalities are a focal, proliferative villitis with necrosis and focal mononuclear cell infiltration; endovascular and perivascular proliferation in villous vessels, leading to vascular obliteration; and focal or diffuse villous immaturity. *T pallidum* is demonstrable in the placenta using immunohistochemical stains; silver staining methods are difficult to perform and easy to misinterpret (321). Polymerase chain reaction (PCR) of placental tissue may confirm the diagnosis of CS, even in some cases that do not have the histopathologic features (322). The focal placental villitis and obliterative arteritis are associated with increased resistance to placental perfusion. Antenatal measurements of uterine and umbilical systolic-to-diastolic ratios using Doppler velocity waveform analysis reveal higher mean ratios in pregnancies complicated by syphilis compared with noninfected controls (323). Necrotizing funisitis, a deep inflammatory process involving the matrix of the umbilical cord and accompanied by phlebitis and thrombosis, is common in syphilitic stillbirths and infants symptomatic at birth (324–325).

Clinical signs of CS appear in approximately two-thirds of affected infants during the third to eighth week of life and in most by 3 months of age (320). Symptoms may be generalized and nonspecific (e.g., fever, lymphadenopathy, irritability, failure to thrive). Alternatively, the highly suggestive triad of snuffles, palmar and plantar bullae, and splenomegaly may be apparent (320). The severity of the clinical illness can vary from mild to fulminant, life-threatening disease (326–329). Premature infants are more likely to have hepatomegaly, respiratory distress, and skin lesions than similarly infected term neonates (330).

Congenitally infected infants may be small for their gestational ages (320). However, a carefully conducted study by Naeye (331) of 36 stillborn and newborn infants with CS revealed that fetal growth was almost normal despite widespread evidence of tissue destruction. The observed growth retardation in some reports may be related to confounding factors such as maternal intravenous drug use or coinfection with other pathogens.

Hepatosplenomegaly occurs in 50% to 90% of infants with early CS (298,320). The enlargement is caused mainly by abundant extramedullary hematopoiesis and by subacute hepatic and splenic inflammation. Jaundice, with direct and indirect hyperbilirubinemia, occurs in about one-third of infants and may be contributed to by hepatitis or hemolysis (298). Syphilitic hepatitis is common and may worsen with penicillin therapy (327,332–334). Alkaline phosphatase elevation is a frequent biochemical abnormality (327). Transaminase and γ-glutamyl transferase concentrations may be high at presentation and increase with antimicrobial therapy to levels approaching 150 times normal (332). Fulminant syphilitic hepatitis can manifest with hypoglycemia, lactic acidosis, encephalopathy, disseminated intravascular coagulation, and shock, mimicking metabolic or other infectious causes of acute liver failure (328,335). Hepatic and splenic abnormalities may persist for as long as 1 year after treatment (320). Liver cirrhosis is uncommon (298).

Generalized lymphadenopathy is found in 20% to 50% of infants with CS (320). The enlarged nodes are firm and nontender.

The mucocutaneous lesions of CS are varied and occur in 30% to 60% of infants (320). The most characteristic are vesiculobullous eruptions that are most pronounced on the palms and soles. The blister fluid abounds with active spirochetes and is highly infectious (320). When a blister ruptures, it leaves behind a macerated red surface that rapidly dries and crusts. The most commonly encountered rash consists of oval, red, maculopapular lesions that are most prominent on the buttocks, back, thighs, and soles; they later change to a copper-brown color with superficial desquamation. Other lesions may be annular, circinate, petechial, or purpuric, or have a blueberry-muffin appearance (320). Mucous patches involving the nares, palate, tongue, lips, and anus can occur; these lesions become deeply fissured and hemorrhagic and subsequently result in rhagades (Parrot radial scars of late CS) (320). Condyloma lata usually are encountered later in infancy in untreated patients. These raised, flat, moist, and wartlike lesions most commonly affect perioral (nares, angles of mouth) and perianal areas (298).

Rhinitis (snuffles) is encountered in 10% to 50% of infected infants and usually precedes the appearance of cutaneous eruptions by 1 to 2 weeks (320,327,336). The extremely contagious discharge initially is watery, but it later becomes thicker, purulent, and even hemorrhagic (320). Without treatment, the nasal cartilage ulcerates with ensuing chondritis, necrosis, and septal perforation leading to the saddle-nose deformity of late CS (298). Throat involvement can produce hoarseness or aphonia (320).

Roentgenographic abnormalities are detected in 20% to more than 95% of infants with early CS (336–341). The lower rates usually are seen in asymptomatic infants (339). Multiple, symmetric bony lesions are common. The metaphyses and diaphyses of long bones, particularly those of the lower extremities, are most commonly affected. Radiologic changes include osteochondritis, periostitis, and osteitis (298). The earliest changes occur in the metaphysis and consist of trans- verse, serrated radiopaque bands (i.e., Wegner sign) alternating with zones of radiolucent osteoporotic bone (320,338). Osteochondritis becomes evident radiographically 5 weeks after fetal infection (320). The metaphysis may become fragmented. Focal erosions involving the proximal medial tibia are referred to as Wimberger's sign. Periosteal reactions may consist of a single layer of new bone formation, multiple layers (i.e., "onion peel periosteum"), or a severe lamellar form (i.e., periostitis of Pehu) (338). Periostitis is radiologically apparent after at least 16 weeks of fetal infection (320). Osteitis can give rise to a celery-stick appearance of longitudinal translucent lines that extend into the diaphysis or lead to a diffuse moth-eaten rarefaction of the shaft. Dactylitis, absence of lower extremity ossification centers, cranial nodules, and pathologic fractures or joint involvement leading to immobility of the affected limb (i.e., pseudoparalysis of Parrot) occasionally are seen (320,338, 342,343).

Hematologic abnormalities are common and include anemia, leukocytosis, leukopenia, and thrombocytopenia (336). Anemia may be as a result of Coombs-negative hemolysis, replacement of bone marrow by syphilitic granulation tissue, or maturation arrest in the erythroblastoid cell line (298). Thrombocytopenia is as a result of shortened peripheral platelet survival.

Clinically silent CNS involvement occurs in as many as 60% of infants with CS (298). Acute syphilitic meningitis may present with neck stiffness, vomiting, bulging anterior fontanelle, and a positive Kernig's sign. CSF examination reveals a normal glucose concentration, modestly elevated protein content, and mononuclear pleocytosis (usually less than 200 cells/μL), a pattern consistent with aseptic meningitis. Chronic meningovascular syphilis develops in untreated infants and manifests in late infancy with progressive, communicating hydrocephalus, cranial nerve palsies, optic atrophy, and cerebral infarctions leading to hemiplegia or seizure disorders (320, 344).

Other less common pathologic changes of early CS involve the eyes (e.g., salt and pepper chorioretinitis, glaucoma, chancres of eyelids, uveitis), lungs (e.g., pneumonia alba, interstitial scarring, extramedullary hematopoiesis), and kidneys (e.g., nephrotic syndrome, glomerulonephritis) (320,345,346). Nonimmune hydrops is found in one-sixth of live born infants with CS (347). Myocarditis, hypopituitarism, pancreatitis, diarrhea, and malabsorption also occur (320,348).

The clinical manifestations of late CS represent residual scars after therapy of early congenital infection or persistent inflammation in untreated persons. Abnormalities of dentition are secondary to early damage incurred by developing tooth buds and can be prevented by penicillin treatment during the neonatal period or in early infancy. Unilateral or bilateral interstitial keratitis occurs in about 10% of patients and usually is diagnosed between 5 and 20 years of age. Saddle-nose deformity, high-arched palate, and poor maxillary growth are late consequences of syphilitic rhinitis. Eighth-nerve deafness occurs infrequently (3% of patients) and is as a result of osteochondritis of the otic capsule and resulting cochlear degeneration. Rhagades are linear scars that radiate from sites of earlier mucocutaneous lesions of the mouth, nares, and anus.

Skeletal manifestations are caused by persistent or recurrent periostitis and its associated bone thickening (320, 349,350).

Diagnosis

Antenatal sonography may reveal placental thickening or fetal abnormalities such as hydrops, hepatomegaly, ascites, or dilated small bowel loops (351–355). Musculoskeletal abnormalities may be visualized on rare occasions with antenatal ultrasonography (356). Spirochetes can be visualized in amniotic fluid samples using darkfield microscopy or indirect immunofluorescent staining (351,353,357). The presence of T pallidum or its deoxyribonucleic acid (DNA) in amniotic fluid can be demonstrated by rabbit infectivity tests or PCR techniques, respectively (358–359). With the availability of umbilical blood sampling, intrauterine infection has been confirmed as early as 24 weeks of gestation by detecting the spirochete or its DNA in fetal blood and by measuring specific IgM antibodies directed against the 47-kilodalton antigen of T. pallidum in fetal serum (351, 354,358). By testing amniotic fluid using the rabbit infectivity test and PCR analysis, some investigators have been able to confirm intrauterine T. pallidum infection antenatally as early as 17 weeks of gestation (359).

At birth, the diagnosis of CS is best established by demonstrating the spirochete or its DNA in tissues or body fluids as previously alluded to. Serologic data obtained from cord blood or neonatal sera are helpful if interpreted with their limitations in mind.

Rapid plasma reagin (RPR) or Venereal Disease Research Laboratory (VDRL) measurements on cord blood samples yield false-positive and false-negative results in 10% and 5% of cases, respectively (360). Serum from the infant, rather than from the umbilical cord, should be used because of lower false-positive and false-negative reactions (361). If an infant's RPR or VDRL titer is at least four-fold higher than a concomitantly obtained maternal titer, the diagnosis of CS is likely. The RPR may be negative in infants whose mothers had acquired syphilis shortly before delivery (327). The FTA-ABS-IgM test yields false-positive and false negative results in 35% and 10% of cases, respectively (298). This is as a result of interference with test performance by rheumatoid factor (fetal IgM antibodies directed against maternal immunoglobin G [IgG]). This problem can be overcome by separating the IgG and IgM fractions of the serum and then testing the IgG-depleted fraction for FTA-ABS-IgM. This assay is known as FTA-ABS-19S-IgM, and it is still investigational (304). The detection of IgM antibodies against specific T. pallidum antigens, especially the 47-kilodalton outer membrane protein antigen, by Western immunoblot assays is diagnostically helpful (298,362–363).

In addition to serologic tests for syphilis, the complete diagnostic evaluation of an infant with CS should include bone radiography, CSF examination, complete blood count, platelet count, liver enzyme concentrations, and HIV-1 antibody determination. However, Moyer and colleagues (341) demonstrated that the results of long-bone radiographs in newborns do not differentiate between active and past infection, and that the results do not alter the management of infants being evaluated for CS.

The diagnosis of congenital neurosyphilis is difficult to ascertain. CSF abnormalities such as mononuclear pleocytosis ($\geq$25 cells/μL), elevated protein concentration (greater than 170 mg/dL), and reactive CSF VDRL are widely used criteria (298). However, the CSF VDRL can be positive in the absence of neurosyphilis because of passive diffusion of nontreponemal IgG antibodies from serum to CSF and in infants with traumatic lumbar punctures (298). The yield of lumbar punctures in asymptomatic newborns with CS is poor (364). A specific IgM response to the *T. pallidum* 47-kilodalton antigen has been detected in the CSF of some infants with congenial syphilis, and this may prove helpful for the diagnosis of neurosyphilis. CSF IgM reactivity can be present in infants with negative CSF VDRL test results (365). The presence of *T. pallidum* in the CSF of some infants with normal CSF cell counts, protein concentrations, and VDRL test results has been demonstrated using sensitive rabbit infectivity tests or PCR methods (298,366).

Treatment

Infants should be treated at birth if they are symptomatic, if maternal therapy was inadequate or unknown, or if follow-up cannot be ensured. Adequate maternal therapy is defined as penicillin treatment at a dose appropriate for the stage of syphilis and started at least 30 days before delivery (367).

One of two dosage regimens can be used for confirmed or presumptive CS:

1. Aqueous crystalline penicillin G at a dose of 100,000 to 150,000 U/kg/d administered intravenously as 50,000 U/kg/dose every 12 hours during the first 7 days of life, and every 8 hours thereafter for a total of 10 days.
2. Procaine penicillin G at a dose of 50,000 U/kg/dose given intramuscularly once daily for 10 days.

If more than 1 day of therapy is missed, the entire course should be restarted (368). Benzathine penicillin G given as a single intramuscular dose of 50,000 U/kg is recommended only for infants whose evaluation (complete blood count and platelets, CSF examination, long bone radiographs) is normal and follow-up is certain. The Jarisch-Herxheimer reaction occurs in some infants within hours of initiation of penicillin therapy.

The VDRL titers should be monitored every 2 to 3 months until they become nonreactive or the titer declines by at least fourfold. Untreated infants should have FTA-ABS tests. Passively acquired maternal antibodies usually disappear by 6 to 12 months of age in uninfected infants (369). If the VDRL titers are stable or rising or if the FTA-ABS test result remains positive beyond 15 months of age, the infant should be thoroughly reexamined and treated. The VDRL titers of adequately treated infants with CS grad-

ually decline, but FTA-ABS reactivities persist. Infants with CSF abnormalities should be retested at 6 months of age. If the CSF VDRL is positive at that time, a second course of penicillin is indicated. Follow-up examinations should emphasize developmental assessment and a careful search for stigmata of CS.

BACTERIAL MENINGITIS

The incidence of bacterial meningitis is 0.4 per 1,000 live births, but rates as high as 1 per 1,000 live births have been reported in a few nurseries (88). The disease is seen more commonly in premature infants (234), male infants, and infants born to mothers with complicated pregnancies or deliveries. In a recent study of 9641 very low birth weight infants, meningitis was diagnosed in 1.4% infants (234).

Etiology

The bacteria causing neonatal meningitis are similar to those causing sepsis neonatorum. Group B β-hemolytic streptococci and *E. coli* presently account for approximately 75% of all cases. The next most common etiologic agent is *L. monocytogenes* (370).

Pathology

The pathologic findings in cases of neonatal meningitis are similar, regardless of the bacterial agent. The most consistent finding at necropsy is a purulent exudate coating the meninges and ependymal surfaces of the ventricles (371). Perivascular inflammation is observed. The inflammatory response of neonates is similar to that in adults with meningitis, with the exception that babies show a relative sparsity of plasma cells and lymphocytes during the subacute stage of meningeal reactions. Hydrocephalus and a noninfectious encephalopathy can be demonstrated in approximately 50% of infants dying of meningitis. Subdural effusions occur rarely in neonates. Various degrees of phlebitis and arteritis of intracranial vessels can be found in all infants. Thrombophlebitis with occlusions of veins may occur in the subependymal zone. Ventriculitis can be demonstrated in virtually all infants dying of meningitis and in approximately 75% of infants at the time of diagnosis.

Clinical Manifestations

The signs and symptoms of central nervous system infection frequently are indistinguishable from those associated with neonatal septicemia. Lethargy, feeding problems, and altered temperature are the most frequent presenting complaints, and respiratory distress, vomiting, diarrhea, and abdominal distention are common findings. Seizures are observed frequently and may be caused by direct central nervous system inflammation or may be associated with hypoglycemia or hypocalcemia. Signs suggesting meningeal involvement, such as a bulging anterior fontanelle, neck stiffness, or opisthotonus, are infrequent.

Pathogenesis

Most cases of meningitis result from bacteremia; spread from a contiguous infected focus is rare. Although there are more than 100 K types of *E. coli*, the K1 type accounts for more than 70% of *E. coli* meningitis cases (60). Most pathogenic *E. coli* carry both the capsular antigen K1 and S fimbria adhesins; the latter promote adherence of *E. coli* to epithelial cells in the choroid plexus and brain ventricles, and to vascular endothelial cells (372). The extracellular polysaccharide capsule allows the organism to avoid host clearance mechanisms. The outer membrane lipopolysaccharide (i.e., endotoxin) is released from dying bacteria and initiates an intense inflammatory reaction. Endotoxin stimulates the production of tumor necrosis factor, interleukin-1β (IL-1β), and other mediators by monocyte-macrophage cells. Tumor necrosis factor and IL-1β induce phospholipase A2 activity, production of other mediators, and receptor-ligand interactions between leukocytes and endothelia. Phospholipase A2 then acts on membrane phospholipids to produce a variety of lipid proinflammatory substances such as platelet-activating factor, leukotrienes, prostaglandins, and thromboxanes. The inflammatory changes result in vascular injury and alterations in the permeability of the blood-brain barrier, with resultant vasogenic edema. The cytokines activate adhesion-promoting receptors on cerebral vascular endothelial cells, which leads to recruitment of leukocytes to sites of stimulation. These polymorphonuclear leukocytes subsequently enter the subarachnoid space, release toxic substances, and cause cytotoxic edema (373). The net pathophysiologic effect is the development of increased intracranial pressure and severe brain edema. Cerebral edema, increased intracranial pressure, systemic hypotension, decreased cerebral perfusion pressure, and a variety of vascular changes result in global or regional reductions of cerebral blood flow and can lead to brain ischemia (374). The pathophysiologic aberrations ultimately cause focal or diffuse neuronal injury, which may be irreversible.

Among the five GBS serotypes, the BIII organisms account for more than 80% of cases of neonatal GBS meningitis. The presence of type-specific antibodies enhances opsonization of the organism in the presence of complement. Cell wall components of the organism can stimulate the inflammatory cascade in a manner similar to that described for endotoxins.

Laboratory Findings

Interpretation of CSF values in newborn infants may be difficult (Table 47-4). The upper limits of "normal" for infants with birth weights of 1,500 g or less are even higher than those for term newborns (375–377).

It is important to examine carefully a stained smear of the CSF of every infant with suspected meningitis. In babies with meningitis caused by GBS or coliform bacteria,

TABLE 47-4

CEREBROSPINAL FLUID VALUES OF NONINFECTED TERM NEWBORNS

CSF Parameter	Age (d)	Mean	SD	Median	Range
WBC count/mm³	0–7	15.3	30.0	6	1–130
	8–14	5.4	4.4	6	0–18
	15–21	7.7	12.1	4	0–62
	22–30	4.8	3.4	4	0–18
ANC/mm³	0–7	4.4	15.2	0	0–65
	8–14	0.1	0.3	0	0–1
	15–21	0.2	0.5	0	0–2
	22–30	0.1	0.2	0	0–1
Protein (mg/dL)	0–7	80.8	30.8	NA	NA
	8–14	69	22.6	NA	NA
	15–21	59.8	23.4	NA	NA
	22–30	54.1	16.2	NA	NA
Glucose (mg/dl)	0–7	45.9	7.5	NA	NA
	8–14	54.3	17	NA	NA
	15–21	46.8	8.8	NA	NA
	22–30	54.1	16.2	NA	NA

ANC, absolute neutrophil count; CSF, cerebrospinal fluid; NA, not available; SD, standard deviation; WBC, white blood cells.
Adapted from Ahmed A, Hickey SM, Ehrett S, et al. Cerebrospinal fluid values in the term neonate. *Pediatr Infect Dis J* 1996;15:298, with permission.

each oil-immersion field usually contains several to many bacteria. This is because there are 10^4 to 10^8 colony-forming units (CFU) per 1 mL of spinal fluid (average 10^7 CFU/mL) present at the time of diagnosis. *Listeria* organisms often are difficult to identify on stained smears because the bacterial counts frequently are on the order of 10^3 CFU/mL. Bacterial antigens can be detected by LPA for GBS, *E. coli* K1, *H. influenzae* type b, *S. pneumoniae*, and non-type B meningococci. Polymerase chain reaction assays for the detection of bacterial DNA in CSF specimens are being developed (378–380). Nonculture methods of diagnosis are most useful for newborns who receive antibiotics before a lumbar puncture is performed.

Blood and urine cultures should be obtained from every infant suspected of meningitis. As many as 33% of infants with positive CSF cultures have sterile blood cultures (229,236).

Treatment

Considerable data have been gathered on the pharmacokinetic properties of antibiotics in neonates with meningitis (381–382). After an intramuscular dose of 2.5 mg/kg of gentamicin, peak levels in lumbar CSF and ventricular fluid are approximately 1 to 2 µg/mL. If lumbar intrathecal gentamicin is added to this regimen, values of 20 to 40 µg/mL or greater several hours after instillation may be observed in the lumbar area. Intraventricular administration of 2.5 mg results in ventricular fluid levels of 20 to 80 µg/mL and in lumbar spinal fluid values of 10 to 50 µg/mL 1 to 4 hours later. With kanamycin, peak CSF values of 6 to 10 µg/mL are observed 4 to 6 hours after an intramuscular dose of 7.5 mg/kg. Peak values of 10 to 30 µg/mL are demonstrated in CSF approximately 2 to 4 hours after a 50 to 70 mg/kg dose of ampicillin.

For the aminoglycosides, the MIC values for the common pathogens frequently are greater than the antibiotic levels achieved in CSF For example, an *E. coli* with a gentamicin MIC value of 2.5 or 5 µg/mL is considered susceptible when bloodstream infection is being treated but may be considered resistant when therapy is for meningitis. This is because peak cerebrospinal and ventricular fluid gentamicin levels after parenteral therapy usually are lower than this MIC value. Alternative therapeutic regimens must be considered, such as adding a second antibiotic, selecting a different antibiotic class, or changing the route of administration. In experimental models of *E. coli* meningitis, the administration of the total daily gentamicin dose undivided results in CSF concentrations of the drug that are three-fold higher than those achieved in animals receiving conventional dosing, and the rate of bacterial killing is greater early on in animals receiving once-daily gentamicin (383).

Ampicillin and gentamicin or ampicillin and cefotaxime are recommended for initial empiric therapy of neonatal meningitis. The dosage of ampicillin or cefotaxime is 200 to 300 mg/kg/d in three divided doses during the first week of life and 200 mg/kg/d in three or four divided doses thereafter. The gentamicin dosage is the same as that used for septicemia. All infants should have repeat spinal fluid examinations and cultures at 48 hours after initiation of therapy. If organisms are seen on a Gram stain of the fluid, the patient should be reevaluated completely regarding making alterations in antimicrobial therapy and to obtaining computed tomography of the head. The radiologic procedures may demonstrate the presence of a subdural empyema, brain abscess, or ventriculitis that requires neurosurgical intervention.

Cefotaxime, with or without an aminoglycoside, can be used for therapy of neonatal meningitis as a result of susceptible gram-negative enteric organisms (384). Although there are no large controlled trials of cefotaxime in neonates, accumulated experience from open studies indicates that this cephalosporin is effective for therapy of neonatal sepsis and meningitis.

The Neonatal Meningitis Cooperative Study group reported that there is no beneficial effect of lumbar intrathecal or intraventricular instillation of gentamicin in the therapy of meningitis caused by gram-negative organism (382). The mortality rate in infants given intraventricular gentamicin was threefold greater than that in infants treated with systemic therapy only. The mean and peak ventricular CSF concentrations of endotoxin and IL-1β were significantly higher for infants treated with intraventricular gentamicin than those receiving intravenous antibiotics alone (385). This difference may have resulted from the enhanced bacterial killing achieved through higher ventricular CSF gentamicin concentrations, with the consequent increased release of damaging inflammatory mediators, which resulted in greater periventricular inflammation.

Therapy for meningitis is continued for a minimum of 2 weeks after sterilization of CSF cultures. This equates to 14 days of therapy for meningitis caused by gram-positive organisms and a minimum of 21 days of therapy for meningitis caused by gram-negative pathogens.

Treatment for *Candida* meningitis is with amphotericin B and flucytosine for a period of 3 to 6 weeks (196). Fluconazole has been used to treat neonatal candidal meningitis, but the optimal dose is not known and the published experience is very limited (279). In an experimental model of *C. albicans* meningitis, amphotericin B was more effective than fluconazole in clearing the infection at the dosage levels that were used (386).

Attention to general supportive therapy is essential in caring for infants with meningitis and is the single most important factor that accounts for the improved outcome during recent years. Disturbances of fluid and electrolyte balance are common, particularly in the first several days of illness when inappropriate antidiuretic hormone secretion may lead to fluid retention and hyponatremia. Hypoglycemia, hypocalcemia, and hyperbilirubinemia are frequent complications. Ventilatory assistance frequently is necessary, and blood pressure should be monitored carefully. During the course of illness, hemoglobin and hematocrit values should be checked frequently because infection may exaggerate and prolong the anemias of infancy, particularly in premature infants. Because of the frequent occurrence of bleeding diathesis, platelet counts, prothrombin time, and partial thromboplastin time should be followed. Neurosurgical evaluation is needed for neonates with a brain abscess to determine the need for abscess decompression.

Prognosis

The mortality from neonatal meningitis is considerable. The overall mortality rate is approximately 10% to 30%, but this varies with etiologic agent, infant population, and the nursery or intensive care unit.

Short- and long-term sequelae of neonatal meningitis are frequent. The acute complications include communicating or noncommunicating hydrocephalus, subdural effusions, ventriculitis, and blindness (387). In 70% of infants with *Citrobacter koseri* (formerly *diversus*) meningitis, there is associated brain abscess (Fig. 47-2) (381,382, 388,389). Jan and colleagues recently reported a study of diffusion weighted imaging in neonates with acute meningitis. In 12 of the 13 infants studied, there was evidence of cortical or deep white-matter infarcts. Magnetic resonance angiography detected vasculitis in 2/5 infants studied. This imaging modality also appears to be sensitive in detecting extra-axial fluid collections representing empyemas (390). Many infants appear relatively normal at the time of discharge. It is only after prolonged and careful follow-up that perceptual difficulties, reading problems, or minimal brain damage is apparent. It is estimated that 30% to 50% of survivors have some evidence of neurologic damage (109, 391–395). Recurrence of gram-negative bacillary meningitis may occur in as many as 10% of patients (387).

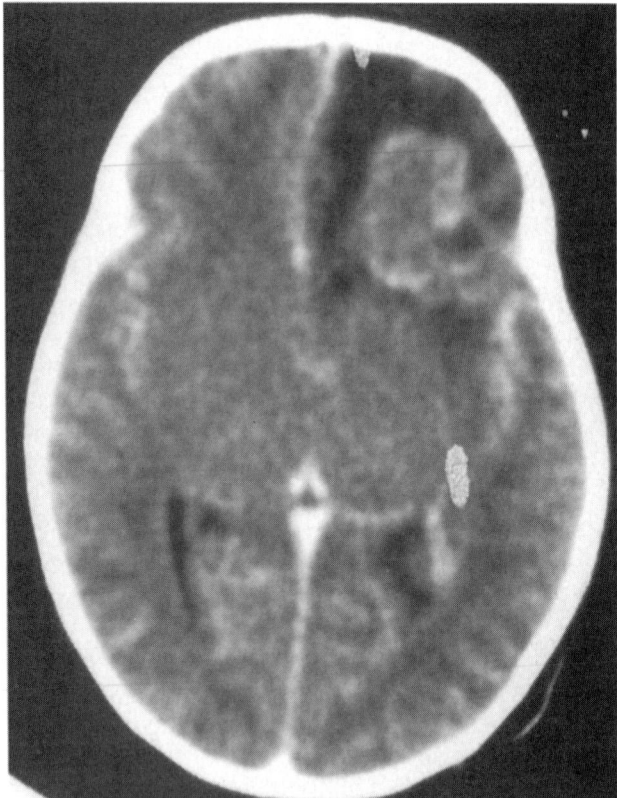

Figure 47-2 Contrast-enhanced computed tomographic scan of the head of a 25-day-old African-American girl with *Citrobacter koseri* infection of the central nervous system. Note the cavitating enhancing lesion abutting the lateral ventricle on the left, with surrounding vasogenic edema.

OSTEOMYELITIS AND SEPTIC ARTHRITIS

Because of the unique nature of the vascular supply of the neonatal skeletal system, osteomyelitis and septic arthritis frequently occur concomitantly. During the first 12 months of life, capillaries perforate the epiphyseal plate of long bones and provide a communication between the metaphysis and the joint space (396). Infections originating in one anatomic location easily spread to the other. This is not true after approximately 1 year of age, when the perforating capillaries disappear.

The capsules of the hip and shoulder attach below the metaphysis of the femur and humerus, respectively. Infection of the epiphyseal cartilage may rupture through the periosteum and enter the joint space, producing purulent arthritis. Because of the capsular articulation of the hip and shoulder, osteomyelitis and septic arthritis may coexist, making the origin of infection difficult to determine.

Infections of the musculoskeletal system are uncommon in the neonate, but incidence figures are not available.

Etiology and Pathogenesis

The infecting organisms in osteomyelitis and septic arthritis vary, but the predominant ones are GBS, *S. aureus*, and gram-negative enteric organisms such as *Klebsiella* spp,

Proteus spp, and *E. coli*. Although gonococcal arthritis and tenosynovitis were encountered commonly in previous decades, they are seen only occasionally today. Other etiologic agents associated with newborn bone and joint infection are *Salmonella* spp, *Pseudomonas* spp, *H. influenzae*, *S. pneumoniae*, coagulase-negative staphylococci and *C. albicans* (397–402). Hospital-acquired methicillin-resistant *S. aureus* (MRSA) osteomyelitis and septic arthritis can develop in sick premature infants after catheter-associated septicemia (401).

Osteomyelitis and arthritis have been reported after several invasive procedures in newborns, including heel puncture, femoral venipuncture, exchange transfusions, fetal monitoring electrode placement, and umbilical artery catheterization (143,397). Osteomyelitis of cranial bones has complicated infected cephalhematomas. In most cases, the origin is unknown and is presumed to be hematogenous.

Clinical Presentation

Nonspecific symptoms of infection, such as lethargy, irritability and poor feeding, may be the initial manifestations of neonatal musculoskeletal infection. Diminished movement of the affected limb, unrelated temporally to birth trauma, is a common clinical sign (403). Warmth, erythema, and swelling are late manifestations. The long bones are affected most commonly. Occasionally, the diagnosis is made unsuspectingly when purulent material is obtained on attempted aspiration of the femoral vein and the needle enters the swollen hip capsule. GBS osteomyelitis is indolent and usually involves a single bone, most commonly the proximal humerus, but can involve the vertebral spine as well (396,404).

Although blood cultures frequently are positive, the infants usually are not clinically toxic. The exception is group A β-hemolytic streptococcal infection, in which the infant may appear gravely ill.

Laboratory Tests and Findings

Blood cultures should be obtained from all infants with suspected infection of the musculoskeletal system. A diagnostic aspiration of the joint or subperiosteal space should be attempted in all patients, and the material obtained should be treated with Gram stain and cultured. Identification of the organism is particularly important, because it may be necessary to treat with more than one potentially nephrotoxic drug until the causative bacterium has been isolated.

The peripheral leukocyte count frequently is elevated, and juvenile forms may be seen. There is little information regarding the erythrocyte sedimentation rate during the neonatal period. In older infants and children, the sedimentation rate is accelerated in osteomyelitis; its return toward normal is a rough indicator of therapeutic success.

Radiographs of the affected bone or joint taken early in illness may be normal or show widening of the articular space. Later in the course of disease, subluxation and destruction of the joint are common. If osteomyelitis is present, the normal fat markings on roentgenograms of the deep tissues may be obliterated, indicating inflammation. Lifting of the periosteum from the bone may be observed, but cortical destruction is unusual before the second week of illness. A complete skeletal survey should be performed because of frequent involvement of multiple sites (403,405). Resolution of bone changes is considerably slower than clinical improvement. Although radioisotope scans (e.g., technetium, gallium) of bone are useful in early diagnosis of osteomyelitis in older infants and children, they may be normal in newborns with proven infection (397). Nevertheless, bone scintigraphy remains more sensitive than plain radiography for the early diagnosis of osteomyelitis (406).

Therapy

Selection of initial antimicrobial therapy should be based on results of the Gram stain of aspirated purulent material and associated clinical findings, such as furuncles or cellulitis. If gram-positive cocci are observed on stained smears, methicillin or nafcillin should be started. Vancomycin may be preferable in nurseries with multiresistant *S. aureus* strains. Cefotaxime or gentamicin is indicated if gram-negative organisms are observed. If no organisms are identified on stained smears, a combination of an antistaphylococcal drug and an aminoglycoside is used. After the organism has been identified and susceptibility studies are available, the most appropriate antibiotic or combination of antibiotics should be used. Direct instillation of an antimicrobial agent into the joint space is unnecessary because most antibiotics penetrate the inflamed synovium, and adequate concentrations are achieved in purulent material (407). This also applies to treatment of osteomyelitis; direct instillation of antibiotics into infected bone is unwarranted.

As a general rule, infection of the joint space and bone should be drained by repeated aspiration or by surgery. Suppurative arthritis of the hip and shoulder is best treated with incision and drainage to prevent vascular compromise or extension of infection into the metaphysis. Orthopedic consultation must be obtained for all patients.

Antimicrobial therapy of neonatal musculoskeletal infections caused by *S. aureus* or coliform organisms should be continued for approximately 3 weeks and, in some patients, for a longer period. For gonococcal or streptococcal infections, 10 days of therapy generally are sufficient with adequate surgical drainage. The duration of therapy must be individualized. In general, systemic symptoms disappear within several days of initiation of therapy and drainage, but local signs such as heat, erythema and swelling may persist for 4 to 7 days. Full range of motion of the involved limb may not return for several months, and physical therapy should be instituted early to prevent contractures. Complete resolution of roentgenographic changes may take several months. The use of large oral dosages of antibiotics for outpatient therapy of neonatal musculoskeletal infections has not been studied systematically and should be undertaken with caution (408).

Prognosis

Death from these diseases is unusual. However, morbidity may be considerable, particularly if weight-bearing joints such as the hip are involved. Bone deformations or shortening, contractures, or muscle damage can be permanent (397,408–411).

CUTANEOUS INFECTIONS

Most infections of the skin and subcutaneous tissues in neonates are caused by *S. aureus*. There are three major presentations of superficial staphylococcal disease. The first and most common are pustules and furuncles, which may be solitary or appear in clusters during the neonatal period. Pustules are frequently in the periumbilical and diaper areas, and they may coalesce gradually and spread to other areas of the body. Bloodstream or organ invasion is unusual unless the cutaneous infection involves extensive areas. Omphalitis usually is caused by staphylococci or streptococci, and infected circumcisions are usually caused by *S. aureus*.

The occurrence of staphylococcal skin infections in several infants from the same nursery should alert the physician to the possibility of nosocomial infection caused by a single, virulent strain of *S. aureus*. If infections are caused by the same strain of *Staphylococcus*, prompt measures should be instituted so that the source of infection can be determined and further colonization and disease can be prevented.

Therapy of cutaneous staphylococcal disease depends on the extent of the lesions and the general condition of the infant. Small, isolated pustules can be managed by local care with a mild cleansing agent or an antiseptic agent such as hexachlorophene or povidone-iodine. Infants with more extensive cutaneous involvement, systemic signs and symptoms of infection, or both should be treated with parenteral antimicrobial agents. The selection of the proper penicillin is based on historic experience and antimicrobial susceptibility studies of staphylococci isolated from the nursery unit.

The second form of neonatal staphylococcal disease has been described as the expanded scalded skin syndrome (122). This group of illnesses includes bullous impetigo, toxic epidermal necrolysis (Ritter disease), and nonstreptococcal scarlatina, usually caused by phage group II staphylococci. The pathogenesis of these entities appears to be related to release of exotoxins (e.g., epidermolytic toxins A and B) that act primarily on the stratum granulosa of the epidermis, causing a generalized erythema, edema, and tenderness, frequently progressing to desquamation and formation of flaccid bullae. The usual sites of staphylococcal infection are conjunctivae, throat, and umbilicus. Infants usually are afebrile. Cultures of blood, nasopharynx, eyes, and other areas should be obtained before therapy. Because phage group II staphylococci frequently are resistant to penicillin, methicillin is the initial drug of choice. Vancomycin should be used for multiresistant strains. *Pseudomonas putida* sepsis presenting as scalded skin syndrome has been described in a 9-day-old newborn (412).

The third form of staphylococcal disease is necrotizing fasciitis, which also can be caused by streptococci, *E. coli*, *Klebsiella*, and anaerobes (413–419). Necrotizing fasciitis, an unusual disease of newborns, is associated with surgical procedures, circumcision, birth trauma, or cutaneous infections. In this condition, subcutaneous tissues, including muscle layers, are invaded, and the organism spreads along the fascial planes. Overlying skin may appear violaceous, and the borders of the lesion usually are indistinct. Extensive surgery to resect the destroyed tissue is imperative in treating necrotizing fasciitis. Blood and tissue cultures should be obtained, and the patient started on methicillin or nafcillin and an aminoglycoside until culture results are available. If necrotizing fasciitis involves the abdomen or perineum, then either clindamycin or metronidazole should be added (418). The necrotic fatty tissue may combine with calcium, resulting in tetany and convulsions. Vigorous fluid resuscitation and correction of electrolyte imbalances are critical.

Breast abscesses most commonly are caused by *S. aureus*, but gram-negative enteric organisms can be causative (420). Anaerobes can be recovered from as many as 40% of samples, one-half of which are in mixed cultures with aerobic bacteria (421). Bacteremia is rare. The physician should attempt to establish an etiologic diagnosis by expressing fluid from the nipple after thorough cleaning or by needle aspiration of the abscess. Treatment is with methicillin, with or without an aminoglycoside, depending on the results of the Gram stain and culture, and it should be continued for 5 to 7 days. For mild infections, antibiotic therapy is adequate; with more severe inflammation, incision and drainage of the abscess are required. Long-term follow-up studies suggest that some girls will have diminished tissue in the affected breast.

Scalp abscesses occur most commonly as a complication of fetal monitoring in which scalp electrodes are used and may occur as localized manifestations of systemic disease (e.g., enterococcal sepsis) (169,422). Etiologic agents include staphylococci, enterococci, gram-negative enteric bacteria, and gonococci (169,422,423). Polymicrobial flora, including anaerobes, are commonly isolated. Treatment consists of incision and drainage. If there is an associated cellulitis, antibiotics are given and continued for 5 to 7 days.

Fungal infections of the neonatal skin can range from localized or widespread candidal dermatitis (424), to localized, discrete follicular pustules, plaques, or nodules caused by *Trichophyton tonsurans*, to rapidly progressive ulceration and necrosis requiring surgical debridement seen with mucormycosis (425–427). The characteristic pathology of mucormycosis is invasion of blood vessels by fungal hyphae resulting in ischemia and infarction of areas supplied by these vessels. Predisposing factors for serious cutaneous fungal disease includes prematurity, disruption of the barrier function of newborn skin associated with adhesive removal, multiple antibiotic treatment courses, and postnatal steroid therapy (425,428). In one study, wooden tongue depressors used to make splints were identified as the source of *Rhizopus microsporus* invasive infection in premature infants (425). The choice of antifungal agent for therapy depends on the specific infection being treated: griseofulvin for superficial dermatophyte infections, topical nystatin for mild-to-moderate candidal dermatitis, fluconazole or amphotericin B for extensive candidal dermatitis, and amphotericin B for mucormycosis.

URINARY TRACT INFECTION

Improved methods for obtaining sterile specimens have made it possible for investigators to define more accurately the incidence of neonatal urinary tract infection. Bacteriuria may be demonstrated in 0.5% to 1.0% of full-term infants and as many as 3% of premature infants in studies using the bladder aspiration technique (429). Urinary tract infections are more common in babies born to bacteriuric mothers and in male neonates, in contrast to the predominance of female infants beyond this period of life.

Etiology

E. coli is the most common etiologic agent of urinary tract infection, as found in older patients. Approximately 50% of causative *E. coli* strains belong to one of eight common O antigen groups. Several polysaccharide capsular antigens (e.g., K1i, K2, K12, K13) are found more often in infants with upper tract disease. This particularly pertains to the K1 antigen (430). Fimbriated *E. coli* can attach to specific receptors on uroepithelial cells. Glycolipids of the P blood group constitute a specific receptor that is believed to be associated with pyelonephritis in patients who do not have reflux. *Klebsiella* and *Pseudomonas* species are encountered less frequently. Gram-positive bacteria, with the exception of enterococci, are rare causes of urinary tract infections. Fungal cystitis and pyelonephritis are encountered in chronically ill premature infants previously treated with multiple broad-spectrum antibiotics and are associated with mucocutaneous candidiasis or invasive disease (194,215,431).

Clinical Manifestations

Many infants with significant bacteriuria are asymptomatic (432). If clinical signs are present, they usually are nonspecific and consist of poor weight gain, altered temperature, cyanosis or gray skin color, abdominal distention, malodorous urine, and poor feeding. In a few patients, jaundice and hepatomegaly may be the presenting features of urinary tract infection (433,434). Thrombocytopenic purpura is found in some of these infants. Localizing signs suggesting urinary tract involvement are unusual; they usually consist of a weak urinary stream or an abdominal tumor from bladder distention or hydronephrosis (434). Gross hematuria has been described as the only presenting symptom, but this is rare (435). The most important predisposing factor is vesicoureteral reflux, which allows easy access for bacteria to ascend to the kidneys and leads to residual urine in the bladder (434–436). Circumcised infants have a lower risk of acquiring a urinary tract infection compared with those who are uncircumcised (437).

Diagnosis

The diagnosis of urinary tract infection is confirmed by examination and culture of urine. The result of these tests depends largely on the method of urine collection. Most pediatricians obtain urine with a sterile, plastic receptacle applied to the cleansed perineum. However, urine obtained by this method may have an elevated cell count because of recent circumcision, vaginal reflux of urine, or contamination from the perineum. Neonatal asphyxia may increase the urinary cell count. Leukocytes must be differentiated from round epithelial cells that appear in the urine in appreciable numbers during the early days of life. Although pyuria commonly accompanies significant bacteriuria, cells can be few or absent in the presence of bacteriuria in as many as one-half of the patients (438). Direct microscopic examination of uncentrifuged, fresh urine is useful. If bacteria are seen readily in each oil-immersion field, there are generally more than 10^5 CFU/mL. Glitter cells are believed by many to be diagnostic of urinary tract infections.

Quantitative urine cultures from infants with documented disease contain more than 50,000 CFU/mL (usually ≥100,000 CFU/mL), but a smaller number of organisms can be found in as many as 20% of patients (439). Any number of bacteria in a urine specimen obtained by percutaneous needle puncture of the bladder should be considered significant. This latter procedure is the single best source of urine for culture and is safe in most newborn infants. Its primary complication is transient gross hematuria lasting less than 24 hours in 0.6% of patients (434,440). Very rare complications of suprapubic bladder aspirations include bowel perforation, peritonitis, hematoma, abdominal wall abscess, and bacteremia (440).

Treatment

There are several approaches to the treatment of neonatal urinary tract infections. Antimicrobial agents initially should be administered parenterally, because septicemia is found in 15% to 30% of infants, and absorption after oral administration may be erratic in neonates (441). The physician should assume that there is infection of renal parenchyma resulting from hematogenous spread.

Antibiotic selection should be based on results of antimicrobial susceptibility studies. Gentamicin is effective against the commonly encountered coliform bacteria. Because urinary concentrations of these drugs are considerably higher than those seen in serum, the usual dosages may be halved. For gentamicin, 2 to 3 mg/kg/d is satisfac-

tory, provided the initial blood cultures are sterile. Ampicillin and gentamicin should be administered to symptomatic infants with pyuria before results of culture and susceptibility tests. Renal candidiasis should be treated systemically with amphotericin B. Bladder irrigation with amphotericin B for infants with uncomplicated *Candida* cystitis has not been properly evaluated, and its use cannot be recommended (442).

A repeat urine culture should be sterile 36 to 48 hours after initiation of appropriate therapy. Infants with persistent bacteriuria must be evaluated for possible abscess formation, with or without urinary obstruction. In the uncomplicated patient, therapy usually is continued for a period of approximately 10 days. Blood urea nitrogen and serum creatinine levels should be determined at the initiation of therapy. If there is evidence of renal compromise, dosage and frequency of administration of the drugs, particularly the aminoglycosides, may need to be reduced. Approximately 1 week after therapy is discontinued, a repeat urine culture is obtained. If the culture is positive, therapy is reinstituted and a thorough investigation of the urinary tract is made to rule out obstruction or abscess formation.

All infants with documented urinary tract infections should have radiologic evaluation of the urinary tract. A renal scan or ultrasound examination is obtained some time during therapy so that the possibility of gross congenital abnormalities of the urinary system can be excluded. Technetium 99m dimercaptosuccinic acid cortical scintigraphy is more sensitive than ultrasound examinations and is abnormal in as many as 73% of infants with pyelonephritis (Fig. 47-3) (443). If obstruction is demonstrated, urologic procedures to ensure proper drainage are mandatory if therapy is to be successful. A voiding cystourethrogram usually is obtained several weeks after therapy has been completed. Radiologic abnormalities, such as vesicoureteral reflux, obstructive uropathy, and renal scars, are found in approximately 45% of infants, especially in girls (434,441,444).

Prognosis

It is the physician's responsibility to be certain that neonates with documented urinary tract infections do not have congenital abnormalities of the urinary system. In such patients, recurrent urinary tract infections are common, and physical growth may be retarded until definitive surgery for stage IV or V vesicoureteral reflux has been performed (445). Renal growth retardation is common after neonatal urinary tract infections, even in patients without reflux (445). Patients with recurrent urinary tract infections may be at increased risk of hypertension or renal insufficiency, but the magnitude of this threat is poorly defined (447). Every patient must have careful long-term follow-up studies to detect recurrent infections, many of which are asymptomatic. Prophylactic antibiotics such as trimethoprim-sulfamethoxazole or nitrofurantoin should be provided for infants with clinically significant reflux to avoid

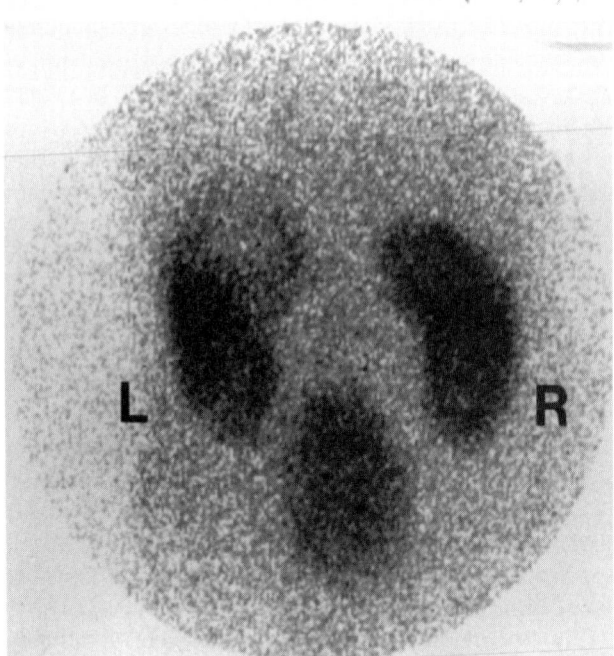

Figure 47-3 Technetium 99m dimercaptosuccinic acid (DMSA) cortical scintigraphy study done on an 11-day-old Caucasian boy with ampicillin-resistant *Escherichia coli* pyelonephritis. This posterior image of the renal beds shows that the left kidney is larger than the right and has a large cold defect involving its superior half.

new scar formation and to ensure normal renal growth. Siblings of infants with urinary tract infection and vesicoureteral reflux should be screened with a voiding cystourethrogram because their risk of having vesicoureteral reflux is 27% to 45% (448).

NEONATAL OPHTHALMIA

Infections of the eye of the newborn may be caused by a variety of microorganisms, including *N. gonorrhoeae*, *C. trachomatis*, *S. aureus*, and *P. aeruginosa*. From a review of 302 cases of eye infections diagnosed in newborns at Grady Memorial Hospital in Atlanta, Georgia, between 1967 and 1973 it was determined that 29% were caused by chlamydiae, 14% by gonococci, 10% by staphylococci, 2% by chemical reactions, and 1% by mixed gonococcal and chlamydial infections (449). The causes of the remaining 44% were uncertain. This frequency distribution of etiologic agents was typical of the experience at large urban general hospitals.

The incidence of ophthalmia neonatorum has not paralleled the significant increase in gonococcal disease rates among adolescents and young adults (450). This almost certainly is a result of universal neonatal gonococcal prophylaxis. The invasive, destructive ophthalmitis described so vividly in old literature is rarely seen today. Several agents have been effective prophylactically against gonococci: 1% silver nitrate, erythromycin or tetracycline ophthalmic ointments, one dose of ceftriaxone administered intramuscularly, and 2.5% solution of povidone-iodine (451–453).

Clinical Manifestations

Gonococcal ophthalmia usually becomes apparent within the first 5 days of life and initially is characterized by a clear, watery discharge. Conjunctival hyperemia and chemosis are associated with a copious discharge of thick, white, purulent material. Both eyes usually are involved but not necessarily to the same degree. Untreated gonococcal ophthalmia may extend to involve the cornea (i.e., keratitis) and the anterior chamber of the eye. Corneal perforation and blindness may occur. Before the introduction of adequate prophylactic measures, ophthalmia neonatorum was the most frequent cause of acquired blindness in the United States.

Differential Diagnosis

Any infant presenting with a conjunctival discharge should be evaluated carefully to determine the cause. Three tests should be performed:

1. Gram stain of the exudate
2. Culture of the exudate
3. Direct immunofluorescent chlamydial stain of scrapings made from the lower palpebral conjunctiva after exudate has been wiped away (454).

Appropriate therapy should be instituted on the basis of the results of the stained smears.

Conjunctivitis occurring in the first days of life can be chemical or bacterial. Chemical irritants, such as silver nitrate, cause transient conjunctival hyperemia and a watery discharge that rarely turns purulent.

If gram-negative rods are seen in the stained exudate, the greatest concern is *P. aeruginosa* because of the virulent, necrotizing endophthalmitis that can result. In this condition, a relatively mild conjunctivitis can progress to infection of the entire globe within 12 to 24 hours. Systemic complications such as bacteremia, meningitis, and brain abscess can occur without evidence of invasive eye disease, especially in VLBW infants (455). Prompt diagnosis and immediate institution of appropriate antimicrobial therapy are mandatory (456). A blood culture should be obtained before antibiotics are started (455).

Conjunctivitis during the second or third week of life may be caused by viral, bacterial, or chlamydial agents. Viral conjunctivitis frequently is associated with other symptoms of respiratory tract disease, such as rhinorrhea, cough, and rash. Several persons in the family or nursery simultaneously may have the disease. The discharge in viral conjunctivitis is watery or mucopurulent but rarely purulent. Preauricular adenopathy is common. Staphylococci, streptococci, *H. influenzae*, *Branhamella (Morexalla) catarrhalis*, and occasionally gonococci cause conjunctivitis in this age group. A smear of purulent material offers some help in differentiating between these bacterial agents. However, the presence of bacteria on a gram-stained smear of exudate is not necessarily related etiologically to the conjunctivitis. Normal inhabitants of the skin and mucous membranes, such as *Staphylococcus*, diphtheroids, and *Neisseria* species may be observed.

Chlamydial eye infection may begin in the first days of life, but it usually does not come to the attention of the physician until the second or third week (457). Clinical manifestations of chlamydial infection vary from mild conjunctivitis to intense inflammation and swelling of the lids, associated with copious purulent discharge. Pseudomembrane formation and a diffuse injection of the tarsal conjunctiva are common. The cornea rarely is affected, and preauricular adenopathy is unusual. In the early stages of disease, one eye may appear more swollen and inflamed than the other, but both eyes usually are involved. The physician establishes the diagnosis by scraping the tarsal conjunctiva and looking for typical cytoplasmic inclusions within epithelial cells or by direct immunofluorescent staining for chlamydial antigens. The scrapings also can be cultured or tested for chlamydial antigens by enzyme immunoassays. Polymerase chain reaction and ligase chain reaction assays for the detection of *C. trachomatis* in ocular and nasopharyngeal specimens appear to be equally specific and more sensitive than culture methods, but the tests are not yet widely used for diagnosis of chlamydial conjunctivitis (458,459,460).

Therapy

Initial therapy is based on the results of stained smears of exudate and epithelial cells. If gonococci are seen, a single dose of ceftriaxone (25 to 50 mg/kg, maximum 125 mg) is given intramuscularly or intravenously (461). If staphylococci are seen, methicillin or another penicillinase-resistant penicillin analog is used. Topical antibiotics are unnecessary, because ample antibiotic to inhibit bacteria exists in the eye secretions (461).

Pseudomonas eye infection should always be treated with parenteral therapy consisting of ceftazidime piperacillin, or ticarcillin and gentamicin. Gentamicin ophthalmic drops are used for simple *Pseudomonas* conjunctivitis, and subconjunctival or sub-Tenon space injections of gentamicin may be needed for endophthalmitis (462).

Ophthalmic solutions containing 1% tetracycline, erythromycin, or sulfacetamide are inferior to oral erythromycin in the treatment of chlamydial conjunctivitis. Topical therapy suppresses chlamydial growth, whereas oral erythromycin eradicates the organism from the eyes and nasopharynx in most infants (463). Erythromycin is used at a dose of 50 mg/kg/d orally divided into four doses for 10 to 14 days. Erythromycin therapy is associated with a 20% to 30% failure rate, which may require second and third courses of therapy. Erythromycin therapy of infants younger than 6 weeks of age has been associated with an increased risk of infantile hypertrophic pyloric stenosis. A shorter course of the azalide antibiotic, azithromycin, may be effective in the treatment of neonatal conjunctivitis, but the optimal dosage and duration of therapy have yet to be determined (464).

Patients with gonococcal ophthalmia should be segregated, and strict hand-washing techniques should be used because of the highly contagious nature of the exudate. The eyes should be irrigated with saline to remove the purulent material. Follow-up examination of infants treated for gonococcal ophthalmia is important to treat subsequent *C. trachomatis* ophthalmia, which can manifest after completion of therapy for gonococcal infection.

DIARRHEAL DISEASE

Although diarrhea disease during the neonatal period usually is brief and self-limited, it can cause significant morbidity in some infants and represents a potential danger to other infants in the nursery unit.

Etiology and Pathogenesis

The most common cause of diarrhea in young infants is alteration of diet and feeding practices, rather than specific bacterial or viral pathogens. Of the infectious causes of diarrhea, rotaviruses are important agents. Both sporadic infections and nursery epidemics have been described. Rotavirus is stable on environmental surfaces and is difficult to eradicate using the usual disinfectants. As a result, it can remain endemic in a nursery for as long as 2 years once established (465). One study from France indicated that 32% of neonates shed rotavirus in their stools; however, of the neonates shedding the virus, 71% had no associated diarrhea (466). Reasons for the asymptomatic nature of most neonatal rotavirus infections are not clear but may include passive protection from transplacentally acquired maternal rotavirus antibodies, the presence of rotavirus antibodies and trypsin inhibitors in breast milk, immaturity of the pancreatic enzymes which may not allow the VP4 protein of the virus to be cleaved (an important step that allows the virus to infect intestinal epithelial cells), and the possibility that rotaviruses that circulate in nurseries may represent attenuated strains of the virus (465). However, neonatal rotavirus diarrhea can be severe and associated with dehydration, hypocalcemia, seizures, and increased frequencies of apnea and bradycardia episodes. It also has been associated with the development of necrotizing enterocolitis (465,468). The finding of rotavirus in the stools of a neonate with diarrhea may be coincidental and not represent the true etiologic agent.

Diarrhea caused by *E. coli* can be mediated through several mechanisms. Some strains are enterotoxigenic (elaborate heat-labile and/or heat-stable toxins), whereas others are enteropathogenic (cause effacement of microvilli and show intimate adherence between the bacterium and the epithelial cell membrane in localized areas), enterohemorrhagic (produce Shiga-like toxin), enteroaggregative (adhere diffusely to intestinal epithelial cells), or enteroinvasive (invade the colonic epithelium and cause ulceration). Enteropathogenic *E. coli* serotypes once were considered the most common bacterial agents responsible for diarrhea in young infants (469). Enterotoxigenic strains of *E. coli* have been identified in nursery outbreaks of diarrheal disease (470). These organisms inhabit the small bowel, in which they attach to, but do not invade, the intestinal mucosa. The enterotoxin produced by these organisms stimulates cyclic adenosine monophosphate, which inhibits sodium and chloride transport across the intestinal wall. These salts are lost into the lumen of the upper bowel, followed passively by water, causing a net loss of stools high in electrolyte content. *Vibrio cholerae, V. parahaemolyticus, Aeromonas,* and some strains of *Campylobacter* and Yersinia are examples of other bacteria that cause diarrhea by this mechanism.

Toxigenic and nontoxigenic *Clostridium difficile* strains commonly are recovered from stool cultures of newborn infants (471). Their significance, however, is unknown because most culture-positive or toxin-positive infants are asymptomatic.

Shigella causes diarrhea through invasion of the intestinal mucosa. Colonic invasion, with subsequent destruction of the mucosa, causes an outpouring of polymorphonuclear cells and mucus. The resultant diarrhea usually is bloody and contains mucus and pus (472). Other organisms causing bloody diarrhea are *Campylobacter, Yersinia,* and *Aeromonas* species (473–476). *Salmonella* species also invade the intestinal mucosa, but extensive destruction does not occur. The epithelial lining is left intact and the organisms reach the lamina propria, in which an inflammatory response is elicited.

Epidemiologic Control

Serotyping of *E. coli* for identification of the traditional enteropathogenic strains no longer is practiced in most hospitals. After an index case of enteropathogenic *E. coli* diarrhea is recognized in a nursery, secondary cases are likely to ensue. This applies to the other etiologic agents of diarrhea in neonates. Any nursery infant with diarrhea should be suspected of having a potentially communicable disease. Ill and healthy colonized infants should be segregated. Infants with diarrhea caused by noninvasive strains of *E. coli* can be treated with nonabsorbable drugs such as oral neomycin (100 mg/kg/d in four divided doses) or colistin sulfate (15 mg/kg/d in three divided doses) for 5 days. Neomycin causes rapid disappearance of the organism and abbreviates the period of diarrhea, but approximately 20% of infants revert to the asymptomatic carrier state after treatment (477). Repeated surveillance of infants is necessary until the pathogenic strain has been eliminated from the nursery.

Clinical Manifestations

The cause of diarrhea cannot be differentiated on clinical grounds in newborn infants. Diarrhea caused by enteropathogenic strains of *E. coli* is insidious in onset, is associated with seven to ten green, watery stools daily, and usually is without blood or mucus. The infants do not appear acutely ill. Complications are rare and are related primarily to dehydration and electrolyte disturbances. *Shigella* infection is uncommon, usually episodic in neonates, and does not spread within nurseries. Shigellosis in the newborn may present as a diarrheic or dysenteric syndrome or may be

evidenced only by a septic or toxic infant (472). Suppurative complications are rare, but dehydration and electrolyte disturbances are common and need immediate and constant attention. *Campylobacter* species can cause bloody diarrhea in otherwise asymptomatic infants (478). Enteritis is the most common manifestation of neonatal *Campylobacter* infection, but more serious disease such as sepsis or meningitis can occur, albeit infrequently (479–480).

Rotavirus infection may be asymptomatic or associated with vomiting and diarrhea. The infants usually are afebrile, but temperature elevation as high as 39°C can occur. Most patients vomit, and the diarrhea is characterized by watery stools containing mucus and no blood. Moderate or severe dehydration may occur, which results in significant electrolyte disturbance in some infants. Fatal disease has been described in a small number of infants. In one report, an outbreak of necrotizing enterocolitis was associated with rotavirus infection (481).

Other viruses can cause neonatal diarrhea. These include enteric adenoviruses, enteroviruses, small round viruses, and coronavirus. The clinical symptoms associated with enteroviruses can vary from a self-limited GI illness to more severe systemic manifestations such as fever, rash, aseptic meningitis, apnea, or myocarditis (480).

Therapy

The most important aspect of therapy for diarrheal disease of newborn infants is maintenance of hydration and electrolyte balance. Parenteral solutions containing appropriate electrolytes should be administered during the time of active diarrhea, and the infant should be examined and weighed frequently so that proper rehydration and prevention of complications are ensured. Estimation of fluid loss from diarrhea and vomiting should be recorded carefully and used as a basis for replacement therapy.

Selection of appropriate antimicrobial therapy depends, in part, on the mechanism of diarrhea. An absorbable antibiotic, such as ampicillin or trimethoprim-sulfamethoxazole, is indicated for disease caused by invasive bacteria (e.g., shigellosis), but orally administered nonabsorbable drugs, such as neomycin or colistin sulfate, are used for noninvasive organisms that produce enterotoxin (e.g., strains of *E. coli*).

Antimicrobial therapy for *Salmonella* gastroenteritis is controversial. Antibiotics do not alter the course of illness and usually prolong intestinal carriage of the organism. Clinical relapse is more common in antibiotic-treated infants. We do not recommend antibiotic therapy for uncomplicated *Salmonella* gastroenteritis if it occurs in older infants and children. Therapy probably is indicated for those with prolonged illness or evidence of colitis, for all neonates, and for infants with systemic symptoms suggesting bloodstream invasion. Ampicillin or amoxicillin usually is satisfactory, as are trimethoprim-sulfamethoxazole, cefotaxime, or ceftriaxone.

Ampicillin was formerly the antibiotic of choice for shigellosis, but significant resistance to this agent has been observed in many areas of the country in recent years. Most strains are susceptible in vitro to trimethoprim-sulfamethoxazole, and infants respond clinically and bacteriologically to a regimen of 10 mg of trimethoprim with 50 mg/kg/d sulfamethoxazole in two divided doses given for 5 days. However, we have limited experience with this agent in newborn infants, and the drug should not be used in those with jaundice. For multiresistant *Shigella* strains, ceftriaxone or cefotaxime may be effective. Erythromycin is the preferred drug for the treatment of symptomatic *Campylobacter* infections.

Any infant with diarrhea must be isolated from other babies in the nursery. Surveillance of all infants in contact with the index case and adoption of strict infection control measures are mandatory.

LOWER RESPIRATORY TRACT INFECTION

Lower respiratory tract infection is an important cause of morbidity in the neonate and is demonstrable on postmortem examination in approximately 20% of neonatal deaths.

Pneumonias can be divided into three categories on the basis of route of acquisition and age at presentation. The first is transplacental pneumonitis, which is acquired *in utero* and presents clinically in the early hours of life. Pneumonia may be part of a generalized congenital infection caused by cytomegalovirus, herpesvirus, rubella virus, *T. gondii*, or *L. monocytogenes*. *T. pallidum* produces a severe, usually fatal pneumonitis (i.e., pneumonia alba), and genital mycoplasmas can cause congenital pneumonia. These infants usually have many organ systems involved, and the pneumonitis may be obscured. Clinical findings may include hepatosplenomegaly, cutaneous manifestations such as rash or petechiae, neurologic abnormalities, and teratogenic effects.

The second category, aspiration pneumonia, is acquired in the immediate perinatal period, and onset of illness occurs within the first hours to days of life. Pathogenesis is by aspiration of amniotic fluid or material from the maternal cervix during the period immediately before or during delivery. Most infants with roentgenographic evidence of aspiration have not swallowed infected material and do not require antimicrobial therapy. This is also true of meconium aspiration, in which the pneumonitis is chemical. The bacterial pathogens most commonly encountered are the group B β-hemolytic streptococci and coliform organisms. Infants with these infections may present in the first 12 hours of life with acute respiratory distress, with or without shock. Mortality is considerable in this condition, even if appropriate antimicrobial therapy is instituted early.

The third category consists of pneumonias acquired during delivery or in the postpartum period, usually beyond the first week of life. Acquired pneumonitis may be caused by viral, chlamydial, or bacterial agents and most

frequently is bronchopneumonic or interstitial. Respiratory syncytial virus (RSV) is the most important pathogen causing lower respiratory tract disease in young infants (482). The parainfluenza viruses, enteroviruses, rhinoviruses, and adenoviruses cause bronchiolitis and pneumonia during early infancy. Herpes simplex virus infection can be acquired at the time of delivery and present in the first week of life. Bronchiolitis, pneumonia, or both usually occur in epidemics among premature and full-term nursery infants or in the community.

Documented nursery outbreaks of lower respiratory tract disease have been associated with RSV, adenovirus, echovirus type 22, influenza A and B viruses, and parainfluenza virus infections. During these outbreaks, many infants are colonized with the epidemic virus strains, but only a few manifest clinical disease.

S. aureus and coliform organisms are the most common bacterial pathogens causing postnatally acquired pneumonia. Disease caused by *S. aureus* and *K. pneumoniae* may occur sporadically or in epidemic fashion during the neonatal period. Pyogenic complications, such as septicemia, osteomyelitis, and meningitis, frequently are associated with the epidemic form of these infections.

Acquisition of *C. trachomatis* in the intrapartum period may result in conjunctivitis (i.e., inclusion blennorrhea) or in pneumonia that usually presents between the fourth and twelfth weeks of life. The pneumonia is associated with a staccato cough, often terminating in vomiting or cyanosis, and with tachypnea; the infants usually are afebrile (483). Rales are heard, and there may be a history of the infant having conjunctivitis in the newborn period. Eosinophilia is seen in approximately half the patients. Chlamydial pneumonia occasionally can occur in the early neonatal period (first 2 weeks of life) (484–485). *C. trachomatis* can cause severe and chronic pneumonia in LBW infants (486–487) *C. trachomatis* pneumonia in otherwise healthy infants has been associated with long-term pulmonary function abnormalities (488).

A considerable body of data indicates that *U. urealyticum* colonization of LBW infants is associated with the subsequent development of chronic lung disease (489–495). *Ureaplasma*-positive infants have much higher ratios of IL-1β to IL-6 and tumor necrosis factor to IL-6 in their tracheal aspirates than do *Ureaplasma*-negative infants (496). Thus, in the preterm lung, *U. urealyticum* may contribute to early injury by inducing the release of inflammatory cytokines. However, treatment of *U. urealyticum* colonization with erythromycin has not been shown to reduce the incidence of chronic lung disease in premature infants (497,498). *Pneumocystis jiroveci* is an uncommon cause of pneumonia in the neonatal period; susceptible infants include malnourished premature newborns living in endemic geographic areas, infants with congenital immunodeficiencies (e.g., severe combined immunodeficiency), and neonates infected with the human immunodeficiency virus type 1 (499–501). *Legionella* pneumonia is uncommon but has been described in newborns, most of whom had underlying problems such as prematurity, chronic lung disease, congenital heart disease, steroid treatment, or hypoxic ischemic encephalopathy. *Legionella* can cause a range of respiratory symptoms from a mild influenza-like illness to severe cavitary pneumonia and death (502,503). *Bordetella pertussis* infection continues to occur and should be suspected in newborns with paroxysmal cough and a parent or sibling with a persistent cough.

Clinical Manifestations

The early signs of lower respiratory tract disease in the neonate and young infant frequently are nonspecific and include change in feeding status, listlessness or irritability, and poor color. More specific findings that may not be present at the onset of illness are tachypnea, dyspnea, cyanosis, hypothermia, cough, and grunting. Accentuation of the normal irregularity of breathing is a common finding in neonates.

The physical findings of pneumonia vary. Flaring of the alae nasi, rapid respirations, and sternal and subcostal retractions frequently are observed. A cough is indicative of lower respiratory tract involvement; a brassy cough frequently is found in viral disease. Percussion dullness is difficult to demonstrate, but it is indicative of consolidation, effusion, or both. Auscultation may reveal diminished breath sounds over the affected area. Rales, wheezes, or both usually can be heard on deep inspiration or when the baby is crying, but may be absent early in the illness. The clinician frequently is surprised by the meager clinical signs in the face of clearly demonstrable and sometimes extensive roentgenographic findings of pneumonia.

Infants with pertussis usually become ill between weeks 2 and 6 of life. The characteristic whoop seen in older infants and children usually is absent. Paroxysmal cough, excessive mucous, and apneic spells are common in these infants. Complications of pertussis are many and include secondary bacterial pneumonia, atelectasis, and asphyxia.

Diagnosis

The leukocyte count may assist in the differentiation of viral from bacterial pneumonia. Infants with early-onset bacterial pneumonia with sepsis may have leukopenia with an increased number of immature neutrophils. Chorioamnionitis has been demonstrated in the mothers of some infants with congenital pneumonia.

Cultures of blood and material from the trachea frequently help to define the etiologic agent of neonatal pneumonia. However, results of cultures from the ear canal, throat, and other external sites are not helpful and may be misleading in newborn and young infants. Thoracentesis or lung puncture should be considered in infants with pleural effusion or consolidated pneumonia, respectively, if the cause is unknown or the infant fails to respond to conventional antimicrobial therapy. Material obtained at puncture should be Gram stained for direct visualization of bacteria and cultured. Chlamydial pneumonia is best diagnosed by culture of nasopharyngeal

secretions or by the polymerase chain reaction (504). Under certain circumstances, the tracheal aspirates or fluid obtained after bronchoalveolar lavage can be examined for *P. jiroveci* cysts, cultured for viruses, fungi, mycoplasmas, *B. pertussis*, acid-fast bacteria, and *Legionella*, and examined by polymerase chain reaction assays for a variety of infectious agents including *U. urealyticum*, *B. pertussis*, and viruses such as herpes simplex virus and cytomegalovirus (501,503,505,506).

A chest radiograph may reveal roentgenographic evidence of pneumonia despite the absence of physical findings. Although it usually is not possible to determine the cause of neonatal pneumonia from chest radiographs, certain roentgenographic patterns may be associated with specific diseases. A consolidating bronchopneumonia with pneumatoceles, with or without empyema, suggests staphylococcal disease. This is particularly true when the radiologic findings advance markedly in a few hours. If a lobar infiltrate is associated with bulging fissures on the radiograph, *K. pneumoniae* infection should be considered. A miliary-type of bronchopneumonia in a septic neonate is characteristic of listeriosis. GBS pneumonia frequently is indistinguishable radiographically from hyaline membrane disease. A bronchopneumonic infiltrate noted on chest roentgenogram during the first postnatal month of life may be caused by aspiration of sterile or infected amniotic fluid or by viral, chlamydial, or bacterial pathogens, or it can represent patchy atelectasis (507).

Staphylococcal pneumonia is found most commonly in young infants; 30% of patients are younger than 3 months of age, and 70% are younger than 1 year of age. Epidemics of staphylococcal disease caused by phage group I organisms are encountered infrequently.

Staphylococci cause a confluent bronchopneumonia characterized by extensive areas of hemorrhagic necrosis and irregular areas of cavitation. The pleural surface is usually covered by a thick layer of fibrinopurulent exudate. Multiple small abscesses are scattered throughout the lungs. Rupture of a small subpleural abscess may result in a pyopneumothorax, which may erode into a bronchus, producing a bronchopleural fistula.

The onset of illness in staphylococcal pneumonia is abrupt, with fever, cough, and respiratory distress as the major manifestations. Tachypnea, grunting respirations, retractions, cyanosis, and anxiety usually are observed. Severe dyspnea and a shock-like state may occur. Rapid progression of symptoms is characteristic. Moist, scattered rales, diminished breath sounds, and rhonchi may be heard early in the illness. With the development of pleural effusion, dullness on percussion is associated with diminished breath sounds.

Most patients with staphylococcal pneumonia have roentgenographic evidence of bronchopneumonia early in the illness. The infiltrate may be patchy and limited in extent or be dense and homogeneous, involving an entire lobe or hemithorax. Pleural effusions or empyema are found in most infants (508). Pneumatoceles of various sizes are common. Although no radiographic change can be considered diagnostic, progression over a few hours from bronchopneumonia to effusion or pyopneumothorax with or without pneumatoceles is highly suggestive of staphylococcal pneumonia.

Treatment

All diagnostic procedures and cultures should be obtained before initiation of therapy. Methicillin is the initial drug of choice for staphylococcal pneumonia and should be administered parenterally in a dosage of 75 mg/kg/d divided in two or three doses for infants younger than 1 week of age and in a dosage of 100 mg/kg/d divided in four doses for older infants.

If infection extends to the pleural surfaces, surgical intervention usually becomes necessary. With small amounts of effusion, repeated pleural taps may be successful in removing fluid, but empyema is best treated by closed drainage with a chest tube of the largest possible caliber.

Vancomycin is preferred for disease as a result of MRSA. For pneumonia caused by *K. pneumoniae* or other coliforms, kanamycin or gentamicin should be used in a total dosage of 15 mg/kg/d or 5 to 7.5 mg/kg/d, respectively. Alternatively, a third-generation cephalosporin, such as cefotaxime, can be used. Treatment for *Listeria* pneumonia is parenteral ampicillin in a dosage of 50 to 100 mg/kg/d divided in two doses for infants younger than 1 week of age and 100 to 150 mg/kg/d divided in three doses for older neonates. Infants with GBS septicemia and pneumonia should be given penicillin as outlined earlier for sepsis neonatorum. Larger doses are required for meningitis. Ampicillin or cefotaxime may be used in place of penicillin.

Pertussis and chlamydial and ureaplasmal pneumonias probably are treated best with orally or intravenously administered erythromycin, depending on the infant's clinical status. This agent has been shown to shorten the course of illness and to eradicate shedding of the organisms from the nasopharynx. *Legionella* pneumonia also is treated with erythromycin; rifampin sometimes is added (503). Trimethoprim-sulfamethoxazole is the initial drug of choice for *P. jiroveci* pneumonia; pentamidine and trimetrexate are reserved for treatment failures.

Pneumonia may be one manifestation of generalized congenital viral infections. It is important to differentiate these infections from CS and bacterial pneumonias resulting from aspiration. Ganciclovir can be used for cytomegalovirus pneumonia, but infants may worsen again on discontinuation of the drug. Vidarabine or acyclovir is effective if given early in disease caused by herpes simplex virus.

Most infants with aspiration pneumonia do not require antimicrobial therapy. It frequently is difficult to differentiate infants with aspiration of sterile amniotic fluid from those aspirating infected materials. If doubt exists, therapy with penicillin and an aminoglycoside should be initiated and continued until results of cultures are available.

OTITIS MEDIA

Otitis media is a frequent finding in premature infants receiving intensive care and an almost universal finding in autopsy studies of infants who died after a period of intensive care (509–512). A principal predisposing factor for otitis media in the newborn is nasotracheal intubation that results in ipsilateral obstruction of the eustachian tube, establishing the conditions eventuating in middle-ear infection. The diagnosis is missed frequently because pneumatic otoscopy is not performed routinely in neonates.

The exact incidence of this condition is unknown. In one prospective study of 70 term infants followed from birth, 34% developed their first episode of otitis media before 2 months of age (513). Symptoms are nonspecific and include irritability, lethargy, fever, cough, diarrhea, vomiting, tachypnea, and anorexia (514). An associated conjunctivitis, pneumonia, or meningitis may be found in as many as half the patients. The diagnosis usually is made by pneumatic otoscopy. Tympanometry is unreliable in neonates.

Pathogenic organisms include *S. pneumoniae*, *H. influenzae*, *S. aureus*, *β. catarrhalis*, *P. aeruginosa*, and coliforms. The predominant isolates vary in different study populations (509–517).

Tympanocentesis should be performed on all newborns with otitis media who develop illness while in the nursery or intensive care unit (518). This may yield an etiologic agent when cultures of other sites are sterile. Some infants have positive blood cultures (517). The choice of antibiotic therapy can be based on the results of the Gram stain and culture of the aspirated middle ear effusion. If no organisms are seen on the smear, treatment should be with methicillin and an aminoglycoside until additional information is available. Infants with otitis media who are seen in the clinic or office usually do not require tympanocentesis for etiologic diagnosis if the illness is mild and can be managed at home. In these infants, amoxicillin is preferred for therapy, and the patients should be reexamined 2 or 3 days after initiation of therapy to ascertain improvement. Infants with onset of otitis media before 2 months of age may need as long as 3 months to clear the effusion, and 33% of them develop chronic otitis media (513).

PERITONITIS

Spontaneous bacterial (i.e., primary) peritonitis without an evident intraabdominal source is rare during the neonatal period (519). It is postulated that bacteria can reach the peritoneal cavity by means of hematogenous, lymphatic, genital, or transmural (i.e., across the gut wall) routes of spread (520). A concurrent omphalitis is common (521). Gram-positive bacteria (e.g., *S. pneumoniae*, groups A and B streptococci) are the predominant pathogens, but gram-negative bacilli such as *Pseudomonas* or *Klebsiella* are responsible for some cases.

Most infants develop peritonitis after perforation of an abdominal viscus, usually as a complication of necrotizing enterocolitis. Other predisposing conditions include spontaneous focal GI perforations, wound infections after abdominal surgery, traumatic perforations (e.g., feeding tube, rectal thermometer), ruptured omphalocele, and meconium peritonitis with subsequent bacterial contamination. Organisms isolated from peritoneal fluid cultures generally mirror the infant's gut flora and include *E. coli*, *Klebsiella* spp, *Enterobacter* spp, *Pseudomonas*, coagulase-positive and coagulase-negative staphylococci, streptococci, enterococci, anaerobic bacteria (e.g., clostridia, *Bacteroides* spp), and *Candida* (522–524).

Clinical signs of peritonitis include vomiting, abdominal distention, abdominal wall edema or discoloration, constipation, diarrhea, grunting, temperature instability (usually hypothermia), shock, and scrotal or vulvar swelling. Abdominal radiographs may reveal free air in the peritoneal cavity, indicating intestinal perforation, or patterns suggesting necrotizing enterocolitis (e.g., pneumatosis intestinalis) or intestinal obstruction. Abdominal ultrasound is helpful in visualizing peritoneal fluid. An abdominal paracentesis may yield pus or reveal a different cause for the illness (e.g., hemoperitoneum, bile peritonitis). Aerobic and anaerobic cultures of the peritoneal fluid and of the blood should be obtained in all cases.

The management of peritonitis consists of supportive measures aimed at reversing hypovolemia, shock, and electrolyte imbalances; surgical correction of underlying conditions; and administration of broad-spectrum antimicrobial agents. Acceptable initial antibiotic regimens include ampicillin, gentamicin and clindamycin, ticarcillin-clavulanate or piperacillin-tazobactam and an aminoglycoside, or vancomycin, ceftazidime, and metronidazole. The broadest antibacterial coverage is attained by the vancomycin, ceftazidime, and metronidazole combination. Treatment can be simplified after the blood and peritoneal fluid culture results become available. Antibiotics are usually administered for a minimum of 10 days. The prognosis depends on several factors, including birth weight and precipitating conditions, and fatality rates range from 10% to 50% (519).

REFERENCES

1. Jason JM. Infectious disease-related deaths of low birth weight infants, United States 1968 to 1982. *Pediatrics* 1989;84:296.
2. Msall ME, Buck GM, Rogers BT, et al. Risk factors for major neurodevelopmental impairments and need for special education resources in extremely premature infants. *J Pediatr* 1991;119:606.
3. Stoll BJ, Hansen N, Fanaroff AA, et al. Late-onset sepsis in very low birth weight neonates: the experience of the NICHD Neonatal Research Network. *Pediatrics* 2002;110:285.
4. Stoll BJ, Hansen N, Fanaroff AA, et al. Changes in pathogens causing early-onset sepsis in very-low-birth-weight infants. *N Engl J Med* 2002;347:240.
5. Inder TE, Wells SJ, Mogridge NB, et al. Defining the nature of the cerebral abnormalities in the premature infant: a qualitative magnetic resonance imaging study. *J Pediatr* 2003;143:171.
6. Murphy DJ, Hope PL, Johnson A. Neonatal risk factors for cerebral palsy in very preterm babies: case-control study. *BMJ* 1997;314:404.
7. Freedman RM, Ingram DL, Gross I, et al. A half century of neonatal sepsis at Yale: 1928 to 1978. *Am J Dis Child* 1981; 135:140.

8. Stoll BJ. The global impact of neonatal infection. *Clin Perinatol* 1997;24:1.
9. Horbar JD, Rogowski J, Plsek PE, et al. Collaborative quality improvement for neonatal intensive care. NIC/Q Project Investigators of the Vermont Oxford Network. *Pediatrics* 2001; 107:14.
10. Gaynes RP, Edwards JR, Jarvis WR, et al. Nosocomial infections among neonates in high-risk nurseries in the United States. National Nosocomial Infections Surveillance System. *Pediatrics* 1996;98:357.
11. Jarvis WR. Benchmarking for prevention: the Centers for Disease Control and Prevention's National Nosocomial Infections Surveillance (NNIS) system experience. *Infection* 2003;31 [Suppl 2]: 44.
12. St. Geme JW III, Harris MC. Coagulase-negative staphylococcal infection in the neonate. *Clin Perinatol* 1991;18:281.
13. Gaynes RP, Edwards JR, Jarvis WR, et al. Nosocomial infections among neonates in high-risk nurseries in the United States. *Pediatrics* 1996;98:357.
14. Back NA, Linnemann CC Jr, Staneck JL, et al. Control of methicillin-resistant Staphylococcus aureus in a neonatal intensive-care unit: use of intensive microbiologic surveillance and mupirocin. *Infect Control Hosp Epidemiol* 1996;17:227.
15. Von Dolinger BD, Matos C, Abdalla VV, et al. An Outbreak of Nosocomial Infection Caused by ESBLs Producing Serratia marcescens in a Brazilian Neonatal Unit. *Braz J Infect Dis* 1999;3:149.
16. Toltzis P, Dul MJ, Hoyen C, et al. Molecular epidemiology of antibiotic-resistant gram-negative bacilli in a neonatal intensive care unit during a nonoutbreak period. *Pediatrics* 2001;108: 1143.
17. Usukura Y, Igarashi T. Examination of severe, hospital acquired infections affecting extremely low birthweight (ELBW) infants. *Pediatr Int* 2003;45:230.
18. Bortolussi R, Thompson TR, Ferrieri P. Early-onset pneumococcal sepsis in newborn infants. *Pediatrics* 1977;60:352.
19. Kaplan M, Rudensky B, Beck A. Perinatal infections with *Streptococcus pneumoniae*. *Am J Perinatol* 1993;10:1.
20. Chugh K, Bhalla CK, Joshi KK. Meningococcal brain abscess and meningitis in a neonate. *Pediatr Infect Dis J* 1988;7:136.
21. Goldmann DA, Leclair J, Macone A. Bacterial colonization of neonates admitted to an intensive care environment. *J Pediatr* 1978;93:288.
22. Eriksson M, Melen B, Myrback KE, et al. Bacterial colonization of newborn infants in a neonatal intensive care unit. *Acta Paediatr Scand* 1982;71:779.
23. Cordero L, Ayers LW, Davis K. Neonatal airway colonization with gram-negative bacilli: association with severity of bronchopulmonary dysplasia. *Pediatr Infect Dis J* 1997;16:18.
24. Goldmann DA. Bacterial colonization and infection in the neonate. *Am J Med* 1981;70:417.
25. Fryklund B, Tullus K, Burman LG. Epidemiology of enteric bacteria in neonatal unit-influence of procedures and patient variables. *J Hosp Infect* 1991;18:15.
26. Goering RV, Ehrenkranz NJ, Sanders CC, et al. Long term epidemiological analysis of *Citrobacter diversus* in a neonatal intensive care unit. *Pediatr Infect Dis J* 1992;11:99.
27. D'Angio CT, McGowan KL, Baumgart S, et al. Surface colonization with coagulase negative staphylococci in premature neonates. *J Pediatr* 1989;114:1029.
28. Kaufman D, Boyle R, Hazen KC, et al. Fluconazole prophylaxis against fungal colonization and infection in preterm infants. *N Engl J Med* 2001;345:1660.
29. Baley JE, Kliegman RM, Boxerbaum B, et al. Fungal colonization in the very low birth weight infant. *Pediatrics* 1986;78:225.
30. Waggoner-Fountain LA, Walker MW, Hollis RJ, et al. Vertical and horizontal transmission of unique *Candida* species to premature newborns. *Clin Infect Dis* 1996;22:803.
31. Aschner JL, Punsalang A Jr, Maniscalco WM, et al. Percutaneous central venous catheter colonization with *Malassezia furfur*: incidence and clinical significance. *Pediatrics* 1987;80:535.
32. Bell LM, Alpert G, Slight PH, et al. *Malassezia furfur* skin colonization in infancy. *Infect Control Hosp Epidemiol* 1988;9:151.
33. Stuart SM, Lane AT. Candida and Malassezia as nursery pathogens. *Semin Dermatol* 1992;11:19.
34. Lane AT, Drost SS. Effect of repeated application of emollient cream to premature neonates' skin. *Pediatrics* 1993;92:415.

35. Edwards WH, Conner JM, Soll RF. The effect of prophylactic ointment therapy on nosocomial sepsis rates and skin integrity in infants with birth weights of 501 to 1000 g. *Pediatrics* 2004;113:1195.

36. Cassell Gil, Waites KB, Crouse DT. Perinatal mycoplasmal infections. *Clin Perinatol* 1991;18:241.

37. Syrogiannopoulos GA, Kapatais-Zoumbos K, Decavalas GO, et al. *Ureaplasma urealyticum* colonization of full term infants: prenatal acquisition and persistence during early infancy. *Pediatr Infect Dis J* 1990;9:236.

38. Hammerschlag MR, Anderka M, Semine DZ, et al. Prospective study of maternal and infantile infection with *Chlamydia trachomatis. Pediatrics* 1979;64:142.

39. Schachter J, Grossman M, Sweet RL, et al. Prospective study of perinatal transmission of *Chiamydia trachomatis. JAMA* 1986; 255:3374.

40. Bell TA, Stamm WE, Wang SP, et al. Chronic *Chlamydia trachomatis* infections in infants. *JAMA* 1992;267:400.

41. Stoll BJ, Holman RC, Schuchat A. Decline in sepsis-associated neonatal and infant deaths in the United States 1979 through 1994. *Pediatrics* 1998;102:e18.

42. Kaftan H, Kinney JS. Early-onset neonatal bacterial infections. *Semin Perinatol* 1998;22:15.

43. Lukacs SL, Schoendorf KC, Schuchat A. Trends in sepsis-related neonatal mortality in the United States 1985–1998. *Pediatr Infect Dis J* 2004;23:599.

44. Peter G, Cashore WJ. Infections acquired in the nursery: epidemiology and control. In: Remington JS, Klein JO, eds. *Infectious diseases of the fetus and newborn infant*, 4th ed. Philadelphia: WB Saunders, 1995:1264.

45. Thompson PJ, Greenough A, Hird ME, et al. Nosocomial bacterial infections in very low birth weight infants. *Eur J Pediatr* 1992;151:451.

46. Moro ML, De Toni A, Stolfi I, et al. Risk factors for nosocomial sepsis in newborn intensive and intermediate care units. *Eur J Pediatr* 1996;155:315.

47. Fanaroff AA, Korones SB, Wright LL, et al. Incidence, presenting features, risk factors and significance of late onset septicemia in very low birth weight infants. *Pediatr Infect Dis J* 1998;17:593.

48. Sáez-Llorens X, McCracken GH Jr. Clinical pharmacology of antibacterial agents. In: Remington JS, Klein JO, eds. *Infectious diseases of the fetus and newborn infant*, 4th ed. Philadelphia: WB Saunders, 1995:1287.

49. Boyer KM, Gotoff SP. Alternative algorithms for prevention of perinatal group B streptococcal infections. *Pediatr Infect Dis J* 1998;17:973.

50. Bada HS, Alojipan LC, Andrews BF. Premature rupture of membranes and its effect on the newborn. *Pediatr Clin North Am* 1977;24:491.

51. St. Geme JW Jr, Murray DL, Carter JA, et al. Perinatal bacterial infection after prolonged rupture of amniotic membranes: an analysis of risk and management. *J Pediatr* 1984;104:608.

52. Sperling RS, Newton E, Gibbs RS. Intraamniotic infection in low birth-weight infants. *J Infect Dis* 1988;157:113.

53. Hillier SL, Krohn MA, Kiviat NB, et al. Microbiologic causes and neonatal outcomes associated with chorioamnion infection. *Am J Obstet Gynecol* 1991;165:955.

54. Belady PH, Farkouh LJ, Gibbs RS. Intra-amniotic infection and premature rupture of the membranes. *Clin Perinatol* 1997;24:43.

55. Marstan G, Wald ER. *Hemophilus influenzae* type b sepsis in infant and mother. *Pediatrics* 1976;58:863.

56. Simpson JM, Patel JS, Ispahani R *Streptococcus pneumaniae* invasive disease in the neonatal period: an increasing problem? *Eur J Pediatr* 1995;154:563.

57. Grossman J, Tompkins RL. Group B beta-hemolytic Streptococcal meningitis in mother and infant. *N Engl J Med* 1974;290:387.

58. Botta GA. Hormonal and type-dependent adhesion of group B *streptococci* to human vaginal cells. *Infect Immun* 1979;25:1084.

59. Braughton RA, Baker CJ. Role of adherence in the pathogenesis of neonatal group B streptococcal infection. *Infect Immun* 1983;39:837.

60. Robbins JB, McCracken GH Jr, Gotschlich EC, et al. *Escherichia coli* K1 capsular polysaccharide associated with neonatal meningitis. *N Engl J Med* 1974;290:1216.

61. Givner LB, Baker CJ. Pooled human IgG hyperimmune far type III *group B streptococci*: evaluation against multiple strains in vitro and in experimental disease. *J Infect Dis* 1991;163:1141.

62. Glade MP, Sutton A, Moxon ER, et al. Pathogenesis of neonatal *Escherichia coli* meningitis: induction of bacteremia and meningitis in infant rats fed E. coli K1. *Infect Immun* 1977;16:75.

63. Larsen JW Jr, London WT, Palmer AE, et al. Experimental group B *Streptococcal* infection in the rhesus monkey: I. Disease production in the neonate. *Am J Obstet Gynecol* 1978;132:686.

64. Martin TR, Ruzinski JT, Rubens CE, et al. The effect of type-specific polysaccharide capsule on the clearance of *group B streptococci* from the lungs of infant and adult rats. *J Infect Dis* 1992;165:306.

65. Baker CJ, Edwards MS, Kasper DL. Role of antibody to native type III polysaccharide of group B Streptococcus in infant protection. *Pediatrics* 1981;68:544.

66. Anderson DC, Edwards MS, Baker CJ. Luminol-enhanced chemiluminescence far evaluation of type III group B Streptococcal opsonins in human sera. *J Infect Dis* 1980;141:370.

67. Vogel LC, Kretschmer RR, Boyer KM, et al. Human immunity to group B Streptococci measured by indirect immunofluorescence: correlation with protection in chick embryos. *J Infect Dis* 1979;140:682.

68. Fischer GW, Hemming VG, Hunter KW Jr, et al. Intravenous immunoglobulin in the treatment of neonatal sepsis: therapeutic strategies and laboratory studies. *Pediatr Infect Dis* 1986;5:S171.

69. Hill HR, Gonzales LA, Knappe WA, et al. Comparative protective activity of human monoclonal and hyperimmune polyclonal antibody against group B Streptococci. *J Infect Dis* 1991;163:792.

70. Baker CJ, Webb BJ, Kasper DL, et al. The natural history of *group B streptococcal* colonization in the pregnant woman and her offspring: II. Determination of serum antibody to capsular polysaccharide from type III, group B Streptococcus. *Am J Obstet Gynecol* 1980;137:39.

71. Anthony BF, Concepcion NE, Concepcion KF. Human antibody to the group-specific polysaccharide of group B Streptococcus. *J Infect Dis* 1985;151:221.

72. Klegerman ME, Boyer KM, Papierniak CK, et al. Estimation of the protective level of human IgG antibody to the type-specific polysaccharide of group B Streptococcus type Ia. *J Infect Dis* 1983;148:648.

73. Boyer KM, Kendall LS, Papierniak CK, et al. Protective levels of human immunoglobulin G antibody to group B Streptococcus type lb. *Infect Immun* 1984;45:618.

74. Gotoff SP, Papierniak CK, Klegerman ME, et al. Quantitation of IgG antibody to the type-specific polysaccharide of group B Streptococcus type lb in pregnant women and infected infants. *J Pediatr* 1984;105:628.

75. Gray BM, Pritchard DG, Dillon HC Jr. Seroepidemiological studies of group B Streptococcus type II. *J Infect Dis* 1985;151:1073.

76. Anthony BF. The role of specific antibody in neonatal bacterial infections: an overview. *Pediatr Infect Dis* 1986;5:S164.

77. Lassiter HA, Tanner JE, Miller RD. Inefficient bacteriolysis of *Escherichia coli* by serum from human neonates. *J Infect Dis* 1992;165:290.

78. Lassiter HA, Watson SW, Seifring ML, et al. Complement factor 9 deficiency in serum of human neonates. *J Infect Dis* 1992;166:53.

79. Edwards MS, Buffone GJ, Fuselier PA, et al. Deficient classical complement pathway activity in newborn sera. *Pediatr Res* 1983;17:685.

80. Máródi L, Leijh PCJ, Braat A, et al. Opsonic activity of cord blood sera against various species of microorganism. *Pediatr Res* 1985;19:433.

81. Edwards MS, Kasper DL, Jennings HJ, et al. Capsular sialic acid prevents activation of the alternative complement pathway by type III, group B Streptococci. *J Immunol* 1982;128:1278.

82. Yoder MC. Therapeutic administration of fibronectins: current uses and potential applications. *Clin Perinatal* 1991;18:325.

83. Gerdes JS, Yoder MC, Douglas SD, et al. Decreased plasma fibronectins in neonatal sepsis. *Pediatrics* 1983;72:877.

84. Domula M, Bykawska K, Wegrzynowicz Z, et al. Plasma fibronectins concentrations in healthy and septic infants. *Eur J Pediatr* 1985;144:49.

85. Butler KM, Baker CJ, Edwards MS. Interaction of soluble fibronectin with group B Streptococci. *Infect Immun* 1987;55:2404.

86. Christensen RD, Rothstein G. Exhaustion of mature marrow neutrophils in neonates with sepsis. *J Pediatr* 1980;96:316.

87. Cairo MS. Neonatal neutrophil host defense: prospects for immunologic enhancement during neonatal sepsis. *Am J Dis Child* 1989;143:40.

88. Klein JO, Marcy SM. Bacterial sepsis and meningitis. In: Remington JS, Klein JO, eds. *Infections diseases of the fetus and newborn infant*, 4th ed. Philadelphia: WB Saunders, 1995:835.

89. Voora S, Srinivasan G, Lilien LD, et al. Fever in full-term newborns in the first four days of life. *Pediatrics* 1982;69:40.

90. McCracken GH Jr. Group B streptococci: the new challenge in neonatal infections. *J Pediatr* 1973;82:703.

91. Franciosi RA, Knostman JD, Zimmerman RA. Group B streptococcal neonatal and infant infections. *J Pediatr* 1973;82:707–718.

92. Gladstone IM, Ehrenkranz RA, Edberg SC, et al. A ten-year review of neonatal sepsis and comparison with the previous fifty-year experience. *Pediatr Infect Dis J* 1990;9:819.

93. Hyde TB, Hilger TM, Reingold A, et al. Trends in incidence and antimicrobial resistance of early-onset sepsis: population-based surveillance in San Francisco and Atlanta. *Pediatrics* 2002;110: 690.

94. Baltimore RS, Huie SM, Meek JI, et al. Early-onset neonatal sepsis in the era of group B streptococcal prevention. *Pediatrics* 2001;108:1094.

95. Boyer KM, Gotoff SP. Prevention of early-onset neonatal group B streptococcal disease with selective intrapartum chemoprophylaxis. *N Engl J Med* 1986;314:1665.

96. American Academy of Pediatrics Committee on Infectious Diseases and Committee on Fetus and Newborn. Guidelines for prevention of group B streptococcal (GBS) infection by chemoprophylaxis. *Pediatrics* 1992;90:775–778.

97. Centers for Disease Control and Prevention. Prevention of perinatal group B streptococcal disease: a public health perspective. *MMWR Recomm Rep* 1996;45:1.

98. Revised guidelines for prevention of early-onset group B streptococcal (GBS) infection. American Academy of Pediatrics Committee on Infectious Diseases and Committee on Fetus and Newborn. *Pediatrics* 1997;99:489.

99. Schrag SJ, Zywicki S, Farley MM, et al. Group B streptococcal disease in the era of intrapartum antibiotic prophylaxis. *N Engl J Med* 2000;342:15.

100. Schrag S, Gorwitz R, Fultz-Butts K, et al. Prevention of perinatal group B streptococcal disease. Revised guidelines from CDC. *MMWR Recomm Rep* 2002;51:1.

101. ACOG Committee Opinion: number 279, December 2002. Prevention of early-onset group B streptococcal disease in newborns. *Obstet Gynecol* 2002;100:1405–1412.

102. Baker CJ, Edwards MS. Group B Streptococcal infections. In: Remington JS, Klein JO, eds. *Infectious diseases of the fetus and newborn infant*, 4th ed. Philadelphia: WB Saunders, 1995:980.

103. Dillon HC Jr, Khare S, Gray BM. Group B Streptococcal carriage and disease: a 6-year prospective study. *J Pediatr* 1987;110:31.

104. Regan JA, Klebanoff MA, Vaginal Infections and Prematurity Study Group, et al. The epidemiology of group B Streptococcal colonization in pregnancy. *Obstet Gynecol* 1991;77:604.

105. Stoll BJ, Schuchat A. Maternal carriage of group B streptococci in developing countries. *Pediatr Infect Dis J* 1998;17:499.

106. Schuchat A. Epidemiology of group B Streptococcal disease in the United States: shifting paradigms. *Clin Microbial Rev* 1998;11:497.

107. Gardner SE, Yow MD, Leeds LJ, et al. Failure of penicillin to eradicate *group B streptococcal* colonization in the pregnant woman: a couple study. *Am J Obstet Gynecol* 1979;135:1062.

108. Jones DE, Kanarek KS, Lim DV. Group B Streptococcal colonization patterns in mothers and their infants. *J Clin Microbial* 1984;20:438.

109. Chin KC, Fitzhardinge PM. Sequelae of early-onset *group B hemolytic streptococcal* neonatal meningitis. *J Pediatr* 1985;106:819.

110. Centers for Disease Control and Prevention. Prevention of perinatal *group B streptococcal* disease: a public health perspective. *MMWR* 1996;45(RR-7):1.

111. Pyati SP, Pildes RS, Ramamurthy RS, et al. Decreasing mortality in neonates with early-onset group B Streptococcal infection: reality or artifact. *J Pediatr* 1981;98:625.

112. Siegel JD, McCracken GH Jr. *Group D streptococcal* infections. *J Pediatr* 1978;93:542.

113. Dyson AE, Read SE. Group G Streptococcal colonization and sepsis in neonates. *J Pediatr* 1981;99:944.

114. Isaacman SH, Heroman WM, Lightsey AL. Purpura fulminans following late-onset group B β-hemolytic Streptococcal sepsis. *Am J Dis Child* 1984;138:915.

115. Howard JB, McCracken GH Jr. The spectrum of group B Streptococcal infections in infancy. *Am J Dis Child* 1974;128:815.

116. Yagupsky P, Menegus MA, Powell KR. The changing spectrum of group B Streptococcal disease in infants: an eleven-year experience in a tertiary care hospital. *Pediatr Infect Dis J* 1991;10:801.

117. Atkins JT, Heresi GP, Coque TM, et al. Recurrent group B Streptococcal disease in infants: who should receive rifampin? *J Pediatr* 1998;132:537.

118. Whitley CB, Thompson LR, Osterholm MT, et al. Toxic shock syndrome in a newborn infant. *Pediatr Res* 1982;16:254A(abst).

119. Chesney PJ, Jaucian RC, McDonald RA, et al. Exfoliative dermatitis in an infant: association with enterotoxin F-producing staphylococci. *Am J Dis Child* 1983;137:899.

120. Peters B, Hentschel J, Mau H, et al. Staphylococcal scalded-skin syndrome complicating wound infection in a preterm infant with postoperative chylothorax. *J Clin Microbiol* 1998;36:3057.

121. Ladhani S, Evans RW. Staphylococcal scalded skin syndrome. *Arch Dis Child* 1998;78:85.

122. Melish ME, Glasgow LA, Turner MD. The staphylococcal scalded skin syndrome: isolation and partial characterization of the exfoliative toxin. *J Infect Dis* 1972;125:129.

123. Dancer SJ, Simmons NA, Poston SM, et al. Outbreak of staphylococcal scalded skin syndrome among neonates. *J Infect* 1988;16:87.

124. Loughead JL. Congenital staphylococcal scalded skin syndrome: report of a case. *Pediatr Infect Dis J* 1992;11:413.

125. Saiman L, Jakob K, Holmes KW, et al. Molecular epidemiology of staphylococcal scalded skin syndrome in premature infants. *Pediatr Infect Dis J* 1998;17:329.

126. Landers S, Moise AA, Fraley JK, et al. Factors associated with umbilical catheter-related sepsis in neonates. *Am J Dis Child* 1991;145:675.

127. Espersen F, Frimodt-Møller N, Rosdahl VT, et al. *Staphylococcus aureus* bacteraemia in children below the age of one year: a review of 407 cases. *Acta Paediatr Scand* 1989;78:56.

128. Pfaller MA, Herwaldt LA. Laboratory, clinical, and epidemiological aspects of coagulase-negative staphylococci. *Clin Microbiol Rev* 1988;1:281.

129. Patrick CC. Coagulase-negative staphylococci: pathogens with increasing clinical significance. *J Pediatr* 1990;116:497.

130. Neumeister B, Kastner S, Conrad S, et al. Characterization of coagulase-negative staphylococci causing nosocomial infections in preterm infants. *Eur J Clin Microbiol Infect Dis* 1995;14:856.

131. Sidebottom DG, Freeman J, Platt R, et al. Fifteen-year experience with bloodstream isolates of coagulase-negative staphylococci in neonatal intensive care. *J Clin Microbiol* 1988;26:713.

132. Freeman J, Epstein MF, Smith NE, et al. Extra hospital stay and antibiotic usage with nosocomial coagulase-negative staphylococcal bacteremia in two neonatal intensive care unit populations. *Am J Dis Child* 1990;144:324.

133. Baumgart S, Hall SE, Campos JM, et al. Sepsis with coagulase negative staphylococci in critically ill newborns. *Am J Dis Child* 1983;137:461.

134. Noel GJ, Edelson PJ. *Staphylococcus epidermidis* bacteremia in neonates: further observations and the occurrence of focal infection. *Pediatrics* 1984;74:832.

135. Hall RT, Hall SL, Barnes WG, et al. Characteristics of coagulase-negative staphylococci from infants with bacteremia. *Pediatr Infect Dis J* 1987;6:377.

136. Yeung C-Y, Lee H-C, Huang F-Y, et al. Sepsis during total parenteral nutrition: exploration of risk factors and determination of the effectiveness of peripherally inserted central venous catheters. *Pediatr Infect Dis J* 1998;17:135.

137. Gruskay J, Harris MC, Costarino AT, et al. Neonatal *Staphylococcus epidermidis* meningitis with unremarkable CSF examination results. *Am J Dis Child* 1989;143:580.

138. Gruskay JA, Abbasi S, Anday E, et al. *Staphylococcus epidermidis*-associated enterocolitis. *J Pediatr* 1986;109:520.

139. Mollitt DL, Tepas JJ, Talbert JL. The role of coagulase-negative Staphylococcus in neonatal necrotizing enterocolitis. *J Pediatr Surg* 1988;23:60.

140. Patrick CC, Kaplan SL, Baker CJ, et al. Persistent bacteremia due to coagulase-negative staphylococci in low birth weight neonates. *Pediatrics* 1989;84:977.

141. Noel GJ, O'Loughlin JE, Edelson PJ. Neonatal *Staphylococcus epidermidis* right-sided endocarditis: description of five catheterized infants. *Pediatrics* 1988;82:234.

142. Wagener MM, Rycheck RR, Yee RB, et al. Septic dermatitis of the neonatal scalp and maternal endomyometritis with intrapartum internal fetal monitoring. *Pediatrics* 1984;74:81.

143. Overturf GD, Balfour G. Osteomyelitis and sepsis: severe complications of fetal monitoring. *Pediatrics* 1975;55:244.
144. Spellerberg B, Steidel K, Lütticken R, et al. Isolation of *Staphylococcus caprae* from blood cultures of a neonate with congenital heart disease. *Eur J Clin Microbiol Infect Dis* 1998;17:61.
145. Freeman J, Goldmann DA, Smith NE, et al. Association of intravenous lipid emulsion and coagulase-negative staphylococcal bacteremia in neonatal intensive care units. *N Engl J Med* 1990;323:301.
146. Matrai-Kovalskis Y, Greenberg D, Shinwell ES, et al. Positive blood cultures for coagulase-negative staphylococci in neonates: does highly selective vancomycin usage affect outcome? *Infection* 1998;26:85.
147. Dunne WM Jr. Effects of subinhibitory concentrations of vancomycin or cefamandole on biofilm production by coagulase-negative staphylococci. *Antimicrob Agents Chemother* 1990;34:390.
148. Gray ED, Peters G, Verstegen M, et al. Effect of extracellular slime substance from *Staphylococcus epidermidis* on the human cellular immune response. *Lancet* 1984;1:365.
149. Johnson GM, Lee DA, Regelmann WE, et al. Interference with granulocyte function by *Staphylococcus epidermidis* slime. *Infect Immun* 1986;54:13.
150. Fleer A, Gerards LJ, Aerts P, et al. Opsonic defense to *Staphylococcus epidermidis* in the premature neonate. *J Infect Dis* 1985;152:930.
151. Schutze GE, Hall MA, Baker CJ, et al. Role of neutrophil receptors in opsonophagocytosis of coagulase negative staphylococci. *Infect Immun* 1991;59:2573.
152. Scheifele DW, Bjornson GL. Delta toxin activity in coagulase-negative staphylococci from the bowels of neonates. *J Clin Microbiol* 1988;26:279.
153. Scheifele DW, Bjornson GL, Dyer RA, et al. Delta-like toxin produced by coagulase-negative staphylococci is associated with neonatal necrotizing enterocolitis. *Infect Immun* 1987;55:2268.
154. Scheifele DW. Role of bacterial toxins in neonatal necrotizing enterocolitis. *J Pediatr* 1990;117:S44.
155. Tappero JW, Schuchat A, Deaver KA, et al. Reduction in the incidence of human listeriosis in the United States: effectiveness of prevention efforts? *JAMA* 1995;273:1118.
156. Gellin BG, Broome CV, Bibb WF, et al. The epidemiology of listeriosis in the United States—1986. Listeriosis Study Group. *Am J Epidemiol* 1991;133:392.
157. Gellin BG, Broome CV. Listeriosis. *JAMA* 1989;261:1313.
158. Southwick FS, Punch DL. Intracellular pathogenesis of listeriosis. *N Engl J Med* 1996;334:770.
159. Becroft DMO, Farmer K, Seddon RJ, et al. Epidemic listeriosis in the newborn. *BMJ* 1971;3:747.
160. Mulder CJJ, Zanen HC. *Listeria monocytogenes* neonatal meningitis in the Netherlands. *Eur J Pediatr* 1986;145:60.
161. Kessler SL, Dajani AS. Listeria meningitis in infants and children. *Pediatr Infect Dis J* 1990;9:61.
162. Schuchat A, Lizano C, Broome CV, et al. Outbreak of neonatal listeriosis associated with mineral oil. *Pediatr Infect Djs J* 1991;10:183.
163. Facinelli B, Varaldo PE, Casolarí C, et al. Cross-infection with *Listeria monocytogenes* confirmed by DNA fingerprinting. *Lancet* 1988;2:1247.
164. Farber JM, Peterkin PI, Carter AO, et al. Neonatal listeriosis due to cross-infection confirmed by isoenzyme typing and DNA fingerprinting. *J Infect Dis* 1991;163:927.
165. Visintine AM, Oleske JM, Nahmias AJ. *Listeria monocytogenes* infection in infants and children. *Am J Dis Child* 1977;131:393.
166. Bavikatte K, Schreiner RL, Lemons JA, et al. Group D Streptococcal septicemia in the neonate. *Am J Dis Child* 1979;133:493.
167. Boulanger JM, Ford-Jones EL, Matlow AG. Enterococcal bacteremia in a pediatric institution: a four-year review. *Rev Infect Dis* 1991;13:847.
168. Coudron PE, Mayhall CG, Facklam RR, et al. *Streptococcus faecium* outbreak in a neonatal intensive care unit. *J Clin Microbiol* 1984;20:1044.
169. Dobson SRM, Baker CJ. Enterococcal sepsis in neonates: features by age at onset and occurrence of focal infection. *Pediatrics* 1990;85:165.
170. Rhinehart E, Smith NE, Wennersten C, et al. Rapid dissemination of β-lactamase producing, aminoglycoside-resistant *Enterococcus faecalis* among patients and staff on an infant-toddler surgical ward. *N Engl J Med* 1990;323:1814.
171. Luginbuhl LM, Rotbart HA, Facklam RR, et al. Neonatal enterococcal sepsis: case-control study and description of an outbreak. *Pediatr Infect Dis J* 1987;6:1022.
172. Klare I, Rodloff AC, Wagner J, et al. Overproduction of a penicillin-binding protein is not the only mechanism of penicillin resistance in *Enterococcus faecium*. *Antimicrob Agents Chemother* 1992;36:783.
173. Patterson JE, Singh KV, Murray BE. Epidemiology of an endemic strain of β-lactamase-producing *Enterococcus faecalis*. *J Clin Microbiol* 1991;29:2513.
174. Sahm DF, Boonlayangoor S, Schulz JE. Detection of high-level aminoglycoside resistance in enterococci other than *Enterococcus faecalis*. *J Clin Microbiol* 1991;29:2595.
175. Kaplan AH, Gilligan PH, Facklam RR. Recovery of resistant enterococci during vancomycin prophylaxis. *J Clin Microbiol* 1988;26:1216.
176. Woodford N. Glycopeptide-resistant enterococci: a decade of experience. *J Med Microbiol* 1998;47:849.
177. Malik RK, Montecalvo MA, Reale MR, et al. Epidemiology and control of vancomycin-resistant enterococci in a regional neonatal intensive care unit. *Pediatr Infect Dis J* 1999;18:352.
178. Toledano H, Schlesinger Y, Raveh D, et al. Prospective surveillance of vancomycin-resistant enterococci in a neonatal intensive care unit. *Eur J Clin Microbiol Infect Dis* 2000;19:282.
179. Chavers LS, Moser SA, Benjamin WH, et al. Vancomycin-resistant enterococci: 15 years and counting. *J Hosp Infect* 2003;53:159.
180. Joseph TA, Pyati SP, Jacobs N. Neonatal early-onset *Escherichia coli* disease: the effect of intrapartum ampicillin. *Arch Pediatr Adolesc Med* 1998;152:35.
181. Towers CV, Carr MH, Padilla G, et al. Potential consequences of widespread antepartal use of ampicillin. *Am J Obstet Gynecol* 1998;179:879.
182. Ghosal SP, Gupta PCS, Mukherjee AK, et al. Noma neonatorum: its aetiopathogenesis. *Lancet* 1978;2:289.
183. Quentin R, Martin C, Musser JM, et al. Genetic characterization of a cryptic genospecies of *Haemophilus* causing urogenital and neonatal infections. *J Clin Microbiol* 1993;31:1111.
184. Quentin R, Runny R, Rosenau A, et al. Genetic identification of cryptic genospecies of *Haemophilus* causing urogenital and neonatal infections by PCR using specific primers targeting genes coding for 16S rRNA. *J Clin Microbiol* 1996;34:1380.
185. Chow AW, Leake RD, Yamauchi T, et al. The significance of anaerobes in neonatal bacteremia: analysis of 23 cases and review of the literature. *Pediatrics* 1974;54:736.
186. Noel GJ, Laufer DA, Edelson PJ. Anaerobic bacteremia in a neonatal intensive care unit: an eighteen-year experience. *Pediatr Infect Dis J* 1988;7:858.
187. Brook I. *Pediatric anaerobic infection: diagnosis and management*, 2nd ed. St. Louis: CV Mosby, 1989:65.
188. Rønnestad A, Abrahamsen TG, Gaustad P, et al. Blood culture isolates during 6 years in a tertiary neonatal intensive care unit. *Scand J Infect Dis* 1998;30:245.
189. Gray J, Gossain S, Morris K. Three-year survey of bacteremia and fungemia in a pediatric intensive care unit. *Pediatr Infect Dis J* 2001;20:416.
190. Spark RP, Wike DA. Nontetanus clostridal neonatal fatality after home delivery. *Ariz Med* 1983;40:697.
191. Likitnukul S, Kusmiesz H, Nelson JD, et al. Role of genital mycoplasmas in young infants with suspected sepsis. *J Pediatr* 1986;109:971.
192. Izraeli S, Samra Z, Sirota L, et al. Genital mycoplasmas in preterm infants: prevalence and clinical significance. *Eur J Pediatr* 1991;150:804.
193. Waites KB, Crouse DT, Philips JB III, et al. Ureaplasmal pneumonia and sepsis associated with persistent pulmonary hypertension of the newborn. *Pediatrics* 1989;83:79.
194. Baley JE. Neonatal candidiasis: the current challenge. *Clin Perinatol* 1991;18:263.
195. Sharp AM, Odds FC, Evans EGV. *Candida* strains from neonates in a special care baby unit. *Arch Dis Child* 1992;67:48.
196. Ng PC. Systemic fungal infections in neonates. *Arch Dis Child* 1994;71:F130.
197. Schwartz DA, Reef S. *Candida albicans* placentitis and funisitis: early diagnosis of congenital candidemia by histopathologic examination of umbilical cord vessels. *Pediatr Infect Dis J* 1990;9:661.

198. Santos LA, Beceiro J, Hernandez R, et al. Congenital cutaneous candidiasis: report of four cases and review of the literature. *Eur J Pediatr* 1991;150:336.

199. Kossoff EH, Buescher ES, Karlowicz MG. Candidemia in a neonatal intensive care unit: trends during fifteen years and clinical features of 111 cases. *Pediatr Infect Dis J* 1998;17:504.

200. Lee BE, Cheung P-Y, Robinson JL, et al. Comparative study of mortality and morbidity in premature infants (birth weight, <1,250 g) with candidemia or candidal meningitis. *Clin Infect Dis* 1998;27:559.

201. Saiman L, Ludington E, Pfaller M, et al. Risk factors for candidemia in Neonatal Intensive Care Unit patients. The National Epidemiology of Mycosis Survey study group. *Pediatr Infect Dis J* 2000;19:319.

202. Makhoul IR, Kassis I, Smolkin T, et al. Review of 49 neonates with acquired fungal sepsis: further characterization. *Pediatrics* 2001;107:61.

203. Faix RG, Kovarik SM, Shaw TR, et al. Mucocutaneous and invasive candidiasis among very low birth weight (<1,500 grams) infants in intensive care nurseries: a prospective study. *Pediatrics* 1989;83:101.

204. Wey SB, Mori M, Pfaller MA, et al. Risk factors for hospital-acquired candidemia: a matched case-control study. *Arch Intern Med* 1989;149:2349.

205. Rowen JL, Atkins JT, Levy ML, et al. Invasive fungal dermatitis in the ≤1000-gram neonate. *Pediatrics* 1995;95:682.

206. Faix RG. Invasive neonatal candidiasis: comparison of albicans and parapsilosis infection. *Pediatr Infect Dis J* 1992;11:88.

207. Sánchez PJ, Siegel JD, Fishbein J. *Candida* endocarditis: successful medical management in three preterm infants and review of the literature. *Pediatr Infect Dis J* 1991;10:239.

208. Zenker PN, Rosenberg EM, Van Dyke RB, et al. Successful medical treatment of presumed Candida endocarditis in critically ill infants. *J Pediatr* 1991;119:472.

209. Annable WL, Kachmer ML, DiMarco M, et al. Long-term follow-up of *Candida* endophthalmitis in the premature infant. *J Pediatr Ophthalmol Strabismus* 1990;27:103.

210. Goldsmith LS, Rubenstein SD, Wolfson BJ, et al. Cerebral calcifications in a neonate with candidiasis. *Pediatr Infect Dis J* 1990;9:451.

211. Baetz-Greenwalt B, Debaz B, Kumar ML. Bladder fungus ball: a reversible cause of neonatal obstructive uropathy. *Pediatrics* 1988;81:826.

212. Rehan VK, Davidson DC. Neonatal renal candidal bezoar. *Arch Dis Child* 1992;67:63.

213. Butler KM, Rench MA, Baker CJ. Amphotericin B as a single agent in the treatment of systemic candidiasis in neonates. *Pediatr Infect Dis J* 1990;9:51.

214. Ward RM, Sattler FR, Dalton AS Jr. Assessment of antifungal therapy in an 800-gram infant with candidal arthritis and osteomyelitis. *Pediatrics* 1983;72:234.

215. Benjamin DK Jr, Fisher RG, McKinney RE Jr, et al. Candidal mycetoma in the neonatal kidney. *Pediatrics* 1999;104:1126.

216. Marcon MJ, Powell DA. Human infections due to *Malassezia* spp. *Clin Microbiol Rev* 1992;5:101.

217. Chang HJ, Miller HL, Watkins N, et al. An epidemic of *Malassezia pachydermatis* in an intensive care nursery associated with colonization of health care workers' pet dogs. *N Engl J Med* 1998;338:706.

218. Henwick S, Hennickson K, Storgion SA, et al. Disseminated neonatal *Trichosporon beigelii*. *Pediatr Infect Dis J* 1992;11:50.

219. Reich JD, Huddleston K, Jorgensen D, et al. Neonatal *Torulopsis glabrata* fungemia. *South Med J* 1997;90:246.

220. Sweet D, Reid M. Disseminated neonatal *Trichosporon beigelii* infection: successful treatment with liposomal amphotericin B. *J Infect* 1998;36:120.

221. Meessen NEL, Oberndorff KMEJ, Jacobs JA. Disseminated aspergillosis in a premature neonate. *J Hosp Infect* 1998; 40:249.

222. Gerdes JS. Clinicopathologic approach to the diagnosis of neonatal sepsis. *Clin Perinatol* 1991;18:361.

223. Schelonka RL, Chai MK, Yoder BA, et al. Volume of blood required to detect common neonatal pathogens. *J Pediatr* 1996; 129:275.

224. Wiswell TE, Hachey WE. Multiple site blood cultures in the initial evaluation for neonatal sepsis during the first week of life. *Pediatr Infect Dis J* 1991;10:365.

225. Phillips SE, Bradley JS. Bacteremia detected by lysis direct plating in a neonatal intensive care unit. *J Clin Microbiol* 1990;28:1.

226. St. Geme JW III, Bell LM, Baumgart S, et al. Distinguishing sepsis from blood culture contamination in young infants with blood cultures growing coagulase-negative staphylococci. *Pediatrics* 1990;86:157.

227. Schelonka RL, Moser SA. Time to positive culture results in neonatal Candida septicemia. *J Pediatr* 2003;142:564–565.

228. Evans ME, Schaffner W, Federspiel CF, et al. Sensitivity, specificity, and predictive value of body surface cultures in a neonatal intensive care unit. *JAMA* 1988;259:248.

229. Visser VE, Hall RT. Lumbar puncture in the evaluation of suspected neonatal sepsis. *J Pediatr* 1980;96:1063.

230. Fielkow S, Reuter S, Gotoff SP. Cerebrospinal fluid examination in symptom-free infants with risk factors for infection. *J Pediatr* 1991;119:971.

231. Weiss MG, Ionides SP, Anderson CL. Meningitis in premature infants with respiratory distress: role of admission lumbar puncture. *J Pediatr* 1991;119:973.

232. Schwersenski J, McIntyre L, Bauer CR. Lumbar puncture frequency and cerebrospinal fluid analysis in the neonate. *Am J Dis Child* 1991;145:54.

233. Kumar P, Sarkar S, Narang A. Role of routine lumbar puncture in neonatal sepsis. *J Paediatr Child Health* 1995;31:8.

234. Wiswell TE, Baumgart S, Gannon CM, et al. No lumbar puncture in the evaluation for early neonatal sepsis: will meningitis be missed? *Pediatrics* 1995;95:803.

235. Joshi P, Barr P. The use of lumbar puncture and laboratory tests for sepsis by Australian neonatologists. *J Paediatr Child Health* 1998; 34:74.

236. Stoll BJ, Hansen N, Fanaroff AA, et al. To tap or not to tap: high likelihood of meningitis without sepsis among very low birth weight infants. *Pediatrics* 2004;113:1181.

237. Manroe BL, Weinberg AG, Rosenfeld CR, et al. The neonatal blood count in health and disease. I. Reference values for neutrophilic cells. *J Pediatr* 1979;95:89.

238. Benuck I, David RJ. Sensitivity of published neutrophil indexes in identifying newborn infants with sepsis. *J Pediatr* 1983; 103:961.

239. Carballo C, Foucar K, Swanson P, et al. Effect of high altitude on neutrophil counts in newborn infants. *J Pediatr* 1991; 119:464.

240. Schelonka RL, Yoder BA, Hall RB, et al. Differentiation of segmented and band neutrophils during the early newborn period. *J Pediatr* 1995;127:298.

241. Greenberg DN, Yoder BA. Changes in the differential white blood cell count in screening for group B Streptococcal sepsis. *Pediatr Infect Dis J* 1990;9:886.

242. Schelonka RL, Yoder BA, desJardins SE, et al. Peripheral leukocyte count and leukocyte indexes in healthy newborn term infants. *J Pediatr* 1994;125:603.

243. Jackson GL, Engle WD, Sendelbach DM, et al. Are complete blood cell counts useful in the evaluation of asymptomatic neonates exposed to suspected chorioamnionitis? *Pediatrics* 2004;113:1173.

244. Kaftan H, Kinney JS. Early-onset neonatal bacterial infections. *Semin Perinatol* 1998;22:15.

245. Schouten-Van Meeteren NYN, Rietveld A, Moolenaar AJ, et al. Influence of perinatal conditions on C-reactive protein production. *J Pediatr* 1992;120:621.

246. Ehl S, Gering B, Bartmann P, et al. C-reactive protein is a useful marker for guiding duration of antibiotic therapy in suspected neonatal bacterial infection. *Pediatrics* 1997;99:216.

247. Lehrnbecher T, Schrod L, Rutsch P, et al. Immunologic parameters in cord blood indicating early-onset sepsis. *Biol Neonate* 1996;70:206.

248. Doellner H, Arntzen KJ, Haereid PE, et al. Interleukin-6 concentrations in neonates evaluated for sepsis. *J Pediatr* 1998; 132:295.

249. Weimann E, Rutkowski S, Reisbach G. G-CSF, GM-CSF, and IL-6 levels in cord blood: diminished increase of G-CSF and IL-6 in preterms with perinatal infection compared to term neonates. *J Perinat Med* 1998;26:211.

250. Küster H, Weiss M, Willeitner AE, et al. Interleukin-1 receptor antagonist and interleukin-6 for early diagnosis of neonatal sepsis 2 days before clinical manifestation. *Lancet* 1998;352:1271.

251. Lacour AG, Gervaix A, Zamora SA, et al. Procalcitonin, IL-6, IL-8, IL-1 receptor antagonist and C-reactive protein as identificators of serious bacterial infections in children with fever without localizing signs. *Eur J Pediatr* 2001;160:95.

252. Resch B, Gusenleitner W, Muller WD. Procalcitonin and interleukin-6 in the diagnosis of early-onset sepsis of the neonate. *Acta Paediatr* 2003;92:243.

253. Chiesa C, Panero A, Rossi N, et al. Reliability of procalcitonin concentrations for the diagnosis of sepsis in critically ill neonates. *Clin Infect Dis* 1998;26:664.

254. Weirich E, Rabin RL, Maldonado Y, et al. Neutrophil CD11b expression as a diagnostic marker for early-onset neonatal infection. *J Pediatr* 1998;132:445.

255. Ascher DP, Wilson S, Fischer GW. Comparison of commercially available group B Streptococcal latex agglutination assays. *J Clin Microbial* 1991;29:2895.

256. Sanchez PJ, Siegel JD, Cushion NB, et al. Significance of a positive urine group B Streptococcal latex agglutination test in neonates. *J Pediatr* 1990;116:601.

257. Ascher DP, Wilson S, Mendiola J, et al. Group B streptococcal latex agglutination testing in neonates. *J Pediatr* 1991;119:458.

258. Mitsutake K, Miyazaki T, Tashiro T, et al. Enolase antigen, mannan antigen, Cand-Tec antigen, and β-glucan in patients with candidemia. *J Clin Microhiol* 1996;34:1918.

259. Avent ML, Kinney JS, Istre GR, et al. Gentamicin and tobramycin in neonates: comparison of a new extended dosing interval regimen with a traditional multiple daily dosing regimen. *Am J Perinatol* 2002;19:413.

260. Schwalbe RS, Stapleton JT, Gilligan PH. Emergence of vancomycin resistance in coagulase-negative staphylococci. *N Engl J Med* 1987;316:927.

261. Tenover FC, Lancaster MV, Hill BC, et al. Characterization of staphylococci with reduced susceptibilities to vancomycin and other glycopeptides. *J Clin Microbiol* 1998;36:1020.

262. Smith TL, Pearson ML, Wilcox KR, et al. Emergence of vancomycin resistance in *Staphylococcus aureus*. *N Engl J Med* 1999;340:493.

263. Siegel JD, Shannon KM, DePasse BM. Recurrent infection associated with penicillin-tolerant group B Streptococci: a report of two cases. *J Pediatr* 1981;99:920.

264. Maugein J, Guillemot D, Dupont MJ, et al. Clinical and microbiological epidemiology of *Streptococcus pneumoniae* bacteremia in eight French counties. *Clin Microbiol Infect* 2003;9:280–288.

265. Eliopoulos GM. Vancomycin-resistant enterococci: mechanism and clinical relevance. *Infect Dis Clin North Am* 1997;11:851.

266. Waites KB, Crouse DT, Cassell GH. Antibiotic susceptibilities and therapeutic options for *Ureaplasma urealyticum* infections in neonates. *Pediatr Infect Dis J* 1992;11:23.

267. Rowen JL, Tate JM, Neonatal Candidiasis Study Group. Management of neonatal candidiasis. *Pediatr Infect Dis J* 1998; 17:1007.

268. Baley JE, Meyers C, Kliegman RM, et al. Pharmacokinetics, outcome of treatment, and toxic effects of amphotericin B and 5-fluorocytosine in neonates. *J Pediatr* 1990;116:791.

269. Koren G, Lau A, Klein J, et al. Pharmacokinetics and adverse effects of amphotericin B in infants and children. *J Pediatr* 1988;113:559.

270. Conly J, Rennie R, Johnson J, et al. Disseminated candidiasis due to amphotericin B-resistant *Candida albicans*. *J Infect Dis* 1992;165:761.

271. Lackner H, Schwinger W, Urban C, et al. Liposomal amphotericin-B (AmBisome) for treatment of disseminated fungal infections in two infants of very low birth weight. *Pediatrics* 1992;89:1259.

272. Weitkamp J-H, Poets CF, Sievers R, et al. *Candida* infection in very low birth-weight infants: outcome and nephrotoxicity of treatment with liposomal amphotericin B (AmBisome®). *Infection* 1998;26:11.

273. Scarcella A, Pasquariello MB, Giugliano B, et al. Liposomal amphotericin B treatment for neonatal fungal infections. *Pediatr Infect Dis J* 1998;17:146.

274. Stocker M, Caduff JH, Spalinger J, et al. Successful treatment of bilateral renal fungal balls with liposomal amphotericin B and fluconazole in an extremely low birth weight infant. *Eur J Pediatr* 2000;159:676.

275. Linder N, Klinger G, Shalit I, et al. Treatment of candidaemia in premature infants: comparison of three amphotericin B preparations. *J Antimicrob Chemother* 2003;52:663.

276. Juster-Reicher A, Flidel-Rimon O, Amitay M, et al. High-dose liposomal amphotericin B in the therapy of systemic candidiasis in neonates. *Eur J Clin Microbiol Infect Dis* 2003; 22:603.

277. Wong-Beringer A, Jacobs RA, Guglielmo BJ. Lipid formulations of amphotericin B: clinical efficacy and toxicities. *Clin Infect Dis* 1998;27:603.

278. Wiest DB, Fowler SL, Garner SS, et al. Fluconazole in neonatal disseminated candidiasis. *Arch Dis Child* 1991;66:1002.

279. Huttova M, Hartmanova I, Kralinsky K, et al. *Candida* fungemia in neonates treated with fluconazole: report of forty cases, including eight with meningitis. *Pediatr Infect Dis J* 1998; 17:1012.

280. Wenzl TG, Schefels J, Hörnchen H, et al. Pharmacokinetics of oral fluconazole in premature infants. *Eur J Pediatr* 1998; 157:661.

281. Krcmery V, Huttova M, Mateicka F, et al. Breakthrough fungaemia in neonates and infants caused by *Candida albicans* and Candida parapsilosis susceptible to fluconazole in vitro. *J Antimicrob Chemother* 2001;48:521.

282. Fishbein JD, Friedman HS, Bennett BB, et al. Catheter-related sepsis refractory to antibiotics treated successfully with adjunctive urokinase infusion. *Pediatr Infect Dis J* 1990;9:676.

283. Raad I. Intravascular-catheter-related infections. *Lancet* 1998; 351:893.

284. Hocker JR, Simpson PM, Rabalais GP, et al. Extracorporeal membrane oxygenation and early-onset group B Streptococcal *sepsis*. *Pediatrics* 1992;89:1.

285. Rouse DJ, Andrews WW, Lin F-YC, et al. Antibiotic susceptibility profile of group B Streptococcus acquired vertically. *Obstet Gynecol* 1998;92:931.

286. Pearlman MD, Pierson CL, Faix RG. Frequent resistance of clinical group B Streptococci isolates to clindamycin and erythromycin. *Obstet Gynecol* 1998;92:258.

287. Crisp BJ, Yancey MK, Uyehara C, et al. Effect of delayed inoculation of selective media in antenatal detection of group B Streptococci. *Obstet Gynecol* 1998;92:923.

288. de Cueto M, Sanchez M-J, Sampedro A, et al. Timing of intrapartum ampicillin and prevention of vertical transmission of group B Streptococcus. *Obstet Gynecol* 1998;91:112.

289. Baker CJ, Paoletti LC, Wessels MR, et al. Safety and immunogenicity of capsular polysaccharide-tetanus toxoid conjugate vaccines for group B Streptococcal types Ia and Ib. *J Infect Dis* 1999;179:142.

290. Baker CJ, Rench MA, Fernandez M, et al. Safety and immunogenicity of a bivalent group B Streptococcal conjugate vaccine for serotypes II and III. *J Infect Dis* 2003;188:66.

291. Baker CJ, Rench MA, McInnes P. Immunization of pregnant women with group B Streptococcal type III capsular polysaccharide-tetanus toxoid conjugate vaccine. *Vaccine* 2003;21:3468.

292. Baker CJ, Paoletti LC, Rench MA, et al. Immune response of healthy women to 2 different group B Streptococcal type V capsular polysaccharide-protein conjugate vaccines. *J Infect Dis* 2004;189:1103–1112.

293. Gutman LT. The spirochetes. In: Joklik WK, Willett HP, Amos DB, Willett CM, eds. *Zinsser microbiology*, 20th ed. Norwalk: Appleton & Lange, 1992:657.

294. Blanco DR, Miller JN, Lovett MA. Surface antigens of the syphilis spirochete and their potential as virulence determinants. *Emerg Infect Dis* 1997;3:11.

295. Hook EW III, Marra CM. Acquired syphilis in adults. *N Engl J Med* 1992;326:1060.

296. Baughn RE. Role of fibronectins in the pathogenesis of syphilis. *Rev Infect Dis* 1987;9:S372.

297. Nelson KE, Vlahov D, Cohn S, et al. Sexually transmitted diseases in a population of intravenous drug users: association with seropositivity to the human immunodeficiency virus (HIV). *J Infect Dis* 1991;164:457.

298. Sánchez PJ. Congenital syphilis. *Adv Pediatr Infect Dis* 1992;7:161.

299. Sánchez PJ, Wendel GD. Syphilis in pregnancy. *Clin Perinatol* 1997;24:71.

300. Dobson SRM, Taber LH, Baughn RE. Recognition of *Treponema pallidum* antigens by IgM and IgG antibodies in congenitally infected newborns and their mothers. *J Infect Dis* 1988;157:903.

301. Wicher V, Zabek J, Wicher K. Pathogen-specific humoral response in *Treponema pallidum*-infected humans, rabbits, and guinea pigs. *J Infect Dis* 1991;163:830.

302. Sánchez PJ, McCracken GH Jr, Wendel GD, et al. Molecular analysis of the fetal IgM response to *Treponema pallidum* antigens: implications for improved serodiagnosis of congenital syphilis. *J Infect Dis* 1989;159:508.
303. Lewis LL, Taber LH, Baughn RE. Evaluation of immunoglobulin M Western blot analysis in the diagnosis of congenital syphilis. *J Clin Microbiol* 1990;28:296.
304. Larsen SA, Steiner BM, Rudolph AH. Laboratory diagnosis and interpretation of tests for syphilis. *Clin Microbial Rev* 1995;8:1.
305. Borenstein LA, Selsted ME, Lehrer RI, et al. Antimicrobial activity of rabbit leukocyte defensins against *Treponema pallidum* subsp. *pallidum*. *Infect Immun* 1991;59:1359.
306. Borenstein LA, Ganz T, Sell S, et al. Contribution of rabbit leukocyte defensins to the host response in experimental syphilis. *Infect Immun* 1991;59:1368.
307. Fitzgerald TJ. The Th$_1$/Th$_2$-like switch in syphilitic infection: is it detrimental? *Infect Immun* 1992;60:3475.
308. Baker-Zander SA, Lukehart SA. Macrophage-mediated killing of opsonized *Treponema pallidum*. *J Infect Dis* 1992;165:69.
309. Baughn RE, Jiang A, Abraham R, et al. Molecular mimicry between an immunodominant amino acid motif on the 47-kDa lipoprotein of *Treponema pallidum* (Tpp47) and multiple repeats of analogous sequences in fibronectins. *J Immunol* 1996;157:720.
310. Wicher K, Abbruscato F, Wicher V, et al. Identification of persistent infection in experimental syphilis by PCR. *Infect Immun* 1998;66:2509.
311. Zenker PN, Berman SM. Congenital syphilis: trends and recommendations for evaluation and management. *Pediatr Infect Dis J* 1991;10:516.
312. Centers for Disease Control and Prevention. Congenital syphilis—New York City 1986–1988. *MMWR* 1989;38:825.
313. Zenker PN, Berman SM. Congenital syphilis: reporting and reality. *Am J Public Health* 1990;80:271.
314. Risser WL, Hwang L-Y. Problems in the current case definitions of congenital syphilis. *J Pediatr* 1996;129:499.
315. Cohen DA, Boyd D, Prabhudas I, et al. The effects of case definition in maternal screening and reporting criteria on rates of congenital syphilis. *Am J Public Health* 1990;80:316.
316. Congenital syphilis—United States 2002. *MMWR* 2004;53:716–719.
317. Fitzgerald TJ, Froberg MK. Congenital syphilis in newborn rabbits: immune functions and susceptibility to challenge infection at 2 and 5 weeks of age. *Infect Immun* 1991;59:1869.
318. Wicher K, Baughn RE, Wicher K, et al. Experimental congenital syphilis: guinea pig model. *Infect Immun* 1992;60:271.
319. Wicher V, Baughn RE, Wicher K. Congenital and neonatal syphilis in guinea-pigs show a different pattern of immune response. *Immunology* 1994;82:404.
320. Schulz KF, Murphy FK, Patamasucon P, et al. Congenital syphilis. In: Holmes KK, Mårdh P-A, Sparling PF, et al, eds. *Sexually transmitted diseases*, 2nd ed. New York: McGraw-Hill, 1990:821.
321. Fox H. *Pathology of the placenta*, 2nd ed. Philadelphia: WB Saunders, 1997:307.
322. Genest DR, Choi-Hong SR, Tate JE, et al. Diagnosis of congenital syphilis from placental examination: comparison of histopathology, Steiner stain, and polymerase chain reaction for *Treponema pallidum* DNA. *Hum Pathol* 1996;27:366.
323. Lucas MJ, Theriot SK, Wendel GD Jr. Doppler systolic-diastolic ratios in pregnancies complicated by syphilis. *Obstet Gynecol* 1991;77:217.
324. Fojaco RM, Hensley GT, Moskowitz L. Congenital syphilis and necrotizing funisitis. *JAMA* 1989;261:1788.
325. Schwartz DA, Larsen SA, Beck-Sague C, et al. Pathology of the umbilical cord in congenital syphilis: analysis of 25 specimens using histochemistry and immunofluorescent antibody to *Treponema pallidum*. *Hum Pathol* 1995;26:784.
326. Boot JM, Oranje AP, Menke HE, et al. Congenital syphilis in the Netherlands: diagnosis and clinical features. *Genitourin Med* 1989;65:300.
327. Dorfman DH, Glaser JH. Congenital syphilis presenting in infants after the newborn period. *N Engl J Med* 1990;323:1299.
328. Wright MS, Tecklenburg FW. Critical illness in congenital syphilis after the newborn period. *Clin Pediatr (Phila)* 1992;31:247.
329. Pieper CH, van Gelderen WFC, Smith J, et al. Chest radiographs of neonates with respiratory failure caused by congenital syphilis. *Pediatr Radiol* 1995;25:198.
330. Liu C-C, So WCM, Lin C-H, et al. Congenital syphilis: clinical manifestations in premature infants. *Scand J Infect Dis* 1993;25:741.
331. Naeye RL. Fetal growth with congenital syphilis: a quantitative study. *Am J Clin Pathol* 1971;55:228.
332. Long WA, Ulshen MH, Lawson EE. Clinical manifestations of congenital syphilitic hepatitis: implications for pathogenesis. *J Pediatr Gastroenterol Nutr* 1984;3:551.
333. Venter A, Pettifor JM, Duursma J, et al. Liver function in early congenital syphilis: does penicillin cause a deterioration? *J Pediatr Gastroenterol Nutr* 1991;12:310.
334. Herman TE. Extensive hepatic calcification secondary to fulminant neonatal syphilitic hepatitis. *Pediatr Radiol* 1995;25:120.
335. Noseda G, Roy C, Phan P, et al. Acute hepatic failure in an infant with congenital syphilis. *Arch Fr Pediatr* 1990;47:445.
336. Berry MC, Dajani AS. Resurgence of congenital syphilis. *Infect Dis Clin North Am* 1992;6:19.
337. Hira SK, Bhat GJ, Patel JB, et al. Early congenital syphilis: clinico-radiologic features in 202 patients. *Sex Transm Dis* 1985;12:177.
338. Rasool MN, Govender S. The skeletal manifestations of congenital syphilis: a review of 197 cases. *J Bone Joint Surg [Br]* 1989;71:752.
339. Brion LP, Manuli M, Rai B, et al. Long-bone radiographic abnormalities as a sign of active congenital syphilis in asymptomatic newborns. *Pediatrics* 1991;88:1037.
340. Greenberg SB, Bernal DV. Are long bone radiographs necessary in neonates suspected of having congenital syphilis? *Radiology* 1992;182:637.
341. Moyer VA, Schneider V, Yetman R, et al. Contribution of long-bone radiographs to the management of congenital syphilis in the newborn infant. *Arch Pediatr Adolesc Med* 1998;152:353.
342. Lim HK, Smith WL, Sato Y, et al. Congenital syphilis mimicking child abuse. *Pediatr Radiol* 1995;25:560.
343. Kocher MS, Caniza M. Parrot pseudoparalysis of the upper extremities. *J Bone Joint Surg [Am]* 1996;78:284.
344. Wolf B, Kalangu K. Congenital neurosyphilis revisited. *Eur J Pediatr* 1993;152:493.
345. Austin R, Melhem RE. Pulmonary changes in congenital syphilis. *Pediatr Radiol* 1991;21:404.
346. Hill LL, Singer DB, Falletta J, Stasney R. The nephrotic syndrome in congenital syphilis: an immunopathy. *Pediatrics* 1972;49:260.
347. Ricci JM, Fojaco RM, O'Sullivan MJ. Congenital syphilis: the University of Miami/Jackson Memorial Medical Center experience 1986–1988. *Obstet Gynecol* 1989;74:687.
348. Daaboul JJ, Kartchner W, Jones KL. Neonatal hypoglycemia caused by hypopituitarism in infants with congenital syphilis. *J Pediatr* 1993;123:983.
349. Fiumara NJ, Lessell S. Manifestations of late congenital syphilis: an analysis of 271 patients. *Arch Dermatol* 1970;102:78.
350. Hendershot EL. Luetic deafness. *Otolaryngol Clin North Am* 1978;11:43.
351. Wendel GD Jr, Sánchez PJ, Peters MT, et al. Identification of *Treponema pallidum* in amniotic fluid and fetal blood from pregnancies complicated by congenital syphilis. *Obstet Gynecol* 1991;78:890.
352. Hill LM, Maloney JB. An unusual constellation of sonographic findings associated with congenital syphilis. *Obstet Gynecol* 1991;78:895.
353. Satin AJ, Twickler DM, Wendel GD Jr. Congenital syphilis associated with dilation of fetal small bowel: a case report. *J Ultrasound Med* 1992;11:49.
354. Hallak M, Peipert JF, Ludomirsky A, et al. Nonimmune hydrops fetalis and fetal congenital syphilis: a case report. *J Reprod Med* 1992;37:173.
355. Nathan L, Twickler DM, Peters MT, et al. Fetal syphilis: correlation of sonographic findings and rabbit infectivity testing of amniotic fluid. *J Ultrasound Med* 1993;12:97.
356. Raafat NA, Birch AA, Altieri LA, et al. Sonographic osseous manifestations of fetal syphilis: a case report. *J Ultrasound Med* 1993;12:783.
357. Glover DD, Winter CA, Charles D, et al. Diagnostic considerations in intra-amniotic syphilis. *Sex Transm Dis* 1985;12:145.
358. Grimprel E, Sanchez PJ, Wendel GD, et al. Use of polymerase chain reaction and rabbit infectivity testing to detect *Treponema*

pallidum in amniotic fluid, fetal and neonatal sera, and cerebrospinal fluid. *J Clin Microbiol* 1991;29:1711.

359. Nathan L, Bohman VR, Sánchez PJ, et al. *In utero* infection with *Treponema pallidum* in early pregnancy. *Prenat Diagn* 1997; 17:119.

360. Rawstron SA, Bromberg K. Comparison of maternal and newborn serologic tests for syphilis. *Am J Dis Child* 1991;145:1383.

361. Chhabra RK, Brion LP, Castro M, et al. Comparison of maternal sera, cord blood, and neonatal sera for detecting presumptive congenital syphilis: relationship with maternal treatment. *Pediatrics* 1993;91:88.

362. Bromberg K, Rawstron S, Tannis G. Diagnosis of congenital syphilis by combining Treponema pallidum-specific IgM detection with immunofluorescent antigen detection for *T. pallidum*. *J Infect Dis* 1993;168:238.

363. Meyer MP, Eddy T, Baughn RE. Analysis of Western blotting (immunoblotting) technique in diagnosis of congenital syphilis. *J Clin Microbiol* 1994;32:629.

364. Beeram MR, Chopde N, Dawood Y, et al. Lumbar puncture in the evaluation of possible asymptomatic congenital syphilis in neonates. *J Pediatr* 1996;128:125.

365. Lewis LL. Congenital syphilis: serologic diagnosis in the young infant. *Infect Dis Clin North Am* 1992;6:31.

366. Sánchez PJ, Wendel GD Jr, Grimprel E, et al. Evaluation of molecular methodologies and rabbit infectivity testing for the diagnosis of congenital syphilis and neonatal central nervous system invasion by Treponema pallidum. *J Infect Dis* 1993;167:148.

367. Centers for Disease Control and Prevention 1998 Guidelines for treatment of sexually transmitted diseases. *MMWR* 1998; 47(RR-1):1.

368. American Academy of Pediatrics. Syphilis. In Pickering LK, ed. Red Book: 2003 Report of the Committee on Infectious Diseases. Elk Grove Village: American Academy of Pediatrics 2003.

369. Chang SN, Chung K-Y, Lee M-G, et al. Seroreversion of the serological tests for syphilis in the newborns born to treated syphilitic mothers. *Genitourin Med* 1995;71:68.

370. Smith AL. Neonatal bacterial meningitis. In: Scheld WM, Whitley RJ, Durack DT, eds. *Infections of the central nervous system*, 2nd ed. Philadelphia: Lippincott-Raven, 1997:313.

371. Bell WE, McGuinness GA. Suppurative central nervous system infections in the neonate. *Semin Perinatol* 1982;6:1.

372. Bingen E, Bonacorsi S, Brahimi N, et al. Virulence patterns of *Escherichia coli* Kl strains associated with neonatal meningitis. *J Clin Microbiol* 1997;35:2981.

373. Sáez-Llorens X, Ramilo O, Mustafa MM, et al. Molecular pathophysiology of bacterial meningitis: current concepts and therapeutic implications. *J Pediatr* 1990;116:671.

374. Ashwal S, Tomasi L, Schneider S, et al. Bacterial meningitis in children: pathophysiology and treatment. *Neurology* 1992;42: 739.

375. Ahmed A, Hickey SM, Ehrett S, et al. Cerebrospinal fluid values in the term neonate. *Pediatr Infect Dis J* 1996;15:298.

376. Sarff LD, Platt LH, McCracken GH Jr. Cerebrospinal fluid evaluation in neonates: comparison of high-risk infants with and without meningitis. *J Pediatr* 1976;88:473.

377. Rodriguez AF, Kaplan SL, Mason EO Jr. Cerebrospinal fluid values in the very low birth weight infant. *J Pediatr* 1990;116:971.

378. Hall LMC, Duke B, Urwin G. An approach to the identification of the pathogens of bacterial meningitis by the polymerase chain reaction. *Eur J Clin Microbiol Infect Dis* 1995;14:1090.

379. Cherian T, Lalitha MK, Manoharan A, et al. PCR-enzyme immunoassay for detection of *Streptococcus pneumoniae* DNA in cerebrospinal fluid samples from patients with culture-negative meningitis. *J Clin Microbiol* 1998;36:3605.

380. Smith K, Diggle MA, Clarke SC. Automation of a fluorescence-based multiplex PCR for the laboratory confirmation of common bacterial pathogens. *J Med Microbiol* 2004;53:115.

381. McCracken GH Jr, Mize SG. A controlled study of intrathecal antibiotic therapy in gram-negative enteric meningitis of infancy: report of the Neonatal Meningitis Cooperative Study Group. *J Pediatr* 1976;89:66.

382. McCracken GH Jr, Mize SG, Threlkeld N. Intraventricular gentamicin therapy in gram-negative bacillary meningitis of infancy: report of the Second Neonatal Meningitis Cooperative Study Group. *Lancet* 1980;1:787.

383. Ahmed A, Paris MM, Trujillo M, et al. Once-daily gentamicin for experimental *Escherichia coli* meningitis. *Antimicrob Agents Chemother* 1997;41:49.

384. Kaplan SL, Patrick CC. Cefotaxime and aminoglycoside treatment of meningitis caused by gram-negative enteric organisms. *Pediatr Infect Dis J* 1990;9:810.

385. Mustafa MM, Mertsola J, Ramilo O, et al. Increased endotoxin and interleukin- 1β concentrations in cerebrospinal fluid of infants with coliform meningitis and ventriculitis associated with intraventricular gentamicin therapy. *J Infect Dis* 1989;160:891.

386. Jafari HS, Sáez-Llorens X, Severien C, et al. Effects of antifungal therapy on inflammation, sterilization, and histology in experimental *Candida albicans* meningitis. *Antimicrob Agents Chemother* 1994;38:83.

387. Unhanand M, Mustafa MM, McCracken GH Jr, et al. Gram-negative enteric bacillary meningitis: a twenty-one-year experience. *J Pediatr* 1993;122:15.

388. Graham DR, Anderson RL, Ariel FE, et al. Epidemic nosocomial meningitis due to *Citrobacter diversus* in neonates. *J Infect Dis* 1981;144:203.

389. Foreman SD, Smith EE, Ryan NJ, et al. Neonatal *Citrobacter* meningitis: pathogenesis of cerebral abscess formation. *Ann Neurol* 1984;16:655.

390. Jan W, Zimmerman RA, Bilaniuk LT, et al. Diffusion-weighted imaging in acute bacterial meningitis in infancy. *Neuroradiology* 2003;45:634.

391. Edwards MS, Rench MA, Haffar AAM, et al. Long-term sequelae of group B Streptococcal meningitis in infants. *J Pediatr* 1985; 106:717.

392. Wald ER, Bergman I, Taylor HG, et al. Long-term outcome of group B Streptococcal meningitis. *Pediatrics* 1986;77:217.

393. Franco SM, Cornelius VE, Andrews BF. Long-term outcome of neonatal meningitis. *Am J Dis Child* 1992;146:567.

394. Bedford H, de Louvois J, Halket S, et al. Meningitis in infancy in England and Wales: follow up at age 5 years. *BMJ* 2001;323: 533.

395. Stevens JP, Eames M, Kent A, et al. Long term outcome of neonatal meningitis. *Arch Dis Child Fetal Neonatal Ed* 2003;88: F179.

396. Ogden JA. Pathophysiology of neonatal osteomyelitis and septic arthritis. In: Polin RA, Fox WM, eds. *Fetal and neonatal physiology*, 2nd ed. Philadelphia: WB Saunders, 1998:2382.

397. Asmar BI. Osteomyelitis in the neonate. *Infect Dis Clin North Am* 1992;6:117.

398. Williams R, Kirkbride V, Corcoran GD. Neonatal osteomyelitis in Down's syndrome due to nonencapsulated *Haemophilus influenzae*. *J Infect* 1994;29:201.

399. Evdoridou J, Roilides E, Bibashi E, et al. Multifocal osteoarthritis due to *Candida albicans* in a neonate: serum level monitoring of liposomal amphotericin B and literature review. *Infection* 1997;25:112.

400. Eisenstein EM, Gesundheit B. Neonatal hand abscess, osteomyelitis and meningitis caused by *Streptococcus pneumoniae*. *Pediatr Infect Dis J* 1998;17:760.

401. Ish-Horowicz MR, Mcintyre P, Nade S. Bone and joint infections caused by multiply resistant *Staphylococcus aureus* in a neonatal intensive care unit. *Pediatr Infect Dis J* 1992;11:82.

402. Eggink BH, Rowen JL. Primary osteomyelitis and suppurative arthritis caused by coagulase-negative staphylococci in a preterm neonate. *Pediatr Infect Dis J* 2003;22:572.

403. Fox L, Sprout K. Neonatal osteomyelitis. *Pediatrics* 1978;62:535.

404. Barton LL, Villar RG, Rice SA. Neonatal group B Streptococcal vertebral osteomyelitis. *Pediatrics* 1996;98:459.

405. Mok PM, Reilly BJ, Ash JM. Osteomyelitis in the neonate. *Radiology* 1982;145:677.

406. Aigner RM, Fueger GE, Ritter G. Results of three-phase bone scintigraphy and radiography in 20 cases of neonatal osteomyelitis. *Nucl Med Commun* 1996;17:20.

407. Nelson JD. Antibiotic concentrations in septic joint effusions. *N Engl J Med* 1971;284:349.

408. Perkins MD, Edwards KM, Heller RM, et al. Neonatal group B Streptococcal osteomyelitis and suppurative arthritis: outpatient therapy. *Clin Pediatr (Phila)* 1989;28:229.

409. Wopperer JM, White JJ, Gillespie R, et al. Long-term follow-up of infantile hip sepsis. *J Pediatr Orthop* 1988;8:322.

410. De Smet L, Gunst P, Fabry G. Acquired ulnar clubhand resulting from neonatal osteomyelitis. *J Pediatr Orthop B* 1998;7:77.

411. Bos CFA, Mol LJCD, Obermann WR, et al. Late sequelae of neonatal septic arthritis of the shoulder. *J Bone Joint Surg [Br]* 1998;80:645.

412. Ladhani S, Bhutta ZA. Neonatal *Pseudomonas putida* infection presenting as staphylococcal scalded skin syndrome. *Eur J Clin Microbiol Infect Dis* 1998;17:642.

413. Weinberger M, Haynes RE, Morse TS. Necrotizing fasciitis in a neonate. *Am J Dis Child* 1972;123:591.

414. Ramamurthy RS, Srinivasan G, Jacobs NM. Necrotizing fasciitis and necrotizing cellulitis due to group B Streptococcus. *Am J Dis Child* 1977;131:1169.

415. Wilson HD, Haltalin KC. Acute necrotizing fasciitis in childhood: report of 11 cases. *Am J Dis Child* 1973;125:591.

416. Bliss DP, Healey PJ, Waldhausen JHT. Necrotizing fasciitis after Plastibell circumcision. *J Pediatr* 1997;131:459.

417. Bodemer C, Panhans A, Chretien-Marquet B, et al. Staphylococcal necrotizing fasciitis in the mammary region in childhood: a report of five cases. *J Pediatr* 1997;131:466.

418. Quinonez JM, Steele RW. Necrotizing fasciitis. *Semin Pediatr Infect Dis* 1997;8:207.

419. Chen JW, Broadbent RS, Thomson IA. Staphylococcal neonatal necrotizing fasciitis: survival without radical debridement. *N Z Med J* 1998;111:251.

420. Rudoy RC, Nelson JD. Breast abscess during the neonatal period: a review. *Am J Dis Child* 1975;129:1031.

421. Brook I. The aerobic and anaerobic microbiology of neonatal breast abscess. *Pediatr Infect Dis J* 1991;10:785.

422. Plavidal FJ, Werch A. Fetal scalp abscess secondary to intrauterine monitoring. *Am J Obstet Gynecol* 1976;125:65.

423. Plavidal FJ, Werch A. Gonococcal fetal scalp abscess: a case report. *Am J Obstet Gynecol* 1977;127:437.

424. Darmstadt GL, Dinulos JG, Miller Z. Congenital cutaneous candidiasis: clinical presentation, pathogenesis, and management guidelines. *Pediatrics* 2000;105:438.

425. Mitchell SJ, Gray J, Morgan MEI, et al. Nosocomial infection with *Rhizopus microsporus* in preterm infants: association with wooden tongue depressors. *Lancet* 1996;348:441.

426. Linder N, Keller N, Huri C, et al. Primary cutaneous mucormycosis in a premature infant: case report and review of the literature. *Am J Perinatol* 1998;15:35.

427. Weston WL, Morelli JG. Neonatal tinea capitis. *Pediatr Infect Dis J* 1998;17:257.

428. Lund CH, Nonato LB, Kuller JM, et al. Disruption of barrier function in neonatal skin associated with adhesive removal. *J Pediatr* 1997;131:367.

429. Nelson JD, Peters PC. Suprapubic aspiration of urine in premature and term infants. *Pediatrics* 1965;36:132.

430. Israele V, Darabi A, McCracken GH Jr. The role of bacterial virulence factors and Tamm-Horsfall protein in the pathogenesis of *Escherichia coli* urinary tract infection in infants. *Am J Dis Child* 1987;141:1230.

431. Hitchcock RJI, Pallett A, Hall MA, et al. Urinary tract candidiasis in neonates and infants. *Br J Urol* 1995;76:252.

432. Nebigil I, Tümer N. Asymptomatic urinary tract infection in childhood. *Eur J Pediatr* 1992;151:308.

433. Bergström T, Larson H, Lincoln K, et al. Studies of urinary tract infections in infancy and childhood: XII. Eighty consecutive patients with neonatal infection. *J Pediatr* 1972;80:858.

434. Leung AKC, Robson WLM. Urinary tract infection in infancy and childhood. *Adv Pediatr* 1991;38:257.

435. Verma RP, Pizzica A. Early neonatal urinary tract infection: a case report and review. *J Perinatol* 1998;18:480.

436. Anderson PAM, Rickwood AMK. Features of primary vesicoureteric reflux detected by prenatal sonography. *Br J Urol* 1991;67:267.

437. Roberts JA. Neonatal circumcision: an end to the controversy? *South Med J* 1996;89:167.

438. Crain EF, Gershel JC. Urinary tract infections in febrile infants younger than 8 weeks of age. *Pediatrics* 1990;86:363.

439. Hansson S, Brandström P, Jodal U, et al. Low bacterial counts in infants with urinary tract infection. *J Pediatr* 1998;132:180.

440. Barkemeyer BM. Suprapubic aspiration of urine in very low birth weight infants. *Pediatrics* 1993;92:457.

441. Ginsburg CM, McCracken GH Jr. Urinary tract infections in young infants. *Pediatrics* 1982;69:409.

442. Wong-Beringer A, Jacobs RA, Guglielmo J. Treatment of funguria. *JAMA* 1992;267:2780.

443. Benador D, Benador N, Slosman DO, et al. Cortical scintigraphy in the evaluation of renal parenchymal changes in children with pyelonephritis. *J Pediatr* 1994;124:17.

444. Bourchier D, Abbott GD, Maling TMJ. Radiological abnormalities in infants with urinary tract infections. *Arch Dis Child* 1984;59:620.

445. Feld LG, Greenfield SP, Ogra PL. Urinary tract infections in infants and children. *Pediatr Rev* 1989;11:71.

446. Hellström M, Jacobsson B, Jodal U, et al. Renal growth after neonatal urinary tract infection. *Pediatr Nephrol* 1987;1:269.

447. Dick PT, Feldman W. Routine diagnostic imaging for childhood urinary tract infections: a systematic overview. *J Pediatr* 1996;128:15.

448. Devriendt K, Groenen P, Van Esch H, et al. Vesico-ureteral reflux: a genetic condition? *Eur J Pediatr* 1998;157:265.

449. Armstrong JH, Zacarias F, Rein MF. Ophthalmia neonatorum: a chart review. *Pediatrics* 1976;57:884.

450. Centers for Disease Control and Prevention. Increasing incidence of gonorrhea—Minnesota 1994. *MMWR* 1995;44:282.

451. Laga M, Naamara W, Brunham RC, et al. Single-dose therapy of gonococcal ophthalmia neonatorum with ceftriaxone. *N Engl J Med* 1986;315:1382.

452. Bell TA, Grayston JT, Krohn MA, et al. Randomized trial of silver nitrate, erythromycin, and no eye prophylaxis for the prevention of conjunctivitis among newborns not at risk for gonococcal ophthalmitis. *Pediatrics* 1993;92:755.

453. Isenberg SJ, Apt L, Wood M. A controlled trial of povidone-iodine as prophylaxis against ophthalmia neonatorum. *N Engl J Med* 1995;332:562.

454. Rapoza PA, Quinn TC, Kiessling LA, et al. Assessment of neonatal conjunctivitis with a direct immunofluorescent monoclonal antibody stain for Chlamydia. *JAMA* 1986;255:3369.

455. Shah SS, Gallagher PG. Complications of conjunctivitis caused by *Pseudomonas aeruginosa* in a newborn intensive care unit. *Pediatr Infect Dis J* 1998;17:97.

456. Burns RP, Rhodes DH Jr. *Pseudomonas* eye infection as a cause of death in premature infants. *Arch Ophthalmol* 1961;65:517.

457. Rowe DS, Aicardi EZ, Dawson CR, et al. Purulent ocular discharge in neonates: significance of *Chlamydia trachomatis*. *Pediatrics* 1979;63:628–632.

458. Talley AR, Garcia-Ferrer F, Laycock KA, et al. Comparative diagnosis of neonatal chlamydial conjunctivitis by polymerase chain reaction and McCoy cell culture. *Am J Ophthalmol* 1994;117:50.

459. Hammerschlag MR, Roblin PM, Gelling M, et al. Use of polymerase chain reaction for the detection of *Chlamydia trachomatis* in ocular and nasopharyngeal specimens from infants with conjunctivitis. *Pediatr Infect Dis J* 1997;16:293.

460. Bird M, Dawson CR, Schachter JS, et al. Does the diagnosis of trachoma adequately identify ocular chlamydial infection in trachoma-endemic areas? *J Infect Dis* 2003;187:1669.

461. Centers for Disease Control and Prevention 1998 Guidelines for treatment of sexually transmitted diseases. *MMWR* 1998;47 (RR-1):65.

462. Golden B. SubTenon injection of gentamicin for bacterial infections of the eye. *J Infect Dis* 1971;124:S271.

463. Patamasucon P, Rettig PJ, Faust KL, et al. Oral v topical erythromycin therapies for chlamydial conjunctivitis. *Am J Dis Child* 1982;136:817.

464. Hammerschlag MR, Gelling M, Roblin PM, et al. Treatment of neonatal chlamydial conjunctivitis with azithromycin. *Pediatr Infect Dis J* 1998;17:1049.

465. Haffejee IE. The epidemiology of rotavirus infections: a global perspective. *J Pediatr Gastroenterol Nutr* 1995;20:275.

466. Champsaur H, Questiaux E, Prevot J, et al. Rotavirus carriage, asymptomatic infection, and disease in the first two years of life: I. Virus shedding. *J Infect Dis* 1984;149:667.

467. Riedel F, Kroener T, Stein K, et al. Rotavirus infection and bradycardia-apnoea-episodes in the neonate. *Eur J Pediatr* 1996;155:36.

468. Foldenauer A, Volbeck, Pohlandt F. Neonatal hypocalcaemia associated with rotavirus diarrhea. *Eur J Pediatr* 1998;157:838.

469. Nataro JP, Kaper JB. Diarrheagenic *Escherichia coli*. *Clin Microbiol Rev* 1998;11:142.

470. Boyer KM, Petersen NJ, Farzaneh I, et al. An outbreak of gastroenteritis due to *E. coli* 0142 in a neonatal nursery. *J Pediatr* 1975;86:919.

471. Lyerly DM, Krivan HC, Wilkins TD. *Clostridium difficile*: its disease and toxins. *Clin Microbiol Rev* 1988;1:1.

472. Haltalin KC. Neonatal shigellosis: report of 16 cases and review of the literature. *Am J Dis Child* 1967;114:603.

473. Wong S-N, Tam AY-C, Yuen K-Y. *Campylobacter* infection in the neonate: case report and review of the literature. *Pediatr Infect Dis J* 1990;9:665.

474. Reina J, Borrell N, Fiol M. Rectal bleeding caused by *Campylobacter jejuni* in a neonate. *Pediatr Infect Dis J* 1992;11:500.

475. Paisley JW, Lauer BA. Neonatal *Yersinia enterocolitica* enteritis. *Pediatr Infect Dis J* 1992;11:331.

476. Freij BJ. *Aeromonas*: biology of the organism and diseases in children. *Pediatr Infect Dis* 1984;3:164.

477. Nelson JD. Duration of neomycin therapy for enteropathogenic *Escherichia coli* diarrheal disease: a comparative study of 113 cases. *Pediatrics* 1971;48:248.

478. DiNicola AF. *Campylobacter jejuni* diarrhea in a 3-day-old male neonate. *Am J Dis Child* 1986;140:191.

479. Berger A, Salzer HR, Weninger M, et al. Septicaemia in an Austrian neonatal intensive care unit: a 7-year analysis. *Acta Paediatr* 1998;87:1066.

480. Kinney JS, Eiden JJ. Enteric infectious disease in neonates: epidemiology, pathogenesis, and a practical approach to evaluation and therapy. *Clin Perinatol* 1994;21:317.

481. Rotbart HA, Levin MJ, Yolken RH, et al. An outbreak of rotavirus-associated neonatal necrotizing enterocolitis. *J Pediatr* 1983;103:454.

482. Abzug MJ, Beam AC, Gyorkos EA, et al. Viral pneumonia in the first month of life. *Pediatr Infect Dis J* 1990;9:881.

483. Tipple MA, Beem MO, Saxon EM. Clinical characteristics of the afebrile pneumonia associated with *Chlamydia trachomatis* infection in infants less than 6 months of age. *Pediatrics* 1979;63:192.

484. Colarizi P, Chiesa C, Pacifico L, et al. *Chiamydia trachomatis*-associated respiratory disease in the very early neonatal period. *Acta Paediatr* 1996;85:991.

485. Niida Y, Numazaki K, Ikehata M, et al. Two full-term infants with *Chlamydia trachomatis* pneumonia in the early neonatal period. *Eur J Pediatr* 1998;157:950.

486. Attenburrow AA, Barker CM. Chlamydial pneumonia in the low birthweight neonate. *Arch Dis Child* 1985;60:1169.

487. Numazaki K, Chiba S, Kogawa K, et al. Chronic respiratory disease in premature infants caused by *Chiamydia trachomatis*. *J Clin Pathol* 1986;39:84.

488. Weiss SG, Newcomb RW, Beem MO. Pulmonary assessment of children after chlamydial pneumonia of infancy. *J Pediatr* 1986;108:659.

489. Walsh WF, Stanley S, Lally KP, et al. *Ureaplasma urealyticum* demonstrated by open lung biopsy in newborns with chronic lung disease. *Pediatr Infect Dis J* 1991;10:823.

490. Wang EEL, Ohlsson A, Kellner JD. Association of *Ureaplasma urealyticum* colonization with chronic lung disease of prematurity: results of a meta-analysis. *J Pediatr* 1995;127:640.

491. Alfa MJ, Embree JE, Degagne P, et al. Transmission of *Ureaplasma urealyticum* from mothers to full and preterm infants. *Pediatr Infect Dis J* 1995;14:341.

492. Pacifico L, Panero A, Roggini M, et al. *Ureaplasma urealyticum* and pulmonary outcome in a neonatal intensive care population. *Pediatr Infect Dis J* 1997;16:579.

493. Bhandari V, Hussain N, Rosenkrantz T, et al. Respiratory tract colonization with mycoplasma species increases the severity of bronchopulmonary dysplasia. *J Perinat Med* 1998;26:37.

494. Castro-Alcaraz S, Greenberg EM, Bateman DA, et al. Patterns of colonization with *Ureaplasma urealyticum* during neonatal intensive care unit hospitalizations of very low birth weight infants and the development of chronic lung disease. *Pediatrics* 2002;110:e45.

495. Kotecha S, Hodge R, Schaber JA, et al. Pulmonary *Ureaplasma urealyticum* is associated with the development of acute lung inflammation and chronic lung disease in preterm infants. *Pediatr Res* 2004;55:61.

496. Patterson AM, Taciak V, Lovchik J, et al. *Ureaplasma urealyticum* respiratory tract colonization is associated with an increase in interleukin 1-beta and tumor necrosis factor alpha relative to interleukin 6 in tracheal aspirates of preterm infants. *Pediatr Infect Dis J* 1998;17:321.

497. Lyon AJ, McColm J, Middlemist L, et al. Randomized trial of erythromycin on the development of chronic lung disease in preterm infants. *Arch Dis Child Fetal Neonatal Ed* 1998;78:F10.

498. Mabanta CG, Pryhuber GS, Weinberg GA, et al. Erythromycin for the prevention of chronic lung disease in intubated preterm infants at risk for, or colonized or infected with *Ureaplasma urealyticum*. *Cochrane Database Syst Rev* 2003;CD003744.

499. Gajdusek DC. *Pneumocystis carinii*-etiologic agent of interstitial plasma cell pneumonia of premature and young infants. *Pediatrics* 1957;19:543.

500. Beach RS, Garcia ER, Sosa R, et al. *Pneumocystis carinii* pneumonia in a human immunodeficiency virus 1-infected neonate with meconium aspiration. *Pediatr Infect Dis J* 1991;10:953.

501. Panero A, Roggini M, Papoff P, et al. *Pneumocystis carinii* pneumonia in preterm infants: report of two cases successfully diagnosed by nonbronchoscopic bronchoalveolar lavage. *Acta Paediatr* 1995;84:1309.

502. Famiglietti RF, Bakerman PR, Saubolle MA, et al. Cavitary legionellosis in two immunocompetent infants. *Pediatrics* 1997;99:899.

503. Levy I, Rubin LG. *Legionella pneumonia* in neonates: a literature review. *J Perinatol* 1998;18:287.

504. Paisley JW, Lauer BA, Melinkovich P, et al. Rapid diagnosis of *Chlamydia trachomatis* pneumonia in infants by direct immunofluorescence microscopy of nasopharyngeal secretions. *J Pediatr* 1986;109:653.

505. Abele-Horn M, Wolff C, Dressel P, et al. Polymerase chain reaction versus culture for detection of *Ureaplasma urealyticum* and *Mycoplasma hominis* in the urogenital tract of adults and the respiratory tract of newborns. *Eur J Clin Microbiol Infect Dis* 1996;15:595.

506. Matlow AG, Nelson S, Wray R, et al. Nosocomial acquisition of pertussis diagnosed by polymerase chain reaction. *Infect Control Hosp Epidemiol* 1997;18:715.

507. Haney PJ, Bohlman M, Sun C-CJ. Radiographic findings in neonatal pneumonia. *AJR Am J Roentgenol* 1984;143:23.

508. Freij BJ, Kusmiesz H, Nelson JD, et al. Parapneumonic effusions and empyema in hospitalized children: a retrospective review of 227 cases. *Pediatr Infect Dis* 1984;3:578.

509. Berman SA, Balkany TJ, Simmons MA. Otitis media in the neonatal intensive care unit. *Pediatrics* 1978;62:198.

510. deSa DJ. Mucosal metaplasia and chronic inflammation in the middle ear of infants receiving intensive care in the neonatal period. *Arch Dis Child* 1983;58:24.

511. Eavey RD. Abnormalities of the neonatal ear: otoscopic observations, histologic observations, and a model for contamination of the middle ear by cellular contents of amniotic fluid. *Laryngoscope* 1993;103[Suppl 58]:1.

512. Burton DM, Seid AB, Kearns DB, et al. Neonatal otitis media: an update. *Arch Otolaryngol Head Neck Surg* 1993;119:672.

513. Marchant CD, Shurin PA, Turczyk VA, et al. Course and outcome of otitis media in early infancy: a prospective study. *J Pediatr* 1984;104:826.

514. Tetzlaff TR, Ashworth C, Nelson JD. Otitis media in children less than 12 weeks of age. *Pediatrics* 1977;59:827.

515. Bland RD. Otitis media in the first six weeks of life: diagnosis, bacteriology, and management. *Pediatrics* 1972;49:187.

516. Shurin PA, Howie VM, Pelton SI, et al. Bacterial etiology of otitis media during the first six weeks of life. *J Pediatr* 1978;92:893.

517. Parker PC, Boles RG. *Pseudomonas* otitis media and bacteremia following a water birth. *Pediatrics* 1997;99:653.

518. Arriaga MA, Bluestone CD, Stool SE. The role of tympanocentesis in the management of infants with sepsis. *Laryngoscope* 1989;99:1048.

519. Bell MJ. Peritonitis in the newborn-current concepts. *Pediatr Clin North Am* 1985;32:1181.

520. Freij BJ, Votteler TP, McCracken GH Jr. Primary peritonitis in previously healthy children. *Am J Dis Child* 1984;138:1058.

521. Duggan MB, Khwaja MS. Neonatal primary peritonitis in Nigeria. *Arch Dis Child* 1975;50:130.

522. Genta VM, Gilligan PH, McCarthy LR. *Clostridium difficile* peritonitis in a neonate: a case report. *Arch Pathol Lab Med* 1984;108:82.

523. Aronoff SC, Olson MM, Gauderer MWL, et al. *Pseudomonas aeruginosa* as a primary pathogen in children with bacterial peritonitis. *J Pediatr Surg* 1987;22:86l.

524. Mollitt DL, Tepas JJ III, Talbert JL. The microbiology of neonatal peritonitis. *Arch Surg* 1988;123:176.

Viral and Protozoal Infections

48

Bishara J. Freij   *John L. Sever*

Microorganisms can reach and infect a fetus or newborn via a number of routes. Vertical spread of a pathogen from an infected mother can occur *in utero*, during delivery, or postnatally (e.g., ingestion of infected breast milk). Horizontal spread of infectious agents to newborns by means of contaminated hands, stethoscopes, blood products, total parenteral nutrition fluid, or respiratory therapy equipment is well documented and can lead to outbreaks of disease in neonatal intensive care units. Iatrogenic fetal infections occasionally occur after invasive procedures such as fetal scalp monitoring or intrauterine transfusions (1). Infection control in the NICU is discussed in detail in Chapter 49.

Maternal infections acquired shortly before conception or during gestation can adversely affect pregnancy outcome indirectly through nonspecific effects of severe maternal illness (e.g., increased rates of spontaneous abortions, stillbirths, or premature births associated with measles infection during pregnancy) or directly through microbial invasion of the fetus or neonate (2). Pathogens can be transmitted from mothers to their infants through hematogenous spread across the placenta (e.g., cytomegalovirus [CMV], *Toxoplasma gondii*), ascension from an infected cervix (e.g., herpes simplex virus [HSV]), or intimate contact between a fetus and infected genital secretions during vaginal delivery (e.g., HSV, hepatitis B virus [HBV], human immunodeficiency virus type 1 [HIV-1], papillomaviruses) (3–5). Maternal coinfection by other microorganisms may enhance the risk of fetal infection by either or both pathogens (6).

The outcome of a fetal or neonatal infection depends on the stage of pregnancy during which infection occurs, virulence of the pathogen, preexisting maternal immunity to the infecting agent, and efficacy of drug therapy for maternal or neonatal disease. Intrauterine infections may lead to resorption of the embryo, fetal demise resulting in a spontaneous abortion or stillbirth, or delivery of an infected neonate. Infected infants who are asymptomatic at birth may develop chronic problems in late infancy or early childhood (e.g., HIV-1, CMV, hepatitis C virus [HCV]) or during adulthood (e.g., rubella, HBV) (7–10). Others suffer from severe acute neonatal disease such as pneumonia or hepatitis (e.g., HSV, syphilis), congenital malformations (e.g., CMV, rubella), intrauterine growth retardation, or prematurity (8,10,11). The number of infants born each year with these conditions is substantial (Table 48-1), and the lifetime expenditures for their medical and educational needs are considerable (12–23).

The acronym TORCH (*T. gondii*, "other," rubella virus, CMV, HSV) has long been used as a reminder that a number of pathogens can cause clinically indistinguishable illnesses in the neonate. These agents originally were grouped together because of shared clinical features (e.g., microcephaly, hepatosplenomegaly, petechiae, ocular abnormalities), their ability to cause asymptomatic infections in the mother and newborn, and their propensity for causing long-term sequelae that may be inapparent at birth (24). Because many other agents (e.g., HIV-1, *Treponema pallidum*, varicella-zoster virus [VZV], coxsackievirus, human parvovirus B19, *Mycobacterium tuberculosis*) are capable of causing similar illnesses, the diagnostic workup of infants suspected of having a TORCH infection should not be restricted to the original four agents, as is common in medical practice (25). The clinical utility of this mnemonic is limited, and its use should be minimized or abandoned altogether (26,27).

The epidemiology, clinical manifestations, diagnosis, and treatment of maternal and fetal infections caused by rubella virus, HSV, CMV, VZV, human parvovirus B19, hepatitis B, hepatitis C, HIV-1, and *T. gondii* is discussed in this chapter. Strategies for the prevention of maternal infection by these organisms or their vertical spread to the fetus or newborn infant are emphasized. Infections caused by other pathogens are addressed in less detail. Respiratory and gastrointestinal viruses that spread horizontally in nursery settings are covered in Chapter 49.

TABLE 48-1

ESTIMATED NUMBER OF INFANTS WITH SELECTED CHRONIC CONGENITAL OR PERINATAL INFECTIONS BORN ANNUALLY IN THE UNITED STATES

Infection	Number of Infants	Year of Estimate
Congenital cytomegalovirus (12)	40,000	1992
Hepatitis B virus (9)		
Exposed	20,000	1999
Chronic carriers[a]	5,500	1999
Hepatitis C virus (13,14)[b]	1,000–3,000	2002
Congenital toxoplasmosis (15)[c]	4,100	2001
Congenital syphilis (16)	451	2002
Perinatal human immunodeficiency		
virus type 1 (17)[d]	390	2001
Neonatal herpes (18)	1,500	2002
Congenital rubella syndrome (19)[e]	1	2002

[a] If not given hepatitis B immune globulin and hepatitis B recombinant vaccine at birth
[b] Some infants will spontaneously clear the virus by two years of age
[c] Rates as low as 1:12,000 live births have been reported from Massachusetts, suggesting a significantly lower estimate for the annual number of infants born with congenital toxoplasmosis in the United States (20)
[d] An additional 140 infected children had no reported or identifiable risk factors for their HIV-1 infection
[e] Due to the passive nature of the reporting system and to missed diagnoses of less severe cases, this figure probably represents an underestimate of the actual cases (21,22).

RUBELLA

Rubella (i.e., German measles, third disease) typically is a subclinical or mild exanthematous infection of children and adults. Gestational rubella can have deleterious effects on the fetus. The infant may have physical and mental abnormalities, such as cataracts, congenital heart disease, deafness, microcephaly, or psychomotor retardation, or present with severe neonatal disease that may include thrombocytopenia, bleeding, hepatosplenomegaly, pneumonia, and myocarditis. Some manifestations of congenital rubella infection may not appear until years or decades later, even among patients asymptomatic at birth (8).

The rubella virus is an enveloped, single positive-stranded ribonucleic acid (RNA) virus that is spherical and has spike-like projections containing hemagglutinin. Only one antigenic type of the virus is known, but there are differences between rubella virus strains in their properties (e.g., hemagglutination, cell tropism), virulence, and teratogenicity. Man is the only natural host for rubella virus, but some animals such as primates, rabbits, and ferrets can be infected under experimental conditions. Rubella virus has three structural polypeptides; two are envelope acylated glycoproteins (E1 and E2) observed as spikes in the form of E1-E2 heterodimers on the virion surface, and one is a nonglycosylated RNA-associated capsid protein (C). E1 contains the domains responsible for binding to host cell receptors and for hemagglutination. The function of E2 is not well defined, but it may carry strain-specific antigens, partial hemagglutination epitopes, and a weak neutralizing domain associated with virus infectivity. The C protein may be involved in the transfer of viral RNA into host cell cytoplasm (28). Rubella virus also possesses a nonstructural polyprotein (p200); this

polyprotein and its cleavage products (p150, p90) have enzymatic activities (e.g., helicase, replicase, protease) and are involved in viral RNA replication (29,30). Molecular techniques such as the polymerase chain reaction (PCR) and nucleotide sequencing allow the differentiation between rubella virus strains. This is useful in the analysis of the molecular epidemiology of the virus and in differentiating between wild-type virus and the RA 27/3 vaccine strain when rubella virus is isolated from individuals with possible vaccine-related adverse effects (31,32).

Person-to-person transmission usually occurs by airborne spread of infected respiratory secretions, and direct contact with virus-containing urine or feces is a less likely route of infection. Although rubella virus can be recovered from the genital tract of infected women, vertical transmission during pregnancy is believed to occur almost exclusively through the placenta (33,34).

On entry into the body in cases of postnatal infection, the rubella virus multiplies in nasopharyngeal epithelial cells and in local lymph nodes. This is followed by a period of viremia and shedding from the throat. It is during this maternal viremic phase that placental and fetal infection occurs. The frequency and nature of fetal involvement depends on the mother's immune status against the virus and the timing during gestation of maternal rubella (8).

The mechanisms by which the virus ravages the fetus are not clearly understood. Necrotic placental vascular endothelial cells can serve as a source of virus-infected emboli. Damage to endothelial cells can lead to thrombosis of small blood vessels, resulting in hypoxic tissue damage (35,36). Rubella-infected cells have diminished mitotic activity as a result of chromosomal breaks. They produce a growth-inhibiting protein and show ultrastructural mitochondrial changes that may interfere with cell metabolism. The virus damages the cytoskeletal microtubular system by altering the arrangement of actin filaments (37). Rubella virus generally establishes a chronic nonlytic infection in the fetus and can potentially infect any organ (29). As with other viruses, it can induce apoptosis of infected cells, but a role for this in its teratogenicity has not been demonstrated. Focal lysis of infected cells can be seen in some organs, but inflammation is not a salient feature of congenital rubella (35). Noninflammatory necrosis in the structures of the heart, eyes, brain, and ears have been seen in aborted rubella-infected fetuses (29). Growth-retarded infants have reduced cell numbers on histopathologic examination (38). Moreover, the virus can modify cell receptors for specific growth factors (39). Late-onset manifestations of congenital rubella may be as a result of viral persistence with ongoing cell destruction or to organ damage by means of a number of immune mechanisms such as circulating rubella-specific immune complexes, defective cytotoxic effector cell function, or the development of autoimmunity (28,40–44). The rubella virus E1 and E2 proteins, but not the C nucleoprotein, appear to be responsible for autoantibody induction (45).

Long-lasting immunity normally develops after recovery from postnatal rubella. Reinfections can occur in persons with low antibody titers, but these are usually asymptomatic. Persons with low antibody levels after rubella vaccination are more prone to reinfections than persons with similarly low titers after natural infection (34).

Circulating antibodies and cell-mediated immune responses are generated after rubella infection. Rubella-specific immunoglobin M (IgM), immunoglobin G (IgG), immunoglobin A (IgA), immunoglobin D (IgD), and immunoglobin E (IgE) antibodies are induced in response to postnatal infection (46). IgM antibodies appear early and are short lived. They usually disappear 5 to 8 weeks after onset of illness, although rubella-specific IgM antibodies rarely can persist for months or years (47). The IgM response after rubella vaccination or natural reinfection generally is weak and of brief duration (48–50). Moreover, rubella-specific IgM antibodies can be detected in acute infections caused by viruses such as parvovirus B19 and Epstein–Barr virus (51). Specific IgD and IgE antibodies appear early and then decline more slowly than specific IgM antibodies (46). Specific IgA antibodies generally emerge within the first 10 days of illness, and they may continue to be measurable for periods ranging from 3 weeks to several years (46,52). Rubella-specific IgG antibodies increase rapidly and persist throughout life; rubella-specific IgG1 has been shown to be the principal IgG subclass (34,53). The most vigorous antibody and lymphocyte proliferative responses in postnatal rubella are directed against glycoprotein E1 (54,55). The avidity of specific IgG to rubella antigens increases with time after primary infection; a low avidity index (less than 40%) can be seen up to 6 weeks after onset of the rubella rash, whereas a high avidity index (greater than 60%) is not seen until after 13 weeks (51). Measurement of rubella IgG avidity can be useful in women

with positive rubella-specific IgM reactions, as it can help distinguish primary infections from unusually prolonged IgM persistence or from reinfection. Rubella-specific IgG also can be detected in the urine, and the results correlate well with serum IgG measurements (56). Men and women appear to differ in the nature and magnitude of their antibody responses to rubella virus structural proteins (57). Men never produce anti-E2 IgA and generate significantly lower levels of IgG antibodies directed against E2 than women. Anti-E1 IgM and IgG antibodies appear earlier in male patients, but female patients have higher levels of rubella-specific IgG antibodies after recovery from the illness. The observed gender differences in antibody responses to viral proteins may be under genetic or hormonal influences and may be related to the increased susceptibility of women to the joint complications of rubella (57).

Immune responses in congenitally infected infants differ from those observed in adults with rubella. Fetal IgM production usually begins after 16 weeks of gestation. Rubella-specific IgM antibodies are detectable until 6 to 12 months of age. Specific IgG antibody levels decrease over time; as many as 20% of affected children have no measurable antibody titers by 5 years of age (34). Circulating antirubella antibodies in infants with intrauterine infection have lower affinities to rubella antigen than antibodies from adults with natural infection (58,59). Serum antibodies to the E2 glycoprotein are quantitatively more abundant than those directed against E1 in some patients with congenital rubella, particularly among older infants. Antibody reactivities against the C protein are poor (54,60). Infants with congenital rubella have diminished cell-mediated immune responses on exposure to rubella antigens compared with children or adults with postnatal infection, and the responses are weakest for infants infected earlier during gestation. The reduction in response is mainly seen with the E1 protein (53,61).

Maternal Rubella

Epidemiology

Major epidemics of rubella formerly occurred at 6- to 9-year intervals in the United States. The last major pandemic took place between 1964 and 1965, at which time 20,000 cases of congenital rubella occurred. Rubella did not become a notifiable disease in the United States until 1966. Since licensure of the rubella vaccine in 1969, the number of postnatal rubella and congenital rubella syndrome (CRS) cases declined by 99% and 97%, respectively. The incidence of reported postnatal rubella cases declined from 0.45 per 100,000 in 1990 to less than 0.02 per 100,000 in 2002. The annual number of reported cases during that same period ranged from a high of 1,412 in 1991 to a low of 18 in 2002, with a median of 192 (19,62).

A significant change in the characteristics of postnatal rubella cases has been noted between 1990 and 2000. Between 1990 and 1992, 50% to 70% of all cases were in children 14 years of age or younger. By 2002, 72% of all cases occurred in individuals 15 to 39 years of age. Only 23% of the 18 postnatal rubella cases in 2002 were in females. Between 1995 and 2000, Hispanics comprised from 56% to 78% of all patients with this infection, most of whom were born outside the United States. Between 1996 and 1999, rubella was reported in 281 women of childbearing age, 26% of whom were pregnant at the time of rash onset (19,62). For the time period from 1990 to 1999, there were 65 outbreaks of rubella (each with five or more epidemiologically linked cases). Common settings for these outbreaks included religious communities, correctional facilities, worksites, and higher education institutions (62). Most affected individuals were either unimmunized or had unknown vaccination status (21,62–64).

Medical students and other health professionals can also serve as vectors for rubella infection, placing susceptible pregnant women to whom they are exposed in a medical setting at significant risk (65). In a study of one hospital system in St. Louis, Missouri, 5.3% of about 6,000 new employees were found to be seronegative for rubella (66).

Approximately 10% to 20% of women of childbearing age in the United States are susceptible to rubella, and the rates are comparable for Hispanics, non-Hispanic whites, and African Americans. Hispanics aged 20 to 29 years are more likely to be seropositive for rubella if born outside the United States (67). Between 1990 and 1999, women delivering infants with CRS tended to be young (median age, 23 years), Hispanic, and foreign-born (62). Rubella susceptibility rates for women of child-bearing age in European countries generally are comparable to those found in the United States, but lower seropositivity rates are encountered among island populations such as those in Hawaii and Jamaica and in certain tropical African countries (34,68–72). Significant regional differences have been found in large countries, such as India and China (73,74).

Clinical Manifestations

Twenty percent to 50% of postnatal rubella infections are subclinical (75). Illness occurs 12 to 23 days (mean 18) after exposure. A prodrome consisting of malaise, low-grade fever that rarely lasts beyond the first day of the exanthem, headache, and conjunctivitis precedes the rash by 1 to 5 days. The exanthem consists of discrete macules or papules that initially appear on the face and behind the ears, spread downward over 1 to 2 days, and usually disappear over 3 to 5 days; rubella virus can be isolated from these skin lesions (76). Postauricular, suboccipital, and posterior cervical lymphadenopathy is common and may persist for several weeks. Complications of rubella develop more frequently in adults. Transient arthralgias may occur in as many as one-third of infected women, but arthritis is uncommon (8). Other complications are rare and include thrombocytopenic purpura, hemolytic anemia, hepatitis, Guillain–Barré syndrome, encephalitis, progressive panencephalitis, myelitis, peripheral neuritis, myocarditis, and pericarditis (8,77–80).

Pregnancy has no effect on the natural course of rubella infection. However, rubella is associated with an increased risk of miscarriages, spontaneous abortions, and stillbirths (8).

Laboratory Diagnosis

The diagnosis of rubella on clinical grounds alone is unreliable, because enteroviruses, measles virus, or parvovirus B19 may produce similar illnesses. Laboratory confirmation by virus isolation or serologic testing thus is essential in pregnant women, for whom an accurate diagnosis of gestational rubella is critical. Shirley and colleagues (81) investigated 627 patients clinically suspected of having rubella, but they could confirm this diagnosis in only 229 (37%). Human parvovirus B19 infection accounted for 7%, measles for 1%, and other infectious agents for 1%; the causes for the remaining 54% could not be determined.

Rubella virus is shed from the nasopharynx for 1 week before and 1 week after onset of the rash. However, the cultures become negative in 50% of patients by the fourth day of the rash. The virus is present in blood and urine during the week preceding the exanthem. Shortly after the rash appears, rubella virus is no longer detectable in the serum but can be found in circulating mononuclear cells for about a week. Rubella virus isolation is impractical for diagnostic purposes because it is expensive, labor intensive, and frequently unavailable to the clinician. The cell line recommended for isolation of rubella virus from clinical specimens is primary African green monkey kidney, but Vero or RK-13 can be used also. Isolation of the virus can take longer than 10 days, especially if present in low titers (82).

Serologic techniques are the most useful methods for diagnosing rubella infection. Available tests include hemagglutination inhibition, enzyme-linked immunosorbent assay (ELISA), immunofluorescence, radioimmunoassay, hemolysis in gel, complement fixation, passive hemagglutination, and latex agglutination tests (50,82). Serum specimens obtained as soon as feasible after the appearance of the exanthem and again 2 weeks later can prove the diagnosis if seroconversion or a fourfold or greater rise in rubella-specific antibody titers can be documented. Paired sera are best tested in unison because of the variability in results of assays done on separate days or by different personnel. If measured by ELISA, hemagglutination inhibition, or radioimmunoassay, rubella-specific IgG antibodies can be found as early as 1 to 2 days before the emergence of the rash; if assayed by the less readily available passive hemagglutination method, these antibodies are not detected until 15 to 50 days after onset of the exanthem and peak approximately 6 to 7 months later. The detection of rubella-specific IgM antibodies within 28 days of the appearance of the rash usually is diagnostic, the caveats being that IgM responses sometimes can persist for a year or more after a primary infection and that they also can be detected in some patients with rubella reinfection (83). Only 50% of postnatal rubella patients have detectable IgM on the day of symptom onset, but more than 90% become IgM positive by the fifth day after the rash appears (82). Newer tests that can be used for the diagnosis of acute postnatal rubella include avidity ELISA in which acutely infected persons have low IgG avidity compared with persons previously immune to rubella who exhibit greater IgG avidity (51). IgG produced in response to rubella vaccination shows low avidity to rubella antigens during the first 2 months after immunization, but this increases significantly over the ensuing months and remains at high levels thereafter (84). Immunoblot techniques have been developed for the sensitive detection of rubella-specific IgG, IgM, and IgA antibodies (85).

Rubella reinfections are confirmed by a fourfold or greater rise in the titer of preexisting rubella-specific IgG antibodies. The specific IgM response is absent or weak, but it is sometimes high enough to be within the range deemed sufficient for the diagnosis of primary rubella (50).

False-positive IgM reactions can occur in sera containing rheumatoid factor, although the IgM capture assay appears to be unaffected by its presence (50). Cross-reactions between rubella and human parvovirus B19, Epstein–Barr virus, or CMV infections in specific IgM tests necessitate caution in interpreting low or equivocal levels of rubella-specific IgM antibodies (75).

Rubella virus RNA can be detected in clinical specimens using a reverse transcription nested PCR assay. This molecular technique has been used on pharyngeal swabs, chorionic villi, amniotic fluid, fetal blood, and lens aspirates (86–88).

Treatment

There is no specific therapy for postnatal rubella. Patients with rubella shed the virus from the nasopharynx for 1 week after appearance of the rash; therefore, these patients should avoid contact with susceptible persons until the exanthem has vanished.

Prevention

The principal goal of rubella immunization programs is the elimination of CRS. The vaccine used in the United States is the RA 27/3 attenuated live rubella virus vaccine. It is available in a monovalent form (i.e., rubella only) and in combination with measles and mumps (i.e., measles–mumps–rubella). The vaccine induces antirubella antibodies in more than 95% of recipients 12 months of age or older, and its protective efficacy is greater than 90% for at least 15 years (89). Immunizing children whose pregnant mothers are susceptible to rubella does not pose a threat to the mother or her fetus. The vaccine is recommended for all susceptible persons 12 months of age or older and usually is given at 15 months of age; a second booster dose is given to children at the time of school entry.

A clinical diagnosis of rubella is considered unreliable and cannot be considered proof of immunity. Persons are deemed protected if they have serologic evidence of immunity or previously had been vaccinated on or after their first birthday. Birth before 1957 is not acceptable evidence of rubella immunity for women who could become pregnant (90).

Pregnant women whose rubella-immune status is not known should be tested for the presence of antirubella antibodies during their first prenatal visit. If a previously unimmunized pregnant woman with unknown antibody status is exposed to rubella, a blood sample should be immediately obtained for rubella antibody testing. If antibody to rubella is found, the woman is considered immune (91). The risk of rubella reinfection after natural disease or vaccination is small, but it is more likely to occur in women with low specific IgG titers (92). Rubella reinfections do not seem to be related to a lack of neutralizing antibodies or to an impaired rubella-specific lymphocyte transformation response (93). Significant fetal pathology after reinfection occurs infrequently, despite rubella virus transmission to the fetus, and is typically not seen if this occurs after the twelfth week of gestation (94–103).

Susceptible women exposed to rubella should be informed of the risks to the fetus if maternal infection occurs. If the woman develops fever, lymphadenopathy, or a rash within the expected incubation period, serum for rubella-specific IgM measurement should be obtained. If a clinical illness does not occur, serum should be obtained 6 to 8 weeks after exposure to exclude a subclinical infection. For women who seroconvert or become positive for rubella-specific IgM, the rate of fetal infection is 81% after maternal rubella during the first 12 weeks of gestation, 54% at 13 to 16 weeks, 36% at 17 to 22 weeks, 30% at 23 to 30 weeks, 60% at 31 to 36 weeks, and 100% at more than 36 weeks of pregnancy. Infants infected before 11 weeks of gestation usually develop congenital defects, most often cardiac anomalies and deafness, but only 35% of infants infected at 13 to 16 weeks of gestation have abnormalities at birth, usually deafness (104). In a study of 106 infants with confirmed CRS in whom the timing of maternal infection was known with reasonable accuracy, Munro and colleagues (105) found deafness in 58% of patients, and it was the sole abnormality in 40% of all infants; infants with congenital cardiac, ocular, or CNS defects almost always were deaf as well. The risk of deafness is small if maternal infection occurs at 17 weeks of gestation or later (104,105). Other investigators have confirmed that rubella virus can be transmitted to the fetus at any stage of pregnancy, and that the earlier the maternal infection during pregnancy, the greater is the severity of congenital defects (106–108).

If maternal rubella occurs during the first 5 months of pregnancy, the option of therapeutic pregnancy termination can be considered. Infections occurring after this time do not produce congenital defects. If available, an attempt at prenatal diagnosis can be made, because fetal involvement after maternal rubella is not universal. The virus has been isolated from amniotic fluid by culture or directly visualized using electron microscopy in a few cases

(109,110). The low sensitivities of these methods limit their usefulness. Amniotic fluid cells in rubella-infected patients are abnormal when examined with a transmission and scanning electron microscope (lack of chromatin, disappearance of electron-dense cytoplasmic layer, membrane damage expressed by a decrease in the size and number of microvilli) (111). Daffos and colleagues studied 18 pregnancies complicated by maternal rubella; fetal blood was obtained at 20 to 26 weeks of gestation, and rubella-specific IgM was detected in 12 fetuses. Contamination of fetal blood specimens by maternal blood was excluded. Of the six fetuses without detectable rubella-specific IgM antibodies, one was found to be infected at birth (112). In another study, investigators were able to detect rubella-specific IgM and IgA as early as 22 weeks of pregnancy (52). Hwa and colleagues performed fetal blood sampling at 22 to 30 weeks gestation (at least 2 weeks after appearance of the rash) on 93 rubella-specific IgM positive pregnant women. Of six infants infected *in utero*, five had rubella-specific IgM in cord blood (113). The drawbacks of this method are that the fetus does not synthesize IgM until the fifth month of gestation, and the quantity produced initially may be meager and below the limits of detection of the assay. Despite these disadvantages, the technique still is helpful in the management of pregnancies complicated by maternal rubella (114).

Terry and associates detected rubella antigens and ribonucleic acid (RNA) sequences in a chorionic villus biopsy specimen obtained at 11 weeks of gestation from a woman with rubella in early pregnancy, and this led to pregnancy termination at week 13 of gestation. Infection was verified in the aborted fetus and placenta by virus isolation, immunoblotting, and hybridization methods (115). However, the detection of rubella virus in chorionic villus samples may not always predict fetal infection (87). PCR has been used successfully to detect rubella virus RNA in fetal and placental tissues, amniotic fluid, chorionic villus samples, and fetal blood (110,116–119). Positive results can be obtained within 24 to 48 hours with PCR, several days to a few weeks earlier than is possible with virus culture methods (87,88,118). In some infected fetuses, rubella virus RNA can be detected in fetal blood but not in concurrently-collected amniotic fluid samples (119). It is generally suggested that the interval between maternal rubella infection and sampling of fetal blood and amniotic fluid should be six to eight weeks to minimize the chance for a false-negative PCR assay result for rubella virus RNA (119).

The administration of immunoglobulin to susceptible pregnant women who are exposed to rubella does not prevent maternal or fetal infection. Its use is confined to women who would not contemplate pregnancy termination under any circumstances (89).

Pregnant women who do not have rubella antibody should be immunized in the immediate postpartum period. However, reports by a group of investigators from Canada have suggested that acute arthritis can occur in as many as 8% of women receiving the rubella RA 27/3 vac-

cine in the postpartum period, and that some subsequently develop chronic arthropathy, neurologic abnormalities such as the carpal tunnel syndrome or paresthesias, and chronic rubella viremia. These women tend to transmit rubella virus to some of their infants through breast-feeding, and a few infected infants go on to develop chronic rubella viremia (120,121). The same research group conducted a prospective, placebo-controlled, double-blind trial of postpartum rubella immunization (using the RA 27/3 vaccine) in 543 seronegative women and showed a higher incidence of acute joint problems, but only a marginally increased risk of chronic or recurrent arthralgias, in vaccine recipients (122). Data from the United States and elsewhere indicate that such complications are rare with the RA 27/3 live rubella vaccine (89,123,124). The mechanisms of rubella vaccine-induced joint disease are poorly understood, but they may include infection of the synovial membrane by vaccine virus or the deposition of rubella antigen-containing immune complexes in the synovium (125–127). Certain human leukocyte antigen class II (HLA-DR) phenotypes may be associated with an increased risk of postpartum arthropathy following rubella vaccination. The relative risk of arthropathy is eightfold higher for persons with both DR1 and DR4 and sevenfold higher for those with both DR4 and DR6 (128). It is advised that all susceptible pregnant women be vaccinated against rubella before hospital discharge (89). About 40% to 55% of CRS cases could be prevented with implementation of postpartum rubella immunization of susceptible women. Although rubella vaccine virus can be shed in breast milk, breast-feeding is not a contraindication to maternal immunization (89,129).

The rubella vaccine should not be knowingly administered during pregnancy because of its small risk of teratogenicity. Data from the Centers for Disease Control and Prevention (CDC) for the period 1979 to 1988 indicate that none of 562 infants born to 683 women inadvertently immunized with the RA 27/3 vaccine within 3 months of conception in the United States had malformations compatible with CRS (130). Between January 1971 and April 1989, 321 known rubella-susceptible women who had been immunized against rubella within 3 months before or after their estimated date of conception with the RA 27/3 or earlier vaccines (Cendehill, HPV-77) were followed by the CDC; none of the 324 infants born to these women had defects consistent with the CRS (89). Combined data from the United States, United Kingdom, Sweden, and Germany on 680 live births to susceptible women who received one of the three rubella vaccines (RA 27/3, Cendehill, HPV-77) 3 months before or during pregnancy showed that none of the infants was born with CRS (131). The RA 27/3 rubella vaccine virus, however, does cross the placenta and produces a subclinical infection in about 3% of infants; the rate of fetal infection was considerably higher (20%) for the earlier rubella vaccines (130). Infection of the fetus by the RA 27/3 rubella vaccine strain can be persistent with virus shedding lasting for several months after birth, even in an otherwise normal infant (132). The possible risk of serious congenital defects after accidental rubella vaccination has been calculated by the CDC to be 0.5%; the observed risk has been zero (131). This risk is considerably lower than the 20% or greater risk of CRS after maternal gestational infection, and it is comparable to the 2% to 3% rate of major birth defects observed in the absence of rubella vaccine exposure (130). Because of the very low, if any, risk of CRS after inadvertent rubella vaccination in pregnancy, the Advisory Committee on Immunization Practices has shortened the interval to avoid pregnancy after receiving a rubella-containing vaccine from three months to 28 days (131).

Congenital Rubella

Epidemiology

The incidence of congenital rubella has shown a consistent decline since the introduction of rubella vaccination programs in the United States. For the period 1990 through 1999, the CDC received reports of 110 confirmed cases of CRS and 7 others that were probable CRS (62). Their mothers were young (median age, 23 years), white (82%), and of Hispanic ethnicity (50%). Hispanic mothers, most of whom were born outside the United States, accounted for 83% of infants with CRS born between 1997 and 1999. Most of the maternal exposures to rubella virus occurred within the United States (62). An additional 13 cases of CRS were reported between 2000 and 2002, but there are no published details about them (19). Because of the passive nature of the CRS reporting system, it is estimated that the reported number of infants with CRS represents only 20% to 30% of actual cases (22).

CRS continues to be a problem in other parts of the world (68). In 1999, the World Health Organization reported that 52% of its member countries offered routine rubella vaccination programs (75). Nevertheless, rubella immunization programs have been successful in reducing the occurrence of CRS wherever implemented (133,134). As an example, the incidence of CRS declined from 3.5 per 100,000 live births in 1980 to 0.41 per 100,000 live births in 1986 in 19 European birth defects registries (133).

Clinical Manifestations

More than one-half of all newborns with congenital rubella are asymptomatic at birth, but most later manifest with one or more signs and symptoms of disease. The most common abnormalities encountered in CRS listed in order of decreasing frequency are sensorineural hearing loss, mental retardation, cardiac malformations, and ocular defects (8). Table 48-2 is a summary of the clinical abnormalities encountered in congenital rubella (37,38,41,42,77,105, 135–174).

If the findings of mental retardation and infection of neurosensory organs such as the eyes or ears are combined, then central nervous system (CNS) involvement occurs in more than 80% of CRS patients (77). Vascular abnormali-

ties, prominent pathologic characteristic of congenital rubella, contribute to the neuropathology by causing ischemic necrosis of adjacent tissues. Microcephaly may be as a result of the generalized organ hypocellularity seen with rubella infection (38).

The development of late-onset CRS manifestations that were inapparent in early infancy may be related to persistence or reactivation of rubella virus infection, the body's immune responses to the infection, or vascular damage. Insulin-dependent diabetes mellitus occurs in about 20% of patients by 35 years of age (174). Rubella virus can infect human fetal pancreatic islet cells and can reduce secretion of insulin (175). About 20% of CRS patients and 50% to 80% of those with glucose intolerance have circulating pancreatic islet cell cytotoxic or surface antibodies (176). These autoantibodies are triggered by rubella virus and cause destruction of pancreatic cells, unmasking the person with a genetic susceptibility to diabetes mellitus (177,178). Thyroid abnormalities develop in about 5%; thyroid microsomal or thyroglobulin antibodies are found more frequently in deaf CRS patients than in those who are hearing impaired from other causes (42). In contrast, none of 25 young adults with CRS from Finland and Poland had detectable islet cell antibodies or insulin autoantibodies, and only 16% had antibodies to thyroid peroxidase (179). Rare cases of growth hormone deficiency of hypothalamic origin have been described (180). About 10% of CRS patients incur additional forms of late-appearing ocular insults, such as glaucoma, keratoconus, corneal hydrops, and spontaneous lens absorption. Permanent damage to the vascular endothelium can induce the formation of obstructive lesions of major vessels such as the pulmonary and renal arteries. Choroidal neovascularization with significant visual loss can complicate CRS retinopathy. Autism and behavioral problems usually are delayed in appearance and can be progressive. Progressive rubella panencephalitis is a rare but ultimately fatal CNS manifestation of CRS that appears late, usually in the second decade of life (174).

Diagnosis

The CDC has established clinical and laboratory criteria for the classification of CRS cases to allow better CRS surveillance (Table 48-3) (181).

The diagnosis of CRS usually is suspected on the basis of the maternal history and the clinical findings. A definitive diagnosis can be achieved by isolating the virus from pharyngeal washings or, less commonly, from urine, cerebrospinal fluid (CSF), conjunctivae, blood, or available organs such as the lens at surgery or autopsy. Although nasopharyngeal shedding of rubella virus may continue for 6 to 12 months, the frequency of its isolation declines from about 85% during the first month of life to approximately 10% at 9 to 12 months of age (182). In children with congenital rubella encephalitis, the virus can be isolated from the CSF for months or even years (151). However, viral isolation seldom is used in clinical practice

TABLE 48-2

CLINICAL ABNORMALITIES IN INFANTS WITH SYMPTOMATIC CONGENITAL RUBELLA

Clinical Abnormality	Remarks
General	
Intrauterine growth retardation	Common (50%–85%); usually have other manifestations of congenital infection; may be due to reduced number of body cells (38)
Postnatal growth retardation	Retarded growth is most severe in infants with multiple congenital defects; long-term follow-up studies indicate that most will have subnormal growth (136,137)
Cardiovascular system	
Patent ductus arteriosus	Most frequently encountered structural defect (30%); may occur with other heart lesions, especially pulmonary valvular or artery stenosis (105)
Pulmonary artery stenosis	Second most common heart defect; results from intimal proliferation (138)
Miscellaneous defects	Individually uncommon; include coarctation of the aorta, atrial and ventricular septal defects, myocarditis, tetralogy of Fallot, ventricular aneurysm, and aneurysms of the arteries of the limbs and viscera (135,138,139)
Hearing loss	The most common congenital defect; almost always present in infants with other malformations; uncommon if maternal rubella occurs at ≥17 weeks of gestation; usually bilateral; may be present at birth or develop later; can be progressive (8,140)
Ocular abnormalities	
Cataract	Found in about 35% of infants; can be unilateral or bilateral; noted at birth or early infancy; virus can be isolated from lens; spontaneous reabsorption of cataracts has been described in rare cases (141–144)
Retinopathy	Common (35%–60%); may be present at birth or appear later in life; often unilateral; salt-and-pepper appearance; does not affect visual acuity (145–148)
Cloudy cornea	Rare; usually present at birth; may coexist with glaucoma; resolves spontaneously; rarely persists (149)
Glaucoma	Occurs in ≤10%; may be bilateral; can be found at birth or appear later in life; leads to blindness if not treated (8,135,148)
Microphthalmia	Common in infants with cataract; concomitant glaucoma common (8,148)
Miscellaneous abnormalities	Uncommon; includes iris hypoplasia, strabismus, and iridocyclitis
Interstitial pneumonia	Occurs in about 5%; probably immunologically mediated; may be acute, subacute, or chronic (41,150)
Central nervous system	
Meningoencephalitis	Occurs in as many as 20%; manifests with bulging anterior fontanelle, hypotonia, irritability, and seizures; cerebrospinal fluid findings include elevated protein concentration, mononuclear pleocytosis, and rubella virus isolation in 30%; transient; most infants have neurodevelopmental deficits; progressive rubella panencephalitis is a delayed manifestation of chronic infection that begins 10 years after the primary infection and characterized by fibrinoid necrosis, severe neuronal loss and demyelination, and old microinfarcts (37,77,135,151,152)
Microcephaly	Uncommon in earlier reports, but more frequently described in recent case series; may be associated with normal intelligence (135)
Intracranial calcifications	May be present in early infancy (103,153,154)
Electroencephalographic abnormalities	Occurs in 36%; usually resolves by 1 year of age (77)
Mental retardation	Occurs in 10%–20%; associated with other stigmata of congenital rubella (135)
Speech defects	Uncommon in absence of hearing impairment
Behavioral disorders	Common; occurs primarily in deaf patients (151,155)
Miscellaneous problems	Autism; central language disorders; spastic quadriparesis; hydrocephalus; cerebral arterial stenosis
Skin	
Blueberry-muffin spots	Transient; infrequent (5%); represents dermal erythropoiesis (156)
Chronic rashes	Generalized; persists for weeks; appears in infancy; virus can be isolated from skin (157,158)
Dermatoglyphic abnormalities	May serve as marker for viral teratogenicity (159)
Miscellaneous abnormalities	Skin dimples; seborrhea; cutis marmorata; patchy pigmentation; circumscribed scleroderma (158,160)
Genitourinary system	Cryptorchidism; testicular agenesis; scrotal calcifications; polycystic kidneys; renal agenesis; renal artery stenosis with hypertension; hypospadias; hydroureter; hydronephrosis; ureteral duplication (161–165)
Skeletal system	
Metaphyseal radiolucencies	Occurs in 10%–20%; most common in distal femur and proximal tibia; usually normalizes by 3 months of age; due to a direct inhibitory effect of rubella virus on bone and cartilage cells (135,166–170)
Large anterior fontanelle	Found in the most severely affected infants (166)
Miscellaneous problems	Micrognathia; pathologic fractures; myositis
Gastrointestinal system	
Hepatosplenomegaly	Common (>50%); transient
Hepatitis	Occurs in 5%–10%; may not be associated with jaundice
Obstructive jaundice	Infrequent (5%)
Miscellaneous problems	Esophageal, jejunal, or rectal atresia; pancreatitis; chronic diarrhea; intraabdominal calcifications (165)

(continued)

TABLE 48-2
(continued)

Clinical Abnormality	Remarks
Blood	
Thrombocytopenic purpura	Occurs in 5%–10%; associated with severe disease; transient (166,171)
Anemia	Transient (171)
Miscellaneous abnormalities	Hemolytic anemia; altered blood group expression (172)
Immune system	
Hypo- or dysgammaglo-bulinemia	Rare; transient (160,173)
Thymic hypoplasia	Rare; fatal
Endocrine glands	Diabetes mellitus; hypothyroidism; hyperthyroidism; thyroiditis; growth hormone deficiency; precocious puberty (8,42,174)

because of its difficulty, expense, and limited availability. Rubella virus RNA can be detected in clinical specimens using PCR, and the results become available sooner than

TABLE 48-3

OUTLINE OF THE CENTERS FOR DISEASE CONTROL AND PREVENTION CRITERIA FOR THE CLASSIFICATION OF CONGENITAL RUBELLA SYNDROME CASES

I. Congenital rubella syndrome confirmed
  Defects present and at least one of the following:
    Isolation of rubella virus
    Detection of rubella-specific IgM antibodies
    Persistence of rubella-specific HI titer beyond the period expected from that of passively transferred maternal antibodies
II. Congenital rubella syndrome compatible
  Incomplete laboratory data for confirmation of diagnosis and any two complications from A or one from A and one from B:
    A. Cataracts or congenital glaucoma, congenital heart disease, hearing loss, pigmentary retinopathy
    B. Purpura, splenomegaly, jaundice, bone radiolucencies, meningoencephalitis, microcephaly, mental retardation
III. Congenital rubella syndrome possible
  Some compatible clinical findings but insufficient criteria for the confirmed or compatible categories
IV. Congenital rubella infection only
  No defects, but laboratory evidence of infection is found
V. Stillbirths
  Stillbirths believed to be a consequence of maternal rubella infection
VI. Congenital rubella syndrome excluded
  At least one of the following inconsistent laboratory findings in a child without evidence of an immunodeficiency disease:
  Absence of rubella-specific HI titer in a child ≤24 months of age
  Absence of rubella-specific HI titer in the mother
  Decrease of rubella-specific HI titer in an infant in a manner consistent with that expected from passively transferred maternal antibodies (i.e., a twofold dilution drop per month)

HI, hemagglutination inhibition.
Adapted from Centers for Disease Control and Prevention. Rubella and congenital rubella syndrome—New York City. *MMWR* 1986;35:770, with permission.

with traditional culture methods; these assays are not widely available (75,82,86).

Rubella-specific IgM usually is present in congenitally infected infants and may persist for 6 to 12 months. It can be used to make a definitive diagnosis of congenital rubella infection; false-positive results may be encountered in sera containing rheumatoid factor. Delays in obtaining serum for IgM measurements can introduce interpretation difficulties because of the possibility that the infant may have acquired rubella infection postnatally. About 20% of infected infants may test negative for rubella-specific IgM at birth but develop detectable titers by a month of age (75,82). Thus, infants suspected of having CRS who test negative for rubella- specific IgM at birth should be re-tested at one month of age. Persistence of rubella-specific IgG antibodies at 6 to 12 months of age, especially in high titers, provides presumptive evidence of congenital or early postnatal infection.

Other techniques for establishing the diagnosis of congenital rubella include negative virus-specific lymphocyte transformation responses in seropositive children younger than 3 years of age, detection of rubella-specific IgM in CSF or saliva, demonstration of low-avidity rubella-specific IgG in seropositive infants, or immunoblotting (58,59,183–186).

Treatment

There is no specific therapy for CRS. A few patients have been treated with amantadine or interferon-α with minimal or no clinical improvement (43,187–189). Intravenous immunoglobulins can be used in infants with hypogamma-globulinemia (160,173). Susceptible pregnant women should avoid contact with CRS patients during their first year of life. The appearance of delayed manifestations of CRS that were not present early in life underscores the importance of close follow-up. CRS patients often require surgical correction of heart or genitourinary defects, removal of dense cataracts, hearing aids, and special schooling. The visual outcome after cataract surgery for infants or children with CRS is generally poor because of the myriad associated ocular abnormalities such as glaucoma, amblyopia, or optic atrophy. In one study, visual acuity after cataract surgery was less than 3/60 in 55% of children with CRS, and 6/24 or better in only 15% (190).

HERPES SIMPLEX VIRUS INFECTIONS

Infections caused by herpes simplex virus (HSV) are common in the United States. Conservative estimates had placed the number of people each year that have their first episode of genital herpes at about 500,000, but recent studies suggest that the actual number is closer to 750,000 to 1,600,000 (191–193). At least 50 million people are living with genital herpes in the United States (194). About 2% of women seroconvert to HSV-2 during pregnancy (195). Neonatal HSV infection occurs in at least 1,500 newborns each year, but other estimates place the minimum number at 2,500 (18,196). It is also estimated that 720,000 cesarean sections are performed annually for the purpose of preventing neonatal herpetic infection (197). The optimal management of women with active or suspected genital HSV infections during pregnancy or at labor continues to generate controversy.

HSV is an enveloped double-stranded deoxyribonucleic acid (DNA) virus that can infect a broad range of hosts. The virus enters the body through mucosal surfaces or abraded skin, and it multiplies in cells of the epidermis or dermis. A number of cellular receptors for HSV have been identified, the most important of which appears to be herpesvirus entry mediator C. Sensory or autonomic nerve endings in the vicinity become infected, and the virus travels intraaxonally in a retrograde fashion to the ganglia. HSV then can continue its multiplication in the ganglia and later spread to other skin and mucous membrane areas through anterograde travel along peripheral sensory nerves, or it can enter a phase of latency in the ganglia. In latently infected ganglia, viral DNA persists as an episome (198). The virus intermittently reactivates and travels to the body surface, in which it can produce clinical disease. Exposure to ultraviolet light, trauma to skin, or immunosuppression can provoke HSV reactivation. Antibody- and cell-mediated immune reactions are generated in response to HSV, both of which are important for control of the infection (191).

The various HSV strains found in the general population can be grouped into two serologic subtypes, HSV-1 and HSV-2. The two subtypes have a high degree of homology but can be differentiated on the basis of their cell culture range, restriction endonuclease analysis, monoclonal antibody-based serologic assays, or polymerase chain reaction (PCR) (198,199).

At least 11 HSV surface glycoproteins (g) have been described (gB, gC, gD, gE, gG, gH, gI, gJ, gK, gL, gM). They mediate attachment and penetration of HSV into cells, play a role in its pathogenesis and spread, and generate host immune responses to the virus (191). Antibodies to the two HSV subtypes cross-react extensively, but two of the glycoproteins (gG and gC) have type-specific antigens and have been found to be helpful in differentiating HSV-1 from HSV-2 antibody responses (200).

Maternal Infection

Epidemiology

Serologic surveys conducted in the United States reveal that the prevalence of antibodies to HSV increases with age, and that it is higher in persons from lower socioeconomic strata and in groups with greater levels of sexual activity. Antibodies to HSV-1 may be present in 90% or more of adults from lower socioeconomic groups but in only about 30% of college students. Antibodies to HSV-2 are present in approximately 21.9% of the United States population 12 years of age or older, and in 27.2% of persons 30 to 49 years of age. African Americans are more likely to have antibodies against HSV-2 than Caucasians or Mexican-Americans (45.9%, 17.6%, and 22.3%, respectively). Among African Americans, women are more likely than men to be seropositive for this virus (55.1% vs. 34.7%, respectively). However, only 2.6% of adults report ever having genital herpes. The seroprevalence of HSV-2 has increased by about 30% during the period from 1988 to 1994 as compared with the years 1976 to 1980 (201). HSV-2 seropositivity is significantly correlated with being female, African American or Hispanic, having a low educational level, income below the poverty line, having ever used cocaine, and the number of lifetime sexual partners (201,202). A 2002 survey of 36 randomly chosen, relatively affluent primary care physician offices surrounding six major United States cities revealed an HSV-2 seroprevalence of 25%; only 12% of seropositive individuals reported a history of genital herpes (203).

Two percent or more of susceptible pregnant women become seropositive for HSV during pregnancy, but only one-third of them will have symptoms consistent with a herpes infection. The risk of transmission from an HSV-seropositive male to a seronegative female is approximately 20% annually. Seroconversion that was completed by the time of onset of labor was not associated with increased neonatal morbidity or cases of congenital herpes infection in one study; however, infants born to mothers who acquired HSV infection shortly before delivery had an almost 50% chance of developing neonatal herpes (195). A study of 35,940 pregnant women in Norway found no association between HSV-2 infection during pregnancy and fetal death (204).

By measuring type-specific antibodies against HSV-2 gG in a group of 190 pregnant women and their husbands, Kulhanjian and colleagues found that 73% of the couples were concordant with respect to their HSV-2 serologies (i.e., both partners were seronegative or seropositive). However, about 9.5% of the pregnant women were seronegative but had seropositive spouses, and therefore they were at risk of gestational primary HSV-2 infection; 56% of these husbands had no history of previous genital

HSV infection. Approximately 5% of pregnant women in this particular study were susceptible to HSV-2 infection but were unaware of their risk of acquiring the virus from their seropositive spouses, who gave no history of prior genital herpes (205).

Asymptomatic shedding of HSV occurs in 0.2% to 7.4% of pregnant women and in 0.2% to 4% of those at or near term. Most HSV infections during pregnancy represent recurrent disease. The frequency of asymptomatic shedding increases as pregnancy advances (10).

Clinical Manifestations

Many primary HSV infections are subclinical. Symptomatic primary HSV disease can include gingivostomatitis, genital herpes, herpetic whitlow, keratitis, chorioretinitis, encephalitis, esophagitis, pneumonia, and hepatitis (10,206).

The most common manifestations of primary HSV-1 infections are gingivostomatitis and pharyngitis, but these occur rarely during pregnancy (207–209). HSV-1 causes from 10% to over 50% of primary genital herpes infections in various populations (192,210). Recurrent episodes of herpes labialis are common, and HSV-1 may be recovered from the pharynx of 1% to 5% of asymptomatic healthy persons (191). One study suggested that the incidence of herpes labialis recurrences was lower during early pregnancy, but that women who did have clinical reactivation had them at higher frequencies than before they became pregnant (211).

The most common clinical illness caused by HSV-2 is genital herpes. Sixty-five percent to 90% of initial HSV-2 infections are subclinical or mild (192). Symptomatic patients can have extensive, painful, vesicular or ulcerative genital lesions with or without associated systemic manifestations (191). Over 75% of patients with symptomatic primary HSV-2 infection will have lesions of the skin and mucous membranes of the genital tract, but another 13% present with cystitis, meningitis, urethritis, or cervicitis (192). Serious complications of HSV infections include pneumonia, hepatitis, disseminated intravascular coagulation, shock, acute retinal necrosis, and encephalitis (191, 212–217). Recent data show that some individuals with no prior history of orolabial or genital herpes and who are seronegative for both HSV-1 and HSV-2 can have T cell responses to HSV suggesting that they may have either undetected infection or acquired immunity to the virus without actual infection (218).

Women with recurrent disease typically have mild or subclinical infections. The likelihood of reactivation of HSV infection is greater for genital than oral–labial disease and for HSV-2 than for HSV-1 (219,220). One-fifth of all patients with primary genital herpes subsequently will have nongenital recurrences; this is most likely to occur on the hands and face for HSV-1 and on the buttocks and legs for HSV-2. Buttock recurrences occur less frequently but last longer than genital lesions (221). Asymptomatic HSV-2 shedding occurs more often during the first 3 months after the primary genital HSV-2 infection than during subsequent periods (220). The overall rate for of cervical or external genital shedding during the first year after primary infection is 1.2% of days for HSV-1 and 4.3% of days for HSV-2 (210). For patients with a documented first episode of genital HSV-2 infection, 90% will have at least one recurrence within a year of diagnosis, 38% will have at least six recurrences, and 20% will have 10 or more recurrences (222). Among women with recurrent genital herpes, 55% of those with HSV-2 and 29% of those with HSV-1 had recurrences during a median follow-up of 105 days in one study (223). HSV-2 shedding (detected by culture) occurred on 2% of all days and usually lasted for 36 hours per recurrence; however, 5.5% of women shed HSV-2 for 4 days or longer. Subclinical shedding is more common in women with frequent symptomatic recurrences (223). When 42 women with no past history of genital herpes, but who were seropositive for HSV-2, were prospectively evaluated with daily swab specimens from their cervicovaginal, vulvar, and perianal areas for about three months, 69% were found to have subclinical shedding of the virus by culture methods at some point; the rate was 80% when a PCR assay was added. Viral shedding was documented on 3% of all days without lesions. For 46 women in the same study who did have a history of genital herpes, the frequency of viral shedding during the follow-up period (symptomatic and asymptomatic) was 91% and they shed the virus on 3.6% of all days with no apparent lesions (224).

Genital herpes infections are categorized according to HSV subtype, serologic evidence of past HSV-1 or HSV-2 infection, and the presence or absence of symptoms. This classification scheme is useful when examining the impact of gestational HSV infection on pregnancy outcome according to the type of maternal genital infection. First episode, primary HSV-1 or HSV-2 infection is considered present if the virus is isolated from the genital tract of a symptomatic or asymptomatic woman who has no serologic evidence of prior infection with HSV-1 or HSV-2 in the acute phase serum, but she subsequently has antibodies to the same HSV subtype when convalescent serum is tested. If the acute-phase serum contains antibodies to the other HSV subtype (e.g., HSV-1 antibodies in a woman with an HSV-2 genital isolate), first episode, nonprimary genital infection is considered present. Recurrent HSV-1 or HSV-2 infection is diagnosed if the patient has antibodies to the same HSV subtype isolated from the genital tract in the acute- and convalescent-phase sera (225). The value of this classification scheme is apparent from a study by Hensleigh and colleagues who evaluated 23 women whose clinical illnesses were consistent with the diagnosis of primary genital herpes. The diagnosis was verified serologically in only one woman with primary HSV-1 infection, whereas three others had nonprimary HSV-2 infection; the remaining 19 women proved to have recurrent disease (226). Wald and her co-investigators found that 62% of HSV-2 seropositive persons with no past history of genital herpes subsequently identified typical herpetic lesions once educated about the infection and its clinical manifestations (224).

Diagnosis

The diagnosis can be made by isolating the virus from tissue cultures of ocular, mucocutaneous, or genital lesions. The best specimen is usually vesicle fluid obtained within 3 days of its appearance. Positive culture results may be obtained within 16 hours to 7 days, depending on the viral load in the clinical specimen. Shell vial cultures may become positive within 16 to 48 hours (227). The enzyme-linked virus-inducible systems (ELVIS tests) have sensitivities comparable to those of standard and shell vial cultures. They are done using genetically-altered cell lines that have a reporter gene β-galactosidase that is driven by the promoter from a specific HSV gene. Once infected by HSV, the cell lines express the reporter gene resulting in a color change (199).

Direct or indirect fluorescent antibody staining, with or without cytospinning, can detect HSV antigens in exfoliated cells within less than two hours. The sensitivity of the direct fluorescent antibody (DFA) stain is higher for specimens from vesicular lesions as compared to healing lesions (199). The Tzanck smear is a rapid and inexpensive method, but it is only 60% sensitive for HSV infections. It involves scraping the base of a fresh vesicle with a scalpel and spreading the cells and debris on a glass slide. The adherent cells are stained with Giemsa, Sedi, or Wright stain. The slide is examined for the presence of virus-induced cytopathic abnormalities, such as multinucleated giant cells, atypical keratinocytes with large nuclei, and ground-glass cytoplasm. A positive Tzanck smear cannot differentiate between VZV and HSV lesions (228).

Serologic methods can be used for the diagnosis of acute HSV infections. Earlier assays did not accurately distinguish HSV-1 from HSV-2 antibodies. Beginning in 1999, type-specific ELISA and immunoblot antibody assays based on gG became available in the United States. The ELISA assay has a sensitivity of 91% to 96% and a specificity of 92% to 95% for HSV-1. For HSV-2, the ELISA assay has a sensitivity of 80% to 98% and a specificity of 96% or higher. The immunoblot assays have higher sensitivities and specifities for HSV-1 and HSV-2 antibodies when compared to ELISA tests. False-negative results can be encountered if testing is done early in the course of an infection. Demonstrating seroconversion is diagnostic of an acute HSV infection. These tests are also useful in distinguishing primary from recurrent infection in pregnant women with their first clinical episodes of genital herpes (194, 199,200). IgM tests based on gG are not commercially available. Western blot assays for HSV antibodies are helpful in patients in which the antibody profiles are not clear for either HSV-1 or HSV-2, but these tests are time-consuming, expensive, and not readily available (199,200).

Molecular biological techniques have been applied for the diagnosis of HSV infection through the detection of viral DNA in clinical specimens (199,228–233). The PCR continues to detect HSV DNA in clinical specimens for several days after the culture becomes negative. The test is relatively rapid and can be completed within a few hours. The yield of PCR in detecting asymptomatic genital shedding is greater when specimens are collected using cervicovaginal lavage instead of a swab (234). The clinical relevance in obstetrical practice of culture-negative, PCR-positive results from genital specimens remains to be elucidated. PCR detection of HSV DNA in CSF specimens helps in the diagnosis of herpes encephalitis (235). Because the PCR technique is sensitive to even minuscule amounts of HSV, contamination from external sources, such as laboratory personnel, physicians, or nurses who may be shedding the virus, can yield false-positive results. The possibility of laboratory contamination is decreased with the use of real-time PCR detection systems (199). Extreme care should be taken while handling the CSF specimen to avoid making an erroneous diagnosis of herpes encephalitis and possibly missing the true culprit (236). False-negative PCR results can occur as a result of problems with the reaction, the presence of inhibitors in the clinical specimens, or because of timing issues such as obtaining the samples too early or too late during the course of the infection (199).

Treatment

Three oral drugs are currently available for the treatment of primary and symptomatic recurrent genital HSV infection: acyclovir, valacyclovir, and famciclovir. The experience with acyclovir is the most extensive, particularly regarding its use in pregnant women.

Acyclovir inhibits the replication of HSV-1, HSV-2, and VZV. Acyclovir is converted in the body to its active triphosphate form, initially through the action of viral thymidine kinase to the monophosphate form and later by cellular enzymes to the diphosphate and triphosphate forms. Acyclovir triphosphate concentrations are 40 to 100 times higher in HSV-infected cells than in uninfected cells. The active form of the drug competes with deoxyguanosine triphosphate as a substrate for viral DNA polymerase and, once incorporated into viral DNA, leads to termination of HSV DNA synthesis (237).

The use of acyclovir during pregnancy is not approved by the Food and Drug Administration and generally is reserved for life-threatening or severe HSV infections such as pneumonia. However, it can be given orally to pregnant women with first episode genital herpes or severe recurrent herpes (194). Maternal antiviral therapy may fail to prevent fetal infection with HSV (238). Acyclovir is teratogenic in rats (239). It crosses the placenta, concentrates in amniotic fluid, and can accumulate in human breast milk (240,241).

A registry of acyclovir use in pregnancy was established on June 1, 1984. As of June 30, 1993, 601 acyclovir-exposed pregnancies from 18 countries had been reported and followed. Of 425 exposures that took place during the first trimester, outcomes included 47 spontaneous fetal losses, 67 legal induced abortions, 298 live births without congenital malformations, and 13 with congenital anomalies. Among 176 second- and third-trimester exposures, three infants were born with anomalies. The reported birth defects were heterogeneous and without a specific pattern.

TABLE 48-4

RECOMMENDED ORAL TREATMENT REGIMENS FOR ADULTS WITH GENITAL HERPES

	Acyclovir	Valacyclovir	Famciclovir
First clinical episode[a]	400 mg three times daily for 7–10 d OR 200 mg orally five times daily for 7–10 d	1 g orally twice a day for 7–10 d	250 mg orally three times a day for 7–10 d
Recurrent infection (HIV-negative)	200 mg orally five times a day for 5 d OR 800 mg orally twice a day for 5 d	1 g orally once a day for 5 d OR 500 mg orally twice a day for 3–5 d	125 mg orally twice a day for 5 d
Recurrent infection (HIV-positive)	200 mg orally five times a day for 5–10 d OR 400 mg orally three times a day for 5–10 d	1 g orally twice a day for 5–10 d	500 mg orally twice a day for 5–10 d
Suppressive therapy (HIV-negative)	400 mg orally twice a day	500 mg orally once a day[b] OR 1 g orally once a day	250 mg orally twice a day
Suppressive therapy (HIV-positive)	400–800 mg orally twice or three times a day	500 mg orally twice a day	500 mg orally twice a day

Abbreviations: d, day; HIV, human immunodeficiency virus.
[a] Treatment can be extended if there is incomplete healing by the tenth day of therapy.
[b] This regimen may be less effective than others for women with 10 or more recurrences per year.
Adapted from Centers for Disease Control and Prevention. Sexually transmitted diseases treatment guidelines 2002. *MMWR* 2002;51(RR-6):1, with permission.

These findings were not different from what was expected for the general population of pregnant women. The size of the cohort in the registry was adequate to detect a teratogenic risk that is twofold higher than expected, but was not large enough to detect smaller increases in risk of birth defects should they exist (242). Similarly, a case-control study performed in Denmark found no association between the use of either systemic or topical acyclovir during pregnancy and adverse outcomes such as congenital malformations, low birth weight, preterm birth, stillbirth, or spontaneous abortion (243).

Acyclovir-resistant HSV strains are uncommon, except in patients with AIDS. The prevailing mechanism of resistance appears to be a mutation that renders the virus deficient in thymidine kinase (237). Infections caused by these acyclovir-resistant HSV strains can be treated with foscarnet, cidofovir, or vidarabine; none is approved by the Food and Drug Administration for use during pregnancy (198,244,245). Foscarnet is an organic analogue of inorganic pyrophosphate and does not require activation by kinases, including thymidine kinase. It has to be administered intravenously and the drug is associated with serious adverse effects such as nephrotoxicity, anemia, and seizures. Foscarnet-resistant HSV strains have been reported (198). Cidofovir is a nucleotide analogue whose main use has been in the treatment of cytomegalovirus retinitis. This drug is active against HSV, including thymidine-kinase deficient strains, but is also nephrotoxic.

Valacyclovir and famciclovir are active against HSV and have been approved for the management of genital herpes in nonpregnant adults. Valacyclovir is the L-valyl ester of acyclovir; it is rapidly absorbed and hydrolyzed in the body to acyclovir and results in much greater bioavailability of the active drug (198,246,247). Famciclovir is a guanosine analogue of the antiviral drug penciclovir (248). Penciclovir, like acyclovir, is phosphorylated to its active metabolite penciclovir triphosphate (198). Acyclovir-resistant HSV mutants usually are resistant to these two drugs as well, although penciclovir may be active against some of these strains (244). Both drugs are classified by the Food and Drug Administration as being in pregnancy category B.

The recommended dosage regimens for the management of genital herpes are summarized in Table 48-4. For severe genital herpes or its extragenital complications (e.g., pneumonia, encephalitis), intravenous acyclovir at a dose of 5 to 10 mg/kg of body weight should be infused every eight hours for 2 to 7 days or until clinical improvement is evident, followed by oral therapy for a total of at least 10 days of antiviral chemotherapy (194). About 70% to 80% of patients with recurrent genital herpes using acyclovir, valacyclovir, or famciclovir for suppressive therapy are recurrence-free after four months. There is also an 80% to 90% reduction in the number of days with subclinical HSV shedding (222). A recent study using different dosage regimens of famciclovir found that the drug reduced both symptomatic and asymptomatic anogenital HSV shedding, and it also delayed the onset of asymptomatic viral shedding in women with frequently recurring genital herpes (249).

Fetal and Neonatal Infection

Epidemiology

Most neonatal HSV infections are acquired during passage through an infected birth canal. Transplacental spread occurs occasionally, with major deleterious fetal effects. About 40% of newborns with herpes are delivered before week 36 of pregnancy (10).

Intrapartum transmission is more likely to occur with primary maternal HSV genital infection. Other risk factors for HSV acquisition by the infant are cervical HSV infection, multiple genital lesions, prematurity, prolonged rupture of maternal membranes, intrauterine instrumentation (e.g., scalp electrodes), and absent or low titers of transplacentally acquired neutralizing HSV antibodies. The risk of vertical transmission is about 33% to 50% for mothers with late term primary herpes and about 1% to 3% for those with recurrent infections (10,18). Postpartum HSV spread to newborns occurs infrequently (191).

The perception at medical centers caring for infants with neonatal HSV infection is that the incidence of the disease is increasing. Data from Seattle had shown a 10-fold increase in the incidence of neonatal HSV infection between 1966 and 1982 (18). However, data for the State of California showed no change in the number of infants (1 to 42 days of age) per 100,000 live births that were discharged from the hospital with a diagnosis of neonatal HSV infection between 1985 and 1995 (250).

Clinical Manifestations

Asymptomatic HSV infections are rare in the newborn. Disease manifestations may be localized or widely disseminated. About 70% to 85% of infants with HSV infections are born to women who are asymptomatic at the time of delivery and who have no history of genital herpes (18). Infants born to asymptomatic women shedding HSV in early labor are ten times more likely to develop neonatal HSV infection if the mother had recently experienced a first episode genital herpes than neonates born to women whose HSV shedding is secondary to reactivated infection (251).

Intrauterine HSV infection is uncommon and accounts for about 5% of all neonatal herpes cases (252–254). Its hallmarks are a vesicular rash that is present at birth or appears shortly thereafter. Associated abnormalities include microcephaly (60%), chorioretinitis (40%–50%), and microphthalmia (25%). The rash is more likely to be generalized than localized. Other skin lesions include bullae and cutaneous scars in 10% to 15% of patients. The intracranial calcifications seen in 15% may be present at birth or evolve later in infancy. Lesions indicative of brain damage, such as hydranencephaly, cerebral necrosis, and brain atrophy, can be seen on computed tomographic (CT) scans or magnetic resonance imaging (MRI) of the head. Other findings can include radiographic bone lucencies, intrauterine growth retardation, limb hypoplasia, aplasia cutis, cutaneous pigmentary abnormalities, skin ulceration, hepatosplenomegaly, optic atrophy, retinal dysplasia, persistent intraocular fetal vasculature, cloudy corneas, and cataracts. About 30% have seizures during the neonatal period. The mortality rate is 40%, and about one-half of the survivors have significant long-term residual problems, such as psychomotor retardation, seizure disorders, spasticity, blindness, or deafness (253–259). Most cases are caused by HSV-2.

The National Institute of Allergy and Infectious Diseases Collaborative Antiviral Study Group (NIAID CASG) reported their experience with 186 acyclovir-treated newborns with HSV infection enrolled between 1981 and 1997. Neonates with HSV were often born at or before 37 weeks of gestation (35%) and had fetal scalp electrodes placed (40%). Their mothers tended to be young (mean age, 22 years) and to have one or no previous children (65%). Their mean birth weight was 2.95 kg, 69% were white, and 52% were boys (260).

About 10% of infants with neonatal HSV infection became sick within the first day of life, and about 30% are ill by the fifth day of life. Because of the nonspecific nature of the initial symptoms, the average time from disease onset to diagnosis is 5 to 7 days. Despite heightened awareness and physician concerns about neonatal herpes infections, the interval from onset of disease symptoms to initiation of antiviral therapy did not become shorter between 1981 and 1997 (260). Thus, a high index of suspicion is needed so that HSV-infected infants can be identified and treated earlier to reduce the risk of progression to more serious disease manifestations. The signs and symptoms of 186 neonates with HSV infection at diagnosis and initiation of therapy are depicted in Fig. 48-1.

Infections resulting from the intrapartum acquisition of HSV may not manifest until about 10 to 12 days of age, with disease localized to the skin, eyes, or mouth (10,260). Cutaneous lesions include discrete vesicles, grouped vesicles, large bullae, or denuded skin (Fig. 48-2). New vesicles typically continue to appear early into therapy. Ulcerative mouth lesions without skin disease may sometimes occur. Eye disease includes keratoconjunctivitis and chorioretinitis. Recurrent mucocutaneous herpes develops in some of these infants. Neurologic abnormalities eventually develop in 25% of infants with recurrent mucocutaneous herpes, even though CNS involvement may not have been evident during the acute illness.

A second group of infants presents at 15 to 19 days of age with localized CNS involvement, with or without skin, mouth, or ocular lesions. Fever may be seen in 44% of infants and, on occasion, it is the sole presenting sign (260,261). Hypothermia in a neonate with irritability, hypotonia, lethargy, apnea, or other neurologic signs and symptoms should raise concerns about HSV CNS disease (262). Skin lesions may be absent in a third of these neonates. The mortality rate is 15% for newborns with HSV-2 CNS disease, and almost none for those with HSV-1 infection. Prematurity and seizures at initiation of therapy are potential risk factors for death. Only 30% of survivors have normal development at one year of age, and this is somewhat worse for infants with HSV-2 infection (260).

A third group presents at 9 to 11 days of age with disseminated disease. CNS involvement is found in about two-thirds of these infants. Other organs that are severely affected are the adrenal glands, gastrointestinal tract, liver, heart, pancreas, and kidneys. Without appropriate therapy, about 80% die. With acyclovir therapy, the mortality rate is about 55%, and about 25% of survivors have severe neurologic impairments (260).

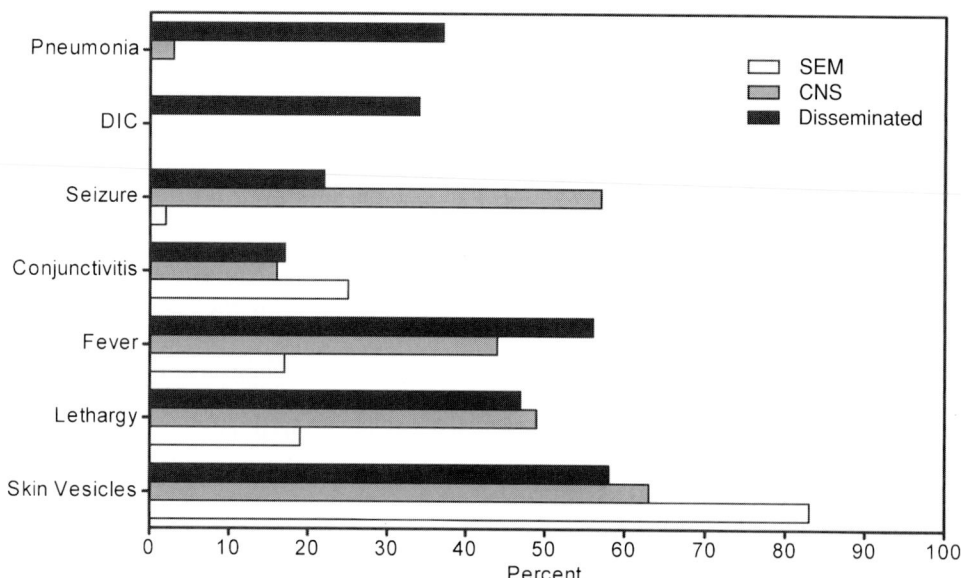

Figure 48-1 Signs and symptoms of neonatal herpes simplex virus infection at diagnosis and initiation of therapy. Abbreviations: SEM, skin, eyes, or mouth; CNS, central nervous system; DIC, disseminated intravacular coagulopathy. Adapted from Kimberlin DW, Lin C-Y, Jacobs RF, et al. Natural history of neonatal herpes simplex virus infections in the acyclovir era. *Pediatrics* 2001;108:223, with permission.

In an earlier trial comparing vidarabine with acyclovir, the NIAID CASG studied 202 infants younger than 1 month of age with HSV infection (263–265). About 4% of infants had congenital HSV infection, and 40% had disease confined to the skin, eyes, or mouth. CNS disease occurred in 34%, and 22% had disseminated infections. Two-thirds of the isolates were HSV-2. In contrast, HSV-1 is the predominant isolate in countries such as the Netherlands where this viral type accounts for 73% of all cases of neonatal herpes (266).

The clinical manifestations of herpes encephalitis in the newborn includes focal or generalized seizures,

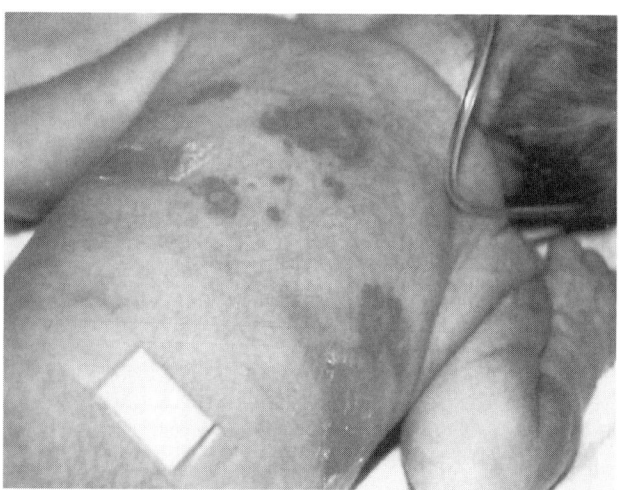

Figure 48-2 Localized cutaneous herpes simplex virus type 2 infection in a neonate. Notice the coalescing vesicular lesions on the back and right arm. The vesicles are surrounded by an erythematous border.

lethargy, hypothermia, apnea, opsoclonus, and pyramidal tract signs (262,267,268). Eventual loss of gag and suck reflexes is common. Skin vesicles may be absent in about 30% to 40% of infants. CSF analysis reveals mononuclear pleocytosis, elevated protein concentrations (as high as 1,000 mg/dL), and either normal or slightly decreased glucose levels (267). Rarely, the CSF may show a predominance of neutrophils or be completely normal (269). Focal or generalized electroencephalographic abnormalities are common (260,267,270). About 8% of surviving infants have CNS relapse within 1 month of completing therapy (263). As many as 40% of infants will have a local skin or CNS relapse within two months of stopping therapy, and this risk is higher for newborns with HSV-2 infection (271).

Ocular herpetic infection may be an isolated problem, but it is more likely to occur in infants with CNS disease. Eye abnormalities include keratitis, conjunctivitis, chorioretinitis, necrotizing retinitis, optic atrophy, and cataracts. Long-term follow-up studies of survivors of neonatal HSV infection indicate that 40% (94% in patients with neurologic impairment; 20% in patients who are neurologically normal) have persistent abnormalities, such as cataracts, corneal scars, optic atrophy, and chorioretinal scars. About 44% have disturbed oculomotor control (272,273).

HSV pneumonia usually presents between days 3 and 14 of life with gradually worsening respiratory distress (274–277). Chest roentgenograms reveal perihilar infiltrates that gradually progress into severe diffuse interstitial and alveolar disease (i.e., "white-out" lungs) (278). Other findings include thrombocytopenia, neutropenia, jaundice, and hyperammonemia (279). The mortality rate of neonatal HSV pneumonia is about 80%, and almost 100% if infants have disseminated intravascular coagulopathy (264).

Diagnosis

Neonatal HSV infections are best diagnosed by isolating the virus from a vesicular lesion. The virus can be recovered from 25% to 40% of CSF specimens obtained from infants with CNS disease. Cultures of urine, feces, blood, nasopharyngeal secretions, and conjunctivae may yield the virus in some patients. Collection of duodenal aspirates may help in the diagnosis of HSV-related hepatitis and necrotizing colitis. Serology is not useful in neonatal HSV infections because of the presence of transplacentally-acquired maternal HSV IgG antibodies. DFA staining of scrapings from the base of fresh vesicles may reveal HSV antigens (254,280,281).

PCR assays for the detection of HSV DNA are valuable diagnostic tools and have become the gold standard for the diagnosis of HSV encephalitis, despite interlaboratory variabilities in assay performance (265,282). In the NIAID CASG trials, HSV DNA was detected in the CSF of 26 (76%) of 34 infants with CNS disease, in 13 (93%) of 14 infants with disseminated infection, and in 7 (24%) of 29 infants with disease seemingly limited to the skin, eyes, or mouth. One of seven PCR-positive patients with disease limited to the skin, eyes, or mouth later developed severe neurologic impairment (283). PCR assays can detect HSV in serum in as many as two thirds of infected patients, including some whose CSF PCR is negative (284). PCR assays on serum and CSF may remain positive for 1 to 2 weeks after starting antiviral therapy (285).

Viral load measurements using a real-time PCR assay has been described for infants with HSV infection. Neonates with disseminated disease had the highest viral loads in their sera and lower levels in their CSF. Newborns with CNS disease had higher viral loads in the CSF than in the serum. Infants who die from their infection have significantly higher viral loads in serum and CSF than those who survive. In one study, CSF viral load did not differ significantly in surviving infants with or without long-term neurologic impairment (286).

Treatment

Antiviral therapy with acyclovir or vidarabine is the mainstay of treatment. In earlier NIAID CASG reports, infants treated with acyclovir (30 mg/kg per day for 10 days) or vidarabine had comparable morbidity and mortality rates (263). No deaths occurred among 85 infants with localized skin, eyes, or mouth disease; about 94% seemed developmentally normal after 1 year. The mortality rates for the encephalitis and the disseminated HSV groups were 14% and 54%, respectively, and 40% to 70% of the survivors were neurologically impaired. Factors influencing mortality included level of consciousness at the start of treatment, prematurity, disease classification, pneumonia, and disseminated intravascular coagulopathy (264). Cutaneous HSV recurrences occurred in 46% of survivors by 6 months after the end of therapy, and the rates were similar for infants treated with acyclovir or vidarabine. Seventy-five percent of survivors with disease caused by HSV-2 were impaired compared with 27% of infants with HSV-1 infection. This is explained partially by the greater *in vitro* susceptibility of HSV-1 to acyclovir (237).

Because of the considerable mortality and long-term neurologic morbidity associated with disseminated or localized CNS HSV disease despite acyclovir therapy, the NIAID CASG studied the impact of higher acyclovir doses on the outcome of these infections. Seventy-two neonates studied between 1990 and 1997 received 60 mg/kg per day of acyclovir for 21 days; 50% had disseminated disease and 35% had localized CNS infections. Acyclovir-induced neutropenia developed in 20% of infants.

The 24-month mortality rate for disseminated disease was 31%, and this beneficial effect was most pronounced for newborns with aspartate aminotransferase (AST) elevations 10 or more times the upper limit of normal. At one year of follow-up, 83% of survivors were developing normally (287).

The 24-month mortality rate for CNS disease was 6%, but this was not statistically different than the outcome of infants who had received the lower acyclovir dose (30 mg/kg per day for 10 days only). Only 30% of infants were developing normally at one year of age, and this was also not statistically different for the infants receiving the higher or lower acyclovir dosage regimens. However, when adjustments were made for the virus type, prematurity, and seizures, there appeared to be 6.6-fold increased likelihood of normal development at one year in infants receiving the higher acyclovir dose (287). HSV has been shown to cause direct injury to neurons leading to apoptotic neuronal death, which may partially explain the frequent development of long-term neurologic dysfunction (288).

Infants receiving acyclovir shed lower virus titers than those on vidarabine. Given its ease of administration compared with vidarabine, its fairly benign toxicity profile, and its efficacy against HSV, intravenous acyclovir (60 mg/kg per day divided in three daily doses) has become the standard regimen for suspected or proven neonatal HSV infections. The duration of therapy is 14 days if the disease is limited to skin, eye, and mouth, and 21 days for disseminated or localized CNS HSV infections. The use of chemical mediators such as bradykinin analogs to increase the permeability of the blood–brain barrier can augment the uptake of acyclovir by two- to three-fold and lower the viral titers in the brains of experimental animals, and this may eventually enhance the efficacy of treatment for neonatal CNS HSV infections (289).

Dosage reductions are needed for infants with renal or hepatic dysfunction (290). The dose of acyclovir should be lowered in infants with reduced creatinine clearance. For serum creatinine levels of 0.8 to 1.1 mg/dL, acyclovir should be administered at a dose of 20 mg/kg every 12 hours. For infants with serum creatinine levels of 1.2 to 1.5 mg/dL, the dose is reduced to 20 mg/kg every 24 hours, and for newborns with creatinine concentrations greater than 1.5 mg/dL or have a urine output less than 1 mL/kg per hour, the dose is lowered to 10 mg/kg every 24 hours (287).

Neonatal infections caused by acyclovir-resistant HSV strains have been encountered, but are very rare (291). Acyclovir resistance in HSV is principally as a result of a mutation that leads to viral thymidine kinase deficiency. Another recognized, but less common, mechanism of resistance is the production by the virus of a thymidine kinase with decreased ability to phosphorylate acyclovir. A third mechanism of resistance is a mutation within the viral gene encoding DNA polymerase. Acyclovir triphosphate is formed but is unable to block viral transcription because of poor affinity for the viral DNA polymerase (292,293).

Topical antiviral agents, such as the ophthalmic preparations of 1% to 2% trifluorothymidine, 3% vidarabine, or 0.1% iododeoxyuridine, should be used in newborns with ocular involvement, in addition to parenteral acyclovir. The use of commercial intravenous γ-globulin preparations for HSV postexposure prophylaxis or treatment of neonates is not recommended, although evidence gleaned from animal studies suggests that the administration of monoclonal or polyclonal neutralizing antibodies given as late as 3 days after HSV infection can decrease mortality and morbidity (294,295).

Seizure control, fluid and electrolyte management, ventilatory support, and treatment of shock and disseminated intravascular coagulation is required for many HSV-infected neonates (292). Contact precautions are needed if mucocutaneous lesions are present (296).

Neuroimaging studies are often utilized in the care of infants with HSV encephalitis, and approximately 65% show abnormalities (260). Ultrasound of the head early in the course of illness may be normal or show areas of increased echogenicity (297). Initial head CT scans may be abnormal in as many as half of newborns with HSV CNS disease. Involved areas of the brain may be hypointense (T1-weighted sequences) or hyperintense (T2-weighted sequences) using MR imaging. Abnormal signal intensities can reflect edema, infarction, or calcifications. In contrast to older children and adults, involvement of the medial temporal or inferior frontal lobes is uncommon (298). Diffusion-weighted imaging appears to be more sensitive than conventional MRI early in the course of HSV encephalitis (299).

A repeat lumbar puncture at the end of 21 days of acyclovir therapy has been recommended by some investigators. If the CSF HSV PCR were still positive, then intravenous acyclovir would be continued until the test becomes negative (254). Whether this approach alters long-term outcome for these infants is unknown.

Given the frequency of cutaneous or CNS recurrences after completion of antiviral therapy, some investigators have tried using oral acyclovir for posttreatment prophylaxis (300,301). The NIAID CASG conducted a phase I/II trial of oral acyclovir prophylactic therapy at a dose of 300 mg/m^2/dose given two or three times daily for 6 months to newborns recovering from HSV-2 infections limited to the skin, eyes, or mouth. Of 16 infants taking the thrice daily acyclovir regimen, 13 (81%) had no recurrences over the

ensuing 6 months. This compared favorably with the 54% rate observed for historic control patients. The number of infants on the twice daily regimen was too small to permit any meaningful conclusions on its effectiveness as prophylaxis. Although acyclovir suppressive therapy appears able to limit cutaneous recurrences, its effectiveness in improving neurologic outcome for these infants is not known. Half the infants became neutropenic (absolute neutrophil counts less than 1,000 cells/μL) while on acyclovir therapy. One infant had an acyclovir-resistant HSV-2 mutant isolated from a skin recurrence that occurred 36 hours after the conclusion of the 6-month suppressive regimen (301). Given the current limitations of available data, it cannot yet be recommended that neonates with HSV infection be routinely placed on oral acyclovir suppressive regimens after completion of their intravenous therapy (302).

Prevention

Because of the enormous morbidity and mortality rates of neonatal HSV infections despite the early initiation of antiviral therapy, the focus of many research groups has been the development of effective prevention strategies. In a detailed decision analysis study, Libman and colleagues used published data to theoretically evaluate nine different obstetric approaches for the prevention of neonatal HSV disease. The investigators concluded that, given the state of technology, physical examination at the time of labor was the most reasonable strategy. This tactic would be expected to reduce the number of neonatal HSV cases by 36% although increasing the rate of cesarean sections by only 3%. The strategy of obtaining genital HSV cultures at weekly intervals from women with a history of recurrent genital herpes and then delivering by cesarean section those whose most recent culture results were positive by onset of labor would result in 547 additional cesarean sections performed to prevent less than one case of neonatal HSV infection (rates per 100,000 deliveries) (303).

Studies on women with histories of recurrent genital herpes have demonstrated that weekly antepartum cultures fail to predict the risks to their infants of HSV exposure at delivery and that most infants exposed to asymptomatic HSV shedding at delivery are born to women without a history of recurrent genital herpes infection (304,305). Garland and co-workers showed that the positive predictive value of a positive antepartum HSV culture for intrapartum viral shedding is only 59% when the interval between visits was two days or less, and dropped to 19% when the days between visits was more than two days (306). Similarly, the practice of screening pregnant women for the presence of type-specific HSV antibodies in an effort to prevent neonatal infection is not recommended (307,308).

Roberts and colleagues were able to reduce the HSV-related cesarean section rate at their institution by 37% (without adverse neonatal consequences) by questioning women in labor about prodromal symptoms of genital HSV infection followed by careful visual inspection of the lower genital tract. Previously, the strategy at their institution had incorporated the use of weekly HSV cultures beginning at 34 weeks of gestation and delivering by cesarean section those whose last genital cultures were positive or unavailable (309).

Cesarean section should be performed on women with signs and symptoms suggesting genital HSV infection at the onset of labor. It is not known whether cesarean delivery can reduce the risk of neonatal herpes when the membranes have been ruptured for longer than 4 to 6 hours, but the American College of Obstetricians and Gynecologists recommends the procedure for women in labor with active HSV genital lesions, irrespective of the duration of premature rupture of membranes (296,310). In a study of 202 women from whom HSV was isolated at time of labor, cesarean delivery reduced the HSV transmission rate by about 85% (311). The same study showed that the risk of transmission of HSV to newborns was increased for first-episode maternal genital infection, for women with no HSV antibodies, when HSV was isolated from the cervix rather from only the vulva, for HSV-1 viral type, when delivery occurred before 38 weeks of gestation, or when invasive monitoring was done (311). Vacuum extraction techniques causing scalp laceration increase the risk of neonatal HSV infection for women who are shedding the virus asymptomatically at delivery (312).

Contact precautions are needed for infants delivered through an infected birth canal, and those delivered by cesarean sections to mothers with herpetic genital lesions (296). The risk of invasive HSV infection is small for infants delivered vaginally to women with recurrent genital herpes who are asymptomatic but shedding the virus at the time of labor (310,313). Cultures of urine, stools, and mucous membranes (e.g., rectum, eyes, mouth, nasopharynx) should be obtained at 24 to 48 hours of life. Earlier positive cultures may reflect transient contamination and not true infection. If the cultures are positive for HSV, antiviral therapy should be started, even if the infant is asymptomatic. Infants who are symptomatic at birth (e.g., scalp lesions, symptoms suggestive of sepsis) should be treated with acyclovir after specimens for HSV culture and PCR (including CSF and blood buffy coat) are obtained. Animal data suggest that acyclovir therapy concomitant with HSV inoculation could inhibit acute viral replication and decrease the number of neurons with latent infection (314).

A number of studies have assessed the potential benefits of suppressive acyclovir therapy for pregnant women with recurrent genital herpes. Various acyclovir doses were tried and started at 36 weeks of gestation. The results of these trials were not in complete agreement, but all showed decreases in viral shedding and clinical recurrences, and a probable decline in the cesarean section rates for these women (315–317). A study of once daily valacyclovir in late pregnancy did not demonstrate any improvements at delivery for any of these parameters (317). Despite the lack of data on whether suppressive therapy in late pregnancy reduces the rate of vertical-fetal HSV transmission, the American College of Obstetricians and Gynecologists has

suggested that antiviral therapy be considered for women at or beyond 36 weeks of gestation who have either a first-episode of genital herpes infection during the pregnancy or are at risk for recurrent HSV (310). For women who are seronegative for HSV-2 but whose sexual partners have recurrent genital herpes, education regarding safer sexual practices and use by the male partner of valacyclovir (500 mg once daily) can reduce the likelihood of infection by approximately 45% (318,319).

The detection of HSV DNA by PCR assays in the amniotic fluid of pregnant women with symptomatic genital HSV may not reflect intrauterine infection (320). Thus, pregnancy termination without other indicators of disease such as an abnormal fetal ultrasound would be unwarranted.

Numerous HSV candidate vaccines (e.g., subunit vaccines, DNA vaccines) are currently at various stages of development. None are available commercially (196,321).

CYTOMEGALOVIRUS INFECTIONS

CMV is the most common congenital viral infection of humans in the United States and is one of the most important opportunistic pathogens causing serious illness and death in immunocompromised patients (322–324). CMV infections are benign for most adults. However, when CMV infection occurs during pregnancy, the virus can be transmitted to the fetus and result in either symptomatic neonatal disease or subclinical congenital infection that may later manifest with hearing loss or learning disabilities.

CMV is an enveloped, double-stranded DNA virus that belongs to the herpes family of viruses (323). It has a restricted host range and only human cells are productively infected by this virus (325). CMV is not eradicated after resolution of the primary infection. It persists in the body in a low-grade chronic infection form or in a latent state with periodic reactivations (325). CMV transmission occurs primarily by direct or indirect person-to-person spread of infected oropharyngeal secretions, sexual intercourse, blood transfusions, or transplacental spread from mother to fetus.

Maternal Infection

Serologic surveys in the United States and Great Britain have shown that antibodies to CMV can be found in the sera of 40% to 60% of adults of middle or upper socioeconomic status, and in as many as 80% of those in lower socioeconomic groups (326). CMV seroprevalence is as high as 90% to 100% in pregnant women from Brazil, Chile, Korea, Japan, and the Ivory Coast (322,327). The higher the prevalence of maternal CMV antibody in a population, the greater is the rate of congenital CMV infection (326). Factors correlating with CMV seropositivity in pregnant women in the United States include non-Caucasian race, unmarried status, lower educational and income levels, and increasing parity (328,329). Sexual activity is an important risk factor for CMV infection in adolescents and young adults, and coinfection with bacterial vaginosis, trichomoniasis, gonorrhea, or other pathogenic organisms increases the odds of intrauterine CMV transmission (330–334).

Intrafamilial CMV transmission from young children to their seronegative pregnant mothers can occur. The risk of CMV seroconversion for a seronegative mother with an infected child is estimated at 10% to 30% per year and is even higher if the child is younger than 20 months of age (326,335). Annual seroconversion rates for seronegative day care providers is about 8% to 12% (336,337). Health care workers with CMV-infected patient contact do not appear to be at increased risk of CMV acquisition compared with persons without patient contact (338).

About 0.7% to 4.1% of susceptible women acquire primary CMV infection during pregnancy, a risk comparable to that of nonpregnant women (322). Seropositive women can reactivate their latent CMV infection during pregnancy or, less commonly, become reinfected by an exogenous CMV strain. Cervical and urinary CMV excretion increases as pregnancy advances from the first to the third trimester (339). Pregnant women may shed CMV from the cervix, urinary tract, throat, and breast milk in the postpartum period (10).

Primary and recurrent maternal CMV infection can result in transmission of the virus to the fetus. This occurs in about 40% (range 24% to 75%) of pregnancies complicated by primary CMV infection (338). The presence of maternal antibodies to CMV in women with recurrent infection does not prevent viral transmission to the fetus, but it does reduce the risk of fetal infection and protects against major fetal damage by CMV (340,341). Severe congenital CMV after maternal reactivation or reinfection by other strains can occur, but is infrequent (342–350). For women who seroconvert between deliveries of successive infants, the risk of transmission of CMV to their offspring is 25%, 10%, and 4.2% when the interval is 24 months or shorter, 25 to 48 months, and more than 48 months, respectively (351).

Most women (90%) with primary CMV infection are asymptomatic, and the rest usually have illnesses resembling infectious mononucleosis (352). In a series of 102 pregnant women with primary cytomegalovirus infection referred to a tertiary care center in Rome, Italy, common symptoms noted were fever (42%), weakness (31%), myalgias (21%), and influenza-like illness (24%). Relative lymphocytosis of 40% or higher was found in 39%, and mild elevations in at least one aminotransferase level was measured in a third of the women (353). Other manifestations are rare but include interstitial pneumonia, myocarditis, aseptic meningitis, encephalopathy, retinitis, hepatitis, colitis, thrombocytopenia, and hemolytic anemia (354,355). Primary CMV infection during the first trimester of pregnancy does not cause fetal loss (356).

Infection can be documented by isolating the virus from urine, saliva, buffy coat, or cervical secretions (357). Viral isolation, however, does not differentiate between primary and recurrent CMV infections. Measurement of CMV-specific IgM antibodies is useful for the diagnosis of pri-

mary infection, but this antibody can persist in serum for 4 to 8 months (358). Furthermore, CMV-specific IgM can appear after primary and reactivated infection (357). CMV-specific IgG antibody levels are helpful if seroconversion or a fourfold titer rise can be demonstrated. The IFA and ELISA are the most practical and reliable methods for detecting CMV antibodies. CMV-specific IgG avidity is low (mean 30%) when measured within the first 14 weeks after seroconversion, and it increases over time (mean 88% for patients with remote infections). This assay may be helpful in the diagnosis of primary CMV infection during pregnancy and may even be able to identify women who would deliver a CMV-infected infant (359,360). Rapid diagnosis of CMV infection is possible using antigen assays or molecular biological techniques such as the PCR (357). One needs to be aware that interlaboratory variability exists in the results of CMV PCR assays, especially for specimens containing lesser quantities of viral DNA (361). In a cohort of asymptomatic adolescents with primary CMV infection, CMV DNA was detected in buffy coat samples by PCR in 75% to 80% within 16 weeks of infection, and this declined to 0% to 25% after 48 weeks; lower recovery rates were noted in plasma specimens (362). Quantitation of CMV DNA in buffy coat, plasma, or serum is available, but this is mostly utilized in the management of immunosuppressed and organ transplant patients (357,363).

Several drugs are currently available for the treatment of CMV infection in the immunocompromised host, but they are almost never used in pregnant women (364–366). The drugs have a number of associated problems such as toxic side effects, poor oral bioavailability, and potential for emergence of drug-resistant virus strains (365). Ganciclovir, an acyclic nucleoside analogue of acyclovir, has excellent inhibitory activity against CMV (367). As with acyclovir, ganciclovir has to be phosphorylated initially by a viral enzyme. It is then eventually converted to the triphosphate form by cellular enzymes. Ganciclovir concentrations are at least ten-fold higher in CMV-infected cells than in uninfected cells (367). Ganciclovir is both mutagenic and teratogenic in pregnant experimental animals. The drug crosses the placenta into the fetal compartment passively without being metabolized (368,369). Valganciclovir is a prodrug of ganciclovir that is given orally (364). Foscarnet (phosphonoformate), another anti-CMV drug, inhibits the DNA polymerase of CMV. Like ganciclovir, foscarnet is used only in the immunosuppressed patient with CMV disease (367). Cidofovir is a nucleotide analogue that inhibits viral DNA polymerase. It has a long intracellular half-life, which allows its administration to adults once every 1 to 2 weeks. It is active against ganciclovir- or foscarnet-resistant CMV isolates. Its use currently is limited to immunocompromised adults, especially those with CMV retinitis (367,370).

Congenital Infection

Congenital infection with CMV occurs in 0.4% to 2.3% of all live births (326). About 10% are symptomatic, and the rest have subclinical infections. It is thought that CMV in women with primary infection is transmitted to the fetus via maternal leukocyte-associated viremia and infection of uterine endothelial cells, with subsequent hematogenous spread to the fetus. Local reactivation of CMV-infected macrophages can lead to infection of placental villi and retrograde spread to the fetus in CMV-seropositive mothers (371). In one study, 30% of placentas from CMV-seropositive women had CMV DNA and this was localized mostly to the villi (372).

Infants with symptomatic congenital CMV have a mortality rate of 15% to 30%, and most survivors have long-term sequelae (10,373–376). Petechiae, jaundice, and hepatosplenomegaly are found in two-thirds of patients, although conjugated hyperbilirubinemia and thrombocytopenia are found in about 80% of cases (340,373). Neurologic abnormalities such as seizures and hypotonia are common, and microcephaly occurs in about 50% to 75% of infants. Intracranial calcifications are seen on the CT scans of one-half of the patients (Fig. 48-3). At autopsy, evidence of multiorgan involvement is apparent (373, 377). Neuropathologic findings include periventricular necrosis, intraventricular hemorrhage, calcifications, cerebellar hypoplasia, periventricular leukomalacia, hydrocephalus, and porencephalic cyst (376,378,379). Hearing loss and neurologic impairment (e.g., psychomotor and mental retardation) develop in one-half of the survivors

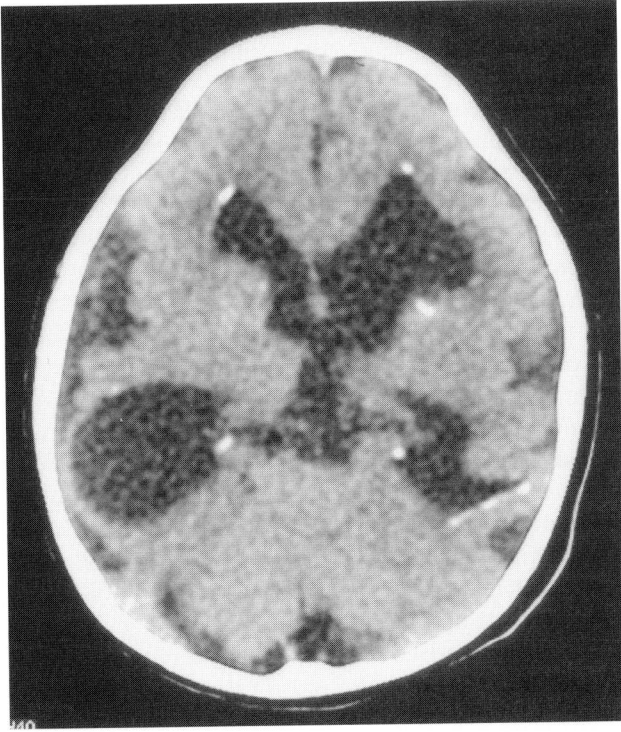

Figure 48-3 Computerized axial tomogram of a microcephalic 3-month-old boy with symptomatic congenital CMV following primary maternal gestational CMV infection. Shown are subepindymal periventricular calcifications, enlarged ventricles and CSF spaces, and loss of periventricular and subcortical white matter volume.

(374,375). Infants whose cranial CT scans are abnormal at birth have a 90% risk of developing at least one long-term sequela such as mental or psychomotor retardation, seizures, cerebral palsy, or hearing loss. In contrast, only 29% of infants with symptomatic congenital CMV infection and normal cranial CT scans at birth have similar long-term residual problems (380).

Chorioretinitis is the most frequent eye abnormality, followed by optic atrophy (10). The chorioretinitis is typically seen in infants with symptomatic congenital CMV, but it can occasionally be the only manifestation of infection. It can also develop several weeks after birth (381,382). Spontaneous resolution of the retinitis has been reported (383). Visual impairment in infants with symptomatic congenital CMV may be as a result of optic atrophy, chorioretinal scars, or damage to the visual cortex (381). Microphthalmia, cloudy cornea, corneal opacities, optic nerve hypoplasia, optic nerve coloboma, nystagmus, strabismus, anophthalmia, and cyclopia also occur. Eye abnormalities are common in infants with intracranial calcifications (10,381,382).

Unilateral or bilateral sensorineural hearing loss that can vary from mild to profound develops in as many as half of infants with symptoms at birth, and in 7% to 13% of those with subclinical infections. Hearing loss may be present at birth in otherwise asymptomatic infants, and it subsequently deteriorates in more than one-half of the patients with a median age at first progression of 18 months (range 2–70) (384–386). In one study, the presence of petechiae or intrauterine growth retardation were predictive of the development of hearing loss; microcephaly and other neurologic abnormalities were not (387). Some patients have normal hearing for the first several years of life, but they subsequently develop sudden or fluctuating hearing loss (385,388). CMV has been shown to be responsible for a substantial percentage of sensorineural hearing loss cases in children. In a study from Italy of 130 children with hearing loss of more than 40 dB, CMV was the culprit for 10% of those detected within the first two months of life, 34% of children with deafness of unidentified cause, and 42% of those with hearing loss more than 70 dB (389).

Intellectual deficits are common, particularly in infants with symptomatic congenital CMV. Microcephaly and an abnormal CT scan are respectively the most specific and sensitive predictors of mental retardation and major motor deficits (390). Some infants with subclinical disease may develop mental or behavioral problems, but a few recent studies have shown no differences in intelligence quotients or neuropsychological test results between patients with asymptomatic congenital CMV and healthy controls or uninfected siblings (391,392). Children with asymptomatic congenital CMV who are developmentally normal at 1 year of age are unlikely to be at increased risk of subsequent neurodevelopmental or intellectual impairments (393).

Dental defects can be found in 40% of the survivors of symptomatic neonatal disease but in only 5% of asymptomatic cases (394). A variety of other congenital anomalies have been described in infants with congenital CMV infection, but these probably reflect coincidental associations rather than true cause-and-effect relationships (395). Reported associations include atrial and ventricular septal defects, tetralogy of Fallot, congenital mitral stenosis, aortic arch thrombosis, congenital lobar emphysema, Mondini deformity of the temporal bone (congenital anomaly of osseus and membranous labyrinth characterized by aplastic cochlea, and deformity of the vestibule and semicircular canal with partial or complete loss of auditory or vestibular function), stuck twin syndrome, renal agenesis, diabetes insipidus, inguinal hernia, hip dislocation, clubfoot, esophageal atresia, megacolon, and extrahepatic biliary atresia (10,396–403).

Maternal CMV antibodies protect the fetus against major CMV-related pathology. Fowler and colleagues found that 18% of 125 infants born to women with primary CMV during pregnancy had symptomatic neonatal disease compared with none of 64 infants born to women with reactivated CMV infection. After a 5-year follow-up period, 13% of infants born to mothers with primary infection had mental impairment (i.e., intelligence quotient ≤70) compared with none in the recurrent infection group. Sensorineural hearing loss was found in 15% and 5% of infants born to mothers with primary and recurrent CMV infections, respectively. Bilateral hearing loss occurred only in the primary infection group (340).

Discordant fetal outcomes are possible after primary maternal CMV infection in twin pregnancies. CMV usually affects both twins if they are monozygotic with a monochorionic placenta. In dizygotic twins with a dichorionic placenta, one twin can be severely affected whereas the other completely escapes infection (404). In one report of a quadruplet pregnancy complicated by primary maternal CMV infection, one infected fetus died antenatally, another died at 3 months of liver failure, one had hearing loss and developmental delay, and the fourth infected infant was normal at his last evaluation at age 18 months (405). CMV viral loads in amniotic fluid of discordant twins have been found to be higher in those born with symptomatic congenital CMV than in their twin with asymptomatic infection (406).

Congenital infection can be diagnosed by isolation of CMV from the urine or saliva within the first 2 weeks of life. Positive cultures from specimens obtained after 3 weeks of age may reflect perinatal CMV acquisition. Congenitally infected infants shed CMV in their urine for many years. The use of shell vial cultures hastens viral isolation. CMV can be also detected in urine by electron microscopy or ELISA. CMV DNA can be detected in clinical specimens such as urine or serum using sensitive hybridization or PCR methods. CMV-specific IgM is detected in many of the infected newborns. IgM detection by radioimmunoassay or ELISA is superior to immunofluorescence (326,357, 407–411). Compared to CMV isolation from urine, Revello and colleagues found that the sensitivities of assays detecting CMV DNA in serum, CMV viremia, antigenemia, and

CMV-specific IgM to be 100%, 28%, 43%, and 71%, respectively (412). CMV viral loads are higher in urine than in cord vein blood or cerebrospinal fluid in congenitally infected infants (413). PCR assays on blood collected on Guthrie cards have been successfully employed in a number of studies to make retrospective diagnoses of congenital CMV infection in infants with unexplained sensorineural hearing loss or CNS malformations (389,414). Guthrie cards are saved in various State Laboratories for periods that range from weeks to years. Storage conditions are highly variable and may allow for cross contamination by blood from other cards.

Ganciclovir has been evaluated as treatment for symptomatic congenital CMV infection. Ganciclovir suppresses viral replication in immunocompromised patients with serious CMV infections. Several problems are associated with ganciclovir use, including the resumption of viral replication on discontinuation of therapy, emergence of ganciclovir-resistant CMV strains after prolonged use in immunosuppressed patients, and drug toxicity (e.g., neutropenia, thrombocytopenia) (367,415). With the exception of one study, information on the utility of ganciclovir for infants with symptomatic congenital CMV infection comes from individual case reports, small case series, and uncontrolled trials utilizing more than one dosage regimen for the drug (326,413,416–429). From these studies, it appears that ganciclovir can lessen or stop viral multiplication and inhibit its shedding; however, viruria resumes on discontinuation of therapy. Regimens that used higher individual doses (7.5 instead of 5 mg/kg) given twice daily and for longer periods (6 to 12 weeks or longer instead of 2 to 3 weeks) were associated with improved short-term outcomes. Drug-related hematologic toxicities (e.g., neutropenia, thrombocytopenia) develop in the majority of treated infants.

A randomized, but not placebo-controlled, trial of intravenous ganciclovir (6 mg/kg per dose every 12 hours) vs. no therapy for 6 weeks enrolled 100 newborns with symptomatic congenital CMV involving the CNS between 1991 and 1999 (415). To be included in the study, infants had to be one month of age or younger, have a gestational age of at least 32 weeks, weigh 1200 grams or more at birth, and be HIV-negative. CNS disease was considered present if infants had one or more of the following: microcephaly, intracranial calcifications, hearing deficits, chorioretinitis, or abnormal CSF findings. A major limitation of the study was that only 42 infants were evaluable at the six-month follow-up. Nevertheless, the investigators found that ganciclovir prevented hearing deterioration at six months. At or beyond one year of age, fewer ganciclovir-treated infants had worsened hearing as compared to baseline (21% vs. 68%). Two-thirds of treated infants developed significant neutropenia requiring dosage adjustment or treatment with granulocyte colony stimulating factor (415).

The optimal treatment for congenital CMV infection remains to be defined. For symptomatic infants with severe disease, ganciclovir needs to be considered. The duration of therapy should be between three and six weeks, depending on clinical response and cessation or reduction of virus replication. Some investigators have suggested treatment durations of 3 months to 3 years. Oral valganciclovir has not yet been studied in newborns, but it might offer options in the future for the treatment of symptomatic congenital CMV or asymptomatic infants with demonstrated hearing deficits (428,430).

Intrauterine therapy for CMV infection was attempted for one fetus at 27 weeks of gestation by infusing ganciclovir once daily into the umbilical vein for 12 days. There was initial improvement in the fetal platelet count and liver enzyme concentrations, and a reduction in the amount of virus in the amniotic fluid and fetal urine, and clearance of CMV from fetal blood. However, viral replication promptly resumed on discontinuation of the drug, and the fetus died in utero at 32 weeks of gestation. Disseminated CMV was demonstrated at autopsy (431). CMV hyperimmune globulin used in conjunction with ganciclovir has improved the survival of bone marrow transplant recipients with CMV pneumonia. The combination was not beneficial in one infant in whom it was tried (418). CMV hyperimmune globulin was injected into the abdominal cavity of another CMV-infected fetus with ascites at 28 and again at 29 weeks of gestation (432). The fetus was delivered at 34 weeks because of fetal distress. The ascites was still evident at that time but disappeared by the fourth day of life. CMV hyperimmune globulin was given intravenously to a mother of twins with only one infected fetus who had intrauterine growth retardation, placental thickening, and umbilical cord edema; a dose of the immunoglobulin was also injected into the amniotic cavity. The affected fetus was developmentally normal at the two-year follow-up, with no visual or auditory impairments (433). There is no published experience with foscarnet or cidofovir in the treatment of congenitally infected infants.

Perinatal Infection

Infants can acquire CMV during passage through an infected birth canal or by ingestion of CMV-positive breast milk (434,435). CMV is found in the milk of 20% to over 90% of seropositive mothers for up to 12 weeks postpartum, and 60% to 80% of infants receiving CMV-containing milk will become infected. However, a report from Japan of 30 preterm infants fed CMV-positive breast milk showed that only three (10%) became infected and none developed symptoms (436). Another study of 22 preterm infants infected with CMV postnatally by breast-feeding found that none had sensorineural hearing loss at 2 to 4.5 years of age, and they did not differ from a CMV-negative preterm comparison group with respect to psychomotor development (437). One of the components of human milk, sialyllactose, has been found to consistently increase the titer of CMV in tissue culture systems at concentrations found in milk. The addition of another component of breast milk, lactoferrin, negates the effects of

sialyllactose on CMV growth (438,439). Pasteurization of breast milk inactivates CMV, although freezing it at $-20°C$ will decrease viral titers.

In contrast to congenital disease, perinatally acquired CMV infection usually is benign. Most infections are subclinical. A self-limited, infantile pneumonitis is the clinical abnormality encountered most commonly among symptomatic term infants. Premature infants, and rarely term babies, may have severe illness, including pneumonia, hepatitis, enteritis, anemia, thrombocytopenia, and neutropenia (429, 440,441). Those born to CMV-seronegative mothers are at risk of acquiring CMV through blood transfusions from CMV-positive donors (440). CMV infection does not appear to be a co-factor for the development of bronchopulmonary dysplasia in preterm infants (442). The long-term prognosis for intellectual abilities and intact hearing for infants with perinatal CMV infection is excellent (443).

Prevention

Termination of the pregnancy can be considered for women who develop a primary CMV infection during gestation. With primary infection, the overall risk of delivering an infant with symptomatic congenital infection is about 5%.

Prenatal diagnosis of fetal CMV infection is feasible and can been accomplished by a variety of invasive methods such as cordocentesis and amniocentesis (371). Fetal blood can be cultured and PCR assays for CMV DNA can be performed. Additionally, fetal blood can be analyzed for the presence of CMV-specific IgM, liver enzyme elevations, anemia, and thrombocytopenia. Amniotic fluid can be tested by culture and PCR assays for evidence of CMV infection. The experiences with hundreds of pregnant women with primary CMV infection in whom prenatal diagnosis was attempted have been described in the literature (371,444–473). In the aggregate, these studies revealed that fetal blood testing is not as sensitive as amniocentesis in establishing the diagnosis of intrauterine CMV infection, and that symptomatic fetuses have higher CMV viral loads and higher CMV-specific IgM levels (371). Patients with positive results with the CMV-specific IgM assay, fetal blood culture, or fetal blood PCR testing also are positive when their amniotic fluid is examined, but the reverse is not true. Fetal blood sampling for CMV infection should only be used for confirmatory tests.

Amniocentesis is easier to perform and carries less risk to the mother and her baby. Studies have shown that neither culture methods nor PCR assays on amniotic fluid are 100% sensitive, and that false-negative results are more likely to be encountered if testing is done shortly after the diagnosis of maternal primary CMV infection is made (454,461,463,466,469). The influence of time between primary CMV infection and prenatal diagnostic tests diminishes when the most sensitive PCR techniques are employed (371). Positive PCR results on amniotic fluid may not necessarily reflect fetal infection. In one study of 82 women with primary CMV infection, PCR detected viral DNA in the amniotic fluid of 27; in only 12 was a congenital infection documented after birth (positive predictive value of 48%) (458). However, other investigators consider the detection of even small amounts of CMV DNA by PCR as an indicator of fetal infection (371). A false-positive amniotic fluid culture or PCR result is possible if contamination occurs with maternal blood or during performance of the assay. In general, higher CMV viral loads are found in the amniotic fluid of fetuses with symptomatic involvement as compared to those with subclinical infection (459,464,470). CMV DNA is not detected by PCR in the amniotic fluid of women who do not have CMV infection (474). Isolation of CMV from the amniotic fluid by culture implies intrauterine infection but does not provide information regarding the severity of fetal disease (454). PCR assays have been used to detect CMV DNA in chorionic villi, but the sensitivity, specificity, and positive and negative predictive values of the method are not known (475).

Ultrasonographic fetal abnormalities in women with gestational primary or recurrent CMV infection generally indicate more severe fetal disease. A variety of sonographic findings have been reported, including microcephaly, ventricular dilation, periventricular pseudocysts, hypoplastic corpus callosum, ascites, hyperechogenic fetal bowel, hepatomegaly, splenomegaly, hydrops, pleural and pericardial effusions, oligohydramnios, intrauterine growth retardation, and intracranial and abdominal calcifications (371,444,457,476–483).

Live attenuated and subunit CMV vaccines are in clinical trials and not yet available in the United States (484,485). Routine CMV serologic screening of pregnant women is not currently recommended (486).

Because blood from seropositive donors contains leukocytes that are latently infected with CMV, many blood banks now screen the blood for CMV antibodies, use leukocyte filters, or use washed erythrocytes. The practice of giving only CMV-negative blood or blood products to ill neonates has greatly reduced or eliminated the occurrence of transfusion-acquired CMV infections in many nurseries. Disseminated CMV infection after extracorporeal membrane oxygenation has been described; CMV screening of blood had not been done (487).

VARICELLA

Varicella (chickenpox) and herpes zoster (shingles) are caused by varicella-zoster virus (VZV). VZV is an enveloped, double-stranded DNA virus. Only one serotype is known, but there are a few genetically distinct strains (488).

Maternal Infection

About 95% of women of childbearing age in the United States have serologic evidence of past VZV infection. The proportion of seropositive women is smaller in those from tropical or semitropical countries (489).

Varicella is a highly communicable and usually benign disease of childhood. Its incubation period is usually 14 to 16 days, with a range of 10 to 21 days. Before licensure of the varicella vaccine in 1995, children younger than 15 years of age accounted for more than 90% of cases and fewer than 2% of reported cases occurred in those 20 years of age or older (490). Vaccination coverage rates were about 80% in U.S. children by the year 2000, but disease activity and hospitalizations had declined by 76% to 87% (491). Although the greatest decrease in incidence has been in children 1 to 4 years of age, cases declined in all age groups including infants and adults (492). The estimated incidence of gestational varicella before vaccine availability was 1 to 7 per 10,000 pregnancies, but there have been no revised estimates to date (493,494). Zoster results from reactivation of latent VZV and is encountered more frequently in elderly or immunosuppressed patients. Its incidence in pregnancy is unknown, but it is probably lower than that of varicella. One estimate placed the incidence at about 0.5 per 10,000 pregnancies (493).

Less than 5% of primary VZV infections are subclinical (495). The typical illness consists of fever, malaise, and a pruritic rash. The exanthem is mostly truncal in distribution and is characterized by crops of maculopapules that rapidly evolve into vesicles. The vesicles gradually crust over. New lesions continue to appear for 3 to 5 days, producing the distinctive finding of cutaneous lesions in various stages of evolution. Complications of varicella include pneumonia, encephalitis, arthritis, bacterial cellulitis, retinal vasculitis, and bleeding diathesis. The risk of incurring complications from varicella in otherwise normal adults may be up to 25-fold greater than that for normal children (490,496,497). Pregnancy is generally not considered a risk factor for maternal complications, but there may be an increased prevalence of varicella pneumonia in the third trimester (497). Immunity after varicella is usually long lasting, but recurrent VZV infections can occur in immunocompetent persons (498,499).

Zoster is characterized by pain localized to the area of distribution of one or more sensory nerve roots. The rash is unilateral in most patients and follows the same evolutionary pattern seen in varicella except for its restricted distribution.

Varicella and herpes zoster usually are diagnosed clinically, and laboratory confirmation is needed infrequently. The virus can be isolated from vesicular fluid by inoculating freshly collected specimens onto human diploid cell lines. The VZV-specific antigens can be detected in vesicular fluid by immunofluorescence staining of smears of cell scrapings collected from the base of fresh vesicles (500). VZV DNA can be detected in vesicle samples, including most crusted lesions, by PCR methodologies (501,502). PCR assays have also been used to detect VZV DNA in CSF, genital lesions, and other clinical specimens (503,504). Quantitative VZV DNA measurements in blood and skin lesions show that viral loads are higher in patients with varicella than in those with herpes zoster (505,506).

Several serologic assays are available for the detection of antibodies to VZV. These include complement fixation, neutralization, IHA, immune adherence hemagglutination, radioimmunoassay, immunoblot, latex agglutination, fluorescent antibody against membrane antigen (FAMA), indirect fluorescent antibody (IFA), and ELISA. These tests can be used to diagnose VZV infections or to ascertain the susceptibility status of an individual (507).

Complement fixation antibodies develop within 10 days of onset of varicella and peak at 2 to 3 weeks. These antibodies appear earlier in herpes zoster. Complement fixation antibodies tend to disappear with time. By 1 year after infection, about two-thirds of persons do not have detectable complement fixation antibody titers. The complement fixation test is relatively insensitive compared with FAMA or ELISA, and it is now rarely used in clinical laboratories. The FAMA test is very sensitive and is considered to be the gold standard for VZV antibody measurements. However, FAMA is arduous to perform and is not readily available. The ELISA test is more frequently used for VZV antibody measurements. The IFA methods appear to be as sensitive as FAMA.

Two serum samples collected 1 to 2 weeks apart can provide a retrospective diagnosis of VZV infection if a fourfold or greater rise in antibody titer is demonstrated. If the first sample is collected late in the course of the illness, a single high titer indicates a recent primary or a reactivated VZV infection.

Measurement of VZV-specific IgM antibodies is useful for documenting a recent infection with this virus. VZV-specific IgM antibodies can be detected in serum for several weeks after varicella and may be transiently found after herpes zoster.

For uncomplicated varicella, symptomatic treatment with antipruritics and cleansing of lesions is adequate. Analgesics are needed for pain control in herpes zoster. Early therapy of varicella within the first day of illness with oral acyclovir (800 mg given orally five times per day for 7 days) or valacyclovir (1000 mg given orally three times daily for 5 days) hastens resolution of fever and shortens the time period to complete crusting of the lesions (508,509). Acyclovir and valacyclovir are not recommended for use during pregnancy, but can be given for the treatment of severe or life-threatening VZV complications such as pneumonia.

There have been several reports of pregnant women with varicella pneumonia who were treated with acyclovir (510–517). The drug was used at doses ranging from 5 to 18 mg/kg every 8 hours, and the treatment results generally have been favorable. It is currently recommended that women who need intravenous acyclovir therapy for varicella pneumonia should get 10 mg/kg every 8 hours for 5 days.

Transmission to the Fetus

VZV transmission to the fetus occurs primarily through the transplacental route. Congenital malformations after maternal infection during the first half of pregnancy occur infrequently. VZV antigens and its DNA have been detected in fetal tissues from pregnancies complicated by varicella using immunohistochemical staining methods and PCR, respectively (518–522).

About one-fourth of newborns delivered to mothers who contract varicella during the last 3 weeks of pregnancy develop clinical infection (516). Paryani and Arvin (523) used several clinical and immunologic criteria to document intrauterine transmission of VZV in 43 pregnancies complicated by varicella and 14 others complicated by herpes zoster. These criteria included malformations consistent with the congenital varicella syndrome, acute varicella of the newborn, detection of VZV-specific IgM in the neonatal period, specific lymphocyte transformation to VZV antigen, persistence of anti-VZV IgG, and the occurrence of herpes zoster in infancy. The rate of intrauterine transmission was 24% after maternal varicella and 0% after maternal herpes zoster (523).

Fetal Infection

Varicella during pregnancy is not associated with an increased incidence of prematurity or fetal death (523–525). Chromosomal abnormalities have occurred after VZV infections in experimentally infected human diploid fibroblasts and in the peripheral leukocytes of patients with acute varicella (526,527). Leukocyte chromosomal breaks were described in one child whose mother had gestational varicella (528). An increased risk of leukemia in the offspring of women with gestational varicella has been found by some investigators, but the numbers are too small to confirm the association (529).

Numerous case reports published over the past 58 years have described the occurrence of congenital malformations in the progeny of women who acquire chickenpox during pregnancy (521,522–524,530–581). With the exception of a few infants with congenital anomalies after maternal varicella at 24 to 32 weeks of gestation, these infections usually occurred during the first half of gestation, and mostly between weeks 8 and 20 of pregnancy (582–585). Abnormalities are primarily cutaneous, musculoskeletal, neurologic, and ocular (Table 48-5).

The risk of fetal or congenital varicella syndrome after maternal chickenpox during pregnancy is low. Pastuszak and colleagues (586) studied 106 women with varicella in their first 20 weeks of pregnancy and found a 1.2% risk (95% confidence interval [CI] of 0%–2.4%) of varicella embryopathy. Enders and associates (587) studied 1,373 women with gestational varicella between 1980 and 1993 and found the risk of fetal varicella syndrome to be 0.4% (95% CI of 0.05%–1.5%) for infections occurring between weeks 0 to 12 of pregnancy, and 2% (95% CI of 0.8%–4.1%) for those occurring between weeks 13 to 20 of pregnancy. Jones and colleagues (588) found that 2 of 146 infants born to women with gestational varicella had abnormalities consistent with the fetal varicella syndrome; four others had a single major malformation. Harger and associates found the frequency of definite congenital varicella syndrome to be 0.4% in a cohort of 347 pregnant women with varicella evaluated between 1993 and 1996 (585). No infants were born with the fetal varicella

TABLE 48-5

ABNORMALITIES IN NEWBORNS AFTER MATERNAL GESTATIONAL VARICELLA

Timing of Maternal Varicella	Neonatal Clinical Abnormalities
Weeks 0 to 20 of pregnancy	Cicatricial skin lesions, denuded skin, herpes zoster, limb hypoplasia, rudimentary digits, muscle atrophy, intrauterine growth retardation, psychomotor retardation, microcephaly, cerebellar and cortical atrophy, hydrocephalus, seizures, intracranial and extracranial calcifications, sensory deficits, Horner syndrome, spinal cord atrophy, anal sphincter dysfunction, dysphagia, intestinal atresia, neurogenic bladder, renal dysplasia, recurrent aspiration pneumonia, clubfoot, microphthalmia, optic atrophy, hypoplasia of optic disc, chorioretinitis, chorioretinal scars, cataract, nystagmus
5 days antepartum to postpartum day 2	Fever, vesicular exanthem, hemorrhagic rash, respiratory distress, cyanosis, pneumonia, widespread necrotic lesions of the viscera (in fatal cases)

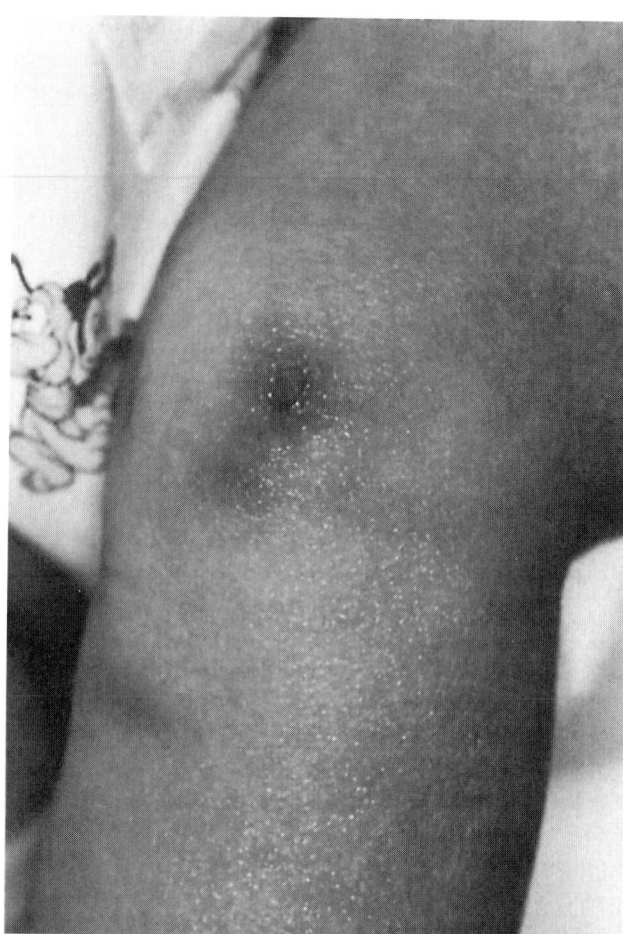

Figure 48-4   Newborn with congenital varicella after maternal infection at about week 13 of pregnancy. Notice the ulcerated area with surrounding scars over the knee; a second scar is visible distally, over the tibia. Despite an otherwise normal physical examination, computerized tomography of the head revealed multiple areas of cerebral infarction and diffuse intracranial calcifications.

syndrome to 57 women described in two other similar studies (589,590).

Cicatricial lesions are the most common skin abnormalities (Fig. 48-4). Cutaneous scars usually occur on hypoplastic extremities, but they can extend to the trunk or opposite extremity. Limb hypoplasia usually is unilateral and most commonly involves the leg. The arm, mandible, or hemithorax can be affected. Rudimentary digits are common on hypoplastic extremities. Detailed clinical and histopathologic studies of some patients suggest that limb abnormalities after intrauterine VZV infection probably is as a result of a neuropathy resulting from damage to dorsal ganglia and anterior columns of the spinal cord (555,557).

CNS pathology is common and includes microcephaly, cortical and cerebellar atrophy, psychomotor retardation, seizures, and focal brain calcifications. Autonomic dysfunction, manifested by loss of bowel and urinary sphincter control, dysphagia, intestinal obstruction, and Horner syndrome, is observed in some patients. Unilateral or bilateral ocular anomalies are common; the eye may be the only organ affected in fetal VZV infection.

The literature contains references to a few infants born with congenital malformations after maternal herpes zoster during pregnancy (591–594). Reported birth defects include microcephaly, microphthalmia, cataracts, and talipes equinovarus. These rare cases probably represent chance occurrences rather than true associations. Paryani and Arvin

(523) prospectively followed 14 pregnancies complicated by herpes zoster and were unable to uncover any clinical or immunologic evidence of intrauterine VZV infection. Enders and associates (587) found no evidence of intrauterine VZV infection in infants of 366 women who developed herpes zoster during the first 36 weeks of pregnancy.

Neonatal Infection

About 25% of newborns become infected when maternal varicella occurs during the last 3 weeks of pregnancy (516). The most important determinant of the severity of neonatal disease is the time of onset of maternal varicella relative to delivery. If maternal infection occurs within 5 days before and 2 days after delivery, varicella lesions in neonates usually appear at 5 to 10 days of age. The illness may be mild, with only a few cutaneous lesions, or may become severe, with fever, hemorrhagic rash, and generalized visceral involvement (see Table 48-5). The mortality rate is about 30%, and death usually is caused by severe pulmonary disease. If maternal varicella occurs 5 to 21 days before delivery, lesions in newborns typically appear in the first 4 days of life and the prognosis is good, with no associated mortality. The mild course probably is as a result of the production and transplacental passage of maternal antibodies, which modify the course of the illness in newborns. Passive transfer of maternal VZV antibodies across the placenta at titers considered to be protective can occur as early as 24 to 28 weeks of gestation (595). Investigators from the Netherlands have shown that the most important determinant of neonatal antibody titers to VZV is the mother's VZV IgG level, and that birth weight or gestational age are less predictive than previously believed (596).

The diagnosis can be confirmed by viral isolation or VZV antigen detection. Infected newborns may have VZV-specific IgM, but these usually disappear shortly after birth. Newborns with varicella should be kept in strict isolation if they require hospitalization. Acyclovir is used for infants with severe disease (597). Although there are no studies to support current practice, the suggested dose of acyclovir is 500 mg/m^2 per dose every 8 hours. Dosage adjustments are needed for premature infants with renal or hepatic dysfunction. If started early in the illness, acyclovir usually leads to more rapid resolution of disease symptoms and signs. Varicella-zoster immune globulin (VZIG) is not beneficial after clinical disease has developed.

Prevention

Management of persons exposed to VZV is critical because varicella is a highly communicable infection that can adversely affect pregnant women and their offspring. Exposed susceptible persons can be protected by passive immunization with VZIG. VZIG is prepared from plasma of normal blood donors found to have high IgG antibody titers to VZV. VZIG can prevent or modify clinical varicella in susceptible persons if given shortly after exposure.

Pregnant women exposed to varicella who have negative or uncertain prior histories of this infection should be tested for VZV susceptibility if sensitive assays are available and the results can be obtained rapidly. About 80% to 95% of these women are immune to varicella, as indicated by positive FAMA, IFA, or ELISA test results (490,598). If a pregnant woman has significant exposure to varicella and is susceptible or if the laboratory test result cannot be obtained in a timely fashion, VZIG should be administered for the purpose of preventing or modifying the infection in the mother to avoid complications. It is not known whether passive maternal immunization can prevent fetal VZV infection (490). VZIG is most efficacious when given as soon after exposure as is feasible, but not later than 96 hours.

A history of previous varicella infection is not always reliable. In a study of 184 military personnel with acute varicella, 20 (10.8%) reported a prior history of chicken-pox. Sera from 19 of these individuals collected 3 days to 34 months earlier and stored at −70° were available for testing; none had VZV-specific IgG (599).

Discordant results with respect to fetal infections are possible in multiple gestation pregnancies. Borzyskowski and collaborators (534) reported a set of female identical twins sharing a single placenta whose mother developed varicella at 10 weeks of gestation. The first twin was normal, and the second had congenital defects consistent with intrauterine VZV infection.

Prenatal diagnosis by detection of VZV-specific IgM in fetal blood was successful in one fetus evaluated at about 32 weeks of gestation, approximately 12 weeks after his mother developed chickenpox (538). Anti-VZV IgM could not be detected in cord blood samples obtained at 27 and 35 weeks of gestation of another fetus whose mother developed chickenpox at 12.5 weeks of gestation; later testing of stored amniotic fluid was positive for VZV DNA by PCR (600). Isada and colleagues (601) attempted to diagnose intrauterine VZV infection in two patients by chorionic villus sampling and PCR. Tissues from both mothers were PCR positive but culture negative. One mother elected to terminate her pregnancy at 23 weeks; examination of the fetal brain by Southern blot hybridization was negative. The second woman continued her pregnancy to term, and her newborn infant was clinically normal. Tests for VZV-specific IgM in cord blood and viral placental cultures were negative. Thus, the detection of VZV DNA sequences in chorionic villus samples did not equate with fetal infection (601). Amniotic fluid viral culture done at 22 weeks of gestation (11 weeks after maternal varicella) confirmed the diagnosis in another infected fetus; concomitant testing of fetal blood failed to detect VZV-specific IgM (602). Amniotic fluid testing using PCR confirmed the diagnosis of fetal varicella infection in 9 of 107 women who had chickenpox before week 24 of gestation; none had detectable VZV-specific IgM in fetal blood (603).

A variety of antenatal sonographic abnormalities have been described for VZV-infected fetuses. These include hypoplastic extremities, clubfoot, flexed limbs, ventriculomegaly, porencephalic cyst, oligohydramnios, polyhydramnios, hydrops, ascites, and calcifications of the lungs, myocardium, liver, and spleen (603–606).

Mattson and colleagues reported on 84 children born to women infected with varicella during pregnancy, only one of whom had features of the congenital varicella syndrome. They were able to show that the children without congenital varicella syndrome were normal when tested with age-appropriate neuropsychological tests at age 3 to 15 years (607).

Children born to mothers who develop varicella within 5 days before and 2 days after delivery should receive 125 U of VZIG as soon as possible. VZIG does not reduce the clinical attack rate in treated newborns, but these infants generally contract milder infections than untreated neonates (490,571,608). Because severe varicella can develop in newborns despite timely administration of

VZIG, some clinicians have advocated the use of acyclovir prophylaxis in these infants (609,610).

Although a few cases of severe neonatal varicella after exposure to mothers who developed the infection more than 2 days after delivery have been described, routine VZIG administration is not recommended, because this group of infants is not regarded as being at increased risk of varicella complications (490,611). Investigators from Taiwan reported on 24 newborns whose mothers developed chickenpox within 14 days before and after delivery. They were able to show that the use of prophylactic intravenous acyclovir (5 mg/kg every 8 hours for 5 days) started 7 days after onset of maternal rash, coupled with one dose of intravenous gammaglobulin either at birth or after postnatal contact, could prevent neonatal varicella infection (612).

Pregnant women with varicella at the time of delivery should be isolated from their newborns until all vesicles have crusted. Neonates with varicella lesions should be isolated from other infants but not from their mothers.

Hospitalized premature infants may be candidates for VZIG if a significant exposure to chickenpox has occurred. All infants less than 28 weeks gestation or with a birth weight of ≥1,000 grams should receive VZIG. Premature infants born at 28 weeks gestation should get VZIG if their mothers have no reliable history of chickenpox or lack serologic evidence of protection (613).

A live, attenuated varicella vaccine (VARIVAX) was licensed in the United States in March 1995. The vaccine should not knowingly be administered to susceptible pregnant women. The vaccine manufacturer established a Pregnancy Registry for VARIVAX (telephone number 1-800-986-8999) to collect data on the pregnancy outcomes of inadvertently immunized women. There were 701 reports of inadvertent exposure to the vaccine from 3 months before or at any time during the pregnancy between March 17, 1995 and March 16, 2000; 362 prospective and 21 retrospective reports were available for analysis. There was no evidence of the congenital varicella syndrome in newborns, including those delivered to seronegative women who received the vaccine during the first or second trimester of pregnancy (614). Seronegative women receiving postpartum varicella vaccination have been shown not to shed the vaccine virus in their breast milk when samples were tested by PCR assays (615).

Screening of pregnant women for varicella susceptibility is not recommended at the present time. Some obstetricians routinely screen their gravid patients who have negative or uncertain histories of past varicella infections, but this approach is felt not to be cost effective (616). One cost-effectiveness analysis concluded that serologic testing of women without prior history of chickenpox, if coupled with postpartum vaccination of susceptibles, could prevent about 43% of adult varicella and at a reasonable cost to the health care system (617). These analyses notwithstanding, the varicella vaccine has already had a major impact on the epidemiology of VZV infections in the United States, and this will inevitably modify our current thinking about the management of this problem in pregnant women and their infants.

OTHER HERPESVIRUS INFECTIONS

Epstein-Barr Virus

Primary Epstein-Barr virus (EBV) infections during pregnancy are rare because ≥95% of adults have serologic evidence of past infection. Estimates place the risk at 0.0% to 0.2% (10). However, the frequency of primary EBV infection was found to be 7% among 46 pregnant women who were susceptible early in gestation (618). Reactivation of latent EBV is common during pregnancy (10).

The majority of primary EBV-infected individuals are asymptomatic. Infectious mononucleosis is the most common clinical manifestation of infection. Complications such as meningoencephalitis, Guillain-Barré syndrome, airway obstruction, or rupture of the spleen are infrequent, but can be severe (10).

Diagnosis typically is made with serologic tests. Hetero-phile antibodies are usually present in most women at onset of symptoms, and decline to undetectable levels within 3 months. Persistence of heterophile antibodies for as long as one year can occur. The measurement of antibodies to the EBV viral capsid antigens (VCA), early antigen (EA), and EBV nuclear antigen (EBNA) can be used to make a specific diagnosis of primary EBV infection. EBV-VCA IgM is usually present at onset of symptoms. It is rarely detected with EBV reactivations. EBV-VCA IgG is generally present early and four-fold titer rises are detected in 20% or fewer patients. Anti-EA is found in 80% of patients with primary EBV, but it can also be detected with virus reactivations. IgG antibodies to EBNA usually appear after 3 or 4 weeks, and remain detectable indefinitely (619).

Transplacental transmission of EBV is rare. Maternal oropharyngeal EBV shedding may increase the risk of maternal-fetal transmission of HIV-1 (620). EBV acquisition during passage through the birth canal is theoretically possible because cervical shedding of this virus has been demonstrated (10). A study of 100 healthy women showed that 46% of women shed EBV in their breast milk, and that the shedding was highest at 3 to 12 weeks postpartum (621).

A variety of congenital defects have been described in the offspring of women with documented EBV infection or infectious mononucleosis. Abnormalities included low birth weight, micrognathia, congenital heart disease, biliary atresia, cataract, microphthalmia, hip dysplasia, and central nervous system malformations. However, there is no specific pattern to these findings and they likely represent chance occurrences (10).

Human Herpesvirus 6

Human herpesvirus 6 (HHV-6) is an enveloped double-stranded DNA virus that is separated into two variants (HHV-6A and HHV-6B) on the basis of differing genetic, immunologic, and biologic properties (622). Most children become infected by two years of age, but seropositivity decreases with age. Transmission is believed to be by infected oral secretions, but the virus is also found in the cervices of some pregnant women in late gestation (622,623).

HHV-6 antibodies were found in 100% of 569 pregnant and nonpregnant women attending a family planning clinic in San Antonio, Texas. HHV-6 genital shedding was found in 2% of the pregnant women, and 3.7% of those who were not pregnant (624). A study of pregnant women in Japan similarly found a 100% prevalence of IgG antibodies to HHV-6, and 1.6% of women had significant increases in these titers suggesting virus reactivation. HHV-6 DNA was found in the genital tract of 3.7% of pregnant women in the first trimester and in 12.2% of the same women in their third trimester (625). Serosurveys of other countries show that the prevalence of HHV-6 antibodies can vary from a low of 50% in Morocco, to 76% in France, and 90% in Ecuador and Congo (626).

Roseola infantum is the clinical illness most often associated with HHV-6 (usually HHV-6B) in children, but most symptomatic HHV-6 infections in infants are non-specific febrile illnesses. Primary infection in healthy adults is rare and may manifest with rash, hepatitis, lymphadenopathy, or encephalitis. In immunosuppressed individuals, especially posttransplantation, HHV-6 (usually HHV-6A) reactivates and is associated with pneumonitis and encephalitis. A variety of unproven disease associations such as Bell's palsy, drug-induced hypersensitivity syndrome, multiple sclerosis, sarcoidosis, and lymphoproliferative disorders have been described for HHV-6 (622).

Diagnosis of HHV-6 is by culture of peripheral blood mononuclear cells or, preferably, by PCR methods. Specimens can include blood cells and other fluids such as CSF. Because of the potential for virus reactivations, the detection of HHV-6 DNA by PCR is only 57% predictive of a primary infection. However, absence of HHV-6 IgG antibodies or the demonstration of a high viral load are strongly suggestive of a primary infection. Positive HHV-6 IgM measurements are suggestive of a primary infection but are subject to cross-reactions with other herpesviruses and can be detected with reactivations. Fourfold rises in HHV-6 IgG titers are also suggestive of a primary infection, but this is more likely to be seen in infants than in adults. Immunohistochemical tests allow the detection of HHV-6 antigens in formalin-fixed, paraffin-embedded tissues (622). HHV-6 antibodies are readily passed through the placenta, and paired mother-infant samples show higher virus titers in cord blood than maternal serum (627).

Treatment of HHV-6 infections is reserved for immunocompromised patients and otherwise healthy individuals with serious complications. Cidofovir is the most active drug against this virus, but ganciclovir is the drug for which there is more clinical experience. Foscarnet is also active against HHV-6, but acyclovir in not. There is no experience with antiviral therapy of pregnant women with serious HHV-6 infections (622).

Maternal-fetal transmission of HHV-6 can occur. HHV-6 antigens were detected in spontaneously aborted villous tissues of 2 of 3 women who were positive for HHV-6 IgM (628). Another study from Japan reported on the detection of HHV-6 DNA in 2 of 8 fetuses with hydrops fetalis but in none of 10 non-hydropic dead fetuses (629). Dunne and Demmler found that 2 of 799 cord blood sera were HHV-6 IgM positive but DNA negative by PCR (630). By contrast, a study of 110 pregnant women in Japan showed that women who had HHV-6 DNA (none of whom had a positive HHV-6 culture result) in vaginal samples collected early in pregnancy did not transmit the virus to their offspring. Infant blood and saliva was collected at birth and again at one month, and all samples were negative by PCR (631). In another study, 7% of HIV-negative infants born to HIV-infected women had HHV-6 DNA in their blood during the first month of life (632). A study of cord blood specimens of 305 babies from Germany found that 1.6% contained HHV-6 DNA suggesting intrauterine infection (633).

Neonatal HHV-6 infections may include severe hepatitis, thrombocytopenia, seizures, aseptic meningitis, fever, or rash (634–636). One newborn with non-febrile seizures was found to have HHV-6B in the CSF; neurologic sequelae such as psychomotor retardation, strabismus, and hypertonia were found at 18 months of age (636). It is not known whether treatment with ganciclovir or other antiviral agents is of any benefit.

Human Herpesvirus 7

Like HHV-6, human herpesvirus 7 (HHV-7) is ubiquitous and can be recovered from the blood and saliva of most adults (637–639). It has been associated with fever, roseola infantum, seizures, hemiplegia, aseptic meningitis, and hepatitis (639–642).

Antibodies to HHV-7 are readily transferred through the placenta, and higher titers are found in cord blood than in maternal sera (627). A study of 72 cervical swabs from pregnant women found 2.7% to be positive for HHV-7 DNA (623). In another study, 2.4% of Japanese women had significant increases in HHV-7 antibody titers (but no HHV-7 IgM) during their pregnancies. HHV-7 DNA was detected in the genital tracts of 2.7% and 9.6% of these women during their first and third trimesters, respectively (625). The clinical relevance of these observations to newborns is not known.

Human Herpesvirus 8

Human herpesvirus 8 (HHV-8), also known as Kaposi sarcoma-associated herpesvirus, has been associated with several tumors including Kaposi sarcoma, multicentric Castleman disease, and one type of non-Hodgkin's lymphoma. In the few known examples of primary HHV-8 infection, clinical presentations included non-specific febrile illnesses, maculopapular rash, splenomegaly, cervical lymphadenopathy, and bone marrow failure in a kidney transplant recipient (643).

Seroprevalence studies from North America show that 0.0% to 20% of the general population have antibodies to

HHV-8, but this is much higher in geographic regions where Kaposi sarcoma is common (643). The seroprevalence of HHV-8 among HIV-infected pregnant women from Italy, Haiti, and Zambia is 39%, 10%, and 51%, respectively (644–646). It is only 11% among Italian women undergoing amniocentesis for genetic screening (647).

It is unclear how HHV-8 is transmitted. Sexual contact appears to be the primary mode in North America, but horizontal transmission is frequent in developing countries (643). It is believed that horizontal spread occurs by infected saliva. Bloodborne transmission is possible, but this is less efficient than for HIV, HCV, or HBV (648). Vertical spread from infected mothers to their offspring is rare (647,649,650). Two of 12 Zambian infants infected with HHV-8 during the first year of life had HHV-8 DNA in their peripheral blood mononuclear cells at birth (650). Preliminary data suggest that there may be a higher risk of abortion among women with high HHV-8 antibody titers (651). The clinical relevance of intrauterine, perinatal, or postnatal HHV-8 infection remains to be elucidated.

PARVOVIRUS B19 INFECTIONS

Human parvovirus B19 was discovered fortuitously in the mid-1970s by British scientists evaluating new laboratory methods for the improved detection of HBsAg in blood donor sera (652). B19 has since been etiologically linked to a variety of conditions, including erythema infectiosum (i.e., fifth disease), aplastic crises in sickle-cell anemia and other hemolytic diseases, chronic anemia in immunocompromised patients, acute arthritis, and fetal hydrops. Less commonly recognized B19-related conditions are myocarditis, hepatitis, aseptic meningitis, and virus-associated hemophagocytosis (653).

B19 is a small, nonenveloped, single-stranded DNA virus. Despite its many genotypes, only one B19 antigenic type is currently recognized. The B19 genome encodes two structural proteins (VP1 and VP2) and one nonstructural protein. The virus does not grow in conventional cell lines, but it can best be propagated in erythroid progenitor cells (653).

B19 causes a lytic infection of human erythroid progenitor cells. The erythroid tropism of B19 is as a result of the tissue distribution of globoside (erythrocyte P antigen), its major cellular receptor. Globoside is a neutral glycophospholipid of red blood cell membranes. Persons who do not have P on their erythrocytes (i.e., p phenotype) are naturally resistant to infection with B19. The frequency of the p phenotype is 1 per 200,000 persons (654). Globoside also can be found on megakaryocytes, endothelial cells, placenta, fetal liver, and heart cells. B19 binds not only to globoside but also to several tissue-specific neutral glycophospholipids, such as those found in granulocytes, kidneys, liver, and bowel tissue (655).

Cessation of erythrocyte production, manifesting as reticulocytopenia, does not cause symptomatic anemia in otherwise healthy persons. However, patients who have reduced erythrocyte lifespans (e.g., sickle-cell anemia, thalassemia major) may develop transient aplastic crises. The nonstructural protein of B19 is cytotoxic and causes the death of erythroid progenitors. Patients with congenital or acquired immunodeficiency disorders may fail to clear the acute infection; a persistent B19 infection ensues, which results in chronic anemia (653). Establishment of a persistent infection sometimes can occur in persons without recognized immune deficiency disorders; a qualitatively or quantitatively aberrant immune response is thought to be responsible for this phenomenon (656). The rash and arthropathy seen in B19 infections are immune-mediated manifestations and are not directly related to the lytic infection of erythrocyte progenitor cells (653).

Maternal Infection

Serologic surveys have found that 30% to 60% of adults in the United States have serum antibodies against B19, indicating prior infection (657,658). Surveys of pregnant women in other countries show B19 seroprevalence rates of 35% in Barcelona, Spain, 40% in Japan, 53% in Kuwait, 64% in Melbourne, Australia, 65% in Denmark, and 81% in Stockholm, Sweden (659–664). The virus is transmitted primarily by B19-infected respiratory secretions. Transmission through transfusions of blood or blood products such as pooled factor VIII or IX concentrates is uncommon. B19 is found in the blood of 1 in 20,000 to 1 in 50,000 donors, but the incidence can be as high as 1 in 260 during epidemic years (665). To reduce the risk of iatrogenic transmission, major producers of plasma derivatives have voluntarily started quantitative measurements of B19 DNA to keep it under 10,000 genome copies per mL in the manufacturing pools (653,665). The incubation period of parvovirus B19 is 4 to 14 days, but it can be as long as 21 days. Infections are more common in late winter and spring in temperate climates, and epidemics usually occur every 4 or 5 years (666).

About 1% of susceptible pregnant women without known exposure to B19-infected persons seroconvert each year in the United States. Rates of 1.5% to 6.8% for acute gestational B19 infections have been reported from other countries (659–661,667). Higher rates are encountered during epidemic periods (661). During a large erythema infectiosum outbreak in Connecticut, pregnant women were tested for serologic evidence of recent B19 infection. Infection rates among exposed susceptible pregnant women were 16% for school teachers, 9% for day care workers, and 9% for homemakers (668). Attack rates of 36% to 38% were documented among susceptible nursing staff who were exposed to patients with sickle-cell anemia and aplastic crisis at a children's hospital (669). However, another study of health care workers under similar circumstances showed no transmission of B19 from patients to susceptible staff members (670).

A study of 30,946 pregnant women from three regions in Denmark conducted between November 1992 and June

1994 found that the presence of B19 IgG correlated with a woman's number of siblings, having a sibling close in age (within 2 years), number of children, and occupational exposure to children. The risk of seroconversion to B19 during pregnancy increased by threefold to sevenfold depending on the number of children at home, and having children 6 to 7 years of age was associated with the highest rate of gestational B19 infection (661).

Half or more of acute B19 infections of adults are subclinical (653,666). Erythema infectiosum is the most commonly identified B19-related condition. This illness is seen primarily in children, and its most characteristic feature is a facial exanthem (i.e., slapped-cheek appearance). The rash is lacy or reticulated, spreads to the trunk and extremities, and fades within 2 weeks. Recrudescence of the rash is observed with stimuli such as temperature changes, sunlight, or emotional stress. Pruritic, petechial, purpuric, vesicular, or erythema multiforme types of rashes are possible with acute B19 infection (653,666,671,672).

In addition to erythema infectiosum, acute B19 infections in otherwise healthy adults can manifest with influenza-type illnesses and symmetric polyarthropathies (e.g., polyarthralgias, polyarthritis). B19-associated joint disease is more common in women, affecting 50% to 80% of those with symptoms (673). The hands are most often involved, but pain, stiffness, and swelling can also involve the wrists, ankles, and knees (653,666). Rheumatoid factor may be positive transiently; therefore the illness could be misdiagnosed as early rheumatoid arthritis (674). B19 infections in compromised patients can result in transient aplastic crises, chronic anemia, and viral-induced hemophagocytic syndrome (653).

A diagnosis of acute or recent B19 infection can be made by detecting B19-specific IgM using enzyme immunoassays. These antibodies are present in the serum of more than 90% of patients by the third day of illness. B19-specific IgM can persist for 4 months or longer in more than 75% of patients, rendering the distinction between acute or recent B19 infection on serologic grounds alone difficult (675). B19-specific IgG usually is formed by the end of the first week of the illness, and it persists for life. The detection of B19-specific IgG antibodies with negative IgM test results is considered evidence of past infection and, probably, immunity to B19 reinfections. There are reports of rare instances of B19 reinfection of women known to be previously seropositive for this virus that have led to hydrops fetalis and fetal demise (676).

B19 DNA can be detected in serum and tissues by nucleic acid hybridization techniques and PCR assays (653). B19 DNA can be found in serum for 2 to 6 months after the onset of illness, but it has persisted for years in a few patients (675,677). B19 antigens can be detected by immunofluorescence, immunoperoxidase, or enzyme immunoassays, but these methods are not widely available (678).

There is no specific treatment for B19-associated illnesses. Immunosuppressed patients with chronic anemia secondary to persistent B19 infections have benefited from the infusion of commercially available intravenous immune globulins (653). Scant evidence suggests that high doses of intravenous immune globulins may be beneficial in preeclamptic B19-infected women with hydropic fetuses (679). Patients with erythema infectiosum are not contagious to others after the rash becomes evident, but those with aplastic crises continue shedding their viruses during the first few days of their hospitalization and require contact isolation.

Fetal Infection

Maternal B19 infection during pregnancy can have an adverse effect on pregnancy outcome, but most fetuses escape infection. Fetal infection can lead to hydrops fetalis or death. B19 is responsible for 8% to 18% of nonimmune hydrops cases (657,663,680–682). Immunohistochemical analysis of placental villous trophoblast cells from women with B19 infection and a poor fetal outcome shows increased apoptosis within these cells (683). The histopathology of fetal B19 infection consists principally of infected erythroblasts with eosinophilic intranuclear inclusions, which are found mostly in the liver, spleen, and bone marrow (680,684).

Gestational B19 infections are associated with a less than 10% risk of pregnancy loss from spontaneous abortion, stillbirth, or delivery of a hydropic infant. In a British prospective study of 190 pregnant women found to be positive for B19-specific IgM during the period 1985 to 1988, the B19-related fetal death rate was estimated at 9% (685). A follow-up study of 274 pregnant women diagnosed between 1992 and 1995 again found the excess rate of B19-related fetal loss to be about 9%, but this risk was confined to the first 20 weeks of gestation. The risk of fetal hydrops in this study was 2.9%, with a 95% CI of 1.2% to 5.9% (686). More recent data from Sweden suggest that B19 may be responsible for 14% and 7.5% of intrauterine fetal deaths occurring at more than or equal to 22 weeks of gestation and the third trimester, respectively (687,688). Most infants with B19-related intrauterine fetal death do not manifest with hydrops fetalis (689). In a case control study conducted in the United States, it was shown that B19 was not a common cause of fetal death in the general population (690).

B19 suppresses fetal bone marrow erythrocyte production, leading to chronic anemia. This is not well tolerated by the fetus because of its rapidly expanding cell volume and its immature immune system, which fails to rapidly contain the B19 infection. Congestive heart failure ensues, usually secondary to the severe anemia. Direct infection of cardiac muscles by B19 can occur and may contribute to cardiac dysfunction (691–693). Using transmission electron microscopy, O'Malley and colleagues were able to demonstrate the presence of intranuclear virions in erythroid precursor cells and in cardiac myocytes of three fetuses with B19-related fatal hydrops fetalis (693).

Koch and colleagues (694) reported on 43 pregnant women with primary B19 infection who were followed to delivery. None of the infants was hydropic. Twenty-two (51%) of the 43 infants had evidence of congenital infection as determined by finding B19 DNA, B19-specific IgM, or B19-specific IgA; one infant tested negative at birth but became positive on all three assays at 6 weeks of age. A 20% rate of intrauterine infection among asymptomatic newborns was noted by Miller and co-workers (686). A study from Japan found an intrauterine B19 transmission rate of about 23% among 57 mother-infant pairs, about two-thirds of whom were asymptomatic (695). Thus, intrauterine B19 infection after primary B19 infection in the mother occurs commonly, but serious complications such as fetal hydrops or stillbirth are infrequent. Congenital anemia and transient erythroblastopenia of the newborn are uncommon manifestations of intrauterine B19 infection (696,697). A few reports of twin pregnancies complicated by maternal B19 infection indicate that it is possible for one fetus to be severely affected by the virus although the other fetus can remain asymptomatic or escape infection altogether (698,699).

Congenital malformations after intrauterine B19 infection rarely have been described, and they may represent chance occurrences rather than a true teratogenic effect of B19. Hartwig and colleagues (700) described a 9-week-old embryo whose tissues were positive for B19 DNA and who had abnormalities of the eyes and damage to skeletal and smooth muscles. Rodis and associates (701) described an electively terminated pregnancy in which the B19-infected fetus had anencephaly. Tiessen and co-workers (702) found B19 DNA in several tissues by PCR in an aborted fetus with cleft lip and palate, micrognathia, webbed joints, and multifocal degenerative changes of skeletal and smooth muscles. Katz and colleagues (703) described two infants with congenital malformations after maternal B19 infection. One infant had myocardial infarction, hepatic and splenic calcifications, and mild hydrocephalus, whereas the second infant had moderate hydrocephalus with dysplasia of the cerebral cortex and glial overgrowth. If B19 were a true teratogen, the associated risk would have to be very small. One case report described a hydropic fetus that died at 24 weeks of gestation after his mother had developed primary B19 infection (704). The fetus had a flat nose and low implanted deformed ears. On detailed examination, these dysmorphic features were found to be as a result of a partial trisomy 3q and a partial monosomy 11q resulting from a balanced translocation between chromosomes 3 and 11 in the mother. This report suggests that some of the rare congenital malformations noted in the offspring of B19-infected women may be related to small chromosomal abnormalities that can be missed unless a careful evaluation is undertaken. Some infants without obvious dysmorphic features had ileal stenosis or atresia with resultant meconium peritonitis after maternal B19 infection (698, 705). Neuropathologic abnormalities consisting of perivascular calcifications and B19-positive multinucleated giant cells were noted in the cerebral white matter of a fetus at postmortem examination (706).

The diagnosis of intrauterine B19 infection in a newly born infant is difficult and rests on detection of B19-specific IgM in serum or B19 DNA in the fetal blood or tissues. Parvovirus particles can be observed in tissues by electron microscopy (682,707–709).

Management of hydropic newborns is supportive and often includes packed erythrocyte transfusions. There are no recognized long-term sequelae for healthy infants born to mothers with gestational B19 infection (686,710). Infants with B19-related hydrops fetalis who recover after treatment with intrauterine transfusion of packed red blood cells do not seem to be at risk for persistent B19 infection, joint problems, or neurodevelopmental delay (711,712). One infant who developed hydrops fetalis at 22 weeks of gestation, with spontaneous resolution by 26 weeks, manifested with angioedema of the face, trunk, and extremities within hours of birth and this faded by the fifth day of life (713).

Prevention

Pregnant women who sustain a significant exposure to a B19-associated illness at home (e.g., erythema infectiosum in a child) and whose B19 antibody status is unknown can be informed that their overall risk of fetal death is at most 2.5%. This figure can be arrived at by multiplying the rate of susceptibility (about 50%), the rate at which exposed susceptible persons acquire B19 infection (maximum of 50%), and the estimated rate of death in documented infection (9%). Had the exposure taken place in a school or day care setting, the risk would decline to less than 1.5%.

Some investigators have suggested the use of intravenous gammaglobulin for postexposure prophylaxis of B19-susceptible pregnant women (666,714). Commercial intravenous gammaglobulin preparations contain anti-B19 IgG antibodies, and they have been shown to be helpful in the treatment of immunosuppressed patients with B19-induced chronic anemia. There are no data to support or refute the use of IGIV for the prevention or amelioration of B19 infection.

If acute or recent B19 infection is confirmed in the pregnant woman by a positive B19-specific IgM assay, serial ultrasound examinations should be performed for the detection of early signs indicative of fetal hydrops or, rarely, meconium peritonitis (698,705,715). Maternal serum alpha-fetoprotein elevations have been observed in pregnancies with B19-related adverse fetal outcomes such as hydrops, but this has been an inconsistent finding (716,717).

Published experience suggests that the prenatal diagnosis of fetal B19 infection is possible and accurate (718–727). B19 can be demonstrated in fetal blood by electron microscopy, molecular biological techniques, or detection of B19-specific IgM antibodies. Török and colleagues (721) used a PCR assay to detect B19 DNA in amniotic fluid and fetal blood. Fifteen mothers who were positive for B19-specific IgM were evaluated. Eight of 15 fetuses were positive for B19 DNA only, and the other seven were positive for B19 DNA and B19-specific IgM. Nine (60%) fetuses had hydrops. Ten infants were born healthy, including four found to have hydrops at 17 to 23 weeks of gestation, which resolved without specific intervention. PCR detected B19 DNA in the sera of 20% of mothers with negative B19-specific IgM assay results, with or without B19-specific IgG; one-half of the fetal specimens corresponding to this group of mothers were B19 DNA positive by PCR (721).

Zerbini and associates (724) studied 18 fetuses with B19-related hydrops fetalis and could detect B19 DNA by nested PCR in nine maternal sera. The less sensitive dot blot hybridization assay failed to detect B19 DNA in any of these specimens. For the 18 hydropic fetuses, B19 DNA was detected in blood obtained at cordocentesis in 62% by PCR and 40% by dot blot hybridization. However, 100% of cell smears prepared from fetal blood were positive for B19 DNA using in situ hybridization. In contrast, only 15% of fetal blood samples were positive for B19-specific IgM. When amniotic fluid was tested for B19 DNA, 83% were found to be positive by PCR, 20% by dot blot hybridization, and 70% by in situ hybridization (724). Thus, a combination of virologic and serologic tests may be needed to ensure an accurate diagnosis of intrauterine B19 infection.

B19 DNA can be detected in chorionic villus samples of some women (726). One study suggested that viral DNA levels are generally higher in the fetus than the mother's blood (727).

Some B19-infected pregnant women may remain negative for B19-specific IgM and IgG antibodies, despite the detection of B19 particles in serum and saliva using electron microscopy or the detection of B19 DNA using PCR or other techniques (721,728). B19 infection of their newborns may or may not be symptomatic.

Fetal therapy with intrauterine blood transfusions has been attempted in many infants, and digitaliztion in a few (657,711,712,718–720,729–734). The indications for intrauterine transfusion are not well defined (666). The degree of fetal anemia can be determined by cordocentesis (732,733). A recent report suggested that noninvasive Doppler ultrasonography showing increased fetal middle cerebral artery peak systolic velocity could predict fetal anemia with good accuracy (735). Fetal hydrops can resolve spontaneously before birth in as many as one-third of patients without specific intervention. These infants typically remain well after birth and during several months of follow-up (721,733,736–739). This indicates that fetal hydrops is not uniformly fatal if not treated and that some fetuses are capable of eventually resolving their B19 infection and reversing the observed pathophysiologic abnormalities. Intrauterine transfusions of packed red blood cells are typically administered into the umbilical vein, but intraperitoneal blood transfusions have been suggested as an alternative (732,734).

Routine screening of pregnant women for B19 infection is not recommended at present (666,740). Candidate B19 vaccines are in development, but none are commercially available (653).

HEPATITIS VIRUS INFECTIONS

Hepatitis A

Hepatitis A virus (HAV) is a small, nonenveloped RNA virus that belongs to the picornavirus family. There are several genotypes of HAV, but only one known serotype. Its incubation period averages four weeks, with a range of 15 to 50 days. HAV replicates in the liver, and then is transported through the biliary tree and shed in the stool. Fecal excretion of the virus begins 1 to 2 weeks before the onset of the illness, and continues for at least 1 week after that. Infants and children can shed HAV in the stools for several months (741,742).

HAV infections are very common in early life in developing countries. In the United States, there were an estimated 90,000 persons with symptomatic hepatitis A and another 90,000 persons with subclinical infection in 1997. A third of reported cases are in children less than 15 years of age. There are geographic variations within the United States with regards to disease incidence, with higher rates in western states such as Arizona, Alaska, Oregon, and New Mexico. HAV infection rates are also highest for American Indians and Alaskan Natives, and lowest for Asian Americans (742).

Transmission of HAV is primarily by person-to-person contact through fecal contamination and oral ingestion of the virus during communitywide outbreaks (742). The virus is highly communicable. Approximately 16% to 30% of an inoculum of HAV can be recovered from infected hands after 4 hours (743). The most commonly reported source of HAV infection in the United States is household or sexual contact with a person with hepatitis A in 12% to 26% of instances. Other sources of exposure are day care attendance or employment, international travel, food or waterborne outbreaks, and injecting or noninjecting drug use (742). A study from Israel found that certain occupations such as yeshiva students, day care center and kindergarten staff, food industry workers, teachers, physicians, and dentists were at increased risk of hepatitis A infection (744).

Neonatal intensive care unit outbreaks of hepatitis A have been described (745–748). The initial infection in some outbreaks occurred through transfusion of neonates with blood or fresh frozen plasma from donors with hepatitis A viremia during the prodromal phase of their illness (746–748). In one nursery outbreak, 20% of infants, 24% of nurses, and several nonnursing staff and household contacts were affected. The study found that having long fingernails, not wearing gloves for certain procedures, smoking, and drinking beverages in the nursery facilitated direct hand-to-mouth contact (747). Other risk factors for spread of hepatitis A to new infants and nursery personnel includes asymptomatic infection, prolonged fecal virus shedding, frequent contact with soiled diapers, and breaks in infection control measures.

Most children younger than 6 years of age have asymptomatic or anicteric HAV infections, whereas most adults have symptomatic disease (742). The typical clinical illness seen in over 80% of symptomatic individuals begins abruptly with fever, malaise, headache, anorexia, nausea, vomiting, and diarrhea; dark urine, clay-colored stool, and jaundice appear a week or two later (741,742). Other disease forms include relapsing hepatitis A, cholestatic hepatitis A, and fulminant hepatitis A. Extrahepatic manifestation such as vasculitis, arthritis, hemolytic anemia, or cryoglobulinemia are infrequent (741). In contrast to hepatitis A and hepatitis B, there is no chronic carrier state for HAV. About 100 persons in the United States die each year as a result of acute liver failure due to hepatitis A (742).

Approximately 33% to 38% of the US population are positive for HAV IgG (741,749). The incidence of acute hepatitis A in pregnancy is 1:1000 or less. Pregnant women are not more susceptible to HAV, nor do they have a worse clinical outcome, than nonpregnant women (749).

Serologic testing is needed to establish a diagnosis of acute hepatitis A. IgM antibodies to HAV are found 5 to 10 days before the onset of symptoms and for 3 to 6 months after that. HAV IgM is measurable for a longer time in patients with symptomatic hepatitis A than in those with asymptomatic infection (750). HAV RNA can be detected by PCR in serum, stool, or other body fluids during the acute phase of infection, but this test is rarely needed and is not readily available (741,742).

Treatment of hepatitis A is supportive. Management of infection usually includes bed rest, nutrition, avoidance of alcohol and hepatotoxic medications (741).

A number of published case reports suggest that intrauterine and perinatal transmission of HAV does occur, with resultant symptomatic disease in the neonate (751–756). In some of these reports, the mothers developed hepatitis A shortly before or immediately after delivery (751–753). Other reports describe women with acute hepatitis A several weeks before parturition. One mother developed hepatitis A at 20 weeks of gestation; an abdominal ultrasound at 27 weeks of gestation showed polyhydramnios and fetal ascites. Cordocentesis allowed the detection of HAV IgM in fetal blood. Meconium peritonitis subsequently developed at 35 weeks of gestation, which required surgical intervention after delivery (754). In another report, a mother developed hepatitis A at week 13 of gestation and her fetus was noted to have ascites at 20 weeks; meconium peritonitis was found at 33 weeks of gestation. The infant was delivered at 35 weeks gestation and a perforated distal ileum was found (755). Another mother whose hepatitis A occurred during her fourth month of pregnancy had protracted jaundice until she delivered at 36 weeks of gestation. The neonate was small for age and subsequently developed acute hepatitis A infection at 4 weeks of age. HAV RNA was detected in the mother's serum obtained at 4 months of pregnancy and the infant's serum at the age of 4 weeks (756).

The prevention of hepatitis A can be accomplished by both passive and active immunization. Intramuscular immune globulin (IGIM) at a dose of 0.02 mL/kg given within 2 weeks of last exposure confers greater than 85% protection. Pregnancy is not a contraindication to IGIM

administration, but only thimerosal-free preparations should be used. Two inactivated hepatitis A vaccines are available in the United States, and one combined inactivated hepatitis A and hepatitis B vaccine. Although the hepatitis A vaccines are not approved for use during pregnancy, the theoretical risk to the fetus should be weighed against the risk of hepatitis A to susceptible women at high risk of exposure to HAV (742). Hepatitis A vaccine is immunogenic in infants, but it is currently approved for use in persons 2 years of age or older. Placental transfer of HAV IgG occurs in both term and preterm newborns, and its presence has been shown to lower the antibody response to the vaccine in these infants (757,758).

Hepatitis B

HBV afflicts nearly 335,000 persons in the United States each year, about 5% of whom become chronic carriers of the virus (759,760). Estimates place the number of chronic, infectious HBV carriers in the United States at more than 1.25 million people (759). Globally, a third of the world population (about 2 billion) have been infected with HBV. The number of chronic HBV carriers worldwide is greater than 400 million, three-quarters of whom are Chinese, according to estimates by the World Health Organization (761). As many as 1 million people die each year from HBV-related acute and chronic hepatic disease (762). More than one-fourth of all carriers develop HBV-related chronic active hepatitis, liver cirrhosis, or hepatocellular carcinoma (759). Women who are chronic carriers of this virus can transmit HBV to their offspring during pregnancy; as many as 90% of perinatally infected infants become chronic carriers themselves (759).

The complete HBV is known as the Dane particle and consists of an outer lipid-containing envelope and an inner core or nucleocapsid. On the surface of the outer coat is the hepatitis B surface antigen (HBsAg), an antigenically complex glycoprotein. HBsAg has many antigenic epitopes that permit the identification of several HBV subtypes; the subtyping scheme is valuable as an epidemiologic tool, but it has no correlation with disease severity. The surface envelope contains three proteins (major, middle, and large S proteins) coded for by the HBV DNA genome. Variations in the major protein account for the subtype determinants, and the middle and large proteins are implicated in receptor-mediated virus uptake by hepatocytes (762).

The virus inner core consists of hepatitis B core antigen (HBcAg), hepatitis B e antigen (HBeAg), hepatitis B x antigen (HBxAg), a partially double-stranded DNA molecule, a DNA-dependent DNA polymerase enzyme with reverse transcription activity, and a protein kinase. HBcAg is found primarily in the nuclei of infected hepatocytes. In serum, HBcAg is found only as a component of circulating Dane particles, but it is never found in free form. HBeAg is a prematurely terminated polypeptide product of the same gene that codes for HBcAg; its presence in serum indicates infectivity. The function of HBeAg is not known. HBxAg directly and indirectly affects host and viral gene expression, and the X protein is essential for *in vivo* replication and spread of HBV. HBV DNA is a partially double-stranded DNA, and HBV DNA polymerase repairs the single-stranded HBV DNA region to form a complete double-stranded molecule (762,763).

With very sensitive assays, HBsAg can be detected in the blood within 1 to 2 weeks of exposure to HBV. However, clinical disease usually occurs 1 to 3 months, and occasionally 6 months, after exposure. HBeAg can be detected late in the incubation period, usually coinciding with or within days of HBsAg appearance. HBV DNA polymerase and HBV DNA are measurable at this stage and generally peak by the latter part of the incubation period. Viral titers during the acute stage of the infection can reach 109 to 1010 virions/mL. In patients who recover, HBsAg usually can no longer be detected at about the time of clinical resolution (764).

The earliest antibodies to appear are those directed against HBcAg (anti-HBc), typically 2 to 4 weeks after HBsAg is first detected. Anti-HBc titers increase during the acute stage of infection and persist for many years. Antibodies to HBeAg (anti-HBe) appear immediately after or within several weeks of HBeAg clearance and usually while HBsAg is still present. A window period that occasionally can be as long as 20 weeks follows HBsAg clearance from the circulation, during which neither HBsAg nor anti-HBs are detectable. However, specific IgM and IgG anti-HBc antibodies usually are present. The patient is contagious during this period. After anti-HBs antibodies become measurable, their titers continue to increase for approximately 6 to 12 months (762,764). Low levels of HBV DNA may persist in the blood for years, despite the appearance of anti-HBs (763). HBV DNA can be found in liver biopsies of patients with self-limited hepatitis B, including those with negative serum HBV assays (765). Anti-HBs antibodies persist for life and protect against future HBV reinfections. Antibodies to HBxAg (anti-HBx) can be detected in only 17% of patients with acute HBV infection and usually appear 3 to 4 weeks after onset of clinical symptoms; their clinical significance is not yet defined (766).

Patients who continue to have detectable serum HBsAg for 20 weeks or longer, or HBeAg for 10 weeks or longer, are likely to become chronic HBsAg carriers. Their serum anti-HBc titers usually are high, and IgM anti-HBc tends to persist for a long time. Approximately 25% to 50% of chronic carriers are HBeAg positive, and the remainder have anti-HBe. Persons who are positive for HBeAg, HBV DNA polymerase, or HBV DNA are highly contagious. Chronically infected patients clear HBV particles from their plasma with a half-life of about 1 day, and about 10^11 virus particles are released daily into the periphery from HBV-infected cells (767). Among persistently infected patients, about 5% to 10% convert each year from being HBeAg-positive to having anti-HBe (763). Over a period of about 10 years, more than 70% will clear HBeAg from their serum (768). Most chronic carriers remain HBV infected for life, but 1.5% to 2% of carriers spontaneously lose their HBsAg each year.

Young age is an important risk factor for developing the chronic carrier state; 70% to 90% of infected newborns become carriers, compared with 25% to 50% of children infected before their fifth birthday and 5% (range of <1%–12%) of adults. Other risk factors include a positive HIV-1 antibody status, hemodialysis, other immunodeficiencies, Down syndrome, and male gender (769). Virus-specific T cell responses in chronic carriers are attenuated in comparison to individuals who clear HBV after their acute infection (763). Reactivation of chronic HBV infection can occur during pregnancy, but this is rare (770).

There are several HBV genotypes (A to H), each with a characteristic geographic distribution and some differences in disease profiles (761). Naturally occurring HBV variants that are unable to produce HBeAg are recognized; these patients have high HBV DNA but no detectable HBeAg during the acute infection, and often have fulminant disease (771).

Clinical Manifestations

Most HBV infections are subclinical, particularly in children. Symptomatic infections can be mild and anicteric or be severe enough to produce encephalopathy, coagulopathy, and death. Fulminant hepatitis is more common in adults than in children and in those infected with certain mutant HBV strains or coinfected with the hepatitis C or D viruses (762,772–774). Extrahepatic disease may manifest as a serum sickness-type illness in patients with acute infections, polyarteritis nodosa, membranous glomerulonephritis, infantile papular acrodermatitis (Gianotti-Crosti syndrome), or cryoglobulinemia (762,775).

Approximately two-thirds of chronic HBsAg carriers develop chronic persistent hepatitis. They usually are healthy but have persistent or recurrent serum transaminase elevations. The remaining third eventually develop chronic active hepatitis, a progressive disorder that ultimately results in postnecrotic liver cirrhosis. Primary hepatocellular carcinoma, a common malignant tumor in certain parts of the world such as southeast Asia, Japan, Greece, and Italy, may be as much as 100 to 400 times more common in HBsAg-positive individuals than in their HBsAg-negative counterparts (776). Patients positive for both HBsAg and HBeAg are at highest risk for developing hepatocellular carcinoma (777). Primary hepatocellular carcinoma develops after an average of 35 years of HBsAg carriage; coexisting cirrhosis is found in 60% to 90%.

Most neonates and infants who acquire HBV from their mothers remain asymptomatic; those with symptoms typically have benign illnesses. Fulminant disease is rare. Most infected infants become chronic carriers and have a 25% or greater lifetime chance of dying of primary hepatocellular carcinoma or liver cirrhosis.

Modes of Transmission

HBsAg has been found in blood, blood products, urine, feces, bile, saliva, tears, sweat, semen, vaginal secretions, gastric contents of newborns, breast milk, cord blood, CSF, synovial fluid, and wound exudate (778). Many routes for

HBV spread are possible, but the most significant are percutaneous or permucosal exposure to infected blood or body fluids during birth or sexual intercourse or by contaminated needles.

HBV-infected blood can enter the body through contaminated needles shared by drug users, if health care providers mistakenly puncture themselves, or if other persons reuse unsterilized devices in medical or dental offices, acupuncture clinics, or tattooing parlors. Contaminated blood can be introduced through mucous membranes, open wounds, or abrasions. Screening of blood and blood products for HBsAg has almost eradicated transfusion-acquired HBV infection.

HBV can spread to sexual partners of chronic HBsAg carriers or patients with acute hepatitis B. HBV infection is more likely in persons with multiple sex partners, more years of sexual activity, and histories of other sexually transmitted diseases. Heterosexual transmission now accounts for 25% of new HBV cases in the United States, a 38% increase from the early 1980s. It is the most important risk factor for women, with parenteral drug abuse in second place. Close, long-term contact with chronic carriers, as happens in households or institutions for the developmentally disabled, is a risk factor. Intrafamilial nonsexual transmission accounts for 2% of new HBV infections in the United States each year. Transplanted organs are uncommon vehicles of HBV spread to susceptible recipients. About 30% to 40% of all patients have no identifiable risk factors (779).

Perinatal Epidemiology

About 0.2% of American Caucasians and 0.9% of African Americans are HBsAg-positive. The prevalence is notably higher in certain high-risk groups, such as immigrants from areas of high HBV endemicity (13%), Alaskan Natives or Pacific Islanders (5% to 15%), clients in institutions for the developmentally disabled (10% to 20%), users of illicit parenteral drugs (7%), household contacts of an HBV carrier (3% to 6%), health care workers with frequent blood contact (1% to 2%), and heterosexuals with multiple partners (0.5%) (780).

The rate of vertical transmission from mother to infant hinges on several factors. For women with acute HBV infection, the risk is about 76% if infection occurs during the third trimester or shortly after delivery, but it is only about 10% if it takes place during the first or second trimester. For HBsAg carrier mothers, the risk of mother-to-infant transmission depends on their HBeAg/anti-HBe status. The rate is estimated to be 70% to 90% for those who are HBeAg-positive, 31% for those who are negative for HBeAg and anti-HBe, and 10% or less for those who are positive for anti-HBe. About one-third of HBsAg-positive pregnant women in the United States also are HBeAg positive. Other variables that enhance vertical transmission are high maternal HBsAg and anti-HBc titers and a high HBV DNA concentration (778,781). In one study of HBsAg-positive pregnant Taiwanese women, the

odds ratio of having a persistently infected infant climbed from 1.0 to 147 as the maternal serum HBV DNA level increased from less than 0.005 to 1.4 ng/mL (782). HBsAg chronic carriers who are HBeAg-positive usually have higher HBV DNA levels than HBeAg-negative women (783). Carrier mothers can transmit HBV to infants born after sequential pregnancies.

Mother-to-infant transmission occurs during delivery in most cases through transplacental microhemorrhages or from ingestion of contaminated maternal secretions. Intrauterine infection is uncommon but may account for 5% to 15% of cases for HBeAg-positive mothers (784). However, a recent study of 59 HBsAg-positive mothers from China found evidence of intrauterine transmission in 40%. These investigators were able to find HBV DNA in 48% of amniotic fluid samples and 52% of vaginal samples, and could detect HBsAg and HBcAg in placentas from these mothers (785). Studies of placentas from HBsAg-positive women have found that HBV infection rates were not the same for all placental layers, and generally decreased from the maternal to the fetal side (785,786). The closer an infected placental cell layer is to the fetal side, the greater the likelihood of intrauterine HBV infection (786). Intrauterine HBV infection has been associated with the development of fetal ascites, abdominal calcifications, and meconium peritonitis in a few infants (787,788). HBsAg is found commonly in breast milk samples from carrier mothers, but no differences in antigenemia rates are found between breast-fed and bottle-fed infants born to infected mothers. There appears to be no added risk of HBV transmission to infants from breast milk, especially in those receiving appropriate immunoprophylaxis at birth (789).

Unimmunized infants who acquire HBV infection from their mothers usually have no detectable serum HBsAg until 1 to 4 months later. Passively acquired low levels of HBsAg may be detected in the peripheral blood of some neonates, and they do not necessarily imply HBV infection. Cord blood should not be used for HBsAg testing because it can be contaminated with maternal blood.

Immunoprophylaxis

Two preparations have been used for passive immunization against HBV: immune serum globulin and hepatitis B immunoglobulin (HBIG). Immune serum globulin has anti-HBs titers of 1:16 to 1:1,000. HBIG, a hyperimmunoglobulin product, has anti-HBs titers of 1:100,000 to 1:250,000. HBIG is prepared from plasma obtained from HIV and HCV antibody-negative donors with a high anti-HBs titer, and its administration does not interfere with the host's immune response to hepatitis B vaccines.

Plasma-derived and recombinant hepatitis B vaccines have been used for active immunization. The plasma-derived vaccine, Heptavax-B, is no longer distributed in the United States. Two recombinant hepatitis B vaccines are available: Recombivax HB and Engerix-B. These vaccines are prepared by insertion of a plasmid containing the HBsAg gene into common baker's yeast, followed by lysis of yeast cells after the intracellular production, assembly, and accumulation of HBsAg polypeptides. HBsAg is later separated from disrupted yeast cell components; less than 5% of the final product is yeast-derived protein. Recombivax HB contains 10 mcg of HBsAg protein per milliliter (a 40 mcg/mL product is available for use in selected adults), and Engerix-B contains 20 mcg/mL (790). A hepatitis A and hepatitis B combined vaccine (Twinrix) is available on the U.S. market, but it is only approved for use in persons 18 years of age or older.

The usual regimen for primary hepatitis B vaccination consists of three intramuscular doses given at 0, 1, and 6 months. The three-dose schedule induces a good antibody response in more than 90% of healthy adults and more than 95% of pediatric patients (newborn through 19 years of age). Hepatitis B vaccines have a protective efficacy of 80% to 95% when given to susceptible recipients. The duration of protection is unknown, but appears to persist even after anti-HBs is no longer detectable (790).

Susceptible pregnant women with accidental percutaneous or permucosal exposure to HBV-infected blood or who had sexual contact with a chronic HBV carrier or an acutely infected man should receive immunoprophylaxis. After exposure to HBV-contaminated blood, immunoprophylaxis should consist of two doses of HBIG (0.06 mL/kg given intramuscularly; maximum 5 mL). The first dose of HBIG should be given as soon as possible or within 24 hours of exposure; its effectiveness when given after 7 days of exposure is unknown. The second dose is given 1 month later. This regimen has not been specifically evaluated in pregnant women, but it is about 75% effective in preventing infection in healthy persons. If the physician decides to use the hepatitis B vaccine, which is the preferred approach, only one HBIG dose needs to be given. The vaccine should be administered intramuscularly at a site different from that used for HBIG, and the first dose can be given concomitantly with HBIG or within 7 days of exposure. For sexual HBV exposure, the prophylactic regimen is similar, except that immunization can begin within 14 days of the last sexual encounter (790).

Pregnancy is not a contraindication to hepatitis B vaccination. However, vaccine manufacturers advise against their use during pregnancy for liability reasons. Avoidance of vaccination in early pregnancy (i.e., period of embryogenesis) is recommended by some experts. No fetal or maternal risks from hepatitis B vaccination are known, and the limited available data suggest that its use in early or late pregnancy is safe (790–793).

Prevention of Perinatal Hepatitis B Virus Transmission

The CDC estimates that 22,000 births per year occur to HBsAg-positive women in the United States and, unless immunoprophylaxis is given at birth, about 6,000 of these newborns would become chronic HBV carriers (778). The administration of HBIG and the initiation of hepatitis B vaccination is 85% to 95% effective in preventing the development of the chronic carrier state in these infants (784).

The CDC initially recommended in 1984 that all high-risk women be screened for HBsAg during pregnancy. However, targeting women in high-risk groups identifies only about 35% to 65% of HBsAg carriers (794,795). The guidelines were later revised, and universal prenatal screening for HBsAg was recommended beginning in 1988 (796). All pregnant women should be routinely screened for HBsAg during an early prenatal visit. HBsAg-negative women at high risk of infection (e.g., those with other sexually transmitted diseases or illicit drug users) should be retested late in pregnancy. Screening of all pregnant women and reporting of the results to health care providers is not complete in many geographic areas, and perinatal screening for women whose HBsAg status is not known is not consistently practiced. This can lead to failure to identify HBsAg-positive women and to administer appropriate immunoprophylaxis to their newborns (797, 798). A year 2000 survey of birthing hospitals in 14 states showed that 96% of pregnant women were screened for HBsAg. Of 10,192 infants born to HBsAg-positive women, 90% had received HBIG and their first dose of the hepatitis B vaccine before discharge from the hospital (794).

Infants born to HBsAg-positive mothers should be bathed as soon as possible to remove HBV-infected blood and other secretions. Suctioning of the stomach contents, if needed, should be performed gently to avoid mucosal trauma that could promote HBV entry into the blood. Delivery by elective cesarean section has been advocated by some as a way to reduce maternal-to-infant HBV transmission; this approach is not recommended because of the lack of evidence to support the practice and because of the efficacy of immunoprophylaxis.

HBIG at a dose of 0.5 mL intramuscularly should be given as soon as possible after birth and no later than 12 hours of life. An HBIG dose given at 12 to 48 hours of life probably is effective, but this has not been proved. The first vaccine dose should be given within the first week of life, preferably within the first 12 hours, and at a different anatomic site; the intramuscular dose is 0.5 mL (5 mg of Recombivax HB or 10 mg of Engerix-B). Later doses are given at 1 and 6 months of age. For preterm infants with a birth weight less than 2000 grams, four vaccine doses are needed (0, 1, 2–3, and 6–7 months of age). Breast-feeding should be allowed for infants who have started immunoprophylaxis (799).

The CDC and the American Academy of Pediatrics (AAP) currently recommend universal hepatitis B vaccination of all infants, regardless of the maternal HBsAg status (794,799). Infants born to HBsAg-positive women are given HBIG and the vaccine as outlined earlier. Infants born to women admitted in labor and whose HBsAg status is unknown should receive the first dose of the vaccine within 12 hours of birth; maternal HBsAg testing should be immediately performed and, if positive, the infant should receive HBIG (0.5 mL) as soon as feasible after birth and no later than 7 days of age. Preterm infants weighing less than 2000 grams at birth should get both HBIG and their first dose of the hepatitis B vaccine by 12 hours of age. Household contacts and sex partners of HBsAg-positive women should be vaccinated against hepatitis B; prevaccination susceptibility testing should be done in adults whenever possible, but is not required in children because of low rates of HBV infection in that age group and the lower costs of smaller individual vaccine doses.

Infants born to HBsAg-negative mothers do not need HBIG administration. They can receive their first dose of vaccine at birth or within the first 2 months of life at routine health maintenance visits. Hepatitis B virus vaccines can be given concurrently but in different syringes with inactivated poliomyelitis, diphtheria-tetanus-pertussis, measles–mumps–rubella, and pneumococcal or *Haemophilus influenzae* type b conjugate vaccines. The use of hepatitis B-containing combination vaccines can begin at the age of 6 to 8 weeks (799).

A study from Taiwan of infants born to HBsAg-positive but HBeAg-negative mothers showed that those receiving both HBIG and the hepatitis B vaccine, as compared to newborns receiving hepatitis vaccine alone, were more likely to have protective anti-HBs titers at 2 months of age (98% vs. 57%, respectively) and their geometric mean titers of this antibody were higher. By 7 months of age, however, just as many infants receiving the hepatitis B vaccine alone had protective anti-HBs levels and the geometric mean titer of anti-HBs in this group was significantly higher than those receiving both HBIG and the vaccine (800). Another study from Italy of 522 children born to HBsAg-positive mothers from 1985 to 1994, and who had received HBIG and the hepatitis B vaccine at birth, found that 79% still had protective anti-HBs levels 5 to 14 years later (801).

Preterm infants generally will respond well to the hepatitis B vaccines if the first dose is given at 1 month of age or at hospital discharge. Anti-HBs titers tend to be lower than those elicited in vaccinated term infants. Very-low-birth-weight infants ($\leq 1,500$ g) who receive their first dose of vaccine within the first 72 hours of life are less likely to have protective anti-HBs levels after the third dose of the vaccine is given than infants of similar weight and gestation who receive their first vaccine dose at 1 month of age (802–805).

Infants who become chronic HBV carriers despite correct immunoprophylaxis may have been infected *in utero*, or their mothers may have had a high virus load or were infected with vaccine-escape virus mutants (801,806–808). Infants who fail immunoprophylaxis do not become HBsAg-positive until 6 to 9 months of age. Immunized infants born to HBsAg-positive mothers should be tested at the age of 9 months or later for HBsAg and anti-HBs. Those who test negative for both should receive a fourth vaccine dose and be tested again 1 month later, and infants found to be HBsAg-positive should be monitored closely to determine whether a chronic carrier state has developed (784).

The United States Public Health Service and the AAP recommended in July 1999 to defer the first dose of hepatitis B vaccine until the age of 2 to 6 months for infants born to mothers who were HBsAg-negative. This stemmed from concerns over mercury exposure contained in thimerosal, a vaccine preservative. Infants born to HBV carrier mother were to continue receiving HBIG and the hepatitis B vaccine as before. The restriction was lifted after preservative-free hepatitis B vaccine became available in September 1999. Hepatitis B vaccination of infants born to women with unknown HBsAg status declined precipitously after the recommendations were issued, but did not rebound to its baseline level until the cohort of infants born 7 to 12 months after the suspension was lifted (809–814). It is estimated that this brief and well-intentioned transient change in recommendations resulted in 750,000 fewer newborns getting vaccinated in 2000 as compared to 1998, and 182,000 children remaining undervaccinated for hepatitis B at 19 months of age (814).

Universal hepatitis B vaccination of newborns has been implemented in over 60% of countries worldwide (815). Dividends from these policies have already become apparent. In Taiwan, the incidence of hepatocellular carcinoma among children 6 to 14 years of age has decreased by 50% and the average mortality from fulminant hepatitis B in infants has declined by 68% (815,816). Other studies have shown that the prevalence of HBsAg among children decreased in Taiwan (10.5% to 1.7%), American Samoa (7.5% to 0%), and The Gambia (10.3% to 0.6%) after programs for universal infant hepatitis B vaccination were started (815,817). It is estimated that perinatal HBV infections in the United States decreased by about 75% between 1987 and 2000 based on existing vaccine coverage rates (794).

Three antiviral agents (alpha interferon, lamivudine, adefovir dipivoxil) are licensed at the present time for the treatment of chronic hepatitis B and numerous others (DNA vaccines, ribozymes, emtricitabine) are under development (818–820). Lamivudine, a nucleoside analogue that inhibits the RNA-dependent DNA polymerase of HBV, is a potent suppressor of HBV replication and leads to a 3 to 4 log reduction in HBV DNA level in a treated chronic carrier (763,818). Its chief limitation is the frequent emergence of lamivudine-resistant HBV strains, although these drug-resistant variants are thought to be less fit than their wild-type counterparts. The rate of resistance approaches 20%, 40%, and 67% after 1, 2, and 4 years of therapy, respectively (763). Lamivudine has been used during pregnancy to reduce maternal viremia in an effort to decrease the rate of perinatal HBV transmission (821,822). In one trial of 8 women with chronic hepatitis B, lamivudine was prescribed during the last month of pregnancy. Additionally, newborns received HBIG and hepatitis B vaccine. Maternal HBV DNA levels decreased with lamivudine treatment. One infant (12.5%) became a chronic hepatitis B carrier compared with 28% of a control group of infants who received immunoprophylaxis at birth but whose mothers did not receive lamivudine (822). The role, if any, of maternal antiviral therapy as a supplement to immunoprophylaxis for the prevention of perinatal HBV infection is unknown at present.

Hepatitis C

Hepatitis C is currently the most common chronic blood-borne infection in the United States. Antibodies to HCV are detected in about 1.8% of the US population, of whom 75% (over 2.7 million people) are believed to have chronic infection (823). Globally, chronic HCV infection afflicts more than 170 million people and was the cause of at least 20% of the 1.4 million deaths from chronic liver disease worldwide in 2001 (824).

HCV is an enveloped, single-stranded RNA virus whose genome encodes for both structural and nonstructural proteins. The structural proteins include two envelope proteins (E1 and E2), which contain neutralizing epitopes, a nucleocapsid core protein (C), and a small protein (P7) whose function is unknown. The nonstructural proteins are essential for viral multiplication and include a helicase (NS2), viral protease (NS3), RNA-dependent RNA polymerase (NS5B), and membrane-binding protein (NS5). There are at least nine known HCV genotypes, which are divided further into more than 90 subtypes; 70% of HCV-infected persons in the United States are infected with genotype 1 (with subtype 1a predominating). Genotypes 1 to 3 circulate in western countries and Asia, genotype 4 in the Middle East and Africa, genotype 5 in South Africa, and genotypes 6, 7, 8, and 9 in Southeast Asia. Viruses circulating within an individual may show nucleotide variability (quasispecies). Quasispecies arise as a result of ongoing host immune surveillance and mutations occurring during viral replication. Antibodies elicited by one virus type may not recognize another HCV type; therefore, patients are not protected against reinfection by either the same or different HCV genotypes. A consequence of the genetic diversity of HCV is its ability to escape host immune surveillance leading to a high rate (greater than 80%) of chronic infections (23,775,825,826).

Epidemiology

The highest incidence of acute HCV infection occurs in persons 20 to 39 years of age. There is great variation in the seroprevalence of HCV within the United States. The highest rates are found in persons with repeated or large percutaneous exposure to blood, such as injecting drug users (72% to 86%) or persons with hemophilia treated with products made before 1987 (74% to 90%). Lower rates are found in other groups, such as chronic hemodialysis patients (10%), persons receiving blood transfusions before 1990 (6%), and persons with a history of a sexually transmitted disease (6%) (23). Approximately 1% to 2% of pregnant women in the United States are positive for HCV antibodies, about 5% of whom pass the virus to their newborns (827).

HCV also can spread via organ transplantation from HCV-infected donors, tattoos, body piercing, sexual activity with an infected person, and nonsexual household contact (23,828). Intrauterine transfusion of HCV-infected blood was shown to be the source of maternal infection in one report (829). These sources account for a very small fraction of all HCV infections in the United States. Only 10% of patients have no identifiable source of infection (23,828). Although HCV RNA can be detected in breast milk from infected mothers (in lower amounts than in maternal serum), infection acquired through breastfeeding has not been documented definitively (830).

Clinical Manifestations

The incubation period of hepatitis C infection is 7 weeks on average, with a range of 2 to 30 weeks. Acute HCV is mostly asymptomatic. Jaundice is seen in 25%, and fulminant hepatitis is rare (825).

Most patients (85%) develop chronic HCV infection. Symptoms are vague and nonspecific (arthralgias, fatigue). Serum aminotransferase concentrations are either persistently or intermittently elevated, and tend to be lower during the third trimester only to return to their prepregnancy levels in the first 3 to 6 months postpartum (14). Aminotransferase concentrations correlate poorly with the degree of liver injury, but individuals with abnormal levels are more likely to have significant hepatic histologic abnormalities (61%) than those with persistently normal ALT levels (19%) (831). Extrahepatic manifestations include mixed cryoglobulinemia, glomerulonephritis, lichen planus, and porphyria cutanea tarda. Cirrhosis develops in as many as 20% within 10 to 20 years of infection. One to four percent of HCV-infected patients are at risk of developing hepatocellular carcinoma (825). Chronic hepatitis C infection does not seem to have adverse pregnancy outcomes such as increased rates of spontaneous abortion, gestational diabetes, or maternal hypertension, or lower birth weight of neonates (14).

Diagnosis

Serologic tests permit the detection of antibodies to HCV (anti-HCV) but do not allow differentiation among acute, chronic, or resolved infections. Two Food and Drug Administration-approved enzyme immunoassays and one enhanced chemiluminescence immunoassay are available in the United States for anti-HCV screening. Sensitivity of these tests is greater than 97% in high-prevalence populations, and the specificity is more than or equal to 99%. Positive results on screening immunoassays usually require confirmation with a supplemental test such as the recombinant immunoblot assay (RIBA) or nucleic acid tests, but this is seldom done by clinical laboratories. RIBA uses both HCV-encoded recombinant antigens and synthetic peptides and can be performed on the same serum sample screened for anti-HCV (832,833).

Very sensitive RNA detection tests are commercially available. Qualitative tests such as the reverse transcriptase PCR (RT-PCR) detect the presence of circulating HCV RNA. These tests are positive as early as 1 to 3 weeks after exposure. Their lower limit for detection is 50 IU/mL. Because some HCV-infected patients are only intermittently HCV RNA-positive, a single negative test result is not considered conclusive. False-positive and false-negative results can occur. Quantitative assays for measuring HCV RNA titers also are available from commercial laboratories. The two most commonly used assays are the quantitative RT-PCR (threshold of 500 viral genome copies per milliliter) and a branched DNA signal amplification assay (threshold of 200,000 genome equivalents per milliliter); both are less sensitive than the qualitative RT-PCR. Patients with chronic hepatitis C infection usually have from 10^5 to 10^7 genome copies per milliliter of circulating virus. The quantitative tests are mostly utilized to assess the response of chronically infected patients to antiviral therapy (23,825,832,833).

It is also possible to group HCV by genotype and subtype using commercially available assays that are not yet approved by the Food and Drug Administration. The clinical utility of these assays is limited at present to possibly altering the length of antiviral therapy, depending on a person's specific HCV genotype (23,832).

Treatment

The goals of treatment are to eradicate HCV and stem the progression of liver injury. Alpha interferons are the mainstay of therapy. These agents have antiviral, antiproliferative, and immunomodulatory effects. Attaching an inert polyethylene glycol (PEG) polymer to interferon leads to a molecule with a longer half-life. At present, the combination of peginterferon-α-2a or peginterferon-α-2b plus ribavirin is the treatment of choice for non-pregnant adults. The dosage and treatment duration depends primarily on the patient's genotype, with the shortest length of treatment (24 weeks) used for genotypes 2 or 3. The overall sustained virologic response is only about 56%, but some patients with good prognostic factors achieve responses of 80% to 95%. Ethnicity is a determinant of treatment outcome, even after adjustment for other factors affecting response to medications. Asians have the best response to therapy, and African Americans the worst. A good response to therapy is seen within 12 weeks (834–837).

Pregnant women with hepatitis C are rarely treated with antiviral agents. Ribavirin is teratogenic in animals. Interferon has not been shown to be teratogenic in humans or experimental animals, possibly because of its large molecular size which limits its ability to cross the placenta (837).

Susceptible HCV-infected women should be vaccinated against both hepatitis A and hepatitis B viruses after delivery of their infants. Superinfection by either virus may lead to a severe illness in HCV-infected persons.

Vertical Transmission

The risk of HCV infection for infants born to women with anti-HCV has been assessed in numerous studies (14,23,838–848). The average transmission rate for HCV-infected but HIV-negative women is 5%, with a range from 0% to 25%. The presence of HCV RNA in the mother at delivery is the most consistent factor associated with vertical transmission. Limited data suggest that women

with higher HCV RNA titers at delivery may be more likely to infect their newborns (14,23,849–852). Infants tend to have less HCV nucleotide variability than their mothers, thus suggesting that not all clones of a quasispecies are vertically transmitted. After several weeks, nucleotide variability in infants increases, but the evolution differs from what occurs in their mothers (852–858).

The average HCV infection rate for infants born to women coinfected with HIV-1 is higher and estimated at 19%, with a range from 5% to 36% (14,23,859). The delivery route (i.e., vaginal or by cesarean section) seems not to have an appreciable impact on the risk of HCV infection for infants. Elective, but not emergency, cesarean section may lower the rate of vertical HCV transmission, but the data are limited and not sufficient to recommend this route of delivery for HCV-infected women (14). Nevertheless, elective cesarean section may be partially protective for infants of HCV-infected women who are coinfected with HIV (860). The specific maternal HCV genotype does not affect the risk of vertical transmission. There is no increased risk of HCV transmission in subsequent pregnancies (861). Invasive procedures such as amniocentesis or fetal scalp monitoring have been examined as potential risk factors for HCV vertical transmission, but the data are inconclusive. They are best avoided unless definitely necessary (14).

Perinatal Management

Routine screening of all pregnant women for HCV infection currently is not recommended. Testing should be limited to women who have high-risk exposure histories. Examples of women for whom screening is suggested are those who are HIV-positive or HBsAg-positive, current or previous intravenous drug users, have current or past sexual partners known to have been intravenous drug users, have a history of transfusion of blood or blood products prior to 1992, were incarcerated, have undergone anonymous donor *in vitro* fertilization, have a history of body piercing or tattooing, have elevated serum aminotransferase levels, or are patients or employees at hemodialysis units (14,861).

Postexposure prophylaxis with immune globulin preparations or antiviral agents for infants born to HCV-infected mothers also is not recommended. Because passively acquired transplacental IgG antibodies against HCV can persist for several months, it is recommended that infants not be tested for anti-HCV before 18 months of age (23,827,861). If earlier diagnosis is desired, RT-PCR for HCV RNA can be performed after the first month of life and repeated at 6 months of age; HCV RNA detected in the first month of life may reflect only transient carriage (861,862). Cord blood should not be used for HCV diagnosis because of the potential for its contamination with maternal blood.

Infants and children found to be infected with HCV require periodic monitoring. Most remain asymptomatic, but half will be persistently viremic and an almost equal number of infants will have HCV RNA intermittently in their sera. Alanine aminotransferase values vary from normal to high. Liver biopsies performed within the first 10 years of life reveal minimal or moderate hepatic inflammation in 20% of perinatally-infected infants (863,864). However, a recent report of a 35-year follow-up of a cohort infected at birth with blood transfusions from a single donor with genotype 1b showed that 89% were HCV RNA-positive, but that the majority of those who underwent liver biopsies had either no or mild portal fibrosis (865,866).

Hepatitis D

Hepatitis D virus (HDV) is a defective RNA virus that causes disease only in persons infected with hepatitis B virus. It can occur as a co-infection with acute hepatitis B or as a superinfection in persons who are chronic HBV carriers. Persons co-infected with HBV and HDV are at high risk for chronic hepatitis, cirrhosis, and liver failure. Diagnosis is made by serologic assays for HDV-specific IgM and IgG. Perinatal transmission is possible, but rare. Measures aimed at prevention of hepatitis B virus infection are effective against HDV (749).

Hepatitis E

Hepatitis E virus (HEV), previously known as enterically transmitted non-A, non-B hepatitis, is a small RNA virus that is transmitted by the fecal-oral route. It causes a self-limited disease that resembles hepatitis A. There is no chronic carrier state associated with HEV infection. Genomic analysis shows that there are several geographically distinct strains of HEV (867).

HEV has caused large outbreaks of disease in India, Nepal, and China, and smaller ones in the Middle East, Africa, and Mexico. The highest attack rates during outbreaks occur among young adults. Pregnant women, especially those in their third trimester, have high mortality rates (15% to 25%). Sporadic HEV infections have been described in numerous countries including Egypt, Italy, Greece, and the United States (867). Seroprevalence studies have shown that HEV antibodies are detectable in as many as 37% in Nepal, 64% in India, 62% in Pakistan, 27% in Bangladesh, 38% in Vietnam, 8% in Nicaragua, 2.2% in Greece, 0.8% in southern Italy, and 0.4% in Ireland (868–872). Studies from the United States showed seroprevalence rates of 5.7% in Iowa and 21% in Baltimore, Maryland (873,874).

Outbreaks are generally related to the ingestion of fecally contaminated drinking water and often follow heavy rains and floods. Person-to-person transmission during outbreaks is uncommon (867). Zoonotic reservoirs (deer, sheep, cows, rodents) for HEV are suspected (872,875,876). In the United States, domestic swine may be the reservoir for HEV (872).

The incubation period is 2 to 10 weeks. Diagnosis of HEV infection is made by detection of HEV-specific IgM in serum or by finding HEV RNA in serum or stools. IgM antibodies disappear after a few months, but specific IgG antibodies can persist for several years (867).

It is not known why pregnant women are at such high risk for death from acute HEV infection. Fulminant hepatitis did not develop in pregnant rhesus monkeys or swine experimentally inoculated with HEV (877).

Vertical transmission of HEV is known to occur at rates of 50% to 100% (878–880). Infected infants can develop either icteric or anicteric hepatitis. Others may suffer from hypothermia and hypoglycemia, and can die within 24 to 48 hours of birth (878,879).

Treatment is supportive. Passive immunoprophylaxis with immune globulin prepared in the United States in not effective. Prevention is best accomplished by use of clean drinking water and proper sanitation (867).

Hepatitis G

Hepatitis G virus (HGV), also known as hepatitis GB virus (GBV-C), is an RNA virus that causes persistent human infection, but no known disease. It appears to be transmitted by blood or blood products, and by sexual contact with infected persons. Vertical transmission occurs in as many as 90%. HGV is associated with decreased mortality among patients co-infected with HIV. The virus appears to replicate in lymphocytes, but not hepatocytes. Its incubation period is not known. Treatment is neither available nor indicated (845,881).

Transfusion-Transmissible Virus

Transfusion-transmissible virus (TTV) is a non-enveloped single stranded DNA virus that has also been associated with posttransfusion hepatitis. Like HGV, it is a virus that causes persistent infection, but no known disease. TTV DNA can be found circulating in the blood of a high percentage (37%–90%) of healthy individuals, but the likelihood of detecting it is higher in those with a history of blood transfusions. Its presence is not associated with liver damage, even in patients who are carriers of HBV or HCV (882,883).

TTV has also been found in feces, saliva, breast milk, and in the cervices of pregnant women. In one study of 100 pregnant Chinese women without a history of blood transfusions, TTV DNA was detected in 66% of the cervical samples (884). Although vertical transmission does occur, it appears that infants are more likely to acquire TTV postnatally. TTV infection becomes persistent in most infants, but without evidence of liver impairment (885–887).

LYMPHOCYTIC CHORIOMENINGITIS VIRUS

Human infections by lymphocytic choriomeningitis virus (LCMV) have been recognized since 1933. LCMV is an RNA virus that belongs to the family Arenaviridae, and its reservoir in nature is rodents such as mice and hamsters. Pregnant wild mice that become viremic can transmit LCMV transplacentally. Mice infected *in utero* are unable to mount an effective immune response to the virus and they remain asymptomatically infected. LCMV is shed in their nasal secretions, saliva, milk, urine, semen, and feces. Horizontal transmission to other rodents such as hamsters further spreads the virus. Humans acquire LCMV by inhaling aerosolized virus or by direct contact with contaminated fomites (888). Although arenaviruses are generally not very pathogenic for rodents, they are capable of causing serious or fatal infections such as aseptic meningitis, liver disease, and hemorrhagic fever in humans, primates, and guinea pigs (888–890).

LCMV infections of humans are asymptomatic or mild in about a third of individuals. Half the symptomatic patients have aseptic meningitis or meningoencephalitis. The typical LCMV infection is biphasic with an initial illness consisting of fever, malaise, headache, photophobia, sore throat, emesis, and cough, followed by defervescence and resolution of symptoms, with subsequent development of CNS symptoms. Mononuclear CSF pleocytosis is noted on the lumbar puncture. Complications of LCMV can include eighth nerve deafness, transverse myelitis, hydrocephalus, Guillain-Barré syndrome, pneumonia, myocarditis, parotitis, and dermatitis. Contact with rodents raises the index of suspicion for LCMV infection. The diagnosis can be established by isolating the virus or by using PCR (serum, CSF), but serologic methods (ELISA, IFA, complement fixation) that detect LCMV-specific IgG and IgM antibodies are generally employed (888,891).

There have been over 50 published cases of congenital LCMV infections from diverse geographic areas, including the United States. Chorioretinitis is the most common findings in infected infants, with peripheral chorioretinal scars next in frequency. Other ocular abnormalities include optic atrophy, nystagmus, conjunctivitis, esotropia, microphthalmos, and cataract. About 40% of the infants are microcephalic, and a third are macrocephalic. Neuroimaging studies reveal hydrocephalus or intracranial calcifications in the majority of affected infants. Other abnormalities such as hearing loss, hepatosplenomegaly, or thrombocytopenia are occasionally noted. Long-term neurologic deficits such as mental retardation, seizures, or decreased visual acuity are expected in the majority. There is no available therapy for LCMV-infected infants, but ribavirin has been used for other arenavirus infections (888,891,892).

WEST NILE VIRUS

West Nile virus (WNV) was first isolated from an infected woman in 1937 in the West Nile district of Uganda, and has since been found to be a fairly common human pathogen in Africa, the Middle East, Asia, Australia, and temperate areas of Europe (893,894). The first documented cases of WNV encephalitis were in New York City in 1952 when patients with advanced malignancies were experimentally inoculated with an Egyptian strain of this virus for its possible oncolytic effect (895). Naturally acquired WNV was initially recognized in North America

in August 1999 when an unusual cluster of cases of meningoencephalitis and muscle weakness in New York City was carefully investigated (896). The virus has since spread throughout much of the United States, and cases in Canada and the Caribbean region have been diagnosed (895,897,898). The number of human WNV infections reported to the CDC peaked at 9,122 (with 223 deaths) in 2003; 2,313 cases (with 79 deaths) were reported for the following year through November 16, 2004 (895,898). Outbreaks of WNV have been described for many countries, including Romania, Russia, Israel, South Africa, and the United States (898).

WNV is a single-stranded RNA virus of the family Flaviviridae, genus Flavirus. It is classified within the Japanese encephalitis virus antigenic complex, which also includes other human pathogens such Japanese encephalitis, Murray Valley encephalitis, Kunjin, and St. Louis encephalitis viruses (899,900). Mosquitoes (primarily *Culex* species) serve as the vector for WNV although birds are the most common amplifying hosts (893,899). Infected birds usually survive WNV infection and become immune, but the infections can be virulent in crows and jays. The virus can be recovered from the oral secretions and feces of birds, and bird-to-bird transmission can occur in the laboratory in the absence of mosquitoes (900). Most vertebrates are susceptible to WNV, and natural infection has been demonstrated in humans, horses, skunks, cats, rabbits, squirrels, chipmunks, and a few bat species (899). The WNV strains isolated in New York in 1999 are most closely related to an isolate obtained from the brain of a dead Chilean flamingo in Israel in 1998, but how this virus was imported into the United States in not known (901).

Human infections are the result of mosquito bites, usually in the summer and early fall (899). Other modes of transmission to humans have also been recognized since the appearance of WNV in the United States. These include intrauterine transmission from mother to fetus, transfusion of blood or blood products, breast feeding, percutaneous inoculation among laboratory workers, receiving an organ-transplant from a viremic donor, and possibly hemodialysis (900,902).

The incubation period is from 2 to 14 days, but can be as long as 21 days after organ transplantation (900). Most infections are asymptomatic (894). In the 1999 New York City outbreak, about 2.6% of the population at the outbreak's epicenter became infected, but only a fifth had exhibited symptoms consisting of mild febrile illnesses (903). The typical WNV illness is mild and lasts 3 to 6 days. Symptoms have a sudden onset, and include fever (usually >39°C), malaise, anorexia, nausea, vomiting, eye pain, headache, myalgias, and rash (899,900). Only about 1 in 150 WNV infections result in meningitis or meningoencephalitis (894). Muscle weakness is common in WNV encephalitis. Other neurologic manifestations encompass poliomyelitis-like acute flaccid paralysis, optic neuritis, cranial nerve abnormalities, seizures, tremor, myoclonus, and parkinsonism (900,904–907). Case-fatality rates of 4% to

18% have been observed among hospitalized patients, with advanced age proving to be the most important risk factor. Persistent abnormalities such as fatigue, memory loss, gait problems, depression, and muscle weakness are common one year after recovery from acute WNV encephalitis (894).

Definitive diagnosis requires the detection of IgM antibodies in serum or CSF using the IgM antibody-capture enzyme-linked immunosorbent assay. CSF IgM is positive by the third to fifth day of the illness, and at least 3 days before serum IgM is detectable. Serum IgG usually appears about 5 days after WNV-specific IgM is detectable (895). False-positive IgM results may be seen in recent recipients of the yellow fever or Japanese encephalitis virus vaccines or persons recently infected with another flavivirus such as St. Louis encephalitis or dengue virus. Plaque reduction neutralization assays can help distinguish cross-reactions from true WNV infection. WNV IgM can be detectable in the blood of most patients for over a year, and this can complicate interpretation of test results. A fourfold or greater increase in WNV-specific neutralizing antibody titers in acute and convalescent phase serum samples confirms acute infection. Viral cultures or detection of WNV RNA in serum and CSF can be helpful, but the sensitivity of these tests is low because of the low magnitude and transient nature of the viremia (894,900,908). Nucleic acid amplification tests in serum and CSF are usually negative by 3 to 5 days of illness (895). WNV nucleic acid amplification tests have been used to screen donated blood in the United States since June 2003 (900,909).

Treatment of WNV infection is supportive. A variety of agents such as ribavirin, interferon-α2b, and steroids have been tried, but none in a controlled trial (900). An intravenous gammaglobulin preparation with high WNV antibody titers obtained from healthy Israeli blood donors was effective both prophylactically and therapeutically in experimentally-infected mice and in anecdotal reports of human infection (895,910). The product is currently being evaluated in human trials in the United States. An inactivated WNV vaccine is available for horses, but not yet for humans. Prevention is best accomplished by applying insect repellents on skin and clothes, draining standing water in which mosquitoes may breed, and avoiding being outdoors during peak mosquito feeding times at dawn and dusk (900,911).

The CDC is compiling data on pregnancy outcomes of over 70 women with WNV infection during pregnancy. In 2002, four cases of WNV infection during pregnancy were investigated. Three infants were born at term and were normal and had no laboratory evidence of WNV infection (911). A fourth infant was delivered at 38 weeks gestation after the 20-year-old mother developed WNV encephalitis at 27 weeks of gestation. The infant had chorioretinal scars and severe white matter loss in the temporal and occipital lobes on brain neuroimaging studies. The infant had positive WNV-specific IgM in the serum and CSF, but the lumbar puncture was traumatic. Nucleic acid amplification assays did not yield consistent results when placental and umbilical cord tissues were tested (912,913). Another infant was delivered at 32 weeks gestation after her mother developed WNV encephalitis at week 16 of gestation. The infant had low birth weight, but no attempt was made to diagnose fetal WNV infection (914).

Probable WNV transmission through breast milk was demonstrated after a woman in Michigan received transfusions in the immediate postpartum period that were later shown to harbor WNV. She developed WNV meningoencephalitis 12 days after delivery. Her breast milk on postpartum day 16 was positive for WNV by nucleic acid amplification methods, and for WNV-specific IgG and IgM. Her term infant had started breast-feeding within a few hours of birth and remained well. However, a serum sample from the infant at 25 days of age was positive for WNV-specific IgM. The infant had minimal outdoor exposures and no known mosquito bites (915). This case was not considered sufficient by the CDC to restrict breast-feeding for women infected with WNV.

The CDC does not recommend screening of pregnant women for WNV infection. Women diagnosed with WNV encephalitis during pregnancy should have a fetal ultrasound within 2 to 4 weeks of disease onset. Amniotic fluid, chorionic villi, or fetal serum can be tested for WNV infection but the sensitivities and specificities of these tests are not established. Infants born to infected women should be examined carefully, and have their sera tested for WNV-specific IgG and IgM. If clinical or serologic evidence of neonatal infection is found, an ophthalmologic examination, lumbar puncture, and CT scan of the brain should be performed. Histopathologic examination and testing for WNV RNA should be done, if available. Hearing screens at birth and again at six months are also encouraged (911).

HUMAN IMMUNODEFICIENCY VIRUS TYPE 1 INFECTION

The global impact of HIV-1 infection is staggering. The WHO has estimated that, as of the end of 2003, approximately 37.8 million people were living with HIV-1 around the world, two thirds of whom resided in Africa. Approximately 20 million people have died of AIDS since the start of the AIDS pandemic. In 2003 alone, 4.8 million people were newly infected with HIV-1, and 2.9 million others died of AIDS. About 1.1% of all persons between 15 and 49 years of age worldwide are now infected with this virus. In some African countries such as Botswana, 37% of adults are HIV-positive (916).

In the United States, the estimated number of persons diagnosed with AIDS between the start of the epidemic and the end of 2002 is 886,575, of whom 501,669 have died (917). About 950,000 people are currently living with HIV-1 in the United States (916). Females account for 29% of persons 13 years of age or older with HIV-1 infection, 66% of whom are African American and 10% Hispanic (918).

There were between 520,000 and 680,000 HIV-1-infected people living in western Europe at the end of 2003. Since the recognition of AIDS, about 259,000 persons had been diagnosed with this condition as of the end of June 2003, of whom 152,000 had died (919).

The region hardest hit is sub-Saharan Africa where most HIV-1-infected persons are found. The median HIV-1 seroprevalence among women attending antenatal clinics there was about 24% in 2002. The highest rates are found in southern African countries such as Botswana, Lesotho, Zimbabwe, Swaziland, and South Africa (920). South Africa, with a total population of about 44 million people, has 5.3 million HIV-1-infected persons living there (916, 920).

Asian countries such as China, Vietnam, and Indonesia are currently experiencing a growing HIV-1 epidemic, largely driven by sex workers and injecting drug use (921). Estimates place the number of people living with HIV-1 at 570,000 in Thailand, 330,000 in Myanmar, and 220,000 in Vietnam. Imprecise estimates suggest that between 430,000 to 1.5 million Chinese are HIV-infected, and that between 2.2 million to 7.6 million individuals in India are HIV-positive (916).

More than 2 million HIV-infected women around the world give birth each year, and 630,000 infants acquire the virus from their mothers. For 2003 alone, the World Health Organization estimates that about 490,000 children 15 years of age or younger died of AIDS, 90% of whom were from sub-Saharan Africa. AIDS as of the end of 2003 had orphaned at least 12 million children in sub-Saharan Africa (916).

There were 9,300 pediatric (children <13 years of age) AIDS cases diagnosed in the United States through the end of 2002. This accounted for 1% of the 886,575 total AIDS cases reported to the CDC between the start of the epidemic and the end of 2002. Perinatal acquisition of HIV-1 was responsible for 8,629 (93%) of these infections. The major maternal risk factors for perinatal HIV-1 infection were injection drug use (38%), having sex with an injection drug user (17%), sex with an HIV-infected person whose risk status is unspecified (17%), sex with a bisexual male (2%), sex with a person with hemophilia (0.4%), and receipt of blood or blood product transfusions (1.8%). The risk factors are not known for 22% of all mothers of children with AIDS (917). Between 1999 and 2002, heterosexual transmission accounted for 64% of all new HIV-1 infections among females 13 years of age or older; 89% of all heterosexually acquired HIV-1 infections in persons 13 to 19 years of age were female (922).

A disproportionate number of children with perinatal AIDS in the United States have been African American (59%) or Hispanic (23%). White children have accounted for 17% of the cumulative number of cases through 2002. With the success of programs for the interruption of mother-to-infant transmission of HIV-1 and the availability of improved antiretroviral drug regimens for HIV-1-infected children, the number of children diagnosed with AIDS in the United States has steadily declined from 952 in 1992 to a low of 92 in 2002. About 55% of all children 13 years of age or younger diagnosed with AIDS since the start of the epidemic have died (917).

HIV-1 is one of several known human retroviruses. It is a single stranded, enveloped RNA virus that is composed of inner core proteins (p18, p24, p27), surface proteins (gp120, gp41), genomic RNA, and enzymes such as reverse transcriptase and protease. The virion contains three structural genes (*gag*, *pol*, and *env*) and regulatory genes (*tat*, *vif*, *nef*, *vpu*, *vpr*, and *rev*). HIV-1 requires a cell-surface glycoprotein known as CD4 for viral entry into cells. CD4 is found on the subset of T lymphocytes referred to as helper T cells, and on macrophages and other cell types (e.g., placenta, CNS cells). Other cell surface molecules (chemokine receptors) serve as co-receptors for HIV-1 entry into cells. Genetic variants of HIV-1 may preferentially bind to different co-receptors. For example, HIV-1 variants that induce syncytium formation depend on the receptor molecule CXCR4, whereas the nonsyncytium-inducing variants use CCR5 co-receptors. The density of receptors on cells, and the relative densities of co-receptors and CD4 in membrane microdomains, are major determinants of infection (923–926). The absence of CCR5 in about 1% of Caucasians, as a result of homozygosity for a 32-nucleotide deletion in the coding region (*CCR5D32* allele), protects against HIV-1 transmission and delays disease progression (927). Other chemokine receptors such as CCR-2b, CCR-3, and CCR-8 are used by HIV-1 as well (925,928). Patients considered to be long-term non-progressors also tend to have lower amounts of circulating HIV-1 RNA, and their activated CD8 lymphocytes may help suppress viral replication through the release of inhibitory chemokines such as RANTES, MIP-1a, and MIP-1b (925).

Although HIV-1 infects a relatively small number of $CD4^+$ T lymphocytes, there is gradual but massive depletion of these cells over time. This renders patients susceptible to a variety of opportunistic infections and malignancies. Studies have suggested that HIV-1 gp120-induced intracellular activation plays a role in inducing apoptosis of uninfected cells as well (926).

Antibody responses to HIV-1 show only weak neutralizing activities against primary HIV-1 isolates. Most of the antibodies produced are non-neutralizing and directed against virion debris. Neutralizing antibodies do not have much impact on HIV-1 replication, but they do exert immune selection pressure. For control of HIV infection, virus-specific $CD8^+$ cytotoxic T lymphocytes (CTL) are pivotal. These cells can be found in a variety of locations including peripheral blood, spleen, lymph nodes, skin, and bronchoalveolar spaces. CTL lyse HIV-1-infected cells and interfere with virus multiplication. However, HIV-1 replication is error-prone and this allows evasion from virus-specific CTL (929,930).

Major strides have been made in the prevention of perinatal HIV-1 infection in the last decade. The most crucial has been the demonstration that the risk of vertical transmission can be reduced significantly by administration of zidovudine during pregnancy, at delivery, and to newborns (931).

As a result, the CDC recommended use of zidovudine to reduce perinatal transmission of the virus (932). Numerous studies followed and showed the feasibility of using alternative regimens of zidovudine, or of other drugs such as nevirapine, to prevent vertical HIV-1 transmission (933). Use of PCR assays has allowed the diagnosis of HIV-1 infection early in infancy, and the availability of antiviral drugs active at various sites in the viral replication cycle has allowed more potent drug combinations to be administered to infected patients. Viral load monitoring now provides a measure of how successful a therapeutic regimen is in suppressing viral replication for an individual patient, and HIV-1 strains can be examined for mutations associated with resistance to specific antiretroviral agents (934–938).

Maternal Infection

Epidemiology

Female adults or adolescents have accounted for 18% of all AIDS cases reported to the CDC through 2002. However, the proportion of women among persons newly diagnosed with AIDS has risen to 25% for the years 1998 through 2002. Heterosexual contact with a high risk person was the route of infection for more than half of these women (917). AIDS incidence and deaths have declined since the mid-1990s across all racial and ethnic groups (918). Of women who were living with AIDS at the end of 2002, 59% were African American and 19% were Hispanic (917). HIV-1 seroprevalence among women of childbearing age varies by state. It ranges from a low of about 0 per 1,000 in Wyoming to highs of 6.9 and 5.2 per 1,000 for the District of Columbia and New York State, respectively. Seroprevalence rates for African American women are 15- to 20-fold higher than for white women, with intermediate rates noted for Hispanic women (939). The risks of HIV-1 infection grow as the number of high-risk behaviors practiced increases. Such behaviors encompass the use of crack cocaine, multiple sexual partners, sexual intercourse with a high-risk partner, having other sexually transmitted diseases, and low level of condom use (940–942).

HIV-1 screening programs targeted at patients who acknowledge high-risk behavior generally fail to identify most HIV-1-infected pregnant women (943,944). It is currently recommended that screening be offered to all pregnant women (4). With proper education, the majority of women offered antenatal HIV-1 testing agree to getting screened for this virus (945,946). It has been suggested that in high-risk populations, pregnant women who were initially HIV-1-negative should be screened again during the third trimester (947). However, 15% of HIV-infected women receive no or minimal prenatal care, and another 20% do not seek care until the third trimester (4). Rapid testing for HIV-1 antibodies for women in labor has been evaluated. These tests take about 20 minutes to perform and can provide results within 45 to 120 minutes of blood collection, thus allowing the identification of HIV-1-

infected women and instituting intrapartum and postpartum zidovudine prophylaxis (948,949). With nondirective counseling about options for terminating or continuing pregnancy, 85% of HIV-1–infected women elect to continue their pregnancies (943,950).

Many studies have examined the effects of HIV-1 infection on pregnancy outcome, and most have found no significant effects of the virus *per se*. Adverse pregnancy outcomes were common in a cohort of 634 HIV-1–infected women who delivered after 24 weeks of gestation. These included preterm birth (20%), low birth weight (19%), and small-for-gestational age newborns (24%) (951). Comparable outcomes have been described in other studies, especially those conducted in resource-poor countries (952). With the increased cesarean delivery rates for HIV-infected women, a rise in postpartum and post-cesarean section complications has been observed (952). Maternal HIV-1 infection may increase the rate of spontaneous fetal loss, but this has not been a consistent finding (924, 953,954). Pregnancy itself has a marginal effect, if any, on accelerating the progression of HIV-1 infection in women (924,955–958). In one study of 160 HIV-1–infected women, HIV-1 RNA viral loads did not change significantly during the pregnancy (957).

Mother-to-Infant Transmission

Vertical transmission of HIV-1 can occur *in utero*, intrapartum, or postpartum (through breast-feeding). Most infants in the United States acquire HIV-1 infection at the time of delivery (959).

Intrauterine transmission accounts for about 30% of all vertically infected infants, and about two thirds of these occur during the last two weeks before delivery (4). Second-trimester fetal blood sampling performed on HIV-1-infected women scheduled for elective pregnancy termination has confirmed the low rate of early *in utero* HIV-1 fetal infections (960,961).

Many studies have examined maternal and obstetric factors that increase the risk of vertical HIV-1 transmission. Not all risk factors have been consistently identified as such in every study, but there are definite patterns that have been observed. Maternal factors that enhance the risk of HIV-1 transmission to infants include advanced stage of maternal infection, low CD4$^+$ absolute cell count or percentage, elevated CD8$^+$ cell count or percentage, high viral load, p24 antigenemia, illicit drug use, co-infection by other sexually transmitted diseases, low titers or avidity of maternal HIV-1 antibodies, and infection by certain HIV-1 genotypes or phenotypes. Maternal vitamin A deficiency is a risk factor for vertical HIV-1 transmission in developing countries. Obstetric factors favoring HIV-1 vertical transmission include premature delivery, vaginal delivery, cervicovaginal HIV-1 viral load, maternofetal blood transfusions, longer (more than 4 hours) durations of membrane rupture, chorioamnionitis, and use of invasive fetal monitoring devices (959,962–974). Maternal plasma HIV-1 viral load is the strongest single predictor of mother-to-child transmission (974). For twins born to HIV-1–infected mothers, the first infant delivered, whether vaginally or by cesarean section, appears to be at least twice as likely to be infected as the second-born twin (975). This may be as a result of more intense exposure of the first born to HIV-1-infected genital secretions. de Martino and associates could not confirm these observations in their studies of twins born to HIV-1–infected mothers. They did observe that, if the first-born twin became infected, 42% of their second-born siblings were infected as well. If the first-born twin escaped HIV-1 infection, only 13% of the second-born siblings got infected (976).

An infant is considered to have early (i.e., *in utero*) infection if the HIV-1 genome is detected by PCR or if HIV-1 is isolated from blood within 48 hours of birth. Positive results should be confirmed with at least one sample obtained after the neonatal period. An infant is considered to have late (i.e., intrapartum) infection if diagnostic studies (e.g., HIV-1 isolation, PCR, serum p24 antigen assays) are negative in blood samples obtained during the first week of life but become positive during the period from day 7 to 90, and the infant has not been breast-fed. Care should be exercised to avoid contaminating cord blood with maternal blood (977).

In the United States, breast-feeding of infants by infected mothers is not recommended. Postnatal HIV-1 transmission rates by breast-feeding are 8% to 18%, but can be as high as 13% to 39% (mean 26%) when mothers acquire their HIV-1 infection while lactating (978,979). Several factors have been associated with higher rates of transmission through breast milk: RNA viral load in milk or plasma, low maternal CD4$^+$ count, breast pathology (mastitis, cracked nipples, abscess), and duration of breast feeding. Because HIV-1 transmission can occur at any time during lactation, longer durations of breast feeding increase the overall risk for HIV-1 infections of infants (979). Both HIV-1–infected cells and cell-free virus are found in breast milk (978–981). Cell-free virus more commonly is found in mature milk than in colostrum (980). The PCR assay can detect HIV-1 RNA in whole milk or its components (breast milk cells, skim milk, lipid fractions), but the sensitivity appears greatest when whole breast milk is used for testing (981,982). After ingestion of infected breast milk, the virus can be transmitted to the infant through gut mucosal surfaces or tonsillar tissues (979).

In 1998, the WHO recommended that HIV-1–infected women in developing countries be provided information about the benefits and risks of breast-feeding so that they can make an informed decision regarding nutrition for their infants. A study of 371 infants born to HIV-1-infected mothers in Nairobi, Kenya, and randomized to breast- or bottle-feeding revealed comparable two-year mortality rates, even after adjusting for HIV-1 status. Both groups had similar rates of diarrhea or pneumonia during their first two years of life. HIV-1–infected infants had a ninefold higher risk of dying by the age of two years when compared to HIV-1-uninfected infants (983).

Vertical HIV-1 transmission has been reported to occur at various rates in different areas of the world. A report by the 19-center European Collaborative Study provided a rate of 14.4% among a cohort of 721 children followed for 18 months or longer (984). A similar rate of 14% to 20% was observed in a nationwide study of a cohort of 286 children born to HIV-1–positive mothers in Switzerland (985). The rate is about 25% to 30% in the United States for women not receiving zidovudine prophylaxis (931, 986). Rates as high as 50% have been reported from African countries such as Zaire and Kenya (987).

Multiple HIV-1 variants exist in infected persons. These variants arise through errors in reverse transcription and by recombination during retroviral replication. Because of the high turnover rate in the HIV-1 population (more than 10 billion virions are generated daily) and the high error frequency during replication, a large number of variants is produced. These variants subsequently undergo selective pressure from cellular tropism, host immune responses, and antiretroviral therapy. Only a small subset of the HIV-1 variants is transmitted from the mother to her infant, but it can include HIV-1 strains that carry specific drug-resistance mutations (988–993). In one study of the first viral isolate from a cohort of 91 HIV-1-infected infants born in New York in 1998 and 1999, 12.1% were shown to harbor zidovudine-resistance mutations (994). There are also concerns that pregnant women with zidovudine resistant HIV-1 strains may transmit the virus more readily to their offspring (993).

Treatment

Women should receive antiretroviral therapy appropriate for their stage of infection without regard to whether or not they are pregnant. Highly active antiretroviral therapy (HAART) is recommended for pregnant women with HIV-1 RNA levels greater than 1,000 copies/mL. However, most experts are of the opinion that HIV-1-infected pregnant women should be treated with potent antiretroviral drugs regardless of their CD4$^+$ count or viral load because of the possibility of vertical transmission, even at relatively low HIV-1 RNA levels (4,995,996). In a review of several European and US prospective studies, Ioannidis and colleagues found 44 instances of HIV-1 transmission from mother to infant among 1,202 pregnant women whose viral load at delivery or one measured closest to delivery was less than 1,000 RNA copies/mL, and observed a 1% transmission rate among treated women compared to 9.8% for the untreated mothers (997). The downside of such a recommendation includes the potential teratogenicity of some of the medications and the risk for emergence of drug-resistant HIV-1 strains, especially among women who do not adhere adequately to the treatment regimen. Circulating resistant strains would impact future treatments for mothers and their infected infants. Women who are in their first trimester of pregnancy and who are not already receiving antiretroviral agents may consider delaying initiation of therapy until after 10 to 12 weeks of gestation (4,995,996). HIV-1–infected women who are already on antiretroviral agents when they become pregnant can expect their HIV-1 viral load to increase, and their CD4$^+$ count to decrease, should they choose to discontinue their medications during the first trimester (998).

At least 20 different drugs have been approved by the Food and Drug Administration for the treatment of adults with HIV-1 infection, but data on their safety in pregnant women is limited for most of these agents (Table 48-6). These antiretrovirals act by inhibiting viral reverse transcriptase or protease, or by interfering with gp41-mediated fusion. Fixed combinations of certain drugs are available in the United States (e.g., zidovudine-lamivudine, emtricitabine-tenofovir disoproxil fumarate) and of others in countries such as India.

Some antiretroviral agents such as zalcitabine, efavirenz, and delavirdine should not be used because of their significant teratogenic potential. Insufficient data exist for tenofovir, amprenavir, fosamprenavir, atazanavir, and enfurvitide to recommend their use in pregnant women. The recommended drugs are zidovudine, lamivudine, nevirapine, nelfinavir, and the saquinavir-ritonavir combination. The remaining medications listed in Table 48-6 are considered alternate agents that can be used when needed (999,1000).

It has been suggested that the use of combination antiretroviral therapy in pregnancy may be associated with preterm birth, but the data are inconclusive. Nevirapine-induced hepatic toxicity associated with rash has been observed in persons on chronic treatment with this medication, but not in those receiving the two-dose regimen for prevention of perinatal HIV-1 transmission. Nucleoside analogues interfere with mitochondrial replication by inhibiting γ DNA polymerase, resulting in mitochondrial DNA depletion and dysfunction. The most potent of these nucleoside analogues is zalcitabine, followed by didanosine, stavudine, zidovudine, lamivudine, abacavir, and tenofovir. Mitochondrial dysfunction can manifest with neuropathy, myopathy, pancreatitis, hepatic steatosis, and lactic acidosis. The frequency of lactic acidosis with microvascular hepatic steatosis in pregnant HIV-1-infected women treated with these drugs is not known, but it has been described in a few infants with intrauterine or neonatal exposures to these drugs (1000).

Zidovudine was the first antiretroviral agent shown to reduce the risk of perinatal HIV-1 transmission. The safety and efficacy of zidovudine as a chemoprophylactic agent against the vertical transmission of HIV-1 was demonstrated in a double-blind, placebo-controlled trial known as the Pediatric AIDS Clinical Trials Group (PACTG) Protocol 076 (931,1000). Pregnant women who were HIV-1 positive and whose CD4$^+$ T-lymphocyte counts were higher than 200 cells per cubic millimeter were enrolled if they had no other indication for antiretroviral therapy and were between 14 and 34 weeks of gestation. Zidovudine (or matching placebo) was given antenatally at a dose of 100 mg orally five times daily followed by intravenous zidovudine during labor (2 mg/kg of body weight given over 1 hour, followed by 1 mg/kg/h until delivery). The

newborns received zidovudine at a dose of 2 mg/kg orally every 6 hours beginning at 8 to 12 hours of age, and this was continued for 6 weeks. The final analysis of this study included 402 mother–infant pairs. The rate of HIV-1 transmission was 7.6% (95% CI of 4.3%–12.3%) with zidovudine treatment and 22.6% (95% CI of 17%–29%) with placebo. The difference was very significant statistically (1001). The study noted that women in the placebo group with large viral burdens were more likely to transmit HIV-1 to their newborns (41% risk for those with more than 15,700 HIV-1 RNA copies per milliliter using the RT-PCR assay or more than 7,530 HIV-1 RNA copies per milliliter using a second-generation branched-chain DNA signal amplification assay). The rate of transmission in the zidovudine-treated cohort was lower than that for the placebo group for women with comparable HIV-1 RNA viral load measurements. Interestingly, the reduced vertical transmission noted with zidovudine was found not be as a result of a reduction of viral RNA from baseline to delivery (1001).

After the results of PACTG 076 became available, zidovudine use during pregnancy and in newborns has steadily increased (946,1002). Several studies have confirmed that pregnant women receiving zidovudine are less likely to transmit HIV-1 to their offspring (1002–1007). A prospective trial (PACTG 185) evaluated pregnant women with advanced HIV-1 infection and low CD4$^+$ count who were already on antiretroviral therapy, a quarter of whom had previously been treated with zidovudine. These women received the same zidovudine regimen used in PACTG 076, plus either standard intravenous immunoglobulin or a hyperimmune HIV-1 immunoglobulin. Although the advantage of one immunoglobulin preparation over the other could not be established, PACTG 185 demonstrated the efficacy of zidovudine for women with advanced disease and low CD4$^+$ count (1007). Further reductions of perinatal HIV-1 transmission rates are possible with the addition of either lamivudine to the maternal and infant zidovudine regimen, or protease inhibitors to the maternal treatment regimen (1000).

The New York State Department of Health examined the risks of perinatal HIV-1 transmission for 939 exposed infants whose mothers received abbreviated zidovudine treatment regimens during pregnancy. The study found that the risk of HIV-1 infection for infants whose mothers received no zidovudine was 26.6% (95% CI of 21.1%–32.7%). When treatment was started antenatally, the risk of perinatal HIV-1 transmission dropped to 6.1% (95% CI of 4.1%–8.9%). When zidovudine was started intrapartum, the rate increased to 10% (95% CI of 3.3%–21.8%), and when it was started within the first 48 hours of life or at 72 hours of age or later, the rates were 9.3% (95% CI of 4.1%–17.5%) or 18.4% (95% CI of 7.7%–34.3%), respectively. Zidovudine should thus be given during labor or the early neonatal period even to women who received no antenatal therapy (1008).

A randomized, placebo-controlled trial of zidovudine prophylaxis for the prevention of perinatal HIV-1 infection was performed in Thailand using a simpler and less

TABLE 48-6

ANTIRETROVIRAL AGENT USE IN PREGNANCY

Drug	FDA Pregnancy Category*	Placental Passage	Breast Milk Passage	Teratogenicity or Carcinogenicity
Nucleoside and nucleotide analogue reverse transcriptase inhibitors:				
Abacavir	C	Yes[1]	Yes[1]	Decreased fetal body weight, fetal anasarca, and skeletal malformations in rats treated with very high doses during organogenesis; malignant tumors of liver, thyroid, and genital tract of rats with high doses of drug
Didanosine	B	Yes (0.35)[2,3]	Yes[1]	None
Emtricitabine	B	Not known	Not known	Not teratogenic in rats or rabbits exposed to 60- to 120-fold higher doses than used in humans; carcinogenicity studies not completed
Lamivudine	C	Yes (1.0)[2,3]	Yes[3]	None
Stavudine	C	Yes (0.5–0.8)[1,3,4]	Yes[1]	Minor skeletal ossification delays in rats; benign and malignant liver and bladder tumors in rats and mice receiving 250-fold to 732-fold usual human doses
Tenofovir DF	B	Yes (0.17)[4]	Yes[1]	Osteomalacia in juvenile animals receiving high doses; carcinogenicity studies not completed
Zalcitabine	C	Yes (0.5–0.6)[4]	Not known	Hydrocephalus in rodents receiving 1,000-fold higher dose than used in humans; decreased fetal weight, skeletal defects, and thymocyte cytotoxicity; thymic lymphoma in rodents
Zidovudine	C	Yes (0.85)[3]	Yes[3]	Vaginal squamous tumors in adult rodents; lung, liver, and female reproductive tumors in offspring of mice treated with 50 times usual human dose; fetal malformations after near-lethal doses (350-fold higher than human dose)
Non-nucleoside reverse transcriptase inhibitors:				
Delavirdine	C	Not known	Yes[1]	Ventricular septal defects in rats given high doses; non-carcinogenic in rats; hepatocellular adenoma and carcinoma in mice; bladder tumors in male mice
Efavirenz	C	Yes (1.0)[1,4,5]	Not known	Anencephaly, cleft palate, anophthalmia, and microphthalmia in monkeys; liver and lung tumors in female mice
Nevirapine	C	Yes (1.0)[3]	Yes[3]	Hepatocellular adenomas and carcinomas in rats and mice; decreased fetal weight in rats receiving high doses
Protease inhibitors:				
Amprenavir	C	Not known	Yes[1]	Hepatocellualr adenomas and carcinomas in male mice and rats at doses 2- to 4-fold higher than for humans; abortion in rabbits; deficient bone ossification in rabbits and rats
Atazanavir	B	Not known	Not known	Carcinogenicity studies not completed; not teratogenic in rabbits or rats exposed to doses comparable to those used in humans
Fosamprenavir	C	Not known	Yes[1]	Benign and malignant liver tumors in male rats and mice; increased rate of abortion in pregnant rabbits
Indinavir	C	Yes[1,6]; minimal in humans	Yes[1]	Thyroid adenomas in male rats; no teratogenicity in rabbits or dogs; extra ribs in rats
Lopinavir + ritonavir	C	Not known	Yes[1]	Carcinogenicity studies not completed; delayed skeletal ossification in rats
Nelfinavir	B	Minimal in humans	Yes[1]	Thyroid follicular adneomas and carcinomas in rats; minor skeletal ossification delay with high doses
Ritonavir	B	Yes[1]; minimal in humans	Yes[1]	Liver adenomas and carcinomas in male mice; cryporchidism in rats; decreased body weight and ossification delays after toxic maternal doses in rats
Saquinavir	B	Minimal[1,3,5]	Yes[1]	Carcinogenicity studies not completed; no teratogenicity in animals studies

TABLE 48-6
(continued)

Drug	FDA Pregnancy Category*	Placental Passage	Breast Milk Passage	Teratogenicity or Carcinogenicity
Fusion inhibitors:				
Enfuvirtide	B	Not known	Yes[1]	Long-term carcinogenicity studies not done; not teratogenic in rats or rabbits at up to 27-fold higher doses than used in humans

Abbreviations: FDA = Food and Drug Administration; DF = disoproxil fumarate
* Pregnancy categories: B = Animal reproduction studies fail to demonstrate a risk to the fetus, but adequate well-controlled studies of pregnant women have not been conducted; C = Safety in human pregnancy has not been determined; animal studies are either positive for fetal risk or have not been conducted, and the drug should not be used unless the potential benefit outweighs the potential risk to the fetus.
[1] Demonstrated in rats
[2] Newborn to mother drug ratio
[3] Demonstrated in humans
[4] Demonstrated in primates
[5] Demonstrated in rabbits
[6] Demonstrated in dogs
Adapted from Public Health Service Task Force. Safety and toxicity of individual antiretroviral agents in pregnancy [online]. Available from http://www.aidsinfo.nih.gov/. Accessed August 28, 2004, Public Health Service Task Force. Recommendations for use of antiretroviral drugs in pregnant HIV-1-infected women for maternal health and interventions to reduce perinatal HIV-1 transmission in the United States, June 23, 2004 [online]. Available from http://www.aidsinfo.nih.gov/. Accessed August 28, 2004, with permission.

expensive protocol. Pregnant women received zidovudine at a dose of 300 mg orally twice daily beginning at 36 weeks of gestation until onset of labor, followed by 300 mg orally every 3 hours from onset of labor to delivery. Women were advised not to breast-feed their infants. Interim analysis of the data on 397 women revealed that the risk of perinatal HIV-1 transmission was 18.6% (95% CI of 13%–24%) in the placebo recipients compared with 9.2% (95% CI of 5%–13.5%) in the zidovudine-treated mothers, representing a 51% decrease in HIV-1 transmission (1009). Another study conducted in Africa (PETRA trial) showed that using a combination of zidovudine and lamivudine starting at 36 weeks gestation, intrapartum, and for one week to the mother and infant in the postpartum period reduced vertical transmission of HIV-1 by 63%, despite breast feeding (1010). The HIVNET 012 study, performed in Uganda, showed that a single 200 mg oral dose of nevirapine given to the mother at onset of labor followed by a single 2 mg/kg oral dose of the same drug administered to the breast-feeding infant at 48 to 72 hours of age was more effective than a short course of zidovudine prophylaxis (600 mg orally at labor onset and 300 mg every 3 hours until delivery, and 4 mg/kg twice daily for 7 days given to the babies). The gain was an estimated 41% reduction in HIV-1 transmission rate, and this was sustained through 18 months of age (1011,1012). However, the benefits of the HIVNET 012 protocol were not realized when it was implemented in Kenya (1013). Another trial (PACTG 316) investigated whether combining the HIVNET 012 and PACTG 076 protocols could further reduce HIV-1 perinatal transmission, but found no difference in outcome compared with the standard zidovudine prophylactic regimen (1014).

A study of 1,844 pregnant HIV-1-infected Thai women who were receiving zidovudine therapy during the third trimester, and conducted between 2001 and 2003, compared three nevirapine regimens: mothers and infants each received a single nevirapine dose, mothers received one nevirapine dose and infants got one dose of placebo, or both mothers and infants were given a placebo. All infants were given zidovudine for one week, and they were formula fed. Women not receiving nevirapine transmitted HIV-1 to 6.3% of their infants, although those getting a single dose of nevirapine transmitted the virus to 1.9% and 2.8% of the infants getting nevirapine or placebo, respectively (1015). The WHO recommends this combination approach (zidovudine beginning at 28 weeks of pregnancy and an intrapartum dose of nevirapine, plus zidovudine for one week and a single dose of nevirapine given soon after birth to infants) for women in resource-limited settings who do not require antiretroviral therapy for themselves (1016). For antiretroviral treatment-naive women who are administered a single intrapartum dose of nevirapine, the use of a single nevirapine dose alone for infants was similar in outcome to one dose of nevirapine plus one week of zidovudine in terms of mother-to-child HIV-1 transmission (1017). Nevirapine should be given to mothers at least one hour before delivery to be effective (1018).

Concerns over the use of nevirapine for prevention of mother-to-child transmission revolve around the emergence of nevirapine-resistance mutations in treated women (1016). In the PACTG 316 protocol, HIV-1-infected pregnant women received a single 200 mg nevirapine dose during labor. Nevirapine-resistance mutations were present in 2.3% of women before receipt of study drug, and in 15% at 6 weeks postpartum (1019). Women receiving intrapartum nevirapine prophylaxis are more likely to have virologic failure if they are subsequently treated with nevirapine-containing antiretroviral drug regimens (1020).

Elective cesarean delivery performed before onset of labor and rupture of membranes has been shown to reduce the rate of mother-to-child HIV-1 transmission. The combined use of elective cesarean delivery and zidovudine provides additive protective effects, reducing the rate of vertical HIV-1 transmission to about 1%. The American College of Obstetricians and Gynecologists recommends that HIV-1-infected pregnant women with HIV-1 RNA levels greater than 1,000 RNA copies/mL near the time of delivery be considered candidates for delivery by elective cesarean section at 38 weeks of gestation. HIV-1-infected women with undetectable viral loads are unlikely to benefit from a scheduled cesarean section, and the morbidity from the procedure outweighs any potential benefits (1000). A Thai study using a combination of zidovudine and lamivudine beginning at 34 weeks of gestation, a scheduled cesarean section at 38 weeks of gestation, preoperative intravenous zidovudine, and 4 weeks of neonatal zidovudine therapy showed that mother-to-child HIV-1 transmission still occurred (1021).

Despite the efficacy of protocols aimed at preventing mother-to-child transmission of HIV-1, there were missed opportunities for perinatal HIV-1 prevention for over half of the infected infants born between 1996 and 2000 at 6 U.S. sites (1022). A survey of 982 U.S. pediatricians found that the maternal HIV-1 status was unknown for 41% of neonates they evaluated in the 3 months before the survey, but that a discussion about screening for this infection was undertaken for only 10% of these infants (1023). Reasons cited for not addressing the need to screen for HIV-1 included low prevalence of disease in a pediatrician's area of practice (65%), parents who do not fit an "at risk" profile (56%), fear of offending the parents (50%), parental lack of understanding about the importance of screening (50%), and lack of sufficient time for counseling (44%). For infants of HIV-1-infected mothers who are prescribed zidovudine, adherence to the neonatal prophylactic regimen is decreased for women who are asymptomatic and lack a social support network (1024).

It is currently recommended that all HIV-1-infected pregnant women be treated with appropriate antiretroviral regimens suitable for their stage of disease. At a minimum, antenatal and intrapartum maternal zidovudine prophylaxis and treatment of newborns with zidovudine for 6 weeks, using the dosage regimens utilized in PACTG 076 as outlined earlier, is recommended (1000). Women who do not receive antenatal zidovudine because of nonlife-threatening serious drug-related toxicity or personal choice should still receive the drug intrapartum and their newborns should be treated. *In utero* exposure of infants to zidovudine has been associated with the occurrence of mild anemia and lower levels of other hematologic parameters, and a possible increased rate of early first febrile seizure (1025–1027). Zidovudine dosing for premature newborns (34 weeks or less of gestation) should be 1.5 mg/kg given intravenously or 2.0 mg/kg given orally every 12 hours, then increased to every 8 hours at 2 weeks of age for those with a gestational age of at least 30 weeks, or at

4 weeks of age for those whose gestational age is 29 weeks or less (1028).

HIV-1-exposed newborns should have a complete blood count done before zidovudine initiation and again at 1 and 2 months of age at a minimum. If anemia develops, a repeat hemoglobin measurement at 12 weeks of age usually shows resolution of zidovudine-related hematologic toxicity. Transient lactic acid elevations have been observed. Mitochondrial dysfunction can occur, but is infrequent. Infants should be assessed at 1, 2, and 6 months for symptoms and signs of mitochondrial toxicity such as encephalopathy, non-febrile seizures, developmental delay, cardiomyopathy, or hepatitis (933,1029).

Prophylaxis for *Pneumocystis jiroveci* (formerly *P. carinii*) should begin at 4 to 6 weeks of life, on completion of zidovudine therapy. The preferred regimen is trimethoprim-sulfamethoxazole (given at a dose of 150 mg/m^2/d of the trimethoprim component in two divided doses, and administered three times per week on consecutive days). The total daily dose of trimethoprim-sulfamethoxazole also can be given as a single dose (instead of two divided doses), or it can be given 7 days per week (instead of on three days of each week), or it can be given in two divided daily doses but administered three times per week on alternate days. Oral dapsone at a dose of 2 mg/kg once daily or 4 mg/kg given once a week, can be prescribed to infants intolerant of trimethoprim-sulfamethoxazole. Intravenous pentamidine (4 mg/kg every 2 to 4 weeks) or atovaquone (30 mg/kg for infants 1 to 3 months of age, or 45 mg/kg for infants 4 to 24 months of age) can be given orally once daily as alternative regimens. These regimens are continued until the diagnosis of perinatal HIV-1 infection is excluded, which usually requires two negative virologic assays done after 1 month of age (933).

HIV-1-exposed infants in the United States should not breast-feed, even if their mothers are on effective antiretroviral drug regimens. Potential exposures to other infectious agents that could be transmitted vertically (e.g., HBV, HCV, HSV, CMV, *T. pallidum*) should be evaluated and managed accordingly.

Fetal and Neonatal Infection

Congenitally infected infants usually are asymptomatic during the neonatal period, although detectable subtle signs such as lymphadenopathy and hepatosplenomegaly have been observed in 2% to 8% of cases, and some infants have been born with evidence of cerebral atrophy (1030,1031). Kaposi sarcoma presenting within the first month of life has been described rarely in HIV-1–infected infants (1032). The clinical latency period to development of AIDS is shorter than that for adults. About one-fourth of all perinatally infected infants develop AIDS by 1 year of age, and 40% to 50% do so by age 3 to 4 years; 33% of all perinatally infected patients remain free of AIDS by 13 years of age. About 10% of all HIV-1-infected infants die by age 1 year, and 25% to 30% by age 5 years (1033–1035). Median survival for perinatally-infected Thai children is estimated at 60 months, but is only 6 months for African infants (1036,1037). The mortality rates for infants infected perinatally with HIV-1 in the United States are 9% and 13% at 12 and 36 months, respectively, after a diagnosis of AIDS is made (917). Higher HIV-1 viral loads and lower CD4$^+$ percentages or absolute counts have been shown to correlate with more rapid progression to AIDS and to death (1038,1039). The slowest progression occurs in infants with low viral loads (plasma RNA levels of less than 10,000 copies per milliliter) and high CD4$^+$ counts (1039–1043). Infants with intrauterine HIV-1 infection are 2.5-fold (95% CI of 1.1–5.8) more likely to progress to AIDS or death than those with intrapartum HIV-1 infection (1044).

The diagnosis of HIV-1 infection during the neonatal period or early infancy can be difficult (933). Measurement of HIV-1–specific IgG is not useful because of passive transplacental passage of this antibody and its persistence for several months. The median age to clearance of passively acquired HIV-1 antibodies is 13 months (range 10 to 16) (1045). Positive HIV-1 antibody test results in those younger than 18 months of age indicate maternal infection but cannot diagnose infection in the infant (933). Although positive HIV-1 antibody test results in toddlers 18 months of age or older generally are considered indicative of infection, the reverse may not be true. Some infants with virologic evidence of HIV-1 infection can have negative or indeterminate serologic test results at 18 to 24 months of age (1046). A few infants who serorevert to an HIV-1–seronegative status in early infancy may actually be HIV-1 infected, and close follow-up is required (1047, 1048). Virus co-culture methods, p24 antigen detection, immune complex dissociation, and HIV-1–specific IgM and IgA measurements are all hampered by low sensitivities in the first weeks of life (1049–1053). Assays for HIV-1–specific IgA during the first month of life detect fewer than 10% of HIV-1-infected infants, but their sensitivities increase to 60% for 3-month-old infants and to 77% to 100% at 6 months of age or later (1051,1052).

The early diagnosis of HIV-1 infection can be accomplished by using DNA or RNA PCR assays (933). HIV-1 DNA PCR has a sensitivity and specificity of 96% and 99%, respectively, by 28 days of age for HIV-1 subtype B (the most common subtype in North America). The assay is less sensitive for non-B subtypes, such as subtype C that predominates in regions of Africa and India or subtype E that predominates in southeast Asia (1039). HIV-1 RNA can be measured in plasma by a variety of assays. HIV-1 RNA assays are at least as sensitive and specific, if not more so, than HIV-1 DNA assays (933,1054). The sensitivity and specificity of PCR is somewhat higher in older infants than in neonates (1054,1055). For infants at low risk of perinatal HIV-1 transmission, the positive predictive value for PCR is about 56% for neonates and 83% for older infants. Approximately 30% to 50% of HIV-1-infected infants are DNA PCR positive at birth, which suggests intrauterine infection, and about 50% to 70% of infected infants have negative DNA PCR results at birth but become positive

after 7 days of age, which suggests intrapartum transmission of the virus (1056). The PCR can be falsely positive if contamination with maternal blood occurs or if there is cross-contamination from other blood specimens in the laboratory.

Infants exposed to HIV-1 should be tested by PCR or other virologic assays at birth, at 4 to 6 weeks of age, and at 2 to 4 months of age. Cord blood should not be used for PCR assays. If either test result is positive for HIV-1, it should be repeated immediately for confirmation. A negative test result at 4 months of age or later provides more than 95% assurance that the infant is not infected with HIV-1. Continued follow-up serologic testing should be performed until disappearance of passively transferred maternal antibodies. An exposed infant is considered uninfected when there are no physical findings suggestive of HIV-1 infection, virologic test results are negative, immunologic test results (CD4$^+$ count and percentage) are normal, and, after the infant is 12 to 18 months of age or older, two or more HIV-1 antibody test results are negative (933). Follow-up of HIV-1–uninfected infants who were exposed *in utero* to maternal zidovudine prophylactic therapy have shown no drug-related ill effects 3 to 5.6 years later (1057).

Antiretroviral treatment should be started in all HIV-1–infected infants younger than 1 year of age as soon as the diagnosis is confirmed, regardless of clinical or immunologic status or viral load results, because they are considered to be at high risk of disease progression. By 12 months of age, about 50% of infants with perinatal HIV-1 infection develop moderate immune suppression, and another 20% have severe immune suppression (1039). Moderate and severe immune suppression for infants less than 12 months of age is defined as absolute CD4$^+$ count (and percentage) of 750 to 1,499 (15%–24%) and less than 750 (<15%), respectively. Treatment with three drugs (preferably two nucleoside reverse transcriptase inhibitors and one protease inhibitor) is recommended, as this affords the infected infant the best opportunity to preserve immune function and delay disease progression by maximally suppressing viral replication, preferably to undetectable levels (1039,1058,1059). Treated infants need close monitoring for medication-related adverse effects and adherence issues, virologic and immunologic responses to therapy, and emergence of drug-resistant HIV-1 strains (938,1029,1039,1060–1062).

The most common AIDS-defining conditions in pediatric patients are *P. jiroveci* pneumonia, lymphoid interstitial hyperplasia, recurrent bacterial infections, HIV-1 wasting syndrome, candidiasis, and HIV-1 encephalopathy (1033,1035–1037,1063). Other problems may include *Mycobacterium avium-intracellulare* infections, tuberculosis, CMV retinitis, disseminated HSV infection, herpes zoster, toxoplasmosis, extrapulmonary cryptococcosis, and cryptosporidiosis. *P. jiroveci* pneumonia can occur at any age, but it is diagnosed most commonly in young infants not receiving appropriate prophylaxis. Lymphoid interstitial hyperplasia is a chronic lung disease that results from the proliferation of lymphoid tissue in the interstitium of the lungs leading to tachypnea, hypoxia, and digital clubbing (1064). Progressive encephalopathy can be the first manifestation of HIV-1 infection in 10% to 15% of patients, and can range in severity from minor developmental delays to severe CNS involvement. Ventricular enlargement is the most common finding, followed by cortical atrophy, attenuation of periventricular white matter, and cerebral calcifications (1065). Cognitive decline sometimes occurs despite viral suppression and immunologic stability (1066). Cardiomyopathy can be present in HIV-1-infected children, and may be reversible with highly active antiretroviral therapy (1067).

Impaired linear growth occurs early and appears to be more pronounced in infants with higher viral loads, and this may not improve after virologic suppression (1068–1071). Altered pancreatic endocrine secretion manifested as increased insulin, glucagon, C-peptide, and glucose measurements is common in HIV-1-infected children not receiving protease inhibitors, and this is associated with growth problems (1072). Parotitis occurs in one-third of children surviving for 5 years or longer (1073).

Children with AIDS are also at increased risk of developing cancer. The most common malignancy is non-Hodgkin lymphoma (Burkitt lymphoma being the most frequent), followed by Kaposi sarcoma, leiomyosarcoma, and Hodgkin lymphoma. Varied proliferative and neoplastic disorders such as papillomavirus-related genital lesions, acute lymphoblastic leukemia, and other sarcomas have also been described. Non-Hodgkin lymphoma develops a median of 14 months after AIDS is diagnosed, but leiomyosarcomas take longer to manifest (1074,1075).

Infusions of IGIV every 4 weeks can reduce the risk of serious and minor viral and bacterial infections (1076). HIV-1–infected infants in the United States should receive all childhood immunizations with the possible exception of the varicella vaccine. However, this vaccine can be considered in those who are asymptomatic or mildly symptomatic and have no evidence of immune suppression. The live, attenuated measles–mumps–rubella vaccine can be given to HIV-1–infected infants who are not severely immunodeficient based on their absolute CD4$^+$ cell count or percentage. The inactivated influenza vaccine, but not the cold-adapted trivalent live vaccine, should be given every season for infants 6 months of age or older (1077).

TOXOPLASMOSIS

Toxoplasmosis is a common zoonosis, afflicting approximately one in three people worldwide. Infections of immunocompetent hosts are typically asymptomatic or benign, but intrauterine infections and illnesses in immunosuppressed patients can be severe or fatal. The causative organism, *T. gondii*, is an obligate intracellular protozoan that can be encountered in the form of a tachyzoite, tissue cyst, or oocyst. In addition to humans, *T. gondii* can infect other warm-blooded animals such as cats, dogs,

sheep, swine, and some birds; cats and other felines are the only known complete hosts for this parasite (15).

The life cycle of *T. gondii* usually is divided into an enteroepithelial sexual phase that occurs only in felines and an extraintestinal asexual phase that takes place in definitive (e.g., cats) and intermediate (e.g., humans) hosts. Susceptible cats can acquire *Toxoplasma* infection by ingesting oocysts or parasite-harboring tissues of other animals. Some of the organisms released in cat intestines invade gut epithelial cells and undergo sexual differentiation into microgametes and macrogametes; the gametocytes later fuse to produce a zygote. After a rigid wall forms around the zygote, it is excreted in feces as an oocyst. Acutely infected cats generally shed millions of oocysts in their feces daily for periods of 1 to 3 weeks. Parasites that do not undergo sexual differentiation may instead penetrate the gut wall and spread to other tissues by way of the blood and lymphatics; this extraintestinal or asexual stage can occur in humans and other susceptible animals as well (1078).

The tachyzoite is the actively proliferating form that is encountered in organs during the acute stage of infection. Tachyzoites gain entry into the cytoplasm of host cells and multiply rapidly. Infected cells subsequently burst and release progeny parasites that go on to attack neighboring host cells, which leads to the formation of necrotic areas that are surrounded by an inflammatory cellular reaction. This process eventually is curtailed by specific cellular and humoral host immune responses. In immunodeficient persons, the acute infection can continue relentlessly and cause serious illnesses.

After the host develops specific immunity against *T. gondii*, the organism can remain in organs in a viable, clinically inapparent tissue cyst form. *T. gondii* tissue cysts most commonly are found in the brain, eyes, myocardium, and skeletal muscles, and can be detected as early as 6 to 12 days postinfection in experimentally infected animals (1079). Each cyst can contain many thousands of slowly propagating or dormant parasites (bradyzoites). Encysted organisms can reactivate and cause serious illnesses, such as encephalitis and pneumonia, in patients who become immunodeficient later in life because of malignancy, AIDS, or immunosuppressive therapy (e.g., organ transplants).

There are three main clonal lineages (or strain types) of *T. gondii*, designated types I to III. Types I and II have generally been recovered from congenitally-infected infants, type II from patients with AIDS, and type III from animals. Sexual recombination between clonal lines occurs in nature (1080,1081).

T. gondii is transmitted to humans primarily through the ingestion of oocyst-contaminated water or food or the consumption of cyst-containing raw or undercooked beef, pork, mutton, or chicken. Unwashed hands can serve as vehicles for the transport of contaminating oocysts from the soil, dust, or cat litter box material into the mouth. Transmission occasionally can occur by eating raw infected eggs, transfusion of infected blood or blood products, or accidental self-inoculation of laboratory workers who are in contact with infected animals, needles, or glassware. Direct human-to-human transmission occurs primarily in the context of transplacental spread of the parasite to a developing fetus and, much less often, after an organ (e.g., heart, kidney) is transplanted from a seropositive donor into a seronegative recipient (1081,1082).

Maternal Toxoplasmosis

Epidemiology

The prevalence of anti-*Toxoplasma* antibodies among women of child-bearing age varies geographically, ranging from none to more than 90%. A seroprevalence of 39% was found in a large study of 22,845 pregnancies from diverse parts of the United States conducted between 1959 and 1966 (1083). Another survey of 17,658 sera from persons 12 years of age or older conducted in the United States between 1988 and 1994 showed that the overall age-adjusted prevalence was 22.5%. The overall prevalence was highest in the Northeast (29%) and lowest in the West (17.5%). Among women between 15 and 44 years of age, 15% had antibodies to *T. gondii*. Risk factors for seropositivity were increased age, birth in a foreign country, lower educational level, living in crowded conditions, and working in soil-related occupations. Current cat ownership did not increase the overall likelihood of having antibodies to this parasite (1084). A study of 4,234 persons 12 years of age or older conducted in 1999 and 2000 in the United States found that 15% of women had antibodies to *T. gondii*, with a higher prevalence among African Americans (1085). Seventh Day Adventists, who follow a diet that contains no meat, have a likelihood of being seropositive for *T. gondii* that is only 20% of that for a control group of other healthy adults living in the same area (1086). The average seroprevalence among HIV-1-infected women from New York, California, Washington, D.C., and Illinois is about 15%. HIV-1-infected women 50 years of age or older and those born outside the United States have seroprevalence rates of 32% to 41% (1087). Examples of seroprevalence figures for women of child-bearing age from other countries are India (Delhi), 2%; Australia (Melbourne), 4%; Taiwan, 9%; China (Lanzhou), 7%; China (Chengdu), 39%; southern Finland, 20%; Saudi Arabia, 30%; France (Strasbourg), 36%; Poland, 36%; Italy, 40%; Belgium, 46%; Germany, 46% to 68%; Greece, 52%; Panama, 63%; and Ethiopia, more than 75% (15,1082).

The incidence of acute *T. gondii* infection during pregnancy varies by locale. Reported frequencies per 1,000 pregnancies include Alabama with 0.6, Finland with 2.4, Australia with 5, New Zealand with 6, Germany with 7.5, and Belgium with 14.3 (15,1088–1090). The risk of infection is greatest for pregnant women leaving a region with a low incidence of toxoplasmosis to reside in an area in which the infection is prevalent (1088). Specific risk factors for acquisition of *T. gondii* infection in pregnancy may include consumption of cured pork and raw meat (including tasting raw meat while preparing food), eating

unwashed raw vegetables or fruits, infrequent washing of hands or kitchen utensils after preparation of raw meat before handling another food item, contact with soil, and cleaning cat litter boxes (1091–1094).

Clinical Manifestations

Acute toxoplasmosis is asymptomatic in 80% to 90% of pregnant women. Individuals with clinically evident illnesses most commonly present with lymphadenopathy, primarily of the head and neck region; a single node is involved in about two-thirds of patients (1095). *T. gondii* causes about 1% to 5% of infectious mononucleosis cases and should be considered a likely etiologic agent in patients with negative heterophile antibody test results (1096). Complications such as hepatitis, pneumonia, myocarditis, encephalitis, and deafness are rare in immunocompetent women (1082,1097,1098). Ocular involvement manifests mainly as retinochoroiditis and retinochoroidal scars, but lesions such as neuroretinitis, retinal vascular occlusions, and scleritis also occur (1099–1101). It is thought that severe ocular disease will occur in the immunocompetent patient if the infecting parasite is type I (1100). Psychiatric complications such as psychoses with schizophreniform features, anxiety, and depression have been encountered on rare occasions (1102,1103). Fulminating illnesses are common in immunosuppressed patients (1098,1104).

T. gondii spreads transplacentally to involve the developing fetus in 25%, 54%, or 65% of pregnant women with untreated primary toxoplasmosis during the first, second, or third trimester, respectively (1082). Proper maternal therapy reduces the overall incidence of fetal infection by more than 50%, and fewer infected infants manifest with severe congenital toxoplasmosis (1105,1106). These data underscore the importance of accurate and timely diagnosis of acute toxoplasmosis in pregnant women.

Diagnostic Tests

A clinical diagnosis of toxoplasmosis should be considered dubious unless supported by appropriate laboratory test results. *T. gondii* can be isolated from infected blood, CSF, aqueous humor, amniotic fluid, or homogenized tissues (e.g., placenta, brain, muscle) by inoculating these specimens into the peritoneal cavities of mice or onto tissue cultures. Tissue culture techniques are faster but less sensitive than intraperitoneal inoculation methods, but neither method is practical for clinical purposes. Tachyzoites can be visualized in tissue sections or smears of body fluids, especially if labeled specific anti-*Toxoplasma* antibodies are used for staining; their presence denotes acute infection. The demonstration of tissue cysts on histopathology can be consistent with an acute or a chronic *Toxoplasma* infection (619).

Other immunologic techniques that have been used for the diagnosis of toxoplasmosis include intradermal skin tests and transformation of lymphocytes on exposure to

Toxoplasma antigens, both of which connote chronic infection (1082). *Toxoplasma* antigens can be detected in CSF, urine, serum, or amniotic fluid using enzyme-linked immunosorbent assays (ELISA) or immunoblotting methods. A positive antigen test result indicates that the infection is recent. This is particularly helpful in newborns and immunodeficient persons in whom antibody responses to infection may be absent or unpredictable (15,1107). The antigen test is not available commercially. The PCR has been used successfully for the direct detection of *T. gondii* DNA in clinical samples by amplification of the *P30* or *B1* genes of the parasite; amplification of TGR1E (a repetitive DNA sequence) and a part of the small subunit ribosomal DNA (rDNA) also have been used (1108–1114).

The diagnosis of toxoplasmosis most often rests on serologic confirmation. The Sabin–Feldman dye test, traditionally the reference test against which newer methods are compared, requires the use of live parasites. Positive titers are usually in the 1:256 to 1:128,000 range. Most laboratories have abandoned the dye test in favor of simpler techniques that use killed antigens, such as the IFA, ELISA, agglutination, and indirect hemagglutination (IHA) tests.

Toxoplasma-specific IgM antibodies can be measured by IFA, ELISA, or IgM immunosorbent agglutination assay (IgM-ISAGA). False-positive IgM-IFA or IgM-ELISA are encountered in sera containing rheumatoid factor or the IgM can be directed against sphingolipids or ceramides that co-migrate with a low molecular weight antigen of the parasite during lipid extraction; these problem are circumvented if a double-sandwich IgM-ELISA (DS-IgM-ELISA) is performed (1111,1115). Specific IgM antibodies usually become positive within 1 to 2 weeks of infection and continue to be detectable for months or years, especially when measured by very sensitive assays such as DS-IgM-ELISA or IgM-ISAGA. The detection of specific IgM antibodies should not be considered proof that an infection is acute. In a British study of 446 *Toxoplasma*-infected women, specific IgM antibodies were detected for median periods of 13 and 10 months using ISAGA or IFA methods, respectively (1116). Persistent IgM responses for longer than 2 years were seen in 27% of women using ISAGA and in 9% using IFA (1116). IgM antibodies have been detected for as long as 12 years after acute infection in rare instances (1111).

High specific IgM titers suggest acute infection, especially if accompanied by high specific IgG titers of about 1:1,000 or greater as measured by IFA or the Sabin–Feldman dye test. Low specific IgM titers measured by DS-IgM-ELISA or IgM-ISAGA generally are encountered in patients whose infections occurred several months earlier. IgM-IFA tests are considerably less sensitive than DS-IgM-ELISA or IgM-ISAGA and are positive in only 60% to 70% of patients with acute infections and 25% to 50% of infants with congenital toxoplasmosis. It is important to know the type of assay used to measure specific IgM antibodies in pregnant women to interpret correctly the significance of positive and negative results (15,619). Commercially available test kits for

Toxoplasma IgM measurements unfortunately are unreliable as the sole determinant of recent *T. gondii* infection during pregnancy, and reliance on a single test result can lead to misdiagnoses and possibly inappropriate interventions (FDA Public Health Advisory: Limitations of *Toxoplasma* IgM Commercial Test Kits, July 25, 1997).

Anti-*Toxoplasma* IgG antibodies usually appear early during an infection. IgG titers peak at about 2 months, gradually drop thereafter, but remain detectable for years. The predominant IgG antibody response is of the IgG1 subclass (1117). A single high specific IgG titer is considered only suggestive of an acute infection. The strength of the binding of specific IgG to multivalent *Toxoplasma* antigens (IgG avidity) has been shown to be low in acute infections and high in chronic infections. Low IgG avidity can persist for as long as a year (1113). This test is being refined with the use of recombinant *Toxoplasma* antigens instead of lysed whole cell antigen, because rates of affinity maturation of IgG antibodies differ for specific parasitic antigens (1118). IgG avidity greater than 20% indicates that the infection occurred at least 20 weeks earlier. Thus, detection of high-avidity IgG antibodies to Toxoplasma antigens in pregnant women during the first half of their pregnancies can provide reassurance that their infections were remote in relation to the pregnancies (1119,1120).

Anti-*Toxoplasma* IgA antibodies directed against the major surface protein of tachyzoites (P30) are present in more than 95% of patients with acute infections (619). These antibodies are detected at the end of the first month of infection and usually disappear within 4 to 7 months, but can last up to 12 months or occasionally longer (619,1111,1121). Specific IgA antibodies are found rarely in patients with chronic infections (1121).

Specific serum IgE antibodies are present in about 86% of women who seroconvert during pregnancy. They appear shortly before or concomitantly with specific IgA antibodies. Specific IgE antibodies usually persist for less than 4 months, but are occasionally detectable for up to 8 months (619,1122).

Antibodies detected by IHA are different from those measured by the dye test, ELISA, or IFA. The titers take several weeks before becoming positive, making the test unsuitable for diagnosis of acute toxoplasmosis during pregnancy (15).

The differential agglutination test (AC/HS test) compares IgG titers obtained using acetone- or methanol-fixed (AC) tachyzoite antigens with those measured using formalin-fixed (HS) tachyzoite antigens. AC antigens detect acute phase-specific IgG antibodies. The AC-to-HS ratio is used to determine the timing of the primary infection. The test can show an acute pattern for up to 14 months (666,1123).

Serologic Diagnosis of Maternal Infection

Acute infection in immunologically normal women can be diagnosed if seroconversion or a fourfold or greater rise in antibody titers occurs when serum samples are collected 3 to 6 weeks apart (1082). The absence of *Toxoplasma*-specific IgM antibodies as measured by the DS-IgM-ELISA or IgM-ISAGA essentially excludes the diagnosis of acute toxoplasmosis. Elevated titers obtained by these assays are considered suggestive of the diagnosis, especially if specific IgG titers are high as well. Positive IgM-IFA results are more likely to represent recent infection. Specific antibodies detected by IgM-ISAGA or DS-IgM-ELISA usually persist at low levels for months or years after infection. High levels measured many years after the acute infection are rare (1111). The detection of *Toxoplasma*-specific serum IgA or IgE antibodies indicates a recent infection; conversely, absence of these antibodies in a seropositive woman suggests that the infection is old (619,1121,1124).

A panel of tests referred to as the Toxoplasma Serological Profile (TSP) is available from the Toxoplasma Serology Reference Laboratory of the Palo Alto Medical Foundation (http://www.pamf.org/serology/). TSP includes DS-IgM-ELISA, ELISA IgA, ELISA IgE, the Sabin-Feldman dye test, and the differential agglutination test (AC/HS test). Of 811 women who had positive *Toxoplasma* IgM test results performed at hospital or commercial laboratories, only 40% were shown to have a recent illness using TSP (1111,1113, 1125).

Immunodeficient women with acute *T. gondii* frequently are unable to mount a specific IgM response, and their IgG responses may be absent or low. Use of the more sensitive antibody assays may be helpful, but direct detection of the parasite or its components (e.g., antigen, DNA) in body fluids or tissues is sometimes the only means of establishing the diagnosis of acute toxoplasmosis (1082, 1111).

Diagnosis of Intrauterine Infection

Estimation of the duration of maternal *T. gondii* infection usually is difficult, and, consequently, assessment of the true risk to the fetus is often fraught with uncertainties. The parasite can be transmitted to the developing fetus at any stage of pregnancy and, in some cases, at or shortly before conception (15,1126,1127). The risk of fetal infection is estimated to be less than 1% if the initial stages of maternal infection occur before conception (1127,1128). This creates considerable anxiety for parents, who may choose an unwarranted end to the pregnancy or unnecessary maternal chemotherapy with potentially toxic drugs.

Prenatal diagnosis of fetal toxoplasmosis can be achieved safely and reliably. Pregnant women shown to have acquired acute *Toxoplasma* infections during the course of their pregnancies can undergo amniocentesis and ultrasound-guided cordocentesis. Parasite isolation studies, if available, include inoculation of these clinical samples into mice or onto tissue cultures. Fetal blood should be shown to be free of maternal blood contamination, using the Kleihauer–Betke stain or hemoglobin electrophoresis, before it is assayed for *Toxoplasma*-specific IgM antibodies or other nonspecific indicators of fetal infection (e.g., leukocyte and differential cell counts, platelet count, total IgM content, lactic dehydrogenase level,

gamma-glutamyltransferase concentration). Serial ultrasound examinations should be done at 2-week intervals to detect ventricular dilation, cerebral or hepatic calcifications, ascites, hydrops, or other fetal abnormalities (1082,1129–1131).

Daffos and colleagues (1132) applied this approach to prenatal diagnosis to 746 women with gestational toxoplasmosis occurring within the first 25 weeks of pregnancy. All mothers were treated with spiramycin. Fetal infection occurred in 42 pregnancies, and 39 (93%) were successfully identified prenatally. The most sensitive test in this study proved to be parasite isolation from amniotic fluid or fetal blood (81%). Despite the use of the sensitive IgM-ISAGA assay, only 21% of infected fetuses tested positive. Serial ultrasound examinations showed abnormalities in 45% of fetuses. Among nonspecific tests, gamma-glutamyl-transferase or total IgM contents of fetal blood were elevated in more than one-half of the patients. Results of prenatal testing led to pregnancy terminations in 62% of cases; the diagnosis was confirmed postnatally in the remainder. No false-positive diagnoses of fetal toxoplasmosis were made in this study, although other investigators have encountered this problem (1132–1134).

Because maternal IgA and IgE antibodies do not cross the placenta, fetal serum IgA and IgE have been explored as possible markers for intrauterine *T. gondii* infection. Decoster and colleagues (1135) were able to detect specific IgA antibodies in fetal blood as early as 23 weeks of gestation. The sensitivity of the assay was only 50%, slightly higher than that for *Toxoplasma*-specific IgM. No false-positive results were obtained. The sensitivity and specificity of *Toxoplasma*-specific fetal serum IgA measurement was 77% and 96%, respectively, in another study of 286 patients (1136). *Toxoplasma*-specific IgA antibodies found in amniotic fluid is probably of maternal origin and is not useful for the diagnosis of fetal toxoplasmosis (1137). Pinon and colleagues were unable to detect specific anti-*Toxoplasma* IgE antibodies in fetal blood (1138).

PCR methods have been used in prenatal diagnosis of fetal toxoplasmosis (1139–1146). Cazenave and colleagues (1140) studied 80 women with documented acute toxoplasmosis during pregnancy. PCR analysis (using *P30* gene amplification) of the amniotic fluid was negative in 70 cases without intrauterine infection and positive for all ten with fetal toxoplasmosis. In this study, the PCR was considerably more sensitive than recovering the parasite from amniotic fluid using culture methods (40%) or detection of specific fetal IgM (40%). Similarly, Grover and associates (1139) amplified the *B1* gene and found the PCR method to be more sensitive than the traditional techniques used for the prenatal diagnosis of toxoplasmosis. Hohlfeld and coinvestigators (1142) evaluated 339 consecutive women with gestational toxoplasmosis using PCR analysis (*B1* gene amplification) of their amniotic fluids and found that 37 of 38 infected fetuses had positive amniotic fluid test results; no false-positive results were encountered. The PCR was more sensitive than the conventional methods used for prenatal diagnosis of fetal toxoplasmosis (97.4% vs. 89.5%, respectively). Other researchers found their PCR assays on amniotic fluid to have lower sensitivities than indicated by these reports (1141,1143). Because the PCR test for *Toxoplasma* DNA is not standardized, interlaboratory variability in test results can be encountered (1147). The PCR can provide results within hours compared with tissue cultures, which require a minimum of 4 days, or animal inoculation techniques, which take at least 5 weeks to complete (1140). A real-time quantitative PCR assay used by Romand and co-workers revealed that high parasite concentrations in the amniotic fluid were associated with more serious fetal outcomes (1146). The sensitivity and versatility of PCR analysis, coupled with its rapidity, has made it valuable as a diagnostic tool (1145).

Treatment

Acute toxoplasmosis in the healthy, nonpregnant woman usually requires no specific therapy because of its benign, self-limited nature. Drugs used to treat toxoplasmosis are active against tachyzoites, but they generally have no effect on the encysted form of the parasite.

The option of pregnancy termination should be confined to women who become infected during the first one-half of their pregnancies. Although the risk of transmission of the parasite to the fetus is at its lowest during this stage, the severity of fetal disease is usually at its greatest. Acutely infected women who elect to proceed with their pregnancies should be treated with spiramycin as soon after diagnosis as possible (1081). Spiramycin is a macrolide antibiotic that is active against *T. gondii* and can cross the placenta to enter the cord blood and amniotic fluid (1148). It achieves high tissue levels, especially in the placenta. However, the measured concentrations of spiramycin and neospiramycin (a major metabolite) in maternal serum, fetal serum, placental tissues, and amniotic fluid appear to be below the levels needed to inhibit the parasite (1149). The main adverse effects of spiramycin are nausea, vomiting, and diarrhea. Although some studies do not confirm benefits from spiramycin, the drug is believed to reduce the risk of intrauterine transmission of the parasite, but it does not alter fetal pathology after infection has developed (1081). Spiramycin is only available by request from the Food and Drug Administration; the adult dose is 1 g per dose, given orally three times daily without food (1150). It is not known whether clarithromycin or azithromycin are effective alternatives to spiramycin in preventing intrauterine *T. gondii* infection.

If prenatal diagnosis is attempted and a fetus is shown to be infected, drugs such as pyrimethamine and sulfadiazine are added. Pyrimethamine, an antimalarial drug, is a folic acid antagonist. Its half-life in adults is about 100 hours, and it achieves tissue concentrations (e.g., brain) that are higher than in serum (1082). The drug causes bone marrow suppression with resultant anemia, granulocytopenia, and thrombocytopenia; severe pancytopenia occasionally occurs (1151). Other side effects include a bad taste in the mouth,

headache, and gastrointestinal discomfort. Pyrimethamine has been shown to be teratogenic in animals receiving massive doses of the drug early in organogenesis, and it should not be used before the fifth month of pregnancy (1082). Sulfadiazine (and its hydroxylated metabolites) or the trisulfapyrimidines act synergistically with pyrimethamine against *Toxoplasma* tachyzoites; other sulfonamides show less synergy and are not used (1152). These drugs are folic acid antagonists. Side effects include bone marrow suppression, rashes, crystalluria, hematuria, and reversible acute renal failure (1082). Treatment protocols vary between medical centers, but a report from the Cochrane Pregnancy and Childbirth Group concluded after reviewing over 3,300 papers that it is still not known whether antenatal treatment of women with toxoplasmosis actually reduces congenital transmission of *T. gondii* (1153). The Cochrane report notwithstanding, one suggested regimen used to treat pregnant women with an infected fetus incorporates monthly courses of a combination of pyrimethamine (100 mg/d in two divided doses for 2 days, then 50 mg/d), sulfadiazine (75 mg/kg per day in two divided doses for 2 days, then 100 mg/kg per day in 2 divided doses, up to a maximum of 4 g/d), and leucovorin supplements (10–20 mg/d), alternating with monthly spiramycin (1 g every 8 hours) (15). Leucovorin (folinic acid) is used to counteract the bone marrow suppressive effects of pyrimethamine and sulfadiazine. This treatment regimen is thought to reduce the occurrence of severe congenital infection and increase the proportion of infants born with asymptomatic toxoplasmosis. A multicenter European study could not demonstrate a beneficial effect of antenatal treatment started less than 4 weeks after diagnosis of maternal toxoplasmosis as compared to therapy prescribed at 4 to 7 weeks or after 8 weeks (1154).

Prevention

A vaccine against *T. gondii* is not yet available. Primary prevention rests on educating susceptible pregnant women on how to avoid becoming infected with this parasite. Cats that are kept indoors and only eat dried, cooked, or canned food are unlikely to get infected and shed oocysts. Contact with cat feces should be avoided; disposable gloves should be worn when handling cat litter boxes or while gardening. Cat litter boxes should be emptied of cat feces daily and disinfected by adding boiling water to the empty box for 5 minutes. Covering children's sandboxes decreases the risk of contamination. Meat should be cooked at 66°C or higher temperatures, smoked, or cured in brine. Hands should not touch the eyes or mouth when handling raw meat, and they must be washed thoroughly afterward. Kitchen surfaces should be cleaned carefully. Fruits and vegetables may have oocysts on their surfaces and should be washed or peeled before being eaten (666). Prenatal health education programs can bring about changes in personal behavior that reduce a susceptible woman's risk of acquiring toxoplasmosis by as much as two-thirds (1155,1156).

Secondary prevention entails the identification and treatment of pregnant women who are acutely infected. Because about 90% of patients with acute toxoplasmosis have minimal or no symptoms, a systematic serologic screening program would be needed. A national prevention program for congenital toxoplasmosis that mandates monthly serologic screening of all seronegative pregnant women has been in place since 1976 in France (1157). A comparable policy for routine screening does not exist in the United States, because it generally is regarded as not being cost effective and can lead to adverse pregnancy outcomes (in view of the difficulties associated with interpreting serologic test results), not the least of which is the termination of several pregnancies with uninfected fetuses per case of congenital toxoplasmosis prevented (1158–1161).

Women found to be seronegative early in pregnancy should be advised to follow the hygienic measures outlined earlier. Retesting at 18 to 22 weeks of gestation can identify women who seroconverted during the first one-half of their pregnancy, affording them the opportunity to consider options such as maternal chemotherapy, prenatal diagnostic procedures, or elective pregnancy termination (1162,1163). Seronegative women gain from testing at the end of pregnancy; this helps to identify asymptomatic newborns with toxoplasmosis that may derive benefit from treatment during the first year of life.

Women found to be seropositive early in gestation should be evaluated further to exclude a recent *Toxoplasma* infection. As a group, infants born to seropositive pregnant women with IHA titers of 1:256 to 1:512 have double the predicted frequency of deafness, a 60% increase in microcephaly, and a 30% increase in the occurrence of intelligence quotients less than 70 (1083). Fetal infections after reactivation of latent toxoplasmosis or following reinfection of immunocompetent seropositive women are known to occur, but are very rare (1164–1168). In twin pregnancies, monozygotic twins are more likely to be concordant with respect to their infection status than dizygotic twins (1169).

Congenital Toxoplasmosis

Epidemiology

The true incidence of congenital toxoplasmosis is unknown. Reported figures underestimate its occurrence. Published rates vary by locale, but they range from 0 to 10 per 1,000 live births. Representative incidence estimates per 1,000 live births include New York City with 0.7, Birmingham, Alabama, with 0.12, Mexico City with 2, Paris with 3, and Austria with 8.3 (1082). Prospectively collected data from Massachusetts and New Hampshire, where all heelstick blood specimens adsorbed onto a filter paper card for routine neonatal screening for metabolic and endocrine disorders also are tested for intrauterine *T. gondii* infection using an IgM capture immunoassay, have shown the rate of congenital toxoplasmosis to be about 1 per 10,000 newborns (1170). Using a similar approach,

Brazilian investigators documented the rate of congenital toxoplasmosis to be 1 per 1,867 newborns (1171).

As treatment of acutely infected pregnant women becomes more commonplace, the occurrence of congenital toxoplasmosis should decline. Trimester-specific *T. gondii* transmission rates decrease with proper maternal chemotherapy from 25% to 8% for the first trimester, from 54% to 19% for the second trimester, and from 65% to 44% for the third trimester (1082).

Clinical Manifestations

At least two-thirds of infants with congenital toxoplasmosis have inapparent disease at birth; however, one-third of all asymptomatic neonates who undergo detailed examinations are found to have abnormalities such as CSF pleocytosis or elevated protein content (20%), chorioretinitis (15%), or intracranial calcifications (10%) (1082,1170). Several weeks or months later, untreated infants develop signs or symptoms of disease.

Symptomatic *Toxoplasma* infection of the newborn can be mild, moderate, or severe. It can involve multiple organ systems or present as isolated abnormalities such as hydrocephalus, hepatosplenomegaly, or prolonged hyperbilirubinemia. Approximately 25% to 50% of symptomatic infants are delivered prematurely. Only 10% of infected infants have severe disease at birth. Systemic manifestations such as fever, jaundice, anemia, hepatomegaly, splenomegaly, or chorioretinitis may predominate in some infants, and neurologic abnormalities such as encephalitis, seizures, hydrocephalus, or intracranial calcifications may be prominent in others. About 10% of congenitally infected infants who have severe disease die, and most surviving infants are left with major neurologic sequelae, such as mental retardation, seizures, spasticity, and visual deficits (15).

CNS involvement is common. Parenchymal lesions may extend to surrounding blood vessels, leading to vasculitis with thrombosis and infarction. Substantial destruction of brain parenchyma can lead to obstruction of the aqueduct of Sylvius with resultant secondary enlargements of the third and lateral ventricles and, ultimately, hydrocephalus. Hydrocephalus can be the sole manifestation of congenital toxoplasmosis. It may be present at birth or develop later in infancy, and it may be static or gradually worsen to the point of requiring shunt placement. Diffuse intracranial calcifications occur in 10% to 20% of infants with congenital toxoplasmosis, but they can be found in 30% to 70% of those with symptomatic disease at birth (Fig. 48-5) (1082,1170,1172). They may increase in number and size over time. However, about 75% of these intracranial calcifications decrease or resolve within 1 year in adequately treated infants (1172). Other neurologic findings encountered in this infection include bulging anterior fontanelle, encephalitis, hydranencephaly, hypotonia or paralysis, spasticity, microcephaly, opisthotonus, swallowing difficulties, or proteinorachia (1173). Radiologic CNS findings may be consistent with an old insult (e.g., hydrocephalus, porencephaly, encephalomalacia,

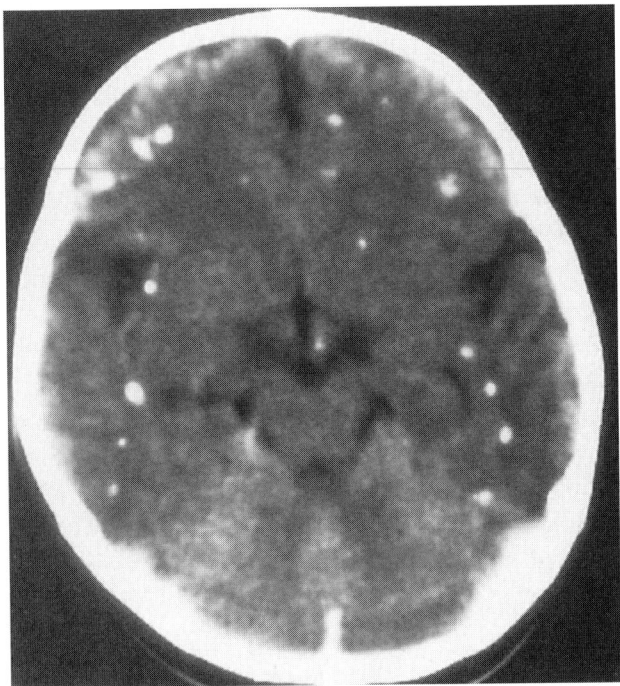

Figure 48-5 Computerized axial head tomogram of a 5-month-old girl with congenital toxoplasmosis. Notice the diffuse parenchymal calcifications and the prominent subarachnoid space bilaterally.

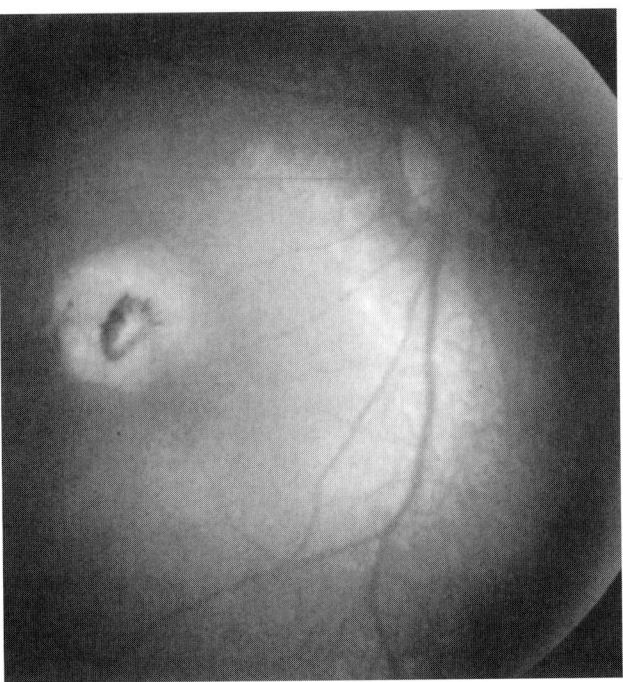

Figure 48-6 Active chorioretinitis in a 5-month-old boy with untreated congenital toxoplasmosis.

cortical atrophy) or, less commonly, with an acute process (e.g., single or multiple hypodense lesions with contrast ring enhancement) (1174,1175).

Manifestations of active congenital ocular toxoplasmosis may include chorioretinal scars, chorioretinitis, iritis, leukocoria, microphthalmia, nystagmus, optic atrophy, optic coloboma, retinal folds and traction detachments, granulomas in the posterior pole, strabismus, small cornea, and cataracts (15,1176–1179). Chorioretinal scars are the most common eye findings and are most likely to be found in the periphery. Macular scars are noted in 75% of untreated infants and are bilateral in about 23%; visual acuity can be markedly reduced in these patients (1178). On ophthalmoscopy, the typical findings are single or multiple yellow-white, fluffy necrotic lesions with indistinct margins that arise at the borders of preexisting, healed, hyperpigmented retinochoroidal scars (Fig. 48-6). Other findings may include retinal hemorrhages, iridocyclitis, vitreous haziness, papillitis, and papilledema. Untreated infants who were asymptomatic at birth are at great risk of subsequent development of chorioretinitis (about 50% for patients older than 10 years) (15).

Sensorineural hearing loss may occur in 15% to 25% of congenitally infected infants, and educationally significant hearing loss afflicts 10% to 15% of infected infants (1180). *T. gondii* has been found in the mastoid and middle ear at autopsy of some infants. Gastrointestinal disturbances such as feeding difficulties, diarrhea, and vomiting are common. The liver and spleen may be enlarged, and hepatic calcifications may be found. Conjugated hyperbilirubinemia sometimes takes months to subside. Biliary atresia associated with congenital toxoplasmosis has been reported (1181). Myocarditis, nephrotic syndrome, hydrops fetalis, interstitial pneumonia, and skeletal metaphyseal lucencies occur infrequently. Cutaneous lesions include ecchymoses, petechiae, purpura, and maculopapular rashes.

Hematologic abnormalities include anemia, eosinophilia, and thrombocytopenia (1182). Transient quantitative (e.g., neutropenia) and qualitative (e.g., enlarged, vacuolated lymphocytes) changes in the leukocytes are common (1182). Total CD4$^+$ lymphocyte counts and CD4$^+$-to-CD8$^+$ ratios usually are depressed (1183). Compared with adults, infants with congenital toxoplasmosis have no or reduced lymphocyte blastogenic responses on exposure to *Toxoplasma* lysate antigens, with failure to produce interferon-γ or interleukin-2; however, they do respond normally to nonspecific stimulators such as concanavalin A (1184). The severe organ damage seen in congenital toxoplasmosis may be as a result of specific deficits in cell-mediated immune responses to *Toxoplasma* antigens.

Diagnosis

Congenital toxoplasmosis is diagnosed if the parasite is recovered from the placenta. *T. gondii* can be isolated from the blood of asymptomatic or symptomatic infants; isolation rates peak at 71% during the first week of life and then decline to 33% at 2 to 4 weeks of age. Attempts at recovering the parasite from the blood of older infants generally are fruitless. The detection of *Toxoplasma* antigens or DNA in body fluids such as urine, CSF, or serum is considered diagnostic (15,1185,1186).

Specific IgM antibodies can be detected in the serum of 25% of congenitally infected infants with the IFA method and in as many as 75% with the DS-IgM-ELISA technique (1082). The sensitivity of the IgM-ISAGA test probably is even greater (1187). Passively transferred maternal anti-*Toxoplasma* IgG antibodies can suppress an infant's specific IgM response. Gross and colleagues (1185,1188) have shown that about 5% of sera have strain-specific immune responses. Unless antigens from more than one *T. gondii* strain are used in the assay, the sera would have no detectable specific antibodies in one test but be positive in another (1188). IgM antibodies can persist for more than 1 year when measured by very sensitive assays (1187). Rarely, intrathecal production of anti-*Toxoplasma* IgM is demonstrable despite the absence of specific antibodies in the serum of congenitally infected infants with CNS involvement (1185).

Levels of anti-*Toxoplasma* IgG antibodies of maternal origin typically drop at a rate of 50% per month in the infant's serum, but they may continue to be detectable for about 1 year. Active congenital infection should be suspected if specific IgG titers do not show the anticipated decline, or if they increase. Untreated infants begin synthesizing their own anti-*Toxoplasma* IgG antibodies by 3 months of age. The intrathecal production of specific IgG is demonstrable in about 2% of infants with CNS involvement (1082).

Toxoplasma-specific serum IgA antibodies are detectable in most congenitally infected infants, significantly more often than IgM antibodies (1121). Specific IgA antibodies were found in the CSF of the few infants in whom it had been measured (1189). Specific serum IgE antibodies can be measured from birth in some patients, especially infants with complications such as hydrocephalus or chorioretinitis (1138).

Research is ongoing to refine existing serologic methods for the diagnosis of congenital toxoplasmosis. Newer techniques that are still considered investigational include IgG, IgA, and IgM immunoblotting which appears to be more sensitive and specific than traditional serologic assays, and serial measurements of IgG avidity to *Toxoplasma* antigens in sera of infants (1113,1190–1194).

Transformation of lymphocytes on exposure to *Toxoplasma* antigens is a sensitive and specific indicator of congenital infection if performed on symptomatic or asymptomatic infants 3 months of age or older (15,1195). The observed blastogenic response is lower in infants than in infected adults (1184).

Treatment

Controlled trials examining the benefits of various treatment protocols are lacking. Drug regimens have been arrived at empirically, and conclusions about their efficacies are based on comparisons with historic data.

The treatment of symptomatic infants during the first 12 months of life usually consists of a combination of pyrimethamine, sulfadiazine, and leucovorin supplements.

After an initial loading dose of 2 mg/kg per day for 2 days, pyrimethamine (1 mg/kg orally in one or two divided doses) is given daily (first 6 months of life) or every other day (at 7 to 12 months of age). Sulfadiazine at 100 mg/kg per day is given in two divided oral doses for 12 months. Leucovorin (10 mg) is injected intramuscularly three times per week (1081). In some medical centers, the regimen is modified after the first 6 months of treatment to include 1-month courses of spiramycin alternating with 1-month courses of pyrimethamine, sulfadiazine, and leucovorin supplements for an additional 6 months. Spiramycin is given daily at a dose of 100 mg/kg per day in two divided oral doses (15,1081,1196,1197).

Corticosteroids such as prednisone or methylprednisolone (1.0–1.5 mg/kg per day orally in two divided doses) are used in infants with chorioretinitis or CSF protein elevations (≥1 g/dL) to reduce the inflammatory response (1082,1198). They should be used concurrently with anti-*Toxoplasma* drugs.

Infants with asymptomatic congenital toxoplasmosis are treated for 1 year. They receive an initial 6-week course of pyrimethamine, sulfadiazine, and leucovorin supplements, followed by alternating courses of spiramycin for 6 weeks and the pyrimethamine, sulfadiazine, and leucovorin combination for 4 weeks.

Healthy infants born to mothers with gestational toxoplasmosis and for whom serologic tests have not provided definitive answers regarding the presence or absence of infection can be treated with a 4-week course of pyrimethamine, sulfadiazine, and leucovorin followed by 4 to 6 weeks of spiramycin. If the diagnosis of congenital toxoplasmosis is later established, chemotherapy is continued as delineated earlier for infants with subclinical *T. gondii* infection. For healthy infants born to mothers with high Sabin–Feldman dye test titers and undetermined timing of maternal infection, a 1-month course of spiramycin usually is prescribed. Therapy is extended if clinical or laboratory evidence of congenital toxoplasmosis is uncovered (15).

Pyrimethamine serum levels do not vary significantly with age during infancy; they are comparable for infants receiving the drug daily or every other day. Pyrimethamine serum concentrations and half-life may be reduced in infants concomitantly treated with phenobarbital. The drug achieves CSF concentrations that are 10% to 25% of concurrently measured serum levels. Seizures have been observed in patients with pyrimethamine overdosage (1199).

Clindamycin and trimethoprim-sulfamethoxazole have been used effectively for the treatment of ocular toxoplasmosis in older patients (1081). There are no data on their efficacies in congenital infection. Photocoagulation of active lesions and of normal retinal tissues immediately bordering chorioretinal scars may be helpful in reducing recurrences (1200). Treatment with pyrimethamine, sulfadiazine, and leucovorin (with corticosteroids during the phase of active inflammation) currently is preferred for ocular toxoplasmosis, primarily because of the limited body of data on the efficacy of alternative regimens. Therapy should be continued for 2 weeks after resolution of active ocular inflammation (1197). Active lesions usually become quiescent after 10 to 14 days of therapy (1178).

Infants treated with pyrimethamine and sulfadiazine should be closely monitored. One or two blood and platelet counts should be done every week for the early detection of pyrimethamine-related adverse effects. The frequency of monitoring can be reduced to one or two times per month for infants receiving pyrimethamine on an every-other-day basis. The leucovorin dose is increased if the absolute neutrophil count falls below 1,000 cells/μL. If the absolute neutrophil count falls below 500 cells/μL, pyrimethamine should be withheld temporarily until the neutropenia resolves (1197).

Prognosis

Most infants with severe symptomatic congenital toxoplasmosis who survive beyond the neonatal period suffer from serious long-term residual problems, such as mental retardation and blindness (15,1088). The majority of those born with subclinical infection who are not treated develop eye problems, and about half will suffer neurologic sequelae (15).

Short-term follow-up studies indicate that maternal therapy during gestation, followed postnatally by treatment of all congenitally infected infants, improves prognosis by reducing the frequency and severity of late-appearing disease sequelae. In the study by Hohlfeld and colleagues (1105), congenital infection remained subclinical in 76%. Almost all treated infants developed normally and were neurologically normal.

Peripheral chorioretinitis that did not impair vision developed in about 10% between 5 and 17 months of age (1105). In another study, early institution of anti-*Toxoplasma* therapy may have prevented the occurrence of sensorineural hearing loss in congenitally infected infants (1180). Guerina and associates (1170) reported that only one of 46 congenitally infected but treated infants identified through their neonatal screening program had a neurologic deficit (hemiplegia), and 10% of those followed for 1 to 6 years had eye lesions.

Long-term follow-up studies of infants with symptomatic or subclinical congenital toxoplasmosis suggest that most patients develop chorioretinitis or chorioretinal scars by 10 to 20 years of age, but treatment may reduce the frequency and severity of adverse sequelae (1201–1206). The prognosis of infants with symptomatic congenital toxoplasmosis treated for 1 year with the pyrimethamine, sulfadiazine, and leucovorin regimen appears to be much better than that of historic untreated controls (1172,1178,1196,1207). All untreated patients develop chorioretinal scars, but this is seen in only 75% of those treated for 1 year. Among treated patients, peripheral chorioretinal scars and macular scarring are seen in 40% to 60% (compared with 82% and 76%, respectively, of untreated historic controls). Thirteen percent of treated infants and 44% of controls later have recurrences of ocular toxoplasmosis. The median time to ocular recurrence is 5 years (range 3 to 10) in treated infants; new lesions can occur in previously normal-appearing retina and contiguous to old scars (1178,1206).

TABLE 48-7

ADVERSE FETAL AND NEONATAL OUTCOMES CAUSED BY OTHER GESTATIONAL VIRAL AND PROTOZOAL INFECTIONS

Pathogen	Fetal and Neonatal Effects
Viruses:	
Cache Valley virus (1208)	Congenital macrocephaly (?)
Measles virus (2,82,1209–1211)	Prematurity; fetal loss; sporadic reports of congenital heart disease, cleft lip, pyloric stenosis, and cyclopia; congenital or perinatal measles; Crohn's disease (?)
Mumps virus (1212–1217)	Fetal loss; endocardial fibroelastosis; multicystic encephalomalacia; hydrocephalus; chorioretinitis; bilateral corneal opacities; malformations of the external ear; urogenital abnormalities; intestinal atresia; neonatal pneumonia; parotitis; splenomegaly; thrombocytopenia
Papillomaviruses (1218–1220)	Juvenile laryngeal papillomatosis; anogenital condylomata; giant cell hepatitis
Smallpox virus (1221)	Congenital smallpox (10%); prematurity; neonatal death; stillbirth
Vaccinia virus (1222)	Fetal vaccinia (skin lesions and internal organ involvement); premature birth; fetal loss
Protozoa:	
Malaria (1223,1224)	Placental infection; stillbirths; low birth weight; prematurity; neonatal death; congenital malaria (fever, anemia, and splenomegaly)
African trypanosomiasis (1225,1226)	Prematurity; abortion; stillbirth; central nervous infection; fever; hepatosplenomegaly
American trypanosomiasis or Chagas' disease (1225,1227)	Placental infection; spontaneous abortion; stillbirth; neonatal death; meningoencephalitis; seizures; anemia; jaundice; hepatosplenomegaly; cataract

Neurologic and developmental outcomes of 36 infants with treated congenital toxoplasmosis were assessed by Roizen and colleagues (1207). Tone and motor abnormalities were present on the initial examinations of 20 infants, and these resolved in 12 of them by 1 year of age. Six infants had perinatal seizures; four could be taken off their anticonvulsant medications within a few months. Low cognitive functioning as measured by a score of less than 50 was found in 21%. Seven children with a score above 50 on the Mental Developmental Index were compared to their siblings who served as controls; patients scored lower than their uninfected siblings (87 vs. 112). Sequential IQ tests done at intervals of at least 1.5 years showed no deterioration over time for congenitally infected children. Seventeen of 18 patients without hydrocephalus, and six of eight children with obstructive hydrocephalus that responded to shunt placement, were neurodevelopmentally normal or near normal; those with more severe CNS involvement did not fare as well. Intracranial calcifications in treated infants may diminish or disappear in as many as 75%, and remain unchanged in the rest (1172).

MISCELLANEOUS VIRAL AND PROTOZOAL PATHOGENS

Table 48-7 is a summary of some known and putative fetal and neonatal ill effects of a few additional viruses and protozoa that can infect pregnant women. Some of the published observations are individual case reports that may represent associations and not necessarily true cause-and-effect relationships (1208–1227).

REFERENCES

1. Gelber SE, Ratner AJ. Hospital-acquired viral pathogens in the neonatal intensive care unit. *Semin Perinatol* 2002;26:346.
2. Atmar RL, Englund JA, Hammill H. Complications of measles during pregnancy. *Clin Infect Dis* 1992;14:217.
3. Zeichner SL, Plotkin SA. Mechanisms and pathways of congenital infections. *Clin Perinatol* 1988;15:163.
4. Minkoff H. Human immunodeficiency virus infection in pregnancy. *Obstet Gynecol* 2003;101:797.
5. Tseng C-J, Liang C-C, Soong Y-K, et al. Perinatal transmission of human papillomavirus in infants: relationship between infection rate and mode of delivery. *Obstet Gynecol* 1998;91:92.
6. Hershow RC, Riester KA, Lew J, et al. Increased vertical transmission of human immunodeficiency virus from hepatitis C virus-coinfected mothers. *J Infect Dis* 1997;176:414.
7. Freij BJ, Sever JL. Congenital viral infections. *Curr Opin Infect Dis* 1992;5:558.
8. Freij BJ, South MA, Sever JL. Maternal rubella and the congenital rubella syndrome. *Clin Perinatol* 1988;15:247.
9. Mast EE, Alter MJ. Viral hepatitis A, B, and C in the newborn infant. *Semin Pediatr Infect Dis* 1999;10:201.
10. Freij BJ, Sever JL. Herpesvirus infections in pregnancy: risks to embryo, fetus, and neonate. *Clin Perinatol* 1988;15:203.
11. Jenson HB. Congenital syphilis. *Semin Pediatr Infect Dis* 1999;10:183.
12. Dobbins JG, Stewart JA, the Collaborating Registry Group, et al. Surveillance of congenital cytomegalovirus disease, 1990–1991. *MMWR* 1992;41(SS-2):35.
13. American Academy of Pediatrics, Committee on Infectious Diseases. Hepatitis C virus infection. *Pediatrics* 1998;101:481.
14. Roberts EA, Yeung L. Maternal-infant transmission of hepatitis C virus infection. *Hepatology* 2002;36:S106.
15. Remington JS, McLeod R, Thulliez P, et al. Toxoplasmosis. In: Remington JS, Klein JO, eds. *Infectious diseases of the fetus and newborn infant*, 5th ed. Philadelphia: WB Saunders, 2001:205.
16. Centers for Disease Control and Prevention. Congenital syphilis—United States, 2002. *MMWR* 2004;53:716.
17. Centers for Disease Control and Prevention. *HIV/AIDS surveillance report*, 2001;13(2):1.
18. Kohl S. The diagnosis and treatment of neonatal herpes simplex virus infection. *Pediatr Ann* 2002;31:726.
19. Centers for Disease Control and Prevention. Summary of notifiable diseases, United States, 2002. *MMWR* 2002;51(53):1.
20. Jara M, Hsu HW, Eaton RB, et al. Epidemiology of congenital toxoplasmosis identified by population-based newborn screening in Massachusetts. *Pediatr Infect Dis J* 2001;20:1132.
21. Lindegren ML, Fehrs LJ, Hadler SC, et al. Update: rubella and congenital rubella syndrome, 1980–1990. *Epidemiol Rev* 1991;13:341.
22. Cochi SL, Edmonds LE, Dyer K, et al. Congenital rubella syndrome in the United States, 1970–1985: on the verge of elimination. *Am J Epidemiol* 1989;129:349.
23. Centers for Disease Control and Prevention. Recommendations for prevention and control of hepatitis C virus (HCV) infection and HCV-related chronic disease. *MMWR* 1998;47(RR-19):1.
24. Kinney JS, Kumar ML. Should we expand the TORCH complex? A description of clinical and diagnostic aspects of selected old and new agents. *Clin Perinatol* 1988;15:727.
25. Alpert G, Plotkin SA. A practical guide to the diagnosis of congenital infections in the newborn infant. *Pediatr Clin North Am* 1986;33:465.
26. Greenough A. The TORCH screen and intrauterine infections. *Arch Dis Child Fetal Neonatal Ed* 1994;70:F163.
27. Cullen A, Brown S, Cafferkey M, et al. Current use of the TORCH screen in the diagnosis of congenital infection. *J Infect* 1998;36:185.
28. Chantler J, Wolinsky JS, Tingle A. Rubella virus. In: Knipe DM, Howley PM, Griffin DE, et al, eds. *Fields virology*, 4th ed. Philadelphia: Lippincott, Williams & Wilkins, 2001:963.
29. Lee J-Y, Bowden DS. Rubella virus replication and links to teratogenicity. *Clin Microbiol Rev* 2000;13:571.
30. Liang Y, Gillam S. Rubella virus RNA replication is cis-preferential and synthesis of negative- and positive-strand RNAs is regulated by the processing of non-structural protein. *Virology* 2001;282:307.
31. Katow S, Minahara H, Fukushima M, et al. Molecular epidemiology of rubella by nucleotide sequences of the rubella virus E1 gene in three East Asian countries. *J Infect Dis* 1997;176:602.
32. Frey TK, Abernathy ES, Bosma TJ, et al. Molecular analysis of rubella virus epidemiology across three continents, North America, Europe, and Asia, 1961–1997. *J Infect Dis* 1998;178:642.
33. Seppälä M, Vaheri A. Natural rubella infection of the female genital tract. *Lancet* 1974;1:46.
34. Holmes SJ, Orenstein WA. Rubella. In: Evans AS, Kaslow RA, eds. *Viral infections of humans: epidemiology and control*, 4th ed. New York: Plenum Publishing, 1997:839.
35. Töndury G, Smith DW. Fetal rubella pathology. *J Pediatr* 1966;68:867.
36. Garcia AGP, Marques RLS, Lobato YY, et al. Placental pathology in congenital rubella. *Placenta* 1985;6:281.
37. Webster WS. Teratogen update: congenital rubella. *Teratology* 1998;58:13.
38. Naeye RL, Blanc W. Pathogenesis of congenital rubella. *JAMA* 1965;194:1277.
39. Yoneda T, Urade M, Sakuda M, et al. Altered growth, differentiation, and responsiveness to epidermal growth factor of human embryonic mesenchymal cells of palate by persistent rubella virus infection. *J Clin Invest* 1986;77:1613.
40. Coyle PK, Wolinsky JS, Buimovici-Klein E, et al. Rubella-specific immune complexes after congenital infection and vaccination. *Infect Immun* 1982;36:498.
41. Boner A, Wilmott RW, Dinwiddie R, et al. Desquamative interstitial pneumonia and antigen-antibody complexes in two infants with congenital rubella. *Pediatrics* 1983;72:835.
42. Clarke WL, Shaver KA, Bright GM, et al. Autoimmunity in congenital rubella syndrome. *J Pediatr* 1984;104:370.

43. Verder H, Dickmeiss E, Haahr S, et al. Late-onset rubella syndrome: coexistence of immune complex disease and defective cytotoxic effector cell function. *Clin Exp Immunol* 1986;63:367.

44. Williams LL, Shannon BT, Leguire LE, et al. Persistently altered T cell immunity in high school students with the congenital rubella syndrome and profound hearing loss. *Pediatr Infect Dis J* 1993;12:831.

45. Yoon J-W, Choi D-S, Liang H-C, et al. Induction of an organ-specific autoimmune disease, lymphocytic hypophysitis, in hamsters by recombinant rubella virus glycoprotein and prevention of disease by neonatal thymectomy. *J Virol* 1992; 66:1210.

46. Salonen E-M, Hovi T, Meurman O, et al. Kinetics of specific IgA, IgD, IgE, IgG, and IgM antibody responses in rubella. *J Med Virol* 1985;16:1.

47. Al-Nakib W, Best JM, Banatvala JE. Rubella-specific serum and nasopharyngeal immunoglobulin responses following naturally acquired and vaccine-induced infection: prolonged persistence of virus-specific IgM. *Lancet* 1975;1:182.

48. Banatvala JE, Best JM, O'Shea S, et al. Persistence of rubella antibodies after vaccination: detection after experimental challenge. *Rev Infect Dis* 1985;7:S86.

49. Zolti M, Ben-Rafael Z, Bider D, et al. Rubella-specific IgM in reinfection and risk to the fetus. *Gynecol Obstet Invest* 1990; 30:184.

50. Cradock-Watson JE. Laboratory diagnosis of rubella: past, present and future. *Epidemiol Infect* 1991;107:1.

51. Böttiger B, Jensen IP. Maturation of rubella IgG avidity over time after acute rubella infection. *Clin Diagn Virol* 1997;8:105.

52. Grangeot-Keros L, Pillot J, Daffos F, et al. Prenatal and postnatal production of IgM and IgA antibodies to rubella virus studied by antibody capture immunoassay. *J Infect Dis* 1988;158:138.

53. Stokes A, Mims CA, Grahame R. Subclass distribution of IgG and IgA responses to rubella virus in man. *J Med Microbiol* 1986;21:283.

54. Katow S, Sugiura A. Antibody response to individual rubella virus proteins in congenital and other rubella virus infections. *J Clin Microbiol* 1985;21:449.

55. Chaye HH, Mauracher CA, Tingle A, et al. Cellular and humoral immune responses to rubella virus structural proteins E1, E2, and C. *J Clin Microbiol* 1992;30:2323.

56. Takahashi S, Machikawa F, Noda A, et al. Detection of immunoglobulin G and A antibodies to rubella virus in urine and antibody responses to vaccine-induced infection. *Clin Diagn Lab Immunol* 1998;5:24.

57. Mitchell LA, Zhang T, Tingle AJ. Differential antibody responses to rubella virus infection in males and females. *J Infect Dis* 1992;166:1258.

58. Fitzgerald MG, Pullen GR, Hosking CS. Low affinity antibody to rubella antigen in patients after rubella infection *in utero*. *Pediatrics* 1988;81:812.

59. Herne V, Hedman K, Reedik P. Immunoglobulin G avidity in the serodiagnosis of congenital rubella syndrome. *Eur J Clin Microbiol Infect Dis* 1997;16:763.

60. de Mazancourt A, Waxham MN, Nicolas JC, et al. Antibody response to the rubella virus structural proteins in infants with the congenital rubella syndrome. *J Med Virol* 1986;19:111.

61. Buimovici-Klein E, Cooper LZ. Cell-mediated immune response in rubella infections. *Rev Infect Dis* 1985;7:S123.

62. Reef SE, Frey TK, Theall K, et al. The changing epidemiology of rubella in the 1990s: on the verge of elimination and new challenges for control and prevention. *JAMA* 2002;287:464.

63. Centers for Disease Control and Prevention. Outbreaks of rubella among the Amish—United States, 1991. *MMWR* 1991;40:264.

64. Mellinger AK, Cragan JD, Atkinson WL, et al. High incidence of congenital rubella syndrome after a rubella outbreak. *Pediatr Infect Dis J* 1995;14:573.

65. Poland GA, Nichol KL. Medical students as sources of rubella and measles outbreaks. *Arch Intern Med* 1990;150:44.

66. Fraser V, Spitznagel E, Medoff G, et al. Results of a rubella screening program for hospital employees: a five-year review (1986–1990). *Am J Epidemiol* 1993;138:756.

67. Dykewicz CA, Kruszon-Moran D, McQuillan GM, et al. Rubella seropositivity in the United States, 1988–1994. *Clin Infect Dis* 2001;33:1279.

68. Assaad F, Ljungars-Esteves K. Rubella—world impact. *Rev Infect Dis* 1985;7:S29.

69. Mingle JAA. Frequency of rubella antibodies in the population of some tropical African countries. *Rev Infect Dis* 1985;7:S68.

70. Prabhakar P, Bailey A, Smikle MF, et al. Seroprevalence of Toxoplasma gondii, rubella virus, cytomegalovirus, herpes simplex virus (TORCH) and syphilis in Jamaican pregnant women. *West Indian Med J* 1991;40:166.

71. Zufferey J, Jacquier P, Chappuis S, et al. Seroprevalence of rubella among women of childbearing age in Switzerland. *Eur J Clin Microbiol Infect Dis* 1995;14:691.

72. Ukkonen P. Rubella immunity and morbidity: impact of different vaccination programs in Finland 1979–1992. *Scand J Infect Dis* 1996;28:31.

73. Seth P, Manjunath N, Balaya S. Rubella infection: the Indian scene. *Rev Infect Dis* 1985;7:S64.

74. Wannian S. Rubella in the People's Republic of China. *Rev Infect Dis* 1985;7:S72.

75. Centers for Disease Control and Prevention. Control and prevention of rubella: evaluation and management of suspected outbreaks, rubella in pregnant women, and surveillance for congenital rubella syndrome. *MMWR* 2001;50(RR-12):1.

76. Heggie AD. Pathogenesis of the rubella exanthem: isolation of rubella virus from the skin. *N Engl J Med* 1971;285:664.

77. Waxham MN, Wolinsky JS. Rubella virus and its effects on the central nervous system. *Neurol Clin* 1984;2:367.

78. Onji M, Kumon I, Kanaoka M, et al. Intrahepatic lymphocyte subpopulations in acute hepatitis in an adult with rubella. *Am J Gastroenterol* 1988;83:320.

79. Thanopoulos BD, Rokas S, Frimas CA, et al. Cardiac involvement in postnatal rubella. *Acta Paediatr Scand* 1989;78:141.

80. Harada T, Ohtaki E, Tobaru T, et al. Rubella-associated perimyocarditis: a case report. *Angiology* 2002;53:727.

81. Shirley JA, Revill S, Cohen BJ, et al. Serological study of rubella-like illnesses. *J Med Virol* 1987;21:369.

82. Bellini WJ, Icenogle JP. Measles and rubella viruses. In: Murray PR, Baron EJ, Jorgensen JH, et al, eds. *Manual of clinical microbiology*, 8th ed. Washington: ASM Press, 2003:1389.

83. Katow S, Sugiura A, Janejai N. Single-serum diagnosis of recent rubella infection with the use of hemagglutination inhibition test and enzyme-linked immunosorbent assays. *Microbiol Immunol* 1989;33:141.

84. Hedman K, Hietala J, Tiilikainen A, et al. Maturation of immunoglobulin G avidity after rubella vaccination studied by an enzyme linked immunosorbent assay (avidity-ELISA) and by haemolysis typing. *J Med Virol* 1989;27:293.

85. Zhang T, Mauracher CA, Mitchell LA, et al. Detection of rubella virus-specific immunoglobulin G (IgG), IgM, and IgA antibodies by immunoblot assays. *J Clin Microbiol* 1992;30:824.

86. Bosma TJ, Corbett KM, O'Shea S, et al. PCR for detection of rubella virus RNA in clinical samples. *J Clin Microbiol* 1995;33:1075.

87. Bosma TJ, Corbett KM, Eckstein MB, et al. Use of PCR for prenatal and postnatal diagnosis of congenital rubella. *J Clin Microbiol* 1995;33:2881.

88. Tanemura M, Suzumori K, Yagami Y, et al. Diagnosis of fetal rubella infection with reverse transcription and nested polymerase chain reaction: a study of 34 cases diagnosed in fetuses. *Am J Obstet Gynecol* 1996;174:578.

89. Centers for Disease Control and Prevention. Rubella prevention: recommendations of the Immunization Practices Advisory Committee (ACIP). *MMWR* 1990;39(RR-15):1.

90. Centers for Disease Control and Prevention. Measles, mumps, and rubella—vaccine use and strategies for elimination of measles, rubella, and congenital rubella syndrome and control of mumps: recommendations of the Advisory Committee on Immunization Practices (ACIP). *MMWR* 1998;47(RR-8):1.

91. American College of Obstetricians and Gynecologists. Rubella and pregnancy: ACOG Technical bulletin number 171-August 1992. *Int J Gynaecol Obstet* 1993;42:60.

92. Wolf JE, Eisen JE, Fraimow HS. Symptomatic rubella reinfection in an immune contact of a rubella vaccine recipient. *South Med J* 1993;86:91.

93. O'Shea S, Corbett KM, Barrow SM, et al. Rubella reinfection; role of neutralising antibodies and cell-mediated immunity. *Clin Diagn Virol* 1994;2:349.

94. Levine JB, Berkowitz CD, St Geme JW Jr. Rubella virus reinfection during pregnancy leading to late-onset congenital rubella syndrome. *J Pediatr* 1982;100:589.

95. Grangeot-Keros L, Nicolas JC, Bricout F, et al. Rubella reinfection and the fetus. *N Engl J Med* 1985;313:1547.

96. Best JM, Banatvala JE, Morgan-Capner P, et al. Fetal infection after maternal reinfection with rubella: criteria for defining reinfection. *BMJ* 1989;299:773.

97. Condon R, Bower C. Congenital rubella after previous maternal vaccination. *Med J Aust* 1992;156:882.

98. Robinson J, Lemay M, Vaudry WL. Congenital rubella after anticipated maternal immunity: two cases and a review of the literature. *Pediatr Infect Dis J* 1994;13:812.

99. Weber B, Enders G, Schlöber R, et al. Congenital rubella syndrome after maternal reinfection. *Infection* 1993;21:118.

100. Braun C, Kampa D, Fressle R, et al. Congenital rubella syndrome despite repeated vaccination of the mother: a coincidence of vaccine failure with failure to vaccinate. *Acta Paediatr* 1994;83:674.

101. Barfield W, Gardner R, Lett S, et al. Congenital rubella reinfection in a mother with anti-cardiolipin and anti-platelet antibodies. *Pediatr Infect Dis J* 1997;16:249.

102. Aboudy Y, Fogel A, Barnea B, et al. Subclinical rubella reinfection during pregnancy followed by transmission of virus to the fetus. *J Infect* 1997;34:273.

103. Bullens D, Smets K, Vanhaesebrouck P. Congenital rubella syndrome after maternal reinfection. *Clin Pediatr (Phila)* 2000;39:113.

104. Miller E, Cradock-Watson JE, Pollock TM. Consequences of confirmed maternal rubella at successive stages of pregnancy. *Lancet* 1982;2:781.

105. Munro ND, Sheppard S, Smithells RW, et al. Temporal relations between maternal rubella and congenital defects. *Lancet* 1987;2:201.

106. Grillner L, Forsgren M, Barr B, et al. Outcome of rubella during pregnancy with special reference to the 17th–24th weeks of gestation. *Scand J Infect Dis* 1983;15:321.

107. Bitsch M. Rubella in pregnant Danish women 1975–1984. *Dan Med Bull* 1987;34:46.

108. Enders G, Nickerl-Pacher U, Miller E, et al. Outcome of confirmed periconceptional maternal rubella. *Lancet* 1988;1:1445.

109. Segondy M, Boulot J, N'Dakortamanda N, et al. Detection of rubella virus in amniotic fluid by electron microscopy. *Eur J Obstet Gynecol Reprod Biol* 1990;37:77.

110. Sandow D, Rosmus K, Karnahl K, et al. Ein Beitrag zur pränatalen Rötelndiagnostik. *Z Geburtshilfe Perinatol* 1991;195:95.

111. Straussberg R, Amir J, Harel L, et al. Ultrastructural alterations of the amniocytes in 2 patients with rubella during the first trimester of pregnancy. *Fetal Diagn Ther* 1995;10:60.

112. Daffos F, Forestier F, Grangeot-Keros L, et al. Prenatal diagnosis of congenital rubella. *Lancet* 1984;2:1.

113. Hwa H-L, Shyu M-K, Lee C-N, et al. Prenatal diagnosis of congenital rubella infection from maternal rubella in Taiwan. *Obstet Gynecol* 1994;84:415.

114. Enders G, Jonatha W. Prenatal diagnosis of intrauterine rubella. *Infection* 1987;15:162.

115. Terry GM, Ho-Terry L, Warren RC, et al. First trimester prenatal diagnosis of congenital rubella: a laboratory investigation. *BMJ* 1986;292:930.

116. Cradock-Watson JE, Miller E, Ridehalgh MKS, et al. Detection of rubella virus in fetal and placental tissues and in the throats of neonates after serologically confirmed rubella in pregnancy. *Prenat Diagn* 1989;9:91.

117. Ho-Terry L, Terry GM, Londesborough P. Diagnosis of foetal rubella virus infection by polymerase chain reaction. *J Gen Virol* 1990;71:1607.

118. Revello MG, Baldanti F, Sarasini A, et al. Prenatal diagnosis of rubella virus infection by direct detection and semiquantitation of viral RNA in clinical samples by reverse transcription-PCR. *J Clin Microbiol* 1997;35:708.

119. Tang JW, Aarons E, Hesketh LM, et al. Prenatal diagnosis of congenital rubella infection in the second trimester of pregnancy. *Prenat Diagn* 2003;23:509.

120. Tingle AJ, Chantler JK, Pot KH, et al. Postpartum rubella immunization: association with development of prolonged arthritis, neurological sequelae, and chronic rubella viremia. *J Infect Dis* 1985;152:606.

121. Losonsky GA, Fishaut JM, Strussenberg J, et al. Effect of immunization against rubella on lactation products. II. Maternal-neonatal interactions. *J Infect Dis* 1982;145:661.

122. Tingle AJ, Mitchell LA, Grace M, et al. Randomised double-blind placebo-controlled study on adverse effects of rubella immunisation in seronegative women. *Lancet* 1997;349:1277.

123. Ray P, Black S, Shinefield H, et al. Risk of chronic arthropathy among women after rubella vaccination. *JAMA* 1997;278:551.

124. Slater PE. Chronic arthropathy after rubella vaccination in women: false alarm? *JAMA* 1997;278:594.

125. Howson CP, Katz M, Johnston RB Jr, et al. Chronic arthritis after rubella vaccination. *Clin Infect Dis* 1992;15:307.

126. Bosma TJ, Etherington J, O'Shea S, et al. Rubella virus and chronic joint disease: is there an association? *J Clin Microbiol* 1998;36:3524.

127. Lund KD, Chantler JK. Mapping of genetic determinants of rubella virus associated with growth in joint tissue. *J Virol* 2000;74:796.

128. Mitchell LA, Tingle AJ, MacWilliam L, et al. HLA-DR class II associations with rubella vaccine-induced joint manifestations. *J Infect Dis* 1998;177:5.

129. Landes RD, Bass JW, Millunchick EW, et al. Neonatal rubella following postpartum maternal immunization. *J Pediatr* 1980;97:465.

130. Centers for Disease Control and Prevention. Rubella vaccination during pregnancy—United States, 1971–1988. *MMWR* 1989;38:289.

131. Centers for Disease Control and Prevention. Revised ACIP recommendation for avoiding pregnancy after receiving a rubella-containing vaccine. *MMWR* 2001;50:1117.

132. Hofmann J, Kortung M, Pustowoit B, et al. Persistent fetal rubella vaccine virus infection following inadvertent vaccination during early pregnancy. *J Med Virol* 2000;61:155.

133. De la Mata I, De Wals P, Dolk H, et al. Incidence of congenital rubella syndrome in 19 regions of Europe in 1980–1986. *Eur J Epidemiol* 1989;5:106.

134. Cheffins T, Chan A, Keane RJ, et al. The impact of rubella immunisation on the incidence of rubella, congenital rubella syndrome and rubella-related terminations of pregnancy in South Australia. *Br J Obstet Gynaecol* 1998;105:998.

135. Schluter WW, Reef SE, Redd SC, et al. Changing epidemiology of congenital rubella syndrome in the United States. *J Infect Dis* 1998;178:636.

136. Tokugawa K, Ueda K, Fukushige J, et al. Congenital rubella syndrome and physical growth: a 17-year, prospective, longitudinal follow-up in the Ryukyu Islands. *Rev Infect Dis* 1986;8:874.

137. Chiriboga-Klein S, Oberfield SE, Casullo AM, et al. Growth in congenital rubella syndrome and correlation with clinical manifestations. *J Pediatr* 1989;115:251.

138. Campbell PE. Vascular abnormalities following maternal rubella. *Br Heart J* 1965;27:134.

139. Rocker MD, Bond SE, McGuinness CL, et al. Multiple aneurysms associated with congenital rubella. *Int J Clin Pract* 2001;55:147.

140. Peckham CS. Clinical and laboratory study of children exposed in utero to maternal rubella. *Arch Dis Child* 1972;47:571.

141. Gregg NM. Congenital cataract following German measles in the mother. *Trans Ophthalmol Soc Aust* 1941;3:35.

142. Romano A, Weinberg M, Bar-Izhak R, et al. Rate and various aspects of eye infection resulting from congenital rubella. *J Pediatr Ophthalmol Strabismus* 1979;16:26.

143. Kanra G, Firat T. Isolation of rubella virus from lens material in cases of congenital cataracts. *J Pediatr Ophthalmol Strabismus* 1979;16:31.

144. Smith GTH, Shun-Shin GA, Bron AJ. Spontaneous reabsorption of a rubella cataract. *Br J Ophthalmol* 1990;74:564.

145. Kresky B, Nauheim JS. Rubella retinitis. *Am J Dis Child* 1967;113:305.

146. Geltzer AI, Guber D, Sears ML. Ocular manifestations of the 1964–1965 rubella epidemic. *Am J Ophthalmol* 1967;63:221.

147. Collis WJ, Cohen DN. Rubella retinopathy: a progressive disorder. *Arch Ophthalmol* 1970;84:33.

148. Givens KT, Lee DA, Jones T, et al. Congenital rubella syndrome: ophthalmic manifestations and associated systemic disorders. *Br J Ophthalmol* 1993;77:358.

149. Deluise VP, Cobo LM, Chandler D. Persistent corneal edema in the congenital rubella syndrome. *Ophthalmology* 1983;90:835.

150. Franklin SL, Kelley R. Congenital rubella and interstitial pneumonitis. *Clin Pediatr (Phila)* 2001;40:101.

151. Desmond MM, Fisher ES, Vorderman AL, et al. The longitudinal course of congenital rubella encephalitis in nonretarded children. *J Pediatr* 1978;93:584.

152. Carey BM, Arthur RJ, Houlsby WT. Ventriculitis in congenital rubella: ultrasound demonstration. *Pediatr Radiol* 1987; 17:415.

153. Yamashita Y, Matsuishi T, Murakami Y, et al. Neuroimaging findings (ultrasonography, CT, MRI) in 3 infants with congenital rubella syndrome. *Pediatr Radiol* 1991;21:547.

154. Chang Y-C, Huang C-C, Liu C-C. Frequency of linear hyperechogenicity over the basal ganglia in young infants with congenital rubella syndrome. *Clin Infect Dis* 1996;22:569.

155. Lim KO, Beal M, Harvey RL Jr, et al. Brain dysmorphology in adults with congenital rubella plus schizophrenialike symptoms. *Biol Psychiatry* 1995;37:764.

156. Hendricks WM, Hu C-H. Blueberry muffin syndrome: cutaneous erythropoiesis and possible intrauterine viral infection. *Cutis* 1984;34:549.

157. Marshall WC, Trompeter RS, Risdon RA. Chronic rashes in congenital rubella: isolation of virus from skin. *Lancet* 1975;1:1349.

158. Ostlere LS, Harris D, Stevens HP, et al. Chronic rash associated with congenital rubella. *J R Soc Med* 1994;87:242.

159. Alter M, Schulenberg R. Dermatoglyphics in the rubella syndrome. *JAMA* 1966;197:685.

160. Español T, Pascual C, Huguet P, et al. Circumscribed scleroderma in congenital rubella syndrome with hypogammaglobulinemia. *Allergy* 1998;53:1005.

161. Menser MA, Dorman DC, Reye RDK, et al. Renal-artery stenosis in the rubella syndrome. *Lancet* 1966;1:790.

162. Menser MA, Robertson SEJ, Dorman DC, et al. Renal lesions in congenital rubella. *Pediatrics* 1967;40:901.

163. Forrest JM, Menser MA. Congenital rubella in school children and adolescents. *Arch Dis Child* 1970;45:63.

164. Kaplan GW, McLaughlin AP III. Urogenital anomalies and congenital rubella syndrome. *Urology* 1973;2:148.

165. Radner M, Vergesslich KA, Weninger M, et al. Meconium peritonitis: a new finding in rubella syndrome. *J Clin Ultrasound* 1993;21:346.

166. Rudolph AJ, Singleton EB, Rosenberg HS, et al. Osseous manifestations of the congenital rubella syndrome. *Am J Dis Child* 1965;110:428.

167. Reed GB Jr. Rubella bone lesions. *J Pediatr* 1969;74:208.

168. London WT, Fuccillo DA, Anderson B, et al. Concentration of rubella virus antigen in chondrocytes of congenitally infected rabbits. *Nature* 1970;226:172.

169. Sekeles E, Ornoy A. Osseous manifestations of gestational rubella in young human fetuses. *Am J Obstet Gynecol* 1975; 122:307.

170. Heggie AD. Growth inhibition of human embryonic and fetal rat bones in organ culture by rubella virus. *Teratology* 1977;15:47.

171. Zinkham WH, Medearis DN Jr, Osborn JE. Blood and bonemarrow findings in congenital rubella. *J Pediatr* 1967;71:512.

172. Sherman LA, Silberstein LE, Berkman EM. Altered blood group expression in a patient with congenital rubella infection. *Transfusion* 1984;24:267.

173. Kawamura N, Okamura A, Furuta H, et al. Improved dysgammaglobulinaemia in congenital rubella syndrome after immunoglobulin therapy: correlation with CD154 expression. *Eur J Pediatr* 2000;159:764.

174. Sever JL, South MA, Shaver KA. Delayed manifestations of congenital rubella. *Rev Infect Dis* 1985;7:S164.

175. Numazaki K, Goldman H, Wong I, et al. Infection of cultured human fetal pancreatic islet cells by rubella virus. *Am J Clin Pathol* 1989;91:446.

176. Ginsberg-Fellner F, Witt ME, Fedun B, et al. Diabetes mellitus and autoimmunity in patients with the congenital rubella syndrome. *Rev Infect Dis* 1985;7:S170.

177. McEvoy RC, Fedun B, Cooper LZ, et al. Children at high risk of diabetes mellitus: New York studies of families with diabetes and of children with congenital rubella syndrome. *Adv Exp Med Biol* 1988;246:221.

178. Ou D, Jonsen LA, Metzger DL, et al. CD4+ and CD8+ T-cell clones from congenital rubella syndrome patients with IDDM recognize overlapping GAD65 protein epitopes: implications for HLA class I and II allelic linkage to disease susceptibility. *Hum Immunol* 1999;60:652.

179. Viskari H, Paronen J, Keskinen P, et al. Humoral β-cell autoimmunity is rare in patients with the congenital rubella syndrome. *Clin Exp Immunol* 2003;133:378.

180. Preece MA, Kearney PJ, Marshall WC. Growth-hormone deficiency in congenital rubella. *Lancet* 1977;2:842.

181. Centers for Disease Control and Prevention. Rubella and congenital rubella syndrome—New York City. *MMWR* 1986;35: 770.

182. Cooper LZ, Krugman S. Clinical manifestations of postnatal and congenital rubella. *Arch Ophthalmol* 1967;77:434.

183. O'Shea S, Best J, Banatvala JE. A lymphocyte transformation assay for the diagnosis of congenital rubella. *J Virol Methods* 1992;37:139.

184. Vesikari T, Meurman OH, Mäki R. Persistent rubella-specific IgM-antibody in the cerebrospinal fluid of a child with congenital rubella. *Arch Dis Child* 1980;55:46.

185. Meitsch K, Enders G, Wolinsky JS, et al. The role of Rubella-Immunoblot and Rubella-Peptide-EIA for the diagnosis of the congenital rubella syndrome during the prenatal and newborn periods. *J Med Virol* 1997;51:280.

186. Eckstein MB, Brown DWG, Foster A, et al. Congenital rubella in south India: diagnosis using saliva from infants with cataract. *BMJ* 1996;312:161.

187. Plotkin SA, Klaus RM, Whitely JP. Hypogammaglobulinemia in an infant with congenital rubella syndrome; failure of l-adamantanamine to stop virus excretion. *J Pediatr* 1966; 69:1085.

188. Larsson A, Forsgren M, Hård af Segerstad S, et al. Administration of interferon to an infant with congenital rubella syndrome involving persistent viremia and cutaneous vasculitis. *Acta Paediatr Scand* 1976;65:105.

189. Arvin AM, Schmidt NJ, Cantell K, et al. Alpha interferon administration to infants with congenital rubella. *Antimicrob Agents Chemother* 1982;21:259.

190. Vijayalakshmi P, Srivastava KK, Poornima B, et al. Visual outcome of cataract surgery in children with congenital rubella syndrome. *J AAPOS* 2003;7:91.

191. Whitley RJ. Herpes simplex viruses. In: Knipe DM, Howley PM, Griffin DE, et al, eds. *Fields virology*, 4th ed. Philadelphia: Lippincott, Williams & Wilkins, 2001:2461.

192. Langenberg AGM, Corey L, Ashley RL, et al. A prospective study of new infections with herpes simplex virus type 1 and type 2. *N Engl J Med* 1999;341:1432.

193. Armstrong GL, Schillinger J, Markowitz L, et al. Incidence of herpes simplex virus type 2 infection in the United States. *Am J Epidemiol* 2001;153:912.

194. Centers for Disease Control and Prevention. Sexually transmitted diseases treatment guidelines 2002. *MMWR* 2002;51(RR-6):1.

195. Brown ZA, Selke S, Zeh J, et al. The acquisition of herpes simplex virus during pregnancy. *N Engl J Med* 1997;337:509.

196. Aurelian L. Herpes simplex virus type 2 vaccines: new ground for optimism? *Clin Diagn Lab Immunol* 2004;11:437.

197. Roizman B. Introduction: objectives of herpes simplex virus vaccines seen from a historical perspective. *Rev Infect Dis* 1991;13:S892.

198. Marques AR, Straus SE. Herpes simplex type 2 infections—an update. *Adv Intern Med* 2000;45:175.

199. Jerome KR, Ashley RL. Herpes simplex viruses and herpes B virus. In: Murray PR, Baron EJ, Jorgensen JH, et al, eds. *Manual of clinical microbiology*, 8th ed. Washington: ASM Press, 2003:1291.

200. Cowan FM. Testing for type-specific antibody to herpes simplex virus—implications for clinical practice. *J Antimicrob Chemother* 2000;45:9.

201. Fleming DT, McQuillan GM, Johnson RE, et al. Herpes simplex virus type 2 in the United States, 1976 to 1994. *N Engl J Med* 1997;337:1105.

202. Siegel D, Golden E, Washington AE, et al. Prevalence and correlates of herpes simplex infections: the population-based AIDS in Multiethnic Neighborhoods Study. *JAMA* 1992;268:1702.

203. Leone P, Fleming DT, Gilsenan AW, et al. Seroprevalence of herpes simplex virus-2 in suburban primary care offices in the United States. *Sex Transm Dis* 2004;31:311.

204. Eskild A, Jeansson S, Stray-Pedersen B, et al. Herpes simplex virus type-2 infection in pregnancy: no risk of fetal death: results from a nested case-control study within 35,940 women. *Br J Obstet Gynaecol* 2002;109:1030.

205. Kulhanjian JA, Soroush V, Au DS, et al. Identification of women at unsuspected risk of primary infection with herpes simplex virus type 2 during pregnancy. *N Engl J Med* 1992; 326:916.

206. Annunziato PW, Gershon A. Herpes simplex virus infections. *Pediatr Rev* 1996;17:415.

207. Taieb A, Body S, Astar I, et al. Clinical epidemiology of symptomatic primary herpetic infection in children: a study of 50 cases. *Acta Paediatr Scand* 1987;76:128.

208. Kuzushima K, Kimura H, Kino Y, et al. Clinical manifestations of primary herpes simplex virus type 1 infection in a closed community. *Pediatrics* 1991;87:152.

209. Pardo J, Yogev Y, Ben-Haroush A, et al. Primary herpes simplex virus type 1 gingivostomatitis during the second and third trimester of pregnancy: foetal and pregnancy outcome. *Scand J Infect Dis* 2004;36:179.

210. Koelle DM, Wald A. Herpes simplex virus: the importance of asymptomatic shedding. *J Antimicrob Chemother* 2000;45:1.

211. Scott D, Moore S, Ide M, et al. Recrudescent herpes labialis during and prior to early pregnancy. *Int J Gynecol Obstet* 2003; 80:263.

212. Jacques SM, Qureshi F. Herpes simplex virus hepatitis in pregnancy: a clinicopathologic study of three cases. *Hum Pathol* 1992;23:183.

213. Glorioso DV, Molloy PJ, Van Thiel DH, et al. Successful empiric treatment of HSV hepatitis in pregnancy: case report and review of the literature. *Dig Dis Sci* 1996;41:1273.

214. Pinna AD, Rakela J, Demetris AJ, et al. Five cases of fulminant hepatitis due to herpes simplex virus in adults. *Dig Dis Sci* 2002;47:750.

215. Frederick DM, Bland D, Gollin Y. Fatal disseminated herpes simplex virus infection in a previously healthy pregnant woman: a case report. *J Reprod Med* 2002;47:591.

216. Godet C, Beby-Defaux A, Agius G, et al. Maternal herpes simplex virus type 2 encephalitis following cesarean section. *J Infect* 2003;47:174.

217. Chiquet C, Thuret G, Poitevin-Later F, et al. Herpes simplex virus acute retinal necrosis during pregnancy. *Eur J Ophthalmol* 2003;13:662.

218. Posavad CM, Wald A, Hosken N, et al. T cell immunity to herpes simplex viruses in seronegative subjects: silent infection or acquired immunity? *J Immunol* 2003;170:4380.

219. Lafferty WE, Coombs RW, Benedetti J, et al. Recurrences after oral and genital herpes simplex virus infection: influence of site of infection and viral type. *N Engl J Med* 1987;316:1444.

220. Koelle DM, Benedetti J, Langenberg A, et al. Asymptomatic reactivation of herpes simplex virus in women after the first episode of genital herpes. *Ann Intern Med* 1992;116:433.

221. Benedetti JK, Zeh J, Selke S, et al. Frequency and reactivation of nongenital lesions among patients with genital herpes simplex virus. *Am J Med* 1995;98:237.

222. Kimberlin DW, Rouse DJ. Genital herpes. *N Engl J Med* 2004;350:1970.

223. Wald A, Zeh J, Selke S, et al. Virologic characteristics of subclinical and symptomatic genital herpes infections. *N Engl J Med* 1995;333:770.

224. Wald A, Zeh J, Selke S, et al. Reactivation of genital herpes simplex virus type 2 infection in asymptomatic seropositive persons. *N Engl J Med* 2000;342:844.

225. Prober CG, Corey L, Brown ZA, et al. The management of pregnancies complicated by genital infections with herpes simplex virus. *Clin Infect Dis* 1992;15:1031.

226. Hensleigh PA, Andrews WW, Brown Z, et al. Genital herpes during pregnancy: inability to distinguish primary and recurrent infections clinically. *Obstet Gynecol* 1997;89:891.

227. Wiedbrauk DL, Johnston SL. *Manual of clinical virology.* New York: Raven Press, 1993:109.

228. Nahass GT, Goldstein BA, Zhu WY, et al. Comparison of Tzanck smear, viral culture, and DNA diagnostic methods in detection of herpes simplex and varicella-zoster infection. *JAMA* 1992;268:2541.

229. Cone RW, Hobson AC, Palmer J, et al. Extended duration of herpes simplex virus DNA in genital lesions detected by the polymerase chain reaction. *J Infect Dis* 1991;164:757.

230. Rogers BB, Josephson SL, Mak SK, et al. Polymerase chain reaction amplification of herpes simplex virus DNA from clinical samples. *Obstet Gynecol* 1992;79:464.

231. Cone RW, Hobson AC, Brown Z, et al. Frequent detection of genital herpes simplex virus DNA by polymerase chain reaction among pregnant women. *JAMA* 1994;272:792.

232. Boggess KA, Watts DH, Hobson AC, et al. Herpes simplex virus type 2 detection by culture and polymerase chain reaction and relationship to genital symptoms and cervical antibody status during the third trimester of pregnancy. *Am J Obstet Gynecol* 1997;176:443.

233. Filun F, Strand A, Allard A, et al. Duplex real-time polymerase chain reaction assay for detection and quantification of herpes simplex virus type 1 and herpes simplex virus type 2 in genital and cutaneous lesions. *Sex Transm Dis* 2004;31:331.

234. Ndjoyi-Mbiguino A, Ozouaki F, Legoff J, et al. Comparison of washing and swabbing procedures for collecting genital fluids to assess cervicovaginal shedding of herpes simplex virus type 2 DNA. *J Clin Microbiol* 2003;41:2662.

235. Tang Y-W, Mitchell PS, Espy MJ, et al. Molecular diagnosis of herpes simplex virus infections in the central nervous system. *J Clin Microbiol* 1999;37:2127.

236. Whitley RJ, Cobbs CG, Alford CA Jr, et al. Diseases that mimic herpes simplex encephalitis: diagnosis, presentation, and outcome. *JAMA* 1989;262:234.

237. Whitley RJ, Gnann JW Jr. Acyclovir: a decade later. *N Engl J Med* 1992;327:782.

238. Berger SA, Weinberg M, Treves T, et al. Herpes encephalitis during pregnancy: failure of acyclovir and adenine arabinoside to prevent neonatal herpes. *Isr J Med Sci* 1986;22:41.

239. Stahlmann R, Klug S, Lewandowski C, et al. Teratogenicity of acyclovir in rats. *Infection* 1987;15:261.

240. Frenkel LM, Brown ZA, Bryson YJ, et al. Pharmacokinetics of acyclovir in the term human pregnancy and neonate. *Am J Obstet Gynecol* 1991;164:569.

241. Lau RJ, Emery MG, Galinsky RE. Unexpected accumulation of acyclovir in breast milk with estimation of infant exposure. *Obstet Gynecol* 1987;69:468.

242. Centers for Disease Control and Prevention. Pregnancy outcomes following systemic prenatal acyclovir exposure—June 1, 1984–June 30, 1993. *MMWR* 1993;42:806.

243. Ratanajamit C, Vinther Skriver M, Jepsen P, et al. Adverse pregnancy outcome in women exposed to acyclovir during pregnancy: a population-based observational study. *Scand J Infect Dis* 2003;35:255.

244. Hodinka RL. What clinicians need to know about antiviral drugs and viral resistance. *Infect Dis Clin North Am* 1997;11:945.

245. Alvarez-McLeod A, Havlik J, Drew KE. Foscarnet treatment of genital infection due to acyclovir-resistant herpes simplex virus type 2 in a pregnant patient with AIDS: case report. *Clin Infect Dis* 1999;29:937.

246. Kimberlin DE, Weller S, Whitley RJ, et al. Pharmacokinetics of oral valacyclovir and acyclovir in late pregnancy. *Am J Obstet Gynecol* 1998;179:846.

247. Tyring SK, Baker D, Snowden W. Valacyclovir for herpes simplex virus infection: long-term safety and sustained efficacy after 20 years' experience with acyclovir. *J Infect Dis* 2002;186(Suppl 1):S40.

248. LaRussa PS. Famciclovir. *Semin Pediatr Infect Dis* 1996;7:138.

249. Sacks SL. Famciclovir suppression of asymptomatic and symptomatic recurrent anogenital herpes simplex virus shedding in women: a randomized, double-blind, double-dummy, placebo-controlled, parallel-group, single-center trial. *J Infect Dis* 2004; 189:1341.

250. Gutierrez KM, Falkovitz Halpern MS, Maldonado Y, et al. The epidemiology of neonatal herpes simplex virus infections in California from 1985 to 1995. *J Infect Dis* 1999;180:199.

251. Brown ZA, Benedetti J, Ashley R, et al. Neonatal herpes simplex virus infection in relation to asymptomatic maternal infection at the time of labor. *N Engl J Med* 1991;324:1247.

252. Baldwin S, Whitley RJ. Teratogen update: intrauterine herpes simplex virus infection. *Teratology* 1989;39:1.

253. Freij BJ, Sever JL. Fetal herpes simplex virus infection. In: Buyse ML, ed. *Birth defects encyclopedia.* Boston: Blackwell Scientific, 1990:713.

254. Kimberlin DW. Neonatal herpes simplex infection. *Clin Microbiol Rev* 2004;17:1.

255. Corey RP, Flynn JT. Maternal intrauterine herpes simplex virus infection leading to persistent fetal vasculature. *Arch Ophthalmol* 2000;118:837.

256. Barefoot KH, Little GA, Ornvold KT. Fetal demise due to herpes simplex virus: an illustrated case report. *J Perinatol* 2002;22:86.
257. Vasileiadis GT, Roukema HW, Romano W, et al. Intrauterine herpes simplex infection. *Am J Perinatol* 2003;20:55.
258. Lee A, Bar-Zeev N, Walker SP, et al. *In utero* herpes simplex encephalitis. *Obstet Gynecol* 2003;102:1197.
259. Johansson A-B, Rassart A, Blum D, et al. Lower-limb hypoplasia due to intrauterine infection with herpes simplex virus type 2: possible confusion with intrauterine varicella-zoster syndrome. *Clin Infect Dis* 2004;38:e57.
260. Kimberlin DW, Lin C-Y, Jacobs RF, et al. Natural history of neonatal herpes simplex virus infections in the acyclovir era. *Pediatrics* 2001;108:223.
261. Filippine MM, Katz BZ. Neonatal herpes simplex virus infection presenting with fever alone. *J Hum Virol* 2001;4:223.
262. Kurtz J, Anslow P. Infantile herpes simplex encephalitis: diagnostic features and differentiation from non-accidental injury. *J Infect* 2003;46:12.
263. Whitley R, Arvin A, Prober C, et al. A controlled trial comparing vidarabine with acyclovir in neonatal herpes simplex virus infection. *N Engl J Med* 1991;324:444.
264. Whitley R, Arvin A, Prober C, et al. Predictors of morbidity and mortality in neonates with herpes simplex virus infections. *N Engl J Med* 1991;324:450.
265. Jacobs RF. Neonatal herpes simplex virus infections. *Semin Perinatol* 1998;22:64.
266. Gaytant MA, Steegers EAP, van Laere M, et al. Seroprevalence of herpes simplex virus type 1 and type 2 among pregnant women in the Netherlands. *Sex Transm Dis* 2002;29:710.
267. Toth C, Harder S, Yager J. Neonatal herpes encephalitis: a case series and review of clinical presentation. *Can J Neurol Sci* 2003;30:36.
268. Krolczyk S, Pacheco E, Valencia P, et al. Opsoclonus: an early sign of neonatal herpes encephalitis. *J Child Neurol* 2003;18:356.
269. Silverman MS, Gartner JG, Halliday WC, et al. Persistent cerebrospinal fluid neutrophilia in delayed-onset neonatal encephalitis caused by herpes simplex virus type 2. *J Pediatr* 1992;120:567.
270. Cameron PD, Wallace SJ, Munro J. Herpes simplex virus encephalitis: problems in diagnosis. *Dev Med Child Neurol* 1992;34:134.
271. Kimura H, Futamura M, Ito Y, et al. Relapse of neonatal herpes simplex virus infection. *Arch Dis Child Fetal Neonatal Ed* 2003;88:F483.
272. el-Azazi M, Malm G, Forsgren M. Late ophthalmologic manifestations of neonatal herpes simplex virus infection. *Am J Ophthalmol* 1990;109:1.
273. Mansour AM, Nichols MM. Congenital diffuse necrotizing herpetic retinitis. *Graefes Arch Clin Exp Ophthalmol* 1993;231:95.
274. Andersen RD. Herpes simplex virus infection of the neonatal respiratory tract. *Am J Dis Child* 1987;141:274.
275. Hubbell C, Dominguez R, Kohl S. Neonatal herpes simplex pneumonitis. *Rev Infect Dis* 1988;10:431.
276. Barker JA, McLean SD, Jordan GD, et al. Primary neonatal herpes simplex virus pneumonia. *Pediatr Infect Dis J* 1990;9:285.
277. Stewart DL, Cook LN, Rabalais GP. Successful use of extracorporeal membrane oxygenation in a newborn with herpes simplex virus pneumonia. *Pediatr Infect Dis J* 1993;12:161.
278. Dominguez R, Rivero H, Gaisie G, et al. Neonatal herpes simplex pneumonia: radiographic findings. *Radiology* 1984;153:395.
279. Schutze GE, Edwards MS, Adham BI, et al. Hyperammonemia and neonatal herpes simplex pneumonitis. *Pediatr Infect Dis J* 1990;9:749.
280. Kohl S. Neonatal herpes simplex virus infection. *Clin Perinatol* 1997;24:129.
281. Stanberry LR, Floyd-Reising SA, Connelly BL, et al. Herpes simplex viremia: report of eight pediatric cases and review of the literature. *Clin Infect Dis* 1994;18:401.
282. Mitchell PS, Espy MJ, Smith TF, et al. Laboratory diagnosis of central nervous system infections with herpes simplex virus by PCR performed with cerebrospinal fluid specimens. *J Clin Microbiol* 1997;35:2873.
283. Kimberlin DW, Lakeman FD, Arvin AM, et al. Application of the polymerase chain reaction to the diagnosis and management of neonatal herpes simplex virus disease. *J Infect Dis* 1996;174:1162.
284. Malm G, Forsgren M. Neonatal herpes simplex virus infections: HSV DNA in cerebrospinal fluid and serum. *Arch Dis Child Fetal Neonatal Ed* 1999;81:F24.
285. Kimura H, Futamura M, Kito H, et al. Detection of viral DNA in neonatal herpes simplex virus infections: frequent and prolonged presence in serum and cerebrospinal fluid. *J Infect Dis* 1991;164:289.
286. Kimura H, Ito Y, Futamura M, et al. Quantitation of viral load in neonatal herpes simplex virus infection and comparison between type 1 and type 2. *J Med Virol* 2002;67:349.
287. Kimberlin DW, Lin C-Y, Jacobs RF, et al. Safety and efficacy of high-dose intravenous acyclovir in the management of neonatal herpes simplex virus infections. *Pediatrics* 2001;108:230.
288. DeBiasi RL, Kleinschmidt-DeMasters BK, Richardson-Burns S, et al. Central nervous system apoptosis in human herpes simplex virus and cytomegalovirus encephalitis. *J Infect Dis* 2002;186:1547.
289. Bidanset DJ, Placidi L, Rybak R, et al. Intravenous infusion of Cereport increases uptake and efficacy of acyclovir in herpes simplex virus-infected rat brains. *Antimicrob Agents Chemother* 2001;45:2316.
290. Englund JA, Fletcher CV, Balfour HH Jr. Acyclovir therapy in neonates. *J Pediatr* 1991;119:129.
291. Nyquist A-C, Rotbart HA, Cotton M, et al. Acyclovir-resistant neonatal herpes simplex virus infection of the larynx. *J Pediatr* 1994;124:967.
292. Kesson AM. Management of neonatal herpes simplex virus infection. *Pediatr Drugs* 2001;3:81.
293. Whitley RJ. Herpes simplex virus infection. *Semin Pediatr Infect Dis* 2002;13:6.
294. Toltzis P. Current issues in neonatal herpes simplex virus infection. *Clin Perinatol* 1991;18:193.
295. Whitley RJ. Neonatal herpes simplex virus infections: is there a role for immunoglobulin in disease prevention and therapy? *Pediatr Infect Dis J* 1994;13:432.
296. American Academy of Pediatrics. Herpes simplex. In: Pickering LK, ed. *Red Book: 2003 report of the Committee on Infectious Diseases*, 26th ed. Elk Grove Village, IL: American Academy of Pediatrics, 2003:344.
297. Coren ME, Buchdahl RM, Cowan FM, et al. Imaging and laboratory investigation in herpes simplex encephalitis. *J Neurol Neurosurg Psychiatry* 1999;67:243.
298. Leonard JR, Moran CJ, Cross DT III, et al. MR imaging of herpes simplex type 1 encephalitis in infants and young children: a separate pattern of findings. *AJR Am J Roentgenol* 2000;174:1651.
299. Teixeira J, Zimmerman RA, Haselgrove JC, et al. Diffusion imaging in pediatric central nervous system infections. *Neuroradiology* 2001;43:1031.
300. Rudd C, Rivadeneira ED, Gutman LT. Dosing considerations for oral acyclovir following neonatal herpes disease. *Acta Paediatr* 1994;83:1237.
301. Kimberlin D, Powell D, Gruber W, et al. Administration of oral acyclovir suppressive therapy after neonatal herpes simplex virus disease limited to the skin, eyes and mouth: results of a Phase I/II trial. *Pediatr Infect Dis J* 1996;15:247.
302. Gutierrez K, Arvin AM. Long term antiviral suppression after treatment for neonatal herpes infection. *Pediatr Infect Dis J* 2003;22:371.
303. Libman MD, Dascal A, Kramer MS, et al. Strategies for the prevention of neonatal infection with herpes simplex virus: a decision analysis. *Rev Infect Dis* 1991;13:1093.
304. Arvin AM, Hensleigh PA, Prober CG, et al. Failure of antepartum maternal cultures to predict the infant's risk of exposure to herpes simplex virus at delivery. *N Engl J Med* 1986;315:796.
305. Prober CG, Hensleigh PA, Boucher FD, et al. Use of routine viral cultures at delivery to identify neonates exposed to herpes simplex virus. *N Engl J Med* 1988;318:887.
306. Garland SM, Lee TN, Sacks S. Do antepartum herpes simplex virus cultures predict intrapartum shedding for pregnant women with recurrent disease? *Infect Dis Obstet Gynecol* 1999;7:230.
307. Mindel A, Taylor J, Tideman RL, et al. Neonatal herpes prevention: a minor public health problem in some communities. *Sex Transm Infect* 2000;76:287.
308. Rouse DJ, Stringer JSA. An appraisal of screening for maternal type-specific herpes simplex virus antibodies to prevent neonatal herpes. *Am J Obstet Gynecol* 2000;183:400.

309. Roberts SW, Cox SM, Dax J, et al. Genital herpes during pregnancy: no lesions, no Cesarean. *Obstet Gynecol* 1995;85:261.

310. American College of Obstetricians and Gynecologists. ACOG practice bulletin. Management of herpes in pregnancy: number 8 October 1999. Clinical management guidelines for obstetrician-gynecologists. *Int J Gynaecol Obstet* 2000;68:165.

311. Brown ZA, Wald A, Morrow RA, et al. Effect of serologic status and Cesarean delivery on transmission rates of herpes simplex virus from mother to infant. *JAMA* 2003;289:203.

312. Kohelet D, Katz N, Sadan O, et al. Herpes simplex virus infection after vacuum-assisted vaginally delivered infants of asymptomatic mothers. *J Perinatol* 2004;24:147.

313. Prober CG, Sullender WM, Yasukawa LL, et al. Low risk of herpes simplex virus infections in neonates exposed to the virus at the time of vaginal delivery to mothers with recurrent genital herpes simplex virus infections. *N Engl J Med* 1987; 316:240.

314. Dobson AT, Little BB, Scott LL. Prevention of herpes simplex virus infection and latency by prophylactic treatment with acyclovir in a weanling mouse model. *Am J Obstet Gynecol* 1998;179:527.

315. Watts DH, Brown ZA, Money D, et al. A double-blind, randomized, placebo-controlled trial of acyclovir in late pregnancy for the reduction of herpes simplex virus shedding and Cesarean delivery. *Am J Obstet Gynecol* 2003;188:836.

316. Sheffield JS, Hollier LM, Hill JB, et al. Acyclovir prophylaxis to prevent herpes simplex virus recurrence at delivery: a systematic review. *Obstet Gynecol* 2003;102:1396.

317. Whitley R. Neonatal herpes simplex virus infection. *Curr Opin Infect Dis* 2004;17:243.

318. Corey L, Wald A, Patel R, et al. Once-daily valacyclovir to reduce the risk of transmission of genital herpes. *N Engl J Med* 2004;350:11.

319. Patel R. Antiviral agents for the prevention of the sexual transmission of herpes simplex in discordant couples. *Curr Opin Infect Dis* 2004;17:45.

320. Alanen A, Hukkanen V. Herpes simplex virus DNA in amniotic fluid without neonatal infection. *Clin Infect Dis* 2000;30:363.

321. Jones CA, Knipe D. Herpes simplex virus vaccines. *Pediatr Infect Dis J* 2003;22:1003.

322. Gaytant MA, Steegers EAP, Semmekrot BA, et al. Congenital cytomegalovirus infection: review of the epidemiology and outcome. *Obstet Gynecol Surv* 2002;57:245.

323. Gehrz RC. Human cytomegalovirus: biology and clinical perspectives. *Adv Pediatr* 1991;38:203.

324. Arribas JR, Storch GA, Clifford DB, et al. Cytomegalovirus encephalitis. *Ann Intern Med* 1996;125:577.

325. Castillo JP, Kowalik TF. HCMV infection: modulating the cell cycle and cell death. *Int Rev Immunol* 2004;23:113.

326. Demmler GJ. Summary of a workshop on surveillance for congenital cytomegalovirus disease. *Rev Infect Dis* 1991;13:315.

327. Spano LC, Gatti J, Nascimento JP, et al. Prevalence of human cytomegalovirus infection in pregnant and non-pregnant women. *J Infect* 2004;48:213.

328. Walmus BF, Yow MD, Lester JW, et al. Factors predictive of cytomegalovirus immune status in pregnant women. *J Infect Dis* 1988;157:172.

329. Tookey PA, Ades AE, Peckham CS. Cytomegalovirus prevalence in pregnant women: the influence of parity. *Arch Dis Child* 1992;67:779.

330. Sohn YM, Oh MK, Balcarek KB, et al. Cytomegalovirus infection in sexually active adolescents. *J Infect Dis* 1991;163:460.

331. Fowler KB, Pass RF. Sexually transmitted diseases in mothers of neonates with congenital cytomegalovirus infection. *J Infect Dis* 1991;164:259.

332. Coonrod D, Collier AC, Ashley R, et al. Association between cytomegalovirus seroconversion and upper genital tract infection among women attending a sexually transmitted disease clinic: a prospective study. *J Infect Dis* 1998;177:1188.

333. Numazaki K, Fujikawa T, Chiba S. Relationship between seropositivity of husbands and primary cytomegalovirus infection during pregnancy. *J Infect Chemother* 2000;6:104.

334. Pereira L, Maidji E, McDonagh S, et al. Human cytomegalovirus transmission from the uterus to the placenta correlates with the presence of pathogenic bacteria and maternal immunity. *J Virol* 2003;77:13301.

335. Adler SP. Cytomegalovirus and child day care: risk factors for maternal infection. *Pediatr Infect Dis J* 1991;10:590.

336. Murph JR, Baron JC, Brown CK, et al. The occupational risk of cytomegalovirus infection among day-care providers. *JAMA* 1991;265:603.

337. Ford-Jones EL, Kitai I, Davis L, et al. Cytomegalovirus infections in Toronto child-care centers: a prospective study of viral excretion in children and seroconversion among day-care providers. *Pediatr Infect Dis J* 1996;15:507.

338. Nelson CT, Demmler GJ. Cytomegalovirus infection in the pregnant mother, fetus, and newborn infant. *Clin Perinatol* 1997;24:151.

339. Shen C-Y, Chang S-F, Yen M-S, et al. Cytomegalovirus excretion in pregnant and nonpregnant women. *J Clin Microbiol* 1993;31:1635.

340. Fowler KB, Stagno S, Pass RF, et al. The outcome of congenital cytomegalovirus infection in relation to maternal antibody status. *N Engl J Med* 1992;326:663.

341. Fowler KB, Stagno S, Pass RF. Maternal immunity and prevention of congenital cytomegalovirus infection. *JAMA* 2003;289:1008.

342. Nigro G, Clerico A, Mondaini C. Symptomatic congenital cytomegalovirus infection in two consecutive sisters. *Arch Dis Child* 1993;69:527.

343. Portolani M, Cermelli C, Sabbatini AMT, et al. A fatal case of congenital cytomegalic inclusion disease following recurrent maternal infection. *New Microbiol* 1995;18:427.

344. Schwebke K, Henry K, Balfour HH Jr, et al. Congenital cytomegalovirus infection as a result of nonprimary cytomegalovirus disease in a mother with acquired immunodeficiency syndrome. *J Pediatr* 1995;126:293.

345. Boppana SB, Fowler KB, Britt WJ, et al. Symptomatic congenital cytomegalovirus infection in infants born to mothers with pre-existing immunity to cytomegalovirus. *Pediatrics* 1999;104:55.

346. Rousseau T, Douvier S, Reynaud I, et al. Severe fetal cytomegalic inclusion disease after documented maternal reactivation of cytomegalovirus infection during pregnancy. *Prenat Diagn* 2000;20:333.

347. Boppana SB, Rivera LB, Fowler KB, et al. Intrauterine transmission of cytomegalovirus to infants of women with preconceptional immunity. *N Engl J Med* 2001;344:1366.

348. Inoue T, Matsumura N, Fukuoka M, et al. Severe congenital cytomegalovirus infection with fetal hydrops in a cytomegalovirus-seropositive healthy woman. *Eur J Obstet Gynecol Reprod Biol* 2001;95:184.

349. Henrich W, Meckies J, Dudenhausen JW, et al. Recurrent cytomegalovirus infection during pregnancy: ultrasonographic diagnosis and fetal outcome. *Ultrasound Obstet Gynecol* 2002; 19:608.

350. Gaytant MA, Rours GIJG, Steegers EAP, et al. Congenital cytomegalovirus infection after recurrent infection: case reports and review of the literature. *Eur J Pediatr* 2003;162:248.

351. Fowler KB, Stagno S, Pass RF. Interval between births and risk of congenital cytomegalovirus infection. *Clin Infect Dis* 2004; 38:1035.

352. Arav-Boger R, Pass RF. Diagnosis and management of cytomegalovirus infection in the newborn. *Pediatr Ann* 2002;31:719.

353. Nigro G, Anceschi MM, Cosmi EV, et al. Clinical manifestations and abnormal laboratory findings in pregnant women with primary cytomegalovirus infection. *BJOG* 2003;110:572.

354. Rawlinson WD. Broadsheet number 50: diagnosis of human cytomegalovirus infection and disease. *Pathology* 1999;31:109.

355. Griffiths PD. The treatment of cytomegalovirus infection. *J Antimicrob Chemother* 2002;49:243.

356. Putland RA, Ford J, Korban G, et al. Investigation of spontaneously aborted concepti for microbial DNA: investigation for cytomegalovirus DNA using polymerase chain reaction. *Aust N Z J Obstet Gynaecol* 1990;30:248.

357. Hodinka RL. Human cytomegalovirus. In: Murray PR, Baron EJ, Jorgensen JH, et al, eds. *Manual of clinical microbiology*, 8th ed. Washington: ASM Press, 2003:1304.

358. Griffiths PD, Stagno S, Pass RF, et al. Infection with cytomegalovirus during pregnancy: specific IgM antibodies as a marker of recent primary infection. *J Infect Dis* 1982;145:647.

359. Grangeot-Keros L, Mayaux MJ, Lebon P, et al. Value of cytomegalovirus (CMV) IgG avidity index for the diagnosis of primary CMV infection in pregnant women. *J Infect Dis* 1997;175:944.

360. Lazzarotto T, Varani S, Spezzacatena P, et al. Maternal IgG avidity and IgM detected by blot as diagnostic tools to identify

pregnant women at risk of transmitting cytomegalovirus. *Viral Immunol* 2000;13:137.

361. Grundy JE, Ehrnst A, Einsele H, et al. A three-center European external quality control study of PCR for detection of cytomegalovirus DNA in blood. *J Clin Microbiol* 1996;34:1166.

362. Zanghellini F, Boppana SB, Emery VC, et al. Asymptomatic primary cytomegalovirus infection: virologic and immunologic features. *J Infect Dis* 1999;180:702.

363. Kalpoe JS, Kroes ACM, de Jong MD, et al. Validation of clinical application of cytomegalovirus plasma DNA load measurement and definition of treatment criteria by analysis of correlation to antigen detection. *J Clin Microbiol* 2004;42:1498.

364. Emery VC, Hassan-Walker AF. Focus on new drugs in development against human cytomegalovirus. *Drugs* 2002;62:1853.

365. De Clercq E. New inhibitors of human cytomegalvirus (HCMV) on the horizon. *J Antimicrob Chemother* 2003;51:1079.

366. Baldanti F, Gerna G. Human cytomegalovirus resistance to antiviral drugs: diagnosis, monitoring and clinical impact. *J Antimicrob Chemother* 2003;52:324.

367. Kimberlin DW. Antiviral therapy for cytomegalovirus infections in pediatric patients. *Semin Pediatr Infect Dis* 2002;13:22.

368. Henderson GI, Hu ZQ, Yang Y, et al. Ganciclovir transfer by human placenta and its effects on rat fetal cells. *Am J Med Sci* 1993;306:151.

369. Brady RC, Schleiss MR, Witte DP, et al. Placental transfer of ganciclovir in a woman with acquired immunodeficiency syndrome and cytomegalovirus disease. *Pediatr Infect Dis J* 2002;21:796.

370. Lea AP, Bryson HM. Cidofovir. *Drugs* 1996;52:225.

371. Revello MG, Gerna G. Pathogenesis and prenatal diagnosis of human cytomegalovirus infection. *J Clin Virol* 2004;29:71.

372. Kumazaki K, Ozono K, Yahara T, et al. Detection of cytomegalovirus DNA in human placenta. *J Med Virol* 2002;68:363.

373. Boppana SB, Pass RF, Britt WJ, et al. Symptomatic congenital cytomegalovirus infection: neonatal morbidity and mortality. *Pediatr Infect Dis J* 1992;11:93.

374. Bale JF Jr, Blackman JA, Sato Y. Outcome in children with symptomatic congenital cytomegalovirus infection. *J Child Neurol* 1990;5:131.

375. Ramsay MEB, Miller E, Peckham CS. Outcome of confirmed symptomatic congenital cytomegalovirus infection. *Arch Dis Child* 1991;66:1068.

376. Perlman JM, Argyle C. Lethal cytomegalovirus infection in preterm infants: clinical, radiological, and neuropathological findings. *Ann Neurol* 1992;31:64.

377. Bissinger AL, Sinzger C, Kaiserling E, et al. Human cytomegalovirus as a direct pathogen: correlation of multiorgan involvement and cell distribution with clinical and pathological findings in a case of congenital inclusion disease. *J Med Virol* 2002;67:200.

378. Nigro G, La Torre R, Sali E, et al. Intraventricular haemorrhage in a fetus with cerebral cytomegalovirus infection. *Prenat Diagn* 2002;22:558.

379. Moinuddin A, McKinstry RC, Martin KA, et al. Intracranial hemorrhage progressing to porencephaly as a result of congenitally acquired cytomegalovirus infection—an illustrative report. *Prenat Diagn* 2003;23:797.

380. Boppana SB, Fowler KB, Vaid Y, et al. Neuroradiographic findings in the newborn period and long-term outcome in children with symptomatic congenital cytomegalovirus infection. *Pediatrics* 1997;99:409.

381. Coats DK, Demmler GJ, Paysse EA, et al. Ophthalmologic findings in children with congenital cytomegalovirus infection. *J AAPOS* 2000;4:110.

382. Mets MB. Eye manifestations of intrauterine infections. *Ophthalmol Clin North Am* 2001;13:521.

383. Noffke AS, Mets MB. Spontaneous resolution of cytomegalovirus retinitis in an infant with congenital cytomegalovirus infection. *Retina* 2001;21:541.

384. Williamson WD, Demmler GJ, Percy AK, et al. Progressive hearing loss in infants with asymptomatic congenital cytomegalovirus infection. *Pediatrics* 1992;90:862.

385. Fowler KB, McCollister FP, Dahle AJ, et al. Progressive and fluctuating sensorineural hearing loss in children with asymptomatic congenital cytomegalovirus infection. *J Pediatr* 1997;130:624.

386. Fowler KB, Dahle AJ, Boppana SB, et al. Newborn hearing screening: will children with hearing loss caused by congenital cytomegalovirus infection be missed? *J Pediatr* 1999;135:60.

387. Rivera LB, Boppana SB, Fowler KB, et al. Predictors of hearing loss in children with symptomatic congenital cytomegalovirus infection. *Pediatrics* 2002;110:762.

388. Huygen PLM, Admiral RJC. Audiovestibular sequelae of congenital cytomegalovirus infection in 3 children presumably representing 3 symptomatically different types of delayed endolymphatic hydrops. *Int J Pediatr Otorhinolaryngol* 1996;35:143.

389. Barbi M, Binda S, Caroppo S, et al. A wider role for congenital cytomegalovirus infection in sensorineural hearing loss. *Pediatr Infect Dis J* 2003;22:39.

390. Noyola DE, Demmler GJ, Nelson CT, et al. Early predictors of neurodevelopmental outcome in symptomatic congenital cytomegalovirus infection. *J Pediatr* 2001;138:325.

391. Kashden J, Frison S, Fowler K, et al. Intellectual assessment of children with asymptomatic congenital cytomegalovirus infection. *J Dev Behav Pediatr* 1998;19:254.

392. Temple RO, Pass RF, Boll TJ. Neuropsychological functioning in patients with asymptomatic congenital cytomegalovirus infection. *J Dev Behav Pediatr* 2000;21:417.

393. Ivarsson S-A, Lernmark B, Svanberg L. Ten-year clinical, developmental, and intellectual follow-up of children with congenital cytomegalovirus infection without neurologic symptoms at one year of age. *Pediatrics* 1997;99:800.

394. Stagno S, Pass RF, Thomas JP, et al. Defects of tooth structure in congenital cytomegalovirus infection. *Pediatrics* 1982;69:646.

395. Morris DJ. Epidemiological evidence is crucial as proof of causation in cytomegalovirus disease. *J Infect* 1991;23:233.

396. Hart MH, Kaufman SS, Vanderhoof JA, et al. Neonatal hepatitis and extrahepatic biliary atresia associated with cytomegalovirus infection in twins. *Am J Dis Child* 1991;145:302.

397. Mena W, Royal S, Pass RF, et al. Diabetes insipidus associated with symptomatic congenital cytomegalovirus infection. *J Pediatr* 1993;122:911.

398. Comas C, Martinez Crespo JM, Puerto B, et al. Bilateral renal agenesis and cytomegalovirus infection in a case of Fraser syndrome. *Fetal Diagn Ther* 1993;8:285.

399. Baker ER, Eberhardt H, Brown ZA. "Stuck twin" syndrome associated with congenital cytomegalovirus infection. *Am J Perinatol* 1993;10:81.

400. Bauman NM, Kirby-Keyser LJ, Dolan KD, et al. Mondini dysplasia and congenital cytomegalovirus infection. *J Pediatr* 1994;124:71.

401. Tarr PI, Haas JE, Christie DL. Biliary atresia, cytomegalovirus, and age at referral. *Pediatrics* 1996;97:828.

402. Carrol ED, Campbell ME, Shaw BNJ, et al. Congenital lobar emphysema in congenital cytomegalovirus infection. *Pediatr Radiol* 1996;26:900.

403. Lanari M, Lazzarotto T, Papa I, et al. Neonatal aortic arch thrombosis as a result of congenital cytomegalovirus infection. *Pediatrics* 2001;108:e114.

404. Ahlfors K, Ivarsson S-A, Nilsson H. On the unpredictable development of congenital cytomegalovirus infection: a study in twins. *Early Hum Dev* 1988;18:125.

405. Schneeberger PM, Groenendaal F, de Vries LS, et al. Variable outcome of a congenital cytomegalovirus infection in a quadruplet after primary infection of the mother during pregnancy. *Acta Paediatr* 1994;83:986.

406. Lazzarotto T, Gabrielli L, Foschini MP, et al. Congenital cytomegalovirus infection in twin pregnancies: viral load in the amniotic fluid and pregnancy outcome. *Pediatrics* 2003;112:e153.

407. Jenson HB, Robert MF. Congenital cytomegalovirus infection with osteolytic lesions: use of DNA hybridization in diagnosis. *Clin Pediatr (Phila)* 1987;26:448.

408. Warren WP, Balcarek K, Smith R, et al. Comparison of rapid methods of detection of cytomegalovirus in saliva with virus isolation in tissue culture. *J Clin Microbiol* 1992;30:786.

409. Chang M-H, Huang H-H, Huang E-S, et al. Polymerase chain reaction to detect human cytomegalovirus in livers of infants with neonatal hepatitis. *Gastroenterology* 1992;103:1022.

410. Nelson CT, Istas AS, Wilkerson MK, et al. PCR detection of cytomegalovirus DNA in serum as a diagnostic test for congenital cytomegalovirus infection. *J Clin Microbiol* 1995;33:3317.

411. Schlesinger Y, Halle D, Eidelman AI, et al. Urine polymerase chain reaction as a screening tool for the detection of congenital cytomegalovirus infection. *Arch Dis Child Fetal Neonatal Ed* 2003;88:F371.

412. Revello MG, Zavattoni M, Baldanti F, et al. Diagnostic and prognostic value of human cytomegalovirus load and IgM antibody in blood of congenitally infected newborns. *J Clin Virol* 1999;14:57.

413. Halwachs-Baumann G, Genser B, Pailer S, et al. Human cytomegalovirus load in various body fluids of congenitally infected newborns. *J Clin Virol* 2002;25(Suppl 3):S81.

414. Zucca C, Binda S, Borgatti R, et al. Retrospective diagnosis of congenital cytomegalovirus infection and cortical maldevelopment. *Neurology* 2003;61:710.

415. Kimberlin DW, Lin C-Y, Sánchez PJ, et al. Effect of ganciclovir therapy on hearing in symptomatic congenital cytomegalovirus disease involving the central nervous system: a randomized, controlled trial. *J Pediatr* 2003;143:16.

416. Zhou X-J, Gruber W, Demmler G, et al. Population pharmacokinetics of ganciclovir in newborns with congenital cytomegalovirus infections. *Antimicrob Agents Chemother* 1996;40:2202.

417. Hocker JR, Cook LN, Adams G, et al. Ganciclovir therapy of congenital cytomegalovirus pneumonia. *Pediatr Infect Dis J* 1990;9:743.

418. Evans DGR, Lyon AJ. Fatal congenital cytomegalovirus infection acquired by an intra-uterine transfusion. *Eur J Pediatr* 1991;150:780.

419. Reigstad H, Bjerknes R, Markestad T, et al. Ganciclovir therapy of congenital cytomegalovirus disease. *Acta Paediatr* 1992;81:707.

420. Attard-Montalto SP, English MC, Stimmler L, et al. Ganciclovir treatment of congenital cytomegalovirus infection: a report of two cases. *Scand J Infect Dis* 1993;25:385.

421. Stronati M, Revello MG, Cerbo RM, et al. Ganciclovir therapy of congenital human cytomegalovirus hepatitis. *Acta Paediatr* 1995;84:340.

422. Halwachs G, Kutschera J, Tiran A, et al. Antiviral treatment of congenitally infected children with a positive cytomegalovirus polymerase chain reaction in the cerebrospinal fluid. *Scand J Infect Dis Suppl* 1995;99:89.

423. Nigro G, Scholz H, Bartmann U. Ganciclovir therapy for symptomatic congenital cytomegalovirus infection in infants: a two-regimen experience. *J Pediatr* 1994;124:318.

424. Whitley RJ, Kimberlin DW. Treatment of viral infections during pregnancy and the neonatal period. *Clin Perinatol* 1997;24:267.

425. Nigro G, Krzysztofiak A, Bartmann U, et al. Ganciclovir therapy for cytomegalovirus-associated liver disease in immunocompetent or immunocompromised children. *Arch Virol* 1997;142:573.

426. Whitley RJ, Cloud G, Gruber W, et al. Ganciclovir treatment of symptomatic congenital cytomegalovirus infection: results of a phase II study. *J Infect Dis* 1997;175:1080.

427. Fischler B, Casswall TH, Malmborg P, et al. Ganciclovir treatment in infants with cytomegalovirus infection and cholestasis. *J Pediatr Gastroenterol Nutr* 2002;34:154.

428. Demmler GJ. Congenital cytomegalovirus infection treatment. *Pediatr Infect Dis J* 2003;22:1005.

429. Rongkavilit C, Bedard MP, Ang JY, et al. Severe cytomegalovirus enterocolitis in an immunocompetent infant. *Pediatr Infect Dis J* 2004;23:579.

430. Prober CG, Enright AM. Congenital cytomegalovirus (CMV) infections: hats off to Alabama. *J Pediatr* 2003;143:4.

431. Revello MG, Percivalle E, Baldanti F, et al. Prenatal treatment of congenital human cytomegalovirus infection by fetal intravascular administration of ganciclovir. *Clin Diagn Virol* 1993;1:61.

432. Negishi H, Yamada H, Hirayama E, et al. Intraperitoneal administration of cytomegalovirus hyperimmunoglobulin to the cytomegalovirus-infected fetus. *J Perinatol* 1998;18:466.

433. Nigro G, La Torre R, Anceschi MM, et al. Hyperimmunoglobulin therapy for a twin fetus with cytomegalovirus infection and growth restriction. *Am J Obstet Gynecol* 1999;180:1222.

434. Alford C. Breast milk transmission of cytomegalovirus (CMV) infection. *Adv Exp Med Biol* 1991;310:293.

435. Bryant P, Morley C, Garland S, et al. Cytomegalovirus transmission from breast milk in premature babies: does it matter? *Arch Dis Child Fetal Neonatal Ed* 2002;87:F75.

436. Yasuda A, Kimura H, Hayakawa M, et al. Evaluation of cytomegalovirus infections transmitted via breast milk in preterm infants with a real-time polymerase chain reaction assay. *Pediatrics* 2003;111:1333.

437. Vollmer B, Seibold-Weiger K, Schmitz-Salue C, et al. Postnatally acquired cytomegalovirus infection via breast milk: effects on

438. Portelli J, Gordon A, May JT. Effect of human milk sialyllactose on cytomegalovirus. *Eur J Clin Microbiol Infect Dis* 1998; 17:66.

439. Portelli J, Gordon A, May JT. Effect of compounds with antibacterial activities in human milk on respiratory syncytial virus and cytomegalovirus in vitro. *J Med Microbiol* 1998;47:1015.

440. de Cates CR, Gray J, Roberton NRC, et al. Acquisition of cytomegalovirus infection by premature neonates. *J Infect* 1994;28:25.

441. Cheong JLY, Cowan FM, Modi N. Gastrointestinal manifestations of postnatal cytomegalovirus infection in infants admitted to a neonatal intensive care unit over a five year period. *Arch Dis Child Fetal Neonatal Ed* 2004;89:F367.

442. Prösch S, Lienicke U, Priemer C, et al. Human adenovirus and human cytomegalovirus infections in preterm newborns: no association with bronchopulmonary dysplasia. *Pediatr Res* 2002;52:219.

443. Gentile MA, Boll TJ, Stagno S, et al. Intellectual ability of children after perinatal cytomegalovirus infection. *Dev Med Child Neurol* 1989;31:782.

444. Lynch L, Daffos F, Emanuel D, et al. Prenatal diagnosis of fetal cytomegalovirus infection. *Am J Obstet Gynecol* 1991;165:714.

445. Hohlfeld P, Vial Y, Maillard-Brignon C, et al. Cytomegalovirus fetal infection: prenatal diagnosis. *Obstet Gynecol* 1991; 78:615.

446. Lamy ME, Mulongo KN, Gadisseux J-F, et al. Prenatal diagnosis of fetal cytomegalovirus infection. *Am J Obstet Gynecol* 1992;166:91.

447. Weber B, Opp M, Born HJ, et al. Laboratory diagnosis of congenital human cytomegalovirus infection using polymerase chain reaction and shell vial culture. *Infection* 1992;20:155.

448. Hogge WA, Buffone GJ, Hogge JS. Prenatal diagnosis of cytomegalovirus (CMV) infection: a preliminary report. *Prenat Diagn* 1993;13:131.

449. Catanzarite V, Dankner WM. Prenatal diagnosis of congenital cytomegalovirus infection: false-negative amniocentesis at 20 weeks gestation. *Prenat Diagn* 1993;13:1021.

450. Donner C, Liesnard C, Content J, et al. Prenatal diagnosis of 52 pregnancies at risk for congenital cytomegalovirus infection. *Obstet Gynecol* 1993;82:481.

451. Achiron R, Pinhas-Hamiel O, Lipitz S, et al. Prenatal ultrasonographic diagnosis of fetal cerebral ventriculitis associated with asymptomatic maternal cytomegalovirus infection. *Prenat Diagn* 1994;14:523.

452. Nicolini U, Kustermann A, Tassis B, et al. Prenatal diagnosis of congenital human cytomegalovirus infection. *Prenat Diagn* 1994;14:903.

453. Watt-Morse ML, Laifer SA, Hill LM. The natural history of fetal cytomegalovirus infection as assessed by serial ultrasound and fetal blood sampling: a case report. *Prenat Diagn* 1995;15:567.

454. Revello MG, Baldanti F, Furione M, et al. Polymerase chain reaction for prenatal diagnosis of congenital human cytomegalovirus infection. *J Med Virol* 1995;47:462.

455. Revello MG, Gerna G. Diagnosis and management of human cytomegalovirus infection in the mother, fetus, and newborn infant. *Clin Microbiol Rev* 2002;15:680.

456. Kyriazopoulou V, Bondis J, Frantzidou F, et al. Prenatal diagnosis of fetal cytomegalovirus infection in seropositive pregnant women. *Eur J Obstet Gynecol Reprod Biol* 1996;69:91.

457. Lipitz S, Yagel S, Shalev E, et al. Prenatal diagnosis of fetal primary cytomegalovirus infection. *Obstet Gynecol* 1997;89:763.

458. Lazzarotto T, Guerra B, Spezzacatena P, et al. Prenatal diagnosis of congenital cytomegalovirus infection. *J Clin Microbiol* 1998;36:3540.

459. Revello MG, Zavattoni M, Furione M, et al. Quantification of human cytomegalovirus DNA in amniotic fluid of mothers of congenitally infected fetuses. *J Clin Microbiol* 1999;37:3350.

460. Nigro G, Mazzocco M, Anceschi MM, et al. Prenatal diagnosis of fetal cytomegalovirus infection after primary or recurrent maternal infection. *Obstet Gynecol* 1999;94:909.

461. Bodéus M, Hubinont C, Bernard P, et al. Prenatal diagnosis of human cytomegalovirus by culture and polymerase chain reaction: 98 pregnancies leading to congenital infection. *Prenat Diagn* 1999;19:314.

462. Antsaklis AJ, Daskalakis GJ, Mesogitis SA, et al. Prenatal diagnosis of fetal primary cytomegalovirus infection. *BJOG* 2000; 107:84.

463. Liesnard C, Donner C, Brancart F, et al. Prenatal diagnosis of congenital cytomegalovirus infection: prospective study of 237 pregnancies at risk. *Obstet Gynecol* 2000;95:881.

464. Guerra B, Lazzarotto T, Quarta S, et al. Prenatal diagnosis of symptomatic congenital cytomegalovirus infection. *Am J Obstet Gynecol* 2000;183:476.

465. Azam A-Z, Vial Y, Fawer C-L, et al. Prenatal diagnosis of congenital cytomegalovirus infection. *Obstet Gynecol* 2001;97:443.

466. Enders G, Bäder U, Lindemann L, et al. Prenatal diagnosis of congenital cytomegalovirus infection in 189 pregnancies with known outcome. *Prenat Diagn* 2001;21:362.

467. Revello MG, Lilleri D, Zavattoni M, et al. Human cytomegalovirus immediate-early messenger RNA in blood of pregnant women with primary infection and of congenitally infected newborns. *J Infect Dis* 2001;184:1078.

468. Gerber S, Vial Y, Hohlfeld P, et al. Prenatal diagnosis of congenital cytomegalovirus infection by detection of immunoglobulin M antibodies to the 70-kd heat shock protein in fetal serum. *Am J Obstet Gynecol* 2002;187:955.

469. Gouarin S, Palmer P, Cointe D, et al. Congenital HCMV infection: a collaborative and comparative study of virus detection in amniotic fluid by culture and by PCR. *J Clin Virol* 2001;21:47.

470. Gouarin S, Gault E, Vabret A, et al. Real-time PCR quantitation of human cytomegalovirus DNA in amniotic fluid samples from mothers with primary infection. *J Clin Microbiol* 2002;40:1767.

471. Lipitz S, Achiron R, Zalel Y, et al. Outcome of pregnancies with vertical transmission of primary cytomegalovirus infection. *Obstet Gynecol* 2002;100:428.

472. Petrikovsky BM, Lipson SM, Kaplan MH. Viral studies on amniotic fluid from fetuses with and without abnormalities detected by prenatal sonography. *J Reprod Med* 2003;48:230.

473. Revello MG, Lilleri D, Zavattoni M, et al. Prenatal diagnosis of congenital human cytomegalovirus infection in amniotic fluid by nucleic acid sequence-based amplification assay. *J Clin Microbiol* 2003;41:1772.

474. Nishimura N, Kimura H, Yabuta Y, et al. Prevalence of maternal cytomegalovirus (CMV) antibody and detection of CMV DNA in amniotic fluid. *Microbiol Immunol* 1999;43:781.

475. Dong Z-W, Yan C, Yi W, et al. Detection of congenital cytomegalovirus infection by using chorionic villi of the early pregnancy and polymerase chain reaction. *Int J Gynaecol Obstet* 1994;44:229.

476. Pletcher BA, Williams MK, Mulivor RA, et al. Intrauterine cytomegalovirus infection presenting as fetal meconium peritonitis. *Obstet Gynecol* 1991;78:903.

477. Mazeron M-C, Cordovi-Voulgaropoulos L, Pérol Y. Transient hydrops fetalis associated with intrauterine cytomegalovirus infection: prenatal diagnosis. *Obstet Gynecol* 1994;84:692.

478. Dogra VK, Menon PA, Poblete J, et al. Neurosonographic imaging of small-for-gestational-age neonates exposed and not exposed to cocaine and cytomegalovirus. *J Clin Ultrasound* 1994;22:93.

479. Muller F, Dommergues M, Aubry M-C, et al. Hyperechogenic fetal bowel: an ultrasonographic marker for adverse fetal and neonatal outcome. *Am J Obstet Gynecol* 1995;173:508.

480. Al-Kouatly HB, Chasen ST, Strelzoff J, et al. The clinical significance of fetal echogenic bowel. *Am J Obstet Gynecol* 2001; 185:1035.

481. Simchen MJ, Toi A, Bona M, et al. Fetal hepatic calcifications: prenatal diagnosis and outcome. *Am J Obstet Gynecol* 2002; 187:1617.

482. Chaoui R, Zodan-Marin T, Wisser J. Marked splenomegaly in fetal cytomegalovirus infection: detection supported by three-dimensional power Doppler ultrasound. *Ultrasound Obstet Gynecol* 2002;20:299.

483. Malinger G, Lev D, Zahalka N, et al. Fetal cytomegalovirus infection of the brain: the spectrum of sonographic findings. *AJNR Am J Neuroradiol* 2003;24:28.

484. Pass RF, Burke RL. Development of cytomegalovirus vaccines: prospects for prevention of congenital CMV infection. *Semin Pediatr Infect Dis* 2002;13:196.

485. Schleiss MR, Bourne N, Stroup G, et al. Protection against congenital cytomegalovirus infection and disease in guinea pigs, conferred by a purified recombinant glycoprotein B vaccine. *J Infect Dis* 2004;189:1374.

486. Collinet P, Subtil D, Houfflin-Debarge V, et al. Routine CMV screening during pregnancy. *Eur J Obstet Gynecol Reprod Biol* 2004;114:3.

487. Tierney AJ, Higa TE, Finer NN. Disseminated cytomegalovirus infection after extracorporeal membrane oxygenation. *Pediatr Infect Dis J* 1992;11:241.

488. Muir WB, Nichols R, Breuer J. Phylogenetic analysis of varicella-zoster virus: evidence of intercontinental spread of genotypes and recombination. *J Virol* 2002;76:1971.

489. Wharton M. The epidemiology of varicella-zoster virus infections. *Infect Dis Clin North Am* 1996;10:571.

490. Centers for Disease Control and Prevention. Varicella-zoster immune globulin for the prevention of chickenpox. *MMWR* 1984;33:84.

491. Vázquez M. Varicella zoster virus infections in children after the introduction of live attenuated varicella vaccine. *Curr Opin Pediatr* 2004;16:80.

492. Seward JF, Watson BM, Peterson CL, et al. Varicella disease after introduction of varicella vaccine in the United States, 1995–2000. *JAMA* 2002;287:606.

493. Sever JL, Ellenberg JH, Ley A, et al. Incidence of clinical infections in a defined population of pregnant women. In: Marois M, ed. *Prevention of physical and mental congenital defects. Part B: epidemiology, early detection and therapy, and environmental factors.* New York: Alan R. Liss, 1985:317.

494. Chapman SJ. Varicella in pregnancy. *Semin Perinatol* 1998; 22:339.

495. Ross AH. Modification of chicken pox in family contacts by administration of gamma globulin. *N Engl J Med* 1962; 267:369.

496. Kuo Y-H, Yip Y, Chen S-N. Retinal vasculitis associated with chickenpox. *Am J Ophthalmol* 2001;132:584.

497. Maupin RT. Obstetric infectious disease emergencies. *Clin Obstet Gynecol* 2002;45:393.

498. Martin KA, Junker AK, Thomas EE, et al. Occurrence of chickenpox during pregnancy in women seropositive for varicella-zoster virus. *J Infect Dis* 1994;170:991.

499. Hall S, Maupin T, Seward J, et al. Second varicella infections: are they more common than previously thought? *Pediatrics* 2002;109:1068.

500. Enders G. Varicella-zoster virus infection in pregnancy. *Prog Med Virol* 1984;29:166.

501. Kido S, Ozaki T, Asada H, et al. Detection of varicella-zoster virus (VZV) DNA in clinical samples from patients with VZV by the polymerase chain reaction. *J Clin Microbiol* 1991;29:76.

502. Koropchak CM, Graham G, Palmer J, et al. Investigation of varicella-zoster virus infection by polymerase chain reaction in the immunocompetent host with acute varicella. *J Infect Dis* 1991;163:1016.

503. Studahl M, Hagberg L, Rekabdar E, et al. Herpesvirus DNA detection in cerebral spinal fluid: differences in clinical presentation between alpha-, beta-, and gamma-herpesviruses. *Scand J Infect Dis* 2000;32:237.

504. Birch CJ, Druce JD, Catton MC, et al. Detection of varicella zoster virus in genital specimens using a multiplex polymerase chain reaction. *Sex Transm Infect* 2003;79:298.

505. Kimura H, Kido S, Ozaki T, et al. Comparison of quantitations of viral load in varicella and zoster. *J Clin Microbiol* 2000;38:2447.

506. de Jong MD, Weel JFL, Schuurman T, et al. Quantitation of varicella-zoster virus DNA in whole blood, plasma, and serum by PCR and electrochemiluminescence. *J Clin Microbiol* 2000; 38:2568.

507. Krah DL. Assays for antibodies to varicella-zoster virus. *Infect Dis Clin North Am* 1996;10:507.

508. Rothe MJ, Feder HM Jr, Grant-Kels JM. Oral acyclovir therapy for varicella and zoster infections in pediatric and pregnant patients: a brief review. *Pediatr Dermatol* 1991;8:236.

509. Wallace MR, Bowler WA, Murray NB, et al. Treatment of adult varicella with oral acyclovir: a randomized, placebo-controlled trial. *Ann Intern Med* 1992;117:358.

510. Broussard RC, Payne DK, George RB. Treatment with acyclovir of varicella pneumonia in pregnancy. *Chest* 1991;99:1045.

511. Esmonde TF, Herdman G, Anderson G. Chickenpox pneumonia: an association with pregnancy. *Thorax* 1989;44:812.

512. Cox SM, Cunningham FG, Luby J. Management of varicella pneumonia complicating pregnancy. *Am J Perinatol* 1990;7:300.

513. Lotshaw RR, Keegan JM, Gordon HR. Parenteral and oral acyclovir for management of varicella pneumonia in pregnancy: a case report with review of literature. *W V Med J* 1991;87:204.

514. Smego RA Jr, Asperilla MO. Use of acyclovir for varicella pneumonia during pregnancy. *Obstet Gynecol* 1991;78:1112.

515. Katz VL, Kuller JA, McMahon MJ, et al. Varicella during pregnancy: maternal and fetal effects. *West J Med* 1995;163:446.

516. Nathwani D, Maclean A, Conway S, et al. Varicella infections in pregnancy and the newborn: a review prepared for the UK Advisory Group on Chickenpox on behalf of the British Society for the Study of Infection. *J Infect* 1998;36(Suppl 1):59.

517. Harger JH, Ernest JM, Thurnau GR, et al. Risk factors and outcome of varicella-zoster virus pneumonia in pregnant women. *J Infect Dis* 2002;185:422.

518. Puchhammer-Stöckl E, Kunz C, Wagner G, et al. Detection of varicella zoster virus (VZV) DNA in fetal tissue by polymerase chain reaction. *J Perinat Med* 1994;22:65.

519. Sauerbrei A, Müller D, Eichhorn U, et al. Detection of varicella-zoster virus in congenital varicella syndrome: a case report. *Obstet Gynecol* 1996;88:687.

520. Oyer CE, Cai R, Coughlin JJ, et al. First trimester pregnancy loss associated with varicella zoster virus infection: histological definition of a case. *Hum Pathol* 1998;29:94.

521. Cooper C, Wojtulewicz J, Ratnamohan VM, et al. Congenital varicella syndrome diagnosed by polymerase chain reaction—scarring of the spinal cord, not the skin. *J Paediatr Child Health* 2000;36:186.

522. Verstraelen H, Vanzieleghem B, Defoort P, et al. Prenatal ultrasound and magnetic resonance imaging in fetal varicella syndrome: correlation with pathology findings. *Prenat Diagn* 2003;23:705.

523. Paryani SG, Arvin AM. Intrauterine infection with varicella-zoster virus after maternal varicella. *N Engl J Med* 1986; 314:1542.

524. Siegel M, Fuerst HT. Low birth weight and maternal virus diseases: a prospective study of rubella, measles, mumps, chickenpox, and hepatitis. *JAMA* 1966;197:680.

525. Siegel M, Fuerst HT, Peress NS. Comparative fetal mortality in maternal virus diseases: a prospective study on rubella, measles, mumps, chickenpox and hepatitis. *N Engl J Med* 1966;274:768.

526. Benyesh-Melnick M, Stich HF, Rapp F, et al. Viruses and mammalian chromosomes. III. Effect of herpes zoster virus on human embryonal lung cultures. *Proc Soc Exp Biol Med* 1964;117:546.

527. Aula P. Chromosomes and viral infections. *Lancet* 1964;1:720.

528. Massimo L, Vianello MG, Dagna-Bricarelli F, et al. Chickenpox and chromosome aberrations. *BMJ* 1965;2:172.

529. Muñoz N. Perinatal viral infections and the risk of certain cancers. *Prog Biochem Pharmacol* 1978;14:104.

530. Alexander I. Congenital varicella. *BMJ* 1979;2:1074.

531. Alkalay AL, Pomerance JJ, Rimoin DL. Fetal varicella syndrome. *J Pediatr* 1987;111:320.

532. Andreou A, Basiakos H, Hatzikoumi I, et al. Fetal varicella syndrome with manifestations limited to the eye. *Am J Perinatol* 1995;12:347.

533. Bennet R, Forsgren M, Herin P. Herpes zoster in a 2-week-old premature infant with possible congenital varicella encephalitis. *Acta Paediatr Scand* 1985;74:979.

534. Borzyskowski M, Harris RF, Jones RWA. The congenital varicella syndrome. *Eur J Pediatr* 1981;137:335.

535. Brice JEH. Congenital varicella resulting from infection during second trimester of pregnancy. *Arch Dis Child* 1976;51:474.

536. Charles NC, Bennett TW, Margolis S. Ocular pathology of the congenital varicella syndrome. *Arch Ophthalmol* 1977;95:2034.

537. Cotlier E. Congenital varicella cataract. *Am J Ophthalmol* 1978;86:627.

538. Cuthbertson G, Weiner CP, Giller RH, et al. Prenatal diagnosis of second-trimester congenital varicella syndrome by virus-specific immunoglobulin M. *J Pediatr* 1987;111:592.

539. Dodion-Fransen J, Dekegel D, Thiry L. Congenital varicella-zoster infection related to maternal disease in early pregnancy. *Scand J Infect Dis* 1973;5:149.

540. Essex-Cater A, Heggarty H. Fatal congenital varicella syndrome. *J Infect* 1983;7:77.

541. Frey HM, Bialkin G, Gershon AA. Congenital varicella: case report of a serologically proved long-term survivor. *Pediatrics* 1977;59:110.

542. Friedman RM, Wood VE. Varicella gangrenosa in the newborn upper extremity: a case report. *J Hand Surg [Am]* 1996;21:487.

543. Hajdi G, Mészner Z, Nyerges G, et al. Congenital varicella syndrome. *Infection* 1986;14:177.

544. Harding B, Baumer JA. Congenital varicella-zoster: a serologically proven case with necrotizing encephalitis and malformation. *Acta Neuropathol (Berl)* 1988;76:311.

545. Higa K, Dan K, Manabe H. Varicella-zoster virus infections during pregnancy: hypothesis concerning the mechanisms of congenital malformations. *Obstet Gynecol* 1987;69:214.

546. Hitchcock R, Birthistle K, Carrington D, et al. Colonic atresia and spinal cord atrophy associated with a case of fetal varicella syndrome. *J Pediatr Surg* 1995;30:1344.

547. Huang Y-C, Lin T-Y, Wong K-S, et al. Congenital anomalies following maternal varicella infection during early pregnancy. *J Formos Med Assoc* 1996;95:393.

548. König R, Gutjahr P, Kruel R, et al. Konnatale Varizellen-Embryo-Fetopathie. *Helv Paediatr Acta* 1985;40:391.

549. Kotchmar GS Jr, Grose C, Brunell PA. Complete spectrum of the varicella congenital defects syndrome in 5-year-old child. *Pediatr Infect Dis* 1984;3:142.

550. LaForet EG, Lynch CL Jr. Multiple congenital defects following maternal varicella: report of a case. *N Engl J Med* 1947; 236:534.

551. McKendry JBJ, Bailey JD. Congenital varicella associated with multiple defects. *CMAJ* 1973;108:66.

552. Randel RC, Kearns DB, Nespeca MP, et al. Vocal cord paralysis as a presentation of intrauterine infection with varicella-zoster virus. *Pediatrics* 1996;97:127.

553. Rigsby CK, Donnelly LF. Fetal varicella syndrome: association with multiple hepatic calcifications and intestinal atresia. *Pediatr Radiol* 1997;27:779.

554. Rinvik R. Congenital varicella encephalomyelitis in surviving newborn. *Am J Dis Child* 1969;117:231.

555. Savage MO, Moosa A, Gordon RR. Maternal varicella infection as a cause of fetal malformations. *Lancet* 1973;1:352.

556. Siegel M. Congenital malformations following chickenpox, measles, mumps, and hepatitis: results of a cohort study. *JAMA* 1973;226:1521.

557. Srabstein JC, Morris N, Bryce Larke RP, et al. Is there a congenital varicella syndrome? *J Pediatr* 1974;84:239.

558. Taranger J, Blomberg J, Strannegård Ö. Intrauterine varicella: a report of two cases associated with hyper-A-immunoglobulinemia. *Scand J Infect Dis* 1981;13:297.

559. Trlifajová J, Benda R, Beneš Č. Effect of maternal varicella-zoster virus infection on the outcome of pregnancy and the analysis of transplacental virus transmission. *Acta Virol* 1986;30:249.

560. Tudehope DI. Two lethal cases of congenital varicella syndrome. *J Paediatr Child Health* 1995;31:259.

561. Unger-Köppel J, Kilcher P, Tönz O. Varizellenfetopathie. *Helv Paediatr Acta* 1985;40:399.

562. Wheatley R, Morton RE, Nicholson J. Chickenpox in mid-trimester pregnancy: always innocent? *Dev Med Child Neurol* 1996;38:462.

563. Williamson AP. The varicella-zoster virus in the etiology of severe congenital defects: a survey of eleven reported instances. *Clin Pediatr (Phila)* 1975;14:553.

564. Lambert SR, Taylor D, Kriss A, et al. Ocular manifestations of the congenital varicella syndrome. *Arch Ophthalmol* 1989; 107:52.

565. Lloyd KM, Dunne JL. Skin lesions as the sole manifestation of the fetal varicella syndrome. *Arch Dermatol* 1990;126:546.

566. Scharf A, Scherr O, Enders G, et al. Virus detection in the fetal tissue of a premature delivery with a congenital varicella syndrome: a case report. *J Perinat Med* 1990;18:317.

567. Da Silva O, Hammerberg O, Chance GW. Fetal varicella syndrome. *Pediatr Infect Dis J* 1990;9:854.

568. Scheffer IE, Baraitser M, Brett EM. Severe microcephaly associated with congenital varicella infection. *Dev Med Child Neurol* 1991;33:916.

569. Magliocco AM, Demetrick DJ, Sarnat HB, et al. Varicella embryopathy. *Arch Pathol Lab Med* 1992;116:181.

570. Liang CD, Yu TJ, Ko SF. Ipsilateral renal dysplasia with hypertensive heart disease in an infant with cutaneous varicella lesions: an unusual presentation of congenital varicella syndrome. *J Am Acad Dermatol* 2000;43:864.

571. Forrest JM, Mego S, Burgess MA. Congenital and neonatal varicella in Australia. *J Paediatr Child Health* 2000;36:108.

572. Choong CS, Patole S, Whitehall J. Congenital varicella syndrome in the absence of cutaneous lesions. *J Paediatr Child Health* 2000;36:184.

573. Bruder E, Ersch J, Hebisch G, et al. Fetal varicella syndrome: disruption of neural development and persistent inflammation of non-neural tissues. *Virch Arch* 2000;437:440.

574. Kent A, Paes B. Congenital varicella syndrome: a rare case of central nervous system involvement without dermatologic features. *Am J Perinatol* 2000;17:253.

575. Schulze A, Dietzsch H-J. The natural history of varicella embryopathy: a 25-year follow-up. *J Pediatr* 2000;137:871.

576. Petignat P, Vial Y, Laurini R, et al. Fetal varicella-herpes zoster syndrome in early pregnancy: ultrasonographic and morphological correlation. *Prenat Diagn* 2001;21:121.

577. Ehrbar T, Arlettaz R, Ersch J, et al. A small-for-dates newborn girl with a mummified left arm. *Eur J Pediatr* 2001;160:395.

578. Mazzella M, Arioni C, Bellini C, et al. Severe hydrocephalus associated with congenital varicella syndrome. *CMAJ* 2003;168:561.

579. Sauve RS, Leung AKC. Congenital varicella syndrome with colonic atresias. *Clin Pediatr (Phila)* 2003;42:451.

580. Sauerbrei A, Pawlak J, Luger C, et al. Intracerebral varicella-zoster virus reactivation in congenital varicella syndrome. *Dev Med Child Neurol* 2003;45:837.

581. Sauerbrei A, Pawlak J, Luger C, et al. Hints of intracerebral varicella-zoster virus reactivation in congenital varicella syndrome. *Eur J Pediatr* 2003;162:354.

582. Asha Bai PV, John TJ. Congenital skin ulcers following varicella in late pregnancy. *J Pediatr* 1979;94:65.

583. Salzman MB, Sood SK. Congenital anomalies resulting from maternal varicella at 25½ weeks of gestation. *Pediatr Infect Dis J* 1992;11:504.

584. Al-Qattan MM, Thomson HG. Congenital varicella of the upper limb: a preventable disaster. *J Hand Surg [Br]* 1995;20:115.

585. Harger JH, Ernest JM, Thurnau GR, et al. Frequency of congenital varicella syndrome in a prospective cohort of 347 pregnant women. *Obstet Gynecol* 2002;100:260.

586. Pastuszak AL, Levy M, Schick B, et al. Outcome after maternal varicella infection in the first 20 weeks of pregnancy. *N Engl J Med* 1994;330:901.

587. Enders G, Miller E, Cradock-Watson J, et al. Consequences of varicella and herpes zoster in pregnancy: prospective study of 1739 cases. *Lancet* 1994;343:1547.

588. Jones KL, Johnson KA, Chambers CD. Offspring of women infected with varicella during pregnancy: a prospective study. *Teratology* 1994;49:29.

589. Figueroa-Damian R, Arredondo-Garcia JL. Perinatal outcome of pregnancies complicated with varicella infection during the first 20 weeks of gestation. *Am J Perinatol* 1997;14:411.

590. Balducci J, Rodis JF, Rosengren S, et al. Pregnancy outcome following first-trimester varicella infection. *Obstet Gynecol* 1992;79:5.

591. Brazin SA, Simkovich JW, Johnson WT. Herpes zoster during pregnancy. *Obstet Gynecol* 1979;53:175.

592. Duehr PA. Herpes zoster as a cause of congenital cataract. *Am J Ophthalmol* 1955;39:157.

593. Klauber GT, Flynn FJ Jr, Altman BD. Congenital varicella syndrome with genitourinary anomalies. *Urology* 1976;8:153.

594. Webster MH, Smith CS. Congenital abnormalities and maternal herpes zoster. *BMJ* 1977;2:1193.

595. Mendez DB, Sinclair MB, Garcia S, et al. Transplacental immunity to varicella-zoster virus in extremely low birthweight infants. *Am J Perinatol* 1992;9:236.

596. van der Zwet WC, Vandenbroucke-Grauls CMJE, van Elburg RM, et al. Neonatal antibody titers against varicella-zoster virus in relation to gestational age, birth weight, and maternal titer. *Pediatrics* 2002;109:79.

597. Arvin AM. Antiviral therapy for varicella and herpes zoster. *Semin Pediatr Infect Dis* 2002;13:12.

598. McGregor JA, Mark S, Crawford GP, et al. Varicella zoster antibody testing in the care of pregnant women exposed to varicella. *Am J Obstet Gynecol* 1987;157:281.

599. Wallace MR, Chamberlin CJ, Zerboni L, et al. Reliability of a history of previous varicella infection in adults. *JAMA* 1997;278:1520.

600. Lécuru F, Taurelle R, Bernard J-P, et al. Varicella zoster virus infection during pregnancy: the limits of prenatal diagnosis. *Eur J Obstet Gynecol Reprod Biol* 1994;56:67.

601. Isada NB, Paar DP, Johnson MP, et al. In utero diagnosis of congenital varicella zoster virus infection by chorionic villus sampling and polymerase chain reaction. *Am J Obstet Gynecol* 1991;165:1727.

602. Pons J-C, Rozenberg F, Imbert M-C, et al. Prenatal diagnosis of second-trimester congenital varicella syndrome. *Prenat Diagn* 1992;12:975.

603. Mouly F, Mirlesse V, Méritet JF, et al. Prenatal diagnosis of fetal varicella-zoster virus infection with polymerase chain reaction of amniotic fluid in 107 cases. *Am J Obstet Gynecol* 1997;177:894.

604. Pretorius DH, Hayward I, Jones KL, et al. Sonographic evaluation of pregnancies with maternal varicella infection. *J Ultrasound Med* 1992;11:459.

605. Hofmeyr GJ, Moolla S, Lawrie T. Prenatal sonographic diagnosis of congenital varicella infection—a case report. *Prenat Diagn* 1996;16:1148.

606. Ong C-L, Daniel ML. Antenatal diagnosis of a porencephalic cyst in congenital varicella-zoster virus infection. *Pediatr Radiol* 1998;28:94.

607. Mattson SN, Jones KL, Gramling LJ, et al. Neurodevelopmental follow-up of children of women infected with varicella during pregnancy: a prospective study. *Pediatr Infect Dis J* 2003;22:819.

608. Hanngren KAJ, Grandien M, Granström G. Effect of zoster immunoglobulin for varicella prophylaxis in the newborn. *Scand J Infect Dis* 1985;17:343.

609. Bakshi SS, Miller TC, Kaplan M, et al. Failure of varicella-zoster immunoglobulin in modification of severe congenital varicella. *Pediatr Infect Dis* 1986;5:699.

610. Haddad J, Simeoni U, Messer J, et al. Acyclovir in prophylaxis and perinatal varicella. *Lancet* 1987;1:161.

611. Rubin L, Leggiadro R, Elie MT, et al. Disseminated varicella in a neonate: implications for immunoprophylaxis of neonates postnatally exposed to varicella. *Pediatr Infect Dis* 1986;5:100.

612. Huang Y-C, Lin T-Y, Lin Y-J, et al. Prophylaxis of intravenous immunoglobulin and acyclovir in perinatal varicella. *Eur J Pediatr* 2001;160:91.

613. American Academy of Pediatrics. Varicella-zoster infections. In: Pickering LK, ed. *Red Book: 2003 report of the Committee on Infectious Diseases*, 26th ed. Elk Grove Village, IL: American Academy of Pediatrics, 2003:672.

614. Shields KE, Galil K, Seward J, et al. Varicella vaccine exposure during pregnancy: data from the first 5 years of the Pregnancy Registry. *Obstet Gynecol* 2001;98:14.

615. Bohlke K, Galil K, Jackson LA, et al. Postpartum varicella vaccination: is the vaccine virus excreted in breast milk? *Obstet Gynecol* 2003;102:970.

616. Glantz JC, Mushlin AI. Cost-effectiveness of routine antenatal varicella screening. *Obstet Gynecol* 1998;91:519.

617. Smith WJ, Jackson LA, Watts DH, et al. Prevention of chickenpox in reproductive-age women: cost-effectiveness of routine prenatal screening with postpartum vaccination of susceptibles. *Obstet Gynecol* 1998;92:535.

618. Fleisher G, Bologonese R. Epstein-Barr virus infections in pregnancy: a prospective study. *J Pediatr* 1984;104:374.

619. Freij BJ, Wiedbrauk DL, Sever JL. Immunologic assessment of infectious diseases. *Immunol Allergy Clin North Am* 1994;14:451.

620. Pitt J, Schluchter M, Jenson H, et al. Maternal and perinatal factors related to maternal-infant transmission of HIV-1 in the P2C2 HIV study: the role of EBV shedding. *J Acquir Immune Defic Syndr Hum Retrovirol* 1998;19:462.

621. Junker AK, Thomas EE, Radcliffe A, et al. Epstein-Barr virus shedding in breast milk. *Am J Med Sci* 1991;302:220.

622. Dockrell DH. Human herpesvirus 6: molecular biology and clinical features. *J Med Microbiol* 2003;52:5.

623. Okuno T, Oishi H, Hayashi K, et al. Human herpesviruses 6 and 7 in cervixes of pregnant women. *J Clin Microbiol* 1995;33:1968.

624. Baillargeon J, Piper J, Leach CT. Epidemiology of human herpesvirus 6 (HHV-6) infection in pregnant and nonpregnant women. *J Clin Virol* 2000;16:149.

625. Ohashi M, Yoshikawa T, Ihira M, et al. Reactivation of human herpesvirus 6 and 7 in pregnant women. *J Med Virol* 2002; 67:354.

626. Ranger S, Patillaud S, Denis F, et al. Seroepidemiology of human herpesvirus-6 in pregnant women from different parts of the world. *J Med Virol* 1991;34:194.

627. Ohashi M, Ihira M, Suzuki K, et al. Transfer of human herpesvirus 6 and 7 antibodies from mothers to their offspring. *Pediatr Infect Dis J* 2001;20:449.

628. Ando Y, Kakimoto K, Ekuni Y, et al. HHV-6 infection during pregnancy and spontaneous abortion. *Lancet* 1992;340:1289.

629. Ashshi AM, Cooper RJ, Klapper PE, et al. Detection of human herpes virus 6 DNA in fetal hydrops. *Lancet* 2000;355:1519.

630. Dunne WM Jr, Demmler GJ. Serological evidence for congenital transmission of human herpesvirus 6. *Lancet* 1992;340:121.

631. Maeda T, Okuno T, Hayashi K, et al. Outcomes of infants whose mothers are positive for human herpesvirus-6 within the genital tract in early gestation. *Acta Paediatr Jpn* 1997;39:653.

632. Kositanont U, Wasi C, Wanprapar N, et al. Primary infection of human herpesvirus 6 in children with vertical infection of human immunodeficiency virus type 1. *J Infect Dis* 1999; 180:50.

633. Adams O, Krempe C, Kögler G, et al. Congenital infections with human herpesvirus 6. *J Infect Dis* 1998;178:544.

634. Kawaguchi S, Suga S, Kozawa T, et al. Primary human herpesvirus-6 infection (exanthem subitum) in the newborn. *Pediatrics* 1992;90:628.

635. Mendel I, de Matteis M, Bertin C, et al. Fulminant hepatitis in neonates with human herpesvirus 6 infection. *Pediatr Infect Dis J* 1995;14:993.

636. Lanari M, Papa I, Venturi V, et al. Congenital infection with human herpesvirus 6 variant B associated with neonatal seizures and poor neurological outcome. *J Med Virol* 2003; 70:628.

637. Sada E, Yasukawa M, Ito C, et al. Detection of human herpesvirus 6 and human herpesvirus 7 in the submandibular gland, parotid gland, and lip salivary gland by PCR. *J Clin Microbiol* 1996;34:2320.

638. Kidd JM, Clark DA, Ait-Khaled M, et al. Measurement of human herpesvirus 7 load in peripheral blood and saliva of healthy subjects by quantitative polymerase chain reaction. *J Infect Dis* 1996;174:396.

639. Pohl-Koppe A, Blay M, Jäger G, et al. Human herpes virus type 7 DNA in the cerebrospinal fluid of children with central nervous system diseases. *Eur J Pediatr* 2001;160:351.

640. Torigoe S, Koide W, Yamada M, et al. Human herpesvirus 7 infection associated with central nervous system manifestations. *J Pediatr* 1996;129:301.

641. Hashida T, Komura E, Yoshida M, et al. Hepatitis in association with human herpesvirus-7 infection. *Pediatrics* 1995; 96:783.

642. Caserta MT, Hall CB, Schnabel K, et al. Primary human herpesvirus 7 infection: a comparison of human herpesvirus 7 and human herpesvirus 6 infections in children. *J Pediatr* 1998; 133:386.

643. Jenson HB. Human herpesvirus 8 infection. *Curr Opin Pediatr* 2003;15:85.

644. Fiore JR, Volpe A, Tosatti MA, et al. High seroprevalence of human herpesvirus 8 (HHV-8) in HIV-1-infected pregnant women of Southeastern Italy: association with injection drug use and hepatitis C virus infection. *J Med Virol* 2004;72:656.

645. Goedert JJ, Kedes DH, Ganem D. Antibodies to human herpesvirus 8 in women and infants born in Haiti and the USA. *Lancet* 1997;349:1368.

646. He J, Bhat G, Kankasa C, et al. Seroprevalence of human herpesvirus 8 among Zambian women of childbearing age without Kaposi's sarcoma (KS) and mother-child pairs with KS. *J Infect Dis* 1998;178:1787.

647. Sarmati L, Carlo T, Rossella S, et al. Human herpesvirus-8 infection in pregnancy and labor: lack of evidence of vertical transmission. *J Med Virol* 2004;72:462.

648. Cannon MJ, Dollard SC, Smith DK, et al. Blood-borne and sexual transmission of human herpesvirus 8 in women with or at risk for human immunodeficiency virus infection. *N Engl J Med* 2001;344:637.

649. Lyall EGH, Patton GS, Sheldon J, et al. Evidence for horizontal and not vertical transmission of human herpesvirus 8 in children born to human immunodeficiency virus-infected mothers. *Pediatr Infect Dis J* 1999;18:795.

650. Brayfield BP, Phiri S, Kankasa C, et al. Postnatal human herpesvirus 8 and human immunodeficiency virus type 1 infection in mothers and infants from Zambia. *J Infect Dis* 2003;187:559.

651. Sarmati L, Ticconi C, Santangelo R, et al. Does the risk of abortion increase in women with high human herpesvirus-8 antibody titers? *J Infect Dis* 2003;188:173.

652. Cossart YE, Field AM, Cant B, et al. Parvovirus-like particles in human sera. *Lancet* 1975;1:72.

653. Young NS, Brown KE. Parvovirus B19. *N Engl J Med* 2004; 350:586.

654. Brown KE, Hibbs JR, Gallinella G, et al. Resistance to parvovirus B19 infection due to lack of virus receptor (erythrocyte P antigen). *N Engl J Med* 1994;330:1192.

655. Cooling LLW, Koerner TAW, Naides SJ. Multiple glycosphingolipids determine the tissue tropism of parvovirus B19. *J Infect Dis* 1995;172:1198.

656. von Poblotzki A, Hemauer A, Gigler A, et al. Antibodies to the nonstructural protein of parvovirus B19 in persistently infected patients: implications for pathogenesis. *J Infect Dis* 1995; 172:1356.

657. Centers for Disease Control and Prevention. Risks associated with human parvovirus B19 infection. *MMWR* 1989;38:81.

658. Harger JH, Adler SP, Koch WC, et al. Prospective evaluation of 618 pregnant women exposed to parvovirus B19: risks and symptoms. *Obstet Gynecol* 1998;91:413.

659. Gratacós E, Torres P-J, Vidal J, et al. The incidence of human parvovirus B19 infection during pregnancy and its impact on perinatal outcome. *J Infect Dis* 1995;171:1360.

660. Skjöldebrand-Sparre L, Fridell E, Nyman M, et al. A prospective study of antibodies against parvovirus B19 in pregnancy. *Acta Obstet Gynecol Scand* 1996;75:336.

661. Valeur-Jensen AK, Pedersen CB, Westergaard T, et al. Risk factors for parvovirus B19 infection in pregnancy. *JAMA* 1999; 281:1099.

662. Maksheed M, Pacsa AS, Essa SS, et al. The prevalence of antibody to human parvovirus B19 in pregnant women in Kuwait. *Acta Trop* 1999;73:225.

663. Yaegashi N, Niinuma T, Chisaka H, et al. Serologic study of human parvovirus B19 infection in pregnancy in Japan. *J Infect* 1999;38:30.

664. Karunajeewa H, Siebert D, Hammond R, et al. Seroprevalence of varicella zoster virus, parvovirus B19 and Toxoplasma gondii in a Melbourne obstetric population: implications for management. *Aust N Z J Obstet Gynaecol* 2001;41:23.

665. Brown KE, Young NS, Alving BM, et al. Parvovirus B19: implications for transfusion medicine. Summary of a workshop. *Transfusion* 2001;41:130.

666. Alger LS. Toxoplasmosis and parvovirus B19. *Infect Dis Clin North Am* 1997;11:55.

667. Koch WC, Adler SP. Human parvovirus B19 infections in women of childbearing age and within families. *Pediatr Infect Dis J* 1989;8:83.

668. Cartter ML, Farley TA, Rosengren S, et al. Occupational risk factors for infection with parvovirus B19 among pregnant women. *J Infect Dis* 1991;163:282.

669. Bell LM, Naides SJ, Stoffman P, et al. Human parvovirus B19 infection among hospital staff members after contact with infected patients. *N Engl J Med* 1989;321:485.

670. Ray SM, Erdman DD, Berschling JD, et al. Nosocomial exposure to parvovirus B19: low risk of transmission to healthcare workers. *Infect Control Hosp Epidemiol* 1997;18:109.

671. Lobkowicz F, Ring J, Schwarz TF, et al. Erythema multiforme in a patient with acute human parvovirus B19 infection. *J Am Acad Dermatol* 1989;20:849.

672. Zerbini M, Musiani M, Venturoli S, et al. Different syndromes associated with B19 parvovirus viraemia in paediatric patients: report of four cases. *Eur J Pediatr* 1992;151:815.

673. Woolf AD, Campion GV, Chishick A, et al. Clinical manifestations of human parvovirus B19 in adults. *Arch Intern Med* 1989;149:1153.

674. Naides SJ, Field EH. Transient rheumatoid factor positivity in acute human parvovirus B19 infection. *Arch Intern Med* 1988;148:2587.

675. Erdman DD, Usher MJ, Tsou C, et al. Human parvovirus B19 specific IgG, IgA, and IgM antibodies and DNA in serum speci-

mens from persons with erythema infectiosum. *J Med Virol* 1991;35:110.

676. Cassinotti P, Schultze D, Wieczorek K, et al. Parvovirus B19 infection during pregnancy and development of hydrops fetalis despite the evidence for preexisting anti-B19 antibody: how reliable are serological results? *Clin Diagn Virol* 1994;2:87.

677. Musiani M, Zerbini M, Gentilomi G, et al. Parvovirus B19 clearance from peripheral blood after acute infection. *J Infect Dis* 1995;172:1360.

678. Gentilomi G, Musiani M, Zerbini M, et al. Dot immunoperoxidase assay for detection of parvovirus B19 antigens in serum samples. *J Clin Microbiol* 1997;35:1575.

679. Selbing A, Josefsson A, Dahle LO, et al. Parvovirus B19 infection during pregnancy treated with high-dose intravenous gammaglobulin. *Lancet* 1995;345:660.

680. Rogers BB, Mark Y, Oyer CE. Diagnosis and incidence of fetal parvovirus infection in an autopsy series. I. Histology. *Pediatr Pathol* 1993;13:371.

681. Yaegashi N, Okamura K, Yajima A, et al. The frequency of human parvovirus B19 infection in nonimmune hydrops fetalis. *J Perinat Med* 1994;22:159.

682. Jordan JA. Identification of human parvovirus B19 infection in idiopathic nonimmune hydrops fetalis. *Am J Obstet Gynecol* 1996;174:37.

683. Jordan JA, Butchko AR. Apoptotic activity in villous trophoblast cells during B19 infection correlates with clinical outcome: assessment by the caspase-related M30 CytoDeath antibody. *Placenta* 2002;23:547.

684. Schwarz TF, Nerlich A, Hottenträger B, et al. Parvovirus B19 infection of the fetus: histology and in situ hybridization. *Am J Clin Pathol* 1991;96:121.

685. Public Health Laboratory Service Working Party on Fifth Disease. Prospective study of human parvovirus (B19) infection in pregnancy. *BMJ* 1990;300:1166.

686. Miller E, Fairley CK, Cohen BJ, et al. Immediate and long term outcome of human parvovirus B19 infection in pregnancy. *Br J Obstet Gynaecol* 1998;105:174.

687. Skjöldebrand-Sparre L, Tolfvenstam T, Papadogiannakis N, et al. Parvovirus B19 infection: association with third-trimester intrauterine fetal death. *BJOG* 2000;107:476.

688. Norbeck O, Papadogiannakis N, Petersson K, et al. Revised clinical presentation of parvovirus B19-associated intrauterine fetal death. *Clin Infect Dis* 2002;35:1032.

689. Tolfvenstam T, Papadogiannakis N, Norbeck O, et al. Frequency of human parvovirus B19 infection in intrauterine fetal death. *Lancet* 2001;357:1494.

690. Kinney JS, Anderson LJ, Farrar J, et al. Risk of adverse outcomes of pregnancy after human parvovirus B19 infection. *J Infect Dis* 1988;157:663.

691. Porter HJ, Quantrill AM, Fleming KA. B19 parvovirus infection of myocardial cells. *Lancet* 1988;1:535.

692. Lambot M-A, Noël J-C, Peny M-O, et al. Fetal parvovirus B19 infection associated with myocardial necrosis. *Prenat Diagn* 1999;19:389.

693. O'Malley A, Barry-Kinsella C, Hughes C, et al. Parvovirus infects cardiac myocytes in hydrops fetalis. *Pediatr Dev Pathol* 2003;6:414.

694. Koch WC, Harger JH, Barnstein B, et al. Serologic and virologic evidence for frequent intrauterine transmission of human parvovirus B19 with a primary maternal infection during pregnancy. *Pediatr Infect Dis J* 1998;17:489.

695. Nunoue T, Kusuhara K, Hara T. Human fetal infection with parvovirus B19: maternal infection time in gestation, viral persistence and fetal prognosis. *Pediatr Infect Dis J* 2002;21:1133.

696. Brown KE, Green SW, de Mayolo JA, et al. Congenital anaemia after transplacental B19 parvovirus infection. *Lancet* 1994;343:895.

697. Tugal O, Pallant B, Shebarek N, et al. Transient erythroblastopenia of the newborn caused by human parvovirus. *Am J Pediatr Hematol Oncol* 1994;16:352.

698. Zerbini M, Musiani M, Gentilomi G, et al. Symptomatic parvovirus B19 infection of one fetus in a twin pregnancy. *Clin Infect Dis* 1993;17:262.

699. Pustilnik TB, Cohen AW. Parvovirus B19 infection in a twin pregnancy. *Obstet Gynecol* 1994;83:834.

700. Hartwig NG, Vermeij-Keers C, van Elsacker-Niele AMW, et al. Embryonic malformations in a case of intrauterine parvovirus B19 infection. *Teratology* 1989;39:295.

701. Rodis JF, Hovick TJ Jr, Quinn DL, et al. Human parvovirus infection in pregnancy. *Obstet Gynecol* 1988;72:733.

702. Tiessen RG, van Elsacker-Niele AMW, Vermeij-Keers C, et al. A fetus with a parvovirus B19 infection and congenital anomalies. *Prenat Diagn* 1994;14:173.

703. Katz VL, McCoy MC, Kuller JA, et al. An association between fetal parvovirus B19 infection and fetal anomalies: a report of two cases. *Am J Perinatol* 1996;13:43.

704. Willekes C, Roumen FJME, van Elsacker-Niele AMW, et al. Human parvovirus B19 infection and unbalanced translocation in a case of hydrops fetalis. *Prenat Diagn* 1994;14:181.

705. Zerbini M, Gentilomi GA, Gallinella G, et al. Intra-uterine parvovirus B19 infection and meconium peritonitis. *Prenat Diagn* 1998;18:599.

706. Isumi H, Nunoue T, Nishida A, et al. Fetal brain infection with human parvovirus B19. *Pediatr Neurol* 1999;21:661.

707. Clewley JP, Cohen BJ, Field AM. Detection of parvovirus B19 DNA, antigen, and particles in the human fetus. *J Med Virol* 1987;23:367.

708. Field AM, Cohen BJ, Brown KE, et al. Detection of B19 parvovirus in human fetal tissues by electron microscopy. *J Med Virol* 1991;35:85.

709. Yamakawa Y, Oka H, Hori S, et al. Detection of human parvovirus B19 DNA by nested polymerase chain reaction. *Obstet Gynecol* 1995;86:126.

710. Rodis JF, Rodner C, Hansen AA, et al. Long-term outcome of children following maternal human parvovirus B19 infection. *Obstet Gynecol* 1998;91:125.

711. Dembinski J, Haverkamp F, Maara H, et al. Neurodevelopmental outcome after intrauterine red cell transfusion for parvovirus B19-induced fetal hydrops. *BJOG* 2002;109:1232.

712. Dembinski J, Eis-Hübinger AM, Maar J, et al. Long term follow up of serostatus after maternofetal parvovirus B19 infection. *Arch Dis Child* 2003;88:219.

713. Miyagawa S, Takahashi Y, Nagai A, et al. Angio-oedema in a neonate with IgG antibodies to parvovirus B19 following intrauterine parvovirus B19 infection. *Br J Dermatol* 2000;143:428.

714. Schwarz TF, Roggendorf M, Hottenträger B, et al. Immunoglobulins in the prophylaxis of parvovirus B19 infection. *J Infect Dis* 1990;162:1214.

715. Bloom MC, Rolland M, Bernard JD, et al. Materno-fetal infection by parvovirus associated with antenatal meconium peritonitis. *Arch Fr Pediatr* 1990;47:437.

716. Carrington D, Gilmore DH, Whittle MJ, et al. Maternal serum alpha-fetoprotein—a marker of fetal aplastic crisis during intrauterine human parvovirus infection. *Lancet* 1987;1:433.

717. Saller DN Jr, Rogers BB, Canick JA. Maternal serum biochemical markers in pregnancies with fetal parvovirus B19 infection. *Prenat Diagn* 1993;13:467.

718. Naides SJ, Weiner CP. Antenatal diagnosis and palliative treatment of non-immune hydrops fetalis secondary to fetal parvovirus B19 infection. *Prenat Diagn* 1989;9:105.

719. Peters MT, Nicolaides KH. Cordocentesis for the diagnosis and treatment of human fetal parvovirus infection. *Obstet Gynecol* 1990;75:501.

720. Sahakian V, Weiner CP, Naides SJ, et al. Intrauterine transfusion treatment of nonimmune hydrops fetalis secondary to human parvovirus B19 infection. *Am J Obstet Gynecol* 1991;164:1090.

721. Török TJ, Wang Q-Y, Gary GW Jr, et al. Prenatal diagnosis of intrauterine infection with parvovirus B19 by the polymerase chain reaction technique. *Clin Infect Dis* 1992;14:149.

722. Iwa N, Yutani C. Cytodiagnosis of parvovirus B19 infection from ascites fluid of hydrops fetalis: report of a case. *Diagn Cytopathol* 1995;13:139.

723. Nikkari S, Ekblad U. A rapid and safe method to detect fetal parvovirus B19 infection in amniotic fluid by polymerase chain reaction: report of a case. *Am J Perinatol* 1995;12:447.

724. Zerbini M, Musiani M, Gentilomi G, et al. Comparative evaluation of virological and serological methods in prenatal diagnosis of parvovirus B19 fetal hydrops. *J Clin Microbiol* 1996;34:603.

725. Musiani M, Pasini P, Zerbini M, et al. Prenatal diagnosis of parvovirus B19-induced hydrops fetalis by chemiluminescence in situ hybridization. *J Clin Microbiol* 1999;37:2326.

726. Dong Z-W, Zhou S-Y, Li Y, et al. Detection of human parvovirus intrauterine infection with the polymerase chain reaction. *J Reprod Med* 2000;45:410.

727. Knöll A, Louwen F, Kochanowski B, et al. Parvovirus B19 infection in pregnancy: quantitative viral DNA analysis using a kinetic fluorescence detection system (TaqMan PCR). *J Med Virol* 2002;67:259.

728. Weiner CP, Naides SJ. Fetal survival after human parvovirus B19 infection: spectrum of intrauterine response in a twin gestation. *Am J Perinatol* 1992;9:66.

729. Odibo AO, Campbell WA, Feldman D, et al. Resolution of human parvovirus B19-induced nonimmune hydrops after intrauterine transfusion. *J Ultrasound Med* 1998;17:547.

730. Fairley CK, Smoleniec JS, Caul OE, et al. Observational study of effect of intrauterine transfusions on outcome of fetal hydrops after parvovirus B19 infection. *Lancet* 1995;346:1335.

731. Duthie SJ, Walkinshaw SA. Parvovirus associated fetal hydrops: reversal of pregnancy induced proteinuric hypertension by in utero fetal transfusion. *Br J Obstet Gynaecol* 1995;102:1011.

732. Schild RL, Bald R, Plath H, et al. Intrauterine management of fetal parvovirus B19 infection. *Ultrasound Obstet Gynecol* 1999;13:161.

733. Forestier F, Tissot J-D, Vial Y, et al. Haematological parameters of parvovirus B19 infection in 13 fetuses with hydrops foetalis. *Br J Haematol* 1999;104:925.

734. Bousquet F, Segondy M, Faure J-M, et al. B19 parvovirus-induced fetal hydrops: good outcome after intrauterine blood transfusion at 18 weeks of gestation. *Fetal Diagn Ther* 2000;15:132.

735. Cosmi E, Mari G, Delle Chiaie L, et al. Noninvasive diagnosis by Doppler ultrasonography of fetal anemia resulting from parvovirus infection. *Am J Obstet Gynecol* 2002;187:1290.

736. Morey AL, Nicolini U, Welch CR, et al. Parvovirus B19 infection and transient fetal hydrops. *Lancet* 1991;337:496.

737. Bhal PS, Davies NJ, Westmoreland D, et al. Spontaneous resolution of non-immune hydrops fetalis secondary to transplacental parvovirus B19 infection. *Ultrasound Obstet Gynecol* 1996;7:55.

738. Rodis JF, Borgida AF, Wilson M, et al. Management of parvovirus infection in pregnancy and outcomes of hydrops: a survey of members of the Society of Perinatal Obstetricians. *Am J Obstet Gynecol* 1998;179:985.

739. Xu J, Raff TC, Muallem NS, et al. Hydrops fetalis secondary to parvovirus B19 infections. *J Am Board Fam Pract* 2003;16:63.

740. Fean WS, Yee CF, Cincotta RB, et al. Human parvovirus B19 infection in pregnancy: should screening be offered to the low-risk population? *Aust N Z J Obstet Gynaecol* 2002;42:347.

741. Kemmer NM, Miskovsky EP. Hepatitis A. *Infect Dis Clin North Am* 2000;14:605.

742. Centers for Disease Control and Prevention. Prevention of hepatitis A through active or passive immunization: recommendations of the Advisory Committee on Immunization Practices (ACIP). *MMWR* 1999;48(RR-12):1.

743. Mbithi JN, Springthorpe VS, Boulet JR, et al. Survival of hepatitis A virus on human hands and its transfer on contact with animate and inanimate surfaces. *J Clin Microbiol* 1992;30:757.

744. Lerman Y, Chodick G, Aloni H, et al. Occupations at increased risk of hepatitis A: a 2-year nationwide historical prospective study. *Am J Epidemiol* 1999;150:312.

745. Klein BS, Michaels JA, Rytel MW, et al. Nosocomial hepatitis A: a multinursery outbreak in Wisconsin. *JAMA* 1984;252:2716.

746. Azimi PH, Roberto RR, Guralnik J, et al. Transfusion-acquired hepatitis A in a premature infant with secondary nosocomial spread in an intensive care nursery. *Am J Dis Child* 1986;140:23.

747. Rosenblum LS, Villarino ME, Nainan OV, et al. Hepatitis A outbreak in a neonatal intensive care unit: risk factors for transmission and evidence of prolonged viral excretion among preterm infants. *J Infect Dis* 1991;164:476.

748. Lee KK, Vargo LR, Lê CT, et al. Transfusion-acquired hepatitis A outbreak from fresh frozen plasma in a neonatal intensive care unit. *Pediatr Infect Dis J* 1992;11:122.

749. Dinsmoor MJ. Hepatitis in the obstetric patient. *Infect Dis Clin North Am* 1997;11:77.

750. Koff RS. Hepatitis A. *Lancet* 1998;351:1643.

751. Tanaka I, Shima M, Kubota Y, et al. Vertical transmission of hepatitis A virus. *Lancet* 1995;345:397.

752. Erkan T, Kutlu T, Çullu F, et al. A case of vertical transmission of hepatitis A virus infection. *Acta Paediatr* 1998;87:1008.

753. Urganci N, Arapoglu M, Akyildiz B, et al. Neonatal cholestasis resulting from vertical transmission of hepatitis A infection. *Pediatr Infect Dis J* 2003;22:381.

754. Leikin E, Lysikiewicz A, Garry D, et al. Intrauterine transmission of hepatitis A virus. *Obstet Gynecol* 1996;88:690.

755. McDuffie RS Jr, Bader T. Fetal meconium peritonitis after maternal hepatitis A. *Am J Obstet Gynecol* 1999;180:1031.

756. Fagan EA, Hadzic N, Saxena R, et al. Symptomatic neonatal hepatitis A disease from a virus variant acquired *in utero*. *Pediatr Infect Dis J* 1999;18:389.

757. Linder N, Karetnyi Y, Gidony Y, et al. Placental transfer of hepatitis A antibodies in full term and preterm infants. *Pediatr Infect Dis J* 1997;16:245.

758. Letson GW, Shapiro CN, Kuehn D, et al. Effect of maternal antibody on immunogenicity of hepatitis A vaccine in infants. *J Pediatr* 2004;144:327.

759. Befeler AS, Di Bisceglie AM. Hepatitis B. *Infect Dis Clin North Am* 2000;14:617.

760. Coleman PJ, McQuillan GM, Moyer LA, et al. Incidence of hepatitis B virus infection in the United States, 1976–1994: estimates from the National Health and Nutrition Examination Surveys. *J Infect Dis* 1998;178:954.

761. Lai CL, Ratziu V, Yuen M-F, et al. Viral hepatitis B. *Lancet* 2003;362:2089.

762. Lee WM. Hepatitis B virus infection. *N Engl J Med* 1997;337:1733.

763. Ganem D, Prince AM. Hepatitis B virus infection—natural history and clinical consequences. *N Engl J Med* 2004;350:1118.

764. Hoofnagle JH, Di Bisceglie AM. Serologic diagnosis of acute and chronic viral hepatitis. *Semin Liver Dis* 1991;11:73.

765. Yuki N, Nagaoka T, Yamashiro M, et al. Long-term histologic and virologic outcomes of acute self-limited hepatitis B. *Hepatology* 2003;37:1172.

766. Levrero M, Stemler M, Pasquinelli C, et al. Significance of anti-HBx antibodies in hepatitis B virus infection. *Hepatology* 1991;13:143.

767. Nowak MA, Bonhoeffer S, Hill AM, et al. Viral dynamics in hepatitis B virus infection. *Proc Natl Acad Sci U S A* 1996;93:4398.

768. McMahon BJ, Holck P, Bulkow L, et al. Serologic and clinical outcomes of 1536 Alaska Natives chronically infected with hepatitis B virus. *Ann Intern Med* 2001;135:759.

769. Hyams KC. Risks of chronicity following acute hepatitis B virus infection: a review. *Clin Infect Dis* 1995;20:992.

770. Rawal BK, Parida S, Watkins RPF, et al. Symptomatic reactivation of hepatitis B in pregnancy. *Lancet* 1991;337:364.

771. Liang TJ, Ghany M. Hepatitis B e antigen—the dangerous endgame of hepatitis B. *N Engl J Med* 2002;347:208.

772. Omata M, Ehata T, Yokosuka O, et al. Mutations in the precore region of hepatitis B virus DNA in patients with fulminant and severe hepatitis. *N Engl J Med* 1991;324:1699.

773. Liang TJ, Hasegawa K, Rimon N, et al. A hepatitis B virus mutant associated with an epidemic of fulminant hepatitis. *N Engl J Med* 1991;324:1705.

774. Romero R, Lavine JE. Viral hepatitis in children. *Semin Liver Dis* 1994;14:289.

775. Hochman JA, Balistreri WF. Chronic viral hepatitis: always be current! *Pediatr Rev* 2003;24:399.

776. Birrer RB, Birrer D, Klavins JV. Hepatocellular carcinoma and hepatitis virus. *Ann Clin Lab Sci* 2003;33:39.

777. Yang H-I, Lu S-N, Liaw Y-F, et al. Hepatitis B e antigen and the risk of hepatocellular carcinoma. *N Engl J Med* 2002;347:168.

778. Shapiro CN, Margolis HS. Impact of hepatitis B virus infection on women and children. *Infect Dis Clin North Am* 1992;6:75.

779. Alter MJ, Hadler SC, Margolis HS, et al. The changing epidemiology of hepatitis B in the United States: need for alternative vaccination strategies. *JAMA* 1990;263:1218.

780. Centers for Disease Control and Prevention. Protection against viral hepatitis: recommendations of the Immunization Practices Advisory Committee (ACIP). *MMWR* 1990;39(S-2):1.

781. Wang Z, Zhang J, Yang H, et al. Quantitative analysis of HBV DNA level and HBeAg titer in hepatitis B surface antigen positive mothers and their babies: HBeAg passage through the placenta and the rate of decay in babies. *J Med Virol* 2003;71:360.

782. Burk RD, Hwang L-Y, Ho GYF, et al. Outcome of perinatal hepatitis B virus exposure is dependent on maternal virus load. *J Infect Dis* 1994;170:1418.

783. Soderstrom A, Norkrans G, Lindh M. Hepatitis B virus DNA during pregnancy and post partum: aspects on vertical transmission. *Scand J Infect Dis* 2003;35:814.

784. Stevens CE. Immunoprophylaxis of hepatitis B virus infection. *Semin Pediatr Infect Dis* 1991;2:135.

785. Zhang S-L, Yue Y-F, Bai G-Q, et al. Mechanism of intrauterine infection of hepatitis B virus. *World J Gastroenterol* 2004;10:437.

786. Xu D-Z, Yan Y-P, Zou S, et al. Role of placental tissues in the intrauterine transmission of hepatitis B virus. *Am J Obstet Gynecol* 2001;185:981.

787. Has R, Yüksel A, Topuz S. Hepatitis B infection in pregnancy: is it really not harmful to the fetus? *Prenat Diagn* 2001;21:701.

788. Su WH, Wang PH, Yuan CC, et al. Fetal meconium peritonitis in the infant of a woman with fulminant hepatitis B: a case report. *J Reprod Med* 2002;47:952.

789. Hill JB, Sheffield JS, Kim MJ, et al. Risk of hepatitis B transmission in breast-fed infants of chronic hepatitis B carriers. *Obstet Gynecol* 2002;99:1049.

790. Grabenstein JD. *ImmunoFacts: vaccines and immunologic drugs.* St. Louis: Wolters Kluwer Health, 2004;170.

791. Levy M, Koren G. Hepatitis B vaccine in pregnancy: maternal and fetal safety. *Am J Perinatol* 1991;8:227.

792. Grosheide PM, Schalm SW, van Os HC, et al. Immune response to hepatitis B vaccine in pregnant women receiving post-exposure prophylaxis. *Eur J Obstet Gynecol Reprod Biol* 1993;50:53.

793. Ingardia CJ, Kelley L, Steinfeld JD, et al. Hepatitis B vaccination in pregnancy: factors influencing efficacy. *Obstet Gynecol* 1999;93:983.

794. Centers for Disease Control and Prevention. Hepatitis B vaccination—United States, 1982–2002. *MMWR* 2002;51:549.

795. Jensen L, Heilmann C, Smith E, et al. Efficacy of selective antenatal screening for hepatitis B among pregnant women in Denmark: is selective screening still an acceptable strategy in a low-endemicity country? *Scand J Infect Dis* 2003;35:378.

796. Centers for Disease Control and Prevention. Prevention of perinatal transmission of hepatitis B virus: prenatal screening of all pregnant women for hepatitis B surface antigen. *MMWR* 1988;37:341.

797. Centers for Disease Control and Prevention. Maternal hepatitis B screening practices—California, Connecticut, Kansas, and United States, 1992–1993. *MMWR* 1994;43:311.

798. Petermann S, Ernest JM. Intrapartum hepatitis B screening. *Am J Obstet Gynecol* 1995;173:369.

799. American Academy of Pediatrics. Hepatitis B. In: Pickering LK, ed. *Red Book: 2003 report of the Committee on Infectious Diseases,* 26th ed. Elk Grove Village, IL: American Academy of Pediatrics, 2003:318.

800. Yang Y-J, Liu C-C, Chen T-J, et al. Role of hepatitis B immunoglobulin in infants born to hepatitis B e antigen-negative carrier mothers in Taiwan. *Pediatr Infect Dis J* 2003;22:584.

801. Mele A, Tancredi F, Romanò L, et al. Effectiveness of hepatitis B vaccination in babies born to hepatitis B surface antigen-positive mothers in Italy. *J Infect Dis* 2001;184:905.

802. Kim SC, Chung EK, Hodinka RL, et al. Immunogenicity of hepatitis B vaccine in preterm infants. *Pediatrics* 1997;99:534.

803. Patel DM, Butler J, Feldman S, et al. Immunogenicity of hepatitis B vaccine in healthy very low birth weight infants. *J Pediatr* 1997;130:641.

804. Blondheim O, Bader D, Abend M, et al. Immunogenicity of hepatitis B vaccine in preterm infants. *Arch Dis Child Fetal Neonat Ed* 1998;79:F206.

805. Arora NK, Ganguly S, Agadi SN, et al. Hepatitis B immunization in low birthweight infants: do they need an additional dose? *Acta Paediatr* 2002;91:995.

806. Marion SA, Pastore MT, Pi DW, et al. Long-term follow-up of hepatitis B vaccine in infants of carrier mothers. *Am J Epidemiol* 1994;140:734.

807. Tang J-R, Hsu H-Y, Lin H-H, et al. Hepatitis B surface antigenemia at birth: a long-term follow-up study. *J Pediatr* 1998;133:374.

808. Ngui SL, Andrews NJ, Underhill GS, et al. Failed postnatal immunoprophylaxis for hepatitis B: characteristics of maternal hepatitis B virus as risk factors. *Clin Infect Dis* 1998;27:100.

809. Centers for Disease Control and Prevention. Availability of hepatitis B vaccine that does not contain thimerosal as a preservative. *MMWR* 1999;48:780.

810. Shete PB, Daum RS. Real versus theoretical: assessing the risks and benefits of postponing the hepatitis B vaccine birth dose. *Pediatrics* 2002;109:701.

811. Oram RJ, Daum RS, Seal JB, et al. Impact of recommendations to suspend the birth dose of hepatitis B virus vaccine. *JAMA* 2001;285:1874.

812. Biroscak BJ, Fiore AE, Fasano N, et al. Impact of the thimerosal controversy on hepatitis B vaccine coverage of infants born to women of unknown hepatitis B surface antigen status in Michigan. *Pediatrics* 2003;111:e645.

813. Thomas AR, Fiore AE, Corwith HL, et al. Hepatitis B vaccine coverage among infants born to women without prenatal screening for hepatitis B virus infection: effects of the Joint Statement on Thimerosal in Vaccines. *Pediatr Infect Dis J* 2004;23:313.

814. Luman ET, Fiore AE, Strine TW, et al. Impact of thimerosal-related changes in hepatitis B vaccine birth-dose recommendations on childhood vaccination coverage. *JAMA* 2004;291:2351.

815. Goldstein ST, Fiore AE. Toward the global elimination of hepatitis B virus transmission. *J Pediatr* 2001;139:343.

816. Kao J-H, Hsu H-M, Shau W-Y, et al. Universal hepatitis B vaccination and the decreased mortality from fulminant hepatitis in infants in Taiwan. *J Pediatr* 2001;139:349.

817. Ni Y-H, Chang M-H, Huang L-M, et al. Hepatitis B virus infection in children and adolescents in a hyperendemic area: 15 years after mass hepatitis B vaccination. *Ann Intern Med* 2001;135:796.

818. Farrell GC. Clinical potential of emerging new agents in hepatitis B. *Drugs* 2000;60:701.

819. Karayiannis P. Hepatitis B virus: old, new and future approaches to antiviral treatment. *J Antimicrob Chemother* 2003;51:761.

820. D'Souza R, Foster GR. Diagnosis and treatment of chronic hepatitis B. *J R Soc Med* 2004;97:318.

821. Kazim SN, Wakil SM, Khan LA, et al. Vertical transmission of hepatitis B virus despite maternal lamivudine therapy. *Lancet* 2002;359:1488.

822. van Zonneveld M, van Nunen AB, Niesters HGM, et al. Lamivudine treatment during pregnancy to prevent perinatal transmission of hepatitis B virus infection. *J Viral Hepat* 2003;10:294.

823. Flamm SL. Chronic hepatitis C virus infection. *JAMA* 2003;289:2413.

824. Poynard T, Yuen M-F, Ratziu V, et al. Viral hepatitis C. *Lancet* 2003;362:2095.

825. Cheney CP, Chopra S, Graham C. Hepatitis C. *Infect Dis Clin North Am* 2000;14:633.

826. Nguyen MH, Keeffe EB. Epidemiology and treatment outcomes of patients with chronic hepatitis C and genotypes 4 to 9. *Rev Gastroenterol Disord* 2004;4(Suppl 1):S14.

827. American Academy of Pediatrics, Committee on Infectious Diseases. Hepatitis C virus infection. *Pediatrics* 1998;101:481.

828. Giles M, Hellard M, Sasadeusz J. Hepatitis C and pregnancy: an update. *Aust N Z J Obstet Gynaecol* 2003;43:290.

829. Geulen O, Hansmann M, Offergeld R, et al. Maternal and fetal hepatitis C virus exposure by intrauterine transfusion. *Lancet* 2000;355:1887.

830. Kumar RM, Shahul S. Role of breast-feeding in transmission of hepatitis C virus to infants of HCV-infected mothers. *J Hepatol* 1998;29:191.

831. Alberti A, Noventa F, Benvegnù L, et al. Prevalence of liver disease in a population of asymptomatic persons with hepatitis C virus infection. *Ann Intern Med* 2002;137:961.

832. Richter SS. Laboratory assays for diagnosis and management of hepatitis C virus infection. *J Clin Microbiol* 2002;40:4407.

833. Centers for Disease Control and Prevention. Guidelines for laboratory testing and result reporting of antibody to hepatitis C virus. *MMWR* 2003;52(RR-3):1.

834. Sarisky RT. Non-nucleoside inhibitors of the HCV polymerase. *J Antimicrob Chemother* 2004;54:14.

835. Fargion S, Fracanzani AL, Valenti L. Treatment choices for people infected with HCV. *J Antimicrob Chemother* 2004;53:708.

836. Hepburn MJ, Hepburn LM, Cantu NS, et al. Differences in treatment outcome for hepatitis C among ethnic groups. *Am J Med* 2004;117:163.

837. Özaslan E, Yilmaz R, Şimşek H, et al. Interferon therapy for acute hepatitis C during pregnancy. *Ann Pharmacother* 2002;36:1715.

838. Fioredda F, Ranieri E, Lorusso C, et al. Vertical transmission of hepatitis C. *Pediatr Infect Dis J* 1996;15:642.

839. Sabatino G, Ramenghi LA, di Marzio M, et al. Vertical transmission of hepatitis C virus: an epidemiological study on 2,980 pregnant women in Italy. *Eur J Epidemiol* 1996;12:443.

840. Polywka S, Feucht H, Zöllner B, et al. Hepatitis C virus infection in pregnancy and the risk of mother-to-child transmission. *Eur J Clin Microbiol Infect Dis* 1997;16:121.

841. Croxson M, Couper A, Voss L, et al. Vertical transmission of hepatitis C virus in New Zealand. *N Z Med J* 1997;110:165.

842. Tanzi M, Bellelli E, Benaglia G, et al. The prevalence of HCV infection in a cohort of pregnant women, the related risk factors and the possibility of vertical transmission. *Eur J Epidemiol* 1997;13:517.

843. La Torre A, Biadaioli R, Capobianco T, et al. Vertical transmission of HCV. *Acta Obstet Gynecol Scand* 1998;77:889.

844. Granovsky MO, Minkoff HL, Tess BH, et al. Hepatitis C virus infection in the Mothers and Infants Cohort Study. *Pediatrics* 1998;102:355.

845. Wejstål R, Månson A-S, Widell A, et al. Perinatal transmission of hepatitis G virus (GB virus type C) and hepatitis C virus infections—a comparison. *Clin Infect Dis* 1999;28:816.

846. Ceci O, Margiotta M, Marello F, et al. High rate of spontaneous viral clearance in a cohort of vertically infected hepatitis C virus infants: what lies behind? *J Hepatol* 2001;35:687.

847. Paternoster DM, Santarossa C, Grella P, et al. Viral load in HCV RNA-positive pregnant women. *Am J Gastroenterol* 2001; 96:2751.

848. Ferrero S, Lungaro P, Bruzzone BM, et al. Prospective study of mother-to-infant transmission of hepatitis C virus: a 10-year survey (1990–2000). *Acta Obstet Gynecol Scand* 2003;82:229.

849. Ohto H, Terazawa S, Sasaki N, et al. Transmission of hepatitis C virus from mothers to infants. *N Engl J Med* 1994;330:744.

850. Dal Molin G, D'Agaro P, Ansaldi F, et al. Mother-to-infant transmission of hepatitis C virus: rate of infection and assessment of viral load and IgM anti-HCV as risk factors. *J Med Virol* 2002;67:137.

851. Steininger C, Kundi M, Jatzko G, et al. Increased risk of mother-to-infant transmission of hepatitis C virus by intrapartum infantile exposure to maternal blood. *J Infect Dis* 2003;187:345.

852. Caudai C, Battiata M, Riccardi MP, et al. Vertical transmission of the hepatitis C virus to infants of anti-human immunodeficiency virus-negative mothers: molecular evolution of hypervariable region 1 in prenatal and perinatal or postnatal infections. *J Clin Microbiol* 2003;41:3955.

853. Aizaki H, Saito A, Kusakawa I, et al. Mother-to-child transmission of a hepatitis C virus variant with an insertional mutation in its hypervariable region. *J Hepatol* 1996;25:608.

854. Ni Y-H, Chang M-H, Chen P-J, et al. Evolution of hepatitis C virus quasispecies in mothers and infants infected through mother-to-infant transmission. *J Hepatol* 1997;26:967.

855. Manzin A, Solforosi L, Debiaggi M, et al. Dominant role of host selective pressure in driving hepatitis C virus evolution in perinatal infection. *J Virol* 2000;74:4327.

856. Rapicetta M, Argentini C, Spada E, et al. Molecular evolution of HCV genotype 2c persistent infection following mother-to-infant transmission. *Arch Virol* 2000;145:965.

857. Sitia G, Cella D, De Mitri MS, et al. Evolution of the E2 region of hepatitis C virus in an infant infected by mother-to-infant transmission. *J Med Virol* 2001;64:476.

858. Pollack H, Hou Z, Hughes AL, et al. Perinatal transmission and viral evolution of hepatitis C virus quasispecies in infants coinfected with HIV. *J Acquir Immune Defic Syndr* 2004;36:890.

859. Pappalardo BL. Influence of maternal human immunodeficiency virus (HIV) co-infection on vertical transmission of hepatitis C virus (HCV): a meta-analysis. *Int J Epidemiol* 2003; 32:727.

860. European Paediatric Hepatitis C Virus Network. Effects of mode of delivery and infant feeding on the risk of mother-to-child transmission of hepatitis C virus. *BJOG* 2001;108:371.

861. Hupertz VF, Wyllie R. Perinatal hepatitis C infection. *Pediatr Infect Dis J* 2003;22:369.

862. Sasaki N, Matsui A, Momoi M, et al. Loss of circulating hepatitis C virus in children who developed a persistent carrier state after mother-to-baby transmission. *Pediatr Res* 1997;42:263.

863. European Paediatric Hepatitis C Virus Network, Tovo P-A, Pembrey LJ, et al. Persistence rate and progression of vertically acquired hepatitis C infection. *J Infect Dis* 2000;181:419.

864. Resti M, Jara P, Hierro L, et al. Clinical features and progression of perinatally acquired hepatitis C virus infection. *J Med Virol* 2003;70:373.

865. Casiraghi MA, De Paschale M, Romanò L, et al. Long-term outcome (35 years) of hepatitis C after acquisition of infection through mini transfusions of blood given at birth. *Hepatology* 2004;39:90.

866. Narkewicz MR. Neonatally acquired hepatitis C—not so risky? *J Pediatr Gatroenterol Nutr* 2004;39:221.

867. Krawczynski K, Aggarwal R, Kamili S. Hepatitis E. *Infect Dis Clin North Am* 2000;14:669.

868. Lynch M, O'Flynn N, Cryan B, et al. Hepatitis E in Ireland. *Eur J Clin Microbiol Infect Dis* 1995;14:1109.

869. Perez OM, Morales W, Paniagua M, et al. Prevalence of antibodies to hepatitis A, B, C, and E viruses in a healthy population in Leon, Nicaragua. *Am J Trop Med Hyg* 1996;55:17.

870. Psichogiou M, Tzala E, Boletis J, et al. Hepatitis E virus infection in individuals at high risk of transmission of non-A, non-B hepatitis and sexually transmitted diseases. *Scand J Infect Dis* 1996;28:443.

871. Pavia M, Iiritano E, Veratti MA, et al. Prevalence of hepatitis E antibodies in healthy persons in southern Italy. *Infection* 1998;26:32.

872. Labrique AB, Thomas DL, Stoszek SK, et al. Hepatitis E: emerging infectious disease. *Epidemiol Rev* 1999;21:162.

873. Karetnyi YV, Gilchrist MJR, Naides SJ. Hepatitis E virus infection prevalence among selected populations in Iowa. *J Clin Virol* 1999;14:51.

874. Thomas DL, Yarbough PO, Vlahov D, et al. Seroreactivity to hepatitis E virus in areas where the disease is not endemic. *J Clin Microbiol* 1997;35:1244.

875. He J, Innis BL, Shrestha MP, et al. Evidence that rodents are a reservoir of hepatitis E virus for humans in Nepal. *J Clin Microbiol* 2002;40:4493.

876. Tei S, Kitajima N, Takahashi K, et al. Zoonotic transmission of hepatitis E virus from deer to human beings. *Lancet* 2003; 362:371.

877. Kasorndorkbua C, Thacker BJ, Halbur PG, et al. Experimental infection of pregnant gilts with swine hepatitis E virus. *Can J Vet Res* 2003;67:303.

878. Khuroo MS, Kamili S, Jameel S. Vertical transmission of hepatitis E virus. *Lancet* 1995;345:1025.

879. Kumar RM, Uduman S, Rana S, et al. Sero-prevalence and mother-to-infant transmission of hepatitis E virus among pregnant women in the United Arab Emirates. *Eur J Obstet Gynecol Reprod Biol* 2001;100:9.

880. Singh S, Mohanty A, Joshi YK, et al. Mother-to-child transmission of hepatitis E virus infection. *Indian J Pediatr* 2003;70:37.

881. Stapleton JT. GB virus type C/hepatitis G virus. *Semin Liver Dis* 2003;23:137.

882. Kelly D, Skidmore S. Hepatitis C-Z: recent advances. *Arch Dis Child* 2002;86:339.

883. Yenice N, Gokden Y, Erdem L, et al. Transfusional transmitted virus seroprevalence in asymptomatic HBsAg (+) hepatitis B carriers. *Scand J Gastroenterol* 2004;39:174.

884. Chan PKS, Tam W-H, Yeo W, et al. High carriage rate of TT virus in the cervices of pregnant women. *Clin Infect Dis* 2001; 32:1376.

885. Kazi A, Miyata H, Kurokawa K, et al. High frequency of postnatal transmission of TT virus in infancy. *Arch Virol* 2000; 145:535.

886. de Martino M, Moriondo M, Azzari C, et al. TT virus infection in human immunodeficiency virus type 1 infected mothers and their infants. *J Med Virol* 2000;61:347.

887. Lin H-H, Kao J-H, Lee P-I, et al. Early acquisition of TT virus in infants: possible minor role of maternal transmission. *J Med Virol* 2002;66:285.

888. Barton LL, Mets MB. Congenital lymphocytic choriomeningitis virus infection: decade of rediscovery. *Clin Infect Dis* 2001; 33:370.

889. Lukashevich IS, Djavani M, Rodas JD, et al. Hemorrhagic fever occurs after intravenous, but not after intragastric, inoculation of rhesus macaques with lymphocytic choriomeningitis virus. *J Med Virol* 2002;67:171.

890. Lukashevich IS, Tikhonov I, Rodas JD, et al. Arenavirus-mediated liver pathology: acute lymphocytic choriomeningitis virus infection of rhesus macaques is characterized by high-level interleukin-6 expression and hepatocyte proliferation. *J Virol* 2003;77:1727.

891. Enders G, Varho-Göbel M, Löhler J, et al. Congenital lymphocytic choriomeningitis virus infection: an underdiagnosed disease. *Pediatr Infect Dis J* 1999;18:652.

892. Barton LL, Mets MB, Beauchamp CL. Lymphocytic choriomeningitis virus: emerging fetal teratogen. *Am J Obstet Gynecol* 2002;187:1715.

893. Rappole JH, Hubálek Z. Migratory birds and West Nile virus. *J Appl Microbiol* 2003;94:47S.

894. Petersen LR, Marfin AA. West Nile virus: a primer for the clinician. *Ann Intern Med* 2002;137:173.

895. Gea-Banacloche J, Johnson RT, Bagic A, et al. West Nile virus: pathogenesis and therapeutic options. *Ann Intern Med* 2004; 140:545.

896. Nash D, Mostashari F, Fine A, et al. The outbreak of West Nile virus infection in the New York City area in 1999. *N Engl J Med* 2001;344:1807.

897. Pepperell C, Rau N, Krajden S, et al. West Nile virus infection in 2002: morbidity and mortality among patients admitted to hospital in southcentral Ontario. *CMAJ* 2003;168:1399.

898. Centers for Disease Control and Prevention. West Nile virus activity—United States, November 9–16, 2004. *MMWR* 2004;53:1071.

899. Campbell GL, Marfin AA, Lanciotti RS, et al. West Nile virus. *Lancet Infect Dis* 2002;2:519.

900. Petersen LR, Marfin AA, Gubler DJ. West Nile virus. *JAMA* 2003;290:524.

901. Lanciotti RS, Roehrig JT, Deubel V, et al. Origin of the West Nile virus responsible for an outbreak of encephalitis in the northeastern United States. *Science* 1999;286:2333.

902. Centers for Disease Control and Prevention. Possible dialysis-related West Nile virus transmission—Georgia, 2003. *MMWR* 2004;53:738.

903. Mostashari F, Bunning ML, Kitsutani PT, et al. Epidemic West Nile encephalitis, New York, 1999: results of a household-based seroepidemiological survey. *Lancet* 2001;358:261.

904. Klein C, Kimiagar I, Pollak L, et al. Neurological features of West Nile virus infection during the 2000 outbreak in a regional hospital in Israel. *J Neurol Sci* 2002;200:63.

905. Li J, Loeb JA, Shy ME, et al. Asymmetric flaccid paralysis: a neuromuscular presentation of West Nile virus infection. *Ann Neurol* 2003;53:703.

906. Sejvar JJ, Haddad MB, Tierney BC, et al. Neurologic manifestations and outcome of West Nile virus infection. *JAMA* 2003; 290:511.

907. Sejvar JJ. West Nile virus and "poliomyelitis". *Neurology* 2004; 63:206.

908. Ratterree MS, Gutierrez RA, Travassos da Rosa APA, et al. Experimental infection of rhesus macaques with West Nile virus: level and duration of viremia and kinetics of the antibody response after infection. *J Infect Dis* 2004;189:669.

909. Centers for Disease Control and Prevention. Update: West Nile virus screening of blood donations and transfusion-associated transmission—United States, 2003. *MMWR* 2004;53:281.

910. Ben-Nathan D, Lustig S, Tam G, et al. Prophylactic and therapeutic efficacy of human intravenous immunoglobulin in treating West Nile virus infection in mice. *J Infect Dis* 2003;188:5.

911. Centers for Disease Control and Prevention. Interim guidelines for the evaluation of infants born to mothers infected with West Nile virus during pregnancy. *MMWR* 2004;53:154.

912. Centers for Disease Control and Prevention. Intrauterine West Nile virus infection—New York, 2002. *MMWR* 2002;51:1135.

913. Alpert SG, Fergerson J, Noël L-P. Intrauterine West Nile virus: ocular and systemic findings. *Am J Ophthalmol* 2003;136:733.

914. Chapa JB, Ahn JT, DiGiovanni LM, et al. West Nile virus encephalitis during pregnancy. *Obstet Gynecol* 2003;102:229.

915. Centers for Disease Control and Prevention. Possible West Nile virus transmission to an infant through breast-feeding—Michigan, 2002. *MMWR* 2002;51:877.

916. Steinbrook R. The AIDS epidemic in 2004. *N Engl J Med* 2004; 351:115.

917. Centers for Disease Control and Prevention. *HIV/AIDS surveillance report*. 2002;14:1.

918. Nakashima AK, Fleming PL. HIV/AIDS surveillance in the United States, 1981–2001. *J Acquir Immune Defic Syndr* 2003; 32:S68.

919. Hamers FF, Downs AM. The changing face of the HIV epidemic in western Europe: what are the implications for public health policies? *Lancet* 2004;364:83.

920. Asamoah-Odei E, Garcia Calleja JM, Boerma JT. HIV prevalence and trends in sub-Saharan Africa: no decline and large subregional differences. *Lancet* 2004;364:35.

921. Ruxrungtham K, Brown T, Phanuphak P. HIV/AIDS in Asia. *Lancet* 2004;364:69.

922. Centers for Disease Control and Prevention. Heterosexual transmission of HIV – 29 states, 1999—2002. *MMWR* 2004; 53:125.

923. Landers DV, Martínez de Tejada B, Coyne BA. Immunology of HIV and pregnancy: the effects of each on the other. *Obstet Gynecol Clin North Am* 1997;24:821.

924. Minkoff HL. Human immunodeficiency virus infection in pregnancy. *Semin Perinatol* 1998;22:293.

925. Garzino-Demo A, Devico AL, Gallo RC. Chemokine receptors and chemokines in HIV infection. *J Clin Immunol* 1998;18:243.

926. Garzino-Demo A, Gallo RC. HIV receptors on lymphocytes. *Curr Opin Hematol* 2003;10:279.

927. Misrahi M, Teglas J-P, N'Go N, et al. CCR5 chemokine receptor variant in HIV-1 mother-to-child transmission and disease progression in children. *JAMA* 1998;279:277.

928. Kostrikis LG, Huang Y, Moore JP, et al. A chemokine receptor CCR2 allele delays HIV-1 disease progression and is associated with a CCR5 promoter mutation. *Nat Med* 1998;4:350.

929. Letvin NL, Walker BD. Immunopathogenesis and immunotherapy in AIDS virus infections. *Nat Med* 2003;9:861.

930. Barouch DH, Letvin NL. HIV escape from cytotoxic T lymphocytes: a potential hurdle for vaccines? *N Engl J Med* 2004;364:10.

931. Connor EM, Sperling RS, Gelber R, et al. Reduction of maternal-infant transmission of human immunodeficiency virus type 1 with zidovudine treatment. *N Engl J Med* 1994; 331:1173.

932. Centers for Disease Control and Prevention. Public Health Service task force recommendations for the use of antiretroviral drugs in pregnant women infected with HIV-1 for maternal health and for reducing perinatal HIV-1 transmission in the United States. *MMWR* 1998;47(RR-2):1.

933. American Academy of Pediatrics. Canadian Paediatric Society. Clinical report: evaluation and treatment of the human immunodeficiency virus-1-exposed infant. *Pediatrics* 2004; 114:497.

934. Hodinka RL. The clinical utility of viral quantitation using molecular methods. *Clin Diagn Virol* 1998;10:25.

935. Cavert W. In vivo detection and quantitation of HIV in blood and tissues. *AIDS* 1998;12(Suppl A):S27.

936. Shaunak S, Teo I. Monitoring HIV disease with new and clinically useful surrogate markers. *Curr Opin Infect Dis* 2003; 16:581.

937. De Luca A, Perno C-F. Impact of different HIV resistance interpretation by distinct systems on clinical utility of resistance testing. *Curr Opin Infect Dis* 2003;16:573.

938. Frenkel LM, Tobin NH. Understanding HIV-1 drug resistance. *Ther Drug Monit* 2004;26:116.

939. Davis SF, Rosen DH, Steinberg S, et al. Trends in HIV prevalence among childbearing women in the United States, 1989–1994. *J Acquir Immune Defic Syndr Hum Retrovirol* 1998;19:158.

940. Cohen M. Natural history of HIV infection in women. *Obstet Gynecol Clin North Am* 1997;24:743.

941. Ellerbrock TV, Lieb S, Harrington PE, et al. Heterosexually transmitted human immunodeficiency virus infection among pregnant women in a rural Florida community. *N Engl J Med* 1992;327:1704.

942. Catania JA, Coates TJ, Stall R, et al. Prevalence of AIDS-related risk factors and condom use in the United States. *Science* 1992;258:1101.

943. Lindsay MK, Peterson HB, Willis S, et al. Incidence and prevalence of human immunodeficiency virus infection in a prenatal population undergoing routine voluntary human immunodeficiency virus screening, July 1987 to June 1990. *Am J Obstet Gynecol* 1991;165:961.

944. Puro V, D'Ubaldo C, Aloisi MS, et al. Women attending human immunodeficiency virus counselling and testing site because of

pregnancy, and prevalence of newly diagnosed infections. *Eur J Obstet Gynecol Reprod Biol* 1998;79:51.

945. Carusi D, Learman LA, Posner SF. Human immunodeficiency virus test refusal in pregnancy: a challenge to voluntary testing. *Obstet Gynecol* 1998;91:540.

946. Centers for Disease Control and Prevention. Prenatal HIV testing and antiretroviral prophylaxis at an urban hospital—Atlanta, Georgia, 1997–2000. *MMWR* 2004;52:1245.

947. Sansom SL, Jamieson DJ, Farnham PG, et al. Human immunodeficiency virus retesting during pregnancy: costs and effectiveness in preventing perinatal transmission. *Obstet Gynecol* 2003;102:782.

948. Forsyth BWC, Barringer SR, Walls TA, et al. Rapid HIV testing of women in labor: too long a delay. *J Acquir Immune Defic Syndr* 2004;35:151.

949. Bulterys M, Jamieson DJ, O'Sullivan MJ, et al. Rapid HIV-1 testing during labor: a multicenter study. *JAMA* 2004;292:219.

950. Stratton P, Mofenson LM, Willoughby AD. Human immunodeficiency virus infection in pregnant women under care at AIDS clinical trials centers in the United States. *Obstet Gynecol* 1992;79:364.

951. Stratton P, Tuomala RE, Abboud R, et al. Obstetric and newborn outcomes in a cohort of HIV-infected pregnant women: a report of the Women and Infants Transmission Study. *J Acquir Immune Defic Syndr Hum Retrovirol* 1999;20:179.

952. McIntyre J. Mothers infected with HIV. *Br Med Bull* 2003;67:127.

953. Langston C, Lewis DE, Hammill HA, et al. Excess intrauterine fetal demise associated with maternal human immunodeficiency virus infection. *J Infect Dis* 1995;172:1451.

954. Massad LS, Springer G, Jacobson L, et al. Pregnancy rates and predictors of conception, miscarriage and abortion in U.S. women with HIV. *AIDS* 2004;18:281.

955. Bessinger R, Clark R, Kissinger P, et al. Pregnancy is not associated with the progression of HIV disease in women attending an HIV outpatient program. *Am J Epidemiol* 1998;147:434.

956. Weisser M, Rudin C, Battegay M, et al. Does pregnancy influence the course of HIV infection? Evidence from two large Swiss cohort studies. *J Acquir Immune Defic Syndr Hum Retrovirol* 1998;17:404.

957. Burns DN, Landesman S, Minkoff H, et al. The influence of pregnancy on human immunodeficiency virus type 1 infection: antepartum and postpartum changes in human immunodeficiency virus type 1 viral load. *Am J Obstet Gynecol* 1998;178:355.

958. Minkoff H, Hershow R, Watts DH, et al. The relationship of pregnancy to human immunodeficiency virus disease progression. *Am J Obstet Gynecol* 2003;189:552.

959. Sullivan JL. Prevention of mother-to-child transmission of HIV—what next? *J Acquir Immune Defic Syndr* 2003;34:S67.

960. Viscarello RR, Cullen MT, DeGennaro NJ, et al. Fetal blood sampling in human immunodeficiency virus-seropositive women before elective midtrimester termination of pregnancy. *Am J Obstet Gynecol* 1992;167:1075.

961. Mandelbrot L, Brossard Y, Aubin J-T, et al. Testing for in utero human immunodeficiency virus infection with fetal blood sampling. *Am J Obstet Gynecol* 1996;175:489.

962. Dickover RE, Garratty EM, Herman SA, et al. Identification of levels of maternal HIV-1 RNA associated with risk of perinatal transmission: effect of maternal zidovudine treatment on viral load. *JAMA* 1996;275:599.

963. Landesman SH, Kalish LA, Burns DN, et al. Obstetrical factors and the transmission of human immunodeficiency virus type 1 from mother to child. *N Engl J Med* 1996;334:1617.

964. Mandelbrot L, Mayaux M-J, Bongain A, et al. Obstetric factors and mother-to-child transmission of human immunodeficiency virus type 1: the French perinatal cohorts. *Am J Obstet Gynecol* 1996;175:661.

965. The European Collaborative Study. Vertical transmission of HIV-1: maternal immune status and obstetric factors. *AIDS* 1996;10:1675.

966. Coll O, Hernandez M, Boucher CAB, et al. Vertical HIV-1 transmission correlates with a high maternal viral load at delivery. *J Acquir Immune Defic Syndr Hum Retrovirol* 1997;14:26.

967. John GC, Nduati RW, Mbori-Ngacha D, et al. Genital shedding of human immunodeficiency virus type 1 DNA during pregnancy: association with immunosuppression, abnormal cervical or vaginal discharge, and severe vitamin A deficiency. *J Infect Dis* 1997;175:57.

968. Ugen KE, Srikantan V, Goedert JJ, et al. Vertical transmission of human immunodeficiency virus type 1: seroreactivity by maternal antibodies to the carboxy region of the gp41 envelope glycoprotein. *J Infect Dis* 1997;175:63.

969. Mayaux MJ, Dussaix E, Isopet J, et al. Maternal virus load during pregnancy and mother-to-child transmission of human immunodeficiency virus type 1: the French perinatal cohort studies. *J Infect Dis* 1997;175:172.

970. Mostad SB, Overbaugh J, DeVange DM, et al. Hormonal contraception, vitamin A deficiency, and other risk factors for shedding of HIV-1 infected cells from the cervix and vagina. *Lancet* 1997;350:922.

971. Montano M, Russell M, Gilbert P, et al. Comparative prediction of perinatal human immunodeficiency virus type 1 transmission, using multiple virus load markers. *J Infect Dis* 2003; 188:406.

972. Renjifo B, Gilbert P, Chaplin B, et al. Preferential *in-utero* transmission of HIV-1 subtype C as compared to HIV-1 subtype A or D. *AIDS* 2004;18:1629.

973. Garcia PM, Kalish LA, Pitt J, et al. Maternal levels of plasma human immunodeficiency virus type 1 RNA and the risk of perinatal transmission. *N Engl J Med* 1999;341:394.

974. Thorne C, Newell M-L. Prevention of mother-to-child transmission of HIV infection. *Curr Opin Infect Dis* 2004;17:247.

975. Goedert JJ, Duliège A-M, Amos CI, et al. High risk of HIV-1 infection for first-born twins. *Lancet* 1991;338:1471.

976. de Martino M, Tovo P-A, Galli L, et al. HIV-I infection in perinatally exposed siblings and twins. *Arch Dis Child* 1991;66:1235.

977. Bryson YJ, Luzuriaga K, Sullivan JL, et al. Proposed definitions for in utero versus intrapartum transmission of HIV-1. *N Engl J Med* 1992;327:1246.

978. Van de Perre P. Postnatal transmission of human immunodeficiency virus type 1: the breast-feeding dilemma. *Am J Obstet Gynecol* 1995;173:483.

979. John-Stewart G, Mbori-Ngacha D, Ekpini R, et al. Breast-feeding and transmission of HIV-1. *J Acquir Immune Defic Syndr* 2004;35:196.

980. Lewis P, Nduati R, Kreiss JK, et al. Cell-free human immunodeficiency virus type 1 in breast milk. *J Infect Dis* 1998;177:34.

981. Hoffman IF, Martinson FEA, Stewart PW, et al. Human immunodeficiency virus type 1 RNA in breast-milk components. *Clin Infect Dis* 2003;188:1209.

982. Ghosh MK, Kuhn L, West J, et al. Quantitation of human immunodeficiency virus type 1 in breast milk. *J Clin Microbiol* 2003;41:2465.

983. Mbori-Ngacha D, Nduati R, John G, et al. Morbidity and mortality in breastfed and formula-fed infants of HIV-1-infected women: a randomized clinical trial. *JAMA* 2001;286:2413.

984. European Collaborative Study. Risk factors for mother-to-child transmission of HIV-1. *Lancet* 1992;339:1007.

985. Kind C, Brändle B, Wyler C-A, et al. Epidemiology of vertically transmitted HIV-1 infection in Switzerland: results of a nationwide prospective study. *Eur J Pediatr* 1992;151:442.

986. Hutto C, Parks WP, Lai S, et al. A hospital-based prospective study of perinatal infection with human immunodeficiency virus type 1. *J Pediatr* 1991;118:347.

987. Van de Perre P, Simonon A, Msellati P, et al. Postnatal transmission of human immunodeficiency virus type 1 from mother to infant: a prospective cohort study in Kigali, Rwanda. *N Engl J Med* 1991;325:593.

988. Wolinsky SM, Wike CM, Korber BTM, et al. Selective transmission of human immunodeficiency virus type-1 variants from mothers to infants. *Science* 1992;255:1134.

989. Lamers SL, Sleasman JW, She JX, et al. Persistence of multiple maternal genotypes of human immunodeficiency virus type 1 in infants infected by vertical transmission. *J Clin Invest* 1994;93:380.

990. Colgrove RC, Pitt J, Chung PH, et al. Selective vertical transmission of HIV-1 antiretroviral resistance mutations. *AIDS* 1998; 12:2281.

991. Pasquier C, Cayrou C, Blancher A, et al. Molecular evidence for mother-to-child transmission of multiple variants by analysis of RNA and DNA sequences of human immunodeficiency virus type 1. *J Virol* 1998;72:8493.

992. Desai N, Mathur M. Selective transmission of multidrug resistant HIV to a newborn related to poor maternal adherence. *Sex Transm Infect* 2003;79:419.

993. Fowler MG, Mofenson L, McConnell M. The interface of perinatal HIV prevention, antiretroviral drug resistance, and antiretroviral treatment: what do we really know? J *Acquir Immune Defic Syndr* 2003;34:308.

994. Parker MM, Wade N, Lloyd RM Jr, et al. Prevalence of genotypic drug resistance among a cohort of HIV-infected newborns. *J Acquir Immune Defic Syndr* 2003;32:292.

995. Loutfy MR, Walmsley SL. Treatment of HIV infection in pregnant women: antiretroviral management options. *Drugs* 2004; 64:471.

996. Yeni PG, Hammer SM, Hirsch MS, et al. Treatment for adult HIV infection: 2004 recommendations of the International AIDS Society-U.S.A. Panel. *JAMA* 2004;292:251.

997. Ioannidis JPA, Abrams EJ, Ammann A, et al. Perinatal transmission of human immunodeficiency virus type 1 by pregnant women with RNA virus loads <1000 copies/mL. *J Infect Dis* 2001;183:539.

998. Bucceri AM, Somigliana E, Matrone R, et al. Discontinuing combination antiretroviral therapy during the first trimester of pregnancy: insights from plasma human immunodeficiency virus-1 RNA viral load and CD4 cell count. *Am J Obstet Gynecol* 2003;189:545.

999. Public Health Service Task Force. Safety and toxicity of individual antiretroviral agents in pregnancy [online]. Available from http://www.aidsinfo.nih.gov/. Accessed August 28, 2004.

1000. Public Health Service Task Force. Recommendations for use of antiretroviral drugs in pregnant HIV-1-infected women for maternal health and interventions to reduce perinatal HIV-1 transmission in the United States, June 23, 2004 [online]. Available from http://www.aidsinfo.nih.gov/. Accessed August 28, 2004.

1001. Sperling RS, Shapiro DE, Coombs RW, et al. Maternal viral load, zidovudine treatment, and the risk of transmission of human immunodeficiency virus type 1 from mother to infant. *N Engl J Med* 1996;335:1621.

1002. Lansky A, Jones JL, Wan P-CT, et al. Trends in zidovudine prescription for pregnant women infected with HIV. *J Acquir Immune Defic Syndr Hum Retrovirol* 1998;18:289.

1003. Phuapradit W, Chaturachinda K, Taneepanichskul S, et al. Vertical transmission of HIV-1 in mid-trimester gestation. *Aust N Z J Obstet Gynaecol* 1995;35:427.

1004. Matheson PB, Abrams EJ, Thomas PA, et al. Efficacy of antenatal zidovudine in reducing perinatal transmission of human immunodeficiency virus type 1. *J Infect Dis* 1995;172:353.

1005. Cooper ER, Nugent RP, Diaz C, et al. After AIDS Clinical Trial 076: the changing pattern of zidovudine use during pregnancy, and the subsequent reduction in the vertical transmission of human immunodeficiency virus in a cohort of infected women and their infants. *J Infect Dis* 1996;174:1207.

1006. Simonds RJ, Steketee R, Nesheim S, et al. Impact of zidovudine use on risk and risk factors for perinatal transmission of HIV. *AIDS* 1998;12:301.

1007. Stiehm ER, Lambert JS, Mofenson LM, et al. Efficacy of zidovudine and human immunodeficiency virus (HIV) hyperimmune immunoglobulin for reducing perinatal HIV transmission from HIV-infected women with advanced disease: results of Pediatric AIDS Clinical Trials Group Protocol 185. *J Infect Dis* 1999; 179:567.

1008. Wade NA, Birkhead GS, Warren BL, et al. Abbreviated regimens of zidovudine prophylaxis and perinatal transmission of the human immunodeficiency virus. *N Engl J Med* 1998;339:1409.

1009. Centers for Disease Control and Prevention. Administration of zidovudine during late pregnancy and delivery to prevent perinatal HIV transmission—Thailand, 1996–1998. *MMWR* 1998; 47:151.

1010. The Petra Study Team. Efficacy of three short-course regimens of zidovudine and lamivudine in preventing early and late transmission of HIV-1 from mother to child in Tanzania, South Africa, and Uganda (Petra study): a randomised, double-blind, placebo-controlled trial. *Lancet* 2002;359:1178.

1011. Guay LA, Musoke P, Fleming T, et al. Intrapartum and neonatal single-dose nevirapine compared with zidovudine for prevention of mother-to-child transmission of HIV-1 in Kampala, Uganda: HIVNET 012 randomised trial. *Lancet* 1999;354:795.

1012. Jackson JB, Musoke P, Fleming T, et al. Intrapartum and neonatal single-dose nevirapine compared with zidovudine for prevention of mother-to-child transmission of HIV-1 in Kampala,

Uganda: 18-month follow-up of the HIVNET 012 randomised trial. *Lancet* 2003;362:859.

1013. Quaghebeur A, Mutunga L, Mwanyumba F, et al. Low efficacy of nevirapine (HIVNET012) in preventing perinatal HIV-1 transmission in a real-life situation. *AIDS* 2004;18:1854.

1014. Dorenbaum A, Cunningham CK, Gelber RD, et al. Two-dose intrapartum/newborn nevirapine and standard antiretroviral therapy to reduce perinatal HIV transmission: a randomized trial. *JAMA* 2002;288:189.

1015. Lallemant M, Jourdain G, Le Coeur S, et al. Single-dose perinatal nevirapine plus standard zidovudine to prevent mother-to-child transmission of HIV-1 in Thailand. *N Engl J Med* 2004;351:217.

1016. Coovadia H. Antiretroviral agents—how best to protect infants from HIV and save their mothers from AIDS. *N Engl J Med* 2004;351:289.

1017. Taha TE, Kumwenda NI, Hoover DR, et al. Nevirapine and zidovudine at birth to reduce perinatal transmission of HIV in an African setting: a randomized controlled trial. *JAMA* 2004; 292:202.

1018. Stringer JSA, Sinkala M, Chapman V, et al. Timing of the maternal drug dose and risk of perinatal HIV transmission in the setting of intrapartum and neonatal single-dose nevirapine. *AIDS* 2003;17:1659.

1019. Cunningham CK, Chaix M-L, Rekacewicz C, et al. Development of resistance mutations in women receiving standard antiretroviral therapy who received intrapartum nevirapine to prevent perinatal human immunodeficiency virus type 1 transmission: a substudy of Pediatric AIDS Clinical Trials Group Protocol 316. *J Infect Dis* 2002;186:181.

1020. Jourdain G, Ngo-Giang-Huong N, Le Coeur S, et al. Intrapartum exposure to nevirapine and subsequent maternal responses to nevirapine-based antiretroviral therapy. *N Engl J Med* 2004; 351:229.

1021. Panburana P, Sirinavin S, Phuapradit W, et al. Elective cesarean delivery plus short-course lamivudine and zidovudine for the prevention of mother-to-child transmission of human immunodeficiency virus type 1. *Am J Obstet Gynecol* 2004;190:803.

1022. Peters V, Liu K-L, Dominguez K, et al. Missed opportunities for perinatal HIV prevention among HIV-exposed infants born 1996–2000, Pediatric Spectrum of HIV Disease Cohort. *Pediatrics* 2003;111:1186.

1023. Kline MW, O'Connor KG. Disparity between pediatricians' knowledge and practices regarding perinatal human immunodeficiency virus counseling and testing. *Pediatrics* 2003;112:e367.

1024. Demas PA, Webber MP, Schoenbaum EE, et al. Maternal adherence to the zidovudine regimen for HIV-exposed infants to prevent HIV infection: a preliminary study. *Pediatrics* 2002;110:e35.

1025. Chotpitayasunondh T, Vanprapar N, Simonds RJ, et al. Safety of late in utero exposure to zidovudine in infants born to human immunodeficiency virus-infected mothers: Bangkok. *Pediatrics* 2001;107:e5.

1026. French Perinatal Cohort Study Group. Risk of early febrile seizure with perinatal exposure to nucleoside analogues. *Lancet* 2002;359:583.

1027. Le Chenadec J, Mayaux M-J, Guihenneuc-Jouyaux C, et al. Perinatal antiretroviral treatment and hematopoiesis in HIV-uninfected infants. *AIDS* 2003;17:2053.

1028. Capparelli EV, Mirochnick M, Dankner WM, et al. Pharmacokinetics and tolerance of zidovudine in preterm infants. *J Pediatr* 2003;142:47.

1029. McComsey GA, Leonard E. Metabolic complications of HIV therapy in children. *AIDS* 2004;18:1753.

1030. Galli L, de Martino M, Tovo P-A, et al. Onset of clinical signs in children with HIV-1 perinatal infection. *AIDS* 1995;9:455.

1031. Mayaux M-J, Burgard M, Teglas J-P, et al. Neonatal characteristics in rapidly progressive perinatally acquired HIV-1 disease. *JAMA* 1996;275:606.

1032. McCarty KA, Bungu Z. Kaposi's sarcoma in a two week old infant born to a mother with Kaposi's sarcoma/AIDS. *Cent Afr J Med* 1995;41:330.

1033. The European Collaborative Study. Natural history of vertically acquired human immunodeficiency virus-1 infection. *Pediatrics* 1994;94:815.

1034. Barnhart HX, Caldwell MB, Thomas P, et al. Natural history of human immunodeficiency virus disease in perinatally infected children: an analysis from the Pediatric Spectrum of Disease project. *Pediatrics* 1996;97:710.

1035. Pliner V, Weedon J, Thomas PA, et al. Incubation period of HIV-1 in perinatally infected children. *AIDS* 1998;12:759.

1036. Chearskul S, Chotpitayasunondh T, Simonds RJ, et al. Survival, disease manifestations, and early predictors of disease progression among children with perinatal human immunodeficiency virus infection in Thailand. *Pediatrics* 2002;110:e25.

1037. Obimbo EM, Mbori-Ngacha DA, Ochieng JO, et al. Predictors of early mortality in a cohort of human immunodeficiency virus type 1-infected African children. *Pediatr Infect Dis J* 2004;23:536.

1038. Abrams EJ, Wiener J, Carter R, et al. Maternal health factors and early pediatric antiretroviral therapy influence the rate of perinatal HIV-1 disease progression in children. *AIDS* 2003;17:867.

1039. Working Group on Antiretroviral Therapy and Medical Management of HIV-Infected Children. Guidelines for the use of antiretroviral agents in pediatric HIV infection, January 20, 2004 [online]. Available from http://www.aidsinfo.nih.gov/. Accessed August 28, 2004.

1040. Shearer WT, Quinn TC, LaRussa P, et al. Viral load and disease progression in infants infected with human immunodeficiency virus type 1. *N Engl J Med* 1997;336:1337.

1041. Zaknun D, Orav J, Kornegay J, et al. Correlation of ribonucleic acid polymerase chain reaction, acid dissociated p24 antigen, and neopterin with progression of disease: a retrospective, longitudinal study of vertically acquired human immunodeficiency virus type 1 infection in children. *J Pediatr* 1997;130:898.

1042. Palumbo PE, Raskino C, Fiscus S, et al. Predictive value of quantitative plasma HIV RNA and CD4$^+$ lymphocyte count in HIV-infected infants and children. *JAMA* 1998;279:756.

1043. Dickover RE, Dillon M, Leung K-M, et al. Early prognostic indicators in primary perinatal human immunodeficiency virus type 1 infection: importance of viral RNA and the timing of transmission on long-term outcome. *J Infect Dis* 1998;178:375.

1044. Kuhn L, Steketee RW, Weedon J, et al. Distinct risk factors for intrauterine and intrapartum human immunodeficiency virus transmission and consequences for disease progression in infected children. *J Infect Dis* 1999;179:52.

1045. Palasanthiran P, Robertson P, Ziegler JB, et al. Decay of transplacental human immunodeficiency virus type 1 antibodies in neonates and infants. *J Infect Dis* 1994;170:1593.

1046. McIntosh K, FitzGerald G, Pitt J, et al. A comparison of peripheral blood coculture versus 18- or 24-month serology in the diagnosis of human immunodeficiency virus infection in the offspring of infected mothers. *J Infect Dis* 1998;178:560.

1047. Borkowsky W, Krasinski K, Pollack H, et al. Early diagnosis of human immunodeficiency virus infection in children <6 months of age: comparison of polymerase chain reaction, culture, and plasma antigen capture techniques. *J Infect Dis* 1992;166:616.

1048. Lepage P, Van de Perre P, Simonon A, et al. Transient seroreversion in children born to human immunodeficiency virus 1-infected mothers. *Pediatr Infect Dis J* 1992;11:892.

1049. Burgard M, Mayaux M-J, Blanche S, et al. The use of viral culture and p24 antigen testing to diagnose human immunodeficiency virus infection in neonates. *N Engl J Med* 1992;327:1192.

1050. Palomba E, Gay V, de Martino M, et al. Early diagnosis of human immunodeficiency virus infection in infants by detection of free and complexed p24 antigen. *J Infect Dis* 1992;165:394.

1051. Landesman S, Weiblen B, Mendez H, et al. Clinical utility of HIV-IgA immunoblot assay in the early diagnosis of perinatal HIV infection. *JAMA* 1991;266:3443.

1052. Quinn TC, Kline RL, Halsey N, et al. Early diagnosis of perinatal HIV infection by detection of viral-specific IgA antibodies. *JAMA* 1991;266:2439.

1053. Miles SA, Balden E, Magpantay L, et al. Rapid serologic testing with immune-complex-dissociated HIV p24 antigen for early detection of HIV infection in neonates. *N Engl J Med* 1993;328:297.

1054. Lambert JS, Harris DR, Stiehm ER, et al. Performance characteristics of HIV-1 culture and HIV-1 DNA and RNA amplification assays for early diagnosis of perinatal HIV-1 infection. *J Acquir Immune Defic Syndr* 2003;34:512.

1055. Bremer JW, Lew JF, Cooper E, et al. Diagnosis of infection with human immunodeficiency virus type 1 by a DNA polymerase chain reaction assay among infants enrolled in the Women and Infants' Transmission Study. *J Pediatr* 1996;129:198.

1056. Luzuriaga K, Sullivan JL. DNA polymerase chain reaction for the diagnosis of vertical HIV infection. *JAMA* 1996;275:1360.

1057. Culnane M, Fowler MG, Lee SS, et al. Lack of long-term effects of in utero exposure to zidovudine among uninfected children born to HIV-infected women. *JAMA* 1999;281:151.

1058. Paediatric European Network for Treatment of AIDS (PENTA). Highly active antiretroviral therapy started in infants under 3 months of age: 72-week follow-up for CD4 cell count, viral load and drug resistance outcome. *AIDS* 2004;18:237.

1059. Luzuriaga K, McManus M, Mofenson L, et al. A trial of three antiretroviral regimens in HIV-1-infected children. *N Engl J Med* 2004;350:2471.

1060. Hermankova M, Ray SC, Ruff C, et al. HIV-1 drug resistance profiles in children and adults with viral load of <50 copies/mL receiving combination therapy. *JAMA* 2001;286:196.

1061. Van Dyke RB, Lee S, Johnson GM, et al. Reported adherence as a determinant of response to highly active antiretroviral therapy in children who have human immunodeficiency virus infection. *Pediatrics* 2002;109:e61.

1062. Fraaij PLA, Rakhmanina N, Burger DM, et al. Therapeutic drug monitoring in children with HIV/AIDS. *Ther Drug Monit* 2004;26:122.

1063. Langston C, Cooper ER, Goldfarb J, et al. Human immunodeficiency virus-related mortality in infants and children: data from the Pediatric Pulmonary and Cardiovascular Complications of Vertically Transmitted HIV (P2C2) Study. *Pediatrics* 2001;107:328.

1064. Scarlatti G. Paediatric HIV infection. *Lancet* 1996;348:863.

1065. Exhenry C, Nadal D. Vertical human immunodeficiency virus-1 infection: involvement of the central nervous system and treatment. *Eur J Pediatr* 1996;155:839.

1066. Tamula MAT, Wolters PL, Walsek C, et al. Cognitive decline with immunologic and virologic stability in four children with human immunodeficiency virus disease. *Pediatrics* 2003;112:679.

1067. Plebani A, Esposito S, Pinzani R, et al. Effect of highly active antiretroviral therapy on cardiovascular involvement in children with human immunodeficiency virus infection. *Pediatr Infect Dis J* 2004;23:559.

1068. Pollack H, Glasberg H, Lee E, et al. Impaired early growth of infants perinatally infected with human immunodeficiency virus: correlation with viral load. *J Pediatr* 1997;130:915.

1069. Carey VJ, Yong FH, Frenkel LM, et al. Pediatric AIDS prognosis using somatic growth velocity. *AIDS* 1998;12:1361.

1070. Nachman SA, Lindsey JC, Pelton S, et al. Growth in human immunodeficiency virus-infected children receiving ritonavir-containing antiretroviral therapy. *Arch Pediatr Adolesc Med* 2002;156:497.

1071. The European Collaborative Study. Height, weight, and growth in children born to mothers with HIV-1 infection in Europe. *Pediatrics* 2003;111:e52.

1072. Rondanelli M, Caselli D, Trotti R, et al. Endocrine pancreatic dysfunction in HIV-infected children: association with growth alterations. *J Infect Dis* 2004;190:908.

1073. Italian Register for HIV Infection in Children. Features of children perinatally infected with HIV-1 surviving longer than 5 years. *Lancet* 1994;343:191.

1074. Biggar RJ, Frisch M, the AIDS-Cancer Match Registry Study Group, et al. Risk of cancer in children with AIDS. *JAMA* 2000;284:205.

1075. Balarezo FS, Joshi VV. Proliferative and neoplastic disorders in children with acquired immunodeficiency syndrome. *Adv Anat Pathol* 2002;9:360.

1076. Mofenson LM, Moye J Jr, Bethel J, et al. Prophylactic intravenous immunoglobulin in HIV-infected children with CD4$^+$ counts of 0.20 x 10^9/L or more: effect on viral, opportunistic, and bacterial infections. *JAMA* 1992;268:483.

1077. American Academy of Pediatrics. Human immunodeficiency virus infection. In: Pickering LK, ed. *Red Book: 2003 report of the Committee on Infectious Diseases*, 26th ed. Elk Grove Village, IL: American Academy of Pediatrics, 2003:360.

1078. Jackson MH, Hutchison WM. The prevalence and source of *Toxoplasma* infection in the environment. *Adv Parasitol* 1989; 28:55.

1079. Wong S-Y, Remington JS. Biology of *Toxoplasma gondii*. *AIDS* 1993;7:299.

1080. Kong J-T, Grigg ME, Uyetake L, et al. Serotyping of *Toxoplasma gondii* infections in humans using synthetic peptides. *J Infect Dis* 2003;187:1484.

1081. Montoya JG, Liesenfeld O. Toxoplasmosis. *Lancet* 2004;363:1965.

1082. Freij BJ, Sever JL. Toxoplasmosis. *Pediatr Rev* 1991;12:227.

1083. Sever JL, Ellenberg JH, Ley AC, et al. Toxoplasmosis: maternal and pediatric findings in 23,000 pregnancies. *Pediatrics* 1988;82:181.

1084. Jones JL, Kruson-Moran D, Wilson M, et al. *Toxoplasma gondii* infection in the United States: seroprevalence and risk factors. *Am J Epidemiol* 2001;154:357.

1085. Jones JL, Kruson-Moran D, Wilson M. *Toxoplasma gondii* infection in the United States, 1999–2000. *Emerg Infect Dis* 2003;9:1371.

1086. Roghmann MC, Faulkner CT, Lefkowitz A, et al. Decreased seroprevalence for *Toxoplasma gondii* in Seventh Day Adventists in Maryland. *Am J Trop Med Hyg* 1999;60:790.

1087. Falusi O, French AL, Seaberg EC, et al. Prevalence and predictors of *Toxoplasma* seropositivity in women with and at risk for human immunodeficiency virus infection. *Clin Infect Dis* 2002;35:1414.

1088. Couvreur J, Desmonts G. Toxoplasmosis. In: MacLeod CL, ed. *Parasitic infections in pregnancy and the newborn*. Oxford: Oxford University Press, 1988:112.

1089. Lappalainen M, Koskela P, Hedman K, et al. Incidence of primary *Toxoplasma* infections during pregnancy in Southern Finland: a prospective cohort study. *Scand J Infect Dis* 1992;24:97.

1090. Moor C, Stone P, Purdie G, et al. An investigation into the incidence of toxoplasmosis in pregnancy in New Zealand. *N Z Med J* 2000;113:29.

1091. Buffolano W, Gilbert RE, Holland FJ, et al. Risk factors for recent *Toxoplasma* infection in pregnant women in Naples. *Epidemiol Infect* 1996;116:347.

1092. Kapperud G, Jenum PA, Stray-Pedersen B, et al. Risk factors for *Toxoplasma gondii* in pregnancy: results of a prospective case-control study in Norway. *Am J Epidemiol* 1996;144:405.

1093. Cook AJC, Gilbert RE, Buffolano W, et al. Sources of *Toxoplasma* infection in pregnant women: European multicentre case-control study. *BMJ* 2000;321:142.

1094. Avelino MM, Campos D Jr, do Carmo Barbosa de Parada J, et al. Pregnancy as a risk factor for acute toxoplasmosis seroconversion. *Eur J Obstet Gynecol Reprod Biol* 2003;108:19.

1095. Wong S-Y, Remington JS. Toxoplasmosis in pregnancy. *Clin Infect Dis* 1994;18:853.

1096. Sayre MR, Jehle D. Elevated *Toxoplasma* IgG antibody in patients tested for infectious mononucleosis in an urban emergency department. *Ann Emerg Med* 1989;18:383.

1097. Katholm M, Johnsen NJ, Siim C, et al. Bilateral sudden deafness and acute acquired toxoplasmosis. *J Laryngol Otol* 1991;105:115.

1098. Evans TG, Schwartzman JD. Pulmonary toxoplasmosis. *Semin Respir Infect* 1991;6:51.

1099. Smith JR, Cunningham ET Jr. Atypical presentations of ocular toxoplasmosis. *Curr Opin Ophthalmol* 2002;13:387.

1100. Holland GN. Ocular toxoplasmosis: a global reassessment. Part II: disease manifestations and management. *Am J Ophthalmol* 2004;137:1.

1101. Lieb DF, Scott IU, Flynn HW Jr, et al. Acute acquired *Toxoplasma* retinitis may present similarly to unilateral acute idiopathic maculopathy. *Am J Ophthalmol* 2004;137:940.

1102. Holliman RE. Toxoplasmosis, behaviour and personality. *J Infect* 1997;35:105.

1103. Torrey EF, Yolken RH. *Toxoplasma gondii* and schizophrenia. *Emerg Infect Dis* 2003;9:1375.

1104. Rabaud C, May T, Amiel C, et al. Extracerebral toxoplasmosis in patients infected with HIV: a French national survey. *Medicine (Baltimore)* 1994;73:306.

1105. Hohlfeld P, Daffos F, Thulliez P, et al. Fetal toxoplasmosis: outcome of pregnancy and infant follow-up after *in utero* treatment. *J Pediatr* 1989;115:765.

1106. Ghidini A, Sirtori M, Spelta A, et al. Results of a preventive program for congenital toxoplasmosis. *J Reprod Med* 1991;36:270.

1107. Hafid J, Tran Manh Sung R, Raberin H, et al. Detection of circulating antigens of *Toxoplasma gondii* in human infection. *Am J Trop Med Hyg* 1995;52:336.

1108. Weiss JB. DNA probes and PCR for diagnosis of parasitic infections. *Clin Microbiol Rev* 1995;8:113.

1109. Dupon M, Cazenave J, Pellegrin J-L, et al. Detection of *Toxoplasma gondii* by PCR and tissue culture in cerebrospinal fluid and blood of human immunodeficiency virus-seropositive patients. *J Clin Microbiol* 1995;33:2421.

1110. Nguyen TD, de Kesel M, Bigaignon G, et al. Detection of *Toxoplasma gondii* tachyzoites and bradyzoites in blood, urine, and brains of infected mice. *Clin Diagn Lab Immunol* 1996;3:635.

1111. Montoya JG. Laboratory diagnosis of *Toxoplasma gondii* infection and toxoplasmosis. *J Infect Dis* 2002;185:S73.

1112. Buchbinder S, Blatz R, Rodloff AC. Comparison of real-time PCR detection methods for B1 and P30 genes of *Toxoplasma gondii*. *Diagn Microbiol Infect Dis* 2003;45:269.

1113. Remington JS, Thulliez P, Montoya JG. Recent developments for diagnosis of toxoplasmosis. *J Clin Microbiol* 2004;42:941.

1114. Hierl T, Reischl U, Lang P, et al. Preliminary evaluation of one conventional nested and two real-time PCR assays for the detection of *Toxoplasma gondii* in immunocompromised patients. *J Med Microbiol* 2004;53:629.

1115. Dao A, Azzouz N, Eloundou Nga C, et al. Unspecific reactivity of IgM directed against the low-molecular-weight antigen of *Toxoplasma gondii*. *Eur J Clin Microbiol Infect Dis* 2003;22:418.

1116. Gras L, Gilbert RE, Wallon M, et al. Duration of the IgM response in women acquiring *Toxoplasma gondii* during pregnancy: implications for clinical practice and cross-sectional incidence studies. *Epidemiol Infect* 2004;132:541.

1117. Huskinson J, Stepick-Biek PN, Araujo FG, et al. *Toxoplasma* antigens recognized by immunoglobulin G subclasses during acute and chronic infection. *J Clin Microbiol* 1989;27:2031.

1118. Beghetto E, Buffolano W, Spadoni A, et al. Use of an immunoglobulin G avidity assay based on recombinant antigens for diagnosis of primary *Toxoplasma gondii* infection during pregnancy. *J Clin Microbiol* 2003;41:5414.

1119. Jenum PA, Stray-Pedersen B, Gundersen A-G. Improved diagnosis of primary *Toxoplasma gondii* infection in early pregnancy by determination of antitoxoplasma immunoglobulin G avidity. *J Clin Microbiol* 1997;35:1972.

1120. Cozon GJN, Ferrandiz J, Nebhi H, et al. Estimation of the avidity of immunoglobulin G for routine diagnosis of chronic *Toxoplasma gondii* infection in pregnant women. *Eur J Clin Microbiol Infect Dis* 1998;17:32.

1121. Decoster A. Detection of IgA anti-P30 (SAG1) antibodies in acquired and congenital toxoplasmosis. *Curr Top Microbiol Immunol* 1996;219:199.

1122. Foudrinier F, Villena I, Jaussaud R, et al. Clinical value of specific immunoglobulin E detection by enzyme-linked immunosorbent assay in cases of acquired and congenital toxoplasmosis. *J Clin Microbiol* 2003;41:1681.

1123. Beazley DM, Egerman RS. Toxoplasmosis. *Semin Perinatol* 1998;22:332.

1124. Gross U, Keksel O, Dardé ML. Value of detecting immunoglobulin E antibodies for the serological diagnosis of *Toxoplasma gondii* infection. *Clin Diagn Lab Immunol* 1997;4:247.

1125. Liesenfeld O, Montoya JG, Tathineni NJ, et al. Confirmatory serologic testing for acute toxoplasmosis and rate of induced abortions among women reported to have positive *Toxoplasma* immunoglobulin M antibody titers. *Am J Obstet Gynecol* 2001;184:140.

1126. Haentjens M, Sacré L, Demeuter F. Congenital toxoplasmosis after maternal infection before or slightly after conception. *Acta Paediatr Scand* 1986;75:343.

1127. Pons JC, Sigrand C, Grangeot-Keros L, et al. Toxoplasmose congénitale: transmission au foetus d'une infection maternelle antéconceptionnelle. *Presse Med* 1995;24:179.

1128. Lynfield R, Eaton RB. Teratogen update: congenital toxoplasmosis. *Teratology* 1995;52:176.

1129. Abboud P, Harika G, Saniez D, et al. Signes échographiques de la foetopathie toxoplasmique: revue de la littérature. *J Gynecol Obstet Biol Reprod (Paris)* 1995;24:733.

1130. Gay-Andrieu F, Marty P, Pialat J, et al. Fetal toxoplasmosis and negative amniocentesis: necessity of an ultrasound follow-up. *Prenat Diagn* 2003;23:558.

1131. Villena I, Bory J-P, Chemla C, et al. Congenital toxoplasmosis: necessity of clinical and ultrasound follow-up despite negative amniocentesis. *Prenat Diagn* 2003;23:1098.

1132. Daffos F, Forestier F, Capella-Pavlovsky M, et al. Prenatal management of 746 pregnancies at risk for congenital toxoplasmosis. *N Engl J Med* 1988;318:271.

1133. Holliman RE, Johnson JD, Constantine G, et al. Difficulties in the diagnosis of congenital toxoplasmosis by cordocentesis: case report. *Br J Obstet Gynaecol* 1991;98:832.

1134. Fricker-Hidalgo H, Pelloux H, Muet F, et al. Prenatal diagnosis of congenital toxoplasmosis: comparative value of fetal blood and amniotic fluid using serological techniques and cultures. *Prenat Diagn* 1997;17:831.

1135. Decoster A, Darcy F, Caron A, et al. Anti-P30 IgA antibodies as prenatal markers for congenital *Toxoplasma* infection. *Clin Exp Immunol* 1992;87:310.

1136. Pratlong F, Boulot P, Villena I, et al. Antenatal diagnosis of congenital toxoplasmosis: evaluation of the biological parameters in a cohort of 286 patients. *Br J Obstet Gynaecol* 1996;103:552.

1137. Cotty F, Descamps P, Body G, et al. Prenatal diagnosis of congenital toxoplasmosis: the role of *Toxoplasma* IgA antibodies in amniotic fluid. *J Infect Dis* 1995;171:1384.

1138. Pinon JM, Toubas D, Marx C, et al. Detection of specific immunoglobulin E in patients with toxoplasmosis. *J Clin Microbiol* 1990;28:1739.

1139. Grover CM, Thulliez P, Remington JS, et al. Rapid prenatal diagnosis of congenital *Toxoplasma* infection by using polymerase chain reaction and amniotic fluid. *J Clin Microbiol* 1990; 28:2297.

1140. Cazenave J, Forestier F, Bessieres MH, et al. Contribution of a new PCR assay to the prenatal diagnosis of congenital toxoplasmosis. *Prenat Diagn* 1992;12:119.

1141. Dupouy-Camet J, Bougnoux ME, Lavareda de Souza S, et al. Comparative value of polymerase chain reaction and conventional biological tests for the prenatal diagnosis of congenital toxoplasmosis. *Ann Biol Clin (Paris)* 1992;50:315.

1142. Hohlfeld P, Daffos F, Costa J-M, et al. Prenatal diagnosis of congenital toxoplasmosis with a polymerase-chain-reaction test on amniotic fluid. *N Engl J Med* 1994;331:695.

1143. Li S, Ding Z, Liang Y, et al. A preliminary study on the antenatal diagnosis and prevention of the fetus toxoplasmosis infection. *Chung Hua Fu Chan Ko Tsa Chih* 1995;30:200.

1144. Knerer B, Hayde M, Gratz G, et al. Direkter Nachweis von *Toxoplasma gondii* mit Polymerase-Kettenreaktion zur Diagnostik einer fetalen *Toxoplasma*-Infektion. *Wien Klin Wochenschr* 1995;107:137.

1145. Antsaklis A, Daskalakis G, Papantoniou N, et al. Prenatal diagnosis of congenital toxoplasmosis. *Prenat Diagn* 2002;22:1107.

1146. Romand S, Chosson M, Franck J, et al. Usefulness of quantitative polymerase chain reaction in amniotic fluid as early prognostic marker of fetal infection with *Toxoplasma gondii*. *Am J Obstet Gynecol* 2004;190:797.

1147. Guy EC, Pelloux H, Lappalainen M, et al. Interlaboratory comparison of polymerase chain reaction for the detection of *Toxoplasma gondii* DNA added to samples of amniotic fluid. *Eur J Clin Microbiol Infect Dis* 1996;15:836.

1148. Couvreur J, Desmonts G, Thulliez P. Prophylaxis of congenital toxoplasmosis: effects of spiramycin on placental infection. *J Antimicrob Chemother* 1988;22(Suppl B):193.

1149. Gratzl R, Sodeck G, Platzer P, et al. Treatment of toxoplasmosis in pregnancy: concentrations of spiramycin and neospiramycin in maternal serum and amniotic fluid. *Eur J Clin Microbiol Infect Dis* 2002;21:12.

1150. St. Georgiev V. Management of toxoplasmosis. *Drugs* 1994; 48:179.

1151. Pajor A. Pancytopenia in a patient given pyrimethamine and sulphamethoxidiazine during pregnancy. *Arch Gynecol Obstet* 1990;247:215.

1152. Schoondermark-van de Ven E, Vree T, Melchers W, et al. In vitro effects of sulfadiazine and its metabolites alone and in combination with pyrimethamine on *Toxoplasma gondii*. *Antimicrob Agents Chemother* 1995;39:763.

1153. Peyron F, Wallon M, Liou C, et al. Treatments for toxoplasmosis in pregnancy. *Cochrane Database Syst Rev* 2000;(2):CD001684.

1154. European Multicentre Study on Congenital Toxoplasmosis. Effect of timing and type of treatment on the risk of mother to child transmission of *Toxoplasma gondii*. *BJOG* 2003;110:112.

1155. Foulon W, Naessens A, Derde MP. Evaluation of the possibilities for preventing congenital toxoplasmosis. *Am J Perinatol* 1994;11:57.

1156. Baril L, Ancelle T, Goulet V, et al. Risk factors for *Toxoplasma* infection in pregnancy: a case-control study in France. *Scand J Infect Dis* 1999;31:305.

1157. Jeannel D, Costagliola D, Niel G, et al. What is known about the prevention of congenital toxoplasmosis? *Lancet* 1990; 336:359.

1158. American College of Obstetricians and Gynecologists. Perinatal viral and parasitic infections: ACOG Technical bulletin number 177-February 1993. *Int J Gynaecol Obstet* 1993;42:300.

1159. Eskild A, Oxman A, Magnus P, et al. Screening for toxoplasmosis in pregnancy: what is the evidence of reducing a health problem? *J Med Screen* 1996;3:188.

1160. Bader TJ, Macones GA, Asch DA. Prenatal screening for toxoplasmosis. *Obstet Gynecol* 1997;90:457.

1161. Mittendorf R, Pryde P, Herschel M, et al. Is routine antenatal toxoplasmosis screening justified in the United States? Statistical considerations in the application of medical screening tests. *Clin Obstet Gynecol* 1999;42:163.

1162. Berrebi A, Kobuch WE, Bessieres MH, et al. Termination of pregnancy for maternal toxoplasmosis. *Lancet* 1994;344:36.

1163. Szénási Z, Ozsvár Z, Nagy E, et al. Prevention of congenital toxoplasmosis in Szeged, Hungary. *Int J Epidemiol* 1997;26:428.

1164. D'Ercole C, Boubli L, Franck J, et al. Recurrent congenital toxoplasmosis in a woman with lupus erythematosus. *Prenat Diagn* 1995;15:1171.

1165. Biedermann K, Flepp M, Fierz W, et al. Pregnancy, immunosuppression and reactivation of latent toxoplasmosis. *J Perinat Med* 1995;23:191.

1166. Gavinet MF, Robert F, Firtion G, et al. Congenital toxoplasmosis due to maternal reinfection during pregnancy. *J Clin Microbiol* 1997;35:1276.

1167. Silveira C, Ferreira R, Muccioli C, et al. Toxoplasmosis transmitted to a newborn from the mother infected 20 years earlier. *Am J Ophthalmol* 2003;136:370.

1168. Kodjikian L, Hoigne I, Adam O, et al. Vertical transmission of toxoplasmosis from a chronically infected immunocompetent woman. *Pediatr Infect Dis J* 2004;23:272.

1169. Peyron F, Ateba AB, Wallon M, et al. Congenital toxoplasmosis in twins: a report of fourteen consecutive cases and a comparison with published data. *Pediatr Infect Dis J* 2003;22:695.

1170. Guerina NG, Hsu H-W, Meissner HC, et al. Neonatal serologic screening and early treatment for congenital *Toxoplasma gondii* infection. *N Engl J Med* 1994;330:1858.

1171. Neto EC, Rubin R, Schulte J, et al. Newborn screening for congenital infectious diseases. *Emerg Infect Dis* 2004;10:1069.

1172. Patel DV, Holfels EM, Vogel NP, et al. Resolution of intracranial calcifications in infants with treated congenital toxoplasmosis. *Radiology* 1996;199:433.

1173. Wallon M, Caudie C, Rubio S, et al. Value of cerebrospinal fluid cytochemical examination for the diagnosis of congenital toxoplasmosis at birth in France. *Pediatr Infect Dis J* 1998;17:705.

1174. Taccone A, Fondelli MP, Ferrea G, et al. An unusual CT presentation of congenital cerebral toxoplasmosis in an 8-month-old boy with AIDS. *Pediatr Radiol* 1992;22:68.

1175. Virkola K, Lappalainen M, Valanne L, et al. Radiological signs in newborns exposed to primary *Toxoplasma* infection *in utero*. *Pediatr Radiol* 1997;27:133.

1176. de Jong PTVM. Ocular toxoplasmosis; common and rare symptoms and signs. *Int Ophthalmol* 1989;13:391.

1177. Brézin AP, Kasner L, Thulliez P, et al. Ocular toxoplasmosis in the fetus: immunohistochemistry analysis and DNA amplification. *Retina* 1994;14:19.

1178. Mets MB, Holfels E, Boyer KM, et al. Eye manifestations of congenital toxoplasmosis. *Am J Ophthalmol* 1996;122:309.

1179. Brady-McCreery KM, Hussein MAW, Paysse EA. Congenital toxoplasmosis with unusual retinal findings. *Arch Ophthalmol* 2003;121:1200.

1180. McGee T, Wolters C, Stein L, et al. Absence of sensorineural hearing loss in treated infants and children with congenital toxoplasmosis. *Otolaryngol Head Neck Surg* 1992;106:75.

1181. Glassman MS, Dellalzedah S, Beneck D, et al. Coincidence of congenital toxoplasmosis and biliary atresia in an infant. *J Pediatr Gastroenterol Nutr* 1991;13:298.

1182. Rajantie J, Siimes MA, Taskinen E, et al. White blood cells in infants with congenital toxoplasmosis: transient appearance of cALL antigen on reactive marrow lymphocytes. *Scand J Infect Dis* 1992;24:227.

1183. Hohlfeld P, Forestier F, Marion S, et al. *Toxoplasma gondii* infection during pregnancy: T lymphocyte subpopulations in mothers and fetuses. *Pediatr Infect Dis J* 1990;9:878.

1184. McLeod R, Mack DG, Boyer K, et al. Phenotypes and functions of lymphocytes in congenital toxoplasmosis. *J Lab Clin Med* 1990;116:623.

1185. Gross U, Müller J, Roos T, et al. Possible reasons for failure of conventional tests for diagnosis of fatal congenital toxoplasmosis: report of a case diagnosed by PCR and immunoblot. *Infection* 1992;20:149.

1186. Fuentes I, Rodriguez M, Domingo CJ, et al. Urine sample used for congenital toxoplasmosis diagnosis by PCR. *J Clin Microbiol* 1996;34:2368.

1187. Skinner LJ, Chatterton JMW, Joss AWL, et al. The use of an IgM immunosorbent agglutination assay to diagnose congenital toxoplasmosis. *J Med Microbiol* 1989;28:125.

1188. Gross U, Roos T, Appoldt D, et al. Improved serological diagnosis of *Toxoplasma gondii* infection by detection of immunoglobulin A (IgA) and IgM antibodies against P30 by using the immunoblot technique. *J Clin Microbiol* 1992;30:1436.

1189. Stepick-Biek P, Thulliez P, Araujo FG, et al. IgA antibodies for diagnosis of acute congenital and acquired toxoplasmosis. *J Infect Dis* 1990;162:270.

1190. Holliman RE, Raymond R, Renton N, et al. The diagnosis of toxoplasmosis using IgG avidity. *Epidemiol Infect* 1994;112:399.

1191. Chumpitazi BFF, Boussaid A, Pelloux H, et al. Diagnosis of congenital toxoplasmosis by immunoblotting and relationship with other methods. *J Clin Microbiol* 1995;33:1479.

1192. Tissot Dupont D, Fricker-Hidalgo H, Brenier-Pinchart MP, et al. Usefulness of Western blot in serological follow-up of newborns suspected of congenital toxoplasmosis. *Eur J Clin Microbiol Infect Dis* 2003;22:122.

1193. Rilling V, Dietz K, Krczal D, et al. Evaluation of a commercial IgG/IgM Western blot assay for early postnatal diagnosis of congenital toxoplasmosis. *Eur J Clin Microbiol Infect Dis* 2003;22:174.

1194. Flori P, Tardy L, Patural H, et al. Reliability of immunoglobulin G antitoxoplasma avidity test and effects of treatment on avidity indexes of infants and pregnant women. *Clin Diagn Lab Immunol* 2004;11:669.

1195. Wilson CB, Desmonts G, Couvreur J, et al. Lymphocyte transformation in the diagnosis of congenital *Toxoplasma* infection. *N Engl J Med* 1980;302:785.

1196. McAuley J, Boyer KM, Patel D, et al. Early and longitudinal evaluations of treated infants and children and untreated historical patients with congenital toxoplasmosis: the Chicago Collaborative Treatment Trial. *Clin Infect Dis* 1994;18:38.

1197. Lynfield R, Guerina NG. Toxoplasmosis. *Pediatr Rev* 1997;18:75.

1198. Wilson CB. Treatment of congenital toxoplasmosis. *Pediatr Infect Dis J* 1990;9:682.

1199. McLeod R, Mack D, Foss R, et al. Levels of pyrimethamine in sera and cerebrospinal and ventricular fluids from infants treated for congenital toxoplasmosis. *Antimicrob Agents Chemother* 1992;36:1040.

1200. Dutton GN. Recent developments in the prevention and treatment of congenital toxoplasmosis. *Int Ophthalmol* 1989;13:407.

1201. Wilson CB, Remington JS, Stagno S, et al. Development of adverse sequelae in children born with subclinical congenital *Toxoplasma* infection. *Pediatrics* 1980;66:767.

1202. Koppe JG, Loewer-Sieger DH, de Roever-Bonnet H. Results of 20-year follow-up of congenital toxoplasmosis. *Lancet* 1986;1:254.

1203. Koppe JG, Rothova A. Congenital toxoplasmosis: a long-term follow-up of 20 years. *Int Ophthalmol* 1989;13:387.

1204. Meenken C, Assies J, van Nieuwenhuizen O, et al. Long term ocular and neurological involvement in severe congenital toxoplasmosis. *Br J Ophthalmol* 1995;79:581.

1205. Brézin AP, Thulliez P, Couvreur J, et al. Ophthalmic outcomes after prenatal and postnatal treatment of congenital toxoplasmosis. *Am J Ophthalmol* 2003;135:779.

1206. Wallon M, Kodjikian L, Binquet C, et al. Long-term ocular prognosis in 327 children with congenital toxoplasmosis. *Pediatrics* 2004;113:1567.

1207. Roizen N, Swisher CN, Stein MA, et al. Neurologic and developmental outcome in treated congenital toxoplasmosis. *Pediatrics* 1995;95:11.

1208. Calisher CH, Sever JL. Are North American Bunyamwera serogroup viruses etiologic agents of human congenital defects of the central nervous system? *Emerg Infect Dis* 1995;1:147.

1209. Ekbom A, Daszak P, Kraaz W, et al. Crohn's disease after *in-utero* measles virus exposure. *Lancet* 1996;348:515.

1210. Ali ME, Albar HM. Measles in pregnancy: maternal morbidity and perinatal outcome. *Int J Gynaecol Obstet* 1997;59:109.

1211. Nakata Y, Nakayama T, Ide Y, et al. Measles virus genome detected up to four months in a case of congenital measles. *Acta Paediatr* 2002;91:1263.

1212. Holowach J, Thurston DL, Becker B. Congenital defects in infants following mumps during pregnancy: a review of the literature and a report of chorioretinitis due to fetal infection. *J Pediatr* 1957;50:689.

1213. Jones JF, Ray CG, Fulginiti VA. Perinatal mumps infection. *J Pediatr* 1980;96:912.

1214. Lyen KR, Lingam S, Butterfill AM, et al. Multicystic encephalomalacia due to fetal viral encephalitis. *Eur J Pediatr* 1981;137:11.

1215. Baumann B, Danon L, Weitz R, et al. Unilateral hydrocephalus due to obstruction of the foramen of Monro: another complication of intrauterine mumps infection? *Eur J Pediatr* 1982;139:158.

1216. Groenendaal F, Rothbarth PH, van den Anker JN, et al. Congenital mumps pneumonia: a rare cause of neonatal respiratory distress. *Acta Paediatr Scand* 1990;79:1252.

1217. Lacour M, Maherzi M, Vienny H, et al. Thrombocytopenia in a case of neonatal mumps infection: evidence for further clinical presentations. *Eur J Pediatr* 1993;152:739.

1218. Tang C-K, Shermeta DW, Wood C. Congenital condylomata acuminata. *Am J Obstet Gynecol* 1978;131:912.

1219. Mounts P, Shah KV. Respiratory papillomatosis: etiological relation to genital tract papillomaviruses. *Prog Med Virol* 1984;29:90.

1220. Freij BJ, Sever JL. Papilloma virus, congenital infection. In: Buyse ML, ed. *Birth defects encyclopedia*. Boston: Blackwell Scientific, 1990:1361.

1221. Suarez VR, Hankins GDV. Smallpox and pregnancy: from eradicated disease to bioterrorist threat. *Obstet Gynecol* 2002;100:87.

1222. Centers for Disease Control and Prevention. Smallpox vaccination and adverse reactions: guidance for clinicians. *MMWR Dispatch* 2003;52(Jan 24):20.

1223. Hulbert TV. Congenital malaria in the United States: report of a case and review. *Clin Infect Dis* 1992;14:922.

1224. Cot M, Deloron P. Malaria prevention strategies. *Br Med Bull* 2003;67:137.

1225. Reinhardt MC. Malaria, trypanosomiasis and Chagas' disease in pregnancy. *J Trop Pediatr* 1980;26:213.

1226. Olowe SA. A case of congenital trypanosomiasis in Lagos. *Trans R Soc Trop Med Hyg* 1975;69:57.

1227. Bittencourt AL. Congenital Chagas disease. *Am J Dis Child* 1976;130:97.

Healthcare-Associated Infections

Jukka K. Korpela   Joyce Campbell   Nalini Singh

Like birth itself, survival of the premature newborn is a miracle. The improved survival of the very low birth weight neonate is possible due to advancement in neonatal intensive care. However, this high-risk population of neonates is also at-risk of nosocomial, or healthcare-associated infections due to invasive monitoring and supportive care (1–6).

The impact of this adverse event is estimated to affect 2 million patients each year in the United States, contributing to 90,000 deaths and adding \$4.5 to \$ 5.7 billion per year to the costs of patient care in the United States (7,8). Twenty five percent of healthcare-associated infections occur in intensive care units, and 70% of these infections are caused by resistant strains of bacteria (9,10). Neonates and young children are among the hospitalized patients at highest risk for acquiring healthcare-associated infections. Infants <1500 g experience a disproportionate share of healthcare-associated infections (~75%) compared to other newborns in the neonatal intensive care unit (NICU) (11). Thus, infection control is a crucial component of patient safety and optimal survival of the newborns hospitalized in the NICU. In this chapter we are attempting to outline the epidemiology of major healthcare-associated infections, the emerging problem of multi-drug resistance organisms, and evidence-based infection control efforts.

EPIDEMIOLOGY

The epidemiology of healthcare-associated infections among neonates in NICUs has been described from the National Nosocomial Infection Surveillance (NNIS) system of the Centers for Disease Control and Prevention (CDC) from January 1992 to June 2004 (12). Device-associated bloodstream infections, followed by ventilator-associated pneumonia, are the most common healthcare-associated infections in the NICU. These infection rates increase with decrease in birth weight and age (13–16). Reports published by the CDC-NNIS provide information on pooled means and percentiles of the distribution of device-associated infection rates by birth weight category and device utilization ratios (Tables 49-1 and 49-2) (12). Pediatric Prevention Network's point prevalence study of NICUs also reports frequency of other infections in the lower respiratory tract (12.9%), urinary tract (8.6%), and ear–nose–throat (8.6%) (11). NICU surveillance is conducted in various methodologies including reporting of site-specific rates by birth weight in the United States (17). The frequency of healthcare-associated infections in individual NICUs varies from 6% to 25% in the United States and 8% to 10% in Europe based upon multicenter studies data (18–22).

In a multicenter study from National Institutes of Child Health and Human Development (NICHD) Neonatal Research Network of 5447 patients, the increased use of intrapartum antimicrobial therapy, for prevention of group B streptococcal disease, was associated with a decrease in the incidence of early-onset (<3 days) group B Streptococcal sepsis (from 5.9 to 1.7 per 1000 live births) but was associated with a proportionate increase in sepsis with ampicillin-resistant *Escherichia coli* isolates (from 3.2 to 6.8 per 1000 live births) (23). In high-risk infants there may also be an increase in the incidence of healthcare-associated infections due to multi-drug resistant gram-negative organisms. This increase in gram negative organisms has been seen in many national and international centers (24–34).

Identifying neonates who are at greatest risk of developing nosocomial sepsis can be complex, but is important so that prompt, accurate diagnosis can be made, appropriate management modalities can be instituted and unnecessary use of broad-spectrum antimicrobial agents can be avoided. Various scoring systems have been developed in an attempt to provide objective criteria to diagnose

TABLE 49-1

MEDIAN NICU BSI AND VAP NI RATES AMONG ALL BIRTH-WEIGHT GROUPS IN PEDIATRIC PREVENTION NETWORK, 1997

Population Survey	Median
All patients NI/1000 patient-days	8.9
BSI/1000 CVC-days	8.6
VAP/1000 ventilator-days	2.5

NICU—Neonatal Intensive Care Unit
BSI—bloodstream infection
VAP—Ventilator associated pneumonia
NI—Nosocomial infection
CVC—Central venous catheter

nosocomial sepsis. Recently, the Nosocomial Sepsis Prediction score for neonates (NOSEP) attempts to do this, based on clinical and laboratory parameters. This model has been validated in five regional NICUs in Europe (35). The NOSEP-NEW- II score includes: (a) body temperature >38.1°C, (b) C-reactive protein ≥30 mg/L, thrombocytopenia, ≤190 × 10^9, and neutrophil fraction >63%, and (c) total parenteral nutrition, ≥15 days. The incorporation of additional factors in this score such as surgery, maternal hypertension, and ventilation at the time of sepsis work up, increased the discriminative performance (A$_z$ of receiver operating characteristic curve from 0.71 to 0.82). The NOSEP-NEW-II score (range 0–19 points) was significantly higher in patients with healthcare associated sepsis (median, 9) than with patients without sepsis (median, 6), $p = 0.008$. The calibration curve of the NOSEP score shows a very good correlation between predicted risk and observed prevalence of nosocomial sepsis (Spearman's

TABLE 49-2

NICU BSI AND VAP NI RATES STRATIFIED BY BIRTH-WEIGHT GROUPS PER 1000 DEVICE DAYS, PEDIATRIC PREVENTION NETWORK (PPN), 1997 AND NATIONAL NOSOCOMIAL INFECTION SURVEILLANCE SYSTEM (NNIS) (2002–2004)

Population Survey		PPN Median	NNIS Median
BSI	<1000 grams	12.8	9.1
BSI	1001–1500 grams	8.9	5.4
BSI	1501–2500 grams	4.7	4.1
BSI	>2500 grams	4.4	3.5
VAP	<1000 grams	3.5	3.5
VAP	1001–1500 grams	4.9	2.4
VAP	1501–2500 grams	1.1	1.9
VAP	>2500 grams	0.9	1.4

BSI—bloodstream infection
VAP—Ventilator associated pneumonia

correlation coefficient $p < .005$). No discrepancy was seen between the predicted and observed outcomes (Hosmer-Lemeshow goodness-of-fit chi square $p = .48$). There was also very good uniformity of fit (similar fit across different strata). A model to predict a future event such as the risk of developing a healthcare associated infection should incorporate both intrinsic and extrinsic risk factors as was done in the pediatric nosocomial infection risk model (36). Limiting factors of these models are applicability differences in case-mix, the diversity of the patient population with varying risk factors (e.g., access to care) and availability to limited laboratory resources developing countries (37).

HEALTHCARE-ASSOCIATED INFECTION RATE

Surveillance of healthcare-associated infection rates is used to evaluate the infection trends in NICUs and to compare different patient populations. These rates are the basic statistical tools for infection control. A comprehensive infection surveillance, prevention, and control program can be a part of the performance-improvement program in the hospital and annual planning for strategies to meet specific hospital needs and priorities (38). Many of the difficulties in comparing intra-hospital and inter-hospital rates can be decreased using standardized definitions and taking risk factors into account (15).

The CDC-NNIS System defines a nosocomial infection as a localized or systemic condition (1) that results from an adverse reaction to the presence of an infectious agent(s) or its toxin(s) and (2) that was not present or incubating at the time of admission to the hospital (39). For determination of the presence and classification of healthcare-associated infections, a combination of clinical findings and results of laboratory tests should be used. These definitions have been developed by CDC to provide uniform criteria to compare infections within hospitals and between different data systems. For infections in infants and neonates, whose clinical manifestations differ from those in older persons, specific criteria are used. These criteria are used according to the listing of major and specific site codes and descriptions. For example laboratory-confirmed primary bloodstream infection in infants or neonates must meet at least one of the following criteria:

1. Patient has a recognized pathogen cultured from one or more blood cultures and the organism cultured from the blood is not related to an infection at another site.

2. Patient ≤1 year of age has at least one of the following signs and symptoms: fever (>38° C), apnea, or bradycardia and at least one of the following:

    (a) common skin contaminant (e.g., diphtheroids, Bacillus species, Propionicbacterium species, coagulase negative staphylococci, or micrococci) cultured from two or more blood cultures drawn on separate occasions

(b) common skin contaminant (e.g., diphtheroids, Bacillus species, Propiobacterum species, coagulase-negative staphylococci—CONS, or micrococci) cultured from at least one blood culture from a patient with an intravascular line, and the physician institutes appropriate antimicrobial therapy

(c) positive antigen test on blood (e.g., *Haemophilus influenzae, Streptococcus pneumoniae, Neisseria meningitidis,* or *group B Streptococcus*) and signs and symptoms and positive laboratory results are not related to an infection at another site.

The evaluations and comparisons of healthcare-associated NICU sepsis caused by CONS have failed partly due to the lack of uniformity in the definition of sepsis (40). Recently using mathematical modeling, the predictive value of a single and two positive blood cultures for CONS was estimated to be 55% and 98% respectively (41). From a surveillance point of view, this may require improving current CDC definitions as follows:

1. Criterion 2 (a) for two positive culture results, should not require clinical signs or symptoms because their diagnostic value is unknown and the positive predictive value when ≥2 cultures are positive is high.
2. Criterion 2 (b) should exclude single positive blood cultures where ≥2 cultures are performed.
3. The definition should account for whether culture was obtained through a central line or a peripheral vein.

Findings from this mathematical modeling are also consistent with recommendations from the Vermont Oxford Neonatal National Evidence-based Quality improvement collaborative for Neonatology (42).

The accuracy of reporting healthcare-associated infections data also varies according to the type of infection (43). In nine participating NNIS hospital intensive-care units, the CDC epidemiologists determined the reported bloodstream infections, pneumonias, surgical-site infections and urinary tract infections. Primary bloodstream infection was the most accurately identified with sensitivity of 85% and specificity of 98.3%, in comparison to the other infections, pneumonia, surgical-site infection and urinary tract infection with a sensitivity of 68%, 67%, and 59% and specificity of 97.8%, 97.7%, and 98.7% respectively. When these CDC-NNIS hospitals reported a healthcare-associated infection, the infection most likely was a true infection.

The CDC-NNIS System collects data from infection control professionals on nosocomial infections in NICU patients. All body sites are included in this data. Site-specific infection rates can be calculated by using as a denominator the number of patients at risk or patient-days, and/or device days (umbilical catheter/central line or ventilator use) for each of the four birth-weight categories (≤1000 g, 1001 to 1500 g, 1501 to 2500 g, and >2500 g) (12). Birth weight specific rates of bloodstream infection

and ventilator-associated pneumonia are shown in Tables 49-1 and 49-2. The incidence of bloodstream infections and ventilator-associated pneumonia is inversely proportional to the birth weight. Birth weight can also be a marker of severity of illness and a predictor of mortality in very low birth weight infants (44).

The device utilization days are widely used in calculating risk-adjusted infection rates in NICU. Device utilization is calculated as follows: Number of umbilical and central line-associated bloodstream infections per number of umbilical and central-line days multiplied by 1000. Another useful measure of device use in a NICU is the device utilization ratio (12). This is calculated as number of device-days per number of patient-days. Device utilization stratified by birth weight group and device utilization ratio are essential for valid inter-hospital NI rate comparisons (17). Increase in device utilization can reflect either higher severity of illness in infants requiring increased use of invasive devices or healthcare provider's patient care practice. Under these circumstances targeted efforts to decrease infection rates may require efforts to decrease use of devices. CDC-NNIS rates can serve as an external benchmark and NICUs can be compared using the percentiles of site-specific infection rate and device utilization ratios. If the infection rates are above the 90th percentile, it may indicate a problem in the infection control or higher severity of illness in patients requiring more device use. If they are below 10th percentile, it may reflect of underreporting of infections or infrequent or/and short duration of device days (12).

The effect of infection control interventions for a NICU should be evaluated at least annually using a risk-adjusted healthcare-associated infection rate. Risk should be adjusted for device use such as central venous catheters and birth weight category (45). Overall impact of an infection control program can be easily estimated within the hospital over a period of time (38). Continuous quality control improvement processes by multidisciplinary teams in a NICU can be evaluated using bloodstream infections rates over the time period in focus (46). Reduction of infection rates will encourage the efforts and show the right direction of control measures.

Many risk factors are not accounted for in the CDC-NNIS High-Risk Nursery surveillance components (47–49). Besides birth weight and use of invasive devices, length of stay in NICU and severity of the co-morbidities and use of total parentral nutrition may contribute to increased incidence of healthcare-associated infections (50,51). Use of dexamethasone and neonatal neutropenia and maternal hypertension should also be considered important risk factors under specific maternal conditions (52,53). High-risk infants acquire nosocomial pathogens either endogenously or exogenously. Exogenously parents can also serve as a vector for transmission of organisms like Pseudomonas aeruginosa and Staphylococcus aureus (54). This vertical and horizontal transmission of microorganisms can be confirmed by use of molecular epidemiological tools (55).

LATE-ONSET SEPSIS

The frequency of healthcare-associated or late-onset sepsis varies from 11% to 30% (56). The number of sepsis episodes increases with decreasing birth weight. Intercenter variability is also seen in the incidence of late onset sepsis in multi-institutional studies (6,57,58). CONS are the most common pathogens responsible for late-onset nosocomial sepsis in the NICU (6). It is still difficult to determine which blood culture isolates of CONS reflect true infections and which are contaminants. CONS are part of the patient's endogenous flora. Oral mucosa and/or skin are colonized with CONS (59). The NICHD Neonatal Research Network reports that Gram-positive organisms specifically CONS were the most common pathogens causing late-onset (>3 days) bloodstream infections in neonates. CONS was isolated from 43.4% of cases with late onset sepsis in very low birth weight infants in the NICHD Neonatal Research Network and 54% in Pediatric Prevention Network (6,60). In a prospective NICU incidence study CONS bacteremia are reported to be 12.4 per 1000 device days (61). Infants with late-onset sepsis have significantly increased length of stay in the hospital (79 days vs 60 days; $p < .001$) and mortality (18% vs 7%; $< .001$) (6). CONS infections usually present between 7 and 14 days of age (62). It is not a significant cause of mortality (less than 1%) (63).

Prolonged hospital stay and complications with prematurity, such as patent ductus arteriosus, prolonged ventilation, prolonged use of intravascular access, bronchopulmonary dysplasia and necrotizing enterocolitis are associated with an increased rate of late-onset sepsis (6). Persistent infections with CONS occur in significantly smaller and less mature infants than with non-CONS, but generally mortality is not higher. Infants with persistent infection should undergo aggressive evaluation for focal complications (64). Primary osteomyelitis and suppurative arthritis with CONS in preterm neonates have been also described in the absence of any indwelling central catheters (65). Most CONS isolates causing sepsis are frequently predominantly antibiotic resistant CONS types (66).

The role of CONS as causative pathogens or contaminants in cultures from blood and cerebrospinal fluid is difficult to determine (67). Procedures to help to differentiate CONS positive blood cultures from CONS contaminants include drawing of at least two blood cultures, using optimal skin antisepsis and catheter disinfection before drawing blood samples, and using adjunctive tests, such as IL-6 and CRP (42,60,68). CONS are the predominant organism, consisting of 44% versus approximately 25% of various Gram-negative bacteria in randomly collected environmental samples in NICU (3). The possible increase of CONS infections after twice-daily petrolatum ointment application indicates that routine ointment practices may colonize skin. Thus ointment routines remain controversial, especially in babies with intact skin (69).

Another cause for possible therapeutic failures in the NICU, is the emergence of vancomycin heteroresistant *Staphylococcus capitis* strains (70). Occurrences of endemic strains require careful evaluation of existing treatment regimens and therapeutic responses. Heteroresistance to vancomycin should be suspected in a NICU where CONS positive bloodstream infections treated with vancomycin and appropriate replacement of intravenous catheters fail to respond to treatment. There is an urgent need for evaluation of clinical practice guidelines for safely decreasing vancomycin use in NICUs (60).

In a recent CDC-NNIS surveillance report 89% of CONS were resistant to methicillin (12). Resistant Staphylococcus epidermidis clones to penicillin, gentamicin and erythromycin with the mecA gene can be significant nosocomial pathogens that can be transmitted between babies in the NICU (71). Usually predominant antibiotic resistant CONS types are detectable in neonates and staff of neonatal units, suggesting cross-contamination (66).

A recent study by NICHD Neonatal Research Network revealed that only one-third of patients with late-onset meningitis had meningitis in the absence of sepsis. Cerebrospinal fluid cultures were performed only half as often as blood cultures, suggesting that meningitis may be under-diagnosed among very low birth weight infants. CONS was recovered from 29% of cases when meningitis occurred (72,77).

Enterococci have also been recognized as clinically important pathogens in high-risk, hospitalized children (73–77). Neonatal nosocomial enterococcal infections are being recognized with increased frequency (78–85). The Pediatric Prevention Network's point prevalence study of NICUs also reports enterococci as the second most frequent (15%) nosocomial pathogen among neonates admitted to the NICU in 1999 and third most common (7.8%) in NICHD Neonatal Research Network studies (11). Most of these were bloodstream infections, but enterococci were isolated in 13.4% of cases with meningitis in NICHD Neonatal Research network studies (86). Enterococci are indigenous to the normal flora in humans and are known to colonize the intestines, gastrointestinal tract, and female genital tract. There are two major species of Enterococci that infect humans, *Enterococcus faecalis* (*E. faecalis*) and *Enterococcus faecium* (*E. faecium*). During the 1980s, *E. faecalis* was responsible for 80% to 90% of all isolates and *E. faecium* had accounted for only 5% to 15% (87).

In one case controlled study risk factors for nosocomial enterococcal infection in neonates are non-umbilical central lines (71% vs 32%), duration of indwelling central lines (26.5 vs 6.5 days), and bowel resection (29% vs 4%) (83). The mean gestational age was 27 weeks and the mean birth weight was 913 grams. Similarly, risk factors in another case-control study of young children also showed that central line and bowel resection are important risk factors, as well as duration of antimicrobial therapy (median duration of use was approximately one week) (88). A mortality of 14 to

17.6% and an attributable mortality of 8.0% were observed with enterococcal bacteremia patients (73,78). To prevent occurrence of nosocomial enterococcal infections, clinicians should carefully monitor the use and duration of antimicrobial agents. Rational delivery of antimicrobial therapy is critical, especially during an era of increasing rates of antimicrobial resistance in enterococci.

Gram-Negative Sepsis

With a significant improvement in the survival of premature and very low birth weight infants, increased incidence of Gram-negative healthcare-associated sepsis is seen in these infants (6,25). The increasing incidence of Gram-negative rods bacteremia has been reported by many NICUs (26,89). The NICHD Research network reported that although Gram-positive organisms caused the majority of late-onset (>3 days) sepsis in very low birth weight neonates (<1500 grams), mortality was highest with Gram-negative sepsis (6). Increase in mortality to 36% and a fulminant clinical course has been reported in these very low birth weight hospitalized infants (6,63,90). Epidemics of multi drug-resistant *Klebsiella pneumoniae* and acinetobacter sepsis have been reported in some nurseries (91–93). Environmental sources, such as cots, incubators and various equipments yield growth of several pathogens, bacteria and fungi. The presence of Gram-negative pathogens, such as *Pseudomonas aeruginosa* and *Serratia marcescens*, varies in different environments and poses a potential threat for infection. In an era of increasing incidence of antimicrobial resistance, the empiric treatment of clinical sepsis in high-risk neonates, should include adequate antimicrobial coverage for resistant Gram-negative rods.

Enterobacter sakazakii has also been reported as a rare cause of invasive infection with high mortality rates in neonates (94). These neonates can present with intestinal colonization, or more invasive disease such as sepsis and meningitis with cerebral infarction (95–97). *E. sakazakii* has neurotropic qualities and should be considered as a part of differential diagnosis of central nervous system abscess and/or infarction along with citrobacter diversus (98–100). Outbreaks of necrotizing enterocolitis have been seen in premature infants (101). This infection has been reported with ingestion of contaminated commercial formula in healthcare settings (102–105). Infection with *E. sakazakii* has also been reported with the use of contaminated spoons or blenders and with ready-made formula kept warm in bottle heaters (106,107). Powdered milk is not sterile and can contain low numbers of *E. sakazakii*. Formula made from powder should be prepared daily and kept in the refrigerator no longer than 30 hours.

Fungal Sepsis

Candida species are the third most common cause of late onset sepsis in NICU patients, affecting approximately

20% of babies weighing <1000 grams (25,108–111). The crude mortality for candidemia has been reported to vary between 15 and 50% (6,86,108). Although Gram-positive organisms caused the majority of late-onset sepsis (>3 days) in very low birth weight neonates (<1500 grams), mortality was highest with Gram-negative and fungal sepsis (6,86). In this multicenter study of 6215 patients, very low birth weight infants were more likely to die if they had infection with fungi (32%; odds ratio fungi vs other organisms 2, $p < .01$).

Prior colonization of body sites (gastrointestinal tract, skin, respiratory tract) is an important risk factor for invasive disease (112,113). The gastrointestinal tract appears to be the earliest, most common site of colonization (108,114). Approximately one-half of very low birth weight infants colonized with $>8 \times 10^6$ colony-forming units of candida species in their gastrointestinal tract developed feeding intolerance and/or bloody stools; 29% of these infants developed candidemia. Colonization of the gastrointestinal tract in NICU patients has been associated with the use of antibiotics, particularly third generation cephalosporins, central catheters, intravenous lipids and H_2 blockers (108). Invasive candida infection in preterm infants has been attributed to intrinsic factors, such as the immaturity of their immune system, increased permeability of skin and mucosal barriers, delayed enteral feedings and extrinsic factors, such as the prolonged use of antimicrobials, mechanical ventilation, parenteral nutrition, and central vascular access (108,115–119). Necrotizing enterocolitis, gastrointestinal tract, respiratory tract or skin colonization of neonates with candida species have also been associated with invasive disease (113,115,120,121). Loss of normal gastrointestinal tract flora secondary to antimicrobial treatment and delayed enteral feedings may facilitate candida species colonization, while skin colonization may occur through horizontal transmission from the hands of health care workers not used again (119,122).

Skin colonization of neonates with candida species, particularly *Candida parapsilosis*, has been shown to occur by horizontal transmission (from person to person) through the hands of health care workers (123–125). Use of molecular typing methods has confirmed horizontal transmission of *Candida parapsilosis candidemia* (122).

Empiric antifungal therapy for at-risk very low birth weight neonates has been proposed based on the clinical predictive model with a sensitivity of 85% and a specificity of 47% (126). In this multicenter study, investigators propose empiric antifungal treatment if neonates are <25 weeks gestational age, have thrombocytopenia or have a history of third-generation cephalosporins or carbapenem exposure in the past 7 days, at the time of obtaining blood culture.

Malasezzia furfur is lipid-dependent yeast that can cause colonization and also systemic infections in neonates (127–129). It is usually seen in neonates receiving intravenous lipid emulsions. Eighty percent of neonates

<1000 grams have been reported to colonize their skin in comparison with 4% of neonates >2000 grams. It appears that 51% of very low birth weight neonates are colonized with *Malasezzia furfur* by two weeks of age (130). Colonization, however, does not predict infection and the predictive value of surveillance cultures is poor (127,130). Peripheral thromboembolism associated with *M. furfur* has been reported in a premature infant (131). Consideration should be given to detection of this liphophilic yeast when neonates receiving intralipids develops signs of catheter related sepsis. The yeasts usually grow slowly in blood culture media but readily when subcultured onto Sabouraud's medium coated with sterile olive oil (129).

VENTILATOR-ASSOCIATED PNEUMONIA

Critically ill, premature neonates in NICUs require ventilator support. The care of these hospitalized neonates contributes to increased rates of ventilator-associated pneumonia (11,13,15,17). Diagnosis of ventilator-associated pneumonia, however, is difficult in neonates with bronchopulmonary dysplasia due to underlying radiographic changes (132). A positive blood culture along with radiographic changes makes diagnosis of ventilator-associated pneumonia with greater specificity and sensitivity (39, 133). The rate of ventilator-associated pneumonia disproportionately affects very low birth weight neonates (Table 49-2) (134). In pediatric intensive care units, ventilator associated pneumonia is also the second most common nosocomial infection and *P. aeruginosa* is the most common cause of these infections, accounting for 22% of the cases (14).

Airway colonization of in-patients begins within 3 days to two weeks of the start of mechanical ventilation and may be due to either endogenous or exogenous organisms. In young children bacterial colonization and infection occurs more frequently in patients ventilated through a tracheotomy. During endotracheal ventilation, lower airway colonization occurs after two weeks of mechanical ventilation (135). Very low birth weight infants are at-risk of airway colonization with Gram-negative bacilli and also bloodstream infections (132,136). Airway colonization with Gram-negative rods may also be associated with severity of brochopulmonary dysplasia (137). Systemic antimicrobial treatment does not eradicate Gram-negative rod airway colonization. This may be in part, to the presence of foreign bodies (tracheal or endotracheal tube), low levels of antimicrobial concentration in respiratory secretions, or translocation of bacteria from the gastrointestinal tract (138). Topical antibiotic combinations of polymyxin E and tobramycin in a 2% paste applied four times a day to the tracheostoma in young children (median age 4 months) were found to be effective in reducing the exogenous route of colonization of the lower respiratory tract (139). High case-fatality rates (30–50%) with *P. aeruginosa* invasive infections has been seen in patients with compromised host defenses and in very low birth weight infants (140,141). Of note, tracheal culture can be negative preceding invasive infections. Ventilator-associated pneumonia is usually present when tracheal culture and blood culture simultaneously grow *P. aeruginosa*. In a retrospective study of 1571 very low birth weight infants, 751 patients were on a ventilator for longer than a week. *P. aeruginosa* colonization occurred in 33 patients and of these, 15 patients also developed bloodstream infections. Thirteen of the 15 infants with bloodstream infections and none of the 33 with tracheal colonization died within two days of positive culture (134).

Care processes in ventilated neonates vary and account for the different rates of ventilator-associated pneumonia. Most neonates are subject to frequent suctioning to maintain patent airways that can easily be blocked by excessive bronchial secretions. There has been increased use of closed endotracheal suctioning systems that permit continuous ventilation of patients instead of open systems that require disconnection from ventilators. In adults, closed endotracheal suctioning systems are associated with increased rates of bacterial colonization without an increased incidence of nosocomial pneumonia (142). Closed endotracheal suctioning systems have a theoretical advantage for use due to fewer physiologic disturbances and suction-induced complications (143). An outbreak of a healthcare–associated acute Gram-negative rod pneumonia suggestive of *P. aeruginosa* on autopsy was seen in one NICU concomitant with the increase use of closed endotracheal suctioning systems with a mortality rate of 33% (10/30) in patients (144). It is possible the catheters of closed endotracheal suctioning systems were not changed every 24 hours in this outbreak, as is recommended. This report differs from that of Cordero et al., who failed to show increased colonization and nosocomial *P. aeruginosa* pneumonia and bloodstream infections among patients undergoing closed endotracheal suctioning systems (145). Guidelines for prevention for nosocomial pneumonia has been recently published (146).

P. aeruginosa is also ubiquitous in the hospital environment and is found on moist surfaces such as sinks, toilets, floor mops and respiratory equipment (141,147,148). Environmental reservoirs have been implicated as sources of transmission of *P. aeruginosa* to patients in NICUs via the use of hand lotion and on contaminated fingernails of health care workers (147,149). Warm tub bath during a term labor was associated with neonatal *P. aeruginosa* meningitis and bacteremia in an 11-day-old neonate in Germany. Genotyping revealed clonal similarity between the blood culture isolate and the shower tubing used to clean the bathtub (150).

URINARY TRACT INFECTIONS

Healthcare-associated urinary tract infection in the neonate continues to be a source of morbidity and prolonged hospital stay. Prevalence of urinary tract infection in the hospitalized neonate ranges from 4 to 25% (151). While the prevalence of urinary tract infections in non-hospitalized infants was only 0.1 to 1% (152). These studies demonstrated that prematurity, low birth weight and male gender contributed to increased risk for urinary tract infection in the hospitalized neonate. With improved survival of low birth weight infants, increased risk of urinary tract infection may also be seen in neonates <1000 grams (153). Incidence of vesicourethral reflux is also low in very low birth weight infants (154). In earlier studies neonatal urinary tract infection often occurred in association with sepsis (151). The exact mechanism of urinary tract infection in the very low birth weight is unknown, as they usually do not have in-dwelling catheters.

INFECTIONS DUE TO MULTI-DRUG RESISTANT ORGANISMS

Multi-drug resistant organisms such as methicillin resistant *Staphylococcus aureus* (MRSA), vancomycin-resistant enterococcus (VRE), and antimicrobial-resistant *Enterobacteriaceae* have emerged as major causes of healthcare-associated infections. According to the CDC-NNIS, recent analysis shows a continuing increase in the incidence of multi-drug resistant organisms in intensive care units in hospitals in the United States. As of 2004, almost 28.5% of enterococcal isolates were VRE, 59% of *Staphylococcus aureus* isolates were MRSA, and 89% of CONS were resistant to methicillin (12). The increase is continuing despite the implementation of standard infection control measures. There are no specific resistance rates for neonates and young children admitted to intensive care units. Clinical manifestations of healthcare-associated infections with multi-drug resistant organisms or susceptible organisms are indistinguishable, which makes it more challenging to diagnose these infections and treat them promptly. The next section discusses the historical perspective of specific multi-drug resistant organisms, epidemiology and interventions.

Methicillin-Resistant *Staphylococcus aureus*

MRSA is an important nosocomial pathogen. It was first reported in the United Kingdom in the 1960s, and in the United States in 1968. In 2004, 59% of *Staphylococcus aureus* isolates causing nosocomial infections among patients hospitalized in intensive care units reporting to the CDC-NNIS System were resistant to methicillin (12). This represented an 11% increase over the average percent of *Staphylococcus aureus* isolates that were resistant to methicillin during the four years from 1998 to 2002. However, a low prevalence of MRSA in NICUs (<3%) was demonstrated in a point prevalence survey conducted by the Pediatric Prevention Network (155). MRSA can cause a high morbidity and mortality in high-risk infants.

Severity of MRSA outbreaks in neonates varies in non-invasive and invasive disease. Some neonates may be colonized, others may acquire superficial infections, such as conjunctivitis and impetigo with high attack rates, but only a few of these patients develop invasive infections(156,157). Others may present with severe, invasive disease, such as bacteremia and meningitis (158–162). An outbreak of MRSA transmitted from a mother to 3 of her preterm quadruplet infants postnatally has been reported (163). Nasal cultures from three of the quadruplets and 2 additional unrelated infants grew the same clone of MRSA. The mother's only identified risk factors for MRSA acquisition were (1) prepartum hospitalizations related to multiple gestation and (2) treatment with ampicillin and erythromycin one week before delivery for ruptured membranes.

Healthcare-associated transmission of community acquired-MRSA infections was also documented in post-partum women in the same NICU (164). The major mode of transmission of MRSA in hospitals is by spread from one patient to another on the hands of hospital personnel (165–167). Asymptomatic patients who carry MRSA can also be a source of infection for other patients because healthcare workers contaminate their hands while caring for these patients and do not adequately disinfect their hands before continuing work in the unit (168). An association between overcrowding and understaffing, and the rate of MRSA infections in a NICU and in an intermediate-care nursery has been reported (169). In this nursery, the outbreak ended when overcrowding and understaffing were temporarily reduced, triple dye was applied to the umbilical cords of all infants, and an infection control nurse was dedicated to the NICU.

Intervention for Control of Methicillin-Resistant *Staphylococcus aureus*

In the NICU baseline prevalence of MRSA should be assessed and efforts should be intensified when there is a case of healthcare-associated infection. Active surveillance for MRSA when epidemiologically appropriate is also proposed in recent guidelines for prevention and control of MRSA (170). Given the seriousness of MRSA infections in the NICU, considerable efforts should be made to identify the reservoir. Active surveillance is cost effective and should be initiated to assess the reservoir of patients who are colonized with MRSA after a single MRSA infection has been identified in a NICU. Cost of weekly active surveillance and isolation of patients with MRSA is 19 to 27-fold less costly than attributable costs of MRSA bacteremia from a new outbreak in the NICU (171). Active surveillance and increased use of alcohol-based hand antiseptic solution for hand hygiene is associated with a significant reduction in the transmission rate of MRSA (172).

Active surveillance and enhanced use of barrier precautions is effective in controlling MRSA (173). When appropriately implemented, contact precautions, weekly surveillance cultures, attempts to eradicate carriage in some patients, and surveillance cultures of personnel who had contact with new cases have decreased the risk of nosocomial transmission in the NICU (174). Use of cohort nursing and intranasal mupirocin may be necessary(158,162,165). Molecular epidemiological tools can be used to assess horizontal transmission. A multifaceted approach to prevent and control of MRSA is often necessary and a variety of interventions may have to be implemented concurrently.

Vancomycin-Resistant *Enterococcus*

In the United States, during late 1989, VRE infections from *E. faecium* were identified in the Northeast and from *E. faecalis* in the Midwest United States (175). In the United States in 2004, CDC-NNIS, analysis shows 12% increase in VRE from the preceding four years (12). Although the rate of VRE colonization among patients in the intensive care units is increasing, the incidence reported from NICUs is low, with relatively few reports related to VRE (144, 176–179). This may be due, in part, to lack of invasive infections with this organism and also to the limited number of pediatric facilities implementing active surveillance programs for detection of multi-drug resistant organisms such as VRE.

VRE has become an important concern in public health because of the strong potential for the *vanA* gene of vancomycin resistance to transfer to virulent pathogens such as *Staphylococcus aureus* (180–184). This is a growing threat to medical facilities (185). Clinical manifestations of vancomycin-resistant and susceptible enterococcal infections are similar. Although prevalence of VRE in NICUs is low, spread is of significant concern, especially in NICUs with a large population of very low birth weight infants requiring longer duration of stay. These neonates are prime targets for the spread of VRE because of lack of bowel control and close proximity of patients; any breach in infection control practices can lead to horizontal spread. Infections due to VRE have been associated with higher health care costs, prolonged morbidity, and greater mortality rates in adults (186,187). Vancomycin-resistant *E. faecium* and vancomycin-resistant *E. faecalis* strains are increasingly being recognized as serious pathogens. *E. faecium* is also more predominant than *E. faecalis* in its resistance to both vancomycin and ampicillin, making it difficult to treat. The risk for developing a VRE infection/colonization is inversely related to birth weight (177). Overall, patients who stay longer in the NICU are at a greater risk for acquiring VRE, which may be due to the increased risk for exposure to a possible carrier and/or prolonged use of antimicrobial therapy (176). Colonized infants are at risk for infections and serve as reservoirs for transmission (144). Multiclonal transmission of VRE strains has occurred in a NICU (178). Active surveillance cultures yielded 65 cases of VRE colonization/infection among the 1820 patients admitted to the NICU. Repetitive sequence PCR was performed on 60 of the VRE isolates

and identified three clusters. Members of cluster one included isolates from 21 patients and four isolates from the environment of the index case. Cluster two and cluster three included isolates from 23 and three patients, respectively. The similarity coefficients among the members of each cluster were ≥93% (Table 49-3). This outbreak illustrates that spread of VRE can occur easily in a NICU setting.

VRE is known to survive in an environment for as long as 5 weeks. Additionally, patients with a compromised immune system are susceptible to other illness, such as gastrointestinal dysfunction, resulting in higher risk for VRE colonization(188,189). VRE can be transferred via hands of health care workers, thermometers, physical therapy equipment, and hospital beds (178,185,190,191). VRE can be transferred from one patient to another via the contaminated gloves of healthcare workers and the environment (176,192).

Patients colonized with VRE do not always acquire infection; however, they do have a greater risk of infection (193). VRE colonized children generally carry the bacteria in their bowel flora for long periods of time without manifesting any clinical signs and symptoms (178,194–196). These infected or colonized patients serve as a reservoir for spread of this organism to other hospitalized patients.

Interventions for Control of Vancomycin-Resistant Enterococci

In 1995, the Hospital Infection Control Practices Advisory Committee (HICPAC) of the Centers for Disease Control and Prevention published guidelines for health institutions to follow in preventing the spread of vancomycin resistance (197). These guidelines include the proper use of vancomycin, education of healthcare workers on the threat of VRE, optimal methods for screening for VRE, and implementation of control measures. However, efforts to prevent VRE colonization and to restrict vancomycin usage in these facilities have been unsuccessful, and the incidence of VRE continues to increase in ICUs in the United States (12). These HICPAC guidelines are being revised (198). The Society of Healthcare Epidemiology has recommended active surveillance for VRE (170). In NICU baseline prevalence of VRE should be assessed and efforts should be intensified when there is a case of healthcare-associated infection.

Hand hygiene should be emphasized at all times. Healthcare workers contaminate their hands after contact with a VRE colonized or infected patient regardless of whether or not gloves are worn (193). In a study, 17 (34%) of 50 healthcare workers had VRE isolates on their gloves; and 5 out of 17 of those workers who wore gloves had VRE on their hands. All health care workers should be trained to enforce appropriate isolation precautions.

As environment plays an important role in transmission of VRE, schedules for routine cleaning of rooms should be strictly adhered (192). Additionally, potentially infectious waste must be disposed of in such a manner to prevent

TABLE 49-3

DENDROGRAM OF VANCOMYCIN RESISTANT ENTEROCOCCI STUDY ISOLATES. REP–PCR WAS PERFORMED ON 60 VRE ISOLATES AND IDENTIFIED THREE GENETICALLY-RELATED CLUSTERS USING THE UPRIME DT PRIMER SET

Pearson correlation (Opt:1.00%) [0.0%-100.0%]
Uprime Dt

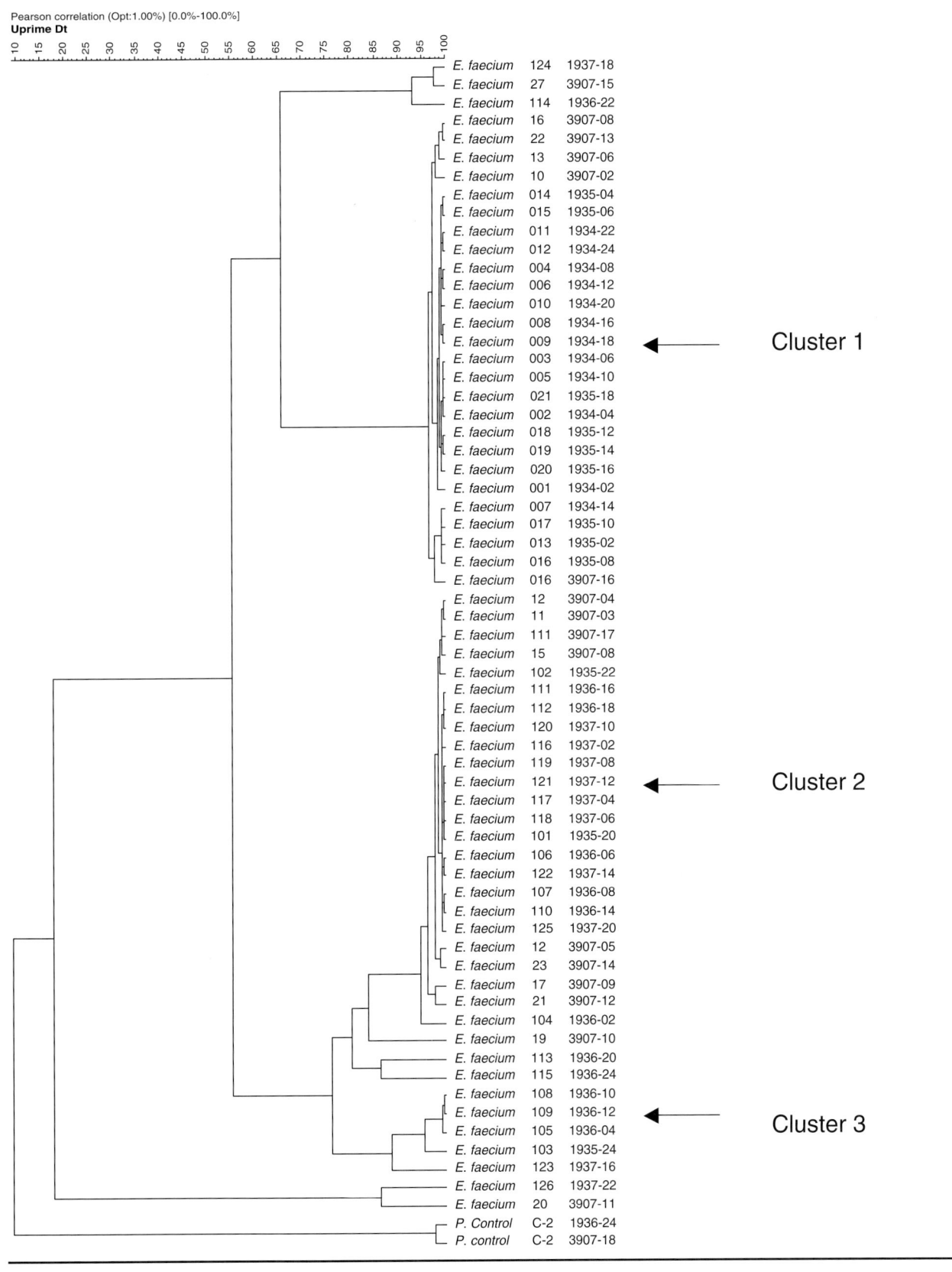

E. faecium	124	1937-18
E. faecium	27	3907-15
E. faecium	114	1936-22
E. faecium	16	3907-08
E. faecium	22	3907-13
E. faecium	13	3907-06
E. faecium	10	3907-02
E. faecium	014	1935-04
E. faecium	015	1935-06
E. faecium	011	1934-22
E. faecium	012	1934-24
E. faecium	004	1934-08
E. faecium	006	1934-12
E. faecium	010	1934-20
E. faecium	008	1934-16
E. faecium	009	1934-18	← Cluster 1
E. faecium	003	1934-06
E. faecium	005	1934-10
E. faecium	021	1935-18
E. faecium	002	1934-04
E. faecium	018	1935-12
E. faecium	019	1935-14
E. faecium	020	1935-16
E. faecium	001	1934-02
E. faecium	007	1934-14
E. faecium	017	1935-10
E. faecium	013	1935-02
E. faecium	016	1935-08
E. faecium	016	3907-16
E. faecium	12	3907-04
E. faecium	11	3907-03
E. faecium	111	3907-17
E. faecium	15	3907-08
E. faecium	102	1935-22
E. faecium	111	1936-16
E. faecium	112	1936-18
E. faecium	120	1937-10
E. faecium	116	1937-02
E. faecium	119	1937-08
E. faecium	121	1937-12	← Cluster 2
E. faecium	117	1937-04
E. faecium	118	1937-06
E. faecium	101	1935-20
E. faecium	106	1936-06
E. faecium	122	1937-14
E. faecium	107	1936-08
E. faecium	110	1936-14
E. faecium	125	1937-20
E. faecium	12	3907-05
E. faecium	23	3907-14
E. faecium	17	3907-09
E. faecium	21	3907-12
E. faecium	104	1936-02
E. faecium	19	3907-10
E. faecium	113	1936-20
E. faecium	115	1936-24
E. faecium	108	1936-10
E. faecium	109	1936-12	← Cluster 3
E. faecium	105	1936-04
E. faecium	103	1935-24
E. faecium	123	1937-16
E. faecium	126	1937-22
E. faecium	20	3907-11
P. Control	C-2	1936-24
P. control	C-2	3907-18

contamination of the environment and minimize the risk of exposure to hospital personnel and patients. For patients colonized or infected with VRE dedicated individual use of non-critical equipment such as thermometers and blood pressure cuffs should be mandatory. Molecular epidemiological tools can be used to assess infant-to-infant transmission.

Antimicrobial-Resistant Enterobacteriaceae

Third generation cephalosporin resistant enteric Gram negative rods are an important cause of healthcare-associated infections in ICUs (24,155). NICU patients frequently acquire intestinal colonization with antimicrobial resistant enterobacteriaceae. Intestinal colonization serves as an important source for transmission to the environment (199). Colonization with these organisms has been detected as early as on the first day of hospitalization (200–202). This colonization may follow transmission from other patients in the unit or may evolve endogenously from the selective pressures afforded by antimicrobial therapy. Approximately 10% of colonized neonates are at risk for development of healthcare-associated systemic infections (203). Clinical manifestations of infants with resistant enterobacteriaceae are similar to the healthcare-associated infections with susceptible pathogens.

Colonization with resistant Gram-negative rods seen in a European NICU was related to empiric use of amoxicillin and cefotaxime (204). In this crossover study, neonates who were given intravenous amoxicillin-cefotaxime therapy were 18 times more likely to harbor resistant Gram-negative rods than neonates who were given penicillin and tobramycin. The combination of amoxicillin and cefotaxime may exert selective pressure encouraging emergence of extended-spectrum beta-lactamase (ESBL) producing bacteria. Cefotaxime may also select for de-repressed *amp C* mutants among the colonizing enterobacteriaceae. The appearance of ESBL-producing Gram-negative rods causes many concerns. These isolates are clinically resistant to all penicillins, cephalosporins, and monobactam agents, making therapeutic intervention difficult. Detection of such isolates is problematic for the clinical microbiology laboratory. Special procedures, such as the triple disk approximation test or the methods described by the National Committee on Clinical Laboratory Standards must be employed by the laboratory to recognize ESBL producers. The spectrum of enterobacteriaceae capable of ESBL production is broadening. In particular, Enterobacter species, Serratia species and Citrobacter species have been found capable of ESBL production (205,206).

Interventions for Control of Antimicrobial-Resistant Enterobacteriaceae

When an endemic problem with antimicrobial resistant enterobacteriaceae exists, multiple interventions are needed.

The focused use of barrier precautions and restricting use of cephalosporins, along with provision of educational programs, helped reduce colonization and healthcare-associated infections with antimicrobial resistance enterobacteriaceae in a Brazilian neonatal unit from 32% to 11% (207,208). Molecular epidemiological tools can be used to assess infant-to infant transmission.

VIRAL INFECTIONS

Viruses account about 5% of all healthcare-associated infections and up to 23% in children (209,210). These viral infections are most common in neonates and young infants. The infections are associated with extended length of hospital stay and have considerable morbidity and mortality. The intensive care environment allows for efficient spread of viral pathogens (211). The spectrum of nosocomial viruses is wide including respiratory, enteric, and blood-borne viruses among others. This section outlines the epidemiology of these viruses and the control measures used to limit exposure.

Respiratory Viruses

This section focuses on the common viruses causing respiratory illness such as respiratory syncytial virus (RSV), influenza virus, adenovirus, and parainfluenza viruses. In a substantial number of cases of respiratory illness when no virus can be cultured, the possibility of metapneumovirus should be considered. Recently, a newly discovered coronavirus associated with severe acute respiratory syndrome (SARS) and metapeumoviruses have also been described in infants and children (212–214).

RSV causes severe morbidity and high mortality in premature infants (215). Nosocomial RSV infections are common when the community is also experiencing a high rate of respiratory viral illness during winter months (216). Neonates acquire these infections from family members and HCWs with mild respiratory illness. Neonates can present with a clinical picture consistent with sepsis, including apnea, lethargy, feeding difficulties and chest x-ray evidence of pulmonary infiltrates. Diagnosis is made by detection of antigen using a rapid viral diagnostic kit. Infections spread by secretions and large droplets. RSV remains infective in fomites for up to 12 hours (215). Prophylactic measures, such as RSV immunoglobulin or humanized monoclonal antibody (palivizumab) are cost-effective only in high-risk patients (215,217). Both of these products are licensed for prevention of RSV disease in infants with brochopulmonary dysplasia or in preterm birth (<35 weeks) (218). Both of these agents can be given once a month, beginning just before the onset of the RSV season, and subsequently 4 more doses given monthly. No safe vaccine is currently available for use in infants. Control measures during the increase in community onset RSV include early identification of patients with respiratory symptoms who are infected with RSV and prompt institution of contact isolation. During large outbreaks cohorting patients and staff may be needed. Exclusion of staff and family members with respiratory tract illness may also be necessary.

Other respiratory viruses, including influenza and parainfluenza, cause healthcare-associated infections less commonly in the NICU (219–222). Although influenza A infection has been rarely described in the neonatal period, it has to be considered one of the possible causes of nosocomial infection during the winter season in the NICU (223). Diagnosis is made by detection of antigen using a rapid viral diagnostic kit. Influenza A is readily transmissible; amantadine has been used to treat symptomatic neonates and for prophylaxis of NICU staff (219). Influenza A prevention by immunization is a priority for those caring for high-risk NICU patients (221). Community acquired influenza A infections are common in children; recommendations for reducing healthcare-associated influenza virus infections include vaccination programs for both healthy children aged 6 to 23 months and health care workers and family members in contact with high-risk patients (224,225).

Parainfluenza viruses are the second most common cause of bronchiolitis and pneumonia in infants. Simultaneous outbreak of RSV and parainfluenza virus 3 has been seen in a newborn nursery (226). Respiratory viral illness due to parainfluenza virus 3 infections in neonates can be seen during summer months. Diagnosis is made by detection of antigen using a rapid viral diagnostic kit. An outbreak of parainfluenza virus 3 was seen in infants with respiratory symptoms and the chest x-ray showed pulmonary infiltrates. Significant morbidity was seen in three of the six neonates requiring ventilator support. Healthcare workers ill with respiratory symptoms were the vehicles of transmission and the nursery was understaffed during this outbreak (220).

Adenoviral pneumonia occurs in approximately 10% of cases and can be more severe than RSV (227–229). Clinical manifestations include findings consistent with clinical sepsis, including decreased feeding, lethargy, apnea, retractions, and progressive pneumonia. Diagnosis is made by detection of antigen using a rapid viral diagnostic kit.

Human coronavirus (HcoV, strains 229E and OC43) has been shown to cause healthcare-associated viral infections in 11% of neonates in a prospective study (230). The incidence rate for other viruses such as RSV, influenza A and B, paramyxoviruses 1,2, and 3 and adenovirus were shown to be less prominent pathogens in the study period (230). Risk factors included prolonged duration of hospitalization, parenteral nutrition, and antibiotic treatment.

SARS, a newly diagnosed respiratory disease caused by a novel coronavirus SARS-CoV, has been seen in a 56-day-old ex-30 week gestation infant in Hong Kong (212,213,231). This infant, upon admission to hospital, presented with hypothermia and respiratory distress. Laboratory and microbiologic results were similar to those found in other pediatric patients with SARS. Lymphopenia and elevation

of enzymes such as AST, ALT, CK and LDH was seen at the time of admission to the critical care unit. Chest radiograph showed focal consolidation. Nasopharyngeal aspirate revealed SARS-CoV by reverse transcriptase-polymerase chain reaction (RT-PCR). This patient was seen during an on going SARS outbreak in regions of China and in Hong Kong.

Human metapneumovirus infection has been recently shown to be one of the leading causes of respiratory tract infections in the first years of life (214). Human metapneumovirus infection produces clinically similar symptoms to RSV infection. In a study using nasal wash samples obtained over a 25-year period, 20 percent of the all previously virus-negative lower respiratory track illnesses were attributable to human metapneumovirus (215). Clinical manifestation included cough (90%), coryza (88%), fever (52%) and other constitutional symptoms. The mean age of human metapneumovirus infected children was 11.6 months. In a substantial proportion of viral infections in NICUs the etiological agent responsible for the disease cannot be found, the possible role of human metapneumovirus remains to be seen.

Parvovirus B19

Parvovirus B19 is the etiologic agent of fifth disease in children. Droplets in household contacts readily spread this virus and infection rates are high (232). Although transmission in healthcare settings has occurred, the risk of healthcare worker transmission is low (233,234). Nosocomial infection has occurred among hospital staff after contact with infected patients with sickle cell disease and aplastic crisis (235). Nosocomial transmission from chronically infected immunocompromised patients can also occur (236). Susceptible healthcare workers are at risk of seroconversion to B19-specific IgM and IgG during community outbreaks of fifth disease (237). Transmission from infected HCWs to patients has been documented, prior to the implementation of standard and isolation precautions practiced for at least past two decades. Transmission of parvovirus in a healthcare setting is less likely to occur with use of stringent infection control practice and good hand hygiene. Pregnant healthcare workers should be informed of the potential risk to the fetus from parvovirus B19 and the preventive measures.

Enteroviruses

Healthcare-associated enteroviral infections are usually associated with community outbreaks during summer and autumn; they spread by the fecal–oral and respiratory routes, and from mother to neonate in the peripartum period. Enteroviruses survive on an environmental surface for a prolonged period of time, with a potential for transfer of infection through fomites. Echovirus type 22 has been identified in nosocomial necrotizing enterocolitis outbreaks (238). Echovirus type 11 was the most common type found in neonatal echovirus infections at a non-mucosal site in the review of 16 outbreaks in nurseries (239,240).

A RT-PCR can detect the presence of enteroviruses-echovirus and coxsackie (241). PCR can be helpful in detecting outbreaks, and in cohorting patients with enteroviruses (*Coxsackie B4*) meningitis and myocarditis (242). Standard and isolation precautions with strict hand hygiene practice after diaper change should minimize exposure to enteroviruses.

Coxsackie B virus infections are also frequent, with attack rates of 22 to 54% (243). They may cause myocarditis, hepatitis and meningitis (242,244). *Coxsackie A* infections are rare, but herpangina and aseptic meningitis have been described (245).

Studies using DNA markers have showed that, in the NICU environment, the most consistently positive sites for Coxsackie B detection included blood gas analyzers, computer mice, telephone receivers, medical charts, ventilator knobs, door handles, radiant warmer control buttons, patient monitors, and the hands of personnel (246). The information revealed by these techniques help in assisting and enforcing cleaning procedures, and educational intervention programs to decrease nosocomial infections.

Other Viruses

Hepatitis A virus (HAV) has been reported to occur as a vertical transmission from a mother with an acute infection (247). Horizontal spread among premature infants by nurses and asymptomatic infected premature infants can be a source of hepatitis A outbreak in nursery infants and personnel and in the community (248). Infants exposed to perinatal HAV may benefit from immunoglobulin, although its efficacy has not been established (249).

Herpes simplex virus (HSV) transmission to the neonate occurs during vaginal delivery from symptomatic or asymptomatic mothers. The incidence of neonatal herpes virus is 1 in 3000 to 20,000 live births. Nosocomial transmission of HSV is very rare (250,251). Interfamilial transmission of HSV infants has been reported and is also rare. Neonates born to mothers with active disease or mucocutaneous lesions should be placed on contact isolation in addition to standard precautions.

Human immunodeficiency virus (HIV) is transmitted vertically, and healthcare-associated transmission of HIV is also reported. Prospective studies of HCWs have estimated that the average risk for HIV transmission after a percutaneous exposure to HIV-infected blood is approximately 0.3% (95% confidence interval = 0.2%–0.5%) and after a mucous membrane exposure is 0.09% (95% CI = 0.006%–0.5%) (252). HIV infection predisposes to neonatal septicemia and congenital infection. Maternal HIV infection has been estimated to increase the stillbirth rate by 1.6 times and neonatal mortality rate by 2.7 times (253). Standard precautions to prevent parenteral, mucous membrane, and non-intact skin exposure to HIV should be used for all patients.

Varicella-zoster virus (VZV) can cause serious morbidity and mortality in neonates if the mother develops varicella from 5 days before to 2 days after delivery. The airborne route readily transmits varicella and prophylactic varicella-zoster immune globulin should be considered for exposed premature infants (254). Indications include: (1) newborn infant whose mother had onset of chicken pox within 5 days before or 48 hours after delivery (2) hospitalized premature infant (≥28 weeks of gestation) whose mother lacks a reliable history of chicken pox or serologic evidence of protection against varicella (3) hospitalized premature infant (≤28 weeks of gestation or ≤1000 grams birth weight), regardless of maternal history of chicken pox. Oral acyclovir has been administered prophylactically to preterm infants in contact with a varicella patient and has been suggested to prevent hospital-acquired VZV infections in situations where VZV immunoglobulin is not available (255). Health-care workers should be screened for VZV immunity and receive vaccine as needed, unless contraindicated (256).

Cytomegalovirus (CMV) infection can occur either vertically from the mother or horizontally from household members or childcare centers. Transfusion-acquired CMV infection of low birth weight neonates of seronegative mothers has been reported (257). Seropositive healthy donors have latent CMV in their leukocytes and blood transfusion can result in viral transmission. Transmission of CMV has been virtually eliminated by the use of CMV antibody negative donors (258). Cells are frozen in glycerol before administration, either the buffy coat is removed, or cells are filtrated to remove the leukocytes. Use of pasteurized milk or freezing of human milk can also decrease the risk of transmission. If human milk is used, infants born to CMV antibody-negative mothers should receive milk only from CMV antibody-negative women. The prevalence of CMV excretion by patients in a neonatal intensive care unit is about 1%. The majority of CMV excreters are symptomatic. Pregnant health care workers are especially concerned, because CMV infection can be associated with significant neurological injury to the fetus. Healthcare-associated transmission from patient to health care worker has not been documented (259). A review of cytomegalovirus excretion in hospitalized patients and prospective evaluations of primary infection in hospital personnel do not support frequent occurrence of cytomegalovirus infection despite ample opportunity for exposure. Adherence to proper isolation techniques and good hand hygiene should be adequate to prevent nosocomial transmission of the cytomegalovirus. However, pregnant healthcare workers should be counseled about the potential risks of acquisition and urged to practice good hand hygiene.

Good hand hygiene, barrier precautions such as gloving, gowning, masks and goggles to prevent person-to-person viral transmission are the key elements in controlling nosocomial spread of viruses in the NICU (260). In specific situations, prophylactic antiviral or specific immunoglobulin is also used, as described above.

INFECTION CONTROL MEASURES

New technologies and better approaches are rapidly changing concepts about infection management. Today, one third of all hospital-acquired infections could be prevented by effective, readily available programs that monitor, prevent and control infections (261,262). Such programs require substantial changes in NICU culture, from the current focus on early detection to a full commitment to prevention and to a multi-step management program that incorporates: (1) surveillance, (2) prevention and control including (i) isolation precautions, (ii) hand hygiene, (iii) oral and skin care, (iv) catheter care, (v) accuracy of diagnosis, and (vi) equipment care, (3) staffing and nursery design, (4) educational and feedback (5) an infection control practitioner (ICP) and availability of a trained infection control physician (hospital epidemiologist) (261,263). In addition, the care of pre-term infants requires specialized knowledge of infectious disease processes and methods to reduce infection.

Surveillance

A key component of infection control is surveillance: the collection, management and organization, analysis (interpretation) and reporting of relevant data. Active surveillance is essential to identify alterable risk factors and detect system problems. Although the patient may be the source of contamination, healthcare workers, invasive devices, and hospital equipment continue to be important vectors promoting the spread of organisms within the nursery. Without effective surveillance, it is not possible to mount effective efforts to prevent infection (9).

Ideally, the progress of each infant would be followed from admission to discharge from an infection control perspective. Methods of active surveillance and detection vary but include clinical case review, review of laboratory results, and retrospective chart review. Patient and environmental risk factors, procedures, and culture results must be recorded and interpreted by the ICP and epidemiologist.

Surveillance also includes monitoring all central lines from insertion to removal. Insertion sites must be inspected. Record the operator's name and the date of catheter insertion, dressing changes and catheter removal, along with signs of infection (fever, hypothermia, apnea, and bradycardia). Surveillance also includes monitoring other risk factors including length of parenteral nutrition and intralipids infusions and device days (Table 49-4).

Not only must the course of each individual infant be followed, but also the entire NICU population must be tracked for multi-drug resistant organisms colonization and infection rates, risks and trends. These observations provide important and practical tools to guide clinical practice and change-efforts as well as measures of quality improvement. Any significant change in the rate of infection or with a particular microbe should be investigated. Identify the microorganism along with its reservoir and risk factors for transmission. Present ICP and epidemiologist recommendations to the NICU staff.

As ICPs monitor each infant's care from the unique perspective of infection control, the practitioner's responsibility is to understand the risk factors identified, and to question closely the characteristics affecting any situation she/he does not understand.

Prevention and Control

Understanding the source of each infection and its mode of transmission is the essential basis for determinations of appropriate control measures (264). Infection risks related to the patient, the personnel, the procedures and devices all must be considered. Neonatal patient risks also include premature rupture of membranes, maternal illness, gut colonization, and mechanical ventilation and each may be important, even those that cannot be modified (58). Often, a combination of strategies to minimize infection can be effective by focusing only on known modifiable risk factors. These include but are not limited to hand hygiene, oral and skin care, catheter care, accurate diagnosis of infection, enhanced isolation precautions, and care of equipment (265).

Successful prevention strategies also include limiting nurse-to-patient ratios and avoiding overcrowding, educating and providing feedback to nursery personnel, and continuously monitoring infection rates.

Isolation Precautions

Guidelines for isolation precautions, revised in 2004/2005, suggest ways control the spread of microorganisms that are transmitted to infants through direct contact with infected or colonized persons, indirect contact with contaminated objects, droplet contact in the air and through contaminated products. It is important to monitor infants for multi-drug–resistant organisms colonization and/or infection and to take appropriate special precautions to prevent transmissions.

Cohorting of patients colonized or infected with multi-drug resistant organisms is appropriate. Treatment for these patients includes aseptic technique, hand hygiene and appropriate antimicrobial usage. Patients colonized with multi-drug–resistant organisms require use of isolation precautions to prevent cross-colonization; a single negative culture does not prove that the infant is no longer colonized with the resistant microorganism.

Hand Hygiene

Lack of hand hygiene is the most frequent (and, most important) source of pathogens in health care facilities, and the institution of strict hand hygiene is the easiest,

TABLE 49-4
SAMPLE SURVEILLANCE SHEET FOR HEALTHCARE ASSOCIATED INFECTION

Name_____DOB_____
Date of Admission_____ Weight_____
Gestation_____Surgery_____

Date	Procedure	T-max	Central line (Site & Dressing change)	Ventilator	Parenteral Nutrition	Intralipids	Culture Site	Culture Results

Comments/date (include clinical signs such as apnea, bradycardia, hypothermia, etc.)

fastest and most effective corrective measure. Although neonatal healthcare workers typically believe that they wash their hands frequently and carefully, they actually are no more compliant than other health care workers. Hand hygiene is a general term that applies to washing with plain soap and water, antiseptic soap and water or an antiseptic waterless product (266). Research findings on hand hygiene is extensive, and provides specific guidelines for healthcare providers. Pathogens are recovered not only from infected wounds, but also from normal intact patient skin, mucous membranes and urine and stool. Bed linen, bedside furniture, and other objects in the immediate environment become contaminated with patient flora, so nurses con-taminate their hands during "clean" activities. Health care workers contaminate their hands or gloves merely by touching inanimate objects in a patient's room. In one study, nurses were instructed to take a femoral pulse for 15 seconds, wash their hands and then touch a catheter. Touching the skin of a patient transferred enough organisms to the nurses' hands to cause subsequent transmission to the catheter, despite hand washing with plain soap and water (267).

Hand antisepsis can reduce the incidence of health-care associated infections significantly, particularly after antiseptic washing using chlorhexidine-containing detergent (266). It is important to wash hands for 30 seconds with conventional antiseptic-containing soap and water or with waterless alcohol-based gel (until dry). These requirements are frequently ignored and most personnel spend less than 15 seconds with each wash (268). Hand hygiene must be enforced between patient contacts, before and after procedures, and after removing gloves.

Alcohol-based waterless hand gels are strongly recommended by the 2002 CDC Guideline for Hand Hygiene in Health-Care Settings. These antiseptic rubs prevent pathogen transmission more effectively than either standard washing or hand antisepsis with antimicrobial soaps (266). Waterless alcohol rubs have excellent activity against Gram-positive and Gram-negative bacteria, including multi-resistant pathogens, most viruses and various fungi. Several products, including 70% ethanol and 70% isopropanol products have been found to reduce titers of an enveloped bacteriophage more effectively than an antimicrobial soap containing 4% chlorhexidine gluconate (269). Alcohol hand rubs are safe, effective, and rapid acting, but are effective only if enough products are applied to wet both the tops and bottoms of each hand, between the fingers and under the nails. It is important to rub the hands together after application until all the alcohol has evaporated. Also, these products are not effective when hands are visibly dirty.

The drying effect of alcohol can be reduced or eliminated by adding 1 to 3% glycerol or other skin conditioning agents (266). Health care workers with respiratory allergies may poorly tolerate alcohol-based products with fragrances. Alcohol-based products cause substantially less skin irritation and dryness than soaps or antimicrobial detergents and are consistently associated with improvements in skin health and improved compliance with hand hygiene when compared with traditional hand washing products (270,271).

Approximately 25% of nurses report symptoms of dermatitis on their hands and 85% give a history of skin problems (272). Frequent and repeated use of hand hygiene products, especially soap and water, is the primary cause (273). Using hot water for hand washing (especially in winter months) also contributes to dermatitis, but allergic dermatitis from alcohol-based hand rubs is uncommon. It is important to provide chlorhexidine-compatible lotion for healthcare workers. Hand lotion can increase skin hydration and replace depleted skin lipids that contribute to the barrier function of normal skin. Skin irritation leads to dryness and cracking of the skin. Skin breakdown can lead to less hand washing and more frequent colonization by staphylococci and Gram-negative bacilli (274). Lotion decreases skin irritation, dryness and cracking, and twice-a-day use of lotion can prevent irritant contact dermatitis caused by hand hygiene products (275). It is important to insure easy access for hand hygiene materials. Sinks must be accessible, along with antiseptic products and paper towels. Dispensers for alcohol-based hand rubs must be accessible and monitored to ensure proper function.

The initial hand wash before entering the NICU should be done with antimicrobial soap and water up to the elbow. Brushes do not seem to be more effective than antiseptic soap alone, are no longer recommended for hand hygiene, and may even be harmful since they lead to sloughing of skin and contribute to dermatitis (276).

The CDC recommends health care workers wear gloves to (1) reduce the risk of personnel acquiring infections from patients, (2) prevent workers' flora from being transmitted to patients and (3) to reduce contamination of the hands of personnel by flora that can be transmitted from one patient to another (277). One study demonstrates that wearing gloves prevented personnel from acquiring VRE on their hands when touching contaminated environmental surfaces (278). Another, involving personnel caring for patients with *C. difficile*, found that gloves effectively prevented hand contamination among a majority of personnel having direct contact with patients (278). However, gloves do not provide complete protection and it is important to wash hands after removing gloves (279).

Artificial nails are a particular hazard. Routine cleaning does not effectively remove bacteria and their use should be banned for direct caregivers in the NICU. There is no longer any question that hand hygiene in health care settings is fundamentally effective. Research findings are abundant on the topic, and they are convincing. Specific guidelines for workers to follow are equally important to help facilitate system improvements and include requirements for detailed monitoring to: (1) periodically record the number of hand-hygiene episodes by personnel compared to the number of hand-hygiene opportunities and provide feedback to personnel regarding their performance, (2) record the volume of alcohol-based hand rub used per 1,000 patient-days, (3) record adherence to policies concerning artificial nails, (4) when outbreaks of infection occur, assess the adequacy of health-care worker hand hygiene. Improvements in compliance tend to be short-lived without ongoing monitoring. The possibility of including parents as partners ensuring compliance with hand decontamination in NICUs needs to be studied.

Skin Care and Oral Hygiene

Very low birth weight infants have inadequate epidermal barriers, so that their risk of infection is elevated. Care should be taken to avoid damage to the newborn skin. While there is no consensus concerning the most effective skin care practice for these infants it is recognized that newborns should be washed with warm water, that may include mild non-medicated soap, immediately after birth (280). Thereafter, whole-body bathing and antiseptic agents are not necessary for routine care but may be indicated during outbreaks. When antiseptic agents are needed, chlorhexidine is a safe choice; it is less toxic than hexachlorophene and cutaneous absorption is negligible (281). Iodophors may not be safe for bathing because of absorption of iodine (282,283). Chlorhexidine cord care has been effective in reducing colonization and infection in some centers. A recent study shows no decreased risk of infection to infants receiving Aquaphor, a topical emollient, in fact there may be an increase in the risk of CONS infection with this practice (284,285).

Recent studies demonstrate that CONS colonize mucosal sites including the gut, nares, and throat of preterm infants. It is possible that mucosal colonization leads to translocation of CONS from mucosal sites to the bloodstream through the mesenteric lymph nodes (59). It is therefore possible that the gut, in addition to the skin, may be an important source of CONS bacteremia. Few studies have been done to support this data, but these findings raise important questions related to infection control practices. Studies in the adult population show that aspiration of oropharyngeal organisms is associated with hospital-acquired pneumonia. Nasogastric tubes, endotracheal tubes, mechanical ventilation, enteral feeds and surgery put patients at risk for hospital-acquired pneumonia. Strategies aimed at decreasing CONS mucosal colonization, including nasal and gut colonization, may help prevent hospital-acquired pneumonia and bloodstream infections.

Probiotic supplements have been suggested to play a role in retaining the normal micro flora in the colon of infants and thus preventing bloodstream infections and late-onset sepsis. The normal intestinal bacterial colonization of very low birth weight infants is disturbed by several factors, such as cesarean section and parenteral nutrition, low modulation of immunity and increased gut permeability allowing bacterial translocation from gut to tissues, and antibiotic treatment (286–288). In a recent prospective double-blind study with lactobacillus treatment no statistical significance in reducing bacterial sepsis was found (289). However, this field remains controversial, and more studies are needed in very low birth weight infants to show possible benefits of probiotics in prevention and control of nosocomial sepsis.

Catheter Care

Most serious catheter-related bloodstream infections (CRBSI) are associated with central venous catheters, especially those placed in ICU patients colonized with hospital-acquired organisms. These catheters are used for extended periods of time and are manipulated several times each day to administer fluids, drugs and blood products. The catheters are also accessed to obtain blood, increasing the potential for contamination and subsequent infection (290). Such infections are both costly and dangerous, with cost per infection ranging from $34,508

to $56,000 and mortality rates between 12% and 15% (291–293).

Migration of skin organisms found at the insertion site into the cutaneous catheter tract, with colonization of the catheter tip, is the most common route of infection for short-term peripherally inserted catheters. Contamination of the catheter hub contributes substantially to intra-lumina colonization of long-term catheters (42). Catheters can also become hematogenously seeded from another focus of infection. Infusate contamination is less common, but leads to catheter-related bloodstream infection.

Extensive research convincingly demonstrates the risk for infection declines following standardization of aseptic catheter care. Specialized IV teams are highly effective in reducing incidence of catheter-related infections (294). Improvements are noted when a limited team of skilled persons consistently performs central line insertions.

Most umbilical and central venous catheters are available with a heparin-bonded coating and impregnated with benzalkonium-chloride, to provide them with both antimicrobial activity and an anti-thrombotic effect (295,296). Other catheters coated or impregnated with antimicrobial or antiseptic agents can decrease the risk for CRBSI. However, these catheters are currently not available for infants weighing less than 3 kg.

The risk of catheter colonization and bloodstream infection for umbilical vein catheters and umbilical artery catheters are similar and high for some newborns. In one study, neonates with very low birth weight receiving antibiotics for >10 days were at an increased risk for umbilical artery CRBSI while those with higher birth weight receiving parenteral nutrition were at increased risk for umbilical vein CRBSI (297). Ideally umbilical catheters should be removed as soon as possible when no longer needed, but umbilical artery catheters can be left in place for 5 days and umbilical venous catheters for 14 days if managed aseptically (290). No relationship has been found between the duration of catheterization and the daily probability of infection, suggesting that routine replacement of most central venous catheters does not reduce the incidence of catheter-related infection (298).

To prevent infection, all central catheters should be inserted using sterile technique including sterile gowns, gloves, masks, large sterile sheets and appropriate skin disinfection (process measure forms Tables 49-5 and 49-6). Avoid small sterile drapes that do not provide an adequate sterile field for catheter insertion in neonates. Maximal sterile precautions (large sheets) help reduce central venous catheter bacteremia in neonates. Two-percent chlorhexidine is the preferred skin antiseptic, but is not yet approved for infants less than two months of age (299). Seventy percent alcohol or ten percent povidone-iodine can be used for these young infants. The skin must be scrubbed for at least 30 to 60 seconds and must be allowed to dry completely. Ten-percent povidone-iodine takes at

---

TABLE 49-5

CENTERS FOR DISEASE CONTROL SAMPLE CENTRAL LINE DATA COLLECTION RECORD

(To be completed by nurse assisting with insertion)

1. **Name of person completing form:** _____
2. **Insertion Date:** _____
3. **Name of inserter:** _____
4. **Inserted by (circle one):** Attending Neo.   Attending Surg.   Housestaff   MD Assistant
   IV Team   Other
5. **Reason for insertion (circle one):**
   New indication for catheter replace malfunctioning/displaced catheter
   Suspected catheter infection other
6. **Is the patient expected to receive total parenteral nutrition (TPN)
   through this catheter? (circle answer)**   **Yes**   **No**
7. **Insertion technique (circle answer for each question):**
   A. Mask worn by inserter?   **Yes**   **No**
   B. Cap worn by inserter?   **Yes**   **No**
   C. Sterile gown worn by inserter?   **Yes**   **No**
   D. Sterile gloves worn by inserter?   **Yes**   *Move up*
   E. Large drape* covering patient?   **Yes**   **No**
8. **Skin prep (circle one):** Chlorhexidine gluconate   Povidone iodine   Alcohol   Other
   8a. **If povidone iodine used, record time (in seconds) from end of application of skin prep
       until first skin puncture:** _____seconds
9*. **Location (circle one):** Jugular   Subclavian   Femoral   Brachial
10. **Antimicrobial coated/catheter used? (circle answer) :**   Yes   No
11. **Was catheter exchanged over a guide wire? (circle answer):**   Yes   No
12. **Was antimicrobial ointment applied to site? (circle answer):**   Yes   No

* Large sterile drape that allows ample sterile field without interfering with clinical assessment of infant well being.

---

least 2 to 3 minutes to air dry, and is not effective until it is thoroughly dry.

The rate of colonization among catheters dressed with transparent dressings (5.7%) is comparable to the colonization of those dressed with gauze (4.6%); there are no substantial differences in the incidence of catheter colonization or phlebitis (300). The catheter-site dressing requires changing when it becomes damp, loose, or visibly soiled. Replace gauze dressings every two days and transparent dressings every seven days except for patients in which the risk of dislodging the catheter outweighs the benefit of changing the dressing (301). Clean or sterile gloves must be used when changing dressings. The chlorhexidine-impregnated sponge (Biopatch) can be used for infants greater than 26 weeks gestation or greater than 7 weeks of age, and cuts infection rates in older children and adults. One study of neonates showed a substantial decrease in colonized catheter tips but no difference in the rates of CRBSI and bloodstream infections without a source (302). Infants in this study with gestational age less than 26 weeks and less than 8 days of age were at increased risk for localized contact dermatitis with the Biopatch dressing. Of the 98 neonates with very low birth weights, 15% developed localized contact dermatitis.

Topical antibiotics or creams at the catheter insertion site are not recommended because they promote fungal infections and antimicrobial resistance (303). Rates of catheter colonization with *candida* species appear to be increased with ointments that have no fungicidal activity (304).

Peripheral venous catheters should be left in place in children until intravenous therapy is completed, unless complications occur (290). Promptly remove any catheter that is no longer essential. Line setups should be designed to limit the number of ports and connections, since each is an independent opportunity for contamination. Hub contamination can be prevented by maintaining catheter sterility during line changes and by effective hand washing, use of a sterile field under the hub, wiping the injection ports with 70% alcohol and friction and allowing the alcohol to dry before accessing the system. Use ports that do not require opening to access. Access ports should be covered with a silicone membrane to reduce risk of contamination. Microorganisms found colonizing the catheter hubs are frequently the same

TABLE 49-6
CENTERS FOR DISEASE CONTROL SAMPLE CVC DAILY INDICATION FOR USE FORM

(Fill out one column each day)
NOTE: Exclude Tunneled Catheters and Ports

Patient ID _____ **Insertion site (circle)** Sub   Jug   Fem   Brach/Ceph   Umbil

Type of line (circle) Surg. placed CVL   PICC   Dialy - Arterial
Other _____

New insertion   ☐
Existing central line ☐   If existing line, date catheter inserted_____

Physician initials:							
Today's date:	/ /	/ /	/ /	/ /	/ /	/ /	/ /
Number of days since catheter has been inserted (insertion day = day0)*:							
Check all that apply:							
Continuous Infusion Vasopressors							
Hemodynamic monitoring							
>Incompatible continuous infusions							
Medications require central venous access (e.g., TPN)							
Rapid fluid administration							
No peripheral access							
None of the above (physician judgment)							

*If catheter was inserted prior to arrival in unit and insertion date is unknown, first day in unit may be used as day 0.

Note: Fill out separate form for every central line inserted in each patient.
Please list comments/questions on use of this form:

organisms as those isolated from the bloodstream in patients with CRBSI (305). Unneeded components and stopcocks should be excluded whenever possible. Replacing intravenous administration sets no more frequently than 72 hours after initiation is safe and cost-effective (306). When a fluid that enhances microbial growth is infused (e.g., lipid emulsions and blood products) more frequent changes of administration sets are indicated, because these products are independent risk factors for CRBSI (305). Exposure to lipids is an independent risk factor for development of coagulase-negative staphylococcal bacteremia, and in very low birth weight infants the risk of infection with *candida* or liphophilic fungus such as *Malasezzia furfur* is also increased (307–310). All tubing used to administer blood, blood products or lipid emulsions should be replaced within 24 hours of administering the infusion. Infusions of lipid-containing solutions should be completed within 24 hours and blood or blood-products within 4 hours.

One port should be designated exclusively for parenteral nutrition if a multi-lumen catheter is used (51,290).

Accuracy of Diagnosis

Accurate diagnoses are essential to support correct remediation. Perhaps the most important step toward accuracy is avoiding false-positive cultures. Antiseptic skin preparation is essential along with aseptic cleansing of the catheter hub. Coagulase negative staphylococcus, a normal skin/oral flora, can lead to false-positive blood cultures. False-negative blood cultures also occur when an inadequate amount of specimen is obtained (311). For example, one mL is the optimal sample volume for blood culture in the NICU. Obtaining two blood cultures with each sepsis evaluation improves the accuracy of diagnosis and allows better antibiotic decisions (41). One culture can be obtained through the central line and the other culture from a peripheral puncture (42).

Equipment Care

Every piece of equipment used in the NICU is a potential source of infection, directly or indirectly. Ventilators, monitor leads, radiology cassettes, thermometers, isolettes, breast pumps and antiseptic solutions are examples (264). All equipment in direct contact with skin or mucous membranes of newborns must be decontaminated with a high-level disinfectant or sterilized between patients. Equipment should be reserved for one patient or decontaminated with alcohol between patients.

Organisms such as *pseudomonas, serratia* and *flavobacterium* are prevalent in the inanimate environment and grow readily at room temperature in water and moist environments such as incubators, humidifier reservoirs and respiratory nebulizers and tubing. Respiratory support equipment such as resuscitation bags, masks, and laryngoscope blades should be decontaminated and replaced periodically according to the Centers for Disease Control's guidelines (www.cdc.gov).

Staffing and Nursery Design

Outbreak investigations clearly associate infection and understaffing or overcrowding, probably because of poor adherence to hand hygiene (170,266). For example, when results are adjusted for confounding factors, the patient-to-nurse ratio remains a significant independent risk factor for bloodstream infection, implying that nursing staff reduction below a critical threshold may jeopardize adequate catheter care (see also Chapter 6) (312).

In one example, during an outbreak of *Enterobacter cloacae* in a neonatal intensive care unit, the daily number of hospitalized neonates was above the maximum capacity of the unit. The number of staff was substantially less than the number recommended and there was a reduced attention to basic infection control measures. Adherence to hand hygiene practices before device contact declined to 25% during the workload peak, but increased to 70% after the end of the understaffing and overcrowding (313). Such results not only demonstrate the link between workload and infection, but they also highlight the intermediate cause of antimicrobial spread: poor adherence to hand hygiene policies.

Understaffing and overcrowding, inexperienced staff and float-pool nurses appear to increase the risk of cross-contamination of organisms (314). Nursery design should provide adequate space for care of the infant and necessary equipment as well as strategically placed sinks. The American Academy of Pediatrics recommends that NICUs have a minimum of 150 net square feet of floor space per infant, with at least 6 feet between incubators and 8-foot aisles (315). There should be at least one sink for every three to four patients. Ventilation in the NICU should provide positive pressure airflow from a ceiling entry to a floor return, pulling dust downward and out. There should be a minimum of 6 to 10 air changes per hour. One nurse for every one to two patients is recommended.

Educational Programs and Feedback to Healthcare Workers

Education of the entire health care team is essential to success in reducing healthcare-associated infection in pre-term infants. To an important degree, preventing hospital-acquired infection depends on influencing and changing the unit culture. Where infection rates are low, the staff tends to be aware and proud of their success. They believe infections are preventable, and are willing to invest the necessary time and effort to insure that result. Where staff do not understand the importance of new procedures, change is not possible. Educational programs teach staff how and why new practices minimize the risk of infection. They include hand washing, catheter care, accurate diagnosis of bloodstream, and standard and enhanced transmission-based precautions. The entire health care team learns the best way to avoid cross-colonization and infection. Educational efforts include developing infection control policies and procedures, staff education modules, skills laboratories and competency tests.

Compliance with the new procedures improves when staff has adequate training, adequate supplies, and ongoing programs to encourage and monitor implementation. Infection control is everyone's responsibility. Staff education must be persistent, but can be offered as infrequently as twice a year for full-time staff and at the beginning of each resident rotation. Feedback needs to be part of all educational activities. Widespread staff involvement and acceptance require frequent communications. Disseminate information through e-mail, in-service sessions, regularly scheduled staff meetings, newsletters, open discussion and posters.

Role of the Infection Control Practitioner

Benchmarking and reliance on well-supported procedures is essential to build institutional confidence in the effectiveness of specific practices that cut infection rates. The ICP and epidemiologist must keep abreast of the most current research and take steps to use those practices that have proved effective. The presence of the infection control practitioner in the NICU increases awareness of the importance of basic infection control principles at the same time it helps control health care related infections and the ICP's presence helps focus medicine, nursing, respiratory therapy and pharmacy on their need to be involved in infection control by providing a line of communication between and among the disciplines. The ICP serves as a resource not only for the medical and nursing staff, but also the consultants, management, ancillary staff and families.

A significant element of effective control of health-care related infections is the understanding that continuing vigilance and effort rather than single interventions are required, and depend on the creation of an effective control system, as well as planned interventions in many disciplines over an extended time frame. Four key habits integral to preventing health-care related infections were identified by the Vermont Oxford National Evidenced-Based Quality Improvement Collaborative for Neonatology in 2003: (1) the habit for change, (2) the habit of systems thinking, (3) the habit of collaborative learning, and (4) the habit of evidenced-based medicine (316).

An additional success factor in infection control is staff conviction regarding the importance of changing practices to improve outcomes. In many cases, small changes can affect the larger process and lead to effective strategies for lowering infection rates. Sharing experiences with other centers (NICUs) is critically important to encourage the team, keep the process exciting and push the improvement process forward. Evidence from randomized trials is not always available. Collaborating with an infection control expert helps place neonatal literature review in the larger framework of healthcare-related infections in medical care. Benchmarking offers the best opportunity to find which practices have the greatest impact. The number one finding common to all benchmark sites in the Vermont Oxford study was the practitioners' attitude regarding their role in lowering infection rates. Practitioners that believe infection rates can be lowered by changes in practice had the most success and the lowest infection rates.

ICPs are able to assist staff in cohorting patients as necessary and to insure that proper isolation precautions are instituted; they review current literature to share with staff members, and are available to give timely feedback related to infection control practice issues in the clinical setting. ICPs play an integral part in reviewing policies and procedures and standardizing patient care, and they help to change the culture of the NICU so that physicians, nurses and other staff members are aware of the vital importance of infection control.

REFERENCES

1. Lopez Sastre JB, Coto Cotallo D and Fernandez Colomer B. Neonatal sepsis of nosocomial origin: an epidemiological study from the "Grupo de Hospitales Castrillo". *J Perinat Med* 2002; 30:149–57
2. Lyytikainen O, Lumio J, Sarkkinen H, Kolho E, Kostiala A and Ruutu P. Nosocomial bloodstream infections in Finnish hospitals during 1999–2000. *Clin Infect Dis* 2002;35:e14–9
3. Newman MJ. Neonatal intensive care unit: reservoirs of nosocomial pathogens. *West Afr J Med* 2002;21:310–2
4. Samanci N, Ovali F, Akdogan Z and Dagoglu T. Neonatal septicemia in a neonatal intensive care unit. Results of four years. *Turk J Pediatr* 1997;39:185–93
5. Sinha A, Yokoe D and Platt R. Epidemiology of neonatal infections: experience during and after hospitalization. *Pediatr Infect Dis J* 2003;22:244–51
6. Stoll BJH, N.Fanaroff, A. A. et. al. Late-onset sepsis in very low birth weight neonates: the experience of the NICHD Neonatal Research Network. *Pediatrics* 2002;110:285–91
7. Public health focus: Surveillance, prevention, and control of nosocomial infections. *Morb Mortal Wkly Rep* 1992;41: 783–787
8. Stone PW LE, Kawar LN. A systematic audit of economic evidence linking nosocomial infections and infection control interventions:1990–2000. *Am J Infect Control* 2002;30:145–152

9. Burke JP. Patient safety: infection control—a problem for patient safety. *N Engl J Med* 2003;348:651–6
10. Eggimann P, Pittet D. Infection control in ICU. *Chest* 2001;120: 2059–2093
11. Sohn AH, Garrett DO, Sinkowitz-Cochran RL, et al. Prevalence of nosocomial infections in neonatal intensive care unit patients: Results from the first national point-prevalence survey. *J Pediatr* 2001;139:821–7
12. National Nosocomial Infections Surveillance (NNIS) System Report, data summary from January 1992 through June 2004, issued October 2004. *Am J Infect Control* 2004;32:470–85
13. Gaynes RP, Edwards, JR, Jarvis, et al. Nosocomial infections in high-risk nurseries in the United States. *Pediatrics* 1996:357–381
14. Richards MJ, Edwards JR, Culver DH and Gaynes RP. Nosocomial infections in pediatric intensive care units in the United States. National Nosocomial Infections Surveillance System. *Pediatrics* 1999;103:e39
15. Gaynes RP, Martone WJ, Culver DH, et al. Comparison of rates of nosocomial infections in neonatal intensive care units in the United States. National Nosocomial Infections Surveillance System. *Am J Med* 1991;91:192S–196S
16. Rodriguez Cervilla J, Fraga JM, Garcia Riestra C, Fernandez Lorenzo JR and Martinez Soto I. [Neonatal sepsis: epidemiologic indicators and relation to birth weight and length of hospitalization time]. *An Esp Pediatr* 1998;48:401–8
17. Stover BH, Shulman ST, Bratcher DF, Brady MT, Levine GL and Jarvis WR. Nosocomial infection rates in US children's hospitals' neonatal and pediatric intensive care units. *Am J Infect Control* 2001;29:152–7
18. Hemming VG, Overall JC, Jr. and Britt MR. Nosocomial infections in a newborn intensive-care unit. Results of forty-one months of surveillance. *N Engl J Med* 1976;294:1310–6
19. Townsend TR, Wenzel RP. Nosocomial bloodstream infections in a newborn intensive care unit: a case-matched control study of morbidity, mortality and risk. *Am J Epidemiol* 1981;114:73–80
20. Ferguson JK, Gill A. Risk-stratified nosocomial infection surveillance in a neonatal intensive care unit: report on 24 months of surveillance. *J Paediatr Child Health* 1996;32:525–31
21. Campins M, Vaque J, Rossello J, et al. Nosocomial infections in pediatric patients: a prevalence study in Spanish hospitals. EPINE Working Group. *Am J Infect Control* 1993;21:58–63
22. Raymond J. [Epidemiology of nosocomial infections in pediatrics]. *Pathol Biol* (Paris) 2000;48:879–84
23. Stoll BJ, Hansen, N, Fanaroff A.A. Changes in pathogens causing early-onset sepsis in very-low-borth weight infants. *N Engl J Med* 2002;347:240–247
24. Fridkin SK, Gaynes RP. Antimicrobial resistance in intensive care units. *Clin Chest Med* 1999;20:303–16, viii
25. Nambiar S, Singh N. Change in epidemiology of health care-associated infections in a neonatal intensive care unit. *Pediatr Infect Dis J* 2002;21:839–42
26. Hervas JA, Ballesteros F, Alomar A, Gil J, Benedi VJ and Alberti S. Increase of Enterobacter in neonatal sepsis: a twenty-two-year study. *Pediatr Infect Dis J* 2001;20:134–40
27. Loiwal V, Kumar A, Gupta P, Gomber S and Ramachandran VG. Enterobacter aerogenes outbreak in a neonatal intensive care unit. *Pediatr Int* 1999;41:157–61
28. Bhutta ZA, Naqvi SH, Muzaffar T and Farooqui BJ. Neonatal sepsis in Pakistan. Presentation and pathogens. *Acta Paediatr Scand* 1991;80:596–601
29. Halder D, Haque ME, Zabidi MH and Kamaruzzaman A. Nosocomial bacterial sepsis in babies weighing 1000–1499 g in Kelantan. *Med J Malaysia* 1999;54:52–7
30. Joshi SG, Ghole VS and Niphadkar KB. Neonatal Gram-negative bacteremia. *Indian J Pediatr* 2000;67:27–32
31. Karpuch J, Goldberg M and Kohelet D. Neonatal bacteremia. A 4-year prospective study. *Isr J Med Sci* 1983;19:963–6
32. Maimon-Greenwald M, Leibovitz E, Maimon N, Peled N and Dagan R. [Gram-negative enteric bacteremia in children in the Negev (1989–1994)]. *Harefuah* 1997;133:275–81, 335
33. Pegues DA, Arathoon EG, Samayoa B, et al. Epidemic Gram-negative bacteremia in a neonatal intensive care unit in Guatemala. *Am J Infect Control* 1994;22:163–71
34. Greenberg D, Shinwell ES, Yagupsky P, et al. A prospective study of neonatal sepsis and meningitis in southern Israel. *Pediatr Infect Dis J* 1997;16:768–73

35. Mahieu LM, De Dooy JJ, Cossey VR, et al. Internal and external validation of the NOSEP prediction score for nosocomial sepsis in neonates. *Crit Care Med* 2002;30:1459–66

36. Singh-Naz N, Sprague BM, Patel KM and Pollack MM. Risk assessment and standardized nosocomial infection rate in critically ill children. *Crit Care Med* 2000;28:2069–75

37. Clinical prediction of serious bacterial infections in young infants in developing countries. The WHO Young Infants Study Group. *Pediatr Infect Dis J* 1999;18:S23–31

38. Weinstein JW, Mazon D, Pantelick E, Reagan-Cirincione P, Dembry LM and Hierholzer WJ, Jr. A decade of prevalence surveys in a tertiary-care center: trends in nosocomial infection rates, device utilization, and patient acuity. *Infect Control Hosp Epidemiol* 1999;20:543–8

39. Garner JS, Jarvis, W.J. Emori, T.G, Horan, T.C, Hughees, J.M. CDC definitions for nosocomial infections. *Am J Infect Control* 1988;15:128–140

40. Craft A, Finer N. Nosocomial coagulase negative staphylococcal (CoNS) catheter-related sepsis in preterm infants: definition, diagnosis, prophylaxis, and prevention. *J Perinatol* 2001;21:186–92

41. Tokars JI. Predictive value of blood cultures positive for coagulase-negative staphylococci: implications for patient care and health care quality assurance. *Clin Infect Dis* 2004;39:333–41

42. Kilbride HW, Powers R, Wirtschafter DD, et al. Evaluation and development of potentially better practices to prevent neonatal nosocomial bacteremia. *Pediatrics* 2003;111:e504–18

43. Emori TG, Edwards JR, Culver DH, et al. Accuracy of reporting nosocomial infections in intensive-care-unit patients to the National Nosocomial Infections Surveillance System: a pilot study. *Infect Control Hosp Epidemiol* 1998;19:308–16

44. Pollack MM, Koch MA, Bartel DA, et al. A comparison of neonatal mortality risk prediction models in very low birth weight infants. *Pediatrics* 2000;105:1051–7

45. Wright J, Stover BH, Wilkerson S and Bratcher D. Expanding the infection control team: development of the infection control liaison position for the neonatal intensive care unit. *Am J Infect Control* 2002;30:174–8

46. Bishop-Kurylo D. The clinical experience of continuous quality improvement in the neonatal intensive care unit. *J Perinat Neonatal Nurs* 1998;12:51–7

47. Jarvis WR, Robles B. Nosocomial infections in pediatric patients. *Adv Pediatr Infect Dis* 1996;12:243–95

48. Auriti C, Maccallini A, Di Liso G, Di Ciommo V, Ronchetti MP and Orzalesi M. Risk factors for nosocomial infections in a neonatal intensive-care unit. *J Hosp Infect* 2003;53:25–30

49. Moro ML, De Toni A, Stolfi I, Carrieri MP, Braga M and Zunin C. Risk factors for nosocomial sepsis in newborn intensive and intermediate care units. *Eur J Pediatr* 1996;155:315–22

50. Guzman JM, Jaraba MP, De La Torre MJ, et al. Parenteral nutrition and immature neonates. Comparative study of neonates weighing under 1000 and 1000–1250 g at birth. *Early Hum Dev* 2001;65 Suppl:S133–44

51. Snydman DR, Murray SA, Kornfeld SJ, Majka JA and Ellis CA. Total parenteral nutrition-related infections. Prospective epidemiologic study using semiquantitative methods. *Am J Med* 1982;73:695–9

52. Gray PH, Rodwell RL. Neonatal neutropenia associated with maternal hypertension poses a risk for nosocomial infection. *Eur J Pediatr* 1999;158:71–3

53. Stoll BJ, Temprosa M, Tyson JE, et al. Dexamethasone therapy increases infection in very low birth weight infants. *Pediatrics* 1999;104:e63

54. Wittrock B, Lavin MA, Pierry D, Thomson R and Wurtz R. Parents as a vector for nosocomial infection in the neonatal intensive care unit. *Infect Control Hosp Epidemiol* 2001;22:472

55. Olive DM, Bean P. Principles and applications of methods for DNA-based typing of microbial organisms. *J Clin Microbiol* 1999;37:1661–9

56. Eduardo S, Augusto, C. Nosocomial infection in neonatology: In search of the best score, in search of an oracle. *Crit Care Med* 2002;2002:1660–1661

57. Carrieri MP, Stolfi I and Moro ML. Intercenter variability and time of onset: two crucial issues in the analysis of risk factors for nosocomial sepsis. *Pediatr Infect Dis J* 2003;22:599–609

58. Kawagoe JY, Segre CA, Pereira CR, Cardoso MF, Silva CV and Fukushima JT. Risk factors for nosocomial infections in critically ill newborns: a 5-year prospective cohort study. *Am J Infect Control* 2001;29:109–14

59. Costa SF, Miceli MH and Anaissie EJ. Mucosa or skin as source of coagulase-negative staphylococcal bacteraemia? *Lancet Infect Dis* 2004;4:278–86

60. Rubin LG, Sanchez PJ, Siegel J, Levine G, Saiman L and Jarvis WR. Evaluation and treatment of neonates with suspected late-onset sepsis: a survey of neonatologists' practices. *Pediatrics* 2002;110:e42

61. Urrea M, Pons M, Serra M, Latorre C and Palomeque A. Prospective incidence study of nosocomial infections in a pediatric intensive care unit. *Pediatr Infect Dis J* 2003;22:490–4

62. Isaacs D. A ten year, multicentre study of coagulase negative staphylococcal infections in Australasian neonatal units. *Arch Dis Child Fetal Neonatal Ed* 2003;88:F89–93

63. Karlowicz MG, Buescher ES and Surka AE. Fulminant late-onset sepsis in a neonatal intensive care unit, 1988–1997, and the impact of avoiding empiric vancomycin therapy. *Pediatrics* 2000;106:1387–90

64. Chapman RL, Faix RG. Persistent bacteremia and outcome in late onset infection among infants in a neonatal intensive care unit. *Pediatr Infect Dis J* 2003;22:17–21

65. Eggink BH, Rowen JL. Primary osteomyelitis and suppurative arthritis caused by coagulase-negative staphylococci in a preterm neonate. *Pediatr Infect Dis J* 2003;22:572–3

66. Krediet TG, Jones ME, Janssen K, Gerards LJ and Fleer A. Prevalence of molecular types and mecA gene carriage of coagulase-negative Staphylococci in a neonatal intensive care unit: relation to nosocomial septicemia. *J Clin Microbiol* 2001;39:3376–8

67. Persson E, Trollfors B, Brandberg LL and Tessin I. Septicaemia and meningitis in neonates and during early infancy in the Goteborg area of Sweden. *Acta Paediatr* 2002;91:1087–92

68. Gonzalez BE, Mercado CK, Johnson L, Brodsky NL and Bhandari V. Early markers of late-onset sepsis in premature neonates: clinical, hematological and cytokine profile. *J Perinat Med* 2003;31:60–8

69. Soll RF, Edwards WH. Emollient ointment for preventing infection in preterm infants. *Cochrane Database Syst Rev* 2000:CD001150

70. Van Der Zwet WC, Debets-Ossenkopp YJ, Reinders E, et al. Nosocomial spread of a Staphylococcus capitis strain with heteroresistance to vancomycin in a neonatal intensive care unit. *J Clin Microbiol* 2002;40:2520–5

71. Raimundo O, Heussler H, Bruhn JB, et al. Molecular epidemiology of coagulase-negative staphylococcal bacteraemia in a newborn intensive care unit. *J Hosp Infect* 2002;51:33–42

72. Stoll BJ, Hansen N, Fanaroff AA, et al. To tap or not to tap: high likelihood of meningitis without sepsis among very low birth weight infants. *Pediatrics* 2004;113:1181–6

73. Das I, Gray J. Enterococcal bacteremia in children: a review of seventy-five episodes in a pediatric hospital. *Pediatr Infect Dis J* 1998;17:1154–8

74. Ashkenazi S, Leibovici L, Churi C, Drucker M, Konisberger H and Samra Z. Childhood bacteremia in Israel: causes, age relation, predisposing factors and source. *Isr J Med Sci* 1994;30:610–6

75. Bilikova E, Babela R and Krcmery V. Nosocomial enterococcal bacteremia in children. *Pediatrics* 2003;111:445–6

76. Vermaat JH, Rosebrugh E, Ford-Jones EL, Ciano J, Kobayashi J and Miller G. An epidemiologic study of nosocomial infections in a pediatric long-term care facility. *Am J Infect Control* 1993;21:183–8

77. Christie C, Hammond J, Reising S and Evans-Patterson J. Clinical and molecular epidemiology of enterococcal bacteremia in a pediatric teaching hospital. *J Pediatr* 1994;125:392–9

78. McNeeley DF, Saint-Louis F and Noel GJ. Neonatal enterococcal bacteremia: an increasingly frequent event with potentially untreatable pathogens. *Pediatr Infect Dis J* 1996;15:800–5

79. Dobson SR, Baker CJ. Enterococcal sepsis in neonates: features by age at onset and occurrence of focal infection. *Pediatrics* 1990;85:165–71

80. Anwer SK, Mustafa S, Pariyani S, Ashraf S and Taufiq KM. Neonatal sepsis: an etiological study. *J Pak Med Assoc* 2000;50:91–4

81. Berger A, Salzer HR, Weninger M, Sageder B and Aspock C. Septicaemia in an Austrian neonatal intensive care unit: a 7-year analysis. *Acta Paediatr* 1998;87:1066–9

82. Chandrashekar MR, Rathish KC and Nagesha CN. Reservoirs of nosocomial pathogens in neonatal intensive care unit. *J Indian Med Assoc* 1997;95:72–4, 77

83. Luginbuhl LM, Rotbart HA, Facklam RR, Roe MH and Elliot JA. Neonatal enterococcal sepsis: case-control study and description of an outbreak. *Pediatr Infect Dis J* 1987;6:1022–6

84. Thompson PJ, Greenough A, Hird MF, Philpott-Howard J and Gamsu HR. Nosocomial bacterial infections in very low birth weight infants. *Eur J Pediatr* 1992;151:451–4

85. Weisman LE, Stoll BJ, Kueser TJ, et al. Intravenous immune globulin prophylaxis of late-onset sepsis in premature neonates. *J Pediatr* 1994;125:922–30

86. Stoll BJ, Gordon T, Korones SB, et al. Late-onset sepsis in very low birth weight neonates: a report from the National Institute of Child Health and Human Development Neonatal Research Network. *J Pediatr* 1996;129:63–71

87. Yuce AK, M; Zeynep, G; Yulug, N. Vancomycin-resistant enterococci in neonates. *Scand J Infect Dis* 2001;33:803–805

88. Singh-Naz N, Rakowsky A, Cantwell E, Patel KM and Campos JM. Nosocomial enterococcal infections in children. *J Infect* 2000;40:145–9

89. Shah SS, Ehrenkranz, R.A, Gallagher, P.G. Increasing incidence of Gram-negative rod bacteremia in a newborn intensive care unit. *Pediatr Infect Dis J* 1999;18:591–595

90. Hughes JR, Newbould M, du Vivier AW and Greenough A. Fatal Pseudomonas septicemia and vasculitis in a premature infant. *Pediatr Dermatol* 1998;15:122–4

91. McKee KT, Jr., Cotton RB, Stratton CW, et al. Nursery epidemic due to multiply-resistant Klebsiella pneumoniae: epidemiologic setting and impact on perinatal health care delivery. *Infect Control* 1982;3:150–6

92. Mishra A, Mishra S, Jaganath G, Mittal RK, Gupta PK and Patra DP. Acinetobacter sepsis in newborns. *Indian Pediatr* 1998;35:27–32

93. Donowitz LG, Marsik FJ, Fisher KA and Wenzel RP. Contaminated breast milk: A source of Klebsiella bacteremia in a newborn intensive care unit. *Rev Infect Dis* 1981;3:716–20

94. Stoll BJ, Hansen N, Fanaroff AA and Lemons JA. Enterobacter sakazakii is a rare cause of neonatal septicemia or meningitis in VLBW infants. *J Pediatr* 2004;144:821–3

95. Enterobacter sakazakii infections associated with the use of powdered infant formula—Tennessee, 2001. *MMWR Morb Mortal Wkly Rep* 2002;51:297–300

96. From the Centers for Disease Control and Prevention. Enterobacter sakazakii infections associated with the use of powdered infant formula—Tennessee, 2001. *Jama* 2002;287:2204–5

97. Arseni A, Malamou-Ladas E, Koutsia C, Xanthou M and Trikka E. Outbreak of colonization of neonates with Enterobacter sakazakii. *J Hosp Infect* 1987;9:143–50

98. Klein MW. Pathogensis of brain abscess caused by citrobacter diversus or enterobacter sakazakii. *Pedi Infect Dis J* 1988;7:891–2

99. Gallagher PG, Ball WS. Cerebral infarctions due to CNS infection with Enterobacter sakazakii. *Pediatr Radiol* 1991;21:135–6

100. Burdette JH, Santos C. Enterobacter sakazakii brain abscess in the neonate: the importance of neuroradiologic imaging. *Pediatr Radiol* 2000;30:33–4

101. van Acker J, de Smet F, Muyldermans G, Bougatef A, Naessens A and Lauwers S. Outbreak of necrotizing enterocolitis associated with Enterobacter sakazakii in powdered milk formula. *J Clin Microbiol* 2001;39:293–7

102. Ries M, Harms D and Scharf J. [Multiple cerebral infarcts with resulting multicystic encephalomalacia in a premature infant with Enterobacter sakazakii meningitis]. *Klin Padiatr* 1994;206:184–6

103. Simmons BP, Gelfand MS, Haas M, Metts L and Ferguson J. Enterobacter sakazakii infections in neonates associated with intrinsic contamination of a powdered infant formula. *Infect Control Hosp Epidemiol* 1989;10:398–401

104. Biering G, Karlsson S, Clark NC, Jonsdottir KE, Ludvigsson P and Steingrimsson O. Three cases of neonatal meningitis caused by Enterobacter sakazakii in powdered milk. *J Clin Microbiol* 1989;27:2054–6

105. Muytjens HL, Kollee LA. Enterobacter sakazakii meningitis in neonates: causative role of formula? *Pediatr Infect Dis J* 1990;9:372–3

106. Block C, Peleg O, Minster N, et al. Cluster of neonatal infections in Jerusalem due to unusual biochemical variant of Enterobacter sakazakii. *Eur J Clin Microbiol Infect Dis* 2002;21:613–6

107. Muytjens HL, Kollee LA. Neonatal meningitis due to Enterobacter sakazakii. *Tijdschr Kindergeneeskd* 1982;50:110–2

108. Saiman L, Ludington E, Pfaller M, et al. Risk factors for candidemia in Neonatal Intensive Care Unit patients. The National Epidemiology of Mycosis Survey study group. *Pediatr Infect Dis J* 2000;19:319–24

109. Leibovitz E, Flidel-Rimon O, Juster-Reicher A, et al. Sepsis at a neonatal intensive care unit: a four-year retrospective study (1989–1992). *Isr J Med Sci* 1997;33:734–8

110. Leibovitz E. Neonatal candidosis: clinical picture, management controversies and consensus, and new therapeutic options. *J Antimicrob Chem* 2002;49,Suppl.S1;.69–73

111. Huang YC, Li CC, Lin TY, et al. Association of fungal colonization and invasive disease in very low birth weight infants. *Pediatr Infect Dis J* 1998;17:819–22

112. el-Mohandes AE, Johnson-Robbins L, Keiser JF, Simmens SJ and Aure MV. Incidence of Candida parapsilosis colonization in an intensive care nursery population and its association with invasive fungal disease. *Pediatr Infect Dis J* 1994;13:520–4

113. Pappu-Katikaneni LD, Rao KP and Banister E. Gastrointestinal colonization with yeast species and Candida septicemia in very low birth weight infants. *Mycoses* 1990;33:20–3

114. Cole GT, Lynn KT and Seshan KR. An animal model for oropharyngeal, esophageal and gastric candidosis. *Mycoses* 1990;33:7–19

115. Johnson DE, Thompson, T.R., Green, T.P., Ferrieri, P. Systemic candidiasis in very low-birth-weight infants (<1500 grams). *Pediatrics* 1984;73:138–143

116. Makhoul IR, Kassis, I., Smolkin, T., Tamir, A, Sujov, P. Review of 49 neonates with acquired fungal sepsis: further characterization. *Pediatrics* 2001;107:61–66

117. El-Masry FAY, Neal, T,J., Subhedar, N,V.,. Risk factors for invasive fungal infection in neonates. *Acta Paediatr* 2002;91:198–202.

118. Faix RG, Kovarik, S.M, Shaw, T.R., Johnson, R.V. Mucocutaneous and invasive candidiasis among very low birth weight (<1500 grams) infants in intensive care nurseries: a prospective study. *Pediatrics* 1989;83:101–117

119. Kennedy MJ VP. Ecology of Candida albicans gut colonization: inhibition of Candida adhesion, colonization, and dissemination from the gastrointestinal tract by bacterial antagonism. *Infect Immun* 1985;49:654–663.

120. Rowen JL, Atkins, J.T, Levy, M.L, Baer, S,C, Baker, C.J. Invasive fungal dermatitis in the =1000-gram neonate. *Pediatrics* 1995;95:682–687

121. Benjamin DK, Jr., Ross K, McKinney RE, Jr., Benjamin DK, Auten R and Fisher RG. When to suspect fungal infection in neonates: A clinical comparison of Candida albicans and Candida parapsilosis fungemia with coagulase-negative staphylococcal bacteremia. *Pediatrics* 2000;106:712–8

122. Lupetti A, Tavanti A, Davini P, et al. Horizontal transmission of Candida parapsilosis candidemia in a neonatal intensive care unit. *J Clin Microbiol* 2002;40:2363–9

123. Saxen H, Virtanen M, Carlson P, et al. Neonatal Candida parapsilosis outbreak with a high case fatality rate. *Pediatr Infect Dis J* 1995;14:776–81

124. Huang YC LT, Leu HS, et al.1999;27:97–102. Outbreak of Candida parapsilosis fungemia in neonatal intensive care units: clinical implication and genotyping analysis. *Infection* 1999;27:97–102

125. Waggoner-Fountain LA, Walker MW, Hollis RJ, et al. Vertical and horizontal transmission of unique Candida species to premature newborns. *Clin Infect Dis* 1996;22:803–8

126. Benjamin DK, Jr., DeLong ER, Steinbach WJ, Cotton CM, Walsh TJ and Clark RH. Empirical therapy for neonatal candidemia in very low birth weight infants. *Pediatrics* 2003;112:543–7

127. Ahtonen P, Lehtonen OP, Kero P, Tunnela E and Havu V. Malassezia furfur colonization of neonates in an intensive care unit. *Mycoses* 1990;33:543–7

128. Bell LM, Alpert G, Slight PH and Campos JM. Malassezia furfur skin colonization in infancy. *Infect Control Hosp Epidemiol* 1988;9:151–3

129. Long JG, Keyserling HL. Catheter-related infection in infants due to an unusual lipophilic yeast—Malassezia furfur. *Pediatrics* 1985;76:896–900

130. Shattuck KE, Cochran CK, Zabransky RJ, Pasarell L, Davis JC and Malloy MH. Colonization and infection associated with Malassezia and Candida species in a neonatal unit. *J Hosp Infect* 1996;34:123–9

131. Kessler AT, Kourtis AP and Simon N. Peripheral thromboembolism associated with Malassezia furfur sepsis. *Pediatr Infect Dis J* 2002;21:356–7

132. Weber S, Wilkinson, A.R, Lindsell, D, Hope, P.L, Dobson, S.R.M, Issacs D.. Neonatal pneumonia. *Arch Dis Child* 1990;65:207–211

133. Cordero L, Coley BD, Hogan MJ and Ayers LW. Radiological pulmonary changes during Gram-negative bacillary nosocomial bloodstream infection in premature infants. *J Perinatol* 1998; 18:291–6

134. Cordero L, Sananes M, Coley B, Hogan M, Gelman M and Ayers LW. Ventilator-associated pneumonia in very low-birth-weight infants at the time of nosocomial bloodstream infection and during airway colonization with Pseudomonas aeruginosa. *Am J Infect Control* 2000;28:333–9

135. Morar P, Singh V, Makura Z, et al. Differing pathways of lower airway colonization and infection according to mode of ventilation (endotracheal vs tracheotomy). *Arch Otolaryngol Head Neck Surg* 2002;128:1061–6

136. Cordero L, Davis, K, Morehead S, Ayers, L.W. Factors affecting microbial colonization of the trachea and specticemia in mechanically ventilated neonates. *Respir Care* 1993;38:1355–1363

137. Cordero L, Ayers LW and Davis K. Neonatal airway colonization with Gram-negative bacilli: association with severity of bronchopulmonary dysplasia. *Pediatr Infect Dis J* 1997;16:18–23

138. Cordero L, Sananes M and Ayers LW. Failure of systemic antibiotics to eradicate Gram-negative bacilli from the airway of mechanically ventilated very low-birth-weight infants. *Am J Infect Control* 2000;28:286–90

139. Morar P, Makura Z, Jones A, et al. Topical antibiotics on tracheostoma prevents exogenous colonization and infection of lower airways in children. *Chest* 2000;117:513–8

140. Leigh L, Stoll BJ, Rahman M and McGowan J, Jr. Pseudomonas aeruginosa infection in very low birth weight infants: a case-control study. *Pediatr Infect Dis J* 1995;14:367–71

141. Moolenaar RL, Crutcher, M, San Joaquin, VH, Sewell, L.V, Hutwagner, L.C, Carson, L.A, Robinson, D.A, Smithee, L.M. K, Jarvis, W.R. A prolonged outbreak of Pesudomonas aeruginosa in a neonate intensive care unit: Did Staff's fingernail's paly a role in disease transmission? *Infec It Control Hosp Epidemiol.* 2000;21:80–65

142. Deppe AS, Kelly, W, thoi, L.L, Chudy, J.H, Longfield, R.N. Ducey, J.P, Truit, C.L. Antopol, M.R. Incidence of colonization, nosocomial pneumonia and mortality in critically ill patients using a trach care closed-suction system versus an open—suction system: propsective, randomized study. *Crit Care Med* 1990;18: 1389–1393

143. Johnson KL, Kearney, P.A, Johson, S.B, Niblett, J.B, MacMillan, N.L, MacClain, R.E. Closed versus open endotracheal suctioning: cots and physiologic consequences. *Crit Care Med* 1994;22: 658–666

144. Singh N, Leger, MML., Campos, C. Use of REP-PCR in Confirming Spread of Vancomycin Resistant Enterococcus faecium among Hospitalized Neonates. *Interscience Conference on Antimicrobial agents and chemotherapy,* 2002

145. Cordero L, Sananes M and Ayers LW. Comparison of a closed (Trach Care MAC) with an open endotracheal suction system in small premature infants. *J Perinatol* 2000;20:151–6

146. Tablan OC, Anderson LJ, Besser R, Bridges C and Hajjeh R. Guidelines for preventing health-care—associated pneumonia, 2003: recommendations of CDC and the Healthcare Infection Control Practices Advisory Committee. *MMWR Recomm Rep* 2004;53:1–36

147. Foca M, Jakob K, Whittier S, et al. Endemic Pseudomonas aeruginosa infection in a neonatal intensive care unit. *N Engl J Med* 2000;343:695–700

148. Grundmann H, Kropec A, Hartung D, Berner R and Daschner F. Pseudomonas aeruginosa in a neonatal intensive care unit: reservoirs and ecology of the nosocomial pathogen. *J Infect Dis* 1993;168:943–7

149. Becks VE, Lorenzoni, N.E. Pseudomonas aeruginosa outbreak in a neonatal intensive care unit: a possible link to contaiminated hand lotion. *Am J Infect Control* 1995;23:396–398

150. Matthias V, Manfred, V, Gerd, D. Sepsis in a newborn due to Pseudomonas aeruginosa from a conatminated tub bath. *N Engl J Med* 2001;345:378–379

151. Maherzi M, Guignard JP and Torrado A. Urinary tract infection in high-risk newborn infants. *Pediatrics* 1978;62:521–3

152. Edelmann CM, Jr., Ogwo JE, Fine BP and Martinez AB. The prevalence of bacteriuria in full-term and premature newborn infants. *J Pediatr* 1973;82:125–32

153. Wahl AM, R., Sprague, B. Singh, N. Predictors of healthcare-associated urinary tract infections in high-risk neonates and the association of antimicrobial resistance. *Society of Pediatric Research* 2004

154. Bauer S, Eliakim A, Pomeranz A, et al. Urinary tract infection in very low birth weight preterm infants. *Pediatr Infect Dis J* 2003; 22:426–30

155. Siegel J, Levine G, Herchline, T, Botelho C, Jarvis W, Goldmann D. Prevalence (PRVE) of antimicrobial resistant bacteria (AMRB) in Prevention Network (PPN) intensive care units. *Infectious Disease Society of America* 2001

156. Back NA, Linnemann CC, Jr., Staneck JL and Kotagal UR. Control of methicillin-resistant Staphylococcus aureus in a neonatal intensive-care unit: use of intensive microbiologic surveillance and mupirocin. *Infect Control Hosp Epidemiol* 1996;17:227–31

157. Zafar AB, Butler RC, Reese DJ, Gaydos LA and Mennonna PA. Use of 0.3% triclosan (Bacti-Stat) to eradicate an outbreak of methicillin-resistant Staphylococcus aureus in a neonatal nursery. *Am J Infect Control* 1995;23:200–8

158. Haddad Q, Sobayo EI, Basit OB and Rotimi VO. Outbreak of methicillin-resistant Staphylococcus aureus in a neonatal intensive care unit. *J Hosp Infect* 1993;23:211–22

159. Noel GJ, Kreiswirth BN, Edelson PJ, et al. Multiple methicillin-resistant Staphylococcus aureus strains as a cause for a single outbreak of severe disease in hospitalized neonates. *Pediatr Infect Dis J* 1992;11:184–8

160. Tan KW, Tay L and Lim SH. An outbreak of methicillin-resistant Staphylococcus aureus in a neonatal intensive care unit in Singapore: a 20-month study of clinical characteristics and control. *Singapore Med J* 1994;35:277–82

161. Reboli AC, John JF, Jr. and Levkoff AH. Epidemic methicillin-gentamicin-resistant Staphylococcus aureus in a neonatal intensive care unit. *Am J Dis Child* 1989;143:34–9

162. Nambiar S, Herwaldt LA and Singh N. Outbreak of invasive disease caused by methicillin-resistant Staphylococcus aureus in neonates and prevalence in the neonatal intensive care unit. *Pediatr Crit Care Med* 2003;4:220–6

163. Morel AS, Wu F, Della-Latta P, Cronquist A, Rubenstein D and Saiman L. Nosocomial transmission of methicillin-resistant Staphylococcus aureus from a mother to her preterm quadruplet infants. *Am J Infect Control* 2002;30:170–3

164. Saiman L, O'Keefe M, Graham PL, 3rd, et al. Hospital transmission of community-acquired methicillin-resistant Staphylococcus aureus among postpartum women. *Clin Infect Dis* 2003;37: 1313–9

165. Liu CC, Hor LI, Wu YH, Huang AH, Lin CH and Chuang YC. Investigation and elimination of epidemic methicillin-resistant Staphylococcus aureus in a neonatal intensive care unit. *Zhonghua Min Guo Xiao Er Ke Yi Xue Hui Za Zhi* 1993;34: 285–93

166. Crossley K. Long-term care facilities as sources of antibiotic-resistant nosocomial pathogens. *Curr Opin Infect Dis* 2001;14:455–9

167. Peacock JE, Jr., Moorman DR, Wenzel RP and Mandell GL. Methicillin-resistant Staphylococcus aureus: microbiologic characteristics, antimicrobial susceptibilities, and assessment of virulence of an epidemic strain. *J Infect Dis* 1981;144:575–82

168. Coello R, Jimenez J, Garcia M, et al. Prospective study of infection, colonization and carriage of methicillin-resistant Staphylococcus aureus in an outbreak affecting 990 patients. *Eur J Clin Microbiol Infect Dis* 1994;13:74–81

169. Haley RW, Cushion NB, Tenover FC, et al. Eradication of endemic methicillin-resistant Staphylococcus aureus infections from a neonatal intensive care unit. *J Infect Dis* 1995;171:614–24

170. Muto CA, Jernigan JA, Ostrowsky BE, et al. SHEA guideline for preventing nosocomial transmission of multidrug-resistant strains of Staphylococcus aureus and enterococcus. *Infect Control Hosp Epidemiol* 2003;24:362–86

171. Karchmer TB, Durbin LJ, Simonton BM and Farr BM. Cost-effectiveness of active surveillance cultures and contact/droplet precautions for control of methicillin-resistant Staphylococcus aureus. *J Hosp Infect* 2002;51:126–32

172. Pittet D, Hugonnet S, Harbarth S, et al. Effectiveness of a hospital-wide programme to improve compliance with hand hygiene. Infection Control Programme. *Lancet* 2000;356:1307–12

173. Boyce JM, Jackson MM, Pugliese G, et al. Methicillin-resistant Staphylococcus aureus (MRSA): a briefing for acute care hospitals and nursing facilities. The AHA Technical Panel on Infections Within Hospitals. *Infect Control Hosp Epidemiol* 1994;15:105–15

174. Jernigan JA, Titus MG, Groschel DH, Getchell-White S and Farr BM. Effectiveness of contact isolation during a hospital outbreak of methicillin-resistant Staphylococcus aureus. *Am J Epidemiol* 1996;143:496–504

175. Prevention. CfDCa. Public health dispatch: vancomycin-resistant Staphylococcus aureus-Pennsylvania. *Morb Mortal Wkly Rep* 2002;51:902

176. Lee HK, Lee WG and Cho SR. Clinical and molecular biological analysis of a nosocomial outbreak of vancomycin-resistant enterococci in a neonatal intensive care unit. *Acta Paediatr* 1999; 88:651–4

177. Malik RK, Montecalvo MA, Reale MR, et al. Epidemiology and control of vancomycin-resistant enterococci in a regional neonatal intensive care unit. *Pediatr Infect Dis J* 1999;18: 352–6

178. Singh N, Léger M-M, Campbell J, Short B, Campos, J. Control of Vancomycin Resistant Enterococci in the Neonatal Intensive Care Unit. *Infec Control Hosp Epidemiol*. 2004;In press

179. Belen O, Campos, J, Singh, N. Multiclonal Dissemination of Vancomycin Resistant Enterococci (VRE) in the Neonatal Intensive Care Unit (NICU). *American Society of Microbiology* 2003

180. Franchi D, Climo MW, Wong AH, Edmond MB and Wenzel RP. Seeking vancomycin resistant Staphylococcus aureus among patients with vancomycin-resistant enterococci. *Clin Infect Dis* 1999;29:1566–8

181. Goldrick B. First reported case of VRSA in the United States. *Am J Nurs* 2002;102:17

182. Vancomycin-resistant Staphylococcus aureus—Pennsylvania, 2002. *MMWR Morb Mortal Wkly Rep* 2002;51:902

183. Bartley J. First case of VRSA identified in Michigan. *Infect Control Hosp Epidemiol* 2002;23:480

184. Staphylococcus aureus resistant to vancomycin—United States, 2002. *MMWR Morb Mortal Wkly Rep* 2002;51:565–7

185. Murray BE. Vancomycin-resistant enterococcal infections. *N Engl J Med* 2000;342:710–21

186. Montecalvo MA, Jarvis WR, Uman J, et al. Costs and savings associated with infection control measures that reduced transmission of vancomycin-resistant enterococci in an endemic setting. *Infect Control Hosp Epidemiol* 2001;22:437–42

187. Edmond MB, Ober JF, Dawson JD, Weinbaum DL and Wenzel RP. Vancomycin-resistant enterococcal bacteremia: natural history and attributable mortality. *Clin Infect Dis* 1996;23:1234–9

188. Singh-Naz N, Sleemi A, Pikis A, Patel KM and Campos JM. Vancomycin-resistant Enterococcus faecium colonization in children. *J Clin Microbiol* 1999;37:413–6

189. Lucas GM, Lechtzin N, Puryear DW, Yau LL, Flexner CW and Moore RD. Vancomycin-resistant and vancomycin-susceptible enterococcal bacteremia: comparison of clinical features and outcomes. *Clin Infect Dis* 1998;26:1127–33

190. Byers KE, Anglim AM, Anneski CJ, et al. A hospital epidemic of vancomycin-resistant Enterococcus: risk factors and control. *Infect Control Hosp Epidemiol* 2001;22:140–7

191. Bonten MJ, Hayden MK, Nathan C, et al. Epidemiology of colonisation of patients and environment with vancomycin-resistant enterococci. *Lancet* 1996;348:1615–9

192. Byers KE, Durbin LJ, Simonton BM, Anglim AM, Adal KA and Farr BM. Disinfection of hospital rooms contaminated with vancomycin-resistant Enterococcus faecium. *Infect Control Hosp Epidemiol* 1998;19:261–4

193. Hayden MK. Insights into the epidemiology and control of infection with vancomycin-resistant enterococci. *Clin Infect Dis* 2000;31:1058–65

194. Henning KJ, Delencastre H, Eagan J, et al. Vancomycin-resistant Enterococcus faecium on a pediatric oncology ward: duration of stool shedding and incidence of clinical infection. *Pediatr Infect Dis J* 1996;15:848–54

195. D'Agata EM, Horn MA and Webb GF. The impact of persistent gastrointestinal colonization on the transmission dynamics of vancomycin-resistant enterococci. *J Infect Dis* 2002;185: 766–73

196. D'Agata EM, Gautam S, Green WK and Tang YW. High rate of false-negative results of the rectal swab culture method in detection of gastrointestinal colonization with vancomycin-resistant enterococci. *Clin Infect Dis* 2002;34:167–72

197. Center for Disease Control and Prvention. Recommendations for preventing the spread of vancomycin resistance: Recommendations of the Hospital Infection Control Practices Advisory Committee (HICPAC). *Morb Mortal Wkly Rep* 1995;44 (RR-12):1–13

198. WWW.CDC.GOV: Guideline for Isolation Precautions: Preventing Transmission of Infectious Agents in Healthcare settings 2004.

199. Donskey CJ. The role of the intestinal tract as a reservoir and source for transmission of nosocomial pathogens. *Clin Infect Dis* 2004;39:219–26

200. Toltzis P, Dul MJ, Hoyen C, et al. Molecular epidemiology of antibiotic-resistant Gram-negative bacilli in a neonatal intensive care unit during a nonoutbreak period. *Pediatrics* 2001;108: 1143–8

201. Almuneef MA BR, Farrel PA, et al. Molecular typing demonstrating transmission of Gram-negative rods in a neonatal intensive care unit in the absence of recognized epidemic. *Clin Infect Dis*. 2001;32:220–227.

202. Venezia RA, Scarano FJ, Preston KE, et al. Molecular epidemiology of an SHV-5 extended-spectrum beta-lactamase in enterobacteriaceae isolated from infants in a neonatal intensive care unit. *Clin Infect Dis* 1995;21:915–23

203. Singh N, Patel KM, Leger MM, et al. Risk of resistant infections with Enterobacteriaceae in hospitalized neonates. *Pediatr Infect Dis J* 2002;21:1029–33

204. de Man P, Verhoeven BA, Verbrugh HA, Vos MC and van den Anker JN. An antibiotic policy to prevent emergence of resistant bacilli. *Lancet* 2000;355:973–8

205. Sanders CC, Barry AL, Washington JA, et al. Detection of extended-spectrum-beta-lactamase-producing members of the family Enterobacteriaceae with Vitek ESBL test. *J Clin Microbiol* 1996;34:2997–3001

206. Tzelepi E, Giakkoupi P, Sofianou D, Loukova V, Kemeroglou A and Tsakris A. Detection of extended-spectrum beta-lactamases in clinical isolates of Enterobacter cloacae and Enterobacter aerogenes. *J Clin Microbiol* 2000;38:542–6

207. Calil R, Marba ST, von Nowakonski A and Tresoldi AT. Reduction in colonization and nosocomial infection by multiresistant bacteria in a neonatal unit after institution of educational measures and restriction in the use of cephalosporins. *Am J Infect Control* 2001;29:133–8

208. Schiff GD, Wisniewski M, Bult J, Parada JP, Aggarwal H and Schwartz DN. Improving inpatient antibiotic prescribing: insights from participation in a national collaborative. *Jt Comm J Qual Improv* 2001;27:387–402

209. Aho LS, Simon I, Bour JB, Morales-Gineste L, Pothier P and Gouyon JB. [Epidemiology of viral nosocomial infections in pediatrics]. *Pathol Biol (Paris)* 2000;48:885–92

210. Wright SA, Bieluch VM. Selected nosocomial viral infections. *Heart Lung* 1993;22:183–7

211. Gelber SE, Ratner AJ. Hospital-acquired viral pathogens in the neonatal intensive care unit. *Semin Perinatol* 2002;26:346–56

212. Ng PC, So KW, Leung TF, et al. Infection control for SARS in a tertiary neonatal centre. *Arch Dis Child Fetal Neonatal Ed* 2003;88:F405–9

213. Hon KL, Leung CW, Cheng WT, et al. Clinical presentations and outcome of severe acute respiratory syndrome in children. *Lancet* 2003;361:1701–3

214. Williams JV, Harris PA, Tollefson SJ, et al. Human metapneumovirus and lower respiratory tract disease in otherwise healthy infants and children. *N Engl J Med* 2004;350:443–50

215. Black CP. Systematic review of the biology and medical management of respiratory syncytial virus infection. *Respir Care* 2003;48:209–31; discussion 231–3

216. Heerens AT, Marshall DD and Bose CL. Nosocomial respiratory syncytial virus: a threat in the modern neonatal intensive care unit. *J Perinatol* 2002;22:306–7

217. Greenough A. Recent advances in the management and prophylaxis of respiratory syncytial virus infection. *Acta Paediatr Suppl* 2001;90:11–4

218. Red book. 2003 Report of the Committee on Infectious Disease. *Respiratory Syncytial virus*. 2003;26th edition: 523–528

219. Cunney RJ, Bialachowski A, Thornley D, Smaill FM and Pennie RA. An outbreak of influenza A in a neonatal intensive care unit. *Infect Control Hosp Epidemiol* 2000;21:449–54

220. Singh-Naz N, Willy M and Riggs N. Outbreak of parainfluenza virus type 3 in a neonatal nursery. *Pediatr Infect Dis J* 1990;9:31–3

221. Munoz FM, Campbell JR, Atmar RL, et al. Influenza A virus outbreak in a neonatal intensive care unit. *Pediatr Infect Dis J* 1999;18:811–5

222. Moisiuk SE, Robson D, Klass L, et al. Outbreak of parainfluenza virus type 3 in an intermediate care neonatal nursery. *Pediatr Infect Dis J* 1998;17:49–53

223. Sagrera X, Ginovart G, Raspall F, et al. Outbreaks of influenza A virus infection in neonatal intensive care units. *Pediatr Infect Dis J* 2002;21:196–200

224. Update: influenza-associated deaths reported among children aged <18 years—United States, 2003–04 influenza season. *MMWR Morb Mortal Wkly Rep* 2004;52:1286–8

225. Glezen WP, Falcao O, Cate TR and Mintz AA. Nosocomial influenza in a general hospital for indigent patients. *Can J Infect Control* 1991;6:65–7

226. Meissner HC, Murray SA, Kiernan MA, Snydman DR and McIntosh K. A simultaneous outbreak of respiratory syncytial virus and parainfluenza virus type 3 in a newborn nursery. *J Pediatr* 1984;104:680–4

227. Singh-Naz N, Brown M and Ganeshananthan M. Nosocomial adenovirus infection: molecular epidemiology of an outbreak. *Pediatr Infect Dis J* 1993;12:922–5

228. Abzug MJ, Beam AC, Gyorkos EA and Levin MJ. Viral pneumonia in the first month of life. *Pediatr Infect Dis J* 1990;9:881–5

229. Abzug MJ, Levin MJ. Neonatal adenovirus infection: four patients and review of the literature. *Pediatrics* 1991;87:890–6

230. Gagneur A, Sizun J, Vallet S, Legr MC, Picard B and Talbot PJ. Coronavirus-related nosocomial viral respiratory infections in a neonatal and paediatric intensive care unit: a prospective study. *J Hosp Infect* 2002;51:59–64

231. Sit SC, Yau EK, Lam YY, et al. A young infant with severe acute respiratory syndrome. *Pediatrics* 2003;112:e257

232. Young NS, Brown KE. Parvovirus B19. *N Engl J Med* 2004;350:586–97

233. Seng C, Watkins P, Morse D, et al. Parvovirus B19 outbreak on an adult ward. *Epidemiol Infect* 1994;113:345–53

234. Ray SM, Erdman DD, Berschling JD, Cooper JE, Torok TJ and Blumberg HM. Nosocomial exposure to parvovirus B19: low risk of transmission to healthcare workers. *Infect Control Hosp Epidemiol* 1997;18:109–14

235. Bell LM, Naides SJ, Stoffman P, Hodinka RL and Plotkin SA. Human parvovirus B19 infection among hospital staff members after contact with infected patients. *N Engl J Med* 1989;321:485–91

236. Liu W, Ittmann M, Liu J, et al. Human parvovirus B19 in bone marrows from adults with acquired immunodeficiency syndrome: a comparative study using in situ hybridization and immunohistochemistry. *Hum Pathol* 1997;28:760–6

237. Dowell SF, Torok TJ, Thorp JA, et al. Parvovirus B19 infection in hospital workers: community or hospital acquisition? *J Infect Dis* 1995;172:1076–9

238. Boccia D, Stolfi I, Lana S and Moro ML. Nosocomial necrotising enterocolitis outbreaks: epidemiology and control measures. *Eur J Pediatr* 2001;160:385–91

239. Modlin JF. Perinatal echovirus infection: insights from a literature review of 61 cases of serious infection and 16 outbreaks in nurseries. *Rev Infect Dis* 1986;8:918–26

240. Rabkin CS, Telzak EE, Ho MS, et al. Outbreak of echovirus 11 infection in hospitalized neonates. *Pediatr Infect Dis J* 1988;7:186–90

241. Takami T, Kawashima H, Takei Y, et al. Usefulness of nested PCR and sequence analysis in a nosocomial outbreak of neonatal enterovirus infection. *J Clin Virol* 1998;11:67–75

242. Austin BJ, Croxson MC, Powell KF and Gunn TR. The successful containment of coxsackie B4 infection in a neonatal unit. *J Paediatr Child Health* 1999;35:102–4

243. Moore M, Kaplan MH, McPhee J, Bregman DJ and Klein SW. Epidemiologic, clinical, and laboratory features of Coxsackie B1–B5 infections in the United States, 1970–79. *Public Health Rep* 1984;99:515–22

244. Helin M, Savola J and Lapinleimu K. Cardiac manifestations during a Coxsackie B5 epidemic. *Br Med J* 1968;3:97–9

245. Chawareewong S, Kiangsiri S, Lokaphadhana K, et al. Neonatal herpangina caused by Coxsackie A-5 virus. *J Pediatr* 1978;93:492–4

246. Oelberg DG, Joyner SE, Jiang X, Laborde D, Islam MP and Pickering LK. Detection of pathogen transmission in neonatal nurseries using DNA markers as surrogate indicators. *Pediatrics* 2000;105:311–5

247. Watson JC, Fleming DW, Borella AJ, Olcott ES, Conrad RE and Baron RC. Vertical transmission of hepatitis A resulting in an outbreak in a neonatal intensive care unit. *J Infect Dis* 1993;167:567–71

248. Klein BS, Michaels JA, Rytel MW, Berg KG and Davis JP. Nosocomial hepatitis A. A multinursery outbreak in Wisconsin. *Jama* 1984;252:2716–21

249. Red book. 2003 Report of the Committee on Infectious Diseases. Hepatitis A. 2003;26th edition:309–318

250. Morand P. [Natural history of HSV1 and HSV2 infection. Asymptomatic viral excretion. Mother-infant transmission. Indirect transmission]. *Ann Dermatol Venereol* 2002;129:577–85

251. Francis DP, Herrmann KL, MacMahon JR, Chavigny KH and Sanderlin KC. Nosocomial and maternally acquired herpesvirus hominis infections. A report of four fatal cases in neonates. *Am J Dis Child* 1975;129:889–93

252. Ippolito G, Puro V and De Carli G. The risk of occupational human immunodeficiency virus infection in health care workers. Italian Multicenter Study. The Italian Study Group on Occupational Risk of HIV infection. *Arch Intern Med* 1993;153:1451–8

253. Aiken CG. HIV-1 infection and perinatal mortality in Zimbabwe. *Arch Dis Child* 1992;67:595–9

254. Red book. 2003 Report of the Committee on Infectious Diseases. Varicella. 2003;26th edition:262

255. Hayakawa M, Kimura H, Ohshiro M, et al. Varicella exposure in a neonatal medical centre: successful prophylaxis with oral acyclovir. *J Hosp Infect* 2003;54:212–5

256. Weber DJ, Rutala WA and Hamilton H. Prevention and control of varicella-zoster infections in healthcare facilities. *Infect Control Hosp Epidemiol* 1996;17:694–705

257. Yeager AS, Grumet FC, Hafleigh EB, Arvin AM, Bradley JS and Prober CG. Prevention of transfusion-acquired cytomegalovirus infections in newborn infants. *J Pediatr* 1981;98:281–7

258. Red book 2003 Report of the Committee on Infectious Diseases. Cytomegalovirus infection. 2003:259–262

259. Demmler GJ, Yow MD, Spector SA, et al. Nosocomial cytomegalovirus infections within two hospitals caring for infants and children. *J Infect Dis* 1987;156:9–16

260. Pursell E. Preventing nosocomial infection in paediatric wards. *J Clin Nurs* 1996;5:313–8

261. Haley RW, Culver DH, White JW, et al. The efficacy of infection surveillance and control programs in preventing nosocomial infections in US hospitals. *Am J Epidemiol* 1985;121:182–205

262. Eggimann P, Harbarth S, Constantin MN, Touveneau S, Chevrolet JC and Pittet D. Impact of a prevention strategy targeted at vascular-access care on incidence of infections acquired in intensive care. *Lancet* 2000;355:1864–8

263. Edwards WH. Preventing nosocomial bloodstream infection in very low birth weight infants. *Semin Neonatol* 2002;7:325–33

264. Adams-Chapman I, Stoll BJ. Prevention of nosocomial infections in the neonatal intensive care unit. *Curr Opin Pediatr* 2002;14:157–64

265. Benjamin DK, Jr., Miller W, Garges H, et al. Bacteremia, central catheters, and neonates: when to pull the line. *Pediatrics* 2001;107:1272–6

266. Boyce JM, Pittet D. Guideline for Hand Hygiene in Health-Care Settings. Recommendations of the Healthcare Infection Control Practices Advisory Committee and the HIPAC/SHEA/APIC/IDSA Hand Hygiene Task Force. *Am J Infect Control* 2002;30:S1–46

267. Ehrenkranz NJ, Alfonso BC. Failure of bland soap handwash to prevent hand transfer of patient bacteria to urethral catheters. *Infect Control Hosp Epidemiol* 1991;12:654–62

268. Gould D, Ream E. Assessing nurses' hand decontamination performance. *Nurs Times* 1993;89:47–50

269. Woolwine JD, Gerberding JL. Effect of testing method on apparent activities of antiviral disinfectants and antiseptics. *Antimicrob Agents Chemother* 1995;39:921–3

270. Larson EL, Aiello AE, Bastyr J, et al. Assessment of two hand hygiene regimens for intensive care unit personnel. *Crit Care Med* 2001;29:944–51

271. Larson EL, Aiello AE, Heilman JM, et al. Comparison of different regimens for surgical hand preparation. *Aorn J* 2001;73:412–4, 417–8, 420 passim

272. Larson E, Friedman C, Cohran J, Treston-Aurand J and Green S. Prevalence and correlates of skin damage on the hands of nurses. *Heart Lung* 1997;26:404–12

273. Tubker R. Detergents and Cleansers. Vol. Chapter 7. New York: CRC Press, 1996 (van der Valk PMH, ed. The Irritant Contact Dermatitis Syndrome)

274. Larson EL, Hughes CA, Pyrek JD, Sparks SM, Cagatay EU and Bartkus JM. Changes in bacterial flora associated with skin damage on hands of health care personnel. *Am J Infect Control* 1998;26:513–21

275. McCormick RD, Buchman TL and Maki DG. Double-blind, randomized trial of scheduled use of a novel barrier cream and an oil-containing lotion for protecting the hands of health care workers. *Am J Infect Control* 2000;28:302–10

276. Loeb MB, Wilcox L, Smaill F, Walter S and Duff Z. A randomized trial of surgical scrubbing with a brush compared to antiseptic soap alone. *Am J Infect Control* 1997;25:11–5

277. Garner JS, Simmons BP. Guideline for isolation precautions in hospitals. *Infect Control* 1983;4:245–325

278. Tenorio AR, Badri SM, Sahgal NB, et al. Effectiveness of gloves in the prevention of hand carriage of vancomycin-resistant enterococcus species by health care workers after patient care. *Clin Infect Dis* 2001;32:826–9

279. Larson EL. APIC guideline for handwashing and hand antisepsis in health care settings. *Am J Infect Control* 1995;23:251–69

280. Munson KA, Bare DE, Hoath SB and Visscher MO. A survey of skin care practices for premature low birth weight infants. *Neonatal Netw* 1999;18:25–31

281. Larson EL. Guideline for use of topical antimicrobial agents. *Am J Inf Cont* 1988;16:253–266

282. Chabrolle JP, Rossier A. Danger of iodine skin absorption in the neonate. *J Pediatr* 1978;93:158–9

283. Chabrolle JP, Rossier A. Goitre and hypothyroidism in the newborn after cutaneous absorption of iodine. *Arch Dis Child* 1978;53:495–8

284. Edwards WH, Conner JM and Soll RF. The effect of prophylactic ointment therapy on nosocomial sepsis rates and skin integrity in infants with birth weights of 501 to 1000 g. *Pediatrics* 2004;113:1195–203

285. Conner JM, Soll RF and Edwards WH. Topical ointment for preventing infection in preterm infants. *Cochrane Database Syst Rev* 2004:CD001150

286. Bennet R, Eriksson M, Nord CE and Zetterstrom R. Fecal bacterial microflora of newborn infants during intensive care management and treatment with five antibiotic regimens. *Pediatr Infect Dis* 1986;5:533–9

287. Isolauri E. Probiotics in human disease. *Am J Clin Nutr* 2001;73:1142S–1146S

288. Zetterstrom R, Bennet R and Nord KE. Early infant feeding and micro-ecology of the gut. *Acta Paediatr Jpn* 1994;36:562–71

289. Dani C, Biadaioli R, Bertini G, Martelli E and Rubaltelli FF. Probiotics feeding in prevention of urinary tract infection, bacterial sepsis and necrotizing enterocolitis in preterm infants. A prospective double-blind study. *Biol Neonate* 2002;82:103–8

290. O'Grady NP, Alexander M, Dellinger EP, et al. Guidelines for the prevention of intravascular catheter-related infections. Centers for Disease Control and Prevention. *MMWR Recomm Rep* 2002;51:1–29

291. Rello J, Ochagavia A, Sabanes E, et al. Evaluation of outcome of intravenous catheter-related infections in critically ill patients. *Am J Respir Crit Care Med* 2000;162:1027–30

292. Dimick JB, Pelz RK, Consunji R, Swoboda SM, Hendrix CW and Lipsett PA. Increased resource use associated with catheter-related bloodstream infection in the surgical intensive care unit. *Arch Surg* 2001;136:229–34

293. Slonim AD, Kurtines HC, Sprague BM and Singh N. The costs associated with nosocomial bloodstream infections in the pediatric intensive care unit. *Pediatr Crit Care Med* 2001;2:170–174

294. Soifer NE, Borzak S, Edlin BR and Weinstein RA. Prevention of peripheral venous catheter complications with an intravenous therapy team: a randomized controlled trial. *Arch Intern Med* 1998;158:473–7

295. Mermel LA, Stolz SM and Maki DG. Surface antimicrobial activity of heparin-bonded and antiseptic-impregnated vascular catheters. *J Infect Dis* 1993;167:920–4

296. Pierce CM, Wade A and Mok Q. Heparin-bonded central venous lines reduce thrombotic and infective complications in critically ill children. *Intensive Care Med* 2000;26:967–72

297. Landers S, Moise AA, Fraley JK, Smith EO and Baker CJ. Factors associated with umbilical catheter-related sepsis in neonates. *Am J Dis Child* 1991;145:675–80

298. Stenzel JP, Green TP, Fuhrman BP, Carlson PE and Marchessault RP. Percutaneous central venous catheterization in a pediatric intensive care unit: a survival analysis of complications. *Crit Care Med* 1989;17:984–8

299. Chaiyakunapruk N, Veenstra DL, Lipsky BA, Sullivan SD and Saint S. Vascular catheter site care: the clinical and economic benefits of chlorhexidine gluconate compared with povidone iodine. *Clin Infect Dis* 2003;37:764–71

300. Maki DG, Ringer M. Evaluation of dressing regimens for prevention of infection with peripheral intravenous catheters. Gauze, a transparent polyurethane dressing, and an iodophor-transparent dressing. *Jama* 1987;258:2396–403

301. Rasero L, Degl'Innocenti M, Mocali M, et al. [Comparison of two different protocols on change of medication in central venous catheterization in patients with bone marrow transplantation: results of a randomized multicenter study]. *Assist Inferm Ric* 2000;19:112–9

302. Garland JS, Alex CP, Mueller CD, et al. A randomized trial comparing povidone-iodine to a chlorhexidine gluconate-impregnated dressing for prevention of central venous catheter infections in neonates. *Pediatrics* 2001;107:1431–6

303. Zakrzewska-Bode A, Muytjens HL, Liem KD and Hoogkamp-Korstanje JA. Mupirocin resistance in coagulase-negative staphylococci, after topical prophylaxis for the reduction of colonization of central venous catheters. *J Hosp Infect* 1995;31:189–93

304. Zinner SH, Denny-Brown BC, Braun P, Burke JP, Toala P and Kass EH. Risk of infection with intravenous indwelling catheters: effect of application of antibiotic ointment. *J Infect Dis* 1969;120:616–9

305. Mueller-Premru M, Gubina M, Kaufmann ME, Primozic J and Cookson BD. Use of semi-quantitative and quantitative culture methods and typing for studying the epidemiology of central venous catheter-related infections in neonates on parenteral nutrition. *J Med Microbiol* 1999;48:451–60

306. Maki DG, Botticelli JT, LeRoy ML and Thielke TS. Prospective study of replacing administration sets for intravenous therapy at 48- vs 72-hour intervals. 72 hours is safe and cost-effective. *Jama* 1987;258:1777–81

307. Avila-Figueroa C, Goldmann DA, Richardson DK, Gray JE, Ferrari A and Freeman J. Intravenous lipid emulsions are the major determinant of coagulase-negative staphylococcal bacteremia in very low birth weight newborns. *Pediatr Infect Dis J* 1998;17:10–7

308. Chang HJ, Miller HL, Watkins N, et al. An epidemic of Malassezia pachydermatis in an intensive care nursery associated with colonization of health care workers' pet dogs. *N Engl J Med* 1998;338:706–11

309. Powell DA, Aungst J, Snedden S, Hansen N and Brady M. Broviac catheter-related Malassezia furfur sepsis in five infants receiving intravenous fat emulsions. *J Pediatr* 1984;105:987–90

310. Saiman L, Ludington E, Dawson JD, et al. Risk factors for Candida species colonization of neonatal intensive care unit patients. *Pediatr Infect Dis J* 2001;20:1119–24

311. Mermel LA, Maki DG. Detection of bacteremia in adults: consequences of culturing an inadequate volume of blood. *Ann Intern Med* 1993;119:270–2

312. Fridkin SK, Pear SM, Williamson TH, Galgiani JN and Jarvis WR. The role of understaffing in central venous catheter-associated bloodstream infections. *Infect Control Hosp Epidemiol* 1996;17:150–8

313. Harbarth S, Sudre P, Dharan S, Cadenas M and Pittet D. Outbreak of Enterobacter cloacae related to understaffing, overcrowding,

and poor hygiene practices. *Infect Control Hosp Epidemiol* 1999;20:598–603

314. Archibald LK, Manning, M.L., Bell, L.M., Banerjee, S., Jarvis, W.R. Patient density, nurse-to-patient ratio and nosocomial infection risk in a peditric cardiac intensive care unit. *Pedi Infect Dis J* 1997;16:1045–1058

315. Oh W, Merenstein G. Fourth edition of the Guidelines for Perinatal Care: summary of changes. *Pediatrics* 1997;100:1021–2

316. Kilbride HW, Wirtschafter DD, Powers RJ and Sheehan MB. Implementation of evidence-based potentially better practices to decrease nosocomial infections. *Pediatrics* 2003;111: e519–33

Neurological and Neuromuscular Disorders

Alan Hill

In the context of dramatic improvements in obstetric care and in the treatment of neonatal respiratory disorders and infection, neurologic problems remain a major cause of morbidity and mortality in the newborn. In this chapter, an approach to the neurologic assessment of the newborn is outlined, and practical aspects of diagnosis and management of the most common neurologic and neuromuscular problems of the newborn are reviewed (e.g., seizures, hypoxic–ischemic cerebral injury, intracranial hemorrhage, traumatic birth injury, spinal muscular atrophy, muscular dystrophies and myopathies). Major bacterial and viral infections, metabolic derangements that affect the central nervous system (CNS), and cerebral dysgenesis are discussed in other chapters.

NEUROLOGIC EVALUATION OF THE NEWBORN

History and Physical Examination

The importance of a detailed history and neurologic examination for assessment of the newborn with suspected neurologic problems cannot be overemphasized (1). Such history must include details of the family history and complications encountered during pregnancy, labor, and delivery, because many neurologic abnormalities that present during the neonatal period actually originate antenatally.

The format of the neurologic examination in the newborn is similar to that used in older patients. However, observations must be interpreted in the context of the level of cerebral maturation at different gestational ages (1,2). The examination should not be prolonged unnecessarily to avoid hypothermia and fluctuations in arterial blood pressure that may be associated even with routine handling, especially in premature newborns.

Neurologic observations also are influenced considerably by the level of alertness of the infant. After 28 weeks of gestation, infants are able to awaken spontaneously or may be roused for several minutes by stimulation. Distinct sleep–wake patterns may be recognized by 40 weeks of gestation.

In an examination of the cranial nerves, pupillary constriction to light and the blink reflex may be elicited as early as 28 weeks of gestation. Pupillary responses are consistent by 31 to 32 weeks. Consistent visual tracking of a bright light and opticokinetic nystagmus can be elicited consistently in the awake infant at term. Fundoscopy may reveal retinal hemorrhages in 20% to 50% of newborns following vaginal delivery, but these rarely indicate significant CNS injury. Dysconjugate and jerky eye movements are common in premature infants and may persist to some extent for several months after term. Full extraocular eye movements to doll's-head maneuver or to caloric stimulation may be elicited after 32 weeks of gestation. Facial muscle weakness may be of central or peripheral origin. Hearing may be difficult to assess, although infants startle to loud noises as early as 28 weeks of gestation. The act of feeding requires coordination of breathing, sucking, and swallowing, which involve principally cranial nerves V, VII, IX, X, and XII. Therefore, observation of feeding provides valuable information regarding function of these cranial nerves and the brainstem in general.

The major features of the motor examination include evaluation of limb posture, spontaneous and elicited movements, muscle power, tendon reflexes, and primitive neonatal reflexes. Muscle tone may be assessed by careful observation of the infant's posture at rest and during various maneuvers of passive manipulation. With increasing gestational age, there is development of predominance of flexor tone in all limbs. Asymmetry of muscle tone and spontaneous limb movements may indicate focal cerebral lesions or peripheral injury, e.g., brachial plexus injury. Tendon reflexes can usually be elicited in the term newborn. Undue emphasis should not be placed on brisk tendon reflexes, ankle clonus, or crossed adductor responses in the absence of corroborative abnormal neurologic signs. Muscle strength may be assessed by gently pinching the infant's distal extremities and eliciting the recoil flexor response.

Careful evaluation of sensory function is particularly important in the evaluation of spinal cord or peripheral nerve injury. A useful aspect of sensory evaluation is the determination of habituation, i.e., the normal dampening of responses to multiple (e.g., 5–10) stimulations. Habituation indicates a high level of response that appears to require input from cerebral hemispheres. It is characteristically absent in anencephalic infants.

Neurodiagnostic Techniques

Because the neurologic examination is often limited by concomitant systemic illness and the requirement for complex life-support systems, a variety of noninvasive neurodiagnostic techniques, e.g., neuroimaging, electroencephalography, evoked potentials, often are used as adjunctive methods for the evaluation of neurologic problems. The clinical applications of various techniques will be discussed in the context of specific neurologic conditions.

NEONATAL SEIZURES

Seizures are the most distinctive manifestation of significant CNS disease in the newborn. Prompt diagnosis and intervention are indicated because not only do seizures often indicate serious underlying disease, they also may interfere with supportive care, e.g., ventilation and alimentation. Repeated seizures are often associated with hypoventilation and apnea which, in turn, may result in cardiovascular collapse and ischemic brain injury. Furthermore, the hypercapnia, in combination with increased lactate and an adaptive

rise in systemic blood pressure, may result in an abrupt rise in cerebral blood flow with associated risk of intracranial hemorrhage especially in premature infants (3). Additionally, experimental animal studies suggest that neonatal seizures may have a deleterious effect on the developing brain by depleting cerebral glucose levels, which, in turn, may interfere with deoxyribonucleic acid (DNA) synthesis, glial proliferation, differentiation, and myelination (4,5). Although the relevance of data from experimental animal studies to the human newborn is not entirely clear, the significance of neonatal seizures has been corroborated by in vivo studies with magnetic resonance spectroscopy (MRS) (6). In terms of management, the possible detrimental effects of neonatal seizures must be balanced against the potentially deleterious effects of anticonvulsants on the developing brain (7).

Clinical Features

Neonatal seizures differ considerably from seizures observed in older children, principally because the immature brain is less capable of propagating generalized or organized electrical discharges. The principal types of neonatal seizures are summarized in Table 50-1 (8). Although individual seizure types are not indicative of specific varieties of brain injury, certain seizure types are associated more commonly with some conditions. For example, generalized tonic seizures, which may represent brainstem release phenomena or posturing, have been observed with major germinal matrix hemorrhage/intraventricular hemorrhage (GMH/IVH). Focal clonic seizures may be associated with focal cerebral infarction or traumatic cerebral contusion.

Differentiation of seizures from nonepileptic movements may be difficult in the newborn. Clonic seizures may be particularly difficult to differentiate clinically from jitteriness or tremulousness, particularly because both occur

TABLE 50-1
CLINICAL FEATURES OF NEONATAL SEIZURES

Seizure Type	Major Clinical Manifestations
Subtle	Repetitive blinking, eye deviation, staring
	Repetitive mouth or tongue movements
	Apnea
	Bicycling–rowing movements
Tonic (i.e., generalized or focal)	Tonic extension of limb or limbs
	Tonic flexion of upper limbs, extension of lower limbs
Clonic (i.e., multifocal or focal)	Multifocal, synchronous, or asynchronous limb movements
	Repetitive, jerky limb movements
	Nonordered progression
	Localized repetitive clonic limb movements with preservation of consciousness
Myoclonic (i.e., generalized, focal, multifocal)	Single or several flexion jerks of upper limbs (common) and lower limbs (rare)

frequently in similar clinical contexts, e.g., hypoxic–ischemic encephalopathy, metabolic derangements, and drug withdrawal. However, jitteriness is classified as a movement disorder that may be associated with good outcome. Benign jitteriness often resolves within weeks. The distinction between jitteriness and seizures may be made clinically as follows:

- Jitteriness is not accompanied by abnormal eye movements.
- Jitteriness may be spontaneous or stimulus sensitive.
- The flexion and extension phases of the tremor are equal in amplitude compared to the unequal phases observed with clonic seizure movements.
- Jitteriness may be stopped by passive flexion or repositioning of the affected body part.

Infants with severe dysfunction of the CNS may have stimulus-sensitive myoclonus, which may be associated with spike or sharp wave discharges on the electroencephalogram (EEG) (9).

Benign neonatal sleep myoclonus occurs during active sleep in healthy premature and term newborns. Myoclonus may be florid and consists of either bilateral synchronous or asynchronous or asymmetric movements that are not stimulus sensitive, but which cease on arousal from sleep. They are not associated with epileptiform or background disturbances on the EEG. Benign sleep myoclonus usually resolves over several months (10,11).

Simultaneous video and EEG monitoring has raised major issues concerning the incidence, classification, pathophysiology, and management of neonatal seizures. Some stereotypic, paroxysmal clinical phenomena, e.g., oral-buccal-lingual movements, generalized tonic, or extensor posturing are not associated consistently with epileptiform discharges on EEG recordings performed using surface electrodes. Subtle clinical phenomena correlate more frequently with simultaneous abnormal EEG discharges in premature than in term newborns (1,8).

Etiology

Neonatal seizures are rarely idiopathic in origin. Thus, when neonatal seizures occur, immediate attention must be directed toward the identification of an underlying etiology to permit rapid and appropriate intervention (when available) and meaningful prediction of outcome (8). Although neonatal seizures may be as a result of numerous underlying causes, most result from a relatively few causes, e.g., hypoxic–ischemic cerebral injury, intracranial hemorrhage, or metabolic derangements. The most important causes of neonatal seizures and their prognostic significance are listed in order of relative frequency in Table 50-2.

Seizures are a distinctly uncommon manifestation of withdrawal from passive addiction to narcotics, e.g., heroin, methadone, or barbiturates. In contrast, maternal cocaine abuse may be associated more commonly with epileptiform EEG abnormalities or seizures in newborns exposed in utero or by breast-feeding. This may relate to direct neuronal excitotoxicity, teratogenic effects, or destructive ischemic and hemorrhagic lesions (1).

Intoxication with local anesthetic after inadvertent injection into the infant's scalp during placement of pudendal, paracervical, or epidural blocks is a rare cause of severe but self-limited neonatal seizures (12). Characteristically, severe, tonic seizures begin during the first hours of life, associated with coma and loss of brainstem reflexes, e.g., apnea and severe hypoventilation, bradycardia, hypotonia, fixed and dilated pupils, and absence of extraocular movements in response to the doll's-head maneuver. The early onset of the latter two features during the first six to eight hours of life is useful for distinguishing such local anesthetic intoxication from hypoxic–ischemic encephalopathy. Evaluation involves careful inspection of the scalp for evidence of injection. Management consists of vigorous support and removal of the drug by diuresis, acidification of urine or exchange transfusion.

Neonatal seizures, which begin after several days of age, are a common manifestation of inborn errors of metabolism.

TABLE 50-2

ETIOLOGY AND PROGNOSIS OF NEONATAL SEIZURES[a]

Etiology	Gestational Age		Time of Onset (d of Age)		Outcome Normal (%)
	Premature	Term	0–3	4–10	
Hypoxic–ischemic encephalopathy	+	+	+		50
Intracranial hemorrhage					
Intraventricular hemorrhage	+	−	+		<10
Subarachnoid hemorrhage	−	+	+		90
Hypoglycemia	+	+	+		50
Infection	+	+		+	<50
Cerebral dysgenesis	+	+		+	0
Hypocalcemia					
Early onset	+	+	+		50
Late onset	−	+		+	100

+, common; −, rare.
[a] From Volpe JJ. *Neurology of the newborn.* Philadelphia: WB Saunders, 2001, with permission.

There is increasing evidence that accurate diagnosis requires analysis of specific metabolites in cerebrospinal fluid and in serum (13).

In addition to the underlying etiologies listed in Table 50-2, there are several recognized epilepsy syndromes that may present during the newborn period. These include two benign syndromes, i.e., "fifth day fits" and benign familial neonatal seizures. The latter often present as frequent seizures on the third day of life and usually are linked to autosomal dominant gene loci on chromosomes 20 or 8 (14,15). Additionally, there are several recognized severe epilepsy syndromes. Early myoclonic encephalopathy (EME) presents within hours of birth with severe, fragmentary, refractory myoclonus, which often is worsened by handling or stimulation. Infants often have a high-arched palate. The initial neuroimaging is normal, but diffuse cerebral atrophy develops and affected infants frequently die in the first 2 years of life. Another entity, early infantile epileptic encephalopathy, also termed "Ohtahara's syndrome," may present with structural cerebral lesions (dysgenesis or destruction) and a severe burst-suppression pattern on the EEG (16).

Diagnosis

Diagnostic evaluation must begin with a careful history and physical examination. Obtaining a maternal history of drug abuse, intrauterine infection, and genetic or metabolic conditions is critical, and it should be obtained directly from the mother whenever possible.

Although the EEG may be useful for confirmation of suspected seizures and for establishment of prognosis, it is rarely helpful for the identification of a specific etiology. Continuous EEG monitoring may be of value for identifying seizures in infants who are paralyzed pharmacologically or those who have electrographic seizures only.

Initial laboratory investigations should address treatable causes (e.g., hypoglycemia, hypocalcemia, hypomagnesemia). Lumbar puncture may identify intracranial infection or hemorrhage. Additionally, cerebrospinal fluid (CSF) analysis may also prove to be critical for identifying inborn errors of metabolism, e.g., folinic-acid responsive seizures and disorders of glucose transport, with low CSF glucose concentration and normal blood glucose concentration which, when treated with the ketogenic diet, may minimize long-term neurologic sequelae (13,17). If the initial screening investigations fail to identify a specific etiology, additional studies should be considered, including neuroimaging, metabolic investigations, e.g., serum amino acids, lactate, ammonia, urine organic acids, screening for drugs, and investigation for congenital viral infections. In some instances, several underlying factors may be operative in the same patient.

Treatment

Treatment of neonatal seizures is directed toward minimizing physiologic and metabolic derangements and preventing the recurrence of seizures. This should involve immediate support of ventilation and perfusion, if required, and correction of hypoglycemia, hypocalcemia, or other metabolic derangements. If seizures persist, a single loading dose of phenobarbital (20 mg/kg) should be administered intravenously, which may be followed by additional doses of 5 mg/kg to a total of 40 mg/kg (including loading dose) as required, if there is no cardiac decompensation. If seizures are still uncontrolled, a single loading dose of phenytoin (20 mg/kg) or possibly fosphenytoin (1.5 mg of fosphenytoin yields 1.0 mg of phenytoin) may be administered slowly with concomitant careful monitoring of cardiac function. If seizures remain refractory to therapy, the use of a benzodiazepine may be considered, e.g., lorazepam (0.05–0.1 mg/kg), or diazepam infusion (0.3 mg/kg/hr). Midazolam may have harmful effects in the newborn and should be avoided. Additionally, there are anecdotal reports of the value of other anticonvulsants for refractory seizures, e.g., primidone, carbamazepine, lamotrigine, and thiopentone (1).

Pyridoxine dependency should be considered if there are recurrent seizures without obvious explanation. This condition may be diagnosed by a therapeutic trial of intravenous pyridoxine (100 mg) with EEG monitoring or oral treatment (100–200 mg daily) which should be continued for approximately 2 weeks.

Several major issues regarding the ongoing treatment of neonatal seizures remain unresolved. These include the optimal maintenance doses and therapeutic ranges of serum levels of anticonvulsants, the importance of eliminating electrographic seizures, and the optimal duration of anticonvulsant therapy. The duration of therapy should be guided by the underlying etiology and the risk of seizure recurrence. Clearly, unnecessary prolongation of therapy should be avoided because of unresolved concerns about possible deleterious effects of anticonvulsants on the immature nervous system (7).

Prognosis

The mortality rate for poorly controlled clinical seizures has decreased to approximately 15% in recent years. The incidence of neurologic sequelae, especially mental retardation and motor deficits (e.g., cerebral palsy), are reported to range from 35% to 55% (1).

Of course, the most important determinant of outcome is the underlying neurologic disease (Table 50-2). Additionally, seizures of early onset, frequent or prolonged seizures, and seizures that are refractory to multiple anticonvulsant treatment are often associated with poor prognosis. Clearly, these features reflect the severity of the underlying cerebral abnormality. Furthermore, in term newborns, normal, background activity on the EEG is rarely associated with neurological sequelae, whereas severe abnormality of background activity, e.g., burst suppression or marked voltage suppression is associated with abnormal outcome in over 90% of cases. However, in a significant proportion of newborns, the EEG is borderline, equivocal, or contains moderate background abnormalities that are associated with an intermediate or uncertain prognosis. Furthermore, the unique features of the neonatal EEG may lead to difficulties in interpretation which, in turn, limits its prognostic value. Also, the number of electrographic seizures and the rate of improvement of serial EEG's is also a useful prognostic factor (18).

HYPOXIC–ISCHEMIC CEREBRAL INJURY

Hypoxic–ischemic cerebral injury results from a combination of hypoxemia and ischemia, which often is associated with impaired cerebrovascular autoregulation and probably exacerbated by diminished cerebral glucose substrates, lactic acidosis, the accumulation of free radicals and excitotoxic amino acids (especially glutamate), and other metabolic derangements. The localization and extent of perinatal hypoxic–ischemic cerebral injury is determined principally by the maturity of the brain at the time of insult and the severity and duration of the insult (1).

Although the importance of antepartum and intrapartum factors have been recognized since 1862, when Little described a relationship between perinatal complications and cerebral palsy, data from large, epidemiologic studies, including the National Collaborative Perinatal Project and the Western Australia Cerebral Palsy Register, suggest that the etiologic role of antepartum factors may have been underestimated in the past (19–21). Review of these large populations of children with cerebral palsy indicate that the incidence of cerebral palsy related to intrapartum asphyxia do not exceed 20% when all factors are considered. Moreover, approximately one-third of these patients had at least one congenital anomaly unrelated to the CNS. This observation raises the possibility that an insult that originated much earlier during gestation may predispose some infants to subsequent hypoxic–ischemic insult at the time of delivery. Nevertheless, there are extensive experimental, clinical, and neuroimaging data that provide compelling evidence that acute, intrapartum hypoxic–ischemic insult is an important etiologic factor for neonatal brain injury (1,22).

Diagnosis

Clinical Features

Term newborns who sustain sufficient intrapartum insult to result in long-term sequelae invariably demonstrate clinical evidence of acute encephalopathy, i.e., altered brain function, during the first days of life (23). In contrast, infants who sustain hypoxic–ischemic cerebral injury earlier in gestation may be asymptomatic during the neonatal period. It is important to consider that the clinical features of hypoxic–ischemic encephalopathy are nonspecific, and similar clinical features may occur in the context of other causes of brain dysfunction, e.g., metabolic derangements, cerebral dysgenesis, and infection. Several aspects of labor and delivery may be used as clinical indicators of probable hypoxic–ischemic insult, e.g., prolonged fetal bradycardia or repetitive late decelerations of the fetal heart rate, low fetal scalp or cord pH, and low extended Apgar scores after 5 minutes of age. However, no single factor or combination of factors can predict accurately the severity or duration of the hypoxic–ischemic insult or the long-term sequelae (22). In the term newborn, the duration and severity of the encephalopathy, the type of EEG abnormality and the neuropathologic patterns of cerebral injury, which may be identified by neuroimaging, may permit determination of outcome with a reasonable degree of accuracy in many instances.

There is a complete spectrum of hypoxic–ischemic encephalopathy in the term newborn. However, classification of the severity of encephalopathy (Table 50-3) is useful for prognostic purposes (23–27). Thus, for example, according to the classification scheme developed by Sarnat and Sarnat (23), mild encephalopathy is characterized by hyperalertness, jitteriness, exaggerated tendon reflexes and Moro response that last only approximately 1 to 2 days. It is generally not associated with long-term neurologic sequelae. Moderate encephalopathy is comprised of lethargy, stupor, hypotonia, diminished spontaneous movements, suppressed tendon reflexes and, in some instances, seizures. Abnormal long-term outcome has been reported in 20% to 40% in this group. Severe encephalopathy is characterized by coma, seizures, brainstem and autonomic dysfunction,

TABLE 50-3
SEVERITY AND OUTCOME OF HYPOXIC–ISCHEMIC ENCEPHALOPATHY IN THE FULL-TERM NEONATE

Severity	Level of Consciousness	Seizures	Primitive Reflexes	Brain Stem Dysfunction	Elevated Intracranial Pressure	Duration	Poor Outcome[a] (%)
Mild	Increased irritability, hyperalertness	−, Jitteriness	Exaggerated	−	−	<24 h	0
Moderate	Lethargy	Variable	Suppressed	−	−	>24 h (variable)	20–40
Severe	Stupor or coma	+	Absent	+	Variable	>5 d	100

[a] Poor outcome is defined as the presence of mental retardation, cerebral palsy, or seizures.
+, common; −, rare.

absent spontaneous movements, and, in some instances, elevated intracranial pressure (28–30). Infants with severe encephalopathy almost invariably die or develop major neurologic sequelae, e.g., microcephaly, spastic quadriplegia, seizures. In severe encephalopathy, the clinical features characteristically worsen during the first 3 days of life. Death occurs most commonly between 24 and 72 hours of life, which corresponds to the time of maximal cerebral edema (1,28). Autopsy studies of infants with increased intracranial pressure demonstrate extensive cerebral necrosis. Thus, increased intracranial pressure appears to be a consequence rather than a cause of extensive hypoxic-ischemic brain injury and interventions to reduce cerebral edema may reduce the intracranial pressure but do not appear to improve the ultimate neurologic outcome (28, 31–33).

Seizures occur in approximately 50% of asphyxiated infants and are indicative of moderate or severe encephalopathy. Seizures, which most commonly are of the subtle and multifocal clonic type, usually begin during the first 24 hours of life. In severe cases, they often occur soon after delivery and are refractory to anticonvulsant therapy. Infants with hypoxic–ischemic encephalopathy who survive beyond 3 or 4 days of age generally demonstrate an improving level of consciousness and gradual resolution of seizures, although impairment of feeding, abnormal muscle tone, and delayed development may persist.

In addition to the neurologic dysfunction, there is often evidence of acute hypoxic–ischemic insult to organs other than brain, e.g., kidneys are particularly vulnerable, but myocardial, GI, hematologic, endocrine and lung complications may also occur (34–36). Such involvement of other organs is often transient and reversible, even in the context of severe encephalopathy, and the extent of systemic abnormalities appears to correlate with the severity of encephalopathy. However, in some instances, especially when intrapartum asphyxia is severe and of short duration, as in the context of uterine rupture or cord prolapse, there may be little or no evidence of injury to organs other than the brain on routine investigations (37,38).

Neuroimaging

In addition to the clinical examination, neuroimaging techniques are of major value for the identification of specific neuropathologic patterns and quantification of extent of cerebral injury (39).

Cranial Ultrasound

In term newborns with severe hypoxic–ischemic injury, abnormalities include diffuse increased echogenicity of parenchyma and effacement of cortical sulci by cerebral edema during the first day of life. Unfortunately, if abnormalities are diffuse, detection may be difficult. This accounts for the disappointing correlation between ultrasound imaging and neurologic outcome in term newborns (39,40).

In term infants who have sustained an hypoxic-ischemic insult, cranial ultrasonography before 24 hours of age has a role for the exclusion of other entities, e.g., hemorrhage or mass lesions, which may produce a clinical picture which may mimic hypoxic–ischemic encephalopathy.

Ultrasound has better predictive value in premature infants with hypoxic–ischemic brain injury, in whom the principal lesions during in the first days of life are increased periventricular echogenicity and intraventricular hemorrhage. The hyperechoic periventricular abnormalities evolve into cystic lesions (cavitations) during the ensuing 2 to 3 weeks in severe cases (41–42). These lesions are transient and if the phase of cyst formation is not documented by serial ultrasound examinations, a later sonogram may show only enlargement of the lateral ventricles with irregular margins.

Current recommendations in many centers are that routine screening with cranial ultrasonography should be performed on all infants of less than 30 weeks gestation at least once between 7 and 14 days of age and should be repeated optimally between 36 and 40 weeks postmenstrual age. Of course, additional scanning may be indicated on the basis of clinical events.

Computed Tomography

In the term newborn, scanning with computed tomography (CT) during the newborn period has excellent prognostic value and may demonstrate diffuse or focal cerebral injury. Optimal timing of CT scans to demonstrate the maximal extent of decreased tissue attenuation is approximately between 2 and 5 days of age, which corresponds to the time of occurrence of maximal extent of cerebral edema (Fig. 50-1A) (28). Accurate interpretation of tissue attenuation on CT requires careful attention to scanning technique to ensure appropriate window and level settings. Two major patterns of hypoxic–ischemic brain injury may be identified on CT. The first pattern in which there is predominantly hypodensity of cortex and subcortical white matter with relative sparing of the deep central grey matter (28), corresponds to a neuropathological pattern which has been documented in experimental animal models following a period of "prolonged, partial asphyxia" usually lasting more than one hour. A second pattern is characterized by low attenuation in thalami and basal ganglia with relative preservation of cortex and subcortical white matter. This pattern occurs in the context of what has been termed an "acute, total" hypoxic–ischemic insult which was identified initially in experimental studies using fetal monkeys. Of course, in the human newborn such an insult should be more correctly termed "acute, near-total" in that the artificially created acute, total insult in the experimental animal studies never occurs even with acute and severe events such as umbilical cord prolapse and uterine rupture (37,43). CT scans performed later in childhood may demonstrate focal or generalized cerebral atrophy, often with multicystic encephalomalacia (Fig. 50-1B).

In contrast to the term newborn, CT is of more limited value for assessment of acute hypoxic–ischemic injury in premature newborns, because the normal high water

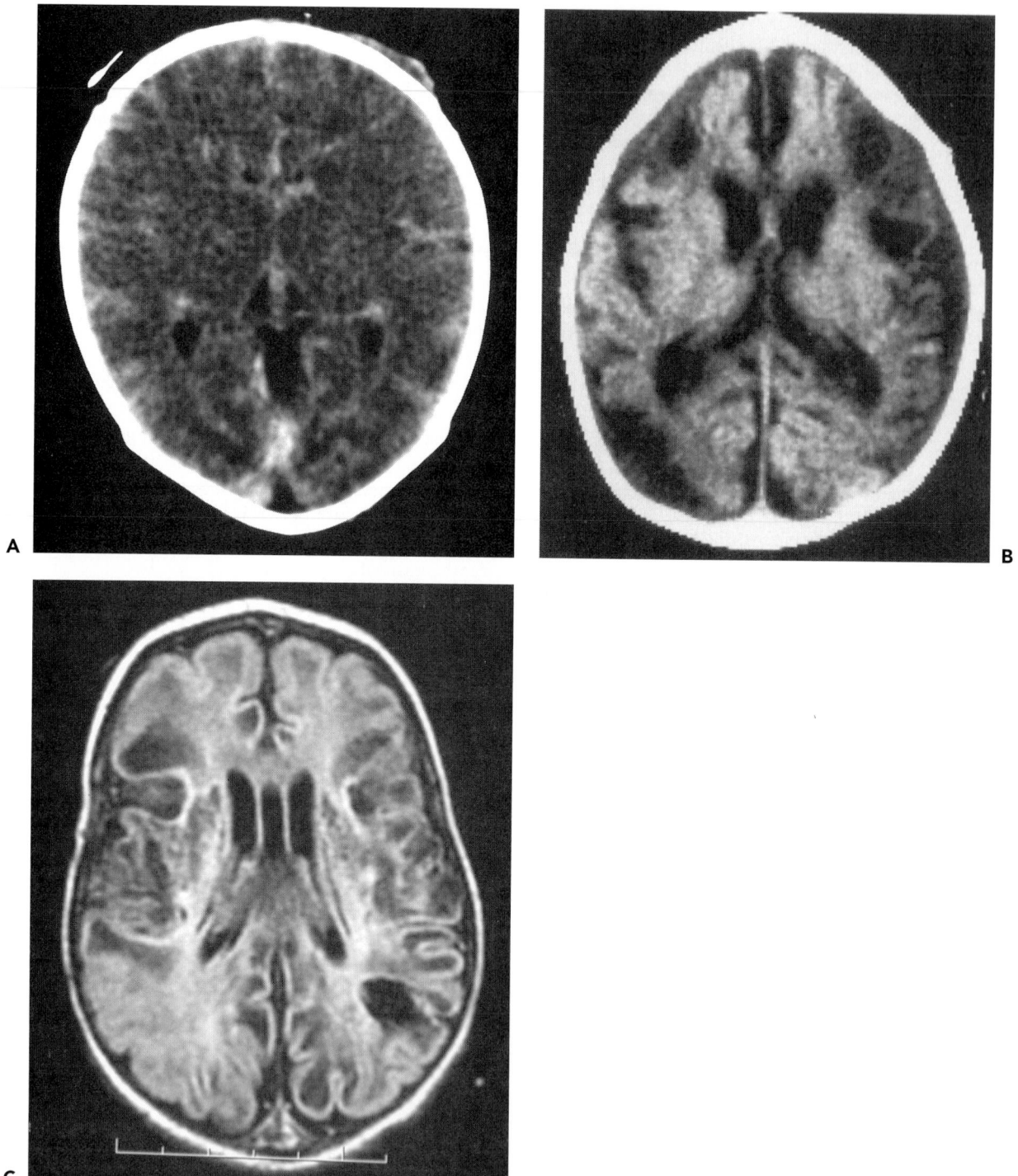

Figure 50-1   A: Computed tomographic scan of a full-term newborn (age 3 days) with severe, acute hypoxic-ischemic encephalopathy shows generalized, decreased tissue attenuation throughout both cerebral hemispheres. **B:** CT scan of the head performed at 4 months of age after hypoxic-ischemic cerebral injury at term demonstrates multicystic encephalomalacia and cerebral atrophy. **C:** Magnetic resonance imaging (T1 weighted image) performed at age 2 years after hypoxic-ischemic brain injury at term shows similar findings to CT, ie., multicystic encephalomalacia and cerebral atrophy.

content of the immature brain results in low tissue attenuation. However, CT scans performed at a later age may demonstrate the characteristic features of end-stage periventricular leukomalacia, which include (a) ventricular dilation with irregular margins of the body and trigone of the lateral ventricles, (b) decreased volume of periventricular white matter, and (c) deep sulci that abut directly on the lateral walls of the ventricles (44).

Magnetic Resonance Imaging

Magnetic resonance imaging (MRI) has the capability to demonstrate specific patterns of injury in both preterm and term newborns that may not be visualized by other imaging techniques (45–51). Thus, T2 prolongation resulting from edema (which may be transient or permanent) may appear as early as 12 to 18 hours after injury, and T1 shortening (high signal on T1-weighted images) appears in injured areas after approximately 3 days. Thus, if CT has been performed and is inconclusive, MRI should be performed between 2 and 10 days of age. Diffusion-weighted MRI appears to be even more sensitive than standard MRI during the first hours following hypoxic–ischemic injury (49,50). However, technical difficulties, e.g., the longer scanning time and difficulty with close monitoring of the sick newborn in the scanner, may limit the routine clinical application of MRI in the context of acute hypoxic–ischemic encephalopathy. At the present time, there are no large studies of CT or MRI to determine the role of MRI for the routine assessment of premature newborns with suspected hypoxic–ischemic brain injury.

Radionuclide Scanning

Radionuclide technetium scanning (52), positron emission tomography (53–55) and single photon emission CT (56), which utilize radionuclides that have the capability to cross the intact blood–brain barrier, can provide insights into regional abnormalities of cerebral perfusion. However, since advances in neuroimaging, especially MRI, have become widely available, these techniques are utilized less frequently in the routine clinical assessment of newborns with hypoxic–ischemic encephalopathy.

Magnetic Resonance Spectroscopy

In severely affected infants studied by phosphorus and proton MRS, a consistent observation has been the development of delayed derangements in cerebral energy metabolism between 12 and 48 hours after resuscitation, despite the maintenance of cardiovascular and respiratory homeostasis, which, in turn, correlates closely with poor neurologic outcome (57,58). However, because of the complexity and cost of the technique, MRS remains essentially a research technique available only on a limited basis at selected centers.

Near-Infrared Spectroscopy

Near-infrared spectroscopy (NIRS), a noninvasive technique that may be used at the bedside, has the capability to provide information concerning cerebral oxygenation and cerebral blood flow in real time. However, the technical limitations of the equipment and complexity of the data analysis have limited its application in critically ill newborns in all but a few centers. In a small number of infants with hypoxic–ischemic encephalopathy, significant cerebral vasodilation and vasoparalysis have been documented using NIRS (59).

Electrodiagnostic Techniques

Electrodiagnostic techniques are used in the evaluation of hypoxic–ischemic cerebral injury, especially in term newborns. On EEG recordings, a discontinuous pattern with voltage suppression or rapid bursts of sharp and slow waves are associated with poor outcome. In contrast, rapid resolution of EEG abnormalities and a normal interictal EEG pattern are associated with a good outcome (23,60–62).

Serial evoked potentials, especially visual evoked responses (63–65), and somatosensory evoked responses (13,66) may provide valuable prognostic information. However, their routine clinical application, especially in premature infants (67,68) has been limited by technical difficulties.

Biochemical Markers

Several enzymes and metabolites (e.g., creatine kinase BB isozyme, hypoxanthine, lactate) in urine, blood, or CSF may be of value as indicators of hypoxic–ischemic cerebral injury (1). In this regard, the measurement of urinary lactate to creatinine ratios appears to be most promising (69). However, further study of the precise sensitivity and specificity of these metabolic parameters is required before they can be recommended for routine use. Furthermore, metabolic derangements that are considered secondary to the hypoxic injury, e.g., acidosis, hypoglycemia, and hyponatremia secondary to inappropriate secretion of antidiuretic hormone, and hyperammonemia may contribute to the cerebral injury.

Pathogenesis and Neuropathology

The pathogenetic mechanisms that determine the major neuropathologic patterns of injury may be explained by a combination of regional circulatory and metabolic factors of the affected brain, especially the regional distribution of excitatory amino acid synapses (e.g., glutamate receptors) and the severity and duration of the hypoxic–ischemic insult. The major neuropathologic patterns of hypoxic–ischemic cerebral injury are listed in Table 50-4.

Circulatory Factors

The initial circulatory response to perinatal asphyxia involves the redistribution of cardiac output with increased perfusion of vital organs, e.g., brain, heart, adrenals and with concomitant decreased blood flow to other organs, e.g., the lungs, kidneys, liver. Prolonged hypoxic–ischemic insult results in systemic hypotension. The significance of hypotension is potentiated by impairment of cerebrovascular autoregulation which may occur even after relatively moderate hypoxic–ischemic insult (70,71). Cerebrovascular autoregulation is the homeostatic mechanism that maintains relatively constant cerebral perfusion over a wide range of systemic arterial blood pressures by means of cerebral arteriolar constriction or dilation. As a consequence of

TABLE 50-4

MAJOR NEUROPATHOLOGIC PATTERNS

Pattern of Injury	Gestational Age		Anatomic Distribution
	Full Term	Premature	
Selective neuronal necrosis	+	+	Cerebral and cerebellar cortex, thalamus, brainstem, hippocampus
Parasagittal	+	−	Parasagittal cortex, subcortical white matter
Focal or multifocal necrosis	+	+	Unilateral or bilateral cerebral cortex
Periventricular leukomalacia	−	+	Periventricular white matter

+, common; −, rare.

the deficiency in the muscular lining of cerebral arterioles in the immature brain, the occurrence of hypercarbia or hypoxemia, or because the normal blood pressure of the newborn is close to the down slope of the normal autoregulatory curve, (or a combination of these factors), the protective mechanism of cerebrovascular autoregulation may be disrupted. This dysfunction of the cerebrovascular autoregulation mechanism results in a direct, linear correlation between cerebral perfusion and systemic blood pressure.

Systemic hypotension, which results in moderate decreases in cerebral perfusion, may result in injury confined principally to the watershed zones of arterial supply. In the term newborn, the watershed zones between the anterior, middle, and posterior cerebral arteries are located in the parasagittal regions of the cerebral cortex. In the premature newborn, the most vulnerable watershed zone is located in the periventricular white matter (72).

Metabolic Factors

Regional differences in the rate of energy metabolism, lactate accumulation, calcium influx, and free-radical formation may explain the increased susceptibility of specific regions, e.g., thalamus, basal ganglia, and brainstem, to acute hypoxic–ischemic insult. Additionally, selective vulnerability may reflect the active myelination in specific locations during the newborn period.

A fundamental process believed to play a critical role in hypoxic–ischemic neuronal damage is excitotoxicity, a term which refers to cell death mediated by excessive stimulation of extracellular excitatory amino acid receptors (73). There is compelling experimental evidence that excitatory neurotransmitters, especially glutamate, play a critical role in the expression of hypoxic–ischemic neuronal injury. Clearly, evolving hypoxic–ischemic injury is accompanied by increased neuronal excitement, e.g., seizures. Furthermore, based on experimental animal models, drugs that block N-methyl-D-aspartate (NMDA) type glutamate channels may protect the brain from severe hypoxic–ischemic insults (74).

Additional processes that are receiving increased attention include mitochondrial failure and delayed programmed cell death or apoptosis (73).

MAJOR NEUROPATHOLOGIC PATTERNS OF INJURY

Selective Neuronal Necrosis

Selective neuronal necrosis of neurons involves specific regions of the cortex, e.g., the Sommer sector of the hippocampus, thalamus, brainstem, cerebellum, and anterior horn cells of the spinal cord. Major pathogenetic factors include circulatory factors and the severity and duration of the insult. Thus, in both experimental animal models (75,76) and human term newborns (28,77,78), "prolonged, partial" hypoxic–ischemic insult results in cerebral injury involving principally the cortex and subcortical white matter. In contrast, "acute, near total" asphyxia, which may occur in the context of events such as umbilical cord prolapse or uterine rupture, results in a pattern of injury affecting predominantly thalami, basal ganglia, and brainstem with relative preservation of cortex and subcortical white matter (37,43). This regional vulnerability relates principally to the differing rates of metabolism and myelination of various locations within the affected brain, including the anatomic distribution of glutamatergic synapses (1,73,79).

The clinical manifestations in the newborn reflect to the specific sites of injury. For example, infants with extensive cortical/subcortical injury may have seizures and possibly raised intracranial pressure (28,78), whereas infants who have predominantly thalamic, basal ganglia and brainstem involvement have characteristic features of irritability, tonic posturing, and lower cranial nerve dysfunction e.g., tongue fasciculations, feeding problems (1,37,43). Although the injury is predominantly central, there is still some cortical injury, albeit less severe, that may result in seizures and other cortical signs.

The late neuropathologic sequelae of selective neuronal necrosis which involves predominantly the cortex and subcortical white matter include cerebral atrophy and, following severe injury, multicystic encephalomalacia (Fig. 50-1B, 50-1C). Clinical features in older children include spastic cerebral palsy, mental retardation, microcephaly, and seizures of varying severity. Injury to thalamus and basal ganglia which may have occurred in the context of an acute, near total type of hypoxic–ischemic insult may result in a striking, marbled appearance of these structures (Fig. 50-2B), and the evolution appears radiologically as shown in Fig. 50-2A,C, which has been termed as "status marmoratus." The characteristic clinical sequelae include choreoathetotic cerebral palsy and bulbar dysfunction (feeding difficulties) and there is relative preservation of function referable to cortex, e.g., cognitive function and absence of seizures.

Parasagittal Cerebral Injury

In the term newborn, the parasagittal cortex and subcortical white matter are located in the watershed zone of arterial supply between the anterior, middle, and posterior cerebral arteries, an area that is vulnerable to ischemic injury (1,77) (Fig. 50-3).

Clinical features of parasagittal injury during the newborn period include hypotonia and weakness, which are more prominent in the proximal upper extremities (shoulder girdle) than in the lower limbs.

Focal and Multifocal Cerebral Necrosis

Focal arterial occlusion by embolus or thrombus is well recognized in the newborn (Fig. 50-4). In premature newborns, such infarction is often multifocal. In the majority of cases, no specific cause can be identified. However, conditions that may predispose to focal ischemic necrosis include coagulation disturbances, e.g., polycythemia, disseminated intravascular coagulation, protein C or S deficiency, antithrombin deficiency, Factor V Leiden deficiency, maternal isoimmune thrombocytopenia, and intrauterine cocaine exposure, vascular maldevelopment, and emboli from punctured or catheterized vessels or involuting placental vessels (80–83).

Newborn infants who develop focal arterial infarction most commonly present with unilateral, focal motor seizures. Alternatively, infants may be asymptomatic or display asymmetric motor function. Long-term sequelae include cerebral palsy (often hemiparesis), seizures, and intellectual impairment (84,85).

Venous sinus thrombosis in the newborn has been diagnosed more frequently because MRI has become more readily available. Predisposing conditions include coagulation disturbances, dehydration, and sepsis (86,87). Clinical features in the newborn include lethargy and seizures that are not necessarily focal. The long-term sequelae are not well defined. Approximately one-third of affected children are reported to have developmental delay.

Periventricular Leukomalacia

This lesion which affects primarily infants born prematurely, involves the arterial end zones within the periventricular white matter in the premature brain (1,72). Two principal components of injury have been recognized: focal and diffuse white matter injury. There is increasing evidence that the pathogenesis of periventricular leukomalacia relates to a variable combination of three major factors: the distribution of arterial vascular end zones within the cerebral white matter, maturation-dependent impairment in cerebrovascular auto-regulation of cerebral blood flow, intrinsic vulnerability of early differentiating oligodendroglial precursors to free radicals and, in some instances, exposure to endotoxemia (71,72,88). Secondary hemorrhage, albeit often of mild severity, has been reported in approximately 25% of autopsy studies in patients with periventricular leukomalacia (89) and in survivors (90).

The severity of white matter injury ranges from minor focal areas of gliosis or necrosis to diffuse involvement (Fig. 50-5). Severe focal lesions may be visualized in vivo by cranial ultrasonography as areas of increased echogenicity in periventricular white matter during the first days of life, which subsequently evolve into cystic lesions after approximately 2 to 3 weeks (41). MRI and diffusion MRI may also permit early visualization of these lesions, but the role of these techniques has not been defined fully (45).

Hemorrhagic periventricular leukomalacia must be distinguished from periventricular hemorrhagic infarction, which is usually unilateral (Fig. 50-6) or strikingly asymmetric (91). This lesion is associated with large GMH or IVH, and it is considered to represent venous infarction resulting from obstruction of the terminal vein by a large GMH (92,93).

The clinical features of periventricular leukomalacia in the premature newborn may be subtle and include weakness or altered muscle tone involving predominantly the lower extremities. Long-term sequelae include spastic diplegia or quadriplegia and, occasionally, visual and auditory impairment related to involvement of the optic and auditory radiations (1). Additionally, periventricular leukomalacia may have a role in the genesis of derangements of cerebral cortical organization because of injury to subplate neurons or interference with late migrating astrocytes, which, in turn, may insult in impaired cognitive function (94).

Management

Awareness of major risk factors during the intrauterine period has promoted prevention of hypoxic–ischemic insult by close monitoring of the high-risk fetus and consideration of urgent delivery in the event of persistent fetal distress. Furthermore, an asphyxiated newborn requires immediate and close surveillance to minimize additional postnatal injury. In this context, provision of adequate ventilation and perfusion, maintenance of normal blood pressure and normoglycemia, and control of seizures are of

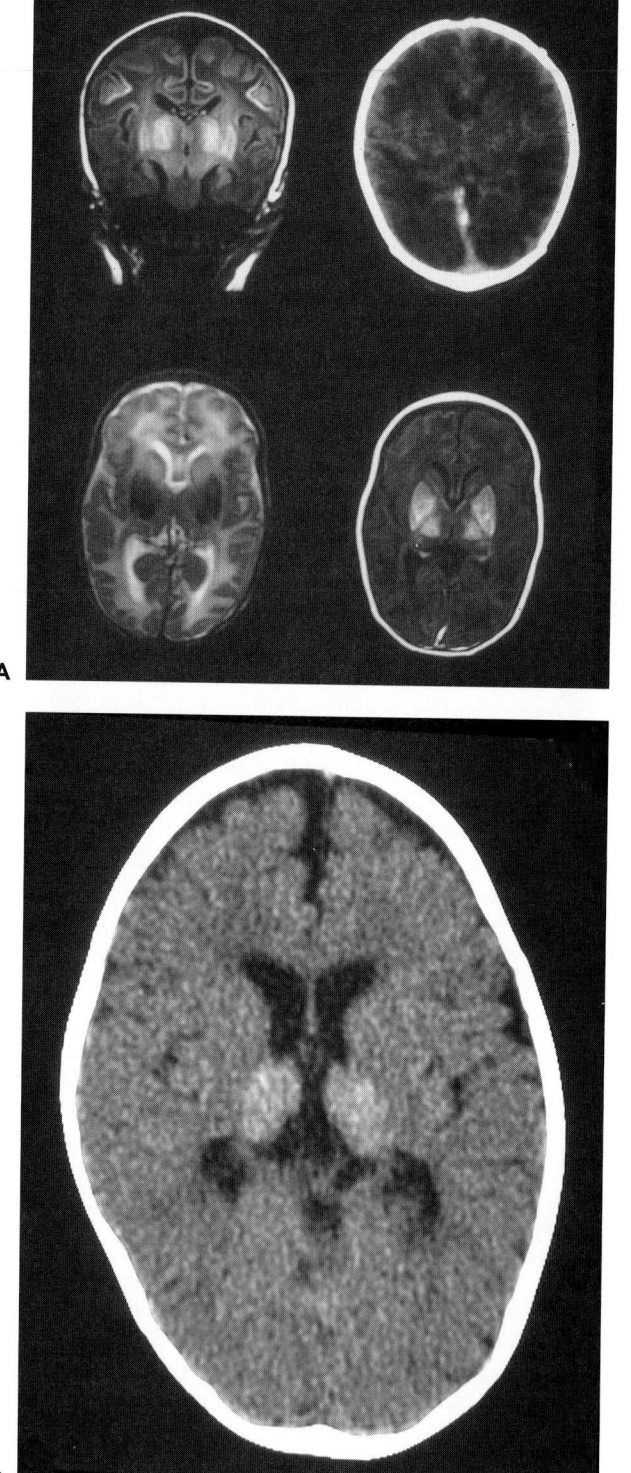

A

B

C

Figure 50-2   A: Composite image demonstrating evolution of central hypoxic-ischemic brain injury (involving thalami and basal ganglia) in term newborn on neuroimaging. Upper right image shows CT at 3 days of age demonstrating decreased tissue attenuation in thalami. Upper left image shows coronal MRI (T1 weighted image) at age 10 days with abnormal signal in thalami, basal ganglia and motor strip of cortex bilaterally. Lower right image shows MRI at age 10 days with abnormal signal in thalami and basal ganglia. Lower left image shows MRI (T2 weighted image) at age 2 years with atrophy and low signal in thalami and basal ganglia. **B:** Status mermoratus of basal ganglia is demonstrated in a coronal section of the cerebral hemispheres stained for myelin from a patient who died years after the insult. The marbled appearance is especially striking in the putamen (courtesy of E.P. Richardson Jr, MD). **C:** CT scan of 4 year old child demonstrates small thalami with gliosis, consistent with status memoratus.

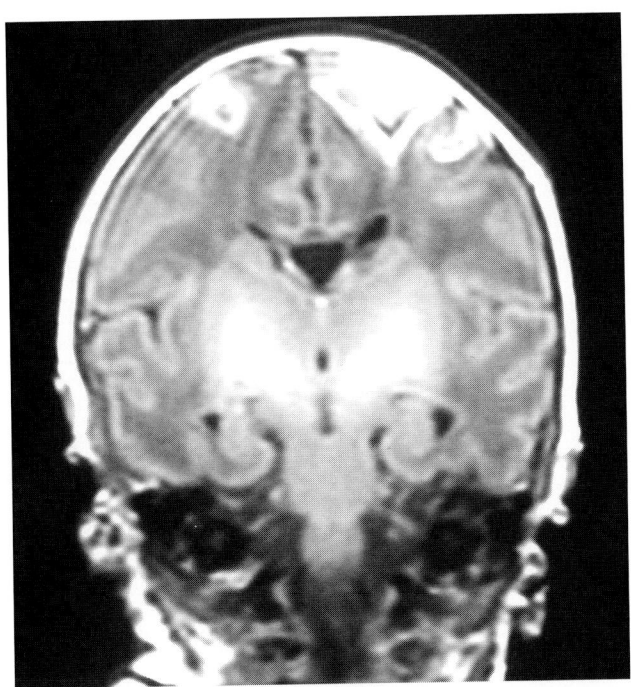

Figure 50-3 Coronal MRI scan (T1-weighted image) of term newborn performed at 10 days of age demonstrates abnormal signal in parasagittal watershed zones and thalami bilaterally.

critical importance. On the other hand it is important to avoid excessive oxygen delivery in that there is increasing concern about the potential deleterious effects of hyperoxia especially in premature newborns (95). There is a high incidence of dysfunction of other organ systems, e.g., heart, kidneys, and gastrointestinal (GI) tract, which must be monitored carefully.

Adequate ventilation and the avoidance of postnatal hypoxemia may be difficult to achieve because of the cardiorespiratory problems associated with severe hyaline membrane disease in the premature newborn and persistent fetal circulation and pulmonary hypertension in the term newborn. Administration of surfactant and nitric oxide, extracorporeal membrane oxygenation and high-frequency ventilation are newer treatment modalities that are discussed in detail elsewhere. Because hypoxemic episodes in the premature newborn may be associated with events such as suctioning or spontaneous crying, minimal handling is recommended for these infants. On the other hand, there is increasing concern that hyperoxia should also be avoided (95).

Because impaired cerebrovascular autoregulation has been documented even in the context of moderate hypoxic– ischemic encephalopathy, maintenance of normal systemic arterial blood pressure and adequate cerebral perfusion are essential. This may require volume replacement and the use of inotropic agents (e.g., dopamine) especially if there is evidence of myocardial dysfunction. In the premature newborn, systemic hypotension may occur in the context of patent ductus arteriosus and recurrent apnea of prematurity. On the other hand, systemic hypertension must also be avoided, especially in the premature newborn,

because it may predispose to GMH/IVH from rupture of the fragile vasculature of the germinal matrix.

Seizures that occur in the context of acute hypoxic–ischemic encephalopathy may be refractory to anticonvulsant therapy. Nevertheless, aggressive treatment is indicated to minimize associated apnea, hypertension, and metabolic derangements, such as depletion of brain glucose and high-energy phosphate compounds.

The optimal levels of blood glucose that should be maintained after hypoxic–ischemic insult have not been established. However, maintenance of normoglycemia is generally recommended. Inappropriate antidiuretic hormone secretion following major hypoxic–ischemic cerebral injury may result in hyponatremia and decreased osmolality, with a consequent risk of cerebral edema and seizures. Fluid overload should be avoided.

Data from human and experimental animal studies suggest that elevated intracranial pressure associated with hypoxic–ischemic encephalopathy in the term newborn reflects extensive cerebral necrosis, which represents a consequence rather than a cause of hypoxic–ischemic brain injury. Maximal elevations of intracranial pressure are observed between 36 and 96 hours after the initial insult and are associated with a poor outcome. Although it is possible to reduce elevated intracranial pressure by antiedema agents (e.g., mannitol and diuretics), there is no evidence that such intervention improves long-term neurologic outcome (28,33).

Potential neuroprotective strategies that are currently under investigation include NMDA receptor antagonists, inhibitors of free radical production, free radical scavengers, nerve growth factors and mild hypothermia. These interventions target either excessive excitotoxic glutamate release or the mitochondrial failure following severe hypoxic–ischemic insult which is associated with disruption of cell membranes and tissue necrosis, or the delayed process of programmed cell death, i.e., apoptosis (73,96,97).

There is increasing understanding of the fact that hypoxic–ischemic insult/reperfusion sets in motion a deleterious cascade of events leading to neuronal death that evolves over many hours and days and which may be interrupted by interventions which are instituted after termination of the insult (96,97). Of the current interventions under consideration, there is extensive experimental evidence from animal studies and promising clinical data in human newborns for the use of mild hypothermia, either whole body hypothermia or head cooling only. Modest hypothermia 34.5°C or 35°C or slightly lower appears to postpone secondary energy failure and may potentially prolong the window for usefulness of other pharmacologic interventions. Observed physiologic changes and complications of hypothermia include fall in heart rate or abnormal cardiac rhythm and coagulation disturbances, none of which are considered to be life-threatening. Preliminary results on the value of hypothermia regarding extent of brain injury based on MRI evaluation and neurological outcome are encouraging. Randomized controlled trials are currently under way to confirm this experience and to establish clinical protocols for the use of hypothermia in human newborns (97–99).

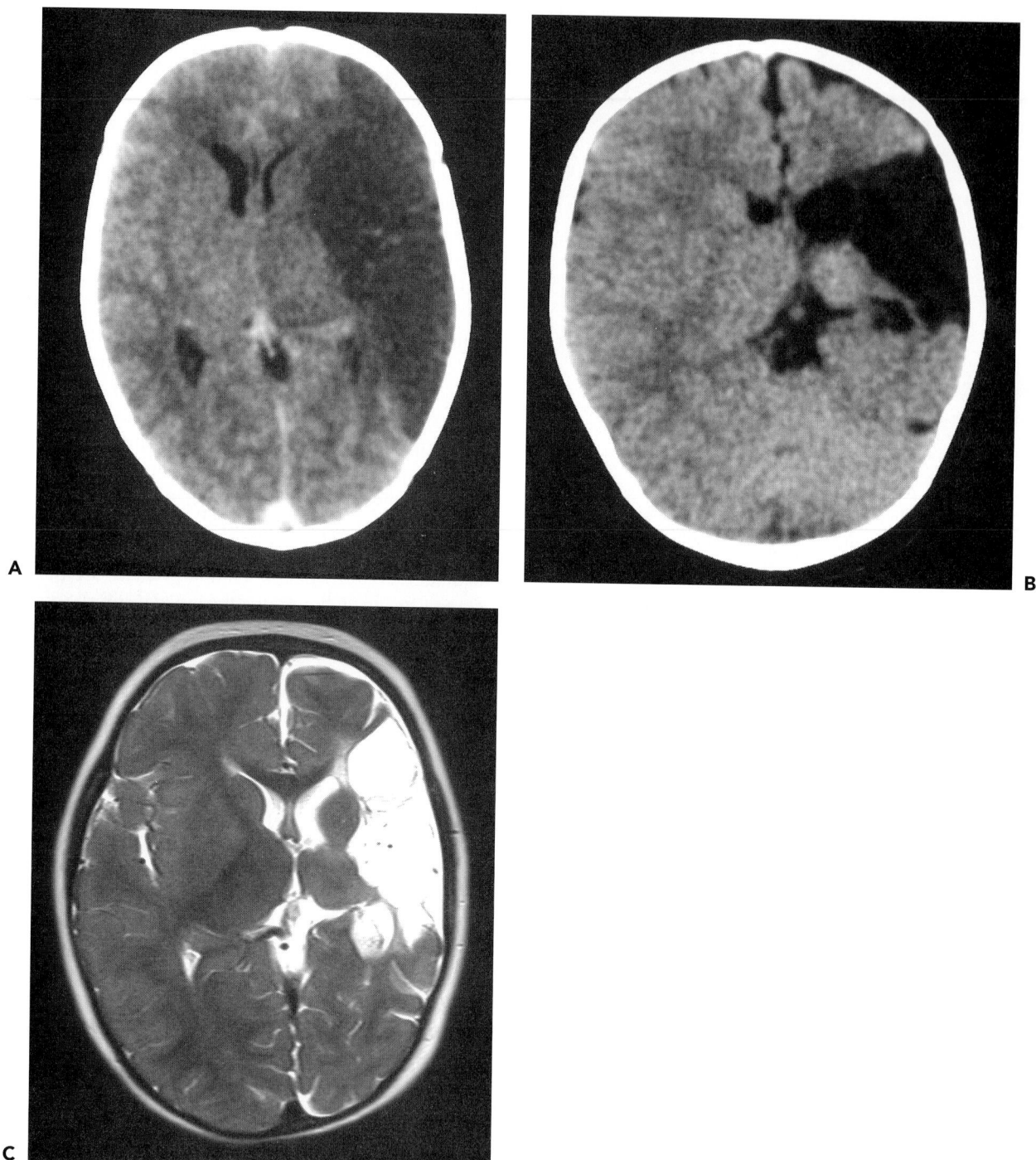

Figure 50-4   A: Computed tomographic scan of a full term newborn with acute, focal infarction involving the territory of the left middle cerebral artery. **B:** CT scan of an infant at 18 months of age showing porencephalic cyst in location of earlier cerebral infarction. **C:** MRI of infant performed at age 2 years with abnormal signal in location of infarction.

Prognosis

In our experience in the term newborn, the severity and duration of the clinical hypoxic–ischemic encephalopathy and severity of the EEG background abnormality, combined with the extent of abnormality on acute neuroimaging, e.g., decreased tissue attenuation visualized on CT scans (performed between 2 and 5 days after the original insult) or abnormal signal on MRI permit reasonably accurate prediction of outcome. The prediction of outcome in the asphyxiated premature newborn is more difficult.

INTRACRANIAL HEMORRHAGE

The incidence of GMH/IVH in premature newborns has declined in recent decades from approximately 40% to less than 20%. Although there has been a significant

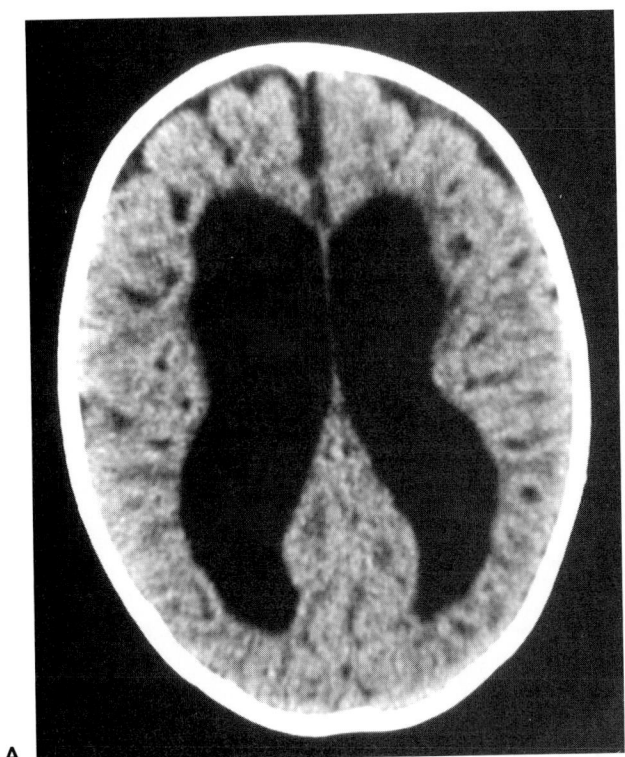
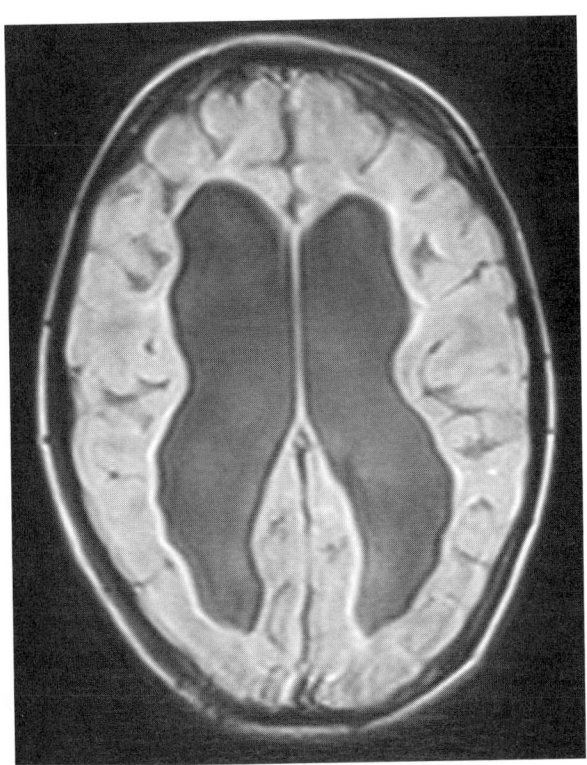

A
B

Figure 50-5 **A:** Computed tomography scan performed at 14 months of age in an infant born prematurely demonstrates periventricular leukomalacia with marked loss of volume of periventricular white matter, with cortex abutting directly onto the ventricles and secondary ventricular enlargement. **B:** MRI scan (T1 weighted image) of infant performed at 2 years of age demonstrating similar findings as CT.

reduction in incidence during recent years, GMH/IVH remains a major concern, principally because of the improved survival rates of very-low-birth-weight infants who are at highest risk for the development of GMH/IVH. In the premature newborn, rupture of fragile vessels in the subependymal germinal matrix occurs relatively frequently (Fig. 50-7). In approximately 80% of cases, there is associated IVH, and in approximately 15% there is associated parenchymal hemorrhagic infarction. Serial cranial ultrasonography has demonstrated that 50% of cases of GMH/IVH originate during the first day of life and 90% occur before 4 days of age. In 20% to 40%, the hemorrhage may extend during the first week of life (1).

Diagnosis

Neuroimaging

Cranial ultrasonography is considered the neuroimaging modality of choice for the diagnosis of GMH/IVH because of its portability, high resolution, and lack of ionizing radiation. Computed tomography and MRI remain superior for the diagnosis of other types of intracranial hemorrhage, including primary subarachnoid, convexity, and posterior fossa subdural or epidural hematomas and for differentiating between hemorrhagic and ischemic parenchymal infarction.

Because of the relatively high risk of GMH/IVH, in many centers cranial ultrasonography is recommended to be performed routinely at least once between 7 and 14 days of age in all infants of less than 30 weeks gestation (100). Ultrasonography should be performed earlier if there are specific clinical concerns. Ultrasound scans are recommended to be done after the first week of life to establish the maximal extent of the lesion. Subsequently, serial scans may be indicated every 1 to 2 weeks after major GMH/IVH for surveillance of ventricular size and possible development of posthemorrhagic hydrocephalus. This is particularly important because of the high degree of compliance of the premature brain and cranium which, together with the relatively large subarachnoid spaces permit considerable increase in ventricular size prior to the onset of excessive head growth.

Clinical Features

The diagnosis of GMH/IVH may be suspected on the basis of clinical signs alone in only approximately 50% of patients. The severity of clinical abnormalities ranges from an asymptomatic state through a saltatory neurologic deterioration over several days to a catastrophic presentation with coma, apnea, tonic extensor posturing, brainstem dysfunction, and flaccid quadriparesis. Associated systemic abnormalities may include hypotension, metabolic acidosis, bradycardia, and disturbances of serum glucose and

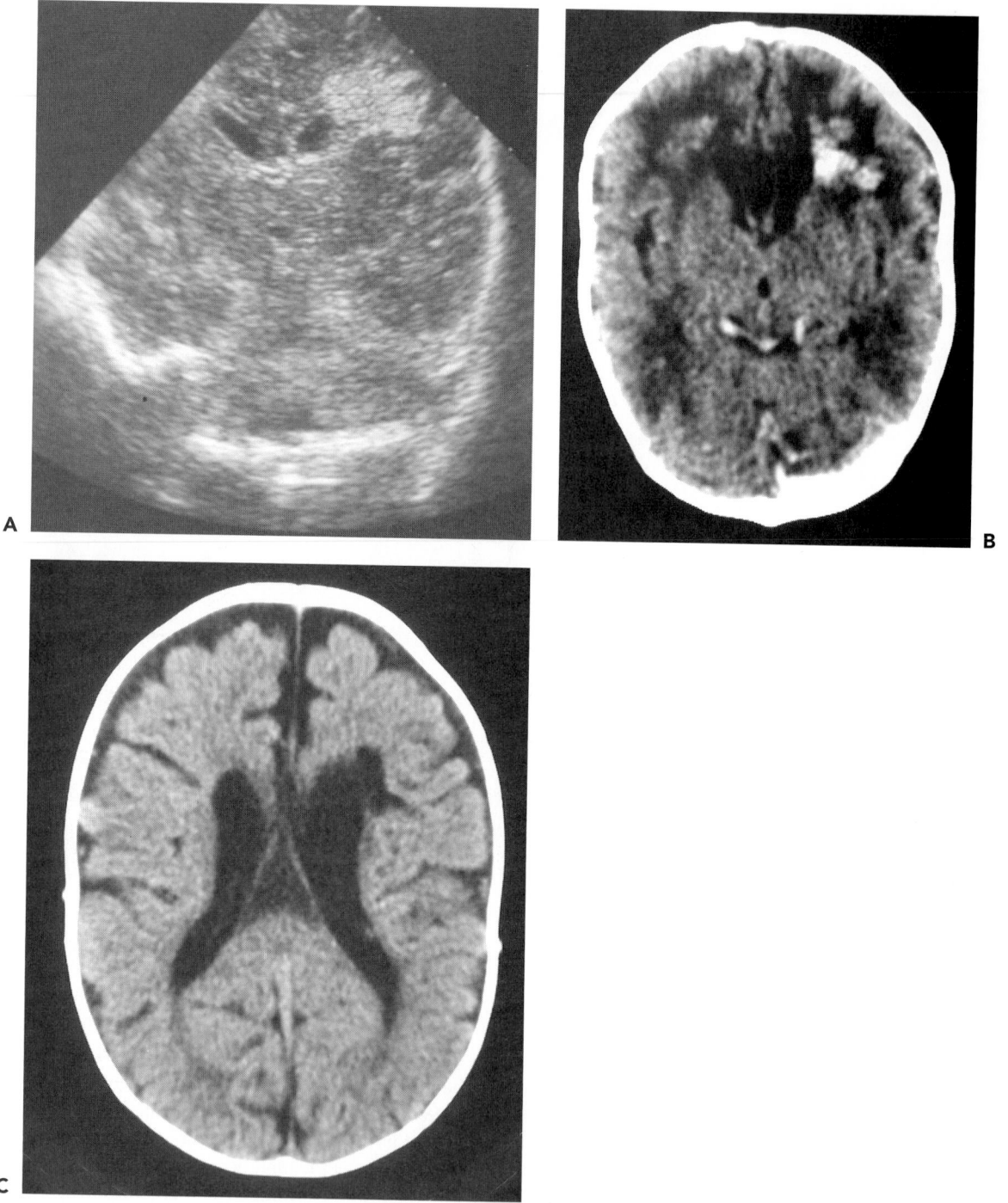

Figure 50-6 **A:** Coronal ultrasound scan of premature infant showing left periventricular hemorrhagic infarction with fan-shaped unilateral increased echoes in periventricular white matter. **B:** CT scan of infant showing unilateral fan-shaped periventricular hemorrhagic infarction. Note absence of intraventricular hemorrhage. **C:** Late CT scan of infant showing fan-shaped cyst in location of previous hemorrhagic infarction.

electrolytes. Bloody or xanthochromic CSF supports a diagnosis of intracranial hemorrhage.

Pathogenesis

The pathogenesis of GMH/IVH is multifactorial and consists of a combination of intravascular, vascular, and extravascular factors (Table 50-5). The importance of individual factors

may vary in different situations. Consideration of these major pathogenetic mechanisms provides a framework for the selection of appropriate interventional strategies.

Intravascular factors involve principally the regulation of cerebral perfusion (e.g., cerebral blood flow and pressure) within the fragile vasculature of the germinal matrix, platelet–capillary interactions and coagulation disturbances. Vascular pathogenetic factors include the fragility of vessels

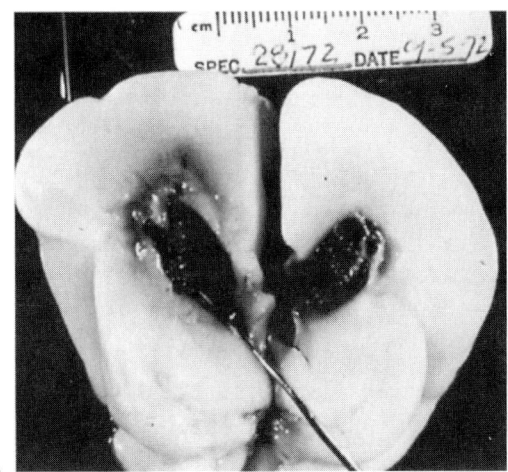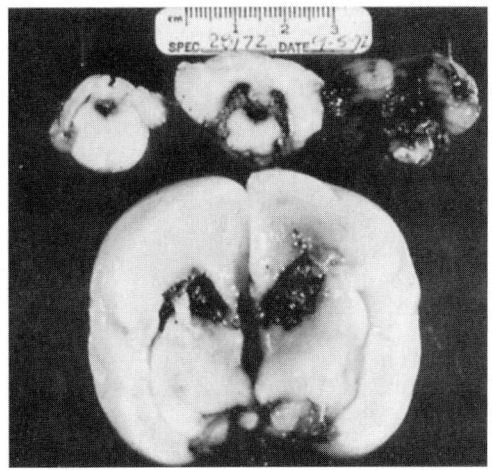

Figure 50-7 **A:** Periventricular hemorrhage with large right subependymal hemorrhage. Blood fills both lateral ventricles. **B:** Hemorrhage can be seen in the lateral ventricles, the aqueduct of Sylvius, the fourth ventricle, and the subarachnoid space around the cerebellum and the base of the brain (courtesy of John Axley, MD).

in the germinal matrix and their vulnerability to hypoxic–ischemic insult. Extravascular factors relate to the characteristics of the supporting tissues, excessive fibrinolytic activity, and a possible decrease in tissue pressure postnatally.

Posthemorrhagic hydrocephalus and periventricular hemorrhagic infarction are the major complications of GMH/IVH. Other mechanisms of cerebral injury associated with GMH/IVH include concomitant or preceding hypoxic–ischemic cerebral injury (e.g., periventricular leukomalacia, neuronal necrosis of the brainstem), and destruction of the germinal matrix with its glial precursors.

Ventriculomegaly and hydrocephalus, i.e., progressive ventriculomegaly associated with disturbed CSF dynamics, occur commonly after major GMH/IVH (Table 50-6). Clearly, massive GMH/IVH may be associated with acute ventriculomegaly. More commonly, communicating hydrocephalus develops gradually over weeks, usually as a consequence of impaired CSF reabsorption secondary to an obliterative arachnoiditis in the posterior fossa. An additional potential mechanism involves the blockage of CSF resorption at the small arachnoid villi by particulate debris floating in CSF after GMH/IVH. Obstructive hydrocephalus may occur secondary to blockage of the flow of CSF especially at the level of the aqueduct of Sylvius by blood clot or other intraventricular debris (1,101).

The characteristic clinical signs of hydrocephalus (e.g., abnormally rapid increase in head circumference, bulging anterior fontanel, suture diastasis) may be delayed for days or weeks after the onset of progressive ventricular dilation is observed on serial ultrasound scans (1).

The delay in clinical manifestation of increased intracranial pressure is related to the high compliance of periventricular tissue in the immature brain, especially after hypoxic–ischemic injury, and the relatively generous subarachnoid space in the premature infant, which allow

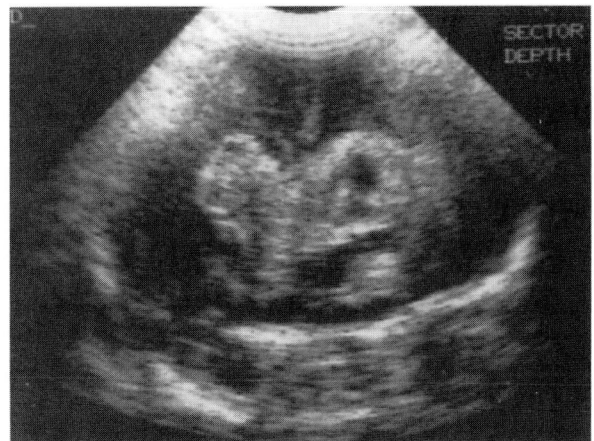

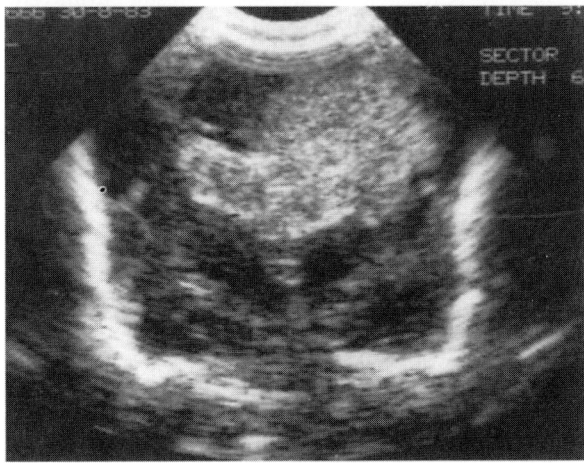

Figure 50-8 **A:** Ultrasonographic scan in the coronal plane of marked intraventricular hemorrhage delineates blood in the dilated frontal borns of the lateral ventricles and central clearing of the hematoma. **B:** Ultrasonographic scan in the coronal plane of marked intraventricular hemorrhage delineates blood in the dilated frontal horns of the lateral ventricles and intraparenchymal hematoma.

TABLE 50-5
PATHOGENESIS OF GERMINAL MATRIX–INTRAVENTRICULAR HEMORRHAGE

Pathogenic Factor

Intravascular
  Alterations in cerebral blood flow
  Alterations in cerebral venous pressure
  Coagulation disturbances
Vascular
  Fragility of vessels in subependymal germinal matrix
Extravascular
  Poor vascular support of germinal matrix
  Decrease in tissue pressure (?)

increase in ventricular size without expansion of head circumference.

Ventriculomegaly after GMH/IVH may become static or resolve spontaneously usually within four weeks of onset in approximately 65% of cases (1). In the remainder, amelioration of increased intracranial pressure by temporary or permanent drainage of CSF or by medical intervention to decrease CSF production is required. Recent data suggest that the natural history of posthemorrhagic ventriculomegaly may be evolving such that the course is more aggressive necessitating intervention in a greater percentage of affected infants (102). In approximately 5% of cases, progressive posthemorrhagic hydrocephalus may be delayed for many months, which necessitates ongoing surveillance of ventricular size by serial cranial ultrasonography during the first year of life (103).

Periventricular hemorrhagic infarction has been documented in approximately 15% of infants with major GMH/IVH. This predominantly unilateral parenchymal lesion is a major determinant of long-term neurologic sequelae (91). Neuropathologic studies indicate that such fan-shaped parenchymal hemorrhage results from venous infarction, usually with secondary hemorrhage related to obstruction of the medullary and terminal veins by large GMH (92,93). This pathogenesis differs from that of hemorrhagic periventricular leukomalacia, which is usually bilateral and represents an arterial ischemic lesion with secondary hemorrhage. Because periventricular hemor-

TABLE 50-6
MAJOR COMPLICATIONS OF GERMINAL MATRIX–INTRAVENTRICULAR HEMORRHAGE

- Ventriculomegaly, posthemorrhagic hydrocephalus
- Periventricular hemorrhagic cerebral infarction
- Acute increased intracranial pressure with major intraventricular hemorrhage
- Destruction of germinal matrix glial precursors
- Focal ischemia (?)
- Concomitant hypoxic–ischemic cerebral injury (i.e., periventricular leukomalacia)

rhagic infarction and periventricular leukomalacia often occur concomitantly, distinction between the two conditions may be difficult.

Management

Clearly, the primary goal is prevention of GMH/IVH. Prevention of premature labor and delivery may be considered to be the optimal management strategy. Alternatively, interventions should address the major pathogenetic mechanisms as outlined previously (104,105).

Antenatal Interventions

Prevention of premature labor and delivery has been attempted with maternal tocolytic therapy, e.g., β-sympathomimetics, indomethacin, or magnesium sulfate. Unfortunately, these medications often succeed in delaying labor for only several days, although even such brief delay may be sufficient to permit administration of a course of antenatal steroids to induce fetal lung maturation, thereby reducing the likelihood of GMH/IVH. Unfortunately, tocolytic medications may have adverse hemodynamic effects in the fetus, which, in turn, may increase the risk of hemorrhagic and ischemic cerebral injury and outweigh potential benefits (106–108). A more encouraging approach to prevention of premature labor in selected women involves antimicrobial treatment (e.g., metronidazole, erythromycin) of bacterial vaginosis, a relatively common condition in which normal vaginal flora is replaced by anaerobic organisms. Such intervention has been shown to decrease the risk for premature rupture of membranes, chorioamnionitis and premature delivery (109,110).

Antenatal corticosteroids which induce fetal lung maturation and lead to maturation and involution of the fragile germinal matrix vasculature, definitely reduce the overall incidence and severity of GMH/IVH. Because even an incomplete course of antenatal corticosteroid has some benefit, prompt treatment is indicated for most women who are at imminent risk for premature delivery (111–113). Additionally, transfer of the high-risk mother to a tertiary perinatal center prior to delivery is recommended.

Intrapartum Management

There is increasing evidence that vaginal delivery, duration of labor longer than 12 hours regardless of the mode of delivery, and a trial of labor before cesarian section are all associated with increased risk of GMH/IVH (111,114). Presumably, risks of labor and vaginal delivery relate principally to deformations of the compliant skull and associated transient increases in cerebral venous pressure. Although earlier studies had suggested that antenatal phenobarbital and Vitamin K may be associated with a reduced incidence of GMH-IVH, recent comprehensive review of combined data from all clinical trials for the Cochrane Database failed to demonstrate a benefit from either medication (115,116).

Postnatal Management

Correction or prevention of major hemodynamic disturbances, including fluctuating cerebral blood flow, systemic hypotension and hypertension, and increases in cerebral venous pressure, may reduce the overall incidence and severity of GMH/IVH. Because of the impaired cerebrovascular autoregulation in the sick premature newborn, alterations in systemic blood pressure are reflected directly in changes in cerebral blood flow. Care must be taken to prevent systemic hypertension associated with excessive handling, suctioning, and rapid infusions of blood or colloid. Additionally, adequate ventilation must be maintained to avoid apnea, pneumothorax, and hypercapnia. Although not available routinely, the noninvasive technique of NIRS has the potential capability of identifying in real time the premature infants with pressure-passive circulation, who are at high risk for developing GMH/IVH (71,72).

Respiratory distress syndrome and its complications, e.g., pneumothorax, bronchopulmonary dysplasia, are associated with a high risk of hemodynamic disturbances and hence, GMH/IVH. Treatment with surfactant is the single most important advance in the management of lung immaturity. Collective data from the Cochrane Database suggests that intratracheal surfactant, either natural or synthetic, administered prophylactically in the delivery room is most efficacious (117). In ventilated infants whose respirations are asynchronous with the ventilator and who are at increased risk of GMH/IVH and pneumothorax, neuromuscular paralysis with pancuronium bromide is associated with significant reduction in GMH/IVH (1). However, at the present time, the routine use of pancuronium in ventilated newborns is not recommended as a result of concerns about long-term pulmonary and neurologic effects (118). Sedation with other agents, e.g., phenobarbital (119), midazolam (120) and the use of high frequency oscillating ventilation (121) have not been shown to be effective for reducing GMH/IVH and may, in fact have deleterious effects.

In addition to hemodynamic disturbances, abnormal coagulation, especially abnormal platelet function, is thought to play a role in the genesis of GMH/IVH in some instances. However, to date, the combined data from all randomized trials do not show a reduction of severe GMH/IVH or mortality with routine use of early volume expansion with normal saline, fresh frozen plasma, albumin or blood substitutes (122).

Indomethacin, which is used for treatment of symptomatic patent ductus arteriosus, appears to be associated with significantly reduced incidence of severe GMH/IVH without adverse long-term effects (123). In addition to altering the hemodynamic status and reduction of cerebral blood flow, indomethacin may have beneficial effects by inhibition of free radical synthesis and acceleration of maturation of the germinal matrix vasculature.

Posthemorrhagic Hydrocephalus

Ventriculomegaly, which has been reported to occur in approximately 25% to 35% of infants with GMH/IVH, may arrest or resolve spontaneously, usually within four weeks of onset. More recent studies suggest that the course of posthemorrhagic hydrocephalus may be evolving such that approximately two thirds of affected infants may require active intervention (102). A major obstacle to developing a rational strategy for the management of posthemorrhagic ventriculomegaly is an inability to diagnose precisely the onset of associated brain injury in premature newborns in whom multiple mechanisms are occurring simultaneously which may predispose to cerebral injury (101).

The situation is complicated further because clinical criteria for the diagnosis of increased intracranial pressure lack sensitivity in the newborn and are often delayed. Serial cranial ultrasonography may identify progressive ventricular dilation which precedes clinical signs. However, to date, there are no standardized measurements of ventricular size. Useful observations of progressive hydrocephalus on ultrasound scans include: rapid progression of ventricular dilation, prominent dilation of the temporal horns of the lateral ventricles, decrease in ventricular size following CSF removal, a periventricular hyperechoic outline (as a result of transependymal CSF accumulation) and echogenicity (signifying subarachnoid hemorrhage) in basal cisterns, sylvian fissure and spinal subarachnoid space.

Temporizing interventions for progressive posthemorrhagic hydrocephalus during the first weeks of life usually involve mechanical removal of CSF by serial lumbar punctures, external ventricular drainage, subcutaneous ventricular access device or ventriculosubgaleal shunt in which fluid is drained from the ventricles into the subgaleal space. These techniques may be effective if it is technically possible to remove sufficient CSF, i.e., 10–15 ml/kg/day, for at least 2 to 3 weeks. The value of early "prophylactic" intervention prior to development of progressive ventriculomegaly with repeated lumbar punctures or ventricular puncture (124) or intraventricular fibrinolytic therapy with streptokinase (125) before the onset of ventriculomegaly to prevent hydrocephalus has revealed no benefit in terms of requirement for permanent shunt placement, death or severity of neurologic sequelae.

The nonsurgical approach to treatment of posthemorrhagic hydrocephalus involves either medications which decrease CSF production, e.g., acetazolamide, furosemide or osmotic agents, e.g., isosorbide, glycerol. Medical therapy is limited by complications which include metabolic acidosis, electrolyte disturbances, hypercalciuria, nephrocalcinosis, glial and myelin toxicity. Comprehensive analysis on medical therapy has concluded that acetazolamide and furosemide are neither effective nor safe for treatment of posthemorrhagic hydrocephalus (126).

The optimal timing for permanent ventriculoperitoneal shunt placement remains controversial. Earlier studies favored early shunt insertion but more recent studies found no correlation between timing of shunt insertion and outcome. In fact, it may be argued that shunt insertion when residual blood clot and debris are present, increases the risk for shunt obstruction and infection which correlate with poor outcome.

Prognosis

The outcome of infants with GMH/IVH is related principally to the size of the hemorrhage, complications of posthemorrhagic hydrocephalus and associated hypoxic–ischemic cerebral injury, e.g., PVL. For infants with small GMH/IVH alone, survival without major neurologic sequelae is the rule. In infants who sustain severe GMH/IVH with ventriculomegaly or parenchymal involvement, the incidence of major neurologic sequelae increases to 30 to 40%. Of course, the most critical determinant of long-term outcome is the extent of parenchymal involvement. Major GMH/IVH occurs frequently in the context of hypoxic–ischemic cerebral insult, and long-term neurologic outcome depends in large part on concomitant or preceding hemorrhagic or nonhemorrhagic hypoxic–ischemic cerebral injury.

There is also a high risk of major neurologic sequelae in infants with posthemorrhagic hydrocephalus, especially those who had placement of a ventriculoperitoneal shunt. In one study, approximately 35% died and 50% had moderate or severe neurologic impairment at 5 years of age (127). In another multicenter, randomized controlled trial of 157 cases of posthemorrhagic hydrocephalus, 20% died and 76% had major motor impairment. Furthermore, early drainage of CSF did not improve outcome significantly compared with controls (128).

SUBDURAL HEMORRHAGE

Improvements in obstetric practice and a decrease in mechanical birth trauma have reduced considerably the incidence of severe subdural hemorrhage. This type of hemorrhage accounts for less than 5% to 10% of intracranial hemorrhage in the newborn (129). However, the data must be interpreted with the recognition that mild subdural hemorrhage which is not uncommon in the posterior fossa may have few associated clinical abnormalities and may remain undiagnosed.

Subdural hemorrhage occurs in premature and term infants and results from laceration of the major veins and sinuses, usually associated with a tear of the dura or dural reflections (e.g., falx, tentorium) overlying the cerebral hemispheres or cerebellum. Excessive molding of the head may play a role in the genesis of subdural hemorrhage. Clinical features include a decreased level of consciousness, seizures, or asymmetry of motor function. Clinical outcome is determined in large part by the extent of associated hypoxic–ischemic injury.

Diagnosis

CT or MRI are the techniques of choice for the identification of subdural hemorrhage. Differentiating subdural from intracerebellar hemorrhage may be difficult in infants who have evidence of hemorrhage in the posterior fossa on CT or MRI scans. Intracerebellar hemorrhage appears to be more common in premature infants (130), and posterior fossa subdural hemorrhage is more common in term newborns (1).

The diagnosis of posterior fossa hemorrhage and small lesions located over the cerebral convexities may be difficult using the traditional cranial ultrasonography approach through the anterior fontanelle. Imaging through the posterolateral fontanelle may improve visualization of the posterior fossa. Supratentorial lesions are usually demonstrated better by CT, whereas MRI is superior for evaluation of posterior fossa hemorrhage. Lumbar puncture is not indicated for diagnostic study in this setting because of the possibility of provoking herniation.

Occipital diastasis and skull fractures are demonstrated best by skull radiographs.

Management

Convexity subdural hemorrhage, particularly if associated with displacement of the midline, should be referred for a neurosurgical opinion for consideration of evacuation by subdural tap or craniotomy, especially if there is clinical deterioration with signs of transtentorial herniation. Massive subdural hemorrhage located in the posterior fossa may require surgical evacuation. Surgical intervention may not significantly improve the long-term outcome if there are no major neurologic signs (1).

Prognosis

The prognosis for infants with major lacerations of the tentorium or falx is poor. The mortality rate is approximately 45%, and survivors frequently develop hydrocephalus and other sequelae. More than 50% of survivors who sustain lesser degrees of hemorrhage are neurologically normal at follow-up. Concomitant hypoxic–ischemic cerebral injury is often the critical factor in determining outcome.

PRIMARY SUBARACHNOID HEMORRHAGE

Primary subarachnoid hemorrhage, which is located most prominently in the subarachnoid space over the cerebral convexities and in the posterior fossa, refers to hemorrhage within the subarachnoid space that is not secondary to extension of subdural hemorrhage, IVH, or cerebellar hemorrhage. Unlike the dramatic arterial hemorrhage in adults, subarachnoid hemorrhage in the newborn is usually self-limited and of venous origin, originating from small vessels in the leptomeningeal plexus or in bridging veins within the subarachnoid space (1). Trauma or hypoxic events may be important antecedents of major degrees of primary subarachnoid hemorrhage, although the pathogenesis usually is uncertain. Long-term sequelae are uncommon. Rarely, hydrocephalus may develop secondary to adhesions at the outflow of the fourth ventricle or over the cerebral convexities.

Clinical Features

Definition of the clinical features related solely to primary subarachnoid hemorrhage has been made difficult by its association with trauma, hypoxic ischemic insult, and other forms of intracerebral hemorrhage that produce abnormal neurologic signs. Nevertheless, three syndromes of primary subarachnoid hemorrhage are generally recognized (1). The first syndrome of minimal or no clinical features is the most common. In the second syndrome, seizures occur most commonly on the second day of life, and the infant is usually well between seizures. The third syndrome, associated with massive subarachnoid hemorrhage, consists of rapid neurologic deterioration and is uncommon. The infant usually has also sustained severe hypoxic–ischemic cerebral injury, with or without trauma, or has a major vascular abnormality, e.g., arteriovenous malformation or aneurysm.

Diagnosis

The diagnosis of primary subarachnoid hemorrhage is based on the finding of uniformly blood-stained CSF on lumbar puncture in an infant in whom other forms of intracranial hemorrhage have been excluded by CT. With primary subarachnoid hemorrhage, CT usually demonstrates blood in the superior longitudinal fissure and in sulci.

Management

Seizures are treated with anticonvulsant medication. Hydrocephalus is managed as described previously in this chapter.

Prognosis

In the absence of preceding severe trauma, hypoxic–ischemic cerebral injury, or ruptured vascular lesion, the outcome is favorable. Outcome correlates well with the neonatal clinical syndrome. In infants with minimal or no clinical signs, the prognosis is excellent. In term infants with seizures, 90% are normal at follow-up. In the rare instance of massive subarachnoid hemorrhage with catastrophic deterioration, death and hydrocephalus are common.

INTRACEREBELLAR HEMORRHAGE

Postmortem studies suggest that primary hemorrhage into the cerebellum is a relatively common lesion, especially in infants born prematurely. The routine use of cranial ultrasonography through the posterolateral fontanelle in premature infants has confirmed that this lesion may have been under diagnosed previously in surviving infants (130).

Neuropathology

Causes of cerebellar hemorrhage include traumatic laceration of the cerebellum or sinuses, venous infarction, or extension of IVH or massive subarachnoid hemorrhage into the cerebellum. Pathogenetic factors include tenuous vascular integrity, skull deformation, occipital diastasis, impaired cerebrovascular autoregulation with hypoxic–ischemic insult, and bleeding from fragile vessels of the germinal external granule cell layer of the cerebellum.

Clinical Features

Most reports of intracerebellar hemorrhage in premature infants are based on autopsy studies. Clinical details are based on retrospective analyses. There is usually a history of hypoxic–ischemic insult or an association with severe respiratory distress syndrome. In most instances, there is a catastrophic deterioration with apnea, bradycardia, and a decrease in hematocrit. Clinical signs appear usually in the first 3 weeks of life, with most beginning within the first 2 days of life. In term infants, there is usually a history of difficult breech delivery, with subsequent development of neurologic signs referable to brainstem compression, e.g., stupor or coma, cranial nerve abnormalities, apnea, bradycardia, and opisthotonus.

Diagnosis

The lesion may be suspected on the basis of the history and physical features as described previously. Definitive diagnosis is made by CT or MRI. Traditional cranial ultrasonography through the anterior fontanelle is of limited value for visualizing intracerebellar hemorrhage (130).

Management

Early detection by CT, MRI, or ultrasound scans is essential. Decisions concerning surgical or conservative management are based on the size of the lesion and the clinical state of the infant. Recovery without surgical intervention has been reported. Fishman and colleagues (131) reported successful conservative management of six full-term infants with intracerebellar hemorrhage and recommend that, if the clinical picture is stable and there is no increase in intracranial pressure, supportive care and serial CT examinations may be all that is necessary. Our ongoing experience with nonsurgical management of selected cases supports this notion. The appropriate management of this lesion in the premature newborn is unclear, although it is unlikely that surgery plays a significant role.

Prognosis

Most reports of intracerebellar hemorrhage in the premature infant are based on autopsy studies. For the premature infant with severe intracerebellar hemorrhage and especially when there are relevant clinical abnormalities, the prognosis is uniformly poor. The outcome of premature newborns with clinically silent presentation and term newborns may be more favorable for survival. However, the majority develop significant long-term motor and cognitive impairment. Hydrocephalus requiring VP shunt insertion occurred in approximately 50% of both surgically treated and untreated infants.

INTRAVENTRICULAR HEMORRHAGE IN THE TERM NEWBORN

Intraventricular hemorrhage is considered to be a condition which occurs principally in premature newborns. However, it occurs also in a small percentage of term newborns, often in the context of prior hypoxic–ischemic or traumatic insults. The sites of origin of IVH in the term newborn are more variable and include residual germinal matrix, choroids plexus, vascular malformations, tumor or hemorrhagic venous infarction of the thalamus. This latter entity often presents somewhat later, after several days or weeks of age (1,132).

The diagnosis and management of IVH and its complications in the term newborn are similar to those described for premature newborns.

The prognosis for IVH in term newborns may be worse than in premature newborns. Approximately 70% of term newborns with IVH develop posthemorrhagic ventriculomegaly, of which only 20% arrest or resolve spontaneously and 50% require placement of a ventriculoperitoneal shunt (1). Long-term neurological sequelae of varying degrees of severity occur in more than 50% of affected children. These relate principally to the associated parenchymal damage, and the underlying etiology, especially trauma and hypoxic–ischemic insult.

BRAIN DEATH IN NEONATES

Current guidelines for the diagnosis of brain death in adults and children do not include preterm or term newborns who are less than 7 days of age because of the lack of sufficient data dealing with this age group (133,134). This topic has been reviewed in detail by Ashwal (125). Clearly, there are fundamental differences between the evolution of brain death in neonates compared to older individuals. In the newborn infant, factors such as the patent sutures and open fontanelle make it unlikely that increased intracranial pressure and consequent decreased cerebral perfusion will develop. Furthermore, brainstem reflexes, which are fundamental for brain-death determination, may be difficult to elicit or they are incomplete especially before 32 weeks' gestation. Apnea testing, which is considered critical for the objective diagnosis of brain death in older individuals, may be invalid especially in infants below 33 weeks of gestational age, who have diminished respiratory drive to CO_2 stimulation (135).

The role of confirmatory neurodiagnostic testing in the newborn, e.g., EEG, cerebral blood flow measurements and radioisotope studies also remains unclear because of the limited data available. Earlier studies of brain-dead neonates have shown significant lack of correlation between EEG and cerebral blood flow (CBF) studies, e.g., one third of neonates who had electrocerebral silence had evidence of CBF and 58% of those with absent CBF had evidence of EEG activity on an initial recording (135). Of the techniques that are currently available for the assessment of cerebral perfusion, four vessel angiography, positron emission tomography and xenon-CT are generally too cumbersome technically for routine use in neonates. Radioisotope flow studies appear to have greater sensitivity and specificity than Doppler CBF velocity measurements. However, this technique does not address the critical issue that blood flow is more likely to persist in brain dead newborns and the lower limits of blood flow required to support the immature brain or brainstem have not been established (136,137).

Although unresolved issues remain, current data suggests that brain death can be diagnosed in the term newborn, provided that there is an awareness of the limitations of the clinical examination and that laboratory investigations, e.g., EEG, CBF studies frequently do not demonstrate the typical confirmatory abnormalities. It is important to perform repeated examinations of infants in whom brain death is suspected to demonstrate the absence of brainstem reflexes more accurately and to perform formal apnea testing that documents loss of respiratory effort when arterial CO_2 tension is greater than 60 torr. An observation period of 48 hours has generally been recommended to establish the diagnosis. This period of time may be shortened to 24 hours if the EEG is isoelectric or if CBF studies demonstrate absence of flow. Although there are few preterm infants who meet these criteria for brain death, it is likely that a similar time frame would be applicable. Using these guidelines, based on the available data, the risk for misdiagnosis appears low. In the rare instances when minimal transient clinical or EEG improvements have been demonstrated, meaningful neurologic function has not been attained and all infants have died after brief periods of time (135).

NEUROMUSCULAR DISORDERS

Neuromuscular disease implies dysfunction of the motor system at a level between the motor cortex and muscle. However, in conventional discussions, this term is often restricted to lower motor neuron and muscle diseases, i.e., disorders at a level between the anterior horn cell and muscle. The most critical task for the physician is to define the anatomic level of the underlying abnormality.

Diagnosis

Lower motor neuron disorders should be considered clinically whenever an alert newborn presents with hypotonia and weakness. However, in many instances, e.g., congenital muscular dystrophy, myotonic dystrophy, and mitochondrial cytopathies, there may be associated CNS involvement. Furthermore, infants with neuromuscular disease may sustain secondary hypoxic–ischemic brain injury related to respiratory muscle weakness or pulmonary hypoplasia.

Because most neuromuscular disorders are inherited and some, e.g., Duchenne muscular dystrophy, may be asymptomatic in the newborn period, a detailed family history is of critical importance. Specific complications of pregnancy, e.g., decreased fetal movements, polyhydramnios, and breech presentation, are a common occurrence. In addition to assessment of muscle bulk, tone, and power, examination for presence of muscle fasciculations, facial diplegia, or ptosis support a diagnosis of neonatal neuromuscular disease.

Laboratory investigations in older children with muscle disease often include elevation of serum creatine phosphokinase levels. Unfortunately, this screening test is of limited value in the newborn, because levels may be increased up to tenfold following normal vaginal delivery. Chest x-ray may demonstrate thin ribs related to decreased fetal respiratory efforts or cardiac enlargement suggestive of cardiomyopathy. Nerve conduction velocities and electromyography may establish the level of involvement of the motor system, but the technical performance and interpretation of data are difficult in the newborn age group (138). Although imaging techniques, e.g., ultrasonography, CT, and MRI, have some role in the investigation of muscle disease, there is limited experience in the newborn. Muscle biopsy, either by open, surgical, or needle biopsy technique, is technically feasible. However, problems with histologic interpretation may arise during the newborn period, as a result of nonspecific abnormalities that exist in the early stages of progressive muscular dystrophies (139).

Molecular genetic techniques have clearly revolutionized the diagnosis of neuromuscular disease and decreased the need for invasive investigations. However, clinical assessment must still direct these genetic investigations (140).

Major Neuromuscular Conditions

Anterior Horn Cell Disease

Anterior horn cell disorders, include type I spinal muscular atrophy (Werdnig–Hoffman disease), type II glycogen storage disease (Pompe's disease), neurogenic arthrogryposis multiplex congenita, and neonatal poliomyelitis. These disorders account for approximately 35% of all cases of neonatal hypotonia of neuromuscular origin. Characteristically, infants are alert but profoundly hypotonic and weak with absent tendon reflexes, paradoxical diaphragmatic respiratory movements, and a majority have prominent fasciculations of the tongue. Electrical studies and muscle biopsy demonstrate severe acute and chronic denervation. The genetic defect of autosomal recessive type I spinal muscular atrophy has been identified on chromosome 5q, which enables molecular diagnostic tests and prenatal testing (141). Although muscle strength may remain relatively static, overall deterioration and decreased survival result from repeated respiratory infections and aspiration, prolonged immobility, and hospitalization (142).

PERIPHERAL NERVE DISORDERS

Disorders of peripheral nerves rarely present in the newborn period. The clinical course is variable and may even be nonprogressive or reversible (1,143). Diagnosis may be confirmed by nerve conduction studies. Adjunctive investigations include measurement of CSF protein, lactate levels, and possibly sural nerve biopsy. Peripheral neuropathy may be one presenting problem of metabolic disorders in the newborn, e.g., Krabbe's disease, mitochondrial disease.

DISORDERS OF THE NEUROMUSCULAR JUNCTION

These conditions present with fluctuating muscle weakness, variable ptosis, ophthalmoplegia, facial weakness, impaired feeding, hypoventilation, and autonomic disturbances. Disorders include myasthenia gravis (transient or congenital) and toxic-metabolic problems, e.g., hypermagnesemia, aminoglycoside toxicity, and infantile botulism.

Transient myasthenia gravis, which is related to circulating maternal antiacetylcholine receptor antibodies, occurs in approximately 20% of infants of mothers with myasthenia. There is no correlation between the disease severity in the mother and that observed in the infant and only poor correlation between maternal antibody titers and disease severity in the infant. The diagnosis may be confirmed by evaluating the infant's response to neostigmine. The advantage of neostigmine in neonates relates to its more prolonged duration of action (1–4 hours) which permits serial assessments. Neostigmine is usually administered intramuscularly or subcutaneously at a dose of 0.15 mg/kg with a maximum dose of 2 mg. The intravenous dose is one third the intramuscular dose and should be accompanied or preceded by atropine, as a result of risk of bronchorrhea, asystole, bradycardia and hypotension.

Management of transient myasthenia gravis includes supportive treatment, anticholinesterase therapy, and possibly exchange transfusion and intravenous immunoglobulin (IVIG) (144) until symptoms resolve, often after several weeks. Congenital myasthenia relates to anatomic defects of the neuromuscular junction, which have variable response to pyridostigmine (139,145).

Early diagnosis of disorders of neuromuscular transmission is critical because many of these conditions respond to treatment and timely intervention may prevent serious complications.

Primary Muscle Disorders

Generalized muscle disorders include the genetically determined progressive muscular dystrophies which have nonspecific histologic features of muscle necrosis, regeneration, fibrosis on muscle biopsy and nonprogressive congenital myopathies, which are characterized by distinctive histologic abnormalities (1,139).

The major muscular dystrophies that present in the newborn include congenital myotonic dystrophy and congenital muscular dystrophy. Congenital myotonic dystrophy is inherited exclusively from the mother. A family history may often not be recognized because the disease is often milder in the mother and may have been undiagnosed prior to the birth of a more severely affected infant. The diagnosis may be confirmed by molecular genetic studies in either the mother or the affected newborn, i.e., demonstration of an increase in trinucleotide repeats (CTG) at the myotonic dystrophy gene locus at chromosome 19q. During pregnancy, there are often decreased fetal movements and a history of polyhydramnios. Often there is failed labor and urgent cesarean section is required. Affected infants are often premature and present at birth with hypotonia, weakness, hypoventilation, impaired sucking and swallowing, facial diplegia, ptosis, and arthrogryposis. Additionally, there is usually significant cognitive impairment, which may be associated with abnormalities on neuroimaging, especially increased risk of intracerebral hemorrhage. Clinical signs of myotonia are absent in neonates but develop later in childhood. However, the EMG of affected newborns may demonstrate myotonic potentials, which are generally higher pitched, quieter and less sustained than those in adults. The mortality rate is high and the long-term clinical course is variable (146). Many affected newborns require ventilator support for respiratory insufficiency. Prognosis is poor for survival if ventilation is required for longer than four weeks. There is risk for recurrent aspiration and persistent feeding difficulties. Orthopedic interventions, e.g., splinting and surgery are required for management of talipes.

The term congenital muscular dystrophy (CMD) comprises several disorders that have an autosomal recessive inheritance pattern and may be classified according to whether there is isolated muscular dystrophy (merosin-positive CMD) or a combination of CNS and skeletal muscle involvement (merosin-deficient CMD). CNS involvement may include cerebral dysgenesis, cerebral white matter, and ocular abnormalities and may be suspected on the basis of seizures, glaucoma, optic nerve abnormalities, or cataracts. The clinical course of patients with a combination of CNS involvement and evidence of merosin deficiency on muscle biopsy is often progressive with decreased survival, whereas in infants who have myopathy alone, (merosin positive CMD) muscle weakness is often static and affected individuals may even attain ambulation (139,147).

Investigations reveal normal or moderate elevation of creatine kinase levels (>1,000 IU) and dystrophic abnormalities on muscle biopsy. Results of neuroimaging studies may be abnormal. In cases with CNS abnormalities, immunocytochemical analysis of the muscle biopsy may reveal deficiency of merosin, an extracellular protein that is associated closely with the muscle membrane. The merosin protein is thought to play a significant role in the pathogenesis of congenital muscular dystrophy.

In addition to the muscular dystrophies, there are numerous congenital myopathies that are classified according to their specific histologic abnormalities. The pathologic process affects exclusively the striated or voluntary muscles. Rarely cardiac muscle may be involved. With the exception of nemaline myopathy and X-linked myotubular myopathy, which may present with respiratory failure in early infancy, hypotonia and weakness are often relatively mild and static.

Nemaline myopathy is the most common type of congenital myopathy, which may have either an autosomal dominant or recessive inheritance pattern. There is a severe neonatal variety` which presents at birth with severe muscle weakness, respiratory insufficiency and difficulties with sucking and swallowing. Pregnancy complications with fetal akinesia may occur. Death as a result of respiratory complications is common during the first weeks or months of life, although some severely involved newborns have survived, with relatively little residual disability. There is a mild, congenital form of nemaline myopathy that presents with mild weakness, feeding difficulties and delayed motor milestones.

Metabolic Myopathies

With the availability of electron microscopy, muscle enzyme assays, and MRS, the diagnosis of muscle conditions in which there is primary derangement of energy metabolism, is being made with increasing frequency, e.g., mitochondrial cytopathies, carnitine deficiency, and disorders of lipid and glycogen. Clinical features in these disorders include hypotonia, weakness, failure to thrive, encephalopathy, hypoglycemia, and cardiomyopathy. Muscle histology and enzyme abnormalities usually are diagnostic. Detailed discussion of the biochemical aspects of metabolic myopathies is beyond the scope of this chapter.

Management

The management of neuromuscular disorders in the newborn is often associated with major genetic and ethical dilemmas, especially regarding a reasonable approach to the initiation and duration of mechanical ventilatory support. Unfortunately, few scientific guidelines exist. Other supportive management strategies include oxygen therapy, nasogastric feeding, and aggressive physiotherapy and orthopedic interventions to minimize joint contractures. Specific therapies exist for some conditions, e.g., pyridostigmine for myasthenia gravis.

Clearly, the prognosis of neuromuscular conditions is variable and depends principally on the specific disorder involved.

REFERENCES

1. Volpe JJ. *Neurology of the newborn.* Philadelphia: WB Saunders, 2001.
2. Dubowitz LMS, Dubowitz V, Mercuri E. *The neurological assessment of the preterm and full term newborn infant.* London: MacKeith Press, 1999.
3. Borch K, Pryds O, Holm S, et al. Regional cerebral blood flow during seizures in neonates. *J Pediatr* 1998;132:431.
4. Wasterlain CG. Recurrent seizures in the developing brain are harmful. *Epilepsia* 1997;38:728.
5. Holmes GL, Gairsa JL, Chevassus-Au-Louis N, et al. Consequences of neonatal seizures in the rat: morphological and behavioural effects. *Ann Neurol* 1998;44:845.
6. Younkin DP, Delivoria-Papadopoulos M, Maris J, et al. Cerebral metabolic effects of neonatal seizures measured with in vivo 31P NMR spectroscopy. *Ann Neurol* 1986;20:513.
7. Holmes GL. Epilepsy in the developing brain: lessons from the laboratory and clinic. *Epilepsia* 1997;38:12.
8. Mizrahi EM, Kellaway P. *Diagnosis and management of neonatal seizures.* Philadelphia: Lippincott-Raven, 1998.
9. Sher MS. Pathological myoclonus of the newborn: electrographic and clinical correlations. Pediatr Neurol 1985;1:342.
10. Paolicchi JM. The spectrum of nonepileptic events in children. *Epilepsia* 2002;43[Suppl 3]:60.
11. Alfonso I, Papazian O, Aicardi J, et al. A simple maneuver to provoke benign neonatal sleep myoclonus. *Pediatrics* 1995;96:1161.
12. Hillman L, Hillman R, Dodson WE. Diagnosis, treatment and follow-up of neonatal mepivacaine intoxication secondary to paracervical and pudendal blocks during labor. *J Pediatr* 1979; 95:472.
13. Hyland K, Arnold LA. Value of lumbar puncture in the diagnosis of infantile epilepsy and folinic acid-responsive seizures. *J Child Neurol* 2002;17(Suppl 3):548.
14. Steinlein O, Haussler M, Fischer C, et al. Benign familial neonatal convulsions: confirmation of genetic heterogeneity and further evidence for a second locus on chromosome 8g. *Hum Genet* 1995;95:411.
15. Berkovic SF, Nicholson GA, Hwang PA, et al. Phenotypic expression of benign familial neonatal convulsions linked to chromosome 20. *Arch Neurol* 1994;51:1125.
16. Wang PJ, Lee WT, Hwu WL, et al. The controversy regarding diagnostic criteria for early myoclonic encephalopathy. *Brain Dev* 1998;20:530.
17. Klepper J, Wang D, Fishberg J, et al. Defective glucose transport across brain tissue barriers: a newly recognized neurological syndrome. *Neurochem Rev* 1995;24:587.
18. Ortibus EL, Sum JM, Hahn JS. Prediction value of EEG for outcome and epilepsy following neonatal seizures. *Electroencephalogr Clin Neurophysiol* 1996;98:175.
19. MacLennan A, the International Cerebral Palsy Task Force, Gunn AJ, et al. A templete for defining a causal relation between acute intrapartum events and cerebral palsy: international consensus statement. *BMJ* 1999;319:1054–1059.
20. Nelson KB, Ellenberg JH. Antecedents of cerebral palsy: multivariate analysis of risk. *N Engl J Med* 1986;315:81.
21. Blair E, Stanley FJ. Intrapartum asphyxia: a rare cause of cerebral palsy. *J Pediatr* 1988;112:515.
22. Roland EH, Hill A. How important is perinatal asphyxia in the causation of brain injury? *MRDD Research Reviews* 1997;3:22.
23. Sarnat HB, Sarnat MS. Neonatal encephalopathy following fetal distress. *Arch Dis Child* 1976;33:696.
24. Robertson CMT, Finer NN. Term infants with hypoxic–ischemic encephalopathy: outcome at 3.5 years. *Dev Med Child Neurol* 1985;27:473.
25. Robertson CMT, Finer NN. Longterm follow-up of term neonates with perinatal asphyxia. *Clin Perinatol* 1993;20:483.
26. Westgate JA, Gunn AJ, Gunn TR. Antecedents of neonatal encephalopathy with fetal acidemia at term. *Br J Obstet Gynecol* 1999; 106:774–782.
27. Robertson CMT, Grace MGA. Validation of prediction of kindergarten-age-school readiness scores of non-disabled survivors of moderate neonatal encephalopathy in term infants. *Can J Public Health* 1992;83[Suppl]:51.
28. Lupton BA, Hill A, Roland EH, et al. Brainswelling in the asphyxiated term newborn: pathogenesis and outcome. *Pediatrics* 1988;82:139.
29. Levene MI, Evans DH, Forde A, et al. Value of intracranial pressure monitoring of asphyxiated newborn infants. *Dev Med Child Neurol* 1987;29:311.
30. Clancy R, Legido A, Newell R, et al. Continuous intracranial pressure monitoring and serial electroencephalographic recordings in severely asphyxiated term newborns. *AJDC* 1988;142:740.
31. Whitelaw A. Intervention after birth asphyxia. *Arch Dis Child* 1989;64:66.
32. Vannucci RC. Current and potentially new management strategies for perinatal hypoxic–ischemic encephalopathy. *Pediatrics* 1990;85:961.
33. Adhikari M, Moodley M, Desai PK. Mannitol in neonatal cerebral oedema. *Brain Dev* 1990;23:349.
34. Perlman JM, Tack ED, Martin T, et al. Acute systemic organ injury in the term infant after asphyxia. *AJDC* 1989; 143:617.
35. Cordes I, Roland EH, Lupton BA, et al. Systemic organ involvement and hypoxic–ischemic encephalopathy in the term newborn. *Ann Neurol* 1992;32:462A.
36. Martin-Ancel A, Garcia-Alix A, Gaya F, et al. Multiple organ involvement in perinatal asphyxia. *J Pediatr* 1995;127:786.
37. Pasternak JF, Gorey MT. The syndrome of acute near-total intrauterine asphyxia in the term infant. *Pediatr Neurol* 1998; 18:391–398.
38. Phelan JP, Ahn MA, Korstl, et al. Intrapartum fetal asphyxial brain injury with absent multiorgan system dysfunction. *J Matern Fetal Med* 1998;7:19–22.
39. Barkovich AJ, Hallam D. Neuroimaging in perinatal hypoxic–ischemic injury. *MRDD Research Reviews* 1997;3:28.
40. Siegel MJ, Schackelford GD, Perlman JM, et al. Hypoxic-ischemic encephalopathy in term infants: diagnosis and prognosis evaluated by ultrasound. *Radiology* 1984;152:395–399.
41. deVries LS, Eken P, Dubowitz LMS. The spectrum of leukomalacia using cranial ultrasound. *Behav Brain Res* 1992;49:1.
42. Goldstein RB, Filly RA, Hechts, et al. Noncystic increased periventricular echogenicity and other mild cranial ultrasonographic abnormalities: predictors of outcome in low birthweight infants. *J Clin Ultrasound* 1989;17:553.
43. Roland EH, Poskitt K, Rodriquez E, et al. Perinatal hypoxic-ischemic thalamic injury: clinical features and neuroimaging. *Ann Neurol* 1998;44:161.
44. Flodmark O, Roland EH, Hill A, et al. Periventricular leukomalacia: radiologic diagnosis. *Radiology* 1987;162:119.
45. Huppi PS. Advances in postnatal neurimaging: relevance to pathogenesis and treatment of brain injury. *Clin Perinatol* 2002;29:827–856.
46. Blankenberg FG, Loh NN, Bracci P, et al. Sonography, CT and MR imaging: a prospective comparisoin of neonates with suspected intracranial ischemia and hemorrhage. *AJNR Am J Neuroradiol* 2000;21:213–218.
47. Krageloh-Mann I, Helber A, Mader I, et al. Bilateral lesions of thalamus and basal ganglia: origin and outcome. *Dev Med Child Neurol* 2002;44:477–484.
48. Mercuri E, Guzzetta F, Baraja L, et al. Neonatal neurological examination in infants with hypoxic-ischemic encephalopathy: correlation with MRI findings. *Neuropediatrics* 1999;(2):83–89.
49. Saul JS, Robertson RL, Tzika AA, et al. Time cause of changes in diffusion-weighted magnetic resonance imaging in a case of neonatal encephalophy with defined onset and duration of hypoxic-ischemic insult. *Pediatrics* 2001;108:1211–1214.
50. Robertson RL, Ben-Sira L, Bajres PD, et al. MR line scan diffusion imaging of term neonates with perinatal brain ischemia. *AJNR Am J Neuroradiol* 1999;20:1658–1670.
51. Flodmark O, Lupton B, Li D, et al. MR imaging of periventricular leukomalacia in childhood. *AJNR Am J Neuroradiol* 1989;10: 111–118.
52. O'Brien MJ, Ash JM, Gilday DL. Radionuclide brain scanning in perinatal hypoxia–ischemia. *Dev Med Child Neurol* 1979;21:161.
53. Volpe JJ, Herscovitch P, Perlman JM, et al. Positron emission tomography in the asphyxiated term newborn: parasagittal impairment of cerebral blood flow. *Ann Neurol* 1985;17:287.

54. Ryding E, Svenningsen NW. Cerebral glucose metabolism measured by positron emission tomography in term newborns with hypoxic-ischemic encephalopathy. *Ped Res* 2001;49:495–501.

55. Chugani HT. Positron emission tomography scanning: applications in newborns. *Clin Perinatol* 1993;20:395–409.

56. Korishi Y, Kuriyama M, Mori I, et al. Assessment of local cerebral blood flow in neonates with N-isopropyl-P[123] iodoamphetamine and single photon emission computed tomography. *Brain Dev* 1995;16:450–453.

57. Barkovich AJ, Baranski K, Vigneron D, et al. Proton MR spectroscopy for the evaluation of brain injury in asphyxiated term neonates. *AJNR Am J Neuroradiol* 1999;20:1399–1405.

58. Martin E, Buchli R, Ritter S, et al. Diagnostic and prognostic value of cerebral magnetic resonance spectroscopy in neonates with perinatal asphyxia. *Pediatr Res* 1996;40:749–458.

59. Adcock LM, Wafelman LS, Hegemier S, et al. Neonatal intensive care applications of near-infrared spectroscopy. *Clin Perinatol* 1999;26:893.

60. Van Lieshout HB, Jacobs JW, Rottevell JJ, et al. The prognostic value of the EEG in asphyxiated newborns. *Acta Neurol Scand* 1995;91:203–207.

61. Morret S, Pavrain N, Menard JF, et al. Prognostic value of neonatal electroencephalography in premature newborns less than 33 weeks of gestational age. *Electroenceph Clin Neurophysiol* 1997;102:178–185.

62. Band D, D'Ailest AM, Lacaze-Mesmonteil T, et al. The early diagnosis of periventricular leukomalacia in premature infants with positive rolandic sharp waves on serial electroencephalography. *J Pediatr* 1998;132:813–817.

63. Eken P, Toet MC, Groenendaal F, et al. Predictive value of early neuroimaging, pulsed Doppler and neurophysiology in full term infants with hypoxic-ischemic encephalopathy. *Arch Dis Child* 1995;73:F75-F80.

64. Muttitt SC, Taylor MJ, Kobayashi JS, et al. Serial visual evoked potentials and outcome in term birth asphyxia. *Pediatr Neurol* 1991;7:86–90.

65. Shepherd AJ, Saunders KW, McCulloch DL, et al. Prognostic value of flash visual evoked potentials in preterm infants. *Dev Med Child Neurol* 1999;41:9–15.

66. Gibson NA, Graham M, Levene MI. Somatosensory evoked potentials and outcome in perinatal asphyxia. *Arch Dis Child* 1992;67:393–398.

67. deVries LS, Eken P, Pierrat V, et al. Prediction of neurodevelopmental outcome in the preterm infant – short latency cortical somatosensory evoked potentials compared with cranial ultrasound. *Arch Dis Child* 1992;67:1177–1181.

68. Pierrat V, Eken P, Duguennay C, et al. Prognostic value of early somatosensory evoked potentials in neonates with cystic leukomalacia. *Dev Med Child Neurol* 1993;35:683–690.

69. Huang GC, Wang ST, Chang YC, et al. Measurement of urinary lactate: creatinine ratio for the early identification of newborn infants at risk for hypoxic-ischemic encephalopathy. *N Engl J Med* 1999;341:328–335.

70. Boylan GB, Young K, Panerai RB, et al. Dynamic cerebral autoregulation in sick newborn infants. *Pediatr Res* 2000;48:12–17.

71. Tsuji M, Saul JP, du Plessis A, et al. Cerebral intravascular oxygenation correlates with mean arterial pressure in critically ill premature infants. *Pediatrics* 2000;106:625–632.

72. Volpe JJ. Neurobiology of periventricular leukomalacia in the premature infant. *Pediatr Res* 2001;50:553–562.

73. Johnston MW, Trescher WH, Isida A, et al. Neurobiology of hypoxic-ischemic injury in the developing brain. *Pediatr Res* 2001;49:735–741.

74. Hapberg H, Gilland E, Diemer NH, et al. Hypoxia-ischemia in the neonatal rat brain: histopathology after post-treatment with NMDA and non-NMDA receptor antagonists. *Biol Neonate* 1994;66:206–213.

75. Myers RE. Four patterns of perinatal brain damage and their conditions of occurrence in primates. *Adv Neurol* 1975;10:223.

76. Myers RE. Two patterns of brain damage and their conditions of occurrence. *Am J Obstet Gynecol* 1972;112:245–276.

77. Rivkin MJ. Hypoxic-ischemic brain injury in the term newborn: neuropathology, clinical aspects and neuroimaging. *Clin Perinatol* 1997;24:607–626.

78. Johnston MV. Selective vulnerability in the neonatal brain. *Ann Neurol* 1998;44:155–156.

79. Johnston MV, Hoon A. Possible mechanisms for selective basal ganglia damage in infants from asphyxia, kernicterus, or mitochondrial encephalopathies. *J Child Neurol* 2000;15: 588–591.

80. Sher MS, Wiznitzer M, Bangert BA. Cerebral infarction in the fetus and neonate: maternal-placental-fetal considerations. *Clin Perinatol* 2002;29:693–724.

81. Andrew ME, Monagle P, de Veber G, et al. Thromboembolic disease and antithrombotic therapy in newborns. *Hematology* 2001;358–374.

82. Miller V. Neonatal cerebral infarction. *Semin Pediatr Neurol* 2000; 7:278–288.

83. Lynch JK, Hirtz DG, de Veber G, et al. Report of the National Institute of Neurological Disorders and Stroke Workshop on perinatal and childhood stroke. *Pediatrics* 2002;109:116–123.

84. Mercuri E. Early diagnostic and prognostic indicators in full term infants with neonatal cerebral infarction: an integrated clinical, neuroradiological and EEG approach. *Minerva Pediatr* 2001; 53:305–311.

85. Sreenan C, Bhargara R, Robertson CM. Cerebral infarction in the term newborn: clinical presentation and long-term outcome. *J Pediatr* 2000;137:351–355.

86. Rivkin MJ, Anderson ML, Kaye EM. Neonatal idiopathic cerebral venous thrombosis: an unrecognized cause of transient seizures or lethargy. *Ann Neurol* 1992;32:51.

87. Wu YW, Miller SP, Chin K, et al. Multiple risk factors in neonatal sinovenous thrombosis. *Neurology* 2002;59:438–440.

88. Back SA, Volpe JJ. Cellular and molecular pathogenesis of periventricular white matter injury. *MRDD Research Reviews* 1997;3:96.

89. Armstrong D, Norman MG. Periventricular leukomalacia in neonates: complications and sequelae. *Arch Dis Child* 1974; 99:367.

90. Kuban K, Sanacka U, Leviton A, et al. White matter disorders of prematurity: association with intraventricular hemorrhage and ventriculomegaly. *J Pediatr* 1999;134;539–546.

91. Guzzetta F, Shackelford GD, Volpe S, et al. Periventricular intraparenchymal echodensities in the premature newborn: critical determinant of neurological status. *Pediatrics* 1986;78:995.

92. Taylor, GA. Effect of germinal matrix hemorrhage on terminal vein position and patency. *Pediatr Radiol* 1995;25:537–540.

93. Takashima S, Mito T, Ando Y. Pathogenesis of periventricular white matter hemorrhages in preterm infants. *Brain Dev* 1986; 8:25.

94. Volpe JJ. Subplate neurons—missing link in brain injury of the premature infant? *Pediatrics* 1996;97:112.

95. Sinha SK, Tin W. The controversies surrounding oxygen therapy in neonatal intensive care units. *Curr Opin Pediatr* 2003;15:161.

96. Volpe JJ. Perinatal brain injury: from pathogenesis to neuroprotection. *MRDD Research Reviews* 2001;7:56.

97. Shankaran S. The postnatal management of the asphyxiated term infant. *Clin Perinatol* 2002;29:675–692.

98. Whitelaw A, Thoreson M. Clinical trials of treatments after perinatal asphyxia. *Curr Opin Pediatr* 2002;14:664.

99. Battin M, Penrice J, Gunn TR, et al. Treatment of term infants with head cooling and mild systemic hypothermia (35°C and 34.5°C) after perinatal asphyxia. *Pediatrics* 2003;111:244.

100. Ment LR, Bada HS, Barnes P, et al. Practice parameter: neuroimaging of the neonate: report of the quality standards subcommittee of the American Academy of Neurology and the practice committee of the Child Neurology Society. *Neurology* 2002;58: 1726–1738.

101. du Plessis AJ. Posthemorrhagic hydrocephalus and brain injury in the preterm Infant Development Program: dilemmas in diagnosis and management. *Pediatr Semin Neurol* 1998;5:161–179.

102. Murphy BP, Inder TE, Rooks V, et al. Posthemorrhagic ventricular dilatation in the premature infant: natural history and predictors of outcome. *Arch Dis Child Fetal Neonatol Ed* 2002;87: F37-F41.

103. Perlman JM, Lynch B, Volpe JJ. Late hydrocephalus after arrest and resolution of neonatal posthemorrhagic hydrocephalus. *Dev Med Child Neurol* 1990;32:725.

104. Hill A. Intraventricular hemorrhage: emphasis on prevention. *Semin Pediatr Neurol* 1998;5:152.

105. Roland EH, Hill A. Germinal matrix intraventricular hemorrhage in the newborn: management and out come. *Neurol Clin N Am* 2003;21:833.

106. Mittendorf R, Dambrosia J, Pryde PG, et al. Association between the use of antenatal magnesium sulfate in preterm labor and adverse health outcomes in infants. *Am J Obstet Gynecol* 2002; 186:1111–1118.
107. Weintraub Z, Solorechick M, Reichman B, et al. Effect of maternal tocolysis on the incidence of severe periventricular intraventricular hemorrhage in very low birthweight infants. *Arch Dis Child Fetal Neonatal Ed* 2001;85:F13-F17.
108. Rosen LJ, Zucher D, Oppenheimer-Gazit J, et al. The great tocolytic debate: some pitfalls in the study of safety. *Am J Obstet Gynecol* 2001;184:1–7.
109. Hillier SL, Nugent RP, Eschenbach DA, et al. Association between bacterial vaginosis and preterm delivery of a low birthweight infant. *N Engl J Med* 1995;333:1737.
110. Hauth JC, Goldlenberg RL, Andrews WW, et al. Reduced incidence of preterm delivery with metranidazole and erythromycin in women with bacterial vaginosis. *N Engl J Med* 1995;333: 1732–1736.
111. Harding JE, Pang J, Knight DB, et al. Do antenatal corticosteroids help in the setting of preterm rupture of membranes. *Am J Obstet Gynecol* 2001;184:131–139.
112. Wright LL, Verter J, Younes N, et al. Antenatal corticosteroid administration and neonatal outcome in very low birthweight infants: the NICHD Neonatal Research Network. *Am J Obstet Gynecol* 1995;173:269.
113. Ment LR, Oh W, Ehrenkranz RA, et al. Antenatal steroids, delivery mode and intraventricular hemorrhage in preterm infants. *Am J Obstet Gynecol* 1995;172:795.
114. Leviton A, Fenton T, Kuban KC, et al. Labor and delivery characteristics and the risk of germinal matrix hemorrhage in low birthweight infants. *J Child Neurol* 1991;6:35.
115. Crowther CA, Henderson-Smart DJ. Phenobarbital prior to preterm birth for preventing neonatal periventricular hemorrhage. *Cochrane Database Syst Rev* 2001;CD000164.
116. Crowther CA, Henderson-Smart DJ. Vitamin K prior to preterm birth for preventing neonatal periventricular hemorrhage. *Cochrane Database Syst Rev* 2000;CD000229.
117. Soll RF, Morley CJ. Prophylactic versus selective use of surfactant in preventing morbidity and mortality in preterm infants. *Cochrane Database of Syst Rev* 2001;CD000510.
118. Cools F, Offinga M. Neurmuscular paralysis for newborn infants receiving mechanical ventilation. *Cochrane Database Syst Rev* 2000;CD002773.
119. Whitelaw A. Postnatal phenobarbitone for the prevention of intraventricular hemorrhage in preterm infants. *Cochrane Database Syst Rev* 2001;CD001691.
120. Ng E, Taddio A, Ohlsson A. Intravenous midazolam infusion for sedation of infants in the neonatal intensive care unit. *Cochrane Database Syst Rev* 2003;CD002052
121. Bhuta T, Henderson-Smart DJ. Rescue high frequency oscillatory ventilation versus conventional ventilation for pulmonary dysfunction in preterm infants. *Cochrane Database Syst Rev* 2000; CD000438.
122. Osborn DA, Evans N. Early volume expansion for prevention of morbidity and mortality in very preterm infants. *Cochrane Database Syst Rev* 2004;CD002055.
123. Fowlie PW, Davis PG. Prophylactic intravenous indomethacin for preventing mortality and morbidity in preterm infants. *Cochrane Database Syst Rev* 2002;CD003483.
124. Whitelaw A. Repeated lumbar or ventricular punctures in newborns with intraventricular hemorrhage. *Cochrane Database Syst Rev* 2000;(2):CD000216.

125. Whitelaw A. Intraventricular streptokinase after intraventricular hemorrhage in newborn infants. *Cochrane Database Syst Rev* 2001;(1):CD000498.
126. Whitelaw A, Kennedy CR, Brian LP. Diuretic therapy for newborn infants with posthemorrhagic ventricular dilatation. *Cochrane Database Syst Rev* 2001;(2):CD 002270.
127. Resch B, Gedermann A, Maurer U, et al. Neurodevelopmental outcome of hydrocephalus following intra/periventricular hemorrhage in preterm infants: short and long term results. *Childs Nerv Syst* 1996;12:27.
128. Ventriculomegaly Trial Group. Randomized trial of early tapping in neonatal posthemorrhagic ventricular dilation: results at 30 months. *Arch Dis Child* 1994;70:F129.
129. Bergman I, Bauer RE, Barmada MA, et al. Intracerebral hemorrhage in the full-term neonatal infant. *Pediatrics* 1985;74:488.
130. Merrill JD, Piecuch RE, Fell SC, et al. A new pattern of cerebellar hemorrhages in preterm infants. *Pediatrics* 1998;102:E62.
131. Fishman MA, Percy AK, Cheek WR, et al. Successful conservative management of cerebellar hematomas in term neonates. *J Pediatr* 1981;98:466.
132. Roland EH, Flodmark O, Hill A. Thalamic hemorrhage with intraventricular hemorrhage in the full-term newborn. *Pediatrics* 1990;85:737.
133. Task Force on Brain Death in Children. Guidelines for the determination of brain death in children. *Ann Neurol* 1987;21:616.
134. Canadian Neurocritical Care Group. Guidelines for the diagnosis of brain death. *Can J Neurol Sci* 1999;26:64.
135. Ashwal S. Brain death in the newborn. Current perspectives. *Clin Perinatol* 1997;24:859.
136. Fishman MA. Validity of brain death criteria in infants. *Pediatrics* 1995;96:513.
137. Altman D, Perlman JM, Powers WJ, et al. Preservation of brainstem ands cerebral blood flow (CCBF) in two asphyxiated newborn infants with clinical brain death. *Pediatr Res* 1987;21:487A.
138. Roland EH. Muscle disease in the newborn. In: Rennie JM, Robertson NRC, eds. *Textbook of neonatology*, 3rd ed. Edinburgh: Churchill-Livingstone, 1999;1284.
139. Royden JH Jr, DeVivo DC, Darras BT. *Neuromuscular disorders of infancy, childhood and adolescence—a clinician's approach.* Philadelphia: Butterworth-Heinemann, 2003.
140. Darras BT, Jones HR. Diagnosis of pediatric neuromuscular disorders in the era of DNA analysis. *Pediatr Neurol* 2000;23:289.
141. Zerres K, Wirth B, Rudnik-Schoeneborn S. Spinal muscular atrophy–clinical and genetic correlations. *Neuromuscul Disord* 1997;7:202.
142. Thomas NH, Dubowitz V. The natural history of type I (severe) spinal muscular atrophy. *Neuromuscul Disord* 1994;4:497.
143. Gabreels-Festen A, Gabreels F. Congenital and Early Infantile Neuropathies. In: *Neuromuscular disorders of infancy, childhood and adolesence—a clinician's approach.* Philadelphia: Butterworth-Heineman, 2003;361.
144. Basson H, Muhlbour Tome A, Spiver Z. High-dose intravenous immunoglobulin in transient neonatal myasthenia gravis. *Pediatr Neurol* 1998;18:181.
145. Engel AG. 73rd ENMC International Workshop: congenital myasthenic syndromes. *Neuromuscul Disord* 2001;11:315.
146. Moxley RT III, Veola G. Myotonic dystrophy. In: Deymeer F, Basal S, Karger AG, eds. *Neuromuscular diseases: from basic mechanisms to clinical management.* 2000;61.
147. Dubowitz V. Proceedings of the 27th ENMC Sponsored Workshop on Congenital Muscular Dystrophy, 1994, The Netherlands. *Neuromuscul Disord* 1995;3:253.

Neurosurgery of the Newborn

Joseph R. Madsen   *David M. Frim*   *Anne R. Hansen*

Treatment of structural and functional abnormalities of the neonatal central nervous system (CNS) provides unique challenges to both the neurosurgeon and neonatologist caring for the infant. Considerations of several interrelated pathophysiologic processes can provide an understanding of the nature of the abnormality and goal of treatment. This understanding forms the basis for a successful interdisciplinary team approach to the management of these infants.

THE PATHOPHYSIOLOGY OF NEONATAL NEUROSURGERY

Almost all neurosurgical interventions in the neonate can be discussed in terms of four categories of technical intervention: (a) drainage or diversion of fluids, (b) closure of openings (including neural tube defects), (c) removal of tissue (including neoplasms and anomalous masses), and (d) opening of fusions (such as craniosynostoses). In the management of many newborn patients, two or more of these inventions may be necessary. Some neonatal nervous system problems, such as vascular disorders, do not yet have a workable neurosurgical intervention.

When applying these inventions to neonatal care, their use must be guided by pathophysiologic mechanisms unique to the neonate, such as (a) the biomechanics of neonatal brain tissue and a distensible skull, (b) recognized and unrecognized congenital anomalies (microscopic and macroscopic), and (c) the plasticity of neonatal CNS tissue and its effects on response to injury. Recent advances in antenatal diagnosis allow unprecedented opportunity to manage these processes even before birth. Frequently, solutions to a neonatal neurosurgical problem must address combinations, or complex interactions, of these pathophysiologic mechanisms.

The biomechanic nature of neonatal brain tissue and a distensible skull accounts for one of the best-known cardinal signs of neurosurgical difficulty in the neonate, namely abnormal head growth. The prodigious ability of the skull to grow and sutures to widen can allow some of the most severe cases of hydrocephalus to result in relatively mild pressure effects, even with an obvious need for cerebrospinal fluid (CSF) shunting for long-term management. These same considerations in the type and nature of response of the tissues to abnormal fluid build-up can result in dramatic structural difficulties once the pressure is relieved. The certainty that the brain and skull biomechanics will change over time adds particular challenge to management of these problems.

Obvious congenital anomalies, especially those involving open neural-tube defects and exposed CNS tissue, may require urgent neurosurgical intervention. A complicating aspect is the potential occurrence of concurrent microscopic abnormalities, such as widespread synaptic miswiring. In many cases, neurologic deficits may be present in a patient with macroscopic structural abnormalities, but major neurologic disability may come from less obvious problems with tissue development, currently not treatable by neurosurgical means.

The details of the plasticity and vulnerability of the neonatal CNS is discussed in Chapter 50. It is well known that the ability to recover function after CNS injury is age dependent and seems to be better in younger individuals. Interaction between the age-dependent variables of CNS plasticity, recoverability, and vulnerability make the task of estimating prognosis after an injury or neurosurgical intervention extremely difficult.

Antenatal diagnosis has changed many aspects of neurosurgical conditions. Obstetric management may be altered, for example, site and mode of delivery in the setting of a known neural-tube defect. In addition, the psychologic issues around the time of neurosurgical therapy for the newborn are altered, as the child's family now has the opportunity to meet the neurosurgeon prenatally and fully discuss and decide upon any contemplated care plan before birth. Antenatal surgery for some neurosurgical conditions (such as neural-tube defects and hydrocephalus) may one day be routine, but at this time these techniques are still available only in experimental, randomized trials.

FLUID COLLECTIONS AND THEIR MANAGEMENT

Disorders of Cerebrospinal Fluid Accumulation

The most common neurosurgical consultation for newborn patients is to evaluate and treat enlargement of the ventricular system. The clinical signs of progressive enlargement of the ventricular system include excessive increase in the head circumference (HC), fullness in the anterior fontanelle (especially when the patient is upright, the venous and fontanelle pressures should be low), episodic apnea and bradycardia, general lethargy, and abnormalities of ocular movement, especially restricted upgaze. Many of these findings are nonspecific and can they be seen with hydrocephalus of any etiology. At a practical level, the most important distinction is between progressive and static abnormalities in ventricular volume. This is relatively easy to determine using serial cranial ultrasound examinations (Fig. 51-1). The recent addition of resistive index (RI) measurements adds a physiologic dimension to the anatomic images gathered by ultrasonography (1). In our experience, the presence of dramatic changes in the Doppler-measured flow signals in the anterior cerebral artery with gentle, brief compression of the anterior fontanelle correlates extremely well with the intracranial pressure by measurement and the probability of eventual need for a ventriculoperitoneal (VP) shunt (1).

The vast majority of hydrocephalus cases seen in neonates are associated with, and traditionally thought to result from, abnormal resorption of CSF. However, Egnor

(2) has persuasively argued the contrasting view that abnormalities in the pulsatile dynamics of the CNS may play a role in the etiology of communicating hydrocephalus. In this view, the purpose of CSF and the ventricular system is to absorb the kinetic energy of the arterial pulsations and transfer this energy out of the skull, primarily via the venous system. After intraventricular hemorrhage (Fig. 51-1), traditional thinking is that partial occlusion of the normal resorptive pathways of CSF through the arachnoid villi causes hydrocephalus. Pulsatile theories suggest that breakdown of the resonance of pulsations could also play a role. Thus, relative blockade of bulk CSF absorption or blockade of absorption of the pulsations could raise the steady state to a relatively higher pressure. In the neonate with open sutures, this results in a larger intracranial volume. It also follows that there would be some cases of mild increase in resistance to absorption of fluid (or pulsations) that would not require specific treatment, whereas higher grades of failure to absorb fluid would cause substantial increases in pressure, leading to neurologic symptoms if not treated.

Placement of a shunt in borderline cases may result in atrophy of physiologic resorption systems and, thereby, cause more permanent obstruction to resorption of CSF. This is conceptualized as atrophy of arachnoid granulations or failure to develop normal resorptive pathways, but the detailed pathology is not well known. A related paradox of shunt physiology, particularly applicable to neonates, is that, with currently available hardware, it is impossible to distinguish between a well-functioning shunt and nonfunctioning shunt in a patient who is no longer shunt dependent. Technologies that accurately measure the flow through the shunt, or through some physiologic pathway such as the aqueduct of Sylvius, or a ratio of these two numbers, could be a reliable descriptor of shunt dependence. It is theoretically possible that such measurements could be made from dynamic magnetic resonance imaging (MRI) studies. So far, such a technique has not been applied reliably.

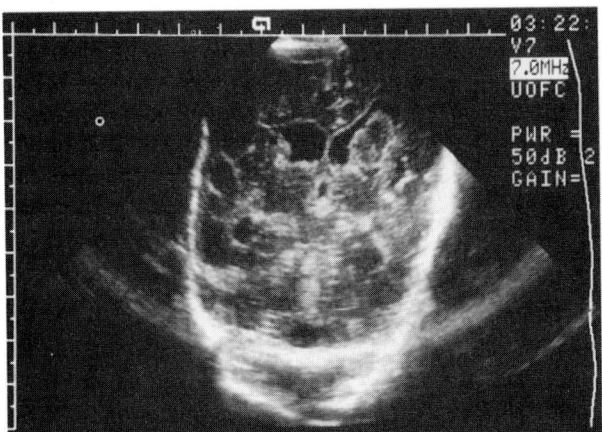
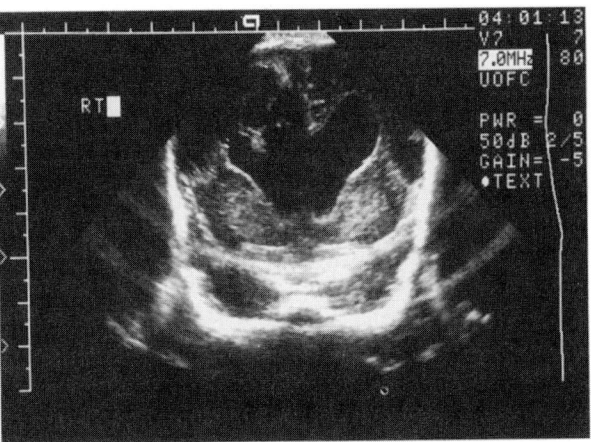

Figure 51-1 Cranial ultrasonography of intraventricular hemorrhage in the coronal plane. **A:** Head ultrasound performed within the first week of life depicts a clot in the left lateral ventricle with mildly dilated ventricles. **B:** Ultrasonography performed 1 month later shows no residual clot, but significant enlargement of the ventricular system, consistent with posthemorrhagic hydrocephalus.

One of the problems with assessing the growth of ventricular size in the neonate is the possibility that the enlargement of the ventricles may at least partially reflect loss of tissue in the brain, rather than increase in pressure. This can become a very complicated situation, as prolonged hydrocephalus itself certainly can cause loss of tissue bulk (3), and the value of shunt placement may be more difficult to determine when the tissue loss is not obviously the result of high pressure. The specific loss of myelin or white matter, called periventricular leukomalacia, is discussed in Chapter 50 . The relationship between periventricular leukomalacia and hydrocephalus is of particular concern in neurosurgical decision making. When a preterm infant, especially one who has sustained an intracranial hemorrhage, shows lateral ventricular enlargement, it is difficult to determine to what extent this is a result of impaired CSF flow or absorption versus diffuse white matter damage or inadequate density of axons. In general, the absence of macrocephaly is an indicator of the atrophy. More specific strategies to rescue white matter in such circumstances probably will evolve and may diminish the call for shunts in some of these patients (4).

Nevertheless, assessing for macrocephaly is complicated by the changing growth rate of the normal neonatal head (5). In general, an HC growth of less than 1 cm/week is acceptable, and an HC growth of more than 1.5 cm/week is considered excessive. Head growth must be interpreted in the context of overall somatic growth measured by weight and length. Babies can have preferential brain catch-up growth, but it is suspicious if the rate of HC increases at the high end of normal while the weight and length remain relatively unchanged. Because major intervention decisions are based on the intrinsically imprecise measurement of HC, any effort to improve its precision is worthwhile. Minimizing the number of care providers obtaining the measurement and overtly standardizing the measurement site and technique improves accuracy. The effect of interpreter variability can be dampened by comparing the HC to the previous day and also to 1 week earlier to calculate average daily growth by dividing by seven. Using a correct and accurate growth curve is also important (6,7).

Fluid in the subarachnoid space outside the brain, sometimes termed "benign external hydrocephalus," is probably a normal variant. The increased collection of extraaxial fluid is generally in the frontal regions. The diagnosis of subdural hygroma frequently has been applied to these cases; this diagnosis must be applied with great caution if it is intended to imply a pathologic collection benefiting from drainage (8).

Treatment of Neonatal Hydrocephalus

Due to the disadvantages and complications of VP shunting, the decision to place a shunt must be made only after all nonsurgical options have failed. The fact that the CSF resorption may change with time, and indeed may improve, provides a rationale for conservatism. As a patient grows and the dynamic relationship between CSF production and resorption changes, the need and indications for diversion of CSF may change over the child's lifetime.

Children born with hydrocephalus due to nonhemorrhagic causes, such as aqueductal stenosis, posterior fossa cysts, holoprosencephaly, or hydranencephaly, can be shunted within 1 to 2 days of birth, pending evaluation of general medical status. Although affected infants usually are born at or near term, a presurgical weight of approximately 1,500 to 2,000 grams is adequate size to support peritoneal drainage of ventricular CSF (9). There are ethic issues that should be raised before placing a VP shunt in a child suffering from hydrocephalus with significantly reduced brain function from either an *in utero* event or developmental anomaly. Frank discussion with the child's parents regarding prognosis is critical. Shunting for affected children without other life-threatening anomalies is certainly reasonable for the purposes of controlling head size in the growing infant. With maximal interventive therapy, most of these children are expected to live beyond a few weeks, and such day-to-day issues as whether the child's head will fit in an infant car seat need to be considered. Shunting at birth is a relatively low-risk method of preventing massive head enlargement and allowing other factors aside from congenital hydrocephalus to determine the child's outcome (10).

Nearly all acquired hydrocephalus in the premature infant is posthemorrhagic (Fig. 51-1). These infants have usually not achieved adequate weight for placement of permanent shunts, and the final determination of lifelong hydrocephalus has not been made. In this situation, medical management (11) is instituted to temporize until surgical management is both clearly indicated and feasible. The mainstays of medical management are serial lumbar punctures and diuretic therapy, though use of the latter is becoming increasingly controversial (12,13). The use of these maneuvers is discussed in Chapter 50. An additional approach that has been tried for posthemorrhagic hydrocephalus (PHH) is the introduction of fibrinolytic therapy directly into the ventricular system. Enzymes such as streptokinase, urokinase, and tissue plasminogen activator all have been proposed and tested with variable success. Some centers have suggested that the risk of VP shunts can be reduced using this technique (14). Others have been unable to show a decrease in the need for VP shunting with this maneuver (15,16). It is possible that the trials which found no helpful effect from fibrinolytic therapy had less favorable results because of patient selection, with a trend toward enrolling the most severe and potentially intractable cases. Infants enrolled in a recent, small trial combining fibrinolytic therapy with continuous drainage and irrigation had a reduced rate of shunt requirement, disability, and mortality compared to historic controls (17). However, larger trials are needed to further delineate the risks and benefits of this high-risk, labor-intensive treatment. At this point, the underlying difficulty with fibrinolytic therapy is the lack of overlap of the safety and efficacy windows. This therapy cannot currently be considered standard therapy.

Another intervention that has been suggested is the use of ventriculoscopic removal of clot, however, based on little published experience, this has not been demonstrated to avert the need for VP shunts. A new technique for the treatment of hydrocephalus caused by obstruction of the aqueduct of Sylvius employs the fiberoptic ventriculoscope to place a fenestration in the floor of the third ventricle to allow the escape of CSF into the subarachnoid space. Indeed, even in such cases of aqueductal stenosis, where eventual therapy using the ventriculoscope works well in older children, most surgeons currently find that the defect in the floor of the third ventricle in the neonate tends to close at a very high rate (18).

The risk of PHH correlates with the severity of intraventricular hemorrhage. Although other grading systems have been described, we use the Papile four-level system of intracranial hemorrhage (19): grade I, subependymal hemorrhage only (no increased risk of PHH); grade II, intraventricular hemorrhage without ventriculomegaly (low risk of progressive PHH); grade III, intraventricular hemorrhage with ventriculomegaly (moderate risk of progressive PHH); and grade IV, intraventricular hemorrhage with intraparenchymal extension (generally at high risk of need for VP shunting, depending on degree of intraventricular component).

There are many published management protocols for children with PHH (9–11,19,20). Evaluation usually includes neurosurgical consultation, ultrasound of the head to assess the size of the ventricles, and lumbar puncture to measure CSF pressure. During a head ultrasound, it can be helpful to measure the RI defined as

$$\frac{\text{systolic} - \text{diastolic blood flow velocity}}{\text{systolic blood flow velocity}}$$

Concern regarding hemodynamic compromise is raised either by an RI above the normal value of 0.5 to 0.7 or a rise in RI with gentle compression of the anterior fontanelle.

Interventions are tailored to maintain the lumbar or ventricular CSF pressure at approximately 5 to 8 cm of water while evaluating the need for permanent shunt placement. The medical approaches to this problem have been described (11,21). The goal of medical management is to decrease CSF volume either by decreasing CSF production via diuretic therapy or removing CSF in bulk.

Mechanical CSF drainage by serial lumbar puncture or direct ventricular access is the mainstay of treatment of elevated intracranial pressure while awaiting the appropriate time for VP shunt insertion. The frequency of CSF drainage procedures is determined by measuring opening CSF pressures during lumbar taps with a goal of less than 10 cm of water (10). For example, if an every third day tapping schedule allows the CSF pressure to rise to greater than 10 cm of water, the frequency of CSF withdrawal should be increased to every other day. Fontanelle tenseness, HC, and ultrasonographic RIs also are acceptable indications of intracranial pressure (1). Approximately 10 to 15 mL/kg

should be removed to leave the closing CSF pressure as low as is feasible, usually less than 3 cm of water. This approach is based on cerebral perfusion management rather than measures of HC or ultrasonographic documentation of ventricular size.

HC, ultrasonographic criteria, and other physical examination criteria provide additional data to guide CSF drainage therapy. Data interpretation and management decisions should be based on the overall goal of maximizing the potential for neuronal development in an environment of low intracranial pressure and minimal periventricular axonal stretch.

Although serial lumbar punctures may be useful in many cases, they often fail because of abnormalities within the spinal system that block CSF flow, particularly common after intraventricular hemorrhage. These have been documented with spinal ultrasound (22).

Acetazolamide and furosemide reduce CSF production. Though theoretically their effects are synergistic, this combination of diuretic therapy is now used with more caution because of concerning studies that found possibly worse neurologic outcome secondary to the use of these medications together (12,13). There are extremely limited data regarding acetazolamide alone. In a sample size of only five, short-term improvement was appreciated in the three patients who did not require the medication to be discontinued secondary to metabolic acidosis (23). Thus, its safety and efficacy as a single agent are essentially unknown. In certain circumstances when serial lumbar punctures are either not possible or not feasible, acetazolamide therapy may play a role. Furosemide should be added with great caution as it adds potential risk with no documented benefit.

Medical treatment with CSF drainage and/or diuretic therapy is continued to determine the natural history of the condition and allow for adequate growth of the infant to permit safe placement of a VP shunt, should that be necessary. During this period, the requirement for CSF drainage will accelerate, remain stable, or decrease. This is ascertained by continuing to measure CSF pressures. If there is no increase in pressure between taps, then it is likely that CSF is being reabsorbed internally. In this situation, the ultrasound image of the ventricles, as well as the HC measurements, is helpful in confirming that the reabsorptive surface is functioning adequately.

Implantation of devices that allow easier intermittent (Fig. 51-2), or continuous CSF drainage, should be considered when the need for drainage accelerates to the point when the neonatal intensivist or neurosurgeon is performing lumbar punctures daily or with such frequency as to endanger an infant's medical stability. Additionally, serial lumbar puncture can cause arachnoid scarring and lead to an inability to obtain adequate CSF drainage from a lumbar approach. In cases of noncommunicating PHH, CSF removal from the lumbar region is not an option. In all of these cases, direct approach to the ventricles either by percutaneous tap or implanted access device is required.

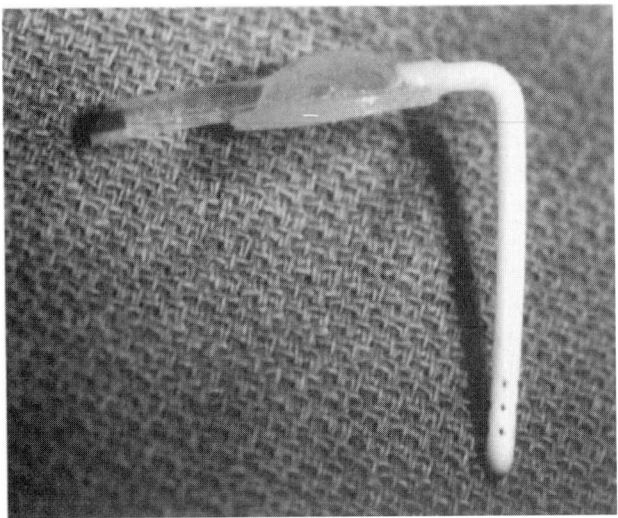

Figure 51-2 Ventricular access device with 30-mm catheter. Implantation allows easy percutaneous access to ventricular fluid.

Though percutaneous ventricular tap in a neonate is a relatively simple procedure, it should only be performed by experienced practitioners. A 20-gauge intravenous catheter is introduced perpendicularly to a plane tangential to the scalp at the lateral edge of the anterior fontanelle.

After penetrating the dura with the inner needle, the soft catheter is advanced over the needle into the ventricle. Drainage then proceeds as with a lumbar puncture.

Ventriculosubgaleal shunts are increasingly being used instead of ventricular access devices to temporize prior to placement of a VP shunt. The device, as well as the surgical implantation technique, is very similar to that of the ventricular access device (Fig. 51-3). The only differences are that the blind end of the catheter is cut off, and the open end is allowed to drain into a subgaleal (essentially subcutaneous) pocket in the infant's head. The major advantage is that the subgaleal pocket may allow some resorption of CSF and certainly can absorb fluid pulsations. Infants with ventriculosubgaleal shunts typically require far less frequent taps, and sometimes no taps at all (24). If necessary, the reservoir or subcutaneous fluid collection can be tapped, just like a ventricular access device . The cosmetic issue of a visible subcutaneous fluid-filled space can be concerning to parents and care providers who are unfamiliar with this technique, but all can be reassured that this will resolve after placement of a VP shunt, which follows in the vast majority of cases. The indications for tapping ventriculosubgaleal shunt devices are the same as for ventricular access devices, and the follow-up assessment tests are identical, including HC, sonographic assessment of ventricular size, and RI.

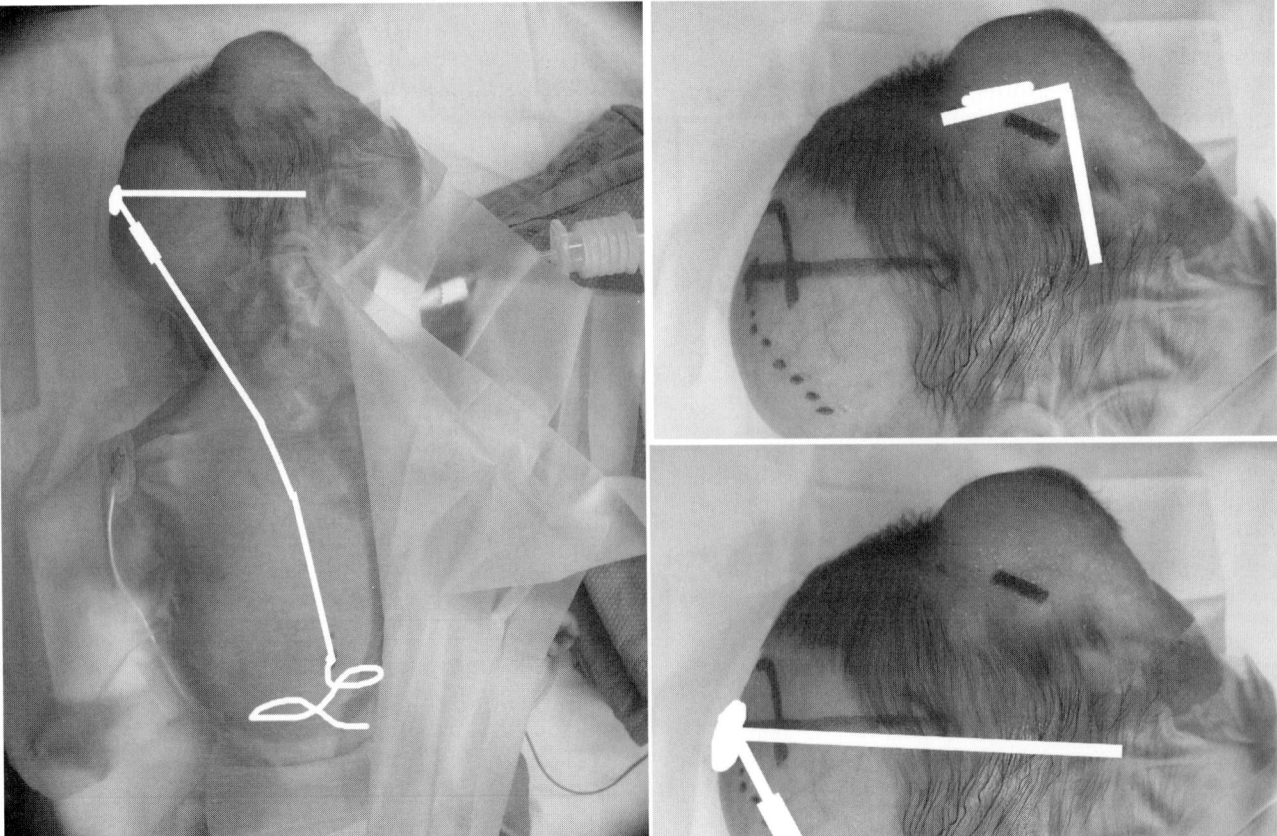

Figure 51-3 1,770-g premature infant, with ventriculosubgaleal shunt (VSGS) and associated subgaleal fluid collection, photographed as positioned for replacement of the VSGS (sketched in the upper right panel) with a ventriculoperitoneal shunt, trajectory shown at left and in the lower right panel.

Though largely replaced by the subgaleal shunt at many institutions, ventricular access devices (Fig. 51-2) are still occasionally placed. These devices allow direct percutaneous access to the ventricle via the subcutaneous reservoir. The protocol for CSF drainage is identical to that for lumber puncture. Infection of these devices is rare despite frequent percutaneous access. Ventricular access devices can be set up for continuous drainage by placement of a Huber needle into the reservoir, which is connected to a ventricular drainage bag. This maneuver is performed when taps are required more than once a day. During periods of continuous drainage, infants should be treated with prophylactic intravenous antibiotics.

After long intervals between CSF removal, if the pressure is unchanged and the ventricles are not enlarging, it is reasonable to continue to follow ventricular size by ultrasound alone. At that point, any diuretic treatment is weaned and then discontinued if tolerated. If the need for CSF drainage remains unchanged or accelerates as the patient grows, then the diagnosis of uncompensated hydrocephalus is made and a VP shunt is inserted. A patient weight of 1,750 grams is usually sufficient to permit implantation of a permanent VP shunt with minimal complications.

The contraindications to implantation of a permanent VP shunt are similar to those found in older children: evidence of CSF infection, significantly elevated CSF protein, presence of a high CSF red blood cell count which may mechanically obstruct the shunt, peritoneal inflammation, or infection such as necrotizing enterocolitis. These problems necessitate a delay in implantation until the child is healthy. CSF glucose parameters are sometimes quite low (less than 20 mg/dL) in neonates with PHH in the absence of infection. The significance of this finding is unclear; however, there is not an increase in shunt infection in these patients. Similarly, patients with intraventricular hemorrhage, whether adult or neonatal, can manifest fever perhaps from the presence of blood in the CSF. The exact cause of this increased temperature in the neonate is unclear; without positive bacteriologic data, it is unlikely to be infection. Therefore, in the absence of positive culture data, shunt placement should not be delayed.

Complications of Ventriculoperitoneal Shunting

Many of the problems of CSF diversion can be managed with simple surgical techniques. For example, since shunts tend to clog with very high protein concentrations, an externally draining system or a ventricular catheter with a tapping reservoir is initially placed (Fig. 51-2). At a later time, it is revised into a VP shunt if the infant requires permanent diversion (10,25). Another potential problem is patients outgrowing their shunts. Initial placement of longer tubing eliminates the need to periodically lengthen the peritoneal catheter because of growth. Catheters up to 90 cm in length are well tolerated, even by neonates.

Prospective studies have not shown any increase in complications, even with tubing up to 120 cm in length (26). Therefore, many centers now place a very long catheter into the peritoneum of even a small baby.

Shunt infection and malfunction are the most serious complications of VP shunting at any age. Neonates are at particularly high risk of these complications because of such factors as their relatively thin skin, nutritional difficulties causing delayed wound healing, and the tendency for CSF to be proteinaceous. Plastic hardware items such as shunts are particularly susceptible to infection, because a small pathogen inoculation, even with a relatively nonpathogenic bacterium, can avoid normal immune surveillance. In several series, the rate of infection correlated significantly with patient's age and often with little else (27).

Another complication of VP shunting sometimes seen in infants, although rarely seen in older individuals, is injury to bowel or other abdominal viscera (28). This is a result of the fragility of these tissues. In addition, migration of the catheter within the infant resulting in penetration into the pleural cavity (Fig. 51-4) has been seen. Migration of ventriculoatrial shunts further into the heart has also been documented (29).

Especially with very large ventricles, rapid decompression of the ventricular system can cause bleeding into the subdural space, ventricles, or parenchyma of the brain. For this reason, only moderate amounts of CSF are typically removed at the time of surgery, and patients are kept flat for the immediate postoperative period, with the elevation of the head titrated gradually based on assessment of the anterior fontanelle. The head can be raised as long as there is not extreme concavity or "ashtray deformity" of the fontanelle. Other authors have suggested the use of higher-pressure valves with very large ventricles (30).

An additional degree of freedom in management of hydrocephalus has come from the introduction of adjustable values. These values have a magnetic rotor that changes the tension on a tiny spring in the valve, thus changing the effective opening pressure of the valve. With such valves, clinicians can "try on" specific valve characteristics without having to surgically revise the valve. Drawbacks include a higher price to purchase the valves, and the possibility of the settings changing with exposure to the strong magnetic field of an MRI scanner. Each individual valve design has a different protocol for ensuring that the setting is as intended; these protocols are well documented in the package inserts from the manufacturers (31).

Ventricular asymmetry occurs with relative frequency. This can be minimized by deliberate placement of catheters across the midline, so that openings on either side of the septum can drain bilateral ventricles (32). Spontaneous resolution of ventricular asymmetry sometimes occurs and therefore, in the absence of an associated asymmetric physical examination, ventricular asymmetry can generally be tolerated with close observation.

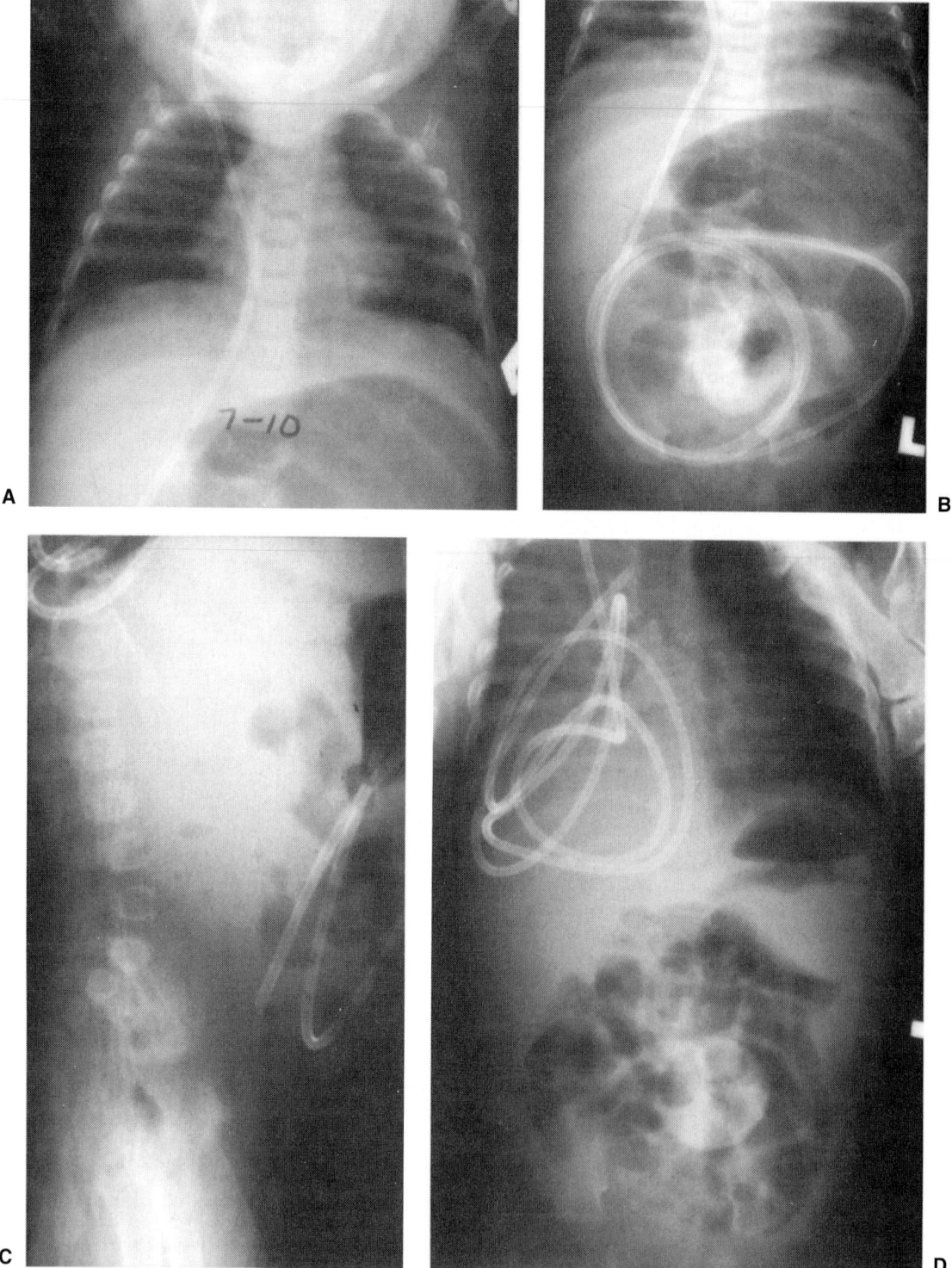

Figure 51-4 Example of an unusual infection-related shunt complication to placement at a very early age—erosion through the chest wall into the pleural cavity. **A, B:** This ventriculoperitoneal shunt was placed in a 1,300-g neonate after treatment of posthemorrhagic hydrocephalous with a ventricular access device and serial taps. Several months later, an umbilical hernia appeared to enlarge, and plain radiographs were obtained of the abdomen. The loops of shunt tubing, which had already migrated into the chest cavity, were not appreciated at that point. Panel **(C)** was obtained only 3 days prior to panel **(D)**. The patient was discharged and returned with a suddenly sunken anterior fontanelle and diminished breath sounds on the right. A plain x-ray demonstrated migration of the shunt tubing into the right pleural cavity **(D)**. The fluid in the chest proved to be purulent. A functioning shunt ultimately was replaced in the peritoneum after removal of hardware, external drainage, and treatment with antibiotics. Presumably a distal catheter infection, although the infant did not present with sepsis, resulted in fluid along the shunt, which erupted into the pleural space, allowing the tubing to retract and coil there with movement of the patient.

Intracranial Cystic Spaces in the Neonate

Interhemispheric, temporal fossa, posterior fossa, and other arachnoid cysts can frequently complicate the treatment of hydrocephalus. There are a variety of techniques for dealing with these entities, including fenestration using either open technique or ventriculoscopy, direct shunting of the cyst, or combined shunting of the cyst and ventricle. Interhemispheric cysts can become quite large, and large arachnoid cysts generally require treatment. Fenestration of the cyst may be the best way to avoid the need for an additional catheter (33). Large interhemispheric cysts can be confused with lobar holoprosencephaly, a diagnosis that confers a considerably worse neurologic prognosis. Frequently, these require placement of a shunt catheter in the cyst, rather than in the ventricle (Fig. 51-5) (34). Dilation of the isolated fourth ventricle is a particularly difficult surgical problem, both because the posterior fossa is a somewhat more technically difficult area into which to place a catheter that will continue to work over a long period of time, and because the neurologic risks are quite high if the catheter draining such a cyst has even a transient failure.

This can result in emergent brainstem symptoms, such as apnea and bradycardia. The risks of fourth ventricular cysts and specific placement of shunts into the cysts to drain them have been documented in several reports (35,36).

MANAGEMENT OF THE INFANT WITH AN OPEN DEFECT OF THE NEURAL AXIS

Abnormal developmental folding of the neural tube and anterior neuropore can result in a wide spectrum of abnormalities. The most benign presentation is spina bifida occulta, a bifid spinal arch seen in up to 30% of the general population with no neurologic sequelae. The most severe presentation is anencephaly or craniospinal raschisis, complete absence of neural-tube closure.

The general guideline is to defer urgent repair of these defects if they are small and truly skin covered, i.e., lipomyelomeningocele. Open defects, such as myelomeningocele, or defects that leak CSF or interfere with airway patency, such as large nasofrontal encephaloceles,

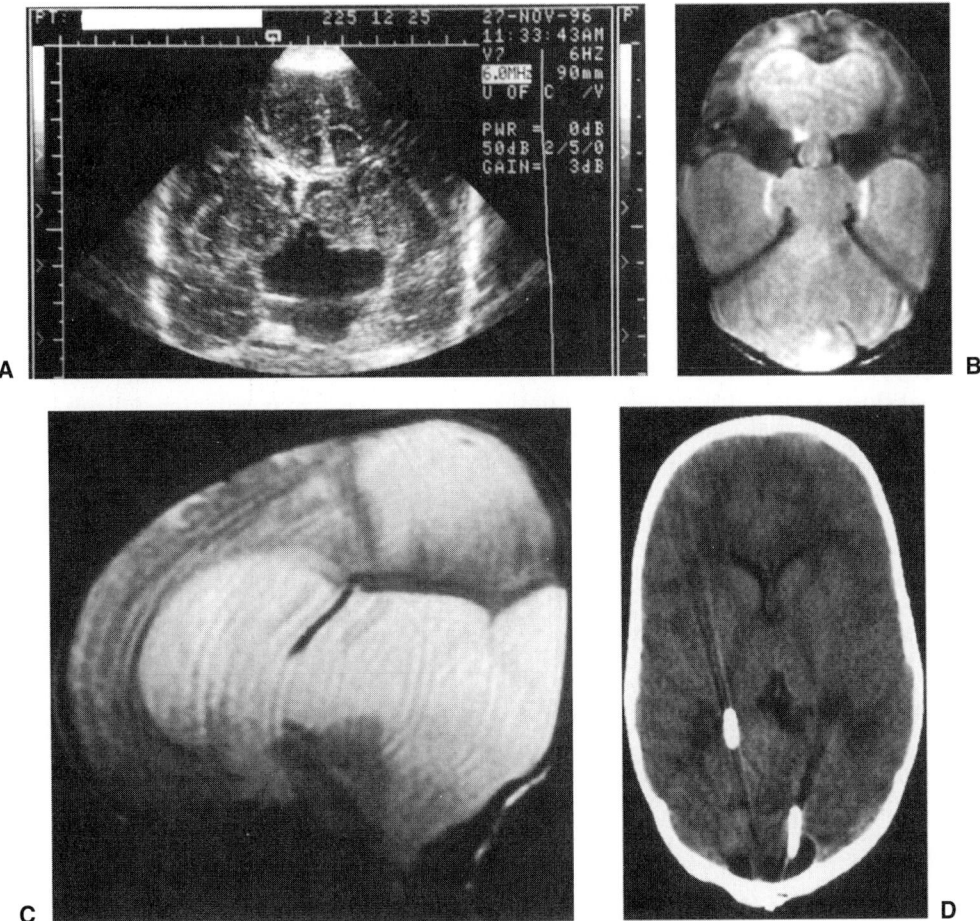

Figure 51-5   Intracranial cysts in the neonate. **A:** Coronal ultrasonography of a suprasellar cyst in a newborn. **B, C:** An intrahemispheric cyst may mimic fluid collection in the posterior fossa, allowing it to be confused with Dandy-Walker malformations. This patient was born with a very severe craniomegaly and compression of brain tissue, and ultimately required a catheter in both the cystic space and residual ventricular system. With these two catheters, the brain configuration eventually returned much more to normal **(D)**, and the patient has had normal developmental milestones subsequently.

require repair within a few days of birth. Infants with enlarging lesions such as occipital encephaloceles are often managed most safely with close observation until they achieve adequate weight to minimize surgical risks.

Neurosurgeons frequently are called upon to evaluate a variety of midline "lumps, bumps, and dimples" along the neural axis from nose to coccyx (Figs. 51-6, 51-7, and 51-8). These lesions often represent myelodysplasia that will require repair. However, in the stable newborn, evaluation and treatment can be deferred until after 3 months of age when surgical intervention is medically safer. Even MRI evaluation can be deferred until that time to obtain a technically superior study. Head and spine ultrasound are useful in the neonatal period for screening these lesions, but a high false-negative rate has been noted. The MRI scan remains the gold standard for preoperative planning of these occult lesions.

Myelomeningocele

Antenatal diagnosis has markedly changed the management of patients with myelomeningoceles. The vast majority of patients with this deformity are diagnosed prenatally on the basis of an elevated serum alpha-fetoprotein, generally followed by an ultrasound study and sometimes an antenatal MRI scan (37,38). Delivery of patients with myelomeningocele by cesarean section prior to labor may improve the functional outcome relative to the anatomic level of the myelomeningocele (39). Elective cesarean section for such patients is recommended as soon as the fetal lungs are known to be sufficiently mature. The technical considerations have been well outlined (40). Because of the associated type II Chiari malformation, as well as some potential obstruction to CSF flow around the incisura and subarachnoid space, more than 90% of these patients require placement of a VP shunt. Most commonly, the shunt does not have to be placed at the time of the initial closure. Placement of the VP shunt can be delayed for at least several days so that the CSF coming in contact with the shunt has not recently had access to the open defect. In some series, the patients with

myelomeningocele manifested high incidences of shunt malfunction within the first year, some in excess of 40% (40). In general, the more severe the ventricular dilatation, the higher the incidence of complications, which also may be a measure of the degree of shunt dependence of individual patients.

Surgery for repair of a myelomeningocele has been well described (40,41). The goal of the surgery is to reconstruct the terminal end of the neuraxis and approximate the topologic relationships that would have occurred if closure of the neural tube had been complete. The neural placode itself is usually plainly visible beneath, or associated with, translucent abnormal tissue stretching from the edge of the skin defect inward to the small island of pinkish tissue, which represents the termination of the spinal cord. It is flat with a groove down the middle. With surgical dissection, it is found to have nerve roots projecting both ventrally through the remnants of the sacrum and lumbar bony elements, as well as some nerve roots projecting more aberrantly out into the soft tissue and skin. Because of the tendency of this placode tissue to dry out in the hours prior to closure, dressing with sterile gauze kept continuously moist with sterile saline is crucial. Antibiotics can be administered as prophylaxis against meningitis until the skin defect is closed.

Once in the operating room, the patient is handled and managed so as to avoid any further trauma to the placode. The patient is usually intubated in the lateral or supine position, with padding very carefully arranged to avoid any pressure on the meningocele sac or placode.

The dissection begins with a circumferential division of the abnormal, thinly epithelialized translucent tissue, which joins the placode to the surrounding skin. The surgeon must carefully remove from the space any remaining dermal elements that may end up inside the dura. Such elements later can cause dermoid tumors that require resection and chronic inflammatory conditions that make later spinal cord untethering difficult.

The tissue of the placode itself is trimmed. Magnification with operating loupes or operating microscope is extremely helpful in preserving all of the neural tissue but

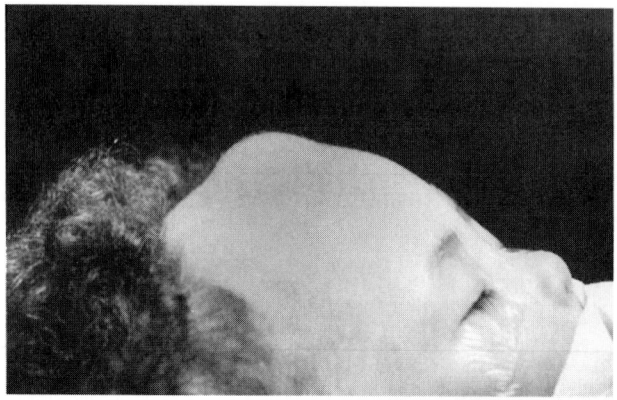
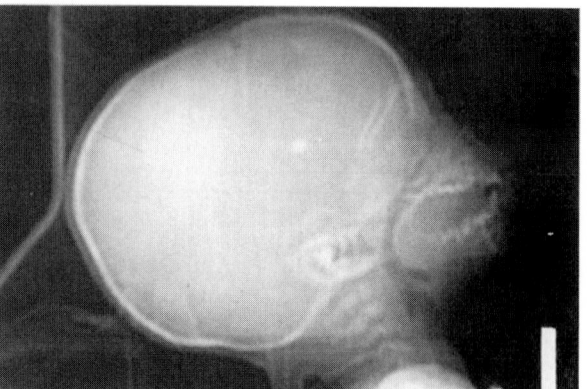

Figure 51-6 Dermoid cyst. External view **(A)** and lateral topogram **(B)** of dermoid cyst arising from the anterior fontanelle. The lesion had eroded the bone around the fontanelle but was removed easily in its entirety.

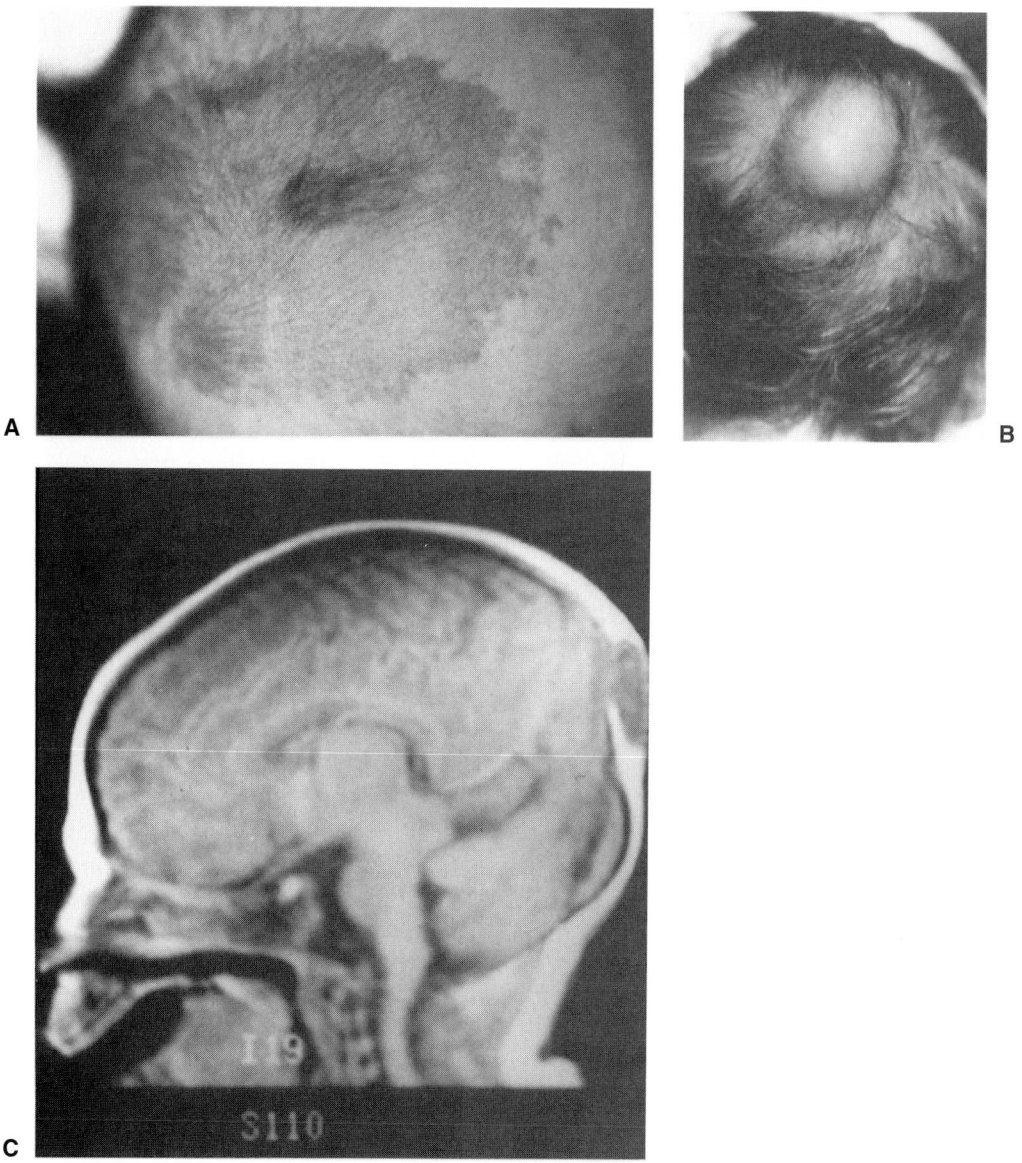

Figure 51-7   **A:** A small hairy patch with surrounding discolored skin noted at birth in the midline occipitally. On exploration, this lesion proved to be a small encephalocele. **B:** A larger occipital encephalocele without a hairy covering was detected easily at birth. **C:** Magnetic resonance scanning of the lesion seen in **(B)** demonstrates the brain tissue outside the confines of the skull as well as anomalous hindbrain anatomy.

removing any possible dermal remnant. The placode then can be rolled into a tubular structure if its shape permits, anchoring pia to pia using very fine sutures. It is important at this stage of the procedure to examine both above and below the placode for other intraspinal pathology, such as a fatty filum or diastematomyelia. Sometimes removal of one lumbar lamina above the area of exposure is necessary to permit full exploration.

Spinal Dysraphism Other Than Myelomeningocele

Although myelomeningocele is the easiest spinal cord defect to identify, the diagnosis of tethered cord syndrome, spinal lipomas, or other related closed malfor-

mations can be made in the newborn period. In general, patients who have hemangiomas, hairy patches, fatty lumps, or deep sinus tracts in the area of the lumbosacral spine deserve investigation within the first few months of life. Spinal ultrasound can be an excellent screening test for determining the level of the conus medullaris, as well as the respiratory excursions of the nerve roots. Ultrasound is also useful in cases of dimples without any other associated findings. As mentioned previously, in the absence of a truly open defect or draining sinus that increases the risk of meningitis or other infection, there is no urgent need to surgically correct these deformities. To diminish the risk of surgical complication, elective repair of tethered spinal cords is typically delayed until the patient is at least 3 months old. Urodynamic

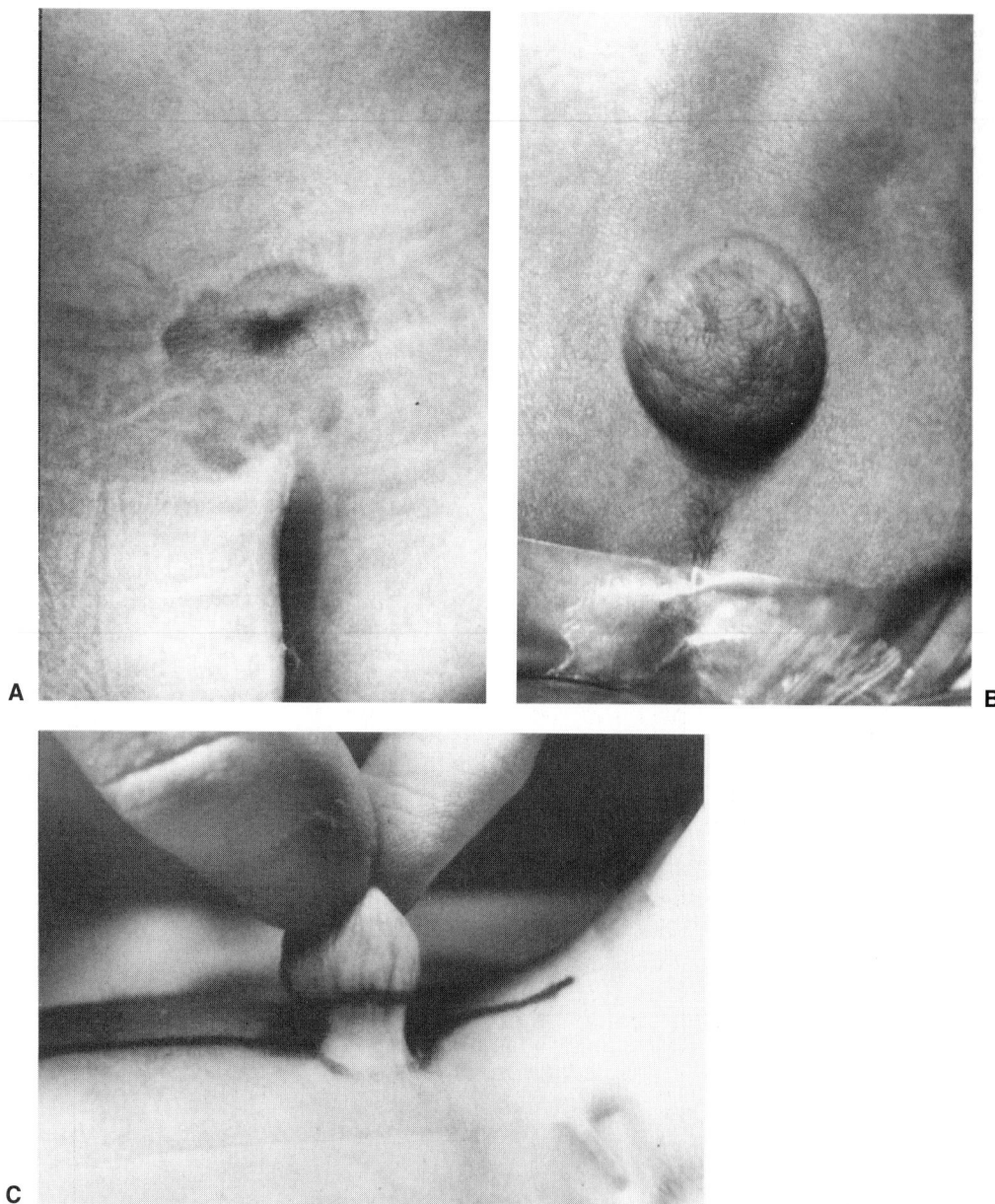

Figure 51-8 A: This small sacral dimple, with encircling reddened patch, was noted at birth. At surgery, it was found to be a dermal sinus tract into the spinal cord. The gluteal cleft is seen below. **B:** This skin-covered lesion noted at birth was found to be an anatomically identifiable myelomeningocele with intact placode and associated meningocele sac. The child had no neurologic deficits at birth. **C:** The skin tag being held up at the cervical area was noted at birth but not referred for evaluation until 3 months of life. Upon surgical exploration, a dermal sinus tract was identified and followed directly into the central canal of the spinal cord. The child had no pre- or postoperative neurologic deficits.

evaluation with electromyographic studies of sphincter function can be useful in comparing the preoperative to postoperative bladder functions in patients too young to be toilet trained. An MRI is extremely useful, preferably obtained at several months of age, shortly before surgery, when the characteristics of the tissue allow better anatomic definition of structures. It is now a generally recommended pediatric neurosurgical practice that all tethered spinal cords be untethered at a relatively early age to prevent the neurologic deterioration that may occur later in life.

Encephaloceles

The cranial analogue of the open myelomeningocele is the encephalocele (Fig. 51-9). Clinically, these vary from small lesions that may cause relatively little disruption of brain structure to large lesions with massive amounts of brain tissue extruded through the cranial opening. Again, the availability of ultrasound and MRI scanning antenatally has allowed improvements in the planning and advice given to prospective parents of babies with these problems. As with open myelomeningocele defects, open cranial

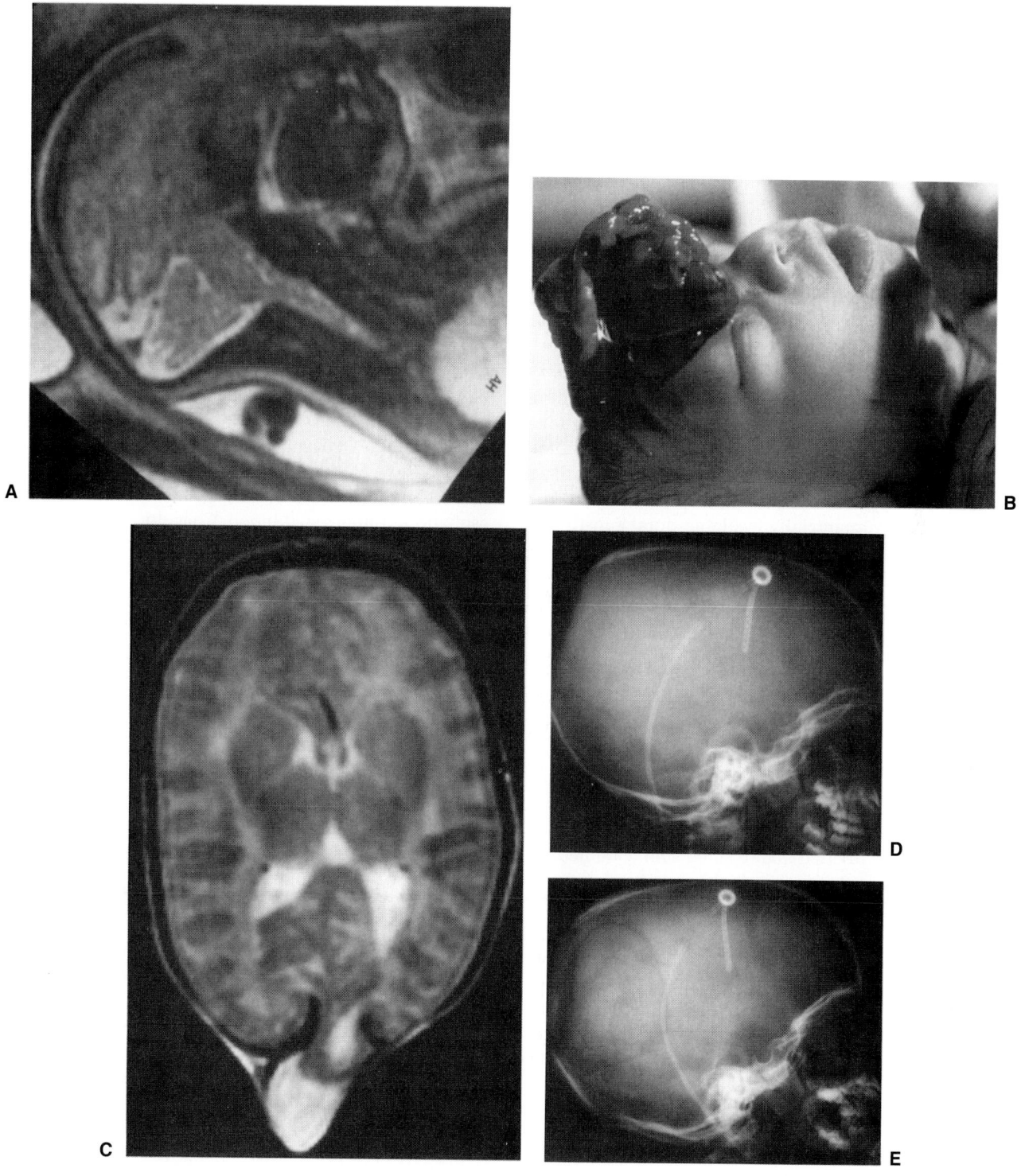

Figure 51-9 Encephaloceles, or open defects of the cranial end of the neuraxis, span a broad range of clinical presentations. A frontal encephalocele with a large extrusion of brain tissue frontally. This was demonstrated on an antenatal magnetic resonance imaging scan **(A)**, which accurately predicted the appearance of the mass at birth **(B)**. A smaller occipital encephalocele **(C)** had much less central nervous system tissue within it and was almost entirely cystic. This required a skull reconstruction to patch the cranial defect **(D, E)**, which healed without any bony defects 1 year after surgery in a neurologically normal child.

defects require acute closure, generally within 24 hours of birth, to minimize the risk of meningitis. Closed lesions can be managed in a variety of ways. If the lesion is large or enlarging, or could potentially cause airway obstruction, early repair is required. As with occult spinal dysraphic states, repair of small lesions can be deferred until radiologic imaging quality is maximized and surgical risks are minimized.

The surgical repair of an encephalocele is very much analogous to myelomeningocele repair. The encephalocele sac is entered and explored for nervous tissue. Generally, extracranial tissue is truncated and discarded because it is nonfunctional. The remainder of the repair is devoted to reconstructing a barrier between brain and subcutaneous tissue by repairing the dural lining and forming a reinforced barrier to CSF leakage through the skin.

The normal skin around the margin of the encephalocele is inspected and trimmed to yield a skin edge that eventually can be closed. There is typically a defect in the cranium as well as in the normal dura. As with myelomeningoceles, there is usually a gradual change from normal tissue to abnormal scar tissue around the edges of the lesion. If the encephalocele is quite large, it is often essentially pedunculated glial material, and it becomes necessary to amputate the excess neural tissue to allow any possibility of a closure. The edges of relatively normal dura are identified and then either closed primarily or with a patched graft, which can be taken from pericranium in some cases, or commercially available dural substitute materials can be used. After a watertight seal is created, the scalp over the dural closure is approximated. In some cases, relaxing incisions or rotational flaps have to be made to allow for a satisfactory closure. Postoperatively, the patient must be carefully observed for the development of symptomatic hydrocephalus, which may have been masked by a gradual leakage of fluid out of the encephalocele. Some encephalocele patients require shunts, but the majority do not.

Children born with encephaloceles, either frontal or occipital, have variable outcomes. In general, frontal nasal encephaloceles that involve the frontal cortex or are purely fluid filled can be resected and repaired with good neurologic and cosmetic outcome. A high percentage of these children will go on to have normal cognitive function. Hydrocephalus is common but certainly not the rule in these children. Occipital encephaloceles, particularly those that involve a significant amount of herniated brain tissue, are predictive of a less robust cognitive outcome. These children have a very high rate of hydrocephalus and often will grow to have developmental delay and other cognitive difficulties.

REMOVAL OF EXCESS INTRACRANIAL MASS

An increase in the contents of the cranial vault can be due to sources other than CSF accumulation. Head trauma and congenital CNS tumors are pathophysiologic categories that cause an increase in intracranial contents that are amenable to neurosurgical intervention. Regardless of the etiology, excess intracranial mass may not present with neurologic symptoms because of the distensibility of the neonatal skull. The fontanelle provides the capacity for constant monitoring of intracranial pressure.

Head Trauma in the Neonate

Mechanical injury to the CNS or peripheral nervous system in the neonate generally is a result of conditions immediately surrounding birth itself. These injuries are dramatically less frequent than they were only a decade or two ago, largely because of improvements in monitoring and imaging that have improved the overall level of obstetric care. The true incidence of head trauma is unknown (42,43) because clinically insignificant injuries are rarely diagnosed. Among diagnosed cases of neonatal head trauma, one in twenty is fatal. Isolated spinal cord or brainstem injury has been observed in 3% to 10% of neonatal autopsies (44).

Extracranial injuries resulting in blood collections in the neonate can be important because of the low circulating blood volume and relatively large capacity for sequestration of blood in infants of this size. An important example is subgaleal hemorrhage, where dramatic blood loss can occur because blood collects below the galea and, therefore, is not bounded by suture lines. Occasionally, these require aspiration of nonclotted blood. Coagulopathies should be excluded.

Cephalohematoma is the collection of blood below the pericranium of the outer surface of the skull. It does not cross suture lines, is unilateral, and is almost always over parietal areas. These clots resolve spontaneously over time. Because these hemorrhages are generally self-limited, the clots are usually not aspirated to avoid the risk of introducing infection. Neurosurgical intervention is largely limited to the occasional cephalohematoma that calcifies and causes an obvious cosmetic deformity.

In the majority of cephalohematomas, there is probably an underlying skull fracture which is never formally diagnosed and reduces spontaneously. These minimally depressed, "ping pong" fractures generally involve the parietal bones. If they do not reduce spontaneously, they can either be elevated by a limited and careful digital manipulation or can be surgically reduced with a very simple procedure in which an instrument is passed through a small hole below the fracture to pop it back into place.

Leptomeningeal cysts, also called growing skull fractures, are usually the result of an underlying brain injury and failure of normal CSF reabsorption, with communication of the leptomeninges through the subarachnoid space. Most frequently, they communicate with the ventricular system through a porencephalic cyst and may be associated with hydrocephalus. In cases of more significant brain injury, it is important to identify these lesions to effect primary closure of the dura, or at least to follow these children closely to ensure that hydrocephalus does not develop.

Although they only rarely require surgical exploration or treatment, the full range of intracranial injuries can occur in the neonate: epidural, subdural, subarachnoid, and parenchymal hemorrhages. An important sign frequently seen on scans is the accumulation of blood within the leaves of the tentorium, which may mimic a tentorial subdural hematoma. It is important to identify this condition because it may look quite dramatic on computed tomographic scan, but surgical exploration can lead to disastrous, uncontrolled bleeding, essentially from the communication of this intradural space with the sinuses. The distensibility of the head and the open sutures and fontanelle provides the neurosurgeon with unique, direct access to the intracranial space. The newborn's head allows for percutaneous aspiration of subdural hematoma or intraparenchymal clot, in a fashion impossible in older children. In many cases, percutaneous aspiration of subdural clot is the procedure of choice for the injured neonate (45).

Spinal Cord Injury

Ligaments are generally lax in the pediatric patient, and in the newborn particularly. However, it is possible to stretch the spinal cord beyond its elastic capacity to the point of injury. Though some patients recover with no observable abnormalities, others will suffer permanent nerve damage that can cause neurologic syndromes with pathophysiologic correlation with the involved nerves. High cervical injury will result in quadriplegia. An extensive lesion of the lower cervical cord would be expected to cause partial dysfunction in the upper extremities, impaired diaphragmatic movement, and paraplegia. The presence or absence of Horner syndrome (failure of sympathetic innervation to the pupil and face on one side) can be an important clue to the structural integrity of the roots emerging from the cervical spinal cord.

Congenital Tumors of the Central Nervous System

There are several types of congenital CNS tumors (Fig. 51-10), all of which are rare. These tumors demonstrate biologic behavior depending on their location and histology (46). Important types of tumors include choroid plexus papillomas (47), teratomas (48,49), and anaplastic lesions such as astrocytomas (50), glioblastomas (51), primary neuroblastomas (52), and astroblastomas (53). Even asymptomatic antenatal tumors have been noted, with one very large intracranial teratoma that caused maternal pain (54).

Although these tumors are extraordinarily rare, their diagnosis is generally rather straightforward because the masses themselves may show up on antenatal ultrasound or postnatal ultrasound obtained to evaluate macrocranium. The initial management of the tumor almost always is neurosurgical, requiring biopsy and generally decompression of tissue, to establish diagnosis and prognosis, as well as to initiate therapy.

OPENING PREMATURE FUSIONS IN THE NEONATE

Craniofacial Anomalies

With the exception of severe synostosis of all of the sutures (Fig. 51-11), treatment of craniosynostosis is aimed at allowing development of a more cosmetically acceptable

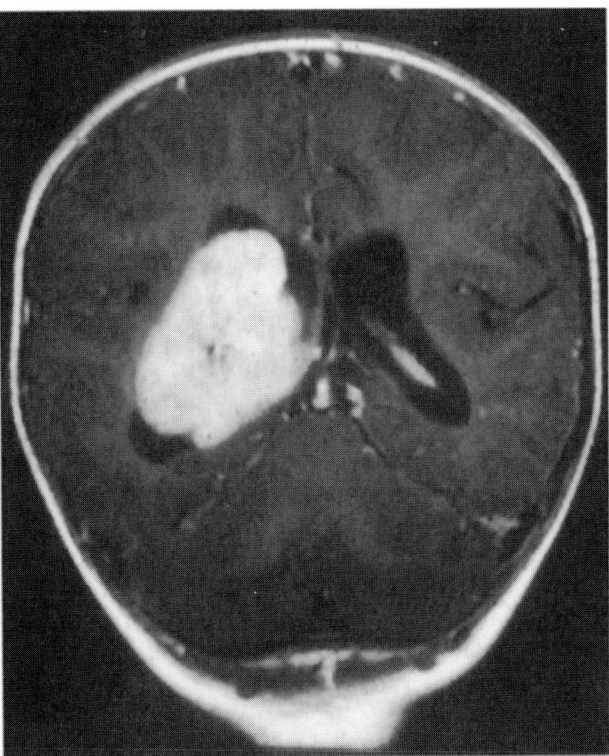

Figure 51-10 Congenital tumors are quite rare, and actual diagnosis during the neonatal period is particularly unusual. This patient proved to have a choroid plexus papilloma, which presented at 4 months of age with a large mass and growing head circumference, although it almost surely was present at birth.

spherically shaped skull. It has minimal or no effect on ultimate neurologic outcome. Generally, the earlier synostosis is treated, the less severe is the surgery. The most common isolated synostosis is sagittal synostosis (Fig. 51-2), which produces a long, narrow cranium, often with a ridge and characteristic lack of movement in the sagittal suture on physical examination. A variety of procedures have been proposed for this condition, but a wide sagittal craniectomy is favored, within the first few months of life. The rounding effect of brain growth is usually adequate for restoring excellent contours. For more complex deformities, particularly the syndromic categories of Crouzon, Apert, and Pfeiffer syndromes, all of which have associated abnormalities of the extremities and other congenital defects, treatment of the brachycephaly is usually deferred for several months beyond the neonatal period so that a more definitive and planned craniofacial approach can be taken, if necessary, with frontal advancement and orbital reshaping.

Treatment of the kleeblattschädel, or cloverleaf deformity, when all sutures are congenitally closed, is the only craniosynostotic syndrome requiring treatment in the neonatal period. Such multisuture synostosis requires early craniectomy, which may involve almost complete removal of the cranial vault to allow early growth. It generally requires one or more frontal advancements, starting several months later, to achieve an acceptable cranial shape.

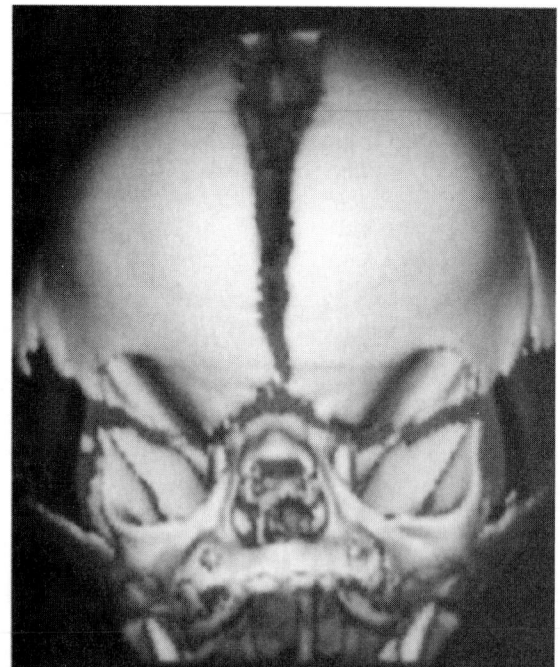

A

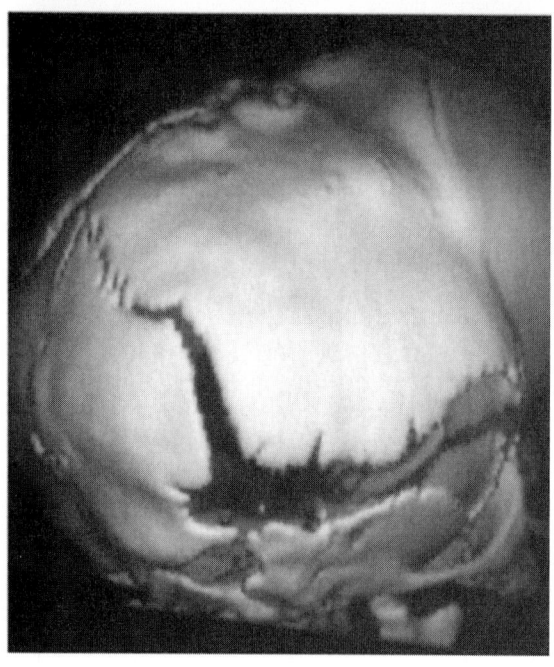

B

Figure 51-11 Closed sutures. Cranial synostosis is a condition that usually is managed several months after birth, but certain conditions, such as kleeblattschädel **(A, B)**, require earlier decompression to diminish the risk of increased intracranial pressure.

CEREBROVASCULAR ANOMALIES OF THE NEWBORN

Although adult-type aneurysms have been demonstrated in children and even newborns, the most common vascular lesions are arteriovenous malformations (55). The characteristic neonatal presentation of an arteriovenous malformation derives from its deep drainage into the vein of Galen system. It can cause a very large dilatation of the vein of Galen, called a vein of Galen aneurysm. Such

lesions frequently present as high output cardiac failure in the neonate, due to the very high flow shunting that occurs. These lesions have an extremely high mortality regardless of interventional efforts. However, there are many lesions with less extensive flow that are amendable to postnatal interventional angiographic techniques to occlude a fistula. The arteriovenous malformations themselves may be identified and respond to resection. Some of these patients do quite well (56).

The angiographic diagnosis and interventional radiographic treatment of arteriovenous malformations, fistulas, and other associated lesions in the neonate have been extensively described (56). These lesions can be subgrouped according to the morphology of the channels comprised (e.g., venous vs. arteriovenous), flow characteristics (low vs. high), and location (galenic, parenchymal, pial, or dural). Antenatal diagnosis has significantly altered the thinking about some of these lesions (56). For high-flow lesions, the flow itself becomes the major symptom, with systemic signs of high-output cardiac state and, in severe cases, cardiac failure with multiple organ dysfunction. Smaller lesions with lower flow may present as macrocephaly and hydrocephalus related to the increased venous pressure and subsequent functional diminution in absorption of CSF. Furthermore, progressive cerebral atrophy may develop.

Vein of Galen aneurysms are believed to occur between 6 and 11 weeks of gestation as a result of arterial communications with the embryologic precursor of the vein of Galen. Circularly, the aneurysm itself becomes symptomatic of the venous hypertension, which results from the abnormal communication.

Transcatheter occlusion of galenic arteriovenous shunts can be accomplished by either a transarterial or transvenous route. Although the transarterial modality is preferred by many endovascular centers, a transvenous approach involving access to the venous drainage by transtorcular, transfemoral, or transjugular catheterization can result in subtotal occlusion of the venous drainage, thereby reducing the shunt volume and cardiac failure. Ultimate cure by thrombosis can potentially be seen in either type of therapy. In cases of severe cardiac failure, however, the cardiac prognosis is poor enough that the outcome is guarded. If possible, these patients should be managed in centers where interventional radiology is available. Antenatal diagnosis makes such postnatal evaluation considerably more feasible.

The management of other arteriovenous malformations and fistulas independent of the vein of Galen also can be undertaken with endovascular or open surgical treatment.

PROGNOSIS AND LONG-TERM OUTLOOK FOR THE NEUROSURGICAL NEONATE

An understanding of the long-term prognosis after any particular type of abnormality is crucial for planning and evaluating therapeutic strategies and for counseling the parents.

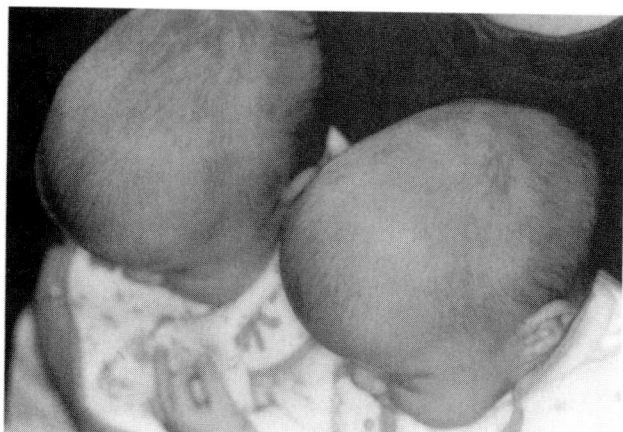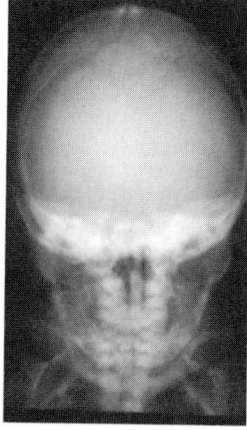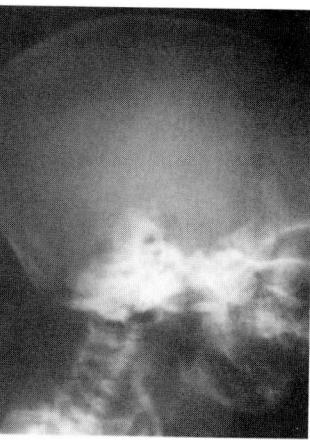

Figure 51-12 Sagittal synostosis, a far more common type of craniosynostosis, can be detected in the nursery and referred for neurosurgical intervention. Definitive treatment may be delayed for several months.

Unfortunately, these weighty decisions must be based on general guidelines that are often not predictive for an individual baby. du Plessis and Volpe (57) have outlined a rational sequence of considerations to use when discussing prognosis in these cases. They emphasize the importance of establishing the etiology of a disease process as the most important predictor. Thus, a particular degree of ventriculomegaly may be associated with a significantly worse cognitive prognosis in Dandy-Walker malformation or aqueductal stenosis than in myelomeningocele or communicating PHH. Such differences can be understood on the basis of major contributions from associated cerebral dysgenesis, earlier called the microanatomic malformations or "wiring" abnormalities. In addition, hydrocephalus resulting from infection will depend, to a very large degree, on the nature of the infection at the cellular level. This will be more predictive of developmental outcome than the degree of secondary ventriculomegaly. From the neurosurgical point of view, it is important to separate the portion of projected disability that is based on hydrodynamic or other neurosurgically solvable problems from that which is intrinsic to the neurons themselves and not remediable by the neurosurgeon. In counseling parents, this distinction should be made quite explicitly, and it should be stated that the disease process involves at least two types of processes: those that can be treated with neurosurgical intervention such as a shunt and those that the intervention will not alter. This enables the neurosurgeon to say, for example, that a shunt may be absolutely necessary to treat a particular infant's condition, but that it may not be sufficient to correct the overall neurologic problem. In effect, this defers part of the issue of prognosis back to the medical and neurologic teams, while enforcing the importance of the proposed neurosurgical intervention. Nevertheless, the general implications of recent literature on the outcome of patients with common neurosurgical conditions should be well understood by neurosurgeons and other clinicians involved at the time of this family counseling.

The outcome for infants with PHH is difficult to ascertain for several reasons. First, long term outcome data lags behind advances in neonatal, neurologic, and neurosurgical care such that the data quickly becomes obsolete. Next, this is a rare condition, making it best suited to multicenter analysis; however, there is also a fairly wide range of practice styles rendering these comparisons of limited value. Finally, these infants often have multiple comorbid complications of prematurity that have a more than additive impact on neurodevelopmental deficits. This makes the exact role of PHH and details of its treatment difficult to tease out.

That said, parents and physicians alike are anxious to understand the prognostic implications of PHH. Though prognosis varies widely by patient population, the majority (from 62% [58] to 88% [59]) of patients who require a temporary ventricular access device progress to need a permanent VP shunt. Direct complications of the temporary ventricular access device and VP shunt include infection (5% to 8%) (57–59) and occlusion (10% to 45%) (58,59), with overall shunt revision rates of approximately 1.5 per patient (60). Long-term neurodevelopment is determined less by shunt mechanics (60) than preexisting parenchymal injuries (58). Expectedly, "grade IV hemorrhage" (parenchymal bleeding), periventricular leukomalacia, shunt infection, and the need for multiple shunt revisions all predict a worse neurodevelopmental outcome (61). A recent study confirmed highly significant predictors for mortality and neurologic outcome on the factors that intuitively are consistent with clinical experience (62). Mortality was best predicted in this study by the extent of intracranial hemorrhage, number of shunt revisions, and birth weight, in that order, with a very high degree of statistic correlation. The grade of hemorrhage, birth weight, and presence of seizure activity were the most important determinants of motor outcome. The grade of hemorrhage itself proved to be the most important variable determining cognitive outcome, motor function, and seizure activity. Because appreciating the long-term outcome of these vulnerable patients is critical to therapeutic improvement, every effort must be made to obtain and interpret outcome data, despite the above difficulties. Clear communication between neurosurgeons and neonatologists will remain a cornerstone of treatment for these small patients.

REFERENCES

1. Taylor GA, Madsen JR. Neonatal hydrocephalus: hemodynamic response to fontanelle compression—correlation with intracranial pressure and need for shunt placement. *Radiology* 1996;201:685–689.
2. Egnor M, Zheng L, Rosiello A, et al. A model of pulsations in communicating hydrocephalus. *Pediatr Neurosurg* 2002;36: 281–303.
3. McAllister JP 2nd, Chovan P. Neonatal hydrocephalus. Mechanisms and consequences. *Neurosurg Clin N Am* 1998;9: 73–93.
4. Leviton A, Gilles F. Ventriculomegaly, delayed myelination, white matter hypoplasia, and "periventricular" leukomalacia: how are they related? *Pediatr Neurol* 1996;15:127–136.
5. Gross SJ, Eckerman CO. Normative early head growth in very-low-birth-weight infants. *J Pediatr* 1983;103:946–949.
6. Sherry B, Mei Z, Grummer-Strawn L, et al. Evaluation of and recommendations for growth references for very low birth weight (≤1500 grams) infants in the United States. *Pediatrics* 2003; 111:750–758.
7. National Institute of Child Health and Human Development Neonatal Research Network. Available at: http://neonatal.rti.org. Accessed November 15, 2004.
8. Fan YF, Chong VF, Tan KP. Subarachnoid spaces in infants and young children. *Ann Acad Med Singapore* 1993;22:732–735.
9. Gurtner P, Bass T, Gudeman SK. Surgical management of posthemorrhagic hydrocephalus in 22 low-birth-weight infants. *Childs Nerv Syst* 1992;8:198–202.
10. Frim DM, Scott MR, Madsen JR. Surgical management of neonatal hydrocephalus. *Neurosurg Clin N Am* 1998;9:105–110.
11. Hansen AR, Snyder EY. Medical management of neonatal posthemorrhagic hydrocephalus. *Neurosurg Clin N Am* 1998;9: 95–104.
12. Kennedy CR, Ayers S, Campbell MJ, et al. Randomized, controlled trial of acetazolamide and furosemide in posthemorrhagic ventricular dilation in infancy: follow-up at 1 year. *Pediatrics* 2001; 108:597–607.
13. International PHVD Drug Trial Group. International randomised controlled trial of acetazolamide and furosemide in posthaemorrhagic ventricular dilatation in infancy. *Lancet* 1998; 352: 433–440.
14. Hudgins RJ, Boydston WR, Hudgins PA, et al. Treatment of intraventricular hemorrhage in the premature infant with urokinase. A preliminary report. *Pediatr Neurosurg* 1994;20:190–197.
15. Hansen AR, Volpe JJ, Goumnerova LC, et al. Intraventricular urokinase for the treatment of posthemorrhagic hydrocephalus. *Pediatr Neurol* 1997;17:213–217.
16. Luciano R, Velardi F, Romagnoli C, et al. Failure of fibrinolytic endoventricular treatment to prevent neonatal post-haemorrhagic hydrocephalus. A case-control trial. *Childs Nerv Syst* 1997;13: 73–76.
17. Whitelaw A, Pople I, Cherian S, et al. Phase 1 trial of prevention of hydrocephalus after intraventricular hemorrhage in newborn infants by drainage, irrigation, and fibrinolytic therapy. *Pediatrics* 2003;111:759–765.
18. Wilcock DJ, Jaspan T, Punt J. CSF flow through third ventriculostomy demonstrated with colour Doppler ultrasonography. *Clin Radiol* 1996;51:127–129.
19. Papile LA, Burstein J, Burstein R, et al. Incidence and evolution of subependymal and intraventricular hemorrhage: a study of infants with birth weights less than 1,500 gm. *J Pediatr* 1978;92:529–534.
20. Marlin AE, Gaskill SJ. The etiology and management of hydrocephalus in the preterm infant. *Concepts Neurosurg* 1990;3:67–78.
21. Hansen A, Puder M, eds. *The manual of surgical neonatal intensive care.* Toronto: BC Decker, 2003.
22. Rudas G, Almassy Z, Varga E, et al. Alterations in spinal fluid drainage in infants with hydrocephalus. *Pediatr Radiol* 1997;27:580–582.
23. Mercuri E, Faundez JC, Cowan F, et al. Acetazolamide without furosemide in the treatment of post-haemorrhagic hydrocephalus. *Acta Paediatr* 1994;83:1319–1321.
24. Fulmer BB, Grabb PA, Oakes WJ, et al. Neonatal ventriculosubgaleal shunts. *Neurosurgery* 2000;47:80–83.
25. Morimoto K, Hayakawa T, Yoshimine T, et al. Two-step procedure for early neonatal surgery of fetal hydrocephalus. *Neurol Med Chir (Tokyo)* 1993;33:158–165.
26. Couldwell WT, LeMay DR, McComb JG. Experience with use of extended length peritoneal shunt catheters. *J Neurosurg* 1996;85:425–427.
27. Dallacasa P, Dappozzo A, Galassi E, et al. Cerebrospinal fluid shunt infections in infants. *Childs Nerv Syst* 1995;11:643–648.
28. Alonso-Vanegas M, Alvarez JL, Delgado L, et al. Gastric perforation due to ventriculo-peritoneal shunt. *Pediatr Neurosurg* 1994; 21:192–194.
29. Kang JK, Jeun SS, Chung DS, et al. Unusual proximal migration of ventriculoperitoneal shunt into the heart. *Childs Nerv Syst* 1996; 12:176–179.
30. Bass T, White LE, Wood RD, et al. Rapid decompression of congenital hydrocephalus associated with parenchymal hemorrhage. *J Neuroimaging* 1995;5:249–251.
31. Scott RM, Madsen JR. Shunt technology: contemporary concepts and prospects. *Clin Neurosurg* 2003;50:256–267.
32. Steinbok P, Poskitt KJ, Cochrane DD, et al. Prevention of postshunting ventricular asymmetry by transseptal placement of ventricular catheters. A randomized study. *Pediatr Neurosurg* 1994;21:59–64.
33. Caldarelli M, Di Rocco C. Surgical options in the treatment of interhemispheric arachnoid cysts. *Surg Neurol* 1996;46:212–221.
34. Lena G, van Calenberg F, Genitori L, et al. Supratentorial interhemispheric cysts associated with callosal agenesis: surgical treatment and outcome in 16 children. *Childs Nerv Syst* 1995;11: 568–573.
35. Eder HG, Leber KA, Gruber W. Complications after shunting isolated IV ventricles. *Childs Nerv Syst* 1997;13:13–16.
36. Rademaker KJ, Govaert P, Vandertop WP, et al. Rapidly progressive enlargement of the fourth ventricle in the preterm infant with post-haemorrhagic ventricular dilatation. *Acta Paediatr* 1995;84:1193–1196.
37. Levine D, Barnes PD, Madsen JR, et al. HASTE MR imaging improves sonographic diagnosis of fetal CNS anomalies. *Radiology* 1997;204:635–642.
38. Madsen JR, Estroff J, Levine D. Prenatal neurosurgical diagnosis and counseling. *Neurosurg Clin N Am* 1998;9:49–61.
39. Luthy DA, Wardinsky T, Shurtleff DB, et al. Cesarean section before the onset of labor and subsequent motor function in infants with meningomyelocele diagnosed antenatally. *N Engl J Med* 1991;324:662–666.
40. McCullough DC, Johnson DL. Myelomeningocele repair: technical considerations and complications. 1988. *Pediatr Neurosurg* 1994;21:83–89.
41. McLone DG. Care of the neonate with a myelomeningocele. *Neurosurg Clin N Am* 1998;9:111–120.
42. Di Rocco C, Verlandi F. Epidemiology and etiology of craniocerebral trauma in the first two years of life. In: Raimondi AJ, Choux M, Di Rocco C, eds. *Head injuries in the newborn and infant.* New York: Springer-Verlag, 1986:125–136.
43. Hovind K. Traumatic birth injuries. In: Raimondi AJ, Choux M, Di Rocco C, eds. *Head injuries in the newborn and infant.* New York: Springer-Verlag, 1986:87–109.
44. Morota N, Sakamoto K, Kobayashi N. Traumatic cervical syringomyelia related to birth injury. *Childs Nerv Syst* 1992;8:234–236.
45. Macdonald RL, Hoffman HJ, Kestle JR, et al. Needle aspiration of acute subdural hematomas in infancy. *Pediatr Neurosurg* 1994;20:73–76.
46. Fort DW, Rushing EJ. Congenital central nervous system tumors. *J Child Neurol* 1997;12:157–164.
47. Tacconi L, Delfini R, Cantore G. Choroid plexus papillomas: consideration of a surgical series of 33 cases. *Acta Neurochir (Wien)* 1996;138:802–810.
48. Ferreira J, Eviatar L, Schneider S, et al. Prenatal diagnosis of intracranial teratoma. Prolonged survival after resection of a malignant teratoma diagnosed prenatally by ultrasound: a case report and literature review. *Pediatr Neurosurg* 1993;19:84–88.
49. Storr U, Rupprecht T, Bornemann A, et al. Congenital intracerebral teratoma: a rare differential diagnosis in newborn hydrocephalus. *Pediatr Radiol* 1997;27:262–264.
50. Heckel S, Favre R, Gasser B, et al. Prenatal diagnosis of a congenital astrocytoma: a case report and literature review. *Ultrasound Obstet Gynecol* 1995;5:63–66.
51. Mazzone D, Magro G, Lucenti A, et al. Report of a case of congenital glioblastoma multiforme: an immunohistochemical study. *Childs Nerv Syst* 1995;11:311–313.

52. Mondkar J, Kalgutkar A, Nalavade Y, et al. Congenital primary cerebral neuroblastoma. *Indian Pediatr* 1994;31:698–702.

53. Pizer BL, Moss T, Oakhill A, et al. Congenital astroblastoma: an immunohistochemical study. Case report. *J Neurosurg* 1995;83: 550–555.

54. Soares FA, Fischer SE, Reis MA, et al. Massive intracranial immature teratoma. Report of a case with polyhidramnios and intense pelvic pain. *Arq Neuropsiquiatr* 1996;54:309–312.

55. Hosotani K, Tokuriki Y, Takebe Y, et al. Ruptured aneurysm of the distal posterior inferior cerebellar artery in a neonate—case report. *Neurol Med Chir (Tokyo)* 1995;35:892–895.

56. Burrows PE, Robertson RL. Neonatal central nervous system vascular disorders. *Neurosurg Clin N Am* 1998;9:155–180.

57. du Plessis A, Volpe JJ. Prognosis for development in the newborn requiring neurosurgical intervention. *Neurosurg Clin N Am* 1998;9:187–197.

58. Berger A, Weninger M, Reinprecht A, et al. Long-term experience with subcutaneously tunneled external ventricular drainage in preterm infants. *Childs Nerv Syst* 2000;16:103–109.

59. Hudgins RJ, Boydston WR, Gilreath CL. Treatment of posthemorrhagic hydrocephalus in the preterm infant with a ventricular access device. *Pediatr Neurosurg* 1998;29:309–313.

60. Reinprecht A, Dietrich W, Berger A, et al. Posthemorrhagic hydrocephalus in preterm infants: long-term follow-up and shunt-related complications. *Childs Nerv Syst* 2001;17:663–669.

61. Resch B, Gedermann A, Maurer U, et al. Neurodevelopmental outcome of hydrocephalus following intra-/periventricular hemorrhage in preterm infants: short- and long-term results. *Childs Nerv Syst* 1996;12:27–33.

62. Levy ML, Masri LS, McComb JG. Outcome for preterm infants with germinal matrix hemorrhage and progressive hydrocephalus. *Neurosurgery* 1997;41:1111–1117.

Orthopedics

William W. Robertson, Jr.

The orthopedic or musculoskeletal examination is a significant part of the neonate evaluation. Normal variations in contour, size, relationships, and range of motion of joints are influenced by genetic factors and by position *in utero*. These normal variations must be distinguished from congenital anomalies and traumatic lesions. The basic principle, that the earlier appropriate treatment is started, the better the correction, makes it incumbent on those caring for the neonate to make an early diagnosis and obtain appropriate consultation promptly.

In current practice, musculoskeletal abnormalities may be detected in the prenatal examination of the fetus. Using ultrasound, conditions such as skeletal dysplasia, spinal malformations, limb length discrepancy, and clubfoot deformities can be detected with some accuracy (1–4). The neonatal examination is vital to the confirmation of such anomalies and to the completion of any prenatal counseling rendered for such problems.

PHYSICAL EXAMINATION

The clinician examines the musculoskeletal system first by inspection, looking for abnormalities in contour, size, and position and observing the spontaneous and reflex movements of the infant, and second by palpation and manipulation to determine whether there are abnormalities of passive motion. This is followed by stimulation, where indicated, so that active motion can be noted. All observations include comparisons between opposite extremities. A routine for examining a newborn should be developed so that each examination will be complete. This routine may vary among physicians, but each part of the musculoskeletal system should be examined systematically.

Head and Neck

The neck is examined passively for rotation, lateral flexion, anterior flexion, and extension. Rotation of 80 degrees and lateral flexion of 40 degrees should be present in a full-term infant. Both these motions are normally symmetric to the right and left. Extension and flexion are difficult to measure, but in flexion the chin should touch or nearly touch the chest wall. Extension should be at least 45 degrees from neutral. When rotation or lateral flexion is asymmetric or when motion is limited, radiographs of the neck should be made.

Upper Extremities

The clavicle and shoulder girdle, including the scapula and proximal humerus, elbow, forearm, and hand, are inspected and palpated, with any anomalies in contour, size, and postural attitudes noted. Range of motion of the shoulder girdle is evaluated. Normal flexion and abduction of the shoulder are 175 to 180 degrees. Extension, internal rotation, and external rotation of the shoulder should be at least 25 degrees, 80 degrees, and 45 degrees, respectively.

The elbow is inspected next, and its motion is evaluated. Normally the newborn's elbow lacks 10 to 15 degrees from going to full extension and flexes 145 degrees. The forearm should pronate and supinate at least 80 degrees. Limitation of these two motions can be missed easily. Supination and pronation are tested by holding the humerus at the side of the trunk with the elbow held flexed 90 degrees with one hand while checking supination and pronation with the other. The wrist flexes 75 to 80 degrees and extends 65 to 75 degrees. The normally clenched fist of the newborn should have full passive extension of the thumb and all fingers. Active finger extension may be elicited, if necessary, by a pinprick to the palm. Extension should be to 0 degrees at the metacarpophalangeal joint, but active extension of the interphalangeal joint usually lacks 5 to 15 degrees from going to 0.

Spine

In the newborn, congenital anomalies of the spine are not readily detectable on physical examination; however, gross anomalies frequently can be recognized by inspection of the spine. Passive flexion and extension and lateral bending of the spine should show smooth contours. Lateral flexion may be slightly asymmetric, secondary to position *in utero*. A hairy tuft, cutaneous vascular pattern, or lipomatous mass may signal underlying axial anomalies.

Lower Extremities

The lower extremities are observed for symmetry and variations in contour, position, and size. The hips of a newborn should flex 145 degrees and generally have flexion contractures, as shown by the Thomas test. This test is performed by fully flexing the infant's hips, and then extending the hip being tested while holding the opposite hip in flexion to lock the pelvis. The number of degrees that the extended thigh lacks from going to 0-degree extension is the degree of flexion contracture present in that hip. It is normal for the term newborn to have a 25- to 30-degree flexion contracture. The hip flexion contracture gradually diminishes during the first 12 weeks after birth, but occasionally will be present longer than 3 months. When hip extension is asymmetric, the more extended hip may be unstable. The stability of the hip always must be evaluated by an Ortolani test (Fig. 52-1A) or the oppositely directed provocative Barlow test (Fig. 52-1B). When there is a difference in the extension of the hips or a positive Ortolani or Barlow test, additional evaluation of the hip by radiography or, preferably, sonography is indicated. The timing of this imaging is discussed later in this chapter.

Internal and external rotation of the newborn's hip should range between 40 and 80 degrees, abduction is between 45 and 75 degrees, and normal abduction is between 10 and 20 degrees. Any asymmetry of motion should be investigated to determine the cause.

Infants who were not in a frank breech fetal position generally will have a knee flexion contracture of 10 to 25 degrees, with additional ability to flex to 120 to 145 degrees. In those positioned in frank breech, the knees usually will hyperextend 10 to 15 degrees and have limitation of flexion.

Examination of the ankles and feet includes observation of resting positions and range of active motion, stimulated by stroking the sole and dorsal, medial, and lateral sides of the foot. The range of passive motion of the ankle in both dorsiflexion and plantarflexion varies depending on the fetal position. Dorsiflexion to above neutral should always be present. Plantarflexion of less than 10 degrees below neutral generally is abnormal. Abduction and adduction of the forefoot is at least 10 to 15 degrees, and the hindfoot has 5 to 10 degrees or more of motion in both varus and valgus.

MUSCULOSKELETAL ANOMALIES

It is not within the scope of this text to discuss all the congenital and acquired abnormalities of the musculoskeletal system seen in the neonate; this chapter does, however, cover most of the more common abnormalities.

Neck

Klippel-Feil syndrome is a defect in segmentation of the cervical vertebrae (5). There is both a decrease in the number of vertebrae and a fusion of two or more vertebrae. The neck appears shorter than normal, and motion is limited in all directions. The limitation of motion depends on the number of fused segments and frequently is asymmetric in both rotation and lateral flexion. The asymmetric motion may simulate muscular torticollis, but radiographic examination of the neck can confirm the presence of the Klippel-Feil deformity. Treatment started early, done several times a day, and consisting of passive stretching of the neck to improve rotation, lateral bending, and flexion–extension, may improve the range of motion of the neck.

Torticollis of the neonate may be one of several types. The typical muscular torticollis (Fig. 52-2A) involves a mass from an intramuscular hematoma that appears in the sternocleidomastoideus at 2 weeks of age and gradually disappears during the next 8 to 10 weeks. This mass may go unnoticed, and the torticollis unrecognized until there is facial asymmetry and limited motion of the neck. The physical findings of muscular torticollis are limited rotation of the neck toward the side of the lesion (Figs. 52-2B and 52-2C) and limited lateral flexion away from the lesion. In well-established, persistent torticollis, there is flattening of the maxillary and frontal bones on the side of the lesion and of the occiput on the opposite side. The asymmetry is not present in the newborn, but may become apparent as early as 2 or 3 weeks and is progressive until

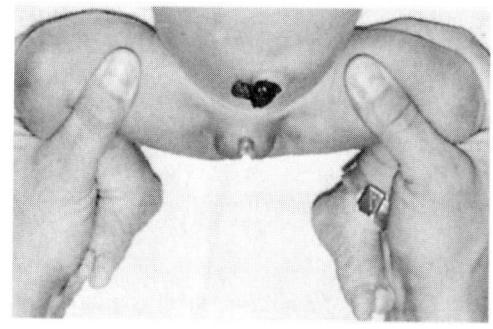
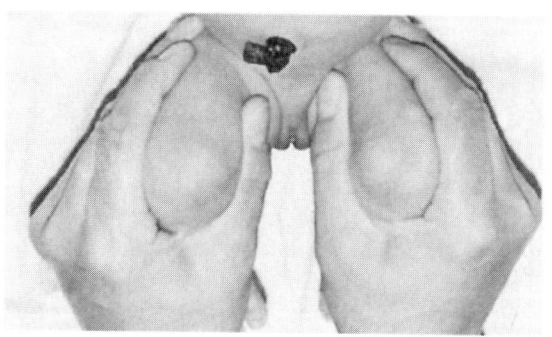

Figure 52-1 A: Ortolani sign. The fingers are on the trochanter and the thumbs grip the femurs as shown. The femurs are lifted forward as the thighs are abducted. If the head is dislocated, it can be felt to reduce. **B:** Barlow maneuver. The thighs are adducted. If the head dislocates, it will be both felt and seen as it suddenly jerks over the acetabulum.

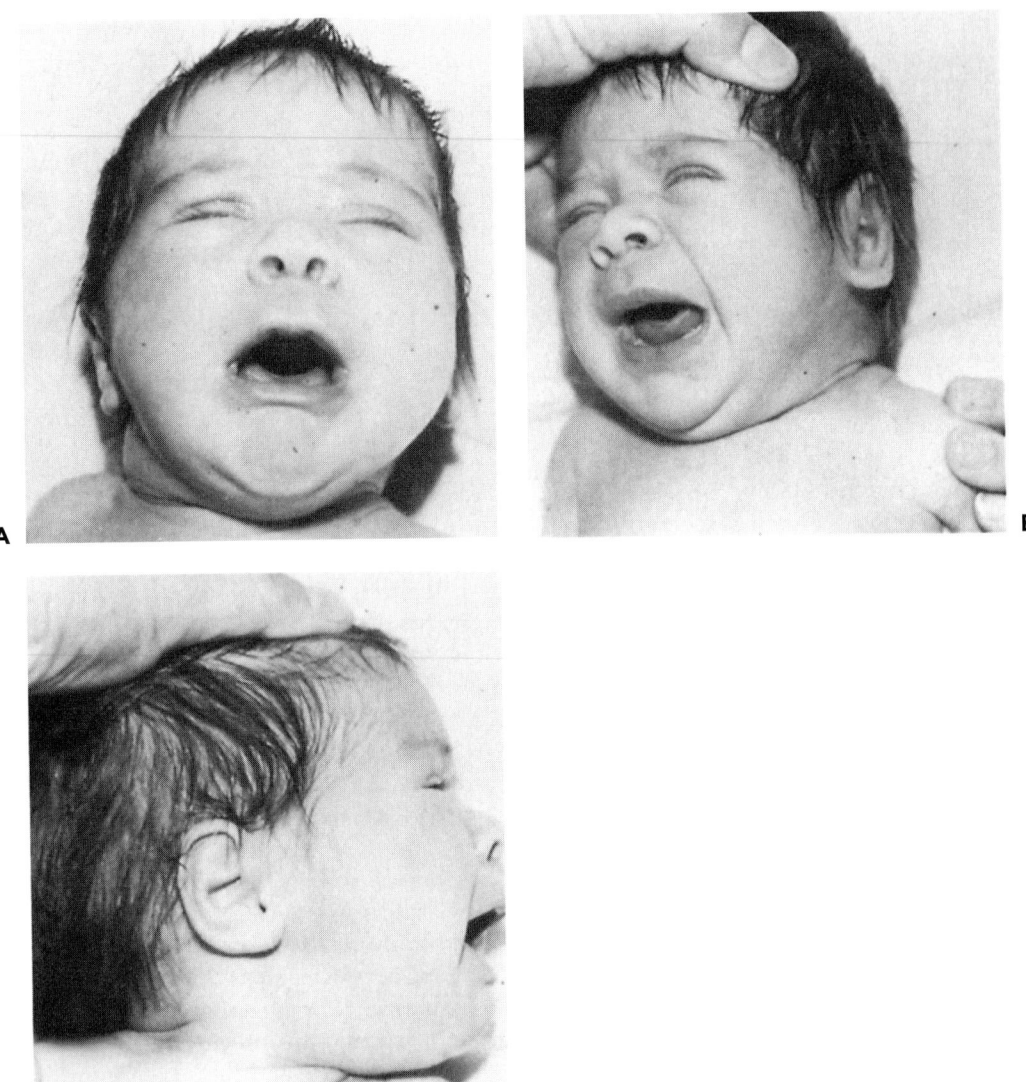

Figure 52-2   A: Congenital muscular torticollis. There is a fibrous mass in the right sternocleido-mastoideus muscle. **B:** Rotation toward the right is limited by the tightness in the right sternocleidomas-toideus muscle. **C:** Rotation toward the left is normal.

the tightness is corrected. Torticollis associated with intrauter-ine deformation may be apparent at birth.

Initial treatment of muscular torticollis is by passive exercise and appropriate positioning of the infant in bed (6). The neck should be gently but firmly stretched four or five times each day toward the direction of limited rotation and lateral flexion. Sandbags or some similar objects may be used to position the baby's head to prevent it from assuming the position that the tight muscle encourages.

There is a type of congenital torticollis that is associated with neither a mass in the sternocleidomastoideus nor cer-vical spine abnormalities. In these infants, there is a myo-static contracture of the sternocleidomastoideus, probably secondary to *in utero* position or compression. This type of torticollis often is associated with scoliosis and abductor contracture of one hip and adductor tightness of the oppo-site hip. The adducted hip may show acetabular dysplasia (Fig. 52-3). The abductor contracture may not be detectable

until the normally present tightness of hip flexors has spontaneously diminished enough that the hip can be extended. Whereas this type of torticollis corrects with lit-tle or no treatment, the associated hip contractions require stretching. The tight hip abductor needs particular atten-tion, with passive stretching and abduction devices such as multiple diaper layers. Rarely, the associated acetabular dysplasia progresses to dislocation.

Spine

Scoliosis

Congenital scoliosis is difficult to recognize at birth unless there is asymmetric movement, a cutaneous lesion (such as aplasia, dimple, dermal sinus tract, flat hemangioma, or hairy tuft), or a lipomatous mass. In the newborn infant, scoliosis is caused by an isolated defect in vertebral body

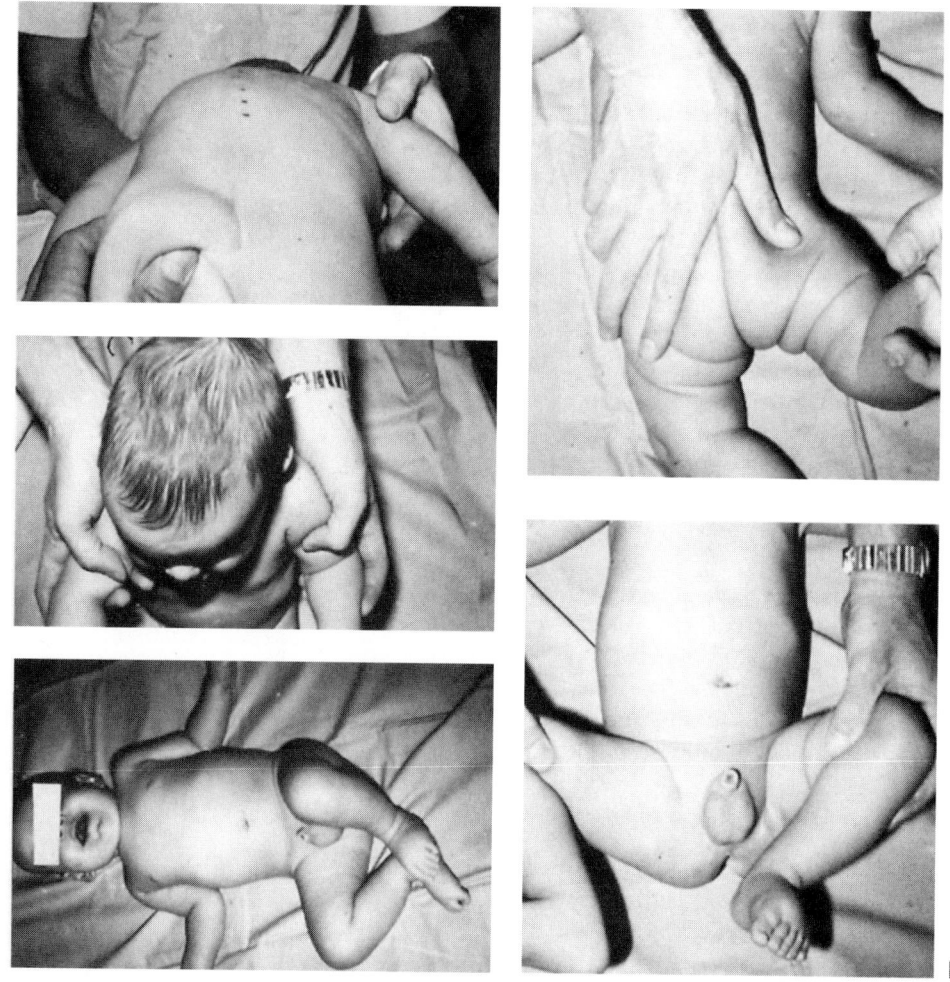

Figure 52-3   A: A 6-month-old infant with left torticollis, left scoliosis, right abductor contracture, and left adductor tightness. **B:** The right abductor and left adductor are tight.

formation or by failure of segmentation. There is little evidence that it is an inherited anomaly, except when it occurs as part of a genetically transmitted syndrome. Because of the cartilaginous nature of much of the spine at birth, only significant anomalies, such as hemivertebrae, can be diagnosed by plain x-ray. Ultrasound is a good alternative for evaluation of suspected cases when magnetic resonance imaging (MRI) is not indicated in the newborn (7,8). For the older infant with significant abnormalities, MRI evaluation is certainly indicated for determination of occult intraspinal pathology, including syringomyelia, diastematomyelia, and tethered cord (9). Because spinal orthoses seldom are of benefit, congenital scoliosis initially is followed only by observation. If a curve is progressive, spinal fusion will be needed and should be done before the curve becomes cosmetically or functionally significant (10). Fusion of a short segment, with or without excision of markedly abnormal bone segments, may be done as early as necessary. Congenital scoliosis is associated with a high incidence of cardiac and related genitourinary anomalies; therefore, the function and anatomy of the cardiovascular and genitourinary systems should be evaluated by MRI and ultrasonic techniques (11).

Congenital kyphosis is a rarer condition that carries a higher risk of progression and the development of neurologic compromise (12). Certain types of deformity require surgical treatment before the age of 5 years (13).

Myelomeningocele

Diagnosis of a myelomeningocele generally poses little problem when there is a skin defect. Because the skin over myelomeningoceles is not always defective, any soft mass in or off the midline must be examined closely to determine its composition. Lipomata always have good skin coverage and tend to be off the midline.

The care of an infant born with myelomeningocele is complex and requires input from several specialties (see Chapter 51). It is important to determine immediately after birth the level of involvement by inspection of the back, careful examination of the muscle function of the lower extremities, and radiographic examination before surgical closure.

The most common abnormalities of the lower extremities associated with myelomeningocele are deformations of the feet, indicating lack of normal fetal muscle activity.

Initial treatment of the deformed foot is with plaster cast correction, followed, if necessary, by surgical releases and transfer of muscle insertions to maintain the correction. These surgeries may be done at almost any age.

Gentle passive exercising and progressive splinting treat flexion or extension deformities of the knee. New splints need to be made frequently as the deformity improves.

Treatment of a dislocated hip in the patient with myelomeningocele is controversial. There is general agreement that in those children with intact hip musculature, the dislocated hip, as in an otherwise normal newborn, reduces easily in flexion and abduction. For those lesions below L-2, hip abduction therapy helps in developing a more stable hip. The flexed, abducted, and externally rotated position achieved in a Pavlik harness should not be used when the lesion is above L-2 because this position may lead to development of contractures that prevent the hip from extending and adducting.

Infants with high lumbar or low thoracic myelomeningoceles have very high mortality and morbidity. The degree of disability correlates well with the level of defect, presence and degree of hydrocephalus, and presence of a bony kyphosis. A lesion above L-1 associated with hydrocephalus and kyphosis indicates, almost without exception, significant mental and motor disability.

Upper Extremities

Duplication and Reduction

Supernumerary parts, absence or reduction anomalies of the extremities, and segmentation defects of the limb should offer no problem in diagnosis. These orthopedic anomalies seldom need immediate attention, but they should be seen early by the orthopedist to plan appropriate therapy and discuss prognosis with the family. This is true for anomalies of both the upper and lower extremities.

Syndactylism, or fusion of any portion of two or more digits, is a common anomaly that is transmitted through an autosomal-dominant gene with varying expressivity. Surgical treatment should be within the first year, with timing dependent on the completeness of the syndactyly and the fingers involved. The thumb and index finger should be separated at 6 months of age, and the little and ring finger separated at 1 year. It is important to determine by radiography if there is a synostosis between fingers because this should be divided by 1 year of age. A delay in surgical separation in synostosis will result in a bowing of the longer finger due to differential growth.

Polydactyly is correctable by surgery, with timing dependent on the extent of duplication. When the duplication does not contain bone or cartilage, it should be removed in infancy. When there is a question about function, surgical correction should be delayed until the degree of function present in each of the duplicated digits can be ascertained.

Absence of the radius, commonly called radial clubhand, is easily recognized (Fig. 52-4). The wrist and hand are deviated 90 degrees or more. Absence of the radius may

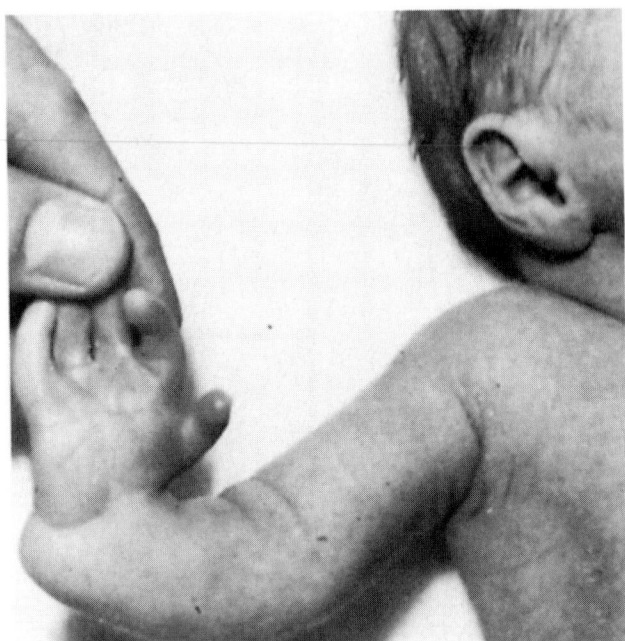

Figure 52-4   Congenital absence of the radius.

be bilateral or unilateral, and the thumb may be present, absent, or hypoplastic. The clubhand is caused by damage to the apical ectoderm or deeper mesenchymal tissue of the limb bud (14). It is not genetically transmitted in the otherwise normal child, but it is associated with several genetically transmitted syndromes and frequently is accompanied by aplastic anemia. Early treatment by corrective splints may be sufficient to correct the radial deviation and prepare the extremity for surgery at a later date.

Congenital absence of the thumb occurs as an isolated anomaly or may be associated with a radial clubhand. When unilateral, little or no treatment is needed, but when the absence is bilateral, pollicization of the index finger of the dominant hand will improve function. When the thumb is rudimentary and nonfunctional, treatment is controversial.

In the extremities, congenital constriction band (Streeter) syndrome is diagnosed at birth by the presence of defects in the soft tissue underlying the skin (that is usually intact). This entity, possibly more accurately called early amnion rupture sequence, has been proposed as an etiologic factor in extremity, truncal, and facial abnormalities, including cleft lip/palate (15). In either the upper or lower extremity, a circumferential band can lead to vascular compromise of the distal part of the extremity (Fig. 52-5). The presentation is one of a visible constriction or, in more extreme cases, cyanosis or extreme edema in the portion of the extremity distal to the band. Surgical treatment to release the band or amputation in severely compromised extremities may be indicated at a relatively early age (16).

Shoulder Girdle

The Sprengel deformity of congenital elevated scapula is one of the more common congenital anomalies of the

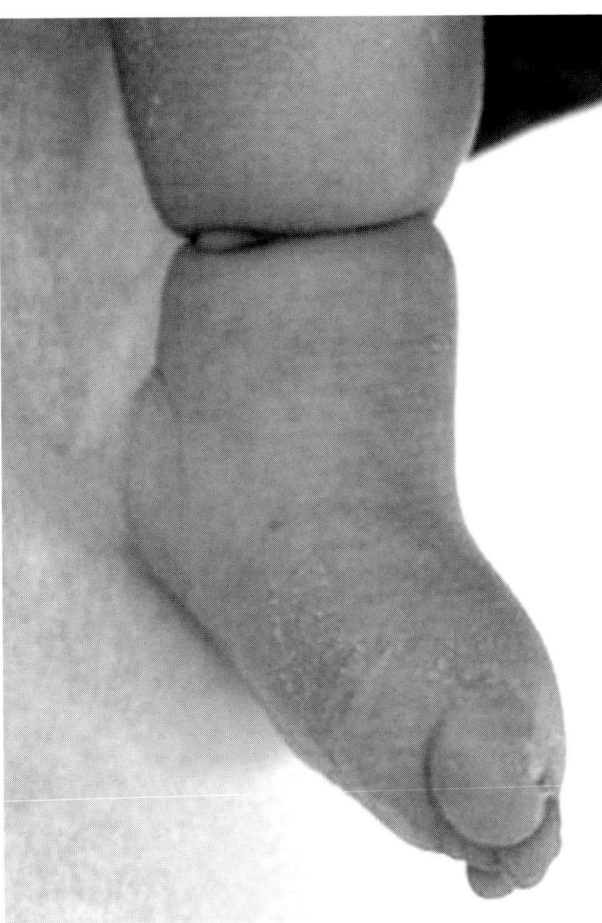

Figure 52-5 Constricting band secondary to amniotic band disruption sequence.

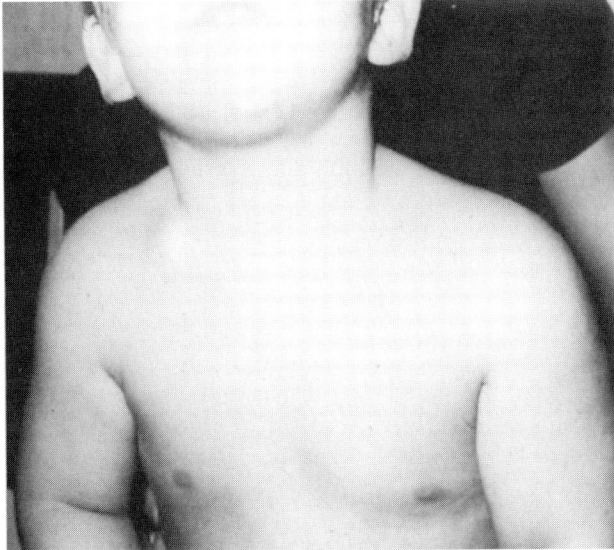

Figure 52-6 A 2-year-old child with pseudoarthrosis of the right clavicle.

shoulder girdle. The deformity may be bilateral or unilateral, and usually it is associated with other abnormalities, such as Klippel-Feil syndrome, congenital anomalies of the upper thoracic vertebrae, or anomalies of the ribs. Asymmetry of the shoulders in unilateral involvement makes recognition easier. On palpation, the affected scapula is high and rotated outward and downward so that its vertebral border lies superiorly and more horizontally than normal. Shoulder abduction and flexion usually, but not always, are limited. The early, conservative treatment is passive range of motion. Surgical correction, at 3 to 4 years or up to 16 years of age, generally improves appearance and function, with the overall improvement from surgery better in the younger child.

Two congenital malformations of the clavicle are congenital pseudoarthrosis and congenital (partial or complete) absence of the clavicle. The physical signs on palpation of congenital pseudoarthrosis are angulation of the clavicle and a painless, bulbar mass in the midclavicular area (Fig. 52-6). The shoulder girdle is hypermobile, with motion in the clavicle at the pseudoarthrosis. Early treatment is not needed before surgical grafting of the defect at 3 to 4 years of age. Because the need for any intervention is controversial, therapy should be individualized. Congenital pseudoarthrosis of the clavicle can be differentiated from

perinatal fracture of the clavicle by abundant callus formation in the healing fracture within 2 to 3 weeks after birth.

Partial or complete absence of the clavicle may be recognized by palpation and the presence of excessive scapulothoracic motion (Fig. 52-7). The completely absent clavicle usually is associated with cranial dysostosis or a widened pubic symphysis. There are no symptoms, and no treatment is needed in complete absence. With partial absence, the end of the clavicle may irritate the brachial plexus, necessitating excision of the fragment. Whereas congenital pseudoarthrosis tends to be an isolated anomaly, partial absence of the clavicle almost always accompanies an axial or appendageal skeletal anomaly.

Defects of Limb Segmentation

Synostosis of the elbow and synostosis of the radius and ulna are two of the more common skeletal anomalies of

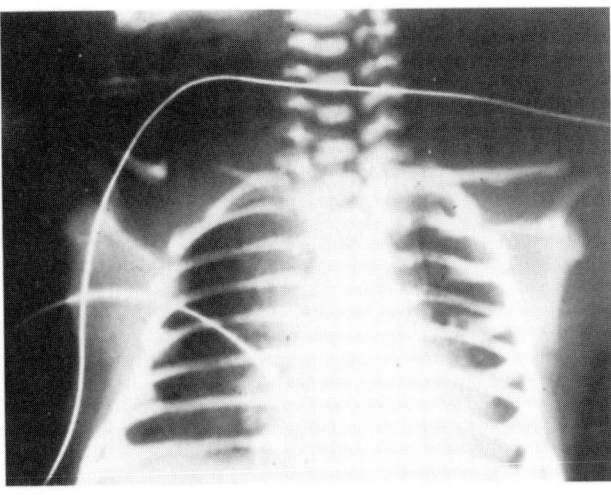

Figure 52-7 Partial absence of the right clavicle.

limb segmentation. Elbow synostosis is easily recognized by the lack of motion and significantly smaller size of the affected extremity. Synostosis of the radius and ulna seldom is diagnosed in the nursery and commonly not diagnosed for several years. This is particularly true if the defect is bilateral because the child himself will not appreciate a difference in his arms. Supinating and pronating the forearm in the initial examination of the newborn should demonstrate this anomaly by lack of range of motion.

Lower Extremities

Variations in contours and postural attitudes of the lower extremities in general and the feet in particular are frequent causes of concern. *In utero*, the feet seldom rest in a neutral position, being dorsiflexed or plantarflexed, inverted or everted, or in a combination of these positions. At times, it may be difficult to determine whether there is a structural abnormality or only a temporary positional deformation.

Feet

Metatarsus adductus (Fig. 52-8) may be either a positional deformity with no bony abnormality or a structural defect, and it is not always easy to distinguish between the two. The distinction becomes easier with time because a positional metatarsus adductus corrects fairly rapidly by passive exercises or even without treatment. A structural deformity does not spontaneously correct completely, becoming more rigid with time.

The differentiation between postural and structural metatarsus adductus is made primarily by physical examination. In structural metatarsus adductus (Fig. 52-8A), the base of the fifth metatarsus and cuboid are prominent, creating an impressive, well-defined skin crease on the medial side of the foot at the first metatarsal–cuneiform joint. In a positional metatarsus adductus, the lateral and medial borders of the foot are curved more gently than in the structural deformity. The most significant physical finding, however, is the presence or absence of rigidity of the forefoot, as determined by its resistance to abduction. In structural deformity, the forefoot usually cannot be abducted beyond the midline (Fig. 52-8B), whereas in positional deformity, the forefoot is more flexible and can be abducted (Fig. 52-8C). The heel of the structural metatarsus adductus foot usually is in valgus, and in positional deformity, it is likely to be in varus or at neutral. The valgus position of the hindfoot can be seen on clinical evaluation and, if necessary, confirmed by radiographic studies.

Treatment of the flexible positional deformity is either observation for spontaneous resolution, or passive stretching of the forefoot into abduction with the foot held as shown in Fig. 52-8B. Structural metatarsus adductus generally needs treatment with repeated cast changes. Surgical treatment may be necessary in the case of more severe structural abnormalities, such as a skew foot.

Talipes calcaneovalgus is not a structural deformity, but rather a reflection of the foot's position *in utero* (Fig. 52-9).

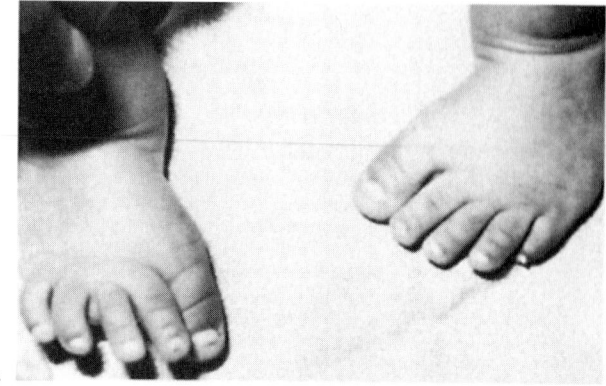

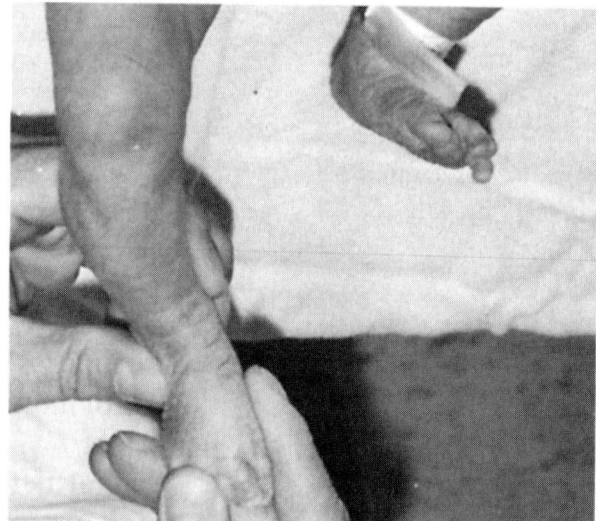

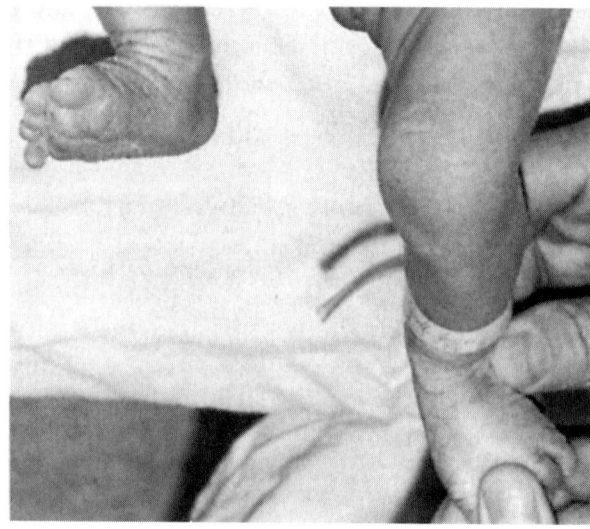

Figure 52-8 **A:** Structural metatarsus adductus. **B:** Structural metatarsus adductus. The forefoot does not abduct beyond neutral. **C:** Positional metatarsus. The forefoot abducts beyond the midline.

The sole lies against the uterine wall, and the foot is dorsiflexed so that its dorsal skin lies against the anterior surface of the tibia. The fibula is prominent and appears to be dislocated posteriorly, being pushed backward by the excessive dorsiflexion. There is a depression over the sinus tarsus. The calcaneovalgus foot is flexible and passively plantarflexes

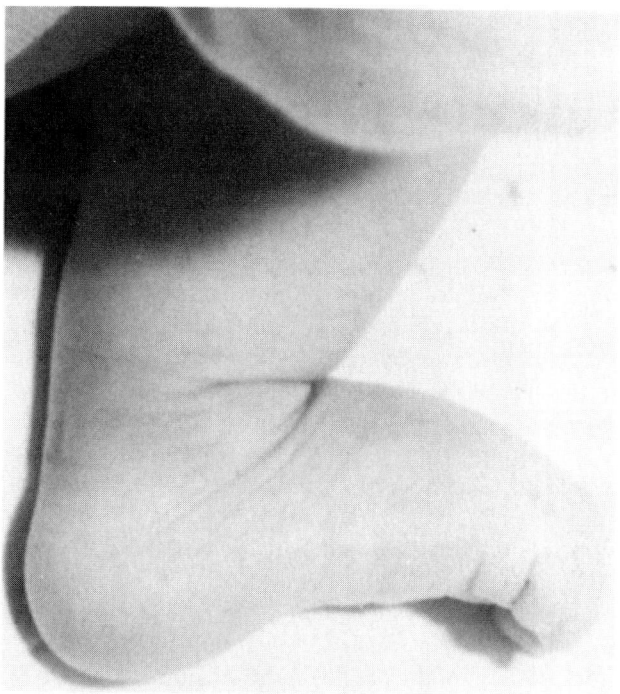

Figure 52-9 Talipes calcaneovalgus.

at least to neutral and, in most instances, to 5 to 10 degrees beyond neutral.

Treatment of the calcaneovalgus foot is by either passive exercises or corrective plaster cast, depending on the sever-

ity of the deformity. Mild cases are treated with exercises that stretch the foot into equinus and varus 15 to 20 times at four to five sessions daily.

The more severely resistant deformities, those that flex only to neutral plantarflexion, are treated by repeated applications of plaster casts for 8 weeks. Casts are changed as needed with growth, and, at each change, the foot is placed in equinus and varus with a mold placed in the arch to relax the plantar ligaments and posterior tibialis muscle. The goal of treatment is to obtain a plantarflexed varus position to allow the plantar ligaments and posterior tibialis tendon that have been stretched *in utero* to shorten.

It is important that the positional calcaneovalgus foot not be confused with congenital vertical talus, a rare but serious anomaly. In congenital vertical talus, the forefoot is dorsiflexed, and the hindfoot is in equinus (Fig. 52-10A). The talus is rigidly fixed in plantarflexion; if the examiner places one thumb on the talus and dorsiflexes and plantarflexes the foot with the other hand, the talus will remain almost stationary as the forefoot moves around it. The forefoot cannot be plantarflexed as much as the calcaneovalgus foot, and seldom can it be plantarflexed more than 5 degrees beyond neutral. A lateral radiographic examination of the foot (Fig. 52-10B) demonstrates the hindfoot equinus and forefoot dorsiflexion. With further dorsiflexion of the forefoot, the lateral radiographic examination (Fig. 52-10C) shows continued equinus of the calcaneus and talus. Serial casting rarely results in correction of this deformity. Although treatment will not create a normal foot, the results are far better when started in the first year of life.

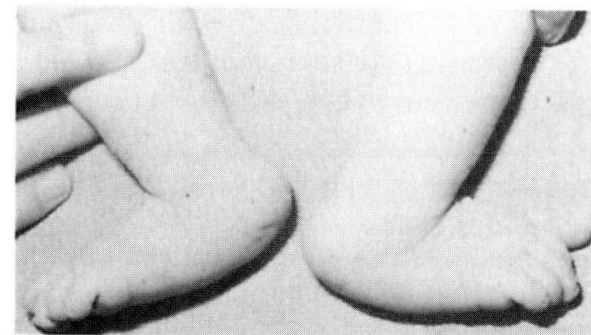

A

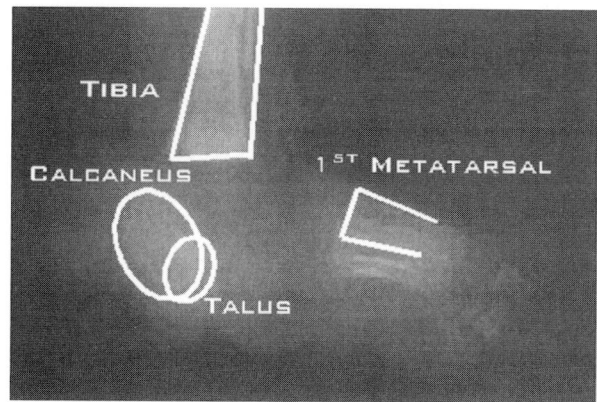

B

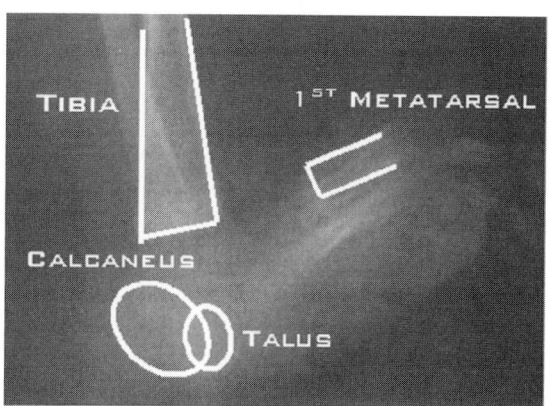

C

Figure 52-10   **A:** Flat foot secondary to congenital vertical talus. **B:** Lateral radiograph demonstrating equinus position of calcaneus and talus with dorsal subluxation of the forefoot. **C:** Lateral radiograph with forefoot dorsiflexion demonstrating persistent equinus position of calcaneus and talus.

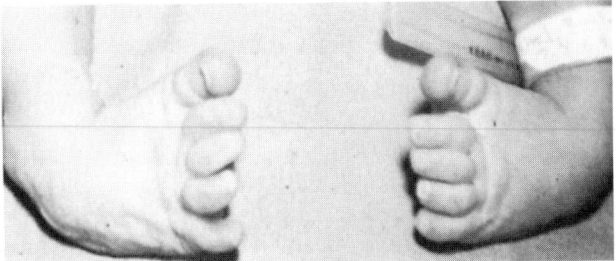

Figure 52-11 Talipes equinocavovarus foot (i.e., clubfoot).

The classic clubfoot is a developmental anomaly of the entire foot (Fig. 52-11). There is varus of the hindfoot, varus and adduction of the forefoot, and equinus that is not apparent until the varus and adduction are corrected to neutral. This is a structural deformity and resists correction; it is easily recognized by its rigidity. There is a positional equinovarus foot that may resemble the true clubfoot, but it is flexible and can be corrected beyond neutral with little difficulty. Treatment of the structural clubfoot is by repeated manipulation and strapping or by manipulation and application of a cast (17). Although early treatment usually is instituted, no studies have demonstrated clearly the advantage of casting newborn as opposed to infants. When conservative measures are unsuccessful in correcting the foot, surgical correction is necessary (18).

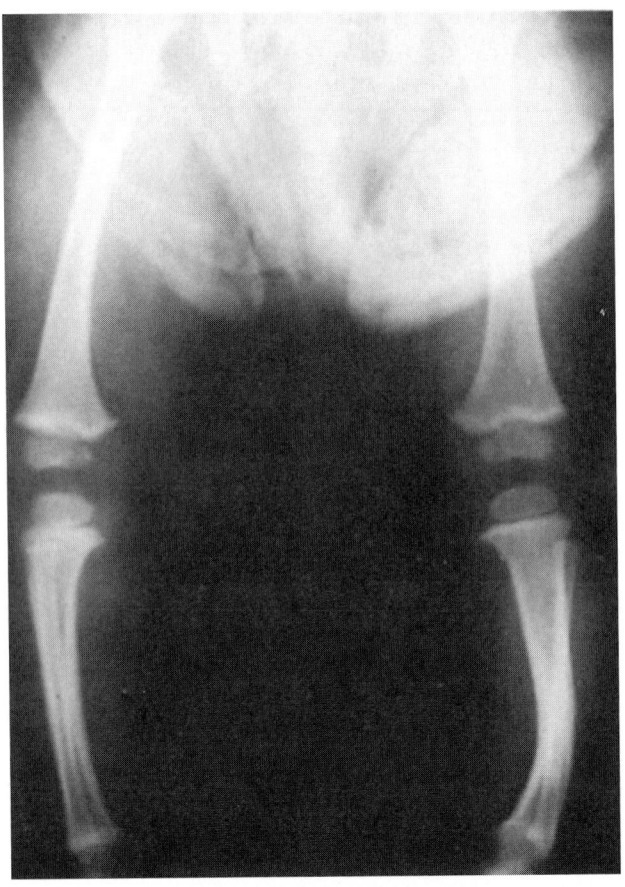

Figure 51-12 Anterior bowed tibia.

Tibia and Fibula

Significant deformities of the tibia and fibula occur infrequently and are not difficult to detect. Congenital absence of the tibia or fibula, congenital amputation, and congenital bowing all are easily recognized. When the tibia is absent, the foot is in varus; when the fibula is absent, the foot has an equinovalgus deformity. These deformities should be seen early by the orthopedist because conservative and supervised treatment of the foot deformities is indicated in some of these children, whereas early amputation is the treatment of choice in others. With newer techniques and knowledge of the biology of bone elongation, more of these limbs are being salvaged.

Anterior bowing of the tibia is a serious deformity (Fig. 52-12). The bone of the tibia is of poor quality, and in most cases, it either is sclerotic with partial or complete obliteration of the intermedullary space or has cystic areas that contain material similar to that in fibrous dysplasia. Pseudoarthrosis may be present at birth; it is always present following a fracture, which is likely within the first 2 years of life. Protection of the tibia by casts and braces is important and may be sufficient to prevent a fracture. Although the case shown in Fig. 52-12 is mild, there is a narrow intramedullary canal, and the bone needs protection for it is unlikely to heal should it fracture. There is no tendency for these cases of anterior bowing to improve spontaneously.

Conversely, a tibia that is posteriorly and medially bowed corrects spontaneously. The posterior-medial bowed tibia needs only to be observed, and any foot deformity treated with manipulation and splinting. There can be subsequent leg length discrepancy as a residual of this deformity (Fig. 52-13).

Most neonates have an inward or medial torsion of the leg distal to the knee and outward rotation above the knee. The medial torsion below the knee may occur in the knee, tibia, ankle, or combination of these, and, except in extreme cases, no treatment is necessary because alignment will improve progressively. The exception to this may be in relatively immobile, premature infants who lie in the same position most of the time.

Knee

Significant deformities of the knee are very rare. Genu recurvatum, a relatively frequent bilateral positional deformity associated with a frank breech position, is not serious and will respond to gentle exercising. The spectrum of knee recurvatum to subluxation or dislocation may reflect congenital hypotonia or Ehlers-Danlos syndrome in the newborn. Recurvatum must be differentiated from the more serious subluxation or dislocation of the knee. When there is doubt as to whether or not a recurvatum represents a subluxation or dislocation, a radiograph should be made. In subluxation, the tibia is forward on the femur but is not completely dislocated, whereas in dislocation, the tibia is completely anterior to the femur. In congenital dislocation, the knee can be hyperextended but not flexed beyond

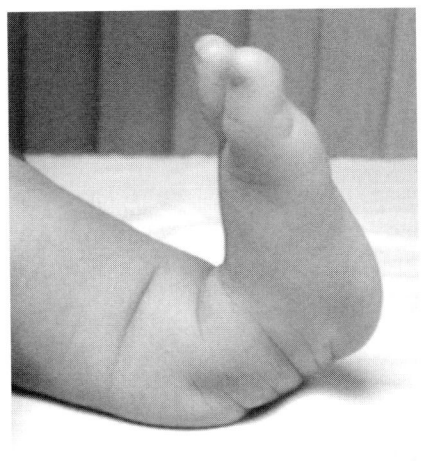
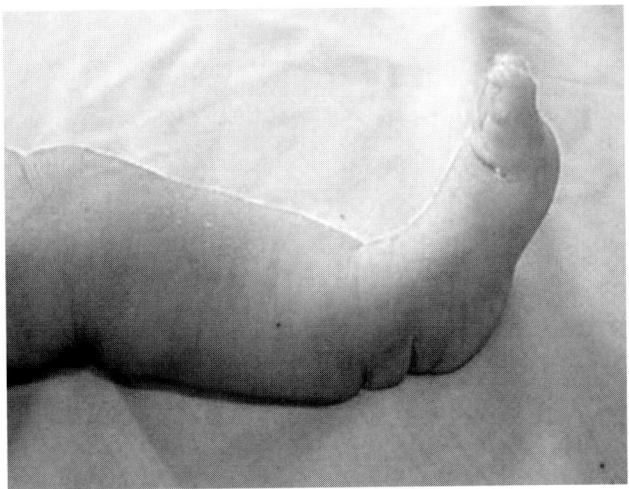

Figure 52-13 **A:** Posterior-medial bowed tibia at 20 days of age. **B:** Marked spontaneous remodeling of posterior-medial bowed tibia at 4 months of age.

neutral, and the tibia is anteriorly displaced on palpation. Both subluxation and dislocation of the knee can be treated with early serial casting. Care must be taken to follow the reduction of the articular surfaces with imaging studies. The subluxed knee reduces with casting, but a dislocated knee may require open reduction.

Unilateral, or more rarely bilateral, congenital fibrosis of part of the quadriceps is an anomaly that prevents knee flexion, causing a more extended posture than normal in neonates. Active and passive flexion is limited and seldom is more than 40 degrees. Treatment is by surgical excision of the fibrous mass.

Hip

Developmental Dysplasia of the Hip

The most common of the neonatal hip abnormalities is developmental dysplasia. This hip is embryologically normal, but as a result of mechanical forces *in utero* and maternal hormones that relax tissues in preparation for parturition, it is dislocated or dislocatable in the perinatal period. The less common type is a teratogenic hip that probably dislocates in the embryologic period of gestation and is associated with malformation of the pelvis and femur.

Developmental dysplasia of the hips occurs more frequently in female infants who present in breech position at term gestation and who have a positive family history. The dysplasia more often is unilateral with the left hip more frequently affected, but it may be bilateral.

In the newborn, the typical dislocated hip may not have the classically described signs of dislocation, such as asymmetric skin folds, limited abduction, and shorter-appearing femur (i.e., Galeazzi sign). These signs are secondary and may not develop until the end of 6 weeks of life as the dislocated hip migrates laterally and superiorly. The clinician diagnoses this condition in the newborn by demonstrating that the femoral head can be lifted into the acetabulum as

the thigh is abducted in flexion (i.e., Ortolani maneuver; Fig. 52-1A) and that it dislocates as the hip is flexed, adducted, and pushed posteriorly (i.e., Barlow maneuver; Fig. 52-1B). The Ortolani test is positive in the dislocated hip until 6 to 8 weeks of age, and sometimes longer. In addition to feeling the dislocation as the thigh is adducted, the examiner should reduce the hip by abduction in flexion and, while maintaining the same degree of abduction, extend the thigh to dislocate the hip. In each instance, whether dislocation is obtained by adducting or extending the thigh, the examiner not only can feel the hip dislocate and relocate but also can see the sudden jerk that occurs as the femoral head rides in and out of the acetabulum.

Hip dislocation usually can be recognized clinically in the first few days of life. However, a large number of hips that are unstable at birth may become stable once the intrauterine environment, both positional and hormonal, is eliminated (19). Unstable hips most at risk for development of dysplasia are those with evidence of uterine packing problems (e.g., first born, breech presentation, torticollis, or metatarsus adductus), female gender, and a positive family history of hip dysplasia. The widespread use of hip ultrasound to evaluate and confirm hip dysplasia makes the quantification of the problem much easier. The question arises as to when to treat an abnormal hip. Some authors advocate the initiation of treatment as soon as any abnormality is discovered (20,21). Other authors feel that this approach may cause overtreatment of as many as one in three hips that would stabilize within 2 to 4 weeks after birth without treatment (22–25). Early treatment is easier on the family and child, with results that are far better than when treatment is started several months or years later.

Hip displacement almost always is reduced in flexion and abduction. The hip is usually, but not always, stable if held flexed 90 degrees or more and then abducted. In the newborn, radiographs of the hip are not necessarily diagnostic, although in some, the hip appears laterally displaced in the anteroposterior projection (Fig. 52-14). Sonography,

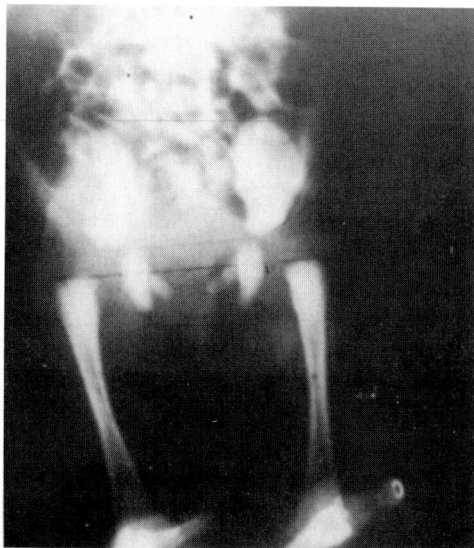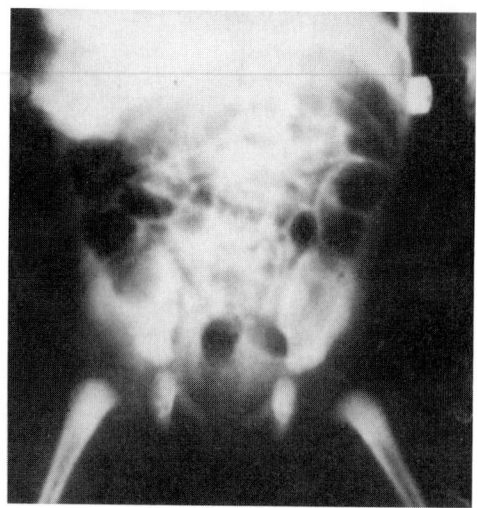

Figure 52-14 Bilateral congenital dislocation of the hip. The metaphyseal–acetabulum distance is wide.

if well done, is the method of choice in the neonate, both to confirm the diagnosis of hip dysplasia and to follow the progress of acetabular development during treatment (26). The greatest advantage of the hip ultrasound is the ability to view the hip when it is stressed in a Barlow-like maneuver.

When sonograms are not available, hip radiographs in both the anteroposterior and horizontal planes should be taken, with the infant in the splint to determine that the hip is held reduced. Rarely, the hip dislocates posteriorly in the splint but appears to be reduced in the anteroposterior view; only the horizontal view will show the dislocation in this instance.

The Pavlik harness is the splint of choice from birth to 6 months of age, but it must be applied properly. Excessive abduction from tight posterior straps can cause avascular necrosis (27).

All infants should have follow-up hip examinations at well-baby checks in the first 3 months. The Ortolani test may be positive for 6 to 12 weeks, but, more commonly, the late physical signs of dislocation are the following:

Asymmetric folds in unilateral dislocation
An apparent discrepancy of leg length caused by pelvic obliquity and a high-riding femoral head
High trochanter
Limited abduction
A palpable defect in the anterior groin where the femoral head normally lies
A piston or telescoping motion

These signs are sufficient to make the diagnosis, but sonography or radiography confirms it. After the development of the ossific nucleus of the femoral head (at 3 to 6 months), the ultrasound no longer is useful, so plain radiographic views are indicated to demonstrate hip displacement.

Developmental hip dislocation is probably the most important condition in the musculoskeletal system in which a delay in diagnosis and treatment has a profound effect on the outcome. The results of treatment in the neonate are far superior to those at any other time, so that special care in diagnosing this condition is warranted.

Teratologic Hip Dislocation

Teratogenic hip dislocation presents with different findings. The hip, which has dislocated early in fetal life, typically will not reduce by flexion and abduction because the femoral head is displaced proximally. Therefore, the Ortolani sign is not present in the teratogenic dislocation. If the dislocation is unilateral, there is asymmetry of abduction of the hips. The dislocated hip will have more extension than the opposite hip and may have limited rotation. When the dislocation is bilateral, the diagnosis is more difficult because there is no asymmetry. Abduction of both hips is limited, the thighs appear short in relation to the lower legs, and the perineum appears wider than normal. Although the diagnosis can be confirmed by ultrasound, plain radiographic examination is always abnormal in teratogenic hip dislocation.

Proximal Femoral Focal Deficiency

Proximal femoral focal deficiency is an anomaly of serious magnitude that may be either unilateral or bilateral. The degree of deficiency is variable and ranges from absence of the diaphysis, upper metaphysis, and femoral head to a very short femur, with coxa vara of the neck and head. It is not uncommon for the fibula to be absent and the foot deformed in the more severely affected infant with proximal femoral focal deficiency. The shortness of the femur is obvious on inspection. Motion of the hip may be limited. Early referral to the orthopedist, who will provide the definitive treatment, is important. Initial treatment may include stretching exercises, traction, or both for correction of contractures about the hip, although these have proven to be of limited value. Definitive surgical management depends on the potential for function in the extremity, and ranges from measures to correct leg length discrepancy to fusion of the knee and amputation of the foot to create a stump for an above-knee prosthesis.

GENERALIZED MUSCULOSKELETAL ANOMALIES

The generalized musculoskeletal disorders/malformations are a diverse group of metabolic diseases and genetic syndromes, including more than 100 recognized forms of skeletal dysplasia (28). In the last 10 years, the classification of these disorders has moved from descriptions of physical and radiographic appearance to genetic etiologies (29). There is little to be done orthopedically for most of these syndromes, but when there is a correctable deformity, treatment should be initiated early.

Some of these entities, such as achondroplasia, chondroectodermal dysplasia (Ellis van Creveld disease), and epiphyseal dysostosis (diastrophic dwarfism), are recognizable at birth and are associated with dwarfism. Infants affected by many skeletal dysplasias or metabolic skeletal abnormalities, however, appear normal at birth, with the skeletal anomalies appearing later in infancy and childhood.

One generalized condition that may require orthopedic evaluation and intervention in the neonatal period is osteogenesis imperfecta. This spectrum of genetic syndromes is manifested by soft, fragile bone. If severe, it is very obvious at birth, but it may be mild enough to go undiagnosed until the child is several years old. Osteogenesis imperfecta involves primarily the skeleton but also affects the skin, ligaments, tendons, sclera, nose, ear, platelet function, and probably other systems (30).

The diagnosis of osteogenesis imperfecta is not difficult when there are multiple fractures, a very soft skull, paradoxic respirations indicating rib fractures, and bluish-gray sclera. For those who survive delivery, gentle handling to prevent additional injuries and skin traction to align the extremities are important considerations. Whether treated with traction, splinting, or observation, the fractures heal rapidly. An important key to the treatment of fractures of osteogenesis imperfecta is to avoid increasing bone fragility with prolonged immobilization.

Arthrogryposis multiplex congenita (Fig. 52-15) is an uncommon but easily recognizable syndrome of the musculoskeletal system. All four extremities and the trunk may be affected, or the abnormalities may be limited to the arms or legs. The hallmark of this entity is the lack of active and passive motion in the affected extremities.

The microscopic picture of the muscle in arthrogryposis shows changes of denervation and fibrofatty replacement. Secondary to the muscle weakness and dysfunction, there is distortion of the joints, as well as limitation of motion. Frequently, these infants have dislocation of the hips, knees, or radial heads, or combinations of the three. In addition, they may have either clubfeet or vertical talus,

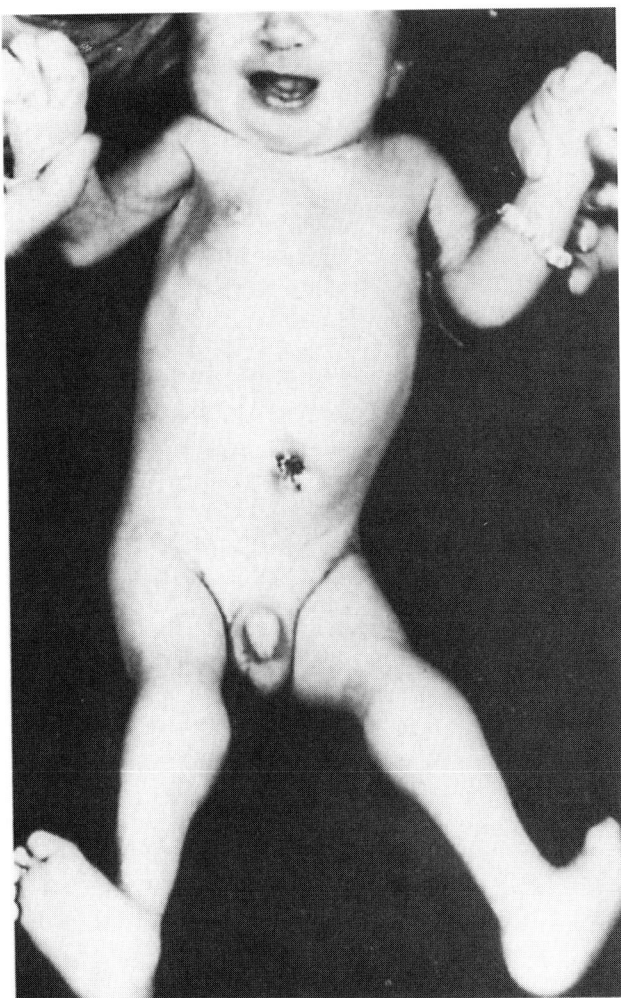

Figure 52-15 Arthrogryposis multiplex congenita.

both of which are more resistant to treatment than those not associated with arthrogryposis. Treatment should begin in the nursery and is directed at increasing the motion of all affected joints by passive exercises done six to eight times each day. Joint dislocation and the hand and foot deformities should be treated early with appropriate plaster splints or casts, or with traction.

BIRTH FRACTURES

Long, difficult labor—particularly with a breech position, large infant, or fetal distress requiring rapid extraction—makes birth injuries in otherwise normal infants more likely. Birth fractures almost always involve clavicle, humerus, or femur. It is rare for birth fractures in a normal infant to occur below the elbow or below the knee. The fracture is more likely to be through either the diaphysis or epiphyseal plate, so that the epiphysis and epiphyseal plate are separated from the metaphysis. At times, the fractures are not noted because pain may be minimal and a deformity may not be apparent. Diagnosis in such cases is made incidental to a radiograph taken for unrelated indications.

In other infants, the fracture is painful and is a cause of pseudoparalysis, with the limb lying limp and not moving on stimulation.

Diaphyseal Fractures

The obstetrician, who hears and feels the snap when the humerus breaks as the baby is being extracted, generally diagnoses fractures of the diaphysis of the humerus. The same can be said about fractures of the femoral shaft and clavicle. A radiograph confirms the fracture.

Fracture of the shaft of the humerus is treated by immobilization of the arm by the side. Soft padding is placed between the arm and chest, and the elbow is held at 90 degrees flexion.

Fractures of the femoral shaft can be held with a posterior splint that extends from below the knee to the waist and is held in place with an elastic bandage for 10 to 14 days.

Fractures of the clavicle may be asymptomatic if undisplaced and need no treatment except care in handling the infant. If the fracture is displaced, it usually is painful. The fracture can be treated either by strapping the arms to the chest, with padding placed in the axilla and the elbow flexed 90 degrees, or by using a figure-of-eight bandage made of stockinette to immobilize the fracture. In 8 to 10 days, the callus is sufficient for immobilization to be discontinued.

Epiphyseal Injuries

An epiphyseal separation or fracture occurs through the hypertrophied layer of cartilage cells in the epiphysis. A fracture through the proximal epiphyseal plate of the humerus is one of the more common skeletal injuries associated with a difficult delivery. The diagnosis has to be based primarily on the clinical findings of swelling about the shoulder and crepitus and pain when the shoulder is moved. Motion is painful, and the arm lies limply. The proximal humeral epiphysis is not ossified at birth and, therefore, is not visible on radiograph. This makes diagnosis by radiography very difficult. If there is complete or almost complete separation of the epiphysis, the metaphysis appears displaced in relation to the glenoid of the scapula, but usually the separation is minimal and there are no radiographic changes noted except soft tissue swelling. After 8 to 10 days, callus appears and is visible on radiographs. Ultrasonic evaluation of suspected epiphyseal injuries is gaining popularity because nonossified epiphyses and hematomas, as well as bony structures, are visible (31).

Treatment for a fracture of the proximal epiphysis of the humerus is immobilization of the arm by the side, with soft padding in the axilla for 8 to 10 days. Healing is rapid, and remodeling is such that even a striking angulation will improve progressively to a point where the bone contour appears normal. If a complete separation is present, reduction by gentle traction probably should be attempted before immobilization.

A fracture separation of the distal humeral epiphysis is very rare. It is difficult to diagnose radiographically because this epiphysis, like the proximal epiphysis, is completely cartilaginous. When an injury is present, there will be swelling about the elbow with pain and crepitus on passive motion. If the epiphysis is displaced, the anteroposterior radiograph will show that the olecranon is displaced medially or laterally in its relationship with the long axis of the humerus. A fracture of the distal epiphysis is more likely to have a significant residual deformity than is a fracture of the proximal humeral epiphysis. Skin traction on the forearm for 9 to 10 days is an option to treat this injury.

Fracture of the proximal femoral epiphysis is an uncommon problem but one that can be confused with a congenital dislocation or with acute pyarthrosis. The epiphyseal plate of the proximal femur is a crescent-shaped line extending from the greater to lesser trochanter and includes the cartilaginous epiphysis of the trochanter, neck, and femoral head. Swelling about the hip is difficult to appreciate, and suspicion of the presence of this injury should be aroused when the baby does not move the extremity on stimulation. Abnormality is confirmed by the presence of pain and crepitus when the hip is moved passively. The radiograph of the hip will show the upper end of the femoral metaphysis to be displaced laterally, and if the separation is complete, the metaphysis is likely to be displaced above the center of the acetabulum as well as displaced laterally. Ultrasonic evaluation will confirm the position of the cartilaginous femoral head in relation to the acetabulum and femoral metaphysis. After several days of incomplete separation, the hip will no longer be painful; most of these fractures will be recognized only after callus formation is seen on an incidental radiograph or after a large callus presents as a firm mass in the groin or upper thigh (Fig. 52-16). If the diagnosis is recognized before healing is underway, the hip should be manipulated gently and immobilized in flexion and abduction for 10 to 14 days.

If ultrasound is not available, aspiration of the joint will help to differentiate a fracture from congenital dislocation and acute pyarthrosis. If a fracture is present, blood should be found in the joint.

Diagnosis of a fracture separation of the distal femoral epiphysis can be made by radiographic studies. Ossification of the distal femoral epiphysis is present at birth, and even slight displacement and angulation can be recognized. If there is swelling around the knee and pain on passive motion, a radiograph will confirm the diagnosis. Treatment is by immobilization in plaster for 10 to 14 days, if displacement is not severe. When displacement or angulation is excessive, reduction by manipulation should be performed and the extremity immobilized in plaster for 14 days.

OBSTETRIC PALSY

Traumatic neuropathy of the brachial plexus is one of the more common birth injuries. It is caused most frequently by traction and lateral flexion of the neck. In

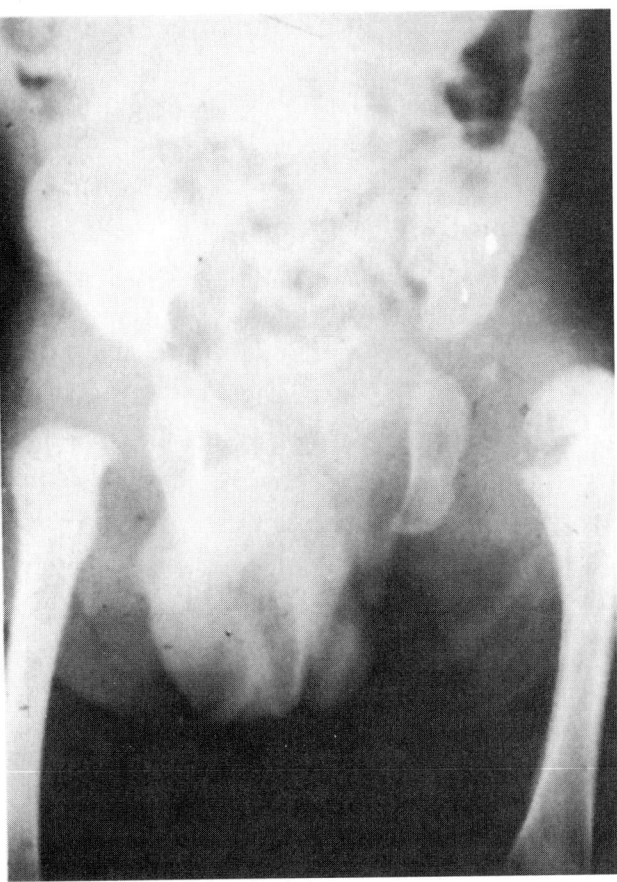

Figure 52-16 A 3-week-old infant with a birth fracture of the proximal epiphysis of the femur.

vertex presentations, the stretch results in traction, and lateral flexion is applied to deliver the shoulder in large babies, and in breech presentations from traction and lateral flexion to deliver the head.

The clinical picture is easily recognized by the absence of active motion of the involved extremity in the Moro reflex. There may be supraclavicular swelling and an associated fractured clavicle.

There are three types of obstetric palsy, and the clinical findings are different in each. The upper plexus type is called Erb-Duchenne (Fig. 52-17), in which the C-5 and C-6 nerve roots are affected, and C-7 roots are less involved. In the lower plexus type, known as Klumpke palsy, the C-8 and T-1 roots are involved. The third type is a total involvement of all roots that make up the plexus. If the C-5 and C-6 roots are affected, the shoulder is held internally rotated with the forearm supinated and the elbow extended and wrist and fingers flexed. A grasp may be present, whereas traction will be absent. When the lower roots, C-8 and T-1, are involved, the hand is flaccid with little or no control. When the entire plexus is affected, the total extremity is flaccid.

The early treatment of obstetric palsy is conservative. Myelography and surgical exploration have little to offer initially in the management of this problem. Recovery of function depends on the degree of injury. When the injury

is a neurapraxia, complete recovery usually takes place over several weeks. When there is a neurotmesis or complete avulsion, no recovery takes place. Loss of sensory function suggests a more severe involvement. Because it is not possible to be certain regarding the severity of injury, all additional injury to the plexus should be prevented in newborns by gentle handling. The arm needs protection for the first 4 to 5 days, until swelling has subsided. After this period, the joints of the arm may be carried through a passive range of motion several times each day for maintenance of flexibility. The paralyzed muscles should be supported in a position of relaxation for part of each day, with care being taken that a contraction of the protected muscles does not occur. Denervated muscles undergo fibrosis; the fibrous tissue can become contracted, producing a fixed deformity. Most obstetric plexus palsy patients recover within 3 months (32). The return of function of the deltoid and biceps are the best clinical parameters of recovery; if these have not shown some recovery by 3 months, return of function is unlikely. When the lesion is limited to the C-5 and C-6 nerve roots without recovery at 3 months, surgical intervention should be considered (33).

In those patients with residual paralysis, passive exercises and progressive active exercises should be continued for months and years, as long as there is some progressive improvement. At 3 to 5 years, certain residual deformities can be improved surgically. Brachial plexus injuries are discussed further in Chapter 50.

BONE AND JOINT INFECTIONS

Osteomyelitis and acute septic arthritis occur in the neonate, although not as frequently as in older infants. Infants with altered immune function or the presence of indwelling vascular lines remain at particular risk for these unusual infections. The priorities of treatment are different in osteomyelitis and septic arthritis, and the differences are of paramount importance.

Osteomyelitis almost always occurs by hematogenous spread, from either a cutaneous or nasopharyngeal lesion, or from other sources such as omphalitis or an indwelling arterial line. *Staphylococcus* (including *Staphylococcus epidermidis* in very premature neonates) and *Streptococcus* species are the most frequent causative organisms, with group B β-hemolytic *Streptococcus* and gram-negative organisms increasing in frequency more recently.

Osteomyelitis begins in the metaphyses of long bones. Bacteria reach the metaphysis through the nutrient artery, which terminates in the sinusoids adjacent to the epiphyseal plate. The rate of blood flow in the sinusoid is slowed, creating an ideal situation for bacterial stasis and multiplication. Edema, vascular engorgement, and cellulitis are followed by thrombosis and abscess formation, with destruction and absorption of trabeculae. The purulent exudate in the metaphysis spreads by way of Volkmann canals to the periosteal space and elevates the loosely attached periosteum, which responds by laying down new

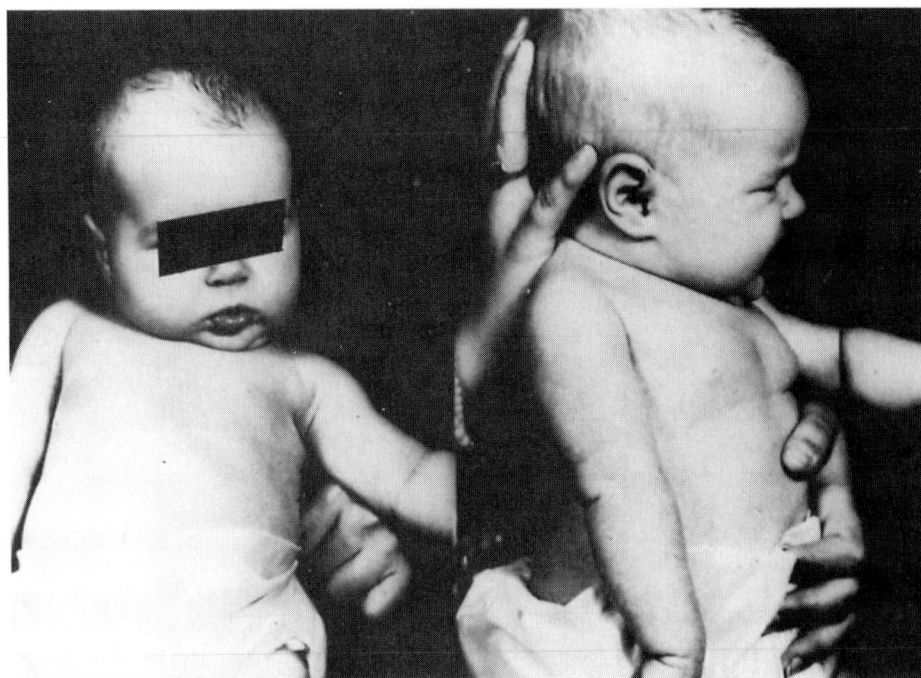

Figure 52-17 An Erb-Duchenne type of brachial plexus injury.

bone over the original cortex. The new bone is the involucrum. In infants, unlike in older children, the exudate perforates the cortex of the metaphysis early and does not spread down the diaphysis, sparing the endosteal and haversian vessels and, therefore, does not cause massive sequestrum in infants as readily as in older children.

In children beyond infancy, the epiphyseal plate acts as a barrier against spread to the epiphysis. Blood vessels cross the infant's epiphyseal plate so that infection of the metaphysis may spread to the epiphysis and cause irreparable damage to the secondary center of the ossification and epiphyseal plate. For this reason, early diagnosis and treatment are very important to prevent destruction of the metaphysis and epiphysis (34).

The neonate with hematogenous osteomyelitis presents with varied complaints and findings. Movement of the affected part may provoke crying. There may be loss of active motion of the affected extremity (i.e., pseudoparalysis), or the baby may have unexplained fever or hypothermia. Palpable swelling of the extremity appears early after the onset of bone infection and is visible in a soft-tissue radiograph. In the newborn, this swelling may be massive, including the entire extremity, before visual changes in the bone are apparent on radiographic evaluation. In a newborn with extensive swelling of an extremity, osteomyelitis must be strongly considered as the diagnosis, until proven otherwise. The infant may be so overwhelmed by infection that he or she responds very little to stimulation. In any infant who is seriously ill or failing to thrive, careful examination of the extremities should be performed, with observation for any evidence of tenderness, pain, and swelling that may indicate the presence of osteomyelitis.

The symptoms of osteomyelitis due to group B β-hemolytic *Streptococcus* are unusual (35). There may be minimal systemic response and little or no local swelling, with a pseudoparalysis or pain on motion as the only symptom of osteomyelitis. When the proximal humerus is involved, the infant holds the affected arm in the same position, as does the infant with an obstetric palsy. Three-phase bone scan has become the diagnostic imaging modality of choice for neonatal osteomyelitis, with a 90% sensitivity in detecting single or multiple lesions (36).

Early treatment with appropriate antibiotics and immobilization usually will control the osteomyelitis. If treatment is started too late, abscesses may form which will require surgical drainage.

Acute septic arthritis has even greater urgency for treatment than osteomyelitis in the neonate, although delayed therapy in either may cause irreparable damage to the secondary centers of ossification. Joint infection is primarily by hematogenous spread, although the hip may be infected by needle inoculation during attempted femoral vein puncture.

The neonate with septic arthritis generally is very ill, but may be so overwhelmed that there are few specific signs. Failure to thrive, as in osteomyelitis, may be the reason for admission. Pseudoparalysis, pain on passive motion, swelling, and increased local warmth are the usual physical findings. Diagnosis is difficult when the hip is affected because visible swelling and palpable warmth are minimal except when there is osteomyelitis associated with the arthritis. Radiographic examination will show a joint effusion and distention, with widening of the joint space. Ultrasound studies may be of significant help in making the diagnosis.

An infected hip joint frequently will be subluxated, and if diagnosis is delayed several days, the intraarticular pressure will cause dislocation of the hip. When dislocation occurs secondary to pyarthrosis, the joint usually is severely and permanently damaged.

Treatment of an infected joint in an infant should be by joint cleaning to remove debris as soon as the diagnosis is confirmed. If the hip is infected, there is no acceptable alternative to arthrotomy for decompression and debridement. A delay in surgical decompression may cause the hip to become dislocated by the increasing accumulation of joint fluid. The blood supply to the femoral head is vulnerable both to the increased pressure and products of the infection, and delay in adequate debridement may cause occlusion of the vessels, which will result in further deterioration of the femoral head. Both these complications can be prevented by early diagnosis, treatment with appropriate antibiotics, and surgical decompression. In other joints, repeated needle aspiration and irrigation may sufficiently debride, but the clinician never knows whether there is pannus covering the joint surface that must be removed to prevent further destruction of the articular cartilage. Because of this risk, open surgical decompression with debridement is a more reliable treatment than needle aspiration.

REFERENCES

1. Burgan HE, Furness ME, Foster BK. Prenatal ultrasound diagnosis of clubfoot. *J Pediatr Orthop* 1999;19:11–13.
2. Dugoff L, Thieme G, Hobbins JC. Skeletal anomalies. *Clin Perinatol* 2000;27:979–1005.
3. Grandjean H, Larroque D, Levi S. The performance of routine ultrasonographic screening of pregnancies in the Eurofetus Study. *Am J Obstet Gynecol* 1999;181:446–454.
4. Treadwell MC, Stanitski CL, King M. Prenatal sonographic diagnosis of clubfoot: implications for patient counseling. *J Pediatr Orthop* 1999;19:8–10.
5. Herman MJ, Pizutillo PD. Cervical spine disorders in children. *Orthop Clin North Am* 1999;30:457–466.
6. Cheng JC, Tang SP, Chen TM. Sternocleidomastoid pseudotumor and congenital muscular torticollis in infants: a prospective study of 510 cases. *J Pediatr* 1999;134:712–716.
7. Dick EA, Patel K, Owens CM, et al. Spinal ultrasound in infants. *Br J Radiol* 2002;75:384–392.
8. Medina LS, Crone K, Kuntz KM. Newborns with suspected occult spinal dysraphism: a cost-effectiveness analysis of diagnostic strategies. *Pediatrics* 2001;108:E101.
9. Prahinski JR, Polly DW Jr, McHale KA, et al. Occult intraspinal anomalies in congenital scoliosis. *J Pediatr Orthop* 2000;20:59–63.
10. Birnbaum K, Weber M, Lorani A, et al. Prognostic significance of the Nasca classification for the long-term course of congenital scoliosis. *Arch Orthop Trauma Surg* 2002;122:383–389.
11. Basu PS, Elsebaie H, Noordeen MH. Congenital spinal deformity: a comprehensive assessment at presentation. *Spine* 2002;27:2255–2259.
12. McMaster MJ, Singh H. Natural history of congenital kyphosis and kyphoscoliosis. A study of one hundred and twelve patients. *J Bone Joint Surg Am* 1999;81:1367–1383.
13. McMaster MJ, Singh H. The surgical management of congenital kyphosis and kyphoscoliosis. *Spine* 2001;26:2146–2154.
14. Lamb DW. Radial club hand. A continuing study of sixty-eight patients with one hundred and seventeen club hands. *J Bone Joint Surg Am* 1977;59:1–13.
15. Bodamer OA, Popek EJ, Bacino C. Atypical presentation of amniotic band sequence. *Am J Med Genet* 2001;100:100–102.
16. Foulkes GD, Reinker K. Congenital constriction band syndrome: a seventy-year experience. *J Pediatr Orthop* 1994;14:242–248.
17. Herzenberg JE, Radler C, Bor N. Ponseti versus traditional methods of casting for idiopathic clubfoot. *J Pediatr Orthop* 2002;22:517–521.
18. Cummings RJ, Davidson RS, Armstrong PF, et al. Congenital clubfoot. *Instr Course Lect* 2002;51:385–400.
19. Barlow TG. Early diagnosis and treatment of congenital dislocation of the hip. *J Bone Joint Surg Br* 1962;44:292–301.
20. Hernandez RJ, Cornell RG, Hensinger RH. Ultrasound diagnosis of neonatal congenital dislocation of the hip. A decision analysis assessment. *J Bone Joint Surg Br* 1994;76:539–543.
21. Herring JA. Conservative treatment of congenital dislocation of the hip in the newborn and infant. *Clin Orthop* 1992;281:41–47.
22. Lorente Molto FJ, Gregori AM, Casas LM, et al. Three-year prospective study of developmental dysplasia of the hip at birth: should all dislocated or dislocatable hips be treated? *J Pediatr Orthop* 2002;22:613–621.
23. Boeree NR, Clarke NMP. Ultrasound imaging and secondary screening for congenital dislocation of the hip. *J Bone Joint Surg Br* 1994;76:525–533.
24. Castelein RM, Sauter AJM, de Vlieger M, et al. Natural history of ultrasound hip abnormalities in clinically normal newborns. *J Pediatr Orthop* 1992;12:423–427.
25. Robertson WW. Treatment of developmental dysplasia of the hip in infancy. Presented at the 1st Balkan Congress of Orthopaedics. Thessaloniki, Greece, 1997.
26. Hangen DH, Kassen JR, Emans JB, et al. The Pavlik harness and developmental dysplasia of the hip: has ultrasound changed treatment patterns? *J Pediatr Orthop* 1995;15:729–735.
27. Mubarak S, Garfin S, Vance R, et al. Pitfalls in the use of the Pavlik harness for treatment of congenital dysplasia, subluxation and dislocation of the hip. *J Bone Joint Surg Am* 1981;63:1239–1248.
28. Unger S. A genetic approach to the diagnosis of skeletal dysplasia. *Clin Orthop* 2002;401:32–38.
29. Boyadijiev SA, Jabs EW. Online Mendelian Inheritance in Man (OMIM) as a knowledge base for human developmental disorders. *Clin Genet* 2000;57:253–266.
30. Cole WG. Advances in osteogenesis imperfecta. *Clin Orthop* 2002;401:6–16.
31. Davidson RS, Markowitz RI, Dormans J, et al. Ultrasonographic evaluation of the elbow in infants and young children after suspected trauma. *J Bone Joint Surg Am* 1994;76:1804–1813.
32. Jackson ST, Hoffer MM, Parrish N. Brachial-plexus palsy in the newborn. *J Bone Joint Surg Am* 1988;70:1217–1220.
33. Waters PM. Obstetrical brachial plexus injuries: evaluation and management. *J Am Acad Orthop Surg* 1997;5:205–214.
34. Peters W, Irving J, Letts M. Long-term effects of neonatal bone and joint infection on adjacent growth plates. *J Pediatr Orthop* 1992;12:806–810.
35. Dormans JP, Drummond DS. Pediatric hematogenous osteomyelitis: new trends in presentation, diagnosis, and treatment *J Am Acad Orthop Surg* 1994;2:333–341.
36. Aigner RM, Fueger GF, Ritter G. Results of three-phase bone scintigraphy and radiography in 20 cases of neonatal osteomyelitis. *Nucl Med Commun* 1996;17:20–28.

Neoplasia

The chapter number 53 is in a circle in the top right.

Robert J. Arceci   *Howard J. Weinstein*

Although neoplasia in infancy is quite rare, it presents important and unique biologic, diagnostic, and therapeutic problems. Such neoplasms often show peculiarities that distinguish them from those occurring later in life. Many tumors in early life are composed of persistent embryonal or fetal tissues, suggesting a failure of proper maturation or cytodifferentiation during intrauterine or early postnatal life. The failure of proper maturation of fetal tissue may be sometimes difficult to distinguish from neoplasia. Additionally, an unexpectedly large number of neoplasms of early life are associated with growth disturbances and congenital anomalies. Spontaneous regression and cytodifferentiation also occur most frequently in tumors of early life.

The unique physiology of the developing neonate provides the clinician with special problems in terms of therapeutic interventions and their long-term sequelae. The neonatal period is also one in which different types of treatment and exposures may affect the long-term risk of secondary malignancies.

EPIDEMIOLOGY

From the data in The Third National Cancer Survey (1969 to 1971), Bader and Miller (1) reported that, in the United States, the annual incidence of malignant neoplasms in infants younger than 1 year of age was 183.4 per 1 million live births and within the first 28 days of life was 36.5 per 1 million live births. They further estimated that approximately 653 infants per year in the United States are diagnosed with cancer and that about 130 (20%) of these patients are neonates. In a later study from Denmark, the incidence of neonatal cancer was calculated to be between 1.88 to 2.98 cases per 100,000 births (2). Approximately one-half of the neonatal malignancies are noted on the first day of life (3). The incidence of childhood cancers also has been observed to show regional differences over time and, over the past 20 years, an absolute increase in childhood cancer has been reported (4,5).

When incidence for all malignancies is compared with mortality as determined from death certificates, the incidence in patients younger than 1 year is 3.5 times greater than mortality, whereas the incidence in patients younger than 29 days old is 4.8 times greater than mortality (1,6). These figures offer an interesting comparison to those reported in children up to 15 years of age, among whom the incidence of malignancy is only about 1.3 to 1.8 times greater than mortality. When individual diseases are considered, there are marked differences in incidence vs. mortality. For example, in neonates, the incidence of neuroblastoma is 10 times greater than the mortality, whereas the incidence of leukemia is only 1.8 times the mortality. The distribution of the types of malignancies found in infants younger than 1 year of age differs from that found in later childhood. In infants younger than 1 year of age, neuroblastoma is the most common malignancy and accounts for about 50% of malignancies in the neonatal period; it is followed by leukemia, renal tumors, sarcomas, central nervous system (CNS) tumors, and hepatic malignancy (2,3,7,8). However, when one considers the total spectrum of neoplastic disorders of infancy, teratoma is usually reported as the most frequently encountered neoplasm, followed by hemangiomas, lymphangiomas, and small nevi lesions (9–12). In older children younger than 15 years of age, leukemia is the most common malignancy (about 30%), followed by CNS tumors, lymphoma, neuroblastoma, sarcoma, and renal tumors. Thus, the incidence and types of neoplastic disorders of infancy contrast greatly compared to later childhood and define the neonatal period as epidemiologically distinct in terms of these disorders.

DEVELOPMENTAL GROWTH DISTURBANCES, GENETIC ABERRATIONS, AND CANCER PATHOGENESIS

Primary, inherited, cytogenetic syndromes usually occur as a result of chromosomal aneuploidy, deletions, translocations, increased fragility or altered epigenetic imprinting, which in turn represent the end result of germline chromosomal defects. An example of aneuploidy is Down syndrome (trisomy 21), in which the frequency of acute leukemia is approximately 15 times the normal. Additionally, an increased incidence of solid tumors has been reported for persons with trisomy 8, 9, 13, and 18 (13). Deletion of part of the long arm of chromosome 13 is associated with psychomotor retardation, microcephaly, cardiac and skeletal defects, and the early development of retinoblastoma. The deletion of the short arm of chromosome 11 results in mental retardation, microcephaly, aniridia, ear and genital anomalies, and an increased incidence of Wilms tumor (WAGR syndrome). These syndromes provided support for the assignment of a retinoblastoma locus to chromosome 13q14 and a Wilms tumor locus (WT1) to 11p13. These mutant genes are heterozygous in constitutional cells and homozygous in retinoblastoma and Wilms tumor cells. WAGR syndrome results from loss of several genes from the 11p13 region. Deletion of one copy of PAX 6 is responsible for aniridia, and loss of one WT1 allele results in genitourinary anomalies. Deletion of the WT1 gene in patients with WAGR syndrome is thought to be the first "genetic hit" in the genesis of a Wilms tumor. The function of WT1 is not clear, but it is an important transcription factor that contributes to the regulation of cell proliferation and differentiation. Homozygosity at the "Wilms tumor locus" on chromosome 11 has also been found in embryonal rhabdomyosarcomas (RMS) and hepatoblastomas, suggesting a common pathogenesis for these embryonal tumors (14). The specific loss of constitutional heterozygosity and its relationship to oncogenesis has been confirmed in studies of transgenic mice that lack a functional tumor suppressor gene, p53. This phenotype, termed Li-Fraumeni Syndrome in humans, is characterized by a higher incidence of embryopathy, and an increased incidence of malignancies developing early in life (15).

A number of inherited syndromes, including Bloom syndrome, Fanconi Anemia, ataxia–telangiectasia, xeroderma pigmentosum, and Werner's syndrome, are characterized by developmental abnormalities and increased incidence of various types of cancer (16,17). These syndromes also demonstrate increased defects in DNA recombination, increased sensitivity to genotoxic agents, increased chromosomal fragility, and abnormal DNA repair (18). Of particular interest is that these syndromes now are known to be caused by defects in genes encoding several novel proteins involved in deoxyribonucleic acid (DNA)/ribonucleic acid (RNA) recombination and repair, such as the DEAD-box helicase of Bloom syndrome or excision repair enzymes associated with some of the complementation groups of xeroderma pigmentosum (18–20). It is intriguing that when these defective genes are inherited through the germline, patients show both developmental abnormalities and an increased incidence of cancer. It will be important to determine whether somatic cell mutations of such genes will increase the chances of a cell becoming malignant, thus showing how the identification of altered genes leading to developmental defects can also increase our understanding of cancer in older individuals.

Malformations (21) and malformation syndromes without obvious cytogenetic abnormalities include hemihypertrophy and Beckwith–Wiedemann syndrome (BWS), which consists of mental retardation, gigantism, macroglossia, omphalocele, and organomegaly; both of these disorders are associated with the development of Wilms tumor, hepatoblastoma, and adrenocortical carcinoma. BWS, which occurs in approximately 1 in 13,000 births, usually is sporadic, although an autosomal dominant inheritance pattern with incomplete penetrance also has been proposed. Patients with BWS have an approximately 7.5% to 10% risk of developing a tumor (22). Sacrococcygeal teratomas and teratocarcinomas are associated with anomalies of the lower spine and urogenital region.

Hamartomas are benign proliferations of cells in their normal anatomic location. Hamartomas in which malignant neoplasms arise include congenital melanotic nevi, which can progress to melanoma, and familial polyposis, which may evolve into colonic carcinoma. Examples of malignancies developing from persistent fetal rests include craniopharyngioma arising from tissue derived embryologically from the Rathke pouch, and persistent neuroblastic cellularity leading to adrenal neuroblastoma.

Naturally occurring DNA sequences homologous to transforming viral oncogenes exist in normal, untransformed cells of all metazoa. Such DNA sequences are called cellular oncogenes and are used in normal cells during growth, development, and differentiation in precise temporal and tissue-specific patterns (23,24). Some of their products function as potent cell growth and death (apoptosis) regulators. The protein products of some cellular oncogenes are quite similar to the products from the homologous viral oncogenes. Because of their expression and critical role during normal development, inherited or acquired mutations affecting cellular oncogene expression can lead to a variety of developmental abnormalities and congenital defects, such as hemihypertrophy syndromes and hamartomas. Additionally, the persistent expression beyond birth of certain growth-related oncogenes may play a role in such proliferative states as the transient myeloproliferative disorder associated with Down syndrome and stage IV-S neuroblastoma found in infants, which both are characterized by subsequent, spontaneous regression.

These predisposing conditions share at least one common element: an inherited or developmental disturbance of cellular growth and/or cell survival, which may be linked to the molecular pathways regulating these genetically determined cellular responses. The finding of these different classes of genes helps to define the molecular links between conditions of abnormal development (i.e., teratogenesis) and neoplastic transformation (25,26).

EXPOSURE TO MATERNAL MALIGNANCY

In addition to the susceptibility of the fetus to adverse effects of chemotherapy during pregnancy, there also is the possibility that the maternal cancer will metastasize to the placenta and fetus. Although many anecdotal reports have documented such involvement, it occurs only very rarely. The types of tumors shown to be transmitted from the mother to the placenta or fetus are quite varied, with melanoma most commonly cited. Although lymphoma and leukemia may involve the placenta, they have usually not been found to be transmitted to the fetus (27–31). The evaluation of infants born to mothers with cancer has not been clearly established, in part because of the rarity of such events. However, recommendations would suggest the utility of close follow-up during the first year of life including physical exams, blood studies such as complete blood count (CBC) and liver function tests, and scans only when indicated. Careful examination of the placenta is an important component of this evaluation.

PRENATAL EXPOSURE TO MATERNAL GENOTOXINS

There are relatively few reports and/or studies of outcome in infants born to mothers undergoing chemotherapy and/or radiation therapy for cancer. Nevertheless, several important lessons can be learned from the available reports. The risk of developmental problems increases with decreased gestational age at the time of maternal treatment (32–34). For example, a recommendation to terminate a pregnancy is often reasonable when significant numbers and doses of anticancer drugs are used during the first trimester because of the increased risk of major birth defects and spontaneous abortions. Outcomes for infants whose mothers are treated during the second and third trimesters are significantly better, although there has been reported some risk of low birth weight, intrauterine growth retardation and stillbirths (32–34). Last, other prenatal drug exposures may lead to increased risk of cancer in offspring. For example, prenatal expsosure to diethyl stilbesterol has been closely linked to the development of clear cell adenocarcinoma of the vagina (35,36), dilantin exposure with neuroblastoma (37,38), nitrosourea compounds with central nervous system tumors (39) and topoisomeras II inhibitors (epipodophyllotoxins, flavonoids, catechins, caffeine) with leukemia associated with mixed lineage leukemia (MLL) gene rearrangements (40–43). Significant use of alcohol and tobacco/marijuana and exposure to pesticides has been reported to be associated with an increased risk of congenital leukemia (44–46). Radiation therapy or significant exposures to radiation through diagnostic testing such as computed tomography (CT) scanning is usually avoided whenever possible in pregnant mothers because of concerns of potential morbidity to the developing fetus (47–50).

TUMORS OF NEUROEPITHELIAL ORIGIN

Neuroectodermal cells of the neural tube differentiate to neuroblasts, which become nervous system tissue and melanocytes; free spongioblasts, which become either astrocytes or oligodendroglia cells; and ependymal spongioblasts, which become ependymal cells. These primitive neuroectodermal cells may be the target for neoplasia, giving rise to a group of morphologically similar tumors involving central and peripheral sites of the nervous system. Neonatal tumors originating from neuroectodermal cells include neuroblastoma, retinoblastoma, peripheral nerve tumors (i.e., neuroepithelioma), medulloblastoma, choroid plexus papilloma, ependymoblastoma, and melanotic neuroectodermal tumors. These tumors show varying degrees of cellular differentiation, have similar histologic features (e.g., small, primitive cells with rosettes or pseudorosettes), and tend to spread along cerebrospinal fluid pathways.

Neuroblastoma

Neuroblastoma is the most common malignant tumor in neonates. It originates from neural crest cells that normally give rise to the adrenal medulla and sympathetic ganglia. Its reported occurrence in siblings and other family members suggests that some cases are hereditary (51,52). In such cases, the tumors usually are diagnosed at an earlier age and often are characterized by having multifocal primary tumors (53,54). An interesting syndrome has been reported in several women who delivered infants diagnosed as having neuroblastoma during the first few months of life (55). The mothers had sweating, pallor, headaches, palpitations, hypertension, and tingling in their hands and feet during the last trimester of pregnancy. These symptoms were relieved after the birth of the affected infants. The authors of that study postulated that this symptom complex is caused by the introduction of fetal tumor catecholamines into the maternal circulation. Although at least half of infants present with an abdominal mass from tumors arising in the adrenal medulla or retroperitoneal sympathetic ganglia, neuroblastoma may arise anywhere along the sympathetic nervous system and present with disseminated disease. An abdominal sonogram or CT scan demonstrates displacement of the kidney without distortion of the calyceal system. The neoplasm also may originate in the posterior mediastinum, neck, or pelvis. Cervical sympathetic ganglion involvement in the neck may result in Horner's syndrome; posterior mediastinal tumors may cause respiratory distress; paravertebral tumors tend to grow through the intervertebral foramina and cause symptoms of spinal cord compression; and presacral neuroblastomas may mimic presacral teratomas. Neuroblastoma also has been detected prenatally by ultrasonography, showing a solid and sometimes cystic suprarenal mass (56–58). Two unusual presentations of neuroblastoma are intractable diarrhea secondary to release of vasoactive intestinal peptide, and the syndrome of opsoclonus, myoclonus, and truncal ataxia (59,60), the etiology of which remains uncertain. The diarrhea secondary to vasoactive intestinal peptide abates after removal of the neuroblastoma. In contrast is the unpredictable improvement after the removal or treatment of neuroblastoma associated with opsoclonus–myoclonus. Nevertheless, survival for children with this syndrome is excellent.

Metastatic lesions are common presenting findings of neuroblastoma, especially in the neonate (60). The primary tumor often cannot be found in infants younger than 6 months of age. These infants present with bluish subcutaneous nodules and extensive hepatomegaly. The liver may be studded with tumor nodules and be so large that it causes respiratory distress secondary to abdominal distention. Clumps of tumor cells often are found in the bone marrow aspirates. Metastases to bones, skull, and orbit, which present as periorbital ecchymoses, are rare in the neonate. The unique metastatic pattern to liver, bone marrow, and skin in infants is classified as stage IV-S neuroblastoma (61–65).

The differential diagnosis for neuroblastoma is limited. The subcutaneous nodules appear similar to those found in congenital leukemia cutis and several congenital infections. The leukoerythroblastosis secondary to bone marrow metastases from neuroblastoma also is observed with congenital infection, severe hemolytic disease, and leukemia. More than 90% of children with neuroblastoma will have elevated urinary excretion of catecholamine metabolites, vanillylmandelic acid or homovanillic acid, or both (66). The diagnosis of neuroblastoma is made by biopsy of the primary tumor or metastatic lesions. The most histologically primitive lesion is neuroblastoma without differentiation and is composed of small, round cells with scant cytoplasm. The ganglioneuroma, its benign counterpart, is composed of large, mature ganglion cells. Ganglioneuroblastoma is intermediate in its degree of cellular differentiation. In the absence of a tissue specimen, the findings of elevated urinary catecholamines and tumor pseudorosettes in a bone marrow specimen usually are sufficient to make a definitive diagnosis.

The prognosis for children with neuroblastoma is inversely correlated to the age of the child at diagnosis and the extent of disease. The infant with stage IV-S disease has a better chance of survival than does the older child with less advanced disease. Evans and associates (61) proposed a clinical staging system for children with neuroblastoma that was prognostically useful (67,68). This system has evolved into an International Staging System, which takes into account many of these basic concepts (63–65).

Infants with stage IV-S have had spontaneous regression of disease, and in other patients malignant neuroblastomas apparently have undergone maturation into mature ganglioneuromas (68). The incidence of spontaneous regression of neuroblastoma may be more common than is clinically evident. Primitive sympathetic neuroblasts, which are derived from neural crest ectoderm, migrate in early embryonic life into the adrenal primordium, in which they arrange themselves in nodules before differentiation into adrenomedullary tissue. These nodules are present in all fetal adrenal glands at 14 to 18 weeks of gestation (69). Beckwith and Perrin (70) detected the presence of microscopic clusters of neuroblastoma cells (i.e., neuroblastoma in situ) in the adrenal glands in a number of autopsies from infants younger than age 3 months who had no clinical evidence of tumor. They estimated that

neuroblastoma in situ occurs in 1 of 250 stillborn infants and infants younger than 3 months of age. Clinically detectable neuroblastoma is noted in only 1 of 10,000 live births. Also pertinent to these data are the observations of the catecholamine screening programs (71–75). These programs demonstrated that this type of screening resulted in an increased incidence of early stage neuroblastoma that, most likely, would not have presented as clinically detectable disease (76–81).

These observations raise the interesting question regarding whether stage IV-S neuroblastoma is not a true malignancy. If stage IV-S neuroblastoma is a classic malignant neoplasm, it should be clonally derived. One such example of clonality in stage IV-S neuroblastoma tumor specimens has been demonstrated by cytogenetic analysis. Although no consistent and specific chromosomal alteration has been found in all stage IV-S specimens, there are increasing numbers of examples of cytogenetic clonality. Additionally, stage IV-S neuroblastoma is often characterized by being hyperdiploid and having variable expression of 1p deletions and N-myc amplification (82–86). The reason(s) for spontaneous regression of stage IV-S disease remains a mystery.

The extent of treatment for neuroblastoma depends on the stage of the disease and biological factors such as histology, N-myc amplification, and DNA ploidy. The infant with stage IV-S disease should be observed for a period of weeks to months before treatment is initiated because of the reasonable likelihood of spontaneous regression (67,79,87,88). Respiratory difficulties, blood vessel (usually vena cava) obstruction, and gastrointestinal compression secondary to rapid tumor expansion can develop and should be considered a medical emergency, with more than 50% mortality in some reports (89). Hsu and associates (90) have described a monitoring and scoring system to follow these patients and predict when, and if, therapeutic interventions should be initiated. This scoring system is based on the presence of the severity of several clinical symptoms, including respiratory compromise, renal insufficiency, extent of lower extremity edema, disseminated intravascular coagulopathy, and the rate of increasing abdominal girth (90). Although both chemotherapy (often single-agent cyclophosphamide) or radiation therapy have been used to effect symptomatic relief for such patients, some reports suggest that 200 to 600 cGy delivered tangentially to the liver to avoid other organs, such as kidneys and gonads, provides for a rapid response and possibly an improved outcome (90,91). Embolization approaches have also been reported to be successful (92).

Complete surgical removal of neuroblastoma is usually accomplished in infants with stage I or II disease. Postoperative treatment generally is not indicated for these patients, and their long-term survival is excellent (93–95). For infants with stage III disease in whom gross residual tumor remains after surgery, postoperative chemotherapy, radiotherapy, or both may be indicated (96). Chemotherapy is the treatment of choice for infants with stage IV disease. The active chemotherapeutic agents against neuroblastoma include alkylating compounds (e.g., cisplatinum, cyclophosphamide, dacarbazine, nitrogen mustard), vincristine, and doxorubicin. Combinations of several of these agents administered for 6 months to 1 year have resulted in greater than 50% long-term survival for children younger than 1 year of age with stage IV neuroblastoma and, in some subgroups up to 90% cure rates (97). This is in contrast to the dismal prognosis for similarly staged children who are older than 1 year.

Retinoblastoma

Retinoblastoma is a congenital malignant tumor arising from the nuclear layer of the retina. Although an extremely rare tumor, it is the most common ocular tumor of childhood. The median age at presentation is 18 months, or 14 months for bilateral cases, but a small percentage of infants are diagnosed during the first few months of life (98). Prenatal diagnosis by sonography of retinoblastoma has been reported (99). Approximately 10% of children with retinoblastoma have a family history of the disease. Approximately 30% with bilateral or multifocal unilateral tumors have a negative family history (100,101). These two groups are capable of transmitting the disease to their offspring in an autosomal dominant fashion. This hereditary tendency is governed by a genetic locus on the long arm of chromosome 13 (i.e., band 13q14), which includes the retinoblastoma (rb) tumor suppressor gene. Retinoblastoma has also been associated with chromosomal 13 deletion mosaicism (102). Preimplantation diagnosis of retinoblastoma has been reported (103). If there is a family history of retinoblastoma, an experienced ophthalmologist should examine the eyes of unaffected siblings regularly although they are under general anesthesia to detect cases early (104). Moll and associates have proposed such screening until age 4 years (105).

The most common initial signs of retinoblastoma include an abnormal white pupil (i.e., leukocoria), known as a cat's-eye reflex and a squint or strabismus. A clinical picture resembling retinoblastoma may result from granulomatosis uveitis, congenital defects, and severe retrolental fibroplasia. Once the diagnosis of retinoblastoma is suspected, both eyes should be examined with the infant under general anesthesia. A bone marrow aspiration and spinal tap for malignant cells should be performed for staging. A staging system for retinoblastoma is based on the size, location, number of tumors in each eye, and distant hematogenous metastases. Vitreous seeding, tumors extending anteriorly to the ora serrata, tumors invading over one-half of the retina, residual orbital disease, and optic nerve or distant metastases are adverse prognostic features.

Retinoblastoma usually is curable when diagnosed early; vision often need not be sacrificed even when bilateral disease is present (106). More recent treatment approaches using cryosurgery in combination with chemotherapy and/or radiation therapy are being developed with the hope of preserving vision and reducing the risk of subsequent in-

field radiation-induced secondary malignancies (106–110). Additionally, stereotactic and proton beam radiation methods are being tested to reduce the amount of normal tissue irradiated and the risk of radiation-induced secondary malignancies (106,111–116). Patients with adverse prognosis features often require enucleation. Children with very advanced and metastatic disease require aggressive chemotherapy regimens.

Brain Tumors and Other Neuroectodermal Tumors

Intracranial tumors presenting in the first year of life are uncommon. In a review from the Hospital for Sick Children in London, 107 of 1,296 children with brain tumors had symptoms before the age of 1 year; 17 were symptomatic within 2 months of birth (117,118). Brain tumors in children in this age group tend to be supratentorial, in contrast to those in older children, which tend to be infratentorial. In infants, the most common presenting symptom is macrocrania, with a bulging fontanelle secondary either to hydrocephalus or tumor volume. Seizures, vomiting, failure to thrive, abnormal eye movement, and irritability also are frequent. The histologic diagnoses of the neuroectodermal tumors are similar to those of tumors in later childhood, with gliomas accounting for most. Of particular interest, a majority of intracranial tumors in neonates have been reported to be teratomas (12,118–121). There is also a high frequency of choroid plexus papillomas in this age group (122). An association of choroid plexus papillomas and the presence of SV40 viral DNA has been reported (123).

Desmoplastic infantile gangliogliomas are rare, but massive, cystic tumors that usually occur supratentorially in the neonatal period (124). They present most commonly with signs of increased intracranial pressure, including seizures. Therapy has included surgery and chemotherapy, but without radiation therapy. For patients who have a complete surgical resection, additional therapy may not be required (125). Prognosis may be better than that observed with other tumors, such as high-grade astrocytoma. In contrast, pineoblastomas are malignant tumors with an extremely poor outcome, even when treated with surgery, chemotherapy, and radiation therapy. Part of the reason for the poor outcome in these infants may be the propensity of pineoblastoma to involve the leptomeninges and extraneural spread (125).

Treatment of infants with brain tumors historically included surgical removal or biopsy followed by radiotherapy (126–128). Operative mortality has been high, and few infants survived for longer than 1 year. In these few, brain radiotherapy resulted in severe intellectual and psychomotor retardation. In attempts to avoid the adverse effects of radiotherapy on the developing brain, more recent therapeutic approaches have evaluated surgery followed by preradiation chemotherapy (119,127–131).

Atypical teratoid/rhabdoid tumors (AT/RT) of the central nervous system, although rare, are usually large, aggressive and have historically had very poor outcomes with the use of conventional therapies used in children with brain tumors (132–134). More aggressive, multidisciplinary approaches have started to show some improvement in patients with this type of brain tumor, although median survival is still estimated to be less than 2 years (134,135). Of particular note is the etiologic role of mutations in the SNF5/INI1 gene in these tumors which encodes for a chromatin remodeling factor (136,137).

Primitive neuroectodermal tumors of peripheral nerve represent a group of soft tissue tumors known as neuro-epitheliomas, medulloepitheliomas, and peripheral neuroblastomas (138,139). They are associated with major branches of peripheral nerves (i.e., tumor of the chest wall arising from intercostal nerve). These are extremely rare tumors, quite aggressive in their biologic behavior, with frequently occurring distant metastases, including to the CNS. Treatment approaches include wide excision, if possible, and chemotherapy modeled after either neuroblastoma or brain tumor protocols.

The melanotic neuroectodermal tumor of infancy has its origin in the neural crest population. Most of these tumors are diagnosed between 1 and 8 months of age and occur in the maxilla, although extremely rare cases have been reported in other sites such as the epididymis (140). They are considered a benign neoplasm, with a local recurrence rate of about 15%. These tumors originate from pluripotential neural crest cells that give rise to both melanoblasts and neuroblasts. The rate of malignancy for this tumor is reported to be approximately 5%. Recommended treatment is wide local excision.

CONGENITAL LEUKEMIA

Leukemia in the newborn is extremely rare with approximately 5 cases reported per million live births (141–143). It has been customary to categorize leukemia as congenital when it is diagnosed within a few days after birth and as neonatal when it manifests itself during the first 4 to 6 weeks of life (144). The kinetics of leukemic cell growth and the estimated leukemic cell burden at the time of diagnosis make it reasonable to assume that clinically detectable leukemia during the first 4 weeks of life originated in utero (145). Molecular studies indicate a prenatal initiation of acute lymphoblastic leukemia (ALL) and some acute myeloid leukemias, in children diagnosed in infancy or even later in life (146–153). In the following discussion, congenital leukemia is considered as leukemia diagnosed from birth to 4 weeks of age.

The etiology and pathogenesis of congenital leukemia, and other leukemias, are unknown. The strongest evidence for a genetic predisposition to acute leukemia is its occurrence in identical twins in which there is a very high concordance (154). If leukemia develops in one of a set of identical twins before 6 years of age, the risk of disease in the other twin is 20%. Leukemia usually develops in the other twin within weeks to months of the first case. In some

of these cases, intrauterine exchange of leukemic cells from one twin to the other has been strongly suggested by the identity of molecular and genetic changes observed postnatally in the leukemias from each twin. For fraternal twins and siblings, the risk of development of leukemia is two and four times higher than in the general population. Congenital leukemia has been associated with trisomy 9, trisomy 13, Turner syndrome, and Down syndrome and rearrangements of the MLL gene (147,155–158). More than 95% of the childhood leukemias, including congenital leukemia, are classified as acute, because they are characterized by a predominance of immature lymphoid or myeloid precursors. In children, the proportion of cases of ALL to acute myelogenous leukemia (AML) is approximately 4 to 1, but this ratio is reversed in the congenital leukemias (141,142). Whereas lymphoblasts from most children with ALL express the common acute lymphoblastic leukemia antigen (CALLA or CD10) on the cell surface and express markers of early B-cell differentiation (e.g., cytoplasmic immunoglobulin or Ig gene rearrangement), the lymphoblasts of congenital and infant ALL are often pre-B, but CD10-negative (159,160). These infants have a higher incidence of CNS leukemia at diagnosis, a higher leukocyte count, increased frequency of hepatosplenomegaly, and a poorer prognosis than older children with ALL. A translocation of the long arms of chromosomes 4 and 11, t(4;11), involving the MLL gene at chromosome 11q23, is commonly observed in infant leukemia. This translocation is associated with greater than 80% of ALL in infancy and carries a poor prognosis (161–166).

The most common subtype of AML in the neonate is acute monocytic leukemia, which accounts for only 20% of AML in older children (167). It is associated with a high incidence of extramedullary leukemia, especially in the CNS. Translocations involving chromosome 11q23 with MLL gene rearrangements are associated with this subtype of AML (167).

Cutaneous manifestations are the most frequent clinical findings noted at birth. In addition to petechiae and purpura, leukemic skin nodules (i.e., leukemia cutis) have been observed in approximately 50% of cases (168–170). These skin nodules may vary in size from a few millimeters to a few centimeters, are bluish to slate gray in color, may appear in all sites, and are palpated as firm tumors of the deep skin (Fig. 53-1). Neonatal leukemia cutis may undergo a spontaneous, temporary regression, but tends to recur in a more generalized form within a few weeks to months.

Hepatosplenomegaly is common, but lymphadenopathy is not. Respiratory distress, secondary to leukostasis within the pulmonary vasculature, may complicate the clinical course. Other nonspecific symptoms of neonatal leukemia include lethargy, pallor, poor feeding, and umbilical, gastrointestinal, or genitourinary bleeding.

In the report of congenital leukemia by Pierce (141), the mean hemoglobin concentration at birth was normal, with a wide range of values (7 to 20 g/dL); the mean leukocyte counts were 150,000 per mm^3 (range 2,000–850,000); and mean platelet counts were 70,000 per mm^3 (range

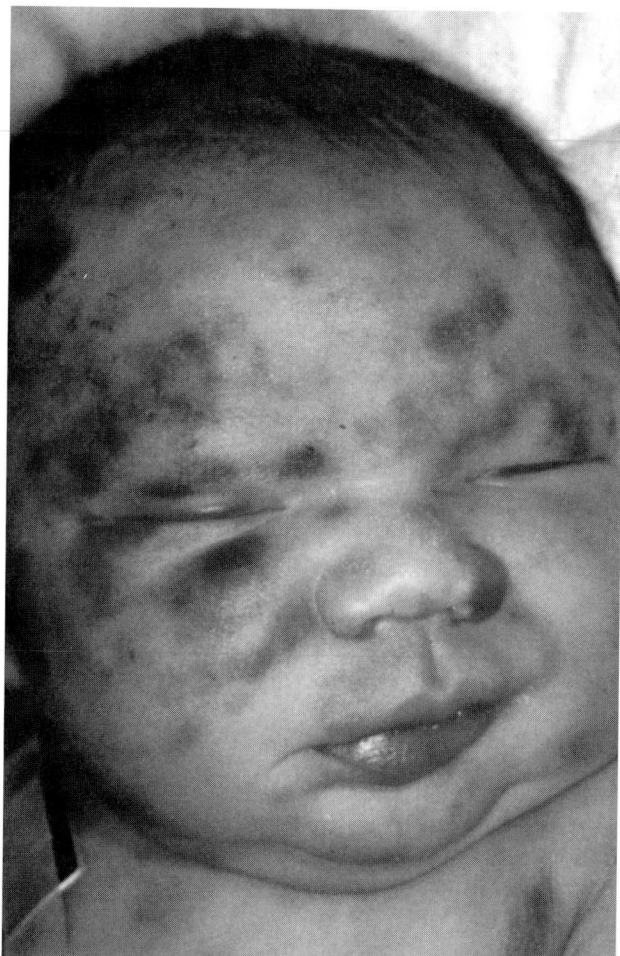

Figure 53-1 Congenital acute monocytic leukemia with skin nodules.

6,000–300,000). The diagnosis of leukemia is confirmed by examination of a bone marrow aspirate obtained from the posterior iliac crest.

A variety of disorders in the newborn imitate leukemia. The newborn bone marrow response to infection, hypoxemia, or severe hemolysis commonly is a leukemoid reaction and an increase in circulating nucleated erythrocytes. These conditions can easily be confused with congenital leukemia.

An enigmatic myeloproliferative disorder described as transient acute leukemia or transient myeloproliferative syndrome occurs primarily in infants with Down syndrome (171–173). This syndrome, noted during the first few days of life, mimics AML. Peripheral leukocyte counts can range from 25,000 to several hundred thousand; bone marrow aspirates reveal 30% to 70% blasts. Hepatosplenomegaly and thrombocytopenia are also common findings. The hematologic status of these neonates usually returns to normal in 1 to 4 months, with only supportive therapy. Several of these children who subsequently died of cardiac or pulmonary disease years after the resolution of their transient myeloproliferative syndrome showed no evidence of leukemia at autopsy. This syndrome has been observed in neonates with stigmata of Down syndrome

and in phenotypically normal infants who have trisomy 21 mosaicism in their hematopoietic cells or skin fibroblasts (174). Molecular studies have identified the presence of truncated GATA1 mutations in essentially all cases of transient myeloproliferative syndrome and the acute megakaryoblastic leukemia associated with Down Syndrome (175–180). GATA1, a critical transcription factor that regulates megakaryopoiesis and erythropoiesis, has thus been etiologically linked in these two hematologic disorders and in the increased drug sensitivity of leukemic megakaryoblasts from children with Down Syndrome (181). There have also been reports of spontaneous remissions of congenital leukemia, even in those children without Down Syndrome (182,183), suggesting that some cases can be initially conservatively managed with observation and/or supportive care (144,184).

In approximately 20 to 30% of these infants, acute leukemia requiring systemic chemotherapy will develop within the first 4 years of life. This leukemia is nearly always acute megakaryoblastic leukemia (M7 subtype). In the setting of constitutional trisomy 21, acute megakaryoblastic leukemia usually has an excellent prognosis, even with less intense therapy than observed for non-Down syndrome children with the same subtype of leukemia (185–188). Although time is still the most definitive indicator of transiency, serial cytogenetic studies may be of value. If there is a chromosome marker in addition to trisomy 21 in spontaneously dividing bone marrow cells, a more aggressive leukemic clone is likely to be present.

Congenital ALL is fatal if untreated and should be managed with systemic chemotherapy. Several national trials are ongoing to improve the outcome of these infants with this poor prognosis leukemia. Age has been an important prognostic variable in childhood ALL, with the most favorable prognosis for patients between 2 and 9 years of age. Prognosis for young infants with ALL remains poor (162,189–192). Because untreated congenital AML also is fatal, aggressive combination chemotherapy in an institution with maximal supportive services is mandatory. One report has described the successful treatment of several neonates with acute monocytic leukemia with either VP-16 or VM-26, but this experience has not been confirmed (193). Aggressive AML treatment regimens have met with considerable success in achieving long-term disease-free survival in neonates with AML (194–199).

NEOPLASMS OF THE KIDNEY

Mesoblastic Nephroma

Most abdominal masses presenting in infancy are renal in origin, and most can be accounted for by cystic disease of the kidney and congenital malformations of the urinary tract leading to hydronephrosis. Although neoplasms of the kidney are rare in infancy, they do occur and have important prognostic implications, making it mandatory that they be included in the evaluation of abdominal masses.

The most common renal tumor found in infants is mesoblastic nephroma, which accounts for nearly 80% of renal tumors in the neonatal period. It also has been called fetal renal hamartoma, mesenchymal hamartoma of infancy, and leiomyomatous hamartoma (200). Mesoblastic nephroma commonly presents as an asymptomatic, enlarging abdominal mass during the first few months of life (201). It is not associated with congenital anomalies and has no race predilection. Of note is the more frequent occurrence of polyhydramnios and premature labor in women whose infants have mesoblastic nephroma (202). The differential diagnosis includes renal cystic disease, congenital malformations of the urinary tract resulting in hydronephrosis, and Wilms tumor. Molecular studies have demonstrated that mesoblastic nephroma shares with most Wilms tumors the expression of insulin-like growth factor II (IGF-II), but, unlike Wilms tumor, does not express the WT1 gene and shows no loss of heterozygosity at 11p13 or 11p15 (203). The bi-allelic expression of the IGF-II has shown that there is a relaxation of the normal epigenetic imprinting pattern of this gene (i.e., the paternal allele is normally expressed with the maternal allele silent) (204). An intriguing finding has been the identification of a chromosomal translocation resulting in a fusion protein, ETV6-NTRK3, in both mesoblastic nephroma and infantile fibrosarcoma (205,206). Of further interest is the requirement of IGF-1 signaling for the transformation potential of the ETV6-NTRK3 to be realized (207).

Most patients with mesoblastic nephroma are cured by surgical excision without adjuvant chemotherapy or radiotherapy (208–210). The addition of chemotherapy has resulted in increased morbidity and, in some instances, fatal complications. In rare cases, such as older infants presenting with metastatic disease or when there is tumor rupture and spillage, chemotherapeutic intervention with regimens containing actinomycin D, vincristine, cyclophosphamide, and doxorubicin have been used effectively. Similar regimens have been used in the rare recurrences (209,211–213). Radiotherapy also has shown efficacy in patients for recurrences, which are relatively uncommon (210,214,215).

Persistent Renal Blastema, Nephroblastomatosis, and Wilms Tumor

The adult or metanephric kidney arises from a complex, inductive interaction between the evaginating uteric bud and its bifurcations with the metanephric, mesodermally derived blastema. By 36 weeks of gestation, normal nephrogenesis is complete, with no residual metanephric blastema. When these metanephric blastemal elements persist, they usually are characterized by microscopic clusters of primitive blastema and occasionally some tubular differentiation (i.e., persistent metanephric blastema). If these fetal rests proliferate, they may develop along several different histologic pathways, each of which has particular relevance to the evolution of Wilms tumor (216–219). Nephroblastomatosis represents the persistence and cellular expansion of metanephric blastema beyond the cessation of nephrogenesis. The proliferation may occur in characteristic patterns, either multifocal or diffuse.

Multifocal nephroblastomatosis refers to the widespread proliferation of blastemal cells, most prominently in the subcapsular cortex and along the penetrating columns of Bertin. Nephromegaly is not always evident. Unlike mesoblastic nephroma, multifocal nephroblastomatosis is associated with congenital malformation syndromes and chromosomal abnormalities. Within the category of multifocal nephroblastomatosis, there are several characteristic lesions. When persistent blastema proliferate in small 100- to 300-mm foci separated by normal renal parenchyma, they are referred to as nodular renal blastema. Nodular renal blastema may regress or evolve into what has been called sclerosing metanephric hamartoma and into Wilms tumorlets, which are 0.3 to 3.5 cm in diameter, noninfiltrating, often multiple, neoplastic tumors separated by normal renal parenchyma. They usually consist of blastema with a monomorphous epithelial pattern of differentiation. Although they resemble true Wilms tumor, they are distinguishable by their smaller size and their noninfiltrating behavior.

A second type of nephroblastomatosis, which is quite rare but found more commonly in infants and young children, is diffuse nephroblastomatosis. The blastemal proliferation may be pan-nephric or superficial, with the latter lesion encasing a normal cortex and medulla. Diffuse nephroblastomatosis presents as bilateral, palpable nephromegaly in association with congenital malformations. Radiographic examination by intravenous pyelogram reveals distortion and elongation of the calyceal system without obstruction (220). On gross inspection, there is an exaggerated pattern of fetal lobulation of the enlarged kidneys.

That these various histologic lesions are related to one another and to the evolution of frank Wilms tumor has been strongly suggested by case studies and by epidemiologic and pathologic correlations (221–223). In about one-third of cases of Wilms tumor, there is suggestive pathologic evidence for the association of nodular renal blastema, nephroblastomatosis, Wilms tumorlets, and Wilms tumor; in bilateral Wilms tumor, this association is nearly always present (224–226).

Management of nephroblastomatosis involves surgery and sometimes chemotherapy, depending on the extent of disease (227,228). Radiation therapy is not very effective. If only one kidney is involved, surgical resection is sufficient, but exploration and biopsy of the contralateral kidney are critical. When both kidneys are extensively involved, nephroblastomatosis usually will respond to the combination chemotherapy used in Wilms tumor (i.e., vincristine and actinomycin). The goal of such treatment is to cause regression of the nephroblastomatosis or cause its development into an end-stage hamartoma. The duration of treatment is based on clinical response. Close follow-up with both radiographic and second-look operations is important in that patients may still progress to the development of true Wilms tumor despite therapy.

True Wilms tumor rarely is seen in the neonatal period (201). It generally presents as an asymptomatic abdominal mass that does not cross the midline but, occasionally, the mass is large enough to cause dystocia at the time of delivery. It is rarely associated with gross hematuria, hypertension, or polycythemia secondary to increased erythropoietin levels. The most common congenital abnormalities associated with Wilms tumor are genitourinary and musculoskeletal anomalies, hemihypertrophy, aniridia, and hamartomas (e.g., hemangiomas, nevi, cafe-au-lait spots). Additionally, there is the Wilms tumor–aniridia syndrome, associated with a deletion of part of the short arm of chromosome 11. CT scan and particularly magnetic resonance imaging (MRI), along with renal ultrasonography, can help define the extent of the tumor.

Pathologically, classic Wilms tumor consists of neoplastic blastemal elements with epithelial and stromal components. In the neonate, Wilms tumor is predominantly epithelial and localized, displaying little invasiveness or metastatic potential. The primary prognostic variables include histology, extent of disease, and age (209,211, 229–231).

The management of a patient with Wilms tumor depends primarily on staging. In the neonate, most patients will be classified as stage I, in that the tumors usually are relatively small (i.e., less than 550 g), localized, noninvasive, and completely resectable. Neonatal Wilms tumor commonly shows favorable histology and appears to metastasize infrequently. At the time of surgery, a frozen section diagnosis is important in ascertaining whether or not nephroblastomatosis is also present. If nephroblastomatosis is present, wedge biopsy of the contralateral kidney is indicated, even if it is grossly normal. The management of bilateral Wilms tumor must often be individualized, with the intent of trying to spare as much normal renal parenchyma as possible (232,233). Careful follow-up in such cases is critical.

For patients with stage I disease, the National Wilms Tumor Study group has recommended 6 months of combination chemotherapy with vincristine and actinomycin; radiation therapy is not given. Disease-free, long-term survival is greater than 90%. Other studies have shown that in infants with localized, noninvasive, nonmetastatic, histologically favorable tumors weighing less than 550 g, are likely to do well with reduced courses of chemotherapy or even no further therapy apart from radical nephrectomy (209,230,234). For advanced stages and for tumors with unfavorable histology, more aggressive therapy, including radiation and intensive chemotherapy, is used (230,235).

Renal Neoplasms Not Associated with Wilms Tumor

Malignant rhabdoid tumor of the kidney, which represents about 2% of primary renal malignancies during childhood and for which the mean age at diagnosis is 13 months, was first described as a rhabdomyosarcomatoid variant of Wilms tumor. Subsequent studies suggested that this tumor is neuroepithelial in origin, possibly from neural crest, and therefore is unrelated to Wilms tumor (236–238). Malignant rhabdoid tumor may also primarily arise in the liver, chest wall, or paravertebral area. There is an association with posterior fossa brain tumors and a predilection for metastasizing to the brain (239). Additionally, the presence of dermal neurovascular hamartomas has been associated with rhabdoid tumors. (240). Despite aggressive therapy, this tumor is associated with a very poor prognosis.

Clear cell sarcoma of the kidney, also originally described as a Wilms tumor variant, is considered a separate entity (241–243). It represents about 2% to 5% of all childhood malignant tumors of the kidney. Age at presentation is similar to that in Wilms tumor. Clear cell renal sarcoma demonstrates a predilection to metastasize to bone and carries a poor prognosis when metastatic but recent studies have demonstrated improved survival for advanced stage III and IV disease (244–247).

TUMORS OF GERM CELL ORIGIN

Germ cell tumors are derived from the stem cells of the embryo that ultimately are determined to differentiate into spermatocytes or ova. Such cells are totipotent and, therefore, are capable of giving rise to tumors containing any fetal, embryonal, or adult tissue. Additionally, their spatial distribution and migration pattern during embryogenesis help explain the various anatomic sites in which such tumors may develop. For example, human primordial germ cells can be recognized first in the 4-week embryo as large cells embedded in a restricted area of the yolk sac. During the fifth week of gestation, the germ cells migrate from the yolk sac to the hindgut wall and along the mesentery to the gonadal ridge, in which they encounter the gonadal anlage. From there they descend into the pelvis or scrotal sac. During their migration from the yolk sac to the definitive gonad, germ cells may be left behind or they may migrate too far along the dorsal wall of the embryo near the midline. Thus, aside from the gonads, germ cell-derived tumors quite commonly arise in locations at or near the midline, anywhere from the sacrum to the head. Depending on their viability, embryonic stage, and anatomic location, they may differentiate along a variety of different cell lineages.

For example, germinomas arise from primitive but developmentally restricted germ cells. When they occur in the testis, they are referred to as seminomas; when they are found in the ovary, they are called dysgerminomas. These neoplasms also may be found outside the gonads, particularly in the mediastinal and pineal regions, and in such cases are referred to as extragonadal germinomas. Germinomas occur only rarely during infancy and develop almost exclusively in older children and adults.

Embryonal carcinoma, which occurs most commonly in individuals from 4 to 28 years of age (median age 15 years), represents a highly malignant tumor of the multipotential germ cells that has the capacity to differentiate further into either extraembryonal or embryonal tissue lineages. Because of this capacity, embryonal carcinoma is considered to arise in the stem cells that can give rise to endodermal sinus (i.e., yolk sac) tumor or choriocarcinoma, both of which are extraembryonal in origin, and to teratomas, which are embryonal in origin.

ENDODERMAL SINUS OR YOLK SAC TUMORS

The endodermal sinus, or yolk sac, tumor represents the most common testicular malignancy occurring in children under the age of 4 years. This tumor also has been called embryonal adenocarcinoma, mesoblastoma, orchioblastoma, and choroid teratoma. At times, it has been confused with embryonal carcinoma. These tumors characteristically form a histologic picture reminiscent of the yolk sac. They may metastasize to the retroperitoneal lymph nodes, which constitute the drainage pathway from the testis, to the liver, to the lung, and to bone, although metastatic disease in the infant is unusual (248–250). Biochemically, yolk sac tumors usually are associated with elevated levels of alpha-fetoprotein, which serves as a useful marker in diagnosis, assessment of treatment response, or of relapse.

The assessment of a patient with the possibility of a germ cell tumor of the testis should include the determination of both alpha-fetoprotein and human chorionic gonadotropin levels; the latter, if positive, suggests a mixed tumor with choriocarcinomatous elements (251). Radiographic workup should include a chest radiograph, chest CT scan, and abdominal CT scan or MRI. A radionuclide scan may be helpful in detecting spread to bone.

After the workup, the operation of choice is a radical orchiectomy with high ligation of the spermatic cord at the level of the internal inguinal ring. A trans-scrotal approach is contraindicated because of the risk of seeding the scrotal sac with tumor cells. Whether or not all children with testicular yolk sac tumors should undergo retroperitoneal dissection as part of further staging remains controversial. Some studies suggest that in infants younger than 12 months of age, only orchiectomy is needed, with close follow-up including radiographic studies, monitoring of α-fetoprotein levels, and physical examination (249,252). In other studies, however, approximately 40% of children younger than age 2 years treated only with orchiectomy die from metastatic disease, compared to only 12% treated with retroperitoneal node dissection and radiation therapy with or without chemotherapy (253–255). These reports suggest that management should include orchiectomy, lymph node dissection, combination chemotherapy, and radiation therapy for those patients with retroperitoneal nodes positive for metastatic disease. Endodermal sinus tumors also may arise in the ovary, usually at a median age of 19 years, and in extragonadal sites such as the pineal body, mediastinum, sacrococcyx, and vagina.

The extraembryonal cell lineage pathway also may lead to a trophoblastic-derived tumor called choriocarcinoma.

Although this neoplasm is extremely rare, when it occurs in infants younger than 12 months of age, it usually is a result of transmission of a placental choriocarcinoma. Patients usually present with pallor, hepatomegaly, and a history of gastrointestinal bleeding with hemoptysis or hematuria. There may be endocrinologic manifestations, with breast enlargement and pubic hair. Chest radiographs may reveal pulmonary metastases; human chorionic gonadotropin levels most often are elevated. Such gestational-related choriocarcinomas are particularly responsive to treatment with methotrexate (256,257).

Teratomas

When germ cell tumors arise from the embryonal compartment, they form teratomas. These are neoplasms that contain cellular or tissue derivatives of more than one of the three primary embryonal germ layers and that are foreign to the anatomic region in which they arise. The name teratoma is derived from the Greek teratos, which literally means monster, plus the ending "-oma," which is used to denote a neoplasm. This name derived from cases in which these tumors contained tissue elements so well organized regarding resemble a deformed fetus.

In early childhood, teratomas primarily occur as extragonadal masses located along the midline axis; about 40% to 50% occur in the sacrococcygeal region, with head and neck, brain, mediastinum, retroperitoneum, abdomen, spinal cord, and other soft tissue locations accounting for 1% to 5% each (258,259). Gonadal teratomas occur more frequently after puberty, particularly in the ovary. About 80% to 90% of early childhood teratomas are benign; malignant teratomas usually are characterized histologically by areas containing embryonal carcinoma or endodermal sinus tumor. Such malignant lesions most often arise in the sacrococcygeal region.

Sacrococcygeal teratoma is the most common teratoma in infancy, with about 67% diagnosed by the age of 1 year. These tumors occur at a rate of 1 in 25,000 to 1 in 40,000 live births and display a significant gender predilection, with girls being affected more than 75% of the time (260,261).

Clinically, these tumors present as a mass protruding between the coccyx and the rectum (Fig. 53-2). They nearly always arise from the tip of the coccyx and vary greatly in the amount of their internal versus external tissue extensions (261). Some lesions can be diagnosed only by rectal examination; however, this examination should be done with extreme care in the neonate to avoid any traumatic damage. The differential diagnosis of a sacrococcygeal teratoma includes meningomyelocele, rectal abscess, pilonidal cyst, bladder neck obstruction, rectal prolapse, duplications of the rectum, imperforate anus, dermoid cyst, angioma, lymphangioma, lipoma, neurogenic tumors of the pelvis and perineum, giant cell tumor of the sacrum, and soft tissue sarcoma.

Benign teratomas usually will produce no functional problems other than obstruction, whereas the presence of

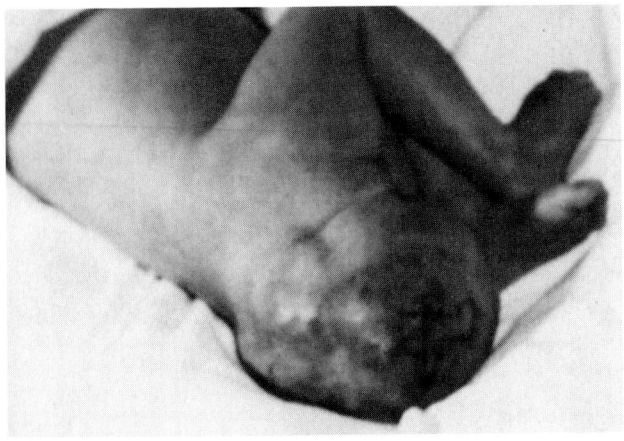

Figure 53-2 Large sacrococcygeal teratoma in a newborn infant.

bowel or bladder dysfunction suggests a malignant lesion. Evidence for venous or lymphatic obstruction or lower leg paralysis is found more commonly in malignant tumors. Approximately 15% of patients with sacrococcygeal teratomas have associated congenital anomalies, including imperforate anus, sacral bone defects, genitourinary abnormalities such as duplication of the uterus or vagina, and occasionally spina bifida and meningomyelocele (262). Radiographic evaluation of the spine can be informative in that meningomyeloceles are associated with characteristic vertebral abnormalities. Abdominal and pelvic ultrasonography along with CT or MRI scanning are useful in assessing the internal extension of the mass. Barium enema may distinguish between a bowel duplication and displacement caused by a tumor mass. Chest radiographs and liver–spleen scans may indicate evidence of metastatic disease. Serum α-fetoprotein and human chorionic gonadotropin levels may be elevated in those teratomas with mixed cellular elements.

The prognosis for a patient with a sacrococcygeal teratoma depends primarily on whether the lesion is benign or malignant (263). For benign lesions, disease-free survival is greater than 90%, whereas for those tumors with malignant components, such as anaplasia or yolk sac histology, associated mortality secondary to tumor may be greater than 90%. The age of the patient at diagnosis appears to be extremely important in determining the likelihood of malignancy. For example, the incidence of malignancy is only 7% to 10% for tumors diagnosed at younger than 2 months of age, whereas this figure increases to about 37% at age 1 year and to 50% by age 2 years. Additionally, there is a significantly higher incidence of malignancy in lesions that show mostly internal tissue extension (261).

The management of a patient with a benign sacrococcygeal teratoma is primarily surgical and includes removal of the coccyx, the site in which the tumor arises. Leaving the coccyx is associated with a 30% to 40% incidence of recurrence, many of which are malignant. Patients with malignant teratomas are managed after surgery with irradiation, if residual disease is present, and always with combination chemotherapy. Some regimens include vincristine, actinomycin D, and cyclophosphamide; others use vinblastine, bleomycin, and cis-platinum (264–268). Regardless of intensive therapy, the prognosis in such patients is poor. The average interval between diagnosis and death usually is less than 10 months, with metastatic disease occurring in lungs, bone, liver, lymph nodes, and peritoneum (269,270). Not surprisingly, survival is poor among patients who develop metastatic disease.

PRIMARY HEPATIC NEOPLASMS

The differential diagnosis of a right upper quadrant mass with hepatomegaly in infants is extensive and includes nonneoplastic lesions and a variety of benign and malignant tumors (271–273). Hemangioendothelioma is the most common tumor found in neonates. Hepatomegaly associated with malignant disease in the infant is secondary much more commonly to leukemia or disseminated neuroblastoma than to a primary hepatic cancer.

Hepatocellular carcinoma, often associated with chronic underlying liver disease, rarely occurs in infancy. This tumor usually is massive, multifocal, and rapid growing, all contributing factors to its frequent unresectability. Despite aggressive combined modality treatment, such patients have a poor prognosis, with up to 90% mortality (274–276).

Hepatoblastoma occurs primarily but not exclusively in children younger than age 3 years, with a mean age of 18 months; it also has been reported in neonates (277–279). There have been anecdotal reports of patients with hepatoblastoma associated with the maternal use of oral contraceptives or with the fetal alcohol syndrome (280,281). Low birth weight also has been associated with the development of hepatoblastoma (282–287). Familial cases of hepatoblastoma have been documented, suggesting an environmental or genetic contribution in some instances (288–292). Hepatoblastoma also has been associated with a variety of congenital anomalies, most notably hemihypertrophy and renal abnormalities, but also with macroglossia, Meckel's diverticulum, tetralogy of Fallot, diaphragmatic hernia, talipes equinovarus, and digital clubbing (293). Wilms tumor and adrenal cortical neoplasms also have been found in patients with hepatoblastoma (294).

Hepatoblastoma presents in most cases with abdominal enlargement and hepatomegaly. In approximately 25% of patients, there also will be associated anorexia, weight loss, pallor, and pain. Less common are vomiting and jaundice. Diarrhea, fever, and precocious puberty are rare. Laboratory studies reveal a mild anemia, a thrombocytosis with bone marrow megakaryocytosis, and, occasionally, thrombocytopenia secondary to platelet trapping (295,296). Increased levels of liver enzyme transaminases and alkaline phosphatase are variable, but mild elevation of bilirubin may be present in up to 15% of cases with hepatoblastoma. A-fetoprotein is elevated many fold in nearly 70% of patients with hepatoblastoma (297). Although not specific for hepatoblastoma, this protein marker, with a half-life of 4 to 6 days, is useful in the assessment of the response to therapy and of tumor recurrence. It should be noted, however, that not all recurring metastatic lesions are positive for alpha-fetoprotein, even though the primary tumor was positive. All values for alpha-fetoprotein should be compared to age-matched values, because levels normally are elevated in the neonatal period and may normalize to adult values for up to 9 months (298,299).

Abdominal radiographs show enlargement of the liver, with right lobe involvement more common. Areas of calcification occur in up to 20% of cases. Chest radiographs may reveal pulmonary metastases, present in about 10% of cases at diagnosis. Abdominal CT or MRI scanning and hepatic angiography are useful in determining tumor size and surgical resectability. Radioisotopic liver scans demonstrate the tumor by its decreased ability to take up the isotope; it appears as a cold lesion when compared with the surrounding, normal hepatic tissue.

The prognosis for patients with hepatoblastoma appears to depend primarily on the lesion's surgical resectability and on histology. Complete surgical excision is possible in 40% to 75% of patients, although perioperative mortality has been reported as high as 10% to 25%. Local and metastatic recurrences after surgical resection usually appear within 36 months, although there have been recurrences as late as 8 years after surgery (277,300).

The histopathology of hepatoblastoma can be viewed as occurring in two major patterns. The first is the pure fetal epithelial type. Several studies have strongly suggested that this type of tumor is associated with a better outcome (301,302). The second type, composed of both epithelial and mesenchymal elements, usually is referred to as a mixed hepatoblastoma and has been associated with a poorer prognosis. Additionally, some hepatoblastomas may have anaplastic or sarcomatous elements that portend a poor prognosis.

Although some reports have demonstrated that approximately 30% to 60% of patients can be cured with complete surgical resection alone, others have shown that adjuvant chemotherapy after tumor resection significantly reduces the risk of development of distant metastases. Chemotherapy should begin about 4 weeks after resection to allow for the adequate regeneration of normal hepatic tissue. For those children with unresectable primary tumors, preoperative embolization or combination chemotherapy may reduce tumor size to allow resection (303–310). Radiation therapy has a limited role, in part because normal liver has a relatively low tolerance to irradiation. The response of both the primary tumor and metastatic disease to chemotherapeutic agents has been best when such agents have been used in combination; they include vincristine, actinomycin D, cyclophosphamide, 5-fluorouracil, doxorubicin, cis-platinum, and methotrexate (311,312). Chemotherapy not only has caused regression of primary tumors, but it also has been associated with a few long-term remissions in patients

with pulmonary metastases. For situations in which the tumor cannot be resected, even after cytoreductive therapy, liver transplantation has been used (313–315).

SOFT TISSUE SARCOMAS

Soft tissue tumors represent a diverse group of neoplasms, all of which share a common cellular origin from mesenchymal elements. In the infant, the spectrum of soft tissue tumor types includes fibrosarcomas, rhabdomyosarcoma (RMS), non-RMS soft tissue sarcomas and fibrous proliferative neoplasms and the rhabdoid tumor (see section on neoplasms of the kidney) (316–319).

RMS accounts for about one-half of soft tissue sarcomas, but is extraordinarily rare in the neonate (320). It may present as an orbital, nasopharyngeal, or sinus tumor; as a truncal or extremity lesion; as a genitourinary tract tumor, usually arising from bladder, prostate, or vagina; or as a paratesticular mass. At the time of diagnosis, about 20% to 40% of patients have evident metastatic disease, usually to lung, lymph nodes, liver, bone marrow, bone, and brain (321,322).

After appropriate assessment of the primary tumor and possible metastatic sites, complete surgical resection with clean margins should be attempted if this can be accomplished with acceptable morbidity. Adjuvant chemotherapy with vincristine, actinomycin D, and cyclophosphamide significantly prolongs disease-free survival. If there is residual microscopic disease as evidenced by involved surgical margins, irradiation usually is used in older children, but should be modified for the neonate or infant because of long-term toxicities (323).

The prognosis for patients with RMS depends on the stage at presentation and histology. In children with the embryonal subtype and early stage tumors, disease-free survival is greater than 80%, whereas in those with more extensive disease or alveolar histology, prognosis remains poor (319,324–330).

Fibrosarcoma represents about 10% of soft tissue sarcomas in patients younger than age 15 years, and more than one-half occur in children younger than age 5 years, with about one-third of these appearing at or shortly after birth (331–333). Congenital infantile fibrosarcoma is a cellular, mitotically active neoplasm with a paradoxically limited biologic potential in most children in contrast to fibrosarcomas in older children (334,335). Molecular studies have linked them to mesoblastic nephromas in that both neoplasias are characterized by a translocation resulting in a ETV6-NTRK3 fusion protein (205,206). Fibrosarcoma most commonly arises in the extremities, with the remaining cases involving the back, retroperitoneum, sacrococcyx, and the head and neck, and occurring as an intracardiac lesion (334,336–339).

For extremity lesions, complete surgical resection is curative in more than 90% of cases, even though local recurrences are common, appearing about 20% to 40% of the time. Occasionally, amputation may be required. Metastatic disease occurs only rarely. For tumors that are not amenable to surgical resection because of size or location, or both, there is some evidence that combination chemotherapy may be quite effective (340,341). Overall survival for infants with fibrosarcoma, RMS, or non-RMS neoplasms has been estimated to be about 60% (316).

Possibly related to fibrosarcoma, but nevertheless distinguishable pathologically, is a group of fibroblastic proliferative disorders that may be seen in the infant and newborn. The digital fibroma is usually found as a soft tissue mass on the medial side of digits, with the exclusion of the thumbs and great toes. As with fibrosarcoma, surgical resection is curative, although recurrence rates may be as high as 75% to 90%. Congenital (i.e., infantile) fibromatosis may occur as solitary or multiple soft tissue lesions (342–346). The solitary lesions occur nearly anywhere on the body. The lesions can involve a wide variety of skeletal sites, and be the cause of significant bone pain in the neonate (347–352). When present as multiple lesions, they involve subcutaneous tissue, muscle, and bones; in some cases, the lesions may become more generalized, producing significant morbidity and mortality from visceral organ involvement (353). These tumors are pathologically benign in appearance. The solitary and multiple lesions are histologically similar, and it has been proposed that they are related to congenital fibrosarcoma and congenital hemangiopericytoma (354).

Treatment of solitary lesions is surgical and curative. There have been several reports of patients with multiple congenital fibromatosis in which spontaneous regression has occurred. After a diagnosis is made, treatment has been primarily supportive, with an excellent prognosis for multiple lesions involving subcutaneous tissue, muscle, and bone, and a poor prognosis when visceral organ involvement is extensive, and especially when involving the central nervous system (355–357). There is little proven benefit from the use of chemotherapy in cases of fibromatosis, although reports of using chemotherapy, including vincristine, actinomycin D, cyclophosphamide and other agents in infants with unresectable fibromatosis have shown some good responses (354,358–360). There are some reports of extensive involvement undergoing spontaneous regression (361).

VASCULAR NEOPLASMS AND MALFORMATIONS

Hemangiomas are the most common tumors found in infancy and childhood and include several different types based on histology, protein expression markers and clinical course (362–365). Most commonly they appear during late fetal or early neonatal life and affect girls more commonly than boys. Skin is the most frequent site of involvement, although they may arise in any organ and often occur in multiple locations. They are soft, compressible, bright red to blue lesions found on a level with, or slightly above, the surface of the skin. They range in size from a few

millimeters to quite massive, occupying large areas of the skin or internal organs.

Their natural course is characterized by rapid growth for the first 4 to 6 months of life, followed by stabilization, then gradual involution over several years. They may be considered true neoplasms in that, during the proliferative phase, they show greatly increased endothelial cell proliferation. They should be distinguished from vascular malformations such as arteriovenous fistulas, which represent anomalous vascular development and do not demonstrate endothelial cell proliferation. Such lesions nearly always are present at birth and increase in size along with the patient, without the usual phase of involution. Lymphatic lesions, such as lymphangioma, are best considered malformations rather than neoplastic growths (366–369).

The clinical complications that arise from hemangiomas are secondary to their size, site of origin, and physiology. They may compromise vision by encroaching on the eye; cause respiratory distress by impinging on the trachea; cause severe and even fatal congestive heart failure when they are very large, as in some liver lesions; cause gastrointestinal or CNS hemorrhage; or cause a consumptive coagulopathy from platelet and fibrinogen trapping, as in Kasabach–Merritt syndrome. Lesions responsible for Kasabach–Merritt syndrome may be a mixture of a proliferative endothelial neoplasm and a malformation sometimes involving lymphatic channels (370).

The first principle of treatment should be to do no harm, because most of these lesions eventually will regress on their own. Nevertheless, when they are the cause of significant morbidity, intervention may be necessary. Corticosteroids can be effective treatment and may accelerate regression (371–374). Radiotherapy may cause undesirable side effects, such as cutaneous scarring, dermatitis, growth disturbances, and possible second tumors (375). Surgery may be difficult for large lesions and may result in unsightly scarring (376). For large lesions of the liver, hepatic artery ligation or embolization occasionally has been successful in controlling high-output cardiac failure, but liver necrosis, renal failure, and other embolic complications may result (377–383). In cases of Kasabach–Merritt syndrome, heparin or aspirin plus dipyridamole, pentoxifylline, and steroids plus epsilon-aminocaproic acid have proven to be useful in treating the associated consumptive coagulopathy (384–388). Laser therapy also has been used effectively (389–393). Subglottic hemangiomas may be life threatening secondary to airway compromise; their treatment has involved laser therapy and surgery, and steroids and alpha-interferon (394–399). The use of a-interferon has demonstrated promising results in cases resistant to corticosteroids (400,401). MRI can be an effective tool for imaging hemangiomas and assessing their response to therapy (402).

Malignant tumors arising from vascular endothelium, such as hemangioendothelioma, hemangiopericytoma, and angiosarcoma, are extremely rare but have been reported in infants (403,404). More information on vascular neoplasms and malformations is given in Chapter 55.

HISTIOCYTOSES

The histiocytoses of childhood represent a heterogeneous group of disorders primarily involving bone marrow derived antigen-presenting cells (405–408). In the late 1980s, the histiocytoses were classified into three separate classes, in part based on the type of histiocyte believed to be pathologically involved (409). This classification schema separated these disorders into: class I—Langerhans cell histiocytosis (LCH); class II—non-LCH; and class III—malignant histiocytosis. Although this classification system has proven useful in delineating these complex disorders, particularly for treatment study purposes, improved understanding of the biology of these diseases is continuing to change the manner in which they are defined, grouped, and treated (405,410,411).

Class I, or the Langerhans cell histiocytoses, includes disorders historically referred to as eosinophilic granuloma, Hand–Christian–Schuller disease, and Letterer–Siwe disease. The diagnosis of the class I histiocytoses is made by biopsy showing characteristic pathologic changes, which include a histologically mixed, reactive infiltrate of cells including eosinophils, neutrophils, lymphocytes, multinucleated giant cells, and proliferation of Langerhans cell histiocytes. Langerhans cell histiocytes are identified by their expression of S-100 and CD1a surface antigens and/or the presence of cytoplasmic Birbeck granules, identifiable by electron microscopy. Birbeck granules most probably represent internalized membrane components and have a characteristic racquet appearance under the electron microscope. Several studies have demonstrated that LCH is a clonal neoplastic disorder (412–417).

Eosinophilic granuloma is found predominantly in older children, teenagers, and young adults, usually presenting as solitary or multiple lytic lesions of bone. Surgical curettage alone is usually curative. The prognosis is excellent. Local recurrences rarely need additional surgery and often can be treated with local injection of steroids if in an easily accessible site (418,419), local radiation therapy with doses in the 400- to 800-cGy range, or even oral, nonsteroidal antiinflammatory agents such as indomethacin (418,420).

Hand–Schuller–Christian disease occurs in younger children from ages 2 to 5 years and often presents with multifocal, lytic bone lesions, particularly of the skull; exophthalmia; oral soft tissue involvement; eczematoid rash; and, sometimes, diabetes insipidus secondary to hypothalamic infiltration. The clinical course is chronic, with multiple recurrences over several years. Therapeutic interventions are indicated for disease that is symptomatic, potentially disfiguring, or likely to result in loss of function, such as loss of vision with proptosis, loss of hearing with extensive mastoid involvement, or paralysis secondary to cord compression (405,406,421). For localized

lesions, surgical curettage, lesional injection of steroids, or low-dose radiation therapy is effective. When there are multifocal bone lesions or multisystem disease, chemotherapy is indicated (422–429). Vinblastine or steroids alone or in combination has been shown to be quite effective (423–431). An international randomized trial compared vinblastine plus steroid with etoposide plus steroid and demonstrated no difference in efficacy of one regimen over the other (432). More intensive, combination chemotherapy is being studied for patients with extensive disease in an attempt to reduce the incidence of recurring disease and long-term sequelae as a result of the disease (429).

Letterer–Siwe disease is the most severe and life-threatening form of LCH (407). It most commonly presents within the first year of life and occasionally in neonates. Cases have been reported among siblings and in twins (433–435). Infants present with scaly, seborrheic, eczematoid, and sometimes maculopapular rashes involving the scalp, face, ear canals, abdomen, and intertriginous areas. Hepatosplenomegaly is common, and there may be signs of hepatic dysfunction with hypoproteinemia and coagulopathy. Draining ears, lymphadenopathy, cough, and tachypnea are common. These infants are commonly irritable and fail to thrive, secondary either to chronic disease and liver dysfunction, or to malabsorption as a result of gastrointestinal infiltration. Lytic bone lesions often are present.

The prognosis for severe Letterer–Siwe disease or systemic involvement with liver, lung, or hematopoietic organ dysfunction is poor despite intensive combination chemotherapy, especially for those patients who show a poor response to initial therapy (425). Hematologic studies reveal anemia, a variable leukocytosis, and thrombocytopenia, with the latter result frequently predicting a fatal outcome. As in the case of Hand–Schuller–Christian disease, vinblastine with prednisone has been shown to be a relatively effective combination, although a more intensive combination chemotherapy regimen is being tested in an international trial (405,429,432,436,437). Small numbers of patients treated with cyclosporine A have been reported (438–441). In refractory cases, allogeneic bone marrow transplantation has been effective in some patients, but the overall results have been disappointing (442–447). Low-dose hemi-body or whole-body radiation therapy has been used, but without prolonged efficacy (448). New agents such as nucleoside inhibitors and more potent immunosuppressive agents are being tested (449–452).

Class II represents the non-Langerhans cell histiocytoses and primarily includes the hemophagocytic lymphohistiocytic (HLH) disorders, some of which are primary (inherited) such as familial erythrophagocytic lymphohistiocytosis (FEL) and or acquired, such as infection-associated hemophagocytic syndrome (453). Primary HLH, which usually presents in early infancy, is inherited as an autosomal recessive condition (454–457). Several gene defects have been shown to be responsible for this disorder and involve pathways in lymphocyte cytolytic granule formation and/or function. Established mutations have been determined in perforin and MUNC-13.4 genes, the former a cytolytic granule and the latter involved in the exocytotic movement of cytolytic granules (458–466). Infants present with failure to thrive, anorexia, fever, and irritability. Seizures and spastic weakness of the limbs may occur secondary to CNS involvement (456). Hepatosplenomegaly usually is prominent. Skin, bones, and lymph nodes, although often affected, are less involved than in Letterer–Siwe disease. Laboratory data characteristically show a hypofibrogenemia and a distinctive hyperlipidemia, with increased triglycerides and decreased high-density lipoproteins (453,467). Pancytopenia develops, and bleeding often becomes a major concern. These patients usually have very low to absent natural killer lymphocyte function, confirming that these disorders are as a result of an underlying immune defect (468–472). Of interest is the observation that otherwise normal parents or siblings of these patients also may show severely depressed natural killer lymphocyte function (468,473). Pathologically, there is extensive lymphohistiocytic infiltration associated with erythrophagocytosis in the visceral organs and leptomeninges, with ultimate depletion of lymphoid tissue.

Prognosis is poor, and most infants will die within weeks of diagnosis from sepsis or hemorrhage, or both unless early treatment is initiated. Plasmapheresis, repeated blood exchange, and high-dose intravenous immunoglobulin have been reported to produce temporary remissions (474). Treatment with the epipodophyllotoxin, VP-16, along with high-dose steroids and intrathecal methotrexate, is an effective regimen that can achieve a temporary remission of disease (475–477). Following the induction of a remission, however, allogeneic stem cell transplantation is the only know curative therapy for primary HLH (476–479).

Congenital self-healing histiocytosis, or self-healing reticulohistiocytosis is characterized by a rash that shows hard, red to dark blue nodules, which occasionally may crust over and often under spontaneous resolution. This condition is part of by a spectrum of disorders known as juvenile xanthogranulomatous disease (480–482). In some instances, lesions can become quite extensive with involvement of visceral organs, including the central nervous system, requiring systemic chemotherapy.

Class III includes malignant disorders of the histiocyte, such as malignant histiocytosis and histiocytic sarcoma, neither of which occurs in the neonatal period (405,430). Additionally, it is now appreciated that most cases described as malignant histiocytosis are really anaplastic large cell lymphomas, which rarely, if ever, appear in infants (483,484).

THERAPEUTIC ISSUES AND LATE EFFECTS OF THERAPY

The issues surrounding the treatment of cancer in infants and young children are unique. Because of their very young age, the balance between therapy and long-term side effects becomes especially important. A close collaboration and

coordination by subspecialists and primary care physicians is critical.

Surgical management must consider the distinctive aspects of neonatal biology (485). Some tumors, such as hemangiomas and stage IV-S neuroblastoma, frequently involute or regress on their own, obviating surgical intervention. With other tumors, such as localized neuroblastomas, a complete resection may be unnecessary, whereas in cases of hepatoblastoma, a complete resection is critical for survival.

The detrimental effects of irradiation to infants are profoundly demonstrated in the treatment of patients with brain tumors, resulting in a high incidence and degree of physical and neurocognitive deficits. Skeletal growth also may be severely affected, with deformities of limbs and scoliosis. Liver, lung, and kidney are major organs whose short- and long-term function can be compromised (215). Additionally, the late appearance of second tumors may be significantly increased as a result of the mutagenic effects of irradiation (215,486).

For many solid tumors, chemotherapy has been effective in the treatment of micrometastatic disease and residual disease after incomplete resection. In cases of disease that is disseminated at the time of diagnosis, such as in leukemia or advanced neuroblastoma, systemic chemotherapy is imperative. The use of chemotherapy in the newborn is complicated by unique differences in absorption, distribution, metabolism, and excretion of such drugs (487, 488). Additionally, these characteristics are constantly changing, as the infant undergoes rapid developmental changes. Dose adjustments are required for certain chemotherapeutic drugs to avoid untoward complications in situations in which decreased drug metabolism occurs, and in cases of increased drug metabolism to achieve effective antitumor drug levels (489–491). Some of the signs and symptoms of drug toxicity may be subtle and must be related to the behavioral repertoire of the infant. Survivors of the successful treatment of malignancy in infancy should be followed closely for long-term sequelae (323, 492,493).

REFERENCES

1. Bader JL, Miller RW. US cancer incidence and mortality in the first year of life. *Am J Dis Child* 1979;133(2):157–159.
2. Borch K, Jacobsen T, Olsen JH, et al. Neonatal cancer in Denmark 1943–1985. *Ugeskr Laeger* 1994;156(2):176–179.
3. Parkes SE, Muir KR, Southern L, et al. Neonatal tumours: a thirty-year population-based study. *Med Pediatr Oncol* 1994; 22(5):309–317.
4. Ross JA, Severson RK, Pollock BH, et al. Childhood cancer in the United States. A geographical analysis of cases from the Pediatric Cooperative Clinical Trials groups. *Cancer* 1996;77(1):201–207.
5. Gurney JG, Davis S, Severson RK, et al. Trends in cancer incidence among children in the U.S. *Cancer* 1996;78(3):532–541.
6. Fraumeni JF Jr, Miller RW. Cancer deaths in the newborn. *Am J Dis Child* 1969;117(2):186–189.
7. Xue H, Horwitz JR, Smith MB, et al. Malignant solid tumors in neonates: a 40-year review. *J Pediatr Surg* 1995;30(4):543–545.
8. Vasilatou-Kosmidis H. Cancer in neonates and infants. *Med Pediatr Oncol* 2003;41(1): 7–9.

9. Martinez-Climent J, Cavalle T, Ferris Tortajada J. Non-malignant tumors that can mimic cancer during the neonatal period. *Eur J Pediatr Surg* 1995;5(3):156–159.

10. Rao S, Azmy A, Carachi R. Neonatal tumours: a single-centre experience. *Pediatr Surg* Int 2002;18(5–6):306–309.

11. Moore SW, Satge D, Sasco AJ, et al. The epidemiology of neonatal tumours. Report of an international working group. *Pediatr Surg Int* 2003;19(7):509–519.

12. Halperin EC. Neonatal neoplasms. *Int J Radiat Oncol Biol Phys* 2000;47(1):171–178.

13. Satge D, Van Den Berghe H. Aspects of the neoplasms observed in patients with constitutional autosomal trisomy. *Cancer Genet Cytogenet* 1996;87(1):63–70.

14. Koufos A, Hansen MF, Copeland NG, et al. Loss of heterozygosity in three embryonal tumours suggests a common pathogenetic mechanism. *Nature* 1985;316(6026):330–334.

15. Donehower LA, Harvey M, Slagle BL, et al. Mice deficient for p53 are developmentally normal but susceptible to spontaneous tumours. *Nature* 1992;356(6366):215–221.

16. Reardon JT, Bessho T, Kung HC, et al. In vitro repair of oxidative DNA damage by human nucleotide excision repair system: possible explanation for neurodegeneration in xeroderma pigmentosum patients. *Proc Natl Acad Sci U S A* 1997;94(17):9463–9468.

17. Ellis NA. DNA helicases in inherited human disorders. *Curr Opin Genet Dev* 1997;7(3):354–363.

18. Rothstein R, Gangloff S. Hyper-recombination and Bloom's syndrome: microbes again provide clues about cancer. *Genome Res* 1995;5(5):421–426.

19. D'Andrea AD. The Fanconi road to cancer. *Genes Dev* 2003; 17(16):1933–1936.

20. Ishikawa T, Zhang SS, Qin X, et al. DNA repair and cancer: lessons from mutant mouse models. *Cancer Sci* 2004;95(2): 112–117.

21. Nishi M, Miyake H, Takeda T, et al. Congenital malformations and childhood cancer. *Med Pediatr Oncol* 2000;34(4): 250–254.

22. Quesnel S, Malkin D. Genetic predisposition to cancer and familial cancer syndromes. *Pediatr Clin North Am* 1997;44(4):791–808.

23. Pavelic K, Slaus NP, Spaventi R. Growth factors and proto-oncogenes in early mouse embryogenesis and tumorigenesis. *Int J Dev Biol* 1991;35(3):209–214.

24. Demant P. Cancer susceptibility in the mouse: genetics, biology and implications for human cancer. *Nat Rev Genet* 2003;4(9): 721–734.

25. Kruslin B, Hrascan R, Manojlovic S, et al. Oncoproteins and tumor suppressor proteins in congenital sacrococcygeal teratomas. *Pediatr Pathol Lab Med* 1997;17(1):43–52.

26. Kruslin B, Visnjic A, Cizmic A, et al. DNA ploidy analysis and cell proliferation in congenital sacrococcygeal teratomas. *Cancer* 2000;89(4):932–937.

27. Tolar J, Coad JE, Neglia JP. Transplacental transfer of small-cell carcinoma of the lung. *N Engl J Med* 2002;346(19):1501–1502.

28. Tolar J, Neglia JP. Transplacental and other routes of cancer transmission between individuals. *J Pediatr Hematol Oncol* 2003;25(6):430–434.

29. Brell J, Kalaycio M. Leukemia in pregnancy. *Semin Oncol* 2000;27(6):667–677.

30. Resnik R. Cancer during pregnancy. *N Engl J Med* 1999; 341(2):120–121.

31. Murray JC, Hill RM, Hegemier S, et al. Lymphoblastic lymphoma following prenatal exposure to phenytoin. *J Pediatr Hematol Oncol* 1996;18(2):241–243.

32. Zuazu J, Julia A, Sierra J, et al. Pregnancy outcome in hematologic malignancies. *Cancer* 1991;67(3):703–709.

33. Zemlickis D, Lishner M, Degendorfer P, et al. Fetal outcome after in utero exposure to cancer chemotherapy. *Arch Intern Med* 1992;152(3):573–576.

34. Zemlickis D, Lishner M, Degendorfer P, et al. Maternal and fetal outcome after breast cancer in pregnancy. *Am J Obstet Gynecol* 1992;166(3):781–787.

35. Hilton C. Carcinoma of the vagina in young adults. *Proc R Soc Med* 1973;66(12):1239.

36. Dolph WA Jr, Lipton A. Female genital tract carcinoma and maternal stilbesterol. *Pa Med* 1972;75(6):61.

37. al-Shammri S, Guberman A, Hsu E. Neuroblastoma and fetal exposure to phenytoin in a child without dysmorphic features. *Can J Neurol Sci* 1992;19(2):243–245.

38. Koren G, Demitrakoudis D, Weksberg R, et al. Neuroblastoma after prenatal exposure to phenytoin: cause and effect? *Teratology* 1989;40(2):157–162.

39. Rice JM, Rehm S, Donovan PJ, et al. Comparative transplacental carcinogenesis by directly acting and metabolism-dependent alkylating agents in rodents and nonhuman primates. *IARC Sci Publ* 1989;(96):17–34.

40. Ross JA. Maternal diet and infant leukemia: a role for DNA topoisomerase II inhibitors? *Int J Cancer Suppl* 1998;11:26–28.

41. Ross JA, Potter JD, Reaman GH, et al. Maternal exposure to potential inhibitors of DNA topoisomerase II and infant leukemia (United States): a report from the Children's Cancer Group. *Cancer Causes Control* 1996;7(6):581–590.

42. Ross JA, Potter JD, Robison LL. Infant leukemia, topoisomerase II inhibitors, and the MLL gene. *J Natl Cancer Inst* 1994;86(22): 1678–1680.

43. Ross JA. Dietary flavonoids and the MLL gene: A pathway to infant leukemia? *Proc Natl Acad Sci U S A* 2000;97(9):4411–4413.

44. Infante-Rivard C, Krajinovic M, Labuda D, et al. Childhood acute lymphoblastic leukemia associated with parental alcohol consumption and polymorphisms of carcinogen-metabolizing genes. *Epidemiology* 2002;13(3):277–281.

45. Alexander FE, Patheal SL, Biondi A, et al. Transplacental chemical exposure and risk of infant leukemia with MLL gene fusion. *Cancer Res* 2001;61(6):2542–2546.

46. Robison LL, Buckley JD, Daigle AE, et al. Maternal drug use and risk of childhood nonlymphoblastic leukemia among offspring. An epidemiologic investigation implicating marijuana (a report from the Childrens Cancer Study Group). *Cancer* 1989;63(10): 1904–1911.

47. Timins JK. Radiation during pregnancy. *N Engl J Med* 2001; 98(6):29–33.

48. Naumburg E, Bellocco R, Cnattingius S, et al. Intrauterine exposure to diagnostic X rays and risk of childhood leukemia subtypes. *Radiat Res* 2001;156(6):718–723.

49. Shu XO, Potter JD, Linet MS, et al. Diagnostic X-rays and ultrasound exposure and risk of childhood acute lymphoblastic leukemia by immunophenotype. *Cancer Epidemiol Biomarkers Prev* 2002;11(2):177–185.

50. Patton T, Olshan AF, Neglia JP, et al. Parental exposure to medical radiation and neuroblastoma in offspring. *Paediatr Perinat Epidemiol* 2004;18(3):178–185.

51. Chatten J, Voorhess ML. Familial neuroblastoma. Report of a kindred with multiple disorders, including neuroblastomas in four siblings. *N Engl J Med* 1967;277(23):1230–1236.

52. Maris JM, Weiss MJ, Mosse Y, et al. Evidence for a hereditary neuroblastoma predisposition locus at chromosome 16p12-13. *Cancer Res* 2002;62(22):6651–6658.

53. Maris JM, Brodeur GM. Are certain children more likely to develop neuroblastoma? *J Pediatr* 1997;131(5):656–657.

54. Maris JM, Kyemba SM, Rebbeck TR, et al. Molecular genetic analysis of familial neuroblastoma. *Eur J Cancer* 1997;33(12): 1923–1928.

55. Voute PA Jr, Wadman SK, van Putten WJ. Congenital neuroblastoma. Symptoms in the mother during pregnancy. *Clin Pediatr (Phila)* 1970;9(4):206–207.

56. Brame M, Masel J, Homsy Y. Antenatal detection and management of suprarenal masses. *Urology* 1999;54(6):1097.

57. Kesrouani A, Duchatel F, Seilanian M, et al. Prenatal diagnosis of adrenal neuroblastoma by ultrasound: a report of two cases and review of the literature. *Ultrasound Obstet Gynecol* 1999;13(6): 446–449.

58. Heling KS, Chaoui R, Hartung J, et al. Prenatal diagnosis of congenital neuroblastoma. Analysis of 4 cases and review of the literature. *Fetal Diagn Ther* 1999;14(1):47–52.

59. Iida Y, Nose O, Kai H, et al. Watery diarrhea with a vasoactive intestinal peptide-producing ganglioneuroblastoma. *Arch Dis Child* 1980;55(12):929–936.

60. D'Angio GJ, Evans AE, Koop CE. Special pattern of widespread neuroblastoma with a favourable prognosis. *Lancet* 1971;1 (7708):1046–1049.

61. Evans AE, D'Angio GJ, Randolph J. A proposed staging for children with neuroblastoma. Children's cancer study group A. *Cancer* 1971;27(2):374–378.

62. Brodeur GM, Pritchard J, Berthold F, et al. Revisions of the international criteria for neuroblastoma diagnosis, staging, and response to treatment. *J Clin Onco* 1993;11(8):1466–1477.

63. Kushner BH, Cheung NK, LaQuaglia MP, et al. International neuroblastoma staging system stage 1 neuroblastoma: a prospective study and literature review. *J Clin Oncol* 1996;14(7): 2174–2180.

64. Cohen MD. International criteria for neuroblastoma diagnosis, staging, and response to treatment. *J Clin Oncol* 1994;12(9): 1991–1993.

65. Castleberry RP, Shuster JJ, Smith EI. The Pediatric Oncology Group experience with the international staging system criteria for neuroblastoma. Member Institutions of the Pediatric Oncology Group. *J Clin Oncol* 1994;12(11):2378–2381.

66. Laug WE, Siegel SE, Shaw KN, et al. Initial urinary catecholamine metabolite concentrations and prognosis in neuroblastoma. *Pediatrics* 1978;62(1):77–83.

67. van Noesel MM, Hahlen K, Hakvoort-Cammel FG, et al. Neuroblastoma 4S: a heterogeneous disease with variable risk factors and treatment strategies. *Cancer* 1997;80(5):834–843.

68. Schwartz AD, Dadash-Zadeh M, Lee H, et al. Spontaneous regression of disseminated neuroblastoma. *J Pediatr* 1974;85(6): 760–763.

69. Ikeda Y, Lister J, Bouton JM, et al. Congenital neuroblastoma, neuroblastoma in situ, and the normal fetal development of the adrenal. *J Pediatr Surg* 1981;16(4 Suppl 1):636–644.

70. Beckwith JB, Perrin EV. In Situ Neuroblastomas: a Contribution to the Natural History of Neural Crest Tumors. *Am J Pathol* 1963;43:1089–1104.

71. Sauvat F, Sarnacki S, Brisse H, et al. Outcome of suprarenal localized masses diagnosed during the perinatal period: a retrospective multicenter study. *Cancer* 2002;94(9):2474–2480.

72. Acharya S, Jayabose S, Kogan SJ, et al . Prenatally diagnosed neuroblastoma. *Cancer* 1997;80(2):304–310.

73. Ho PT, Estroff JA, Kozakewich H, et al. Prenatal detection of neuroblastoma: a ten-year experience from the Dana-Farber Cancer Institute and Children's Hospital. *Pediatrics* 1993;92(3):358–364.

74. Kerbl R, Urban CE, Ambros IM, et al. Neuroblastoma mass screening in late infancy: insights into the biology of neuroblastic tumors. *J Clin Oncol* 2003;21(22):4228–4234.

75. Schilling FH, Spix C, Berthold F, et al. Neuroblastoma screening at one year of age. *N Engl J Med* 2002;346(14):1047–1053.

76. Law C. Neuroblastoma screening test may do more harm than good. *J Natl Cancer Inst* 1997;89(4):276–277.

77. Esteve J, Parker L, Roy P, et al. Is neuroblastoma screening evaluation needed and feasible? *Br J Cancer* 1995;71(6):1125–1131.

78. Woods WG, Tuchman M, Robison LL, et al. Screening for neuroblastoma is ineffective in reducing the incidence of unfavourable advanced stage disease in older children. *Eur J Cancer* 1997;33(12):2106–2112.

79. Levitt GA, Platt KA, De Byrne R, et al. 4S neuroblastoma: the long-term outcome. *Pediatr Blood Cancer* 2004;43(2):120–125.

80. Woods WG. Screening for neuroblastoma: the final chapters. *J Pediatr Hematol Oncol* 2003;25(1):3–4.

81. Tsubono Y, Hisamichi S. A halt to neuroblastoma screening in Japan. *N Engl J Med* 2004;350(19):2010–2011.

82. Vettenranta K, Aalto Y, Wikstrom S, et al. Comparative genomic hybridization reveals changes in DNA-copy number in poor-risk neuroblastoma. *Cancer Genet Cytogenet* 2001;125(2):125–130.

83. Caron H, van Sluis P, de Kraker J, et al. Allelic loss of chromosome 1p as a predictor of unfavorable outcome in patients with neuroblastoma. *N Engl J Med* 1996;334(4):225–230.

84. Bourhis J, Dominici C, McDowell H, et al. N-myc genomic content and DNA ploidy in stage IVS neuroblastoma. *J Clin Oncol* 1991;9(8):1371–1375.

85. Naito M, Iwafuchi M, Ohsawa Y, et al. Flow cytometric DNA analysis of neuroblastoma: prognostic significance of DNA ploidy in unfavorable group. *J Pediatr Surg* 1991;26(7):834–837.

86. Cohn SL, Herst CV, Maurer HS, et al. N-myc amplification in an infant with stage IVS neuroblastoma. *J Clin Oncol* 1987;5(9): 1441–1444.

87. Evans AE, Chatten J, D'Angio GJ, et al. A review of 17 IV-S neuroblastoma patients at the children's hospital of Philadelphia. *Cancer* 1980;45(5):833–839.

88. Nickerson HJ, Matthay KK, Seeger RC, et al. Favorable biology and outcome of stage IV-S neuroblastoma with supportive care or minimal therapy: a Children's Cancer Group study. *J Clin Oncol* 2000;18(3):477–486.

89. Hain RD, Rayner L, Weitzman S, et al. Acute tumour lysis syndrome complicating treatment of stage IVS neuroblastoma in infants under six months old. *Med Pediatr Oncol* 1994;23(2): 136–139.

90. Hsu LL, Evans AE, D'Angio GJ. Hepatomegaly in neuroblastoma stage 4s: criteria for treatment of the vulnerable neonate. *Med Pediatr Oncol* 1996;27(6):521–528.

91. Blatt J, Deutsch M, Wollman MR. Results of therapy in stage IV-S neuroblastoma with massive hepatomegaly. *Int J Radiat Oncol Biol Phys* 1987;13(10):1467–1471.

92. Weintraub M, Bloom AI, Gross E, et al. Successful treatment of progressive stage 4s hepatic neuroblastoma in a neonate with intra-arterial chemoembolization. *Pediatr Blood Cancer* 2004; 43(2):148–151.

93. Suita S, Zaizen Y, Sera Y, et al. Neuroblastoma in infants aged less than 6 months: is more aggressive treatment necessary? A report from the Pediatric Oncology Study Group of the Kyushu area. *J Pediatr Surg* 1995;30(5):715–721.

94. Tsuchida Y, Ikeda H, Iehara T, et al. Neonatal neuroblastoma: incidence and clinical outcome. *Med Pediatr Oncol* 2003;40(6): 391–393.

95. Hosoda Y, Miyano T, Kimura K, et al. Characteristics and management of patients with fetal neuroblastoma. *J Pediatr Surg* 1992;27(5):623–625.

96. Matthay KK, Perez C, Seeger RC, et al. Successful treatment of stage III neuroblastoma based on prospective biologic staging: a Children's Cancer Group study. *J Clin Oncol* 1998;16(4):1256–1264.

97. Schmidt ML, Lukens JN, Seeger RC, et al. Biologic factors determine prognosis in infants with stage IV neuroblastoma: a prospective Children's Cancer Group study. *J Clin Oncol* 2000;18(6):1260–1268.

98. Ellsworth RM, Retinoblastoma. *Mod Probl Ophthalmol* 1977;18: 94–100.

99. Salim A, Wiknjosastro GH, Danukusumo D, et al. Fetal retinoblastoma. *J Ultrasound Med* 1998;17(11):717–720.

100. Murphree AL, Benedict WF. Retinoblastoma: clues to human oncogenesis. *Science* 1984;223(4640):1028–1033.

101. Knudson AG Jr. Retinoblastoma: a prototypic hereditary neoplasm. *Semin Oncol* 1978;5(1):57–60.

102. Kivela T, Tuppurainen K, Riikonen P, et al. Retinoblastoma associated with chromosomal 13q14 deletion mosaicism. *Ophthalmology* 2003;110(10):1983–1988.

103. Xu K, Rosenwaks Z, Beaverson K, et al. Preimplantation genetic diagnosis for retinoblastoma: the first reported liveborn. *Am J Ophthalmol* 2004;137(1):18–23.

104. Raizis A, Clemett R, Corbett R, et al. Improved clinical management of retinoblastoma through gene testing. *N Z Med J* 2002; 115(1154):231–234.

105. Moll AC, Imhof SM, Meeteren AY, et al. At what age could screening for familial retinoblastoma be stopped? A register based study 1945–1998. *Br J Ophthalmol* 2000;84(10):1170–1172.

106. Shields CL, Mashayekhi A, Demirci H, et al. Practical approach to management of retinoblastoma. *Arch Ophthalmol* 2004; 122(5):729–735.

107. Rodriguez-Galindo C, Wilson MW, Haik BG, et al. Treatment of intraocular retinoblastoma with vincristine and carboplatin. *J Clin Oncol* 2003;21(10):2019–2025.

108. Bellaton E, Bertozzi AI, Behar C, et al. Neoadjuvant chemotherapy for extensive unilateral retinoblastoma. *Br J Ophthalmol* 2003;87(3):327–329.

109. Shields CL, Honavar SG, Meadows AT, et al. Chemoreduction for unilateral retinoblastoma. *Arch Ophthalmol* 2002;120(12): 1653–1658.

110. Lumbroso L, Doz F, Urbieta M, et al. Chemothermotherapy in the management of retinoblastoma. *Ophthalmology* 2002;109(6): 1130–1136.

111. Chantada G, Fandino A, Davila MT, et al. Results of a prospective study for the treatment of retinoblastoma. *Cancer* 2004; 100(4):834–842.

112. Wilson MW, Rodriguez-Galindo C, Haik BG, et al. Multiagent chemotherapy as neoadjuvant treatment for multifocal intraocular retinoblastoma. *Ophthalmology* 2001;108(11):2106–2114, discussion 2114–2115.

113. Levy C, Doz F, Quintana E, et al. Role of chemotherapy alone or in combination with hyperthermia in the primary treatment of intraocular retinoblastoma: preliminary results. *Br J Ophthalmol* 1998;82(10):1154–1158.

114. Sauerwein W, Hopping W, Bornfeld N. Radiotherapy for retinoblastoma. Treatment strategies. *Front Radiat Ther Oncol* 1997;30:93–96.

115. Gallie BL, Budning A, DeBoer G, et al. Chemotherapy with focal therapy can cure intraocular retinoblastoma without radiotherapy. *Arch Ophthalmol* 1996;114(11):1321–1328.

116. Chan HS, DeBoer G, Thiessen JJ, et al. Combining cyclosporin with chemotherapy controls intraocular retinoblastoma without requiring radiation. *Clin Cancer Res* 1996;2(9):1499–1508.

117. Jooma R, Hayward RD, Grant DN. Intracranial neoplasms during the first year of life: analysis of one hundred consecutive cases. *Neurosurgery* 1984;14(1):31–41.

118. Jooma R, Kendall BE, Hayward RD. Intracranial tumors in neonates: a report of seventeen cases. *Surg Neurol* 1984;21(2):165–170.

119. Isaacs H Jr. II. Perinatal brain tumors: a review of 250 cases. *Pediatr Neurol* 2002;27(5):333–342.

120. Isaacs H Jr. I. Perinatal brain tumors: a review of 250 cases. *Pediatr Neurol* 2002;27(4):249–261.

121. Canan A, Gulsevin T, Nejat A, et al. Neonatal intracranial teratoma. *Brain Dev* 2000;22(5):340–342.

122. Matson DD. Hydrocephalus in a premature infant caused by papilloma of the choroid plexus; with report of surgical treatment. *J Neurosurg* 1953;10(4):416–420.

123. Bergsagel DJ, Finegold MJ, Butel JS, et al. DNA sequences similar to those of simian virus 40 in ependymomas and choroid plexus tumors of childhood. *N Engl J Med* 1992;326(15):988–993.

124. Duffner PK, Burger PC, Cohen ME, et al. Desmoplastic infantile gangliogliomas: an approach to therapy. *Neurosurgery* 1994;34(4):583–589, discussion 589.

125. Duffner PK, Cohen ME, Sanford RA, et al. Lack of efficacy of postoperative chemotherapy and delayed radiation in very young children with pineoblastoma. Pediatric Oncology Group. *Med Pediatr Oncol* 1995;25(1):38–44.

126. Allen JC, Siffert J. Contemporary issues in the management of childhood brain tumors. *Curr Opin Neurol* 1997;10(2):137–141.

127. Rivera-Luna R, Medina-Sanson A, Leal-Leal C, et al. Brain tumors in children under 1 year of age: emphasis on the relationship of prognostic factors. *Childs Nerv Syst* 2003;19(5–6):311–314.

128. Duffner P. Brain tumors in children under 1 year of age: emphasis on the relationship of prognostic factors. *Childs Nerv Syst* 2003;19(5–6):315.

129. Ater JL, van Eys J, Woo SY, et al. MOPP chemotherapy without irradiation as primary postsurgical therapy for brain tumors in infants and young children. *J Neurooncol* 1997;32(3):243–252.

130. Geyer JR, Finlay JL, Boyett JM, et al. Survival of infants with malignant astrocytomas. A Report from the Childrens Cancer Group. *Cancer* 1995;75(4):1045–1050.

131. Duffner PK, Krischer JP, Burger PC, et al. Treatment of infants with malignant gliomas: the Pediatric Oncology Group experience. *J Neurooncol* 1996;28(2–3):245–256.

132. Hirth A, Pedersen PH, Wester K, et al. Cerebral atypical teratoid/rhabdoid tumor of infancy: long-term survival after multimodal treatment, also including triple intrathecal chemotherapy and gamma knife radiosurgery—case report. *Pediatr Hematol Oncol* 2003;20(4):327–332.

133. Lee YK, Choi CG, Lee JH. Atypical teratoid/rhabdoid tumor of the cerebellum: report of two infantile cases. *AJNR Am J Neuroradiol* 2004;25(3):481–483.

134. Hilden JM, Meerbaum S, Burger P, et al. Central nervous system atypical teratoid/rhabdoid tumor: results of therapy in children enrolled in a registry. *J Clin Oncol* 2004;22(14):2877–2884.

135. Zuccoli G, Izzi G, Bacchini E, et al. Central nervous system atypical teratoid/rhabdoid tumour of infancy. CT and MR findings. *Clin Imaging* 1999;23(6):356–360.

136. Biegel JA, Fogelgren B, Zhou JY, et al. Mutations of the INI1 rhabdoid tumor suppressor gene in medulloblastomas and primitive neuroectodermal tumors of the central nervous system. *Clin Cancer Res* 2000;6(7):2759–2763.

137. Kusafuka T, Miao J, Yoneda A, et al. Novel germ-line deletion of SNF5/INI1/SMARCB1 gene in neonate presenting with congenital malignant rhabdoid tumor of kidney and brain primitive neuroectodermal tumor. *Genes Chromosomes Cancer* 2004;40(2):133–139.

138. Das L, Chang CH, Cushing B, et al. Congenital primitive neuroectodermal tumor (neuroepithelioma) of the chest wall. *Med Pediatr Oncol* 1982;10(4):349–358.

139. Seemayer TA, Thelmo WL, Bolande RP, et al. Peripheral neuroectodermal tumors. *Perspect Pediatr Pathol* 1975;2:151–172.

140. Cutler LS, Chaudhry AP, Topazian R. Melanotic neuroectodermal tumor of infancy: an ultrastructural study, literature review, and reevaluation. *Cancer* 1981;48(2):257–270.

141. Pierce MI, Leukemia in the newborn infant. *J Pediatr* 1959;54(5):691–706.

142. Ross JA, Davies SM, Potter JD, et al. Epidemiology of childhood leukemia, with a focus on infants. *Epidemiol Rev* 1994;16(2):243–272.

143. Shu XO. Epidemiology of childhood leukemia. *Curr Opin Hematol* 1997;4(4):227–232.

144. Sande JE, Arceci RJ, Lampkin BC. Congenital and neonatal leukemia. *Semin Perinatol* 1999;23(4):274–285.

145. Bayoumy M, Wynn T, Jamil A, et al. Prenatal presentation supports the in utero development of congenital leukemia: a case report. *J Pediatr Hematol Oncol* 2003;25(2):148–152.

146. Mahmoud HH, Ridge SA, Behm FG, et al. Intrauterine monoclonal origin of neonatal concordant acute lymphoblastic leukemia in monozygotic twins. *Med Pediatr Oncol* 1995;24(2):77–81.

147. Bayar E, Kurczynski TW, Robinson MG, et al. Monozygotic twins with congenital acute lymphoblastic leukemia (ALL) and t(4;11)(q21;q23). *Cancer Genet Cytogenet* 1996;89(2):177–180.

148. Megonigal MD, Rappaport EF, Jones DH, et al. t(11;22) (q23;q11.2) In acute myeloid leukemia of infant twins fuses MLL with hCDCrel, a cell division cycle gene in the genomic region of deletion in DiGeorge and velocardiofacial syndromes. *Proc Natl Acad Sci U S A* 1998;95(11):6413–6418.

149. Ng KC, Tan AM, Chong YY, et al. Congenital acute megakaryoblastic leukemia (M7) with chromosomal t(1;22)(p13;q13) translocation in a set of identical twins. *J Pediatr Hematol Oncol* 1999;21(5):428–430.

150. Taub JW, Ge Y. The prenatal origin of childhood acute lymphoblastic leukemia. *Leuk Lymphoma* 2004;45(1):19–25.

151. Taub JW, Konrad MA, Ge Y, et al. High frequency of leukemic clones in newborn screening blood samples of children with B-precursor acute lymphoblastic leukemia. *Blood* 2002;99(8):2992–2996.

152. Gale KB, Ford AM, Repp R, et al. Backtracking leukemia to birth: identification of clonotypic gene fusion sequences in neonatal blood spots. *Proc Natl Acad Sci U S A* 1997;94(25):13950–13954.

153. Greaves M. Prenatal origins of childhood leukemia. *Rev Clin Exp Hematol* 2003;7(3):233–245.

154. Greaves MF, Maia AT, Wiemels JL, et al. Leukemia in twins: lessons in natural history. *Blood* 2003;102(7):2321–2333.

155. Rosner F, Lee SL. Down's syndrome and acute leukemia: myeloblastic or lymphoblastic? Report of forty-three cases and review of the literature. *Am J Med* 1972;53(2):203–218.

156. Krivit W, Good RA. Simultaneous occurrence of mongolism and leukemia; report of a nationwide survey. *Am J Dis Child* 1957;94(3):289–293.

157. Djernes BW, Soukup SW, Bove KE, et al. Congenital leukemia associated with mosaic trisomy 9. *J Pediatr* 1976;88(4 Pt 1):596–597.

158. Miller RW. Persons with exceptionally high risk of leukemia. *Cancer Res* 1967;27(12):2420–2423.

159. Spier CM, Kjeldsberg CR, O'Brien R. Pre-B cell acute lymphoblastic leukemia in the newborn. *Blood* 1984;64(5):1064–1066.

160. Crist W, Boyett J, Pullen J, et al. Clinical and biologic features predict poor prognosis in acute lymphoid leukemias in children and adolescents: a Pediatric Oncology Group review. *Med Pediatr Oncol* 1986;14(3):135–139.

161. Eguchi M, Eguchi-Ishimae M, Greaves M. The role of the MLL gene in infant leukemia. *Int J Hematol* 2003;78(5):390–401.

162. Kosaka Y, Koh K, Kinukawa N, et al. Infant acute lymphoblastic leukemia with MLL gene rearrangements: outcome following intensive chemotherapy and hematopoietic stem cell transplantation. *Blood* 2004.

163. Borkhardt A, Wuchter C, Viehmann S, et al. Infant acute lymphoblastic leukemia—combined cytogenetic, immunophenotypical and molecular analysis of 77 cases. *Leukemia* 2002;16(9):1685–1690.

164. Heerema NA, Sather HN, Ge J, et al. Cytogenetic studies of infant acute lymphoblastic leukemia: poor prognosis of infants with t(4;11)—a report of the Children's Cancer Group. *Leukemia* 1999;13(5):679–686.

165. Uckun FM, Herman-Hatten K, Crotty ML, et al. Clinical significance of MLL-AF4 fusion transcript expression in the absence of a cytogenetically detectable t(4;11)(q21;q23) chromosomal translocation. *Blood* 1998;92(3):810–821.

166. Behm FG, Raimondi SC, Frestedt JL, et al. Rearrangement of the MLL gene confers a poor prognosis in childhood acute lymphoblastic leukemia, regardless of presenting age. *Blood* 1996;87(7):2870–2877.

167. Sorensen PH, Chen CS, Smith FO, et al. Molecular rearrangements of the MLL gene are present in most cases of infant acute myeloid leukemia and are strongly correlated with monocytic or myelomonocytic phenotypes. *J Clin Invest* 1994;93(1):429–437.

168. Reimann DL, Clemmens RL, Pillsbury WA. Congenital acute leukemia; skin nodules, a first sign. *J Pediatr* 1955;46(4):415–418.

169. Yen A, Sanchez R, Oblender M, et al. Leukemia cutis: Darier's sign in a neonate with acute lymphoblastic leukemia. *J Am Acad Dermatol* 1996;34(2 Pt 2):375–378.

170. Millot F, Robert A, Bertrand Y, et al. Cutaneous involvement in children with acute lymphoblastic leukemia or lymphoblastic lymphoma. The Children's Leukemia Cooperative Group of the European Organization of Research and Treatment of Cancer (EORTC). *Pediatrics* 1997;100(1):60–64.

171. Engel RR, Hammond D, Eitzman DV, et al. Transient Congenital Leukemia in 7 Infants with Mongolism. *J Pediatr* 1964;65:303–305.

172. Zipursky A, Brown E, Christensen H, et al. Leukemia and/or myeloproliferative syndrome in neonates with Down syndrome. *Semin Perinatol* 1997;21(1):97–101.

173. Zipursky A. Transient leukaemia—a benign form of leukaemia in newborn infants with trisomy 21. *Br J Haematol* 2003;120(6):930–938.

174. Brodeur GM, Dahl GV, Williams DL, et al. Transient leukemoid reaction and trisomy 21 mosaicism in a phenotypically normal newborn. *Blood* 1980;55(4):691–693.

175. Wechsler J, Greene M, McDevitt MA, et al. Acquired mutations in GATA1 in the megakaryoblastic leukemia of Down syndrome. *Nat Genet* 2002;32(1):148–152.

176. Mundschau G, Gurbuxani S, Gamis AS, et al. Mutagenesis of GATA1 is an initiating event in Down syndrome leukemogenesis. *Blood* 2003;101(11):4298–4300.

177. Hitzler JK, Cheung J, Li Y, et al. GATA1 mutations in transient leukemia and acute megakaryoblastic leukemia of Down syndrome. *Blood* 2003;101(11):4301–4304.

178. Rainis L, Bercovich D, Strehl S, et al. Mutations in exon 2 of GATA1 are early events in megakaryocytic malignancies associated with trisomy 21. *Blood* 2003;102(3):981–986.

179. Ahmed M, Sternberg A, Hall G, et al. Natural history of GATA1 mutations in Down syndrome. *Blood* 2004;103(7):2480–2489.

180. Groet J, McElwaine S, Spinelli M, et al. Acquired mutations in GATA1 in neonates with Down's syndrome with transient myeloid disorder. *Lancet* 2003;361(9369):1617–1620.

181. Ge Y, Jensen TL, Stout ML, et al. The role of cytidine deaminase and GATA1 mutations in the increased cytosine arabinoside sensitivity of Down syndrome myeloblasts and leukemia cell lines. *Cancer Res* 2004;64(2):728–735.

182. Dinulos JG, Hawkins DS, Clark BS, et al. Spontaneous remission of congenital leukemia. *J Pediatr* 1997;131(2):300–303.

183. Weintraub M, Kaplinsky C, Amariglio N, et al. Spontaneous regression of congenital leukaemia with an 8;16 translocation. *Br J Haematol* 2000;111(2):641–643.

184. Lampkin BC. The newborn infant with leukemia. *J Pediatr* 1997;131(2):176–177.

185. Creutzig U, Ritter J, Ludwig WD, et al. Acute myeloid leukemia in children with Down syndrome. *Klin Padiatr* 1995;207(4):136–144.

186. Creutzig U, Ritter J, Vormoor J, et al. Transient myeloproliferation and acute myeloid leukemia in infants with Down's syndrome. *Klin Padiatr* 1990;202(4):253–257.

187. Ravindranath Y, Abella E, Krischer JP, et al. Acute myeloid leukemia (AML) in Down's syndrome is highly responsive to chemotherapy: experience on Pediatric Oncology Group AML Study 8498. *Blood* 1992;80(9):2210–2214.

188. Gamis AS, Woods WG, Alonzo TA, A et al. Increased age at diagnosis has a significantly negative effect on outcome in children with Down syndrome and acute myeloid leukemia: a report from the Children's Cancer Group Study 2891. *J Clin Oncol* 2003;21(18):3415–3422.

189. Bresters D, Reus AC, Veerman AJ, et al. Congenital leukaemia: the Dutch experience and review of the literature. *Br J Haematol* 2002;117(3):513–524.

190. LeClerc JM, Billett AL, Gelber RD, et al. Treatment of childhood acute lymphoblastic leukemia: results of Dana-Farber ALL Consortium Protocol 87-01. *J Clin Oncol* 2002;20(1):237–246.

191. Schrappe M. Evolution of BFM trials for childhood ALL. *Ann Hematol* 2004;83(Suppl 1):S121-S123.

192. Isoyama K, Eguchi M, Hibi S, et al. Risk-directed treatment of infant acute lymphoblastic leukaemia based on early assessment of MLL gene status: results of the Japan Infant Leukaemia Study (MLL96). *Br J Haematol* 2002;118(4):999–1010.

193. Odom LF, Gordon EM. Acute monoblastic leukemia in infancy and early childhood: successful treatment with an epipodophyllotoxin. *Blood* 1984;64(4):875–882.

194. Creutzig U, Ritter J, Zimmermann M, et al. Improved treatment results in high-risk pediatric acute myeloid leukemia patients after intensification with high-dose cytarabine and mitoxantrone: results of Study Acute Myeloid Leukemia-Berlin-Frankfurt-Munster 93. *J Clin Oncol* 2001;19(10):2705–2713.

195. Arnaout MK, Radomski KM, Srivastava DK, et al. Treatment of childhood acute myelogenous leukemia with an intensive regimen (AML-87) that individualizes etoposide and cytarabine dosages: short- and long-term effects. *Leukemia* 2000;14(10):1736–1742.

196. Hann IM, Webb DK, Gibson BE, et al. MRC trials in childhood acute myeloid leukaemia. *Ann Hematol* 2004;83(Suppl 1):S108-S112.

197. Neudorf S, Sanders J, Kobrinsky N, et al. Allogeneic bone marrow transplantation for children with acute myelocytic leukemia in first remission demonstrates a role for graft versus leukemia in the maintenance of disease-free survival. *Blood* 2004;103(10):3655–3661.

198. Creutzig U, Berthold F, Boos J, et al. Improved treatment results in children with AML: Results of study AML-BFM 93. *Klin Padiatr* 2001;213(4):175–185.

199. Creutzig U, Reinhardt D, Zimmermann M. Prognostic relevance of risk groups in the pediatric AML-BFM trials 93 and 98. *Ann Hematol* 2004;83(Suppl 1):S112–S116.

200. Bolande RP, Brough AJ, Izant RJ Jr. Congenital mesoblastic nephroma of infancy. A report of eight cases and the relationship to Wilms' tumor. *Pediatrics* 1967;40(2):272–278.

201. Hrabovsky EE, Othersen HB Jr, deLorimier A, et al. Wilms' tumor in the neonate: a report from the National Wilms' Tumor Study. *J Pediatr Surg* 1986;21(5):385–387.

202. Blank E, Neerhout RC, Burry KA. Congenital mesoblastic nephroma and polyhydramnios. *JAMA* 1978;240(14):1504–1505.

203. Tomlinson GE, Argyle JC, Velasco S, et al. Molecular characterization of congenital mesoblastic nephroma and its distinction from Wilms' tumor. *Cancer* 1992;70(9):2358–2361.

204. Becroft DM, Mauger DC, Skeen JE, et al. Good prognosis of cellular mesoblastic nephroma with hyperdiploidy and relaxation of imprinting of the maternal IGF2 gene. *Pediatr Pathol Lab Med* 1995;15(5):679–688.

205. Adem C, Gisselsson D, Cin PD, et al. ETV6 rearrangements in patients with infantile fibrosarcomas and congenital mesoblastic nephromas by fluorescence in situ hybridization. *Mod Pathol* 2001;14(12):1246–1251.

206. McCahon E, Sorensen PH, Davis JH, et al. Non-resectable congenital tumors with the ETV6-NTRK3 gene fusion are highly responsive to chemotherapy. *Med Pediatr Oncol* 2003;40(5):288–292.

207. Morrison KB, Tognon CE, Garnett MJ, et al. ETV6-NTRK3 transformation requires insulin-like growth factor 1 receptor signaling and is associated with constitutive IRS-1 tyrosine phosphorylation. *Oncogene* 2002;21(37):5684–5695.

208. Levie NS, de Kraker J, Bokkerink JP, et al. SIOP treatment guidelines for renal tumours in small infants: fact or fantasy? *Eur J Surg Oncol* 2000;26(6):567–570.

209. Reinhard H, Semler O, Burger D, et al. Results of the SIOP 93-01/GPOH trial and study for the treatment of patients with unilateral nonmetastatic Wilms' Tumor. *Klin Padiatr* 2004;216(3):132–140.

210. Howell CG, Othersen HB, Kiviat NE, et al. Therapy and outcome in 51 children with mesoblastic nephroma: a report of the National Wilms' Tumor Study. *J Pediatr Surg* 1982;17(6):826–831.

211. D'Angio GJ, Evans A, Breslow N, et al. The treatment of Wilms' tumor: results of the Second National Wilms' Tumor Study. *Cancer* 1981;47(9):2302–2311.

212. Gonzalez-Crussi F, Sotelo-Avila C, Kidd JM. Malignant mesenchymal nephroma of infancy: report of a case with pulmonary metastases. *Am J Surg Pathol* 1980;4(2):185–190.

213. Varsa EW, McConnell TS, Dressler LG, et al. Atypical congenital mesoblastic nephroma. Report of a case with karyotypic and flow cytometric analysis. *Arch Pathol Lab Med* 1989;113(9):1078–1080.

214. Arensman RM, Belman AB. Ruptured congenital mesoblastic nephroma: chemotherapy and irradiation as adjuvants to nephrectomy. *Urology* 1980;15(4):394–396.

215. Littman P, D'Angio GJ. Radiation therapy in the neonate. *Am J Pediatr Hematol Oncol* 1981;3(3):279–285.

216. Laberge JM. Nephroblastomatosis update. *Med Pediatr Oncol* 2003;41(1):96–97.

217. Machin GA. Persistent renal blastema (nephroblastomatosis) as a frequent precursor of Wilms' tumor; a pathological and clinical review. Part 2. Significance of nephroblastomatosis in the genesis of Wilms' tumor. *Am J Pediatr Hematol Oncol* 1980; 2(3):253–261.

218. Machin GA. Nephroblastomatosis and multiple bilateral nephroblastomata. Histologic, therapeutic, and theoretical aspects. *Arch Pathol Lab Med* 1978;102(12):639–642.

219. Machin GA, McCaughey WT. A new precursor lesion of Wilms' tumour (nephroblastoma): intralobar multifocal nephroblastomatosis. *Histopathology* 1984;8(1):35–53.

220. Gylys-Morin V, Hoffer FA, Kozakewich H, et al. Wilms' tumor and nephroblastomatosis: imaging characteristics at gadolinium-enhanced MR imaging. *Radiology* 1993;188(2):517–521.

221. Kulkkarni R, Bailie MD, Bernstein J, et al. Progression of nephroblastomatosis to Wilms' tumor. *J Pediatr* 1980;96(1):178.

222. Bove KE. Nephroblastomatosis. An overview. *Arch Pathol Lab Med* 1989;113(7):723–724.

223. Bove KEMcAdams AJ. The nephroblastomatosis complex and its relationship to Wilms' tumor: a clinicopathologic treatise. *Perspect Pediatr Pathol* 1976;3:185–223.

224. Dimmick JE, Johnson HW, Coleman GU, et al. Wilms' tumorlet, nodular renal blastema and multicystic renal dysplasia. *J Urol* 1989;142(2 Pt 2):484–485, discussion 489.

225. Steenman M, Redeker B, de Meulemeester M, et al. Comparative genomic hybridization analysis of Wilms' tumors. *Cytogenet Cell Genet* 1997;77(3–4):296–303.

226. Beckwith JB. Precursor lesions of Wilms' tumor: clinical and biological implications. *Med Pediatr Oncol* 1993;21(3):158–168.

227. Coopes MJ, Ritchey ML. Managing nephroblastomatosis. *Med Pediatr Oncol* 2000;35(4):433.

228. Prasil P, Laberge JM, Bond M, et al. Management decisions in children with nephroblastomatosis. *Med Pediatr Oncol* 2000; 35(4):429–432, discussion 433.

229. Bown N, Cotterill SJ, Roberts P, et al. Cytogenetic abnormalities and clinical outcome in Wilms' tumor: a study by the U.K. cancer cytogenetics group and the U.K. Children's Cancer Study Group. *Med Pediatr Oncol* 2002;38(1):11–21.

230. Green DM. The treatment of stages I-IV favorable histology Wilms' tumor. *J Clin Oncol* 2004;22(8):1366–1372.

231. Kalapurakal JA, Dome JS, Perlman EJ, et al. Management of Wilms' tumour: current practice and future goals. *Lancet Oncol* 2004;5(1):37–46.

232. Regalado JJ, Rodriguez MM, Toledano S. Bilaterally multicentric synchronous Wilms' tumor: successful conservative treatment despite persistence of nephrogenic rests. *Med Pediatr Oncol* 1997;28(6):420–423.

233. Delgado G, Viluce C, Fletcher E, et al. Bilateral Wilms' tumor. Current treatment. *Rev Med Panama* 1996;21(3):93–101.

234. Green DM. Treatment of stage I Wilms' tumor. *J Clin Oncol* 1995;13(6):1530.

235. Green DM, Breslow NE, Evans I, et al. Treatment of children with stage IV favorable histology Wilms' tumor: a report from the National Wilms' Tumor Study Group. *Med Pediatr Oncol* 1996;26(3):147–152.

236. Beckwith JB, Palmer NF. Histopathology and prognosis of Wilms tumors: results from the First National Wilms' Tumor Study. *Cancer* 1978;41(5):1937–1948.

237. Haas JE, Palmer NF, Weinberg AG, et al. Ultrastructure of malignant rhabdoid tumor of the kidney. A distinctive renal tumor of children. *Hum Pathol* 1981;12(7):646–657.

238. Palmer NF, Sutow W. Clinical aspects of the rhabdoid tumor of the kidney: a report of the National Wilms' Tumor Study Group. *Med Pediatr Oncol* 1983;11(4):242–245.

239. Bonnin JM, Rubinstein LJ, Palmer NF, et al. The association of embryonal tumors originating in the kidney and in the brain. A report of seven cases. *Cancer* 1984;54(10):2137–2146.

240. Perez-Atayde AR, Newbury R, Fletcher JA, et al. Congenital "neurovascular hamartoma" of the skin. A possible marker of malignant rhabdoid tumor. *Am J Surg Pathol* 1994;18(10):1030–1038.

241. Gonzalez-Crussi F, Baum ES. Renal sarcomas of childhood. A clinicopathologic and ultrastructural study. *Cancer* 1983;51(5): 898–912.

242. Carcassonne M, Raybaud C, Lebreuil G. Clear cell sarcoma of the kidney in children: a distinct entity. *J Pediatr Surg* 1981;16(4 Suppl 1):645–648.

243. Newbould MJ, Kelsey AM. Clear cell sarcoma of the kidney in a 4-month-old infant: a case report. *Med Pediatr Oncol* 1993; 21(7):525–528.

244. Mazzoleni S, Vecchiato L, Alaggio R, et al. Clear cell sarcoma of the kidney in a newborn. *Med Pediatr Oncol* 2003;41(2):153–155.

245. Grundy RG, Hutton C, Middleton H, et al. Outcome of patients with stage III or inoperable WT treated on the second United Kingdom WT protocol (UKWT2); a United Kingdom Children's Cancer Study Group (UKCCSG) study. *Pediatr Blood Cancer* 2004;42(4):311–319.

246. Argani P, Perlman EJ, Breslow NE, et al. Clear cell sarcoma of the kidney: a review of 351 cases from the National Wilms' Tumor Study Group Pathology Center. *Am J Surg Pathol* 2000;24(1):4–18.

247. Kusumakumary P, Mathews A, James FV, et al. Clear cell sarcoma kidney: clinical features and outcome. *Pediatr Hematol Oncol* 1999;16(2):169–174.

248. Ise T, Ohtsuki H, Matsumoto K, et al. Management of malignant testicular tumors in children. *Cancer* 1976;37(3):1539–1545.

249. Exelby PR. Testis cancer in children. *Semin Oncol* 1979;6(1): 116–120.

250. Isaacs H Jr. Perinatal (fetal and neonatal) germ cell tumors. *J Pediatr Surg* 2004;39(7):1003–1013.

251. Labdenne P, Heikinheimo M. Clinical use of tumor markers in childhood malignancies. *Ann Med* 2002;34(5):316–323.

252. Liu HC, Liang DC, Chen SH, et al. The stage I yolk sac tumor of testis in children younger than 2 years, chemotherapy or not? *Pediatr Hematol Oncol* 1998;15(3):223–228.

253. Drago JR, Nelson RP, Palmer JM. Childhood embryonal carcinoma of testes. *Urology* 1978;12(5):499–503.

254. Colodny AH, Hopkins TB. Testicular tumors in infants and children. *Urol Clin North Am* 1977;4(3):347–358.

255. Metcalfe PD, Farivar-Mohseni H, Farhat W, et al. Pediatric testicular tumors: contemporary incidence and efficacy of testicular preserving surgery. *J Urol* 2003;170(6 Pt 1):2412–2415, discussion 2415–2416.

256. Belchis DA, Mowry J, Davis JH. Infantile choriocarcinoma. Re-examination of a potentially curable entity. *Cancer* 1993;72(6): 2028–2032.

257. Witzleben CL, Bruninga G. Infantile choriocarcinoma: a characteristic syndrome. *J Pediatr* 1968;73(3):374–378.

258. Tapper D, Lack EE. Teratomas in infancy and childhood. A 54-year experience at the Children's Hospital Medical Center. *Ann Surg* 1983;198(3):398–410.

259. Gobel U, Calaminus G, Engert J, et al. Teratomas in infancy and childhood. *Med Pediatr Oncol* 1998;31(1):8–15.

260. Wakhlu A, Misra S, Tandon RK, et al. Sacrococcygeal teratoma. *Pediatr Surg Int* 2002;18(5–6):384–387.

261. Altman RP, Randolph JG, Lilly JR. Sacrococcygeal teratoma: American Academy of Pediatrics Surgical Section Survey-1973. *J Pediatr Surg* 1974;9(3):389–398.

262. Fraumeni JF Jr, Li FP, Dalager N. Teratomas in children: epidemiologic features. *J Natl Cancer Inst* 1973;51(5):1425–1430.

263. Hawkins E, Issacs H, Cushing B, et al. Occult malignancy in neonatal sacrococcygeal teratomas. A report from a Combined Pediatric Oncology Group and Children's Cancer Group study. *Am J Pediatr Hematol Oncol* 1993;15(4):406–409.

264. Raney RB Jr, Chatten J, Littman P, et al. Treatment strategies for infants with malignant sacrococcygeal teratoma. *J Pediatr Surg* 1981;16(4 Suppl 1):573–577.

265. Einhorn LH, Donohue J. Cis-diamminedichloroplatinum, vinblastine, and bleomycin combination chemotherapy in disseminated testicular cancer. *Ann Intern Med* 1977;87(3):293–298.

266. Herrmann ME, Thompson K, Wojcik EM, et al. Congenital sacrococcygeal teratomas: effect of gestational age on size, morphologic pattern, ploidy, p53, and ret expression. *Pediatr Dev Pathol* 2000;3(3):240–248.

267. Hedrick HL, Flake AW, Crombleholme TM, et al. Sacrococcygeal teratoma: prenatal assessment, fetal intervention, and outcome. *J Pediatr Surg* 2004;39(3):430–438, discussion 430–438.

268. Huddart SN, Mann JR, Robinson K, et al. Sacrococcygeal teratomas: the UK Children's Cancer Study Group's experience. I. Neonatal. *Pediatr Surg Int* 2003;19(1–2):47–51.

269. Noseworthy J, Lack EE, Kozakewich HP, et al. Sacrococcygeal germ cell tumors in childhood: an updated experience with 118 patients. *J Pediatr Surg* 1981;16(3):358–364.

270. Valdiserri RO, Yunis EJ. Sacrococcygeal teratomas: a review of 68 cases. *Cancer* 1981;48(1):217–221.

271. Edmondson HA. Differential diagnosis of tumors and tumor-like lesions of liver in infancy and childhood. *Am J Dis Child* 1956;91(2):168–186.

272. von Schweinitz D. Neonatal liver tumours. *Semin Neonatol* 2003;8(5):403–410.

273. von Schweinitz D, Gluer S, Mildenberger H. Liver tumors in neonates and very young infants: diagnostic pitfalls and therapeutic problems. *Eur J Pediatr Surg* 1995;5(2):72–76.

274. Lack EE, Neave C, Vawter GF. Hepatocellular carcinoma. Review of 32 cases in childhood and adolescence. *Cancer* 1983;52(8):1510–1515.

275. Perilongo G, Shafford EA. Liver tumours. *Eur J Cancer* 1999;35(6):953–958, discussion 958–959.

276. Weinberg AG, Finegold MJ. Primary hepatic tumors of childhood. *Hum Pathol* 1983;14(6):512–537.

277. Ein SH, Stephens CA. Malignant liver tumors in children. *J Pediatr Surg* 1974;9(4):491–494.

278. Randolph JG, Altman RP, Arensman RM, et al. Liver resection in children with hepatic neoplasms. *Ann Surg* 1978;187(6):599–605.

279. Clatworthy HW Jr, Schiller M, Grosfeld JL. Primary liver tumors in infancy and childhood. 41 cases variously treated. *Arch Surg* 1974;109(2):143–147.

280. Khan A, Bader JL, Hoy GR, et al. Hepatoblastoma in child with fetal alcohol syndrome. *Lancet* 1979;1(8131):1403–1404.

281. Otten J, Smets R, De Jager R, et al. Hepatoblastoma in an infant after contraceptive intake during pregnancy. *N Engl J Med* 1977;297(4):222.

282. Feusner J, Plaschkes J. Hepatoblastoma and low birth weight: a trend or chance observation? *Med Pediatr Oncol* 2002;39(5):508–509.

283. Kisato Y, Nishikubo T, Uchida Y, et al. Hepatoblastoma in a low-birthweight infant complicated with cleft palate, Dandy-Walker malformation and chronic lung disease. *Pediatr Int* 2002;44(6):698–701.

284. Jaing TH, Hung IJ, Lin JN, et al. Hepatoblastoma in a child of extremely low birth weight. *Am J Perinatol* 2002;19(3):149–153.

285. Latini G, Gallo F, De Felice C. Birth characteristics and hepatoblastoma risk in young children. *Cancer* 2004;101(1):210.

286. Donma MM, Donma O. Low birth weight: a possible risk factor also for liver diseases in adult life? *Med Hypotheses* 2003;61(4):435–438.

287. Oue T, Kubota A, Okuyama H, et al. Hepatoblastoma in children of extremely low birth weight: a report from a single perinatal center. *J Pediatr Surg* 2003;38(1):134–137, discussion 134–137.

288. Thomas D, Pritchard J, Davidson R, P et al. Familial hepatoblastoma and APC gene mutations: renewed call for molecular research. *Eur J Cancer* 2003;39(15):2200–2204.

289. Herzog CE, Andrassy RJ, Eftekhari F. Childhood cancers: hepatoblastoma. *Oncologist* 2000;5(6):445–453.

290. Bernstein IT, Bulow S, Mauritzen K. Hepatoblastoma in two cousins in a family with adenomatous polyposis. Report of two cases. *Dis Colon Rectum* 1992;35(4):373–374.

291. Riikonen P, Tuominen L, Seppa A, et al. Simultaneous hepatoblastoma in identical male twins. *Cancer* 1990;66(11):2429–2431.

292. Surendran N, Radhakrishna K, Chellam VG. Hepatoblastoma in siblings. *J Pediatr Surg* 1989;24(11):1169–1171.

293. Berry CL, Keeling J, Hilton C. Coincidence of congenital malformation and embryonic tumours of childhood. *Arch Dis Child* 1970;45(240):229–231.

294. Fraumeni JF Jr, Miller RW. Adrenocortical neoplasms with hemihypertrophy, brain tumors, and other disorders. *J Pediatr* 1967;70(1):129–138.

295. Nickerson HJ, Silberman TL, McDonald TP. Hepatoblastoma, thrombocytosis, and increased thrombopoietin. *Cancer* 1980;45(2):315–317.

296. Yamaguchi H, Ishii E, Hayashida Y, et al. Mechanism of thrombocytosis in hepatoblastoma: a case report. *Pediatr Hematol Oncol* 1996;13(6):539–544.

297. Exelby PR, Filler RM, Grosfeld JL. Liver tumors in children in the particular reference to hepatoblastoma and hepatocellular carcinoma: American Academy of Pediatrics Surgical Section Survey—1974. *J Pediatr Surg* 1975;10(3):329–337.

298. Tsuchida Y, Honna T, Fukui M, et al. The ratio of fucosylation of alpha-fetoprotein in hepatoblastoma. *Cancer* 1989;63(11):2174–2176.

299. Tsuchida Y, Terada M, Honna T, et al. The role of subfractionation of alpha-fetoprotein in the treatment of pediatric surgical patients. *J Pediatr Surg* 1997;32(3):514–517.

300. Moazam F, Talbert JL, Rodgers BM. Primary tumors of the liver in infancy and childhood. *J Fla Med Assoc* 1982;69(12):991–996.

301. Lack EE, Neave C, Vawter GF. Hepatoblastoma. A clinical and pathologic study of 54 cases. *Am J Surg Pathol* 1982;6(8):693–705.

302. Kasai M, Watanabe I. Histologic classification of liver-cell carcinoma in infancy and childhood and its clinical evaluation. A study of 70 cases collected in Japan. *Cancer* 1970;25(3):551–563.

303. Chan KL, Tam PK. Successful right trisegmentectomy for ruptured hepatoblastoma with preoperative transcatheter arterial embolization. *J Pediatr Surg* 1998;33(5):783–786.

304. Tashjian DB, Moriarty KP, Courtney RA, et al. Preoperative chemoembolization for unresectable hepatoblastoma. *Pediatr Surg Int* 2002;18(2–3):187–189.

305. Evans AE, Land VJ, Newton WA, et al. Combination chemotherapy (vincristine, adriamycin, cyclophosphamide, and 5-fluorouracil) in the treatment of children with malignant hepatoma. *Cancer* 1982;50(5):821–826.

306. Munro FD, Simpson E, Azmy AF. Resectability of advanced liver tumours in children after combination chemotherapy. *Ann R Coll Surg Engl* 1994;76(4):253–256.

307. Reynolds M, Douglass EC, Finegold M, et al. Chemotherapy can convert unresectable hepatoblastoma. *J Pediatr Surg* 1992;27(8):1080–1083, discussion 1083–1084.

308. Filler RM, Ehrlich PF, Greenberg ML, et al. Preoperative chemotherapy in hepatoblastoma. *Surgery* 1991;110(4):591–596, discussion 596–597.

309. Fuchs J, Rydzynski J, Hecker H, et al. The influence of preoperative chemotherapy and surgical technique in the treatment of hepatoblastoma—a report from the German Cooperative Liver Tumour Studies HB 89 and HB 94. *Eur J Pediatr Surg* 2002;12(4):255–261.

310. Choudhury SR, Singh D. Advanced hepatoblastoma: successful liver resection following preoperative chemotherapy. *Trop Gastroenterol* 2004;25(1):32–33.

311. Suita S, Tajiri T, Takamatsu H, et al. Improved survival outcome for hepatoblastoma based on an optimal chemotherapeutic regimen—a report from the study group for pediatric solid malignant tumors in the Kyushu area. *J Pediatr Surg* 2004;39(2):195–198, discussion 195–198.

312. Nishimura S, Sato T, Fujita N, et al. High-dose chemotherapy in children with metastatic hepatoblastoma. *Pediatr Int* 2002;44(3):300–305.

313. Cillo U, Ciarleglio FA, Bassanello M, et al. Liver transplantation for the management of hepatoblastoma. *Transplant Proc* 2003;35(8):2983–2985.

314. Srinivasan P, McCall J, Pritchard J, et al. Orthotopic liver transplantation for unresectable hepatoblastoma. *Transplantation* 2002;74(5):652–655.

315. Molmenti EP, Wilkinson K, Molmenti H, et al. Treatment of unresectable hepatoblastoma with liver transplantation in the pediatric population. *Am J Transplant* 2002;2(6):535–538.

316. Dillon PW, Whalen TV, Azizkhan RG, et al. Neonatal soft tissue sarcomas: the influence of pathology on treatment and survival. Children's Cancer Group Surgical Committee. *J Pediatr Surg* 1995;30(7):1038–1041.

317. Filston HC. Common lumps and bumps of the head and neck in infants and children. *Pediatr Ann* 1989;18(3): 180–182, 184,186.

318. Koscielniak E, Harms D, Schmidt D, et al. Soft tissue sarcomas in infants younger than 1 year of age: a report of the German Soft Tissue Sarcoma Study Group (CWS-81). *Med Pediatr Oncol* 1989;17(2):105–110.

319. Salloum E, Flamant F, Rey A, et al. Rhabdomyosarcoma in infants under one year of age: experience of the Institut Gustave-Roussy. *Med Pediatr Oncol* 1989;17(5):424–428.

320. Ragab AH, Heyn R, Tefft M, et al. Infants younger than 1 year of age with rhabdomyosarcoma. *Cancer* 1986;58(12):2606–2610.

321. King DR, Clatworthy HW Jr. The pediatric patient with sarcoma. *Semin Oncol* 1981;8(2):215–221.

322. Grosfeld JL, Weber TR, Weetman RM, et al. Rhabdomyosarcoma in childhood: analysis of survival in 98 cases. *J Pediatr Surg* 1983;18(2):141–146.

323. Piver MS, Rose PG. Long-term follow-up and complications of infants with vulvovaginal embryonal rhabdomyosarcoma treated with surgery, radiation therapy, and chemotherapy. *Obstet Gynecol* 1988;71(3 Pt 2):435–437.

324. Anderson JR, Meyer WH, Wiener ES. Favorable outcome for children with paratesticular alveolar history rhabdomyosarcoma. *Pediatr Blood Cancer* 2004;43(2):180.

325. Meyer WH, Spunt SL. Soft tissue sarcomas of childhood. *Cancer Treat Rev* 2004;30(3):269–280.

326. Herzog CE, Stewart JM, Blakely ML. Pediatric soft tissue sarcomas. *Surg Oncol Clin N Am* 2003;12(2):419–447, vii.

327. Ferrari A, Casanova M, Bisogno G, et al. Rhabdomyosarcoma in infants younger than one year old: a report from the Italian Cooperative Group. *Cancer* 2003;97(10):2597–2604.

328. Zagars GK, Ballo MT, Pisters PW, et al. Prognostic factors for patients with localized soft-tissue sarcoma treated with conservation surgery and radiation therapy: an analysis of 225 patients. *Cancer* 2003;97(10):2530–2543.

329. Coffin CM, Dehner LP. Soft tissue tumors in first year of life: a report of 190 cases. *Pediatr Pathol* 1990;10(4):509–526.

330. Nag S, Martinez-Monge R, Ruymann F, et al. Innovation in the management of soft tissue sarcomas in infants and young children: high-dose-rate brachytherapy. *J Clin Oncol* 1997;15(9): 3075–3084.

331. Chung EB, Enzinger FM. Infantile fibrosarcoma. *Cancer* 1976; 38(2):729–739.

332. Soule EH, Mahour GH, Mills SD, et al. Soft-tissue sarcomas of infants and children: a clinicopathologic study of 135 cases. *Mayo Clin Proc* 1968;43(5):313–326.

333. Soule EH, Pritchard DJ. Fibrosarcoma in infants and children: a review of 110 cases. *Cancer* 1977;40(4):1711–1721.

334. Kynaston JA, Malcolm AJ, Craft AW, et al. Chemotherapy in the management of infantile fibrosarcoma. *Med Pediatr Oncol* 1993;21(7):488–493.

335. Coffin CM, Jaszcz W, O'Shea PA, et al. So-called congenital-infantile fibrosarcoma: does it exist and what is it? *Pediatr Pathol* 1994;14(1):133–150.

336. Morerio C, Rapella A, Rosanda C, et al. Differential diagnosis of congenital fibrosarcoma. *Cancer Genet Cytogenet* 2004;152(2): 167–168.

337. Asgari M, Rubin BP, Hornung RL. Neonate with a fibrosarcoma and consumptive coagulopathy. *J Am Acad Dermatol* 2004; 50(Suppl 2):S23–S25.

338. Takach TJ, Reul GJ, Ott DA, et al. Primary cardiac tumors in infants and children: immediate and long-term operative results. *Ann Thorac Surg* 1996;62(2):559–564.

339. Boon LM, Fishman SJ, Lund DP, et al. Congenital fibrosarcoma masquerading as congenital hemangioma: report of two cases. *J Pediatr Surg* 1995;30(9):1378–1381.

340. Ferguson WS. Advances in the adjuvant treatment of infantile fibrosarcoma. *Expert Rev Anticancer Ther* 2003;3(2):185–191.

341. Cofer BR, Vescio PJ, Wiener ES. Infantile fibrosarcoma: complete excision is the appropriate treatment. *Ann Surg Oncol* 1996;3(2): 159–161.

342. Kanwar AJ, Kaur S, Thami GP, et al. Congenital infantile digital fibromatosis. *Pediatr Dermatol* 2002;19(4):370–371.

343. Rimareix F, Bardot J, Andrac L, et al. Infantile digital fibroma—report on eleven cases. *Eur J Pediatr Surg* 1997;7(6):345–348.

344. Falco NA, Upton J. Infantile digital fibromas. *J Hand Surg (Am)* 1995;20(6):1014–1020.

345. Parker RK, Mallory SB, Baker GF. Infantile myofibromatosis. *Pediatr Dermatol* 1991;8(2):129–132.

346. Hartig G, Koopmann C Jr, Esclamado R. Infantile myofibromatosis: a commonly misdiagnosed entity. *Otolaryngol Head Neck Surg* 1993;109(4):753–757.

347. Duffy MT, Harris M, Hornblass A. Infantile myofibromatosis of orbital bone. A case report with computed tomography, magnetic resonance imaging, and histologic findings. *Ophthalmology* 1997;104(9):1471–1474.

348. Linder JS, Harris GJ, Segura AD. Periorbital infantile myofibromatosis. *Arch Ophthalmol* 1996;114(2):219–222.

349. Atar D, Tenenbaum Y, Lehman WB, et al. Hip dislocation caused by infantile myofibromatosis. *Am J Orthop* 1995;24(10):774–776.

350. Dautenhahn L, Blaser SI, Weitzman S, et al. Infantile myofibromatosis: a cause of vertebra plana. *AJNR Am J Neuroradiol* 1995;16(Suppl 4):828–830.

351. Queralt JA, Poirier VC. Solitary infantile myofibromatosis of the skull. *AJNR Am J Neuroradiol* 1995;16(3):476–478.

352. Jenkins EA, Cawley MI. Infantile myofibromatosis: a cause of severe bone pain in a neonate. *Br J Rheumatol* 1993;32(9):849–852.

353. Chung EB, Enzinger FM. Infantile myofibromatosis. *Cancer* 1981;48(8):1807–1818.

354. Variend S, Bax NM, van Gorp J. Are infantile myofibromatosis, congenital fibrosarcoma and congenital haemangiopericytoma histogenetically related? *Histopathology* 1995;26(1):57–62.

355. Tamburrini G, Gessi M, Colosimo C Jr, et al. Infantile myofibromatosis of the central nervous system. *Childs Nerv Syst* 2003;19(9):650–654.

356. Kaplan SS, Ojemann JG, Grange DK, et al. Intracranial infantile myofibromatosis with intraparenchymal involvement. *Pediatr Neurosurg* 2002;36(4):214–217.

357. Soylemezoglu F, Tezel GG, Koybasoglu F, et al. Cranial infantile myofibromatosis: report of three cases. *Childs Nerv Syst* 2001;17(9):524–527.

358. Gandhi MM, Nathan PC, Weitzman S, et al. Successful treatment of life-threatening generalized infantile myofibromatosis using low-dose chemotherapy. *J Pediatr Hematol Oncol* 2003; 25(9):750–754.

359. Williams W, Craver RD, Correa H, et al. Use of 2-chlorodeoxyadenosine to treat infantile myofibromatosis. *J Pediatr Hematol Oncol* 2002;24(1):59–63.

360. Day M, Edwards AO, Weinberg A, et al. Brief report: successful therapy of a patient with infantile generalized myofibromatosis. *Med Pediatr Oncol* 2002;38(5):371–373.

361. Hatzidaki E, Korakaki E, Voloudaki A, et al. Infantile myofibromatosis with visceral involvement and complete spontaneous regression. *J Dermatol* 2001;28(7):379–382.

362. Mulliken JB, Enjolras O. Congenital hemangiomas and infantile hemangioma: missing links. *J Am Acad Dermatol* 2004;50(6): 875–882.

363. Frischer JS, Huang J, Serur A, et al. Biomolecular markers and involution of hemangiomas. *J Pediatr Surg* 2004;39(3):400–404.

364. Berenguer B, Mulliken JB, Enjolras O, et al. Rapidly involuting congenital hemangioma: clinical and histopathologic features. *Pediatr Dev Pathol* 2003;6(6):495–510.

365. Silverman RA. Hemangiomas and vascular malformations. *Pediatr Clin North Am* 1991;38(4):811–834.

366. Mulliken JB, Zetter BR, Folkman J. In vitro characteristics of endothelium from hemangiomas and vascular malformations. *Surgery* 1982;92(2):348–353.

367. Mulliken JB, Fishman SJ, Burrows PE. Vascular anomalies. *Curr Probl Surg* 2000;37(8):517–584.

368. Edgerton MT, Hiebert JM. Vascular and lymphatic tumors in infancy, childhood and adulthood: challenge of diagnosis and treatment. *Curr Probl Cancer* 1978;2(7):1–44.

369. Williams EF 3rd, Stanislaw P, Dupree M, et al. Hemangiomas in infants and children. An algorithm for intervention. *Arch Facial Plast Surg* 2000;2(2):103–111.

370. Enjolras O, Wassef M, Mazoyer E, et al. Infants with Kasabach-Merritt syndrome do not have "true" hemangiomas. *J Pediatr* 1997;130(4):631–640.

371. Akyuz C, Yaris N, Kutluk MT, et al. Management of cutaneous hemangiomas: a retrospective analysis of 1109 cases and comparison of conventional dose prednisolone with high-dose

methylprednisolone therapy. *Pediatr Hematol Oncol* 2001;18(1): 47–55.

372. Sharma LK, Dalal SS. Corticosteroid therapy in the treatment of cutaneous hemangioma of infancy and childhood. *Indian J Pediatr* 1983;50(403):153–156.

373. Sadan N, Wolach B. Treatment of hemangiomas of infants with high doses of prednisone. *J Pediatr* 1996;128(1):141–146.

374. Padalkar JA, Bapat VS, Phadke MA, et al. Successful treatment of hepatic hemangiomas with corticosteroids. *Indian Pediatr* 1992;29(6):769–770.

375. Schild SE, Buskirk SJ, Frick LM, et al. Radiotherapy for large symptomatic hemangiomas. *Int J Radiat Oncol Biol Phys* 1991; 21(3):729–735.

376. Belli L, De Carlis L, Beati C, et al. Surgical treatment of symptomatic giant hemangiomas of the liver. *Surg Gynecol Obstet* 1992;174(6):474–478.

377. Boon LM, Burrows PE, Paltiel HJ, et al. Hepatic vascular anomalies in infancy: a twenty-seven-year experience. *J Pediatr* 1996;129(3):346–354.

378. Burrows PE, Rosenberg HC, Chuang HS. Diffuse hepatic hemangiomas: percutaneous transcatheter embolization with detachable silicone balloons. *Radiology* 1985;156(1):85–88.

379. Warmann S, Bertram H, Kardorff R, et al. Interventional treatment of infantile hepatic hemangioendothelioma. *J Pediatr Surg* 2003;38(8):1177–1181.

380. Firth PG, Ahmed MI. Systemic embolism in an infant following haemangioma embolization: a two-step process. *Paediatr Anaesth* 2003;13(8):728–732.

381. Kullendorff CM, Cwikiel W, Sandstrom S. Embolization of hepatic hemangiomas in infants. *Eur J Pediatr Surg* 2002;12(5): 348–352.

382. Hosono S, Ohno T, Kimoto H, et al. Successful transcutaneous arterial embolization of a giant hemangioma associated with high-output cardiac failure and Kasabach-Merritt syndrome in a neonate: a case report. *J Perinat Med* 1999;27(5):399–403.

383. Daller JA, Bueno J, Gutierrez J, et al. Hepatic hemangioendothelioma: clinical experience and management strategy. *J Pediatr Surg* 1999;34(1):98–105, discussion 105–106.

384. Carnelli V, Bellini F, Ferrari M, et al. Giant hemangioma with consumption coagulopathy: sustained response to heparin and radiotherapy. *J Pediatr* 1977;91(3):504–505.

385. Koerper MA, Addiego JE Jr, deLorimier AA, et al. Use of aspirin and dipyridamole in children with platelet trapping syndromes. *J Pediatr* 1983;102(2):311–314.

386. de Prost Y, Teillac D, Bodemer C, et al. Successful treatment of Kasabach-Merritt syndrome with pentoxifylline. *J Am Acad Dermatol* 1991;25(5 Pt 1):854–855.

387. Dresse MF, David M, Hume H, et al. Successful treatment of Kasabach-Merritt syndrome with prednisone and epsilon-aminocaproic acid. *Pediatr Hematol Oncol* 1991;8(4):329–334.

388. Neubert AG, Golden MA, Rose NC. Kasabach-Merritt coagulopathy complicating Klippel-Trenaunay-Weber syndrome in pregnancy. *Obstet Gynecol* 1995;85(5 Pt 2):831–833.

389. Maier H, Donath P, Neumann R. Early pulsed-dye laser treatment of childhood haemangiomas. *Lancet* 2003;361(9354):348, author reply 349.

390. Hohenleutner U, Landthaler M. Laser treatment of childhood haemangioma: progress or not? *Lancet* 2002;360(9332):502–503.

391. Chatrath P, Black M, Jani P, et al. A review of the current management of infantile subglottic haemangioma, including a comparison of CO(2) laser therapy versus tracheostomy. *Int J Pediatr Otorhinolaryngol* 2002;64(2):143–157.

392. Batta K, Goodyear HM, Moss C, et al. Randomised controlled study of early pulsed dye laser treatment of uncomplicated childhood haemangiomas: results of a 1-year analysis. *Lancet* 2002; 360(9332):521–527.

393. Glassberg E, Lask G. Laser treatment of proliferating cutaneous hemangiomas. *Dermatol Surg* 1995;21(2):185.

394. Froehlich P, Seid AB, Morgon A. Contrasting strategic approaches to the management of subglottic hemangiomas. *Int J Pediatr Otorhinolaryngol* 1996;36(2):137–146.

395. Marler JJ, Rubin JB, Trede NS, et al. Successful antiangiogenic therapy of giant cell angioblastoma with interferon alfa 2b: report of 2 cases. *Pediatrics* 2002;109(2):E37.

396. Deb G, Donfrancesco A, Ilari I, et al. Hemangioendothelioma: successful therapy with interferon-alpha: a study in Association

with the Italian Pediatric Haematology/Oncology Society (AIEOP). *Med Pediatr Oncol* 2002;38(2):118–119.

397. Tryfonas GI, Tsikopoulos G, Liasidou E, et al. Conservative treatment of hemangiomas in infancy and childhood with interferon-alpha 2a. *Pediatr Surg Int* 1998;13(8):590–593.

398. Anger J, Carneiro RG, Pinus J, et al. The rebound effect in the treatment of complex hemangioma with interferon alpha 2A. *Rev Paul Med* 1998;116(5):1826–1828.

399. Barlow CF, Priebe CJ, Mulliken JB, et al. Spastic diplegia as a complication of interferon Alfa-2a treatment of hemangiomas of infancy. *J Pediatr* 1998;132(3 Pt 1):527–530.

400. Ezekowitz A, Mulliken J, Folkman J. Interferon alpha therapy of haemangiomas in newborns and infants. *Br J Haematol* 1991;79(Suppl 1):67–68.

401. Ezekowitz RA, Mulliken JB, Folkman J. Interferon alfa-2a therapy for life-threatening hemangiomas of infancy. *N Engl J Med* 1992;326(22):1456–1463.

402. Chung T, Hoffer FA, Burrows PE, et al. MR imaging of hepatic hemangiomas of infancy and changes seen with interferon alpha-2a treatment. *Pediatr Radiol* 1996;26(5):341–348.

403. Falk H, Herbert JT, Edmonds L, et al. Review of four cases of childhood hepatic angiosarcoma—elevated environmental arsenic exposure in one case. *Cancer* 1981;47(2):382–391.

404. Bedros AA, Munson J, Toomey FE. Hemangioendothelioma presenting as posterior mediastinal mass in a child. *Cancer* 1980;46(4):801–803.

405. Arceci RJ.. The histiocytoses: the fall of the Tower of Babel. *Eur J Cancer* 1999;35(5):747–767, discussion 767–769.

406. Arceci RJ, Longley BJ, Emanuel PD. Atypical cellular disorders. *Hematology (Am Soc Hematol Educ Program)* 2002;297–314.

407. Huang F, Arceci R. The histiocytoses of infancy. *Semin Perinatol* 1999;23(4):319–331.

408. Egeler RM, Nesbit ME. Langerhans cell histiocytosis and other disorders of monocyte-histiocyte lineage. *Crit Rev Oncol Hematol* 1995;18(1):9–35.

409. Chu T, D'Angio GJ, Favara BE, et al. Histiocytosis syndromes in children. *Lancet* 1987;2(8549):41–42.

410. Laman JD, Leenen PJ, Annels NE, et al. Langerhans-cell histiocytosis 'insight into DC biology'. *Trends Immunol* 2003;24(4):190–196.

411. Favara BE, Feller AC, Pauli M, et al. Contemporary classification of histiocytic disorders. The WHO Committee On Histiocytic/Reticulum Cell Proliferations. Reclassification Working Group of the Histiocyte Society. *Med Pediatr Oncol* 1997;29(3):157–166.

412. Willman CL, Busque L, Griffith BB, et al. Langerhans'-cell histiocytosis (histiocytosis X)—a clonal proliferative disease. *N Engl J Med* 1994;331(3):154–160.

413. Yu RC, Chu C, Buluwela L, et al. Clonal proliferation of Langerhans cells in Langerhans cell histiocytosis. *Lancet* 1994;343(8900):767–768.

414. Cotter FE, Pritchard J. Clonality in Langerhans' cell histiocytosis. *BMJ* 1995;310(6972):74–75.

415. Egeler RM. Clonality in Langerhan's cell histiocytosis. *BMJ* 1995;310(6982):804–805.

416. Willman CL, McClain KL. An update on clonality, cytokines, and viral etiology in Langerhans cell histiocytosis. *Hematol Oncol Clin North Am* 1998;12(2):407–416.

417. Willman CL. Detection of clonal histiocytes in Langerhans cell histiocytosis: biology and clinical significance. *Br J Cancer Suppl* 1994;23:S29–S33.

418. Libicher M, Roeren T, Troger J. Localized Langerhans cell histiocytosis of bone: treatment and follow-up in children. *Pediatr Radiol* 1995;25(Suppl 1):S134–S137.

419. Bernstrand C, Bjork O, Ahstrom L, et al. Intralesional steroids in Langerhans cell histiocytosis of bone. *Acta Paediatr* 1996;85(4):502–504.

420. Cassady JR. Current role of radiation therapy in the management of histiocytosis-X. *Hematol Oncol Clin North Am* 1987; 1(1):123–129.

421. Webb DK. Histiocyte disorders. *Br Med Bull* 1996;52(4):818–825.

422. Greenberger JS, Crocker AC, Vawter G, et al. Results of treatment of 127 patients with systemic histiocytosis. *Medicine (Baltimore)* 1981;60(5):311–338.

423. Song A, Johnson TE, Dubovy SR, et al. Treatment of recurrent eosinophilic granuloma with systemic therapy. *Ophthal Plast Reconstr Surg* 2003;19(2):140–144.

424. Ghanem I, Tolo VT, D'Ambra P, et al. Langerhans cell histiocytosis of bone in children and adolescents. *J Pediatr Orthop* 2003; 23(1):124–130.

425. Minkov M, Grois N, Heitger A, et al. Response to initial treatment of multisystem Langerhans cell histiocytosis: an important prognostic indicator. *Med Pediatr Oncol* 2002;39(6):581–585.

426. Minkov M, Grois N, Heitger A, et al. Treatment of multisystem Langerhans cell histiocytosis. Results of the DAL-HX 83 and DAL-HX 90 studies. DAL-HX Study Group. *Klin Padiatr* 2000; 212(4):139–144.

427. Ladisch S. Langerhans cell histiocytosis. *Curr Opin Hematol* 1998;5(1):54–58.

428. Ladisch S, Gadner H. Treatment of Langerhans cell histiocytosis—evolution and current approaches. *Br J Cancer Suppl* 1994; 23:S41-S46.

429. Gadner H, Heitger A, Grois N, et al. Treatment strategy for disseminated Langerhans cell histiocytosis. DAL HX-83 Study Group. *Med Pediatr Oncol* 1994;23(2):72–80.

430. Arceci RJ, Grabowski G. Histiocytoses and Disorders of the Reticuloendothelial System. In: Handin RI, Lux SE, Stossel TP, et al, eds. *Blood: principles and Practice of hematology.* Philadelphia: Lippincott Williams & Wilkins, 2003:921–957.

431. Martinez-Perez, D, Mulliken JB, Arceci RJ. Langerhans cell histiocytosis: an uncommon disease commonly manifesting in the craniofacial skeleton. *Plast Reconstr Surg* 1996;98(2):211–216.

432. Ladisch S, Gadner H, Arico M, et al. LCH-I: a randomized trial of etoposide vs. vinblastine in disseminated Langerhans cell histiocytosis. The Histiocyte Society. *Med Pediatr Oncol* 1994;23(2): 107–110.

433. Glass AG, Miller RW. U.S. mortality from Letterer-Siwe disease, 1960–1964. *Pediatrics* 1968;42(2):364–367.

434. Juberg RC, Kloepfer HW, Oberman HA. Genetic determination of acute disseminated histiocytosis X. *Pediatrics* 1970;45(5): 753–765.

435. Arico M, Nichols K, Whitlock JA, et al. Familial clustering of Langerhans cell histiocytosis. *Br J Haematol* 1999;107(4):883–888.

436. Arceci RJ, Brenner MK, Pritchard J. Controversies and new approaches to treatment of Langerhans cell histiocytosis. *Hematol Oncol Clin North Am* 1998;12(2):339–357.

437. Arceci RJ. Treatment options—commentary. *Br J Cancer Suppl* 1994;23:S58–S60.

438. Arico M. Cyclosporine therapy for refractory Langerhans cell histiocytosis. *Blood* 1991;78(11):3107.

439. Arico M, Colella R, Conter V, et al. Cyclosporine therapy for refractory Langerhans cell histiocytosis. *Med Pediatr Oncol* 1995;25(1):12–16.

440. Mahmoud HH, Wang WC, Murphy SB. Cyclosporine therapy for advanced Langerhans cell histiocytosis. *Blood* 1991;77(4): 721–725.

441. Sawamura M, Yamaguchi S, Marayama K, et al. Cyclosporine therapy for Langerhans cell histiocytosis. *Br J Haematol* 1993; 83(1):178–179.

442. Nagarajan R, Neglia J, Ramsay N, et al. Successful treatment of refractory Langerhans cell histiocytosis with unrelated cord blood transplantation. *J Pediatr Hematol Oncol* 2001;23(9): 629–632.

443. Ringden O, Ahstrom L, Lonnqvist B, et al. Allogeneic bone marrow transplantation in a patient with chemotherapy-resistant progressive histiocytosis X. *N Engl J Med* 1987;316(12):733–735.

444. Ringden O, Lantz B, Bolme P, et al. Bone marrow transplantation at Huddinge Hospital: more and more successful therapy in malignant disease—the indications are gradually increasing. *Lakartidningen* 1985;82(24):2239–2242.

445. Hale GA, Bowman LC, Woodard JP, et al. Allogeneic bone marrow transplantation for children with histiocytic disorders: use of TBI and omission of etoposide in the conditioning regimen. *Bone Marrow Transplant* 2003;31(11):981–986.

446. Conter V, Reciputo A, Arrigo C, et al. Bone marrow transplantation for refractory Langerhans' cell histiocytosis. *Haematologica* 1996;81(5):468–471.

447. Greinix HT, Storb R, Sanders JE, et al. Marrow transplantation for treatment of multisystem progressive Langerhans cell histiocytosis. *Bone Marrow Transplant* 1992;10(1):39–44.

448. Richter MP, D'Angio GJ. The role of radiation therapy in the management of children with histiocytosis X. *Am J Pediatr Hematol Oncol* 1981;3(2):161–163.

449. Goh NS, McDonald CE, MacGregor DP, et al. Successful treatment of Langerhans cell histiocytosis with 2-chlorodeoxyadenosine. *Respirology* 2003;8(1):91–94.

450. Pardanani A, Phyliky RL, Li CY, et al. 2-Chlorodeoxyadenosine therapy for disseminated Langerhans cell histiocytosis. *Mayo Clin Proc* 2003;78(3):301–306.

451. Rodriguez-Galindo C, Kelly P, Jeng M, et al. Treatment of children with Langerhans cell histiocytosis with 2-chlorodeoxyadenosine. *Am J Hematol* 2002;69(3):179–184.

452. Weitzman S, Wayne AS, Arceci R, et al. Nucleoside analogues in the therapy of Langerhans cell histiocytosis: a survey of members of the histiocyte society and review of the literature. *Med Pediatr Oncol* 1999;33(5):476–481.

453. Henter JI, Arico M, Elinder G, et al. Familial hemophagocytic lymphohistiocytosis. Primary hemophagocytic lymphohistiocytosis. *Hematol Oncol Clin North Am* 1998;12(2):417–433.

454. Farquhar JW, Claireaux AE. Familial haemophagocytic reticulosis. *Arch Dis Child* 1952;27(136):519–525.

455. Macmahon HE, Bedizel M, Ellis CA. Familial Erythrophagocytic Lymphohistiocytosis. *Pediatrics* 1963;32:868–879.

456. Henter JI, Nennesmo I. Neuropathologic findings and neurologic symptoms in twenty-three children with hemophagocytic lymphohistiocytosis. *J Pediatr* 1997;130(3):358–365.

457. Imashuku S, Hlbi S, Todo S. Hemophagocytic lymphohistiocytosis in infancy and childhood. *J Pediatr* 1997;130(3):352–357.

458. zur Stadt U, Pruggmayer M, Jung H, et al. Prenatal diagnosis of perforin gene mutations in familial hemophagocytic lymphohistiocytosis (FHLH). *Prenat Diagn* 2002;22(1):80–81.

459. Zipursky A. Perforin deficiency and familial hemophagocytic lymphohistiocytosis. *Pediatr Res* 2001;49(1):3.

460. Ueda I, Morimoto A, Inaba T, et al. Characteristic perforin gene mutations of haemophagocytic lymphohistiocytosis patients in Japan. *Br J Haematol* 2003;121(3):503–510.

461. Suga N, Takada H, Nomura A, et al. Perforin defects of primary haemophagocytic lymphohistiocytosis in Japan. *Br J Haematol* 2002;116(2):346–349.

462. Stepp SE, Dufourcq-Lagelouse R, Le Deist F, et al. Perforin gene defects in familial hemophagocytic lymphohistiocytosis. *Science* 1999;286(5446):1957–1959.

463. Grunebaum E, Roifman CM. Gene abnormalities in patients with hemophagocytic lymphohistiocytosis. *Isr Med Assoc J* 2002; 4(5):366–369.

464. Feldmann J, Le Deist F, Ouachee-Chardin M, et al. Functional consequences of perforin gene mutations in 22 patients with familial haemophagocytic lymphohistiocytosis. *Br J Haematol* 2002;117(4):965–972.

465. Feldmann J, Callebaut I, Raposo G, et al. Munc13-4 is essential for cytolytic granules fusion and is mutated in a form of familial hemophagocytic lymphohistiocytosis (FHL3). *Cell* 2003;115(4): 461–473.

466. Arico M, Imashuku S, Clementi R, S et al. Hemophagocytic lymphohistiocytosis due to germline mutations in SH2D1A, the X-linked lymphoproliferative disease gene. *Blood* 2001;97(4): 1131–1133.

467. Ansbacher LE, Singsen BH, Hosler MW, et al. Familial erythrophagocytic lymphohistiocytosis: an association with serum lipid abnormalities. *J Pediatr* 1983;102(2):270–273.

468. Egeler RM, Shapiro R, Loechelt B, et al. Characteristic immune abnormalities in hemophagocytic lymphohistiocytosis. *J Pediatr Hematol Oncol* 1996;18(4): 340–345.

469. Filipovich AH. Hemophagocytic lymphohistiocytosis: a lethal disorder of immune regulation. *J Pediatr* 1997;130(3):337–338.

470. Schneider EM, Lorenz I, Walther P, et al. Natural killer deficiency: a minor or major factor in the manifestation of hemophagocytic lymphohistiocytosis? *J Pediatr Hematol Oncol* 2003;25(9): 680–683.

471. Schneider EM, Lorenz I, Muller-Rosenberger M, et al. Hemophagocytic lymphohistiocytosis is associated with deficiencies of cellular cytolysis but normal expression of transcripts relevant to killer-cell-induced apoptosis. *Blood* 2002;100(8): 2891–2898.

472. Osugi Y, Hara J, Tagawa S, et al. Cytokine production regulating Th1 and Th2 cytokines in hemophagocytic lymphohistiocytosis. *Blood* 1997;89(11):4100–4103.

473. Sullivan KE, Delaat CA, Douglas SD, et al. Defective natural killer cell function in patients with hemophagocytic lymphohistiocytosis and in first degree relatives. *Pediatr Res* 1998;44(4):465–468.

474. Ladisch S, Ho W, Matheson D, et al. Immunologic and clinical effects of repeated blood exchange in familial erythrophagocytic lymphohistiocytosis. *Blood* 1982;60(4):814–821.

475. Henter JI, Elinder G, Finkel Y, et al. Successful induction with chemotherapy including teniposide in familial erythrophagocytic lymphohistiocytosis. *Lancet* 1986;2(8520):1402.

476. Henter JI, Arico M, Egeler RM, et al. HLH-94: a treatment protocol for hemophagocytic lymphohistiocytosis. HLH study Group of the Histiocyte Society. *Med Pediatr Oncol* 1997;28(5):342–347.

477. Arico M, Allen M, Brusa S, et al. Haemophagocytic lymphohistiocytosis: proposal of a diagnostic algorithm based on perforin expression. *Br J Haematol* 2002;119(1):180–188.

478. Bolme P, Henter JI, Winiarski J, et al. Allogeneic bone marrow transplantation for hemophagocytic lymphohistiocytosis in Sweden. *Bone Marrow Transplant* 1995;15(3):331–335.

479. Baker KS, DeLaat CA, Steinbuch M, et al. Successful correction of hemophagocytic lymphohistiocytosis with related or unrelated bone marrow transplantation. *Blood* 1997;89(10):3857–3863.

480. Marsh WL Jr, Lew SW, Heath VC, et al. Congenital self-healing histiocytosis-X. *Am J Pediatr Hematol Oncol* 1983;5(3):227–233.

481. Hashimoto K, Bale GF, Hawkins HK, et al. Congenital self-healing reticulohistiocytosis (Hashimoto-Pritzker type). *Int J Dermatol* 1986;25(8):516–523.

482. Jaffe R. The Other Histiocytosis. *Pediatr Dev Pathol* 2004;7(1).

483. Egeler RM, Schmitz L, Sonneveld P, et al. Malignant histiocytosis: a reassessment of cases formerly classified as histiocytic neoplasms and review of the literature. *Med Pediatr Oncol* 1995;25(1):1–7.

484. Bucsky P, Egeler RM. Malignant histiocytic disorders in children. Clinical and therapeutic approaches with a nosologic discussion. *Hematol Oncol Clin North Am* 1998;12(2):465–471.

485. de Lorimier AA, Harrison MR. Surgical treatment of tumors in the newborn. *Am J Pediatr Hematol Oncol* 1981;3(3):271–277.

486. Pastore G, Antonelli R, Fine W, et al. Late effects of treatment of cancer in infancy. *Med Pediatr Oncol* 1982;10(4):369–375.

487. Morselli PL. Clincial pharmacokinetics in neonates. *Clin Pharmacokinet* 1976;1(2):81–98.

488. Siegel SE, Moran RG. Problems in the chemotherapy of cancer in the neonate. *Am J Pediatr Hematol Oncol* 1981;3(3):287–296.

489. McLeod HL, Evans WE. Pediatric pharmacokinetics and therapeutic drug monitoring. *Pediatr Rev* 1992;13(11):413–421.

490. McLeod HL, Relling MV, Crom WR, et al. Disposition of antineoplastic agents in the very young child. *Br J Cancer Suppl* 1992;18:S23–S29.

491. Woods WG, O'Leary M, Nesbit ME. Life-threatening neuropathy and hepatotoxicity in infants during induction therapy for acute lymphoblastic leukemia. *J Pediatr* 1981;98(4):642–645.

492. Mulhern RK, Kovnar E, Langston J, et al. Long-term survivors of leukemia treated in infancy: factors associated with neuropsychologic status. *J Clin Oncol* 1992;10(7):1095–1102.

493. Pinter AB, Hock A, Kajtar P, et al. Long-term follow-up of cancer in neonates and infants: a national survey of 142 patients. *Pediatr Surg Int* 2003;19(4):233–239.

Eye Disorders

Sherwin J. Isenberg

The eye is possibly the fastest developing organ in the body. As soon as 4 to 6 months after birth, some ocular functions are permanently set and if impaired, cannot be fully restored to normalcy. The neonate with a serious ophthalmic disorder may be compared to a time bomb. It is not adequate to simply reverse or cure the problem. The treatment must be conducted rapidly, effectively, and reconstruction (amblyopia) must be commenced. Thus, the neonatologist has some responsibility to recognize ocular abnormalities and quickly begin the process of healing.

GENERAL CONSIDERATIONS

Amblyopia

Amblyopia can be defined as a reduction in vision in the absence of, or beyond that explained by, an apparent organic cause. Amblyopia can be divided into a few etiologic classes. Strabismic amblyopia results from a child preferring one eye when the visual axes are misaligned. Reversal, generally with occlusion of the preferred eye, can only be achieved by age 7 to 9 years; the earlier treatment begins, the better. Refractive amblyopia generally results from significant inequality of the refractive errors in each eye. This form of amblyopia also should be reversed by 7 to 9 years of age, with treatment usually consisting of spectacles (or contact lenses) and occlusion of the sound eye. Either of these two forms of amblyopia can begin within the first few postnatal months.

The form of amblyopia that is most feared in infants is deprivation amblyopia. It usually arises before 3 months of age. The cause is blockage of clear images from reaching the retina. It may be unilateral or bilateral and may be caused by a cataract, corneal opacity, or severe eyelid ptosis. There is considerable urgency in reversing this form of amblyopia because good vision can only be attained within the first 3 to 6 months after birth. This timetable coincides with the "critical period" of ocular development in humans (1). Thus, for example, if a significant unilateral congenital cataract is discovered after 6 months of age, one would not expect excellent visual recovery, even after surgery and optical (usually contact lens or intraocular lens) therapy.

Growth and Development of the Eye

At birth, the sagittal (axial) diameter of the eye is 16 mm in full-term neonates (2). It is less in preterm infants at birth. In the first year, this dimension grows 3.8 mm, with half the expected lifetime increase achieved by 12 months of age. With this information, one can appreciate the early anatomic maturity of the eye.

The corneal diameter often is used as an indicator of the size of the entire eye. At term, the corneal diameter averages 10.0 mm. The diagnosis of microcornea (less than 9 mm) or megalocornea (greater than 11 mm) (Fig. 54-1) suggests a similar abnormality in size of the entire globe, which should lead to an appropriate workup (see following). Ultrasonography can be utilized to determine precisely the size of the entire eye. The tactile corneal reflex is absent in 90% of infants at birth, but develops in all by 3 months of age (3).

Three developmental markers exist in the preterm eye that can help the neonatologist define a neonate's postconceptional age. The tunica vasculosa lentis is a plexus of vessels, which is visible prior to 32 to 34 weeks postconception, crossing the pupil anterior to the lens. The lens surface is covered by these vessels at 27 to 28 weeks postconception, at which time they begin to disintegrate (4). Except for a few vessels at the lens periphery, they should be gone by 34 weeks (Fig. 54-2).

The status of the pupil follows a relatively predictable developmental pattern (Fig. 54-3) (5). At 26 to 31 weeks' postconception, the pupillary diameter in relative darkness is quite large (up to 5.0 mm), and the pupil does not respond to light. By 31 weeks, the pupil diameter has decreased to a stable size of 3.5 mm, and the pupil begins to react to light. The light reaction increases in magnitude until reaching stability at term.

The appearance of the macula in the retina is easily appreciated with the ophthalmoscope after the pupil is dilated. The examiner can determine the infant's postconceptional age by observing the development of three land-

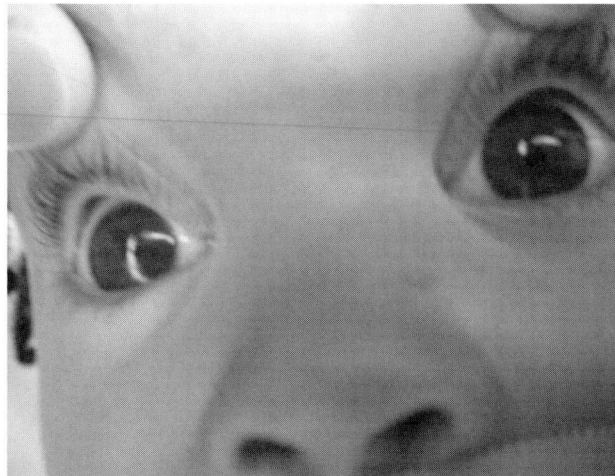

Figure 54-1 When the corneal diameter exceeds 11 mm in a neonate, a differential diagnosis must be considered.

marks in the macula: pigmentation, annular reflex, and foveola (Table 54-1) (6). With these three anatomic findings, a neonate's postconceptional age can be estimated from 27 weeks' postconception to term.

EXAMINATION TECHNIQUES

Visual Acuity

In the neonatal period, there is seldom a reason to even attempt to determine the infant's visual acuity. In the first 2 months after birth, the visual acuity is no better than 20/400 because of immaturity of the retina. The retinal periphery, however, can be stimulated with horizontal optokinetic targets to produce nystagmus. This will prove that the infant is developing some vision. Vertical nystagmus responses develop later. Laboratory techniques can be utilized, if necessary, to more precisely determine the visual acuity. These techniques include preferential forced looking and pattern electroretinograms. A blink response to light confirms the presence of light perception.

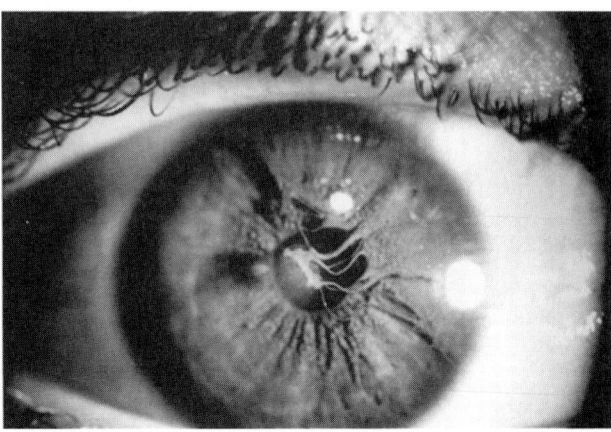

Figure 54-2 Persistent pupillary membranes, remaining from tunica vasculosa lentis vessels, are the most common embryonic remnants found in adults.

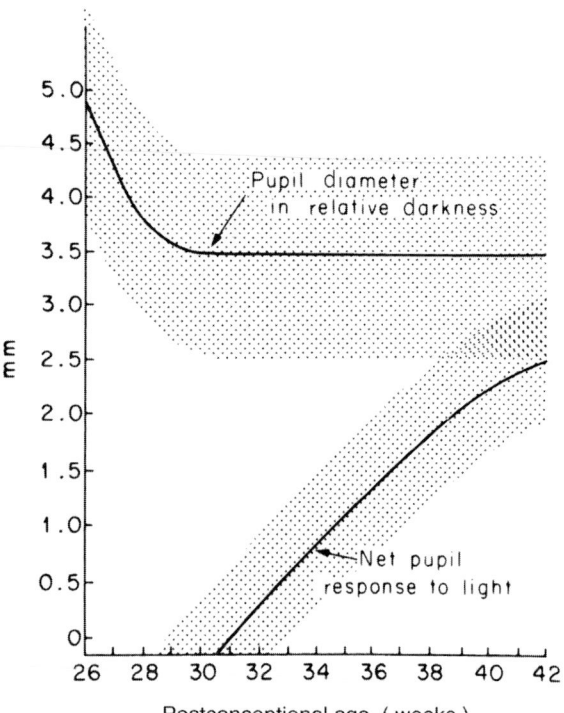

Figure 54-3 Diameter of the pupil (mean ± standard deviation) in term and preterm neonates in relative darkness (less than 10 ft-c) and after light stimulation (600 ft-c). (From Isenberg SJ. Examination methods. In: Isenberg SJ, ed. *The eye in infancy*, 2nd ed. St. Louis: Mosby-Year Book, 1994:47, with permission.)

Anterior Segment

The anterior segment can be examined using a strong penlight, with magnification as provided with loupes. Alternatively, a direct ophthalmoscope with a setting of about +5 can be utilized. The examiner should observe the eyelids, conjunctiva, cornea, iris, and lens. The corneal diameter can be measured. As described previously, the pupil diameter initially should be observed with a dim light, followed by evaluation of the reactivity to a bright light.

Posterior Segment

Prior to examining the vitreous and retina, it is usually necessary to dilate the pupil. The choice of dilating agents is important because retinal examinations often are indicated in low-weight preterm infants to rule out retinopathy of prematurity (ROP). Sympathomimetic eyedrops can raise a low-weight neonate's blood pressure (7), whereas anticholinergic eyedrops that are thought to be of low concentration can significantly increase gastric acid (8). A safe and effective combination mydriatic eyedrop is 1.0% phenylephrine/0.2% cyclopentolate. One drop should be applied to both eyes and then repeated 5 to 10 minutes later. A third set occasionally may be required if the iris is darkly pigmented.

Although the eyelids can be held open by an assistant if the examination will be brief, usually an eyelid speculum specifically designed for neonatal use is utilized after application of an anesthetic eyedrop. When the examiner is

TABLE 54-1	
DEVELOPMENT OF THE MACULA	
Observations in the Macula	**Postconceptional Age (weeks)**
No pigmentation exists	31.5 ± 1.5
Dark red pigmentation appears	34.8 ± 1.0
Part of the annular reflex is evident	34.7 ± 2.4
Annular reflex is complete	36.3 ± 2.2
Foveolar pit is difficult to appreciate	37.6 ± 3.3
Foveolar light reflex is easily observed	41.7 ± 4.0

From Isenberg SJ. Macular development in the premature infant. *Am J Ophthalmol* 1986;101:74–80.

manipulating the eye, infants have been shown to display an oculocardiac reflex, defined as any dysrhythmia or a bradycardia of 10% or more, in as many as 31% of cases (9). Therefore, the assistant should monitor the baby, as well as the eye, as the retinal examination progresses. During the retinal examination, the cornea tends to become dry and opacify somewhat because of the heat of the light, exposure, evaporation, and the recent finding that neonates, especially preterm infants, produce both basal and reflex tears at a reduced rate (10). Thus, while ensuring the stability of the speculum, the assistant also will need to lubricate the cornea.

CONGENITAL ANOMALIES

Ocular Size and Shape

Enlarged Eyes

An enlarged eye is suspected when the corneal diameter exceeds 11.0 mm in a term newborn. For confirmation, an A-scan ultrasound can be obtained easily to measure the ocular axial length, which is normally 16 mm at birth (2). If the eye is enlarged, infantile glaucoma caused by an elevated intraocular pressure should be suspected immediately. Infantile glaucoma also often will present with tearing, squinting, photosensitivity, and a cloudy cornea (Fig. 54-4). The cornea often is found to have horizontal lines called Haab striae, which result from a disruption of Descemet membrane. The optic nerve is noted to have an enlarged cup on fundus examination. To differentiate the tearing of glaucoma from that of the much more common nasolacrimal duct obstruction, the examiner should look at, or into, the nostrils. If tears emanate from the nostrils, the nasolacrimal apparatus is patent and glaucoma is possible. If no tears are found in the nostril, a nasolacrimal duct obstruction is likely.

The treatment of glaucoma is fairly urgent because uncontrolled infantile glaucoma will cause opacification of the cornea, enlargement of the eye, creation of significant myopia, and damage to the optic nerve. If unilateral, the myopia engendered can cause amblyopia, even if the cornea is fairly clear. The corneal opacification can cause deprivation amblyopia.

The infant must be examined while under anesthesia to confirm the diagnosis. After confirmation, the treatment is surgical. The ophthalmologist must open the trabecular meshwork filtration system either internally (goniotomy) or externally (trabeculotomy). If those approaches fail, the ophthalmologist may create an external filtration area (trabeculectomy) or implant an artificial drainage device.

Infantile glaucoma has been associated with other ocular problems, such as aniridia; goniodysgeneses (or mesodermal dysgeneses), which include Axenfeld and Rieger syndromes; and persistent fetal vasculature (see following). It has been associated with a number of systemic disorders and syndromes, including Sturge-Weber, neurofibromatosis, Marfan, Pierre Robin, homocystinuria, Lowe, rubella, Rubenstein-Taybi, and chromosomal abnormalities.

The cornea also may be enlarged on a structural basis without glaucoma. However, in this case, the rest of the eye has a normal shape, as can be demonstrated by ultrasonographic examination. Megalocornea is uncommon and usually has an X-linked inheritance pattern.

Small Eyes

A small eye will present with a corneal diameter less than 9 mm in a term birth. Confirmation of an axial length less

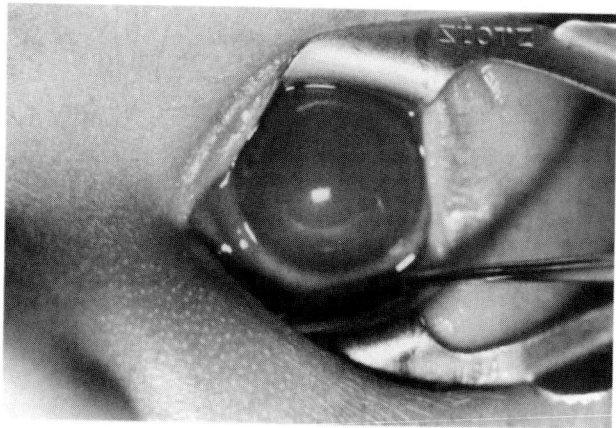

Figure 54-4 This cornea is diffusely opacified and enlarged from infantile glaucoma.

than the normal 16 mm, as shown by ultrasound, is desirable. Microphthalmos can range from an eye that is slightly smaller than normal but otherwise intact to an eye that is so small that it cannot be found on routine examination (anophthalmos). In cases of anophthalmos, a small, often cystic, eye sometimes can be demonstrated by MRI, CT, or ultrasound. It may be associated with Klinefelter syndrome or trisomy 13.

There are two, not infrequent, ophthalmic disorders associated with microphthalmos. A coloboma is a developmental gap generally located inferiorly in the eye. It can be recognized externally as an inferior notch in the pupil caused by missing iris tissue, which by itself does not affect vision. More ominously, the defect also can include the optic nerve, macula, and other parts of the retina, which can result in legal blindness (Fig. 54-5). With experience, ophthalmologists now are recognizing the frequent combination of systemic findings called the CHARGE association. It consists of coloboma (C), heart defects (H), atresia choanae (A), retarded growth and development (R), genital hypoplasia (G), and ear anomalies and deafness (E). Facial palsy also is common. At least four of these findings must be present to make the diagnosis.

A second ophthalmic disorder commonly associated with microphthalmos is persistent hyperplastic primary vitreous. It has recently been renamed persistent fetal vasculature, a more encompassing name (11). This disorder often is associated with microphthalmos and hypoplasia of the fovea, as it represents an arrest of ocular development. Many of the sequelae result from abnormal vessels in the vitreous, anterior lens, and equator, causing persistent pupillary membranes, pigmented star-shaped structures on the anterior lens capsule, fibrovascular remnants on the optic nerve (Bergmeister papilla), and nonattachment of the retina. Serious secondary events can ensue, including cataract, glaucoma, lens subluxation, corneal opacities, intraocular hemorrhages, retinal detachments, and chronic inflammation. Because some of these mani-

festations are treatable, the neonatologist should seek an ophthalmic consultation for any infant with a small eye.

Eyelid Abnormalities

Congenital eyelid ptosis is readily apparent to the parents and all who observe a baby. Therefore, its presence often generates an examination within a few weeks of birth. Although the ptosis can be surgically corrected at any time in the baby's life, two considerations will indicate the proper timing of surgery. If the ptosis threatens the infant's vision, it should be corrected early—even within the first few postnatal months. The vision can be threatened in two ways. If the ptosis is total or near total, the visual axis will be obstructed and the child may develop deprivation amblyopia. This is unusual because ptosis is seldom total, which allows the child, once head control is established, to elevate the chin to see under the ptotic eyelid. A more likely mechanism of potential visual loss is by an astigmatism induced by the ptotic eyelid applying subtle pressure to the cornea. This unilateral astigmatism can cause refractive amblyopia, even in a young infant. If vision is not threatened, the surgery can be deferred until 4 or 5 years of age.

A number of eyelid tumors can present at birth. Most frequent is the capillary hemangioma (Fig. 54-6), which generally continues to grow after birth. The skin overlying the mass can be dimpled and red, resembling a strawberry, or it can assume a diffuse purple color if the lesion is deeper. The lesion does not transilluminate and feels spongy. Left untreated, most of these tumors will spontaneously involute after 1 to 2 years of age. Treatment is indicated if vision is threatened by obstruction of the visual axis or induction of astigmatism, as noted previously. Treatment is by injection of a combination of corticosteroids directly into the tumor or by systemic corticosteroids. The direct route may be safer. Favorable results recently have been reported with subcutaneous injections of interferon alfa-2b (12). Lymphangiomata and dermoid cysts of the eyelid also can present at birth.

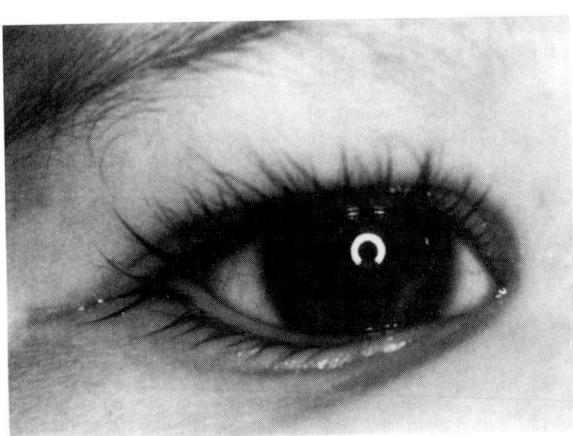
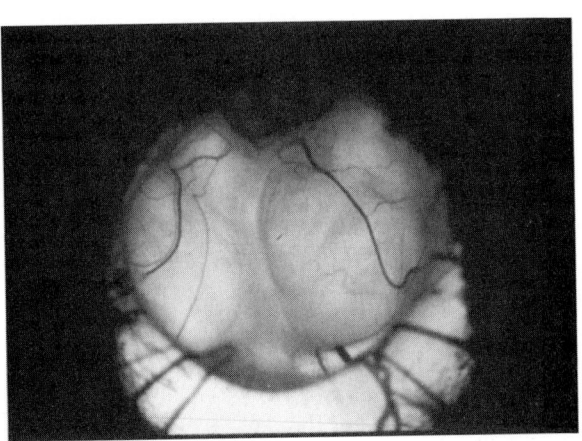

A   B

Figure 54-5   **A:** The inferior iris defect, which resembles a keyhole, does not by itself affect vision.
B: In this coloboma of the posterior pole of the fundus, the optic nerve is seen at the *top*. A defect as large as this will compromise vision, especially if fibers to the macula are deficient.

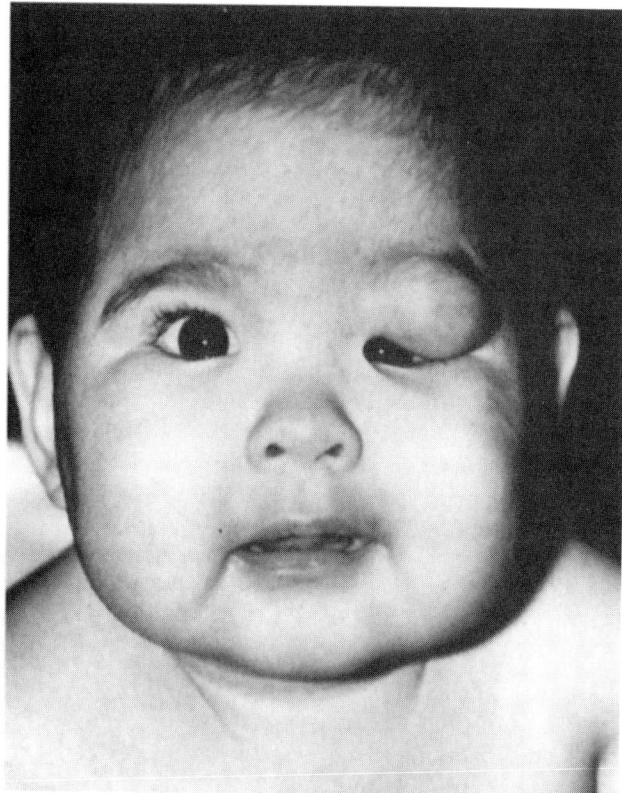

Figure 54-6 A hemangioma of the eyelid may not affect vision, even if it is large.

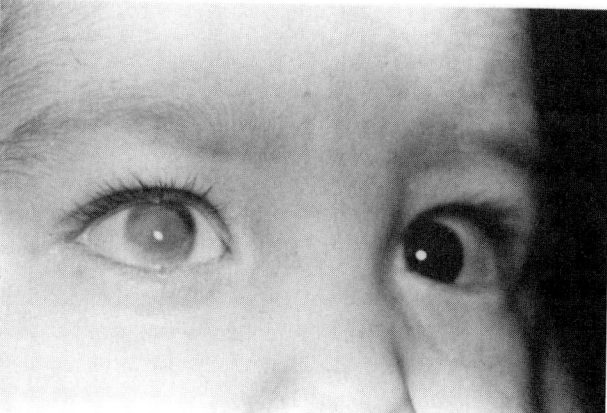

Figure 54-7 In this unilateral case of Peters anomaly, the cornea is opaque centrally and clear peripherally.

Corneal Opacities

A number of congenital anomalies can cause corneal opacities at birth. Congenital glaucoma and persistent fetal vasculature have been discussed and must always be ruled out; however, other diagnoses also should be considered.

Birth trauma, usually induced by a forceps placed at or near the eye during delivery, can cause opacities of the cornea. These opacities usually clear within a few days but may leave corneal scars. The corneal damage can leave scarring in the visual axis or induce significant refractive error, which can result in poor vision.

Sclerocornea is a nonprogressive, usually bilateral, anomaly in which the cornea is replaced by opaque sclera-like tissue. Central or total sclerocornea usually is devastating to a child's vision.

Dermoid tumors of the cornea may affect vision similarly if located centrally. A peripheral corneal tumor can affect vision by inducing refractive error. The tumor may be isolated or part of Goldenhar syndrome.

Peters anomaly, characterized by a central corneal opacity and variable iris-corneal or lens-corneal adhesions, is uncommon but a frequent cause of corneal transplant in infants (Fig. 54-7). The periphery of the cornea usually is normal. It has been associated with fetal alcohol syndrome. Corneal surgery often is reserved for bilateral cases because the prognosis for good vision following even initially successful corneal transplantation is guarded. In unilateral cases, poor vision is almost inevitable because of amblyopia in the affected eye. The amblyopia may result from a number of causes, including a possible graft rejection, significant refractive errors, recurrent opacities, and secondary glaucoma.

Aniridia

Aniridia, in which much or even the entire iris visible to the examiner is missing, can be compatible with good vision (Fig. 54-8). However, vision can be quite compromised by other ocular associations, including cataracts, peripheral corneal opacities, foveal hypoplasia, glaucoma and nystagmus. If the vision is quite reduced in infancy, nystagmus usually is found.

These children must be followed closely because some of the problems, such as glaucoma and central corneal pannus, may arise later in childhood. The glaucoma is particularly difficult to treat because it often is refractory to medical management. Surgical treatment of the glaucoma can induce a cataract because there may be no iris to protect the lens during and after the operation.

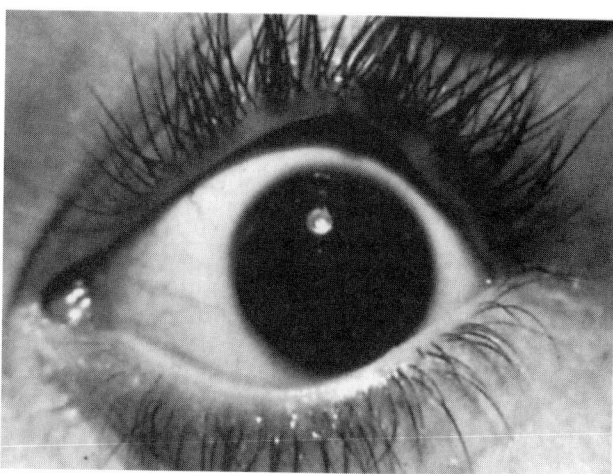

Figure 54-8 Aniridia is evident by the largely missing iris.

Wilms tumor has been reported to occur in up to one third of all sporadic aniridia cases. Therefore, periodic abdominal ultrasonography of children with aniridia is justified. An 11p deletion has been associated with the complex of aniridia, ambiguous genitalia, and mental retardation. Wilms tumor also may occur with this deletion.

Cataracts

Lens opacities in infants may be isolated or associated with a systemic condition. The morphology of infantile cataracts often is distinctive, which differentiates the infantile from other forms of cataract (Fig. 54-9). The location of the opacity within the baby's lens permits a classification of polar, zonular (or lamellar), nuclear, sutural, or total cataract.

About 25% of infantile cataracts are hereditary, especially if bilateral. Therefore, in the workup of infantile cataracts, it is important to examine the parents and siblings. If an asymptomatic cataract that resembles an infantile cataract is found in a family member, the etiology is attributed to heredity and an extensive workup can be avoided. The most frequent mode of inheritance is autosomal dominant with variable expressivity but almost complete penetrance.

Metabolic problems have been noted to cause cataracts in infants. Among these are hypoglycemia, mannosidosis, hypoparathyroidism, maternal diabetes, and galactosemia. Galactosemia, inherited as an autosomal-recessive trait, should be diagnosed on neonatal screening of urinary-reducing substances. But a child with a galactosemia cataract may still present to the pediatrician if he or she was born abroad or has the galactokinase deficiency type, which usually presents after 5 months of age. The cataract resembles a typical oil droplet. Early intervention with a lactose-free diet may reduce the lens level of dulcitol and reverse some or all of the lens opacity. Medications, such as corticosteroids, may cause cataracts but seldom in neonates.

A number of systemic conditions are associated with cataracts. In rubella, cataracts are characteristically total or near total opacities in a smaller than normal lens. In addition, the eye in rubella often is small, has abnormalities of the retinal pigment epithelium (noted as "salt and pepper" changes), and may be glaucomatous. Live rubella virus can survive in the lens for years. Therefore, at surgery, care should be taken with the lens aspirates, especially if personnel in the operating room may be pregnant. Cataracts have been described in other congenital infections, including herpes simplex and varicella.

The presence of a cataract should initiate an appropriate workup with the many causes and associations in mind. The list of other conditions associated with infantile cataract is very long and have been discussed elsewhere (13). To rule out familial cataract, both a family history, including any consanguinity, and an examination of the lenses of the parents and siblings should be undertaken. The history should include questions regarding low-birth weight, ROP, hypoglycemia, serum calcium abnormalities, syndromes, or any systemic disorders. A maternal history of infections while pregnant, diabetes, drug ingestion, and toxin exposure should be sought. Laboratory evaluation should include serum for glucose, blood urea nitrogen, calcium, phosphorus, galactose, and "TORCH" titers (toxoplasmosis, rubella, cytomegalovirus, varicella, and herpes simplex). A newly described fetal teratogen, lymphocytic choriomeningitis virus, may also be responsible for some cataracts in families exposed to rodents (14). Urine should be sent for amino acid levels and hematuria. Other tests should be ordered as indicated by the nonocular findings.

An ophthalmologist should judge if the cataract(s) are vision threatening. If so and if the child is less than about 4 months old in unilateral cases or 4 to 6 months old in bilateral cases, surgery is urgent to avoid legal blindness from deprivation amblyopia. The surgeon will remove the cataract using an intraocular suction-cutting device (lensectomy) and remove the anterior vitreous (vitrectomy) to avoid the postoperative development of posterior opacified membranes. It should be emphasized that many of the techniques used for cataract surgery in adults are not applicable to children. Compared with adults, a baby's sclera is more elastic, which can allow an eye to collapse during surgery; the lens itself is softer; the lens capsule is stiffer; and the vitreous is more

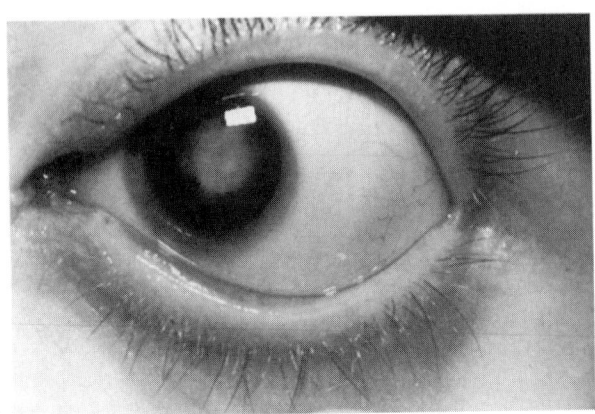
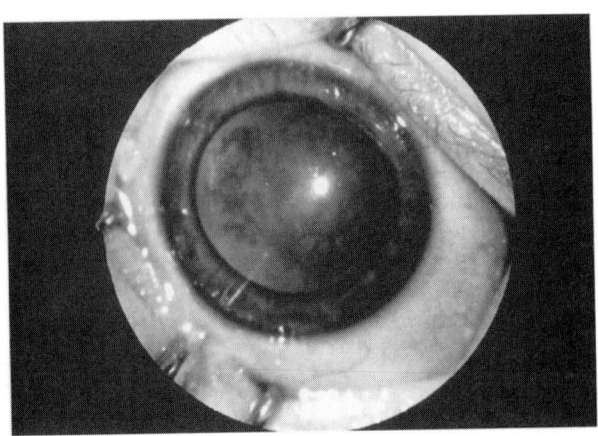

A   **B**

Figure 54-9   **A:** This zonular (or lamellar) lens opacity occupies a central area of the lens with small satellite opacities. **B:** The red retinal light reflex is disrupted by a cataract.

solid. For these reasons, special training and experience is desirable prior to operating on the cataracts of babies.

The end of the surgery is far from the end of the infant's visual rehabilitation. An optical device must be used to provide focus after loss of the lens. Spectacles could work, but few infants will keep spectacles in place while in the crib or toddling later. Intraocular lenses, as commonly utilized in adults, generally are not used in infants in developed countries. Current intraocular lenses have one fixed power (focal length), which the surgeon must choose at the time of surgery. The refractive power of the baby's eye will decrease up to eight diopters by 12 months of age and decrease even more later (15). Thus, a lens properly powered for a 1-month-old infant will make the baby highly myopic by 1 year of age. Conversely, a lens placed in an infant's eye with a power appropriate for later in life will leave him quite hyperopic in infancy, when good focus is crucial to developing vision and avoiding amblyopia. For these reasons and because of the concern of leaving a "plastic" lens in an eye for perhaps more than 80 years, intraocular lenses generally are not used by ophthalmologists in infants, unless under a special protocol. New studies are underway to investigate the use of different types of intraocular lenses in infants (16). In underdeveloped countries where no alternative exists, intraocular lenses are being implanted in infants.

The current method of choice to rehabilitate infant's eyes after cataract surgery is contact lenses. The parents are taught to insert the lens in the morning and remove it in the evening. Certain types of contact lenses may be left in overnight, but some ophthalmologists avoid them because of the increased risk of ocular infection. With contact lenses, the eye doctor can easily change the power as the eye grows and the hyperopic prescription decreases.

In all unilateral cases and some bilateral cases, the optical rehabilitation must be accompanied by occlusion of the better seeing eye to reverse amblyopia. Whether to occlude many hours a day to best improve visual acuity or fewer hours to maximize binocularity is a controversial subject (17).

Optic Nerve Hypoplasia

Optic nerve hypoplasia is a frequent cause of unsuspected visual loss. It results in a diminished number of axons in the optic nerve. The number can be low enough to cause legal or complete blindness, or sufficiently reduced vision to cause peripheral field loss with normal visual acuity. The appearance of the nerve can vary from a subtle reduction in size in one segment to a grossly small nerve surrounded by a pigment ring and yellow halo known as the "double ring sign" (Fig. 54-10). If bilateral and vision reducing, this entity often will cause nystagmus in infancy. If unilateral and vision reducing, it may present as a unilateral strabismus in the first 5 years of life. The diagnosis can be made with the direct ophthalmoscope by comparing features of the two optic nerves or with other instruments.

Although this disorder is associated with a number of other entities, two deserve the special interest of neonatologists. Fetal alcohol syndrome appears to be a major cause

of optic nerve hypoplasia. In Scandinavia, optic nerve hypoplasia was found to occur in almost half the cases of fetal alcohol syndrome (18). It may be the most frequently encountered ocular teratogenic event.

Another association with optic nerve hypoplasia is septooptic dysplasia (de Morsier syndrome), in which the child has a number of midline central nervous disorders, such as absence of the septum pellucidum, agenesis of the corpus callosum, and dysplasia of the third ventricle. Hypopituitarism, most commonly evident by dwarfism, occurs frequently. Hypothyroidism, neonatal hypoglycemia, sexual infantilism or precocity, hypoadrenalism, hyperprolactinemia, and diabetes insipidus also have been reported. This diagnosis, suggested by the presence of optic nerve hypoplasia, can lead to early treatment to modify these endocrinopathies. Therefore, all infants with bilateral optic nerve hypoplasia should have imaging to look for abnormalities of the septum pellucidum, corpus callosum, and third ventricle. Endocrine abnormalities are especially likely if the posterior pituitary is ectopic or bright on MRI or the infundibulum is absent (19). The same workup may also be warranted for unilateral hypoplasia of the optic nerve.

Strabismus

In the first few months after birth, infants usually display a variable intermittent exotropia. This divergence decreases with time, as visual acuity and binocularity develop, until the eyes are generally straight by 3 to 6 months of age. Even infants who develop infantile esotropia are initially exotropic after birth (20). Unless the eye position is constantly abnormal in the first 3 postnatal months, observation is appropriate until the baby is 4 months old. Babies with small or variable angles of esotropia may spontaneously improve (21). A constant unilateral strabismus may suggest an examination for the strabismus and the presence of amblyopia, possibly caused by an organic lesion such as retinoblastoma. Neonatologists and pediatricians should

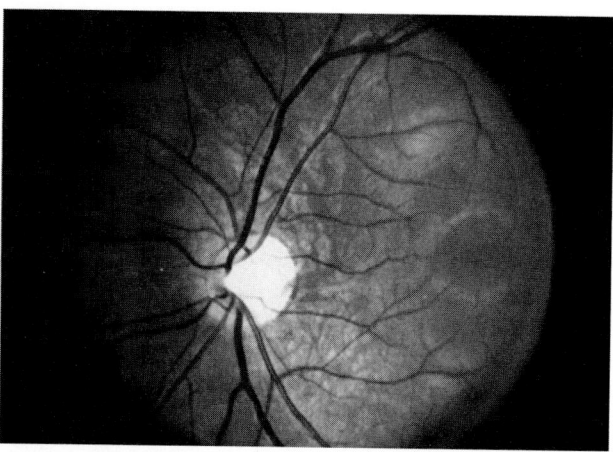

Figure 54-10 The diagnosis of optic nerve hypoplasia, although not extremely small, is revealed by the rings of white representing sclera and pigmentation representing retinal pigment epithelium.

can be intubated with silicone tubing. The tubes are removed in 3 to 6 months. A new and quite successful method of treating cases that fail an initial simple probing is to dilate the nasolacrimal duct with a balloon catheter (26).

Systemic Infections

Acquired Immunodeficiency Syndrome

Most infants with human immunodeficiency virus (HIV) infection are asymptomatic. Young HIV-positive children have been reported to have retinal vascular sheathing, optic atrophy, and dry eye syndrome, but these are unusual. They may have a mildly increased risk to develop strabismus and amblyopia. Opportunistic infections of the eye, such as ocular toxoplasmosis and cytomegalovirus retinitis, are less common than in adults and often develop later in childhood. Bacterial infections of the ocular adnexa may be more common than in adults (27).

Rubella

Ocular manifestations of congenital rubella syndrome include pigmentary retinopathy, cataracts, glaucoma, shallowing of the anterior chamber, anterior uveitis, microphthalmos, and corneal clouding with or without glaucoma. About half of all children with rubella will have ocular symptoms, which are bilateral in 70% of cases.

Rubella retinopathy, characterized by pigmentary changes secondary to damage to the retinal pigment epithelium, may be the most common ocular manifestation. The appearance has led to the term "salt and pepper" retinopathy. It usually is concentrated in the posterior pole and can be seen with the direct ophthalmoscope if the media are clear. Despite the appearance, visual acuity is seldom affected by the retinal involvement alone.

Cataracts occur in 30% to 75% of cases (Fig. 54-12). The morphology of the cataract is fairly typical, being either a total opacification or dense nuclear opacities. About half of

the cataracts develop and worsen after birth. Because live virus can still be cultured from the lens up to 3 years after birth, it is wise to exclude from the surgical suite during lensectomy any surgical personnel who could potentially be pregnant, even if rubella is only suspected. The surgeon must obsessively remove all the lens protein and much of the capsule. Residual lens particles in rubella can cause a severe inflammation that itself can lead to blindness.

Cytomegalovirus

The cytomegalovirus reaches the eye hematogenously. It essentially affects only the retina and choroid. The retinopathy presents as patches of retinal whitening, generally in the periphery. The borders of the lesions are indistinct, and retinal hemorrhages with vascular sheathing may be found. The retinopathy occurs in about 5% of infected infants either at birth or later.

Toxoplasmosis

Seventy-five percent of all patients with congenital toxoplasmosis will have ocular involvement. In 10%, the ocular lesions will be present with no evidence of infection in other organs. *Toxoplasma gondii* causes a focally destructive retinal lesion, with severe inflammation that also affects the choroid. The overlying vitreous becomes hazy with inflammatory cells and exudate. The infection often is unappreciated when it is acute, but is recognized later as a discrete yellow-white atrophic scar with hyperpigmented borders and smaller satellite scars (Fig. 54-13). The macula, which is involved in approximately 46% of cases, will reduce vision and may cause a secondary strabismus (28). This is the single major cause of pediatric blindness in South America and other regions of the world. Peripheral retinal lesions are generally asymptomatic. Although lesions may look quiescent, live organisms may survive within them for years. This is probably the cause of recurrent inflammation in children and adults.

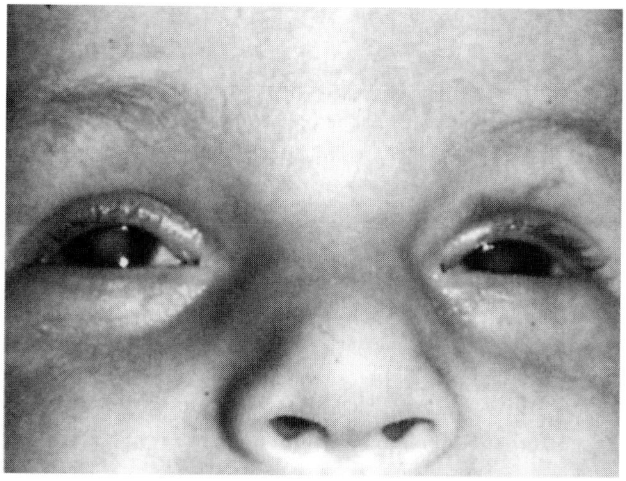

Figure 54-12 Rubella cataracts in a 7-week-old infant.

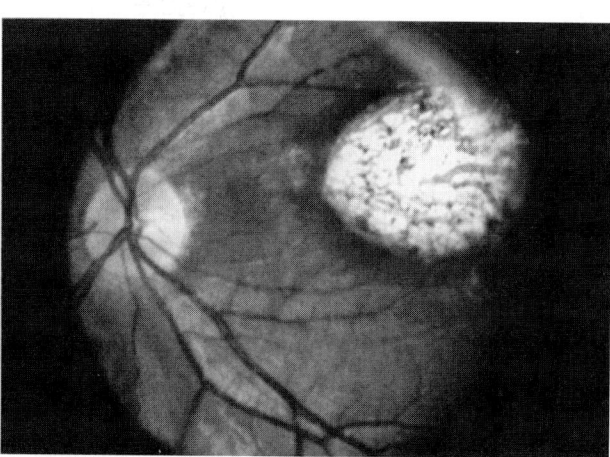

Figure 54-13 A large chorioretinal scar has destroyed the fovea in this child with toxoplasmosis.

Local treatment with subconjunctival corticosteroid injections usually is reserved for severely inflamed eyes in conjunction with systemic therapy, as with pyrimethamine and sulfonamides (29). Treatment may not prevent late recurrence.

TRAUMA

Birth Trauma

Any portion of the eye or adnexa can be injured in the birth process in up to 50% of difficult deliveries. The eyelids may be swollen and ecchymotic. Rarely, the eyelids may be everted totally, with the conjunctiva exposed to the environment. If everted, the exposed surfaces should be kept moist with lubricants until reversion is achieved spontaneously or with manual or surgical measures.

The eyeball may be subluxated, usually by delivery forceps. Orbital fractures and hemorrhages may be reported. The conjunctiva may have hemorrhages in at least 13% of births.

A cloudy cornea may result from forceps injury. It almost always is unilateral. Glaucoma, which also presents with a cloudy cornea, must be ruled out (see glaucoma section). Following birth, the cornea trauma often is accompanied by eyelid edema and ecchymosis, as well as conjunctival hemorrhage. Corneal examination may reveal linear opacities, usually oriented vertically, caused by Descemet membrane rupture. Although the overall corneal opacity clears within 2 weeks, healing of the Descemet membrane rupture can create a severe astigmatism or myopia, which can lead to amblyopia and strabismus.

A hyphema (hemorrhage within the anterior chamber) may result from forceps delivery, especially if residual fetal vessels are present. These hyphemas clear in a few weeks with no specific treatment. Vitreous hemorrhages, however, can cause amblyopia and severe myopia, especially if they persist for more than 3 weeks (30). They have been associated with protein C deficiency. Vitrectomy ultimately may be necessary if the hemorrhage does not spontaneously clear. Compression of the head in the course of a vaginal delivery often results in retinal hemorrhages (Fig. 54-14). The incidence has been reported to be 40% within 1 hour of birth, which decreases to 11% by 72 hours (31). They can occur in any area or layer of the retina. Retinal hemorrhages appear flame shaped in the nerve fiber layer, dot shaped in the inner plexiform layer, and dome shaped beneath the internal limiting membrane. The domes may look like Roth spots, with a white center surrounded by an elevated red hemorrhage. Even extensive hemorrhage will resorb within 6 weeks after birth. Rarely, hemorrhages in the fovea resorb slower, resulting in amblyopia in a normal-appearing eye.

Nonaccidental Trauma

Amniocentesis has been reported to damage eyes, usually in the midtrimester of pregnancy. Although most cases have

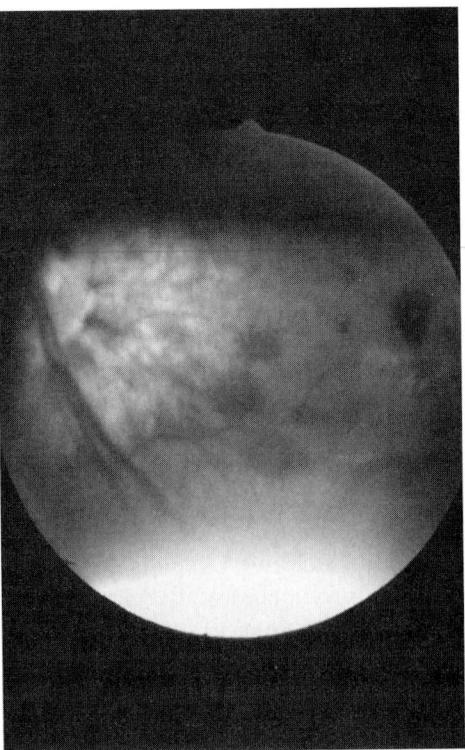

Figure 54-14   Retinal hemorrhages in an infant 1 day after birth.

resulted in blindness with frequent loss of the eye, early repair may salvage vision (32). The presence of segmental edema of the conjunctiva or corneal edema in a neonate should raise the possibility of an amniocentesis injury.

Child abuse often will affect the eye. There are many possible ocular effects of abuse, but intraocular hemorrhage is the most specific sign. Buys and colleagues (33) reported no retinal hemorrhages in a series of 75 children with documented accidental head trauma; however, their nonaccidental trauma cases all had retinal hemorrhages. Thus, any case of suspected child abuse should have an ophthalmology consultation (34).

A different sort of "child abuse" also should be considered. The self-abusing mother may affect ocular development. The most frequent teratogenic effect is probably optic nerve hypoplasia in fetal alcohol syndrome, as described previously. Cocaine abuse has been noted to affect the eye by inducing hypervascularization of the iris (Fig. 54-15) (35). The dilated and tortuous vessels, which run from the pupil to the periphery, usually are gone 1 week after birth. If these vessels are noted shortly after birth, a toxicity screen, which includes cocaine, is indicated.

PHOTOTHERAPY FOR HYPERBILIRUBINEMIA

Light has the ability to photooxidize bilirubin from the skin and subcutaneous tissue. Although useful to reduce hyperbilirubinemia, animal studies have shown that very intense light damages the outer retinal layers irreversibly. In human

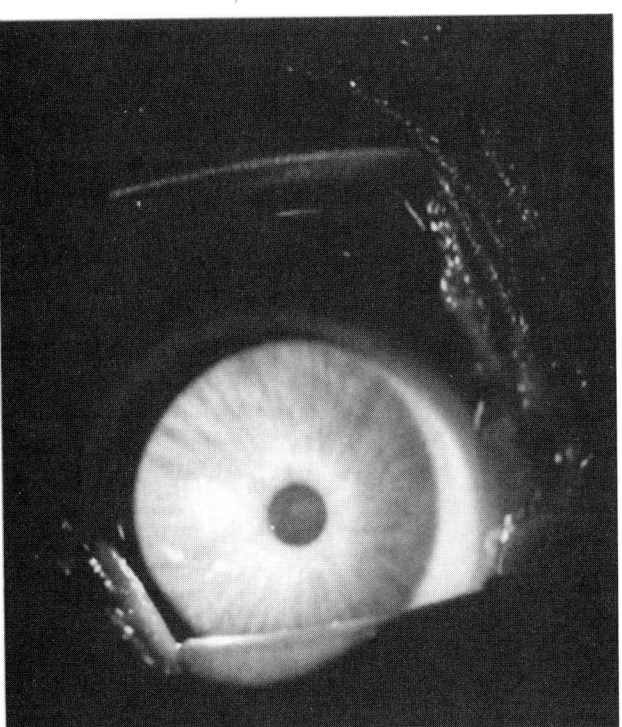

Figure 54-15 Tortuous and dilated iris vessels run peripherally to and from the pupil in this cocaine-intoxicated newborn.

infants, however, there has been little evidence of long-term damage from these lights (36). Nonetheless, it is prudent to occlude both eyes with an opaque mask or eye patches during this therapy. To prevent the possibility of amblyopia, both eyes should be occluded equally and securely.

RETINOPATHY OF PREMATURITY

In developed countries, ROP is one of the major causes of blindness in infants. This disorder of abnormal vascularization of the retina, formerly called retrolental fibroplasia, tends to occur in low-weight neonates often exposed to large amounts of oxygen. The more premature the child, the more likely is the disease. Of infants with a birth weight under 1 kg, 82% will develop ROP, with 9.3% progressing to vision-threatening sequelae (37). Of infants with a birth weight between 1 and 1.5 kg, 47% will develop ROP, and 2% will be in danger of losing vision.

Prevention

Infants who develop ROP often have other morbidities of the very preterm infant, as well as a complicated hospital course. This makes clinical correlations between ROP and other clinical entities difficult to interpret. Nonetheless, measures have been taken to prevent ROP. Oxygen use is often minimized because hyperoxemia has been shown to be associated or causative in many but not all studies (38). Although it has been recommended to keep arterial oxygen levels between 50 and 80 mm Hg, studies have not defini-

tively determined that this range is safe. Pulse oximetry can be useful, but when the saturation reaches 98% or 99%, the arterial oxygen tension can be very elevated, which may be conducive to the development of ROP. Monitoring the oxygen tension from the conjunctiva may prove to better control hyperoxemia (39).

A number of studies have investigated the use of vitamin E to prevent ROP. Despite early enthusiasm, especially in infants born beyond 27 postconceptional weeks (40), more recent studies have been less supportive. Any benefit from high doses of vitamin E has been overshadowed by the morbidity it has produced in clinical trials, including sepsis, necrotizing enterocolitis, intraventricular hemorrhage, and increased mortality (41–43).

The bright lights often found in nurseries have been considered as possibly contributing to ROP. Glass and associates (44) found less ROP in two nurseries utilizing lower ambient light levels. However, problems with controls, randomization, and masking in this study have left the topic of bright lights still in doubt. Studies in humans and animals have yielded conflicting results regarding the effects of bright lights on ROP (45). A subsequent prospective study of 409 neonates found that reducing ambient light exposure in the nursery did not affect the incidence of ROP (46).

Pathogenesis

The pathogenesis of ROP is thought to begin from a combination of prematurity, supplemental oxygen, and other possible factors causing vasoconstriction of immature retinal vessels. This vasoconstriction interrupts the normal developmental migration of the blood vessels from the optic nerve peripherally to the ora serrata. Vascular closure may cause localized ischemia. Endothelial proliferation adjacent to the vessels extends within the retina and into the vitreous. Fibrous and glial tissue grows, producing hemorrhage, traction, and retinal detachment.

Others feel that the neovascularization is induced by oxidative insult to spindle cells, resulting in gap junctions. If correct, antioxidants would help prevent the disease. The lack of strong evidence for the role of antioxidants, as tocopherol (vitamin E), has limited the acceptance of this theory.

Examination

The decision of which babies to screen is somewhat controversial. Most nurseries desire an examination of any infant with a birth weight below 1,250 g, whereas others use a weight as high as 1,600 g. A University of Pittsburgh study found that above a birth weight of 1,500 g, ROP developed only in infants exposed to at least 6 weeks of continuous oxygen (47).

The examination should be performed as soon as the media is clear enough to permit ophthalmoscopy and the neonate can tolerate the "trauma" of a retinal examination. The use of proper dilating eyedrops was discussed previously.

A number of centers advise the first examination be performed 6 weeks after birth. Because vision-threatening ROP has been shown to arise at 33 to 41 weeks postconception, it would be wise to time the first examination at approximately 32 weeks, if possible. Larger preterm newborns may need their first examination sooner after birth than smaller ones.

The subsequent examinations should be conducted as indicated by the findings of the first examination. If no ROP is found but the retina is still being vascularized, the examination should be repeated every 1 to 2 weeks. If ROP is found, the examinations should be repeated weekly. If "plus disease" (tortuosity and dilation of the blood vessels in the posterior pole of the fundus) is noted, the disease may be progressing faster, justifying a repeat evaluation in 3 to 4 days. The examinations are continued until the retinal vascularization has reached zone III (see following), the threshold for treatment (see following) is achieved, or the disease has definitely regressed. There are some rare cases in which regression was followed by reactivation.

Classification

The internationally established classification of acute ROP is meant to characterize accurately the extent of the disorder in a particular eye. Three dimensions or criteria are used—stage, location (anterior to posterior), and extent.

The staging scheme is presented in Table 54-2. In stage 1, the normal progression of vascularization of the retina toward the periphery is halted at a thin demarcation line found by an abrupt change in color of the retina. The line divides the vascularized from the nonvascularized retina. Importantly, the vessels multibranch or arcade at the line. The latter appearance differentiates early ROP from normal vascularization because in the normal state, the advancing vessels usually bifurcate and do not break into an arcade. In stage 2, the demarcation line extends up out of the retinal plane toward the vitreous. This ridge may change color from white or tan to red. In stage 3, extraretinal fibrovascular tissue grows either on the top of the ridge, yielding a ragged appearance, or just posterior. As it grows, it reaches into the vitreous (Fig. 54-16). Stage 4 is reached when the retina begins to detach from traction exerted by the extraretinal fibrovascular tissue condensing (analogous to a purse string) or, less commonly, from serous fluid elevating

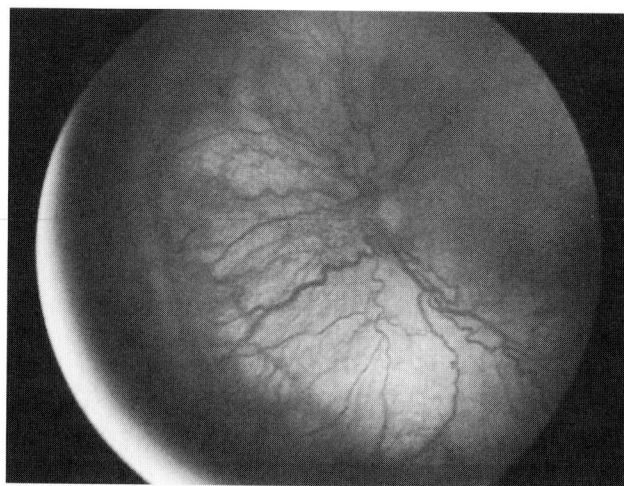

Figure 54-16 In stage 3 retinopathy of prematurity, laser or cryotherapy is applied when all criteria are met. Note the dilation and tortuosity of the retinal vessels in "plus disease."

the retina. The macula still is spared from detachment in stage 4A, and the visual prognosis is still hopeful. The visual prognosis decreases markedly in stage 4B as the macula detaches. In stage 5, the retinal detachment is total and shaped like a funnel or tulip. In describing the stage, one also should indicate if "plus disease" is present. "Plus disease" is the presence of tortuosity and dilation of the blood vessels in the posterior pole of the fundus. These posterior vascular changes usually indicate that an arteriovenous shunt is occurring in the extraretinal fibrovascular tissue on top of the ridge. "Plus disease" is a worse prognostic sign and may indicate that the disease is progressing faster.

The location is described in zones (Fig. 54-17). Zone I, the most posterior, is a circle centered on the optic nerve, with a radius twice the distance from the optic nerve to the fovea. Zone II extends from the edge of zone I all the way to the ora serrata on the nasal side and, on the temporal side, to the anatomic equator. This leaves zone III, which is a peripheral crescent on the temporal side. ROP in zone I is potentially the most dangerous, whereas disease in zone III is seldom of any concern. The circumferential extent of the disease is noted in clock hours, with an entire eye composed of 12 clock hours. One clock hour equals 30 degrees.

This classification pertains to the acute changes of ROP. There also are cicatricial changes that should be considered. Classification of the cicatricial changes is not yet universally accepted. Usually these changes arise in eyes that have reached acute stage 3 but did not progress to a significant retinal detachment. In these eyes, the vessels are drawn to the lateral side by cicatrization distorting the optic nerve and dragging the fovea laterally (Fig. 54-18). A retinal fold may form. These developments often reduce vision significantly.

Treatment

Many eyes that develop ROP will improve without treatment to the point that few or no remnants of the disorder are evident later. The point at which the prognosis for

TABLE 54-2
STAGES OF RETINOPATHY OF PREMATURITY

Stage	Character
1	Demarcation line
2	Ridge
3	Extraretinal fibrovascular proliferation
4A	Partial retinal detachment, macula still attached
4B	Partial retinal detachment, macula detached
5	Total retinal detachment
Plus	Dilation and tortuosity of posterior retinal vessels

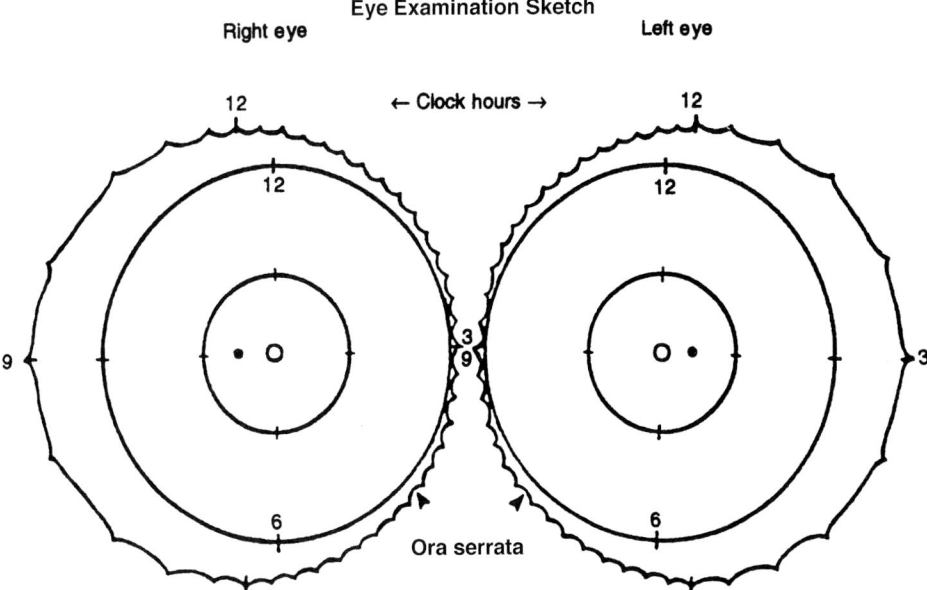

Figure 54-17 The scheme of zones and clock hours in the classification of acute retinopathy of prematurity.

regression is below 50% is considered the threshold level for treatment. The multicenter trial of cryotherapy defined the threshold level as stage 3 in five adjacent or eight cumulative clock hours in combination with "plus disease" (48). This definition has proven appropriate for disease in zone II. But the results of treatment using this threshold have not been as favorable for disease in zone I. It is very likely that a lower threshold for treatment will be established for zone I disease in the next few years.

The rationale behind this treatment is to ablate the peripheral avascular retina for 360 degrees in the affected eye(s). This approach has been shown in numerous studies to improve diabetic retinopathy, presumably by reducing or eliminating the signal from the ischemic or avascular tissue to the retina to produce neovascular vessels. Initially, cryotherapy was used to destroy areas of the peripheral retina by freezing. Cryotherapy had a number of both triv-

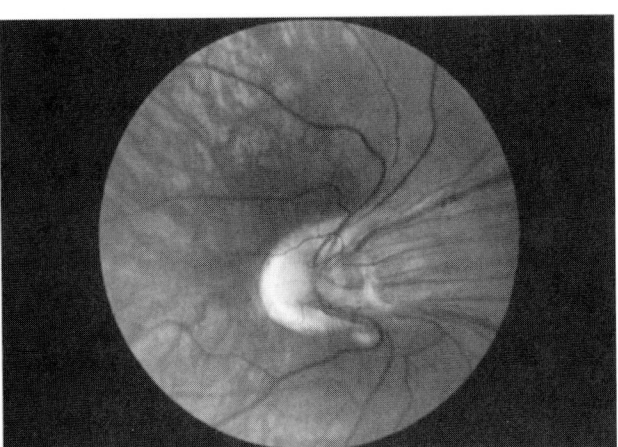

Figure 54-18 The macula is dragged laterally amidst the retinal folds in cicatricial retinopathy of prematurity.

ial and important complications, including subconjunctival hematoma, vitreous hemorrhage, bradycardia or dysrhythmia, and conjunctival laceration.

Currently, cryotherapy has been replaced for most applications by the use of lasers, which usually are mounted on an indirect ophthalmoscope worn on the head of the surgeon (49). There are some specific instances in which cryotherapy is still the method of choice. However, laser therapy has a number of advantages over cryotreatment. Laser surgery can be performed in the nursery with mild sedation and only topical anesthesia because it probably causes less pain than cryotherapy. The treatment session is faster with laser. The eyelids, conjunctiva, and cornea look normal after laser, whereas, after cryotherapy, they easily become edematous and inflamed. The latter consideration often is important to parents concerned about the fate of their premature child. In some studies, laser therapy was reported to produce better visual and structural results than cryotherapy (50). With laser, the incidence of subconjunctival hematoma, conjunctival laceration, and other complications seen with cryotherapy has been reduced to almost zero. However, cataracts have been reported to occur after laser treatment in less than 1% of cases.

The long-term beneficial effects demonstrated by cryotherapy were evaluated in a large multicenter trial. The frequency of the potentially blinding ROP sequelae of retinal detachment and retinal fold was reduced by half after cryotherapy (51). At about 6 years of age, poor visual acuity (20/200 or worse) was found in 62% of untreated eyes compared with 47% of treated eyes (52). Despite the destruction of parts of the peripheral retina by cryotherapy, long-term follow-up has found only a six-degree loss of peripheral visual field (53). Whether their infant is treated with laser or cryotherapy, the parents must be informed that although the treatment will reduce the possibility of blindness, blindness may still result despite treatment. Too often, parents assume that, with treatment, blindness definitely will be avoided.

If retinal detachment occurs, all is not lost. Modern vitreoretinal surgery can reattach a detached retina with ROP more than 30% of the time. Once the macula detaches, however, the visual prognosis decreases markedly, even if the retina is reattached successfully. For stage 4A, visual acuity results as good as 20/20 have been reported with the macula still attached. Stage 4B results have been in the 20/80 to 20/200 range. With a total detachment (stage 5), the results decrease considerably to the 20/600 to 20/1600 range or even lower (54). This low level of vision may allow the child to ambulate independently and certainly is better than the blindness that would occur without surgery.

Long-Term Problems

Aside from the problems of poor vision from a detached retina or retinal folds, there are other sequelae that can arise in the eyes of infants with regressed ROP. Even with an attached retina and intact macula, children with regressed ROP have been shown to be more susceptible to a number of visual disorders, including myopia, amblyopia, strabismus, and nystagmus. Children who develop cicatricial retinal changes, even with good vision, are at risk for future retinal problems, including detachment. Therefore, these children should be examined at least annually throughout their life, or at least until they are mature and literate enough to rule out amblyopia and strabismus.

COMMON DIFFERENTIAL DIAGNOSTIC PROBLEMS

Leukocoria

When faced with an infant with a white pupil or unusual retinal light reflex, the neonatologist or pediatrician should consider the differential diagnosis and begin a workup (Fig. 54-19). The first obligation is to rule out the potentially fatal retinoblastoma, even in a neonate (Fig. 54-20). The most common lesions that may, to some extent, simulate a retinoblastoma by presenting with leukocoria in infancy include cataract, persistent fetal vasculature, Coats disease, large retinal coloboma, and retinal detachment resulting from ROP. Toxocariasis is not a disease of infants. Coats disease is caused by anomalous telangiectatic retinal vessels that cause massive exudation and retinal detachment. It is important to realize that behind an opaque cataract can lie other problems, such as retinal detachment or a mass.

The history should reveal the presence of prematurity, oxygen use, illnesses during pregnancy (such as rubella, toxoplasmosis, and cytomegalovirus), possible child abuse,

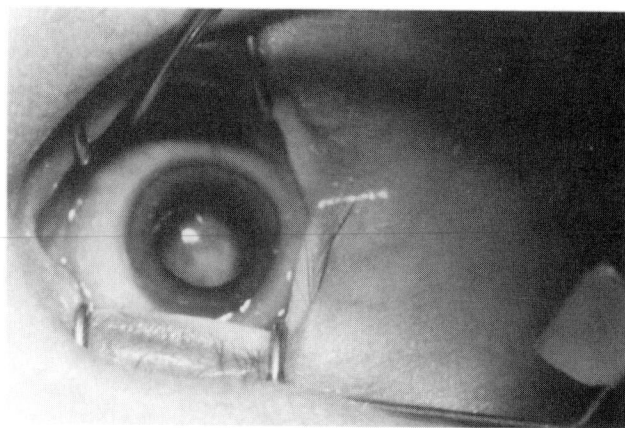

Figure 54-19 Bilateral leukocoria was found in this neonate. A family history of Norrie disease simplified the diagnosis.

or traumatic birth. The nonocular history may help. Deafness suggests the possibility of rubella or Norrie disease (cataract with retinal detachment). Toxoplasmosis or tuberous sclerosis may present with seizures. Incontinentia pigmenti or tuberous sclerosis may have skin lesions. Bilateral leukocoria would favor the diagnoses of ROP, Norrie disease, child abuse, and retinal dysplasias. Unilateral leukocoria is more consistent with Coats disease, persistent fetal vasculature, and intraocular foreign body. Although Norrie and Coats diseases are more common in males, incontinentia pigmenti is more frequent in females.

The examination may actually begin with the eyes of the parents. Parents have been found to have an asymptomatic congenital cataract, regressed retinoblastoma, unappreciated coloboma, and findings of familial exudative retinopathy, which closely resembles ROP. Any of these findings in a parent, who usually cooperates better in the examination, generally establishes the diagnosis for the baby. Examination of the child may reveal microphthalmos, which is consistent with coloboma or persistent fetal vasculature. The level of the opacity may be evident with a light or portable slit lamp. If there is a defect in the inferior iris, coloboma should be considered. Lens opacity, of course, constitutes a cataract, but

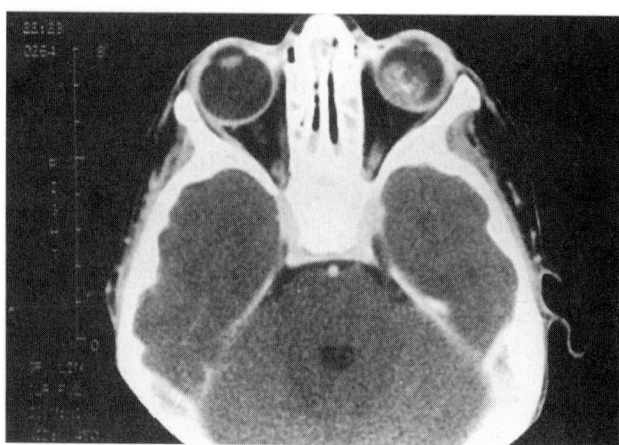

Figure 54-20 A calcified intraocular mass in an infant with retinoblastoma.

additional examinations, perhaps with ultrasound or radiologic tests, may reveal pathology in the vitreous or retina. A detailed retinal examination is crucial, if the media are sufficiently clear, to diagnose many entities that present with leukocoria.

Cloudy Cornea

Profound amblyopia will result from an opacified cornea, especially if it is unilateral. Although some opacities clear with time, others remain. The history, associated findings, and examination will clarify the prognosis.

The history should include illnesses during pregnancy to rule out rubella, syphilis, and herpes, which can cause keratitis. Delivery by forceps of a large neonate suggests birth trauma (Fig. 54-21). Conjunctival hemorrhages suggest a traumatic etiology. The presence of conjunctival inflammation implies infection or pupillary block glaucoma as an etiology.

Systemic physical abnormalities may imply an etiology as an umbilic hernia suggests glaucoma associated with Rieger syndrome. Glaucoma also is suggested by a history of photosensitivity and tearing. Family history is important. On examination, the eyelids may reveal evidence of phakomatoses as the angiomatosis of Sturge-Weber syndrome or a neurofibroma.

Most important is the corneal examination. The corneal diameter should be measured as accurately as possible. An enlarged cornea strongly indicates glaucoma, whereas a small opacified cornea may result from sclerocornea, microphthalmos, trisomy 13, or rubella. Striae in the cornea are often helpful. Horizontally oriented striae are compatible with glaucoma, whereas vertical or oblique ones often result from birth trauma. A mass overlying the cornea may be a dermoid tumor.

Measurement of the intraocular pressure in these cases often is imperative to rule in glaucoma. Examination of the iris may reveal adhesions to the cornea. This can result from trauma or may indicate a mesodermal dysgenesis

syndrome. This syndrome encompasses a number of developmental disorders, such as Peters anomaly—the most frequent reason to perform corneal transplants in infants. A cataractous lens behind an opacified cornea may be caused by rubella, birth trauma, Lowe syndrome, or mesodermal dysgenesis. If the eye and intraocular pressure are otherwise normal, the opacified cornea may result from a hereditary corneal dystrophy.

REFERENCES

1. Rakic P. Development of visual centers in the primate brain depends on binocular competition before birth. *Science* 1981;214: 928–931.
2. Isenberg SJ, Neumann D, Cheong PY, et al. Growth of the internal and external eye in term and preterm infants. *Ophthalmology* 1995;102:827–830.
3. Snir M, Axer-Siegel R, Bourla D, et al. Tactile corneal reflex development in full-term babies. *Ophthalmology* 2002;109:526–529.
4. Hittner HM, Hirsch NJ, Rudolph AJ. Assessment of gestational age by examination of the anterior vascular capsule of the lens. *J Pediatr* 1977;91:455–458.
5. Isenberg SJ. Clinical application of the pupil examination in neonates. *J Pediatr* 1991;118:650–652.
6. Isenberg SJ. Macular development in the premature infant. *Am J Ophthalmol* 1986;101:74–80.
7. Isenberg SJ, Everett S. Cardiovascular effect of mydriatics in low-birth-weight infants. *J Pediatr* 1984;105:111–112.
8. Isenberg SJ, Abrams C, Hyman PE. Effect of cyclopentolate eyedrops on gastric secretory function in pre-term infants. *Ophthalmology* 1985;92:698–700.
9. Clarke WN, Hodges E, Noel LP, et al. The oculocardiac reflex during ophthalmoscopy in premature infants. *Am J Ophthalmol* 1985; 99:649–651.
10. Isenberg SJ, Apt L, McCarty JA, et al. Development of tearing in preterm and term neonates. *Arch Ophthalmol* 1998;116:773–776.
11. Goldberg MF. Persistent fetal vasculature (PFV): an integrated interpretation of signs and symptoms associated with persistent hyperplastic primary vitreous (PHPV). LIV Edward Jackson Memorial Lecture. *Am J Ophthalmol* 1997;124:587–626.
12. Hastings MM, Milot J, Barsoum-Homsy M, et al. Recombinant interferon alfa-2b in the treatment of vision-threatening capillary hemangiomas in childhood. *J AAPOS* 1997;1:226–230.
13. Hiles DA, Kilty LA. Disorders of the lens. In: Isenberg SJ, ed. *The eye in infancy,* 2nd ed. St. Louis: Mosby-Year Book, 1994:336–373.
14. Barton LL, Mets MB, Beauchamp CL. Lymphocytic choriomeningitis virus: emerging fetal teratogen. *Am J Obstet Gynecol* 2002; 187:1715–1716.
15. Neumann D, Weissman BA, Isenberg SJ, et al. The effectiveness of daily wear contact lenses for the correction of infantile aphakia. *Arch Ophthalmol* 1993;111:927–930.
16. Lambert SR, Lynn M, Drews-Botsch C, et al. A comparison of grating visual acuity, strabismus, and reoperation outcomes among children with aphakia and pseudophakia after unilateral cataract surgery during the first six months of life. *J AAPOS* 2001;5:70–75.
17. Wright KW. Pediatric cataracts. *Curr Opin Ophthalmol* 1997;8:50–55.
18. Stromland K. Ocular abnormalities in the fetal alcohol syndrome. *Acta Ophthalmol Suppl* 1985;171:1–50.
19. Phillips PH, Spear C, Brodsky MC. Magnetic resonance diagnosis of congenital hypopituitarism in children with optic nerve hypoplasia. *J AAPOS* 2001;5:275–280.
20. Archer SM, Sondhi N, Helveston EM. Strabismus in infancy. *Ophthalmology* 1989;96:133–137.
21. Birch E, Stager D, Wright K, et al, for the Pediatric Eye Disease Investigator Group. The natural history of infantile esotropia during the first six months of life. *J AAPOS* 1998;2:325–328.
22. Hammerschlag MR, Cummings C, Roblin PM, et al. Efficacy of neonatal ocular prophylaxis for the prevention of chlamydial and gonococcal conjunctivitis. *N Engl J Med* 1989;320:769–772.
23. Isenberg SJ, Apt L, Yoshimori R, et al. Povidone-iodine for ophthalmia neonatorum prophylaxis. *Am J Ophthalmol* 1994;118: 701–706.

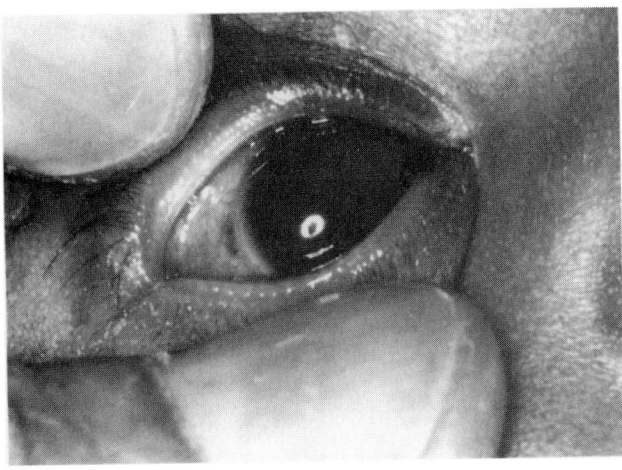

Figure 54-21 One week after birth, the corneal opacity caused by a forceps injury is fading.

24. Isenberg SJ, Apt L, Wood M. A clinical trial of povidone-iodine as prophylaxis against ophthalmia neonatorum. *N Engl J Med* 1995; 332:562–566.

25. Petersen RA, Robb RM. The natural course of congenital obstruction of the nasolacrimal duct. *J Pediatr Ophthalmol Strabismus* 1978;15:246–250.

26. Lueder GT. Balloon catheter dilation for treatment of persistent nasolacrimal duct obstruction. *Am J Ophthalmol* 2002:133:337–340.

27. Dennehy PJ, Warman R, Flynn JT, et al. Ocular manifestations in pediatric patients with acquired immunodeficiency syndrome. *Arch Ophthalmol* 1989;107:978–982.

28. Hogan MJ, Kimura SJ, O'Connor GR. Ocular toxoplasmosis. *Arch Ophthalmol* 1964;72:592–600.

29. Engstrom RE Jr, Holland GN, Nussenblatt RB, et al. Current practices in the management of ocular toxoplasmosis. *Am J Ophthalmol* 1991;111:601–610.

30. Mohney BG. Axial myopia associated with dense vitreous hemorrhage of the neonate. *J AAPOS* 2002;6:348–353.

31. Jain IS, Singh YP, Grupta SL, et al. Ocular hazards during birth. *J Pediatr Ophthalmol Strabismus* 1980;17:14–16.

32. Naylor G, Roper JP, Willshaw HE. Ophthalmic complications of amniocentesis. *Eye* 1990;4:845–849.

33. Buys YM, Levin AV, Enzenauer RW, et al. Retinal findings after head trauma in infants and young children. *Ophthalmology* 1992; 99:1718–1723.

34. Morad Y, Kim YM, Armstrong DC, et al. Correlation between retinal abnormalities and intracranial abnormalities in the shaken baby syndrome. *Am J Ophthalmol* 2002;134:354–359.

35. Isenberg SJ, Spierer A, Inkelis SH. Ocular signs of cocaine intoxication in neonates. *Am J Ophthalmol* 1987;103:211–214.

36. Kalina RE, Forrest GL. Ocular hazards of phototherapy for hyperbilirubinemia. *J Pediatr Ophthalmol* 1971;8:116.

37. Palmer EA, Flynn JT, Hardy RJ, et al, for the Cryotherapy for Retinopathy of Prematurity Cooperative Group. Incidence and early course of retinopathy of prematurity. *Ophthalmology* 1991; 98:1628–1640.

38. Flynn JT, Bancalari E, Snyder ES, et al. A cohort study of transcutaneous oxygen tension and the incidence and severity of retinopathy of prematurity. *N Engl J Med* 1992;326:1050–1054.

39. Isenberg SJ, Neumann D, Fink S, et al. Continuous oxygen monitoring of the conjunctiva in neonates. *J Perinatol* 2002;22:46–49.

40. Phelps DL. Vitamin E and retinopathy of prematurity. In: Silverman WA, Flynn JT, eds. *Contemporary issues in fetal and neonatal medicine 2: retinopathy of prematurity.* Boston: Blackwell, 1985:181–205.

41. Johnson L, Bowen FW Jr, Abassi S, et al. Relationship of prolonged pharmacologic serum levels of vitamin E to incidence of sepsis and necrotizing enterocolitis in infants with birth weights 1,500 grams or less. *Pediatrics* 1985;75:619–638.

42. Martone WJ, Williams WW, Mortensen ML, et al. Illness with fatalities in premature infants: association with an intravenous vitamin E preparation, E-Ferol. *Pediatrics* 1986;78:591–600.

43. Phelps DL, Rosenbaum AL, Isenberg SJ, et al. Tocopherol efficacy and safety for preventing retinopathy of prematurity: a randomized, controlled, double-masked trial. *Pediatrics* 1987;79: 489–500.

44. Glass P, Avery GB, Subramanian KN, et al. Effect of bright light in the hospital nursery on the incidence of retinopathy of prematurity. *N Engl J Med* 1985;313:401–404.

45. Ackerman B, Sherwonit E, Williams J. Reduced incidental light exposure: effect on the development of retinopathy of prematurity in low birth weight infants. *Pediatrics* 1989;83:958–962.

46. Reynolds JD, Hardy RJ, Kennedy KA, et al, for the Light Reduction in Retinopathy of Prematurity (LIGHT-ROP) Cooperative Group. Lack of efficacy of light reduction in preventing retinopathy of prematurity. *N Engl J Med* 1998;338:1572–1576.

47. Brown DR, Biglan AW, Stretavsky MAM. Screening criteria for the detection of retinopathy of prematurity in patients in a neonatal intensive care unit. *J Pediatr Ophthalmol Strabismus* 1987;24:212–215.

48. Cryotherapy for Retinopathy of Prematurity Cooperative Group. Multicenter trial of cryotherapy for retinopathy of prematurity: Preliminary results. *Arch Ophthalmol* 1988;106:471–479.

49. Hunter DG, Repka MX. Diode laser photocoagulation for threshold retinopathy of prematurity. A randomized study. *Ophthalmology* 1993;100:238–244.

50. Ng EY, Connolly BP, McNamara JA, et al. A comparison of laser photocoagulation with cryotherapy for threshold retinopathy of prematurity at 10 years: part 1. Visual function and structural outcome. *Ophthalmology* 2002;109:928–934.

51. Cryotherapy for Retinopathy of Prematurity Cooperative Group. Multicenter trial of cryotherapy for retinopathy of prematurity. One-year outcome—structure and function. *Arch Ophthalmol* 1990;108:1408–1416.

52. Cryotherapy for Retinopathy of Prematurity Cooperative Group. Multicenter trial of cryotherapy for retinopathy of prematurity: Snellen acuity and structural outcome at $5^1/_2$ years after randomization. *Arch Ophthalmol* 1996;114:417–424.

53. Quinn GR, Dobson V, Hardy RJ, et al, for the CRYO-Retinopathy of Prematurity Cooperative Group. Visual fields measured with double-arc perimetry in eyes with threshold retinopathy of prematurity from the cryotherapy for retinopathy of prematurity trial. *Ophthalmology* 1996;103:1432–1437.

54. Maguire AM, Trese MT. Visual results of lens-sparing vitreoretinal surgery in infants. *J Pediatr Ophthalmol Strabismus* 1993;30:28–32.

Dermatologic Conditions

James G. H. Dinulos Gary L. Darmstadt

INTRODUCTION

As an organ, the skin provides essential functions for survival and can be an indicator of overall health. At no other time in life are these roles more evident than in a newborn infant who is adjusting to life outside the uterus. Abnormalities in the skin may be extremely distressing to parents and it is important for medical providers to be able to distinguish a worrisome from a banal newborn skin disorder. To assist in this process, this chapter reviews basics of skin structure and development, techniques of skin examination and recognition and management of important newborn skin disorders.

SKIN DEVELOPMENT, STRUCTURE, AND FUNCTION

The skin is composed of three anatomic layers, epidermis, dermis, and fat; and three adnexal structures, hair, nails, and glands. The formation of these skin layers and structures from primitive embryonic tissues occurs in a predicable and sequential manner. Most structural development is complete by 24 weeks of gestation, however, complete functional activity of the skin, such as epidermal barrier development, is not achieved until after birth (1).

The epidermis plays critical functions in fluid homeostasis and in protection from infections, toxins, and adverse effects of ultraviolet radiation (2). The outermost layer, the stratum corneum, provides most of this protection. Lamellar bilayers composed of hydrophobic lipids, principally fatty acids, cholesterol and ceramides, are "cemented" between multiple layers of tightly knit protein- and keratin-rich cornified cells (2,3). These lipids and proteins protect by creating an impermeable barrier and by providing an acidic and xeric environment that impedes microbial invasion. The epidermis is not merely a static barrier, however, as keratinocytes actively produce antibacterial products, including cytokines, lipid breakdown products and cationic antimicrobial peptides that provide an important link between the innate and adaptive immune systems (4,5).

Prematurity and a number of skin disorders disrupt epidermal permeability barrier function and may allow for massive transepidermal water loss (TEWL) (6). Premature infants can lose up to 30% of their total body weight in 24 hours, as their rate of TEWL may be 10 to 15 times greater than in a full-term infant (7). Such significant fluid losses can cause hypotension, electrolyte imbalance, increased caloric demands, and may contribute to intraventricular hemorrhage (IVH) and necrotizing enterocolitis. Epidermal barrier development is accelerated by exposure to the dry, extra-uterine environment (7,8). This barrier maturation typically takes 2 to 4 weeks and may be delayed for 8 weeks in extremely premature infants. Thus, premature infants are particularly vulnerable to infections and toxins, particularly during the first week of life when approximately two thirds of all neonatal deaths worldwide occur.

During development, skin and its structures are thought to migrate along the "lines of Blaschko" (9). Most authorities believe that Blaschko lines are an expression of epidermal and not dermal migration. Conditions that follow these lines are thought to result from a single postzygotic mutation of a single clone of cells or from a mutation on the X chromosome that is brought about by X-inactivation (10). Incontinentia pigmenti and linear epidermal nevi are two examples of conditions that occur along lines of Blaschko.

Newborn skin may look and feel different depending on the newborn's gestational age. Premature infants less than 32 weeks estimated gestational age (EGA), have skin that appears thin and transparent. Infants born after 40 weeks EGA have thicker skin with wrinkles and peeling. Most term infants have a pasty substance on their skin, referred to as vernix caseosa. Vernix caseosa is a substance composed of sloughed corneocytes, shed lanugo hair and lipids (11). The role of this substance is not fully understood, although it is thought to assist in passage through the birth canal and have an important role in skin hydration and innate immune defense (12). Most premature and postmature infants have little vernix.

Skin adnexal structures (hair, nails, and glands) can provide valuable clues to the overall well-being of the newborn. Most infants are born with hair on the scalp and some have hair on the body. Typically, hair in the newborn

TABLE 55-1

STEPS IN A NEWBORN SKIN EXAMINATION

1. Assess skin integrity.
   a. Skin breakdown
   b. Texture
   c. Hydration
   d. Swelling
2. Determine primary and secondary skin lesions (See Table 2).
3. Determine the location, configuration and distribution of the skin lesions.
4. Evaluate mucous membranes, palms, soles, hair and nails.
5. If there is a rash, determine whether it is fixed or evolving.
6. Develop a differential diagnosis.
7. Perform appropriate diagnostic tests.
8. Consider referral to a specialist.

undergoes "physiologic" shedding at approximately 3 months of age.

EXAMINATION OF NEWBORN SKIN

Newborns should be examined with an adequate light source, preferably natural sunlight. Side-lighting and magnification are helpful to accentuate surface topography. Handheld devices applied directly to the skin such as a dermatoscope can be helpful, especially to examine pigmented lesions. The environment should be kept warm to minimize reactive vascular changes as a result of temperature. Table 55-1 summarizes the steps of a newborn skin examination and an approach to dermatological diagnosis. Table 55-2 lists primary lesions, secondary lesions, special configurations and distributions of skin lesions.

SCALY RASHES

Rashes are common in the first month of life, affecting 80% of newborns (13). During the first week of life, the vast majority of term and postterm infants will have superficial peeling or desquamation of skin; it rarely occurs in those under 35 weeks of gestation. Deeper skin peeling that results in denuded skin or continuous peeling for longer than 1 week are potential warning signs of an underlying systemic process. Scales should be examined for quality (firm, adherent), color (white, yellow), and associated inflammation (redness), features which help in identification of a variety of skin diseases.

Inflammatory Rashes

Diaper Dermatitis

Diaper dermatitis is common in newborns. It is characterized by a pink to red scaly rash localized to the diaper area and is caused by prolonged exposure to urine and stool combined with the frictional forces of the diaper. This irri-

tant contact dermatitis should be distinguished from numerous other dermatological conditions affecting the diaper area. Irritant contact dermatitis affects skin contacting the diaper, such as the pubis, penis, labia majora, scrotum, upper thighs, and buttocks. Generally, the creases are spared. Continued irritant exposure may produce painful fissures and ulcerations (Jacquet's erosive dermatitis), especially in premature infants (Fig. 55-1). Involved skin is susceptible to secondary infection, primarily with Candida albicans, Staphylococcus aureus and Streptococcus pyogenes. Candida albicans causes pustules on a red base ("beefy-red") that, after rupture, form erosions surrounded by fine superficial white scale. Frequently, the inguinal and gluteal folds are involved. *Staphylococcus aureus* and *S. pyogenes* cause a superficial skin infection called impetigo, which is characterized by pustules on a red base that form yellow crusts when ruptured. Certain types of *S. aureus* produce an epidermolytic toxin, causing superficial bullae. However, secondary bacterial infection with *S. aureus* and *S. pyogenes* may be characterized primarily by superficial erosions and crusting.

TABLE 55-2

PRIMARY AND SECONDARY SKIN LESIONS, CONFIGURATIONS, AND LOCATIONS

1. Primary lesions
   a. Macule (<0.5 cm) and Patch (>0.5 cm) – well-circumscribed flat lesion
   b. Papule (<0.5 cm) and Plaque (>0.5 cm) – well-circumscribed raised lesion
   c. Vesicle (<0.5 cm) and Bullae (>0.5 cm) – fluid-filled raised lesion
   d. Pustule – well-circumscribed raised fluid-filled lesion containing leukocytes
   e. Nodule (>0.5 cm) – deep-seated raised lesion
   f. Tumor – a large nodule
   g. Wheal (hive) – raised transient (<24 hours) lesion
   h. Cyst – fluid-filled nodule
   i. Telangiectasia – dilated dermal blood vessel
   j. Petechiae – areas of extravasated red blood cells resulting from broken capillaries
2. Secondary lesions
   a. Atrophy – depressed lesion
   b. Erosion – superficial break in the skin
   c. Ulceration – full-thickness (i.e., break in the skin through the dermis)
   d. Scale – flakes of skin
   e. Crust – scale with serum
   f. Fissure – linear erosion
   g. Scar – fibrosis of the dermis
3. Configuration
   a. Blaschko – embryologic lines of skin cell migration (i.e. whorled)
   b. Linear – straight
   c. Annular – round with normal skin in central "ring"
   d. Iris – round with a dark center
   e. Nummular – round, 'coin-shaped'
4. Location
   a. Symmetric – both sides of the body
   b. Localized – one area
   c. Widespread – generalized

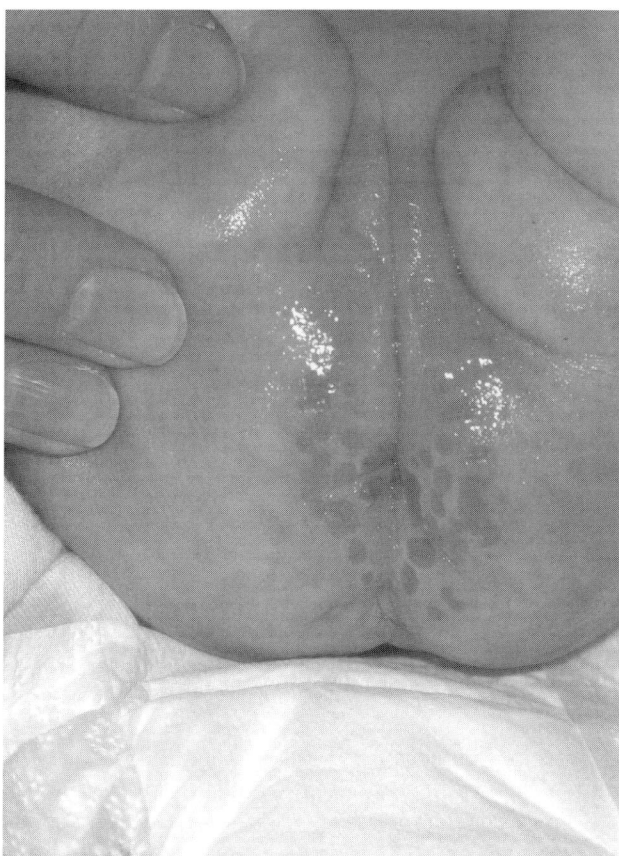

Figure 55-1 Erosive dermatitis.

Factors involved in the genesis of diaper dermatitis include increased skin wetness (e.g., sweat, urine and stool) of the stratum corneum (14), which makes the skin more susceptible to friction from the diaper material; and irritation from elevated pH caused by urinary ammonia and from activation of fecal proteases and lipases in the alkaline milieu (15,16). When alkaline urine combines with feces, the potential for irritation is compounded. Breast-fed infants have been noted to have stools with lower pH, which may account for their decreased incidence of diaper dermatitis.

The differential diagnosis of irritant diaper dermatitis includes psoriasis, seborrheic dermatitis, secondary syphilis, histiocytosis, acrodermatitis enteropathica, and cystic fibrosis. In those conditions, however, unlike diaper dermatitis, skin outside the diaper area is usually involved.

Treatment of diaper dermatitis should be targeted toward reducing skin wetness, minimizing contact of the skin with urine and feces, and eradicating infectious organisms. Skin wetness and irritation can be minimized in several ways. Ultra-absorbent diapers have been shown to be superior to cloth diapers in decreasing skin wetness and maintaining an acidic skin pH (17,18). Frequent diaper changes also help to minimize wetness. Barrier ointments (e.g., containing petrolatum) help keep urine and feces from contacting the skin. Other commercial products containing zinc, vitamin A and D also may be effective. The skin should be gently cleansed with water, or if necessary, a mild nonalkaline

soap before barrier ointment re-application. Complete removal of barrier ointment with diaper changes is not necessary, however if attempted, may further exacerbate skin injury. When diaper dermatitis is unusually severe, recalcitrant, or when risk factors are likely to be ongoing (e.g., malabsorption syndromes), a thick layer of pectin-based paste without alcohol, followed by a barrier ointment or zinc oxide ointment, may prove efficacious. Commercially available diaper wipes can exacerbate irritation, and should be reserved for healthy appearing skin or for circumstances in which soap and water is not available.

Mild, low-potency topical corticosteroids such as 1% hydrocortisone ointment can be applied if inflammation is significant; however, higher potency topical steroids should be avoided because of the risk of cutaneous atrophy, striae, adrenal suppression, and Cushing syndrome. Combination antifungal-steroid compounds such as Lotrisone® and Mycolog II® have no use in treating neonatal skin conditions involving the diaper area. Each contains a potent topical corticosteroid (betamethasone dipropionate, and triamcinolone 0.1%, respectively) that when placed under diaper occlusion can cause cutaneous and systemic side effects. Use of powders also should be avoided. Fungal or bacterial superinfection can be managed with appropriate topical antimicrobial agents (19). Topical antifungal agents such as nystatin, clotrimazole, miconazole or ketoconazole can be safely applied to newborn skin. Bacterial infection generally responds to mupirocin or bacitracin. Neomycin carries a higher risk of allergic contact sensitization and should be avoided.

Intertrigo

Intertrigo is a symmetric, red, moist, macerated eruption that occurs in the skin folds. It is thought to be as a result of excessive sweating and close approximation of the skin surfaces. Yeast and bacterial super-infection is common (see diaper dermatitis). The most effective treatment is exposure of skin to air. Barrier creams and occlusive ointments can exacerbate intertrigo. A light application of 0.5% to 1% hydrocortisone cream two to three times a day, pimecrolimus or tacrolimus can help. Concurrent bacterial and/or yeast infections must be treated in a manner similar to irritant contact diaper dermatitis.

Seborrheic Dermatitis

Seborrheic dermatitis is characterized by red skin with white-yellow waxy scale, occurring on the scalp, eyebrows and in the intertriginous areas, especially in the posterior auricular, neck, axillary and inguinal folds (Fig. 55-2). Typical scale is absent in the intertriginous areas. The eruption begins at 2 to 3 weeks of age and in some infants becomes widespread over the ensuing months. The vast majority of patients with seborrheic dermatitis improve significantly during the first year of life. Persistent and severe seborrheic dermatitis may be associated with human immunodeficiency virus (HIV) infection and other underlying systemic diseases.

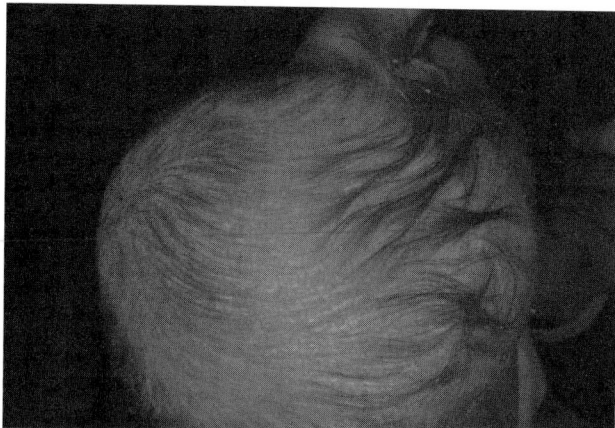

Figure 55-2 Seborrheic dermatitis.

Alterations in fatty acid metabolism, nutrition, and/or immunity, and infection with Pityrosporum ovalae have been thought to contribute to seborrheic dermatitis, but no firm cause has been established.

Atopic dermatitis, psoriasis, Langerhans cell histiocytosis, scabies, and dermatophyte infections are the principle conditions that must be excluded. In general, atopic dermatitis produces itching and psoriasis is more difficult to control than seborrheic dermatitis. Sometimes, several visits with careful observation and assessment of the therapeutic response are required to establish the proper diagnosis; skin biopsy sometimes becomes necessary for diagnosis.

When infants have limited involvement, no specific therapy is required other than mild shampoo and/or mineral oil to gently remove the scale. For more adherent, thick scalp scale, selenium sulfide shampoo or 2% ketoconazole shampoo may be helpful. Ketoconazole 2% cream, hydrocortisone 0.5% to 1% (lotion, cream, ointment), pimecrolimus cream and tacrolimus ointment applied once to twice daily are alternative therapies.

Psoriasis

Psoriasis can produce various cutaneous patterns such as guttate (tear drop), papules, pustules, and plaques. Most infants with psoriasis develop thick, pink plaques with firmly adherent thick white (micaceous) scale in a distribution similar to seborrheic dermatitis. Psoriasis in the newborn period is uncommon and congenital psoriasis is rare. When newborns are affected, they tend to have localized plaques, either on the scalp, diaper area, or hands. One can also see isolated nail and nail-fold involvement. Rarely, newborns develop generalized pustular erythroderma with fever.

The cause of psoriasis is unknown, but genetic influences play an important role because children with two psoriatic parents have an approximately 50% lifetime risk (20). Infection (S. pyogenes), cold weather, emotional stress, medications (antimalarials), and withdrawal from systemic corticosteroids have all been shown to provoke psoriatic flares. Psoriasis improves with therapies targeting T-lymphocytes (cyclosporine), suggesting that psoriasis is a T-lymphocyte mediated disease (21). T-lymphocytes comprise most of the psoriatic inflammatory cell infiltrate, further supporting the central role of T-lymphocytes (22).

A family history of psoriasis and "soft signs" of psoriasis (e.g., pink skin in the gluteal cleft, nail pitting, geographic tongue) are useful aids to diagnoses.

Medium-strength topical corticosteroids, tacrolimus, and pimecrolimus are the mainstay of therapy for infantile psoriasis. Short contact therapy (application for less than 30 minutes, followed by washing) with anthralin is a safe therapy, but may be limiting because of skin irritation. Calcipotriol may be applied, but to limited areas because of risk of vitamin D toxicity. Tar ointments are effective, but have an unpleasant odor, and stain the skin, and may not be well accepted by caregivers. Treatments targeting T-lymphocytes and associated cytokines are showing promising results in adults, but have not been studied in infants.

Atopic Dermatitis

Newborns with atopic dermatitis develop red, itchy, papules and plaques involving the forehead, cheeks and flexural surfaces, with relative sparing of the diaper area; there may be widespread generalized redness and scaling. Well-defined criteria exist to diagnose atopic dermatitis (23). In the newborn, atopic dermatitis is recognized when an infant has the typical rash and a family history of atopy, asthma or atopic dermatitis. In the young infant, pruritus may not be evident because of lack of scratching. Many infants are colonized with S. aureus and all are susceptible to viral infections (e.g., herpes simplex virus, small pox virus, molluscum contagiosum virus, and human papilloma virus).

Although up to 30% of infants have concurrent food hypersensitivity, atopic dermatitis is not thought to be caused simply by allergies. Rather, atopic dermatitis is a complex disorder subject to genetic, immunological, and environmental influences (24). Atopic dermatitis must be differentiated from seborrhea, psoriasis, fungal infection and scabies, and the treatment is similar to other noninfectious inflammatory conditions. Moisturizers, low-potency topical steroids, tacrolimus, pimecrolimus, avoidance of cutaneous irritation, and treatment of secondary infections are the fundamental elements of therapy.

Erythroderma

Erythroderma is a generalized red eruption as a result of a number of inherited and acquired conditions. Inflammatory conditions (atopic dermatitis, seborrheic dermatitis, mastocytosis), infectious conditions (syphilis, herpes, S. aureus), metabolic conditions (methylmalonic aciduria, maple syrup urine disease, cobalamine deficiency), genetic skin diseases (ichthyosis, Netherton syndrome, nonbullous ichthyosiform erythroderma) immunodeficiency (severe combined immunodeficiency, common variable hypogammaglobulinemia) are examples of conditions that can result in erythroderma. These infants have a compromised epidermal permeability barrier and are at risk for hypothermia, dehydration and sepsis. Diagnostic evaluation should be directed by history and physical examination. Typically, a skin biopsy is not helpful during acute erythroderma. Management focuses on fluid and temperature homeostasis, utilizing intravenous fluids, emollients and placing infants in isolettes with warm humidified air. The caloric requirements of the infant are dramatically increased and parenteral nutrition is sometimes required. Emollients applied two to three times daily assist in healing the skin barrier. Fissures should be treated with topical antibiotics such as mupirocin or bacitracin. Infants with signs of skin infection (e.g., crusting, oozing, malodorous areas) and sepsis should be cultured and treated with appropriate systemic antibiotics.

Neoplastic

Langerhans Cell Histiocytosis

Langerhans cell histiocytosis (LCH) is a malignant condition as a result of abnormal clones of Langerhans cells. Langerhans cells are skin antigen presenting cells, derived from the bone marrow. Infants with LCH can develop a range of cutaneous findings, including crusted papules, pustules, vesicles, bullae, petechiae, purpura and nodules. Lesions can occur in the "seborrhea areas" (scalp, face, and flexural areas), and extremities, including the palms and soles. Many infants with LCH develop lesions limited to the skin. Cutaneous features of LCH often precede systemic signs (e.g., fever, hepatosplenomegaly, lymphadenopathy, anemia), however, making early diagnosis in more aggressive forms of LCH more difficult.

Acral vesicles and bullae must be differentiated from bullous impetigo, scabies and syphilis. LCH in the seborrheic areas can mimic benign inflammatory conditions such as intertrigo, seborrhea, psoriasis and atopic dermatitis.

All infants with LCH should have an evaluation for systemic involvement (hematologic, pulmonary, hepatic, renal, and skeletal) and they should be followed closely, because extracutaneous relapses may occur months to years after diagnosis. Topical corticosteroids and moisturizers can be used for cutaneous lesions, however, the rash typically responds poorly. Patients with systemic signs of disease should also be followed by pediatric hematology and/or oncology specialists.

Genetic Skin Diseases

Collodion Baby

Infants born with a thick "saran-wrap" covering of skin (collodion membrane) are referred to as collodion babies (Fig. 55-3). In the early newborn period, this covering can produce respiratory distress, painful cracks and fissures, temperature and fluid instability. Newborns frequently

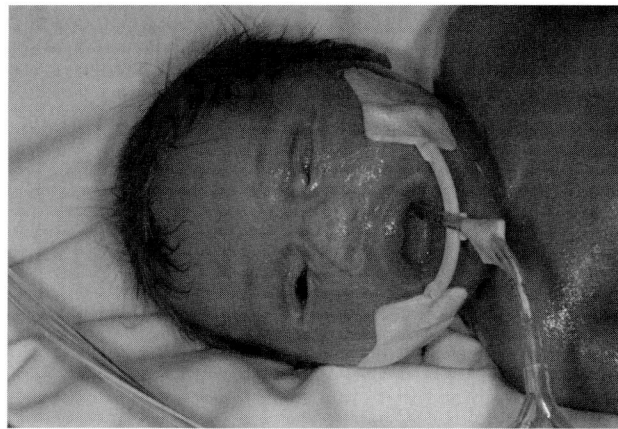

Figure 55-3   Collodion baby.

require oxygen, a humidified air isolette, and liberal applications of emollients. The eyes should be meticulously cared for because desiccation may cause corneal scarring. The collodion membrane sloughs over a period of 2 to 4 weeks. The vast majority of infants who present with a collodion membrane have lamellar ichthyosis. Other causes of collodion membrane include trichothiodystrophy, Sjogren-Larsson syndrome, Conradi-Hunermann syndrome, Gaucher's disease (Type IIB), and Refsum disease. Ten percent to 15% of infants have no underlying disorder and have normal skin when the collodion membrane resolves.

Harlequin Ichthyosis

Infants with harlequin ichthyosis are born with an extremely thick and cracked, armor-like covering with pronounced eclabium and ectropion. Harlequin infants are exceedingly rare and usually die during infancy; however, there are some long term survivors. This condition is inherited in an autosomal recessive manner and the underlying genetic defect remains unknown. Treatment with a systemic retinoid may increase survival of these infants.

Ichthyosis

Ichthyosis is a term utilized to describe inherited and acquired conditions that produce "fish-like" scales. There are different clinical forms, including ichthyosis vulgaris, X-linked ichthyosis, and lamellar ichthyosis. Ichthyosis vulgaris, the most common form is inherited in an autosomal dominant manner and usually manifests after 3 months of age. Ichthyosis vulgaris can be associated with atopic dermatitis. Infants with ichthyosis vulgaris often have fine light-colored scale that becomes thicker on the lower extremities. X-linked ichthyosis occurs with an incidence of 1:6,000 males. Most infants show signs of this form of ichthyosis by 3 months of age. The skin develops thick brown firmly adherent scale with relative sparing of the flexural regions. X-linked ichthyosis is caused by a mutation in the steroid sulfatase gene, resulting in decreased shedding of keratinocytes. Infants with X-linked ichthyosis are frequently born after prolonged labor, because absence of steroid sulfatase can lead to increased fetal productions of DHEAS and decreased placental estrogen. Undescended testes, testicular cancer, and cataracts are associated with X-linked ichthyosis. Lamellar ichthyosis is rare and inherited in an autosomal recessive manner, although autosomal dominant forms have been described. Most infants with lamellar ichthyosis have mutations in the transglutaminase 1 gene. Transglutaminase is important in keratinocyte differentiation. Alterations in this protein produce the thick plate-like scale seen in infants with lamellar ichthyosis. Sometimes, infants with lamellar ichthyosis are born with a saran-wrap covering of skin referred to as a collodion membrane (see section on collodion membrane). Newborns with ichthyosis are primarily managed with emollients, such as vaseline and aquaphor. A thinner lotion may be preferable, if a thicker emollient is difficult to apply. Keratolytic emollients containing lactic and salicylic acid should be avoided, because they can be systemically absorbed. Infants with severe forms of ichthyosis can benefit from topical and/or systemic retinoids, but these medications should be used in consultation with a dermatologist. Genetic counseling is essential for families of infants with ichthyosis.

Ectodermal Dysplasia

Ectodermal dysplasia is a term that refers to conditions resulting in abnormalities of the skin and adnexal structures (teeth, hair, and nails). There are many different forms of ectodermal dysplasia. Hypohidrotic ectodermal dysplasia, hidrotic ectodermal dysplasia, keratosis ichthyosis and deafness (KID) are examples. Infants with ectodermal dysplasia are difficult to diagnose in the newborn period, because teeth are rarely present at birth, and most infants have sparse hair and thin nails. Unexplained fevers may be the first clue to hypohidrotic ectodermal dysplasia. There is no specific therapy for ectodermal dysplasia. Skin health should be maintained with mild soaps and meticulous applications of bland emollients. Families should be referred to a dermatologist and geneticist to assist in diagnosis and genetic counseling.

Netherton Syndrome

Netherton syndrome is a condition that causes progressive and diffuse cutaneous findings (Fig. 55-4). Newborns are frequently born prematurely and fail to thrive. Typically, there is erythroderma in the newborn period. Newborns with extensive skin barrier compromise are at risk for dehydration and sepsis. The rash can appear very similar to atopic dermatitis with significant involvement of the face and scalp. Infants develop sparse scalp hair as a result of hair fragility. Netherton syndrome is diagnosed after finding a characteristic hair shaft abnormality referred to as trichorrhexis invaginata ("bamboo hair" or "ball-and-socket hair"). Only 30% of hairs many be involved and typically

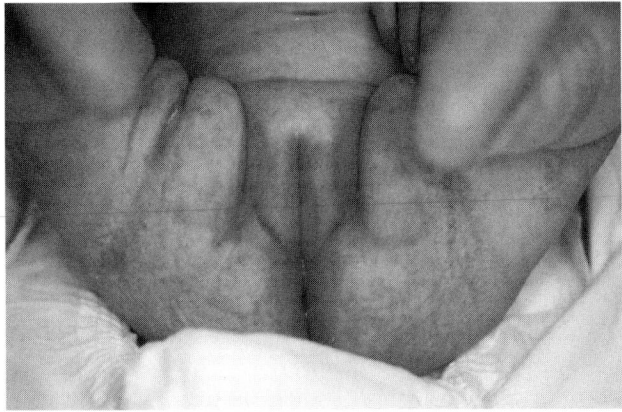

Figure 55-4 Netherton syndrome.

trichorrhexis invaginata occurs after 3 months of age, making early diagnosis of Netherton syndrome difficult. There are no specific laboratory abnormalities, except most infants have elevated levels of immunoglobulin E (IgE). A mutation in SPINK5, encoding a serine protease inhibitor, (LEKTI) has been shown to cause Netherton syndrome in some patients (25). Patients are managed with topical corticosteroids, emollients and antihistamines. Tacrolimus and pimecrolimus should be used with caution in infants with Netherton syndrome, because high serum levels of tacrolimus have been detected in some infants. Serum levels of tacrolimus should be checked in infants treated with this medication. Special attention should be given to nutrition, because these patients tend to have problems with growth.

Metabolic and Nutritional Disorders

There are a number of metabolic diseases and nutritional deficiencies that can cause diffuse red dry flaky skin in the newborn period (26). Examples include maple syrup urine disease, carbamoyl phosphate synthetase deficiency, argininosuccinic aciduria, propionic acidemia, methylmalonic aciduria, cystic fibrosis, biotinidase deficiency (multiple carboxylase deficiency), and essential fatty acid deficiency. Acrodermatitis enteropathica (zinc deficiency) produces a unique rash and will be discussed in more detail.

Acrodermatitis Enteropathica

Acrodermatitis enteropathica (AE) is caused by zinc deficiency. This condition results from decreased zinc intake, poor gastrointestinal absorption and/or increase metabolic needs. Infants develop a tetrad of diarrhea, periorificial and acral vesiculobullous dermatitis, alopecia, and apathy (Fig. 55-5). Autosomal recessive AE is as a result of an altered gastrointestinal zinc transport mechanism and develops within the first several months of life. Usually, the dermatitis is the first sign. Acquired forms of AE are more common and result from low or absent levels of zinc in the breast milk, decreased gastrointestinal absorption (as a result of diarrhea), or increased metabolic requirements.

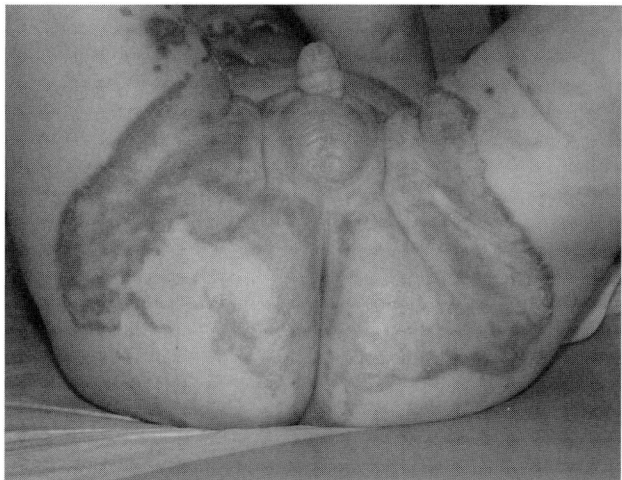

Figure 55-5 Acrodermatitis enteropathica.

Absent or low zinc in the breast milk occurs because of altered transfer of zinc from maternal serum. Mothers usually have normal serum zinc levels. Breast-fed premature infants can develop symptoms when their nutritional requirements rise. Premature infants and those with HIV infection develop more severe disease. A low plasma zinc level (<65 mg/dL) is diagnostic, although AE can occur in the setting of normal zinc levels. Administration of zinc gluconate or sulfate at a dose of 5 mg/kg per day divided into two doses results in rapid improvement of symptoms in 2 to 4 days and may prevent death. Metabolic disorders such as cystic fibrosis may also produce a similar rash (27,28).

Connective Tissue Disorders

Neonatal Lupus Erythematosus

Neonatal lupus erythematosus (NLE) is a connective tissue disorder resulting in an annular, red, scaly rash and/or congenital heart block in newborns. Except for the rash, most infants thrive and appear well. Affected newborns develop sharply demarcated plaques with central atrophy and peripheral white scale. The rash can be purpuric and appear lacy. Typically the head, neck, and periorbital areas (raccoon eyes) are involved. Skin biopsy shows vacuolar interface dermatitis with perivascular and perifollicular lymphocytes. Increased mucin is found within the superficial and deep dermis. Less than 5% of newborns develop involvement of other organ systems. Mothers with systemic lupus erythematosus (SLE) have a 30% chance of delivering a newborn with NLE. Infants born to mothers with SLE should be followed closely for congenital heart block, because not all infants develop cutaneous findings. Anti–Ro antibody is found in 98% of infants with NLE. Newborns with NLE should receive special protection from ultraviolet radiation. Topical corticosteroids are effective for skin lesions. Infants with NLE have an excellent prognosis with most symptoms resolving by 1 year of age.

Infections

Staphylococcal Scalded Skin Syndrome

Newborns can acutely develop widespread red skin referred to as erythroderma (see erythroderma section). Bacterial exotoxins are an important cause of diffuse erythroderma in the newborn period (29). These extracellular toxin(s) can be produced at a focus of infection or colonization, and oftentimes the site of bacterial replication is inconspicuous. Toxins can act locally, as in bullous impetigo; or can cause widespread clinical signs as a result of hematogenous spread, as in scalded skin syndrome.

Staphylococcal scalded skin syndrome (SSSS) is a staphylococcal epidermolytic toxin-mediated disease characterized by painful, diffuse redness of the skin with accentuation in flexural and periorificial areas (Fig. 55-6). In 2 to 5 days, the skin develops fine flaky desquamation, especially in the flexural surfaces. Severely affected newborns can develop widespread sterile, flaccid blisters that easily rupture with gentle shear forces (Nikolsky sign), leaving large areas of open, weeping skin. Many newborns develop a distinctive radial crusting and fissuring around the eyes, mouth, and nose. Widespread skin break-down compromises the epidermal permeability barrier, putting newborns at risk for sepsis, fluid and electrolyte imbalance, and temperature instability.

SSSS is caused predominantly by phage group II staphylococci, particularly strains 71 and 55; occasionally, a group I or III isolate is involved. Foci of infection include the nasopharynx, umbilicus, urinary tract, a cutaneous wound, and the conjunctivae. Bacteria produce epidermolytic (i.e., exfoliative or exfoliatin) toxins A or B, which enter the bloodstream. Rarely, disease has also been transmitted through breast feeding. The disease severity is related to the toxin load in the blood, rather than the site of infection or colonization. Reduced renal clearance of the toxin is thought to put newborns at risk for SSSS. The epidermolytic toxins produce superficial blisters by binding to an epidermal cadherin called desmoglein I. SSSS may be mistaken for a number of other disorders, including scarlet

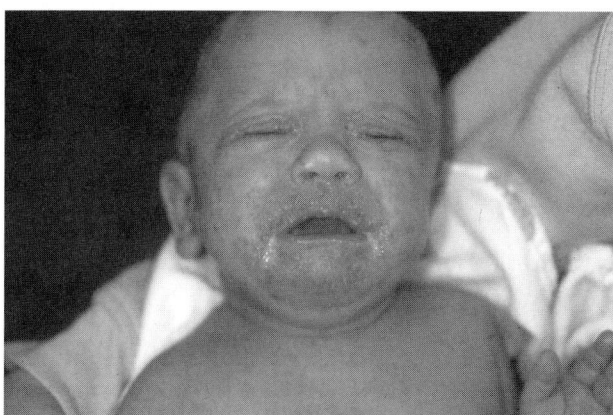

Figure 55-6 Staphylococcal scalded skin syndrome.

fever, bullous impetigo, epidermolysis bullosa, diffuse cutaneous mastocytosis, familial peeling skin syndrome with eosinophilia, epidermolytic hyperkeratosis, drug eruption, erythema multiforme, and drug-induced toxic epidermal necrolysis (TEN; Lyell's Disease). TEN often can be distinguished by a history of drug ingestion, presence of the Nikolsky sign only at sites of erythema, and absence of perioral crusting. The differentiation of TEN from SSSS may occasionally require a skin biopsy: TEN results in full-thickness epidermal necrosis, with a blister cleavage plane in the lowermost epidermis. Distinguishing between these conditions is particularly important because mortality rates are relatively higher with TEN and avoidance of the offending drug is crucial to preventing a recurrence.

Recovery usually is rapid once appropriate antibiotic therapy is begun. Parenteral therapy with nafcillin or methicillin should be given promptly. General principles include minimizing handling of the infant and use of emollients (e.g., petrolatum and vaseline gauze) and semi-occlusive dressings to provide lubrication and minimize pain. Healing occurs without scarring in 10 to 14 days.

VESICLES AND PUSTULES

Commonly, newborns develop transient noninfectious vesicles and pustules. Infectious causes must be investigated by history, physical examination and laboratory tests.

Idiopathic

Erythema Toxicum Neonatorum

Erythema toxicum neonatorum is a common benign transient eruption characterized by evanescent macules that become pink papules and pustules on an erythematous base. Occasionally, only small pink macules develop. Erythema toxicum is most prominent on the face, torso, and extremities, with sparing of the palms and soles. Typically, lesions are not present at birth, but develop within 2 days of life and continue to appear for the first 3 to 4 weeks of life. The appearance can be striking, especially when the pustules coalesce to form large pustular plaques (Fig. 55-7). When the diagnosis is in question, a smear of a pustule shows abundant eosinophils, a few neutrophils and no bacteria and yeast. Cultures should be done for bacteria and yeast to rule out infections. The cause of erythema toxicum is unknown and treatment is not necessary.

Acropustulosis of Infancy

Acropustulosis of infancy is a benign recurrent pustular eruption, occurring from birth to 1 or sometimes 2 years of age. Infants develop pruritic pink papules that quickly evolve into vesicles and pustules. Most infants are irritable and have pruritus. Pustules resolve in 7 to 14 days, leaving white scale, but tend to recur in crops in 2- to 4-week cycles. The lesions occur on acral sites such as the palms and soles;

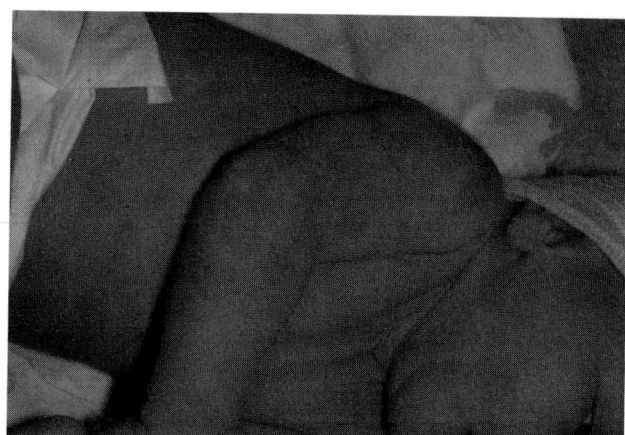

Figure 55-7   Erythema toxicum neonatorum.

however, this condition can involve other areas of the body. The cause of acropustulosis is unknown. Many infants with suspected acrodermatitis of infancy have scabies. Diagnostic evaluation should include a scabies preparation, bacterial and fungal cultures. Topical corticosteroids and oral antihistamines are effective to control symptoms.

Eosinophilic Pustular Folliculitis

Infants with eosinophilic pustular folliculitis develop recurrent crops of very pruritic papules and pustules on the head and neck, especially the scalp (30). The scalp can have yellow scale, similar to seborrheic dermatitis. Usually, the rash is not present at birth, and occurs during the first year of life. Diagnosis is established with a Giemsa or Wright stain of the contents of a pustule and a skin biopsy. A smear of the pustule contents shows abundant eosinophils and lacks bacterial and fungal organisms. Skin biopsy shows a dense infiltrate of eosinophils (primarily), lymphocytes, and histiocytes, involving the dermis and hair follicle outer root sheath. Like acropustulosis of infancy the cause of eosinophilic pustular folliculitis is unknown; however, both conditions have a similar clinical course, suggesting these two conditions lie on the same disease spectrum. Infants should be treated with low potency topical corticosteroids and selenium sulfide or zinc pyrethrin shampoo. Unlike adults, eosinophilic pustular folliculitis of infancy is not associated with HIV infection. The eruption typically resolves within the first year of life.

Miliaria

Miliaria is a rash that occurs as a result of blocked eccrine ducts and retention of sweat. There are four types: (a) miliaria crystallina is composed of small superficial clear vesicles as a result of blockage in the stratum corneum (i.e., sudamina), (b) miliaria rubrum has small pink papules and vesicles as a result of blockage at the dermal-epidermal junction (i.e., prickly heat), (c) miliaria pustulosa includes pustules on an erythematous base as a result of blockage at the mid-dermal level, and (d) miliaria profunda is characterized by pink nodules as a result of blockage at the deep dermal level. Miliaria is more common in intertriginous areas, but can occur on any body surface. This disorder tends to occur in the setting of increased temperature and humidity (e.g., heat lamps, bundling) and resolves in a cool dry environment. Miliaria crystallina and rubrum resolve quickly with environmental cooling. Lesions of miliaria pustulosa and profunda are not quick to resolve as they involve blockage of eccrine ducts at deeper levels, creating a more intense inflammatory response within the skin. Affected infants may benefit from low potency topical corticosteroids.

Transient Neonatal Pustular Melanosis

Transient neonatal pustular melanosis is a benign eruption occurring at birth in healthy newborns. Approximately 5% of African American and 0.6% of Caucasian newborns are affected. The rash is characterized by superficial pustules that easily rupture, forming fine collarettes of scale and hyperpigmented macules. The pustules may rupture before birth and may not be seen. The most common sites are the head and neck folds. Pustules and scales resolve over 1 to 3 weeks, however, hyperpigmented macules can persist for several years. Fluid from a pustule shows neutrophils and is sterile. No treatment is necessary.

Acne Neonatorum

Acne neonatorum develops within the first 2 months of life and is more common in boys and breast-fed infants. Like acne seen in adolescents, the rash is characterized by comedones (open and closed), and erythematous papules and pustules on the cheeks, chin and forehead. Rarely, cysts and scars develop (Fig. 55-8). Most cases resolve within 2 years. Neonatal acne is thought to be caused by blocked sebaceous ducts, increased sebum production, inflammation and Propionibacterium acnes infection. Most infants respond to low-strength salicylic acid, sodium sulfacetamide and/or low strength benzoyl peroxide washes. For moderate neonatal acne, topical antibiotics such as erythromycin or clindamycin in combination with topical retinoids can be effective. Severe nodulocystic and scarring acne should be treated aggressively with oral erythromycin or amoxicillin and, rarely, isotretinoin. Tetracycline antibiotics should be avoided because of the risk of staining permanent teeth. Petrolatum, baby oils, and lotions can block sebaceous pores, making neonatal acne worse, and should be avoided. Neonates with severe acne should be referred to a dermatologist for management.

Neonatal cephalic pustulosis is a variant of neonatal acne that is thought to be as a result of Malassezia spp. This condition manifests as monomorphic appearing pustules without comedones. Infants with pustules should be cultured for bacteria and fungus to evaluate for resistant organisms. Topical antifungal creams can be helpful for more severely affected newborns. Generally, neonatal cephalic pustulosis spontaneously remits.

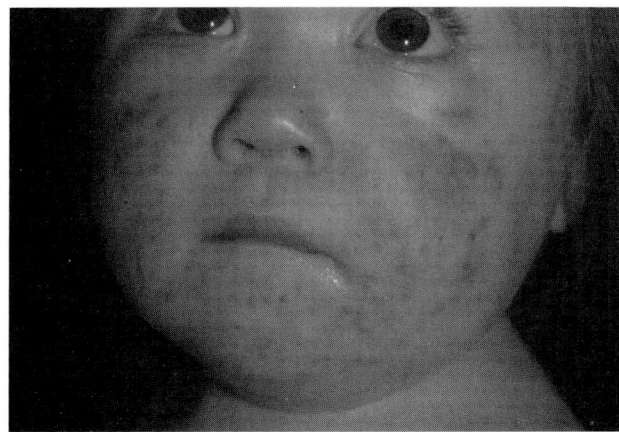

Figure 55-8   Acne neonatorum.

Genetic Skin Disease

Genetic skin conditions are rare, but important causes of blisters and bullae in the newborn period. Bullous congenital *ichthyosiform erythroderma*, *epidermolysis bullosa*, and *incontinentia pigmenti* are examples.

Bullous Congenital Ichthyosiform Erythroderma (*Epidermolytic Hyperkeratosis*)

Bullous congenital ichthyosiform erythroderma (BCIE) is an autosomal dominant condition as a result of mutations in keratin 1 and 10 genes. Keratin 1 and 10 are intermediate filament proteins found in the superficial layers of the epidermis (granular cell and upper spinous layers). Alterations in these proteins weaken the epidermis and affected newborns develop widespread areas of denuded skin with superficial blisters. These infants are at risk for secondary cutaneous infection with Staphylococcus aureus and sepsis. Later in infancy and early childhood, blistering becomes less evident and the skin develops verrucous appearing scale that is prominent in the flexures. Typically, involved areas are heavily colonized with bacteria, producing an odor. Newborns should have topical emollients such as vaseline and aquaphor applied to assist with skin barrier function and be monitored closely for sepsis.

Epidermolysis Bullosa

Epidermolysis bullosa (EB) as its name suggests represents a large group of inherited skin disorders characterized by blisters and breakdown of the epidermis. This condition is caused by mutations in genes responsible for structural proteins important in maintaining the skin integrity, especially the epidermis. Minimal skin friction can produce extensive erosions in the skin. Although classifications schemes may change as new genes are identified, traditionally, epidermolysis bullosa has been classified as EB simplex, junctional EB, and dystrophic EB. EB simplex is due alterations in proteins found in the epidermis (Weber-Cockayne: keratin 5/14), junctional EB is as a result of altered proteins at the dermo-epidermal junction (Herlitz: laminin 5), and dystrophic EB is as a result of altered proteins below the dermoepidermal junction (dominant dystrophic EB: collagen type VII). It is thought that the severity of EB is determined by the location of the mutation within the gene; mutations in highly conserved regions produce more severe disease. These phenotypic-genotypic correlations will become more apparent in the future. Some of the proteins involved in EB are important for the proper function of other organ systems. For instance, autosomal recessive junctional EB associated with pyloric atresia is as a result of abnormal plectin. These patients also have muscle disease, indicating that this protein is also important in muscle as well. In the newborn period, distinguishing between subtypes on clinical appearance alone can be extremely difficult, because all forms of EB can present with widespread blisters. Skin biopsies taken for routine histology, transmission electron microscopy, immunofluorescence mapping, and deoxyribonucleic acid (DNA) mutational analysis assist in properly classifying newborns with EB.

A newborn who presents with blisters and erosions as a result of friction should be suspected as having EB. The blisters of EB simplex are more superficial than those of junctional and dystrophic EB. Groups of blisters can be seen in EB simplex Dowling Meara variant. This form of EB can be severe in the newborn period (Fig. 55-9). Significant mucosal erosions suggest junctional or dystrophic EB, although newborns with EB simplex can develop mild mucosal blisters. Laryngeal, urological and gastrointestinal involvement is seen in the more severely affected infants. This extracutaneous involvement is more commonly seen in the junctional and dystrophic variants.

Managing newborns with severe EB is difficult. Friction should be minimized as much as possible and wounds should be carefully dressed with a nonadherent dressing (vaseline gauze, Mepitel, exu-dry). Gauze wrap is then placed, followed by tube wrap. Tape should not be applied directly to the skin. Extra petrolatum added to the vaseline gauze can keep the vaseline gauze from adhering to the skin. Topical antibiotics such as bacitracin can be helpful to prevent wound infection. Bacterial resistance (*S. aureus*) to bactroban has occurred and this topical antibiotic should only be used for cutaneous infection in EB patients. The skin is the portal of entry for bacteria that result in sepsis, thus the skin should be assessed daily. Prophylactic oral or intravenous antibiotics should be avoided. Like burn patients, dressings should be gently removed; removal can be facilitated by soaking off the dressing in a tub with warm water. Blisters should be opened in a sterile manner and the roof left in place. Tense blisters easily spread in EB patients because of the inherent skin fragility. Newborns with EB have increased nutritional and fluid requirements. If intravenous catheters are required, they can be sutured in place. Nasogastric tube feedings can be used sparingly to assist in the early newborn period. Percutaneous gastrostomy tubes should be placed early, if feeding and nutrition are problematic. The Haberman feeder (www.melela.com) is a nipple with a valve that allows for delivery of breast milk or formula without having to exert too much negative pressure.

The diagnosis of EB is psychologically distressing for parents and families. Addressing these issues is an essential part of EB management. Advocacy groups such as Dystrophic Epidermolysis Bullosa Research and Advocacy (DebRA of America, Inc. 5 West 36th Street, Suite 404; New York, NY 10018) are invaluable resources for families.

Incontinentia Pigmenti (Bloch-Sulzberger Syndrome)

Incontinentia pigmenti (IP) is an autosomal dominant skin disease characterized by linear streaks and whorls of blisters. The blisters pass through stages and become verrucous or warty, then flatten forming hyperpigmented patches and finally hypopigmented patches. Typically, these four stages occur in sequence, although patients can "skip" stages and different stages can be seen together. (Fig. 55-10) The vesicles that are seen in stage one can be confused in the newborn period for infection such as herpes simplex, varicella, or impetigo. Females with IP

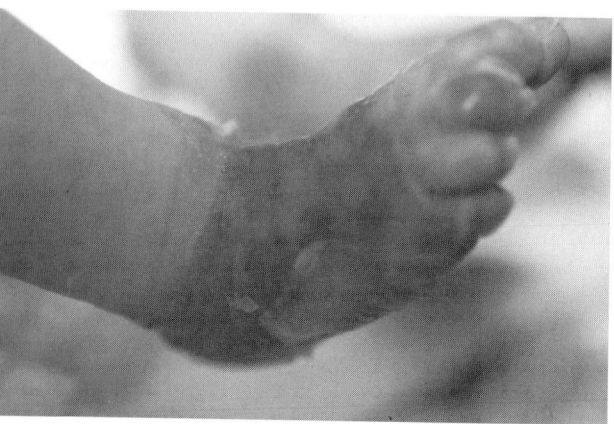

Figure 55-9 Epidermolysis bullosa.

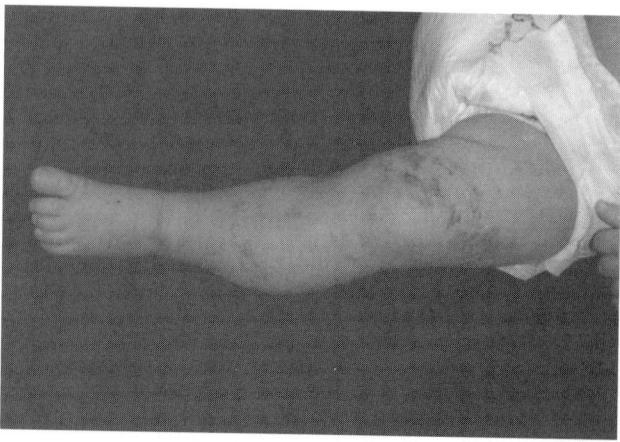

Figure 55-10 Incontinentia pigmenti.

develop characteristic skin lesions within the first 2 to 3 weeks of life. This condition is lethal in males and is as a result of mutations in the NEMO gene on Xq28.

Early on in the condition, peripheral eosinophilia can be seen. Other extracutaneous findings seen in association with IP include: central nervous system (CNS) abnormalities (seizures), ocular defects (retinal changes), immunological abnormalities (elevated IgE) skeletal anomalies (spina bifida). Newborns suspected of having IP should have a skin biopsy and appropriate bacterial and viral cultures performed. Parents should be referred to a geneticist for genetic counseling.

Immunologic

Mastocytosis

Mast cell disease is rare in the newborn period. Like older affected infants and children, newborns can develop solitary mastocytomas, urticaria pigmentosa, systemic mastocytosis and mast cell leukemia. Cutaneous signs of mast cell disease include hyperpigmented macules, papules and nodules which form wheals with rubbing (Darier's sign) (Fig. 55-11). In some instances, frank bullae develop, especially on the palms and soles. More commonly, infants develop single to multiple hyperpigmented macules on the torso, extremities and scalp that show Darier's sign. Although this sign is characteristic of mast cell disease, other conditions such as leukemia cutis can form wheals when rubbed. Thus, skin biopsy should be done if the diagnosis is in doubt. In the vast majority of cases, cutaneous involvement resolves within several years. Systemic mastocytosis occurs in less than 2% of patients with cutaneous mastocytosis and most infants present with diffuse cutaneous involvement with blisters. However, systemic mastocytosis can occur with minimal cutaneous involvement. When affected infants show signs of systemic disease such as flushing, diarrhea, respiratory distress,

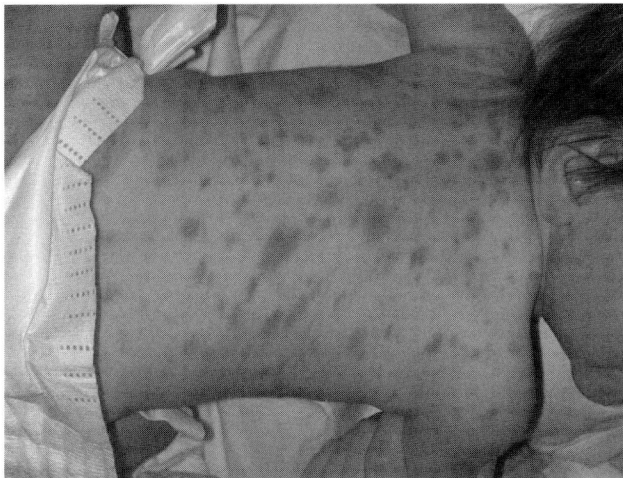

Figure 55-11 Mastocytosis.

tachycardia, hypotension and/or hepatosplenomegaly, they should be evaluated for systemic mastocytosis. Serum tryptase levels (to assess overall mast cell burden), abdominal ultrasound, and bone marrow biopsy should be considered.

Parents of infants with mast cell disease should carry an Epi-pen and should be aware of medicines that cause spontaneous degranulation of mast cells such as opiates, radiocontrast dyes, and bee stings. Antihistamines such as hydroxyzine (Atarax) and diphenhydramine (Benadryl) can help control symptoms as a result of histamine release.

Traumatic

Sucking Blisters

Blisters and erosions can occur at sites of *in utero* sucking, especially the thumb, index finger, wrist, or lip. Sucking blisters should be differentiated from mechanobullous eruptions such as epidermolysis bullosa, bacterial and viral infections.

Infectious

Herpes Simplex Infection

Herpes simplex virus 1 and 2 (HSV-1 and HSV-2) infections can be seen in the neonatal period and have different patterns of disease. Congenitally acquired HSV presents differently depending on when the infection was acquired. Infection acquired within the first two trimesters can result in intrauterine growth retardation and microcephaly. HSV acquired just before or at the time of delivery presents within the first month of life, most commonly within the first week. Up to 30% of infants can have symptoms on the first day of life. Symptoms can be varied and include cutaneous signs involving skin and mucous membranes and systemic signs involving multiple organ systems, but especially the CNS.

The primary cutaneous lesion of HSV is a vesicle with a central dell. The vesicles are grouped. Within 1 to 2 days the vesicles develop into pustules and form crusts (Fig. 55-12). The edge of a group of herpes vesicles appears as a scalloped border. The mucous membranes are typically involved and can appear as blepharitis, conjunctivitis, stomatitis, and urethritis. Infants with eczema are at risk for disseminated herpes infection referred to as eczema herpeticum (Figure 55–13). Children with neonatally acquired HSV can have reactivation of their herpes later in life, often as recurrent localized eruptions of crops of vesicles.

HSV infections can be diagnosed with direct immunofluorescence and viral culture of the lesions. Direct immunofluorescence is performed by unroofing a vesicle and scrapping the base of the vesicle. Skin biopsy can show signs of viral cytopathic effect in the epidermis. Neonatal HSV should be treated with acyclovir (see Chapter 48).

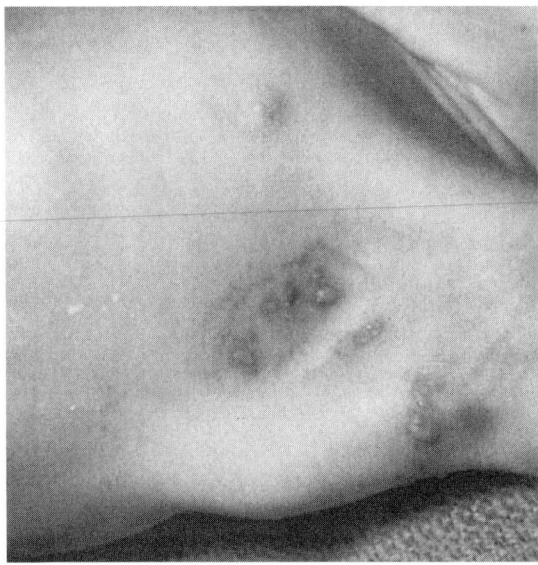

Figure 55-12   Herpes simplex.

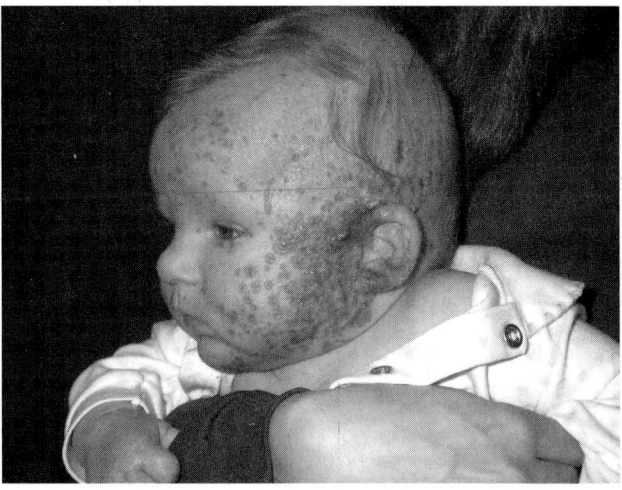

Figure 55-13   Eczema herpeticum.

DISORDERS OF PIGMENTATION (BROWN SPOTS/WHITE SPOTS)

Most irregularities in pigmentation are normal; however, pigment alterations can be the first indicator of an underlying inherited genetic skin condition. Hyperpigmentation or hypopigmentation occurring in whorls or in straight lines is thought to be as a result of genetic mosaicism. Newborns with alterations in skin pigment following the lines of Blaschko should be evaluated closely for associated extracutaneous defects. Examples of genetic conditions with hyperpigmentation following the lines of Blaschko include: incontinentia pigmenti, Conradi-Hunermann disease, and segmental neurofibromatosis. Examples of genetic conditions with hypopigmentation following the lines of Blaschko include: piebaldism, and hypomelanosis of Ito.

BROWN SPOTS

Café Au Lait Macules

Café-au-lait macules (CALMS) are small, oval, and tan to brown macules. They can be quite large and involve a large surface area of the body (giant CALMS). They are more common in heavily pigmented children and are as a result of increased melanin content of the basal melanocytes and keratinocytes. The number and size of CALMS increase during infancy and early childhood. Although 19% of normal children have CALMS, they are seen in increased numbers in several inherited conditions such as neurofibromatosis, proteus syndrome, and McCune-Albright syndrome. Six or more CALMS larger than 0.5 cm (they may be smaller in infancy) is one of the diagnostic criteria for neurofibromatosis type I. Crowe's sign (axillary and inguinal freckling) is another clinical feature of neurofibromatosis type I.

Congenital Melanocytic Nevi

Congenital melanocytic nevi (CMN) are tan to brown hyperpigmented macules, papules and plaques, consisting of increased numbers of melanocytes. Typically, they contain increased numbers of hairs (vellus and terminal) and have been termed "hairy nevi." Congenital melanocytic nevi are classified with respect to the largest diameter that they would achieve in adulthood (small: <1 to 1.5 cm; intermediate: 1 to 1.5–20 cm; large: >20 cm) (Fig. 55-14). The size of the CMN is relevant for future melanoma risk. Patients with large CMN have a 5% to 8% lifetime risk of developing a malignant melanoma. This risk is highest in prepubertal children; approximately 50% of the melanomas occur by age 5. The prognosis of melanoma, occurring within large CMN is poor with many infants developing early metastasis. Large CMN involving the scalp and midline back are associated with neurocutaneous melanosis or involvement of the leptomeninges. Magnetic resonance imaging can be helpful to evaluate for leptomeningeal involvement. Other malignant tumors arising within large CMN include neuroblastoma, rhabdomyosarcoma,

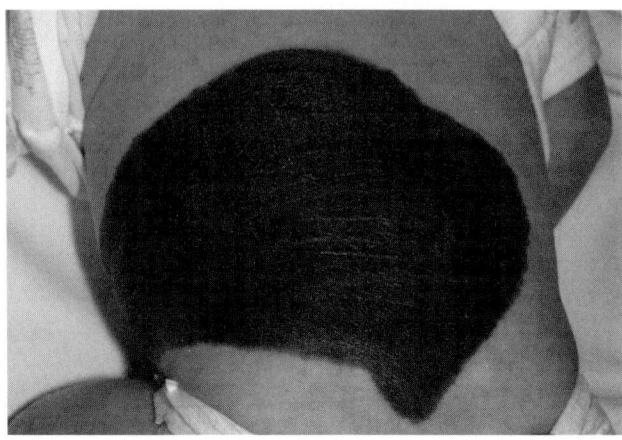

Figure 55-14   Large congenital nevus.

primitive neuroectodermal tumors, liposarcoma and mixed neoplasms. The risk of malignant melanoma in association with small and intermediate CMN is unknown, but probably increased in the postpubertal child. Other factors such as family history of melanoma and ultraviolet radiation exposure are important to determine melanoma risk for these lesions. High risk CMN are prophylactically excised. When considering surgical excision, lesions should be evaluated for size, location, color, border, family history and evolution of the lesion. Infants with CMN should be referred to a dermatologist for management.

Other Types of Melanocytic Nevi

A blue nevus is a blue to black macule or papule, consisting of spindle-shaped dermal melanocytes. A Spitz nevus is a pink to brown papule, consisting of spindle-shaped melanocytes at the dermal-epidermal junction and in the dermis. A nevus spilus is a hyperpigmented macule studded with darker brown macules. All three nevi are considered benign, although malignant variants have been described.

Dermal Melanocytosis

Dermal melanocytosis (Mongolian spot) arises as a result of increased numbers of melanocytes within the dermis (Fig. 55-15). They are very common in newborns of color, and should not be confused with child abuse. Mongolian spots have a tendency to fade over a number of years. Extensive dermal melanocytosis has been described as an early sign of GM1 gangliosidosis.

Epidermal Nevi

Epidermal nevi are papules and plaques that develop as a result of hyperplasia of keratinocytes. Typically the lesions are solitary, however, they can be linear (linear epidermal nevus), inflamed (inflammatory epidermal nevus), widespread (systematized epidermal nevus), and associated with

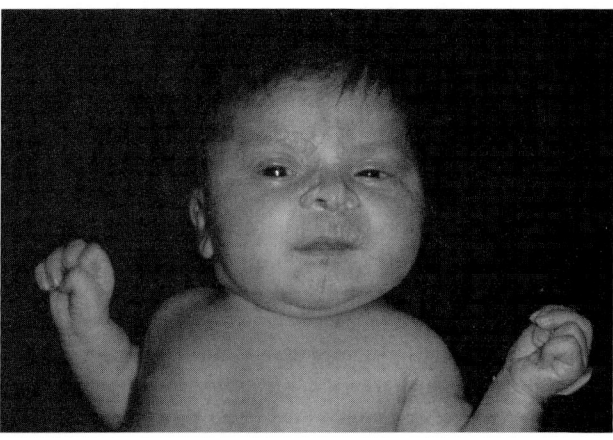

Figure 55-16   Epidermal nevus syndrome.

underlying neurological deficits, blindness, and skeletal abnormalities (epidermal nevus syndrome) (Fig. 55-16). Epidermal nevi are thought to occur as a result of somatic mutations in keratinocytes. Some epidermal nevi show a characteristic microscopic finding called epidermolytic hyperkeratosis. These nevi arise as a result of mutations in keratins 1 and/or 10, and females with gonadal tissue involvement can give birth to infants with bullous congenital ichthyosiform erythroderma, a rare congenital form of ichthyosis.

Disorders of Pigmentation—White Spots

White spots occur when there is either a decreased number or function of melanocytes. The exception is nevus anemicus, which is caused by blood vessel constriction. Hypopigmentation or decreased pigment should be distinguished from depigmentation or absence of pigment. With natural lighting, this distinction may be difficult. Fluorescent light (Wood's light) shows pure white in depigmentation and off-white in hypopigmentation. Nevus anemicus loses its border with diascopy (pressure) and does not show a color change with Wood's light examination.

Ash Leaf Macules

Ash leaf macules are small oval areas of decreased pigmentation. They are seen in 3% to 5% of the normal population, but can be an indicator of tuberous sclerosis. Other cutaneous signs of tuberous sclerosis include connective tissue nevus (shagreen patch), periungual fibromas, confetti hypopigmentation, gingival fibromas and facial angiofibromas (adenoma sebaceum).

Hypomelanosis of Ito

Hypomelanosis of Ito consists of whirls of hypopigmentation following Blaschko lines that can be seen in association with seizures, developmental delay, and ocular and/or skeletal anomalies.

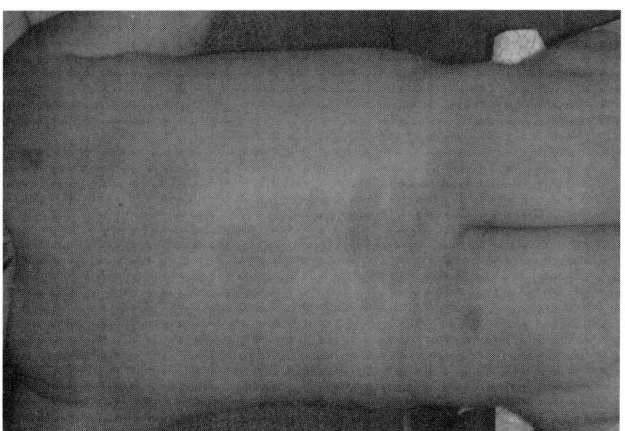

Figure 55-15   Dermal melanocytosis (Mongolian spot).

Nevus Achromicus

Nevus achromicus or depigmentosus is a hypopigmented patch occurring as long linear streaks or as well circumscribed isolated patches. Affected areas are usually unilateral and may be small or they may be very broad affecting a large part of the body. Nevus achromicus is not associated with extra-cutaneous organ involvement.

Diffuse Hypopigmentation/Depigmentation

Generalized hypopigmentation or pigment dilution is seen in newborns with Chediak-Higashi syndrome and phenylketonuria. Generalized depigmentation is seen in the different forms of oculocutaneous albinism.

ATROPHIC LESIONS

Atrophic skin or thinned skin results from an underdevelopment of one of the components of the skin. Atrophic lesions can occur in isolation or they can be seen as part of syndromes with multiple malformations.

Aplasia Cutis Congenita

Aplasia cutis congenita (ACC) is absence of the skin. (Fig. 55-17) There are nine different groups of the condition: (a) ACC of the scalp without multiple systemic anomalies, (b) ACC with associated limb abnormalities, (c) ACC with organoid and epidermal nevi, (d) ACC with overlying embryologic abnormalities, (e) ACC with associated fetus papyraceus or placental infarcts, (f) ACC associated with epidermolysis bullosa, (g) ACC localized to the extremities without blistering, (h) ACC caused by teratogens, and (i) ACC associated with malformation syndromes (31). Most infants have isolated scalp ACC (Group 1). Eighty percent of the lesions are near the parietal scalp whorl and 76% are single lesions. Up to one-third of cases of ACC have underlying defects in the

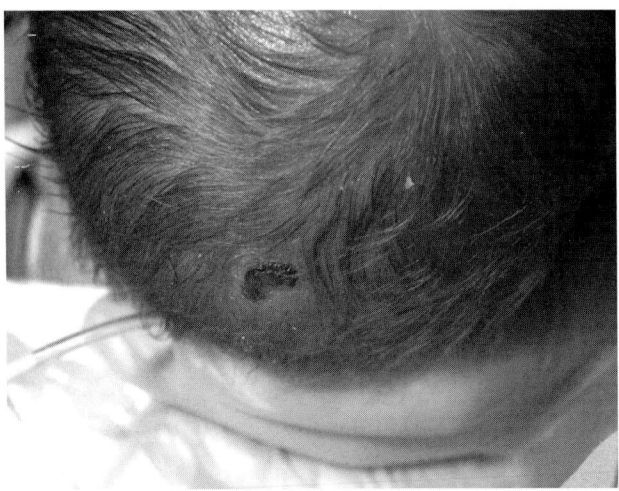

Figure 55-17 Aplasia cutis congenita.

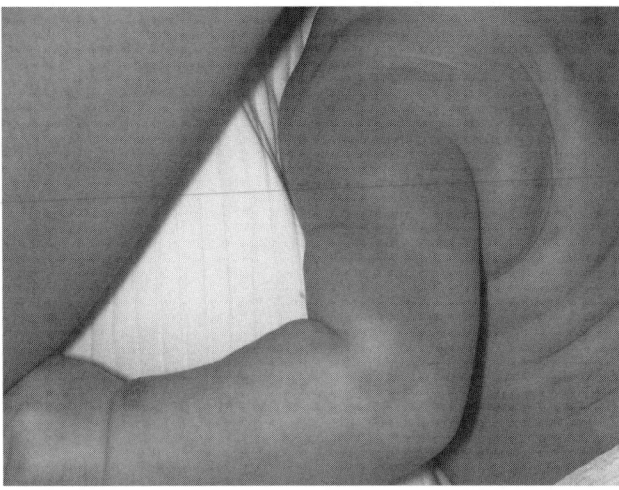

Figure 55-18 Subcutaneous fat necrosis.

bone. Sometimes ACC is partially healed at birth, giving variable morphologies from a small patch of alopecia to full thickness ulceration with an underlying bony defect.

Subcutaneous Fat Necrosis

Subcutaneous fat necrosis presents as red-purple, indurated subcutaneous nodules or plaques on the extremities, trunk, or buttocks during the first weeks of life (Fig. 55-18) (32). It has been attributed to trauma, shock, cold, and asphyxia. Infants appear healthy, although subcutaneous fat necrosis has been associated with hypercalcemia. Lesions spontaneously resolve over a period of weeks to months. Rarely, sterile abscesses form with attendant atrophy and scarring. The sterile abscesses should not be drained.

Sclerema Neonatorum

Extensive subcutaneous fat necrosis occurring in preterm or severely ill term infants is referred to as sclerema neonatorum. The extremities may be involved at first, but generalized involvement occurs quickly within 3 to 4 days. If the infant survives, sclerometers skin changes resolve within about 3 weeks. The cause is unknown, but because the microscopic appearance is identical to subcutaneous fat necrosis, similar etiological factors are likely involved. Other than treating the associated illness, no specific therapy is indicated.

Focal Dermal Hypoplasia of Goltz

Focal dermal hypoplasia (Goltz syndrome) is an X-linked dominant condition characterized by thinned or absent dermis with fat herniation, following the lines of Blaschko. Other cutaneous signs include alopecia, nail dystrophy, atrophic scars, ACC, telangiectasias, dermatographism, and red papillomas (perioral, intraoral, perianal, vulvar). Infants with Goltz syndrome can have skeletal, ocular, dental, and neurological defects. Patients suspected of having focal dermal hypoplasia should be referred to a dermatologist and geneticist.

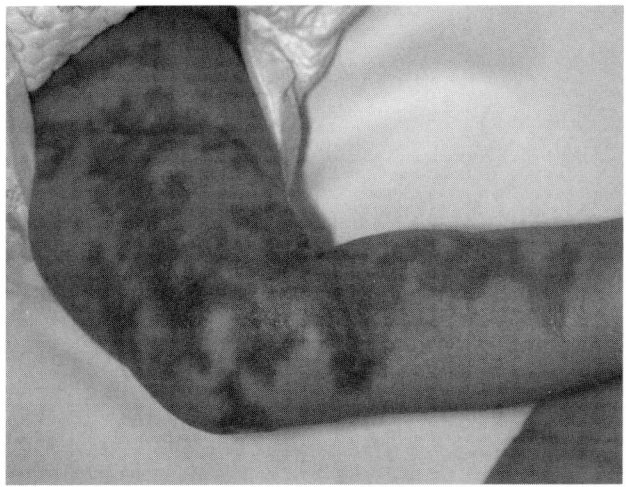

Figure 55-19 Cutis marmorata telangiectatica congenita.

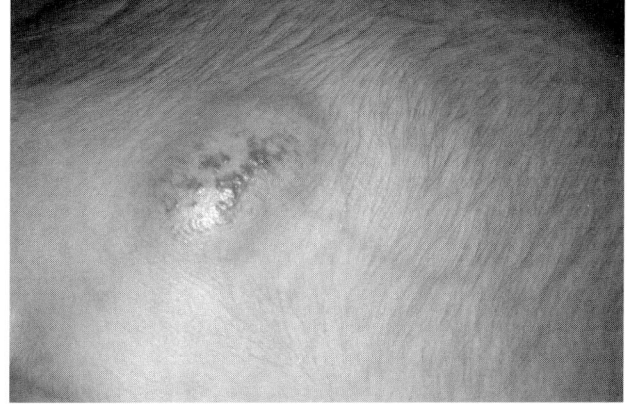

Figure 55-20 Deep hemangioma.

TRANSIENT VASCULAR LESIONS

Cutis Marmorata

Cutis marmorata is a transient net-like erythema, occurring in newborns exposed to cooler temperatures. This reaction pattern is caused by constriction of the capillaries and venules and usually disappears quickly with rewarming. Persistent and extensive cutis marmorata can be seen in association with trisomy 18 and 21 and Cornelia De Lange syndrome. Cutis marmorata should not be confused with a vascular malformation referred to as cutis marmorata telangiectatica congenita (CMTC) (Fig. 55-19). Infants with CMTC are born with atrophic net-like red-blue patches in a dermatomal pattern. Lesions have a tendency to become less noticeable by adulthood (33). Rarely, CMTC is associated with underlying ocular, skeletal and cardiac malformations.

Halequin Color Change

Harlequin color change describes a sharply demarcated erythema that develops on the dependent half of an infant who is in the lateral decubitus position. This interesting phenomenon occurs in both healthy and ill newborns (especially low birth weight infants), lasts 1 to 30 minutes, and reverses if the infant is placed on the opposite side. The underlying mechanism for harlequin color change is unknown. This reaction may last up to 3 weeks and is not associated with long term sequelae.

VASCULAR GROWTHS

Hemangioma of Infancy

Hemangiomas of infancy (HOI) are benign growths of endothelial cells (34). They represent the most common vascular tumor of childhood, affecting 1% of all newborns and 10% of 1-year-olds. Only 30% are noticeable at birth; most are noted within the first month of life. Deeper lesions may not be detected until later in infancy. Characteristically, HOI have a growth phase lasting up to a year; then a stabilization phase, followed by an involution phase. Approximately 50% of HOI are completely involuted by age 5 years, 60% by age 6 and involution is usually complete by age 10. HOI are more common in female and premature infants and have a predilection for the head and neck. Most infants have solitary HOI; however, 10% to 15% have multiple HOI. Nascent or early HOI may appear as pale macules or patches, and contain a few dilated blood vessels. The color of HOI is determined by the depth and phase of growth. Growing HOIs are firm, rubbery, and their color can range from red (superficial) to blue (deep) (Fig. 55-20). When a HOI begins to involute, it softens and develops centrally located fibrotic grey bands (Fig. 55-21).

The vast majority of HOI follow a benign course. Local complications include infection, ulceration, and scarring. HOIs can be life threatening by obstructing the airway or by interrupting feeding. They can also compromise vision.

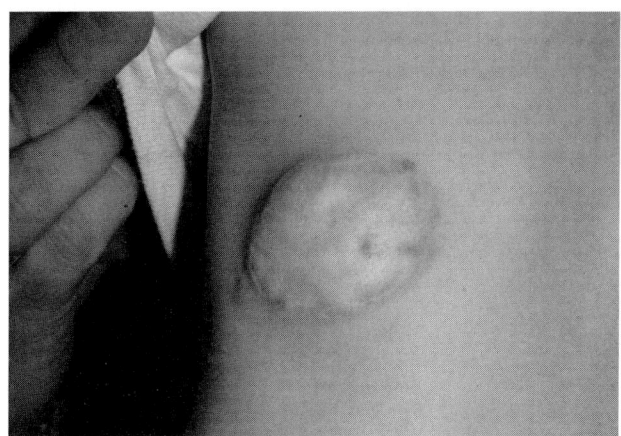

Figure 55-21 Involuting hemangioma.

HOIs located near or on the mandible ("beard distribution") can be associated with glottic involvement. Multiple HOIs or visceral hemangiomas can cause a consumptive coagulopathy (Kassebach-Merritt syndrome); however, this complication occurs more frequently with other vascular tumors such as tufted angioma and hemangioendothelioma. Midline HOI can be associated with underlying occult cranial and vertebral anomalies; midline sacral hemangiomas have been associated with a tethered spinal cord (Cobb syndrome). Large plaque-like hemangiomas involving the face can be associated with multiple anomalies (PHACES syndrome—posterior fossa malformations, hemangioma, arterial anomalies, coarctation of the aorta and cardiac defects, eye anomalies, and sternal defects)35. Multiple cutaneous HOI can be an indicator of internal involvement, however, visceral hemangiomas can occur without cutaneous HOIs, and the vast majority of infants with multiple cutaneous HOIs do not have involvement of the viscera.

Pyogenic Granuloma

Pyogenic granulomas or lobular capillary hemangiomas are small pink to red papules occurring on the head, neck, torso and mucous membranes. They are collections of endothelial cells that are thought to arise from trauma. They are rare in the newborn period.

Vascular Malformations

Vascular malformations are anomalies in blood and lymphatic vessels as a result of altered morphogenesis. As such, they are all congenital; however, they may not be noticed until sometime after birth. Unlike HOI, they exhibit normal endothelial cell growth and grow with the somatic growth of the patient. Vascular malformations can undergo apparent rapid increase in size as they fill up with blood or lymph fluid. They are classified by the vessel type (capillary, venous, arterial, lymphatic, mixed and arteriovenous) and the flow characteristics (high and low flow). Almost all vascular malformations are sporadic, although new genes are being discovered in some familial cases. Blue rubber bleb nevus syndrome and multiple glomovenous malformations have autosomal dominant inheritance.

Capillary Malformations

Capillary malformations can appear as "macular stains" of the nape ("stork bite"), eyelids ("angel kisses"), and glabella. They are found in at least 50% of newborns, and fade with time. Many nuchal patches and some glabellar patches persist into adulthood and are more noticeable with crying or anger. Capillary malformations can be more substantial and involve diffuse segments of skin, particularly segments of skin innervated by the trigeminal nerve (Fig. 55-22). Approximately 10% of newborns with V1 involvement will also have ocular and CNS involvement. This triad is referred to as Sturge-Weber syndrome (SWS).

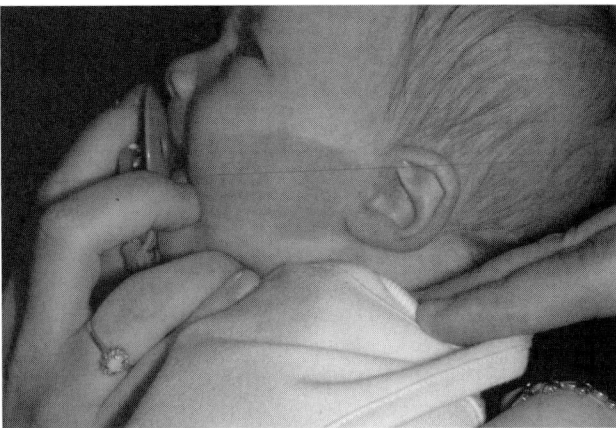

Figure 55-22   Capillary malformations.

Patients with SWS can develop glaucoma, seizures, and facial asymmetry as a result of overgrowth of facial bones. Imaging of the CNS should be delayed until after infancy in an asymptomatic infant, because radiographic changes sometimes occur later. Almost all capillary malformations occur as isolated defects. They have been described, however, in association with trisomy 13, Rubenstein–Taybi, Beckwith–Weidemann, and Klippel–Trenaunay–Weber syndromes. Some lesions lighten with age, and some darken. Vascular laser therapy is an excellent modality and may be more effective if used in infancy. Green tinted cosmetics (e.g., Covermark, Retouch) effectively conceal most capillary malformations.

Venous Malformations

Malformations of the veins are slow-flow vascular malformations, taking on a variety of clinical appearances: varicosities, isolated local spongy nodules, or large complex infiltrating channels. The vast majority of venous malformations are sporadic, although they can be inherited in autosomal dominant and recessive manners. Multiple lesions are more likely to be inherited. Patients with venous malformations often complain of pain and swelling, especially in the morning with ambulation. Venous stasis, intravascular thrombosis and calcifications (phleboliths) are thought to be responsible for the pain. Extensive venous thrombosis can result in widespread coagulopathy.

Lymphatic

Lymphatic malformations (lymphangiomas) are uncommon lesions resulting from dilated lymphatic channels and abnormal flow of lymph fluid. They can be classified broadly as microcystic (small channels), macrocystic (large channels) or mixed.

Microcystic lymphatic malformations have been referred to as lymphangioma circumscriptum. Lymphangioma circumscriptum appear as small translucent pseudovesicles

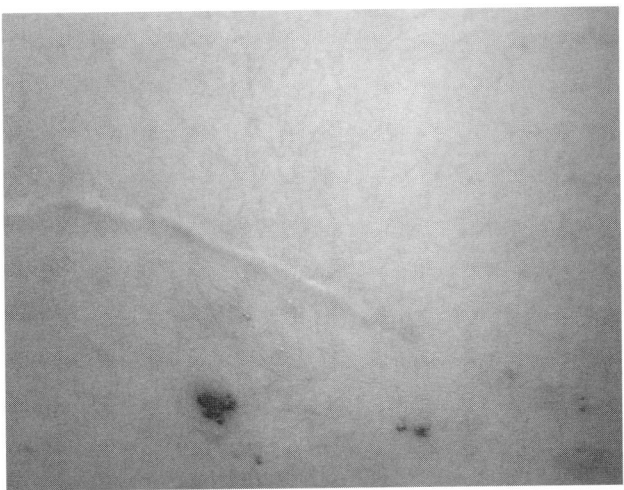

Figure 55-23   Lymphangioma circumscriptum.

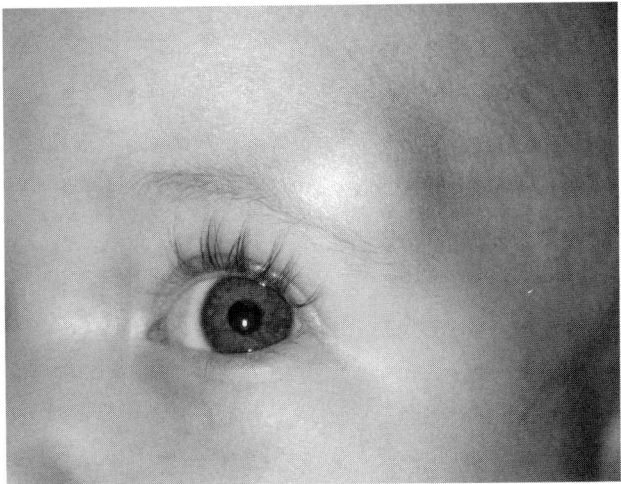

Figure 55-24   Dermoid.

that resemble "frogs spawn" (Fig. 55-23). Commonly, some of the vesicles are hemorrhagic and there may be an underlying deep component giving a blue hue. Microcystic lymphatic malformations can occur on any site, however, axillary folds, neck, shoulders, proximal limbs, perineum, tongue, and buccal mucous membranes are more commonly involved. These malformations have been mistaken for warts and can be confused with sexual abuse (36). They may be small (<1 cm) or very large, covering an extensive surface area. Patients can develop cellulitis in the involved areas and lymphatic malformations commonly recur around previously excised sites.

Macrocystic lymphatic malformations (cystic hygroma) are large single or multiple masses occurring on the neck, axillae, groin and/or chest. Most commonly, these malformations are detected within the first 2 years of life and can cause significant morbidity and even death as a result of airway compromise and infection. They may be detected en utero by ultrasound and increased α-fetoprotein levels and may be associated with Down syndrome or Turner syndrome. The lesions are persistent and can expand, although spontaneous remission has been described, usually after infection. Treatment measures have included sclerotherapy and surgical excision.

Arteriovenous Malformations

Arteriovenous malformations (AVM) are most common in the head and neck region, but also occur on the extremities. These fast-flow malformations are dangerous and can produce cardiovascular instability. Increased warmth, swelling, bruits and thrills are signs of an AVM. A warm swollen extremity with an associated capillary malformation can be a sign of an underlying AVM. Doppler ultrasound and MRI with angiography are helpful to assess the extent of an AVM. These malformations are difficult to manage and may require surgery and/or endovascular embolization.

CYSTS AND NODULES

Dermoid Cysts

Dermoid cysts are common cysts composed of tissue of all three embryonic tissues along lines of fusion. They can occur in any cutaneous site, but are more common on the scalp, especially on the lateral eyebrow. Dermoid cysts can be superficial or they can have a deeper component that involves muscle and bone (Fig. 55-24). Midline cysts should raise concern for a possible underlying connection with the CNS. An imaging study such as an MRI should be performed before operating on a midline lesion. Newer techniques utilizing endoscopy can be performed, minimizing scar formation.

Developmental Anomalies

Skin abnormalities in the form of cysts and nodules can occur as a result of abnormalities in embryonic development. Branchial cleft abnormalities can produce pits, nodules, and cysts along closure lines on the corresponding branchial arch of the face and neck. Common abnormalities include accessory tragus (1st branchial arch) in the preauricular region (Fig. 55-25), midline clefts (1st branchial arch), preauricular cysts (1st branchial arch), lateral cervical cysts, sinuses, and fistulae (2nd branchial arch) (Fig. 55-26). Thyroglossal duct cysts occur in the midline neck and are as a result of failure of fusion of the thyroglossal duct. Bronchogenic cysts occur on the chest, and develop as a result of abnormal development of the primitive foregut. They can drain mucous fluid. Median raphe cysts occur along the ventral surface of the penis and scrotum (Fig. 55-27). They are thought to occur because of entrapped epidermal or urethral cells. If median raphe cysts enlarge or become infected, they can be surgically removed.

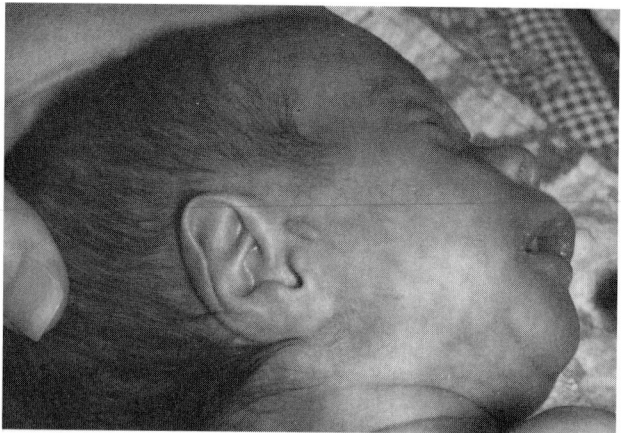

Figure 55-25   Accessory tragus.

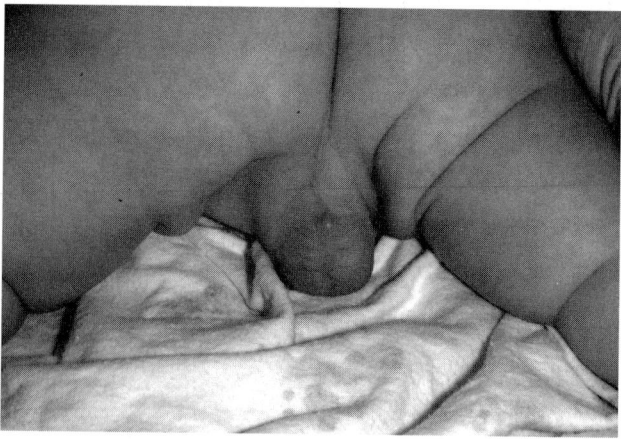

Figure 55-27   Median raphe cyst.

Multiple Red-Blue Nodules ("Blueberry Muffin Baby")

A number of conditions produce cutaneous infiltrates in the skin. When infants develop multiple nodules, they have been described as having the "blueberry muffin" phenotype. Leukemia cutis, extramedullary hematopiesis, Langerhans cell histiocytosis, neuroblastoma, congenital syphilis, congenital toxoplasmosis, and erythroblastosis fetalis are several of the conditions capable of causing multiple red-blue nodules in the newborn period.

EDEMA

Congenital lymphedema can be primary or secondary. Milroy disease describes primary congenital lymphedema that is primarily located distally on the lower legs and feet. Initially the edema is pitting, but later becomes firm and nonpitting. Turner syndrome and Noonan syndrome are two important conditions associated with congenital lymphedema.

Caput Succedaneum

Caput succedaneum develops during delivery as marked swelling of the presenting part of the scalp and can be especially pronounced with a prolonged second stage of labor (37). Pressures from the uterus and vacuum extraction have been shown to cause caput succedaneum. Swelling crosses bony sutures and can be noted at birth or within the first hours of life. Scalp molding is usually noted after the swelling subsides. Rarely, caput succedaneum is associated with skin necrosis and alopecia. No treatment is necessary.

Cephalohematoma

Cephalohematoma is as a result of bleeding, which occurs at the subperiosteal level. Typically, the swelling is unilateral and does not extend beyond the respective suture lines. Cephalohematomas are thought to be as a result of rupture of diploic veins. Bleeding is slow and can take several days to become apparent. Like caput succedaneum, prolonged labor and vacuum extraction are risk factors. Cephalohematomas can be complicated by skull fracture and bacterial infection. They resolve over a period of months and can be associated with cutaneous calcifications.

PURPURA

Purpuric Light Eruption

Purpuric light eruption is a transient purpuric generalized eruption occurring in newborns who received blood transfusions and phototherapy for hyperbilirubinemia. The purpura appears within 4 days of the light therapy and clears within one week of stopping phototherapy. The underlying cause of this eruption is unknown, but in some infants it may be related to a transient increase in porphyrins.

Purpura Fulminans

In the newborn period, purpura fulminans appears as widespread purpura as a result of congenital deficiencies of

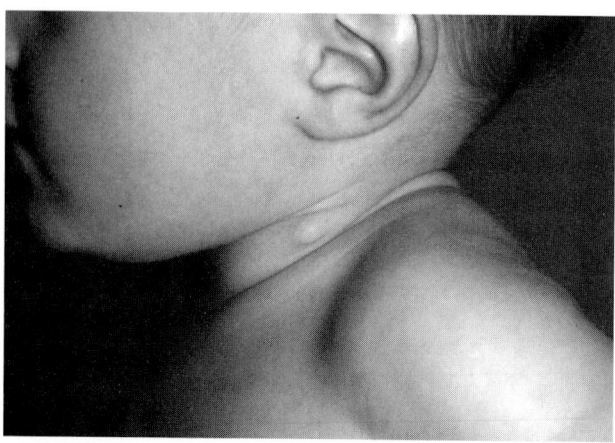

Figure 55-26   Lateral cervical cyst.

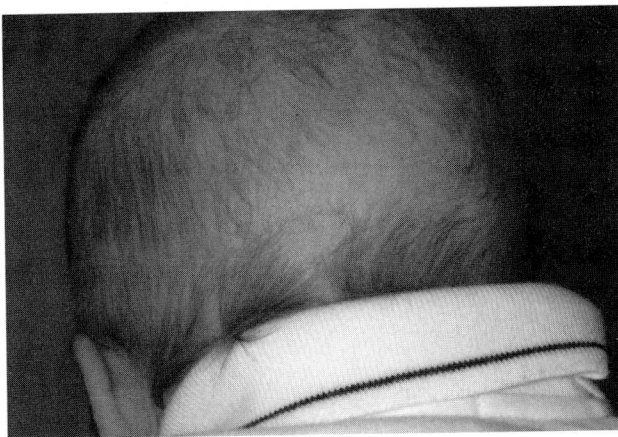

Figure 55-28   Nevus sebaceus.

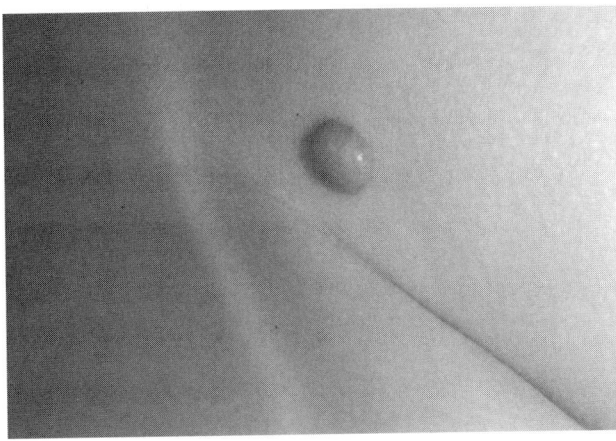

Figure 55-29   Juvenile xanthogranuloma.

proteins C and S38. It can also occur in the setting of overwhelming sepsis.

YELLOW-ORANGE LESIONS

Nevus Sebaceus

Nevus sebaceous is a common congenital hamartoma consisting of increased numbers of sebaceous glands. Most lesions occur on the head and neck and are isolated, although larger facial, especially midline lesions can be associated with underlying bony, brain, ocular, and palatal abnormalities. In some instances, benign (trichoblastoma, syringocystadenoma papilliferum) and malignant (basal cell carcinoma, squamous cell carcinoma) tumors arise within sebaceus nevi, prompting prophylactic surgical excision of these lesions before puberty (Fig. 55-28). The incidence of tumors arising within sebaceus nevi is subject to some controversy and not all sebaceus nevi need to be prophylactically removed. Lesion size and location should be considered when determining timing of surgical excision. Large scalp lesions should be removed in infancy because the skin of the scalp is more elastic and the scalp is easier to close at a younger age. Other treatment methods include carbon dioxide laser and liquid nitrogen.

Juvenile Xanthogranuloma

Juvenile xanthogranuloma (JXG) is a common tumor seen in infants and children. JXG consist of dermal lipid-laden histiocytes with scattered Touton giant cells (wreath-like) and eosinophils. Typically, JXG appear as single or multiple discrete yellow-brown papules on the head and trunk (especially flexural areas) (Fig. 55-29). Lichenoid, plaque and subcutaneous variants have been described. JXG lesions resolve spontaneously over a period of months to several years, leaving few cutaneous sequelae. Hyperpigmentation and atrophic scars remain in some patients. Periocular JXG should raise the suspicion of intraocular

lesions and glaucoma, and these patients should be examined by an ophthalmologist. Rarely, JXG can be associated with neurofibromatosis type I, and juvenile chronic myeloid leukemia.

Sebaceous Gland Hyperplasia

Sebaceous gland hyperplasia appears as numerous small pinpoint yellow to white papules involving the nose, upper lip, and malar areas. Maternal androgens enlarge the pilosebaceous glands. The vast majority of term infants are affected and, occasionally, preterm infants are affected. This condition resolves by 2 to 6 months of age.

Milia

Milia are common discrete yellow-white papules that are slightly larger than those seen in sebaceous gland hyperplasia, and represent tiny epidermal inclusion cysts. They occur on the forehead, nose, cheeks, chin and forehead. They resolve within the first several months of life. Larger milia can be persistent. Most milia arise spontaneously (primary milia) and can affect 40% of newborns. Milia can result from trauma (secondary milia) and be associated with genetic conditions (epidermolysis bullosa, pachyonychia congenita).

Disorders of Hair and Nails

Hair

Newborns are covered with very fine hair referred to as lanugo. This hair is normally shed and replaced with vellus hair within the first several months of life. Scalp hair undergoes repeated patterns of shedding with regrowth from front to back within the first year of life. Hair can be abundant (hypertrichosis) or absent (alopecia). Examples of genetic conditions associated with hypertrichosis include congenital hypertrichosis lanuginosa, Cornelia de Lange syndrome and Rubenstein-Taybi syndrome. Congenital alopecia can be an isolated inherited condition or it can be associated with a number of the ectodermal dysplasias.

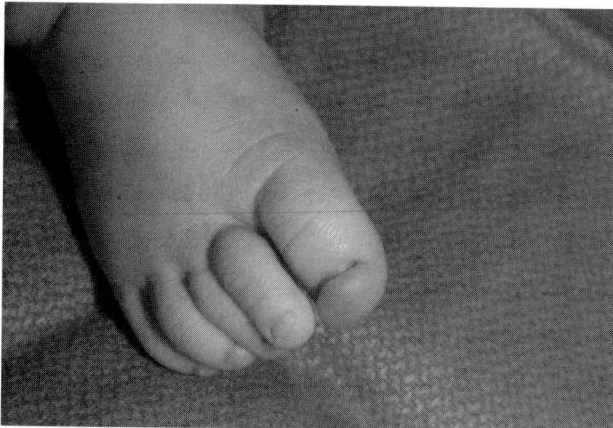

Figure 55-30   Congenital ingrown toenail.

Congenital Ingrown Nails

Toenails that grow into the surrounding skin are referred to as ingrown toenails (onychocryptosis). Infants develop painful, red, swollen skin as the distal free edge of the nail becomes embedded into the skin. It is not clear if the distal free edge embeds into the skin because of misalignment of the nail plate or because of underlying thickening of the tissue surrounding the nail (Fig. 55-30). Toenails and fingernails can develop spicules that ingrow into the lateral nail folds. This type of onychocryptosis is thought to be as a result of clipping the nails too short. Rarely, the nail plate can be deviated on the long axis of the nail (congenital misalignment of the hallux nail) and can be inherited in an autosomal dominant manner. Most ingrown toenails spontaneously involute within the first year of life and require no treatment. With significant paronychia, antibiotics and surgical nail avulsion may be required. Infants with bulbous nail folds without signs of infection may respond to daily application of high potency topical steroids.

Anonychia and Micronychia

Anonychia (complete nail absence) and micronychia (small nail) are rare and can be sporadic or associated with a number of underlying genetic conditions such as ectodermal dysplasia, teratogen exposure (hydantoins, alcohol), Coffin-Siris syndrome, amniotic bands, trisomy 13 or 18, and dyskeratosis congenita. In many instances, there are deformities of the underlying phalanx.

REFERENCES

1. Behne MJ, Barry NP, Hanson KM, et al. Neonatal development of the stratum corneum pH gradient: localization and mechanisms leading to emergence of optimal barrier function. *J Invest Dermatol* 2003;120:998–1006.
2. Madison KC. Barrier function of the skin: "la raison d'etre" of the epidermis. *J Invest Dermatol* 2003;121:231–241.
3. Rassner U, Feingold KR, Crumrine DA, et al. Coordinate assembly of lipids and enzyme proteins into epidermal lamellar bodies. *Tissue Cell* 1999;31:489–498.
4. Darmstadt GL, Mentele L, Fleckman P, et al. Role of keratinocyte injury in adherence of Streptococcus pyogenes. *Infect Immun* 1999;67:6707–6709.
5. Miller SJ, Aly R, Shinefeld HR, et al. In vitro and in vivo anti-staphylococcal activity of human stratum corneum lipids. *Arch Dermatol* 1988;124:209–215.
6. Grubauer G, Elias PM, Feingold KR. Transepidermal water loss: the signal for recovery of barrier structure and function. *J Lipid Res* 1989;30:323–333.
7. Rutter N. The immature skin. *Br Med Bull* 1988;44:957–970.
8. Williams ML, Hanley K, Elias PM, et al. Ontogeny of the epidermal permeability barrier. *J Investig Dermatol Symp Proc* 1998;3:75–79.
9. Blaschko A. Die Nervenverteilung in der Haut ihrer Beziehung zu den Erkrankungen der Haut Wien: Wilhelm Braumuller. 1901.
10. Bolognia JL, Orlow SJ, Glick SA. Lines of Blaschko. *J Am Acad Dermatol* 1994;31:157–190, quiz 90–92.
11. Hoeger PH, Schreiner V, Klaassen IA, et al. Epidermal barrier lipids in human vernix caseosa: corresponding ceramide pattern in vernix and fetal skin. *Br J Dermatol* 2002;146:194–201.
12. Yoshio H, Tollin M, Gudmundsson GH, et al. Antimicrobial polypeptides of human vernix caseosa and amniotic fluid: implications for newborn innate defense. *Pediatr Res* 2003;53:211–216.
13. Cetta F, Lambert GH, Ros SP. Newborn chemical exposure from over-the-counter skin care products. *Clin Pediatr (Phila)* 1991;30:286–289.
14. Warner RR, Boissy YL, Lilly NA, et al. Water disrupts stratum corneum lipid lamellae: damage is similar to surfactants. *J Invest Dermatol* 1999;113:960–966.
15. Berg RW, Buckingham KW, Stewart RL. Etiologic factors in diaper dermatitis: the role of urine. *Pediatr Dermatol* 1986;3:102–106.
16. Buckingham KW, Berg RW. Etiologic factors in diaper dermatitis: the role of feces. *Pediatr Dermatol* 1986;3:107–112.
17. Campbell RL. Clinical tests with improved disposable diapers. *Pediatrician* 1987;14[Suppl 1]:34–38.
18. Campbell RL, Seymour JL, Stone LC, et al. Clinical studies with disposable diapers containing absorbent gelling materials: evaluation of effects on infant skin condition. *J Am Acad Dermatol* 1987;17:978–987.
19. Darmstadt GL, Dinulos JG. Neonatal skin care. *Pediatr Clin North Am* 2000;47:757–782.
20. Traupe H, van Gurp PJ, Happle R, et al. Psoriasis vulgaris, fetal growth, and genomic imprinting. *Am J Med Genet* 1992;42:649–654.
21. Umezawa Y, Oh-i T, Koga M. Relationship between lymphocyte cyclosporin sensitivity and clinical progress of psoriasis. *J Dermatol Sci* 2001;26:94–99.
22. Krueger JG. The immunologic basis for the treatment of psoriasis with new biologic agents. *J Am Acad Dermatol* 2002;46:1–23.
23. Williams HC, Burney PG, Hay RJ, et al. The U.K. Working Party's Diagnostic Criteria for Atopic Dermatitis: I. Derivation of a minimum set of discriminators for atopic dermatitis. *Br J Dermatol* 1994;131:383–396.
24. Leung DY, Jain N, Leo HL. New concepts in the pathogenesis of atopic dermatitis. *Curr Opin Immunol* 2003;15:634–638.
25. Chavanas S, Bodemer C, Rochat A, et al. Mutations in SPINK5, encoding a serine protease inhibitor, cause Netherton syndrome. *Nat Genet* 2000;25:141–142.
26. Darmstadt GL. The skin and nutritional disorders in the newborn. *Eur J Pediatr Dermatol* 1997;8:221–228.
27. Darmstadt GL, McGuire J, Ziboh VA. Malnutrition-associated rash of cystic fibrosis. *Pediatr Dermatol* 2000;17:337–347.
28. Darmstadt GL, Schmidt CP, Wechsler DS, et al. Dermatitis as a presenting sign of cystic fibrosis. *Arch Dermatol* 1992;128:1358–1364.
29. Darmstadt G. Skin and Soft Tissue Infections. In: Long S, Pickering LK, Prober CG, eds. *Principals and Practice of Pediatric Infectious Disease*, 2nd. New York: Churchill Livingstone, 2003:424–457.
30. Darmstadt GL, Tunnessen WW Jr, Swerer RJ. Eosinophilic pustular folliculitis. *Pediatrics* 1992;89:1095–1098.
31. Frieden IJ. Aplasia cutis congenita: a clinical review and proposal for classification. *J Am Acad Dermatol* 1986;14:646–660.
32. Darmstadt GL, Kanzler MH. Pathological case of the month. Subcutaneous fat necrosis of the newborn. *Arch Pediatr Adolesc Med* 1994;148:61–62.

33. Fujita M, Darmstadt GL, Dinulos JG. Cutis marmorata telangiectatica congenita with hemangiomatous histopathologic features. *J Am Acad Dermatol* 2003;48:950–954.

34. Metry DW, Hebert AA. Benign cutaneous vascular tumors of infancy: when to worry, what to do. *Arch Dermatol* 2000;136:905–914.

35. Frieden IJ, Reese V, Cohen D. PHACE syndrome. The association of posterior fossa brain malformations, hemangiomas, arterial anomalies, coarctation of the aorta and cardiac defects, and eye abnormalities. *Arch Dermatol* 1996;132:307–311.

36. Darmstadt GL. Perianal lymphangioma circumscriptum mistaken for genital warts. *Pediatrics* 1996;98:461–463.

37. Pachman DJ. Massive hemorrhage in the scalp of the newborn infant: hemorrhagic caput succedaneum. *Pediatrics* 1962;29:907–910.

38. Darmstadt GL. Acute infectious purpura fulminans: pathogenesis and medical management. *Pediatr Dermatol* 1998;15:169–183.

Pharmacology

Drug Therapy in the Newborn

Robert M. Ward   *Ralph A. Lugo*

The developmental uniqueness of the neonate has tremendous impact on drug therapy. This uniqueness and the potential for dramatic and rapid developmental changes beginning shortly after birth defy accurate generalizations, and illustrate the need for age-specific studies in the increasingly premature patients surviving today. These developmental changes affect all aspects of drug action, from absorption and protein binding to receptor interaction and elimination. The impact of these developmental changes on drug action and the use of pharmacokinetics to adjust drug dosages will be outlined to guide the clinician between the Charybdis of ineffective therapy and the Scylla of drug overdose and toxicity (see also Appendix H).

PRINCIPLES OF PHARMACOLOGY APPLIED TO NEONATES

Free-Drug Theory and Protein Binding

Most clinical drug assays measure both bound and unbound drug; however, it is only the nonprotein-bound or free-drug molecules that are active i.e., cross membranes, bind to receptors to exert pharmacologic action, undergo metabolism and excretion (1). Serum protein binding usually is a rapidly reversible process, so that additional drug is released to replace the unbound drug removed by distribution into tissue or by elimination. The rate of release from serum protein binding usually is much faster than the rate of transfer across membranes. Seldom is the rate of release from serum proteins so slow that it limits the availability of drug molecules for transfer across membranes to exert pharmacologic effects (2).

For most drugs in premature infants, the percentage of unbound drug in the circulation is greater than in adults, because both the amount and the binding affinity of circulating proteins are decreased (3). For example, the albumin of term newborns, compared to that of adults, binds less

theophylline, warfarin and sulfonamides but similar amounts of diazepam (4,5). Because the effects of a drug are related to the amount of unbound drug reaching the site of action, some drug effects in newborns may be explained only by measuring circulating concentrations of free drug. Furthermore, circulating total drug concentrations that are in the therapeutic range for adults or older children may represent free-drug concentrations that are in a toxic range in the premature neonate (5).

Absorption

In drug treatment, absorption refers to the transfer of drug from the site of administration into the circulation. The rates of drug absorption are related to several factors, beginning with the route of administration and including the same characteristics that influence transfer of any substance across lipid bilayers: degree of ionization, molecular weight, lipid solubility, concentration gradient, and active transport.

Enteral

Enteral drug treatment of neonates may not produce reliable and reproducible circulating drug concentrations for a variety of reasons. Although most studies of enteral drug therapy have been conducted in adults, many of the problems of enteral drug administration identified from these studies are likely to occur in neonates.

Intestinal villi and microvilli increase the surface area of the gastrointestinal tract, so that rates of drug absorption are usually much greater from the intestine than from the stomach. Delayed gastric emptying slows passage of drug into the intestine, which prolongs the absorption phase of many drugs. Elimination begins during this absorption phase, so that delayed gastric emptying reduces the area under the curve (AUC) for circulating drug concentration vs. time. This reduces the desired therapeutic effect for many drugs whose effects are directly proportional to the AUC. Gastroesophageal reflux is common in neonates and may be associated with delayed gastric emptying that reduces the therapeutic effects of drugs administered orally. Few studies have addressed this aspect of drug treatment of newborns (6).

Additional problems, unique to the immature patient, may affect enteral drug treatment of newborns. Neonates, especially premature neonates, malabsorb fat which may alter enteral drug absorption. Elevated right atrial pressure, leading to passive congestion of hepatic and mesenteric circulations, often reduces enteral drug absorption in adults. Prolonged enteral drug administration often is necessary for treatment of infants with chronic disorders. These include bronchopulmonary dysplasia (BPD) and congestive heart failure, which may increase right atrial pressure and cause intestinal venous congestion that decreases enteral drug absorption and bioavailability. Therefore, larger doses may be required to achieve the desired therapeutic response. This phenomenon has been reported with furosemide in an infant with BPD, who required a six-fold higher enteral dose to reach plasma concentrations comparable to a 1 mg/kg dose administered intravenously (i.v.) (6).

Intramuscular

Intramuscular drug absorption is directly proportional to blood flow and the surface area of the drug deposited in the muscle (7). Although intramuscular drug administration is often considered more reliable than enteral, the sick or hypothermic neonate with limited muscle mass and poor perfusion of muscle may not absorb intramuscular doses rapidly or completely. As a result of limited amounts of muscle, injections intended for the muscle may enter subcutaneous tissue, from which absorption is slow and unpredictable. Caustic drugs (e.g., phenytoin, pH = 12) damage surrounding tissues and isolate the dose of drug from blood flow, or precipitate to a chemical form that is absorbed very slowly in what has been described as a depot effect (7). Intramuscular injection sites in neonates may leave sterile abscesses that later require surgical repair. In general, prolonged intramuscular administration of drugs in neonates should be avoided.

Intravenous

Intravenous drug administration is most likely to ensure effective drug therapy in neonates. Although this route of drug treatment is the most reliable, certain problems must be recognized that are unique to neonates. The infusion rate for i.v. fluids in extremely small neonates is so slow that drug doses injected distant from where the i.v. enters the vessel or up the i.v. tubing away from the patient, may not reach the circulation for several hours (8).

The most reliable method for administering medications intravenously to neonates is to use a small-volume syringe pump and micro-bore tubing connected as close to the patient as possible. If the syringe is prepared to contain the exact dose, the tubing must be flushed following drug administration to ensure complete drug delivery. Alternatively, it may be preferable to include overfill in the syringe so that the tubing may be primed prior to drug administration. Thus, once the drug is infused, the tubing will contain extra drug that may be discarded without the necessity of flushing.

Distribution

Distribution is the partitioning of drug from the circulation into various body fluids, organs, and tissues (9). At equilibrium, this distribution is related to organ blood flow; pH and composition of body fluids and tissues; physical and chemical properties of the drug including lipid solubility, polarity, and size; and the extent of binding to plasma and tissue proteins.

Dramatic developmental changes in body composition of newborns influence the distribution of polar and nonpolar drugs within the body. At 24 weeks of gestation, water comprises about 89% of body weight, with 0.1% to 0.5% as fat (10,11). Thus, water-soluble drugs that distribute primarily into extracellular fluid will have larger distribution volumes in premature neonates. By 40 weeks of gestation, the body is approximately 75% water and 15% fat, compared to adults in whom the body is about 65% water and the fat content is variable. The low fat content of the brain of the extremely premature newborn may affect the distribution and effects of centrally active drugs, such as barbiturates and gaseous anesthetics (12).

Metabolism

Many drugs require biotransformation to more polar forms before they can be eliminated from the body. Biotransformation reactions are designated phase I reactions that make the drug more polar through oxidation, reduction, or hydrolysis; or phase II, conjugation reactions, such as glucuronidation, sulfation, and acetylation (9). The liver is the primary site for biotransformation, however other organs are also involved. As early as 9 to 22 weeks gestation, metabolic enzyme activities of the fetal liver vary from 2% to 36% of adult activity (13). This variation precludes broad generalizations regarding hepatic drug metabolism in premature newborns. Over the past decade, intense research into the biochemistry of drug metabolism has revealed multiple forms of cytochrome P450 with different substrate specificities and different activities during development from the fetus to the adult (14–17). Clinicians should have an understanding of P450 nomenclature in addition to understanding which isoforms are responsible for metabolism of commonly used drugs. Both induction and inhibition of specific isoforms may require more frequent therapeutic drug monitoring and dosage adjustments.

Cytochromes P450

Quantitatively, the most important of the phase I enzymes are the cytochromes P450, a superfamily of heme-containing proteins that catalyze the metabolism of many lipophilic substances. The cytochrome P450 isozymes are designated as CYPs that are grouped by the degree of identity in their amino acid sequences. CYP is followed in order by (a) an Arabic number representing the gene family for enzymes with greater than 40% identity; (b) a letter which indicates the subfamily for enzymes with greater than 55% identity; and (c) sequential numbering of the P450 enzymes for different isoforms within each subfamily (9,16). Isozymes which are important in human drug metabolism are found mostly in the CYP1, CYP2, and CYP3 gene families. Table 56-1 outlines the P450 isozymes and their common substrates in the newborn.

Research in the early 1970s revealed that newborn infants have significantly reduced total quantities of cytochrome P450 in liver microsomes (18). This hemoprotein increases with gestational age but reaches only 50% of adult values at term (18). Reduced cytochrome P450 in neonates explains the low clearance and significantly prolonged half-lives of theophylline, caffeine, phenytoin, phenobarbital and other substances that are metabolized via cytochrome P450 (5,19–21). Although newborns are poor metabolizers of many xenobiotics, specific P450 cytochromes exhibit unique developmental patterns during gestation and postnatal life that invalidate broad generalizations about drug metabolism. Table 56-1 outlines important developmental patterns for many of these enzymes.

Ontogeny of Important P450 Cytochromes

Cytochrome P4501A2 is extensively involved in the metabolism of caffeine (1,3,7-trimethylxanthine) (22,23) and theophylline (1,3-dimethylxanthine) (24,25), drugs that are commonly used to treat neonatal apnea and bradycardia (see methylxanthines). CYP1A2 is not significantly expressed in human fetal liver and expression is very low in neonates reaching only 50% of adult activity by 1 year of age (25,26). Metabolically, this limits N-3- and N-7-demethylation of caffeine in the newborn period (23). Caffeine elimination in both preterm and term infants is significantly prolonged (27). Maturation of this pathway to adult levels occurs between four and six months postnatally (28,29). A similar pharmacokinetic trend is noted with theophylline in which 3-demethylation and 8-hydroxylation are catalyzed by CYP1A2 (24,25). Clinically, theophylline clearance and urine metabolite patterns reach adult values by 55 weeks postconceptional age or approximately 4 to 5 months postnatally (30).

Other P450 enzymes which appear to be reduced or absent in the fetus include CYP2D6 and CYP2C9 (14,15,31). The former is responsible for the metabolism of numerous important therapeutic compounds including β-blockers, antiarrhythmics, antidepressants, antipsychotics, and codeine. Although CYP2D6 is absent in the fetal liver and appears to be expressed postnatally (15), activity remains low for an extended period (see Table 56-1) (32). In contrast to the slow development of CYP1A2 and CYP2D6, other enzymes such as CYP2C9 (responsible for the metabolism of nonsteroidal antiinflammatory drugs,

TABLE 56-1

DEVELOPMENTAL PATTERNS FOR IMPORTANT CYTOCHROME P450 ENZYMES IN THE NEONATE

Enzymes	Selected Substrates	Developmental Pattern
CYP1A2	acetaminophen, caffeine, theophylline, warfarin	Not present to an appreciable extent in human fetal liver. Adult levels reached by 4 months of age and may be exceeded in children 1–2 years of age. Inhibited by cimetidine and erythromycin. Induced by cigarette smoke, phenobarbital, and phenytoin.
CYP2C9 CYP2C19	phenytoin, torsemide, S-warfarin phenytoin, diazepam, omeprazole, propranolol	Not apparent in fetal liver. Inferential data using phenytoin disposition as a nonspecific pharmacologic probe suggest low activity during first week of life, with adult activity reached by 6 months of age and peak activity reached by 3–4 years of age. Metabolism induced by rifampin and phenobarbital and inhibited by cimetidine.
CYP2D6	captopril, codeine, propranolol ondansetron	Low to absent in fetal liver but uniformly present at 1-week postnatal age. Poor activity (approximately 20% of adults) at 1 month postnatal age. Adult competence reached by approximately 3–5 years of age. Metabolism inhibited by cimetidine.
CYP3A4 CYP3A7	acetaminophen, alfentanil, amiodarone, budesonide, carbamazepine, diazepam, erythromycin, lidocaine, midazolam, nifedipine, omeprazole, cisapride, theophylline, verapamil, R-warfarin Dehydroepiandrosterone, ethinylestradiol, various dihydropyridines.	CYP3A4 has low activity in the first month of life, with approach toward adult levels by 6–12 months postnatally. CYP3A7 is functionally active in fetus; approximately 30% to 75% of adult levels of CYP3A4. Induced by carbamazepine, dexamethasone, phenobarbital, phenytoin, and rifampin. Enzyme inhibitors include azole antifungals, erythromycin, and cimetidine.

Adapted from Leeder et al. *Pediatr Clin North Am* 1997;44:55–77, with permission.

warfarin, and phenytoin) develop more rapidly after birth. For example, although CYP2C9 is not significantly present during fetal life (31), phenytoin pharmacokinetic data in newborns suggest rapid enzyme maturation within the first weeks of life (20,33).

For drug metabolism, the most important of the cytochromes P450 is CYP3A, because of the large number of therapeutic substrates for this subfamily of enzymes (see Table 56-1). Additionally, CYP3A accounts for the majority of P450 cytochromes present in the adult human liver (9). Unlike most of the other important cytochromes, CYP3A is functionally present during embryogenesis, primarily as CYP3A7 (34). CYP3A activity is detectable in large amounts as early as 17 weeks gestation, and reaches 75% of adult activity at 30 weeks gestation (15). *In vivo*, CYP3A activity appears to be mature at birth (17,35). Postnatally, there is a poorly understood transition from the fetal CYP3A7 to the predominant adult isoform CYP3A4.

Phase II Reactions

The phase II reactions are known as synthetic or conjugation reactions and function to increase the hydrophilicity of drug molecules which facilitates renal elimination (9). The phase II enzymes include glucuronosyltransferase, sulfotransferase, N-acetyltransferase, glutathione S-transferase, and methyl transferase. Although the ontogeny of phase II reactions as a group is not well studied, developmental changes during infancy influence drug clearance (see Table 56-2).

Most conjugation reactions show low activity during fetal development, although sulfation is relatively active in the fetus (16,36,37). One of the most common synthetic reactions involves conjugation with uridine diphosphoglucuronosyltransferases (UDP-GT). This enzyme system which is comprised of numerous isoforms is also responsible for glucuronidation of endogenous compounds such as bilirubin (38). Although UDP-GT activity for bilirubin develops relatively rapidly after birth (36), the ability of the infant to glucuronidate

xenobiotics is significantly limited during the newborn period. Thus, without dosage adjustments, drugs may accumulate to toxic concentrations during the newborn period. A tragic example occurred in the early 1960s when newborns received standard pediatric doses of chloramphenicol and developed fatal circulatory collapse, a condition known as the gray baby syndrome (39–41). The clearance of chloramphenicol is low during the neonatal period and dosage adjustments are necessary in preterm and full-term infants to avoid chloramphenicol toxicity (42).

Other drugs used in the newborn period that undergo glucuronidation include morphine, acetaminophen, and lorazepam. The major metabolic pathway of morphine in children and adults is glucuronidation in the 3- and 6-position (43,44). However, neonates have limited ability to glucuronidate morphine and thus require dosage adjustment (45–47). Morphine clearance (45,48), in particular 3- and 6-glucuronide formation, are depressed at birth and increase with birth weight (47), gestational age (49), and postnatal age (43,46). Morphine's clearance and half-life begin to approach adult values after the age of 1 month (46,50), although other reports indicate that adult values are not reached until at least 5 to 6 months (45,51). Overall, the maturation of glucuronosyltransferase enzymes is isoform-specific; however, adult activity is usually achieved by 6 to 18 months of age (16).

In contrast to glucuronosyltransferase, the sulfotransferase enzyme system is well developed in the newborn and may compensate for limited glucuronidation, as is the case with the metabolism of acetaminophen. Although acetaminophen is primarily glucuronidated in adults, the half-life of acetaminophen is only moderately prolonged in term newborns as compared to older infants and adults (52–54). In the neonate, this is explained by a relatively large formation rate constant for the acetaminophen-sulfate leading to a greater percent of the dose excreted as the acetaminophen-sulfate conjugate (52,53). Preferential sulfation of acetaminophen continues into childhood (53,55).

TABLE 56-2

DEVELOPMENTAL PATTERNS FOR IMPORTANT CONJUGATION REACTIONS IN THE NEONATE

Enzymes	Selected Substrates	Developmental Pattern
Uridine diphosphoglucuronosyltransferase (UDP-GT)	chloramphenicol, morphine, acetaminophen, valproic acid, lorazepam	Ontogeny is isoform specific. In general, adult activity is achieved by 6–18 months of age. May be induced by cigarette smoke and phenobarbital.
Sulfotransferase	bile acids, acetaminophen, cholesterol, polyethylene glycols, dopamine, chloramphenicol	Ontogeny seems to be more rapid than UDP-GT; however, it is substrate specific. Activity for some isoforms may exceed adult values during infancy and childhood (e.g. that responsible for acetaminophen metabolism)
N-Acetyl Transferase 2	hydralazine, procainamide, clonazepam, caffeine, sulfamethoxazole	Some fetal activity present by 16 weeks. Virtually 100% of infants between birth and 2 months of age exhibit the slow metabolizer phenotype. Adult activity present by approximately 1–3 years of age.

Adapted from Leeder et al. *Pediatr Clin North Am* 1997;44:55–77, with permission.

Alterations in Biotransformation

Biotransformation reactions, especially those involving certain forms of cytochrome P450, are often inducible before birth through maternal exposure to drugs, cigarette smoke, or other xenobiotic inducing agents. Biotransformation reactions may also be induced by postnatal drug exposure (see Tables 56-1 and 56-2) and may be slowed postnatally by hypoxia/asphyxia, organ damage, and/or critical illness. Additional postnatal changes in hepatic blood flow, protein binding, and/or biliary function may also significantly alter drug elimination. Additional studies in premature neonates are required to generate the population pharmacokinetic data necessary to design safe and effective pharmacotherapeutic regimens.

Excretion

Excretion involves elimination of drug from the body by several potential routes, including the biliary tract, lungs, and kidneys. Both unchanged and metabolized forms of drug may be excreted, but only unbound drug undergoes filtration and tubular transport. Glomerular and tubular function are decreased at birth, both in absolute terms and after normalization to body mass (56,57). Glomerular filtration in newborns averages 30% of the adult rate after normalization to body surface area. Birth accelerates maturation of glomerular filtration through an increase in cardiac output, decreased renal vascular resistance, redistribution of intrarenal blood flow, and changes in the intrinsic function of the glomerular basement membrane (56). Renal tubular maturation seems to proceed more slowly than glomerular maturation after birth (56). This produces an imbalance in glomerular and tubular function that persists for several months. Because most low molecular weight unbound molecules are filtered, tubular reabsorption exerts a profound influence on the elimination rate for many drugs. Additionally, hypoxemia, nephrotoxic drugs, and underperfusion may alter renal function of newborns, which prevents accurate prediction of the rates of drug elimination after birth.

PHARMACOKINETICS

Pharmacokinetics describes the changes in drug concentrations within the body with time. These concepts are presented as a general overview to assist the clinician with dose adjustments and practical interpretation of therapeutic drug monitoring (58–60). The more rigorous mathematical intricacies of pharmacokinetics are covered elsewhere (61–64). Although a drug may penetrate several body fluids and tissues at different rates, the change in its circulating concentration is used to characterize its kinetics and to guide dosages. The rate of removal of drug from the circulation usually fits either first-order or zero-order exponential mathematical equations. These two types of equations describe two different processes that have important implications for dosage regimes.

Rates and Distribution

First-Order Kinetics

Most drugs are cleared from the body with first-order exponential rates. Exponential clearance indicates that a constant fraction or constant proportion of drug is removed per unit of time. This means that the higher the concentration, the greater the amount of drug removed from the body. Such changes in concentration fit exponential equations of the following form:

$$C_t = C_0 - e^{kt} \qquad [1]$$

where C_t is the concentration at a particular time t, C_0 is the starting concentration, which is a constant, and k is the elimination rate constant with units of 1/time. First-order indicates that the exponent is raised to the first power ($-kt$ in Eq. 1). First-order exponential equations, such as Eq. 1, may be solved by taking the natural logarithm of both sides.

$$\ln C_t = \ln C_0 + -kt \qquad [2]$$

This transforms the equation to that of a straight line ($y = mx + b$). If ln (i.e., natural logarithm) C is graphed vs. time, the slope is $-k$, and the intercept is $\ln C_0$. If log i.e., common logarithm C is graphed vs. time, the slope is $-k/2.303$, because ln x equals 2.303 log x. When graphed on linear-linear axes, exponential rates are curvilinear and on semilogarithmic axes, they produce a straight line.

Half-Life

One of the more familiar exponential rates used clinically is the half-life, i.e., the time for a drug concentration to decrease by one-half. Half-life is a first-order kinetic process, because the same proportion or fraction of the drug is removed during equal time periods. At higher concentrations, a greater amount is removed during a single half-life than when the concentration is lower. For example a drug concentration may decrease by 200 from 400 to 200 in one half-life, and decrease by 100 from 200 to 100 in the next half-life (Fig. 56-1).

Half-life can be determined by several methods. If concentration is converted to the natural logarithm of concentration and graphed vs. time, as described in Eq. 2, the slope of this graph is the elimination rate constant, k. Usually at least three concentration-time points are needed to determine the slope accurately; however, in clinical practice, k is often determined from just two concentrations obtained during the terminal elimination phase. To increase the accuracy of the latter, at least one half-life should elapse between concentration-time points. With multiple data points, the slope of ln C vs. time may be calculated easily by least-squares linear regression analysis. Half-life ($t_{1/2}$) may be calculated from the elimination rate constant, k (1/time), as follows:

$$t_{1/2} = \frac{\text{natural logarithm (2)}}{k} = \frac{0.693}{k} \qquad [3]$$

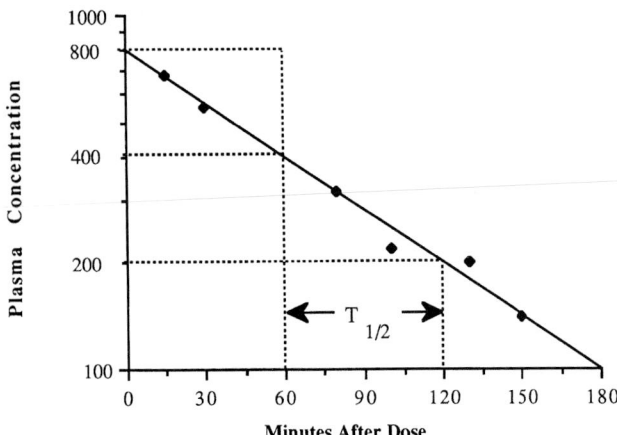

Figure 56-1   Graph method for estimation of half-life. From Ward RM. Pharmacologic principles and practicalities. In: Taeusch HW, Ballard RA, Avery ME, eds. *Shaffer and Avery's diseases of the newborn.* 6th ed. Philadelphia: WB Saunders, 1991:289, with permission.

Half-life may be determined graphically from a series of drug concentrations graphed on semilogarithmic axes. With multiple data points, the best-fit line is determined either visually or by linear regression analysis. The times corresponding to carefully chosen concentrations are then used to estimate the interval required for the concentration to decrease by one-half. In Fig. 56-1, this is illustrated by the times corresponding to concentrations of 400, 200, and 100, estimated by the horizontal broken line intercepts with the concentration line and the intercepts with the time axis indicated by the vertical broken lines. Note that the concentrations decrease by 50% every 60 minutes, so that $t_{1/2}$ equals 60 minutes.

First-Order Single-Compartment Kinetics

The number of compartments refers to the number of exponential equations required to describe the observed changes in concentration. These compartments theoretically represent a group of similar tissues, fluids, and/or organs and may be correlated with different anatomic fluids and tissues. Although multiple transfers of drug among tissues and body fluids may be occurring, a drug's clearance may fit first-order, single-compartment kinetics if it distributes rapidly and homogeneously within the circulation from which it is removed through metabolism or excretion. This may be judged visually, if a semilogarithmic graph of a series of concentrations fits a single straight line. Kinetics may falsely appear to be single-compartment if drug concentrations are not measured quickly enough after i.v. administration to detect the initial distribution phase.

First-Order Multicompartment Kinetics

If drug clearance from the circulation is studied carefully, with measurement of concentration several times within the first 15 to 30 minutes after i.v. administration and dur-

ing the next several hours, two or more rates of clearance often are detected by a change in slope of a semilogarithmic graph of concentration vs. time (Fig. 56-2). The number and nature of the compartments for the clearance of a drug do not necessarily correspond to specific body fluids or tissues. When two first-order exponential equations are required to describe the clearance of drug from the circulation, the kinetics are designated first-order and two-compartment i.e., central and peripheral compartments and are represented by the following equation (58):

$$C = Ae^{-\alpha t} + Be^{-\beta t} \qquad [4]$$

In Eq. 4, C is concentration, t is time after the dose, A is the concentration at time 0 for the distribution rate represented by the broken line graph with the steepest slope, is the rate constant for distribution, B is the concentration at time 0 for the terminal elimination rate, and β is the rate constant for terminal elimination. Rate constants indicate the rate of change in concentration and correspond to the slope of the line divided by 2.303 for logarithm concentration vs. time.

Such biphasic kinetics are observed commonly for drugs that rapidly distribute out of the central compartment (blood volume + extracellular fluid of highly perfused organs) after i.v. administration (58). For such drugs, the initial rapid decrease in concentration is referred to as the alpha distribution phase and represents primarily distribution to the peripheral (tissue) compartments in addition to drug elimination. After the inflection point in the slope and during the terminal (beta) phase of the curve, elimination accounts for most of the change in drug concentration. The alpha distribution rate constant (α) (see Fig. 56-2) can be determined from the slope of the line generated by subtracting concentrations from the beta elimination phase from those during the alpha distribution phase. A more detailed mathematical discussion may be found elsewhere (58,61).

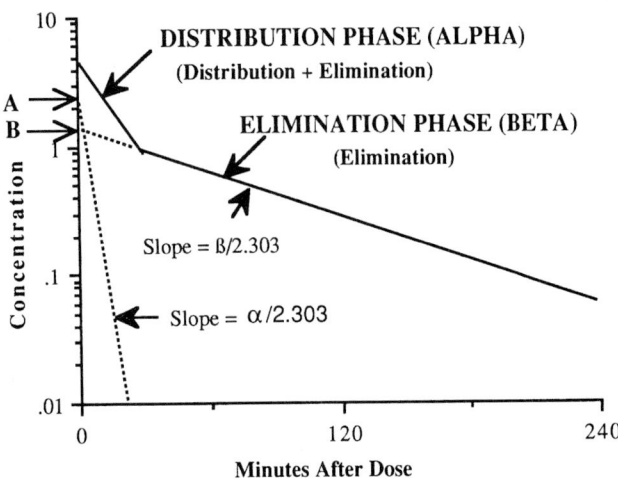

Figure 56-2   Multicompartment first-order exponential kinetics. From Ward RM. Pharmacologic principles and practicalities. In: Taeusch HW, Ballard RA, Avery ME, eds. *Shaffer and Avery's diseases of the newborn.* 6th ed. Philadelphia: WB Saunders, 1991:289, with permission.

Although many drugs demonstrate multicompartment kinetics, the intensive blood sampling required to fit data to more than one compartment is not clinically feasible, particularly in newborns. Furthermore, the mathematical complexity of two compartment models makes this kinetic approach clinically impractical. To minimize cost and simplify pharmacokinetic calculations, only two plasma concentrations (peak and trough) are usually obtained for therapeutic monitoring of commonly used drugs, e.g., gentamicin and vancomycin. Accordingly, a one-compartment model is assumed and the elimination rate constant (k) is determined from the slope of these points plotted on a semi-logarithmic scale. Because the elimination rate constant should be determined from the terminal elimination phase, it is important that peak concentrations of multicompartment drugs not be drawn prematurely, i.e., during the initial distribution phase. If drawn too early, the concentrations will be higher than those during the terminal elimination phase (see Fig. 56-2), which will overestimate the slope and the terminal elimination rate constant. Clinically, this is not usually problematic with gentamicin because the initial distribution phase commonly occurs during the 30- to 60-minute infusion (65). Thus, a peak concentration obtained 30 to 60 minutes after the end of infusion usually reflects the terminal phase of elimination. However, with vancomycin, the half-life of the initial distribution phase is approximately 0.5 hours (66). Thus, a peak vancomycin concentration drawn prematurely may lead to error in estimating the pharmacokinetic parameters.

Zero-Order Kinetics

Some drugs are eliminated by a constant amount per unit time, rather than a constant fraction. Such rates are zero-order and the following equation can be used to calculate the change in the amount of drug in the body (61):

$$-dA/dt = k_0 \qquad [5]$$

in which dA is the change in the amount of drug in the body (mg), dt is the change in time, and k_0 is the elimination rate constant with units of amount/time. After solving this equation, it has the following form:

$$A = A_0 - k_0 t \qquad [6]$$

in which A_0 is the initial amount in body and A is the amount of drug in the body (mg) at time t.

Zero-order kinetics also is referred to as saturation kinetics, because it may occur when excess amounts of drug saturate the capacity of metabolic enzymes or transport systems so that only a constant amount of drug is metabolized or transported per unit of time. This may be detected graphically from a serum concentration vs. time plot in which zero-order elimination is linear on linear-linear axes and is curved when graphed on logarithmic-linear (i.e., semilogarithmic) axes. Clinically, zero-order elimination may be observed after administration of excessive doses, or during dysfunction of the organ of elimination without a decrease in dosage. Certain drugs administered

TABLE 56-3

DRUGS THAT DEMONSTRATE ZERO-ORDER (SATURATION) KINETICS WITH THERAPEUTIC DOSES IN NEWBORNS

Caffeine
Chloramphenicol
Diazepam
Furosemide
Indomethacin
Phenytoin

From Ward RM. Pharmacologic principles and practicalities. In: Taeusch HW, Ballard RA, Avery ME, eds. *Schaffer and Avery's Diseases of the Newborn*, 6th ed. Philadelphia: WB Saunders, 1991, 285, with permission.

to newborns exhibit zero-order kinetics at therapeutic doses, and may accumulate to excessive concentrations (Table 56-3). Some drugs, e.g., phenytoin, may exhibit Michaelis-Menten kinetics, i.e., first-order at low concentrations and zero-order after enzymes are saturated at higher concentrations. For these drugs, a small increment in dose may cause disproportionately large increments in serum concentrations (Fig. 56-3).

Apparent Volume of Distribution

Volume of distribution does not necessarily correspond to a physiologic body fluid or tissue volume, hence the designation "apparent." The apparent volume of distribution (Vd) is a mathematical term that relates the dose to the circulating concentration observed immediately after intravenous administration. It might be viewed as the volume of dilution. For drugs such as digoxin, Vd in neonates may reach 10 L/kg, a physical impossibility. Such a large Vd occurs when drug concentrates outside of the plasma compartment, for example bound to red blood cells or in tissue. This emphasizes the mathematical nature of Vd. The units used to express concentration are amount/volume and may help to remind the reader of the following equation that expresses the relation between dose in amount/kg and the Vd in volume/kg that dilutes the dose to produce the concentration:

$$\text{Concentration change (mg/L)} = \frac{\text{Dose (mg/kg)}}{\text{Vd(L/kg)}} \qquad [7]$$

To facilitate canceling units, concentration is expressed with the unconventional units of milligrams per liter rather than micrograms per milliliter, because they are equivalent. This equation serves as the basis for most of the pharmacokinetic calculations, because it is easily rearranged to solve for Vd and Dose. It is also important to note that this equation represents the change in concentration following a rapidly administered intravenous dose. Following an intravenous infusion, e.g., vancomycin or gentamicin, a more complex exponential equation may be required to account for drug elimination during the time of infusion (61).

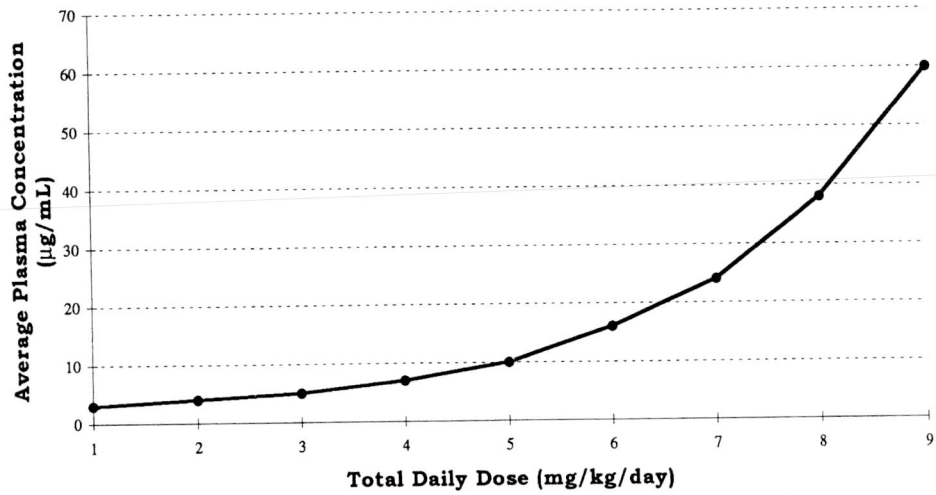

Figure 56-3 Nonlinear (Michaelis-Menten) kinetics illustrated for a hypothetical drug. As dosage increases above 3 mg/kg/day, there is a disproportionate increase in average plasma concentration as elimination changes from a first-order to a zero-order process.

However, such equations are needed only when the drug is rapidly eliminated, i.e., the duration of infusion approaches the drug's half-life. In neonates, who have relatively slow drug elimination, only a small fraction of drug is eliminated during the time of infusion, and such adjustments can be omitted. Accordingly, we may use the simpler and more practical equation to estimate pharmacokinetic parameters.

Knowledge of the apparent distribution volume is essential for dosage adjustments. Vd may be calculated by rearranging Eq. 7.

$$Vd\ (L/kg) = \frac{Dose\ (mg/kg)}{C\ (postdose) - C\ (predose)\ (mg/L)} \quad [8]$$

The concentration after drug infusion, C (postdose), must be measured after the distribution phase to avoid overestimating the peak concentration that would result in an erroneously low Vd. For the first dose, the predose concentration is zero.

Pharmacokinetic Example

To illustrate the practical application of the principles outlined above, we recommend a simple four-step approach: (a) calculate Vd; (b) calculate half-life; (c) calculate a new dose and dosing interval based on a desired peak and trough; (d) check the peak and trough of the new dosage regimen.

For example, gentamicin 2.5 mg/kg every 12 hours was administered i.v. over 30 minutes. The following plasma concentrations were measured on the third day of treatment (presumed steady-state). The predose or trough concentration was 1.8 mg/L; the peak concentration, measured 30 minutes after the end of the infusion, was 4.8 mg/L.

Step 1: Substituting the data into Eq. 8, we calculate Vd.

$$Vd\ (L/kg) = \frac{2.5\ mg/kg}{4.8\ mg/L - 1.8\ mg/L} = \frac{2.5\ mg/kg}{3.0\ mg/L}$$
$$= 0.83\ L/kg.$$

Step 2: At steady-state, trough concentrations remain unchanged from one dose to the next. Therefore, for the

purpose of these calculations, steady-state trough concentration may be understood to follow the peak concentration. Thus, the time between the peak and trough concentrations is 11 hours, i.e., 12 hours minus 0.5 hour infusion, minus 0.5 hour to peak concentration. The plasma concentration decreased from 4.8 to 2.4 mg/L in one half-life, and then from 2.4 to 1.2 mg/L in a second half-life. The trough of 1.8 was reached approximately half way between the first and second half-lives. Because 1.5 half-lives elapsed during the 11 hours between the peak and trough, the half-life is approximately 11 hours/1.5 half-lives, or 7.3 hours.

Step 3: A new dosage regimen must be calculated if the concentrations are unsatisfactory. Accordingly, one must decide on a desired peak and trough concentration. If, for example, the desired gentamicin peak and trough concentrations were 6.5 mg/L (5–10 mg/L) and 1.5 mg/L (1–2 mg/L), respectively, then Eq. 8 may be rearranged to solve for the new dose.

$$Dose\ (mg/kg) = Vd\ (L/kg) \times [C\ (peak\ desired) \quad [9]$$
$$- C\ (post\ desired)\ (mg/L)]$$
$$Dose\ (mg/kg) = 0.83\ L/kg \times [6.5\ mg/L - 1.5\ mg/L]$$
$$Dose\ (mg/kg) = 4.15\ mg/kg$$

Increasing the dose to 4.15 mg/kg (66% increase) will lead to a higher trough if the dosage interval is kept at 12 hours. Because trough concentrations above 2 mg/L are associated with ototoxicity and nephrotoxicity, the dosage interval needs to be increased. Aminoglycosides, in general, are dosed every 2 to 2.5 half-lives for neonates. However, to reduce the risk of administration errors, one should choose a conventional dosage interval that approximates 2 to 2.5 half-lives, i.e., every 8, 12, 18, 24, or 36 hours. In the above example, dosing every two half-lives would require a 15-hour dosage interval that might lead to administration errors. Thus, the dosage interval should be increased to 18 hr, an interval that corresponds to approximately 2.5 half-lives.

Step 4: Mathematically estimating peak and trough concentrations with the new regimen provides a good double check against a math error. Because 18 hours was chosen as the new interval, waiting 18 hours after the previous dose to begin the new regimen is reasonable. At that time, approximately 2.5 half-lives after the measured peak of 4.8 mg/L, we would expect the trough concentration to be approximately 0.9 mg/L (half-life #1: 4.8 mg/L → 2.4 mg/L; half-life #2: 2.4 mg/L → 1.2 mg/L, half-life #3: 1.2 mg/L → 0.6 mg/L, with half of this third half-life occurring at 0.9 mg/L). Using Eq. 7, we calculate that the plasma concentration will increase by 5 mg/L after each 4.15 mg/kg dose. Accordingly, the measured peak concentration will be 5.9 mg/L after the first dose and will decrease to 1.1 mg/L over the next 2.5 half-lives (5.9 mg/L → 2.95 mg/L → 1.48 mg/L → 0.74 mg/L in 3 half-lives, or → 1.1 mg/L in 2.5 half-lives). After the second dose of 4.15 mg/kg, the measured peak concentration will be 6.1 mg/L and will decrease to 1.15 mg/L in 2.5 half-lives. Because the trough has not changed from the previous trough, one can conclude that this dosage schedule will meet the desired therapeutic levels. Estimation of concentrations after a fraction of a half-life assumes a linear rather than logarithmic decline in concentrations and is not mathematically correct for first-order, exponential rates in which the amount of drug eliminated decreases as the concentration decreases. However, this approach is suitable for clinical applications, in which only a reasonable estimate of plasma concentration is needed for dosage adjustments.

Therapeutic Drug Monitoring

Circulating concentrations of drugs should be measured primarily to ensure that the treatment regime achieves concentrations that are effective in clinical situations in which drug treatment is critical, response is not immediately apparent (e.g., for culture-proven sepsis), and a good correlation exists between circulating drug concentration and desired effect. Drug concentrations should be measured to avoid toxicity when they clearly correlate with toxicity in newborns (e.g., for chloramphenicol), to verify toxicity when symptoms correspond to a known drug toxicity, or to investigate symptoms that are unexplained by the disease process. Extrapolation of toxic and therapeutic ranges from adults to neonates has led to some recommendations about therapeutic drug monitoring in newborns (e.g., for gentamicin) that are not well supported by subsequent experience (67).

Several basic requirements must be met to justify therapeutic drug monitoring in newborns and to modify drug treatment accurately based on measured circulating drug concentrations (68).

- Drug analysis using small blood volumes must be accurate.
- Circulating drug concentrations must correlate with both effective and toxic pharmacologic effects. This implies that the circulating total (i.e., free plus protein-bound) drug concentration correlates with the free-drug

concentration at the site of drug action, such as the drug receptor or tissue site.
- The therapeutic index, the concentration range between efficacy and toxicity, should be narrow.
- Clinical studies should have established a concentration range for efficacy and toxicity in the population being monitored.
- Pharmacokinetics are variable and unpredictable in newborns.

In the extremely premature newborn, decreased protein binding may significantly affect therapeutic drug monitoring. As a result of unpredictable decreases in protein binding associated with organ dysfunction or immaturity, free-drug concentrations may be much higher than would be predicted from the total drug concentration that usually is measured clinically. Higher percentages of free drug in the newborn may account for signs of toxicity or adequate therapeutic response at paradoxically low total drug concentrations. When available and when therapeutic concentration ranges have been established, as for phenytoin, measurement of free-drug concentrations may be helpful in newborns demonstrating signs of drug toxicity with therapeutic or subtherapeutic circulating total drug concentrations.

Effective drug therapy is measured by response, not by achieving a particular circulating drug concentration. Concentration ranges described as therapeutic are statistical ranges for drug levels that usually are effective and nontoxic. Individual patients may require drug concentrations outside these ranges to achieve optimal drug treatment.

Repetitive Dosing and Drug Accumulation

During most courses of repetitive drug therapy, the doses are administered before complete elimination of the previous one. This leads to accumulation of drug, with increasing peak and trough concentrations until a steady state concentration is reached (Fig. 56-4). The average Css can be calculated as follows (59):

$$\text{Avg Css} = \frac{1}{\text{Clearance}} \times \frac{f \times D}{\tau}, \qquad [10]$$

$$= \frac{1}{k \times \text{Vd}_{(area)}} \times \frac{f \times D}{\tau},$$

$$= \frac{1.44 \times t_{1/2}}{\text{Vd}_{(area)}} \times \frac{f \times D}{\tau}, \qquad [11]$$

In Eq. 10 and 11, f is the fraction of the dose that is absorbed, D is the dose, τ is the dosing interval in the same units of time as the elimination half-life, k is the elimination rate constant, and 1.44 equals 1/0.693 (see Eq. 56-3). The magnitude of the average Css is directly proportional to a ratio of τ/half-life and D. (59)

Steady State

Steady-state occurs when the amount of drug removed from the body between doses equals the amount of the dose

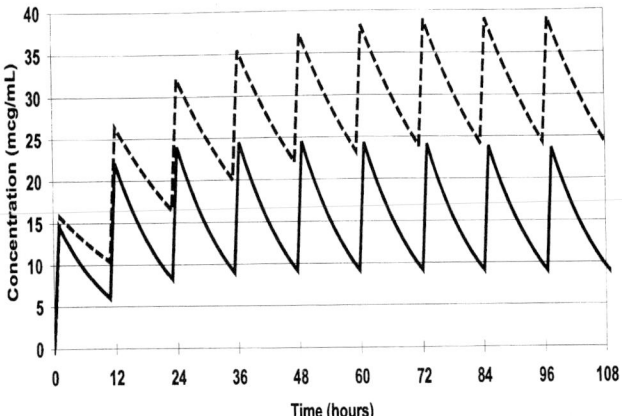

Figure 56-4 The effect of 2 different half-lives on the steady state concentrations of vancomycin during repetitive dosing with the same dose (15 mg/kg and a Vd of 0.9 L/kg). The solid line represents a half-life of 8 hours and the broken line represents a half-life of 16 hours. Peak and trough concentrations increase until steady-state is achieved, but steady-state is achieved by the fourth dose (36 hrs) with the 8 hour half-life, but not until the 7th dose (72 hours) with the 16 hour half-life.

(64,69). Five half-lives are usually required for drug elimination and distribution among tissue and fluid compartments to reach an equilibrium. When all tissues are at equilibrium, i.e., steady-state, the peak and trough concentrations are the same after each dose. However, prior to this time, constant peak and trough concentrations after intermittent doses, or constant concentrations during drug infusions, do not prove that a steady-state has been achieved because drug may still be entering and leaving deep tissue compartments. During continuous infusion, the fraction of steady state concentration that has been reached can be calculated in terms of multiples of the drug's half-life (59). After 3 half-lives, the concentration is 88% of that at steady state. The effect of dosage changes on drug concentrations during chronic treatment usually should not be rechecked until several half-lives have elapsed, unless elimination is impaired or toxic symptoms occur. Drug concentrations may not need to be checked if symptoms improve.

Loading Dose

If the time to reach a constant concentration by continuous or intermittent dosing is too long, a loading dose may be used to reach a higher constant concentration more quickly. This frequently is applied to initial treatment with digoxin, which has a 35- to 69-hour half-life in term neonates and an even longer half-life in preterm newborns (70). Use of a loading dose produces a higher circulating drug concentration earlier in the therapeutic course, but the equilibration to reach a true steady-state still requires treatment for five or more half-lives. Loading doses must be used cautiously, because they increase the likelihood of drug toxicity, as has been observed with digoxin digitalizing doses (70).

Special Considerations for Neonates

Intravenous Administration

Intravenous administration of drugs is considered the most reliable route. In neonates, especially those who weigh 500 to 1000 g and receive small volumes of i.v. fluids, i.v. drug administration may not reliably deliver the dose into the circulation (8,69). Because some types of i.v. tubing may contain 12- to 15-mL of fluid and the i.v. infusion rates for 500- to 1,000-g neonates may be 1.5 to 2.5 mL/hour, infusion of a drug into the i.v. tubing several cm from the patient will markedly delay drug administration. This may confound therapeutic drug monitoring by causing the peak concentration to be less than the trough, because the dose has not reached the patient. For this reason, microbore tubing, which has a volume of 0.5 mL should be used whenever possible and should be connected to a port closest to the patient. Slow delivery of drug to the circulation may prevent the attainment of an adequate peak concentration to enhance drug diffusion into tissue down a concentration gradient. Lastly, filters present potential obstacle to effective i.v. drug treatment. Drugs may adsorb to the filter or settle to the bottom of a reservoir in the filter, out of the main flow of the infusing solution (71).

Exchange Transfusion

Because few studies have evaluated the amount of drug actually removed from neonates during an exchange transfusion, theoretical estimates have been developed (69,72). The amounts removed vary with the individual drug's volume of distribution, rate of distribution, and circulating concentration at the time of the exchange, and the volume of blood exchanged and the rate of the exchange.

CLINICAL TOXICOLOGY

Newborn infants, both full-term and premature, present an alarmingly wide spectrum of susceptibilities to unanticipated, adverse effects from exposure to exogenous chemicals. New drugs, together with unrecognized chemicals ranging from tape remover to plasticizers, are introduced into the care of neonates each year. Prescription drug exposure of the extremely preterm neonate is extensive. In the late 1970s, neonates admitted to a neonatal intensive care unit (NICU) received 1 to 26 drugs, averaging 6.2 drugs per infant (73). This drug exposure was not innocuous, because 30% of infants in the NICU manifested an adverse drug reaction, of which 15% were considered fatal or life-threatening (74). Similar drug exposure of newborns was documented in Boston from 1974 to 1977, in which infants in the intensive care nursery received more drugs (10.4/patient) than any other hospitalized children (75).

Several factors increase the susceptibility of newborns and preterm newborns to chemical toxicities. Immaturity of liver and renal function frequently delays drug elimination, which prolongs the exposure of the newborn to a drug and predisposes to drug accumulation during repeated administration. New therapeutic agents often are introduced into treatment of critically ill neonates when all other therapy has failed, although pharmacokinetic data to guide dose and dosing intervals are lacking. Without the guide of pharmacokinetic or concentration-response studies, treatment failure may be considered an indication to increase the dose, rather than the result of administering excess amounts of the drug (76).

Specific enzyme immaturities of the newborn also may place them at risk. Inadequate function of the glucuronosyltransferase system predisposes the newborn to inadequate elimination of chemicals requiring glucuronide conjugation, such as bilirubin. Circulating albumin binds bilirubin at the levels encountered in physiologic jaundice and protects the newborn from bilirubin encephalopathy as long as the blood–brain barrier remains intact (77,78). Failure to recognize the competition of drugs for bilirubin's albumin-binding sites has led to displacement of bound bilirubin and kernicterus (79–81). Large doses of chloramphenicol were associated with unexplained cardiovascular collapse in infants in 1959 (40). That same year, a randomized, controlled study of antibiotics for neonatal sepsis revealed that the groups treated with chloramphenicol alone or in combination had a 60% mortality, threefold higher than neonates receiving no antibiotics (41). The no-treatment control group, however, showed the same survival as the alternate antibiotic treatment group. Inadequate glucuronide conjugation of chloramphenicol and decreased tubular secretion of conjugated chloramphenicol combined to reduce chloramphenicol elimination and led to accumulation to toxic concentrations (39). Acute intoxication with high serum chloramphenicol concentrations manifested with jaundice, vomiting, anorexia, respiratory distress, abdominal distention, cyanosis, green stools, lethargy, and ashen color (41).

The preservative, benzyl alcohol, has been implicated in a fatal syndrome in premature infants of cardiovascular collapse and death associated with metabolic acidosis, gasping respirations, thrombocytopenia, hepatic and renal failure, and progressive central nervous system (CNS) depression (82). The minimal intake to produce toxicity was estimated at 130 mg/kg/day (82). Removal of benzyl alcohol as a preservative in the fluid frequently used to flush i.v. catheters in neonates essentially has eliminated this problem. Although many nurseries and pharmacies have excluded all solutions and medications containing benzyl alcohol, the major problem seemed to lie with i.v. solutions and flush solutions. Considering the dose estimated for toxicity, exposure to the small amounts in medications (which can be estimated from the benzyl alcohol concentration and dosing volume) might pose an acceptable risk compared to the benefit of the drug treatment. Propylene glycol (PG), a solvent frequently used with water-insoluble drugs, has also been associated with toxicity in neonates (83,84). At high doses, propylene glycol is partly metabolized to lactic acid and may cause serum hyperosmolality with a marked osmolar gap, lactic acidosis, seizures, and cardiac arrhythmias (83–86). Because up to 45% of PG is eliminated renally, patients with poor renal function (including preterm neonates) may be predisposed to PG toxicity. Lorazepam, which is commonly used in neonates, contains propylene glycol and caution must be exercised in prescribing large scheduled doses of lorazepam for sedation of sick neonates.

Dermal exposure to a variety of chemical agents, including isopropyl alcohol, may be hazardous to the newborn (87,88). Toxic epidermal necrolysis was reported in a neonate after prolonged exposure to a commonly used distillate-containing adhesive remover (89). Unintended percutaneous absorption of toxic substances through the permeable skin of neonates has recurred with several substances. This has led to toxicity from methanol (90), isopropanol (91,92), hexachlorophene (93), iodine-containing topical disinfectants (94,95), aniline dye in diapers (96), and topical antibiotics such as neomycin (97). Advantageous and disadvantageous transcutaneous drug absorption by newborns has been reviewed (98). Chemical intoxication of the fetus and newborn has been reviewed in detail (70).

Inadvertent exposure of the neonate to a variety of chemicals may occur with little notice. Phthalate plasticizers accumulate in the myocardial and gastrointestinal tissue of neonates with umbilical catheters and those who receive blood products (99). Although phthalates probably produce minimal acute toxicity, they accumulate in tissues and may exert effects that are not recognized. Since the report by Hillman and colleagues (99), the extent of exposure of NICU patients to plastic products appears to have increased, causing greater exposure to soluble chemicals in the plastic, such as phthalates.

SPECIFIC CLASSES OF DRUGS

Antiarrhythmics

Treatment of cardiac arrhythmias has advanced with increased understanding of the transmembrane ion currents that control both normal and abnormal myocardial depolarization (100–102). Developmental changes in these channels are described using both electrophysiological techniques and molecular biological means of investigation (103). Careful interpretation of various studies is needed, however, as a result of species differences in the timing of innervation and in the development of various channels (103,104).

Antiarrhythmic drugs have been classified and reclassified according to the mechanisms responsible for arrhythmias, including effects on ion channels, duration of repolarization, and receptor interaction (Table 56-4) (100,105–107). A discussion of the various subtypes of

TABLE 56-4
ANTIARRHYTHMIC DRUGS BY MECHANISM OF ACTION

Class	Action/Structure	Drugs
IA	Sodium ± potassium channel blockade Phase 0 dV/dt – slowed Conduction slowed (prolonged PR, QRS, and QT) Repolarization usually delayed Anticholinergic	Quinidine Procainamide Dysopyramide
IB	Sodium channel blockade Phase 0 dV/dt,-minimal change Repolarization usually shortened (QT shortened) Fibrillation thresholds elevated	Lidocaine Mexilitine Moricizine
IC	Sodium channel blockade Phase 0 dV/dt,-markedly slowed Repolarization minimally changed, PR and QRS markedly prolonged	Flecainide Propafenone
II	Beta-adrenergic blockade, variable selectivity	Propranolol Atenolol Esmolol
III	Repolarization and Action Potential Prolonged	Amiodarone Sotalol
IV	Calcium Channel Blockade	Verapamil
V	Digitalis Glycosides	Digoxin Ouabain
VI	Purinergic Agonists	Adenosine

Adapted from Grant AO. Mechanisms of action of antiarrhythmic drugs: From ion channel blockage to arrhythmia termination. *Pacing Clin Electrophysiol* 1997;20:432–444; Perry JC. Pharmacologic therapy of arrhythmias. In Deal B, Wolff G, Gelband H (eds). *Current Concepts in Diagnosis and Management of Arrhythmias in Infants and Children.* Armonk, NY: Futura Publishing Co., 1998:267–305, with permission.

ion channels is beyond the scope of this chapter (100–102,108,109). Such classification systems help with analysis of the effects of individual antiarrhythmic drugs and selection of treatment for specific arrhythmias, but drugs and their metabolites may interact with multiple ion channels and more than one antiarrhythmic mechanism (106,110). Drugs within a given class, however, may differ in their effectiveness for an individual patient's arrhythmia. Dosages for drugs used frequently for resuscitation of newborns are listed (see Table 56-5) (111).

Drug selection for treatment of arrhythmias should be guided, whenever possible, by more precise identification of the type of arrhythmia. The most frequent arrhythmia requiring management in neonates is supraventricular tachycardia (SVT) (112). In general, SVT arises from either an aberrant conduction pathway or abnormal automaticity in a discrete focus that captures the ventricle (112). Reentrant mechanisms are the most common cause of SVT in neonates and usually involve retrograde conduction from the ventricle via the accessory conduction pathway to the atrium which then depolarizes prematurely. This has been designated orthodromic reciprocating tachycardia (ORT). A variant of ORT arises from a posterior accessory conducting pathway that causes a slower, but incessant form of SVT, permanent junctional reciprocating tachycardia (PJRT). PJRT, left untreated, may cause a cardiomyopathy and CHF. In the Wolff-Parkinson-White syndrome

(WPW), the accessory conduction pathway can be identified during sinus rhythm from early depolarization that creates a beginning shoulder (delta wave) on the QRS complex with a shortened PR interval (112). Unfortunately, almost 50% of reentrant SVT in infants does not show preexcitation overtly during sinus rhythm. When the depolarization returns from the ventricle through the atrioventricular node to cause SVT, it is termed antidromic reentrant tachycardia, and causes a wide complex tachycardia. Reentrant tachycardias, either overt or concealed, can be identified during electrophysiologic studies by being able to be initiated and terminated by atrial or ventricular extrastimulation (110,112).

Nonreentrant SVT is rare in infancy and difficult to treat pharmacologically. SVT caused by a nonsinus node focus of abnormal automaticity is designated Automatic Atrial Tachycardia (AAT) and is difficult to treat medically (110). AAT must be distinguished from sinus tachycardia because the heart rate may gradually speed up and slow down. The p-wave morphology during AAT differs from that during sinus rhythm and the PR interval of conducted beats may lengthen, rather than shorten as the rate increases (110). SVT may also arise from a site of abnormal automaticity within or near the AV node, designated junctional ectopic tachycardia (JET) (110). JET is also quite difficult to treat with the usual antiarrhythmics (113,114). Treatment of SVT may be required in two situations, acute termination

TABLE 56-5
DRUGS FOR NEWBORN RESUSCITATION AND ACUTE TREATMENT OF ARRHYTHMIAS

Drug and Formulation	Final Concentration	Dose (Amount/kg)	Dose (mL/kg)
Adenosine 6 mg/2 mL	3 mg/mL	Start: 50 μg/kg rapid IV push, followed by flush of IV catheter; if no response within 0.5–2 minutes, increase dose by 50 μg/kg and repeat until conversion of SVT or AV block, to maximum single dose of 250–500 μg/kg	Dilute 0.5 ml with 2.5 ml saline, infuse 0.1 mL/kg IV for every 50 μg/kg dose
Atropine 10.0%	0.1 mg/mL	IV dosage: 0.01–0.02 mg/kg (minimum dose 0.1 mg); may repeat in 10 min to maximum of 0.04 mg/kg; IT dosage: 0.02–0.04 mg/kg	0.1–0.2 mL/kg IV 0.2–0.4 mL/kg IT
Bicarbonate 0.05 mEq/mL	0.5 mEq/mL	1–2 mEq/kg; treat measured metabolic acidosis; avoid 1.0 mEq/mL formulation in newborns; maintain ventilation	1–2 mL/kg IV
Calcium Gluconate 10%	100 mg/mL (9.3 mg Ca^{++}/mL)	60 mg/kg infused slowly and stop infusion for symptomatic bradycardia; repeat as needed for clinical effect; extravasation causes tissue necrosis	0.6 mL/kg IV
Calcium Chloride 10%	100 mg/mL (27 mg Ca^{++}/mL)	20 mg/kg infused slowly and stop infusion for symptomatic bradycardia; repeat as needed for clinical effect; extravasation causes tissue necrosis	0.2 mL/kg IV
Direct Current Defibrillation		1 Watt-sec/kg; increase by 1 Watt-sec/kg if unsuccessful	
Epinephrine 1:10,000	0.1 mg/mL	0.01–0.03 mg/kg IV or IO 0.1 mg/kg IT	0.1–0.3 mL/kg i.v., i.o. 1.0 mL/kg IT
Glucose 10%	100 mg/mL	200–500 mg/kg	2–5 mL/kg IV
Lidocaine 2%	20 mg/mL	0.5–1.0 mg/kg; repeat every 5–10 minutes to maximum of 3 mg/kg	Dilute 0.5 mL + 9.5 mL D5W Infuse: 0.5-1.0 mL/kg IV, IT
Naloxone 0.4 mg/mL	0.4 mg/mL	0.1 mg/kg; dose may be repeated to maintain opioid reversal. This dose is indicated for acute opiate intoxication. Titration to effect with lower initial doses (0.01 mg/kg or 10 μg/kg) should be considered for respiratory depression during pain management. **WARNING: May induce acute withdrawal in opioid dependent patients.**	0.25 mL/kg IV, IM
Procainamide 100 mg/mL	100 mg/mL	3–6 mg/kg over 5 minutes, repeat to a titrated maximum of 15 mg/kg loading dose, infuse slowly with myocardial dysfunction	Dilute 1 mL + 9 mL D5W, Infuse: 0.3–0.6 mL/kg IV

* i.v. = intravenous
IT = through endotratracheal tube and dose should be diluted in saline or tube flushed with saline after dose
Adapted from Moak JP. Pharmacology and electrophysiology of antiarrhythmic drugs. In: Gillette PC, Garson Jr A, eds. *Pediatric Arrhythmias: Electrophysiology and Pacing*. Philadelphia: WB Saunders, 1990:37–115; Roberts RJ. *Drug Therapy in Infants. Pharmacologic Principles and Clinical Experience*. Philadelphia: WB Saunders, 1984. American Academy of Pediatrics Committee on Drugs. Drugs for pediatric emergencies. *Pediatrics* 1998;101:e13, with permission.

of a symptomatic tachycardia and chronic suppression of SVT that has recurred or is likely to recur. Synchronized direct current electrocardioversion terminated SVT in about 50% of cases, but was more successful if P waves were not present (115). Vagal maneuvers, such as stimulation of the diving reflex through ice applied to the face, are still frequently used for the acute termination of SVT, although bilateral carotid massage or pressure on the eyes should be avoided.

For the acute treatment of SVT, adenosine has been used with moderate success. Adenosine slows spontaneous heart rate, prolongs the PR interval, and decreases the slope of phase 4 repolarization through activation of A1-purinoceptors coupled to sarcolemmal potassium channels. In one report, electroconversion was not required for conversion of infant onset SVT during the 6 years after the introduction of

adenosine (116). The ventricle is minimally affected by adenosine whose action begins within seconds of administration. With a 9-second half-life, it must be administered as a rapid i.v. infusion over seconds, but it has been administered successfully by intraosseus infusion (117). Its short half-life limits its usefulness to the acute treatment of SVT. Adenosine treatment may be started with 50 to 150 μg/kg doses, with increases in the dose by 50 μg/kg every minute to a maximum of 300 to 350 μg/kg (106,118,119). Because theophylline is a competitive antagonist of adenosine (120), higher adenosine dosages may be required in infants treated with theophylline (121). Adenosine may precipitate bronchoconstriction and wheezing and hypotension as a result of vasodilatation (122).

SVT that has not responded to adenosine may be managed with an infusion of procainamide, a class 1A drug that blocks both sodium and potassium channels (106). Rapid infusion may precipitate hypotension, whereas chronic treatment produces antinuclear antibodies in 50% to 90% of patients associated with a systemic lupus erythematosus-type syndrome (106,122). High concentrations of procainamide may depress myocardial contractility and predispose to congestive heart failure (106). Although more than half of a procainamide dose is excreted unchanged, it is metabolized in the liver to N-acetylprocainamide (NAPA), an active metabolite which acts through a different (class III) antiarrhythmic mechanism (106). Acetylation to NAPA involves the N-acetyltransferase enzyme system, which is involved in the metabolism of isoniazid. Adults may be phenotyped as fast or slow acetylators (123), however infants between birth and 2 months of age are uniformly slow acetylators as a result of the immaturity of the enzyme system (16). Both NAPA and procainamide accumulate with renal insufficiency. Procainamide levels of 4 to 8 mcg/ml are generally effective for control of arrhythmias.

Lidocaine, a class 1B antiarrhythmic, primarily blocks the fast inward sodium channel, like other local anesthetic antiarrhythmic drugs (106,122). Its effects are much greater on the conducting system and the ventricular muscle than on the atrium. It has active metabolites that also block the sodium channel. Plasma concentrations should be maintained between 2 and 5 μg/mL, because concentrations exceeding 6 μg/mL may produce seizures or respiratory arrest (106,122). Drugs known to decrease hepatic blood flow, such as cimetidine, will decrease hepatic clearance of lidocaine and increase concentrations unless the dose is reduced.

Chronic treatment of SVT is not needed in every patient (110). If the frequency of SVT is rare, not associated with cardiovascular compromise, and is easily terminated with vagal maneuvers, chronic treatment may not be required provided that the child can be monitored adequately at home (110). The presence of WPW, however, is a significant predictor of recurrence of SVT after stopping medications (124). Digoxin treatment of WPW is controversial, because it has been associated with sudden death in 1% to 5% of patients (110,125). In another series of patients with SVT, digoxin treatment was successful in 65% regardless of whether or not they showed preexcitation (116). A review of patients treated for SVT at Texas Children's Hospital revealed no difference in the success rate for treatment of SVT with digitalis among patients with and without WPW (115).

Propranolol is frequently used to treat neonates with SVT, if digoxin is contraindicated because of the presence of WPW (106). It has special pharmacokinetic features that must be considered in its administration. When administered enterally, propranolol is cleared largely through first-pass extraction by the liver. It is metabolized extensively to an active metabolite, 4-hydroxypropranolol (126). During repetitive doses, hepatic extraction decreases, and plasma concentrations may vary widely at steady-state. If administered i.v., the propranolol dose must be reduced at least tenfold because it bypasses hepatic extraction and pro-

duces a dose- and concentration-related decrease in heart rate and cardiac contractility. Propranolol has been used most frequently to treat supraventricular and ventricular arrhythmias. It also has a role in treatment of sinus tachycardia related to hypermetabolic states such as thyrotoxicosis (122). Data on dosing, kinetics, and efficacy in neonates for other beta-adrenergic blocking drugs such as atenolol, nadolol, sotalol, and esmolol are limited.

Verapamil has been used for treatment of SVT with moderate success, but its use in infants younger than 12 months of age has been discouraged (106,127). As a result of its negative inotropic activity and ability to decrease sinus function, verapamil should not be used with beta-adrenergic blocking drugs in infants and children (122). They have been used together successfully in adults.

Amiodarone is a benzofuran compound with structural similarity to thyroxine that was originally synthesized in 1962 and released in the United States in 1985. Because of the associated toxicities, it was approved as a "last resort" drug that should be reserved for refractory, life-threatening arrhythmias (128). During the last few years, much more information has accumulated about both its efficacy and its toxicity. Amiodarone illustrates the limitations of a classification system for antiarrhythmics. It inhibits both the fast sodium channel and the slow calcium channel, has noncompetitive antisympathetic effects, and modulates thyroid function (129). Amiodarone has a relatively low negative inotropic effect and therefore may be the preferred antiarrhythmic treatment for infants and children with depressed myocardial function as a result of incessant tachycardias or perioperative tachycardias following surgery for congenital heart disease (130). Acutely, amiodarone slows AV node conduction with little effect on the QTc, although during chronic therapy, it lengthens QTc and prolongs the refractory period (129). Although reports are limited in neonates, the following adverse effects have been observed after amiodarone treatment of infants and children: photosensitivity (131,132), corneal deposits (132), gray skin color (132), abnormal liver function tests (132), hypothyroidism (131,132), hyperthyroidism (131,132), accelerated bone maturation (131), delayed longitudinal growth (131), excess weight gain (131), headaches (131), pulmonary infiltrates (133), and sleep disturbances (132). Amiodarone increases the concentration of several drugs, usually by decreasing clearance and volume of distribution, including digoxin, quinidine, procainamide, phenytoin, and flecainide. Decreased clearance of warfarin by amiodarone may precipitate hemorrhage. Overall, the frequency of adverse effects is greater in adults than in children and greater in older children than in infants.

Amiodarone treatment of refractory and serious arrhythmias in infants and children has been successful with limited acute toxicity. In a multi-center trial, Perry reported a 93% rate of improvement with the compassionate use of amiodarone for life-threatening arrhythmias in 40 patients from 8 centers (134). Several serious and refractory arrhythmias have been successfully treated with amiodarone, including: multifocal atrial tachycardia (chaotic atrial tachycardia) (135,136), ventricular tachycardia as a result of intracardiac tumor (137), and refractory SVT (138,139). In a study by Burri and associates, i.v. amiodarone was reported to be safe and effective therapy for life-threatening incessant tachycardias in infants (130). Twenty-three hemodynamically unstable infants (median age 8 days) with life-threatening tachycardias (17 supraventricular, 6 ventricular) were treated with i.v. amiodarone 5 mg/kg administered over 1 hour followed by 5 µg/kg/min with stepwise increase to 25 µg/kg/min (130). Amiodarone was effective in 83% of infants. Median time to arrhythmia control was 24 h and the median maintenance dose was 15 µg/kg/min (range 5–26 µg/kg/min). Adverse effects were not significant: sinus bradycardia in 2 patients and hypotension in one infant, which resolved after dose reduction. Choreoathetotic movements and elevated liver enzymes occurred in two patients.

Dosages of amiodarone have varied widely from study to study. Initial treatment with amiodarone usually begins with a loading dose (5 mg/kg) followed by an infusion of 10 to 15 mg/kg/day (134) to 7.5 to 13.5 mg/kg/day for 9 to 10 days (140). Larger dosages were required for infants less than 1 year of age in one study (132). Oral treatment alone has been successful in some studies (132,141). In a study by Etheridge and associates, 44 neonates and infants (1.0 ± 1.5 months) with difficult to control tachycardias were treated with oral amiodarone using a 7- to 10-day load of amiodarone at either 10 or 20 mg/kg/day in two divided doses (141). The higher loading dose was used for more difficult to control tachycardias. Oral propranolol (2 mg/kg/d) was added for sustained or symptomatic episodes of tachycardia (n = 25). Rhythm control was achieved in all patients. Infants were discharged on maintenance amiodarone dose of 5 to 10 mg/kg/day (mean dose 7 ± 2 mg/kg/day) and drugs were discontinued as tolerated. Sixty-eight percent of patients remained free of arrhythmias at one year, despite discontinuation of propranolol and amiodarone. There were no side effects necessitating drug withdrawal.

The prolonged loading dose likely relates to amiodarone's extremely long half-life that has been estimated in adults to exceed 50 days (128). Levels of amiodarone are kept between 0.8 and 2.0 mg/L in adults (132), but there is no clear relationship between levels of amiodarone or its metabolite desethylamiodarone and toxicity or efficacy (142,143).

Newborns with fetal arrhythmias may be treated with amiodarone and require evaluation of potential adverse effects in the nursery. A healthy fetus whose mother was treated with amiodarone for sick sinus syndrome delivered and breast fed with no changes in thyroid function (144). Both neonatal hyperthyroidism and hypothyroidism with or without a goiter have been observed after fetal exposure to amiodarone (145–148).

Anticonvulsants

Seizures remain a frequent therapeutic problem for neonates admitted to an intensive care unit. They may be caused by a variety of disorders, such as meningitis, inadequate pyridoxal-5-phosphate binding, i.e., pyridoxine dependency, hypoglycemia, hypocalcemia, inborn errors of metabolism, neonatal abstinence from narcotics, or intracranial hemorrhage (149). Because treatment differs according to etiology, causes for seizures outside the brain should always be considered and evaluated. Some noncerebral causes of seizures may produce recurrent seizures that require prolonged anticonvulsant drug treatment, in addition to treatment of the primary metabolic or infectious disorder. Because prolonged seizures per se may harm the brain, treatment should not be delayed (149).

Phenobarbital remains the mainstay of treatment and is effective in approximately one-third of cases; babies who respond tend to have a smaller seizure burden and a relatively normal background electroencephalogram (150,151). Phenobarbital is often ineffective as a first line anticonvulsant in neonates with seizures in whom the background electroencephalogram (EEG) is significantly abnormal (151,152). Although seizures are controlled in some patients with phenobarbital levels of 15 µg/mL, the minimal effective therapeutic concentration should be regarded as 20 µg/mL and many patients may require concentrations as high as 40 µg/mL to achieve seizure control (153). As a result of a volume of distribution of approximately 0.9 L/kg in neonates, a loading dose of 15 to 20 mg/kg is required to reach a minimum concentration of 20 µg/mL (154). A total loading dose of up to 40 mg/kg rapidly achieves therapeutic levels (150). Caution is advised in nonventilated infants because a single loading dose of 40 mg/kg can result in apnea (150). Accordingly, splitting the loading dose into two 20 mg/kg doses is advised.

The half-life of phenobarbital is prolonged at birth, ranging from 43 to 217 hours (155). Consequently, lower doses of phenobarbital (2–3 mg/kg/day) should be used during the first week of life. Phenobarbital clearance increases significantly during the neonatal period and the half-life decreases to approximately 45 hours at 28 days of life (154). Thus, maintenance doses will often need to be increased within the first several weeks after birth (3–5 mg/kg/day). A good correlation has been demonstrated between plasma and brain concentrations of both phenobarbital and phenytoin, so that increasing plasma concentrations should increase the anticonvulsant concentration at the site of action (12).

Concerns have increased about the effects of long-term phenobarbital treatment on cognitive development. When phenobarbital was compared to placebo in two randomized groups of children treated for 2 years for febrile seizures, the phenobarbital-treated group had significantly lower intelligent quotients (IQs) (156). In a randomized, crossover trial of three anticonvulsants, phenobarbital produced more impairment of neuropsychological performance than did carbamazepine or phenytoin (157). The American Academy of Pediatrics (AAP) Committee on Drugs summarized concerns about the cognitive effects of phenobarbital (158).

Phenytoin has served as the second line anticonvulsant for neonates. Phenytoin and phenobarbital have been shown to be equally but incompletely effective as anticonvulsants in neonates.(151) The severity of the seizure is a stronger predictor of successful treatment than the agent. Painter and associates evaluated phenytoin (15 mg/kg) as an alternative to phenobarbital. Of the 29 babies administered phenytoin as first-line treatment, 45% responded (151). Phenytoin and lidocaine are probably more effective than any of the benzodiazepines as second line, but very few evaluation studies have been reported (150). Disadvantages of phenytoin are its highly variable and nonlinear pharmacokinetics, i.e., exponential elimination decreases with increasing serum concentrations. The latter phenomenon requires considerable caution because small increases in maintenance dose may result in disproportionately large increases in plasma concentrations. The initially prolonged half-life of phenytoin decreases rapidly during the neonatal period from 57.3 ± 48.2 hours during the first days of life to 19.7 ± 1.3 hours during the fourth week (33). In term infants between 2 and 21 weeks of age, the half-life ranged from 6.6 hours to 15.1 hours (20). However, preterm infants often exhibit prolonged half-lives (15.6 to 160 hours) up to 18 days after birth (20).

Phenytoin is a water-insoluble base and the commercially available injection formulation is prepared using 40% propylene glycol at a final pH of 12. Side effects associated with parenteral phenytoin, caused primarily by its high pH and the propylene glycol content, include burning at the infusion site and severe local cutaneous reactions following infiltration into surrounding tissue (159). Many of these side effects can be avoided in children with the use of fosphenytoin, a phosphorylated prodrug of phenytoin which has few cardiac and local irritation adverse effects (160). The accepted therapeutic serum concentration range for phenytoin (or fosphenytoin converted to phenytoin) is 10 to 20 µg/mL and a loading dose of 15 to 20 mg/kg will achieve a therapeutic concentration (161). To avoid hypotension, arrhythmias, and precipitation during administration, phenytoin should be administered slowly (maximum 0.5–1 mg/kg/min) into an i.v. line containing only saline. Because the drug is caustic to tissues, intramuscular administration should be avoided and intravenous doses should be infused through as large a vein as is available taking care to avoid extravasation.

Interpretation of phenytoin plasma concentrations requires consideration of protein binding. In adults, the unbound concentration of phenytoin is approximately 10% of the total concentration (162). Thus, the therapeutic range for unbound (free) phenytoin is 1 to 2 µg/mL. Because plasma protein concentrations and binding affinity of albumin are low in newborns, plasma protein binding of phenytoin is reduced in infants. In normobilirubinemic newborns, the free (unbound) fraction of phenytoin is 15% to 20% and in hyperbilirubinemic infants, the free fraction may reach 30% (20,163,164). Thus, despite apparent subtherapeutic total concentrations (<10 µg/mL) free concentrations may be within the therapeutic range of 1 to 2 µg/mL. Monitoring free phenytoin concentrations may

be useful in this circumstance to determine if concentrations are within the therapeutic range. If free concentrations of phenytoin are not available, targeting total concentrations of 6 to 14 µg/mL are appropriate in the immediate neonatal period (20). However, as protein binding normalizes in the weeks to months after birth, the therapeutic range will require readjustment to 10 to 20 µg/mL.

As a result of the significant variability in pharmacokinetics during the first weeks of life, a standard dose of phenytoin cannot be recommended and plasma concentrations must be monitored. During the first week of life, doses of 4–8 mg/kg/day may be required (20). However, chronic oral phenytoin therapy in infants often requires much higher doses (161). By the second week after birth, most infants will require at least 8 mg/kg/day divided every 6 to 8 hours (20), however oral doses as high as 17.7 ± 4.3 mg/kg/day and intravenous doses of 25 mg/kg/day have been required to maintain therapeutic concentrations (161,165). Although some have attributed these dose requirements to poor absorption of the oral formulation (161), high doses are also required after intravenous administration (165). Other investigators have demonstrated complete absorption in infants receiving oral doses (166). High oral dosage requirements in infants likely reflects several pharmacokinetic events, including poor and erratic absorption, increased phenytoin metabolism during the first year of life, and hepatic enzyme induction by concomitant treatment with phenobarbital (161,165,166).

Recently, the introduction of fosphenytoin has significantly reduced the potential for the adverse effects usually associated with phenytoin, including pain on administration, extravasation injury, propylene glycol-associated hyperosmolality (83), CNS changes (85,86), acidosis (167), and cardiovascular compromise (168) following rapid intravenous injection (159). Fosphenytoin is a water-soluble prodrug that is rapidly hydrolyzed to phenytoin via blood and tissue phosphatases (169). Because it is an aqueous solution and contains no propylene glycol, it has few pharmaceutical compatibility problems and may be administered by intravenous injection or by intramuscular injection (169). Because fosphenytoin is converted to phenytoin, issues regarding protein binding, therapeutic concentrations, and drug interactions associated with phenytoin must still be considered. There is limited published experience of its use in newborn infants (160).

Benzodiazepines can be used for additional drug therapy beyond phenobarbital and phenytoin to control seizures in the newborn. Diazepam has been used to treat refractory seizures in neonates, but its efficacy is limited by its short duration of action, respiratory depression, prolonged half-life, and metabolism to active metabolites (170). Lorazepam, in a dose of 0.05 to 0.1 mg/kg has been effective for controlling refractory seizures in neonates and has a duration of action up to 24 hours (84,170). Total doses up to 0.15 mg/kg may be necessary to control neonatal seizures that are refractory to phenobarbital (171). Because metabolism of lorazepam requires glucuronidation, which is poorly developed in newborns, the half-life of lorazepam in newborns is prolonged (mean 40 hours) and correlates with gestational age (172). The dose of benzyl alcohol associated with lorazepam treatment is low enough not to represent a risk for toxicity (173). Some have reported "seizure-like" stereotypic movements after lorazepam administration (174,175). The cause of this movement disorder is not known.

Recently midazolam has been used in adults and children for treatment of epileptic episodes of various types, including status epilepticus (176,177). A study was conducted in six neonates (aged 1–9 days; gestation, 30–41 weeks) with persistent seizures despite a mean phenobarbital concentration of 50.5 mg/L (178). Seizures were controlled in all patients within one hour of administering continuous intravenous infusions of midazolam (0.1–0.4 mg/kg/hour). Because neonatal seizures are sometimes refractory to high-dose phenobarbital, midazolam may be a valuable adjunctive therapy (178). Care must be taken to avoid rapid bolus doses of midazolam over 1 to 2 minutes that may cause hypotension in infants receiving fentanyl infusions (15) or tonic-clonic movements similar to those reported in older children following lorazepam (179).

Neonatal seizures refractory to phenobarbital have recently been shown to respond to oral administration of carbamazepine (180). Carbamazepine is a first-line anticonvulsant in the treatment of partial seizures with or without secondary generalization in children and adults. Ten preterm infants (gestational age 23 to 34) with neonatal seizures refractory to phenobarbital (plasma concentration ranging from 50–64 mg/L) received 7–15 mg/kg/day in 2 to 3 divided doses to achieve a plasma concentration of 3–12 mg/L. Nine out of the ten patients had excellent results without adverse effects. In another report, 10 full-term neonates with two or more seizures as a result of hypoxic-ischemic encephalopathy were administered 10 mg/kg of carbamazepine as a loading dose (via nasogastric tube) followed by a maintenance regimen of 15 to 21 mg/kg/day (181). Absorption of carbamazepine was excellent and therapeutic levels were reached in 2 to 4 hours with peak levels achieved in 9.2 ± 4.2 hours. The elimination half-life was 24.5 hours. Levels dropped precipitously around 8 to 15 days and declined slowly over the next 3 months. Seizure control was excellent and there were no adverse effects (181).

Of the newer anticonvulsants, lamotrigine is effective in adults and children with generalized and partial seizures. Lamotrigine is a phenyltriazine structurally unrelated to conventional antiepileptic drugs (AEDs). Recently, lamotrigine has been shown to be a useful agent for treatment of refractory seizures, partial seizures, and infantile spasms (182,183). Thirteen infants (<1 year) with a mean age of 3.7 months (five were 2–4 weeks) had either partial seizures or infantile spasms or both (182). Both were significantly reduced ($p < 0.05$) and lamotrigine was well tolerated. The mean apparent clearance was 82% lower in the infants less than 2 months of age compared with those that were 2 to 12 months of age. Lamotrigine is mainly eliminated by hepatic metabolism to an inactive metabolite

through glucuronidation (184). Co-medication with enzyme inducers increases metabolism (184), and although not studied in neonates, one would expect a drug interaction with phenobarbital. The adverse effect which often leads to drug discontinuation is skin reactions. Overall, rash develops in 12% of patients and the risk of rash is approximately 3 times greater in children as compared to adults (184). Other reported adverse effects include leucopenia, agranulocytosis, and hepatic failure.

Topiramate, another one of the newer antiepileptic drugs, is currently approved for adjunctive therapy for the treatment of generalized tonic-clonic seizures and partial seizures, and Lennox-Gastaut syndrome. It differs both structurally and pharmacologically from other classes of AEDs. Topiramate is a sulfamate-substituted monosaccharide D-fructose derivative with limited protein binding (9%–17%) (185). It is primarily eliminated by renal excretion with a small portion metabolized by hydrolysis, hydroxylation, and glucuronidation (185). No studies have been conducted in neonates, although a report of 5 infants (4 term and one born at 36 weeks) exposed to topiramate in utero indicated extensive transplacental transfer and a half-life of approximately 24 hours, which is close to the 20 to 30 hours reported in adults (185).

The decision to continue or to stop treatment with anticonvulsant medications before discharge from the NICU remains controversial. Scher and Painter suggest that anticonvulsants may be discontinued for infants who show no abnormalities of the brain on imaging studies, have an age-appropriate neurologic examination, and have a normal interictal electroencephalogram (186). Up to 30% of neonates with seizures later have epilepsy, but frequently the later seizure pattern takes the form of infantile spasms or minor motor seizures that are not very responsive to phenobarbital and phenytoin (186).

Antihypertensives

The relationship between blood pressure, gestational age, birth weight and postconceptional age was defined by Zubrow and associates in 695 neonates studied over a period of 3 months (187). Based on these data, hypertension in term and preterm infants may be defined as blood pressure above the upper limit of the 95% confidence interval for infants of similar gestational or postconceptual age and size (188). Drug treatment for hypertension should start with a single drug from one of the following classes, angiotensin-converting enzyme (ACE) inhibitors, vasodilators, beta-receptor antagonists, calcium channel blockers, or diuretics (189).

For severe hypertension in the neonate, a continuous intravenous infusion is advantageous because blood pressure fluctuations observed with intermittent dosing are eliminated and the dose may be titrated to keep blood pressure within narrow parameters. Antihypertensive agents that have been used in neonates or infants by continuous infusion include esmolol (190), nitroprusside, and nicardipine (191,192). Small studies have found that intravenous nicardipine may be effective in treating hypertensive neonates (191,192). Milou and associates studied 20 neonates (15 preterm) who were administered intravenous nicardipine 0.5 μg/kg/min (maximum 0.74 ± 0.41 μg/kg/min) for 14.6 ± 11.6 days (192). Blood pressure significantly decreased (approximately 20%) after 3, 6, 12, 24, and 48 hours of nicardipine treatment. No hypotension was observed. Gouyon et al. studied 8 preterm infants with systemic hypertension and treated them with intravenous nicardipine 0.5 μg/kg/min ($n = 2$) or 1.7 μg/kg/min ($n = 6$) (191). The maximum infusion rate was 1.56 ± 0.45 μg/kg/min and the treatment duration was 15.9 ± 10.3 days. Systolic blood pressure significantly decreased after 12 and 24 hours of nicardipine treatment ($-17 ± 17\%$ and $-21 ± 10\%$, respectively) and diastolic blood pressure decreased after 24 hours of treatment ($-22 ± 16\%$) No hypotension or other side effects were noted. Hypertensive emergencies are infrequent in neonates, but can be treated with esmolol, hyralazine, labetalol, sodium nitroprusside if renal function is normal, fenoldopam, isradipine, and minoxidil (189). As observed in older patients, thiocyanate and cyanide may accumulate during sodium nitroprusside treatment. Severe prolonged hypotension has been reported in severely hypertensive neonates treated with enalaprilat (189).

Intermittently administered intravenous agents may be useful for patients with mild-to-moderate hypertension. These agents include hydralazine, labetalol, and enalaprilat, (193) although enalaprilat should be used with great caution as a result of the potential for significant and prolonged hypotension (188).

Oral antihypertensives may be used in infants with mild-to-moderate hypertension or in patients being transitioned from intravenous therapy. Angiotensin-converting enzyme inhibitors (e.g., captopril) have a special role in the treatment of neonatal renovascular hypertension that is caused by markedly elevated renin and angiotensin (194). Aortic catheters may distribute microemboli to the kidneys, which increase secretion of renin and angiotensin in response to focal underperfusion. Although captopril may be relatively specific treatment for many cases of renovascular hypertension in neonates, dosage adjustments are difficult because a liquid dosage form is not commercially available. An extemporaneously compounded dosage form containing ascorbate has been shown to be stable for 14 days at room temperature (195). Captopril treatment of neonates should start with doses of 0.01 mg/kg, rather than the earlier recommendations of 0.1 to 0.3 mg/kg/dose, to avoid hypotension and acute renal insufficiency (196). Doses should be increased daily if hypertension persists. Initial captopril treatment may cause a triphasic reaction of hypotension with renal failure, managed by dose reduction, followed by a rise in blood pressure despite increasing doses above the original dose (197). At the start of captopril treatment, hypotension is exaggerated in salt and water-depleted patients (198). As in adults, captopril may be useful for afterload reduction in the treatment of chronic congestive heart failure in newborns (198). Other

oral agents that have been used include the vasodilators hydralazine and minoxidil, and the calcium channel blocker isradipine (188). Isradipine can be compounded into a suspension and its successful and safe use has been reported in infants and children (199,200). The use of isradipine suspension allows infants and young children to be treated as readily as older children.

Antimicrobials

Beta-Lactams

Historically, the selection of antibiotics for the treatment of sepsis and infections in neonates has been empiric based on the most frequent pathogens observed in the clinical setting. Ampicillin and an aminoglycosides have been the mainstay for treatment of presumed sepsis and meningitis in the newborn (201). The advantages of this combination include low cost, relatively few problems with resistance (202,203), and a combined spectrum of activity that covers the majority of neonatal pathogens, including Group B *Streptococcus*, *E. coli*, and *Listeria monocytogenes* (201). However, resistance to antimicrobial agents and changes in the pathogens causing neonatal infections must be the focus of ongoing surveillance to respond with the most appropriate antibiotic combination. As antepartum antibiotic use for the prevention of group B streptococcal disease increases, organisms recovered in early onset disease may shift toward *Escherichia coli* resistant to ampicillin (204,205). In a study of 5447 very-low-birth-weight (VLBW) infants born between 1998 and 2000, there was a marked reduction in group B streptococcal sepsis (from 5.9 to 1.7 per 1,000 live births, $p < 0.001$) and an increase in Escherichia coli sepsis (from 3.2 to 6.8 per 1,000 live births, $p = 0.004$) as compared to VLBW infants born between 1991 and 1993 (205). Most *E. coli* isolates from the recent birth cohort (85%) were resistant to ampicillin. Ampicillin-resistant strains of *Morganella morganii* have also been reported to cause early onset sepsis in babies born to mothers who received intrapartum ampicillin (206).

The use of third-generation cephalosporins (e.g., cefotaxime, ceftriaxone, and ceftazidime) continues to proliferate, primarily as a result of their excellent penetration into cerebrospinal fluid, minimal nephrotoxicity, and broad gram-negative activity, including *Klebsiella sp.* and many gentamicin-resistant isolates (207). When *L. monocytogenes* or *Enterococci* are potential causes of infection, initial empiric therapy with third generation cephalosporins must be combined with ampicillin because the cephalosporins are not active against these pathogens. The choice of third generation cephalosporins over an aminoglycoside will depend on institutional susceptibility patterns. However, because excessive use of extended spectrum cephalosporins is associated with selection for highly resistant, extended spectrum β-lactamase (ESBL) producing organisms (208–211), many experts favor a regimen of a penicillin and aminoglycoside for primary therapy of suspected sepsis (208). It has been proposed that the biliary excretion of broad spectrum antibiotics promotes overgrowth of resistant strains (especially *Enterobacter* and *Enterococcus*) which can translocate from the intestines into the bloodstream to causeinfection (212,213).

Among the cephalosporins, there is considerable experience using cefotaxime in severe neonatal infections (214). Cefotaxime has often replaced gentamicin for coverage of gram-negative bacilli during outbreaks of sepsis caused by gentamicin-resistant gram-negative bacteria (209,215). Although this combination may increase the relative number of enterobacter isolates and their resistance (209,211, 216,217). The incidence of serious gram-negative infections decreased during a 5-year period when cefotaxime was substituted for gentamicin (215). Ceftriaxone has a very similar spectrum of activity as cefotaxime, with the primary difference being its pharmacokinetic profile. Ceftriaxone was well tolerated in 80 neonates (mean gestational age 34 weeks), although six patients had sonographic findings consistent with 'biliary sludge' which resolved spontaneously within 2 weeks (218). It is believed that ceftriaxone forms a complex with calcium that is poorly soluble in bile resulting in biliary sludge, which appears to be a transient phenomenon (219). Ceftriaxone may also displace bilirubin from albumin binding sites (220,221). An *in vivo* study demonstrated the potential significance of this interaction and the investigators recommended that ceftriaxone be withheld from jaundiced neonates or premature newborns with acidosis, hypoxia, or sepsis who are at increased risk for developing bilirubin encephalopathy (221).

Certain cephalosporins have unique properties that fit clinical problems encountered frequently in neonates, e.g., ceftazidime is considered the drug of choice to treat Pseudomonas infections. It should be combined with an aminoglycoside for synergy and to avoid emergence of resistant strains (222,223). A recent study of 1316 cases of suspected cases of sepsis in the newborn (median age ≤ 3 days) found that ceftazidime in combination with ampicillin had a significantly higher cure rate (97%) than ampicillin and an aminoglycoside (66%) (224). No problems with ceftazidime resistance were encountered. Pharmacokinetic data in preterm infants indicate that the ceftazidime dose during the first 2 weeks of life should be based on gestational age and postnatal age-related changes in glomerular filtration rate (225,226). Additionally, exposure of preterm infants to indomethacin or asphyxia in term infants may reduce ceftazidime's clearance and dosage requirements (225).

The ureidopenicillins, ticarcillin and piperacillin, provide broader gram-negative coverage than ampicillin and are particularly suitable for the treatment of late-onset sepsis (227). For treatment of *Pseudomonas* sp. infections, piperacillin is more active in vitro than ticarcillin and may be combined with an aminoglycoside for synergy and to decrease the emergence of resistant organisms (228–230). When piperacillin is combined with an aminoglycoside such as gentamicin, the combination provides excellent activity against aerobic and anaerobic bacteria encountered after intestinal perforation. Piperacillin dosage requirements are based on both gestational and postnatal age (231).

The most common mechanism for resistance to beta-lactam antibiotics is production of inactivating beta-lactamases (232). Beta-lactamase inhibitors, including clavulanate and tazobactam, were developed to bind irreversibly to enzyme substrate, thereby blocking this mode of resistance and preserving activity of the penicillins against many organisms. As a result, ticarcillin-clavulanate and piperacillin-tazobactam have significantly improved spectra of activity, including beta-lactamase producing strains of gram-positive organisms, methicillin-sensitive *Staphylococcus* aureus, many *Enterobacteriaceae*, fastidious gram-negative bacteria such as *H. influenzae* and *M. catarrhalis*, and many anaerobes (233–235). This makes the combination of a beta-lactam and a beta-lactamase inhibitor an excellent therapeutic alternative for providing broad spectrum antimicrobial coverage in the treatment of late-onset sepsis (236). Furthermore, combination beta-lactam/beta-lactamase inhibitors are less likely to promote development of resistance because of their decreased potency for inducing beta-lactamases and their minimal effect on gastrointestinal flora (236). Generally, piperacillin-tazobactam is more active than ticarcillin-clavulanate against *Enterococcus faecalis* and gram-negative bacilli, including *Pseudomonas aeruginosa* (235). Piperacillin-tazobactam may be a useful combination in the treatment of *Klebsiella pneumoniae* infections in neonates (237).

The carbapenems, imipenem-cilastatin and meropenem, have an extremely broad spectrum of activity, including gram-positive, gram-negative, and anaerobic organisms (238). Both agents are beta-lactamase stable and have activity against penicillin-resistant pneumococci, *E. faecalis*, *L. monocytogenes*, *P. aeruginosa*, and multi-resistant strains of gram-negative organisms (239). Imipenem is combined with cilastatin, a renal dehydropeptidase I inhibitor, which prevents metabolic activation of imipenem to a nephrotoxic compound. Meropenem is more active against gram-negative bacilli and less active against gram-positive cocci (including *Enterococcus* sp) than is imipenem (239). Both agents penetrate into cerebral spinal fluid in the presence of inflammation associated with meningitis (240). Meropenem and cefotaxime were equally efficacious in the treatment of meningitis in 190 children (median age 1 year) (241).

Carbapenems, through their epileptogenic activity, are potentially more neurotoxic than the penicillins and cephalosporins (242). A study of imipenem-cilastatin treatment of bacterial meningitis in 21 infants and children was terminated when 33% developed seizures after antibiotic administration (243). Seizures with imipenem have often been associated with high plasma concentrations associated with renal dysfunction and high doses, or increased susceptibility, such as underlying central nervous system abnormality (239). An additive risk with concomitant theophylline treatment has been reported (244). The safety margin of meropenem appears to be higher and meropenem can be used at higher doses than imipenem-cilastatin (242). More than 1,200 children (ages 3 months–12 years) have been treated in prospective, randomized, clinical trials of meropenem (238). A promising finding is that meropenem does not cause seizures with greater frequency than other antibiotics used to treat meningitis (238,245).

The published experience of imipenem in neonates and in particular in preterm neonates is limited. Nalin and associates assessed the safety of imipenem in 61 children up to 6 months old and noted that 15% developed seizures; however, neonates weighing less than 750 g or those who were critically ill were excluded (246). Stuart and colleagues investigated the safety of imipenem (20–80 mg/kg/day) in 80 neonates at 32 weeks postconceptional age and noted that only 2 patients developed seizures (2.5%), both of whom had documented seizures before commencing imipenem (247). Overall, adverse effects were minimal and no neonate was withdrawn as a result of toxicity. There are currently no studies evaluating the efficacy or safety of meropenem in neonates.

Both imipenem and meropenem are primarily excreted in the urine (239). Both agents demonstrate age-related pharmacokinetics; thus, the longest half-lives are in premature neonates (248). Although the carbapenems are administered every 6 to 8 hours in adults, plasma concentrations in neonates should exceed the minimum inhibitory concentrations (MICs) for most organisms for 12 hours after a single dose, suggesting that q12h dosing may be appropriate; however, additional studies are required to determine the optimal dose and interval (248).

Aztreonam is a monobactam and shows excellent activity against aerobic gram-negative bacilli, including *P. aeruginosa*, but it is devoid of activity against gram-positive or anaerobic bacteria (249). A limited evaluation of its efficacy and pharmacokinetics has been conducted in neonates (250,251). Ampicillin plus aztreonam was compared to ampicillin plus amikacin in 147 neonates, 60 with documented gram-negative bacterial infections (251). Clinical response was noted in 90% of those who received aztreonam as compared with 72% those who received amikacin. Because aztreonam does not have the nephrotoxic potential of aminoglycosides, it may be considered as an alternative in the treatment of serious gram-negative infections, particularly when there is a concern regarding concomitant treatment with several nephrotoxic agents.

The antistaphylococcal penicillin, nafcillin, has largely replaced methicillin for the treatment of *S. aureus* infections because it has a lower risk of adverse reactions. Nafcillin is eliminated primarily through biliary excretion, which may be impaired in neonates as a result of cholestasis related to prolonged hyperalimentation (252). To reduce vancomycin resistance in hospitals, the antistaphylococcal penicillins should be used whenever possible.

E. cloacae, *Enterococcus* sp., and *K. pneumoniae* are emerging in neonatal patients as multiply resistant organisms, possibly as a result of the increased use of cephalosporin antibiotics in NICUs (125,253–255). This growing problem of bacterial resistance requires that new classes of antibacterial agents be evaluated for the treatment of severe infections in neonates. Because potent and broad spectrum antibiotics have received less study in neonates, they should be used judiciously and with guidance from a specialist in infectious diseases.

Vancomycin

Patterns of antimicrobial use in neonatology have evolved with the changing spectrum of infections and development of new antimicrobial agents. Emergence of infections with beta-lactam-resistant *S. epidermidis*, *S. aureus*, and *Enterococcus* sp., has led to the frequent use of vancomycin in neonates (256). Reports of the increasing prevalence of enterococcal infections in newborns is of significant concern (257), particularly in view of the nationwide 20-fold increase in the percentage of nosocomial enterococci resistant to vancomycin (258). Among vancomycin-resistant strains of enterococci isolated in a pediatric center, the prevalence of *E. faecium* has increased dramatically (259). Forty-two percent of isolates were from the NICU (259). This trend suggests that future enterococcal infections in neonates may become far more difficult to treat. Although recent studies in newborns demonstrate that prophylactically administered vancomycin reduces infections with coagulase negative staphylococcus (260,261), clinicians must be cognizant of the dangers of overusing (and misusing) antibiotics, particularly vancomycin. One study reported that gram-negative bacteremia was positively associated with the use of vancomycin (odds ratio, 8.1; 95% confidence interval, 3.1 to 20.9), thus reiterating the importance of minimizing the inappropriate and unnecessary use of vancomycin (262). In response to the increasing prevalence of vancomycin-resistant *Enterococcus* (VRE), the Hospital Infection Control Practices Advisory Committee of the Centers for Disease Control and Prevention (CDC) drafted guidelines to prevent the spread of VRE. These guidelines address, among other things, the appropriate use of vancomycin (263). To minimize the pressure for selecting antibiotic-resistant organisms, vancomycin should generally be reserved for methicillin-resistant staphylococci and ampicillin-resistant enterococcal infections (263).

There appears to be a widely held belief that vancomycin is a nephrotoxin. Consequently, a significant amount of resources are allocated to monitoring serum vancomycin concentrations. Although early preparations of vancomycin were impure and high peaks and troughs were associated with nephro- and ototoxicity (264), these toxicities are now relatively uncommon; however, concomitant administration with aminoglycosides or other nephrotoxins may increase this risk (265,266). Despite a poor correlation between vancomycin plasma concentrations and efficacy and toxicity, medical care has evolved to include the monitoring of vancomycin concentrations. The currently accepted therapeutic range for vancomycin was not derived from rigorous scientific evaluation. Because

MICs for most *Staphylococcus* sp. were less than or equal to 5 µg/mL and early toxicities most often occurred at serum concentrations less than 30 to 40 µg/mL, desired trough concentrations were designated as 5 to 10 µg/mL and peak concentrations 20 to 40 µg/mL (267). These somewhat arbitrary ranges have become the standard for "therapeutic" vancomycin concentrations, however there are a paucity of data to substantiate these recommendations (268). In the last decade, clinicians have questioned the utility and cost-effectiveness of measuring peak and trough concentrations (268–271). Because the association between peak concentrations and toxicity is poor, some have recommended measuring trough concentrations only (272), although others have suggested not measuring any concentrations in the majority of children with normal renal function (271). However, in critically ill neonates, one must consider the inherently poor glomerular filtration rate associated with prematurity and compromised cardiovascular function, and the large intrapatient variation in the pharmacokinetics of vancomycin (273). Limited data in neonates support adjusting vancomycin dosages in premature or term infants on the basis of trough concentration monitoring alone (274); however, until more data are published, it remains prudent to measure both peak and trough concentrations, particularly in those with poor or changing renal function and those receiving multiple nephrotoxic agents.

Vancomycin clearance in premature infants is directly proportional to postconceptional age, body weight, and surface area (275). Its half-life and volume of distribution range from 3 hours and 0.38 L/kg, respectively, in infants whose postconceptional age is more than 43 weeks to 9.8 hours and 0.74 L/kg in premature infants of 32 weeks gestation (276,277). The reader is referred to a review for a more in-depth discussion of vancomycin pharmacokinetics and dosage recommendations (278).

Adverse effects of vancomycin include thrombophlebitis and infusion-related histamine release, hypotension, and red-man syndrome. Doses of vancomycin should be infused over at least 1 hour, and never in a rapid i.v. bolus dose, to avoid this reaction (279).

Aminoglycosides

Aminoglycosides continue to play an important role in the treatment of severe gram-negative sepsis. Clearance of aminoglycosides is directly related to the glomerular filtration rate, which is quite low and variable in premature and sick newborns; thus, plasma concentration monitoring is essential to maximizing efficacy and minimizing toxicity. Desired peak gentamicin concentrations are between 5 to 10 µg/mL and trough concentrations should be kept 1 to 2 µg/mL (65,280). Therapeutic drug monitoring may be unnecessary during the first 2 to 3 days of therapy while cultures are pending, unless the patient exhibits overt renal dysfunction (67). To reach appropriate peak concentrations, larger initial doses are necessary in premature infants as compared with infants and children (281,282). This is

because aminoglycosides distribute primarily into the extracellular fluid compartment, which is larger in premature infants. Accordingly, a 4 mg/kg gentamicin loading dose has been recommended to reach therapeutic peaks more expeditiously (282). Although gentamicin trough concentrations should always be kept less than 2 (µg/mL, gentamicin-induced renal toxicity and ototoxicity are uniquely less frequent in neonates than in adults (67).

In recent years, the use of a single, large, daily dose of an aminoglycoside, i.e., "once-daily aminoglycosides" has become commonplace both in adult medicine and in pediatrics. The rationale for this regimen is based on concentration-dependent bactericidal activity of aminoglycosides (283,284). Thus, a peak concentration:MIC ratio of at least 8:1 to 10:1 optimizes bactericidal activity (285). Secondly, the postantibiotic effect (PAE) of aminoglycosides against gram-negative bacteria is longer at increasingly higher serum concentrations (286,287). PAE refers to the continued suppression of bacterial growth after antibiotic exposure, thus permitting trough concentrations to fall below the MIC with reduced risk of bacterial regrowth (287). Aminoglycosides demonstrate a PAE of 1–8 hours when tested against gram-negative organisms at concentrations of 2 to 10 times the MIC (280). Thirdly, longer dosing intervals permit drug-free periods, which may limit the development of adaptive resistance, a phenomenon which occurs when an organism is constantly exposed to aminoglycosides (285). Lastly, the uptake of aminoglycoside into the renal cortex is saturable, resulting in reduced renal accumulation and a ceiling effect regarding nephrotoxicity (280,288).

Several dozen studies, primarily in adults, have evaluated the efficacy and toxicity of once-daily aminoglycoside. The majority of studies demonstrate no difference in efficacy or toxicity between dosage regimens (280). The remainder suggest that once-daily aminoglycoside treatment is superior in either efficacy or toxicity. The reader is referred to extensive reviews and meta-analyses on the subject (280,285,289–291).

In neonates, the use of the phrase "once-daily gentamicin" is potentially confusing, because preterm newborns often receive gentamicin every 24 hours, albeit at a much lower dose than the usual 4.5 to 7 mg/kg reported for once-daily dosing of gentamicin in children. Thus, it may be less confusing to use the phrase "extended-interval dosing" to refer to the single, large, daily dose of aminoglycoside. Nonetheless, this dosing regimen has not been well studied in neonates or infants. In a study that compared 4 mg/kg as a single daily dose to 2 mg/kg every 12 hours in 20 term newborns, the mean peak concentration was 10.9 µg/mL for the single daily dose and 7.4 µg/mL for the twice daily dosing (292). Mean trough concentrations were 0.8 µg/mL and 1.0 µg/mL for the two groups, respectively. *In vitro*, the 4 mg/kg once daily dose was significantly superior in bactericidal activity against isolates with high MICs, including *P. aeruginosa*, *E. faecalis*, and *L. monocytogenes*. In another study of 302 term infants, 3.5 to 4 mg/kg administered once daily produced peak concentrations (>6 µg/mL) in 100% of infants as compared with only 45% of those who received 2 to 2.5 mg/kg every 12 hours (292). In the single daily dose group, only one patient (1.2%) had a trough concentration above 2 µg/mL as compared to 4.5% of those receiving the twice daily regimen. In a study of gentamicin 5 mg/kg in predominantly term infants, peak and trough concentrations averaged 10.7 µg/mL and 1.7 µg/mL, respectively (293). As compared to peak concentrations achieved with conventional aminoglycoside dosing, the peak concentrations in this study were more suitable for optimizing bactericidal activity. However, the mean trough concentration was higher than that reported in most adult studies (<1 µg/mL). Because patients with renal dysfunction were excluded from most clinical studies of once-daily aminoglycosides, the toxic effects of these higher troughs are unknown. Furthermore, it is not known whether these trough concentrations are low enough to prevent the development of adaptive resistance.

Although the majority of neonatal studies of extended interval dosing of aminoglycosides has been conducted in neonates of 34 weeks gestation or older (294–297), recent data have been published in preterm infants as well (298–300). Premature neonates have significantly larger aminoglycoside distribution volumes and longer half-lives than infants and children. Thus, achieving serum concentration-time curves consistent with once-daily gentamicin in adults, i.e., peak concentrations more than 10 to 15 µg/mL and trough concentrations less than 1 µg/mL in a 24-hour period, is impossible in most preterm infants less than 34 weeks gestation. This was demonstrated in a study of predominantly preterm infants (gestational age of 14 of 21 infants ≤34 weeks) who received netilmicin 6 mg/kg per day (301). One-third of the infants had 24-hour trough concentrations that exceeded 2 µg/mL and only 2 of 21 infants had trough concentrations less than 1 µg/mL (301). These high trough concentrations may increase the potential for nephrotoxicity; however, increasing the dosing interval to 36 or 48 hours may permit these larger doses to be given although allowing the trough concentrations to fall to less than 1 µg/mL. Such a strategy was published by Rastogi and associates who compared 4.5 to 5.0 mg/kg q48h with 2.5–3.0 mg/kg q24h in 58 very low birth weight infants (300). Ninety percent of peak concentrations in the q48h group were in the therapeutic range (6–12 µg/mL) as compared to 55% in the q24h group (*p* = 0.0005). None of the q48h infants had subtherapeutic peak concentrations after the first dose vs. 36% of q24h infants (*p* < 0.005). Furthermore, 18% of the q24h infants continued to have subtherapeutic peak concentrations even after the third dose. Although this strategy of administering larger doses less frequently was more effective in achieving therapeutic peak concentrations, it is noteworthy that 30% of infants in the q48h group had trough concentrations less than 0.5 µg/mL. This raises concerns regarding the potential for bacterial growth during prolonged periods of extremely low serum concentrations.

In another study, which included 52 VLBW and ELBW neonates, 5 mg/kg q36–48h of gentamicin resulted in higher peak concentrations than 2.5 mg/kg q18 to 24h (8.0 ± 1.7 vs. 5.8 ± 2.2 µg/mL, respectively, *p* < 0.01). Almost one-third of patients in the 2.5 mg/kg group had subtherapeutic peak concentrations (<5 µg/mL) and the mean trough concentration was higher than in the 5 mg/kg group, 1.2 ± 0.74 vs. 0.7 ± 0.5 µg/mL, respectively.

In summary, preliminary data suggest that therapeutic peak concentrations may be more effectively achieved in preterm and term neonates by administering larger doses of aminoglycosides less frequently as compared with the traditional dosing regimens. The potential advantages of this therapeutic approach are numerous, including increased bactericidal activity, longer postantibiotic effects, and reduced potential for developing adaptive resistance. However, more studies must be conducted in preterm infants and those with renal dysfunction to determine the optimal dosage regimen. The endpoints of such studies need to include both safety and efficacy before they are widely adopted.

Antireflux and Promotility Medications

Reflux may occur when the lower esophageal sphincter transiently relaxes and liquid enters the esophagus. A critical review of the evidence for potential sequelae of gastroesophageal reflux (GER) in preterm infants demonstrates that (a) apnea is unrelated to GER in preterm infants (302); (b) failure to thrive does not occur with GER; (c) although GER may cause aspiration, a relationship between GER and chronic airway problems has not been confirmed in preterm infants (303). Certain infants with BPD clearly reflux, aspirate, and have apnea (304–306). Many other infants regurgitate feeds without a clear association with symptoms of chronic lung disease or apnea (307). GER is more frequent in more premature neonates (308) and correlates with reduced lower esophageal sphincter tone and inadequate lower esophageal clearance (309,310). Some of the controversy may relate to measurement of GER by pH probe and the buffering effect of formula on gastric acid that would prevent detection of reflux by a drop in pH. A recent study using impedance found that 34% of reflux episodes were not detected by pH probe measurements (311). Although gastric emptying may be delayed in premature infants, it does not correlate with GER (312).

Despite the debate about whether clinical signs such as gagging and bradycardia and apnea relate to GER, treatment for GER in neonates is frequent in NICUs (304,313,314). Pharmacologic treatment has included cholinomimetics, such as bethanechol, prokinetic drugs, such as metoclopramide and erythromycin, and drugs to reduce gastric acid, such as H2-antagonists and proton pump inhibitors. Prokinetic agents reduce regurgitation by affecting lower esophageal sphincter, esophageal peristalsis, and gastric emptying time (315). H_2-antagonists available for use in neonates include ranitidine (316), famotidine (317), and cimetidine; although the use of cimetidine is limited by the potential of significant drug interactions by inhibition of hepatic cytochrome P450 isoenzymes and the availability of safer agents.

There are limited studies evaluating the efficacy and adverse effects of these agents in the neonatal population. A blinded, placebo-controlled, crossover trial evaluated bethanechol treatment of GER in 30 infants aged 3 weeks to 12 months with careful manometric measurements (318). Bethanechol improved lower esophageal sphincter tone, decreased vomiting, decreased the number and duration of reflux episodes and improved weight gain. One study confirmed these observations (319) although another study did not (320). As a cholinomimetic, bethanechol may increase bronchial secretions and bronchoconstriction. Reactive airway disease is a relative contraindication to treatment with bethanechol (318).

Metoclopramide, a derivative of procainamide that antagonizes dopamine, stimulates gastrointestinal motility (321) and has been used to treat GER in preterm neonates (322). Through its cholinergic effects, metoclopramide increases gastric fundal and lower esophageal sphincter tone and peristalsis in the esophagus, gastric antrum, and small intestine (321). Consistent with its central dopamine antagonist activities, it may precipitate extrapyramidal symptoms and stimulate prolactin secretion. Facial spasms, opisthotonos, and oculogyric crisis have been observed in children treated with metoclopramide (321). In an uncontrolled study of 6 preterm infants with signs of GER and impaired gastric emptying, metoclopramide (0.1 mg/kg/day) decreased gastric residual volume, improved feeding tolerance, and improved weight gain without dystonic reactions (322). When compared to placebo in a well-designed, prospective, blinded, crossover trial, metoclopramide decreased the length of time that the esophageal pH was less than 4.0 without changing the total number of reflux episodes or the number of prolonged episodes (323). A significant placebo effect was observed on symptom scores reported by parents. Greater efficacy was observed in infants older than 3 months. In a dosage of 0.1 mg/kg/dose four times daily, no side effects were noted (323). In dosages of 0.5 mg/kg/day divided into four doses, metoclopramide actually increased the number of reflux episodes and the time during which the esophageal pH was less than 4. (324) Hyams and colleagues suggested that infants (mean 3.2 months) with GER may require metoclopramide dose escalation to 1.2 mg/kg/day (325). Although these higher dosages improved efficacy in some studies (325), higher dosages caused more irritability to the point of patients dropping out of the study (324). These higher doses must be used very cautiously, if at all, in preterm infants. Kearns and colleagues found that 30% of preterm infants (31–40 weeks postconceptional age) had delayed metoclopramide clearance (326). Thus, high doses may result in unacceptable toxicity in some preterm infants, particularly as a result of the propensity of metoclopramide to cause dystonic reactions in children (327). Although clearance did not correlate with age, the investigators recommended that oral metoclopramide therapy be initiated at a dose of 0.15 mg/kg

every 6 hours in preterm infants more than 31 weeks postconceptional age (326).

As a prokinetic agent, there is considerable evidence that erythromycin exerts its pharmacological effect via direct activation of motilin receptors in the gastrointestinal tract (328). Although there are numerous published reports of erythromycin's use as a prokinetic agent in neonates, the quality of these data are limited by the paucity of randomized placebo-controlled trials (328). The majority of these studies evaluated the effect of erythromycin on feeding intolerance, gastrointestinal transit time, and time to full feeds (328). Costalos and associates studied 21 preterm infants at 32.5 weeks postconceptional age with feeding intolerance in a double blind, placebo-controlled, randomized, crossover study. Treatment with low oral doses of erythromycin (1.5 mg/kg every 6 hours) for 7 days significantly decreased whole gastrointestinal transit time (WGTT) from 15. 9 $\pm$ 7.2 hr to 10.2 $\pm$ 4.6 hr ($p < 0.01$) (329). In a double-blind, placebo-controlled, study of 56 preterm infants ($<1,500$ g), erythromycin treatment of 12.5 mg/kg every 6 hours orally reduced the time to reach full feeds by 10 days and reduced cholestatic jaundice (presumably because of less parenteral nutrition) (330). In a study of the gastrointestinal effects of erythromycin, Costalos and associates treated 20 preterm infants (median gestational age of 32 weeks; range 26–34 weeks) with erythromycin (10 mg/kg orally every 8 hours for 7 days) in a double-blind randomized, crossover design (331). Erythromycin treatment shortened antral contractility from 70 $\pm$ 13 minutes to 31 $\pm$ 9.9 minutes ($p < 0.01$) and WGTT was from 49.3 $\pm$ 29 hours to 23.1 $\pm$ 12.9 hours ($p < 0.01$). In contrast to these studies, Patole et al did not find that erythromycin shortened the time to full feeds in a controlled trial of oral erythromycin treatment using 12 mg/kg/dose every 6 hours administered for 14 days (332). No adverse effects of pyloric stenosis or arrhythmias or sepsis with resistant organisms have been reported in these controlled studies.

An association between erythromycin treatment of infants and pyloric stenosis was first reported in 1976 (333), but more recent cases have supported this association. Following a pertussis exposure in a community hospital, erythromycin prophylaxis was recommended for around 200 neonates born during one month (334–336). Erythromycin treatment increased the relative risk by 7-fold for developing infantile hypertrophic pyloric stenosis (IHPS). Using Medicaid or TennCare records in Tennessee from 1985 to 1997 with a cohort of 314,029 enrolled births, erythromycin treatment increased the risk of pyloric stenosis by 8-fold (337). Others have reported the same association with neonatal erythromycin treatment during the first 2 weeks after birth (338). This association has also been observed with maternal treatment with macrolide antibiotics during breast feeding in a case report (339) and in a population-based cohort study from Denmark (340). Because IHPS has a distinct developmental timing of presentation with a later onset in premature newborns (341), the ELBW infant may not be as susceptible as the term neonate, but treatment of all infants with erythromycin must weigh the risks and benefits.

In summary, there is a lack of published evidence relating to the efficacy of pharmacologic management of GER and additional data are needed regarding the optimal treatment of gastrointestinal dysmotility. Potentially significant side effects are associated with pharmacologic treatment, and debate persists about the efficacy and indications for pharmacologic treatment of these conditions.

Bronchodilators

The use of bronchodilators has increased with the survival of more immature newborns with greater susceptibility to development of BPD. Histologic studies in infants with BPD confirm bronchiolar smooth muscle hypertrophy, which can lead to airway narrowing.(342) Consistent with these anatomic changes, infants with BPD demonstrate bronchodilatation, increased dynamic airway compliance, and reduction in airway resistance in response to β-adrenergic agents and ipratropium, an anticholinergic drug (343–356). Airway responsiveness to bronchodilators develops by two weeks postnatal age in most neonates requiring mechanical ventilation and as early as 26 weeks postconceptional age (357). Consequently, bronchodilator treatment is frequently used in the management of BPD in preterm neonates.

The method of administering bronchodilators may influence efficacy. Aerosolized albuterol may be administered by either nebulizer or metered dose inhaler (MDI) and spacer. Until recently, the former was commonly used in mechanically ventilated patients. Nebulized albuterol (2.5 mg) increased respiratory system compliance (Crs/kg) by 35.3% as compared with a 2.8% improvement following saline placebo ($p < 0.001$) in ventilator-dependent, ELBW infants as early as 5 to 31 days after birth (352). A significant decrease in pCO_2 (>10 mm Hg) was noted in 47% of measurements. As expected, heart rate increased an average of 17.5 beats/min and persisted for 30 to 120 minutes after albuterol administration. In a study by Wilkie and colleagues, both nebulized salbutamol (albuterol) and ipratropium bromide, improved lung mechanics in ventilator-dependent neonates who were progressing into chronic lung disease (355). These infants, whose gestational ages ranged from 25 to 29 weeks with birthweights of 560 to 1,050 g, demonstrated bronchodilatation as early as 19 days after birth. These findings were confirmed in ventilator-dependent preterm infants who demonstrated dose-related bronchodilatation to nebulized ipratropium alone, and in combination with salbutamol (albuterol), by 18 to 34 days after birth (358). No synergistic bronchodilatation in neonates between an anticholinergic agent and albuterol has been reported (347). Oral administration of albuterol has also been noted to improve lung function in infants with BPD (354,359).

Nebulization of albuterol has several undesirable effects, including cooling of the inspired gas, higher cost of administration as compared with metered dose inhaler,

loss of drug by continuous flow, and inefficient delivery. Previous studies in ventilator models revealed that only 1–3% of nebulized drug is delivered to the patient (250,360,361). Our data in a neonatal ventilator-lung model indicate that only 0.2% of nebulized albuterol is delivered to the lungs of the ventilated neonate (362). Delivery of aerosolized albuterol is markedly improved when it is administered by MDI and spacer (362). When administered by MDI and spacer, both 72 μg of ipratropium and 400 μg of albuterol improved oxygenation and ventilation in 1 week-old, 880 gm neonates by 30 minutes after administration and increased heart rate an average of 23 beasts/min (350). In 2 week-old, average 28-week gestation, ventilator-dependent newborns, albuterol improved pulmonary mechanics in 9 of 10 patients (344). Seven of 10 patients responded after one MDI actuation (100 μg), and two of the remaining three patients after 200 μg (344). Improvement in pulmonary resistance was maximal at 30 minutes and lasted three hours. Albuterol treatment was associated with a significant tachycardia (mean 180 beats/min).

Beta agonists also improve pulmonary function of nonventilated infants with BPD. Nebulized isoproterenol markedly improved airway resistance and specific airway conductance in nonventilated infants with BPD at 41 weeks postconceptional age (348). Today, albuterol is the preferred agent over isoproterenol as a result of its greater selectivity for β2 receptors. Gappa and colleagues reported a significant reduction in airway resistance following albuterol administration by either nebulizer or MDI in spontaneously breathing infants (postconceptional age 37.1 ± 2.3 weeks) with BPD (345). Administration of the latter was facilitated by attaching the MDI to a holding chamber and face mask and allowing the infant to breathe for 30 seconds between puffs.

Choosing between albuterol delivery by nebulizer or MDI requires careful consideration of the differences in delivery efficiency, convenience and ease of use, disturbance to the patient, and adverse effect profile. In a recent survey of NICUs, 57% of centers administer albuterol by MDIs at least some of the time, although 19% of centers use MDIs exclusively (363). In most cases, MDIs are the preferred method of administration as a result of their greater efficiency in drug delivery (345), short delivery time, and reduced administration costs. Additionally, MDIs obviate the need to change ventilator flow rates and do not cause potentially troublesome cooling of ventilator gas. On the other hand, MDI dosages can only be changed in fixed increments.

Diuretics

Several classes of diuretic drugs are available, including osmotic agents such as mannitol, carbonic anhydrase inhibitors such as acetazolamide, thiazides such as chlorothiazide, high-ceiling or loop diuretics such as furosemide, and potassium-sparing diuretics such as spironolactone (364). The last three classes are used frequently in the treatment of neonates, both for acute fluid overload and for chronic therapy of BPD and congestive heart failure. Distinct differences in mechanisms of action and potency should guide selection of specific drugs (365,366).

Thiazides are sulfonamide diuretics whose major action is to block sodium and chloride cotransport in the first portion of the distal tubule, which causes a natriuresis (364–366). Thiazide-induced diuresis produces a greater loss of sodium and potassium per urine volume than does a diuresis induced by loop diuretics, although only a moderate amount of sodium is excreted (364). Among diuretics, thiazides are relatively unique in that they decrease the renal excretion of calcium, although magnesium excretion is increased. In high doses, thiazides may inhibit carbonic anhydrase with a potency equal to that of acetazolamide. They also may induce hypoglycemia, hypercholesterolemia, and hypertriglyceridemia (364). Thiazide elimination occurs through the renal tubular organic acid transport system, and may be inhibited by other organic acids such as probenecid. The diuretic action of thiazides depends on secretion into the renal tubular fluid, so that competitive inhibition of the transport of a thiazide by another organic acid may blunt its diuretic effect.

Spironolactone, the potassium-sparing diuretic commonly used for treatment of newborns, is a 17-spironolactone steroid that competitively antagonizes mineralocorticoids, predominantly aldosterone (364,366). Because aldosterone increases sodium reabsorption and potassium secretion, increased aldosterone secretion may be suspected by the ratio of urine sodium to potassium. Similarly, effective antagonism of aldosterone by spironolactone may be detected by an increasing urine sodium to potassium ratio. The appropriate dose of spironolactone relates to the concentration of aldosterone, because it acts through competitive inhibition. Spironolactone is available only for enteral administration and undergoes extensive first-pass hepatic metabolism to an active metabolite, canrenone.

The most serious toxicity of spironolactone is hyperkalemia during cotreatment with potassium supplements (366). Spironolactone increases calcium excretion and, in older males, may produce gynecomastia as a result of an antiandrogen effect. In rats exposed to high doses of spironolactone for prolonged periods, tumors may develop, but this has not been reported in humans to date (364). Other side effects include rashes, diarrhea, and vomiting.

Alternate potassium-sparing diuretics that do not work through aldosterone inhibition, such as triamterene and amiloride, rarely are administered to neonates. Their potassium-sparing action probably occurs through inhibition of the electrogenic sodium transport in the distal nephron (364).

Among the three loop diuretics in clinical use in the United States, bumetanide, ethacrynic acid, and furosemide, furosemide is the best studied in neonates. All three are organic acids, but furosemide and bumetanide are sulfonamides. All three diuretics induce diuresis by inhibiting the chloride pump in the ascending limb of the loop of Henle. Their diuretic effects require secretion into the tubular fluid by the organic acid transport system that may be competitively inhibited by other organic acids such as probenecid or penicillin (365,367). Because of these similarities in action, there is almost no reason to use two loop diuretics simultaneously. Patients who are resistant to furosemide, however, may still respond to bumetanide likely as a result of its greater potency (366). Loop diuretics produce excretion of dilute urine, with an increase in free-water excretion compared to sodium excretion (368).

Calcium excretion is increased by furosemide (366). This contributes to renal parenchymal calcification, nephrolithiasis, and osteopenia during chronic treatment of neonates with furosemide. Cholelithiasis has also been observed during chronic furosemide treatment. Although furosemide is highly protein bound, it appears unlikely that doses administered to neonates produce high enough concentrations to displace bilirubin (365).

As might be expected for a drug eliminated by renal tubular secretion, the half-life of furosemide in neonates is long and variable, ranging from 4.7 to 44.9 hours (369). During repetitive dosing, Vert and colleagues demonstrated an inverse relationship between postconceptional age and furosemide half-life (369). Petersen and colleagues have confirmed this prolonged half-life for furosemide in preterm neonates during the first few weeks after birth (6). They also noted that some neonates have poor absorption of orally administered furosemide, leading to an inadequate diuretic response. The prolonged half-life does not support the current clinical practice of administering furosemide every 6 to 8 hours in neonates.

The effects of furosemide on lung function, both acutely and chronically, have been studied in neonates with BPD (370) and in neonates recovering from hyaline membrane disease (371). In patients with BPD, pulmonary compliance improved after a single dose of furosemide. Prolonged treatment improved pulmonary compliance, pulmonary resistance, and oxygenation without an effect on transcutaneous PCO_2 (370). In a controlled study of preterm neonates recovering from hyaline membrane disease, furosemide improved pulmonary compliance by 2 hours after administration (371). This improvement persisted for 4 hours and then returned to baseline by 6 hours. Chronic furosemide treatment for 4 days produced a further improvement in alveolar–arterial difference in partial pressure of oxygen ($AaDO_2$).

One prospective, controlled study of newborns has found that furosemide treatment increases the frequency of patent ductus arteriosus, presumably as a result of the release of prostaglandin (PG) E_2 that accompanies diuresis (372). Other investigators have administered furosemide with indomethacin to blunt the oliguric response to indomethacin without loss of indomethacin-induced ductal closure (373). Indomethacin blocks the natriuretic response to furosemide and the increase in renal blood flow that furosemide produces (374).

Both furosemide and ethacrynic acid may produce ototoxicity (364). Furosemide-induced hearing loss occurs after large doses (1,000 mg in adults) administered i.v., especially to patients with renal failure who would be expected to have poor clearance of the drug (375). This transient ototoxicity correlates with changes in electrolyte concentrations in the middle ear fluids, endolymph and perilymph, that reduce endocochlear potentials (375). Compared to furosemide, bumetanide caused a similar frequency of adverse effects, except for ototoxicity, which appeared to be less with bumetanide (376).

Both thiazides and furosemide may produce allergic interstitial nephritis (364). The most frequent adverse effects associated with treatment of newborns with loop diuretics reflect their actions that frequently lead to hypochloremic, hypokalemic alkalosis. Electrolyte monitoring is needed at the start of treatment to detect excessive sodium depletion to serum values less than 120 mEq/L.

Although seldom used as a diuretic, methylxanthines may produce significant diuresis, natriuresis, and choliuresis (377).

Histamine$_2$ Receptor Antagonists

Acid suppressant therapy is commonly used in critically ill patients to prevent acute gastric mucosal damage (AGMD) and its severe complications, such as hemorrhage or perforation (378–380). Studies evaluating the risk of AGMD in critically ill infants and children are few in number and discrepant in results, thus making the issue of stress ulcer prophylaxis controversial (381,382). A small study in critically ill preterm infants (median gestational age 29.7 weeks) endoscopically demonstrated a high prevalence (94%) of asymptomatic esophageal and gastric lesions, including macroscopic esophagitis and gastritis together with ulceration (383). In children, a histamine$_2$-antagonist, in particular ranitidine, has been the agent of choice to treat these lesions and prevent the development of gastric hemorrhage (384).

Histamine$_2$ receptor antagonists inhibit histamine-induced gastric acid secretion (385). A series of structurally related compounds have been developed to block the histamine$_2$ receptor, including cimetidine, ranitidine, and famotidine. Although all of these drugs are used clinically, patients report adverse effects more often with cimetidine than ranitidine (386). Adverse effects most commonly reported by adults include diarrhea, nausea, vomiting, and constipation. In newborns, the most important undesired effect of cimetidine is its inhibition of the elimination of numerous drugs metabolized by cytochrome P450 (CYP) isoenzymes, including those metabolized by CYP1A2, CYP2C9, and CYP2D6 (387). Cimetidine, like other drugs with an imidazole structure, such as ketoconazole and metronidazole, binds to cytochrome P450 and reduces its activity (388). In newborns, one of the most frequently encountered and troublesome drug-drug interactions during cimetidine therapy is its inhibition of theophylline metabolism (CYP1A2) (389). This drug interaction requires vigilance and careful monitoring of theophylline concentrations to prevent toxicity. Other potential interactions include decreased clearance of propranolol, phenytoin, lidocaine, nifedipine, and diazepam (388). Drugs such as lorazepam, which require conjugation for elimination, are not affected by cimetidine treatment. Ranitidine, in which the imidazole ring is replaced with a furan ring, binds much less to liver microsomes and cytochrome P450 with approximately one tenth the affinity of cimetidine (388). Because of its greater potency and longer duration of effect, ranitidine is administered less frequently than cimetidine. Because ranitidine has at least three to four times the molar potency of cimetidine, it has minimal effects on cytochrome P450 in usual clinical doses (390,391). Accordingly, it is often the preferred agent in newborns and infants for suppression of histamine$_2$ receptor mediated acid secretion.

In a randomized, controlled study of 23 mechanically ventilated, preterm and full-term newborns (mean gestational age 32 weeks), 5 mg/kg/day of ranitidine markedly decreased the risk for endoscopically proven gastric mucosal lesions (384). In a case report, ranitidine provided effective treatment for a preterm neonate with a life-threatening upper gastrointestinal hemorrhage after indomethacin (392). In this preterm newborn, an infusion of 0.2 mg/kg/hour resulted in high concentrations with a half-life of approximately 5.5 hours, which is greater than twice the elimination half-life reported in older children (248).

To determine the optimal dosage requirement of ranitidine, many investigators have used gastric pH as a surrogate endpoint. The validity of this endpoint is based on adult data that demonstrate that maintaining gastric pH above 4 reduces the risk of stress ulceration and gastric hemorrhage in critically ill patients (393). Kuusela and associates studied intraluminal gastric pH in 16 preterm and term infants who received three different bolus doses of ranitidine: 0.5 mg, 1.0 mg, and 1.5 mg per kg of body weight to keep the intraluminal gastric pH greater than 4 on a 24-hour basis (316). Preterm infants needed significantly smaller doses of ranitidine than term neonates to keep their gastric pH greater than 4. The required optimal dose of ranitidine for preterm infants was 0.5 mg/kg/body weight twice a day and 1.5 mg/kg three times a day for term infants (316). Kelly and associates found that ranitidine infused at 0.0625 mg/kg/hour was sufficient to increase and maintain gastric pH above 4 in 10 premature neonates (median gestational age 27.5 weeks) who were receiving dexamethasone (394). Fontana and associates studied the pharmacokinetics of ranitidine in 27 term infants during the first day after birth and reported that concentrations greater than 100 ng/mL and 200 ng/mL could be expected for at least 12 hours after a single intravenous bolus dose of 1.6 mg/kg and 3.3 mg/kg, respectively (395). The same average concentration could be maintained at steady-state with an intravenous infusion rate between 0.03 and 0.06 mg/kg/hour based on their reported mean half-life of 207 minutes (395).

Famotidine is an H$_2$-antagonist that is not well studied in neonates and infants. Advantages over ranitidine and cimetidine include its potency, relatively longer elimination half-life, and lack of interaction with the cytochrome P450 isoforms. The pharmacokinetics and pharmacodynamics of intravenous famotidine were evaluated in 10 infants (5–19 days of age) (396). After a 0.5 mg/kg infusion of famotidine, the terminal elimination half-life was 10.5 ± 5.4 hours. Six of the nine infants who had intragastric pH monitoring maintained a gastric pH > 4 until the final 24-hour sampling point. Orenstein and associates evaluated the safety and efficacy of famotidine in 35 infants (1.3–10.5 months of age) in a randomized, placebo-controlled trial evaluating famotidine 0.5 mg/kg and 1.0 mg/kg once daily for up to 8 weeks in the treatment of GERD (317). No serious adverse events were reported. Eleven of 16 patients had nonserious, possibly drug-related adverse experiences. The investigators concluded that a possibly efficacious famotidine dose for infants is 0.5 mg/kg, however dosage individualization may be required based on response. Larger placebo-controlled evaluations of famotidine in infants are warranted.

Inotropes

Although inotropy refers specifically to myocardial contractility, inotropic drugs improve cardiac contractility, increase cardiac rate, and alter vascular tone (397,398). Cardiac output is determined by preload, contractility, and afterload and represents stroke volume × heart rate. The inotrope should be selected according to its specific pharmacologic properties and the specific cardiovascular abnormality to be corrected. Despite frequent administration of inotropes to newborns, they have received limited study in this population.

Shock occurs when blood flow and oxygen supply are inadequate to meet tissue demands. The same principles apply to the myocardium. Increasing cardiac wall stiffness increases myocardial oxygen consumption and may decrease flow during diastole. Inotropic drug treatment for the failing heart must balance increasing myocardial oxygen consumption against the increase in cardiac output that provides more oxygenated blood through the coronary circulation to the myocardium. Disproportionate increases in myocardial wall stiffness from increased contractility and increased afterload may impede coronary flow and worsen myocardial ischemia. Conversely, excess peripheral vasodilation may reduce the blood pressure to a level in which there is too little pressure to maintain coronary flow during diastole.

Specific receptor interactions, cardiovascular effects, and controlled clinical trials of inotropic drugs in newborns should guide their clinical use (Table 56-6) (398–400). Dosages for drugs used frequently in newborn resuscitation are indicated in Table 56-5. All the inotropes should be dosed to effect. Prolonged infusion of catecholamines has been shown to down-regulate receptors which reduces their effects.

Isoproterenol is a direct-acting, potent, pure beta-adrenergic agonist whose usefulness is limited by tachycardia and peripheral vasodilation. Tachycardia and diversion of blood flow to the extensive vasculature in muscle may steal perfusion away from more vital organs and extend myocardial infarction (401). Isoproterenol is most effective for raising heart rate, for instance in the treatment of complete heart block. Epinephrine stimulates all adrenergic receptors directly, but its vascular effects vary among organs, with β_2 stimulation usually exceeding β_1 vasoconstriction so that peripheral vascular usually falls (398). The effects of epinephrine infusions of 0.05 to 2.6 µg/kg/min were described in thirty-one 23 to 30 week gestation, hypotensive newborns who had not responded to treatment with three 10 to 15 ml/kg infusions of crystalloid and 15 µg/kg/min infusions of dopamine (402). Epinephrine normalized blood pressure in all, increased heart rate an average of 10 beats/min, improved urine output in 5 of 6 patients with oliguria, but it increased the base deficit an average of 3 mEq/L. No controlled trials have compared epinephrine treatment of hypotensive premature newborns to dopamine or dobutamine as initial treatment.

Dopamine, the immediate precursor of norepinephrine, is unique among inotropes because it dilates renal, coronary, and mesenteric vascular beds of adults at low doses through activation of the D_1-dopaminergic receptors (398). Dopamine exerts some of its effects through release of endogenous norepinephrine, which may become depleted during prolonged infusions (398). Peripheral infusions of dopamine do not cross the blood–brain barrier to interact with CNS dopamine receptors. Extravasation of dopamine may cause severe ischemic tissue damage, which may be treated by local infiltration of diluted phentolamine (403).

The dose-response in neonates for dopamine to raise blood pressure appears to start at 2 µg/kg/min, but the upper limit of its dose response in neonates has not been defined. At high concentrations, dopamine's alpha$_1$ receptor activity is reported to cause vasoconstriction to predominate in all circulations (397). This effect appears to vary with development and clinical condition. Studies of renal vascular resistance in newborn animals infused with 32 to 50 µg/kg/minute of dopamine have not detected this effect (404,405). Similarly high-dose (30–50 µg/kg/min) infusions in oliguric, hypotensive, near-term newborns improved urine output and increased heart rate suggesting that the alpha$_1$ vasoconstrictor effects that are expected at high dosages may not predominate and reduce renal perfusion in all newborns (406).

The regional blood flow effects of dopamine have been studied in premature newborns using Doppler measures of blood flow velocity to derive a pulsatility index (PI) that provides indirect evidence of vascular tone. The greater the degree of initial vasoconstriction in the renal arteries, the greater the degree of vasodilation by dopamine, measured as a decrease in PI (407). Although dopamine did not change flow in the cerebral or mesenteric arteries, it increased aortic blood pressure without changing aortic PI suggesting this occurred through peripheral vasoconstriction. A related study of dopamine in hypotensive preterm

TABLE 56-6

RELATIVE CARDIOVASCULAR RECEPTOR INTERACTIONS OF INOTROPES AND THE ASSOCIATED EFFECTS

CARDIOVASCULAR RECEPTOR INTERACTIONS AND EFFECTS

Catecholmine	α_1 Vasoconstriction; ↑Cardiac Contractility	α_2 Vasoconstriction; ↓Norepinephrine Release	β_1 ↑Contractility, ↑Conduction Velocity	β_2 Vasodilation, Bronchodilation	Dopamine, D_1 Renal, Mesenteric and Coronary Vasodilation	Indirect Release of Endogenous Norepinephrine
Dobutamine	1+	0	3+	1+	0	0
Dopamine	0 to 3+	1+	2+ to 3+	2+	3+	1+
Epinephrine	2+	2+	3+	3+	0	0
Isoproterenol	0	0	3+	3+	0	0

0 = lowest to 3+ = highest interaction

Adapted from Zaritsky, A and Chernow, B. Use of catecholamines in pediatrics. *J Pediatr* 1984;105:341–350; Lefkowitz RJ, Hoffman BB, Taylor P. Neurotransmission. The autonomic and somatic motor nervous systems. In Hardman JG, Limbird LE, Molinoff PB, Ruddon RW, Gilman AG (eds): *Goodman & Gilman's The Pharmacological Basis of Therapeutics*, 9th ed. New York: McGraw-Hill. 1996:105–139, with permission.

newborns with PDA's estimated both pulmonary and systemic blood pressures after dopamine treatment using Doppler blood flow velocities (408). In this study of 18 neonates, pulmonary/systemic artery mean blood pressure ratio decreased or remained the same in 9 and increased in 9. In 2 patients with lower baseline PA BP, the rise in PA pressure was sufficient to reverse ductal flow and create a right to left shunt. For the 9 neonates whose mPAP/mSBP increased, the increase was similar in magnitude to the decrease in the other 9 (+17% vs. −19%). This unpredictability of PA responses implies that dopamine needs to be used carefully with frequent reevaluation of its effects.

Dobutamine is the product of directed structural manipulation of dopamine and isoproterenol to produce hydroxyphenyl–isobutyl–dopamine (dobutamine), an inotrope designed to increase contractility with a minimum of tachycardia and vasodilation (409). Initially, dobutamine was thought to possess balanced vascular α_1 and β_2 activities. Later study demonstrated that dobutamine exists in two enantiomorphic forms, with different receptor activities (410). The. (−) isomer is a potent α_1-agonist that increases cardiac contractility, whereas the (+) isomer is a potent α_2-antagonist. The (+) isomer is several-fold more potent for β receptors than the (−) isomer. Overall, dobutamine is more selective for β_1 than for β_2 receptors. With infusions at less than 20 μg/kg/minute, dobutamine increases cardiac output and contractility with minimal changes in peripheral resistance and modest increases in heart rate (411). In neonates, dosages of 5 and 7.5 μg/kg/minute increased cardiac output without changing heart rate or blood pressure (412). The lack of vasoconstriction may limit dobutamine's usefulness in patients with severe hypotension, but may be useful in patients with cardiogenic failure in whom cardiac function may worsen with increased afterload.

The effectiveness of dopamine and dobutamine to raise blood pressure have been studied in hypotensive, premature newborns with RDS (413–416). In this specific group of neonates without asphyxia or sepsis, dopamine is more effective than dobutamine for treatment of hypotension unresponsive to volume expansion. This likely relates to the peripheral vasodilating effects of dobutamine and the vasoconstricting effects of dopamine.

The effects of dobutamine and dopamine on systemic blood flow were compared using SVC blood flow velocity (416). Dobutamine increased SVC blood flow velocity more than dopamine, although dopamine raised blood pressure to a greater degree. This would be consistent with effects of dobutamine in adults in whom it lowers systemic vascular resistance although increasing cardiac output.

Phosphodiesterase inhibitors represent a relatively new class of inotropic drugs for newborns, although they have been used extensively since the 1980s to treat adults and older children, especially following cardiac surgery (417–419). These drugs increase cardiac output through a combination of increased contractility and decreased afterload without receptor interactions. In contrast to catecholamines that increase intracellular cyclic adenosine monophosphate (cAMP) through activation of adenyl cyclase, these newer bipyridine compounds increase cAMP by inhibition of cyclic nucleotide phosphodiesterase.

The first of these drugs approved and used in the United States was amrinone which has been studied in neonates and infants (420–424). Rapid redistribution of amrinone after cardiac surgery creates complex pharmacokinetics in adults that require a higher loading and infusion dosages to maintain therapeutic concentrations (425). Neonates have a smaller distribution volume and lower clearance of amrinone than infants, despite equal rates of n-acetylation, leading to a half-life of 10.7 hr vs. 6.1 hr for infants (426). In infants, amrinone increases cardiac index more than nitroprusside alone likely as a result of the combination of increased cardiac contractility and vasodilation (421). The use of amrinone has been limited, however, as a result of reversible thrombocytopenia with a frequency of 20% (417) to 44% in a pediatric study (427). The latter study found that thrombocytopenia correlated with the AUC of N-acetylamrinone, but not that of amrinone (427).

Milrinone represents the next generation of bipyridine phosphodiesterase inhibitor to be marketed in the United States to augment cardiac output. In an open-labeled study of 10 neonates with low cardiac output after cardiac surgery, milrinone treatment with a 50 μg/kg loading dose and infusion of 0.50 μg/kg/min for 30 minutes increased heart rate, decreased average atrial pressures, systemic and pulmonary arterial pressures and increased cardiac index more than 205 in 9/10 patients by an average of 48% (428). As would be predicted systemic and pulmonary vascular resistances decreased, as well. A more definitive, multi-centered, placebo-controlled, dose-response study of milrinone was conducted in 238 infants greater than 35 weeks postconceptual age undergoing cardiac surgery (419). In this study, high-dose milrinone (75 μg/kg over 60 minutes followed by 0.75 μg/kg/min for 35 hours) was superior to low dose milrinone (25 μg/kg over 60 minutes followed by 0.25 mcg/kg/min for 35 hours) and to placebo for prevention of low cardiac output state (9.6% in high dose, 17.7% in low dose, and 26.7% in placebo) (419). In a comparison of milrinone and amrinone treatment of adults during cardiopulmonary to prevent low cardiac output state, no differences were noted (429). As with amrinone, milrinone has a lower clearance in infants than in children (430). As with amrinone, milrinone has been associated with the development of thrombocytopenia in infants and children (430). Before adopting widespread treatment of premature neonates with milrinone, the kinetics must be studied in this population. The phosphodiesterase inhibitors, however, may provide an important new treatment for low cardiac output in neonates that avoids adrenergic receptor down-regulation, and depletion of endogenous catecholamines.

Digoxin, despite its long history, remains a useful drug for the chronic enteral treatment of congestive heart failure, although the phosphodiesterase inhibitors may take its place. The efficacy of digitalis for the treatment of congestive heart failure varies according to myocardial dynamics (431). In a study of 21 infants with congestive heart failure as a result of ventricular septal defects, digoxin improved 12 clinically, but only 6 improved by echocardiographic measurements (432). The digoxin serum half-life averages 35 hours (range 17–52 hours) in term newborns and 57 hours (range 38 to 88 hours) in premature (birth weight range of 1,150–2,230 gm) newborns (433). This likely reflects the dependence on renal excretion for most of the elimination of digoxin (434) and suggests that premature neonates require a smaller digoxin maintenance dose (435).

Digoxin toxicity, like efficacy, is not defined by a specific concentration, but by signs and symptoms such as emesis, arrhythmias, or conduction abnormalities, such as complete heart block (436). Various drugs may increase digoxin concentrations, such as antibiotics that reduce inactivation by gut flora (437), spironolactone that reduces its clearance (438), and amiodarone that may either reduce the clearance or increase the bioavailability of digoxin (128). Life-threatening arrhythmias as a result of excessive digitalis concentrations may be treated successfully with antidigoxin Fab antibody fragments (439).

Older assays for therapeutic monitoring of digoxin cross-reacted with an endogenous molecule, digoxin-like immunoreactive substance (DLIS), which was increased in the circulation of preterm newborns, pregnant women, and patients with renal failure (440,441). DLIS has been identified as having both the structure (442) and function of ouabain (443). The cross-reactivity of the newer assays has been eliminated.

Methylxanthines

Methylxanthines, including caffeine, theophylline, and aminophylline (an ethylenediamine complex of theophylline) are commonly administered to preterm neonates to treat apnea of prematurity and to aid in weaning from mechanical ventilation. The proposed mechanisms of actions of methylxanthines include (444): (a) increased central neural drive; (b) adenosine receptor blockade, thereby inhibiting adenosine's potent respiratory depressant effects (445); (c) improved respiratory muscle function, particularly diaphragmatic contraction (446); and (d) natriuresis. The often cited mechanism of increased cyclic AMP through phosphodiesterase inhibition does not explain the *in vivo* effects of theophylline because this mechanism requires concentrations which are usually toxic (>20 μg/mL) (447). Other factors which may contribute to the action of methylxanthines include catecholamine release that increases cardiac output and improves oxygenation, and increased blood glucose which may reduce the frequency of apneic spells (444).

Theophylline

The effectiveness of theophylline in the treatment of neonatal apnea was first documented over two decades ago (448–450). Theophylline increases minute ventilation, reduces $PaCO_2$, increases central respiratory drive, and significantly reduces the frequency of apnea (444,449,

451–453). Additionally, theophylline may promote extubation of infants recovering from respiratory distress syndrome (454).

The desired plasma concentration of theophylline in the treatment of apnea is approximately 5 to 15 μg/mL (455), although concentrations as low as 2.8 to 3.9 μg/mL have been reported to be effective (456). To achieve and maintain therapeutic concentrations, a loading dose of 5 to 6 mg/kg of theophylline is administered followed by a maintenance dose of 2 to 4 mg/kg/day in two to four divided doses (444). Note that the therapeutic range to treat apnea is lower than the commonly accepted therapeutic range to treat asthma in older patients (10–20 μg/mL). This is as a result of reduced protein binding and higher free concentrations of theophylline in neonates as compared to adults (5). Because the unbound fraction of drug in plasma is considered pharmacologically active, a greater response may be expected in the newborn than in the adult, despite the same plasma concentrations. For example, at a total theophylline plasma concentration of 17 μg/mL, approximately 44% is unbound and pharmacologically active in the adult as compared to 64% in the full-term infant (5). Thus, 17 μg/ml of theophylline in a newborn would be equivalent to 24.7 μg/ml total theophylline concentration in the adult. Despite achieving therapeutic concentrations of theophylline, about 25% of infants with apnea may not respond (444).

Metabolism of theophylline (1,3-dimethylxanthine) and caffeine (1,3,7-trimethylxanthine) via demethylation is primarily mediated by cytochrome P4501A2 (CYP1A2) (22–25). However, because expression of CYP1A2 is low in neonates, clearance of these agents is significantly reduced, especially in preterm infants (23,34). Newborns, unlike adults, are able to hepatically methylate theophylline to caffeine, and plasma caffeine/theophylline ratios may reach 0.3 to 0.4 at steady-state (457–459). Thus, both compounds may contribute to theophylline's therapeutic effects (459,460). Changes in theophylline kinetics during maturation of infants born at gestations of 25 to 30 weeks were studied with stable isotopes (461). This technique allows more accurate determination of the elimination phase by monitoring concentrations for prolonged periods although continuing administration of the unlabeled medication. Theophylline half-life correlated best with postnatal age, rather than postconceptional age. As would be expected, the theophylline half-life varied inversely with postnatal age as follows:

$$\log t_{1/2} \text{ (hours)} = 1.72 - 0.00565 \times \text{postnatal age (days).} \quad (12)$$

Clinically, theophylline clearance and urine metabolite patterns reach adult values by 55 weeks postconceptional age or approximately 4 to 5 months after birth (30). As a result of the significant interindividual variability in clearance and protein binding, theophylline plasma concentrations should be monitored and doses should be adjusted to maintain therapeutic concentrations.

When monitoring theophylline concentrations, one must consider factors that alter theophylline clearance. Theophylline's metabolism is increased and its half-life shortened by inducing agents, such as anticonvulsants (462). Metabolism is delayed by viral infections, such as influenza (359), and numerous interacting drugs, including erythromycin and cimetidine (463). Ranitidine was also noted to reduce theophylline clearance, although this interaction is less significant and less predictable than with cimetidine (464,465).

Adverse effects of theophylline include irritability, sleeplessness, natriuresis, hyperglycemia, hyperreflexia, tremor, seizures, hypertension, tachycardia, and cardiac arrhythmias (466,467). Tachycardia is the most common side effect associated with aminophylline. Theophylline relaxes the gastroesophageal sphincter of adults and probably has the same effect in newborns. If apnea occurs as a result of gastroesophageal reflux, theophylline treatment may worsen this problem.

Caffeine

Caffeine and theophylline have similar efficacy in treating or preventing apnea and bradycardia in premature infants (468–470). However, caffeine has fewer associated adverse effects and a more favorable therapeutic index than aminophylline (466,467,471). Additionally, caffeine has a longer half-life, thus permitting a convenient once or twice daily dosage schedule.

Apnea was reduced by administering caffeine citrate 20 mg/kg followed by 5 to 10 mg/kg/day once or twice daily to 18 preterm infants with a mean gestational age of 27.5 weeks (472). The average number of episodes were reduced from 13.6 to 2.1 episodes per day. Note that caffeine citrate doubles the weight of the administered drug, so that 20 mg/kg is equivalent to 10 mg/kg of caffeine base. Subsequent pharmacokinetic studies from the same group led to the current dosing recommendation of 10 mg/kg of caffeine base, followed by a maintenance dose of 2.5 mg/kg/day given as a single daily dose (27). More recently, Scanlon and associates reported that "high dose" caffeine (50 mg/kg caffeine citrate loading dose followed by 12 mg/kg/day) improved apnea more rapidly than the standard dose (25 mg/kg loading dose followed by 6 mg/kg/day) without increasing adverse effects (473).

Effective caffeine concentrations for the treatment of apnea of prematurity range from 5 to 25 µg/mL (467). Previous reports suggest that caffeine plasma concentrations of up to 50 µg/mL may be tolerated without significant adverse effects (27,473). Caffeine is noted to have minimal metabolic effects in the newborn infant (474). In a study of 12 premature neonates, 20 mg/kg caffeine citrate did not increase excretion of electrolytes or catecholamine metabolites, however glucose concentrations were lower in formula fed infants after caffeine administration (474). Infants who received continuous glucose infusions had no change in plasma glucose concentrations. Caffeine's wide therapeutic index reduces the necessity for the close plasma concentration monitoring that is required with theophylline. Similar to theophylline, approximately one-third of patients do not respond to treatment with caffeine (444).

As a result of limited biotransformation, caffeine elimination in the neonate is dependent on renal clearance. Unchanged caffeine comprised about 86% of the methylated xanthines and methyluric acids in the urine of infants less than 1 month of age (466). As a consequence of limited biotransformation, the half-life of caffeine is significantly prolonged and may exceed 200 hours in preterm infants (27). Similar to theophylline, the half-life of caffeine in preterm infants decreases after birth (475,476). In 34 preterm infants 25 to 32 weeks gestation with a mean postnatal age of 4.8 ± 0.7 days, the half-life of caffeine was markedly reduced from 129.8 hours to 93.5 hours ($p < 0.005$) by treatment day 7 (476). Even full-term infants, who were exposed to caffeine transplacentally, have prolonged half-lives, ranging from 31 to 132 hours (477). In general, adult values for the caffeine half-life are reached at approximately 60 weeks postconception or 4 to 6 months postnatally (28,29).

Muscle Relaxants

Muscle relaxants are commonly administered to neonates during mechanical ventilation and anesthesia for surgical procedures (478). Nondepolarizing muscle relaxants, which competitively inhibit acetylcholine at the motor end-plate, have become the mainstay for neuromuscular (NM) blockade in the NICU. Although pancuronium has been used extensively in treatment of neonates, the use of the shorter acting nondepolarizing agents, vecuronium and atracurium, has increased in recent years.

Pancuronium is a long-acting neuromuscular blocker with an average duration of action in neonates of 60 to 120 minutes following a 0.05 mg/kg dose (478). Pancuronium is primarily excreted by the kidney (60–80%) with approximately 15% hepatically metabolized to an active metabolite (479). Its predominant renal elimination requires that caution be used to avoid accumulation in premature neonates or infants with poor renal function. Pancuronium does not cause histamine release, however tachycardia and increased systolic blood pressure as a result of vagal blockade are characteristic (480,481).

Pancuronium dosage requirements for neonates increase with postnatal age, and decrease with prematurity (482). Treatment during the first week after birth required a dose of 0.03 mg/kg, compared to 0.09 mg/kg by 2 to 4 weeks after birth. Dose reductions were required not only for prematurity, but also for acidosis and hypothermia. By monitoring muscle twitch to determine neuromuscular blockade, others have shown that newborns have widely variable dosage requirements of pancuronium (483). Generally, larger doses of pancuronium are required for muscle relaxation in infants than in adults, presumably as a result of a larger volume of distribution. Repeated administration of pancuronium to neonates may lead to prolonged neuromuscular blockade, possibly as a result of its pharmacologically active metabolite and long half-life, which is related to immaturity of liver and renal function.

Vecuronium and atracurium are intermediate-acting neuromuscular blockers with a shorter duration of effect than pancuronium. In contrast to pancuronium, vecuronium, and in large part atracurium, have little to no cardiovascular effects (481). In neonates, 0.03 mg/kg of vecuronium produces a 30 to 40 minute duration of action as compared to 20 to 30 minutes after 0.15 to 0.3 mg/kg of atracurium (478). Vecuronium's effects are much longer in neonates and infants than in children and adolescents (484). A 0.1 mg/kg dose maintained neuromuscular blockade by analysis of muscle twitch for more than 58 minutes in infants and 18 minutes in children, aged 3 to 10 years (484).

Vecuronium is 20% renally excreted unchanged and the remainder is excreted in the bile (485). Vecuronium's limited renal excretion has often led to its choice in patients with renal dysfunction; however, its active metabolite (3-desacetylvecuronium) may accumulate in renal failure and result in prolonged neuromuscular blockade (480). Although repeated administration of vecuronium carries a lower risk than pancuronium of prolonged neuromuscular blockade, this phenomenon has been reported in neonates both with and without renal failure (486,487). The latter occurred in a 2-month old infant as a result of vecuronium accumulation at doses of 1.67 μg/kg/min for 5 days followed by 0.83 μg/kg/min for 2 days. The infant required 48 hours to regain full neuromuscular function. Lower doses may be required in some neonates and infants and monitoring of the neuromuscular junction may reduce the use of excessive doses.

Atracurium does not rely on renal or hepatic elimination and undergoes a spontaneous, nonenzymatic, ester hydrolysis at the pH of body fluids (Hoffmann elimination). The breakdown products are not pharmacologically active, making this an excellent agent for use in patients with renal and/or hepatic dysfunction (488). Unlike pancuronium and vecuronium, atracurium has the potential for histamine release that may result in cutaneous flushing and/or hypotension. Neonates appear to be more sensitive to atracurium than older children (489) and infusion requirements are approximately 25% lower than older children to maintain 90% to 95% neuromuscular blockade (490).

Neuromuscular blockade for several days may produce prolonged muscle weakness. Several metabolic factors and other drugs may enhance neuromuscular blockade, including acidosis and hypokalemia, and treatment with magnesium and aminoglycoside antibiotics (478). The contribution of drug accumulation at the myoneural junction or alteration of the myoneural junction requires more study. Monitoring of muscle fiber twitch during prolonged paralysis may be helpful for evaluating and avoiding this side effect.

Prostaglandins and Prostaglandin Inhibitors

During the last 25 years, understanding of the pharmacology and physiology of the eicosanoids has expanded dra-

matically from PGE_1 and $PGF_1\alpha$ to thromboxane and prostacyclin, products of the cyclooxygenase pathway, and leukotrienes, noncyclized products of the lipoxygenase pathway. Better understanding of leukotrienes has helped to account for previously recognized biologic mediators such as slow-reacting substance A, which is the same as leukotriene C. Despite the enormous variety of functions mediated through the eicosanoids, PGE_1 and PGE_2 are the most frequently used eicosanoids in newborn medicine (491). They have been used primarily to maintain patency of the ductus arteriosus, and occasionally, for pulmonary vasodilation in the treatment of persistent pulmonary hypertension of the newborn (PPHN). The effectiveness of PGE_1 for maintaining ductal patency has been confirmed in various studies, including a multicenter collaborative investigation (492).

Prostaglandin E_1 usually has been administered by continuous venous or arterial infusion (493). Dosages generally have started at 0.1 μg/kg/minute and have been associated with a variety of adverse reactions, including cutaneous vasodilation, edema, hypotension, apnea, fever, irritability, seizures, hypoglycemia, diarrhea, disseminated intravascular coagulation, osteolysis, hypercalcemia, and thrombocytopenia (493). By reducing starting dosages to 0.05 μg/kg/minute, side effects, in particular apnea, are reduced. If oxygenation is maintained, dosages can be tapered to 0.01 μg/kg/minute (494).

Prolonged treatment with PGE_2 is needed for patients with ductal-dependent cardiac malformations awaiting transplantation. Oral PGE_2 also is effective for maintaining ductal patency and oxygenation (494). Patients who were changed from the i.v. to the oral route, however, did have a significant decrease in PaO_2. Oral treatment utilized doses of 35 to 65 μg/kg/hour by gastric drip, with a slow increase in dosing intervals from 1 to 4 hours during the second and third week of treatment. This is consistent with recent reports of treatment of adults with PGE analogues for healing of ulcers (495).

Closure of the patent ductus arteriosus with cyclooxygenase inhibitors also is an integral part of neonatal pharmacology. Ductal patency after birth is maintained by PGE_2, the secretion of which is inhibited by rising oxygen tension (491). Ductal closure was first achieved with oral indomethacin in large dosages (2.5–5 mg/kg) (496). Since that report, indomethacin has been formulated in an i.v. preparation and used in a multicenter collaborative trial that demonstrated the efficacy of treatment with a 0.2 mg/kg loading dose, followed by 0.1 to 0.25 mg/kg/doses every 12 hours for a total of three doses (497). This study also illustrated the side effects of cyclooxygenase inhibition in neonates, including oliguria, increased serum creatinine, and transient mild bleeding.

Infants with intracranial hemorrhage were excluded from the collaborative study (497). Subsequent studies have found that early indomethacin treatment actually decreases the risk of intracranial hemorrhage (498). When the presence of an intracranial hemorrhage was not a contraindication to indomethacin treatment, it has not been shown to cause extension of intracranial hemorrhages (499,500). These studies do not indicate that intracranial hemorrhage should be a contraindication for indomethacin treatment, although some physicians follow the approach used in the multicenter collaborative trial and avoid administration of indomethacin to neonates with intracranial hemorrhages (497).

Developmental changes in the pharmacokinetics of indomethacin have been defined for preterm infants (501). Lower average indomethacin concentrations were noted in patients who did not sustain ductal closure after treatment with indomethacin. Indomethacin clearance increased with both postnatal age and body weight. A correlation between individual indomethacin levels and ductal closure was not found, however, possibly relating to variation in rates of PGE2 production among patients.

The optimal length of indomethacin treatment for low-birth-weight neonates has not been settled. After initial treatment with two doses of indomethacin, once-daily doses of indomethacin have been continued for 5 additional days in 22 infants with birth weight under 1,500 g (502). The group that was treated for a sustained period of time had no patent ductus 3 days after ending treatment and fewer intraventricular hemorrhages. The ductus reopened eventually in almost one-half of this group, but at a much older age. Longer courses of indomethacin need more study, but may be more effective for ductal closure.

The neonate who is several weeks old and has a symptomatic patent ductus arteriosus presents a therapeutic dilemma. McCarthy and colleagues reported failure of ductal closure in infants who were 37 to 40 weeks postconceptional age at the time of indomethacin treatment (503). Efforts to maintain effective indomethacin concentrations in older patients with patent ductus arteriosus, by higher doses administered more frequently, have not ensured ductal closure (504).

The renal effects of indomethacin in premature infants are quite similar to those observed in symptomatic adults (505). In premature infants, indomethacin decreases urine flow, glomerular filtration rate, and free-water clearance, which combine to decrease renal electrolyte excretion (506). Oliguria during indomethacin treatment of premature infants has been improved with dopamine (507) and with furosemide (371). In adults, salt depletion and hypovolemia accentuate the adverse effects of nonsteroidal anti-inflammatory drugs on renal function (505,508,509). Seri and colleagues found that dopamine prevented a decrease in urine flow and increased sodium excretion (507).

The rate of indomethacin infusion has a significant effect on its cardiovascular effects. When indomethacin was infused over 0.2 to 4 minutes, cerebral blood flow velocity decreased 48% to 75% (510). When indomethacin was infused over 20 minutes, cerebral blood flow velocity was not reduced (511). A similar reduction in mesenteric blood flow occurs when indomethacin is administered over 20 seconds or less, and this can be prevented by slow infusion over 30 to 35 minutes (512). It is too early to determine whether the common practice of discontinua-

tion of feeds during indomethacin treatment is unnecessary when doses are administered more slowly.

Pulmonary Vasodilators

Because the pulmonary vasculature of many neonates is in parallel with the systemic vasculature, through patency of the ductus arteriosus and foramen ovale, an effective pulmonary vasodilator must dilate the pulmonary vasculature more than the systemic vasculature (513). Endothelium-derived relaxing factor (EDRF) was shown to be involved in control of the perinatal pulmonary circulation as it dilates after birth (514,515). EDRF was shown to have the same properties as nitric oxide (NO) (516). NO dilates pulmonary arteries selectively through release of cyclic guanosine monophosphate (cGMP) (517,518). Infants with persistent pulmonary hypertension of the newborn (PPHN) have lower circulating cGMP likely as a result of inadequate NO production needed to dilate the pulmonary vasculature after birth.(519) The selectivity of NO for the pulmonary vasculature derives from its administration by inhalation and inactivation by binding to hemoglobin as soon as it enters the blood stream. This same binding, however, may induce methemoglobinemia at higher doses of NO (520). NO is a highly reactive compound whose dose must be carefully monitored to avoid potentially severe or even lethal toxicity (517).

Improved oxygenation and a reduced need for ECMO have been demonstrated in randomized, controlled trials of NO treatment of near term neonates with respiratory failure (521–525). A meta-analysis of 12 controlled trials found that NO improves oxygenation in about 50% of term and near-term neonates and significantly reduced the need for ECMO (525). No improvement in outcome was demonstrated for infants with diaphragmatic hernia. Although NO has been used to treat a variety of disorders (526), when respiratory failure is accompanied by pulmonary disease and severe infiltrates, NO treatment is less successful, possibly because inhalational delivery does not reach the pulmonary vasculature (527). Dose-response studies indicate that neonates achieve maximum improvement in oxygenation at 20 ppm (528) to 40 ppm (529–531). Prolonged treatment longer than 10 days has been associated with pulmonary toxicity demonstrated by detection of nitrotyrosine (532). Platelet function has been reduced during NO treatment of adults, likely through increased cGMP, and this may represent a risk for neonates (533). In the critically ill, neonatal population treated with NO, long-term outcome should be evaluated in comparison to control, comparably sick infants not exposed to NO. From a randomized, controlled study of NO treatment in 248 neonates, evaluation at 1 year showed no increase in mortality, reactive airway disease, chronic lung disease, or developmental delay in the NO treated group (534).

Although NO was approved for the near term neonate with pulmonary hypertension, preterm neonate less than 32 weeks gestation have been treated with NO (535). A group of 70 infants born at 23 to 31 weeks gestation with hypoxic respiratory failure defined by aAO$_2$ less than 0.22, were randomized to treatment with 5 ppm NO or no treatment and pulmonary blood flow velocity was measured by Doppler. NO treatment increased pulmonary blood flow and significantly improved oxygenation with a 71% increase in aAO$_2$.

Several other drugs have been used for treatment of PPHN, including tolazoline, PGE$_1$, PGI$_2$, PGD$_2$, acetylcholine, isoproterenol, chlorpromazine, nitroprusside, and sildenafil (536). None of these have proven to be selective for the pulmonary vasculature. Although tolazoline has been reported to improve oxygenation in approximately 60% of patients, high mortality persisted, and adverse effects occurred at an unacceptably high rate (76). Improvement in oxygenation was recently reported in 72% of forty-three ELBW neonates with birth weight less than 750 gm treated with slow bolus tolazoline infusions of 0.5 to 2.0 mg/kg (537). Inappropriately high prolonged infusion doses of tolazoline, used without the guidance of kinetic studies, may have contributed to the high rate of adverse effects associated with tolazoline treatment (76). Despite this recent report of efficacy of tolazoline in ELBW neonates, it has been removed from production.

Investigations of the mechanisms through which NO controls neonatal pulmonary vascular tone and which control NO production in the pulmonary vasculature point to potential, new alternatives for treatment of PPHN (515,517). Inhibition of phosphodiesterase 5 increases cGMP and dilates pulmonary arteries. Despite hopes that sildenafil, a phosphodiesterase 5 inhibitor, would be a specific pulmonary vasodilator, a small randomized study in infants following cardiac surgery found that sildenafil reduced systemic and pulmonary vascular resistance and worsened oxygenation and the aAO$_2$ gradient (538). Studies of prostacyclin administered via the airway have shown promise in a small number of neonates with PPHN, but controlled studies are needed to evaluate the efficacy of this prostanoid (539,540). For now, inhaled NO remains the only selective pulmonary vasodilator in neonates. Alternate drug treatment may still be successful at improving pulmonary perfusion in patients with PPHN, but their effectiveness must be confirmed in appropriate controlled trials.

Respiratory Stimulants

Doxapram has been administered to newborns both i.v. and orally, to treat apnea that was unresponsive to methylxanthines (see Methylxanthines) (541). Doxapram is a general stimulant of the CNS respiratory center, along with the entire cerebrospinal axis. Originally, doxapram was administered by continuous i.v. infusion for treatment of apnea of prematurity (542,543). When administered enterally, only 10% to 12% of the doxapram dose is absorbed (544). Despite poor absorption when administered enterally, doxapram decreases apnea of the newborn (545). Side effects observed during enteral administration included occult blood in stools, necrotizing enterocolitis,

and premature teeth buds. Seizures have been associated with high circulating concentrations, although Alpan and colleagues suggest that the ratio of effective to convulsive concentration is 1:70 (542). Seizures have been observed in two neonates treated with doxapram, but these were thought most likely to reflect intraventricular hemorrhages (543).

Steroids

The use of dexamethasone for the prevention and treatment of BPD in ventilator-dependent neonates increased for several years until concerns about neurologic damage began to emerge (546–550). Treatment was based on efforts to reduce pulmonary inflammation associated with the pathogenesis of chronic lung disease (547,551–555). Randomized, placebo-controlled studies have documented that dexamethasone reduces ventilator settings, oxygen requirement, and facilitates extubation of ventilator-dependent neonates at 14 to 35 days of age (556–563). Although the beneficial respiratory effects of dexamethasone have usually been attributed to its antiinflammatory activity, other factors may contribute to respiratory improvement such as increases in vitamin A and retinol binding protein.(564) The most common dexamethasone dosage regimen used was 0.5 mg/kg/day divided into two daily doses and tapered over a period of 7 to 42 days (556–560). These dosages, however, were not based on pharmacokinetic studies in premature newborns.

Dexamethasone is a pure glucocorticoid, without mineralocorticoid activity, but with approximately 25 times more antiinflammatory potency than cortisol (565). Such comparisons, however, do not consider pharmacokinetic differences in the elimination rates between endogenous corticosteroids, such as cortisol, and the halogenated steroid, dexamethasone, that has a very low clearance in ELBW neonates (566,567). This reduced clearance is likely to produce much greater areas under the concentration-time curve and progressive accumulation with repetitive dosing at intervals less than one half-life.

The onset and duration of treatment of preterm neonates has varied widely with initiation of treatment within hours of birth (547,563,568) within the first week (561,569) or after 3 weeks (562). The duration of treatment has ranged from less than 48 hours to 42 days. As more randomized studies were completed, meta-analyses have shown that early treatment for less than 48 hours did not reduce death or BPD (570) although treatment for longer periods reduces duration of intubation, BPD, death or BPD at 36 weeks, PDA and severe ROP (563). Similar findings but without an effect on ROP were noted with later treatment at 7 to 14 postnatal days (561).

Early reports of adverse effects of dexamethasone treatment of neonates showed poor growth and weight gain during treatment (558,560,571–575), hypertension (572, 573,576–580), hypothalamic-pituitary-adrenal (HPA) axis suppression (581–586), hypertrophic cardiomyopathy (587–589), gastrointestinal hemorrhage and perforation

(579,590–592), and hyperglycemia (572,576,579). Many adverse effects are reversible on drug discontinuation, however some may be severe or even life-threatening. Some degree of HPA-axis suppression is often evident following dexamethasone regimens of 14 to 42 days (581–586). Adrenal suppression may persist for months, so this population may require a prolonged steroid taper (581). During this period, Byyny found that stresses such as surgery or infection may require temporary administration of exogenous glucocorticoids at two to three times the maintenance dose (593). The effect of a short course of dexamethasone on the HPA-axis is more controversial. Some investigators reported that 7 days of dexamethasone had no effect on adrenal responsiveness to ACTH (594, 595). Others reported hyporesponsiveness to both ACTH and corticotropin releasing hormone following as little as a 7-day course of dexamethasone (596–598), although this effect appears short-lived and not clinically significant (596). A sufficient number of controlled trials of postnatal dexamethasone treatment are now published to allow meta-analysis of adverse effects that show significant increases in: gastrointestinal bleeding and perforation, hyperglycemia, hypertension, growth delay and hypertrophic cardiomyopathy (561–563).

The beneficial respiratory effects of postnatal treatment of preterm neonates with dexamethasone are offset by concerns about neurologic impairment. Stark and associates reported reduced head sizes at 36 weeks postmenstrual age in a controlled trial of dexamethasone treatment beginning within 12 hours of birth with a relatively low dose (0.15 mg/kg/day) for 3 days followed by a 7 day taper (599). The controlled trial of early dexamethasone treatment by Yeh et al showed developmental delay at school age (550). Concern was also raised by Shinwell in a multicenter, controlled study of dexamethasone treatment beginning within 12 hours after birth that showed a significant increase in neurologic injury associated with dexamethasone treatment, even in preterm newborns with normal cranial ultrasound studies (549). Animal studies have shown that prolonged dexamethasone treatment may adversely affect brain growth (600–602). Other controlled trials, however, beginning within 3 to 10 days after birth have not shown an increase in neurologic damage (569,603). Cummings and associates reported an improved neurological outcome with a 42-day dexamethasone regimen as compared with an 18-day treatment regimen or placebo (557). One-year and three-year follow-up studies have not demonstrated any long-term neurological benefits or adverse effects associated with steroid treatment during infancy (229,604). The largest meta-analyses of controlled studies of postnatal steroid treatment of neonates with long term follow-up have not found a significant correlation between treatment and adverse neurologic outcomes (561–563).

The National Institute of Child Health and Human Development Neonatal Network retrospectively correlated postnatal steroid treatment with reduced Bayley II scales of motor and mental development at 18 to 22 months adjusted age (605). Such correlations point to the need for, and the importance of, controlled studies because postnatal steroid treatment may simply be a marker for the extremely ill neonates with severe hypotension, severe lung disease, or other conditions or treatments that lead to neurologic damage. Opinions about the adverse effects of dexamethasone treatment of neonates have lead to significant debate (606–608) and even a policy statement of warning by the AAP (609).

Accurately attributing long-term neurologic impairment to treatment with a single drug, dexamethasone, is difficult in this critically ill, immature population that is treated with a plethora of medications during their months of NICU care. The study must be large enough to achieve equipoise in acuity between the control and treated groups, include similar rates of elective steroid treatment contamination outside the study assignments, and similar distributions of other factors that can cause brain injury, such as sepsis and hypotension.

Continued dexamethasone treatment requires better pharmacokinetic study to determine the optimal dosing interval, because current empiric schedules are likely to cause significant drug accumulation. Regardless of the difficulties with study of this issue, enough concern has been expressed that treatment with dexamethasone should be reserved for significantly ill infants in whom treatment benefits are carefully weighed against potential neurologic harm and the adverse effects indicated above.

Recognition of the contribution of low cortisol secretion to chronic lung disease in extremely preterm neonates (610–612) and to adrenal insufficiency with hypotension and oliguria (613–616), have led to studies of steroid treatment of neonates with hydrocortisone (cortisol). In a randomized, placebo-controlled study of 40 extremely premature neonates, prophylactic hydrocortisone treatment (1.0 mg/kg/day) increased survival without supplemental oxygen at 36 weeks adjusted age, decreased days on the ventilator and need for oxygen at discharge (617). The effects seemed to be greater in infants with chorioamnionitis. None of the adverse effects associated with systemic steroid treatment were increased by hydrocortisone treatment. Specifically, there was no increase in sepsis, IVH, ROP, GI perforation, NEC, hyperglycemia, hypertension, or PDA.

Hydrocortisone and prednisolone treatment of premature neonates have been compared to dexamethasone. The hydrocortisone study was a retrospective controlled study conducted in 2 neonatal centers to determine short and long-term outcomes of hydrocortisone treatment, started at 5 mg/kg, at one center and dexamethasone treatment, started at 0.5 mg/kg, at the other center (618). Doses were then tapered over 21 to 22 days Both steroid treatments reduced the need for oxygen. Dexamethasone, but not hydrocortisone, increased blood urea concentrations and blood pressure and reduced weight gain. Long-term outcome evaluated at 5 to 7 years showed that dexamethasone, but not hydrocortisone, was associated with a greater frequency of needing special education. If the potency of dexamethasone is at least 25-fold that of hydrocortisone and if it persists longer in the circulation, the steroid equivalent dosage of dexamethasone is much larger than that of hydrocortisone which may explain its greater toxicity (565). In the prednisolone study, 45 consecutively delivered premature newborns at gestational age less than 30 weeks who were at risk of developing CLD were treated with methylprednisolone and the outcomes compared to historical dexamethasone-treated, matched controls (619). Doses were tapered from 0.6 to 0.2 mg/kg q6h with each dose maintained for 72 hours. No differences in CLD were noted, but the methylprednisolone-treated group had faster weight gain, less frequent glucose intolerance, and less frequent cystic periventricular leucomalacia. Again, just as in the hydrocortisone study, the dosages in cortisol equivalents are much greater in the dexamethasone treated group without considering probable differences in rates of clearance and areas under the concentration-time curve (565).

This assumes that hydrocortisone is effectively cleared in extremely premature neonates by the usual endogenous enzymes. This needs more study, because current treatment with 2 to 3 doses/day is based on that assumption. This will also help to determine the lowest hydrocortisone dose needed to achieve the desired effects.

Inhaled Steroids

Concern for the adverse effects associated with intravenous dexamethasone has prompted study of treatment of neonates with aerosolized topical corticosteroids, such as beclomethasone, budesonide and fluticasone to prevent BPD. In theory, administration of topical steroids to the lung should minimize systemic drug exposure, thus reducing the potential for systemic adverse effects, but it may also reduce efficacy. Controlled treatment trials have analyzed success of extubations, indices of lung inflammation, measures of lung function, and need for additional steroid treatment. In a placebo-controlled study of 161 ventilated neonates, beclomethasone reduced airway inflammation after 8 and 15 days of treatment assessed by measurement of interleukin-8 levels in tracheal aspirates (620). An earlier study by Groneck and associates in 7 beclomethasone-treated patients did not find a significant decrease in IL-8A levels compared to 9 patients treated with systemic dexamethasone (621). A meta-analysis of 12 randomized, controlled trials of inhaled steroid treatment of preterm neonates to reduce chronic lung disease helps to resolve some of these differences (622). In this meta-analysis, Halliday found that inhaled steroid treatment begun within 2 weeks of birth reduced the need for later dexamethasone treatment (622). More importantly treatment begun after 2 weeks of age was associated with more successful extubations and measurable improvements in lung function. Adverse effects of inhaled steroids appeared to be minimal.

The effects of systemic steroids and inhaled steroid were compared in an earlier meta-analysis that found only 2 randomized studies with a total of 294 subjects that met their criteria for inclusion (623). The frequency of death or chronic lung disease at 36 weeks adjusted age was not different between the two modes of steroid administration. The need for supplemental oxygen was longer in the inhaled steroid group indicating lower efficacy. As might be expected, adverse effects of hyperglycemia, gastrointestinal hemorrhage and perforation were less in the inhaled steroid group. The authors caution that neither inhaled steroids, nor systemic steroids, can be recommended as standard practice for ventilated preterm infants without additional study. The lower rate of adverse effects associated with inhaled steroids treatment supports such study. If higher doses of inhaled steroids are tested, potential toxicities from chlorofluorocarbon propellants, including bronchospasm and cardiac toxicity, must be evaluated (624–626).

Vitamin E

Vitamin E refers to several chemically related compounds, differing in degrees of methylation, desaturation, and oxygen content, classified generically as tocopherols (627). The oxygen molecules and aromatic ring conjugation allow interconversion between hydroxyl and quinone forms, so that vitamin E functions as an antioxidant. Alpha-tocopherol is the primary, naturally occurring member of this group.

The clinical administration of vitamin E to premature neonates is based on its antioxidant activity, low vitamin E concentrations in many preterm neonates at birth, and animal studies suggesting that vitamin E protects against oxidant injury to the lung and eye. Initial favorable effects of vitamin E on BPD (628) were not confirmed in a subsequent randomized, double-blind study by the same investigators (629).

For prevention of retinopathy of prematurity (ROP), a prospective, double-blind, randomized trial reported that 100 mg of vitamin E per day reduced the severity, but not frequency of ROP (630). Studies of tocopherol in a kitten model of ROP, in doses of 50 to 1000 mg/kg/day, revealed a high frequency of mortality with lethargy, weight loss, and seizures (631). Livers were enlarged and extensively vacuolated with fat in the vitamin E-treated animals.

In 1984, the CDC and Bodenstein separately described infants with a new symptom complex that included pulmonary deterioration, thrombocytopenia, liver failure, ascites, and renal failure leading to death in some cases (632,633). These symptoms were attributed to a specific brand of alpha-tocopherol acetate, E-Ferol, which had begun to be administered i.v. to prevent oxidant injury to eyes and lungs. This syndrome ceased after the use of E-Ferol was discontinued. It was never completely clear whether the toxicity was a result of alpha-tocopherol, the polysorbate emulsifiers, or an unknown contaminant (634,635). Sepsis, necrotizing enterocolitis, and intraventricular hemorrhage also have been attributed to treatment of neonates with vitamin E (627). The AAP Committee on Fetus and Newborn (COFN) concluded that pharmacologic doses of vitamin E should be regarded as experimental, and not routinely indicated for infants weighing under 1,500 g

(636). The COFN recommends 5 to 10 IU of vitamin E per day for preterm infants, provided through supplemented formulas or supplemental vitamins (348).

DRUG EXCRETION IN BREAST MILK

Over 50% of newborn infants are breast-feeding at the time of discharge (637). Although almost all drugs and chemicals present in the maternal circulation may enter human milk, the extent of transfer is quite variable. Maternal intake of prescription medications, over-the-counter medications, illicit drugs, and exposure to a multitude of environmental substances may expose the breast-feeding infant to a complex mixture of potentially harmful chemicals.

The nature of human milk influences its drug content. Human milk has been described as a suspension of fat in a protein–mineral–carbohydrate solution (638). The lactose secreted in milk is synthesized from glucose by the alveolar cells of the breast, in a process that requires alpha-lactalbumin. Milk contains a variety of proteins, including alpha-lactalbumin, lactoferrin albumin, lysozyme, and immunoglobulin A, all of which may bind drugs during transport into milk (638). The lipid within milk is maintained in the aqueous phase in milkfat globules surrounded by lipoprotein membranes. Milk is iso-osmotic to plasma, with an average pH of 7.2.

Several factors affect drug transfer into milk, including molecular weight, lipid solubility, maternal plasma protein binding, and extent of ionization. These are similar factors to those that influence transfer of molecules across any lipid bilayer membrane. Because milk usually is acidic to maternal plasma, and non–protein-bound, nonionized molecules are free to cross membranes, the Henderson–Hasselbach equation may be used to estimate drug distribution between maternal plasma and milk (639). This predicts that organic bases (pKa > 7.4) will reach a higher concentration in milk than in maternal serum. Many quantitative studies of human milk drug excretion have estimated that approximately 1% to 2% of a maternal drug dose will appear in milk (640).

The AAP Committee on Drugs has written policy statements about the transfer of drugs and chemicals into humans since 1983. The latest revision in 2001 updated information about transfer of chemicals into milk and included sections that address smoking, the presence of breast implants, and the use of psychoactive drugs during breast feeding (641). The information is presented in tables that indicate the relative risk to the breast feeding infant. The full text of this statement is available at http://aapolicy.aapublications.org.

REFERENCES

1. Wilkinson GR. Pharmacokinetics. The dynamics of drug absorption, distribution, and elimination. In: Hardman JG, Limbird LE, Gilman AG, eds. *Goodman & Gilman's the pharmacological basis of therapeutics*, 10th ed. New York: McGraw-Hill, 2001:3–29.
2. Oellerich M. Influence of protein binding commentary. In: Evans WE, Schentag JJ, Jusko WJ, eds. *Applied pharmacokinetics*, 2nd ed. Spokane: Applied Therapeutics, 1986:220–228.
3. Boreus LO. *Principles of pediatric pharmacology.* New York: Churchill-Livingston; 1982.
4. Brodersen R, Honore B. Drug binding properties of neonatal albumin. *Acta Paediatr* Scand 1989;78(3):342–346.
5. Aranda JV, Sitar DS, Parsons WD, et al. Pharmacokinetic aspects of theophylline in premature newborns. *N Engl J Med* 1976; 295(8):413–416.
6. Peterson RG, Simmons MA, Rumack BH, et al. Pharmacology of furosemide in the premature newborn infant. *J Pediatr* 1980; 97(1):139–143.
7. Evans EF, Proctor JD, Fratkin MJ, et al. Blood flow in muscle groups and drug absorption. *Clin Pharmacol Ther* 1975;17(1): 44–47.
8. Leff RD, Roberts RJ. Methods of intravenous drug administration in the pediatric patient. *J Pediatr* 1981;98(4):631–635.
9. Wilkinson G. Pharmacokinetics. The dynamics of drug absorption, distribution, and elimination. In: Hardman J, Limbird L, Gilman A, ed. *Goodman & Gilman's the pharmacological basis of therapeutics*, 10th ed. New York: McGraw-Hill, 2001:3–29.
10. Friis-Hansen B. Body composition during growth. In vivo measurements and biochemical data correlated to differential anatomical growth. *Pediatrics* 1971;47(1)[Suppl 2]:264.
11. Ziegler EE, O'Donnell AM, Nelson SE, et al. Body composition of the reference fetus. *Growth* 1976;40(4):329–341.
12. Painter MJ, Pippenger C, Wasterlain C, et al. Phenobarbital and phenytoin in neonatal seizures: metabolism and tissue distribution. *Neurology* 1981;31(9):1107–1112.
13. Pelkonen O, Kaltiala EH, Larmi TK, et al. Comparison of activities of drug-metabolizing enzymes in human fetal and adult livers. *Clin Pharmacol Ther* 1973;14(5):840–846.
14. Ladona MG, Lindstrom B, Thyr C, et al. Differential foetal development of the O- and N-demethylation of codeine and dextromethorphan in man. *Br J Clin Pharmacol* 1991;32(3): 295–302.
15. Jacqz-Aigrain E, Cresteil T. Cytochrome P450-dependent metabolism of dextromethorphan: fetal and adult studies. *Dev Pharmacol Ther* 1992;18(3–4):161–168.
16. Leeder JS, Kearns GL. Pharmacogenetics in pediatrics. Implications for practice. *Pediatr Clin North Am* 1997;44(1): 55–77.
17. de Wildt SN, Kearns GL, Leeder JS, et al. Cytochrome P450 3A: ontogeny and drug disposition. *Clin Pharmacokinet* 1999; 37(6):485–505.
18. Aranda JV, MacLeod SM, Renton KW, et al. Hepatic microsomal drug oxidation and electron transport in newborn infants. *J Pediatr* 1974;85(4):534–542.
19. Aldridge A, Aranda JV, Neims AH. Caffeine metabolism in the newborn. *Clin Pharmacol Ther* 1979;25(4):447–453.
20. Loughnan PM, Greenwald A, Purton WW, et al. Pharmacokinetic observations of phenytoin disposition in the newborn and young infant. *Arch Dis Child* 1977;52(4):302–309.
21. Pitlick W, Painter M, Pippenger C. Phenobarbital pharmacokinetics in neonates. *Clin Pharmacol Ther* 1978;23(3):346–350.
22. Kalow W, Tang BK. The use of caffeine for enzyme assays: a critical appraisal. *Clin Pharmacol Ther* 1993;53(5):503–514.
23. Cazeneuve C, Pons G, Rey E, et al. Biotransformation of caffeine in human liver microsomes from foetuses, neonates, infants, and adults. *Br J Clin Pharmacol* 1994;37(5):405–412.
24. Zhang ZY, Kaminsky LS. Characterization of human cytochromes P450 involved in theophylline 8-hydroxylation. *Biochem Pharmacol* 1995;50(2):205–211.
25. Ha HR, Chen J, Freiburghaus AU, et al. Metabolism of theophylline by cDNA-expressed human cytochromes P-450. *Br J Clin Pharmacol* 1995;39(3):321–326.
26. Sonnier M, Cresteil T. Delayed ontogenesis of CYP1A2 in the human liver. *Eur J Biochem* 1998;251(3):893–898.
27. Aranda JV, Cook CE, Gorman W, et al. Pharmacokinetic profile of caffeine in the premature newborn infant with apnea. *J Pediatr* 1979;94(4):663–668.
28. Pons G, Carrier O, Richard MO, et al. Developmental changes of caffeine elimination in infancy. *Dev Pharmacol Ther* 1988;11(5): 258–264.

29. Carrier O, Pons G, Rey E, et al. Maturation of caffeine metabolic pathways in infancy. *Clin Pharmacol Ther* 1988;44(2): 145–151.

30. Kraus DM, Fischer JH, Reitz SJ, et al. Alterations in theophylline metabolism during the first year of life. *Clin Pharmacol Ther* 1993;54(4):351–359.

31. Shimada T, Yamazaki H, Mimura M, et al. Characterization of microsomal cytochrome P450 enzymes involved in the oxidation of xenobiotic chemicals in human fetal liver and adult lungs. *Drug Metab Dispos* 1996;24(5):515–522.

32. Treluyer JM, Jacqz-Aigrain E, Alvarez F, et al. Expression of CYP2D6 in developing human liver. *Eur J Biochem* 1991;202(2): 583–588.

33. Bourgeois BF, Dodson WE. Phenytoin elimination in newborns. *Neurology* 1983;33(2):173–178.

34. Yang HY, Lee QP, Rettie AE, et al. Functional cytochrome P4503A isoforms in human embryonic tissues: expression during organogenesis. *Mol Pharmacol* 1994;46(5):922–928.

35. Vauzelle-Kervroedan F, Rey E, Pariente-Khayat A, et al. Non invasive in vivo study of the maturation of CYP IIIA in neonates and infants. *Eur J Clin Pharmacol* 1996;51(1):69–72.

36. Coughtrie MW, Burchell B, Leakey JE, et al. The inadequacy of perinatal glucuronidation: immunoblot analysis of the developmental expression of individual UDP-glucuronosyltransferase isoenzymes in rat and human liver microsomes. *Mol Pharmacol* 1988;34(6):729–735.

37. Richard K, Hume R, Kaptein E, et al. Sulfation of thyroid hormone and dopamine during human development: ontogeny of phenol sulfotransferases and arylsulfatase in liver, lung, and brain. *J Clin Endocrinol Metab* 2001;86(6):2734–2742.

38. de Wildt SN, Kearns GL, Leeder JS, et al. Glucuronidation in humans. Pharmacogenetic and developmental aspects. *Clin Pharmacokinet* 1999;36(6):439–452.

39. Weiss C, Glazko A, Weston J. Chloramphenicol in the newborn infant: a physiologic explanation of its toxicity when given in excessive doses. *N Engl J Med* 1960;262:787–794.

40. Sutherland JM. Fatal cardiovascular collapse of infants receiving large amounts of chloramphenicol. *Am J Dis Child* 1959;97: 761–767.

41. Burns LE, Hodgeman JE, Cass AB. Fatal and circulatory collapse in premature infants receiving chloramphenicol. *N Engl J Med* 1959;261:1318–1321.

42. Mulhall A, Berry DJ, de Louvois J. Chloramphenicol in paediatrics: current prescribing practice and the need to monitor. *Eur J Pediatr* 1988;147(6):574–578.

43. Choonara IA, McKay P, Hain R, et al. Morphine metabolism in children. *Br J Clin Pharmacol* 1989;28(5):599–604.

44. Sawe J, Kager L, Svensson Eng JO, et al. Oral morphine in cancer patients: in vivo kinetics and in vitro hepatic glucuronidation. *Br J Clin Pharmacol* 1985;19(4):495–501.

45. McRorie TI, Lynn AM, Nespeca MK, et al. The maturation of morphine clearance and metabolism. *Am J Dis Child* 1992; 146(8):972–976.

46. Pokela ML, Olkkola KT, Seppala T, et al. Age-related morphine kinetics in infants. *Dev Pharmacol Ther* 1993;20(1–2):26–34.

47. Hartley R, Green M, Quinn MW, et al. Development of morphine glucuronidation in premature neonates. *Biol Neonate* 1994;66(1):1–9.

48. Mikkelsen S, Feilberg VL, Christensen CB, et al. Morphine pharmacokinetics in premature and mature newborn infants. *Acta Paediatr* 1994;83(10):1025–1028.

49. Bhat R, Chari G, Gulati A, et al. Pharmacokinetics of a single dose of morphine in preterm infants during the first week of life. *J Pediatr* 1990;117(3):477–481.

50. Lynn AM, Slattery JT. Morphine pharmacokinetics in early infancy. *Anesthesiology* 1987;66(2):136–139.

51. Olkkola KT, Maunuksela EL, Korpela R, et al. Kinetics and dynamics of postoperative intravenous morphine in children. *Clin Pharmacol Ther* 1988;44(2):128–136.

52. Levy G, Khanna NN, Soda DM, et al. Pharmacokinetics of acetaminophen in the human neonate: formation of acetaminophen glucuronide and sulfate in relation to plasma bilirubin concentration and D-glucaric acid excretion. *Pediatrics* 1975;55(6): 818–825.

53. Miller RP, Roberts RJ, Fischer LJ. Acetaminophen elimination kinetics in neonates, children, and adults. *Clin Pharmacol Ther* 1976;19(3):284–294.

54. Autret E, Dutertre JP, Breteau M, et al. Pharmacokinetics of paracetamol in the neonate and infant after administration of propacetamol chlorhydrate. *Dev Pharmacol Ther* 1993;20(3–4): 129–134.

55. Alam SN, Roberts RJ, Fischer LJ. Age-related differences in salicylamide and acetaminophen conjugation in man. *J Pediatr* 1977;90(1):130–135.

56. Aperia A, Broberger O, Elinder G, et al. Postnatal development of renal function in pre-term and full-term infants. *Acta Paediatr Scand* 1981;70(2):183–187.

57. Engle WD. Evaluation of renal function and acute renal failure in the neonate. *Pediatr Clin North Am* 1986;33(1):129–151.

58. Greenblatt DJ, Kock-Weser J. Drug therapy. Clinical Pharmacokinetics (first of two parts). *N Engl J Med* 1975;293(14): 702–705.

59. Greenblatt DJ, Koch-Weser J. Clinical pharmacokinetics (second of two parts). *N Engl J Med* 1975;293(19):964–970.

60. Roberts RJ. Pharmacokinetics: basic principles and clinical applications. In: *Drug therapy in infants. Pharmacologic principles and clinical experience.* Philadelphia: WB Saunders, 1984:13–24.

61. Galinsky RE, Svvensson CK. Basic pharmacokinetics. In: Gennaro AR, Chase GD, Mardersonian AD, et al, eds. *Remington: the science and practice of pharmacy,* 19th ed. Easton: Mack, 1995: 724–760.

62. Gibaldi M, Perrier D. *Pharmacokinetics,* 2nd ed. New York: Marcel Dekker, 1982.

63. Jusko WJ. Guidelines for collection and analysis of pharmacokinetic data. In: Evans WE, Schentag JJ, Jusko WJ, eds. Applied Therapeutics. *Principles of therapeutic drug monitoring,* 2nd ed. Spokane: Applied Therapeutics, 1986:9–54.

64. Notari RE. Principles of pharmacokinetics. In: *Biopharmaceutics and clinical pharmacokinetics,* 3rd ed. New York: Marcel Dekker, 1980:45–106.

65. Zaske DE. Aminoglycosides. In: Evans WE, Schentag JJ, Jusko WJ, eds. *Applied pharmacokinetics: principles of therapeutic drug monitoring,* 3rd ed. Vancouver: Applied Therapeutics, 1992:1–14.

66. Matzke G. Vancomycin. In: Evans W, Schentag J, Jusko W, eds. *Applied Pharmacokinetics: principles of therapeutic drug monitoring,* 3rd ed. Vancouver: Applied Therapeutics, 1992:15.

67. McCracken GH Jr. Aminoglycoside toxicity in infants and children. *Am J Med* 1986;80(6B):172–178.

68. Spector R, Park GD, Johnson GF, et al. Therapeutic drug monitoring. *Clin Pharmacol Ther* 1988;43(4):345–353.

69. Roberts RJ. Special considerations in drug therapy in infants. In: *Drug therapy in infants. pharmacologic principles and clinical experience.* Philadelphia: WB Saunders, 1984:25–34.

70. Roberts RJ. Cardiovascular drugs. In: *Drug therapy in infants. pharmacologic principles and clinical experience.* Philadelphia: WB Saunders, 1984:138–225.

71. Wagman GH, Bailey JV, Weinstein MJ. Binding of aminoglycoside antibiotics to filtration materials. *Antimicrob Agents Chemother* 1975;7(3):316–319.

72. Lackner TE. Drug replacement following exchange transfusion. *J Pediatr* 1982;100(5):811–814.

73. Aranda JV, Collinge JM, Clarkson S. Epidemiologic aspects of drug utilization in a newborn intensive care unit. *Semin Perinatol* 1982;6:148–154.

74. Aranda JV, Portuguez-Malavasi A, Collinge JM, et al. Epidemiology of adverse drug reactions in the newborn. *Dev Pharmacol Ther* 1982;5(3–4):173–184.

75. Mitchell AA, Goldman P, Shapiro S, et al. Drug utilization and reported adverse reactions in hospitalized children. *Am J Epidemiol* 1979;110(2):196–204.

76. Ward RM. Pharmacology of tolazoline. *Clin Perinatol* 1984; 11(3):703–713.

77. Hansen TW, Bratlid D. Bilirubin and brain toxicity. *Acta Paediatr Scand* 1986;75(4):513–522.

78. Maisels MJ. Jaundice in the newborn. *Pediatr Rev* 1982;3:305.

79. Odell GB. The distribution and toxicity of bilirubin. E. Mead Johnson address 1969. *Pediatrics* 1970;46(1):16–24.

80. Rose AL, Wisniewski H. Acute bilirubin encephalopathy induced with sulfadimethoxine in Gunn rats. *J Neuropathol Exp Neurol* 1979;38(2):152–164.

81. Silverman WA, Andersen DH, Blanc WA, et al. A difference in mortality rate and incidence of kernicterus among premature infants allotted to two prophylactic antibacterial regiments. *Pediatrics* 1956;18:614–624.

82. Brown WJ, Buist NR, Gipson HT, et al. Fatal benzyl alcohol poisoning in a neonatal intensive care unit. *Lancet* 1982;1(8283): 1250.

83. Glasgow AM, Boeckx RL, Miller MK, et al. Hyperosmolality in small infants due to propylene glycol. *Pediatrics* 1983;72(3): 353–355.

84. MacDonald MG, Getson PR, Glasgow AM, et al. Propylene glycol: increased incidence of seizures in low birth weight infants. *Pediatrics* 1987;79(4):622–625.

85. Arulanantham K, Genel M. Central nervous system toxicity associated with ingestion of propylene glycol. *J Pediatr* 1978;93(3): 515–516.

86. Martin G, Finberg L. Propylene glycol: a potentially toxic vehicle in liquid dosage form. *J Pediatr* 1970;77(5):877–878.

87. Schick JB, Milstein JM. Burn hazard of isopropyl alcohol in the neonate. *Pediatrics* 1981;68(4):587–588.

88. Weintraub Z, Iancu TC. Isopropyl alcohol burns. *Pediatrics* 1982;69(4):506.

89. Ittmann PI, Bozynski ME. Toxic epidermal necrolysis in a newborn infant after exposure to adhesive remover. *J Perinatol* 1993;13(6):476–477.

90. Wenzl JE, Mills SD, McCall JT. Methanol poisoning in an infant. Successful treatment with peritoneal dialysis. *Am J Dis Child* 1968;116(4):445–447.

91. Moss MH. Alcohol-induced hypoglycemia and coma caused by alcohol sponging. *Pediatrics* 1970;46(3):445–447.

92. Vicas IM, Beck R. Fatal inhalational isopropyl alcohol poisoning in a neonate. *J Toxicol Clin Toxicol* 1993;31(3):473–481.

93. Shuman RM, Leech RW, Alvord EC Jr. Neurotoxicity of hexachlorophene in humans. II. A clinical pathological study of 46 premature infants. *Arch Neurol* 1975;32:320–325.

94. l'Allemand D, Gruters A, Heidemann P, et al. Iodine-induced alterations of thyroid function in newborn infants after prenatal and perinatal exposure to povidone iodine. *J Pediatr* 1983; 102(6):935–938.

95. Linder N, Davidovitch N, Reichman B, et al. Topical iodine-containing antiseptics and subclinical hypothyroidism in preterm infants. *J Pediatr* 1997;131(3):434–439.

96. Fisch RO, Beglund EB, Bridge AG, et al. Methemoglobinemia in a hospital nursery. *J Am Med Assoc* 1963;185:760–763.

97. Morrell P, Hey E, Mackee IW, et al. Deafness in preterm baby associated with topical antibiotic spray containing neomycin. *Lancet* 1985;1(8438):1167–1168.

98. Rutter N. Percutaneous drug absorption in the newborn: hazards and uses. *Clin Perinatol* 1987;14(4):911–930.

99. Hillman LS, Goodwin SL, Sherman WR. Identification and measurement of plasticizer in neonatal tissues after umbilical catheters and blood products. *N Engl J Med* 1975;292(8):381–386.

100. Grant AO. Mechanisms of action of antiarrhythmic drugs: from ion channel blockage to arrhythmia termination. *Pacing Clin Electrophysiol* 1997;20(2 Pt 2):432–444.

101. Roden DM, George AL Jr. The cardiac ion channels: relevance to management of arrhythmias. *Annu Rev Med* 1996;47:135–148.

102. Whalley DW, Wendt DJ, Grant AO. Basic concepts in cellular cardiac electrophysiology: part I: ion channels, membrane currents, and the action potential. *Pacing Clin Electrophysiol* 1995;18 (8):1556–1574.

103. Wetzel GT, Klitzner TS. Developmental cardiac electrophysiology recent advances in cellular physiology. *Cardiovasc Res* 1996;31 [Spec No]:E52–E60.

104. Robinson RB. Autonomic receptor-effector coupling during postnatal development. *Cardiovasc Res* 1996;31[Spec No]:E68–E76.

105. Task Force of the Working Group on Arrhythmias of the European Society of Cardiology. The Sicilian Gambit. A new approach to the classification of antiarrhythmic drugs based on their actions on arrhythmogenic mechanisms. *Circulation* 1991; 84:1831–1851.

106. Perry JC. Pharmacologic therapy of arrhythmias. In: Deal BJ, Wolff G, Gelband H, eds. *Current concepts in diagnosis and management of arrhythmias in infants and children.* Armonk, NY: Futura, 1998:267–305.

107. Vaughan Williams EM. *Classification of antiarrhythmic drugs.* In: Sandoe E, Flensted-Jensen E, Olsen EH, eds. Symposium on Cardiac Arrhythmias. Denmark: Astra, 1970:449–501.

108. Barry DM, Nerbonne JM. Myocardial potassium channels: electrophysiological and molecular diversity. *Annu Rev Physiol* 1996;58:363–394.

109. Deal KK, England SK, Tamkun MM. Molecular physiology of cardiac potassium channels. *Physiol Rev* 1996;76(1):49–67.

110. Young M-L, Deal BJ, Wolff GS. Supraventricular tachycardia-electrophysiologic evaluation and treatment. In: Deal BJ, Wolff G, Gelband H, eds. *Current concepts in diagnosis and management of arrhythmias in infants and children.* Armonk, NY: Futura , 1998: 145–179.

111. American Academy of Pediatrics Committee on Drugs. Drugs for pediatric emergencies. *Pediatrics* 1998;101:e13.

112. Deal BJ. Supraventricular tachycardia mechanisms and natural history. In: Deal BJ, Wolff G, Gelband H, eds. *Current concepts in diagnosis and management of arrhythmias in infants and children.* Armonk, NY: Futura , 1998:117–143.

113. Cilliers AM, du Plessis JP, Clur SA, et al. Junctional ectopic tachycardia in six paediatric patients. *Heart* 1997;78(4):413–415.

114. Garson A Jr, Gillette PC. Junctional ectopic tachycardia in children: electrocardiography, electrophysiology and pharmacologic response. *Am J Cardiol* 1979;44(2):298–302.

115. Ludomirsky A, Garson A Jr. Supraventricular tachycardia. In: Gillette PC, Garson A Jr, eds. *Pediatric arrhythmias: electrophysiology and pacing.* Philadelphia: WB Saunders, 1990:380–426.

116. Pfammatter JP, Stocker FP. Re-entrant supraventricular tachycardia in infancy: current role of prophylactic digoxin treatment. *Eur J Pediatr* 1998;157(2):101–106.

117. Friedman FD. Intraosseous adenosine for the termination of supraventricular tachycardia in an infant. *Ann Emerg Med* 1996; 28(3):356–358.

118. Luedtke SA, Kuhn RJ, McCaffrey FM. Pharmacologic management of supraventricular tachycardias in children. Part 2: atrial flutter, atrial fibrillation, and junctional and atrial ectopic tachycardia. *Ann Pharmacother* 1997;31(11):1347–1359.

119. Paret G, Steinmetz D, Kuint J, et al. Adenosine for the treatment of paroxysmal supraventricular tachycardia in full-term and preterm newborn infants. *Am J Perinatol* 1996;13(6):343–346.

120. Smits P, Lenders JW, Thien T. Caffeine and theophylline attenuate adenosine-induced vasodilation in humans. *Clin Pharmacol Ther* 1990;48(4):410–418.

121. Berul CI. Higher adenosine dosage required for supraventricular tachycardia in infants treated with theophylline. *Clin Pediatr (Phila)* 1993;32(3):167–168.

122. Moak JP. Pharmacology and electrophysiology of antiarrhythmic drugs. In: Gillette PC, Garson A Jr, eds. *Pediatric arrhythmias: electrophysiology and pacing.* Philadelphia: WB Saunders, 1990: 37–115.

123. Reidenberg MM, Drayer DE, Levy M, et al. Polymorphic acetylation procainamide in man. *Clin Pharmacol Ther* 1975;17(6): 722–730.

124. Lemler MS, Schaffer MS. Neonatal supraventricular tachycardia: predictors of successful treatment withdrawal. *Am Heart J* 1997;133(1):130–131.

125. Byrum CJ, Wahl RA, Behrendt DM, et al. Ventricular fibrillation associated with use of digitalis in a newborn infant with Wolff-Parkinson-White syndrome. *J Pediatr* 1982;101(3):400–403.

126. Nies AS, Shand DG. Clinical pharmacology of propranolol. *Circulation* 1975;52(1):6–15.

127. Epstein ML, Kiel EA, Victorica BE. Cardiac decompensation following verapamil therapy in infants with supraventricular tachycardia. *Pediatrics* 1985;75(4):737–740.

128. Mason JW. Amiodarone. *N Engl J Med* 1987;316(8):455–466.

129. Kodama I, Kamiya K, Toyama J. Cellular electropharmacology of amiodarone. *Cardiovasc Res* 1997;35(1):13–29.

130. Burri S, Hug MI, Bauersfeld U. Efficacy and safety of intravenous amiodarone for incessant tachycardias in infants. *Eur J Pediatr* 2003;162(12):880–884.

131. Ardura J, Hermoso F, Bermejo J. Effect on growth of children with cardiac dysrhythmias treated with amiodarone. *Pediatr Cardiol* 1988;9(1):33–36.

132. Keeton BR, Bucknall CA, Curry PV, et al. Use of amiodarone in childhood. *Br J Clin Pract Suppl* 1986;44:115–120.

133. Daniels CJ, Schutte DA, Hammond S, et al. Acute pulmonary toxicity in an infant from intravenous amiodarone. *Am J Cardiol* 1997;80(8):1113–1116.

134. Perry JC, Fenrich AL, Hulse JE, et al. Pediatric use of intravenous amiodarone: efficacy and safety in critically ill patients from a multicenter protocol. *J Am Coll Cardiol* 1996;27(5):1246–1250.

135. Dodo H, Gow RM, Hamilton RM, et al. Chaotic atrial rhythm in children. *Am Heart J* 1995;129(5):990–995.

136. Fish FA, Mehta AV, Johns JA. Characteristics and management of chaotic atrial tachycardia of infancy. *Am J Cardiol* 1996;78(9): 1052–1055.

137. Bouillon T, Schiffmann H, Bartmus D, et al. Amiodarone in a newborn with ventricular tachycardia and an intracardiac tumor: adjusting the dose according to an individualized dosing regimen. *Pediatr Cardiol* 1996;17(2):112–114.

138. Chen RP, Ignaszewski AP, Robertson MA. Successful treatment of supraventricular tachycardia-induced cardiomyopathy with amiodarone: case report and review of literature. *Can J Cardiol* 1995;11(10):918–922.

139. Rosenberg EM, Elbl F, Solinger RE, et al. Neonatal refractory supraventricular tachycardia: successful treatment with amiodarone. *South Med J* 1988;81(4):539–540.

140. Fenrich AL Jr, Perry JC, Friedman RA. Flecainide and amiodarone: combined therapy for refractory tachyarrhythmias in infancy. *J Am Coll Cardiol* 1995;25(5):1195–1198.

141. Etheridge SP, Craig JE, Compton SJ. Amiodarone is safe and highly effective therapy for supraventricular tachycardia in infants. *Am Heart J* 2001;141(1):105–110.

142. Kannan R, Yabek SM, Garson A Jr, et al. Amiodarone efficacy in a young population: relationship to serum amiodarone and desethylamiodarone levels. *Am Heart J* 1987;114(2):283–287.

143. Vrobel TR, Miller PE, Mostow ND, et al. A general overview of amiodarone toxicity: its prevention, detection, and management. *Prog Cardiovasc Dis* 1989;31(6):393–426.

144. Strunge P, Frandsen J, Andreasen F. Amiodarone during pregnancy. *Eur Heart J* 1988;9(1):106–109.

145. De Wolf D, De Schepper J, Verhaaren H, et al. Congenital hypothyroid goiter and amiodarone. *Acta Paediatr Scand* 1988;77(4):616–618.

146. Laurent M, Betremieux P, Biron Y, et al. Neonatal hypothyroidism after treatment by amiodarone during pregnancy. *Am J Cardiol* 1987;60(10):942.

147. Magee LA, Downar E, Sermer M, et al. Pregnancy outcome after gestational exposure to amiodarone in Canada. *Am J Obstet Gynecol* 1995;172(4 Pt 1):1307–1311.

148. Tubman R, Jenkins J, Lim J. Neonatal hyperthyroxinaemia associated with maternal amiodarone therapy: case report. *Ir J Med Sci* 1988;157(7):243.

149. Volpe JJ. Neonatal seizures. In: *Neurology of the newborn*, 2nd ed. Philadelphia: WB Saunders, 1987:129–157.

150. Rennie JM, Boylan GB. Neonatal seizures and their treatment. *Curr Opin Neurol* 2003;16(2):177–181.

151. Painter MJ, Scher MS, Stein AD, et al. Phenobarbital compared with phenytoin for the treatment of neonatal seizures. *N Engl J Med* 1999;341(7):485–489.

152. Boylan GB, Rennie JM, Pressler RM, et al. Phenobarbitone, neonatal seizures, and video-EEG. *Arch Dis Child Fetal Neonatal Ed* 2002;86(3):F165–F170.

153. Gilman JT, Gal P, Duchowny MS, et al. Rapid sequential phenobarbital treatment of neonatal seizures. *Pediatrics* 1989;83(5): 674–678.

154. Painter MJ, Pippenger C, MacDonald H, et al. Phenobarbital and diphenylhydantoin levels in neonates with seizures. *J Pediatr* 1978;92(2):315–319.

155. Fischer JH, Lockman LA, Zaske D, et al. Phenobarbital maintenance dose requirements in treating neonatal seizures. *Neurology* 1981;31(8):1042–1044.

156. Farwell JR, Lee YJ, Hirtz DG, et al. Phenobarbital for febrile seizures—effects on intelligence and on seizure recurrence. *N Engl J Med* 1990;322(6):364–369.

157. Meador KJ, Loring DW, Huh K, et al. Comparative cognitive effects of anticonvulsants. *Neurology* 1990;40(3 Pt 1):391–394.

158. American Academy of Pediatrics Committee on Drugs. Behavioral and cognitive effects of anticonvulsant therapy. *Pediatrics* 1985;76:644–647.

159. Wheless JW. Pediatric use of intravenous and intramuscular phenytoin: lessons learned. *J Child Neurol* 1998;13[Suppl 1]:S11–S14, discussion S30–S32.

160. Kriel RL, Cifuentes RF. Fosphenytoin in infants of extremely low birth weight. *Pediatr Neurol* 2001;24(3):219–221.

161. Albani M, Wernicke I. Oral phenytoin in infancy: dose requirement, absorption, and elimination. *Pediatr Pharmacol (New York)* 1983;3(3–4):229–236.

162. Tozer TN, Winter ME. Phenytoin. In: Evans W, Schentag J, Jusko W, ed. *Applied pharmacokinetics: principles of therapeutic drug monitoring*, 3rd ed. Vancouver: Applied Therapeutics, 1992: 1–44.

163. Fredholm BB, Rane A, Persson B. Diphenylhydantoin binding to proteins in plasma and its dependence on free fatty acid and bilirubin concentration in dogs and newborn infants. *Pediatr Res* 1975;9:26–30.

164. Ehrnebo M, Agurell S, Jalling B, et al. Age differences in drug binding by plasma proteins: studies on human foetuses, neonates and adults. *Eur J Clin Pharmacol* 1971;3(4):189–193.

165. Whelan HT, Hendeles L, Haberkern CM, et al. High intravenous phenytoin dosage requirement in a newborn infant. *Neurology* 1983;33(1):106–108.

166. Leff RD, Fischer LJ, Roberts RJ. Phenytoin metabolism in infants following intravenous and oral administration. *Dev Pharmacol Ther* 1986;9(4):217–223.

167. Cate JC 4th, Hedrick R. Propylene glycol intoxication and lactic acidosis [Letter]. *N Engl J Med* 1980;303:1237.

168. Louis S, Kutt H, McDowell F. The cardiocirculatory changes caused by intravenous Dilantin and its solvent. *Am Heart J* 1967;74(4):523–529.

169. Fierro LS, Savulich DH, Benezra DA. Safety of fosphenytoin sodium. *Am J Health Syst Pharm* 1996;53(22):2707–2712.

170. Deshmukh A, Wittert W, Schnitzler E, et al. Lorazepam in the treatment of refractory neonatal seizures. A pilot study. *Am J Dis Child* 1986;140(10):1042–1044.

171. Maytal J, Novak GP, King KC. Lorazepam in the treatment of refractory neonatal seizures. *J Child Neurol* 1991;6(4):319–323.

172. McDermott CA, Kowalczyk AL, Schnitzler ER, et al. Pharmacokinetics of lorazepam in critically ill neonates with seizures. *J Pediatr* 1992;120(3):479–483.

173. Roberts RJ. Fetal and infant intoxication. In: *Drug therapy in infants. Pharmacologic principles and clinical experience.* Philadelphia: WB Saunders, 1984:322–383.

174. Chess PR, D'Angio CT. Clonic movements following lorazepam administration in full-term infants. *Arch Pediatr Adolesc Med* 1998;152(1):98–99.

175. Sexson WR, Thigpen J, Stajich GV. Stereotypic movements after lorazepam administration in premature neonates: a series and review of the literature. *J Perinatol* 1995;15(2):146–149, quiz 50–51.

176. Kumar A, Bleck TP. Intravenous midazolam for the treatment of refractory status epilepticus. *Crit Care Med* 1992;20(4):483–488.

177. Lahat E, Aladjem M, Eshel G, et al. Midazolam in treatment of epileptic seizures. *Pediatr Neurol* 1992;8(3):215–216.

178. Sheth RD, Buckley DJ, Gutierrez AR, et al. Midazolam in the treatment of refractory neonatal seizures. *Clin Neuropharmacol* 1996;19(2):165–170.

179. Grawe G, Ward RM. Seizure-like activity following bolus administration of midazolam to neonates. *Clin Res* 1994;42:16A.

180. Hoppen T, Elger CE, Bartmann P. Carbamazepine in phenobarbital-nonresponders: experience with ten preterm infants. *Eur J Pediatr* 2001;160(7):444–447.

181. Singh B, Singh P, al Hifzi I, et al. Treatment of neonatal seizures with carbamazepine. *J Child Neurol* 1996;11(5):378–382.

182. Mikati MA, Fayad M, Koleilat M, et al. Efficacy, tolerability, and kinetics of lamotrigine in infants. *J Pediatr* 2002;141(1):31–35.

183. Barr PA, Buettiker VE, Antony JH. Efficacy of lamotrigine in refractory neonatal seizures. *Pediatr Neurol* 1999;20(2):161–163.

184. Sabers A, Gram L. Newer anticonvulsants: comparative review of drug interactions and adverse effects. *Drugs* 2000;60(1):23–33.

185. Ohman I, Vitols S, Luef G, et al. Topiramate kinetics during delivery, lactation, and in the neonate: preliminary observations. *Epilepsia* 2002;43(10):1157–1160.

186. Scher MS, Painter MJ. Controversies concerning neonatal seizures. *Pediatr Clin North Am* 1989;36(2):281–310.

187. Zubrow AB, Hulman S, Kushner H, et al. Determinants of blood pressure in infants admitted to neonatal intensive care units: a prospective multicenter study. Philadelphia Neonatal Blood Pressure Study Group. *J Perinatol* 1995;15(6):470–479.

188. Flynn JT. Neonatal hypertension: diagnosis and management. *Pediatr Nephrol* 2000;14(4):332–341.

189. The fourth report on the diagnosis, evaluation, and treatment of high blood pressure in children and adolescents. *Pediatrics* 2004;114:555–576.

190. Wiest DB, Garner SS, Uber WE, et al. Esmolol for the management of pediatric hypertension after cardiac operations. *J Thorac Cardiovasc Surg* 1998;115(4):890–897.

191. Gouyon JB, Geneste B, Semama DS, et al. Intravenous nicardipine in hypertensive preterm infants. *Arch Dis Child Fetal Neonatal Ed* 1997;76(2):F126-F127.

192. Milou C, Debuche-Benouachkou V, Semama DS, et al. Intravenous nicardipine as a first-line antihypertensive drug in neonates. *Intensive Care Med* 2000;26(7):956-958.

193. Wells TG, Bunchman TE, Kearns GL. Treatment of neonatal hypertension with enalaprilat. *J Pediatr* 1990;117(4):664-667.

194. Bauer SB, Feldman SM, Gellis SS, et al. Neonatal hypertension. A complication of umbilical-artery catheterization. *N Engl J Med* 1975;293(20):1032-1033.

195. Nahata MC, Morosco RS, Hipple TF. Stability of captopril in three liquid dosage forms. *Am J Hosp Pharm* 1994;51(1):95-96.

196. O'Dea RF, Mirkin BL, Alward CT, et al. Treatment of neonatal hypertension with captopril. *J Pediatr* 1988;113(2):403-406.

197. Tack ED, Perlman JM. Renal failure in sick hypertensive premature infants receiving captopril therapy. *J Pediatr* 1988;112(5):805-810.

198. Romankiewicz JA, Brogden RN, Heel RC, et al. Captopril: an update review of its pharmacological properties and therapeutic efficacy in congestive heart failure. *Drugs* 1983;25(1):6-40.

199. Strauser LM, Groshong T, Tobias JD. Initial experience with isradipine for the treatment of hypertension in children. *South Med J* 2000;93(3):287-293.

200. Flynn JT, Warnick SJ. Isradipine treatment of hypertension in children: a single-center experience. *Pediatr Nephrol* 2002;17(9):748-753.

201. Starr SE. Antimicrobial therapy of bacterial sepsis in the newborn infant. *J Pediatr* 1985;106(6):1043-1048.

202. Krediet TG, Fleer A, Gerards LJ. Development of resistance to aminoglycosides among coagulase-negative staphylococci and enterobacteriaceae in a neonatal intensive care unit. *J Hosp Infect* 1993;24(1):39-46.

203. Powell KR, Pincus PH. Five years of experience with the exclusive use of amikacin in a neonatal intensive care unit. *Pediatr Infect Dis J* 1987;6(5):461-466.

204. Hyde TB, Hilger TM, Reingold A, et al. Trends in incidence and antimicrobial resistance of early-onset sepsis: population-based surveillance in San Francisco and Atlanta. *Pediatrics* 2002;110(4):690-695.

205. Stoll BJ, Hansen N, Fanaroff AA, et al. Changes in pathogens causing early-onset sepsis in very-low-birth-weight infants. *N Engl J Med* 2002;347(4):240-247.

206. Rowen JL, Lopez SM. Morganella morganii early onset sepsis. *Pediatr Infect Dis J* 1998;17(12):1176-1177.

207. Braveny I, Dickert H. In-vitro activity of cefotaxime against gentamicin and mezlocillin resistant strains. *Lancet* 1979;2(8150):1023-1024.

208. Boyle RJ, Curtis N, Kelly N, et al. Clinical implications of inducible beta-lactamase activity in Gram-negative bacteremia in children. *Pediatr Infect Dis J* 2002;21(10):935-940.

209. Bryan CS, John JF Jr, Pai MS, et al. Gentamicin vs cefotaxime for therapy of neonatal sepsis. Relationship to drug resistance. *Am J Dis Child* 1985;139(11):1086-1089.

210. McCracken GH Jr. Use of third-generation cephalosporins for treatment of neonatal infections. *Am J Dis Child* 1985;139(11):1079-1080.

211. Modi N, Damjanovic V, Cooke RW. Outbreak of cephalosporin resistant Enterobacter cloacae infection in a neonatal intensive care unit. *Arch Dis Child* 1987;62(2):148-151.

212. Bourrillon A, Brackman D, Boussougant Y, et al. Cefotaxime effects on the intestinal flora of the newborn. *Dev Pharmacol Ther* 1984;7[Suppl 1]:144-149.

213. Mathieu H, Lambert-Zechovsky N, Bourrillon A, et al. Antibiotic therapy and bacterial overgrowth in intestinal microbial ecosystem: a major risk of secondary infections in newborns. *Dev Pharmacol Ther* 1984;7[Suppl 1]:158-163.

214. Kafetzis DA, Brater DC, Kapiki AN, et al. Treatment of severe neonatal infections with cefotaxime. Efficacy and pharmacokinetics. *J Pediatr* 1982;100(3):483-489.

215. Spritzer R, vd Kamp HJ, Dzoljic G, et al. Five years of cefotaxime use in a neonatal intensive care unit. *Pediatr Infect Dis J* 1990;9(2):92-96.

216. Heusser MF, Patterson JE, Kuritza AP, et al. Emergence of resistance to multiple beta-lactams in Enterobacter cloacae during treatment for neonatal meningitis with cefotaxime. *Pediatr Infect Dis J* 1990;9(7):509-512.

217. Finnstrom O, Isaksson B, Haeggman S, et al. Control of an outbreak of a highly beta-lactam-resistant Enterobacter cloacae strain in a neonatal special care unit. *Acta Paediatr* 1998;87(10):1070-1074.

218. Van Reempts PJ, Van Overmeire B, Mahieu LM, et al. Clinical experience with ceftriaxone treatment in the neonate. *Chemotherapy* 1995;41(4):316-322.

219. Schaad UB, Tschappeler H, Lentze MJ. Transient formation of precipitations in the gallbladder associated with ceftriaxone therapy. *Pediatr Infect Dis* 1986;5(6):708-710.

220. Gulian JM, Gonard V, Dalmasso C, et al. Bilirubin displacement by ceftriaxone in neonates: evaluation by determination of 'free' bilirubin and erythrocyte-bound bilirubin. *J Antimicrob Chemother* 1987;19(6):823-829.

221. Martin E, Fanconi S, Kalin P, et al. Ceftriaxone—bilirubin-albumin interactions in the neonate: an in vivo study. *Eur J Pediatr* 1993;152(6):530-534.

222. Barriere SL. Bacterial resistance to beta-lactams, and its prevention with combination antimicrobial therapy. *Pharmacotherapy* 1992;12(5):397-402.

223. Gerceker AA, Gurler B. In-vitro activities of various antibiotics, alone and in combination with amikacin against Pseudomonas aeruginosa. *J Antimicrob Chemother* 1995;36(4):707-711.

224. de Louvois J, Dagan R, Tessin I. A comparison of ceftazidime and aminoglycoside based regimens as empirical treatment in 1316 cases of suspected sepsis in the newborn. European Society for Paediatric Infectious Diseases—Neonatal Sepsis Study Group. *Eur J Pediatr* 1992;151(12):876-884.

225. van den Anker JN, van der Heijden BJ, Hop WCJ, et al. The effect of asphyxia on the pharmacokinetics of ceftazidime in the term newborn. *Pediatr Res* 1995;38:808-811.

226. van den Anker JN, Hop WCJ, Shoemaker RC, et al. Ceftazidime pharmacokinetics in preterm infants: effect of postnatal age and postnatal exposure to indomethacin. *Br J Clin Pharmacol* 1995;40:439-443.

227. Placzek M, Whitelaw A, Want S, et al. Piperacillin in early neonatal infection. *Arch Dis Child* 1983;58(12):1006-1009.

228. Eichenwald HF. Antimicrobial therapy in infants and children: update 1976-1985. Part II. *J Pediatr* 1985;107(3):337-345.

229. Jones R, Wincott E, Elbourne D, et al. Controlled trial of dexamethasone in neonatal chronic lung disease: a 3-year follow-up. *Pediatrics* 1995;96(5 Pt 1):897-906.

230. Jones RN, Packer RR, Barry AL, et al. Piperacillin (T-1220), a new semisynthetic penicillin. II. In vitro antimicrobial activity and synergy comparison with carbenicillin and gentamicin. *J Antibiot (Tokyo)* 1979;32(1):29-35.

231. Kacet N, Roussel-Delvallez M, Gremillet C, et al. Pharmacokinetic study of piperacillin in newborns relating to gestational and postnatal age. *Pediatr Infect Dis J* 1992;11(5):365-369.

232. Sanders CC. beta-Lactamases of gram-negative bacteria: new challenges for new drugs. *Clin Infect Dis* 1992;14(5):1089-1099.

233. Clarke AM, Zemcov SJ. Clavulanic acid in combination with ticarcillin: an in-vitro comparison with other beta-lactams. *J Antimicrob Chemother* 1984;13(2):121-128.

234. Hickey SM, McCracken GH Jr. Antibacterial therapeutic agents. In: Feigin RD, Cherry JD, eds. *Textbook of pediatric infectious diseases*, 4th ed. Philadelphia: WB Saunders, 1998.

235. Sanders WE Jr, Sanders CC. Piperacillin/tazobactam: a critical review of the evolving clinical literature. *Clin Infect Dis* 1996;22(1):107-123.

236. Rubino CM, Gal P, Ransom JL. A review of the pharmacokinetic and pharmacodynamic characteristics of beta-lactam/beta-lactamase inhibitor combination antibiotics in premature infants. *Pediatr Infect Dis J* 1998;17(12):1200-1210.

237. Pillay T, Pillay DG, Adhikari M, et al. Piperacillin/tazobactam in the treatment of Klebsiella pneumoniae infections in neonates. *Am J Perinatol* 1998;15(1):47-51.

238. Bradley JS. Meropenem: a new, extremely broad spectrum beta-lactam antibiotic for serious infections in pediatrics. *Pediatr Infect Dis J* 1997;16(3):263-268.

239. Craig WA. The pharmacology of meropenem, a new carbapenem antibiotic. *Clin Infect Dis* 1997;24[Suppl 2]:S266-S275.

240. Klugman KP, Dagan R. Carbapenem treatment of meningitis. *Scand J Infect Dis Suppl* 1995;96:45-48.

241. Klugman KP, Dagan R. Randomized comparison of meropenem with cefotaxime for treatment of bacterial meningitis.

Meropenem Meningitis Study Group. *Antimicrob Agents Chemother* 1995;39(5):1140–1146.

242. Norrby SR. Neurotoxicity of carbapenem antibacterials. *Drug Saf* 1996;15(2):87–90.

243. Wong VK, Wright HT Jr, Ross LA, et al. Imipenem/cilastatin treatment of bacterial meningitis in children. *Pediatr Infect Dis J* 1991;10(2):122–125.

244. Semel JD, Allen N. Seizures in patients simultaneously receiving theophylline and imipenem or ciprofloxacin or metronidazole. *South Med J* 1991;84(4):465–468.

245. Arrieta A. Use of meropenem in the treatment of serious infections in children: review of the current literature. *Clin Infect Dis* 1998;24[Suppl 2]:S207–S212.

246. Nalin DR, Jacobsen CA. Imipenem/cilastatin therapy for serious infections in neonates and infants. *Scand J Infect Dis Suppl* 1987;52:46–55.

247. Stuart RL, Turnidge J, Grayson ML. Safety of imipenem in neonates. *Pediatr Infect Dis J* 1995;14(9):804–805.

248. Blumer JL. Pharmacokinetic determinants of carbapenem therapy in neonates and children. *Pediatr Infect Dis J* 1996;15(8):733–737.

249. Stutman HR. Clinical experience with aztreonam for treatment of infections in children. *Rev Infect Dis* 1991;13[Suppl 7]:S582–S585.

250. Cuzzolin L, Fanos V, Zambreri D, et al. Pharmacokinetics and renal tolerance of aztreonam in premature infants. *Antimicrob Agents Chemother* 1991;35(9):1726–1728.

251. Umana MA, Odio CM, Castro E, et al. Evaluation of aztreonam and ampicillin vs. amikacin and ampicillin for treatment of neonatal bacterial infections. *Pediatr Infect Dis J* 1990;9(3):175–180.

252. Banner W Jr, Gooch WM 3rd, Burckart G, et al. Pharmacokinetics of nafcillin in infants with low birth weights. *Antimicrob Agents Chemother* 1980;17(4):691–694.

253. Reish O, Ashkenazi S, Naor N, et al. An outbreak of multiresistant Klebsiella in a neonatal intensive care unit. *J Hosp Infect* 1993;25(4):287–291.

254. Snelling S, Hart CA, Cooke RW. Ceftazidime or gentamicin plus benzylpenicillin in neonates less than forty-eight hours old. *J Antimicrob Chemother* 1983;12[Suppl A]:353–356.

255. Weinstein RA. Endemic emergence of cephalosporin-resistant Enterobacter: relation to prior therapy. *Infect Control* 1986;7[Suppl 2]:120–123.

256. Isaacs D. Rationing antibiotic use in neonatal units. *Arch Dis Child Fetal Neonatal Ed* 2000;82(1):F1–F2.

257. McNeeley DF, Saint-Louis F, Noel GJ. Neonatal enterococcal bacteremia: an increasingly frequent event with potentially untreatable pathogens. *Pediatr Infect Dis J* 1996;15(9):800–805.

258. Centers for Disease Control and Prevention. Nosocomial enterococci resistant to vancomycin-United States, 1989–1993. *MMWR Morbid Mortal Wkly Rep* 1993;42:597–599.

259. McNeeley DF, Brown AE, Noel GJ, et al. An investigation of vancomycin-resistant Enterococcus faecium within the pediatric service of a large urban medical center. *Pediatr Infect Dis J* 1998;17(3):184–188.

260. Baier RJ, Bocchini JA Jr, Brown EG. Selective use of vancomycin to prevent coagulase-negative staphylococcal nosocomial bacteremia in high risk very low birth weight infants. *Pediatr Infect Dis J* 1998;17(3):179–183.

261. Moller JC, Nachtrodt G, Richter A, et al. Prophylactic vancomycin to prevent staphylococcal septicaemia in very-low-birth-weight infants. *Lancet* 1992;340(8816):424.

262. Van Houten MA, Uiterwaal CS, Heesen GJ, et al. Does the empiric use of vancomycin in pediatrics increase the risk for Gram-negative bacteremia? *Pediatr Infect Dis J* 2001;20(2):171–177.

263. Centers for Disease Control and Prevention. Recommendations for preventing the spread of vancomycin resistance. *MMWR Morb Mortal Wkly Rep* 1995;44:1–19.

264. Bailie GR, Neal D. Vancomycin ototoxicity and nephrotoxicity. A review. *Med Toxicol Adverse Drug Exp* 1988;3(5):376–386.

265. Farber BF, Moellering RC Jr. Retrospective study of the toxicity of preparations of vancomycin from 1974 to 1981. *Antimicrob Agents Chemother* 1983;23(1):138–141.

266. Rybak MJ, Albrecht LM, Boike SC, et al. Nephrotoxicity of vancomycin, alone and with an aminoglycoside. *J Antimicrob Chemother* 1990;25(4):679–687.

267. Wilhelm MP. Vancomycin. *Mayo Clin Proc* 1991;66(11):1165–1170.

268. Freeman CD, Quintiliani R, Nightingale CH. Vancomycin therapeutic drug monitoring: is it necessary? *Ann Pharmacother* 1993;27(5):594–598.

269. Cantu TG, Yamanaka-Yuen NA, Lietman PS. Serum vancomycin concentrations: reappraisal of their clinical value. *Clin Infect Dis* 1994;18(4):533–543.

270. Moellering RC Jr. Monitoring serum vancomycin levels: climbing the mountain because it is there? *Clin Infect Dis* 1994;18(4):544–546.

271. Thomas MP, Steele RW. Monitoring serum vancomycin concentrations in children: is it necessary? *Pediatr Infect Dis J* 1998;17(4):351–353.

272. Saunders NJ. Why monitor peak vancomycin concentrations? *Lancet* 1994;344(8939–8940):1748–1750.

273. Gous AG, Dance MD, Lipman J, et al. Changes in vancomycin pharmacokinetics in critically ill infants. *Anaesth Intensive Care* 1995;23(6):678–682.

274. Tan WH, Brown N, Kelsall AW, et al. Dose regimen for vancomycin not needing serum peak levels? *Arch Dis Child Fetal Neonatal Ed* 2002;87(3):F214–F216.

275. Reed MD, Kliegman RM, Weiner JS, et al. The clinical pharmacology of vancomycin in seriously ill preterm infants. *Pediatr Res* 1987;22(3):360–363.

276. Naqvi SH, Keenan WJ, Reichley RM, et al. Vancomycin pharmacokinetics in small, seriously ill infants. *Am J Dis Child* 1986;140(2):107–110.

277. Schaad UB, McCracken GH Jr, Nelson JD. Clinical pharmacology and efficacy of vancomycin in pediatric patients. *J Pediatr* 1980;96(1):119–126.

278. Wandstrat TL, Phleps SJ. Vancomycin dosing in neonatal patients: the controversy continues. *Neonatal Netw* 1994;13(3):33–39.

279. Levy M, Koren G, Dupuis L, et al. Vancomycin-induced red man syndrome. *Pediatrics* 1990;86(4):572–580.

280. Barclay ML, Begg EJ, Hickling KG. What is the evidence for once-daily aminoglycoside therapy? *Clin Pharmacokinet* 1994;27(1):32–48.

281. Gal P, Ransom JL, Weaver RL. Gentamicin in neonates: the need for loading doses. *Am J Perinatol* 1990;7(3):254–257.

282. Isemann BT, Kotagal UR, Mashni SM, et al. Optimal gentamicin therapy in preterm neonates includes loading doses and early monitoring. *Ther Drug Monit* 1996;18(5):549–555.

283. Kapusnik JE, Hackbarth CJ, Chambers HF, et al. Single, large, daily dosing versus intermittent dosing of tobramycin for treating experimental pseudomonas pneumonia. *J Infect Dis* 1988;158(1):7–12.

284. Vogelman B, Craig WA. Kinetics of antimicrobial activity. *J Pediatr* 1986;108(5 Pt 2):835–840.

285. Freeman CD, Nicolau DP, Belliveau PP, et al. Once-daily dosing of aminoglycosides: review and recommendations for clinical practice. *J Antimicrob Chemother* 1997;39(6):677–686.

286. Isaksson B, Nilsson L, Maller R, et al. Postantibiotic effect of aminoglycosides on gram-negative bacteria evaluated by a new method. *J Antimicrob Chemother* 1988;22(1):23–33.

287. Zhanel GG, Craig WA. Pharmacokinetic contributions to postantibiotic effects. Focus on aminoglycosides. *Clin Pharmacokinet* 1994;27(5):377–392.

288. Verpooten GA, Giuliano RA, Verbist L, et al. Once-daily dosing decreases renal accumulation of gentamicin and netilmicin. *Clin Pharmacol Ther* 1989;45(1):22–27.

289. Munckhof WJ, Grayson ML, Turnidge JD. A meta-analysis of studies on the safety and efficacy of aminoglycosides given either once daily or as divided doses. *J Antimicrob Chemother* 1996;37(4):645–663.

290. Kraus DM, Pai MP, Rodvold KA. Efficacy and tolerability of extended-interval aminoglycoside administration in pediatric patients. *Paediatr Drugs* 2002;4(7):469–484.

291. Fisman DN, Kaye KM. Once-daily dosing of aminoglycoside antibiotics. *Infect Dis Clin North Am* 2000;14(2):475–487.

292. Skopnik H, Heimann G. Once daily aminoglycoside dosing in full term neonates. *Pediatr Infect Dis J* 1995;14(1):71–72.

293. Hayani KC, Hatzopoulos FK, Frank AL, et al. Pharmacokinetics of once-daily dosing of gentamicin in neonates. *J Pediatr* 1997;131:76–80.

294. Lundergan FS, Glasscock GF, Kim EH, et al. Once-daily gentamicin dosing in newborn infants. *Pediatrics* 1999;103(6 Pt 1):1228–1234.

295. Agarwal G, Rastogi A, Pyati S, et al. Comparison of once-daily versus twice-daily gentamicin dosing regimens in infants > or = 2500 g. *J Perinatol* 2002;22(4):268–274.

296. Hayani KC, Hatzopoulos FK, Frank AL, et al. Pharmacokinetics of once-daily dosing of gentamicin in neonates. *J Pediatr* 1997;131(1 Pt 1):76–80.

297. Thureen PJ, Reiter PD, Gresores A, et al. Once- versus twice-daily gentamicin dosing in neonates >/=34 weeks' gestation: cost-effectiveness analyses. *Pediatrics* 1999;103(3):594–598.

298. Avent ML, Kinney JS, Istre GR, et al. Gentamicin and tobramycin in neonates: comparison of a new extended dosing interval regimen with a traditional multiple daily dosing regimen. *Am J Perinatol* 2002;19(8):413–420.

299. Ohler KH, Menke JA, Fuller L. Use of higher dose extended interval aminoglycosides in a neonatal intensive care unit. *Am J Perinatol* 2000;17(6):285–290.

300. Rastogi A, Agarwal G, Pyati S, et al. Comparison of two gentamicin dosing schedules in very low birth weight infants. *Pediatr Infect Dis J* 2002;21(3):234–240.

301. Ettlinger JJ, Bedford KA, Lovering AM, et al. Pharmacokinetics of once-a-day netilmicin (6 mg/kg) in neonates. *J Antimicrob Chemother* 1996;38(3):499–505.

302. Peter CS, Sprodowski N, Bohnhorst B, et al. Gastroesophageal reflux and apnea of prematurity: no temporal relationship. *Pediatrics* 2002;109(1):8–11.

303. Poets CF. Gastroesophageal reflux: a critical review of its role in preterm infants. *Pediatrics* 2004;113(2):e128-e132.

304. Hampton FJ, MacFadyen UM, Beardsmore CS, et al. Gastro-oesophageal reflux and respiratory function in infants with respiratory symptoms. *Arch Dis Child* 1991;66(7):848–853.

305. Leape LL, Holder TM, Franklin JD, et al. Respiratory arrest in infants secondary to gastroesophageal reflux. *Pediatrics* 1977;60(6):924–928.

306. Spitzer AR, Boyle JT, Tuchman DN, et al. Awake apnea associated with gastroesophageal reflux: a specific clinical syndrome. *J Pediatr* 1984;104(2):200–205.

307. Paton JY, Macfadyen U, Williams A, et al. Gastro-oesophageal reflux and apnoeic pauses during sleep in infancy—no direct relation. *Eur J Pediatr* 1990;149(10):680–686.

308. Sutphen JL, Dillard VL. Effects of maturation and gastric acidity on gastroesophageal reflux in infants. *Am J Dis Child* 1986;140(10):1062–1064.

309. Cucchiara S, Staiano A, Di Lorenzo C, et al. Pathophysiology of gastroesophageal reflux and distal esophageal motility in children with gastroesophageal reflux disease. *J Pediatr Gastroenterol Nutr* 1988;7(6):830–836.

310. Weihrauch TR. Gastro-oesophageal reflux—pathogenesis and clinical implications. *Eur J Pediatr* 1985;144(3):215–218.

311. Skopnik H, Silny J, Heiber O, et al. Gastroesophageal reflux in infants: evaluation of a new intraluminal impedance technique. *J Pediatr Gastroenterol Nutr* 1996;23(5):591–598.

312. Ewer AK, Durbin GM, Morgan ME, et al. Gastric emptying and gastro-oesophageal reflux in preterm infants. *Arch Dis Child Fetal Neonatal Ed* 1996;75(2):F117–F121.

313. Marcon MA. Advances in the diagnosis and treatment of gastroesophageal reflux disease. *Curr Opin Pediatr* 1997;9(5):490–493.

314. Ward RM, Lemons JA, Molteni RA. Cisapride: a survey of the frequency of use and adverse events in premature newborns. *Pediatrics* 1999;103(2):469–472.

315. Cezard JP. Managing gastro-oesophageal reflux disease in children. *Digestion* 2004;69 [Suppl 1]:3–8.

316. Kuusela AL. Long-term gastric pH monitoring for determining optimal dose of ranitidine for critically ill preterm and term neonates. *Arch Dis Child Fetal Neonatal Ed* 1998;78(2):F151–F153.

317. Orenstein SR, Shalaby TM, Devandry SN, et al. Famotidine for infant gastro-oesophageal reflux: a multi-centre, randomized, placebo-controlled, withdrawal trial. *Pharmacol Ther* 2003;17(9):1097–1107.

318. Euler AR. Use of bethanechol for the treatment of gastroesophageal reflux. *J Pediatr* 1980;96(2):321–324.

319. Strickland AD, Chang JH. Results of treatment of gastroesophageal reflux with bethanechol. *J Pediatr* 1983;103(2):311–315.

320. Sondheimer JM, Mintz HL, Michaels M. Bethanechol treatment of gastroesophageal reflux in infants: effect on continuous esophageal pH records. *J Pediatr* 1984;104(1):128–131.

321. Schulze-Delrieu K. Drug therapy. Metoclopramide. *N Engl J Med* 1981;305(1):28–33.

322. Sankaran K, Yeboah E, Bingham WT, et al. Use of metoclopramide in preterm infants. *Dev Pharmacol Ther* 1982;5(3–4):114–119.

323. Tolia V, Calhoun J, Kuhns L, et al. Randomized, prospective double-blind trial of metoclopramide and placebo for gastroesophageal reflux in infants. *J Pediatr* 1989;115(1):141–145.

324. Machida HM, Forbes DA, Gall DG, et al. Metoclopramide in gastroesophageal reflux of infancy. *J Pediatr* 1988;112(3):483–487.

325. Hyams JS, Leichtner AM, Zamett LO, et al. Effect of metoclopramide on prolonged intraesophageal pH testing in infants with gastroesophageal reflux. *J Pediatr Gastroenterol Nutr* 1986;5(5):716–720.

326. Kearns GL, van den Anker JN, Reed MD, et al. Pharmacokinetics of metoclopramide in neonates. *J Clin Pharmacol* 1998;38(2):122–128.

327. Leary PM. Adverse reactions in children. Special considerations in prevention and management. *Drug Saf* 1991;6(3):171–182.

328. Curry JI, Lander TD, Stringer MD. Review article: erythromycin as a prokinetic agent in infants and children. *Aliment Pharmacol Ther* 2001;15(5):595–603.

329. Costalos C, Gavrili V, Skouteri V, et al. The effect of low-dose erythromycin on whole gastrointestinal transit time of preterm infants. *Early Hum Dev* 2001;65(2):91–96.

330. Ng PC, So KW, Fung KS, et al. Randomised controlled study of oral erythromycin for treatment of gastrointestinal dysmotility in preterm infants. *Arch Dis Child Fetal Neonatal Ed* 2001;84(3):F177–F182.

331. Costalos C, Gounaris A, Varhalama E, et al. Erythromycin as a prokinetic agent in preterm infants. *J Pediatr Gastroenterol Nutr* 2002;34(1):23–25.

332. Patole SK, Almonte R, Kadalraja R, et al. Can prophylactic oral erythromycin reduce time to full enteral feeds in preterm neonates? *Int J Clin Pract* 2000;54(8):504–508.

333. SanFilippo A. Infantile hypertrophic pyloric stenosis related to ingestion of erythromycine estolate: a report of five cases. *J Pediatr Surg* 1976;11(2):177–180.

334. Honein MA, Paulozzi LJ, Himelright IM, et al. Infantile hypertrophic pyloric stenosis after pertussis prophylaxis with erythromcyin: a case review and cohort study. *Lancet* 1999;354(9196):2101–2105.

335. The Centers for Disease Control and Prevention. Hypertrophic pyloric stenosis in infants following pertussis prophylaxis with erythromycin—Knoxville, Tennessee, 1999. *JAMA* 2000;283(4):471–472.

336. Hoey J. Hypertrophic pyloric stenosis caused by erythromycin. *CMAJ* 2000;162(8):1198.

337. Cooper WO, Griffin MR, Arbogast P, et al. Very early exposure to erythromycin and infantile hypertrophic pyloric stenosis. *Arch Pediatr Adolesc Med* 2002;156(7):647–650.

338. Mahon BE, Rosenman MB, Kleiman MB. Maternal and infant use of erythromycin and other macrolide antibiotics as risk factors for infantile hypertrophic pyloric stenosis. *J Pediatr* 2001;139(3):380–384.

339. Stang H. Pyloric stenosis associated with erythromycin ingested through breastmilk. *Minn Med* 1986;69(11):669–670,682.

340. Sorensen HT, Skriver MV, Pedersen L, et al. Risk of infantile hypertrophic pyloric stenosis after maternal postnatal use of macrolides. *Scand J Infect Dis* 2003;35(2):104–106.

341. Schechter R, Torfs CP, Bateson TF. The epidemiology of infantile hypertrophic pyloric stenosis. *Paediatr Perinat Epidemiol* 1997;11(4):407–427.

342. Bonikos DS, Bensch KG, Northway WH Jr, et al. Bronchopulmonary dysplasia: the pulmonary pathologic sequel of necrotizing bronchiolitis and pulmonary fibrosis. *Hum Pathol* 1976;7(6):643–666.

343. Cabal LA, Larrazabal C, Ramanathan R, et al. Effects of metaproterenol on pulmonary mechanics, oxygenation, and ventilation in infants with chronic lung disease. *J Pediatr* 1987;110(1):116–119.

344. Denjean A, Guimaraes H, Migdal M, et al. Dose-related bronchodilator response to aerosolized salbutamol (albuterol) in ventilator-dependent premature infants. *J Pediatr* 1992;120(6):974–979.

345. Gappa M, Gartner M, Poets CF, et al. Effects of salbutamol delivery from a metered dose inhaler versus jet nebulizer on dynamic

lung mechanics in very preterm infants with chronic lung disease. *Pediatr Pulmonol* 1997;23(6):442–448.

346. Gomez-Del Rio M, Gerhardt T, Hehre D, et al. Effect of a beta-agonist nebulization on lung function in neonates with increased pulmonary resistance. *Pediatr Pulmonol* 1986;2(5):287–291.

347. Kao LC, Durand DJ, Nickerson BG. Effects of inhaled metaproterenol and atropine on the pulmonary mechanics of infants with bronchopulmonary dysplasia. *Pediatr Pulmonol* 1989;6(2):74–80.

348. Kao LC, Warburton D, Platzker AC, et al. Effect of isoproterenol inhalation on airway resistance in chronic bronchopulmonary dysplasia. *Pediatrics* 1984;73(4):509–514.

349. Kirpalani H, Koren G, Schmidt B, et al. Respiratory response and pharmacokinetics of intravenous salbutamol in infants with bronchopulmonary dysplasia. *Crit Care Med* 1990;18(12):1374–1377.

350. Lee H, Arnon S, Silverman M. Bronchodilator aerosol administered by metered dose inhaler and spacer in subacute neonatal respiratory distress syndrome. *Arch Dis Child Fetal Neonatal Ed* 1994;70(3):F218–F222.

351. Pfenninger J, Aebi C. Respiratory response to salbutamol (albuterol) in ventilator-dependent infants with chronic lung disease: pressurized aerosol delivery versus intravenous injection. *Intensive Care Med* 1993;19(5):251–255.

352. Rotschild A, Solimano A, Puterman M, et al. Increased compliance in response to salbutamol in premature infants with developing bronchopulmonary dysplasia. *J Pediatr* 1989;115(6):984–991.

353. Sosulski R, Abbasi S, Bhutani VK, et al. Physiologic effects of terbutaline on pulmonary function of infants with bronchopulmonary dysplasia. *Pediatr Pulmonol* 1986;2(5):269–273.

354. Stefano JL, Bhutani VK, Fox WW. A randomized placebo-controlled study to evaluate the effects of oral albuterol on pulmonary mechanics in ventilator-dependent infants at risk of developing BPD. *Pediatr Pulmonol* 1991;10(3):183–190.

355. Wilkie RA, Bryan MH. Effect of bronchodilators on airway resistance in ventilator-dependent neonates with chronic lung disease. *J Pediatr* 1987;111(2):278–282.

356. Yuksel B, Greenough A. Effect of nebulized salbutamol in preterm infants during the first year of life. *Eur Respir J* 1991;4(9):1088–1092.

357. Motoyama EK, Fort MD, Klesh KW, et al. Early onset of airway reactivity in premature infants with bronchopulmonary dysplasia. *Am Rev Respir Dis* 1987;136(1):50–57.

358. Brundage KL, Mohsini KG, Froese AB, et al. Bronchodilator response to ipratropium bromide in infants with bronchopulmonary dysplasia. *Am Rev Respir Dis* 1990;142(5):1137–1142.

359. Kraemer R, Birrer P, Schoni MH. Dose-response relationships and time course of the response to systemic beta adrenoreceptor agonists in infants with bronchopulmonary disease. *Thorax* 1988;43(10):770–776.

360. Grigg J, Arnon S, Jones T, et al. Delivery of therapeutic aerosols to intubated babies. *Arch Dis Child* 1992;67(Spec No 1):25–30.

361. MacIntyre NR, Silver RM, Miller CW, et al. Aerosol delivery in intubated, mechanically ventilated patients. *Crit Care Med* 1985;13(2):81–84.

362. Lugo RA, Kenney JK, Keenan J, et al. Albuterol delivery in a neonatal ventilated lung model: nebulization versus chlorofluorocarbon- and hydrofluoroalkane-pressurized metered dose inhalers. *Pediatr Pulmonol* 2001;31(3):247–254.

363. Ballard J, Lugo RA, Salyer JW. A survey of albuterol administration practices in intubated patients in the neonatal intensive care unit. *Respir Care* 2002;47(1):31–38.

364. Jackson EK. Diuretics. In: Hardman JG, Limbird LE, Molinoff PB, et al, eds. *Goodman and Gilman's the pharmacological basis of therapeutics*, 9th ed. New York: McGraw-Hill, 1996:685–713.

365. Chemtob S, Kaplan BS, Sherbotie JR, et al. Pharmacology of diuretics in the newborn. *Pediatr Clin North Am* 1989;36(5):1231–1250.

366. Green TP. The pharmacologic basis of diuretic therapy in the newborn. *Clin Perinatol* 1987;14(4):951–964.

367. Brater DC. Determinants of the overall response to furosemide: pharmacokinetics and pharmacodynamics. *Fed Proc* 1983;42(6):1711–1713.

368. Schrier RW, Lehman D, Zacherle B, et al. Effect of furosemide on free water excretion in edematous patients with hyponatremia. *Kidney Int* 1973;3(1):30–34.

369. Vert P, Broquaire M, Legagneur M, et al. Pharmacokinetics of furosemide in neonates. *Eur J Clin Pharmacol* 1982;22(1):39–45.

370. Engelhardt B, Elliott S, Hazinski TA. Short- and long-term effects of furosemide on lung function in infants with bronchopulmonary dysplasia. *J Pediatr* 1986;109(6):1034–1039.

371. Najak ZD, Harris EM, Lazzara A Jr, et al. Pulmonary effects of furosemide in preterm infants with lung disease. *J Pediatr* 1983;102(5):758–763.

372. Green TP, Thompson TR, Johnson DE, et al. Furosemide promotes patent ductus arteriosus in premature infants with the respiratory-distress syndrome. *N Engl J Med* 1983;308(13):743–748.

373. Yeh TF, Wilks A, Singh J, et al. Furosemide prevents the renal side effects of indomethacin therapy in premature infants with patent ductus arteriosus. *J Pediatr* 1982;101(3):433–437.

374. Brater DC. Resistance to loop diuretics. Why it happens and what to do about it. *Drugs* 1985;30(5):427–443.

375. Rybak LP. Furosemide ototoxicity: clinical and experimental aspects. *Laryngoscope* 1985;95(9 Pt 2)[Suppl 38]:1–14.

376. Flamenbaum W, Friedman R. Pharmacology, therapeutic efficacy, and adverse effects of bumetanide, a new "loop" diuretic. *Pharmacotherapy* 1982;2(4):213–222.

377. Shannon DC, Gotay F. Effects of theophylline on serum and urine electrolytes in preterm infants with apnea. *J Pediatr* 1979;94(6):963–965.

378. Cook D, Guyatt G, Marshall J, et al. A comparison of sucralfate and ranitidine for the prevention of upper gastrointestinal bleeding in patients requiring mechanical ventilation. Canadian Critical Care Trials Group. *N Engl J Med* 1998;338(12):791–797.

379. Cook DJ, Fuller HD, Guyatt GH, et al. Risk factors for gastrointestinal bleeding in critically ill patients. Canadian Critical Care Trials Group. *N Engl J Med* 1994;330(6):377–381.

380. Cook DJ, Witt LG, Cook RJ, et al. Stress ulcer prophylaxis in the critically ill: a meta-analysis. *Am J Med* 1991;91(5):519–527.

381. Lacroix J, Nadeau D, Laberge S, et al. Frequency of upper gastrointestinal bleeding in a pediatric intensive care unit. *Crit Care Med* 1992;20(1):35–42.

382. Lopez-Herce J, Dorao P, Elola P, et al. Frequency and prophylaxis of upper gastrointestinal hemorrhage in critically ill children: a prospective study comparing the efficacy of almagate, ranitidine, and sucralfate. The Gastrointestinal Hemorrhage Study Group. *Crit Care Med* 1992;20(8):1082–1089.

383. Maki M, Ruuska T, Kuusela AL, et al. High prevalence of asymptomatic esophageal and gastric lesions in preterm infants in intensive care. *Crit Care Med* 1993;21(12):1863–1867.

384. Kuusela AL, Ruuska T, Karikoski R, et al. A randomized, controlled study of prophylactic ranitidine in preventing stress-induced gastric mucosal lesions in neonatal intensive care unit patients. *Crit Care Med* 1997;25(2):346–351.

385. Black JW, Duncan WA, Durant CJ, et al. Definition and antagonism of histamine H2-receptors. *Nature* 1972;236(5347):385–390.

386. Smith K, Crisp C. Clinical comparison of H2-antagonists. *Conn Med* 1986;50(12):815–817.

387. Hansten PD. *Drug interactions and updates.* Vancouver: Applied Therapeutic, 1990.

388. Powell JR, Donn KH. Histamine H2-antagonist drug interactions in perspective: mechanistic concepts and clinical implications. *Am J Med* 1984;77(5B):57–84.

389. Fenje PC, Isles AF, Baltodano A, et al. Interaction of cimetidine and theophylline in two infants. *Can Med Assoc J* 1982;126(10):1178.

390. Peterson WL, Richardson CT. Intravenous cimetidine or two regimens of ranitidine to reduce fasting gastric acidity. *Ann Intern Med* 1986;104(4):505–507.

391. Zeldis JB, Friedman LS, Isselbacher KJ. Ranitidine: a new H2-receptor antagonist. *N Engl J Med* 1983;309(22):1368–1373.

392. Rosenthal M, Miller PW. Ranitidine in the newborn. *Arch Dis Child* 1988;63(1):88–89.

393. Zinner MJ, Zuidema GD, Smith P, et al. The prevention of upper gastrointestinal tract bleeding in patients in an intensive care unit. *Surg Gynecol Obstet* 1981;153(2):214–220.

394. Kelly EJ, Chatfield SL, Brownlee KG, et al. The effect of intravenous ranitidine on the intragastric pH of preterm infants receiving dexamethasone. *Arch Dis Child* 1993;69(1 Spec No):37–39.

395. Fontana M, Massironi E, Rossi A, et al. Ranitidine pharmacokinetics in newborn infants. *Arch Dis Child* 1993;68(5 Spec No): 602–603.

396. James LP, Marotti T, Stowe CD, et al. Pharmacokinetics and pharmacodynamics of famotidine in infants. *J Clin Pharmacol* 1998;38(12):1089–1095.

397. Driscoll DJ. Use of inotropic and chronotropic agents in neonates. *Clin Perinatol* 1987;14(4):931–949.

398. Hoffman BB. Catecholamines, sympathomimetic drugs, and adrenergic receptor antagonists. In: Hardman JG, Limbird LE, Gilman AG, eds. *Goodman & Gilman's the pharmacological basis of therapeutics*, 10th ed. New York: McGraw-Hill, 2001:215–268.

399. Zaritsky A, Chernow B. Use of catecholamines in pediatrics. *J Pediatr* 1984;105(3):341–350.

400. Hoffman BB, Taylor P. Neurotransmission: the autonomic and somatic motor nervous systems. In: Hardman JG, Limbird LE, Gilman AG, eds. *Goodman and Gilman's the pharmacological basis of therapeutics*, 10th ed. New York: McGraw-Hill, 2001:115–153.

401. Rude RE, Bush LR, Izquierdo C, et al. Effects of inotropic and chronotropic stimuli on acute myocardial ischemic injury. III. Influence of basal heart rate. *Am J Cardiol* 1984;53(11): 1688–1694.

402. Heckmann M, Trotter A, Pohlandt F, et al. Epinephrine treatment of hypotension in very low birthweight infants. *Acta Paediatr* 2002;91(5):566–570.

403. Siwy BK, Sadove AM. Acute management of dopamine infiltration injury with Regitine. *Plast Reconstr Surg* 1987;80(4): 610–612.

404. Driscoll DJ, Gillette PC, Lewis RM, et al. Comparative hemodynamic effects of isoproterenol, dopamine, and dobutamine in the newborn dog. *Pediatr Res* 1979;13(9):1006–1009.

405. Fiser DH, Fewell JE, Hill DE, et al. Cardiovascular and renal effects of dopamine and dobutamine in healthy, conscious piglets. *Crit Care Med* 1988;16(4):340–345.

406. Perez CA, Reimer JM, Schreiber MD, et al. Effect of high-dose dopamine on urine output in newborn infants. *Crit Care Med* 1986;14(12):1045–1049.

407. Seri I, Abbasi S, Wood DC, et al. Regional hemodynamic effects of dopamine in the sick preterm neonate. *J Pediatr* 1998;133(6): 728–734.

408. Liet JM, Boscher C, Gras-Leguen C, et al. Dopamine effects on pulmonary artery pressure in hypotensive preterm infants with patent ductus arteriosus. *J Pediatr* 2002;140(3):373–375.

409. Tuttle RR, Mills J. Dobutamine: development of a new catecholamine to selectively increase cardiac contractility. *Circ Res* 1975;36(1):185–196.

410. Ruffolo RR Jr, Yaden EL. Vascular effects of the stereoisomers of dobutamine. *J Pharmacol Exp Ther* 1983;224(1):46–50.

411. Hoffman BB, Lefkowitz RJ. Catecholamines and sympathomimetic drugs, and adrenergic receptor antagonists. In: Hardman JG, Limbird LE, Molinoff PB, et al, eds. *Goodman and Gilman's the pharmacological basis of therapeutics*, 9th ed. New York: McGraw-Hill, 1996:199–248.

412. Martinez AM, Padbury JF, Thio S. Dobutamine pharmacokinetics and cardiovascular responses in critically ill neonates. *Pediatrics* 1992;89(1):47–51.

413. Roze JC, Tohier C, Maingueneau C, et al. Response to dobutamine and dopamine in the hypotensive very preterm infant. *Arch Dis Child* 1993;69(1 Spec No):59–63.

414. Greenough A, Emery EF. Randomized trial comparing dopamine and dobutamine in preterm infants. *Eur J Pediatr* 1993; 152(11):925–927.

415. Klarr JM, Faix RG, Pryce CJ, et al. Randomized, blind trial of dopamine versus dobutamine for treatment of hypotension in preterm infants with respiratory distress syndrome. *J Pediatr* 1994;125(1):117–122.

416. Osborn D, Evans N, Kluckow M. Randomized trial of dobutamine versus dopamine in preterm infants with low systemic blood flow. *J Pediatr* 2002;140(2):183–191.

417. Ward A, Brogden RN, Heel RC, et al. Amrinone. A preliminary review of its pharmacological properties and therapeutic use. *Drugs* 1983;26(6):468–502.

418. Bottorff MB, Rutledge DR, Pieper JA. Evaluation of intravenous amrinone: the first of a new class of positive inotropic agents with vasodilator properties. *Pharmacotherapy* 1985;5(5):227–237.

419. Hoffman TM, Wernovsky G, Atz AM, et al. Efficacy and safety of milrinone in preventing low cardiac output syndrome in infants

420. Williams GD, Sorensen GK, Oakes R, et al. Amrinone loading during cardiopulmonary bypass in neonates, infants, and children. *J Cardiothorac Vasc Anesth* 1995;9(3):278–282.

421. Bailey JM, Miller BE, Kanter KR, et al. A comparison of the hemodynamic effects of amrinone and sodium nitroprusside in infants after cardiac surgery. *Anesth Analg* 1997;84(2):294–298.

422. Laitinen P, Happonen JM, Sairanen H, et al. Amrinone versus dopamine-nitroglycerin after reconstructive surgery for complete atrioventricular septal defect. *J Cardiothorac Vasc Anesth* 1997;11(7):870–874.

423. Laitinen P, Happonen JM, Sairanen H, et al. Amrinone versus dopamine and nitroglycerin in neonates after arterial switch operation for transposition of the great arteries. *J Cardiothorac Vasc Anesth* 1999;13(2):186–190.

424. Levy JH, Bailey JM. Phosphodiesterase inhibitors: the inotropes of choice for the new millennium? *J Cardiothorac Vasc Anesth* 2000;14(4):365–366.

425. Bailey JM, Levy JH, Rogers HG, et al. Pharmacokinetics of amrinone during cardiac surgery. *Anesthesiology* 1991;75(6):961–968.

426. Laitinen P, Ahonen J, Olkkola KT, et al. Pharmacokinetics of amrinone in neonates and infants. *J Cardiothorac Vasc Anesth* 2000;14(4):378–382.

427. Ross MP, Allen-Webb EM, Pappas JB, et al. Amrinone-associated thrombocytopenia: pharmacokinetic analysis. *Clin Pharmacol Ther* 1993;53(6):661–667.

428. Chang AC, Atz AM, Wernovsky G, et al. Milrinone: systemic and pulmonary hemodynamic effects in neonates after cardiac surgery. *Crit Care Med* 1995;23(11):1907–1914.

429. Hamada Y, Kawachi K, Yamamoto T, et al. Effects of single administration of a phosphodiesterase III inhibitor during cardiopulmonary bypass: comparison of milrinone and amrinone. *Jpn Circ J* 1999;63(8):605–609.

430. Ramamoorthy C, Anderson GD, Williams GD, et al. Pharmacokinetics and side effects of milrinone in infants and children after open heart surgery. *Anesth Analg* 1998;86(2):283–289.

431. Smith TW. Digitalis. Mechanisms of action and clinical use. *N Engl J Med* 1988;318(6):358–365.

432. Berman W Jr, Yabek SM, Dillon T, et al. Effects of digoxin in infants with congested circulatory state due to a ventricular septal defect. *N Engl J Med* 1983;308(7):363–366.

433. Lang D, von Bernuth G. Serum concentration and serum half-life of digoxin in premature and mature newborns. *Pediatrics* 1977;59(6):902–906.

434. Steiness E. Renal tubular secretion of digoxin. *Circulation* 1974;50(1):103–107.

435. Hastreiter AR, van der Horst RL, Voda C, et al. Maintenance digoxin dosage and steady-state plasma concentration in infants and children. *J Pediatr* 1985;107(1):140–146.

436. Ingelfinger JA, Goldman P. The serum digitalis concentration—does it diagnose digitalis toxicity? *N Engl J Med* 1976;294(16):867–870.

437. Lindenbaum J, Rund DG, Butler VP Jr, et al. Inactivation of digoxin by the gut flora: reversal by antibiotic therapy. *N Engl J Med* 1981;305(14):789–794.

438. Waldorff S, Andersen JD, Heeboll-Nielsen N, et al. Spironolactone-induced changes in digoxin kinetics. *Clin Pharmacol Ther* 1978;24(2):162–167.

439. Smith TW, Butler VP Jr, Haber E, et al. Treatment of life-threatening digitalis intoxication with digoxin-specific Fab antibody fragments: experience in 26 cases. *N Engl J Med* 1982;307(22): 1357–1362.

440. Seccombe DW, Pudek MR, Whitfield MF, et al. Perinatal changes in a digoxin-like immunoreactive substance. *Pediatr Res* 1984; 18(11):1097–1099.

441. Valdes R Jr. Endogenous digoxin-immunoactive factor in human subjects. *Fed Proc* 1985;44(12):2800–2805.

442. Mathews WR, DuCharme DW, Hamlyn JM, et al. Mass spectral characterization of an endogenous digitalislike factor from human plasma. *Hypertension* 1991;17(6 Pt 2):930–935.

443. Bova S, Blaustein MP, Ludens JH, et al. Effects of an endogenous ouabainlike compound on heart and aorta. *Hypertension* 1991; 17(6 Pt 2):944–950.

444. Aranda JV, Lopes JM, Blanchard P, et al. Drug treatment of neonatal apnea. In: Yaffe SJ, Aranda JV, eds. *Pediatric pharmacology: therapeutic principles in practice*, 2nd ed. Philadelphia: WB Saunders, 1992:193–204.

445. Runold M, Lagercrantz H, Fredholm BB. Ventilatory effect of an adenosine analogue in unanesthetized rabbits during development. *J Appl Physiol* 1986;61(1):255–259.

446. Aubier M, De Troyer A, Sampson M, et al. Aminophylline improves diaphragmatic contractility. *N Engl J Med* 1981;305(5):249–252.

447. Serafin WE. Drug used in the treatment of asthma. In: Hardman JG, Limbird LE, Molinoff PB, et al, eds. *Goodman & Gilman's the pharmacological basis of therapeutics*, 10th ed. New York: McGraw-Hill, 1996:659–682.

448. Kuzemko JA, Paala J. Apnoeic attacks in the newborn treated with aminophylline. *Arch Dis Child* 1973;48(5):404–406.

449. Shannon DC, Gotay F, Stein IM, et al. Prevention of apnea and bradycardia in low-birthweight infants. *Pediatrics* 1975;55(5):589–594.

450. Uauy R, Shapiro DL, Smith B, et al. Treatment of severe apnea in prematures with orally administered theophylline. *Pediatrics* 1975;55(5):595–598.

451. Barrington KJ, Finer NN. A randomized, controlled trial of aminophylline in ventilatory weaning of premature infants. *Crit Care Med* 1993;21(6):846–850.

452. Cordoba E, Gerhardt T, Rojas M, et al. Comparison of the effects of acetazolamide and aminophylline on apnea incidence and on ventilatory response to CO_2 in preterm infants. *Pediatr Pulmonol* 1994;17(5):291–295.

453. Roberts JL, Mathew OP, Thach BT. The efficacy of theophylline in premature infants with mixed and obstructive apnea and apnea associated with pulmonary and neurologic disease. *J Pediatr* 1982;100(6):968–970.

454. Harris MC, Baumgart S, Rooklin AR, et al. Successful extubation of infants with respiratory distress syndrome using aminophylline. *J Pediatr* 1983;103(2):303–305.

455. Peabody JL, Neese AL, Philip AG, et al. Transcutaneous oxygen monitoring in aminophylline-treated apneic infants. *Pediatrics* 1978;62(5):698–701.

456. Myers TF, Milsap RL, Krauss AN, et al. Low-dose theophylline therapy in idiopathic apnea of prematurity. *J Pediatr* 1980;96(1):99–103.

457. Aranda JV, Louridas AT, Vitullo BB, et al. Metabolism of theophylline to caffeine in human fetal liver. *Science* 1979;206(4424):1319–1321.

458. Bada HS, Khanna NN, Somani SM, et al. Interconversion of theophylline and caffeine in newborn infants. *J Pediatr* 1979;94(6):993–995.

459. Bory C, Baltassat P, Porthault M, et al. Metabolism of theophylline to caffeine in premature newborn infants. *J Pediatr* 1979;94(6):988–993.

460. Boutroy MJ, Vert P, Royer RJ, et al. Caffeine, a metabolite of theophylline during the treatment of apnea in the premature infant. *J Pediatr* 1979;94(6):996–998.

461. Dothey CI, Tserng KY, Kaw S, et al. Maturational changes of theophylline pharmacokinetics in preterm infants. *Clin Pharmacol Ther* 1989;45(5):461–468.

462. Marquis JF, Carruthers SG, Spence JD, et al. Phenytoin-theophylline interaction. *N Engl J Med* 1982;307(19):1189–1190.

463. Prince RA, Wing DS, Weinberger MM, et al. Effect of erythromycin on theophylline kinetics. *J Allergy Clin Immunol* 1981;68(6):427–431.

464. Fernandes E, Melewicz FM. Ranitidine and theophylline. *Ann Intern Med* 1984;100(3):459.

465. Gardner ME, Sikorski GW. Ranitidine and theophylline. *Ann Intern Med* 1985;102(4):559.

466. Aranda JV, Grondin D, Sasyniuk BI. Pharmacologic considerations in the therapy of neonatal apnea. *Pediatr Clin North Am* 1981;28(1):113–133.

467. Roberts RJ. Methylxanthine therapy: caffeine and theophylline. In: *Drug therapy in infants. pharmacologic principles and clinical experience*. Philadelphia: WB Saunders, 1984:119–137.

468. Bairam A, Boutroy MJ, Badonnel Y, et al. Theophylline versus caffeine: comparative effects in treatment of idiopathic apnea in the preterm infant. *J Pediatr* 1987;110(4):636–639.

469. Brouard C, Moriette G, Murat I, et al. Comparative efficacy of theophylline and caffeine in the treatment of idiopathic apnea in premature infants. *Am J Dis Child* 1985;139(7):698–700.

470. Larsen PB, Brendstrup L, Skov L, et al. Aminophylline versus caffeine citrate for apnea and bradycardia prophylaxis in premature neonates. *Acta Paediatr* 1995;84(4):360–364.

471. Raval DS, Yeh TF. Apnea. In: Yeh T, ed. *Drug therapy in the neonate and small infant*. Chicago: Year Book Medical 1985:57–71.

472. Aranda JV, Gorman W, Bergsteinsson H, et al. Efficacy of caffeine in treatment of apnea in the low-birth-weight infant. *J Pediatr* 1977;90(3):467–472.

473. Scanlon JE, Chin KC, Morgan ME, et al. Caffeine or theophylline for neonatal apnoea? *Arch Dis Child* 1992;67(4 Spec No):425–428.

474. Rothberg AD, Marks KH, Ward RM, et al. The metabolic effects of caffeine in the newborn infant. *Pediatr Pharmacol (New York)* 1981;1(3):181–186.

475. Le Guennec JC, Billon B, Pare C. Maturational changes of caffeine concentrations and disposition in infancy during maintenance therapy for apnea of prematurity: influence of gestational age, hepatic disease, and breast-feeding. *Pediatrics* 1985;76(5):834–840.

476. Wakamatsu A, Umetsu M, Motoya H, et al. Change of plasma half-life of caffeine during caffeine therapy for apnea in premature infants. *Acta Paediatr Jpn* 1987;29(4):595–599.

477. Parsons WD, Neims AH. Prolonged half-life of caffeine in healthy term newborn infants. *J Pediatr* 1981;98(4):640–641.

478. Costarino AT, Polin RA. Neuromuscular relaxants in the neonate. *Clin Perinatol* 1987;14(4):965–989.

479. Larijani GE, Gratz I, Silverberg M, et al. Clinical pharmacology of the neuromuscular blocking agents. *DICP* 1991;25(1):54–64.

480. Gronert BJ, Brandom BW. Neuromuscular blocking drugs in infants and children. *Pediatr Clin North Am* 1994;41(1):73–91.

481. Miller RD, Rupp SM, Fisher DM, et al. Clinical pharmacology of vecuronium and atracurium. *Anesthesiology* 1984;61(4):444–453.

482. Bennett EJ, Ramamurthy S, Dalal FY, et al. Pancuronium and the neonate. *Br J Anaesth* 1975;47(1):75–78.

483. Goudsouzian NG, Crone RK, Todres ID. Recovery from pancuronium blockade in the neonatal intensive care unit. *Br J Anaesth* 1981;53(12):1303–1309.

484. Meretoja OA. Is vecuronium a long-acting neuromuscular blocking agent in neonates and infants? *Br J Anaesth* 1989;62(2):184–187.

485. Bencini AF, Scaf AH, Sohn YJ, et al. Disposition and urinary excretion of vecuronium bromide in anesthetized patients with normal renal function or renal failure. *Anesth Analg* 1986;65(3):245–251.

486. Haynes SR, Morton NS. Prolonged neuromuscular blockade with vecuronium in a neonate with renal failure. *Anaesthesia* 1990;45(9):743–745.

487. Sinclair JF, Malcolm GA, Stephenson JB, et al. Prolonged neuromuscular blockade in an infant. *Anaesthesia* 1987;42(9):1020.

488. Hilgenberg JC. Comparison of the pharmacology and vecuronium and atracurium with that of other currently available muscle relaxants. *Anesth Analg* 1983;62(5):524–531.

489. Meakin G, Shaw EA, Baker RD, et al. Comparison of atracurium-induced neuromuscular blockade in neonates, infants and children. *Br J Anaesth* 1988;60(2):171–175.

490. Kalli I, Meretoja OA. Infusion of atracurium in neonates, infants and children. A study of dose requirements. *Br J Anaesth* 1988;60(6):651–654.

491. Coceani F, Olley PM. Role of prostaglandins, prostacyclin, and thromboxanes in the control of prenatal patency and postnatal closure of the ductus arteriosus. *Semin Perinatol* 1980;4(2):109–113.

492. Freed MD, Heymann MA, Lewis AB, et al. Prostaglandin E1 infants with ductus arteriosus-dependent congenital heart disease. *Circulation* 1981;64(5):899–905.

493. Lewis AB, Takahashi M, Lurie PR. Administration of prostaglandin E1 in neonates with critical congenital cardiac defects. *J Pediatr* 1978;93(3):481–485.

494. Thanopoulos BD, Andreou A, Frimas C. Prostaglandin E2 administration in infants with ductus-dependent cyanotic congenital heart disease. *Eur J Pediatr* 1987;146(3):279–282.

495. Monk JP, Clissold SP. Misoprostol. A preliminary review of its pharmacodynamic and pharmacokinetic properties, and therapeutic efficacy in the treatment of peptic ulcer disease. *Drugs* 1987;33(1):1–30.

496. Friedman WF, Hirschklau MJ, Printz MP, et al. Pharmacologic closure of patent ductus arteriosus in the premature infant. *N Engl J Med* 1976;295(10):526–529.

497. Gersony WM, Peckham GJ, Ellison RC, et al. Effects of indomethacin in premature infants with patent ductus arteriosus:

results of a national collaborative study. *J Pediatr* 1983;102(6): 895–906.

498. Bandstra ES, Montalvo BM, Goldberg RN, et al. Prophylactic indomethacin for prevention of intraventricular hemorrhage in premature infants. *Pediatrics* 1988;82(4):533–542.

499. Maher P, Lane B, Ballard R, et al. Does indomethacin cause extension of intracranial hemorrhages: a preliminary study. *Pediatrics* 1985;75(3):497–500.

500. Merritt TA, Bejar R, Corazza M, et al. Clinical trials of intravenous indomethacin for closure of the patent ductus arteriosus. *Ped Cardiol* 1983;4(Suppl II):71–79.

501. Wiest DB, Pinson JB, Gal PS, et al. Population pharmacokinetics of intravenous indomethacin in neonates with symptomatic patent ductus arteriosus. *Clin Pharmacol Ther* 1991;49(5): 550–557.

502. Rhodes PG, Ferguson MG, Reddy NS, et al. Effects of prolonged versus acute indomethacin therapy in very low birth-weight infants with patent ductus arteriosus. *Eur J Pediatr* 1988;147(5): 481–484.

503. McCarthy JS, Zies LG, Gelband H. Age-dependent closure of the patent ductus arteriosus by indomethacin. *Pediatrics* 1978; 62(5):706–712.

504. Achanti B, Pyati S, Yeh TF. Indomethacin therapy in premature infants of advanced postnatal age. *J Perinatol* 1987;7(3): 235–237.

505. DiBona GF. Prostaglandins and nonsteroidal anti-inflammatory drugs. Effects on renal hemodynamics. *Am J Med* 1986;80(1A): 12–21.

506. Cifuentes RF, Olley PM, Balfe JW, et al. Indomethacin and renal function in premature infants with persistent patent ductus arteriosus. *J Pediatr* 1979;95(4):583–587.

507. Seri I, Tulassay T, Kiszel J, et al. The use of dopamine for the prevention of the renal side effects of indomethacin in premature infants with patent ductus arteriosus. *Int J Pediatr Nephrol* 1984;5(4):209–214.

508. Clive DM, Stoff JS. Renal syndromes associated with nonsteroidal antiinflammatory drugs. *N Engl J Med* 1984;310(9): 563–572.

509. Walshe JJ, Venuto RC. Acute oliguric renal failure induced by indomethacin: possible mechanism. *Ann Intern Med* 1979; 91(1):47–49.

510. Cowan F. Indomethacin, patent ductus arteriosus, and cerebral blood flow. *J Pediatr* 1986;109(2):341–344.

511. Colditz P, Murphy D, Rolfe P, et al. Effect of infusion rate of indomethacin on cerebrovascular responses in preterm neonates. *Arch Dis Child* 1989;64(1 Spec No):8–12.

512. Coombs RC, Morgan ME, Durbin GM, et al. Gut blood flow velocities in the newborn: effects of patent ductus arteriosus and parenteral indomethacin. *Arch Dis Child* 1990;65(10 Spec No):1067–1071.

513. Ward RM. Persistent pulmonary hypertension. In: Nelson NM, ed. *Current therapy in neonatal-perinatal medicine-2.* Toronto: BC Decker, 1990:331–338.

514. Abman SH, Chatfield BA, Hall SL, et al. Role of endothelium-derived relaxing factor during transition of pulmonary circulation at birth. *Am J Physiol* 1990;259(6 Pt 2):H1921–H1927.

515. Shaul PW. Ontogeny of nitric oxide in the pulmonary vasculature. *Semin Perinatol* 1997;21(5):381–392.

516. Palmer RM, Ferrige AG, Moncada S. Nitric oxide release accounts for the biological activity of endothelium-derived relaxing factor. *Nature* 1987;327(6122):524–526.

517. McAndrew J, Patel RP, Jo H, et al. The interplay of nitric oxide and peroxynitrite with signal transduction pathways: implications for disease. *Semin Perinatol* 1997;21(5):351–366.

518. Steinhorn RH, Morin FC 3rd, Fineman JR. Models of persistent pulmonary hypertension of the newborn (PPHN) and the role of cyclic guanosine monophosphate (GMP) in pulmonary vasorelaxation. *Semin Perinatol* 1997;21(5):393–408.

519. Christou H, Adatia I, Van Marter LJ, et al. Effect of inhaled nitric oxide on endothelin-1 and cyclic guanosine 5′-monophosphate plasma concentrations in newborn infants with persistent pulmonary hypertension. *J Pediatr* 1997;130(4):603–611.

520. Nakajima W, Ishida A, Arai H, et al. Methaemoglobinaemia after inhalation of nitric oxide in infant with pulmonary hypertension. *Lancet* 1997;350(9083):1002–1003.

521. Finer NN, Barrington KJ. Nitric oxide in respiratory failure in the newborn infant. *Semin Perinatol* 1997;21(5):426–440.

522. Kinsella JP, Truog WE, Walsh WF, et al. Randomized, multicenter trial of inhaled nitric oxide and high-frequency oscillatory ventilation in severe, persistent pulmonary hypertension of the newborn. *J Pediatr* 1997;131(1 Pt 1):55–62.

523. Roberts JD Jr, Fineman JR, Morin FC 3rd, et al. Inhaled nitric oxide and persistent pulmonary hypertension of the newborn. The Inhaled Nitric Oxide Study Group. *N Engl J Med* 1997; 336(9):605–610.

524. Cornfield DN, Maynard RC, deRegnier RA, et al. Randomized, controlled trial of low-dose inhaled nitric oxide in the treatment of term and near-term infants with respiratory failure and pulmonary hypertension. *Pediatrics* 1999;104(5 Pt 1):1089–1094.

525. Finer NN, Barrington KJ. Nitric oxide for respiratory failure in infants born at or near term. *Cochrane Database Syst Rev* 2001(4):CD000399.

526. Nelin LD, Hoffman GM. The use of inhaled nitric oxide in a wide variety of clinical problems. *Pediatr Clin North Am* 1998;45(3):531–548.

527. Day RW, Lynch JM, White KS, et al. Acute response to inhaled nitric oxide in newborns with respiratory failure and pulmonary hypertension. *Pediatrics* 1996;98(4 Pt 1):698–705.

528. Demirakca S, Dotsch J, Knothe C, et al. Inhaled nitric oxide in neonatal and pediatric acute respiratory distress syndrome: dose response, prolonged inhalation, and weaning. *Crit Care Med* 1996;24(11):1913–1919.

529. Lonnqvist PA. Inhaled nitric oxide in newborn and paediatric patients with pulmonary hypertension and moderate to severe impaired oxygenation: effects of doses of 3–100 parts per million. *Intensive Care Med* 1997;23(7):773–779.

530. Nakagawa TA, Morris A, Gomez RJ, et al. Dose response to inhaled nitric oxide in pediatric patients with pulmonary hypertension and acute respiratory distress syndrome. *J Pediatr* 1997;131(1 Pt 1):63–69.

531. Tworetzky W, Bristow J, Moore P, et al. Inhaled nitric oxide in neonates with persistent pulmonary hypertension. *Lancet* 2001;357(9250):118–120.

532. Hallman M, Bry K, Turbow R, et al. Pulmonary toxicity associated with nitric oxide in term infants with severe respiratory failure. *J Pediatr* 1998;132(5):827–829.

533. Cheung PY, Salas E, Schulz R, et al. Nitric oxide and platelet function: implications for neonatology. *Semin Perinatol* 1997;21(5):409–417.

534. Clark RH, Huckaby JL, Kueser TJ, et al. Low-dose nitric oxide therapy for persistent pulmonary hypertension: 1-year follow-up. *J Perinatol* 2003;23(4):300–303.

535. Desandes R, Desandes E, Droulle P, et al. Inhaled nitric oxide improves oxygenation in very premature infants with low pulmonary blood flow. *Acta Paediatr* 2004;93(1):66–69.

536. Kulik TJ, Lock JE. Pulmonary vasodilator therapy in persistent pulmonary hypertension of the newborn. *Clin Perinatol* 1984;11(3):693–701.

537. Nuntnarumit P, Korones SB, Yang W, et al. Efficacy and safety of tolazoline for treatment of severe hypoxemia in extremely preterm infants. *Pediatrics* 2002;109(5):852–856.

538. Stocker C, Penny DJ, Brizard CP, et al. Intravenous sildenafil and inhaled nitric oxide: a randomised trial in infants after cardiac surgery. *Intensive Care Med* 2003;29(11):1996–2003.

539. Ehlen M, Wiebe B. Iloprost in persistent pulmonary hypertension of the newborn. *Cardiol Young* 2003;13(4):361–363.

540. Kelly LK, Porta NF, Goodman DM, et al. Inhaled prostacyclin for term infants with persistent pulmonary hypertension refractory to inhaled nitric oxide. *J Pediatr* 2002;141(6):830–832.

541. Peliowski A, Finer NN. A blinded, randomized, placebo-controlled trial to compare theophylline and doxapram for the treatment of apnea of prematurity. *J Pediatr* 1990;116(4): 648–653.

542. Alpan G, Eyal F, Sagi E, et al. Doxapram in the treatment of idiopathic apnea of prematurity unresponsive to aminophylline. *J Pediatr* 1984;104(4):634–637.

543. Barrington KJ, Finer NN, Peters KL, et al. Physiologic effects of doxapram in idiopathic apnea of prematurity. *J Pediatr* 1986;108(1):124–129.

544. Bairam A, Akramoff-Gershan L, Beharry K, et al. Gastrointestinal absorption of doxapram in neonates. *Am J Perinatol* 1991;8(2): 110–113.

545. Tay-Uyboco J, Kwiatkowski K, Cates DB, et al. Clinical and physiological responses to prolonged nasogastric administration of

doxapram for apnea of prematurity. *Biol Neonate* 1991;59(4): 190–200.

546. Avery GB, Fletcher AB, Kaplan M, et al. Controlled trial of dexamethasone in respirator-dependent infants with bronchopulmonary dysplasia. *Pediatrics* 1985;75:106–111.

547. Yeh TF, Lin YJ, Lin CH, et al. Early postnatal (<12 hours) dexamethasone therapy for prevention of BPD in preterm infants with RDS—a two year follow-up study. *Pediatr Res* 1997;41:188A.

548. Yeh TF, Lin YJ, Huang CC, et al. Early dexamethasone therapy in preterm infants: a follow-up study. *Pediatrics* 1998;101(5):E7.

549. Shinwell ES, Karplus M, Reich D, et al. Early postnatal dexamethasone treatment and increased incidence of cerebral palsy. *Arch Dis Child Fetal Neonatal Ed* 2000;83(3):F177–F181.

550. Yeh TF, Lin YJ, Lin HC, et al. Outcomes at school age after postnatal dexamethasone therapy for lung disease of prematurity. *N Engl J Med* 2004;350(13):1304–1313.

551. Bagchi A, Viscardi RM, Taciak V, et al. Increased activity of interleukin-6 but not tumor necrosis factor-alpha in lung lavage of premature infants is associated with the development of bronchopulmonary dysplasia. *Pediatr Res* 1994;36(2):244–252.

552. Groneck P, Goetze-Speer B, Speer CP. Inflammatory bronchopulmonary response of preterm infants with microbial colonisation of the airways at birth. *Arch Dis Child Fetal Neonatal* Ed 1996;74(1):F51–F55.

553. Groneck P, Gotze-Speer B, Oppermann M, et al. Association of pulmonary inflammation and increased microvascular permeability during the development of bronchopulmonary dysplasia: a sequential analysis of inflammatory mediators in respiratory fluids of high-risk preterm neonates. *Pediatrics* 1994;93(5):712–718.

554. Merritt TA, Cochrane CG, Holcomb K, et al. Elastase and alpha 1-proteinase inhibitor activity in tracheal aspirates during respiratory distress syndrome. Role of inflammation in the pathogenesis of bronchopulmonary dysplasia. *J Clin Invest* 1983;72(2): 656–666.

555. Ogden BE, Murphy SA, Saunders GC, et al. Neonatal lung neutrophils and elastase/proteinase inhibitor imbalance. *Am Rev Respir Dis* 1984;130(5):817–821.

556. Avery GB, Fletcher AB, Kaplan M, et al. Controlled trial of dexamethasone in respirator-dependent infants with bronchopulmonary dysplasia. *Pediatrics* 1985;75(1):106–111.

557. Cummings JJ, D'Eugenio DB, Gross SJ. A controlled trial of dexamethasone in preterm infants at high risk for bronchopulmonary dysplasia. *N Engl J Med* 1989;320(23):1505–1510.

558. Harkavy KL, Scanlon JW, Chowdhry PK, et al. Dexamethasone therapy for chronic lung disease in ventilator- and oxygen-dependent infants: a controlled trial. *J Pediatr* 1989;115(6): 979–983.

559. Kazzi NJ, Brans YW, Poland RL. Dexamethasone effects on the hospital course of infants with bronchopulmonary dysplasia who are dependent on artificial ventilation. *Pediatrics* 1990; 86(5):722–727.

560. Ohlsson A, Calvert SA, Hosking M, et al. Randomized controlled trial of dexamethasone treatment in very-low-birth-weight infants with ventilator-dependent chronic lung disease. *Acta Paediatr* 1992;81(10):751–756.

561. Halliday HL, Ehrenkranz RA, Doyle LW. Moderate early (7–14 days) postnatal corticosteroids for preventing chronic lung disease in preterm infants. *Cochrane Database Syst Rev* 2003;1: CD001144.

562. Halliday HL, Ehrenkranz RA, Doyle LW. Delayed (>3 weeks) postnatal corticosteroids for chronic lung disease in preterm infants. *Cochrane Database Syst Rev* 2003;1:CD001145.

563. Halliday HL, Ehrenkranz RA, Doyle LW. Early (<96 hours) corticosteroids for preventing chronic lung disease in preterm infants. *Cochrane Database Syst Rev* 2003;1:CD001146.

564. Shenai JP, Mellen BG, Chytil F. Vitamin A status and postnatal dexamethasone treatment in bronchopulmonary dysplasia. *Pediatrics* 2000;106(3):547–553.

565. Schimmer BP, Parker KL. Adrenocorticotropic hormone; adrenocortical steroids and their synthetic analogs; inhibitors of the synthesis and actions of the adrencortical hormones. In: Hardman JG, Limbird LE, Gilman AG, eds. *Goodman and Gilman's the pharmacological basis of therapeutics*, 10th ed. New York: McGraw-Hill, 2001:1649–1677.

566. Charles B, Schild P, Steer P, et al. Pharmacokinetics of dexamethasone following single-dose intravenous administration to extremely low birth weight infants. *Dev Pharmacol Ther Vermont Oxford Network Study Group.* 1993;20(3–4):205–210.

567. Lugo RA, Nahata MC, Menke JA, et al. Pharmacokinetics of dexamethasone in premature neonates. *Eur J Clin Pharmacol* 1996;49(6):477–483.

568. Early postnatal dexamethasone therapy for the prevention of chronic lung disease. *Pediatrics* 2001;108(3):741–748.

569. Romagnoli C, Zecca E, Luciano R, et al. Controlled trial of early dexamethasone treatment for the prevention of chronic lung disease in preterm infants: a 3-year follow-up. *Pediatrics* 2002;109(6):e85.

570. Banks BA. Postnatal dexamethasone for bronchopulmonary dysplasia: a systematic review and meta-analysis of 20 years of clinical trials. *NeoReviews* 2002;3:e24-e34.

571. Noble-Jamieson CM, Regev R, Silverman M. Dexamethasone in neonatal chronic lung disease: pulmonary effects and intracranial complications. *Eur J Pediatr* 1989;148(4):365–367.

572. Papile LA, Tyson JE, Stoll BJ, et al. A multicenter trial of two dexamethasone regimens in ventilator-dependent premature infants. *N Engl J Med* 1998;338(16):1112–1118.

573. Rastogi A, Akintorin SM, Bez ML, et al. A controlled trial of dexamethasone to prevent bronchopulmonary dysplasia in surfactant-treated infants. *Pediatrics* 1996;98(2 Pt 1):204–210.

574. Skinner AM, Battin M, Solimano A, et al. Growth and growth factors in premature infants receiving dexamethasone for bronchopulmonary dysplasia. *Am J Perinatol* 1997;14(9): 539–546.

575. Yeh TF, Torre JA, Rastogi A, et al. Early postnatal dexamethasone therapy in premature infants with severe respiratory distress syndrome: a double-blind, controlled study. *J Pediatr* 1990; 117(2 Pt 1):273–282.

576. Durand M, Sardesai S, McEvoy C. Effects of early dexamethasone therapy on pulmonary mechanics and chronic lung disease in very low birth weight infants: a randomized, controlled trial. *Pediatrics* 1995;95(4):584–590.

577. Marinelli KA, Burke GS, Herson VC. Effects of dexamethasone on blood pressure in premature infants with bronchopulmonary dysplasia. *J Pediatr* 1997;130(4):594–602.

578. Sanders RJ, Cox C, Phelps DL, et al. Two doses of early intravenous dexamethasone for the prevention of bronchopulmonary dysplasia in babies with respiratory distress syndrome. *Pediatr Res* 1994;36(1 Pt 1):122–128.

579. Shinwell ES, Karplus M, Zmora E, et al. Failure of early postnatal dexamethasone to prevent chronic lung disease in infants with respiratory distress syndrome. *Arch Dis Child Fetal Neonatal Ed* 1996;74(1):F33–F37.

580. Smets K, Vanhaesebrouck P. Dexamethasone associated systemic hypertension in low birth weight babies with chronic lung disease. *Eur J Pediatr* 1996;155(7):573–575.

581. Alkalay AL, Pomerance JJ, Puri AR, et al. Hypothalamic-pituitary-adrenal axis function in very low birth weight infants treated with dexamethasone. *Pediatrics* 1990;86(2):204–210.

582. Arnold JD, Leslie GI, Williams G, et al. Adrenocortical responsiveness in neonates weaned from the ventilator with dexamethasone. *Aust Paediatr J* 1987;23(4):227–229.

583. Ford LR, Willi SM, Hollis BW, et al. Suppression and recovery of the neonatal hypothalamic-pituitary-adrenal axis after prolonged dexamethasone therapy. *J Pediatr* 1997;131(5):722–726.

584. Ng PC, Blackburn ME, Brownlee KG, et al. Adrenal response in very low birthweight babies after dexamethasone treatment for bronchopulmonary dysplasia. *Arch Dis Child* 1989;64(12): 1721–1726.

585. Ng PC, Wong GW, Lam CW, et al. Pituitary-adrenal suppression and recovery in preterm very low birth weight infants after dexamethasone treatment for bronchopulmonary dysplasia. *J Clin Endocrinol Metab* 1997;82(8):2429–2432.

586. Sauder SE, Powers WF, Wise JE. Suppression of pituitary-adrenal axis in very low birth weight infants after dexamethasone therapy for bronchopulmonary dysplasia. *Clin Res* 1987;35: 913A(abst).

587. Brand PL, van Lingen RA, Brus F, et al. Hypertrophic obstructive cardiomyopathy as a side effect of dexamethasone treatment for bronchopulmonary dysplasia. *Acta Paediatr* 1993;82(6–7): 614–617.

588. Israel BA, Sherman FS, Guthrie RD. Hypertrophic cardiomyopathy associated with dexamethasone therapy for chronic lung disease in preterm infants. *Am J Perinatol* 1993;10(4):307–310.

589. Ohning BL, Fyfe DA, Riedel PA. Reversible obstructive hypertrophic cardiomyopathy after dexamethasone therapy for bronchopulmonary dysplasia. *Am Heart J* 1993;125(1): 253–256.

590. Ng PC, Fok TF, So KW, et al. Lower gastrointestinal tract perforation in preterm infants treated with dexamethasone for bronchopulmonary dysplasia. *Pediatr Surg Int* 1997;12(2–3): 211–212.

591. O'Neil EA, Chwals WJ, O'Shea MD, et al. Dexamethasone treatment during ventilator dependency: possible life threatening gastrointestinal complications. *Arch Dis Child* 1992;67(1 Spec No):10–11.

592. Werner JC, Sicard RE, Hansen TW, et al. Hypertrophic cardiomyopathy associated with dexamethasone therapy for bronchopulmonary dysplasia. *J Pediatr* 1992;120(2 Pt 1):286–291.

593. Byyny RL. Withdrawal from glucocorticoid therapy. *N Engl J Med* 1976;295(1):30–32.

594. Brundage KL, Mohsini KG, Froese AB, et al. Dexamethasone therapy for bronchopulmonary dysplasia: improved respiratory mechanics without adrenal suppression. *Pediatr Pulmonol* 1992;12(3):162–169.

595. Wilson DM, Baldwin RB, Ariagno RL. A randomized, placebo-controlled trial of effects of dexamethasone on hypothalamic-pituitary-adrenal axis in preterm infants. *J Pediatr* 1988;113(4): 764–768.

596. Kari MA, Heinonen K, Ikonen RS, et al. Dexamethasone treatment in preterm infants at risk for bronchopulmonary dysplasia. *Arch Dis Child* 1993;68(5 Spec No):566–569.

597. Kari MA, Raivio KO, Stenman UH, et al. Serum cortisol, dehydroepiandrosterone sulfate, and steroid-binding globulins in preterm neonates: effect of gestational age and dexamethasone therapy. *Pediatr Res* 1996;40(2):319–324.

598. Rizvi ZB, Aniol HS, Myers TF, et al. Effects of dexamethasone on the hypothalamic-pituitary-adrenal axis in preterm infants. *J Pediatr* 1992;120(6):961–965.

599. Stark AR, Carlo WA, Tyson JE, et al. Adverse effects of early dexamethasone in extremely-low-birth-weight infants. National Institute of Child Health and Human Development Neonatal Research Network. *N Engl J Med* 2001;344(2):95–101.

600. Cotterrell M, Balazs R, Johnson AL. Effects of corticosteroids on the biochemical maturation of rat brain: postnatal cell formation. *J Neurochem* 1972;19(9):2151–2167.

601. Gumbinas M, Oda M, Huttenlocher P. The effects of corticosteroids on myelination of the developing rat brain. *Biol Neonate* 1973;22(5):355–366.

602. Weichsel ME Jr. The therapeutic use of glucocorticoid hormones in the perinatal period: potential neurological hazards. *Ann Neurol* 1977;2(5):364–366.

603. Romagnoli C, Zecca E, Luciano R, et al. A three year follow up of preterm infants after moderately early treatment with dexamethasone. *Arch Dis Child Fetal Neonatal Ed* 2002;87(1): F55–F58.

604. O'Shea TM, Kothadia JM, Klinepeter KL, et al. Follow-up of preterm infants treated with dexamethasone for chronic lung disease. *Am J Dis Child* 1993;147(6):658–661.

605. Vohr BR, Wright LL, Dusick AM, et al. Neurodevelopmental and functional outcomes of extremely low birth weight infants in the National Institute of Child Health and Human Development Neonatal Research Network, 1993–1994. *Pediatrics* 2000; 105(6):1216–1226.

606. Thebaud B, Lacaze-Masmonteil T, Watterberg K. Postnatal glucocorticoids in very preterm infants: "the good, the bad, and the ugly"? *Pediatrics* 2001;107(2):413–415.

607. Barrington KJ. Postnatal steroids and neurodevelopmental outcomes: a problem in the making. *Pediatrics* 2001;107(6): 1425–1426.

608. Jacobs HC, Chapman RL, Gross I. Premature conclusions on postnatal steroid effects. *Pediatrics* 2002;110(1 Pt 1):200–201, author reply 201.

609. Postnatal corticosteroids to treat or prevent chronic lung disease in preterm infants. *Pediatrics* 2002;109(2):330–338.

610. Watterberg KL, Scott SM. Evidence of early adrenal insufficiency in babies who develop bronchopulmonary dysplasia. *Pediatrics* 1995;95(1):120–125.

611. Korte C, Styne D, Merritt TA, et al. Adrenocortical function in the very low birth weight infant: improved testing sensitivity and association with neonatal outcome. *J Pediatr* 1996;128(2):257–263.

612. Watterberg KL, Gerdes JS, Cook KL. Impaired glucocorticoid synthesis in premature infants developing chronic lung disease. *Pediatr Res* 2001;50(2):190–195.

613. Colasurdo MA, Hanna CE, Gilhooly JT, et al. Hydrocortisone replacement in extremely premature infants with cortisol insufficiency. *Clin Res* 1989;37(1):180A.

614. Ward RM, Kimura RE, Rich-Denson C. Addisonian crisis in extremely premature neonates. *Clin Res* 1991;39(1):11A.

615. Ng PC, Lam CW, Fok TF, et al. Refractory hypotension in preterm infants with adrenocortical insufficiency. *Arch Dis Child Fetal Neonatal Ed* 2001;84(2):F122–F124.

616. Ng PC, Lee CH, Lam CW, et al. Transient adrenocortical insufficiency of prematurity and systemic hypotension in very low birthweight infants. *Arch Dis Child Fetal Neonatal Ed* 2004; 89(2):F119-F126.

617. Watterberg KL, Gerdes JS, Gifford KL, et al. Prophylaxis against early adrenal insufficiency to prevent chronic lung disease in premature infants. *Pediatrics* 1999;104(6):1258–1263.

618. van der Heide-Jalving M, Kamphuis PJ, van der Laan MJ, et al. Short- and long-term effects of neonatal glucocorticoid therapy: is hydrocortisone an alternative to dexamethasone? *Acta Paediatr* 2003;92(7):827–835.

619. Andre P, Thebaud B, Odievre MH, et al. Methylprednisolone, an alternative to dexamethasone in very premature infants at risk of chronic lung disease. *Intensive Care Med* 2000;26(10): 1496–1500.

620. Gupta GK, Cole CH, Abbasi S, et al. Effects of early inhaled beclomethasone therapy on tracheal aspirate inflammatory mediators IL-8 and IL-1ra in ventilated preterm infants at risk for bronchopulmonary dysplasia. *Pediatr Pulmonol* 2000;30(4): 275–281.

621. Groneck P, Goetze-Speer B, Speer CP. Effects of inhaled beclomethasone compared to systemic dexamethasone on lung inflammation in preterm infants at risk of chronic lung disease. *Pediatr Pulmonol* 1999;27(6):383–387.

622. Halliday HL. Postnatal steroids and chronic lung disease in the newborn. *Paediatr Respir Rev* 2004;5[Suppl A]:S245–S248.

623. Shah SS, Ohlsson A, Halliday H, et al. Inhaled versus systemic corticosteroids for the treatment of chronic lung disease in ventilated very low birth weight preterm infants. *Cochrane Database Syst Rev* 2003(2):CD002057.

624. Graff-Lonnevig V. Diurnal expiratory flow after inhalation of Freons and fenoterol in childhood asthma. *J Allergy Clin Immunol* 1979;64(6 Pt 1):534–538.

625. Taylor GJ, Harris WS. Cardiac toxicity of aerosol propellants. *JAMA* 1970;214(1):81–85.

626. Yarbrough J, Mansfield LE, Ting S. Metered dose inhaler induced bronchospasm in asthmatic patients. *Ann Allergy* 1985;55(1): 25–27.

627. Roberts RJ, Knight ME. Pharmacology of vitamin E in the newborn. *Clin Perinatol* 1987;14(4):843–855.

628. Ehrenkranz RA, Bonta BW, Ablow RC, et al. Amelioration of bronchopulmonary dysplasia after vitamin E administration. A preliminary report. *N Engl J Med* 1978;299(11): 564–569.

629. Ehrenkranz RA, Ablow RC, Warshaw JB. Prevention of bronchopulmonary dysplasia with vitamin E administration during the acute stages of respiratory distress syndrome. *J Pediatr* 1979;95(5 Pt 2):873–878.

630. Hittner HM, Godio LB, Rudolph AJ, et al. Retrolental fibroplasia: efficacy of vitamin E in a double-blind clinical study of preterm infants. *N Engl J Med* 1981;305(23):1365–1371.

631. Phelps DL. Local and systemic reactions to the parenteral administration of vitamin E. *Dev Pharmacol Ther* 1981;2 (3):156–171.

632. Centers for Disease Control. Unusual syndrome with fatalities among premature infants: association with a new intravenous vitamin E product. *MMWR Morb Mortal Wkly Rep* 1984;33: 198–199.

633. Bodenstein CJ. Intravenous vitamin E and deaths in the intensive care unit. *Pediatrics* 1984;73(5):733.

634. Balistreri WF, Farrell MK, Bove KE. Lessons from the E-Ferol tragedy. *Pediatrics* 1986;78(3):503–506.

635. Martone WJ, Williams WW, Mortensen ML, et al. Illness with fatalities in premature infants: association with an intravenous vitamin E preparation, E-Ferol. *Pediatrics* 1986;78 (4):591–600.

636. American Academy of Pediatrics Committee on Fetus and Newborn. Vitamin E and the prevention of retinopathy of prematurity. *Pediatrics* 1985;76:315–316.

637. American Academy of Pediatrics Committee on Drugs. Transfer of drugs and other chemicals into human milk. *Pediatrics* 1994;93:137–150.

638. Berlin CM Jr. Pharmacologic considerations of drug use in the lactating mother. *Obstet Gynecol* 1981;58[Suppl 5]:17S–23S.

639. Berlin CM. The excretion of drugs in human milk. *Prog Clin Biol Res* 1980;36:115–127.

640. Berlin CM Jr. Drugs and chemicals: exposure of the nursing mother. *Pediatr Clin North Am* 1989;36(5):1089–1097.

641. American Academy of Pediatrics Committee on Drugs. Transfer of drugs and other chemicals into human milk. *Pediatrics* 2001;108:776–789.

57

Anesthesia and Analgesia in the Neonate

Sally H. Vitali   Anthony J. Camerota   John H. Arnold

Despite the widespread use of potent analgesic agents in adult patients and older children, it is remarkable that, until recently, systemic analgesia and sedation were rarely administered to neonates. An analysis of neonatal anesthetic practice published in 1985 revealed that only 23% of preterm infants undergoing patent ductus arteriosus ligation received adequate intraoperative anesthesia (1). In a retrospective survey of opioid use in a single institution, only 14% of 933 neonates received opioid analgesia after a variety of surgical procedures (2). However, in a 1995 questionnaire, all neonates received either systemic opioids and/or regional anesthesia for major surgery (3). Although appreciation and management of operative and postoperative pain in neonates has improved, use of analgesia for nonoperative painful procedures remains limited. Despite evidence that premedication reduces the pain and physiologic instability associated with awake direct laryngoscopy and endotracheal intubation in neonates, surveys in the United States, Canada, and Great Britain indicate that premedication is rare even in nonemergent intubations in neonatal intensive care units (4–7). Circumcision is another known source of neonatal pain that can be reduced with premedication, but a 1998 survey of residency programs teaching circumcision training practices indicated that 26% of programs teaching circumcision provided no training in anesthesia and analgesia for the procedure (8). A recent consensus statement by the American Academy of Pediatrics and Canadian Pediatric Society recognizes the recent improvement in neonatal pain assessment and management but concludes that "prevention and treatment of unnecessary pain attributable to anticipated noxious stimuli remain limited" (9).

Although adequate anesthesia and analgesia were not given to neonates in the past because of the belief that they could not feel pain, there is overwhelming evidence that pain perception and physiologic responses to stress occur in neonates of all gestational ages (10). It is broadly accepted that anesthesia and analgesia in the neonatal population have important clinical and physiologic consequences and may have long-term psychologic impact. Control of the stress response in the perioperative period may improve the outcome of infants after cardiac surgery (11,12). Appropriate analgesia and sedation are proven means of reducing catabolism associated with surgery and recovery from surgery, illness, and injury (13). Human and animal studies have found compelling evidence that early pain and stress affect nociception and behavioral responses to pain later in life, but the conflicting results of these studies leave the nature and mechanism of these long-term effects largely unexplained (14,15). Given that critically ill preterm neonates have been reported to experience as many as 488 painful procedures during their stay in neonatal intensive care units, pain and its management may have profound implications for the health of these children (16).

As these data are assimilated and accepted, there is often a discrepancy between the growing understanding of neonatal pain and actual clinical practice. A survey of British pediatric anesthetists found that only 5% routinely prescribed systemic opioids to neonates postoperatively, although 80% of the respondents believed that neonates feel pain (17). There are probably several reasons for the lag in changing clinical practice to match current knowledge, but a crucial element may be the lack of standard guidelines for the use of drugs, doses, and schedules that can be applied to various clinical situations by the practitioner at the bedside. The International Evidence-Based Group for Neonatal Pain summarized the current evidence for a set of standard guidelines in 2001; the impact of these guidelines on clinical practice remains to be studied (18).

This chapter reviews the rapidly developing field of neonatal anesthesia and analgesia, summarizes the relevant pharmacokinetic and pharmacodynamic data, and highlights practical considerations for the most commonly used agents.

PAIN PERCEPTION

In addition to the ethic arguments for preventing needless human suffering, the risks and benefits of using anesthesia and analgesia to prevent pain and stress must be physiologically evaluated. Pivotal aspects of this physiologic rationale are based on one question: Does the neonate feel pain?

Components of the pain system may be traced from sensory receptors in the skin to sensory areas in the cerebral cortex and used as a framework to study its development (4). The density of nociceptive nerve endings in newborn skin, labeling of specific proteins (e.g., GAP-43) produced by axonal growth cones, reflex activity and receptive fields of primary afferent neurons, and development of synapses between primary afferents and interneurons in the dorsal horn of the spinal cord indicate the anatomic and functional maturity of the peripheral pain system during fetal life (19,20). Cellular and subcellular organization in the dorsal horn, with maturation of primary afferent terminations, occur during later in gestation and postnatally (21,22). In the dorsal horn, various neurotransmitter and neuromodulatory substances associated with pain (e.g., substance P, somatostatin, calcitonin gene-related peptide, vasoactive intestinal peptide, met-enkephalin, glutamate) appear during early gestation (23).

Lack of myelination in neonatal nerves or central nerve tracts is offset completely by the shorter interneuronal and neuromuscular distances traveled by the impulses. Quantitative neuroanatomic data show that nociceptive nerve tracts in the spinal cord and central nervous system undergo complete myelination during the second and third trimesters of gestation (10). Subcortical foci associated with nociception are characterized by a high density of opioid receptors during the middle of gestation, with a differential reduction in binding capacities during the third trimester (24). Development of the fetal neocortex begins at 8 weeks of gestation; by 20 weeks, each cortex has a full complement of 109 neurons. Arborization of dendritic processes in the cortical neurons is followed by synaptogenesis with incoming thalamocortical fibers by 24 to 26 weeks of gestation. Functional maturity of the cerebral cortex is suggested by fetal and neonatal electroencephalographic patterns, cortical somatosensory-evoked potentials, studies of regional cerebral metabolism, early behavioral development, and the specific behavioral responses of neonates to painful stimuli (10,25).

Endorphinergic cells in the anterior pituitary are responsive to corticotrophin-releasing factor stimulation *in vitro* and show increased β-endorphin production during fetal and neonatal life. Endogenous opioids and other hormones (e.g., catecholamines, steroid hormones, glucagon, growth hormone) are secreted by the human fetus in response to stress, leading to catabolism and other complications (12,26). Significant changes in cardiovascular parameters, transcutaneous partial pressure of oxygen, and palmar sweating have been observed in neonates undergoing painful clinical procedures. These physiologic changes are closely associated with behavioral responses of newborns to pain. Neonatal behavioral responses are characterized by simple motor responses, precise changes in facial expression associated with pain, highly specific patterns of crying activity, and a variety of complex behavioral changes. These neonatal responses suggest integrated emotional and behavioral changes correlated with pain, and they are retained in memory long enough to modify subsequent behavior patterns (10).

The surgical stress responses of neonates can be inhibited by potent anesthesia, as demonstrated by randomized trials of halothane anesthesia in term neonates, fentanyl anesthesia in preterm neonates, and sufentanil anesthesia in neonates undergoing cardiac surgery (12,27,28). These results imply that the nociceptive stimuli during surgery are at least partially responsible for the marked stress responses of neonates and are prevented by the provision of adequate anesthesia. In these trials, the reduction in surgical stress responses was associated with significant improvements in clinical outcome, supporting the use of potent anesthetic agents for newborns undergoing surgery. In contrast, a recent randomized, double-blind study of fentanyl bolus, fentanyl infusion, and fentanyl-midazolam infusion in infants less than 6 months old undergoing cardiac surgery found that these anesthetic regimens did not blunt the metabolic and hormonal responses to surgical stress, yet no adverse postoperative outcomes were observed. These findings indicate that improvements in clinical outcome observed in previous trials may have been related to factors other than reduction in surgical stress (29).

In recent years, the concept of blunting the pain response in neonates to improve physiologic parameters has been extended from the operating room to the intensive care unit. High-dose narcotic anesthesia for the first postoperative night after complex cardiac surgery reduces mortality (6,30,31). Using narcotics during painful procedures, such as tracheal suctioning, has been shown to reduce concomitant hypoxemia (32). Fentanyl infusions have been shown to decrease plasma stress hormone levels in preterm infants (33). A multicenter pilot study of 67 premature infants randomized to midazolam (0.2 mg/kg loading dose followed by 0.02 to 0.06 mg/kg/hour infusion), morphine (0.1 mg/kg loading dose followed by 0.01 to 0.03 mg/kg/hour infusion), or 10% dextrose for up to 14 days of mechanic ventilation showed improvement in pain scores and neurologic outcome in the morphine-treated infants, but a much larger trial will be required before this practice can be universally recommended (34).

ANESTHESIA

Anesthesia is classically defined as a drug-induced state that includes analgesia, amnesia, and muscle relaxation.

The provision of anesthesia to infants undergoing surgical procedures has gone through a remarkable transition coincident with the development of new intravenous agents and more sophisticated monitoring techniques. As recently as 1985, there was considerable debate about whether neonates feel pain, and sophisticated researchers advocated the use of minimal anesthesia in neonates undergoing surgical procedures, citing the dangers of anesthetic administration to this population (35–37). Beginning with the landmark paper of Robinson and Gregory (38), practitioners of neonatal and pediatric anesthesia have proclaimed the importance of providing adequate anesthesia, particularly to ill preterm infants (38,39). In modern anesthetic practice, adequate anesthetic depth and control of the neonatal stress response can be achieved without undue risk to the infant.

The appropriate anesthetic technique is dictated by the preoperative condition of the patient, planned surgical procedure, and skills of the anesthetist. The encounter between the anesthesiologist and neonate usually occurs in the setting of a surgical emergency, and a general anesthetic with control of the airway is most often the technique of choice. General anesthesia is provided using a combination of inhaled and intravenous agents and muscle relaxants. The inhaled agents include an inorganic gas (e.g., nitrous oxide) and volatile liquids (e.g., halothane, enflurane, isoflurane, sevoflurane, and desflurane). Delivery of potent inhaled agents by means of the respiratory system offers a reliable route of administration and excretion with the ability to rapidly alter anesthetic concentrations in the central nervous system.

Inhaled Anesthetics

Each of the inhaled anesthetic agents has unique effects on the cardiovascular, respiratory, and central nervous systems, which are not exhaustively reviewed here (Table 57-1). The volatile anesthetics produce dose-dependent decreases in mean arterial blood pressure, particularly in premature infants, due to direct myocardial depression, and decreases in systemic vascular resistance due to exaggerated depression of the baroreceptor reflex (40–42). Nitrous oxide produces minimal alterations in myocardial performance or

systemic vascular resistance, due in part to direct stimulation of the sympathetic nervous system (43). However, if combined with a potent volatile agent or opioids, nitrous oxide significantly depresses myocardial contractility (44). If ventilation is carefully controlled, nitrous oxide has insignificant effects on pulmonary vascular resistance (45).

All inhaled agents increase the respiratory rate, reduce tidal volume and functional residual capacity, decrease the ventilatory responses to hypoxemia and hypercapnia, and decrease bronchial smooth muscle reactivity. These agents produce a dose-dependent increase in cerebral blood flow despite simultaneous depression of cerebral metabolic oxygen requirement. At high concentrations, isoflurane and desflurane induce an isoelectric electroencephalographic pattern; this property is not shared by the other inhaled anesthetic agents.

Although halothane is most frequently associated with perioperative hepatic dysfunction, other inhaled agents and intravenous anesthetics may result in hepatic necrosis (46). True halothane-induced hepatitis is a rare event, occurring in approximately 1 of 30,000 patients. It is seen most commonly after repeated administration and is probably mediated by an immune mechanism involving an intermediate oxidative metabolite (47,48). The inhaled agents produce dose-related decreases in renal blood flow and urine output due to effects on cardiac output and systemic vascular resistance. Fluoride-induced nephrotoxicity is a potential complication of prolonged exposure to the fluorinated hydrocarbons (e.g., enflurane, isoflurane), although it is of practical concern only during prolonged administration of enflurane and sevoflurane (49,50).

Two newer inhaled anesthetics, sevoflurane and desflurane, are gaining popularity due to their low lipid solubility (51). This property allows for rapid induction of anesthesia as well as a short recovery time. Sevoflurane has the advantage of providing a smooth, less irritating induction of anesthesia that rivals that of halothane, with less risk of hepatitis and fewer hemodynamic effects (52,53). The drawbacks are the biotransformation of sevoflurane into potentially toxic Compound A (2-fluoromethoxy-1,1,3, 3,3-pentafluoro-1-propene) and the accumulation of fluoride ions (54,55). As in adults, inhaled sevoflurane has been shown to prolong the QTc interval in infants, an

TABLE 57-1
SYSTEMIC EFFECTS OF INHALED ANESTHETICS

	Myocardial Function	Heart Rate	Systemic Vascular Resistance	Cerebral Blood Flow
Halothane	– –	– –	+/–	++
Enflurane	–	+	–	+
Isoflurane	–	++	– –	+/– [a]
N₂O	+/–	+/–	–/–	+/–
Desflurane	–	++	– –	+/– [a]
Sevoflurane	–	+/–	+/–	+/– [a]

[a] In doses <1.0 minimum alveolar concentration.
++, greatly increased; +, moderately increased; +/– no consistent effect; –, moderately decreased; – –, greatly decreased.

effect that lasts at least 60 minutes into the postoperative period (56). Desflurane does not undergo biodegradation *in vivo* or *in vitro*, but its irritating effects on the airway prevent its role as an induction agent (57,58).

Opioid Anesthesia

Morphine and the synthetic opioids have been a consistent adjunct to the volatile agents throughout the history of anesthesia. High-dose opioids have become the preferred anesthetic technique for cardiac surgical procedures in adults and children (59,60). The virtues of opioids include minimal effects on myocardial performance, ablation of pulmonary vascular responses to nociceptive stimuli, and preservation of hypoxic pulmonary vasoconstriction (61–63).

Because of their wide margin of safety in ill infants with congenital heart disease, opioid anesthesia is often effective in ill preterm infants with cardiopulmonary instability undergoing surgical stress. Fentanyl, sufentanil, and remifentanil are the most popular agents due to their negligible effect on cardiovascular function, but if combined with other anesthetic agents, these opioids may be associated with significant hemodynamic instability. Morphine anesthesia may increase plasma histamine concentrations and decrease vascular resistance, and it is not recommended as a primary anesthetic for ill neonates (64).

The elimination half-lives of most opioids are variable but significantly prolonged in the neonate (Table 57-2) and may be further prolonged by any compromise of hepatic blood flow (65–70). The exception to this rule is the synthetic opioid remifentanil; a recent study in children showed that clearance was as much as twice as rapid in infants from birth to 2 years than in older children, and half-life was similar in all age groups studied (71). Premature infants have an even more prolonged morphine clearance than term newborns that shortens with postconceptual age (72). Prolonged postoperative respiratory depression may occur if these important pharmacokinetic variables are ignored in the perioperative period.

Regional, Neuraxial, and Local Anesthesia

Regional anesthetic techniques have become increasingly popular in the pediatric and neonatal populations (73). General anesthesia may be associated with an increased incidence of postoperative apnea in the preterm infant (74). This may be a particularly difficult issue in the day-surgery setting, where former preterm neonates commonly present for minor surgical procedures (e.g., circumcision, herniorrhaphy). It is in this population that regional or local anesthetic techniques may be particularly advantageous. The use of spinal anesthesia for herniorrhaphy decreases the need for postoperative mechanic ventilation in former preterm infants matched for gestational age at birth and incidence of bronchopulmonary dysplasia (75). Epidural anesthesia has been shown to reduce the need for postoperative ventilation after both esophageal atresia repair and Nissen fundoplication (76,77).

Spinal anesthesia consists of injection of an anesthetic agent into the subarachnoid space. The technique is easy to perform and safe (78,79). The most frequent local anesthetic agents are hyperbaric lidocaine, tetracaine, and bupivacaine. Side effects of spinal anesthesia, such as dural puncture headaches and hemodynamic compromise, are common in adults but surprisingly uncommon in infants or children (78,80).

Epidural anesthesia consists of a single injection or repeated injections through an epidural catheter of an anesthetic agent into the potential space between the dura mater and ligamentum flavum. The advantage epidural has over spinal anesthesia is the potential for long-term, continuous, or intermittent administration of anesthetics. Although the epidural space can be approached at any level, for most infants, a lumbar or caudal epidural blockade is used. Caudally inserted epidural catheters can also be advanced to the thoracic region and dilute local anesthetic solutions applied for thoracic-level anesthesia in infants, but radiographic confirmation of tip placement has been shown to be important for safety (81). Caudal epidural blockade with bupivacaine is used most frequently for postoperative pain relief after lower abdominal and lower extremity procedures. Compared with older children and adults, infants and toddlers require higher doses of local anesthetic and demonstrate a shorter duration of effect. Combining local anesthetics with an epidural opioid (fentanyl, hydromorphone), clonidine, or ketamine prolongs the duration of analgesia (82). Several case reports have suggested that epidural clonidine may contribute to postoperative apnea in the former preterm infant (83–85). Caudal anesthesia has been sufficient as

---

TABLE 57-2

ELIMINATION HALF-LIVES OF OPIOIDS

	Opioid Relative Dose	Preterm	Neonate	Child
Morphine	0.1 mg	9–10 h	6.8 h	2.2 h
Fentanyl	1–5 μg	6–32 h	4.2 h	3.5 h
Sufentanil	0.2–1 μg	N/A	12.3 h	2.3 h
Alfentanil	5–25 μg	N/A	8.8 h	1.4 h
Remifentanil	0.25–1 μg	N/A	3–10 min	3–10 min

N/A, unknown.

the sole anesthetic technique for lower abdominal procedures (86). Caudal epidural blockade may be used in combination with general anesthesia in infants during abdominal procedures. Complications rarely result from improper placement of the needle and injection of the anesthetic agent into a vein, the dura, the subarachnoid space, or sacral marrow.

Local anesthetics may be used to block peripheral nerves in infants undergoing limited surgical procedures (e.g., orchiopexy, herniorrhaphy, circumcision). These techniques are simple to perform, have limited complications, and significantly decrease the need for postoperative analgesia (87–89).

Local anesthetic toxicity is manifested by effects on the cardiovascular system (e.g., myocardial depression, arrhythmias) and central nervous system (e.g., delirium, seizures) (90,91). In premature infants, the subtle behavioral changes that precede cardiovascular collapse and generalized seizures may be difficult to recognize. The reduced protein binding and prolonged elimination of local anesthetics in this population make the neonate susceptible to toxic effects at lower doses, decreasing the therapeutic index. Careful attention to total administered dose (particularly with field blocks) and monitoring of cardiovascular parameters during the administration of any local anesthetic are essential.

The topical anesthetic EMLA, a eutectic mixture of 2.5% lidocaine and 2.5% prilocaine, has shown efficacy in neonatal circumcisions (92,93), but two randomized, controlled trials have shown that dorsal penile nerve block is more effective than EMLA (94,95). EMLA is not effective in reducing pain with heel sticks, perhaps owing to the incidental vasoconstriction associated with EMLA which may require more vigorous squeezing to obtain a blood sample (96). Oral sucrose has been shown to be more effective than EMLA as analgesia for neonatal venipuncture in two randomized, controlled trials (97,98). Although methemoglobinemia is a potential side effect of EMLA, it appears to be safe even in preterm infants (99,100). A newer topical agent, amethocaine, in a 4% gel, avoids the possibility of methemoglobinemia, and its vasodilatory effects on the skin may facilitate blood sampling (101).

Propofol

Propofol, as a loading dose of 2 to 4 mg/kg, acts as a complete anesthetic with a short recovery period, similar to or even briefer than the lipid-soluble pentothal. A continuous infusion of 50 to 100 mg/kg/minute maintains anesthesia and may, when discontinued, have a shorter recovery time than that of inhalation agents. However, prolonged infusions lead to lipid deposition and persistent anesthetic effects of propofol, even with discontinuation. A recent study of propofol infusions in neonates, infants, and children showed that most newborns and children have similar propofol pharmacokinetics as adults, but that elimination is prolonged in children after cardiac surgery and in low-birth-weight infants (102). Postoperative emesis and

analgesic requirements may be reduced with propofol versus pentothal–halothane. Pain at the infusion site has limited the enthusiasm for propofol. Pain can be alleviated by adding 0.2 mg/kg of lidocaine for every 3 mg/kg of propofol. The incidence of hypotension with propofol is comparable to similar agents.

Prolonged propofol infusion (3 to 5 days) has been linked to metabolic acidosis, heart failure, and death in critically ill children. Associated with these have been lipemic serum and fatty infiltration of the liver (103). Propofol may be used during the course of some anesthetics, but a recent, unpublished clinical trial showed a significantly increased mortality in children sedated with propofol, and as a result, its use for sedation of children younger than 16 years is contraindicated (104).

ANALGESIA

Opioids

The provision of adequate analgesia for painful diseases and procedures should be of utmost concern to the neonatologist (105). Despite widespread misgivings about their potential side effects, systemic therapy with opioid analgesics remains the mainstay of treatment for severe pain in neonates. The administration of opioids produces profound analgesia and sedation through specific activity on μ_1, δ, and other opioid receptors in the brain and spinal cord (106).

The dosage and mode of administration of opioids should be carefully titrated to avoid undertreatment of pain or oversedation (Fig. 57-1). Continuous intravenous infusion of opioids provides an effective alternative to intermittent intravenous doses, with constant blood levels and minimal fluctuations in analgesia. Nearly all opioids have prolonged half-lives in neonates (Table 57-2), and continuous infusions can result in a slow accumulation of the drug over time, with high blood levels that may not be considered or detected immediately. In addition, morphine has an active metabolite that can accumulate in renal insufficiency, compounding the narcotic effect. Despite this disadvantage, continuous intravenous infusion is ideal for providing a constant level of analgesia if appropriate precautions are observed.

A newer agent, remifentanil, is quickly degraded by red cell and tissue esterases, giving it an elimination half-life of about 3 minutes. Unlike the other opioids, its brief duration of action is maintained, even after prolonged continuous infusions (107). A study of remifentanil pharmacokinetics in neonates showed a similar half-life as in older children (71).

Alternative modes of administration are rarely indicated in neonates. Subcutaneous morphine or fentanyl, given as a lozenge or transdermally, is not routinely used in neonates because precise documentation of their efficacy and safety is not available. The transdermal route may be an attractive future alternative to intravenous infusions in premature neonates, particularly because the permeability

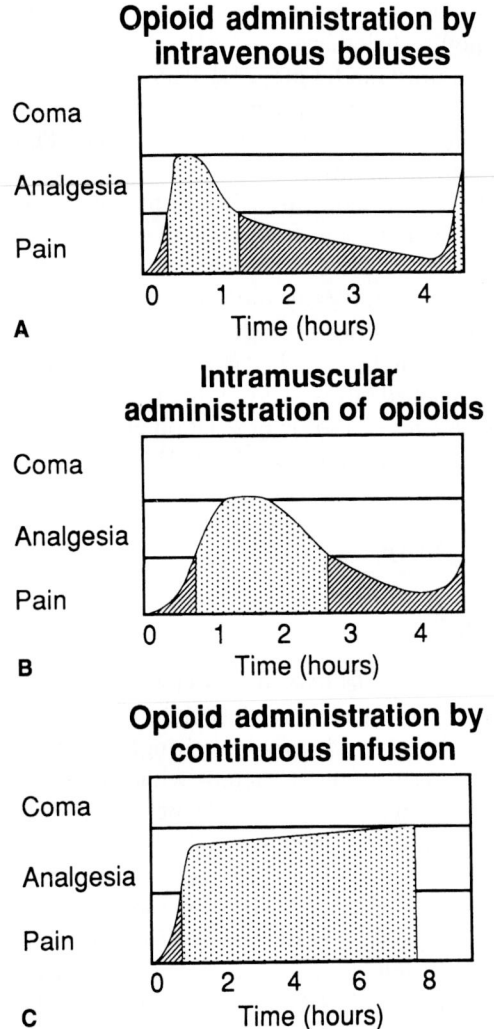

Opioid administration by intravenous boluses

Coma

Analgesia

Pain

0   1   2   3   4

Time (hours)

A

Intramuscular administration of opioids

Coma

Analgesia

Pain

0   1   2   3   4

Time (hours)

B

Opioid administration by continuous infusion

Coma

Analgesia

Pain

0   2   4   6   8

Time (hours)

C

Figure 57-1 Modes of opioid administration. **A:** Patients given intermittent intravenous boluses every 4 hours experience deep sedative effects at peak levels after a dose, with prolonged periods of pain between doses. **B:** Patients given intramuscular injections experience less fluctuation in opioid effects but undergo alternate periods of pain and analgesia. **C:** Patients receiving continuous infusions of opioids experience constant analgesia but are at risk for a slow build-up in plasma levels, resulting in sedation or toxicity. (Adapted from Berde CB. Pediatric postoperative pain management. *Pediatr Clin North Am* 1989;36:921–940, with permission.)

of preterm skin is 102 to 103 times greater than the skin of term neonates (108). Oral or rectal opioids can be used in the neonate, but only if the same close monitoring provided for intravenous opioid analgesia can be given to these patients. The oral bioavailabilities of commonly used opioids are listed in Table 57-3, although these data have been derived mostly from older children and adults. The pharmacokinetics of oral opioids have not been studied in neonates, but the onset and duration of action are likely to be delayed, and close monitoring should continue for at least 24 hours after the last dose.

Opioid side effects include respiratory depression, tolerance and dependence, alterations in chest wall compliance, decreased gastrointestinal motility, and nausea. Exogenously administered opioids may alter endogenous

opioid receptor physiology and possibly influence subsequent behavioral development (24,109,110). Chronic opioid administration also has immunosuppressive effects through both direct (immune cell receptors) and indirect (centrally mediated) mechanisms (111). However, these agents are probably the most suitable and effective analgesics currently available for treatment of severe pain in neonates.

All opioids produce dose-related respiratory depression characterized by decreased ventilatory and behavioral responses to hypoxemia and hypercarbia. The carbon dioxide response curve is displaced to the right and resting partial pressure of carbon dioxide rises. Clinically, the respiratory rate decreases with an incomplete compensatory increase in tidal volume. It is not widely appreciated that standard doses of morphine (0.1 mg/kg) almost abolish the ventilatory response to hypoxemia. In patients with airway obstruction or atelectasis after surgery, blunting of hypoxic drive can lead to dangerous hypoventilation. Opioid-induced respiratory depression can be reversed with naloxone, but the effect of this drug diminishes within 30 minutes, and repeated dosing may be required, particularly after the use of morphine or methadone (112). It was long believed that newborn infants were more prone than older children or adults to opioid-induced respiratory depression, perhaps because of an immature blood–brain barrier (113). It has been shown that opioid-induced apnea is less common in neonates than in older infants and children at similar plasma concentrations (114,115). Neonates conjugate morphine into morphine-6-glucuronide and morphine-3-glucuronide. Compared with infants and older children, however, the neonate produces less of the 6-glucuronide metabolite. Morphine-6-glucuronide is a more potent analgesic than morphine itself, and it induces less apnea. The more plentiful metabolite in the neonate, morphine-3-glucuronide, may actually antagonize the effects of its parent molecule, morphine (116,117). This may partially explain the susceptibility of the neonate to morphine-induced apnea.

Tolerance occurs if there is a reduction in the clinical effects of a drug with repeated administration. The rate of development of tolerance to the analgesic effects of opioids is extremely variable. There is evidence that tolerance may develop more rapidly in the absence of nociceptive stimulation (118). Dependence is the requirement for continued drug administration to prevent withdrawal symptoms, including agitation, dysphoria, tachycardia, tachypnea, piloerection, nasal congestion, temperature instability, and feeding intolerance. Tolerance and dependence have been described in neonatal and pediatric patients during the therapeutic use of opioids (119–122). Although tolerance to opioids may appear to develop more rapidly in neonates than at other ages, it is likely that tolerance to the sedative and cardiovascular effects of opioids may precede a tolerance to their analgesic effects (123). The predominance of the antagonistic morphine-3-glucuronide metabolite in infants may help explain their more rapid development of tolerance to morphine (124). Opioid

TABLE 57-3

RECOMMENDED DOSAGES AND ORAL/PARENTERAL RATIOS FOR OPIOIDS

Drug	Routes of Administration	Parental Dosage (mg/kg)	Frequency (Parenteral)	Oral/Parenteral Ratio	Frequency (Oral/Rectal)
Morphine	IM, IV,[a] SQ, po, pr, neuraxial[b]	0.05–0.2	q 1–2 h IV; q 2–4 h IM or SQ	3–6	q 4–6 h[c]; q 8–12 h[d]
Meperidine	IM, IV, SQ, po	0.5–1.5	q 1–2 h IV; q 2–4 h IM or SQ	4	q 4–6 h
Codeine	IM, IV,[a] SQ, po	0.5–1.0	q 2–4 h	1.5–2	q 4–6 h
Hydromorphone	IM, IV, SQ, po, pr	0.02–0.04	q 2–4 h	2–4	q 4–6 h po; q 6–8 h PR
Methadone	IM, IV, SQ, po	0.05–0.2	q 12–24 h	2	q 24 h
Fentanyl	IM, IV, TM/TD,[e] neuraxial[b]	0.0005–0.003	q 1–2 h		

IM, intramuscular; IV, intravenous; po, oral; pr, rectal; SQ, subcutaneous; TM/TD, transmucosal/transdermal.
[a] IV administration may be associated with significant histamine release and possible hypotension.
[b] Neuraxial (i.e., epidural, subarachnoid) administration can be performed only by qualified and experienced anesthesiologists.
[c] Pertains to regular oral preparations (e.g., MSIR, Roxanal; tablets and oral solutions).
[d] Pertains to slow-release oral or rectal preparations (e.g., MS Contin, Duramorph, Roxanol SR).
[e] TM/TD preparations have not been standardized for use in full-term or preterm neonates.

tolerance may develop more rapidly with continuous infusions as compared with intermittent dosing (123,125). The development of physical dependence is quite variable, and withdrawal symptoms have been observed in infants in whom opioid administration was discontinued abruptly after periods of administration as short as 5 days (121). Fear of precipitating the abstinence syndrome should not inhibit the appropriate administration of opioids because withdrawal symptoms can be effectively managed by gradually tapering the opioid dosage over 5 to 7 days (Fig. 57-2).

Dependence is a set of physiologic responses that should be differentiated from addiction, which is a behavioral syndrome of compulsive drug seeking. Addiction is extremely rare in patients of all ages receiving opioids for pain or sedation, and fear of addiction should not affect the appropriate treatment of acute pain or agitation in neonatal intensive care.

Opioids increase airway resistance, and there is much debate about the effect of histamine release on bronchial

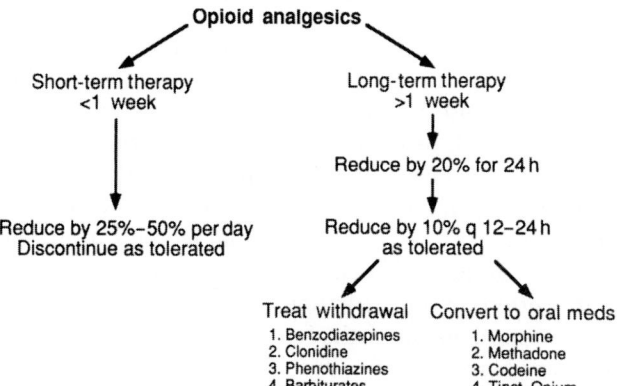

Figure 57-2 Suggested algorithm for weaning a patient from opioid analgesics after short- and long-term therapy. These pharmacologic approaches can be applied in conjunction with nonpharmacologic therapies to decrease the duration of therapy for the opioid abstinence syndrome.

smooth muscle and whether histamine-releasing agents such as morphine are contraindicated in patients with reactive airway disease (126). Although intravenous morphine releases greater amounts of histamine than fentanyl, precipitation of bronchospasm has not been reported after the administration of morphine (64). Intravenous morphine has been used frequently in patients with severe asthma requiring mechanic ventilation, based on evidence that it might inhibit bronchoconstriction and mucous hypersecretion (127–129).

Chest-wall rigidity is a well-described complication of opioid administration and has been documented in patients receiving large doses of fentanyl, sufentanil, or alfentanil (44,130,131). The administration of 30 mg/kg of fentanyl in tracheostomized patients produced a minor increase in total lung compliance, suggesting that inability to maintain a mask airway during fentanyl administration is due to supraglottic obstruction and not chest-wall rigidity (132,133). Rigidity has occurred at an average dose of 15 to 17 mg/kg of fentanyl (132,133). There are no controlled data available in term or preterm neonates receiving fentanyl. However, clinical experience indicates that chest-wall rigidity may occur at significantly lower opioid doses in the neonate. The mechanism that mediates this phenomenon may involve μ_1 opioid receptor modulation of gamma-aminobutyric acid pathways in the spinal cord. Rigidity on induction of anesthesia is avoided by pretreatment with a subrelaxant dose of pancuronium (0.01 to 0.02 mg/kg) and by slow intravenous infusion of the opioid (130, 134,135).

All opioids delay gastric emptying, decrease intestinal motility, produce nausea by direct stimulation of the chemoreceptor trigger zone, and increase common bile duct pressure. Impaired absorption of enteral nutrients is undesirable in neonates, and opiate-induced ileus may increase the risk of regurgitation and aspiration of gastric contents. One case report described a newborn given morphine who developed a reversible and nonobstructive dilation of the common hepatic duct that resolved after morphine was discontinued (136). Although such side effects are mediated by means of μ_2 opioid receptors, they may occur with high doses of opioids devoid of μ_2 activity (e.g., fentanyl) as a result of nonspecific effects on all opioid receptors.

Nonopioid Agents

There are many nonopioid agents available for the treatment of mild pain or use as adjuvants for decreasing the doses and potential side effects of opioid drugs. Various other analgesic agents can be used systemically for providing sedation or in combination with regional and topical analgesia to produce effective analgesia while minimizing the side effects of any single agent.

Acetaminophen

Acetaminophen (N-acetyl-p-aminophenol) is used commonly in all age groups as an antipyretic and analgesic. Its use in neonates has been limited by misconceptions about its metabolism, excretion, and potential for hepatotoxicity. Experimental data and clinical experience have supported the relative safety and analgesic efficacy of acetaminophen in newborn infants, without the significant side effects on platelet aggregation, the ductus arteriosus, or the gastric mucosa, commonly seen with aspirin or other nonsteroidal antiinflammatory drugs (NSAIDs) (137).

The hepatic metabolism of acetaminophen occurs primarily by sulfation or glucuronidation, but a small fraction is oxidized by the cytochrome P450 mixed-function oxidase system into an arene compound (i.e., a reactive metabolite), which is conjugated with glutathione before excretion (138,139). In acute toxicity, the hepatic stores of glutathione are depleted rapidly, and this reactive metabolite binds irreversibly to membrane proteins, leading to liver cell necrosis. In the newborn or fetal liver, this metabolic pathway is seven to ten times slower than in the adult liver and occurs well after the development of glutathione synthesis, mediating a protective effect in fetal hepatocytes (140). These experimental data have been substantiated by the absence of hepatic dysfunction in clinical reports of neonatal poisoning with acetaminophen (141,142). The clinical use of acetaminophen in term or preterm neonates should not be overly restrained by concerns about its potential hepatotoxicity.

Acetaminophen has many potential advantages as an analgesic in neonates. It has approximately the same analgesic efficacy as 0.5 to 1.0 mg/kg of codeine, and the analgesia is generally thought to be additive to that provided by opioids. It is effective at reducing pain after circumcision but does not reduce the pain with heel stick (143,144). Recent data from a randomized, double-blind, controlled trial indicate that prophylactic use of rectal acetaminophen up to 40 mg/kg for elective cleft-palate repair had no opioid-sparing effect in the immediate postoperative period

and failed to produce therapeutic serum acetaminophen levels, calling into question both the dosing of rectal acetaminophen in the operative period and its additive effects with the opioids (145). Acetaminophen produces no respiratory depression, and tolerance to acetaminophen-induced analgesia has not been reported. It can be given rectally in doses of 20 to 25 mg/kg, avoiding the need for intravenous lines in infants who cannot be given oral medications.

Nonsteroidal Antiinflammatory Drugs

The NSAIDs are a group of drugs with many actions, including potent analgesic and antiinflammatory properties. The antiinflammatory effects are mediated through inhibition of prostaglandin synthesis by means of the cyclooxygenase pathway. Several NSAIDs have been used in pediatric patients, although data pertaining to neonates are scarce and come from uncontrolled clinical reports (146). Indomethacin and ibuprofen are the most commonly prescribed NSAIDs, but drugs such as ketorolac tromethamine, tolmetin, and naproxen are being used with increasing frequency.

The toxicity of NSAIDs limits their potency and clinical usefulness as analgesics (147). Major toxicity is related to gastrointestinal bleeding, hepatotoxicity, blood dyscrasias, decreased renal and splanchnic perfusion, and severe skin reactions. Because of the chemical diversity of NSAIDs, adverse reactions to a particular NSAID do not predict similar reactions to other drugs in the class. Significant advantages include the low incidence of side effects in judicious analgesic doses (Table 57-4), absence of respiratory depression or sedative effects, relatively long duration of analgesia, and lack of tolerance or potential for abuse. Selective cyclooxygenase-2 (COX-2) inhibitors are designed to avoid the gastrointestinal and antiplatelet side effects of the classic NSAIDs, but these have not been studied in infants or children.

NONPHARMACOLOGIC TECHNIQUES

Neonatal pain may be reduced by using a variety of nonpharmacologic methods. Several studies have shown that intraoral sucrose or glucose is effective for reducing pain associated with procedures such as heel stick, circumcision, venipuncture, and subcutaneous injection in term and preterm infants (148–152). The antinociceptive effects of sucrose appear to be opioid receptor mediated. Sucrose's antinociceptive properties in rats can be reversed with naltrexone administration (153). However, neonates born to mothers on methadone do not appear to derive analgesic benefits from sucrose (154). Infant formula and its components (protein, fat, sucrose, but not lactose) also have shown antinociceptive properties (155). In a randomized, controlled trial, breastfeeding has been shown to reduce pain associated with newborn heel stick as much as sucking glucose on a pacifier (156).

TABLE 57-4
RECOMMENDED DOSES FOR NONSTEROIDAL ANTIINFLAMMATORY DRUGS

Drug	Dosage (mg/kg)	Routes of Administration	Frequency
Acetaminophen	10–15	po, pr	q 4–6 h
Aspirin	10–15	po	q 4 h
Choline-magnesium trisalicylate	10–15	po	q 6–8 h
Ibuprofen	5–15	po, pr	q 6–8 h
Naprosyn	5–7	po	q 8–12 h
Tolectin	5–7	po	q 8–12 h
Ketorolac tromethamine	0.3–0.6	po, IM, IV	q 6–8 h

IM, intramuscular; IV, intravenous; po, oral; pr, rectal.

Facilitated tucking, by holding the neonate's extremities flexed and close to the trunk, lowered the heart rate and produced less crying (157). Nonnutritive sucking, enhanced by the use of a pacifier, reduces the physiologic response to circumcision pain and is synergistic with the effects of intraoral glucose or sucrose (151,158). Clearly, nonpharmacologic techniques to reduce pain should be sought whenever possible because of their effectiveness coupled with a rarity of side effects.

SEDATION

The goals of sedation in the intensive care unit include analgesia for painful diseases and procedures and compliance with controlled ventilation and routine care. The ideal agent would not have hemodynamic or pulmonary side effects and would not be associated with the production or accumulation of toxic metabolites. It would have a short duration of action and a high therapeutic index. The wide variety of medications and combinations of agents that have been used suggests that no single agent meets this ideal standard. Opioids have become exceeding popular due to their relatively high toxic-to-therapeutic ratio, reported lack of side effects, and potent analgesic properties. Although opioids are considered the mainstay of sedation in the intensive care setting, tolerance to their sedating effects may occur rapidly, and adequate sedation for prolonged periods can be ensured only by administration of adjuvant sedative agents (121,159).

Benzodiazepines

The benzodiazepines have a variety of desirable clinical effects that include hypnosis, anxiolysis, anticonvulsant activity, anterograde amnesia, and muscle relaxation. The amnestic properties of benzodiazepines may be affected by the clinical status of the patient before administration. In the presence of a painful stimulus, the benzodiazepines

may produce hyperalgesia and agitation (159–162). These problems usually do not occur if benzodiazepines are combined with opioids.

Benzodiazepines act on specific receptors, located mainly in the cerebral cortex, hypothalamus, cerebellum, corpus striatum, and medulla oblongata, which are coupled to gamma-aminobutyric acid receptors by means of a common chloride channel in synaptic membranes (163). Early pharmacokinetic data showed that the half-lives of diazepam and its active metabolites were markedly prolonged in neonates (164). Diazepam is used commonly for sedation in neonates, with doses of 0.1 to 0.3 mg/kg given every 4 to 6 hours. Doses as high as 50 mg/kg/day have been used to treat neonatal tetanus, with a low incidence of side effects (165). Diazepam has no analgesic effects, and it causes respiratory depression and mild hypotension, both of which are potentiated by opioids and other sedatives. Prolonged use may produce tolerance and withdrawal. In preterm neonates, doses as high as 0.5 mg/kg were associated with cardiovascular stability and no alteration in cerebral blood flow (166).

Lorazepam is five to ten times more potent than diazepam. In doses of 0.05 to 0.1 mg/kg, therapeutic levels may persist for 24 to 48 hours. Oral administration results in reliable absorption, with maximal plasma concentrations in 2 to 4 hours. Although lorazepam is insoluble unless combined with an organic solvent, it is suitable for intramuscular or intravenous injection and causes much less tissue irritation than diazepam (167). Lorazepam is glucuronidated to form inactive metabolites. Its elimination half-life is 10 to 20 hours, but clinical effects may be prolonged because of its pharmacodynamic differences from the other benzodiazepines. The cardiovascular and respiratory effects of lorazepam are similar to those of diazepam. Lorazepam should be used judiciously for sedation in the intensive care setting because of prolonged effects on mental status and respiratory drive. Unlike the other benzodiazepines, it contains polyethylene glycol 400 in propylene glycol, which causes an elevated osmolar gap, metabolic acidosis, and can be nephrotoxic when large amounts of lorazepam are given as a continuous infusion, particularly in patients susceptible to renal injury (168). Lorazepam infusions can lead to significant metabolic acidosis and acute renal insufficiency in term and preterm infants, and some guidelines advise to avoid these infusions in infants under 6 months of age. There have been case reports of lorazepam triggering myoclonus and seizures in neonates (169).

Midazolam, a water-soluble and shorter-acting benzodiazepine, has been used in neonates requiring sedation, alone or combined with opioid analgesics such as fentanyl. Loading doses of 0.2 mg/kg and continuous infusions of 0.4 mg/kg/minute of midazolam were used in patients weighing as little as 3 kg and provided good sedation without any apparent adverse effects (170). At the benzodiazepine receptor, midazolam has twice the binding affinity of diazepam and inhibits gamma-aminobutyric acid reuptake. The pharmacokinetics of midazolam in neonates are characterized by rapid redistribution, plasma clearance of 6.9 mL/kg/minute, and elimination half-life of 6.5 hours, which is significantly longer than the elimination half-life reported for older infants and children (171,172).

After prolonged intravenous therapy with midazolam, a withdrawal syndrome has been described in infants, which is characterized by agitation, poor visual tracking, constant choreoathetoid and dyskinetic movements of the face, tongue, and limbs, and depression of consciousness (173–175). Midazolam may be used intermittently as premedication for specific invasive procedures in doses of 0.05 to 0.2 mg/kg, for short-term sedation by continuous infusion (less than 12 hours) at rates of 0.025 to 0.05 mg/kg/hour, or for longer term sedation of the intubated patient at rates starting at 0.05 mg/kg/hour. After 12 hours, the 1- and α-hydroxymidazolam metabolites that have longer half-lives begin to accumulate, and midazolam's duration of action is prolonged. The respiratory depression and hypotension caused by benzodiazepines are synergistic with the similar effects of potent opioids. Midazolam and fentanyl given by rapid intravenous injection may cause severe, life-threatening hypotension and cardiorespiratory arrest (176). This combination should be used with extreme caution in neonates and only with close monitoring in an intensive care unit.

Flumazenil, a short-acting benzodiazepine antagonist, can be used as a bolus of 10 mg/kg followed by an infusion (5 mg/kg/minute) to reverse the effects of the benzodiazepines. Rapid reversal of the benzodiazepines can trigger seizures in susceptible patients.

Barbiturates

Phenobarbital has long been used as an anticonvulsant in newborns and children, although its routine use for sedation has been discouraged because of several drawbacks. Phenobarbital has hyperalgesic effects and may increase the requirement for analgesia, and rapid tolerance to its sedative action invariably occurs (177). It has a prolonged elimination half-life in neonates (5 to 6 days), and it may increase the risk of intraventricular hemorrhage in premature neonates (178,179). Phenobarbital has no specific antagonist, and prolonged use is associated with microsomal induction of hepatic enzymes and with a withdrawal syndrome. Its advantages in neonates include increased bilirubin metabolism, relatively mild cardiovascular and respiratory depression, and familiarity with its usage in preterm and term neonates. In ventilated preterm neonates, the changes in mean arterial pressure and intracranial pressure associated with endotracheal suctioning were blunted with phenobarbital therapy (180). A neonatal dose-response study found increasing degrees of sedation and feeding difficulties with increasing serum phenobarbital concentrations. These responses were greater in preterm neonates than in term neonates (181). Loading doses of 5 to 20 mg/kg and maintenance doses of 2.5 mg/kg every 12 hours, given orally or intravenously, are generally used for sedation.

Pentobarbital is a shorter-acting barbiturate than phenobarbital with a half-life of 19 to 34 hours in adults. It is useful as an adjunct for sedation of the intubated infant and child, particularly when tolerance has led to rapid escalations of narcotic and benzodiazepine infusions to continue an appropriate and safe level of sedation. One clinical practice guideline for sedation of the intubated infant and child suggests adding intermittent doses of 2 to 6 mg/kg of pentobarbital every 4 hours when infusions of morphine and midazolam begin to exceed 0.5 mg/kg/hour each. Pentobarbital is associated with both tolerance and withdrawal and is generally discontinued in a "last-on, first-off" fashion when sedation is being weaned. Pentobarbital causes more hypotension than most other sedatives used in the infant and child; slower infusions over 15 to 30 minutes reduce this side effect. Like lorazepam, pentobarbital is mixed in propylene glycol, and continuous infusions may precipitate metabolic acidosis and nephrotoxic effects, particularly in patients susceptible to renal injury.

Chloral Hydrate

Chloral hydrate is used frequently as a sedative in doses of 25 to 50 mg/kg or as a hypnotic in doses of 50 to 100 mg/kg for short procedures in neonates and for infants with chronic lung disease (182). Higher doses may be required after repeated use in neonates because of the slow development of tolerance. The advantages of chloral hydrate include ease of administration (e.g., oral syrup, rectal suppositories), although repeated doses can be irritating to the enteral mucosa; lack of respiratory depression; lack of other side effects (e.g., emesis, changes in vital signs or behavior) with usual therapeutic doses; and familiarity with its use in newborns and older infants (183,184). However, an infant who received 165 mg/kg of chloral hydrate over 16 hours developed the toxic reactions of respiratory depression and lethargy (185). Other reports have documented complications such as direct hyperbilirubinemia, decreased tidal volume, hypertriglyceridemia, acute laryngeal edema, and cardiac arrhythmias (e.g., supraventricular tachycardia) in neonates and infants (186–190). One of its metabolites, trichloroethylene, has been described as carcinogenic with chronic exposure (191).

The sedative action of chloral hydrate may be mediated by generalized neuronal depression, similar to other halogenated hydrocarbons. A precise mechanism of action is unknown, and there is no specific antagonist. The pharmacokinetics of chloral hydrate are not clearly defined in neonates. Onset of clinical effects after oral dosage occurs at 30 minutes, and its duration of action is usually 2 to 4 hours, depending on the exact doses used.

Ketamine

Ketamine is a dissociative anesthetic that has been used as an induction agent for anesthesia, analgesic for conscious sedation, premedication before induction of anesthesia, and sedative for critically ill patients. There is a broad range of experience with this agent in older patients, but limited experience in infants and newborns (192,193). Ketamine has been used to provide anesthesia in the spontaneously breathing, nonintubated newborn and causes less neonatal neurobehavioral depression than thiopental after maternal administration for vaginal delivery (194,195). Ketamine produces reliable serum levels within 1 minute when administered intravenously or within 5 minutes when administered intramuscularly, and it is rapidly redistributed, with awakening occurring in 10 to 15 minutes. In neonates, the elimination half-life is significantly longer than 130 minutes, which has been reported in older children and adults (196,197). Extensive hepatic biotransformation necessitates higher doses when administered orally or rectally.

Tolerance and hepatic enzyme induction have been demonstrated during chronic administration of ketamine. Cross-tolerance with opiates has been demonstrated in animals, but convincing evidence from human studies is lacking (198,199). The precise site of action of ketamine is unknown, despite suggestions that ketamine may interfere with excitatory transmission by means of N-methyl-D-aspartate receptors (200). The anesthetic effects of ketamine have been attributed to electrophysiologic dissociation between the thalamoneocortical and limbic systems. Other clinical effects at anesthetic plasma concentrations include catalepsy, nystagmus, hypertonicity, and nonpurposeful movements. Ketamine is a potent stimulator of the cardiovascular system, presumably by means of central sympathetic effects and inhibition of catecholamine reuptake (201). Compared with isoflurane, halothane, and fentanyl, ketamine had the least effects on mean arterial pressure in ill preterm neonates undergoing surgery (202). Pulmonary vascular resistance does not appear to be altered in infants with or without preexisting pulmonary hypertension (203). For critically ill patients with moderate hypovolemia, low doses of ketamine (i.e., 0.5 to 1 mg/kg) are safer than barbiturates as rapid induction agents before tracheal intubation.

CLONIDINE

Clonidine is an α2-adrenoreceptor agonist, and its receptor activation in the locus coeruleus of the brain leads to decreased sympathetic outflow and a resulting antihypertensive effect. In addition to its antihypertensive actions, clonidine has both sedative and antinociceptive effects as well. The mechanisms for these effects are less well understood, but both appear to be mediated through α2-receptor action because they are blocked by α2-antagonist drugs (204). Animal data has shown that the same potassium channels activated by μ opioid receptor agonists are also activated by α agonists, and these effects seem to be mediated via different G-proteins (124). Clonidine has been used as a component of epidural anesthesia because of its synergistic effects with local anesthetics. In addition, oral or transdermal administration at initial doses of 5 μg/kg/day is useful as an adjunct for sedation of the critically ill infant and child. Transdermal delivery is limited in the neonate because the smallest patch (TTS-1 providing 100 μg/day) can be halved for the 10-kg child but cannot easily be quartered. An oral suspension of clonidine is not commercially available but can be prepared by guidelines in the literature; dosing of 5 μg/kg/day divided into two or three times per day is effective. Doses which provide sedative and analgesic effects without accompanying hypotension are easily achievable (205). The mild antihypertensive effect contributes to the usefulness of clonidine in combating narcotic, benzodiazepine, and barbiturate withdrawal syndromes.

SUMMARY

The proper approach to sedation includes an individualized regimen, which ensures analgesia with careful consideration of the important pharmacokinetic and pharmacodynamic differences in the neonatal population. Analgesia and sedation are needed for neonates undergoing stressful or painful procedures required for essential monitoring and therapy in intensive care. Safe and effective techniques are available that can be used in a variety of clinical circumstances. As the International Evidence-Based Group for Neonatal Pain concluded in their recent consensus statement, universal attention to standard guidelines for neonatal pain control "will not only improve the clinical care provided to all neonates, but may also have a positive impact on their subsequent health and behaviors during childhood and adolescence" (18).

REFERENCES

1. Anand KJ, Aynsley Green A. Metabolic and endocrine effects of surgical ligation of patent ductus arteriosus in the human preterm neonate: are there implications for improvement of postoperative outcome? *Mod Probl Pediatr* 1985;23:143–157.
2. Purcell-Jones G, Dormon F, Sumner E. The use of opioids in neonates. A retrospective study of 933 cases. *Anaesthesia* 1987;42:1316–1320.

3. de Lima J, Lloyd-Thomas AR, Howard RF, et al. Infant and neonatal pain: anaesthetists' perceptions and prescribing patterns. *BMJ* 1996;313:787.

4. Duncan HP, Zurick NJ, Wolf AR. Should we reconsider awake neonatal intubation? A review of the evidence and treatment strategies. *Paediatr Anaesth* 2001;11:135–145.

5. Ziegler JW, Todres ID. Intubation of newborns. *Am J Dis Child* 1992;146:147–149.

6. Fernandez CV, Rees EP. Pain management in Canadian level 3 neonatal intensive care units. *CMAJ* 1994;150:499–504.

7. Whyte S, Birrell G, Wyllie J. Premedication before intubation in UK neonatal units. *Arch Dis Child Fetal Neonatal Ed* 2000;82:F38–F41.

8. Howard CR, Howard FM, Garfunkel LC, et al. Neonatal circumcision and pain relief: current training practices. *Pediatrics* 1998;101:423–428.

9. American Academy of Pediatrics, Committee on Fetus and Newborn, Committee on Drugs, Section on Anesthesiology, Section on Surgery, and Canadian Pediatric Society. Prevention and management of pain and stress in the neonate. *Pediatrics* 2000;105:454–461.

10. Anand KJ, Hickey PR. Pain and its effects in the human neonate and fetus. *N Engl J Med* 1987;317:1321–1329.

11. Anand KJ, Hansen DD, Hickey PR. Hormonal-metabolic stress responses in neonates undergoing cardiac surgery. *Anesthesiology* 1990;73:661–670.

12. Anand KJS, Hickey PR. Halothane-morphine compared with high-dose sufentanil for anesthesia and postoperative analgesia in neonatal cardiac surgery. *N Engl J Med* 1992;326:1–9.

13. Agus MS, Jaksic T. Nutritional support of the critically ill child. *Curr Opin Pediatr* 2002;14:470–481.

14. Lidow MS. Long-term effects of neonatal pain on nociceptive systems. *Pain* 2002;99:377–383.

15. Anand KJS. Pain, plasticity, and premature birth: a prescription for permanent suffering? *Nature Med* 2000;6:971.

16. Barker DP, Rutter N. Exposure to invasive procedures in neonatal intensive care unit admissions. *Arch Dis Child Fetal Neonatal Ed* 1995;72:F47–F48.

17. Purcell-Jones G, Dormon F, Sumner E. Paediatric anaesthetists' perceptions of neonatal and infant pain. *Pain* 1988;33:181–187.

18. Anand KJS, for the International Evidence-Based Group for Neonatal Pain. Consensus statement for the prevention and management of pain in the newborn. *Arch Pediatr Adolesc Med* 2001;155:173–180.

19. Reynolds ML, Fitzgerald M, Benowitz LI. GAP-43 expression in developing cutaneous and muscle nerves in the rat hindlimb. *Neuroscience* 1991;41:201–211.

20. Fitzgerald M. A physiological study of the prenatal development of cutaneous sensory inputs to dorsal horn cells in the rat. *J Physiol* 1991;432:473–482.

21. Rizvi TA, Wadhwa S, Mehra RD, et al. Ultrastructure of marginal zone during prenatal development of human spinal cord. *Exp Brain Res* 1986;64:483–490.

22. Pignatelli D, Ribeiro-da Silva A, Coimbra A. Postnatal maturation of primary afferent terminations in the substantia gelatinosa of the rat spinal cord. An electron microscopic study. *Brain Res* 1989;491:33–44.

23. Anand KJ, Carr DB. The neuroanatomy, neurophysiology, and neurochemistry of pain, stress, and analgesia in newborns and children. *Pediatr Clin North Am* 1989;36:795–822.

24. Kinney HC, Ottoson CK, White WF. Three-dimensional distribution of ^{3}H-naloxone binding to opiate receptors in the human fetal and infant brainstem. *J Comp Neurol* 1990;291:55–78.

25. Klimach VJ, Cooke RW. Maturation of the neonatal somatosensory evoked response in preterm infants. *Dev Med Child Neurol* 1988;30:208–214.

26. Anand KJ. Hormonal and metabolic functions of neonates and infants undergoing surgery. *Curr Opin Cardiol* 1986;1:681–689.

27. Anand KJ, Sippell WG, Schofield NM, et al. Does halothane anaesthesia decrease the metabolic and endocrine stress responses of newborn infants undergoing operation? *Br Med J (Clin Res Ed)* 1988;296:668–672.

28. Anand KJ, Sippell WG, Aynsley Green A. Randomised trial of fentanyl anaesthesia in preterm babies undergoing surgery: effects on the stress response. *Lancet* 1987;1:62–66.

29. Gruber EM, Laussen PC, Casta A, et al. Stress response in infants undergoing cardiac surgery: a randomized study of fentanyl bolus, fentanyl infusion, and fentanyl-midazolam infusion. *Anesth Analg* 2001;92:882–890.

30. Newburger JW, Jonas RA, Wernovsky G, et al. A comparison of the perioperative neurologic effects of hypothermic circulatory arrest versus low-flow cardiopulmonary bypass in infant heart surgery. *N Engl J Med* 1993;329:1057–1064.

31. Wessel DL. Hemodynamic responses to perioperative pain and stress in infants. *Crit Care Med* 1993;21(Suppl):S361–S362.

32. Pokela ML. Pain relief can reduce hypoxemia in distressed neonates during routine treatment procedures. *Pediatrics* 1994;93:379–383.

33. Orsini AJ, Leef KH, Costarino A, et al. Routine use of fentanyl infusions for pain and stress reduction in infants with respiratory distress syndrome. *J Pediatr* 1996;129:140–145.

34. Anand KJS, Barton BA, McIntosh N, et al. Analgesia and sedation in premature neonates who require ventilatory support: results from the NOPAIN trial. Neonatal Outcome and Prolonged Analgesia in Neonates. *Arch Ped Adol Med* 1999;153:331–338.

35. Richards T. Can a fetus feel pain? *Br Med J (Clin Res Ed)* 1985;291:1220–1221.

36. Lippmann M, Nelson RJ, Emmanouilides GC, et al. Ligation of patent ductus arteriosus in premature infants. *Br J Anaesth* 1976;48:365–369.

37. Shearer MH. Surgery on the paralyzed, unanesthetized newborn. *Birth* 1986;13:79.

38. Robinson S, Gregory GA. Fentanyl-air-oxygen anesthesia for ligation of patent ductus arteriosus in preterm infants. *Anesth Analg* 1981;60:331–334.

39. Yaster M. Analgesia and anesthesia in neonates. *J Pediatr* 1987;111:394–396.

40. Friesen RH, Lichtor JL. Cardiovascular effects of inhalation induction with isoflurane in infants. *Anesth Analg* 1983;62:411–414.

41. Friesen RH, Lichtor JL. Cardiovascular depression during halothane anesthesia in infants: study of three induction techniques. *Anesth Analg* 1982;61:42–45.

42. Gregory GA. The baroresponses of preterm infants during halothane anaesthesia. *Can Anaesth Soc J* 1982;29:105–107.

43. Eisele JH, Smith NT. Cardiovascular effects of 40 percent nitrous oxide in man. *Anesth Analg* 1972;51:956–963.

44. Lunn JK, Stanley TH, Eisele J, et al. High dose fentanyl anesthesia for coronary artery surgery: plasma fentanyl concentrations and influence of nitrous oxide on cardiovascular responses. *Anesth Analg* 1979;58:390–395.

45. Hickey PR, Hansen DD, Strafford M, et al. Pulmonary and systemic hemodynamic effects of nitrous oxide in infants with normal and elevated pulmonary vascular resistance. *Anesthesiology* 1986;65:374–378.

46. Shingu K, Eger EI II, Johnson BH, et al. Effect of oxygen concentration, hyperthermia, and choice of vendor on anesthetic-induced hepatic injury in rats. *Anesth Analg* 1983;62:146–150.

47. Summary of the National Halothane Study. Possible association between halothane anesthesia and postoperative hepatic necrosis. *JAMA* 1966;197:775–788.

48. Hubbard AK, Roth TP, Gandolfi AJ, et al. Halothane hepatitis patients generate an antibody response toward a covalently bound metabolite of halothane. *Anesthesiology* 1988;68:791–796.

49. Mazze RI, Calverley RK, Smith NT. Inorganic fluoride nephrotoxicity: prolonged enflurane and halothane anesthesia in volunteers. *Anesthesiology* 1977;46:265–271.

50. Conzen PF, Nuscheler M, Melotte A, et al. Renal function and serum fluoride concentrations in patients with stable renal insufficiency after anesthesia with sevoflurane or enflurane. *Anesth Analg* 1995;81:569–575.

51. Young CJ, Apfelbaum JL. Inhalational anesthetics: desflurane and sevoflurane. *J Clin Anesth* 1995;7:564–577.

52. Harkin CP, Pagel PS, Kersten JR, et al. Direct negative inotropic and lusitropic effects of sevoflurane. *Anesthesiology* 1994;81:156–167.

53. Russell IA, Miller Hance WC, Gregory G, et al. The safety and efficacy of sevoflurane anesthesia in infants and children with congenital heart disease. *Anesth Analg* 2001;92:1152–1158.

54. Holaday DA, Smith FR. Clinical characteristics and biotransformation of sevoflurane in healthy human volunteers. *Anesthesiology* 1981;54:100–106.

55. Kharasch ED, Karol MD, Lanni C, et al. Clinical sevoflurane metabolism and disposition. I. Sevoflurane and metabolite pharmacokinetics. *Anesthesiology* 1995;82:1369–1378.

56. Loeckinger A, Kleinsasser A, Maier S, et al. Sustained prolongation of the QTc interval after anesthesia with sevoflurane in infants during the first 6 months of life. *Anesthesiology* 2003;98:639–642.

57. Eger EI II. Desflurane animal and human pharmacology: aspects of kinetics, safety, and MAC. *Anesth Analg* 1992;75(Suppl):S3–S7.

58. Walker TJ, Chakrabarti MK, Lockwood GG. Uptake of desflurane during anaesthesia. *Anaesthesia* 1996;51:33–36.

59. Bovill JG, Sebel PS, Stanley TH. Opioid analgesics in anesthesia: with special reference to their use in cardiovascular anesthesia. *Anesthesiology* 1984;61:731–755.

60. Koren G, Goresky G, Crean P, et al. Pediatric fentanyl dosing based on pharmacokinetics during cardiac surgery. *Anesth Analg* 1984;63:577–582.

61. Hickey PR, Hansen DD, Wessel DL, et al. Pulmonary and systemic hemodynamic responses to fentanyl in infants. *Anesth Analg* 1985;64:483–486.

62. Hickey PR, Hansen DD, Wessel DL, et al. Blunting of stress responses in the pulmonary circulation of infants by fentanyl. *Anesth Analg* 1985;64:1137–1142.

63. Bjertnaes L, Hauge A, Kriz M. Hypoxia-induced pulmonary vasoconstriction: effects of fentanyl following different routes of administration. *Acta Anaesthesiol Scand* 1980;24:53–57.

64. Rosow CE, Moss J, Philbin DM, et al. Histamine release during morphine and fentanyl anesthesia. *Anesthesiology* 1982;56:93–96.

65. Lynn AM, Slattery JT. Morphine pharmacokinetics in early infancy. *Anesthesiology* 1987;66:136–139.

66. Gauntlett IS, Fisher DM, Hertzka RE, et al. Pharmacokinetics of fentanyl in neonatal humans and lambs: effects of age. *Anesthesiology* 1988;69:683–687.

67. Greeley WJ, de Bruijn NP, Davis DP. Sufentanil pharmacokinetics in pediatric cardiovascular patients. *Anesth Analg* 1987;66:1067–1072.

68. Greeley WJ, de Bruijn NP. Changes in sufentanil pharmacokinetics within the neonatal period. *Anesth Analg* 1988;67:86–90.

69. Killian A, Davis PJ, Stiller RL, et al. Influence of gestational age on pharmacokinetics of alfentanil in neonates. *Dev Pharmacol Ther* 1991;15:82–85.

70. Mather LE. Clinical pharmacokinetics of fentanyl and its newer derivatives. *Clin Pharmacokinet* 1983;8:422–446.

71. Ross AK, Davis PJ, Dear GD, et al. Pharmacokinetics of remifentanil in anesthetized pediatric patients undergoing elective surgery or diagnostic procedures. *Anesth Analg* 2001;93:1393–1401.

72. Scott CS, Riggs KW, Ling EW, et.al. Morphine pharmacokinetics and pain assessment in premature newborns. *J Pediatr* 1999;135:423–429.

73. Dalens B. Regional anesthesia in children. *Anesth Analg* 1989;68:654–672.

74. Liu LM, Cote CJ, Goudsouzian NG, et al. Life-threatening apnea in infants recovering from anesthesia. *Anesthesiology* 1983;59:506–510.

75. Huang JJ, Hirschberg G. Regional anaesthesia decreases the need for postoperative mechanical ventilation in very low birth weight infants undergoing herniorraphy. *Paediatr Anaesth* 2001;11:705–709.

76. Bosenberg AT, Hadley GP, Wiersma R. Esophageal atresia; caudo-thoracic epidural anesthesia reduces the need for postoperative ventilatory support. *Paediatr Surg Int* 1992;7:289–291.

77. McNeely JK, Farber NE, Rusy LM, et al. Epidural analgesia improves outcome following pediatric fundoplication. A retrospective analysis. *Reg Anesth* 1997;22:16–23.

78. Abajian JC, Mellish RW, Browne AF, et al. Spinal anesthesia for surgery in the high-risk infant. *Anesth Analg* 1984;63:359–362.

79. Shenkman Z, Hoppenstein D, Litmanowitz I, et al. Spinal anesthesia in 62 premature, former-premature or young infants—technical aspects and pitfalls. *Can J Anaesth* 2002;49:262–269.

80. Mahe V, Ecoffey C. Spinal anesthesia with isobaric bupivacaine in infants. *Anesthesiology* 1988;68:601–603.

81. Valairucha S, Seefelder C, Houck CS. Thoracic epidural catheters placed by the caudal route in infants: the importance of radiographic confirmation. *Paediatr Anaesth* 2002;12:424–428.

82. Cook B, Doyle E. The use of additives to local anesthetic solutions for caudal epidural blockade. *Paediatr Anaesth* 1996;6:353–359.

83. Fellmann C, Gerber AC, Weiss M. Apnoea in a former preterm infant after caudal bupivacaine with clonidine for inguinal herniorraphy. *Paediatr Anaesth* 2002;12:637–640.

84. Bouchut JC, Dubois R, Godard J. Clonidine in preterm-infant caudal anesthesia may be responsible for postoperative apnea. *Reg Anesth Pain Med* 2001;26:83–85.

85. Breschan C, Krumpholz R, Likar R, e .al. Can a dose of 2 μg/kg caudal clonidine cause respiratory depression in neonates? *Paediatr Anaesth* 1999;9:81–83.

86. Spear RM, Deshpande JK, Maxwell LG. Caudal anesthesia in the awake, high-risk infant. *Anesthesiology* 1988;69:407–409.

87. Shandling B, Steward DJ. Regional analgesia for postoperative pain in pediatric outpatient surgery. *J Pediatr Surg* 1980;15:477–480.

88. Broadman LM, Hannallah RS, Belman AB, et al. Post-circumcision analgesia—a prospective evaluation of subcutaneous ring block of the penis. *Anesthesiology* 1987;67:399–402.

89. Hannallah RS, Broadman LM, Belman AB, et al. Comparison of caudal and ilioinguinal/iliohypogastric nerve blocks for control of post-orchiopexy pain in pediatric ambulatory surgery. *Anesthesiology* 1987;66:832–834.

90. Reiz S, Nath S. Cardiotoxicity of local anaesthetic agents. *Br J Anaesth* 1986;58:736–746.

91. Scott DB. Toxic effects of local anaesthetic agents on the central nervous system. *Br J Anaesth* 1986;58:732–735.

92. Benini F, Johnston CC, Faucher D, et al. Topical anesthesia during circumcision in newborn infants. *JAMA* 1993;270:850–853.

93. Taddio A, Ohlsson K, Ohlsson A. Lidocaine-prilocaine cream for analgesia during circumcision in newborn boys. *Cochrane Database Syst Rev* 2000;2:CD000496.

94. Butler-O'Hara M, LeMoine C, Guillet R. Analgesia for neonatal circumcision: a randomized, controlled trial of EMLA cream versus dorsal penile nerve block. *Pediatrics* 1998;101:E5.

95. Howard CR, Howard FM, Fortune K, et al. A randomized, controlled trial of a eutectic mixture of local anesthetic cream (lidocaine and prilocaine) versus penile nerve block for pain relief during circumcision. *Am J Obstet Gynecol* 1999;181:1506–1511.

96. McIntosh N, van Veen L, Bramayer H. Alleviation of the pain of heelstick in preterm infants. *Arch Dis Child* 1994;70:F177.

97. Abad F, Diaz-Gomez NM, Domenech E, et al. Oral sucrose compares favourably with lidocaine-prilocaine cream for pain relief during venepuncture in infants. *Acta Paediatr* 2001;90:160–165.

98. Gradin M, Eriksson M, Holmqvist G, et al. Pain reduction at venipuncture in newborns: oral glucose compared with local anesthetic cream. *Pediatrics* 2002;110:1053–1057.

99. Taddio A, Shennan AT, Stevens B, et al. Safety of lidocaine-prilocaine cream in the treatment of preterm neonates. *J Pediatr* 1995;127:1002–1005.

100. Gourrier E, Karoubi P, el Hanache A, et al. Safety of EMLA cream in a department of neonatology. *Pain* 1996;68:431–434.

101. Lawson RA, Smart NG, Gudgeon AC, et al. Evaluation of an amethocaine gel preparation for percutaneous analgesia before venous cannulation in children. *Br J Anaesth* 1995;75:282–285.

102. Rigby-Jones AE, Nolan JA, Priston MJ, et al. Pharmacokinetics of propofol infusions in critically ill neonates, infants, and children in an intensive care unit. *Anesthesiology* 2002;97:1393–1400.

103. Parke TJ, Stevens JE, Rice AS, et al. Metabolic acidosis and fatal myocardial failure after propofol infusion in children: five case reports. *BMJ* 1992;305:613–616.

104. Committee on Safety of Medicines/Medicines Control Agency. Propofol (Diprivan) infusion: sedation in children aged 16 years or younger contraindicated. *Curr Problems Pharmacovigilance* 2001;27:10.

105. Truog R, Anand KJ. Management of pain in the postoperative neonate. *Clin Perinatol* 1989;16:61–78.

106. Callahan P, Pasternak GW. Opiates, opioid peptides, and their receptors. *J Cardiothorac Anesth* 1987;569:576.

107. Davis PJ, Ross A, Stiller R, et al. Pharmacokinetics of remifentanil in anesthetized children 2–12 years of age. *Anesth Analg* 1995;80:S93.

108. Barker N, Hadgraft J, Rutter N. Skin permeability in the newborn. *J Invest Dermatol* 1987;88:409–411.

109. Hess GD, Zagon IS. Endogenous opioid systems and neural development: ultrastructural studies in the cerebellar cortex of infant and weanling rats. *Brain Res Bull* 1988;20:473–478.

110. Bardo MT, Hughes RA. Single-dose tolerance to morphine-induced analgesic and hypoactive effects in infant rats. *Dev Psychobiol* 1981;14:415–423.

111. Roy S, Loh HH. Effects of opioids on the immune system. *Neurochem Res* 1996;21:1375–1386.

112. Evans JM, Hogg MIJ, Rosen M. Reversal of narcotic depression in the neonate by naloxone. *Br Med J* 1976;2:1098–1100.

113. Way WL, Costley EC, Leong-Way EL. Respiratory sensitivity of the newborn infant to meperidine and morphine. *Clin Pharmacol Ther* 1965;11:454–461.

114. Hertzka RE, Gauntlett IS, Fisher DM, et al. Fentanyl-induced ventilatory depression: effects of age. *Anesthesiology* 1989;70:213–218.

115. Olkkola KT, Maunuksela E-L, Korpela R, et al. Kinetics and dynamics of postoperative intravenous morphine in children. *Clin Pharmacol Ther* 1991;44:128–136.

116. Chay PC, Duffy BJ, Walker JS. Pharmacokinetic-pharmacodynamic relationships of morphine in neonates. *Clin Pharmacol Ther* 1992;51:334–342.

117. Hartley R, Green M, Quinn MW, et al. Development of morphine glucuronidation in premature neonates. *Biol Neonate* 1994;66:1–9.

118. Colpaert FC, Niemegeers CJ, Janssen PA, et al. The effects of prior fentanyl administration and of pain on fentanyl analgesia: tolerance to and enhancement of narcotic analgesia. *J Pharmacol Exp Ther* 1980;213:418–424.

119. Hasday JD, Weintraub M. Propoxyphene in children with iatrogenic morphine dependence. *Am J Dis Child* 1983;137:745–748.

120. Miser AW, Chayt KJ, Sandlund JT, et al. Narcotic withdrawal syndrome in young adults after the therapeutic use of opiates. *Am J Dis Child* 1986;140:603–604.

121. Arnold JH, Truog RD, Orav EJ, et al. Tolerance and dependence in neonates sedated with fentanyl during extracorporeal membrane oxygenation. *Anesthesiology* 1990;73:1136–1140.

122. Tobias JD, Schleien CL, Haun SE. Methadone as treatment for iatrogenic narcotic dependency in pediatric intensive care unit patients. *Crit Care Med* 1990;18:1292–1293.

123. Arnold JH, Truog RD, Scavone JM, et al. Changes in the pharmacodynamic response to fentanyl in neonates during continuous infusion. *J Pediatr* 1991;119:639–643.

124. Suresh S, Anand KJS. Opioid tolerance in neonates: a state-of-the-art review. *Paediatr Anaesth* 2001;11:511–521.

125. Horav E, Weinstock M. Temporal factors influencing the development of acute tolerance to opiates. *J Pharmacol Exp Ther* 1987;242:251–256.

126. Yasuda I, Hirano T, Yusa T, et al. Tracheal constriction by morphine and by fentanyl in man. *Anesthesiology* 1978;49:117–119.

127. Soleymani Y, Weiss NS, Sinnott EC, et al. Management of life-threatening asthma in children. A preliminary study of the use of morphine in respiratory failure. *Am J Dis Child* 1972;123:533–540.

128. Eschenbacher WL, Bethel RA, Boushey HA, et al. Morphine sulfate inhibits bronchoconstriction in subjects with mild asthma whose responses are inhibited by atropine. *Am Rev Respir Dis* 1984;130:363–367.

129. Rogers DF, Barnes PJ. Opioid inhibition of neurally mediated mucus secretion in human bronchi. *Lancet* 1989;1:930–932.

130. Comstock MK, Carter JG, Moyers JR, et al. Rigidity and hypercarbia associated with high dose fentanyl induction of anesthesia. *Anesth Analg* 1981;60:362–363.

131. Kentor ML, Schwalb AJ, Lieberman RW. Rapid high-dose fentanyl induction for CABG. *Anesthesiology* 1980;53:S95.

132. Scamman FL. Fentanyl-O$_2$-N$_2$O rigidity and pulmonary compliance. *Anesth Analg* 1983;62:332–334.

133. Hill AB, Nahrwold ML, de Rosayro AM, et al. Prevention of rigidity during fentanyl–oxygen induction of anesthesia. *Anesthesiology* 1981;55:452–454.

134. Bailey PL, Wilbrink J, Zwanikken P, et al. Anesthetic induction with fentanyl. *Anesth Analg* 1985;64:48–53.

135. Freye E, Hartung E, Buhl R. [Lung compliance in man is impaired by the rapid injection of alfentanyl.] *Anaesthesist* 1986;35:543–546.

136. Schlesinger AE, Null DM. Enlarged common hepatic duct secondary to morphine in a neonate. *Pediatr Radiol* 1988;18:235–236.

137. Peterson RG. Consequences associated with nonnarcotic analgesics in the fetus and newborn. *Fed Proc* 1985;44:2309–2313.

138. Levy G, Khanna NN, Soda DM, et al. Pharmacokinetics of acetaminophen in the human neonate: formation of acetaminophen glucuronide and sulfate in relation to plasma bilirubin concentration and D-glucaric acid excretion. *Pediatrics* 1975;55:818–825.

139. Miller RP, Roberts RJ, Fischer LJ. Acetaminophen elimination kinetics in neonates, children, and adults. *Clin Pharmacol Ther* 1976;19:284–294.

140. Collins E. Maternal and fetal effects of acetaminophen and salicylates in pregnancy. *Obstet Gynecol* 1981;58(Suppl):57S–62S.

141. Beattie JO, Chen CP, MacDonald TH. Neonatal distalgesic poisoning. *Lancet* 1981;2:49.

142. Roberts I, Robinson MJ, Mughal MZ, et al. Paracetamol metabolites in the neonate following maternal overdose. *Br J Clin Pharmacol* 1984;18:201–206.

143. Howard CR, Howard FM, Weitzman ML. Acetaminophen analgesia in neonatal circumcision: the effect on pain. *Pediatrics* 1994;93:641–646.

144. Shah V, Taddio A, Ohlsson A. Randomised controlled trial of paracetamol for heel prick pain in neonates. *Arch Dis Child Fetal Neonatal Ed* 1998;79:F209–F211.

145. Bremerich DH, Neidhart G, Heimann K, et al. Prophylactically-administered rectal acetaminophen does not reduce postoperative opioid requirements in infants and small children undergoing elective cleft palate repair. *Anesth Analg* 2001;92:907–912.

146. Stiehm ER. Nonsteroidal anti-inflammatory drugs in pediatric patients. *Am J Dis Child* 1988;142:1281–1282.

147. Brogden RN. Nonsteroidal anti-inflammatory analgesics other than salicylates. *Drugs* 1986;32(suppl 4):27–45.

148. Bucher H, Moser T, von Siebenthal K, et al. Sucrose reduces pain reaction to heel lancing in preterm infants: a placebo-controlled, randomized and masked study. *Pediatr Res* 1995;38:332–335.

149. Haouari N, Wood C, Griffiths G, et al. The analgesic effect of sucrose in full term infants: a randomised controlled trial. *BMJ* 1995;310:1498–1500.

150. Blass EM, Shah A. Pain-reducing properties of sucrose in human newborns. *Chem Senses* 1995;20:29–35.

151. Carbajal R, Chauvet X, Couderc S, et al. Randomized trial of analgesic effects of sucrose, glucose, and pacifiers in term neonates. *BMJ* 1999;319:1393–1397.

152. Carbajal R, Lenclen R, Gajdos V, et al. Crossover trial of analgesic efficacy of glucose and pacifier in very preterm neonates during subcutaneous injections. *Pediatrics* 2002;110:389–393.

153. Shide DJ, Blass EM. Opioidlike effects of intraoral infusions of corn oil and polycose on stress reactions in 10-day-old rats. *Behav Neurosci* 1989;103:1168–1175.

154. Chasnoff IJ, Hatcher R, Burns WJ. Early growth patterns of methadone-addicted infants. *Am J Dis Child* 1980;134:1049–1051.

155. Blass EM. Milk-induced hypoalgesia in human newborns. *Pediatrics* 1997;99:825–829.

156. Carbajal R, Veerapen S, Couderc S, et al. Analgesic effect of breast feeding in term neonates: randomised controlled trial. *BMJ* 2003;326:13.

157. Corff KE, Seideman R, Venkataraman PS, et al. Facilitated tucking: a nonpharmacologic comfort measure for pain in preterm neonates. *J Obstet Gynecol Neonatal Nurs* 1995;24:143–147.

158. Stevens B. Management of painful procedures in the newborn. *Curr Opin Pediatr* 1996;8:102–107.

159. Norton SJ. Aftereffects of morphine and fentanyl analgesia: a retrospective study. *Neonatal Netw* 1988;7:25–28.

160. Desai N, Taylor-Davies A, Barnett DB. The effects of diazepam and oxprenolol on short term memory in individuals of high and low state anxiety. *Br J Clin Pharmacol* 1983;15:197–202.

161. Niv D, Davidovich S, Geller E, et al. Analgesic and hyperalgesic effects of midazolam: dependence on route of administration. *Anesth Analg* 1988;67:1169–1173.

162. Rattan AK, McDonald JS, Tejwani GA. Differential effects of intrathecal midazolam on morphine-induced antinociception in the rat: role of spinal opioid receptors. *Anesth Analg* 1991;73:124–131.

163. Reves JG, Fragen RJ, Vinik HR, et al. Midazolam: pharmacology and uses. *Anesthesiology* 1985;62:310–324.

164. Morselli PL, Principi N, Tognoni G. Diazepam elimination in premature and full term infants, and children. *J Perinat Med* 1973;1:133–141.

165. Tekur U, Gupta A, Tayal G, et al. Blood concentrations of diazepam and its metabolites in children and neonates with tetanus. *J Pediatr* 1983;102:145–147.
166. Jorch G, Rabe H, Rickers E, et al. Cerebral blood flow velocity assessed by Doppler technique after intravenous application of diazepam in very low birth weight infants. *Dev Pharmacol Ther* 1989;14:102–107.
167. Hegarty JE, Dundee JW. Sequelae after the intravenous injection of three benzodiazepines—diazepam, lorazepam, and flunitrazepam. *Br Med J* 1977;2:1384–1385.
168. Laine GA, Hossain SM, Solis RT, et al. Polyethylene glycol nephrotoxicity secondary to prolonged high-dose intravenous lorazepam. *Ann Pharmacother* 1995;29:1110–1114.
169. Lee DS, Wong HA, Knoppert DC. Myoclonus associated with lorazepam therapy in very-low-birth-weight infants. *Biol Neonate* 1994;66:311–315.
170. Silvasi DL, Rosen DA, Rosen KR. Continuous intravenous midazolam infusion for sedation in the pediatric intensive care unit. *Anesth Analg* 1988;67:286–288.
171. Jacqz-Aigrain E, Wood C, Robieux I. Pharmacokinetics of midazolam in critically ill neonates. *Eur J Clin Pharmacol* 1990;39:191–192.
172. Byatt CM, Lewis LD, Dawling S, et al. Accumulation of midazolam after repeated dosage in patients receiving mechanical ventilation in an intensive care unit. *Br Med J (Clin Res Ed)* 1984;289:799–800.
173. Boisse NR, Quaglietta N, Samoriski GM, et al. Tolerance and physical dependence to a short-acting benzodiazepine, midazolam. *J Pharmacol Exp Ther* 1990;252:1125–1133.
174. McLellan I, Douglas E. Midazolam withdrawal syndrome. *Anaesthesia* 1991;46:420.
175. Bergman I, Steeves M, Burckart G, et al. Reversible neurologic abnormalities associated with prolonged intravenous midazolam and fentanyl administration. *J Pediatr* 1991;119:644–649.
176. Burtin P, Daoud P, Jacqz-Aigrain E, et al. Hypotension with midazolam and fentanyl in the newborn. *Lancet* 1991;337:1545–1546.
177. Kissin I, Mason JO III, Bradley EL Jr. Morphine and fentanyl interactions with thiopental in relation to movement response to noxious stimulation. *Anesth Analg* 1986;65:1149–1154.
178. Grasela TH Jr, Donn SM. Neonatal population pharmacokinetics of phenobarbital derived from routine clinical data. *Dev Pharmacol Ther* 1985;8:374–383.
179. Kuban KCK, Leviton A, Krishnamoorthy KS. Neonatal intracranial hemorrhage and phenobarbital. *Pediatrics* 1986;77:443–450.
180. Ninan A, O'Donnell M, Hamilton K, et al. Physiologic changes induced by endotracheal instillation and suctioning in critically ill preterm infants with and without sedation. *Am J Perinatol* 1986;3:94–97.
181. Gilman JT, Gal P, Duchowny MS, et al. Rapid sequential phenobarbital treatment of neonatal seizures. *Pediatrics* 1989;83:674–678.
182. Franck LS. A national survey of the assessment and treatment of pain and agitation in the neonatal intensive care unit. *J Obstet Gynecol Neonatal Nurs* 1987;16:387–393.
183. Lees MH, Olsen GD, McGilliard KL, et al. Chloral hydrate and the carbon dioxide chemoreceptor response: a study of puppies and infants. *Pediatrics* 1982;70:447–450.
184. Rumm PD, Takao RT, Fox DJ, et al. Efficacy of sedation of children with chloral hydrate. *South Med J* 1990;83:1040–1043.
185. Laptook AR, Rosenfeld CR. Chloral hydrate toxicity in a preterm infant. *Pediatr Pharmacol (New York)* 1984;4:161–165.
186. Lambert GH, Muraskas J, Anderson CL, et al. Direct hyperbilirubinemia associated with chloral hydrate administration in the newborn. *Pediatrics* 1990;86:277–281.
187. Turner DJ, Morgan SE, Landau LI, et al. Methodological aspects of flow-volume studies in infants. *Pediatr Pulmonol* 1990;8:289–293.
188. Gonzalez JL, Lambert GH, Muraskas J, et al. Hypertriglyceridemia in infants with bronchopulmonary dysplasia. *J Pediatr* 1989;115:506.
189. Farber B, Abramow A. Acute laryngeal edema due to chloral hydrate. *Isr J Med Sci* 1985;21:858–859.
190. Hirsch IA, Zauder HL. Chloral hydrate: a potential cause of arrhythmias. *Anesth Analg* 1986;65:691–692.
191. Salmon AG, Kizer KW, Zeise L, et al. Potential carcinogenicity of chloral hydrate—a review. *J Toxicol Clin Toxicol* 1995;33:115–121.
192. Reich DL, Silvay G. Ketamine: an update on the first twenty-five years of clinical experience. *Can J Anaesth* 1989;36:186–197.
193. Tashiro C, Matsui Y, Nakano S, et al. Respiratory outcome in extremely premature infants following ketamine anaesthesia. *Can J Anaesth* 1991;38:287–291.
194. Chatterjee SC, Syed A. Ketamine and infants. *Anaesthesia* 1983;38:1007.
195. Hodgkinson R, Marx GF, Kim SS, et al. Neonatal neurobehavioral tests following vaginal delivery under ketamine, thiopental, and extradural anesthesia. *Anesth Analg* 1977;56:548A.
196. Grant IS, Nimmo WS, McNicol LR, et al. Ketamine disposition in children and adults. *Br J Anaesth* 1983;55:1107–1111.
197. Cook DR. Newborn anaesthesia: pharmacological considerations. *Can Anaesth Soc J* 1986;33:S38–S42.
198. Winters WD, Hance AJ, Cadd GG, et al. Ketamine- and morphine-induced analgesia and catalepsy. I. Tolerance, cross-tolerance, potentiation, residual morphine levels and naloxone action in the rat. *J Pharmacol Exp Ther* 1988;244:51–57.
199. Finck AD, Samaniego E, Ngai SH. Morphine tolerance decreases the analgesic effects of ketamine in mice. *Anesthesiology* 1988;68:397–400.
200. Thomson AM, West DC, Lodge D. An N-methylaspartate receptor-mediated synapse in rat cerebral cortex: a site of action of ketamine? *Nature* 1985;313:479–481.
201. Lundy PM, Lockwood PA, Thompson G, et al. Differential effects of ketamine isomers on neuronal and extraneuronal catecholamine uptake mechanisms. *Anesthesiology* 1986;64:359–363.
202. Friesen RH, Henry DB. Cardiovascular changes in preterm neonates receiving isoflurane, halothane, fentanyl, and ketamine. *Anesthesiology* 1986;64:238–242.
203. Hickey PR, Hansen DD, Cramolini GM, et al. Pulmonary and systemic hemodynamic responses to ketamine in infants with normal and elevated pulmonary vascular resistance. *Anesthesiology* 1985;62:287–293.
204. Drew GM, Gower AJ, Marriott AS. Alpha 2-adrenoceptors mediate clonidine-induced sedation in the rat. *Br J Pharmacol* 1979;67:133–141.
205. Ambrose C, Sale S, Howells R, et al. Intravenous clonidine infusion in critically ill children: dose-dependent sedative effects and cardiovascular stability. *Br J Anaesth* 2000;84:794–796.
206. Berde CB. Pediatric postoperative pain management. *Pediatr Clin North Am* 1989;36:921–940.

The Infant of the Drug-Dependent Mother

58

Enrique M. Ostrea, Jr.   J. Edgar Winston Cruz Posecion
Maria Esterlita-Uy   T. Villanueva

The problem of drug abuse has reached epidemic proportions during the past two decades, with increases not only in the number of drug users but also in the types of drugs abused. Equally alarming is the increase in the proportion of drugs users among women of childbearing age or are pregnant, because the effects of drugs on the pregnancy and fetus can be far reaching. In this chapter, the latter will be addressed. Existing information in the literature on the maternal, neonatal, and long-term complications in infants of drug use during pregnancy will be consolidated plus a brief historical and epidemiologic perspective of the problem. There will be many instances in which the data presented are conflicting. This reflects the limitations of studies on human population, because of the influence of many confounding factors especially multiple drug use, socioeconomic status, environmental factors, parental education and psychopathology.

EPIDEMIOLOGY

In 2001, the National Household Survey on Drug Abuse estimated that 15.9 million (7.1%) Americans of age 12 years or older were current illicit drug users (1). This represents an increase from 6.3 percent in 1999 and 2000 (Table 58-1). Between 2000 and 2001, statistically significant increases were also noted for the current use of marijuana (4.8%–5.4%), cocaine (0.5%–0.7%), psychotherapeutic drugs (1.7%–2.1%) and hallucinogens (0.4–0.6%). Current heroin use was estimated at 0.1%. Marijuana was the most commonly used illicit drug. Approximately 56% consumed only marijuana, 20% used marijuana and another illicit drug, and the remaining 24% used an illicit drug but not marijuana in the past month. Thus, about 44 percent of current illicit drug users in 2001 (7 million Americans) used illicit drugs other than marijuana and hashish, with or without using marijuana as well.

The rate of drug use substantially varied by age. Among youths 12 to 17 years of age, 10.8% were current illicit drug users which tended to increase with age and peaked at age 18 to 20 years (22.4%). By race, the rate of current illicit drug use was 7.4% for blacks, 7.2% for whites (6.1%), and 6.4% for Hispanics. The rate was highest among American Indians/Alaskan natives (9.9%). As in prior years, men continue to have a higher rate of current illicit drug use than women (8.7% vs. 5.5%). Illicit drug use remains highly correlated with educational status and employment. Those who did not complete a high school education had the highest rate of use (7.6%) compared to college graduates (4.3%). Similarly, the rate of illicit drug use was 17.1% among unemployed adults (18 years of older) compared to 6.9% of full time employed adults. Among pregnant women, aged 15 to 44 years, 3.7% reported using illicit drugs. The rate was highest among pregnant women aged 15 to 17 years (15.1%). Rates of illicit drug use among pregnant women aged 18 to 25 and 26 to 44 years were 5.6% and 1.6%, respectively. The rates of current illicit drug use were similar for white (4.0%), black (3.7%), and Hispanic (3.3%) pregnant women. However, the true prevalence of illicit drug use among pregnant women is difficult to determine, as a result of significant underreporting of drug use by these women. One study, based on a survey using maternal history, urine toxicology, or both, of predominantly urban hospitals, gave an estimate of drug use among pregnant women as 0.4% to 27%; cocaine use ranged from 0.2% to 17%. With the use of a more sensitive drug screening method (e.g., meconium drug test), a 44% prevalence of illicit drug use was found among pregnant women in a high risk center in contrast to 11% by maternal self-report and 30% of the infants were positive for cocaine (2). The association of illicit drug use with HIV infection in pregnant women is high. Use of hard drugs was 42% in a cohort of HIV-infected pregnant women and was further associated

TABLE 58-1

ILLICIT DRUG USE AMONG PERSONS 12 YEARS OR OLDER BY DRUG (1999–2001)

	1999	2000	2001
Any illicit drug	6.3%	6.3%	7.1%
Marijuana	4.7%	4.8%	5.4%
Psychotherapeutic	1.8%	1.7%	2.1%
Cocaine	0.7%	0.5%	0.7%
Hallucinogen	0.4%	0.4%	0.6%
Inhalants	0.3%	0.3%	0.2%

From *National Household Survey on Drug Abuse 2001.* Substance Abuse and Mental Health Services Administration, Washington: US Government Printing Office, with permission.

with positive maternal HIV culture at delivery and perinatal transmission (3).

NARCOTICS

The term "opiate" or "narcotic" refers to any natural or synthetic drug that has morphine like pharmacologic actions. The natural opiates include morphine and codeine, whereas the synthetic opiates include heroin, methadone, propoxyohene (Darvon), pentazocine (Talwin), meperidine (Demerol), oxycodone (Percodan, Tylox, Vecodine, Percocet), hydromorphone (Dilaudid), and fentanyl (Immovar, Sublimaze). Chronic use of narcotics, even in therapeutic doses, results in addiction, which is characterized by psychological and physical dependence on the drug.

HISTORY

Opium use probably dates back to about 6,000 years. One of the earliest references to opiate complications in the perinatal period was made by Hippocrates, who mentioned "uterine suffocation" as possibly secondary to opium use. By the late nineteenth and early twentieth century, reference to the passively addicted neonate is evident from reports describing the diffusion of morphine through the placenta and transmission through the breast milk (4). The naturally occurring opiates, morphine and codeine, are derived from the seeds of the unripe poppy plant, Papaver somniferum, and were consumed for their narcotic and analgesic properties. Heroin (diacetylmorphine), a semisynthetic opioid, was first introduced in 1874. It became popular because of the rapid onset of its central nervous system (CNS) effects. By 1950, heroin had supplanted morphine as the drug of choice among abusers (5). It is available illicitly in bags containing up to 40 to 50 mg of the active ingredient, cut or diluted variably with quinine, lactose, starch, lidocaine, or even powdered milk. Methadone was first synthesized in 1945. It is longer-acting than heroin, and can be administered orally. These properties render it the drug of choice for replacement

therapy of heroin addicts undergoing detoxification. Because Dole and Nyswander (6) advocated the use of methadone in maintenance treatment programs, it has become the most widely used and studied opiate in pregnancy. However, methadone treatment of the opioid dependent pregnant woman has also led to significant withdrawal in the infant (7).

Almost all narcotics taken by the pregnant woman cross the placenta and enter the fetal circulation. Thus, the fetus is chronically exposed to these drugs and can develop problems in utero and after birth. Although the development of passive addiction is the most commonly known fetal complication of morphine, many other important problems are encountered (Table 58-2).

ANTENATAL PROBLEMS

Intrauterine asphyxia is perhaps the single greatest risk to the fetus of a drug-dependent woman based on reports of a high incidence of stillbirths, meconium-stained amniotic fluid, fetal distress, non reactive stress test, low Apgar score, and neonatal aspiration pneumonia (8–12). The predisposition of the fetus to asphyxia underscores the need for repeated evaluation of fetal well-being during the course of the pregnancy of the drug dependent woman. Fetal asphyxia may be secondary to a number of factors. Studies using methadone in a fetal lamb model suggest that opiates affect both quiet and rapid-eye-movement (REM) sleep, which lead to a hyperactive state that causes a 20% increase in fetal oxygen consumption (13). Sleep disturbances, consisting of more REM and less quiet sleep, have been observed in newborn infants chronically exposed in utero to low doses of methadone with or without concomitant heroin usage (14–15). Another possible cause of fetal asphyxia is fetal withdrawal, which usually coincides with the mother's withdrawal. Fetal withdrawal leads to fetal hyperactivity, increase in catecholamine release, increase in oxygen consumption and, if not adequately compensated for, fetal asphyxia (16). In a lamb model, withdrawal was induced in the morphine-exposed fetal lamb by the administration of naloxone, an opiate antagonist. Manifestations included immediate bradycardia associated with transient increases in systolic and diastolic blood pressure, rapid, continuous deep breathing movements, increased total body movements, eye movements and neck tone, and desynchronization of electrocortical activity (15). A high incidence of preeclampsia, abruptio placentae and placenta previa in the pregnant addict also predispose to placental insufficiency and fetal distress (7).

Meconium-stained amniotic fluid is frequently encountered in the pregnant addict and is a manifestation of fetal distress (7). Aspiration of meconium as a result of fetal distress may account for the increased frequency of meconium aspiration syndrome and persistent pulmonary hypertension of the newborn after birth.

Intrauterine infection is another risk in the fetus of a drug addict. Because of the life-style of the pregnant addict of

TABLE 58-2
SUMMARY OF PERINATAL AND LONG TERM COMPLICATIONS ASSOCIATED WITH FETAL EXPOSURE TO DRUGS

Drugs	Antenatal	Intrapartum	Neonatal	Long Term
Narcotics (morphine, heroin, methadone)	Stillbirth Spontaneous abortion Fetal asphyxia Maternal infection Premature rupture of membranes (PROM)	Fetal distress Low Apgar score Neonatal depression Meconium stained fluid	Prematurity Low birth weight Small-for-gestational-age (SGA) Aspiration pneumonia Meconium aspiration Persistent pulmonary hypertension (PPHN) Transient tachypnea Hyaline membrane disease Minor congenital anomalies Altered sleep pattern Thrombocytosis Abstinence syndrome Abnormal Brazelton Neonatal Assessment Scale (BNAS)	Persistence of withdrawal Child neglect and abuse Sudden infant death Syndrome (SIDS) Psychomotor delay Strabismus/nystagmus Behavior problems, e.g., hyperactivity, aggression, inattention, impulsiveness, short attention span Language problems Preschool – problems in perception, short term memory and organization
Nonnarcotic hypno-sedatives			Abstinence syndrome Omphalocoele-exstrophy (diazepam) Hyperphagia	
Cocaine	Stillbirth Spontaneous abortion Increased uterine vascular resistance Maternal infection Placental infarcts Intrauterine growth retardation (IUGR) Abnormal fetal breathing	Abruptio placenta Premature labor PROM Shortened duration of labor Meconium stained fluid	Prematurity Low birth weight Small for gestation Small head circumference Multiorgan dysfunction Abnormal EEG Abnormal auditory brain stem responses (ABR) Transient hypertonia Subependymal cysts Cerebral infarction Mobius syndrome Heart rate/rhythm abnormalities Increased apnea density Increased serum creatine kinase and myoglobin Abnormal breathing pattern Necrotizing enterocolitis Intestinal perforation Abnormal BNAS Retinal hemorrhage and tortuous of iris vessels	Strabismus/nystagmus Problem in expressive and receptive language Low verbal comprehension Poor recognition, memory and information processing Low Fagan score Low Bayley score Poor cognitive functions Decreased visual attention Behavior problems, e.g., distractibility, attention deficit SIDS Passive cocaine intoxication
Alcohol	Spontaneous abortion Aneuploidy Stillbirth Breech presentation IUGR Abnormal fetal heart rate pattern Decreased fetal breathing, eye and body movement	Abruptio placenta Premature labor	Prematurity Low birth weight SGA, symmetric Abstinence syndrome Facial dysmorphism Fetal alcohol syndrome Fetal alcohol effect Abnormal BNAS Abnormal EEG in sleep state	Growth deficits in weight, length, head circumference Low Bayley scores Low Fagan scores Hyperactivity and attention deficit Language problem Behavior problem Poor academic achievement (low aptitude score) Adolescent: difficulty in tasks involving manipulation of information, goal management, attention, memory, calculation, estimation test

TABLE 58-2
(continued)

Drugs	Antenatal	Intrapartum	Neonatal	Long Term
Marijuana		Precipitous or dysfunctional labor Meconium stained fluid	Prematurity Increase in male births Abnormal BNAS	Fine tremors Disrupted sleep patterns Poor abstract/visual reasoning, poor memory and verbal skills at age 3–4 yrs Poor motor skills, short length of play at age 3 years Abnormal attention behavior Small risk for SIDS
Nicotine	Spontaneous abortion Stillbirth Placental decidual necrosis and calcification	Abruptio placenta Premature labor	Decrease in birth weight, length, head circumference Congenital heart defect, aortopulmonary septum defect, cheilognathopalatoschisis, deformities of the extremities, polycystic kidney, gastroschisis, skull deformities Persistent pulmonary hypertension Abnormal BNAS	Low test scores in cognitive, psychomotor, language and general academic achievement, including reading, mathematics Risk for prepubertal onset conduct disorder and adolescent onset drug dependence Sudden infant death syndrome
Phencyclidine	Intrauterine growth retardation,	Precipitous labor Meconium stained fluid	Drug intoxication (irritability, tremors, hypertonicity, poor attention, bizarre eye movements, staring spells, hypertonic ankle reflexes, depressed grasp and rooting reflexes. Sudden, rapid change in level of consciousness, with lethargy alternating with irritability)	Temperament and sleep problems
Amphetamine, methamphetamine	Fetal death Retroplacental hemorrhage		Prematurity Neonatal death Drug intoxication (abnormal sleep patterns, tremors, poor feeding, hypertonia, sneezing, high-pitched cry, frantic fist sucking, loose stools, fever, yawning, tachypnea, hyperreflexia and excoriation)	Decrease in IQ at 4 years (Terman Merrill method) Aggressive behavior and peer-related problems Poor academic performance and various behavioral problems in adolescent children
Caffeine	Small risk for spontaneous abortion Reduced fetal growth		Cardiac arrhythmias Potential abstinence syndrome, (jitteriness, irritability, vomiting)	

trading sex for drugs, she is predisposed to infections, particularly of sexually transmitted diseases such as syphilis, gonorrhea, hepatitis and HIV infection, all of which can be transmitted to her fetus (2,17–18). During delivery or before labor, the increased incidence of premature membrane rupture in the pregnant addict further exposes the fetus to the risk of nonspecific infections (7). Opiates may also compromise immune functions in the fetus through its adverse effect on cell-mediated and humoral immune responses (19,20).

NEONATAL PROBLEMS

Prematurity and Low Birth Weight

Infants born to mothers on heroin have a higher incidence of prematurity, low birth weight, small for gestation, and small head circumference (between the 3rd and 5th percentile) than drug-free control subjects (20–25). One mechanism for the fetal growth restriction in narcotic addiction may be the effect of opiates stimulating opiate kappa receptors which inhibit acetylcholine release in the placenta. Acetylcholine is responsible for increasing placental blood flow through vasodilatation and facilitating the transport of amino acids across the placenta (26).

On the other hand, the birth weight of infants whose mothers were on methadone have varied from being higher (27) or lower (24) than the infants of untreated pregnant addicts, or not significantly different from the general newborn population (22). Higher birth weights probably reflect the good prenatal care that the woman receives in a methadone program. On the other hand, studies on pregnant rats exposed to methadone have shown their offspring to have significantly lower body weight, length, head diameter, and organ weight (28), and impaired brain development (29) and thermoregulation (30) compared to non–methadone-exposed pups. Women who reduced their methadone dose during pregnancy delivered infants of significantly higher birth weight than those whose methadone dose remained the same or were increased (31). A meta-analyses of opiate use and birth weight showed a mean reduction of 489 g associated with heroin use, 279 g with methadone use and 557 g on combined heroin and methadone use. These findings suggest that concurrent use of heroin although on methadone treatment counteracts the birth weight advantage gained from methadone alone (32).

Low Apgar Score

There is a high incidence of low Apgar score in infants of drug-dependent mothers. This may be related to intrauterine asphyxia (see Antenatal Problems) or to the effects of narcotics which the mother received before delivery. Not infrequently, the pregnant addict will obtain a heroin fix before entering the hospital, which can depress the infant.

Significantly large amounts of morphine have been found in the urine and cord blood of infants born to these women (6). Caution must therefore be exercised with the use of narcotic antagonists to reverse the respiratory depression in drug-dependent infants, because the narcotic antagonists can precipitate an acute withdrawal in the infant.

Others

In addition to withdrawal, other problems are seen with increased frequency in the infant of a drug-dependent mother: jaundice, aspiration pneumonia, meconium aspiration, persistent pulmonary hypertension of the newborn, transient tachypnea, hyaline membrane disease, congenital malformations, and infections (7). These problems are significant because they are the principal causes of death in these infants.

Aspiration pneumonia, hyaline membrane disease, and transient tachypnea are the leading pulmonary problems in the infant of the drug-dependent mother. About 30% of aspiration pneumonia is as a result of meconium aspiration (7). Transient tachypnea may be secondary to the inhibitory effects of narcotics on the reflex clearing of fluid by the lungs (33). The high incidence of hyaline membrane disease among infants of drug-dependent mothers is likely as a result of prematurity. What has been reported as a protection among premature, drug-dependent infants from hyaline membrane disease is due primarily to the increased incidence of small-for-gestational-age infants in this group (7,34). Thus, the factors that cause a fetus to be small for gestational age are probably more important determinants of the infant's risk for developing hyaline membrane disease than is the direct action of narcotics (e.g., heroin) in accelerating pulmonary maturation (35). Meconium aspiration, persistent pulmonary hypertension of the newborn and hyaline membrane disease account for more than 50% of the deaths among infants of drug-dependent mothers (7).

In general, opiates are not teratogenic to the fetus. Most reports do not show an increase in the frequency of congenital anomalies (11,30), and in one study, although an increased frequency of malformations was found (7,36), the malformations were minor (e.g., skin tag) and no consistent pattern of malformation was observed. Animal studies, however, have shown a dose-related teratogenic effect of narcotics on the CNS of the developing hamster, which can be blocked by narcotic antagonists (37). *In vitro* studies have also shown opiates to impair deoxyribonucleic acid (DNA) repair and cause chromosome aberration with hyperdiploidy (38).

There is an altered sleep pattern in infants of drug dependent mothers, characterized by more rapid eye movement associated sleep than quiet sleep (39,40). In term infants exposed to opiates, abnormal auditory brainstem evoked response show decreased conductance time for waves I-III (41,42). Abnormal heart rate and breathing patterns have also been observed (43,44). The respiratory rates are higher with low end tidal volume PCO_2 and a shift to the left in their breathing response to CO_2 (45). These abnormalities have been suggested to increase their predisposition to the sudden infant death syndrome (see Long-Term Outcome).

There is an increased incidence of jaundice in the infants of drug-dependent mothers, which is likely related to the high incidence of prematurity in this group (7). Although induction of liver enzymes by morphine has been demonstrated in animals (45), the dose of morphine used was exceedingly high (250 mg/kg); a situation unlikely to be paralleled in a clinical setting. A significant thrombocytosis, occasionally exceeding 1,000,000 platelets per mm^3, was reported in infants of mothers receiving maintenance doses of 40 to 90 mg of methadone per day. Onset was by the second week of life, with counts remaining high for over 16 weeks. The thrombocytosis, and associated increased circulating platelet aggregates, may play a role in the development of the focal cerebral infarctions and germinal matrix and subarachnoid hemorrhages which were encountered in some postmortem examinations of the infants (46). The incidence of intraventricular hemorrhage in the opiate exposed infant is not increased (47). Cranial ultrasound have shown slit like ventricles and small intracranial diameter (48).

Along with the high incidence of infection in the pregnant addict is a correspondingly high incidence of infection in her infant. Although some of the neonatal infections are nonspecific in nature, such as sepsis, omphalitis, necrotizing enterocolitis, and gastroenteritis, many are related to the life style of the mother and include hepatitis and venereal diseases, e.g., syphilis, gonorrhea, herpes simplex, group B streptococcal, and HIV infections (2,7,17,18).

Neonatal Narcotic Withdrawal or Abstinence Syndrome

The onset of withdrawal usually occurs within the first 72 hours after birth, commonly within the first 24 to 48 hours. In a few instances, the onset may appear soon after birth, particularly if the mother has begun to experience withdrawal before delivery. Reports of withdrawal occurring after the first or second week may be secondary to withdrawal from other drugs, e.g., phenobarbital, beside the narcotics (49). Many factors, such as amount of narcotics used by the mother, timing of the last dose before delivery, character of the labor, type and amount of anesthesia or analgesia given to the mother, and the maturity and nutritional status of the infant, influence the onset of withdrawal (7).

Withdrawal in the infant usually peaks by about the third day of postnatal life and decreases in intensity by the fifth to seventh day. The duration of withdrawal is related to its severity. When drugs are used to treat the withdrawal, relapse may occur if treatment is discontinued abruptly. The withdrawal manifestations, although they may improve within a week, do not completely disappear until about 8 to 16 weeks of age (see Long-Term Outcome).

The severity of the withdrawal is influenced by several factors. It is less severe in the preterm infants as a result of their neurologic immaturity or reduced total exposure to narcotics (50). Withdrawal is significantly related to the amount of narcotics that the mother used during pregnancy. With methadone, a high maintenance maternal methadone dose during pregnancy or the dose at the last methadone intake is associated with more intense withdrawal (7,51–53). Almost half (46%) of these infants were treated for narcotic withdrawal; with the methadone dosage correlating both to the duration of hospitalization and neonatal abstinence score (32). Buprenorphine, a potentially safer, opioid, maintenance drug than methadone, has been shown to lead to lower incidence of abstinence syndrome in both the mother and infant and lower mean weight reduction in the infant (54–58). Neither the infant's gender, race, and Apgar score nor the mother's age, parity, and duration of heroin intake correlated to the severity of withdrawal (7). Similarly, manipulation of the environment such as reducing the amount of light or noise in the nursery did not ameliorate the severity of withdrawal in the infants (7). Adults experience abdominal cramps, palpitation, nausea, and other discomforts while undergoing withdrawal. It is likely that similar discomforts are also experienced by the infant which may nullify any potential benefits from light or noise reduction in the nursery.

Neonatal narcotic withdrawal is associated with noradrenergic hyperactivity and the manifestations involve the central nervous system, the respiratory, gastrointestinal, vasomotor and cutaneous systems (Table 58-3).

Central Nervous System Signs. Neurologic signs predominate and appear early. The findings are those of CNS excitability, such as hyperactivity, irritability, tremors, sneezing and hypertonicity. Occasionally, fever may accompany these increased neuromuscular activities.

Hyperactivity manifests almost as incessant movements of the extremities. When the infant is supine and unrestrained, the movements assume a jerky, purposeless, en masse nature, apparently perpetuated by unchecked, proprioceptive stimuli. When placed in the prone position, the motor behavior becomes more organized. There are crawling movements, which may actually lead to the infant's displacement from the crib, and other motions such as chin lifting, head movement from side to side, chest elevation, and hand-to-mouth facility. The latter usually soothes the infant, indicating the usefulness of pacifiers. Hyperirritability manifests almost as incessant crying with shrill, high-pitched outcries. The infant's muscle tone is exaggerated and sometimes, an opisthotonic position is assumed. This makes the infant difficult to hold as a result of its failure to mold to the body of the holder. Sleep is also disturbed. Tremors and myoclonic jerks are frequent, and are sometimes sustained. To distinguish tremors from seizures, the former can be abolished by restraint of the tremulous extremities. The reflexes of the infant (e.g., Moro, traction response, weight bearing, placing, stepping, crawling, and Landau) are all exaggerated. The infant's

TABLE 58-3

MANIFESTATIONS OF NEONATAL NARCOTIC WITHDRAWAL

Central nervous system
  Hyperactivity
  Hyperirritability-excess crying, high-pitched outcry
  Increased muscle tone
  Exaggerated reflexes
  Tremors
  Sneezing, hiccups, yawning
  Short, nonquiet sleep
  Fever
Respiratory system
  Tachypnea
  Excess secretions
Gastrointestinal system
  Disorganized sucking with reduced pressure
  Vomiting
  Drooling
  Sensitive gag
  Hyperphagia
  Diarrhea
  Abdominal cramps
Vasomotor system
  Stuffy nose
  Flushing
  Sweating
  Sudden, circumoral pallor
Cutaneous system
  Excoriated buttocks
  Facial scratches
  Pressure-point abrasions

From Ostrea EM, Chavez CJ, Stryker JS. The care of the drug dependent woman and her infant. Lansing, MI: Michigan Department of Public Health, 1978:30, with permission.

responses to stimuli, such as sound and light, are also increased disproportionately. In premature infants, the neural hyperexcitability is more episodic. The infants appear restless and overactive for short periods and then lapse into periods of lethargy and inactivity. Sustained tremors usually are not seen in premature infants until they mature to a point when sufficient tone is present in the upper and lower extremities. Electroencephalographic (EEG) tracings on the addicted neonate may be abnormal and show high-frequency dysynchronous activity suggestive of CNS irritability.

Respiratory Signs. Infants in withdrawal may be tachypneic, with irregular respirations. Alkalosis as a result of hyperventilation may result. Fluid loss may also be increased.

Gastrointestinal Signs. The suck of the infant is disorganized, reduced in rate and sucking pressure (59) and poorly coordinated with swallowing. Consequently, milk frequently drools around the corners of the infant's mouth. The infant appears incessantly hungry, which, when unfulfilled, leads to mounting agitation, persistent crying, hyperactivity, and exhaustion. Proper positioning of the infant to enhance hand-to-mouth facility may be extremely soothing. Vomiting and diarrhea are often observed. This may

lead to dehydration, electrolyte imbalance, and excoriations around the buttocks (see Complications).

Vasomotor Signs. Significant vasomotor instability manifests as stuffy nose, flushing, mottling, sweating, and episodes of sudden, circumoral pallor.

Cutaneous Signs. Because of hyperactivity, facial scratches and abrasions on pressure points may be observed on the infant's skin. Excoriations of the buttocks can occur if diarrhea is present.

Complications

The complications associated with neonatal drug withdrawal are related to its severity. Abnormalities in serum electrolytes and pH and dehydration may occur secondary to vomiting and diarrhea. Weight loss may be profound, not only as a result of increased fluid loss and hyperactivity, but also to poor and ineffective oral intake. Aspiration pneumonia may occur, as a result of vomiting, incoordinate sucking and swallowing. Respiratory alkalosis can result from tachyp- nea. In some instances, convulsion may be observed. However, it should be noted that convulsion is a more frequent manifestation of narcotic compared to nonnarcotic withdrawal (see Nonnarcotic Abstinence Syndrome).

Mortality

The mortality rate among infants born to drug-dependent mothers used to be as high as 50%. With early recognition and treatment of the withdrawal syndrome and prevention of its complications, the mortality from neonatal withdrawal is almost negligible. Nonetheless, overall mortality among infants of drug-dependent mothers remains high. In one report, mortality rate was 27 per 1,000 live births compared to 12 per 1,000 live births in the general population (7). The causes of death were related to immaturity, prematurity, hyaline membrane disease, meconium aspiration, persistent pulmonary hypertension of the newborn (PPHN) and major congenital malformations. Pulmonary problems (e.g., meconium aspiration, PPHN, hyaline membrane disease) accounted for more than 50% of the deaths.

Neonatal Neurobehavioral Abnormalities

By the Brazelton Neonatal Assessment Scale, the manifestations of neonatal withdrawal such as hypertonicity, hyperirritability, hyperactivity, and increased hand-to-mouth facility can be demonstrated. Some other fine behavioral abnormalities are also found that could affect early infant–caregiver interaction (60). For instance, congenital addiction seems to affect those behavior systems which are associated with arousal and early development of mother–infant bonding. Although the addicted infant is more likely to elicit caregiver consolation because it cries more often, it is less easy to cuddle, because of increased tone. It is also less readily maintained in an alert state through handling and less responsive to visual stimuli, although auditory evoked responses are better integrated. Because cuddliness, alertness, and visual regard are the primary means by which the infant initiates and maintains interaction with its mother, the impairment of these behavior patterns may have a profound effect on the early infant–mother bonding (61).

Long-Term Outcome

Persistence of Withdrawal. The withdrawal of infants from narcotics may persist for 8 to 16 weeks (62,63), but are usually milder than the initial course and consist of mild irritability, tremors, hypertonicity, sneezing, hiccups, and regurgitation. The persistence of withdrawal is related directly to its initial severity and is more prolonged in those infants who had severe withdrawal and were treated with drugs for withdrawal. Thus, although drug treatment may ameliorate the manifestations of withdrawal, it does not shorten its duration. It is important therefore that the mother is made aware that the infant's withdrawal may persist for sometime, albeit manageable, once the infant is discharged from the nursery. Otherwise, she may become alarmed when the infant continues to manifest withdrawal at home. The unwarned mother may also misinterpret the infant's irritability as hunger and over feed the infant which can then lead to diarrhea and vomiting. The mother also should be instructed on how to reduce the infant's discomfort by swaddling and cuddling the infant. Additionally, she should be reassured that the infant's withdrawal will eventually subside without the use of medications. In most instances, the mother who is well informed can cope with the situation successfully.

Child Abuse and Neglect and Sudden Infant Death Syndrome. The high incidence of child abuse and neglect constitutes one of the serious problems in the infants of drug addicted mothers (64,65). Thermal burns, usually from cigarette burns, traumatic ecchymoses, and hematoma have been observed in 8% of infants during the first 8 months of life (58). About 8.3% of the infants have to be placed in alternative care environment because of maternal neglect, abandonment or maternal death. Many factors contribute to the risk of child abuse. The persistence of withdrawal for some weeks, feeding problems, abnormal sleep patterns and periods of restlessness in the infant can generate undue tension in the mother, whose tolerance for frustration is already low. Thus, the mother, unable to cope with the situation, may simply withdraw from her infant and avoid any contact or may abandon or injure the infant.

There is a four to fivefold increase in the incidence of sudden death syndrome in infants of opiate-dependent mothers (66,67). This complication is observed whether the infant is cared for by the mother or in an extended family or foster home. The cause is not clear, although its occurrence is significantly higher in those infants who had moderate to severe than mild withdrawal after birth (66,67). Abnormal breathing patterns, control of breath-

ing and exposure of the infant to maternal smoking have been implicated as contributory causes to sudden infant death syndrome (SIDS) (44).

Growth and Psychomotor Development

In general, the physical growth of the congenitally addicted infant has shown a catch up in growth when adjusted for sex, race, maternal education and smoking. At 12 months of age, the growth in terms of weight, head circumference and length of the infants have been observed to fall within the 10th to the 90th percentile on the growth chart. Similarly, the percentage of addicted infants whose growth parameters were below the 10th percentile did not differ significantly from the nonaddict group (68). However, some studies have reported retardation in the weight, length, and head circumference at age 3 to 6 years (69–73). A high incidence of transient or minor motor deficits, poor motor coordination, and abnormal eye findings, such as nystagmus and strabismus have also been observed in these infants in the first year of life (71,74,75).

The mental and cognitive performance of the opiate exposed infants have been shown to be comparable to the control, non drug exposed group (63,68,76,77). Within the first year, infants of narcotic addicts have been shown to manifest some difficulty in regulating their behavior, but otherwise had normal developmental scores except in early language development (69–71,78). However, at preschool age, compared to controls, i.e., children at similar environmental risk and sociodemographic background, the addicted children performed less well in terms of perception, short-term memory, and organization, but did just as well on objective tests of activity and attention (70).

Behavioral problems have been observed among the opiate exposed infant and have persisted even in late childhood. These consisted of hyperactivity, aggressiveness, inattention, impulsiveness, short attention span and lack of concentration and inhibition (63,78–82). This leads to learning problems in school, truancy and suspension (64). However, these problems are probably more the result of environmental and emotional deprivation of the infant than from the effects of in utero drug exposure. These include significant psychopathology in the mother (or parents) with or without comorbid alcohol abuse, and negative parenting behavior which contribute to poor infant rearing. The problems are further compounded by arrest or incarceration of the mother and her treatment for emotional disorders (64,65,83,84). The mother is also more socially isolated and less likely to pursue vocational or educational attainment. Thus, the addicted mother needs assistance in parenting. Someone should be available to help her in the care of her child (often the maternal grandmother) and that a visiting or public health nurse and a social and protective service worker should actively participate in the follow up of the mother and her infant (85–87). Alternative measures of placement of the child into a more favorable home environment have sometimes resulted in better behavioral functions of the child (81).

NONNARCOTIC HYPNOSEDATIVES

Nonnarcotic Abstinence Syndrome

Infants born to women who have used nonnarcotic hypnosedatives during pregnancy (Table 58-4) can become addicted to the drugs and manifest withdrawal, as well. The manifestations of nonnarcotic withdrawal in the neonate are similar to those of narcotic withdrawal (88). In a few instances (e.g., with barbiturate withdrawal or ethchlorvynol withdrawal), hyperphagia has been described as a prominent manifestation.

Although the manifestations of withdrawal from narcotic and nonnarcotic drugs are similar, major differences exist (58).

In adults, the rate of developing physical dependence to the nonnarcotic hypnosedatives does not increase with the drug dose, as it does with narcotics. Rather, prolonged and continuous administration of large and partially incapacitating doses are necessary, over months or years, to produce addiction to nonnarcotics, especially if the drugs are taken orally. The situation is different in the newborn infant. Passive addiction in the fetus and infant have been observed even with therapeutic doses of nonnarcotic drugs used by the mother during pregnancy. For instance, a pregnant woman who is treated with phenobarbital for epilepsy can induce serious addiction in her fetus, although she herself, may not be addicted to the drug (49).

The manifestations of the nonnarcotic abstinence syndrome are more frequently intense and life threatening compared to narcotic withdrawal. The occurrence of convulsion is also more frequent.

Most of the withdrawal from narcotics is seen within the first 3 days of postnatal life, as a result of the short half-life of most narcotics. In contrast, withdrawal from the nonnarcotics, particularly phenobarbital, may be observed at 7 to 10 days after birth as a result of the slow clearance of the drug in the infant.

TABLE 58-4
NONNARCOTIC DRUGS

Hypnosedatives
   Barbiturate
Nonbarbiturate sedatives and tranquilizers
   Bromide
   Chloral hydrate
   Chlordiazepoxide (Librium)
   Diazepam (Valium)
   Ethchlorvynol (Placidyl)
   Glutethimide (Doriden)
   Ethanol

Unlike the narcotics, neonatal addiction to many of the nonnarcotic hypnosedatives has been induced by physicians who prescribe the drug to the mother, totally unaware of its addicting potential on the fetus (58).

BARBITURATES

Barbiturates have been used in clinical medicine for many years, but its addiction potential has only been recently recognized. In adults, the frequent association of barbiturate use with alcohol may have contributed to the delayed recognition of its addicting potential because of the ability of barbiturates to control the withdrawal from alcohol (89,90).

Barbiturates are classified, based on their duration of their action, as ultrashort, intermediate, and long acting. The intermediate-acting barbiturates are most frequently abused (e.g., secobarbital [Seconal], pentobarbital [Nembutal], amobarbital [Amytal], butabarbital [Butisol]). The abuse of the long-acting barbiturates (e.g., phenobarbital) is not as common as the abuse of the shorter-acting forms. Phenobarbital, however, is more frequently involved in withdrawal syndrome in the newborn because it is used frequently by the mother for insomnia, for the relief of anxiety, as an anticonvulsant, or for sedation when toxemia of pregnancy occurs.

Passive addiction of the fetus to barbiturates can occur after its prolonged exposure to the drug *in utero* (49,91). Barbiturates cross the placenta readily and establish high levels in both the maternal and cord blood. Relatively high levels of barbiturates have been found in the fetal brain, liver and adrenal glands (92). The manifestations of barbiturate withdrawal in the neonate are similar, regardless of the type of barbiturate used by the mother; however, the onset of withdrawal may differ. Withdrawal typically occurs within a day after birth with intermediate-acting barbiturates (93), and from 3 to 7 days after birth with the long-acting barbiturates (91).

Barbiturates are metabolized principally by the liver, although a significant portion may be excreted unchanged by the kidney. In adults, up to 30% of the total dose of phenobarbital ingested is excreted unchanged in the urine (94). The half-life of phenobarbital prenatally administered to infants is almost twice that in the adult, and varies inversely with the extent of the prenatal exposure to the drug (95). Phenobarbital levels in the arterial cord blood have ranged from 77% to 100% of maternal levels depending on the duration of maternal treatment, gestational age and cord pH in the infant (96).

The signs of withdrawal from barbiturates in neonates are similar to those described in adults. The infants are overactive and restless, with excessive crying, twitching, hyperactive reflexes and hypertonicity. They also manifest diarrhea, vomiting, and poor sucking ability. When tonic-clonic convulsions occur, the EEG patterns show diffuse, paroxysmal, high-voltage, slow-wave bursts, similar to those seen in adults (91). A subacute phase of hyperphagia, episodes of prolonged crying, episodic irritability, hyperacusis, and sweating have been described (91). These manifestations may last from 2 to 6 months. A combination of phenobarbital-phenytoin treatment of the mother has also been observed to predispose to smaller occipitofrontal circumference in the infants compared to phenobarbital monotherapy alone (97). Cognitive functions in infants exposed to phenobarbital, in utero, did not differ from controls, except for a higher incidence of learning problems (98).

Recognition of the abstinence syndrome from phenobarbital is essential for the proper management of the infant. An awareness of late onset withdrawal in infants exposed in utero to long-acting barbiturates should alert the clinician to follow these infants closely during the first 2 weeks of life.

CHLORDIAZEPOXIDE AND DIAZEPAM

Chlordiazepoxide (Librium) and diazepam (Valium) are widely used for their hypnosedative effects. Abuse and dependence on these drugs have been reported in adults. During pregnancy, benzodiazepines cross the placenta with relative ease, resulting in significant drug levels in the serum and tissues of the fetus (99). Placental transfer of diazepam can occur from the sixth week of gestation and accumulate in the fetal tissues during organogenesis (100). Mean levels of diazepam were found to be markedly higher in the umbilical cord serum than in the maternal serum after a single intravenous injection of 10 mg of diazepam (101).

An acute withdrawal syndrome from chlordiazepoxide or diazepam was observed in the newborn infant (102,103). A presumptive diagnosis of chlordiazepoxide withdrawal was made in a set of twins born to a mother who used chlordiazepoxide (20 mg per day) during the second and third trimesters of her pregnancy (102). The withdrawal occurred on day 21 of life, and consisted of severe irritability and coarse tremors. However, in three reports of neonatal withdrawal from diazepam, the onset of withdrawal occurred within 2.5 to 6 hours after birth and consisted of tremors, irritability, hypertonicity, vigorous sucking, vomiting, and diarrhea (103). The dose of diazepam used by the mother up to the time of birth ranged from 15 to 20 mg per day. In all three cases, phenobarbital was effective in controlling the withdrawal in the infant, although the drug had to be administered for a prolonged period (13–25 days). In another report, a mother used narcotics and diazepam during pregnancy. There was an initial good response of the infant to treatment for narcotic withdrawal but the withdrawal manifestations intensified at 7 to 14 days of life. The late withdrawal was attributed to prenatal diazepam exposure (104). Late third trimester use and exposure to diazepam during labor has been associated with the floppy infant syndrome, or marked neonatal withdrawal. The manifestations varied from mild sedation, hypotonia and reluctance to suck, to apneic spells, cyanosis and impaired metabolic responses to cold stress. These signs may persist from a few hours to months after birth (105). High dose,

intravenous administration or prolonged duration of diazepam therapy in mothers has also caused significant depression in the newborn with poor muscle tone (101,106). In one report, infants prenatally exposed to diazepam had lower birth weight compared to controls, but eventually showed catch up growth by eight months of age (107). Congenital malformations are uncommon with antenatal diazepam exposure although a case has been reported of an omphalocoele-exstrophy-imperforate anus-spina bifida complex occurring in a infant whose mother took 30 mg of diazepam daily for affective disorder during the entire pregnancy (108). Offspring of rats who were treated with chlordiazepoxide during the critical period of neural development showed significant deficits in learning acquisition and retention (109). In general, most studies involving first trimester use of benzodiazepines have shown the majority of infants to be normal at birth and have normal postnatal development (105).

OTHER HYPNOSEDATIVES

Hypnosedatives, which used to be popular in the past, have been associated with adverse effects in the newborn infants. These include chloral hydrate (110), bromide (111–113), etchlorvynol (114–119), and gluthetimide (120). A withdrawal syndrome and growth retardation have been reported in newborn infants after the use of bromides by the mother during pregnancy (111,112). Studies on rat pups whose dams were given sodium bromide, ad libitum, showed significant delay in postnatal development, permanent deficits in body weight, brain weight and protein content of brain tissue but with an increased size of the olfactory glomeruli (113). Etchlorvynol (Placidyl) was introduced in 1955 as a nonbarbiturate, non addicting hypnotic for the treatment of insomnia (114,118). However, subsequent reports of addiction to ethchlorvynol have been reported (115–117). An abstinence syndrome from ethchlorvynol was observed in a newborn infant, which consisted of extreme jitteriness, irritability, and hyperphagia (119). The drug that was taken by the mother was within the recommended therapeutic dose. The onset of withdrawal in the infant occurred during the second day of life. No convulsions were noted because the infant received phenobarbital treatment early in the course of the abstinence syndrome. Gluthetimide (Doriden) was first introduced in 1954 as a nonbarbiturate hypnosedative, allegedly free of addicting properties. As in the case of most nonbarbiturate hypnosedatives, this led to its widespread use, particularly as a substitute drug for the treatment of alcohol addiction (120). Since then, numerous reports of acute and sometimes fatal intoxication with the drug in adults and the occurrence of physical dependence have been reported (120–122). Gluthetimide is structurally related to phenobarbital.

A possible case of neonatal withdrawal to gluthetimide was reported in a pregnant heroin addict who supplemented her habit with 2 to 3 g of gluthetimide three or four times a week to get a desired euphoric effect (123). Within 8 hours of birth, the infant exhibited signs of withdrawal from narcotics that were readily controlled with chlorpromazine. However, on the tenth day of life, while on a tapering dose of chlorpromazine, the infant suddenly manifested diarrhea, fever, tachypnea, irritability, hypertonicity, and diaphoresis. It was presumed that the unusual recurrence of withdrawal on the tenth day of life may have been secondary to withdrawal from glutethimide.

DIFFERENTIAL DIAGNOSIS

Withdrawal from the narcotic and nonnarcotic hypnosedatives should be distinguished from hypoglycemia, hypocalcemia, hypomagnesemia, sepsis, meningitis, subarachnoid hemorrhage, infectious diarrhea, and intestinal obstruction. Blood chemistry, white cell count and differential, cerebrospinal fluid examination, radiographic examination, and cultures should be performed as indicated by the clinical circumstances.

Infants whose mothers were on tricyclic antidepressants and lithium during pregnancy for psychiatric conditions may manifest toxicity similar to withdrawal, such as irritability, tachycardia, respiratory distress, sweating, and convulsions (124–128). Likewise, maternal intake of phenothiazines (e.g., chlorpromazine) may induce extrapyramidal dysfunctions in the newborn infant, such as tremors, facial grimacing, increased muscle tone, cogwheel rigidity, increased reflexes, and torticollis, all of which can resemble the withdrawal syndrome (129,130). The prenatal history and the identification of the corresponding drug in the infant's serum or urine are necessary to establish the diagnosis.

COCAINE

Types

Cocaine is an alkaloid that is extracted from the leaves of the Erythroxylon coca bush. Its chemical name is methylbenzoylecgonine, and is the only known, naturally occurring local anesthetic. Cocaine was first extracted and identified by the German chemist, Albert Niemann in 1860. The drug is extracted from the leaves of the coca plant by a series of solvent extractions. Coca paste is the first extraction product of cocaine and contains about 80% cocaine (131,132). The paste can be smoked by applying it to tobacco or marijuana. Cocaine hydrochloride is the most common available form of cocaine. In its acid state, cocaine HCl is a white powder that is soluble in water and can be snorted or injected. Cocaine HCl usually is adulterated with starch, glucose, phencyclidine (PCP), heroin, or amphetamines, and its purity ranges from 20% to 80% (131–132).

An alkaloidal base of cocaine can be obtained from cocaine HCl ("free-basing") by alkalinizing the aqueous solution of cocaine HCl and then extracting the cocaine alkaloid base using volatile organic solvents, such as ether. The gummy cocaine residue, called "rock," has a lower melting point than cocaine HCl and can be smoked using a special pipe. Crack cocaine is the most popular, abused form of the drug. Crack cocaine is produced when cocaine HCl is mixed with ammonia, water, and baking soda and heated. The resulting paste, once dried, forms a hard, rocklike substance that can be smoked. The term "crack" is derived from the crackling sound that is produced when crack cocaine is prepared or smoked.

When taken orally, cocaine HCl has a peak effect at between 45 minutes and 90 minutes. Intranasal administration of cocaine, i.e., snorting has a peak effect in 15 to 30 minutes, and lasts from 60 to 90 minutes. Smoking cocaine ("crack" cocaine) provides the most rapid delivery of the drug to the body. Peak effect is within 60 to 90 seconds, but the high lasts only for about 5 to 10 minutes. The intense high is followed by a down period as the effect of the drug wears off. The down period may be so unpleasant that more of the drug is used to re-experience the high, or other drugs, e.g., alcohol are used. Thus, cocaine use promotes the abuse of other drugs (131).

Cocaine is metabolized by plasma and hepatic esterases into three major water-soluble metabolites, ecgonine methyl ester, benzoylecgonine, and ecgonine, although other minor metabolites are also present. The half-life of cocaine in adults depends on the route of administration—an average of 0.6 hour after intravenous administration, 0.9 hour after oral use, and 1.3 hours after intranasal use. The metabolites can be found in the urine 72 hours after administration. In infants, metabolites can be found for up to 2 weeks after administration (132,133).

Pharmacology

The neuropharmacologic effect of cocaine is secondary to its effect on three neurotransmitters: norepinephrine, dopamine, and serotonin. Cocaine inhibits the reuptake of norepinephrine and dopamine (134), which accumulate at the synaptic cleft, leading to prolonged stimulation of their corresponding receptors. Therefore, the effects of norepinephrine stimulation (e.g., tachycardia, hypertension, arrhythmia, diaphoresis, tremors) and dopamine stimulation (e.g., increased alertness, euphoria or enhanced feeling of well-being, sexual excitement, heightened energy) are experienced. Cocaine also decreases the uptake of tryptophan, which affects serotonin biosynthesis. A diminished serotonin level is associated with diminished need for sleep, because serotonin regulates the sleep–wake cycle (132).

Adverse Effects on Pregnancy

Studies in pregnant sheep have shown that maternal blood pressure becomes elevated within 5 minutes after cocaine infusion (135–137), coupled with an increase in uterine vascular resistance and decrease in uterine blood flow. Fetal heart rate and blood pressure also increase, but fetal partial pressure of oxygen (PO_2) and oxygen (O_2) content decrease as a consequence of the reduced uterine blood flow. Thus, oxygen availability to the fetus is impaired. The cocaine-induced uterine vasoconstriction is mediated solely by adrenergic stimulation because adrenergic blockade by phentolamine does not ablate the response. Pregnancy can potentiate the toxic effects of cocaine, because progesterone can increase the adrenergic sensitivity of the receptors or delay cocaine metabolism (137).

At serum levels found in humans, cocaine per se has no effect on human and animal umbilical arteries, However, cocaine enhances the umbilical artery vasoconstrictor action of catecholamines and serotonin, presumably by increasing the sensitivity of the α-adrenergic receptors of arterial smooth muscle (138).

Overall, the cardiovascular effect of cocaine on the materno-fetal circulation is maternal hypertension, increase in uterine vascular resistance, decrease in uterine blood flow, decrease in oxygen transport to the fetus, and fetal hypoxemia.

Obstetric Effects

A characteristic profile has been observed in the pregnant women who abuse cocaine: multigravid, multiparous, service patient and with little to no prenatal care (3). The lifestyle of prostitution, with little attention to personal health care, contributes to these attributes. The women are also older (mean age of 33 years), of low income and are more likely to smoke cigarettes, drink alcohol and use another drug, beside cocaine. In the United States, the majority of cocaine users are Afro-American, with a high incidence of suicidal ideation and emergency room visits (139–141). The pregnant addict is generally of poor health, as a result of poor nutrition and vitamin deficiency, and is at high risk for infection, particularly hepatitis, syphilis gonorrhea and HIV infection (142,143). Cocaine use and HIV infection have also noted to be significant risk factors for maternal pneumonia (144).

Maternal use of cocaine has been associated with a number of obstetric complications. Spontaneous abortion occurs in 25% to 38% of pregnancies of cocaine-using women (145–147). The rate of stillbirth is five to ten times higher among pregnant women who continue to use cocaine late in the third trimester. This may be secondary to placental abruptio, placental infarcts or hemorrhage (145,148). Fetal anuria, anasarca and neonatal gastrointestinal hemorrhage were reported in association with maternal use of cocaine and indomethacin during pregnancy (149,150).

There is a tenfold increase in the incidence of abruptio placenta and vaginal bleeding with cocaine use during pregnancy (17,145–148,151–153), although some studies do not show this association (2,154,155). One of the latter was a study based on a large obstetric population and the use of a more sensitive test to detect cocaine exposure in the infants (3).

An increased occurrence of premature labor and premature rupture of the membranes have been observed among pregnant women who use cocaine (145,156–158). There is a belief among these women that cocaine will shorten the duration of their labor. Although one study does not support this belief (159), another has shown a significant decrease in the duration of labor in women who used cocaine compared to nonusers or to those who only used opiates during the pregnancy (3).

There has been no observed increase in the incidence of amnionitis, abnormal presentation, eclampsia, preeclampsia, or placenta praevia in pregnant women who abuse cocaine (145).

Placental Transfer

Because of its low molecular weight and high lipid solubility, cocaine crosses the placenta by simple diffusion (147). However, the fetal concentration of cocaine is only one-fourth to one ninth that of the mother. Nonetheless, the elimination of cocaine and its metabolites is much slower in the fetus than in the mother; thus, the risk of cocaine toxicity in the fetus is increased.

Effects on the Neonate

The cocaine-exposed infant is at risk for a number of complications. Cocaine decreases placental perfusion, which leads to poor gas exchange and fetal oxygenation (135–137). Fetal hypoxemia in turn leads to fetal distress, meconium staining of the amniotic fluid, and low Apgar score. Meconium staining has been observed in 23% of the births in cocaine-abusing women—approximately twice the incidence among nondrug users (3,145). There is also an increased incidence of premature birth (145,156,157,160–165) and intrauterine growth retardation (147,155,158,161,166). These rates are about three to four times higher than in nonusers. Numerous studies have also reported lower birth weights and smaller body length and head circumference in infants exposed to cocaine during pregnancy compared to controls (17,147,150,152,157,160,161,163,164,167,168–174). Somatic growth deceleration seems to be evident after 32 weeks of gestation (171). In a meta-analysis study, maternal cocaine use was not only associated with low birth weight in the infants but that the effect is increased with heavier drug use (175). The dose related, negative effect of cocaine on head circumference may reflect specific central nervous system insult that interferes with prenatal brain growth (176). Again, maternal smoking, alcohol and opiate use (177) and lead exposure (178) are important contributing factors for these reduced growth parameters in the infant.

Cocaine use during pregnancy has been associated with an increased incidence of the congenital malformations in animals, such as neural tube defects, skeletal deficits (e.g., camptodactyly, bradydactyly) and hydrocephalus (145, 158,179,180). It is suggested that fetal vascular disruption secondary to vasoconstriction may lead to these defects (181). On the other hand, congenital malformation is not increased among cocaine exposed newborn infants. A previously reported increase in the rate of genitourinary malformations was not subsequently substantiated by renal ultrasound study of 100 term infants who were exposed to cocaine during pregnancy (182). In a large, blinded, prospective and systemative study of infants, an increased incidence of congenital abnormalities was not observed among prenatally cocaine exposed infants (183,184).

Maternal cocaine use during pregnancy has been associated with a number of multiorgan dysfunctions in the infant (185) (Table 58-5). Neurologic abnormalities have included seizures (186), transient dystonia (187), hypertonia/hyperreflexia and tremors (188–190), and transient abnormal EEG suggestive of CNS irritability (191). Problems of low arousal, poor quality of movement, high excitability, poor attention, hypertonia, jitteriness and non optimal reflexes have also been observed (192–196). The infant's cry is characterized as few, short and less crying in the hyperphonation mode (197). These acoustic cry characteristics which reflect reactivity, respiratory and neural control have also been found to be compromised in marijuana, opiate and alcohol exposed newborn infants (192). The sleep pattern of the infant shows more wakefulness, more frequent arousals and a higher proportion of active compared to quiet sleep (198–200).

Abnormal hearing tests have been consistently observed among prenatally cocaine exposed infants. The auditory brainstem evoked response shows prolonged interpeak and absolute latencies suggesting abnormal neural trans-mission (201,202,203,204). There is also impaired auditory information processing with impaired habituation to novel stimulus (205).

The incidence of severe intraventricular hemorrhage among preterm infants is not increased with cocaine exposure (206). Recent studies however, have shown dose-related increase in the incidence of mild periventricular-intraventricular hemorrhage, specifically in the caudothalamic groove, echolucencies in the basal ganglia and caudate nucleus, ventricle dilatation and germinal matrix or subependymal cysts (207–210). An increased flow velocity in the anterior cerebral artery has been shown in these infants and is consistent with the vasoconstrictive effects of cocaine (211). Although high resolution single photon emission computed tomographic scans have shown normal cerebral blood flow in 21 infants with confirmed cocaine exposure (212), cerebral infarction and hemorrhage has been reported in an infant whose mother had taken a large amount of cocaine during the intrapartum period. A Mobius syndrome was observed in an infant born to a mother with heavy use of cocaine and alcohol. It was suggested that cocaine-induced vasoconstriction at a critical time of cerebrovascular development produced a vascular disruption sequence leading to the syndrome (213). The vasoconstrictive effect of cocaine on the cerebral circulation is prominent in utero because the fetus is more consistently exposed to the drug. Postnatally, this may no longer be observed as cocaine exposure is discontinued and is evidenced by a significant drop in arterial blood pressure and cerebral blood flow velocities in the second compared to the first day of the infant (214).

In the cardiovascular system, asymptomatic cocaine exposed infants showed either decreased (215,216) or increased (217,218) heart rate variability after birth and are related to the effect of cocaine on the autonomic nervous system either through sympathetic stimulation or vagal suppression. However, the effect is transient and the vagal tone eventually recovers as cocaine exposure ceases after birth (215,216). A decrease in cardiac output and stroke volume and increase in arterial blood pressure have been reported in cocaine exposed infants (219,220) and atrial and ventricular arrhythmias (221) and transient ST segment elevation (221,222). In children, sustained arrhythmias which may result from an increased number of potential initiating premature beats, may be associated with congestive heart failure, cardiopulmonary arrest and death (223).

In the respiratory system, abnormal breathing patterns have been observed in the cocaine exposed infants, e.g., high respiratory rate, decreased end tidal PCO_2 and shift to the left of the breathing response curve to CO_2 (44). There have also been described increased apnea density and periodic breathing (219). The failure in animals to ventilate adequately in the presence of hypoxia, after prenatal exposure to cocaine, may indicate retardation of development of their ventilatory control system (224). In preterm infants with respiratory distress syndrome, cocaine exposure was associated with less frequent use and fewer doses of surfactant and with less frequent intubation (225).

TABLE 58-5

REPORTED COMPLICATIONS INVOLVING SPECIFIC ORGAN SYSTEMS IN COCAINE EXPOSED NEWBORN INFANTS

Central nervous system
  Cerebral infarction
  Mobius syndrome
  Seizures, tremors
  Hypertonicity/hypereflexia and transient dystonia
  Abnormal head ultrasound, e.g., echolucencies in basal ganglia,
    ventricles, periventricular and germinal matrix cyts
  Abnormal EEG
  Abnormal sleep pattern
  Abnormal cry
Sensory organs
  Abnormal brainstem auditory evoked response
  Increased auditory startle response
  Retinal hemorrhage and tortuosity and dilatation of iris vessels
Cardiovascular system
  Transient tachycardia
  Hypertension and diminished stroke volume and cardiac output
  Atrial and ventricular arrthythmia
Respiratory system
  Apnea
  Abnormal breathing pattern, e.g., periodic breathing
Genitourinary system
  Renal ectopia

Other findings in the neonate which are attributed to in utero cocaine exposure include: elevation in serum myoglobin and creatine kinase secondary to tremors (226) and decreased jaundice because cocaine is a strong inducer of the glutathione-S transferase family of enzymes that is closely associated with bilirubin transport (ligandin) in the liver (227). An increased incidence of early onset necrotizing enterocolitis and intestinal perforation, not related to necrotizing enterocolitis, have been observed which may be secondary to the vasoconstrictive and ischemic effect of cocaine on the gastrointestinal tract (228,229). Eye findings of retinal hemorrhages (230) and dilated and tortuous iris vessels have been reported (231). Retinal, vascular, disruptive lesions which consisted of blot full-thickness hemorrhages with rounded domed contours suggestive of venous occlusion and retinal ischemia have been described (230,231,232). These lesions took longer to resolve compared with those hemorrhages as a result of birth trauma.

Neonatal Neurobehavoiral Assessment

By the Neonatal Brazelton Assessment Scale (NBAS), cocaine-exposed newborns exhibited significantly depressed performance on the habituation clusters, including lower state regulation and greater depression. During sleep-wake behavior observations, the infants showed difficulty in maintaining alert states and self-regulating their behavior, and spent more time in indeterminate sleep and had decreased periods of quiet sleep and increased levels of agitated behavior, including tremulousness, mouthing, multiple limb movements, and clenched fists. (233–239). There is a dose-response relationship between cocaine fetal exposure and performance on the NBAS (233–239,192). High urinary norepinephrine, dopamine, and cortisol levels were noted during these conditions (239). A significant negative correlation was observed between serum norepinephrine concentration and orientation cluster score for the cocaine-exposed newborns (240). Similarly, a significant negative effect was observed between cocaine concentration in meconium and the cluster scores on motor and regulation state (234). An increase in the infant's auditory startle response has also been observed (241). Two neurobehavioral syndromes have been described in these infants: an excitable state, which may be as a result of the direct neurotoxic effects of the drug and a depressed state that may be indirect effects of intrauterine growth retardation (242).

Cocaine use during pregnancy has not only caused significant medical problems in the infant, but has been an economic burden, as well. Increased hospitalization costs have resulted from prematurity and adverse birth outcome, prolonged stay while awaiting home and social evaluation of foster care placement and laboratory fees (243–248). Cocaine exposed infants had longer length of hospital stay (249), more likely to be admitted to a neonatal intensive care unit, be treated for congenital syphilis and discharged to a person other than the mother (250).

An abstinence syndrome has not been commonly observed with cocaine exposure. Reports of withdrawal-like manifestations with cocaine may be related to polydrug abuse, particularly opiates or cocaine toxicity.

Long-Term Outcome

In terms of physical growth, the infants prenatally exposed to cocaine showed catch up in weight and length (251), although head circumference still tended to be smaller (252,253) than control infants. Strabismus, high blood pressure and hypertonicity were noted particularly during the first year of life (188,254,255). Hypertonia, both symmetrical and peripheral, were also noted during infancy but disappeared by 24 months (188,256).

Difficulties in early language development, lower verbal comprehension and reasoning and poor recognition memory and information process have been more consistently reported (251,252,257–260). The infants also showed lower scores in the Fagan Intelligence tests (261), Bayley Scales of Infant Development (262,263), language skills (264,265,266), cognitive functions (267), and visual attention (268). Behavior problems dealing with attention deficits and distractability have been noted (269). The adverse effect of cocaine on the child's attention processing (270) and expressive language (271) were noted even up to school age. These may indicate the long lasting disruption of the brain systems subserving arousal and attention as noted in the neonatal period (270,272). Cocaine exposure is not associated with differences in play behavior of the infant at 18 and 24 months (273) despite previous report to the contrary (274). However, behavior problems dealing with attention deficits and distractability have been noted (269).

Many of the adverse long term outcome in the infants are not exclusively the effects of prenatal cocaine exposure alone but the influence of other important factors as well, such as aberrant parental behavior and interaction with the child (275), poor home environment (255,276), poor caregiving skills (276–280), abnormal maternal psychological functions (279), and low socio-economic status (280–284). In a meta-analysis study, which controlled for many of these confounding factors, many of the reported adverse effects of cocaine on the growth and development of infants were not observed except for decreased attentiveness and emotional expressivity (285).

As in the opiate exposed infant, there is increased risk to SIDS and child abuse with prenatal cocaine exposure (198). The risk however, is not specific for cocaine exposure alone but to intrauterine exposure to illicit drugs in general (286). The chaotic home environment and a high incidence of depression, emotional and physical neglect, inadequate skills and poor self esteem in the mother are important contributing factors for child abuse and neglect (255). Perinatal drug abuse including cocaine, opiate and cannabinoid has not been associated with increased infant mortality within the first two years of life except among the low birth weight infants (287).

Cocaine Exposure During Infancy and Childhood

The exposure of the infant to cocaine can be ongoing after birth through breastfeeding, intentional administration of the drug by caregivers, accidental ingestion of cocaine or cocaine contaminated household dust via normal hand to mouth activity or passive inhalation of cocaine smoke during freebasing activities of adults (288). Cocaine and benzoylecgonine have been found in the hair, saliva, skin and urine of these children (258,289). The incidence of passive cocaine exposure in ill infants younger than 1 year old seeking medical care through the emergency services may be as high as 1 in 3 to 6 infants (290). Morbidity from postnatal cocaine exposure have included seizures, drowsiness and unsteady gait, diarrhea and shock from intoxication and sometimes, death (291–294). Two major age-related patterns have been observed: in children less than 5 years of age, seizures (focal or generalized) and obtundation and in older children, delirium, dizziness, drooling, and lethargy (295). Thus, afebrile seizures in infants and young children should include a consideration of cocaine intoxication. The development of upper and lower respiratory tract symptoms also correlate significantly with cocaine exposure (290).

ALCOHOL

The use or abuse of alcohol during pregnancy has serious effects on the fetus and newborn. The adverse effects of alcohol on the offspring have been observed for centuries, although the fetal alcohol syndrome (FAS) was not defined as a medical entity until 1973 (296,297). Infants born to alcoholic parents may have dysmorphic features and are subsequently observed to have a higher than expected incidence of delayed growth and development and of neurologic disorders (298,299). Excellent reviews on this topic have been written (300–302).

Epidemiology

Almost half of Americans aged 12 or older (48.3%) reported being current drinkers of alcohol in a recent survey of the National Household Survey on Drug Abuse (1). This is equivalent to an estimated 109 million people. The rate of alcohol use and the number of drinkers have increased from 2000, when 104 million, or 46.6% of people aged 12 or older reported drinking in the past 30 days. Approximately one fifth (20.5%) of persons aged 12 or older participated in binge drinking at least once in the 30 days prior to the survey. Although the number of current drinkers increased between 2000 and 2001, the number of those reporting binge drinking have not changed significantly. Heavy drinking was reported by 5.7 percent of the population aged 12 or older, or 12.9 million people. These 2001 estimates are similar to the 2000 estimates.

Alcohol use during pregnancy is a significant public health problem. Among pregnant women aged 15 to 44 years in 2000 and 2001 combined, 12.9 percent used alcohol and 4.6% were binge drinkers (1). These rates were significantly lower than the rates for nonpregnant women of that age (49.8 and 20.5%, respectively). A variety of programs have been developed to prevent drinking during pregnancy, such as public service announcements and beverage warning labels, which strive to increase public knowledge about fetal alcohol effects. Selective prevention approaches to women of reproductive age involve screening all pregnant women for alcohol consumption and counseling for those who drink (303). It has been shown that knowledge among pregnant adolescents about drinking especially those with specific knowledge of FAS drank less before pregnancy (304). Among drinkers, general knowledge was significantly related to a decrease in drinking between prepregnancy and first trimester, and between first trimester and third trimester (303).

Widely used terms such as "light," "moderate," and "heavy" alcohol consumption are unstandardized. Attempts to standardize these terms resulted in considerable agreement for the following operational definitions: "light" drinking as 1.2 drinks/day; "moderate" as 2.2 drinks/day and heavy drinking as 3.5 drinks/day (305).

Although most of the women who report alcohol use are light drinkers, those who drink heavily are more likely young, white, single, to have higher education and income and to be employed outside the home (306,307). However, women who drink during pregnancy, and particularly those who continue to drink through the third trimester are different. They are older, more likely black, have higher rates of illicit drug use, less education and lower social status (306). They also have higher levels of psychopathology such as depression, psychopathic deviance, schizophrenia and social introversion (308). In one survey, almost half (45%) of all pregnant women drank alcohol during the first three months before finding out they were pregnant (307).

Alcohol consumption and pregnancy in the adolescent group has also been increasing the past years (308). Although adults have significantly higher average daily volume of alcohol prior to pregnancy than adolescents, this was no longer significant during pregnancy. The rate of binge drinking (5+ drinks/occasion) during the first trimester was higher in pregnant teenagers (309,310). Binger drinkers are more likely to be young, white and with heavier use of tobacco, marijuana and cocaine compared with nonbinge drinker (309,311). Offsprings of these binge drinkers may be at higher risk for intermittent high peak alcohol exposure further into the pregnancy than those of adult drinkers (310).

The concept of moderate consumption of ethanol has evolved over time from considering this level as nonintoxicating and noninjurious, to encompassing levels defined as statistically normal in particular populations (312). Moderate consumption of alcohol may be defined as >2 drinks/week to 2 drinks per day (313). A meta-analysis showed no association between moderate alcohol intake during the first trimester of pregnancy and increased risk of fetal malformation (313). It was also not noted to be associated with intrauterine growth retardation (314) and abnormal child development at 18 and 42 months of age (315). On the other hand, one study has shown a 7-point decrease in the general cognitive index on the McCarthy scales at preschool age in offspring of women with moderate alcohol consumption during pregnancy (316).

Metabolism and Placental Transfer

Ethanol is an anxiolytic analgesic with a depressant effect on the central nervous system (301). It is absorbed rapidly by diffusion across the mucosa of the stomach (20%) and intestines (80%). The absorption rate is not affected by pregnancy, but blood alcohol levels may be higher in pregnancy (300). Alcohol is usually cleared from the bloodstream within 1 hour in adults and 2 hours in newborns. Approximately 95% is metabolized by the liver and 5% is eliminated by the kidneys and lungs. Ethanol is metabolized to acetaldehyde and then to acetate. Acetaldehyde is more toxic than ethanol itself. Acetaldehyde levels are frequently elevated in chronic alcoholics and in children with alcohol related birth defects (317). Genetic predisposition to alcohol and its effects may be present. The alcohol dehydrogenase 2 genotype (ADH2–1/3) is found to be more prevalent among black women who reported high alcohol use during pregnancy. There is also subsequent higher percentage of affected infants carrying this genotype (318). There is an unimpeded bidirectional placental transfer of ethanol during pregnancy. Alcohol is distributed rapidly and nearly equally in maternal and fetal tissues (319). Fetal ethanol is eliminated by maternal hepatic biotransformation. Ethanol has been detected in amniotic fluid and constitutes an additional reservoir for fetal exposure (301,320,321).

Maternal alcohol abuse is difficult to assess by laboratory tests. Biological markers which have been studied include: increased levels of mean cell volume, gamma-glutamyl transferase, carbohydrate deficient transferrin, hemoglobin acetaldehyde adducts (322,323,324) and decreased hepatic levels of glutathione (325). In the infant, fatty acid ethyl esters in meconium are promising biomarkers of fetal exposure to alcohol (326,327,328,329).

Ethanol has been implicated in the impairment of normal placental function. It affects or interferes with the transport of amino acids across the placenta to the fetus (330). Placental expression of epidermal growth factor and placental growth factor is also altered in alcohol abusing women (331). Ethanol has also been found to inhibit DNA synthesis, protein synthesis (332), inhibit phospholipase A2 (333), decrease PGI2 production (334), and increase HCG production in the placenta (335).

Effects on Pregnancy

An increased incidence of spontaneous abortion, abruptio placentae, and breech presentation have been observed among women who abuse alcohol during pregnancy.

The incidence of spontaneous abortion among alcoholic pregnant women ranges between 18.8% to 52% of pregnancies (300). In a large, prospective study of 12,127 pregnant women, alcoholic women were found to have a 2.3 times higher incidence of three or more spontaneous abortions than nonalcoholics (336). The single variable that correlated highly with spontaneous abortion was an extremely heavy episode of drinking during the early first trimester. In another cohort of 24,768 singleton pregnancies, the risk ratio for stillbirth among women who consumed more than 5 drinks/week during pregnancy was 2.96. The increased risk of stillbirth was independent of other alcohol effects like prematurity, low birthweight, or malformations (336). Other reports, however, do not show an association of alcohol consumption with an increased risk for spontaneous abortions in nonheavy drinkers (338) nor an increased risk of stillbirths even among women classified as problem or heavy drinkers (336, 338–340). However, the risk of abruptio placenta is increased (341,342).

Studies in nonhuman primates have shown that an increase in spontaneous abortion occurred only when blood alcohol levels reached approximately 200 mg/dL (343–348).

An increase in the frequency of aneuploidy was found in abortuses of women who consumed two or more drinks per week (347). Although in mice, preovulatory alcohol exposure did not increase the incidence of abortion (348) or aneuploidy, (349), alcohol administration shortly after ovulation resulted in a 7.5% incidence of aneuploidy. Ingestion shortly after mating also resulted in a 15% incidence of aneuploidy (350). Alcohol administration to mating female mice 2 hours after ovulation resulted in a significant increase in fetal death associated with aneuploidy. Another study showed that successful fertilization of such eggs after a single "binge," consequently resulted in the production of aneuploid embryos, which had a very high chance of being spontaneously aborted during the first trimester. Those relatively few aneuploid conceptuses that survived to term invariably showed moderate to severe degrees of mental retardation, craniofacial and other abnormalities and having a significantly reduced life expectancy (351). These studies raise the possibility that the high rate of spontaneous abortions among alcoholic women may be as a result of a single episode of heavy drinking around the time of conception (352).

Fetal alcohol syndrome is strongly associated with breech presentation. Seventy percent of infants with FAS were breech births (300). In other studies, 9 of 23 (39%) infants born to heavy drinkers were delivered as breech (353); however, only 3 of 59 infants of moderate drinkers had breech presentation (354). Thus, it appears that heavy consumption of alcohol increases the incidence of breech births.

Effects on the Fetus

Animal studies have shown that in utero alcohol exposure may cause fetal malnutrition and chronic fetal hypoxia by inducing hypoglycemia at high blood alcohol levels (301). Alcohol decreases adrenergic receptors on the hepatic plasma membrane, resulting in reduced epinephrine-induced stimulation of glycogen phosphorylase activity and interference with carbohydrate metabolism and prenatal and postnatal growth. Low concentrations of somatomedin C and high growth hormone levels have been noted in infants of alcoholic mothers (355). A dose dependent contraction of the human umbilical cord, in vitro, and decreased fetal placental flow, *in vivo*, have been demonstrated with alcohol exposure and may further contribute to fetal hypoxia (356). Abnormal fetal heart rate patterns (357), decreased fetal breathing (358), decreased fetal eye movements, disorganized behavioral state organization (359) and decreased fetal movements (360) have all been described with alcohol use during pregnancy. There also is a reduction in the amount of neurotransmitters in the human brain, a decrease in the myelination process and decreases in fetal hippocampal nitric oxide synthase activity (361–366).

Effects on the Newborn Infant

Prematurity

The incidence of prematurity ranges from 46% to 52% in infants with FAS (365,367). The relationship between alcohol exposure and preterm birth in which FAS is not a factor is not as clear. Several reports indicate increased preterm delivery in alcohol abusers (368–372). This may be as a result of an associated increase in congenital anomalies, rather than directly to alcohol itself. Nonetheless, heavy alcohol consumption during pregnancy (i.e., six or more drinks per day) has been associated with an approximately threefold increased risk of preterm delivery (373).

Growth and Morphology

Maternal alcohol consumption has been associated with an increased risk for infants with low birth weight and with length and head circumference below the tenth percentile, if the mother's drinking took place during the early first trimester of pregnancy (302,375). Similarly, birth weight, length, and head circumference have been reported to be significantly reduced in the offspring of women who drank continuously throughout pregnancy (376,377,372,374). Abnormalities in fetal brain development have also been described (378,379). In rat pups, an increased vulnerability of brain development was observed (decreased brain to body weight ratio) when the pups were exposed to alcohol especially in the third trimester compared with other times in the pregnancy (380). The low birth weight was influenced both by dose and duration of alcohol exposure. Moderate or light drinking has been associated with a decrease in the birth weight of the infants (381). The birth weights, however, are within the range of normal, have no biologic significance, and often cease to achieve statistical significance when other risk factors, such as smoking, are taken into account. There are also a few reports that show no association between alcohol use and the infant's birth weight. In a group of healthy, full-term infants, no growth difference was noted between those exposed and those not exposed to alcohol (381–383).

Some minor morphologic malformations in the infant have been observed with alcohol use during pregnancy (382–386). On the other hand, other reports have failed to demonstrate this phenomenon (381,387–389). In a large prospective birth defects study involving 32,870 women, light and moderate drinkers were not found to have an increased rate of malformations in their offspring compared to nondrinkers (390).

Newborn Withdrawal

Withdrawal from alcohol occurs in infants but is rarely observed, because the withdrawal may be confused with withdrawal from narcotics or other drugs that are used together with alcohol. The withdrawal from ethanol has been described to occur within 12 hours of birth and may manifest as abdominal distention, opisthotonus, convulsions, tremors, hypertonia, apnea, and cyanosis. The infants are irritable, have restless sleep, and engage in exaggerated mouthing behavior (391,392).

Neurobehavioral Effects

Alcohol-exposed infants have been found to habituate less well to aversive stimuli as measured by the Neonatal Behavioral Assessment Scale (393,394), exhibit changes in their reflexive behavior, state control, and motor behavior,(381,395), and have increased irritability (396) and depressed range of state (397). These effects, however, have not been universally observed (386). Timing of prenatal exposure to alcohol, especially in early gestation, also had deleterious effects on neurobehavioral tests (398).

Sleep cycling and arousal have been studied as a measure of neurophysiologic development, integrity, and maturation. Infants of mothers who drank heavily throughout pregnancy showed a greater amount of restless sleep and more bodily movements (399,400). Electroencephalographic power spectra analyses of the infants showed hypersynchrony of the EEG and an increase in the integrated power in all sleep states, particularly with active sleep (401,402). Electroencephalographic maturation also was affected by maternal binge drinking (403).

Animal studies have shown that the deleterious effect of ethanol on brain development is a result of ethanol's potential to interfere with neuronal migration, trigger widespread neuronal apoptosis by blockade of NMDA glutamate receptors and excessive activation of GABA (404) and induce loss of myelinated axons in the CNS (405).

Breast-Feeding and Alcohol

Alcohol is distributed in breast milk; however, the amount ingested by the infant is only a small fraction of the amount consumed by the mother (300). Short-term alcohol consumption by lactating women had an immediate effect on the odor of their milk and the feeding behavior of their infant (406). The infants sucked more frequently during the first minute after their mothers had consumed alcohol, but consumed significantly less milk. The postnatal growth was not affected in breastfed infants whose mothers consumed alcohol during lactation (407). In animal studies, ethanol has been shown to block the secretion of oxytocin, thereby preventing milk ejection (408). A similar effect has been observed in normal women (409).

Long-Term Effects of Prenatal Alcohol Use

Growth

Growth deficits were found in infants at 6.5 to 18 months of age and were related to alcohol use during the second and third trimesters of pregnancy (410,411). These children continued to be smaller in weight, length, and head circumference at 3 years of age, even after controlling for nutrition, current environment, exposure to alcohol during lactation, and other significant covariates. Variations in growth retardation have been observed. Growth retardation at 8 months of age, but not at subsequent evaluations (412), and significant effects on height and head circumference in children at 6 years of age have been reported (386). Some catch up growth after 8 months of age have been observed whether the children were exposed to alcohol in the first and second trimester or throughout gestation (413–415). However, head circumference remained smaller among children who were exposed throughout pregnancy (416). On the other hand, there are reports which show no effects of prenatal alcohol exposure on the infants' growth at 1 and 2 years of age (417,418).

Behavioral and Cognitive Effects

Infants of mothers who drank throughout pregnancy showed less improvement in reflexes and autonomic regulation over the first month of life than infants of women who stopped drinking or who never drank (419). At 6 to 8 months of age, these infants had significantly lower Bayley mental and motor scores (420–422) slower reaction time, longer fixation time, lower scores in elicited play and longer periods of toy exploration which may indicate slower cognitive processing (423,424,425). At 13 months of age, infants of women who drank during pregnancy did less well on the mental index and on the verbal comprehension and spoken language cluster scores derived from the Bayley Scales (417,426,427). Antenatal reports of alcohol use was a reliable predictor of poorer cognitive performance on Bayley Scales and symbolic play, slower processing speed on the Fagan Test of Infant intelligence and slower reaction time in infants tested from 6 to 13 months of age (428). Fried and Watkinson found that infants exposed to alcohol prenatally evidenced no deficits at 12 months of age (429). However, at 24 months of age, they performed more poorly than non-alcohol-exposed controls on the Bayley Mental Scale and

the Reynell Language Scale. At 36 months of age, the language development of the exposed children continued to be affected, but at 48 months of age no significant relationships were found (430). Again, others have found that prenatal alcohol use did not significantly predict Bayley mental or motor scores at either 8 or 18 months of age (431).

Alcohol use during pregnancy was associated negatively with IQ at 4 years of age (432). At 4 years of age, children who were exposed prenatally to moderate drinking were less attentive and more active during naturalistic observations at home (433), and were less attentive and had longer reaction times on a vigilance task in a laboratory setting (434). Prepregnancy alcohol exposure also was related to increased fine motor errors, increased time to correct the errors, and poorer gross motor balance (435). Preschool children who were exposed to alcohol throughout gestation (with a range of 2–9 drinks per day) were more likely to show hyperactivity, language problems and motor deficits compared with those whose mothers stopped drinking by the second trimester (436). Difficulty in management, tantrums and eating problems were reported in 3 year old children prenatally exposed to alcohol. In children evaluated between 2 to 12 years of age, alcohol exposure during any part of pregnancy appeared to be associated with poorer academic achievement, although exposure during the third trimester appeared to be associated with lower aptitude scores (416).

Attention, distraction, and reaction time on a continuous performance task at 7 years of age continued to be negatively related to alcohol exposure during pregnancy (437). Children with any prenatal alcohol exposure were more likely to have higher scores on Externalizing (aggressive and delinquent) and Internalizing (anxious/depressed and withdrawn) compared with non exposed controls (372). Intelligence quotient effects persisted at 7.5 years, with a decrement of 7 IQ points with exposure to more than 1 ounce of alcohol per day during pregnancy (438). Achievement scores were related to binge drinking before pregnancy. Evaluation during adolescence showed difficulties in tasks which involve manipulation of information, goal management (439), attention, memory (414), calculation, and estimation tests with intact reading and writing ability (430). Again, the inconsistencies regarding the long-term effects of prenatal alcohol exposure on the child's development may lie in the difficulty in separating the teratogenic effects of alcohol from the effects of the disordered environments, both interpersonal and structural, that often accompany alcohol and drug use (440,441).

With regards to alcohol ingestion by the infant through breast feeding, a slight but significant negative effect was observed in these infants on their motor development as measured by the Bayley scales psychomotor developmental index (PDI) but not on the mental developmental index (410).

Fetal Alcohol Syndrome

The Fetal Alcohol Study Group of the Research Society on Alcoholism defined three specific criteria for the diagnosis of FAS (300). An infant must exhibit an abnormality from each category to qualify for a diagnosis of FAS:

Prenatal or postnatal growth retardation, i.e., weight, length, or head circumference < the 10th percentile when corrected for gestational age.

CNS involvement, which includes signs of neurologic abnormalities (e.g., irritability in infancy, hyperactivity during childhood), developmental delay, hypotonia or intellectual impairment (e.g., mental retardation)

Characteristic facial dysmorphology (at least two of the three must be present)

Microcephaly, i.e., head circumference < 3rd percentile
Microphthalmia or short palpebral fissures
Poorly developed philtrum, thin upper lip, i.e., vermillion border, and flattening of the maxilla.

Physical findings of smooth philtrum, thin upper lip and short palpebral fissure have a 100% sensitivity in diagnosing FAS (442,443). Presence of some, but not all, of these features is defined as alcohol-related birth defects (ARBD), or fetal alcohol effects (Table 58-6). Current criteria for diagnosis of FAS depend on recognition of subtle physical anomalies, growth retardation and nonspecific developmental aberrations which may change with time and varying degrees of severity which is affected by patient's age, or racial background. Under diagnosis of FAS usually occurs when complete patterns of abnormalities cannot be substantiated or when there is clinician's fear of stigmatizing the mother and child (444).

Incidence

The incidence of FAS has been estimated at 1 to 3 per 1000 live births. Fetal Alcohol Spectrum Disorders (FASD) (which include FAS) are estimated to occur in about 1 in 100 births (445). The reported rate in the United States is 2.2 per 1000 live births (300). Prevalence estimates vary, depending on geographic location and specific population studied (446). The highest reported incidence of FAS occurs in the Native American and black population and those with low socioeconomic status. In a review of North Dakota FAS registry, 80.6% of FAS cases were native Americans and 18.2% were Caucasians and with more female than male infants (61.4% vs. 38.6%). Maternal characteristics include older maternal age, lower educational level, fewer months of prenatal care, fewer prenatal visits and less prenatal weight gain (447). Sokol and associates, in a prospective study of 8,331 pregnancies, identified 25 cases of FAS (448). Four significant prenatal risk factors were identified: black race, high parity, percentage drinking days, and positive Michigan Alcoholism Screening Test. In the absence of any of these factors, the probability of a child being afflicted with FAS was 2%; in the presence of all four, the probability was 85.2%.

Among alcohol-abusing women, the incidence of FAS in the world literature is 71 per 1000 live births, and in the United States, from 24 to 42 per 1000 live births

(299). The National Institute on Drug Abuse (NIDA) estimated that approximately 7.62 million babies (18.6%) were exposed to alcohol during gestation (449). One factor that has been associated with an increase in the risk of FAS is the history of previous siblings with FAS in the family. It is estimated that the risk of a younger sibling having FAS, given an older sibling diagnosed as having FAS, is increased by 406 times, so that the incidence of FAS occurring in this group is 771 per 1,000 live births (300). Older siblings are not as likely to be severely affected as younger siblings (300). There is a higher risk of FAS with increasing maternal age and parity. This may be as a result of increase in maternal body fat-to-water ratio and a faster rate of alcohol metabolism in chronic drinking women (450).

Alcohol has the most teratogenic effect during organogenesis and development of nervous system (451). Teratogenesis is grossly dose related (394,452) although threshold dose is still not known. Estimates of 21 ounces of absolute alcohol per week around the time of conception may be a critical dose (422,452).

Alcohol-Related Birth Defects

Alcohol-related birth defects may account for as many as 5% of all congenital anomalies (301). Alcohol-related birth defects result from variable dose exposures at variable gestational times, and are offset by the genetic background. These determinants place the fetus at a higher risk for possible adverse outcome. The frequency of ARBD is 3 to 5 per 1000 live births. Table 58-6 shows the various dysmorphic features that may be observed in the infant after prenatal alcohol exposure.

Follow-Up of Infants with Fetal Alcohol Syndrome

Postnatal growth retardation and retarded motor performance are hallmarks of prenatal alcohol exposure, especially of FAS. A 10-year follow-up of patients diagnosed to have FAS showed that the children continued to be growth retarded with respect to weight, height, and head circumference. Weight-for-height was especially decreased (453,454). Long-term study of children with FAS showed that the characteristic craniofacial malformations of FAS diminished with time but the microcephaly and, to a lesser degree, short stature, and underweight persisted in boys. In female adolescents, body weight normalized (455–457). Significant differences in facial features between exposed and nonexposed infants were mostly evident only up to 3 months of age (457). However, mental retardation persisted ranging from near normal to severe (458,459). The long-term neurobehavioral effects of FAS, which consisted of attention and memory deficits, poor adaptability and organization did not improve with age (460). Significant adaptive behavior defects in adolescent and adults with FAS and FAE particularly in areas of socialization and communicative skills also persisted (456). Behavioral prob-

TABLE 58-6

ALCOHOL AND FETAL DYSMORPHOGENESIS[c]

Central nervous system	
Neurobehavioral	Intellectual impairment (i.e., mild to moderate mental retardation),[a] low IQ (65–70), hypotonia,[b] developmental delay, poor coordination, cognitive and sensory deficits, attention deficits, hyperactivity and irritability in infancy, hyperactivity in childhood,[c] language disabilities and sleep–wake cycle disturbances, electroencephalogram hypersynchrony, delayed or deficient myelination, corpus callosum hypoplasia, echolalia, cerebral palsy
Craniofacial	
Head	Microcephaly,[a] Dandy–Walker malformation, anencephaly, porencephaly, meningomyelocele, spasmus nutans
Eyes	Ocular retinal tortuosity, ptosis, strabismus, epicanthal folds, myopia, retinal coloboma, astigmatism, steep corneal curvature, anterior chamber anomalies, sensorineural hearing loss
Ears	Poorly formed conchae and posterior rotation of the ear and eustachian tube
Nose	Short, upturned[b] hypoplastic philtrum[a]
Mouth	Dental malalignments, small teeth with faulty enamel, retrognathia in infancy[a] or relative prognathia in adolescence, cleft lip or cleft palate, malocclusions, prominent palatine ridges, thinned upper vermillion,[a] poor suck reflex
Maxilla	Hypoplastic[b]
Cardiovascular	
Heart	All cardiac defects (57%), particularly ventricular septal defect, atrial septal defects, murmurs, tetralogy of Fallot, double-outlet right ventricle, dextrocardia, patent ductus arteriosus, and great vessel anomalies
Pulmonary	
Chest	Pectus excavatum, bifid xiphoid
Lungs	Pulmonary atresia, atelectasis, upper respiratory infections
Gastrointestinal	
Abdomen	Inguinal and abdominal hernias, diastasis recti, gastroschisis, hepatic fibrosis, childhood cirrhosis, extrahepatic biliary atresia, hyperbilirubinemia in childhood
Urogenital	
Renal	Hydronephrosis; small rotated kidneys; aplastic, dysplastic, or hypoplastic kidneys; horseshoe kidneys; ureteral duplications; megaloureter, cystic diverticula; vesicovaginal fistula, pyelonephritis
Dermatologic	
Dermatogliphic	Aberrant fingerprint and palmar creases, hemangiomas in one-half of the cases, disproportionately diminished adipose tissue,[b] abnormal whorls on scalp, hirsutism in infancy, nail hypoplasia, poor proprioception
Orthopedic	
Skeletal	Polydactyly, radioulnar synostosis, talipes equinovarus, dislocated hip, scoliosis, Klippel–Feil syndrome, limited joint movement, lumbosacral lipoma, shortened fifth digit, syndactyly, camptodactyly, clinodactyly, flexion contractures
Endocrinology	
Congenital	DiGeorge syndrome

[a] Feature seen in 80% of patients.
[b] Feature seen in more than 50% of patients.
[c] From Pietrantoni M, Knuppel RA. Alcohol in pregnancy. *Clin Perinatol* 1991;18:93.

lems included general spatial memory deficit and distorted spatial arrangement (461), profound verbal and learning deficits (462), stereotyped behaviors, irritability, hyperactivity, attention deficits tremulousness, and hyperdistractibility (367,461–466). The excess psychopathology (hyperkinetic disorders, emotional disorders, sleep disorders, abnormal habits and stereotypes) strongly persisted over time (466). Speech may be delayed or impaired and may be partly as a result of hearing impairments (464–471).

Slow growth of the head circumference indicates slow brain growth in children with moderate to severe FAS (443). Neurologic findings by MRI showed significant reduction in the cerebellar vermis (472), cerebral vault, basal ganglia and diencephalon. The basal ganglia changes

may relate to behavioral findings seen in these children (473). Another study has shown mildline anomalies such as complete callosal agenesis, hypoplastic corpus callosum, cavum septum pellucidum and cavum vergae which are associated with greater number of facial anomalies (408,474).

Ophthalmologic abnormalities are also found in children with FAS. These consist primarily of fundus anomalies and optic nerve hypoplasia (475–477). These defects have been attributed to competition of ethanol with retinol at the same ADH-binding sites (478). Other eye findings include strabismus, blepharoptosis, epicanthus, cataract, glaucoma, persistent hyperplastic primary vision and increased tortuosity of retinal vessels with smaller number of vascular branching (476,479).

Four types of hearing disorders are associated with FAS: (a) developmental delay in auditory maturation, (b) sensorineural hearing loss, (c) intermittent conductive hearing loss as a result of recurrent serous otitis media, and (d) central hearing loss (480). Seventy-seven percent of children with FAS have conductive hearing loss secondary to recurrent, serous otitis media. Twenty-seven percent have sensorineural hearing loss and 100% have central hearing function injuries. Majority of the patients have associated speech pathology, expressive language defects and receptive language defects (481). The craniofacial abnormalities may also increase the susceptibility to peripheral hearing disorders (482).

MARIJUANA

Marijuana is the most widely used illicit drug among women of childbearing age in the United States (483). In 2001, marijuana was used by 76% of current illicit drug users, 56% of whom consumed marijuana exclusively. The number of new users continues to rise with about 2.4 million new users reported in 2000 (1). In 1999 and 2000 about 2% to 2.8% of pregnant women in the United States were current marijuana users. The majority were young mothers between the ages of 15 and 25 years old. The incidence of marijuana use during pregnancy is notably lower than that of non pregnant women of the same age group. This trend seems to persist amongst new mothers up to one year after the delivery.

There are some common terminology pertaining to marijuana: (a) cannabis refers to the crude material from the plant, *c. sativa*, (b) marijuana refers to a mixture of crushed leaves, twigs, seeds, and sometimes flowers of the plant, (c) sinsemilla is a variety of high-potency marijuana originally grown in northern California, and (d) hashish is a resin obtained by pressing, scraping, and shaking the plant in hash oil, to produce a potent extract (484,485). Cannabis contains more than 400 chemicals, of which 61 are unique to cannabis and are referred to collectively as cannabinoids. The primary psychoactive component is δ-9-tetrahydrocannabinol (THC). Other cannabinoids, however, such as cannabidiol and cannabinol, also have biologic activity and potentially can affect the fetus (486,487).

Placental Transfer

Tetrahydrocannabinol is highly bound to the lipoprotein fraction in blood. Studies using radiolabeled THC have shown that tissues with high blood flow show a rapid uptake of the drug. Tetrahydrocannabinol gets into the placenta within minutes of administration; however, the placenta may retard THC passage to the fetus. In rats, the placenta contained ten times more radiolabeled THC than fetal serum (488), and fetal rat THC serum levels were well below the maternal serum levels (489). In humans, however, the concentrations of THC in maternal and fetal sera essentially are identical (490).

Effects on Pregnancy

Based on a large perinatal study, no significant differences were observed between marijuana users and control subjects matched for amount of alcohol consumption, cigarette use, and family income regarding several birth outcome measures, such as miscarriage rate, presentation at birth, Apgar status, and the frequency of complications at birth (491,492). In another prospective, multicenter, cohort study no significant association was found between marijuana use during pregnancy and preterm delivery or abruptio placenta (493). Severe nausea and vomiting have often been observed in pregnant women who discontinued marijuana during the first trimester (494), which is consistent with the known antiemetic effect of the drug. Higher levels of blood carboxyhemoglobin and tar have been reported with marijuana smoking compared to regular cigarettes. Low blood levels of folate and ferritin have also been reported in pregnant women with high serum levels of PCP, cocaine, and cannabinoids (494). Studies on marijuana use during pregnancy have shown infrequent adverse pregnancy outcomes except for a higher incidence of precipitous or dysfunctional labor and meconium staining compared to controls (494).

Effects on the Fetus and Newborn Infant

A reduction by 0.8 weeks was observed in the gestational age of infants of heavy marijuana users (six or more times/week) compared to infants of nonusers although in some studies, a 25% prematurity rate was reported (492,495). However, this effect was not consistently observed (496–499).

Most studies did not show an increase in the incidence of major or minor malformations in the offspring with prenatal marijuana exposure (498–500). In the few reported cases of malformations, the confounding variables of poor nutrition, little prenatal care, low socioeconomic status, and other factors that may have interacted to produce these abnormalities were not controlled for (501).

There seems to be an increase in the gender ratio of male–female offspring in marijuana users. In animals, litters from dams fed 50 mg/kg of THC showed a significant increase in the proportion of male offspring, ranging from 57% to 61% (411,412). In a study of women who smoked marijuana during pregnancy, heavy use similarly was associated with a significant increase in male over female births (497).

Most studies do not show a significant effect of prenatal marijuana use on fetal growth and weight. In animal studies, reduced birth weights among the drug-exposed offspring were observed (489), but appeared to have resulted largely from the reduced maternal food and water intake rather than the effect of the drug (502).

There is equivocal relationship between prenatal marijuana use and neurobehavioral outcome of the offspring (503). Prenatal marijuana exposure has been associated with increased fine tremors in the infant, accompanied by exaggerated and prolonged startles, both spontaneous and in response to mild stimulation. Poor visual but not auditory stimuli habituation (503) and decreased ability to regulate state and disrupted sleep patterns (504) have also been noted. Elevated serum norepinephrine levels were observed among these infants (505). Again, there are also reports that have not found altered neurobehavioral patterns in marijuana-exposed offspring (399, 497,506).

Long-Term Outcome

After controlling for confounding variables, prenatal marijuana use was found to be associated with increased infant weight at 12 months and increased height at 24 months of age (429). One report, however, found no effect on infant growth at 12 months of age (497). Assessment of growth from birth up to 6 years failed to demonstrate any independent effect of marijuana (507). In general, there has been no observed adverse effect of antenatal marijuana exposure on infant motor and mental development at 12 months of age, as determined by the Bayley Scales of Infant Development (429,497). Global IQ was not also affected (508). However, women who used marijuana prenatally were found to be less involved with their children at 24 months of age and provided less stimulating home environment. From a preschool sample, no effect of prenatal marijuana use on IQ scores was found at 4 years of age. However, contrasting observations have also been published. There are reports, among infants at age 36 to 48 months, of poor abstract/ visual reasoning and poor memory and verbal outcome in association with heavy prenatal marijuana use (257,429, 430,503). Follow-up studies on children with prenatal exposure to marijuana also showed increased fearfulness, poorer motor skills, and shorter length of play at age 3 years (509). Additionally, attention behavior and visual analysis/hypothesis testing appeared to be negatively associated with in utero cannabis exposure (508). No effects on language development have been reported. Abnormal sleep patterns in infants which persisted at 3 years of age have raised concerns about potential neural alterations or disruptions (509). Others have reported frequent maternal cannabis intake as a small risk factor for SIDS (511). Drug interactions may play a role in the effect of marijuana exposure. There is an increased risk for FAS if the mother reported marijuana use in addition to alcohol (512).

NICOTINE AND SMOKING

Cigarette smoke contains about 4,000 chemical compounds. Most are found in the gas phase of cigarette smoke and include carbon monoxide, carbon dioxide, nitrogen oxide, ammonia, hydrogen cyanide, and other compounds. A smaller number of undesirable compounds are in the particulate phase of cigarette smoke (e.g., nicotine and tar). Tar is what remains after the moisture and nicotine are subtracted. It consists primarily of polycyclic aromatic hydrocarbons (e.g., nitrosamines, aromatic amines, polycyclic hydrocarbons) and numerous other compounds, including metallic ions and radioactive compounds (513).

Absorption and Metabolism

Nicotine is the most studied compound in cigarette smoke, and is primarily responsible for the pharmacologic effects of smoking. It is absorbed readily from the lungs, almost with the same efficiency as intravenous administration. Blood nicotine levels vary depending on the amount of nicotine delivered. The amount of nicotine delivered depends on the duration and intensity of inhalation, the number of inhalations per cigarette, the presence or absence of filters, the brand of the cigarette (which affects the composition of the tobacco), how densely the tobacco is packed, and the length of the column of tobacco (513).

Nicotine is distributed rapidly throughout the body. It reaches the brain within 8 seconds after inhalation. Peak concentrations of nicotine in plasma after a cigarette is smoked are typically between 25 to 50 ng/mL. The course of elimination of nicotine is multiexponential. After a single cigarette, concentrations decline rapidly, i.e., over 5–10 minutes, primarily reflecting distribution. After long-term smoking, the elimination half-life of nicotine is approximately 2 hours (513).

Nicotine is metabolized mainly in the liver but also in the kidneys and lungs. The two main metabolites are cotinine and nicotine-1'-N-oxide. Cotinine has few or no cardiovascular or subjective effects. It is cleared more slowly than nicotine, with a half-life of about 19 hours. Cotinine concentrations in the plasma and breast milk of mothers and in the urine of their infants have been reported to reflect the smoking habits of the mothers during pregnancy (514). Thus, it is a better measure of overall intake than nicotine itself. Nicotine crosses the placenta and also is excreted in the milk of lactating women (513). There is a close correlation between nicotine concentration in the mother's plasma and milk after smoking (514). Cotinine, the principal metabolite of nicotine, has been detected in breast milk, particularly in the colostrums in women who smoked actively during pregnancy. Cotinine has also been detected in amniotic fluid and placenta (515).

Incidence

An estimated 66.5 million Americans reported current use of tobacco products in 2001, representing a smoking rate of 29.5% for the population age 12 and older (1). Tobacco is still widely used by women of childbearing age. Based on 2000 and 2001 combined data of the National Household Survey on Drug Abuse, 19.8% of pregnant women aged 15 to 44 smoked cigarettes in the past month compared with 29.5% of nonpregnant women of the same age group. The trend has increased from 1999 and 2000 in which 17% of pregnant women were current smokers (1). Pregnant women aged 15 to 25 were twice as likely to have smoked cigarettes in the last month compared to women aged 26 to 44. Most of those who smoked during pregnancy were Caucasian. About 23.6% of current smokers smoked during the first trimester, 23.8% continued to smoke during the second trimester and 17% up to third trimester (1).

Spontaneous Abortion

The relationship between cigarette smoking and spontaneous abortion has been documented in both animal and human studies. When other risk factors are controlled, women who smoke cigarettes during pregnancy are 1.2 to 2 times more likely to have a spontaneous abortion than those who do not smoke (516). The higher rate of abortion was noted in women who smoke one-half of a pack per day compared to nonsmokers. The mechanism for this association has not been completely elucidated, although studies support the theory that this may be as a result of the vasoactive effects of nicotine on the umbilical arteries (517). Nicotine decreases prostacyclin production in the umbilical artery and reduces its capacity for vasodilatation, thereby affecting fetal nutrition and oxygen transport especially in conditions causing asphyxia (518). Other studies attribute the higher rate of abortion to abnormalities in placental development, and dysfunction of hormones that sustain pregnancy (519,520).

Placental Effects

An increased incidence of placental abruption, and an increase in fetal death as a result of abruption, were seen among women who smoke more than ten cigarettes per day (521). Maternal smoking was associated with the finding of decidual necrosis on pathologic examination. Extensive placental calcification occurred significantly more often in smokers than in nonsmokers (46% vs. 14%) (518). Intervillous blood flow was reported to be reduced acutely during smoking, and for 15 minutes afterward (520).

Apgar Scores

Several studies have noted that maternal cigarette smoking during pregnancy is associated with low Apgar score; however, other risk factors were not controlled for (522). When potentially confounding factors were controlled for, no significant independent association was noted between cigarette smoking and Apgar score (523).

Preterm Birth

Maternal smoking has been reported to be a risk factor for preterm labor and delivery (524). The incidence of preterm labor and birth increases with the number of cigarettes smoked per day (525,526). or nicotine levels in maternal hair (524). However, other studies have shown no effect of smoking on length of gestation (527).

Fetal Death and Neonatal Mortality

Epidemiologic studies have shown a significant effect of smoking on late fetal death and neonatal mortality. Among first-born infants, there was a 25% greater risk for fetal death and neonatal mortality for less than one-pack-per-day smokers and a 56% greater risk for more than one-pack-per-day smokers, compared to the nonsmokers (528). For second or higher births, a 30% greater risk of late fetal death and neonatal mortality was noted in maternal smokers compared to nonsmokers. Maternal smoking had a relative risk for late fetal death of 1.4 and a relative risk for early neonatal mortality of 1.2 (529).

Effects on Fetus and Newborn

Animal models have been designed to prove that nicotine is a neuroteratogen. Nicotine targets specific neurotransmitter receptors in the fetal brain, leading to a decrease in the number of cells and subsequently to altered synaptic activity. The adverse effects of nicotine involve multiple neurotransmitter pathways that alter not only immediate developmental events but also the eventual programming of synaptic competence. These defects may eventually lead to disabilities in learning and cognition which appear later in childhood or adolescence. Alterations in the development of the autonomic nervous system may lead to increased susceptibility to hypoxic-ischemic brain injury, stillbirth and SIDS (530).

Numerous studies have examined the association between smoking prior to or during pregnancy and birth weight and have consistently demonstrated a decrease in birth weight (531) of approximately 200 g, and an increased percentage of low-birth-weight (LBW) infants. (423,526,532–534). Additionally, a dose–response relationship has been demonstrated between the number of cigarettes smoked and the decrease in birth weight (535,536) and the percentage of LBW infants (537). These findings remain consistent after controlling for confounding variables (423). Race is an important factor. In Caucasian mothers, the incidence of LBW babies ranged from 4.8% for women who did not smoke, to 8% for women who smoked 1 to 10 cigarettes per day, and to 13.4% for women who smoked more than 20 cigarettes per day. For black women, the incidence of LBW babies ranged from 8.3% for women who did not smoke, to 13.5% for women who smoked 1 to 10 cigarettes per day, to 22.7% for women who smoked more than 20 cigarettes per day (537). One study demonstrated that serum nicotine levels were more strongly correlated with reduced birth weight than with smoking history (538). This indicates the importance of using biochemical markers in studies of pregnancy outcome.

Studies comparing infant birth weights showed that mothers who quit smoking during pregnancy have infants with higher birth weights than do mothers who continued to smoke during pregnancy, although the overall birth weight was still about 179 g lower compared to nonsmoking mothers (537). The difference in birth weight was highly significant when smoking was discontinued by as late as 16 weeks of gestation, compared to persistent smokers. However, even beyond 16 weeks of gestation, cessation of smoking was still found to be associated with infants with higher birth weights than the offspring of persistent smokers (536). Pregnant women who switched to low tar or low nicotine containing cigarettes continue to have increased risk of having a small for gestational age infant (539).

Attention has been recently focused on the role of environmental tobacco smoke exposure (ETS) as a potential risk factor for low birth weight infants. In one review, infants with ETS exposure in utero were 1.5 to 4 times more likely to be born with low birth weight. ETS was associated with a 25 to 90 g reduction in birth weight and infants born to mothers with ETS exposure were 2 to 4 times more likely to be born small for gestational age (540).

The nature of the growth deficit in terms of newborn body composition, was assessed by examining the anthropometric indices of subcutaneous fat deposition and lean body mass in infants of smokers and nonsmokers. There was no difference between the two groups of infants in the skinfold measurements or in the calculated cross-sectional fat area of the upper arm. These results suggest that the reduction in birth weight of infants whose mothers smoke is due primarily to a decrease in the lean body mass of the newborn, whereas deposition of subcutaneous fat is relatively unaffected (541,542).

Besides birth weight, length and head circumference were also found to be smaller for infants of smoking mothers (533,543), especially among those who continued to smoke to the third trimester (544).

Various studies assessing the association between cigarette smoking during pregnancy and congenital malformations have shown conflicting results. The British Perinatal Mortality Survey, in a study of 17,418 subjects, demonstrated that maternal smoking was associated with congenital heart defects, even after maternal age, parity, and social class were controlled for (545). Other reported deformities included cheilognathopalatoschisis, deformities of the extremities, polycystic kidney, aortopulmonary septum defect, gastroschisis, and skull deformities (546). However, the United States Collaborative Perinatal Project, in a study of 50,282 subjects, did not observe these findings (547, 548). The inconsistency of reports suggests that cigarette smoking per se may not be a cause of congenital malformations in infants (549).

Active, and passive, smoking during pregnancy has recently been reported as an independent risk factor for the development of persistent pulmonary hypertension of the newborn (550).

Neurobehavioral Effects

Several studies have investigated the impact of cigarette smoking during pregnancy on newborn behavior and on later child development (550,551). Offspring of mothers who smoked during pregnancy have been observed to perform less well on the Brazelton Neonatal Behavioral Assessment Score in items such as habituating to sound or orienting to a voice, compared to offspring of nonsmoking mothers. Other studies indicate poorer performance with head turning and sucking, lower visual alertness, more crying, tremors and startles, and increased lability of color and problems with arousal and behavioral regulation (552,553). Most of the studies, however, do not demonstrate a clinically significant effect on neonatal behavior that can be attributed independently to maternal cigarette smoking alone.

Long-Term Outcome

Long-term follow-up evaluation of children's cognitive and developmental functions indicate that when sociodemographic factors were controlled for, children exposed to cigarette smoke in utero performed less in tests of cognitive, psychomotor, language, and general academic achievement, including reading and mathematics. Although the differences were statistically significant between the two groups, they were small compared to other factors that affected the children's performance (509,554–557). Children of mothers who smoked during pregnancy have been shown to be at a higher risk for prepubertal onset conduct disorder and, adolescent onset drug dependence (558).

Sudden Infant Death Syndrome

Several studies have reported that maternal cigarette smoking significantly increases the likelihood of sudden infant death syndrome (559–562). It is proposed that nicotine affects catecholamine metabolism in the brain causing an attenuated response to hypoxia which later causes disturbances in respiratory and cardiovascular control mechanisms (560). Maternal smoking has also been associated with increased incidence of central apnea among infants (561). Mothers of infants who died from the sudden infant death syndrome were more likely to smoke cigarettes either during pregnancy or after their baby was born.

PHENCYCLIDINE

Phencyclidine (PCP) was first introduced in 1957 as a dissociative anesthetic. Despite its wide margin of safety in humans, its clinical use was discontinued after reports of adverse effects that include agitation, confusion, delirium, and persistent hallucinations. Other untoward effects noted with its use were feelings of paranoia, impending death, outbursts of bizarre, agitated, or violent behavior, and a psychosis mimicking schizophrenia. It remains popular as a drug of abuse as a result of its sedative and hallucinogenic effects, its synthesis from readily available precursors, low cost, and variety of routes of administration. Most users smoke PCP; others sniff or snort the powder, drink the liquid form mixed with lemonade or alcohol, or inject it intravenously (563–566).

Placental Transfer and Metabolism

Placental transfer of PCP has been studied in the pig, mouse, rabbit, and humans. In piglets, serum levels of PCP were ten times higher than in the sow (567,568); in fetal rabbits, similar high serum levels were found that reached a peak 2 hours after parenteral administration of the drug to the doe (569). In the mouse, there was almost a tenfold higher concentration of PCP in fetal tissue than in maternal blood (569), and PCP appeared in the pup's brain as early as 15 minutes after subcutaneous injection to the dam (564). Phencyclidine also has been detected in amniotic fluid and umbilical cord blood at high concentrations (570).

Phencyclidine appears rapidly in breast milk, appearing within 15 minutes of maternal administration. By 3 hours, the ratio of levels in milk to those in plasma is approximately ten to one (569).

Phencyclidine is lipophilic. It is stored in body fat and in the CNS for a prolonged period and is released slowly into the bloodstream. The major routes of elimination involve metabolism of PCP in the liver and excretion in the urine and feces (571). The half-life of the drug in the body usually is about 3 days, although it has been found in the urine as long as 8 days after last use (572). The half-life of PCP in the fetus is approximately twice that in the mother (569).

Mode of Action

Phencyclidine has strong, centrally mediated effects in animals and humans, and influences many different neuronal systems. It inhibits the uptake and increases the release of monoamines in the brain, interacts with cholinergic and serotonergic systems, and antagonizes the neuronal stimulation caused by the excitatory amino acid, N-methyl aspartate (563). Phencyclidine may produce a general enhancement of neurotransmitter release by blocking voltage-sensitive potassium channels, and thus might act at several different loci (573).

Incidence

The abuse of PCP first occurred in 1970, peaked in 1979, and then declined by 1981 (574). National surveys, however, have indicated that PCP abuse is again on the rise, especially in large urban areas.

The prevalence of PCP abuse during pregnancy has not been firmly established, because most reports have come from urban areas and could not be generalized to a national level.

Between 1981 and 1982 in Cleveland, 7.5% of 2327 pregnant women gave a history of PCP use, although only 0.8% could be confirmed by maternal urine screening (575,576). In 1983, a study from Los Angeles reported

that 12% of a random sample of 200 newborns had measurable quantities of PCP in their cord blood (570). In 1995 and 1996 about 2.6% of pregnant women admitted having used PCP in their lifetime although 0.2% admitted having used it in the last year. In 2000 and 2001, there were 16,000 women of reproductive age (aged 15 to 44) who were current users of PCP (1). Although the number of new users of hallucinogens continues to rise, it is due largely to the use of methylenedioxymethamphetamine (MDMA) or ecstasy, a member of the so called club drugs.

Growth and Morphology

Animal studies indicate that maternal weight gain is lower in PCP-exposed mice. The birth weights of exposed pups were approximately 7% lower than those of nonexposed pups (564). In most human studies, no significant difference in the birth weight and length and head circumference was observed in PCP-exposed newborns compared to matched controls (577,469,5). In another study, two of five preterm and none of seven term PCP-exposed newborns were small for gestational age. All 12 newborns were normocephalic (579). However, in other studies, intrauterine growth retardation, precipitous labor and neonatal drug withdrawal/intoxication and longer hospital stay were observed among PCP-exposed newborns that were comparable, if not less pronounced (580,581) than cocaine effects (581).

There was also a higher incidence of meconium stained amniotic fluid and less incidence of premature delivery (581). In both animal and human studies, PCP has not been shown to be teratogenic, and no reports of congenital malformations attributable to PCP have as yet been made. Some animal studies have shown either neurodegenerative or antiapoptotic changes in various regions of the brain which resulted in decreased motor coordination and hyperactivity in newborn pups (582). Drugs like PCP have also been shown to produce widespread apoptotic neurodegeneration throughout the developing brain when administered to immature rodents during the period of synaptogenesis which is known as the growth spurt period in the developing brain. This eventually resulted in decreased brain mass and perhaps may also account for the neurobehavioral disturbances seen in the postnatal period (583).

Neurobehavioral Effects

Early case reports of PCP-exposed newborns showed abnormal neurobehavioral findings in the infants. These included irritability, tremors, hypertonicity, poor attention, bizarre eye movements, staring spells, hypertonic ankle reflexes, and depressed grasp and rooting reflexes (576,577,584). One of the most characteristic features in infants is a sudden and rapid change in level of consciousness, with lethargy alternating with irritability. The behavioral outcome of these newborns has been attributed to PCP intoxication, rather than to withdrawal (580). The very low threshold of stimulation, coarse, flapping tremors, and rapid changes in state are similar to behavior reported in children and adults intoxicated with PCP (577).

Long-Term Outcome

The Bayley psychomotor and mental development indices of PCP-exposed infants at 3 months and at 1 year (585) of age were not statistically different from those of controls (577). In one study however, temperament and sleep problems were noted at 12 months of age (585). At 9 and 18 months of age, fine motor development, adaptive or playing behavior, language skills, and personal–social development as determined by the Gesell Developmental Evaluation were within normal range. PCP exposure reportedly, does not affect Bailey Scores during the first 2 years of life (586). These findings are consistent with the interpretation that the observed PCP effects on infants at birth result from acute intoxication rather than from morphologic CNS damage.

AMPHETAMINES

The amphetamines are a group of chemically related sympathomimetic amines that have both CNS stimulant and peripheral α and β actions (587). Since their synthesis in the 1880s, therapeutic uses have included the treatment of exogenous obesity, narcolepsy, hyperkinesis, and depression. There is a very strong abuse potential because of their psychic effects, which include a decreased sense of fatigue, wakefulness, alertness, mood elevation, self-confidence, and often euphoria and elation.

Epidemiology

After initial epidemics of abuse of speed in the 1950s and 1960s, there was a decline in the abuse of amphetamines with the emergence of other drugs of abuse (e.g., heroin, crack cocaine). Lately, a resurgence of amphetamine use in epidemic proportions has occurred, particularly in Japan and parts of Asia, Hawaii, and areas of the West Coast. Of the estimated 356,000 women of reproductive age who were current users of stimulants in 1999–2000 about 4000 (1.12%) of these women were pregnant (1).

Methamphetamine

Methamphetamine is the methylated derivative of amphetamine, and is prepared through the reduction of ephedrine or pseudoephedrine. The ease of its synthesis, its availability and affordability, and a state of prolonged high have made it an increasingly popular drug of abuse. Ice, the form of methamphetamine that can be smoked, is claimed to produce an intense euphoria. High doses may cause aggressive behavior, arrhythmias, severe anxiety, seizures,

shock, strokes, abdominal cramps, insomnia, and death. Chronic use can produce paranoid psychosis.

Effects on Pregnancy

Outcomes of pregnancies in 52 self-reported intravenous methamphetamine abusers were studied; these patients used other drugs as well (588). The infants had significantly lower birth weight, length, and head circumference than infants of non–drug-users. There was no significant difference, however, in the frequency of pregnancy complications such as pregnancy-induced hypertension, peripartal hemorrhage, chorioamnionitis, syphilis, and hepatitis.

No significant increase in the frequency of major congenital anomalies has been associated with methamphetamine use during pregnancy (588,589), although clefting and cardiac anomalies have been reported (590).

Higher incidence of prematurity, intrauterine growth retardation, and smaller head circumference have been reported in infants of mothers who abused cocaine and methamphetamine (591,592). A higher incidence of retroplacental hemorrhage also was noted (591). Fetal and neonatal deaths from maternal methamphetamine abuse have been reported (593).

Effects on Neonates

An infant of a known amphetamine addict manifested after birth with diaphoresis, episodes of agitation alternating with lassitude, meiosis, and vomiting (594). Infants exposed to both cocaine and methamphetamine were described as having abnormal sleep patterns, tremors, poor feeding, hypertonia, sneezing, a high-pitched cry, frantic fist sucking, tachypnea, loose stools, fever, yawning, hyperreflexia, and excoriation (591). Cranial ultrasound performed on term neonates exposed to cocaine, methamphetamine (or cocaine and a narcotic) showed a higher incidence of cranial abnormalities similar to the incidence of infants at risk for hypoxic ischemic injury. The abnormalities include intraventricular hemorrhage, cavitary lesions, echodensities associated with necrosis, mostly found in basal ganglion, frontal lobes and posterior fossa. This is probably related to the vasoconstrictive property of these drugs (595). Brain proton magnetic resonance spectroscopy of children with in utero exposure to methamphetamines showed abnormal energy metabolism but no visible structural abnormalities (596).

Long-Term Effects

Long-term, prospective follow-up of 65 children of women who abused amphetamines and also used alcohol and smoked cigarettes during pregnancy revealed that, at 1 year of age, somatic growth was normal, although illness and accident rates were increased (597). At 4 and 8 years of age, somatic growth and general health still were normal (598,599). Prenatal amphetamine and or cocaine exposure has been reported as a risk factor for later subtle neurologic abnormalities. Developmental screening at 4 years of age, using the Terman Merrill method, revealed significantly lower IQs (484,598), but IQ and psychomotor development were within normal limits by 8 years of age (599). Aggressive behavior and peer-related problems also were noted (599). Poor academic performance and various behavioral problems have been reported among adolescent children who were exposed to amphetamines *in utero* (600).

CLUB DRUGS (ECSTASY, GHB, KETAMINE)

The illicit use and abuse of club drugs such as methylene-dioxymethamphetamine or MDMA (ecstasy), gamma hydroxybutyrate (GHB) and ketamine hydrochloride have increased during the past decade. These club drugs are chemical substances used recreationally by young people during all-night dance parties. In 2001, an estimated 8.1 million (3.6%) of Americans aged 12 or older had tried ecstasy at least once in their lifetime compared to 6.5 million with the highest percentage occurring in the 18 to 25 age group. Use of this drug has been rising steadily since 1992 (1). There is growing concern about its potential toxicity and their effects on human pregnancy because it is being used by a significant number of women of child bearing age. Only a few data are available regarding the effects of these drugs on the fetus.

An animal study on the effect of exposure to ecstasy in utero during the maturation phase suggest that it does not produce damage to 5-HT nerve terminals in the fetal rat brain in contrast to the damage seen on the brain of the mother. This may be as a result of ecstasy being metabolized into free radical producing entities in the adult brain but not in the immature brain or, alternatively, this may be as a result of more effective or more active free radical scavenging mechanisms being present in the immature brain (601). In a prospective follow-up of 136 babies exposed to ecstasy in utero one study indicated that the drug may be associated with a significantly increased risk of congenital defects predominantly cardiovascular and musculoskeletal anomalies (602). There is still much to be learned about the effects of these club drugs on the fetus and the newborn, much less is known about its long-term effects in children. Clinical and basic science research data have remained limited.

CAFFEINE

Caffeine (1,3,7 trimethylxanthine) is a mild CNS stimulant, which is the most widely used psychoactive drug in the world. It is found in coffee (the most important source of caffeine in the American diet), tea, chocolate, cocoa and in numerous prescription and over-the-counter medications (603).

Caffeine is readily absorbed from the digestive tract and is rapidly distributed to all tissues. It easily crosses the placenta and is found in breast milk. Caffeine has several proposed mechanisms of action. One is that it inhibits phosphodiesterase thereby causing intracellular accumulation of cyclic adenosine monophosphate (cAMP). It may also block adenosine receptors and cause increased release of calcium ions from the terminal cisternae of the sarcoplasmic reticulum (604). The major effects of caffeine, as with other xanthine derivatives, are: CNS stimulation, emesis, cardiovascular effects, diuresis, and smooth muscle effects leading to vasodilatation or bronchodilatation (604).

Teratogenicity, Spontaneous Abortion, and Prematurity

Caffeine is teratogenic when given in high concentrations to experimental animals causing limb and facial anomalies. However, no correlation exists between caffeine consumption in humans and birth defect (605). In rodents, caffeine causes malformations usually at high doses not seen in humans. Maternal caffeine consumption during gestation affects the hematologic parameters in both rat and human infants (605,606). Overwhelming evidence indicates that caffeine is not a human teratogen and that caffeine appears to have no effect on preterm labor and delivery (527,607–609). However, there is a small but statistically significant increase in the risk for spontaneous abortion and low birth weight infants in pregnant women consuming more than 150 mg caffeine per day. However, the possible contribution of maternal age, smoking and ethanol, however, could not be excluded (610).

Fetal and Neonatal Effects

Most of the reported effects of maternal caffeine consumption on fetal growth and development are on their adverse effects on birth weight and IUGR. Caffeine ingested in large amounts (>7 cups of coffee/day or >300 g of caffeine/day) during pregnancy causes a dose dependent decrease in birth weight of about 6.5% (606–608,611–612). The risk for low birth weight is further increased by concomitant use of alcohol, nicotine and illicit drugs (612). Other studies however have reported no adverse effects especially with moderate maternal consumption (614) or when other confounding variables like maternal smoking (615), cannabis (417), alcohol (616), and other socioeconomic factors are controlled for. Pregnant mothers are therefore advised to consume coffee or caffeinated beverages in moderation. Elevated levels of maternal third trimester serum paraxanthine, which reflects caffeine consumption, was associated with a higher risk of reduced fetal growth, particularly among women who smoked (617).

Neurobehavioural Effects

Maternal caffeine consumption has been reported to induce long term effects on sleep, locomotion, learning abilities and anxiety among experimental animals. More studies are needed to confirm these observations among human infants (606). Other effects reported include cardiac arrhythmias (618,619) and a possible withdrawal syndrome, characterized by jitteriness, irritability and vomiting (620). It is postulated that these withdrawal signs are caused by a tripling of the half life of caffeine during the last 2 trimesters of pregnancy resulting in a much higher caffeine blood levels in both the mother and the fetus. This is further aggravated by the neonate's inability to metabolize caffeine efficiently (606,621).

Caffeine, during or after pregnancy was not found to be an independent risk factor for SIDS after adjustment for maternal age, education, parity, and smoking during pregnancy (622).

DIAGNOSIS OF DRUG EXPOSURE

Methods to Detect Drug Exposure in the Mother and Infant

The identification of drug exposure in the mother or her neonate is not easy. Mothers rarely fully admit to the use of drugs, because of fear of the consequences stemming from such an admission. Even with maternal cooperation, information on the type and extent of drug use often is inaccurate (3). Similarly, many of the drugs to which the fetus is exposed in utero do not produce immediate or recognizable effects in neonates (623). There are a number of methods used to detect prenatal drug exposure.

Methods to detect substance abuse in a pregnant woman or intrauterine drug exposure in a neonate ideally should address not only the types of drug abused, but also the amount, frequency, and duration of drug exposure. Two general methods are used to achieve this: maternal interview and laboratory tests.

Maternal Interview

Maternal interview has the greatest potential for providing comprehensive information on the type, amount, frequency, and duration of drug use. Two types of maternal interview generally are used.

Routine Interview. The routine interview forms an integral part of the obstetric history, which is obtained either prenatally or when a woman is admitted in labor. The accuracy of the data obtained by this method depends on the attention devoted to the interview. Cursory interview often results in underreporting of drug use, whereas the incidence increases threefold to fivefold if a more organized protocol is used (17,624). There are many elements inherent to routine history taking that affect its accuracy. Maternal fear of the consequences of admission, underestimation of drug use even by those who admit to the use of drugs, and physical discomfort experienced by the woman, particularly if in labor, all affect the accuracy of her self-report. Under these circumstances, the reporting of drug

abuse by the mother can be as low as one fourth of the true incidence (3).

Structured Interview. A structured interview is a highly organized interview, frequently using a standard questionnaire. Examples of this are the Khavari Alcohol Test (625), or its modification (626), and the Cahalan Volume Variability Scale (627). The structured interview is more accurate because more time is spent with the patient and the interview frequently is conducted in a more favorable environment than is the routine interview, i.e., it is not conducted when the mother is in labor. Structured interviews frequently are used as research tools. On the other hand, structured interviews are expensive and time-consuming to conduct, and are not practical for routine clinical use when dealing with patients who present in labor and have received little or no prenatal care. Interview directed at drug use at the time of conception (or when the woman first learned that she was pregnant) has a higher degree of accuracy and correlates more to pregnancy and neonatal outcome than interview on drug use during pregnancy as a result of the stigma associated with the latter (628).

Laboratory Tests

Most of the laboratory tests for drug detection are used simply for screening purposes. Confirmation with the use of another, unrelated procedure is usually needed if results are to withstand further scrutiny. It is apparent that as more confirmatory tests are done, the testing process becomes more expensive. Thus, the extent to which further tests are carried out after the initial screen is determined by the reasons that initiated the test.

Various analytical procedures are used for drug detection: thin-layer chromatography, immunoassays, high-performance liquid chromatography (HPLC) and gas chromatography for screening and gas chromatography–mass spectrometry (GCMS) for confirmation. A good review of the use and limitations of these procedures has been published (629).

Specimens for Drug Testing

Urine. The testing of biologic fluids for drugs is by far the most common method used to detect drug abuse in a pregnant woman, or intrauterine drug exposure in a neonate. There are several limitations to this method, however. Identification of drugs in biologic fluids will differentiate only those who have been exposed to drugs vs. those who were not. The test cannot provide information on the amount, frequency, duration, or the time of last drug use. Among the biologic fluids, urine has been most often tested owing to several advantages (630): urine collection is easy and noninvasive; drug metabolites in urine usually are found in higher concentrations than in serum, as a result of the concentrating ability of the kidneys; large volumes of urine can be collected; urine is easier to analyze than blood because it usually is devoid of protein and other cellular constituents; the metabolites in urine usually are stable, especially if frozen; and urine is amenable to all of the drug-testing methods mentioned above.

However, there are several drawbacks to the use of urine for testing. Foremost is the high rate of false-negative results (14,509). In the mother, unless collection is watched closely, urine easily can be substituted with a clean specimen. Urine samples can be tampered with by dilution or by the addition of ions, such as salt, which may interfere with the testing methods. Drug metabolites in urine also reflect only very recent use of the drug, so that negative results may occur if the woman abstains from the use of the drug a few days before testing (630). In the infant, the incidence of false-negative urine tests also is high, ranging from 32% to 63% (631–634). Urine specimens must be obtained as close to birth as possible to reflect the infant's intrauterine exposure to drugs. The later after birth that urine is collected and tested, the higher is the likelihood of a false-negative test. Collection of the requisite volume of urine for both the screening test and the confirmatory test from an extremely small or very sick infant may also be difficult. The cutoff concentration for positivity used by the laboratory can also influence the detection rate (635). Recent abstention by the mother from the use of drugs may result in a negative urine test in the infant. The detection rate for drugs in the urine also can improve if a battery rather than a single test is used (634).

Meconium. The concept behind meconium drug testing was based on studies in pregnant rhesus monkeys which received morphine throughout gestation; a high concentration of morphine and its metabolites were found in the gastrointestines or "meconium" of their fetuses (636). It was postulated that the drug accumulated in meconium as a consequence of fetal swallowing of amniotic fluid which contained drugs originating from fetal urine or from the excretion of drug metabolites through the bile. Subsequent studies in pregnant rats further showed that the concentration of morphine and cocaine in meconium were related to the dose, timing and duration of drug administration to the dam (637,638).

Meconium drug testing has been adapted to various analytical methods which included radioimmunoassay, EMIT, FPIA, HPLC and GCMS (639). The original analysis of meconium for drugs was by radioimmunoassay and the recovery of morphine and benzoylecgonine which were spiked in meconium ranged from 84% to 97% and 70% to 100%, respectively (640). The use of radioimmunoassays, which can detect both parent drug and its metabolites, e.g., Coat-a-Count (DPC, Los Angeles, CA) result in a higher detection rate compared to those tests which are specific only for the metabolites. A radioimmunoassay-based meconium drug testing kit, called Mectest (Meco Industries, Walnut, CA) is approved by the FDA for the testing of cocaine, opiate and cannabinoid in meconium and exhibits high sensitivity, specificity and precision. The detection limit is 7.62 ng/mL for cocaine, 27.8 ng/mL for opiate and 5.3% ng/mL for cannabinoid.

The concentration of drugs in meconium can change if meconium is left at room temperature for 24 hours: 25%

decrease in cocaine, 62% increase in morphine and 30% decrease in cannabinoid. The increase in morphine is as a result of the endogenous hydrolysis of morphine glucuronide into morphine in meconium from the action of β glucuronidase and the higher sensitivity of the radioimmunoassay for morphine compared to its glucuronide. On the other hand, drugs are stable in meconium, if frozen, for as long as 9 months.

Meconium drug testing has also been adapted to other drug testing methods such as EMIT or enzyme multiplied immunoassay technique and FPIA or fluorescence polarization immunoassay (641). However, when compared to radioimmunoassay, the sensitivity of enzyme immunoassay for cocaine, opiate and cannabinoid detection is lower, although its specificity is still 100%. With EMIT and FPIA, the cutoff concentrations for meconium drug testing are 50 ng/mL for cocaine, 100 ng/mL for morphine and 25 ng/mL for cannabinoid (642). Meconium has also been tested for methamphetamine and phencyclidine using EMIT and the detection limits are 730 and 100 ng/g meconium, respectively (642). Meconium drug testing has been adapted to HPLC (642–645), and GC/MS analysis (646–650) and the detection limit by HPLC is 50 ng/g meconium for benzoylecgonine and 500 ng/g meconium for morphine and amphetamine. By GCMS, the limit of detection is 11 ng/mL for cocaine and its metabolites, 5 ng/g meconium for morphine, codeine, hydromorphine, and hydrocodone and 2 ng/g meconium for cannabinoids. Fatty acid esters of ethanol have also been analyzed in meconium by GCMS and their concentrations have correlated well to maternal alcohol use during pregnancy (326–329). Likewise, nicotine metabolites (cotinine and trans 3'-hydroxycotinine) have been measured in meconium by radioimmunoassay and GCMS (651).

A number of clinical studies using the meconium drug test have demonstrated major advantages of meconium drug testing over urine testing in newborn infants. These include the ease and noninvasiveness of meconium collection which is particularly useful in anonymous, drug prevalence study; high sensitivity and specificity of the test; large window for detecting intrauterine drug exposure to as early as the 16th week of gestation, reliability of testing meconium samples even for those obtained beyond 24 hours after birth and positive correlation between concentration of drugs in meconium and the amount of drug use by the mother during gestation (141,638,651–657). The main disadvantage of meconium drug testing is the nonhomogeniety of meconium which requires preparative procedures to produce the analyte. In, one report using GCMS for drug analysis, maternal urine, infant urine and meconium analysis yielded equivalent results (658).

Hair. Hair analysis has been one of the recent additions to drug testing (659). The test is based on the principle that illicit substances and their metabolic products are incorporated from the serum into the hair follicle and grow into the cuticle and hair shaft. The drug, once deposited in the hair shaft, remains for an indefinite period. As the hair grows at the rate of 1 to 2 cm month, the deposited drugs follow the growth of the hair shaft. The section of the hair closest to the scalp is the most recently exposed portion. Sectional analysis can be performed by month to provide information on the duration and time of drug use. The information on the chronicity of drug use makes hair analysis advantageous compared with urine or other body fluid testing. Furthermore, quantitative detection of drugs in hair has been correlated with the amount of drug use in the past.

Hair has been analyzed to detect opiates (660), cocaine (661), PCP (662), methamphetamine, antidepressants, and nicotine (663) by radioimmunoassay (659), GCMS (664), HPLC (665), and collisional spectroscopy (666).

The validity of hair analysis for drug detection has been demonstrated both in the mother and her neonate (664). Although hair analysis has exciting potential, there are some significant drawbacks to the use of hair for testing in women (667). Patients who are not chronic drug users may not be detected by this technique, because drug deposition in hair relies on serum levels during hair growth. The expense of the test mounts with the number of drugs being screened for, and has limited its usefulness in prenatal clinics. The quantity of hair necessary to perform the drug screen, i.e., a pencil-sized diameter plug of hair from the posterior scalp, may be difficult to collect in some newborn infants. Use of hair dye, bleach, and other cosmetic agents by the woman may modify the amount of drug in hair, but should not totally eliminate its presence because the drug is incorporated into the hair shaft. Some ethnic groups weave hair from other individuals into their own hair, and this creates the potential for false test results. Because of misconceptions about cosmetic effects, some patients may refuse hair testing. Hair can also be passively exposed to drugs that can be smoked (e.g., cocaine, marijuana).

Others. Other types of specimens have been tested for drugs. These include perspiration, nail clippings, menstrual blood, gastric juice, semen, and saliva (668–670). The use of these specimens for drug detection has been uncommon, however.

TREATMENT

Initial management of the infant is directed toward the antenatal and neonatal complications that are associated with maternal drug abuse such as asphyxia, fetal distress, prematurity, meconium aspiration, and congenital malformation. Additionally, the infant should be routinely tested for syphilis and HIV disease, be assessed for drug withdrawal, undergo drug testing and receive social service referral.

Narcotic Withdrawal

The infant of an opiate-dependent mother should be observed closely for withdrawal. The severity of the withdrawal can be assessed by several clinical scoring systems (671,672). We use a system that evaluates the infant specifically on manifestations that are life-threatening: vomiting, diarrhea, weight loss, irritability, tremors, and tachypnea (Table 58-7). With this system, drugs are used to treat the withdrawal if there is moderate vomiting, diarrhea, or weight loss; or any severe criterion.

Both narcotic and nonnarcotic drugs have been used to treat narcotic withdrawal (673) (Table 58-8). Narcotics are preferred, however, because their action is more physiologic for an abstinence state. Although the neurologic manifestations of withdrawal may be controlled successfully by nonnarcotic drugs, narcotics are more effective in relieving the non-CNS manifestations (e.g., diarrhea).

Among the narcotic drugs, paregoric, laudanum, and sometimes methadone are used. We prefer to use tincture

TABLE 58-7

ASSESSMENT OF THE CLINICAL SEVERITY OF NEONATAL NARCOTIC WITHDRAWAL

Sign	Mild	Moderate	Severe
Vomiting	Spitting up	Extensive vomiting for three successive feedings	Vomiting associated with imbalance of serum electrolytes
Diarrhea	Watery stools < four times per day	Watery stools five to six times per day for 3 days; no electrolyte imbalance	Diarrhea associated with imbalance of serum electrolytes
Weight loss	<10% of birth weight	10%–15% of birth weight	>15%
Irritability	Minimal	Marked but relieved by cuddling or feeding	Unrelieved by cuddling or feeding
Tremors	Mild tremors when twitching	Marked tremors or stimulated	Convulsions twitching when stimulated
Tachypnea	60–80 breaths/min	80–100 breaths/min	>100 breaths/min; associated with respiratory alkalosis

TABLE 58-8

TREATMENT OF NEONATAL WITHDRAWAL SYNDROME[a]

Drug	Dosage
Paregoric	0.1–0.4 mL/kg (2–6 drops) every 4 to 6 h, PO
Laudanum (0.4%)	0.1–0.4 mL/kg (2–6 drops) every 4 to 6 h, PO
Chlorpromazine	0.55 mg/kg every 6 h, PO or IM
Phenobarbital	Loading dose: 16 mg/kg/day PO
	Maintenance dose: 2–8 mg/kg/day PO
Methadone	0.05–1.0 mg/kg every 6 hours, PO with increases of 0.05 mg/kg until signs are controlled.

[a] From Osborn DA, Cole MJ, Jeffrey HE. Opiate treatment for opiate withdrawal in newborn infants. *Cochrane Database Syst Rev* 2002; CD002059, with permission.

of opium or laudanum, United States Pharmacopeia (USP) over paregoric, because paregoric contains camphor, a CNS stimulant. Laudanum USP is available in a standard 10% solution, contains 1.0% morphine, and must be used with caution. Laudanum USP must be diluted 25-fold to a concentration of 0.4% to reduce its morphine content to a level equivalent to the amount present in paregoric. Laudanum USP (0.4%) can be given at the same dose as paregoric, i.e., 3–6 drops every 4–6 hours.

The aim of treatment with drugs is to render the infant comfortable, but not obtunded. Thus, the drug should be titrated, starting with the smallest recommended dose and increased accordingly until the desired effect is achieved. Once the infant is asymptomatic, the drug can be tapered slowly until it is completely discontinued which usually takes between 4 to 6 days. The infant should be observed for a day or two after discontinuance of the drug for possible recurrence of withdrawal manifestations ("rebound" phenomenon). Overall, it will normally take between 10 to 14 days from the time that pharmacologic treatment is initiated up to the time that the infant is discharged home without the need for medication. When the infant is discharged from the nursery, the mother should be instructed to anticipate some mild jitteriness and irritability that may persist in the infant for 8 to 16 weeks, depending on the initial severity of the withdrawal.

In view of their hyperirritability, infants manifesting withdrawal should be swaddled, placed in a prone position, and cuddled more often. Swaddling, particularly with the infant's extremities flexed and hands placed in front of its mouth, enhances the infant's hand-to-mouth facility and is soothing. A similar soothing action can be achieved with a pacifier.

The frequency of diarrhea and vomiting should be noted, and the infant's weight checked at least every 8 hours. Temperature, heart rate, and respiratory rates should be recorded every 4 hours. Laboratory examinations to detect serum electrolyte or pH imbalance should be done as indicated.

There are only a few studies which have compared the efficacy of the different pharmacologic agents for the treatment of neonatal opiate withdrawal and these are reviewed in a meta-analysis study (674). The conclusion is that opiates, as compared to supportive care only, appear to reduce the time to regain birth weight and reduce the duration of supportive care, but increase the duration of hospital stay. There was no treatment failure. When compared to phenobarbital, opiates reduced the incidence of seizures, but overall, no evidence of treatment failure. When compared to diazepam, opiates reduced the incidence of treatment failure.

Nonnarcotic Withdrawal

A cross reaction exists between the different drugs belonging to the alcohol–hypnosedative group (see Table 58-4). Each drug is effective in treating withdrawal from any of the drugs belonging to this group (1). Thus, barbiturates can be used to treat withdrawal from nonbarbiturates, including alcohol, or vice versa.

The two drugs that have been used commonly during the neonatal period for this purpose are phenobarbital, 3 to 5 mg/kg/day in divided doses every 6 hours, and chlorpromazine, 1 to 2 mg intramuscularly every 8 hours. Chlorpromazine also has been used successfully at a dose of 2 to 3 mg/kg/day in divided doses every 6 hours (12). Although chlorpromazine does not belong to the group of nonnarcotic drugs that can cause withdrawal manifestations, its ability to ameliorate the signs and symptoms of withdrawal may be secondary to its capacity to suppress REM sleep, which is exaggerated during the state of withdrawal (14).

During the treatment of withdrawal, attention also should be focused on the nutrition and the fluid and electrolyte balance of the infants, particularly if vomiting, diarrhea, hyperpyrexia, and hyperhidrosis occur. Appropriate intravenous fluids may be required to correct deficits or prevent the occurrence of fluid and electrolyte imbalances in the patients.

Maternal Support

The addicted woman has some serious impediments to a successful mothering role. She has meager past mothering experience to rely on; often there is little or no support from a father or husband because frequently she is single, and, finally, the neurobehavioral abnormalities and withdrawal in her infant may hamper the gratifying feedback that she wishes to experience from her infant.

Thus, the mother and child should have early and repeated contacts. A staff member also should have repeated and relatively brief contacts with the mother, to describe the status of the child and to reassure her that, with the disappearance of withdrawal, the infant will feed more vigorously and will respond better to maternal ministrations.

On the other hand, should it be decided that the infant will be placed in a foster care home, it should be remembered that the infant will need human contact for its normal growth and development. As part of its care in the nursery, the child should be stimulated appropriately through frequent handling or fondling by the staff professionals.

Breast-Feeding

Most drugs taken by the mother will cross into her breast milk. The concentration of illicit drug in the breast milk will depend on the amount and time of drug intake by the mother. In general, breastfeeding is discouraged in the pregnant addict who has not been compliant in her attendance in her drug treatment program because of the potential presence of multiple drugs of abuse in her breast milk. On the other hand, compliant mothers, even on methadone treatment, can safely breast-feed because the amount of methadone in breast milk is less than 5% of the maternal dose (675). If the mother is HIV positive, there is the danger of HIV transmission through the breast milk and breast-feeding is not recommended.

DRUG-ADDICTED WOMEN AS INFANT CAREGIVERS

The ability of the drug-addicted woman to perform her functions as a mother and provide adequate care for her infant has been seriously questioned on many occasions. Frequently, these women have been denied their maternal rights and responsibilities soon after the infant's birth on the basis of their unstable homes, life-styles, and their emotional and psychological weaknesses. Evidence suggests that this practice may be unnecessary and counterproductive in many cases. A study that determined outcome of infants on the basis of the type of caregiver showed that the outcome, measured by growth, development, frequency of medical illnesses, and child abuse, for infants cared for by the mother with the help of a caregiver (e.g., either a husband or relative) was better than the outcome for infants in foster home care (74). Thus, with proper guidance and supervision, the addict mother may be capable of providing adequate care for her infant, particularly because most of these women desire to fulfill their mothering functions. It has been reported that mothers who had full time responsibility for child care had significantly higher levels of maternal adaptation than part time mothers (676). Similarly, although a high incidence of problems suggestive of child abuse (e.g., cigarette burns, hematoma) were noted in infants who were cared for exclusively by the mother, very few of these complications were noted in infants whose mother had help available. Thus, it is important that when allowing the mother to care for her infant, someone should help her at home (often the maternal grandmother) in the care of the infant to ensure its better care and protection. Likewise, the drug dependent mother needs assistance in parenting which can be given through a regular follow up of the mother and infant by a visiting or public health nurse and the social and protective service worker. Such interventions have been proven to be beneficial (85–87). In appropriate circumstances, alternative measures of placement of the child into known favorable home environment have also resulted in better behavioral functions of the child (81).

Social Service Referral

All infants of drug-dependent mothers should have a social service referral to assess the adequacy of parenting and care at home. The discharge of the infant to the mother's care is the primary objective, unless serious conditions dictate otherwise. The care of the infant by the mother, with the help of a support person, usually a grandmother or other relative, has, in our experience, been the best arrangement for a favorable outcome for the infant. The discharge of the infant to a person other than the mother (e.g., foster parent) or an agency should be resorted to only when it is apparent that the infant will be neglected, poorly cared for, or abused. Most mothers hesitate to admit to the use of drugs during pregnancy because of fear that their infants will be taken away from them. They should be assured otherwise; in fact, they should be encouraged to be responsible for the primary care of their infants. The social worker and physician also should advise the mother about available medical and social services in the community, such as substance abuse counseling and family planning services.

Potential Child Abuse

As part of child protection laws that are operative in many states, infants born to drug-dependent mothers are considered as potentially abused and are required by law to be reported to child protection agencies. Many of these agencies require a positive drug screen in the infant before they will take action on the reports. The precautionary measure intended in the referral of the infant to the child protection agencies is useful if the intent is to ensure the adequacy of care of the infant at home. It is when punitive measures are taken against the mother that the outcome may become counterproductive.

FOLLOW-UP

The infant of the drug-dependent mother is at risk to many long-term problems (see Drug Addicted Women as Infant Caregiver and Potential Child Abuse) and to ongoing exposure to drugs in the household as a result of accidental ingestion or passive exposure, particularly to crack cocaine (see above). Follow-up of these infants should be planned not only to assess their medical well-being but to ascertain that further risks to drug exposure are prevented and that appropriate interventions are initiated.

REFERENCES

1. *National Household Survey on Drug Abuse 2001*. Substance Abuse and Mental Health Services Administration, Washington: US Government Printing Office.
2. Ostrea EM, Brady M, Gause S, et al. Drug screening of newborn infants by meconium analysis: a large scale prospective, epidemiologic study. *Pediatrics* 1992;89:107.
3. Rodriguez EM, Mofenson LM, Chang BHm Rich KC, et al. Association of maternal drug use during pregnancy with maternal HIV culture positivity and perinatal transmission. *AIDS* 1996;10:273–282.
4. Zagon IS. Opioids and development: new lessons from old problems. *NIDA Research Monograph* 1985;60:58.
5. Goodfriend MJ, Shey IA, Klein MD. The effect of maternal narcotic addiction on the newborn. *Am J Obstet Gynecol* 1956;71:29.
6. Dole VP, Nyswander MA. Medical treatment for diacetyl-morphine (heroin) addiction. *J Am Med Assoc* 1965;193:646.
7. Ostrea EM, Chavez CJ, Strauss ME. A study of the factors that influence the severity of neonatal narcotic withdrawal. *J Pediatr* 1976; 88:642.
8. Anyaegbunam A, Tran T, Jadali D, et al. Assessment of fetal well-being in methadone-maintained pregnancies: abnormal non-stress tests. *Gynecol Obstet Invest* 1997;43(1):25–28.
9. Connaughton JF, Finnegan LP, Schur J, et al. Current concepts in the management of the pregnant opiate addict. *Addict Dis* 1975; 2:21.
10. Naeye RL, Blanc W, Leblanc W, et al. Fetal complications of maternal heroin addiction: abnormal growth, infections, and episodes of stress. *J Pediatr* 1973;83:1055.
11. Zelson C. Infant of the addicted mother. *N Engl J Med* 1973; 288:1393.
12. Ostrea EM, Chavez CJ. Perinatal problems (excluding neonatal withdrawal) in maternal drug addiction: a study of 830 cases. *J Pediatr* 1979;94:292.
13. Szeto HH. Effects of narcotic drugs on fetal behavioral activity: acute methadone exposure. *Am J Obstet Gynecol* 1983;146:211.
14. Dinges DF, Davis MM, Glass P. Fetal exposure to narcotics: neonatal sleep as a measure of nervous system disturbance. *Science* 1980;209:619.
15. Umans JG, Szeto HH. Precipitated opiate abstinence in utero. *Am J Obstet Gynecol* 1985;151:441.
16. Zuspan FB, Gumpel JA, Mejia-Zelaya A, et al. Fetal stress from methadone withdrawal. *Am J Obstet Gynecol* 1975;122:43.
17. Bauer CR, Shankaran S, Bada HS, et al. The Maternal Lifestyle Study: drug exposure during pregnancy and short-term maternal outcomes. *Am J Obstet Gynecol* 2002;186:487–495.
18. Perlmutter JF. Heroin addiction and pregnancy. *Obstet Gynecol Surv* 1974;29:439.
19. Donahoe R. Opiates as immunocompromising drugs: the evidence and possible mechanisms. *NIDA Research Monograph* 1988; 90:105.
20. Shafer DA, Falek A, Donahoe RM, et al. Biogenetic effects of opiates. *Int J Addict* 1990–1991;25:1.
21. Harper RG, Solish GI, Purow HM, et al. The effect of a methadone treatment program upon pregnant heroin addicts and their newborn infants. *Pediatrics* 1974;54:300.
22. Chasnoff I, Hatcher R, Burns WJ. Early growth patterns in methadone-addicted infants. *Am J Dis Child* 1980;134:1049.
23. Chasnoff I, Hatcher R, Burns WJ. Polydrug and methadone addicted newborns: a continuum of impairment. *Pediatrics* 1982;70:210.
24. Kaltenbach K, Finnegan LP. Children exposed to methadone in utero. *Ann NY Acad Sci* 1989;562:360.
25. Doberczak TM, Thornton JC, Bernstein J, et al. Impact of maternal drug dependency on birth weight and head circumference of offspring. *Am J Dis Child* 1987;141:1163.
26. Sastry BV. Placental toxicology: tobacco smoke, abused drugs, multiple chemical interactions, and placental function. *Reprod Fertil Dev* 1991;3:355.
27. Rosen TS, Johnson HL. Children of methadone-maintained mothers: follow-up to 18 months of age. *J Pediatr* 1982;101:192.
28. McLaughlin PJ, Zagon IS, White WJ. Perinatal methadone exposure in rats: effects on body and organ development. *Biol Neonate* 1978;34:48.
29. Zagon IS, McLaughlin PJ. Effect of chronic maternal methadone exposure on perinatal development. *Biol Neonate* 1977;31:271.
30. Thompson CI, Zagon IS. Long-term thermoregulatory changes following perinatal methadone exposure in rats. *Pharmacol Biochem Behav* 1980;14:653.
31. Hulse GK, Milne E, English DR, et al. The relationship between maternal use of heroin and methadone and infant birth weight. *Addiction* 1997;92:1571–1579.
32. Dashe JS, Sheffield JS, Olscher DA, et al. Relationship between maternal methadone dosage and neonatal withdrawal. *Obstet Gynecol* 2002;100:1244–1249.
33. Sundell H, Garrot J, Blakenship WJ, et al. Studies on infants with type II respiratory distress syndrome. *J Pediatr* 1971;78:754.
34. Glass L, Rajegowda BK, Evans HE. Absence of respiratory distress syndrome in premature infants of heroin-addicted mothers. *Lancet* 1971;2:685.
35. Taeusch HM Jr, Carson SH, Wang NS, et al. Heroin induction of lung maturation and growth retardation in fetal rabbits. *J Pediatr* 1973;82:869.
36. Rothstein P, Gould JB. Born with a habit: infants of drug-addicted mothers. *Pediatr Clin North Am* 1974;21:307.
37. Geber WF, Schramm LC. Congenital malformations of the central nervous system produced by narcotic analgesics in the hamster. *Am J Obstet Gynecol* 1975;123:705.
38. Amarose AP. Chromosome aberrations in the mother and the newborn from drug-addiction pregnancies. *J Reprod Med* 1978; 20:323.
39. Dinges DF, Davis MM, Glass P. Fetal exposure to narcotics: neonatal sleep as a measure of nervous system disturbance. *Science* 1980;209:619.
40. Pinto F, Torrioli MG, Casella G, et al. Sleep in babies born to chronically heroin addicted mothers. A follow up study. *Drug Alcohol Depend* 1988;21:43.
41. McPherson DL, Madden JD, Payne TF. Auditory brainstem-evoked potentials in term infants born to mothers addicted to opiates. *J Perinatol* 1989;9:262.
42. Trammer RM, Aust G, Koster K, et al. Narcotic and nicotine effects on the neonatal auditory system. *Acta Paediatr* 1992;81:962.
43. Ostrea EM Jr, Kresbach P, Knapp DK, et al. Abnormal heart rate tracings and serum creatine phosphokinase in addicted neonates. *Neurotoxicol Teratol* 1987;9:305.
44. McCann EM, Lewis K. Control of breathing in babies of narcotic- and cocaine-abusing mothers. *Early Hum Dev* 1991;27:175.
45. Nathenson G, Cohen M, Litt I, et al. The effect of maternal heroin addiction on neonatal jaundice. *J Pediatr* 1972;81:899.
46. Burstein Y, Giardina PJV, Rausen AR, et al. Thrombocytosis and increased circulating platelet aggregates in newborn infants of polydrug users. *J Pediatr* 1979;94:895.
47. Cepeda EE, Lee MI, Mehdizadeh B. Decreased incidence of intra-ventricular hemorrhage in infants of opiate dependent mothers. *Acta Paediatr* 1987;76:16.
48. Pasto ME, Graziani LJ, Tunis SL, et al. Ventricular configuration and cerebral growth in infants born to drug-dependent mothers. *Pediatr Radiol* 1985;15:77.
49. Desmond MM, Schwanecke RP, Wilson GS, et al. Maternal barbiturate utilization and neonatal withdrawal symptomatology. *J Pediatr* 1972;80:190.
50. Doberczak TM, Kandal SR, Wilets I. Neonatal opiate abstinence syndrome in term and preterm infants. *J Pediatr* 1991;118(6): 933.
51. Hagopian GS, Wolfe HM, Sokol RJ, et al. Neonatal outcome following methadone exposure in utero. *J Matern Fetal Med* 1996;5:348.
52. Strauss ME, Andresko M, Stryker JC, et al. Relationship of neonatal withdrawal to maternal methadone dose. *Am J Drug Alcohol Abuse* 1976;3:339.
53. Rosen TS, Pippenger CE. Pharmacologic observations on the neonatal withdrawal syndrome. *J Pediatr* 1976;88:1044.
54. Fischer G, Etzersdorfer P, Eder H, et al. Buprenorphine maintenance in pregnant opiate addicts. *Eur Addict Res* 1998;4 [Suppl 1]:32.
55. Fischer G, Johnson RE, Eder H, et al. Treatment of opioid-dependent pregnant women with buprenorphine. *Addiction* 2000: 95:239.
56. Eder H, Rupp I, Peternell A, et al. Buprenorphine in pregnancy. *Psychiatr Prax* 2001;28:267.
57. Schindler SD, Eder H, Ortner R, et al. Neonatal outcome following buprenorphine maintenance during conception and throughout pregnancy. *Addiction* 2003;98:103.

58. Ostrea EM, Chavez CJ, Stryker JS. *The care of the drug dependent women and her infant.* Lansing, MI: Michigan Department of Public Health, 1978:28.

59. Kron RE, Finnegan LP, Kaplan SL, et al. The assessment of behavioral change in infants undergoing narcotic withdrawal: comparative data from clinical and objective methods. *Addict Dis* 1975;2:257.

60. Strauss ME, Lessen-Firestone JK, Starr RH, et al. Behavior of narcotic addicted newborns. *Child Dev* 1975;46:887.

61. Coppolillo HP. Drug impediments to mothering behavior. *Addict Dis Int J* 1975;2:201.

62. Chavez CJ, Ostrea EM, Strauss ME, et al. Prognosis of infants born to drug dependent mothers: its relation to the severity of the withdrawal during the neonatal period. *Pediatr Res* 1976;10:328A.

63. Hutchings DE. Methadone and heroin during pregnancy: a review of behavioral effects in human and animal offspring. *Neurobehav Toxicol* 1982;4:429.

64. Kolar AF, Brown BS, Haertzen CA, et al. Children of opiate abusers: the life experiences of children of opiate addicts in methadone maintenance. *Am J Drug Alcohol Abuse* 1994;20:159.

65. Casado-Flores J, Bano-Rodrigo A, Romero E. Social and medical problems in children of heroin-addicted parents. A study of 75 patients. *Am J Dis Child* 1990;144:977.

66. Chavez CJ, Ostrea EM, Stryker JS, et al. Sudden infant death syndrome among infants of drug dependent mothers. *J Pediatr* 1979;95:407.

67. Pierson PS, Howard P, Kleber HD. Sudden deaths in infants born to methadone maintained addicts. *J Am Med Assoc* 1972;220: 1933.

68. Strauss ME, Starr RH, Ostrea EM, et al. Behavior concomitants of prenatal addiction to narcotics. *J Pediatr* 1976;89:842.

69. Wilson GS, Desmond MM, Verniaud WW. Early development of infants of heroin addicted mothers. *Am J Dis Child* 1973;126: 457.

70. Wilson, GS, McCreary R, Kean J, et al. The development of preschool children of heroin-addicted mothers: a controlled trial study. *Pediatrics* 1979;63:135.

71. Wilson GS, Desmond MM, Wait RB. Follow-up of methadone-treated and untreated narcotic-dependent women and their infants: health, developmental and social implications. *J Pediatr* 1981;98:716.

72. van Baar A. Development of infants of drug dependent mothers. *J Child Psychol Psychiatry* 1990;31:911.

73. Rosen TS, Johnson HL. Children of methadone-maintained mothers: follow-up to 18 months of age. *J Pediatr* 1982;101:192.

74. Chavez CJ, Ostrea EM. Outcome of infants of drug dependent mothers based on the type of caregiver. *Pediatr Res* 1977;11:375A.

75. Nelson LB, Ehrlich S, Calhoun JH, et al. Occurrence of strabismus in infants born to drug-dependent women. *Am J Dis Child* 1987;141:175.

76. Kaltenbach K, Finnegan LP. Perinatal and developmental outcome of infants exposed to methadone in-utero. *Neurotoxicol Teratol* 1987;9:311.

77. Strauss ME, Lessen-Firestone JK, Chavez CJ, et al. Children of methadone-treated women at five years of age. *Pharmacol Biochem Behav* 1979;11(Suppl):3.

78. van Baar A. Development of infants of drug dependent mothers. *J Child Psychol Psychiatry* 1990;31:911.

79. Herjanic BM, Barredo VH, Herjanic M, et al. Children of heroin addicts. *Int J Addict* 1979;14:919.

80. Marcus J, Hans SL, Jeremy RJ. Differential motor and state functioning in newborns of women on methadone. *Neurobehav Toxicol* 1982;4:459.

81. Ornoy A, Michailevskaya V, Lukashov I, et al. The developmental outcome of children born to heroin-dependent mothers, raised at home or adopted. *Child Abuse Negl* 1996;20:385.

82. Olofsson M, Buckley W, Andersen GE, et al. Investigation of 89 children born by drug-dependent mothers. I. Neonatal course. *Acta Paediatr* 1983;72:403.

83. Miles DR, Svikis DS, Kulstad, et al. Psychopathology in pregnant drug-dependent women with and without comorbid alcohol dependence. *Alcohol Clin Exp Res* 2001;25:1012.

84. Hans SL, Bernstein VJ, Henson LG. The role of psychopathology in the parenting of drug-dependent women. *Dev Psychopathol* 1999;11:957.

85. Butz AM, Pulsifer M, Marano N, et al. Effectiveness of a home intervention for perceived child behavioral problems and par-

enting stress in children with in utero drug exposure. *Arch Pediatr Adolesc Med* 2001;155:1029.

86. Schuler ME, Nair P, Black MM. Ongoing maternal drug use, parenting attitudes, and a home intervention: effects on mother-child interaction at 18 months. *J Dev Behav Pediatr* 2002;23:87.

87. Schuler ME, Nair P, Kettinger L. Drug-exposed infants and developmental outcome: effects of a home intervention and ongoing maternal drug use. *Arch Pediatr Adolesc Med* 2003;157:133.

88. Levy M, Spino M. Neonatal withdrawal syndrome: associated drugs and pharmacologic management [Review]. *Pharmacotherapy* 1993;13:202.

89. Essig CF. Addiction to barbiturate and non barbiturate sedative drugs. *Res Publ Assoc Res Nerv Ment Dis* 1968;46:188.

90. Isbell H. Addiction to barbiturates and the barbiturate abstinence syndrome. *Ann Intern Med* 1950;33:108.

91. Bleyer W, Marshall RE. Barbiturate withdrawal syndrome in a passively addicted infant. *J Am Med Assoc* 1972;221:185.

92. Ploman L, Persson BH. On the transfer of barbiturates to the human fetus and their accumulation in some of its vital organs. *Br J Obstet Gynaecol* 1957;64:706.

93. Ostrea EM Jr. Neonatal withdrawal from intrauterine exposure to butalbital. *Am J Obstet Gynecol* 1982;143:597.

94. Harvey SC. Hypnotics and sedatives: barbiturates. In: Gilman A, Rall TW, Goodman LS, et al, eds. *Goodman and Gilman's the pharmacological basis of therapeutics.* 8th ed. New York: Pergamon Press, 1990:358.

95. Jalling B, Boreus LO, Kallberg N, et al. Disappearance from the newborn of circulating prenatally administered phenobarbital. *Eur J Clin Pharmacol* 1973;6:234.

96. De Carolis MP, Romagnoli C, Frezza S, et al. Placental transfer of phenobarbital: what is new? *Dev Pharmacol Ther* 1992;19:19.

97. Dessens AB, Cohen-Kettenis PT, Mellenbergh GJ, et al. Association of prenatal Phenobarbital and phenytoin exposure with small head size at birth and with learning problems. *Acta Paediatr* 2000;89:533.

98. Shankaran S, Papile LA, Wright LL, et al. Neurodevelopmental outcome of premature infants after antenatal phenobarbital. *Amer J Obstet Gynecol* 2002;187:171.

99. Erkkola R, Kangas L, Pekkarinen A. The transfer of diazepam across the placenta during labour. *Acta Obstet Gynecol Scand* 1973;52:167.

100. Jauniaux E, Jurjovic D, Lees C, et al. In-vivo study of diazepam transfer across the first trimester human placenta. *Hum Reprod* 1996;11:8899.

101. Pan B, Lu Y, Wang D. Determination of diazepam concentration in maternal and fetal serum after intravenous administration during active phase of labor and its effects in neonates [Chinese]. *Chinese J Obstet Gynecol* 1995;30:707.

102. Athinarayanan P, Pierog SH, Nigam SK, et al. Chlordiazepoxide withdrawal in the neonate. *Am J Obstet Gynecol* 1976;124:212.

103. Rementeria JL, Bhatt K. Withdrawal symptoms in neonates from intrauterine exposure to diazepam. *J Pediatr* 1977;90:123.

104. Sutton LR, Hinderliter SA. Diazepam abuse in pregnant women on methadone maintenance. Implications for the neonate. *Clin Pediatr* 1990;29:108.

105. McElhatton PR. The effects of benzodiazepine use during pregancy and lactation. *Reprod Toxicol* 1994;8:461.

106. Kanjilal S, Pan NR, Chakraborty DP, et al. Cord blood diazepam: clinical effects in neonates of ecclamptic mothers. *Indian J Pediatr* 1993;60:257.

107. Czeizel AE, Szegal BA, Joffe JM, et al. The effect of diazepam and promethazine treatment during pregnancy on the somatic development of human offspring. *Neurotoxicol Teratol* 1999;21:157.

108. Liscano-Gil LA, Garcia-Cruz D, Sanchez-Corona J. Omphalocele-exstrophy-imperforate-anus-spina bifida (OEIS) complex in a male prenatally exposed to diazepam [Letter]. *Arch Med Res* 1995;26:95.

109. Jaiswal AK, Bhattacharya SK. Effect of gestational undernutrition and chlordiazepoxide treatment on black/white discrimination learning and retention in young rats. *Indian J Expl Biol* 1884; 32:184.

110. Margetts EL. Chloral delirium. *Psychiatry* 1950;24:278.

111. Opitz JM, Grosse FR, Heneberg B. Congenital effects of bromism. *Lancet* 1972;1:91.

112. Rossiter EJR, Rendle-Short TJ. Congenital effects of bromism. *Lancet* 1972;2:705.

113. Disse M, Joo F, Schulz H, et al. Prenatal exposure to sodium bromide affects the postnatal growth and brain development. *J Hirnforsch* 1996;37:127.

114. Garetz FD. Ethchlorvynol: addiction hazard. *Minn Med* 1969; 52:1131.

115. Magness JL. Ethchlorvynol intoxication and severe abstinence reaction. *Lancet* 1965;1:80.

116. Aycrigg JB. Two cases of withdrawal from ethchlorvynol. *Am J Psychiatry* 1964;120:1201.

117. Hudson HS, Walker HI. Withdrawal symptoms following ethchlorvynol dependence. *Am J Psychiatry* 1961;118:361.

118. Hume AS, Williams JM, Douglas BG. Disposition of ethchlorvynol in maternal blood, amniotic fluid and chorionic fluid. *J Reprod Med* 1971;6:229.

119. Rumack BH, Walravens PA. Neonatal withdrawal following maternal ingestion of ethchlorvynol (Placidyl). *Pediatrics* 1973;52:714.

120. Sadwin A, Glen RS. Addiction to glutethimide (Doriden). *Am J Psychiatry* 1958;115:469.

121. Kanter DM. The acute toxicity of Doriden overdosage. *Conn Med J* 1957;21:314.

122. Bay AJ, Katsas GG. Glutethimide poisoning: a report of four fatal cases. *N Engl J Med* 1957;257:97.

123. Pildes RS. Neonatal withdrawal symptoms associated with glutethimide (Doriden) addiction in the mother during pregnancy. *Clin Pediatr* 1977;16:424.

124. Eggermont E. The adverse influence of imipramine on the adaptation of the newborn infant to extrauterine life. *Acta Pediatr Belg* 1972;26:197.

125. Sothers J. Lithium toxicity in the newborn. *Br Med J* 1973;3:233.

126. Tunnessen W. Toxic effects of lithium in newborn infants. *J Pediatr* 1972;81:804.

127. Webster PAC. Withdrawal symptoms in neonates associated with maternal antidepressant therapy. *Lancet* 1973;2:318.

128. Wilbanks B. Toxic effects of lithium carbonate in a mother and newborn infant. *J Am Med Assoc* 1970;213:865.

129. Hill RM, Desmond MM, Kay JL. Extrapyramidal dysfunction in an infant of a schizophrenic mother. *J Pediatr* 1966;69:589.

130. Levy W, Wisniewski K. Chlorpromazine causing extrapyramidal dysfunction in newborn infant of psychotic mother. *NY State J Med* 1974;74:684.

131. Krug S. Cocaine abuse: historical epidemiologic and clinical perspectives for pediatricians. *Adv Pediatr* 1989;36:369.

132. Farrar HC, Kearns GL. Cocaine: clinical pharmacology and toxicology. *J Pediatr* 1989;115:665.

133. Udell B. Crack cocaine: crack vs. cocaine. In: *Special currents: cocaine babies.* Columbus, OH: Ross Laboratories, 1989:5.

134. Tarr JE, Macklin M. Cocaine. *Pediatr Clin North Am* 1987;34:319.

135. Woods JR, Plessinger MA, Clark KE. Effect of cocaine on uterine blood flow and fetal oxygenation. *J Am Med Assoc* 1987;257:957.

136. Moore TR, Sorg J, Miller L, et al. Hemodynamic effects of intravenous cocaine on the pregnant ewe and fetus. *Am J Obstet Gynecol* 1986;155:883.

137. Woods JR, Plessinger MA. Pregnancy increases cardiovascular toxicity to cocaine. *Am J Obstet Gynecol* 1990;162:529.

138. Cejtin HE, Parsons MT, Wilson L. Cocaine use and its effects on umbilical artery prostacyclin production. *Prostaglandins* 1990;40:249.

139. Richardson GA, Hamel SC, Goldschmidt L, et al. Growth of infants prenatally exposed to cocaine/crack: comparison of a prenatal care and a no prenatal care sampled. *Pediatrics* 1999;104:18.

140. Dudish SA, Hatsukami DK. Gender differences in crack users who are research volunteers. *Drug Alcohol Depend* 1996;42(1):55.

141. Lester BM, ElSohly M, Wright LL, et al. The Maternal Lifestyle Study: drug use by meconium toxicology and maternal self-report. *Pediatrics* 2001;107:2309.

142. Sison CG, Ostrea EM Jr, Reyes MP, et al. The resurgence of congenital syphilis: a cocaine-related problem. *J Pediatr* 1997; 130:289.

143. Rodriguez EM, Mofenson LM, Chang BH, et al. Association of maternal drug use during pregnancy with maternal HIV culture positivity and perinatal HIV transmission. *AIDS* 1997;10:273.

144. Berkowitz K, LaSala A. Risk factors associated with the increasing prevalence of pneumonia during pregnancy. *Am J Obstet Gynecol* 1990;163:981.

145. Church MW, Kaufmann RA, Keenan JA, et al. Effect of prenatal cocaine exposure. In: Watson R, ed. *Biochemistry and physiology of substance abuse.* vol. 3. Boca Raton, FL: CRC Press, 1990:179.

146. Chasnoff IJ, Burns WJ, Schnoll SH, et al. Cocaine use in pregnancy. *N Engl J Med* 1985;313:666.

147. Hadeed AJ, Siegel SR. Maternal cocaine use during pregnancy: effect on the newborn infant. *Pediatrics* 1989;84:205.

148. Meeker JE, Reynolds PC. Fetal and newborn death associated with maternal cocaine use. *J Anal Toxicol* 1990;14:379.

149. Carlan SJ, Stromquist C, Angel JL, et al. Cocaine and indomethacin: fetal anuria, neonatal edema, and gastrointestinal bleeding. *Obstet Gynecol* 1991;78:501.

150. Bingol N, Fuchs M, Diaz V, et al. Teratogenicity of cocaine in humans. *J Pediatr* 1987;110:93.

151. Chasnoff IJ, Burns KA, Burns WJ. Cocaine use in pregnancy: perinatal morbidity and mortality. *Neurotoxicol Teratol* 1987;9:291.

152. Addis A, Moretti ME, Ahmed Syed F, et al. Fetal effects of cocaine: an updated meta-analysis. *Reprod Toxicol* 2001;15:341.

153. Burkett G, Yasin SY, Palow D, et al. Patterns of cocaine binging: effect on pregnancy. *Am J Obstet Gynecol* 1994;171:372.

154. Chouteau M, Namerow PB, Leppert P. The effect of cocaine abuse on birth weight and gestational age. *Obstet Gynecol* 1988; 72:351.

155. Doberczak TM, Shanzer S, Senie RT, et al. Neonatal neurologic and electroencephalographic effects of intrauterine cocaine exposure. *J Pediatr* 1988;113:354.

156. Neerhof M, MacGregor S, Retzky S, et al. Cocaine abuse during pregnancy: peripartum prevalence and perinatal outcome. *Am J Obstet Gynecol* 1989;161:633.

157. Cerukuri R, Minkoff H, Feldman J, et al. A cohort study of alkaloidal cocaine ("crack") in pregnancy. *Obstet Gynecol* 1988;72:147.

158. Fulroth R, Phillips B, Durand D. Perinatal outcome of infants exposed to cocaine and or heroin in utero. *Am J Dis Child* 1989; 143:905.

159. Dombrowski MP, Wolfe HM, Welch RA, et al. Cocaine abuse is associated with abruptio placentae and decreased birth weight, but not shorter labor. *Obstet Gynecol* 1991;77:139.

160. Little B, Snell L, Klein V, et al. Cocaine abuse during pregnancy: maternal and fetal complications. *Obstet Gynecol* 1989;73:157.

161. Oro A, Dixon S. Perinatal cocaine and methamphetamine exposure: maternal and neonatal correlates. *J Pediatr* 1987;117:571.

162. Chasnoff I, Griffith D, MacGregor S, et al. Temporal patterns of cocaine use in pregnancy. *J Am Med Assoc* 1989;261:1741.

163. Leblar P, Parekh A, Naso B, et al. Effects of intrauterine exposure to alkaloidal cocaine (crack). *Am J Dis Child* 1987;141:937.

164. Zuckerman B, Frank D, Hingson R, et al. Effects of maternal marijuana and cocaine use on fetal growth. *N Engl J Med* 1989; 320:762.

165. Kliegman RM, Madura D, Kiwi R, et al. Relation of maternal cocaine use to the risks of prematurity and low birth weight. *J Pediatr* 1994;124:751.

166. Hume R Jr, O'Donnell K, Stanger C, et al. In utero cocaine exposure: observations of fetal behavioral state may predict neonatal outcome. *Am J Obstet Gynecol* 1989;161:685.

167. Ryan L, Ehrlich S, Finnegan L. Cocaine abuse in pregnancy: effects on the fetus and newborn. *Neurotoxicol Teratol* 1987;9:295.

168. Chouteau M, Namerow P, Leppert P. The effects of cocaine abuse on birth weight and gestational age. *Obstet Gynecol* 1988;72:351.

169. Anday E, Cohen M, Kelly N, et al. Effect of in utero cocaine exposure on startle and its modifications. *Dev Pharmacol Ther* 1989;12:137.

170. Bandstra ES, Morrow CE, Anthony JC, et al. Intrauterine growth of full-term infants: impact of prenatal cocaine exposure. *Pediatrics* 2001;108:1309–1319.

171. Bada HS, Das A, Bauer CR, et al. Gestational cocaine exposure and intrauterine growth: maternal lifestyle study. *Obstet Gynecol* 2002;100:916.

172. Datta-Bhutada S, Johnson HL, Rosen TS. Intrauterine cocaine and crack exposure:neonatal outcome. *J Perinatol* 1999;18:183.

173. Shiono PH, Klebanoff MA, Nugent RP, Cotch M, et al. The impact of cocaine and marijuana use on low birth weight and preterm birth: a multicenter study. *Am J Obstet Gynecol* 1995;172:19.

174. Mirochnick M, Frank DA, Cabral H, et al. Relation between meconium concentration of the cocaine metabolite benzoylecgonine and fetal growth. *J Pediatr* 1995;126:636.

175. Hulse GK, English DR, Milne E, et al. Maternal cocaine use and low birth weight newborns: a meta-analysis. *Addiction* 1997; 92:1561–1570.

176. Bateman DA, Chiriboga CA. Dose-response effect of cocaine on newborn head circumference. *Pediatrics* 2000;106:E33.

177. Jacobson JL, Jacobson SW, Sokol RJ. Effects of prenatal exposure to alcohol, smoking, and illicit drugs on postpartum somatic growth. *Alcohol Clin Exp Res* 1994;18:317.

178. Neuspiel DR, Markowitz M, Drucker E. Intrauterine cocaine, lead, and nicotine exposure and fetal growth. *Am J Public Health* 1994;84:1492.

179. Chasnoff I, Burns K, Burns W. Cocaine use in pregnancy: perinatal morbidity and mortality. *Neurotoxicol Teratol* 1987;9:291.

180. Chasnoff I, Chisum G, Kaplan W. Maternal cocaine use and genitourinary tract malformations. *Teratology* 1988;37:201.

181. Hoyme HE, Jones KL, Dixon SD, et al. Prenatal cocaine exposure and fetal vascular disruption. *Pediatrics* 1990;85:743.

182. Rosenstein BJ, Wheeler JS, Heid PL. Congenital renal abnormalities in infants with in utero cocaine exposure. *J Urol* 1990;144:110.

183. Behnke M, Eyler FD, Garvan CW, et al. The search for congenital malformations in newborns with fetal cocaine exposure. *Pediatrics* 2001;107:E74.

184. Little BB, Wilson GN, Jackson G. Is there a cocaine syndrome? Dysmorphic and anthropometric assessment of infants exposed to cocaine. *Teratol* 1996;54:145.

185. Bandstra E, Burkett G. Maternal–fetal and neonatal effects of in utero cocaine exposure. *Semin Perinatol* 1991;15:288.

186. Kramer LD, Locke GE, Qgunyemi A, et al. Neonatal cocaine-related seizures. *J Child Neurol* 1990;(Jan);5:60.

187. Beltran RS, Coker SB. Transient dystonia of infancy, a result of intrauterine cocaine exposure? *Pediatr Neurol* 1995;12:354.

188. Chiriboga CA, Vibbert M, Malouf R, et al. Neurological correlates of fetal cocaine exposure: transient hypertonia of infancy and early childhood. *Pediatrics* 1995;96:1070.

189. Chiriboga CA, Bateman DA, Brust JC, et al. Neurologic findings in neonates with intrauterine cocaine exposure. *Pediatr Neurol* 1993;9:115.

190. Tsay CH, Partridge JC, Villarreal SF, et al. Neurologic and ophthalmologic findings in children exposed to cocaine in utero. *J Child Neurol* 1996;11:25.

191. Doberczak TM, Shanzer S, Senie RT, et al. Neonatal neurologic and electroencephalographic effects of intrauterine cocaine exposure. *J Pediatr* 1988;113:354.

192. Lester BM, Tronick EZ, LaGasse L, et al. The maternal lifestyle study: effects of substance exposure during pregnancy on neurodevelopmental outcome in 1-month-old infants. *Pediatrics* 2002;110:1182.

193. Kasofsky BE. Cocaine-induced alterations in neurodevelopment. *Semin Speech Lang* 1998;19:102–121.

194. Eyler FD, Behnke M, Conlon M, et al. Birth outcome from a prospective, matched study of prenatal cocaine/crack use. II. Interactive and dose effects on neurobehavioral assessment. *Pediatrics* 1998;101:237.

195. Chiriboga CA, Vibbert M, Malouf R, et al. Neurological correlates of fetal cocaine exposure: transient hypertonia of infancy and early childhood. *Pediatrics* 1995;96:1070.

196. Singer LT, Arendt R, Minnes S, et al. Neurobehavioral outcomes of cocaine-exposed infants. *Neurotoxicol Teratol* 2000;22:653.

197. Corwin MJ, Lester BM, Sepkoski C, et al. Effects of in utero cocaine exposure on newborn acoustical cry characteristics. *Pediatrics* 1992;89:1199.

198. Chasnoff IJ, Hunt CE, Kletter R, et al. Prenatal cocaine exposure is associated with respiratory pattern abnormalities. *Am J Dis Child* 1989;143:583.

199. Gingras JL, Feibel JB, Dalley LB, et al. Maternal polydrug use including cocaine and postnatal infant sleep architecture: preliminary observations and implications for respiratory control and behavior. *Early Hum Dev* 1995;43:197.

200. Karmel BZ, Gardner JM. Prenatal cocaine exposure effects on arousal-modulated attention during the neonatal period. *Dev Psychobiol* 1996;29:463.

201. Salamy A, Eldredge L. Risk for ABR abnormalities in the nursery. *Electroencephalogr Clin Neurophysiol* 1994;92:392.

202. Shih L, Cone-Wesson B, Reddix B. Effects of maternal cocaine abuse on the neonatal auditory system. *Int J Pediatr Otorhinolaryngol* 1988;15:245.

203. Lester BM, Lagasse L, Seifer R, et al. The Maternal Lifestyle Study (MLS): effects of prenatal cocaine and/or opiate exposure on auditory brain response at one month. *J Pediatr* 142:279

204. Tan-Laxa MA, Sison-Switala C, Rintelman W, et al. Abnormal auditory brainstem response among infants with prenatal cocaine exposure. *Pediatrics* 2003; (In press).

205. Potter SM, Zelazo PR, Stack DM, et al. Adverse effects of fetal cocaine exposure on neonatal auditory information processing. *Pediatrics* 2000;105:E40.

206. McLenan DA, Ajayi PA, Rydmn RJ, et al. Evaluation of the relationship between cocaine and intraventricular hemorrhage. *J Natl Med Assoc* 1994;86:281.

207. Dogra VS, Shyken JM, Menon PA, et al. Neurosonographic abnormalities associated with maternal history of cocaine use in neonates of appropriate size for their gestational age. *AJNR Am J Neuroradiol* 1994;15:697.

208. Singer LT, Yamashita TS, Hawkins S, et al. Increased incidence of intraventricular hemorrhage and developmental delay in cocaine-exposed, very low birth weight infants. *J Pediatr* 1994;124:765.

209. Frank DA, McCArten KM, Robson CD, et al. Level of in utero cocaine exposure and neonatal ultrasound findings. *Pediatrics* 1999;104:1101.

210. Smith LM, Qureshi N, Renslo R, et al. Prenatal cocaine exposure and cranial sonographic findings in preterm infants. *J Clin Ultrasound* 2001;29:72.

211. King TA, Perlman JM, Laptook AR, et al. Neurologic manifestation of in utero cocaine exposure in near-term and term infants. *Pediatrics* 1995;96:259.

212. Konkol RJ, Tikofsky RS, Wells R, et al. Normal high-resolution cerebral 99mTc-HMPAO SPECT scans in symptomatic neonates exposed to cocaine. *J Child Neurol* 1994;9:278.

213. Kankirawatana P, Tennison MB, D'Cruz O, et al. Mobius syndrome in infant exposed to cocaine in utero. *Pediatr Neurol* 1993; 9:71.

214. van de Bor M, Walther FJ, Sims ME. Increased cerebral blood flow velocity in infants of mothers who abuse cocaine. *Pediatrics* 1990;85:733.

215. Mehta SK, Super DM, Connuck D, et al. Autonomic alterations in cocaine-exposed infants. *Am Heart J* 2002;144:1109.

216. Garde S, Regalado MG, Schechtman VL, et al. Nonlinear dynamics of heart rate variability in cocaine-exposed neonates during sleep. *Am J Physiol Heart Circ Physiol* 2001;280:H2920.

217. Regalado MG, Schechtman VL, Del Angel AP, et al. Cardiac and respiratory patterns during sleep in cocaine-exposed neonates. *Early Hum Dev* 1996;44:187.

218. Bard KA, Coles CD, Platzman KA, et al. The effects of prenatal drug exposure, term status and caregiving on arousal and arousal modulation in 8-week-old infants. *Dev Psychobiol* 2000; 36:194.

219. Silvestri JM, Long JM, Weese-Mayer DE, et al. Effect of prenatal cocaine on respiration, heart rate, and sudden infant death syndrome. *Pediatr Pulmonol* 1991;11:328.

220. Horn PT. Persistent hypertension after prenatal cocaine exposure. *J Pediatr* 1992;121:288.

221. Mehta SK, Finkelhor RS, Anderson RL, et al. Transient myocardial ischemia in infants prenatally exposed to cocaine. *J Pediatr* 1993;122:945.

222. Regalado MG, Schechtman VL, Khoo MC, et al. Spectral analysis of heart rate variability and respiration during sleep in cocaine-exposed neonates. *Clin Physiol* 2001;21:428.

223. Frassica JJ, Orav EJ, Walsh EP, et al. Arrhythmias in children prenatally exposed to cocaine. *Arch Pediatr Adolesc Med* 1994;148:1163.

224. St-John WM. Maternal cocaine alters eupneic ventilation but not gasping of neonatal rats. *Neurosci Lett* 1998;246:137.

225. Hand IL, Noble L, McVeigh TJ, et al. The effects of intrauterine cocaine exposure on the respiratory status of the very low birth weight infants. *J Perinatol* 2001;21:372.

226. Roby PV, Glenn CM, Watkins SL, et al. Association of elevated umbilical cord blood creatine kinase and myoglobin levels with the presence of cocaine metabolites in maternal urine. *Am J Perinatol* 1996;13:453.

227. Wennberg RP, Yin J, Miller M, Maynard A. Fetal cocaine exposure and neonatal bilirubinemia. *J Pediatr* 1994;125:613.

228. Lopez SL, Taeusch HW, Findlay RD, et al. Time of onset of necrotizing enterocolitis in newborn infants with known prenatal cocaine exposure. *Clin Pediatr* 1995;34:424.

229. The TG, Young M, Rosser S. In-utero cocaine exposure and neonatal intestinal perforation: a case report. *J Natl Med Assoc* 1995; 87:889.

230. Silva-Araujo A, Tavares MA. Development of the eye after gestational exposure to cocaine. Vascular disruption in the retina of rats and humans. *Ann N Y Acad Sci* 1996;31;801:274.

231. Silva-Araujo A, Tavares MA, Patacao MH, et al. Retinal hemorrhages associated with in utero exposure to cocaine. Experimental and clinical findings. *Retina* 1996;16:411.

232. Isenberg SJ, Spierer A, Inkelis SH. Ocular signs of cocaine intoxication in neonates. *Am J Ophthalmol* 1987;15;103:211.

233. Held JR, Riggs ML, Dorman C. The effect of prenatal cocaine exposure on neurobehavioral outcome: a meta-analysis. *Neurotoxicol Teratol* 1999;21:619.

234. Delaney-Black V, Covington C, Ostrea E Jr, et al. Prenatal cocaine and neonatal outcome: evaluation of dose-response relationship. *Pediatrics* 1996; 98:735.

235. Morrow CE, Bandstra ES, Anthony JC, et al. Influence of prenatal cocaine exposure on full-term infant neurobehavioral functioning. *Neurotoxicol Teratol* 2001;23:533.

236. Eyler Fd, Behnke M, Garvan CW, et al. Newborn evaluation of toxicity and withdrawal related to prenatal cocaine exposure. *Neurotoxicol Teratol* 2001;23:399.

237. Mayes LC, Granger RH, Frank MA, et al. Neurobehavioral profiles of neonates exposed to cocaine prenatally. *Pediatrics* 1993;91:778.

238. Eisen LN, Field TM, Bandstra ES, et al. Perinatal cocaine effects on neonatal stress behavior and performance on the Brazelton Scale. *Pediatrics* 1991;88:477.

239. Scafidi FA, Field TM, Wheeden A, et al. Cocaine-exposed preterm neonates show behavioral and hormonal differences. *Pediatrics* 1996;97:851.

240. Mirochnick M, Meyer J, Cole J, et al. Circulating catecholamine concentrations in cocaine-exposed neonates: a pilot study. *Pediatrics* 1991;88:481.

241. Anday E, Cohen M, Kelly N, et al. Effect of in utero cocaine exposure on startle and its modificaions. *Dev Pharmacol Ther* 1989; 12:137.

242. Lester BM, Corwin MJ, Sepkoski C, et al. Neurobehavioral syndromes in cocaine-exposed newborn infants. *Child Dev* 1991;62:694.

243. Chiu TT, Vaughn AJ, Carzoli RP. Hospital costs for cocaine-exposed infants. *J Fla Med Assoc* 1990;77:897.

244. Joyce T, Racine AD, McCalla S, et al. The impact of prenatal exposure to cocaine on newborn costs and length of stay. *Health Serv Res* 1995;30:341.

245. Phibbs CS, Bateman DA, Schwartz RM. The neonatal costs of maternal cocaine use. *J Am Med Assoc* 1991;266:1521.

246. Calhoun BC, Watson PT. The cost of maternal cocaine abuse: I. Perinatal costs. *Obstet Gynecol* 1991;78:731.

247. Ostrea EM Jr, Lizardo E, Tanafranca M. The prevalence of illicit drug exposure in infants in the NICU as determined by meconium drug screen: its medical and economic impact. *Pediatr Res* 1992;31:215A.

248. Behnke M, Eyler FD, Conlon M, et al. How fetal cocaine exposure increases neonatal hospital costs. *Pediatrics* 1997;99:204.

249. Nair P, Rothblum S, Hebel R. Neonatal outcome in infants with evidence of fetal exposure to opiates, cocaine and cannabinoids. *Clin Pediatr (Phila)* 1994;33:280.

250. Hurt H, Brodsky NL, Betancourt L, et al. Cocaine-exposed children: follow-up through 30 months. *J Dev Behav Pediatr* 1995; 16:29–35.

251. Fetters L, Tronick EZ. Neuromotor development of cocaine-exposed and control infants from birth through 15 months: poor and poorer performance. *Pediatrics* 1996;98:938.

252. Hurt H, Brodsky NL, Braitman LE, et al. Natal status of infants of cocaine users and control subjects: a prospective comparison. *J Perinatol* 1995;15:297.

253. Azuma SD, Chasnoff IJ. Outcome of children prenatally exposed to cocaine and other drugs: a path analysis of three-year data. *Pediatrics* 1993;92:396.

254. Jacobson SW, Jacobson JL, Sokol RJ. Effects of fetal alcohol exposure on infant reaction time. *Alcohol Clin Exp Res* 1994;18:1125.

255. Hawley TL, Halle TG, Drasin RE, et al. Children of addicted mothers: effects of the 'crack epidemic' on the caregiving environment and the development of preschoolers. *Am J Orthopsychiatry* 1995;(Jul);65:364.

256. Nulman I, Rovet J, Altmann D, et al. Neurodevelopment of adopted children exposed in utero to cocaine. *Can Med Assoc J* 1994;151:1591.

257. Griffith DR, Azuma SD, Chasnoff IJ. Three-year outcome of children exposed prenatally to drugs. *J Am Acad Child Psychiatry* 1994;33:20.

258. Rosenberg NM, Meert KL, Marino D, et al. Occult cocaine and opiate exposure in children and associated physical findings. *Pediatr Emerg Care* 1995;11:167.

259. Block SS, Moore BD, Scharre JE. Visual anomalies in young children exposed to cocaine. *Optom Vis Sci* 1997;74:28.

260. Belcher HM, Shapiro BK, Leppert M, et al. Sequential neuromotor examination in children with intrauterine cocaine/polydrug exposure. *Dev Med Child Neurol* 1999;41:240–246.

261. van Baar A. Development of infants of drug dependent mothers. *J Child Psychol Psychiatry* 1990;31:911.

262. Mentis M, Lundgren K. Effects of prenatalexposure to cocaine and associated risk factors on language development. *J Speech Hear Res* 1995;1303.

263. Bender SL, Word CO, DiClemente RJ, et al. The developmental implications of prenatal and/or postnatal crack cocaine exposure in preschool children: a preliminary report. *J Dev Behav Pediatr* 1995;16:418.

264. Angelilli ML, Fischer H, Delaney-Black V, et al. History of in utero cocaine exposure in language-delayed children. *Clin Pediatr* 1994;33:514.

265. Jacobson SW, Jacobson JL, Sokol RJ, et al. New evidence for neurobehavioral effects of in utero cocaine exposure. *J Pediatr* 1996;129:581.

266. Jacobsen SW. Specificity of neurobehavioral outcomes associated with prenatal alcohol exposure. *Alcohol Clin Exp Res* 1998;22: 313–320.

267. Alessandri SM, Bendersky M, Lewis M. Cognitive functioning in 8- to 18-month-old drug-exposed infants. *Dev Psychol* 1998; 34:565.

268. Morrow CE, Bandstra ES, Anthony JC, et al. Influence of prenatal cocaine exposure on full-term infant neurobehavioral functioning. *Neurotoxicol Teratol* 2001;23:533.

269. Singer LT, Arendt R, Minnes S, et al. Developing language skills of cocaine-exposed infants. *Pediatrics* 2001;107:1057.

270. Thyssen Van Beveren T, Little BB, Spence MJ. Effects of prenatal cocaine exposure and postnatal environment on child development. *Am J Human Biol* 2000;12:417.

271. Heffelfinger AK, Craft S, White DA, et al. Visual attention in preschool children prenatally exposed to cocaine:Implications for behavioral regulation. *J Int Neuropsychol Soc* 2002;8:12.

272. Struthers JM, Hansen RL. Visual recognition memory in drug-exposed infants. *J Dev Behav Pediatr* 1992;13:108.

273. Bandstra ES, Morrow CE, Anthony JC, et al. Longitudinal investigation of task persistence and sustained attention in children with prenatal cocaine exposure. *Neurotoxicol Teratol* 2001;23:545.

274. Delaney-Black V, Covington C, Templin T, et al. Expressive language development of children exposed to cocaine prenatally: literature review and a report of a prospective cohort study. *J Comun Disord* 2000;33:463.

275. Kasofsky BE. Cocaine-induced alterations in neuro-development. *Semin Speech Lang* 1998;19:102.

276. Hurt H, Brodsky NL, Betancourt L, et al. Play behavior in toddlers with in utero cocaine exposure: a prospective, masked, controlled study. *J Dev Behav Pediatr* 1996;17:373.

277. Rodning C, Beckwith L, Howards J. Characteristics of attachment organization and play organization in prenatally drug exposed toddlers. *Dev Psychopathol* 1990;1:277.

278. Singer LT, Hawkins S, Huang J, et al. Developmental outcomes and environmental correlates of very low birthweight, cocaine-exposed infants. *Early Hum Dev* 2001;64:91.

279. Hurt H, Malmud E, Betancourt LM, et al. A prospective comparison of developmental outcome of children with in utero cocaines exposure and controls using the Battelle Developmental Inventory. *J Dev Behav Pediatr* 2001;22:27.

280. Frank DA, Jacobs RR, Beeghly M, et al. Level of prenatal cocaine exposure and scores on the Bayley Scales of Infant Development: modifying effects of caregiver, early intervention and birth weight. *Pediatrics* 2002;110:1143.

281. Howard J, Beckwith L, Espinosa M, et al. Development of infants born to cocaine-abusing women: biologic/maternal influences. *Neurotoxicol Teratol* 1995;17:403–411.

282. Accornero VH, Morrow CE, Bandstra ES, et al. Behavioral outcome of preschoolers exposed prenatally to cocaine: role of maternal behavioral health. *J Pediatr Psychol* 2002;27:259.

283. Hurt H, Malmud E, Betancourt L, et al. Children with in utero cocaine exposure do not differ from control subjects on intelligence testing. *Arch Pediatr Adolesc Med* 1997;151:1237.

284. Frank DA, Augustyn M, Knight WG, et al. Growth, development, and behavior in early childhood following prenatal cocaine exposure: a systematic review. *JAMA* 2001;285:1613.

285. Fares I, McCulloch KM, Raju TN. Intrauterine cocaine exposure and the risk for sudden infant death syndrome: a meta-analysis. *J Perinatol* 1997;17:179.

286. Ostrea EM Jr, Ostrea AR, Simpson PM. Mortality within the first 2 years in infants exposed to cocaine, opiate, or cannabinoid during gestation. *Pediatrics* 1997;100:79.

287. Kharasch SJ, Glotzer D, Vinci R, et al. Unsuspected cocaine exposure in young children. *Am J Dis Child* 1991;145:204.

288. Smith FP, Kidwell DA. Cocaine in hair, saliva, skin swabs, and urine of cocaine users' children. *Forensic Sci Int* 1996;83;179.

289. Lustbader AS, Nayes LC, McGee BA, et al. Incidence of passive exposure to crack/cocaines and clinical findings in infants seen in an outpatient service. *Pediatrics* 1998;102:e5.

290. Bateman DA, Heagarty MC. Passive freebase cocaine ('crack') inhalation by infants and toddlers. *Amer J Dis Child* 1989; 143:25.

291. Riggs D, Weibley RE. Acute hemorrhagic diarrhea and cardiovascular collapse in a young child owing to environmentally acquired cocaine. *Pediatr Emerg Care* 1991;7:154.

292. Ernst AA, Sanders WM. Unexpected cocaine intoxication presenting as seizures in children. *Ann Emerg Med* 1989;18:774.

293. Mirchandani HG, Mirchandani IH, Hellman F, et al. Passive inhalation of free-base cocaine ('crack') smoke by infants. *Arch Path Lab Med* 1991;115:494.

294. Mott SH, Packer RJ, Soldin SJ. Neurologic manifestations of cocaine exposure in childhood. *Pediatrics* 1994:557.

295. Jones KL, Smith DW. Recognition of the fetal alcohol syndrome in early infancy. *Lancet* 1973;2:999.

296. Jones KL, Smith DW, Ulleland CN, et al. Pattern of malformation in offspring of chronic alcoholic mothers. *Lancet* 1973; 1:1267.

297. Christiaens L, Mizon JP, Delmarie G. Sur la descendance des alcooliques (On the offspring of alcoholics). *Ann Pediatr* 1960;36:37.

298. Heuyer H, Mises R, Dereux JF. La descendance les alcooliques (The offspring of alcoholics). *Nouvelle Press Medicale (Paris)* 1957;29:657.

299. Abel EL. *Fetal alcohol syndrome.* Oradell, NJ: Med Econ Company, 1990.

300. Pietrantoni M, Knuppel RA. Alcohol in pregnancy. *Clin Perinatol* 1991;18:93.

301. Day NL, Richardson GA. Prenatal alcohol exposure: a continuum of effects. *Semin Perinatol* 1991;15:271.

302. Hankin Jr, Fetal alcohol syndrome prevention research. *Alcohol Res Health* 2002;26:58–65.

303. Cornelius MD, Lebow HA, Day NL. Attitudes and knowledge about drinking: relationships with drinking behavior among pregnant teenagers. *J Drug Educ* 1997;27:231.

304. Abel EL, Kruger ML, Friedl J. How do physicians define "light", "moderate" and "heavy" drinking? *Alcohol Clin Exp Res* 1998; 22:979.

305. Day NL, Cottreau CM, Richardson GA. The epidemiology of alcohol, marijuana and cocaine use among women of childbearing age and pregnant women. *Clin Obstet Gynecol* 1993;36:232.

306. Floyd RL, Decoufle P, Hungerford DW. Alcohol use prior to pregnancy recognition. *Am J Prev Med* 1999;17:101.

307. Mile DR, Svikis DS, Kulstad, et al. Psychopathology in pregnant drug-dependent women with or without comorbid alcohol dependence. *Alcohol Clin Exp Res* 2001;25:1012.

308. Cornelius MD, Day NL, Cornelius JR, et al. Drinking patterns and correlates of drinking among pregnant teenagers. *Alcohol Clin Exp Res* 1993;17:290.

309. Cornelius MD, Richardson GA, Day NL, et al. A comparison of prenatal drinking in two recent samples of adolescents and adults. *J Study Alcohol* 1994;55:412.

310. Gladstone J, Levy M, Nulman I, et al. Characteristics of pregnant women who engae in binge alcohol consumption. *CMAJ* 1997; 156:789.

311. Eckardt MJ, File SE, Gessa GL, et al. Effects of moderate alcohol consumption on the central nervous system. *Alcohol Clin Ex Res* 1998;2:998.

312. Polygenis D, Wharton S, Malmberg C, et al. Moderate alcohol consumption during pregnancy and the incidence of fetal malformations: a meta-analysis. *Neurotoxicol Teratol* 1998;20:61.

313. Yang Q, Withiewicz BB, Olney RS, et al. A case-control study of maternal alcohol consumption and intrauterine growth retardation. *Ann Epidemiol* 2001;11:497.

314. Olsen J. Effects of moderate alcohol consumption during pregnancy on child development at 18 and 42 months. *Alcohol Clin Exp Res* 1994;18:1109.

315. Larroque B, Kaminski M. Prenatal alcohol exposure and development at preschool age: main results of a French study. *Alcohol Clin Exp Res* 1998;22:295.

316. Hard ML, Einarson TR, Koren G. The role of acetaldehyde in pregnancy outcome after prenatal exposure. *Ther Drug Monit* 2001;23:427.

317. Stoler JM, Huntington KS, Peterson CM, et al. The prenatal detection of significant alcohol exposure with maternal blood markers. *J Pediatr* 1998;133:346.

318. Brien JF, Loomis CW, Trammer J, et al. Disposition of ethanol in human maternal venous blood and amniotic fluid. *Am J Obstet Gynecol* 1983;181.

319. Day NL, Richardson GA, Geva D, et al. Alcohol, marijuana and tobacco: effects of prenatal exposure on offspring growth and morphology at age six. *Alcohol Clin Exp Res* 1994;18: 786.

320. Brien J, Clark D, Smith G, et al. Disposition of acute, multiple-dose ethanol in the near-term pregnant ewe. *Am J Obstet Gynecol* 1987;157:204.

321. Halmesmaki, E, Roine R, Salaspuro N. Gamma-glutamyltransferase, aspartate and alanine aminotransferase and their ratio, mean cell volume and urinal dolichol in pregnant alcohol abuser. *Br J Obstet Gynaecol* 1992;99:287.

322. Sarkola T, Ericksson CJ, Niemala O,et al. Mean cell volume and gamma-glutamyl transferase are superior to carbohydrate-deficient transferring and hemoglobin-acataldehyde adducts in the follow-up of pregnant women with alcohol abuse. *Acta Obstet Gynecol Scand* 200;79:359.

323. Stoler JM, Huntington KS, Peterson CM, et al. The prenatal detection of significant alcohol exposure with maternal blood markers. *J Pediatr* 1998;133:346.

324. Reyes E, Ott S. Effects of buthionine sulfoximine on the outcome of the in utero adminstration of alcohol on fetal development. *Alcohol Clin Exp Res* 1996;207:1243.

325. Mac E, Pacis M, Garcia G, et al. A marker of fetal exposure to alcohol by meconium analysis. *Pediatr Res* 1994;35:238A.

326. Klein, J, Karaskov T, Korent G. Fatty acid ethyl esters: a novel biologic marker for heavy in utero ethanol exposure: a case report. *Ther Drug Monit* 1999;21:644.

327. Bearer CF, Lee S, Salvator AE, et al. Ethyl linoleate in meconium: a biomarker for prenatal ethanol exposure. *Alcohol Clin Exp Res* 1999;3:487.

328. Kan J, Hernandez J, Leonardo G, et al. Fatty acid ethyl esters (FAEE) in meconium: potential biomarker of fetal exposure to alcohol. *Pediatr Res* 2002;50:140A.

329. Fisher ES. Selective fetal malnutrition: the fetal alcohol syndrome. *J Am Coll Nutr* 1988;7:101.

330. Vuorela P, Sarkola T, Alfthan H, et al. Hepatocyte growth factor, epidermal growth factor, and placental growth factor concentrations in peripheral blood of pregnant women with alcohol abuse. *Alcohol Clin Exp Res* 2002;26:682–687.

331. Weston WM, Greene RM, Uberti M, et al. Ethanol effects on embryonic craniofacial growth & development: implications for study of the fetal alcohol syndrome. *Alcohol Clin Exp Res* 1994; 18:177.

332. Ylikorkala O, Halmesmaki E, Viinikka L. Effect of ethanol on thromboxane and prostacyclin synthesis by fetal platelets and umbilical artery. *Life Sci* 1987;41:371.

333. Randall CL, Saulnier JL. Effect of ethanol on prostacyclin, thromboxane, and prostaglandin E production in human umbilical veins. *Alcohol Clin Exp Res* 1995;19:741.

334. Karl PI, Harvey B, Fisher SE. Ethanol and mitotic inhibitors promote differentiation of trophoblastic cells. *Alcohol Clin Exp Res* 1996;20:1269.

335. Sokol RJ, Miller SI, Reed G. Alcohol abuse during pregnancy: an epidemiologic study. *Alcohol Clin Exp Res* 1980;4:135.

336. Kesmodel U, Wisborg K, Olsen SF, et al. Moderate alcohol intake during pregnancy and the risk of stillbirth and death during the first year of life. *Am J Epidemiol* 2002;15;155:305.

337. Plant M. *Women, drinking and pregnancy.* London: Tavistock Publications, 1985.

338. Clarren SK. Fetal alcohol syndrome: a new primate model for binge drinking and its relevance to human ethanol teratogenesis. *J Pediatr* 1982;101:819.

339. Scott WJ, Fradkin R. The effects of prenatal ethanol in cynomolgus monkeys Macaca fascicularis. *Teratology* 1984;29:49.

340. Altshuler HL, Shippenberg TS. A subhuman primate model for fetal alcohol syndrome research. *Neurotoxicol Teratol* 1981;3:121.

341. Abel EL. Maternal alcohol consumption and spontaneous abortion. *Alcohol Alcohol* ____;32:211.

342. Kline J, Shrout P, Stein Z, et al. Drinking during pregnancy and spontaneous abortion. *Lancet* 1980;2:176.

343. Machemer L, Lorke D. Experiences with the dominant lethal test in female mice: effects of alkylating agents and artificial sweeteners on pre-ovulatory oocyte stages. *Mutat Res* 1975;29:209.

344. Koike M. Cytogenetic effects of maternal alcohol uptake on F1 mouse fetuses. *Japanese J Hyg* 1985;40:575.

345. Kaufman MH. Ethanol-induced chromosomal abnormalities at conception. *Nature* 1983;302:258.

346. Kaufman MH. The teratogenic effects of alcohol following exposure during pregnancy, and its influence on the chromosome constitution of the pre-ovulatory egg. *Alcohol* 1997;32:113.

347. Washington WJ, Cain KT, Cacheiro NLA, et al. Ethanol-induced late fetal death in mice exposed around the time of fertilization. *Mutat Res* 1985;147:205.

348. Marbury MC, Linn S, Monson RP, et al. The association of alcohol consumption with outcome of pregnancy. *Am J Public Health* 1983;73:1165.

349. Prager K, Malin H, Graves C, et al. Maternal smoking and drinking behavior before and during pregnancy. In: *Health and prevention profile*. Hyattsville, MD: US Department of Health and Human Services, National Center for Health Statistics, 1983:19.

350. National Institute on Alcohol Abuse and Alcoholism. *Program strategies for preventing fetal alcohol syndrome and alcohol-related birth defects*. Washington: US Department of Health and Human Services, Public Health Service, Alcohol, Drug Abuse, and Mental Health Administration, 1986.

351. Randall CL, Taylor WJ, Walker DW. Ethanol-induced malformations in mice. *Alcohol Clin Exp Res* 1977;1:219.

352. Halliday HC, MacReid M, MacClure G. Results of heavy drinking in pregnancy. *Br J Obstet Gynaecol* 1982;89:892.

353. Staisey N, Fried P. Relationships between moderate maternal alcohol consumption during pregnancy and infant neurological development. *J Stud Alcohol* 1983;44:262.

354. Halmesmaki E, Valimaki M, Karonen S. Low somatomedin C and high growth hormone levels in newborns damaged by maternal alcohol abuse. *Obstet Gynecol* 1989;74:366.

355. Savoy-Moore RT, Dombrowski MP, Cheng A, et al. Low dose alcohol contracts the human umbilical artery in vitro. *Alcohol Clin Exp Res* 1989;13:40.

356. Silva PD, Miller KD, Madden J, et al. Abnormal fetal heart rate pattern associated with severe intrapartum maternal ethanol intoxication. A case report. *J Reprod Med* 1987;32:144.

357. Akay M, Mulder EJ. Investigating the effect of maternal alcohol intake on human fetal breathing rate using adaptive time-frequency analysis methods. *Early Hum Dev* 1996;46:153.

358. Mulder EJ, Morssink LP, van der Schee T, et al. Acute maternal alcohol consumption disrupts behavioral state organization in the near-term fetus. *Pediatr Res* 1998;44:774–779.

359. McLeod WJ, Brien C, Loomis L, et al. Effect of maternal ingestion on fetal breathing movements, gross body movements and heart rate at 37 to 40 weeks gestational age. *Am J Obstet Gynecol* 1983;145:251.

360. Druse MJ, Hoffeig JH. The effect of chronic maternal alcohol consumption on the development of the central nervous system myelin subfractions in rat offspring. *Drug Alcohol Depend* 1977;2:421.

361. Hoff S. Synaptogenesis in the hippocampal dentae gyrus: effects of in utero ethanol exposure. *Brain Res Bull* 1988;21:47.

362. Kennedy LA. The pathogenesis of brain abnormalities in the fetal alcohol syndrome: an intergrading hypothesis. *Teratology* 1984;29:263.

363. Shoemaker WJ, Baetge G, Azad R, et al. Effects of prenatal alcohol exposure on amine and peptide neurotransmitter systems. *Monogr Neural Sci* 1983;9:130.

364. Dehaene PH, Crepin G, Delahousse G, et al. Aspects epidemiologiques du syndrome d'alcoolisme foetal: 45 observations en 3 ans (Epidemiological aspects of the foetal alcoholism syndrome: 45 cases). *Nouvelle Press Medicale* 1981;10:2639.

365. Kimura KA, Parr AM, Brien JF. Effect of chronic maternal ethanol administration on nitric oxide synthase activity in the hippocampus of the mature fetal guinea pig. *Alcohol Clin Exp Res* 1996;20:948.

366. Ollegard R, Sabel K, Aronsson M, et al. Effects on the child of alcohol abuse during pregnancy: retrospective and prospective studies. *Acta Paediatr Scand* 1979;275:112.

367. Dehaene PH, Samaille-Villette CH, Samaille P, et al. Le syndrome d'alcoolisme foetal dans le nord de la France (The fetal alcohol syndrome in the north of France). *Revue de l'Alcoolisme (Paris)* 1977;23:145.

368. Ouellette EM, Rosett HL, Rosman NP, et al. Adverse effects on offspring of maternal alcohol abuse during pregnancy. *N Engl J Med* 1977;297:528.

369. Jesse DE, Alligood MR. Holistic Obstetrical Problem Evaluation (HOPE): testing a theory to predict birth outcomes in a group of women from Appalachia. *Health Care Women Int* 2002;23: 587–599.

370. Kesmodel U, Olsen SF, Secher NJ. Does alcohol increase the risk of preterm delivery? *Epidemiology* 2000;12:512–518.

371. Sood B, Delaney-Black V, Covington C, et al. Prenatal alcohol exposure and cildhood behavior at age 6 to 7 years: I. dose-response effect. *Pediatrics* 2001;108:E34.

372. Wilsnack SC, Klassen AD, Wilsnack RW. Drinking and reproductive dysfunction among women in a 1981 national survey. *Alcohol Clin Exp Res* 1984;8:451.

373. Backstrand JR, Allen LH, Martinez E, et al. Maternal consumption of pulque, a traditional Mexican alcoholic beverage: relationship to infant growth and development. *Public Health Nutr* 2001;4:882–891.

374. Day NL, Jasperse D, Richardson G, et al. Prenatal exposure to alcohol: effect on infant growth and morphologic characteristics. *Pediatrics* 1989;84:536.

375. Smith IE, Coles CD, Lancaster J, et al. The effect of volume and duration of prenatal ethanol exposure on neonatal physical and behavioral development. *Neurotoxicol Teratol* 1986;8:375.

376. Coles CD, Platzman KA, Rashkind-Hood Cl, et al. A comparison of children affected by prenatal alcohol exposure and attention deficit, hyperactivity disorder. *Alcohol Clin Exp Res* 1997;21:150.

377. Konovalov HV, Kovetsky NS, Bobryshev YV, et al. Disorders in brain development in the progeny of mothers who use alcohol during pregnancy. *Early Hum Dev* 48(1–2):153.

378. Holzman C, Paneth N, Little R, et al. Perinatal brain injury in premature infants born to mothers using alcohol in pregnancy. Neonatal Brain Hemorrhage Study Team. *Pediatrics* 1995; 95:66.

379. Maier SE, Chen WJ, Miller JA, et al. Fetal alcohol exposure and temporal vulnerability regional differences in alcohol-induced microencephaly as a function of binge-like alcohol exposure during rat brain development. *Alcohol Clin Exp Res* 1997; 21:1418.

380. Coles CD, Smith I, Fernhoff PM, et al. Neonatal neurobehavioral characteristics as correlates of maternal alcohol use during gestation. *Alcohol Clin Exp Res* 1985;9:454.

381. Ernhart CB, Wolf AW, Linn PL, et al. Alcohol-related birth defects: syndromal anomalies, intrauterine growth retardation, and neonatal behavioral assessment. *Alcohol Clin Exp Res* 1985; 9:447.

382. Anderson RC, Anderson KE. The effects of alcohol consumption during pregnancy. *AAOHN Journal* 1986;34:88.

383. Sokol RJ, Miller SI, Debanne S, et al. The Cleveland NIAAA prospective alcohol in-pregnancy study: the first year. *Neurotoxicol Teratol* 1981;3:203.

384. Hanson J, Streissguth AP, Smith D. The effects of moderate alcohol consumption during pregnancy on fetal growth and morphogenesis. *J Pediatr* 1978;92:457.

385. Russell M. Clinical implications of recent research on the fetal alcohol syndrome. *Bull NY Acad Med* 1991;67:207.

386. Kaminski M, Rumeau C, Schwartz D. Alcohol consumption in pregnant women and the outcome of pregnancy. *Alcohol Clin Exp Res* 1978;2:155.

387. Tennes K, Blackard C. Maternal alcohol consumption, birth weight and minor physical anomalies. *Am J Obstet Gynecol* 1980;138:774.

388. Hingson R, Alpert J, Day NL, et al. Effects of maternal drinking and marijuana use on fetal growth and development. *Pediatrics* 1982;70:539.

389. Mills JL, Graubard BI. Is moderate drinking during pregnancy associated with an increased rate of malformations? *Pediatrics* 1987;80:309.

390. Robe LB, Gromisch DS, Iosub S. Symptoms of neonatal ethanol withdrawal. *Curr Alcohol* 1981;8:485.

391. Coles CD, Smith I, Fernhoff PM, et al. Neonatal ethanol withdrawal: characteristics in clinically normal, nondysmorphic neonates. *J Pediatr* 1984;105:445.

392. Streissguth A, Barr H, Martin D. Maternal alcohol use and neonatal habituation assessed with the Brazelton Scale. *Child Dev* 1983;545:1109.

393. Streissguth AP, Sampson PD, Barr HM, et al. Studying alcohol teratogenesis from the perspective of the fetal alcohol syndrome: methodological and statistical issues. *Ann NY Acad Sci* 1986;477:63.

394. Smith IE, Coles CD, Lancaster J, et al. The effect of volume and duration of prenatal ethanol exposure on neonatal physical and behavioral development. *Neurobehav Toxicol Teratol* 1986;8:375.

395. Fried PA, Makin JE. Neonatal behavioral correlates of prenatal exposure to marijuana cigarettes and alcohol in a low-risk population. *Neurotoxicol Teratol* 1987;9:1.

396. Jacobson SW, Fein GG, Jacobson JL, et al. Neonatal correlates of prenatal exposure to smoking, caffeine, and alcohol. *Infant Behav Dev* 1984;7:253.

397. Schneider ML, Moore CF, Becker EF. Timing of moderate alcohol exposure during pregnancy and neonatal outcome in rhesus monkeys (Macaca mulatta). *Alcohol Clin Exp Res* 2001;25:1238.

398. Richardson GA, Day NL, Taylor P. The effect of prenatal alcohol, marijuana and tobacco exposure on neonatal behavior. *Infant Behav Dev* 1989;12:199.

399. Rosett H, Snyder P, Sander LW, et al. Effects of maternal drinking on neonate state regulation. *Dev Med Child Neurol* 1979; 21:464.

400. Chernick V, Childiaeva R, Ioffe S. Effects of maternal alcohol intake and smoking on neonatal electroencephalogram and anthropometric measurements. *Am J Obstet Gynecol* 1983; 146:41.

401. Ioffe S, Childiaeva R, Chernick V. Prolonged effects of maternal alcohol ingestion on the neonatal encephalogram. *Pediatrics* 1984;74:330.

402. Ioffe S, Chernick, V. Development of the EEG between 30 and 40 weeks gestation in normal and alcohol-exposed infants. *Dev Med Child Neurol* 1988;30:797.

403. Olney JW, Wozniak DF, Jevtovic-Todorovic V, et al. Glutamate signaling and the fetal alcohol syndrome. *Ment Retard Dev Disabil Res Rev* 2001;7:267.

404. Parson SH, Sojitra NM. Loss of myelinated axons is specific to the central nervous system in a mouse model of the fetal alcohol syndrome. *J Anat* 1995;187:739.

405. Mennella JA, Beauchamp GK. The transfer of alcohol to human milk. *N Engl J Med* 1991;325:981.

406. Flores-Huerta S, Hernandez-Montes H, Argote RM, et al. Effects of ethanol consumption during pregnancy and lactation on the outcome and postnatal growth of the offspring. *Ann Nutr Metab* 1992;36:121.

407. Kiessling KH, Pilstrom L. Effects of ethanol on rat liver: the influence of vitamins, electrolytes and amino acids on the structure and function of mitochondria from rats receiving ethanol. *Br J Nutr* 1967;21:547.

408. Cobo E. Effect of different doses of ethanol on the milk-ejecting reflex in lactating women. *Am J Obstet Gynecol* 1973;115:817.

409. Little RE, Anderson KW, Ervin CH, et al. Maternal alcohol use during breast-feeding and infant mental and motor development at one year. *N Engl J Med* 1989;321:425.

410. Day NL, Robles N, Richardson G, et al. The effects of prenatal alcohol use on the growth of children at three years of age. *Alcohol Clin Exp Res* 1991;15:67.

411. Barr HM, Streissguth AP, Martin DC, et al. Infant size at 8 months of age: relationships to maternal use of alcohol, nicotine and caffeine during pregnancy. *Pediatrics* 1984;74:336.

412. Sampson PD, Bookstein FL, Barr HM, et al. Prenatal alcohol exposure, birthweight, and measures of child size from birth to age 14 years. *Am J Public Health* 1994;84:1421.

413. Streissguth AP, Barr HM, Olson HC, et al. Drinking during pregnancy decreases word attack and arithmetic scores on standardized tests: adolescent data from a population-based prospective study. *Alcohol Clin Exp Res* 1994;18:248.

414. Greene T, Ernhart CB, Sokol RJ, et al. Prenatal alcohol exposure and preschool physical growth: a longitudinal analysis. *Alcohol Clin Exp Res* 1991;15:905.

415. Coles CD, Brown RT, Smith LE, et al. Effects of prenatal alcohol exposure at school age: I. Physical and cognitive development. *Curr Alcohol* 1991;13:1.

416. O'Connor MJ, Brill NJ, Sigman M. Alcohol use in primiparous women older than 30 years of age: relation to infant development. *Pediatrics* 1986;78:444.

417. Fried, PA, O'Connell CM. A comparison of effects of prenatal exposure to tobacco, alcohol, cannabis and caffeine on birth size and subsequent growth. *Neurotoxicol Teratol* 1987;9:79.

418. Coles CD, Smith IE, Lancaster JS, et al. Persistence over the first month of neurobehavioral differences in infants exposed to alcohol prenatally. *Infant Behav Dev* 1987;10:23.

419. Coles CD, Smith IE, Falek A. Prenatal alcohol exposure and infant behavior: immediate effects and implications for later development. In: Bean-Bayog M, ed. *Children of alcoholics.* New York: Hayworth Press, 1987:87.

420. Streissguth AP, Barr HM, Martin DC, et al. Effects of maternal alcohol, nicotine and caffeine use during pregnancy on infant mental and motor development at eight months. *Alcohol Clin Exp Res* 1980;4:152.

421. Jacobson JL, Jacobson SW, Sokol RJ, et al. Teratogenic effects of alcohol on infant development. *Alcohol Clin Exp Res* 1993;17:174.

422. Jacobson JL, Jacobson SW, Sokol RJ, et al. Effects of alcohol use, smoking, and illicit drug use on fetal growth in black infants. *J Pediatr* 1994;124:757.

423. Jacobson SW, Jacobson JL, Sokol RJ, et al. Prenatal alcohol exposure and infant information processing ability. *Child Dev* 1993;64:1706.

424. Jacobson SW. Specificity of neurobehavioral outcomes associated with prenatal alcohol exposure. *Alcohol Clin Exp Res* 1998; 22:313.

425. Gusella J, Fried P. Effects of maternal social drinking and smoking on offspring at 13 months. *Neurotoxicol Teratol* 1984;6:13.

426. O'Connor MJ, Brill NJ, Sigman M. Alcohol use in primiparous women older than 30 years of age: relation to infant development. *Pediatrics* 1986;78:444.

427. Jacobson SW, Chiodo LM, Sokol RJ, et al. Validity of maternal report of prenatal alcohol, cocaine and smoking in relation to neurobehavioral outcome. *Pediatrics* 2002;109:815.

428. Fried PA, Watkinson B. 12- and 24-month neurobehavioral follow-up of children prenatally exposed to marijuana, cigarettes and alcohol. *Neurotoxicol Teratol* 1988;10:305.

429. Fried PA, Watkinson B. 36- and 48-month neurobehavioral follow-up of children prenatally exposed to marijuana, cigarettes and alcohol. *J Dev Behav Pediatr* 1990;11:49.

430. Richardson GA, Day NL. *Prenatal exposure to alcohol, marijuana and tobacco: effect on infant mental and motor development.* Presented at the meeting of the Society for Research in Child Development. Seattle, Washington. April 1991.

431. Streissguth AP, Barr HM, Sampson PD, et al. IQ at age 4 in relation to maternal alcohol use and smoking during pregnancy. *Dev Psychol* 1989;25:3.

432. Landesman-Dwyer S, Ragozin A, Little R. Behavioral correlates of prenatal alcohol exposure: a four-year follow-up study. *Neurotoxicol Teratol* 1981;3:187.

433. Streissguth AP, Martin DC, Barr HM, et al. Intrauterine alcohol and nicotine exposure: attention and reaction time in 4-year-old children. *Dev Psychol* 1984;20:533.

434. Barr HM, Streissguth AP, Darby BL, et al. Prenatal exposure to alcohol, caffeine, tobacco and aspirin: effects on fine and gross motor performance in 4-year-old children. *Dev Psychol* 1990; 26:339.

435. Larsson G, Bohlin AB, Tunnell R. Prospective study of children exposed to variable amounts of alcohol in utero. *Arch Dis Child* 1985;60:315.

436. Streissguth AP, Barr HM, Sampson PD, et al. Attention distraction and reaction time at seven years and prenatal alcohol exposure. *Neurotoxicol Teratol* 1986;8:717.

437. Streissguth AP, Barr HM, Sampson PD. Moderate prenatal alcohol exposure: effects on child IQ and learning problems at age 7 1/2 years. *Alcohol Clin Exp Res* 1990;14:662.

438. Kodituwakku PW, Handmaker NS, Cutler SK, et al. Specific impairments in self-regulation in children exposed to alcohol prenatally. *Alcohol Clin Exp Res* 1995;19:1558.

439. Kolata GB. Fetal alcohol advisory debated. *Science* 1981;214:642.

440. Kopera-Frye K, Dehaene S, Streissguth AP. Impairments of number processing induced by prenatal alcohol exposure. *Neuropsychologia* 1996;32:1187.

441. Astley SJ, Clarren SK. A fetal alcohol syndrome screeing tool. *Alcohol Clin Exp Res* 1995;19:1565.

442. Astley SJ, Clarren SK. A case definition and photographic screening tool for the facial phenotype of fetal alcohol syndrome. *J Pediatr* 1996;129:33.

443. Aase JM, Clinical Recognition of FAS: difficulties of Detection and Diagnosis. *Alcohol World* 1994;18:5.

444. Barr HM, Streissguth AP. Identifying maternal self-reported alcohol use associated with fetal alcohol spectrum disorders. *Alcohol Clin Exp Res* 2001;25:283.

445. Spagnolo A. Teratogenesis of alcohol [Review]. *Ann Ist Super Sanita* 1993;29:89.

446. Bagheri MM, Burd L, Martsolf JT, et al. Fetal alcohol syndrome: maternal and neonatal characteristics. *J Perinat Med* 1998; 26:263.

447. Sokol RJ, Ager J, Martier S, et al. Significant determinants of susceptibility to alcohol teratogenicity. *Ann NY Acad Sci* 1986;77:87.

448. Young NK. Effects of alcohol and other drugs on children. *J Psychoactive Drugs* 1997;29:23.

449. Jacobson JL, Jacobson SW, Sokol RJ. Increased vulnerability to alcohol-related birth defects in the offspring of mothers over 30. *Alcohol Clin Exp Res* 1996;20:359.

450. Armant DR, Saunders DE. exposure of embryonic cells to alcohol: contrasting effects during preimplantation and postimplantation development. *Semin Perinatol* 1996;20:127.

451. Ernhart CB, Sokol RJ, Martier S, et al. Alcohol teratogenicity in the human: a detailed assessment of specificity, critical period, and threshold. *Am J Obstet Gynecol* 1987;156:33.

452. Streissguth AP, Clarren SK, Jones KL. Natural history of the fetal alcohol syndrome: a ten-year follow-up of eleven patients. *Lancet* 1985;2:85.

453. Kyllerman M, Aronson M, Sabel KG, et al. Children of alcoholic mothers (growth and motor performance compared to matched controls). *Acta Paediatr Scand* 1985;70:20.

454. Spohr HL, Willms J, Steinhahusen HC. Prenatal alcohol exposure and long-term developmental consequences. *Lancet* 1993; 341(8850):907.

455. Streissguth AP. Fetal alcohol syndrome in older patients. *Alcohol Alcohol* 1993;2[Suppl]:209.

456. Van Der Leeden M, Van Dongen K, Kleinhout M, et al. Infants exposed to alcohol prenatally: outcome at 3 and 7 months of age. *Ann Trop Paediatr* 2001;21:127.

457. Landesman-Dwyer S. The relationship of children's behavior to maternal alcohol consumption. In: Abel EL, ed. *Fetal alcohol syndrome: human studies.* vol. 2. Boca Raton, FL: CRC Press, 1982:127.

458. Streissguth AP, Herman C, Smith D. Stability of intelligence in the fetal alcohol syndrome: a preliminary report. *Alcohol Clin Exp Res* 1978;2:165.

459. Loebstein R, Koren G. Pregnancy outcome and neurodevelopment of children exposed in utero to psychoactive drugs: the Motherisk experience. *J Psychiatry Neurosci* 1997;22:192.

460. Ueker A. Nadel L. Spatial locations gone awry: object and spatial memory deficits in children with fetal alcohol syndrome. *Neuropsychologia* 1996;34:209.

461. Mattson SN, Riley EP, Delis DC, et al. Verbal learning and memory in children with fetal alcohol syndrome. *Alcohol Clin Exp Res* 1996;20:810.

462. Shaywitz S, Cohen D, Shaywitz B. Behavior and learning difficulties in children of normal intelligence born to alcoholic mothers. *J Pediatr* 1980;96:978.

463. Steinhausen HC, Nestler V, Spohr HL. Development and psychopathology of children with the fetal alcohol syndrome. *J Dev Behav Pediatr* 1982;3:49.

464. Caruso K., ten Bensel R. Fetal alcohol syndrome and fetal alcohol effects. The University of Minnesota experience. *Minn Med* 1993;76:25.

465. Coles CD, Platzman KA, Rashkind-Hood CL, et al. A comparison of children affected by prenatal alcohol exposure and attention deficit, hyperactivity disorder. *Alcohol Clin Exp Res* 1997;21: 150.

466. Steinhausen HC, Spohr H. Long term outcome of children with fetal alcohol syndrome: psychopathology, behavior and intelligence. *Alcohol Clin Exp Res* 1998;22:334.

467. Church MW, Gerkin KP. Hearing disorders in children with fetal alcohol syndrome: findings from case reports. *Pediatrics* 1988; 82:147.

468. Flint EF. Severe childhood deafness in Glasgow, 1965–1979. *J Laryngol Otol* 1983;97:421.

469. Thiringer K, Kankkunen A, Liden G, et al. Perinatal risk factors in the etiology of hearing loss in preschool children. *Dev Med Child Neurol* 1984;26:799.

470. Aronson M, Kyllerman M, Sabel KG, et al. Children of alcoholic mothers (developmental, perceptual and behavioral characteristics as compared to matched controls). *Acta Paediatr* 1985;74:27.

471. Sowell ER, Jernigan TL, Mattson SN, et al. Abnormal development of the cerebellar vermis in children prenatally exposed to alcohol size reduction in lobules I–V. *Alcohol Clin Exp Res* 1996;20:31.

472. Mattson SN, Riley EP, Delis DC, et al. Verbal learning and memory in children with fetal alcohol syndrome. *Alcohol Clin Exp Res* 1996;20:810.

473. Swayze VW 2nd, Johnson VP, Hanson JW, et al. Magnetic resonance imaging of brain anomalies in fetal alcohol syndrome. *Pediatrics* 1997;99:232.

474. Johnson VP, Swayze VW 2nd, Sato Y, et al. Fetal alcohol syndrome: craniofacial and central nervous system manifestations. *Amer J Med Genet* 1996;61:329.

475. Hellstrom A, Chen Y, Stromland K. Fundus morphology assessed by digital analysis in children with fetal alcohol syndrome. *J Pediatr Ophthalmol Strabismus* 1997;34:17.

476. Stromland K. Hellstrom A. Fetal alcohol syndrome—an ophthalmologic and socioeducational prospective study. *Pediatrics* 1996;97:845.

477. Duester G. Retinoids and the alcohol dehydrogenase gene family. *EXS* 1994;71:279.

478. Stromland K. Pinazo-Duran MD. Optic nerve hypoplasia: comparative effects in children and rats exposed to alcohol during preganancy. *Teratology* 1994;50:100.

479. Church MW, Eldis F, Blakley BW, et al. Hearing, language, speech, vestibular and dentofacial disorders in fetal alcohol syndrome. *Alcohol Clin Exp Res* 1997;21:227.

480. Church MW, Kaltenbach JA. Hearing, Speech, Language and Vestibular Disorders in the Fetal Alcohol Syndrome: a literature review. *Alcohol Clin Exp Res* 1997;21:495.

481. Rossig C, Wasser S, Oppermann P. Audiologic manifestations in fetal alcohol syndrome assessed by brainstem auditory-evoked potentials. *Neuropadiatrie* 1994;25:245.

482. Khalsa JH, Gfroerer JC. Epidemiology and health consequences of drug abuse among pregnant women. *Semin Perinatol* 1991;15: 265.

483. Abel EL. *Marijuana, the first twelve thousand years.* New York: Plenum Press, 1980.

484. Marijuana and Health. Report of a study by the Committee of the Institute of Medicine, Division of Health Sciences Policy. Washington, DC: National Academy Press, 1982.

485. Dewey WL. Cannabinoid pharmacology. *Pharmacol Rev* 1986; 38:151.

486. Martin BR. Cellular effects of cannabinoids. *Pharmacol Rev* 1986;38:45.

487. Harbison RD, Mantilla-Plata B. Prenatal, toxicity, maternal distribution and placental transfer of tetrahydrocannabinol. *J Pharmacol Exp Ther* 1972;180:446.

488. Abel EL, Rockwood GA, Riley EP. The effects of early marijuana exposure. In: Riley EP, Vorhees CV, eds. *Handbook of behavioral teratology.* New York: Plenum Press, 1986:267.

489. Ostrea EM, Subramanian MG, Abel EL. Placental transfer of cannabinoids in humans: comparison between meconium, maternal and cord blood sera. In: Chesner G, Consroe P, Musty R, eds. *Marijuana: an international research report: proceedings of the Melbourne Symposium on Cannabis.* Series 7. Canberra: Australian Government Publishing Service, 1987:103.

490. Fried PA, Buckingham M, Von Kulmiz P. Marijuana use during pregnancy and perinatal risk factors. *Am J Obstet Gynecol* 1983; 144:22.

491. Fried PA, Watkinson B, Willan A. Marijuana use during pregnancy and decreased length of gestation. *Am J Obstet Gynecol* 1984;150:23.

492. Shiono PH, Klebanoff MA, Nugent RP, et al. The impact of cocaine and marijuana use on low birth weight and preterm birth: a multicenter study. *Am J Obstet Gynecol* 1995;172:19.

493. Bishai R, Koren G. Maternal and obstetric effects of prenatal drug exposure. *Clin Perinatol* 1999;26:75.

494. Gibson GT, Baghurst PA, Colley DP. Maternal alcohol, tobacco and cannabis consumption and the outcome of pregnancy. *Aust N Z J Obstet Gynaecol* 1983;23:15.

495. Day NL, Richardson, GA. Prenatal marijuana use: epidemiology, methodologic issues, and infant outcome. *Clin Perinatol* 1991; 18:77.

496. Tennes K, Avitable N, Blackard C, et al. Marijuana: prenatal and postnatal exposure in the human. *NIDA Research Monograph* 1985;59:48.

497. Linn S, Schoenbaum S, Monson R, et al. The association of marijuana use with outcome of pregnancy. *Am J Public Health* 1983; 73:1161.

498. Zuckerman B, Frank D, Hingson R, et al. Effects of maternal marijuana and cocaine use on fetal growth. *N Engl J Med* 1989;320:762.

499. O'Connell CM, Fried PA. An investigation of prenatal cannabis exposure and minor physical anomalies in a low risk population. *Neurotoxicol Teratol* 1984;6:345.

500. Qazi QH, Mariano E, Milman DH, et al. Abnormalities in offspring associated with prenatal marijuana exposure. *Dev Pharmacol Ther* 1985;8:141.

501. Hutchings DE, Dow-Edwards D. Animal models of opiate, cocaine and cannabis use. *Clin Perinatol* 1991;18:1.

502. Fried PA. Marijuana use during pregnancy: consequences for the offspring. *Semin Perinatol* 1991;15:280.

503. Scher MS, Richardson GA, Coble PA, et al. The effects of prenatal alcohol and marijuana exposure: disturbances in neonatal sleep cycling and arousal. *Pediatr Res* 1988;24:101.

504. Mirochnick M, Meyer J, Frank DA, et al. Elevated plasma norepinephrine after in utero exposure to cocaine and marijuana. *Pediatrics* 1997;99:555.

505. Hayes JS, Dreher MC, Nugent JK. Newborn outcomes with maternal marihuana use in Jamaican women. *Pediatr Nurs* 1988;14:107.

506. Bauer CR, Shankaran S, Bada HS, et al. Maternal Lifestyles Study (MLS). Effects of substance abuse exposure during pregnancy on acute maternal outcomes. *Pediatr Res* 1996;39:257A.

507. Fried PA, Smith AM. A literature review of the consequences of prenatal marijuana exposure. An emerging theme of a deficiency in aspects of executive function. *Neurotoxicol Teratol* 2001; 23:1–11.

508. Faden VB, Graubard BI. Maternal substance use during pregnancy and developmental outcome at age three. *J Subst Abuse* 2000;12:329.

509. Dahl RE, Scher MS, Williamson DE, et al. A longitudinal study of prenatal marijuana use. *Arch Pediatr Adolesc Med* 1995;149:145.

510. Scragg RK, Mitchell EA, Ford RP, et al. Maternal cannabis use in the sudden death syndrome. *Acta Paediatr* 2001;90:57.

511. Hingson R, Alpert JJ, Day N, et al. Effects of maternal drinking and marijuana use on fetal growth and development. *Pediatrics* 1982;70:539.

512. Taylor P. Agents acting at the neuromuscular junction and autonomic ganglia: nicotine. In: Gilman A, Goodman LS, Rall TW, et al, eds. *Goodman and Gilman's the pharmacologic basis of therapeutics.* 8th ed. New York: Pergamon Press, 1990:180.

513. Dahlstrom A, Lundell B, Curvall M, et al. Nicotine and cotinine concentrations in the nursing mother and her infant. *Acta Paediatr* 1990;79:142.

514. Dobek D, Karmowski A, Sobiech KA, et al. Average quantitative concentration of cotinine within the system pregnant woman-baby. *Arch Immunol Ther Exp (Warsz)* 1998;46:59.

515. Kline J, Stein ZA, Susser M. Smoking as a risk factor for spontaneous abortion. *N Engl J Med* 1977;297:793.

516. Milart P, Kauffels W, Schneider J. Vasoactive effects of nicotine in human umbilical arteries. *Zentralbl Gynakol* 1994;116:217.

517. Ahlsten G, Ewald U, Tuvemo T. Maternal smoking reduces prostacyclin formation in human umbilical arteries. A study on strictly selected pregnancies. *Acta Obstet Gynecol Scand* 1986; 65:645.

518. Brown HL, Miller JM, Khawli O, et al. Premature placental calcification in maternal cigarette smokers. *Obstet Gynecol* 1988;71:914.

519. Lehtovirta P, Forss M. The acute effect of smoking on intervillous blood flow of the placenta. *Br J Obstet Gynaecol* 1978;85:729.

520. Naeye RL, Harkness WL, Utts J. Abruptio placentae and perinatal death: a prospective study. *Am J Obstet Gynecol* 1977;128,740.

521. Garn SM, Johnson M, Ridella SA, et al. Effects of maternal cigarette smoking on Apgar scores. *Am J Dis Child* 1981;135:503.

522. Hingson R, Gould JR, Morelock S, et al. Maternal cigarette smoking, psychoactive substance use and infant Apgar scores. *Am J Obstet Gynecol* 1982;144:959.

523. Jaakkola JJ, Jaakkola N, Zahlsen K. Fetal growth and length of gestation in relation to prenatal exposure to environmental tobacco smoke assessed by hair nicotine concentration. *Environ Health Perspect* 2001;109:557.

524. Meyer MB, Tonascia JA. Maternal smoking, pregnancy complications, and perinatal mortality. *Am J Obstet Gynecol* 1977;128:494.

525. Wen SW, Goldenberg RL, Cutter GR, et al. Smoking, maternal age, fetal growth, and gestational age at delivery. *Am J Obstet Gynecol* 1990;162:53.

526. Peacock JL, Bland JM, Anderson HR. Preterm delivery: effects of socioeconomic factors, psychological stress, smoking, alcohol, and caffeine. *Brit Med J* 1995;311:531.

527. Kleinman JC, Pierre MB, Madans JS, et al. The effects of maternal smoking on fetal and infant mortality. *Am J Epidemiol* 1988; 127:274.

528. Cnattingius S, Haglund B, Meirik O. Cigarette smoking as risk factor for late fetal and early neonatal death. *Br Med J* 1988; 297:258.

529. Slotkin TA. Fetal nicotine or cocaine exposure: which one is worse? *J Pharmacol Exp Ther* 1998;285:931.

530. Ernst M, Moolchan ET, Robinson ML. Behavioral and neural consequences of prenatal exposure to nicotine. *J Amer Acad Child Adolesc Psych* 2001;40:630.

531. Miller HC, Hassanein K. Maternal smoking and fetal growth of full term infants. *Pediatr Res* 1974;8:960.

532. Beaulac-Baillargeon L, Desrosiers C. Caffeine-cigarette interaction on fetal growth. *Am J Obstet Gynecol* 1987;157:1236.

533. Brooke OG, Anderson HR, Bland JM, et al. Effects on birth weight of smoking, alcohol, caffeine, socioeconomic factors, and psychosocial stress. *Br Med J* 1989;298:795.

534. MacArthur C, Knox EG. Smoking in pregnancy: effects of stopping at different stages. *Br J Obstet Gynaecol* 1988;95:551.

535. Shu XO, Hatch MC, Mills J, et al. Maternal smoking, alcohol drinking, caffeine consumption, and fetal growth: results from a prospective study. *Epidemiol* 1995;6:115.

536. Abel EL. *Marijuana, tobacco, alcohol and reproduction.* Boca Raton, FL: CRC Press, 1983.

537. Mitchell EA, Thompson JM, Robinson E, et al. Smoking, nicotine and tar and risk of small for gestational age babies. *Acta Paediatr* 2002;91:323.

538. Misra DP, Nguyen RH. Environmental tobacco smoke and low birth weight; a hazard in the workplace? *Environ Health Perspect* 1999;107[Suppl 6]:897.

539. Haddow JE, Knight GJ, Palomaki GE, et al. Cigarette consumption and serum cotinine in relation to birth weight. *Br J Obstet Gynaecol* 1987;94:678.

540. Harrison GG, Ranson RS, Vaugher YE. Association of maternal smoking with body composition of the newborn. *Am J Clin Nutr* 1983;38:757.

541. Fried PA, Watkinson B, Gray R. Growth from birth to early adolescence in offspring of prenatally exposed to cigarettes and marijuana. *Neurotoxicol Teratol* 1999;21:513.

542. Fried PA, O'Connell CM. A comparison of the effects of prenatal exposure to tobacco, alcohol, cannabis and caffeine on birth size and subsequent growth. *Neurotoxicol Teratol* 1987;9:79.

543. Fedick J, Alberman E, Goldstein H. Possible teratogenic effect of cigarette smoking. *Nature* 1971;231:530.

544. Hausrein KO. Cigarette smoking, nicotine and pregnancy. *Intern J Pharmacol Ther* 1999;37:417.

545. Heinonen OP. Risk factors for congenital heart disease: a prospective study. In: Kelly S, Hook EB, Janerich DT, eds. *Birth defects: risks and consequences.* New York: Academic Press, 1976:221.

546. Martin JC, Martin DC, Lund C. Maternal alcohol ingestion and cigarette smoking and their effect upon newborn conditioning. *Alcohol Clin Exp Res* 1973;1:243.

547. Chiriboga CA. Fetal effects [Review]. *Neurol Clin* 1993;11:707.

548. Bearer C, Emerson RK, O'Riordan M, et al. Maternal tobacco smoke exposure and persistent pulmonary hypertension of the newborn. *Environ Health Perspect* 1997;105:202.

549. Saxton DW. The behavior of infants whose mothers smoke in pregnancy. *Early Hum Dev* 1978;2:363.

550. Landesman-Dwyer S, Keller LS, Streissguth AP. Naturalistic observations of newborns: effects of maternal alcohol intake. *Alcohol Clin Exp Res* 1978;2:171.

551. Bard KA, Coles CD, Platzman KA, et al. The effects of prenatal drug exposure, term status and caregiving on arousal and arousal modulation in 8-week old infants. *Dev Psychobiol* 2000; 36:194.

552. Woodson EM, DaCosta P, Woodson RH. *Maternal smoking and newborn behavior.* Presented at the International Conference on Infant Studies, New Haven, Conn, 1980.

553. Butler NR, Goldstein H. Smoking in pregnancy and subsequent child development. *Br Med J* 1973;4:573.

554. Dunn HG, McBurney AK, Ingram S, et al. Maternal cigarette smoking during pregnancy and the child's subsequent development: II. Neurological and intellectual maturation to the age of 6.5 years. *Can J Public Health* 1977;68:43.

555. Zuckerman B. Marijuana and cigarette smoking during pregnancy: neonatal effects. In: Chasnoff IJ, ed. *Drugs, alcohol, pregnancy and parenting.* Lancaster, UK: Kluwer Academic Publishers, 1988:73.

556. Weisman MM, Warner V, et al. Maternal smoking during pregnancy and psychopathology in offspring followed to adulthood. *J Amer Acad Child Adolesc Psychiat* 1999;38:892.

557. Bergman AB, Wiesner LA. Relationship of passive cigarette smoking to sudden infant death syndrome. *Pediatrics* 1976;58:665.

558. Milerad J, Sundell H. Nicotine exposure and the risk of SIDS. *Acta Paediatr Suppl* 1993;82[Suppl 389]:70.

559. Toubas PL, Duke JC, McCaffree MA, et al. Effects of maternal smoking and caffeine habits on infantile apnea: a retrospective study. *Pediatrics* 1986;78:159.

560. Milerad J, Vege A, Opdal SH, et al. Objective measurements of nicotine exposure in victims of sudden infant death syndrome and in other unexpected child deaths. *J Pediatr* 1998;133:232.

561. Johnston M, Evans V, Baigel S. Phencyclidine. *Br J Anaesth* 1959; 31:433.

562. Marwah J, Pitts DK. Psychopharmacology of phencyclidine. *NIDA Research Monograph* 1986;64:127.

563. Fico TA, Vanderwende C. Phencyclidine during pregnancy: behavioral and neurochemical effects in the offspring. *Ann NY Acad Sci* 1989;562:319.

564. McCarron M. Phencyclidine intoxication. *NIDA Research Monograph* 1986;64:209.

565. Cummings AJ. Transplacental disposition of phencyclidine in the pig. *Xenobiotica* 1979;9:447.

566. Cooper JE, Cummings AJ, Jones H. The placental transfer of phencyclidine in the pig, plasma levels in the sow and its piglets. *J Physiol* 1977;267:17.

567. Nicholas JM, Lipshitz J, Schreiber E. Phencyclidine: its transfer across the placenta as well as into breast milk. *Am J Obstet Gynecol* 1982;143:143.

568. Kaufman KR, Petrucha RA, Pitts FN, et al. Phencyclidine in umbilical cord blood: preliminary data. *Am J Psychiatr* 1983; 140:450.

569. Aniline O, Pitts FN. Phencyclidine (PCP): a review and perspectives. *Crit Rev Toxicol* 1982;10:145.

570. Domino ET, Wilson AE. Effects of urine acidification on plasma and urine phencyclidine levels in overdosage. *Clin Pharmacol Ther* 1977;22:421.

571. Blaustein MP, Bartschat DK, Sorensen RG. Phencyclidine (PCP) selectively blocks certain presynaptic potassium channels. *Natl Inst Drug Abuse Res Monogr Ser* 1986;64:37.

572. Crider R. Phencyclidine: changing abuse patterns. *Natl Inst Drug Abuse Res Monogr Ser* 1986;64:163.

573. Golden NL, Kuhnert BR, Sokol RJ, et al. Phencyclidine use during pregnancy. *Am J Obstet Gynecol* 1984;148:254.

574. Golden NL, Kuhnert BR, Sokol RJ, et al. Neonatal manifestations of maternal phencyclidine exposure. *J Perinat Med* 1987; 15:185.

575. Chasnoff IJ, Burns WJ, Hatcher RP, et al. Phencyclidine: effects on the fetus and neonate. *Dev Pharmacol Ther* 1983;6:404.

576. Mvula MM, Miller JM Jr, Ragan FA. Relationship of phencyclidine and pregnancy outcome. *J Reprod Med* 1999;44:1021.

577. Howard J, Kropenske V, Tyler R. The long-term effects on neurodevelopment in infants exposed prenatally to PCP. *Natl Inst Drug Abuse Res Monogr Ser* 1986;64:237.

578. Rahbar F, Fomufod A, White D, et al. Impact of intrauterine exposure to phencyclidine (PCP) and cocaine on neonates. *J Natl Med Assoc* 1993;85:349.

579. Tabor BL, Smith-Wallace T, Yonekura ML. Perinatal outcome associated with PCP versus cocaine use. *Am J Drug Alcohol Abuse* 1990;16:337.

580. Jebelli AK, Doan N, Ellison G. Prenatal phencyclidine induces heightened neurodegeneration in rats in some brain regions, especially during 2nd trimester, but possible anti-apoptotic effects in others. *Pharmacol Toxicol* 2002;90:20.

581. Olney JW, Wozniak DF, Jevtovic-Todorovic V, et al. Drug-induced apoptotic neurodegeneration in the developing brain. *Brain Pathol* 2002;12:488.

582. Strauss AA, Modanlou D, Bosu SK. Neonatal manifestations of maternal phencyclidine (PCP) abuse. *Pediatrics* 1981;68:550.

583. Wachsman L, Schuetz S, Chan LS, et al. What happens to babies exposed to phencyclidine (PCP) in utero? *Am J Drug Alcohol Abuse* 1989;15:31.

584. Chasnoff IJ , Burns KA, Burns WJ, et al. Prenatal drug exposure: effects on neonatal and infant growth and development. *Neurobehav Toxicol Teratol* 1986;8:357.

585. Hoffman BB, Lefkowitz RJ. Catecholamines and sympathomimetics. In: Gilman AG, Rall TW, Nies AS, et al, eds. *Goodman and Gilman's the pharmacological basis of therapeutics.* 8th ed. New York: Pergamon Press, 1990:187.

586. Little BB, Snell LM, Gilstrap LC III. Methamphetamine abuse during pregnancy: outcome and fetal effects. *Obstet Gynecol* 1988;72:541.

587. Milkovich L, Van den Berg BJ. Effects of antenatal exposure to anorectic drugs. *Am J Obstet Gynecol* 1977;129:637.

588. Plessinger MA. Prenatal exposure to amphetamines. Risks and adverse outcomes in pregnancy. *Obstet Gynecol Clin North Am* 1998;25:119.

589. Oro AS, Dixon SD. Perinatal cocaine and methamphetamine exposure: maternal and neonatal correlates. *J Pediatr* 1987;111:571.

590. Dixon SD. Effects of transplacental exposure to cocaine and methamphetamine on the neonate. *West J Med* 1989;150:436.

591. Stewart JL, Meeker JE. Fetal and infant deaths associated with maternal methamphetamine abuse. *J Anal Toxicol* 1997;21:515.

592. Ramer CM. The case history of an infant born to an amphetamine-addicted mother. *Clin Pediatr* 1974;13:596.

593. Dixon SD, Bejar R. Echoencephalographic findings in neonates associated with maternal cocaine and methamphetamine use: incidence and clinical correlates. *J Pediatr* 1989;115:770.

594. Smith LM, Chang L, Yonekura ML, et al. Brain proton magnetic resonance spectroscopy in children exposed to methamphetamine in utero. *Neurology* 2110;57:255.

595. Eriksson M, Larsson G, Winbladh B, et al. The influence of amphetamine addiction on pregnancy and the newborn infant. *Acta Paediatr Scand* 1978;67:95.

596. Billing L, Eriksson M, Steneroth G, et al. Pre-school children of amphetamine-addicted mothers: I. Somatic and psychomotor development. *Acta Paediatr Scand* 1985;74:179.

597. Eriksson M, Billing L, Steneroth G, et al. Health and development of 8 year-old children whose mother abused amphetamines during pregnancy. *Acta Paediatr Scand* 1989;78:944.

598. Eriksson M, Jonsson B. Amphetamine abuse during pregnancy: environmental factors and outcome after 14–15 years. *Scand J Public Health* 2000;28:154.

599. Colado MI, O'Shea E. A study of the neurotoxic effect of MDMA (ecstasy) on 5-HT neurons in the brains of mothers and neonates following administration of the drug during pregnancy. *Br J Pharmacol* 1997;121:827.

600. Melhatton PR, Bateman DN, et al. Congenital anomalies after prenatal Ecstasy exposure. *Lancet* 1999;23:354:1141

601. O'Brien CP. Drug Addiction and Drug Abuse. In: Gilman AG, Hardman JG, et al, eds. *Goodman and Gilman's the pharmacologic basis of therapeutics.* 9th ed. New York: McGraw Hill, 1996:557.

602. Rall TW. CNS stimulants: the Methylxanthenes. In: Gilman AG, Goodman LS, Rall TW, et al, eds. *Goodman and Gilman's the pharmacological basis of therapeutics.* 7th ed. New York: McMillan Press, 1985:589.

603. Schardein JL. Current status of drugs as teratogens in man. *Progr Clin Biol Res* 1985;163C:181.

604. Nehlig A, Debry G. Potential teratogenic and neurodevelopmental consequences of coffee and caffeine exposure: a review on human and animal data. *Neurotoxicol Teratol* 1994;16:531.

605. Martin TR, Bracken MB. The association between low birth weight and caffeine consumption during pregnancy. *Am J Epidemiol* 1987;126:813.

606. Fenster L, Eskenazi B, Windham GC, et al. Caffeine consumption during pregnancy and fetal growth. *Am J Public Health* 1991; 81:458.
607. Christian MS, Brent RL. Teratogen update: evaluation of the reproductive and developmental risks of caffeine. *Teratology* 2001;64:51.
608. Fernandes O, Sabharwal M, Smiley T, et al. Moderate to heavy caffeine consumption during pregnancy and relationship to spontaneous abortion and abnormal fetal growth: a meta-analysis. *Reprod Toxicol* 1998;12:435.
609. Caan BJ, Goldhaber MK. Caffeinated beverages and low birthweight: a case-control study. *Am J Public Health* 1989;79:1299.
610. Bland JM , Anderson HR . Effects on birthweight of alcohol and caffeine consumption in smoking women. *J Epidemiol Com Health* 1991;45:159.
611. Fortier I, Marcoux S, Beaulac-Baillargeon L. Relation of caffeine intake during pregnancy to intrauterine growth retardation and preterm birth. *Am J Epidemiol* 1993;137:931.
612. Leviton A. Caffeine consumption and the risk of reproductive hazards. *J Reprod Med* 1988;33:175.
613. Larroque B, Kaminski M , Lelong N, et al. Effects of birth weight of alcohol and caffeine consumption during pregnancy. *Am J Epidemiol* 1993;1:137:941.
614. Shu XO, Hatch MC, Mills J, et al. Maternal smoking, alcohol drinking, caffeine consumption, and fetal growth: results from a prospective study. *Epidemiol* 1995;6:115.
615. Klebanoff MA, Levine RJ, Clemens DJ, et al. Maternal serum caffeine metabolites and small for gestational age birth. *Amer J Epidemiol* 2002;1;155:32.
616. Hadeed A, Siegel S. Newborn cardiac arrhythmias associated with maternal caffeine use during pregnancy. *Clin Pediatr* 1993; 32:45.
617. Oei SG, Vosters RP, van der Hagen NL. Fetal arrhythmia caused by excessive intake of caffeine by pregnant women. *Brit Med J* 1989;298:568.
618. McGowan JD, Altman RE, Kanto WP Jr. Neonatal withdrawal symptoms after chronic maternal ingestion of caffeine. *South Med J* 1988;81:1092.
619. McKim EM. Caffeine and its effects on pregnancy and the neonate. *J Nurse Midwifery* 1991;36:226.
620. Alm B, Wennergren G, Norvenius G, et al. Caffeine and alcohol as risk factors for sudden infant death syndrome. Nordic epidemiological SIDS study. *Arch Dis Child* 1999;81:107
621. Kandall SR, Gartner LM. Late presentation of drug withdrawal symptoms in newborns. *Am J Dis Child* 1974;127:58.
622. Chasnoff IJ. Drug use and women: establishing a standard of care. *Ann NY Acad Sci* 1989;562:208.
623. Khavari K, Farber P. A profile instrument for the quantification and assessment of alcohol consumption. *J Stud Alcohol* 1978; 39:1525.
624. Khavari KA, Douglass FM. The drug use profile (DUP): an instrument for clinical and research evaluations for drug use patterns. *Drug Alcohol Depend* 1981;8:119.
625. Cahalan D, Cisin I, Crossley H. *American drinking practices.* Monograph No. 6. New Brunswick, NJ: Rutgers Center of Alcohol Studies, 1969.
626. Streissguth AP, Barr HM, Martin DC. Offspring effects and pregnancy complications related to self reported maternal alcohol use. *Dev Pharmacol Ther* 1982;5:21.
627. Ostrea EM Jr, Welch RR. Detection of prenatal drug exposure in the pregnant woman and her newborn infant. *Clin Perinatol* 1991;18:629.
628. Schonberg SK, Blasinsky M, eds. Substance abuse: a guide for health professionals. *Am Acad Pediatr Ctr Adv Heath Stud* 1988;48.
629. Ostrea EM, Martier S, Welch R, et al. Sensitivity of meconium drug screen in detecting intrauterine drug exposure of infants. *Pediatr Res* 1990;27:219A.
630. Ostrea EM, Brady MJ, Parks PM, et al. Drug screening of meconium in infants of drug dependent mothers: an alternative to urine testing. *J Pediatr* 1989;115:474.
631. Halstead AC, Godolphin W, Lockitch G, et al. Timing of specimens is crucial in urine screening of drug dependent mothers and infants. *Clin Biochem* 1988;21:59.
632. Osterloh JD, Lee BL. Urine drug screening in mothers and infants. *Am J Dis Child* 1989;143:791.
633. Hicks, JM, Morales A, Soldin SJ. Drugs of abuse in a pediatric outpatient population. *Clin Chem* 1990;36:1256.

634. Ostrea EM, Lynn SN, Wayne RH, et al. Tissue distribution of morphine in the newborns of addicted monkeys and humans. *Dev Pharmacol Ther* 1980;1:163.
635. Silvestre MA, Lucena J, Ostrea EM. The effect of timing, dosage and duration or morphine intake during pregnancy on the amount of morphine in meconium in a rat model. *Biol Neonate* 1997;72:112.
636. Ostrea EM Jr, Romero A, Knapp DK, et al. Postmortem analysis of meconium in early gestation human fetuses exposed to cocaine: clinical implications. *J Pediatrics* 1994;124:477.
637. Ostrea EM. Detection of prenatal drug exposure in the pregnant woman and her newborn infant. In: Kilbey MM, Asghar KK, eds. Methodological issues in epidemiological, prevention and treatment of research on drug exposed women and their children. US Department of Health and Human Services. *Natl Inst Drug Abuse Res Monogr Ser* 1992;96–121.
638. Ostrea EM, Parks P, Brady M. Rapid isolation and detection of drugs in meconium of infants of drug dependent mothers. *Clin Chem* 1988;34:2372.
639. Ostrea EM Jr, Romero A, Yee H. Adaptation of the meconium drug test for mass screening. *J Pediatr* 1993;122:152.
640. Mac E, Matias O, Ostrea EM, et al. Clinical adaptation of HPLC to meconium drug testing. *Pediatric Res* 1995;37:221A.
641. Murphey LJ, Olsen GD, Konkol RJ. Quantitation of benzoylnorecgonine and other cocaine metabolites in meconium by high-performance liquid chromatography. *J Chromatography* 1993;12;330.
642. Browne SP, Moore CM, Negrusz A, et al. Detection of cocaine norcocaine and cocaethylene in the meconium of premature neonates. *J Forensic Sci* 1994;39:1515.
643. Browne SP, Tebbett IR, Moore CM, et al. Analysis of meconium for cocaine in neonates. *J Chromatogr* 1992;75:158.
644. Montes N, Romero A, Ostrea EM, et al. Improved method of GC/MS analysis of meconium for opiate, cocaine and cannabinoid. *Pediatric Res* 1993;33:66A.
645. Wingert WE, Feldman MS, Kim MH, et al. A comparison of meconium, maternal urine and neonatal urine for detection of maternal drug use during pregnancy. *J Forensic Sci* 1994;39:150.
646. Moriya F, Chan KM, Noguchi TT, et al. Testing for drugs of abuse in meconium of newborn infants. *J Anal Toxicol* 1994; 18:41.
647. Clark GD, Rosenzweig B, Raisys VA. Analysis of cocaine and benzoylecgonine in meconium of infants born to cocaine dependent mothers. *Clin Chem* 1990;36:1022A.
648. Lombardero N, Casanova O, Behnke M, et al. Measurement of cocaine and metabolites in urine, meconu, and, and diapers by gas chromatography/mass spectrometry. *Ann Clin Lab Sci* 1993;23:385.
649. Ostrea EM, Knapp DK, Romero A, et al. Meconium analysis to assess fetal exposure to access fetal exposure to active and passive maternal smoking. *J Pediatr* 1994;15:474.
650. Ostrea EM, Brady MJ, Parks PM, et al. Drug screening of meconium in infants of drug-dependent mothers: An alternative to urine testing. *J Pediatr* 1989;15:474.
651. Ryan RM, Wagner CL, Schultz JM, et al. Meconium analysis for improved identification of infants exposed to cocaine in utero. *J Pediatr* 1994;125:435.
652. Maynard E, Amoroso LP, W. Osteopathic Hospitals w. Meconium for drug testing. *Am J Dis Child* 1991;45:650.
653. Callahan CM, Grant TM, Phipps P, et al. Measurement of gestational cocaine exposure: sensitivity of newborn hair, meconium, and urine. *J Pediatr* 1992;120:763.
654. Lewis DE, Moore CM, Leikin JB, et al. Meconium analysis for cocaine: a validation study and comparison with paired urine analysis. *J Anal Toxicol* 1995;19:148.
655. Bandstra E, Steele B, Chitwood D. Detection of in utero cocaine exposure: a comparative methodologic study. *Pediatr Res* 1992; 31:58A.
656. Casanova OQ, Lombardero N, Behnke M, et al. Detection of cocaine exposure in the neonate. Analyses of urine, meconium, and amniotic fluid from mothers and infants exposed to cocaine. *Arch Path Lab Med* 1994;118:988.
657. Baumgartner A, Jones P, Black C. Detection of phencyclidine in hair. *J Forensic Sci* 1981;26:576.
658. Baumgartner A, Jones P, Baumgartner W, et al. Radioimmunoassay of hair for determining opiate abuse histories. *J Nucl Med* 1979;2:748.

659. Baumgartner W, Black C, Jones P, et al. Radioimmunoassay of cocaine in hair: a concise communication. *J Nucl Med* 1982; 23:790.

660. Baumgartner A, Jones P, Black C. Detection of phencyclidine in hair. *J Forensic Sci* 1981;26:576.

661. Ishiyama I. Detection of basic drugs (methamphetamine, antidepressants and nicotine) from human hair. *J Forensic Sci* 1983; 28:380.

662. Balabanova S, Homoki J. Determination of cocaine in human hair by gas chromatography/mass spectrometry. *Z Rechtsmed* 1987;98:235.

663. Marigo M, Tagliaro F, Poiesi C, et al. Determination of morphine in the hair of heroin addicts by high performance liquid chromatography with fluorimetric detection. *J Anal Toxicol* 1986;10:158.

664. Pelli B, Traldi P, Tagliaro F, et al. Collisional spectroscopy for unequivocal and rapid determination of morphine at ppb level in the hair of heroin addicts. *Biomed Environ Mass Spectrum* 1987;14:63.

665. Bailey DN. Drug screening in an unconventional matrix: hair analysis. *J Am Med Assoc* 1989;262:3331.

666. Smith FP, Liu RH. Detection of cocaine metabolites in perspiration stain, menstrual bloodstain and hair. *J Forensic Sci* 1986; 31:1269.

667. Smith FP. Detection of phenobarbital in bloodstains, semen, seminal stains, saliva stains, saliva, perspiration stains and hair. *J Forensic Sci* 1981;26:582.

668. Garcia D, Romero A, Garcia G, et al. Gastric fluid analysis for determining gestational cocaine exposure. *J Pediatr* 1996;98: 291–293.

669. Finnegan LP. Neonatal abstinence. In: Nelson NM, ed. *Current therapy in neonatal perinatal medicine.* Philadelphia: BC Decker, 1990:314.

670. Lipsitz PJ. A proposed narcotic withdrawal score for use with newborn infants. *Clin Pediatr* 1975;14:592.

671. Neonatal drug withdrawal. American Academy of Pediatrics Committee on Drugs. *Pediatrics* 1998;101:1079.

672. Osborn DA, Cole MJ, Jeffrey HE. Opiate treatment for opiate withdrawal in newborn infants. *Cochrane Database Syst Rev* 2002;CD002059.

673. Begg EJ, Malpas TJ, Hackett LP, et al. Distribution of R- and S-methadone into human milk during multiple, medium to high oral dosing. *Br J Clin Pharmacol* 2001;52:681.

674. Jackson MR, Berry GL. Motherhood and drug-dependency: the attributes of full-time versus part-time responsibility for child care. *Int J Addict* 1994;29:1519.

Beyond the Nursery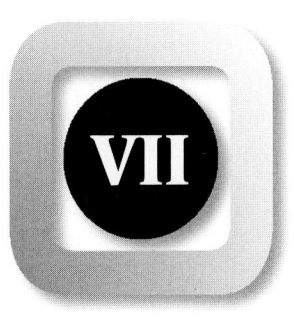

Medical Care After Discharge

59

Judy Bernbaum

Once the high-risk infant is discharged from the hospital, his or her many special care needs do not cease. Although they still require well-child care, many of these infants have needs that are far from routine. Special attention must be given to their growth and nutrition, immunizations, vision and hearing, and sequelae of illnesses experienced during the neonatal period. While premature infants have a higher likelihood for long-term sequelae and continuing medical problems than term infants do, many of the issues discussed specifically about prematurity apply to term infants as well.

EXPECTATIONS OF GROWTH

Growth patterns are a valuable indicator of an infant's well being. Aberrant growth may reflect the presence of chronic illness, feeding difficulties, inadequate nutrition, or social–emotional difficulties. Preterm infants are at particular risk for growth disorders. Many infants with chronic illness, while at an age when rapid growth is expected, have high caloric requirements but are unable to meet them because they have impaired feeding abilities. It is crucial to monitor nutritional intake closely and to interpret growth rates with a complete understanding of the infant's past history, current problems, and expectations for growth.

Many factors affect the growth of a preterm infant, including gestational age, birth weight, severity of neonatal illness, caloric intake, current illnesses, environmental factors in the home, and heredity. Caloric requirements for a healthy preterm infant generally exceed those of a term, normal-birth-weight infant, especially during rapid catch-up growth. Chronic illnesses that increase caloric expenditure add to an infant's daily requirements. Malabsorption after necrotizing enterocolitis (NEC) or chronic emesis from gastroesophageal reflux disease (GERD) may impair growth through increased losses. In contrast, decreased intake may be caused by fatigue, hypoxemia, oral motor dysfunction, or reflux esophagitis. Finally, infants with intrauterine growth retardation caused by congenital infections, chromosomal abnormalities, or other syndromes may never achieve normal growth (1–4).

Patterns of Growth

When the growth of a low-birth-weight (LBW) infant is evaluated, the gestational age should be considered. Growth parameters should be plotted on growth curves that have been developed using low-birth-weight preterm infants exclusively (5). Measurements should be plotted according to the infant's adjusted age until approximately 2.5 years of age, when the age difference becomes insignificant. Various patterns of growth emerge from different groups of patients.

Healthy, LBW, appropriate-for-gestational-age (AGA) infants generally experience catch-up growth during the first 2 years of life, with maximal growth rates between 36 and 40 weeks of gestational age. Little catch-up growth occurs after 3 years of age. Head circumference usually is the first parameter to demonstrate catch-up growth and often plots at a higher percentile than do weight and length. Increases in weight are followed within several weeks by increases in length. Rapid catch-up head growth must be distinguished from pathologic growth associated with hydrocephalus. An imaging study may be indicated if the infant's history or symptoms suggest hydrocephalus. Insufficient brain growth, a head circumference falling more than two standard deviations below the mean, indicates that the infant is at risk for significant developmental disability.

Growth velocities for weight and height vary considerably. Some preterm infants show growth on curves between the 75th and 97th percentiles by 3 months adjusted age, whereas others remain on low curves well beyond the child's first year. It is helpful to evaluate an infant's weight gain in comparison to gains in length. Low weight for length or a decline in all growth parameters suggests inadequate nutrition. Weight percentiles significantly greater than length percentiles indicate obesity. Obesity may occur in a preterm infant whose parents overfeed their previously underweight baby. It is common to see an infant who was formerly failing to thrive rather abruptly become obese when the medical problems resolve but the diet remains high in calories.

Growth of the small-for-gestational-age (SGA) infant is influenced strongly by the cause of the intrauterine growth retardation. Overall, LBW–SGA infants demonstrate less catch-up growth than LBW–AGA infants, but if they do, acceleration starts by 8 to 12 months of adjusted age (2). Approximately 50% of LBW–SGA infants are below average in weight at 3 years of age, whereas only 15% of LBW–AGA infants remain below average weight at the same age (4). Symmetric SGA infants with birth head circumference similar in percentile to birth weight are less likely to demonstrate catch-up growth than are those asymmetric SGA infants whose birth head circumference was at a significantly higher percentile than their weight. As with AGA infants, head circumference is normally the first parameter to demonstrate catch-up, followed by weight and then by length.

Because of the wide range of growth that is considered normal during the first several years of life, it is best to analyze trends in growth rather than make assumptions based on single measurements. When abnormalities are noted in growth trends, investigation of the infant's nutritional status during hospitalization, the results of cranial sonography studies, and the status of continuing illnesses should be undertaken to identify a possible cause.

Nutritional Requirements

Traditionally, although somewhat controversial, the goal for preterm infants is to achieve a growth rate approximating that expected while *in utero* had they not been born prematurely (4). Because weight gain is suboptimal during acute illness, all efforts should be made to promote catch-up growth once the medical condition is stable. The nutritional needs of the preterm infant during the first few months of life exceed those of a term neonate and may continue for the entire first year of life even if there are no exceptional medical or feeding problems. Appropriate choices for many preterm infants include breast milk and routine infant formulas, but because many preterm infants continue to have increased caloric requirements, breast milk and routine formulas often need to be supplemented with either carbohydrates or fats. Formulas can be concentrated somewhat to increase their caloric density, allowing the infant to consume more calories per unit volume. There are now commercially available premature growth formulas tailored to address the unique protein, fat and caloric needs of the growing preterm infant for the first year of life (6,7,8). Most infants do not tolerate feedings with caloric densities greater than 30 kcal/oz. Infants given feedings concentrated beyond 24 kcal/oz should be monitored for symptoms of intolerance such as vomiting and diarrhea and for hyperosmolar dehydration secondary to insufficient free water intake. Whole cow's milk is poorly tolerated and should be avoided. When caloric additives or concentrated formulas are used, care should be taken to maintain an appropriate caloric distribution of nutrients with a ratio among carbohydrates–fats–protein of approximately 40–50–10 (6).

Caloric requirements for adequate growth vary. Healthy preterm infants generally require 110 to 130 kcal/kg per day, but some infants with chronic disease may require up to 150 kcal/kg per day (9). Caloric intake should be increased as tolerated until weight gain is satisfactory.

Often infants with ongoing illness or those just recovering from their long hospitalization will be unable to consume the volume of formula or breast milk needed to provide them with the calories they need for catch-up or even maintenance of their ideal growth rate. It is not uncommon to suggest offering up to one-half of their daily calculated needs by continuous feedings (by tube) through the night and allowing them to feed the remainder orally during the day. Taking that approach often decreases the need to consume large volumes by oral feeding and allows the infant to increase volumes as tolerated during the day, after which nighttime volumes can begin to be decreased.

FEEDING PROBLEMS

Although unusual in term infants, feeding disorders are relatively common in preterm infants. Most feeding problems occur in the neonatal period, but many infants demonstrate recurrent or chronic problems with sucking and swallowing (10). Unrecognized, these problems may lead to significantly impaired nutritional intake and negatively affect the parent–infant relationship. Infants at risk for development of feeding problems include those with a delay in initiating oral feedings during the neonatal period and those with immature oral motor skills related to prematurity. Additionally, those with transient neurologic immaturity or more permanent neurologic deficits are at highest risk. Additional risk factors for development of feeding dysfunction include chronic lung disease, tracheostomy, gastroesophageal reflux, and repeated exposure to noxious, albeit life-sustaining, equipment secured around the area of the nose and mouth. These include suction catheters, endotracheal tubes, naso- or orogastric tubes, and oxygen cannulas. Frequently, many feeding difficulties can be avoided and transition to all oral feedings can be enhanced by offering nonnutritive sucking opportunities during gavage feedings (10).

Oral reflexes that allow normal feeding and protect the airway from aspiration may be hypoactive or hyperactive in preterm infants. Abnormal reflexes such as a tongue thrust or hyperactive gag can further complicate successful and pleasurable feeding. A hyperactive gag is particularly troublesome because the infant may manifest oral hypersensitivity and be unable to tolerate the nipple or spoon on the tongue and resist any oral stimulation. Other causes of hypersensitivity or tactile defensiveness include the noxious stimuli mentioned above.

The evaluation of a possible feeding disorder includes a detailed history of feeding behaviors and nutritional intake, a physical examination with assessment of oral motor reflexes, and observation of a feeding. If an infant with chronic lung disease desaturates during feeding, increasing the supplemental oxygen during feeding can improve feeding behavior (11,12). Evaluation of the type of nipple and the size of its hole may show that the hole is too small, causing fatigue, or too large, making it difficult to control the flow. There are now a large variety of nipples available that can specifically be chosen for the individual infant's needs. Indications for radiologic evaluation include suspected aspiration during feeding or an anatomic abnormality such as a tracheoesophageal fistula.

All of these conditions are amenable to therapy if identified early. Treatment of underlying medical problems, the most common of which is gastroesophageal reflux, often helps ameliorate the feeding problems. A pediatric speech pathologist or occupational therapist trained in feeding techniques can assess an infant and develop an appropriate feeding program once a problem has been defined.

Feeding an infant is normally a relaxing, nurturing act that plays a role in parent–infant bonding. In the presence of a feeding disorder, feedings may become a major source of stress, frustration, and anxiety for the infant, parents, and physicians.

IMMUNIZATIONS

Most preterm infants should receive the same immunizations as the term infant and on similar schedules. However, special consideration should be given to the preterm infant with the following vaccines or regarding certain infectious diseases (13,14).

Diphtheria, Tetanus, Pertussis

The American Academy of Pediatrics (AAP) recommends that full doses of DtaP vaccine be administered to prematurely born infants at the appropriate postnatal i.e., chronologic age. A large percentage of preterm infants demonstrate inadequate protection if given a reduced dosage of DTaP vaccine at the routine intervals. Fewer side effects occur in preterm infants who receive full-dose vaccine than in their full-term counterparts, and the use of acellular pertussis vaccine should obviate any concerns in this regard. The same contraindications to immunizing full-term infants against pertussis apply to preterm infants. Most importantly, infants with bronchopulmonary dysplasia (BPD) are at highest risk for serious sequelae if they contract pertussis. Therefore, the pertussis component of this vaccine should not be withheld. Similarly, the pertussis component should also be given to any child with cerebral palsy or other muscle tone abnormalities. If an infant has an underlying seizure disorder, the decision to withhold pertussis should be reviewed with the individual's neurologist.

Polio, Haemophilus Influenzae Type b, Pneumococcal, Varicella, and Measles-Mumps-Rubella Vaccines

The AAP Committee on Immunization Practices recommends that full-dose inactivated, enhanced potency polio (IPV), haemophilus influenzae type b (Hib), pneumococcal, varicella, and measles-mumps-rubella (MMR) vaccines be administered at the appropriate chronologic age.

Influenza

Infants with chronic pulmonary disease (e.g., BPD) or cardiac disease with pulmonary vascular congestion are at high risk for the development of serious illness if infected with an influenza virus (14). Infants with influenza have presented with symptoms of sepsis, apnea, and lower airways disease. To protect vulnerable infants, immunization with influenza vaccine is indicated for household contacts, including siblings, primary caretakers, and home care nurses and hospital personnel. For infants older than 6 months chronological age, two doses of split virus vaccine should be given 1 month apart between October and December, followed by an annual dose. It is now recommended that influenza vaccine be given to all infants under 2 years of age (13,14). Older siblings under 9 years of age who have not received previous influenza vaccines also require two doses initially. However, adults and older siblings with natural immunity or who have received previous immunizations need only one yearly dose.

Respiratory Syncytial Virus

Preterm infants, especially those with underlying chronic lung disease, are particularly at high risk for serious sequelae after becoming infected with respiratory syncytial virus (RSV) during the late fall and winter months. Many will require re-hospitalization and re-intubation for respiratory failure and are often left with worsening lung disease requiring increased support with supplemental oxygen, bronchodilators, or and/or diuretics. Attempts at developing a vaccine to protect against RSV have been unsuccessful; however, an anti-RSV monoclonal antibody (Synagis®) has been approved for use in high-risk infants (15,16). Monthly intramuscular injections are necessary to provide passive protection throughout the RSV season. Synagis® is expensive; thus, its use should be limited to those infants most at risk. According to the guidelines set forth by the AAP (14), those who should be considered to receive monthly injections include the following:

- Children under 24 months with BPD who require:
  - Supplemental oxygen
  - Have required oxygen within 6 months of RSV season
  - Are currently requiring mechanical ventilation
  - Are being treated with bronchodilators or diuretics

- Premature infants without BPD may benefit if gestational age is:
  - Between 29 and 32 weeks until they are 6 months of age
  - Less than 28 weeks until they are 12 months of age.
- Premature infants between 32 and 35 weeks of age who are at high risk for developing severe sequelae if they develop RSV disease including:
  - multiple births, attendance in daycare, exposure to older siblings (especially if in day care or school), and living in crowded conditions.

Hepatitis B

For infants with birth weights below 2,000 g born to hepatitis B surface antigen–negative women, it is advised to delay the initiation of hepatitis B vaccine until just before initial hospital discharge, provided the infant weighs more than 2,000 g or until 2 months of age when other immunizations are given (13).

SPECIALIZED CARE

In addition to routine well-child care, the preterm infant may require specialized follow-up for the monitoring, detection, and management of sequelae from neonatal problems. The remainder of this chapter is devoted to a discussion of these special needs.

Retinopathy of Prematurity

Retinopathy of prematurity (ROP) (see Chapter 54) is a disorder that interrupts the normal vascularization of the developing retina. Although it has been reported in term infants, ROP is mainly a disease associated with prematurity and, in particular, with those less than 32 weeks gestation. The incidence and severity of ROP increase with decreasing gestational age. Most cases of ROP resolve spontaneously, but even with complete resolution, scarring of the retina may occur. Generally, the more severe the disease, the longer it takes for resolution. An infant with ROP affecting Zone 1, however, is at a much greater risk for permanent visual sequelae than one who has the disease affecting Zone 2 or 3 (17,18). According to recommendations in the AAP Guidelines for Perinatal Care (19), infants with a birth weight of less than 1,500 g or with a gestational age of 28 weeks or less, and selected infants between 1,500 and 2,000 g with an unstable clinical course who are believed to be at high risk by their attending pediatrician or neonatologist should have an ophthalmologic examination for ROP. The initial examination should not take place before 4 to 6 weeks chronologic age or, alternatively, within the 31st to 33rd week of postconceptional age, whichever is later. Prior to this, the yield for identifying ROP is low. If only one examination is possible, it should be at 7 to 9 weeks of age to catch the peak period of occurrence. A schedule of follow-up visits is based on the retinal findings and should be determined by the examining ophthalmologist. All infants with immature fundi or any stage of ROP require close monitoring until the eyes have matured or the ROP has completely resolved. Thereafter, follow-up to assess for refractive errors should be at 1 year of age and before kindergarten, or earlier for any clinical concerns. Infants with resolving (incompletely resolved) ROP need careful follow-up because some revert to active disease.

Sequelae of ROP depend largely on the extent of retinal scarring. As much as 80% of stage 3 ROP resolves spontaneously without significant scarring, but, even in infants with fully regressed ROP, there may be subtle retinal changes resulting in refractive errors, strabismus, or amblyopia. Additionally, an infant left with moderate scarring can experience retinal tears, late retinal detachment, nystagmus, glaucoma, cataracts, vitreous hemorrhage or membranes, and severe scarring that can lead to blindness (19). Services for visually impaired children are available on county and state levels. Early identification of a child with visual handicaps to such programs is essential to provide the child and family with the services and resources they need.

Hearing Problems

The incidence of sensorineural hearing loss in preterm infants is generally reported to be between 1% and 3%. Several factors place these infants at particular risk for hearing loss, including hypoxia, hyperbilirubinemia, infections, unstable blood pressure, environmental noise, and ototoxic drugs. According to the Joint Committee on Infant Hearing, Year 1999 Position Statement where the Universal Newborn Hearing Screening (UNHS) Program is described, all infants should have access to hearing screening using a physiologic measure before hospital discharge or have access to and be referred for screening before one month of age (20). However, all newborns or infants who require neonatal intensive care should receive hearing screening before discharge from the hospital. All infants who do not pass the initial screen or any subsequent rescreening should begin appropriate audiologic and medical evaluations to confirm the presence of hearing loss before 3 months of age. All infants with confirmed permanent hearing loss should receive services before 6 months of age in interdisciplinary intervention programs that recognize and build on strengths, informed choice, traditions, and cultural beliefs of the family. All infants who pass newborn hearing screening but who have risk indicators for other auditory disorders and/or speech and language delay should receive ongoing audiologic and medical surveillance and monitoring for communication development. Infants with indicators associated with late-onset, progressive, or fluctuating hearing loss and auditory neural conduction disorders and/or brainstem auditory pathway dysfunction should be monitored.

Depending on the screening technology selected, infants with hearing loss less than 30 dB or with hearing loss related to auditory neuropathy or neural conduction disorders may not be detected in a universal newborn hearing screening program.

All infants, regardless of newborn hearing screening outcome, should receive ongoing monitoring for development of age-appropriate auditory behaviors and communication skills. Passing an initial hearing screening does not preclude the possibility of a later, acquired hearing loss. Absent or abnormal responses to auditory stimulation, delays in speech development, poor articulation, or inattentiveness should raise the suspicion of a hearing loss that requires a more thorough evaluation. All infants who do not pass an initial hearing screen should be referred to an audiologist for further testing and intervention. In general, an infant with a sensorineural hearing loss should have a repeat audiologic evaluation performed every 3 months for 1 year after initial diagnosis, every 6 months during the preschool period, and yearly while in school.

In hearing tests, zero-decibel (dB) represents the level at which response to a sound should occur 50% of the time. If sound is not heard at this level, the decibel level is raised until the sound is audible 50% of the time. Responses above 15 dB are indicative of some degree of hearing loss (Table 59-1).

Children with moderate to profound hearing loss are at high risk for delayed onset of language, problems with articulation, language impairment, and alterations in voice quality. Cognitive delays may be encountered as a result of a loss of auditory input or a language delay. Behavior problems often are experienced and include inattentiveness, overactive or aggressive behaviors, and immature peer relations.

Hearing aids can be fitted early in infancy to avoid acoustic deprivation. With auditory stimulation being provided, language acquisition may proceed more normally. Along with hearing amplification, language stimulation therapy (sign language) should be provided.

For those children whose hearing loss cannot be improved by hearing aids, different modes of communication are necessary. These include sign language, alternate methods of gesturing or word spelling, language boards, or computer-assisted communication devices. The latter two methods are particularly useful for a child who is limited motorically as a result of cerebral palsy.

TABLE 59-1
CLASSIFICATION OF HEARING LOSS

Hearing Loss (dB)	Description
0–15	Normal
16–25	Borderline–mild
26–40	Mild
41–55	Mild–moderate
56–70	Moderate–severe
71–90	Severe
91 and above	Profound

Necrotizing Enterocolitis

Survivors of NEC, especially those who required surgical intervention, may have problems after discharge. The most common complications include strictures or adhesions and short bowel syndrome (SBS).

Strictures or adhesions of the small or large intestines may develop within 2 weeks to 2 months after the acute episode of NEC. Symptoms of complete or, more commonly partial, intestinal obstruction include vomiting, abdominal distention, constipation or obstipation, or hematochezia. Lower gastrointestinal bleeding may be the only symptom of stricture formation without any other symptoms of obstruction being evident. Intermittent or persistent problems with constipation or obstipation are the more common symptoms that an infant may experience well into the first year of life. Management of significant strictures or adhesions generally involves surgical resection, but those with minimal symptoms may be treated conservatively. Stool softeners are useful in preventing obstipation or constipation.

Short bowel syndrome often results from decreased intestinal length or function. Necrotizing enterocolitis requiring significant bowel resection is one of the most common causes of SBS. The associated symptoms are caused by decreased digestion and absorption of nutrients by a smaller intestinal surface area and a more rapid transit time. Most often, evidence is seen of carbohydrate, protein, fat, vitamin, and mineral malabsorption and an increase in colonic water secretion. Occasionally, SBS is associated with a decreased enterohepatic circulation and gallstones. The resultant problems of SBS constitute a syndrome of chronic diarrhea, malabsorption, growth retardation, and vitamin and mineral deficiencies. The prognosis of SBS is reasonably good if more than 25 cm of small bowel without an ileocecal valve, or more than 15 cm of small bowel with an ileocecal valve, remains after surgery (21). If long-term total parenteral nutrition (TPN) is needed, complications with its use will affect the child's prognosis.

Gastroesophageal Reflux

Gastroesophageal reflux (GER) refers to a condition in which gastric contents reflux into the esophagus and cause subtle or overt signs and symptoms. Although it can develop in full-term infants, GER occurs more commonly in preterm infants. Symptoms develop from incompetence of the lower esophageal sphincter often complicated by poor stomach emptying. Recurrent, nonprojectile emesis is the most common presenting symptom of GER. Usually, an infant will vomit within 1 to 2 hours after a feeding. An infant may experience several small-volume emeses after a feeding or only one or two large-volume emeses. Some children, however, have no significant emesis but reflux into the esophagus or mouth and then re-swallow. Many infants will present with arching of the trunk during or after a feeding. Infants also may present with Sandifer's syndrome, a condition in which an infant cranes his or her neck in various directions, attempting to stretch the esophagus and reduce the discomfort associated with reflux. An infant with this presentation may be misdiagnosed as having dystonia or a neurologic abnormality.

Failure to thrive or dehydration may result from chronic vomiting. Additionally, many of these infants avoid or refuse feedings because they quickly learn to associate feeding with the discomfort of GER and its related esophagitis.

Apnea and bradycardia are complications of GER. Occasionally, GER will worsen if an attempt is made to treat apnea and bradycardia with caffeine because this medication tends to decrease lower esophageal tone, exacerbating symptoms of GER. The physician should consider an evaluation for GER in an infant when his or her apnea or bradycardia worsens, fails to respond to, or worsens with, traditional medical therapy, other causes are ruled out, or if symptoms persist beyond 44 weeks of adjusted age (22).

Aspiration pneumonia is a serious sequela of GER. If acute in onset, symptoms are overt, so GER-related aspiration is more likely to be suspected and diagnosed. If chronic, unrecognized aspiration may cause or exacerbate underlying reactive airways disease. The possibility of GER should be considered in infants with BPD whose disease worsens or fails to improve even in the absence of other signs and symptoms of GER (23).

The evaluation of GER should be individualized. A clinical assessment is sufficient if the history and observation of a feeding present a classic picture of reflux. A technetium-labeled milk scan is helpful to document suspected aspiration and will be able to assess gastric emptying. A pH–thermistor study is useful to document the amount and the degree of acid reflux and any associated apnea or bradycardia. Because of the high false-positive and false-negative rates, a barium swallow and upper gastrointestinal series are of limited value except for documenting underlying anatomic abnormalities (24).

Management of GER depends on the severity of the reflux and its associated symptoms. Simple medical management, successful in 80% of patients, includes thickening formula with cereal, keeping the infant in a semiupright position after meals, and avoiding any increase in abdominal pressure such as may occur when the infant is placed in an infant seat after meals. Medications may be considered for infants who do not respond to conservative management or who have more severe symptoms. Medications are used to increase lower esophageal sphincter tone and improve gastric emptying. These include metoclopramide (Reglan®) and bethanechol (Urecholine®). Bethanechol should be used with caution in infants with chronic lung disease because it may induce or worsen bronchospasm. Another agent, cisapride (Propulsid®), is a prokinetic agent that increases transit time throughout the entire GI tract. As a result of reports of fatal cardiac arrhythmias or sudden death, cisapride was restricted to a limited access by gastroenterologists for use in this entity (25). Antacids, histamine H2-receptor antagonists, or proton pump inhibitors can be used as adjunct therapy to treat or prevent secondary esophagitis.

Surgical management, most often a Nissen fundoplication, is necessary in about 10% of patients with GER. Surgery should be reserved for infants who either fail to respond to medical management or manifest recurrent pulmonary infections from suspected chronic aspiration pneumonia, chronic esophagitis, unremitting apnea, or failure to thrive despite aggressive medical management.

Intraventricular Hemorrhage

Intraventricular hemorrhage (IVH) is one of the most serious neurologic events encountered by neonates. It occurs in up to 50% of infants born weighing under 1,500 g (26). There is an inverse relationship between gestational age and the incidence of hemorrhage. With the increase in survival of infants at lower gestational ages, an increase in the number of infants with IVH may be expected as well. Follow-up imaging studies should be performed to demonstrate resolution of hemorrhage and to diagnose any anatomic sequelae. The most common complications of IVH include hemorrhagic infarction, posthemorrhagic hydrocephalus, porencephalic cyst, and ventriculomegaly without hydrocephalus (e.g., hydrocephalus ex vacuo).

In clinical practice, a common problem when an infant's head circumference crosses percentiles is distinguishing the onset of hydrocephalus from catch-up head growth. Clinically, all premature infants with and without IVH should be monitored with at least monthly measurements of head circumference and documentation of neurodevelopmental progress. If a child has a weekly increase in head circumference greater than 2 cm or demonstrates any symptoms of increased intracranial pressure or a change in neurologic status, hydrocephalus should be considered and evaluated by cranial imaging studies. In general, most ventriculomegaly following IVH occurs within 2 weeks of the initial insult, and radiographic appearance rarely changes after 3 months unless a shunt was required.

Most often, when a ventriculoperitoneal shunt is placed for progressive hydrocephalus, it continues to work without complication according to the principle of volume dependence. If complications occur, they usually are caused by mechanical malfunction or infection. Mechanical malfunctions may result from disconnections at any point along the shunt apparatus or from an obstruction either proximally, along the length of the tubing, or distally within the peritoneum. Signs of malfunction are those associated with an increase in intracranial pressure.

If symptoms suggest malfunction, ultrasonography or a computed tomographic (CT) scan is recommended to evaluate the size of the ventricles compared to baseline, as is a simple roentgenogram of the entire length of shunt tubing to determine its integrity. Pumping the reservoir, if one is present, should be performed only by a physician familiar with the procedure. The information obtained can help determine the location of a blockage but could be misinterpreted by those unfamiliar with the technique. An obstructed or malfunctioning shunt dictates immediate neurosurgical evaluation.

Symptoms of an infected shunt include signs of increased intraventricular pressure associated with an obstruction plus fever and irritability. Shunt infections result in ventriculitis more often than meningitis. Infection may represent colonization of the apparatus only. Diagnosis is made by performing a needle aspiration of cerebrospinal fluid (CSF) from the reservoir using aseptic technique and obtaining a Gram stain and culture. Treatment usually includes appropriate intravenous antibiotics. Removing or externalizing the shunt tubing may also be required. If it is still felt to be necessary, the shunt tubing can be replaced once the CSF remains sterile for at least 72 hours (27).

If a shunt functions properly, follow-up usually is based on the individual neurosurgeon's recommendations. A routine imaging study for baseline usually is obtained when the infant is medically stable before hospital discharge. The clinician following the infant as an outpatient should use the same imaging technique so that a comparison can be made with the baseline study for any change suggestive of an obstruction. If the brain appears normal, and no symptoms of obstruction or infection develop, a follow-up scan may be avoided.

Periventricular Leukomalacia

Periventricular leukomalacia (PVL) is caused by ischemic infarction of the white matter adjacent to the lateral ventricles. A weakening in the integrity of the white matter in this area occurs, followed by either repair or the development of cysts. The reported incidence of PVL in infants with birth weights under 1,500 g varies from 2% to 22% (28–31). Infants at risk for PVL are those whose perinatal course was complicated by severe hypoxia, ischemia, or both. Additionally, infants of early gestational age are particularly susceptible to the development of PVL because of their poorly developed cerebral vascular system, especially after sepsis, seizures, meningitis, IVH, cardiorespiratory (CR) arrest, or life-threatening apnea.

In the weeks that follow a major insult leading to PVL, phagocytosis of the necrotic material occurs with development of fluid-filled periventricular cysts. Periventricular leukomalacia and, subsequently, the presence and size of cysts can be determined using cranial ultrasonography, CT, or magnetic resonance imaging scan. Resolution of the cysts is highly variable, and some never completely resolve (29).

Beyond the neonatal period, screening for the presence of PVL should be considered in any child with cerebral palsy without an apparent cause (31). Because there are no symptoms specific for PVL, it can easily be missed during the neonatal period if routine screening is not performed.

If PVL is associated with the loss of vital areas of neural tissue as with the formation of cysts greater than 3 mm in diameter, the infant so affected is at increased risk for cerebral palsy, developmental delay, and visual or auditory impairments. If PVL is not associated with residual cysts, few if any sequelae develop. When cysts persist, an infant's motor development is most affected. Cerebral palsy, manifested as moderate to severe quadriplegia or diplegia, is reported to develop in a large proportion of children with cystic residua after PVL. The intellectual capacities of children with PVL and cyst formation are more variable. Mental retardation is more common in infants with residual cysts but ranges from mild to severe. If the cysts develop in the occipital region, visual impairment may result (31).

All infants with PVL, especially those with cysts, should be monitored closely for neurodevelopmental sequelae. Periodic cranial imaging, preferably an MRI study, will determine stability, resolution of the cysts or the degree of residual damage. Parents of infants with PVL should be counseled on the importance of periodic neurodevelopmental assessments for early detection of any sequelae and intervention when appropriate.

Seizures

Seizures during the newborn period may be subtle or overt and may occur singly or repetitively. Diagnosis usually is made while the infant still is hospitalized. Medical staff often will document motor activity or behavioral changes consistent with seizure activity that can then be confirmed by electroencephalography (EEG). Although the normal immature cortex has a relatively high seizure threshold, cortical injury enhances the brain's susceptibility to seizures. Most neonatal seizures are provoked by a significant neurologic insult such as intracranial hemorrhage, hypoxic–ischemic insult (e.g., asphyxia), cerebral infarct, metabolic disturbances, or central nervous system (CNS) infections (32).

The primary determinant of the outcome of neonatal seizures is correlated closely with the underlying cause. Infants with relatively harmless conditions such as hypocalcemia do well with appropriate treatment of the underlying disturbance. Those with an intracranial hemorrhage or an anoxic insult experience greater morbidity. Infants with seizures associated with asphyxia that was noted at younger than 24 hours of age have a poorer outcome than those with later onset of seizures. Similarly, those with more severe seizures (e.g., status epilepticus, frequent seizures) fare worse (33).

The decision to treat seizures with anticonvulsants usually is made early in the evolution of the infant's evaluation. If a transient metabolic abnormality is identified and corrected, seizure activity should cease, usually without anticonvulsant therapy. Recommendations regarding the duration of long-term anticonvulsant therapy for neonatal seizures vary. In some cases, medications may be discontinued before initial hospital discharge. Most often, however, once seizures are well controlled, a seizure-free interval of at least 3 months passes before anticonvulsants are withdrawn. Before making a decision to withdraw medications, the physician should make certain that the infant has no further clinical seizure activity and no epileptiform discharges on EEG. A neurologist should evaluate any infant with seizures that persist, to help in their long-term management.

Apnea and Bradycardia

Infants may continue to experience episodes of apnea or bradycardia after initial hospital discharge. Apnea of infancy is defined as "an unexplained episode of cessation of breathing for 20 seconds or longer, or a shorter respiratory pause associated with bradycardia, cyanosis, pallor, and/or marked hypotonia" (34). The incidence of apnea and bradycardia and its chronicity are inversely proportional to the gestational age of the infant and often parallel the severity of problems the infant had during the neonatal period. Although CNS immaturity is the most common cause for apnea in preterm infants, it is important to rule out medical problems that may cause apnea even after hospital discharge. If clinically indicated, the symptomatic infant with apnea should be evaluated for the possibility of underlying anemia, sepsis, meningitis or other infections, seizures, upper airway obstruction, GER, hypoxia, or bronchospasm as possible inciting factors (35).

Once it has been determined that no remediable factors exist, a decision should be made whether to monitor a child at home. The need for home memory event CR monitoring with or without medication is determined before hospital discharge based on clinical judgment or results of specialized evaluations. The use of CR monitoring, however, remains somewhat controversial. The American Academy of Pediatrics Panel on Apnea, Sudden Infant Death Syndrome, and Home Monitoring established medical indications for use of CR monitoring (36). These include the following recommendations:

1. Premature infants who are at high risk of recurrent episodes of apnea, bradycardia, and hypoxemia after hospital discharge. The use of home cardiorespiratory monitoring in this population should be limited to approximately 43 weeks' postmenstrual age or after the cessation of extreme episodes, whichever comes last.
2. Infants who are technology dependent (tracheostomy, continuous positive airway pressure), have unstable airways, have rare medical conditions affecting regulation of breathing, or have symptomatic chronic lung disease.

If home cardiorespiratory monitoring is prescribed, the monitor should be equipped with an event recorder. However, the AAP also recommends that parents should be advised that home cardiorespiratory monitoring has not been proven to prevent sudden unexpected deaths in infants. Pediatricians should continue to promote proven practices that decrease the risk of sudden infant death syndrome (SIDS)—supine sleep position, safe sleeping environments, and elimination of prenatal and postnatal exposure to tobacco smoke.

Alarm settings usually are placed at a low heart rate of 80 beats per minute with or without a 5 second delay and a high heart rate at 240 to 250 beats per minute with a maximum respiratory pause of 15 seconds. These may be changed depending on the infant's age or specific clinical circumstances. In most infants, resting heart rate decreases with increasing age, changing to 70 bpm at 3 months and 60 bpm at 6 months of age.

Often, preterm infants require caffeine in addition to or in lieu of home monitoring (37). Unless dosage is adjusted as the infant gains weight, the blood level of medication gradually will fall, but it rarely is necessary to recheck levels after discharge as long as apnea and/or bradycardia episodes are infrequent. If episodes continue or increase in frequency despite therapeutic xanthine levels, an evaluation for other possible causes is indicated. In most cases, the infant should be allowed to outgrow and discontinue the medication when there are no more episodes of apnea for 2 months either clinically or by monthly CR monitor downloads (37).

Once the infant is symptom-free for 4 to 6 weeks, medication most often can be safely stopped. If there are no subsequent episodes identified by the monitor, a home pneumocardiogram recording or monitor download can be performed 1 to 2 weeks after stopping the medication to determine the need for continued monitoring. If no further episodes are documented, the monitor can be safely discontinued one month after the medication has been discontinued (Fig. 59-1).

Chronic Lung Disease

Bronchopulmonary dysplasia is the most frequently diagnosed chronic lung disease in preterm infants. Usually it develops as a sequel to the acute lung injury experienced during the first few weeks of life. The definition of BPD has changed over the years. A traditional diagnosis covered lung disease resulting from respiratory distress shortly after birth that required more than 28 days of oxygen exposure with representative findings noted on chest roentgenogram (38). Because many infants with a gestational age younger than 30 weeks require oxygen for more than 28 days without developing chronic lung disease, a more restrictive definition of BPD is more appropriate: BPD in a preterm infant less than 30 weeks of gestation is now defined as lung disease for which supplemental oxygen is still required beyond 36 weeks corrected gestational age (39). Although the diagnosis of BPD is given before initial hospital discharge, some infants with mild or minimal residual lung disease may come to the primary care provider's attention with their first viral respiratory tract infection. Those with more severe disease often will be discharged with medications, nebulized bronchodilator treatments, and supplemental oxygen. Clinical manifestations are similar to those in the nursery and include tachypnea, tachycardia, retractions, rhonchi, bronchospasm, and poor air movement into the lungs bilaterally. More subtle signs of chronic respiratory distress include poor weight gain, feeding intolerance, decreased activity, and a reduced exercise tolerance. Medical management of infants with BPD often includes any combination of the following: fluid restriction, diuretic

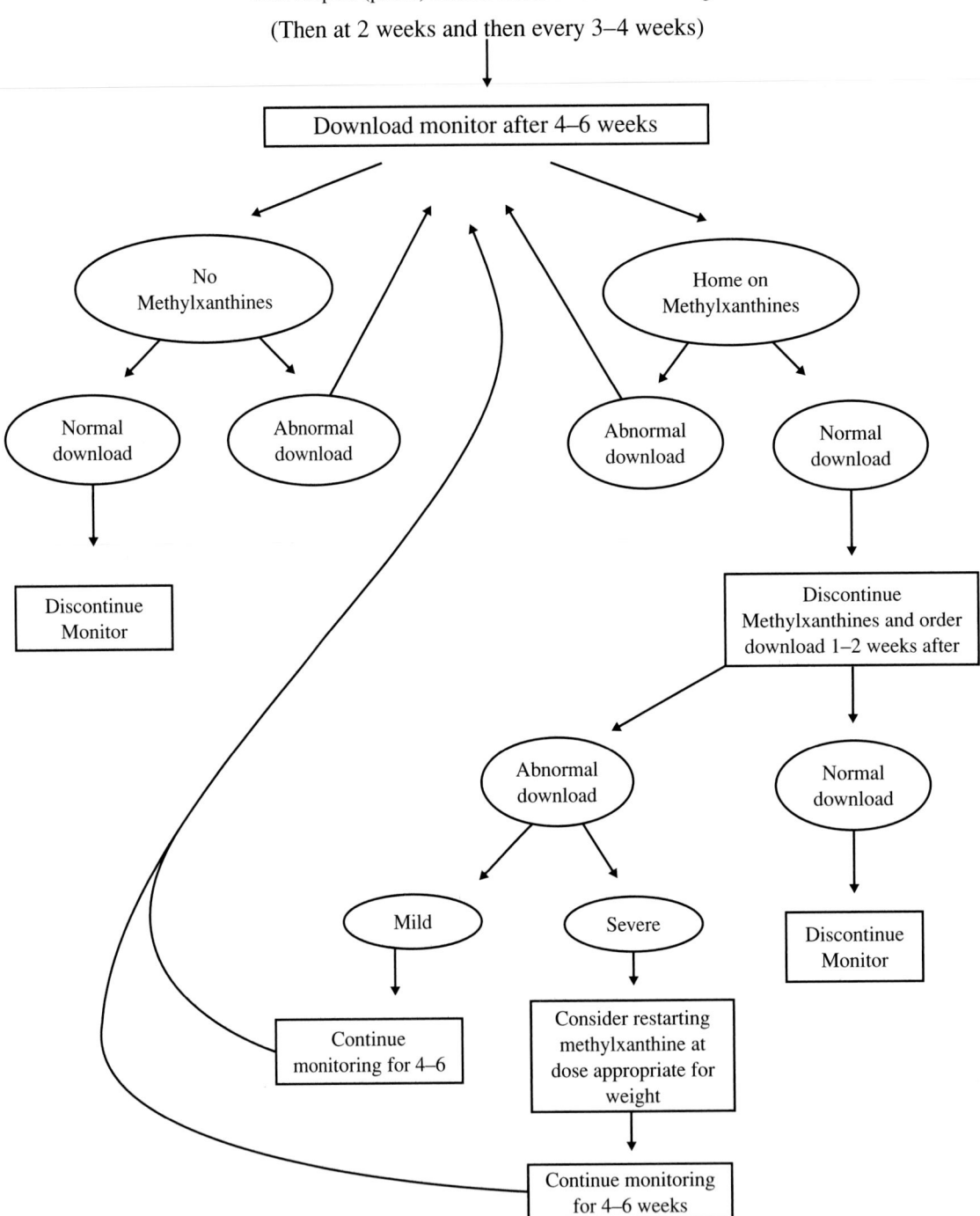

Figure 59-1   Schema for home monitor management.

therapy, bronchodilator medications, steroids, and supplemental oxygen, even after initial hospital discharge. These therapies are altered depending on the infant's clinical status and are eventually withdrawn as the infant matures and improves. How early withdrawal can begin depends on both the severity of lung disease at the time of discharge and its resolution over time. Additionally, BPD may worsen after discharge so that infants who tolerated either no medication or lower doses may begin to require aggressive inter-

vention after discharge. This occurs most often if the infant contracts a serious respiratory tract infection such as RSV pneumonia or less serious but more frequent intercurrent respiratory-related illnesses.

Diuretics

Most often diuretic therapy supplements fluid restriction in an attempt to decrease the fluid retention typical of

BPD. Although rarely initiated after discharge, diuretic usage requires monitoring of oral intake, urine output, weight gain, and, less frequently, electrolytes. Normally, one spot-check of serum electrolytes a few weeks after discharge is sufficient and, if normal, need not be rechecked as long as the infant remains medically stable with no significant dietary changes or increase in their diuretic dosage. Infants can outgrow their diuretic doses if there is no worsening of respiratory distress, evidence of peripheral or pulmonary edema, or clinical signs or symptoms of right ventricular strain or failure.

Bronchodilators

Many infants with BPD are discharged on maintenance bronchodilator medications. Unlike diuretics, these medications may need to be modified and continued as part of an aggressive medical regimen. Bronchodilators are used for outpatient therapy of BPD primarily to help maintain the infant's airways maximally dilated and in a bronchospasm-free state. They are used either as maintenance therapy or during intercurrent illnesses. Although the mechanisms of action of the different medications vary, all cause bronchodilation by relaxation of the smooth muscles of the small airways, allowing better oxygenation and prevention of recurrent bronchospasm. Many clinicians have been prescribing inhaled, aerosolized bronchodilators with increasing frequency because of its ease of administration and its direct effect on small airways without much in the way of systemic effect. Bronchodilators can be withdrawn if there has been adequate weight gain, medical stability, good activity level and continued developmental progress, and no exacerbation of underlying bronchospasm. Usually, weaning is not attempted until the infant is off supplemental oxygen. Bronchodilators may be needed either as maintenance therapy or intermittently for acute intercurrent illnesses that precipitate bronchospasm.

Supplemental Oxygen

The decision to continue an infant on supplemental oxygen relates to the severity of underlying lung disease. The need for supplemental oxygen that can be administered via a nasal cannula should not necessarily interfere with hospital discharge. Some of the more common indications for the use of supplemental oxygen include the following: evidence of desaturation while breathing room air; poor oral feeding because of air hunger, apnea, or bradycardia associated with hypoxia; poor growth associated with borderline hypoxia; poor exercise tolerance lethargy; and tachycardia or tachypnea that improves with the use of supplemental oxygen. If possible, it is best to determine the adequacy of oxygenation during sleep, feedings, and periods of activity. Pulse oximetry should indicate saturations of in the mid to high 90's. This level of saturation has been shown to result in a significant increase in pulmonary vasodilation, which may preclude the development of pulmonary hypertension and resultant right heart strain

(41). Although many centers begin weaning infants with lower oxygen saturations, studies have shown that infants with chronic lung disease who are optimally oxygenated demonstrate better weight gain, attain corrected age-appropriate milestones more readily, and have fewer intercurrent respiratory illnesses than do infants with lower saturations (42).

Before an infant is weaned from supplemental oxygen, its medical stability must be assured, as must adequacy of weight gain, exercise tolerance, and caloric intake. It is preferable to wean a child off oxygen slowly and in a stepwise fashion (43). A period of several weeks should pass during which the infant remains medically stable, gains adequate weight, demonstrates good exercise tolerance, and maintains adequate oxygen saturations before a move to the next step is considered. If the child is sent home without a pulse oximeter, many home care services can perform intermittent oximetry in the home to assist in making management decisions. It is easier to wean an infant off oxygen if he or she is kept maximally bronchodilated with supplemental medications. During an illness, it is common to have to increase the amount of supplemental oxygen or to restart it temporarily if the child has been recently weaned.

To compensate for increased energy expenditures, the infant with BPD often requires a high caloric intake, between 120 and 150 kcal/kg per day (44). Increased caloric needs complicated by poor nutritional intake often result in poor growth. Poor nutritional intake in this population may be caused by hypoxemia, anorexia, tachypnea, exercise intolerance, oral motor dysfunction, or GER. Additionally, it often is difficult to maximize caloric intake in the face of fluid restriction and exercise intolerance related to feeding. Caloric intake can be maximized by adding supplements, concentrating formulas, or using isocaloric formulas. A list of common supplements can be found in Table 59-2.

Even when supplemental calories are provided, there are times when growth is not adequate because the infant either tires easily or refuses any additional increased oral intake. It is then that supplemental nasogastric feedings should be considered, to be given either after each bottle-feeding or continuously during the night. Each method has its own advantages and disadvantages and must be considered within the context of individual family and patient needs. It is crucial to offer sucking opportunities routinely to any child who is tube-fed to stimulate the development of the sucking reflex (45). A feeding therapist may need to begin working early with an infant with BPD who demonstrates feeding difficulties to prevent the poor quality suck/swallow coordination frequently encountered in these children.

Intercurrent Illnesses

Bronchospasm with viral or bacterial respiratory illnesses will develop in many infants with BPD. When the infant is not already on maintenance therapy, bronchodilators can

TABLE 59-2

CALORIC SUPPLEMENTS[c]

Supplement	Caloric Density	Advantages	Disadvantages
Polycose[a]	2 kcal/mL	Well tolerated	Low caloric density
Karo syrup[a]	4 kcal/mL	Well tolerated; readily available; inexpensive	May cause loose stools
Microlipids[b]	4.5 kcal/mL	Well tolerated	Limited availability; high cost
Medium-chain triglyceride oil[b]	7.6 kcal/mL	High caloric density; usually well tolerated	May cause diarrhea; does not mix well with formula
Vegetable oil[b]	9 kcal/mL	Easily available and low cost	Does not mix well with formula
Avocado			
(1/2 avocado/26 oz formula)		High caloric density;	Season availability; expensive
(brown, Calif. Variety)	7.4 kcal/oz		
(Florida variety, green)	5.7 kcal/oz		
Dry baby cereal	10 kcal/Tbsp	Readily available; inexpensive; may help with gastroesophageal reflux	May cause constipation
Powdered skim milk	27 kcal/Tbsp	Readily available; mixes well with formula	
Duocal	42 kcal/Tbsp	CHO and Fat mixture/well tolerated	Adding 1 tsp/8 oz. Formula adds 1.75 kcal/oz

[a] Often not used as a suppplementation for infants with BPD, because those infants have been shown to have increased work of breathing when receiving a high-carbohydrate load, compared to those supplemented with fat.
[b] Use of oil supplements is contraindicated in cases where aspiration is suspected.
[c] From Bernbaum J. *Preterm Infants in Primary Care: A guide to office management.* Columbus, Ohio: 2000: Chapter 3, with permission.

be initiated during acute illnesses. If the infant is on maintenance bronchodilator therapy, synergistic medications can be added during acute exacerbations and withdrawn as the acute symptoms resolve, returning to maintenance therapy.

Minimizing the exposure of infants with BPD to environmental irritants and communicable diseases will help decrease the frequency of intercurrent episodes of bronchospasm and allow more time for the lung to heal. Some environmental irritants include cigarette or fireplace smoke, pet fur or dander, kerosene heaters, perfumes, paint, and infectious agents. The less irritation the lung is exposed to, the quicker the recovery process will be. All infants with chronic lung disease should receive RSV prophylaxis if they fall into one of the at risk categories listed previously under immunizations.

Rehospitalization is a common occurrence in children with BPD, especially during the first year of life. Parents of these infants should be advised of this possibility before the initial hospital discharge. Every effort should be made to treat intercurrent illnesses and associated bronchospasm on an outpatient basis, but if the infant does not respond readily, hospitalization is appropriate for more aggressive treatment. If, however, the child requires an elective surgical procedure such as a hernia repair, admission should be avoided during epidemics of respiratory-related illnesses.

Managing infants with BPD is one of the greatest clinical challenges for the practicing physician. The many facets of their care require a complete understanding of how their lung disease affects their physical well-being. Fortunately, most of their medical problems occur during the first year or two of life, and improvement can be expected in each subsequent year.

DISCHARGE PLANNING

Discharge of the intensive care graduate either to home or back to the referral hospital is frequently viewed as one of the most challenging tasks for the hospital staff and can be equally stressful and time-consuming for the family and the child's primary care physician. This transition can be made more smoothly and with less stress if a method is established for an organized discharge planning process (46). Discharge planning is a method whereby the needs of the patient and family are identified and a plan of care is designed and communicated to the appropriate people who will be providing care to the infant and family in the community. The process is intended to lessen the impact on the family of having to care for an infant without the support of the neonatal intensive care unit (NICU) staff on whom they have come to rely 24 hours a day. The discharge planning team usually consists of the physician caring for the infant, the patient's primary care nurse, social worker, therapist(s), and discharge planner (involved in obtaining home nursing, equipment and therapy needs, and coordinating this with insurance provider). Once a plan is determined, it must be communicated with the community agencies that will be involved in providing care. It is crucial that a primary care physician be identified well in advance of discharge not only so that they can continue to be updated on the child's progress while in the hospital but also that the discharge plan is reviewed to insure a seamless transition to home.

Preparation of the child for discharge begins with a thorough assessment of all aspects of the child's management with the goal of minimizing the disruption in the level of care being provided in the transition from hospital to home. One must first determine the feasibility for discharge. The following criteria should be met:

- Medical stability must be present, with minimal fluctuation in the day-to-day level of care.
- The child must tolerate a nutritional regimen that can be provided in a home setting, resulting in consistent weight gain.
- Level of care needed is practical for home.
- Parents are emotionally and technically competent in providing medical care themselves and appropriate support systems are identified when necessary.
- Funding must be available for equipment, medications, formula, and support services.
- Alternative discharge sites (chronic care facility, foster care, or relatives) should be considered for infants whose families are unable to provide the necessary care.

A thorough chart review close to the time of discharge will assist in the determination of outstanding issues. In particular, a list can be generated of pending medical test results, evaluations that are necessary before or after discharge, the types of equipment, medications, and nutritional supplements that will be needed for home care, and any unmet parental teaching needs. Additionally, a list of predischarge tests should be developed at each institution and should be reviewed before each child's discharge. Guidelines may vary from institution to institution, and the tests performed should be individualized based on the

patient's history and clinical course. Tests listed in Table 59-3 can function as a guideline for the predischarge examination.

When it is decided that discharge is medically feasible, all aspects of the child's care should be assessed for ways to minimize home care needs. Attempts should be made to withdraw medications that are in the subtherapeutic range based on weight or blood levels. Medications that are no longer needed should be discontinued. Once the medication needs are established, dosage should be adjusted to an amount appropriate for the infant's weight with a buffer for weight gain included. Repeat blood levels at the new dosage should be obtained when appropriate to confirm therapeutic adequacy (e.g., Phenobarbital or caffeine). Additionally, medication schedules should be streamlined to avoid middle-of-the-night doses and to decrease the frequency of administration when possible. Many pediatric medications are difficult to obtain in some communities. To minimize these difficulties, prescriptions should be written and given to the parents several days before discharge to allow time for the local pharmacy to obtain the medications. To avoid confusion, the concentration and dosage of each medication should be written. Parents should be encouraged to bring the filled prescriptions to the hospital before discharge for a final medication teaching session.

Determination of postdischarge nutritional needs should be based on the following:

TABLE 59-3

SUGGESTED TESTS IN PREPARATION FOR DISCHARGE AFTER COMPLICATED NEONATAL COURSE[a]

Test	<1,000	<1,500	>1,500 g	Other Considerations
Ophthalmologic exam	Yes	Yes	See other	1. 1500–2000 grams with an unstable clinical course or received supplemental oxygen 2. ECMO
Audiologic evaluation	Yes	Yes	Yes	Universal screening for all infants regardless of birth wt.
Thermistor/pneumogram	See other	See other	See other	Perform if clinically indicated; consider if: 1. Recent clinical A's and B's 2. Gastroesophageal reflux
Car seat evaluation	Yes	Yes	<37 weeks	1. First hospital discharge 2. At risk of apnea or oxygen desaturation in car seat
CBC with reticulocyte count	See other	See other	See other	All infants approaching discharge
Drug levels	See other	See other	See other	All infants receiving medications requiring monitoring or blood levels
Rickets screening	Yes	See other	See other	1. Prolonged use of TPN 2. GI malabsorption 3. Cholestatic liver disease
Nephrocalcinosis	Yes	See other	See other	Any preterm infant receiving chronic furosemide therapy
Chest radiograph	See other	See other	See other	A recent chest radiograph should be obtained for those with chronic lung disease and a copy provided to the family to keep with infant records.

[a] From Bernbaum JC. Transition Care of The Preterm Infant: Essential Elements of Neonatal Discharge. Columbus, Ohio: 1999.

- Expected as opposed to actual rate of growth:
  - The infant's tolerance of the present feeding regimen just before discharge
  - The infant's ability to feed orally or the need for supplemental NG feedings
  - The presence of underlying illness that may increase metabolic demands, require fluid restriction, predispose to malabsorption, or require special nutritional formulations

When possible, fluid intake should be liberalized several days before discharge to assess the child's ability to feed orally and tolerate larger volumes of formula. If possible several days before discharge, the child should be switched to a commercially available formula that can be concentrated or have supplements added when additional calories are needed to assess tolerance of the formulation and rate of growth. If a special formula or nutritional supplements are needed, arrangements must be made far enough in advance of discharge to allow for procurement of these items. The infant who is a borderline oral feeder may avoid the need for nasogastric supplementation after discharge through the use of concentrated formula or nutritional supplements.

A careful assessment of appointments that are needed after discharge can avoid fragmentation of care. A thorough chart review can identify any services that have been involved during the hospitalization, and some of these services may have suggested continued involvement immediately before or after discharge. These appointments should be set up before discharge, and attempts made to coordinate as many as possible on the same day without overstressing the child. Remind parents that some insurance policies do not cover many of the outpatient visits or they may need a referral for the visit from the infant's primary care physician. If the child requires oxygen, CPAP, or mechanical ventilation, these needs should be identified so that support can be provided during the outpatient visit.

A comprehensive discharge summary aids in providing continuity of care between the hospital and the primary care provider. The summary should include the following:

- Birth weight, gestational age, Apgar scores, and date of birth
- Significant prenatal and delivery history
- Summary of hospital course, including
  - Severity of respiratory illness
  - Type and length of ventilatory support
  - Significant neurologic insults
  - Any surgical procedures
  - Complete list of diagnoses
- Results of screening tests
- Immunizations given and dates
- List of problems remaining at the time of discharge
- Discharge medications and dosages and recent blood levels when applicable
- Relevant social history
- Need for therapeutic interventions (physical, occupational, speech/feeding, or educational services)

- Home equipment needs
- Need for specialized nursing interventions

Careful planning and coordination of all aspects of an infant's care form the most challenging part of a successful discharge. When health care providers anticipate postdischarge needs and work in collaboration with the child's family to meet those needs, the quality of care should remain unchanged during the transition from hospital to home.

REFERENCES

1. Hack M, Weissman B, Borawski-Clark E. Catch-up growth during childhood among very low-birth-weight children. *Arch Pediatr Adolesc Med* 1996;150:1122.
2. Seminara S, Rapisardi G, La Cauza F, et al. Catch-up growth in short-at-birth NICU graduates. *Horm Res* 2000;53:139.
3. Saigal S, Stoskopf BL, Streiner DL, et al. Physical growth and current health status of infants who were of extremely low birth weight and controls at adolescence. *Pediatrics* 2001;108:407.
4. Friedman SA, Bernbaum JC. Growth outcome of critically-ill neonates. In: Polin RA, Fox WW, eds. *Fetal and neonatal physiology*. Philadelphia: WB Saunders, 1998:394.
5. Casey P, Bernbaum JC, Kraemer HC, et al. *Growth curves for preterm infants*. Columbus, OH: Ross Products Division, Abbott Laboratories, 1995.
6. *Pediatric Nutrition Handbook*. Committee on Nutrition, American Academy of Pediatrics. Elk Grove Village, IL: American Academy of Pediatrics, 1998.
7. Innis SM, Adamkin KH, Hall RT, et al. Docosahexaenoic acid and arachidonic acid enhance growth with no adverse effects in preterm infants fed formula. *J Pediatr* 2002;140:547.
8. Fewtrell MS, Morley R, Abbott RA, et al. Double-blind, randomized trial of long-chain polyunsaturated fatty acid supplementation in formula fed to preterm infants. *Pediatrics* 2002;110:73.
9. Reimers KJ, Carlson SJ, Lombard KA. Nutritional management of infants with bronchopulmonary dysplasia. *Nutr Clin Pract* 1992;7:127.
10. Bernbaum J, Hoffman-Williamson M. *Primary care of the preterm infant*. St. Louis: Mosby Year Book, 1991.
11. Poets CF, Langner MU, Bohnhorst B. Effects of bottle feeding and two different methods of gavage feeding on oxygenation and breathing patterns in preterm infants. *Acta Paediatr* 1997; 86:419.
12. Shiao SY, Brooker J, DiFiore T. Desaturation events during oral feedings with and without a nasogastric tube in very low birth weight infants. *Heart Lung* 1996;25(3):236–245.
13. Advisory Committee on Immunization Practices (ACIP); 2002 Recommendations. *Morb Mortal Wkly Rep* 2002;51(RR02):1.
14. American Academy of Pediatrics, Committee on Infectious Diseases. In: Peter G, ed. *2000 Redbook: Report of the Committee on Infectious Diseases*, 26th ed. Elk Grove Village, IL: American Academy of Pediatrics, 2001.
15. Groothuis JR, King SJ, Hogerman DA, et al. Safety and immunogenicity of a purified F protein respiratory syncytial virus (PFP-2) vaccine in seropositive children with bronchopulmonary dysplasia. *J Infect Dis* 1998;177:467.
16. The IMpact-RSV Study Group. *Pediatrics* 1998;102:531.
17. Cryotherapy for Retinopathy of Prematurity Cooperative Group. The natural ocular outcome of premature birth and retinopathy. Status at 1 year. *Arch Ophthalmol* 1994;112:903.
18. Multicenter trial of cryotherapy for retinopathy of prematurity. The natural history ROP: ocular outcome at 5(1/2) years in premature infants with birth weights less than 1251 g. *Arch Ophthalmol* 2002;120:595.
19. Policy Statement: Screening Examination of Premature Infants for Retinopathy of Prematurity. A joint statement of the American Academy of Pediatrics, Section on Ophthalmology, American Association for Pediatric Ophthalmology and Strabismus and the American Academy of Ophthalmology. *Pediatrics* 2001; 108:809.

20. Joint Committee on Infant Hearing. Year 2000 Position Statement: principles and guidelines for early hearing detection and intervention programs. *Pediatrics* 2000;106:798–817.

21. Rescorla FJ. Surgical management of pediatric necrotizing enterocolitis. *Curr Opin Pediatr* 1995;7:335.

22. Gorrotxategi I, Eizaguirre A, Saenz de Ugarte MJ, et al. Contintinuous esophageal pH-metering in infants with gastroesophageal reflux and apparent life threatening events. *Neonatal Intensive Care* 1997;(Jan-Feb):29.

23. Orenstein SR. An overview of reflux-associated disorders in infants: apnea, laryngospasm, and aspiration. *Am J Med* 2001; 111:60S.

24. Hillemeier AC. Gastroesophageal reflux. Diagnostic and therapeutic approaches. *Pediatr Clin North Am* 1996;43:197.

25. Augood C, Gilbert R, Logan S, et al. Cisapride treatment for gastro-oesophageal reflux in children. *Cochrane Database Syst Rev* 2002;(3):CD002300.

26. Vohr B, Ment LR. Intraventricular hemorrrhage in the preterm infant. *Early Hum Dev* 1996;44:1.

27. Hanekom WA, Yageu R. Cerebrospinal fluid shunt infections. *Adv Pediatr Infect Dis* 1994;11:29.

28. Allen MC, Donohue PK, Dusman AE. The limits of viability–neonatal outcome of infants born at 22–25 weeks gestation. *N Engl J Med* 1993;329:1597.

29. Wilkinson I, Bear J, Smith J, et al. Neurological outcome of severe cystic periventricular leukomalacia. *J Pediatr Health* 1996; 32:445.

30. Olsen P, Paakko E, Vainlopa L, et al. MR imaging of periventricular leukomalacia and its clinical correlation in children. *Ann Neurol* 1997;41:754.

31. Graziani LJ, Pasto M, Stanley C, et al. Neonatal neurosonographic correlates of cerebral palsy in preterm infants. *Pediatrics* 1986; 78:88.

32. Clancy RR. Neonatal seizures. In: Stevenson DL, Sunshine P, eds. *Fetal and neonatal brain injury: mechanisms, management and the risk of practice.* Philadelphia: BC Decker, 1989:123.

33. Mizrah, EM. Neonatal seizures and neonatal epileptic syndromes. *Neurol Clin* 2001;9:427.

34. National Institutes of Health, Consensus Development Conference on Infantile Apnea and Home Monitoring, Sept 29 to Oct 1, 1986. *Pediatrics* 1987;79:292.

35. Theobald K, Botwinski C, Albanna S, et al. Apnea of prematurity: diagnosis, implications for care, and pharmacologic management. *Neonatal Netw* 2000;19:17.

36. AAP Committee on Fetus and Newborn Pediatrics. *Apnea, sudden infant death syndrome, and home monitoring.* American Academy of Pediatrics Policy Statement. Organizational principles to guide and define the child health care system and/or improve the health of all children. 2003;111:914.

37. Bhatia J. Current options in the management of apnea of prematurity. *Clin Pediatr* 2000;39:327.

38. Avery ME, Tooley WH, Keller JB, et al. Is chronic lung disease in LBW infants preventable? A survey of 8 centers. *Pediatrics* 1987; 79:26.

39. Shennan AT, Dunn MS, Ohlsson A, et al. Abnormal pulmonary outcomes in premature infants: prediction from oxygen requirement in the neonatal period. *Pediatrics* 1988;82:327.

40. Abman SH, Woolfe RR, Acccurso FJ, et al. Pulmonary vascular response to oxygen in infants with severe BPD. *Pediatrics* 1985;75:80.

41. Poets CF. When do infants need additional inspired oxygen? A review of the current literature. *Pediatr Pulmonol* 1998;26:424.

42. Chronic Lung Disease. In: Bernbaum J, ed. *Preterm infants in primary care: a guide to office management.* Columbus, OH. 2000:3:4.

43. Yeh TF, McClenan DA, Ajayi OA, et al. Metabolic rate and energy balance in infants with BPD. *J Pediatr* 1989;114:448.

44. Bernbaum JC, Pererra GR, Watkins JB, et al. Non-nutritive sucking during gavage feeding enhances growth and maturation in premature infants. *Pediatrics* 1983;71:41.

45. Bernbaum JC. *Transition care of the preterm infant: essential elements of neonatal discharge.* Columbus, OH, 1999.

Developmental Outcome

Forrest C. Bennett

More than 300,000 low-birth-weight infants (LBW; ≤2,500 grams) are born each year in the United States, constituting approximately 7.5% of all live births. Of these infants, approximately 60,000 annually are of very low birth weight (VLBW; ≤1,500 grams), constituting approximately 1.5% of all births. Because the estimated LBW incidence has remained relatively stable over the past 40 years and actually increased over the past 15 years (Fig. 60-1), contemporary reductions in neonatal mortality are steadily increasing the prevalence of biologically vulnerable infants and children in the overall population (1).

Although much medical, legal, ethical, and economic debate continues to occur over the effects of neonatal intensive care on the long-term developmental status of LBW survivors, most investigators are in agreement that the single clearest outcome of this technically enhanced care has been a dramatic and continuing reduction in neonatal mortality since the early 1960s, particularly for VLBW infants since the mid-1970s (Fig. 60-1) (2,3). With current standards of practice in the neonatal intensive care unit (NICU), many more LBW premature infants are surviving to be discharged home after extended hospitalizations than was the case even 5 to 10 years ago. The major factors responsible for this increased survival include the more widespread use of antenatal steroids in situations of anticipated premature birth; the technical ability to provide assisted mechanical ventilation to the smallest of LBW infants; the regionalization of perinatal-neonatal care, with greater numbers of maternal transports to and infants born in tertiary centers; and the widespread use of exogenous surfactant.

Remarkable improvements in the birth-weight–specific mortality rates accounted for 90% of the overall decline in neonatal mortality between 1960 and 1980 (4). During these two decades, decreases in the mortality rates of infants weighing between 1,500 and 2,500 grams contributed more than any other weight group because of both greater proportional decreases and higher absolute declines in mortality; however, there has been steady and statistically significant reduction in mortality rates among VLBW infants throughout the last 20 to 25 years. Mortality for infants with birth weights of 1,001 to 1,500 grams has fallen from more than 50% in 1961 to less than 10% today. Moreover, the most substantial improvement of the 1980s over the 1970s in neonatal mortality rates was in the 751 to 1,000-gram birth-weight group (5). This improvement continued between 1995 and 2000 with these infants having greater than an 85% chance of surviving today if they are admitted to an NICU (6). Finally, in the 1990s and beyond, 40% to more than 60% survival for infants between 500 and 750 grams is being accomplished even though the percent change between 1995 and 2000 was less than that for infants between 751 and 1,000 grams (6–9). The intact survival of a 380-g infant has been described (10).

Although survival continues to increase in all LBW categories, the greatest impact of neonatal intensive care technology clearly has been on the smallest, sickest, and most medically fragile infants. The success in achieving these improved survival rates for LBW premature infants raises obvious concerns about the subsequent development of such vulnerable infants. It mandates an organized neurodevelopmental follow-up approach to carefully and continuously monitor the quality of survival of the NICU graduate.

ORGANIZATION OF A HIGH-RISK INFANT FOLLOW-UP PROGRAM

Objectives

There are a number of compelling reasons for conducting longitudinal neurodevelopmental surveillance of survivors of neonatal intensive care. There also are practical problems

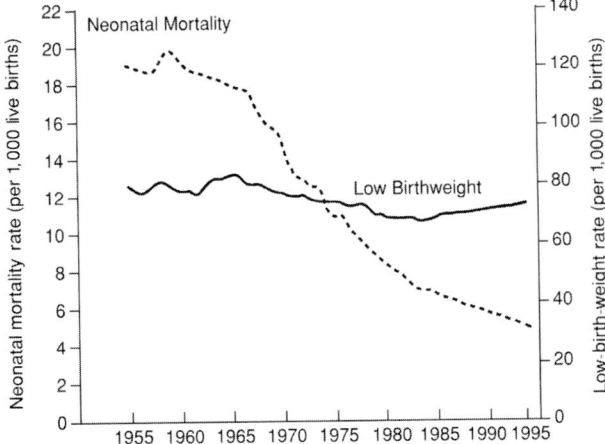

Figure 60-1 United States annual rates of neonatal mortality and low-birth-weight births from 1955 to 2000. (Adapted from Lee KS, Paneth N, Gartner LM, et al. Neonatal mortality: an analysis of the recent improvement in the United States. *Am J Public Health* 1980;70:15–21, with permission.)

encountered in providing comprehensive follow-up services. Individual follow-up programs must clearly define their own goals and objectives and then organize their roles and activities accordingly. A community hospital's follow-up efforts likely will be determined by a different set of expectations than those of a university-affiliated tertiary care center. Furthermore, ideal follow-up care in the United States frequently is constrained by limited resources. In general, follow-up programs are designed to meet one or more of the following objectives.

Quality Control

Regular, periodic follow-up of a large proportion of survivors can provide one type of audit of an individual NICU's performance. Because intensive care nurseries differ in such critical management areas as neonatal resuscitation, modes of assisted ventilation, treatment of ventriculomegaly, and use of parenteral nutrition, and also in such neonatal outcomes as mortality and prevalence of medical complications (e.g., bronchopulmonary dysplasia [BPD], intracranial hemorrhage), units may wish to compare their neurodevelopmental morbidity with the contemporary experience of similar nurseries (11). They also may wish to monitor their major disabling morbidities from year to year to detect any significant differences that might accompany further reductions in mortality or the introduction of new intensive care procedures or treatments. It must be recognized that follow-up at 1 or 2 years of age, although providing much useful information about the prevalence of major neurosensory impairment among survivors, is of insufficient duration to identify changes over time in more subtle aspects of brain function, such as learning and behavior.

Developmental Services

Neurodevelopmental follow-up can provide important ongoing subspecialty care to at-risk children and families.

Follow-up clinic personnel with a multidisciplinary approach will likely have the most experience and expertise in a given community concerning the unique developmental patterns of LBW premature infants. In general, the follow-up program should complement and serve as secondary or tertiary developmental consultants to the primary health care providers. The program will encourage and facilitate the establishment of a community-based medical home (e.g., private practitioner, public health clinic) for every medically complex survivor. Experience with biologically and environmentally vulnerable indigent populations, however, suggests that actual provision of primary health care, in addition to evaluation and case management services, may be necessary in some situations to prevent attrition and maintain contact with those children and families at greatest long-term risk (12). Although the appropriate approach to this issue of role definition is likely to vary with different populations and access to medical care in different settings, it obviously is of fundamental importance to the organization of follow-up clinics and also to the maintenance of mutual trust relationships with the primary care community.

The specific objectives of follow-up neurodevelopmental assessment activities may be grouped conveniently as follows: to provide cautious reassurance to anxious parents; to ensure early identification and intervention for persistent developmental abnormalities; and to recognize the natural history of transient developmental abnormalities and thereby avoid unnecessary, costly interventions. Maintaining an appropriate balance of diagnostic and reassurance functions is one of the greatest challenges for the contemporary high-risk follow-up program.

Developmental Training

The follow-up clinic provides a marvelous setting for interdisciplinary developmental training. It is a clinical laboratory for the observation of the gradual recovery and normalization over time of most at-risk infants and, in other cases, the gradual evolution of a wide variety of permanent neurodevelopmental dysfunctions. Thus, the at-risk population offers a longitudinal training experience that spans the normal-abnormal development continuum. In many pediatric training programs, the follow-up clinic is the sole opportunity for pediatric residents to observe the outcomes of their own intensive care efforts. It would seem virtually impossible for physicians to be informed adequately about the ethical debates and dilemmas surrounding neonatal intensive care without a first-hand follow-up experience. Likewise, other child development professionals (e.g., psychologists, physical therapists, communication disorders specialists) can use the follow-up clinic profitably as a diverse training base, particularly to broaden the range of normative development for their students. Obviously, these training objectives will apply primarily to university-affiliated tertiary care centers, with their numerous and varied trainee availability.

Outcome Research

The university-affiliated follow-up program should be engaged actively in clinical research that contributes to the understanding of the neurodevelopmental and neurobehavioral outcomes of children who experienced neonatal intensive care. These studies may take the form of either descriptive observational reports or clinical trials of specific perinatal-neonatal interventions. For example, the University of Washington's High-Risk Infant Follow-Up Program has published studies describing the outcome of infants weighing less than 800 g at birth (13–15), as well as studies evaluating the utility of procedures such as electronic fetal monitoring of premature labor and delivery (16) and treatments such as high-frequency mechanical ventilation (17). Although tremendous variability exists in the target populations, methodologies, and general scientific quality of the accumulated high-risk follow-up research, a growing consensus of valid outcome observations gradually has emerged over the last 30 years, and informative summary conclusions can be synthesized. Even though the ideal, population-based, nonrisk-controlled, longitudinal to school age study rarely is accomplished for a variety of practical reasons (e.g., cost, subject mobility, investigator discontinuity), individual follow-up investigations, carefully performed with a limited scope, continue to modify and refine overall knowledge and, in some cases, challenge assumptions.

This is not to say that broad, well-funded, collaborative follow-up efforts should not be pursued vigorously on both regional and national, and even international, levels. A recognized need for uniform population descriptions, standardized assessment protocols, common disability definitions, and adequate numbers of pooled subjects still exists. Threats to the interpretability and generalizability of small, local studies include population demographic bias, neonatal treatment differences, attrition of highest-risk (i.e., doubly vulnerable) subjects, and cross-sectional data analysis combining multiple age end points. A great deal has been learned about the short- and long-term prognoses of NICU survivors from hundreds of independent follow-up studies, but much more has yet to be clarified by enhanced research approaches (18).

Personnel

The size and complexity of the neurodevelopmental follow-up team depend on the scope of the program and size of the patient population. For example, a level II to III community hospital with primarily developmental service objectives will likely employ a smaller team, follow for a shorter period of time, and administer fewer standardized measures than a university-affiliated tertiary care center with training and research responsibilities. In either case, certain key tasks must be accomplished. Probably the most critical role in terms of maximizing follow-up compliance and minimizing attrition is that of the follow-up coordinator, usually a program nurse. This person is the liaison

between the NICU and follow-up clinic. The nurse coordinator can identify and meet eligible infants and families before they leave the nursery, participate in the discharge conference and transition plans, and, in some cases, make preliminary contact with the family by means of a home visit before the initial follow-up evaluation. This liaison function is particularly important in those programs that conduct high-risk follow-up at a separate site away from the intensive care nursery and in which none of the follow-up personnel is actively involved in the NICU.

Overall program direction is typically provided by a physician or psychologist. This person ultimately is responsible both for meeting the broad programmatic objectives and also for day-to-day operations. The director of a university-affiliated follow-up program frequently must balance competing service, training, and research obligations while eclectically maintaining sufficient funding sources to ensure long-term program viability. The director certainly should be knowledgeable in terms of current follow-up literature and contemporary models of program structure and function.

Other follow-up roles of the interdisciplinary team include the following:

Medical-neurologic assessment. This may be provided by a neonatologist, developmental pediatrician, or child neurologist. In some programs, a pediatric nurse practitioner or the nurse coordinator may provide health, nutritional, and behavioral guidance pertaining especially to such issues as feeding, sleeping, temperament, and discipline.

Developmental-intellectual-academic achievement assessment. This often will be performed by a physical therapist during infancy and by a clinical psychologist or psychometrist thereafter. Some tertiary centers may use a neuropsychologist at school age. In some programs, an early childhood educator or infant developmental specialist participates in early assessments.

Neuromotor assessment. This usually will be done by a physical therapist during the first years of life when gross motor concerns are paramount, and then by an occupational therapist during the preschool and school years when fine motor concerns predominate.

Language-speech assessment. In many follow-up programs, this responsibility is assumed by the psychologist. Some programs have the necessary personnel and funding resources to use a communication disorders specialist on a regular basis.

Family assessment. The increasingly important task of evaluating and monitoring the home parenting environment may be performed by a social worker, clinical nurse specialist, or both. As the number of dysfunctional families in the NICU setting steadily increases because of such prevalent influences as poverty, single parenthood, and prenatal substance abuse, so does the requirement of follow-up programs increase for qualified psychosocial personnel.

Hearing assessment. The adequate ability to assess hearing at any age by a clinical audiologist is imperative for tertiary follow-up programs. Both electrophysiologic and behavioral audiometric procedures should be available.

Visual assessment. A pediatric ophthalmologist should be readily accessible for consultation to the follow-up program, particularly for extremely low-birth-weight (ELBW; ≤1,000 grams birth weight) infants.

Patient Selection

Once again, the goals, objectives, personnel, and resources of an individual follow-up program will combine to determine the proportion and nature of at-risk survivors who can be served. Since it usually is impossible for a program to follow all infants receiving neonatal intensive care, somewhat arbitrary risk criteria generally are established to provide broad follow-up guidelines (19). In light of the variation and imperfection of assigned risk factors in accurately predicting neurodevelopmental outcome, a follow-up program is wise to adopt a flexible, rather than rigid, approach to the issue of eligibility. In general, a follow-up program will target the smallest and sickest NICU graduates to maximize the likely necessity of its services. Different levels of follow-up priority (e.g., high, medium, low) frequently are used to structure the selection and longitudinal monitoring process. University-affiliated follow-up programs conducting specific clinical research will tailor patient selection according to study requirements.

Common risk criteria for follow-up include the following factors:

- VLBW: In smaller programs with limited personnel and resources, the birth weight criterion may, by necessity, be arbitrarily lowered to 1,250, 1,200, or even 1,000 grams.
- Small for gestational age (SGA): Most programs strive to include infants whose weight or head circumference at birth was more than two standard deviations below the mean for gestational age.
- BPD: Programs will vary on the required duration of mechanic ventilation and oxygen administration.
- Neuroimaging abnormalities: This criterion typically will include such findings as severe intracranial hemorrhage (e.g., large intraventricular hemorrhage, intraparenchymal hemorrhage), severe ventriculomegaly, or extensive cystic periventricular leukomalacia.
- Prolonged seizures or other abnormal neurologic behavior: This includes those infants who continue to demonstrate an atypical neurologic examination at the time of nursery discharge.
- Central nervous system infection: The targeted infection may have occurred during the intrauterine, intrapartum, or neonatal time period.
- Miscellaneous perinatal-neonatal events of potential neurodevelopmental significance: Most programs will prioritize infants who have experienced to a severe degree such complications as asphyxia, hyperbilirubinemia, hypoglycemia, or polycythemia. Specific threshold determinations will vary from program to program. Table 60-1

TABLE 60-1

RISK FACTORS FOR MAJOR NEUROLOGIC AND COGNITIVE SEQUELAE IN SURVIVING INFANTS REQUIRING NEONATAL INTENSIVE CARE

Birth Weight (g)	Risk Factor	Category (%)
>2,500	All admissions	<5
	Respiratory distress syndrome	5
	Postasphyxia seizure	30–50
	Meningitis	30–50
1,501–2,500	All admissions	10
	Small for gestational age	<10
	Respiratory distress syndrome	<10
	Bronchopulmonary dysplasia	20–30
	Postasphyxia seizure	30–50
	Meningitis	30–50
1,000–1,500	All admissions	10–30
	Appropriate for gestational age, nonventilated	10–15
	Appropriate for gestational age, ventilated	30–40
	Small for gestational age	30–50
	Seizures, decerebrate posture	75–80
<1,000	All admissions	10–40

Adapted from Fitzhardinge PM. Follow-up studies of the high-risk newborn. In: Avery Gb, ed. *Neonatology: pathophysiology and management of the newborn,* 2nd ed. Philadelphia: JB Lippincott, 1981:353–370, with permission

quantifies the major neurodevelopmental risk associated with many of these follow-up inclusion criteria.

Many states use or are developing some type of comprehensive high-risk tracking or screening system to monitor the growth and development of biologically vulnerable infants (20). In some states (e.g., Iowa, North Carolina, Washington), this broadly based tracking system serves as an initial screen to identify those infants and toddlers who merit complete, tertiary developmental assessment. This coordinated approach to follow-up offers the advantages of tracking many more at-risk infants and families while also increasing the efficiency and appropriate use of the formal follow-up clinic.

Clinic Schedule

The schedule of evaluations conducted by the University of Washington's High-Risk Infant Follow-up Program is outlined in Table 60-2. This plan is illustrated as an example of a follow-up program with combined clinical service, training, and research objectives. Smaller hospital-based programs without training or research requirements often will be able to meet their clinical needs with different formats, shorter duration of follow-up, and fewer standardized assessments. Basic monitoring concepts applicable to all follow-up programs, however, include special attention to neuromotor development the first year, language and cognitive development the second and third years, school readiness skills between 4 and 5 years of age, and academic achievement during the early school years. In addition, attention to family function ideally should be an integral part of each clinic visit. With this developmental sequence of evaluations, timely identification of delays and dysfunctions as well as appropriate referral to community-based intervention services are optimized (21).

A frequent topic of debate concerns the calculation of assessment age for premature infants (22). Whereas most follow-up programs plan their clinic visit schedule and score their evaluation measures on the basis of fully corrected age (i.e., chronologic age minus the number of weeks premature), a number of others continue to use unadjusted chronologic age or even, in a few cases, one-half correction (i.e., chronologic age minus one-half the number of weeks premature). The reluctance to use full gestational age correction stems from a concern over the potential artificial inflation of developmental test scores and coincident underuse of early intervention services during the first several years of life. Although these are valid clinical concerns to consider when providing parental feedback and making referral decisions, the weight of the evidence in terms of the neuromaturation of premature infants favors the practice of gestational age correction, at least to 3 years of age, when monitoring the growth and development of NICU survivors.

Regardless of the scheduling mode used, all follow-up personnel must appreciate the imprecisions and variabilities of early developmental assessment. LBW premature infants may demonstrate improving developmental performance during the first years of life as they recover from perinatal-neonatal insults and chronic health impairments (e.g., BPD, necrotizing enterocolitis). Conversely, they also may demonstrate additional developmental dysfunction over time as more subtle disabilities become increasingly apparent and testable. In light of these patterns of development, health and developmental professionals who work with premature infants and their families must be aware of the hazards implicit in the high-risk concept. Parents may permanently regard their child as vulnerable, once so labeled, and contribute to a self-fulfilling prophecy. There can be an overzealous tendency in well-intended follow-up programs to presume the presence of abnormality rather than normality, despite the evidence of more optimistic outcome data to the contrary. In fact, most high-risk infants do not develop the conditions for which they are at increased statistical risk, and there frequently is a poor correlation between the severity of the neonatal course and specific neurodevelopmental outcomes for individual premature infants. There is a need for monitoring of this population with a keen awareness of, but not an expectation of, adverse sequelae. Documented developmental dysfunction certainly should not be ignored, but an initial follow-up posture of cautious optimism is appropriate in most cases.

TABLE 60-2
HIGH-RISK INFANT FOLLOW-UP CLINIC SCHEDULE

Corrected Age	Test
4 months	BSID
	MAI
	Physical and neurologic examinations
8 months[a]	BSID
	MAI
	Audiologic evaluation by visual reinforcement audiometry
	Physical and neurologic examinations
12 months	BSID
	Physical and neurologic examinations
24 months	BSID
	Physical and neurologic examinations
36 months	Stanford-binet intelligence scale
	Peabody picture vocabulary test
	Expressive language sample
	Physical and neurologic examinations
4.5 years	Wechsler preschool and primary scale of intelligence
	Peabody developmental motor scales
	Physical and neurologic examinations
6 and 8 years	Wechsler intelligence scale for children
	Peabody individual achievement test
	Physical and neurologic examinations

BSID, Bayley Scales of Infant Development; MAI, Movement Assessment of Infants.
[a] Scheduled selectively for those infants with possible neuromotor abnormalities at 4 months of age.

NEURODEVELOPMENTAL OUTCOME OF LOW-BIRTH-WEIGHT PREMATURE INFANTS

Despite contemporary reductions in LBW morbidity compared to disability rates before the introduction of neonatal intensive care, permanent neurodevelopmental problems are seen in many survivors. Such problems include major neurosensory impairments, cognitive and language delays, specific neuromotor deficits, neurobehavioral and socio-emotional abnormalities, and school dysfunction (23).

Major Neurosensory Impairments

The major neurosensory impairments associated with prematurity are cerebral palsy, particularly of the spastic diplegia type; mental retardation (i.e., intelligence quotient [IQ] more than two standard deviations below the standardized test mean; sensorineural hearing loss; and visual impairment, primarily the consequences of retinopathy of prematurity (ROP) (24). These major developmental disabilities may occur together in the same child and occasionally are complicated by progressive hydrocephalus or a chronic seizure disorder. They usually are clinically apparent by 2 years of age and vary in severity from mild to profound. Children with one or more of these major impairments generally require special educational programming and individual therapeutic intervention throughout childhood. These conditions occur two to five times more frequently in LBW compared to normal birth weight (NBW) infants. As a group, their prevalence increases with decreasing birth weight and gestational age; the disability rate in boys consistently exceeds that in girls (25). Table 60-3 provides combined prevalence estimates and ranges by birth weight group and gestational age for these chronic neurosensory impairments. The actual numbers represent a synthesis from reporting tertiary care centers in the United States, Canada, Australia, and Western Europe.

Such major morbidity statistics may be viewed either positively or negatively, or in both ways. On the one hand, the occurrence of these major sequelae is far less than initially predicted at the beginning of the NICU era, and many more nondisabled than disabled survivors (approximately 8:1) are being added to the population (26). Conversely, epidemiologic investigations appear to docu-

TABLE 60-4

PREVALENCE OF MAJOR IMPAIRMENTS IN SURVIVORS WEIGHING LESS THAN 800 G AT BIRTH AT THE UNIVERSITY OF WASHINGTON

	Major Impairment (%)
1991–1995	8/74 (11)
1986–1990	17/78 (22)
1983–1985	8/38 (21)
1977–1980	3/16 (19)

From LaPine TR, Jackson JC, Bennett FC. Outcome of infants weighing less than 800 grams at birth: 15 years' experience. *Pediatrics* 1995;96:479–483 and LaPine TR, Felix SD, Tarczy-Hornoch P, et al. Outcome trends of infants weighing less than 800 grams at birth. *J Invest Med* 1999;47:7A, with permission.

ment that reductions in LBW major morbidity have not paralleled or kept pace with reductions in LBW mortality and that the major impairment rate has changed little over the past 20 to 25 years. Actual increases in both the incidence and prevalence of major disabilities among the smallest and sickest survivors have been reported by some (27,28). Others, however, have reported a stable major morbidity rate for infants weighing less than 800 grams at birth (Table 60-4), a subgroup whose survival has dramatically increased during this time period (13–15). This encouraging observation that the overall incidence of serious neurodevelopmental deficits is remaining stable while survival continues to increase has been repeatedly corroborated even for those ELBW infants who weighed less than 750 grams at birth (9,29.32). A recent population-based study from the United Kingdom and Ireland reported a severe disability rate of almost 25% in children born at 25 or fewer weeks of gestation; nevertheless, almost 50% had no evidence of disability at a median age of 30 months (33).

Cerebral Palsy

Cerebral palsy, of varying types and severities, remains the most prevalent major developmental disability encountered in premature infants; the prevalence in VLBW infants varies between 6% and 10%, and approximately 40% of all children with cerebral palsy were born prematurely (i.e., less than 37 weeks of gestation) (34). Although both spastic (i.e., pyramidal) and athetoid (i.e., extrapyramidal) types of cerebral palsy may be encountered in NICU graduates, the spastic cerebral palsy syndromes (i.e., diplegia, hemiplegia, and quadriplegia) are the neuromuscular disorders most commonly seen in LBW infants. One specific type, spastic diplegia, in which the legs are much more affected than arms, is so strongly associated with prematurity (i.e., at least two-thirds of all children with this disorder are born before 37 weeks of gestation) that for over a century it has been referred to as "the disease of immaturity" (35). Figure 60-2 illustrates the relationship between spastic

TABLE 60-3

LOW-BIRTH-WEIGHT INFANTS WHO SURVIVE WITH ONE OR MORE MAJOR IMPAIRMENTS

Birth Weight (Gestational Age) (g)	Percent with Major Impairments (Range)
1,501–2,500 (32–36)	8 (5–20)
1,001–1,500 (28–31)	15 (5–30)
≤1,000 (<28)	25 (8–40)

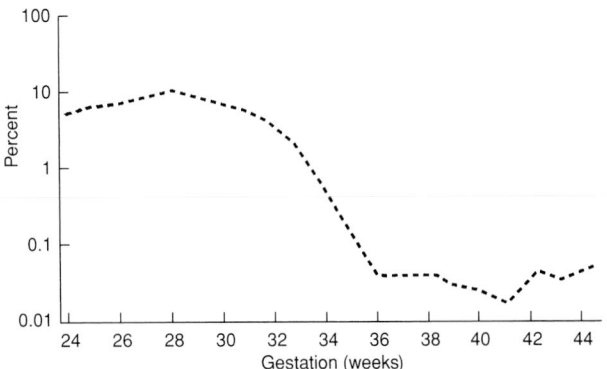

Figure 60-2 Occurrence of spastic diplegia as related to gestational age.

diplegia and gestational age. Most cases occur in a window of vulnerability in infants born between 28 and 34 weeks of gestation.

Despite the long consistency of the spastic diplegia-prematurity association, the exact etiologic factors involved often have been elusive and difficult to identify precisely prospectively (36). Neither the severity of perinatal-neonatal illness nor the presence or severity of intracranial hemorrhage reliably predicts spastic diplegia. Data derived primarily from studies correlating ultrasonographic, neuropathologic, and clinical information led to the conclusion that spastic diplegia is the clinical expression of periventricular leukomalacia and its variants (37). Periventricular leukomalacia appears to be caused, in large part, by hypoxic-ischemic injury to the periventricular white matter. The demonstration on serial cranial ultrasounds of initial extensive periventricular echodensities followed in days to weeks by large, bilateral cyst formation (i.e., periventricular white matter infarction) is highly predictive (80% to 85%) of permanent cerebral palsy, especially the spastic diplegia type (38,39). Many cases of symmetric cystic periventricular leukomalacia occur in infants with relatively benign clinical courses and are detected only by routine ultrasound screening. Premature infants born to mothers with prolonged rupture of membranes and/or chorioamnionitis seem to be at an increased risk in some studies (40) but not in others (41). Several investigators have implicated prenatal factors (e.g., intrauterine growth retardation) in the etiology of some cases of spastic diplegia. Hagberg (42) has postulated that the complex interaction of prenatal abnormalities (i.e., "fetal deprivation of supply") with perinatal difficulties in the birth process and the adjustment to the extrauterine environment may constitute a common pathogenetic mechanism of spastic diplegia. Accordingly, the etiology of spastic diplegia frequently is multifactorial, and all LBW infants merit close neuromotor monitoring during the first 2 years of life, regardless of the severity of their nursery course.

In contrast, development of the more severe spastic quadriplegia type of cerebral palsy, in which all four extremities are equally affected, often can be predicted better in NICU graduates on the basis of specific perinatal or neonatal events, including asphyxia, marked bilateral

intraventricular hemorrhage with ventriculomegaly, prolonged neonatal seizures, and central nervous system infection. Although most premature children with spastic diplegia have average or near average mental abilities, children with spastic quadriplegia are far more likely also to have serious cognitive impairments. Spastic hemiplegia, in which only one side is affected, with the arm usually more than the leg, often is heralded by the ultrasonographic appearance of a unilateral, periventricular hemorrhagic infarction with subsequent cystic transformation that occurs in association with and presumably as a result of substantial asymmetric intraventricular hemorrhage (37).

Cerebral palsy typically presents over time in a developmental manner. Thus, very early neurologic signs and symptoms may prove to be transient in nature and not indicative of eventual cerebral palsy. Conversely, infants may initially appear asymptomatic with a relatively normal neurologic examination at the time of nursery discharge and even for several months thereafter, particularly in the cases of spastic diplegia and spastic hemiplegia, only to manifest clearly evident cerebral palsy by 1 year of age. Premature infants with evolving cerebral palsy reveal increasing neuromotor abnormalities of muscle tone, movement, posture, and reflex activity, particularly between 6 and 18 months of corrected age, in combination with increasingly delayed motor milestones.

Mental Retardation

Mental retardation, as defined by a standardized intelligence or developmental quotient consistently more than two standard deviations below the test mean for corrected age, often occurs in conjunction with one or more of the other major handicaps, especially cerebral palsy. In fact, severe mental retardation and severe cerebral palsy share associated perinatal-neonatal risk factors. Evidence suggests some increase in the prevalence of severely multihandicapped children after increased VLBW survival (28). Mental retardation occurs in 4% to 5% of VLBW infants followed longitudinally to school age. Isolated mental retardation, without cerebral palsy, is a reported consequence of severe BPD, particularly in cases of greatly prolonged duration of mechanic ventilation and oxygen administration (43,44).

Hearing Impairment

NICU graduates are at increased risk for both sensorineural and conductive hearing loss. Although the risk of sensorineural loss sufficient to require hearing aids, special education, and nonvocal communication strategies (60 to 100 dB) usually is estimated to be 2% to 3% for VLBW infants, some investigators have reported prevalence estimates between 5% and 9% coincident with the increased survival of more vulnerable infants (45). Exposure to ototoxic drugs, infections, hypoxia/ischemia, and hyperbilirubinemia are among the interacting and cumulative factors contributing to the risk of sensorineural loss. The duration and extent of hyperbilirubinemia in VLBW infants has been examined carefully. de Vries and colleagues (46) found bilirubin levels in excess of 14 mg/dL to be associated with a high risk of deafness in VLBW infants but not in healthy premature infants with a birth weight greater than 1,500 grams. Others also have emphasized the potential ototoxicity of hyperbilirubinemia in VLBW infants in combination with hypoxia, acidosis, and prolonged administration of multiple ototoxic medications such as the aminoglycoside antibiotics and furosemide. These investigators conclude that the additive effects of protracted illness plus its associated treatments, independent of specific diagnostic categories, constitute important risk factors for permanent hearing loss in this population (47).

There is ample evidence that infants of all birth weights who sustain severe persistent pulmonary hypertension of the newborn comprise a particularly high-risk subgroup for sensorineural hearing loss, with prevalence estimates ranging from 20% to 40% (48). In some cases, the loss is progressive during the first 3 years of life. The exact mechanism of insult remains unclear in this population of infants who typically experience prolonged hypoxia, severe acute and chronic lung disease, and multiple aggressive interventions. Another concern has been the potential deleterious effect of prolonged incubator noise on hearing function. Abramovich and associates (49) found no evidence for this hypothesis in VLBW infants. Many of the risk factors associated with hearing impairment also are associated with cerebral palsy, and these two disabilities often occur together in the same child.

Mild and moderate (25 to 59 dB) sensorineural hearing losses, sufficient to contribute to delayed language development but compatible with oral communication, also occur with increased frequency (6% to 8%) in LBW infants. Previously unrecognized unilateral sensorineural hearing losses, with adverse language and learning consequences, may become apparent in the older child (50). A high prevalence (20% to 30%) of chronic otitis media with middle ear effusion and fluctuating, conductive hearing loss greater than 25 dB is reported in LBW premature infants (51). Suggested mechanisms for this relationship focus on probable eustachian tube dysfunction initiated by a combination of dolichocephalic head shape, muscular hypotonia, and prolonged nasotracheal intubation.

There have been important advances in the hearing assessment of LBW infants. Two techniques in particular, electrophysiologic auditory brainstem response (ABR) audiometry and behavioral visual reinforcement audiometry, have made early, reliable detection of hearing loss in the NICU graduate clinically feasible. Centers that routinely screen high-risk, LBW infants with ABR before nursery discharge report a false-positive rate of 8% to 10% compared to follow-up testing at 4 months of age (52). Conversely, the unanticipated appearance of severe sensorineural hearing loss in high-risk survivors of neonatal intensive care after having passed an initial ABR screening test in the newborn period has been reported (53). It also must be recognized that ABR tests only the high sound

frequencies (i.e., 2,000 Hz and above) and will not detect hearing losses confined to the lower frequencies. Thus, clinicians must remember that determinations of the adequacy of hearing made only with ABR test data before nursery discharge are subject to error. Visual reinforcement audiometry is an operant conditioning technique that reliably can provide auditory thresholds for infants who are functioning at a developmental age of approximately 6 months or older. It has great utility in the high-risk follow-up clinic. A third and newer audiologic procedure, evoked otoacoustic emissions, is of use in newborn screening in conjunction with ABR (54).

Visual Impairment

The major cause of visual loss in LBW infants is retrolental fibroplasia, now included under the rubric of ROP. With controlled oxygen administration, ROP was relatively rare until the last 15 years or so, when significant numbers of extremely premature infants began to survive. The name ROP recognizes that immaturity at birth is the single largest risk factor for this disease. For all practical purposes, this is a disorder of the VLBW infant. Virtually no retinal detachment and little retinal scarring is described in larger premature infants. For the entire VLBW population, current prevalence estimates range from 20% to 25% with early-stage, regressed ROP; 5% to 10% with more advanced-stage, scarred ROP; and 2% to 4% with major visual impairments, including legal blindness and requiring special educational assistance. The distribution of visually impaired infants, however, is skewed heavily toward those weighing 1,000 grams or less at birth. In these ELBW infants, regressed ROP occurs in 40% to 50% of survivors, scarred ROP in 10% to 25%, and major visual impairments in 5% to 10%. Figure 60-3 shows the overall prevalence of ROP by birth weight. These estimates continue to apply with a greater than 80% prevalence for infants of 26 or fewer weeks' gestational age.

Alteration of normal retinal vascular development is the hallmark of ROP. Although a great deal of effort has been

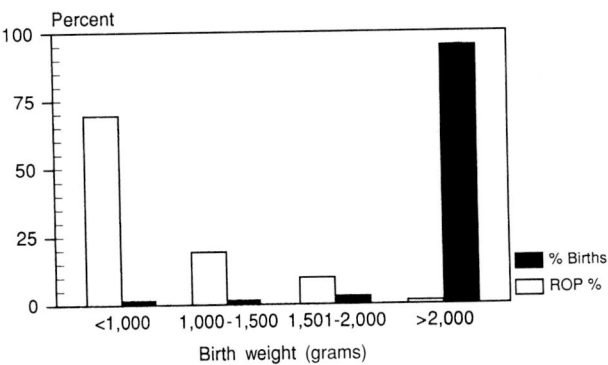

Figure 60-3 Percentage of retinopathy of prematurity (ROP) by birth weight versus proportion of births by birth weight. (From Glass P, Avery GB, Subramanian KNS, et al. Effect of bright light in the hospital nursery on the incidence of retinopathy of prematurity. *N Engl J Med* 1985;313:401–404, with permission.)

invested in clinical and animal studies of ROP, there remains an etiologic maze in which no single factor stands alone (55). It appears that the embryonic retina of the small premature infant, developing outside the uterus, is vulnerable to many sources that can disrupt orderly differentiation and vascularization. In addition to the well-known impact of hyperoxia, it seems that hypoxia, variations in arterial carbon dioxide pressure, pH, retinal oxygen consumption, light exposure, and other factors that affect retinal perfusion all may play a role. A formula for ROP could be: immaturity (always) + oxygen (often) + other factors (variably) = ROP (56). Simply stated, the smallest and sickest newborns have the most complications that potentially can impede retinal function, and they also have the most ROP.

Even regressed ROP is associated with an increased risk for refractive errors, amblyopia, and strabismus. "Myopia of prematurity," even without ROP, has been described to occur in approximately one-third of surviving ELBW infants (57). It is considered to be mostly lenticular in origin and to improve slowly, but not completely, throughout childhood, with slight visual acuity differences still apparent in early adulthood. Strabismus may represent an isolated problem or, in some cases, may be an initial indication of a generalized neuromotor problem such as cerebral palsy. Visual and hearing impairments may coexist, and prematurity is the leading cause of children with both deficits. Monitoring of eye muscle balance and alignment and visual acuity should be part of routine follow-up of the premature infant, particularly during the preschool years. Required interventions may include eye muscle surgery, antisuppression patching, or corrective lenses.

Progressive Hydrocephalus

Depending on the reporting center, between 20% and 40% of VLBW infants have neonatal ultrasonographic evidence of intracranial hemorrhage, frequently including intraventricular hemorrhage with ventriculomegaly (11). Whereas older reports indicated discouragingly high rates of posthemorrhagic hydrocephalus, subsequent reports described a much lower prevalence (2% to 4%) of progressive hydrocephalus requiring ventriculoperitoneal shunting in VLBW infants (58,59). Serial scanning with cranial ultrasonography has revealed that most cases of early ventriculomegaly either spontaneously resolve or arrest. Interventions (e.g., repeated lumbar puncture, ventricular taps) to prevent the transition from relatively asymptomatic ventriculomegaly to progressive hydrocephalus appear to be unnecessary. Surgical ventriculostomy drainage is frequently employed as a temporizing procedure in more advanced cases.

For the infant in whom posthemorrhagic progressive hydrocephalus does develop, it generally becomes clinically evident between 2 and 8 weeks of age; however, appearance during late infancy occasionally has been reported. Vigilance in measurement of the head circumference at each follow-up examination of the infant is important, and obtaining a cranial ultrasound, if head growth becomes substantially out of proportion to the other growth parameters, may be indicated. Although the initial months of life are the time when progressive hydrocephalus is most likely to develop in premature infants, it also is the period of time when the normal phenomenon of catch-up head growth in these recovering infants becomes most apparent. Thus, increase in head circumference relative to weight and length usually is an anticipated sign rather than a pathologic one, and such awareness should guide clinical investigative decisions. When progressive hydrocephalus does occur, neurodevelopmental outcome is frequently, although not invariably, abnormal, complicated by one or more of the major disabilities (e.g., cerebral palsy, mental retardation, sensory impairments) (60).

Minor Impairments

Although major disabling sequelae are by far the easiest to quantify and report, a large and persuasive body of long-term follow-up studies clearly indicates that a broad spectrum of cognitive, behavioral, and other minor neurodevelopmental and neurobehavioral sequelae are substantially more prevalent in surviving LBW, premature infants. These morbidities become increasingly apparent in a variety of clinical manifestations with increasing age, particularly during the first 6 years of life. These early, often subtle, developmental and behavioral delays and differences are not necessarily outgrown but frequently portend future school dysfunction and may therefore become major impediments to normal academic and social progress. Collectively, these problems often are referred to as the "new morbidity" of prematurity, reflecting their more insidious nature and more intense scrutiny in recent years (24). Recent studies have documented the persistence of these differences into adolescence and young adulthood (61,62).

Specific types of developmental morbidities described in LBW cohorts include cognitive delays (i.e., lower IQ), speech and language disorders, persistent neuromotor abnormalities, including difficulties with balance and coordination, and perceptual problems. Specific areas of suboptimal behavioral style and performance include neonatal behavior, infant and toddler temperament, emotional maturity, social competence, and selective attention. As with major impairments, the overall prevalence of these minor sequelae increases with decreasing birth weight and gestational age and also is greater in male survivors. Prevalence estimates in VLBW infants vary between 15% and 25%. Accordingly, when the 15% to 20% major disability rate is combined, between 35% and 45% of VLBW survivors demonstrate a residual developmental or behavioral problem that compromises their anticipated function (63). Recent estimates for ELBW infants are in excess of 50% (64). As with major impairments, most of the minor developmental morbidities associated with LBW and prematurity also are related to the severity of perinatal-neonatal illness. That is, LBW infants who experience a prolonged hospital course with many medical complications have an increased likelihood of developing some type of developmental dysfunction. Thus, the smallest and sickest infants, particularly those ELBW new survivors of the 1990s, are the most vulnerable to experience these problems.

In the hundreds of outcome studies across multiple developmental and behavioral domains, a consistent finding is that, regardless of the measures used, groups of premature children are less competent and score less well than groups of full-term children (26). However, this does not mean that individual premature children will invariably be less capable than individual full-term children. Despite the large number of significant group associations in follow-up studies, individual developmental outcome remains very difficult to predict prospectively with accuracy in the NICU, and infants with apparently similar neonatal courses may develop entirely differently.

Cognitive and Perceptual Development

Consistent deficits in performance on intelligence measures repeatedly have been observed and reported in LBW premature children compared to NBW full-term children (65,66). Furthermore, these differences in cognitive development become apparent in the first years of life and then persist and increase during the preschool and early school years even when the single most powerful predictor of IQ—socioeconomic status—is adequately controlled. In other words, significant deficits in cognitive and perceptual functions occur frequently even in middle to upper-middle social class children born prematurely, particularly compared to their full-term peers. This important and academically relevant group difference exists despite the fact that most LBW children will have measured IQs within the average range (23). Encouragingly, improvement in verbal and IQ test scores throughout early and middle childhood has recently been reported in a large cohort of VLBW infants followed over time (67).

Cognitive developmental differences between premature and full-term infants have been reported in early infancy. Rose (68) investigated the effect of increasing familiarization time on the visual recognition memory of 6- and 12-month-old premature and full-term infants. Whereas the older infants showed evidence of recognition memory after less familiarization time than the younger ones, premature infants at both ages required considerably longer familiarization times (i.e., more practice) than did full-term infants. These results suggest that there are persistent differences between premature and full-term infants throughout at least the first year of life in a very fundamental aspect of cognition, namely, visual information processing.

Because manipulative exploration of objects may be important to the infant's perception and conceptualization of objects, Ruff and colleagues (69) studied this developmental function in both premature and full-term 9-month-old infants by means of coded and scored videotapes. The videotapes were scored for behaviors such as looking, handling, mouthing, turning the object around, transferring the object from hand to hand, and banging. A high-risk subgroup of premature infants, based on neonatal compli-cations, manipulated the objects significantly less than either the low-risk premature or full-term infants. There was a relationship between manipulative exploration at 9 months and later cognitive functioning at 24 months.

LBW cognitive deficits have been described from the earliest days of neonatal intensive care and even before. Using a sample of approximately 600 children born in two hospitals in Edinburgh, Scotland, in 1953 to 1955, Drillien (70) demonstrated that IQ scores decline with decreasing birth weight in the first 4 years of life. The percentage of children with IQ scores below 80 at 4 years was 29% for those under 4.5 pounds (2.0 kg), 13% for those between 4.5 and 5.5 pounds (2.5 kg), and 4% for those above 5.5 pounds. Wiener and colleagues (71), reporting on a sample of 417 eight- to ten-year-old LBW children who had been tested with the Wechsler Intelligence Scale for Children, found that the verbal IQ, which consists of predominantly cognitive and language items; performance IQ, which consists of predominantly motor-perceptual items; and full-scale IQ, which consists of a combination of the verbal and performance scales, all showed increasing impairment with decreasing birth weight even though all subtest means remained within the average range of intelligence. Moreover, approximately twice as large a proportion of LBW children as NBW control children fell into the borderline IQ category (70 to 84), which usually is associated with special educational needs. Visual-motor-perceptual skills, as measured independently by the Bender Gestalt Test, also varied directly with birth weight. Hunt and colleagues (72) reported the following cognitive outcome proportions in a cohort of 108 VLBW children at 8 years of age: 4.6% had a very low IQ (less than 70), 13.9% had a low IQ (70 to 84), and, for those with an IQ greater than 84, 12.0% had language disability, 12.0% had performance disability, 21.4% had visual-motor disability, and 36.1% were apparently normal.

In a Vancouver, British Columbia, study of 501 LBW and 203 NBW children born between 1958 and 1965, the IQ difference between LBW and NBW groups on the Stanford-Binet Intelligence Scale was 9 points at 30 months of age and 15 points at 48 months, even after exclusion of children with major cerebral deficit or IQ scores under 50 or significant visual problems (65). In both the Edinburgh and Vancouver studies, the poor functioning of LBW children is convincingly exacerbated in socioeconomically disadvantaged subgroups. Table 60-5 illustrates this interaction of both biologic and environmental risk factors in the determination of measured IQ of the Vancouver study children. At both 2.5 and 4 years of age, NBW, highest-social-class children earned the highest subgroup mean IQ score, whereas LBW, lowest-social-class children earned the lowest. Both NBW and LBW groups demonstrated an IQ score continuum from the highest social class, which had the highest mean IQ, to the lowest social class, which had the lowest mean IQ, with the NBW subgroup always higher than the LBW regardless of social class; at 4 years of age, even NBW, lowest-social-class children scored higher than their LBW, highest-social-class peers.

TABLE 60-5

COMPARISON OF INTELLIGENCE QUOTIENT MEANS FOR LOW-BIRTH-WEIGHT CHILDREN VERSUS NORMAL-BIRTH-WEIGHT CONTROLS WITHIN SOCIAL CLASS GROUPS

Hollingshead Social Class	Statistic	30 Months of Age		48 Months of Age	
		IQ	Number	IQ	Number
I, II, III	LBW mean ± SD	97.0 ± 15.1	48	99.5 ± 13.7	67
	Control mean ± SD	108.8 ± 8.2	19	118.3 ± 11.4	26
	Difference ± SE	11.8 ± 2.9		18.8 ± 2.8	
	p	<0.001		<0.001	
IV	LBW mean ± SD	91.7 ± 10.7	59	94.3 ± 11.3	100
	Control mean ± SD	102.9 ± 12.6	43	110.0 ± 16.8	58
	Difference ± SE	11.2 ± 2.4		15.7 ± 2.5	
	p	<0.001		<0.001	
V	LBW mean ± SD	89.5 ± 13.9	52	90.6 ± 15.8	79
	Control mean ± SD	96.0 ± 9.7	32	102.3 ± 12.9	42
	Difference ± SE	6.5 ± 2.6		11.7 ± 2.7	
	p	<0.01		<0.001	

LBW, low birth weight; IQ determined from Stanford-Binet tests.
Adapted from McBurney AK, Eaves LC. Evolution of developmental and psychological test scores. In: Dunn HG, ed.
Sequelae of low birthweight: the Vancouver Study. Philadelphia: JB Lippincott, 1986:61, with permission.

The cognitive performance of ELBW preschool children has been the subject of more recent attention. Halsey and colleagues (73) compared predominantly white, middle-class ELBW 4-year-olds with matched full-term children and also with matched LBW children (1,500 to 2,500 grams at birth) and found both comparison groups to be 2.5 times more likely to have optimal development. Comparison children had mean cognitive scores 15 to 18 points higher than ELBW children. The investigators concluded that weaker performance on all study measures (i.e., language, motor, memory, visual-motor, perceptual) exists before school entry among nondisabled ELBW children compared with their peers. Breslau and colleagues (74) confirmed these cognitive concerns for ELBW survivors in describing a gradient relationship between LBW and IQ at age 6 years. They found the largest deficit in full-scale IQ in those children born weighing 1,500 grams or less, an intermediate deficit in those born weighing 1,501 through 2,000 grams, and the least pronounced deficit in those born weighing 2,001 through 2,500 grams.

Language Development

Communication skills involving auditory and visual perception, learning and conceptualizing of a verbal symbol system (i.e., language), and actual production of speech are critical to academic learning and social adjustment. Several investigations have focused exclusively on this important area of development in premature infants. Zarin-Ackerman and colleagues (75) noted both receptive and expressive language deficiencies at 2 years of age in a group of children born as at-risk (i.e., predominantly premature) infants compared to others born as healthy, full-term infants. They emphasized that these deficits could not be a function of social class, which is a major factor influencing language development, because this variable was controlled. In Switzerland, Largo and associates (76) compared 114 premature children to 97 healthy, full-term children throughout the first 5 years of life. Most stages of language development occurred at slightly later ages among the premature children than among those born at term. Birth weight and gestational age were negatively correlated with language development at all ages. Perinatal-neonatal complications also were significantly negatively correlated with the ages at which the stages of language development were reached, and also with final language performance at 5 years of age. There were no significant differences in socioeconomic status between the premature and full-term groups. The particular demographics of this unique study allowed the authors to conclude that biomedical factors exert a considerable effect on the early language development of premature children and that this effect is greater than previously had been recognized (76).

Several smaller studies have confirmed the existence of linguistic dysfunctions among premature children, particularly those with complicated neonatal courses (77,78). On the basis of a wide variety of measures, inferior performance has been reported consistently in receptive language or comprehension, expressive language parameters such as vocabulary and word finding, and speech qualities such as articulation and fluency.

Motor Development

Numerous studies from several continents repeatedly have documented that the neuromotor development of LBW premature infants during the first 2 years of life is different, more delayed, and generally more worrisome than that of healthy, full-term infants. Premature developmental scores, using such measures as the Bayley Scales of Infant Development, are consistently and significantly below those of full-term infants at 12 months of corrected age, and premature motor scores also usually are 10 to 15 points (i.e., practically one standard deviation) below premature mental scores at this age (79).

This phenomenon of transiently abnormal neuromotor signs in the first years of life was described initially by Drillien (80), in a 1972 report from Scotland, as "transient dystonia of low birth weight infants.". Drillien reported that its prevalence during the first half of infancy varied inversely with birth weight, involving approximately 35% of infants weighing 1,501 to 2,000 grams at birth and 60% to 70% of infants weighing 1,500 grams or less at birth, and that its prevalence also varied directly with perinatal-neonatal complications (i.e., more frequent among sick premature infants). Transient dystonia includes such neurologic findings as increased or decreased muscle tone, diminished volitional movement, retention and accentuation of primitive reflex patterns, delayed appearance of normal infantile automatic reactions, and asymmetric neuromotor development. Because these neuromotor signs also are the very signs seen in infants in whom cerebral palsy is developing, it is not surprising that a reliable diagnosis of cerebral palsy is quite difficult in most premature infants throughout early infancy. As described by Amiel-Tison (81), however, by 8 to 10 months of corrected age, most LBW infants with transient dystonia are gradually and spontaneously normalizing on examination, whereas those relatively few infants in whom permanent cerebral palsy is developing appear increasingly abnormal. With the knowledge of this common evolution of neuromotor signs, every VLBW infant can be assigned to one of three diagnostic and prognostic groups at 12 months of age: those who were always neurologically normal throughout infancy (25% to 30%); those who showed transient dystonia with subsequent normalization (65% to 70%); and those with cerebral palsy (5% to 10%).

Coolman and colleagues (82) and others have extended these observations to 24 months of age, albeit most neuromotor changes occur in the first year of life. They found that some infants with transient dystonia retained subtle, persistent neuromotor differences that would not be labeled as cerebral palsy but that represented qualitative deviations from the norm. Longitudinal studies indicate that infants who have experienced transient dystonia are far more likely to have language, learning, and behavioral problems (i.e., minimal brain dysfunction) in later childhood than are infants who never demonstrated these abnormalities (83,84). This would indicate that although transient dystonia largely resolves, these neuromotor signs in early infancy may be predictive markers for later manifestations of central nervous system disorganization.

Differences in the motor development of premature infants throughout the preschool years have been reported. Burns and Bullock (85) found premature children at 5 years of age to be significantly different from their full-term peers in terms of tremulous involuntary hand movements, less competent gross motor ability, and difficulties in postural control and balance. Crowe and associates (86) described ELBW infants as a group to have significantly inferior skills in all motor functions at 4 years of age. Symptomatic intracranial hemorrhage was associated with poorer motor performance.

Neurobehavioral Development

As LBW premature survivors are assessed more critically and at older ages, a variety of potential behavioral dysfunctions throughout infancy and childhood become evident. Numerous studies have compared the neonatal neurobehavioral performance of LBW infants to that of NBW infants. These studies typically compare premature infants at their corrected age and also tend to use premature infants with relatively uncomplicated neonatal courses. Nevertheless, despite these sampling features that might obscure group differences, premature infants consistently perform less optimally than healthy, full-term infants on these early measures.

Ferrari and colleagues (87) compared low-risk premature infants to healthy, full-term infants using the Brazelton Neonatal Behavioral Assessment Scale. They found the premature infants to be significantly inferior in sensory orientation, regulation of behavioral state (i.e., quiet-active status), and autonomic regulation. Additionally, the clustering of neurobehavioral items was more heterogeneous among premature infants. The authors concluded that prematurity itself is associated with a behavioral repertoire that is different, more variable, and on the average less competent than that of full-term infants (87). Friedman and colleagues (88), also comparing low-risk premature infants and healthy, full-term infants, found that the premature infants fussed and cried more, were less soothable, and tended to change behavioral state more frequently. They suggested that these neonatal neurobehavioral differences are potential contributors to suboptimal interaction between premature infants and their caregivers. Aylward and colleagues (89), in a report from the National Institutes of Health (NIH) Collaborative Study on Antenatal Steroid Therapy, reported significant effects of both gestational age and severity of perinatal-neonatal illness on the neurobehavioral responses of premature infants. Specifically, at 40 weeks of corrected age, premature infants born at younger gestational ages and with greater medical complications demonstrated altered behavior in terms of diminished spontaneous activity and vigor, inability to maintain and modulate responses, and poorer visual orientation capabilities.

A number of studies using a wide variety of electrophysiologic techniques have supported the results of these clinical behavioral investigations. Compared to full-term infants, premature infants have shown delayed maturation of both cortical and brainstem auditory-evoked potentials, more variable and labile behavioral state organization as measured by time-lapse videosomnography, and decreased resting heart rate variability and vagal tone (i.e., an indirect measure of overall autonomic nervous system activity) (90–93). Several of these functions, particularly state organization and autonomic regulation, have been related positively to longer-term developmental outcome (94,95).

Several studies have explored the related behavioral areas of temperament, social interaction and competence, and emotional expression and affect. Most of these studies have examined mother-infant interactions, and there is an overall consensus of findings that indicates an imbalance in LBW premature dyads compared to NBW full-term dyads, with LBW infants typically less responsive and low in communicative signaling behavior, and their mothers compensating for this relative inactivity by displaying high levels of stimulating and engaging activity. Investigations of LBW infants with complicated perinatal-neonatal courses have indicated that these infants exhibit high levels of gaze aversion, avoidance of interaction, and low levels of vocalizing and playing (96–98). Field (99) has reported these interactional differences in depth and succinctly summarizes the problem: "High-risk infants and their parents 'have less fun' than normal infants and their parents during their early interactions together." In a study comparing premature-mother dyads with full-term-mother dyads at approximately 4 months of corrected age, Field found the premature infants to be less alert and attentive, less responsive, less interested in game playing, less contingent, less smiling and content, and more affectively negative and irritable than the matched full-term infants. Correspondingly, the mothers of premature infants exhibited fewer happy expressions than the mothers of full-terms but were more vocal as they attempted to elicit social and communicative responses from their infants.

Crnic and associates (100) and Malatesta and colleagues (101) have replicated and extended these observations throughout the entire first year of life; LBW/NBW differences in expressive behavior and affect were persistent and continued to affect maternal behavior. Malatesta and colleagues emphasized that in their primarily middle to upper-middle social class sample, these differences were seen even in the absence of confounding neonatal medical complications. They speculate that the observed LBW/NBW differences probably are even more pronounced with less advantaged, more stressed, or sicker premature infants. Of long-term importance and concern is the increasing evidence of continuity between early interactional disturbances and later behavioral dysfunctions.

School Function

Finally, as increasing numbers of studies have followed LBW premature infants into the school years, the full spectrum of these children's learning and behavioral performance is emerging and becoming clearer. Although prevalence estimates of school problems vary between reports, almost all investigators agree that LBW survivors have a distinctly increased risk for school dysfunction in some form (24). A disturbing four-fold greater likelihood

than NBW children of not graduating from high school by age 19 has been reported (102). The most recent reports have focused on school-age ELBW children and consistently describe the most problematic school function of all. Again, these new survivors, although relatively small in overall number, are disproportionately represented in regard to academic and social failure. There also is general agreement that although this substantial risk exists independently of socioeconomic status, the combination and interaction of biologic and environmental risks produces an especially worrisome doubly vulnerable milieu and a highly appropriate target population for early developmental intervention efforts because of the documented importance of psychosocial variables in the ultimate prognosis for LBW premature infants (103).

Dunn and colleagues (104), in one of the most extensive longitudinal follow-up studies published, reported minimal cerebral dysfunction (i.e., minor developmental and behavioral abnormalities) to be the single most prevalent (20%) disabling syndrome at school age in a population of more than 300 LBW premature children. Furthermore, the authors stress the difficulty in adequately predicting or identifying such dysfunctions before school entry at the age of 5 years (104). This important group of sequelae consequently is liable to be missed when the outcome of NICU graduates is assessed before that age. Figure 60-4 illustrates this diagnostic evolution and increase in developmental-behavioral problems over time. As in other studies, this study found a disproportionate number of boys compared to girls who experienced school dysfunction and required remedial assistance. This investigation was continued into adolescence (105). Although several of the LBW children with earlier problems no longer were demonstrating all of them, an almost equal number of previously unrecognized children had manifested academic and social problems, thus resulting in a relatively stable number of such problems over time.

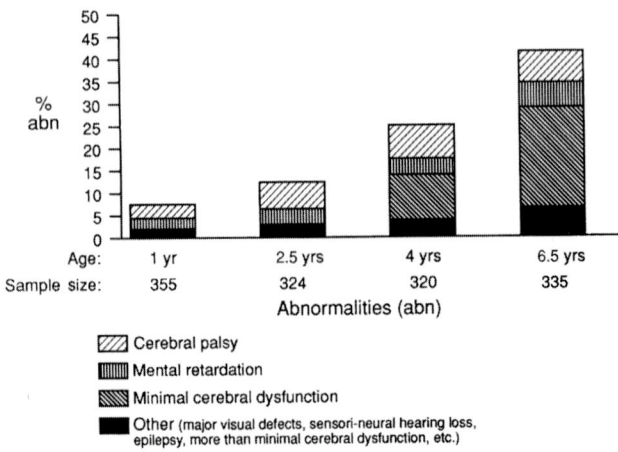

Figure 60-4 Evolution of developmental dysfunction in low-birth-weight, premature children. (Adapted from Anders TF, Keener M, Kraemer H. Sleep-wake state organization, neonatal assessment and development in premature infants during the first year of life: II. *Sleep* 1985;8:193–206, with permission.)

Additionally, whereas behaviors such as overactivity, temper tantrums, and perseveration had greatly subsided, symptoms of neuropsychiatric disturbance, including distractibility, irritability, unhappiness, low frustration tolerance, fears, disobedience, poor motivation, and sleep difficulties, persisted or increased.

Other studies have confirmed these observations in VLBW children at 8 to 15 years of age and have documented, in such areas as verbal expression, academic achievement, social competence, and emotional maturity, continued problems that cannot be attributed primarily to social class or differences in the quality of parenting (106,107). Nickel and colleagues (108) evaluated the school performances at a mean age of 10 years of 25 ELBW children who were cared for at a time (1960–1972) when only very premature infants who had little or no neonatal illness survived. Despite an overall mean IQ of 90 (range 50 to 141), 16 (64%) of these children had been or currently were in special educational programs. Only seven (28%) were rated by their teachers to be achieving at or above grade level. Arithmetic reasoning, mathematics achievement, reading comprehension, balance, fine motor coordination, and perceptual function were specific and common weaknesses for these children.

Klein and associates (109) compared 65 nine-year-old children born in Cleveland, Ohio, in 1976, who were VLBW and free of neurologic impairment, to 65 NBW children who had been matched for age, gender, race, and social class on measures of IQ, visual-motor and fine motor abilities, and academic achievement. The following were the major findings:

- The VLBW children scored significantly lower than the NBW children on tests that measured general intelligence, even though both group means were within the average range.
- The VLBW children scored significantly lower than the NBW children on tests that measured academic achievement.
- The VLBW children had particular deficits in mathematics achievement.
- The VLBW children had particular deficits on tests that involved visual or spatial skills.
- These results were independent of social class.

In a similarly controlled and longitudinal New York City study, Ross and colleagues (110) showed that a much higher proportion of 8-year-old VLBW children required special educational interventions (48%) than either NBW children (15%) or the New York State public elementary school population (10%). VLBW children scored significantly lower than NBW children on tests of IQ, verbal ability, academic achievement, and auditory memory. There was an interaction of prematurity and social class on IQ, verbal tests, academic achievement, and attention, with premature children of lower socioeconomic status scoring lowest on these measures. Rickards and associates (61) compared the academic and social function of VLBW and NBW children at 14 years of age. VLBW children continued

to perform at a significantly lower level on tests of intelligence, arithmetic, visual processing, visual memory, and overall problem solving. In addition, significantly more VLBW children were rated by teachers as socially rejected and by their parents as having learning problems at school.

A number of more recent reports emphasize the school problems of ELBW children. From an analysis by birth-weight subgroups, Klebanov and colleagues (111) indicated that as birth weight decreases, the prevalence of grade failure, placement in special classes, and classification as impaired increases, even when maternal education and neonatal length of stay are controlled for. The ELBW children scored lower than all other birth-weight groups on math and reading achievement tests. Even among children with IQ scores above 85, ELBW children still obtained lower math scores than the other children. Even with optimal socioeconomic environments, approximately one of every two ELBW children requires special educational services (112). In a Scottish population-based sample of 8-year-old children, ELBW children placed heavy demands on regular schools, with 52% requiring learning support compared with 16% of NBW comparison children (113). Hack and colleagues (64) have delineated school-age outcomes in ELBW children with birth weights under 750 grams (Fig. 60-5). Compared with VLBW children weighing 750 to 1,499 grams at birth and also with NBW children, these markedly ELBW children were inferior in cognitive ability, psychomotor skills, and academic achievement. They had poorer social skills and adaptive behavior and more behavioral and attention problems. In all assessed areas, the functioning of VLBW children was intermediate between that of ELBW and NBW children. Saigal et al. (114) recently reported that ELBW teens aged 12 to 16 years, who were born in Ontario, Canada, scored 13 to 18 points lower on cognitive and academic achievement tests than an NBW comparison group. more than half (58%) of ELBW teens were receiving special educational assistance and/or had repeated a grade compared with 13% of NBW teens. Even apparently normal ELBW teens were having significantly more school difficulties

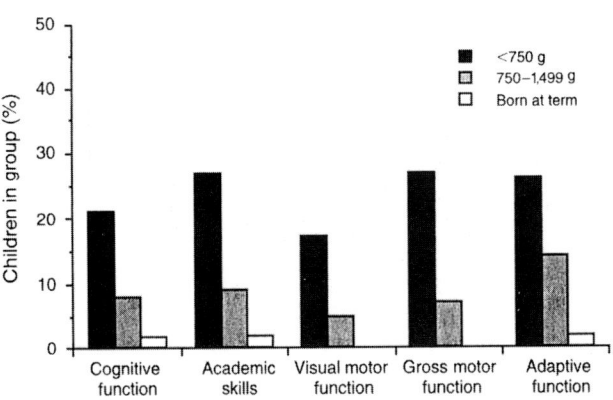

Figure 60-5 Percentage of children in each study group with subnormal functioning. (From Avery GB, Glass P. Retinopathy of prematurity: what causes it? *Clin Perinatol* 1988;15:917–928, with permission.)

than NBW teens. ELBW teens who weighed less than 750 grams at birth fared worst in all areas.

Although data on the prevalence of behavior problems in older LBW children are somewhat sparse, it is likely that the prevalence is substantially higher than in NBW children. For example, Escalona (115) found that 30% of a primarily disadvantaged premature sample exhibited major behavior problems before the age of 4 years. The most comprehensive investigation of long-term behavioral function in this population comes from the same Cleveland, Ohio cohort described in terms of academic achievement (109). Breslau and colleagues (116) compared 65 nine-year-old VLBW children to 65 NBW children, matched for age, gender, race, social class, and school, on parents' ratings on the Child Behavior Checklist and teachers' ratings on the Teacher's Report Form. Results from parents and teachers converged on key findings. The major findings were the following:

The VLBW boys manifested significantly more behavioral disturbances and poorer social competence than NBW boys.

The excess in behavior problems in VLBW boys spanned a wide range of behavioral domains, including both internalizing (e.g., depressive-anxious) and externalizing (e.g., hyperactive, aggressive, conduct problems) syndromes.

The effect of VLBW on behavior problems and social adjustment in boys was not a function of IQ.

These results were independent of social class.

Although VLBW girls did not differ significantly from NBW girls, suggestive trends in the same direction as the boys may indicate that there is an increased risk for behavior problems in both genders but that these sequelae become evident at an earlier age in boys than in girls.

As in other neurodevelopmental and neurobehavioral domains, Klebanov and colleagues (117) found that ELBW children had lower attention, language skills, overall social competence, scholastic competence, and athletic ability than all other birth-weight groups (very low, low, and normal) as measured by classroom teachers, even when neonatal length of stay, child's gender and ethnicity, and maternal education were controlled for. The classroom behavior of ELBW children was rated by teachers as poor, even for children who had not failed a grade. More recently Hille and associates (118) reported that, in spite of cultural differences, ELBW children in the Netherlands, Germany, Canada, and the United States had very similar difficulties in thought, social interactions, and attention compared with NBW children. They tended to have trouble making friends, be immature, be impulsive, and have trouble with concentration leading to the diagnosis of attention deficit hyperactivity disorder. The investigators concluded that biologic mechanisms are major contributors to the behavior problems of ELBW children.

A number of recent studies have attempted to quantify "quality of life" outcomes. Direct measures of self-reported health status and overall functionality scores indicated that, as a group, ELBW adolescents suffer from a greater burden of morbidity and rate their health-related quality of life as significantly lower than NBW adolescents (119). Nevertheless, the vast majority of ELBW respondents view their quality of life as quite satisfactory and are difficult to distinguish from controls. Likewise, interviews of parents of ELBW teens revealed that they were fully aware that their children were more disabled than their age-matched peers but still believed that their children's quality of life was fairly high (120). Msall and Tremont (121) conclude that the measurement of long-term functional outcomes including higher education attainment, independent living, and job success will elucidate the full risks and resiliencies of low birth weight/prematurity and is the ultimate challenge of future studies.

SPECIFIC PERINATAL-NEONATAL COMPLICATIONS IN HIGH-RISK INFANTS

Intrauterine Growth Retardation

The SGA infant has a higher mortality rate, higher incidence of perinatal-neonatal complications, and higher prevalence of chronic neurologic impairments than the appropriate-for-gestational-age (AGA) infant of similar gestational age (122). The diagnosis of SGA is useful in identifying a high-risk population needing careful follow-up; however, the population of SGA infants is a heterogeneous one with multiple etiologies. Intrauterine growth pattern, associated congenital anomalies, mortality rate, risk of perinatal-neonatal complications, and long-term outcome reflect the nature of the insult and the timing as well. Drillien and colleagues (83) have stressed the need to differentiate early-pregnancy-onset SGA infants, many of whom demonstrate intrinsic defects such as congenital anomalies, from late-pregnancy-onset SGA infants, who may have antenatal histories of placental insufficiency or maternal chronic illness. Long-term developmental prognosis, in terms of major and minor impairments and school function, is significantly worse for early-pregnancy-onset SGA infants.

Most SGA outcome studies also distinguish between full-term and premature SGA infants because of marked differences in mortality and morbidity rates, both of which are significantly higher for premature SGA infants. For both groups of SGA infants, great variability among outcome studies is the norm, again reflecting the inevitable heterogeneity of the SGA diagnosis. Many studies report few major neurologic disabilities in full-term SGA infants followed from birth. In 96 full-term SGA infants followed to the age of 5 years, Fitzhardinge and Stevens (123) reported only a 1% prevalence of cerebral palsy and 6% prevalence of seizures. In a cerebral-palsied population in Sweden, full-term SGA infants had a somewhat higher risk for cerebral palsy than full-term AGA infants but a much lower risk than premature AGA and premature SGA infants (42). Most full-term SGA infants are of average intelligence, whether tested during the preschool or school years, even though the mean IQ of the SGA population usually has been somewhat lower than that of control groups (124). Fitzhardinge and Stevens, however, found that, despite average intelligence, 50% of the SGA boys and 36% of the SGA girls were doing poorly in school. One-third of the SGA children with IQs above 100 were failing consistently at school. A history of perinatal asphyxia was an important contributing risk factor. Other studies provide good evidence of an increased prevalence of speech and language problems, minor neurologic findings, and attention deficits in this subgroup (125).

More recently, several long-term studies have added further information to our understanding of this important risk group. Hollo and associates (126), reporting on a Finnish cohort, confirmed multiple academic deficiencies at age 10 years. Of particular interest, a 26-year follow-up of the 1970 British Birth Cohort found that adults who were born SGA had significant reductions in academic achievement and professional attainment compared with adults who were NBW (127). However, there were no long-term social or emotional consequences of being SGA; these adults were as likely to be employed, married, and satisfied with life.

Relatively few studies evaluate the outcome of premature SGA infants, and the results are contradictory. The prevalence of reported impairments varies from nearly 50% to as low as 10%. Commey and Fitzhardinge (128) found that 15% of premature SGA infants had cerebral palsy at the age of 2 years, twice the prevalence encountered in premature AGA infants. In the Swedish cerebral palsy study, premature SGA infants had the highest risk for cerebral palsy, 15 times greater than full-term AGA infants and significantly more than full-term SGA and premature AGA infants (42). Commey and Fitzhardinge found a high prevalence of subnormal intelligence in premature SGA infants tested at the age of 2 years. Drillien (129) reported that, in all birth-weight subgroups, fewer premature SGA infants were average cognitively, and more had borderline intelligence or mental retardation, especially those born to parents of low socioeconomic status.

There is little specific information about school function in this subgroup, but premature SGA infants certainly must be presumed to be at substantial risk in this area as well. A recent report compared the cognitive and neurologic outcomes of 129 premature SGA infants with 300 premature AGA infants through 6 years of age (130). The SGA infants had significantly poorer cognitive scores at each assessment age than AGA infants of similar gestational ages. Normal neurologic status was more likely at all assessments for the AGA than for SGA infants of comparable gestational age. Nevertheless, there was a significant effect of SGA on cognitive outcome at school age independent of neurologic status.

Asphyxia

Hypoxic-ischemic brain injury is the single most important neurologic problem occurring in the perinatal period

(131). This variety of brain injury accounts for many, although not the majority, of the severe, nonprogressive neurologic deficits seen in children. This is particularly the case for full-term infants but also is of etiologic significance for premature infants. The neurodevelopmental deficits of concern are principally the triad of cerebral palsy, mental retardation, and epilepsy, often occurring together in varying degrees. In addition, more subtle developmental and behavioral dysfunctions in the areas of language, fine motor coordination, socioemotional competence, attention, and school learning are increasingly recognized in the relatively few studies designed to investigate these long-term sequelae. The common denominator of this form of brain injury is deprivation of the supply of oxygen to the central nervous system. The developing brain can be deprived of oxygen by two major pathogenetic mechanisms—hypoxemia (i.e., diminished amount of oxygen in the blood supply) or ischemia (i.e., diminished amount of blood perfusing the tissue). These two overlapping mechanisms typically coexist clinically, are virtually impossible to isolate and delineate precisely in the individual infant, and together constitute the basis of the syndrome of asphyxia (132).

As noted by Paneth and Stark (133), the fundamental problem in assessing the exact relationship between asphyxia and subsequent neurodevelopmental outcome has been the difficulty in assessing the degree of asphyxia. Various techniques have been used to identify the asphyxiated infant, including the time to initiate spontaneous respiration (less than 1 minute), the time that positive-pressure ventilation was required to sustain the infant (less than 1 minute), and the use of the neonatal scoring system developed by Apgar (134). This scoring system originally was created to identify infants who were physiologically depressed at birth and who required resuscitative efforts. It has been shown to have limited utility in premature infants (135). Although Apgar did not design the scoring system to be used as a tool to predict long-term neurologic status, it has been used by many for correlation with ultimate outcome because of the paucity of alternative asphyxial markers. Fetal scalp blood and umbilic cord blood sampling for pH and other acid–base parameters have been recommended as potentially providing more objective perinatal data.

Although the Apgar scoring system is not perfect, it continues to be the standard by which almost all neonates are evaluated immediately after birth, and, as such, was the perinatal measure used in the NIH National Collaborative Perinatal Project between 1959 and 1966. This multisite prospective study of more than 50,000 pregnant woman and their children remains the largest single resource for investigating the associations between perinatal asphyxia and neurodevelopmental outcome, particularly cerebral palsy. Several main conclusions emerged (136):

Cerebral palsy does not develop in most (95%) asphyxiated full-term infants with an Apgar score less than or equal to 3 at 5 minutes.

As the duration of severe asphyxia increases from 5 to 20 minutes, the likelihood of neonatal death or permanent cerebral palsy also increases in parallel fashion; approximately 60% cerebral palsy prevalence exists in full-term survivors with Apgar scores of less than or equal to 3 at 20 minutes.

The more premature the infant, the greater the incidence (i.e., approximately 30% at 28 weeks of gestational age), severity, and mortality associated with perinatal asphyxia.

Most infants in whom cerebral palsy develops were not asphyxiated at birth.

Although perinatal asphyxia certainly is an important cause of severe psychomotor retardation, especially during the intrapartum period, its relative contribution to these adverse outcomes has, in the past, frequently been overstated. It is estimated that between 10% and 20% of all cases of cerebral palsy are attributable to intrapartum asphyxia. Many of these cases are complicated by mental retardation of variable severity. Freeman and Nelson (137) correctly emphasize the four necessary criteria to link causally intrapartum asphyxia and neurodevelopmental disability in full-term infants:

1. Intrapartum abnormalities (e.g., nonreassuring fetal heart rate patterns, passage of meconium, hemorrhage)
2. Depression at birth (e.g., low Apgar scores, need for resuscitation)
3. Neonatal hypoxic ischemic encephalopathy (e.g., seizures in the first 48 hours, hypotonia and lethargy, metabolic acidosis, apnea)
4. Anticipated outcomes (e.g., cerebral palsy with associated deficits, not severe mental retardation or epilepsy by themselves)

Outcome studies in full-term infants have identified the neonatal factors most predictive of neurodevelopmental disability after an episode of intrapartum asphyxia. The key predictors include failure to establish spontaneous respiration by 5 minutes, onset of seizures within the first 12 hours and refractory to treatment, prolonged deep encephalopathy (i.e., Sarnat stage 3) (138), failure of the electroencephalogram to normalize by 5 to 7 days, and inability to establish adequate oral feedings by 1 week of age (139). Fitzhardinge and colleagues (140) described the predictive utility of the computed tomography scan between 1 and 2 weeks after birth. The most ominous findings were diffuse hypodensities throughout both the white and gray matter and extensive intraparenchymal or intraventricular hemorrhage. Byrne and associates (141) reported that 8 months of age appears to be the earliest time at which magnetic resonance imaging findings (e.g., delayed myelination, acquired structural abnormalities) correlate well with later adverse neurodevelopmental outcome in this population. Finally, Robertson and colleagues (142) compared 145 asphyxiated full-term children who had experienced neonatal encephalopathy with a similar number of nonasphyxiated peer children at 8 years of age.

The prevalence of major impairment, which included cerebral palsy, mental retardation, epilepsy, cortical blindness, and severe hearing loss, was 16%. Intellectual, visual-motor integration, and receptive vocabulary scores, as well as reading, spelling, and arithmetic grade levels for those children with moderate or severe encephalopathy were significantly below those in the mild encephalopathy or peer comparison groups. Thus, children who survive moderate or severe neonatal asphyxial encephalopathy are at increased risk for both major neurosensory impairment and reduced school performance.

REFERENCES

1. McCormick MC. The contribution of low birth weight to infant mortality and childhood morbidity. *N Engl J Med* 1985;312:82–90.
2. Philip AGS, Little GA, Polivy DR, et al. Neonatal mortality risk for the eighties: the importance of birth weight/gestational age groups. *Pediatrics* 1981;68:122–130.
3. Paneth N, Kiely JL, Wallenstein S, et al. Newborn intensive care and neonatal mortality in low-birth-weight infants: a population study. *N Engl J Med* 1982;307:149–155.
4. Buehler JW, Kleinman JC, Hogue CJR. Birth weight-specific infant mortality, United States, 1960 and 1980. *Public Health Rep* 1987;102:151–161.
5. Herdman RC, Behney CJ, Wagner JL, et al. *Neonatal intensive care for low birthweight infants: costs and effectiveness. Health Technology Case Study 38*, publication OTA-HCS-38. Washington: Office of Technology Assessment, 1987.
6. MacDorman MF, Minino AM, Strobino DM, et al. Annual summary of vital statistics—2001. *Pediatrics* 2002;110:1037–1052.
7. Hack M, Fanaroff AA. Outcomes of extremely-low-birth-weight infants between 1982 and 1988. *N Engl J Med* 1989;321:1642–1647.
8. Phelps DL, Brown DR, Tung B, et al. 28-day survival rates of 6676 neonates with birth weights of 1250 grams or less. *Pediatrics* 1991;87:7–17.
9. Hack M, Friedman H, Fanaroff AA. Outcomes of extremely low birth weight infants. *Pediatrics* 1996;98:931–937.
10. Ginsberg HG, Goldsmith JP, Stedman CM. Intact survival and 20 month follow-up of a 380-gram infant. *J Perinatol* 1990;10:330–333.
11. Hack M, Horbar JD, Malloy MH, et al. Very low birth weight outcomes of the National Institute of Child Health and Human Development Neonatal Network. *Pediatrics* 1991;87:587–597.
12. Lasky RE, Tyson JE, Rosenfeld CR, et al. Disappointing follow-up findings for indigent high-risk newborns. *Am J Dis Child* 1987;141:100–105.
13. Bennett FC, Robinson NM, Sells CJ. Growth and development of infants weighing less than 800 grams at birth. *Pediatrics* 1983;71:319–323.
14. Hoffman EL, Bennett FC. Birthweight less than 800 grams: changing outcomes and influences of gender and gestation number. *Pediatrics* 1990;86:27–34.
15. LaPine TR, Jackson JC, Bennett FC. Outcome of infants weighing less than 800 grams at birth: 15 years' experience. *Pediatrics* 1995;96:479–483.
16. Shy KK, Luthy DA, Bennett FC, et al. Effects of electronic fetal heart-rate monitoring, as compared with periodic auscultation, on the neurologic development of premature infants. *N Engl J Med* 1990;322:588–593.
17. The HIFI Study Group. High-frequency oscillatory ventilation compared with conventional intermittent mechanical ventilation in the treatment of respiratory failure in preterm infants: neurodevelopmental status at 16 to 24 months of postterm age. *J Pediatr* 1990;117:939–946.
18. Aylward GP, Pfeiffer SI, Wright A, et al. Outcome studies of low birth weight infants published in the last decade: a metaanalysis. *J Pediatr* 1989;115:515–520.

19. Blackman J. *Warning signals: basic criteria for tracking at-risk infants and toddlers.* Washington: National Center for Clinical Infant Programs, 1986.

20. Blackman JA, Hein HA. Iowa's system for screening and tracking high-risk infants. *Am J Dis Child* 1985;139:826–831.

21. Tekolste KA, Bennett FC. The high risk infant: transitions in health, development, and family during the first years of life. *J Perinatol* 1987;7:368–377.

22. Barrera ME, Rosenbaum PL, Cunningham CE. Corrected and uncorrected Bayley scores: longitudinal developmental patterns in low and high birthweight infants. *Infant Behav Dev* 1987;10:337–346.

23. McCormick MC. Long-term follow-up of infants discharged from neonatal intensive care units. *JAMA* 1989;261:1767–1772.

24. Bennett FC. Neurodevelopmental outcome in low birthweight infants: the role of developmental intervention. In: Guthrie R, ed. *Clinics in critical care medicine, 13: neonatal intensive care.* New York: Churchill Livingstone, 1988:221–249.

25. Brothwood M, Wolke D, Gamsu H, et al. Prognosis of the very low birthweight baby in relation to gender. *Arch Dis Child* 1986;61:559–564.

26. Bennett FC, Scott DT. Long-term perspective on premature infant outcome and contemporary intervention issues. *Semin Perinatol* 1997;21:190–201.

27. Paneth N, Kiely JL, Stein Z, et al. Cerebral palsy and newborn care. III. Estimated prevalence rates of cerebral palsy under differing rates of mortality and impairment of low-birthweight infants. *Dev Med Child Neurol* 1981;23:801–806.

28. Hagberg B, Hagberg G, Olow I, et al. The changing panorama of cerebral palsy in Sweden. V. The birth year period 1979–82. *Acta Paediatr Scand* 1989;78:283–290.

29. Blaymore-Bier J, Pezzullo J, Kim E, et al. Outcome of extremely low-birth-weight infants: 1980–1990. *Acta Paediatr* 1994;83:1244–1248.

30. Robertson CMT, Hrynchyshyn GJ, Etches PC, et al. Population-based study of the incidence, complexity, and severity of neurologic disability among survivors weighing 500 through 1250 grams at birth: a comparison of two birth cohorts. *Pediatrics* 1992;90:750–755.

31. O'Shea TM, Klinepeter KL, Goldstein DJ, et al. Survival and developmental disability in infants with birth weights of 501 to 800 grams, born between 1979 and 1994. *Pediatrics* 1997;100:982–986.

32. Lemons JA, Bauer CR, Oh W, et al, for the NICHD Neonatal Research Network. Very low birth weight outcomes of the National Institute of Child Health and Human Development Neonatal Research Network, January 1995 through December 1996. *Pediatrics* 2001;107:E1.

33. Wood NS, Marlow N, Costeloe K, et al, for the EPICure Study Group. Neurologic and developmental disability after extremely preterm birth. *N Engl J Med* 2000;343:378–384.

34. Pharoah PO, Cooke T, Cooke RW, et al. Birthweight specific trends in cerebral palsy. *Arch Dis Child* 1990;65:602–606.

35. Freud S. *Infantile cerebral paralysis.* Coral Gables, FL: University of Miami Press, 1968. Russin LA, translator.

36. Bennett FC, Chandler LS, Robinson NM, et al. Spastic diplegia in premature infants. Etiologic and diagnostic considerations. *Am J Dis Child* 1981;135:732–737.

37. Volpe JJ. Cognitive deficits in premature infants. *N Engl J Med* 1991;325:276–278.

38. Graziani LJ, Pasto M, Stanley C, et al. Neonatal neurosonographic correlates of cerebral palsy in preterm infants. *Pediatrics* 1986;78:88–95.

39. Bozynski ME, Nelson MN, Genaze D, et al. Cranial ultrasonography and the prediction of cerebral palsy in infants weighing less than or equal to 1200 grams at birth. *Dev Med Child Neurol* 1988;30:342–348.

40. Perlman JM, Risser R, Broyles RS. Bilateral cystic periventricular leukomalacia in the premature infant: associated risk factors. *Pediatrics* 1996;97:822–827.

41. Grether JK, Nelson KB, Walsh E, et al. Intrauterine exposure to infection and risk of cerebral palsy in very preterm infants. *Arch Pediatr Adolesc Med* 2003;157:26–32.

42. Hagberg B. Epidemiological and preventive aspects of cerebral palsy and severe mental retardation in Sweden. *Eur J Pediatr* 1979;130:71–78.

43. Gibson RL, Jackson JC, Twiggs GA, et al. Bronchopulmonary dysplasia. Survival after prolonged mechanical ventilation. *Am J Dis Child* 1988;142:721–725.

44. Singer L, Yamashita T, Lilien L, et al. A longitudinal study of developmental outcome of infants with bronchopulmonary dysplasia and very low birth weight. *Pediatrics* 1997;100:987–993.

45. Bradford BC, Baudin J, Conway MJ, et al. Identification of sensory neural hearing loss in very preterm infants by brainstem auditory evoked potentials. *Arch Dis Child* 1985;60:105–109.

46. de Vries LS, Lary S, Dubowitz LMS. Relationship of serum bilirubin levels to ototoxicity and deafness in high-risk low-birthweight infants. *Pediatrics* 1985;76:351–354.

47. Salamy A, Eldredge L, Tooley WH. Neonatal status and hearing loss in high-risk infants. *J Pediatr* 1989;114:847–852.

48. Leavitt AM, Watchko JF, Bennett FC, et al. Neurodevelopmental outcome following persistent pulmonary hypertension of the neonate. *J Perinatol* 1987;7:288–291.

49. Abramovich SJ, Gregory S, Slemick M, et al. Hearing loss in very low birthweight infants treated with neonatal intensive care. *Arch Dis Child* 1979;54:421–426.

50. Bess FH, Tharpe AM. Unilateral hearing impairment in children. *Pediatrics* 1984;74:206–216.

51. Thompson G, Folsom R. Hearing assessment of at-risk infants. Current status of audiometry in young infants. *Clin Pediatr* 1981;20:257–261.

52. Marshall RE, Reichert TJ, Kerley SV, et al. Auditory function in newborn intensive care unit patients revealed by auditory brainstem potentials. *J Pediatr* 1980;96:731–735.

53. Nield TA, Schrier S, Ramos AD, et al. Unexpected hearing loss in high-risk infants. *Pediatrics* 1986;78:417–422.

54. Norton SJ, Gorga MP, Widen JE, et al. Identification of neonatal hearing impairment: transient evoked otoacoustic emissions during the perinatal period. *Ear Hear* 2000;21:425–442.

55. Avery GB, Glass P. Retinopathy of prematurity: progress report. *Pediatr Ann* 1988;17:528–533.

56. Avery GB, Glass P. Retinopathy of prematurity: what causes it? *Clin Perinatol* 1988;15:917–928.

57. Scharf J, Zonis S, Zeltzer M. Refraction in premature babies: a prospective study. *J Pediatr Ophthalmol Strabismus* 1978;15:48–50.

58. Camfield PR, Camfield CS, Allen AC, et al. Progressive hydrocephalus in infants with birthweights less than 1500 grams. *Arch Neurol* 1981;38:653–655.

59. Shinnar S, Molteni RA, Gammon K, et al. Intraventricular hemorrhage in the premature infant. *N Engl J Med* 1982;306:1464–1468.

60. Chaplin ER, Goldstein GW, Myerberg DZ, et al. Posthemorrhagic hydrocephalus in the preterm infant. *Pediatrics* 1980;65:901–909.

61. Rickards AL, Kelly EA, Doyle LW, et al. Cognition, academic progress, behavior and self-concept at 14 years of very low birth weight children. *J Dev Behav Pediatr* 2001;22:11–18.

62. Hack M, Flannery DJ, Schluchter M, et al. Outcomes in young adulthood for very low birth weight infants. *N Engl J Med* 2002;346:149–157.

63. Saigal S, Rosenbaum P, Stoskopf B, et al. Follow-up of infants 501 to 1500 gm birthweight delivered to residents of a geographically defined region with perinatal intensive care facilities. *J Pediatr* 1982;100:606–613.

64. Hack M, Taylor HG, Klein N, et al. School-age outcomes in children with birth weights under 750 g. *N Engl J Med* 1994;331:753–759.

65. McBurney AK, Eaves LC. Evolution of developmental and psychological test scores. In: Dunn HG, ed. *Sequelae of low birthweight: the Vancouver study.* Philadelphia: JB Lippincott, 1986:54–67.

66. Hoy EA, Bill JM, Sykes DH. Very low birthweight: a long-term developmental impairment? *Int J Behav Dev* 1988;11:37–67.

67. Ment LR, Vohr B, Allan W, et al. Change in cognitive function over time in very low birth weight infants. *JAMA* 2003;289:705–711.

68. Rose SA. Differential rates of visual information processing in full-term and preterm infants. *Child Dev* 1983;54:1189–1198.

69. Ruff HA, McCarton C, Kurtzberg D, et al. Preterm infants' manipulative exploration of objects. *Child Dev* 1984;55:1166–1173.

70. Drillien CM. *The growth and development of the prematurely born infant.* Edinburgh: Livingstone, 1964.

71. Wiener G, Rider RV, Oppel WC, et al. Correlates of low birthweight: psychological status at eight to ten years of age. *Pediatr Res* 1968;2:110–118.

72. Hunt JV, Cooper BAB, Tooley WH. Very low birthweight infants at 8 and 11 years of age: role of neonatal illness and family status. *Pediatrics* 1988;82:596–603.

73. Halsey CL, Collin MF, Anderson CL. Extremely low birth weight children and their peers: a comparison of preschool performance. *Pediatrics* 1993;91:807–811.

74. Breslau N, DelDotto JE, Brown GG, et al. A gradient relationship between low birth weight and IQ at age 6 years. *Arch Pediatr Adolesc Med* 1994;148:377–383.

75. Zarin-Ackerman J, Lewis M, Driscoll JM. Language development in 2-year-old normal and risk infants. *Pediatrics* 1977;59:982–986.

76. Largo RH, Molinari L, Comenale-Pinto L, et al. Language development of term and preterm children during the first five years of life. *Dev Med Child Neurol* 1986;28:333–350.

77. Michelsson K, Noronen M. Neurological, psychological and articulatory impairment in five year old children with a birthweight of 2000 g or less. *Eur J Pediatr* 1983;141:96–100.

78. Hubatch LM, Johnson CJ, Kistler DJ, et al. Early language abilities of high-risk infants. *J Speech Hear Disord* 1985;50:195–207.

79. Bennett FC, Robinson NM, Sells CJ. Hyaline membrane disease, birthweight, and gestational age: effects on development in the first two years. *Am J Dis Child* 1982;136:888–891.

80. Drillien CM. Abnormal neurologic signs in the first year of life in low birthweight infants: possible prognostic significance. *Dev Med Child Neurol* 1972;14:575–584.

81. Amiel-Tison C. A method for neurologic evaluation within the first year of life. *Curr Probl Pediatr* 1976;7:1–50.

82. Coolman RB, Bennett FC, Sells CJ, et al. Neuromotor development of graduates of the neonatal intensive care unit: patterns encountered in the first two years of life. *J Dev Behav Pediatr* 1985;6:327–333.

83. Drillien CM, Thomson AJM, Burgoyne K. Low birthweight children at early school age: a longitudinal study. *Dev Med Child Neurol* 1980;22:26–47.

84. Ross G, Lipper EG, Auld PAM. Consistency and change in the development of premature infants weighing less than 1501 grams at birth. *Pediatrics* 1985;76:885–891.

85. Burns YR, Bullock MI. Comparison of abilities of preterm and mature born children at 5 years of age. *Aust Paediatr J* 1985;21:31–38.

86. Crowe TK, Deitz JC, Bennett FC, et al. Preschool motor skills of children born prematurely and not diagnosed as having cerebral palsy. *J Dev Behav Pediatr* 1988;9:189–193.

87. Ferrari F, Grosoli MV, Fontana G, et al. Neurobehavioral comparison of low-risk preterm and full-term infants at term conceptional age. *Dev Med Child Neurol* 1983;25:450–458.

88. Freidman SL, Jacobs BS, Werthmann MW. Preterms of low medical risk: spontaneous behaviors and soothability at expected date of birth. *Infant Behav Dev* 1982;5:3–10.

89. Aylward GP, Hatcher RP, Leavitt LA, et al. Factors affecting neurobehavioral responses of preterm infants at term conceptional age. *Child Dev* 1984;55:1155–1165.

90. Kurtzberg D, Hilpert PL, Kreuzer JA, et al. Differential maturation of cortical auditory evoked potentials to speech sounds in normal full-term and very low birthweight infants. *Dev Med Child Neurol* 1984;26:466.

91. Anders TF, Keener M. Developmental coarse of nighttime sleep-wake patterns in full-term and premature infants during the first year of life: I. *Sleep* 1985;8:173.

92. Fox NA, Porges SW. The relation between neonatal heart period patterns and developmental outcome. *Child Dev* 1985;56:28.

93. Kaga K, Hashira S, Marsh RR. Auditory brainstem responses and behavioral responses in preterm infants. *Br J Audiol* 1986;20:121.

94. Anders TF, Keener M, Kraemer H. Sleep-wake state organization, neonatal assessment and development in premature infants during the first year of life: II. *Sleep* 1985;8:193–206.

95. Cohen SE, Parmelee AH, Beckwith L, et al. Cognitive development in preterm infants: birth to eight years. *J Dev Behav Pediatr* 1986;7:102–110.

96. DiVitto B, Goldberg S. The effects of newborn medical status on early parent-infant interactions. In: Field TM, ed. *Infants born at risk.* New York: Spectrum, 1979:311–332.

97. Field TM. Interaction patterns of preterm and term infants. In: Field TM, Sostek AM, Goldberg S, et al, eds. *Infants born at risk.* New York: Spectrum, 1979:333–356.

98. Watt J. Interaction and development in the first year: I. The effects of prematurity. *Early Hum Dev* 1986;13:195–210.

99. Field TM. High-risk infants "have less fun" during early interactions. *Top Early Child Spec Educ* 1983;3:77–87.

100. Crnic KA, Ragozin AS, Greenberg MT, et al. Social interaction and developmental competence of preterm and full-term infants during the first year of life. *Child Dev* 1983;54:1199–1210.

101. Malatesta CZ, Grigoryev P, Lamb C, et al. Emotion socialization and expressive development in preterm and full-term infants. *Child Dev* 1986;57:316–330.

102. Conely D, Bennett NG. Is biology destiny? Birth weight and life chances. *Am Sociol Rev* 2000;65:458–467.

103. Kopp CB. Risk factors in development. In: Haith MM, Campos JJ, eds. *Handbook of child psychology,* vol 2. *Infancy and developmental psychobiology.* New York: John Wiley & Sons, 1983:1081–1098.

104. Dunn HG, Crichton JU, Grunau RVE, et al. Neurological, psychological and educational sequelae of low birthweight. *Brain Dev* 1980;2:57–67.

105. Dunn HG, ed. *Sequelae of low birthweight: the Vancouver Study.* Clinics in Developmental Medicine series. London: MacKeith, 1986.

106. Wright FH, Blough RR, Chamberlin A, et al. A controlled follow-up study of small prematures born from 1952 through 1956. *Am J Dis Child* 1972;124:506–521.

107. Caputo DV, Goldstein KM, Taub HB. The development of prematurely born children through middle childhood. In: Field TM, Sostek AM, Goldberg S, et al, eds. *Infants born at risk.* New York: Spectrum, 1979:219–247.

108. Nickel RE, Bennett FC, Lamson FN. School performance of children with birthweights of 1000 g or less. *Am J Dis Child* 1982;136:105–110.

109. Klein NK, Hack M, Breslau N. Children who were very low birthweight: development and academic achievement at nine years of age. *J Dev Behav Pediatr* 1989;10:32–37.

110. Ross G, Lipper EG, Auld PAM. Educational status and school related abilities of very low birthweight premature children. *Pediatrics* 1991;88:1125–1134.

111. Klebanov PK, Brooks-Gunn J, McCormick MC. School achievement and failure in very low birth weight children. *J Dev Behav Pediatr* 1994;15:248–256.

112. Halsey CL, Collin MF, Anderson CL. Extremely low-birth-weight children and their peers: a comparison of school-age outcomes. *Arch Pediatr Adolesc Med* 1996;150:790–794.

113. Hall A, McLeod A, Counsell C, et al. School attainment, cognitive ability and motor function in a total Scottish very-low-birthweight population at eight years: a controlled study. *Dev Med Child Neurol* 1995;37:1037–1050.

114. Saigal S, Hoult LA, Streiner DL, et al. School difficulties at adolescence in a regional cohort of children who were extremely low birth weight. *Pediatrics* 2000;105:325–331.

115. Escalona SK. Babies at double hazard: early development of infants at biologic and social risk. *Pediatrics* 1982;70:670–676.

116. Breslau N, Klein N, Allen L. Very low birthweight: behavioral sequelae at nine years of age. *J Am Acad Child Adolesc Psychiatry* 1988;27:605–612.

117. Klebanov PK, Brooks-Gunn J, McCormick MC. Classroom behavior of very low birth weight elementary school children. *Pediatrics* 1994;94:700–708.

118. Hille A, den Ouden L, Saigal S, et al. Behavioral problems in children who weigh 1000 grams or less at birth in four countries. *Lancet* 2001;357:1641–1643.

119. Saigal S, Feeny D, Rosenbaum P, et al. Self-perceived health status and health-related quality of life of extremely low birth weight infants at adolescence. *JAMA* 1996;276:453–459.

120. Saigal S, Rosenbaum PL, Feeny D, et al. Parental perspectives of the health status and health-related quality of life of teen-aged children who were extremely low birth weight and term controls. *Pediatrics* 2000;105:569–574.

121. Msall ME, Tremont MR. Measuring functional outcomes after prematurity: developmental impact of very low birth weight and extremely low birth weight status on childhood disability. *Ment Retard Dev Disabil Res Rev* 2002;8:258–272.

122. Allen MC. Developmental outcome and follow-up of the small for gestational age infant. *Semin Perinatol* 1984;8:123–156.

123. Fitzhardinge PM, Stevens EM. The small-for-date infant: II. Neurological and intellectual sequelae. *Pediatrics* 1972;50:50–57.

124. Westwood M, Kramer MS, Munz D, et al. Growth and development of full-term nonasphyxiated small-for-gestational-age newborns: follow-up through adolescence. *Pediatrics* 1983;71:376–382.

125. Neligan GA, Kolvin I, Scott DM, et al, eds. *Born too soon or born too small: a follow-up study to seven years of age.* Clinics in Developmental Medicine series. Philadelphia: JB Lippincott, 1976.

126. Hollo O, Rautava P, Korhonen T, et al. Academic achievement of small-for-gestational-age children at age 10 years. *Arch Pediatr Adolesc Med* 2002;156:179–187.

127. Strauss RS. Adult functional outcome of those born small for gestational age. *JAMA* 2000; 283:625–632.

128. Commey JO, Fitzhardinge PM. Handicap in the preterm small-for-gestational-age infant. *J Pediatr* 1979;94:779–786.

129. Drillien CM. Aetiology and outcome in low birthweight infants. *Dev Med Child Neurol* 1972;14:563–574.

130. McCarton CM, Wallace IF, Divon M, et al. Cognitive and neurologic development of the premature, small for gestational age infant through age 6: comparison by birth weight and gestational age. *Pediatrics* 1996;98:1167–1178.

131. Shaywitz BA. The sequelae of hypoxic ischemic encephalopathy. *Semin Perinatol* 1987;11:180–190.

132. Volpe JJ. Perinatal hypoxic ischemic brain injury. *Pediatr Clin North Am* 1976;23:383–397.

133. Paneth N, Stark RI. Cerebral palsy and mental retardation in relation to indicators of perinatal asphyxia: an epidemiologic overview. *Am J Obstet Gynecol* 1983;147:960–966.

134. Apgar V, James LS. Further observations on the newborn scoring system. *Am J Dis Child* 1962;104:419–428.

135. Hegyi T, Carbone T, Anwar M, et al. The Apgar score and its components in the preterm infant. *Pediatrics* 1998;101:77–81.

136. Nelson KB, Ellenberg JH. Apgar scores as predictors of chronic neurologic disability. *Pediatrics* 1981;68:36–44.

137. Freeman JM, Nelson KB. Intrapartum asphyxia and cerebral palsy. *Pediatrics* 1988;82:240–249.

138. Sarnat HB, Sarnat MS. Neonatal encephalopathy following fetal distress: a clinical and electroencephalographic study. *Arch Neurol* 1976;33:696–705.

139. Finer NN, Robertson CM, Richards RT, et al. Hypoxicischemic encephalopathy in term neonates: perinatal factors and outcome. *J Pediatr* 1981;98:112–117.

140. Fitzhardinge PM, Flodmark O, Fitz CR, et al. The prognostic value of computed tomography as an adjunct to assessment of the term infant with postasphyxial encephalopathy. *J Pediatr* 1981;99:777–781.

141. Byrne P, Welch R, Johnson MA, et al. Serial magnetic resonance imaging in neonatal hypoxicischemic encephalopathy. *J Pediatr* 1990;117:694–700.

142. Robertson CM, Finer NN, Grace MG. School performance of survivors of neonatal encephalopathy associated with birth asphyxia at term. *J Pediatr* 1989;114:753–760.

143. Fitzhardinge PM. Follow-up studies of the high-risk newborn. In: Avery GB, ed. *Neonatology: pathophysiology and management of the newborn*, 2nd ed. Philadelphia: JB Lippincott, 1981:353–370.

144. LaPine TR, Felix SD, Tarczy-Hornoch P, et al. Outcome trends of infants weighing less than 800 grams at birth. *J Invest Med* 1999;47:7A.

145. Lee KS, Paneth N, Gartner LM, et al. Neonatal mortality: an analysis of the recent improvement in the United States. *Am J Public Health* 1980;70:15–21.

146. Glass P, Avery GB, Subramanian KNS, et al. Effect of bright light in the hospital nursery on the incidence of retinopathy of prematurity. *N Engl J Med* 1985;313:401–404.

The Healthcare Matrix

A. The Healthcare Matrix is a response to the challenge of linking all six competencies with the realities of medical education. It is a framework that accurately projects the complexity of an "episode of care" yet uncovers the interaction between quality outcomes (*IOM Aims for Improvement*) and the skills, knowledge and attitudes (*ACGME Core Competencies*) necessary to affect those outcomes. The first row, "Patient Care," is evaluated against the six IOM Aims. If care fails to meet (or in some instances exceeds) these Aims, the learner drills down through the remaining four competencies to analyze deficiencies or to learn why the system worked well. Finally, suboptimal performance is synthesized into the implementation of improvement strategies (practice-based learning and improvement). The intent is to create a new organizational culture by imbedding the Matrix in the daily work of the residents. This new culture acknowledges that residents are learning *in* and *about* the system of care. The Matrix provides a common framework for evaluating patient care across all disciplines and for all specialties (Reference: Joint Commission on Accreditation of Hospitals, *Journal of Quality and Safety*, February 2005).

APPENDIX A
HEALTHCARE MATRIX: CARE OF PATIENT(S) WITH....

ACGME* \ IOM[†]	SAFE[1]	TIMELY[2]	EFFECTIVE[3]	EFFICIENT[4]	EQUITABLE[5]	PATIENT-CENTERED[6]
Assessment of Care						
I. PATIENT CARE[7] (Overall Assessment) Yes/No						
II. A MEDICAL KNOWLEDGE[8] (What must I know)						
II. B INTERPERSONAL AND COMMUNICATION SKILLS[9] (What must I say)						
II. C PROFESSIONALISM[10] (How must I act)						
II. D SYSTEM-BASED PRACTICE[11] (On whom do I depend and who depends on me)						
Improvement						
III. PRACTICE-BASED LEARNING AND IMPROVEMENT[12] (How must we improve)						
Information Technology						

© 2004 Bingham, Quinn Vanderbilt University. All rights reserved.

[1] Safe: Avoiding injuries to patients from the care that is intended to help them.

[2] Timely: reducing waits and sometimes harmful delays for both those who receive and those who give care.

[3] Effective: providing services based on scientific knowledge to all how could benefit and refraining from providing services to those not likely to benefit (avoiding underuse and overuse, respectively).

[4] Efficient: avoiding waste, including waste of equipment, supplies, ideas, and energy.

[5] Equitable: providing care that does not vary in quality because of personal characteristics such as gender, ethnicity, geographic location, and socio-economic status.

[6] Patient-Centered: providing care that is respectful of and responsive to individual patient preferences, needs and values and ensuring that patient values guide all clinical decisions.

[7] Patient care that is compassionate, appropriate, and effective for the treatment of health problems and the promotion of health.

[8] Medical Knowledge about established and evolving biomedical, clinical, and cognate sciences (e.g. epidemiological and social-behavioral) and the application of this knowledge to patient care.

[9] Interpersonal and communication skills that result in effective information exchange and teaming with patients, their families and other health professionals.

[10] Professionalism, as manifested through a commitment to carrying out professional responsibilities, adherence to ethical principles, and sensitivity to a diverse patient population.

[11] System-based practice, as manifested by actions that demonstrate an awareness of and responsiveness to the larger context and system of health care and the ability to effectively call on system resources to provide care that is of optimal value.

[12] Practice-based learning and improvement that involves investigation and evaluation of their own patient care, appraisal and assimilation of scientific evidence, and improvement in patient care.

[†] IOM; Institute of Medicine

[*] ACGME; Accreditation Council for Graduate Medical Education

Hemoglobin–Oxygen Dissociation Curves

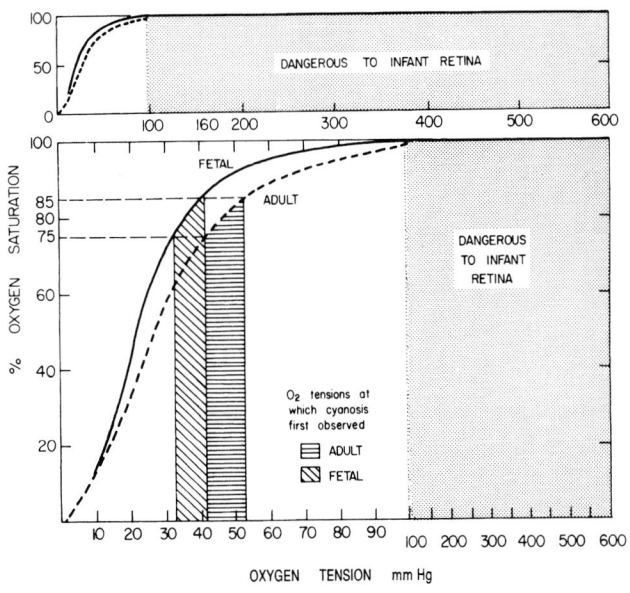

APPENDIX B

OXYGEN DISSOCIATION CURVES OF FETAL AND ADULT HEMOGLOBINS AT A pH OF 7.4 AND TEMPERATURE OF 37°C

Cyanosis is observed at 5 g unsaturated hemoglobin, which corresponds to different arterial tensions in the adult and the infant. From Klaus MH, Fanaroff AA. Care of the high risk neonate. Philadelphia: WB Saunders, 1973.

Breast Milk in the NICU

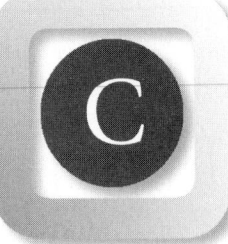

APPENDIX C-1
GALACTOGOGUES: AUGMENTING MATERNAL MILK SUPPLY[a]

Galactogogues are medications or other substances believed to assist initiation or maintenance of maternal milk production. Low milk supply is one of the most common reasons given for discontinuing breastfeeding so both mothers and physicians have sought help for this problem. Common indications for galactogogues are adoptive nursing, relactation, and improving a faltering milk supply. Before using any medication to increase the supply, attention should be directed to improving the supply by evaluation of frequency and thoroughness of milk removal. The mother should be given information on any medication and be followed up by the prescribing physician. Short-term use of these medications may have been studied but long-term use has not. Below is a brief table of galactogogues.

Modified from the Academy of Breast Feeding Medicine, clinical protocol #9. More information may be obtained at *www.bfmed.org*.

Medications	Mechanism of Action	Side Effects in Mother	Effects in Infant	Dose
Metoclopramide	dopamine antagonist; ↑prolactin	restlessness, fatigue, headache, depression, confusion, anxiety. Acute dystonic reactions rare.	none noted	30–45 mg/day in 3 or 4 divided doses for 7–14d then taper over 5–7d
Domperidone*	dopamine antagonist	dry mouth, headache, abdominal cramps	none noted	10–20 mg 3–4 times/day for 3–8 wks
Human growth hormone**			none noted	0.1 IU/kg/day subcutaneously for 7d
Thyrotrophin-releasing*** hormone	releases prolactin from pituitary		none noted	1 spray qid.
Herbal remedies				
Fenugreek		odor of sweat & urine, lower blood glucose	none noted	1–4 capsules 3–4 times/day
Goat's rue		none noted	lethargy in 2 infants	1 tsp dried leaves in 8 oz water as tea tid
Milk thistle		none noted	none noted	1 tsp crushed seeds in 8 oz water as tea tid

* Not available in US except from compounding pharmacists
** Expensive, usefulness appears limited
*** Long-term use not evaluated. Not commonly used.

APPENDIX C-2

HUMAN MILK FOR THE HOSPITALIZED ILL BABY[a]

Below are the important points about assisting mothers with supplying human milk for their hospitalized infant.

A. **Expression (collection) of human milk in the hospital:** Use a pumping kit suitable for double breast pumping, instruct the mother in the correct use of the pump and hygiene.
Use a single-use clean hard-plastic milk storage container for collection.
Medications the mother is taking should be noted and contraindicated medications discussed with mother's physician for a change to allow mother to continue to safety breastfeed.
Signs and symptoms of infections should be monitored and treated as necessary. Extremely few maternal illnesses require stopping breastfeeding.

B. **Handling human milk:** Hospital staff should follow Standard Precautions when handling expressed human milk.

C. **Labeling human milk:** Label with a human milk label, a patient name and ID, and date/time milk expressed and date/time thawed if previously frozen. Place in a bin labeled with the patient's name in refrigerator and/or freezer dedicated for that purpose. Milk intended for use within a 24–48 hour period should be refrigerated. Milk containing supplements or additives can be refrigerated for 24 hours. Human milk can be stored in a self-contained freezer in a refrigerator, i.e., separate door, at $>0°$ Celsius for 3 months; or in a deep freezer ($\leq 0°$ Celsius) for 6 months.

E. **Transportation of human milk:** Use an insulated container with a freezer gel pack.

F. **Identifying human milk:** Verify correct patient label by two RNs before use or addition of additives.

G. **Thawing frozen milk:** Check expiration date and use oldest first. Thaw in patient's own basin with lukewarm water and label with time and date. Do not allow water to touch lid. Do not microwave. Swirl container to distribute milk components.

[a] Modified from The Academy of Breastfeeding Medicine clinical protocol number #10. *www.bfmed.org*

APPENDIX C-3

PROCESS OF OBTAINING DONOR HUMAN MILK FOR THE HOSPITALIZED PATIENT

Donor human milk may be important for the treatment of various medical conditions.

A. Consent for use of donor human milk is obtained by using a standard hospital consent form.

B. The patient's insurance company must be informed that donor human milk has been prescribed. Hospital Purchasing is contacted to obtain a PO number that is used when ordering the milk.

C. Donor milk is obtained from a milk bank belonging to the Human Milk Banking Association of North America (HMBANA) *www.hmbana.org*.

D. A prescription for a week's worth of milk is sent/faxed to the Milk Bank, along with any required documentation. Donor milk is usually shipped on a weekly basis. Donor milk specifically from mothers of premature infants can be ordered and will be shipped when available.

E. Donor milk is shipped to hospital receiving area and should be labeled with the patient's name following Milk Banks' request. Any milk that has completely defrosted must be used in the next 24 hours or discarded. If milk arrives defrosted, notify the sending Donor Milk Bank.

APPENDIX C-4

TRANSITIONING THE BREASTFEEDING/ BREASTMILK-FED PREMATURE INFANT FROM THE NEONATAL INTENSIVE CARE UNIT TO HOME[a]

This protocol addresses the care of premature infants <37 weeks gestation and <2500 grams at birth, who are being transitioned from the hospital to home. Most slow growth in these babies, with the exception of the extremely low birth weight infant is a function of absolute intake rather than milk composition such that every effort to ensure optimal milk volume should be exhausted prior to switching feedings to formula.

[a] Modified from The Academy of Breastfeeding Medicine clinical protocol number #12. *www.bfmed.org*

General support of mothers of prematures wishing to breastfeed includes encouraging kangaroo care early, expression of milk soon after delivery and continuing every 3 hours. Mothers should understand that early feeding attempts are gradual, and not expected to result in full feedings. Sustained suckling with swallowing for five minutes is an indicator that the infant may be ready to transition from nasogastric tube to breastfeeding. Trained breastfeeding personnel should help evaluate the breastfeeding on a regular basis.

I. Pre-discharge: Discharge Planning

A. The clinician should work with the mother to devise a feeding plan well before the actual date of discharge. The plan may include a combination of breastmilk (directly from the breast and/or expressed) or breast milk and formula.

B. The following aspects of the current feeding plan should be assessed: type of feeding, amount of feeding, method of feeding, adequacy of growth and adequacy of nutrition.

1. Optimal nutrition includes: entire intake orally, normal growth, and normal biochemical indices. (Table 1)
2. Sub-optimal nutrition includes ANY of the following: intake is <160 cc/kg/day, cannot consume all feedings orally, growth is inadequate, and/or biochemical indices are abnormal.

C. For infants with optimal nutritional assessment: change diet to unfortified human milk ad libitum, by breastfeeding and/or alternative feeding methods, one week before anticipated discharge. Add iron, 2 mg/kg/day and a complete multivitamin preparation. Monitor milk intake and growth (weight and length) during this week. If intake and growth are adequate, continue this diet after discharge.

D. For infants with sub-optimal assessment: change diet to unfortified human milk, plus a minimum of 2 to 3 feedings of enriched post-discharge formula prepared per manufacturer instructions (~22 kcal/oz) at least one week before anticipated discharge. The mother should continue pumping or expressing milk at least three times/day. Assess adequacy of breastfeeding and address problems with latch, milk volume, frequency of feeds, maternal satisfaction, and consider a feeding device such as a shield or feeding tube device. If intake and growth are adequate during this week after switching, add iron and multivitamin preparation (1/2 to full dose depending upon how much formula is fed).

II. Post-Discharge Assessment

A. Nutrition should be monitored one week after discharge with growth assessment and biochemical indices of status. Reassess nutritional status as optimal or sub-optimal. If optimal re-evaluate in one month. If sub-optimal assessment, consider the issues with the adequacy of breastfeeding such as latch, volume, frequency etc.

APPENDIX C-5

BIOCHEMICAL[a] AND GROWTH MONITORING FOR PREMATURE INFANTS IN THE POST-DISCHARGE PERIOD[b]

Parameter	Action Values
Growth	
Weight gain	<20 g/day
Length increase	<0.5 cm/wk
Head circumference increase	<0.5 cm/wk
Biochemical Markers	
Phosphorus	<4.5 mg/dL
Alkaline phosphatase	>450 IU/L
Blood Urea Nitrogen	<5 mg/dL

[a] It is recognized that biochemical monitoring is not feasible in all settings; presence or absence of clinical rickets then becomes a substitute parameter.
[b] Modified from Hall RA. Nutritional follow-up of the breastfeeding premature infant after hospital discharge. Pediatr Clin North Amer 2001;48:453–460 and Schanler RJ. Nutrition support of the low birth weight infant. IN: Walker WA, Watkins JB, Duggan CP (eds): Nutrition in Pediatrics, 3rd edition, BC Decker Inc, Hamilton, ON, Canada, 2003;392–412.

Growth Parameters

1. INTRAUTERINE GROWTH CURVES

APPENDIX D-1
THE COLORADO INTRAUTERINE GROWTH CHARTS

The Colorado curves give percentiles of intrauterine growth for weight, length, and head circumference. From Lubchenco LO, Hansman C, Boyd E, *Pediatrics* 1966;37:403. Copyright © American Academy of Pediatrics, 1966.

APPENDIX D-2

INTRAUTERINE GROWTH CHART FOR MONOCHORIONIC TWINS, BOTH GENDERS

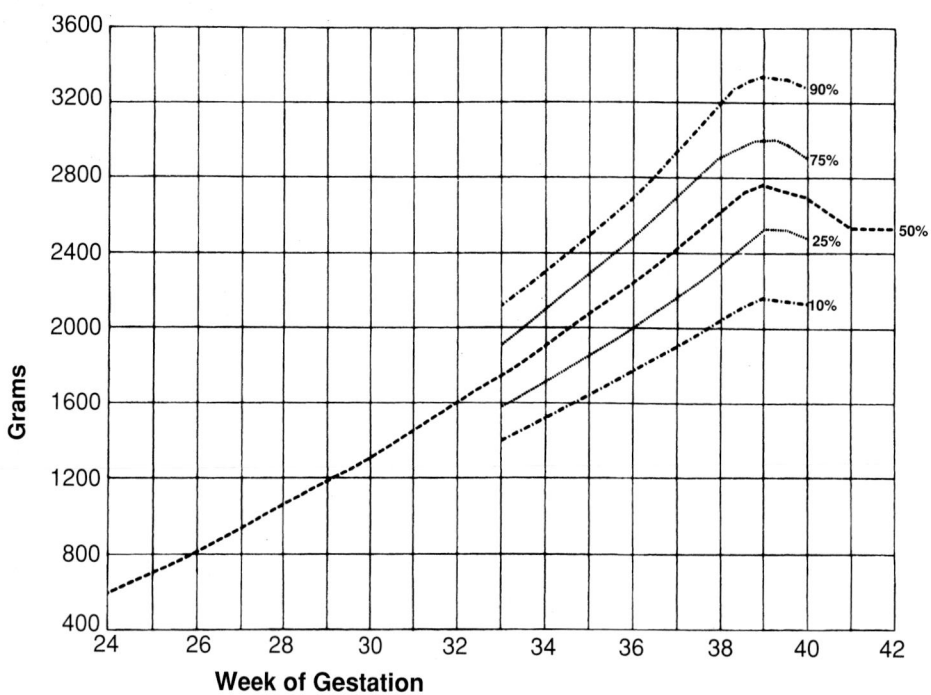

The weights of liveborn monochorionic twins at 24 to 42 weeks gestational ages are graphed as per centages.

From Naeye R, Bernirschke K, Hagstrom J, et al. *Pediatrics* 1966:37:409. Copyright © American Academy of Pediatrics, 1966.

APPENDIX D-3

INTRAUTERINE GROWTH CHART FOR DICHORIONIC TWINS, BOTH GENDERS

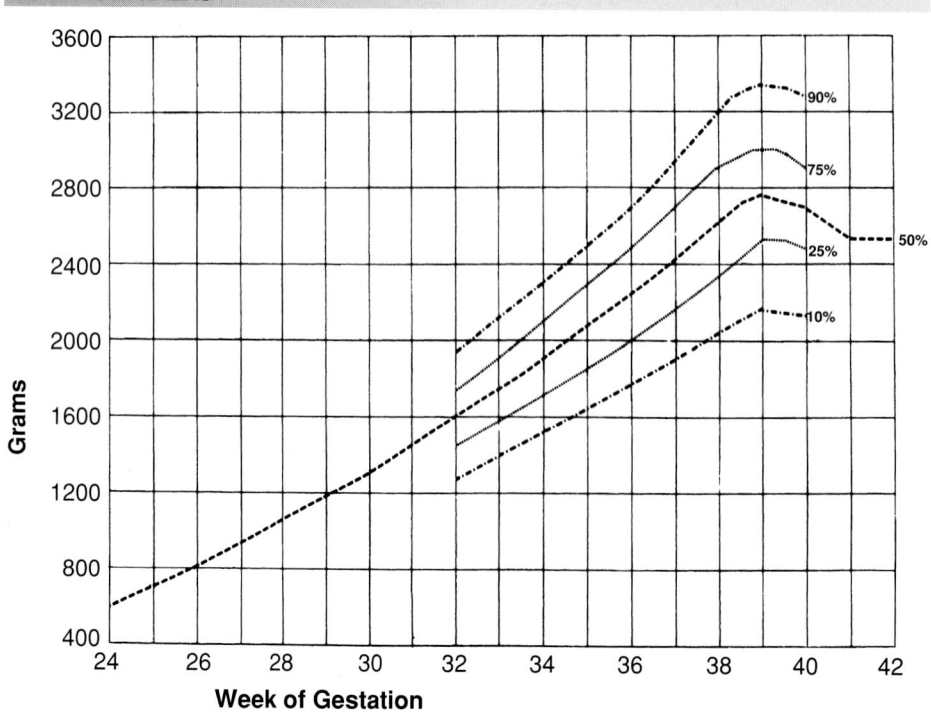

From Naeye R, Bernirschke K, Hagstrom J, et al. *Pediatrics* 1966:37:409. Copyright © American Academy of Pediatrics, 1966.

2. WEIGHT CONVERSION

APPENDIX D-4
CONVERSIONS OF POUNDS AND OUNCES TO GRAMS

Pounds	0	1	2	3	4	5	6	7	8	9	10	11	12	13	14	15
														Ounces		
0		28	57	85	113	142	170	198	227	255	283	312	340	369	397	425
1	454	482	510	539	567	595	624	652	680	709	737	765	794	822	850	879
2	907	936	964	992	1021	1049	1077	1106	1134	1162	1191	1219	1247	1276	1304	1332
3	1361	1389	1417	1446	1474	1503	1531	1559	1588	1616	1644	1673	1701	1729	1758	1786
4	1814	1843	1871	1899	1928	1956	1984	2013	2041	2070	2098	2126	2155	2183	2211	2240
5	2268	2296	2325	2353	2381	2410	2438	2466	2495	2523	2551	2580	2608	2637	2665	2693
6	2722	2750	2778	2807	2835	2863	2892	2920	2948	2977	3005	3033	3062	3090	3118	3147
7	3175	3203	3232	3260	3289	3317	3345	3374	3402	3430	3459	3487	3515	3544	3572	3600
8	3629	3657	3685	3714	3742	3770	3799	3827	3856	3884	3912	3941	3969	3997	4026	4054
9	4082	4111	4139	4167	4196	4224	4252	4281	4309	4337	4366	4394	4423	4451	4479	4508
10	4536	4564	4593	4621	4649	4678	4706	4734	4763	4791	4819	4848	4876	4904	4933	4961
11	4990	5018	5046	5075	5103	5131	5160	5188	5216	5245	5273	5301	5330	5358	5386	5415
12	5443	5471	5500	5528	5557	5585	5613	5642	5670	5698	5727	5755	5783	5812	5840	5868
13	5897	5925	5953	5982	6010	6038	6067	6095	6123	6152	6180	6209	6237	6265	6294	6322
14	6350	6379	6407	6435	6464	6492	6520	6549	6577	6605	6634	6662	6690	6719	6747	6776
15	6804	6832	6860	6889	6917	6945	6973	7002	7030	7059	7087	7115	7144	7172	7201	7228
16	7257	7286	7313	7342	7371	7399	7427	7456	7484	7512	7541	7569	7597	7626	7654	7682
17	7711	7739	7768	7796	7824	7853	7881	7909	7938	7966	7994	8023	8051	8079	8108	8136
18	8165	8192	8221	8249	8278	8306	8335	8363	8391	8420	8448	8476	8504	8533	8561	8590
19	8618	8646	8675	8703	8731	8760	8788	8816	8845	8873	8902	8930	8958	8987	9015	9043
20	9072	9100	9128	9157	9185	9213	9242	9270	9298	9327	9355	9383	9412	9440	9469	9497
21	9525	9554	9582	9610	9639	9667	9695	9724	9752	9780	9809	9837	9865	9894	9922	9950
22	9979	10007	10036	10064	10092	10120	10149	10177	10206	10234	10262	10291	10319	10347	10376	10404

3. GROWTH CHARTS

APPENDIX D-5A
BIRTH TO 36 MONTHS: BOYS LENGTH-FOR-AGE AND WEIGHT-FOR-AGE PERCENTILES

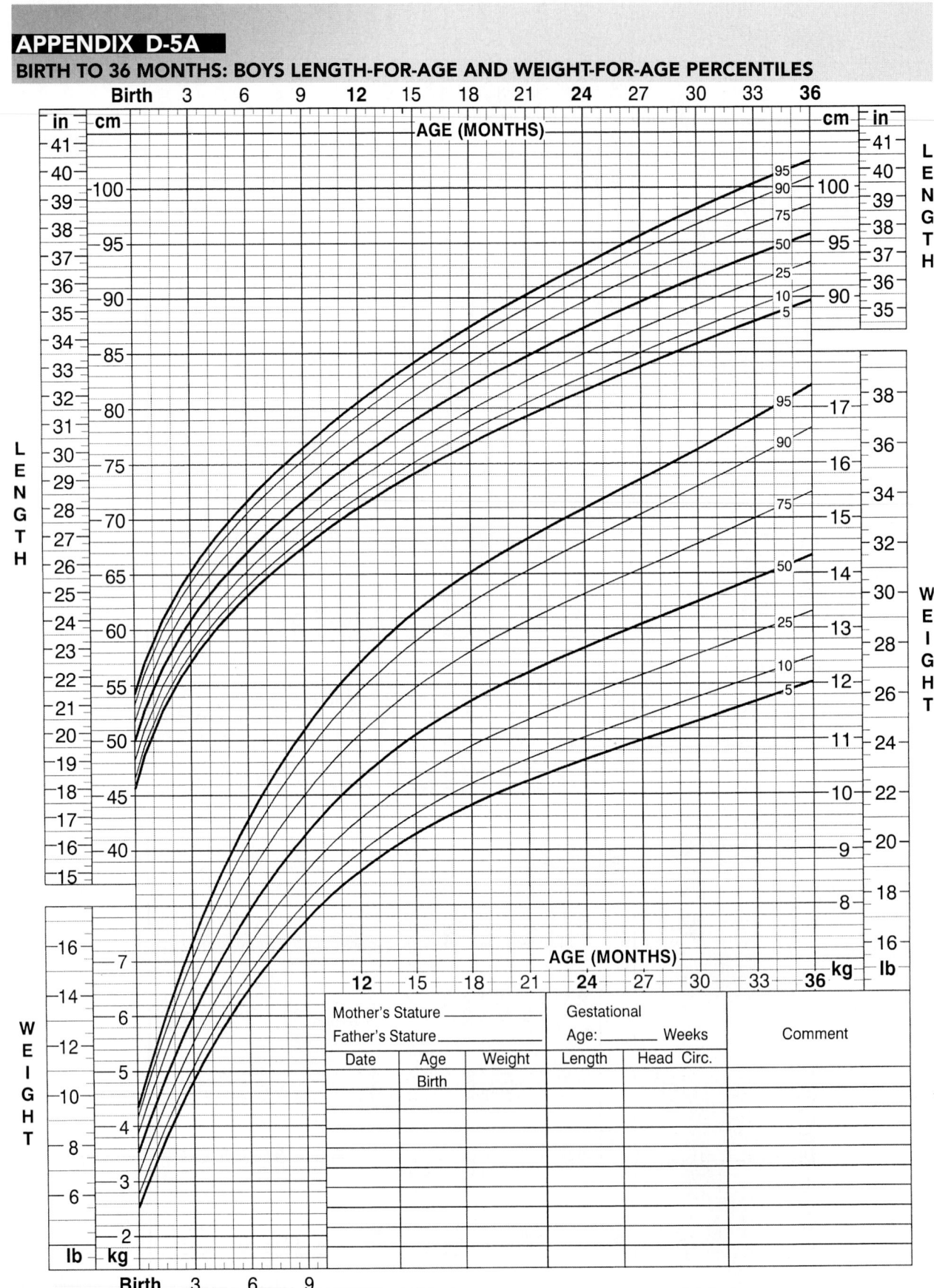

Published May 30, 2000 (modified 4/20/01).
SOURCE: Developed by the National Center for Health Statistics in collaboration with
the National Center for Chronic Disease Prevention and Health Promotion (2000).
http://www.cdc.gov/growthcharts

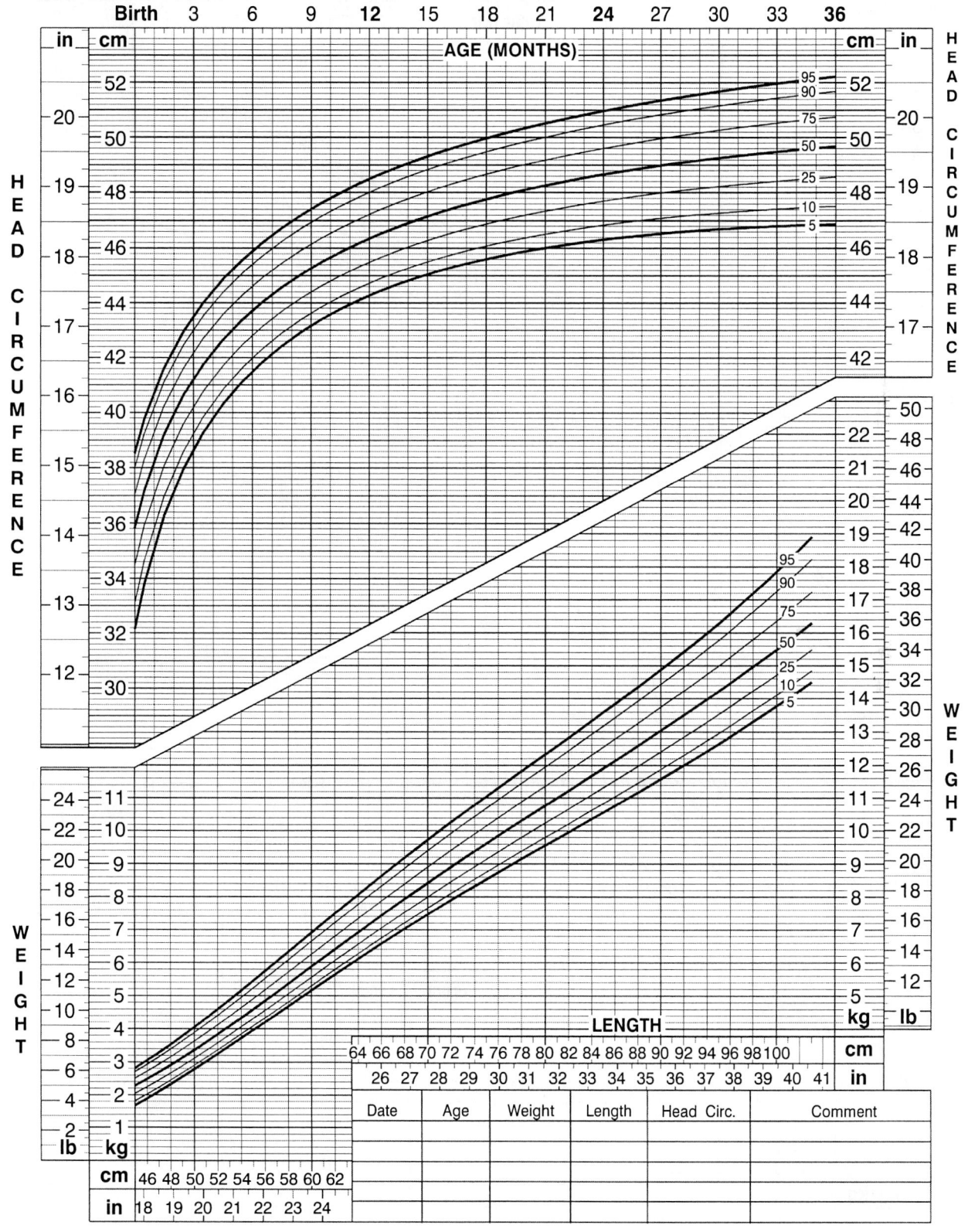

Published May 30, 2000 (modified 10/16/00).

SOURCE: Developed by the National Center for Health Statistics in collaboration with
the National Center for Chronic Disease Prevention and Health Promotion (2000).
http://www.cdc.gov/growthcharts

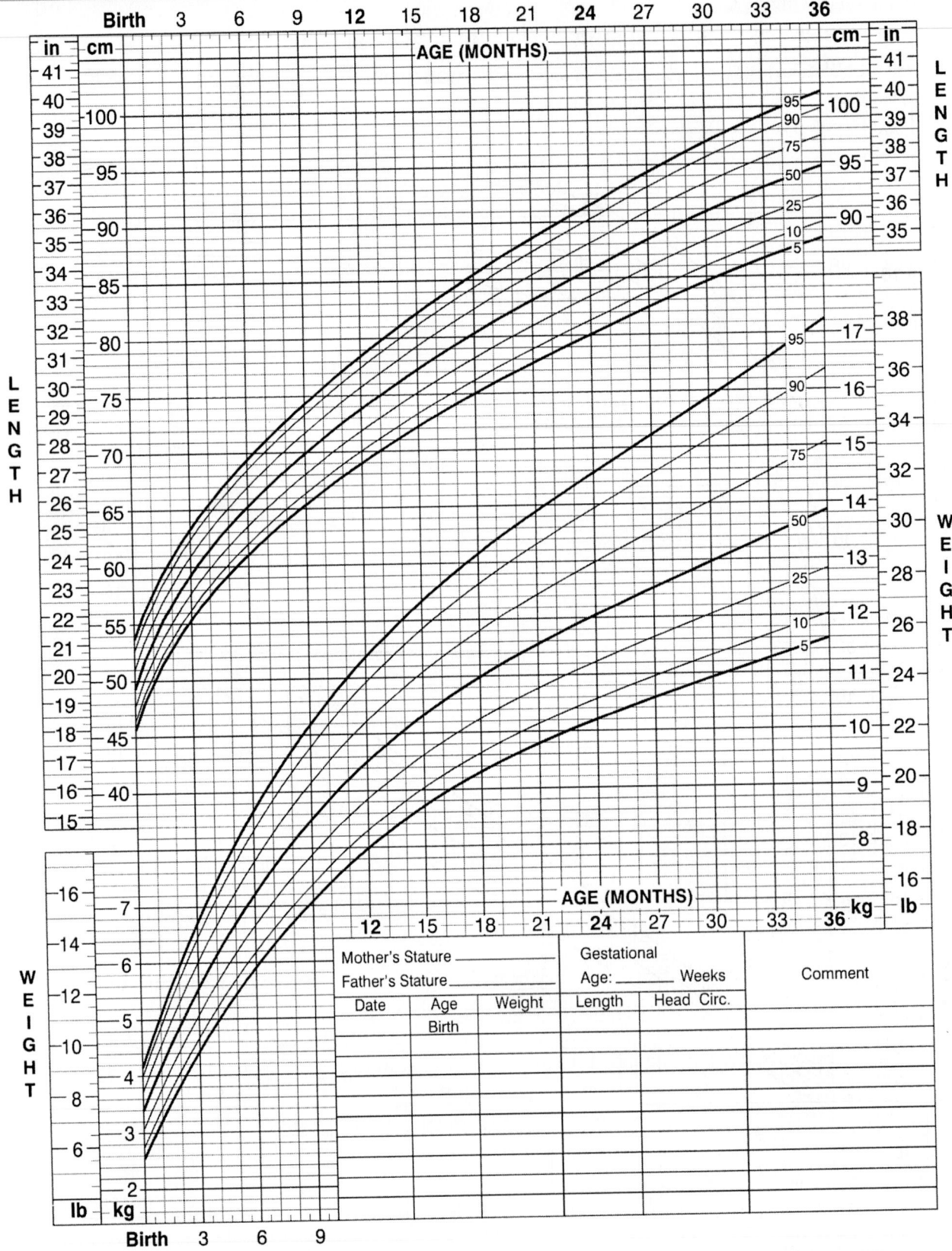

Published May 30, 2000 (modified 4/20/01).

SOURCE: Developed by the National Center for Health Statistics in collaboration with the National Center for Chronic Disease Prevention and Health Promotion (2000).

http://www.cdc.gov/growthcharts

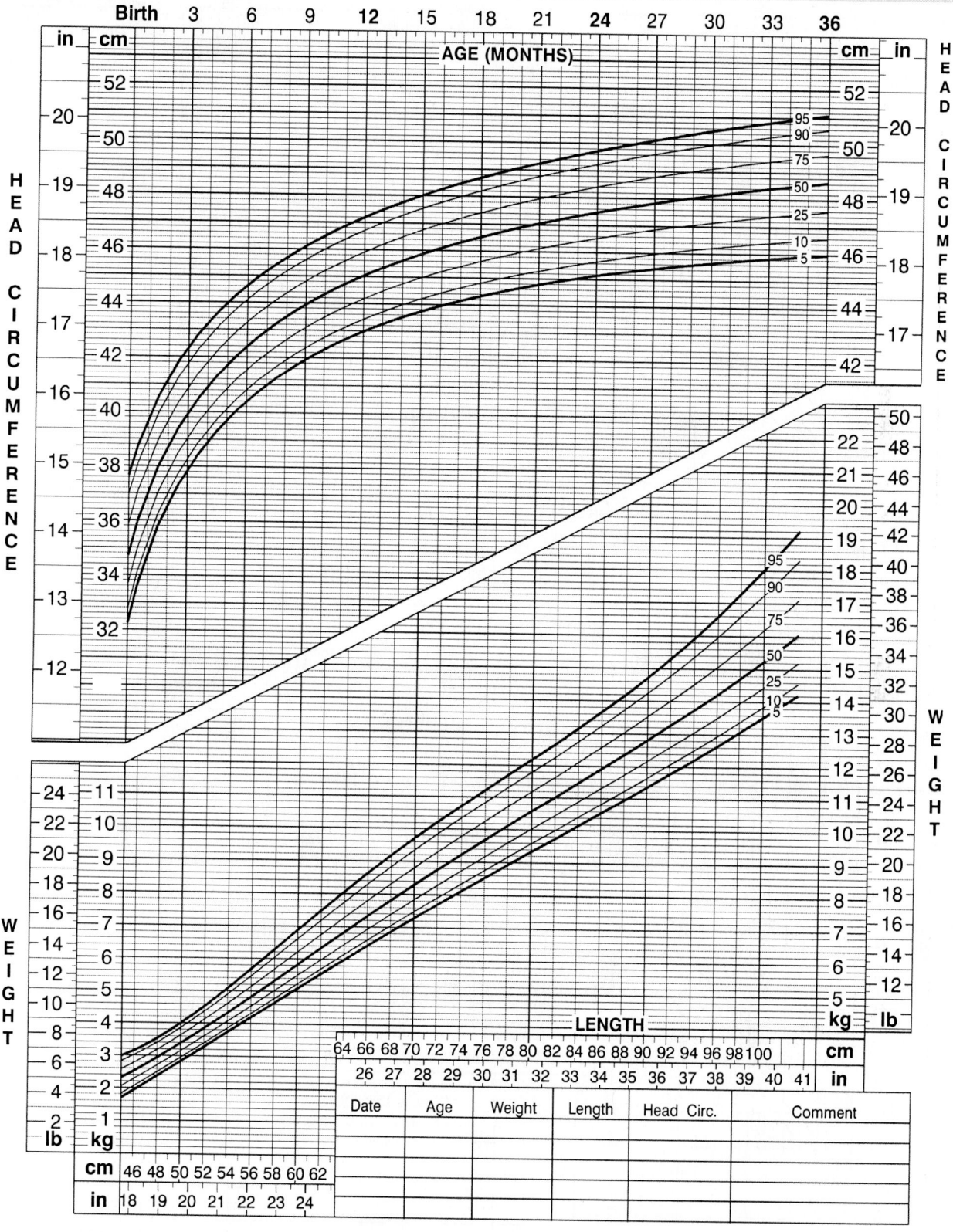

Published May 30, 2000 (modified 10/16/00).
SOURCE: Developed by the National Center for Health Statistics in collaboration with
the National Center for Chronic Disease Prevention and Health Promotion (2000).
http://www.cdc.gov/growthcharts

IHDP* GROWTH PERCENTILES: VLBW PREMATURE BOYS[1,2]
(≤1800 g BW, ≤37 wk GA)

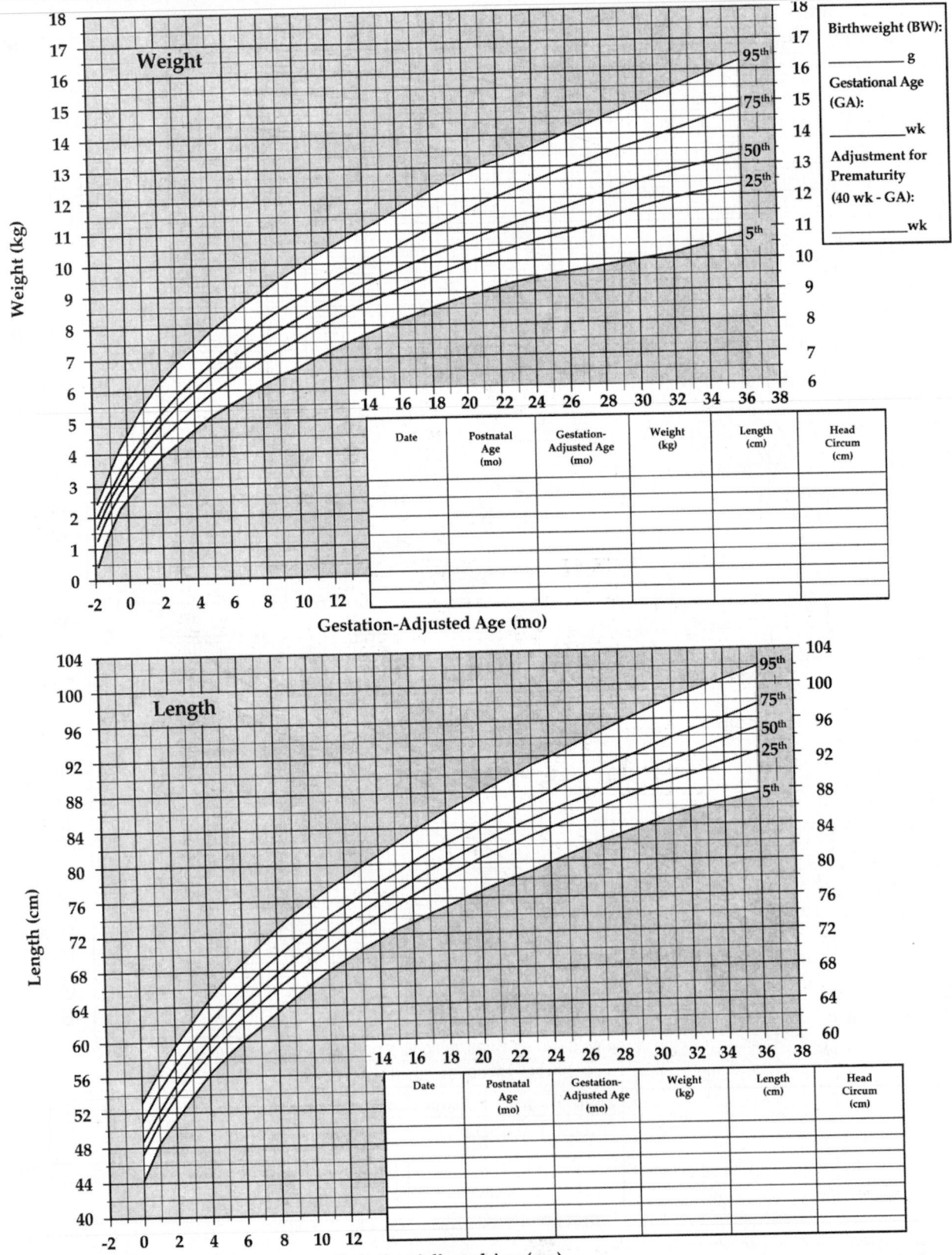

* Infant Health and Development Program

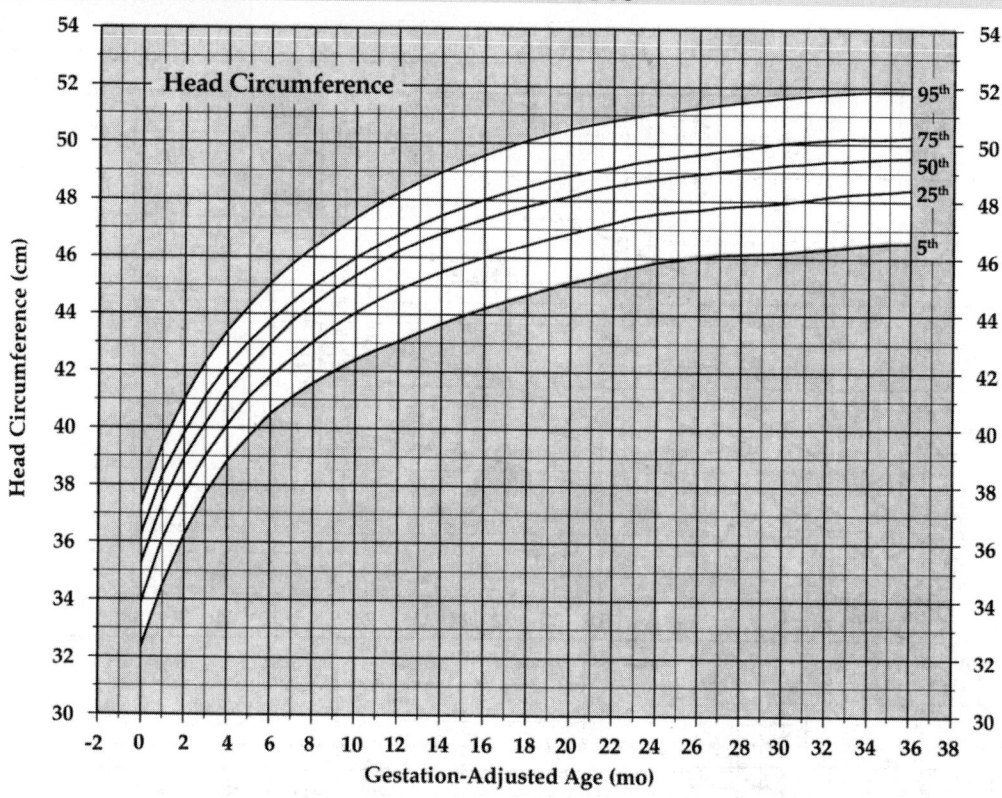

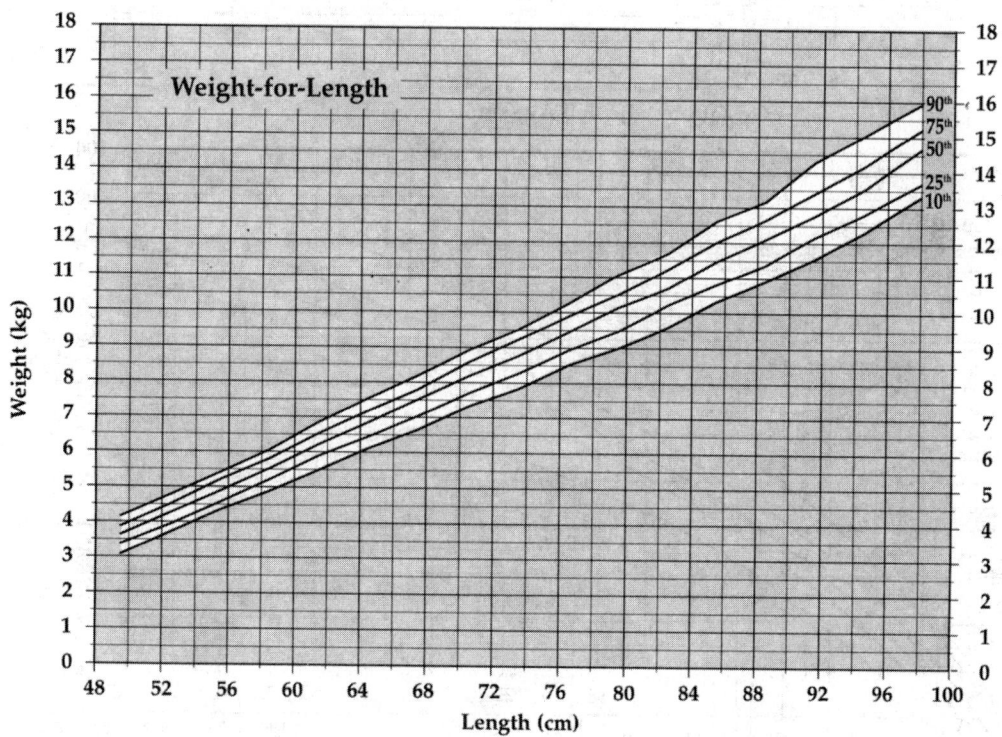

References

1. Guo SS, Roche AF, Chumlea WC, et al: Growth in weight, recumbent length, and head circumference for preterm low-birthweight infants during the first three years of life using gestation-adjusted ages. *Early Hum Dev* 1997;47:305-325.

2. Guo SS, Wholihan K, Roche AF, et al: Weight-for-length reference data for preterm, low-birth-weight infants. *Arch Pediatr Adolesc Med* 1996;150:964-970. Copyright: 1996, American Medical Association.

Acknowledgment

IHDP studies were supported by grants from the Robert Wood Johnson Foundation, Pew Charitable Trusts, and the Bureau of Maternal and Child Health, US Department of Health and Human Services. The IHDP growth percentile graphs were prepared by S.S. Guo and A.F. Roche, Wright State University, Yellow Springs, Ohio. IHDP, its sponsors and the investigators do not endorse specific products.

Provided by Ross Products Division of Abbott Laboratories Inc.

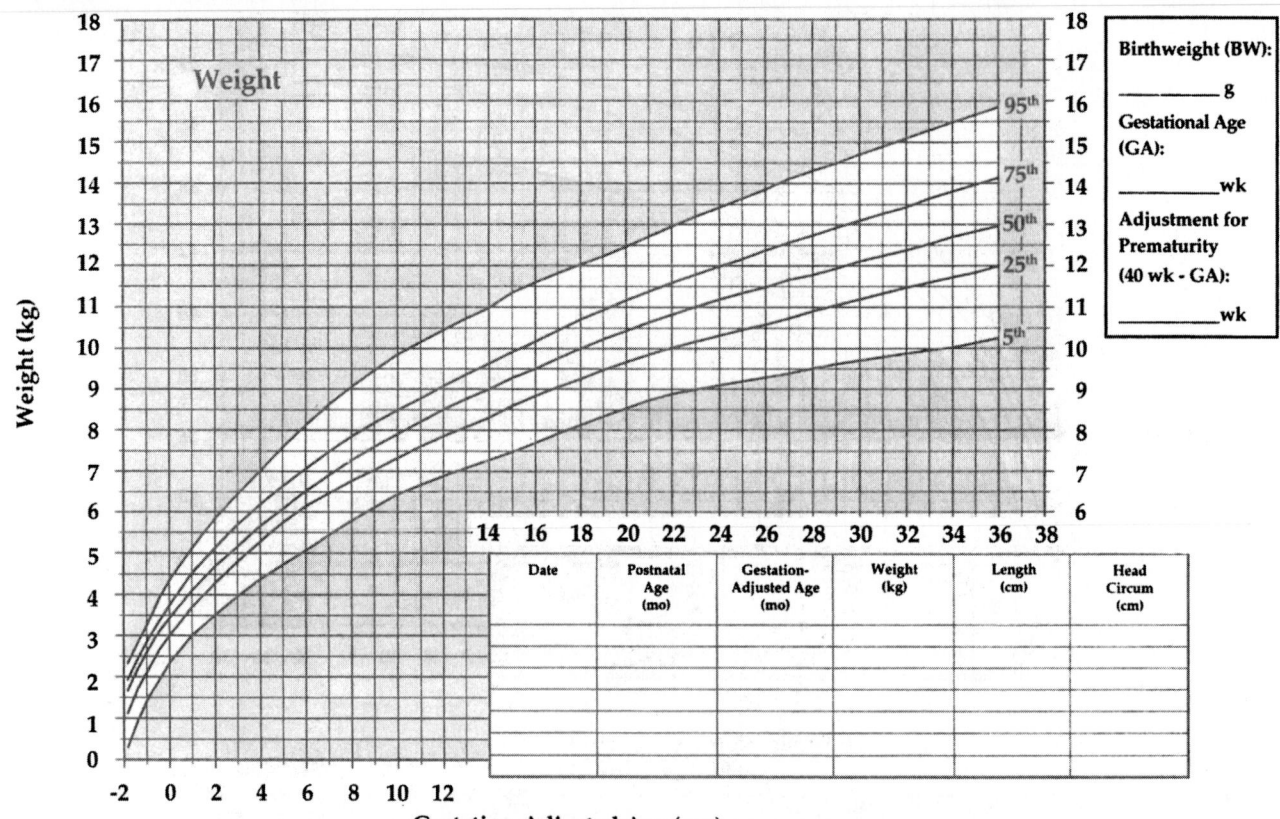

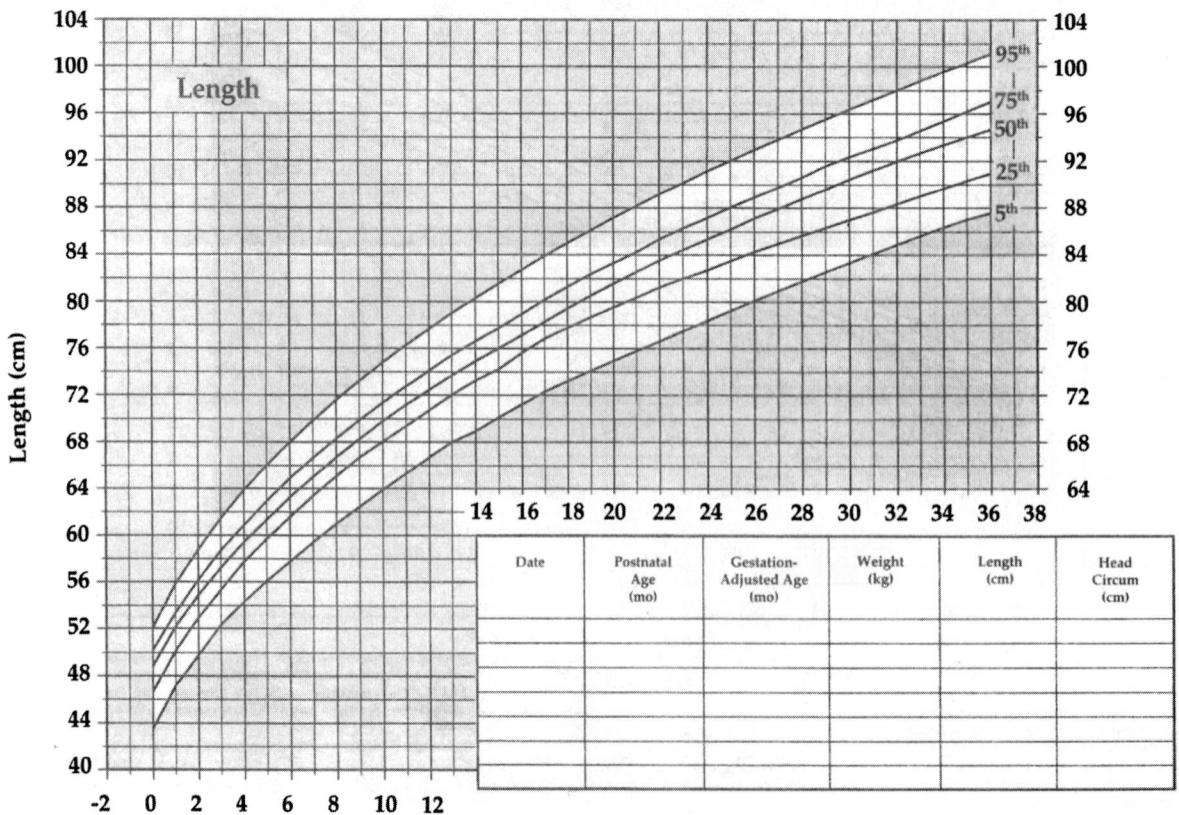

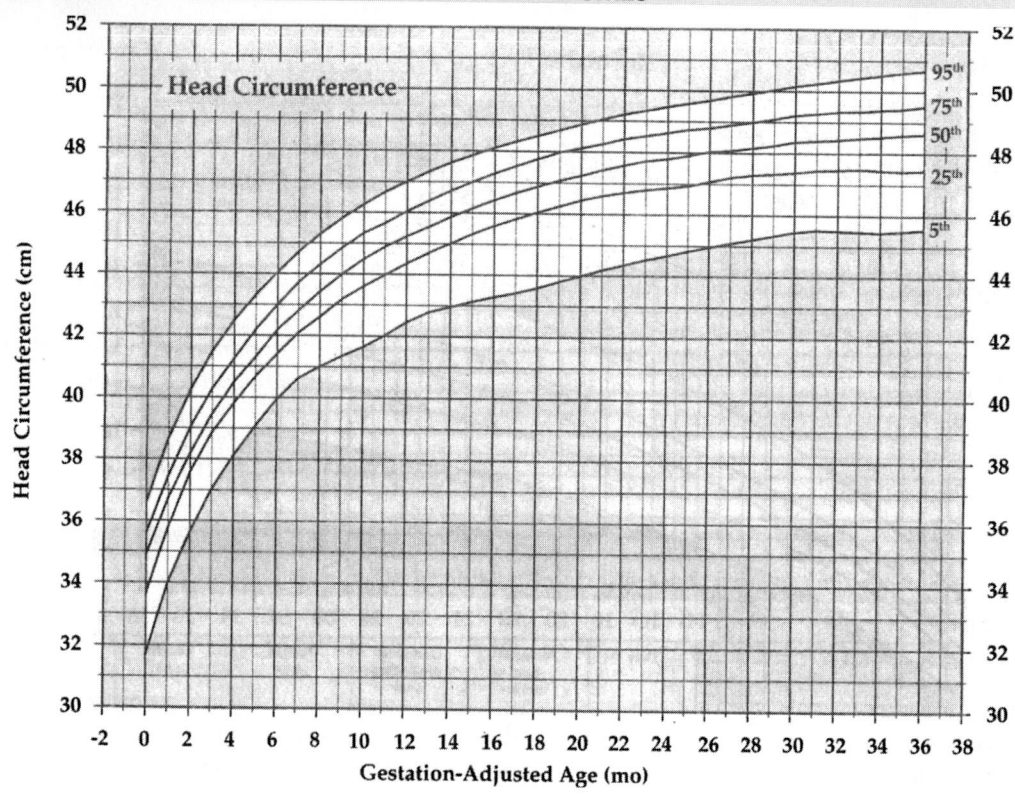

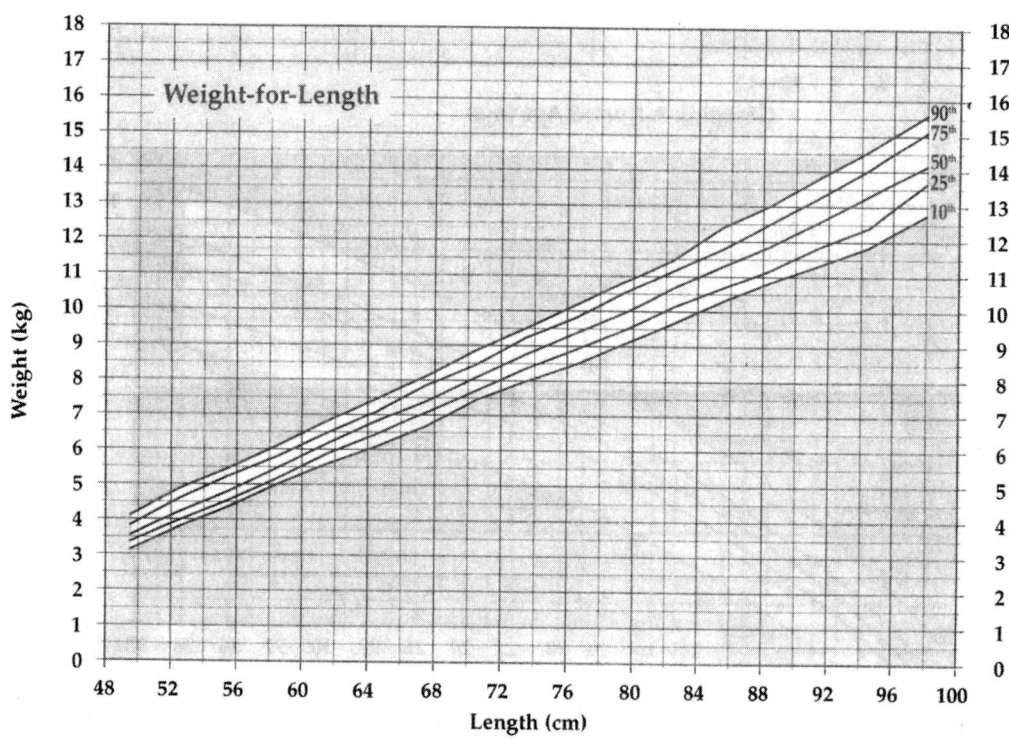

References

1. Guo SS, Roche AF, Chumlea WC, et al: Growth in weight, recumbent length, and head circumference for preterm low-birthweight infants during the first three years of life using gestation-adjusted ages. *Early Hum Dev* 1997;47:305-325.

2. Guo SS, Wholihan K, Roche AF, et al: Weight-for-length reference data for preterm, low-birth-weight infants. *Arch Pediatr Adolesc Med* 1996;150:964-970. Copyright: 1996, American Medical Association.

Acknowledgment

IHDP studies were supported by grants from the Robert Wood Johnson Foundation, Pew Charitable Trusts, and the Bureau of Maternal and Child Health, US Department of Health and Human Services. The IHDP growth percentile graphs were prepared by S.S. Guo and A.F. Roche, Wright State University, Yellow Springs, Ohio. IHDP, its sponsors and the investigators do not endorse specific products.

Provided by Ross Products Division of Abbott Laboratories Inc.

Jaundice

Appendix E. The following Frequently Asked Questions" (FAQs) are from the American Academy of Pediatrics (AAP). Feel free to excerpt these FAQs or use them in their entirety for distribution to your families. Please attribute these FAQs to the American Academy of Pediatrics.

Congratulations on the birth of your new baby!
To make sure your baby's first week is safe and healthy, it is important that:

Your baby is checked for jaundice in the hospital.
If you are breastfeeding, you get the help you need to make sure it is going well.
Your baby is seen by a doctor or nurse at 3 to 5 days of age.

Q: What is jaundice?

A: Jaundice is the yellow color seen in the skin of many newborns. It happens when a chemical called bilirubin builds up in the baby's blood. Jaundice can occur in babies of any race or color.

Q: Why is jaundice common in newborns?

A: Everyone's blood contains bilirubin, which is removed by the liver. Before birth, the mother's liver does this for the baby. Most babies develop jaundice in the first few days after birth because it takes a few days for the baby's liver to get better at removing bilirubin.

Q: How can I tell if my baby is jaundiced?

A: The skin of a baby with jaundice usually appears yellow. The best way to see jaundice is in good light, such as daylight or under fluorescent lights. Jaundice usually appears first in the face and then moves to the chest, abdomen, arms, and legs as the bilirubin level increases. The whites of the eyes may also be yellow. Jaundice may be harder to see in babies with darker skin color.

Q: Can jaundice hurt my baby?

A: Most infants have mild jaundice that is harmless, but in unusual situations the bilirubin level can get very high and might cause brain damage. This is why newborns should be checked carefully for jaundice and treated to prevent a high bilirubin level.

Q: How should my baby be checked for jaundice?

A: If your baby looks jaundiced in the first few days after birth, your baby's doctor or nurse may use a skin test or blood test to check your baby's bilirubin level. A bilirubin level is always needed if jaundice develops before the baby is 24 hours old. Whether a test is needed after that depends on the baby's age, the amount of jaundice, and whether the baby has other factors that make jaundice more likely or harder to see.

Q: Does breastfeeding affect jaundice?

A: Jaundice is more common in babies who are breastfed than babies who are formula-fed, but this occurs mainly in infants who are not nursing well. If you are breastfeeding, you should nurse your baby at least 8 to 12 times a day for the first few days. This will help you produce enough milk and will help to keep the baby's bilirubin level down. If you are having trouble breastfeeding, ask your baby's doctor or nurse or a lactation specialist for help. Breast milk is the ideal food for your baby.

Q: When should my newborn get checked after leaving the hospital?

A: It is important for your baby to be seen by a nurse or doctor when the baby is between 3 and 5 days old, because this is usually when a baby's bilirubin level is highest. The timing of this visit may vary depending on your baby's age when released from the hospital and other factors.

Q: Which babies require more attention for jaundice?

A: Some babies have a greater risk for high levels of bilirubin and may need to be seen sooner after discharge from the hospital. Ask your doctor about an early follow-up visit if your baby has any of the following:

A high bilirubin level before leaving the hospital
Early birth (more than 2 weeks before the due date)
Jaundice in the first 24 hours after birth
Breastfeeding that is not going well
A lot of bruising or bleeding under the scalp related to labor and delivery
A parent or brother or sister who had high bilirubin and received light therapy

Q: When should I call my baby's doctor?

A: Call your baby's doctor if:

Your baby's skin turns more yellow.
Your baby's abdomen, arms, or legs are yellow.
The whites of your baby's eyes are yellow.
Your baby is jaundiced and is hard to wake, fussy, or not nursing or taking formula well.

Q: How is harmful jaundice prevented?

A: Most jaundice requires no treatment. When treatment is necessary, placing your baby under special lights while he or she is undressed will lower the bilirubin level. Depending on your baby's bilirubin level, this can be done in the hospital or at home. Jaundice is treated at levels that are much lower than those at which brain damage is a concern. Treatment can prevent the harmful effects of jaundice.

Putting your baby in sunlight is not recommended as a safe way of treating jaundice. Exposing your baby to sunlight might help lower the bilirubin level, but this will only work if the baby is completely undressed. This cannot be done safely inside your home because your baby will get cold, and newborns should never be put in direct sunlight outside because they might get sunburned.

Q: When does jaundice go away?

A: In breastfed infants, jaundice often lasts for more than 2 to 3 weeks. In formula-fed infants, most jaundice goes away by 2 weeks. If your baby is jaundiced for more than 3 weeks, see your baby's doctor.

The information contained in this publication should not be used as a substitute for the medical care and advice of your pediatrician. There may be variations in treatment that your pediatrician may recommend based on individual facts and circumstances.

© COPYRIGHT AMERICAN ACADEMY OF PEDIATRICS, ALL RIGHTS RESERVED. Site map | Contact us | Privacy statement | About us | Home
American Academy of Pediatrics, 141 Northwest Point Blvd., Elk Grove Village, IL, 60007, 847-434-4000

Blood Pressure

APPENDIX F-1
BLOOD PRESSURE BY GESTATIONAL AGE

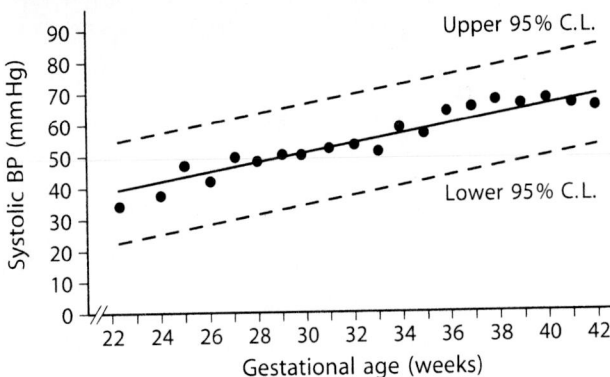

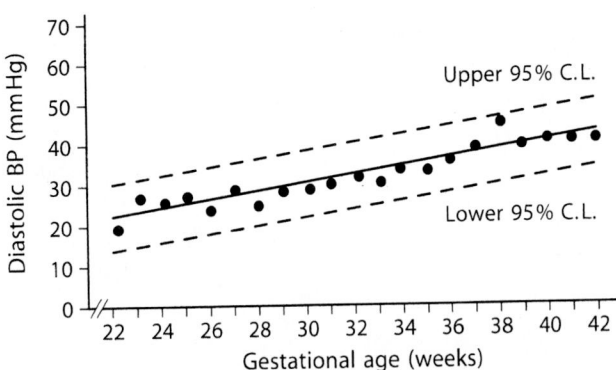

Appendix F-1 Linear regression between gestational age and mean systolic (A) and diastolic (B) blood pressure, along with the upper and lower 95% confidence limits, which approximate mean ± 2 standard deviations (Reprinted with permission from Zubrow AB, Hulman S, Kushner H, Falkner B. Determinants of blood pressure in infants admitted to neonatal intensive care units: A prospective multicenter study. J Perinatol 1995;15:470–479).

APPENDIX F-2
BLOOD PRESSURE BY BIRTHWEIGHT

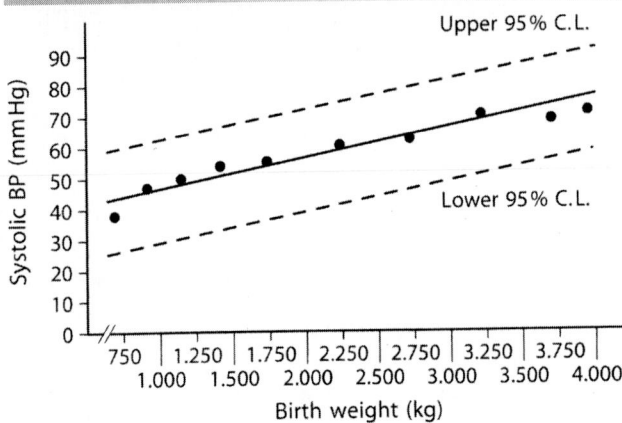

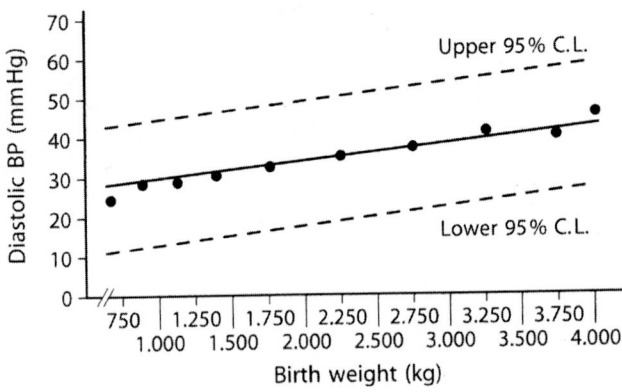

Appendix F-2 Linear regression between birth weight and mean systolic (A) and diastolic (B) blood pressure, along with the upper and lower 95% confidence limits, which approximate mean ± 2 standard deviations (Reprinted with permission from Zubrow AB, Hulman S, Kushner H, Falkner B. Determinants of blood pressure in infants admitted to neonatal intensive care units: A prospective multicenter study. J Perinatol 1995;15:470–479).

APPENDIX F-3
BLOOD PRESSURE BY POST CONCEPTIONAL AGE

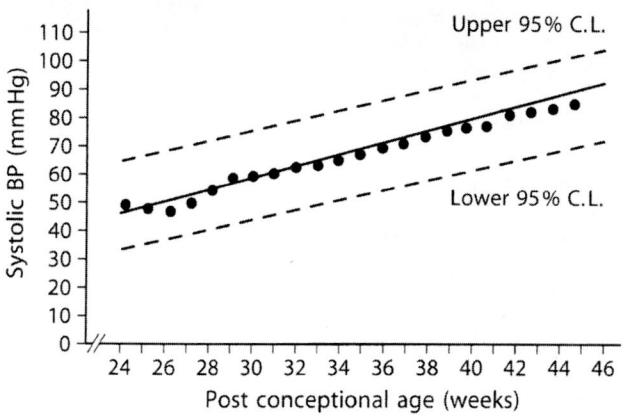

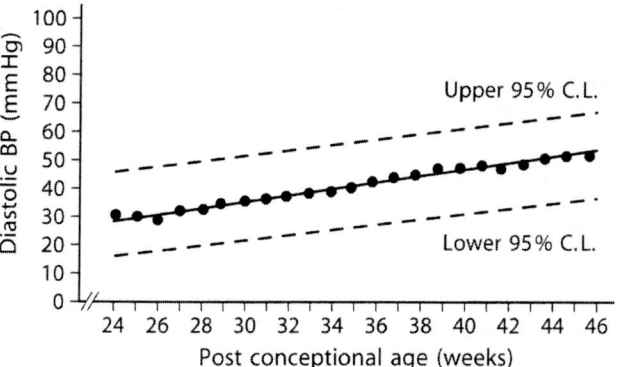

Appendix F-3   Linear regression between post-conceptual age and mean systolic (A) and diastolic (B) blood pressure, along with the upper and lower 95% confidence limits, which approximate mean ±2 standard deviations (Reprinted with permission from Zubrow AB, Hulman S, Kushner H, Falkner B. Determinants of blood pressure in infants admitted to neonatal intensive care units: A prospective multicenter study. J Perinatol 1995;15:470–479).

APPENDIX F-4
AGE-SPECIFIC BLOOD PRESSURE BY SEX UP TO 1 YEAR

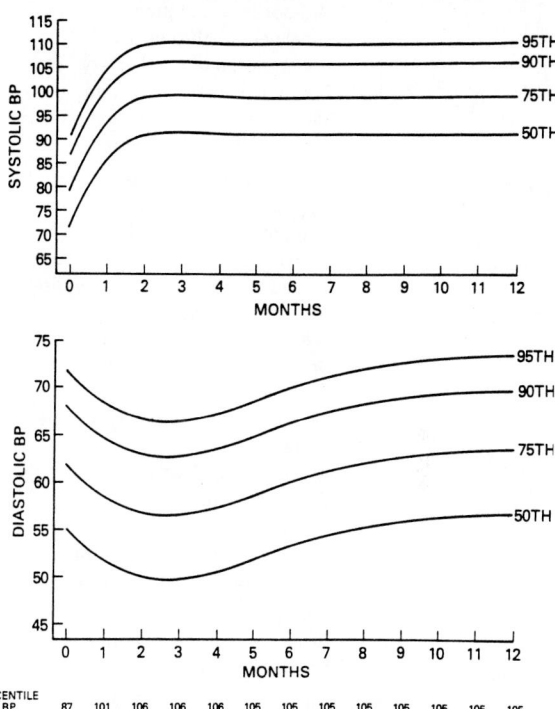

90TH PERCENTILE													
SYSTOLIC BP	87	101	106	106	106	105	105	105	105	105	105	105	105
DIASTOLIC BP	68	65	63	63	63	65	66	67	68	68	69	69	69
HEIGHT CM	51	59	63	66	68	70	72	73	74	76	77	78	80
WEIGHT KG	4	4	5	5	6	7	8	9	9	10	10	11	11

Appendix F-4   Age-specific distributions of systolic and diastolic blood pressure for male (A) and female (B) infants between birth and 12 months of age (Reprinted with permission from National Heart, Lung and Blood Institute Task Force on Blood Pressure Control in Children. Report of the Second Task Force on blood pressure control in children–1987. National Institutes of Health, January 1987).

APPENDIX F-5
CAUSES OF HYPERTENSION IN INFANCY

Renovascular
- Thromboembolism
- Renal artery stenosis (FMD)
- Mid-aortic coarctation
- Renal venous thrombosis
- Compression of renal artery
- Abdominal aortic aneurysm
- Idiopathic arterial calcification
- Congenital rubella syndrome

Renal Parenchymal Disease
- Congenital
  - Autosomal Dominant PKD
  - Autosomal Recessive PKD
  - Multicystic-dysplastic kidney disease
  - Tuberous Sclerosis
  - Ureteropelvic junction obstruction
  - Unilateral renal hypoplasia
  - Primary megaureter
  - Congenital Nephrotic Syndrome
- Acquired
  - Acute Tubular Necrosis
  - Cortical Necrosis
  - Interstitial Nephritis
  - Hemolytic-Uremic Syndrome
  - Obstruction (stones, tumors)

Pulmonary
- Bronchopulmonary Dysplasia
- Pneumothorax

Cardiac
- Thoracic aortic coarctation

Genetic
- Single-gene disorders
  - Glucocorticoid-Remediable Aldosteronism
  - Liddle's Syndrome
  - Pseudohypoaldosteronism type II
    (Gordon's Syndrome)
- Malformation syndromes
  - Williams Syndrome
  - Turner Syndrome
  - Neurofibromatosis
  - Cockayne Syndrome

Endocrine
- Congenital Adrenal Hyperplasia
  - 11β-hydroxylase deficiency
  - 17α-hydroxylase deficiency
  - 11β-hydroxysteroid dehydrogenase deficiency
- Hyperaldosteronism
- Hyperthyroidism

Medications/Intoxications
- Infant
  - Dexamethasone/corticosteroids
  - Adrenergic agents
  - Vitamin D Intoxication
  - Theophylline/aminophylline
  - Caffeine
  - Pancuronium
  - Phenylephrine eye drops
- Maternal
  - Cocaine
  - Heroin

Neoplasia
- Wilms tumor
- Mesoblastic nephroma
- Neuroblastoma
- Pheochromocytoma

Neurologic
- Pain
- Intracranial hypertension
- Seizures
- Familial dysautonomia
- Subdural hematoma
- Opiate withdrawal

Miscellaneous
- Fluid overload
- Total Parenteral Nutrition (TPN)
- Closure of abdominal wall defect
- Adrenal hemorrhage
- Hypercalcemia
- Traction
- ECMO
- Birth asphyxia

Abbreviations used in Appendix F-5
ECMO, extracorporeal membrane oxygenation; FMD, fibromuscular dysplasia; PKD, polycystic kidney disease.

APPENDIX F-6
DIAGNOSTIC STUDIES FOR EVALUATION OF HYPERTENSIVE INFANTS

Generally Useful	Useful in Selected Infants
BUN, Creatinine	Abdominal/pelvic ultrasound
Calcium	Aldosterone
CBC & platelet count	Aortography
Chest x-ray	Cortisol (morning)
Electrolytes	Echocardiogram
Plasma renin	Nuclear scan (DTPA/MAG-3)
Renal Ultrasound with Doppler	Renal angiography
Urinalysis ($+/-$ culture)	Thyroid studies
	Urine VMA/HVA
	VCUG

Abbreviations used: BUN, blood urea nitrogen; CBC, complete blood count; DTPA, diethylenetriaminepentaacetic acid; HVA, homovanillic acid; MAG, mercaptoacetyltriglycine; VMA, vanillylmandelic acid; VCUG, voiding cystourethrogram.

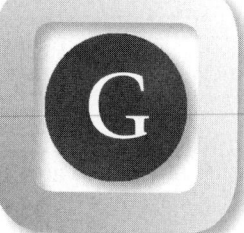

Renal and Urinary Tract Anomalies

APPENDIX G-1

ASSOCIATIONS BETWEEN RENAL-URINARY TRACT ANOMALIES AND OTHER STRUCTURAL DEFECTS

Diagnosis (Mode of Genetic Transmission)	Frequency of Anomalies	Renal Anomalies	Urologic Anomalies	Other Associations
Hereditary associations				
Acrorenal syndrome, or radial ray aplasia and renal anomalies (AD)*	100%	Agenesis, ectopia		Absence of radius and thumb
Acrorenocular syndrome (AD/sporadic)	100%	Malrotation, ectopia	VUR, bladder diverticula	Thumb hypoplasia preaxial polydactyly, coloboma, ptosis
Acrorenomandibular syndrome (AR)†	Frequent	Agenesis, ectopia		Split hand/split foot, cataracts ear and genital anomalies
Adams-Oliver syndrome (AD)	Occasional		Duplicated collecting system	Aplasia cutis congenita, terminal transverse defects of limbs
Alport syndrome (AD, but fully expressed only in males; X-linked)	Frequent	Nephritis; recurrent hematuria		Deafness cataracts, myopia lenticonus
Antley-Bixler syndrome (AR?)	Occasional	Displaced kidney, accessory renal artery		Craniosynostosis, choanal atresia, radiohumeral synostosis
Arthrogryposis multiplex congenita with renal and hepatic abnormalities (AR/X-linked?)	100%	Glycosuria, polyuria, nephrocalcinosis hypercalciuria, hyperposphaturia		Arthrogryposis multiplex congenita, rarefaction of motor neurons in anterior horn, cholestasis, all reported patients died before 4 months of age
Baller-Gerold syndrome, or Craniosynostosis-radial aplasia syndrome (AR)	Occasional	Pelvic kidney		MR (50%), growth deficiency, craniosynostosis, radial aplasia, CHD
Branchiootoureteral syndrome (AD)	50%	Bifid renal pelvis	Bifid ureters	Preauricular pit/tag, bilateral hearing loss
Campomelic dysplasia (AR)	30%	Usually hydronephrosis, MKD		Bowed tibiae, hypoplastic scapulae, flat facies growth deficiency, CNS disorganization, most die of respiratory failure as neonates or in infancy
Carpenter syndrome (AR)	Occasional		Ureteral dilatation	Acrocephaly, polydactyly—syndactyly of feet, lateral displacement of inner canthi, hypogenitalism
CHILD syndrome (X-linked?, lethal in hemizygotic male)	Occasional	Unilateral agenesis		Unilateral hypomelia, ichthyosis, CHD, mild SGA

* AD-autosomal dominant
† AR-autosomal recessive

APPENDIX G-1

ASSOCIATIONS BETWEEN RENAL-URINARY TRACT ANOMALIES AND OTHER STRUCTURAL DEFECTS
(*continued*)

Diagnosis (Mode of Genetic Transmission)	Frequency of Anomalies	Renal Anomalies	Urologic Anomalies	Other Associations
COFS syndrome (AR)	Occasional	Agenesis		Neurogenic arthrogryposis, microcephaly, microphthalmia/cataract/blepharophimosis, large ear pinnae, prominent nasal bridge, no growth, usually die before 5 years of age
Cohen syndrome (AR)	Occasional		UPJ obstruction	Hypotonia, obesity, prominent incisors, moderate MR
Deal syndrome (AR)	100%	Fanconi syndrome		Ichthyosis, jaundice, musculoskeletal deformities, diarrhea, failure to thrive, death in infancy
Digitorenocerebral syndrome (AR)	Frequent	Agenesis, hypoplasia, dysplasia		Facial dysmorphism, seizures, malformed fingers and toes
EEC syndrome (AD, variable penetrance)	Occasional	Agenesis, hydronephrosis medullary dysplasia	Ureterocele	Ectrodactyly, ectodermal dysplasia, cleft lip/palate, defective lacrimal duct
Fanconi-pancytopenia syndrome (AR)	Frequent	Hypoplastic/malformed	Hypospadias, ureter duplication	Radial hypoplasia, hyperpigmentation, pancytopenia, short stature, microcephaly, MR
FG syndrome (X-linked R)	Occasional		Dilation	Prominent forehead, hypotonia, MR, imperforate anus
Fraser or cryptophthalmos syndrome (AR)	Frequent	Agenesis or hypoplasia		Cryptophthalmos, ear anomalies, genital anomaly, laryngeal stenosis/atresia, anal atresia, CHD
Frontometaphyseal dysplasia (X-linked, severe in male)	Occasional		Obstruction	Coarse facies, prominent supraorbital ridges, joint limitations, splayed metaphyses
Hereditary renal aplasia (AD, 50%—90% penetrance)	50%—90%	Unilateral or bilateral agenesis		Potter (oligohydramnios) sequence if bilateral agenesis, uterine anomaly
Jarcho-Levin syndrome, or spondylothoracic dysplasia (AR)	Occasional	Hydronephrosis	Urethral atresia Ureteral obstruction, bilobate bladder	Prominent occiput, short neck, most die in infancy due to lung hypoplasia, short thorax, diminished ribs, vertebral defects, most Puerto Rican origin
Johanson-Blizzard syndrome (AR)	Frequent	Caliectasis, hydronephrosis		Hypoplasia alae nasi, hypothyroidism, deafness
LEOPARD syndrome; or multiple lentigines syndrome (AD)	Occasional	Agenesis or hypoplasia		Lentigines, hypertelorism, deafness, pulmonary stenosis, obstructive cardiomyopathy, mild growth failure, variable expression in individual patient
Lethal multiple pterygium syndrome (AR)	Occasional	Hydronephrosis	Megaureter	SGA, hypertelorism, epicanthal folds, joint contractures, pterygia, early death due to lung hypoplasia
Levy-Hollister syndrome, or lacrimo-auriculo-dento-digital syndrome (AD)	Occasional	Agenesis, nephrosclerosis		Nasolacrimal duct obstruction, ear anomalies, hearing loss, variable anomalies of upper limbs
Melnick-Fraser syndrome, or branchio-oto-renal syndrome (AD)	Frequent	Dysplasia, hypoplasia, agenesis, ectopia		Hearing loss, preauricular pits, anomalous pinna, branchial fistula
Melnick-Needles syndrome (AD?; lethal in male or X-linked)	Occasional	Hydronephrosis	Ureteral stenosis	Prominent eyes, bowing of long bones, ribbonlike ribs

(*continued*)

APPENDIX G-1
ASSOCIATIONS BETWEEN RENAL-URINARY TRACT ANOMALIES AND OTHER STRUCTURAL DEFECTS
(*continued*)

Diagnosis (Mode of Genetic Transmission)	Frequency of Anomalies	Renal Anomalies	Urologic Anomalies	Other Associations
Menke's Kinky Hair syndrome (X-linked R)	Occasional		Bladder diverticula	Sparse, brittle hair, short stature wormian bones
Neu-Laxova syndrome (AR)	Occasional	Agenesis		Microcephaly, lissencephaly, exophthalmos, syndactyly and edema, polyhydramnios, short umbilical cord, early death
Opitz-Frias syndrome, G syndrome; or hyper-telorism-hypospadias syndrome (AD)	Occasional	Renal defect	Hypospadias, crytorchidism, bifid scrotum	Hypertelorism, swallowing difficulties
Perlman syndrome (AR?)		Nephromegaly, nephro-blastomatosis	Cryptorchidism, hypospadias	Macrosomia, visceromegaly, polyhydramnios, diaphragmatic hernia, interrupted aortic arch, polysplenia
Polycystic Kidney Disease Adult-AD, infantile-AR	100%	Polycystic kidneys		Cysts in liver and other organs
Rutledge syndrome (AR?)	100%	Oligopapillary renal hypoplasia	Urethral anomalies	Joint contractures, cerebellar hypoplasia, tongue cysts, short limbs, eye and ear anomalies, CHD, gallbladder agenesis
Saethre-Chotzen syndrome (AD)	Occasional	Renal anomaly		Craniosynostosis, brachycephaly, maxillary hypoplasia, abnormal ear, syndactyly
Schinzel-Giedion syndrome (AR)	Frequent	Hydronephrosis	Hydroureter, hypospadias	Severe growth failure, profound MR, midface retraction, cardiac and skeletal anomalies
TAR syndrome (AR)	Occasional	Ectopia, dysplasia	Hypospadias	Thrombocytopenia, granulocytosis, eosinophilia, anemia, radial absence or hypoplasia with thumbs present, CHD
Townes syndrome (AD)	Frequent	Hypoplasia	Ureterovesical reflux, urethral valves	Thumb, ear, and anal anomalies
Weyers oligodactyly syndrome (AR)	Frequent	Bilateral hydronephrosis		Deficient ulnar and fibular rays, oligodactyly
Chromosomal anomalies				
4p—syndrome	Occasional	Agenesis		Hypertelorism, broad or beaked nose, microcephaly, cranial asymmetry, low-set ears, dimple, CHD, severe MR, seizures
5p—syndrome, or cri du chat syndrome	Occasional	Agenesis		SGA, slow growth, catlike cry, MR, hypotonia, CHD, microcephaly, downslanting palpebral fissures, hypertelorism, round face, epicanthal folds, strabismus, low set ears
9p—syndrome	Occasional	Hydronephrosis		Craniostenosis, trigonocephaly, upslanting palpebral fissures, hypoplastic supraorbital ridges
13q—syndrome	Occasional	Agenesis or hypoplasia, PKD, hydronephrosis		Microcephaly, high nasal bridge, MR, CHD, hypertelorism, coloboma, microphthalmia, retinoblastoma
18q—syndrome	Occasional	Horseshoe kidney		Poor growth, microcephaly, hypotonia, midfacial hypoplasia, abnormal ears, cleft palate, thumb hypoplasia

APPENDIX G-1
ASSOCIATIONS BETWEEN RENAL-URINARY TRACT ANOMALIES AND OTHER STRUCTURAL DEFECTS
(*continued*)

Diagnosis (Mode of Genetic Transmission)	Frequency of Anomalies	Renal Anomalies	Urologic Anomalies	Other Associations
Cat-eye syndrome[a]	Frequent	Horseshoe kidney, agenesis, hydronephrosis		Coloboma of the iris, downslanting palpebral fissures, anal atresia
Kleinfelter's syndrome, or XXY, XXXY	Frequent		Testes small, undescended	Delayed puberty
Partial trisomy 10q syndrome	Frequent			Ptosis, short palpebral fissures, campodactyly, marked MR
Penta X syndrome, or XXXXX syndrome	Occasional	Dysplasia		Microcephaly, growth deficiency, upward slanting palpebral fissures, low nasal bridge, short neck, small hands, clinodactyly of fifth fingers, PDA
Triploidy syndrome	Frequent	Cystic kidney, hydronephrosis, dysplasia		Large placenta and hydatiform changes; poor growth; brain, facies, and cardiac anomalies; syndactyly
Trisomy 4p syndrome	Occasional	Atresia, horseshoe kidney, hypoplasia, hydronephrosis	VUR	Microcephaly, severe MR, hypertonia in infancy, seizures, SGA, bulbous nose, prominent forehead, clinodactyly
Trisomy 8 syndrome, or mosaic syndrome	Occasional	Hydronephrosis, horseshoe kidney, agenesis	Bifid pelvis	Prominent forehead and ears, deep-set eyes, hypertelorism, micrognathia, MR, CHD, vertebral anomalies, campodactyly
Trisomy 9 mosaic syndrome	Frequent			Joint contractures; heart, CNS, and ear anomalies
Trisomy 9p syndrome	Occasional	Malformations		SGA, macrocephaly, hypertelorism, downslanting palpebral fissures, distal phalangeal hypoplasia, skeletal anomalies
Trisomy 13 syndrome	Occasional	PKD, glomerular cysts, duplication	Ureter duplication, hydroureter	Holoprosencephaly, occipital scalp defect, polydactyly, microphthalmia, narrow hyperconvex fingernails
Trisomy 18 syndrome	Frequent	Horseshoe kidney, ectopic, PKD, hypoplasia or agenesis, duplication	Ureter duplication	Polyhydramnios, single UA, poor growth, prominent occiput, clenched hand
Trisomy 20p syndrome	Occasional	Malformations		Blepharophimosis, brachycephaly, large ears, MR, cubitus valgus, vertebral defects, CHD
Turner syndrome, or XO syndrome	60%	Horseshoe kidney, hypertension	Double or cleft pelvis	Short broad chest, widely spaced nipples, lymphedema, webbed neck, cubitus valgus
Sporadic associations				
Aniridia-Wilms tumor association[b]	50%	Bilateral Wilms tumor		Microcephaly, growth deficiency, MR, prominent lips, cataracts, ptosis, nystagmus, ambiguous genitalia
Beckwith-Wiedemann syndrome, or exomphalos-"macroglossia-gigantism syndrome	Frequent	Large kidneys, medullary dysplasia, Wilms tumor	Hypospadias	Omphalocele, macroglossia, gigantism, ear creases, polyhydramnios, prematurity, hypoglycemia, polycythemia, apnea
Caudal dysplasia sequence, or caudal regression sequence	Occasional	Agenesis	Neurogenic bladder	Abnormal vertebrae and lower limbs, neurologic defects, R/O maternal diabetes, imperforate anus

(*continued*)

APPENDIX G-1
ASSOCIATIONS BETWEEN RENAL-URINARY TRACT ANOMALIES AND OTHER STRUCTURAL DEFECTS
(*continued*)

Diagnosis (Mode of Genetic Transmission)	Frequency of Anomalies	Renal Anomalies	Urologic Anomalies	Other Associations
CHARGE association	5%	Agenesis, hypoplasia, hydronephrosis, heterotopic kidneys		Coloboma (iris, retina, anophthalmos), CHD, choanal atresia, growth retardation (postnatal), mental deficiency, genital hypoplasia (in males), ear anomalies, deafness
Goldenhar syndrome, facioauriculovertebral spectrum, first and second branchial arch syndrome	Occasional	Renal anomalies		Hemifacial microsomia, hemivertebrae, occasional abnormal ears and eyes, deafness, CHD, MR, SGA
Klippel-Feil syndrome	Frequent	Renal anomalies		Short neck, abnormal cervical vertebrae, deafness, CHD
Klippel Trenauny syndrome	Occasional		Hemangiomas of urinary tract	Multiple arterio venous fistulae, limb overgrowth
Laterality sequences Ivemark syndrome, or bilateral right-sidedness	Frequent	Renal anomalies		Situs inversus, asplenia, CHD and vessel anomalies,
Bilateral left-sidedness	Occasional	Renal anomalies		Situs inversus, CHD, polysplenia
Meningomyelocele, spina bifida and occult spinal dysraphism sequence	Frequent	Hydronephrosis, UTI, renal failure, horseshoe kidney, hypoplasia, agenesis, ectopia, duplication	Neurogenic bladder	Neurologic defect, hydrocephalus
Megacystis-microcolon-intestinal hypoperistalsis syndrome	100%	Hydronephrosis	Massive bladder distention (100%), VUR	Neonatal bowel obstruction, hypoperistalsis, microcolon, frequently early death
Mullerian aplasia, Rokitansky sequence, or Rokitansky-Kustner-Hauser syndrome	30%–50%	Unilateral renal aplasia, hypoplasia, ectopia	Ureter duplication	Vaginal atresia, rudimentary uterus
MURCS association	>50%	Agenesis or ectopia (88%)		Absence of vagina, hypoplasia of uterus, abnormal cervico-thoracic vertebrae
Monozygote twinning	Occasional		Exstrophy of the cloaca	Sacrococcygeal teratoma, sirenomelia, VATER, holo-prosencephaly, anencephaly
Pallister-Hall syndrome	Frequent	Dysplasia		Hypothalamic hamartoblastoma, hypopituitarism, imperforate anus, polydactyly
Poland anomaly	Occasional	Renal anomaly		Variable unilateral features: absence of pectoralis muscle, upper limb hypoplasia, syndactyly
Potter sequence, or oligohydramnios sequence	100%	Hypoplasia, aplasia, agenesis, PKD, dysplasia	Urethral valves	Amnion nodosum, oligohydramnios, lung hypoplasia, limb malposition, facies compression
Prune-belly syndrome, or early urethral obstruction sequence	100%	Dysplasia, hypoplasia, horseshoe kidney, hydronephrosis	Urethral valves, persistent urachus, bladder agenesis, ectopic ureter	Prune belly, cryptorchidism, abnormal genitalia, Potter GI malformation (anal, hepatobiliary, mesentery, esophageal, pancreas), talipes equinovarus, scoliosis, thorax deformities, cardiac anomalies, iliac vessel compression
Rubinstein-Taybi syndrome	Frequent	Duplication	Ureter duplication	Broad thumbs and toes, hypoplastic maxilla, MR, slanted palpebral fissures
Sirenomelia sequence	Frequent	Agenesis, dysplasia	Bladder agenesis	Fusion of lower limbs, single UA, absence of genitalia except gonads, absence of sacrum and rectum, imperforate anus

APPENDIX G-1

APPENDIX G-1

ASSOCIATIONS BETWEEN RENAL-URINARY TRACT ANOMALIES AND OTHER STRUCTURAL DEFECTS (continued)

Diagnosis (Mode of Genetic Transmission)	Frequency of Anomalies	Renal Anomalies	Urologic Anomalies	Other Associations
Thanatophoric dysplasia	Occasional	Horseshoe kidney, hydronephrosis		Short limbs, flat vertebrae, large cranium, low nasal bridge, severe SGA, hypotonia, polyhydramnios, lung hypoplasia, early death
Tracheal agenesis association[c]	50%	Agenesis, hydronephrosis, dysplasia	Duplication	Laryngeal/tracheal atresia, GI anomalies (e.g., duodenal atresia), CHD, limb reduction defect (i.e., radial hypoplasia)
VATER/VACTERL association	50%–74%	Agenesis, hydronephrosis, cystic dysplasia	Duplication, urethral atresia	TEF, vertebral and anal atresia, CHD, limb anomalies (i.e., radial dysplasia)
Renal cystic disease[d]				
Alagille syndrome, or arteriohepatic dysplasia (AD)	Occasional	Cystic tubular dilatations, CRF, tubulointerstitial disease		Facies: deep-set eyes, prominent forehead, cholestasis, PPS, butterfly vertebrae
Apart syndrome, or acrocephalosyndactyly (AD; fresh mutation common)	Occasional	MKD, hydronephrosis		Craniosynostosis, midfacial hypoplasia, syndactyly, broad distal phalanx (i.e., thumb and big toe), occasional CHD, GI tract and lung anomalies
Congenital nephrotic syndrome, Finnish type (AR)	100%	CNF, tubular cystic dilatations		Polyhydramnios, elevated a-fetoprotein in amniotic fluid
Cystic hamartomata of lung and kidney	100%	Multilocular cysts		Hamartomatous pulmonary cysts
Dandy-Walker malformation	Occasional	MKD		Congenital hepatic fibrosis
Ehler-Danlos syndrome (AD, AR, X-linked)	Occasional	RTA		Skin and joint hyperextensibility, poor wound healing
Elejalde syndrome (AR)		Cystic dysplasia		Short-limb dwarfism, acrocephaly, polysyndactyly, subcutaneous hypertrophy, cholestasis, pancreatic dysplasia
Ellis-van Creveld syndrome, or chondroectodermal dysplasia (AR)	Occasional	Agenesis, cystic/medullary dysplasia	Epispadias	Short distal extremities, polydactyly, nail hypoplasia CHD (50%), SGA and short eventual stature, cholestasis
Familial juvenile nephronophthisis with hepatic fibrosis (AR)	Frequent	Glomerular cysts		Congenital hepatic fibrosis
Familial renal-retinal dystrophy (AR)	Common	Nephronophthisis-medullary cystic kidney disease		Pigmentary retinal dystrophy
Femoral hypoplasia-unusual facies syndrome		PKD, agenesis	Abnormal collecting system	Femoral hypoplasia, short nose, cleft palate
Fryns syndrome (AR)	50%	MKD, cortical cysts		Facial dysmorphism, microretrognathia, diaphragm defects, lung hypoplasia, neonatal death, bicornuate uterus or scrotum anomaly, distal limb hypoplasia
Glutaric aciduria syndrome, type II, or multiple acyl-coA dehydrogenase deficiency (AR)	Frequent	Cystic dysplasia, ultrastructural anomaly of glomerular basement membrane		Cerebral dysplasia, macrocephaly, facial dysmorphism, fatty liver, genital defects, hypoglycemia, metabolic acidosis
Ivemark syndrome, or renal-hepatic-pancreatic dysplasia (AR)	Frequent	Glomerular cysts, cystic dysplasia		Hepatic and pancreatic dysplasia, occasional splenic anomalies, may be associated with homogenous syndrome (Bernstein)

(continued)

Diagnosis (Mode of Genetic Transmission)	Frequency of Anomalies	Renal Anomalies	Urologic Anomalies	Other Associations
Jeune asphyxiating thoracic dystrophy (AR)	Frequent	Glomerular sclerosis, tubular cysts, renal failure		Small chest, lung hypoplasia, short limbs, cholestasis
Lowe syndrome, or oculocerebrorenal syndrome (X-linked)	100% (male)	Fanconi syndrome, CRF		Cataracts, mental deficiency, hypotonia
Meckel-Gruber syndrome, or dysencephalia splanchnocystica (AR)	100%	MKD, PKD, dysplasia, hypoplasia		Encephalocele, holoprosencephaly, polydactyly, Potter sequence, cholestasis
Nail-patella syndrome, or hereditary osteoonychodystrophy	Frequent	Proteinuria, hematuria, casts, CRF, PKD	Ureter duplication	Nail dysplasia, patella hypoplasia, iliac spurs
Orofacial digital syndrome, type 1 (D, lethal in male)	Frequent	Glomerular cysts		Oral frenula and clefts, hypoplasia of alae nasi, digital asymmetry
Roberts-SC phocomelia syndrome, hypomelia-hypotrichosis-facial hemangioma syndrome, or pseudothalidomide (AR)	Occasional	MKD, horseshoe kidney		Hypomelia, midfacial defect, cleft palate and lip, severe growth deficiency, cholestasis
Short-rib polydactyly, type I (Saldino-Noonan type)	Frequent	MKD, hypoplastic		Short-limb dwarfism, severe lung hypoplasia, early death, short ribs, with or without polydactyly, CHD, imperforate anus
Short rib-polydactyly syndrome, type II (Majewski type) (AR)	Frequent	Glomerular cysts, focal dilatation of distal tubules		Short-limb dwarfism, severe lung hypoplasia, early death, short ribs, with or without polydactyly, CHD, ambiguous genitalia
Smith-Lemli-Opitz syndrome (AR)	Occasional	MKD		MR, growth retardation, microcephaly, micrognathia, anteverted nostrils, ptosis of eyelids, syndactyly of second-third toes, ambiguous genitalia
Tuberous sclerosis (AD)	50%—80%	Glomerular and tubular cysts (rarely neonatal), angiomyolipomas, CRF		Seizures, skin lesions, tumors
Von Hippel-Lindau syndrome (AD)	Occasional	PKD		Retinal angioma, cerebellar hemangioblastoma
Zellweger syndrome, or cerebrohepatorenal syndrome (AR)	100%	Glomerular cysts, albuminuria		Hypotonia, abnormal brain, seizures, flat facies, peroxisomal deficiency, cholestasis
Metabolic diseases				
Hyperoxaluria type I, or oxalosis (AR)	100%	Nephrocalcinosis/lithiasis, CRF		Anorexia, failure to thrive, vomiting, dehydration and fever, liver failure, acidosis
Galactose-1-phosphate uridyl transferase deficiency, or galactosemia (AR)	Frequent	Fanconi syndrome		Hypoglycemia, anorexia, liver failure, sepsis, cataracts, MR
Hereditary fructose intolerance, fructose-l-phosphate aldolase deficiency (AR)	Frequent	Fanconi syndrome		Hypoglycemia, anorexia, liver failure, failure to thrive
Tyrosinemia type I, tyrosinosis, or hepatorenal tyrosinemia (AR)	Frequent	Fanconi syndrome		Growth failure, cabbagelike odor, vomiting, diarrhea, metabolic acidosis, liver failure, edema, fever
Glycogenosis with Fanconi syndrome, or Fanconi-Bickel syndrome (AR)	100%	Fanconi syndrome		Fever, vomiting, growth failure, rickets, hypoglycemia, hepatomegaly

APPENDIX G-1

ASSOCIATIONS BETWEEN RENAL-URINARY TRACT ANOMALIES AND OTHER STRUCTURAL DEFECTS
(continued)

Diagnosis (Mode of Genetic Transmission)	Frequency of Anomalies	Renal Anomalies	Urologic Anomalies	Other Associations
Cystinosis (AR)	100%	Fanconi syndrome		Light skin and hair, failure to thrive, anorexia, fussiness, episodes of acidosis, dehydration and fever, rickets
Teratogens				
Fetal alcohol syndrome	18%	Renal agenesis, hypoplasia, hydronephrosis	Ureteral duplication	SGA, microcephaly, facial dysmorphism, MR
Fetal hydantoin syndrome	Occasional	Various malformations		Poor growth; microcephaly; craniofacial dysmorphism; brain, limb, and GI anomalies; CHD
Thalidomide embryopathy	Occasional	Various malformations		Phocomelia; polydactyly; syndactyly; hydrocephalus; facial capillary hemangioma; CHD; ear, eye, and GI anomalies
Fetal trimethadione syndrome	Occasional	Various malformations		Poor growth, craniofacial anomalies, CHD
Angiotensin converting enzyme inhibitors	Frequent(?)	Nephron dysgenesis		Hypocalvaria
Congenital infections				
Congenital syphilis	Occasional	Nephrotic syndrome		Snuffles, meningitis, bone changes
Congenital toxoplasmosis	Rare	Nephrotic syndrome		Microcephaly, deafness, chorioretinitis, SGA
Renal failure[e]				
Bardet-Biedl syndrome, or Laurence-Moon-Biedl syndrome (AR)	Frequent	Dysplasia, nephrosclerosis, interstitial scarring, cyst, HTN	Hydroureter	Retinitis pigmentosa, obesity, polydactyly
Drash syndrome, or nephropathy associated with gonadal dysgenesis and Wilms tumor	100%	Glomerulonephritis, interstitial changes, nephrotic syndrome, hematuria, HTN, ESRD, often Wilms tumor		Ambiguous genitalia (often male pseudohermaphroditism)
Fabry syndrome, or angiokeratoma corporis diffusum (X-linked)	Frequent	Proteinuria, hematuria, casts, leukocyturia		Dark nodular angiectases, corneal opacities, seizures, CNS symptoms
Russell-Silver syndrome (AD)	Sporadic	Wilms syndrome	Posterior urethral valves, hypospadias	Small stature, skeletal asymmetry, small fifth finger, small triangular facies
Williams syndrome	Occasional	Hypertension	Bladder diverticula	Decreased growth, hyper-calcemia, subaortic stenosis, prominent lips, hoarse voice

This table has been made by selecting well-defined associations, described in at least three patients, in whom renal manifestations may develop before 1 year of age.
[a] Extra chromosome corresponding to segments of chromosome 22.
[b] May have partial deletion of chromosome 1 p.
[c] Overlaps with VATER association.
[d] See also trisomy 13 and 18, VATER, cocaine, and other subheadings (i.e., renal dysplasia).
[e] See also other headings.
AD, autosomal dominant; AR, autosomal recessive; CHD, congenital heart disease; CHARGE, coloboma, heart disease, atresia of the choanae, retarded mental development and growth, genital hypoplasia, ear anomalies; CHILD, congenital hemidysplasia with ichthyosiform erythroderma and limb defects; COFS, cerebrooculofacioskeletal; CNS; central nervous system; CRF, chronic renal failure; D, dominant; EEC, ectrodactyly-ectodermal dysplasia-clefting; EKG, electrocardiogram; ESRD, end-stage renal disease; GI, gastrointestinal; HTN, hypertension; LEOPARD, lentigenes, EKG anomalies, ocular anomalies, pulmonary stenosis, abnormal genitalia, retardation of growth, and deafness; MKD, multicystic kidney disease; MR, mental retardation; MURCS, Mullerian duct, renal, cervical somite; PDA, patent ductus arteriosus; PKD, polycystic kidney disease; PPS, peripheral pulmonic stenosis; R, recessive; R/0, rule out; RTA, renal tubular acidosis; SGA, small for gestational age; TAR, radial aplasia-thrombocytopenia; TEF, tracheoesophageal fistula; UA, umbilical artery; UPJ, ureteropelvic junction; UTI, urinary tract infection; VACTERL, vertebrae, anus, cardiac, tracheoesophageal, renal, limb; VATER, vertebrae, anus, tracheoesophageal, renal; VUR, vesicoureteral reflux.

APPENDIX G-2
RELATIONSHIP BETWEEN SINGLE SIGNS AND RENAL-URINARY TRACT MALFORMATIONS

Sign	Criteria for Entry into the Study	Method used to Detect Renal-Urinary Tract Malformations	Type of Malformations	Minimum Incidence[a] of Patients with Renal-Urinary Tract Anomalies	Incidence of Patients with Renal-Urinary Tract Anomalies Who had no Evidence of Other Malformations at Birth[b]
Abnormal Vertebrae					
Kohler 1982 (1)	Abnormal vertebrae or vertebrae	IVU	Agenesis, ectopic, horseshoe kidney, duplication	8/46 (17%)	NA
Macewen 1972 (2)	Congenital scoliosis, without suspicion of neurogenic bladder	IVU	Agenesis, duplication, ectopia, obstruction, VUR, horseshoe kidney	42/231 (18%)	NA
Anorectal Anomalies					
Munn 1983 (3)	Imperforation or atresia	IVU	Agenesis, duplication, VUR, hypospadias, UPJ obstruction, neurogenic bladder	20/28 (71%)	NA
Hoekstra 1983 (4)[c]	Congenital anomalies	Autopsy; IVU excess in 3/126	VUR, agenesis, hypoplasia, ectopia, PKD UPJ obstruction, horseshoe kidney, hypospadias	95/150 (63%)	NA
Khuri 1981 (5)[d]	Imperforate anus and hypospadias	IVU	NA (part of study on hypospadias)	6/13 (46%)	NA
Congenital Diaphragmatic Hernia					
Siebert 1990 (6)	Autopsy	Autopsy	Agenesis, dysplasia or hypoplasia, UPJ/ureterovesical obstruction	16/27 (59%)	4/16 (25%)
Cunniff 1990 (7)	Chart review	Surgery or autopsy	Agenesis, hydronephrosis, cysts, ectopic or duplicated ureter	5/103 (5%)	0%
Hypospadias					
Khuri 1981 (5)	Hypospadias	IVU in 460/1076	Agenesis, UPJ obstruction, VUR, Wilms, PKD, ectopic kidney, horseshoe kidney	48/1076 (4%)	15/48 (31%)[e]
Shelton 1985 (8)	Asymptomatic hypospadias	IVU, VCUG	Agenesis, duplication, pelvic kidney, VUR	27/102 (27%)	0%
Pulmonary Hypoplasia					
Page 1982 (9)	Neonatal autopsy	Autopsy	Agenesis, dysgenesis, dysplasia, PKD	16/77 (21%)	NA
Single Umbilical Artery					
Bourke (10)	Isolated single UA, examination of umbilical cord	US with VCUG if persistently abnormal	VUR, megaureter, agenesis, dilation of collecting system	8/112 (7%)	8/112 (7%)
Spontaneous Air Leak Syndrome					
Bashour 1977 (11)	Symptomatic pneumothorax	IVU	hypoplasia or agenesis, PKD, dysplasia, urethral valves, Potter facies (n = 3)	12/47 (26%)	3/12 (25%)

APPENDIX G-2
RELATIONSHIP BETWEEN SINGLE SIGNS AND RENAL-URINARY TRACT MALFORMATIONS (*continued*)

Sign	Criteria for Entry into the Study	Method used to Detect Renal-Urinary Tract Malformations	Type of Malformations	Minimum Incidence[a] of Patients with Renal-Urinary Tract Anomalies	Incidence of Patients with Renal-Urinary Tract Anomalies Who had no Evidence of Other Malformations at Birth[b]
Supernumerary Nipples					
Mehes 1983 (12)	Hospitalized	Clinical examination and IVU	Hydronephrosis, megaureter, duplication	9/37 (24%)	NA
Mimouni 1983 (13)	Neonatal (Israel)	Physical examination US (11/42)		0/43 (0%)	0%
Varsano 1984 (14)	ER/pediatric clinic (Israel)	IVU	PKD, hydronephrosis (UPJ obstruction), duplicated ureter, ureteral prolapse	6/26 (23%)	6/6 (100%)[g]
Robertson 1986 (15)	Neonatal (African-Americans)	US		0/32 (0%)	0%
Hersh 1987 (16)	Genetic/developmental clinic; 10 controls (United States, mostly Caucasian)	US or IVU	MKD, agenesis, Hydronephrosis, horseshoe kidney	7/65 (11%)	2/7 (29%)[h]
Urbani 1996 (17)	Adult subjects	US, urinalysis	ADPKD, unilateral renal agenesis MKD, familial cysts, UPJ stenosis	NA	NA

[a] Hypospadias excluded.
[b] Except for minor anomalies such as pes equinovarus.
[c] Eighty-one of 150 patients in the study had no congenital abnormalities of the other organs (54%).
[d] Among patients with first-degree hypospadias, the incidence of upper urinary tract malformations was 1.3%.
[e] Also 3 patients with undescended testes.
[f] One patient had epilepsy; two patients had pyloric stenosis.
[g] One patient had Niemann-Pick disease.
[h] Three patients had anomalies.
ER, emergency room; IVU, intravenous urography; MKD, multicystic kidney dysplasia; NA, not available; PKD, polycystic kidney disease; UA, umbilical artery, UPJ/UV, ureteropelvic junction-ureterovesical; US, ultrasound; VUR, vesicoureteral reflex.

APPENDIX G-3
CLASSIFICATION OF CYSTIC KIDNEY DISEASE

Genetic Diseases
AR polycystic kidney disease: associated with congenital hepatic fibrosis
AD polycystic kidney disease: associated with central nervous system aneurysms
  Type I – chromosome 16
  Type II – chromosome 4
Juvenile nephronophthisis—medullary cystic disease complex
  Juvenile nephronophthisis with hepatic fibrosis (AR)
  Medullary cystic disease complex (AD)
Glomerulocystic kidney disease:
  AD glomerulocystic kidney disease
  Familial hypoplastic glomerulocystic kidney disease
Malformation syndromes
  Multicystic kidney disease
    Apert syndrome, or acrocephalosyndactyly (AD, new mutation common)
    Elejalde syndrome (AR)
    Ellis-van Creveld syndrome, or chondroectodermal dysplasia (AR)
    Fryns syndrome (AR)
    Joubert syndrome (AR)
    Meckel-Gruber syndrome, or dysencephalia splanchnocystica (AR)
    Roberts phocomelia, hypomelia—hypotrichosis—facial hemangioma syndrome or
      pseudothalidomide syndrome (AR)
    Short rib-polydactyly syndrome, Saldino-Noonan type (AR)
    Smith-Lemli-Optiz syndrome (AR)
  Glomerulocystic disease
    Short rib-polydactyly syndrome, Majewski type (AR)
    Tuberous sclerosis (AD): glomerular and tubular cysts
    Zellweger cerebrohepatorenal syndrome (AR)
    Ivemark syndrome, or renal-hepatic-pancreatic dysplasia (AR): cystic dysplasia
    Orofacial digital syndrome, type 1 (X-linked D, lethal in males)
  Nephronophthisis-medullary cystic disease
    Familial renal-retinal dystrophy (AR)
  Other
    Von Hippel-Lindau syndrome (AD)
    Jeune syndrome, or asphyxiating thoracic dystrophy (AR)
    Alagille syndrome, or arteriohepatic dysplasia (AD)
    Trisomy 13
    Trisomy 18
    Ehlers-Danlos syndrome (AD, AR, X-linked)
    Glutaric aciduria syndrome, type II, or multiple acyl-coA dehydrogenase deficiency
      (AR)
    Lowe syndrome, or oculo-cerebro-renal syndrome (X-linked)
    Nail-patella syndrome, or hereditary osteoonychodystrophy (AD)
  Congenital hypernephronic nephromegaly with tubular dysgenesis syndrome (AR)
  Congenital nephritic syndrome, Finnish type, or infantile microcystic disease (AR)
Sporadic and Acquired Diseases
Multicystic kidney disease, or multicystic dysplasia
  Dandy-Walker malformation
Sporadic glomerulocystic kidney disease
Nephron dysgenesis: glomerular or tubular immaturity
Brachymesomelia-renal syndrome (only one case described)
Femoral hypoplasia-unusual facies syndrome
Multilocular cystic nephroma, or cystadenoma
Simple cyst (benign)

APPENDIX G-3
CLASSIFICATION OF CYSTIC KIDNEY DISEASE (*continued*)

Medullary sponge kidney (<5% inherited; no renal failure)
Cystic hamartoma of lung and kidney (multilocular cysts)
Acquired renal cystic disease in chronic hemodialysis patients
Caliceal diverticulum, or pyelogenic cyst

AD, autosomal dominant; AR, autosomal recessive; D, dominant.
See Appendix G-1 for description of associated malformations.

1. Kohler R, Dodat H, Charollais Y. Malformations congénitales vertébrales et urinaires. Fréquence de leur association et conduite à tenir. *Pediatrie* 1982;37:91.
2. Macewen GD, Winter RB, Hardy JH. Evaluation of kidney anomalies in congenital scoliosis. *J Bone Joint Surg* 1972;54:1451.
3. Munn R, Schillinger JF Urologic abnormalities found with imperforate anus. *Urol* 1983;21:260.
4. Hoekstra WJ, Scholtmeijer RJ, Molenar JC, Schreeve RH, Schroeder FH. Urogenital tract abnormalities associated with congenital anorectal anomalies. *J Urol* 1983;130:962.
5. Khuri FJ, Hardy BE, Churchill BM. Urologic anomalies associated with hypospadias. *Urol Clin North Am* 1981;8:565.
6. Siebert JR, Benjamin DR, Juul S, Glick PL. Urinary tract anomalies associated with congenital diaphragmatic defects. *Am J Med Genet* 1990;37:1.
7. Cunniff C, Jones KL, Jones MC. Patterns of malformation in children with congenital diaphragmatic defects. *J Pediatr* 1990;116:258.
8. Shelton TB, Noe HN. The role of excretory urography in patients with hypospadias. *J Urol* 1985;134:97.
9. Page DV, Stocker JT. Anomalies associated with pulmonary hypoplasia. *Am Rev Resp Dis* 1982;125:216.
10. Bourke WG, Clarke TA, Mathews TG, O'Halpin D, Donoghue VB. Isolated single umbilical artery—the case for routine renal screening. *Arch Dis Child* 1993;68(5Spec No):600.
11. Bashour BN, Balfe JW. Urinary tract anomalies in neonates with spontaneous pneumothorax and/or pneumomediastinum. *Pediatr* 1977;59 (Suppl):1048.
12. Mehes K. Association of supernumerary nipples with other anomalies (letter). *J Pediatr* 1983;102:161.
13. Mimouni F, Merlob P, Reisner SH. Occurrence of supernumerary nipples in newborns. *Am J Dis Child* 1983;137:952.
14. Varsano IB, Jaber L, Garty BZ, Mukamel MM, Grunebaum M. Urinary tract abnormalities in children with supernumerary nipples. *Pediatrics* 1984;73:103.
15. Robertson A, Sale P, Sathyanarayan. Lack of association of supernumerary nipples with renal anomalies in black infants. *J Pediatr* 1986;109:502.
16. Hersh JH, Bloom AS, Cromer AO, Harrison HL, Weisskopf B. Does a supernumerary nipple/renal field defect exist? *Am J Dis Child* 1987;141:989.
17. Urbani, CE, Betti R. Accessory mammary tissue associated with congenital and hereditary nephrourinary malformations. *Int J Dermatol* 1996;35:349.

Drug Formulary

1. MEDICATIONS IN BREAST MILK

APPENDIX H-1a
CYTOTOXIC DRUGS THAT MAY INTERFERE WITH CELLULAR METABOLISM OF NURSING INFANT

Drug	Reason for Concern, Reported Sign or, Symptom in Infant, or Effect on Lactation
Cyclophosphamide	Possible immune suppression; unknown effect on growth or association with carcinogenesis neutropenia
Cyclosporine	Possible immune suppression; unknown effect on growth or association with carcinogenesis
Doxorubicin*	Possible immune suppression; unknown effect on growth or association with carcinogenesis
Methotrexate	Possible immune suppression; unknown effect on growth or association with carcinogenesis; neutropenia

* Drug is concentrated in human milk

APPENDIX H-1b
DRUGS OF ABUSE FOR WHICH ADVERSE EFFECTS ON THE INFANT DURING BREAST-FEEDING HAVE BEEN REPORTED*

Drug	Reported Effect or Reason for Concern
Amphetamine†	Irritability, poor sleeping pattern
Cocaine	Cocaine Intoxication: irritability, vomiting, diarrhea, tremulousness, seizures
Heroin	Tremors, restlessness, vomiting, poor feeding
Marijuana	Only 1 report in literature; no effect mentioned; very long half-life of some components
Phencyclidine	Potent hallucinogen

* The Committee on Drugs strongly believes that nursing mothers should not ingest drugs of abuse, because they are hazardous to the nursing infant and to the health of the mother
† Drug is concentrated in Human milk

APPENDIX H-1c

RADIOACTIVE COMPOUNDS THAT REQUIRE TEMPORARY CESSATION OF BREASTFEEDING*

Compound	Recommended Time for Cessation of Breastfeeding
Copper 64 (^{65}Cu)	Radioactivity in milk present at 50 h
Gallium 67 (^{67}Ga)	Radioactivity in milk present for 2 wk
Indium 111 (^{111}In)	Very small amount present at 20 h
Iodine 123 (^{123}I)	Radioactivity in milk present up to 36 h
Iodine 125 (^{125}I)	Radioactivity in milk present for 12 d
Iodine 131 (^{131}I)	Radioactivity in milk present 2–14 d, depending on study
Iodine 131	If used for treatment of thyroid cancer, high radioactivity may prolong exposure to infant
Radioactive Sodium	Radioactivity in milk present at 96 h
Technetium 99m (^{99m}Tc), ^{99m}Tc Macroaggregates, ^{99m}TcO$_4$	Radioactivity in milk present at 15 h to 3 d

* Consult nuclear medicine physician before performing diagnostic study so that radionuclide that has the shortest excretion time in breast milk can be used. Before study, the mother should pump her breast and store enough milk in the freezer for feeding the infant; after the study, the mother should pump her breast to maintain milk production but discard all milk for the required time that radioactivity is present in milk. Milk samples can be screened by radiology departments for radioactivity before resumption of nursing.

APPENDIX H-1d

DRUGS FOR WHICH THE EFFECT ON NURSING INFANTS IS UNKNOWN BUT MAY BE OF CONCERN

Drug	Reported or Possible Effect
Anti-anxiety	
Alprazolam	None
Diazepam	None
Lorazepam	None
Midazolam	
Perphenazine	None
Prazepam†	None
Quazepam	None
Temazepam	
Antidepressants	
Amitriptyline	None
Amoxapine	None
Bupropion	None
Clomipramine	None
Desipramine	None
Dothiepin	None
Doxepin	None
Fluoxetine	Colic, irritability, feeding and sleep disorders, slow weight gain
Fluvoxamine	
Imipramine	None
Nortriptyline	None
Paroxetine	None
Sertraline†	None
Trazadone	None
Antipsychotic	
Chlorpromazine	Galactorrhea in mother; drowsiness and lethargy in infant; decline in developmental scores
Chlorprothixene	None
Clozapine†	None
Haloperidol	Decline in developmental scores
Mesoridazine	None
Trifluoperazine	None

(continued)

APPENDIX H-1d

DRUGS FOR WHICH THE EFFECT ON NURSING INFANTS IS UNKNOWN BUT MAY BE OF CONCERN (continued)

Drug	Reported or Possible Effect
OTHERS	
Amiodarone	Possible hypothyroidism
Chloramphenicol	Possible idiosyncratic bone marrow suppression
Clofazimine	Potential for transfer of high percentage of maternal dose; possible increase in skin pigmentation
Lamotrigine	Potential therapeutic serum concentrations in infant
Metroclopramide†	None described; dopaminergic blocking agent
Metronidazole	In vitro mutagen; may discontinue breastfeeding for 12–24 h to allow excretion of dose when single- therapy given to mother
Tinidazole	See Metronidazole

* Psychotropic drugs, the compounds listed under anti-anxiety, antidepressant, and antipsychotic categories, are of special concern when given to nursing mothers for long periods. Although there are very few case reports of adverse effects in breastfeeding infants, these drugs do appear in human milk, and thus, could conceivable alter short-term and long-term central nervous system functions.[56] See discussion in text of psychotropic drugs.
† Drug is concentrated in human milk relative to simultaneous maternal plasma concentrations

APPENDIX H-1e

DRUGS THAT HAVE BEEN ASSOCIATED WITH SIGNIFICANT EFFECTS ON NURSING INFANTS AND SHOULD BE GIVEN TO NURSING MOTHERS WITH CAUTION*

Drug	Reason for Concern
Acebutolol	Hypotension; bradycardia; tachypnea
5-Aminosalicylic Acid	Diarrhea (1 case)
Atenolol	Cyanosis; bradycardia
Bromocriptine	Suppresses lactation; may be hazardous to the mother
Aspirin (salicylates)	Metabolic acidosis (1 case)
Clemastine	Drowsiness, irritability, refusal to feed, high-pitched cry, neck stiffness (1 case)
Ergotamine	Vomiting, diarrhea, convulsions (doses used in migraine medications)
Lithium	1/3 to ½ therapeutic blood concentrations in infants
Phenindione	Anticoagulang; increased prothrombin and partial Thromboplastin time in one infant; not used in U.S.
Phenobarbital	Sedation; infantile spasms after weaning from milk containing Phenobarbital, methamoglobinemia (1 case)
Primidone	Sedation, feeding problems
Sulfasalizine	Bloody diarrhea (1 case) (salicylazosulfapyridine)

* Blood concentration in the infant may be of critical importance.
Modified from American Academy of Pediatrics, Committee on Drugs. Transfer of drugs and other chemicals into human milk. *Pediatrics* 2001;108:776–789

2. PHARMACOPOEIA

APPENDIX H-2
PHARMACOPOEIA

Drug	Dose/kg	Route and Frequency	Comments
Abelcet	See Amphotericin B lipid complex		
Acetazolamide	Diuretic: 5 mg	PO, IV, qd	May cause acidosis, hypokalemia, and GI irritation
	Hydrocephalus: 5 mg (increase each day by 25 mg/kg/day up to a max of 100 mg/kg/day)	q6h	
Acyclovir	neonatal HSV 20 mg	IV; over 1 h Term, normal renal function q8h <30 wk or mod. decrease renal function: q12h dec renal function and dec u/o (Cr > 1.2): q24h	Treat for 14–21 d Adequate hydration required to avoid crystalline nephropathy
Adenosine	0.05 mg	IVP Titrate dose in increments of 0.05 mg/kg every 2 min to a max of 0.25 mg/kg or until termination of PSVT	Push over 1–2 seconds flush with NS Higher doses may be needed for peripheral administration vs, central administration
Albumin 5%	0.5–1 g (1 g/20 mL)	IV over 30–60 min	Contains 0.13–0.16 mEq of sodium per ml Avoid circulatory overload
Albuterol	0.05–0.25 mg per dose	Inhalation for bronchodilation q2h to q6h	Tachycardia, arrhythmias, tremor, hypokalemia, and irritable behavior have been reported
Amikacin	<1.2 kg (0–4 wks) 7.5 mg	IM, IV, over 30 min q24h	Therapeutic levels: Pk = 20–30 mcg/ml Tr = 5–10 mcg/ml
	1.2–2 kg (0–7 days) 7.5 mg	q12h	Dose adjustment required in renal dysfunction
	>7 days 7.5 mg	q8–12h	Risk of ototoxicity increases when given concurrently with loop diuretics
	>2 kg (0–7days) 10 mg	q12h	
	>7 days 10 mg	q8h	
Aminophylline	loading dose 6 mg	IV once	Therapeutic level Bronchospasm: 10–20 mcg/ml Neonatal apnea: 6–13 mcg/ml
	maintenance dose <1000 g 2 mg/kg/dose	Infuse over 20–30 min IV q8h give first maintenance dose 8 h after the loading dose	Signs of toxicity include irritability, GI upset and arrhythmias. When switching to theophylline, remember that aminophylline is 80% theophylline
	>1000 g 2.5–3 mg/kg/dose	q8h	
Ammonium chloride	Metabolic alkalosis 1–2 mEq	PO, IV × 1	GI Irritation-administer oral doses after meals Hyperventilation Pain at injection site if infused too rapidly Maximum concentration for injection is 0.4 mEq/ml Maximum infusion rate is 1 mEq/kg/h
	Urinary acidification 0.25–0.37 mEq	PO, IV q6h	
Amoxicillin	10–15 mg	PO q12h	See comments for Ampicillin
Amphotericin B	Test dose for infants and children: 0.1 mg (maximum total dose: 1 mg) test dose is optional in neonates	IV once infuse over 1 h	Total dose for treatment: Disseminated infection: 25–30 mg/kg Catheter-associated infection: 10–15 mg/kg Not to exceed 1.5 mg/kg/day Max concentration: 0.1 mg/ml
	Initial dose: 0.5 mg	On the first day of treatment, subtract the test dose from the initial dose and give the remainder over 3 h if there is no adverse reaction	Max dextrose concentration: 20% Incompatible with saline solution and TPN Monitor electrolytes, renal and hematological status
	Maintenance dose: 0.5–1 mg (increase dose in increments of 0.25 mg/kg/d)	IV qd over 2–4 h	Avoid additional nephrotoxic drugs

(continued)

Drug	Dose/kg	Route and Frequency	Comments
Amphotericin B Lipid complex	2.5–5 mg (increase dose daily in 1 mg/kg increments)	Infuse over 2 h	Use higher doses for meningitis, osteoarthritis, cryptococcal infections, and aspergillosis Mix to a 1–2 mg/ml dilution with D5W only Do not mix with saline or any other drug Flush line with D5W
Ampicillin	Sepsis: 25 mg Meningitis: 50 mg	Infusion 15–30 min IV, IM ≤7 d: ≤2 kg: q12h ≤7 d: ≥2 kg: q8h >7 d: <1.2 kg: q12h >7 d: 1.2–2 kg q8h >7 d: >2 kg q6h ≤7 d: ≤2 kg: q12h ≤7 d: >2 kg: q8h >7 d: <1.2 kg q12h >7 d: 1.2–2 kg q8h >7 d: >2 kg q6h	May cause rash, interstitial nephritis, hemolytic anemia, and pseudomembranous colitis Lengthen interval in renal dysfunction Not to exceed 100 mg/min infusion
Atracurium	Initial dose 0.3–0.5 mg Maintenance dose: 0.3–0.4 mg	IV; once As needed to maintain paralysis	Hypertension associated with histamine release Ventilatory rate may need to be adjusted to compensate for loss of spontaneous ventilation Aminoglycoside antibiotics prolong duration of action Preservative Free now available Elimination not substantially altered by renal or hepatic dysfunction
Atropine	Bradycardia: 0.02 mg Bronchospasm: 0.03–0.05 mg	IV over 1 min; min single dose 0.1 mg, max single dose 0.5 mg May repeat every 5 min to a max total dose of 1 mg or 0.04 mg/kg Via inhalation q8h–q6h; min single dose 0.25 mg, max single dose 1 mg	Infants with down syndrome have both increased sensitivity to cardiac effects and mydrias May cause hyperthermia, urinary retention, tachycardia, and elevated WBC count Antidote: physostigmine
Bumetanide	0.01–0.05 mg	IV, IM, PO qod-qd	Push IV doses over 1–2 min 40 times more potent than furosemide Monitor serum electrolytes Ototoxic
Caffeine base	Loading dose 5–10 mg Maintenance daily dose 2.5 mg–5 mg	IV, PO once Infuse over 30 min qd Administer first maintenance dose 24 h after the loading dose	Therapeutic levels: 5–20 mcg/ml Do Not skip scheduled doses when giving a bolus Toxicity (CV, neurological and GI) rarely occurs at levels <50 mcg/ml
Calcium chloride 10% (27 mg elemental Calcium/ml)	Hypocalcemia: 10–20 mg elemental Ca Cardiac arrest: 5 mg elemental Ca	IV PO q6h IV slow push over 10 min max rate 1 mg/kg/min	Use IV solution with extreme caution severe necrosis occurs in extravasation Monitor serum Ca levels Use with caution in digitalized patients
Calcium Glubionate (Neo-Calglucon) (23 mg elemental calcium/ml)	Hypocalcemia: 10–20 mg elemental Ca	PO q6h	Give prior to feeds for best absorption High osmotic load: large doses may cause diarrhea Dilute 1:1 with sterile water to have osmolarity Monitor serum Ca level

APPENDIX H-2
PHARMACOPOEIA (continued)

Drug	Dose/kg	Route and Frequency	Comments
Calcium Gluconate 10% (9.4 mg elemental calcium/ml)	Hypocalcemia: 10–20 mg elemental Ca	IV, PO q6–q12h	
	Cardiac arrest: 10 mg elemental Ca	IV may repeat every 10 min	May cause bradycardia and potentiation of digitalis
			Extravasation causes necrosis of subcutaneous tissues
			Do not use scalp veins
			Precipitates with Na Bicarb and phosphate salts
			Monitor serum Ca levels
Captopril	0.05–0.1 mg; may titrate up to 0.5 mg/kg/dose	PO q6h–q24h	Give 1 h prior to feeds
			Adjust dose in renal dysfunction
			Monitor blood pressure; severe hypotension may occur in patients who are sodium or volume depleted
			May cause rash, proteinuria, neutropenia
Cefazolin	20 mg	IV, IM ≤7 d: q12h >7 d, ≤2 kg: q12h >7 d >2 kg: q8h	First generation cephalosporin Adjust dose and or interval in renal dysfunction May cause rash and elevated liver enzymes
Cefotaxime	50 mg	IV, IM <1.2 kg, <7 d: q12h ≥1.2 kg, >7 d: q8h	Third generation cephalosporin Good CNS penetration Adjust dose and/or interval in renal dysfunction
Ceftazidime	50 mg	IV, IM <1.2 kg 0–4 wk: q12h ≥1.2 kg ≤7d: q12h ≥1.2 kg >7d: q8h	Third generation cephalosporin Adjust dose and/or interval in renal dysfunction Rash, false positive Coomb's test
Ceftriaxone	50 mg 50–75 mg	IV, IM ≤7 d: q24h >7 d ≤2 kg: q24h >7 d >2 kg: qd or may divide into two daily doses	Third generation cephalosporin No adjustment in renal dysfunction
	Meningitis: LD 75–100 mg MD 50 mg	IV × 1 IV q12–24hr begin maintenance dose 12–24 h after loading dose	Painful IM injection. The use of lidocaine for reconstitution of ceftriaxone doses for very small babies is not recommended due to possible lidocaine-related cardiac adverse effects Not recommended for use in neonates with hyperbilirubinemia
Cefuroxime	25–50 mg	IV, IM q12h	Second generation cephalosporin Adjust dose in renal dysfunction May cause transient elevation in BUN/Cr, pseudomembranous colitis and rash
Chloral Hydrate	Sedative: 25–40 mg	PO, PR q6–8h prn	May cause paradoxical excitement and accumulation of toxic metabolites Use with caution in hepatic and/or renal failure May cause GI distress and indirect hyperbilirubinemia
	Hypnotic: 25–50 mg	PO, PR once	
Chloramphenicol	25 mg	IV, PO >2 kg ≤7 d: qd ≤2 kg >7 d: qd >2 kg >7 d: q12h	Therapeutic levels: 10–25 mcg/ml "Gray baby": syndrome with levels >50 mcg/ml May cause bone marrow depression Increases phenytoin blood levels
Chlorothiazide	10–20 mg Max 375 mg/day	PO q12h	Use with caution in liver and severe renal failure May cause fluid and electrolyte imbalance, hyperbilirubinemia, and hyperglycemia
	1–4 mg	IV q12h	

(continued)

APPENDIX H-2
PHARMACOPOEIA (*continued*)

Drug	Dose/kg	Route and Frequency	Comments
Cholestyramine	80 mg of the active resin	PO; tid with feeds	May cause constipation, diarrhea, malabsorption of fat soluble vitamins, and metabolic acidosis Alters absorption of drugs when given concurrently. Give oral meds 1 h prior to or 4–6 h after cholestyramine
Cimetidine	5–10 mg/kg/day in neonates	IV, IM, PO q8–12h	May cause diarrhea, rash, neutropenia, and gynecomastia Increases blood levels of theophylline, phenytoin, and other drugs Decrease dose in renal dysfunction
	10–20 mg/kg/day in infants	IV, IM, PO q6–12h	
Cisapride	0.15–0.3 mg	PO, tid-qid 15–30 min prior to feeds	available only by limited access protocol
Clindamycin	5 mg	<7 d: <2 kg: q12h IV, IM ≤7 d: ≤2 kg; q12h ≤7 d: >2 kg: q8h <7 d: 1.2–2 kg: q8h >7 d: >2 kg: q6h	Not indicated for meningitis GI disturbance Pseudomembraneous colitis (rare in children)
Cromolyn	20 mg /dose	Inhalation q6–q8h	Bronchospasm, cough, nasal congestion, and pharyngeal irritation have been reported
Dexamethasone	Anti-inflammatory: 0.025–0.05 mg Airway edema: 0.25 mg	IV, IM, PO q6–q12h IV, IM, PO For extubation: Give first dose 4 h prior to extubation. Then repeat q8h × 3 doses. Max 1 mg/kg/day. A longer duration of therapy may be needed with more severe cases.	May increase risk of infection May cause hypertension, salt retention, adrenal suppression, hyperglycemia, and leukocytosis Consider steroid coverage for periods of stress after therapy for BPD, and in intercurrent illness (see BPD section) Give hydrocortisone stress doses for surgery up to six months after stopping taper See hydrocortisone for stress dosing guidelines All calculations must use the same body weight
	BPD	IV, IM, PO (numerous tapers have proposed) Day Daily dose 1–2 0.2–0.3 mg/kg 3–4 0.1–0.15 mg/kg 5–6 0.05 mg/ kg divided q12h with max exposure of 7–10 days	Recent AAP statement recommends use in VLBW only for the most serious chronic lung disease due to long-term neurologic sequellae associated with therapy.
Diazepam	Status epilepticus: 0.1–0.5 mg	Slow IV push (over 3 min) every 15–30 min for two to three doses; may repeat in 4 h to a max of 2 mg per 24 hr	Not a first line agent for neonates Lorazepam is a better choice for maintenance therapy May cause hypotension and respiratory depression Displacement of bilirubin by sodium benzoate may occur
	Sedation: 0.04–0.3 mg	IV q2–4h prn Maximum of 0.6 mg/kg within 8 h period	
Diazoxide	Hypertension 1–3 mg	IV push every 5–15 min until blood pressure is controlled, then q4–24h	May cause hyperglycemia, ketoacidosis, GI irritation, salt and water retention, hypotension
	Hypoglycemia 2–5 mg	PO q8–q12h	Use only if refractory to glucose infusion
Digoxin	Total digitalizing dose (TDD) oral Premie: 20–30 mcg Term: 25–35 mcg 1–24 mo: 35–60 mcg	Give 1/2 of the TDD initially, then 1/4 of the TDD q8h–q24h × 2 doses	May cause bradycardia, PVC's, vomiting, poor feeding, and arrhythmias Check ECG trace during digitalization and periodically

APPENDIX H-2
PHARMACOPOEIA (*continued*)

Drug	Dose/kg	Route and Frequency	Comments
	Oral maintenance (25% of TDD) Premie: 5–7.5 mcg Term 6–10 mcg 1–24 mo: 10–15 mcg TDD injectable: Premie: 15–25 mcg Term 20–30 mcg 1–24 mo: 30–50 mcg Injectable maintenance dose (25% of TDD) Premie: 4–6 mcg Term: 5–8 mcg 1–24 mo: 7.5–12 mcg	q12h IV, IM follow same guidelines as for oral administration IV, IM q12h	Adjust dose per clinical response and renal function Bioavailability of elixir is 70–85% of the injectable preparation
Dobutamine	1–20 mcg/kg/min; max dose: 40 mcg/min	IV infusion	Titrate according to patient's response Use same precautions as with dopamine
Dopamine	1–5 mcg/kg/min	IV infusion, mostly dopaminergic effect and some beta- adrenergic;	Monitor blood and pulse pressures Observe for pulmonary hypertension
	5–15 mcg/min	Mostly beta-adrenergic; some dopaminergic effect at lower end of this range; some alpha- adrenergic at higher end of dosage range	Tissue necrosis may occur with extravasation May cause ectopic beats
	>20 mcg/min; max dose 50 mcg/min	Mostly alpha-adrenergic effect	
Doxapram	Loading dose 2.5–3 mg	IV infusion over 1 h	Maintain therapeutic caffeine or theophylline levels while on doxapram Taper drug to avoid rebound apneic episodes Increases oxygen consumption and may cause hypertension, tachycardia, and seizures
	Maintenance dose 1–2.5 mg/kg/h	Continuous IV infusion; start at 1 mg/kg/h and titrate up to mininum effective dose Max dose 2.5 mg/kg/hr Maximum concentration; 2 mg/ml	
Edrophonium	Myasthenia gravis test: Neonates: 0.1 mg (single dose, not per kg) Infants: 0.04 mg/kg/ dose ×1 (max of 1 mg for body weight) <34 kg and 2 mg ≥34 kg	IV once If no IV access availabe, may give IM or SC	Keep atropine and resuscitation equipment available Antidote: Atropine 0.01–0.04 mg/kg/dose
Enalapril (PO)	0.05–0.1 mg	PO qd titrate to max of 0.5 mg/kg	Adjust dose in renal impairment: CrCl 10–50 ml/min: give 75% of dose
Enalaprilat (IV)	5–10 mcg	IV q8–24 h administer over 5 min	CrCl < 10 ml/min: give 50% of dose May cause hypoglycemia, hyperkalemia, neutropenia, anemia, and deterioration of renal function
Epinephrine 1:10,000	0.1–0.3 ml	IV, Intratracheal Every 3–5 min as needed	IV drip used for hypotension refractory to dopamine and dobutamine Higher end of dosage range used for cardiac resuscitation; intracardiac route should be last resort Dilute intratracheal doses to 1–2 ml with saline soln
	0.1–1 mcg/kg/min	Continuous IV infusion; titrate up as needed	
Epinephrine (racemic) 2.25% solution	0.25 ml total dose	Inhalation via nebulizer over 15 min q4h prn Dilute with NS to total volume of 2.5–3 ml	May cause tachycardia and arrhythmias

(*continued*)

Drug	Dose/kg	Route and Frequency	Comments
Epoetin	see	Erythropoietin	
Erythromycin	anti-infective: 10 mg	IV, PO	Decreases clearance of theophylline,
		≤7 d: q12h	digoxin, carbamazepine, and others
		>7 d <1.2 kg: q12h	
		>7 d ≥1.2 kg: q8h	
	Prokinetic agent: 3 mg then 5 mg	IV ×1 infuse over 60 min	Causes GI distress
		Po q6h	
Erythropoietin	Anemia of prematurity:	SC three times weekly	Must give iron supplementation
	50–100 units or 200 units		
		Titrate dose up based on clinical	
		response IV/SC qd/qod for	
		2–6 wk	
Exosurf	(see Surfactant)		
Fentanyl	1–3 mcg	IV, IM q2–q4h prn pain	Causes muscle rigidity, respiratory
	0.5–2 mcg/kg/h	Continuous IV infusion; titrate up	depression and dependence; causes less
			CV effect than morphine
Ferrous sulfate	Iron deficiency anemia: 2–3 mg	PO q12–24h (max dose:	Do not give concurrently with antacids,
	elemental Fe/kg/day	15 mg/day)	milk, or cereal
			Cimetidine decreases absorption of Iron
			May cause GI irritation; colors stools black
	With Erythropoietin: 3–6 mg	PO q12–q8h	
	elemental Fe	Max 15 mg/kg/day	
	Premature supplement: 1 mg	PO q12h or give formula with Fe	
Fluconazole	5–6 mg	PO/IV	Monitor renal and liver functions;
		Infuse over 1–2h	Renal dosing
		<29 wks gestation 0–14 days:	CrCl 21–50 ml/min 50% of dose
		q72h	CrCl 11–20 ml/min 25% of dose
	5–6 mg	>14 days: q48h	
	3–6 mg	30–36 wks gestation 0–14 days:	
		q48h	
	6 mg	>14 days: qd	
Flucytosine	25–50 mg	PO q12–24h	May cause GI irritation, bone marrow
			depression, elevated liver enzymes,
			elevated BUN, and creatinine
			Used in combination with amphotericin B or
			fluconazole
Furosemide	1–2 mg	IV, IM q12h– q24h	Causes sodium and potassium depletion:
	2–4 mg	PO q12h–q24h	dehydration
			Additive ototoxicity with aminoglycosides
Gentamicin	3 mg	<1.2 kg <30 days: qd	Monitor renal function
	2.5 mg	<1.2 kg >30 days: q12h	Ototoxicity is related to length of therapy
	2.5 mg	≥1.2 kg 0–14 days:q12h	Therapeutic range:
			Peak 5–12 mcg/ml
	2.5 mg	≥1.2 kg >14 days: q8h	Trough <2 mcg/ml
Gentian violet	1% topical solution	Dilute to 0.5% solution 3–4 drops	Stains skin and clothing; apply with cotton
		under the tongue or apply to	tip applicator
		lesions after feedings bid-tid	Do not apply to face
Glucagon	Hypoglycemia or insulin shock:	IV push, SC, IM	1 unit = 1 mg
	0.03–0.3 mg	Every 30 min prn	May cause rebound hypoglycemia
	Max dose 1 mg/dose		
Heparin	For maintenance of central	IV	See protamine sulfate for treatment of
	catheters: 0.5–2 units/ mL		overdose
	of IV fluid		Monitor clotting time; titrate dose to
			achieve 1.5–2.5 times normal physiologic
			values
	Anticoagulation: bolus	IV	
	50 units/kg	Once	
	Maintenance: 10–25 units/kg/h	IV continuous infusion titrate up	
		based on APTT/PTT	
	Intermittent dosing: 50–100 units/	IV q4h	Not preferred
	kg/dose		

APPENDIX H-2
PHARMACOPOEIA (*continued*)

Drug	Dose/kg	Route and Frequency	Comments
Hydralazine	Parenteral Initial: 0.1–0.8 titrate up not, to exceed 2 mg/kg/dose	IV, IM q4–q6h	Adjust dose in renal impairment: CrCl = 10–50 ml/min: give q8h CrCl < 10 ml/min; give q12–q24h
	Oral Initial 0.2–0.3 mg titrate up, Max daily dose 5 mg/kg	PO, NG q8–q12h	May cause tachycardia and sodium and water retention
Hydrocortisone	Congenital adrenal hyperplasia 20–35 mg/m2/d Maintenance: 12.5–37.5 mg/m2/d	PO divided as follows: 1/4 dose in morning and at noon, 1/2 dose at night	Increases chance of infection May cause hypertension, salt and water retention, adrenal suppression, and hyperglycemia
	Shock: Initial 35–50 mg/kg Maintenance: 12.5–37.5 mg/kg	IV Once IV q6h × 48–72 h	Approximate weight to body surface area conversion table:

Weight kg	M^2	
0.5	0.5	
1	0.1	
2	0.15	
3	0.2	
4	0.25	

Drug	Dose/kg	Route and Frequency	No. 1	No. 2	No. 3
Hydrocortisone	Stress dose: 50 mg/m²/d	IV, IM Divided q12–q6h			
Indomethacin	Dose (mg/kg) PDA (see comments)	IV q8–q12 h × 3 doses <48 h of life 2–7 d >7 d	0.2 0.2 0.2	0.1 0.2 0.25	0.1 0.2 0.25
	Extended treatment 0.2 mg	IV qd × 5 days following standard three dose regimen may decrease recurrence of PDA			
	Prevention of IVH: 0.1 mg/kg	q24h for three doses, beginning at 6–12 h of age			

Drug	Dose/kg	Route and Frequency	Comments
Insulin	Hyperglycemia: Initial: 0.1 unit	IV Once over 15–20 min	Monitor blood glucose and titrate dose accordingly: may cause rebound hyperglycemia if discontinued abruptly
	Maintenance: 0.02–0.1 unit/kg/h	IV, continuous infusion	Use only human regular insulin for IV infusions
	Intermittent: 0.1–0.2 units	SC, q6–q12h	
	Hyperkalemia: 0.3 units/g of glucose	IV with dextrose: 500 mg/kg/dose	
Iron	See Ferrous sulfate		
Isoniazid	5–10 mg	PO, IM q12–24h	May cause vitamin B6 (pyridoxine) depletion; monitor liver function
Kayexalate (sodium polystyrene)	1 g	PO, PR q6h prn	Hyperosmotic; monitor serum electrolytes
Labetalol	Bolus: 0.25 mg	IV over 2 min Dose can be doubled and repeated every 10 min until desired clinical response or total dose of 4 mg/kg is reached	Absolute contraindication: CHF, heart block, sinus tachycardia
	Maintenance: 0.25–1 mg	IV q4h	May cause bradycardia, edema, and bronchospasm
	1.5–2 mg 0.25–1.5 mg/kg/h	PO q12h Continuous IV infusion Max conc 1 mg/ml	
Levothyroxine	5–8 mcg	IV push over 30–60 sec; q24h	Monitor serum T4 and TSH levels Do not mix with any other IV fluids; mix immediately prior to administration
	8–14 mcg Alternate dose: 25–50 mcg total	PO q24h PO q24h	Increases effects of oral anticoagulants
Lidocaine	0.5–1 mg 10–50 mcg/kg/min	IV every 5–10 min × 2 doses Continuous IV infusion Max conc 8 mg/ml	May cause bradycardia and hypotension; decrease dose in CHF; contraindicated in severe heart block Therapeutic levels 1.5–5 mcg/ml

(continued)

APPENDIX H-2
PHARMACOPOEIA (continued)

Drug	Dose/kg	Route and Frequency	Comments
Lorazepam	Status epilepticus: 0.05 mg Sedation: 0.05–0.1 mg	IV may repeat every 15–20 min × 2 doses IV q4–8h Max dose 2 mg	Contains benzyl alcohol; may cause respiratory depression, hypotension, and bradycardia Do not give intraarterially Administer over 2–5 min
Magnesium sulfate	Hypomagnesemia: 0.2–0.4 mEq	Infuse over 2–4 h IV 2–3 doses q8–12h	Monitor serum levels May cause hypotension and respiratory depression Max concentration 1.6 mEq/ml
Mannitol	0.25–1 g (15%–20% solution) Oliguria test dose: 0.2 g	IV once over 2–6 h IV over 3–5 min	Always use a 5 micron filter May cause rebound edema and circulatory overload
Methylene blue	1–2 mg	IV slow push over 5 min (1% soln)	Methylene blue is a reducing agent; it may decrease hemoglobin O2 capacity
Metoclopramide	0.1–0.2 mg Renal dose adjustment: C/Cr % of dose 20–50 75 <40 50 <10 25–50	May repeat in 1 h IV, IM, PO q6h	Dilute to 0.2 mg/ml and infuse over 15–30 min May cause extrapyramidal symptoms with higher doses; may lower seizure thershold
Metolazone	0.2 mg	PO q12–q24h	May cause metabolic alkalosis and hyperuricemia; monitor serum electrolytes
Metronidazole	7.5 mg 15 mg	IV, PO 0–4 wk <1.2 kg q48h ≤7 d 1.2–2 kg q24h ≤7 d >2 kg q12h >7 d 1.2–2 kg q12h >7 d>2 kg q12h	Penetrates effectively into CSF; may cause leukopenia, rash, phlebitis, and seizures
Midazolam	0.03–0.1 mg 0.05 mg/h	IV, IM, q2–4h prn Continuous IV infusion; titrate up based on clinical response	May cause respiratory depression, hypotension, and dependence
Morphine	0.05–0.1 mg 10–20 mcg/kg/h	IV, IM, SC q2–q4h prn Continuous IV infusion: titrate up based on clinical response	May cause respiratory and CNS depression, hypotension, and dependence Nalxone reverses acute overdose Use preservative free formulation
Nafcillin	25 mg	IV, IM <1.2 kg <1 mo: q12h 1.2–2 kg ≤7 d: q12h >2 kg ≤7 d: q8h 1.2–2 kg >7 d: q8h >2 kg >7 d: q6h	Consider changing dosing interval in patients with hepatic dysfunction Cases of granulocytopenia or agranulocytosis have been reported
Naloxone	Maternal opiate exposure 0.1mg Reversal of opiate analgesia 0.01 mg	IV, IM, SC endotracheally every 2–3 min prn	For ET administration dilute to 1–2 ml with NS Max conc for IV infusion: 4 mcg/ml; undiluted drug may be pushed over 30 sec May precipitate withdrawal symptoms in patients with physical dependence
Neo-calglucon	See Calcium glubionate		
Neomycin	12.5–25 mg	PO q6h	May cause nephrotoxicity and ototoxicity
Neostigmine	Myasthenia gravis test: 0.025–0.04 mg Treatment: 0.01–0.04 mg 0.25–0.3 mg	IM Once IV, IM, SC q2–q4h prn PO q3–q4h prn	May cause cholinergic crisis Antidote: atropine 0.01–0.4 mg/kg
Nitroprusside	Initial 0.3–0.5 mcg/kg/min Maintenance: 3–4 mcg/kg/min Max 8–10 mcg/min	IV continuous infusion	Monitor for cyanide toxicity May cause hypotension and tachyphylaxis Protect from light
Nystatin	100,000–200,000 units total dose	PO q6h Apply 1/2 of the dose to each side of the mouth for oral thrush	Poor oral absorption

APPENDIX H-2
PHARMACOPOEIA (continued)

Drug	Dose/kg	Route and Frequency	Comments
Octreotide	1–10 mcg	IV, SC q12–q24h	Start treatment using lower end of dosage range
			Causes growth hormone suppression
Oxacillin	25 mg	IV, IM ≤2 kg <7 d q12h ≤2 kg >7 d q8h >2 kg ≤7 d q8h >2 kg >7 d q6h	Contraindicated in patients allergic to penicillins May cause thrombophlebitis and clostridium difficile colitis Monitor liver function
Palivizumab	See Synagis		
Pancuronium	0.04–0.1 mg	IV q1–4h prn movement	Short half-life; titrate dose based on clinical response Aminoglycosides increase the action of pancuronium Monitor for CNS depression
Paregoric	Initial dose: 0.2–0.3 ml total dose subsequent doses: increase by 0.05 ml up to max of 0.7 ml total dose	PO q3–4h	Give with feeds to minimize GI irritation; same adverse effects as morphine
Penicillin-G K	Congenital syphillis: 50,000 units	IV, IM ≤7 d: q12h >7 d: q8	May cause hypersensitivity reactions, thrombophlebitis, and acute intersitial nephritis
	Meningitis: group B strep: 75,000–100,000 units	IV, IM ≤2 kg ≤7 d: q12h ≤2 kg >7 d: q8h	
	Other infections: 25,000–50,000 units	>2 kg <7 d q8h >2 kg >7 d: q6h	
Phenobarbital	Loading dose: 20 mg	IV, IM once	Monitor levels weekly or as clincally indicated Induces the metabolism of other drugs, may cause respiratory and CNS depression at higher doses Therapeutic levels: seizures: 20–40 mcg/ml hyperbilirubinemia: 15 mcg/ml
	Maintenance dose: 3–4 mg/kg/day	IV, IM, PO qd	
Phenytoin	Loading dose: 20 mg	IV once	Rapid infusion may precipitate cardiovascular collapse; do not exceed 0.5 mg/kg/min infusion
	Maintenance dose: 2–4 mg	IV, PO q12h Some patients may need q8h intervals	Toxicity may lead to seizures and CNS depression Therapeutic range: 15–20 mcg/ml
Phytonadione (vitamin K$_1$)	Neonatal hemorrhagic disease: Prophylaxis: 0.5–1 mg total dose	IM, SC once within 1 hour of birth; may repeat 6–8 h later	IV route should be used only when other routes are not available; infuse at a max rate of 1 mg/min; severe reactions resembling anaphylaxis may occur with IV administration
	Treatment: 1–2 mg total dose	IV, SC once	
Piperacillin	50 mg	IV ≤7 d q8h >7 d q6h	Used in combination with aminoglycosides Eosinophilia, hyperbilirubinemia, elevations in ALT, AST, BUN, and serum creatinine have been observed
Prednisolone	Antiinflammatory: 0.5–1 mg	PO q12h	May cause hypertension, GI irritation, and adrenal suppression
Propranolol	0.01–0.1 mg maximum 0.25 mg	IV push over 10 min q6–q8h dose: 1 mg PO q6–q8h titrate up to maximum of 5 mg/kg/day	May cause hypotension, bronchospasm, and heart block
Prostaglandin E$_1$	0.05–0.4 mcg/kg/min	IV continuous infusion; use lowest effective dose	May cause apnea, fever, hypotension, and cutaneous vasodilation
Protamine	Dose of protamine in mg to neutralize 100 units of heparin	Protamine / Time elapsed 1–1.5 / immediate 0.5–0.75 / 30–60 min 0.25–0.375 / >2 h	May cause hypotension and bradycardia Max conc: 10 mg/ml

(continued)

APPENDIX H-2
PHARMACOPOEIA (continued)

Drug	Dose/kg	Route and Frequency	Comments
Pyridoxine (vitamin B$_6$)	Deficiency: 5–25 mg × 3 weeks then 1.5–2.5 mg	PO, IV, IM Q24h	Decreases serum levels of phenobarbital, phenytoin, and folic acid; may cause hypersensitivity reactions, respiratory distress, and burning at site of injection
	pyridoxine dependent seizure: 50–100 mg total dose	PO, IV, IM Q24h	
Pyrimethamine	Toxoplasmosis: LD: 2 mg/kg/day	PO q12h for 2 days	Supplementation with folic acid is recommended
		PO; qd for 2–6 months, then 3× per week to complete 12 months treatment	May cause glossitis, seizures, and rash Given with sulfadiazine
Ranitidine	0.75–1.5 mg	IV, IM q6–q8h max 6 mg/kg/d	Renal dosing: CrCl < 50 ml/min oral give q24h IV, IM: give q18–q24h Monitor serum creatinine
	1.25–2.5 mg	PO q12h	
RSV immune globulin	750 mg (15 ml)	IV, monthly during RSV season	Not recommended for use in patients with cyanotic heart disease. Some patients may develop respiratory distress due to excessive fluid
		Administration guidelines: 1.5 ml/kg/h × 15 min 3 ml/kg/h × 15 min 6 ml/kg/h until finished	Live vaccines should be delayed for 9 mo after administration
Spironolactone	0.5–1.5 mg	PO q8–q12h	Avoid in hyperkalemia; may cause rash, vomiting, and diarrhea; contraindicated in renal failure
Surfactant	Curosurf (poractant alfa) initial: 2.5 ml subsequent: 1.25 ml	One dose as soon as RDS diagnosis is confirmed intratracheally. Subsequent dose × 2 q12h after first dose if baby is still ventilator dependent.	Adverse effects include pulmonary hemorrhage, apnea, and mucous plugging Adjust ventilatory parameters to prevent hyperoxia and hypocarbia May open ductus
Surfactant	Infasurf (calfactant) 3 ml	Endotracheal: one dose q12h up to a total of 3 doses	Adverse effects include pulmonary hemorrhage, apnea, and mucous plugging Adjust ventilatory parameters to prevent hyperoxia and hypocarbia May open ductus
Surfactant	Survanta (beractant) 4 ml	Endotracheal rescue treatment: one dose as soon as RDS diagnosis is confirmed. May repeat q6h to a total of four doses Prophylaxis: First dose given as soon as possible after birth; may give a total of four doses during first 48 hours of life, no more frequently than 6 h apart	Adverse effects include pulmonary hemorrhage, apnea, and mucous plugging Adjust ventilatory parameters to prevent hyperoxia and hypocarbia May open ductus
Survanta	See Surfactant		
Synagis	15 mg	IM; monthly during RSV season	Typically RSV season begins in November and last through April Inject in the anterolateral aspect of the thigh. Gluteal injections may damage the sciatic nerve
Tham	See Tromethamine		
Ticarcillin + Clavulanic acid (Timentin)	75 mg	IV, IM ≤2 kg 0–7 d q12h ≤2 kg > 7 d q8h >2 kg 0–7 d q8h >2 kg > 7 d q6h	May cause hypersensitivity reactions, phlebitis, pseudomembranous colitis, hypernatremia, and inhibition of platelet aggregation
Tobramycin	3 mg 2.5 mg 2.5 mg 2.5 mg	<2 kg < 30 days qd <1.2 kg > 30 days q12h ≥2 kg 0–14 days q12h ≥1.2 kg > 14 days q8h	Monitor renal function Therapeutic range: Peak 5–10 mcg/ml Trough <2 mcg/ml

APPENDIX H-2
PHARMACOPOEIA (*continued*)

Drug	Dose/kg	Route and Frequency	Comments
Tromethamine	3 ml	IV slow infusion Max rate: 1ml/h	1 ml = 0.3 mEq;1mM = 1 Meq Infuse preferably in large blood vessel; may cause hypoglycemia, hyperkalemia, apnea, and fluid overload
Vancomycin	15 mg	IV infused over 90–120 min <1.2 kg q24h	Therapeutic range:
	15 mg	≤7 days 1.2–2 kg: q12h	Peak 20–40 mcg/ml
	15 mg	≤7 days >2 kg: q12h	Trough <10 mcg/ml
			May cause renal and ototoxicity, redman syndrome may occur with rapid in fusion; some patients may require 2 h infusion
	15 mg	>7 days > 1.2–2 kg: q8–12h	
	15 mg	>2 kg: q8h	
Vasopressin (aqueous)	Diabetes insipidus 2.5–10 units total dose	IM, SC q12–q16h	May cause bronchoconstriction, diarrhea and electrolyte imbalance
Vecuronium	0.03–0.15 mg 0.05–0.1 mg/kg/h	IV q1–2 h prn movement IV continuous infusion Max concentration:1 mg/ml	Neuromuscular effects may be prolonged after continuous infusion and when aminoglycosides are administered concurrently
			May need to adjust for renal dysfunction
Vitamin K$_1$	See phytonadione		

Dosages in this table are single dose per kilogram. Frequency is suggested in the third column but may vary with maturity and rate of metabolism. In most cases, the most conservative dosage is given.

ACTH, adrenocorticotropic hormone; AV, atrioventricular; BP, blood pressure; BUN, blood urea nitrogen; CNS, central nervous system; CSF, cerebrospinal fluid; ECG, electrocardiogram; ET, endotracheal; GI, gastrointestinal; IT, intrathecal; NS, normal saline; PO, by mouth; PR, per rectum; prn, as needed; PVC, premature ventricular contraction; SC, subcutaneous; TDD, total digitalizing dose; TSH, thyroid stimulating hormone; WBC, leukocyte.

Reviewed and updated by Diana Joachim, Pharm D and Kelsey Briggs, Pharm D, West Virginia University Hospitals, Morgantown, WV.

Nutritional Values

APPENDIX I-1

COMPARISON OF ENTERAL INTAKE RECOMMENDATIONS FOR GROWING PRETERM NEONATES IN STABLE CLINICAL CONDITION[a]

Nutrients per 100 kcal*	Consensus Recommendations		AAPCON[†]	ESPGAN-CON[†]
	<1,000 g	>1,000 g		
Water, mL	125–167	125–167	—	115–154
Energy, kcal	100	100	100	100
Protein, g	3–3.16	2.5–3	2.9–3.3	2.25–3.1
Carbohydrate, g	—	—	9–13	7–14
Lactose, g	3.16-9.5	3.16–9.8	—	—
Oligomers, g	0–7	0–7	—	—
Fat, g	—	—	4.5–6	3.6–7
Linoleic acid, g	0.44–1.7	0.44–1.7	0.4+	0.5–1.4
Linolenic acid, g	0.11–0.44	0.11–0.44	—	>0.055
$C_{18:2}/C_{18:3}$	>5	>5	—	5–15
Vitamin A, IU	583–1,250	583–1,250	75–225	270–450
With lung disease	2,250–2,333	2,250–2,333	—	—
Vitamin D, IU	125–333	125–333	270	800–1,600/d
Vitamin E, IU	5–10	5–10	>1.1	0.6–10
Supplement, human milk	2.9	2.9	—	—
Vitamin K, µg	6.66–8.33	6.66–8.33	4	4–15
Ascorbate, mg	15–20	15–20	35	7–40
Thiamine, µg	150–200	150–200	>40	20–250
Riboflavin, µg	200–300	200–300	>60	60–600
Pyridoxine, µg	125–175	125–175	>35	35–250
Niacin, mg	3–4	3–4	>0.25	0.8–5
Pantothenate, mg	1–1.5	1–1.5	>0.3	>0.3
Biotin, µg	3–5	3–5	>1.5	>1.5
Folate, µg	21–42	21–42	33	>60
Vitamin B_{12}, µg	0.25	0.25	>0.15	>0.15
Sodium, mg	38–58	38–58	48–67	23–53
Potassium, mg	65–100	65–100	66–98	90–152
Chloride, mg	59–89	59–89	—	57–89
Calcium, mg	100–192	100–192	175	70–140
Phosphorus, mg	50–117	50–117	91.5	50–87
Magnesium, mg	6.6–12.5	6.6–12.5	—	6–12

(continued)

APPENDIX I-1
Continued

Nutrients per 100 kcal*	Consensus Recommendations			
	<1,000 g	>1,000 g	AAPCON[†]	ESPGAN-CON[†]
Iron, mg	1.67	1.67	1.7–2.5	1.5
Zinc, μg	833	833	>500	550–1,100
Copper, μg	100–125	100–125	90	90–120
Selenium, μg	1.08–2.5	1.08–2.5	—	—
Chromium, μg	0.083–0.42	0.083–0.42	—	—
Manganese, μg	6.3	6.3	>5	1.5–7.5
Molybdenum, μg	0.25	0.25	—	—
Iodine, μg	25–50	25–50	5	10–45
Taurine, mg	3.75–7.5	3.75–7.5	—	—
Carnitine, mg	2.4	2.4	—	>1.2
Inositol, mg	27–67.5	27–67.5	—	—
Chlorine, mg	12–23.4	12–23.4	—	—

* Based on a need for 120 mg/kg per day
[†] AAPCON indicates American Academy of Pediatrics. Committee on Nutrition; ESPGAN-CON, European Society of Paediatric Gastroenterology and Nutrition, Committee on Nutritioin of the Preterm infant.
[a] Guidelines for Perinatal Care. 5th Ed. 2002. American academy of Pediatrics. American College of Obstetrics and bynecologists. P. 261.

APPENDIX I-2
IRON AND CALORIC CONTENT OF COMMERCIALLY PREPARED STRAINED AND JUNIOR FOODS

Food	Mean Iron Content (mg per jar)	Caloric Content (kcals per jar)
Dry Cereals		
1tbsp = 2.4 g	1.14	9
Cereal with Fruit, Strained Rice	6.72	53
Strained Food		
Juices (4oz)	0.1–0.9	50–60
Fruits (jar)	0.2–0.3	52–73
Plain vegetables	0.4–1.06	26–73
Creamed vegetables	0.36–0.8	54–73
Meats	1.19–1.46	106–129
Egg yolks/cereal	0.6	65
Dinners	0.35–0.76	55–87
Desserts	0.11–0.27	67–96
Junior Foods†		
Meat Sticks	1.0	109–131

† Other foods similar to strained foods.
From Pennington, JAT. *Bowes and Church's food values of portions commonly used*, 17th ed. Philadelphia: JB Lippincott, 1998.

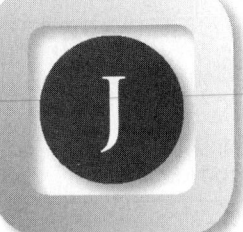

Technical Procedures

1. PLACEMENT OF UMBILICAL CATHETERS

APPENDIX J-1A

THE LENGTH OF CATHETER INSERTED INTO THE UMBILICAL ARTERY IN ORDER TO REACH THE BIFURCATION OF THE AORTA, THE DIAPHRAGM, OR THE AORTIC VALVES VERSUS THE TOTAL BODY LENGTH OF AN INFANT

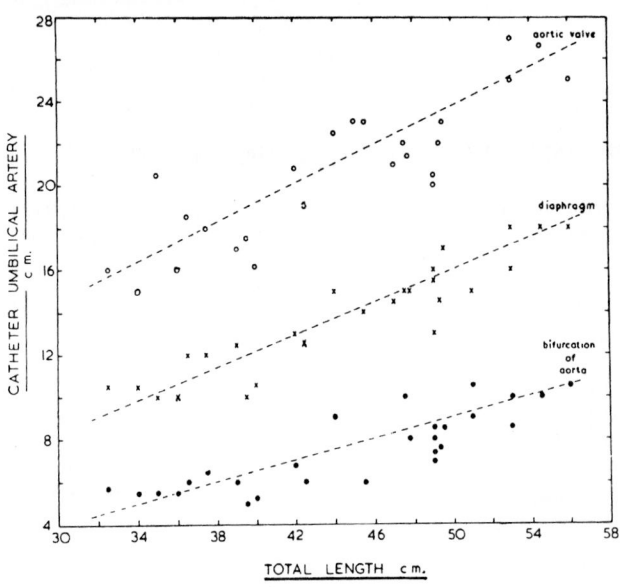

From Dunn PM. *Arch Dis Child* 1966;41:71

APPENDIX J-1B

THE LENGTH OF CATHETER INSERTED INTO THE UMBILICAL VEIN IN ORDER TO REACH THE DIAPHRAGM (X) AND THE LEFT ATRIUM (O) VERSUS THE SHOULDER—UMBILICUS LENGTH OF AN INFANT

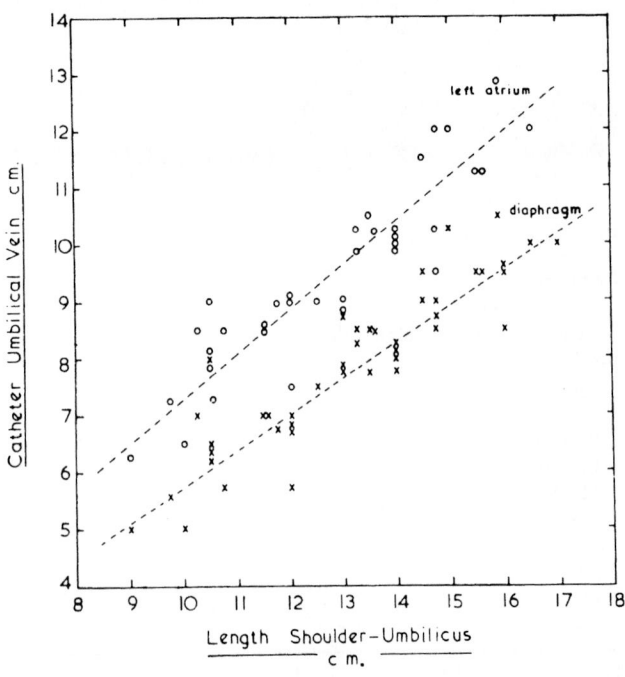

From Dunn PM. *Arch Dis Child* 1966;41:71

2. DETERMINING ENDOTRACHEAL TUBE SIZE

ESTIMATES OF INSERTIONAL LENGTH OF UMBILICAL CATHETERS BASED ON BIRTH WEIGHT, WITH 95% CONFIDENCE INTERVALS

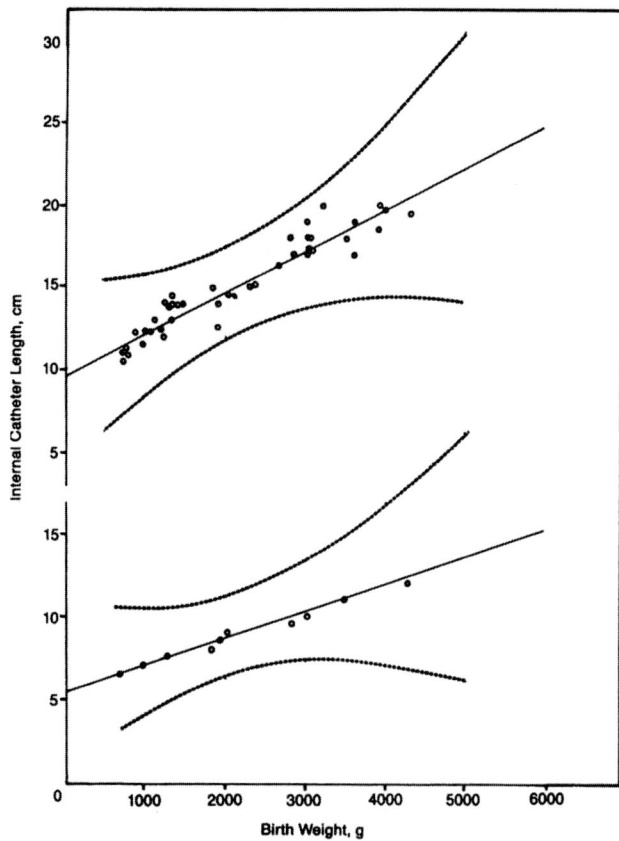

APPENDIX J-2
ENDOTRACHEAL TUBE SIZE

| Infant weight (g) | Tube Diameter | |
	Inside	Outside
<1000	2.5 mm	12 Fr
1000–1500	3 mm	14 Fr
1500–2200	3.5 mm	16 Fr
2200+	4 mm	18 Fr

Umbilical artery catheter tip inserted between T6 and T10; umbilical vein catheter tip inserted above diaphragm in inferior vena cava near the right atrium. Modified estimating equations using birth weight (BW) are as follows: umbilical artery length = 2.5 × BW + 9.7 (top) and umbilical vein length = 1.5 × BW + 5.6 (bottom), where BW is measured in kilograms and lengths in centimeters.

From Shukla H, Ferrara A. *Am J Dis Child* 1986;140:786.

Index

A

Abacavir, 1319
  pregnancy, 1320t
Abdomen
  auscultation, 344
  examination, 341–344, 347t
  palpation, 343–344
  size of, 341–342
  symmetry of, 341–342
Abdominal circumference, 168
Abdominal injury
  ventriculoperitoneal shunt, 1414
Abdominal masses, 994, 1083
  of renal origin, 1084t
Abdominal muscles
  congenital deficiency, 1129
Abdominal surgery, 1113–1123
Abdominal wall
  abnormalities, 1126–1127
Abdominal wall defects, 945
  fluids and electrolytes, 374
Abelcet, 1690
Abnormal placentation
  abortions with, 226
Abnormal thyroglobulin, 934
ABO hemolytic disease, 801–803,
      1180–1181
  diagnosis, 802–803
Abortions, 232
  with normal chromosomes,
      225–226
Abruptio placentae
  with intrapartum asphyxia, 308t
  with maternal drugs, 1583
  maternal drug use, 1573
Absent pulmonary valve syndrome,
      719–720
Abstinence syndrome
  with cocaine, 1585
Acardiac twinning, 528
Accelerated ventricular rhythm,
      701–703
Accessory tragus, 1501, 1502f
Accountability, 90
  vs. blame, 106
Acebutolol
  breast milk, 1689
Acetaldehyde, 1587
Acetaminophen, 1564
  breast feeding, 279
  doses, 1565t
  glucuronidation, 1510
Acetazolamide, 1690
  for hydrocephalus, 1413
Achondroplasia, 906, 906f

Acid base, 988
  balance, 372
    ELBW, 471–472
  mineral deposits, 1006
Acid peptic disease, 948
Acinetobacter sepsis, 1361
Acne neonatorum, 1493
Acquired disorders, 1476–1478
Acquired hemorrhagic diathesis, 1193
Acquired immunodeficiency syndrome
      (AIDS), 1315–1316, 1477
  with granulocyte transfusion, 1216
Acquired renal failure, 1008
Acrodermatitis enteropathica, 1490–1491,
      1491f
Acropustulosis of infancy, 1492
Acrorenal syndrome, 1675
Acrorenocular syndrome, 1675
Acrorenomandibular syndrome, 1675
Active euthanasia, 14
Active transport
  placenta, 152–153
Activity, Pulse, Grimace, Appearance, and
      Respiration (APGAR) scores, 562
ACUTE (acute, critical, unexpected,
      treatable, easily diagnosed), 20
Acute bilirubin encephalopathy, 783–784
  classification, 785t
  clinical features of, 784t
Acute care in-hospital costs, 27–28
Acute infection, 1235–1264
  epidemiology, 1235–1236
Acute lymphoblastic leukemia (ALL),
      1449
Acute medical care post discharge
  costs, 30
Acute metabolic encephalopathy, 965–968,
      971t
  emergency treatment of, 971–972
Acute myelogenous leukemia (AML),
      1449
Acute pyelonephritis, 1024
Acute renal failure
  fluid and electrolytes, 1005
  oligoanuria, 1000–1010
    diagnosis, 1000
  prevention and early diagnosis, 1002
  SGA, 512t
  treatment, 1004–1005
Acute respiratory disorders, 553–575
Acute respiratory failure
  hereditary causes, 556–557
Acute tubular necrosis
  hematuria with, 1083
  pathophysiology, 1000

Acyanotic anomalies
  with abnormal cardiac function,
      691–700
  with left-to-right shunt, 682–684
  with systemic outflow obstruction,
      678–680
Acyanotic lesions, 678–691
Acyanotic neonates
  cardiac examination
    differential diagnosis, 643f, 645f
Acyclovir, 1012, 1690
  for fetal herpes simplex virus, 1287
  for herpes simplex virus, 1285–1286,
      1286t
  for neonatal HSV, 1289
  for recurrent genital herpes in pregnancy,
      1291
Adams-Oliver syndrome, 1675
Adaptive immune mechanisms, 1144
Adefovir dipivoxil
  for hepatitis B, 1310
Adenine phosphoribosyltransferase
  deficiency, 1028
Adenosine, 696t, 1690
  for arrhythmias, 1519, 1519t
  neonates, 1518t
  for supraventricular tachycardia,
      704
Adenosine-deaminase (ADA)
  deficiency, 198
Adenoviral pneumonia, 1366–1367
ADH
  DDAVP, 991
Adhesion molecules, 1140–1141
Adipose tissue
  SGA, 499–500
Adrenal cortex, 926
Adrenal gland
  development, 926
  function, 926
Adrenal gland disorders, 926
Adrenal hemorrhage, 1082–1083
Adrenal hyperplasia, 1088f
Adrenal insufficiency, 927–931
  diagnosis, 930
  treatment, 930–931
Adrenal steroid
  biosynthetic pathway, 928f
Adrenocorticotropic hormone deficiency,
      924, 927
Adult disease
  fetal origins of, 162
Advanced care planning, 95
Advanced practice nurses
  NICU, 77–78

Adverse sentinel events, 105–106
Advisory board
    neonatal transport, 41–42
African Americans
    perinatal health outcomes, 24
African trypanosomiasis, 1332t
After load, 740
Agammaglobulinemia, 1158t, 1206,
    1206t
Age
    ECMO, 623–624
Agency for Healthcare Research and
    Quality, 85t
Agonist antagonist opioids
    fetal and neonatal effects, 267
Air leaks, 574–575
    pathophysiology, 574
    risk factors, 574–575
Airway resistance
    assisted mechanical ventilation, 610
Alagille arteriohepatic dysplasia, 636t,
    1680
Albumin, 1690
    binding, 778
    transfusion, 1217
Albuterol, 1005, 1530, 1690
    for BPD, 590, 590t
Alcohol, 233
    adverse effects, 1574t
    fetal dysmorphogenesis, 1591t
    fetal effects, 234t, 1588
    maternal exposure to, 1446
    neonatal effects, 1588
    pregnancy, 1587–1588
    related birth defects, 1590–1592
    use, 36
        epidemiology, 1586–1587
        during pregnancy, 1586
Alcohol-based waterless hand gels, 1370
Aldosterone, 366–367, 926
Aldosterone deficiency, 929
Alimentum
    for formula protein induced
        enterocolitis, 955
    for intractable diarrhea of infancy, 955
    for short bowel syndrome, 951–952
Alkaline phosphatase
    TPN, 397
Allantoin
    BPD, 581
Allele specific oligonucleotide
    hybridization, 134
Alopecia, 1503–1504
Alpha1-antitrypsin
    BPD, 582
    deficiency, 974t, 975
Alpha-fetoprotein (AFP), 172, 1090
    placental transfer, 151
9alpha-fludrocortisone (Florinef)
    for adrenal insufficiency, 931
11alpha-hydroxylase deficiency, 929t
17alpha-hydroxylase deficiency, 929t
Alpha interferon
    for hepatitis B, 1310
Alpha methyldopa
    during pregnancy, 207

5alpha-reductase deficiency, 918
Alphoid DNA, 131
Alport syndrome, 1675
Altitude
    bilirubin, 797
    neonatal transport, 45
Aluminum
    toxicity, 396
Alu sequences, 131
Alveolar duct, 608f
Alveoli, 608f
    cysts, 340t
    lymphangioma, 340t
Ambiguous genitalia, 1087–1088,
    1124–1125
    etiology, 920t
    evaluation, 919–923, 920t
        with mullerian structures, 921f
        without mullerian structures, 922f
Amblyopia, 1469, 1483
Ambulances
    neonatal transport, 46
American Academy of Pediatrics (AAP)
    exchange transfusion guidelines, 824f
    neonatal hyperbilirubinemia guidelines,
        812t
    resuscitation guidelines, 17
American Heart Association
    resuscitation guidelines, 17
American trypanosomiasis, 1332t
Amikacin, 1690
Amino acid, 991
    metabolism
        SGA, 514
    metabolism disorders, 966t
    IUGR, 505–506
Amino acidurias, 1037
Aminoglycosides, 1011, 1524, 1527–1528
    bilirubin albumin binding, 779
    fetal effects, 240
    for meningitis, 1253
    for sepsis neonatorum, 1244, 1245
Aminophylline, 1536, 1690
    for AOP, 479
    bilirubin albumin binding, 781
    for BPD, 590t
Aminopterin
    fetal effects, 234t, 238–239
5-aminosalicylic acid
    breast milk, 1689
Amiodarone, 697t
    for arrhythmias, 1520–1521
    breast milk, 1689
    for JET, 742
    neonates, 1518t
Ammonium chloride, 1690
Amniocentesis, 142f
    cytomegalovirus, 1295–1296
    technical aspects of, 142
Amnion
    fetus, 157
Amnioninfusion
    MAS, 564
Amniotic band
    constricting band secondary to,
        1433f

Amniotic fluid, 156–157
Amniotic liquid
    fetal lambs, 285f
Amoxicillin, 1690
    for diarrhea, 1260
    fetal effects, 241
Amphetamine
    adverse effects, 1575t
    breast milk, 1687
Amphetamines, 26
Amphotericin B, 1012, 1690, 1691
    for sepsis neonatorum, 1245
Ampicillin, 1524, 1691
    for diarrhea, 1260–1261
    fetal effects, 241
    for Listeria pneumonia, 1263
    for meningitis, 1253
    for sepsis neonatorum, 1244, 1245
Amprenavir
    pregnancy, 1320t
    teratogenic potential, 1319
Amrinone, 657t, 1535
Amylase
    carbohydrate absorption, 941
Analgesia, 1561–1562
Ancillary costs
    VLBW, 30t
Androgen insensitivity syndrome (AIS), 918
Androgen resistance syndrome, 918–919
Androgens, 926
    fetal effects, 234t, 239
4-androstenedione, 926
Anemia, 1169–1190
    from blood loss, 1172
    with congenital rubella, 1282t
    in ELBW, 474–475
    erythroid development, 1169
    iatrogenic from blood sampling,
        1174–1175, 1175f
    internal hemorrhage, 1174
    neonates, 1187
    in newborns, 1170–1172
    obstetric accidents and complications,
        1174
    secondary to blood loss, 1175–1176
    with syphilis, 1250
Anemia of prematurity, 1169–1170
Anencephaly
    decision making, 18
Anesthesia, 1558–1561
Anesthetics
    effect on newborn neurobehavioral
        evaluation, 261–262
    for fetal surgery, 273–274
    for surgery during pregnancy, 272–274
Aneuploidy, 1444–1445
    with maternal alcohol, 1587
    sonographic markers, 137f
Angelman syndrome, 141, 907
Angiotensin converting enzyme (ACE)
    inhibitors, 1008, 1013, 1682
    fetal effects, 234t, 239–240
    during pregnancy, 207
Aniridia, 1474, 1474f
Aniridia-Wilms tumor, 1678
Ankyloglossia, 340t, 341

Annular pancreas, 1117–1118

Anomalous left coronary artery from pulmonary artery (ALCAPA), 733

Anonychia, 1504

Antenatal care, 351–352
  immunization information, 352
  infant feeding information, 352
  information, 351
  informed care, 352
  risk, 351
  vitamin K information, 352

Antenatal steroids
  for BPD, 593

Anterior bowed tibia, 1436f

Anterior horn cell disease, 1405

Anterior nasal stenosis, 1101

Anterior pituitary disorders, 923–924

Anterior segment
  examination of, 1470

Antiarrhythmics
  neonates, 1517–1518, 1518t, 1519t

Antibiotics
  fetal effects, 234t, 240
  for neonatal infection, 1161–1162
  for preterm delivery, 204

Antibodies, 1141–1144
  transplacental transfer, 1155t

Antibody replacement therapy, 1162–1163

Anticoagulants, 1220–1221
  adverse effects, 1220

Anticonvulsants
  causing neonatal hypocalcemia, 859
  neonates, 1521–1523

Anti-D
  fetal erythrocytes
    destruction, 1178

Antidiuretic hormone (ADH), 924–925, 991
  causes of elevated levels in newborn, 926t

Antihypertensive agents
  fetal effects, 234t, 241–243
  intravenous, 1020t
  neonates, 1523–1524
  oral, 1021t
  during pregnancy, 207

Antiinfective effects
  human milk, 418, 421t

Antimicrobial-resistant enterobacteriaceae, 1364–1366

Antimicrobial therapy
  neonates, 1524–1528
  pharmacologic basis, 1236

Antioxidant enzymes
  BPD, 583

Antioxidants
  with BPD, 581–582
  changes during gestation, 581f

Antiphospholipid antibodies, 211
  abortions with, 226
  pregnancy complications with, 211t

Antiphospholipid syndrome, 211

Antireflux, 1528–1530

Antiretroviral treatment
  HIV-1 infected infants, 1323

Antithyroid medications
  fetal effects, 238t, 250

Antitrypsin
  BPD, 582
  deficiency, 974t, 975

Antituberculosis therapy
  fetal effects, 235t, 240

Antley-Bixler syndrome, 1675

Anus
  examination, 347t

Aorta
  coarctation and interruption, 678–680, 680f
  complex coarctation and interruption, 680–681, 681f

Aortic stenosis, 681–682, 682f

Aortic thrombosis, 1221

Aortic valve stenosis, 712

Aortocaval compression
  left lateral tilt relieving, 273f

Aortopulmonary collateral arteries, 720–721, 752–753

Aortopulmonary window, 689–690, 732–733, 760

Apart syndrome, 1680

Apert acrocephalosyndactyly, 636t

Apert syndrome, 907, 908f, 1423

Apgar score, 260–261
  in infants of drug-dependent mothers, 1576
  smoking, 23

Aplasia cutis congenita, 1498, 1498f

Apnea, 539
  etiology, 540t
  with gastroesophageal reflux, 1623
  postdischarge medical care, 1625
  premature infants, 539t

Apnea of prematurity (AOP), 539–545, 540f
  diagnosis, 541
  discharge planning, 543–544
  in ELBW, 478–479
  feeding related symptoms, 543
  GER, 543
  home care, 543–544
  idiopathic ALTE, 545
  incidence, 541
  neurodevelopmental outcome, 544–545
  treatment, 541

Apparent life threatening events (ALTE)
  idiopathic, 545

Aquaphor, 455

Arachidonic acid (ARA), 384

Arginine
  for urea cycle defects, 972

Arginine vasopressin (AVP), 366, 984

Arnold-Chiari malformation, 172

Aromatase deficiency, 918

Arrhythmias, 642, 700–701
  following congenital heart surgery, 741–742

Arterial blood gas, 316f

Arterial catheters, 1221

Arterial ischemic stroke, 1221

Arterioles
  vasoconstriction, 1000

Arteriovenous malformations (AVM), 690, 1501

Arthrogryposis multiplex congenita, 1439f, 1675

Artificial airway, 607–608

Artificial nipples, 433

Artificial nutrition, 18

Ashkenazi Jews, 132

Ash leaf macules, 1497

Asphyxia
  multiple gestation, 528–529
  resuscitation, 308–316
    clinical assessment, 310
    equipment and supplies, 309–310
    initial steps, 310
    SGA, 512–513, 512t

Aspiration pneumonia, 1261, 1263
  with gastroesophageal reflux, 1623
  in infants of drug-dependent mothers, 1576

Aspirin
  breast milk, 1689
  fetal effects, 235t, 242

Asplenia syndrome, 677t, 678f

Assisted mechanical ventilation, 606, 612t
  indications for, 610
  lung volume measurements, 611
  modes, 612–613
  new forms, 611–612
  physiologic considerations, 610–611

Assisted reproductive technology (ART), 136, 524

Assisted ventilation
  airway associated problems, 618
  AOP, 543
  complications, 618
  pulmonary air leak complications, 618–619

Asthma medications, 594f

Asynchronous data transmission, 55

Ataxia-telangiectasia, 1211, 1445

Atazanavir
  pregnancy, 1320t
  teratogenic potential, 1319

Atelectasis
  with BPD, 586, 586f

Atenolol
  breast milk, 1689
  neonates, 1518t
  for supraventricular tachycardia, 705

Atopic dermatitis, 1488

Atopic disease
  industrialized countries, 1149–1150

Atracurium, 1538, 1691

Atrial fibrillation, 703–704

Atrial flutter, 703–704, 704f

Atrial natriuretic factor (ANF), 367, 984–985

Atrial premature depolarization, 701

Atrial septal defect, 731, 759

Atrioventricular block, 706–707

Atrioventricular canal defect, 732, 759–760

Atrioventricular cushion septal defect, 687g

Atrioventricular reentrant tachycardia
  following congenital heart surgery, 741

Atrophic lesions, 1498–1499

Atropine, 1691
  for arrhythmias, 1519t
  for BPD, 590

Atypical teratoid/rhabdoid tumors (AT/RT)
central nervous system, 1448–1449
Audiometric evoked response
hyperbilirubinemia, 790
Auditory brainstem response (ABR), 778
Auditory system, 118–121
deficits, 119
development, 118–119
intrauterine experience, 119–120
NICU, 120–121
Australia
NICU resources, 9
Autoimmune disorders, 209–210
Autoimmune lymphoproliferative
syndrome (ALPS), 1206t, 1207
Automatic Atrial Tachycardia (AAT), 1518
Autosomal dominant hypophosphatemic
rickets, 1036
Autosomal recessive polycystic kidney
disease (ARPCKD), 1069, 1069f
Azathioprine
with heart transplantation, 760
Aztreonam, 1526

B

Baby Doe, 10t, 12, 18
Baby Doe regulations, 10t, 15
Baby Houle, 10t
Baby Jane Doe, 10t
Baby K, 10t
Bacillus Calmette-Guerin (BCG), 1149
Back transport, 51–52
Back transport pack, 50t
Bacterial meningitis, 1251–1253
Bacterial overgrowth
with short bowel syndrome, 952
Bacterial vaginosis
preterm delivery, 205
Bacteriuria
preterm delivery, 205
and urinary tract infections, 1023–1026
Baird, Dugald, 1
Baller-Gerold syndrome, 1675
Balloon septostomy catheter, 662f
Band neutrophil, 1200f
Barbiturates, 1566, 1580–1581
Bardet-Biedl syndrome, 1682
Barlow test, 1429, 1437
Barotrauma
with BPD, 579–580
Barter syndrome, 1033
Barth syndrome, 1205–1207
Basal ganglia
status marmoratus, 1393f
Baths
for labor pain, 266
Battery, 92
Battery theory, 94
Bayley Mental Scale, 1589
Bayley Scales of Infant Development, 1585
B-cell system, 1150–1153
maturation, 1150f
Beckwith-Wiedemann syndrome, 636t,
882, 909, 909f, 1445, 1678
associated with congenital heart disease,
717t

Beds
determining appropriate number of, 65
Behavioral disorders
in cocaine exposed infants, 1585
with congenital rubella, 1281t
with infants of drug addicts, 1579–1580
Behavioral effects
with prenatal alcohol use, 1589
Benchmarking, 81–82
Benign cystic nephroma, 1082
Benign external hydrocephalus, 1412
Benign neonatal sleep myoclonus, 1386
Benzoate
bilirubin albumin binding, 779
Benzodiazepines, 1565–1566
fetal effects, 235t, 242
for pulmonary hypertension, 743
for seizures, 1522
Benzothiazides, 882
Benzyl alcohol
bilirubin albumin binding, 779
neonates, 1517
Best interests standards, 14–15
Beta adrenergic agents
pulmonary maturation, 559
Beta blockers
during pregnancy, 207
Beta glucuronidase, 797
11 beta hydroxyandrostenedione, 926
3 beta-hydroxysteroid dehydrogenase
deficiency, 929t
Beta-lactamase inhibitors, 1525
Beta-lactams, 1524–1526
Betamethasone
fetal effects, 245–246
Betamimetic agents
complications of, 204t
Bethanechol
for gastroesophageal reflux, 946
Bethanechol (UrecholineR)
for gastroesophageal reflux, 1623
Bicarbonate
for arrhythmias, 1519t
plasma, 988
Bi-directional Glenn or hemi-Fontan
operation, 750–751, 751f
Bifid uvula, 340t
Bile
composition, 958
Bile acids
fat absorption, 941–942
Bile pigment metabolism
neonate, 770f
Biliary hypoplasia, 1125
BiliBlanket phototherapy system,
835
BiliChek, 814, 815
Bilirubin
antepartum excretion of, 153f
biosynthesis of, 769f
birth weight, 795f
brain, 781–783
chemical structure of, 769f
chemistry of, 776–778
conformation of, 769
conjugation and excretion of, 771

Coombs test, 802t
decreased clearance, 806–808
decreased clearance from plasma, 773
effects on neurons, 777f
entering brain, 782f, 783
enterohepatic circulation of
inhibition of, 839
excretion, 152, 153f
formation of, 768
increased load, 799–800
increased load on liver cell, 773
interpreting level of, 816–817
intestinal transport, 772
intramolecular cyclization of, 831f
laboratory measurements of, 815–817
mean total daily, 796f
measuring production of, 819–820
meconium, 797
metabolism, 768–769
neonatal jaundice natural history,
798–799
neurotoxicity of, 776–778
noninvasive measurements of, 814
physiologic role of, 839
predischarge measurement of, 819
production of, 770
inhibition of, 838–839
properties of, 768
structure of, 768
toxicity of, 774–783
transfer into bile, 772
transport and hepatic uptake of,
770–771, 771f
umbilical cord, 798
Bilirubin albumin binding, 779–780
competing anions, 781
drugs effect on, 779, 780t
Bilirubin encephalopathy
clinical features of, 783–785
comorbidity, 789t
hemolytic disease, 828
terminology, 783
Bilirubin induced neurologic dysfunction
(BIND), 783
Bilirubin metabolism
neonate, 770–772
Bilirubin photochemistry, 831
Bilirubin toxicity
pathophysiology of, 776–779
Bioconversion
maternal medications, 230
Biophysical profile score, 181t
electronic fetal monitoring, 263
Biophysical profile score (BPS), 169
Biotin
fetal effects, 238t, 251
Birth
cardiorespiratory adjustments at, 284–299
circulatory adjustments, 639–640
pulmonary adaptation, 285–288
respiratory adaptation, 288–294
Birth defects
past, present, future, 5t
Birth fractures, 1439–1440
Birth injury
resuscitation, 325

Birth weights
    bilirubin, 795f
    coronary heart disease, 162–163
    decision making, 17
    diabetes mellitus, 163
    factors determining variance in, 502t
    gestation duration, 492f
    hypertension, 163
    impact on outcome, 461t
    neonatal jaundice, 794
Bladder
    agenesis of, 1071–1072
    anomalies of, 1071–1072
Bladder exstrophy, 1077–1079, 1077f
Bladder outlet obstruction, 177
Blame
    vs. accountability, 106
Bleeding
    following congenital heart surgery,
        745–746
Bleeding diathesis
    in ELBW, 475
Bleeding disorders, 1190–1195
Blood
    opsonic capacity, 1144
Blood brain barrier (BBB)
    bilirubin, 781–783
    factors affecting permeability,
        783
    lipid solubility, 783
    maturity effect on, 783
Blood cerebrospinal fluid barriers
    bilirubin, 781–783
Blood circulation
    fetus, 294f
Blood gas analysis
    fetal scalp, 261
    umbilical cord, 261
Blood plasma
    ion distribution, 364f
Blood pressure, 335, 346t, 1669–1670
    neonatal period, 994
        abdomen, 994–995
        chest, 994
        hydration, 994–995
        limbs, 994–995
Blood sampling
    capillary vs. venous, 816
    parenteral fluid therapy, 375
Bloodspot screening, 355
Blood transfusion, 1212–1217
    estimated risks, 1215t
Blood urea nitrogen, 997
Blooming Baby, 10t
Blueberry-muffin spots
    with congenital rubella, 1281t
Blue diaper syndrome, 864
Blue nevus, 1497
Blunt trauma, 1478
Board certified
    neonatal and perinatal specialists, 26f
Body fluids
    electrolyte content, 370t
    solute distribution, 363–364
Body surface area, 981–982
    calculated, 449t

Body temperature
    physiologic control of, 455
Body water
    changes, 363t
    distribution, 363f
Body weight
    endocrine deficiencies, 507t
    organs contribution to, 506t
Bone and joint infections, 1441–1443
Bone marrow transplantation (BMT), 195
Bone mineralization
    TPN, 397
Bone mineralization status
    newborn monitoring, 406
Boston Circulatory Arrest Study, 749
Bottle feeding, 357
Bowel injury
    ventriculoperitoneal shunt, 1414
Bowel loops
    MRI, 176f
Brachial plexus injury, 349
Bradycardia
    with gastroesophageal reflux, 1623
    postdischarge medical care, 1625
Brain
    bilirubin, 781–783
Brain death, 13, 17
    neonates, 1404–1405
Brain derived neurotrophic factor (BDNF),
        536
Brain injury
    past, present, future, 5t
Brainstem
    serotonergic receptors, 536
Brainstem auditory evoked response,
        790f
Brainstem muscarinic cholinergic
        pathways, 536
Brain tumors, 1448–1449
BranchAmine, 394
Branchial cleft anomalies
    surgery, 1099
Branchial cleft cyst, 1099f
Branchial cyst
    surgery, 1099
Branchiootoureteral syndrome, 1675
Brazelton Neonatal Behavioral Assessment
        Scale (NBAS), 261–262, 790–791,
        1578
Breast abscess, 1256
Breast cancer
    phototherapy, 826–827
    during pregnancy, 216
Breast feeding, 356–357, 413–439. See also
        Human milk
    advantages of, 416–419, 416t
    alternative methods, 433–434
    assessment of readiness for, 430
    contraindications to, 401, 438
    cross-cradle position, 432f
    decision to, 423–424
    developmental progression toward,
        429–433
    discharge planning, 435–436
    epidural analgesia, 272
    football hold, 432f

human immunodeficiency virus (HIV),
        1318
    incidence of, 414–416
    jaundice prevention and treatment, 827t
    with maternal alcohol, 1589
    maternal drugs, 32
    medications, 439
    neonatal hyperbilirubinemia, 812–813
    neonatal jaundice, 795–797, 797f
    NICU
        supporting, 436–437
    on-cue, 432
    ongoing sessions, 433–435
    pain medications, 278–279
    premature infant
        transitioning from NICU to home,
            1656
    premature infants
        latching, 431
    prevalence, 401
    space for, 70
    supplementary feedings impact on
        bilirubin, 813f
    terminology, 415, 415t
Breast massage
    human milk production, 425–426
Breast milk
    drug excretion in, 1543
    medications, 1687–1689
    NICU, 1655–1657
    preterm, 398
Breast pumps, 424–425
Breathing
    clinical disorders in control of, 539–545
    genetic influences, 536
    initiation at birth, 537–538
    normal control of, 535–539
    patterns
        with cocaine exposed infants,
            1584–1585
    preterm infants, 538
Breath sounds
    auscultation, 342
Breech presentation
    hemorrhage, 1174
    safest route of delivery, 463
Bretylium, 697t
Broad thumb hallux syndrome, 636t
Bromide, 1581
Bromocriptine
    breast feeding, 439
    breast milk, 1689
Bronchodilators, 1530
    for chronic lung disease, 477
    home care, 1626
Bronchogenic cyst, 1105
Bronchopulmonary dysplasia (BPD), 373,
        578–595, 585f, 1017, 1625–1628
    bronchodilators, 590–591
    cardiopulmonary function, 592
    cardiovascular changes, 585
    clinical assessment, 584
    corticosteroids for, 590
    CT, 584–585
    defined, 578–579, 579t
    diuretics, 589–590

Bronchopulmonary dysplasia (BPD)
  (*contd.*)
  effect on nutritional status, 392
  growth, 593
  incidence, 578–579
  infection, 592–593
  intercurrent illness, 1628
  mechanical ventilation, 588
  medications, 589, 590t
  mortality, 592
  MRI, 584–585
  neurologic development, 593
  nutrition, 589
  outcome, 591–593
  pathogenesis, 579–584, 579f
  pathologic changes, 586–587, 587f
  pathophysiologic changes, 584–587
  physical therapy, 590
  prevention, 593–595
  pulmonary changes, 585–586
  radiographic abnormalities, 584–585
  radiographic progression, 584, 584t
  rehospitalization, 1628
  treatment, 587–591
Bronze baby syndrome, 835
Brown fat, 446
Brown spots, 1496–1497
Budin, Pierre, 1
Bullous congenital ichthyosiform
    erythroderma (epidermolytic
    hyperkeratosis), 1493
Bumetanide, 1531, 1691
Bupivacaine
  electronic fetal monitoring, 262–263
Buprenorphine, 1577
Business plan
  telehealth, 62

C
Cache Valley virus, 1332t
Caffeine, 27, 1536, 1537
  adverse effects, 1575t
  for AOP, 479
  for BPD, 590–591, 590t
  fetal effects, 28, 235t, 243
  maternal exposure to, 1446
  neonatal effects, 28
  neurobehavioral effects, 28
  teratogenicity, 27–28
Cahalan Volume Variability Scale, 28
Calcipotriol
  for psoriasis, 1488
Calcitonin, 367
  calcium and magnesium control,
    851–853
  hypocalcemia, 857t
Calcium, 989
  absorption, 942
  circulating concentration, 848
  ELBW, 471
  homeostasis nonclassic control, 855–856
  hypocalcemia, 857t
  with IDM, 887f
  for osteopenia, 870
  physiologic control, 849–855
  requirements, 387

tissue distribution, 847
  TPN, 395, 397
Calcium channel blockers
  during pregnancy, 207
Calcium channel inhibitors
  complications of, 204t
Calcium chloride, 1691
  for arrhythmias, 1519t
  for hypocalcemia, 860
Calcium glubionate, 1691
Calcium gluconate, 1692
  for arrhythmias, 1519t
  for hypocalcemia, 860
Calcium-sensing receptor, 989
Calcium status
  newborn monitoring, 406
Caloric intake
  neonatal jaundice, 795
Caloric supplements, 1627t
Calories
  SGA, 500–501
Campomelic dysplasia, 1675
Campylobacter jejuni
  infectious diarrhea, 954
Canada
  NICU resources, 9
Canadian Collaborative Study, 461t
Canadian Paediatric Society
  resuscitation guidelines, 17
Canadian Task Force on the Periodic
    Health Examination, 85t
Cancer
  pathogenesis, 1444–1445
  during pregnancy, 216–217
Candida albicans, 1236, 1243
  rashes, 1486
Candida glabrata, 1243
Candida lusitaniae, 1243
Candida parapsilosis, 1243
Candida tropicalis, 1236, 1243
Cannabis, 1592
Capillary hemangiomas, 1473
Capillary hematocrit
  total erythrocyte mass, 1187–1188, 1187f,
    1188f
Capillary hemoglobin, 1187
Capillary leak
  with cardiopulmonary bypass, 735
Capillary malformation, 1500, 1500f
Captopril, 1692
  fetal effects, 239–240
  for hypertension, 1524
Captopril (Capoten), 656t
Caput succedaneum, 338, 1502
Carbamazepine
  fetal effects, 235t, 243
Carbamyl phosphate synthetase
  for urea cycle defects, 972
Carbapenems, 1525
Carbimazole
  for drug-induced neonatal goiter, 934
Carbohydrate
  absorption, 940–941
Carbohydrate homeostasis, 876–888
Carbohydrate metabolism disorders,
    966t

Carbohydrates
  digestion, 382
  human milk, 418
  in infant formula, 402
  in preterm discharge formulas, 405
  sources, 383–384
Carbon dioxide
  fetal breathing, 289
Cardiac anatomy, 641
Cardiac arrest
  following congenital heart surgery, 746
Cardiac contractility
  following congenital heart surgery, 740
Cardiac disease, 633–707
  acute lung disease, 649–650
  age of presentation, 645
  chest radiography, 650
  clinical features, 643–650, 647f
  diagnosis, 634t, 635t, 649t, 650–653
  diagnostic catheterization and
    angiography, 653–654
  echocardiography, 652–653, 653f, 654f
  electrocardiography, 650–652, 651f,
    651t
  etiology, 634–638
  incidence, 633
  infant mortality, 633
  long-term survival, 633–634
  magnetic resonance imaging, 653
  management, 654–659
  noncardiac anomalies, 638t, 650
  physical examination, 645–646
  respiratory symptoms, 645–646
  systemic perfusion and pressure, 646
Cardiac examination, 346t
Cardiac fibroma, 700
Cardiac function, 641–642
Cardiac malposition, 677–678
Cardiac massage
  EKG, 312f
Cardiac output
  following congenital heart surgery,
    739–740, 739f
Cardiac physiology, 641
Cardiac rhabdomyoma, 700
Cardiac stun
  ECMO, 629–630
Cardiac surgery
  during pregnancy, 215
Cardiac tumors, 700
Cardiomyopathy, 691–692
  with IDM, 887f
Cardiopulmonary bypass
  adverse effects, 735
Cardiopulmonary disease
  ECMO, 624
Cardiotocogram (CTG), 262
Cardiovascular system
  examination, 344–345
Care au lait macules (CALMS), 1496
Care of family, 3
Care practices team, 65–66
Carnitine, 384–385
Carpenter acrocephalopolsndactyly type 2,
    636t
Carpenter syndrome, 1675

Car safety, 360
Cartilage-hair hypoplasia, 1206t, 1207
Casein hydrolysate formula, 402
Case manager
    NICU, 76
Cataracts, 1474–1475
    with congenital rubella, 1281t
    with inborn errors of metabolism, 977t
Catch 22, 1158t
Catechins
    maternal exposure to, 1446
Catecholamines
    changes after birth, 878f
Cat eye syndrome, 637t, 1678
Catheter related bloodstream infections
    (CRBSI), 1371–1372
Catheter-related infections
    with short bowel syndrome, 953
Catheters
    care of, 1371–1372
Cat's eye reflex, 1448
Caudal dysplasia sequence, 1678
Cause effect diagram, 86
CAVH, 1004
CDH
    ventilation, 618f
CD40 ligand (CD40L), 1151
CD40 receptor (CD40-R), 1150
Cefaclor (Ceclor)
    fetal effects, 240
Cefazolin, 1692
Cefixime (Suprax)
    fetal effects, 240
Cefotaxime, 1524, 1525, 1692
    for meningitis, 1253
    for osteomyelitis, 1255
    for sepsis neonatorum, 1245
Ceftazidime, 1524, 1525, 1692
Ceftriaxone, 1524, 1692
    fetal effects, 234t, 241
    for neonatal ophthalmia, 1259
Cefuroxime, 1692
Cell-mediated immune system
    evaluation of, 26161
Cell-mediated immunity (CMI), 1144,
        1156–1157
    neonates
        diagnostic tests, 1160t
Cellular immunodeficiency with abnormal
        immunoglobulins, 1158t
Centers for Disease Control (CDC)
    sample central line data collection
            record, 1372t
    sample CVC daily indication, 1373t
Central airways
    following congenital heart surgery, 747
Central diabetes insipidus
    etiology, 925t
Centrally placed catheters
    thrombosis, 395
Central nervous system
    congenital tumors, 1423
    injury
        fluids and electrolytes, 374
    resuscitation, 316
Central vein thrombosis, 1130

Central venous catheters, 1130, 1221
    infection, 1371–1372
Cephalexin (Keflex)
    fetal effects, 240
Cephalhematoma, 338, 1422, 1502
Cephalic index, 168
Cephalosporins, 1524, 1525
    fetal effects, 240
Cerebral palsy, 1637–1638
Cerebral venous thrombosis, 1221
Cerebrospinal fluid
    newborns, 1252t
Cerebrospinal fluid accumulation,
        1411–1412
Cerebrovascular anomalies, 1424
Cervical cancer
    during pregnancy, 216
Cervical cutaneous tabs
    surgery, 1099
Cervical cyst, 1502f
Cervical fistulas
    surgery, 1099
Cervical incompetence
    abortions with, 226
Cervix
    examination of, 205
Cesarean section
    anesthetic techniques for, 275–278
Cesarean section rate, 463t
Chagas' disease, 1332t
CHARGE association, 637t, 1679
Charge nurse
    NICU, 77
Chediak-Higashi syndrome, 1206t, 1207
Chemical senses, 116–118
    disorders, 117
    intrauterine experience, 117–118
    NICU, 118
Cherry red spot
    with inborn errors of metabolism, 977t
Chest
    auscultation, 344
    examination, 341–344
    palpation, 344
    retractions, 341
    size of, 341–342
    symmetry of, 341–342
Chest compressions
    resuscitation, 311–312
Child abuse, 1479
    with drug addicts, 1579
Child Abuse Protection Act, 10t
Child neglect
    with infants of drug addicts, 1579
Children
    perinatal acquired immunodeficiency
            syndrome (AIDS), 1316
CHILD syndrome, 1675
Chlamydia trachomatis, 1236, 1476
    lower respiratory tract, 1261
    with pneumonia, 570
    preterm delivery, 205
Chloral hydrate, 1566–1567, 1581, 1692
    hyperbilirubinemia with, 797, 809
Chloramphenicol, 1692
    breast milk, 1689

    glucuronidation, 1510
Chlordiazepoxide (Librium), 1581
    fetal effects, 235t, 242
Chlorhexidine, 1371, 1372
Chloride
    maintenance requirements of, 369–370
    requirements, 387
    TPN, 395
Chlorothiazide (Diuril), 656t, 1692
Chlorpromazine
    for nonnarcotic withdrawal, 32
Chlorpropamide, 882
Chlorthiazide
    for BPD, 590t
Choanal atresia, 1101
Cholecystokinin (CCK), 943–944
    fat absorption, 941
Choledochal cysts, 1125
Cholelithiasis, 1125–1126
    with short bowel syndrome, 953
Cholestasis, 396
    etiology, 959–960
    evaluation, 959t
Cholestasis syndrome, 1030
Cholestatic liver disease, 958
Cholesterol-ester storage disease
    with liver disease, 960
Cholestyramine, 1693
Chondrodysplasia punctata
    rhizomelic type, 906–907, 908f
Chorion
    fetus, 157
Chorionic gonadotropins
    multiple gestations, 524
Chorionic villus sampling, 138–139, 139f
    vs. early amniocentesis, 140–141
    technical aspects, 139–140
Chorionic villus sampling (CVS), 192
Chorioretinitis, 1330f
    cytomegalovirus, 1293
Chromium
    recommended intake for preterm infants,
            400t
Chromosomal anomalies, 900, 905t
    abortions with, 226t
    decision making, 17–18
    with maternal drugs, 224
Chromosomal mosaicism, 138
Chromosomal sex disorders, 916
Chromosomal syndrome
    cardiac disease, 634–638
Chronic bilirubin encephalopathy. *See*
        Kernicterus
Chronic congenital infection
    infants born with, 1275t
Chronic granulomatous disease (CGD),
        1139, 1158t
Chronic idiopathic intestinal
        pseudoobstruction syndrome, 957
Chronic lung disease (CLD)
    CPAP for, 605–606
    in ELBW, 475–477
    postdischarge medical care, 1625–1626
Chronic mucocutaneous candidiasis, 1158t
Chronic perinatal infection
    infants born with, 1275t

Chronic postkernicteric bilirubin
  encephalopathy
  clinical features of, 785t
Chronic pulmonary hypertension, 699–700
Chronic renal disease
  with intrapartum asphyxia, 308t
Chronic renal failure, 1013
Chylothorax, 395
Cidofovir
  cytomegalovirus, 1292
  for herpes simplex virus, 1286
Cigarette smoking, 36
  SIDS, 548
Cimetidine, 1528–1529, 1532–1533, 1693
  for gastroesophageal reflux, 946
Ciprofloxacin
  fetal effects, 241
Circulation
  placenta, 299
  transition from fetal to neonatal, 295f
Circulatory adaptation, 294–299, 305
Circulatory status
  monitoring, 319–321
Circumcision, 1088, 1089f, 1090f
Cisapride (PropulsidR), 1693
  for gastroesophageal reflux, 1623
Citrobacter koseri, 1254f
Citrulline
  for urea cycle defects, 972
CKD
  infancy management, 1013–1015
  infant dialysis, 1015
  infants, 1014t
Clarithromycin (Biaxin)
  fetal effects, 240–241
Classification, 327–349
Clavicle
  fractures, 1440
  partial absence of, 1433f
Clavicles
  examination, 342
  physical examination, 1428
Clavulanate, 1525
Clavulanic acid (timentin), 1699
Clear cell sarcoma
  kidney, 1452
Cleft lip, 1098f
  surgery, 1098
Cleft palate
  surgery, 1098
Clemastine
  breast milk, 1689
Click
  examination, 346t
Clicky hip, 358
Clindamycin, 1693
  for toxoplasmosis, 1331
Clinical dietitians
  NICU, 77
Clinical nurse specialist
  NICU, 76, 77
Clinicians
  decision making, 16
Cloaca
  abnormalities of, 1092, 1092f
  exstrophy of, 1078, 1078f

Clofazimine
  breast milk, 1689
Clomiphene citrate (Clomid,
  Serophene)
  multiple gestations, 523–524
Clonidine, 1567
  fetal effects, 234t, 241–242
Clostridium difficile
  diarrhea, 1260
  infectious diarrhea, 954
Clothing, 114
Clotrimazole
  for diaper dermatitis, 1487
Cloudy cornea
  with congenital rubella, 1281t
Cloverleaf deformity, 1423
Club drugs, 27
Clubfoot, 1436f
Clusters of differentiation (*Clostridium
  difficile*), 1146t
Coagulase-negative staphylococci (CONS),
  1359–1360
Coagulation tests
  reference values, 1707
    newborn, 1191t
    premature infants, 1192t
Coarctation of the aorta, 712
Coast disease, 1483
Cocaine, 1479f, 1582
  adverse effects, 1574t
  breast feeding, 439
  breast milk, 1687
  epidemiology, 1572, 1573t
  fetal effects, 235t, 243–244
  infant exposure, 1586
  neonatal effects, 1583–1585,
    1584t
    long-term outcome, 1585–1586
  obstetric effects, 1583
  pharmacology, 1582
  placental transfer, 1583–1585
  pregnancy, 1582–1583
Cocaine abuse, 1479
Cochrane Group, 1016
Codeine
  dosage, 1563t
  history, 1573t
Coffin-Sirs fifth digit syndrome, 636t
COFS syndrome, 1676
Cognition
  human milk, 422
Cognitive effects
  with prenatal alcohol use, 1589
Cohen syndrome, 1676
Cold
  newborn, 358
Colipase
  fat absorption, 941
Collaborative Perinatal Project (CPP),
  786
Collagenase
  BPD, 582
Collecting system
  bilateral duplication of, 1072f
Collodion baby, 1489, 1489f
Coloboma, 1472, 1472f

Colon
  anatomic lesions, 956
  congenital anomalies, 956
  motility disorders, 956–957
Colonic duplication, 956
Colonic stenosis, 956
Color
  examination, 334, 346t
Colorado Air National Guard, 40
Colorado Collective for Medical Decisions
  resuscitation guidelines, 17
Colorectal cancer
  during pregnancy, 216
Colostomy, 1115
Colostrum oral care, 429
Comfort care, 18
Commission on Accreditation of Medical
  Transport Systems (CAMTS), 48
Commissural lip pits, 340t
Common variable immunodeficiency,
  1206t
Communication
  with consultants, 109
  within health care team, 108–109
  neonatal transport, 43
  with parents and guardians, 107–108
Communication systems, 71
Community health centers, 33
Comparative databases, 81–82
Complement system, 1140
Complete AIS (CAIS), 918
Complete DiGeorge anomaly, 1147
Complete gonadal dysgenesis, 917
Complete heart block
  following congenital heart surgery, 742
Compliance program, 102
Compromised fetus
  intrauterine resuscitation of, 274
Computer based patient records, 97
Conception stimulants
  multiple gestations, 523
Conductive heat loss
  warming mattresses, 450
Congenital acute monocytic leukemia, 1450f
Congenital adrenal hyperplasia, 192–193,
  927
  clinical findings, 929t
  with hypoglycemia, 883
  prenatal diagnosis and treatment, 930
Congenital adrenal hyperplasia (CAH), 917
Congenital aganglionic megacolon, 956
Congenital amegakaryocytic
  thrombocytopenia, 1212
Congenital anomalies, 892–911
  adjunctive investigations, 896
  cardiac disease, 636t–637t
  chromosomal analysis, 896–897
  classification, 892–894
  common to Trisomy 13 and Trisomy 18,
    903t
  data, 897–898
  defined, 892–894
  etiology, 893t
  examples, 899–910
  family history, 894–895
  history, 894

integrated treatment, 896f
metabolic studies, 897
multiple gestation, 529–530
physical examination, 895–896
terminology, 893t
treatment, 894–898
Congenital asplenia, 1158t
Congenital Bochdalek hernia, 1105–1107
Congenital constriction band syndrome, 1432
Congenital cystic adenomatoid malformation (CCAM), 189–190
Congenital diagnosis, 1106f
Congenital diaphragmatic hernia surgery, 1105–1107
Congenital diaphragmatic hernia (CDH), 173–174, 174f, 622
Congenital duodenal obstruction, 1118f
Congenital dwarfism, 332
Congenital dyserythropoietic anemia, 1186
Congenital erythropoietic porphyria contraindicating phototherapy effects on, 834
Congenital eyelid ptosis, 1472–1473
Congenital heart block, 210
Congenital heart disease, 174–175
chest radiography, 713
Doppler, 175
echocardiogram, 175
electrocardiogram, 713
initial evaluation and stabilization, 713–714
risk factors warranting fetal echocardiography, 711–712, 711t
teratogens, 638t
Congenital heart surgery
early postoperative physiology and management, 749–751
gastrointestinal complications, 748
infectious complications, 748
mechanical cardiac support, 746–747
neurologic complications, 748–749
postoperative complications, 739–749
pulmonary complications, 747–748
renal insufficiency, 748
Congenital hemorrhagic disorders neonates, 1194–1195
Congenital hypopituitarism with hypoglycemia, 883
Congenital hypothyroidism, 932
incidence, 936t
Congenital hypotonia, 1436
Congenital infections, 359–360, 1040
Congenital ingrown toenail, 1504, 1504f
Congenital leukemia, 1449–1450
infants, 1207–1208
Congenital lipoid hyperplasia, 929–930, 929t
Congenital lobar emphysema, 1104
Congenital malformations, 226–228
decision making, 17–18
etiology, 226t
Congenital melanocytic nevi, 1496–1497
Congenital microgastria, 948
Congenital midline nasal masses, 1101–1102

Congenital nephrotic syndrome, 1038–1043, 1680
differential diagnosis, 1039
Congenital nevus, 1496f
Congenital rubella, 1280–1283
clinical manifestations, 1280, 1281t–1282t
diagnosis, 1280–1281
treatment, 1282–1283
Congenital rubella syndrome
CDC classification, 1282t
Congenital sideroblastic anemia, 1186
Congenital syphilis, 1248
Congenital thyrotoxicosis, 937
Congenital toxoplasmosis, 1329, 1330f
clinical manifestations, 1329–1330
diagnosis, 1330–1331
epidemiology, 1329
prognosis, 1332–1333
Congenital tumors, 1423f
Congenital urinary tract malformations, 1008
Congenital varicella syndrome, 1297–1298
Congenital vascular anomalies, 1016
Congestive heart failure
acyanotic neonates, 679t
effect on nutritional status, 392
treatment, 656t–657t
Conjugated bilirubin, 816
elevated, 817, 828
Connective tissue disorders, 1491–1492
Conotruncal anomaly face syndrome, 905–906
Constrained parental autonomy, 16
Consultants
communication with, 109
Consultation, 109t
Consulting neonatologist
neonatal transport, 41
Consumptive hypothyroidism
secondary to giant hemangioma, 936–937
Continuing education, 93
telehealth, 61
Continuous breathing
establishment at birth, 290–292
Continuous labor support, 266
Continuous positive airway pressure (CPAP), 605
AOP, 542–543, 542f
indications for, 605–606
RDS, 561
Continuous quality improvement (CQI), 80–83
measurement, 81
Contraction stress test (CST), 180
Contracts, 92
Convection warmed incubators, 448–451
evaporation, 449
incubator humidification, 450
partitional calorimetry, 448f
radiant heat loss, 450
servocontrolled incubator homeothermy, 451
skin surface servocontrol temperature, 451

Conventional ventilation, 612–613
Coombs test
bilirubin, 802t
Copper
absorption, 942
recommended intake for preterm infants, 400t
Cord blood mononuclear cells (CBPM), 1148
Cordocentesis, 143–145
indications for, 143t
parental counseling, 144
Cornea
cloudy, 1483–1484
diameter, 1470f
examination, 1484, 1484f
opacified, 1471f
opacity, 1473
Corneal clouding
with inborn errors of metabolism, 977t
Cornelia de Lange syndrome, 909–910, 909f, 1503–1504
Coronary heart disease
birth weights, 162–163
Cor pulmonale, 699–700
with BPD, 585
Corpus luteum deficiency
abortions with, 226t
Cortical necrosis
medullary necrosis, 1010
Corticomedullary gradient, 991
Corticosteroids
for diaper dermatitis, 1487
with heart transplantation, 760
for low cardiac output, 741
for preterm delivery, 203–204
for toxoplasmosis, 1331
Cortisol, 926
Cortisone
for adrenal insufficiency, 930
Cosmids, 135
Costs
acute medical care post discharge, 30
discharge diagnoses, 29t
VLBW, 29t
Coumarin
fetal effects, 236t, 244
Couney, Martin, 40
Coupling defect, 934
CPAP
for BPD, 588
complications, 606
effectiveness, 606
Crack cocaine, 1582
Cranial nerves
assessment, 349t
Cranial sutures, 337f
Cranial synostosis, 1424f
Craniofacial anomalies, 1423–1424
Craniosynostosis (CS), 332, 337–338, 337f
C-reactive protein (CRP), 1244
Creatine
postnatal evolution, 996f

Cribs, 115
Cri-du-Chat syndrome, 637t, 904, 904f
  associated with congenital heart disease,
    717t
Crigler-Najjar syndrome, 784f, 806–808,
    807t, 975
  phototherapy, 836
  phototherapy complications with, 835
Critical aortic valve stenosis, 722, 753
Critical coarctation of aorta, 722–723
Critical complications, 723f, 753–754
Critical congenital heart block, 718
Critical congenital heart disease
  cardiomyopathy, 733
  cardiopulmonary bypass, 734–735
  cardiopulmonary management, 716–717
  congenital heart centers, 715–716
  genetic syndrome associated with, 717t
  heart transplantation, 733–734, 734t
  left ventricular outflow tract obstruction,
    722–727
  mixing lesions, 727–731
  nutrition, 718
  postoperative care, 734–738
  prematurity, 717–718
  preoperative care, 711–712, 716–718
  preoperative physiology and
    management, 718–721
  presentation of, 712–713
  surgery
    arterial access, 736–737
    central venous access, 736
    chest tubes, 737
    ICU stabilization following, 735–737
    invasive hemodynamic monitoring, 736
    physical examination, 737
    pulmonary artery lines, 736
    temperature, 737
  transitional circulation, 712
Critical pulmonary valve stenosis, 718,
    719f, 751–752
Cromolyn, 1693
Crouzon syndrome, 1423
Crown heel length, 332
Crown rump length, 332
Cry analysis
  hyperbilirubinemia, 790
Cryoprecipitates
  transfusion, 1217
Cryotherapy
  for ROP, 1482
Cryptorchidism, 359, 919, 1084
Cuba
  infant mortality, 24
Cultural diversity, 11–14
Cup feeding, 434, 434f
Cutaneous infection, 1255–1256
Cutis marmorata telangiectatica congenita,
    1499, 1499f
Cyanocobalamin
  fetal effects, 238t
Cyanosis, 649, 666f
  cardiac anatomy, 663f, 666f
  following congenital heart surgery, 745
Cyanotic heart disease
  differential diagnosis, 658t

Cyanotic lesions, 659–678
  clinical findings, 660–661, 663
  differential diagnosis, 661, 663–664
  pathophysiology, 662–663
  treatment, 661–662, 664–665
Cyanotic neonates
  cardiac examination
    differential diagnosis, 644f
  chest radiographs
    differential diagnosis, 646f
  diagnosis, 648f
Cyclic neutropenia, 1205
Cyclooxygenase, 984
  prenatal administration, 1008
Cyclophosphamide
  breast milk, 1687
  fetal effects, 236t, 244–245
Cyclosporine
  breast milk, 1687
  with heart transplantation, 760
Cyclosporine A
  during pregnancy, 215
Cystic adenomatoid malformation (CAM),
    173, 1104–1105
  MRI, 173f
Cystic fibrosis, 132, 957–958
  with liver disease, 960
Cystic hamartoma of lung and kidney,
    1680
Cystic hygroma, 341, 1100f
  surgery, 1099–1100
Cystic kidney disease
  classification, 1685–1686
Cystic kidneys, 1083
Cystic lymphangioma, 341
Cystic renal disease, 177–178
Cystinuria, 1037
Cystourethrogram, 998–999
Cysts, 1501–1502
Cytochromes P450, 1509
  enzymes
    developmental patterns, 1509t
    ontogeny, 1509–1510
Cytokines, 1136, 1141, 1142t–1143t, 1147f
Cytomegalovirus (CMV) infection, 213t,
    571, 1291–1292, 1368, 1478
  breast feeding, 438
  CMI, 1156
  congenital infection, 1292–1294
  with granulocyte transfusion, 1216
  intrafamilial transmission, 1292
  maternal infection, 1291–1292
  perinatal infection, 1295–1296
    prevention, 1295–1296
  PMN transfusion, 1164
  with pneumonia, 570
  prevention, 1217
Cytopenia
  related to metabolic disorders, 1212
Cytotoxic chemotherapy
  during pregnancy, 217

D

Dacryocystoceles, 340
Damus-Kaye-Stansel procedure, 749, 750
Dandy-Walker malformations, 244, 1680

Dane particle, 1306
Danville Twins, 10t
Dapsone, 1322
Data acquisition, 81
Dax-1, 915
DDAVP
  ADH, 991
Deaf-mutism
  with endemic goitrous hypothyroidism,
    933
Deal syndrome, 1676
Death by neurological criteria, 13
Debilitating maternal disease
  abortions with, 226
Decision making, 9–11, 12–16
  standards for, 14–15
Deep hypothermic circulatory arrest
    (DHCA), 749
Defensive medicine, 90
Dehalogenase defect, 934
Dehydration
  with gastroesophageal reflux, 1623
Dehydroepiandrosterone (DHEA), 926
De Lange syndrome, 636t
Delavirdine
  pregnancy, 1320t
  teratogenic potential, 1319
Delayed hypersensitivity, 1150
Delayed pushing
  fetal and neonatal effects, 271
DeLee, Joseph, 40
DeLee suctioning
  MAS, 564
Deletion syndrome, 905–906
Delivery room, 304–325
Delivery suite
  thermal balance, 445–446
Dental dysplasia
  kernicterus, 785
Denys-Drash syndrome, 1039
Depigmentation, 1498
Depigmentosus, 1498
Dermal melanocytosis (Mongolian spot),
    1497, 1497f
Dermatologic conditions, 1485–1504
Dermoid cyst, 1418f, 1501, 1501f
Dermoid tumors
  cornea, 1473
Desflurane, 1559, 1559t
  fetal and neonatal effects, 276
Design team, 66
Desmoplastic infantile gangliogliomas,
    1448
Desmopressin
  for DI, 925
Developmental growth disturbances,
    1444–1445
Developmental outcomes, 1632–1648
Developmental stages
  maternal medications, 228–229
Developmental toxicants
  evaluating misconceptions, 232–233
  factors influencing susceptibility to,
    228t
Deviated nasal septum, 1101
Dewey, John, 9

Dexamethasone, 1540–1541, 1693
  for BPD, 590, 590t
  for CPB adverse effects, 735
  fetal effects, 245–246
Dextrose
  TPN, 394
DHA
  in preterm human milk, 403
Diabetes
  plasma glucose changes, 877f
Diabetes insipidus, 925
  treatment, 925
Diabetes mellitus
  birth weights, 163
  with intrapartum asphyxia, 308t
  maternal medications, 230–231
  placenta, 159–160
  during pregnancy, 207–209
Diabetic mothers
  hypertrophic cardiomyopathy, 698, 699f
Dialysis
  during pregnancy, 215
Diamond-Blackfan syndrome, 1185
Diaper dermatitis, 1486–1487
  differential diagnosis, 1487
  treatment, 1487
Diaphragm
  eventration of, 1107
Diaphyseal fractures, 1440
Diarrhea, 1259–1261
  with acquired immunodeficiency
      syndrome (AIDS), 954
  clinical manifestations, 1260
  epidemiologic control, 1260
  etiology, 1259–1260
  fluids and electrolytes, 374–375
  hormonal changes in, 954
  pathogenesis, 1259–1260
  phototherapy, 836
  treatment, 1260–1261
Diastrophic dwarfism, 1439
Diazepam (Valium), 1565, 1581, 1693
  fetal effects, 235t, 242
  for seizures, 1522
Diazoxide, 1693
Didanosine, 1319
  pregnancy, 1320t
Diet
  neonatal jaundice, 795
Dietary protein
  and urea cycle defects, 972
Diethylstilbestrol (DES)
  fetal effects, 236t, 245
  maternal exposure to, 1446
Differential cyanosis, 713
Diffuse hypopigmentation, 1498
Diffuse mesangial sclerosis, 1039
Diffuse nephroblastomatosis, 1451
Diffusion
  placenta, 150–152, 151t
DiGeorge syndrome, 141, 636t, 905–906,
      1146, 1211
  associated with congenital heart disease,
      717t
  cardiac disease, 634–635

Digital echocardiography, 59
Digital fibroma, 1456
Digital subscriber lines (DSL), 56
Digitorenocerebral syndrome, 1676
Digoxin (Lanoxin), 656t, 696t,
      1535–1536, 1693
  fetal effects, 236t, 245
  neonates, 1518t
  for supraventricular tachycardia, 705
Dihydrotestosterone (DHT), 915
Diiodotyrosine (DIT), 931
Dilantin
  maternal exposure to, 1446
Dilated bladder, 187f
Dilated cardiomyopathy, 692–694, 692t
Dinitrochlorobenzene
  contact sensitization, 1160
Dipalmitoylphosphatidylcholine (DPPC),
      558f
Diphenylhydantoin
  fetal effects, 236t, 245
Diphosphoglycerate, 1190
Diphtheria immunization, 1620
Direct current defibrillation
  for arrhythmias, 1519t
Direct fluorescent antibody (DFA)
  for herpes simplex virus, 1285
Direct reacting bilirubin
  elevated, 828
Discharge diagnoses
  cost, 29t
  length of stay, 29t
Discharge planning, 1628–1629
  AOP, 543–544
  tests preparing for, 1629t
Discharge teaching
  NICU, 79
Disopyramide, 696t
Dispatch center
  vehicle operator
      communication during neonatal
          transport, 43–44
Disseminated intravascular coagulation
      (DIC), 1193–1194
Distal humeral epiphysis, 1440
Distal renal tubular acidosis, 1035
Diuretics, 1021–1023, 1530–1532
  home care, 1626
  during pregnancy, 207
Dizygotic twins, 523
DNA
  alphoid, 131
Dobutamine, 657t, 1535, 1694
  for low cardiac output, 739–740
Docosahexaenoic acid (DHA), 384
  human milk, 422–423
Documentation
  neonatal transport, 47
Domperidone, 426, 1655
Donor human milk, 426–427
Dopamine, 657t, 1004, 1533, 1535, 1582,
      1694
  for low cardiac output, 739–740
  with resuscitation, 314
Dopamine inhibitors, 426
Dopamine receptors, 984

Doppler echocardiography, 652
Doppler velocity rations
  umbilical artery, 169
Double aortic arch, 691, 691f
Double-outlet right ventricle, 676–677
Double walled incubators, 450–451
Down syndrome, 1450
  atrioventricular canal, 686f
  cardiac disease, 635
  decision making, 18
  integrated test, 136
  major anomalies with, 901t
  and maternal age, 902t
  minor anomalies with, 901t
Doxapram, 1540, 1694
  AOP, 543
Doxorubicin
  breast milk, 1687
Doxycycline
  fetal effects, 241
D-penicillamine
  fetal effects, 237t, 247
Drash syndrome, 1682
Drug(s)
  adsorption, 1507–1508
  apparent volume of distribution
      neonates, 1513
  biotransformation
      neonates, 1511
  clinical toxicology
      neonates, 1516–1517
  conjugation reactions, 1510, 1510t
  distribution
      neonates, 1508
  exchange transfusion
      neonates, 1516
  excretion
      neonates, 1511
  first-order kinetics
      neonates, 1511
  first-order multicompartment
      kinetics
      neonates, 1512–1513
  first-order single-compartment
      kinetics
      neonates, 1512
  half-life
      neonates, 1511–1512
  intravenous administration
      neonates, 1516
  loading dose
      neonates, 1516
  metabolism
      neonates, 1508
  newborn resuscitation, 1519t
  pharmacokinetic example
      neonate, 1514
  pharmacokinetics
      neonates, 1511–1516
  phase II reactions, 1510
  rates and distribution
      neonates, 1511–1512
  repetitive dosing and accumulation
      neonates, 1515–1516
  steady state
      neonates, 1515–1516

Drug(s) (*contd.*)
  synthetic reactions, 1510
  use
    laboratory tests, 29–30
  zero-order kinetics
    neonates, 1513, 1513t
Drug-addicted women
  as infant caregivers, 32
  potential child abuse, 33
  social service referral, 32–33
Drug-induced female
    pseudohermaphroditism,
    917–918
Drug-induced neonatal goiter, 934
Drying
  thermal balance, 447
D-transposition of the great arteries
    (d-TGA), 659, 660f, 710, 712–714,
    727–728
Ductus arteriosus
  oxygenated blood, 639
Ductus venosus
  oxygenated blood, 639
Due care, 90
Duff & Campbell, 10t
Duodenal atresia, 175, 1117–1118
Duodenal stenosis, 1117–1118
Duodenum
  congenital anomalies, 948–949
Duplications, 1120
Duty to act, 90–91
Dyskeratosis congenita, 1206t, 1212
Dysmorphic syndromes, 976
Dysmorphism, 993
Dysopyramide
  neonates, 1518t

E
Ear cartilage
  assessment of, 331
Early amniocentesis, 140
  vs. chorionic villus sampling, 140–141
Early death syndrome, 1030
Early discharge
  jaundice, 810–811
Early Neonatal Neurobehavioral Scale
    (ENNS), 261–262
Early prenatal care, 25f
  expenditures, 31
Early response cytokines
  BPD, 582
Ears
  examination, 339
Ebstein's anomaly of tricuspid valve,
    670–671, 670f, 721, 722f, 753
EBV
  PMN transfusion, 1164
ECMO
  following congenital heart surgery,
    746–747
  with HFOV, 617
  for PPHN, 569
Economics and evaluation
  telehealth, 57–58
Economic success, 8
Ectodermal dysplasia, 1490

Ectopia lentis
  with inborn errors of metabolism, 977t
Ectopic atrial tachycardia, 703
  following congenital heart surgery,
    741–742
Ectopic ureter, 1073f
  development of, 1072f
  orifices, 1073f
Ectopic ureterocele, 1074f
Eczema herpeticum, 1496f
Edema, 1502
  examination, 347t
Edrophonium, 1694
EEC syndrome, 1676
EEV
  ventilation model, 614f
Efavirenz
  pregnancy, 1320t
  teratogenic potential, 1319
Effective renal plasma flow (ERPF), 982f
Ehlers-Danlos syndrome, 1436, 1680
18q-syndrome, 1677
Elastase
  BPD, 582
Elastase inhibitors, 4
Elbow
  physical examination, 1428
  synostosis, 1433–1434
Electrolyte deficits, 368
Electrolytes
  body fluids, 370t
Electrolyte status
  newborn monitoring, 406
Electrolyte therapy, 367–372
Electronic fetal monitoring
  biophysical profile score, 263
  fetal Doppler, 264
  fetal pulse oximetry, 263
  maternal analgesia, 262–263
  static charge sensitive bed, 264
Elejalde syndrome, 1680
Elemental formula, 402
11alpha-hydroxylase deficiency, 929t
11beta hydroxyandrostenedione, 926
ELISA
  for herpes simplex virus, 1285
Ellis van Creveld disease, 636t, 1439, 1680
Embden-Meyerhof pathway disorders, 805
Embolism, 1217–1222
Embryonal carcinoma, 1452–1453
EMLA, 1561
Emollients, 455
Employee Retirement Income Security Act
    of 1974 (ERISA), 100
Emtricitabine
  pregnancy, 1320t
Enalapril, 1694
Enalaprilat, 1694
Encephalocele, 172, 1419f, 1421f
  surgery, 1422
Encephaloceles, 1420–1422
Encephalopathy, 17
Endemic goitrous hypothyroidism, 933
End-expiratory volume (EEV)
  assisted mechanical ventilation, 610
Endocardial cushion defects, 685–687

Endocrine regulation
  fetus, 878–879
Endocrinopathy
  maternal medications, 230–231
Endodermal sinus tumors, 1453–1454
Endothelin 1 (ET 1), 296
Endothelium-derived relaxing factor
    (EDRF), 1539
Endotracheal intubation, 608–609
  laryngoscopy, 609f
  positioning, 609
  resuscitation, 312–313
  route, 608
  technique, 608–609
Endotracheal tube
  assisted ventilation via, 613t
  care of, 609–610
Energy
  human milk, 418
  metabolism
    disorders, 1031
    SGA, 514
  requirements, 383
  sources, 383–385
  tissue components, 502t
Enflurane, 1559t
  fetal and neonatal effects, 276
Enfurvirtide
  pregnancy, 1321t
  teratogenic potential, 1319
Enteral drug treatment
  neonates, 1507–1508
Enteral nutrition, 398–399
  in ELBW, 470–471
  for short bowel syndrome, 951–952
Enteric neuropeptides, 943–944
Enterobacter
  with pneumonia, 570
Enterobacter sakazakii, 1361
Enteroglucagon, 944
  with diarrhea, 954
Enterohepatic circulation, 797
Enterokinase
  protein absorption, 942
Enteromammary circulation, 1153
Enteromammary immune system, 420f
Enterostomal therapist
  with short bowel syndrome, 951
Environment
  immune system, 1135–1136, 1136t
Environmental agents
  threshold dose-response relationships,
    230t
Environmental factors
  neonatal transport, 44, 44t
Environmental risk factors
  SIDS, 546–548, 546t
Environmental temperature
  IWL, 365
Environmental teratogens
  abortions with, 226
Enzyme-linked virus-inducible systems
    (ELVIS) tests
  for herpes simplex virus, 1285
Eosinophilic granuloma, 1457
Eosinophilic pustular folliculitis, 1492

Eosinophils
    premature infants, 1211f
EPICure study, 482
Epidemiological risk factors
    SIDS, 547t
Epidermal barrier protection, 454–455
Epidermal growth factor (EGF)
    human milk, 418
    pulmonary maturation, 559
Epidermal nevi, 1497
Epidermal nevus syndrome, 1497f
Epidermis
    function, 1485
Epidermolysis bullosa, 1493–1494, 1494f
Epidural analgesia
    breast feeding, 272
    fetal and neonatal effects, 277
    instrumental vaginal delivery, 271
Epidural anesthesia, 1560–1561
Epiglottis
    newborn, 1100
Epilepsy
    maternal medications, 230–231
Epinephrine, 657t, 1694
    for arrhythmias, 1519t
    for hypoglycemia, 884
    with resuscitation, 313–314
Epiphyseal injuries, 1440
Epipodophyllotoxins
    maternal exposure to, 1446
Epispadias, 1086–1087, 1087f
Epoetin, 1695
Epstein-Barr virus, 1300
Epstein pearls, 341
Epulis, 340t
Equipment
    neonatal transport, 46
    with respiratory problems, 619
Erb-Duchenne, 1441, 1442f
Ergotamine
    breast feeding, 439
    breast milk, 1689
Erosive dermatitis, 1487f
Erythema toxicum neonatorum, 1492,
        1492f
Erythroblastosis
    placenta, 160
Erythroblastosis fetalis, 882
    MRI, 786f
Erythrocyte membrane
    abnormalities of, 1183–1184
Erythrocytes, 1176–1177, 1176f
    acquired defects of, 1185
    differential counts, 1177t
    glycolytic enzyme defects, 1183
    inherited defects of, 1181
    normal values during gestation, 1170t
    oxidative stress, 1182f
Erythrocyte sedimentation rate, 1244
Erythrocytes transfusion, 1212–1214, 1213t
Erythroderma, 1488–1489
Erythromycin, 1529, 1695
    fetal effects, 234t
    for neonatal ophthalmia, 1259
Erythropoiesis, 1169
Erythropoietin, 1695

Escherichia coli, 571–572
    diarrhea, 1259
    infectious diarrhea, 954
    with pneumonia, 570
Esmolol, 696t
    for JET, 742
    neonates, 1518t
    for supraventricular tachycardia, 704
Esophageal atresia, 947, 1109f, 1110f
    delayed primary repair, 1110–1111
    genetics, 1107
    immediate operative repair, 1110
    staged repair, 1110–1111
    surgery, 1107–1110
        complications, 1111
    with tracheoesophageal fistula,
        1107–1108
    without fistula, 1111–1112
Esophageal lesions
    surgery, 1107–1113
Esophageal stricture, 1111
Esophagus
    disorders, 945–946
Estrogens
    breast feeding, 439
    placenta, 155, 156f
    pulmonary maturation, 559
Ethacrynic acid, 1531
Ethanol
    with congenital anomalies, 899
    metabolism, 1587
    placental transfer, 1587
Ethchlorvynol (Placidyl), 1581
Ethical problems
    working through, 11–14
Ethics, 3, 9–11
Ethionamide
    fetal effects, 240
Ethnicity
    neonatal jaundice, 793–794
Etrentinate
    fetal effects, 237t, 248–249
Euploidy, 225–226, 226t
Euthanasia, 13–14
Euthyroid sick syndrome, 936
Evaporation
    convection warmed incubators, 449
Evidence based medicine, 83–85
Evidence grading systems, 84–85, 85t
Examination, 333–349
    abdomen, 341–344, 347t
    cardiovascular system, 344–345
    chest, 341–344
    color, 334, 346t
    ears, 339
    eyes, 338–339
    facies, 335
    general assessment, 333
    genitalia, 345, 347t
    genitourinary system, 345
    hair and scalp, 336
    head and neck, 335–336
    heart rate, 346t
    inspection, 333
    lymph nodes, 341
    musculoskeletal system, 345–347

nervous system, 347–349
    nose, 339–340
    posture, 334
    pulse, 346t
    respiratory effort, 334
    skin, 341
    spontaneous activity, 334
    state, 333–334
    vital signs, 335
Examination utero intrapartum treatment
        (EXIT), 274
Excess intracranial mass
    removal of, 1422–1423
Exchange transfusion, 825f, 837–838
    AAP guidelines for, 824f
    bilirubin dynamics, 838
    guidelines for, 821t, 822t
    readmitted for, 826t
    repeat, 838
    risks of, 837–838, 837t
Exclusive breast milk
    defined, 415t
Exosurf, 1695
Expanded Ballard score, 330f
Expenditures
    early prenatal care, 31
    for obstetric and neonatal care, 24
Extracellular body water (EBW), 362–363
Extracorporeal Life Support Organization
        (ELSO)
    database, 565
Extracorporeal membrane oxygenation
    historical development, 2
Extracorporeal membrane oxygenation
        (ECMO), 622–631, 623t
    age, 623–624
    cardiopulmonary disease, 624
    coordinator
        NICU, 76
    daily medical management, 628–630
    equipment, 627f, 627t
    equipment and systems, 626–628
    hematologic limitations, 624
    indications for, 623–625
    MAS, 629f
    for MAS, 565
    mortality criteria, 624–625, 624t
    outcome data, 630
    patient care after, 630
    patient management, 628–630
    prior mechanical ventilation, 624
    procedure, 625–626
    risk assessment, 624–625
    venoarterial circuit, 625f
    venoarterial method, 625
    venovenous method, 625–626
    weight, 623–624
Extrauterine breaths
    pressure volume curves, 293f
Extrauterine circulation
    transition to, 297
Extravascular blood, 805
Extremely low birth weight infant (ELBW),
        332, 459–484
    cardiovascular support, 467–469
    cognitive function, 483t

Extremely low birth weight infant (ELBW)
(*contd.*)
  cost benefit ratio, 31
  decision making, 16–17
  delivery room, 464–465
  developmental care, 480–481
  epidemiology, 460–462
  ethical issues, 483–484
  first sixty minutes of life, 464t
  fluids and electrolytes, 469–472
  followup, 481–483
  future directions, 483–484
  health improvement, 483t
  hematologic disorders, 474–475
  hospital discharge, 481
  impending delivery, 463–464
  major morbidities of, 472–481
  major problems in, 460t
  neonatal infections, 479–480
  neurologic disorders, 472
  NICU admission, 465
  nutrition, 470–471
  pain control, 480–481
  perinatal management, 462–469
  population profile, 461t
  predictors of, 461
  prenatal management, 462–463
  prevention of, 31
  prophylactic phototherapy, 834
  respiratory support, 465–467
  sensory overload, 480–481
Extreme prematurity
  fluids and electrolytes, 372–373
Exutero Intrapartum Treatment (EXIT), 173
  procedure, 191
Eye
  congenital anomalies, 1471–1476
  crusting, 339
  disorders, 1469–1484
  enlarged, 1471
  examination, 338–339
  examination techniques, 1470–1471
  growth and development of, 1469–1470
  prophylaxis
    newborn, 355
  size and shape
    anomalies, 1471–1472
Eyebrows
  examination, 338–339
Eyelids
  abnormalities, 1472–1473
  maturation of, 121t
  tumors, 1473

F

Fabry syndrome, 1682
Facies, 335
Facilitated diffusion
  placenta, 152
Factor VIII concentrates
  transfusion, 1217
Fagan Intelligence tests, 1585
Failure to thrive
  with gastroesophageal reflux, 1623
Famciclovir
  for herpes simplex virus, 1286, 1286t

Familial erythrophagocytic
    lymphohistiocytosis (FEL), 1457
Familial hypocalciuric hypercalcemia, 1028
Familial juvenile nephronophthisis with
    hepatic fibrosis, 1680
Familial renal-retinal dystrophy, 1680
Family
  centered care
    NICU, 78–79, 78t, 79f
  education
    NICU, 79
  information transfer to, 90
  neonatal transport psychological impact,
    49
  satisfaction measures, 81
Famotidine, 1528–1529, 1532–1533
Fanconi anemia, 1212
Fanconi-pancytopenia syndrome, 1676
Fanconi syndrome, 1029
  glycogen storage disease, 1030
  infancy, 1029t
Fat
  absorption, 941–942
  digestion, 381–382
  in human milk, 401
  with IDM, 886
  in infant formula, 402
  in preterm human milk, 403
  in preterm infant formulas, 404
  soluble vitamins
    requirements, 390–391
  sources, 384–385
Fatty acids
  bilirubin albumin binding, 779
  oxidation defects, 966t
  in preterm human milk, 403
Fecal flora
  human milk, 419
Feeding
  poor, 357
  tube device, 435, 435f
Feet
  abnormalities, 1434–1435
Female genital abnormalities, 1091
Female pseudohermaphroditism, 917
Femoral hypoplasia-unusual facies
    syndrome, 1680
Femur length, 168
  fractures, 1440
Fentanyl, 1695
  chest-wall rigidity, 1563
  dosage, 1563t
  electronic fetal monitoring, 262–263
  fetal and neonatal effects, 267
  following congenital heart surgery, 738
  for pain, 1558
  for pulmonary hypertension, 743
Fenugreek, 1655
Ferrous sulfate, 1695
Fetal abdomen
  MRI, 170f
Fetal acidosis, 305
Fetal age
  assessment of, 166–168
Fetal alcohol syndrome (FAS), 233, 899,
    976, 1586, 1587–1588, 1590, 1682

  incidence, 1590
  structural anomalies in, 900t
Fetal anatomy
  MRI, 170
  ultrasound, 169–179
Fetal asphyxia
  detection of, 179–181
  in infants with drug-dependent mother,
    1573
Fetal bilirubin metabolism, 770t
Fetal biophysical profile, 180, 180t
Fetal biparietal diameter (BPD), 167–168,
    167f
Fetal blood
  normal oxygen values in, 152t
Fetal bowel
  MRI, 175
Fetal brain
  MRI, 170f, 172f
  sonogram, 171f
  transvaginal scan, 170f
Fetal breathing, 288–289, 289f, 290f, 291f,
    536–537
  carbon dioxide, 289
  neurochemical, 289
  oxygen, 289
  placenta, 292f
Fetal cardiac intervention, 642
Fetal cardiology, 638–642
  myocardial function, 640
  pulmonary vasculature, 640
  ventricular work, 640
Fetal central nervous system abnormalities,
    170–171
Fetal chest
  MRI, 170f, 173f, 174f
Fetal chest abnormalities
  MRI, 173f
Fetal circulation, 638–639, 639f
  circulatory adaptation, 294–295
Fetal death
  smoking, 23
Fetal distress, 274
  in infants with drug-dependent mother,
    1573
  safest route of delivery, 463
Fetal Doppler
  electronic fetal monitoring, 264
Fetal drug exposure
  complications, 1574t–1575t
Fetal echocardiography, 640, 641f, 642f
  for critical congenital heart disease, 711,
    711t
  indications for, 641f
Fetal esophagus
  imaging, 175
Fetal eye
  third trimester
    maturation of, 121t
Fetal fibronectin (fFN), 204–205
Fetal gastrointestinal tract, 175
Fetal goiterous hypothyroidism, 193
Fetal growth
  assessment of, 166, 169
  normal variations and assessment of,
    491

Fetal growth curves
  interpretation of, 492–494
Fetal heart rate (FHR)
  with fetal and neonatal distress, 308t
  maternal analgesia, 262–263
Fetal hemoglobin, 1190
Fetal herpes simplex virus, 1286–1291
  clinical manifestations, 1287–1288
  diagnosis, 1289
  epidemiology, 1286–1287
  prevention, 1290–1291
  treatment, 1289–1290
Fetal hydantoin syndrome, 1682
Fetal imaging, 166–182
Fetal infection, 144
Fetal kidneys
  imaging, 177
Fetal leg
  MRI, 170f
Fetal lung fluid, 285–287
  clearance at birth, 287–288
Fetal maturity
  assessment of, 166
  ultrasound, 169
Fetal mediastinum, 173
Fetal platelet counts, 1706
Fetal pulmonary vascular resistance
  regulation of, 295–297
Fetal pulse oximetry
  electronic fetal monitoring, 263
Fetal pyelectasis, 177
Fetal red blood cell assay, 801
Fetal scalp
  blood gas analysis, 261
Fetal shunts
  closure, 299
Fetal stomach
  imaging, 175
Fetal surgery
  anesthetics for, 273–274
Fetal therapy, 186–199
  open surgery, 188
  surgery, 186–191
  in utero closed fetal surgery, 186–188
Fetal thermal regulation, 445
Fetal thorax
  MRI, 173
Fetal thyrotoxic goiter, 193
Fetal thyrotoxicosis, 193
Fetal trachea
  surgical isolation of, 189f
Fetal trimethadione syndrome, 1682
Fetal vessels
  Doppler assessment of blood velocities,
    181–182
Fetal weight estimates, 168
Fetal withdrawal
  in infants with drug-dependent mother,
    1573
Fetendo Clip Procedure, 189
Feto-maternal hemorrhage, 1173
Feto-maternal interactions, 149–163
Fetus
  adrenal disorders, 192–194
  amnion, 157
  blood circulation, 294f

body composition, 362–364
body weight and fat content, 500f
chemical composition of, 0t
chorion, 157
congenital diaphragmatic hernia, 188–189
endocrine disorders, 192–194
glucose producing and regulatory
    capabilities, 877–879
growth, 496–501
growth regulation, 501–505
immune system
    development, 1144t
immunology, 1135–1164
membranes, 157
nutrients, 499t
sacrococcygeal teratoma (SCT), 190, 190f
thyroid disorders, 193–194
water content, 495f
Fever
  mechanisms producing, 455–456
  thermal regulation, 455
FFA
  changes after birth, 878f
FG syndrome, 1676
Fiberoptic systems
  phototherapy, 832–833
Fibrin
  ECMO, 629
Fibronectin, 1140–1141
Fibrosarcoma, 1455
Fibula
  anomalies, 1436
Finances
  neonatal transport, 43–44
Financial planning team, 65
Finger feeding, 434
Fingers
  physical examination, 1428
First trimester
  assessment of, 166
  prenatal diagnosis, 138–140
5alpha-reductase deficiency, 918
5-aminosalicylic acid
  breast milk, 1689
5 hydroxytryptophan
  fetal breathing, 537
5p-syndrome, 1677
Fixed wing aircraft
  neonatal transport, 46–47
Fixed wing transport, 40
Flat foot, 1435f
Flavonoids
  maternal exposure to, 1446
Flecainide, 696t
  neonates, 1518t
  for supraventricular tachycardia, 704
Flexible nasopharyngoscopy and
    laryngoscopy, 1100–1101
Flight for Life, 40
Flowcharting, 86
Fluconazole, 1695
  for sepsis neonatorum, 1245, 1246
Flucytosine, 1695
  for sepsis neonatorum, 1245
Fludrocortisone (Florinef)
  for adrenal insufficiency, 931

Fluid and electrolyte therapy
  monitoring effectiveness of, 370–372
Fluid collection, 1411–1417
Fluid deficit, 367–368
Fluid requirements
  ECMO, 629
Fluid retention
  following congenital heart surgery, 738
Fluids and electrolytes
  abdominal wall defects, 374
  abnormal losses of, 370
  bronchopulmonary dysplasia, 373
  calculation of, 370
  calculation of requirements, 368–369
  central nervous system injury, 374
  diarrhea, 374–375
  extreme prematurity, 372–373
  intake calculation, 371t
  maintenance of, 369
  necrotizing enterocolitis, 374
  neuroendocrine control, 366–367
  pyloric stenosis, 374
  RDS, 373
  renal function, 367
  resuscitation, 315–316
  sepsis, 374
Fluids and growth
  newborn, 355–356
Flumazenil, 1566
Fluorescence in situ hybridization (FISH),
    145, 897
  microdeletions, 141
Fluorescent tubes
  phototherapy, 832
Fluorquinolones
  fetal effects, 241
Focal cerebral necrosis, 1393
Focal dermal hypoplasia of Goltz (Goltz
    syndrome), 1498–1499
Folate, 191
Folic acid
  fetal effects, 238t
  maternal nutrition, 206
Follicle stimulating hormone (FSH)
  multiple gestations, 523
Fontanelles, 338
Foods
  iron and caloric content of, 1702
Foramen ovale, 639–640
Forearm
  physical examination, 1428
For lower respiratory tract infection, 1263
Formula protein induced enterocolitis, 955
Formula protein intolerance, 954–955
Fosamprenavir
  pregnancy, 1320t
  teratogenic potential, 1319
Foscarnet
  cytomegalovirus, 1292
  for herpes simplex virus, 1286
Fosphenytoin
  for seizures, 1522
4-androstenedione, 926
4p-syndrome, 1677
4Z, 15E bilirubin isomer, 831, 831f
Fragile x syndrome, 637t

France
  active euthanasia, 13
Franconi anemia, 1445
Fraser syndrome, 1676
Free bilirubin, 778
  measurement of, 778–779
Free-drug theory, 1507
Free fatty acids, 396
Free radicals, 581t
  BPD, 581
Frequency-specific auditory environment, 119f
Fresh frozen plasma
  transfusion, 1217
Frontometaphyseal dysplasia, 1676
Fryns syndrome, 1680
FTA-ABS-IgM test, 1250
Full term infants
  phototherapy, 833
Functional residual capacity (FRC), 293
  with BPD, 586
Fungal sepsis, 1361
Furosemide, 1023, 1530–1531, 1532, 1695
  for hydrocephalus, 1413
  for hypercalcemia, 865
Furosemide (Lasix), 656t
  for BPD, 589–590, 590t
Fusion inhibitors
  pregnancy, 1321t
Futility, 16

G
Galactogogues, 1655
Galactopoiesis, 424–425
Galactose
  carbohydrate absorption, 940
Galactose-L-phosphate uridyltransferase (GALT), 195
Galactosemia, 195, 401, 402, 809, 974t
  carbohydrate absorption, 940
  with liver disease, 960
Galactose-1-phosphate uridyl transferase
  deficiency, 1030
Galeazzi sign, 1437
Galen aneurysm, 1424
Galenic arteriovenous shunt
  transcatheter occlusion, 1424
Galloway-Mowat syndrome, 1039
Gamma hydroxybutyrate (GHB), 27
Ganciclovir
  cytomegalovirus, 1292, 1294–1295
Gartner's duct, 1072
Gas exchange
  arterial CO2, 604–605
  assessment of, 602–605
  blood gas tension measurements, 602
  cannulation, 602–603, 603f
  clinical assessment of, 602
  end tidal CO2 monitoring, 604
  measurement, 602
  near infrared spectroscopy, 604
  pulse oximetry, 604
  transcutaneous PO2 and PCO2, 603
Gastric aspirate stains, 1244
Gastric emptying
  human milk, 418

positioning, 116
Gastric perforation, 1114
Gastrin, 943–944
Gastroesophageal reflux (GER), 943, 945–947, 1111, 1112–1113, 1528–1530, 1622–1623
  AOP, 543
  Nissen fundoplication, 1113f
Gastrointestinal disease, 940–961
Gastrointestinal function
  resuscitation, 316
Gastrointestinal hormones, 943–944
Gastrointestinal perforation
  SGA, 512t
Gastrointestinal tract
  abnormalities, 945–961
  development of, 940–943
  motility, 381
Gastrointestinal tract motility
  following congenital heart surgery, 738
Gastroschisis, 175–176, 945, 1128–1129, 1128f
  fluids and electrolytes, 374
Gastrostomy, 1114–1115
Gaucher disease
  with liver disease, 960
Gavage feedings, 399–400
  transition to nipple feeds, 398–399
Gaze abnormalities
  kernicterus, 785
G-CSF, 1143t
Gender
  neonatal jaundice, 795
Gender assignment, 1087
Gene function
  past, present, future, 5t
General anesthesia
  fetal and neonatal effects, 275–276
General assessment, 333
Genetic aberrations, 1444–1445
Genetic abnormalities
  abortions with, 225
Genetic counseling, 910–912
  books, 911–912
  decisions, 910–911
  Internet resources, 911
  resources, 911–912
Genetics
  BPD, 583–584
  neonatal jaundice, 793–794
Genetic skin diseases, 1489, 1493
Genetic testing, 19–20
Genital abnormalities, 1084–1090
Genital herpes, 1284
Genitalia
  abnormalities, 1123–1125
  examination, 345, 347t
  maturity of, 331–332
Genital phenotype inconsistent with
  genotype, 919
  etiology, 919t
Genital tract
  screening, 205
Genitourinary system, 176–177
  Doppler imaging, 1066
  examination, 345

imaging, 1066
  structural abnormalities of, 1066–1093
  ultrasonography, 1066
  voiding cystourethrography, 1066
Genotype
  maternal medications, 231
Gentamicin, 1527–1528, 1695
  fetal effects, 240
  for meningitis, 1252, 1253
  for osteomyelitis, 1255
  for sepsis neonatorum, 1244, 1245
  for short bowel syndrome, 952
  for urinary tract infection, 1257
Gentian violet, 1695
Gentleness, 1
Genu recurvatum, 1436
Germ cell tumors, 1452–1453
Germinal matrix-intraventricular
  hemorrhage
  complications, 1400t
  pathogenesis, 1400t
Germinomas, 1452
Gestational age
  assessment, 329–332
  birth weight percentiles for, 493f
  dry weight and fat content, 500f
  impact on survival, 461t
  influences on, 332
  neuromuscular maturity, 331
  physical maturity, 331–332
  survival rate by, 462t
  techniques, 329–330
Gestational criteria
  decision making, 17
Gestational diabetes, 207–209
Gestational diabetes mellitus, 209
  fetal assessment, 209
Gilbert promoter abnormality, 808f
Gilbert syndrome, 807–808, 807t
Gingiva
  cysts, 340t
Gingivostomatitis
  with HSV, 1284
Gitelman syndrome, 1033
Glans
  duplication of, 1086f
Glans penis, 1089f
Glaucoma, 1471, 1472
  with congenital rubella, 1281t
Glomerular filtration, 985
  rate, 985f
Glossoptosis, 1102
Gloves, 1370
Glucagon, 1695
  changes after birth, 878f
  fetus, 878
  for hypoglycemia, 884
Glucoamylase
  carbohydrate absorption, 941
Glucocorticoids, 926, 987
  fetal effects, 236t, 245–246
  fetal growth, 508
  immune system, 1136
  pulmonary maturation, 558–559
Gluconeogenesis
  fetus, 877–878

inadequate glucose production, 881
Gluconeogenic capability
  congenital absence of, 881
Glucose, 990
  for arrhythmias, 1519t
  carbohydrate absorption, 940
  changes after birth, 878f
  ELBW, 471
  for hypoglycemia, 884
  inadequate
    consequences, 885–888
  IUGR, 505
  resuscitation, 315
Glucose challenge
  insulin secretion fetus, 878f
Glucose-dependent insulinotropic peptide
  (GIP), 943–944
Glucose 6 phosphate dehydrogenase
  deficiency, 803–805, 804t, 1181–1183
    clinical course, 804
    etiology, 1182t
    with neonatal jaundice, 1182–1183
    pathogenesis, 804
    treatment, 805
Glucose phosphate isomerase deficiency,
  805
Glucose production
  glucose utilization, 880f
Glucose status
  newborn monitoring, 406
Glucose transporters
  fetus, 879
Glucose turnover
  body mass, 880f
  neonates, 879
Glucosuria, 1036
Glucuronidase, 797
Glucuronosyltransferase system, 1517
Glutaric acidemia type II
  abnormal odors, 976
Glutaric aciduria syndrome, 1680
Glutethimide, 1581
Glutethimide (Doriden), 1581
Glycogen
  changes after birth, 878f
  fetus, 877
  glucose production, 880–881
  SGA, 498–499
Glycogen storage disease (GSD), 881, 970f,
  974t, 975, 1205
Glycosuria
  ELBW, 471
Glyoxylate aminotransferase, 1027
GM-CSF
  T cells, 1148
Goat's rue, 1655
Goldenhar hemifacial microsomia, 636t
Goldenhar syndrome, 1473, 1679
  associated with congenital heart disease,
    717t
Gonadal determination disorders, 916–917
Gonadal stromal tumors, 1089
Gonadotropin deficiency, 924
Gonococcal ophthalmia neonatorum,
  1476f
Gordon's syndrome, 1018

GRA, 1018
Graft-*versus*-host disease
  with granulocyte transfusion, 1216–1217
Gram-negative sepsis, 1360–1361
Granulocyte-macrophage cerebrospinal
  fluid (GM-CSF), 559
Granulocyte transfusion, 1215–1216
Graves disease, 193, 937
Gray baby syndrome, 1510
Griscelli disease, 1206t, 1207
Group B beta hemolytic *Streptococcus*, 1236,
  1238–1239, 1442
  with pneumonia, 570
  prevention, 1247t
  risk factors for, 1239t
Group B beta streptococcal (GBS)
  pneumonia, 572–573, 572f
Group B beta *Streptococcus* pneumonia,
  571f
Group B streptococcal disease, 214t
  multiple gestation, 530
  preterm delivery, 205
Groups B streptococcal infection, 1162
Growth, 332–333
  birth weight classification of, 490–491
  expectations of, 1618–1619
  in infants exposed to alcohol, 1588
  with infants of drug addicts, 1579
  interpretation of parameters, 332–333
  measurement techniques, 332–333
  multiple gestation, 529
  nutritional requirements for, 1619
  patterns of, 1618–1619
  phencyclidine, 25–26
  with prenatal alcohol use, 1589
Growth charts, 1661–1668
Growth curves
  based on fetal measurements, 493–494
  based on neonatal measurements,
    492–493
Growth hormone deficiency, 923–924
Growth hormones
  fetal growth, 508
Growth parameters, 1658–1668
  interpretation of, 332–333
Growth retardation
  with congenital rubella, 1281t
Guardians
  communication with, 107–108
Gut
  malrotation, 948
  motility, 942–943
  nonrotation, 948
Gut-associated lymphoid tissues (GALT),
  1153

H

Haemophilus influenzae, 571
Haemophilus influenzae type b
  immunization, 1620
Hair, 1503–1504
  development of, 1485–1486
  drug testing, 30
Hair and scalp
  examination, 336
Hairy nevi, 1496

Halequin color changes, 1499
Hallucinogens
  epidemiology, 1573t
Halogen lamps
  phototherapy, 832
Halothane, 1559, 1559t
  fetal and neonatal effects, 276
Hamartomas, 1445
Hand
  examination, 345–347
  physical examination, 1428
Hand ambulance, 40
Hand-Christian-Schuller disease, 1457
Hand gels
  alcohol-based waterless, 1370
Handwritten communications
  medical confidentiality, 96–98
Harlequin ichthyosis, 1489
Hashimoto thyroiditis, 193, 937
HCA *vs.* Miller, 10t
Head
  circumference of, 332
  palpation of, 336–337
  physical examination, 1428
Head and neck
  examination, 335–336
Head and neck lesions
  surgery, 1097–1099
Head size
  SGA, 517
Head trauma, 1422–1423
Healthcare-associated enteroviruses, 1367
Healthcare-associated infections,
  1357–1375
  diagnosis accuracy, 1373–1374
  educational programs, 1374
  epidemiology, 1357–1358
  equipment care, 1374
  expanded isolation precautions,
    1369–1370
  hand hygiene, 1370–1371
  infection control, 1368–1371
  nursery design, 1374–1375
  prevention and control, 1369
  sample surveillance sheet, 1369t
  staffing, 1374–1375
  surveillance, 1368–1369
  viral infection, 1366–1368
Healthcare-associated multidrug-resistant
    organisms, 1362–1363
Healthcare-associated urinary tract
    infection, 1362
Healthcare Matrix, 1652–1653
Health care quality
  IOM, 109
Health care team
  communication within, 108–109
Health Insurance Portability and Acco-
    untability Act of 1996 (HIPAA), 90, 98
Health maintenance organization (HMO),
  99
Health professionals
  licensing, 56–57
Hearing
  with cocaine exposed infants, 1584
  postdischarge medical care, 1621–1622

Hearing disorders
  with fetal alcohol syndrome, 1592
Hearing impairment, 1638–1639
  in ELBW, 474
Hearing loss
  classification of, 1622f
  with congenital rubella, 1281t
  hyperbilirubinemia, 790
  kernicterus, 792
Heart disease
  during pregnancy, 215–216
Heart rate, 335
  with cocaine exposed infants, 1584
  examination, 346t
Heart sounds, 648–649
Heart transplantation, 760–761
Heat loss
  neonatal transport, 45
Heat shielding, 454–455
Heel to ear maneuver, 331
Height, 517f
  SGA, 517
Heinz bodies
  hemolytic anemia, 1182f
Heinz body hemolytic anemia,
    1185
Hemangioma, 1456, 1499f
  eyelids, 1473f
  incidence, 1444
Hemangioma of infancy (HOI),
    1499–1500
Hematologic disturbances, 1007
Hematology, 1169–1223
  resuscitation, 315
Hematopoietic differentiation, 1144
Hematuria, 1040–1043, 1083–1084
  differential diagnosis, 1041f
  etiology, 1040–1042
  evaluation, 1040–1042
Hemodialysis
  during pregnancy, 215
Hemodynamic formulations, 655t
Hemoglobin, 600
  normal levels, 1169–1170, 1169f
  oxygen equilibrium curves, 602f
  premature infants, 1170f
  sampling site, 1187
  synthesis disorders, 1184–1185
Hemoglobinopathy, 805
Hemoglobin-oxygen dissociation curves,
    1654
Hemolysis
  heritable causes of, 803–805
Hemolytic anemia, 1176
  infections, 1185
Hemolytic disease, 799–800
  bilirubin encephalopathy, 828
  from minor blood group
    incompatibility, 1181
Hemophagocytic lymphohistiocytic (HLH)
    disorders, 1207, 1457
Hemophilia
  molecular diagnosis, 144
Hemorrhage
  aortic blood pressure, 319f
  with cocaine exposed infants, 1584

neonate, 1172t
  obstetric accidents and complications,
    1174
Hemorrhagic disorders
  newborn, 1193–1194
Hemostasis
  in ELBW, 475
Heparin, 1695
  ECMO, 629
HepatAmine, 394
Hepatic glucose production, 884f
Hepatic glycogenolysis
  fetus, 878
Hepatic toxicity, 398
Hepatic transplantation, 975
Hepatitis
  with congenital rubella, 1281t
  with granulocyte transfusion, 1215–1216
Hepatitis A, 960, 1304–1305, 1367
  neonatal intensive care unit outbreaks,
    1304
  perinatal transmission, 1306
  prevention, 1306
  transmission, 1304
  vaccine, 1306
  virus, 1304–1305
Hepatitis B, 213t, 360, 1306–1307
  clinical manifestations, 1307
  with hepatocellular carcinoma, 959–960
  immunoprophylaxis, 1308–1309
  mother-to-infant transmission, 1308
  perinatal epidemiology, 1308
  perinatal transmission prevention,
    1309–1310
  prevention, 1217
  transmission, 1307–1308
  vaccine, 1621
Hepatitis B immunoglobulin (HBIG),
    1308–1309
Hepatitis B vaccine (HBV), 1306–1307
Hepatitis C, 960, 1311–1312
  clinical manifestations, 1311
  diagnosis, 1311–1312
  epidemiology, 1311–1312
  perinatal management, 1312–1313
  treatment, 1312
  vertical transmission, 1303
Hepatitis D, 1313
Hepatitis E, 1313
Hepatitis G, 1313
Hepatitis virus
  PMN transfusion, 1164
Hepatoblastoma, 1454–1455
Hepatocellular carcinoma, 1454
Hepatomegaly, 343
Hepatorenal tyrosinemia, 1031
Hepatosplenomegaly
  with congenital rubella, 1281t
  with syphilis, 1249
Hereditary elliptocytosis, 1184
Hereditary fructose intolerance, 974, 1031
  with liver disease, 960
Hereditary hemorrhagic telangiectasia,
    636t
Hereditary renal aplasia, 1676
Hereditary SP-B deficiency, 556

Hereditary spherocytosis, 1183–1184
  erythrocytes, 1181f
Hereditary tyrosinemia, 974t, 975
Hernia, 1126
Heroin
  adverse effects, 1574t
  breast feeding, 439
  breast milk, 1687
  history, 1573t
Herpes encephalitis
  neonate, 1288
Herpes simplex
  with pneumonia, 570
Herpes simplex infection
  skin, 1495–1496
Herpes simplex pneumonia, 573
Herpes simplex virus (HSV), 213t,
    1283–1291
  maternal infection, 1283–1284
    clinical manifestations, 1284–1285
    diagnosis, 1285
    epidemiology, 1283–1284
    treatment, 1285–1286
Herpes virus, 1367
  CMI, 1156
Herpes zoster, 1296–1297
Hess, Julius, 1
Heterochromatin, 130–131
Hexokinase deficiency, 805
Hexose monophosphate pathway (HMP),
    1138
High-frequency flow interrupters (HFFI),
    617–618
  indications for, 616
High-frequency jet ventilators (HFJV),
    616–617
  indications for, 616
High frequency oscillatory ventilation
    (HFOV), 467, 615
  vs. conventional ventilator, 617–618
  by disease, 618f
  indications for, 616
  for MAS, 565
  for PPHN, 568–569
High frequency ventilation (HFV)
  advantage, 615
  for BPD, 593
  gas transport mechanisms, 615f
  principles, 615
High-frequency ventilators, 616t
Highly active antiretroviral therapy
    (HAART)
  pregnancy, 1318–1319
High-risk infant followup program,
    1632–1636
  clinic schedule, 1636, 1636t
  developmental-intellectual-academic
    assessment, 1634
  developmental services, 1633
  developmental training, 1633
  family assessment, 1634
  hearing assessment, 1634–1635
  language-speech assessment, 1634
  medical-neurologic assessment, 1634
  neuromotor assessment, 1634
  objectives, 1632–1634

outcomes research, 1634
patient selection, 1635–1636
personnel, 1634–1635
quality control, 1633
High-risk infants
asphyxia, 1647–1648
IURG, 1646–1647
High risk pregnancies
intrapartum asphyxia, 308
High technology home care, 18–19
Hind milk, 427–428
Hip
anomalies, 1437–1439
developmental dysplasia of, 1437–1438
dislocation of, 1438f
examination, 347
infection, 1442
physical examination, 1429
teratologic dislocation, 1438
Hirschsprung's disease, 956, 1120–1121
diagnosis, 957
treatment, 957
Histamine-2 (H2) receptor antagonists,
1532–1533
for gastroesophageal reflux, 946
Histiocytoses, 1457–1458
HIV screening, 19
HLHS, 712
Hoarseness
with assisted ventilation, 618
Hodgkin disease
during pregnancy, 216
HOFV
principle, 617f
Holocarboxylase synthetase gene (HCS), 194
Holt-Oram syndrome, 636t
associated with congenital heart disease,
717t
Home care, 3–4
AOP, 543–544
Home monitors, 1626f
Home oxygen therapy
for ELBW, 477
Home parenteral nutrition
for short bowel syndrome, 952
Home phototherapy, 836
Home uterine activity monitoring
(HUAM), 204
Homocystinuria, 972
Hopkins Baby, 10t
Hormones
changes after birth, 878f
Horseshoe kidneys, 1068
Hospital administration
neonatal transport, 41
Hospital costs
newborns greater than 1500 g birth
weight, 30f
Hospital policies, 90
Host defenses
deficiencies, 1137t
HSV, 571
HSV pneumonia
neonate, 1288
Human chorionic gonadotropic (hCG),
154–155

Human coronavirus, 1366
Human growth hormone, 1655
Human herpesvirus 6, 1300–1301
Human herpesvirus 7, 1301
Human herpesvirus 8, 1301–1302
Human immunodeficiency virus (HIV),
213t, 360, 954, 1367–1368
breast feeding, 438
illicit drug use, 1572
neonatal immune response to,
1157–1159
treatment, 1318–1319
Human immunodeficiency virus (HIV)
type 1 infection, 1315–1316
epidemiology, 1317
fetal and neonatal infection,
1322–1323
maternal infection, 1317–1318
mother-to-infant transmission, 1317
Human leukocyte antigen (HLA), 192
Human metapneumovirus, 1367
Human milk, 401, 413–439. *See also* Breast
feeding
advantages of, 416–419
challenges of, 423–426
commercial fortifiers, 428–429
expression of, 423–424
optimal, 425t
vs. formula, 401
fortification for VLBWB, 427–429
gastrointestinal advantages of, 418–419
host defense advantages, 419–422
neurodevelopmental advantages,
422–423
in NICU, 426–427
nutritional advantages of, 416–417
obtaining, 1656
physiological advantages, 423
preterm infant impact on, 425
for preterm infants, 402–403
problems, 403
production of
skin-to-skin care, 425–426
supply of, 425–426
Human Milk Banking Association of North
America (HMBANA), 427
Human neutrophil antigens (HNA), 1205t
Human placentation, 149
Human T-cell lymphotropic virus (HTLV-1)
breast feeding, 438
Humerus
fractures, 1440
physical examination, 1428
Humidity
IWL, 366, 366t
neonatal transport, 45
Humoral immune systems
evaluation of, 1159
neonates
diagnosis, 1160t
Huntington disease locus, 132
Hyaline membrane disease
effect on nutritional status, 392
in infants of drug-dependent mothers,
1576
multiple gestation, 530

Hyaline membrane disease (HMD), 294
Hybrid incubator radiant warmer design,
455
Hydralazine, 1696
fetal effects, 234t, 242
Hydration, 18
Hydrocele, 1126
Hydrocephalus, 1411
with cocaine use, 1584
MRI, 171–172
treatment, 1412–1415
Hydrochlorothiazide
for BPD, 590t
Hydrocolpos, 1091
Hydrocortisone, 1541–1542, 1696
for adrenal insufficiency, 930
fetal effects, 245–246
for hypoglycemia, 884
Hydrometrocolpos, 1091
Hydromorphone
dosage, 1563t
Hydronephrosis, 1075f, 1076f, 1083,
1090
Hydrops
resuscitation, 323–324
Hydrops fetalis, 801
etiology, 1178t
jaundice, 828
parvovirus B 19, 1304
Hydroxyandrostenedione, 926
Hydroxylase deficiency, 929t
Hydroxyprogesterone, 192
17-hydroxyprogesterone (17-OHP), 192
Hydroxysteroid dehydrogenase deficiency,
929t
5 hydroxytryptophan
fetal breathing, 537
Hygiene hypothesis, 1149–1150
Hyperactivity
with narcotic withdrawal, 1577
Hyperammonemia, 968–969, 969f
Hyperbilirubinemia, 396
audiometric evoked response, 790
bilirubin binding capacity, 788–790
clinical risk factors, 818–819
clinical sequelae of, 786–792
cry analysis, 790
decreasing gestation, 819
discharge diagnosis, 802t
duration of, 790
followup, 820, 820t
hearing loss, 790
with IDM, 887f
incidence of, 803f, 805f
infant behavior, 790–791
kernicterus, 788–790
LBW, 827–828
pharmacologic treatment, 838–839
phototherapy for, 1479
preventing, 817–820
prolonged indirect
causes of, 809t
pulmonary hemorrhage, 792
risk assessment, 818, 818t, 819t
treatment of, 820–828
without hemolysis, 787–790

Hypercalcemia, 862–866
  diagnosis, 864–865, 864t
  pathophysiology, 862–864, 863f
  treatment, 865
Hypercalcinuria, 1026–1027
Hypercalciuria, 1036
Hypercarbia
  risks of, 605t
Hypercyanotic episodes, 719
  treatment, 720t
Hypergastrinemia
  with short bowel syndrome, 951
Hyperglycemia
  consequences of, 885
  ELBW, 471
  with intrapartum asphyxia, 307
  SGA, 512t, 514
  surfactant secretion, 559
Hyper IgM syndrome, 1206–1207, 1206t
Hyperimmune serum globulin, 1217
Hyperinsulinemia
  surfactant secretion, 559
Hyperinsulinism, 881–882
Hyperirritability
  with narcotic withdrawal, 1577
Hyperkalemia, 1005
  in ELBW, 469
  with intrapartum asphyxia, 307–308
  with spironolactone, 1531
Hypermagnesemia, 868–869, 868t
Hypermethioninemia, 809
Hyperoxia
  with BPD, 589
Hyperoxia test, 713
Hyperphosphaturic syndromes, 1036
Hypertension, 206–212, 929, 1016–1023
  birth weights, 163
  causes, 1018
  clinical feature and investigation, 1019
  clinical presentation, 1024
  genetic causes, 1018
  infants
    etiology, 1673
  with intrapartum asphyxia, 308t
  neonates, 1523–1524
  renal causes, 1017
  types, 1017
Hypertensive infants
  diagnosis, 1674
  physical exam, 1019t
Hypertensive mothers
  infants of, 1205
Hyperthyroidism, 193, 212
  fetus, 193
  maternal, 1156t
Hypertrichosis, 1503–1504
Hypertrophic cardiomyopathy, 693t, 698
Hypertrophic pyloric stenosis, 1116–1117
Hyperviscosity
  with IDM, 887f
  SGA, 512t
Hypocalcemia, 856–862, 1006
  diagnosis, 859–860, 860t
  pathophysiology of, 856–859, 857t
  risk factors, 856t
  treatment, 860–862, 861t

Hypocapnia
  brain effects, 605f
Hypocarbia
  risks of, 605t
Hypoglycemia, 973
  breast feeding, 437–438
  consequences of, 885
  diagnosis, 884
  ELBW, 471
  with IDM, 886
  infants at risk for, 881t
  with intrapartum asphyxia, 307
  newborn, 358
  SGA, 512t, 513, 513f
  symptoms of, 880t
  treatment, 884
Hypokalemia, 1023
Hypokalemic alkalosis, 1032
  differential diagnosis, 1033t
Hypokalemic Salt LOSING tubulopathies,
    1032–1033
Hypomagnesemia, 866–868, 866t
  diagnosis, 867
  hypocalcemia, 858
  with IDM, 886
  treatment, 867–868
Hypomelanosis of Ito, 1497
Hyponatremia, 1023
  with preterm human milk, 403
Hypophosphatemia, 1036
Hypophosphatemic rickets, 1036
Hypopituitarism, 810
Hypoplastic left heart syndrome (HLHS),
    658t, 671–673, 672f, 710, 723–724,
    724f, 725f, 726f, 727f
  clinical findings, 671
  differential diagnosis, 671
  hospital survival, 727f
  pathophysiology, 671
  surgery, 754–757
  treatment, 671–673
Hypospadiac meatal position, 1086f
Hypospadias, 919, 1085–1086
  classification of, 1086f
Hypothalamic-pituitary axis
  development of, 923
Hypothalamic-pituitary axis disorders
  etiology, 923t
Hypothalamus disorders, 923
  diagnosis, 924
  treatment, 924
Hypothermia
  with hypoglycemia, 883
Hypothyroidism, 193–194, 212, 809
  diagnosis, 935–936
  fetus, 193–194
  prognosis, 936
  symptoms of, 935
  treatment, 936
Hypoxemia
  diagnosis, 568t
Hypoxia, 396
Hypoxic-ischemic cerebral injury,
    1388–1392
  biochemical markers, 1391
  circulatory factors, 1391–1392

clinical features, 1388–1389
computed tomography, 1389–1390, 1390f
cranial ultrasound, 1389
diagnosis, 1388–1389
electrodiagnostic techniques, 1391
magnetic resonance imaging, 1390–1391
magnetic resonance spectroscopy, 1391
metabolic factors, 1392
near-infrared spectroscopy, 1391
neuroimaging, 1389
neuropathology, 1391
outcome, 1388t
pathogenesis, 1391
prognosis, 1398
radionuclide scanning, 1391
treatment, 1395–1398

I
Iatrogenic adrenal insufficiency, 931
Iatrogenic airway injury, 1105
Ibuprofen
  doses, 1565t
  for PDA, 468
Ichthyosis, 1489–1490
ICU
  carpet
    vs. hard flooring, 71
  ceiling materials, 71
  communication systems, 72–73
  equipment, 73–74
  headwalls, 72
  heating and cooling systems, 72
  infection control, 71
  maintenance, 73
  noise abatement, 71
  renovations, 73
  sinks, 71
  wall finishes, 71
ICU design
  review and approval, 74–75
ICU renovation
  human dynamics for moving, 75
Idiopathic female
    pseudohermaphroditism, 918
Idiopathic neonatal hepatitis, 958
Idiopathic thrombocytopenia
  maternal, 1156t
IDM, 886f
  IV glucose challenge, 886f
IDS
  congenital abnormalities, 888
  MRI, 888f
  postnatal problems, 888
IgA deficiency, 1206t
IgG
  placental transport, 153
Ileal atresia, 949
Ileostomy, 1115
Illicit drug use, 36–37
  epidemiology, 1573t
Illicit drug users
  epidemiology, 1572
Imipenem, 1526
Imipenem-cilastatin, 1525
Immature lung
  assisted mechanical ventilation, 606–607

Immature neutrophil count, 1704
Immune mediated hemolytic disease, 799–800
Immune response
  development, 1135
  ontogeny, 1145f
Immune shifting, 1149
Immune system
  cellular components, 1137
  development, 1135–1136
  humoral component, 1140
Immune systems
  neonates
    clinical evaluation of, 1159t
Immunization
  human milk, 419
Immunization information
  antenatal care, 352
Immunization schedule, 352t
Immunodeficiency disorders
  diagnosis, 1157, 1158t
  neonates
    diagnostic clues, 1159t
Immunodeficiency with ataxia and telangiectasia, 1158t
Immunodeficiency with eczema and thrombocytopenia, 1158t
Immunoglobulin (Ig) M, 144
Immunologic evaluation, 1157
Immunologic therapy, 1161
Immunology
  applications, 1136t
Immunosuppression
  with heart transplantation, 760
Imperforate anus, 1122–1123, 1123f, 1124f
  urologic implications of, 1091
Imperforate hymen, 1091f
Inborn errors of metabolism, 194–195, 966t–967t, 968t
  abnormal eye findings, 976–977, 977t
  with neonatal liver disease, 974t
  samples, 977
Incomplete masculinization, 928–929
Incontinentia pigmenti, 1494f
Incontinentia pigmenti (Bloch-Sulzberger syndrome), 1494–1495
Incubation
  thermodynamics of, 448
Incubator
  IWL, 366, 366t
Incubator humidification
  convection warmed incubators, 450
Indinavir
  pregnancy, 1320t
Indirect reacting hyperbilirubinemia, 799–801
  causes of, 799t
Individualized prognosis, 13
Individual practice association (IPA), 99
Indomethacin, 1012, 1539, 1696
  fetal breathing, 537
  fetal effects, 236t, 246
  for PDA, 468
Infant bioethics review committees, 12
Infant drug exposure
  detection, 28

Infant feeding
  parental decisions about, 424
Infant feeding information
  antenatal care, 352
Infantile polycystic kidney disease, 178f
Infant mortality, 24, 34f
  by country, 25t
  race, 34f
Infant mortality rate, 33
Infants
  digestive functions relative to adults, 941t
  normal hematologic values, 1703
Infants of diabetic mother (IDM)
  hypoglycemia, 881
Infants of diagnosis
  consequences of, 885–886
Infants with drug-dependent mother, 1572–1604
  antenatal problems, 1573–1576
  epidemiology, 1572–1573
Infection, 1476–1478
  BPD, 582–583
  breast feeding, 438
  following heart transplantation, 760
  industrialized countries, 1149–1150
  multiple gestation, 530–531
  neonates
    treatment, 1161–1162
  past, present, future, 5t
  prevention
    LBW, 1161
  VLBW
    formula *vs.* breast feeding, 429f
Infection control practitioner
  NICU, 1374–1375
Infectious diarrhea, 954
  screening stood studies, 954t
Infectious disease
  human milk, 419–420
Inflammation
  BPD, 582
Inflammatory rashes, 1486–1487
Inflammatory response, 1137
Influenza
  vaccine, 1620
Influenza A
  immunization, 1366–1367
Information and communications technology (ICT), 54
Information transfer
  to patients and families, 90
Informed care
  antenatal care, 352
Informed consent, 94–95
Infravesical obstruction
  voiding cystogram, 1081
Ingram Icterometer, 814
Inguinal hernias
  in ELBW, 478
Inhalants
  epidemiology, 1573t
Inhalation anesthetics
  fetal and neonatal effects, 276
Inhaled anesthetics, 1559–1560
  systemic effects of, 1559t

Inhaled NO (INO)
  for BPD, 595
Inhaled steroids, 1542
Inherited metabolic disorders, 965–978
  clinical manifestations of, 965–968
  newborn screening for, 977–978
Inherited thrombocytopenia, 1198
In-hospital neonatal care, 25–27
Injury
  neuropathologic patterns of, 1392–1398, 1392t
Innominate artery
  anomalous origin, 691
INO
  by disease, 618f
  with HFOV, 617
Inotropes, 1533–1534
  cardiovascular receptor interactions, 1534t
Insensible water loss
  phototherapy, 835
Insensible water loss (IWL), 364–366, 364f, 364t, 365f, 365t
  factors increasing, 365–367
  factors reducing, 366
Inspection, 333
Institute of Healthcare Improvement Breakthrough Series, 83
Institute of Medicine
  quality of care defined, 79–80
Institute of Medicine (IOM)
  health care quality, 109
Institutional collaboration
  quality improvement, 83
Instrumental vaginal delivery
  epidural analgesia, 271
  fetal and neonatal effects, 271
Insulin, 1696
  changes after birth, 878f
  fetus, 878
  growth, 507f
  IUGR, 506–507
Insulin-like growth factor binding protein-2
  fetal growth, 508
Insulin-like growth factor binding protein-3
  fetal growth, 508
Insulin-like growth factor I
  fetal growth, 508
Insulin-like growth factor II
  fetal growth, 508
Insurance, 32f
Intellectual deficits
  cytomegalovirus, 1293
Intensive care bed
  total births, 28f
Intensive care nursery (ICN), 2
  as space station, 4
Intensive phototherapy, 833
Intercellular adhesion molecule-1 (ICAM-1), 1138
Interferon
  for hepatitis B, 1310
Interferon alpha (IFN alpha), 1143t
Interferon beta (IFN beta), 1143t

Interferon gamma (IFN gamma), 1143t
  T cells, 1148
  Th2, 1149
Interinstitutional transfer
  decision making, 20
Interleukin-1 (IL-1), 1142t
Interleukin-1 (IL-2), 1142t
Interleukin-2 (IL-2)
  T cells, 1148
Interleukin-3 (IL-3), 1142t
  T cells, 1148
Interleukin-4 (IL-4), 1142t
  T cells, 1148
Interleukin-5 (IL-5), 1142t
  T cells, 1148
Interleukin-6 (IL-6), 1142t
  T cells, 1148
Interleukin-7 (IL-7), 1142t
Interleukin-8 (IL-8), 1142t
Interleukin-9 (IL-9), 1142t
Interleukin-10 (IL-10), 1142t
Interleukin-11 (IL-11), 1142t
Interleukin-12
  Th2, 1149
Interleukin-12 (IL-12), 1142t
Interleukin-13 (IL-13), 1142t
Interleukin-14 (IL-14), 1142t
Interleukin-15 (IL-15), 1142t
Interleukin-16 (IL-16), 1142t
Interleukin-17 (IL-17), 1143t
Interleukin-18 (IL-18), 1143t
Interleukin-19 (IL-19), 1143t
Interleukin-20 (IL-20), 1143t
Interleukin-21 (IL-21), 1143t
Interleukin-22 (IL-22), 1143t
Interleukin-23 (IL-23), 1143t
Interleukin-24 (IL-24), 1143t
Interleukin-25 (IL-25), 1143t
International practice, 91–92
Internet drug prescriptions
  FDA, 92
Interrupted aortic arch (IAA), 727, 757, 1146
  types of, 727f
Intersex abnormality
  diagnosis, 1125t
Interstate practice, 91–92
Interstitial pneumonia
  with congenital rubella, 1281t
Interstitial pneumonitis, 572
Intertrigo, 1487
Intervillous pool flow system, 151f
Intestinal tract
  temporary diversion of, 1114–1115
Intestinal transplantation
  for short bowel syndrome, 953
Intestine
  localized perforation, 950–951
Intimate family, 16
Intoxication
  with intrapartum asphyxia, 308t
Intracellular body water (IBW), 362–363
Intracerebellar hemorrhage, 1403–1404
Intracranial cystic spaces, 1417, 1417f
Intracranial hemorrhage, 1398–1402
  antenatal intervention, 1400–1401
  clinical features, 1399

diagnosis, 1398–1399
  intrapartum management, 1401
  neuroimaging, 1398–1399
  pathogenesis, 1399–1400
  posthemorrhagic hydrocephalus,
    1401–1402
  postnatal management, 1401
  prognosis, 1402
  treatment, 1400
Intracranial tumors, 1448–1449
Intractable diarrhea of infancy, 955–956
Intradermal water blocks
  for labor pain, 266
Intramuscular drug adsorption
  neonates, 1508
Intramuscular immune globulin (IGIM)
  for hepatitis A, 1306
Intrapartum asphyxia
  cardiopulmonary changes with, 306, 306f
  pathophysiology of, 305–308
  resuscitation of, 308–316
  risk factors, 308t
Intrapartum care, 353
Intraperitoneal air collection, 1114f
Intrauterine death
  SGA, 512t
Intrauterine growth curves, 1658–1659
Intrauterine growth restriction, 1008
Intrauterine growth restrictions
  defined, 490
  preterm birth, 494–496, 496t
  SGA, 490–519
Intrauterine growth retardation, 169
  with IDM, 886
Intrauterine infection
  immunologic consequences, 1156–1157
  maternal drug use, 1573
Intrauterine resuscitation
  of compromised fetus, 274
Intravascular catheters
  thrombosis, 1217–1218
Intravenous alimentation
  phototherapy, 836
Intravenous drug administration
  neonates, 1508
Intravenous fats, 394
Intravenous fluid infusion
  parenteral fluid therapy, 375–376
Intravenous gamma globulin
  for parvovirus B 19, 1304
Intravenous immunoglobulin
  inhibiting hemolysis, 839
Intravenous lipids, 396
Intraventricular hemorrhage, 1399f, 1411f,
    1485
  with ELBW, 472
  postdischarge medical care, 1623–1624
  term newborn, 1404
Introital masses, 1093
Intubation
  AOP, 543
In utero environment
  fetal origins of adult disease, 162
In vitro fertilization (IVF), 145
Iodides
  fetal effects, 238t

Iodide trap defect, 933
Iodine
  recommended intake for preterm infants,
    400t
Iododeoxyuridine
  for neonatal HSV, 1290
Ion distribution
  blood plasma, 364f
Ionized calcium (iCa), 848
Ipratropium bromide
  for BPD, 590t
IP (Internet Protocol) videoconferencing,
    56
Iris
  color, 339
  dilated vessels, 1479f
Iron, 1696
  absorption, 942
  in human milk, 401
  requirements, 387–389
Iron status
  newborn monitoring, 406
Irradiance
  phototherapy, 830–831, 830f
ISDN (Integrated Services Digital
    Network), 56
Islet cells
  fetus, 878
Isoflurane, 1559t
  fetal and neonatal effects, 276
Isoimmunization
  maternal, 1156t
Isoimmunization screening
  neonatal hyperbilirubinemia,
    812–813
Isolated tracheoesophageal fistula, 1112
Isoniazid, 1696
  fetal effects, 240
Isopropyl alcohol
  neonates, 1517
Isoproterenol, 657t, 1530, 1533
  for low cardiac output, 739
Isotretinoin
  fetal effects, 237t, 248–249
Isovaleric acidemia
  abnormal odors, 976
Isradipine
  amlodipine, 1020
  for hypertension, 1524
IUGR
  adult disorders resulting from,
    518–519
  antenatal care, 508–509
  diagnosis, 508–509
  epidemiology, 501–502
  fetal endocrine and autocrine/paracrine-
    acting growth factor effects, 506
  fetal nutrient uptake, 505–510
  genetics, 502
  insulin, 506–507
  maternal chronic disease, 503
  maternal drugs, 503–504, 503t
  maternal nutrition, 503
  metabolism, 505–510
  nongenetic maternal factors, 502–503
  placenta, 504–505, 504f, 504t

Ivemark syndrome, 1680
IVIG
  for neonatal infection, 1161–1162
IWL, 369–370

J

Jaundice, 359, 768–839, 973–976,
    1669–1670
  beyond three weeks, 817
  breast feeding, 438
  cause of, 816
  in ELBW, 472
  in healthy newborn, 798–799
  in infants of drug-dependent mothers,
    1577
  kernicterus, 810–811
  laboratory evaluation of, 817t
  mixed forms of, 809–810
  pathologic causes of, 799–810
  prevention and treatment
    with breast feeding, 827t
  sepsis, 809–810
  visual assessment of, 814
Jejunal atresia, 949, 1118–1119, 1118f
Jeune asphyxiating thoracic dystrophy,
    1681
Jitteriness, 349
JM-103, 814, 815
Johanson-Blizzard syndrome, 1676
Joint Commission on the Accreditation of
    Healthcare Organizations (JCAHO),
    105–106
Junctional ectopic tachycardia (JET),
    703–706, 1518
  following congenital heart surgery, 742
Juvenile myelomonocytic leukemia,
    1208–1209
Juvenile xanthogranuloma, 1503, 1503f

K

Kanamycin
  fetal effects, 240
  for meningitis, 1252
Kangaroo Care, 425–426, 429
Kangaroo care, 447–448
Kaposi sarcoma, 1322–1323
Karo syrup, 1627t
Karyotyping, 187
Kayexalate, 1696
Kernicterus, 774–776, 783, 784–786
  auditory abnormalities, 785
  clinical and pathologic correlations, 776
  clinical features of, 785
  comorbidity, 789t
  comparative neuropathology of, 774t,
    777t
  cytology, 775–776
  dental dysplasia, 785
  extrapyramidal disturbances, 785
  gaze abnormalities, 785
  gross anatomy, 775
  hearing loss, 792
  histology, 775–776
  hyperbilirubinemia, 788–790
  jaundice, 810–811
  MRI, 785

neuropathologic findings of, 775f
  pathology, 774
  preventing, 817–820
  temporal evolution, 784–785
  topography, 774–775
Ketamine, 1567
  fetal and neonatal effects, 276
Ketamine hydrochloride, 27
Ketoconazole
  for diaper dermatitis, 1487
Ketones
  oxidation, 877f
Ketorolac
  doses, 1565t
Khavari Alcohol Test, 28
Kidneys, 1067f
  abnormalities of position, 1068
  anomalies of, 1066–1071
  ascent failure, 1068
  blood flow, 981–983
  developmental physiology, 981–991
  embryology, 981
  fusion anomalies, 1068
  neoplasms, 1450–1452
  palpation, 343
Kinin system, 983, 983f
Klebsiella
  with pneumonia, 570
Klebsiella pneumoniae, 571–572, 1361
Kleeblattschadel, 1423
Kleihauer Betke assay, 801
Kleinfelter's syndrome, 1678
Klinefelter syndrome, 903
Klippel-Feil syndrome, 636t, 1429, 1433,
    1679
Klippel Trenauny syndrome, 1679
Knee
  anomalies, 1436–1437
KNOT (known, not treatable), 20
Kostmann syndrome, 1205

L

Labetalol, 1696
  during pregnancy, 207
Labor analgesic techniques
  fetal and newborn effects,
    266–272
  nonpharmacologic methods, 266
  systemic opioids, 266–268
Labor and delivery
  multiple gestation, 526
  neonatal jaundice, 794
Labor and delivery pain
  maternal implications, 265–266
Labor epidurals
  fetal and neonatal effects, 270–271
  outcome, 270–271
Labor pain
  fetal implications, 264–265
Lactase
  carbohydrate absorption, 940–941
  human milk, 418
Lactase deficient, 402
Lactation
  breast pumps, 424–425
Lactic acidemias, 966t–967t

Lactic acidosis, 970
  following congenital heart surgery, 738
Lactobacillus bifidus, 419
Lactogen
  placenta, 155
Lactogenesis, 424
Lactose, 382, 401
  carbohydrate absorption, 940
Ladd bands, 948
Lamivudine, 1319
  for hepatitis B, 1310
  pregnancy, 1320t
Lamotrigine
  breast milk, 1689
  for seizures, 1523
LAN (local area network), 56
Langerhans cell histiocytoses, 1457, 1489
Language disorders, 119
  in cocaine exposed infants, 1585
Lanugo, 331
Laryngeal atresia/web, 1102–1103
Laryngeal obstruction
  surgery, 1102–1103
Laryngomalacia, 1102
  with assisted ventilation, 618
Laryngotracheoesophageal cleft, 1112
Lasers
  for ROP, 1482
Late anemia, 801
Late chorionic villus sampling (CVS),
    142–143
Late-onset sepsis, 1359–1360
Laterality sequences Ivemark syndrome,
    1679
Laudanum
  for narcotic withdrawal, 30–31
Lazy colon syndrome
  with IDM, 888
LBW
  cognitive development, 1641–1642
  intelligence quotients, 1642t
  language development, 1642
  motor development, 1642–1643
  perceptual development, 1641–1642
L-carnitine, 972
Learning
  past, present, future, 5t
Left pulmonary artery
  anomalous origin, 691
Left to right shunts, 731–732, 759–760
Left ventricular hypertrophy (LVH)
  with BPD, 585
Left ventricular outflow tract obstruction,
    753–757
Legal considerations
  historical overview, 89–90
  neonatal transport, 50–51, 51f
Legal issues
  managed care, 98–100
Leiner disease, 1160
Length of stay
  discharge diagnoses, 29t
  VLBW, 29t
Lens
  maturation of, 121t
  opacity, 1474–1475

LEOPARD syndrome, 1676
Leptomeningeal cysts, 1422
Lethal multiple pterygium syndrome, 1676
Letterer-Siwe disease, 1457
Leucovorin
  for toxoplasmosis, 1328, 1331
Leukemia
  incidence, 1444
  during pregnancy, 216
Leukocoria, 1483, 1483f
Leukocyte adhesion deficiency 1 (LAD-1), 1138, 1158t
Leukocytes, 1200–1212
  neonates
    normal count, 1200–1201
Leukoedema, 340t
Levothyroxine, 1696
Levy-Hollister syndrome, 1676
Leydig cells, 915
LGA
  with transient hypoglycemia, 882
Liability, 90
Licensure, 91–92
Liddle's syndrome, 1018
Lidocaine, 696t, 1696
  for arrhythmias, 1519t, 1520
  neonates, 1518t
  for seizures, 1522
Lifestyle choices
  pregnancy, 36–37
Li-Fraumeni syndrome, 1445
Light
  behavior, 124
  photobiological effects in NICU, 123–124
Light emitting diodes (LED)
  phototherapy, 832
Lighting
  neonatal transport, 45
Light spectrum
  phototherapy, 829–830
Limb reduction defects (LRD), 139
Limb segmentation
  defects of, 1433–1434
Lines of Blaschko, 1485
Lipase
  fat absorption, 941
Lipid
  metabolism
    SGA, 514
Lipids
  human milk, 417–418
Lipid storage diseases
  with liver disease, 960
Liquid ventilation, 619
Listeriosis
  with hepatitis, 960
  multiple gestation, 530
Lithium carbonate
  breast milk, 1689
  fetal effects, 236t, 246
Liver
  development, 958
  glycogen, 498f
  palpation, 343

Liver disease, 958
Liver dysfunction, 973–976
Local anesthesia, 1560–1561
Localized intravascular coagulation (Kasabach-Merritt syndrome), 1194
Logarithm of the odds (LOD), 133
Long chain fatty acids, 382
Long chain polyunsaturated fatty acid (LC-PUFA), 384
Long chain polyunsaturated fatty acids (LC-PUFA)
  human milk, 422
Long QT syndrome, 638, 705–706
Long term costs, 30–31
Lopinavir
  pregnancy, 1320t
Lorazepam, 1532–1533, 1565–1566, 1697
  glucuronidation, 1510
  for seizures, 1523
Lotrisone
  for diaper dermatitis, 1487
Low bilirubin kernicterus
  premature infants, 791–792
Low birth weight (LBW), 332
  developmental dysfunction, 1644f
  expected hemoglobin values, 1703
  hyperbilirubinemia, 827–828
  incidence, 35, 35f
  in infants of mothers on heroin, 1576
  with major impairments, 1637t
  neurobehavioral development, 1643–1644
  neurodevelopmental outcome, 1637–1646
  oral feeding schedule, 389t
  oral hygiene, 1371–1373
  school function, 1644–1646
  skin care, 1371–1373
  smoking, 24
  trends, 36f
Low density lipoprotein (LDL) cholesterol
  receptor mediated endocytosis, 154
Low dose aspirin
  prevention preeclampsia, 207
Lower extremities
  anomalies, 1434–1437
  physical examination, 1429
Lower respiratory tract infection, 1261–1263
  clinical manifestations, 1262
  diagnosis, 1262–1263
  treatment, 1263
Lower urinary tract obstruction (LUTO), 186
Lowe syndrome, 1681
  abnormal eye findings, 976–977
Low molecular weight heparin (LMWH), 1220–1221
L-transposition of the great arteries, 677
Lundeen, Evelyn, 1
Lung compliance
  assisted mechanical ventilation, 610
  with BPD, 586
Lung development, 553–555, 554f
  alveolar stage, 555
  anomalies, 555–557

  canalicular stage, 555
  pseudoglandular stage, 555
  saccular stage, 555
Lung function
  past, present, future, 5t
Lung liquid absorption, 287f
Lung liquid secretion, 286f
Lung luminal liquid
  fetal lambs, 285f
Lungs
  air vs. liquid expansion
    pressure volume curves, 293f
  opening pressure at birth, 293
  ventilation of, 297–298
Lupus
  with intrapartum asphyxia, 308t
Lupus erythematosus
  maternal, 1156t
Luteinizing hormone (LH)
  multiple gestations, 523
Lymphangioma
  incidence, 1444
Lymphangioma circumscriptum, 1501f
Lymphangiomas, 1500–1501
Lymphatic malformations, 1500–1501
Lymph nodes
  examination, 341
Lymphocyte surface molecules
  classification, 1146t
Lymphocytic choriomeningitis virus (LMCV), 1313–1314
Lymphopenia, 1209–1210
  neonates, 1210t
Lymphopoietic differentiation, 1144–1145
Lysinuric protein intolerance, 1037–1038
Lysosomal storage disorders, 967t

M
Macrocrania, 1448
Macrocystic lymphatic malformation (cystic hygroma), 1501
Macroglossia, 1102
Macrolides
  fetal effects, 240–241
Macrophages, 1136, 1139–1140
  BPD, 582
Macrosomia, 208
  with IDM, 885–886, 885f
Macula
  development of, 1471t
Magnesium, 990
  absorption, 942
  homeostasis nonclassic control, 855–856
  hypocalcemia, 857t
  physiologic control, 849–855
  requirements, 387
  tissue distribution, 847
Magnesium sulfate, 1697
  complications of, 204t
Magnetic resonance imaging
  historical development, 2
Malaria, 1332t
Malassezia furfur, 1243
Malassezia furfur, 1361
Malassezia pachydermatis, 1243
Male pseudohermaphroditism, 918

Malformation sequences, 907
Malignant infantile osteopetrosis, 859
Malignant rhabdoid tumor
  kidney, 1452
Malpractice insurance
  telehealth, 57
Malrotation, 945, 1115–1116
  with midgut volvulus, 1116
Mammalian B-cell differentiation model,
  1151f
Managed care
  legal issues, 98–100
Manganese
  recommended intake for preterm infants,
  400t
Mannitol, 1697
  for CPB adverse effects, 735
Maple sugar urine disease, 971t
Maple syrup urine disease
  abnormal odors, 976
Marfan's syndrome, 636t
  associated with congenital heart disease,
  717t
  cardiac disease, 635
Marijuana, 1592
  adverse effects, 1575t
  breast feeding, 439
  breast milk, 1687
  epidemiology, 1572, 1573t
  fetus, 1592–1593
  infants, 1592–1593
  maternal exposure to, 1446
  pregnancy, 1592
MAS
  ventilation, 618f
Masculinization, 347t
Massage
  for labor pain, 266
Mastocytosis, 1495, 1495f
Maternal alcohol abuse, 1587
Maternal analgesia
  electronic fetal monitoring, 262–263
Maternal antibodies
  harmful effects, 1156t
Maternal blood
  normal oxygen values in, 152t
Maternal cardiac arrest, 274–275
Maternal congenital heart lesions
  during pregnancy, 216t
Maternal corpus luteum
  abortions with, 225
Maternal diabetes mellitus, 876
  abortions with, 225
  hyperbilirubinemia, 806
  neonatal jaundice, 794
Maternal drugs, 224–251
  adverse reproductive outcomes,
  224–228
Maternal drug use
  detection, 28
  neonatal treatment, 30
  SIDS, 548
Maternal factors
  neonatal jaundice, 794
Maternal fasting
  fetus, 876–877

Maternal-fetal histocompatibility
  abortions with, 226
Maternal fetal interactions, 1153–1156
Maternal fever
  fetal and neonatal effects, 271–272
Maternal genotoxins
  prenatal exposure, 1446
Maternal gestational varicella
  newborn abnormalities, 1298f, 1298t
Maternal history, 328
Maternal hyperbilirubinemia, 769
Maternal hyperthyroidism
  abortions with, 225
Maternal hypothyroidism
  abortions with, 225
Maternal illness, 202–217, 206–217
Maternal immunoglobulin
  placental transport, 153–154
Maternal-Infant Bonding, 3
Maternal infection
  abortions with, 225–226, 226t
Maternal insulin secretion
  pregnancy, 876
Maternal interview, 28
Maternal malignancy, 1445–1446
Maternal malnutrition
  maternal medications, 230–231
Maternal medications
  active metabolites, 229
  developmental risks, 231–232
  dose-response relationship, 229
  drug interaction, 229
  exposure magnitude, 229
  fat solubility, 229
  fetal period, 229
  maternal disease, 230–231
  pharmacokinetics and metabolism,
  229–230
  potential developmental toxicity, 232t
  potential toxicity, 233
  self-administered, 234t–238t
  susceptibility, 228–251
  threshold phenomena, 229
Maternal metabolic disorders, 978
Maternal milk supply
  augmenting, 1655
Maternal movement and positioning
  for labor pain, 266
Maternal neonatal interactions,
  1153–1156
Maternal nutrition, 205–206
Maternal oxygen
  fetal effects of, 277–278
Maternal pain
  adverse fetal effects, 265f
Maternal phenylketonuria
  congenital anomalies with, 899t
Maternal placental progesterone
  abortions with, 225
Maternal rubella, 1276–1280
  epidemiology, 1276–1277
Maternal serum alpha-fetoprotein
  (MSAFP), 191
Maternal smoking
  neonatal jaundice, 794
  SIDS, 548

Maternal toxoplasmosis, 1325–1326
  clinical manifestations, 1325
  diagnosis, 1325–1326
  epidemiology, 1325
  serologic diagnosis, 1326–1327
Maternal virilizing disorders, 918
Maternofetal transport, 150f
  patterns of, 150f
Mature circulation, 640f
McCune-Albright syndrome, 1496
M-CSF, 1143t
MDMA (ecstasy), 27
Mean arterial blood pressure, 982
Mean arterial blood pressure (MAP),
  982
Mean arterial pressure, 994
Measles-mumps-rubella vaccine, 1620
Measles virus, 1332t
Mechanical ventilation
  birth weight, 607f
  for ELBW, 466
Mechanic uterine problems
  abortions with, 226
Meckel-Gruber, 172
Meckel-Gruber syndrome, 1681
Meconium, 354
  bilirubin, 797
  drug testing, 29–30
Meconium aspiration syndrome (MAS),
  562–565, 622
  clinical presentation, 563
  pathogenesis of, 563f
  pathology, 563
  pathophysiology of, 563–564
  prevention of, 564
  SGA, 512t
  surfactant treatment, 564–565
  treatment, 564
  ventilatory support, 565
Meconium ileus, 949, 1119–1120, 1119f
Meconium peritonitis, 949, 1119
Meconium plug syndrome, 956, 1119
Meconium stained amniotic fluid,
  321–322
Meconium-stained amniotic fluid (MSAF),
  562
  maternal drug use, 1573
Median alveolar notch, 340t
Median raphe cyst, 1502f
Medicaid, 32
Medical confidentiality
  communications, 96–98
Medical director
  neonatal transport, 41
Medical errors
  classification of, 80, 80t
Medical malpractice, 92–93
  elements of, 93–94
Medical records, 95–96
Medical torts, 92
Medications
  resuscitation, 313–314
Medicolegal and regulatory issues
  telehealth, 56–57
Medium chain acyl CoA dehydrogenase
  deficiency, 973

Megacystis microcolon intestinal hypoperistalsis syndrome (MMIHS), 1079

Megacystitis-microcolon-intestinal hypoperistalsis syndrome, 1679

Melanoma
during pregnancy, 216

Melanotic neuroectodermal tumor, 1449

Melnick-Fraser syndrome, 1676

Melnick-Needles syndrome, 1676

Memorial University of Newfoundland (MUN)
Telemedicine Centre, 55

Memory cells, 1135

Meningitis, 1251–1253
prognosis, 1253–1254

Meningocele, 172

Meningoencephalitis
with congenital rubella, 1281t

Meningomyelocele, spina bifida, and occult spinal dysraphism sequence, 1679

Meningomyeloceles, 172, 191

Menkes (kinky hair) disease, 135

Menke's Kinky Hair syndrome, 1677

Menotropins
multiple gestations, 524

Mental retardation, 1638
with congenital rubella, 1281t

Meperidine
breast feeding, 439
dosage, 1563t
fetal and neonatal effects, 267

Meprobamate
fetal effects, 235t, 242

Mercaptoacetyl triglycine, 999

Meropenem, 1525, 1526

Mesoblastic nephroma, 1082, 1450–1451

Messenger, 10t

Metabolic acidosis, 374, 969–971
following congenital heart surgery, 738

Metabolic fuels
changes after birth, 878f

Metabolic function
past, present, future, 5t

Metabolic myopathies, 1406–1407

Metal metabolism disorders, 967t

Metanalyses, 84

Metanephros, 981

Metaphyseal radiolucencies
with congenital rubella, 1281t

Metatarsus adductus, 1434, 1434f

Methadone
adverse effects, 1574t
dosage, 1563t
history, 1573t
for narcotic withdrawal, 30–31

Methamphetamine, 26
adverse effects, 1575t
long-term effects, 27
neonates, 27
pregnancy, 26–27

Methicillin
for lower respiratory tract infection, 1263
for sepsis neonatorum, 1245

Methicillin resistant *Staphylococcus aureus* (MRSA), 1362–1364

Methimazole, 212
for drug-induced neonatal goiter, 934

Methohexital
fetal and neonatal effects, 276

Methotrexate
breast milk, 1687
fetal effects, 234t, 238–239

Methyldopa
fetal effects, 234t, 242
during pregnancy, 207

Methylene blue, 1697
fetal effects, 236t, 246–247

Methylmalonic acidemia, 194, 970, 972

Methylprednisone
fetal effects, 245–246
for toxoplasmosis, 1331

Methylxanthines, 1536
AOP, 542, 542t
for AOP, 479
for BPD, 590–591

Metoclopramide, 426, 1529, 1655, 1697
for gastroesophageal reflux, 947, 1623

Metolazone, 1697

Metroclopramide
breast milk, 1689

Metronidazole (Flagyl), 1697
breast milk, 1689
fetal effects, 241
for short bowel syndrome, 952

Mexilitine
neonates, 1518t

Meyer-Rokitansky-Kuster-Hauser syndrome, 1091

Micellar solubilization, 941

Michigan Alcoholism Screening Test, 1590

Miconazole
for diaper dermatitis, 1487

Micorlipidsb, 1627t

Microcephaly
with congenital rubella, 1281t

Microchemistry tests, 2

Microcolon
with IDM, 888

Microcystic congenital cystic adenomatous malformation, 190f

Microcystic lymphatic malformation, 1501

Microdeletions
FISH, 141

Microdeletion syndrome, 905–906, 905t

Microencephaly
cytomegalovirus, 1293, 1293f

Micronutrient
absorption, 942

Micronychia, 1504

Micropenis, 919

Microphallus, 1084–1085

Microphthalmia
with congenital rubella, 1281t

Microphthalmos, 1472

Microvillus brush border membrane, 150

Midazolam, 1566, 1697
fetal and neonatal effects, 276
for pain, 1558
for seizures, 1523

Midtrimester amniocentesis, 141–142

Migrant health centers, 33

Milia, 1503

Miliaria, 1492–1493

Milk thistle, 1655

Milrinone, 1535
for low cardiac output, 740

Mineral
requirements, 387–391

Mineral homeostasis disturbances
skeletal manifestations of, 869–870

Mineralocorticoid insufficiency, 929

Mineralocorticoids, 926

Minerals
absorption, 942
fetal growth, 497

Mineral status
newborn monitoring, 406

Minimal observed metabolic rate (MOMR), 452–453

Minolta Air Shields jaundice meter, 814

Misoprostol
fetal effects, 237t, 247

Mission statement
developing, 64

Mobius syndrome
with cocaine exposed infants, 1584

Moderately repetitive DNA, 131

Modified Blalock-Taussig shunt, 749–750, 749f

Modified ultrafiltration (MUF)
for CPB adverse effects, 735

Molecular genetics, 131–135

Molybdenum
recommended intake for preterm infants, 400t

Molybdenum cofactor deficiency, 971, 971t

Monitor artifacts, 45

Monocytes, 1136, 1139–1140

Monoiodotyrosine (MIT), 931

Monosomy X (Turner syndrome)
associated with congenital heart disease, 717t

Monozygote twinning, 1679

Moral deliberation, 9–11

Morbidities, 35–37

Moricizine
neonates, 1518t

Moro reflex
examination, 348t

Morphine, 1560, 1697
adverse effects, 1574t
breast feeding, 278–279
dosage, 1563t
fetal breathing, 537
following congenital heart surgery, 738
glucuronidation, 1510
for pain, 1558

Mortality
decline by birth weight, 460t

Motilin, 943–944
with diarrhea, 954

Motion sickness
transport team, 45

Motor activity
examination, 348t

MRI
  computed tomography, 999
Mucopolysaccharidosis type 1, 636t
Mucormycosis, 1256
Mucosa-associated lymphoid tissues,
      1152–1153
Mucosa-associated lymphoid tissues
      (MALT), 1152f
Mucosal immunity, 1153f
Mucosal injury disorders, 953–954
Mullerian aplasia, 1679
Müllerian duct aplasia, renal aplasia, and
      cervicothoracic somite
      malformations (MURCS
      association), 1091
Mullerian inhibiting substance (MIS),
      915
Multicystic dysplastic kidneys, 178, 1070f,
      1071f
Multicystic kidney disease, 1069–1070
Multifactoral model of inheritance,
      899–900, 900t
Multifetal pregnancies, 9
Multifocal cerebral necrosis, 1393
Multifocal nephroblastomatosis, 1451
Multiple births
  incidence, 36
  resuscitation, 324–325
Multiple carboxylase deficiency, 194, 972
Multiple congenital malformations, 893
  treatment, 895t
Multiple gestation
  antepartum complications, 525
  antepartum management, 525–526
  asphyxia, 528–529
  birth statistics, 529t
  congenital anomalies, 529–530
  growth, 529
  labor and delivery, 526
  mortality, 526–527
  neonatal disorders, 530–531
  placentation, 525
  postnatal care, 531
  stuck twin, 528
Multiple gestations, 523–531
  epidemiology, 523–524
  reproductive technology, 524
Multiple red-blue nodules (blueberry
      muffin baby), 1502
Mumps virus, 1332t
MURCS association, 1679
Murmurs, 344, 647–648
  examination, 346t
Muscle relaxants, 1537–1538
Musculoskeletal system
  anomalies of, 1429–1439
  examination, 345–347
  generalized anomalies, 1439
Myasthenia gravis
  maternal, 1156t
Mycolog II
  for diaper dermatitis, 1487
Mycophenolate
  with heart transplantation, 760
Mycoplasma hominis, 1243
Mydriasis, 339

Myelodysplasia
  urologic aspects of, 1090
Myelomeningocele, 1418–1419, 1420f,
      1431–1432
  dislocated hip with, 1432
Myocardial infarction
  during pregnancy, 215–216
Myocardial systolic dysfunction
  with cardiopulmonary bypass, 735
Myoglobinuria-hemoglobinuria, 1013

N
N-acetylprocainamide (NAPA), 1520
N-acetyl transferase 2, 1510t
Nafcillin, 1526, 1697
Nail-patella syndrome, 1681
Nails
  development of, 1485–1486
Nalbuphine
  fetal and neonatal effects, 267
Naloxone hydrochloride (Narcan), 1697
  for arrhythmias, 1519t
  fetal and neonatal effects, 268
  with resuscitation, 314
Naphthalene
  causing hemolytic anemia, 1185
Naprosyn
  doses, 1565t
Narcotics, 1573t
  adverse effects, 1574t
  history, 1573t
  withdrawal
    infants, 30–31
Nasal continuous positive airway pressure
      (NCPAP), 542, 580
  for ELBW, 465
Nasal obstruction
  surgery, 1101–1102
Nasal pyriform aperture stenosis, 1101
Nasal ventilation
  for ELBW, 465
Nasolacrimal obstruction, 1477
National Aeronautics and Space Agency
      (NASA), 55
National Health Planning and Resources
      Development Act (Public Law
      93064), 3
National Health Service Corps, 33
National Institute of Child Health and
      Development Neonatal Research
      Network, 82, 472
National Institute of Child Health and
      Human Development (NICHD),
      189
National Practitioner Data Bank, 100
Natural monozygotic twins, 523
NCPAP
  for BPD, 588, 593
Near term infants
  breast feeding, 437
  phototherapy, 833
Neck
  anomalies of, 1429–1430
  physical examination, 1428
Neck masses
  surgery, 1099–1100

Necrotizing enterocolitis, 949–950,
      1121–1122, 1121f, 1485, 1622
  in ELBW, 477–478
  fluids and electrolytes, 374
  human milk, 421–422
  multiple gestation, 530
  postsurgical complications, 950
Necrotizing fasciitis, 1256
Negligence
  elements of, 93f
Neisseria gonorrhoeae, 214t
  preterm delivery, 205
Nelfinavir
  pregnancy, 1320t
Nellcor N-400/FS 14 fetal pulse oximeter,
      263
Neo-calglucon, 1697
Neocate
  for short bowel syndrome, 952
Neomycin, 1697
Neonatal alloimmune neutropenia,
      1203–1205
Neonatal alloimmune thrombocytopenia,
      1195–1197
Neonatal and perinatal specialists
  board certified, 26f
Neonatal antiarrhythmic drugs, 696t–697t
Neonatal autoimmune neutropenia, 1205
Neonatal autoimmune thrombocytopenia,
      1197–1198
Neonatal Behavioral Assessment Scale, 1588
Neonatal biliary atresia, 958–959
Neonatal Brazelton Assessment Scale
      (NBAS), 1585
Neonatal care, 353–359
  delivery costs, 27–33
  physician and hospital capacity, 26t
Neonatal cholestasis
  etiology of, 800t
Neonatal cholestatic syndrome, 1125
Neonatal diabetes mellitus, 883–884
Neonatal endocrine disorders, 914–937
Neonatal erythrocytes, 1190
Neonatal ethics
  landmark cases, 10t
Neonatal glucose requirements, 879–884
Neonatal hemochromatosis, 974t, 975
  with liver disease, 960
Neonatal hepatitis, 958–959
  vs. biliary atresia, 958–959
Neonatal herpes simplex virus
  localized cutaneous, 1288f
  signs and symptoms, 1288f
Neonatal hospital bed capacity, 25–26
Neonatal hyperbilirubinemia
  AAP guidelines for, 812t
  breast feeding, 812–813
  diagnosis, 802t
  epidemiology of, 792–793
  identification, 811–815
  prenatal testing, 812–813
  prevention, 811–815
  primary prevention, 812–813
  treatment of, 811–815
Neonatal hyperglycemia, 883–884
Neonatal hyperthyroidism, 193

Neonatal hypoglycemia, 879–880
Neonatal illness
    effect on nutrition requirements,
        391–392
Neonatal immune thrombocytopenia,
    1195–1199
Neonatal intensive care unit (NICU), 4
    care organization, 76–79
    global comparison, 9
Neonatal iron storage disease
    with liver disease, 960
Neonatal jaundice
    cephalocaudal progression of, 813–814
    clinical approach to, 792–798
    clinical assessment, 813–814
    epidemiology of, 793t
    ethnicity, 793–794
    genetics, 793–794
    hospital policy, 818
    identification of, 813–814
    labor and delivery, 794
    maternal factors, 794
    natural history of, 798–799
    parental information, 820
    phototherapy, 832f
    physiologic mechanisms of, 773–774
    physiology, 773t
    treatment of, 825–826
Neonatal leukemoid reactions, 1209
Neonatal lupus erythematosus (NLE), 1491
Neonatal lupus syndrome, 210
Neonatal medicine pack, 49t
Neonatal mortality, 34f
    race, 34f
    rates of, 1633f
    smoking, 23
Neonatal mortality rate (NMR), 33–34
Neonatal narcotic withdrawal
    severity assessment of, 31t
    treatment, 31t
Neonatal narcotic withdrawal or
        abstinence syndrome, 1577–1578
    complications, 1578
    long term outcome, 1579–1580
    manifestations, 1578t
    mortality, 1578
    neurobehavioral abnormalities,
        1578–1579
Neonatal nurse practitioners
    neonatal transport, 42
Neonatal nurse practitioners (NNP)
    NICU, 76
Neonatal ophthalmia, 1258–1259
Neonatal-perinatal medicine (NPM)
    goals, 8
Neonatal-perinatal tree, 2f
Neonatal pharmacology, 1507–1511
Neonatal respiratory effort
    patterns of, 334t
Neonatal respiratory therapy pack, 48t
Neonatal Resuscitation Program guidelines,
    18
Neonatal seizures, 1385–1388
    clinical features, 1385–1386, 1385t
    diagnosis, 1387
    etiology, 1386–1387, 1386t

prognosis, 1386t, 1387–1388
    treatment, 1387
Neonatal sensory systems
    maturation, 112
Neonatal small left colon
    with IDM, 888
Neonatal surgery, 2
Neonatal thrombocytopenia
    etiology, 1195t
Neonatal thyrotoxicosis, 193, 937
Neonatal transport, 40–52
    administrative personnel, 40–44, 41f
    communication, 43
    documentation, 47
    eliminating physician attendance, 42–43
    environmental factors, 44, 44t
    finances, 43–44
    history of, 40
    legal considerations, 50–51, 51f
    nursing pack, 47t
    organization and administration, 40
    personnel proficiencies, 43
    psychosocial considerations, 49
    quality assurance, 48
    referring hospital personnel, 49
    return, 51–52
    technical aspects, 44–47
    vehicles, 46–47
Neonatal tricuspid valve regurgitation,
    699
Neonatal viral myocarditis, 694–695
Neonate
    bile pigment metabolism, 770f
    bilirubin metabolism, 770–772
    neurobehavioral assessment, 1585–1586
Neonates
    glucose turnover, 879f
Neonatologist
    birth per, 27t
    total births, 28f
Neonatologist workforce
    size and effectiveness of, 26–27
Neonatology
    branches, 2–3
    future, 4–6, 5t
    past, 1–2, 5t
    present, 2, 3–4, 5t
    scope and organization, 24–38
Neoplasia, 1444–1459
    epidemiology, 1444
    treatment, 1458
Neostigmine, 1697
    for neuromuscular junction disorders,
        1406
NephrAmine, 394
Nephroblastomatosis, 1082, 1451–1452
Nephrocalcinosis, 1026–1027
    premature infants, 1027
Nephrogenesis, 1067
Nephrogenic defect
    urinary concentration
        etiology, 1032t
Nephrogenic diabetes insipidus, 1032
Nephrolithiasis, 1026–1027
Nephrotoxicity, 1010–1012
Nephrotoxins, 1011

Nervous system
    examination, 347–349, 348t
Nesidioblastosis, 882
Netherlands
    active euthanasia, 13
Netherton syndrome, 1490, 1490f
Neu-Laxova syndrome, 1677
Neural axis open defect
    treatment, 1417–1422
Neural tube defects, 172
    with cocaine use, 1583–1584
Neural tube defects (NTD), 190–191,
    900
Neuraminidase deficiency, 1038
Neuraxial analgesia
    fetal and neonatal effects, 267–270
Neuraxial anesthesia, 1560–1561
Neuraxial local anesthetics
    fetal and neonatal effects, 270
Neuraxial opioids
    fetal and neonatal effects, 269–270
Neuroblastoma, 1446–1448
    differential diagnosis, 1447
    incidence, 1444
    metastases, 1447
    prognosis, 1447
    surgery, 1447–1448
    treatment, 1447–1448
Neurochemical
    fetal breathing, 289
Neurodevelopmental sequelae, 37
Neurofibromatosis, 636t, 1496
Neurological and neuromuscular disorders,
    1384–1407
Neurologic and Adaptive Capacity Score
    (NACS), 261–262
Neuromuscular blocking drugs
    fetal and neonatal effects, 276
Neuromuscular disorders, 1405
Neuromuscular junction
    disorders, 1405–1407
Neuromuscular maturity
    gestational age assessment, 331
Neuronal necrosis, 776
Neurosurgery, 1410–1425
    pathophysiology of, 1410–1411
Neurosurgical neonate
    prognosis, 1424–1425
Neurotensin, 944
Neutropenia, 1158t, 1201–1202
    associated with immunodeficiency
        syndrome, 1206, 1206t
    infants
        evaluation, 1209
    neonate
        etiology, 1202
    rare causes of, 1203–1205
Neutropenia of prematurity, 1202–1203
Neutrophil disorders, 1200
Neutrophilia, 1209
Neutrophils
    bacterial infection, 1202
    BPD, 582
    decreased production of, 1205
    immature to total, 1705
    increased destruction of, 1203–1204

infants, 1201f
  VLBW, 1201f
Neutrophil transfusion therapy, 1164
Nevirapine, 1321
  with hepatic toxicity, 1319
  pregnancy, 1320t
Nevus achromicus, 1498
Nevus sebaceus, 1503, 1503f
Nevus spilus, 1497
New Ballard Score (NBS), 329
Newborn
  anemia
    workup, 1188–1189, 1189f
  body composition, 362–364
  bonding, 354
  clinical examination, 355
  cold, 358
  digestive and absorptive capabilities,
    381–382
  drying, 354
  eye prophylaxis, 355
  fluids and growth, 355–356
  history of, 328–329
  HIV screening, 19
  hypoglycemia, 358
  identification, 354
  immunology, 1135–1164
  infection control, 354–355
  local bleeding problems, 1193
  moral status of, 12
  neurobehavioral evaluation, 261–262
  neurodiagnostic techniques, 1385
  neurological maturity, 380–381
  neurologic evaluation of, 1384–1385
    history, 1384–1385
    physical examination, 1384–1385
  nutritional capabilities of, 380–382
  nutritional monitoring, 405–406
  screening tests, 355
  security, 354
  skin appearance, 358
  temperature control, 354
Newborn drug therapy, 1507–1543
Newborn ICU design, 64–75
Newborn individualized developmental
    care and assessment program
    (NIDCAP), 480
Newborn mass
  inverse relationship of, 493f
Newborns
  nomogram, 811f
  what to feed, 400–405
Newborn withdrawal
  in infants exposed to alcohol, 1588
New York Heart Association (NYHA)
    functional classification of heart
    disease, 215t
Nicardipine, 1020
Nicotine, 1593
  absorption, 1593
  adverse effects, 1575t
  fetal effects, 237t, 249
  metabolism, 1593
NIC/Q Quality Improvement
    Collaborative, 83
  Vermont Oxford Network, 80t

NICU
  design issues, 67–68
  direct patient care, 68–69
  family centered care, 78–79, 78t, 79f
  family support space, 70
  floor space requirements, 67
  general support space, 69
  infections, 1358t
  lighting, 70, 123f
  location within hospital, 67–68
  outcome variability, 82–83
  quality improvement, 79–87
  reception area, 68
  security, 68
  staff support space, 69–70
  surface finishes, 71
  tactile intervention, 113–114
  touch and handling, 113
  vestibular experience, 115
NICU staff nurses
  neonatal transport, 42
Niemann-Pick disease
  with liver disease, 960
Niemann-Pick disease type C, 974t, 975
Nifedipine
  complications of, 204t
  fetal effects, 235t, 242
  during pregnancy, 207
Nightingale, Florence, 1
Nijmegen breakage syndrome, 1211
9alpha-fludrocortisone (Florinef)
  for adrenal insufficiency, 931
9p-syndrome, 1677
Nipples
  examination, 342
  nonnutritive sucking, 114–115
Nipple shield, 433, 435
Nissen fundoplication, 1113f
  esophageal anomalies
    for gastroesophageal r8eflux, 947
Nitric oxide, 984
Nitric oxide (NO), 295, 296f, 1539
  for PPHN, 568–569
  for pulmonary hypertension, 743
  RDS, 562
Nitric oxide synthase (NOS), 295
Nitroblue tetrazine test, 1160
Nitroblue tetrazolium test, 1244
Nitrogen
  fetal growth, 497–498
  SGA, 498
Nitroglycerin, 657t
Nitroprusside, 657t, 1697
Nitrosourea
  maternal exposure to, 1446
Nitrous oxide
  fetal and neonatal effects, 267
No breast milk
  defined, 415t
Nodules, 1501–1502
Noises
  neonatal transport, 45
Nonfat dry weight
  gestational age, 494f
Nonionizing radiant energy
  IWL, 365

Nonketotic hyperglycinemia (NKH), 139,
    971, 971t
Nonlinear (Michaelis-Menten) kinetics,
    1514f
Nonnarcotic abstinence syndrome, 1580
  differential diagnosis, 1582
Nonnarcotic drugs, 1580t
Nonnarcotic hypnosedatives, 1580
Nonnarcotic withdrawal
  neonates, 32
Non-nucleoside reverse transcriptase
    inhibitors
  pregnancy, 1320t
Nonnutritive sucking, 114–115
Nonoliguric renal failure, 1004
Nonphysician personnel
  neonatal transport, 42
Nonphysician personnel director
  neonatal transport, 41
Nonphysician providers (NPP)
  physician liability arising from, 100, 101t
Nonsteroidal anti-inflammatory agents,
    1012–1015
Nonsteroidal antiinflammatory drugs
    (NSAIDs), 1564
  breast feeding, 279
  doses, 1565t
Nonstress test (NST), 180
Nonviral perinatal infections, 214t
Noonan syndrome, 636t
  associated with congenital heart disease,
    717t
Norepinephrine, 447f, 1582
Norfloxacin
  fetal effects, 241
Normeperidine
  fetal and neonatal effects, 267
North American Pediatric Renal Transplant
    Cooperative Study, 1013
Northern blotting, 132, 134
Norwood operation, 749, 754–757, 754f
  arterial oxygen saturation, 755f
  pulmonary to systemic flow ratio, 756f
  superior vena cava saturation, 756f
Nose
  examination, 339–340
Nosocomial infections
  rate of, 1358–1359
Nosocomial Sepsis Prediction (NOSEP),
    1358
Nucleoside analogues, 1319
Nurse educator
  NICU, 76
Nurse manager
  NICU, 76–77
Nurses
  with respiratory problems, 619
Nursing work area
  lighting, 70
Nutramigen
  for formula protein induced
    enterocolitis, 955
Nutrient delivery, 392–400
Nutrition, 380–406
  BPD, 583
  past, present, future, 5t

Nutritional values, 1701–1702
Nystatin, 1697
  for diaper dermatitis, 1487
Nystatin (Mycostatin)
  for necrotizing enterocolitis, 1121–1122

O

Obesity
  with IDM, 888
Obstetric and neonatal care
  expenditures for, 24
Obstetric palsy, 1440–1441
Obstructive jaundice, 1125–1126
  with congenital rubella, 1281t
Obstructive uropathy, 177
Occipital frontal circumference (OFC), 332
Occlusive plastic blankets, 454, 454f
Occult hemorrhage
  before birth, 1172–1173
Ochoa urofacial syndrome, 1079
Octreotide, 1698
Ocular herpetic infection
  neonate, 1288
Oculocerebrorenal Lowe syndrome, 1031
Odors
  abnormal, 976
Ofloxacin
  fetal effects, 241
Olfaction
  development of, 117
Oligoanuria, 1010
  and acute renal failure, 1000–1010
  general approach, 1002
Oligohydramnios, 168f, 169, 173, 179, 187f
Oligonucleotide probes, 132
Omenn's syndrome, 1211
Omeprazole
  for gastroesophageal reflux, 946
Omphalocele, 176f, 177f, 945, 1127–1128,
    1128f
  fluids and electrolytes, 374
Omphaloceles, 175–176
Ophthalmia neonatorum, 1476–1477
Opiates, 1573t
Opioid anesthesia, 1560
Opioids, 1561–1562
  administration modes, 1562f
  airway resistance, 1563
  chest-wall rigidity, 1563
  dependence, 1563
  dosage, 1563t
  elimination half-lives, 1560t
  side effects, 1562
  tolerance, 1562, 1563
  weaning from, 1563f
Opitz-Frias syndrome, 1677
Opium
  history, 1573t
Optic nerve
  hypoplasia, 1475–1476, 1475f
Oral aversion, 399
Oral communications
  medical confidentiality, 96–98
Oral examination, 340t
Oral feeding, 398–399
Organic acidemia, 966t, 971t

Organic acids, 990
Organification defect, 933–934
Organogenesis, 229, 554f
Ornithine transcarbamylase deficiency
  with liver disease, 960
Orofacial digital syndrome, 1681
Oropharyngeal obstruction
  surgery, 1102
Orotracheal tube
  depth of insertion, 609t
Orthodromic reciprocating tachycardia
    (ORT), 1518
Orthopedics, 1428–1443
  physical examination, 1428–1429
Ortolani Barlow test, 1429, 1429f, 1437,
    1438
Osler-Weber-Rendu, 636t
Osteoclasts
  hypocalcemia, 857t
Osteogenesis imperfecta, 179f, 1439
Osteomyelitis, 1254–1255, 1441, 1442
Osteopenia, 869
  with preterm human milk, 403
  prevention, 870–871
  risk factors, 869t
  treatment, 870–871
Ostomy devices
  with short bowel syndrome, 951
Otitis media, 1263
Oubain
  neonates, 1518t
Outcome measures, 33–35, 81, 81t
Ovarian cancer
  during pregnancy, 216
Ovarian cysts, 1092–1093
Ovarian masses, 1124
Overheating, 455
Overmature gametes
  abortions with, 226
Oxacillin, 1698
Oxazolidine
  fetal effects, 237t, 247
Oxifirst Fetal Pulse Oximetry, 263f
Oxygen
  administration, 602
  for BPD, 588–589
  with BPD, 581–582
  delivery, 601–602
  fetal breathing, 289
  in maternal and fetal blood, 152t
Oxygenation
  optimal levels of, 600–601
  pulmonary vascular conductance, 299
Oxygen consumption
  metabolic rate of, 453f
Oxygen dissociation curve
  normal adult blood, 1190f
Oxygen extraction ratio (OER)
  following congenital heart surgery, 738f
Oxygen therapy, 600–602
Oxytocin, 424, 924–925

P

Pain
  nonpharmacologic techniques, 1564–1565
  perceptionFIRST page, 1558

Pain control, 18, 264–266
Pain medications
  breast feeding, 278–279
Palate
  cysts, 340t
Palivizumab, 1698
Palliative care, 18
Pallister-Hall syndrome, 1679
Pancake kidneys, 1068
Pancreatic disorders, 957–958
Pancuronium, 1537–1538, 1698
  hyperbilirubinemia with, 797, 809
Pancytopenia, 1211–1212
Papillomaviruses, 1332t
Paracervical block
  fetal and neonatal effects, 267
Parainfluenza viruses, 1366–1367
Parasagittal cerebral injury, 1393
Parathormone
  with IDM, 887f
Parathyroid hormone, 989
Parathyroid hormone (PTH), 367
  calcium and magnesium control,
    849–851
  hypocalcemia, 857t, 858
Paregoric, 1698
  for narcotic withdrawal, 30–31
Parental counseling
  cordocentesis, 144
Parental information
  neonatal jaundice, 820
Parental permission, 14
Parent education and counseling
  space for, 70
Parenteral amino acids
  toxicity, 396
Parenteral fluid therapy
  blood sampling, 375
  intravenous fluid infusion,
    375–376
  technical aspects of, 375–376
Parenteral nutrition, 393–394
  delivery routes, 393–394
  indications for, 393
  with liver disease, 960
Parenteral nutrition hepatobiliary tract
    disease
  with short bowel syndrome, 953
Parent-Infant Bonding, 3
Parents
  communication with, 107–108
  decision making, 14
  with respiratory problems, 619–620
Pareto analysis, 86
Partial aneusomies, 904–905
Partial breast milk
  defined, 415t
Partial gonadal dysgenesis, 917
Partial thickness burns
  from phototherapy, 834–835
Partial trisomy 10q syndrome, 1678
Partitional calorimetry
  convection warmed incubators, 448f
  preterm infants, 451f
  servocontrolled radiant warmers,
    452f

Parvovirus B 19, 213t, 1186, 1302–1303, 1367
  fetal infection, 1303–1304
  maternal infection, 1302–1303
  prevention, 1304–1305
Passive euthanasia, 13
Patent ductus arteriosus (PDA), 688–689, 723, 732, 760
  with congenital rubella, 1281t
  with ELBW, 467–468
Patent omphalomesenteric duct, 1127
Patent urachus, 1079, 1127
Patient dumping, 91
Patient education
  NICU, 79
Patients
  information transfer to, 90
Patient satisfaction measures, 81, 81t
Patient-triggered ventilation, 612–613
Pavlik harness, 1438
Payers
  of perinatal care, 31
PCA narcotic administration
  factors influencing fetal drug levels, 267f
PCR
  for herpes simplex virus, 1285
  for neonatal HSV, 1289
Pediatric acquired immunodeficiency syndrome, 1158t
Pediatricians
  birth per, 27t
PEEP
  for FRC, 580
Peginterferon
  for hepatitis C, 1312
Penicillin, 1698
  fetal effects, 241
Penicillin G, 1236
  fetal effects, 234t
  for syphilis, 1251
Penile agenesis, 1084, 1085f
Penile duplication, 1084
Penta x syndrome, 1678
Pentobarbital, 1566
Percutaneous central venous catheter
  for ELBW, 465
Percutaneous umbilical blood sampling (PUBS), 143
Perfluorocarbon-filled ventilator circuit, 619
Performance improvement, 101–109
Perimortem Cesarean section, 275
Perinatal asphyxia, 373–374, 1002
Perinatal care
  major payers of, 31
Perinatal health outcomes
  racial and ethnic disparities, 24
Perinatal infections, 212–213
Perinatal mortality rate, 34–35
  race, 35f
Perinatal pneumonia
  with PPHN, 570–571
Perinatal viral infections, 213t
Perinatology, 2–3
Periodic breathing, 538–539
Peripheral leukocyte count, 1244

Peripherally inserted central catheter (PICC), 393
Peripheral nerve disorders, 1405
Peritoneal dialysis, 1007
Peritonitis, 1263–1264
Periventricular hemorrhage, 1398f
Periventricular leukomalacia (PVL), 1393–1394, 1396f, 1397f, 1624
  in ELBW, 473–474
Perlman syndrome, 1677
Permanent junctional reciprocating tachycardia (PJRT), 1518
Peroxidase defect, 933–934
Peroxisomal disorders, 967t
Persistent hyperinsulinemic hypoglycemia of infancy, 882
Persistent hyperplastic primary vitreous, 1472
Persistent junctional reciprocating tachycardia, 703
Persistent pulmonary hypertension (PPHN), 565–574, 622, 658t
  classification, 567t
  clinical presentation, 566–567
  etiology, 566
  fast phase, 566
  final phase, 566
  immediate phase, 565
  pathophysiology, 565
  respiratory and metabolic alkalosis, 568
  SGA, 512t
  treatment, 567–568
  in utero circulation, 565
Persistent pulmonary hypertension of the newborn (PPHN), 1539
Persistent pupillary membranes, 1470f
Persistent renal blastema, 1451–1452
Personal information privacy
  telehealth, 57
Pertussis
  treatment, 1263
Pertussis immunization, 1620
Pesticides
  maternal exposure to, 1446
Peters anomaly, 1473
Pfeiffer syndrome, 1423
PGE1
  for congenital heart disease, 713–715
  side effects, 714t
Phagocytic tests, 1160
Phagocytosis, 1138–1139, 1144
  oxygen-dependent systems, 1138–1139
  oxygen-independent systems, 1139
Pharmacists
  NICU, 77–78
Pharyngitis
  with HSV, 1284
Phasic tone
  examination, 348t
Phencyclidine
  adverse effects, 1575t
  breast feeding, 439
  breast milk, 1687
  long-term outcome, 26
  neurobehavioral effects, 26

Phencyclidine (PCP), 25
  incidence, 25
  mode of action, 25
  placental transfer, 25
Phenindione
  breast milk, 1689
Phenobarbital, 1566, 1698
  breast milk, 1689
  causing neonatal hypocalcemia, 859
  fetal effects, 237t, 248
  for hyperbilirubinemia, 838
  for neonatal seizures, 1387
  for nonnarcotic withdrawal, 32
  for seizures, 1521
Phenobarbital-phenytoin, 1581
Phenolic detergents
  bilirubin, 797
Phenotypic sex disorders, 917–919
Phenylephrine, 657t
Phenylketonuria, 977
  maternal medications, 230–231
Phenytoin, 696t, 1698
  causing neonatal hypocalcemia, 859
  Michaelis-Menten kinetics, 1513
  for seizures, 1521–1522
Phenytoin (Dilantin)
  congenital anomalies with, 899t
Phosphate, 989–990
  for adrenal insufficiency, 930
Phosphodiesterase inhibitors, 1535
Phosphofructokinase deficiency, 805
Phospholipase
  fat absorption, 941
Phospholipid
  synthesis, 558
Phospholipids
  fat absorption, 941
Phosphorous
  absorption, 942
Phosphorus
  ELBW, 471
  hypocalcemia, 857t, 858
  for osteopenia, 870
  requirements, 387
  TPN, 395
Photooxidation, 831
Phototherapy, 828–836
  biologic effects of, 834–835
  blood flow, 835–836
  breast cancer, 826–827
  cell damage, 836
  clinical use of, 832
  complications of, 834–835
  Crigler-Najjar syndrome, 836
  determining dose, 828t
  diarrhea, 836
  efficacy of, 832
  eye damage, 835
  factors affecting dose and efficacy, 829t
  full term infants, 833
  guidelines for, 821t, 823t
  hydration and feeding, 834
  insensible water loss, 835
  intermittent *vs.* continuous, 834
  intravenous alimentation, 836

Phototherapy (*contd.*)
  irradiance, 830–831, 830f
  light sources, 832–833
  light spectrum, 829–830
  measuring dose of, 833–834
  mechanism of action, 831
  near term infants, 833
  neonatal jaundice, 832f
  preterm delivery, 834
  radiometric quantities, 829t
  readmitted for, 826t
  risks, 823–828
  spectral power, 830
  sunlight exposure, 836
  terminology, 829–830
  thermal regulation, 835
Phototoxicity
  in animals, 123
Phrenic nerves
  following congenital heart surgery, 747
Phthalate plasticizers necrolysis
  neonates, 1517
Physical assessment, 327–349
Physical maturity
  gestational age assessment, 331–332
Physician and hospital capacity
  neonatal care, 26t
Physicians
  liability arising from NPP, 100, 101t
Physiologic hypogammaglobulinemia,
    1155
Physiologic jaundice, 773–774
Physiology, 1
Physiology of the Newborn Infant, 1
Phytonadione, 1698
Picture archiving and communication
    systems (PACS), 55
Pierre Robin sequence, 637t, 907
  surgery, 1098–1099
Pierre Robin sequence (PRS)
  surgery, 1102
Pigmentary retinopathy
  with inborn errors of metabolism, 977t
Pigmentation disorders, 1496–1497
Pilocarpine
  fetal breathing, 537
Pilonidal sinus, 345
Pimecrolimus
  for psoriasis, 1488
Pink tets, 719
Piperacillin, 1525, 1698
Pitressin
  for DI, 925
Pituitary disorders, 923
  diagnosis, 924
  treatment, 924
PKU, 978
Placenta, 149, 150f
  active transport, 152–153
  barrier, 150f
  circulation, 299
  clues for gestational history, 328–329
  continuous breathing, 290–292
  diabetes mellitus, 159–160
  diffusion, 150–152, 151t
  as endocrine organ, 154–156

erythroblastosis, 160
estrogen, 155, 156f
facilitated diffusion, 152
fetal breathing, 292f
flow, 151f
hormones produced during pregnancy,
    155f
lactogen, 155
maternal blood supply to, 158f
maternal medications, 230, 231
metabolism, 154
physiology in disease states, 158–162
preeclampsia, 158–159
progesterone, 155–156, 156f
receptor mediated endocytosis, 153–154
with syphilis, 1249
transfer, 149–154
TTTS, 160–162
weights, 501f
Placental insufficiency
  maternal drug use, 1573
Placental metabolism, 154
Placental progesterone deficiency
  abortions with, 226t
Placental transfer, 149–154
  active transport, 152–153
  diffusion, 150–152, 151f
  facilitated diffusion, 152
  receptor-mediated endocytosis, 153–154
Placenta previa
  with intrapartum asphyxia, 308t
Placentation
  multiple gestation, 525
Plan do study act (PDSA), 87
Plantar surface
  assessment of, 331
Plasma aldosterone, 987
Plasma component transfusion, 1164
Plasma creatinine
  fetal lambs, 285f
  premature infants, 372f
Plasma derivatives
  transfusion, 1217
Plasma renin activity, 997
Plasmids, 135
Plastic blankets
  IWL, 366
Plastic heat shields, 454
Platelet-activating factor (PAF)
  human milk, 422
Platelet disorders, 1195–1200
Platelets
  decreased production of, 1198–1199
Platelet-specific alloantigens, 1196t
Platelet transfusion, 1214–1215, 1215t
Plexiglass heat shields
  IWL, 366
Pluralistic democracy, 9
PMI, 346t
Pneumococcal
  immunization, 1620
Pneumocystis carinii, 1261
Pneumocystis carinii, 1322, 1323
Pneumocystis jiroveci, 1322, 1323
Pneumonia
  pathogens of, 570t

pathologic findings, 571
  with PPHN, 569
  treatment, 1263
Pneumopericardium
  with assisted ventilation, 618–619
Pneumoperitoneum, 1114
Pneumothorax
  with assisted ventilation, 618–619
Point of maximal impulse (PMI), 344
Poland anomaly, 1679
Polio immunization, 1620
Polycosea, 1627t
Polycystic kidney disease, 1017, 1677
Polycythemia, 805–806
  neonate, 1189, 1189t
  SGA, 512t
Polycythemia hyperviscosity syndrome
  with hypoglycemia, 883
Polycythemia-hyperviscosity syndrome
  SGA, 515
Polydactyly, 1432
Polyhydramnios, 175, 525, 528, 1108
  with diabetic pregnancies, 208
Polymerase chain reaction (PCR), 132,
    134, 134f
Polymorphonuclear leukocytes
  adherence, 1137–1138
  chemotaxis, 1137–1138
  motility, 1137–1138
  neonates
    diagnostic tests, 1161t
Polymorphonuclear leukocyte storage
    pools, 1137
Polymorphonuclear leukocyte transfusion,
    1164
Polypeptide (PP), 957
Polysplenia syndrome, 677t
Polyuric phase, 1007
Popliteal angle
  determination of, 331
Positional calcaneovalgus foot, 1435
Positional cloning, 135
Positive end-expiratory pressure (PEEP), 562
Positive pressure ventilation (PPV)
  RDS, 561
  resuscitation, 310–311
Positive support
  examination, 348t
Possetting, 357
Postdischarge, 360–361
  timing and planning, 360–361
Postdischarge medical care, 1618–1629
  feeding problems, 1619–1620
  immunization, 1620–1621
  specialized care, 1621–1622
Posterior laryngeal cleft, 1103
Posterior pituitary disorders, 924–926
Posterior segment
  examination of, 1470–1471
Posterior urethral valves, 1079–1080, 1081f
Posthemorrhagic hydrocephalus (PHH),
    1399, 1412–1413
Postnatal breaths
  mechanics of, 292–294
Postnatal care
  multiple gestation, 531

Postnatal pneumonia, 571
Postnatal serum evolution, 996f
Postneonatal mortality, 34f
Postneonatal mortality rate (PNMR), 33
Postpartum pain management, 278–279
Postrenal failure, 1010
Postural tone
  examination, 348t
Posture, 334
Potassium, 371, 987–988
  maintenance requirements of, 369–370
  in preterm infant formulas, 404
  requirements, 387
POTS (plain old telephone system), 56
Potter sequence, 1679
Poverty, 8
PPHN
  long term outcome, 569
Prader Willi syndrome, 141, 907
Prealbumin, 396
Preauricular tabs and sinuses
  surgery, 1099
Prednisolone, 1541–1542, 1698
Prednisone
  for hypoglycemia, 884
  for toxoplasmosis, 1331
Predominant breast milk
  defined, 415t
Preeclampsia, 206
  fetal effects of, 207
  with intrapartum asphyxia, 308t
  maternal drug use, 1573
  placenta, 158–159
  prostaglandins, 159
  risk factors associated with, 207f
Preferred provider organization (PPO), 99
Pregestational diabetes mellitus, 208–209
Pregestimil
  for formula protein induced
      enterocolitis, 955
  for intractable diarrhea of infancy, 955
  for short bowel syndrome, 951–952
Pregnancy
  active immunization, 1163
  antihypertensive agents during, 207
  antiretrovirals, 1320t
  diabetes mellitus during, 207–209
  hepatitis A, 1306
  HIV screening, 19
  lifestyle choices, 36–37
  maternal metabolism during, 876–877
  medications
    adverse effects, 228
  outcome vs. time from conception, 225t
  RA 27/3 attenuated live rubella virus
      vaccine, 1279
  resuscitation, 274–275
  rubella, 1277
  substance abuse, 19
  surgery during, 272–274
Pregnancy associated plasma protein A
    (PAPP-A), 136
Pregnancy induced hypertension (PIH)
  clinical manifestations of, 206t
Pregnancy Risk Assessment and Monitoring
    System (PRAMS), 414

Preimplantation genetic diagnosis (PGD),
    145
Premature arterial complexes (PAC)
  following congenital heart surgery, 741
Premature fusions
  opening, 1423
Premature infants
  aortic blood pressure, 318f
  apnea, 539t
  breast feeding, 431f
  effect on human milk, 425
  glycogen
    glucose production, 880–881
  low bilirubin kernicterus, 791–792
  multiple gestation, 530
  plasma creatinine, 372f
  postdischarge
    monitoring, 1657
  transepidermal water evaporation, 449f
Premature rupture of membranes (PROM),
    202–203
Premature ventricular contractions (PVC)
  following congenital heart surgery, 742
Prematurity
  caffeine, 27–28
  circulation, 642–643
  in infants of mothers on heroin, 1576
  in neonates exposed to alcohol, 1588
Prenatal alcohol use
  long-term effects of, 1589–1590
Prenatal diagnosis, 130–146, 135–146
  first trimester, 138–140
  gene organization, 130–131
  indications for, 136t
  second trimester, 141–142
  third trimester, 141–142
Prenatal hematopoietic stem cell
      transplantation, 195–198
  diseases amenable to, 196
  donor cells, 196
  hemoglobinopathies, 196–197
  immunodeficiency diseases, 197–198
  inborn errors of metabolism, 198–199
  in utero transplantation, 196, 197t
Prenatal marijuana, 1593
Prenatal testing
  neonatal hyperbilirubinemia, 812–813
Preoperative pulmonary hypertension
  factors contributing to, 743t
Prepuce, 1088
President's Commission, 10t
Pressure regulation vs. volume guidance,
    614
Preterm delivery, 8, 202–205
  incidence, 35, 35f
  multiple gestation, 525
  pharmacologic tocolysis for, 203–204
  phototherapy, 834
  predisposing factors for, 203
  resuscitation, 322–323
  screening for, 204
  smoking, 23
  underlying conditions associated with,
    203t
Preterm discharge formulas, 405
Preterm infant formulas, 403–404

Preterm infants
  breathing, 538
  carbon dioxide response curves, 538f
  nutrient requirements, 382–392
  partitional calorimetry, 451f
  recommended micromineral intakes, 400t
  transfusion guidelines, 1704
  what to feed, 402–405
Preterm milk
  nutrient and mineral content, 386f
  vs. term milk, 416–417, 417t
Primary muscle disorders, 1406
Primary nurses
  NICU, 77
Primary subarachnoid hemorrhage, 1403
Primidone
  breast milk, 1689
Principlism, 11–12
Private health insurance, 31–32
Probiotics
  for short bowel syndrome, 952
Procainamide, 696t
  for arrhythmias, 1519, 1519t
  for JET, 742
  neonates, 1518t
  for supraventricular tachycardia, 704
Process control chart, 86
Process measures, 81t
Professional issues, 8–9
Professional negligence, 92–93
Progesterone
  placenta, 155–156, 156f
Progestins
  fetal effects, 237t, 248
Progressive hydrocephalus, 1640
Proinflammatory cytokines
  BPD, 582
Prolactin, 424
  pulmonary maturation, 559
Prolactin enhancers, 426
Prolonged indirect reacting
      hyperbilirubinemia, 809
Prolonged rupture of membranes
  with intrapartum asphyxia, 308t
Promotility medications, 1528–1530
Propafenone
  neonates, 1518t
Prophylactic phototherapy
  ELBW, 834
Propofol, 1561
  fetal and neonatal effects, 276
Propranolol, 696t, 1698
  for arrhythmias, 1520
  fetal effects, 235t, 242
  neonates, 1518t
  for supraventricular tachycardia, 704, 705
Propylthiouracil (PTU), 212
  for drug-induced neonatal goiter, 934
  for fetal thyrotoxicosis, 193
Prostacycline
  for pulmonary hypertension, 745
Prostaglandin E1, 1538, 1698
Prostaglandin inhibitors, 1538–1539
Prostaglandins, 983–984, 1538
  fetal breathing, 291
  preeclampsia, 159

Prostaglandin synthetase inhibitor, 983
Prostaglandin synthetase inhibitors
  complications of, 204t
Protamine, 1698
Protazoan infection, 1274–1333
Protease inhibitors
  pregnancy, 1320t
Protein
  absorption, 942
  fetal growth, 497–498
  human milk, 417
  in infant formula, 402
  metabolism
    SGA, 514
  in preterm human milk, 403
  in preterm infant formulas, 404
  requirements, 385–387
  SGA, 498
  TPN, 394
Protein binding, 1507
Protein digestion, 381
Protein-energy status
  newborn monitoring, 405–406
Protein synthesis
  gestation, 506f
Proteinuria, 995t, 1040–1043
  differential diagnosis, 1042f
  etiology, 1040–1042
  evaluation, 1040–1042
Proteus
  with pneumonia, 570
Proteus syndrome, 1496
Proton pump antagonists
  for gastroesophageal reflux, 946
Proximal femoral epiphysis fracture, 1440,
  1441f
Proximal femoral focal deficiency,
  1438–1439
Proximal renal tubular acidosis,
  1034–1035
Prune-belly syndrome, 1083, 1090–1091,
  1129f, 1679
Pseudoarthrosis, 1433f
Pseudoephedrine
  breast feeding, 439
Pseudohypoaldosteronism,
  1035–1036
Pseudohypoparathyroidism, 859
Pseudomonas, 571–572
Pseudomonas aeruginosa, 1362
Pseudomonas eye infection, 1259
Pseudomonas septicemia, 1242
Psoriasis, 1488
Psychomotor development
  with infants of drug addicts,
  1579–1580
Psychotherapeutic drugs
  epidemiology, 1572, 1573t
4p-syndrome, 1677
5p-syndrome, 1677
9p-syndrome, 1677
Pulmonary adaptation
  at birth, 285–288
Pulmonary artery band, 750, 750f
Pulmonary artery stenosis, 667
  with congenital rubella, 1281t

Pulmonary atresia, 658t, 667f, 712,
  720–721, 752–753
  clinical findings, 667–668
  differential diagnosis, 668
  with intact ventricular septum, 667, 721,
    753
  pathophysiology, 667
  treatment, 668
Pulmonary hemorrhage, 573–574
  clinical findings, 574
  hyperbilirubinemia, 792
  treatment, 574
Pulmonary hypertension, 396
  with BPD, 585
  following congenital heart surgery and
    treatment strategies, 742–745,
    744t
  following heart transplantation,
    760
Pulmonary interstitial emphysema (PIE),
  466
Pulmonary stenosis, 658t, 665–667
Pulmonary valve and subvalvar stenosis,
  665–667
Pulmonary valve stenosis, 712
Pulmonary vascular conductance, 297f
  oxygenation, 299
  shear stress, 299
Pulmonary vascular resistance (PVR)
  with BPD, 585
Pulmonary vasodilatation, 297–298
Pulmonary vasodilators, 1539–1540
Pulse
  examination, 346t
Pulse oximetry
  for BPD, 588–589
  for ELBW, 466
  historical development, 2
Pupil
  maturation of, 121t
Pupillary response to light, 339
Purine metabolism disorders, 1028
Purpura, 1502–1503
Purpura fulminans, 1502–1503
Purpuric light eruption, 1502
Pustules, 1492–1493
Pyelonephritis, 1258f
  bacteriuria, 1025
Pyloric stenosis, 947–948
  with erythromycin, 1529
  fluids and electrolytes, 374
Pyogenic granuloma, 1500
Pyridoxine, 1699
  for neonatal seizures, 1387
Pyrimethamine, 1699
  for toxoplasmosis, 1328, 1331
Pyruvate kinase deficiency, 805
PYY
  with diarrhea, 954

Q

22q11.s deletion syndrome, 905–906
13q-syndrome, 1677
18q-syndrome, 1677
Quality
  defined, 15

Quality assurance, 90, 101–109
  neonatal transport, 48
  telehealth, 62–63
Quality improvement
  institutional collaboration, 83
  NICU, 79–87
  tools for, 86
  typical measures of, 81t
Quality monitoring
  risk reduction, 103–104
Quality of care
  defined, 79–80
Quality of life standards, 15
Quinidine, 696t
  neonates, 1518t
Quinolones
  fetal effects, 241

R

RA 27/3 attenuated live rubella virus
  vaccine, 1278
Race
  infant mortality, 34f
  neonatal mortality, 34f
  perinatal mortality rate, 35f
Racial and ethnic disparities
  perinatal health outcomes, 24
Radial artery line, 1130
Radial clubhand, 1432
Radiant heat loss
  convection warmed incubators, 450
Radiant warmer
  IWL, 366, 366t
Radiant warmer bed, 451–454
Radiation exposure
  during pregnancy, 217
Radioactive compounds
  breast milk, 1688
Radiocontrast agents, 1012–1013
Radius
  absence of, 1432
  synostosis, 1433–1434
Ramstedt-Fredet pyloromyotomy, 1117,
  1117f
Randomized controlled trials (RCT), 79, 84
Ranitidine, 1528–1529, 1532–1533, 1699
  for gastroesophageal reflux, 946
Ranula, 340t
Rapid cycle continuous quality
  improvement, 86–87, 87f
RDS
  with IDM, 887f
  ventilation, 618f
Reasonableness standards, 15
Rebound phenomenon, 31t
Rebuck skin-window technique, 1160
Receptor mediated endocytosis, 154f
  placenta, 153–154
Recombinant growth factors
  newborn
    randomized trials, 1204t
Recombinant human copper zinc SOD
  (rhSOD)
  for BPD, 594
Recombinant human granulocyte-colony
  stimulating factor (rhG-CSF), 1163

Recombinant human granulocyte-macrophage-colony-stimulating factor (rhGM-CSF), 1163
Recombination fraction, 133
Recombivax HB, 1309
Recurrent apnea
    CPAP for, 606
Recurrent fistulas, 1111
Red cell enzyme deficiency, 803–805
Red cell membrane defects, 803
Red reflex, 339
Reducing substances
    urine testing for, 971
Reductase deficiency, 918
Referring hospital personnel
    neonatal transport, 49
Regional anesthesia, 1560–1561
    fetal and neonatal effects, 276–277
Regional connections, 3
Regionalization, 37–38
Regulatory considerations
    historical overview, 89–90
Religious
    diversity, 11–14
Remifentanil, 1561
    fetal and neonatal effects, 267
Renal agenesis, 1067–1068
    incidence of, 1068
Renal and urinary tract anomalies, 993, 1675–1686
Renal and urinary tract malformations, 992
    infancy, 992t
Renal artery thrombosis, 1009–1010
Renal blood flow, 981–983, 1001
    glomerular filtration rate
        autoregulation, 985–986
Renal blood flow (RBF), 981–983
Renal calculi
    hematuria with, 1083
Renal cystic disease, 1069–1071
    classification of, 1069t
Renal disease, 981–1043, 981–1043
    developmental physiology, 981–991
    embryology, 981
Renal disorders
    during pregnancy, 214–215
Renal ectopia and fusion, 1068
Renal failure
    children, 1014t
Renal function
    imaging and treatment, 1025–1026
Renal function and disease
    clinical evaluation, 992–999
    clinical observations, 995
    genetic, biochemical, and molecular
        diagnosis, 997
    laboratory evaluation, 995–997
    physical examination, 993–999
        vital signs, 993
    pregnancy, 993
    urinalysis, 995
    urine output, 995
Renal malrotation, 1068
Renal nerves
    adrenergic system, 984

Renal obstruction, 1017
Renal pathology, 999–1000
Renal physiology, 981
Renal radionuclide scan, 999
Renal replacement therapy, 1007
Renal response
    acid, 988
Renal thromboembolism, 1016
Renal transplantation, 1015
Renal tubular acidosis, 1033–1034
    infancy, 1034t
    mixed, 1035
Renal tubular dysfunction, 1030
Renal tumors, 1082
Renal-urinary tract malformations
    single signs, 1683–1684
Renal vascular resistance, 982
Renal vascular resistance (RVR), 982
Renal vein thrombosis, 1082, 1221
    hematuria with, 1083
Renal venous thrombosis, 1010
Renin-angiotensin system, 983, 983f
Renovascular hypertension, 1016
Reproductive risks, 225t
Reproductive technology
    multiple gestations, 524
Res ipsa loquitur, 94
Respiration
    detecting onset, 613t
Respiratory acidosis, 372
Respiratory adaptation, 304–305
    at birth, 288–294
Respiratory alkalosis, 372
Respiratory burst, 1138
Respiratory control, 536f
Respiratory distress, 320
Respiratory distress syndrome (RDS), 322, 466, 560–562, 561f
    clinical presentation, 560
    complications, 562
    fluids and electrolytes, 373
    pathology, 560
    pathophysiology, 560–561
    prevention, 561
    surfactant replacement, 559
    treatment, 561–562
Respiratory effort, 334
    examination, 334
Respiratory pattern, 346t
Respiratory problems
    in ICU, 619–620
    treatment, 600–620
Respiratory rate, 335
Respiratory rate vs. tidal volume, 616f
Respiratory specialists
    NICU, 77
Respiratory stimulants, 1540
Respiratory support, 605–619
Respiratory syncytial virus (RSV), 543
    vaccine, 1620–1621
Respiratory syncytial virus immune
    globulin (RSV-IVIG), 1163
Respiratory viruses, 1366–1367
Respondeat superior, 50
Respondeat superior, 99–100
Responsibility, 90

Resting posture
    examination, 348t
Restriction fragment length polymorphism
    (RFLP), 132, 132f
Resuscitation, 353–354
    arterial blood gas, 318f
    asphyxia, 308–316
        clinical assessment, 310
        equipment and supplies, 309–310
        initial steps, 310
    birth injury, 325
    discontinuation of, 316–321
    EKG, 312f
    endotracheal intubation, 312–313
    guidelines for, 17
    hydrops, 323–324
    lowest gestational age, 463
    medications, 313–314
    multiple births, 324–325
    of newborn with airway compromise, 323
    of newborn with surgical condition, 323
    PPV, 310–311
    pregnancy, 274–275
    preterm delivery, 322–323
    reasonable noninitiation, 317
    respiratory status monitoring, 317–318
    supportive care, 317
RetCamII, 60f
Reticular dysgenesia, 1206t, 1207
Retina
    maturation of, 121t
Retinal detachment, 1482
Retinal hemorrhage, 1479f
Retinal telephotoscreening, 59–60
Retinoblastoma, 1448, 1483f
    signs, 1448
    treatment, 1448
Retinoic acid (Accutane)
    congenital anomalies with, 899t
Retinoids
    fetal effects, 237t, 248–249, 249
Retinopathy
    with congenital rubella, 1281t
Retinopathy of prematurity (ROP), 59–60, 61f, 122, 1479–1483, 1481f, 1482f, 1639–1640, 1639f
    classification, 1480–1482
    in ELBW, 478
    examination, 1480
    long term problems, 1482–1483
    pathogenesis, 1480
    postdischarge medical care, 1621
    prevention, 1480
    stages, 1480t
    treatment, 1482
Reverse genetics, 135
Reynell Language Scale, 1589
Rhabdomyosarcoma (RMS), 1455
Rh erythroblastosis fetalis, 799–800
Rheumatoid arthritis, 210–211
Rheumatologic disorders, 209–210
Rh hemolytic disease of the newborn, 786–787, 1177–1180
    clinical manifestations, 1178

Rh hemolytic disease of the newborn (*contd.*)
  intrauterine diagnosis and treatment, 1179–1180
  laboratory findings, 1179
  pathogenesis, 1177–1178
  prevention, 1179
  treatment, 1180
Rh immune globulin
  fetal effects, 237t, 249
Rhinitis
  with syphilis, 1249
Rh isoimmunization, 144
Ribavirin
  for hepatitis C, 1312
Ribosomal RNA (rRNA), 134
Rickets, 869, 870
  monitoring of, 871
  prevention, 870–871
  risk factors, 869t
  treatment, 870–871
Rifampin
  fetal effects, 240
  for GBS, 1240
Right aortic arch
  with anomalous left subclavian artery, 690–691
Right ventricular outflow tract obstruction, 718, 751–753
Risk communication, 106–108
Risk management, 90, 101–109
  establishing program, 102–106
  growth of, 101–102
  plan, 104
  staff education, 104–105
Risk reduction
  quality monitoring, 103–104
Ritonavir
  pregnancy, 1320t
Ritter disease, 1240
Roberts-SC phocomelia syndrome, 1681
Rock, 1582
Rocking chairs, 115
Rooming in
  space for, 70
Ross Laboratories Mothers Survey, 414, 415
Rotational abnormalities, 1115–1116
Rotor wing aircraft
  neonatal transport, 46
RSV immune globulin, 1699
Rubella, 213t, 1477–1478, 1477f
  clinical manifestations, 1277
  congenital anomalies with, 899t
  laboratory diagnosis, 1277–1278
  prevention, 1278–1280
  reinfection, 1278
  treatment, 1278
Rubella (German measles, third disease), 1275–1276
Rubinstein-Taybi, 636t, 1679
Rubinstein-Taybi syndrome, 1503–1504
Rules of evidence, 93
Ruptured membranes
  between 18 and 22 weeks, 463
Russell-Silver syndrome, 907, 1682
Rutledge syndrome, 1677

S
Sabin-Feldman dye test, 1326
Sacrococcygeal teratoma, 1129–1130, 1454f
Saethre-Chotzen syndrome, 636t, 1677
Sagittal synostosis, 1425f
Salicylates
  with hypoglycemia, 883
Salt loss, 929
Sano modification, 756
Saquinavir
  pregnancy, 1320t
SARS, 1367
Satellite DNA, 131
Saturation kinetics, 1513
Scalp
  abscess, 1256
  rugae, 336
Scaly rashes, 1486–1487
Scapula
  physical examination, 1428
Scarf sign, 331
Schaffer, Alexander, 1
Schinzel-Giedion syndrome, 1677
Scintiscan
  for gastroesophageal reflux, 946
Sclerema neonatorum, 1498
Sclerocornea, 1473
Scleroderma, 211
Scoliosis, 1430–1431, 1431f
Scope of practice
  past, present, future, 5t
Screening tests
  Down syndrome, 136
  newborn, 355
Sebaceous gland hyperplasia, 1503
Seborrheic dermatitis, 1487–1488, 1488f
Secondary hypothyroidism, 935
Second trimester
  assessment of, 167–168
  prenatal diagnosis, 141–142
Secretin, 943–944
Secretory diarrhea
  with short bowel syndrome, 953
Secretory IgA, 1155
Secundum venosus atrial septal defects, 684–685, 685f
Sedation, 1565–1566
Seizures
  in ELBW, 474
  neonates, 1521–1523
  postdischarge medical care, 1624–1625
Selective neuronal necrosis, 1392–1393
Selenium
  recommended intake for preterm infants, 400t
  requirements, 389
Self-abusing mother, 1479
Self-healing histiocytosis, 1458
Self-healing reticulohistiocytosis, 1458
Semiocclusive artificial skin, 454
Sensorineural hearing loss
  cytomegalovirus, 1293
  with toxoplasmosis, 1330
Sepsis
  effect on nutritional status, 392
  fluids and electrolytes, 374

  human milk, 420
  jaundice, 809–810
  neonates
    hematologic scoring system, 1230f
Sepsis neonatorum, 1236–1247
  anaerobic infection, 1242–1243
  clinical manifestations, 1238–1240
  coagulase-negative staphylococcal disease, 1240–1241
  coagulase-positive staphylococcal disease, 1240
  enterococcal infection, 1242
  fungal infection, 1243
  genital mycoplasmas, 1243
  gram-negative bacterial infection, 1242
  laboratory tests, 1243–1244
  listeria monocytogenes disease, 1241–1242
  pathogenesis, 1236–1238
  prevention, 1246–1247
  streptococcal disease, 1238–1239
  treatment, 1244–1246
Septic arthritis, 1254–1255, 1441, 1442
Septooptic dysplasia (de Morsier syndrome), 1476
Serotonergic receptors
  brainstem, 536
Serotonin, 1582
Sertoli cells, 915
Sertoli cell tumors, 1089
Serum immunoglobulins
  development of, 1154f
Serum mineral concentrations
  disturbances in, 856–869
Service area
  defining, 65
Servocontrolled incubator homeothermy
  convection warmed incubators, 451
Servocontrolled radiant warmers
  partitional calorimetry, 452f
17alpha-hydroxylase deficiency, 929t
17-hydroxyprogesterone (17-OHP), 192
Severe combined immunodeficiency syndrome (SCID), 197–198, 1158t, 1210
Sevoflurane, 1559, 1559t
Sex chromosomes
  abnormalities of, 903–904
Sex differentiation pathway, 915f
Sexual differentiation
  normal, 914–915
Sexual differentiation disorders, 914–920
SGA
  behavioral observation, 511
  clinical evaluation, 510–511
  clinical problems of, 511–516, 512t
  delivery room evaluation, 510
  delivery room physical examination, 510
  gestational age assessment, 510
  growth and developmental outcomes, 516
  hospitalization, 516
  immune function, 515–516
  inadequate glucose production, 881
  infectious disease, 515–516
  mortality, 511
  neurologic examination, 511

NICU physical examination, 511
under nutrition, 518t
nutritional problems, 514–535
outcomes, 516–519
postnatal neurodevelopmental
outcomes, 517–518
postnatal physical growth, 516–517
vs. preterm birth, 511–512
symmetric and asymmetric growth
restriction, 491
temperature regulation, 515
Shared vision, 64
Shear stress, 296
pulmonary vascular conductance, 299
Shigella
diarrhea, 1260
Short bowel syndrome, 951–952, 1622
complications, 952
Short-rib polydactyly, 1681
Shoulder dystocia, 208
Shoulder girdle
anomalies, 1432–1433
physical examination, 1428
Shprintzen syndrome, 905–906, 1146
Shprintzen velocardiofacial syndrome, 636t
Shwachman syndrome, 957, 1206t,
1211–1212
SIADH, 1004
Sickle cell disease
molecular diagnosis, 144
SIDS
epidemiological risk factors, 547t
Signs, 70
Silicone membrane lung, 626f
Silicone nipple shield, 435f
Single cell diagnosis, 145–146
Single ventricle
palliation, 749
Single ventricle anomalies, 675–676
Sinus arrhythmia, 701
Sinus tachycardia, 701
Sinus venosus atrial septal defects,
684–685
Sirenomelia sequence, 1679
Site visits, 66–67
planning, 66
sample questionnaire, 66–67
Sjogren syndrome, 211
Skeletal dysplasia, 178–179
Skin
development, 1485–1486
developmental anomalies, 1501
in ELBW, 470
examination, 341, 1486, 1486t
function
1-2, 1485–1486
fungal infection, 1256
IWL, 365
metabolic disorders, 1490
nutritional disorders, 1490
phototherapy effects on, 834–835
structure, 1485–1486
Skin appearance
newborn, 358
Skin-associated lymphoid tissues (SALT),
1153

Skins lesions, 1486t
Skin surface servocontrol temperature
convection warmed incubators, 451
Skin to skin care. *See* Kangaroo care
Skin-to-skin care, 425–426, 429, 430f
Sleep cycling
with maternal alcohol, 1588
Sleep disturbances
in infants of drug-dependent mothers,
1576–1577
in infants with drug-dependent mother,
1573
Slovakia
infant mortality, 24
Small eyes, 1472
Small for gestational age (SGA), 169
defined, 490
intrauterine growth restrictions,
490–519
Small intestine
congenital anomalies, 948–949
maturation, 381
Smallpox virus, 1332t
Smith, Clement, 1
Smith-Lemli-Opitz syndrome, 637t, 906,
907f, 976, 1681
Smith-Lemli-Opitz syndrome (SLOS), 195
Smith-Magenis syndrome, 141
Smoking, 1593
fetal effects, 237t, 249
fetus effects, 23–24
incidence, 1594
long-term outcome, 24
neurobehavioral effects, 24
newborn effects, 23–24
placental effects, 23
SIDS, 25
Societal issues, 8–9
Society of Obstetricians and Gynaecologists
of Canada
resuscitation guidelines, 17
Sodium, 986–987
in human milk, 401
maintenance requirements of, 369–370
in preterm infant formulas, 404
requirements, 387
urinary excretion of, 370f
Sodium bicarbonate, 1005
with resuscitation, 314
Sodium deficit
calculation of, 368t
Sodium loss, 929
Sodium thiopental
fetal and neonatal effects, 275
Soft tissue sarcomas, 1455–1456
Somatostatin, 943–944
Sonographic markers
aneuploidy, 137f
Sopite syndrome
transport team, 45
Sotalol, 697t
neonates, 1518t
for supraventricular tachycardia, 704
Southern blot, 132, 133, 133f
SOX9, 914–915
Soy formulas, 402

Space
neonatal transport, 46
Spastic diplegia, 1638f
Special demonstration projects, 33
Spectral irradiance, 451f
Spectral power
phototherapy, 830
Speech defects
with congenital rubella, 1281t
Spina bifida, 172
decision making, 18
Spinal anesthesia, 1560
fetal and neonatal effects, 277
Spinal cord injury, 349, 1423
Spine
congenital anomalies, 1430–1432
examination, 345
physical examination, 1428
Spiramycin
for toxoplasmosis, 1328
Spironolactone (Aldactone), 656t,
1530–1531, 1699
for BPD, 590, 590t
Spitz nevus, 1497
Spleen
palpation, 343
Spontaneous abortion
caffeine, 27–28
etiology, 226t
with maternal alcohol, 1587
with maternal drugs, 224–225, 1583
smoking, 23
Spontaneous activity, 334
Spontaneous errors of development, 227
Sprengel deformity, 1432
SRY, 914–915
S.T.A.B.L.E. (sugar, temperature, artificial
breathing, blood pressure, lab work,
and emotional support), 61
Staff education
risk management, 104–105
Staffing patterns, 65
Staff nurses
NICU, 77
Standard of care, 93
Staphylococcal pneumonia, 1262–1263
Staphylococcal scalded skin syndrome,
1240f, 1255–1256, 1491–1492,
1491f
Staphylococcus, 1441, 1476
Staphylococcus aureus, 571, 1255–1256
lower respiratory tract, 1261
rashes, 1486
Staphylococcus epidermidis, 1235–1236
Staphylococcus pyogenes
rashes, 1486
StAR protein, 929
State
examination, 348t
Static charge sensitive bed
electronic fetal monitoring, 264
Statistical prognosis, 13
Stavudine, 1319
pregnancy, 1320t
Steroidogenic factor 1 (SF-1), 914
Steroidogenic pathway, 192f

Steroids, 1540–1542
Stillbirth
with maternal drugs, 1583
Stinson baby, 10t
Stomach
congenital anomalies, 947–948
maturation, 381
Stooling, 356t
Storage disease
findings suggestive of, 975–976
Store and forward data transmission, 55
Strabismus, 1476
Strategic planning team, 64–65
Streeter syndrome, 1432
Streptococcus, 1441, 1476
Streptomycin
fetal effects, 234t, 240
Stridor
with assisted ventilation, 618
Stuck twin, 325, 528
Subconjunctival hemorrhages, 339
Subcutaneous fat necrosis, 1498, 1498f
Subdural hemorrhage, 1402–1403
Subgaleal hematoma, 338
Subglottic hemangioma, 1103
Subglottic stenosis, 1103
Substance abuse
pregnancy, 19
Succinylcholine
fetal and neonatal effects, 276
Sucking blisters, 1495
Sucking reflex, 380, 943
Sudden infant death syndrome, 244
with infants of drug addicts, 1579
multiple gestation, 531
Sudden infant death syndrome (SIDS),
536, 545–550
ages, 547t
environmental risk factors, 546–548
gene environment interactions, 548–549
maternal drug use, 548
maternal smoking, 548
pathology, 546
physiologic studies, 549, 549t
reducing risk for, 549–550
Sufentanil
fetal and neonatal effects, 267
Sulfacetamide
for neonatal ophthalmia, 1259
Sulfadiazine
for toxoplasmosis, 1328, 1331
Sulfasalazine
breast milk, 1689
Sulfonamides
breast feeding, 439
fetal effects, 241
Sulfotransferase, 1510, 1510t
Sunlight
phototherapy, 836
Superior mesenteric artery
apple peel deformity of, 949
Christmas tree deformity of, 949
Superior vena cava
clotting, 395
Superior venous catheters, 1130
Supernumerary kidneys, 1068

Supernumerary nipples, 342
Supernumerary parts, 1432
Supplemental oxygen
home care, 1626–1627
Suppurative pneumonia, 571–572
Supraventricular tachycardia (SVT),
702–703, 702f, 1518
treatment, 704–705
Surfactant, 558f, 1699
catabolism, 559
composition of, 557–558
lung disease, 559
recycling, 559
replacement, 559–560
secretion, 558, 559
synthesis, 558
Surfactant phospholipids, 557f
Surfactant protein A (SP-A), 557
Surfactant protein B (SP-B), 557
Surfactant protein D (SP-D), 557
Surfactant replacement therapy, 580
Surfactant system, 557–560
Surfactant therapy
for ELBW, 466
Surgery, 1097–1130
fluids and electrolytes, 375
during pregnancy, 272–274
Survanta, 1699
Surviving infants
risk factors for neurologic and cognitive
sequelae, 1635t
Swaddling, 114, 455
for narcotic withdrawal, 31
Swallowing reflex, 943
Swings, 115
Synchronized intermittent mechanical
ventilation (SIMV), 580
Syndactylism, 1432
Syndrome of inappropriate antidiuretic
hormone secretion (SIADH), 925–926
Synophrys, 338–339
Syphilis, 359–360, 1247–1251
clinical manifestations, 1248–1250
diagnosis, 1250–1251
with hepatitis, 960
treatment, 1251
Systemic hypertension
with BPD, 585
ECMO, 629
following heart transplantation, 760
Systemic infection, 1477–1478
Systemic lupus erythematosus (SLE),
209–210
Systemic opioids
labor analgesic techniques, 266–268
Systemic to pulmonary artery shunt,
749–750
Systolic murmur, 358–359

T
Tachyarrhythmia, 701–702
diagnosis, 695t
treatment, 695t
Tacrolimus
with heart transplantation, 760
for psoriasis, 1488

Tactile system, 112–114
development, 112
disturbances, 112–113
intrauterine experience, 113
Talipes calcaneovalgus, 1435f
Talipes equinocavovarus foot, 1436f
Tandem mass spectroscopy, 977
Tandem repeat sequences, 131
TAR syndrome, 1677
Taste
development of, 116–117
Taurine, 153
Tazobactam, 1525
T cells, 1147–1150
T cell system, 1145–1147
maturation, 1148f
^{99}Tc scintiscan
for gastroesophageal reflux, 946
Teams
creating, 64–66
Tearing, 339
Teen birth rates, 25f
Telecardiology, 59
Telehealth
antepartum, 58
business plan, 62
continuing education, 61
economics and evaluation, 57–58
evaluation, 62–63
future implications, 63
history of, 55
implementation, 61–63
malpractice insurance, 57
medicolegal and regulatory issues,
56–57
needs assessment, 62
neonatal applications, 58–61
personal information privacy, 57
program management, 62
quality assurance, 62–63
readiness assessment, 62
technology, 55–56
Telehomecare, 61
Telemedicine, 91–92
Telephone linked care (TLC), 91
Televisitation, 60–61
Temperature
examination, 335
past, present, future, 5t
Temperature control
newborn, 354
Tenofovir, 1319
pregnancy, 1320t
teratogenic potential, 1319
Tension pneumothorax, 317–318
Teratogenesis
mechanisms of, 227t
Teratogens, 899, 899t
Teratology of Fallot, 658t, 662f
Teratoma
incidence, 1444
Teratomas, 1453–1454
Term infants
caloric distribution, 502t
nutrient requirements, 382–392
what to feed, 401–402

Terminology
  bilirubin encephalopathy, 783
  phototherapy, 829–830
Tertiary hypothyroidism, 935
Testicular torsion, 1089
Testicular tumors, 1089
Testis
  examination, 347t
Testosterone, 915
Testosterone biosynthesis defects, 918
Tetanus immunization, 1620
Tetracycline
  fetal effects, 234t
  for neonatal ophthalmia, 1259
Tetracyclines
  fetal effects, 241
Tetrahydrocannabinol, 1592
  placental transfer, 1592
Tetralogy of Fallot, 664f, 665f, 712,
      718–720, 752
  with absent pulmonary valve, 720f
Th1, 1149f
Th2, 1149f
Thalassemia
  molecular diagnosis, 144
Thalidomide
  fetal effects, 238t, 249–250
Thalidomide embryopathy, 1682
Thalidomide induced limb reduction
      defects, 228t
Thanatophoric dysplasia, 1680
Theophylline, 1536–1537
  for AOP, 479
  for BPD, 590–591, 590t
Therapeutic drug monitoring
  neonates, 1515
Therapeutic trials, 1–2
Thermal balance
  delivery suite, 445–446
  drying, 447
  early intervention, 447
  kangaroo care, 447–448
Thermal neutral environment, 445
Thermal neutral environmental
      temperature, 446f
Thermal neutral radiant warming,
      452–453
Thermal regulation, 445–455
  body temperature, 455
  epidermal barrier protection, 454–455
  fever, 455
  heat shielding, 454–455
  historical perspective, 445
Thermal response
  physiology of, 446–447
Thiazides, 1023, 1531, 1532
  for BPD, 590
Thioamides
  fetal effects, 250
Third trimester
  assessment of, 167–168
  prenatal diagnosis, 141–142
13q-syndrome, 1677
Thomas test, 1429
Thoracic lesions
  surgery, 1104–1107

Thoracostomy tube
  with pneumothorax, 619
3beta-hydroxysteroid dehydrogenase
      deficiency, 929t
Thrombocytopenia
  neonates
      evaluation, 1199–1200, 1199f
      premature infants, 1198–1199
      with syphilis, 1250
Thrombocytopenia absent radius, 637t
Thrombocytopenic purpura
  with congenital rubella, 1282t
Thromboembolic disorders, 213–214
  newborn
      clinical presentation, 1219t
Thrombosis, 1217–1222
Thrush, 340t
Thumb
  congenital absence of, 1432
Thymopoietin, 1146
Thyroglossal duct cysts, 1501
Thyroglossal duct remnants
  surgery, 1099
Thyroid
  development of, 931
  function of, 931
Thyroid disorders, 193–194, 211–212,
      931
Thyroid function tests, 931–934
Thyroid gland
  agenesis, 932–933 (See also
      Hypothyroidism)
  dysgenesis, 932–933
Thyroid hormone
  fetal growth, 508
  mean values, 932t, 933t
  resistance to, 934–935
  synthesis, 932f
Thyroid hormones
  pulmonary maturation, 559
Thyroid-stimulating hormone
  mean values, 932t, 933t
  measurements, 933t
  unresponsiveness to, 935
Thyroid stimulating hormone deficiency,
      924
Thyroid stimulating immunoglobulins
      (TSI), 931
Thyrotrophin-releasing hormone, 1655
Thyrotropin-releasing hormone (TRH)
  pulmonary maturation, 559
Thyroxine
  for hypothyroidism, 936
  inborn synthesis errors, 933
Thyroxine-binding globulin (TBG), 931
  deficiency, 936
Tibia
  anomalies, 1436
  anterior bowing, 1436
  bowed, 1437f
Ticarcillin, 1525, 1699
Ticarcillin-clavulanate
  for sepsis neonatorum, 1245
Tidal volume tracings, 614f
Tinidazole
  breast milk, 1689

Tin mesoporphyrin (SnMP)
  for hyperbilirubinemia, 838–839
Title V Maternal and Child Health Block
      Grant Program, 32–33
Tobacco
  maternal exposure to, 1446
Tobramycin, 1699
  fetal effects, 240
Tocolytic agents
  complications of, 204t
  fetal effects, 238t, 250
  for preterm delivery, 203–204
TOF spells, 719
  treatment, 720t
Tolazoline, 1540
Tolectin
  doses, 1565t
Toluene
  fetal effects, 238t, 250
Tongue tie, 341
Tonic neck reflex
  examination, 348t
Topiramate
  for seizures, 1523
Topoisomeras II inhibitors
  maternal exposure to, 1446
TORCH, 1274
Torticollis, 1429, 1430f, 1431f
Torulopsis glabrata, 1243
Total anomalous pulmonary venous return
      (TAPVR), 658t, 673–674, 673f,
      730–731, 757–758
  clinical findings, 674
  differential diagnosis, 674
  pathophysiology, 673–674
  treatment, 674
Total births, 28f
Total body water (TBW)
  growth changes, 363–364
Total breast milk
  defined, 415t
Total liquid ventilation, 619
Total parental nutrition, 1007
Total parenteral nutrition (TPN), 18
  complications, 395–396
  daily requirements of, 395t
  monitoring efficacy and toxicity,
      396–398
  monitoring for, 397t
Total serum bilirubin (TSM), 799f
  laboratory measurements of, 815–826
Touch
  for labor pain, 266
Townes syndrome, 1677
Toxic epidermal necrolysis
  neonates, 1517
Toxic megacolon, 956
Toxoplasma gondii, 214t, 1324–1325, 1325,
      1330
Toxoplasmosis, 144, 1324–1325, 1478, 1478f
      54, 1328
  with hepatitis, 960
  intrauterine infection diagnosis,
      1327–1328
  prevention, 1328–1329
  treatment, 1331–1332

TPA, 1221
Trace elements
    BPD, 583
    requirements, 389
    TPN, 395
Trace minerals
    TPN, 398
Trachea
    occlusion, 189
Tracheal agenesis, 1680
Tracheal obstruction
    surgery, 1103–1104
Tracheal stenosis, 1103–1104
Tracheobronchial ischemia
    following congenital heart surgery, 747
Tracheoesophageal fistula, 947
Tracheomalacia, 1104, 1111
Traction response
    examination, 348t
Traffic patterns, 71
Tranquilizers
    fetal effects, 250–251
Trans-Canada rounds, 61
Transcutaneous bilirubin (TcB) index, 814
Transcutaneous electrodes
    historical development, 2
Transdermal fentanyl, 1561
Transdermal morphine, 1561
Transepidermal water evaporation
    premature infants, 449f
Transepidermal water loss (TEWL), 1485
Transferrin iron complex
    placental transport, 154
    receptor mediated endocytosis, 154
Transfer RNA (tRNA), 134
Transfusion-transmissible virus (TIV),
    1313
Transient acute leukemia, 1450
Transient congenital hypoparathyroidism
    (TCHP), 857
Transient dystonia, 1643
Transient hyperammonemia of the
    newborn (THAN), 968
    with liver disease, 960
Transient hypomotility, 957
Transient leukemia
    Down syndrome, 1208–1209
Transient microscopic hematuria, 1041
Transient myasthenia gravis, 1406
Transient myeloproliferative syndrome,
    1450
    Down syndrome, 1208–1209
Transient neonatal pustular melanosis,
    1493
Transient tachypnea of the newborn (TTN),
    573, 574f
    in infants of drug-dependent mothers,
    1576
Transient vascular lesions, 1499
Translation, 131
Transplacental bacterial pneumonia
    with PPHN, 570
Transplacental viral pneumonia
    with PPHN, 569–570
Transport coordinator
    NICU, 76

Transport disorders, 967t
Transport team
    neonatal transport, 42
    vibration effects, 45
Transposition of the great arteries (TGA),
    658t, 727–729, 728f, 729f, 757,
    758f
Transpyloric tube, 399–400
Transthyretin, 396
Trauma, 1478
Treacher Collins syndrome, 636t, 907, 908f
Treponema pallidum, 214t, 359, 1247–1251
Tretinoin
    fetal effects, 237t
Trichomonas vaginalis
    preterm delivery, 205
Trichosporon beigelii, 1243
Tricuspid atresia, 658t, 669, 669f, 670f,
    729–730, 757
    classification system for, 730t
    clinical findings, 669–670
    pathophysiology, 669
    treatment, 670
Trifluorothymidine
    for neonatal HSV, 1290
Trigger delay, 613f
Trimethoprim-sulfamethoxazole (Bactrim),
    1322
    fetal effects, 241
    for short bowel syndrome, 952
    for toxoplasmosis, 1331
Triploidy syndrome, 1678
Trisomy 13, 902–903, 903f, 903t
    associated with congenital heart disease,
    717t
Trisomy 13
    decision making, 18
Trisomy 18, 903t
Trisomy 18
    decision making, 18
Trisomy 18 (Edwards syndrome), 901–902,
    902f
    associated with congenital heart disease,
    717t
Trisomy 21
    decision making, 18
Trisomy 21 (Down syndrome), 900–901,
    901f
    aneuploidy, 1444–1445
    associated with congenital heart disease,
    717t
    with atrioventricular canal defect,
    732
Trisomy 21 Down syndrome, 637t
Trisomy 18 Edwards syndrome, 637t
Trisomy 13 mosaicism
    with hypoglycemia, 883
Trisomy 9 mosaic syndrome, 1678
Trisomy 13 Patau syndrome, 637t
Trisomy 4p syndrome, 1678
Trisomy 8p syndrome, 1678
Trisomy 9p syndrome, 1678
Trisomy 20p syndrome, 1678
Trisomy 13 syndrome, 1678
Trisomy 18 syndrome, 1678
Tromethamine, 1700

Trophic feedings
    for preterm infants, 400
True hermaphroditism, 917
Truncus arteriosus, 658t, 674–675, 675f,
    731, 759
Tuberous sclerosis, 636t, 1069, 1681
Tubular dysfunction, 1026–1038
Tubular function, 986
Tubuloglomerular feedback, 986
Tumor necrosis factor alpha (TNF alpha),
    1143t
    T cells, 1148
Tumor necrosis factor beta (TNF beta),
    1143t
Tumors
    of neuroepithelial origin, 1446–1447
Turner syndrome, 637t, 903–904, 904f,
    916, 1678
Twenty-four hour potential of hydrogen
    monitoring
    for gastroesophageal reflux, 946
22q11.s deletion syndrome, 905–906
Twin placenta, 160f
Twin presentation, 526t
Twinrix, 1309
Twin-to-twin transfusion, 1173–1174
Twin to twin transfusion syndrome (TTTS),
    525, 527–528
    placenta, 160–162
Tympanocentesis, 1263
Tyrosinemia, 809
    with liver disease, 960

U
U. urealyticum, 1243
    lower respiratory tract, 1261
Ultrasonography
    historical development, 2
Ultrasound
    cytomegalovirus, 1296
Ultrasound fetal indices
    menstrual weeks gestational age, 167t
Umbilical artery catheter
    for ELBW, 465
    mean aortic blood pressure, 319f
Umbilical catheterization
    complications, 604t
Umbilical cord
    bilirubin, 798
    blood gas analysis, 261
    continuous breathing, 290
Umbilical cord clamping, 157–158, 354
Umbilical vessel catheterization
    with resuscitation, 314–315
Umbilical vessels
    Doppler assessment of blood velocities,
    181–182
Umbilic artery catheter
    malposition of, 882
Umbilicus
    abnormalities, 1126–1127
    examination, 343
    granuloma, 1127–1129
    hernia, 1126
    infection, 1126–1127
    opening, 1127f

Uncertain prognosis
strategies for, 13
Unexpected fetal death
with IDM, 887f
Unexplained neonatal hyperinsulinemia, 882
Unexplained neonatal hypoglycemia, 882
Unfractionated heparin, 1220
Uninsured, self-paying patients, 33
United Kingdom
NICU resources, 9
UNSURE (unknown disease, suspected responses), 20
Upper airway obstruction
surgery, 1100–1104
Upper extremities
anomalies, 1432–1433
duplication, 1432
physical examination, 1428
reduction, 1432
Upright suspension
examination, 348t
Urea cycle disorders, 966t, 971t
Ureaplasma urealyticum
with BPD, 582–583
with pneumonia, 570
UrecholineR
for gastroesophageal reflux, 1623
Ureidopenicillin, 1525
Ureteral bud, 1066
Ureteral ectopia, 1072–1073
Ureteral obstruction, 1017
Ureterocele, 1073–1075
Ureteropelvic junction obstruction, 1075–1076
with hydronephrosis, 1075f
Ureterosigmoidostomy, 1078
Ureterovesical junction, 1077f
Ureterovesical obstruction, 1076, 1076f
Ureters
anomalies of, 1071–1083
duplication of, 1071
triplication of, 1071
Urethral duplication, 1087
Urethral valves, 1080
classification of, 1080f
Uric acid, 997, 1037
Uridine diphosphoglucuronosyl transferase (UDPGT), 769, 770f, 1510t
1A1 gene
structure and function of, 771–772, 772f, 772t
inherited unconjugated hyperbilirubinemia inborn errors, 806–808
Urinary acidification, 997
Urinary ascites, 178f, 1080
Urinary concentration and dilution, 991
Urinary infection
hematuria with, 1083
Urinary obstruction
prenatal intervention, 187t
Urinary potassium excretion, 988
Urinary sodium, 987
Urinary tract
kidney imaging, 998
prenatal ultrasonography, 1083

Urinary tract abnormalities, 177
Urinary tract infection, 1090, 1256–1258
clinical manifestations, 1256–1257
diagnosis, 1257
etiology, 1256
jaundice, 809–810
preterm delivery, 205
prognosis, 1257–1258
treatment, 1257
Urinary tract infections
and bacteriuria, 1023–1026
Urinary tract obstruction
hematuria with, 1083
Urination
characteristics, 995
Urine
blood analysis, 1002–1004
drug testing, 29
electrolytes and osmolality, 997
microscopic examination, 997
nonglucose reducing substances in, 971t
Urine and solute excretion
various effect types, 1022t
Urine culture, 1024
Urine output, 1001–1002
Urobilinogen, 797
Urogenital sinus, 1092
US Food and Drug Administration (FDA)
Internet drug prescriptions, 92
Uterine anomalies, 1123–1125
Uterus
duplication of, 1092
UTI
acute stage, 1025

V
Vaccinia virus, 1332t
VACTERL association, 637t
VACTER/VACTERL
associated with congenital heart disease, 717t
Vagina
duplication of, 1092
Vaginal agenesis, 1091
Vaginal anomalies, 1123–1125
Valacyclovir
for herpes simplex virus, 1286, 1286t
for recurrent genital herpes in pregnancy, 1291
Valgancyclovir
cytomegalovirus, 1292
Valproic acid
fetal effects, 238t, 251
Vancomycin, 1526–1527, 1700
bilirubin albumin binding, 781
for lower respiratory tract infection, 1263
Vancomycin-resistant enterococcus (VRE), 1362–1363, 1363–1364, 1526–1527
dendrogram, 1365t
treatment, 1364–1366
Varicella, 1296–1297
congenital anomalies with, 899t
fetal infection, 1297–1298
maternal infection, 1296–1297

neonatal infection, 1298–1299
prevention, 1299–1300
Varicella zoster, 213t
Varicella-zoster immune globulin (VZIG), 1299–1300
Varicella zoster virus (VZV), 1296–1297, 1368
fetal transmission, 1297
immunization, 1620
VARIVAX, 1300
Vascular access, 1130
Vascular compression, 1104
Vascular disruption, 227
Vascular endothelial growth factor (VEGF), 4
Vascular growth, 1499–1500
Vascular malformation, 1456–1457, 1500
Vascular neoplasms, 1456–1457
Vascular resistance
following congenital heart surgery, 740
Vascular rings and slings, 690
Vasoactive intestinal polypeptide
fetal growth, 508
Vasopressin, 924–925, 1700
VATER/VACTERL association, 1680
VE
ventilation model, 614f
Vecuronium, 1538, 1700
Velocardiofacial syndrome, 141, 905–906. *See* DiGeorge syndrome
cardiac disease, 635
Velocardiofacial syndrome (VCF), 1146
Venous malformation, 1500
Venous pulse, 347t
Venovenous catheter, 626f
Ventilation
hybrid patterns of, 617
resuscitation, 315f
Ventilation devices
indications for, 616
Ventilator-associated pneumonia, 1361–1362
Ventral abdominal wall defects, 175–176
Ventral suspension
examination, 348t
Ventricular access device, 1414f
Ventricular hemorrhages, 2
Ventricular premature depolarization, 701
Ventricular septal defect, 682–684, 683f, 684f, 759
Ventricular septal defect (VSD), 358, 710, 720–721, 731–732, 752–753
Ventricular system
enlargement of, 1411–1412
Ventricular tachycardia, 705–706
following congenital heart surgery, 742
Ventricular tap, 1414
Ventriculoamniotic shunts, 188
Ventriculomegaly, 171, 172
Ventriculoperitoneal shunt, 1416f
complications of, 1414
infection, 1414
Ventriculosubgaleal shunt (VSGS), 1414, 1414f
Verapamil, 697t
for arrhythmias, 1520
neonates, 1518t

Vermont Oxford Network
  NIC/Q Quality Improvement
    Collaborative, 80t
Vermont Oxford Network (VON), 81–82,
    85
  outcomes and interventions, 82t
Vermont Oxford Trial Network, 467
Vertebral, anorectal, cardiac,
    tracheoesophageal, renal, radial, and
    limb abnormalities (VACTERRL),
    1091
Very low birth weight infants (VLBW), 332,
    459
  ancillary costs, 30t
  costs, 29t
  glucose infusion rates, 885f
  human milk fortification for, 427–429
  incidence, 35f
  length of stay, 29t
  pathogens, 1237t
Very premature infant
  hyperglycemia, 883
Vesicles, 1492–1493
Vesicoamniotic catheter shunt, 187
Vesicoamniotic shunt, 187f
Vesicoureteral reflux, 1071, 1076–1077
Vestibular system, 115–116
  development, 115
  disturbance, 115
  intervention, 115–116
  intrauterine experience, 115
  kangaroo care, 116
  positioning, 116
Vibration
  equipment, 45
  neonatal transport, 45
Vidarabine
  for herpes simplex virus, 1286
  for neonatal HSV, 1289, 1290
Videoconferencing, 59f
Viral infection, 1274–1333
Virilization, 927–928
Visual acuity, 1470
Visual cortex
  maturation of, 121t
Visual impairment, 1639–1640
Visual system, 121–124
  deficits, 122
  development of, 121–122
  intrauterine environment, 122
  NICU, 122–123, 124
Vital signs, 335
Vitamin A
  BPD, 583
  fetal effects, 238t, 251
  maternal nutrition, 206
  in preterm infant formulas, 404
  TPN, 398
Vitamin A deficiency, 390
Vitamin B12
  fetal effects, 251
  maternal nutrition, 205–206
  for organic acidemia, 972
Vitamin C
  BPD, 583

Vitamin D
  calcium and magnesium control,
    853–855
  fetal effects, 238t, 251
  in human milk, 401
  hypocalcemia, 857t
  maternal nutrition, 205
  for osteopenia, 870
  in preterm infant formulas, 404
Vitamin D deficiency, 390
Vitamin D dependent rickets type I,
    1036
Vitamin deficiencies, 1186–1187
Vitamin E, 1542–1543
  in preterm infant formulas, 404
Vitamin E deficiency, 390
  TPN, 398
Vitamin K, 1700
Vitamin K deficiency, 390, 1193
Vitamin K information
  antenatal care, 352
Vitamins
  fetal effects, 238t, 251
  requirements, 389–390
Vocal cord paralysis, 1102
Voiding, 356t
Volutrauma
  with BPD, 579–580
Vomiting, 357
  with inborn errors of metabolism,
    968
Von Hippel-Lindau syndrome, 1681
Vulnerable neonate, 111–125
Vulvar cancer
  during pregnancy, 216

W
WAGR syndrome, 1445
WAN (wide area network), 56
Warfarin (Coumadin), 1221
  congenital anomalies with, 899t
Warming mattresses
  conductive heat loss, 450
Water
  fetal growth, 496–497
Water soluble vitamins
  requirements, 390
Weight
  ECMO, 623–624
  SGA, 517
Weight conversion, 1660
Weight loss
  neonatal jaundice, 795
Well being
  evaluation of, 260–264
Werner's syndrome, 1445
West Nile virus, 1314–1315
Weyers oligodactyly syndrome, 1677
WHIM syndrome, 1206t
WHIM (warts, hypogammaglobulinemia,
    infections, myelokathexis)
    syndrome, 1207
White blood cell counts, 1705
White-out lungs, 1288
White spots, 1497

Williams-Beuren syndrome, 636t
Williams syndrome, 141, 1682
  associated with congenital heart disease,
    717t
  cardiac disease, 635
  hypercalcemia, 864
Wilms tumor, 1451–1452
Wiskott-Aldrich syndrome, 1206t,
    1207
Withdrawal reflex
  examination, 348t
Withdrawing, 13–14
Withholding, 13–14
Wnt-4, 915
Wolfe syndrome, 637t
Wolffian duct, 1067f
Wolff-Parkinson-White syndrome
  atrioventricular reciprocating
    tachycardia, 702–703
  following congenital heart surgery, 741
Wolf-Hirschhron syndrome
  associated with congenital heart disease,
    717t
Wolf-Parkinson-White syndrome, 638
Wolman disease
  with liver disease, 960
Wrist
  physical examination, 1428

X
Xanax
  fetal effects, 242
Xanthinuria, 1028
Xeroderma pigmentosum, 1445
X-linked hypophosphatemia, 1036
X-linked recessive inheritance severe
    combined immunodeficiency
    syndrome (X-SCID), 197–198

Y
Yellow orange lesions, 1503–1504
Yolk sac tumors, 1453–1454

Z
4Z, 15E bilirubin isomer, 831, 831f
Zalcitabine, 1319
  pregnancy, 1320t
  teratogenic potential, 1319
Zellweger syndrome, 637t, 974t, 975,
    1681
  abnormal eye findings, 976–977
  with liver disease, 960
Zidovudine, 1319, 1321, 1322
  active transport, 153
  placental transport, 153
  pregnancy, 1320t
Zinc
  absorption, 942
  maternal nutrition, 205–206
  recommended intake for preterm infants,
    400t
Zonular lens opacity, 1474f
Zygosity, 524, 525t